WILDERNESS MEDICINE

FOURTH EDITION

WILDERNESS
MEDICINE

PAUL S. AUERBACH, MD, MS

Clinical Professor of Surgery,
Division of Emergency Medicine,
Stanford University School of Medicine,
Stanford, California;
Venture Partner,
Delphi Ventures,
Menlo Park, California

with 1248 illustrations

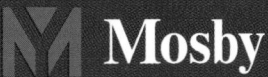

Mosby

A Harcourt Health Sciences Company

St. Louis   London   Philadelphia   Sydney   Toronto

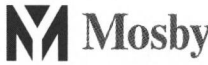

A Harcourt Health Sciences Company

Acquiring Editor: Judith Fletcher
Senior Managing Editor: Kathy Falk
Project Manager: Carol Sullivan Weis
Senior Production Editor: Rick Dudley
Designer: Mark A. Oberkrom
Cover Photograph: Paul S. Auerbach

FOURTH EDITION

Mosby, Inc.
A Harcourt Health Sciences Company
11830 Westline Industrial Drive
St. Louis, Missouri 63146

Printed in the United States of America

International Standard Book Number ISBN 0-323-00950-6

01   02   03   04   05   TG/KPT   9   8   7   6   5   4   3   2   1

Contributors

Javier A. Adachi, MD
Fellow, Department of Infectious Diseases,
Center for Infectious Disease,
The University of Texas–Houston Medical School and
    School of Public Health,
Houston, Texas;
Universidad Peruana Cayetano Heredia,
Lima, Peru

**Michele Adler, BPharm, Cert. Hoft. Hons. Post.
Grad. Dip. Ed.**
Lecturer in Horticulture,
Horticultural Consultant,
University of Melbourne–Burnley College,
Richmond, Victoria, Australia

Robert C. Allen, DO, FACEP
Lt. Col. USAF,
Group Surgeon,
720th Special Tactics Group,
Air Force Special Operations Command,
Hurlburt Field, Florida

**Christopher J. Andrews, BE, MBBS, MEngSc, PhD,
DipCSc, EDIC**
Clinical Associate Lecturer,
University of Queensland,
St. Lucia, Queensland, Australia;
Registrar in Anaesthesia,
The Mater Hospital,
South Brisbane, Queensland, Australia

Betsy R. Armstrong, MA
Chief Operating Officer,
Women of the West Museum,
Denver, Colorado

Richard L. Armstrong
Senior Research Scientist,
Cooperative Institute for Research in Environmental
    Sciences,
National Snow and Ice Data Center,
University of Colorado,
Boulder, Colorado

E. Wayne Askew, PhD
Professor, Division of Foods and Nutrition,
College of Health,
University of Utah,
Salt Lake City, Utah

Dale Atkins, BA Geography
Avalanche Scientist and Forecaster,
Colorado Avalanche Information Center,
Boulder, Colorado

Paul S. Auerbach, MD, MS
Clinical Professor of Surgery,
Division of Emergency Medicine,
Stanford University School of Medicine,
Stanford, California;
Venture Partner,
Delphi Ventures,
Menlo Park, California

Howard D. Backer, MD, MPH
Emergency Department,
Kaiser Permanente Medical Center,
Hayward, California;
Currently, Medical Consultant and Epidemiologist,
Immunization Branch,
Division of Communicable Disease Control,
California Department of Health Services

James P. Bagian, BSME, MD
Clinical Assistant Professor of Preventive Medicine
    and Community Health,
University of Texas Medical Branch,
Galveston, Texas;
Adjunct Assistant Professor of Military and
    Emergency Medicine,
Uniformed Services University of the Health
    Sciences,
F. Edward Hebert School of Medicine,
Bethesda, Maryland;
Director, National Center for Patient Safety,
Veterans Health Administration,
Ann Arbor, Michigan;
Colonel, U.S. Air Force Reserve 920th Rescue Group,
Patrick Air Force Base, Florida

H. Bernard Bechtel, MD
Staff, South Georgia Medical Center,
Valdosta, Georgia

Greta J. Binford, PhD
Research Associate,
Department of Biochemistry and Center for Insect
    Sciences,
University of Arizona,
Tucson, Arizona

Warren D. Bowman, Jr., MD, FACP
Clinical Associate Professor of Medicine Emeritus,
University of Washington School of Medicine,
Seattle, Washington;
National Medical Director Emeritus,
National Ski Patrol System,
Denver, Colorado;
Past President,
Wilderness Medical Society,
Colorado Springs, Colorado

Leslie V. Boyer, MD
Assistant Professor,
Department of Pediatrics,
University of Arizona Health Sciences Center;
Medical Director,
Arizona Poison and Drug Information Center,
Tucson, Arizona

George Braitberg, MBBS, FACEM
Senior Fellow,
Department of Medicine,
Director of Emergency Medicine,
Consultant Medical Toxicologist,
University of Melbourne,
Parkville, Victoria, Australia;
Consultant Medical Toxicologist,
National Poison Centre,
Austin and Repatriation Medical Centre,
Heidelberg, Victoria, Australia

Robert K. Bush, MD
Professor of Medicine,
University of Wisconsin–Madison;
Chief of Allergy,
William S. Middleton VA Hospital,
Madison, Wisconsin

Sean P. Bush, MD, FACEP
Staff Emergency Physician and Venom Specialist,
Associate Professor of Emergency Medicine,
Loma Linda University Medical Center and School of
    Medicine,
Loma Linda, California

Frank K. Butler, Jr., MD
Director of Biomedical Research,
U.S. Naval Special Warfare Command;
Attending Ophthalmologist,
Naval Hospital Pensacola,
Pensacola, Florida

Michael L. Callaham, MD, FACEP
Chief, Division of Emergency Medicine,
Professor of Emergency Medicine,
University of California, San Francisco,
San Francisco, California

Steven C. Carleton, MD, PhD
Assistant Professor,
Department of Emergency Medicine,
University of Cincinnati College of Medicine;
Medical Director,
University Air Care,
University Hospital, Inc.,
Cincinnati, Ohio

Betty Carlisle, MD
Emergency Physician,
South Bend, Washington

Richard F. Clark, MD
Associate Professor of Medicine,
University of California, San Diego;
Director, Division of Medical Toxicology,
Department of Emergency Medicine,
University of California, San Diego Medical Center,
San Diego, California

Loui H. Clem
Littleton, Colorado

David A. Connor, MD
Clinical Toxicologist,
Department of Medical Toxicology,
Good Samaritan Regional Medical Center,
Phoenix, Arizona

Donald C. Cooper, BS, MS, MBA, NREMT-P
Deputy Fire Chief,
Cuyahoga Falls Fire Department,
Cuyahoga Falls, Ohio

Mary Ann Cooper, MD
Associate Professor,
Department of Emergency Medicine,
University of Illinois at Chicago,
Chicago, Illinois

Larry I. Crawshaw, PhD
Professor, Department of Biology,
Portland State University;
Professor, Behavioral Neuroscience,
Oregon Health Sciences University,
Portland, Oregon

Barbara D. Dahl, MD
Attending Physician,
Kaiser Santa Clara Emergency Department,
Stanford/Kaiser Emergency Medicine Residency
    Program,
Santa Clara, California;
Department of Emergency Medicine,
St. Rose Hospital,
Hayward, California

Daniel F. Danzl, MD
Professor and Chair,
Department of Emergency Medicine,
University of Louisville School of Medicine,
Louisville, Kentucky

Richard C. Dart, MD, PhD
Associate Professor of Surgery, Medicine and
    Pharmacy,
University of Colorado Health Sciences Center;
Director, Rocky Mountain Poison and Drug Center,
Denver Health Authority,
Denver, Colorado

Kathleen Mary Davis, BS Forestry, MS Forestry
Chief, Natural Resources,
Southern Arizona Office,
National Park Service,
Phoenix, Arizona

Kevin Jon Davison, ND, LAc
Maui East-West Clinic, Ltd.,
Haiku, Maui, Hawaii

Anne E. Dickison, MD
Clinical Associate Professor of Anesthesiology and
    Pediatrics,
University of Florida College of Medicine;
Faculty Pediatric Intensivist and Anesthesiologist,
Shands Teaching Hospital at the University of
    Florida,
Gainesville, Florida

Mark Donnelly, MD
Resident,
Department of Emergency Medicine,
University of Rochester Medical Center,
Rochester, New York

Howard J. Donner, MD
Clinic Physician,
Telluride Medical Center,
Telluride, Colorado

Herbert L. DuPont, MD
Chief, Internal Medicine Service,
St. Luke's Episcopal Hospital;
H. Irving Schweppe, Jr., M.D. Chair in Internal
    Medicine;
Vice Chairman,
Department of Internal Medicine,
Baylor College of Medicine;
Mary W. Kelsey Professor of Medical Sciences,
The University of Texas Health Sciences Center at
    Houston,
Houston, Texas

Thomas J. Ellis, MD
Director of Orthopedic Trauma,
Assistant Professor,
Oregon Health Sciences University,
Portland, Oregon

John H. Epstein, MD, MS
Clinical Professor of Dermatology,
Department of Dermatology,
University of California, San Francisco,
San Francisco, California

William L. Epstein, MD
Professor of Dermatology, Emeritus,
University of California, San Francisco,
San Francisco, California

Blair D. Erb, MD
Past President,
Wilderness Medical Society,
Colorado Springs, Colorado;
The Study Center;
Jackson–Madison County General Hospital,
Jackson, Tennessee

Timothy B. Erickson, MD
Director, Emergency Medicine Residency Program,
Director, Division of Clinical Toxicology,
Associate Professor,
University of Illinois at Chicago,
Chicago, Illinois

Murray E. Fowler, DVM
Professor Emeritus,
Zoological Medicine,
University of California School of Veterinary
    Medicine,
Davis, California

Mark S. Fradin, MD
Clinical Associate Professor,
Department of Dermatology,
University of North Carolina School of Medicine,
Chapel Hill, North Carolina

Bryan L. Frank, MD
Senior Clinical Instructor,
Medical Acupuncture for Physicians Program,
Continuing Education Office,
University of California, Los Angeles School of
    Medicine;
President,
American Academy of Medical Acupuncture,
Los Angeles, California;
President, Integrated Medicine Seminars, L.L.C.,
Richardson, Texas

Luanne Freer, MD
Clinical Assistant Professor of Emergency Medicine,
George Washington University,
Washington, D.C.;
Chief of Staff,
Yellowstone Park Medical Services,
Yellowstone National Park, Wyoming;
Emergency Physician,
Bozeman, Montana,
Idaho Falls, Idaho

Steven P. French, MD
Research Director,
Yellowstone Grizzly Foundation,
Jackson Hole, Wyoming;
Member,
Bear Specialists Group,
World Conservation Union;
ER Medical Director (Retired)

Stephen L. Gaffin, PhD
Research Physiologist,
Thermal and Mountain Medicine,
U.S. Army Research Institute of Environmental
    Medicine,
Natick, Massachussetts

Douglas A. Gentile, MD, MBA
Attending Physician,
University of Vermont College of Medicine,
Burlington, Vermont

Gordon G. Giesbrecht, PhD
Professor,
Health, Leisure and Human Performance Research
    Institute;
Associate Professor,
Department of Anesthesia,
Faculty of Medicine,
University of Manitoba,
Winnipeg, Manitoba, Canada

Philip H. Goodman, MD, MS, FACP
Professor of Medicine,
Chief, Division of General Internal Medicine and
    Health Care Research,
University of Nevada School of Medicine,
Reno, Nevada

John Gookin
Curriculum Manager,
Senior Staff Instructor,
The National Outdoor Leadership School (NOLS),
Lander, Wyoming;
Associate Faculty,
University of Utah,
Salt Lake City, Utah

Kimberlie A. Graeme, MD
Clinical Assistant Professor,
Section of Toxicology,
Division of Emergency Medicine,
Department of Surgery,
University of Arizona College of Medicine,
Tucson, Arizona;
Fellowship Director,
Department of Medical Toxicology,
Good Samaritan Regional Medical Center,
Phoenix, Arizona;
Attending Physician,
Mayo Clinic Hospital,
Scottsdale, Arizona

Peter H. Hackett, MD
Affiliate Associate Professor,
Department of Medicine,
University of Washington School of Medicine,
Seattle, Washington;
Emergency Department,
St. Mary's Medical Center,
Grand Junction, Colorado

Murray P. Hamlet, DVM
Chief, Research Programs and Operations Division,
U.S. Army Research Institute of Environmental
    Medicine,
Natick, Massachusetts

Susan L. Hefle, PhD
Assistant Professor,
Department of Food Science and Technology,
University of Nebraska,
Lincoln, Nebraska

John P. Heggers, PhD, FAAM, CWS (AAWM)
Professor, Surgery (Plastic),
ILT-UTMB Medical School,
University of Texas Medical Branch;
Director of Clinical Microbiology,
Directory of Microbiology Research,
Shriners Burns Institute,
Galveston, Texas

David Heimbach, MD
Professor of Surgery,
University of Washington School of Medicine,
Seattle, Washington

Henry J. Herrmann, DMD, FAGD
Private Practice,
Falls Church, Virginia

Ronald L. Holle, MS
Meteorologist,
Global Atmospherics, Inc.,
Tucson, Arizona

Rivkah S. Horowitz, MD, PhD
Clinical Assistant Professor of Medicine,
Brown University School of Medicine,
Providence, Rhode Island;
Attending Physician,
Lawrence and Memorial Hospital,
New London, Connecticut

Frank R. Hubbell, DO
Clinical Instructor,
University of New England College of Osteopathic
    Medicine,
Biddeford, Maine

Steve Hudson
President,
Pigeon Mountain Industries, Inc.,
LaFayette, Georgia

Kenneth V. Iserson, MD, MBA
Professor of Surgery,
University of Arizona College of Medicine;
Director, Arizona Bioethics Program,
University of Arizona,
Tucson, Arizona

Michael E. Jacobs, MD
Private Practice in Internal Medicine and
    Gastroenterology;
United States Coast Guard Licensed Captain;
Professional Sailor,
Martha's Vineyard, Massachussetts

Elaine C. Jong, MD
Clinical Professor of Medicine,
Director, Hall Health Primary Care
    Center/University of Washington Student Health
    Service,
University of Washington School of Medicine,
Seattle, Washington

Lee A. Kaplan, MD
Associate Clinical Professor of
    Medicine/Dermatology,
University of California, San Diego,
San Diego, California;
Private Practice in Dermatology,
Dermatologist Medical Group,
La Jolla, California

James W. Kazura, MD
Professor, Division of Geographic Medicine,
Case Western Reserve University School of Medicine,
Cleveland, Ohio

Barbara C. Kennedy, MD
Assistant Professor,
University of Vermont College of Medicine;
Attending Physician,
Fletcher Allen Health Care,
Burlington, Vermont

Sean Keogh, MRCP, FRCSEd, FACEM, FFAEM
Consultant, Emergency Medicine,
Auckland Hospital,
Auckland, New Zealand

Kenneth W. Kizer, MD, MPH
Distinguished Professor of Military and Emergency
    Medicine,
Uniformed Services University of the Health
    Sciences,
Bethesda, Maryland;
President and Chief Executive Officer,
The National Quality Forum,
Washington, D.C.

Judith R. Klein, MD
Resident,
Emergency Medicine,
Stanford University,
Stanford, California

Donald B. Kunkel, MD (deceased)
Associate in Pharmacology and Toxicology,
Health Sciences Center,
University of Arizona,
Tucson, Arizona;
Medical Director, Samaritan Regional Poison Center,
Samaritan Regional Medical Center,
Phoenix, Arizona

Jason E. Lang, MD
Clinical Instructor,
University of Vermont College of Medicine;
Chief Resident in Pediatrics,
Fletcher Allen Health Care;
Burlington, Vermont

Carolyn S. Langer, MD, JD, MPH
Instructor in Occupational Medicine,
Lecturer in Occupational Health Law,
Harvard School of Public Health,
Boston, Massachusetts

Patrick H. LaValla
President,
ERI International,
Olympia, Washington

Raúl E. López, PhD
Research Meteorologist (Retired),
National Severe Storms Laboratory,
National Oceanic and Atmospheric Administration,
Norman, Oklahoma

Roberta A. Mann, MD
Medical Director,
Torrance Memorial Burn Center and Wound Healing
  Center,
Torrance Memorial Medical Center,
Torrance, California

Ariel D. Marks, MD, MS, FACEP
Staff Physician,
Emergency Department,
Sequoia Hospital,
Redwood City, California

Vicki Mazzorana, MD, FACEP
Clinical Assistant Professor of Emergency Medicine,
Department of Surgery,
Stanford University School of Medicine,
Stanford, California

Robert L. McCauley, MD
Professor of Surgery and Pediatrics,
University of Texas Medical Branch;
Chief, Plastic and Reconstructive Surgery,
Shriners Burns Institute,
Galveston, Texas

Jude T. McNally, RPh, ABAT
Managing Director,
Arizona Poison and Drug Information Center,
University of Arizona College of Pharmacy,
Tucson, Arizona

James Messenger
Lieutenant, EMT-P,
Cuyahoga Falls Fire Department,
Cuyahoga Falls, Ohio;
Rescue Specialist,
F.E.M.A. Ohio Task Force 1 (OH TF-1)

Timothy P. Mier, BA
Lieutenant,
Cuyahoga Falls Fire Department,
Cuyahoga Falls, Ohio

Sherman A. Minton, MD (deceased)
Professor Emeritus,
Microbiology & Immunology,
Indiana University School of Medicine,
Indianapolis, Indiana;
Research Associate,
Department of Herpetology,
American Museum of Natural History,
New York, New York

James K. Mitchell, PhD
Professor of Geography,
Rutgers University,
Piscataway, New Jersey

Daniel S. Moran, PhD
Visiting Lecturer,
Sackler Faculty of Medicine,
Tel Aviv University,
Tel Aviv, Israel;
Head, Physiology Unit,
Heller Institute of Medical Research,
Chaim Sheba Medical Center,
Tel Hashomer, Israel

John A. Morris, Jr., MD
Professor of Surgery,
Director, Division of Trauma,
Vanderbilt University School of Medicine,
Nashville, Tennessee

Robert W. Mutch, BA, MSF
Fire Management Consultant,
Fire Management Applications,
Missoula, Montana

Andrew B. Newman, MD, FCCP
Clinical Associate Professor of Medicine,
Stanford University School of Medicine,
Stanford, California

Eric K. Noji, MD, MPH
Chief, Epidemiology, Surveillance and Emergency
  Response Branch,
Bioterrorism Preparedness and Response Program,
National Center for Infectious Diseases,
Centers for Disease Control and Prevention (CDC),
Atlanta, Georgia

Robert L. Norris, Jr., MD
Associate Professor of Surgery/Emergency Medicine,
Stanford University School of Medicine;
Chief, Division of Emergency Medicine,
Stanford University Hospital,
Stanford, California

Edward J. Otten, MD, FACMT
Professor of Emergency Medicine and Pediatrics,
Director, Division of Toxicology,
University of Cincinnati,
Cincinnati, Ohio

Naresh J. Patel, DO
Fellow, Allergy/Immunology,
Department of Medicine,
University of Wisconsin–Madison,
Madison, Wisconsin

Claude A. Piantadosi, MD
Professor,
Department of Medicine (Pulmonary),
Duke University Medical Center,
Durham, North Carolina

Richard N. Rausch, PhD
Postdoctoral Fellow,
Department of Biology,
Portland State University,
Portland, Oregon

Sheila B. Reed, MS Education
Consultant, International Disaster Management,
Middleton, Wisconsin

Robert C. Roach, PhD
Research Associate Professor,
New Mexico Highlands University,
Las Vegas, New Mexico;
Director, The Hypoxia Institute,
Montezuma, New Mexico

Martin C. Robson, MD
Professor of Surgery,
Division of Plastic Surgery, Department of Surgery,
University of South Florida,
Tampa, Florida

Sandra Schneider, MD
Professor and Chair,
Department of Emergency Medicine,
University of Rochester;
Strong Memorial Hospital,
Rochester, New York

Bern Shen, MD, MPhil
Institute for Health Policy Studies,
University of California, San Francisco,
San Francisco, California

David J. Smith, Jr., MD
Professor and Section Head,
Department of Plastic Surgery,
University of Michigan Medical Center,
Ann Arbor, Michigan

Alan M. Steinman, MD, MPH
Fellow, American College of Preventive Medicine;
Board of Directors, Marine Safety Foundation

Robert C. Stoffel
President, Emergency Response International, Inc.,
Cashmere, Washington

Jeffrey R. Suchard, MD
Assistant Clinical Professor of Medicine,
Division of Emergency Medicine,
University of California, Irvine Medical Center,
Orange, California

Mark F. Swiontkowski, MD
Professor and Chairman,
Department of Orthopaedics,
University of Minnesota,
Minneapolis, Minnesota

Eric A. Toschlog, MD
Division of General Surgery,
Department of Surgery,
East Carolina University,
The Brody School of Medicine,
Greenville, North Carolina

Kenneth F. Trofatter, Jr., MD, PhD
3M Clinical Professor,
Department of Obstetrics, Gynecology, and Women's
  Health,
University of Minnesota Medical School,
Minneapolis, Minnesota

Karen B. Van Hoesen, MD
Assistant Clinical Professor,
Department of Emergency Medicine;
Director, Diving Medicine Center;
Director, Hyperbaric Medicine Fellowship,
University of California, San Diego,
San Diego, California

John Walden, MD, DTM&H
Professor and Associate Dean for Development and
  Outreach,
Marshall University Joan C. Edwards School of
  Medicine,
Huntington, West Virginia

Kimberley P. Walker, MA, NREMT-P, CHT
Manager of Corporate Systems Education,
Department of Information Technology,
Duke University Medical Center;
Trainer, Divers Alert Network,
Durham, North Carolina

Helen L. Wallace, BS
Research Associate,
Department of Biology,
Portland State University,
Portland, Oregon

Eric A. Weiss, MD
Assistant Professor of Emergency Medicine,
Stanford University School of Medicine;
Associate Director of Trauma,
Stanford University Medical Center,
Stanford, California

Eric L. Weiss, MD, DTM&H
Assistant Professor,
Emergency Medicine and Infectious Diseases,
Director, Stanford Travel Medicine Service,
Stanford University School of Medicine,
Stanford, California;
Chief Medical Officer,
Medicine Planet, Inc.

Knox Williams, MS Atmospheric Science
Fort Collins, Colorado

Sarah R. Williams, MD
Emergency Medicine Ultrasound Fellow,
Chief Resident,
Clinical Instructor of Surgery,
Attending Physician,
Division of Emergency Medicine,
Stanford University Medical Center,
Stanford, California;
Attending Physician,
Emergency Department,
Kiaser Santa Clara Medical Center,
Santa Clara, California

Ian J. Woolley, MBBS, FRACP
Senior Lecturer,
Department of Medicine,
Senior Staff Specialist,
Infectious Diseases Unit,
Alfred Hospital,
Monash University;
Director, Infection Control Units,
Senior Staff Specialist, Infectious Diseases,
Peninsula Health,
Melbourne, Victoria, Australia

Steven C. Zell, MD
Professor of Medicine,
Division of General Internal Medicine and Health
    Care Research,
University of Nevada School of Medicine,
Reno, Nevada

Foreword

"Everything to hope, with but little to fear"

Food was scarce and the hunter was determined to bring back meat for his hungry friends. Thousands of bison swarmed over the prairie, and it did not take him long to shoot a fat male. As he watched the animal die, blood pouring from its mouth, he failed to see the grizzly bear until it was 20 steps away. He had no time to reload his clumsy gun, but could only retreat. There was no good place to hide—no trees, no bushes, only the nearby river. As soon as he turned, the bear charged after him, roaring open-mouthed and covering the ground with frightening speed. Fortunately, the riverbank was low and the hunter plunged into the water and turned to face the bear, hoping it would not follow. The bear rushed to within 20 feet, sized up the situation, turned away and ran off as fast as it had charged. Meriwether Lewis had just escaped with his life.

The Lewis and Clark Expedition had been 11 months on the trail and was more than a thousand miles from its base. There was no contact with the outside world and no possibility of help. Supplies of food had run low, and the group depended on their hunters for meat. The native population had not always been friendly. The explorers could not speak the local languages and relied on interpreters. Attacks by ferocious animals were a daily danger.

On June 16, 1804, 2 days after the bear attack, a critical point was reached in their journey. The outcome would not depend on their hunting skills and luck but on their medical knowledge. The leaders described the situation later in their diaries:

June 12, 1805: The interpreter's woman very sick. One man has a felon rising on his hand; the other, with the toothache, has taken a cold in the jaw, &c. (Clark)

June 13, 1805: A fair morning. Some dew this morning. The Indian woman very sick. I gave her a dose of salts. We set out early. (Clark)

June 14, 1805: A fine morning. The Indian woman complaining all night, and excessively bad this morning. Her case is somewhat dangerous. Two men with the toothache, two with tumors, and one with a tumor and light fever. (Clark)

June 15, 1805: Our Indian woman sick and low spirited. I gave her the bark and applied it externally to her region, which revived her much. (Clark)

June 16, 1805: Found the Indian woman extremely ill and much reduced by her indisposition. This gave me some

concern, as well for the poor object herself—then with a young child in her arms—as from the consideration of her being our only dependence for a friendly negotiation with the Snake Indians, on whom we depend for horses to assist us in our portage from the Missouri to the Columbia River. (Lewis)

Sacagawea, a 17-year-old Shoshone Indian with a 6-month-old baby, was married to one of the interpreters, Toussaint Charbonneau. She had been critically ill for several days and was not responding to treatment.

Meriwether Lewis, who was in modern terms the "trip doctor" and the leader, took over her care. He had studied medicinal botany and had sought advice from America's leading physician, Dr. Benjamin Rush, before taking command of the group, but he was not a physician. Nonetheless, his knowledge of medical problems in the wilderness was not much different from that of many doctors of the time. Few doctors had medical degrees, and many were only apprenticed to an older physician for a few years before practicing on their own. The decision not to have a physician on the trip was made with the agreement of President Thomas Jefferson, who was the moving force behind the expedition.

Sacagawea was suffering from abdominal pain and vomiting. She was febrile and nearly unconscious. Clark had treated her empirically with bleeding, salts, and abdominal poultices. In taking control of the case, Lewis did everything that a modern doctor would do under the same circumstances. He took a history, examined the patient, came to a diagnosis, and prescribed such treatment as was available. He concluded that her problem was due to "an obstruction of the mensis in consequence of taking could"—a diagnosis strange to our thinking but one that suggests a careful and detailed history. At that time, men did not naturally discuss such intimate details of the lives of women. He prescribed poultices and doses of mineral waters and laudanum.

Sacagawea improved greatly and was able to get up and take a walk. Within 2 days she was back to normal. Her recovery was vital for the expedition because she was the key to opening the route to the Pacific Ocean. She had been captured while a child, taken hundreds of miles to the East, and was now on the verge of returning to her own country. Without her ability to interpret the language of the Shoshones, the expedition might have failed. When they finally met the Shoshones, Sacagawea found that her brother, now grown to manhood, was the chief of the tribe. Further progress of the expedition was assured. Lewis had achieved his two aims: recovery of his patient and salvage of the expedition.

For many years, President Jefferson had visions of opening a water route to the West Coast, wresting the lucrative fur trade from the British and French, and finding the mythical Northwest Passage. The Spanish and British had similar aspirations to send explorers to the West Coast. In 1793, Alexander Mackenzie crossed the spine of the Rocky Mountains farther north, through an area so inhospitable that it was useless for trade. In the same year, a French botanist, André Michaux, supported by the American Philosophical Society, tried to travel up the Missouri River but failed. Two obstacles prevented further American attempts from coming to fruition: Congress would not appropriate money, and France and Spain controlled the land west of the Mississippi River.

Knowledge of the geography of the country was limited and naïve. No one—British, French, Canadian, Spanish, or American—understood the vastness and complexity of the land. They were all blind men feeling a continental elephant. The British and Spanish had superficially explored the West Coast as far as Alaska. In 1792, Captain Gray, an adventurous American sailor, had discovered and named the Columbia River, which obviously flowed from the distant peaks. Exploration was confined to the coast, and people could only guess at what lay beyond the mountains that divided the country. Since fur traders had long used the lower reaches of the Missouri River to bring their trophies to St. Louis and New Orleans, Jefferson thought, why not an expedition that would ascend the Missouri, make a short portage across the mountains, and continue down the Columbia to the coast?

Until 1800, Spain controlled the territory west of the Mississippi through which an expedition would have to move. Rule of the land passed to France from 1800 to 1803, until Napoleon sold the territory to the United States in the Louisiana Purchase. Suddenly the United States had dominion over a vast expanse of land from the Missouri to the Pacific.

In 1802, Jefferson secretly persuaded Congress to appropriate $2500 for an expedition "for the purpose of extending the external commerce of the U.S." The expedition was also called a "literary pursuit," slim camouflage for an act of commercial imperialism that amazingly achieved its objectives with almost no loss of life, and without starting a war with Britain, Spain, or the Indians.

President Jefferson chose his private secretary, Captain Meriwether Lewis, to lead the expedition. Lewis was an experienced army officer with knowledge of wilderness travel and a proven record of leadership. In addition, he was a member of a distinguished Virginia family and a close friend of the President. Lewis, in turn, chose his former commanding officer, William Clark, to be his co-leader. Time proved them to be the perfect team, as leaders, scientists, observers, and diarists—and occasionally as physicians.

President Jefferson organized the preparations meticulously. Lewis was dispatched to Philadelphia by Jefferson to learn celestial navigation, botany, and zoology, and become proficient in the preservation of biologic specimens. He visited Benjamin Rush, the leading physician of his day and physician to President Jefferson, to find out what medications he should take and how to treat the diseases he might encounter.

Rush prepared a list of 14 questions for Lewis to answer and gave him 10 pieces of advice on how to maintain his own health. The questions to be answered concerned the health, morals, and religious practices of the Indians. Rush wanted Lewis to inquire about the diseases of these people and how they were cured. When did their women start and stop menstruating? How long were their children suckled? What were their sexual mores and habits? Rush was particularly interested in knowing if any of the religious ceremonies of the Indians were similar to those of Judaism because there was a belief, in some circles, that the lost tribe of Israel had ended up in the American West.

Rush advised rest after strenuous exercise, moderation in drink and food, and the liberal use of purges, to both prevent and cure ailments. He told them to wear flannel next to the skin, especially in cold and wet weather, and advised that the men wear shoes without heels, since they would be less fatiguing than shoes with higher heels. The advice about purging, bleeding, and sweating conformed with the current theories of medical practice. Rush outspokenly believed that blood, bowel contents, and sweat contained the causes of disease that could be removed.

Based on advice from Rush, the medical dispensary of the expedition contained a liberal supply of Rush's Pills, a potent mixture of calomel and jalap, both laxatives strong enough to empty the bowels of the hardiest frontiersman. Numerous drugs, herbs, and instruments, including laudanum for pain, medications for eye problems, four penis syringes for treating venereal disease, and lancets for bleeding, were packaged in a specially constructed wooden chest. The total cost of the medical supplies was $96.69.

The Corps of Discovery, as the expedition was called, spent the winter of 1803-1804 in Camp Dubois, north of St. Louis, on the east bank of the Mississippi River (the west bank was not yet in the United States) and opposite the mouth of the Missouri River, training and equipping for the long and uncertain journey.

Captain Clark, 23 army privates, four sergeants, Drouillard (a French-Indian hunter), York (William Clark's slave), and Lewis' Newfoundland dog Seaman pushed out onto the Missouri River on May 14, 1804. Lewis joined the group a few days later. They sailed in a 55-foot keel boat and two smaller pirogues. They struggled upstream, poling, rowing, sailing, and hauling the boats by hand. The weather was hot, with frequent summer storms. Thick clouds of mosquitoes were a constant plague. The food was bad and often scarce. Although generous supplies of some foods had been taken, the prime source of meat was obtained by hunting. At first they were lucky. There were vast herds of buffalo, deer, and elk. Game could often be shot within a short distance of camp. Such profusion would not last long after the opening of the West.

The men were young, strong, and chosen for their wilderness skills. There were hunters, boatmen, carpenters, interpreters, and French voyageurs, as healthy and adventurous a group of young men as could be found. However, despite their strength, diseases plagued them constantly: diarrhea, fevers, near starvation, skin infections and boils, cuts from knives, sunburn, snakebites, dislocated shoulders, and feet lacerated from cactus spines. Only luck saved them from being killed by grizzly bears. A sleeping sergeant was bitten on the hand by a wolf. Sacagawea had a difficult labor but gave birth 10 minutes after receiving a concoction of rattlesnake rattles. Diarrhea and intestinal infections came to be expected. The men took few sanitary precautions, although the army knew that troops that remained on the move and dug latrines far from camp remained healthier than did those that stayed in one camp for a long time. Perhaps their mobility saved them from some problems. During the two periods they stayed in camps, medical problems were more common than when they were on the move.

On August 17, 1804, Sergeant Charles Floyd developed abdominal pain that progressed over the next 3 days. During that time, he continued to work on the boat, but the pain became worse, shock developed, and on August 20, he died. Before he died, he said to Captain Clark, "I am going to leave you. I want you to write me a letter." He died "with composure" and was buried with military honors on a bluff overlooking the river, where there is now a monument to his memory. He was the only fatality in the Corps and the first U.S. soldier to die west of the Mississippi. The diagnosis is uncertain, although his symptoms suggest a ruptured appendix. Lewis described the symptoms as "bilious cholic," but there was no record of an examination. We do not know if Floyd's abdomen was tense, distended, or painful. Neither Lewis nor Clark was a doctor, and although Lewis was knowledgeable about herbs and probably knew how to treat wounds and accidents, he was not trained to diagnose illnesses or to make a phys-

ical examination. If the diagnosis was, indeed, a ruptured appendix, Sergeant Floyd would not have survived, even had he been in Philadelphia under Benjamin Rush's care.

The first winter was spent in a collection of huts surrounded by a wooden stockade, near a Mandan Indian village. The weather was bitterly cold, and the supply of food ran low. The Indians were friendly, but they too had very little food; some members of the expedition helped them by going out on hunting excursions. Although the temperature dropped to −38° F, none of the Corps members sustained damaging frostbite. A Mandan boy, stranded out overnight and left for dead, was brought in with frozen feet. After a few days, the boy's toes became gangrenous and Clark "sawed off his toes." The endurance of another Indian amazed the soldiers. Stranded overnight in freezing weather, with no food and only the clothes on his back, he had neither frostbite nor hypothermia. The Mandans slept with their feet towards the campfire, to prevent frostbite during the night, but could not stave off frostbite while hunting with only thin moccasins on their feet.

Prairie plums, cherries, and gooseberries supplemented the protein diet and contained enough vitamin C to prevent scurvy. As winter gave way to spring, thousands of buffalo returned and meat became available. The strength and health of the men improved. When they were about to set out again on the river on April 7, 1805, Lewis was able to write to Jefferson, "I can foresee no material or probable obstruction to our progress, and entertain therefore the most sanguine hopes of complete success. . . . With such men I have everything to hope, and but little to fear." At the same time he wrote to his mother, ". . . not a whisper of discontent or murmur is to be heard among them, but all act in unison, and with the most perfect harmony." The Corps, which had experienced disciplinary problems, a desertion, and the need for floggings, was now a tough, unified group, confident in their officers and prepared to embark on an endeavor more difficult than they could ever imagine.

The journey westward through the Bitterroot Mountains was a constant struggle. Food was scarce; sometimes there was none. After days of pushing their way through fallen timber, along barely discernible trails, they staggered, half starved, into the territory of the Nez Perce Indians. At first, the Nez Perce wanted to kill the strange intruders, but an old woman, who had been befriended by a white person while a prisoner in the East, persuaded them to spare their lives. The Indians became loyal friends, supplying and guiding the expedition.

Like many others of his day, Jefferson thought the portage from the Missouri River to the Columbia River would be short; perhaps there would be a direct connection between the two rivers. The "connection" was, in fact, 340 miles long, with 60 of them over "tremendious mountains" covered with snow. The journey down the Snake River and into the valley of the Columbia River was a relief, drifting downstream instead of hauling supplies on reluctant, stumbling horses, up mountains and through forests. Salmon became part of the diet and, in place of deer or elk, dogs became a common and, for many, a favorite food.

On November 7, 1805, Clark saw the sea. "Ocian in view! O! the joy!," he wrote in his diary. The explorers searched a long time for a good campsite until choosing what became Fort Clatsop, their log cabin camp for the winter. Like Fort Mandan, it was built to keep out inquisitive Indians. Lewis had been ordered by Jefferson to take every precaution against fighting with the Indians and had been very successful in avoiding trouble. The Clatsop Indians were not aggressive and had already traded with western sailors; but in some ways, they were too friendly, bringing girls to the camp, a temptation the men could not resist. They paid for their indulgence with the acquisition of venereal disease, repeating their experiences of the previous winter at the Mandan village.

The winter at Fort Clatsop was cold and wet. Between November 4 and March 25, only 12 days were free of rain and only six were sunny. The diet was often nothing but spoiled elk, alternated with pounded fish and a handful of roots. A whale washed up on the shore, and the blubber and oil provided a pleasant new taste. There was the usual toll of accidents. One man cut his leg badly with a knife. Another developed severe low back pain that crippled him for weeks until he was cured by a sweat bath, alternating heat with cold.

In March 1806 the Corps of Discovery launched their canoes on the river and set their course for home. Their delight was great but their troubles were not over. Crossing the mountains at first proved to be impossible because of deep, lingering snows. The expedition had to wait for several weeks, bargaining and competing with the Nez Perce in athletic contests and horse races. The trinkets they had brought as trade goods had been used up. One service remained that could be traded for food or horses—medical aid. Clark proved to be a popular doctor with the Indians. He treated their sore eyes, set their fractures, and tried to cure a chief who was paralyzed by treating him in a sweat bath. However, he did not always treat with grace, calling one patient "a sulky bitch." Lewis had twinges of conscience in allowing the Indians to think that Clark was a doctor but excused the mild deception as necessary to get the horses and food they needed to continue.

After the expedition finally crossed the mountains and left the Nez Perce guides behind, they divided into two groups—one to explore the Yellowstone River, and the other, led by Lewis, to go north along the Marias River.

All went well with Lewis and the three men with him until they met a party of Blackfoot Indians, the most warlike tribe in the area. After nervous greetings, the two groups spent the night around the same campfire. The next morning, the braves tried to steal a gun and horses. One of Lewis' men ran after the thief who had stolen his gun and stabbed him to death, and Lewis shot and killed the horse thief. It was the first time anyone in the Corps of Discovery had killed an Indian. Lewis and his men mounted their horses and made a dramatic escape, riding more than 100 miles in 24 hours before joining up with the rest of the expedition.

A few weeks later, one of the hunters, Cruzatte, who had bad eyesight, and Lewis were hunting a wounded elk in thick willows and riverside brush. Cruzatte thought he saw an elk, shot, and hit the buckskinclothed Lewis in the buttock. The treatment Lewis gave himself was as good as might be given today under similar circumstances. Drains were inserted into the entrance and exit wounds, which were dressed. The bullet was found in Lewis' clothing, so no attempt had to be made to find it in the wound, which was the standard treatment of the day. Fortunately, the wound did not become infected, and within a few weeks, before the end of the voyage, Lewis was completely healed.

On September 23, 1806, the expedition reached St. Louis. They had been away for 2 years and 4 months and had journeyed more than 8000 miles. Lewis reported to the President:

> In obedience to your orders we have penitrated the Continent of North America to the Pacific Ocean, and sufficiently explored the interior of the country to affirm with confidence that we have discovered the most practicable rout which does exist across the continent by means of the navigable branches of the Missouri and Columbia Rivers.

Looking back, one can only be amazed at the medical success of the expedition, which returned with the loss of only one man. Was it skill? Was it luck? Was the trip a tribute to the endurance and resistance of the human body to cold, heat, starvation, insects, injuries, and medications that could have done more harm than good? The bear that attacked Meriwether Lewis turned away at the end of a bluff charge. The wolf that bit the sleeping sergeant was not rabid. When rattlesnakes struck, no serious injuries resulted. The cuts by knives and wounds from prickly pears caused no major infections. No man became blind. No limbs were lost to frostbite. The lead ball shot into Lewis was recovered in his clothing, so there was no dirty surgery. Sacagawea recovered, perhaps because the water that Lewis gave her from a mineral spring restored her electrolyte losses. Pompey, Sacagawea's son, recovered from a lifethreatening abscess in his neck without the benefit of antibiotics. When Lewis used his penknife to bleed a man, septicemia did not follow.

The medicine chest contained little of therapeutic value except opium and laudanum. Peruvian bark, related to quinine, could have been useful for malaria, but there is no evidence that malaria was a problem. The ferocious laxatives fortunately caused little but discomfort. Tartar emetic was not needed because no man ingested poison. The lancets for bleeding were, mercifully, used sparingly.

Could a modern doctor have done better? Not much. Some illnesses might have been shortened, some pain relieved, but many more medications would have been dispensed, more lacerations sutured, and perhaps even snakebite antivenom administered. Sergeant Floyd might only have been saved by a heroic operation under imperfect circumstances. So, the expedition would still probably have returned with the loss of one man and the medical bill would have been much greater than 96 dollars and 69 cents.

REFERENCES

1. Elliott Coues, editor: *The history of the Lewis and Clark expedition,* vols I-III, New York, 1893, Francis P Harper; unabridged reprint by Dover Publications, 1998.
2. Ambrose SE: *Undaunted courage: Meriwether Lewis, Thomas Jefferson and the opening of the American West,* New York, 1996, Simon and Schuster.
3. Dillon R: *Meriwether Lewis, a biography,* Santa Cruz, Calif, 1988, Western Tanager Press.

Bruce C. Paton, MD
Emeritus Clinical Professor of Surgery,
University of Colorado Health Sciences Center,
Denver, Colorado

Preface

This fourth edition of *Wilderness Medicine* is designed to be a great improvement over the previous edition. It is necessarily expanded in girth in order to accommodate additional topics of relevance to medical professionals called upon to rescue, diagnose, and treat victims in outdoor environments. The specialty of wilderness medicine continues to mature, as most of the active participants in its progress come to agree on the body of knowledge that must be mastered to promote its science and create effective practitioners.

Outdoor pursuits comprise the fastest growing segment of recreational life in the United States, and perhaps the world. Men and women of all nationalities have become travelers and adventurers in unprecedented numbers, and the related encounters with risk and danger have kept pace. The widely publicized tragedies that afflict climbers on Mount Everest, victims of avalanches, and explorers in hazardous seas regularly heighten our awareness of the powerful natural forces that prevail despite our best intentions and preventive efforts. As we climb into rarified air, sled over thin ice, eschew safety ropes and helmets, and stretch the limits of our diving decompression algorithms, we will be reminded of our vulnerability and limitations on a planet that shows no mercy in its most terrifying moments. Therein lies the relevance, challenge, and opportunity for wilderness medicine.

In seeking to understand the pathophysiology of high altitude, we witness the beauty of pristine rock faces and summits. While we learn to repel sharks, we marvel at the rainbow colors of the barrier reefs. In the quest for a cure for malaria, the tropical scientist gazes into the emerald canopy of the rainforest. As we battle forest fires and survive the lightning and fierce winds of a thunderstorm, our attention is drawn to a herd of bison stampeding across a grass prairie that stretches as far as the imagination. No medical specialty or healthcare-related avocation is more connected to this planet than is wilderness medicine. My colleagues and I, and everyone else involved in outdoor health and wilderness medicine, could not be more fortunate.

Wilderness medicine is presented here by experts and devotees. For example, the integration of basic science and clinical art is blended brilliantly in the chapters on heat-related illness. In recognition of our aging population, a new chapter is devoted to elders. A significant upgrade to the content is embodied by the non-medical topics, such as the information on navigation, clothing, backcountry equipment, and ropes and knot tying. Wilderness medicine practitioners have long recognized that essential survival skills may need to be deployed by healers when outfitters and guides cannot function at full capacity. The physician who can recite everything there is to know about exposure to the sun and treatment of dehydration must also be able to pitch in and gather water; knowing how to avoid a shark attack is just as important as knowing how to treat a shark attack victim.

A new information age is upon us. The Internet allows us to link "many to many," and to collect information from disparate locations in a hugely expedited fashion. However, it isn't yet a perfect filter for the reliability of the content, and so there is still much to be said for sitting down with a good book. *Wilderness Medicine* is meant to be a reference, but also to be a stimulus for inquiry and adventure. The publisher and I have worked hard to keep it to a manageable size, and the addition of color images throughout the book and emphasis on practical matters make this the most complete and relevant edition to date.

Wilderness Medicine has become a life's work, and will continue to grow. In addition, the Wilderness Medical Society; the journal *Wilderness and Environmental Medicine* (recently accepted into the *Index Medicus*); a plethora of continuing medical education programs in wilderness medicine, diving medicine, adventure and travel medicine, and outdoor health; *Field Guide to Wilderness Medicine*; the book for laypersons *Medicine for the Outdoors*; and all of the opportunities yet to come by virtue of television and the Internet have propelled this 20-year effort into an established medical discipline for as long as there will be wilderness.

I am grateful for Kathy Falk and Rick Dudley, my editors for this fourth edition. The contributors, some of whom have been with this book since its inception and who continue to learn, teach, and enhance this field, share my enormous thanks and respect. With great pleasure, I can now observe the activities of my children, and the children of many of the contributors, as they continue to increase their appreciation for the wilderness and outdoor health. In the continuing endeavor of *Wilderness Medicine,* I am in many ways the luckiest editor on Earth.

Paul S. Auerbach

Contents

WILDERNESS
MEDICINE

Mountain Medicine

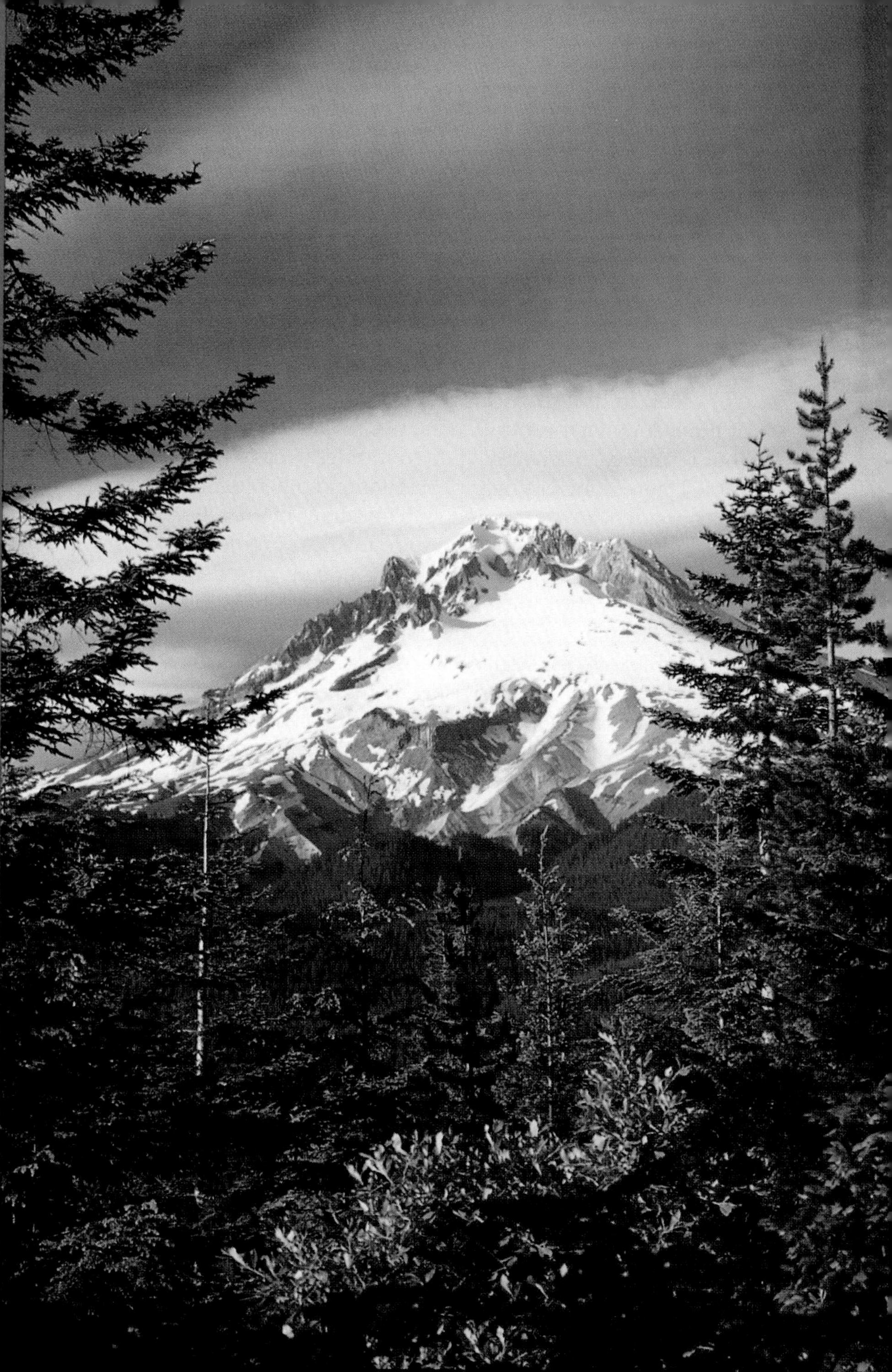

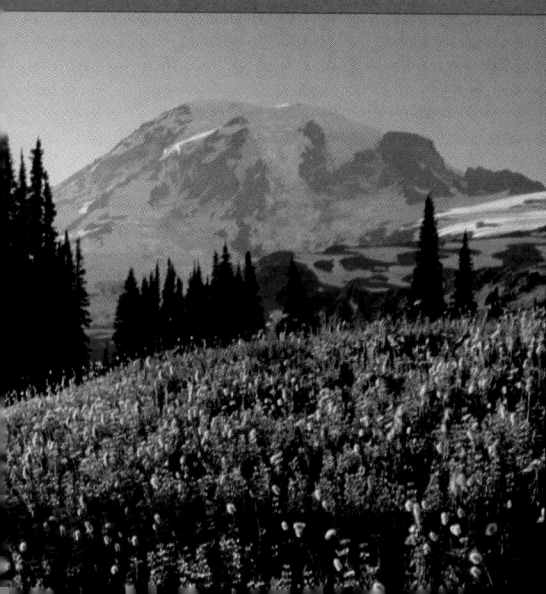

1

1 High-Altitude Medicine

Peter H. Hackett and Robert C. Roach

Millions of persons visit recreation areas above 2400 m (7874 feet) in the American West each year. Hundreds of thousands visit central and south Asia, Africa, and South America, many traveling to altitudes over 4000 m (13,124 feet).[234] Increasingly, physicians and other health care providers are confronted with questions of prevention and treatment of high-altitude medical problems (Box 1-1), as well as the effects of altitude on preexisting medical conditions. Despite advances in high-altitude medicine, significant morbidity and mortality persist (Table 1-1). Clearly, better education of the population at risk and those advising them is essential. This chapter reviews the basic physiology of ascent to high altitude, as well as the pathophysiology, recognition, and management of medical problems associated with high altitude. Much of the information presented in this chapter is drawn from major high-altitude physiology and medical studies of the last 40 years, with an emphasis on the last decade (see the recent reviews by Houston,[139] Nakashima,[246] Richalet,[272] and West[355]).

DEFINITIONS

High Altitude (1500 to 3500 m [4921 to 11,483 feet])

The onset of physiologic effects of diminished P_{IO_2} includes decreased exercise performance and increased ventilation (lower arterial P_{CO_2}) (Box 1-2). Minor impairment exists in arterial oxygen transport (Sa_{O_2} at least 90%), but high-altitude illness is common with rapid ascent above 2500 m (8202 feet) (Table 1-2).

Very High Altitude (3500 to 5500 m [11,483 to 18,045 feet])

Maximum arterial oxygen saturation falls below 90% as the arterial P_{O_2} falls below 60 torr (Table 1-3; Figure 1-1). Extreme hypoxemia may occur during exercise, sleep, and high-altitude illness. This is the most common range for severe altitude illness.

Extreme Altitude (over 5500 m [18,045 feet])

Marked hypoxemia and hypocapnia manifest at extreme altitude. Progressive deterioration of physiologic function eventually outstrips acclimatization. As a result, no permanent human habitation is above 5500 m (18,045 feet). A period of acclimatization is necessary when ascending to extreme altitude; abrupt ascent without supplemental oxygen for other than brief exposures invites severe altitude illness.

ENVIRONMENT AT HIGH ALTITUDE

Barometric pressure falls with increasing altitude in a logarithmic fashion (see Table 1-2). Therefore the partial pressure of oxygen (21% of barometric pressure) also decreases, resulting in the primary insult of high altitude: hypoxia. At approximately 5800 m (19,030 feet), barometric pressure is one half that at sea level, and on the summit of Mt. Everest (8848 m [29,029 feet]) the inspired pressure of oxygen is approximately 28% that at sea level (see Figure 1-1 and Table 1-2).

The relationship of barometric pressure to altitude changes with the distance from the equator. Thus polar regions afford greater hypoxia at high altitude, as well as extreme cold. West[354] has calculated that the barometric pressure on the summit of Mt. Everest (27° N latitude) would be about 222 torr instead of 253 torr if Everest were located at the latitude of Mt. McKinley (62° N). Such a difference, he claims, would be sufficient to render an ascent without supplemental oxygen impossible.

In addition to the role of latitude, fluctuations related to season, weather, and temperature affect the pressure-altitude relationship. Pressure is lower in winter than in summer. A low-pressure trough can reduce pressure 10 torr in one night on Mt. McKinley, making climbers awaken "physiologically higher" by 200 m (656 feet). The degree of hypoxia, then, is directly related to the barometric pressure and not solely to geographic altitude.[354]

Temperature decreases with altitude (average of 6.5° C per 1000 m [3281 feet]), and the effects of cold and hypoxia are generally additive in provoking both cold injuries and altitude problems.[269,351] Ultraviolet light penetration increases approximately 4% per 300-m (984-foot) gain in altitude, increasing the risk of sunburn, skin cancer, and snowblindness. Reflection of sunlight in glacial cirques and on flat glaciers can cause intense radiation of heat in the absence of wind. We have observed temperatures of 40° to 42° C in tents on both Mt. Everest and Mt. McKinley. Heat problems, primarily heat exhaustion, are often unrecognized in this usually cold environment. Physiologists have not yet examined the consequences of heat stress or rapid, extreme changes in environmental temperature combined with the hypoxia of high altitude.

Above the snow line is the "high-altitude desert," where water can be obtained only by melting snow or ice. This factor, combined with increased water loss

Box 1-1 POTENTIAL MEDICAL PROBLEMS OF LOWLANDERS ON ASCENT TO HIGH ALTITUDE

Acute hypoxia
High-altitude headache
Acute mountain sickness
High-altitude cerebral edema
Cerebrovascular syndromes
High-altitude pulmonary edema
High-altitude deterioration
Organic brain syndrome

Peripheral edema
Retinopathy
Disordered sleep
Sleep periodic breathing
High-altitude pharyngitis and bronchitis
Ultraviolet keratitis (snowblindness)
Exacerbation of preexisting illness

TABLE 1-1. Incidence of Altitude Illness in Various Groups

STUDY GROUP	NUMBER AT RISK PER YEAR	SLEEPING ALTITUDE (m)	MAXIMUM ALTITUDE REACHED (m)	AVERAGE RATE OF ASCENT*	PERCENT WITH AMS	PERCENT WITH HAPE AND/OR HACE	REFERENCE
Western State visitors	30 million	~2000	3500	1-2	18-20	0.01	134
		~2500			22		
		~≥3000			27-42		68
Mt. Everest trekkers	6000	3000-5200	5500	1-2 (fly in)	47	1.6	106
				10-13 (walk in)	23	0.05	
9				Not specified	30-50		243
Mt. McKinley climbers	1200	3000-5300	6194	3-7	30	2-3	111
Mt. Rainier climbers	10,000	3000	4392	1-2	67	—	188
Mt. Rosa, Swiss Alps	†	2850	2850	1-2	7	—	201
		4559	4559	2-3	27	5	64,201
Indian soldiers	Unknown	3000-5500	5500	1-2	†	2.3-15.5	320, 321

AMS, Acute mountain sickness; HACE, high-altitude cerebral edema; HAPE, high-altitude pulmonary edema.
*Days to sleeping altitude from low altitude.
†Reliable estimate unavailable.

Box 1-2 GLOSSARY OF PHYSIOLOGIC TERMS

P_B Barometric pressure (torr)
P_{O_2} Partial pressure of oxygen
P_{IO_2} Inspired P_{O_2} [$0.21 \times P_B - 47$ torr (vapor pressure of H_2O at $37°$ C)]
P_{AO_2} P_{O_2} in alveolus
P_{ACO_2} P_{CO_2} in alveolus
P_{aO_2} P_{O_2} in arterial blood

P_{aCO_2} P_{CO_2} in arterial blood
$S_{aO_2}\%$ Arterial oxygen saturation % (HbO_2/total Hb $\times$ 100)
R Respiratory quotient (CO_2 produced/O_2 consumed)

Alveolar gas equation: $P_{aO_2} = P_{IO_2} - P_{aCO_2}/R$

TABLE 1-2. Altitude Conversion, Barometric Pressure, Estimated Partial Pressure of Inspired Oxygen, and the Related Oxygen Concentration at Sea Level*

m	ft	P_B	P_{IO_2}	F_{IO_2} at SL	m	ft	P_B	P_{IO_2}	F_{IO_2} at SL
Sea Level		759.6	149.1	0.209	5486	18000	394.6	72.8	0.102
1000	3281	678.7	132.2	0.185	5500	18045	393.9	72.6	0.102
1219	4000	661.8	128.7	0.180	5791	19000	379.5	69.6	0.098
1500	4921	640.8	124.3	0.174	6000	19685	369.4	67.5	0.095
1524	5000	639.0	123.9	0.174	6096	20000	364.9	66.5	0.093
1829	6000	616.7	119.2	0.167	6401	21000	350.7	63.6	0.089
2000	6562	604.5	116.7	0.164	6500	21325	346.2	62.6	0.088
2134	7000	595.1	114.7	0.161	6706	22000	337.0	60.7	0.085
2438	8000	574.1	110.3	0.155	7000	22966	324.2	58.0	0.081
2500	8202	569.9	109.4	0.154	7010	23000	323.8	57.9	0.081
2743	9000	553.7	106.0	0.149	7315	24000	310.9	55.2	0.077
3000	9843	536.9	102.5	0.144	7500	24606	303.4	53.7	0.075
3048	10000	533.8	101.9	0.143	7620	25000	298.6	52.6	0.074
3353	11000	514.5	97.9	0.137	7925	26000	286.6	50.1	0.070
3500	11483	505.4	95.9	0.135	8000	26247	283.7	49.5	0.069
3658	12000	495.8	93.9	0.132	8230	27000	275.0	47.7	0.067
3962	13000	477.6	90.1	0.126	8500	27887	265.1	45.6	0.064
4000	13123	475.4	89.7	0.126	8534	28000	263.8	45.4	0.064
4267	14000	460.0	86.4	0.121	8839	29000	253.0	43.1	0.060
4500	14764	446.9	83.7	0.117	8848	29029	252.7	43.1	0.060
4572	15000	442.9	82.9	0.116	9000	29528	247.5	42.0	0.059
4877	16000	426.3	79.4	0.111	9144	30000	242.6	40.9	0.057
5000	16404	419.7	78.0	0.109	9500	31168	230.9	38.5	0.054
5182	17000	410.2	76.0	0.107	10000	32808	215.2	35.2	0.049

*Barometric pressure is approximated by the equation $P_B = Exp(6.6328 - \{0.1112 \times altitude - [0.00149 \times (altitude^2)]\})$, where altitude = terrestrial altitude in (meters/1000 or km). P_{IO_2} is calculated as the $P_B - 47$(water vapor pressure at body temperature) × fraction of O_2 in inspired air. The F_{IO_2} at sea level related to the given altitude is calculated as $P_{IO_2}/(760 - 47)$. Similar calculations for F_{IO_2} at different altitudes may be made by substituting ambient P_B for 760 in the equation.

TABLE 1-3. Blood Gases and Altitude

| POPULATION | ALTITUDE | | P_B (torr) | PaO_2 (torr) | SaO_2 (%) | $PaCO_2$ (torr) |
	METERS	FEET				
Altitude residents*	1646	5400	630	73.0 (65.0-83.0)	95.1 (93.0-97.0)	35.6 (30.7-41.8)
Acute exposure†	2810	9200	543	60.0 (47.4-73.6)	91.0 (86.6-95.2)	33.9 (31.3-36.5)
	3660	12020	489	47.6 (42.2-53.0)	84.5 (80.5-89.0)	29.5 (23.5-34.3)
	4700	15440	429	44.6 (36.4-47.5)	78.0 (70.8-85.0)	27.1 (22.9-34.0)
	5340	17500	401	43.1 (37.6-50.4)	76.2 (65.4-81.6)	25.7 (21.7-29.7)
	6140	20140	356	35.0 (26.9-40.1)	65.6 (55.5-73.0)	22.0 (19.2-24.8)
Chronic exposure	6500‡	21325	346	41.1±3.3	75.2±6	20±2.8
	7000‡	22966	324			
	8000‡	26247	284	36.6±2.2	67.8±5	12.5±1.1
	8848‡	29029	253	30.3±2.1	58±4.5	11.2±1.7
	8848§	29029	253	30.6±1.4		11.9±1.4

*Data for altitude residents from Loeppky JA, Caprihan A, Luft UC: VA/Q inequality during clinical hypoxemia and its alterations. In Shiraki K, Yousef MK, editors: *Man in stressful environments,* Springfield, Ill, 1987, Charles C Thomas.
†Data for acute exposure from McFarland RA, Dill DB: *J Aviat Med* 9:18, 1938.
‡Data for chronic exposure during Operation Everest II data are from Sutton JR et al: *J Appl Physiol* 64:1309, 1988.
§The second data set for acclimatized subjects studied during acute exposure to the simulated summit of Everest is from Richalet JP et al: Operation Everest III (COMEX '97), *Adv Exp Med Biol* 474:297, 1999.
Data are mean values and (range) or ±SD, where available. All values are for subjects age 20 to 40 years who were acclimatizing well.

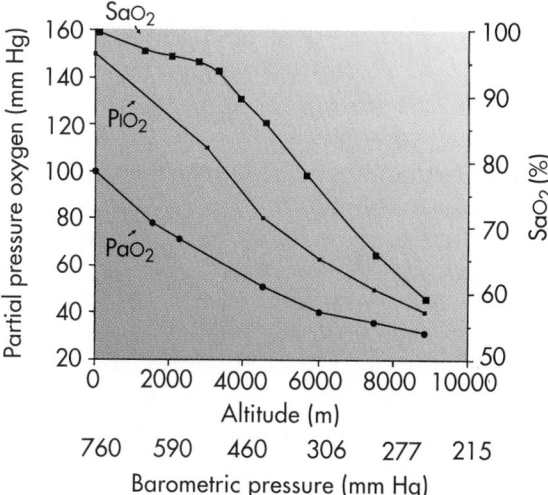

Figure 1-1 Increasing altitude results in decrease in inspired Po_2 (Pio_2), arterial Po_2 (Pao_2), and arterial oxygen saturation (Sao_2). Note that the difference between Pio_2 and Pao_2 narrows at high altitude because of increased ventilation and that Sao_2 is well maintained while awake until over 3000 m (9840 feet). (*Data from Morris A: Clinical pulmonary function tests: a manual of uniform lab procedures, Intermountain Thoracic Society, 1984; and Sutton JR et al: J Appl Physiol 64:1309, 1988.*)

through the lungs from increased respiration and through the skin, commonly results in dehydration that may be debilitating. Thus the high-altitude environment imposes multiple stresses, some of which may contribute to or be confused with the effects of hypoxia.

ACCLIMATIZATION TO HIGH ALTITUDE

Rapid exposure to the altitude at the summit of Mt. Everest causes loss of consciousness in a few minutes and death shortly thereafter. However, climbers ascending Mt. Everest over a period of weeks without supplemental oxygen have experienced only minor symptoms of illness. The process by which individuals gradually adjust to hypoxia and enhance survival and performance is termed *acclimatization*. A complex series of physiologic adjustments increases oxygen delivery to cells and improves their hypoxic tolerance. The severity of hypoxic stress, rate of onset, and individual physiology determine whether the body successfully acclimatizes or is overwhelmed.

Individuals vary in their ability to acclimatize, no doubt reflecting certain genetic polymorphisms. Some adjust quickly, without discomfort, whereas acute mountain sickness (AMS) develops in others, who go on to recover. A small percentage fail to acclimatize even with gradual exposure over weeks. The tendency to acclimatize well or to become ill is consistent on re-

peated exposure if rate of ascent and altitude gained are similar. Successful initial acclimatization protects against altitude illness and improves sleep. Longer-term acclimatization (weeks) primarily improves aerobic exercise ability. These adjustments disappear at a similar rate on descent to low altitude. A few days at low altitude may be sufficient to render a person susceptible to altitude illness, especially high-altitude pulmonary edema (HAPE), on reascent. The improved ability to do physical work at high altitude, however, persists for weeks.[198] Persons who live at high altitude during growth and development appear to realize the maximum benefit of acclimatization changes; for example, their exercise performance matches that of persons at sea level.[237] No genetic adaptation to high altitude in humans has yet been confirmed, but recent reports of normal pulmonary artery pressures and normal birth weights in Tibetans suggest selection of genetic traits for life at high altitude.[100,238,372]

Ventilation

By reducing alveolar carbon dioxide, increased ventilation raises alveolar oxygen, improving oxygen delivery (see Figure 1-1). This response starts at an altitude as low as 1500 m (4921 feet) (Pio_2 = 124 torr; see Table 1-2) and within the first few minutes to hours of high-altitude exposure. The carotid body, sensing a decrease in arterial Po_2, signals the central respiratory center in the medulla to increase ventilation. This carotid body function (hypoxic ventilatory response [HVR]) is genetically determined[352] but influenced by a number of extrinsic factors. Respiratory depressants, such as alcohol and soporifics, as well as fragmented sleep, depress the HVR. Agents that increase general metabolism, such as caffeine and coca, as well as specific respiratory stimulants, such as progesterone[182] and almitrine,[114] increase the HVR. (Acetazolamide, a respiratory stimulant, acts on the central respiratory center rather than on the carotid body.) Physical conditioning apparently has no effect on the HVR. Numerous studies have shown that a good ventilatory response enhances acclimatization and performance and that a very low HVR may contribute to illness[277] (see Acute Mountain Sickness and High-Altitude Pulmonary Edema).

Other factors influence ventilation on ascent to high altitude. As ventilation increases, hypocapnia produces alkalosis, which acts as a braking mechanism on the central respiratory center and limits a further increase in ventilation. To compensate for the alkalosis, within 24 to 48 hours of ascent the kidneys excrete bicarbonate, decreasing the pH toward normal; ventilation increases as the negative effect of the alkalosis is removed. Ventilation continues to increase slowly, reaching a maximum only after 4 to 7 days at the same altitude (Figure 1-2). The plasma bicarbonate concentration continues to drop and ventilation continues to increase with each successive increase in altitude. This process is greatly facilitated by acetazolamide (see Acetazolamide Prophylaxis).

A way to appreciate the importance of the ventilatory pump at increasing altitude is to plot values for alveolar oxygen and carbon dioxide on the Rahn-Otis diagram (Figure 1-3). This approach clearly contrasts the effects of acute and chronic hypoxic exposure and can be used to assess the degree of ventilatory acclimatization.[265] As ventilation increases, the decrease in alveolar carbon dioxide allows an equivalent increase in alveolar oxygen. The level of ventilation ($\sim$PACO$_2$) is therefore what determines alveolar oxygen for a given inspired oxygen tension, according to the alveolar gas equation: $P_{AO_2} = P_{IO_2} - P_{ACO_2}/R$. The paramount importance of hyperventilation is readily apparent from the following calculation: the alveolar PO$_2$ on the summit of Mt. Everest (about 33 torr) would be reached at only 5000 m (16,404 feet) if alveolar PCO$_2$ stayed at 40 torr, limiting an ascent without supplemental oxygen to near this altitude. Table 1-3 gives the measured arterial blood gases resulting from acclimatization to various altitudes.

Circulation

The circulatory pump is the next step in the transfer of oxygen, moving oxygenated blood from the lungs to the tissues.

Systemic Circulation. Increased sympathetic activity on ascent causes an initial mild increase in blood pressure, moderate increase in heart rate and cardiac output, and increase in venous tone. Stroke volume is low because of decreased plasma volume, which drops as much as 12% over the first 24 hours[365] as a result of the bicarbonate diuresis, a fluid shift from the intravascular space, and suppression of aldosterone.[25] Resting heart rate returns to near sea level values with acclimatization, except at extremely high altitude. Maximum heart rate follows the decline in maximal oxygen uptake with increasing altitude. As the limits of hypoxic acclimatization are approached, maximum and resting heart rates converge. During Operation Everest II (OEII), cardiac function was appropriate for the level of work performed and cardiac output was not a limiting factor for performance.[268,331] Interestingly, myocardial ischemia at high altitude has not been reported in healthy persons, despite extreme hypoxemia. This is partly because of the reduction in myocardial oxygen demand from reduced maximal heart rate and cardiac output. Pulmonary capillary wedge pressures are low, and there has been no evidence of left ventricular dysfunction or abnormal filling pressures in humans at rest.[101,158] On echocardiography, the left ventricle is smaller than normal because of de-

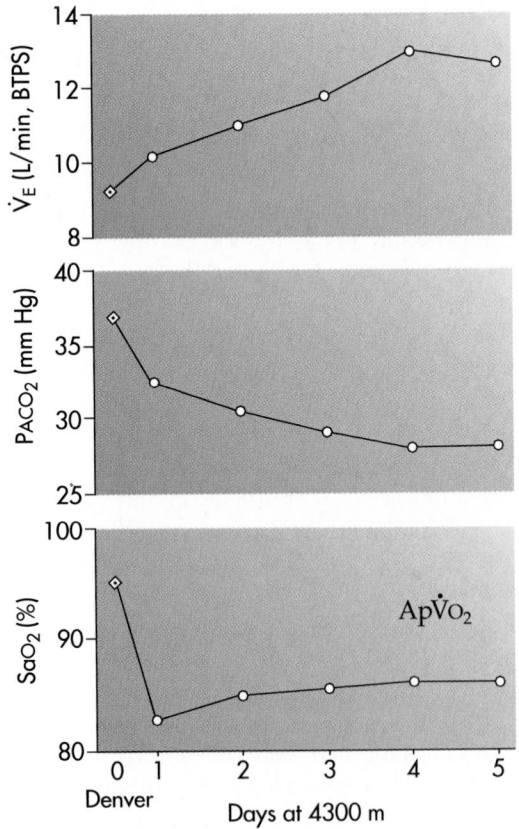

Figure 1-2 Change in minute ventilation, ($\dot{V}_E$) end-tidal carbon dioxide (PACO$_2$), and arterial oxygen saturation (SaO$_2$) during 5 days' acclimatization to 4300 m (14,104 feet). (*Modified from Huang SY et al: J Appl Physiol 56:602, 1984.*)

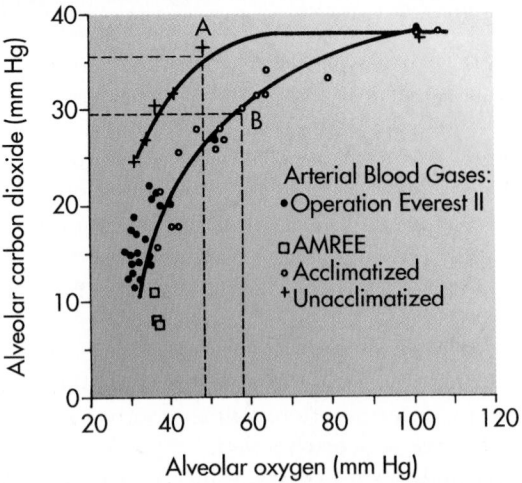

Figure 1-3 Rahn-Otis diagram, with recent data from extreme high altitude. Note that after acclimatization, alveolar oxygen is higher because of lower alveolar carbon dioxide. Point A is average alveolar gases in unacclimatized subjects (1 hour's exposure) to 3800 m (12,464 feet). Point B is after acclimatization to 3800 m (12,464 feet). (*Data from Malconian MK et al: Aviat Space Environ Med 64:37, 1993; Rahn H, Otis AB: Am J Physiol 157:445, 1949; and West JB et al: J Appl Physiol 55:688, 1983.*)

creased stroke volume, whereas the right ventricle may become enlarged.[331]

Pulmonary Circulation. A prompt but variable increase in pulmonary vascular resistance occurs on ascent to high altitude as a result of hypoxic pulmonary vasoconstriction, which increases pulmonary artery pressure. Mild pulmonary hypertension is greatly augmented by exercise, with pulmonary pressure reaching near-systemic values,[101] especially in persons with a previous history of HAPE. During OEII, Groves et al[101] demonstrated that even when associated with a mean pulmonary artery pressure of 60 torr, cardiac output remained appropriate and right atrial pressure did not rise above sea level values. This suggested that right ventricular function was intact in spite of extreme hypoxemia and hypertension.

Administration of oxygen at high altitude does not completely restore pulmonary artery pressure to sea level values, an indication that increased pulmonary vascular resistance does not result solely from hypoxic vasoconstriction.[101,156] The explanation is likely vascular remodeling with medial hypertrophy. See Stenmark et al[328] for a recent review of molecular and cellular mechanisms of the pulmonary vascular response to hypoxia, including remodeling.

Cerebral Circulation. Cerebral oxygen delivery is the product of arterial oxygen content and cerebral blood flow (CBF) and depends on the net balance between hypoxic vasodilation and hypocapnia-induced vasoconstriction. CBF increases, despite the hypocapnia, when PaO_2 is less than 60 torr (altitude greater than 2800 m [9187 feet]). In a classic study, CBF increased 24% on abrupt ascent to 3810 m (12,501 feet) and then returned to normal over 3 to 5 days.[312] More recent studies have shown considerable individual variation,[30,31,166] but overall, cerebral oxygen delivery and global cerebral metabolism are well maintained with moderate hypoxia.[67]

Blood

Hematopoietic Responses to Altitude. Ever since the observation in 1890 by Viault[345] that hemoglobin concentration was higher than normal in animals living in the Andes, scientists have regarded the hematopoietic response to increasing altitude as an important component of the acclimatization process. On the other hand, hemoglobin concentration has no relationship to susceptibility to high-altitude illness on initial ascent.

In response to hypoxemia, erythropoietin is secreted and stimulates bone marrow production of red blood cells.[309] The hormone is detectable within 2 hours of ascent, nucleated immature red blood cells can be found on a peripheral blood smear within days, and new red blood cells are in circulation within 4 to 5 days. Over a period of weeks to months, red blood cell mass increases in proportion to the degree of hypoxemia. Iron supplementation can be important: women who take supplemental iron at high altitude approach the hematocrit values of men at altitude[122] (Figure 1-4).

Overshoot of the hematopoietic response causes excessive polycythemia, which may actually impair oxygen transport because of increased blood viscosity. Although the "ideal" hematocrit at high altitude is not established, phlebotomy is often recommended when hematocrit values exceed 60% to 65%. During the American Medical Research Expedition to Mt. Everest (AMREE), hematocrit was reduced by hemodilution from 58% ± 1.3% to 50.5% ± 1.5% at 5400 m (17,717 feet) with no decrement in maximum oxygen uptake and an increase in cerebral functioning.[299] The increase in hemoglobin concentration seen 1 to 2 days after ascent is due to hemoconcentration secondary to decreased plasma volume rather than a true increase in red blood cell mass. This results in a higher hemoglobin concentration at the cost of decreased blood volume, a trade-off that might impair exercise performance. Longer-term acclimatization leads to an increase in plasma volume, as well as in red blood cell mass, thereby increasing total blood volume.

Oxyhemoglobin Dissociation Curve. The oxyhemoglobin dissociation curve plays a crucial role in oxygen transport. Because of the sigmoidal shape of the curve, $SaO_2\%$ is well maintained up to 3000 m (9843 feet) despite a significant decrease in arterial PO_2 (see Figure 1-1). Above that altitude, small changes in arterial PO_2 result in large changes in arterial oxygen saturation (Figure 1-5).

In 1936, Keys et al[173] demonstrated an in vitro right shift in the position of the oxyhemoglobin dissociation curve at high altitude, a shift that favors the release of oxygen from the blood to the tissues. This change occurs because of the increase in 2,3-diphosphoglycerate

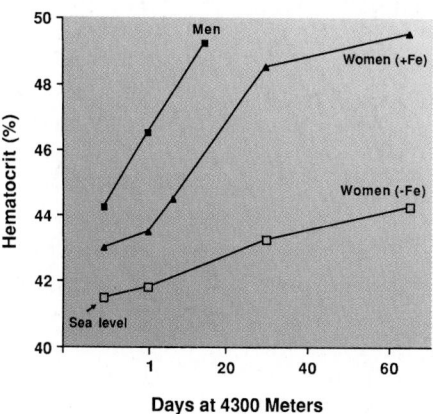

Figure 1-4 Hematocrit changes on ascent to altitude in men and in women with and without supplemental iron. (*Modified from Hannon JP, Chinn KS, Shields JL: Fed Proc 28:1178, 1969.*)

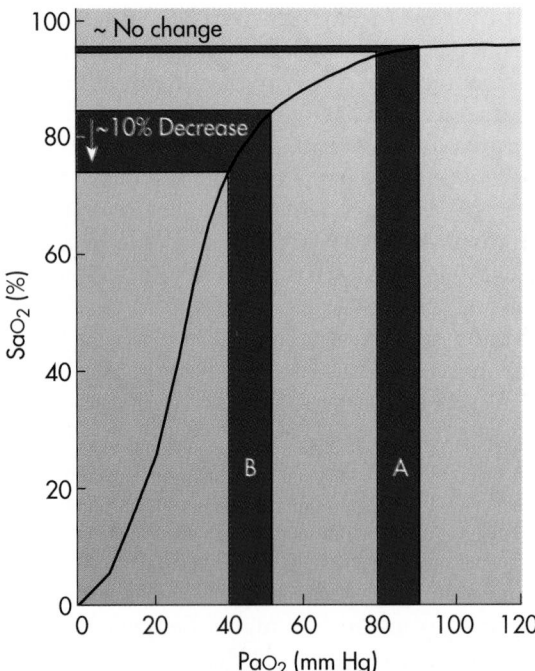

Figure 1-5 Oxyhemoglobin dissociation curve showing effect of 10-torr decrement in Pao$_2$ *(shaded areas)* on arterial oxygen saturation at **A,** sea level, and **B,** near 4400 m (14,432 feet). Note the much larger drop in Sao$_2$ at high altitude. *(Modified from Severinghaus JW et al: Circ Res 19:274, 1966.)*

(2,3-DPG), which is proportional to the severity of hypoxemia. In vivo, however, this is offset by alkalosis, and at moderate altitude little net change occurs in the position of the oxyhemoglobin dissociation curve. On the other hand, the marked alkalosis of extreme hyperventilation, as measured on the summit and simulated summit of Mt. Everest (Pco$_2$ 8 to 10 torr, pH greater than 7.5), shifts the oxyhemoglobin dissociation curve to the left, which facilitates oxyhemoglobin binding in the lung, raises Sao$_2$%, and is thought to be advantageous.[297] This concept is further supported by observing that when persons with a very left-shifted oxygen-hemoglobin curve, caused by an abnormal hemoglobin (Andrew-Minneapolis), were taken to moderate (3100 m [10,171 feet]) altitude, they had less tachycardia and dyspnea and remarkably had no decrease in exercise performance.[127]

Tissue Changes

The next link in the oxygen transport chain is tissue oxygen transfer, which depends on capillary perfusion, diffusion distance, and driving pressure of oxygen from the capillary to the cell. The final link, then, is use of oxygen within the cell. Banchero[13] has shown that capillary density in dog skeletal muscle doubled in 3 weeks at a barometric pressure of 435 torr. A recent study in humans noted higher-than-normal muscle capillary density, although it was impossible to determine whether this was an adaptation to high altitude or to physical training.[253] Ou and Tenney[256] revealed a 40% increase in mitochondrial number but no change in mitochondrial size, whereas the study of Oelz et al[253] showed that high-altitude climbers had normal mitochondrial density. During OEII, a significant reduction in muscle size was noted, and although no de novo synthesis of capillaries or mitochondria occurred, capillary density and the ratio of mitochondrial volume to contractile protein fraction increased, primarily as a result of the atrophy.[199] Nevertheless, this change decreased the diffusion distance for oxygen.

Sleep At High Altitude

Disturbed sleep is common at high altitude. Reite et al[270] studied six men during a 12-day stay at 4300 m (14,108 feet). All subjects complained of disturbed sleep. Compared with sea level control studies, stages 3 and 4 sleep were reduced, stage 1 time increased, and stage 2 did not change. More time was spent awake, with a significant increase in arousals and slightly less rapid eye movement (REM) time. The subjective complaints of poor sleep were out of proportion to the small reduction in total sleep time. Five of the six had periodic breathing. Interestingly, the arousals were not necessarily related to periodic breathing. One subject had periodic breathing for 90% of the night and no recorded arousals. With more extreme hypoxia, sleep time was dramatically shortened and arousals increased, without a change in ratio of sleep stages but with a reduction in REM sleep.[5] Presumably, the mechanism of the arousals is cerebral hypoxia. Periodic breathing appears to play only a minor role in altering sleep architecture at high altitude.[296]

Periodic Breathing. Periodic breathing is primarily a nocturnal phenomenon, characterized by hyperpnea followed by apnea (Figure 1-6). Respiratory alkalosis during hyperpnea acts on the central respiratory center, causing apnea. During apnea, Sao$_2$% decreases, carbon dioxide level increases, and the carotid body is stimulated, causing a recurrent hyperpnea and apnea cycle. Persons with a high HVR have more periodic breathing, with mild oscillations in Sao$_2$%,[184] whereas persons with a low HVR have more regular breathing overall but may suffer periods of apnea with extreme hypoxemia distinct from periodic breathing.[114] As acclimatization progresses, periodic breathing lessens but does not disappear and Sao$_2$% increases (Figure 1-7).[5,333] Periodic breathing has not been implicated in the etiology of high-altitude illness, but a chaotic pattern without apparent periodicity was found in HAPE-susceptible subjects.[91] Eichenberger et al[81] have also reported greater periodic breathing in those with HAPE, secondary to lower Sao$_2$%.

Acetazolamide, 125 mg at bedtime, diminishes peri-

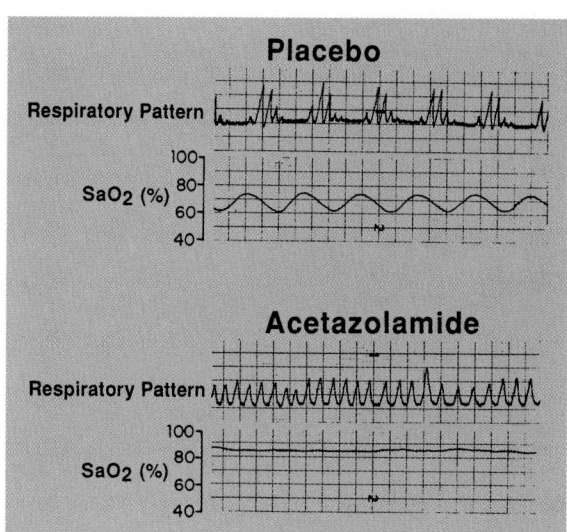

Figure 1-6 Respiratory patterns and arterial oxygen saturation (SaO₂) with placebo and acetazolamide in two sleep studies of a subject at 4200 m (13,776 feet). Note pattern of hyperpnea followed by apnea during placebo treatment, which is changed with acetazolamide. (*Modified from Hackett PH et al: Am Rev Respir Dis 135:896, 1987.*)

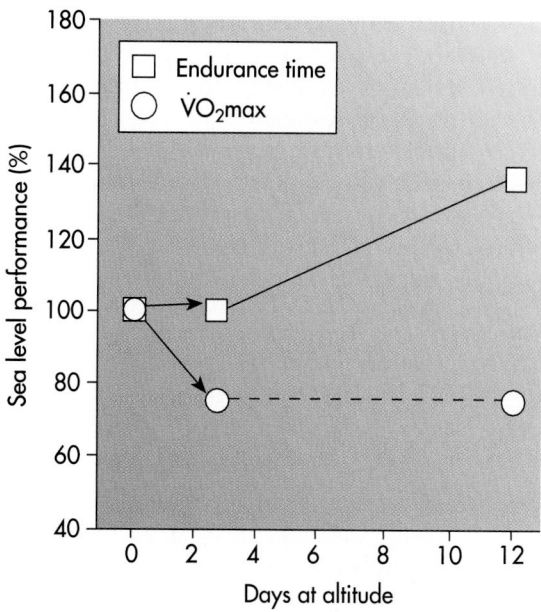

Figure 1-8 On ascent to altitude, $\dot{V}O_2$ max decreases and remains suppressed. In contrast, endurance time (minutes to exhaustion at 75% of altitude-specific $\dot{V}O_2$ max) increases with acclimatization. (*Modified from Maher JT, Jones LG, Hartley LH: J Appl Physiol 37:895, 1974.*)

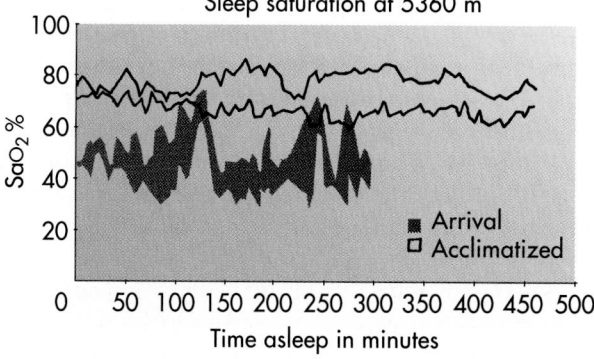

Figure 1-7 Sleep oxygenation improves with acclimatization to same altitude. Top line is maximum and bottom line is minimum SaO₂ in an acclimatized person. Shaded area is maximum and minimum SaO₂ values for new arrival at 5360 m (17,581 feet). (*Modified from Sutton JR et al: N Engl J Med 301:1329, 1979.*)

odic breathing, improves oxygenation, and is a safe and superior agent to use as a sleeping aid (see Figures 1-6 and 1-7). If insomnia is due to causes other than periodic breathing, diphenhydramine (Benadryl, 50 to 75 mg) or the short-acting benzodiazepines, such as triazolam (Halcion, 0.125 to 0.25 mg) and temazepam (Restoril, 15 mg), can be used. However, these are potentially dangerous in ill persons at high altitude because of resulting respiratory depression, and they may decrease oxygenation even in persons who are accli-

matizing well. Bradwell et al[44] showed that acetazolamide (500 mg slow-release orally) given with temazepam (10 mg orally) improved sleep and maintained SaO₂%, counteracting a 20% decrease in SaO₂% when temazepam was given alone. A new, nonbenzodiazapine hypnotic, zolpidem (Ambien, 10 mg) was recently shown to improve sleep at 4000 m (13,123 feet) without adversely affecting ventilation.[32]

Exercise

Maximal oxygen consumption drops dramatically on ascent to high altitude (see references 92 and 278 for recent reviews). Maximal oxygen uptake ($\dot{V}O_2$ max) falls approximately 10% for each 1000 m (3281 feet) of altitude gained above 1500 m (4921 feet). Those with the highest sea level $\dot{V}O_2$ max values have the largest decrement in $\dot{V}O_2$ max at high altitude, but overall performance at high altitude is not consistently related to sea level $\dot{V}O_2$ max.[253,273,356] In fact, many of the world's elite mountaineers have quite average $\dot{V}O_2$ max values, in contrast to other endurance athletes.[253] Acclimatization at moderate altitudes enhances submaximal endurance time but not $\dot{V}O_2$ max (Figure 1-8).[92] Preliminary recent work suggests that genetic factors may play a role in determining exercise performance in mountaineers at high altitude. Montgomery et al identified a polymorphism in the gene encoding angiotensin converting enzyme (ACE) that was strongly related to mountaineering performance in 25 British mountaineers.[233] The mechanism by which an ACE gene polymorphism could enhance exercise performance at high altitude is unknown but provides interesting and important direction for further investigations.

Oxygen transport during exercise at high altitude becomes increasingly dependent on the ventilatory pump. The marked rise in ventilation produces a sensation of breathlessness, even at low work levels. The following quotation is from a high-altitude mountaineer:

> After every few steps, we huddle over our ice axes, mouths agape, struggling for sufficient breath to keep our muscles going. I have the feeling I am about to burst apart. As we get higher, it becomes necessary to lie down to recover our breath.[222]

In contrast to the increase in ventilation with exercise, at increasing altitudes in OEII, cardiac function and cardiac output were maintained at or near sea level values for a given oxygen consumption (workload).[268] Although related to decreased oxygen transport, the exact limiting factors to exercise at high altitude remain elusive. Wagner[350] has proposed that the pressure gradient for diffusion of oxygen from capillaries to the working muscle cells may be inadequate. Another concept is that increased cerebral hypoxia from exercise-induced desaturation is the limiting factor.[57] Mountaineers, for example, become lightheaded and their vision dims when they move too quickly at extreme altitude (Figure 1-9).[353]

Training at High Altitude. Optimal training for increased performance at high altitude depends on the altitude of residence and the athletic event. For aerobic activities (events lasting more than 3 or 4 minutes) at altitudes above 2000 m (6562 feet), acclimatization for 10 to 20 days is necessary to maximize performance.[202] For events occurring above 4000 m (13,123 feet), acclimatization at an intermediate altitude is recommended. Highly anaerobic events at intermediate altitudes require only arrival at the time of the event, although mountain sickness may become a problem.

The benefits of training at high altitude for subsequent performance at or near sea level depend on choosing the training altitude that maximizes the benefits and minimizes the "detraining" inevitable when maximal oxygen uptake is limited (altitude greater than 1500 to 2000 m [4921 to 6562 feet]). Hence, data from training above 2400 m (7874 feet) have shown no increase in subsequent sea level performance. Balke, Nagle, and Daniels[12] returned subjects to sea level after 10 days' training at 2000 m (6562 feet) and demonstrated an increase in aerobic power, plasma volume, and hemoglobin concentration, with faster running times. More recent work suggests training benefits from intermittent altitude exposure[192] and from training at low altitude while sleeping at high alti-

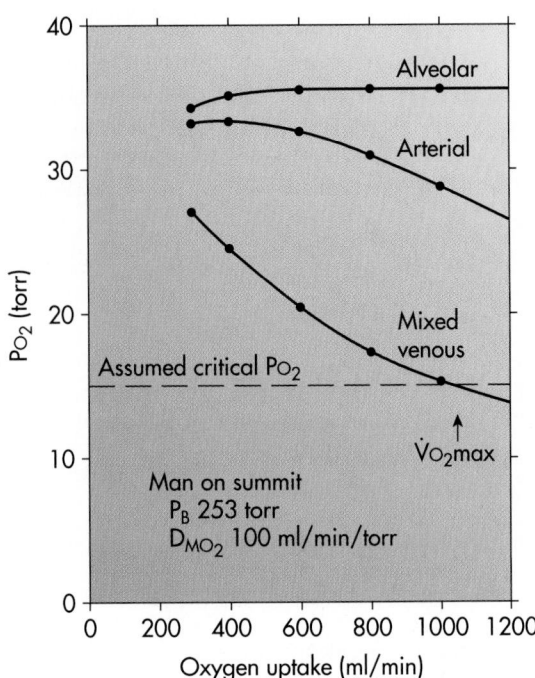

Figure 1-9 Calculated changes in the P_{O_2} of alveolar gas and arterial and mixed venous blood as oxygen uptake is increased for a climber on the summit of Mt. Everest. Unconsciousness develops at a mixed venous P_{O_2} of 15 torr. DM_{O_2}, Muscle O_2 diffusing capacity. (*Modified from West JB: Respir Physiol 52:265, 1983.*)

tude.[11,194,329] Coaches and endurance athletes from around the world are convinced of the benefits of training and/or sleeping at moderate altitude to improve sea level performance.[10,40,71] The benefit appears to be due to enhanced erythropoietin production and increased red cell mass, which requires adequate iron stores, and thus usually iron supplementation.[204,285,330]

HIGH-ALTITUDE SYNDROMES

High-altitude syndromes are illnesses attributed directly to hypobaric hypoxia. Exact mechanisms, however, are unclear. For example, all persons at a given high altitude are hypoxic and those with AMS are barely more hypoxemic than those who are well.[99,132] Also, there is a delay from the onset of hypoxia to the onset of high-altitude illness. These two facts have led to the conclusion that hypoxia induces time-dependent processes that are responsible for AMS, in contrast to the syndrome of acute hypoxia.

Considerable overlap exists among the high-altitude syndromes, and terminology and classification of high-altitude illness remain somewhat confusing. Sudden exposure to extreme altitude may result in death from acute hypoxia (asphyxia), whereas more gradual ascent to the same altitude may result in AMS or no illness at all. Where symptoms of acute hypoxia end and AMS begins is vague, as reflected in the classic experiments of Bert.[37] In terms of altitude illness, the general concept of a spectrum of illness with a common underlying pathogenesis is well accepted and provides a useful framework for discussion. We find it useful to separate the syndrome into neurologic and pulmonary components. For the neurologic syndromes, the spectrum progresses from AMS to high-altitude cerebral edema (HACE). In the lung, the spectrum includes pulmonary hypertension, interstitial edema, and HAPE. These problems all occur within the first few days of ascent to a higher altitude, have many common features, and respond to descent and oxygen. Longer-term problems of altitude exposure include high-altitude deterioration and chronic mountain sickness.

Neurologic Syndromes

The numerous neurologic syndromes at high altitude reflect the nervous system's sensitivity to hypoxia. The spectrum of clinical effects ranges from subtle cognitive changes to death from gross cerebral edema. Acute hypoxia is also included here because it is essentially a neurologic insult. We consider AMS and HACE as manifestations of a common underlying pathophysiology of vasogenic edema, but we give special consideration to high-altitude headache, which might have a number of mechanisms. Acute hypoxia and cognitive dysfunction are related to neurotransmitter dysfunction, whereas the focal neurologic syndromes, such as transient ischemic attack (TIA) and stroke, are related to secondary ischemia.

Acute Hypoxia

Acute, profound hypoxia, although of greatest interest in aviation medicine, may also occur on terra firma when ascent is too rapid or when hypoxia abruptly worsens. Carbon monoxide poisoning, pulmonary edema, overexertion, sleep apnea, or a failed oxygen delivery system may rapidly exaggerate hypoxemia. In an unacclimatized person, loss of consciousness from acute hypoxia occurs at an SaO_2 of 40% to 60% or at an arterial Po_2 of less than about 30 torr.[36] Tissandier, the sole survivor of the flight of the balloon Zenith in 1875, gave a graphic description of the effects of acute hypoxia:

But soon I was keeping absolutely motionless, without suspecting that perhaps I had already lost use of my movements. Towards 7,500 m, the numbness one experiences is extraordinary. The body and the mind weakens little by little, gradually, unconsciously, without one's knowledge. One does not suffer at all; on the contrary. One experiences inner joy, as if it were an effect of the inundating flood of light. One becomes indifferent; one no longer thinks of the perilous situation or of the danger; one rises and is happy to rise. Vertigo of the lofty regions is not a vain word. But as far as I can judge by my personal impression, this vertigo appears at the last moment; it immediately precedes annihilation—sudden, unexpected, irresistible. I wanted to seize the oxygen tube, but could not

raise my arm. My mind, however, was still very lucid. I was still looking at the barometer; my eyes were fixed on the needle which soon reached the pressure number of 280, beyond which it passed. I wanted to cry out "We are at 8,000 meters." But my tongue was paralyzed. Suddenly I closed my eyes and fell inert, completely losing consciousness.[37]

The ascent to over 8000 m (26,247 feet) took 3 hours, and the descent less than 1 hour. When the balloon landed, Tissandier's two companions were dead.

The prodigious work that Paul Bert conducted in an altitude chamber during the 1870s showed that lack of oxygen, rather than an effect of isolated hypobaria, explained the symptoms experienced during rapid ascent to extreme altitude:

There exists a parallelism to the smallest details between two animals, one of which is subjected in normal air to a progressive diminution of pressure to the point of death, while the other breathes, also to the point of death, under normal pressure, an air that grows weaker and weaker in oxygen. Both will die after having presented the same symptoms.[37]

Bert goes on to describe the symptoms of acute exposure to hypoxia:

It is the nervous system which reacts first. The sensation of fatigue, the weakening of the sense perceptions, the cerebral symptoms, vertigo, sleepiness, hallucinations, buzzing in the ears, dizziness, pricklings . . . are the signs of insufficient oxygenation of central and peripheral nervous organs. . . . The symptoms. . . disappear very quickly when the balloon descends from the higher altitudes, very quickly also . . . the normal proportion of oxygen reappears in the blood. *There is an unfailing connection here.*[37]

Bert was also able to prevent and immediately resolve symptoms by breathing oxygen.

Acute hypoxia can be quickly reversed by immediate administration of oxygen; rapid pressurization or descent; or correction of an underlying cause, such as relief of apnea, removal of a carbon monoxide source, repair of an oxygen delivery system, or cessation of overexertion. Hyperventilation increases time of useful consciousness.

High-Altitude Headache

Headache is generally the first unpleasant symptom consequent to altitude exposure and is sometimes the only symptom.[134] It may or may not be the harbinger of AMS, which is defined as the presence of headache plus at least one of four other symptoms, in the setting of an acute altitude gain.[281] One could argue that it is the headache itself that causes other symptoms, such as anorexia, nausea, lassitude, and insomnia, as is commonly seen in migraine or tension headaches, and that mild AMS is essentially due to headache. Whether an

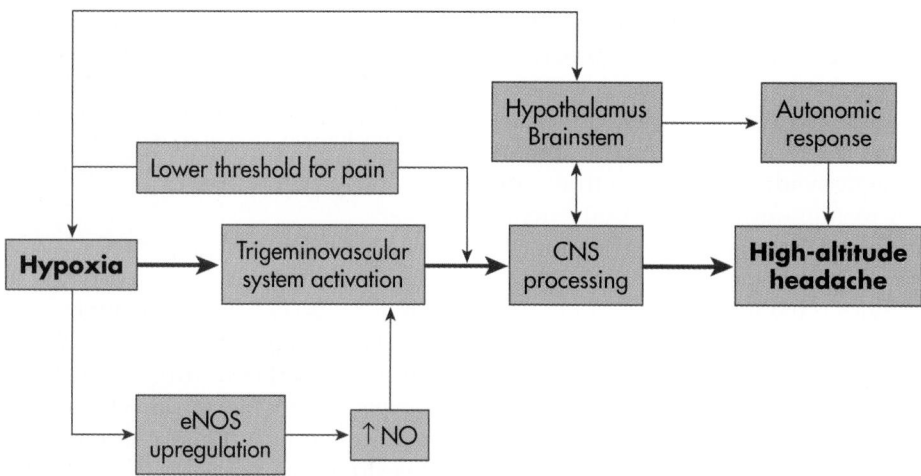

Figure 1-10 Proposed pathophysiology of high-altitude headache. *CNS,* Central nervous system; *eNOS,* endogenous nitric oxide synthase; *NO,* nitric oxide. *(Modified from Sanchez del Rio M, Moskowitz MA: High altitude headache,* Adv Exp Med Biol *474:145, 1999.)*

isolated headache is any different from the headache of moderate to severe AMS is unsettled until we have a better understanding of the pathophysiology. Because moderate to severe AMS is associated with vasogenic edema, and because headache by itself might not be, we choose to consider high-altitude headache as a separate category, pending further investigation. The term *high-altitude headache* (HAH) has been used in the literature for decades, and studies directed toward the pathophysiology and treatment of HAH have been reported.* Obviously, these are to an extent studies of AMS as well. Headache lends itself to investigation better than some other symptoms; headache scores have been well validated.[164]

In general, the literature suggests that HAH can be prevented by the use of nonsteroidal antiinflammatory drugs,[46,50] as well as the drugs commonly used for prophylaxis of AMS, acetazolamide and dexamethasone. Some agents appear more effective than others, with ibuprofen and aspirin apparently superior to naproxen.[46,49,51] A serotonin agonist (sumatriptan, a 5-HT$_1$ receptor agonist) was reported to be effective for HAH prevention and/or treatment in some studies[48,343] but not in others.[27] Interestingly, oxygen is often immediately effective for HAH in subjects with and without AMS, indicating a rapidly reversible mechanism of the headache.[22,108]

The response to many different agents might reflect multiple components of the pathophysiology or merely the nonspecific nature of analgesics in some studies. As Sanchez del Rio and Moskowitz[298] have pointed out, different inciting factors for headache may result in a final common pathway, such that the response to different therapies is not necessarily related to the initial cause of the headache. They recently provided a useful multifactorial concept of the pathogenesis of HAH, based on current understanding of headaches in general.[298] They suggest that the trigeminovascular system is activated at altitude by both mechanical and chemical stimuli (vasodilation, nitric oxide and other noxious agents), and in addition, the threshold for pain is likely altered at high altitude (Figure 1-10).[298] If AMS and especially HACE ensue, altered intracranial dynamics may also play a role, via compression or distension of pain-sensitive structures.

Acute Mountain Sickness

Although the syndrome of AMS has been recognized for centuries, modern rapid transport and the proliferation of participants in mountain sports have increased the number of victims and therefore public awareness (see Table 1-1). The incidence and severity of AMS depend on the rate of ascent and the altitude attained (especially the sleeping altitude), length of altitude exposure, level of exertion,[283] and inherent physiologic susceptibility. For example, AMS is more common on Mt. Rainier because of the rapid ascent, whereas HAPE is uncommon because of the short stay (less than 36 hours). Age has a small influence on incidence,[106] with the elderly somewhat less vulnerable.[282] Women apparently have the same[280] or a slightly greater incidence of AMS[106,134] but may be less susceptible to pulmonary edema.[64,323] It is useful clinically to classify AMS as mild or moderate to severe on the basis of symptoms (Table 1-4). Importantly, AMS can herald the beginning of life-threatening cerebral edema.

Diagnosis. The diagnosis of AMS is based on setting, symptoms, physical findings, and exclusion of other illnesses. The setting is generally rapid ascent of unaccli-

---

*References 27, 46, 48-50, 108, 267, 343.

TABLE 1-4. Classification of Acute Mountain Sickness

	HAH	MILD AMS	MODERATE TO SEVERE AMS	HACE
			CLINICAL CLASSIFICATION	
Symptoms	Headache only	Headache + 1 more symptom (nausea/vomiting, fatigue/lassitude, dizziness or difficulty sleeping) All symptoms of mild severity	Headache + 1 or more symptoms (nausea/vomiting, fatigue/lassitude, dizziness or difficulty sleeping) Symptoms of moderate to severe intensity	±Headache Worsening of symptoms seen in moderate to severe AMS
LL-AMS score*	1-3, headache only	2-4	5-15	
Physical signs	None	None	None	Ataxia, altered mental status
Findings	None	None	Antidiuresis, slight increase in temperature, slight desaturation, widened A-a gradient, elevated ICP, white matter edema (CT, MRI)	HAPE common: +chest x-ray, rales, dyspnea at rest; elevated ICP; white matter edema (CT, MRI)
Pathophysiology	Cerebral vasodilation, activation of trigeminovascular system†	Same as HAH, plus early vasogenic edema	Vasogenic edema	Advanced vasogenic cerebral edema

*The self-report Lake Louise AMS score.
†See Figure 1-10 and a recent review (reference 298).

matized persons to 2500 m (8202 feet) or higher from altitudes below 1500 m (4921 feet). For partially acclimatized persons, abrupt ascent to a higher altitude, overexertion, use of respiratory depressants, and perhaps onset of infectious illness[243] are common contributing factors.

The cardinal symptom of early AMS is headache, followed in incidence by fatigue, dizziness, and anorexia.[106,134,321] The headache is usually throbbing, bitemporal or occipital, typically worse during the night and on awakening, and made worse by Valsalva's maneuver or stooping over. A good appetite is distinctly uncommon. Nausea is common. These initial symptoms are strikingly similar to an alcohol hangover. Frequent awakening may fragment sleep, and periodic breathing often produces a feeling of suffocation. Although sleep disorder is nearly universal at high altitude, these symptoms may be exaggerated during AMS. Affected persons commonly complain of a deep inner chill, unlike mere exposure to cold temperature, accompanied by facial pallor. Other symptoms may include vomiting, dyspnea on exertion, and irritability. Lassitude can be disabling, with the victim too apathetic to contribute to his or her own or the group's basic needs. Any symptom suggestive of AMS should be considered caused by altitude unless proven otherwise.

Pulmonary symptoms vary considerably. Everyone experiences dyspnea on exertion at high altitude; it may be difficult to distinguish normal from abnormal. Dyspnea at rest is distinctly abnormal, however, and presages HAPE rather than AMS. Cough is also extremely common at high altitude and not particularly associated with AMS. Recent work suggests that altitude hypoxia actually lowers the cough threshold, as measured with an inhaled citric acid stimulus.[209] However, any pulmonary symptom mandates careful examination for pulmonary edema.

Specific physical findings are lacking in mild AMS. Early authors described tachycardia, but Singh et al[321] noted bradycardia (heart rate less than 66 beats/min) in two thirds of 1975 soldiers with AMS. Blood pressure is normal, but postural hypotension may be present. Rales localized to one area of the chest are common (5% to 20% incidence)[201] and probably represent pulmonary vascular congestion. A slight increased body temperature with AMS was recently reported.[200] Funduscopic examination reveals venous tortuosity and dilation; retinal hemorrhages may or may not be present and are not diagnostic; they are more common in AMS than non-AMS subjects at 4243 m (13,921 feet).[105] Absence of the normal altitude diuresis, evidenced by lack of increased urine output and retention of fluid, is an early finding in AMS although not always present.[25,110,284,321,335]

More obvious physical findings develop if AMS progresses to HACE. Typically, with onset of HACE, the victim wants to be left alone; lassitude progresses to inability to perform perfunctory activities, such as eating and dressing; ataxia develops; and finally, changes in consciousness appear, with confusion, disorientation, and impaired judgment. Coma may ensue within 24 hours of the onset of ataxia. Ataxia is the single most useful sign for recognizing the progression from AMS to HACE; all persons proceeding to high altitudes should be aware of this fact.

Differential Diagnosis. AMS is most commonly misdiagnosed as a viral flulike illness, hangover, exhaustion, dehydration, or medication or drug effect. Unlike an infectious illness, uncomplicated AMS is not associated with fever and myalgia. Hangover is excluded by the history (see Alcohol and Altitude). Exhaustion may cause lassitude, weakness, irritability, and headache and may therefore be difficult to distinguish from AMS. Dehydration, which causes weakness, decreased urine output, headache, and nausea, is commonly confused with AMS. Response to fluids helps differentiate the two. AMS is not improved by fluid administration alone; body hydration does not influence susceptibility to AMS (contrary to conventional wisdom).[7] Hypothermia may manifest as ataxia and mental changes. Sleeping medication can cause ataxia and mental changes, but soporifics may also precipitate high-altitude illness because of increased hypoxemia during sleep.

Carbon Monoxide. Carbon monoxide poisoning is a danger at high altitude, where field shelters are designed to be small and windproof. Cooking inside closed tents and snow shelters during storms is a particular hazard.[342] The effects of carbon monoxide and high-altitude hypoxia are additive. A reduction in oxyhemoglobin caused by carbon monoxide increases hypoxic stress, rendering a person at a "physiologically higher" altitude, which may precipitate AMS. Because of preexisting hypoxemia, smaller amounts of carboxyhemoglobin produce symptoms of carbon monoxide poisoning. These two problems may coexist. Immediate removal of the victim from the source of carbon monoxide and forced hyperventilation, preferably with supplemental oxygen, rapidly reverse carbon monoxide poisoning. Persistent unconsciousness in the setting of carbon monoxide exposure at high altitude can be due to either severe carbon monoxide poisoning or high-altitude cerebral edema. The management is nearly the same and includes coma care, oxygen, descent, and evacuation to a hospital.

Pathophysiology. Although the basic cause of AMS is hypobaric hypoxia, the syndrome is different from acute hypoxia. Because of a lag time in onset of symptoms after ascent and lack of immediate reversal of all symptoms with oxygen, AMS is thought to be secondary to the body's responses to modest hypoxia. In addition, even though an altitude of 2500 to 2700 m (8202 to 8859 feet) presents only a minor decrement in arterial oxygen transport (SaO_2 is still above 90%), AMS is common and certain individuals may become desperately ill. An acceptable explanation of pathophysiology must therefore address lag time, individual susceptibility to even modest hypoxia, and how acclimatization prevents the illness.

Findings documented in mild to moderate AMS that relate to pathophysiology include relative hypoventilation,[212,236] impaired gas exchange (interstitial edema),[99,188] fluid retention and redistribution,[25,284,335] and increased sympathetic activity.[19,23] In mild to moderate AMS, limited data suggest that intracranial pressure (ICP) is not elevated.[125,366] In contrast, increased ICP and cerebral edema are documented in moderate to severe AMS, reflecting the continuum from AMS to HACE.[140,180,213,321,361]

Relative hypoventilation may be due primarily to a decreased drive to breathe (low HVR) or may be secondary to ventilatory depression associated with AMS.[236,277] Persons with quite low HVR are more likely to suffer AMS than are those with a high ventilatory drive.[131,212,236] For persons with intermediate HVR values (most people), ventilatory drive probably has no predictive value.[225,277] The protective role of a high HVR most likely results from overall increased oxygen transport, especially during sleep and exercise.

Pulmonary dysfunction in AMS includes decreased vital capacity and peak expiratory flow rate,[321] increased alveolar-arterial oxygen difference,[99,132] decreased transthoracic impedance,[163] and a high incidence of rales.[201] These findings are compatible with interstitial edema, that is, increased extravascular lung water, most likely related to fluid retention and an increased interstitial water compartment. The fact that exercise can contribute to interstitial edema at altitude was recently confirmed.[6] Whether this can be considered a mild form of HAPE is unclear. The fact that nifedipine effectively prevents HAPE but does not prevent AMS or the increased A-a oxygen gradient observed in AMS[132] speaks against the increased lung water of AMS being related to HAPE, but the issue deserves further study.

The mechanism of fluid retention may be multifactorial. Renal responses to hypoxia are variable and depend on plasma arginine vasopressin (AVP) concentration and sympathetic tone.[128,335] Persons with AMS had elevated plasma or urine AVP levels in some studies,[23,321] but cause and effect could not be established. Other studies showed no AVP elevation.[25] The usual decrease in aldosterone on ascent to altitude does not occur in persons with AMS, and this may contribute to the antidiuresis.[25] The renin-angiotensin system, although suppressed compared with its activity at sea level in both AMS and non-AMS groups, was more active in persons with AMS.[19] Atrial natriuretic peptide (ANP) is elevated in AMS. Although this is most likely compensatory, elevated plasma ANP levels may contribute to vasodilation and increased microvascular permeability.[19,359] One factor that can explain many of these changes is increased sympathetic activity, which reduces renal blood flow, glomerular filtration rate, and urine output, and suppresses renin.[335] Increased sympathetic nervous system activity is also consistent with the greater rise in norepinephrine noted in subjects with AMS.[23] See Krasney[177] for a discussion of the critical role of central sympathetic activation on the kidney and its role in the pathophysiology of AMS. Whatever the exact mechanism, it seems that renal water handling switches from net loss or no change to net gain of water as persons become ill with AMS. The effectiveness of diuretics in treating AMS also supports a pivotal role for fluid retention and fluid shifts in the pathology of AMS.[99,321]

Persons with moderate to severe AMS or HACE display white matter edema on brain imaging and elevated ICP.* Possible mechanisms include cytotoxic edema with a shift of fluid into the cells, or vasogenic (interstitial) edema from increased permeability of the blood-brain barrier (BBB), or both. The classic view that hypoxia causes failure of the adenosine triphosphate (ATP)–dependent sodium pump and subsequent intracellular edema[137] is untenable, given the newer understanding of brain energetics; ATP levels are maintained even in severe hypoxemia.[315] The evidence now favors vasogenic brain edema as the cause of AMS/HACE. Hackett et al[118] point out that reversible white matter edema, with sparing of the gray matter, is characteristic of vasogenic edema (see Figure 1-13). The fact that dexamethasone is so effective for AMS also suggests vasogenic edema because this is the only steroid-responsive brain edema. In addition, a model of AMS in conscious sheep exposed to 10% oxygen for several days supports the vasogenic brain-swelling hypothesis. Krasney et al[179] have shown that cerebral capillary pressure rises, which causes filtration of fluid across the BBB and an increase in wet-to-dry cerebral tissue ratio. The pathophysiology may be similar to hypertensive encephalopathy, in which loss of vascular autoregulation results in increased pressures transmitted to the capil-

laries with resultant white matter edema.[189,190] Because prolonged cerebral vasodilation by itself, however, is not sufficient to induce vasogenic edema, Hackett[104] and Krasney[178] have proposed the additional factor of increased BBB permeability in the pathophysiology of AMS. Possible mechanisms of altered BBB permeability in AMS/HACE include vascular endothelial growth factor (VEGF), inflammatory cytokines, products of lipid peroxidation, endothelium-derived products, such as nitric oxide, and direct neural and humoral factors known to affect the BBB. For a complete discussion of the mechanisms of BBB permeability and their possible role in altitude illness, see the recent reviews by Drewes,[77] Hackett,[104] Hossman,[135] and Schilling[304] (Figure 1-11).

The question of whether mild AMS, especially headache alone, is due to vasogenic cerebral edema is not yet answered (see High-Altitude Headache). Recent magnetic resonance imaging (MRI) studies demonstrated brain swelling in all subjects ascending rapidly to moderate altitude, regardless of the presence of AMS.[162,244] The change in brain volume was greater than that expected from increased cerebral blood volume alone (resulting from vasodilation), but the individual components of blood and brain parenchyma could not be determined with MRI. Therefore whether edema was present was not established. Regardless, the changes in the ill and the well groups were similar. Interestingly, Kilgore et al[174] did show a small but significant increase in T2 signal of the corpus callosum, hinting that vasogenic edema was starting, and the increase in the AMS group was twice that of the non-AMS group, though not quite statistically significant. Although still very much an open question, the literature to date does not confirm that mild AMS or headache alone is related to brain edema.

To summarize, moderate to severe AMS and HACE represent a continuum from mild to severe vasogenic cerebral edema. Headache alone, or the earliest stages of AMS, might be related to edema or could be related to other factors, such as cerebral vasodilation or a migraine mechanism; further research is needed to clarify this issue.

INDIVIDUAL SUSCEPTIBILITY AND INTRACRANIAL DYNAMICS. What might explain individual susceptibility to AMS? Correlations of AMS with HVR, ventilation, fluid status, lung function, and physical fitness have been weak at best. Ross[294] hypothesized in 1985 that the apparent random nature of susceptibility might be explained by random anatomic differences. Specifically, he suggested that persons with smaller intracranial and intraspinal cerebrospinal fluid (CSF) capacity would be disposed to develop AMS because they would not tolerate brain

---

*References 118, 140, 180, 194, 213, 321.

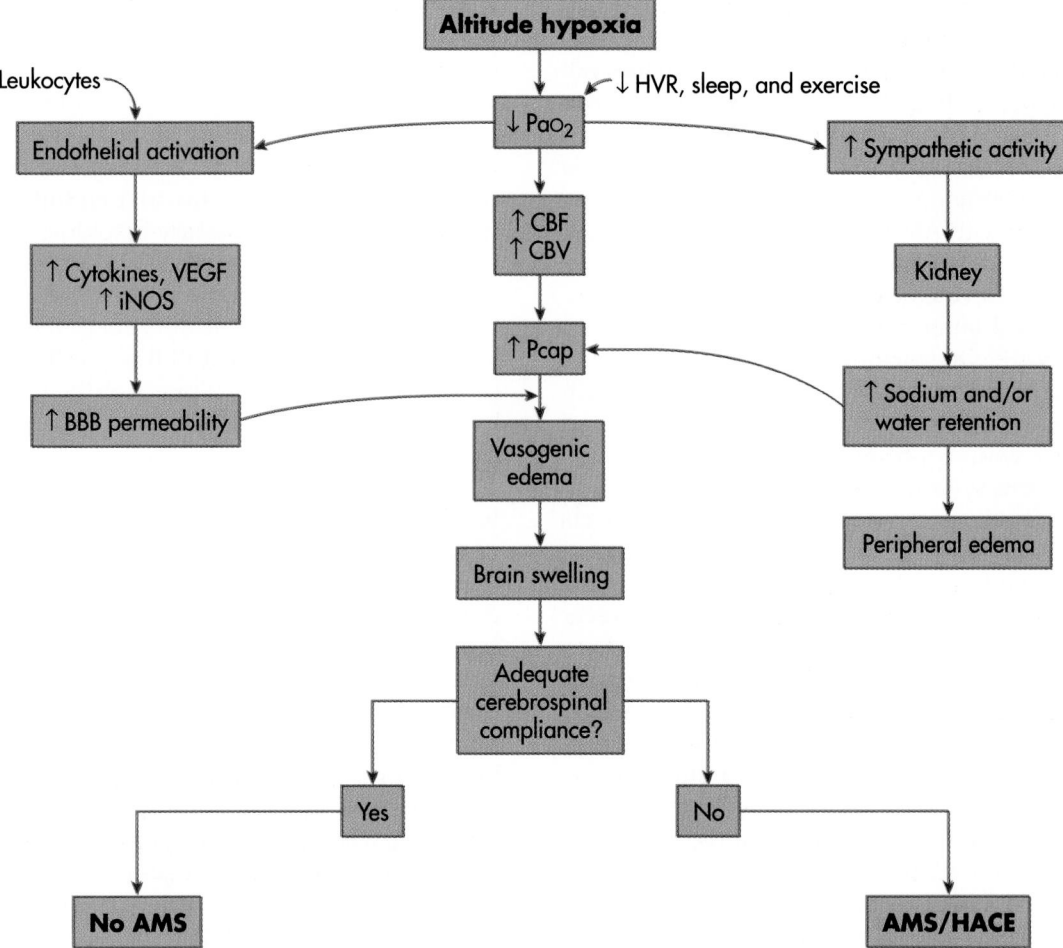

Figure 1-11 Proposed pathophysiology of acute mountain sickness. *BBB*, Blood-brain barrier; *CBF*, cerebral blood flow; *CBV*, cerebral blood volume; *HVR*, hypoxic ventilatory response; *iNOS*, inducible nitric oxide synthase; *Pcap*, capillary pressure; *VEGF*, vascular endothelial growth factor.

swelling as well as those with more "room" in the craniospinal axis. The displacement of CSF through the foramen magnum into the spinal canal is the first compensatory response to increased brain volume, followed by increased CSF absorption and decreased CSF formation. Studies have shown that the increase in ICP for a given increase in brain volume is directly related to the "tightness" of the brain in the cranium (the brain volume:intracranial volume ratio) and to the volume of the spinal canal.[313] Thus the greater the initial CSF volume, the more accommodation that can take place in response to brain edema. Increases in volume are "buffered" by CSF dynamics. In light of our present understanding of increased brain volume on ascent to altitude, his hypothesis is very attractive. Preliminary data that showed a relationship of preascent ventricular size or brain volume:cranial vault ratios and susceptibility to AMS support this hypothesis, and the idea deserves further study.[104,373] Figure 1-11 incorporates this concept into the pathophysiology.

Natural Course of Acute Mountain Sickness. The natural history of AMS varies with initial altitude, rate of ascent, and clinical severity. Singh et al[321] followed the illness in soldiers airlifted to altitudes of 3300 to 5500 m (10,827 to 18,045 feet). Incapacitating illness lasted 2 to 5 days, but 40% still had symptoms after 1 week and 13% after 1 month. Nine soldiers failed to acclimatize in 6 months and were considered unfit for duty at high altitude.[321] Chinese investigators report that a percentage of lowland Han Chinese stationed on the Tibet Plateau cannot tolerate the altitude because of persistent symptoms and must be relocated to the plains.[367] Persistent anorexia, nausea, and headache may afflict climbers at extreme altitude for weeks and can be considered a form of persistent AMS. The natural history of AMS in tourists who sleep at more moderate altitudes is much more benign. Duration of symptoms at 3000 m (9840 feet) was 15 hours, with a range of 6 to 94 hours.[68] Most individuals treat or tolerate their symptoms as the illness resolves over 1 to 3 days while acclimatization improves, but some persons with AMS seek medical treatment or are forced to descend if symptoms persist. A small percentage of those with AMS (8% at 4243 m [13,921 feet])[106] go on to develop cerebral edema, especially if ascent is continued in spite of illness.

Treatment. The proper management of AMS is based on early diagnosis and acknowledgment that initial clinical presentation does not predict eventual severity (Box 1-3). Therefore proceeding to a higher sleeping altitude in the presence of symptoms is contraindicated. The victim must be carefully monitored for progression of illness. If symptoms worsen despite an extra 24 hours of acclimatization or treatment, descent is indicated. The two indications for immediate descent are neurologic changes (ataxia or change in consciousness) and pulmonary edema.

Mild AMS can be treated by halting the ascent and waiting for acclimatization to improve, which can take from 12 hours to 3 or 4 days. Acetazolamide (125 to 250 mg twice a day orally) speeds acclimatization and thus terminates the illness if given early.[99] Symptomatic therapy includes analgesics such as aspirin (650 mg), acetaminophen (650 to 1000 mg), ibuprofen[46] or other nonsteroidal antiinflammatory drugs, or codeine (30 mg) for headache. Prochlorperazine (Compazine, 5 to 10 mg intramuscularly) can be given by an appropriate route for nausea and vomiting and has the advantage of augmenting the HVR.[255] Promethazine (Phenergan, 50 mg by suppository or ingestion) is also useful. Persons with AMS should avoid alcohol and other respiratory depressants because of the danger of exaggerated hypoxemia during sleep.

Descent to an altitude lower than where symptoms began effectively reverses AMS. Although the person should descend as far as necessary for improvement, descending 500 to 1000 m (1640 to 3281 feet) is usually sufficient. Exertion should be minimized. Oxygen, if available, is particularly effective (and supply is conserved) if given in low flow (0.5 to 1 L/min by mask or cannula) during the night. Hyperbaric chambers, which simulate descent, have been used to treat AMS and aid acclimatization. They are effective and require no supplemental oxygen. Lightweight (less than 7 kg) fabric pressure bags inflated by manual air pumps are now being used on mountaineering expeditions and in mountain clinics (Figure 1-12). An inflation of 2 psi is roughly equivalent to a drop in altitude of 1600 m (5250 feet); the exact equivalent depends on initial altitude.[168,279] A few hours of pressurization result in symptomatic improvement and can be an effective temporizing measure while awaiting descent or the benefit of medical therapy.[168,242,258,286,338] Long-term (12 hours or more) use of these portable devices would be necessary to resolve AMS completely.

Box 1-3 FIELD TREATMENT OF HIGH-ALTITUDE ILLNESS

HIGH-ALTITUDE HEADACHE AND MILD ACUTE MOUNTAIN SICKNESS

Stop ascent, rest, acclimatize at same altitude
Acetazolamide, 125 to 250 mg bid, to speed acclimatization
Symptomatic treatment as necessary with analgesics and antiemetics
or Descend 500 m or more

MODERATE TO SEVERE ACUTE MOUNTAIN SICKNESS

Low-flow oxygen, if available
Acetazolamide, 125 to 250 mg bid, with or without dexamethasone, 4 mg po, IM, or IV q6h
Hyperbaric therapy
Or Immediate descent

HIGH-ALTITUDE CEREBRAL EDEMA

Immediate descent or evacuation
Oxygen, 2 to 4 L/min
Dexamethasone, 4 mg po, IM, or IV q6h
Hyperbaric therapy

HIGH-ALTITUDE PULMONARY EDEMA

Minimize exertion and keep warm
Oxygen, 4 to 6 L/min until improving, then 2 to 4 L/min
Nifedipine, 10 mg po q4h by titration to response, or 10 mg po once, followed by 30 mg extended release q12 to 24h
Hyperbaric therapy
or Immediate descent

PERIODIC BREATHING

Acetazolamide, 62.5 to 125 mg at bedtime as needed

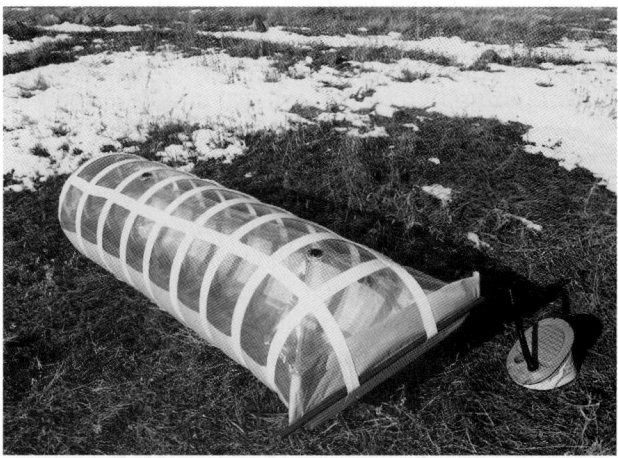

Figure 1-12 The HELP System (Live High, Boulder, Colo.) uses breathing bladder technology to minimize the pumping necessary to circulate air in the hyperbaric compartment.

The use of diuretics has a sound basis because of fluid retention associated with AMS. Acetazolamide is of unquestionable prophylactic value and is now commonly and successfully used to treat AMS as well. Acetazolamide may be helpful in part because of its diuretic action; its multiple modes of action are discussed later. Singh et al[321] successfully used furosemide (80 mg twice a day for 2 days) to treat 446 soldiers with all degrees of AMS; it has not since been studied for treatment. Furosemide induced a brisk diuresis, relieved pulmonary congestion, and improved headache and other neurologic symptoms. Spironolactone, hydrochlorothiazide, and other diuretics have not yet been evaluated for treatment.

The steroid betamethasone was initially reported by Singh et al[321] to improve symptoms of soldiers with severe AMS. Since then, dexamethasone was found to be very effective for treatment of all degrees of AMS. Dexamethasone is effective for treatment of moderate to severe AMS.[86,116,171] Hackett et al[116] used 4 mg orally or intramuscularly every 6 hours, and Ferrazinni et al[86] gave 8 mg initially, followed by 4 mg every 6 hours. Both studies reported marked improvement within 12 hours, with no significant side effects. Symptoms increased when dexamethasone was discontinued after 24 hours.[289] Dexamethasone should be started in conjunction with descent or hyperbaric treatment,[171] if possible, and continued until the victim is down to low altitude. Although the mechanism of action of dexamethasone is not clear, it probably acts by improving brain capillary integrity and diminishing vasogenic edema.[65] Dexamethasone seems not to improve acclimatization because symptoms recur when the drug is withdrawn. Therefore an argument could be made for using dexamethasone to relieve symptoms and acetazolamide to speed acclimatization.[35]

Prevention. Graded ascent is the surest and safest method of prevention, although particularly susceptible individuals may still become ill. Current recommendations for persons without altitude experience are to avoid abrupt ascent to sleeping altitudes greater than 3000 m (9843 feet) and to spend 2 to 3 nights at 2500 to 3000 m (8202 to 9843 feet) before going higher, with an extra night for acclimatization every 600 to 900 m (1969 to 2953 feet) if continuing ascent. Abrupt increases of more than 600 m (1969 feet) in sleeping altitude should be avoided when over 2500 m (8202 feet). Day trips to higher altitude, with a return to lower altitude for sleep, aid acclimatization. Alcohol and sedative-hypnotics are best avoided on the first 2 nights at high altitude. Whether a diet high in carbohydrates reduces AMS symptoms is controversial.[62,124,337] Exertion early in altitude exposure contributes to altitude illness,[283] whereas limited exercise seems to aid acclimatization.

ACETAZOLAMIDE PROPHYLAXIS. Acetazolamide is the drug of choice for prophylaxis of AMS. A carbonic anhydrase (CA) inhibitor, acetazolamide slows the hydration of carbon dioxide:

$$CO_2 + H_2O \leftrightarrow H_2CO_3 \leftrightarrow H^+ + HCO_3^-$$
$$CA$$

The effects are protean, involving particularly the red blood cells, brain, lungs, and kidneys. By inhibiting renal carbonic anhydrase, acetazolamide reduces reabsorption of bicarbonate and sodium and thus causes a bicarbonate diuresis and metabolic acidosis starting within 1 hour after ingestion. This rapidly enhances ventilatory acclimatization. Perhaps most important, the drug maintains oxygenation during sleep and prevents periods of extreme hypoxemia (see Figure 1-6).[114,332,336] Because of acetazolamide's diuretic action, it counteracts the fluid retention of AMS. It also diminishes nocturnal antidiuretic hormone (ADH) secretion[56] and decreases CSF production and volume and possibly CSF pressure.[310] Which of these effects is most important in preventing AMS is unclear. Numerous studies taken together indicate that acetazolamide is approximately 75% effective in preventing AMS in persons rapidly transported to altitudes of 3000 to 4500 m (9843 to 14,764 feet).[84]

Indications for acetazolamide prophylaxis include rapid ascent (1 day or less) to altitudes over 3000 m (9843 feet); a rapid gain in sleeping altitude, for example, moving camp from 4000 m (13,123 feet) to 5000 m (16,404 feet) in a day; and a past history of recurrent AMS or HAPE. Numerous dosage regimens have been effective.[74,80] Smaller doses (125 to 250 mg twice a day) starting 24 hours before ascent work as well as higher doses started earlier.[223] A 500-mg sustained action capsule of Diamox taken every 24 hours is probably equally effective and results in fewer side effects because of lower peak serum levels.[363] Most authors recommend continuing for the first day or two at high altitude, and some suggest daily acetazolamide the entire time at high altitude.[43] This hardly seems necessary once acclimatization is established and the danger of AMS has passed. Spironolactone[165,186] and other diuretics have shown equivocal results for AMS prevention.

Acetazolamide has side effects, most notably peripheral paresthesias and polyuria, and less commonly nausea, drowsiness, impotence, and myopia. Because it inhibits the instant hydration of carbon dioxide on the tongue, acetazolamide allows carbon dioxide to be tasted and can ruin the flavor of carbonated beverages, including beer. A sulfa drug, acetazolamide carries the usual precautions about hypersensitivity, crystalluria, and bone marrow suppression.

DEXAMETHASONE. Dexamethasone is also useful for prevention of AMS. The initial chamber study in 1984 was with sedentary subjects.[167] The drug reduced the incidence of AMS from 78% to 20%, comparable with previous studies with acetazolamide. Dexamethasone was not as effective in exercising subjects on Pike's Peak,[289] but subsequent work has shown effectiveness comparable with acetazolamide.[84,195,374] The combination of acetazolamide and dexamethasone proved superior to dexamethasone alone.[374] Because of potential serious side effects and the rebound phenomenon, dexamethasone is best reserved for treatment rather than for prevention of AMS, or used for prophylaxis when necessary in persons intolerant of or allergic to acetazolamide.

High-Altitude Cerebral Edema

HACE is characterized clinically by a progression to encephalopathy in the setting of AMS or HAPE. As discussed previously, AMS is essentially a neurologic disorder, probably related to brain swelling, and HACE appears to be the extreme form of AMS; the distinction between AMS and HACE is therefore inherently blurred.

Clinical Presentation. The hallmarks of HACE are ataxic gait, severe lassitude, and altered consciousness, including confusion, impaired mentation, drowsiness, stupor, and coma. Headache, nausea, and vomiting are frequently, but not always, present. Hallucinations, cranial nerve palsy, hemiparesis, hemiplegia, seizures, and focal neurologic signs have also been reported.[120,140,321] Retinal hemorrhages are common but not diagnostic. The progression from mild AMS to unconsciousness may be as fast as 12 hours but usually requires 1 to 3 days. Cyanosis or a gray pallor is common. Arterial blood gas study or pulse oximetry reveals exaggerated hypoxemia. Clinical examination, chest radiography, and autopsy have often demonstrated pulmonary edema; indeed, isolated HACE without HAPE is uncommon.[103,118]

The following case report from Mt. McKinley illustrates a clinical course of HACE, in conjunction with HAPE:

H.E. was a 26-year-old German lumberjack with extensive mountaineering experience. He ascended to 5200 m (17,061 feet) from 2000 m (6562 feet) in 4 days and attempted the summit (6194 m [20,323 feet]) on the fifth day. At 5800 m (19,030 feet) he turned back because of severe fatigue, headache, and malaise. He returned alone to 5200 m (17,061 feet), stumbling on the way because of loss of coordination. He had no appetite and crawled into his sleeping bag too weak, tired, and disoriented to undress. He recalled no pulmonary symptoms. In the morning H.E. was unarousable, slightly cyanotic, and noted to have Cheyne-Stokes respirations. After 10 minutes on high-flow oxygen H.E. began to regain consciousness, although he was com-

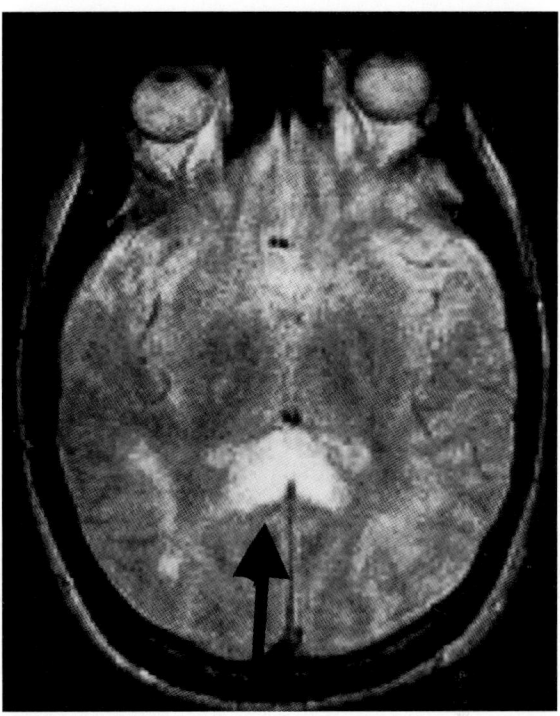

Figure 1-13 Magnetic resonance image of patient with high-altitude cerebral edema. Increased T2 signal in splenium of corpus callosum *(arrow)* indicates edema.

pletely disoriented and unable to move. A rescue team lowered him down a steep slope, and on arrival at 4400 m (14,436 feet) 4 hours later he was conscious but still disoriented, able to move extremities but unable to stand. Respiratory rate was 60 breaths/min and heart rate was 112 beats/min. Papilledema and a few rales were present. SaO₂% was 54% on room air (normal is 85% to 90%). On a nonrebreathing oxygen mask with 14 L/min oxygen, the SaO₂% increased to 88% and the respiratory rate decreased to 40 breaths/min. Eight milligrams of dexamethasone were administered intramuscularly at 4:20 PM and continued orally, 4 mg every 6 hours. At 5:20 PM H.E. began to respond to commands. The next morning H.E. was still ataxic but was able to stand, take fluids, and eat heartily. He was evacuated by air to Anchorage (sea level) at 12:00 PM. On admission to the hospital at 3:30 PM, roughly 36 hours after regaining consciousness, H.E. was somewhat confused and mildly ataxic. Arterial blood gas studies on room air showed a PO₂ of 58 torr, pH of 7.5, and PCO₂ of 27 torr. Bilateral pulmonary infiltrates were present on the chest radiograph. Magnetic resonance imaging of the brain revealed white matter edema, primarily of the corpus callosum (Figure 1-13). On discharge the next morning H.E. was oriented, bright, and cheerful and had very minor ataxia and clear lung fields.

Pathophysiology. The pathophysiology of HACE is a progression of the same mechanism as AMS (see Acute Mountain Sickness, Pathophysiology and Figure 1-11). The early brain swelling of AMS becomes much more severe. In cases similar to this, lumbar punctures have revealed elevated CSF pressures, often more than 300 mm H_2O[140,361]; evidence of cerebral edema on CT scan and MRI[118,176]; and gross cerebral edema on necropsy.[72,73] Small petechial hemorrhages were also consistently found on autopsy, and venous sinus thromboses were occasionally seen.[72,73] Well-documented cases have often included pulmonary edema that was not clinically apparent.

Whereas the mild brain swelling of AMS and reversible HACE is most likely vasogenic, as the spectrum shifts to severe, end-stage HACE, gray matter (presumably cytotoxic) edema develops as well, culminating in death. As Klatzo[175] has pointed out, as vasogenic edema progresses, the distance between brain cells and their capillaries increases, so that nutrients and oxygen eventually fail to diffuse and the cells are rendered ischemic, leading to intracellular (cytotoxic) edema. Raised ICP produces many of its effects by decreasing cerebral blood flow, and brain tissue becomes ischemic on this basis also.[219] Focal neurologic signs caused by brainstem distortion and by extraaxial compression, as in third and sixth cranial nerve palsies, may develop,[291] making cerebral edema difficult to differentiate from primary cerebrovascular events. The most common clinical presentation, however, is change in consciousness associated with ataxia, without focal signs.

Treatment. Successful treatment of HACE requires early recognition. At the first sign of ataxia or change in consciousness, descent should be started, dexamethasone (4 to 8 mg intravenously, intramuscularly, or orally initially, followed by 4 mg every 6 hours) administered, and oxygen (2 to 4 L/min by vented mask or nasal cannula) applied if available (see Box 1-3). Oxygen can be titrated to maintain SaO_2 at greater than 90% if oximetry is available. Comatose patients require additional airway management and bladder drainage. Attempting to decrease ICP by intubation and hyperventilation is a reasonable approach, although these patients are already alkalotic and overhyperventilation could result in cerebral ischemia. Loop diuretics, such as furosemide (40 to 80 mg) or bumetanide (1 to 2 mg), may reduce brain hydration, but an adequate intravascular volume to maintain perfusion pressure is critical. Hypertonic solutions of saline, mannitol, or oral glycerol have been suggested but rarely are used in the field. Controlled studies are lacking, but empirically the response to steroids and oxygen seems excellent if they are given early in the course of the illness and disappointing if they are not started until the victim is unconscious. Coma may persist for days, even after evacuation to low altitude, but other causes of coma must be considered and ruled out by appropriate evaluation.[140] Sequelae lasting weeks are common[118,140]; longer-term follow-up has been limited. Prevention of HACE is the same as for AMS.

Focal Neurologic Conditions without Cerebral Edema

Various localizing neurologic signs, transient in nature and not necessarily occurring in the setting of AMS, suggest migraine, cerebrovascular spasm, TIA, local hypoxia without loss of perfusion (watershed effect), or focal edema. Cortical blindness is one such condition. Hackett et al[113] reported six cases of transient blindness in climbers or trekkers with intact pupillary reflexes, which indicated that the condition was due to a cortical process. Treatment with breathing of either carbon dioxide (a potent cerebral vasodilator) or oxygen resulted in prompt relief, suggesting that the blindness was due to inadequate regional circulation or oxygenation. Descent effected relief more slowly. Other conditions that could be attributed to spasm or "transient ischemic attack" have included transient hemiplegia or hemiparesis, transient global amnesia, unilateral paresthesia, aphasia, and scotomas.[41,196,274,364]

The occurrence of stroke in a young, fit person at high altitude is uncommon but tragic. A number of case reports have described climbers with resultant permanent dysfunction.[55,138,322] Factors contributing to stroke may include polycythemia, dehydration, and increased ICP if AMS is present; increased cerebrovenous pressure; cerebrovascular spasm; and perhaps coagulation abnormalities. Stroke may be confused with HACE. Neurologic symptoms, especially focal abnormalities without AMS or HAPE, suggest a cerebrovascular event and mandate careful evaluation.

Clinical Presentation

E.H., a 42-year-old male climber on a Mt. Everest expedition, awoke at 8000 m (26,247 feet) with dense paralysis of the right arm and weakness of the right leg. On descent the paresis cleared, but at base camp (5000 m [16,404 feet]) severe vertigo developed, along with extreme ataxia and weakness. Neurologic consultation on return to the United States resulted in a diagnosis of multiple small cerebral infarcts, but none was visible on CT scan of the brain. The hematocrit value 3 weeks after descent from the mountain was 70%. Over the next 4 years, signs gradually improved, but mild ataxia, nystagmus, and dyslexia persist. The focal and persistent nature of the cerebral symptoms and signs, although multiple, indicates a cerebrovascular, rather than an ICP, cause. The hematocrit value on the mountain was greater than 70%, high enough for increased viscosity and microcirculatory sludging to contribute to ischemia and infarction.

Treatment of stroke is supportive. Oxygen and steroids may be worthwhile to treat any AMS or HACE component. Immediate evacuation to a hospital is indicated. Persons with TIAs at high altitude should probably be started on aspirin therapy and proceed to a lower altitude. Oxygen may quickly abort cerebrovascular spasm and will improve watershed hypoxic events. When oxygen is not available, rebreathing to raise alveolar P_{CO_2} may be helpful by increasing cerebral blood flow.

Cognitive Changes at High Altitude

If cerebral oxygen consumption is constant, what causes the well-documented, albeit mild, cognitive changes at high altitude? The cognitive changes may be related to specific neurotransmitters that are affected by mild hypoxia. For example, tryptophan hydroxylase in the serotonin synthesis pathway has a high requirement for oxygen (Km = 37 torr).[61,94] Tyrosine hydroxylase, in the dopamine pathway, is also oxygen-sensitive. Gibson[94] suggested that a decrease in acetylcholine activity during hypoxia might explain the lassitude. In a fascinating study, Banderet[14] showed that increased dietary tyrosine reduced mood changes and symptoms of environmental stress in subjects at simulated altitude. Further work with neurotransmitter agonists and antagonists will help shed light on their role in cognitive dysfunction at altitude and could lead to new pharmacologic approaches to improve neurologic function.

High-Altitude Pulmonary Edema

The most common cause of death related to high altitude, HAPE, is completely and easily reversed if recognized early and treated properly. Undoubtedly HAPE was misdiagnosed for centuries, as evidenced by frequent reports of young, vigorous men suddenly dying of "pneumonia" within days of arriving at high altitude. The death of Dr. Jacottet, "a robust, broad-shouldered young man," on Mt. Blanc in 1891 (he refused descent so that he could "observe the acclimatization process" in himself) may have provided the first autopsy of HAPE. Angelo Mosso wrote,

> From Dr. Wizard's post-mortem examination . . . the more immediate cause of death was therefore probably a suffocative catarrh accompanied by acute edema of the lungs. . . . I have gone into the particulars of this sorrowful incident because a case of inflammation of the lungs also occurred during our expedition, on the summit of Monte Rosa, from which, however, the sufferer fortunately recovered.[241]

On an expedition to K2 (Karakorum Range, Pakistan) in 1902, Crowley[66] described a climber "suffering from edema of both lungs and his mind was gone." In the Andes, physicians were familiar with pulmonary edema peculiar to high altitude,[160] but it was not until Hultgren[147] and Houston[136] that the English-speaking world became aware of high-altitude pulmonary edema (see Rennie[271] for a recent review). Hultgren[157] then published hemodynamic measurements in persons with HAPE, demonstrating that it was a noncardiogenic type of edema. Since that time, many studies and reviews have been published,[16,93] and HAPE is still the subject of intense investigation.

The incidence of HAPE varies from less than 1 in 10,000 skiers in Colorado to 1 in 50 climbers on Mt. McKinley and was higher (15%) in some regiments in the Indian Army (see Table 1-1). Individual susceptibility, rate of ascent, altitude reached, degree of cold,[269] physical exertion, and use of sleeping medications are all factors implicated in its occurrence. Younger persons seem more susceptible.[324] Although HAPE occurs in both genders, it is perhaps less common in women.[64,153,323]

Clinical Presentation

D.L., a 34-year-old man, was in excellent physical condition and had been on numerous high-altitude backpacking trips, occasionally suffering mild symptoms of AMS. He drove from sea level to the trailhead and hiked to a 3050-m (10,007-foot) sleeping altitude the first night of his trip in the Sierra Nevada. He proceeded to 3700 m (12,140 feet) the next day, noticing more dyspnea on exertion when walking uphill, a longer time than usual to recover when he rested, and a dry cough. He complained of headache, shivering, dyspnea, and insomnia the second night. The third day the group descended to 3500 m (11,483 feet) and rested, primarily for D.L.'s benefit. That night D.L. was unable to eat, noted severe dyspnea, and suffered coughing spasms and headache. On the fourth morning, D.L. was too exhausted and weak to get out of his sleeping bag. His companions noted that he was breathless, cyanotic, and ataxic but had clear mental status. A few hours later he was transported by helicopter to a hospital at 1200 m (3937 feet). On admission he was cyanotic, oral temperature was 37.8° C (100° F), blood pressure 130/76 torr, heart rate 96 beats/min, and respiratory frequency 20 breaths/min. Bilateral basilar rales were noted up to the scapulae. Findings of the cardiac examination were reported as normal. Romberg's and finger-to-nose tests revealed 1+ ataxia. Arterial blood gas studies on room air revealed P_{O_2} 24 torr, P_{CO_2} 28 torr, and pH 7.45. The chest radiograph showed extensive bilateral patchy infiltrates (Figure 1-14, C). D.L. was treated with bed rest and supplemental oxygen. On discharge to his sea level home 3 days later, his pulmonary infiltrates and rales had cleared, although his blood gas values were still abnormal: P_{O_2} 76 torr, P_{CO_2} 30 torr, and pH 7.45. He had an uneventful, complete recovery at home. D.L. was advised to ascend more slowly in the future, staging his ascent with nights spent at 1500 m and 2500 m (4921 feet and 8202 feet). He was taught the early signs and symptoms of HAPE and was advised about pharmacologic prophylaxis.

This case illustrates a number of typical aspects of HAPE. Victims are frequently young, fit men who ascend rapidly from sea level and may not have previously suffered HAPE even with repeated altitude exposures.

HAPE usually occurs within the first 2 to 4 days of ascent to higher altitudes (above 2500 m [8202 feet]), most commonly on the second night.[103] The earliest indications of the illness are decreased exercise performance and increased recovery time from exercise. The victim usually notices fatigue, weakness, and dyspnea on exertion, especially when he or she is trying to walk

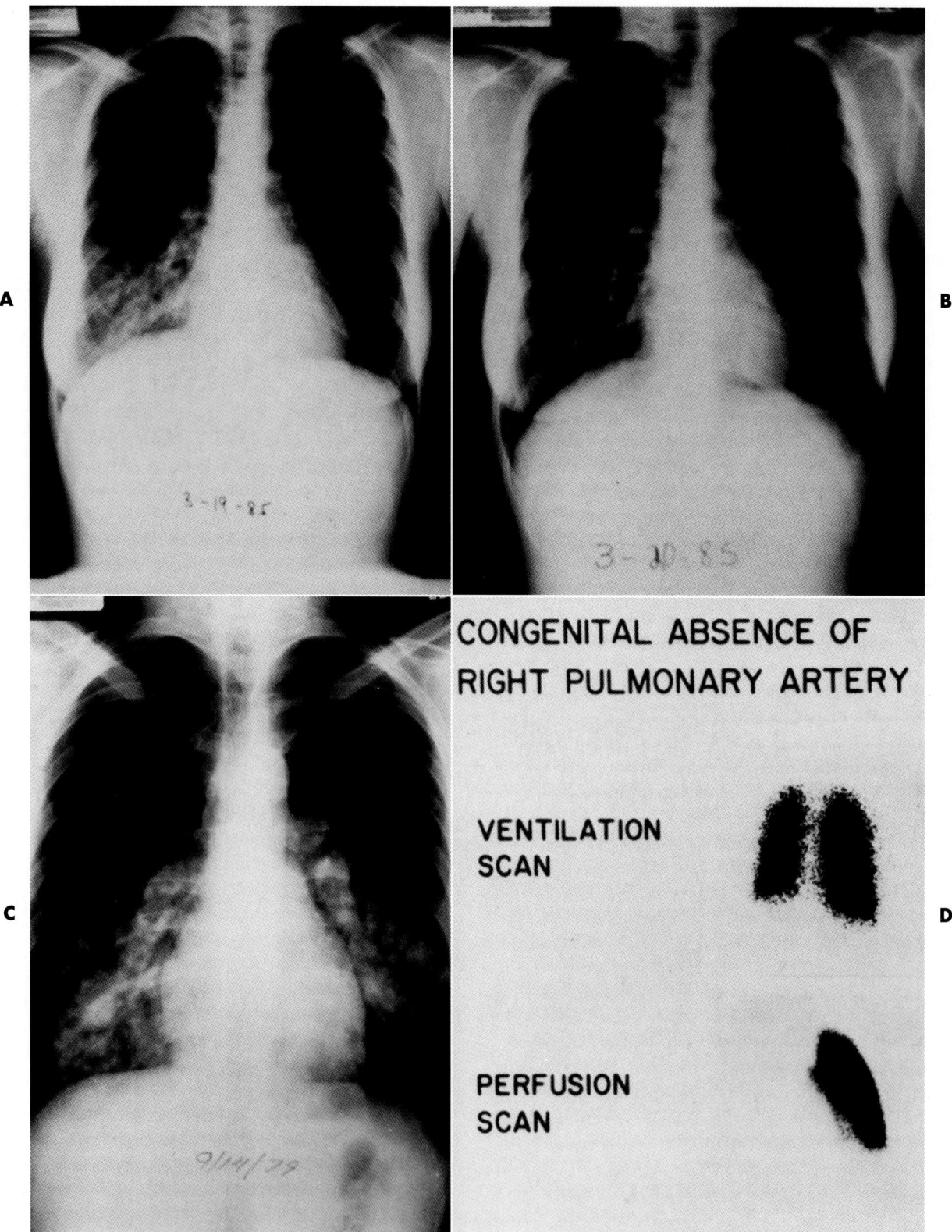

Figure 1-14 **A,** Typical radiograph of high-altitude pulmonary edema (HAPE) in 29-year-old female skier at 2450 m (8036 feet). **B,** Same patient 1 day after descent and oxygen administration, showing rapid clearing. **C,** Bilateral pulmonary infiltrates on radiograph of patient with severe HAPE after descent (case presented in text). **D,** Ventilation and perfusion scans in person with congenital absence of right pulmonary artery after recovery from HAPE.

TABLE 1-5. Severity Classification of High-Altitude Pulmonary Edema

GRADE	SYMPTOMS	SIGNS	CHEST FILM
1 Mild	Dyspnea on exertion, dry cough, fatigue while moving uphill	HR (rest) < 90-100; RR (rest) < 20; dusky nail beds; localized rales, if any	Minor exudate involving less than 25% of one lung field
2 Moderate	Dyspnea, weakness, fatigue on level walking; raspy cough; headache; anorexia	HR 90-100; RR 16-30; cyanotic nail beds; rales present; ataxia may be present	Some infiltrate involving 50% of one lung or smaller area of both lungs
3 Severe	Dyspnea at rest, productive cough, orthopnea, extreme weakness	Bilateral rales; HR > 110; RR > 30; facial and nail bed cyanosis; ataxia; stupor; coma; blood-tinged sputum	Bilateral infiltrates > 50% of each lung

Modified from Hultgren HN: High altitude pulmonary edema. In Staub NC, editor: *Lung water and solute exchange*, New York, 1978, Marcel Dekker. *HR*, Heart rate; *RR*, respiratory rate.

uphill; he or she often ascribes these nonspecific symptoms to various other causes. Signs of AMS, such as headache, anorexia, and lassitude, are present about 50% of the time.[153] A persistent dry cough develops. Nail beds and lips become cyanotic. The condition typically worsens at night, and tachycardia and tachypnea develop at rest. Dyspnea at rest and audible congestion in the chest herald to the victim the development of a serious condition. In contrast to the usual 1- to 2-day gradual onset, HAPE may strike abruptly, especially in a sedentary person who may not notice the early stages.[347] Orthopnea is uncommon (7%). Pink or blood-tinged, frothy sputum is a very late finding. Hemoptysis was present in 6% in one series.[159] Severe hypoxemia may produce cerebral edema with mental changes, ataxia, decreased level of consciousness, and coma. Hultgren[159] reported an incidence of HACE of 14% in those with HAPE at ski resorts.

On admission to the hospital, the victim does not generally appear as ill as would be expected based on arterial blood gas and radiographic findings. Elevated temperature of up to 38.5° C (101.3° F) is common. Tachycardia correlates with respiratory rate and severity of illness (Table 1-5).[157] Rales may be unilateral or bilateral and usually originate from the right middle lobe. Concomitant respiratory infection is sometimes present.

Pulmonary edema sometimes presents with predominantly neurologic manifestations and minimal pulmonary symptoms and findings. Cerebral edema, especially with coma, may obscure the diagnosis of HAPE.[107] Pulse oximetry or chest radiography confirms the diagnosis. The differential diagnosis includes pneumonia, pulmonary embolism or infarct, and sometimes asthma. Complications include infection, cerebral edema, pulmonary embolism or thrombosis, and such injuries as frostbite or trauma secondary to incapacitation.[16,107,154]

TABLE 1-6. Hemodynamic Measurements during High-Altitude Pulmonary Edema (HAPE) and after Recovery in Two Subjects and in a Group of 31 Control Subjects

	HAPE*	RECOVERY*	CONTROLS†
SaO$_2$%	58.0	84.0	89.0
Mean pulmonary artery pressure (mm Hg)	63.0	18.0	21.3
Wedge pressure (mm Hg)	1.5	3.5	7.1
Cardiac index (L/m^2)	2.5	4.4	4.1
Pulmonary vascular resistance (dyne/cm^{-5})	1210.0	169.0	169.0
Mean arterial blood pressure (mm Hg)	82.0	—	96.0

*HAPE and recovery values from Penaloza D, Sime F: *Am J Cardiol* 23:369, 1969.
†Mean values from 31 normal subjects studied at 3700 m; from Hultgren HN, Grover RF: *Annu Rev Med* 19:119, 1968.

Hemodynamics. Hemodynamic measurements show elevated pulmonary artery pressure and pulmonary vascular resistance, low to normal pulmonary wedge pressure, and low to normal cardiac output and systemic arterial blood pressure (Table 1-6).[155,260] Echocardiography demonstrates high estimated pulmonary artery pressures, tricuspid regurgitation, normal left ventricular function, and variable right-sided heart findings of increased atrial and ventricular size.[117,254]

The electrocardiogram usually reveals sinus tachycardia. Changes consistent with acute pulmonary hypertension have been described, such as right axis deviation, right bundle branch block, voltage for right ventricular hypertrophy, and P wave abnormalities.[16,153] Atrial flutter has been reported, but ventricular arrhythmias have not.

Laboratory Studies. Kobayashi et al[176] reported clinical laboratory values in 27 patients with HAPE. This report confirms typical mild elevations of hematocrit and hemoglobin, probably secondary to intravascular volume depletion and perhaps plasma leakage into the lung. Elevation of the peripheral white blood cell count is common, but rarely is it above 14,000 cells/ml[3]. The serum concentration of creatine phosphokinase (CPK) is increased. Most of the rise in CPK has been attributed to skeletal muscle damage, although in two patients, CPK isoenzymes showed brain fraction levels of 1% of the total, which according to the authors may have indicated brain damage.[176]

Arterial blood gas studies consistently reveal respiratory alkalosis and marked hypoxemia, more severe than expected for the patient's clinical condition. Respiratory or metabolic acidosis related to hypoxemia has not been reported. Therefore arterial blood gas studies are not essential if noninvasive pulse oximetry is available to measure arterial oxygenation. At 4200 m (13,780 feet) on Mt. McKinley, the mean value of arterial PO_2 in HAPE was 28 ± 4 torr. Values as low as 24 torr in HAPE are not unusual. Arterial oxygen saturation values in our HAPE subjects ranged from 40% to 70%, with a mean of $56\% \pm 8\%$.[307] Arterial acid-base values may be misleading in patients taking acetazolamide because this drug produces significant metabolic acidosis.

Radiologic Findings. The radiologic findings in HAPE have been described in original reports.[157,206,348,349] Findings are consistent with noncardiogenic pulmonary edema, with generally normal heart size and left atrial size and no evidence of pulmonary venous prominence, such as Kerley's lines. The pulmonary arteries increase in diameter.[348] Infiltrates are commonly described as fluffy and patchy with areas of aeration between infiltrates, and in a peripheral location rather than central. Infiltrates may be unilateral or bilateral, with a predilection for the right middle lung field, which corresponds to the usual area of rales. Pleural effusion is quite rare. The x-ray findings generally correlate with the severity of the illness and degree of hypoxemia. A small right hemithorax, absence of pulmonary vascular markings on the right, and edema confined to the left lung are the basis for a diagnosis of unilateral absent pulmonary artery syndrome.[109] The x-ray findings of HAPE are presented in Figure 1-14.

Clearing of infiltrates is generally rapid once treatment is initiated. Depending on severity, complete clearing may take from one to several days. Infiltrates are likely to persist longer if the patient remains at high altitude, even if confined to bed and receiving oxygen therapy. Radiographs taken within 48 hours of return to low altitude may confirm a diagnosis of HAPE.

Pathologic Findings. More than 20 autopsy reports of persons who died of HAPE have been published.* Of those whose cranium was opened, more than half had cerebral edema. All lungs showed extensive and severe edema, with bloody, foamy fluid in the airways. Lung weights were two to four times normal. The left side of the heart was normal. The right atrium and main pulmonary artery were often distended. Proteinaceous exudate with hyaline membranes was characteristic. All lungs had areas of inflammation with neutrophil accumulation. The diagnosis of bronchopneumonia was common, although bacteria were not noted. Pulmonary veins, the left ventricle, and the left atrium were generally not dilated, in contrast to the right ventricle and atrium. Most reports mention capillary and arteriolar thrombi and alveolar fibrin deposits, as well as microvascular and gross pulmonary hemorrhage and infarcts. The autopsy findings thus suggest a protein-rich, permeability type of edema, with thrombi or emboli. Confirmation of HAPE as a permeability edema was obtained by analysis of alveolar lavage fluid by Schoene et al.[306,307] These authors found a 100-fold increase in lavage fluid protein levels in patients with HAPE compared with well control subjects and patients with AMS.[307] The lavage fluid also had a low percentage of neutrophils, in contrast to findings in adult respiratory distress syndrome. Further evidence for a permeability edema was a 1:1 ratio of aspirated edema fluid protein to plasma protein level found by Hackett et al.[112] In addition, the lavage fluid contained vasoactive eicosanoids and complement proteins, indicative of endothelium-leukocyte interactions.

Mechanisms of High-Altitude Pulmonary Edema. The search continues for the mechanism triggering the pulmonary vascular leak. An acceptable explanation for HAPE must take into account three well-established facts: excessive pulmonary hypertension; high-protein permeability leak; and normal function of the left side of the heart. One mechanism that is consistent with the facts is failure of capillaries secondary to overperfusion edema (Figure 1-15).

ROLE OF PULMONARY HYPERTENSION. Excessive pulmonary artery pressure (PAP) is the sine qua non of

---

*References 8, 72, 247, 319, 321, 361.

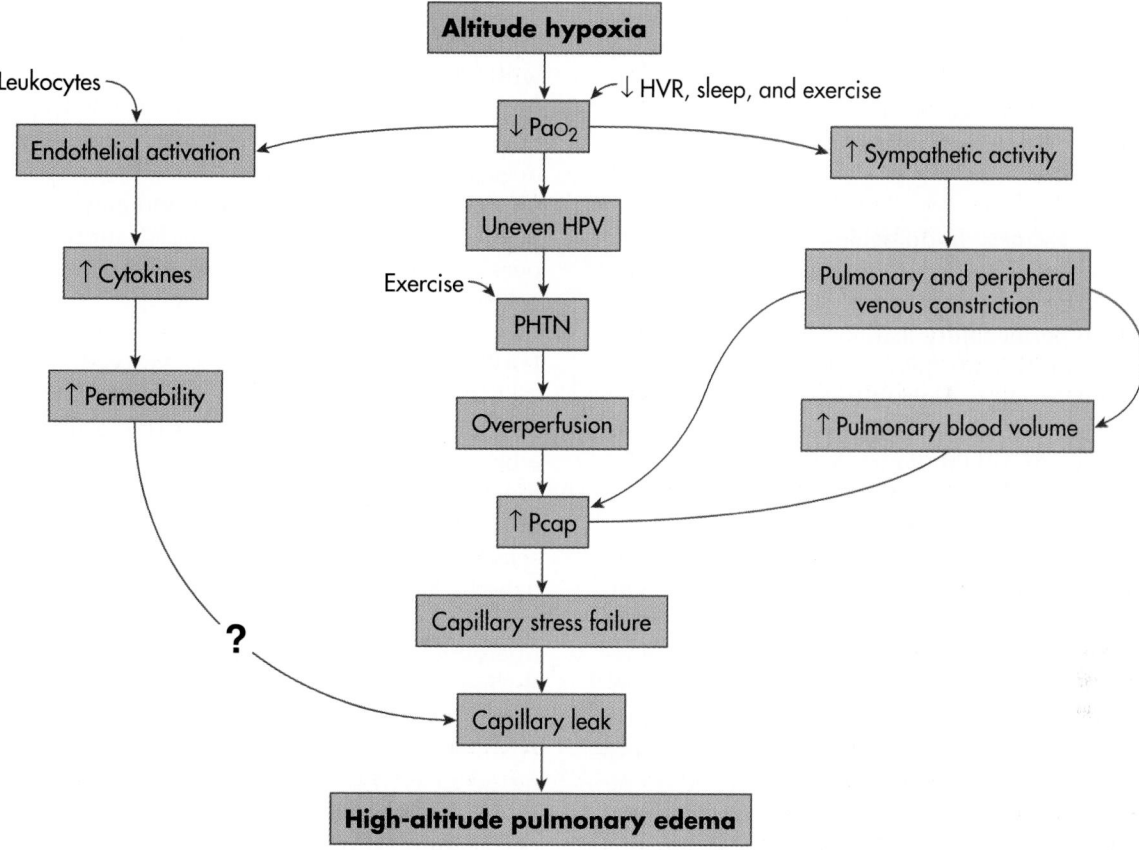

Figure 1-15 Proposed pathophysiology of high-altitude pulmonary edema. *HPV,* Hypoxic pulmonary vaso-constriction; *HVR,* hypoxic ventilatory response; *Pcap,* capillary pressure; *PHTN,* pulmonary hypertension.

HAPE; no cases of HAPE have been reported without pulmonary hypertension. All persons ascending to high altitudes or otherwise enduring hypoxia, however, have some elevation of PAP. The hypoxic pulmonary vasoconstrictor response (HPVR) is thought to be useful in humans at sea level because it helps match perfusion with ventilation. When local areas of the lung are poorly ventilated because of infection, atelectasis, or some other cause, the HPVR directs blood away from those areas to well-ventilated regions. In the setting of global hypoxia as occurs with ascent to high altitude, HPVR is presumably diffuse and all areas of the lung constrict, causing a restricted vascular bed and an increase in PAP, which is of little if any value for ventilation-perfusion matching at high altitude. The degree of HPVR varies widely among individuals (as well as among species). Presumably those with a greater HPVR have a greater percentage of muscularized arterioles, constrict more units (a greater amount) of the circulation, and have a more restricted vascular bed and a greater rise in PAP. Although other factors, such as the vigor of the ventilatory response and subsequent arterial PO$_2$, may help determine the ultimate degree of pulmonary hypertension, HPVR appears to be the dominant factor. Because all persons with HAPE have excessive pulmonary hypertension, but not all those with excessive pulmonary hypertension have HAPE, it appears that pulmonary hypertension is a necessary factor but in itself is not the cause of HAPE.

OVERPERFUSION. Hultgren[148] suggested that in those who develop HAPE, the hypoxic pulmonary vasoconstriction is uneven and the microcirculation in an unconstricted (relatively dilated) area is subjected to high pressure and flow, leading to edema. The unevenness could be due to anatomic characteristics, such as distribution of muscularized arterioles, or to functional factors, such as loss of HPVR in severely hypoxic regions.[148] Uneven perfusion is suggested clinically by the typical patchy x-ray appearance and is supported by lung scans during acute hypoxia that show uneven perfusion in persons susceptible to HAPE.[346] Persons born without a right pulmonary artery are highly susceptible to HAPE (see Figure 1-14, *D*),[109] supporting the concept of overperfusion of a restricted vascular bed as a cause of edema, because the entire cardiac output flows into one lung. Staub,[326] in an accompanying editorial, supported the concept of overperfusion edema but pointed out that hydrostatic edema generally produces a low-protein transudate. Other causes of overperfusion of the pulmonary circulation include left-to-right shunts, such as atrial septal defect (ASD), ventricular septal defect (VSD), and patent ductus arteriosus (PDA).

PERMEABILITY FACTORS. Endothelial damage from shear forces,[287] as well as stress failure of the capillary membrane,[357,358] has therefore been invoked to explain the high-protein permeability leak from overperfusion. A recent preliminary study has found activity of adhesion molecules on ascent to high altitude,[82] which indicates interaction of leukocytes and endothelium. The lavage fluid findings of inflammatory mediators also point to the possible endothelial involvement, as do a number of animal studies that failed to produce permeability edema with overperfusion alone but succeeded when the pulmonary vascular bed was embolized with microspheres.[98]

The overperfusion hypothesis is consistent with recent clinical trials of vasodilators intended for prevention and treatment of HAPE. Presumably, when pulmonary vasoconstriction is relieved, flow becomes more homogeneous, and because overall PAP is reduced, microvascular pressure also drops. The rapid reversibility of the illness is also consistent with this mechanism.

Other factors contributing to increased hydrostatic pressure, such as exercise or a high salt load with subsequent hypervolemia, could also play a role in HAPE. The effective use of diuretics and vasodilators also supports a rationale for reducing hydrostatic pressure. A recent study found that an intravenous α-adrenergic blocker, phentolamine, was effective in reducing PAP in HAPE,[117] which raises the possibility that pulmonary venous constriction, which is sympathetically mediated, could be a factor. Any degree of venous constriction could significantly contribute to increased microvascular pressure. Experiments that convincingly demonstrate the validity of the preceding hypotheses are obviously difficult to perform in humans and await a successful animal model of HAPE. For now, the exact site and mechanism of the leak in HAPE remain enigmatic.

CONTROL OF VENTILATION. As in AMS, control of ventilation may play a role in the pathophysiology of HAPE. Victims have been shown to have a lower HVR than persons who acclimatized well,[115,211] but not all persons with a low HVR become ill. Thus low HVR appears to play a permissive, rather than causative, role in the development of HAPE. A brisk HVR, and therefore a large increase in ventilation, appears to be protective. Persons who tend to hypoventilate are more hypoxemic and presumably suffer greater pulmonary hypertension. Possibly more important, a low HVR may permit episodes of extreme hypoxemia during sleep (see Figure 1-6). Supporting this concept is the frequency with which the onset of HAPE occurs during sleep, especially in persons who have ingested sleep medications.[103,115] In addition, a HAPE victim with a low HVR does not mount an adequate ventilatory response to the severe hypoxemia of the illness and may suffer further ventilatory depression through CNS suppression. Such persons, when given oxygen, show a "paradoxical" increase in ventilation.[115]

HAPE Susceptibility. Persons susceptible to HAPE (HAPE-s) show an abnormal rise of PAP and pulmonary vascular resistance during a hypoxic challenge at rest[169,370] and during exercise, and even during exercise in normoxia.[83,169] The response of PAP in HAPE-s may be related to greater alveolar hypoxemia secondary to lower HVR.[115,133,214] Recent work established a direct link in HAPE-s between the rise in PAP and greater sympathetic activation (as measured by microneurographic recordings in the peroneal nerve during hypoxia).[78] The authors concluded that sympathetic overactivation might contribute to HAPE. Also, smaller and less distensible lungs have been noted in HAPE-s.[83,133,327] Another characteristic of HAPE-s is reduced nitric oxide synthesis during hypoxia, suggesting impaired endothelial function.[302] Additional preliminary studies suggest that HAPE-s subjects are characterized by impairment of respiratory transepithelial sodium and water transport, which in mice is related to a genetic defect in the amiloride-sensitive sodium channel (αEnaC).[300,303] Further evidence for a genetic component to HAPE susceptibility comes from study of major human leukocyte antigen (HLA) alleles in 28 male and 2 female subjects with a history of HAPE compared with HLA alleles in 100 healthy volunteers.[121] The HLA-DR6 and HLA-DQ4 antigens were associated with HAPE, and HLA-DR6 with pulmonary hypertension. These preliminary findings suggest that an immunogenetic susceptibility may underlie the development of HAPE, at least in some cases. In summary, overactivation of the sympathetic nervous system in response to hypoxia, a low HVR, small lungs, and impaired pulmonary nitric oxide synthesis apparently combine to render a person susceptible to HAPE. The role of genetically determined impairment of respiratory epithelial sodium and water transport and the link between components of the major histocompatibility complex and HAPE provide exciting avenues for further investigation into the pathophysiology of HAPE.

TREATMENT. Early recognition is the key to successful outcome, as with other high-altitude illnesses (see Box 1-3). The therapy for HAPE depends on the severity of the illness and on the environment. In the wilderness, where oxygen and medical expertise may not be available, persons with HAPE should be evacuated to a lower altitude as soon as possible. However, because of augmented pulmonary hypertension and greater hypoxemia with exercise, exertion must be minimized. If the disorder is diagnosed early, recovery is rapid with a descent of only 500 to 1000 m (1640 to 3281 feet) and the victim may be able to reascend slowly 2 or 3 days later. In high-altitude locations with oxygen supplies, bed rest with supplemental oxygen may suffice,[208] but severe HAPE may require high-flow oxygen (4 to 6 L/min or more) for more than 24 hours. Hyperbaric therapy is equivalent to low-flow oxygen and can help conserve oxygen supplies.[279]

Oxygen immediately increases arterial oxygenation and reduces PAP, heart rate, respiratory rate, and symptoms. When descent is not possible, oxygen (or a hyperbaric bag) can be lifesaving. Rescue groups should make delivery of oxygen to the victim, by airdrop if necessary, the highest priority if descent is slow or delayed. If oxygen is not available, immediate descent is lifesaving. Waiting for a helicopter or rescue team has too often proved fatal. Because cold stress elevates PAP, the victim should be kept warm.[54] The use of a mask providing pressure (resistance) on expiration (EPAP) was shown to improve gas exchange in HAPE, and this may be useful as a temporizing measure.[187,305] The same is accomplished with pursed-lip breathing. An unusual case report suggested that a climber may have saved his partner's life by postural drainage to expel airway fluid.[38]

Drugs are of limited necessity in HAPE because oxygen and descent are so effective. Medications that reduce pulmonary blood volume, PAP, and pulmonary vascular resistance are physiologically rational to use when oxygen is not available or descent delayed. Singh et al[321] reported good results with furosemide (80 mg every 12 hours), and greater diuresis and clinical improvement occurred when 15 mg parenteral morphine was given with the first dose of furosemide. Their use, however, has been eclipsed by recent results with vasodilators. The calcium channel blocker nifedipine (30 mg slow release every 12 to 24 hours or 10 mg orally repeated as necessary) has proved effective in reducing pulmonary vascular resistance and PAP,[24] as have hydralazine and phentolamine.[117,254] The vasodilators can cause hypotension, but they avoid the danger of CNS depression from morphine and possible hypovolemia from diuretics. Nifedipine does not quickly improve oxygenation, however, and clinical improvement is much better with oxygen and descent than with any of these drugs. Nifedipine and perhaps other vasodilators appear to be useful adjunctive therapy but are no substitute for definitive treatment (see Box 1-3).

After evacuation of the victim to a lower altitude, hospitalization may be warranted for severe cases. Treatment consists of bed rest and oxygen (sufficient to maintain SaO_2% greater than 90%), and rapid recovery is the rule. A rare instance of progression to adult respiratory distress syndrome has been reported, but it was impossible to exclude other diagnoses completely.[376] Antibiotics are indicated for infection when present. Occasionally, pulmonary artery catheterization or Doppler echocardiography is necessary to differentiate cardiogenic from high-altitude pulmonary edema. Endotracheal intubation and mechanical ventilation are rarely needed. A HAPE victim demonstrating unusual susceptibility, such as onset of HAPE despite adequate acclimatization, or onset below 2750 m (9023 feet), might require further investigation, such as echocardiography, to rule out an intracardiac shunt. In children, undiagnosed congenital heart disease is worth considering (Figure 1-16). Hospitalization until blood gases are completely normal is not warranted; all persons returning from high altitude are at least partially acclimatized to hypoxemia, and hypocapnic alkalosis persists for days after descent. Distinct clinical improvement, radiographic improvement over 24 to 48 hours, and an arterial PO_2 of 60 torr or an SaO_2% greater than 90% are adequate discharge criteria. Patients are advised to resume normal activities gradually and are warned that they may require up to 2 weeks to recover complete strength. Physicians should recommend preventive measures, including graded ascent with adequate time for acclimatization, and should provide instruction on the use of acetazolamide or nifedipine for future ascents. An episode of HAPE is not a contraindication to subsequent high-altitude exposure, but education to ensure proper preventive measures and recognition of early symptoms is critical.

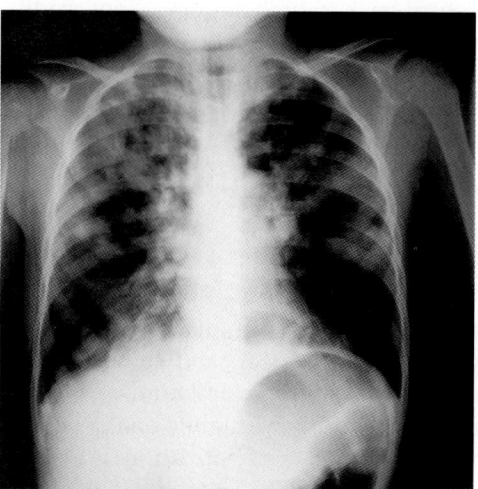

Figure 1-16 Chest x-ray of severe HAPE in a 4-year-old girl with a small previously undiagnosed patent ductus arteriosus that predisposed her to HAPE.

PREVENTION. The preventive measures previously described for AMS also apply to HAPE: graded ascent, time for acclimatization, low sleeping altitudes, and avoidance of alcohol and sleeping pills. The role of exertion in HAPE may be overemphasized. Reports from North America have included hikers, climbers, and skiers, all of whom were exercising vigorously. Menon et al[221] clearly showed that sedentary men taken abruptly to high altitude were just as likely to become victims of HAPE. Nonetheless, because PAP rises with increasing level of exercise, prudence dictates no overexertion for the first day or two at altitude. Considerable clinical experience (but no data) suggests that acetazolamide prevents HAPE in persons with a history of recurrent episodes. Nifedipine (20 mg slow release every 8 hours) prevented HAPE in subjects with a history of repeated episodes.[24] The drug should be carried by such individuals and started at the first signs of HAPE or, for an abrupt ascent, started when leaving low altitude.

Reentry Pulmonary Edema

In some persons who have lived for years at high altitude, HAPE develops on reascent from a trip to low altitude.[79] Authors have suggested that the incidence of HAPE on reascent may be higher than that during initial ascent by flatlanders,[19,150] but data on true incidence are difficult to obtain. Children and adolescents are more susceptible than adults.[79] Hultgren[149] found a prevalence of HAPE in Peruvian natives of 6.4 per 100 exposures in the 1-to-20 age group, and 0.4 per 100 exposures in persons over 21 years. The phenomenon has been observed most often in Peru, where high-altitude residents can return from sea level to high altitude quite rapidly. Cases have also been reported in Leadville, Colorado,[308] but reports are conspicuously absent from Nepal and Tibet, perhaps because such rapid return back to high altitude is not readily available.[368] Severinghaus[311] has postulated that increased muscularization of pulmonary arterioles that develops with chronic high-altitude exposure generates an inordinately high PAP on reascent, causing the edema.

OTHER MEDICAL CONCERNS AT HIGH ALTITUDE

High-Altitude Deterioration

The world's highest human habitation is at approximately 5500 m (18,045 feet), and above this deterioration outstrips the ability to acclimatize.[172] The deterioration is more rapid the higher one goes above the maximum point of acclimatization. Above 8000 m (26,247 feet), deterioration is so rapid that, without supplemental oxygen, death can occur in a matter of days. Life-preserving tasks, such as melting snow for water, may become too difficult, and death may result from dehydration, starvation, hypothermia, and especially neurologic and psychiatric dysfunction.[295]

Loss of body weight is a prominent feature of high-altitude deterioration. Body weight is progressively lost because of anorexia and malabsorption during expeditions to extreme high altitude. Pugh[262] reported a 14- to 20-kg body weight loss in climbers on the 1953 British Mt. Everest Expedition. Nearly 30 years later, with improvement in food and cooking techniques, climbers on AMREE still lost an average of 6 kg.[42] This was due in part to a 49% decrease in fat absorption and a 24% decrease in carbohydrate absorption. During OEII, in which the "climbers" were allowed to eat foods of their choosing ad libitum, they still suffered large weight losses: 8 kg overall, including 3 kg of fat and 5 kg of lean body weight (muscle).[141,292] At 4300 m (14,108 feet), weight loss was attenuated by adjusting caloric intake to match caloric expenditure.[52] Thus significant weight loss with prolonged exposure to high altitude may be overcome with adequate caloric intake, but decreased appetite is a problem.[170,341] At very high altitudes, an increase in caloric intake may not be sufficient to completely counteract the severe anorexia and weight loss.

At extreme altitude, Ryn[295] reported an incidence of acute organic brain syndrome in 35% of climbers going above 7000 m (22,966 feet), in association with high-altitude deterioration. This syndrome, which includes impaired judgment or frank psychosis, could directly threaten survival.

Children at High Altitude

Children born at high altitude in North America appear to have a higher incidence of complications in the neonatal period than do their lower-altitude counterparts.[250] In populations better adapted to high altitude over many generations, neonatal transition has not been as well scrutinized, but there does appear to be some morbidity.[360] High-altitude residence does not clearly affect eventual stature, but growth and development are slowed.[69,235] In the developing world, confounding factors such as nutrition and socioeconomic status make these issues difficult to assess.[145] Children residing at high altitude are more likely to develop pulmonary edema on return to their homes from a low-altitude sojourn than are lowland children on induction to high altitude.

Lowland children traveling to high altitude are just as likely to suffer AMS as are adults. No data indicate that children are more susceptible to altitude illness, although diagnosis can be more difficult in preverbal children.[371] Despite this somewhat reassuring fact, very conservative recommendations are made regarding taking children to high altitude; it should be made clear that these opinions are not based on the science.[28,261] Durmowicz et al[79] showed that children with respiratory infections were more susceptible to HAPE.

Children can be given acetazolamide or dexamethasone as necessary for AMS/HACE. The dosage of acetazolamide for prevention or treatment of AMS in children is 5 mg/kg/day in divided doses.

High-Altitude Syncope

Syncope within the first 24 hours of arrival appears to be common at moderate altitude[248] but is rarely observed in mountaineers at higher altitudes; it is a problem of acute induction to altitude. The mechanism is an unstable cardiovascular control system, and it is considered a form of neurohumoral (or neurocardiogenic) syncope.[89] An unstable state of cerebral autoregulation may also play a role.[375] These events appear to be random and seldom occur a second time. Preexisting cardiovascular disease is not a factor in most cases. Postprandial state and alcohol ingestion might be contributing factors. Altitude syncope has no direct relationship to high-altitude illness.

Alcohol at High Altitude

Two questions regarding alcohol are frequently asked: (1) does alcohol affect acclimatization, and (2) does altitude potentiate the effects of alcohol? A recent epidemiologic study indicated that 64% of tourists ingested alcohol during the first few days at 2800 m (9187 feet).[134] The effect of alcohol on altitude tolerance and acclimatization might therefore be of considerable relevance. Roeggla et al[290] determined blood gases 1 hour after ingestion of 50 g of alcohol (equivalent to 1 liter of beer), at 171 m (561 feet) and again after 4 hours at 3000 m (9843 feet). A placebo-controlled, double-blind paired design was used. For the 10 subjects, alcohol had no effect on ventilation at the low altitude, but at high altitude it depressed ventilation, as gauged by a decreased arterial PO_2 (from 69 to 64 mm Hg) and increased PCO_2 (from 32.5 to 34 mm Hg).[290] Whether this degree of ventilatory depression would contribute to AMS, and whether repeated doses would have greater effect, was not tested. Nonetheless, the authors argue that alcohol might impede ventilatory acclimatization and should be used with caution at high altitude.

Conventional wisdom proffers an additive effect of altitude and alcohol on brain function. McFarland,[216] who was concerned about the interaction in aviators, wrote ". . . the alcohol in two or three cocktails would have the physiological action of four or five drinks at altitudes of approximately 10,000 to 12,000 ft." Also, "Airmen should be informed that the effects of alcohol are similar to those of oxygen want and that the combined effects on the brain and the CNS are significant at altitudes even as low as 8,000 to 10,000 ft."[216] His original observations were made on two subjects in the Andes in 1936. He found that blood alcohol levels rose more rapidly and reached higher values at altitude but noted no interactive effect of alcohol and altitudes of

3810 and 5335 m (12,501 and 17,504 feet).[217] Most subsequent studies refuted the increased blood alcohol concentration data except at the highest altitudes, over 5450 m (17,881 feet). Higgins et al,[129,130] in a series of chamber studies, found blood alcohol levels were similar at 392 m (1286 feet) and 3660 m (12,008 feet), and they noted no synergistic effects of alcohol and altitude. Lategola et al[191] found that blood alcohol uptake curves were the same at sea level and 3660 m (12,008 feet), and performance on math tests showed no interaction between alcohol and altitude. In another study of 25 men, performance scores were similar at sea level and at a simulated 3810-m (12,501-foot) altitude, with blood alcohol level of 88 mg%.[59] Performance was not affected by hypoxia, only by alcohol, and older subjects were more affected. When more demanding tasks were tested, Collins[58] found that a blood alcohol level of 91 mg% affected performance, as did an altitude of 3660 m (12,008 feet) during night sessions when the subjects were sleep deprived, but there was no significant altitude/alcohol interaction. In the one study in which Collins et al[60] were able to discern some altitude effect, there was a simple additive interaction of altitude (hypoxic gas breathing) and alcohol. He concluded that performance decrements resulting from alcohol may be increased by altitudes of 3660 m (12,008 feet) if subjects are negatively affected by that altitude without alcohol. All of these aviation-oriented studies used acute hypoxia equivalent to no more than 3500 m (11,483 feet). Perhaps the highest altitude (without supplemental oxygen) at which alcohol was studied was 4350 m (14,272 feet), on the summit of Mt. Evans in Colorado. Freedman et al[88] found that alcohol affected auditory evoked potentials the same as in Denver; that is, no influence of altitude was detectable.

In summary, the possibility of interactions between alcohol and altitude deserves study. The limited data on blood gases at altitude after alcohol ingestion support the popular notion that alcohol could slow ventilatory acclimatization. Considerable data, however, refute the belief that at least up to 3660 m (12,008 feet), altitude potentiates the effect of alcohol. How altitude and alcohol might interact during various stages of acclimatization in individuals at higher altitudes is still unknown.

Thrombosis: Coagulation and Platelet Changes

Autopsy findings of widespread thrombi in the brain and lungs have led to investigations of the clotting mechanism at high altitude. Changes in platelets and coagulation have been observed in rabbits, mice, rats, calves, and humans on ascent to high altitude.[126] A report from OEII found no changes in concentration or inhibition of coagulation factors; significant altitude illness did not develop in OEII subjects. A remarkable case illustrating coagulation abnormalities at high altitude was reported by O'Brodovich et al.[252] In one of the women in this chamber study, disseminated intravascular coagulation developed within 1½ hours of exposure to hypobaric hypoxia (PB = 410 torr, about 4600 m [15,092 feet]). The platelet count had decreased by 93,000/mm³, and the activated partial thromboplastin time (aPTT) had shortened by 10 seconds. When symptoms of AMS developed, the study was discontinued. The exact mechanism is unknown. The woman and other subjects showed a shortening of the aPTT, perhaps secondary to the increase in procoagulant VII:C.

Singh et al[318] reported that patients with HAPE had increased fibrinogen levels and prolonged clot lysis times, attributed to a breakdown of fibrinolysis. These authors also reported thrombotic, occlusive hypertensive pulmonary vascular disease in soldiers who had recently arrived at high altitude.[317] These findings, plus autopsy data, prompted Dickinson et al[72] to conclude that "hypercoagulability of the blood and sequestration of platelets in the pulmonary vascular bed provoke pulmonary thrombosis, and may contribute to the pathogenesis of HAPE."

A series of experiments by Bärtsch et al[17,18,20,21] however, carefully examined this issue in well subjects and in those with AMS and HAPE. They concluded that HAPE is not preceded by a prothrombotic state and that only in "advanced HAPE" is there fibrin generation, which abates rapidly with oxygen treatment. They considered the coagulation and platelet activation as an epiphenomenon rather than as an inciting pathophysiologic factor. Fibrin formation would, however, contribute to worsening of edema because of vascular obstruction, increased vascular permeability, and derangement of surfactant function.[26]

Thrombotic and embolic events in mountaineers may be explained on the basis of dehydration, polycythemia, cold, constrictive clothing, and venous stasis from prolonged periods of weather-imposed inactivity. A role for hypoxia-induced abnormal clotting in the pathogenesis of these events, especially stroke, is not established.

Peripheral Edema

Edema of the face, hands, and ankles at high altitude is common, especially in females. Incidence of edema in at least one area of the body in trekkers at 4200 m (13,780 feet) was 18% overall, 28% in females, 14% in males, 7% in asymptomatic trekkers, and 27% in those with AMS.[105] Although not a serious clinical problem, edema can be bothersome. The presence of peripheral edema demands an examination for pulmonary and cerebral edema. In the absence of AMS, peripheral edema is effectively treated with a diuretic. Treatment of accompanying AMS by descent or medical therapy also results in diuresis and resolution of peripheral edema.

The mechanism is presumably similar to fluid retention in AMS but may also be merely due to exercise.[224]

Immunosuppression

Mountaineers have observed that infections are common at high altitude, slow to resolve, and often resistant to antibiotics.[243] On AMREE in 1981, serious skin and soft tissue infections developed. "Nearly every accidental wound, no matter how small, suppurated for a period of time and subsequently healed slowly."[299] A suppurative hand wound and septic olecranon bursitis did not respond to antibiotics but did respond to descent to 4300 m (14,108 feet) from the 5300-m (17,389-foot) base camp. Nine of 21 persons had significant infections not related to the respiratory tract. Most high-altitude expeditions report similar problems.

Data from OEII indicated that healthy individuals are more susceptible to infections at high altitude because of impaired T lymphocyte function; this is consistent with previous Russian studies in humans and animals.[220] In contrast, B cells and active immunity are not impaired. Therefore resistance to viruses may not be impaired, whereas susceptibility to bacterial infection is increased. The degree of immunosuppression is similar to that seen with trauma, burns, emotional depression, and space flight. The mechanism may be related, at least in part, to release of adrenocorticotropic hormone, cortisone, and β-endorphins, all of which modulate the immune response. Intense ultraviolet exposure has also been shown to impair immunity. Persons with serious infections at high altitude may need oxygen or descent for effective treatment. Impaired immunity because of altitude should be anticipated in situations in which infection could be a complication, such as trauma, burns, and surgical and invasive procedures.

High-Altitude Pharyngitis and Bronchitis

Sore throat, chronic cough, and bronchitis are nearly universal in persons who spend more than 2 weeks at an extreme altitude (over 5500 m [18,045 feet]).[209] All 21 members of AMREE suffered these problems.[299] Only two of eight subjects in OEII (where the temperature was greater than 21° C [70° F] and relative humidity was greater than 80%) developed cough, and only above 6500 m (21,325 feet). Only four had sore throat. Obviously, factors other than hypoxia are involved. In the field, these problems usually appear without fever or chills, myalgias, lymphadenopathy, exudate, or other signs of infection. Whether these are infections is debatable. The increase in ventilation, especially with exercise, forces obligate mouth breathing at altitude, bypassing the warming and moisturizing action of the nasal mucous membranes and sinuses. Movement of large volumes of dry, cold air across the pharyngeal mucosa can cause marked dehydration, irritation, and pain, similar to pharyngitis. Vasomotor rhinitis, quite common in cold temperatures, aggravates this condition by necessitating mouth breathing during sleep. For this reason, decongestant nasal spray is one of the most coveted items in an expedition medical kit. Other countermeasures include forced hydration, hard candies, lozenges, and steam inhalation.

High-altitude bronchitis can be disabling because of severe coughing spasms. Cough fractures of one or more ribs are not rare; two climbers on AMREE had such fractures. Purulent sputum is common. Response to antibiotics is poor; most victims resign themselves to taking medications such as codeine and do not expect a cure until descent. A recent study of high-altitude bronchitis on Aconcagua revealed that bronchitis developed in 13 of 19 climbers above 4300 m (14,108 feet).[264] Mean sputum production was 6 teaspoons per day. All reported that onset was after a period of excessive hyperventilation associated with strenuous activity. Although an infectious etiology is possible, experimental evidence suggests that respiratory heat loss results in purulent sputum and sufficient airway irritation to cause persistent cough.[215] This is supported by the beneficial effect of steam inhalation and lack of response to antibiotics. Many climbers find that a silk balaclava or similar material that is porous enough for breathing but that traps some moisture and heat effectively prevents or ameliorates the problem.

Chronic Mountain Polycythemia

In 1928, Carlos Monge[231] described a syndrome in Andean high-altitude natives that was characterized by headaches, insomnia, lethargy, plethoric appearance, and polycythemia greater than expected for the altitude. Known variously as Monge's disease, chronic mountain polycythemia, or chronic mountain sickness, the condition has now been recognized in all high-altitude areas of the world.[183,229,259] Both lowlanders who relocate to high altitude and native residents are susceptible. Chinese investigators reported that 13% of lowland Chinese males and 1.6% of females who had relocated to Tibet developed excessive polycythemia (hemoglobin level greater than 20 g/dl blood).[369] The incidence in Leadville, Colorado, is also high in men over 40 and distinctly low in women.[181] The increased hematopoiesis is apparently related to greater hypoxic stress, which may be due to a number of causes, such as lung disease, sleep apnea syndromes, and idiopathic hypoventilation. A diagnosis of "pure" chronic mountain polycythemia excludes lung disease and is characterized by relative alveolar hypoventilation and respiratory insensitivity to hypoxia.[229] Some studies suggest that even for the degree of hypoxemia, the red blood cell mass is excessive, implying excessive amounts or

overactivity of erythropoietin.[362] Increasing age is also an important factor.[230]

Regardless of the exact mechanism, therapy is routinely successful. Descent to a lower altitude is the definitive treatment. Supplemental oxygen during sleep is valuable. Phlebotomy is a common practice, provides subjective improvement (without significant objective changes), and is generally recommended when hematocrit is greater than 60% or hemoglobin level is greater than 20 g/dl blood.[362] The respiratory stimulants medroxyprogesterone acetate (20 to 60 mg/day) and acetazolamide (250 mg twice a day) have also been shown to reduce the hematocrit value by improving oxygenation.[182] The response to respiratory stimulants emphasizes the contribution of hypoventilation to chronic mountain polycythemia.

High-Altitude Flatus Expulsion

High-altitude flatus expulsion (HAFE) is the unwelcome spontaneous passage of colonic gas at altitudes above 3000 m (9843 feet).[9a] The mechanism has been postulated to relate to the expansion of intraluminal bowel gas at the decreased atmospheric pressure of altitude. Affected individuals may benefit from the oral administration of digestive enzymes or simethicone and a preferential carbohydrate diet.

High-Altitude Retinopathy and Ultraviolet Keratitis

See Chapter 22.

Fingernail Changes

A white transverse band visible across the fingernail plates may correspond to duration of altitude-related hypoxia. This has been observed (Figure 1-17) in a 34-year-old climber who spent approximately 6 weeks at or above 5500 m (18,045 feet) climbing on Mt. Everest.[161] It

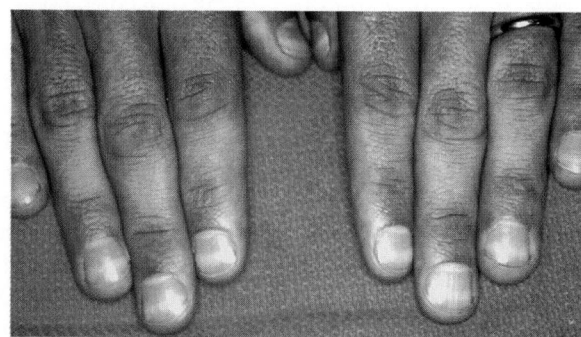

Figure 1-17 This photograph was taken 3 months after return to low altitude. A white transverse band grew out from the nail beds and was due to exposure to extremely high altitude. (*From Hutchison SJ, Amin S: N Engl J Med 336:229, 1997.*)

was hypothesized that the white band may have been an effect of hypoxia and catabolic stress.

COMMON MEDICAL CONDITIONS AND HIGH ALTITUDE

Persons with certain preexisting illnesses might be at risk for adverse effects upon ascent to high altitude, either because of exacerbation of their illnesses or because these illnesses might affect acclimatization and susceptibility to altitude illness. Certain populations also require special consideration, such as the pregnant and the elderly. This section presents an overview of current knowledge regarding these issues. Despite the importance of the interaction of altitude and common medical conditions, research has so far been limited. See the recent review by Hackett[102] for a more complete discussion. Conditions that can be aggravated by high-altitude exposure are listed in Box 1-4.

Respiratory Diseases

Chronic Lung Disease. Although oxygen saturation remains above 90% in a normally acclimatizing, healthy, awake person until at an altitude over 3000 m (9843 feet) (see Figure 1-1), persons with hypoxemic lung disease reach this threshold at a lower altitude that depends on the baseline blood oxygen values. As a result, these persons might have altitude-related problems at lower altitudes than would healthy individuals. In terms of their lung disease, improved airflow will result from decreased air density at high altitude, but hypoxemia, pulmonary hypertension, disordered control of ventilation, and sleep-disordered breathing could all become worse. Unfortunately, few data are available to guide the clinician advising such a person undertaking a trip to altitude. Hypoxic gas breathing at sea level can predict oxygenation at high altitude, but this does not always correlate with symptoms and is not convenient. Sea level P_{O_2} values of 68 and 72 torr successfully classified more than 90% of the subjects with a Pa_{O_2} greater than 55 torr at simulated altitudes of 1525 m (5004 feet) and 2440 m (8006 feet), respectively.[95,96] Such predictions have been further refined with the addition of spirometry.[76] A Pa_{O_2} of 55 torr results in a saturation of 90% at high altitude, where there is slight alkalosis. These data suggested that persons with Pa_{O_2} values lower than these at sea level might require supplemental oxygen at modest altitudes. However, in the only clinical study to date, Graham and Houston[97] found that eight subjects with chronic obstructive pulmonary disease (COPD) tolerated 1920-m (6300-foot) altitude quite well. Persons with cor pulmonale or angina were excluded. The subjects had only minor symptoms on ascent, despite the fact that mean Pa_{O_2} declined from 66 at sea level to 51 mm Hg while at rest and from 63 to 47 mm Hg with exercise. The patients did acclimatize, with a drop in

Box 1-4 ADVISABILITY OF EXPOSURE TO HIGH AND VERY HIGH ALTITUDE FOR COMMON CONDITIONS (WITHOUT SUPPLEMENTAL OXYGEN)

PROBABLY NO EXTRA RISK

Young and old
Fit and unfit
Obesity
Diabetes
After coronary artery bypass grafting (without angina)
Mild chronic obstructive pulmonary disease (COPD)
Asthma
Low-risk pregnancy
Controlled hypertension
Controlled seizure disorder
Psychiatric disorders
Neoplastic diseases
Inflammatory conditions

CAUTION

Moderate COPD
Compensated congestive heart failure (CHF)
Sleep apnea syndromes
Troublesome arrhythmias
Stable angina/coronary artery disease
High-risk pregnancy
Sickle cell trait
Cerebrovascular diseases
Any cause for restricted pulmonary circulation
Seizure disorder (not on medication)
Radial keratotomy

CONTRAINDICATED

Sickle cell anemia (with history of crises)
Severe COPD
Pulmonary hypertension
Uncompensated CHF

Pco_2, and a corresponding increase in Pa_{O_2} over 4 days, the same response as seen in healthy persons. The authors concluded that travel to this moderate altitude is safe for such patients. They speculated that these persons might have been partially acclimatized because of their hypoxic lung disease and were therefore less likely to develop AMS. Unfortunately, no further investigations with sicker patients or at higher altitudes have yet been reported.

Persons with COPD who become uncomfortable at altitude should be treated with oxygen therapy. Oxygen should also be considered for those predicted to become severely hypoxemic.[33] To adjust oxygen therapy at altitude for persons already on supplemental oxygen, Fi_{O_2} is increased by the ratio of higher to lower barometric pressure (see Table 1-2). Oxygen also improved hemodynamics (lowered blood pressure) and decreased pulsus paradoxus and pulse pressure in COPD patients at a simulated altitude of 2438 m (7999 feet).[34] With the advent of simple and inexpensive pulse oximetry, patients can be counseled to monitor their oxygen saturation, determine the need for oxygen, and titrate their own oxygen use.

Interestingly, reports of persons with COPD developing altitude illness are absent from the literature. On the other hand, the issue has not been specifically addressed. Any degree of pulmonary hypertension might be expected to increase the likelihood of HAPE, and although this has been clearly demonstrated in other conditions (see High-Altitude Pulmonary Edema), it has not yet been reported with pulmonary hypertension associated with COPD. No research has yet addressed the use of medications such as acetazolamide or medroxyprogesterone in these patients, to determine if respiratory stimulants might improve altitude tolerance.

Cystic Fibrosis. Children with cystic fibrosis have been reported to do poorly at high altitude,[325] and hypoxic testing has also tried to predict the need for supplemental oxygen upon ascent in this condition.[251] As with COPD, such tests are not particularly useful and tend to underestimate the oxygen requirements because they are done only during rest and while awake. Supplemental oxygen should be available for these children, and oxygen saturation monitoring might be desirable in certain circumstances. The physician should be liberal with the use of antibiotics and adjunctive therapy for exacerbations at high altitude, given the likely danger of greater hypoxemia and greater difficulty treating infections at high altitude.

Asthma. The available literature suggests that asthmatics do well at high altitude, both residents and sojourners, primarily because of decreased allergens and pollution.[39,316,344] Indeed, high altitude as a treatment for asthma has been popular in Europe for many decades. However, because altitude exposure often includes exercise (and cold), asthmatics with exercise-induced bronchospasm rather than allergic asthma might have problems at altitude. Matsuda et al[210] investigated the effect of altitude on 20 asthmatic children with exercise-induced bronchospasm in a hypobaric chamber simulating 1500 m (4921 feet) but with the temperature and humidity held constant. Except for the increased respiratory rate during exercise, as expected, all other physiologic variables were unchanged compared with sea level. The authors concluded that the modest altitude of 1500 m (4921 feet) does not exacerbate exercise-induced asthma. Future work will hopefully evaluate asthmatics at higher altitudes and in the field, where humidity and temperature are lower.

In the presence of bronchoconstriction at high altitude, however, hypoxemia is likely to be greater than at low altitude, and for this reason there could be an association between asthma and HAPE or AMS. Reassuringly, no such relationship has yet been reported. Mirrakhimov[227] investigated the effect of acetazolamide in 16 asthmatic patients taken to 3200 m (10,499 feet). Acetazolamide showed the same benefits as in nonasthmatics, with higher oxygen saturation and fewer AMS symptoms compared with the placebo control group. Seven of the eight asthmatics in the control group developed symptoms of AMS, a rather high incidence, but without a nonasthmatic control group for comparison, whether this incidence was abnormal is unknown.

Persons with asthma ascending to high altitude should be advised to be at maximum function before ascent; to continue on their usual medications, including steroids; and to have steroids and bronchodilators with them in the event of an exacerbation. Because airway heat loss can be a trigger for bronchospasm, the use of an airway warming mask might be helpful but is unproven.[293] In summary, the available data, although limited, suggest that high altitude does not exacerbate asthma, and it actually improves allergic asthma. Further work needs to determine if asthma might have any influence on susceptibility to AMS and HAPE; anecdotally, this does not seem to be the case. Although it seems likely that a severe asthma attack at high altitude would be more dangerous than at low altitude, no data are available to answer this question. Although caution and adequate preparation are necessary, asthma is not a contraindication to high-altitude travel.

Sleep Apnea and Sleep-Disordered Breathing

Persons with snoring, sleep apnea syndrome, and sleep-disordered breathing (SDB) who become mildly hypoxemic at sea level may become severely hypoxemic at high altitude. This could contribute to high-altitude illness and aggravate attendant problems, such as polycythemia, pulmonary hypertension, cardiac arrhythmia, or insomnia. On the other hand, changes in ventilatory control and breathing secondary to altitude hypoxia might conceivably improve certain apnea syndromes. Fujimoto et al[91] suggested that SDB at high altitude was related to altitude illnesses, including HAPE, but whether the SDB was present before altitude exposure was not determined. The chaotic breathing pattern during sleep that these investigators found in HAPE-s subjects was clearly different from the usual periodic breathing of high altitude. In fact, periodic breathing (Cheyne-Stokes) is considered benign, has not been related to AMS or HAPE, and is associated with a brisk HVR, which is generally considered beneficial at altitude.[114] Patients with SDB being treated with continuous positive airway pressure (CPAP) should be aware that the hypobaria of high altitude decreases the delivered pressure of CPAP machines that do not have pressure-compensating features. Therefore they might need to adjust their machines. The error is greater the higher the altitude and the higher the initial pressure setting.[90] For those not being treated with CPAP but who exhibit hypoxemia during sleep at low altitude, the physician might want to consider supplemental nocturnal oxygen during an altitude sojourn.

Cardiovascular Conditions

Hypertension. In healthy persons rapidly ascending to high altitude, the change in blood pressure, if any, is variable, depending on magnitude of hypoxic stress, cold, diet, exercise, and genetic factors. Most studies report a slight increase in blood pressure, associated with increased catecholamine activity and increased sympathetic activity.[266] One well-controlled study showed an increase in blood pressure at 3500 m (11,483 feet) from a mean of 105/66 mm Hg at sea level to 119/77 mm Hg at 3 days, 111/75 mm Hg at 3 weeks, and back to 102/65 mm Hg on return to sea level.[207] Pugh[263] reported transient increases in blood pressure in athletes at the 1968 Olympics in Mexico City. Certain individuals, however, appear to have a pathologic response upon induction to high altitude. For example, arterial hypertension develops in 10% of lowland Chinese who move to Tibet.[314] The authors consider this a form of altitude maladaptation and treat the condition by returning the affected individuals to low altitude. After a period of at least months, however, down-regulation of adrenergic receptors results in attenuation of the initial blood pressure response. This mechanism is thought to be the reason that long-term residents of high altitude have lower blood pressure than their sea level counterparts.[151,288] Apparently for the same reason, chronic altitude exposure has also been shown to inhibit progression of hypertension.[228]

As for the effect of short-term altitude exposure on preexisting hypertension, studies have generated mixed results. In general, the response in hypertensives is similar to those without hypertension, that is, a small increase in blood pressure, with an exaggerated response in some individuals. The greater the hypoxic stress (the higher the altitude), the greater the change in blood pressure. Altitudes less than 3000 m (9843 feet) seem to result in little if any change.[282] Palatini et al[257] studied 12 normotensives and 12 untreated mild hypertensives with 24-hour ambulatory blood pressure monitoring at sea level, after 12 hours at 1210 m (3970 feet), and after 1½ to 3 hours at 3000 m (9843 feet). The authors concluded that the increase of blood pressure in both normotensives and hypertensives was not important at 1210 m (3970 feet) but could become so at 3000 m (9843 feet). However, individual variability was great; the maximum change was 17.4 mm Hg for systolic and 16.3 for diastolic blood pressures. Two other studies were able to demonstrate a slightly greater blood pressure response in hypertensives compared with normotensives upon ascent to 2572 m (8439 feet) and 3460 m (11,352 feet).[69a,301] Again, these authors also noted important individual variation, with some subjects increasing their systolic blood pressure by as much as 25 mm Hg at rest and 40 mm Hg during exercise, compared with sea level measurements. The important question of whether the blood pressure would continue to increase over the first 2 weeks at high altitude, as it does in normotensives, has not yet been addressed. At a more modest altitude, Halhuber[119] claimed a significant reduction in the blood pressure of 593 persons with hypertension after 14 days at 1700 to 2000 m (5578 to 6562 feet) in the Alps. A similar study of hypertensives at higher altitude will hopefully be accomplished.

Patients receiving antihypertensive treatment should continue their medications while at high altitude. Because some persons may unpredictably become markedly hypertensive acutely,[152] blood pressure monitoring should be considered, especially in those with labile hypertension or those who become symptomatic at altitude. Hypertension in short-term high-altitude sojourners for the most part should be considered transient and should not be treated because it rarely reaches dangerously high levels and will resolve on descent. Given the large number of hypertensive patients visiting ski resorts and trekking at high altitude, however, the occasional person with an exaggerated response will require treatment.[152] Because the mechanism appears to be increased α-adrenergic activity, an α-blocker might be the best choice of therapy for these individuals. A preliminary report also suggested that nifedipine might useful and superior to atenolol.[70] There is no evidence to date to suggest that hypertensive patients are more likely to develop high-altitude illnesses. Although requiring some caution, hypertension does not seem to be a contraindication to high-altitude exposure.

Arteriosclerotic Heart Disease. Lifelong residence at high altitude appears to offer some protection from coronary artery disease (CAD) and the attendant acute coronary artery events,[226] perhaps in part resulting from increased myocardial vascularity.[53] Other factors that might explain this finding, such as genetics, fitness, and diet, have not been adequately evaluated. The effect of acute, transient exposure to high altitude on the healthy heart also appears to be benign. Various avenues of research have indicated that the healthy heart tolerates even extreme hypoxia quite well, all the way to the summit of Mt. Everest (PaO_2 less than 30 torr). Numerous electrocardiograms (ECGs), echocardiograms, heart catheterizations, and exercise tests have failed to demonstrate any evidence of cardiac ischemia or cardiac dysfunction in healthy persons at high altitudes. This could partly be due to the marked reduction in maximal exercise with increasing altitude, which reduces maximal heart rate and myocardial oxygen demand, and also due to the increased coronary blood flow. A person with CAD, however, may not have the same adaptive capacities. For example, diseased coronary arteries might have limited ability to vasodilate and might actually constrict because of unopposed sympathetic activation.[193] What, then, are the risks, and what to advise those with CAD considering a visit to high altitude?

Surprisingly little literature is available to help the physician advise such persons. Does high altitude provoke acute coronary events or sudden death? In the United States, no evidence from state or county mortality statistics suggests an increased prevalence of acute coronary events in visitors to high-altitude locations. In Europe, Halhuber[119] reported an incidence of only 0.2% for myocardial infarction in 434 patients with CAD taken to altitudes between 1700 and 3200 m (5578 and 10,499 feet) for 4 weeks in the Alps. He also reported a very low incidence of sudden death in 151,000 vacationers in the Alps, 69,000 of whom were over age 40. In contrast are data from Austria claiming a higher rate of sudden cardiac death in the mountains, compared with the overall risk of sudden cardiac death.[47] However, the altitudes were rather low (1000 to 2100 m [3281 to 6890 feet]), and no increased risk was evident in men who participated regularly in sports. The authors suggested that abrupt onset of exercise in sedentary men combined with altitude stress might induce cardiac sudden death, but whether altitude contributed at all is unclear. In summary, limited data suggest no increased risk for sudden cardiac death or myocardial infarction at altitudes up to 2500 m (8202 feet).

Another important question is whether altitude will exacerbate stable ischemia. The slight increase in heart rate and blood pressure on initial ascent to altitude might exacerbate angina in those with coronary artery disease, as described by Hultgren.[152] One study evaluated nine men with stable exercise-induced angina by exercise treadmill test at 1600 m (5250 feet; Denver), and within the first hour of arrival at 3100 m (10,171 feet).[239] Cardiac work was slightly higher for a given workload at high altitude compared with low altitude, and as a result, the onset of angina was at a slightly lower workload. They found that a heart rate of 70% to 85% of the rate that produced ischemia at low altitude was associated with angina-free exercise at 3100 m (10,171 feet), and they suggested that angina patients at altitude adjust their activity level based on heart rate, at least on the day of arrival.[239] Brammel et al[45] reported similar results and also suggested that those with angina need to reduce their activity at high altitude to avoid angina episodes. In a more recent study, Levine et al[193] investigated 20 men who were much older than those in the previous investigations (mean age 68 ± 3 years) and performed symptom-limited exercise tests. With acute exposure to 2500 m (8202 feet), the double product (heart rate times systolic blood pressure) required to induce 1 mm ST depression was decreased about 5%, but after 5 days of acclimatization at 2500 m (8202 feet), this value was unchanged from sea level. The degree of ischemia (maximal ST segment depression) was the same at sea level, with acute altitude exposure, and after 5 days at 2500 m (8202 feet). Also, no new wall motion abnormalities on echocardiography were seen at high altitude. Only one subject exhibited increased angina at altitude, and one person with severe CAD developed a myocardial infarction after maximal exercise at 2500 m (8202 feet). The authors concluded that CAD patients who are well compensated at sea level do well at a moderate altitude after a few days of acclimatization, but that acutely angina threshold may be lower and activity should be reduced.[193] Finally, a study of 97 elderly persons visiting 2500 m (8202 feet), many with CAD and abnormal ECGs, found no new ECG changes and no events suggestive of ischemia. In contrast to the Levine study, these subjects did not do exhaustive exercise tests but merely their usual activities, which included walking in the mountains.[282] Taken altogether, these various investigations indicate that those with CAD, including the elderly, generally do well at the modest altitude of 2500 m (8202 feet), but that reducing their activities the first few days at altitude is wise.

To address the question of whether altitude might provoke cardiac arrhythmia, Levine et al,[193] in their study mentioned above, found that premature ventricular contractions (PVCs) increased 63% on acute ascent but returned to baseline after 5 days of acclimatization. A simultaneous rise in urine norepinephrine in these subjects indicated that sympathetic activation was the cause of the increased ectopy. They observed no increase in higher-grade ectopy, however, and no changes in signal-averaged ECG suggestive of a change in fibrillation threshold; in other words, the PVCs appeared benign. Halhuber[119] also found increased ectopy in his subjects and also no serious adverse events. In addition, Alexander[2] described asymptomatic PVCs and ventricular bigeminy in himself while trekking to 5900 m (19,358 feet). Subsequent evaluation found no evidence of heart disease, and the event prompted him to thoroughly review the subject of altitude, age, and arrhythmia. Although no dangerous arrhythmias have ever been reported in high-altitude studies, persons with troublesome or high-grade arrhythmia have not been evaluated upon ascent to high altitude. The available evidence would suggest that patients whose arrhythmias are well controlled on medication should continue the medication at altitude, whereas those with poorly controlled arrhythmias might do better to avoid visiting high altitude.

In terms of advising persons with CAD or high likelihood of CAD about altitude exposure, the stress of high altitude on the coronary circulation appears to be minimal at rest but significant in conjunction with exercise. Ideally, no one with known CAD or even risk factors for CAD should undertake unaccustomed exercise at any altitude and especially at high altitude. Therefore advising an exercise program at sea level before exercising at altitude is prudent. The same technique of risk stratification that is commonly used at sea level can be applied for providing advice for high altitude.[146] Using the standard recommendations, asymptomatic men over age 50 with no risk factors require no testing. For asymptomatic men over age 50 with risk factors, an exercise test is recommended to determine risk status before exercising at high altitude and then further evaluation as indicated. Patients with previous myocardial ischemia, bypass surgery, or angioplasty are considered high risk only if they have a strongly positive exercise treadmill test. Patients with multiple-vessel bypass grafts who were asymptomatic and with normal exercise tests at sea level have successfully visited altitudes over 5000 m (16,404 feet). High-risk patients may require coronary angiography to establish appropriate management. Alexander[1] has proposed different criteria for those with CAD at high risk at altitude: an ejection fraction less than 35% at rest, a fall in exercise systolic blood pressure, ST segment depression greater than 2 mm at peak heart rate, and high-grade ventricular ectopy. For these persons, he recommends ascent to no more than 2500 m (8202 feet) and proximity to medical care. Both sets of recommendations, although reasonable, need to be validated with outcome studies.

HEART FAILURE. Although information on the effect of high altitude on heart failure is scant, physicians in resort areas have noted a tendency toward acute decompensation in those with a history of heart failure within 24 hours of arrival. Those with CAD and low ejection fractions (less than 45%), but without active heart failure, actually did quite well, as gauged by exercise tests during acute exposure to 2500 m (8202 feet).[85] Compared with 23 control subjects, the decrement in exercise performance was similar, and no complications or signs of ischemia developed. Although these results are encouraging for such patients, they made no observations past the first few hours at altitude. One concern is that those with heart failure might be more likely to retain fluid at altitude, especially if AMS were to develop, and that this could aggravate failure. Supporting this notion, Alexander et al[3] found that ejection fraction declined at altitude during an exercise study in patients with angina, with an increase in end-diastolic and systolic volume as measured by two-dimensional echo. Ventricular contractility was not depressed, however, and these changes were attributed to fluid overload. Patients with heart failure need to be informed about possible consequences of high-altitude exposure. In particular, they need to avoid AMS, which is associated with fluid retention, and they need to continue their regular medications and be prepared to increase their diuretic should symptoms of failure exacerbate. Acetazolamide prophylaxis may be useful to consider in terms of speeding acclimatization, inducing a diuresis, and preventing AMS, but its efficacy in these patients remains untested.

PULMONARY VASCULAR DISORDERS. Because of the danger of HAPE, pulmonary hypertension (of any etiology) is at least a relative contraindication to high-altitude exposure. In addition, hypoxic pulmonary vasoconstriction will most likely exaggerate preexisting pulmonary hypertension and could lead to greater symptomatology in those with congenital cardiac defects, primary pulmonary hypertension (PPH), and related disorders. This caution also applies to unilateral absent pulmonary artery, granulomatous mediastinitis, and restrictive lung diseases, all of which have been associated with HAPE.[109,275,340] As Hultgren[152] has observed, however, some patients with PPH are able to tolerate high altitude, and hypoxic gas breathing can be used to identify an individual's response to hypoxia if clinically indicated. Persons with PPH who must travel to high altitude might benefit from calcium channel blockers, isoproterenol, and/or low-flow oxygen. A recent report highlighted the increased susceptibility to HAPE in those with pulmonary hypertension; a lowland woman with pulmonary hypertension secondary to fenfluramine developed two episodes of HAPE.[245] The first episode was at 2300 m (7546 feet) and the second one at only 1850 m (6070 feet), with skiing up to 2350 m (7710 feet). Other conditions warranting caution include bronchopulmonary dysplasia, recurrent pulmonary emboli, mitral stenosis, and kyphoscoliosis. Whether pulmonary hypertension is primary or secondary, patients should be made aware of the potential hazards of high altitude, including right heart failure and HAPE.

Sickle Cell Disease

Sickle cell crisis is a well-recognized complication of high-altitude exposure.[87] Even the modest altitude of a pressurized aircraft (1500 to 2000 m [4921 to 6562 feet]) causes 20% of persons with hemoglobin SC and sickle-thalassemia genetic configuration to have a vasoocclusive crisis.[203] High-altitude exposure may precipitate the first vasoocclusive crisis in persons previously unaware of their condition. Persons with sickle cell anemia and a history of vasoocclusive crises are advised to avoid altitudes over 1800 m (5906 feet) unless they are taking supplemental oxygen. Persons with sickle cell disease who live at high altitude in Saudi Arabia have twice the incidence of crises, hospitalizations, and complications as do Saudis at low altitude. Splenic infarction syndrome has been reported more commonly in those with sickle cell trait than in those with sickle cell anemia, probably because sickle cell disease produces autosplenectomy early in life. Frequent reports in the literature emphasize the need to consider splenic syndrome caused by sickle cell trait in any person with left upper quadrant pain, even at an altitude of only 1500 m (5921 feet).[185,203] A number of authors have suggested that nonblack persons with the trait may be at greater risk for splenic syndrome at high altitude than are black persons.[185] Treatment of splenic syndrome consists of intravenous hydration, oxygen, and removal to a lower altitude.[339] The overall incidence of problems in persons with the trait is low, however, and no special precaution other than recognition of the splenic syndrome is recommended. The U.S. Army, for example, does not consider soldiers with the trait unfit for duty at high altitude.[75]

Pregnancy

In high-altitude natives, pregnancy-induced hypertension is four times more common than in low-altitude pregnancies, preeclampsia is more common, and full-term infants are small for gestational age.[234,235] These problems raise the issue of whether short-term altitude exposure may also pose a risk. So far, there is no evidence that these problems, or others such as spontaneous abortion, abruptio placentae, or placenta previa, can result from a sojourn to high altitude.[249] Unfortunately, however, few data exist on the influence of a high-altitude visit during pregnancy on the mother and the fetus. For moderate altitude, the research to date has been reassuring.[143,144] Artal et al[9] studied seven sedentary women at 34 weeks gestation. Maximal and submaximal exercise tests were completed at sea level and 6000 feet (1829 m) after 2 to 4 days of acclimatization. They reported the expected decrease in maximal aerobic work but found no difference from sea level in fetal heart rate responses, or in maternal lactate, epinephrine, and norepinephrine levels. In a small number of subjects, the authors considered it safe for women in their third trimester of pregnancy to engage in brief bouts of exercise at moderate altitude. A similar conclusion was reached in a study of 12 pregnant subjects who exercised after ascent to 2225 m (7300 feet). The authors found no abnormal fetal heart rate responses and considered the exercise at altitude benign for both mother and fetus.[29] Huch[143] also concluded that short-term exposure, with exercise, was safe during pregnancy. In summary, the available data, though limited, indicate that short-term exposure to altitudes up to 2500 m (8202 feet), with exercise, is safe for a lowland woman with a normal pregnancy.

Another avenue of research has been alteration of blood gases during pregnancy. Human and animal studies with acute hypoxic challenge, as well as oxygen-breathing studies, have drawn two conclusions: (1) that a compromised placental-fetal circulation could be unmasked at high altitude, and (2) that a fetus with a normal placental-fetal circulation seems to tolerate a level of acute hypoxia far exceeding a moderate altitude exposure.[15,63,276]

Based on the available research, it seems prudent to recommend that only women with normal, low-risk pregnancy undertake a sojourn to altitude. For these women, exposure to an altitude at which SaO_2 will remain above 85% most of the time (up to 3000 m [9843 feet] altitude) appears to pose no risk of harm, but further study is needed to place these recommendations on a more solid scientific footing. An ultrasound or other assessment may be useful to rule out the more common complications before travel. Of course, it is not the altitude per se that determines whether the fetus becomes stressed but rather the maternal (and fetal) arterial oxygen transport. A woman with HAPE at 2500 m (8202 feet), for example, is much more hypoxemic than a healthy woman at 5000 m (16,404 feet). Therefore a strategy for preventing altitude illness, especially pulmonary edema, must be explained and implemented. Similarly, carboxyhemoglobin from smoking, lung disease, and other problems of oxygen transport will render the pregnant patient at altitude more hypoxemic and physiologically at a higher altitude. Consideration of a high-altitude sojourn in the developing world, or in a wilderness setting, raises other issues that may be more important than the modest hypoxia. These include remoteness from medical care should a problem arise, the quality of available medical care, the use of medications for such important things as malaria and traveler's diarrhea (many of which are contraindicated in pregnancy), and the risks of trauma.

REFERENCES

1. Alexander J: Coronary heart disease at altitude, *Tex Heart Inst J* 21:261, 1994.
2. Alexander J: Age, altitude and arrhythmia, *Tex Heart Inst J* 22:308, 1995.
3. Alexander J et al: Left ventricular function in coronary heart disease at high altitude, *Circulation* 78:II, 1988 (abstract).
4. Andrew M, O'Brodovich H, Sutton J: Operation Everest II: coagulation system during prolonged decompression to 282 torr, *J Appl Physiol* 63:1262, 1987.
5. Anholm JD et al: Operation Everest II: Arterial oxygen saturation and sleep at extreme simulated altitude, *Am Rev Respir Dis* 145:817, 1992.
6. Anholm JD et al: Radiographic evidence of interstitial pulmonary edema after exercise at altitude, *J Appl Physiol* 86:503, 1999.
7. Aoki VS, Robinson SM: Body hydration and the incidence and severity of acute mountain sickness, *J Appl Physiol* 31:363, 1971.
8. Arias-Stella J, Kryger H: Pathology of high altitude pulmonary edema, *Arch Pathol* 76:43, 1963.
9. Artal R et al: A comparison of cardiopulmonary adaptations to exercise in pregnancy at sea level and altitude, *Am J Obstet Gynecol* 172:1170, 1995.
9a. Auerbach PS, Miller EY: High altitude flatus expulsion (HAFE), *West J Med* 134:173, 1981 (letter).
10. Bailey DM, Davies B: Physiological implications of altitude training for endurance performance at sea level: a review, *Br J Sports Med* 31:183, 1997.

11. Bailey DM et al: Implications of moderate altitude training for sea-level endurance in elite distance runners, *Eur J Appl Physiol* 78:360, 1998.

12. Balke B, Nagle FJ, Daniels JT: Altitude and maximum performance in work and sports activity, *JAMA* 194:176, 1965.

13. Banchero N: Capillary density of skeletal muscle in dogs exposed to simulated altitude, *Proc Soc Exp Biol Med* 148:435, 1975.

14. Banderet LE, Lieberman HR: Treatment with tyrosine, a neurotransmitter precursor, reduces environmental stress in humans, *Brain Res Bull* 22:759, 1989.

15. Bartnicki J, Saling E: Influence of maternal oxygen administration on the computer-analysed fetal heart rate patterns in small-for-gestational-age fetuses, *Gynecol Obstet Invest* 37:172, 1994.

16. Bärtsch P: High altitude pulmonary edema, *Med Sci Sports Exerc* 31:S23, 1999.

17. Bärtsch P, Schmidt EK, Straub PW: Fibrinopeptide A after strenuous physical exercise at high altitude, *J Appl Physiol* 53:40, 1982.

18. Bärtsch P et al: Enhanced fibrin formation in high-altitude pulmonary edema, *J Appl Physiol* 63:752, 1987.

19. Bärtsch P et al: Atrial natriuretic peptide in acute mountain sickness, *J Appl Physiol* 65:1929, 1988.

20. Bärtsch P et al: Coagulation and fibrinolysis in acute mountain sickness and beginning pulmonary edema, *J Appl Physiol* 66:2136, 1989.

21. Bärtsch P et al: Contact phase of blood coagulation is not activated in edema of high altitude, *J Appl Physiol* 67:1336, 1989.

22. Bärtsch P et al: Comparison of carbon-dioxide enriched, oxygen-enriched and normal air in treatment of acute mountain sickness, *Lancet* 336:772, 1990.

23. Bärtsch P et al: Enhanced exercise-induced rise of aldosterone and vasopressin preceding mountain sickness, *J Appl Physiol* 71:136, 1991.

24. Bärtsch P et al: Prevention of high-altitude pulmonary edema by nifedipine, *N Engl J Med* 325:1284, 1991.

25. Bärtsch P et al: Aldosterone, antidiuretic hormone and atrial natriuretic peptide in acute mountain sickness. In Sutton JR, Coates G, Houston CS, editors: *Hypoxia and mountain medicine*, Burlington, Vt, 1992, Queen City Press.

26. Bärtsch P et al: High altitude pulmonary edema: blood coagulation. In Sutton JR, Houston CS, Coates G, editors: *Hypoxia and molecular medicine*, Burlington, Vt, 1993, Queen City Press.

27. Bärtsch P et al: Sumatriptan for high-altitude headache, *Lancet* 344:1445, 1994 (letter).

28. Basnyat B et al: Children in the mountains. Advice given was too conservative, *BMJ* 317:540, 1998 (letter; comment).

29. Baumann H et al: Reaktion von mutter und fetus auf die Koperliche belastung in oler hohe, *Geburtshilfe Frauenheilkd* 45:869, 1985.

30. Baumgartner RW et al: Enhanced cerebral blood flow in acute mountain sickness, *Aviat Space Environ Med* 65:726, 1994.

31. Baumgartner RW et al: Acute mountain sickness is not related to cerebral blood flow: a decompression chamber study, *J Appl Physiol* 86:1578, 1999.

32. Beaumont M et al: Effect of zolpidem on sleep and ventilatory patterns at simulated altitude of 4,000 meters, *Am J Respir Crit Care Med* 153:1864, 1996.

33. Berg B et al: Oxygen supplementation during air travel in patients with chronic obstructive lung disease, *Chest* 101:638, 1992.

34. Berg BW et al: Hemodynamic effects of altitude exposure and oxygen administration in chronic obstructive pulmonary disease, *Am J Med* 94:407, 1993.

35. Bernhard WN et al: Acetazolamide plus low-dose dexamethasone is better than acetazolamide alone to ameliorate symptoms of acute mountain sickness, *Aviat Space Environ Med* 69:883, 1998.

36. Berry CA: Aerospace medicine: the vertical frontier. In Auerbach P, Gheer E, editors: *Management of wilderness and environmental emergencies*, New York, 1983, Macmillan.

37. Bert P: *Barometric pressure*, Bethesda, Md, 1978, Undersea Medical Society.

38. Bock J, Hultgren HN: Emergency maneuver in high altitude pulmonary edema, *JAMA* 255:3245, 1986 (letter).

39. Boner A et al: Bronchial reactivity in asthmatic children at high and low altitude: effect of budesonide, *Am J Respir Crit Care* 151:1194, 1995.

40. Boning D: Altitude and hypoxia training—a short review, *Int J Sports Med* 18:565, 1997.

41. Botella de Maglia J, Garrido Marin E, Catala Barcelo J: Transient motor aphasia at high altitude, *Rev Clin Esp* 193:296, 1993.

42. Boyer SJ, Blume FD: Weight loss and changes in body composition at high altitude, *J Appl Physiol* 57:1580, 1984.

43. Bradwell AR, Burnett D, Davies F: Acetazolamide in control of acute mountain sickness, *Lancet* 1:180, 1981.

44. Bradwell AR et al: The effect of temazepam and Diamox on nocturnal hypoxia at altitude (abstract). In Sutton JR, Houston CS, Coates G, editors: *Hypoxia and cold*, New York, 1987, Praeger.

45. Brammell HL et al: Exercise tolerance is reduced at altitude in patients with coronary artery disease, *Circulation* 66:II, 1982.

46. Broome JR et al: High altitude headache: treatment with ibuprofen, *Aviat Space Environ Med* 65:19, 1994.

47. Burtscher M, Philadelphy M, Likar R: Sudden cardiac death during mountain hiking and downhill skiing, *N Engl J Med* 329:1738, 1993.

48. Burtscher M et al: Ibuprofen versus sumatriptan for high-altitude headache *Lancet* 346:254, 1995 (letter).

49. Burtscher M et al: Aspirin for prophylaxis against headache at high altitudes: randomised, double blind, placebo controlled trial, *BMJ* 316:1057, 1998.

50. Burtscher M et al: Aspirin versus Diamox plus aspirin for headache prevention during physical activity at high altitude, *Adv Exp Med Biol* 474:370, 1999 (abstract).

51. Burtscher M et al: Naproxen for therapy of high-altitude headache, *Adv Exp Med Biol* 474:372, 1999 (abstract).

52. Butterfield GE: Increased energy intake minimizes weight loss in men at high altitude, *J Appl Physiol* 72:1741, 1992.

53. Carmelino M: *Man at high altitude*, Edinburgh, 1981, Churchill Livingstone.

54. Chauca D, Bligh J: An additive effect of cold exposure and hypoxia on pulmonary artery pressure in sheep, *Res Vet Sci* 21:123, 1976.

55. Clarke CR: Cerebral infarction at extreme altitude (abstract). In Sutton JR, Houston CS, Jones NL, editors: *Hypoxia, exercise and altitude*, New York, 1983, AR Liss.

56. Claybaugh JR, Brooks DP, Cymerman A: Hormonal control of fluid and electrolyte balance at high altitude in normal subjects. In Sutton JR, Coates G, Houston CS, editors: *Hypoxia and mountain medicine*, Burlington, Vt, 1992, Queen City Press.

57. Colier WNJM et al: Cerebral de-oxygenation during peak exercise at 5260 m in well acclimatized sea level subjects, *FASEB J* 14:A82, 2000.

58. Collins WE: Performance effects of alcohol intoxication and hangover at ground level and at simulated altitude, *Aviat Space Environ Med* 51:327, 1980.

59. Collins WE, Mertens HW: Age, alcohol, and simulated altitude: effects on performance and breathalyzer scores, *Aviat Space Environ Med* 59:1026, 1988.

60. Collins WE, Mertens HW, Higgins EA: Some effects of alcohol and simulated altitude on complex performance scores and breathalyzer readings, *Aviat Space Environ Med* 58:328, 1987.

61. Cone JB: Cellular oxygen utilization. In Snyder JV, Pinsky MR, editors: *Oxygen transport in the critically ill*, St Louis, 1987, Mosby.

62. Consolazio CF et al: Effects of a high-carbohydrate diet on performance and clinical symptomology after rapid ascent to high altitude, *Fed Proc* 28:937, 1969.

63. Copher DE, Huber CP: Heart rate response of the human fetus to induced maternal hypoxia, *Am J Obstet Gynecol* 98:320, 1967.

64. Cremona G et al: High altitude pulmonary edema at 4559 m: a population study, *Adv Exp Med Biol* 474:375, 1999 (abstract).

65. Criscuolo GR, Balledux JP: Clinical neurosciences in the decade of the brain: hypotheses in neuro-oncology. VEG/PF acts upon the actin cytoskeleton and is inhibited by dexamethasone: relevance to tumor angiogenesis and vasogenic edema, *Yale J Biol Med* 69:337, 1996.

66. Crowley A: *The confessions of Alistair Crowley: an autobiography*, New York, 1971, Bantam Books.

67. Curran-Everett DC, Iwamoto J, Krasney JA: Intracranial pressures and O_2 extraction in conscious sheep during 72 h of hypoxia, *Am J Physiol* 261:H103, 1991.

68. Dean AG, Yip R, Hoffman RE: High incidence of mild acute mountain sickness in conference attendees at 10,000 foot altitude, *J Wilderness Med* 1:86, 1990.

69. de Meer K, Heymans HS, Zijlstra WG: Physical adaptation of children to life at high altitude, *Eur J Pediatr* 154:263, 1995.

69a. D'Este D, Mantovan R, Martino A, et al: Blood pressure changes at rest and during effort in normotensive and hypertensive subjects in response to altitude acute hypoxia, *G Ital Cardiol* 21:643, 1991.

70. Deuber HJ: Treatment of hypertension and coronary heart disease during stays at high altitude, *Aviat Space Environ Med* 60:119, 1989 (abstract).

71. Dick FW: Training at altitude in practice, *Int J Sports Med* 13:S203, 1992.

72. Dickinson J et al: Altitude-related deaths in seven trekkers in the Himalayas, *Thorax* 38:646, 1983.

73. Dickinson JG: High altitude cerebral edema: cerebral acute mountain sickness, *Semin Respir Med* 5:151, 1983.

74. Dickinson JG: Acetazolamide in acute mountain sickness, *BMJ* 295:1161, 1987.

75. Diggs L: The sickle cell trait in relation to the training and assignment of duties in the Armed Forces: IV. Considerations and recommendations, *Aviat Space Environ Med* 55:487, 1984.

76. Dillard T et al: The preflight evaluation—a comparison of the hypoxia inhalation test with hypobaric exposure, *Chest* 107:352, 1995.

77. Drewes LR: What is the blood-brain barrier? A molecular perspective, *Adv Exp Med Biol* 474:111, 1999.

78. Duplain H et al: Augmented sympathetic activation during short-term hypoxia and high-altitude exposure in subjects susceptible to high-altitude pulmonary edema, *Circulation* 99:1713, 1999.

79. Durmowicz AG et al: Inflammatory processes may predispose children to high-altitude pulmonary edema, *J Pediatr* 130:838, 1997.

80. Editorial: Acetazolamide prophylaxis for acute mountain sickness, *Drug Ther Bull* 25:45, 1987.

81. Eichenberger U et al: Nocturnal periodic breathing and the development of acute high altitude illness, *Am J Respir Crit Care Med* 154:1748, 1996.

82. Eldridge MW et al: Evidence of immunological mediator activation with exposure to high altitude, *ALA/ATS Intl Conference*, 1994 (abstract).

83. Eldridge MW et al: Pulmonary hemodynamic response to exercise in subjects with prior high-altitude pulmonary edema, *J Appl Physiol* 81:911, 1996.

84. Ellsworth AJ, Meyer EF, Larson EB: Acetazolamide or dexamethasone use versus placebo to prevent acute mountain sickness on Mount Rainier, *West J Med* 154:289, 1991.

85. Erdmann J et al: Effects of exposure to altitude on men with coronary artery disease and impaired left ventricular function, *Am J Cardiol* 81:266, 1998.

86. Ferrazzini G et al: Successful treatment of acute mountain sickness with dexamethasone, *BMJ* 294:1380, 1987.

87. Franklin V: Sickle cell crisis. In Sutton JR, Jones NL, Houston CS, editors: *Hypoxia: man at altitude*, New York, 1982, Thieme-Stratton.

88. Freedman R et al: Electrophysiological effects of low dose alcohol on human subjects at high altitude, *Alcohol Drug Res* 6:289, 1985.

89. Freitas J et al: High altitude-related neurocardiogenic syncope, *Am J Cardiol* 77:1021, 1996.

90. Fromm RE Jr et al: CPAP machine performance and altitude, *Chest* 108:1577, 1995.

91. Fujimoto K et al: Irregular nocturnal breathing patterns at high altitude in subjects susceptible to high-altitude pulmonary edema (HAPE): a preliminary study, *Aviat Space Environ Med* 60:786, 1989.

92. Fulco CS, Rock PB, Cymerman A: Maximal and submaximal exercise performance at altitude, *Aviat Space Environ Med* 69:793, 1998.

93. Gibbs JSR: Pulmonary hemodynamics: implications for high altitude pulmonary edema (HAPE), *Adv Exp Med Biol* 474:81, 1999.

94. Gibson GE, Blass JP: Impaired synthesis of acetylcholine in brain accompanying mild hypoxia and hypoglycemia, *J Neurochem* 27:37, 1976.

95. Gong H Jr: Exposure to moderate altitude and cardiorespiratory diseases, *Cardiologia* 40:477, 1995.

96. Gong HJ et al: Hypoxia-altitude simulation test: evaluation of patients with chronic airway obstruction, *Am Rev Respir Dis* 130:980, 1984.

97. Graham WG, Houston CS: Short-term adaptation to moderate altitude: patients with chronic obstructive pulmonary disease, *JAMA* 240:1491, 1978.

98. Gray GW: High altitude pulmonary edema, *Semin Respir Med* 5:141, 1983.

99. Grissom CK et al: Acetazolamide in the treatment of acute mountain sickness: clinical efficacy and effect on gas exchange, *Ann Intern Med* 116:461, 1992.

100. Groves B et al: Minimal hypoxic pulmonary hypertension in normal Tibetans at 3,658 m, *J Appl Physiol* 74:312, 1993.

101. Groves BM et al: Operation Everest II: elevated high altitude pulmonary resistance unresponsive to oxygen, *J Appl Physiol* 63:521, 1987.

102. Hackett P: High altitude and common medical conditions. In Hornbein T, Schoene R, editors: *High altitude*, New York, 2000, Marcel Dekker.

103. Hackett PH: *Mountain sickness: prevention, recognition and treatment*, New York, 1980, American Alpine Club.

104. Hackett PH: High altitude cerebral edema and acute mountain sickness: a pathophysiology update. *Adv Exp Med Biol* 474:23, 1999.

105. Hackett PH, Rennie ID: Rales, peripheral edema, retinal hemorrhage and acute mountain sickness, *Am J Med* 67:214, 1979.

106. Hackett PH, Rennie ID, Levine HD: The incidence, importance, and prophylaxis of acute mountain sickness, *Lancet* 2:1149, 1976.

107. Hackett PH, Roach RC: High altitude pulmonary edema, *J Wilderness Med* 1:3, 1990.

108. Hackett PH, Roach RC, Greene ER: Oxygenation, but not increased cerebral blood flow, improves high altitude headache (abstract). In Sutton JR, Coates G, Remmers JE, editors: *Hypoxia: the adaptations*, Philadelphia, 1990, BC Dekker.

109. Hackett PH et al: High altitude pulmonary edema in persons without the right pulmonary artery, *N Engl J Med* 302:1070, 1980.

110. Hackett PH et al: Fluid retention and relative hypoventilation in acute mountain sickness, *Respiration* 43:321, 1982.

111. Hackett PH et al: The Denali Medical Research Project, 1982-1985, *Am Alpine J* 28:129, 1986.

112. Hackett PH et al: Pulmonary edema fluid protein in high altitude pulmonary edema, *JAMA* 256:36, 1986 (letter).

113. Hackett PH et al: Cortical blindness in high altitude climbers and trekkers—a report on six cases (abstract). In Sutton JR, Houston CS, Coates G, editors: *Hypoxia and cold,* New York, 1987, Praeger.

114. Hackett PH et al: Respiratory stimulants and sleep periodic breathing at high altitude: almitrine versus acetazolamide, *Am Rev Respir Dis* 135:896, 1987.

115. Hackett PH et al: Abnormal control of ventilation in high-altitude pulmonary edema, *J Appl Physiol* 64:1268, 1988.

116. Hackett PH et al: Dexamethasone for prevention and treatment of acute mountain sickness, *Aviat Space Environ Med* 59:950, 1988.

117. Hackett PH et al: The effect of vasodilators on pulmonary hemodynamics in high altitude pulmonary edema: a comparison, *Int J Sports Med* 13:S68, 1992.

118. Hackett PH et al: High-altitude cerebral edema evaluated with magnetic resonance imaging: clinical correlation and pathophysiology, *JAMA* 280:1920, 1998.

119. Halhuber M et al: Does altitude cause exhaustion of the heart and circulatory system? *Med Sport Sci* 19:192, 1985.

120. Hamilton AJ, Cymmerman A, Black PM: High altitude cerebral edema, *Neurosurgery* 19:841, 1986.

121. Hanaoka M et al: Association of high-altitude pulmonary edema with the major histocompatibility complex, *Circulation* 97:1124, 1998.

122. Hannon JP: Comparative altitude adaptability of young men and women. In Folinsbee LJ et al, editors: *Environmental stress: individual human adaptations*, New York, 1978, Academic Press.

123. Hannon JP, Chinn KS, Shields JL: Effects of acute high altitude exposure on body fluids, *Fed Proc* 28:1178, 1969.

124. Hansen JE, Hartley LH, Hogan RPI: Arterial oxygen increase by high-carbohydrate diet at altitude, *J Appl Physiol* 33:441, 1972.

125. Hartig GS, Hackett PH: Cerebral spinal fluid pressure and cerebral blood velocity in acute mountain sickness. In Sutton JR, Coates G, Houston CS, editors: *Hypoxia and mountain medicine*, Burlington, Vt, 1992, Queen City Press.

126. Heath D: *Man at high altitude*, Edinburgh, 1989, Churchill Livingstone.

127. Hebbel RP et al: Human llamas: adaptation to altitude in subjects with high hemoglobin oxygen affinity, *J Clin Invest* 62:593, 1978.

128. Heyes MP, Sutton JR: High altitude ills: a malady of water, electrolyte, and hormonal imbalance? *Semin Respir Med* 5:207, 1983.

129. Higgins E, Vaughn J, Funkhauser G: *Blood alcohol concentrations as affected by combinations of alcoholic beverage dosages and altitude*, Washington, DC, 1970, Federal Aviation Administration Office of Aviation Medicine.

130. Higgins E et al: *The effects of alcohol at three simulated aircraft cabin conditions*, Washington, DC, 1968, Federal Aviation Administration Office of Aviation Medicine.

131. Hoefer M et al: Ventilatory response and associated heart rate change predict the severity of acute mountain sickness, *Adv Exp Med Biol* 474:391, 1999 (abstract).

132. Hohenhaus E et al: Nifedipine does not prevent acute mountain sickness, *Am J Respir Crit Care Med* 150:857, 1994.

133. Hohenhaus E et al: Ventilatory and pulmonary vascular response to hypoxia and susceptibility to high altitude pulmonary oedema, *Eur Respir J* 8:1825, 1995.

134. Honigman B et al: Acute mountain sickness in a general tourist population at moderate altitudes, *Ann Intern Med* 118:587, 1993.

135. Hossmann KA: The hypoxic brain: Insights from ischemia research. In Roach RC, Wagner PD, Hackett PH, editors: Hypoxia: into the next millennium, *Advances in experimental medicine and biology*, New York, 1999, Plenum/Kluwer Academic Publishing.

136. Houston CS: Acute pulmonary edema of high altitude, *N Engl J Med* 263:478, 1960.

137. Houston CS: Altitude illness: manifestations, etiology and management. In Loeppky JA, Riedesel ML, editors: *Oxygen transport to human tissue*, New York, 1982, Elsevier/North Holland.

138. Houston CS: *Going higher: the story of man at high altitude*, Boston, 1987, Little, Brown.

139. Houston CS: History of high altitude medicine. In Hornbein TF, Schoene RB, editors: *High altitude*, New York, 2000, Marcel Dekker.

140. Houston CS, Dickinson JG: Cerebral form of high altitude illness, *Lancet* 2:758, 1975.

141. Houston CS, Sutton JR, Cymerman A: Operation Everest II: man at extreme altitude, *J Appl Physiol* 63:877, 1987.

142. Huang SY et al: Hypocapnia and sustained hypoxia blunt ventilation on arrival at high altitude, *J Appl Physiol* 56:602, 1984.

143. Huch R: Physical activity at altitude in pregnancy, *Semin Perinatol* 20:303, 1996.

144. Huch R et al: Physiologic changes in pregnant women and their fetuses during jet air travel, *Am J Obstet Gynecol* 154:996, 1986.

145. Huijbers PM et al: Nutritional status and mortality of highland children in Nepal: impact of sociocultural factors, *Am J Phys Anthropol* 101:137, 1996.

146. Hultgren H: Coronary heart disease and trekking, *Journal of Wilderness Medicine* 1:154, 1990.

147. Hultgren H, Spickard W: Medical experiences in Peru, *Stanford Medical Bulletin* 18:76, 1960.

148. Hultgren HN: High altitude pulmonary edema. In Hegnauer A, editor: *Biomedical problems of high terrestrial elevations*, Springfield, Va, 1967, Federal Scientific and Technical Information Service.

149. Hultgren HN: High altitude pulmonary edema, *Adv Cardiol* 5:24, 1970.

150. Hultgren HN: High altitude pulmonary edema. In Staub NC, editor: *Lung water and solute exchange*, New York, 1978, Marcel Dekker.

151. Hultgren HN: Reduction of systemic arterial blood pressure at high altitude, *Adv Cardiol* 5:49, 1979.

152. Hultgren HN: Effects of altitude upon cardiovascular diseases, *Journal of Wilderness Medicine* 3:301, 1992.

153. Hultgren HN: High-altitude pulmonary edema: current concepts, *Annu Rev Med* 47:267, 1996.

154. Hultgren HN: *High altitude medicine*, Stanford, Calif, 1997, Hultgren Publications.

155. Hultgren HN, Grover RF: Circulatory adaptations to high altitude, *Annu Rev Med* 19:119, 1968.

156. Hultgren HN, Grover RF, Hartley LH: Abnormal circulatory responses to high altitude in subjects with a previous history of high altitude pulmonary edema, *Circulation* 54:759, 1971.

157. Hultgren HN et al: High altitude pulmonary edema, *Medicine* 40:289, 1961.

158. Hultgren HN et al: Physiologic studies of pulmonary edema at high altitude, *Circulation* 29:393, 1964.

159. Hultgren HN et al: High-altitude pulmonary edema at a ski resort, *West J Med* 164:222, 1996.

160. Hurtado A: *Aspectos fisiologicos y patologicos de la vida en las Alturas*, Lima, Peru, 1937, Imprenta Rimac.

161. Hutchison SJ, Amin S: Everest nails, *N Engl J Med* 336:229, 1997 (letter).

162. Icenogle M et al: Cranial CSF volume (cCSF) is reduced by altitude exposure but is not related to early acute mountain sickness (AMS), *Adv Exp Med Biol* 474:392, 1999 (abstract).

163. Jaeger JJ et al: Evidence for increased intrathoracic fluid volume in man at high altitude, *J Appl Physiol* 47:670, 1979.

164. Jahanshahi M, Hunter M, Philips C: The headache scale: an examination of its reliability and validity, *Headache* 26:76, 1986.

165. Jain SC et al: Amelioration of acute mountain sickness: comparative study of acetazolamide and spironolactone, *Int J Biometeorol* 30:293, 1986.

166. Jensen JB et al: Augmented hypoxic cerebral vasodilation in men during 5 days at 3,810 m altitude, *J Appl Physiol* 80:1214, 1996.

167. Johnson TS et al: Prevention of acute mountain sickness by dexamethasone, *N Engl J Med* 310:683, 1984.

168. Kasic JF et al: Treatment of acute mountain sickness: hyperbaric versus oxygen therapy, *Ann Emerg Med* 20:1109, 1991.

169. Kawashima A et al: Hemodynamic responses to acute hypoxia, hypobaria, and exercise in subjects susceptible to high-altitude pulmonary edema, *J Appl Physiol* 67:1982, 1989.

170. Kayser B: Nutrition and high altitude exposure, *Int J Sports Med* 13:S129, 1992.

171. Keller HR et al: Simulated descent v dexamethasone in treatment of acute mountain sickness: a randomised trial, *BMJ* 310:1232, 1995.

172. Keys A: The physiology of life at high altitude, *Science Monthly* 43:289, 1936.

173. Keys A, Hall FG, Barron ES: The position of the oxygen dissociation curve of human blood at high altitude, *Am J Physiol* 115:292, 1936.

174. Kilgore D et al: Corpus callosum (CC) MRI: early altitude exposure, *Adv Exp Med Biol* 474:396, 1999 (abstract).

175. Klatzo I: Pathophysiological aspects of brain edema, *Acta Neuropathol (Berl)* 72:236, 1987.

176. Kobayashi T et al: Clinical features of patients with high altitude pulmonary edema in Japan, *Chest* 92:814, 1987.

177. Krasney JA: A neurogenic basis for acute altitude illness, *Med Sci Sports Exerc* 26:195, 1994.

178. Krasney JA: Cerebral hemodynamics and high altitude cerebral edema. In Houston CS, Coates G, editors: *Hypoxia: women at altitude*, Burlington, Vt, 1997, Queen City Publishers.

179. Krasney JA, Jensen JB, Lassen NA: Cerebral blood flow does not adapt to sustained hypoxia, *J Cereb Blood Flow Metab* 10:759, 1990.

180. Kronenberg RS et al: Pulmonary artery pressure and alveolar gas exchange in man during acclimatization to 12,470ft, *J Clin Invest* 50:827, 1971.

181. Kryger M et al: Excessive polycythemia of high altitude: role of ventilatory drive and lung disease, *Am Rev Respir Dis* 118:659, 1978.

182. Kryger M et al: Treatment of excessive polycythemia of high altitude with respiratory stimulant drugs, *Am Rev Respir Dis* 117:455, 1978.

183. Kryger MH, Grover RF: Chronic mountain sickness, *Semin Respir Med* 5:164, 1983.

184. Lahiri S, Data PG: Chemosensitivity and regulation of ventilation during sleep at high altitude, *Int J Sports Med* 13:S31, 1992.

185. Lane PA, Githens JH: Splenic syndrome at mountain altitudes in sickle cell trait: its occurrence in nonblack persons, *JAMA* 253:2252, 1985.

186. Larsen RF et al: Effect of spironolactone on acute mountain sickness (abstract). In Sutton JR, Houston CS, Coates G, editors: *Hypoxia and cold*, New York, 1987, Praeger.

187. Larson EB: Positive airway pressure for high altitude pulmonary edema, *Lancet* 1:371, 1985.

188. Larson EB et al: Acute mountain sickness and acetazolamide: clinical efficacy and effect on ventilation, *JAMA* 288:328, 1982.

189. Lassen NA: Increase of cerebral blood flow at high altitude: its possible relation to AMS, *Int J Sports Med* 13:S47, 1992.

190. Lassen NA, Harper AM: High altitude cerebral oedema, *Lancet* 2:1154, 1975 (letter).

191. Lategola M, Lyne P, Burr M: *Alcohol-induced physiological displacements and their effects on flight-related functions*, Washington, DC, 1982, Federal Aviation Administration.

192. Leadbetter G et al: *The effect of intermittent altitude exposure on acute mountain sickness*, San Diego, 1992, Southwestern Chapter of American College of Sports Medicine (abstract).

193. Levine B, Zuckerman J, deFilippi C: Effect of high altitude exposure in the elderly: the 10th Mountain Division Study, *Circulation* 96:1224, 1997.

194. Levine BD, Stray-Gundersen J: "Living high-training low": effect of moderate-altitude acclimatization with low-altitude training on performance, *J Appl Physiol* 83:102, 1997.

195. Levine BD et al: Dexamethasone in the treatment of acute mountain sickness, *N Engl J Med* 321:1707, 1989.

196. Litch JA, Bishop RA: Transient global amnesia at high altitude, *N Engl J Med* 340:1444, 1999 (letter).

197. Loeppky JA, Caprihan A, Luft UC: VA/Q inequality during clinical hypoxemia and its alterations. In Shiraki K, Yousef MK, editors: *Man in stressful environments*, Springfield, Ill, 1987, Charles C Thomas.

198. Lyons TP et al: The effect of altitude pre-acclimatization on acute mountain sickness during reexposure, *Aviat Space Environ Med* 66:957, 1995.

199. MacDougall JD et al: Operation Everest II: structural adaptations in skeletal muscle in response to extreme simulated altitude, *Acta Physiol Scand* 142:421, 1991.

200. Maggiorini M, Bartsch P, Oelz O: Association between raised body temperature and acute mountain sickness: cross sectional study, *BMJ* 315:403, 1997.

201. Maggiorini M et al: Prevalence of acute mountain sickness in the Swiss Alps, *BMJ* 301:853, 1990.

202. Maher JT, Jones LG, Hartley LH: Effects of high altitude exposure on submaximal endurance capacity of men, *J Appl Physiol* 37:895, 1974.

203. Mahoney BS, Githens JH: Sickling crisis and altitude: occurrence in the Colorado patient population, *Clin Pediatr* 18:431, 1979.

204. Mairbaurl H: Red blood cell functions at high altitude, *Ann Sport Med* 4:189, 1989.

205. Malconian MK et al: Operation Everest II: gas tensions in expired air and arterial blood at extreme altitude, *Aviat Space Environ Med* 64:37, 1993.

206. Maldonado D: High altitude pulmonary edema, *Radiol Clin North Am* 16:537, 1978.

207. Malhotra MS et al: Responses of the autonomic nervous system during acclimatization to high altitude in man, *Aviat Space Environ Med* 47:1076, 1976.

208. Marticorena E, Hultgren HN: Evaluation of therapeutic methods in high altitude pulmonary edema, *Am J Cardiol* 43:307, 1979.

209. Mason NP et al: Cough frequency and cough receptor sensitivity to citric acid challenge during a simulated ascent to extreme altitude, *Eur Respir J* 13:508, 1999.

210. Matsuda S, Onda T, Iikura Y: Bronchial responses of asthmatic patients in an atmosphere-changing chamber, *Int Arch Allergy Immunol* 107:402, 1995.

211. Matsuzawa Y et al: Blunted hypoxic ventilatory drive in subjects susceptible to high-altitude pulmonary edema, *J Appl Physiol* 66:1152, 1989.

212. Matsuzawa Y et al: Low hypoxic ventilatory response and relative hypoventilation in acute mountain sickness, *Jpn J Mountain Med* 10:151, 1990.

213. Matsuzawa Y et al: Cerebral edema in acute mountain sickness. In Ueda G, Reeves JT, Sekiguchi M, editors: *High altitude medicine,* Matsumoto, Japan, 1992, Shinshu University Press.

214. Matsuzawa Y et al: Hypoxic ventilatory response and pulmonary gas exchange during exposure to high altitude in subjects susceptible to high altitude pulmonary edema (HAPE). In Sutton JR, Houston CS, Coates G, editors: *Hypoxia and the brain,* Burlington, Vt, 1995, Queen City Press.

215. McFadden ER: The lower airway. In Sutton JR, Houston CS, Coates G, editors: *Hypoxia and cold,* New York, 1987, Praeger.

216. McFarland R: *Human factors in air transportation,* New York, 1953, McGraw-Hill.

217. McFarland R, Forbes W: The metabolism of alcohol in man at altitude, *Hum Biol* 8:387, 1936.

218. McFarland RA, Dill DB: A comparative study of the effects of reduced oxygen pressure on man during acclimatization, *J Aviat Med* 9:18, 1938.

219. McGillicudy JE: Cerebral protection: pathophysiology and treatment of increased intracranial pressure, *Chest* 87:85, 1985.

220. Meehan RT: Immune suppression at high altitude, *Ann Emerg Med* 16:974, 1987.

221. Menon ND: High altitude pulmonary edema, *N Engl J Med* 273:66, 1965.

222. Messner R: *Everest: expedition to the ultimate,* London, 1979, Kay and Ward.

223. Meyer BH: The use of low-dose acetazolamide to prevent mountain sickness, *S Afr Med J* 85:792, 1995 (letter).

224. Milledge JS: Salt and water control at altitude, *Int J Sports Med* 13:S61, 1992.

225. Milledge JS et al: Acute mountain sickness susceptibility, fitness and hypoxic ventilatory response, *Eur Respir J* 4:1000, 1991.

226. Mirrakhimov M, Winslow R: The cardiovascular system at high altitude. In Fregly M, Blatteis C, editors: *Handbook of physiology,* Oxford, 1996, Oxford University Press (American Physiological Society).

227. Mirrakhimov M et al: Effects of acetazolamide on overnight oxygenation and acute mountain sickness in patients with asthma, *Eur Respir J* 6:536, 1993.

228. Mirrakhimov MM: Biological and physiological characteristics of the high-altitude natives of Tien Shan and the Pamirs. In Baker PT, editor: *The biology of high-altitude peoples,* London, 1978, Cambridge University Press.

229. Monge CC, Arregui A, Leon-Velarde F: Pathophysiology and epidemiology of chronic mountain sickness, *Int J Sports Med* 13:S79, 1992.

230. Monge CC, Leon-Velarde F, Arregui A: Increasing prevalence of excessive erythrocytosis with age among healthy high-altitude miners, *N Engl J Med* 321:1271, 1989 (letter).

231. Monge CM: La enfermedad de los Andes: sindromes eritremicos, *Ann Fac Med (Lima)* 11:75, 1928.

232. Montgomery AB, Mills J, Luce JM: Incidence of acute mountain sickness at intermediate altitude, *JAMA* 261:732, 1989.

233. Montogomery HE et al: Human gene for physical performance, *Nature* 393:221, 1999.

234. Moore LG: Altitude aggravated illness: examples from pregnancy and prenatal life, *Ann Emerg Med* 16:965, 1986.

235. Moore LG, Niermeyer S, Zamudio S: Human adaptation to high altitude: regional and life-cycle perspectives, *Am J Phys Anthropol* 27(suppl):25, 1998.

236. Moore LG et al: Low acute hypoxic ventilatory response and hypoxic depression in acute altitude sickness, *J Appl Physiol* 60:1407, 1986.

237. Moore LG et al: Are Tibetans better adapted? *Int J Sports Med* 13:S86, 1992.

238. Moore LG et al: Genetic adaptations to high altitude. In Wood SC, Roach RC, editors: *Sport and exercise medicine,* New York, 1994 Marcel Dekker.

239. Morgan BJ et al: The patient with coronary heart disease at altitude: observations during acute exposure to 3100 meters, *Journal of Wilderness Medicine* 1:147, 1990.

240. Morris A: *Clinical pulmonary function tests: a manual of uniform lab procedures,* Salt Lake City, 1984, Intermountain Thoracic Society.

241. Mosso A: *Life of man in the high Alps,* London, 1898, T Fisher Unwin.

242. Murdoch D: The portable hyperbaric chamber for the treatment of high altitude illness, *N Z Med J* 105:361, 1992.

243. Murdoch DR: Symptoms of infection and altitude illness among hikers in the Mount Everest region of Nepal, *Aviat Space Environ Med* 66:148, 1995.

244. Muza SR et al: Effect of altitude exposure on brain volume and development of acute mountain sickness (AMS), *Adv Exp Med Biol* 474:414, 1999 (abstract).

245. Naeije R et al: High-altitude pulmonary edema with primary pulmonary hypertension, *Chest* 110:286, 1996.

246. Nakashima M: The Japanese Himalayan Expeditions. In Ohno H et al, editors: *Progress in mountain medicine and high altitude physiology,* Matsumoto, Japan, 1998, Japanese Society of Mountain Medicine.

247. Nayak NC, Roy S, Narayaran TK: Pathologic features of altitude sickness, *Am J Pathol* 45:381, 1964.

248. Nicholas R, O'Meara PD, Calonge N: Is syncope related to moderate altitude exposure? *JAMA* 268:904, 1992.

249. Niermeyer S: The pregnant altitude visitor, *Adv Exp Med Biol* 474:65, 1999.

250. Niermeyer S et al: Neonatal cardiopulmonary transition at high altitude (abstract). In Sutton JR, Coates G, Houston CS, editors: *Hypoxia and mountain medicine,* Burlington, Vt, 1992, Queen City Press.

251. Oades PJ, Buchdahl RM, Bush A: Prediction of hypoxaemia at high altitude in children with cystic fibrosis, *BMJ* 308:15, 1994.

252. O'Brodovich H et al: Hypoxia alters blood coagulation during acute decompression in humans, *J Appl Physiol* 56:666, 1984.

253. Oelz O et al: Physiological profile of world-class high altitude climbers, *J Appl Physiol* 60:1734, 1986.

254. Oelz O et al: Nifedipine for high altitude pulmonary edema, *Lancet* 2:1241, 1989.

255. Olson LG, Hensley MJ, Saunders NA: Augmentation of ventilatory response to asphyxia by prochlorperazine in humans, *J Appl Physiol* 53:637, 1982.

256. Ou LC, Tenney SM: Properties of mitochondria from hearts of cattle acclimatized to high altitude, *Respir Physiol* 8:151, 1970.

257. Palatini P et al: Effects of low altitude exposure on 24-hour blood pressure and adrenergic activity, *Am J Cardiol* 64:1379, 1989.

258. Parker SJ et al: Treatment of acute mountain sickness in Himalayan trekkers: a preliminary prospective randomized trial of hyperbaria versus dexamethasone (abstract). In Sutton JR, Houston CS, Coates G, editors: *Hypoxia and the brain,* Burlington, Vt, 1995, Queen City Press.

259. Pei SX et al: Chronic mountain sickness in Tibet, *QJM* 71:555, 1989.

260. Penaloza D, Sime F: Circulatory dynamics during high altitude pulmonary edema, *Am J Cardiol* 23:369, 1969.

261. Pollard AJ, Murdoch DR, Bartsch P: Children in the mountains, *BMJ* 316:874, 1998 (editorial; comment).

262. Pugh LG: Metabolic problems of high altitude operations. In Vaughan L, editor: *Proceedings Symposia Arctic Biology and Medicine V: nutritional requirements for survival in the cold and at altitude,* Ft Wainwright, Alaska, 1966, Arctic Aeromedical Laboratory.

263. Pugh LG: Report of medical research project into effects of altitude in Mexico City. In Astrand PO, Rodahl K, editors: *Textbook of work physiology,* New York, 1977, McGraw-Hill.

264. Rabold MB: *High altitude bronchitis on Cerro Aconcagua,* Aspen, Colo, 1987, Wilderness Medical Society (abstract).

265. Rahn H, Otis AB: Man's respiratory response during and after acclimatization to high altitude, *Am J Physiol* 157:445, 1949.

266. Reeves JT: Sympathetics and hypoxia: a brief overview. In Sutton JR, Houston CS, Coates G, editors: *Hypoxia and molecular medicine,* Burlington, Vt, 1993, Queen City Press.

267. Reeves JT et al: Headache at high altitude is not related to internal carotid arterial blood velocity, *J Appl Physiol* 59:909, 1985.

268. Reeves JT et al: Operation Everest II: preservation of cardiac function at extreme altitude, *J Appl Physiol* 63:531, 1987.

269. Reeves JT et al: Seasonal variation in barometric pressure and temperature in Summit County: effect on altitude illness. In Sutton JR, Houston CS, Coates G, editors: *Hypoxia and molecular medicine,* Burlington, Vt, 1993, Queen City Press.

270. Reite M et al: Sleep physiology at high altitude, *Electroencephalogr Clin Neurophysiol* 38:463, 1975.

271. Rennie D: Herb Hultgren in Peru: what caused high altitude pulmonary edema? *Adv Exp Med Biol* 474:1, 1999.

272. Richalet JP: Joseph Vallot and the history of altitude physiology on Mont Blanc. In Ohno H et al, editors: *Progress in mountain medicine and high altitude physiology,* Matsumoto, Japan, 1998, Japanese Society of Mountain Medicine.

273. Richalet JP et al: Physiological characteristics of high altitude climbers, *Sci Sport* 3:89, 1988.

274. Richalet JP et al: Operation Everest III (COMEX '97), *Adv Exp Med Biol* 474:297, 1999.

275. Rios B, Driscoll DJ, McNamara DG: High-altitude pulmonary edema with absent right pulmonary artery, *Pediatrics* 75:314, 1985.

276. Ritchie J, Lakhani K: Fetal breathing movements and maternal hyperoxia, *Br J Obstet Gynaecol* 87:12, 1980.

277. Roach RC: The role of the hypoxic ventilatory response in performance at high altitude. In Wood SC, Roach RC, editors: *Modern topics in sports medicine*, New York, 1994, Marcel Dekker.

278. Roach RC: Cardiovascular regulation during hypoxia. In Ohno H et al, editors: *Progress in mountain medicine and high altitude physiology*, Matsumoto, Japan, 1998, Japanese Society of Mountain Medicine.

279. Roach RC, Hackett PH: Hyperbaria and high altitude illness. In Sutton JR, Coates G, Houston CS, editors: *Hypoxia and mountain medicine*, Burlington, Vt, 1992, Queen City Press.

280. Roach RC, Loeppky JA, Icenogle M: AMS in women, *J Appl Physiol* (in press).

281. Roach RC et al: The Lake Louise acute mountain sickness scoring system. In Sutton JR, Houston CS, Coates G, editors: *Hypoxia and molecular medicine*, Burlington, Vt, 1993, Queen City Press.

282. Roach RC et al: How well do older persons tolerate moderate altitude? *West J Med* 162:32, 1995.

283. Roach RC et al: Exercise exacerbates acute mountain sickness at simulated high altitude, *J Appl Physiol* 88:581, 2000.

284. Roach RC et al: Fluid redistribution and acute mountain sickness (AMS) *FASEB J* 14:A82, 2000 (abstract).

285. Roberts D, Smith DJ: Erythropoietin: induction of synthesis to signal transduction, *J Mol Endocrinol* 12:131, 1994.

286. Robertson JA, Shlim DR: Treatment of moderate acute mountain sickness with pressurization in a portable hyperbaric (GamowTM) bag, *Journal of Wilderness Medicine* 2:268, 1991.

287. Robin ED: Permeability pulmonary edema. In Fishman AP, Renkin EM, editors: *Pulmonary edema*, Bethesda, Md, 1979, American Physiological Society.

288. Roca Cusachs A: Pattern of blood pressure among high and low altitude residents of southern Arabia, *J Hum Hypertens* 9:293, 1995 (letter).

289. Rock PB et al: Effect of dexamethasone on symptoms of acute mountain sickness at Pike's Peak, Colorado (4,300), *Aviat Space Environ Med* 58:668, 1987.

290. Roeggla G et al: Effect of alcohol on acute ventilatory adaptation to mild hypoxia at moderate altitude, *Ann Intern Med* 122:925, 1995.

291. Ropper AH: Raised intracranial pressure in neurologic diseases, *Semin Neurol* 4:397, 1984.

292. Rose MS et al: Operation Everest II: nutrition and body composition, *J Appl Physiol* 65:2545, 1988.

293. Rosen A, Rosen J: Effect of a face mask on respiratory water loss during sleep in cold conditions, *Wilderness and Environmental Medicine* 6:189, 1995.

294. Ross RT: The random nature of cerebral mountain sickness, *Lancet* 1:990, 1985.

295. Ryn Z: Psychopathology in mountaineering—mental disturbances under high-altitude stress, *Int J Sports Med* 9:163, 1988.

296. Salvaggio A et al: Effects of high-altitude periodic breathing on sleep and arterial oxyhaemoglobin saturation, *Eur Respir J* 12:408, 1998.

297. Samaja M, di Prampero PE, Cerretelli P: The role of 2,3-DPG in the oxygen transport at altitude, *Respir Physiol* 64:191, 1986.

298. Sanchez del Rio M, Moskowitz MA: High altitude headache, *Adv Exp Med Biol* 474:145, 1999.

299. Sarnquist FH: Physicians on Mount Everest: a clinical account of the 1981 American medical research expedition to Everest, *West J Med* 139:480, 1983.

300. Sartori C et al: Impairment of amiloride-sensitive sodium transport in individuals susceptible to high altitude pulmonary edema, *Adv Exp Med Biol* 474:426, 1999 (abstract).

301. Savonitto S et al: Effects of acute exposure to altitude (3,460 m) on blood pressure response to dynamic and isometric exercise in men with systemic hypertension, *Am J Cardiol* 70:1493, 1992.

302. Scherrer U et al: Inhaled nitric oxide for high-altitude pulmonary edema, *N Engl J Med* 334:624, 1996.

303. Scherrer U et al: High-altitude pulmonary edema: from exaggerated pulmonary hypertension to a defect in transepithelial sodium transport, *Adv Exp Med Biol* 474:93, 1999.

304. Schilling L, Wahl M: Mediators of cerebral edema, *Adv Exp Med Biol* 474:123, 1999.

305. Schoene RB et al: High altitude pulmonary edema and exercise at 4400 meters on Mt. McKinley: effect of expiratory positive airway pressure, *Chest* 87:330, 1985.

306. Schoene RB et al: High altitude pulmonary edema: characteristics of lung lavage fluid, *JAMA* 256:63, 1986.

307. Schoene RB et al: The lung at high altitude: bronchoalveolar lavage in acute mountain sickness and pulmonary edema, *J Appl Physiol* 64:2605, 1988.

308. Scoggin CH et al: High-altitude pulmonary edema in the children and young adults of Leadville, Colorado, *N Engl J Med* 297:1269, 1977.

309. Semenza GL: Regulation of erythropoietin production: new insights into molecular mechanisms of oxygen homeostasis, *Hematol Oncol Clin North Am* 8:863, 1994.

310. Senay LC, Tolbert DL: Effect of arginine vasopressin, acetazolamide and angiotensin II on CSF pressure at simulated altitude, *Aviat Space Environ Med* 55:370, 1984.

311. Severinghaus JW: Transarterial leakage: a possible mechanism of high altitude pulmonary edema. In Porter R, Knight J, editors: *High altitude physiology: cardiac and respiratory aspects*, London, 1971, Churchill Livingstone.

312. Severinghaus JW et al: Cerebral blood flow in man at high altitude: role of cerebrospinal fluid pH in normalization of flow in chronic hypoxia, *Circ Res* 19:274, 1966.

313. Shapiro K, Marmarou A, Shulman K: Characterization of clinical CSF dynamics and neural axis compliance using the pressure volume index. I. The normal pressure volume index, *Ann Neurol* 7:508, 1980.

314. Shinfu S: Epidemiology of hypertension on the Tibetan plateau, *Hum Biol* 58:507, 1986.

315. Siesjo BK, Ingvar M: Ventilation and brain metabolism. In Cherniack NS, Widdicombe JG, editors: *Handbook of physiology: the respiratory system*, Bethesda, Md, 1986, American Physiological Society.

316. Simon H et al: High altitude climate therapy reduces peripheral blood T lymphocyte activation, eosinophilia, and bronchial obstruction in children with house-dust mite allergic asthma, *Pediatr Pulmonol* 17:304, 1994.

317. Singh I: Pulmonary hypertension in new arrivals at high altitude, *Proceedings of World Health Organization Meeting on Primary Pulmonary Hypertension*, Geneva, 1974, 1973.

318. Singh I, Chohan IS, Mathew NT: Fibrinolytic activity in high altitude pulmonary oedema, *Ind J Med Res* 57:210, 1969.

319. Singh I, Roy SB: High altitude pulmonary edema: clinical, hemodynamic, and pathologic studies. In Hegnauer A, editor: *Biomedical problems of high terrestrial elevations*, Springfield, Va, 1962, Federal Scientific and Technical Information Service.

320. Singh I et al: High altitude pulmonary oedema, *Lancet* 1:229, 1965.

321. Singh I et al: Acute mountain sickness, *N Engl J Med* 280:175, 1969.

322. Song S-Y et al: Cerebral thrombosis at altitude: its pathogenesis and the problems of prevention and treatment, *Aviat Space Environ Med* 57:71, 1986.

323. Sophocles AM: High-altitude pulmonary edema in Vail, Colorado, 1975-1982, *West J Med* 144:569, 1986.

324. Sophocles AM, Bachman J: High altitude pulmonary edema among visitors to Summit County, Colorado, *J Fam Pract* 17:1015, 1983.

325. Speechly-Dick M, Rimmer S, Hodson M: Exacerbations of cystic fibrosis after holidays at high altitude—a cautionary tale, *Respir Med* 86:55, 1992.

326. Staub NC: Pulmonary edema—hypoxia and overperfusion, *N Engl J Med* 302:1085, 1980 (editorial).

327. Steinacker JM et al: Lung diffusing capacity and exercise in subjects with previous high altitude pulmonary oedema, *Eur Respir J* 11:643, 1998.

328. Stenmark KR et al: Hypoxia induces cell-specific changes in gene expression in vascular wall cells: implications for pulmonary hypertension, *Adv Exp Med Biol* 474:231, 1999.

329. Stray-Gundersen J, Levine BD: "Living high and training low" can improve sea level performance in endurance athletes, *Br J Sports Med* 33:150, 1999.

330. Stray-Gundersen J et al: Failure of red cell volume to increase to altitude exposure in iron deficient runners, *Med Sci Sports Exerc* 24:S90, 1992 (abstract).

331. Suarez J, Alexander JK, Houston CS: Enhanced left ventricular systolic performance at high altitude during Operation Everest II, *Am J Cardiol* 60:137, 1987.

332. Sutton JR et al: Effect of acetazolamide on hypoxemia during sleep at high altitude, *N Engl J Med* 301:1329, 1979.

333. Sutton JR et al: Effects of acclimatization on sleep hypoxemia at altitude. In West JB, Lahiri S, editors: *High altitude and man*, Bethesda, Md, 1984, American Physiological Society.

334. Sutton JR et al: Operation Everest II: oxygen transport during exercise at extreme simulated altitude, *J Appl Physiol* 64:1309, 1988.

335. Swenson ER: High altitude diuresis: fact or fancy. In Houston CS, Coates G, editors: *Hypoxia: women at altitude*, Burlington, Vt, 1997, Queen City Publishers.

336. Swenson ER et al: Renal carbonic anhydrase inhibition reduces high altitude sleep periodic breathing, *Respir Physiol* 86:333, 1991.

337. Swenson ER et al: Acute mountain sickness is not altered by a high carbohydrate diet nor associated with elevated circulating cytokines, *Aviat Space Environ Med* 68:1, 1997.

338. Taber RL: Protocols for the use of a portable hyperbaric chamber for the treatment of high altitude disorders, *Journal of Wilderness Medicine* 1:181, 1990.

339. Tiernan C: Splenic crisis at high altitude in 2 white men with sickle cell trait, *Ann Emerg Med* 33:230, 1999.

340. Torrington KG: Recurrent high-altitude illness associated with right pulmonary artery occlusion from granulomatous mediastinitis, *Chest* 96:1422, 1989.

341. Tschöp M et al: Raised leptin concentrations at high altitude associated with loss of appetite, *Lancet* 352:1119, 1998 (letter).

342. Turner WA et al: Carbon monoxide exposure in mountaineers on Denali, *Alaska Med* 30:85, 1988.

343. Utiger D et al: Transient improvement of high altitude headache by sumatriptan in a placebo controlled trial, *Adv Exp Med Biol* 474:435, 1999 (abstract).

344. Vervolet D et al: Asthma-allergy. Altitude: a study model, *Presse Med* 23:1684, 1994 (editorial).

345. Viault F: On the large increase in the number of red cells in the blood of the inhabitants of the high plateaus of South America. In West JB, editor: *High altitude physiology*, Stroudsberg, Penn, 1981, Hutchinson Ross.

346. Viswanathan R, Subramanian S, Radha TG: Effect of hypoxia on regional lung perfusion, by scanning, *Respiration* 37:142, 1979.

347. Viswanathan R et al: Further studies on pulmonary oedema of high altitude, *Respiration* 36:216, 1978.

348. Vock P et al: High-altitude pulmonary edema: findings at high-altitude chest radiography and physical examination, *Radiology* 170:661, 1989.

349. Vock P et al: Variable radiomorphologic data of high altitude pulmonary edema: features from 60 patients, *Chest* 100:1306, 1991.

350. Wagner PD: Gas exchange and peripheral diffusion limitation, *Med Sci Sports Exerc* 24:54, 1992.

351. Ward MP, Milledge JS, West JB: *High altitude medicine and physiology*, London, 1995, Chapman and Hall Medical.

352. Weil JV et al: Hypoxic ventilatory drive in normal man, *J Clin Invest* 49:1061, 1970.

353. West JB: Climbing Mt. Everest without oxygen: an analysis of maximal exercise during extreme hypoxia, *Respir Physiol* 52:265, 1983.

354. West JB: "Oxygenless" climbs and barometric pressure, *Am Alpine J* 226:126, 1984.

355. West JB: *High life: a history of high-altitude physiology and medicine*, New York, 1998, Oxford University Press.

356. West JB et al: Maximal exercise at extreme altitudes on Mount Everest, *J Appl Physiol* 55:688, 1983.

357. West JB et al: Pulmonary gas exchange on the summit of Mount Everest, *J Appl Physiol* 55:678, 1983.

358. West JB et al: Stress failure in pulmonary capillaries, *J Appl Physiol* 70:1731, 1991.

359. Westendorp RG et al: Atrial natriuretic peptide improves pulmonary gas exchange in subjects exposed to hypoxia, *Am Rev Respir Dis* 148, 1993.

360. Wiley AS: Neonatal size and infant mortality at high altitude in the Western Himalaya, *Am J Phys Anthropol* 94:289, 1994.

361. Wilson R: Acute high altitude illness in mountaineers and problems of rescue, *Ann Intern Med* 78:421, 1973.

362. Winslow RM: High altitude polycythemia. In West JB, Lahiri S, editors: *High altitude and man*, Bethesda, Md, 1984, American Physiological Society.

363. Wistrand PJ: The use of carbonic anhydrase in ophthalmology and clinical medicine, *Ann NY Acad Sci* 429:609, 1984.

364. Wohns RN: Transient ischemic attacks at high altitude, *Crit Care Med* 14:517, 1986.

365. Wolfel EE et al: Oxygen transport during steady-state submaximal exercise in chronic hypoxia, *J Appl Physiol* 70:1129, 1991.

366. Wright AD et al: Intracranial pressure at high altitude and acute mountain sickness, *Clin Sci (Colch)* 89:201, 1995.

367. Wu TY: An epidemiological study on high altitude disease, *Chung Hua Liu Hsing Ping Hsueh Tsa Chih* 8:65, 1987.

368. Wu TY et al: Low incidence of reascent high altitude pulmonary edema in Tibetan native highlanders, *Acta Andina* 5:39, 1996.

369. Xie CF, Pei SX: Some physiological data on sojourners and native highlanders at three different altitudes on Xizang, *Proceedings of Symposium on Tibet Plateau*, New York, 1981, Gordon & Breach.

370. Yagi H et al: Doppler assessment of pulmonary hypertension induced by hypoxic breathing in subjects susceptible to high altitude pulmonary edema, *Am Rev Respir Dis* 142:796, 1990.

371. Yaron M et al: The diagnosis of acute mountain sickness in preverbal children, *Arch Pediatr Adolesc Med* 152:683, 1998.

372. Zamudio S et al: Protection from intrauterine growth retardation in Tibetans at high altitude, *Am J Phys Anthropol* 91:215, 1993.

373. Zavasky D, Hackett P: Cerebral etiology of acute mountain sickness: MRI findings, *Wilderness and Environmental Medicine* 6:229, 1995.

374. Zell SC, Goodman PH: Acetazolamide and dexamethasone in the prevention of acute mountain sickness, *West J Med* 148:541, 1988.

375. Zhang R, Zuckerman JH, Levine BD: Deterioration of cerebral autoregulation during orthostatic stress: insights from the frequency domain, *J Appl Physiol* 85:1113, 1998.

376. Zimmerman GA, Crapo RO: Adult respiratory distress syndrome secondary to high altitude pulmonary edema, *West J Med* 133:335, 1980.

2 Avalanches

Knox Williams, Betsy R. Armstrong, Richard L. Armstrong, and Dale Atkins

An avalanche is a mass of snow that slides down a mountainside. In the United States, approximately 100,000 avalanches occur annually, of which about 100 cause injury, death, or destruction of property. Based on reported incidents in the 1990s, about 200 people a year are caught in avalanches (that is, they are bodily involved in the moving snow or its effects). Of these, 75 are partly or wholly buried, 18 sustain injury, and 24 are killed. Average annual property damage is approximately $520,000. This chapter describes the properties of the mountain snowpack that contribute to avalanche formation and describes avalanche safety techniques.

PROPERTIES OF SNOW

Physical Properties

Although snow cover appears to be nothing more than a thick, homogeneous blanket covering the ground, it is in fact one of the most complex materials found in nature. It is highly variable and goes through significant changes in relatively short periods of time.

In nature, snow cover is variable on both the broad geographic scale (Antarctic snow is quite different from snow found in the Cascade Mountains of North America) and on the microscale (where snow conditions may vary greatly from one side of a rock or tree to the other). All snow crystals are made of the same substance, the water molecule, but local environmental conditions control the type and character of snow found at a given location. At a single site the snow cover varies from top to bottom, resulting in a complex layered structure.

Individual layers may be quite thick or very thin. In general, thicker layers represent consistent conditions during one storm, when new snow crystals falling are of the same type, wind speed and direction vary little, and temperature and precipitation are fairly constant. Thinner layers, perhaps only millimeters in thickness, often reflect conditions between storms, such as the formation during fair weather of a melt-freeze crust, a period of strong winds creating a wind crust, or the occurrence of surface hoar, the winter equivalent of dew. Delicate feather-shaped crystals of surface hoar deposited from the moist atmosphere onto the cold snow surface overnight offer a beautiful glistening sight as they reflect the sun of the following day. However, they are very fragile and weak, and once buried by subsequent snowfalls, they may be major contributors to avalanche formation.

One property of snow is strength, or hardness, which is of great importance in terms of avalanche for-mation. Snow can vary from light and fluffy, easy to shovel, and especially delightful to ski through, to heavy and dense, impossible to penetrate with a shovel, and hard enough to make it very difficult for a skier to carve a turn, even with sharp metal edges. The arrangement of the ice skeleton and the changing density (mass per unit volume) produce this wide range of conditions. In the case of snow, density is determined by the volume mixture of ice crystals and air. The denser the snow layer, the harder and stronger it becomes, as long as it is not melting.

The density of new snow can have a wide range of values. This depends on how closely the new snow crystals pack together, which is controlled by the shape of the crystals. The initial crystals have a variety of shapes, and some pack more closely together than others (Figure 2-1). For example, needles pack more closely than stellars and as a consequence may possess a density 3 to 4 times that of stellars.

Wind can alter the shape of new snow crystals, breaking them into much smaller pieces that pack very closely together to form wind slabs. These in turn may possess a density 5 to 10 times that of new stellars falling in the absence of wind. Because these processes occur at different times and locations at the surface of the snow cover and are buried by subsequent snowfalls, a varied, nonhomogeneous layered structure results. Therefore what may seem to the casual observer to be minor variations in atmospheric conditions can have an important influence on the properties of snow.

After snow has been deposited on the ground, the density increases as the snow layer settles vertically or shrinks in thickness. Because an increase in density equals an increase in strength, the rate at which this change occurs is important with respect to avalanche potential. Snow can settle simply because of its own weight. It is highly compressible because it is composed mostly of empty airspace within an ice skeleton of snow crystals. In a typical layer of new snow, 85% to 95% of the volume is empty airspace. Individual ice crystals can move and slide past each other, and because the force of gravity causes them to move slowly downward, the layer shrinks. The heavier the snow above and the warmer the temperature, the faster this settlement proceeds.

At the same time, the complex, intricate shapes that characterize the new snow crystals begin to change. They become rounded and suitable for closer packing. Intricate crystals change because they possess a shape

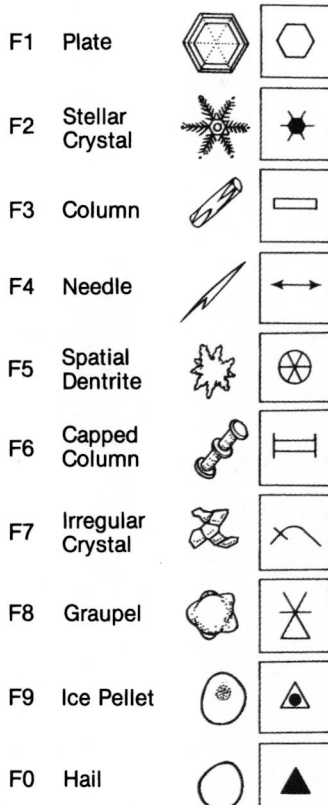

F1	Plate
F2	Stellar Crystal
F3	Column
F4	Needle
F5	Spatial Dentrite
F6	Capped Column
F7	Irregular Crystal
F8	Graupel
F9	Ice Pellet
F0	Hail

Figure 2-1 International classification of solid precipitation. *(From the International Association of Scientific Hydrology.)*

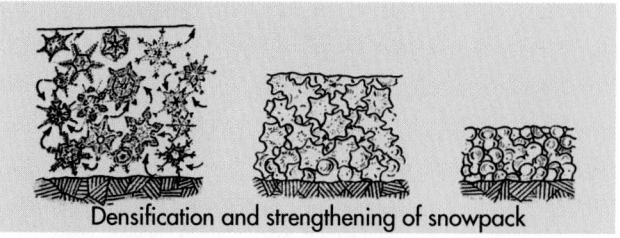

Densification and strengthening of snowpack

Figure 2-2 Settlement. As the crystal shapes become more rounded, they can pack more closely together and the layer settles or shrinks in thickness.

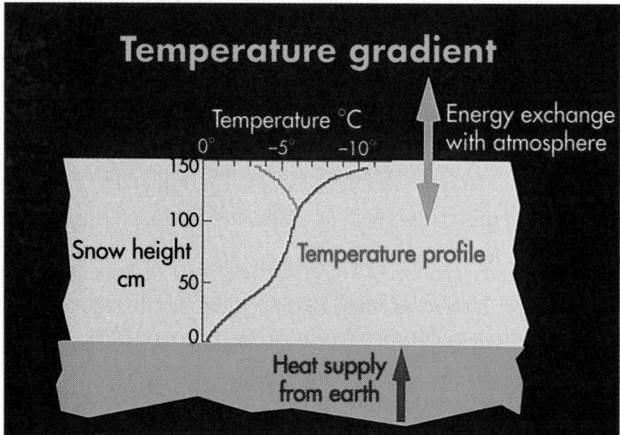

Figure 2-3 When an insulating layer of snow separates the warm ground from the cold air, a temperature gradient develops across the snow layer.

that is naturally unstable. New snow crystals have a large surface area/volume ratio and are composed of crystalline solid close to its melting point. In this aspect, snow crystals are almost unique among materials found in nature. Surface energy physics dictates that this unstable condition will change; the warmer the temperature, the faster the change. Under very cold conditions, the original shapes of the snow crystals are recognizable after they have been in the snow cover for several days or even a week or two. As temperatures warm and approach the melting point, such shapes disappear within a few hours to a day. Changes in the shape or texture of snow crystals are examples of initial metamorphism. The geologic term *metamorphism* defines changes that result from the effects of temperature and pressure. As the crystal shapes simplify, they can pack more closely together, enhancing further settlement (Figure 2-2).

The changes generally occur within hours to a few days. The structure of snow cover changes over a period of weeks to months via other processes. Settlement, which may initially have been rapid, continues at a much slower rate. Other factors begin to exert dominant influences on metamorphism. These factors include the difference in temperature measured upward

or downward in the snow layer, called the *temperature gradient.*

Averaged over 24 hours, snow temperatures generally are coldest near the surface and warmest near the ground at the base of the snow cover, creating a temperature gradient across a snow layer sandwiched between cold winter air and relatively warm ground (Figure 2-3). The temperature gradient crosses both ice and large void spaces filled with air. Within the ice skeleton, the temperature adjacent to the ground is warmer than that of the snow layer just above, and this pattern continues through the snow cover in the direction of the colder surface.

Warm air contains more water vapor than does cold air; this holds true for the air trapped within the snow cover. The greater the amount of water vapor, the greater the pressure. Therefore both a pressure gradient and a temperature gradient exist through the snow cover. When a pressure difference exists, the difference naturally tends to equalize, just as adjacent high and low atmospheric pressure centers cause movement of air masses. Pressure differences within snow cause va-

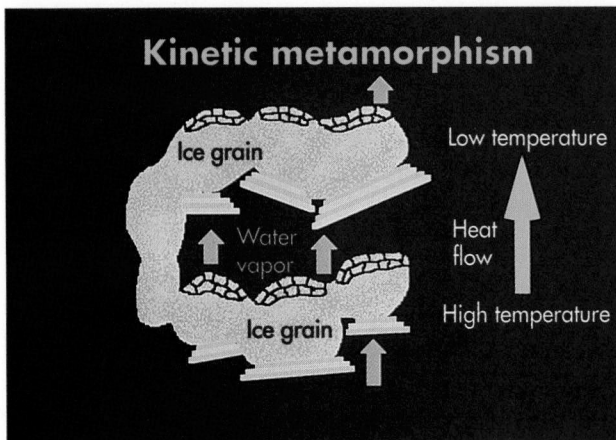

Figure 2-4 In the temperature-gradient process, ice sublimates from the top of one grain, moves upward as water vapor, and then is deposited on the bottom surface of the grain above. If conditions allow this process to continue long enough, all of the original grains are lost as the recrystallization produces a layer of totally new crystals.

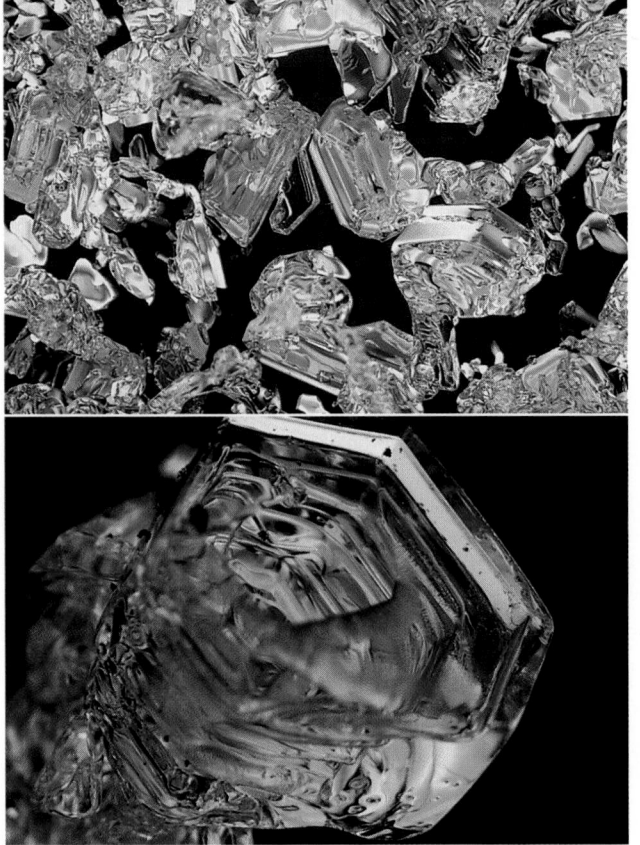

Figure 2-5 **A,** Mature depth hoar grains. Facets and angles are visible. Grain size: 3 to 5 mm. **B,** Advanced temperature-gradient grains attain a hollow cup-shaped form. Size: 4 mm. (**A** and **B,** *Polarized-light photos by Doug Driskell.*)

por to move upward through the snow layers. The air within the layers of the snow cover is saturated with water vapor, with a relative humidity of 100%. When air moves upward to a colder layer, the amount of water vapor that can be supported in the airspace diminishes. Some vapor changes to ice and is deposited on the surrounding ice grains. We witness a similar process when warm, moist air in a heated room comes in contact with a cold windowpane. The invisible water vapor is cooled to its ice point, and some of the vapor changes state and is deposited as frost on the window.

Figure 2-4 shows how the texture of the snow layer changes during this temperature-gradient process. Water molecules sublimate from the upper surfaces of a grain. The vapor moves upward along the temperature (and vapor) gradient and is deposited as a solid ice molecule on the underside of a colder grain above. If this process continues long enough (it continues as long as a strong temperature gradient exists), all grains in the snow layer are transformed from solid to vapor and back to solid again; that is, they totally recrystallize. New crystals are completely different in texture from their initial form. They become large, coarse grains with facets and sharp angles and may eventually evolve into a hollow cup form. Examples of these crystals are shown in Figure 2-5. The process is called *temperature-gradient metamorphism,* or kinetic metamorphism, and well-developed crystals are commonly known as *depth hoar.*

Depth hoar is of particular importance to avalanche formation. It is very weak because there is little or no cohesion or bonding at the grain contacts. Depth hoar or temperature-gradient snow layers can be compared to dry sand. Each grain may possess significant strength, but a layer composed of grains is very weak and friable because the grains lack connections. Thus depth hoar is commonly called "sugar snow." Depth hoar usually develops whenever the temperature gradient is equal to or greater than about 10° C (18° F) per meter. In the cold, shallow snow covers of a continental climate, such as that of the Rocky Mountains, a gradient of this magnitude is common within the first snow layers of the season. Therefore a layer of depth hoar is frequently found at the bottom of the snow cover, and the resulting low strength becomes a significant factor for future avalanches.

In the absence of a strong temperature gradient, a totally different type of snow texture develops. When the gradient is less than about 10° C per meter, there is still a vapor pressure difference and upward movement of vapor through the snow layers, but at a much slower rate. As a result, water vapor deposited on a colder grain tends to cover the total grain in a more homogeneous manner, rather than showing the preferential deposition characteristic of depth hoar. This process produces a grain with a smooth surface of more rounded or oblong shape. Over time, vapor is deposited at the

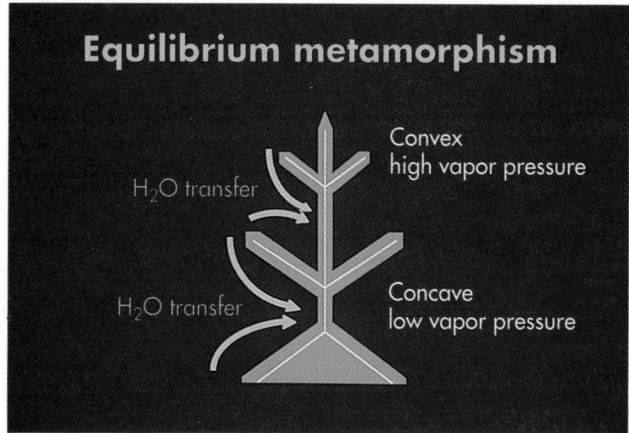

Figure 2-6 In the equilibrium metamorphism process, ice molecules sublimate from crystal points (convexities) and redeposit on flat or concave areas of the crystal.

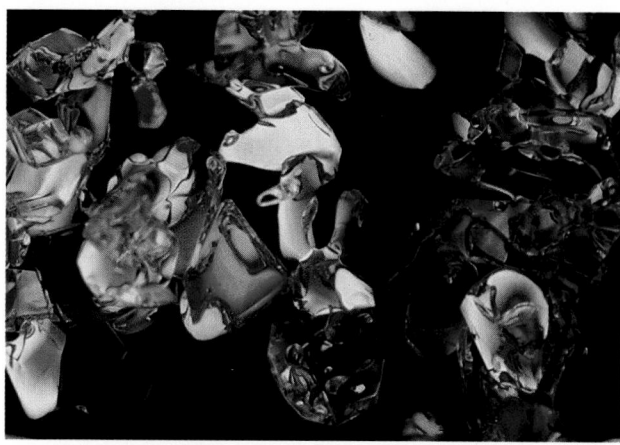

Figure 2-8 Bonded or sintered grains resulting from equitemperature metamorphism. Grain size: 0.5 to 1 mm. *(Polarized-light photo by Doug Driskell.)*

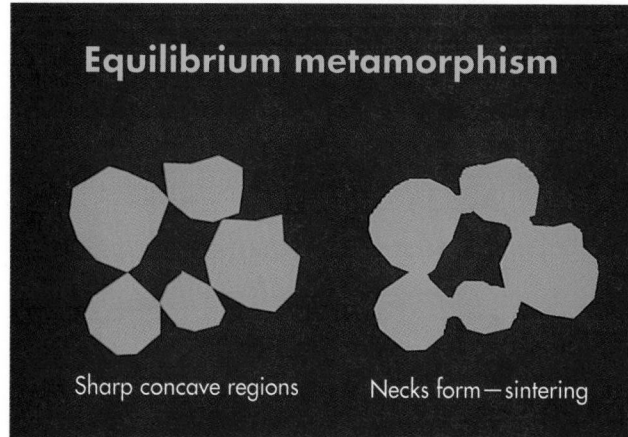

Figure 2-7 Equitemperature grain growth. In the presence of weak temperature gradients, bonds grow at the grain contacts.

grain contacts (concavities), as well as over the remaining surface of the grain (convexity) (Figure 2-6). Connecting bonds formed at the grain contacts give the snow layer strength over time (Figure 2-7). Bond growth, called *sintering,* yields a cohesive texture, in complete contrast to the cohesionless texture of depth hoar. This type of grain has been referred to by various terms (destructive metamorphism, equitemperature metamorphism, and equilibrium metamorphism) but can generally be described as fine-grained or well-sintered (bonded) snow. Rounded and interconnected grains are shown in Figure 2-8.

The preceding paragraphs describe the "big picture" in terms of what happens to snow layers after they have been buried by subsequent snowfalls. If the layer is subfreezing (i.e., if no melt is taking place), one of the two processes described previously is occurring, or per-

haps a transition exists between the two. Within the total snow cover, these processes may occur simultaneously, but only one can take place within a given layer at a given time. Both processes accelerate with warmer snow temperature because water vapor is involved. The temperature gradient across the layer determines whether the process involves the growth of weak depth hoar crystals or the development of a stronger snow layer with a sintered, interconnected texture.

Slab Avalanche Formation

There are two basic types of avalanche release. The first is point-release, or loose snow, avalanche (Figure 2-9). A loose snow avalanche involves cohesionless snow and is initiated at a point, spreading out laterally as it moves down the slope to form a characteristic inverted V shape. A single grain or a clump of grains slips out of place and dislodges those below on the slope, which in turn dislodge others. The avalanche continues as long as the snow is cohesionless and the slope is steep enough. This type of avalanche usually involves only small amounts of near-surface snow.

The second type of avalanche, the slab avalanche, requires a cohesive snow layer poorly anchored to the snow below because of the presence of a weak layer. The cohesive blanket of snow breaks away simultaneously over a broad area (Figure 2-10). A slab release can involve a range of snow thicknesses, from the near-surface layers to the entire snow cover down to the ground. In contrast to a loose snow avalanche, a slab avalanche has the potential to involve very large amounts of snow.

To understand the conditions in snow cover that contribute to slab avalanche formation, it is essential to reemphasize that snow cover develops layer by layer. Although a layered structure can develop by metamor-

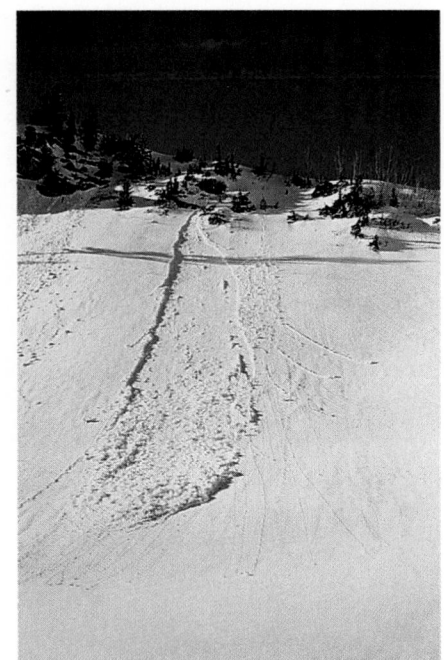

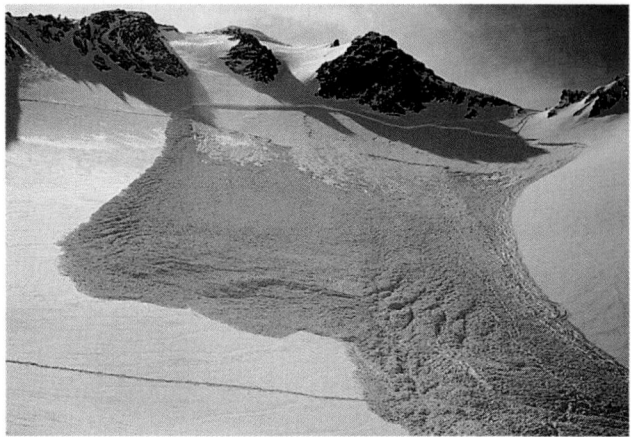

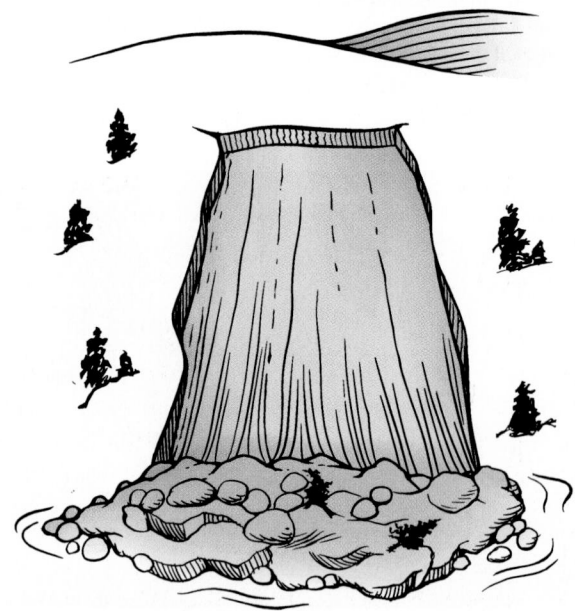

Figure 2-10 Slab avalanche. (*From USDA Forest Service:* The snowy torrents. *Photo by Alexis Kelner.*)

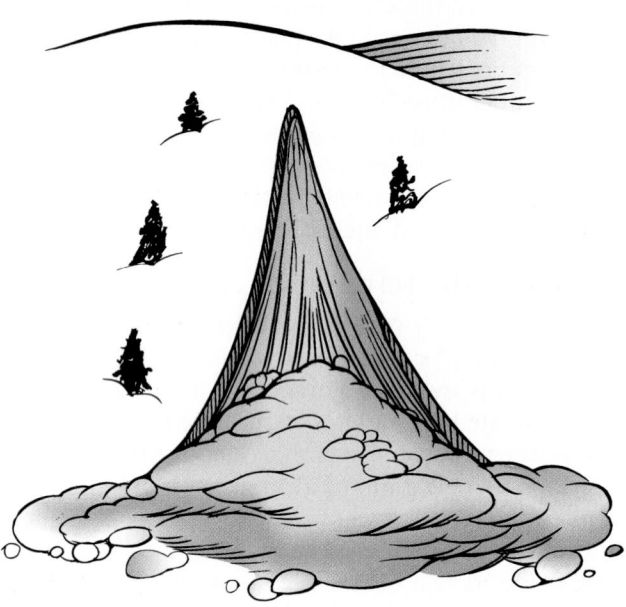

Figure 2-9 Loose snow or point-release avalanche. (*USDA Forest Service photo.*)

phic processes, distinct layers develop in numerous other ways, most of which have some influence on avalanche formation. The layered structure is directly tied to the two ingredients essential to the formation of slab avalanches: the cohesive layer of snow and the weak layer beneath. If the snow cover is homogeneous from the ground to the surface, there is no danger of slab avalanches, regardless of the snow type. If the entire snow layer is sintered, dense, and strong, stability is very high. Even if the entire snow cover is composed of a very weak layer of depth hoar, there is still no hazard from slab avalanches because the cohesionless character does not allow propagation of the cracks necessary for slab avalanches to form. However, the combination of a basal layer of depth hoar with a cohesive layer above, for example, provides exactly the ingredients for slab avalanche danger. For successful evaluation of slab avalanche potential, information is needed about the entire snowpack, not just the surface. A hard wind slab at the surface may seem strong and safe to the uninitiated, but when it rests on a weaker layer, which may be well below the surface, it may fail under the weight of a skier and be released as a slab avalanche.

Many snow structure combinations can contribute

to slab formation. One scenario involves thick layers of weak snow, which result from development of depth hoar early in the season. The typical combination of climatic factors that produce these layers is early winter snowfalls followed by several weeks of clear, cold weather. Even at higher elevations in the mountains, snow cover on the slopes with a southerly aspect may melt off during a period of fair weather. However, in October and early November, the sun angle is low enough that steep slopes with a northerly aspect receive little or no direct heating from the sun. Snow remains on the ground but not without change. Snow on north-facing slopes experiences optimal conditions for depth hoar formation; a thin, low-density snow cover (maximum opportunity for vapor flow) is sandwiched between the warm ground, still retaining much of its summer heat, and the cold air above. This snow layer recrystallizes over a period of weeks. When the first large storm of winter arrives in November, cohesive layers of wind-deposited snow accumulate on a very weak base, setting the scene for a widespread avalanche cycle. Figure 2-11 describes other combinations that result in brittle or cohesive layers of snow on a weak layer.

Mechanical Properties

How Snow Deforms on a Slope. Almost all physical properties of snow can be easily seen or measured. A snowpit provides a wealth of information regarding these properties, layer by layer, throughout the thickness of the snow cover. However, even detailed knowledge of these properties does not provide all the information necessary to evaluate avalanche potential. The current mechanical state of the snow cover must be considered. Unfortunately, for the average person these properties are virtually impossible to measure directly.

Mechanical deformation occurs within the snow cover just before its failure and the start of a slab avalanche. Snow cover has a tendency to settle simply from its own weight. When this occurs on level ground, the settlement is perpendicular to the ground and the snow layer densities and gains in strength. The situation is not so simple when snow rests on a slope. The force of gravity is divided into two components, one tending to cause the snow layer to shrink in thickness, and a new component acting parallel to the slope, which tends to pull the snow down the slope. Downslope movement within the snow cover occurs at all times, even on gentle slopes. The speed of movement is slow, generally on the order of a few millimeters per day up to millimeters per hour within new snow on steep slopes. The evidence of these forces is often clearly visible in the bending of trees and damage to structures built on snow-covered slopes. Although the movement is slow, when deep

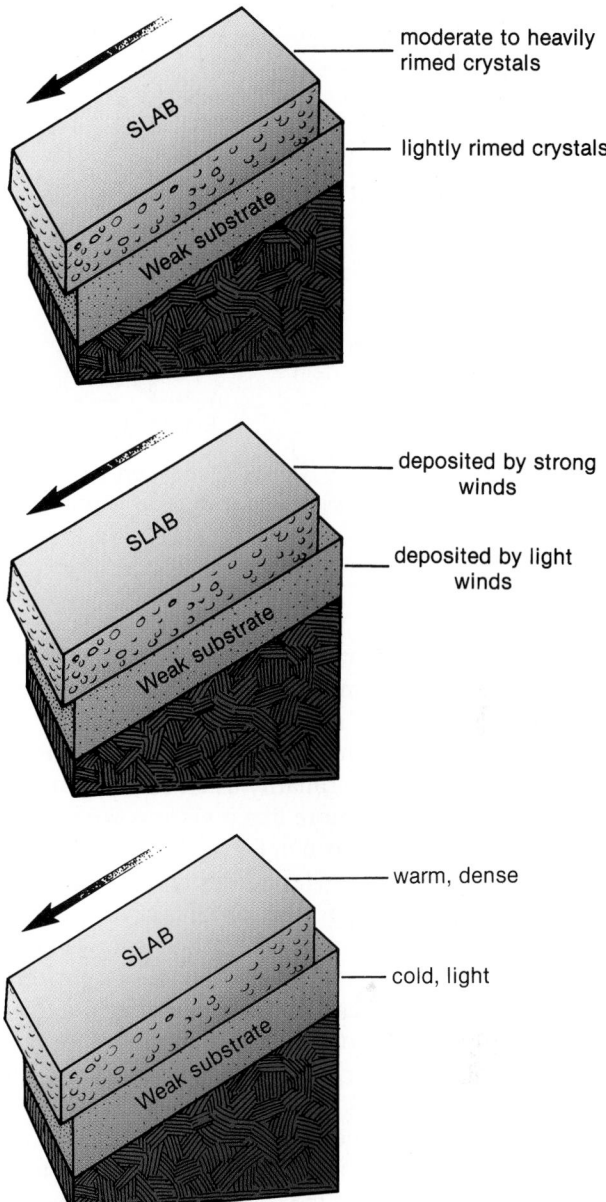

Figure 2-11 Snow layer combinations that often contribute to avalanche formation.

snow pushes against a rigid structure, the forces are significant and even large buildings can be pushed off their foundations.

Snow deforms in a highly variable fashion. It is generally described as a viscoelastic material. Sometimes it deforms as if it were a liquid (viscous) and at other times it responds more like a solid (elastic). Viscous deformation implies continuous and irreversible flow. Elastic deformation implies that once the force causing the deformation is removed, some small part of the initial deformation is recovered. The elasticity of snow is

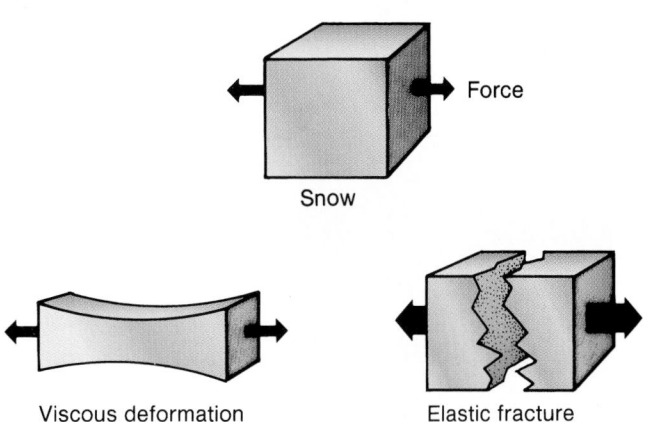

Figure 2-12 Depending on prevailing conditions, snow may deform and stretch in a viscous or flowing manner, or it may respond more like a solid and fracture.

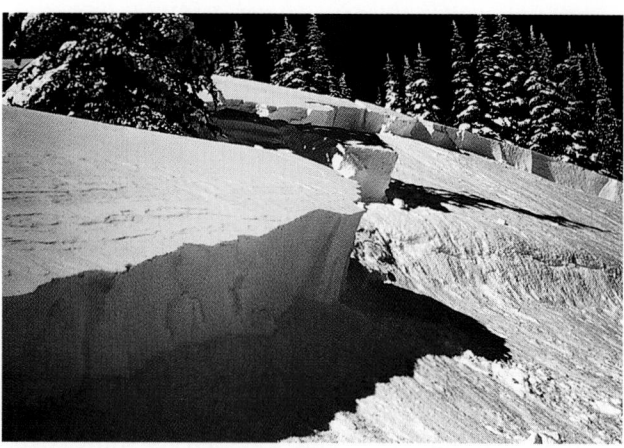

Figure 2-13 The consistent 90-degree angle between crown face and bed surface of the avalanche shows that slab avalanches result from an elastic fracture. *(Photo by A. Judson.)*

not so obvious, primarily because the amount of rebound is very small compared with that of more familiar materials.

In regard to avalanche formation, it is important to know when snow acts primarily as an elastic material and when it responds more like a viscous substance. These conditions are shown in Figure 2-12. Laboratory experiments have shown that conditions of warm temperatures and slow application of force favor viscous deformation. We see examples of this as snow slowly deforms and bends over the edge of a roof or sags from a tree branch. In such cases, the snow deforms but does not crack or break. In contrast, when temperatures are very cold or when force is applied rapidly, snow reacts like an elastic material. If enough force is applied, it fractures. We think of such a substance as brittle; the release of stored elastic energy causes fractures to move through the material. In the case of snow cover on a steep slope, forces associated with accumulating snow or the weight of a skier may increase until the snow fails. At that point, stored elastic energy is released and is available to drive brittle fractures over great distances through the snow slab.

The slab avalanche provides the best example of elastic deformation in snow cover. Although the deformation cannot actually be seen, evidence of the resultant brittle failure is clearly present in the form of the sharp, linear fracture line and crown face of the slab release (Figure 2-13). The crown face is almost always perpendicular to the bed surface, evidence that snow has failed in a brittle manner.

To fully understand the slab avalanche condition or the stability of the snow cover, its mechanical state must be considered. Snow is always deforming downslope, but throughout most of the winter the strength of the snow is sufficient to prevent an avalanche. The snow cover is layered, and some layers are weaker than others. During periods of snowfall, blowing snow, or both, an additional load, or weight, is being applied to the snow in the starting zone, the snow is creeping faster, and these new stresses are beginning to approach the strength of the weakest layers. The weakest layer has a weakest point somewhere within its continuous structure. If the stresses caused by the load of the new snow or the weight of a skier reach the level at which they equal the strength of the weakest point, the snow fails completely at that point (Figure 2-14). This means that the strength at that point immediately goes to zero. This is analogous to what would happen if someone on a tug-of-war team were to let go of the rope. If the remainder of the team were strong enough to make up for the lost member, not much would change immediately. The same situation exists with the snow cover. If the surrounding snow has sufficient strength to make up for the fact that the strength at the weakest point has now gone to zero, nothing happens beyond perhaps a local movement or settlement in the snow. If, however, the surrounding snow is not capable of doing this, the area of snow next to the initial weak point fails, and then the area next to it, and the chain reaction begins.

As the initial crack forms in the now unstable snow, the elastic energy is released, which in turn drives the crack further, releasing more elastic energy, and so forth. The ability of snow to store elastic energy is essentially what allows large slab avalanches to occur. As long as the snow properties are similar across the avalanche starting zone, the crack will continue to propagate, allowing entire basins, many acres in area, to be set in motion within a few seconds.

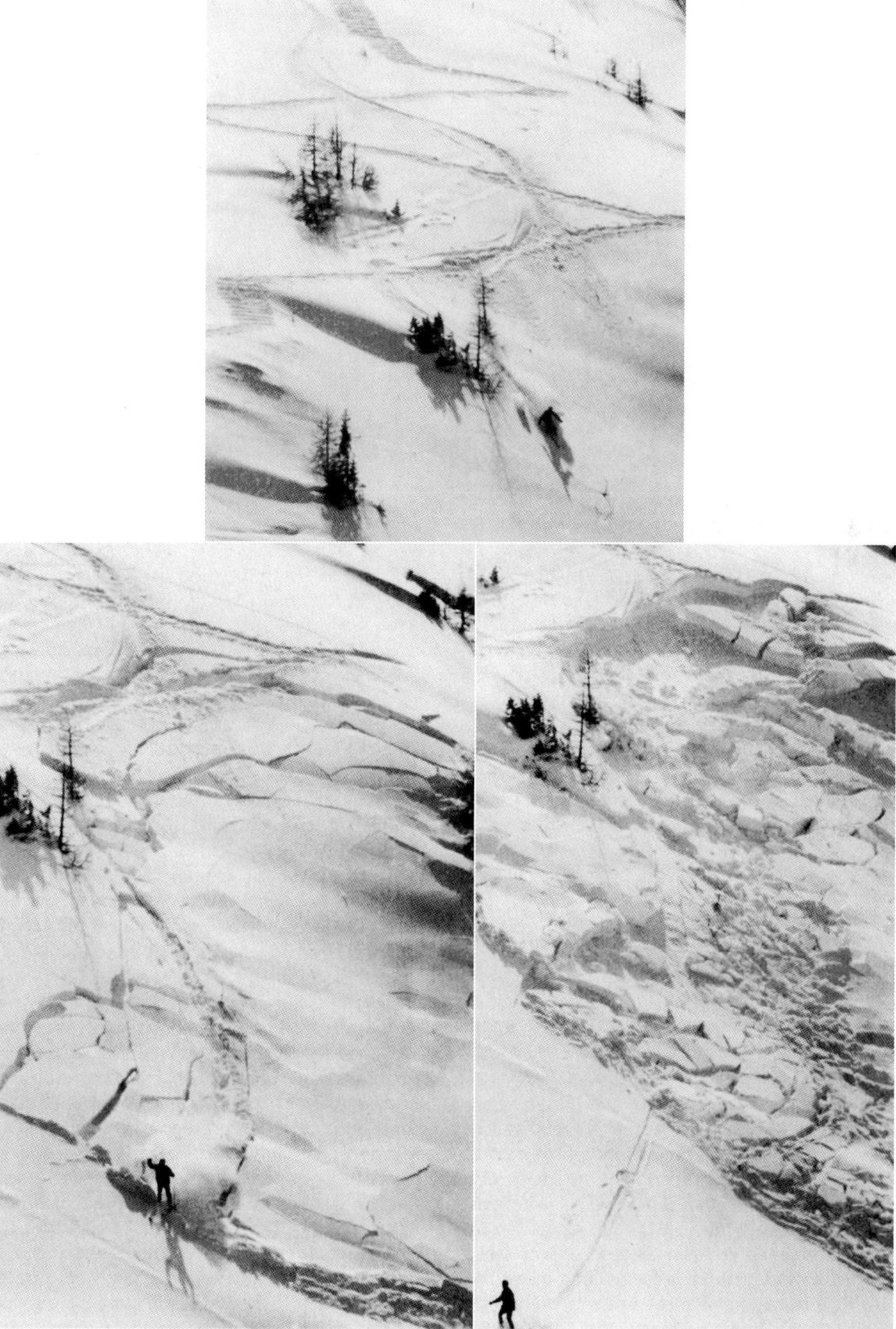

Figure 2-14 Slab avalanche released by a skier. *(Photo by R. Ludwig.)*

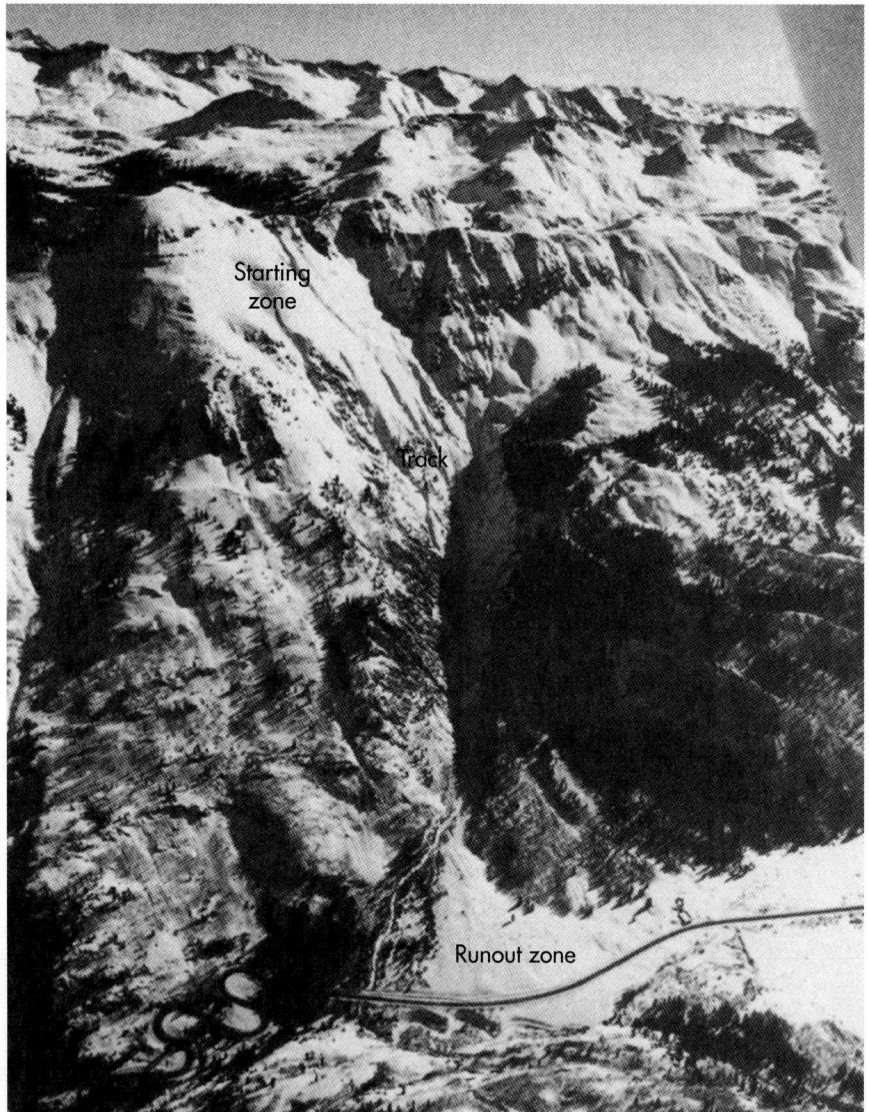

Figure 2-15 The three parts of an avalanche path: starting zone, track, and runout zone. *(Photo by B. Armstrong.)*

AVALANCHE DYNAMICS

The topic of avalanche dynamics includes how avalanches move, how fast they move, and how far and with how much destructive power they travel. The science of avalanche dynamics is not well advanced, although much has been learned in the past few decades. Measured data for avalanche velocity and impact pressure are still lacking. Although any environmental measurement presents its own set of problems, it is obvious that opportunities for making measurements inside a moving avalanche are extremely limited. Although avalanche paths exist in a variety of sizes and shapes, they all have three distinct parts with respect to dynamics (Figure 2-15). In the starting zone,

usually the steepest part of the path, the avalanche breaks away, accelerates down the slope, and picks up additional snow. From the starting zone the avalanche proceeds to the track, where it remains essentially constant and picks up little or no additional snow as it moves; the average slope angle has become less steep and frequently the snow cover is more stable than in the starting zone. (However, a study from Switzerland in 2000 showed that a significant amount of snow could be entrained into the avalanche from the track.) Small avalanches often stop in the track. After traveling down the track, the avalanche reaches the runout zone. Here the avalanche motion ends, either slowly as it decelerates across a gradual slope, such as an alluvial fan, or abruptly as it crashes into the bottom of a gorge or ravine. As a general rule, the slope angle of starting zones is 30 to 45 degrees, of the track is 20 to 30 degrees, and of the runout zone is less than 20 degrees.

Few actual measurements of avalanche velocities have been made, but enough data have been obtained to provide some typical values for the various avalanche types. For the highly turbulent dry-powder avalanches, the velocities are commonly in the range of 75 to 100 mph, with rare examples in the range of 150 to 200 mph. Such speeds are possible for powder avalanches because large amounts of air in the moving snow greatly reduce the forces resulting from internal friction. As snow in the starting zone becomes dense, wetter, or both, movement becomes less turbulent and a more flowing type of motion reduces typical velocities to the range of 50 to 75 mph. During spring conditions when the snow contains large amounts of liquid water, speeds may reach only about 25 mph (Figure 2-16).

In most cases, the avalanche simply follows a path down the steepest route on the slope while being guided or channeled by terrain features. However, the higher-speed avalanche may deviate from this path. Terrain features, such as the side walls of a gully, which would normally direct the flow of the avalanche around a bend, may be overridden by a high-velocity powder avalanche (Figure 2-17). The slower-moving avalanches, which travel near the ground, tend to follow terrain features, giving them somewhat predictable courses.

Because avalanches can travel at very high speeds, the resultant impact pressures can be significant. Smaller and medium-sized events (impact pressures of 1 to 15 kilopascals [kPa]) have the potential to heavily damage wood frame structures. Extremely large avalanches (impact pressures of more than 150 kPa) possess the force to uproot mature forests and even destroy structures built of concrete.

Some reports of avalanche damage describe circumstances that cannot be easily explained simply by the impact of large amounts of fast-moving dense snow. Some observers have noted that as an avalanche passed, some buildings actually exploded, perhaps from some form of vacuum created by the fast-moving snow. Other reports indicate that a structure was destroyed by the "air blast" preceding the avalanche because there was no evidence of large amounts of avalanche debris in the area. However, this is more likely to be damage resulting from the powder cloud, which may only comprise a few inches of settled snow yet contributes significantly to the total impact force. The presence of snow crystals can increase the air density by a factor of three or more. A powder cloud traveling at a moderate dry avalanche speed of 60 mph could have the impact force of a 180-mph wind, well beyond the destructive capacity of a hurricane.

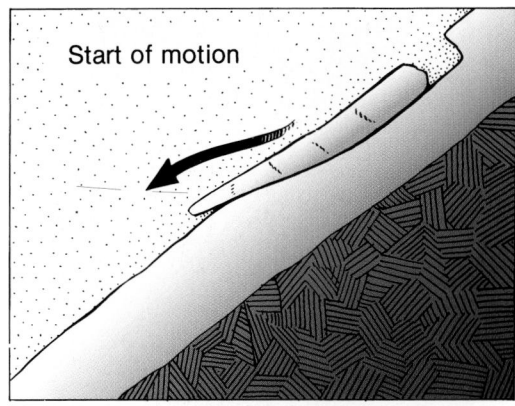

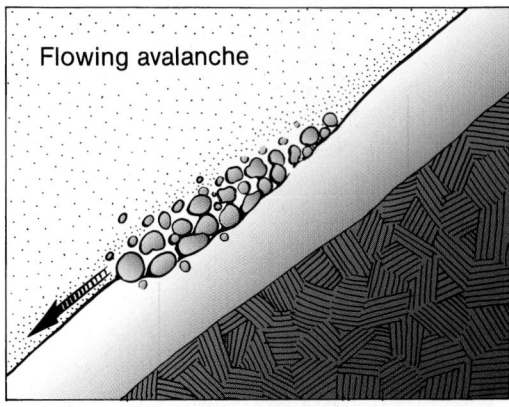

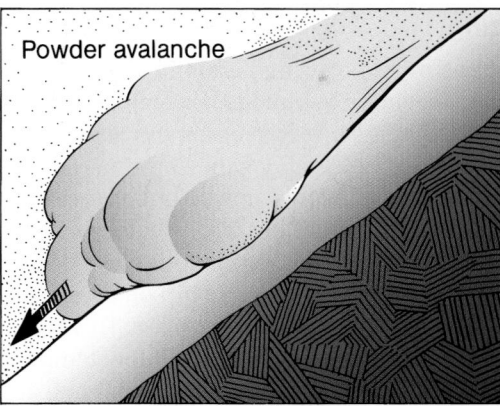

Figure 2-16 A dry-snow avalanche may have a slowing motion and travel near the surface or, with lower density snow and higher velocities, the turbulent dust cloud of the powder avalanche develops.

IDENTIFYING AVALANCHE PATH CHARACTERISTICS

Characteristics such as elevation, slope profiles, and weather determine whether a mountain can produce avalanches. The ingredients of an avalanche, snow and a steep enough slope, are such that any mountain can produce an avalanche if conditions are exactly right. To

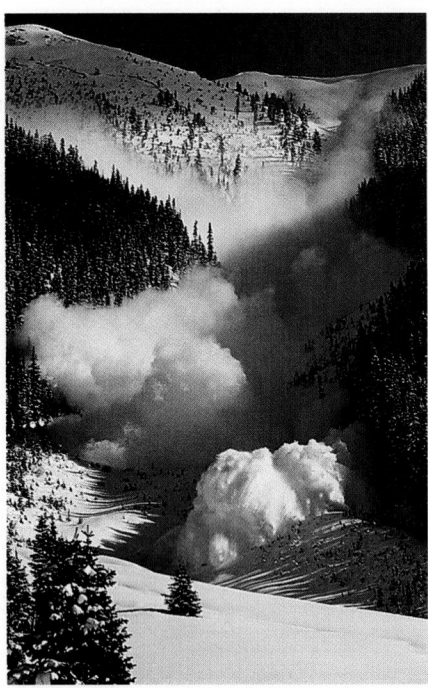

Figure 2-17 The large powder cloud associated with a fast-moving dry-snow avalanche. *(Photo by R. Armstrong.)*

be a consistent producer of avalanches, a mountain and its weather must work in harmony.

Elevation

Mountains must be at high enough latitudes or high enough in elevation to build and sustain a winter snow cover before their slopes can become avalanche threats. Temperature drops steadily with elevation. This has the obvious effect of allowing snow to build up deeper and remain longer at higher elevations before melting depletes the snow cover. A less obvious effect of the temperature and elevation relationship on avalanche formation is the demarcation called *treeline*. This is the level above which the combined effects of low temperature, strong winds, and heavy snowfall prevent tree growth.

The treeline can be quite variable in any mountain range, depending on the microclimates. On a single mountain, treeline is generally higher on south slopes than on north slopes (in the northern hemisphere) because more sunshine leads to warmer average temperatures on southern exposures. Latitudinal variation in the elevation of treeline ranges from sea level in northern Alaska to almost 3658 m (12,000 feet) in the Sierras of southern California and the Rockies of New Mexico.

Mountains that rise above treeline are more likely to produce avalanches. Dense timber anchors the snowpack so avalanches can seldom start. Below treeline, avalanches can start on slopes having no trees or only scattered trees, a circumstance arising either from natural causes, such as a streambed or rockslide area, or

from human-made causes, such as clearcuts. Above treeline, avalanches are free to start, and once set in motion, they can easily cut a swath through the trees below. The classic avalanche path is one having a steep bowl above treeline to catch the snow and a track extending below treeline. Avalanches run repeatedly down the track and ravage whatever vegetation grows there, leaving a scar of small or stunted trees that cuts through larger trees on either side.

Slope Angle

In snow that is thoroughly saturated with water, so that a slush mixture is formed, the slope needs only to have a slight tilt to produce an avalanche. For example, a wet-snow avalanche in Japan occurred on a beginner slope at a ski area. The slope was only 10 degrees, but the avalanche was big enough to kill seven skiers. This extreme applies only to a water-saturated snowpack, which behaves more like a liquid than a solid.

A more realistic slope is 22 degrees, the "angle of repose" for granular substances, such as sand and dry, unbonded snow. Round grains will not stack up in a pile having sides much steeper than 22 degrees before gravity rearranges the pile. Dry-snow avalanches have occurred on slopes of 22 to 25 degrees; these are rare because snow grains are seldom round and seldom touch without forming bonds. A useful minimum steepness for producing avalanches is 30 degrees. Avalanches occur with the greatest frequency on slopes of 30 to 45 degrees. These are the angles in which the balance between strength (the bonding of the snow trying to hold it in place) and stress (the force of gravity trying to pull it loose) is most critical. On even steeper slopes, the force of gravity wins; snow continually rolls or sloughs off, preventing buildup of deep snowpacks. Exceptions exist, such as damp snow plastered to a steep slope by strong winds.

Orientation

Avalanches occur on slopes facing every point of the compass. Steep slopes are equally likely to face east or west, north or south. There are factors, however, that cause more avalanches to fall on slopes facing north, northeast, and east than those facing south through west. These relate to slope orientation with respect to sun and wind. The sun angle in northern hemisphere winters causes south slopes to get much more sunshine and heating than do north slopes, which frequently leads to radically different snow covers. North slopes have deeper and colder snow covers, often with a substantial layer of depth hoar near the ground. South slopes usually carry a shallower and warmer snow cover, laced with multiple ice layers formed on warm days between storms. Most ski areas are built on predominantly north-facing slopes to take advantage of deeper and longer-lasting snow cover. At high latitudes, such as in Alaska, the winter sun is so low on the horizon and heat input to south slopes is so small that there are few differences in the snow covers of north and south slopes.

The effect of the prevailing west wind at midlatitudes is important. Storms most often move west to east, and storm winds are most frequently from the western quadrant: southwest, west, or northwest. The effect is to pick up fallen snow and redeposit it on slopes facing away from the wind, that is, onto northeast, east, and southeast slopes. These are the slopes most often overburdened with wind-drifted snow. The net effect of sun and wind is to cause more avalanches on north- through east-facing slopes.

Avalanche Terrain

The frequency with which a path produces avalanches depends on a number of factors, with slope steepness a major factor. The easiest way to create high stress is to increase the slope angle; gravity works that much harder to stretch the snow out and rip it from its underpinnings. A slope of 45 degrees produces many more avalanches than one of 30 degrees. However, specific terrain features are also important.

Broad slopes that are curved into a bowl shape and narrow slopes that are confined to a gully efficiently collect snow. Those having a curved horizontal profile, such as a bowl or gully, trap blowing snow coming from several directions; the snow drifts over the top and settles as a deep pillow. On the other hand, the plane-surfaced slope collects snow efficiently only if it is being blown directly from behind. A side wind scours the slope more than it loads it.

The surface conditions of a starting zone often dictate the size and type of avalanche. A particularly rough ground surface, such as a boulder field, will not usually produce avalanches early in the winter, since it takes considerable snowfall to cover the ground anchors. Once most of the rocks are covered, avalanches will pull out in sections, the area between two exposed rocks running one time, and the area between two other rocks running another. A smooth rock face or grassy slope provides a surface that is too slick for snow to grip. Therefore full-depth avalanches are distinctly possible; if the avalanche does not run during the winter, it is likely to run to ground in the spring, once melt water percolates through the snow and lubricates the ground surface.

Vegetation has a mixed effect on avalanche releases. Bushes provide anchoring support until they become totally covered; at that point they may provide weak points in the snow cover, since air circulates well around the bush, providing an ideal habitat for the growth of depth hoar. It is common to see that the fracture line of an avalanche has run from a rock to a tree to a bush, all places of healthy depth hoar growth.

A dense stand of trees can easily provide enough anchors to prevent avalanches. Reforestation of slopes de-void of trees because of logging, fire, or avalanche is an effective means of avalanche control. Scattered trees on a gladed slope offer little if any support to hold snow in place. Isolated trees may do more harm than good by providing concentrated weak points on the slope.

FACTORS CONTRIBUTING TO AVALANCHE FORMATION

The factors that contribute to avalanche release are terrain, weather, and snowpack. Terrain factors are fixed; however, the state of the weather and snowpack changes daily, even hourly. Precipitation, wind, temperature, snow depth, snow surface, weak layers, and settlement are all factors determining whether an avalanche will occur.

Snowfall

New snowfall is the event that leads to most avalanches; more than 80% of all avalanches fall during or just after a storm. Fresh snowfall adds weight to existing snow cover. If the snow cover is not strong enough to absorb this extra weight, avalanche releases occur. The size of the avalanche is usually related to the amount of new snow. Snowfalls of less than 6 inches seldom produce avalanches. Snows of 6 to 12 inches usually produce a few small slides, and some of these harm skiers who release them. Snows of 1 to 2 feet produce avalanches of larger size that present a considerable threat to skiers and pose closure problems for highways and railways. Snows of 2 to 4 feet are much more dangerous, and snowfalls greater than 4 feet produce major avalanches capable of large-scale destruction. These figures are guidelines based on data and experience and must be considered with other factors to arrive at the true hazard. For example, a snowfall of 10 inches whipped by strong winds may be serious; a fall of 2 feet of feather-light snow in the absence of wind may produce no avalanches.

Snowfall Intensity

The rate at which snowfall accumulates is almost as important as the amount of snow. A snowfall of 3 feet in one day is far more hazardous than 3 feet in 3 days. As a viscoelastic material, snow can absorb slow loading by deforming or compressing. Under a rapid load, the snow cannot deform quickly enough and is more likely to crack, which is how slab avalanches begin. A snowfall rate of 1 inch per hour or greater sustained for 10 hours or more is generally a red flag indicating danger. The danger worsens if snowfall is accompanied by wind.

Rain

Light rain falling on a cold snowpack invariably freezes into an ice crust, which adds strength to the snow cover. At a later time, the smooth crust could become a sliding layer beneath the new fall of snow. Heavy rain (usually an inch or more) greatly weakens the snow cover. First, it adds weight. An inch of rain is the equivalent in weight to 10 to 12 inches of snow. Second, it adds no internal strength of its own (in the form of a skeleton of ice, as new snow would), while it dissolves bonds between snow grains as it percolates through the top snow layers, reducing strength even further.

New Snow Density and Crystal Type

A layer of fresh snow contains only a small amount of solid material (ice); the large majority of the volume is occupied by air. It is convenient to refer to snow density as a percentage of the volume occupied by ice. New snow densities usually range from 7% to 12%. In the high elevations of Colorado, 7% is an average value; in the more maritime climates of the Sierras and Cascades, 12% is a typical value. Density becomes an important factor in avalanche formation when it varies from average values.

Wet snowfalls or falls of heavily rimed crystals, such as graupel, may have densities of 20% or greater. A layer of heavier-than-normal snow presents a danger because of excess weight. Snowfall that is much lighter than normal, 2% to 4% for example, can also present a dangerous situation. If the low-density layer quickly becomes buried by snowfall of normal or high density, a weak layer has been introduced into the snowpack. By virtue of low density, the weak layer has marginal ability to withstand the weight of layers above, making it susceptible to collapse. Storms that begin with low temperatures but then warm up produce a layer of weak snow beneath a stronger, heavier layer.

Density is closely linked to crystal type. Snowfalls consisting of graupel, fine needles, and columns can accumulate at high densities. Snowfalls of plates, stellars, and dendritic forms account for most of the lower densities.

Wind Speed and Direction

Wind drives fallen snow into drifts and cornices from which avalanches begin. Winds pick up snow from exposed, windward slopes and drive it onto adjacent, leeward slopes, where it is deposited into sheltered hollows and gullies.

A speed of 15 mph is sufficient to pick up freshly fallen snow. Higher speeds are required to dislodge older snow. Speeds of 20 to 50 mph are the most efficient in transporting snow into avalanche starting zones. Speeds greater than 50 mph can create spectacular banners of snow streaming from high peaks, but much of this snow is lost to evaporation in the air or is deposited far down the slope away from the avalanche starting zone.

Winds play a dual role in increasing avalanche potential. First, wind scours snow from a large area (of a windward slope) and deposits it in a smaller area (of a starting zone). Wind can thus turn a 1-foot snowfall into a 3-foot drift in a starting zone. The rate at which blowing snow collects in bowls and gullies can be impressive. In one test at Berthoud Pass, Colorado, the wind deposited snow in a gully at a rate of 18 inches per hour. Another wind effect is that blowing snow is denser after deposit than before. This is because snow grains are subjected to harsh treatment in their travels; each collision with another grain knocks off arms and sharp angles, reducing size and allowing the pieces to settle into a denser layer. The net result of wind is to fill avalanche starting zones with more and heavier snow than if the wind had not blown.

Temperature

The role of temperature in snow metamorphism is played over a period of days, weeks, and even months. The influence of temperature on the mechanical state of the snow cover is more acute, with changes occurring in minutes to hours. The actual effect of temperature is not always easy to interpret; whereas an increase in temperature may contribute to stabilization of the snow cover in one situation, it might at another time lead to avalanche activity.

In several situations an increase in temperature clearly produces an increase in avalanche potential. In general, these include a rise in temperature during a storm or immediately after a storm, or a prolonged period of warm, fair weather such as occurs with spring conditions. In the first example, the temperature at the beginning of snowfall may be well below freezing, but as the storm progresses, the temperature increases. As a result, the initial layers of new snow are light, fluffy, low density, and relatively low in strength, whereas the later layers are warmer, denser, and stiffer. Thus the essential ingredients for a slab avalanche are provided within the new snow layers of the storm: a cohesive slab resting on a weak layer. If the temperature continues to rise, the falling snow turns to rain, a situation not uncommon in lower-elevation coastal mountain ranges. Once this happens, avalanches are almost certain because as the rain falls, additional weight is added to the avalanche slope, but no additional strength is provided as it is whenever a layer of snow accumulates.

The second example may occur after an overnight snowstorm that does not produce an avalanche on the slope of interest. By morning, the precipitation stops and clear skies allow the morning sun to shine directly on the slopes. The sun rapidly warms the cold, low-density new snow, which begins to deform and creep downslope. The new snow layer settles, becomes more dense, and gains strength. At the same time, it is stretched downhill and some of the bonds between the grains are pulled apart; thus the snow layer becomes weaker. If more bonds are broken by stretching than are formed by settlement, there is not enough strength to hold the snow on the slope and an avalanche occurs.

In these first two examples, the complete snow cover generally remains at temperatures below freezing. A third example occurs when a substantial amount of the winter's snow cover is warmed to the melting point. During winter, sun angles are low, days are short, and air temperatures are cold enough that the small amount of heat gained by the snow cover during the day is lost during the long cold night. As spring approaches, this pattern changes, and eventually enough heat is available at the snow surface during the day to cause some melt. This melt layer refreezes again that night, but the next day more heat may be available, so that eventually a substantial amount of melting occurs and melt water begins to move down through the snow cover. As melt water percolates slowly downward, it melts the bonds that attach the snow grains and the strength of the layers decreases. At first the near-surface layers are affected, with the midday melt reaching only as far as the uppermost few inches, with little or no increase in avalanche hazard. If warm weather continues, the melt layer becomes thicker and the potential for wet snow avalanches increases. The conditions most favorable for wet slab avalanches occur when the snow structure provides the necessary layering. When melt water encounters an ice layer or impermeable crust, or in some cases a layer of weak depth hoar, wet slab avalanches are likely to occur.

Depth of Snow Cover

Of the snowpack factors contributing to avalanche formation, this is the most basic. When the early-winter snowpack covers natural anchors, such as rocks and bushes, the start of the avalanche season is at hand. North-facing slopes are usually covered before other slopes. A scan of the terrain usually suffices to weigh this clue, but another method can be used to determine the time of the first significant avalanches. Long-term studies show a relationship between snow depth at a study site and avalanche activity. For example, along Red Mountain Pass, Colorado, it is unlikely that an avalanche large enough to reach the highway will run until close to 3 feet of snow covers the ground at the University of Colorado's snow study site. At Alta, Utah, once 52 inches of snowpack have built up, the first avalanche to cover the road leading from Salt Lake City can be expected.

Nature of the Snow Surface

How well new snow bonds to the old snow surface is a key factor in determining whether an avalanche will release within the layer of new snow or deeper in the snowpack. A poor bond, usually new snow resting on a smooth, cold surface with snowfalls of 1 foot or more, almost always produces a new-snow avalanche. A strong bond, usually onto a warm, soft, or rough surface, may produce nothing at all, or if weaknesses lie at deeper layers of the snow cover, a large snowfall will cause avalanches to pull out older layers of snow in addition to the new snow layer. These avalanches have more potential for destruction. A cold, hard snow surface offers little grip to fresh, cold snow. Ice crusts are commonly observed to be avalanche-sliding surfaces. The crust could be a sun crust, rain crust, or a hardened layer of firm snow that has survived the summer. Firm layers are especially dangerous in early winter when first snows fall.

Weak Layers

Any layer susceptible to collapse or failure because of the weight of the overburden is a weak link. Of the snowpack contributory factors, this is the most important, since a weak layer is essential to every avalanche. The weak layer releases along what is called the failure plane, sliding surface, or bed surface.

One common weak layer is an old snow surface that offers a poor bond for new snow. Another weak layer that forms on the snow surface is hoar frost, or surface hoar. This is the solid equivalent of dew. On clear, calm nights, it forms a layer of feathery, sparkling flakes that grow on the snow surface. The layer can be a major contributor to avalanche formation when buried by a snowfall. Many avalanches have been known to release on a buried layer of surface hoar, sometimes a layer more than 1 month old and 6 feet or more below the surface.

A weak layer that is almost always found in the snowpacks that blanket the Rocky Mountains and occasionally the Cascades and Sierra Nevadas is temperature-gradient snow, or depth hoar. The way to decide whether a temperature-gradient layer is near its collapse point is to test the strength of the overlying layers and the support provided around the edges of the slope. This is no easy task. One method is to try jumping on your skis while standing on a shallow slope. Collapse is a good indication that similar snow cover on a steeper slope will produce an avalanche. Often skiers and climbers cause inadvertent collapses while skiing or walking on a depth hoar–riddled snowpack. The resulting "whoomf" sound is a warning of weak snow below.

Finally, a weak layer can be created within the snow cover when surface melting or rain causes water to percolate into the snow and then fan out on an impermeable layer, thereby lubricating that layer and destroying its shear strength. Combining the contributory factors on a day-by-day basis is the avalanche forecaster's art. Every avalanche must have a weak layer to release on, so knowledge of snow stratigraphy, or layering, and what sort of applied load will cause a layer to fail is the essence of forecasting.

SAFE TRAVEL IN AVALANCHE TERRAIN

The first major decision often faced in backcountry situations is whether to avoid or confront a potential avalanche hazard. A group touring with no particular goal in mind will probably not challenge avalanches. For this group, being able to recognize and avoid avalanche terrain is sufficient education. In the other extreme, mountaineering expeditions that have specific goals and are willing to wait out dangerous periods or take severe risks to succeed need considerably more information.

The ability to travel safely in avalanche terrain requires special preparations, including education and possession of safety and rescue equipment. The group should have the skills required to anticipate and react to an avalanche.

Identifying Avalanche Terrain

Because most avalanches release on slopes of 30 to 45 degrees of pitch, judging angle is a prime skill in recognizing potential avalanche areas. An inclinometer is an instrument used to measure slope angles. Some compasses are also equipped for this purpose; a second needle and a graduated scale in degrees can be used to measure slope angles. A ski pole may be used to judge approximate slope angle. When dangled by its strap, the pole becomes a plumb line from which the slope angle can be "eyeballed."

Evidence of fresh avalanche activity identifies avalanche slopes: the presence of fracture lines and the rubble of avalanche snow on the slope or at the bottom. Other clues are swaths of missing trees or trees that are bent downhill or damaged, especially with the uphill branches removed. Above treeline, steep bowls and gullies are almost always capable of producing avalanches.

Route Finding

Good route-finding techniques are necessary for safe travel in avalanche terrain (Figure 2-18). The object of a good route in avalanche country is more than avoiding avalanches. It should also be efficient and take into account the abilities and desires of the group when choosing a route that is not overly technical, tiresome, or time consuming. The safest way to avoid avalanches is to travel above or below and well away from them. When taking the high route, the traveler should choose a ridgeline that is above the avalanche starting zones. It is safest to travel the windward side of the ridge. The snow cover is usually thinner and windpacked, with rocks sticking through: not the most pleasant skiing, but safe. Cornice collapses present a very real hazard; they should be avoided by staying on the roughened snow more to windward.

Skiers taking the low route in the valley should not linger in the runouts of avalanche paths. Even though it is unlikely that a skier traveling along the valley could trigger an avalanche high up on the slope, the skier should not boost the odds of getting caught in an avalanche released by natural forces far above. Slopes of 30 degrees or more should be avoided. By climbing, descending, and traversing only in gentle terrain, avalanche terrain can be avoided.

Stability Evaluation Tests

Skiers can perform several tests of stability. On a small slope that is not too steep (and therefore will not avalanche), the skier can try a ski test by skiing along a shallow traverse and then setting the ski edges in a hard check. Any cracks or settlement noises indicate that the same slope, if steeper, would have probably avalanched, and on the steeper slope it would have taken less weight or jolt to cause the avalanche.

Another test is to push a ski pole into the snow, handle end first. This helps to feel the major layering of the snowpack. For example, the skier may feel the layer of new snow, midpack stronger layers, and depth hoar layers, if the pole is long enough. Hard-snow layers and ice lenses resist penetration altogether. This test reveals only the gross layers; thin weak layers, such as buried surface hoar or a poor bond between any two layers, cannot be detected. Thus the ski pole test has limited value.

A much better way to directly observe and test snowpack layers is to dig a hasty snowpit. (This is an excellent use of the shovel that, in the next section, we recommend the skier carry.) In a spot as near as possible to a suspected avalanche slope without putting the traveler at risk, a pit 4 to 5 feet deep and 3 feet wide should be dug. With the shovel, the uphill wall is shaved until it is smooth and vertical. Now the layers of snow can be observed and felt. The tester can see where the new snow touches the layer beneath, poke the pit wall with a finger to test hardness, and brush the pit wall with a paintbrush to see which layers are soft and fall away and which are hard and stay in place after being brushed. By grabbing a handful of depth hoar, the skier can see how large the grains are and how poorly they stick together.

The shovel shear test gauges the shear strength between layers and thus locates weak layers. First a column of snow is isolated from the vertical pit wall. Both sides and the back of the column are cut with the shovel or a ski, so that the column is free standing. The dimensions are a shovel's width on all sides. The tester inserts the shovel blade at the back of the column and gently pulls forward on the handle. An unstable slab will shear loose on the weak layer, making a clean break; the poorer the bond, the easier the shear. A five-point scale is used to rate the shear: "very easy" if it

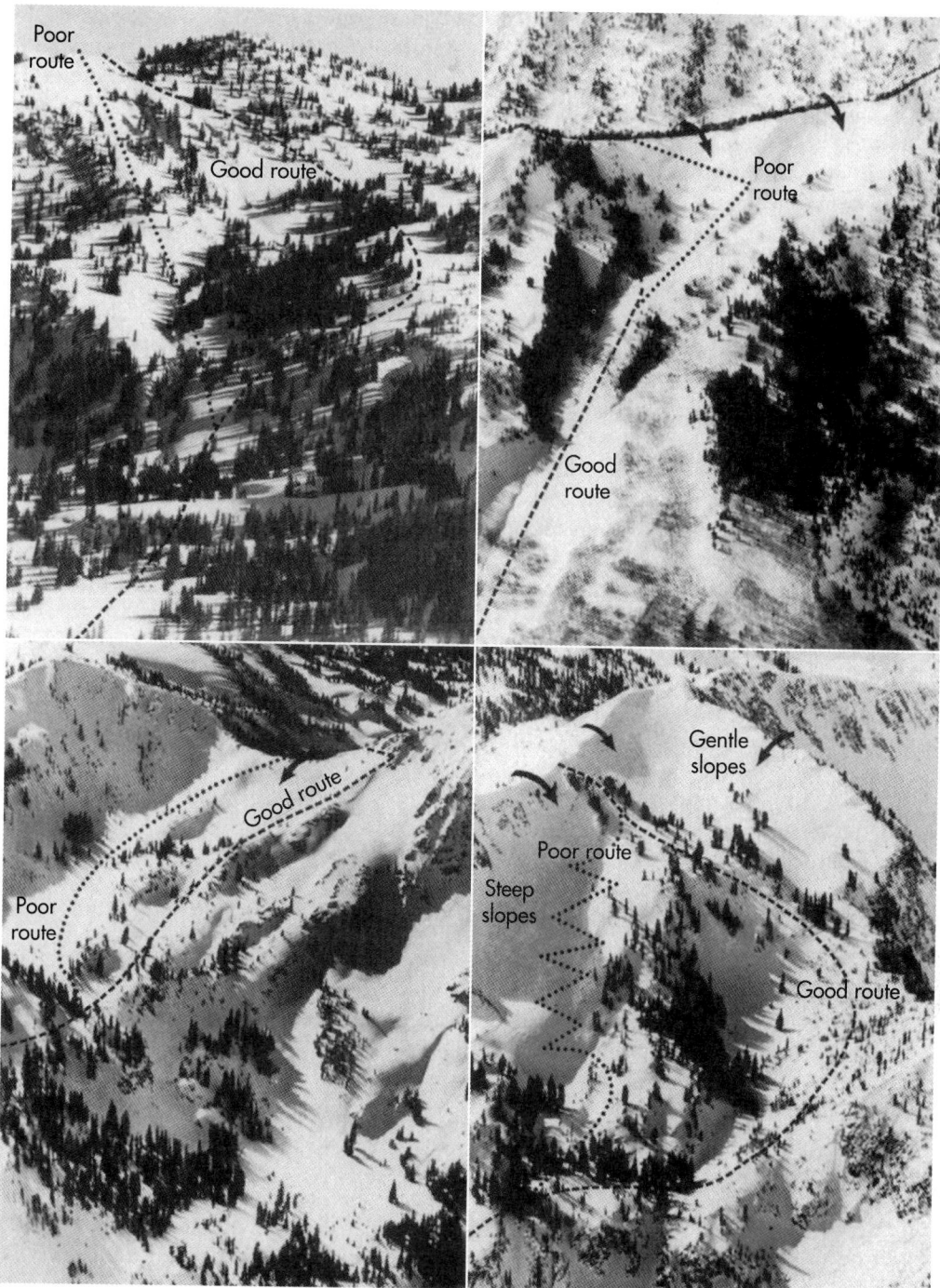

Figure 2-18 Four ski-touring areas showing the safer routes *(dashed lines)* and the more hazardous routes *(dotted lines)*. Arrows indicate areas of wind loading. *(From USDA Forest Service:* Avalanche handbook, *Agricultural Handbook 489, USDA. Photo by Alexis Kelner.)*

breaks as the column is being cut or the shovel is being inserted; "easy" if a gentle pull on the shovel does the job; "moderate" if a slightly stronger shovel-pry is required; "hard" if a solid tug is required; "very hard" if a major effort is needed to break the snow. Generally, "very easy" and "easy" shears indicate unconditionally unstable snow, "moderate" means conditionally unstable, and "hard" and "very hard" mean stable.

The value of the shovel shear test is that it can find thin weak layers undetectable by any other method. Its shortcoming is that it is not a true test of stability, since it does not indicate the amount of weight required to cause shear failure.

A test that does a better job of indicating actual stability is the Rutschblock, or shear block, test. This test is calibrated to the skier's weight and the stress he or she would put on the snow. Again, a snowpit is dug with a vertical uphill wall, but the pit must be about 8 feet wide. By cutting into the pit wall, the skier isolates a block of snow that is about 7 feet wide (a ski length) and goes back 4 feet (a ski pole length) into the pit wall. Both sides and the back are cut with a shovel or ski so that the block is free standing. Wearing skis, the skier climbs around and well uphill from the isolated block and carefully approaches it from above. With skis across the fall line, the skier gently steps onto the block, first with the downhill ski and then the uphill ski, so that he or she is standing on the isolated block of snow. If the slab of snow has not yet failed, gently flexing the knees applies a little more pressure. Next some gentle jumps are tried. The stress should be by jumping harder until the block eventually shears loose or crumbles apart.

The interpretation of the results is: "extremely unstable" if the block fails while the skier is cutting it, approaching it from above, or merely standing on it; "unstable" if it fails with a knee flex or one gentle jump; "moderately stable" if it fails after repeated jumps; and "very stable" if it never fails but merely crumbles. These are objective results that help answer the bigger question—will it slide?—and help the mountain traveler decide how much risk to take.

Avalanche Rescue Equipment

Shovel. The first piece of safety equipment the skier or climber should own is a shovel. It can be used to dig snowpits for stability evaluation and snow caves for overnight shelter. A shovel is also needed for digging in avalanche debris, since such snow is far too hard for digging with the hands or skis.

The shovel should be sturdy and strong enough to dig in avalanche debris, yet light and small enough to fit into a pack. There is no excuse for not carrying a shovel. Shovels are made of aluminum or high-strength plastic and can be collapsible. Many good types are available in mountaineering stores.

Probe. Several pieces of equipment are designed specifically for finding buried avalanche victims. The first is a collapsible probe pole. Organized rescue teams keep rigid poles in 10- or 12-foot lengths as part of their rescue caches. The recreationist can buy probe poles of tubular steel that come in 2-foot sections that fit together to make a full-length probe. Ski poles with removable grips and baskets can be screwed together to make an avalanche probe. Survivors of an accident use probes to search for buried victims.

Avalanche Cord. An avalanche cord is orange or red rope, approximately 50 feet long, that can be coiled and attached to a belt. When traveling in avalanche terrain, a skier or climber strings the cord out behind. The idea is that if an avalanche releases and the victim is buried, the cord will float and some portion of it will come to rest on the surface. Rescuers follow the cord, or probe in the immediate area, to locate the victim.

Avalanche cords have saved many lives in the past, but now they are obsolete and have virtually disappeared from use. They have been replaced as personal rescue devices by avalanche beacons, which are far more reliable. Avalanche cords always had severe limitations: tests done in the early 1970s by the International Vanni Eigenmann Foundation of Milan, Italy, showed that avalanche cords were only marginally effective. In tests performed by attaching an avalanche cord to a sandbag dummy tossed onto an avalanche path, a portion of the avalanche cord was visible on the surface only 40% of the time.

Avalanche Rescue Beacon. Avalanche rescue beacons, or transceivers, have become the most-used personal rescue devices worldwide. When used properly, they are a fast and effective way to locate buried avalanche victims. In the United States, these have become standard issue for ski area patrollers involved in avalanche work and for helicopter-skiing guides and clients. They are also commonly used by highway departments, search and rescue teams, and an increasing number of winter recreationists. Since beacons were introduced in the United States, they have saved at least 30 lives. Beacons save at least two or three lives per winter.

Transceivers act as transmitters that emit a signal on a frequency of 457 kHz. (This is now the world-standard frequency. The old frequency of 2.275 kHz is no longer used, and all beacons using this frequency have been—or should be—retired.) A buried victim's unit emits this signal, while the rescuers' units receive the signal. The signal carries 30 to 46 m (100 to 150 feet) and, once picked up, guides searchers specifically to the buried unit.

Beacon technology is evolving rapidly and improving the beacons on the market. Two types of beacon have emerged: analog, which processes the signal in the traditional way to allow for a stronger (louder) signal as the receiving beacon approaches the sending beacon; and digital, which uses a computer chip to process the signal to display a digital read-out of the range to the buried unit.

Both types operate on the same frequency and therefore are compatible with one another. However, different search techniques may be necessary to use each type most efficiently. Therefore special training and practice are required before the user attains proficiency. The main brands available in the United States are Ortovox, Pieps, Tracker, and SOS.

Merely possessing a beacon does not ensure its life-saving capability. Frequent practice is required to master a beacon-guided search, which may not be straight-forward. Skilled practitioners can find a buried unit in less than 5 minutes once they pick up the signal. Since speed is of the essence in avalanche rescue, beacons are obvious lifesavers. The best proven rescue equipment is a beacon for a quick find and a shovel for a quick recovery (Box 2-1).

Box 2-1 AVALANCHE TRANSCEIVER SEARCH

INITIAL SEARCH

1. Have everyone switch their transceivers to "receive" and turn the volume on "high."
2. If enough people are available, post a lookout to warn others of further slides.
3. Should a second slide occur, have rescuers immediately switch their transceivers to "transmit."
4. Have rescuers space themselves no more than 30 m (100 feet) apart and walk along the slope parallel to one another.
5. For a single rescuer searching within a wide path, zigzag across the rescue zone. Limit the distance between crossings to 30 m.
6. For multiple victims, when a signal is picked up, have one or two rescuers continue to locate the victim while the remainder of the group carries out the search for additional victims.
7. For a single victim, when a signal is picked up, have one or two rescuers continue to locate the victim while the remainder of the group prepares shovels, probes, and medical supplies for the rescue.

LOCATING THE VICTIM

With practice, the induction line search is more efficient than the conventional grid search. An induction line search requires a 457 kHz transceiver.

Induction line search (preferred method)

When an induction line search is used, the rescuer may initially follow a line that leads away from victim (Figure 2-19). Remember to lower transceiver volume if it is too loud because the ear detects signal strength variations better at lower volume settings.

1. After picking up a signal during the initial search, hold the transceiver horizontally (parallel with the ground) with the front of the transceiver pointing forward (see Figure 2-19, A).
2. Holding the transceiver in this position, turn until the signal is maximal (maximum volume), then walk five steps (about 5 m [16 feet]), stop, and turn again to locate the maximum signal (see Figure 2-19, B). When locating the maximum signal, do not turn yourself (or the transceiver) more than 90 degrees in either direction. If you rotate more than 90 degrees to locate the maximum signal, you will become turned around and follow the induction line in the reverse direction.

3. Walk another five steps, as described above, and then stop and orient the transceiver toward the maximum signal. Reduce the volume.
4. Continue repeating the above steps. You should be walking in a curved path along the "induction line" toward the victim (see Figure 2-19, C).
5. When the signal is loud at minimum volume setting, you should be very close to the victim and can begin the pinpoint search (see below).

Grid search

1. When a signal is picked up, stand and rotate the transceiver, which is held horizontally (parallel with the ground), to obtain the maximum signal (loudest volume). Maintain the transceiver in this orientation during the remainder of the search.
2. Turn the volume control down until you can just hear the signal. Walk in a straight line, down the fall line from the victim's last-seen location, until the signal fades.
3. When the signal starts to fade, turn 180 degrees and walk back toward the starting position. The signal will increase in volume and then fade again. Walk back to the point of loudest volume/maximum signal, which should be in the middle of two fade points.
4. At this point, turn 90 degrees in one direction or the other. From that position, reorient the transceiver (held parallel with the ground) to locate the maximum signal. After orienting the transceiver to the maximum signal, reduce the volume, and begin walking forward. If the signal fades, turn around 180 degrees and begin walking again.
5. As the signal volume increases, repeat steps 3 and 4 until you have reached the lowest volume control setting on the transceiver. This time, when you return to the middle of the fade points (maximum signal strength), you should be very close to the buried victim and can now begin pinpointing him or her.
   a. While stationary, orient the transceiver to receive the maximum signal (loudest volume). At this point, turn the volume control all the way down.
   b. Maintain the transceiver in this orientation and sweep the transceiver from side to side and back and forth just above the surface of the snow.
   c. Find the signal position halfway between fade points (i.e., the loudest signal). At this point, you should be very close to the victim's position and can begin to mechanically probe. Speed is essential.

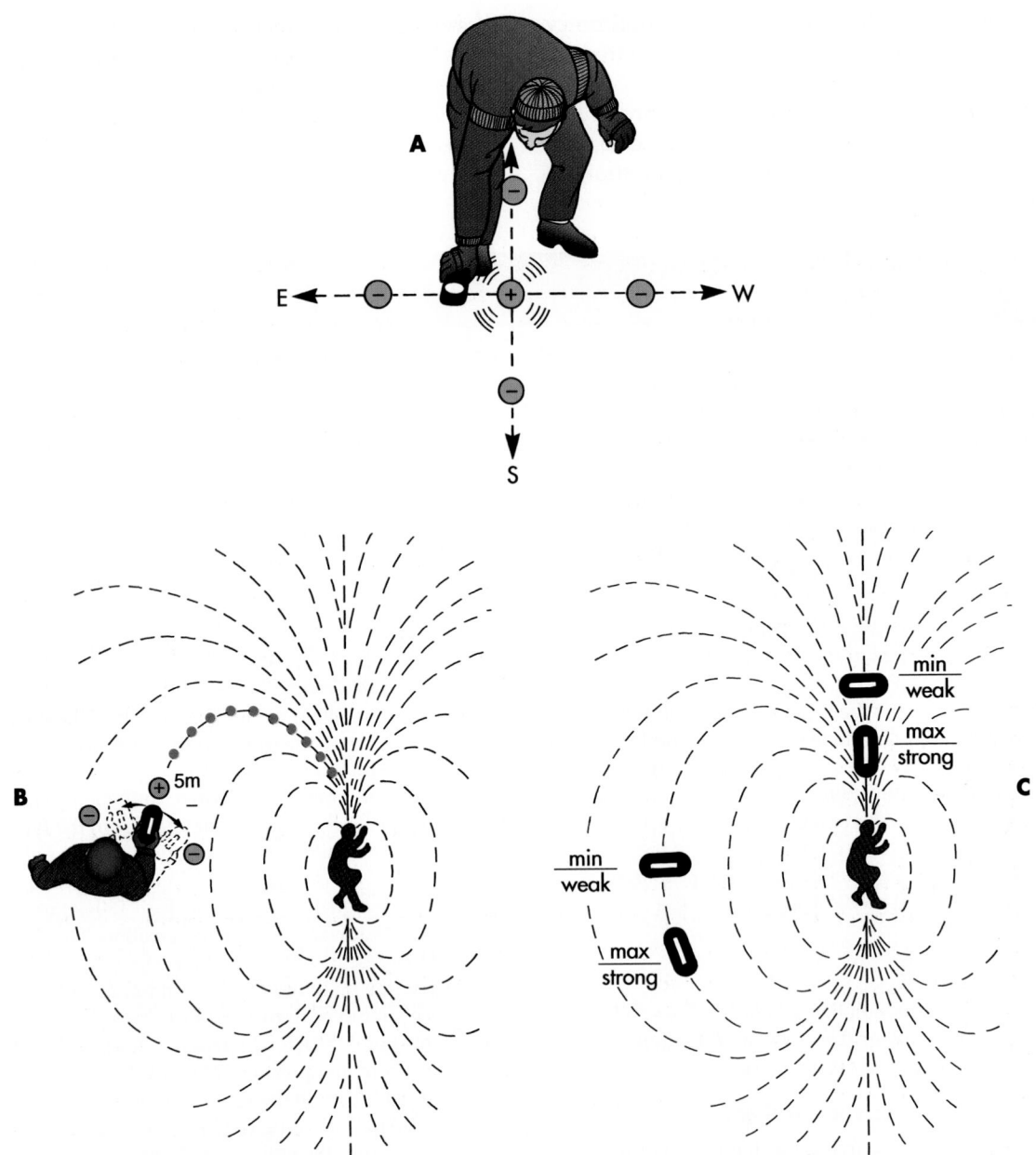

Figure 2-19 Induction line search. (*From Auerbach PS et al:* Field guide to wilderness medicine, *St Louis, 1999, Mosby.*)

Airbag. In 1995 a new rescue device made in Germany was introduced in Europe. It was the ABS Avalanche Airbag System and was designed specifically for guides and ski patrollers. The user wears the airbag in a pack and deploys it by pulling a rip cord. This releases a cartridge of nitrogen gas that escapes at high velocity and draws in outside air through jets; it is capable of inflating two 75-L airbags in 2 seconds. This gives the avalanche victim buoyancy and cushioning against impact with trees or rocks. To operate the device, the user must be able to grab and pull the rip cord.

By 1999, there had been 18 documented avalanche incidents in the Alps that involved 31 people equipped with airbags. In one case the airbag failed to work, and three other people failed to pull the rip cord, but all four survived anyway. There were 27 people with inflated airbags, and of these, 14 were not buried, 9 were partially buried, and 4 were bodily buried but a portion of the airbag remained on the surface, allowing for a quick recovery. All 27 survived.

Airbags will be available in the United States by 2000. They are an additional rescue device available to the backcountry adventurer and someday may become a viable alternative to beacons, although they should never replace good judgment.

AvaLung. In 1996, Dr. Thomas Crowley received a patent for an emergency breathing device to extract air from the snow surrounding a buried avalanche victim. Called the AvaLung, it is worn as a vest by the user. If buried, the victim can breathe through a mouthpiece and flex-tube connected to the vest. The victim can inhale oxygenated air coming from the surrounding snow, which passes through a membrane in the vest. The exhaled air, rich in carbon dioxide, passes through a one-way valve and into another area of the snow surrounding the victim to slow the effects of carbon dioxide narcosis caused by contaminating the air space.

The AvaLung will be marketed by Black Diamond Equipment, Ltd., in 2000. It has worked well in simulated burials, allowing the victim to breathe for 1 hour in tightly packed snow. It has yet to be proven in an actual avalanche burial. In time, the AvaLung may prove to be a lifesaver among avalanche professionals, but only as an instrument of last resort.

Crossing Avalanche Slopes

Travel through avalanche country always involves risk, but certain travel techniques can minimize that risk. Proper travel techniques might not prevent an avalanche release but can improve the odds of surviving. The timing of a trip has a lot to do with safety. Most avalanches occur during and just after storms. Waiting a full day after a storm has ended can allow the snowpack to react to the new snow load and gain strength.

Before crossing a potential avalanche slope, the skier or hiker should get personal gear in order by tightening up clothing, zipping up zippers, and putting on hat, gloves, and goggles. A person should be padded and insulated if trapped. If a heavy mountaineering pack is carried, the straps should be loosened or slung over one shoulder only so that the pack can be easily discarded if the person is knocked down. A heavy pack makes a person top-heavy, making it difficult to swim with the avalanche. The skier should remove pole wrist straps and ski runaway straps because poles and skis attached to a victim hinder swimming motions and only serve to drag the victim under. Finally, a person wearing a rescue beacon should be certain it is transmitting.

If possible, the person should cross low on the slope, near the bottom or in the runout zone. Crossing rarely causes a release in the starting zone far above. The greater risk is getting hit by an untimely natural release from above. If crossing high without reaching the safety of the ridge is necessary, the starting zone should be traversed as high as possible and close to rocks, cliff, or cornice. Should the slope fracture, most of the sliding snow will be below and the chance of staying on the surface of the moving avalanche will be better. Invariably, the person highest on the slope runs the least risk of being buried.

A person who must climb or descend an avalanche path should keep far to the sides. Should the slope fracture, escaping to the side improves the chance of surviving. Only one person at a time should cross, climb, or descend an avalanche slope; all other members should watch from a safe location. Two commonsense principles lie behind this advice. First, only one group member is exposed to the hazard, leaving the others available as rescuers. Second, less weight is put on the snow. All persons should traverse in the same track. This not only reduces the amount of work required but also disturbs less snow, which lowers the chance of avalanche release.

Skiers and climbers should never drop their guard on an avalanche slope. They should not stop in the middle of a slope, but only at the edge or beneath a point of protection, such as a rock outcropping. It is possible for the second, third, or even tenth person traversing or skiing down a slope to trigger the avalanche. Trouble should always be anticipated, and an escape route, such as getting out to the side or grabbing a tree, should be kept in mind.

Survival of Victims

Escaping to the Side. The moment the snow begins to move around the person, he or she has a split second to make a decision or make a move. Whether on foot, skis, or snowmobile, the person should first try to escape to the side of the avalanche or try to grab onto a tree. Staying on one's feet or snow machine gives some control and keeps the head up. Escaping to the side gets the person out altogether or to a place where the forces and speeds are less. Turning skis or the snow machine downhill in an effort to outrun the avalanche is a bad move, since the avalanche invariably overtakes its victims.

The person should shout and then close the mouth. Shouting alerts companions to what is happening. Clamping the mouth shut and breathing through the nose prevents inhalation of a mouthful of snow.

Swimming. A person knocked off his or her feet should attempt to swim with the avalanche. Cumbersome or heavy gear should be discarded. Ski poles should be tossed away; with luck, the avalanche will strip away the skis. The victim should get away from the snow machine. Swimming motions with the arms and legs increase the freedom to maneuver the body. The purpose is to maintain a position near the surface. Any swimming motions will do, but if the person has been thrown forward and is being carried head first downhill, the breast stroke with the arms (similar to body surfing) should be used; if being carried down feet first, the person should try to roll onto his or her back and attempt to "tread water" with the arms and legs.

Reaching the Surface. Avalanches come to a stop when they flow out onto more gentle terrain. A victim may have a second or two when he or she feels the sensation of slowing down. This is a crucial point in the ordeal, the best chance to reach the surface. The person should thrust upward with swimming motions and try to burst through to the surface. Unless very deeply buried at this time, the person will probably know which way is up. All possible strength should be exerted to get the head, an arm, or even a hand above the surface. Even if the person cannot get his or her head out, being near the surface greatly improves the odds for survival. If any clue is on the surface, it gives the rescuers something to see. A hand should be used to clear a breathing space over the mouth.

Rescue by Survivors

Marking the Last-Seen Point. A survivor or eyewitness to an accident needs to act quickly and positively. The rescuer's actions over the next several minutes may mean the difference between life and death for the victim. First, the victim's last-seen point should be fixed and marked with a piece of equipment, clothing, a tree branch, or anything that can be seen from a distance downslope. It is most often safe to move out onto the bed surface of the avalanche that has recently run. It is dangerous when the fracture line has broken at midslope, leaving a large mass of snow still hanging above the fracture.

Searching for Clues. The fall line should be searched below the last-seen point for any clues of the victim. The snow should be scuffed by kicking and turning over loose chunks to look for anything that might be attached to the victim or that will give the victim's trajectory and narrow the search area. Shallow probes should be made into likely burial spots with an avalanche probe, ski, ski pole, or tree limb. Likely spots are the uphill sides of trees and rocks, and benches or bends in the slope where snow avalanche debris is concentrated. The toe of the debris should be searched thoroughly; many victims are found in this area.

Rescue Beacons. If the group was using beacons, all survivors must immediately switch their units to receive mode. While making the fast scuff-search for visual clues, survivors should at the same time search the debris, listening for the beeping sound coming from the buried beacon. When they pick up the signal, they will be able to narrow the search area quickly. If skilled in this kind of search, they will pinpoint the burial site in a few minutes.

Probing. Probing avalanche debris is a simple but slow method for searching for buried victims. A probe line is composed of up to a dozen rescuers with avalanche probes, or sounding rods, who stand elbow to elbow on the avalanche debris. Ideally, probes should be 3 to 4 m (10 to 13 feet) long. Once the whole area is probed without a find, the proper decision is to do it again. In rescues with enough manpower, shovelers stand nearby to check out any possible strike. The line does not stop in such an event but continues to march forward with its methodical "down, up, step" cadence.

Coarse probing is 4 to 5 times faster than the more thorough technique called fine probing. For a coarse probe, probers straddle a distance of 50 cm and are spaced 75 cm apart (Figure 2-20). This leaves 25 cm between the toes of adjacent probers. Probes are pushed into the center of the straddled span. Upon command from the leader, the line advances one step, about 70 cm. (Where terrain is steep or probers are few, an alternative is to stand "fingertip-to-fingertip." Probers probe first on one side of their body, then on the other.) This method gives about a 70% chance of finding the victim.

After several passes of coarse probing with no results, a fine probe is done, usually when the objective is body recovery. For this method the line is arranged as for coarse probing. Each searcher probes in front of the left foot, in the center of the straddled position, and in front of the right foot. On signal the line advances 30 cm and repeats the three probes. This method gives a 100% probability of finding a victim. The probe holes are spaced 25 by 30 cm, or 13 probes per square meter. On average, 20 searchers can fine probe an area 100 × 100 m (328 × 328 feet) in 16 to 20 hours.

Avalanche Guard. If the threat of a second avalanche exists, one person should stand in a safe location to shout out a warning. This gives the searchers a few seconds to flee to safety. Rescues are often carried out in dangerous conditions, and self-preservation should be a major consideration.

Going for Help. A difficult question in rescues is when to seek outside help. If the accident occurs in or near a ski area and there are several rescuers, one person can be sent to notify the ski patrol immediately. If only one rescuer is present, the correct choice becomes harder. The best advice is to search the surface hastily but thoroughly for clues before leaving to notify the patrol. If a patrol phone is close, the rescuer should notify the patrol and then return immediately to resume the search.

If the avalanche occurs in the backcountry far from any organized body of rescuers, all party members should remain at the site. The guiding principle in backcountry rescues is that survivors search until they

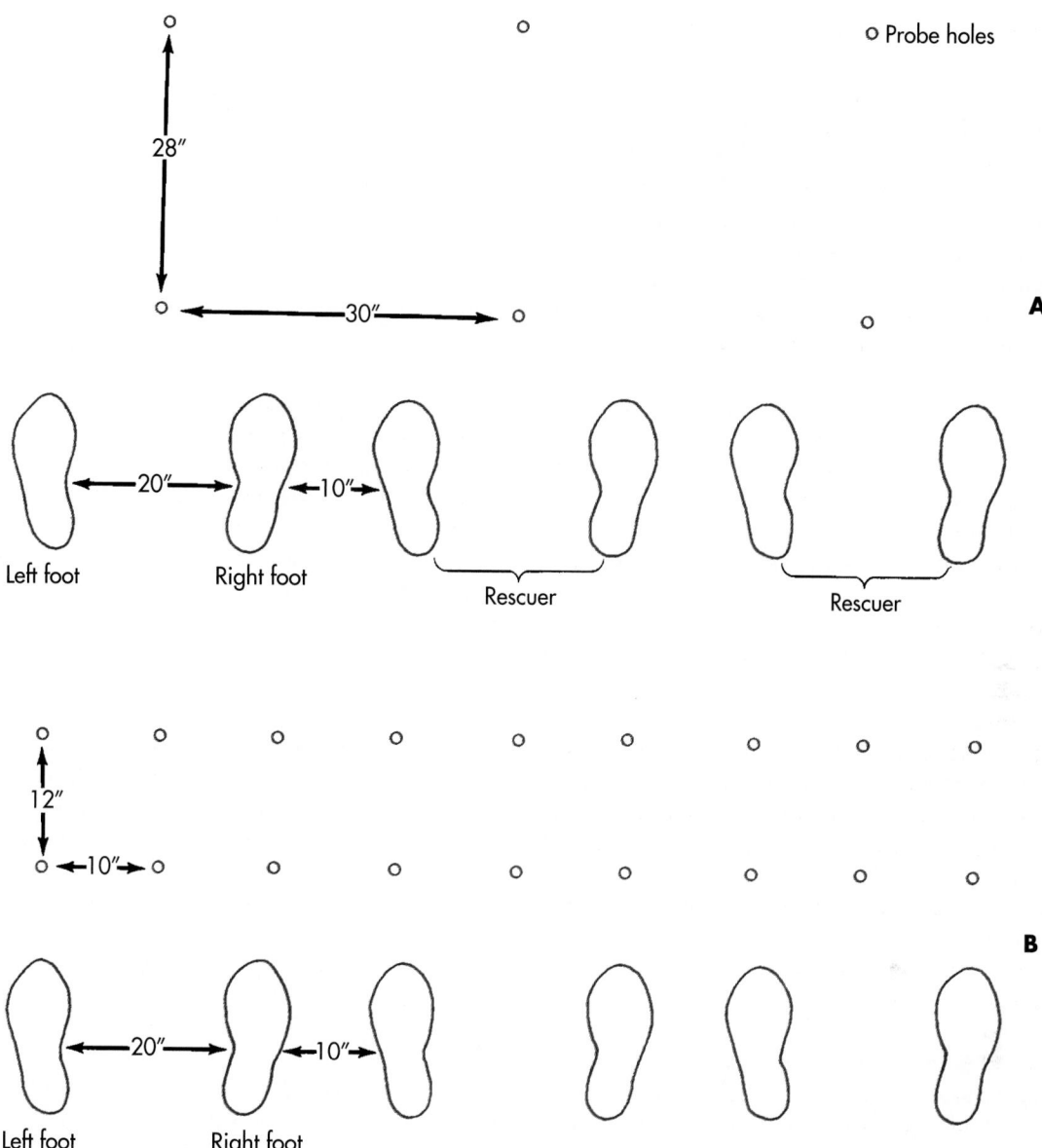

○ Probe holes

A

28″

30″

20″   10″

Left foot   Right foot   Rescuer   Rescuer

12″

10″

B

20″   10″

Left foot   Right foot

Figure 2-20 A, Coarse, and **B,** fine avalanche probing.

cannot or should not continue. When deciding when to stop searching, the safety of the search party must be weighed against the decreasing survival chances of the buried victim.

One exception exists to the rule of all party members staying to search. When there are a large number of survivors, two people can go out to secure help and the search party will still have a sizable rescue force on hand.

Three-Stage Rescue. A full-scale operation is divided into three stages. The first stage is the hasty search column. This group, composed of as many people as are on hand, heads swiftly to the site carrying probes, shovels, and first-aid equipment. They scuff the ava-

lanche for clues and probe likely areas in hopes of making a quick find. The person reporting the avalanche often accompanies this column back to the site.

The second stage brings the main body of rescuers to the site. They carry bulkier equipment needed for search, resuscitation, and evacuation: more probes and shovels, toboggans, sleeping bags, resuscitation equipment, medical supplies, and a trained avalanche dog and handler, if available. Ideally, stage two should begin 10 to 15 minutes after stage one.

The third stage brings in support for stages one and two, in the case of a prolonged rescue. Included are fresh rescuers to take over for cold and tired searchers, hot food and drink, tents, warm clothing, and lights.

Avalanche dogs and handlers can provide additional search power.

THE MODERN AVALANCHE VICTIM

Avalanche deaths have increased in the United States each decade since 1950. Figure 2-21 shows annual deaths; Figure 2-22 shows these numbers averaged over 5-year periods. From 1950 to 1999, 571 people have died in avalanches. Of these, 471 (82%) were men and 54 (10%) were women. (Interestingly, not all accident reports list the gender of the victim.) The average age of all victims is 28 years. The youngest was 6; the oldest, 66.

Figure 2-23 shows the activity groups for the victims. Most victims (83%) were pursuing some form of recreation at the time of their accident, with climbers, ski tourers, snowmobilers, and lift skiers heading the list. The distinction between ski tourers and lift skiers is that lift skiers pursue their sport in and around developed ski areas and rely on lifts to get them up the hill. This category includes skiers who leave the area boundary or ski into "closed" areas within the ski area boundary. The ski tourers category includes ski mountaineers, backcountry skiers, helicopter skiers, and snowcat skiers. Miscellaneous recreation includes hikers, snowshoers, and persons playing in the snow. Among nonrecreation groups, avalanches strike houses (residents), highways (motorists and plow drivers), and the workplace (ski patrollers and others whose job puts them at risk). Since 1950, 15 states have registered avalanche fatalities (Figure 2-24).

Statistics of Avalanche Burials

Numerous factors affect a buried victim's chances for survival: time buried, depth buried, clues on the surface, safety equipment, injury, ability to swim with the avalanche, body position, snow density, presence of airspace, and size of airspace. A victim who is uninjured and able to fight and swim on the downhill ride usually has a better chance of ending up only partly buried, or if completely buried, a better chance of creating an airspace for breathing. A victim who is severely injured or knocked unconscious is like a ragdoll being rolled, flipped, and twisted. Being trapped in an avalanche is a life-and-death struggle, with the upper hand going to those who fight the hardest.

Avalanches kill in two ways. First, serious injury is always possible in a tumble down an avalanche path. Trees, rocks, cliffs, and the wrenching action of snow in motion can do horrible things to the human body. About one third of all avalanche deaths are caused by trauma, especially to the head and neck. Second, snow burial causes suffocation in two thirds of avalanche deaths. The problem of breathing in an avalanche does not start with being buried. A victim being carried down in the churning maelstrom of snow has an extraordinarily hard time breathing. Inhaled snow clogs the mouth and nose; suffocation occurs quickly if the victim is buried with the airway already blocked. Snow

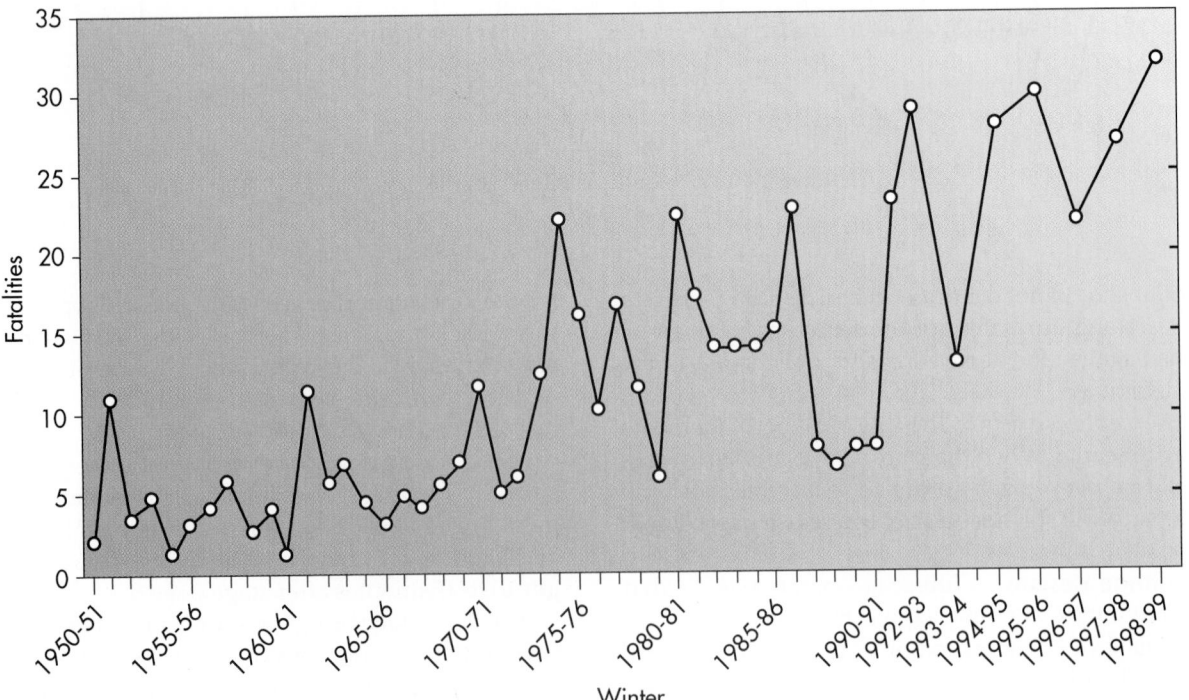

Figure 2-21 Avalanche fatalities in the United States from the winters of 1950-1951 to 1998-1999.

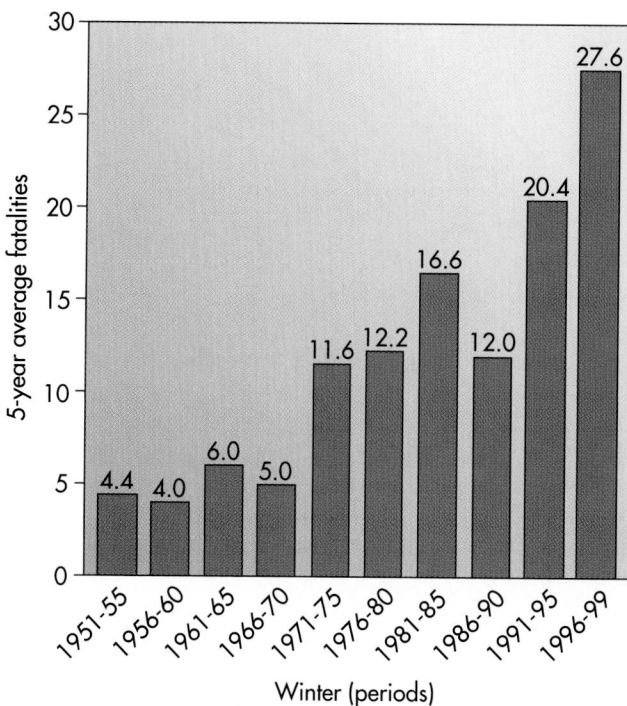

Figure 2-22 Avalanche fatalities in the United States averaged by five-winter periods, 1950-1951 to 1998-1999.

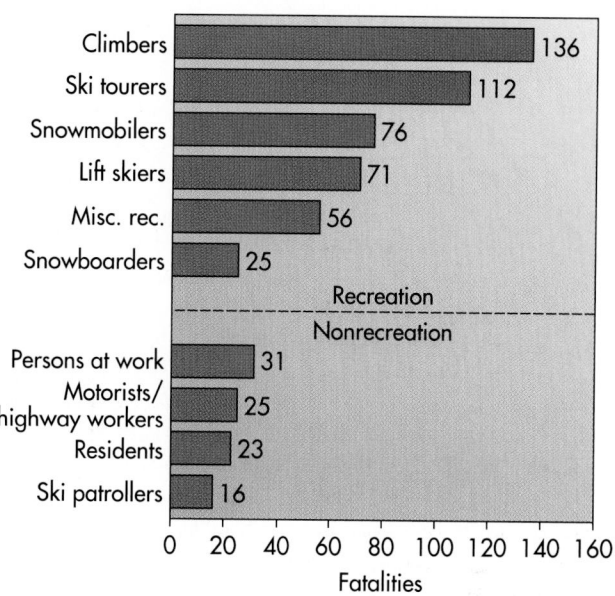

Figure 2-23 Avalanche fatalities in the United States from 1950-1951 to 1998-1999 by activity categories.

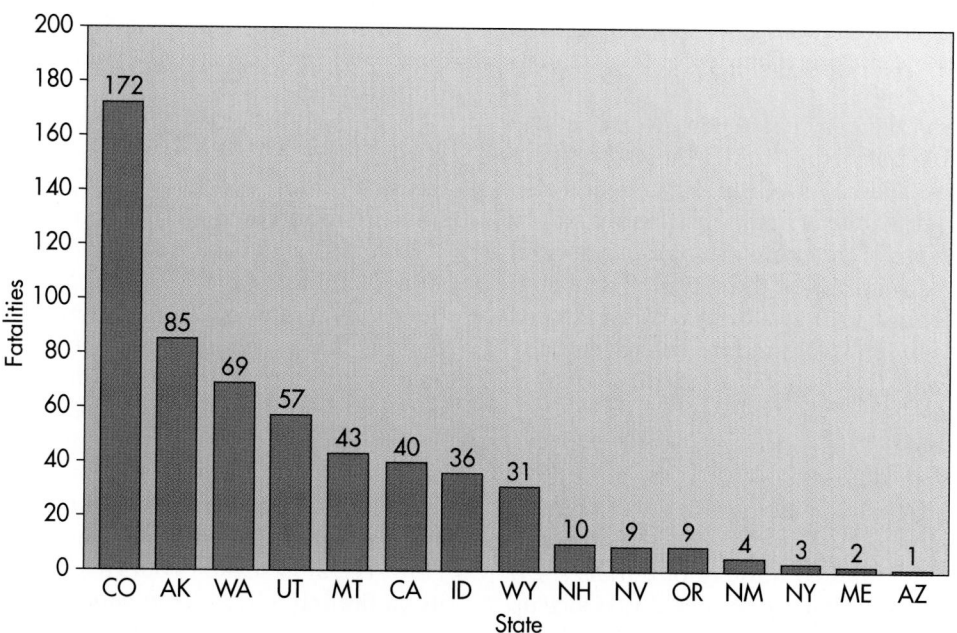

Figure 2-24 Avalanche fatalities in the United States from 1950-1951 to 1998-1999 by state.

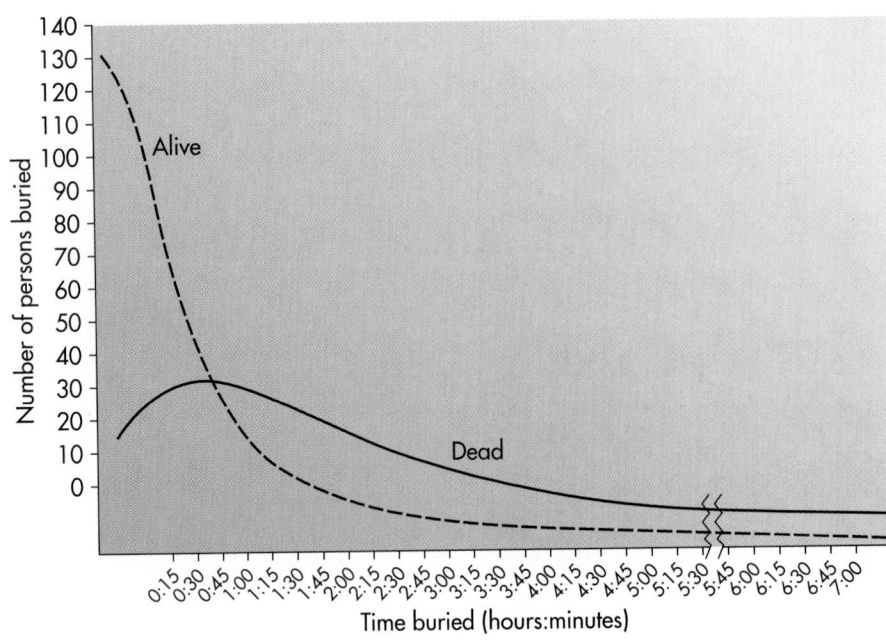

Figure 2-25 Length of time buried for U.S. avalanche fatalities and survivors in direct contact with the snow (not in a structure or vehicle) from 1950-1951 through 1998-1999.

that was light and airy when a skier carved turns in it becomes viselike in its new form. Where the snow might have been 80% air to begin with, it might be less than 50% air after an avalanche. The snow is much less permeable to airflow, making it harder for the victim to breathe.

Snow sets up hard and solid after an avalanche. It is almost impossible for victims to dig themselves out, even if buried less than a foot deep. Hard debris also makes recovery very difficult in the absence of a sturdy shovel. The pressure of the snow in a burial of several feet sometimes is so great that the victim is unable to expand his or her chest to draw a breath. Warm exhaled breath freezes on the snow around the face, eventually forming an ice lens that cuts off all airflow. It takes longer than snow-clogged airways, but the result is still death by suffocation.

Another factor that affects survival is the position of the victim's head; that is, whether they were buried face up or face down. The most favorable position is face up. Data from a limited number of burials show the victim is twice as likely to survive if buried face up rather than face down. If buried face up, an airspace forms around the face as the back of the head melts into the snow; if buried face down, an airspace cannot form as the face melts into the snow.

The statistics on survival are derived from a large number of avalanche burials. In compiling these figures, we have included only persons who were totally buried in direct contact with the snow. We have not included victims buried in the wreckage of buildings or vehicles, since such victims can be shielded from the snow to allow sizable airspaces. Under favorable circumstances such as this, some victims have been able to live for days. In 1982, Anna Conrad lived for 5 days at Alpine Meadows, California, in the rubble of a demolished building, the longest survival on record in the United States.

A completely buried victim has a poor chance of survival. Figure 2-25 shows decreasing survival with increasing burial time. In the first 15 minutes, more persons are found alive (87%) than dead. Between 16 to 30 minutes, an equal number are found dead and alive. After 30 minutes, more are found dead than alive and the survival rate continues to diminish. The important point is that speed is essential in the search. In favorable circumstances, buried victims can live for several hours beneath the snow; therefore rescuers should never abandon a search prematurely. A miner in Colorado who was buried by an avalanche near a mine portal was able to dig himself out after being buried for approximately 22 hours and nearly 1.8 m (6 feet) deep. However, after several hours the diminishing probability of finding a live victim should be weighed against the safety of the search party.

Survival is interrelated with both time and depth of burial, as shown in Figure 2-26. Survival probabilities diminish with increasing burial depth. To date, no one in the United States who has been buried deeper than 2.1 m (7 feet) has been recovered alive.

Statistics of Rescue

A buried victim's chance of survival directly relates not only to depth and length of time of burial but also to

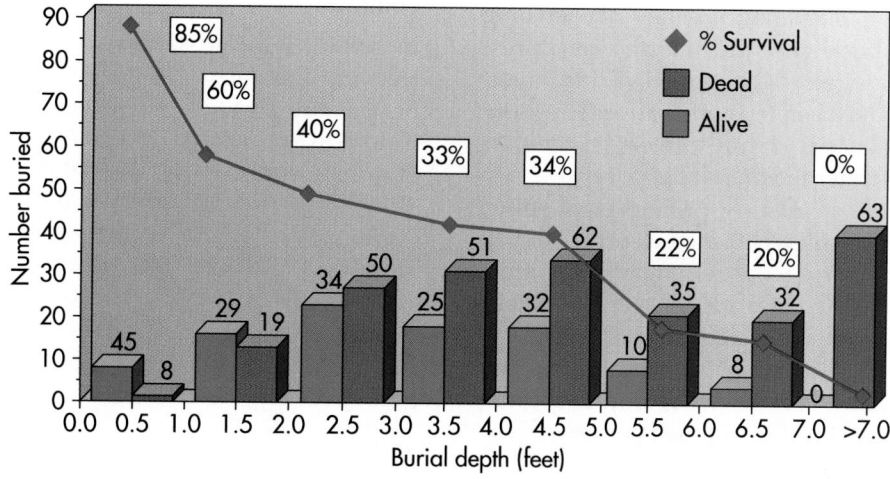

Figure 2-26 Depth of burial for U.S. avalanche fatalities and survivors and percentage survival for victims in direct contact with the snow (not in a structure or vehicle) from 1950-1951 through 1998-1999.

TABLE 2-1. Type of Rescue for Buried Avalanche Victims in Direct Contact with Snow, Based on a Sample of 682 Burials in the United States from 1950-1951 to 1998-1999

	SELF-RESCUE	RESCUE BY PARTY MEMBERS	RESCUE BY ORGANIZED TEAM	TOTAL
Found alive	49 (16%)	186 (64%)	57 (20%)	292
Found dead	—	84 (22%)	306 (78%)	390

TABLE 2-2. Method of Locating (First Contact) Buried Avalanche Victims, Based on a Sample of 748 Avalanche Burials in the United States from 1950-1951 to 1998-1999

METHOD	FOUND ALIVE	FOUND DEAD	TOTAL
Attached object or body part	108	39	147
Hasty search or spot probe	26	38	64
Coarse or fine probe	22	139	161
Rescue transceiver	36	58	94
Avalanche cord	1	0	1
Acoustic contact	26	1	27
Avalanche dog	6	34	40
Other (digging, bulldozer)	17	14	31
Found after long time span	0	41	41
Inside vehicle	30	10	40
Inside structure	22	28	50
Method not known	19	33	52
TOTAL	313	435	748

type of rescue. Table 2-1 compiles the statistics on survival as a function of type of rescue. Buried victims rescued by party members or groups at the accident site have a much better chance of survival than those rescued by organized rescue groups, time being the major influencing factor. Of those found alive, 64% were rescued by party members and 20% by an organized rescue party.

Table 2-2 describes methods of rescue for buried avalanche victims. Seventy-three percent of victims (108 of 147) who were buried with a body part (such as a hand) or an attached object (such as a ski tip) protruding from the snow were found alive. In some cases this was simply good luck, but in many cases it was the result of actively fighting or swimming with the avalanche or of thrusting a hand upward when the avalanche began to slow down. Either way, this statistic shows the advantages of a shallow burial: less time required to search, shorter digging time, and the possibility of attached objects or body parts being visible on the debris. Of the fatalities in this category, many were skiing alone, with no one to spot the hand or ski tip and provide rescue.

Organized probe lines have found more victims than any other method, but because of the time required, most victims (86%) are recovered dead. Only 22 people were found alive by this method, with 139 recovered dead.

Rescue transceivers are an efficient method to locate victims, but two problems have limited the number of survivors who were wearing beacons. First, few who wear beacons are well practiced in the art of using them instantly and efficiently to save a life; and second, even with a quick pinpointing of the burial location, extricating the victim from deeper burials may take too long to save a life. Therefore, since the first transceiver rescue in 1974, only 38% (36 of 94) of buried victims found with transceivers have been recovered alive. The more practice and experience with transceivers on the part of the rescuers, the faster the find and recovery.

Despite the sound-insulating properties of snow, 26 victims who were shallowly buried were able to yell and be heard by rescuers (acoustic contact). An unfortunate case was the man whose moans were heard but who was dead when uncovered 20 minutes later.

Trained search dogs are capable of locating buried victims very quickly, but because they are often brought to the scene only after extended periods of burial, there have been few live rescues. In the March 1982 avalanche disaster at Alpine Meadows, California, a dog made the first live recovery of an avalanche victim in the United States. Since then, dogs have effected five additional live recoveries.

A trained avalanche dog can search more effectively than can 30 searchers. Search dogs move rapidly over avalanche debris, using their sensitive noses to scan for human scent diffusing up through the snowpack. Dogs have found bodies buried 10 m (33 feet) deep but have also passed over some buried only 2 m (6½ feet) deep. They are not 100% effective. Search and rescue teams and law enforcement agencies work closely with search dog handlers, and trained avalanche dogs are becoming common fixtures at several ski areas in the western United States.

These statistics point out the extreme importance of rescue skills. Organized rescue teams, such as ski patrollers, must be highly practiced. They must have adequate training, manpower, and equipment to perform a hasty search and probe of likely burial spots within a minimum time span. For backcountry rescues the message is clear that a buried victim's best hope for survival is to be found by his or her companions. The need to seek outside rescue units practically ensures a body recovery mission.

APPENDIX A

Public Information

Twenty-four-hour regional avalanche information is available, generally from November through April, by calling the following Internet web sites or recorded telephone messages.

California

Internet: www.r5.fs.fed.us/tahoe/avalanche/
Truckee   530-587-2158
Mammoth Lakes   760-924-5500

Colorado

Internet: www.caic.state.co.us
Denver/Boulder   303-275-5360
Fort Collins   970-482-0457
Colorado Springs   719-520-0020
Summit County   970-668-0600
Vail   970-479-4652
Aspen   970-920-1664
Durango   970-247-8187

Idaho

Internet: www.avalanche.org/~ciac/bulletin.txt
Sun Valley   208-788-1200 x8027

Montana

Internet: www.gomontana.com/avalanche
Bozeman   406-587-6981
Cooke City   406-838-2341

New Hampshire

Internet: www.mountwashington.org/avalanche

Utah

Internet: www.avalanche.org/~uafc/
Salt Lake City   801-364-1581
Provo   801-378-4333
Ogden   801-626-8600
Park City   435-658-5512
Logan   801-797-4146
Alta   801-742-0830
Moab   801-259-7669

Washington and Oregon

Internet: www.nwac.noaa.gov
Seattle   206-526-6677
Portland   503-808-2400

Wyoming

Internet: www.untracked.com/forecast
Jackson   307-733-2664

Canada

Internet: www.avalanche.ca

APPENDIX B

Avalanche Education

Several organizations teach basic and advanced avalanche awareness and training courses. Beyond those listed here, many local colleges and universities, ski patrols, and recreation departments offer courses.

Adventures to the Edge
Box 91
Crested Butte, CO 81224
970-349-5219

Alaska Avalanche School
Alaska Mountain Safety Center
9140 Brewsters Drive
Anchorage, AK 99516
907-345-3566

American Avalanche Institute
Box 308
Wilson, WY 83014
307-733-3315

Canadian Avalanche Association Training Schools
Box 2759
Revelstoke, BC, Canada V0E 2S0
250-837-2435

Canadian Ski Patrol System
8 Vartown Place NW
Calgary, AB, Canada T3A 0B5
403-938-2101

Federation of Mountain Clubs of British Columbia
336-1367 West Broadway
Vancouver, B.C., Canada V6H 4A9
604-739-7175

National Avalanche School
National Avalanche Foundation
133 South Van Gordon St., Suite 100
Lakewood, CO 80228
303-988-1111

National Outdoor Leadership School
Box 345
Victor, ID 83455
208-354-8443

National Ski Patrol
133 South Van Gordon St., Suite 100
Lakewood, CO 80228
303-988-1111

Northwest Avalanche Institute
39238 258th Ave., SE
Enumclaw, WA 98022
360-825-9261

Sierra Ski Touring
Box 176
Gardnerville, NV 89410
702-782-3047

Silverton Avalanche School
Box 178
Silverton, CO 81433

Summit County Rescue Group
Box 1794
Breckenridge, CO 80424

Telluride Avalanche School
Box 261
Telluride, CO 81435
970-728-3829

Colleges and universities that offer avalanche and snow related courses (mostly graduate level) and the E-mail contact:

University of Arizona
Department of Hydrology and Water Resources
Dr. Roger Bales: roger@hwr.arizona.edu

Arizona State University
Department of Geography
Dr. Andrew Ellis: andrew.w.ellis@asu.edu
University of California, Santa Barbara
Donald Bren School of Environmental Science
    and Management
Dr. Jeff Dozier: dozier@bren.ucsb.edu

University of British Columbia (Vancouver)
Department of Geography & Civil Engineering
Dr. Dave McClung: mcclung@geog.ubc.ca

University of Calgary (Calgary)
Department of Geology and Geophysics
Department of Civil Engineering
Dr. Bruce Jamieson: jbjamies@ucalgary.ca

University of Colorado (Boulder)
Department of Geography
Institute of Arctic and Alpine Research (INSTAAR)
Dr. Mark W. Williams: markw@snobear.colorado.edu

Colorado State University (Fort Collins)
Department of Earth Resources
Dr. Kelly Elder: kelder@cnr.colostate.edu

Montana State University (Bozeman)
Department of Civil Engineering
Dr. Ed Adams: eda@ce.montana.edu
Department of Earth Sciences
Dr. Katherine Hansen: ueskh@montana.edu

Northern Arizona University (Flagstaff)
Department of Geography
Dr. Lee Dexter: Lee.Dexter@nau.edu

University of Oregon (Eugene)
Department of Geography
Dr. Cary Mock: cmock@oregon.uoregon.edu

Rutgers University (Piscataway, NJ)
Department of Geography
Dr. David A. Robinson: drobins@rci.rutgers.edu

Sierra College
Tahoe-Truckee Extension Center
Box 2467
Truckee, CA 96161
530-587-3849

University of Utah (Salt Lake City)
Department of Civil Engineering
Dr. Rand Decker: rdecker@civil.utah.edu

Utah State University (Logan)
Department of Forest Resources
Dr. Michael J. Jenkins: mjenkins@cc.usu.edu

University of Washington (Seattle)
Geophysics Program
Dr. Howard Conway:
    conway@geophys.washington.edu

APPENDIX C

Avalanche Safety Equipment Manufacturers and Suppliers

Backcountry Access, Inc.
2820 Wilderness Place, Unit H
Boulder, CO 80301
303-417-1345
Backcountry ski equipment, Tracker rescue beacons

Black Diamond Equipment, Ltd.
2084 East 3900 South
Salt Lake City, UT 84124
801-278-5552
Backcountry ski equipment, clothing, survival gear, rescue beacons, AvaLung

Cascade Toboggan
25802 West Valley Highway
Kent, WA 98032
206-852-0182
Shovels, probes, rescue beacons, other rescue equipment

Climb High
1861 Shelburne Road
Shelburne, VT 05482
802-985-5055
Backcountry ski and expedition equipment, rescue beacons, shovels, probes, and clothing

Eastern Mountain Sports
1 Vose Farm Road
Peterborough, NH 03458
603-924-9571
(or local retail store)
Backcountry ski equipment, clothing, survival gear, rescue beacons

Life Link International
P.O. Box 2913
Jackson Hole, WY 83001
307-733-2266
Snowpit instruments, shovels, probes, rescue beacons, other rescue equipment

Mountain Safety Research
4225 2nd Avenue South
Seattle, WA 98134
206-624-857
Survival gear, probes, other rescue equipment

Mt. Tam Sports
Box 111
Kentfield, CA 94914
415-461-8111
Snowpit instruments, rescue equipment, first aid equipment

Ortovox USA, Inc.
455 Irish Hill Road
Hopkinton, NH 03229
603-746-3176
Ortovox rescue beacons, shovels, rescue equipment

Recreational Equipment, Inc.
P.O. Box 88125
Seattle, WA 98138-2125
206-323-8333
(or local retail store)
Backcountry ski equipment, clothing, survival gear, rescue beacons

Survival on Snow, Inc.
Box 1, Site 218 RR2
St. Albert, AB, Canada T8N 1M9
403-973-5412
SOS rescue beacons, rescue equipment

Wasatch Touring
702 East 100 South
Salt Lake City, UT 84102
801-359-9361
Snowpit instruments, probes, shovels, rescue beacons

SUGGESTED READINGS

Armstrong BR, Williams K: *The avalanche book*, Golden, Colo, 1992, Fulcrum, Inc.

The Avalanche Review, P.O. Box 1032, Bozeman, MT 59771-1032 (official publication of the American Association of Avalanche Professionals).

Daffern T: *Avalanche safety for skiers and climbers*, ed 2, Seattle, Wash, 1992, Cloudcap.

Fraser C: *Avalanches and snow safety*, New York, 1978, Charles Scribner.

Fredston J, Fesler D: *Snow sense: a guide to evaluating avalanche hazard*, ed 4, Anchorage, 1994, Alaska Mountain Safety Center.

LaChapelle E: *The ABC's of avalanche safety*, ed 2, Seattle, Wash, 1985, The Mountaineers Books.

Logan N, Atkins D: *The snowy torrents: avalanche accidents in the United States 1980-86*, Denver, Colo, 1996, Colorado Geological Survey Spec Pub 39.

McClung D, Schaerer P: *The avalanche handbook*, Seattle, Wash, 1993, The Mountaineers Books.

3 Lightning Injuries

Mary Ann Cooper, Christopher J. Andrews, Ronald L Holle, and Raúl E López

HISTORICAL OVERVIEW

Humans have always viewed lightning with awe and trepidation. Priests, the earliest astronomers and meteorologists, became proficient at weather prediction, interpreting changes in weather as omens of good or bad fortune, sometimes to the advantage of their political mentors. As a spectacular celestial event, lightning was often depicted in ancient cultures and religions.[52] A roll seal from Akkadian times (2200 BC) portrays a goddess holding sheaves of lightning bolts in each hand.[52] Next to her, a weather god drives a chariot and creates lightning bolts by flicking a whip at his horses, while priests offer libations. A relief found on a castle gate in northern Syria (900 BC) depicts the weather god Teshub holding a three-pronged thunderbolt.

Beginning around 700 BC, Greek artists began to incorporate lightning symbols representing Zeus's tool of warning or favor. Aristotle noted that lightning resulted from the ignition of telluric fumes that made up storm clouds. Roman mythology saw lightning as more ominous than did the Greeks, with Jupiter using thunderbolts as tools of vengeance and condemnation so that Romans who were struck were denied burial rituals. Several Roman emperors wore laurel wreaths or sealskin to ward off lightning strikes. Important matters of state were often decided on observations of lightning and other natural phenomena. Both Seneca and Titus Lucretius discussed lightning in their treatises on natural events, and Plutarch noted that sleeping persons, having no spirit of life, were immune to lightning strikes.[52] The Norsemen named their thunder god Thor. Thursday is named for him.

In Chinese mythology the goddess of lightning, Tien Mu, used mirrors to direct bolts of lightning. She was one of the deities of the "Ministry of Thunderstorms" of ancient Chinese religion. Lightning also played a role in Buddhist symbolism.

Although lightning is most frequently rendered as fire, it has also been represented as stone axes hurled from the heavens. French peasants carry a *pierre do tonnerre*, or lightning stone, to ward off lightning strikes. The Yakuts of eastern Asia regard rounded stones found in fields hit by lightning as thunder axes and often use the powdered stones in medicines and potions. In Africa the Basuto tribe views lightning as the great thunderbird Umpundulo, flashing its wings in the clouds as it descends to Earth.

Some Native American cultures had the Thunderbird in their religions. The Navajo have a story about the hero Twins who used "the lightning that strikes straight" and "the lightning that strikes crooked" to kill several mythical beasts that were plaguing the People (Navajo) and in the process created the Grand Canyon.[13] The art of the native Australians incorporates lightning symbols as well.

MYTHS, SUPERSTITIONS, AND MISCONCEPTIONS[33]

The Roman Pliny noted that a man who heard thunder was safe from the lightning stroke. In general this is true because the light and strike precede the noise, depending on the distance from the lightning strike. However, some victims of direct hits report a sledgehammer-like effect of the force while seeing a bright light and occasionally hearing a loud noise. Others who receive side flashes or ground current report both seeing the flash and hearing the stroke, indicating that the main stroke was some distance away.

Many myths about lightning still persist today, including the notion that lightning strikes are invariably fatal. According to an American study of cases reported in the lightning literature since 1900, lightning strike carries a mortality of 30% and morbidity of 70%.[29] A slightly different statistical interpretation of the same data yielded a mortality figure of 20%.[2,8] Because literature reports are usually biased toward the severe or interesting cases, a review of cases will tend to overestimate the mortality rate. In reality, mortality may be as low as 5% to 10%.[25]

Most people suspect that the major cause of death would be from burns. However, the only cause of immediate death is from cardiac arrest.[29] Persons who are stunned or lose consciousness without cardiopulmonary arrest are highly unlikely to die, although they may still have serious sequelae.[31] Unfortunately, delayed causes of death include suicide induced by the life changes from disabilities wrought by lightning.

Most people know to seek shelter when storm clouds roll overhead. Few realize that one of the most dangerous times for a fatal strike is before the storm.[35] Lightning may travel nearly horizontally as far as 10 miles or more in front of the thunderstorm and seem to occur "out of a clear blue sky," or at least when the day is still sunny. The faster the storm is traveling and the more violent it is, the more likely that a fatal strike will occur. Another time underestimated for the potential danger of lightning is the end of a thunderstorm, which has been shown to be as dangerous as the start of the storm.

The "30-30 rule" is now recommended for lightning safety.[37] If you see lightning and can count to 30 seconds before you hear the thunder, you are already in danger and should be seeking shelter. Activities should not be resumed for at least 30 minutes after the last lightning is seen and the last thunder heard.[37,117] To calculate your distance from lightning, take the number of seconds between the "flash" and the "bang" (flash-to-bang method) and divide by 5 to find the number of miles.[116] The problem with the flash-to-bang method is that it is sometimes difficult to match the correct thunder to the correct lightning flash in an active storm. In addition, many people forget to divide by 5 and so overestimate the miles (and their safety factor) by a factor of five.

The distance between successive lightning flashes may be as little as a few yards or as much as 5 miles plus or minus another 5 miles (a count of 50 seconds) depending on the terrain and other local geographic factors.[86] One way to teach children lightning safety is to use the following phrase: "If you see it, flee it; if you hear it, clear it."

Winter lightning (thunderblizzard), although rare, is usually more dangerous because it tends to be much more powerful than summer lightning.

Most people believe that they are immune from lightning strikes when inside a building. Unfortunately, a significant proportion of injuries occurs to persons who are in their homes or places of employment.[1a,6,43,105,110] Side flashes strike people through plumbing fixtures, telephones, and other appliances attached to the outside of the house by metal conductors.[1a] Portable cellular phones offer protection from the electrical effects, although victims may suffer acoustic damage from the static in the earpiece similar to having a firecracker go off next to their ear.[6] With a hard-wired phone, they may suffer neurocognitive deficits,[32,36,103] death, or a myriad of other lightning-related problems because the phone system in most houses is not grounded to the house's electrical system and acts as a conduit for lightning either to come into the home or to exit from it. Telephone companies include warnings in their directories against using telephones during thunderstorms.

Taking shelter in small sheds, such as hikers' lean-tos or those on golf courses, especially above tree level on a mountain, can be especially dangerous when lightning splashes onto the inhabitants. Unfortunately, the most recently published *NFPA Journal* (National Fire Protection Association) discusses protection that may be effective for the shelter but may actually increase the lightning risk to any inhabitants who seek shelter in them.

The "crispy critter" myth is the belief that the victim struck by lightning bursts into flames or is reduced to a pile of ashes.[35] In reality, lightning often flashes over the outside of a victim, sometimes blowing off the clothes but leaving few external signs of injury and few if any burns.

Two other myths held by the public and many physicians are: "If you're not killed by lightning, you'll be OK," and, "If there are no outward signs of lightning injury, the damage can't be serious."[35] Medical literature, because of lack of follow-up case reports, also implies that there are few permanent sequelae of lightning injury. However, in the last few years it has become apparent that several permanent sequelae may occur.* In addition, many lightning victims with significant sequelae had no evidence acutely of burns. Peripheral neuropathy, chronic pain syndromes, and neuropsychologic symptoms, including severe short-term memory difficulty, difficulty processing new information, depression, and posttraumatic stress disorder, may be debilitating.[36,102,103] Further study is needed to elucidate how malingerers may be distinguished from real victims of lightning injury.[60,61]

Occasionally, lighting victims show pathognomonic skin changes that are not true burns but have a fernlike pattern. At one time, these patterns were thought to be imprints of the surrounding vegetation transferred onto the victim's skin by the lightning. Actually these fernlike patterns resemble fractals or the kind of pattern that can be obtained from placing a photographic plate in a strong electromagnetic field, which is what lightning produces for a short time around the victim.[62,121] They do not follow the distribution of nerves or blood vessels. Although they have been photographed and well described in the literature, no histologic study has been reported to explain the structure of the marking. It has been postulated that the pattern is caused by the forceful extravasation of red blood cells from the capillaries as they contract, similar to a bruise, which would also explain the evanescent nature of the markings.

A myth still prevalent is that the lightning victim retains the charge and is dangerous to touch, since he or she is still "electrified." This myth has led to unnecessary deaths by delaying resuscitation efforts.[35]

Medical literature and practice are plagued by myths that grew out of misread, misquoted, or misinterpreted data and continue to be propagated without further investigation. Not the least of these is the tenet that lightning victims who have resuscitation for several hours may still successfully recover. This belief seems to be grounded in the old idea of suspended

---

*References 1, 5, 28, 30, 33, 36, 47, 98, 102, 103, 110, 115, 122, 123.

animation—the concept that lightning is capable of shutting off systemic and cerebral metabolism, allowing rescuers a longer period in which to resuscitate the patient. This concept, credited to Taussig,[113] actually appeared some time before her article. In addition, the case recounted by Taussig that is the basis for this myth, when searched to its source, was a case report by Morikawa and Steichen.[94] The case does show a somewhat longer resuscitation period than usual, but not as miraculous as reported in Taussig's paper or as propagated in subsequent references to her paper.

In a study of lightning survivors, Andrews, Colquhoun, and Darveniza[4] have shown increasing prolongation of the QT interval, bringing up the theoretic possibility of torsades as a mechanism for the suspended animation reports. There is new evidence from animal experiments to support the teaching that respiratory arrest may persist longer than cardiac arrest.[2,38,39] One study, in which Australian sheep were hit with simulated lightning strokes, showed histologic evidence of greater damage to the respiratory centers than to the cardiac center in the fourth ventricle.[2] Prolonged assisted ventilation may in some cases be successful after cardiac activity has returned.

Another series of animal experiments by Cooper and Kotsos[38,39] with hairless rats has shown that it is possible to obtain the skin changes (keraunographic markings), primary and secondary arrest with prolonged respiratory arrest, and temporary lower extremity paralysis with simulated lightning strike.

Several booklets listing precautions for personal lightning protection appeared in the late 1700s and early 1800s. One of the superstitions listed was that humans, by their presence, could attract lightning to a nearby object. A book of the times, *Catechism of Thunderstorms*, illustrated other myths. Lightning was said to follow the draft of warm air behind a horse-drawn cart, so that coachmen were cautioned to walk their horses slowly through a storm. Other precautions listed included seeking shelter away from tall trees and sheaves of corn if caught in the open and installing lightning rods for the protection of buildings and ships.

Historically, many remedies for resuscitation of lightning victims have been offered. On July 15, 1889, Alfred West testified in a New York court that he was revived by "drawing out the electricity" when his feet were placed in warm water while his rescuer pulled on Mr. West's toes with one hand and milked a cow with the other.[10]

Other early attempts at resuscitation included friction to the bare skin, dousing the victim with a bucket of cold water, and chest compression. An early attempt at cardiopulmonary resuscitation was given in 1807 when mouth-to-mouth ventilation was used for lightning victims and it was proposed that gentle electric shocks from galvanic batteries passed through the chest

might be successful in resuscitating a victim of lightning.[16] Before that, Benjamin Franklin had purposely electrocuted a chicken during a lightning experiment and reported successful resuscitation with mouth-to-beak ventilation.[50]

A myth in current treatment is that lightning injuries should be treated like other high-voltage electric injuries. Although lightning as an electric phenomenon follows the same laws of physics, the injuries seen with lightning are very different from high-voltage injuries and should be treated differently if iatrogenic morbidity and mortality are to be avoided.[9,34]

"Lightning never strikes the same place twice." In reality, the Empire State Building and the Sears Tower are hit dozens of times a year, as are mountaintops and radio-television antennas. If the circumstances facilitating the original lightning strike are still in effect in an area, the laws of nature will encourage further lightning strikes.

Other myths[35]:

1. Victims may have "internal burns": There may be cellular damage and certainly nervous system damage but rarely, if ever, internal burns such as those suffered with high-voltage electrical injuries. However, some physicians use this euphemism with patients to explain their pain and neurologic injuries.

2. Wearing rubber-soled shoes, raincoats, etc., will protect a person: If lightning has burned its way a mile or more through the air, which is a superb insulator, it is foolish to believe that a fraction of an inch of rubber or composite material will serve as an adequate insulator.

3. The rubber tires on an auto are what protects a person from lightning injury: See entry 2 above. Electrical energy goes along the outside of a metal conductor (the car body) and dissipates through the rainwater to the ground or off the axles or bumper of the car.

4. Wearing metal around the head or as cleats on shoes will increase the risk or "attract lightning": There is no evidence to support this. Secondary burns on the soles of the feet where metal cleats or grommets heat up have been reported, but there is no evidence that a person increases his or her risk by wearing these.

5. Carrying an umbrella increases the risk: This is true if a person's height becomes greater by holding an umbrella.

6. Lightning always hits the highest object: False. Lightning only "sees" objects about 30 to 50 meters from its tip. In addition, several pictures exist of lightning hitting halfway down a flagpole or at the bottom of the space shuttle gantry.

7. There is no danger of lightning injury unless it is raining: False. Although lightning only occurs as

a result of thunderstorms, it can travel 10 or more miles in front of the thundercloud and seem to "come out of the blue" to strike a person or object long before the rain comes down in their area. Nearly 10% of lightning occurs when there is no rain falling in the area of the strike. It has also been known to reach over a mountain ridge and "hit out of the blue" from the thunderstorm that was on the other side of the peak and was neither visible nor audible to the victim.

8. Lightning may occur without thunder: Whenever there is lightning, there is thunder, and vice versa. Sometimes it will appear that there is lightning without thunder because thunder is seldom heard more than 10 miles from the lightning stroke or may be blocked by buildings or mountains.

INCIDENCE OF INJURY

Spatial Distribution of Lightning in the United States

The distribution of cloud-to-ground lightning across the United States is known because of deployment and operation for the last decade of automatic real-time lightning detection networks. On the average, over 20 million cloud-to-ground flashes are detected each year in the United States.[69] On a shorter time scale, more than 50,000 flashes per hour are sometimes detected during summer afternoons over the United States.[40]

A multiyear climatology of lightning from detection network data shows that central Florida always has the greatest number of flashes per area in a given year (Figure 3-1, A). Flash density decreases to the north and west from there. Flash densities over Missouri, Iowa, and Illinois during the 1993 Mississippi River flood rivaled Florida.[93] In addition to the general features in Figure 3-1, important local variations occur along the coast of the Gulf of Mexico, where sea breezes enhance lightning frequency.[81,119]

Additional important maxima and minima are found in and around the regions in the western United States with mountains and large slopes in terrain.[81,89]

Temporal Distribution of Lightning in the United States

Lightning is most common in summer months (Figure 3-2, A). About two thirds of the flashes occur in June, July, and August. In the southeastern states, lightning occurs quite often during all months of the year. A primary ingredient for lightning formation is a significant amount of moisture in the lower and middle levels of the atmosphere; this fuel for thunderstorms is consistently found in humid subtropical and tropical regions. Mechanisms to lift the moisture into thunderstorms are

necessary. Especially along coastlines and mountain slopes, updrafts are produced almost daily that provide favored locations for thunderstorms.

Lightning is most common in the afternoon (Figure 3-2, B). Nearly half of all lightning occurs from 1500 through 1800 local standard time (LST). Figure 3-2, B, combines regional results during the summer for Arizona,[120] northeast Colorado and central Florida,[81] and central Georgia.[80] There is no publication to date showing diurnal variation of lightning over the entire United States with detection network data. Lightning is at a maximum in the afternoon because the updrafts necessary for thunderstorm formation are strongest during the hours of the day when surface temperatures are highest, which results in the greatest vertical instability.

Lightning Around the World

Lightning detection systems similar to the U.S. network have been installed over part or all of about two dozen countries on every continent except Antarctica. Some have been in operation for up to a decade. At this time, there is no compilation of cloud-to-ground lightning flashes from such networks covering more than one country. Instead, Figure 3-1, B, shows the worldwide map of total lightning developed from the satellite-borne Optical Transient Detector (OTD), which measures both cloud-to-ground and cloud flashes.[26] Flash densities have been calculated statistically using OTD data to estimate that there are over 1.2 billion lightning flashes of all types around the world every year.

Most lightning is over tropical and subtropical continents, and there is far more lightning over land than the oceans. Some of the highest frequencies are much greater than found in the United States over Florida and other Gulf Coast locations.

Lightning is an afternoon phenomenon nearly everywhere, as was shown for the United States. At higher latitudes, most lightning occurs during the summer months. In Southeast Asia and surrounding regions toward the equator, maximum lightning activity during the year is influenced primarily by the monsoon and coincides generally with the months of heaviest rainfall.

U.S. Lightning Casualties in Storm Data

Every month, each National Weather Service (NWS) office in the United States compiles a list of damaging or notable weather phenomena occurring within the office's area of responsibility. This list is sent to National Oceanic and Atmospheric Administration (NOAA) headquarters, then to NOAA's National Climatic Data Center (NCDC) in Asheville, NC. These lists are combined at NCDC and *Storm Data* is published.

From 1959 to 1994, *Storm Data* had 3239 deaths, 9818 injuries, and 19,814 property-damage reports caused by

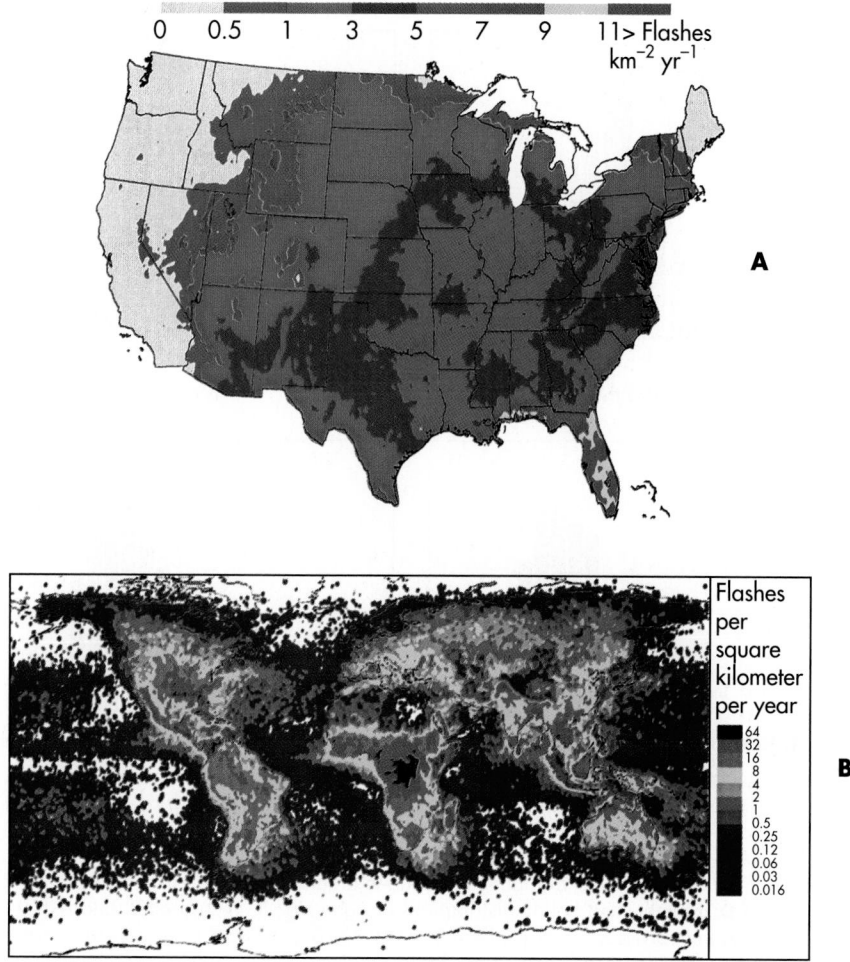

Figure 3-1 A, Cloud-to-ground flashes per square kilometer per year in the United States from a network of lightning detection antennas from 1989-1996. **B,** Total flashes per square kilometer per year for the world from May 1995 to April 1999 from the Optical Transient Detector. (**A** *from Huffines GR, Orville RE: J Appl Meteor 38:1013, 1999;* **B** *courtesy Hugh Christian, NASA/Marshall Space Flight Center.*)

lightning. Each report has some or all of the following: year, month, day, time, state and county, as well as number, gender, and location of fatalities and injuries, and amount and type of damage.

Lightning-related casualties and damages are often less spectacular and more dispersed in time and space than other weather phenomena. Therefore lightning deaths, injuries, and damages have been found to be underreported.[66,88,92,111] Factors contributing to the underreporting include the fact that most casualty events involve only one person or object, the fact that *Storm Data* relies on newspaper clipping services for lightning events, internal inconsistency within *Storm Data* in tabulation of individual occurrences into summary tables, lack of an accepted definition of lightning vs. "lightning-related" deaths, and inconsistency in the listing of medical diagnoses.[84,92,111] Regardless, *Storm Data* is the only consistent national data source for sev-

eral decades. Table 3-1 shows that lightning is second only to flash floods and floods in weather-related deaths during the 30-year record.

Spatial Distributions of Lightning Casualties

The lightning casualty distribution (deaths and injuries combined) is shown from 1959 to 1994 in Figure 3-3, *A.* The general pattern has similarities to the distribution of lightning in Figure 3-1, but Florida has twice as many casualties as any other state. Many of the other high numbers of casualties are from populous eastern states. It is preferable to use casualties for these results because the number of deaths is not very large and there is no obvious reason to expect differences in the geographic distribution of deaths vs. injuries.

The lightning hazard is shown better when population is taken into account (Figure 3-3, *B*). The maximum rate of lightning casualties shifts from populous east-

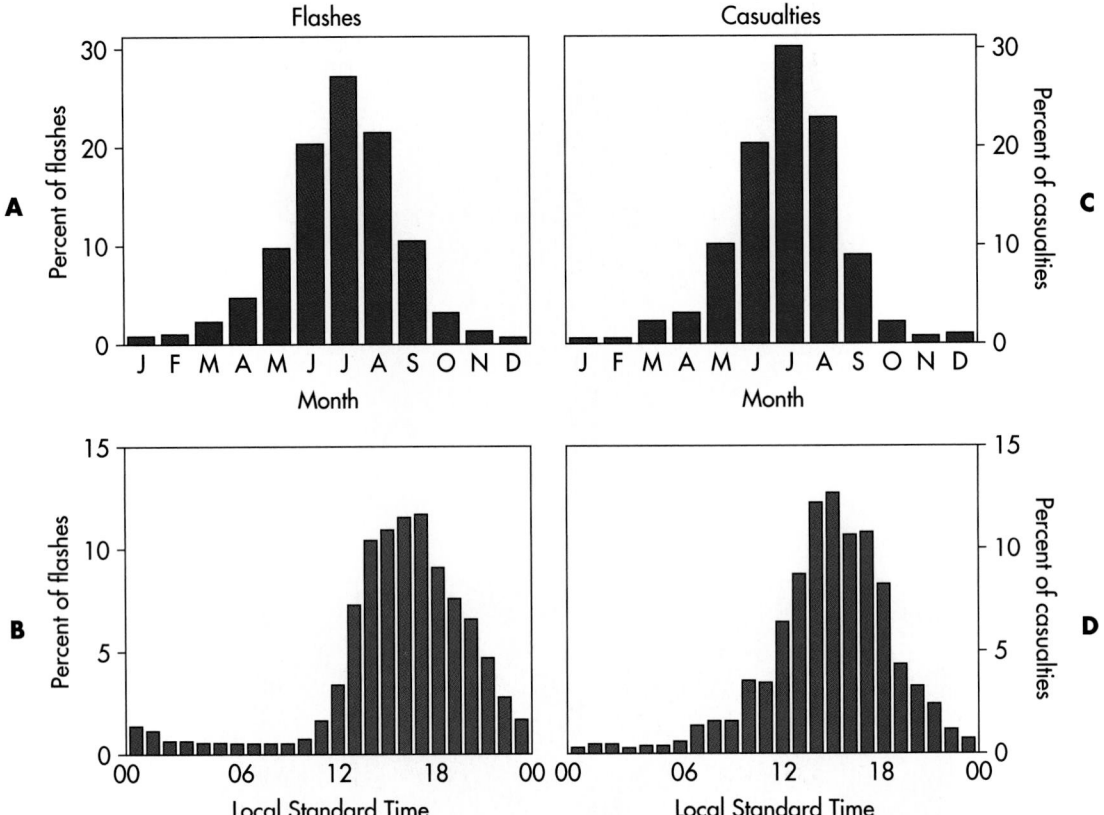

Figure 3-2 A, Monthly distribution of U.S. cloud-to-ground lightning from 1992 to 1995 from a lightning detection network. **B,** Hourly distribution of cloud-to-ground lightning from networks in four U.S. locations. **C** and **D,** Monthly and hourly distributions of lightning casualties from 1959 to 1994 in the United States. (**A** *from Orville RE, Silver AC: Mon Wea Rev 125:631, 1997;* **B** *from López RE, Holle RL: Mon Wea Rev 114:1288, 1986;* **C** *and* **D** *from Curran EB, Holle RL, López RE: Lightning fatalities, injuries, and damage reports in the United States from 1959-1994, NOAA Tech Memo NWS SW-193, 1997.*)

TABLE 3-1. Weather-Related 30-Year Average Deaths (1965-1994), and 1994 Weather Casualties; Order is by 30-Year Average Deaths, Then 1994 Deaths

WEATHER TYPE	DEATHS PER YEAR	1994 DEATHS	1994 INJURIES
Flash flood	139	59	33
River flood		32	14
Lightning	87	69	484
Tornado	82	69	1067
Hurricane	27	9	45
Extreme temperatures		81	298
Winter weather		31	2690
Thunderstorm wind		17	315
Other high wind		12	61
Fog		3	99
Other		6	99
TOTALS		388	5165

ern states to Rocky Mountain and plains states. The top two rates are from Wyoming and New Mexico; these states were 35th and 21st in number of casualties. Wyoming had most of its casualties in the 1960s and 1970s, and almost none since then. Southeastern states often have high rankings in both casualties and casualty rates (Figure 3-4, *A* and *B*). The only states in the top 10 of both casualties and casualty rate are Florida, Colorado, and North Carolina. Detailed listings of deaths and injuries by state, as well as death and injury rates per state, are in Curran et al.[41] This reference also contains information on the distribution of lightning damage reports, which has a high concentration over the plains states.

Two lightning fatality studies for the United States had substantially similar results to Figure 3-3. Duclos and Sanderson[44] used data from the National Center for Health Statistics, and Mogil et al[92] used *Storm Data.* Single-state maps by county were compiled for Florida,[44] North Carolina,[75] Michigan,[48] and Colorado.[82,87] In other countries, fatalities divided by political boundaries were

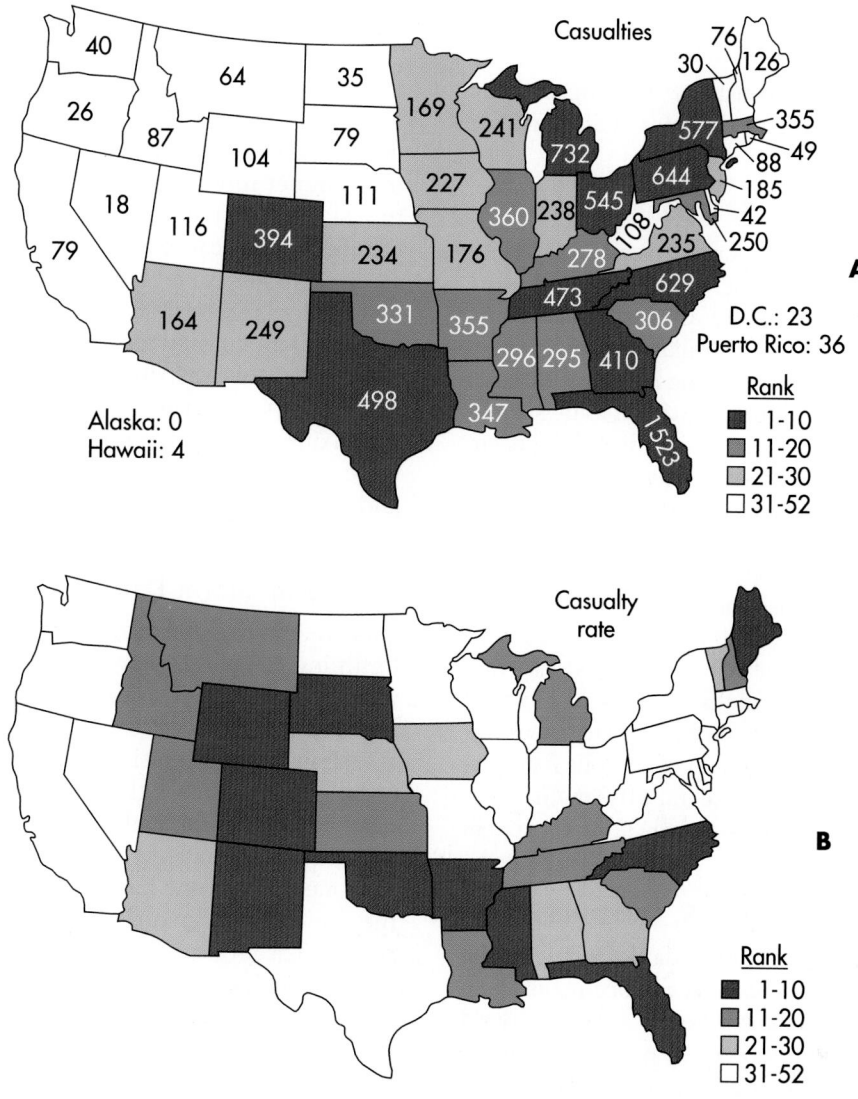

Figure 3-3 Rank of each state in lightning casualties (deaths and injuries combined) from 1959 to 1994. **A,** Casualties per state. **B,** Casualties weighted by state population. (*From Curran EB, Holle RL, López RE:* Lightning fatalities, injuries, and damage reports in the United States from 1959-1994, *NOAA Tech Memo NWS SW-193, 1997.*)

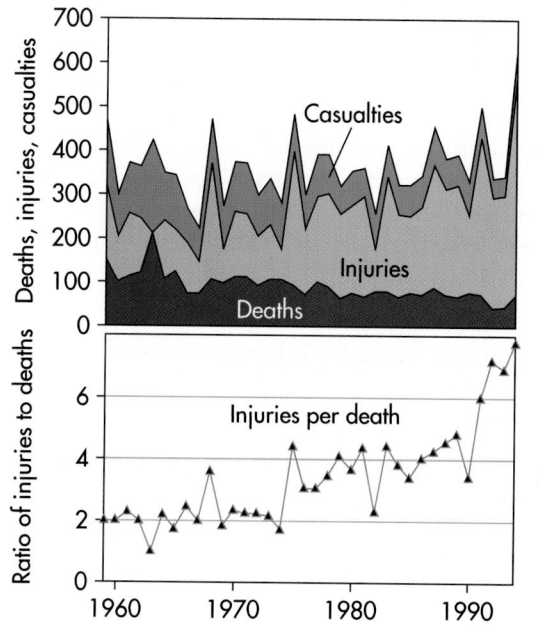

Figure 3-4 **A,** Number of casualties, deaths, and injuries. **B,** Ratio of injuries to deaths from 1959 to 1994 in the United States. (*From Curran EB, Holle RL, López RE:* Lightning fatalities, injuries, and damage reports in the United States from 1959-1994, *NOAA Tech Memo NWS SW-193, 1997.*)

developed for Canada by Hornstein,[68] for Singapore by Pakiam et al,[101] for Australia by Coates et al,[27] and for France by Gourbière et al.[55]

Monthly Variations of U.S. Casualties

By month, lightning casualties peak during July (Figure 3-2, C). The percentages increase gradually before July, then decline more quickly after the maximum. Cloud-to-ground flashes show similar features (Figure 3-2, A). Seasonal maps of lightning casualty rates in Curran et al[41] show the summer patterns to be similar to annual maps. During other seasons, lightning casualty rates are higher in southern states. Casualty rates in the northeast are low except during the summer, whereas they are highest on the West Coast during autumn and winter.

A July maximum was also found in prior *Storm Data* studies, as well as a slower increase before and a faster decrease after July.[44,48,82,87,92] August maxima were found in Florida by Duclos et al[44] and Holle et al.[64] January has the largest number of Australian fatalities, resulting from the reversal of seasons from the United States.[27] The Singapore fatality maxima in November and April are similar to the annual cycle of local thunderstorms.[101]

Time of Day Variations of U.S. Casualties

By time of day, most lightning casualties occur in the afternoon (Figure 3-2, D); two thirds occur between 1200 and 1800 LST. They show a steady increase toward a maximum at 1600 LST, followed by a slower decrease after the maximum. Lightning flashes in Figure 3-2, B, showed a faster increase to the afternoon maximum than shown here for casualties. Lightning occurs most often in the afternoon because the ground is heated most strongly by the sun during that time period. As a result, vertical cumulus clouds form and produce lightning when they are tall enough to have tops colder than freezing temperatures. Narrower distributions of casualties centered in the afternoon are apparent in the Rockies, Southeast, and Northeast compared with the broader time series in the plains and Midwest.[41]

In the evening and at night (1800 to 0559 LST), casualties are most frequent in the plains, upper midwest, and some populous eastern states.[41] Of the 29 deaths from 0000 to 0559 LST, 59% occurred when people were in a house set on fire by lightning, and 21% occurred when people were camping in tents. Casualties in the morning are spread widely across the country. Casualties during the afternoon resemble Figure 3-2, D, since these are the most frequent hours for deaths (67%) and injuries (63%).

In winter, casualties are spread erratically through the day.[41] Spring casualties occur during nearly the same afternoon hours as for the year, but there is a secondary peak before noon. Summer casualties follow the annual cycle. Autumn casualties have a broad afternoon peak and a secondary morning peak. The casualties are spread more widely through the day outside of the summer months. This spread can be attributed to two factors. First, lightning is less concentrated during the afternoon because the ground is not heated as much as in summer. As a result, more thunderstorms are formed by large-scale traveling disturbances. Second, the number of casualties, especially in winter, is much smaller, so that distributions are affected more by a small number of cases.

Maximum lightning impacts from 1400 to 1600 LST were documented by Duclos and Sanderson,[44] Ferrett and Ojala,[48] and López and Holle.[87] Duclos and Sanderson[44] found an 1800 LST peak in North Carolina deaths.

Additional Storm Data Information

Table 3-2 shows that males were much more frequent lightning casualties than were females. Similar ratios were found in the United States,[44,45,64,75] Singapore,[101] and England and Wales.[46]

The most common situation was for only one victim to be involved in a lightning incident. This is an important contributor to the underreporting of lightning casualties. For incidents involving deaths only, 91% had just one fatality; the largest single case resulted from the 1963 crash of an airliner in Maryland that killed 81 people. The largest number of injuries at one event was 90 at a Michigan campground.[48] The same tendency for single victims was noted in the United States,[87] Singapore,[101] and Australia.[27]

According to *Storm Data*, nearly half of all lightning damages are between $5000 and $50,000.[41] However, these amounts are much larger than insured losses paid for claims by homeowners and small businesses.[66,73]

Storm Data Trends in Lightning Casualties

From 1959 to 1994, *Storm Data* shows a slow decrease in lightning deaths, while injuries increase (Figure 3-4). As a result, the ratio of injuries to deaths steadily increases. The typical ratio of injuries to deaths had been between 2:1 and 4:1. However, an uncertainty exists, since more injuries are missed than are deaths.[66,88,92] Cherington et al[25] found that a ratio of 10 injuries to one death applied in a thorough search of Colorado hospital and emergency room visits. There are additional in-

TABLE 3-2. Casualty Information in Storm Data from 1959 to 1994

TOPIC	DEATHS	INJURIES	CASUALTIES
Males	84%	82%	83%
One victim per event	91%	68%	68%

juries to persons whose visits are not documented by a medical clinic or if they are not treated. As a result, it is likely that a 10:1 ratio of injuries to deaths is the better estimate.

After population growth was taken into account (normalization), several major trends were identified.[83,84] A 30% decrease in the number of deaths per million persons was attributed to improved forecasts and warnings, better awareness of the lightning threat, more substantial buildings available for safe refuge, and/or other socioeconomic changes. An additional 40% reduction in normalized deaths may be due to improved medical care and emergency communications. The injury rate decreased only 8%; this lowered rate may be due to transfer of some potential deaths into injuries as a result of better emergency communications, medical attention, and other factors.

Notable decreases in deaths were documented with long-term data sets in England and Wales,[46] England and Wales compared with Australia,[53] and Singapore.[101] Australian deaths increased during the years 1825 to 1918, then decreased through 1991.[27]

Twentieth-Century Trends in Lightning Deaths

Another difficulty in determining the number of casualties and deaths is changes in reporting systems since the turn of the last century. Beginning in 1900, the Bureau of the Census established a national registration of vital statistics for deaths that included states, Washington, D.C., and large cities; annual death statistics, including lightning as a cause of death, have been compiled and published by the U.S. government. Although only 10 states and several cities reported to the Bureau of the Census in 1900, the number of states increased gradually until all states and Washington, D.C., were covered by 1935. *Mortality Statistics* was published be-

fore 1937 and the series *Vital Statistics of the United States* was published after that. Starting with the 1945 records published in 1947, data collection was changed from the Bureau of the Census to the Public Health Service. Since then, data have come from the National Center for Health Statistics, Centers for Disease Control and Prevention, Public Health Service, of the Department of Health and Human Services.[85,104]

The number of lightning deaths reported since 1900 is shown in Figure 3-5, *A*. During the first 20 years, annual deaths increased from less than 100 to about 450 because of an increase in reporting states. In comparing the increase in deaths with the increased reporting population, the fatality increase appears exceptionally large. During the 1920s and 1930s there were about 400 lightning deaths per year, whereas recently it has been less than 100 per year. There has been a persistent drop in deaths since 1944. The same dramatic decline since 1940 was noted by others.[12,44,92]

The effect of changes in population can be taken into account by dividing by the population. Figure 3-5, *B*, shows the number of lightning deaths per million people per year. In the earlier part of the series, year-to-year fluctuations are relatively large, probably because of random inclusion of reporting states with different demographic and climatic conditions. However, since 1925, the fluctuations are consistently smaller and more regular, and they decrease as the death rate decreases. The normalized time series and an exponential curve fitted to the data indicate a decrease during the twentieth century from more than 6 to a low of 0.4 deaths per million people.

Effect of Rural-to-Urban Migration

Before the turn of the last century, lightning deaths appeared to occur often in rural settings.[63] Since then, the

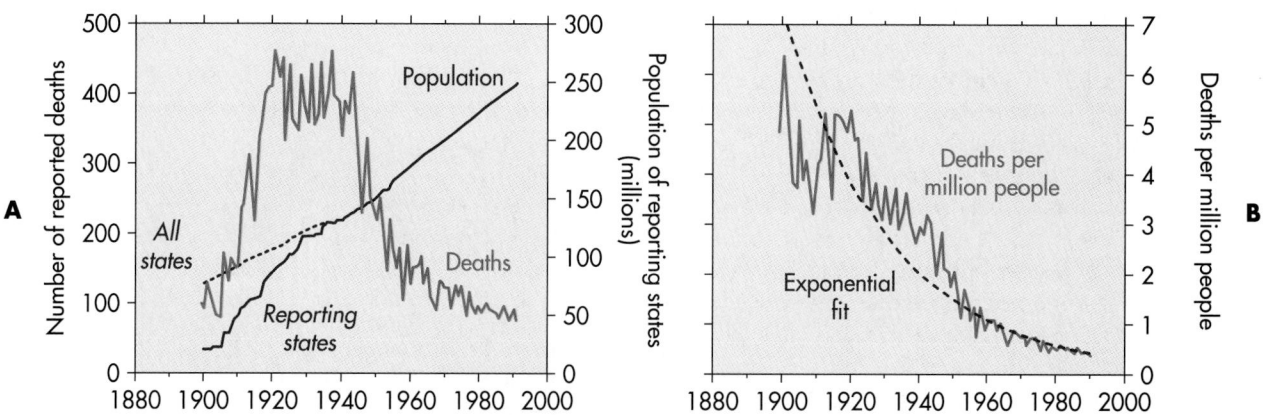

Figure 3-5 **A,** Annual lightning deaths reported by Bureau of the Census and Public Health Service from 1900 to 1991 *(red)*. Solid blue line is population of reporting states and District of Columbia; dashed is total population of contiguous United States and District of Columbia. **B,** Time series of lightning deaths normalized by population of reporting states *(red)* and exponential function *(blue)* fitted to data. *(From López RE, Holle RL: J Climate 11:2070, 1998.)*

percentage of the U.S. population in rural areas (but not the actual population) has dramatically decreased. Figure 3-6, *A*, shows that the percentage of the population living in rural areas since 1890 decreased from 60% in 1900 to 25% in 1990. The only significant departures from the exponential decrease were a slowing in the 1930s and early 1940s during the Great Depression, and an acceleration of the trend in the 1950s and 1960s with increased urbanization after World War II and the Korean War.

The rural population curve is superimposed on the adjusted normalized lightning-death plot in Figure 3-6, *B*. The remarkable agreement leads to a conclusion that the secular exponential decrease in population-adjusted deaths is closely related to the relative reduction in rural population. This long-term decrease has been noted by several authors, and a decrease in rural population has been hypothesized as a factor, together with improved home electrical systems, which include substantial grounding, as well as medical treatment, education, and meteorologic warnings.[12,44,83,87,92] These factors are also linked to the decrease in rural population resulting from emigration to cities or enhanced urbanization of rural areas.

Similar decreases in lightning death rates have been found in two other countries. Figure 3-7, *A*, shows the decrease for the last century in Canada compared with the United States. The Canadian death rate is probably less because of the lower flash rate for this higher-latitude country. Both the United States and Canada had a proportional shift of people from rural to urban regions. In contrast, the shift to urban population for Spain was delayed by several decades (Figure 3-7, *B*) because of a national policy of maintaining rural populations. However, when industrialization began, the lightning death rate plunged.

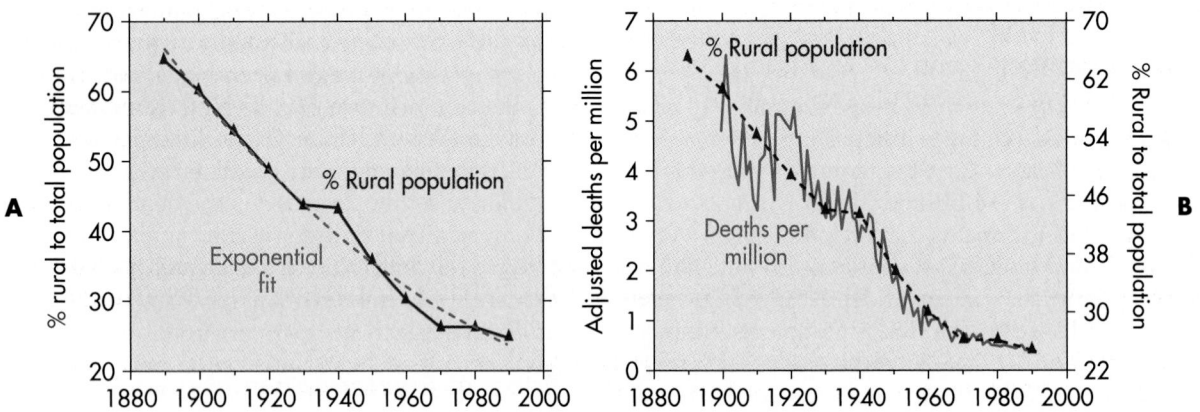

Figure 3-6 A, Percent of contiguous U.S. population living in rural areas since 1890 *(solid line)*, and an exponential function fitted to data *(dashed line)*. **B,** Adjusted yearly lightning deaths normalized by population, as in **A.** *Dashed line,* Percent of population in rural areas. *(From López RE, Holle RL: J Climate 11:2070, 1998.)*

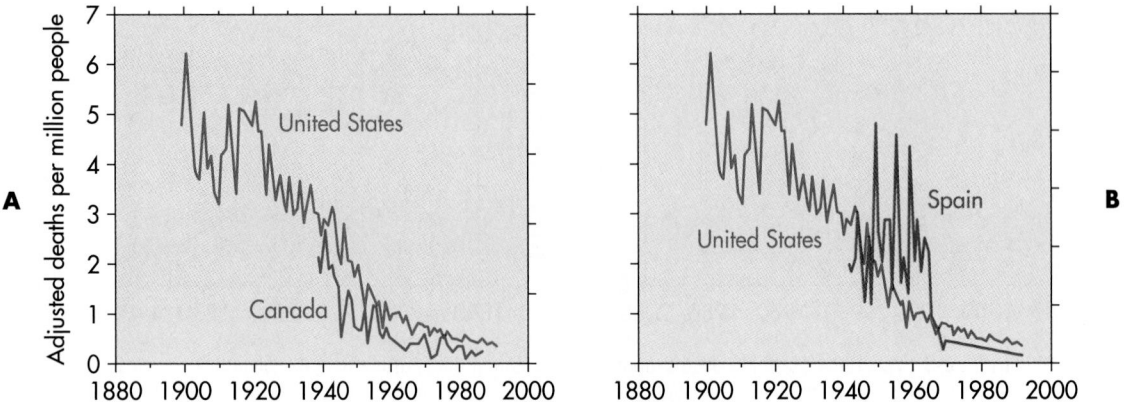

Figure 3-7 Time series of yearly lightning deaths normalized by population for United States and Canada **(A)** and Spain **(B).**

Types of Lightning Casualty Incidents

The preceding analyses suggest a link between the shift from rural to urban settings and the number of lightning casualties. *Storm Data* has the location of lightning victims since 1959, but the categories are not especially helpful because 40% of its locations are unknown. It is necessary to go beyond location to discover a person's activity to better identify the type of incident.

A key to understanding the influence of the urban migration can be found in analysis of Kretzer (1895), who documented 1043 lightning deaths and injuries from 1891 to 1894. An overall impression was developed for each entry as to whether the situation was rural or urban.[63] It was not possible to make this determination in roughly one third of the cases. The verbal narratives in *Storm Data* from 1991 to 1994 were used in a similar analysis. Events were subdivided by type of incident based on both activity and location.[63]

In the 1890s, rural deaths were much more frequent than urban (Figure 3-8, *A*). Indoor fatalities were the most frequent; 23% of all deaths were inside houses. The next largest types were outdoors and agricultural incidents, whereas recreation and sports incidents were virtually nonexistent.

In the 1990s, rural settings account for a much smaller proportion of casualties (Figure 3-8, *B*), and agricultural incidents are much less frequent than 100 years ago. Only 2% of modern deaths were to people inside houses, one tenth of the percentage a century earlier. Outdoors has become the largest type of incident, with the most frequent incidents occurring under or near trees (15% of all deaths) and in the yard or garden of a house. A high percentage of incidents occurs during recreation; these cases are dominated by beach, water, and camping situations. Sports incidents involve participating in and observing sporting events; many involved golf.[63]

These comparisons agree with the influence of the rural-to-urban migration on lightning casualties in the United States. Rural casualties are now half as frequent as urban cases. The inside of a house is no longer as dangerous as it was. This trend is most likely a result of grounding by modern wiring and plumbing. Recreation and sports have become relatively greater contributors to the population at risk from lightning.[27,82,87]

Worldwide Lightning Fatalities

Cautious extrapolation of U.S. results to the world can be considered. There were over 400 lightning deaths a year early in the twentieth century in the United States, at a rate exceeding 6 deaths per million people (see Figs. 3-5 and 3-7). These often occurred in agricultural incidents in rural settings or inside buildings before widespread installation of wiring and plumbing.

Since the rates and trends are similar in Canada and Spain, they can be considered typical of much of Europe and other industrialized, urbanized countries. However, many people around the world rely on labor-intensive agriculture and live in dwellings with minimal grounding. The earlier rates from the United States could be appropriate for populous tropical and subtropical areas of Africa, South America, and Southeast Asia, where there is frequent lightning.

About 100 lightning deaths per year currently occur in the United States. This number would be approximately 1000 if the U.S. population was still rural, practiced labor-intensive agriculture, and lived in dwellings with minimal lightning protection. So it might be reasonable to expect that the worldwide lightning death rate is at least 10,000 per year, since a large number of people live in such situations. A ratio of 5 to 10 injuries per death gives a worldwide total of 50,000 to 100,000 injuries a year from lightning.

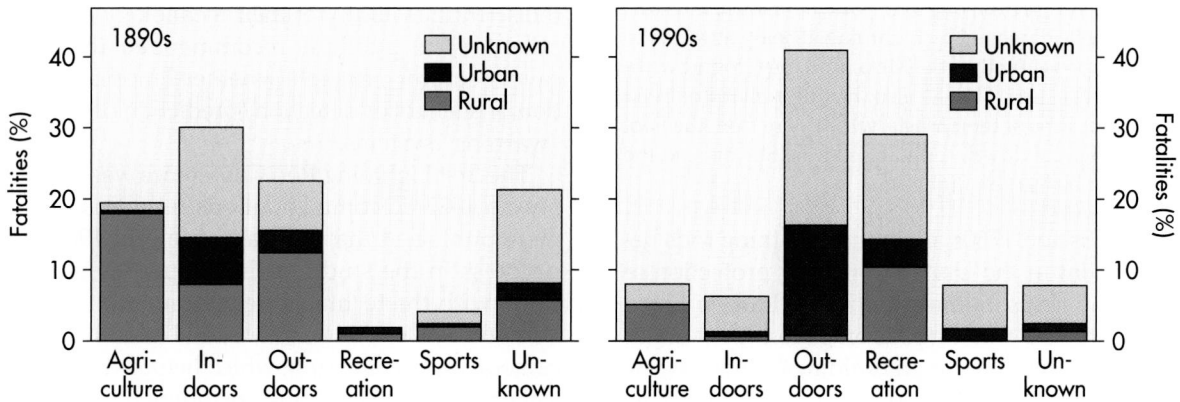

Figure 3-8 Types of U.S. lightning casualty incidents (%) from 1891 to 1894 compared with 1991-1994. (*From Holle RL, López RE, Navarro BC: U.S. lightning deaths, injuries, and damages in the 1890s compared to the 1990s, National Oceanic and Atmospheric Administration Tech Memo, ERL pending, 2000.*)

EARLY SCIENTIFIC STUDIES AND INVENTION OF THE LIGHTNING ROD[49,50]

The study of electric phenomena is often traced to the publication of Gilbert's *De Magnete* in London in 1600. Experiments in France and Germany and by members of the Royal Society of London led to the invention of the Leyden jar in 1745.

Benjamin Franklin is generally regarded as the father of electric science and during his lifetime was known as the American Newton. The reason he was accepted into the French and English courts around the time of the American Revolution was not because he was an ambassador from America but because he was considered to be one of the foremost scientists of his time. Franklin was elected to every major scientific society at the time and received medals of honor from France and England for his scientific contributions.

Before his work, it was thought that two distinct types of electric phenomena existed. Franklin's work unified these two forces, and he is responsible for renaming them as positive and negative charges.[50] He also proved with numerous experiments that lightning was an electric phenomenon and that thunderclouds are electrically charged, as demonstrated by the famous kite and key experiment.[49] He invented the lightning rod and announced its use in 1753 in *Poor Richard's Almanack*:

It has pleased God in his Goodness to Mankind, at length to discover to them the Means of securing their Habitation and other Buildings from Mischief by Thunder and Lightning. The Method is this: Provide a small Iron Rod (It may be made of the Rod-iron used by the Nailers) but of such a Length, that one End being three or four Feet in the moist Ground, the other may be six or eight Feet above the highest Part of the Building. To the upper End of the Rod fasten a Foot of brass Wire the Size of a common Knitting-needle, sharpened to a fine Point; the Rod may be secured to the House by a few small Staples. If the House or Barn be long, there may be a Rod and Point at each End, and a middling Wire along the Ridge from one to the other. A House thus furnished will not be damaged by Lightning, it being attracted to the Points, and passing thro the Metal into the Ground without hurting any Thing. Vessels also, having a sharp pointed rod fix'd on the Tops of their Masts, with a Wire from the Foot of the Rod reaching down, round one of the Shrouds, to the Water, will not be hurt by Lightning.

In the 1750s and 1760s, the use of lightning rods became prevalent in the United States for protection of buildings and ships. Some scientists in Europe urged the installation of lightning rods on government buildings, churches, and other high buildings. However, religious advocates maintained that it would be blasphemy to install such devices on church steeples, since the churches received divine protection. Because of this divine protection, some towns chose to store munitions in their churches, leading on more than one occasion to significant destruction and loss of life when the churches were hit by lightning.

Part of the delay in installing lightning rods in England may have been due to British distrust of the scientific theories of the upstart, newly independent United States. Years and numerous unsuccessful trials with English designs were required before the Franklin rod became accepted on Her Majesty's ships and buildings.[16]

At one time, lightning rods were theorized to be diffusers of electric charges that could neutralize a storm cloud passing overhead, thus averting a lightning stroke. This theory was in part an outgrowth of the observation of St. Elmo's fire, an aura appearing around the tip of lightning rods and ships' masts during a thunderstorm. This phenomenon is caused by an electron discharge that results from the strong electromagnetic field induced around the glowing object.

Properly installed lightning rods and lightning protection systems do not "attract" lightning, but protect a building by allowing the current from a lightning strike that would have occurred, regardless of the protection system, to flow harmlessly through the system to the ground instead of into or through the building, which often causes more extensive damage.[51] It has not been uncommon for charlatans to take advantage of the fear of lightning and the danger of lightning-caused fires. In the past, they drove from farm to farm offering to "discharge" the lightning rods on the barns and homes for a fee. Lightning protection still remains an area of great controversy, with few of the lightning codes verified by true research. Some of the recent codes (written by the lightning protection industry) now do more to protect buildings and shelters but unfortunately may actually increase the risk for those seeking "shelter" in bus, pool, rain, or golf types of structures, not only by increasing the sheltering person's effective height but also by increasing the chances of side-flash from the lightning protection wiring. Systems that claim to "predict" lightning rather than detect it have yet to prove the scientific validity of their technology by achieving patents. The public is recommended to follow the caveat emptor principle whether it applies to protection of shelters or detection/prediction of lightning by "warning" systems.

The first Lightning Rod Conference was held in London in 1882. Recommendations from this conference were published that year and again in 1905. Further progress in the study of the properties of lightning came with the technical development of Sir Charles Vernon Boy's rotating camera and Dufour's high-speed cathode ray oscillograph, which helped delineate physical properties of lightning, including the direction and speed of the strokes.

Certain countries developed codes of practice for lightning protection (Germany 1924, United States

1929, Britain 1943, British colonies 1965). A variety of materials, including copper, aluminum, and iron, are recommended by these codes, which also specify the measurements and construction of the protective system, depending on the height, location, and construction of the structure to be protected. The most recent U.S. code revision was the National Fire Protection Act of 1993, written by lightning protection practitioners.

Lightning strokes vary in power and frequency, depending on the terrain and geographic location.[90] Complicated formulas have been devised to take into account the relative frequency of strikes in an area; the height, construction, and design of the building; and the degree of protection desired, depending on whether it is a storage shed, house, school, hospital, or munitions factory.[73]

A lightning protection system should be designed to take into account these factors plus the economic considerations of construction. Including a system in the initial design and construction is always easier and less expensive than modifying a completed building. In addition, except where prohibited by code, the owner may decide that a lightning protection system is not worth the expense, for example, for a mountain retreat that is seldom visited.[73,90] An excellent noncommercial source for discussion of these risks is www.lightningsafety.com.

PHYSICS OF LIGHTNING STROKE

Lightning Discharge[51-53,90,114,118]

The study of lightning discharge and formation is extremely complex and involves an entire branch of physics and meteorology. We therefore illustrate here the simplified and most common mechanism of thundercloud formation and lightning strike.

Thunderstorms can be created by a number of factors that produce vertical updrafts. These ingredients are usually caused by cold fronts, large-scale upward motions, sea and lake breezes, lifting by mountains, and afternoon heating of warm, moist air (Figure 3-9, B).[52,114]

As warm air rises, turbulence and induced friction cause complex redistribution of charges within the cloud (Figure 3-9, C). Water droplets and ice crystals within the cloud acquire and increase their individual charges. A complex layering of charges, with large potential differences between the layers, results from the interaction between charged particles and internal and external electrical fields within the cloud.

Generally lower layers of the thundercloud become negatively charged relative to the earth, particularly when the storm occurs over a flat surface. The earth, which normally is negatively charged relative to the atmosphere, has a strong positive charge induced as the negatively charged thunderstorm passes overhead. The induced positive charge tends to flow as an upward current into trees, tall buildings, or people in the area of the thunderstorm cloud and may actually course upward as "upward streamers."

Normally, discharge of the potential difference is discouraged by the strong insulatory nature of air. However, when the potential difference between charges within the clouds or between the thundercloud and ground becomes sufficient, the charge may be dissipated as lightning.

A lightning stroke begins as a relatively weak and slow downward leader from the cloud (Figure 3-9, D). Although the tip of the leader may be luminous, the stepped leader itself is barely discernible with the unassisted eye. The leader travels at about one-third the speed of light (1×10^8 m/sec), and the potential difference between the tip and the earth ranges from 10 to 200 million volts. The leader ionizes a pathway that contains superheated ions, both positive and negative, thus forming a plasma column of very low resistance. It travels with relatively short branched steps, going down about 50 m (164 feet) and then retreating upwards. The next time it goes down, it fills the original ionized path but branches at the end to go down another 50 m and then retreat again. This up-and-down, poly-branching process continues until the leader comes to within 30 to 50 m (98 to 164 feet) of the ground. Since lightning follows this ionized path, its tip "sees" only objects within about a 30- to 50-m radius, meaning that the hill or tower 200 feet (61 m) away from a person will not be "seen" by the lightning as a potential target.

As the tip of the lightning gets closer to the earth with the large potential at its tip, more concentrated areas of induced charge accumulate up on earth, particularly at the peaks of tall, relatively sharp objects. Several upward streamers (Figure 3-9, E) may rise vertically from these objects toward the downward leader head. Ultimately one, or a small number, of the upward streamers will contact the downward leader, thus completing a lightning channel of low resistance between cloud and ground. The process of the downward leader joining with the upward streamer(s) is called *attachment*. There is often more than one point of attachment to the ground.[107]

As the low-resistance channel is formed by attachment, the potential difference between cloud and ground effectively disappears and the energy available is dissipated in an avalanche of charge between cloud and ground. This avalanche is referred to as the *return stroke* (Figure 3-9, F) and is highly luminous. Subsequent to the discharge through the return stroke, the channel remains attached for a small amount of time, and with quick redistribution of charge from other regions of the cloud to the top of the channel (via J- and K-intracloud streamers), further return strokes may occur. Thus a lightning flash may be made up of multiple

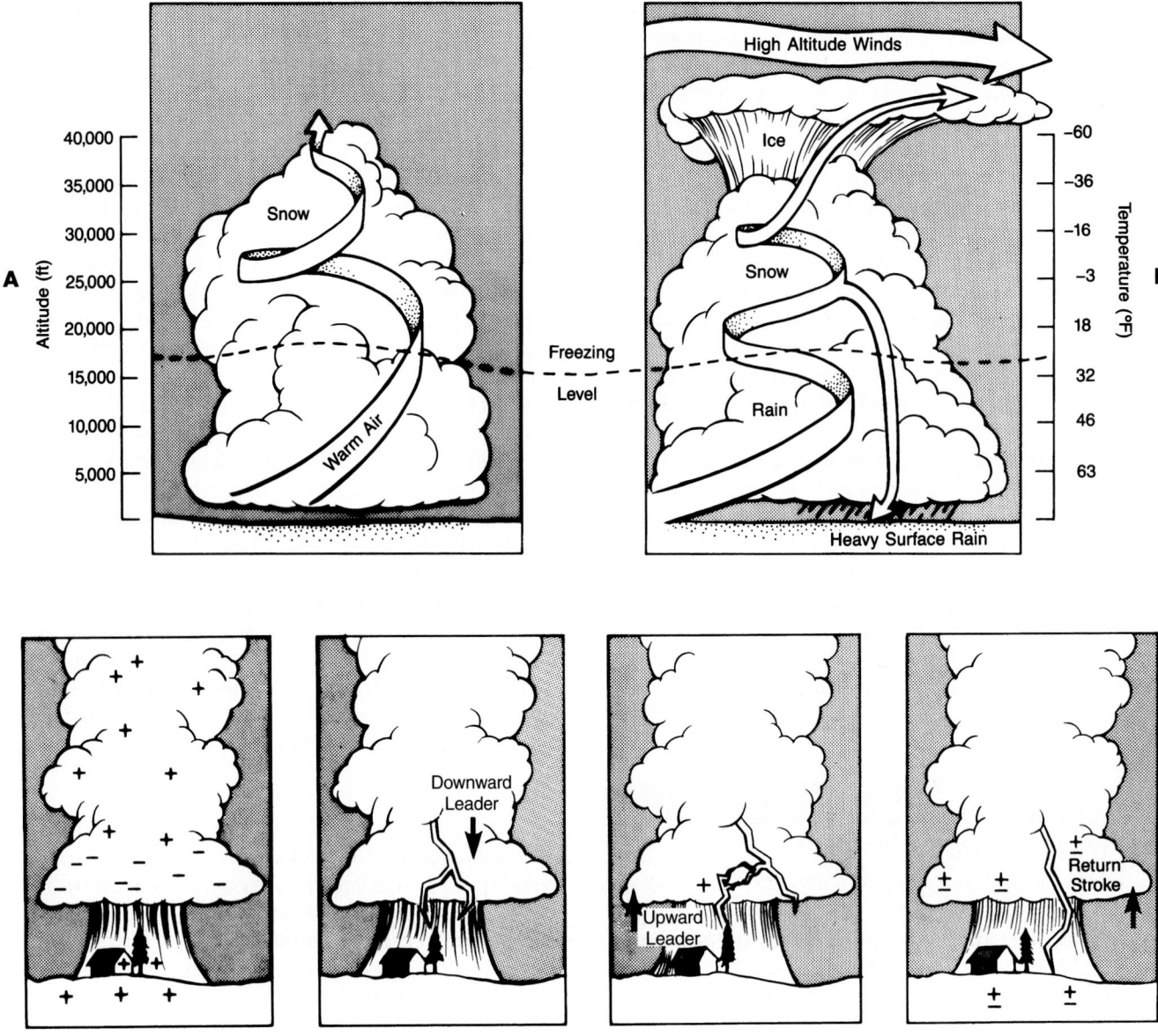

Figure 3-9 **A,** Warm, low-pressure air rises and condenses into a cumulonimbus cloud. **B,** Typical anvil-shaped thundercloud. **C,** Water droplets within the cloud accumulate and layer changes. **D,** Relatively weak and slow-stepped downward leader initiates the lightning strike. **E,** Positive upward streamer rises from the ground to meet the stepped leader. **F,** Return stroke rushes from the ground to the cloud.

strokes (1 to 30, mean 4 to 5) and is perceived by the eye as flickering of the main channel.

When a very tall building is involved, or when high mountains rise into the clouds, the leader stroke may initiate from the building or mountain rather than from the cloud. In such cases, a joining stroke is rarely seen initiating from the cloud. The channel of ions formed by the leader stroke is maintained as a continuous stroke as the return stroke (misnamed in this instance) travels in the same direction from the ground or object to the cloud, dissipating the charge difference.

The tip of the downward leader is the most luminous of the sequence of strokes in each lightning discharge, since a huge amount of energy must be expended to overcome air resistance and ionize a channel. Because of the relative slowness and brilliance of the leader, lightning is perceived as traveling from the cloud to the earth, although the vast majority of energy is actually dissipated in the opposite direction with the return strokes. The direction of the return stroke is not visually perceived because of its tremendous speed and is recognized merely as an instantaneous brightening or flickering of the ionized pathway. Lightning may vary in color, either from the excitation of nitrogen atoms in the atmosphere (radiant light energy released as a bluish or reddish afterglow), or because the particles of dust through which the lightning passes are high in ion or mineral content.

Diameter and Temperature of Lightning[52,114]

Many techniques could be used to measure the diameter or temperature of the lightning stroke. Unfortunately, all measurement techniques have artifact problems. Visual measurement of the stroke using standard photography usually shows the diameter of the main body of the stroke to be about 2 to 3 cm.

The diameter of the arc channel is sometimes measured indirectly, using measurements of holes and strips of damage that lightning produces when it hits aluminum airplane wings, buildings, or trees. Measurements vary from 0.003 to 8 cm, depending on the material destroyed, with hard metallic structures sustaining smaller punctures than do relatively softer objects, such as trees. The ionized sheath around the tip of the bright leader stroke has never been measured but is estimated to be 3 to 20 m (10 to 66 feet) in diameter.

The temperature of the lightning stroke varies with the diameter of the stroke and has been calculated to be about 8000° C (14,432° F). Others estimate the temperature to be as high as 50,000° C (90,032° F). In a few milliseconds the temperature falls to 2000° to 3000° C (3632° to 5432° F), that of a normal high-voltage electric arc.

Forms of Lightning

Lightning occurs in many forms. As described previously, the most common is streak lightning (Figure 3-10). Sheet lightning is a shapeless flash of light that represents lightning discharges within and between clouds. Sheet lightning may also be seen when lightning occurs over the horizon. Ribbon lightning is streak lightning driven by winds of the thunderstorm; the ionized air channel moves so rapidly across the earth that the successive secondary or return strokes seem to parallel one another. Bead lightning occurs when different areas of ionization and charge persist, lending a bead-like appearance to the afterstrokes. Another possible explanation of bead lightning may be perception of the bright end-on appearance of portions of a very jagged stroke.

The most unusual, least understood, and least predictable type of lightning is ball lightning. Ball lightning is usually described as a softball-sized orange to white globe. It may enter a plane, ship, or house, travel down the hallway, injure some people and objects and not others that it encounters, and exit out another door, chimney, or window, explode with a loud bang, or exhibit other bizarre behavior.[9,16]

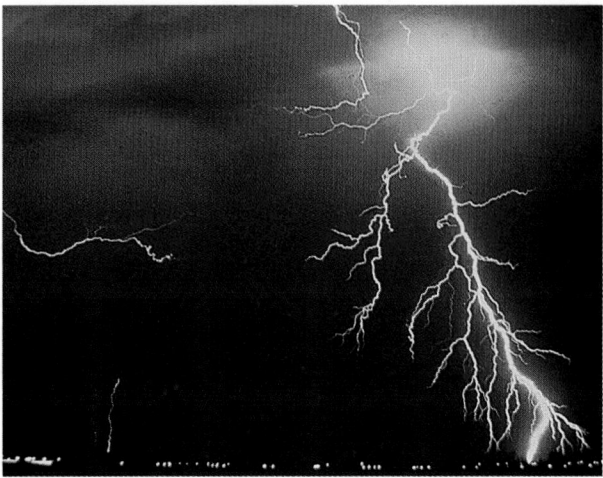

Figure 3-10 Example of classic streak lightning.

Lightning may be either positive or negative in charge. Negative lightning is the more common. Positive lightning tends to occur during the winter, at the beginning of very violent thunderstorms, and with tornadoes, and may have a very different injury profile from negative lightning. Positive lightning may be more likely to occur when there is particulate matter in the air.

Thunder

Thunder is formed when shock waves result from the almost explosive expansion of air heated and ionized by the lightning stroke.[52,114] The following are accepted statements:

1. Cloud-to-ground lightning flashes produce the loudest thunder.
2. Thunder is seldom heard over distances greater than 10 miles (16 km).
3. The time interval between the perception of lightning and the first sound of thunder can be used to estimate distance from the lightning stroke.
4. Atmospheric turbulence reduces audibility of the thunder.
5. The intensity of a pattern of thunder in one geographic location appears different from the pattern in another location.
6. The pitch of thunder deepens as the rumble persists.

The thunder clap from a lightning flash that is close by is heard as a sharp crack. Distant thunder rumbles as the sound waves are refracted and modified by the thunderstorm's turbulence.[114] Using the difference in speeds between light and sound gives an estimate of the distance to the lightning stroke. To obtain the approximate distance to the flash in miles, a person can take the difference in seconds between the perception of the flash and the rumble and divide by five (flash-to-bang method).[65,116]

MECHANISMS OF INJURY BY LIGHTNING[8,9,17,34]

Lightning is directly dangerous for three reasons: electrical effects, heat production, and concussive force. In addition, lightning may injure indirectly via forest fires, house fires, and explosions or by felling objects such as trees onto occupied homes and automobiles. Only injuries directly caused by lightning are discussed here: direct hit, splash, contact, step voltage, blunt trauma,[34] and the newly described upward streamer.[1]

A direct strike is most likely to hit a person in the open who has been unable to find a safe location.

A more frequent cause of injury is a splash. Splash injuries occur when lightning that has hit a tree or building splashes onto a victim who may have found shelter nearby.[53] The current, seeking the path of least resistance, may jump to a person whose body has less resistance than the tree or object that the lightning had initially contacted. There are multiple reports of side flashes indoors from metal objects, including plumbing and telephones.[1a,105,110] Splashes may also occur from person to person when several people are standing close together. On occasion, splashes occur from a fence or other long conductive object that was hit by lightning some distance away. Groups of animals have been killed as they stood near a fence or sought shelter under trees.[53]

Contact injury occurs when the person is holding onto an object that is either directly hit or splashed by lightning.

Step voltage, also called stride voltage or ground current, is produced when lightning hits the ground or an object nearby.[10] The current spreads like a wave in a pond, diminishing as the radius from the strike increases. Contrary to the public's belief that the Earth's surface is a decent "ground" (a good absorber of electrical energy), in reality, it is an excellent resistor of electrical energy. As walking bags of saltwater, animals and humans often have less resistance than the ground. If a person has one foot closer to the strike and one foot further away, a large potential difference may exist between them. Often the current will pass up and through the lower resistance circuit made by the victim's legs and body rather than stay in the ground. Swimmers may also be affected by this mechanism as the current passes through them in the water. Four-legged animals with longer distances between their front and back legs are at even greater risk.

Although ground current is less likely to produce fatalities than are direct hits or splashes, multiple victims and injuries are frequent. Large groups have been injured on baseball fields, at racetracks, while hiking, and during military maneuvers.[16]

Persons may suffer blunt injury either by being close to the concussive force of the shock wave produced as lightning strikes nearby or if ground current or some other mechanism induces an opisthotonic contraction. Victims have been witnessed to have been thrown tens of yards by either mechanism. In addition, some have theorized that the person who is struck by lightning may suffer from explosive and implosive forces created by the thunderclap, with resulting contusions and pressure injuries, including tympanic membrane rupture.

Injury caused by being the conduit for an upward leader, even though it may not contact a downward leader to complete a lightning pathway, has recently been described.[35a]

PATHOPHYSIOLOGY OF LIGHTNING INJURY*

It is necessary to distinguish between lightning and generator-produced high-voltage electrical injuries, since there are significant differences between the mechanisms of injuries and their treatment. Although lightning is an electrical phenomenon and is governed by the laws of physics, it accounts for a unique spectrum of induced diseases that are best understood relative to specific physical properties of lightning.

Kouwenhoven determined six factors that affect the type and severity of injury encountered with electrical accidents (Box 3-1): frequency, duration of exposure, voltage, amperage, resistance of the tissues, and pathway of the current. The factor that seems most important in distinguishing lightning from high-voltage electric injuries is the duration of exposure to the current.

Frequency

Lightning is neither a direct nor an alternating current. At best, lightning is a unidirectional massive current impulse. The cloud-to-ground impulse results from breakdown of a large electric field between cloud and ground, measured in millions of volts. Once connection is made with the ground, the voltage difference between cloud and ground disappears and a large current flows impulsively in a very short time. The study of massive electrical discharges of such short duration, particularly their effects on the human body, is not well

---

*References 7, 9, 30, 31, 34, 70, 76, 77.

Box 3-1 FACTORS AFFECTING SEVERITY OF ELECTRICAL BURNS

Frequency	Resistance
Voltage	Pathway
Amperage	Duration

advanced. Lightning is said to be a "current" phenomenon rather than a "voltage" phenomenon.

Voltage, Amperage, and Resistance

Lightning, being a current phenomenon, is not easily considered in terms of Ohm's law ($V = I \times R$) and power calculation ($P = V \times I$) terms. Because the voltage between cloud and ground disappears after lightning attachment, examining the particular voltage in these equations becomes difficult. Thus we must resort to alternative formulations of the equations.

The energy dissipated in a given tissue is determined by the current flowing through the tissue and its resistance by:

$$\text{Energy (heat)} = \text{Current}^2 \times \text{Resistance} \times \text{Time}$$

where a current flows through a resistance for time t.

As resistance goes up, so does the heat generated by passage of the current. In humans when low energy levels are encountered, much of the electric energy may be dissipated by the skin, so that superficial burns are often not accompanied by internal injuries.

Although lightning occasionally creates discrete entry and exit wounds, these are rare. Lightning more commonly causes only superficial streaking burns. The exception to this is when "hot lightning," or long continuous current (LCC), occurs. LCC is a prolonged stroke lasting up to 0.5 second that delivers a tremendous amount of energy, capable of exploding trees, setting fires, and acting like high-voltage electricity to produce injuries. Other factors not understood may contribute to the formation of deep burns, although deep burns similar to those of high-voltage electric injuries generally are quite rare with lightning.

Pathway, Duration of Current, and Flashover Effect

It takes a finite amount of time for the skin to break down when exposed to heat or energy. Generally, lightning is not around long enough to cause this skin breakdown. Probably a large portion travels along the outside of the skin as "flashover."[100] There is some experimental evidence that a portion of the current may enter the cranial orifices—eyes, ears, nose, and mouth.[2,3,7] This pathway would help explain the myriad eye and ear symptoms that have been reported with lightning injury.

Andrews[2] further examined the functional consequences of lightning on cardiorespiratory function and concluded that entry of current into cranial orifices leads to passage of current directly to the brainstem. In a sheep study, he was able to demonstrate specific damage to neurons at the floor of the fourth ventricle in the location of the medullary cardiorespiratory control centers. It is postulated that current travels from there cau-

dad via cerebrospinal fluid (CSF) and blood vessel pathways to impinge directly on the myocardium. Andrews[2] also showed histologic damage to the myocardium, consistent with a number of autopsy reports of inferior myocardial necrosis.[6]

An alternative hypothesis can be tested with mathematical modeling.[2,9] Certain assumptions are made in any model, usually based on principles accepted in the literature.[11,76] Figure 3-11, *A*, shows a model for skin resistance, and its connection to the internal body milieu is shown in Figure 3-11, *B*. It will be noted that the internal body structures are regarded as purely resistive, whereas the skin contains significant elements of capacitance.[11,76]

The sequence of events during the strike started with the postulate that the stroke attached initially to the head of the victim. For a small fraction of time, current flowed internally as the skin capacitance elements became charged. At a voltage taken as 5 kV, the skin was assumed to break down. It is worth noting in the context of time scale that a lightning stroke is modeled as a current wave building to a maximum value in around 8 msec, although this may be "modulated lightning"— lightning that has passed through other structures, such as wiring. Others have measured the rise time of direct lightning as 1.2 to 1.5 msec. Once the internal current increased, the voltage across the body to earth built up, and external flashover across the body occurred when the field reached the breakdown strength of air.

The results of mathematical modeling of these events are shown in Figure 3-12, and the relative magnitudes of the various voltage components can be seen with their time scale. On this time scale the times to breakdown are short and most events occur early in the course of the stroke. In summary, in this model, lightning applies a current to the human body. This current initially is transmitted internally, following which skin breaks down. Ultimately, external flashover occurs. Andrews[2] draws support for this model from measurements made in the experimental application of lightning impulses to sheep. Further modeling of step voltage injury verified that for the erect human, this mechanism is less dangerous than is a direct strike.

Experimental evidence suggests that "a fast flashover appreciably diminishes the energy dissipation within the body and results in survival."[100] In addition, Ishikawa obtained experimental results with rabbits similar to the human data found by Cooper's study.[29] Cooper[38,39] has carried her studies to animals in developing an animal model of lightning injury and has successfully shown primary cardiac arrhythmias, prolonged ventilatory arrest, secondary cardiac arrest, keraunographic skin changes, and temporary lower extremity paralysis.

As current flashes over the outside of the body, it may vaporize moisture on the skin and blast apart

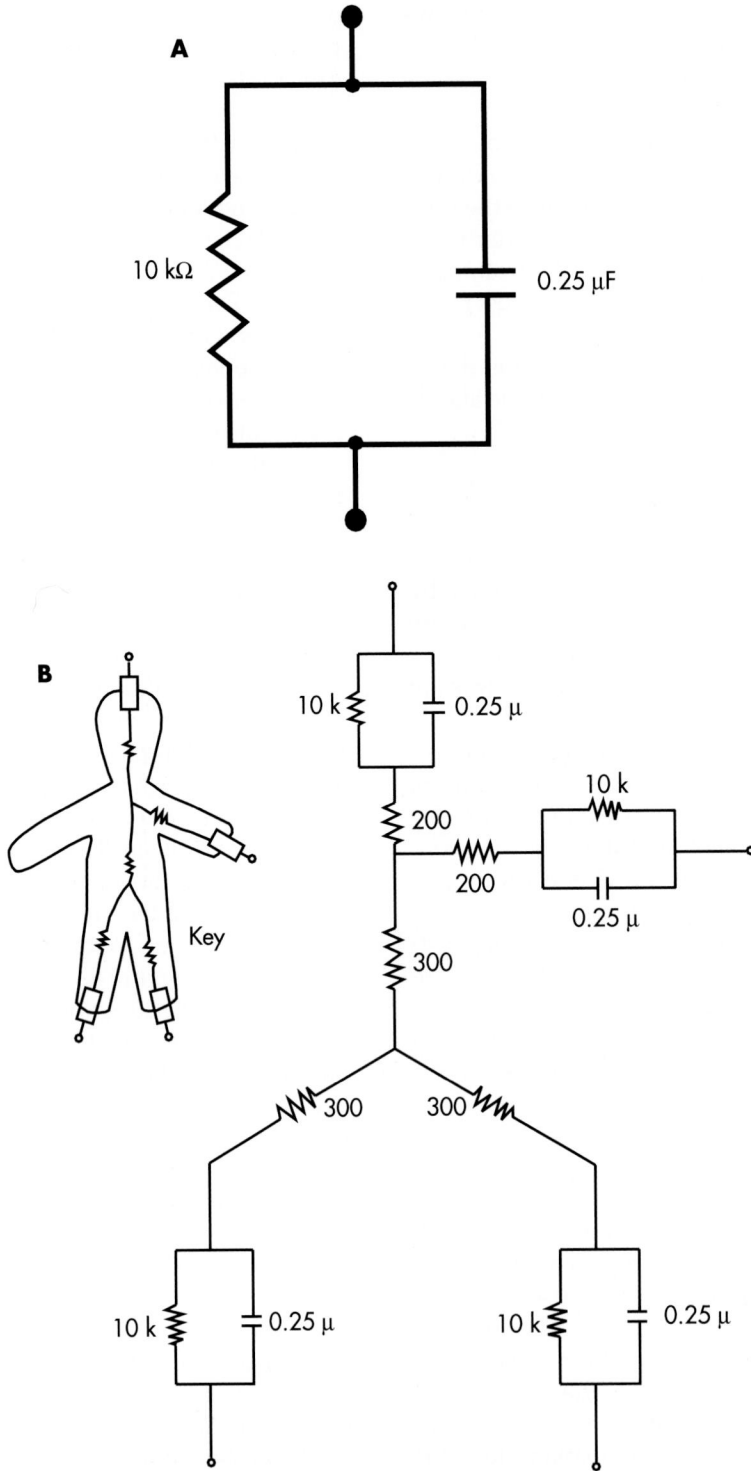

Figure 3-11 **A,** Electrical model for human skin impedance. **B,** Model of human body for the purposes of examination of currents flowing during lightning strike.

clothes and shoes, leaving the victim nearly naked, as noted by Hegner[58] in 1917:

The clothing may not be affected in any way. It may be stripped or burned in part or entirely shredded to ribbons. Either warp or woof may be destroyed leaving the outer gar-

ments and the skin intact. . . . Metallic objects in or on the clothing are bent, broken, more or less fused or not affected. The shoes most constantly show the effects of the current. People are usually standing when struck, the current then enters or leaves the body through the feet. The shoes, especially when dry or only partially damp, interpose a substance of in-

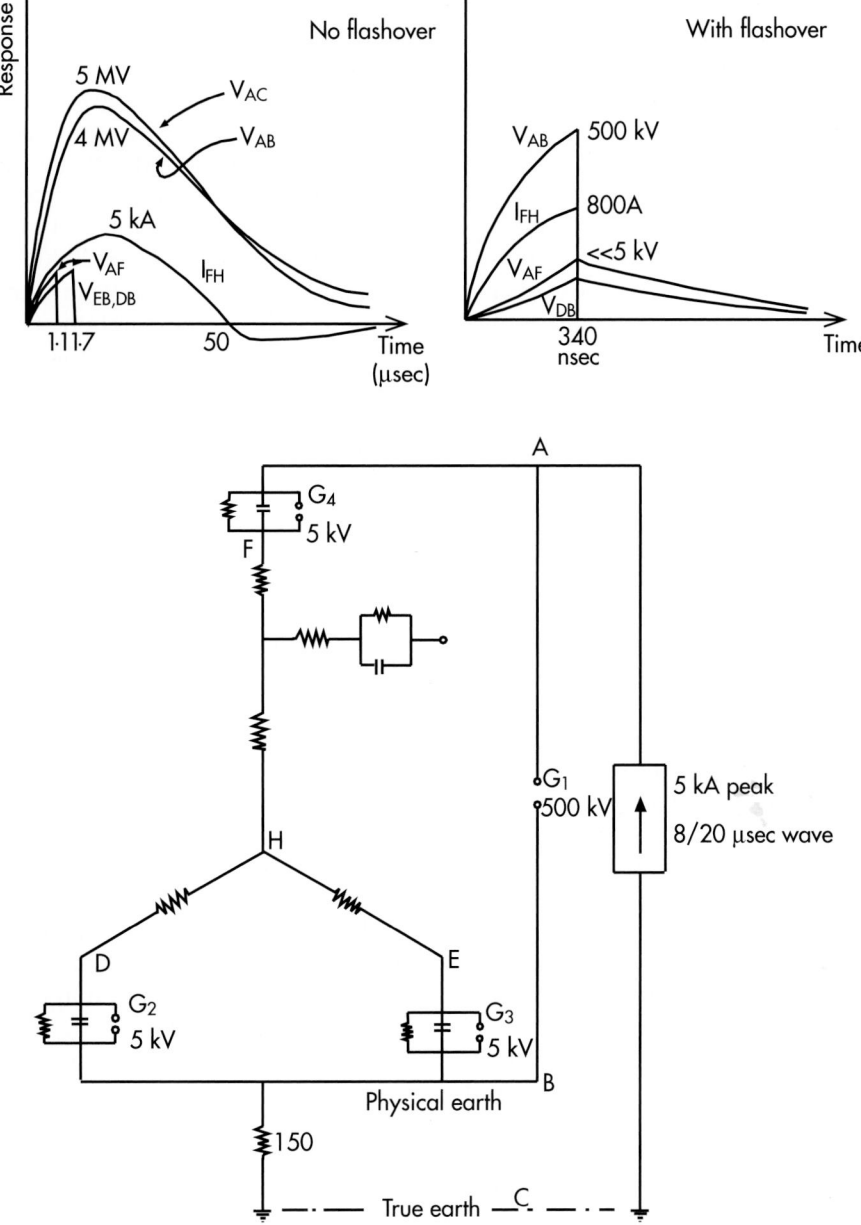

Figure 3-12 Model of human body adapted for the circumstance of direct lightning strike. Responses of the body model are shown for cases of direct strike with and without subsequent flashover.

creased resistance. One or both shoes may be affected. They may be gently removed, or violently thrown many feet, be punctured or have a large hole torn in any part, shredded, split, reduced to lint or disappear entirely. The soles may disappear with or without the heels. Any of the foregoing may occur and the person not injured or only slightly shocked.

The amount of damage to clothing or to the surface of the body is not an index to the severity of injuries sustained within a human. Either may be disproportionately great or small. However, in unwitnessed situations, the first author (MAC) and others have found that forensic evidence of damage to shoes and clothing

may be the most important and reliable indicator in determining if lightning caused a person's death.[72]

Behavior of Current in Tissue

High- or low-voltage electric current may be carried through tissue in a direct conduction fashion, obeying simple linear equations such as Ohm's law. The result is heating of tissues under Joule's law, with thermally induced cellular death and dysfunction. Simple passage of current may interfere with neural and muscular function.[76]

Earlier in the previous century, electric injury was thought to occur not only because of thermal effects but also because of some mysterious cellular effects.[10,70] Unfortunately, the technology was not available to investigate these effects and this idea was largely forgotten. In the last few years, the theory of electroporation has been proposed. Cell wall integrity, enzyme reactions, protein shape and structure, and cell membrane "gates" and pumps operate by changes on the order of microvolts. It is not beyond the realm of imagination that passage of an electric current too small to produce significant thermal damage still may cause irreversible changes in these functions, leading to cell death or dysfunction.[76] Induction of electric charges by external electromagnetic fields has been shown to force water molecules into cell walls, causing the occurrence of fatal "pores."

Magnetic Field Effects

Some persons contend that the injurious effects of lightning can in part be magnetically mediated.[24] The case cited in support of this contention was a golfer under a tree in company with three other persons. It was stated that death occurred without evidence of current entering or leaving the index case. On the other hand, one accompanying golfer showed evidence of current traversal but survived. It is stated that three methods of shock exist—direct strike, side flash, and ground potential—but no evidence of any was seen. It was apparently considered that contact potential was not relevant, and this may have been historically so. In this case, with persons under a tree, it would seem possible to explain deleterious effects without resort to a magnetic hypothesis, but nonetheless the hypothesis bears examination, since it is a recurrent question.

In the case under consideration, the stroke was considered a line current 1 m distant from the victim, and calculation of peak fields and their effects were given. It is useful to consider the stroke as a single line current as referenced; however, we must also gain a feeling for how far from a victim such a stroke will act. If the stroke is close to a victim, then attachment to the victim will take place and electrical effects will apply. If further away, the magnetic field will be operative without attachment and magnetic effects need to be examined. Ground potential at this distance will also exist.

To determine the magnitude of this effect, it is necessary to find the minimum distance away from a victim that a stroke reaches ground without attachment to the victim, to give the worst-case distance from (that closest to) a victim at which pure magnetic field acts.

The standard striking distance formula gives such a distance.[42] The formula is:

$$d_s = 10I^{0.65}$$

where d_s (m) is the striking distance and I is the stroke current in kA. This represents the distance at the last turn of the downward stepped leader, such that if an object lies inside this distance, attachment of the leader to the object will take place.

For illustrative purposes, let a stroke have a peak current of 20,000 A. This gives d_s of 70.09 m (230 feet). Pure magnetic effects are applicable at this distance and beyond. Inside this distance, the victim will be subject to electrical current effects. By comparison, the ground potential between two points 1 m (3 feet) apart at 60 m (197 feet) from a stroke of 20 kA is about 60 volts, assuming earth resistivity of 100 ohm-meters.

In examining the magnetic fields involved at this distance, assume a 20 kA stroke at 70 m distance from an individual. The peak magnetic B field (the "magnetic induction," formally quantifying the force on a moving charge in its influence) is:

$$B = \mu 0I/2\pi d_s = 57 \times 10^{-6}$$

$$w/m^2 = 57\ \mu T$$

For comparison, the earth's magnetic field is about 1 μT, and the magnetic fields causing concern for power line fields are around the 1 to 100 μT range. The magnetic fields used in magnetic resonance imaging (MRI) scanning are around 2,000,000 to 5,000,000 times these levels. Thus, if concern is realistically held for power line fields in terms of field level, then the field of a lightning stroke must be regarded as dangerous. However, magnetic problems of the acute kind are not seen in this circumstance, and the major concern (if any exists) would only be in terms of chronic exposure. Similarly, if one is concerned about a lightning stroke magnetic field, he or she should be entirely concerned about MRI fields. Again, the concern is not seen in the same terms.

Certainly, the time varying nature of any B field is important, both in terms of the rate of change of the field and of movement of a conductor within this field. If one assumes that the above B field is generated in about 2 μsec, then the time rate of change for the B field is about 30 T/sec. Suppose this is applied to an aorta of cross section 8 cm^2 ($8 \times 10^{-4}\ m^2$). Then the magnitude of the induced electric field in this region is approximately 0.024 V/m. If the resistivity of blood is taken as 1 ohm-meter, then the current induced in the aorta has density of 0.024 A/m^2. The corresponding current is therefore approximately 20 μA in the cross section under consideration. It is stated elsewhere that the blood vessels represent the most likely conducting medium in the body, and the most likely danger of arrhythmia exists in the current-passing media around the heart, the ventricle being of the same order in dimension as the aorta. This current in the aorta broadly approximates that within the ventricle.

This current is calculated under quite ideal circumstances, and if myocardial effects are to occur, then the current must penetrate into a tissue of considerably higher resistivity with good coupling. This is unlikely, and the current in itself is of arguable danger in any case.

One therefore concludes that magnetic field danger in normal circumstances is slight. Certainly special circumstances might exist, such as the presence of a pacemaker or the presence of an arrhythmic pathway, but in normal terms, magnetic effects would not seem to be clinically significant during occurrences of lightning strike.

INJURIES FROM LIGHTNING

Severity of Injury

Some of the most common signs and symptoms are listed in Box 3-2. Lightning is almost instantaneous in its action and seemingly unpredictable in its physical effects. Each case report of lightning injury has unique characteristics, and symptoms may vary from trivial to fatal. For prognostic purposes, victims generally can be placed in one of three groups.

Minor Injury. These victims are awake and may report dysesthesia in the affected extremity from a lightning splash or, in more serious strokes, a feeling of having been hit on the head or having been in an explosion. They may or may not have perceived lightning or thunder. They often suffer confusion, amnesia, temporary deafness or blindness, or temporary unconsciousness at the scene.[16] They seldom demonstrate cutaneous burns or paralysis but may complain of paresthesias, muscular pain, confusion, and amnesia lasting from hours to days. Victims may suffer tympanic membrane rupture from the explosive force of the lightning shock wave. Vital signs are usually stable, although occasional victims demonstrate transient mild hypertension. Recovery is usually gradual and may or may not be complete. Permanent neurocognitive damage may occur.

Box 3-2   LIGHTNING INJURIES

IMMEDIATE

Ventricular asystole
Neurologic signs
    Seizures
    Deafness
    Confusion, amnesia
    Blindness
Contusion from shock wave
Chest pain, muscle aches
Tympanic membrane rupture

DELAYED

Dysesthesias, peripheral neuropathy
Neuropsychologic changes

Moderate Injury. Moderately injured victims may be disoriented, combative, or comatose. They frequently exhibit motor paralysis, particularly of the lower extremities, with mottled skin and diminished or absent pulses. Nonpalpable peripheral pulses may indicate arterial spasm and sympathetic instability, which should be differentiated from hypotension. If true hypotension occurs and persists, the victim should be scrutinized for fractures and other signs of blunt injury. Spinal shock from cervical or other spinal fractures, although rare with lightning, also may account for hypotension.

Occasionally, victims have suffered temporary cardiopulmonary standstill, although it is seldom documented. Spontaneous recovery of the pulse is attributed to the heart's inherent automaticity. However, respiratory arrest that often occurs with lightning injury may be prolonged and lead to secondary cardiac arrest from hypoxia or some other yet-to-be-elucidated cause. Seizures may also occur.

First-and second-degree burns not prominent on admission may evolve over the first several hours. Rarely, third-degree burns may occur. Tympanic membrane rupture should be anticipated[44] and, along with hemotympanum, may indicate a basilar skull fracture.

Whereas the clinical condition often improves within the first few hours, victims are prone to have permanent sequelae, such as sleep disorders, irritability, difficulty with fine psychomotor functions, paresthesias, generalized weakness, sympathetic nervous system dysfunction, and sometimes posttraumatic stress syndrome. A few cases of atrophic spinal paralysis have been reported.

Severe Injury. Victims with severe injury may be in cardiac arrest with either ventricular standstill or fibrillation when first examined. Cardiac resuscitation may not be successful if the victim has suffered a prolonged period of cardiac and central nervous system (CNS) ischemia. Direct brain damage may occur from the lightning strike or blast effect. Tympanic membrane rupture with hemotympanum and CSF otorrhea is common in this group.

Victims with other signs of blunt trauma are likely to have endured direct hits, although sometimes no burns are noted.

The prognosis is usually poor in the severely injured group because of direct lightning damage, often complicated by a delay in initiating cardiopulmonary resuscitation with resultant anoxic injury to the brain and other organ systems.

Differences between Injuries from High-Voltage Electricity and Lightning[9,34]

There are marked differences in injuries caused by high-voltage electric accidents and lightning (Table 3-3). Lightning contact with the body is almost instantaneous, often leading to flashover. Exposure to high-voltage

TABLE 3-3. Lightning Injuries

FACTOR	LIGHTNING	HIGH VOLTAGE
Energy level	30 million volts, 50,000 Å	Usually much lower
Time of exposure	Brief, instantaneous	Prolonged
Pathway	Flashover, orifice	Deep, internal
Burns	Superficial, minor	Deep, major injury
Cardiac	Primary and secondary arrest, asystole	Fibrillation
Renal	Rare myoglobinuria or hemoglobinuria	Myoglobinuric renal failure common
Fasciotomy	Rarely if ever necessary	Common, early, and extensive
Blunt injury	Explosive thunder effect	Falls, being thrown

generated electricity tends to be more prolonged because the victim often freezes to the circuit. With skin breakdown, electric energy surges through the tissues with little resistance to flow, causing massive internal thermal injury that sometimes necessitates major amputations. Myoglobin release may be pronounced, and renal failure may occur. In addition, compartment syndromes requiring fasciotomy may occur. This is not the case with lightning injuries, in which burns and deep injury are uncommon and fluid restriction and expectant care are usually the rule.

Cardiopulmonary Arrest

The most common cause of death in a lightning victim is cardiopulmonary arrest. In fact, a victim is highly unlikely ($p < .0001$) to die unless cardiopulmonary arrest is suffered as an immediate effect of the strike.[29] In the past, nearly 75% of those who suffered cardiopulmonary arrest from lightning injuries died, many because cardiopulmonary resuscitation was not attempted.

Primary and secondary cardiac arrests had previously been hypothesized and were recently confirmed in animal studies.[2,6,7,34,113] Injury first occurs with immediate asystolic cardiac arrest and respiratory standstill. Because of the heart's automaticity, an organized series of contractions generally resumes within a short time. Unfortunately, respiratory arrest caused by paralysis of the medullary respiratory center may last far longer than cardiac arrest. Unless the victim receives immediate ventilatory assistance, attendant hypoxia may induce arrhythmias and secondary cardiac arrest. Alternatively, the respiratory arrest and secondary cardiac arrest may be from more severe injury and not cause and effect.

The course has been verified experimentally in sheep, with initial asystole, followed by resumption of a short run of bradycardia, then tachycardia, followed by an eventual block or bradycardia, and finally with second asystolic arrest.[2] Figure 3-13 shows the result on respiratory rhythm of an impulse applied to the cranium of a sheep. Initial muscle spasm is seen, followed by cessation of natural rhythm. Figure 3-14 shows the

progress of myocardial activity of another sheep, from impulse through asystole to secondary arrest. Prolonged respiratory arrest has also been confirmed in hairless rats by the first author (unpublished report).

Both asystole and ventricular fibrillation[3] have been reported with lightning strike. As noted in the animal work, asystole seems to be both the first and last response to the strike, as the secondary arrest rhythm of ventricular fibrillation deteriorates.[2] Premature ventricular contractions, ventricular tachycardia, and atrial fibrillation have been reported.[79]

It is not uncommon to find electrocardiographic (ECG) ST changes consistent with ischemia and damage in subepicardial, posterior, inferior, or anterior patterns.[6,79] Creatine phosphokinase MB isoenzyme elevation has been reported. Documentation of troponin levels in lightning patients has not been published. Elevations of serum glutamic oxaloacetic transaminase and lactate dehydrogenase may reflect concomitant trauma to other tissues.

ECG changes may not occur until the second day, making the initial ECG a poor screening tool for ischemia. In addition, several authors stress that cardiac symptomatology may be inapparent on initial presentation. Premature ventricular contractions were reported to begin in one patient nearly 1 week after presentation. Whereas most ECG changes resolve within a few days, some may persist for months.[10]

The QT interval may be prolonged following lightning strike.[4] This has been verified in animal experiments (Figure 3-15) in which the ischemic form of the ECG complexes gave way to normalization of morphology, followed by prolongation of the QT interval at 270 seconds after lightning strike in sheep that did not suffer respiratory arrest. Another hypothesis is that QT prolongation may have implications for the cessation of metabolism hypothesis if torsades des pointes is involved.[4]

Some authors have theorized that vascular spasm is a cause of cardiac damage.[161] However, ECG changes are not always consistent with cardiac vascular supply patterns.[83] Areas of focal cardiac necrosis have been re-

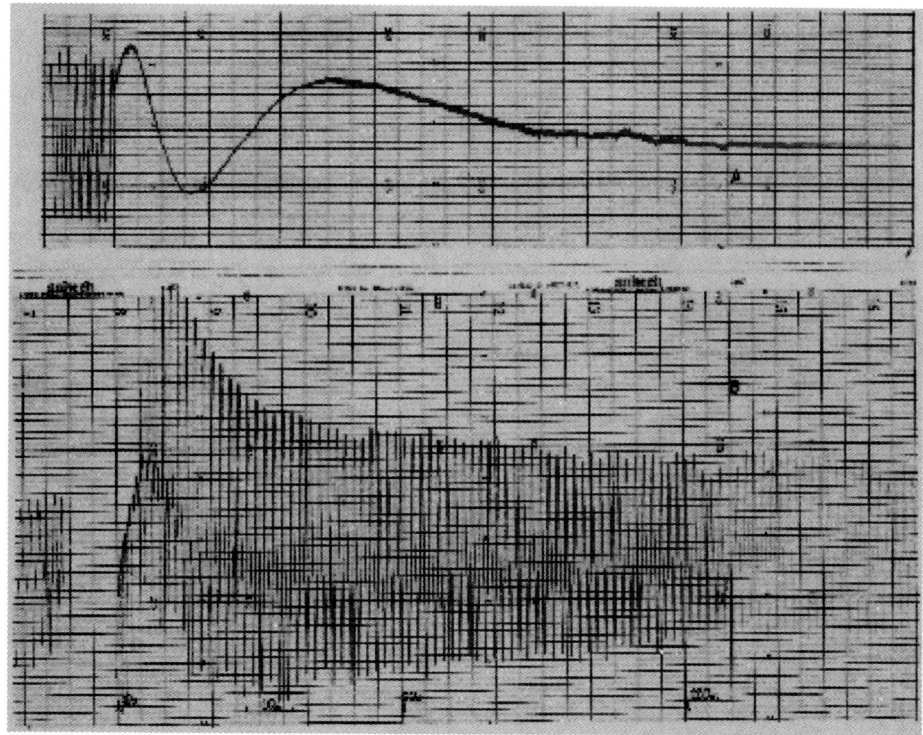

Figure 3-13 Respiratory activity tracing in sheep struck by laboratory-generated lightning. *Top,* Where respiratory arrest did not occur. *Bottom,* Where respiratory muscle spasm occurred followed by respiratory arrest.

ported in autopsies, and histologic changes have been shown in sheep hearts.[2]

Pulmonary edema may accompany severe cardiac damage. Pulmonary contusion, with severe hemoptysis and pulmonary hemorrhage, may result from blunt injury or direct lung damage.[112]

Neurologic Injuries

Although cardiac arrest may be the only immediate cause of death, lightning is primarily a neurologic insult with damage possible to central, peripheral, and sympathetic nervous systems. Injury to the nervous system far and away causes the greatest number of long-term problems to survivors. Tools commonly used in evaluation and treatment include functional scans, such as single photon emission computed tomography (SPECT) (often positive); anatomic scans, such as computed tomography (CT) and MRI (usually negative); neuropsychologic assessment and tracking; cognitive retraining; pharmacotherapy as already mentioned; psychotherapy; and computed body tomography (CBT). Electroencephalography (EEG) is often mentioned in other literature but is of variable utility and may be normal.[6,34]

Central Nervous System Injury. When current traverses the brain, there can be coagulation of brain sub-

stance, formation of epidural and subdural hematomas, paralysis of the respiratory center, and intraventricular hemorrhage. Autopsy findings include meningeal and parenchymal blood extravasation, petechiae, dural tears, scalp hematomas, and skull fractures. CT of the brain may show diffuse edema or intracranial hemorrhage but is more commonly normal.[20-22] Direct brain damage from blunt head injury occurs in a limited number of victims, particularly those whose mental status deteriorates over time.[20,22] There have been reports of MRI findings in a few acutely injured victims.[21] Unfortunately, for victims with more chronic complaints, CT and MRI examinations are usually unremarkable.[6,34] Transient elevation of creatine phosphokinase BB has been reported.

Direct cellular damage to the respiratory and cardiac centers in the fourth ventricle, as well as the anterior surface of the brainstem, has been shown in animals.[2] If current enters through the orifices of the head, passes through the area of the pituitary and hypothalamus, and through the CSF into the retropharyngeal area, it is reasonable to expect signs and symptoms consistent with damage to these areas, including endocrine dysfunction, respiratory or cardiac arrest, and sleep disturbances.

Seizures may accompany initial cardiorespiratory arrest as a result of hypoxia or intracranial damage.

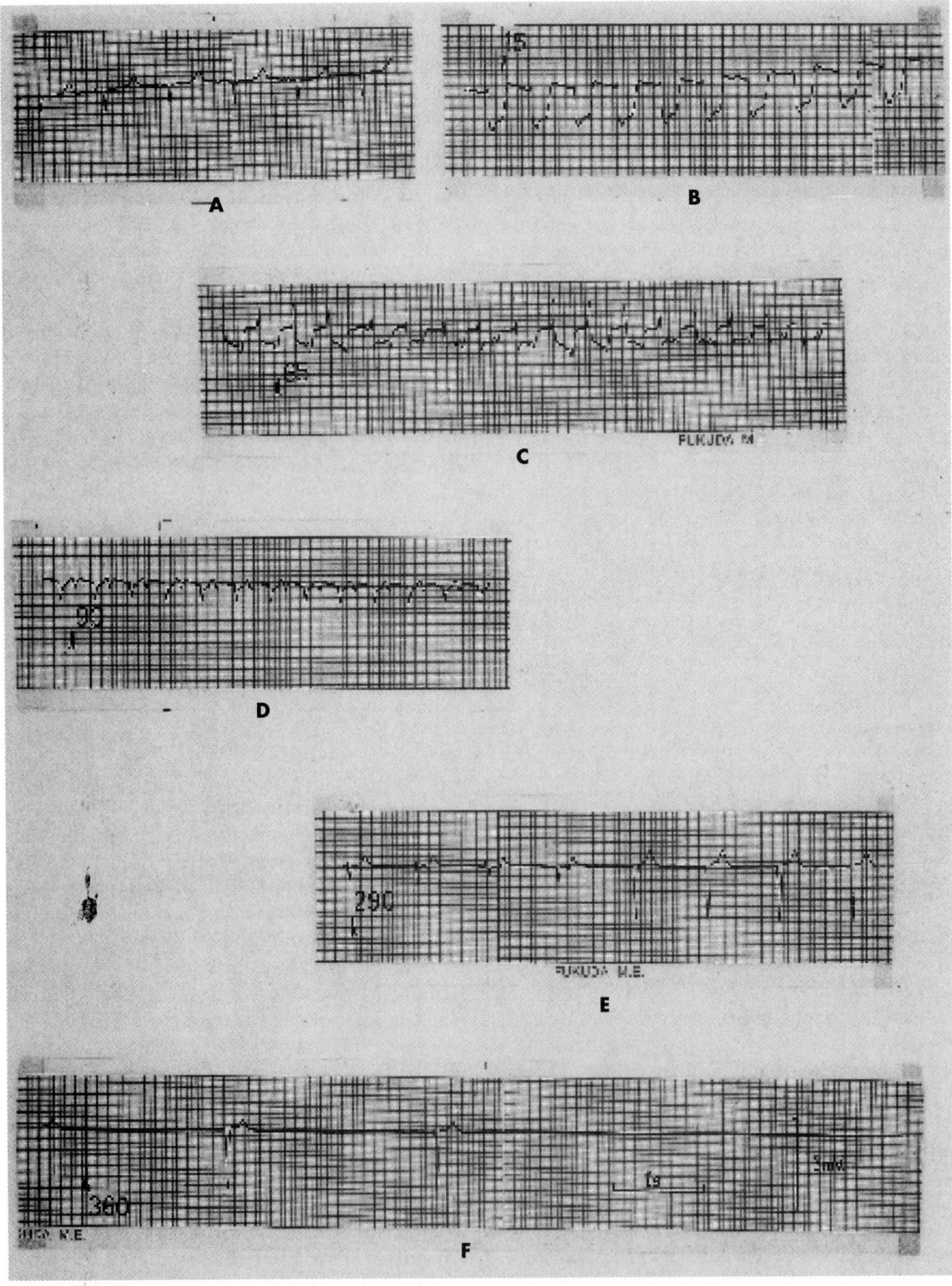

Figure 3-14 Cardiac response in sheep (nonstandard leads) subjected to laboratory-generated lightning strike. **A,** Baseline. **B,** Initial morphology change, followed by, **C** to **E,** normalization of morphology, **C** and **D,** tachycardia, **E** and **F,** bradycardia, and, **F,** hypoxic secondary arrest. A short period of asystole was initially seen before tracing **B.**

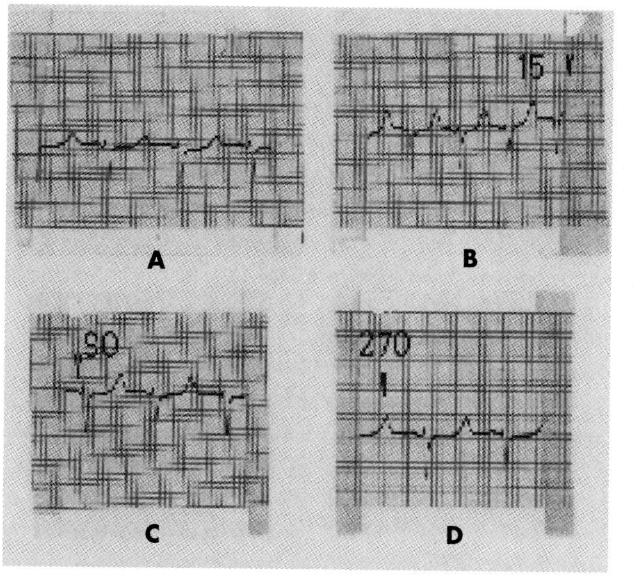

Figure 3-15 Electrocardiogram (nonstandard leads) for sheep struck by laboratory-generated lightning. Asystolic arrest did not occur. QT was prolonged by 270 seconds after the strike

These are usually transient but may continue for the first few days.

EEG changes may isolate an epileptogenic focus in the acute phase in many lightning victims. These patterns may be focal or diffuse, varying with the site and type of injury. Many patients do not experience seizures during hospitalization, and most usually have normalization of their EEG within a few months. Other victims, including children, develop delayed seizures, some of which present as "absence spells," memory losses, or blackouts that are often diagnosed as "pseudoseizures." One severely injured patient was reported to have continued seizures after discharge to a nursing home.[95]

Obviously, if the victim has prolonged cardiopulmonary arrest, there may be anoxic brain injury that is not specific to lightning injury.

In Cooper's study[29] of severely injured victims, nearly two thirds had some degree of lower extremity paralysis (keraunoparalysis), usually demarcating around the waist or pelvis. Almost one third of victims incur upper extremity paralysis.[29] The affected extremities appear cold, clammy, mottled, insensate, and pulseless.[9] This is the result of sympathetic instability and intense vascular spasm, which has been likened to Raynaud's phenomenon in appearance, and which usually clears after several hours.[9,34] Fasciotomies are almost never indicated for lightning injuries, since any signs of compartment syndrome or distal ischemia usually clear with patient observation. Pulses can sometimes be elicited with a Doppler examination. Atrophic spinal paralysis has been reported, as have persistent

paresis, paresthesias, incoordination, delayed and acute cerebellar ataxia, hemiplegia, and aphasia. There is one report of quadriplegia developing 36 hours after injury and one of progressive muscle atrophy of the upper extremities.

Nearly 72% of the victims in Cooper's study suffered loss of consciousness,[29] which may be an ominous sign, since nearly three fourths of these persons also suffered a cardiopulmonary arrest.[29] Those with cranial burns are two to three times more likely to suffer immediate cardiopulmonary arrest and have a three to four times greater probability of death.[29] Persons who are stunned or lose consciousness without cardiopulmonary arrest are highly unlikely to die,[29] although they may still suffer serious sequelae.

Whether or not victims have suffered loss of consciousness, they almost universally demonstrate anterograde amnesia and confusion, which may last for several days. Retrograde amnesia is less common. Often, the victim appears to be well oriented and remembers his or her actions before the strike but may not be able to assimilate new experiences for several days, even when there is no external evidence of lightning burns on the head or neck. Victims often act like persons who have experienced electroconvulsive therapy.[36]

Survivors may have persistent sleep disturbances, difficulty with fine mental and motor functions, dysesthesias, headaches, mood abnormalities, emotional lability, storm phobias, decreased exercise tolerance, and posttraumatic stress disorder.[36,110]

The basal ganglia and cerebellum may also be affected.[21,22] This agrees with older reports of localization. CNS damage may also eventually present as parkinsonism or an extrapyramidal syndrome, signs of intracranial hematomata and hemorrhage, infarction, hypoxia, edema, cerebellar signs of infarction, dysfunction and atrophy, and centrally derived pain and psychologic syndromes.[19]

Peripheral Injury. The peripheral nervous system is often affected. Pain and paresthesias are prominent features of the injury, particularly in the line of the current passage. It would seem that the majority of ongoing pain and dysfunction may be explained in peripheral terms. On the other hand, much of the ongoing psychologic disturbance may be seen in central terms.

There is some suspicion that the peripheral nerves may be preferentially injured because of their lower resistance to electricity, although this may be more important in electrical than lightning injuries.[122] There may also be possible mechanical damage to the nerves from electroporation.[76,77] Certainly, damage is noted by threshold alteration in chronic injury, which although usually reversible, can become persistent.

Symptoms may be delayed by weeks to years. Paraesthesias are frequently seen, often mirroring the area of keraunoparalysis. There is also evidence of autonomic neuropathy.

Autonomic Dystrophy.* Chronic pain syndromes may occur. Autonomic dystrophy, also called sympathetic dystrophy or sympathetically mediated pain syndrome (SMPS), may occur. The victim may exhibit perfusion alterations in affected limbs, altered temperature control, and altered skin appearance and reactions, most commonly in the path of the current, although these may later extend to other areas of the body. Autonomic dystrophies may have associated pain and movement disorders.

Reflex sympathetic dystrophy (RSD), a deep peripheral nerve disorder caused by injury to nerve, is a long-term neural sequela to damage characterized by pain, edema, autonomic dysfunction, and movement disorder. Schwartzman[108] and Hendler[59] provide equally excellent reviews with good summaries and useful diagnostic testing protocols,[6] although the diagnosis is primarily clinical.

Damage to injured nerves containing sympathetic components is likely to yield an "injury picture." A partial nerve injury presents as "causalgia." Causalgia does not follow complete nerve transection and requires some form of intact, while damaged, sympathetic function.

There are three stages of RSD. The diagnosis is clinical; certain aspects of the stages may overlap or never appear. Much of the pain in lightning injury fits variants of these patterns, and the autonomic component cannot be ignored. In the first stage, the condition is sympathetically maintained. The second stage becomes independent. The third stage can involve spread to initially uninjured tissue, as well as to contralateral areas. Early in its course (first stage), induced sympathetic blockade will be diagnostic and may effectively break the pain cycle. Testing with local anesthetic blockade or intravenous phentolamine can be used as a screening test. Cure can sometimes be effected at the early stage, and sympathectomy may be considered.

Clinically, stage 1 follows quickly after injury, sometimes in a matter of hours. Autonomic instability may precede the picture and continue through this stage. The pain is described as burning, diffuse, deep, and usually distal. It is exacerbated by movement, emotion, and dependency. There may also be hyperalgesia, allodynia, and hyperpathia. Adrenergic blockade can relieve the syndrome. This stage is also characterized by edema, nail and hair growth, and temperature change with or without hyperemia. The stage may last up to about 6 months after injury.

In stage 2 (the dystrophic stage), pain spreads and has significant psychologic overtones. Whereas stage 1 requires maintenance by the sympathetic nervous system, stage 2 becomes independent of it. Edema becomes indurated, and cool hyperhidrosis is present.

Cystic bone change may be seen, and hair and nail loss often develops. Cyanotic change may be seen secondary to autonomic vascular alterations.

In stage 3, pain spreads further and becomes dominant, with the pathologic changes of allodynia, hyperalgesia, and hyperpathia. Reversed plantar reflexes are seen, and small finger flexion is tight. Movement disorder is marked and often ascribed to hysteria. This stage includes initiation difficulty, weakness, spasms, tremor, and dystonia.

Posttraumatic Headache.[30] Many victims of lightning injury exhibit severe, unrelenting headaches for the first several months after lightning injury. The first author (MAC) has found acupuncture to be effective for at least some of the headaches. Many victims complain of nausea and unexpected, frequent vomiting spells early on in their recovery period. Dizziness and tinnitus are also common complaints, especially with telephone-transmitted lightning strikes.

Burns

Most people assume that, because of the tremendous energy discharge involved, a lightning victim will be flash cooked.[16,35] Fortunately, the flashover effect saves most victims from more than minor burns. Although extensive third-and fourth-degree burns may occur in combination with skeletal disruption, these are quite rare. Often there are no burns, especially with ground current effects.

As shown in mathematical models, a portion of the lightning current may travel through the tissues.[2] If the electric field in the tissue becomes too large, electrons can be freed from their atoms. Referred to as *dielectric breakdown*,[76] this can cause a large increase in the flow of current and become manifest as an electric arc. This may occur internal to the body or external to the body when the breakdown strength of air (2×10^6 V/m) is exceeded. Arclike burns can result. This happens more often with high-voltage electrical injury but may also occasionally occur with lightning.

Discrete entry and exit points are rare with lightning. The burns most commonly seen may be divided into five categories: linear burns; punctate, full-thickness burns; feathering or flowers; thermal burns from ignited clothing or heated metal; and combinations.

Linear burns (Figure 3-16) often begin at the victim's head and progress down the chest, where they split and continue down both legs. The burns generally are 1 to 4 cm wide and tend to follow areas of heavy sweat concentration, such as beneath breasts, down the midchest, and in the midaxillary line.[9,34] Linear burns are usually first-and second-degree burns that may be present initially or develop as late as several hours after the lightning strike. They are probably not primary lightning injuries but are steam burns secondary to vaporization of sweat or rainwater on the victim's skin.

---

*References 28, 59, 67, 106, 108, 109.

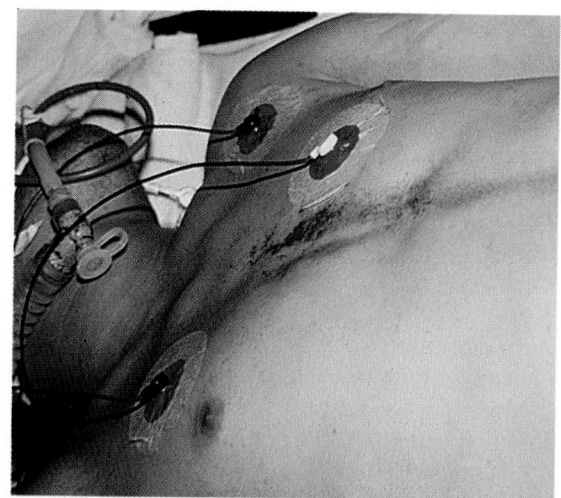

Figure 3-16 Linear burns from lightning injury.

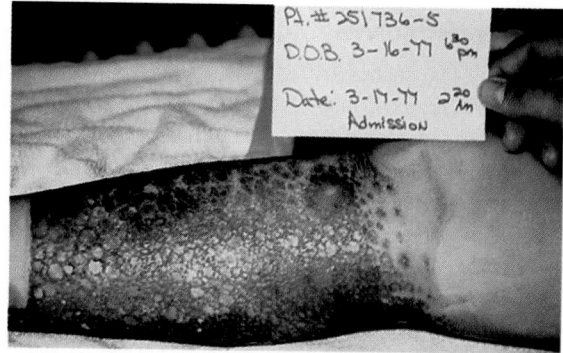

Figure 3-17 Punctate burns from lightning injury. *(Courtesy Art Kahn, M.D.)*

Punctate burns (Figure 3-17) are multiple, closely spaced, and discrete circular burns that individually range from a few millimeters to a centimeter in diameter. They may be full thickness and resemble cigarette burns but are usually too small to require grafting.

Feathering burns (Figure 3-18) are pathognomonic of lightning and known by such names as Lichtenberg's flowers, filigree burns, arborescent burns, ferning, and keraunographic markings.[53,62] There are references to these markings in the Bible, where they were described to represent photographic imprints of vegetation surrounding the victim. These markings are not true burns but appear as usually transient pink to brownish, sometimes lightly palpable, arborescent marks that follow neither the vascular pattern nor the nerve pathways. The pattern found is similar to that on a photographic plate exposed to a strong electric field and has been compared to fractals. Sometimes the most superficial skin over the areas will slough or flake off after a few days. Although many pictures exist of these marks, they have never been described histologically. They may represent blood cells extravasated into the superficial layers of the skin from capillaries. At least experimentally, they follow the current lines seen in flashover in Cooper's animal model.[38,39]

On rare occasions, clothing is ignited by lightning, causing severe thermal burns.[9,34] A victim wearing metal, such as a necklace or belt buckle, or carrying coins in his or her pocket may suffer second-and third-degree burns to adjacent skin as the objects become heated by the electric energy. Figure 3-19 shows the burn resulting from a metal belt buckle or athletic supporter worn by a young man who was struck while playing softball.

Victims of lightning may exhibit a combination of burns.

One author has related the prognosis of the victim

Figure 3-18 Feathering burns. *(Courtesy Mary Ann Cooper.)*

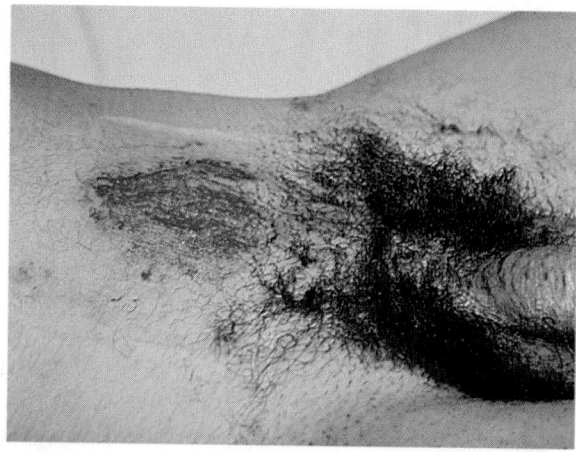

Figure 3-19 Burn resulting from metal belt buckle or athletic supporter worn by a man struck by lightning.

to the location of the burns.[29] Persons who suffer cranial burns are four times more likely to die than those who do not have cranial burns ($p < .25$). Victims with cranial burns are two and a half times more likely to have a cardiopulmonary arrest than those who do not exhibit burns around the head and neck (p <.025).[29] Persons with leg burns are five times more likely to die than those who have no leg burns, perhaps because of a ground current etiology ($p < .05$).[29]

Blunt and Explosive Injuries

The recipient of a lightning strike may be injured directly from the explosive force of lightning or from a fall (as from a horse or mountain ledge, out of a vehicle, or being hurled by endogenous opisthotonic force). Lightning victims incur a variety of fractures, including skull, ribs, extremities, and spine. Rarely, a burst-like injury of soft tissue occurs and discloses extensive underlying injuries, especially in the feet, where boots or socks may come apart (Figure 3-20).

Hemoglobinuria and myoglobinuria are seldom reported. When they occur, they are usually transient. Myoglobinuric renal failure has not yet been reported, although one case has been verbally relayed to the first author.

Persistent hypotension should alert the physician to blunt injuries to the chest, spine, lungs, heart, and intestines, which may lead to complications of prolonged coma, pulmonary contusions,[112] heart failure, and ischemic bowel.

Several victims have complained of jaw pain. At least one was found to have a styloid process fracture. Many recovering victims believe that premature arthritis may be a result of their injury, although this has never been proven.

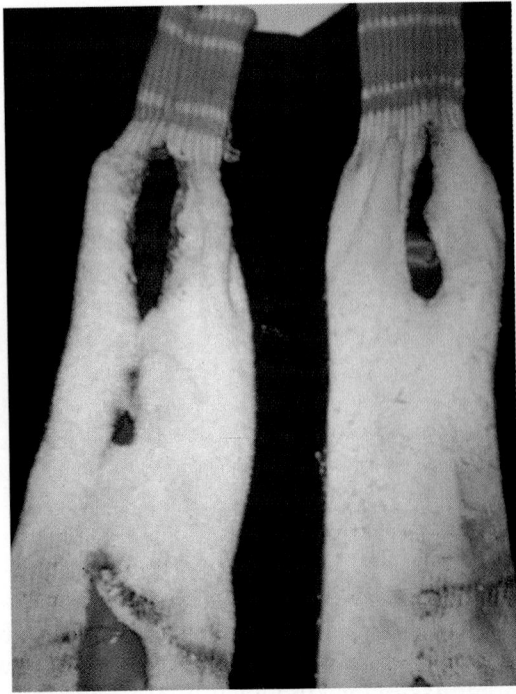

Figure 3-20 Socks blown off during explosive lightning stroke.

Eye Injuries*

Ocular injuries may occur in as many as 55% of persons struck by lightning and may be due to direct thermal or electrical damage, intense light, contusion from the shock wave, or combinations of these factors.

Although cataracts most commonly develop within the first few days, they may occur as late as 2 years after the strike and are often bilateral.[15,43] Whereas the cataracts may be the typical anterior midperipheral type, posterior subcapsular opacities and vacuolization seem to occur more often with lightning injuries.[15] Corneal lesions, hyphema, uveitis, iridocyclitis, and vitreous hemorrhage occur with greater frequency than do choroidal rupture, chorioretinitis, retinal detachment, macular degeneration, and optic atrophy.[15] Diplopia, loss of accommodation, and decreased color sense have also been reported.

Autonomic disturbances of the eye, including mydriasis, Horner's syndrome, anisocoria, and loss of light reflexes, may be transient or permanent. Transient bilateral blindness of unknown etiology is not uncommon. Intense photophobia may be present as the victim recovers.

Dilated or unreactive pupils should never be used as a prognostic sign or as a criterion for brain death in a lightning victim until all anatomic and functional lesions have been ruled out.[18]

Ear Injuries[56,94,99,105]

Temporary deafness is not uncommon.[71] It has been postulated that the intense noise and shock wave accompanying thunder may be responsible for sensorineural hearing loss. Newer work shows that entry of lightning current through cranial orifices could also account for some of the injuries.[2,7] Telephone-transmitted lightning strikes may also account for otologic damage.[1a,6]

Between 30% and 50% of lightning victims have rupture of one or both tympanic membranes, which may be from the shock wave effect, concomitant basilar skull fracture, or direct burn damage because of current flow into this orifice.[29] CSF otorrhea or hemotympanum may occur. Disruption of the ossicles and mastoid has been reported. Many cases of permanent deafness are noted in older literature. Facial palsies, both acute and delayed, may occur from direct nerve damage by lightning. Nystagmus, vertigo, tinnitus, and ataxia may follow otologic damage.

Fetal Survival

The fetus of a pregnant woman who has been struck by lightning has an unpredictable prognosis.[29] Of 11 cases reported, nearly one half of the pregnancies ended in full-term live births, with no recognizable abnormality in the child. Approximately one fourth resulted in live births with subsequent neonatal death; the remainder

---

*References 43, 54, 56, 57, 71, 97.

were stillbirths or deaths in utero. There has been one report of ruptured uterus after lightning strike.

Hematologic Abnormalities

Several unusual hematologic complications have been attributed to lightning injuries. These include disseminated intravascular coagulation, transiently positive Coombs' test, and Di Guglielmo's syndrome, a type of erythroleukemia characterized by erythroblastosis, thrombocytopenia, and hepatosplenomegaly. There have been anecdotal reports of increased hypersensitivity, development of allergies, and increased risk of cancer in lightning victims, perhaps indicating an immunologic component to lightning injury, although this has not been studied.

Endocrine and Sexual Dysfunction

One 32-year-old victim reported amenorrhea and premature menopause as a result of her injury. Others have reported menstrual irregularities lasting for 1 to 2 years. Impotence and decreased libido are common complaints. A report of male hypersexuality after a lightning strike has not been authenticated.

Psychologic Dysfunction

It is not uncommon for a person hit by lightning to rest at home for a few days, assuming that he or she is supposed to feel "bad" after being hit by lighting. The victim may not see a physician until family members insist or symptoms do not abate. Often, the person will attempt to return to work after the injury, but because of decreased work tolerance, short-term memory problems, and difficulty assimilating new information, he or she will be unable to continue in the prestrike occupation. Neurocognitive deficits may not become apparent until a victim attempts skilled mental functions.

Although some medical authors were historically suspicious of victims' complaints of psychologic and neurocognitive dysfunction, evaluation of many such patients appears to have confirmed a vast commonality of psychologic symptomatology. This should begin to reverse a regrettable tendency, both medically and legally, to discount complaints as evidence of malingering, excessive reaction, conversion reaction, personality problems, or manifestations of "weak" coping strategies.

The syndrome is described first from a clinical viewpoint and then discussed in light of the extant literature.

The experience of the authors demonstrates the following components of the syndrome:

Functional Issues

1. *Memory disturbance.* Individuals show marked diminution of short-term memory ability. They require shopping lists and reminder lists. Memory for recent names and places is diminished to the point of disability. In consequence, individuals do not mix socially or go into new circumstances. Study becomes impossible, and retraining for new facets of employment is difficult.
2. *Concentration disturbance.* Individuals are unable to focus attention for more than a short period and are easily distracted. In particular, reading and understanding are poor. Job training is detrimentally affected. This is coupled with sleep disturbance, indicated below.
3. *Cognitive powers.* Individuals report diminished ability with mental agility. The keeping of accounts is a noteworthy example. Calculation and estimation become erratic and affect work performance. Ability at mental manipulation and problem solving is markedly decreased.
4. *Higher executive functioning.* Individuals are neither able to coordinate multiple tasks simultaneously nor to follow orders for complex tasks they used to perform easily before the injury. One victim described it as if "the office manager of my brain had quit."

Behavioral Issues

1. *Emotional lability and aggression.* Individuals find that they are more aggressive than before. They are liable to outbursts and uncontrolled displays of temper and are easily frustrated. They state they hurt the people who they love and who provide care for "no good reason." The strains on a partnership are significant, and marital and relationship dysfunction are common. An increased state of arousal and anxiety may further complicate distractibility, as well as the proper recognition and assimilation of new learning.
2. *Sleep disturbance.* Extreme fatigue, sleep disturbance, or hypersomnolence is common and may last for years. Flashbacks and nightmares may be experienced.
3. *Phobic behavior.* Avoidance of the precipitant circumstances is demonstrated, in some cases to phobic proportion tantamount to posttraumatic stress disorder.

Depression is almost always present in quite classical biologic form and should be anticipated. Although the above symptoms can certainly arise secondary to a depressive state, it would also be quite reasonable for a victim to react with depression to the decrements in work power and lifestyle engendered by chronic pain or decreased personal performance. A third reasonable possibility is concurrent neuropsychologic syndrome and biologic endogenous depression. It is the view of the authors that the psychologic disturbance exists as an organic entity, and that part of that syndrome is also depressive as a primary organic entity. Both elements "feed" each other, compounding to a mixed picture.

Antidepressant medication is useful, reinforcing the view that a biologic component is present. Formal neuropsychologic testing is used to attempt to establish the injury pattern and quantify a functional baseline. Very few studies have formally examined the syndrome.[102,103,115] Primeau et al point to research difficulties, including sample bias and heterogeneity, methodology (cross-sectional rather than longitudinal or prospective), and the essential difficulties of determining premorbid status or current independent psychiatric status. It is also noted that the magnitude of insult does not correlate with psychologic disability. Duration, type, and severity of the syndrome are therefore unpredictable.

Disturbances of verbal memory, attention, concentration, and new learning are very frequently identified.[102] This commonality among victims is noteworthy.

Primeau et al also draw attention to the similarity of some facets of the disorder and that in other etiologies. They generally find the head injury model a useful one that can guide treatment. Other syndromes of which the lightning and electrical injury syndrome shows similarities include PTSD. They also examine depression, anxiety, obsessional, and adjustment disorders. Features of these are seen to be present, although the disorder is not simply an example of these dysfunctions per se.

We have considered somatoform disorders as a cause, noting the tendency to be preoccupied with the injury and to overattribute subsequent symptoms to the lightning injury. This may be due, in part, to the general lack of knowledge by physicians of the problems and likely outcomes of the injury, so that victims do not know what to expect in the future.

Conversion reaction may also be considered, although it cannot account for the symptomatology of lightning and electrical disability. Good neuropsychologic testing can detect this facet. One difficulty with neurocognitive testing is the use and interpretation of the Minnesota Multiphasic Personality Inventory (MMPI), which, although it was not developed to characterize patients with chronic problems, has been applied to them, often resulting in erroneous conclusion of conversion reaction or preoccupation with physical complaints. It should be a surprise to no one that anyone who has chronic pain and neurologic injury hampering their normal preinjury activities will rank higher on the "preoccupation with physical complaints" and "conversion" scales than uninjured normal individuals.

Ultimately the authors conclude that a prototype of the disorder does not exist. It seems that a description, such as "postelectric shock syndrome," is warranted. Andrews et al[5] recognized three postinjury syndromes and correlated these with the postinjury periods of 1 week, 1 week to 3 months, and 3 months to 3 years. Primeau et al[102] add a fourth—those persons experiencing longer and perhaps lifetime dysfunction.[56]

The first 12 months after injury are crucial to recovery. It is in this period that the most recovery is seen, with possible mild improvement up to 3 years after injury. Beyond this time, chronic dysfunction may be assumed.

Van Zomeren et al[115] provide one of the few thorough examinations of the syndrome in lightning-injured patients. Fatigue and energy loss were the main complaints; poor concentration, irritability, and emotional lability were other common themes. Impairment of memory, attention, and visual reaction times were documented. Depression and "convincing signs of PTSD" were seen. The syndrome was highly differentiable from normal ($p < .001$) and no parallel model was available for comparison. They stated that the lasting complaints and mild cognitive impairments could not be explained on the basis of anxiety reactions or depression. The summarized their findings under the heading of "vegetative dystonia."

RECOGNITION AND TREATMENT OF LIGHTNING INJURIES

Diagnosis

The diagnosis of lightning injury may be difficult. A history of a thunderstorm, witnesses who can report having seen the strike, and typical physical findings in the victim make diagnosis easier.

However, lightning can strike on a relatively sunny day, or thunder may not be appreciated. If the victim is struck while working alone in a field, the diagnosis may be initially confused with other entities (Box 3-3). In the past, persons have been suspected to have been the victims of assault because of the disarray of clothing and belongings.

A diligent historical effort and careful physical examination at the earliest opportunity may help determine the true cause. Any person found with linear burns and clothes exploded off should be treated as a victim of lightning strike. Feathering marks are pathognomonic of lightning strike and occur in no other type

---

BOX 3-3 DIFFERENTIAL DIAGNOSIS OF LIGHTNING INJURY

Cerebrovascular accident
   Subarachnoid hemorrhage
   Intraventricular hemorrhage
   Stroke
Seizure disorder
Spinal cord injury
Closed head injury
Hypertensive encephalopathy
Cardiac arrhythmia
Myocardial infarction
Toxic ingestion (heavy metals)
Malingering, conversion reaction

of injury. Unfortunately, burns of any kind are not always present.

Another sign/symptom complex that is diagnostic of lightning strike includes linear or punctate burns, tympanic membrane rupture, confusion, and outdoor location, whether or not there is history of a thunderstorm. Because there have been several cases of lightning sideflashes from indoor plumbing and telephones, the physician should suspect lightning strike in persons found confused and unconscious indoors after or during a thunderstorm.[1a,5,9,34]

Initial First Aid and Triage of Victims[9,34]

As in any other emergency, the first steps are the ABCs: airway, breathing, and circulation. If the victim has suffered a cardiac arrest, cardiopulmonary resuscitation should be started immediately and a rescue vehicle called for transportation.

If the strike occurs far from civilization and evacuation is improbable, the victim will probably die unless pulse and respirations resume spontaneously in a short period of time. The heart may resume activity but may slip into secondary arrest. It is unknown whether the secondary cardiac arrest is due to primary brain damage, hypoxia from prolonged respiratory arrest, primary cardiac damage, or autonomic nervous system damage. If the rescuer is successful in obtaining a pulse with cardiopulmonary resuscitation, ventilation should be continued until spontaneous adequate respirations resume, the victim is pronounced dead, continued resuscitation is deemed unfeasible owing to rescuers' exhaustion, or there is danger to rescuers' survival.

When lightning strike involves multiple victims, resources and rescuers may not meet the demand and triage must be instituted. Normally the rules of triage in multiple-casualty situations dictate bypassing dead persons for those who are moderately or severely injured and can benefit from resuscitation efforts. However, "resuscitate the dead" is the rule in lightning incidents, since victims who show some return of consciousness or who have spontaneous breathing are already on the way to recovery. Survivors should be routinely stabilized and transported to the hospital for more thorough evaluation. In the field, the most vigorous attempts at cardiopulmonary resuscitation should be directed to the victims who appear to be dead because they may ultimately recover if properly resuscitated.

The probability that lightning victims can recover after prolonged cardiopulmonary resuscitation (several hours) is not high. Other than for a few anecdotal reports, there is no reason to believe that these victims will respond to prolonged efforts. If the victim has not regained a pulse after 20 to 30 minutes of resuscitation, the chances of recovery are slim and the rescuer should not feel guilty about stopping resuscitation. Often in a remote setting, the rescuer is emotionally tied to the victim by age and friendship and may tend to continue resuscitation past the point of futility. In pronouncing a victim dead, the rescuer must be sure that other problems, such as hypothermia, are not clouding the victim's response to resuscitation efforts.

Other stabilization procedures, including splinting of fractures, endotracheal intubation, spinal precautions, and institution of intravenous fluids and oxygen, should be accomplished whenever indicated and feasible before transport.

History and Physical Examination

An eyewitness report is helpful, since victims are often confused and amnestic. The history should include a description of the event and the victim's behavior following the strike.

Like any other trauma victim, the victim must be completely undressed to facilitate examination. Special note should be taken of the vital signs, temperature, and level of consciousness. Because many victims are struck during a thunderstorm, they may be wet and cold. Hypothermia should be anticipated and treated appropriately (see Chapter 6).

The awake patient should be assessed for orientation and short-term memory. A cursory mental status examination of the lightning victim may reveal good ability to carry on a "social conversation" that easily hides deficits in fine neurocognitive skills. It is easy to discover deficits when they are so severe that the victim cannot assimilate information, perseverates, or asks repetitive questions. Continuing confusion or a deteriorating level of consciousness mandates CT of the head to rule out an intracranial injury.

Examination of the victim's eyes is essential to establish pupillary reactivity and ocular injury. Tympanic membrane rupture is an important indicator of lightning strike. Ossicular disruption may be one explanation for a victim's lack of appropriate response to verbal stimuli.

Although the pulmonary system may be affected by cardiac arrest, pulmonary edema, or adult respiratory distress syndrome, it is uncommon to witness these initially. The cardiovascular examination should include distal pulses in all extremities, appreciation of arrhythmias, and evaluation of cardiac damage, including isoenzymatic and ECG changes.

The victim's abdominal examination occasionally demonstrates absent bowel sounds, which suggests ileus or indicates acute traumatic injury, such as contusion of the liver, bowel, or spleen.

The examiner should document any skin changes. The victim's skin may show mottling, especially below the waist. Burns are not universally present or may take a period of hours to evolve. Notation of pulses, color, and movement and sensory examination of the victim's extremities are important.

The physical findings and mental state of minimally and moderately injured victims tend to change considerably over the first few hours; careful observation and documentation delineate the course so that therapy can be appropriate. The minimally injured victim can almost always be discharged to a responsible person or require only overnight observation, whereas the severely injured person may require intensive care with mechanical ventilation, antiarrhythmic medications, and invasive interventions and monitoring techniques.

Laboratory and X-ray Tests

Minimum laboratory examinations include complete blood cell count and urinalysis (including a test for myoglobin on fresh urine). Blood tests indicated for the more severely injured victim include electrolyte screen, blood urea nitrogen (BUN), and creatinine. Serial cardiac enzymes, isoenzyme tests, and troponin may be indicated in some cases. If the victim is to be placed on a ventilator, arterial blood gases will be necessary; if intracranial pressure monitoring is used, serum osmolality may be required.

An ECG is essential for all lightning victims and frequently shows QT prolongation, even when otherwise normal.

Radiographs and other imaging studies may be obtained, depending on the presentation and history. Cervical spine imaging should occur if there is any evidence of cranial burns, contusions, loss of consciousness, or change in mentation that would make the physical examination unreliable, or if there are other historical considerations, such as a fall. The victim who is unconscious, confused, or has a deteriorating level of consciousness requires a CT or MRI scan of the brain to identify trauma or ischemic injury. X-ray studies to rule out fractures, dislocations, and other bony injuries are ordered as indicated.

Treatment

Fluid Therapy. An intravenous lifeline is mandatory for the victim who shows unstable vital signs, unconsciousness, or disorientation. If the victim is hypotensive, fluid resuscitation with normal saline or Ringer's lactate solution is required, with the caution that significant cerebral edema may develop. Fluid restriction in normotensive or hypertensive victims is recommended because of this risk.

Arterial and/or central venous pressure monitoring may be indicated. Careful intake and output measurement is necessary in the severely injured patient and requires placement of an indwelling urinary catheter. Myoglobinuria is rare and usually transient, so that the mannitol diuresis, alkalinization, and aggressive fluid loading used with high-voltage electric injuries are rarely necessary. However, if burns are severe and extensive, which is rarely the case, resuscitation such as is necessary for high-voltage electrical injuries may be required.

Fasciotomy. The presence of keraunoparalysis, paralyzed and pulseless extremities seen with lightning injuries, should not be treated like similar-appearing traumatized extremities caused by high-voltage electric injury. Intense vascular spasm with lightning usually is caused by sympathetic instability. The victim's extremities should be treated expectantly.[9,34,91] Steady improvement in the mottled, cool extremity, with return of pulses in a few hours, is the rule rather than the exception. Fasciotomies are rarely indicated unless the extremity shows no signs of recovery and raised intracompartmental tissue pressures are documented. Only one case necessitating fasciotomy has been reported as of this writing.

Antibiotics and Tetanus Prophylaxis. Prophylactic antibiotics are not indicated. Standard therapy should follow culture and identification of pathogens. Exceptions to this rule include open extremity fracture or cranial fracture that violates the dura. In the latter situation, many neurosurgeons recommend antibiotic prophylaxis. Appropriate tetanus prophylaxis is mandatory if burns or lacerations are present.

Cardiovascular Therapy. Management of cardiac arrest is standard. In the victim who is not in a state of cardiac arrest, vasospasm may still make peripheral pulses difficult to palpate. Usually, femoral, brachial, or carotid pulses may be appreciated. A Doppler examination may be necessary to locate peripheral pulses and record blood pressure.

If a victim remains hypotensive on Doppler examination, fluid resuscitation may be necessary to establish adequate blood pressure and tissue perfusion. Causes of hypotension include major fractures, blood loss from abdominal or chest injuries, spinal shock, cardiogenic shock, and occasionally deep burns similar to high-voltage electric burns. As soon as an adequate central blood pressure is obtained, fluids should probably be restricted because of the high incidence of cranial injuries and cerebral edema.

The victim who is without spontaneous or adequate respirations should be mechanically ventilated until brain death is declared, he resumes adequate ventilation, or the physician and family decide to cease efforts.

All lightning victims, regardless of their condition, should have an ECG. Cardiac monitoring, serial isoenzyme, and troponin measurements are indicated if there is any sign of ischemia or arrhythmia or if the victim complains of chest pain. Injury patterns, as well as arrhythmias, have been reported.[34] The indications for antiarrhythmic drugs and pressor agents are the same as for a suspected myocardial infarction.[34]

Prolongation of the QT interval has been proposed, when part of a torsades des pointes phenomenon, as a possible explanation for the reports of suspended animation with recovery.[4]

Transient hypertension may be so short-lived as to require no acute therapy. However, several cases of hypertension have occurred 12 to 72 hours after lightning strike and seemed to respond well to β-blockers and other antihypertensive medications. Use of newer antihypertensive agents with lightning injuries has not been reported but would probably be equally effective.

Central Nervous System Injury.* Every lightning victim should have a complete neurologic examination. If there is a history of loss of consciousness or if the victim exhibits confusion, hospital admission is necessary. The victim with tympanic membrane rupture, cranial burns, or loss of consciousness, or who shows a decreasing level of consciousness, should undergo cervical spine imaging, brain CT, and possibly brain MRI. Serial CT scans may be useful in assessing ventricular hemorrhage and edema.

In the victim with persistent loss of consciousness, slight hyperventilation may be useful to control cerebral edema. If there are no other contraindications, the head should be elevated.

Intracranial pressure monitoring may be a useful adjunct in persons with elevated intracranial pressure.[78] Cerebral edema may be managed with mannitol, furosemide, fluid restriction, and other standard therapies.[78] Although hypothermia was reported to contribute to complete recovery in one victim with prolonged cardiac arrest before resuscitation efforts, there is no firm evidence that this would benefit all victims.

Early seizures are probably due to anoxia. If there is evidence of CNS damage or if seizures continue after adequate oxygenation and perfusion have been restored, standard pharmacologic intervention with diazepam, phenytoin, or phenobarbital should be considered.

If paralysis does not improve, causes other than lightning, including blunt injury from a fall, may be responsible. In addition, spinal artery syndrome has been reported, perhaps caused by arterial spasm. A physical therapy program should be initiated before discharge. Unfortunately, in a number of patients, peripheral neuropathies develop with continuing dysesthesias and weakness. These may respond to chronic pain management techniques, including combinations of nonsteroidal antiinflammatory drugs, carbamazepine, and tricyclic antidepressants.[5,9,47,110]

In recent years, neuropsychologic deficits from lightning have become better appreciated.[36,102,103,115] Heightened anxiety states, hyperirritability, memory deficits, aphasia, sleep disturbance, posttraumatic stress disorder, and other evidence of brain damage should be assessed.[5,47] Some of these deficits are much like those suffered by victims of blunt head trauma. A rehabilitation program should be instituted early for these patients to return them to as functional a state as possible.

Often, the victim's family and co-workers have difficulty understanding the change in personality that affects many of these victims. Neuropsychologic testing with appropriate therapy may be necessary. Certain personality types may predispose victims to more pronounced neuropsychologic symptoms.

The feeling of isolation and change that victims sometimes experience may lead to depression, substance abuse, and thoughts of suicide. Because of unfamiliarity with lightning injuries and their sequelae, many physicians are ill equipped to manage long-term care of lightning victims, leading the victim and the family to become angry.

Referral to Support Groups and Other Information Sources. Referral to Lightning Strike and Electric Shock Survivors International (LSESSI), a support group founded in the late 1980s, can be of substantial help to victims and families. LSESSI is located at PO Box 1156, Jacksonville, NC 28541-1156, telephone 910-346-4708, E-mail lightnin@nternet.net, http://lightningstrike.home.mindspring.com. Some local chapters have been formed in areas with a high incidence of lightning strikes. Other useful websites are http://www.uic.edu/labs/lightninginjury and http://www.thehub.com.au/~candy/rsch.htm.

Burns. Lightning burns may be apparent at the time of admission but more commonly develop within the first few hours. They are generally superficial, unlike high-voltage electrical burns, and seldom cause massive muscle destruction. Vigorous fluid therapy and mannitol diuresis are not indicated. The patient's urine should be tested for myoglobin, although it is infrequently seen. In the rare instance of myoglobinuria, intravenous mannitol and alkalinization of the urine with bicarbonate may be used. Overhydration with resultant cerebral edema probably has killed more lightning victims than has myoglobinuric renal failure.

Lightning burns are generally so superficial that they do not require treatment with topical agents. In the unusual instance of deep injury, topical therapy should be standard. The findings that lightning burns are superficial and do not require active surgical intervention is reinforced by Matthews et al.[91] Their paper provides a useful guide to the remote need for surgical intervention in lightning injury.

Eye Injuries.[43,99] Visual acuity should be measured and the victim's eyes thoroughly examined. Cataracts are not uncommon. Eye injuries should be treated in

---

*References 9, 19, 21-23, 34, 78, 123.

standard fashion and may require referral to an oph-thalmologist. Dinakaran et al[43] report a case in which cataract can be ascribed to a telephone-transmitted lightning strike.

Ear Injuries.[56,94,99] Simple tympanic membrane rupture is usually handled conservatively with observation until the victim's tissues heal. Sensorineural damage to the auditory nerve and facial nerve palsies are not uncommon. Loss of hearing mandates otologic evaluation. Ossicular disruption or more severe damage may necessitate surgical repair. Otorrhea and hemotympanum are not uncommon and suggest basilar skull fracture. Complaints of pain around the angle of the victim's jaw should lead the physician to a search for occult fracture of the styloid process and other musculoskeletal damage. Gordon et al[54] hypothesize that the injury must include components other than blast and consider burns the most likely. The present authors concur and cite the possibility of the cranial orifices being portals of entry for current.[3] Mora-Magana et al[93] provide a review of the otic effects of lightning.

Pregnant Victims. If a pregnant woman is struck, fetal viability must be assessed, including fetal heart tones and ultrasonography to observe fetal activity. Fetal death is treated with evacuation of the uterus.

Other Considerations. Gastric irritation is occasionally seen. Histamine-2 antagonists or antacid therapy may be indicated. A nasogastric tube is appropriate if ileus or hematemesis occurs. An abdominal CT scan may be indicated in comatose patients who remain hypotensive, since intestinal contusions and hemorrhage have been reported.

Endocrine dysfunction, perhaps as a result of pituitary or hypothalamic damage, including amenorrhea, impotence, and decreased libido, has occurred in some victims.

Pronouncing the Victim Dead.[14,18] The question of when to declare a lightning victim dead has always been controversial. Dilated pupils should not be taken as a sign of brain death in the lightning victim. It is always necessary to exclude other causes of dysfunction and eliminate them before death is declared. Hypothermia with lightning injury is possible, so normothermia should first be established if possible. Charleton[18] states that lightning injury carries a high survival, so persistence in resuscitation should be the norm. His notion seems sensible, but his statement has drawn substantial correspondence. Campbell-Hewson et al,[14] for example, raise the notion that it is a falsehood to claim that resuscitation after prolonged arrest is more likely with lightning-induced arrest. We entirely agree with this and agree that the notion arose from one misreported case.

PRECAUTIONS FOR AVOIDING LIGHTNING INJURY[37,74,96,117]

A multidisciplinary group of internationally recognized lightning experts met and reviewed new safety guidelines, which, along with the names of the participants, are available at http://www.uic.edu/labs/lightninginjury. These guidelines are the first to address different size groups and evacuation times. Most lightning accidents are isolated events. It is impractical for the National Weather Service to warn of every potentially dangerous lightning event, so the key to safety is individual education and responsibility.

The exceptions to this are when adults are in charge of groups of children and for large planned events, such as professional sporting or entertainment events.[96] In the former, the adult must assume responsibility for the children and have a plan for evacuation. A simple motto to teach children is, "If you *see* if, *flee* it; if you *hear* it, *clear* it."

Promoters of large events carry the responsibility to be aware of threatening weather, determine when events should be cancelled, and have a plan of action that includes proper warning, shelter guidelines, and all-clear signals.

Everyone should be aware of weather predictions and conditions before undertaking excursions or working in the open. If a person cannot avoid being outdoors, he or she should carry a small radio to monitor weather reports. Be prepared to seek a safe location if a severe thunderstorm watch or warning is announced. If bad weather is expected, someone should appoint a spotter whose duty it is to watch the weather and provide appropriate warning.

Based on new meteorologic data, the "30-30 rule" states that when the time between seeing lightning and hearing the thunder is 30 seconds or shorter (the first 30 of the 30-30 rule), persons are in danger and should be seeking shelter. Persons who have a long evacuation time, such as those on golf courses or who are responsible for many others, should use an even longer count. It is not uncommon for a portion of the sky to be blue when lightning hits, and at least 10% of lightning strikes occur with no rain at the site of the strike, so that people should not delay until the rain sets in. Lightning often hits more than one spot on the ground.

It is easy to underestimate the danger at the end of a storm. Outdoor activities should not be resumed until at least 30 minutes (the second 30 in the 30-30 rule) after the last lightning is seen or the last thunder heard. Although there is still risk after the 30 minutes, this measure offers about a 90% chance of safety from lightning injury.

If a storm strikes, seek safety in a substantial building or in an all-metal vehicle, such as a car, but avoid convertibles. Small buildings, such as golf shelters, bus shelters, and rain shelters, may actually increase the person's risk, depending on the size and height of the building, since side flashes can occur to the occupants. Tents offer little protection because the metal support poles actually may act as lightning rods. Occupants of the tents should stay as far away from the poles and wet cloth as possible. Ground pads seem to offer increased protection against ground potential but are not foolproof.

All-metal vehicles (not a cloth-top convertible or Jeep) provide a safe haven because the automobile will diffuse the current around the occupants to the ground. It is a myth that rubber tires provide insulation, but it is true that the metal body generally affords protection. Golf tournament promoters often place a number of rented school buses around the course for lightning protection. A series of minivans around a soccer field can provide the same type of safety to a more limited number of people. Another alternative is to assure access to public buildings where the playing fields are located. If a safe location is not available and a group of people is exposed, they should spread out and stay several yards apart, so that in the event of a strike, the fewest number is injured seriously by ground current and by side flashes between persons.

All of the recommendations of decisions about "safer places" that follow should not be necessary if you have taken the proper initial precautions: known the weather, had an evacuation-safety plan, and followed the plan. Those persons who are "caught" by a storm have usually not used appropriate prudence and have already made too many bad decisions to remedy in any substantial way with the following advice.

Stay away from metal objects, such as motorcycles, tractors, fences, and bicycles, and any that are taller than you. Avoid areas near power lines, pipelines, fences, ski lifts, and other structural steel fabrications. If you are wearing a backpack that protrudes above your head, increasing your height and risk, it may be worth the time to shed it, if only because you can run faster to a safer area. Otherwise, throwing off metal wastes time and is useless because it is a myth that wearing metal attracts lightning.

If you are unable to find a safe location, do not stand near tall, isolated trees, on hilltops, or at a lookout or other exposed area. In a forest, seek a low area under a thick growth of saplings or small trees. Seeking a clearing to avoid trees makes a person the tallest object in the clearing and more likely to be struck. Avoid cornstalks, haystacks, or other objects that project above the ground. Caves of substantial size, ditches, and valleys may provide some protection unless they are saturated with water, which may conduct current. Sheltering under a small outcropping or overhang may actually increase a person's risk of injury, since lightning energy that has hit a hill tends to flow through the heavy downpour and literally "drip" onto the person with the rain.

If you are totally in the open, stay far away from single trees to avoid lightning splashes. The "lightning position," recommended by the Lightning Safety Group, requires squatting with both feet close together and the ears covered by the hands to avoid acoustic trauma. This position minimizes a person's height, the area touching the ground, and the possibility of ground current effect. However, it is difficult for anyone over 35 years of age to achieve this position or for anyone to hold it for more than a few minutes. It is our best educated guess without scientific evidence that it is also acceptable to kneel on the ground or sit cross-legged, positions that are both much easier to achieve and maintain, and that increase the ground contact only minimally. One of these positions also puts the person in the position of supplication to a Higher Authority for Divine Intervention, which is highly recommended by all of the authors at this point.

If indoors during a thunderstorm, avoid open doors and windows, fireplaces, and metal objects, such as pipes, sinks, radiators, and plug-in electrical appliances. Avoid using the telephone or computer. Clothesline poles and fences may act as lightning rods and transmit lightning along the line or wire.

If you are on the water, seek the shore. Avoid swimming, boating, or being the tallest object near a large, open body of water. Lightning will usually preferentially strike the metal masts or other objects projecting above the surface of the water and flows well through the water to injure swimmers, on the same principle as ground current injuries. Moving under a bridge or cliff while in the boat may provide some protection. Sailboats and powerboats should be protected with lightning rods and grounding equipment attached to a metal keel or understructure of the boat.

INDUSTRIAL ELECTRICAL INJURIES

Direct current (DC) causes only one third as much damage as alternating current (AC) of the same voltage and amperage. High-voltage commercial electricity usually alternates at about 60 cycles per second, just the right frequency to cause muscle tetany. Because the victim is often working with the electrical source, the hands are the most frequently injured part of the body. The tetanic force triggered by the electricity causes the hand to freeze to the circuit, since the flexors of the forearm are stronger than the extensors. The current also arcs across flexed joints, producing kissing burns at each flexion point, including the wrist, elbow, and axilla.

The presence of water or sweat on the skin can lower resistance as much as 25 to 100 times. When the resistance of the dermis is lowered by moisture or diminished thickness, the applied energy preferentially courses through the inside of the body via lower resistance tissues. As a result, high-voltage electrical burns are characterized by deep muscle, nerve, and vascular damage, with variable overlying skin damage.

Both entry and exit wounds are usually seen with high-voltage electrical injuries, with diffuse, unpredictable damage occurring in between, similar to that of gunshot wounds.

If, as often happens, the victim clasps the current source in his or her hand, the exposure becomes prolonged and the victim's skin breaks down, allowing the current to pass internally through the excellent electrolyte media of the blood and muscles. The external wound may appear fairly benign, hiding the extensive damage that may have occurred in deeper structures. After high-voltage injuries, fasciotomies may be needed to maintain the circulation and viability of distal structures. Extensive amputations are not infrequent with high-voltage electrical injuries. Fluid loading, mannitol diuresis, and alkalinization may be necessary to prevent myoglobinuric renal failure.

PRECAUTIONS FOR AVOIDING ELECTRICAL INJURY

Protection against the effects of electric current appears easy. Prevention is better than cure, and contact with any conductor should be avoided at all costs, on the assumption that the conductor is live. In the wilderness, high-voltage transmission lines are more likely to be encountered, with attendant increased danger. All intentional contact with conductors should be avoided.

Persons should not climb pylons, swing from lines, or otherwise touch power lines. Insulation of electrical lines is for the sole protection of the lines from the weather and should not be assumed to be adequate to protect living things that touch or grab the line.

Nonetheless, nonintentional contact with electrical conductors can occur. They may be hidden from view; insulation on normally touched apparatus may have been damaged or have aged; lines may have fallen; and any one of many other scenarios of accidental contact may occur. As a general principle, any item unidentifiable from a safe distance should be assumed harmful and not investigated until safety is ensured. This applies no less to electrical objects.

Persons working on electrical equipment should follow the procedures in Box 3-4.

Residual current devices (RCDs), also known as ground fault circuit interrupters, sense any difference between current entering and leaving the line to which they are connected. Any difference must represent current conducted to the earth, and the circuit is immediately deenergized on the assumption the leak may be through a person. Because roughly 80% of accidents occur in this way, the RCD's importance is notable. RCDs are now required by code in new installations, particularly domestic ones, but they may be absent in older construction.

REFERENCES

1. Anderson RB: A fifth mechanism to explain injuries due to close lightning flashes? Submitted to the *Journal of the IEEE Engineering in Medicine and Biology Society*, 2000.
1a. Andrews CJ: Telephone-related lightning injury, *Med J Aust* 157:823, 1992.
2. Andrews CJ: *Studies in aspects of lightning injury*, doctoral dissertation, Brisbane, Australia, 1993, University of Queensland.
3. Andrews CJ: Structural changes after lightning strike, with special emphasis on special sense orifices as portals of entry, *Semin Neurol* 15:296-303, 1995.
4. Andrews CJ, Colquhoun DM, Darveniza M: The QT interval in lightning injury with implications for the "cessation of metabolism" hypothesis, *J Wilderness Med* 4:155, 1993.
5. Andrews CJ, Darveniza M: Telephone mediated lightning injury: an Australian survey, *J Trauma* 29:665, 1989.
6. Andrews CJ, Darveniza M: *Determination of acoustic insult in telephone mediated lightning strike*, unpublished material, 1992.
7. Andrews CJ, Darveniza M: New models of the electrical insult in lightning strike. In Proceedings of the 9th International Conference on Atmospheric Physics, St Petersburg, Russia, 1992.
8. Andrews CJ, Darveniza M, Mackerras D: Lightning injury: a review of clinical aspects, pathophysiology and treatment, *Adv Trauma* 4:241, 1989.
9. Andrews CJ et al: *Lightning injuries: electrical, medical, and legal aspects*, Boca Raton, Fla, 1992, CRC Press.
10. Bernstein T: Theories of the causes of death from electricity in the late 19th century, *Med Instum* 9:267, 1975.
11. Biegelmeier G: New knowledge of the impedance of the human body. In Bridges J et al, editors: *Electric shock safety criteria*, New York, 1985, Pergamon Press.
12. Bridges J et al, editors: *Electric shock safety criteria*, New York, 1985, Pergamon Press.
13. Bruhac J: *How the hero twins found their father, flying with the eagle, racing with the great bear*, Mexico, 1993, BridgeWater Books.
14. Campbell-Hewson, G: Death after electric shock and lightning strike is more clear cut than suggested, *BMJ* 314:442, 1997.
15. Campo RV, Lewis RS: Lightning-induced macular hole, *Am J Otolaryngol* 97:792, 1984.

16. Cannel H: Struck by lightning: the effects upon the men and the ships of H M Navy, *J R Nav Med Serv* 65:165, 1979.

17. Chai JC: Human body responses to step voltages due to ground currents in lightning attachments. In *Proceedings of the International Conference on Lightning and Static Electricity*, October 6-8, 1992, Atlantic City, NJ, FAA Report No DOT/FAA/CT-92/20, pp P21-P2-10.

18. Charlton R: Diagnosing death, *BMJ* 313:956, 1996.

19. Cherington M: Central nervous system complications of lightning and electrical injuries, *Semin Neurol* 15:233, 1995.

20. Cherington M, Vervalin C: Lightning injuries: who is at greatest risk? *Phys Sportsmed* 18:58, 1990.

21. Cherington M, Yarnell P, Hallmark D: MRI in lightning encephalopathy, *Neurology* 43:1437, 1993.

22. Cherington M, Yarnell P, Lammereste D: Lightning strikes: nature of neurological damage in patients evaluated in hospital emergency departments, *Ann Emerg Med* 21:575, 1992.

23. Cherington M et al: A bolt from the blue: lightning strike to the head, *Neurology* 48:683, 1997.

24. Cherington M et al: Could lightning injury be magnetically induced? *Lancet* 351:1788, 1998.

25. Cherington M et al: Closing the gap on the actual numbers of lightning casualties and deaths. *Preprints, 11th Conference on Applied Climatology*, Dallas, January 10-15, Boston, American Meteorological Society, 1999.

26. Christian HJ et al: Global frequency and distribution of lightning as observed by the Optical Transient Detector (OTD). In *Proceedings of the 11th International Conference on Atmospheric Electricity*, Guntersville, Ala, June 7-11, 1999.

27. Coates L, Blong R, Siciliano F: Lightning fatalities in Australia, 1824-1991, *Natural Hazards* 8:217, 1993.

28. Cohen JA: Autonomic nervous system disorders and reflex sympathetic dystrophy in lightning and electrical injuries, *Semin Neurol* 15:387, 1995.

29. Cooper MA: Lightning injuries: prognostic signs for death, *Ann Emerg Med* 9:134, 1980.

30. Cooper MA: Medical aspects of lightning injury. Proceedings of the 9th International Conference on Atmospheric Physics, St. Petersburg, Russia, June 1992.

31. Cooper MA: Physiological aspects of lightning injury. Proceedings of the 9th International Conference on Atmospheric Electricity, St. Petersburg, Russia, June 1992.

32. Cooper MA: Post electrocution syndrome—long term effects of lightning injury. Proceedings of the Foudre et Montagne, Chamonix-Mont Blanc, France, June 1994.

33. Cooper MA: Chronic pain syndrome in a lightning victim. In *Proceedings of the International Aerospace and Ground Conference on Lightning and Static Electricity*, Williamsburg, Va, September 1995, US Navy NAWCADPAX-95-306-PRO.

34. Cooper MA: Emergent care of lightning and electrical injuries, *Semin Neurol* 15:268, 1995.

35. Cooper MA: *Myths, miracles, and mirages*, Semin Neurol 15:358, 1995.

35a. Cooper MA: *Lightning injury from upward leaders*, in preparation.

36. Cooper MA, Andrews CJ, ten Duis HJ: Neuropsychological aspects of lighting injury. Proceedings of the 9th International Conference on Atmospheric Physics, St. Petersburg, Russia, June 1992.

37. Cooper MA, Holle R, Lopez R: Recommendations for lightning safety, *JAMA* 282:1132, 1999.

38. Cooper MA, Kotsos TP: Development of an animal model of lightning injury with flashover utilizing a table-top lightning generator. Proceedings of the Foudre et Montagne '97, Chamonix-Mont Blanc France, June 4, 1997.

39. Cooper MA, Kotsos TP: Development of an animal model of lightning injury—an update. Proceedings of the International Scientific Meeting on Electromagnetics in Medicine, Chicago, November 1997.

40. Cummins KL et al: A combined TOA/MDF technology upgrade of the U.S. National Lightning Detection Network, *J Geophys Res* 103:9035, 1998.

41. Curran EB, Holle RL, López RE: *Lightning fatalities, injuries, and damage reports in the United States from 1959-1994*, National Oceanic and Atmospheric Administration Technical Memo NWS SR-193, 1997.

42. Darveniza M et al: Critical review of claimed enhanced lightning protection characteristics of early streamer emission air terminals for lightning protection of buildings, in press.

43. Dinakaran S et al: Telephone mediated lightning injury causing cataract, *Injury* 29:645, 1998.

44. Duclos PJ, Sanderson LM: An epidemiological description of lightning-related deaths in the United States, *Int J Epidemiol* 19:673, 1990.

45. Duclos PJ, Sanderson LM, Klontz KC: Lightning-related mortality and morbidity in Florida, *Public Health Rep* 105:276, 1990.

46. Elsom DM: Deaths caused by lightning in England and Wales, 1852-1990, *Weather* 48:83, 1993.

47. Engelstatter GH: *Psychological effects of lightning strike and electric shock injuries*. In lecture notes, Third Annual International Meeting of Lightning Strike and Electric Shock Victims, Maggie Valley, NC, 1993.

48. Ferrett RL, Ojala CF: The lightning hazard in Michigan, *Michigan Academician* 24:427, 1992.

49. Franklin B: *Experiments and observations on electricity made at Philadelphia*, London, 1774, E Cave.

50. Franklin B: *The autobiography of Benjamin Franklin*, New Haven, Conn, 1973, Yale University Press.

51. Golde RH: *Lightning protection*, New York, 1973, Chemical Publishing.

52. Golde RH: *Lightning*, vols 1 and 2, London, 1977, Academic Press.

53. Golde RH, Lee WR: Death by lightning, *Proc Inst Elec Eng* 123:1163, 1976.

54. Gordon M et al: *Lightning injury of the tympanic membrane*, Am J Otolaryngol 16:373, 1995.

55. Gourbière E et al: Lightning injured people in France, the first French national inquiry with regard to the striking of people—objectives, methods, first results. Proceedings, Conference on Lightning and Mountains '97, Chamonix Mont Blanc, France, 1997.

56. Grossman A et al: Auditory and neuropsychiatric behavior patterns after electrical injury, *J Burn Care Rehabil* 14:169, 1993.

57. Grover S, Goodwin J: Lightning and electrical injuries: neuro-ophthalmologic aspects, *Semin Neurol* 15:335, 1995.

58. Hegner CF: Lightning—some of its effects, *Ann Surg* 65:401, 1917.

59. Hendler N, Raja SN: Reflex sympathetic dystrophy and causalgia. In Tollison CD et al, editors: *Handbook of pain management*, Baltimore, 1994, Williams & Wilkins.

60. Hendler N, Talo S: Chronic pain patient versus the malingering patient. In *Current therapy of pain*, Philadelphia, 1989, BC Decker.

61. Hendler NH et al: A comparison between the Minnesota Multiphasic Personality Inventory and the "Mensana Clinic Back Pain Test" for validating the complaint of chronic back pain, *J Occup Med* 30:98, 1988.

62. Hocking B, Andrews CJ: Fractals and lightning injury, *Med J Aust* 150:409, 1989.

63. Holle RL, López RE, Navarro BC: *U.S. lightning deaths, injuries, and damages in the 1890s compared to the 1990s*, National Oceanic and Atmospheric Administration Technical Memo, ERL pending, 2000.

64. Holle RL et al: The local meteorological environment of lightning casualties in central Florida. In Preprints, 17th Conference on Severe Local Storms and Conference on Atmospheric Electricity, St Louis, American Meteorological Society, October 4-8, 1993.

65. Holle RL et al: Safety in the presence of lightning, *Semin Neurol* 15:375, 1995.

66. Holle RL et al: Insured lightning-caused property damage in three western states, *J Appl Meteorol* 35:1344, 1996.

67. Hooshmand H: *Chronic pain*, Boca Raton, Fla, 1993, CRC Press.

68. Hornstein RA: *Canadian lightning deaths and damage*, Meteorological Branch, Department of Transport, Canada, CIR-3719, TEC-423, 1962.

69. Huffines GR, Orville RE: Lightning ground flash density and thunderstorm duration in the contiguous United States: 1989-1996, *J Appl Meteorol* 38:1013, 1999.

70. Jex-Blake AJ: Death by electric currents and by lightning, The Ghoulstonian Lectures, Lecture III, *BMJ*, p 548, 1906.

71. Jones DT et al: Lightning and its effects on the auditory system, *Laryngoscope* 101:830, 1992.

72. Jumbelic MI: Forensic perspectives of electrical and lightning injuries, *Semin Neurol* 15:342, 1995.

73. Kithill R: Results of investigations into annual USA lightning costs and losses. International Conference on Atmospheric Electricity, Huntsville, Ala, June 1999.

74. Kitigawa N, Ohashi M, Ishikawa T: Safety guide against lightning hazards, *Res Lett Atmosph Electr* 10:37, 1990.

74a. Kretzer HF: *Lightning record, a book of reference and information*, St Louis, 1895.

75. Langley RL, Dunn KA, Esinhart JD: Lightning fatalities in North Carolina 1972-1988, *NC Med J* 52:281, 1991.

76. Lee RC, Cravalho EG, Burke JF: *Electrical trauma: the pathophysiology, manifestations and clinical management*, Cambridge, UK, 1992, Cambridge University Press.

77. Lee RC et al: Biophysical mechanisms of cell membrane damage in electrical shock, *Semin Neurol* 15:367, 1995.

78. Lehman LB: Successful management of an adult lightning victim using intracranial pressure monitoring, *Neurosurgery* 28:907, 1991.

79. Lichtenberg R et al: Cardiovascular effects of lightning strikes, *J Am Coll Cardiol* 21:531, 1993.

80. Livingston ES, Nielsen-Gammon JW, Orville RE: A climatology, synoptic assessment, and thermodynamic evaluation for cloud-to-ground lightning in Georgia: a study for the 1996 summer Olympics, *Bull Am Meteorol Soc* 77:1483, 1996.

81. López RE, Holle RL: Diurnal and spatial variability of lightning activity in northeastern Colorado and central Florida during the summer, *Mon Wea Rev* 114:1288, 1986.

82. López RE, Holle RL: Demographics of lightning casualties, *Semin Neurol* 15:286, 1995.

83. López RE, Holle RL: Fluctuations of lightning casualties in the United States: 1959-1990, *J Climate* 9:608, 1996.

84. López RE, Holle RL: Changes in the number of lightning deaths in the United States during the twentieth century, *J Climate* 11:2070, 1998.

85. López RE, Holle RL: Climate related trends in the number of lightning deaths during the twentieth century. Preprints, 11th Conference on Applied Climatology, Dallas, American Meteorological Society, 1999.

86. López RE, Holle RL: *The distance between successive lightning flashes*, National Oceanic and Atmospheric Administration Technical Memo NWS ERL NSSL-105, National Severe Storms Laboratory, Norman, Okla, 1999.

87. López RE, Holle RL, Heitkamp TA: Lightning casualties and property damage in Colorado from 1950 to 1991 based on Storm Data, *Weather and Forecasting* 10:114, 1995.

88. López RE et al: The underreporting of lightning injuries and deaths in Colorado, *Bull Am Meteorol Soc* 74:2171, 1993.

89. López RE et al: Spatial and temporal distributions of lightning over Arizona from a power utility perspective, *J Appl Meteorol* 36:825, 1997.

90. Krider EP, Uman MA: Cloud-to-ground lightning: mechanisms of damage and methods of protection, *Semin Neurol* 15:227, 1995.

91. Matthews M et al: Plastic surgical considerations in lightning injuries, *Ann Plast Surg* 39:561, 1997.

92. Mogil HM, Rush M, Kutka M: *Lightning—An update*, Preprints, 10th Conference on Severe Local Storms, Omaha, Neb, 1997, American Meteorological Society.

93. Mora-Magana I et al: Acoustic trauma caused by lightning, *Int J Pediatr Otorhinolaryngol* 35:59, 1996.

94. Morikawa S, Steichen F: Successful resuscitation after death from lightning, *Anesthesia* 21:222, 1960.

95. National Collegiate Athletic Association: Guideline 1D: Lightning Safety. *In 1998-99 NCAA Sports Medicine Handbook*, 1998.

96. Norman ME, Younge BR: Association of high-dose intravenous methylprednisolone with reversal of blindness from lightning in two patients, *Ophthalmology* 106:743, 1999.

97. O'Brien CF: Involuntary movement disorders following lightning and electrical injuries, *Semin Neurol* 15:263, 1995.

98. Ogren FP, Edmunds AL: Neuro-otologic findings in the lightning-injured patient, *Semin Neurol* 15:256, 1995.

99. Ohashi M, Kitagawa N, Ishikawa T: Lightning injury caused by discharges accompanying flashover—a clinical and experimental study of death and survival, *Burns* 12:496, 1986.

100. Orville RE, Silver AC: Lightning ground flash density in the contiguous United States: 1992-95, *Mon Wea Rev* 125:631, 1997.

101. Pakiam JE, Chao TC, Chia J: Lightning fatalities in Singapore, *The Meteorological Magazine* 110:175-187, 1981.

102. Primeau M, Engelstetter G, Bares K: Behavioral consequences of lightning and electrical injury, *Semin Neurol* 15:279, 1995.

103. Primeau M, Engelstetter G, Cooper MA: Psychological sequelae of lightning injury. *Proceedings of the International Aerospace and Ground Conference on Lightning and Static Electricity*, Williamsburg Va, September 1995, US Navy NAWCADPAX-95-306-PRO.

104. *Public Health Service, 1947 to present: vital statistics of the United States*, Washington, DC, US Government Printing Office.

105. Qureshi N: Indirect lightning strike via telephone wire, *Injury* 26:629,1995.

106. Raja SN: Sympathetically maintained pain, *Curr Pract Anaesth* 2:421, 1990.

107. Rakov VA, Uman MA: Some properties of negative cloud-to-ground lightning flashes versus stroke order, *J Geophys Res* 95:5447, 1990.

108. Schwartzman RJ: The movement disorder of reflex sympathetic dystrophy, *Neurology* 40:57, 1990.

109. Schwartzman RJ: Causalgia and reflex sympathetic dystrophy. In Feldmann E, editor: *Current diagnosis in neurology*, St Louis, 1994, Mosby.

110. Shantha TR: Causalgia induced by telephone-mediated lightning electrical injury and treated by interpleural block, *Anesth Analg* 73:507, 1991.

111. Shearman KM, Ojala CF: Some causes for lightning data inaccuracies: the case of Michigan, *Bull Am Meteorol Soc* 80:1883, 1999.

112. Solterman B, Frutiger A, Kuhn M: Lightning injury with lung bleeding in a tracheotomized patient, *Chest* 99:240, 1991.

113. Taussig H: "Death" from lightning and the possibility of living again, *Ann Intern Med* 68:1345, 1968.

114. Uman MA: *Understanding lightning*, Carnegie, Pa, 1971, Bek Technical Publications (reissued as *All about lightning*, New York, 1986, Dover).

115. Van Zomeren A et al: Lightning stroke and neuropsychological impairment: cases and questions, *J Neurol Neurosurg Psychiatry* 64:763, 1998.

116. Vavrek J, Holle RL, Allsopp J: Flash to bang, *The Earth Scientist* 4:3, 1993.

117. Vavrek RJ, Holle RL, López RE: *Updated lightning safety recommendations*, Preprints, 8th symposium on Education, January 10-15, Dallas, Boston, American Meteorological Society.

118. Viemeister RE: *The lightning book*, Boston, 1972, MIT Press.

119. Watson AI, Holle RL: An eight-year lightning climatology of the southeast United States prepared for the 1996 summer Olympics, *Bull Am Meteorol Soc* 77:883, 1996.

120. Watson AI, López RE, Holle RL: Diurnal cloud-to-ground lightning patterns in Arizona during the southwest monsoon, *Mon Wea Rev* 122:1716, 1994.

121. Webb J et al: Unusual skin injury from lightning, *Lancet* 347:321, 1996.

122. Wilbourn AJ: Peripheral nerve disorders in electrical and lightning injuries, *Semin Neurol* 15:241, 1995.

123. World Health Organization: *Manual of the international statistical classification of diseases, injuries and causes of death, sixth revision of the international lists of diseases and causes of death*, Adopted 1948. Geneva, vol 1, 352 pp.

124. Yarnell PR, Lammertse DP: Neurorehabilitation of lightning and electrical injuries, *Semin Neurol* 15:391, 1995.

125. Zegel FH: Lightning deaths in the United States: a seven-year survey from 1959 to 1965, *Weatherwise* 20:169, 1967.

Cold and
Heat

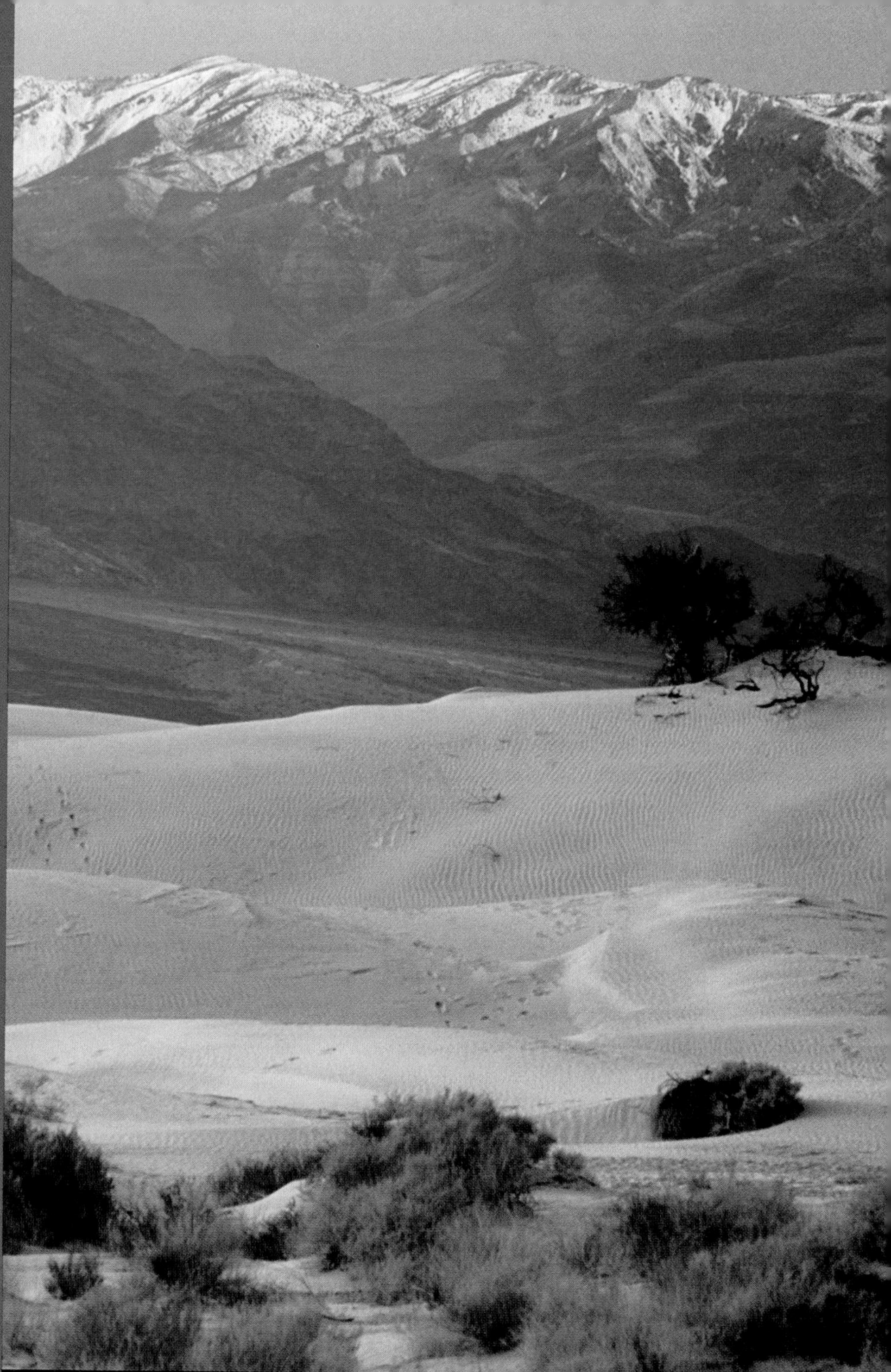

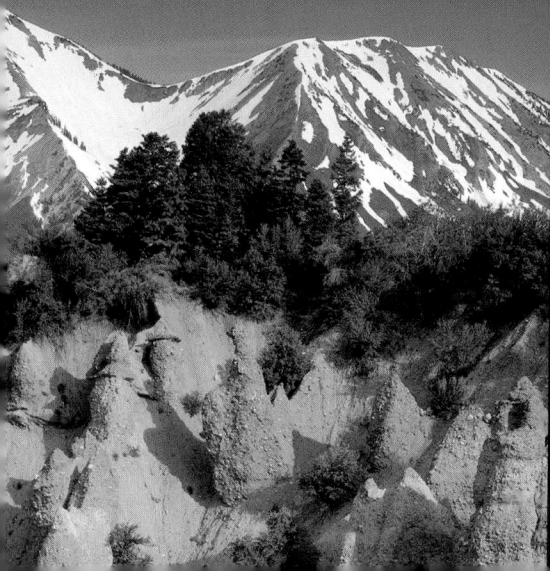

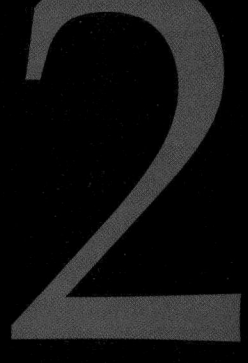

2

4 Thermoregulation

Larry I. Crawshaw, Richard N. Rausch, and Helen L. Wallace

A warm body has long been recognized as a primary condition for and sign of life. Faced with primitive circumstances, maintaining body temperature can require both ingenuity and physiologic knowledge. Three thousand years ago, an aged King David suffered hypothermia. Ministrations included covering him with clothes and finding a "fair damsel" to keep him warm. Unfortunately, these attempts to achieve a positive heat balance were unsuccessful.[56] More recently, the efficacy of body-to-body contact was assessed quantitatively when immersion hypothermia "victims" were placed in a sleeping bag alone or with male or female "heat donors." Surprisingly, the "victims" who were supplied with "donors" exhibited a blunted shivering thermogenesis and rewarmed at a lower rate.[40]

Because the thermal environment can be extremely complicated and the human thermoregulatory system is similarly complex and only partially understood, decisions about body temperature maintenance in the field can be difficult. This chapter is designed to aid the decision process by providing a basic understanding of the relationships among the ambient thermal environment, the body's thermal characteristics, and the thermoregulatory system. First, the heat balance equation is used to quantify the thermal relationship between the body and the environment. Second, peripheral neuronal inputs, the nature of the central regulator, and methods for assessing core temperature are elucidated. Third, the various organ systems that the body uses as effectors to regulate body temperature are outlined. Finally, a number of special circumstances that affect temperature regulation are noted.

PHYSICAL FACTORS GOVERNING HEAT EXCHANGE—THE HEAT BALANCE EQUATION[23,48,86,93,108]

The physical laws governing heat transfer determine the net energy flux into or out of the body. The heat balance equation is a convenient method for partitioning and quantifying the flow of energy between the environment and the body. A high rate of metabolic heat production is critical for maintaining a constant body temperature in mammals. This is represented by total heat production (H_{tot}) on the left side of the equation. For a person whose body is at thermal equilibrium,

$$H_{tot} = \pm H_d \pm H_c \pm H_r \pm H_e$$

where

H_{tot} = total metabolic heat production
H_d = conductive heat exchange
H_c = convective heat exchange
H_r = radiative heat exchange
H_e = evaporative heat exchange

H_{tot} is always positive, although the various channels of heat exchange can be positive or negative, depending on the situation. Positive values refer to net heat loss from the body. If the sum of the net heat exchange through the various channels exceeds H_{tot}, heat content of the body will decrease and mean body temperature will fall. On the other hand, if H_{tot} is greater than the net heat exchange, heat content of the body will increase and mean body temperature will rise.

Conductive Heat Exchange (H_d)

Heat transfer between objects in direct contact is termed *conduction*. The direction of heat flow is always from the higher to the lower temperature. Since conduction involves a direct interaction between molecules (contact), this type of heat transfer is minimal except under certain circumstances, such as sitting on a cold rock with little insulation. Under these conditions, the heat loss to the rock would be similar to that lost from the remainder of the body surface by radiation and convection.[85] The equation governing heat exchange by conduction is

$$H_d = \frac{kA(T_{sk} - T_a)}{1}$$

where

k = thermal conductivity
A = area of contact
T_{sk} = skin temperature
T_a = ambient temperature
1 = distance between the two surfaces

The thermal conductivity of a number of substances is given in Table 4-1. Note that water has 25 times the conductivity of air, but only one fifth that of granite. Muscle tissue has about twice the conductivity of fat. The conduction of heat through a tissue is termed *thermal diffusivity*. This expression is obtained by dividing the thermal conductivity by the product of the density and the

TABLE 4-1. Thermal Characteristics of Selected Substances

SUBSTANCE	CONDUCTIVITY $(cal \cdot s^{-1} \cdot cm^{-1} \cdot {}^\circ C^{-1})$	SPECIFIC HEAT $(cal \cdot g^{-1} \cdot {}^\circ C^{-1})$	VOLUMETRIC HEAT CAPACITY $(cal \cdot l^{-1} \cdot {}^\circ C^{-1})$
Air	0.000057	0.24	0.29
Water	0.0014	1.0	1000
Granite	0.007	0.2	540
Muscle tissue	0.0011	0.8	850
Fat	0.00051	0.5	460

Data from Schmidt-Nielsen K: *Animal physiology: adaptation and enviroment*, ed 4, Cambridge, 1990, Cambridge University Press; Cossins AR, Bowler K: *Temperature biology of animals*, New York, 1987, Chapman & Hall; and Hodgman CD, editor: *Handbook of chemistry and physics: a ready-reference book of chemical and physical data*, ed 43, Cleveland, 1962, Chemical Rubber.

specific heat. The specific heat of various substances is also given in Table 4-1. Water and muscle tissue (mostly water) have particularly high values. Specific heats can be misleading, however, so the volumetric heat capacities are also listed in Table 4-1. Although the specific heat of water is four times that of air, it takes about 3500 times as much heat to raise the temperature of a given volume of water by 1° C (1.8° F) as it does to accomplish the same feat with a similar volume of air. For someone in the water, the consequence of these properties is that skin temperature is within 1° C of water temperature, and heat transfer to or from the environment is greatly facilitated. In cool water, during rest, skin blood flow will be minimized because of peripheral vasoconstriction. Heat loss will, importantly, be determined by the subcutaneous fat layer; an average-sized fat person (36% body fat by weight) will begin shivering at a water temperature of about 27° C (81° F), whereas a lean person (below 10% body fat) will start shivering at about 33° C (91° F).[92]

Convective Heat Exchange (H$_c$)

Convection can be seen as a facilitation of conduction caused by the movement of molecules in a gas or liquid. This movement decreases the functional value of 1, the denominator in the conduction equation. Convection can be either forced or natural (free). Forced convection results from gas or liquid movement caused by the application of an external force, such as the movement of a fan or the pumping of a heart. Natural convection results from density changes that are produced by heating or cooling molecules adjacent to the body. These density changes cause the molecules to move with respect to the body surface. For humans, natural convection predominates at air speeds below 0.2 m sec^{-1}, whereas forced convection is more important at air speeds above this level.[86]

The relationships defining heat exchange as a result of convection can be complicated and depend on surface temperature profiles, surface shape, flow dynamics, density, conductivity, and specific heat. Any factor that impedes movement of the boundary layer (the

molecules immediately adjacent to the body) greatly retards convective heat transfer.

Brengelmann and Brown[8] have noted that under relatively neutral conditions (T$_a$ = 29° C [84.2° F], wind velocity = 0.9 msec^{-1}), about 40% of the heat loss from a nude human is mediated by convection. Increases in air or fluid velocity greatly increase convective heat transfer.

Radiative Heat Exchange (H$_r$)

All objects at temperatures above absolute zero emit electromagnetic radiation. This energy transfer occurs through space and does not require an intervening medium. In any given situation, the object is both transmitting and receiving infrared thermal radiation. In some cases, the object also receives solar radiation. The net heat transfer depends on the absolute temperatures, the nature of the surfaces involved, and solar input. Surfaces that are effective absorbers of radiation are also effective emitters of radiation. The idealized "black body" illustrates this property; such bodies absorb all and reflect none of the incident radiation. Conversely, poor absorbers (such as a polished silver surface) are also poor emitters. Heat transfer resulting from infrared (first-term) and solar (second-term) radiation is given by the following equations:

$$H_r = \sigma \epsilon_{sk} \epsilon_a (T_{sk}^4 - T_a^4) + a(1 + r)s$$

where

σ = Stefan-Boltzmann proportionality constant
ϵ_{sk} = emissivity of the skin
ϵ_a = emissivity of the environment
T_{sk} = skin temperature (K)
T_a = ambient temperature (K)
a = absorptance
r = reflectance
s = solar radiation

For temperatures in the physiologic range, and where $(T_{sk} - T_a)$ is less than 20° C (36° F), several authors have noted that infrared radiation heat exchange is roughly proportional to $T_{sk} - T_a$.[9,108] Also of note is that the spectrum of emitted radiation depends on the temperature of the object. At physiologic temperatures, the wavelengths of emitted radiation are longer (infrared), whereas at higher temperatures, like that of the sun's surface, the wavelengths are shorter (visible radiation) and can be detected by the human eye. This difference leads to some important consequences. The middle infrared radiation that is emitted by mammals is maximal regardless of skin pigmentation or the color of clothing. Solar radiation, however, peaks in the visible portion of the spectrum and is absorbed to a significantly greater extent by darker clothes or skin.

Incident radiation can vary drastically under different environmental conditions and may severely tax the body's ability to respond. Heat input from solar radiation on a cloudless day may exceed by several times the heat produced by basal metabolism; on a cloudless night there is a significant net loss of radiation to the sky. Under the relatively thermoneutral conditions noted earlier by Brengelmann and Brown,[8] radiant heat loss accounted for about 45% of the total.

Evaporative Heat Exchange (H_e)

When water changes state, a large amount of energy is either absorbed or given off. Evaporation of 1 g of water at 35° C (95° F), the usual skin temperature of a person sweating,[108] requires the input of 0.58 kcal of thermal energy. In a neutral thermal environment, sweating does not occur and evaporation accounts for only 15% of the total heat loss. Of this, slightly more than half is due to evaporation from the respiratory tract, with the remainder coming from water that passively diffuses through the skin and evaporates.[8]

Although it is unusual, the evaporation term (H_e) of the heat balance equation can become negative (meaning that heat is being introduced into the body). This occurs during airway rewarming when water-saturated oxygen is introduced into the respiratory system at about 43° C (109° F). Since the victim's body is considerably colder than 43° C, water condenses in the airways. For every gram of liquid water that is formed, the body heat content increases by 0.58 kcal.

THERMOREGULATORY NETWORK

A regulatory system requires sensing the controlled variable, comparing it with an ideal value, and producing an appropriate output signal. In this section, the role of the nervous system in the maintenance of a stable body temperature is outlined.

Peripheral Thermal Sensors

The entire outer surface of the body is well supplied with sensitive thermoreceptive structures. Because one destination of information from these receptors is the sensory cortex, many properties of the receptors can be gleaned from direct experience. Afferent thermal information produces both hot and cold sensations and is particularly rate sensitive. In addition to cortical input that arrives via the medial lemniscus and ventrobasal thalamus, the brain receives a large amount of thermal information from pathways that synapse in the reticular area.[13] Although cortical thermal input is part of the sensory information used to reconstruct the external thermal environment, reticular inputs are more important in behavioral and autonomic regulation of body temperature.[27] This distinction was pointed out by Cabanac,[17] who found that internal body temperature determined whether a particular surface temperature was perceived as pleasant or unpleasant. However, altered body temperature did not affect the discriminative (cortically mediated) aspects of the thermal stimulus; subjects had no problem correctly identifying the actual peripheral temperature. This study also confirms the intimate relationship between the thermoregulatory network and the pleasure-pain system.[96]

Although the structure, location, and properties of peripheral thermoreceptors are well documented, the transduction mechanism is poorly understood. Thermal sensors are free nerve endings and are categorized as either warm or cold. Cold receptors are found immediately beneath the epidermis, whereas warm receptors are located slightly deeper in the dermis. The hallmark of both types of receptors is their extremely high rate sensitivity (Figure 4-1).[51] Although the static firing rate of cold receptors is usually less than 10 impulses per second, firing rates are often an order of magnitude higher under conditions of rapid temperature change. Cold receptors are excited by cooling, inhibited by warming, and have static maxima at about 25° C (77° F). These receptors are active from about 10° to 40° C (50° to 104° F). Warm receptors are excited by warming, inhibited by cooling, and have static maxima above 40° C. They are active from about 30° to 45° C (86° to 113° F).[50] Studies on the mechanism underlying peripheral cold sensitivity have implicated thermal effects on the electrogenic Na^+/K^+ pump.[6]

Psychophysical and physiologic studies indicate that thermal receptors are not uniformly distributed across the body surface and that there are far more cold receptors.[50] Since peripheral thermal input is intimately involved in the regulation of body temperature, which body site is heated or cooled can have a definite effect on the magnitude of the response produced. In one study, for example, cooling the forehead was more than three times as effective (per unit area) in decreasing ongoing sweating as was cooling the lower leg.[26] A separate study evaluated regional trunk and appendage sensitivity to cooling by assessing the magnitude of the gasping response that occurs at the onset of immersion.

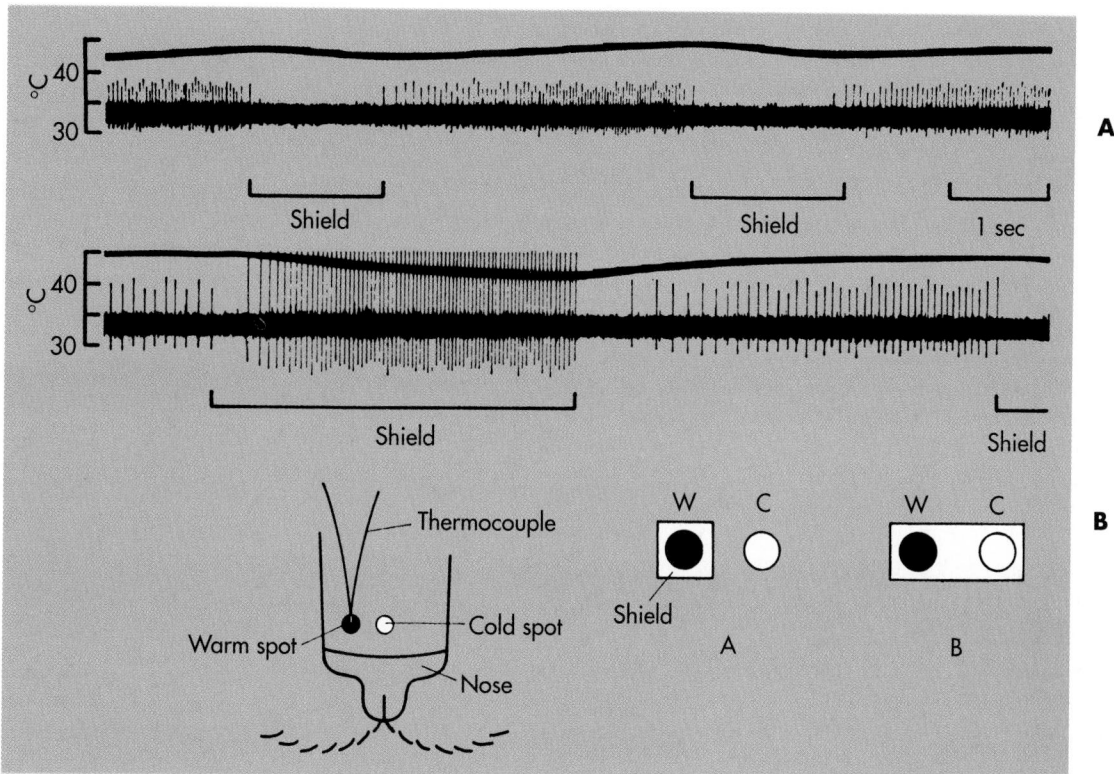

Figure 4-1 Impulses from a recording of peripheral neurons that includes a single warm fiber and a single cold fiber. In recording **A,** a shield was periodically placed in front of and then moved away from the skin site that was innervated by the warm fiber. The discharge stops immediately when the skin is shielded from the radiation source. In recording **B,** the shield was simultaneously placed in front of the skin site innervated by both the warm fiber and the cold fiber. This caused excitation of the cold fiber and inhibition of the warm fiber. (*From Hensel H, Kenshalo DR:* J Physiol [Lond] *204:99, 1969.*)

In this case, exposing various parts of the body to 15° C (59° F) water indicated that the upper torso had the greatest cold receptor density or sensitivity, or both. The lower torso was somewhat less sensitive, with the arms and legs exhibiting similar but considerably lower sensitivity.[16]

The extremes of the thermal spectrum are sensed by a separate set of receptors, the hot-pain and cold-pain endings.[44] Evidence provided by intradermal and intravenous temperature profiles, as well as intravenous nerve block, indicates that cold-pain receptors may be the nociceptors of the cutaneous veins.[70]

Central Thermal Sensors

Many sites within the body are capable of eliciting generalized thermoregulatory responses. Such areas include the abdominal viscera, spinal cord, hypothalamus, and lower portions of the brainstem.[6,48] The genesis of input to the regulator resulting from heating or cooling these areas is poorly understood. Some of the effects may be due to modulation of synaptic connections, rather than stimulation of specific thermodetectors per se. Input from central detectors is not rate sensitive but is rather a direct reflection of the absolute temperature. The area with the highest thermal sensitivity, and that has received the greatest amount of experimental attention, is the preoptic nucleus–anterior hypothalamic area (PO/AH). Heating or cooling this portion of the brainstem elicits the entire array of autonomic and behavioral heat loss and heat gain responses, respectively.[45] Neurons in this portion of the brain exhibit both warm sensitivity and cold sensitivity.[6] Recent work on hypothalamic slice preparations using synaptic blockers has indicated that warm sensitivity may be an inherent property of some of the PO/AH neurons, whereas cold sensitivity in this area of the brain requires synaptic input.[6,28] Figure 4-2 illustrates the effect of temperature on firing rates of three representative types of hypothalamic neurons. The high level of temperature sensitivity shown by one of the cells (labeled *C*) is due to the temperature-dependent characteristic of the prepotential. Voltage clamp experiments indicate that the altered rate of depolarization is most likely due to an effect on hyperpolarizing (K^+) conductances.[42] Work using hypothalamic slices has also established that about half of the thermosensitive neurons also respond to nonthermal stimuli, such as osmotic pressure, glucose concentration, or steroid hor-

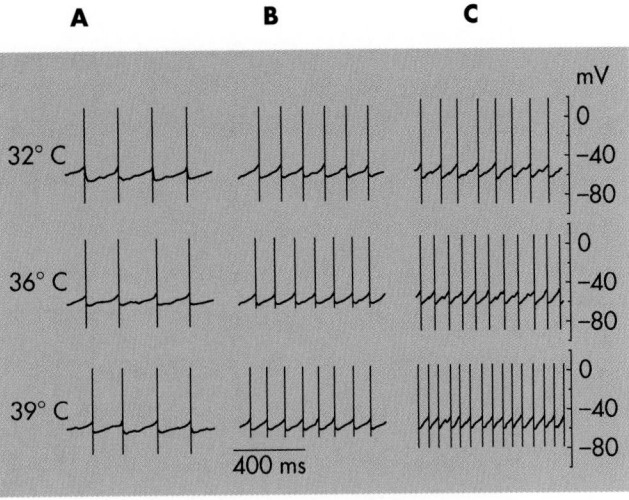

Figure 4-2 Effect of temperature on intracellular activity of three different types of hypothalamic neurons. Each vertical column represents the same neuron at the three temperatures shown. **A,** Low-slope temperature-insensitive neuron; **B,** moderate-slope temperature-insensitive neuron; **C,** warm-sensitive neuron. The thermosensitivity in each case was 0.06 **(A),** 0.5 **(B),** and 1.1 impulses $s^{-1} ° C^{-1}$ **(C).** All three types of neurons displayed depolarizing prepotentials, and action potentials occurred when the prepotentials reached threshold. As exemplified in **C,** putative postsynaptic potentials (especially IPSPs) were often observed in all neuronal types. (*From Griffin JD, Kaple ML, Chow AR, Boulant JA:* J Physiol *492:231, 1996.*)

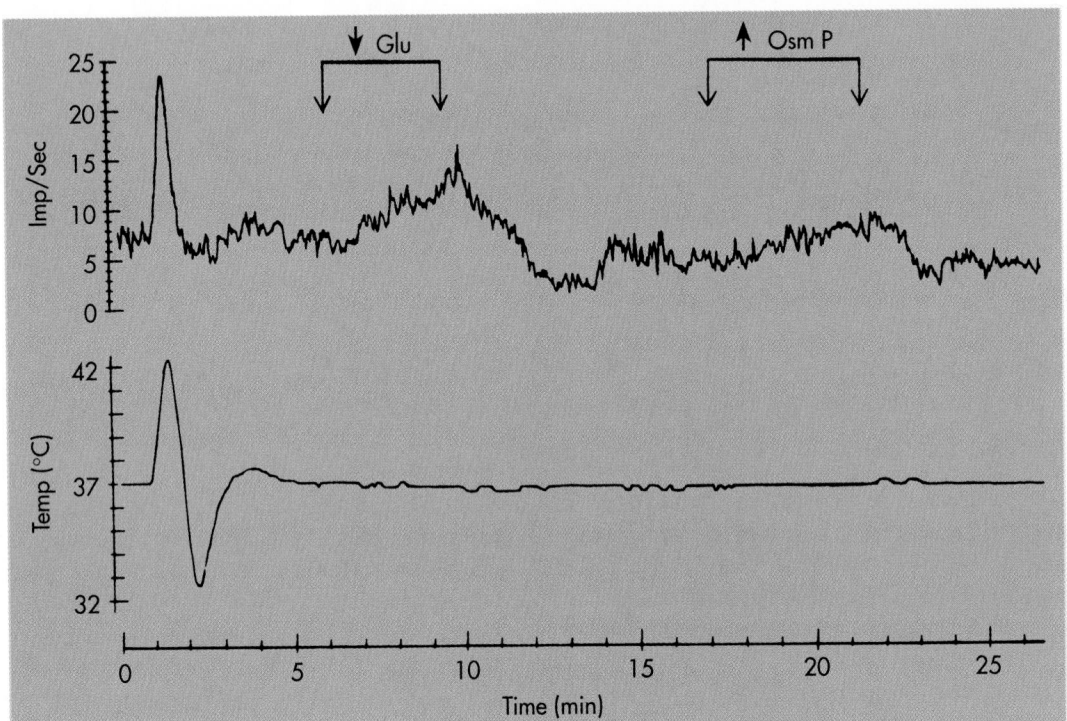

Figure 4-3 The response of a warm-sensitive preoptic nucleus–anterior hypothalamic area neuron to changes in temperature, glucose concentration, and osmotic pressure. The large downward arrows indicate changes in the media bathing the neurons. (*From Boulant JA, Silva NL:* Brain Res Bull *20:871, 1988.*)

mone concentration. Such neurons could form the basis for the interactions between homeostatic systems described subsequently. Figure 4-3 illustrates the response of a warm-sensitive PO/AH neuron in a slice preparation. This cell is excited by increased temperature, low glucose, or increased osmotic pressure.[7]

Regulator

The neuroanatomic structures that establish the regulated body temperature include portions of the spinal cord, lower brainstem, hypothalamus, and septum. The PO/AH and the caudal hypothalamus, in particular, are recognized as important integrating areas.[47] The PO/AH has been assigned a unique role as the center of central nervous thermosensitivity and thermointegration,[45] but other sites are also involved. As noted by Blatteis,[5]

Autonomic thermoregulatory functions may be attributed to brain areas outside of the PO/AH. These mechanisms appear to be subsidiary controls, may have their own (direct?) links to thermoeffectors, and are capable of operating independently of the PO/AH, although they normally may be influenced by it through ascending and/or descending connections. Thus, the role of the PO/AH in temperature regulation may be seen as not essential, but nevertheless pre-eminent in

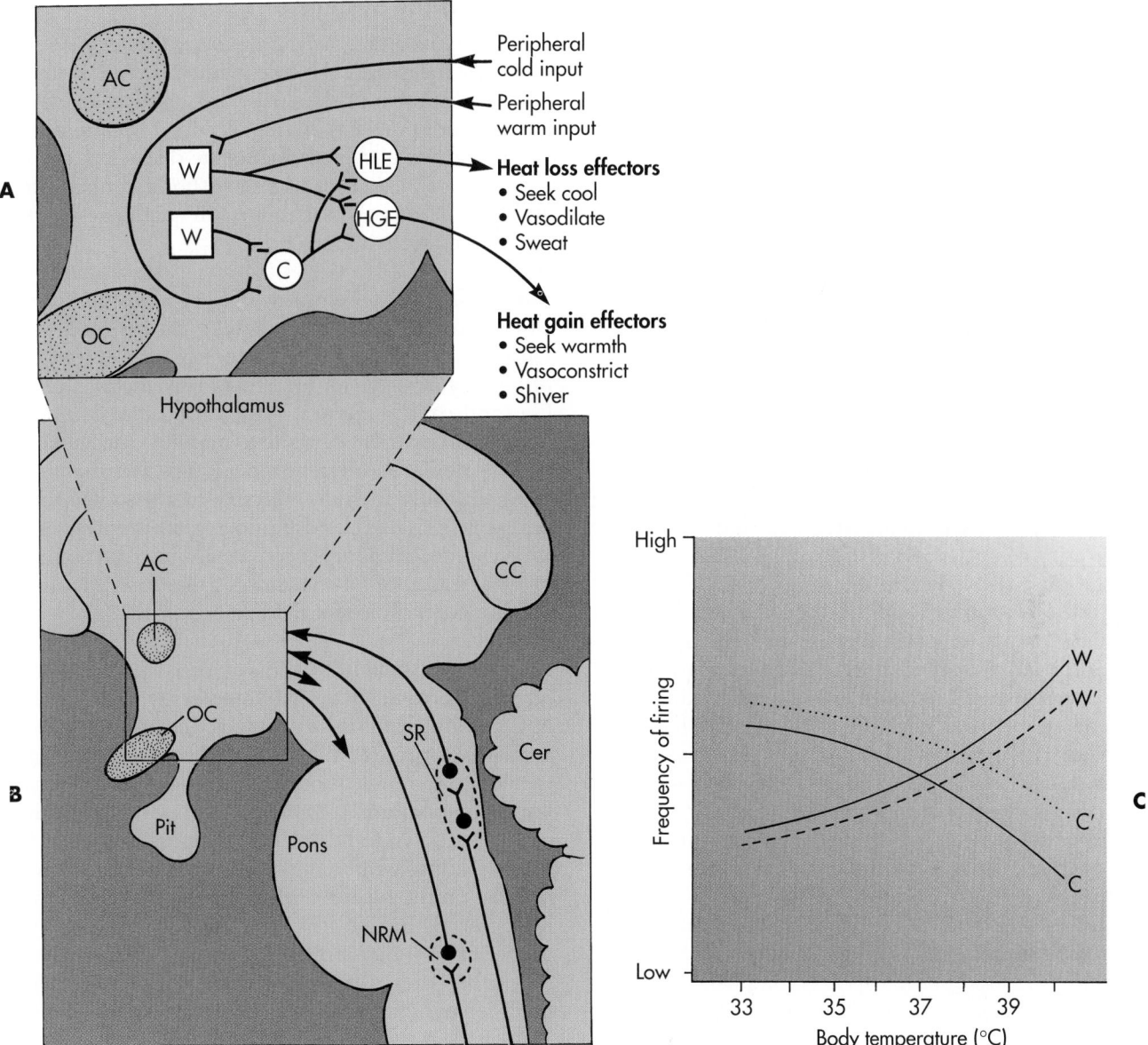

Figure 4-4   A schematic diagram denoting a suggested neuronal network to account for thermoregulation. **A,** The peripheral inputs and the site of the preoptic nucleus–anterior hypothalamic area (PO/AH)—the rectangle. **B,** Neuronal connections in the PO/AH. **C,** The firing rates of the warm-sensitive *(W)* and cold-sensitive *(C)* PO/AH neurons at different body (brain) temperatures. Synapses not shown as inhibitory are assumed to be excitatory. Details about the functioning of this system are in the text. *AC,* Anterior commissure; *CC,* corpus callosum; *Cer,* cerebellum; *C,* relays input from peripheral cold receptor; *NRM,* nucleus raphe magnus; *OC,* optic chiasm; *Pit,* pituitary; *SR,* subceruleus region; *W,* relays input from peripheral warm receptor. *(Concepts and information for this figure from Boulant JA, Curras MC, Dean JB: Neurophysiological aspects of thermoregulation. In Wang LCH, editor:* Advances in comparative and environmental physiology, *vol 4, Berlin, 1989, Springer-Verlag; Brück K, Hinckel P: Thermoafferent networks and their adaptive modifications. In Schönbaum E, Lomax P, editors:* Thermoregulation: physiology and biochemistry, *New York, 1990, Pergamon Press; and Hammel HT:* Annu Rev Physiol *30:641, 1968.)*

the control of appropriate, coordinated, and low-threshold thermoregulatory responses. In this role, it receives afferent information from thermosensitive regions throughout the body, and is connected with all the thermoeffectors.

A model for the regulation of body temperature is depicted in Figure 4-4. Such models have the advan-

tage of clearly depicting how the regulatory system could work, but, as has been emphasized,[125] they greatly oversimplify the complexity and dynamic balance of the elements of the system. Some of the many inputs to this system include those illustrated in Figure 4-3 (glucose concentration and osmotic pressure), as well as factors covered later in this chapter (e.g., time of day, hormone levels, pyrogen titer, and oxygen concentration in the blood).

The network in Figure 4-4 is based on the work of Hammel[45] but also incorporates other sources.[6,13] This system depends on input from peripheral warm and cold receptors and central thermodetectors. Input arising from cold-sensitive peripheral neurons impinges on cells that excite noradrenergic neurons in the subceruleus region projecting to cold-sensitive neurons in the PO/AH. Peripheral warm-sensitive neurons provide input to serotonergic cells in the nucleus raphe magnus, which project to warm-sensitive cells in the PO/AH. The warm-sensitive (W in Figure 4-4) and cold-sensitive (C in Figure 4-4) neurons of the PO/AH provide reciprocal innervation that forms the basis for the thermostat. In this scheme, central cold sensitivity is postulated to be derived from inhibitory input via inherently warm-sensitive PO/AH cells. The interconnections of these neurons are shown in Figure 4-4, B.

The firing characteristics of the warm (W) and cold (C) cells are illustrated in Figure 4-4, C. At 37° C (98.6° F), the firing rates of warm and cold cells are balanced and there is no net output to either the heat loss or the heat gain effectors. If internal temperature increases, the warm cells fire faster, and vasodilation, sweating, and seeking of a cool environment are stimulated. On the other hand, if the internal temperature falls below 37° C, cold cells predominate, and vasoconstriction, shivering, and seeking of a warm environment are stimulated.

Without the aforementioned peripheral input, body temperature would have to change considerably to create the error signal needed to compensate for varying ambient thermal conditions. This does not occur; core temperature remains remarkably constant under most climatic conditions. This is accomplished by incorporating information from the peripheral thermodetectors. As illustrated in Figure 4-4, C, if an animal moves into a cold environment, peripheral cold receptors are stimulated and peripheral warm receptors are inhibited. This produces the altered firing rates shown by the W' and C' curves. Now, even though body temperature is still 37° C, hypothalamic cold cells are firing faster than hypothalamic warm cells. This leads to activation of the heat gain effectors. If the system is properly designed (it is), augmentation of vasoconstriction and metabolism is just sufficient to match increased heat loss caused by the new, cooler thermal environment. The reverse occurs when a warmer environment is encountered. Peripheral warm receptors are stimulated and peripheral cold receptors are inhibited; the greater firing rate of the hypothalamic warm cells initiates sweating and vasodilation even though body temperature remains at 37° C. In this way, the regulator can maintain a remarkably constant internal temperature despite wide variations in ambient temperature.

Assessing the System

Overall status of the thermoregulatory system is determined by measuring the core temperature. This can be done at a number of sites with several types of instruments (thermometers). In this section, the relative merits of locations and instruments are discussed, and an overview of the causes of altered body temperatures and the consequences of abnormally high and low tissue temperatures are given.

Monitoring Core Temperature. A recent history of clinical thermometry is available,[80] as are good overviews of the assessment of core temperature.[4,20,124] Minimally invasive measurement sites include the axilla, oral cavity, rectum, tympanum, and forehead. There is no clear-cut best site to monitor; particular situations demand different techniques. Thermometers used clinically include mercury-in-glass, electronic, tympanic radiation, and liquid crystal thermometers. Whatever instrument is used should have an accuracy of ±0.1° C (0.18° F). The handheld electronic thermometer is a good choice for field emergencies.

MEASURING INSTRUMENTS. Clinical mercury-in-glass thermometers are widely available and easily used, but they have a number of disadvantages. In some situations, breakage can pose a problem, and the equilibration time is at least 3 minutes. These thermometers read the maximum temperature. It is therefore important that they be shaken down fully, or a core temperature below the initial reading will be missed. In addition, the lowest reading on the typical clinical mercury-in-glass thermometer (34.5° C [94.1° F]) is insufficient when hypothermia is a possibility.[4,78] Although typically accurate when new, mercury thermometers may lose precision over time. In one evaluation, after 10 months, 24% of the thermometers failed to meet the accuracy standard referred to above.[20]

The handheld electronic thermometer has replaced the mercury-in-glass thermometer in many applications. These instruments can use either thermistors or thermocouples as sensors, have the requisite degree of accuracy, and are very flexible in application. Although an equilibration time of 1 minute is specified for the typical probe, this is due largely to the need for a stiff casing for ease of insertion. Smaller probes are available that can equilibrate in seconds. The digital display of these instruments reduces errors, and the probes can be left in place for continuous monitoring. A quality instrument with a wide range of interchangeable probes is important. Even then, these devices are subject to the usual problems inherent with electronic instruments. A mercury thermometer for backup and calibration, an alternate probe, and a spare battery are essential.

Tympanic infrared radiometers are often used in hospital settings, but even in this relatively predictable environment, controversy exists over their ability to accurately assess core temperature. These instruments monitor electromagnetic radiation emanating from the ear canal, and various manufacturers use different, complicated electronic circuitry to produce a temperature display. An advantage is that the reading takes only a few seconds.[20] Questions still remain, however, about the overall accuracy of the measurement displayed. In a laboratory situation in which the auditory canal is plugged with a sponge and the probe measures only radiation emanating from the tympanum, infrared tympanic thermometry provides an excellent estimate of the core temperature.[115] In clinical settings, however, the results are less consistent. In one study, infrared tympanic thermometry produced core temperatures that were much more variable than rectal temperatures. Even after correcting for the higher rectal values (0.5° C [0.9° F]), tympanic measurements still inaccurately displayed one third of the temperatures above 37.7° C (99.° F). An extended training program did not significantly alter the accuracy of the readings.[98]

In one instance, a child arriving at an emergency department presented with tachycardia and skin vasoconstriction. Separate tympanic infrared thermometers gave core temperatures of 36.4° and 37.6° C (97.5° and 99.7° F). The rectal temperature was determined to be 42.2° C (108° F).[103] On the other hand, in a hospital setting with a trained operator and immobile patients, two brands of infrared tympanic thermometers produced readings that were closer to pulmonary artery readings than were those of the axilla or rectum.[102]

The potential benefits of a continuous, easily applied core temperature monitor has led to repeated attempts to validate liquid-crystal thermometers, typically placed on the head or neck surface. Unfortunately, the temperature readings produced by this methodology are not reliable.[4,80] Since these measurements are compromised by thermoregulatory vascular changes associated with heat conservation and heat dissipation, as well by as changes in ambient temperature,[58] they are particularly unsuited for field emergency measurements.

MEASUREMENT SITES. Although the deep internal temperatures of normothermic humans are reasonably similar, no specific anatomic site represents *the* core temperature. The temperature at each location is a consequence of a combination of local metabolic rate, local perfusion rate, proximity to the outer shell, and proximity to other locations with differing rates of metabolism and perfusion. Nevertheless, because of the generally high overall rates of tissue perfusion in mammals, deep core temperatures rarely differ by more than 0.5° C (0.9° F). The temperature of the pulmonary artery is a good reference temperature for the overall status of the thermal core. At steady state, accepted sites for assessing core temperature differ in varying amounts from

this temperature. Esophageal and tympanic temperatures are essentially the same as the temperature of the pulmonary artery,[102,106] whereas rectal temperature averages about 0.4° C (0.7° F) higher and axillary and oral temperatures about 0.2° and 0.4° C (0.4° and 0.7° F) lower, respectively.[4,78,102]

Although the esophageal temperature is somewhat difficult to obtain, this is the site most likely to accurately reflect the temperature of the pulmonary artery. Measurement at this location accurately follows changes in core temperature and is reasonably noninvasive. For placement, the probe is lubricated and a small amount of local anesthetic is applied. It is then passed via a nasal passage into the distal portion of the esophagus at the level of the heart. The probe can be moved up and down slightly to obtain the highest temperature. Although somewhat unpleasant for conscious persons, this procedure is routinely used in physiology experiments. Esophageal temperature is transiently (30 sec) affected by swallowing.

Tympanic temperature as an estimation of core temperature has long been controversial. Since the tympanic membrane is highly vascular and supplied by branches of the external and internal carotid arteries, it should be an ideal site. Nevertheless, many studies have indicated that tympanic temperature is affected by ambient temperature and local facial cooling.[106] The conditions under which these complications can be avoided have now been clarified. If (1) the ear canal is insulated, (2) the thermocouple is made of fine wire and insulated except at the active junction, and (3) the thermocouple is in direct contact with the tympanum (which causes the subject to "hear" a continuous low-pitched sound), then alterations in core temperature are detected more rapidly than by an esophageal probe, are not affected by facial skin temperature, and are otherwise identical to esophageal temperature.[106] Very similar results were obtained when an insulated probe was used in conjunction with an optical sensor to detect infrared radiation from the tympanum.[115] Whether the conditions met in these two carefully controlled studies can be duplicated in the field is doubtful.

In steady-state conditions, rectal temperature is a good index of core temperature. However, when the heat content of the body or of the internal thermal compartments is in flux, rectal temperature changes more slowly than temperatures measured in other commonly used sites.[102] There is a thermal gradient along the rectum, so all measurements should be made at a standard depth; 4 cm is recommended.[4] The higher temperatures recorded in this region may be due to a combination of low perfusion rates, digestive reactions, and bacterial activity, but there is no clear evidence in this regard.[79]

Oral temperature is an excellent index of core temperature, provided the mouth is kept closed. The sublingual pocket is well perfused and responds quite rapidly to alterations in core temperature. Mastication, smoking, fluid intake, and mouth breathing can affect sublingual temperature and should be avoided in the period immediately preceding measurement.[4,78,79] Use of an electronic thermometer with a rapidly responding sensor will make this measurement considerably more accurate and rapid than when performed with a mercury-in-glass thermometer.

Although axillary temperature reflects core temperature, it has a number of negative characteristics and should be used only as a last resort. The axillary temperature is affected by local blood flow, as well as by thermal and nonthermal sweating.[4] Changes in core temperature are slow to affect the axillary temperature, and there is high interpatient variability.[102] This measurement, however, has proven particularly useful for assessing core temperature in infants.[4,79]

Heterothermy. Core temperature, as assessed in the previous section, provides a good estimate of the temperature of critical internal organs. This temperature is vigorously defended by the body. At low temperatures, regional heterothermy resulting from peripheral vasoconstriction forms an important aspect of this defense, increasing insulation by decreasing skin temperature. This decreases the thermal gradient for heat loss from the skin to the environment. Thus, at cooler temperatures, there can be a large amount of tissue that is well below core temperature, and as a consequence, the overall heat content of the body is greatly decreased. A nude human resting at 35° C (95° F) or 20° C (68° F) will exhibit similar temperatures at various locations within the core. However, because of decreased temperatures in the outer shell, the same person resting at 20° C will have a total heat content that is about 200 kcal lower than the same person resting at 35° C.[108] If the peripheral vessels were suddenly dilated, an immediate drop in core temperature of about 3.5° C (6.3° F) would result. In a hypothermic individual, the discrepancy between core and shell temperatures could be considerably greater. The temperature of the outer shell can be estimated by measuring skin temperature at a number of sites, with the sensor in contact with the skin on one side and insulated on the other.[4] An equation has been developed to estimate the mean temperature of the body using measurements of ambient temperature, several skin temperatures, and core temperature.[38] Although this approach is not feasible in the field, several measurements along the distal extremities give an estimate of outer shell cooling.

A different type of heterothermy may be present in hyperthermic humans. As the brain temperature reaches high levels, blood flow that is normally outward from the intracranium to the face via the ophthalmic vein is redirected and flows from the face inward.[54] This results in the brain being cooler than the remainder of the core. Although brain cooling is clearly documented and accepted in many mammals,[3] it remains controversial in humans.[10,18] Nevertheless, the head is an extremely important area for heat loss.[10,18] Thus, for hyperthermic patients, it is important to optimize the heat loss from that region and, when necessary, to augment cranial heat dissipation by fanning and moistening.

Reasons for Altered Core Temperature. Various conditions can lead to an abnormal core temperature. Under some circumstances, the regulator may be defending an altered core temperature for reasons to be described. Alternatively, the thermal load posed by the environment or by heavy exercise may be too great for the capacity of the effectors. Finally, the regulator could be deranged as a result of substance abuse, extreme temperatures, side effects of prescription drugs, or other factors. When interpreting a particular core temperature, it is important to evaluate all of the above alternatives.

Consequences of Altered Body Temperatures. When tissue temperatures change, there are immediate and important effects on metabolism, as well as on other physiologic mechanisms. With a 10° C (18° F) increase in temperature, the typical human tissue increases metabolism by a factor (the Q_{10}) of about 2.7. The metabolic rate of the entire organism (apart from thermoregulatory responses) responds similarly. Within the normal range of body temperatures, higher temperatures favor speed at the expense of tissue resources, whereas lower temperatures conserve resources. Although both high and low temperature extremes pose a threat to humans, increased temperatures greatly accelerate the development of serious complications and pose a much more immediate danger. Although a deviation of about 2° C (3.6° F) above or below the normal core temperature is well tolerated by the various regulatory systems of the body, a discrepancy of about 3° C (5.4° F) begins to disrupt these systems, including those involved in temperature regulation. At this level of deviation, if there is no intervention, physiologic problems compound very rapidly.

EFFECTOR RESPONSES

This section examines the properties of the response systems that heat or cool the body according to the output demands of the regulator. These effectors are influenced both by the output of the thermoregulatory network and by the temperature of the effector organ itself. Since patients away from medical facilities often exhibit whole body or regional hyperthermia or hypothermia, both central outputs and local effects are relevant; these factors are discussed separately.

Vascular Adjustments

Excellent overviews on the role of the vasculature in coping with thermal stresses are available.[41,62] One function of the circulatory system is to maintain a relatively homogeneous internal body temperature. Heat from metabolically active organs is convectively distributed to portions of the body where less heat is produced. More commonly appreciated are the alterations of blood flow patterns that increase or decrease the body's overall thermal conductivity during exposure to hot or cold environments, respectively. Some of these alterations in conductivity result from preferentially shunting peripheral blood flow superficial or deep to the subcutaneous fat layer. Indeed, fat has about half the tissue conductivity of muscle. Nevertheless, shunting of blood away from major portions of the body is at least as important in determining overall conductivity as is the conductive property of the tissue itself. For example, during immersion in cold water, muscle accounts for about 90% of the total tissue insulation of the forearm.[30] Thus directing blood away from poorly insulated (more highly conductive) regions reduces heat loss and preserves core temperature.

In addition to capillaries, microcirculatory units contain arterioles, metarterioles, and arteriovenous anastomoses. Flow through all of these vessels is under the control of smooth muscle. The smooth muscle of precapillary sphincters is largely influenced by local factors, whereas the other vessels are well supplied with receptors that respond to both neuronal and endocrine inputs. Active vasoconstrictor and vasodilator systems are both present. The vasoconstrictor system acts primarily through α_1 and α_2 adrenoceptors,[67] whereas the active vasodilator system appears to use both acetylcholine and nitric oxide. About 90% of the elevation in skin blood flow during heat stress is due to input from the active vasodilator system.[66] Thermoregulatory skin blood flow can reach up to 8 L per minute and involve 60% of cardiac output.[67]

Operation of the vasomotor effector system is affected by excessive exposure to ultraviolet B radiation. A moderate sunburn impairs the vasoconstrictor response to cold; an associated, uncontrolled increase in thermal conduction is still present 1 week after exposure, although the original erythema has disappeared.[95]

Central Signal. Vascular changes are bioenergetically the least costly thermoregulatory autonomic effector responses. Because of the vasomotor system's high sensitivity, ambient temperatures between the thresholds for sweating and shivering are often referred to as being in the zone of vasomotor regulation. If a particular vascular bed is kept at a relatively constant temperature, output from the central nervous regulator can be assessed. Under these conditions, in dogs, manipulations of hypothalamic temperature confirm a high level of vasomotor activity between the thresholds for the activation of panting and shivering.[49] In humans, forearm blood flow increases rapidly as core temperature rises; a sixfold increase in blood flow can occur with a core temperature that has risen to only 38° C (100.4° F).[121] Within the vasomotor zone (skin temperatures of 33° to 35° C [91.4° to 95° F]), core and skin temperatures linearly combine to control skin blood flow. Skin blood flow responds very accurately and rapidly to changes in skin temperature, which leads to a very stable core temperature.[11]

Although most peripheral arterioles are well supplied with adrenergic receptors, output from the thermoregulatory centers is not homogeneously distributed. Extensive nervous inputs from the thermoregulatory centers occur only in the lips, ears, and distal extremities. Thus immersing the feet in cold water leads to marked vasoconstriction in the hands and forearms but not in the abdomen or upper arms.[41]

Local Modulation. Local temperature has a great effect on the vasomotor status of peripheral vessels, and in some cases it may be largely responsible for the observed thermal conductivities. Although heat is generally considered a vasodilator,[41] this is true only for cutaneous vascular beds; many other vascular beds dilate when cooled.[33] The specific response to cold shown by cutaneous vessels follows from the observed distribution and properties of the α-adrenergic vascular receptors. Although in most of the vasculature α_1 receptors predominate, in the superficial cutaneous areas α_2 receptors constitute a clear majority. The usual predominance of α_1 receptors is found in the deeper blood vessels. Local temperature affects α_2 and α_1 receptors in a reciprocal manner. Although cooling augments the response of α_2 receptors, it either inhibits or does not affect the response of α_1 receptors. Cooling the skin, then, not only constricts the superficial vessels but also concomitantly dilates many underlying vessels. The ensuing flow pattern increases tissue insulation and augments countercurrent exchange between incoming cool blood and outgoing warm blood.[33,34] Although initial work was done on canine vessels, subsequent studies using α-adrenergic agonists and antagonists have demonstrated that a similar mechanism exists in human fingers.[31,36]

Evaporative Responses

At high workloads and at environmental temperatures approaching 37° C (98.6° F), the only way to maintain thermal balance is to augment evaporative cooling by mobilizing the eccrine sweat glands. This sympathetic, cholinergically innervated organ system is spread over the entire body surface but is more profuse in some areas than in others. High rates of sweating occur on the forehead, neck, anterior and posterior portions of the trunk, and the dorsal surfaces of the hand and forearm. Low rates occur on the medial femoral regions, lateral trunk areas, palms, and soles.[91] Sweat is secreted in these latter two areas in response to emotional but not thermal inputs.[8] Sweat gland activity interacts with the regional vasculature; both cholinergic receptors on local vessels and metabolic products of active sweat glands increase blood flow in areas of active sweating.[41]

Central Signal. By controlling the local milieu at different skin sites, it has been possible to separate the central thermoregulatory drive to sweat glands from local effects on the glands themselves. The central thermoregulatory system provides proportional output that is influenced by both internal and whole body skin temperatures. Per degree increase above thermoneutral values, internal temperature is about 10 times as important as mean skin temperature in eliciting an output to the sweat glands.[87,89]

Local Modulation. Local effects are important in determining the output of sweat glands. Temperature exerts a multiplicative effect on sweat secretion; the Q_{10} for this augmentation is about 3.70. Skin wetness also has an important local effect on sweat glands. The wetter the skin, the greater the suppression of sweating.[88]

A moderate sunburn disrupts evaporative cooling. This effect is locally mediated and involves decreases in both the responsiveness and the capacity of the sweat glands.[94]

Metabolic Responses

Heat is an inevitable by-product of the inefficiencies in the body's metabolic reactions. In oxidizing foodstuffs to carbon dioxide and water during adenosine triphosphate (ATP) production and transferring the ATP produced to the functional systems of the cells, about 75% of the original chemical potential energy appears as heat. Excepting that energy excreted or used to perform physical work, the remaining 25% of the original energy is also converted to heat when ATP is used in the body's numerous metabolic reactions.[109] Mammals, relative to poikilotherms such as reptiles or fish, use much more ATP to maintain ionic and electrochemical balance of the cells,[117] as well as for many other functions. This leads to greatly increased metabolic heat production, which forms the basis for homeothermy. It also creates the need to maintain a substantial thermal gradient between the body and the environment to dissipate the high levels of heat that are produced.

An increased rate of metabolism above basal levels is critical for maintenance of body temperature in cold environments. Elevated heat production is derived largely from simultaneous rhythmic excitation of agonistic and antagonistic skeletal muscles (shivering), but other domains, such as the gastrointestinal tract or adipose tissue,[41,116] may be involved to some degree. There is evidence that both epinephrine and thyroid hormones are released in humans after cold exposure.[37] Since these hormones augment overall tissue metabolism, they are components of the response to cold environments.

Central Signal. Of the various thermoregulatory outputs, metabolism is the easiest to evaluate quantitatively. The most complete documentation is available for this response, and most models of the thermoregulatory system are based on this information. Experiments on medium-sized mammals have allowed separate thermal manipulation of various parts of the brain, body core, and skin. This work has made it clear that the thermoregulatory centers act as proportional controllers and that skin temperature provides a feedforward input to the system.[45,60] Thus greater decreases in either core or skin temperature, or both, below neutral values elicit proportionally larger compensatory increases in metabolism.

Evidence indicates that humans have a similar control system. In a summary of their data and of that collected previously, Hong and Nadel[57] noted that the central output for shivering is augmented by an increased rate of skin cooling. They also concluded that a given decrease in core temperature elicits 10 to 20 times the metabolic response of an equivalent decrease in mean skin temperature. Exercise is not incompatible with shivering, but increased levels of exercise exert increasing degrees of suppression on the shivering response, possibly as a consequence of an increased arousal response.[57]

Hypothyroid states are associated with impaired metabolic thermogenesis. It has recently been shown that hypothyroidism (in rats) leads to a decrease in regulated core temperature of about 1° C (1.8° F).[123]

Local Modulation. Although the central and local effects of decreased core temperature on shivering have not been directly partitioned, both inputs are important. Slight decreases in core temperature create large compensatory responses, as delineated previously. However, even moderate hypothermia decreases the metabolic response to cold, and at about 30° C (86° F), the shivering response is lost.[9] This decrement must involve nervous system malfunction, since the muscles themselves are quite responsive below 30° C. For example, limb muscles and diaphragm muscles develop peak tensions that are not greatly affected by temperatures down to 25° C (77° F), and fatigue resistance is considerably increased at 25° C.[99,110]

Behavioral Responses

In most wilderness situations, various ambient temperatures are available, and external insulation is easily adjusted. Under these conditions, the choice of thermal microenvironment and clothing provides a far higher gain than do any of the autonomic effector systems discussed previously. Whole body adjustments are achieved by all motile animals and are particularly well developed in vertebrates.[24] In addition to moving the body, the somatic effectors are important for optimizing the autonomic responses to thermal stress. Thus spreading out the arms and legs during heat stress increases the surface area available for autonomic augmentation of conductive, convective, evaporative, and radiative heat losses.

Central Signal. Available evidence indicates that behavioral responses are elicited by the thermoregulatory controller through outputs similar to those delivered to the autonomic effector organs.[24,27] Severe deviations of core temperature disrupt this system; when this occurs, the person no longer feels too hot or too cold and the desire to take corrective action is lost.

Local Modulation. As with shivering, most problems involving behavioral temperature regulation probably emanate from disruption of the centrally generated output. The muscles used to move the body are fairly resistant to thermal incapacitation (see previous discussion), but if this occurs, a major disruption of the body's thermal defenses ensues.

IMPORTANT MODIFICATIONS OF THERMOREGULATORY RESPONSES

Core temperature measurements typically provide information about whether body temperature is within the range for optimal physiologic function. Monitoring body temperature also provides a significant diagnostic indicator for many pathologic conditions. Whether the goal is to stabilize or to monitor body temperature, it is necessary to understand the many conditions that affect both the regulated temperature and the effectiveness of the thermoregulatory system. In this section, these circumstances are elucidated.

Normal Variation in the Regulated Temperature and in the Ability to Maintain Body Temperature

The same body temperature can represent a different state of affairs even under regularly encountered circumstances. Some of these conditions are noted in the following paragraphs.

Level of Activity. Activity normally leads to increases in body temperature. Unlike peripheral temperature, the level of activity does not appear to provide direct input to the regulator of body temperature. Rather, the magnitude of the error signal for increased heat dissipation is determined simply by the increase in body temperature.[118] Thus someone exercising heavily (or having just exercised) in a neutral environment has an unusually high body temperature, whereas someone sleeping or resting quietly has a relatively low body temperature. At a given level of exercise, core temperature will plateau 30 to 40 minutes after the exercise is initiated; higher levels of exercise will result in higher plateau levels of core temperature. For someone working at 50% of their maximal aerobic capacity, the increase in core temperature will be about 1° C (1.8° F).[92]

Circadian Changes. Body temperature shows cyclic changes throughout the day. Some of this variation is due to the daily cycle of activity, as described previously. However, there also exists a circadian rhythm for the body temperature set point. This sinusoidal rhythm accounts for much of the observed variation in body temperature. In a study involving 700 observations on 148 healthy individuals, the daily mean oral reading was 36.8° C (98.2° F). However, this was only a midpoint; the mean early morning low was 36.4° C (97.6° F) and the mean late afternoon high was 36.9° C (98.4° F).[81] These diurnal changes definitely reflect alterations in the controller, since the body temperature thresholds for eliciting sweating and peripheral vasodilation are significantly lower in the early morning than in the afternoon or evening, while the sensitivities and maximal response levels remain unchanged.[1,2] Melatonin may be an important factor in the rhythm of body temperature; light exposure produces similar shifts in both temperature and melatonin rhythms,[114] and artificial reductions in melatonin levels attenuate the circadian decline in body temperature.[19] A thorough, current review of body temperature cycles is available.[101]

Interindividual Differences. Normally, there is surprisingly little interindividual variability in core body temperature. In the study involving 700 observations described earlier, 90% of the early morning values were between 36.0° and 37.1° C (96.9° and 98.9° F); corresponding values for the late afternoon were 36.3° and 37.4° C (97.4° and 99.4° F). Based on these interindividual differences, as well as the diurnal changes described above, it has been suggested that the upper limit for a normal oral temperature should be 37.2° C (98.9° F) in early morning, increase gradually to 37.8° C (99.9° F) by early afternoon, and remain at that level until the early evening.[81] These values delineate the 99th percentile for body temperature observed during the respective time periods.

On the other hand, it is important to be aware that the normal body temperature of some individuals will fall outside of population norms. In one person we encountered, core temperature was consistently 35.5° to 36° C (95.9° to 96.8° F). He mentioned that on one occasion he had felt chills and malaise but was told by his physician that his temperature of 37° C (98.6° F) was normal. It was not; for this person a core temperature of 37° C represented a febrile state. Many individuals with atypical body temperatures are aware of their condition; it is prudent to ask about this possibility.

Age. The circadian rhythm of body temperature develops soon after birth. Although newborns display small-amplitude rhythms, the patterns are not circadian. Circadian rhythmicity begins to develop during the second and third weeks of life, and after progressive increases in amplitude, typical adult temperature rhythms are reached at 2 years of age.[101] Under thermoneutral conditions, rectal temperatures for the elderly are similar to those of younger people, whereas oral and axillary temperatures are slightly lower.[65]

Of the major regulatory systems, temperature regulation is unique in the extent to which effector organs are "borrowed" from other systems. This makes developmental assessments difficult, since functional changes may be secondary to changes in primary systems, such as skeletal muscles or blood vessels. Other difficulties, detailed by Cooper,[22] include inconsistencies between chronologic age and physiologic viability, and the increased incidence of interfering disease states and cerebral microinfarcts as aging progresses.

Thermoregulatory capacities of the young show progressive increases but are not fully developed until after puberty. Effectors more important to infants than adults include certain behavioral responses (call for help) and the ability to activate thermogenic brown adipose tissue. Although brown adipose tissue is of little consequence in adults, it may aid in the production of heat in infants; adults may have the capacity to develop brown adipose tissue if subjected to chronic cold stress.[53] Shivering is not present in infants and develops fully only after several years as the nervous system matures. Metabolism in infants is increased to some degree by an increase in motor activity, which accompanies cold stress.[69]

Sweating is present and effective in children, but increases in sweat gland output during puberty lead to the typical high capacity for evaporative heat loss present in adults.[32] For the adult years, factors affecting the loss of body heat during cold stress have been investigated by using a multiple regression analysis to evaluate fitness, fatness, and age (from the twenties to the early fifties). Fitness has no effect, whereas fatness retards heat loss. Aging during this period is correlated with a progressive weakening of the vasoconstrictor response to cold.[14]

Individuals in their late sixties and beyond have a definite decrease in thermoregulatory capacity. Sweating is lessened in response to passive heating,[59] vascular responses to heating and cooling are significantly reduced,[67,68] and a distinct shivering tremor is rarely observed.[69]

Gender. Although less work has been done on thermoregulation in females, evidence indicates that their thermoregulatory responses are qualitatively similar to those of males.[43] Taken as a group, females have a number of physiologic and morphologic characteristics that produce subtle differences in the regulation of body temperature. Such attributes include smaller blood volume, lower hemoglobin concentration, smaller heart, smaller lean body mass, greater percent of subcutaneous and total body fat, greater surface area–to–mass ratio, higher set point for cutaneous vasodilation and sweating onset, greater resting vasoconstriction in hands and feet, geometrically thinner extremities, and cyclic hormonal changes.[83]

When age, thermal acclimation, body size, maximal aerobic capacity, and relative workload are matched, thermoregulatory gender differences are negligible. Nevertheless, in situations such as those encountered in the U.S. Navy, men and women do not tend to be matched for such nonthermoregulatory factors, and different thermal exposure standards may be required for the genders.[43]

The menstrual cycle, menopause, and pregnancy are all associated with important effects on the thermoregulatory system. Relative to the early follicular phase of the menstrual cycle, core temperature is typically 0.3° C (0.5° F) higher in the late follicular phase and 0.7° C (1.3° F) higher in the luteal phase.[74] Postmenopausal hot flashes are experienced by most women and involve increases in sweating, vasodilation, and heart rate. Heat and exercise may be particularly stressful during and after these episodes. The proximate mechanism appears to involve central noradrenergic activation.[35] Some information about hormonal effects on thermoregulation has been gained by studying postmenopausal women undergoing hormone replacement therapy. Administered estrogen acts to lower the core temperature at which heat loss effector mechanisms are activated and results in a lowered core temperature. The addition of exogenous progestins blocks these effects.[12]

During pregnancy, the thermoregulatory system is far more sensitive to the heat produced by continuous exercise. The effector responses are initiated sooner and are more vigorous, so that toward the end of pregnancy, the steady-state core temperature during exercise is about 1° C (1.8° F) lower than before conception. This adjustment is seen as an adaptation that reduces possible thermal stress on the embryo and fetus.[21]

Induced Alterations of the Regulated Temperature

The optimal body temperature is not always the same. In certain conditions of stress or vulnerability, the regulated temperature of the body may be altered. This is often an adaptive response to a particular physiologic crisis. Some of these situations are delineated in the following paragraphs. In such circumstances, altered body temperature may be beneficial and should not necessarily be manipulated until the underlying condition is improved.

Fever. Increased body temperatures have been associated with illness for thousands of years. Based on the population data presented previously, febrile body temperatures for resting, young adults would include morning temperatures equal to or exceeding 37.3° C (99.2° F), increasing gradually to 37.8° C (100° F) for early afternoon and evening. Such elevated temperatures would need to reflect a regulated increase to be considered a true fever. Pathogens and cancers are the usual causes of such increases in regulated temperature but are not directly responsible for increased body temperature. Rather, they interact with components of the immune system, such as macrophages, T cells, monocytes, and Kupffer's cells, as well as with glial, epithelial, and many other types of cells. This interaction stimulates the cells to produce pyrogenic cytokines.[81] Such cytokines include interleukin-1, interleukin-6, and macrophage inflammatory protein-1. Cytokines act on cells in the vicinity of the anterior hypothalamus, inducing them to release prostaglandin E_2, which leads to an increase in the regulated temperature.[73] Important avenues by which cytokine-mediated pyrogenic signals reach the brain include peripheral inputs from the abdominal vagus nerve[105] and central inputs via the subfornical organs.[119] Aspirin and related drugs block fever by inhibiting prostaglandin synthesis.[73] Interleukin-1 and other cytokines have many effects in addition to causing fever. These include decreased appetite, hypoferremia, activation of B and T lymphocytes, and increased slow-wave sleep.[71]

The increase in body temperature during fever aids many immune functions: neutrophil migration, antibacterial chemical secretion, and interferon production. It has been suggested that the most important aspect of fever is to greatly increase the temperatures of the peripheral tissues via selection of a warmer microclimate, increased insulation, and postural changes. As temperatures increase from typical peripheral tissue temperatures (29° to 33° C [84.2° to 91.4° F]) to those approximating core temperature, activation, proliferation, and effector production in cells involved in cell-mediated and humoral immunity show temperature coefficients (calculated for a 10° C [18° F] interval) of 100 to 1000. In contrast, the temperature coefficients for the effectiveness of the newly created effectors themselves, as well as for antigen-nonspecific defense systems, are much lower—about 1.5 to 5.36.

The presence and beneficial effects of fever have been documented in a variety of cold- and warmblooded vertebrates, and even in some invertebrates. Under most conditions it is probably not advisable to alleviate a fever. Obvious exceptions include malignant hyperthermia, particularly high fevers during pregnancy, and any situation in which weakness makes the thermally induced increase in metabolic demands dangerous.[71,72]

Alcohol, Anesthetics, and Toxins. Increases in the blood concentrations of ethanol, anesthetics, and a number of toxic substances lead to substantial decreases in body temperature.[25,112] In many cases, this fall is due to a decrease in the regulated temperature. In the case of high concentrations of alcohol and certain toxins, the reduction appears to be an adaptive adjustment that promotes survival. These chemicals disrupt protein structures within the cell membrane, an effect that is counteracted by a lower temperature.[25] Indeed, studies of mice have shown that decreased body temperature counteracts ethanol toxicity.[82] However, the lower blood ethanol levels associated with moderate consumption in humans, although causing some increase in vasodilation, have minimal, inconsistent effects on thermal balance of the whole body.[29,63]

Excellent overviews of the effects of general anesthetics on perioperative thermoregulation are available.[111,113] In anesthetic doses, many of these substances (halothane, fentanyl–nitrous oxide, enflurane, and isoflurane) act in a similar manner. Heat loss thresholds are increased by about 1° C (1.8° F), and heat maintenance thresholds are lowered by approximately 2.5° C (4.5° F). Interestingly, in the typical clinical dose range, the gain (sensitivity) of the effector responses is nearly normal. In the conditions under which general anesthetics are normally administered, body temperature decreases significantly. An initial rapid drop is due to redistribution of heat; cool blood from the periphery lowers central core temperature. A second, slower decrease results from a fall in body heat content. Finally, a plateau is reached, either because heat production and heat loss are passively balanced or because heat maintenance thresholds are reached. During postanesthetic recovery, there is vigorous shivering. Cutaneous warming before and during anesthesia prevents development of hypothermia and decreases the incidence of infectious complications.[75,111]

Severe Hypoxia and Endotoxin Shock. When inspired oxygen concentration falls to 10% to 12%, a substantial decrease in the regulated temperature occurs. This reaction has been documented, using behavioral responses, in fish, amphibians, reptiles, and mammals.[39,122] For humans exercising in 28° C (82.4° F) water under eucapnic conditions, decreasing inspired oxygen to 12% lowers core temperature thresholds for vasoconstriction and shivering and increases the rate of core cooling by 33%.[64] The value of the resultant lowered body temperature is clear: the affinity of hemoglobin for oxygen is increased and overall metabolic rate is decreased. The mechanism underlying the change in the regulated temperature may involve differential sensitivities of central neurons; hypoxia specifically increases activity of the warm-sensitive neurons (denoted by *W* in Figure 4-4) in the PO/AH.[120]

A somewhat similar regulated hypothermic response occurs when an animal is exposed to very high levels of pyrogens; the same response occurs under less extreme conditions in weak or malnourished animals. The lowered body temperature may serve to decrease the energetic costs of maintaining a high body temperature for a severely compromised animal.[103]

Altered System Responsiveness

A number of situations alter responsiveness of the thermoregulatory system. An awareness of these conditions is important in assessing the thermoregulatory capabilities of a particular person and in determining possible causes for hyperthermia or hypothermia.

Thermal Acclimation.
Thermoregulation is affected by chronic exposure to very cold environments, as well as by chronic exercise in cool or warm environments. Such exercise in a cool environment greatly increases responsiveness of the sweat glands; if exercise is in the heat, the central temperature at which sweating is initiated is also lowered. The net consequence of these adjustments is that a heat- and exercise-acclimated individual can work at a given level with far less increase in core temperature.[90] Exercise in humid heat appears to decrease resting core temperature in acclimated individuals.[15] Physical training also increases skin blood flow at any given increase in core temperature.[61] Increases in both core and skin temperatures contribute to various changes involved in heat acclimation.[100]

Conversely, repeated exposure to very cold environments (for example, 80 30-minute sessions at 5° C [41° F]) decreases the metabolic response to a standard cold air test, often leading to lower internal temperatures in cold-acclimated individuals.[52]

Competition with Other Homeostatic Systems.
In addition to a constant core temperature, the body has many other requirements. When certain of these other needs are not met, thermoregulatory response can be compromised. For heat production and heat conservation, an adequate energy supply, patent nervous system, and functional effector organs are critical. Hypoglycemia decreases the core temperature at which shivering is initiated while leaving the thresholds for sweating and vasodilation unaffected.[97] For maintaining exercise performance and body temperature in a warm environment, body water status is critical.[84,107] It is common for a person working in the heat to lose 1 L of water per hour, and even when fluids are readily available, maintaining a euhydrated state may be difficult. For hypohydration during activity, each percent decrease in body weight leads to a core temperature increase of about 0.15° C (0.27° F). This decreased heat dissipation is mediated by two mechanisms. At a given core temperature, hypertonicity decreases the sweating response and hypovolemia reduces skin blood flow.[107] Hyperhydration has no effect on thermoregulation during compensable exercise-heat stress.[76] During uncompensable exercise-heat stress, hyperhydration slightly increases the time to exhaustion, but only by delaying hypohydration; thermoregulation is not affected.[77]

Alcohol, Drugs, Anesthetics, and Toxins.
Although moderate doses of many substances elicit adaptive changes in the regulated body temperature, elevated doses impair or abolish both autonomic and behavioral aspects of thermoregulation. Body temperature then changes passively, depending on the thermal environment. This can be particularly dangerous when elevated levels of alcohol or similar substances are combined with heat stress. An impaired ability to dissipate heat is then combined with the enhanced toxicity of increased tissue temperature.

ACKNOWLEDGMENTS

During the preparation of this chapter, the first author was partially supported by NIAAA Grant P50-AA10760. Helpful suggestions were made by Dr. Stanley Hillman, Dr. Randy Zelick, and Mark Haffner. Jackie Parker, Kim-Dung Tran, and Mirella Henderson are thanked for their work on the manuscript.

REFERENCES

1. Aoki K et al: Circadian variation of sweating responses to passive heat stress, *Acta Physiol Scand* 161:397, 1997.
2. Aoki K et al: Circadian variation in skin blood flow responses to passive heat stress, *Physiol Behav* 63:1, 1998.
3. Baker MA: Brain cooling in endotherms in heat and exercise, *Annu Rev Physiol* 44:85, 1982.
4. Blatteis CM: Functional anatomy of the hypothalamus from the point of view of temperature. In Szelényi Z, Székely M, editors: *Contributions to thermal physiology*, Budapest, 1980, Akademiai Kiado.
5. Blatteis CM: Methods of body temperature measurement. In Blatteis CM, editor: *Physiology and pathophysiology of temperature regulation*, Singapore, 1998, World Scientific.
6. Boulant JA, Curras MC, Dean JB: Neurophysiological aspects of thermoregulation. In Wang LCH, editor: *Advances in comparative and environmental physiology*, vol 4, Berlin, 1989, Springer-Verlag.
7. Boulant JA, Silva NL: Neuronal sensitivies in preoptic tissue slices: interactions among homeostatic systems, *Brain Res Bull* 20:871, 1988.
8. Brengelmann G, Brown AC: Temperature regulation. In Ruch TC, Patton HD, editors: *Physiology and biophysics*, ed 19, Philadelphia, 1965, WB Saunders.
9. Brengelmann GL: Body temperature regulation. In Patton HD et al, editors: *Textbook of physiology: circulation, respiration, body fluids, metabolism, and endocrinology*, ed 21, Philadelphia, 1989, WB Saunders.
10. Brenglemann GL: Specialized brain cooling in humans? *FASEB J* 7:1148, 1993.
11. Brengelmann GL, Savage MV: Temperature regulation in the neutral zone, *Ann NY Acad Sci* 813:39, 1997.
12. Brooks EM et al: Chronic hormone replacement therapy alters thermoregulatory and vasomotor function is postmenopausal women, *J Appl Physiol* 83:477, 1997.
13. Brück K, Hinckel P: Thermoafferent networks and their adaptive modifications. In Schönbaum E, Lomax P, editors: *Thermoregulation: physiology and biochemistry*, New York, 1990, Pergamon Press.

14. Budd GM et al: Effects of fitness, fatness, and age on men's responses to whole body cooling in air, *J Appl Physiol* 71:2387, 1991.

15. Buono J, Heaney JH, Canine KM: Acclimation to humid heat lowers resting core temperature, *Am J Physiol* 274:R1295, 1998.

16. Burke WEA, Mekjavić IB: Estimation of regional cutaneous cold sensitivity by analysis of the gasping response, *J Appl Physiol* 71:1933, 1991.

17. Cabanac M: Physiological role of pleasure, *Science* 173:1103, 1971.

18. Cabanac M: *Human selective brain cooling*, Heidelberg, Germany, 1995, Springer-Verlag.

19. Cagnacci A, Elliott JA, Yen SSC: Melatonin: a major regulator of the circadian rhythm of core temperature in humans, *J Clin Endocrinol Metab* 75:447, 1992.

20. Cetas TC: Thermometers. In Mackowiak PA, editor: *Fever: basic mechanisms and management*, ed 2, Philadelphia, 1997, Lippincott-Raven.

21. Clapp JF III: The changing thermal response to endurance exercise during pregnancy, *Am J Obstet Gynecol* 165:1684, 1991.

22. Cooper KE: Thermoregulation in the elderly. In Blatteis CM, editor: *Physiology and pathophysiology of temperature regulation*, Singapore, 1998, World Scientific.

23. Cossins AR, Bowler K: *Temperature biology of animals*, New York, 1987, Chapman & Hall.

24. Crawshaw LI: Temperature regulation in vertebrates, *Annu Rev Physiol* 42:473, 1980.

25. Crawshaw LI, Wallace H, Crabbe J: Ethanol, body temperature and thermoregulation, *Clin Exp Pharmacol Physiol* 25:150, 1998.

26. Crawshaw LI et al: Effect of local cooling on sweating rate and cold sensation, *Pflügers Arch* 354:19, 1975.

27. Crawshaw LI et al: Body temperature regulation in vertebrates: comparative aspects and neuronal elements. In Schönbaum E, Lomax P, editors: *Thermoregulation: physiology and biochemistry*, New York, 1990, Pergamon Press.

28. Dean JB, Boulant JA: Effects of synaptic blockade on thermosensitive neurons in rat diencephalon in vitro, *Am J Physiol* 257:R65, 1989.

29. Desruelle A-V, Boisvert P, Candas V: Alcohol and its variable effect on human thermoregulatory response to exercise in a warm environment, *Eur J Appl Physiol* 74:572, 1996.

30. Ducharme MB, Tikuisis P: In vivo thermal conductivity of the human forearm tissues, *J Appl Physiol* 70:2682, 1991.

31. Ekenvall L et al: α-Adrenoceptors and cold-induced vasoconstriction in human finger skin, *Am J Physiol* 255:H1000, 1988.

32. Falk B et al: Sweat gland response to exercise in the heat among pre-, mid-, and late-pubertal boys, *Med Sci Sports Exerc* 24:313, 1992.

33. Flavahan NA: The role of vascular α_2-adrenoreceptors as cutaneous thermosensors, *New Physiol Sci* 6:251, 1991.

34. Flavahan NA et al: Cooling and α_1- and α_2-adrenergic responses in cutaneous veins: role of receptor reserve, *Am J Physiol* 249:H950, 1970.

35. Freedman RR: Biochemical, metabolic, and vascular mechanisms in menopausal hot flashes, *Fertil Steril* 70:332, 1998.

36. Freedman RR et al: Local temperature modulates α_1- and α_2-adrenergic vasoconstriction in men, *Am J Physiol* 32:H1197, 1992.

37. Fregly M: Activity of the hypothalamic-pituitary-thyroid axis during exposure to cold. In Schönbaum E, Lomax P, editors: *Thermoregulation: physiology and biochemistry*, New York, 1990, Pergamon Press.

38. Gagge AP, Gonzales RR: Mechanisms of heat exchange: biophysics and physiology. In Fregly ML, Blatteis CM, editors: *Handbook of physiology*, vol 1, Bethesda, Md, 1996, Oxford University Press.

39. Gautier H et al: Effects of hypoxia and cold acclimation on thermoregulation in the rat, *J Appl Physiol* 71:1355, 1991.

40. Giesbrecht GK et al: Treatment of immersion hypothermia by direct body-to-body contact, *FASEB J* 7:A441, 1993.

41. Grayson J: Responses of the microcirculation to hot and cold environments. In Schönbaum E, Lomax P, editors: *Thermoregulation: physiology and biochemistry*, New York, 1990, Pergamon Press.

42. Griffin JD et al: Cellular mechanisms for neuronal thermosensitivity in the rat hypothalamus, *J Physiol* 492:231, 1996.

43. Grucza R: Thermoregulatory responses to heat loads in men and women. In Johannsen BN, Nielsen R, editors: *Thermal physiology*, Copenhagen, 1997, August Krogh Institute.

44. Guyton AC: *Medical physiology*, Philadelphia, 1981, WB Saunders.

45. Hammel HT: Regulation of internal body temperature, *Annu Rev Physiol* 30:641, 1968.

46. Hanson DF: Fever, temperature, and the immune response, *Ann NY Acad Sci* 813:453, 1997.

47. Hardy JD: Physiology of temperature regulation, *Physiol Rev* 41:521, 1961.

48. Hardy JD: Body temperature regulation. In Mountcastle VB, editor: *Medical physiology*, vol 2, ed 2, St Louis, 1980, Mosby.

49. Hellstrom B, Hammel HT: Some characteristics of temperature regulation in the unanesthetized dog, *Am J Physiol* 213:547, 1967.

50. Hensel H: Cutaneous thermoreceptors. In Iggo A, editor: *Handbook of sensory physiology*, vol 2, Berlin, 1973, Springer-Verlag.

51. Hensel H, Kenshalo DR: Warm receptors in the nasal region of cats, *J Physiol (Lond)* 204:99, 1969.

52. Hesslink RL Jr et al: Human cold air habituation is independent of thyroxine and thyrotropin, *J Appl Physiol* 72:2134, 1992.

53. Himms-Hagen S: Brown adipose tissue thermogenesis: role in thermoregulation, energy regulation and obesity. In Schönbaum E, Lomax P, editors: *Thermoregulation: physiology and biochemistry*, New York, 1990, Pergamon Press.

54. Hirashita M, Shido O, Tanabe M: Blood flow through the ophthalmic veins during exercise in humans, *Eur J Appl Physiol* 64:92, 1992.

55. Hodgman CD, editor: *Handbook of chemistry and physics: a ready-reference book of chemical and physical data*, ed 43, Cleveland, 1962, Chemical Rubber.

56. *Holy Bible (King James Version)*, 1 Kings 1:1-4, Boston, Whittemore Associates.

57. Hong S, Nadel ER: Thermogenic control during exercise in a cold environment, *J Appl Physiol* 47:1084, 1979.

58. Ikeda T et al: Influence of thermoregulatory vasomotion and ambient temperature variation on the accuracy of core-temperature estimates by cutaneous liquid-crystal thermometers, *Anesthesiology* 86:603, 1997.

59. Inoue Y et al: Regional differences in the sweating responses of older and younger men, *J Appl Physiol* 71:2453, 1991.

60. Jessen C: Thermal afferents in the control of body temperature. In Schönbaum E, Lomax P, editors: *Thermoregulation: physiology and biochemistry*, New York, 1990, Pergamon Press.

61. Johnson JM: Physical training and the control of skin blood flow, *Med Sci Sports Exerc* 30:382, 1998.

62. Johnson JM, Proppe DW: Cardiovascular adjustments to heat stress. In Fregly ML, Blatteis CM, editors: *Handbook of physiology*, vol 1, Bethesda, Md, 1996, Oxford University Press.

63. Johnston CE et al: Alcohol lowers the vasoconstriction threshold in humans without affecting core cooling rate during mild cold exposure, *Eur J Appl Physiol* 74:293, 1996.

64. Johnston CE et al: Eucapnic hypoxia lowers human cold thermoregulatory response thresholds and accelerates core cooling, *J Appl Physiol* 80:422, 1996.

65. Jones SR: Fever in the elderly. In Mackowiak PA, editor: *Fever: basic mechanisms and management*, ed 2, Philadelphia, 1997, Lippincott-Raven.

66. Kellogg DL et al: Nitric oxide and cutaneous active vasodilation during heat stress in humans, *J Appl Physiol* 85:824, 1998.

67. Kenney WL: Control of skin vasodilation: mechanisms and influences. In Johannsen BN, Nielsen R, editors: *Thermal physiology*, Copenhagen, 1997, August Krogh Institute.

68. Khan F, Spence VA, Belch JJF: Cutaneous vascular responses and thermoregulation in relation to age, *Clin Sci* 82:521, 1992.

69. Kleinebeckel D, Klussman FW: Shivering. In Schönbaum E, Lomax P, editors: *Thermoregulation: physiology and biochemistry*, New York, 1990, Pergamon Press.

70. Klement W, Arndt JO: The role of nociceptors of cutaneous veins in the mediation of cold pain in man, *J Physiol* 449:73, 1992.

71. Kluger MJ: Is fever beneficial?, *Yale J Biol Med* 59:89, 1986.

72. Kluger MJ et al: The adaptive value of fever. In Mackowiak PA, editor: *Fever: basic mechanisms and management*, ed 2, Philadelphia, 1997, Lippincott-Raven.

73. Kluger MJ et al: Fever and antipyresis. In Sharma HS, Westman J, editors: *Brain function in hot environment*, New York, 1998, Elsevier Science.

74. Kolka MA, Stephenson LA: Resetting the thermoregulatory set-point by endogenous estradiol or progesterone in women, *Ann NY Acad Sci* 813: 204, 1997.

75. Kurz A, Sessler DI, Lenhardt R: Perioperative normothermia to reduce the incidence of surgical-wound infection and shorten hospitalization, *N Engl J Med* 334:1209, 1996.

76. Latzka WA et al: Hyperhydration: thermoregulatory effects during compensable exercise-heat stress, *J Appl Physiol* 83:860, 1997.

77. Latzka WA et al: Hyperhydration: tolerance and cardiovascular effects during uncompensable exercise-heat stress, *J Appl Physiol* 84:1858, 1998.

78. MacKenzie MA: *Poikilothermia in man. Pathophysiological aspects and clinical implications*, master's thesis, Nijmegen, Netherlands, 1996, University of Nijmegen.

79. Mackowiak PA: Clinical thermometric measurements. In Mackowiak PA, editor: *Mechanisms and management*, ed 2, Philadelphia, 1997, Lippincott-Raven.

80. Mackowiak PA: History of clinical thermometry. In Mackowiak PA, editor: *Mechanisms and management*, ed 2, Philadelphia, 1997, Lippincott-Raven.

81. Mackowiak PA et al: Concepts of fever: recent advances and lingering dogma, *Clin Infect Dis* 25:119, 1997.

82. Malcolm RD, Alkana RL: Temperature dependence of ethanol depression in mice, *J Pharmacol Exp Ther* 35:306, 1983.

83. Mitchell JH et al: Acute response and chronic adaptation to exercise in women, *Med Sci Sports Exerc* 24(suppl 6):S258, 1992.

84. Morimoto T, Itoh T, Takamata A: Thermoregulation and body fluid in hot environment. In Sharma HS, Westman J, editors: *Progress in brain research*, vol 115, New York, 1998, Elsevier.

85. Mount LE: *The climatic physiology of the pig*, London, 1968, Edward Arnold.

86. Mount LE: *Adaptation to thermal environment: man and his productive animals*, Baltimore, 1979, University Park Press.

87. Nadel ER, Bullard RW, Stolwijk JAJ: Importance of skin temperature in the regulation of sweating, *J Appl Physiol* 31:80, 1971.

88. Nadel ER, Stolwijk JAJ: Effect of skin wettedness on sweat gland response, *J Appl Physiol* 35:689, 1973.

89. Nadel ER et al: Peripheral modifications to the central drive for sweating, *J Appl Physiol* 31:828, 1971.

90. Nadel ER et al: Mechanisms of thermal acclimation to exercise and heat, *J Appl Physiol* 37:515, 1974.

91. Newburgh LH: *Physiology of heat regulation and the science of clothing*, Philadelphia, 1949, WB Saunders.

92. Nielsen B, Kaciuba-Uscilko H: Temperature regulation in exercise. In Blatteis CM, editor: *Physiology and pathophysiology of temperature regulation*, Singapore, 1998, World Scientific.

93. Nobel PS: *Biophysical plant physiology and ecology*, New York, 1983, WH Freeman.

94. Pandolf KB et al: Human thermoregulatory responses during heat exposure after artificially induced sunburn, *Am J Physiol* 262:R610, 1992.

95. Pandolf KB et al: Human thermoregulatory responses during cold water immersion after artificially induced sunburn, *Am J Physiol* 262:R617, 1992.

96. Panksepp J: Hypothalamic integration of behavior: rewards, punishments, and related psychological processes. In Morgane PJ, Panksepp J, editors: *Handbook of the hypothalamus*, vol 3, New York, 1980, Marcel Dekker.

97. Passias TC, Meneilly GS, Mekjavić IB: Effect of hypoglycemia on thermoregulatory responses, *J Appl Physiol* 80:1021, 1996.

98. Petersen MH, Hauge HN: Can training improve the results with infrared tympanic thermometers? *Acta Anaesthesiol Scand* 41:1066, 1997.

99. Prezant DJ et al: Temperature dependence of rat diaphragm muscle contractility and fatigue, *J Appl Physiol* 69:1740, 1990.

100. Regan JM, Macfarlane DJ, Taylor NAS: An evaluation of the role of skin temperature during heat adaptation, *Acta Physiol Scand* 158:365, 1996.

101. Reinberg A, Smolensky M: Chronobiology and thermoregulation. In Schönbaum E, Lomax P, editors: *Thermoregulation: physiology and biochemistry*, New York, 1990, Pergamon Press.

102. Robinson J et al: Oesophageal, rectal, axillary, tympanic and pulmonary artery temperatures during cardiac surgery, *Can J Anaesth* 45:317. 1998.

103. Romanovsky AA et al: Endotoxin shock: thermoregulatory mechanisms, *Am J Physiol* 39:R693, 1996.

104. Romanovsky AA et al: A difference of 5° C between ear and rectal temperatures in a febrile patient, *Am J Emerg Med* 15:383, 1997.

105. Romanovsky AA et al: The vagus nerve in the thermoregulatory response to systemic inflammation, *Am J Physiol* 273:R407, 1997.

106. Sato KT et al: Reexamination of tympanic membrane temperature as a core temperature, *J Appl Physiol* 80:1233, 1996.

107. Sawka MN: Physiological consequences of hypohydration: exercise performance and thermoregulation, *Med Sci Sports Exerc* 24:657, 1992.

108. Schmidt-Nielsen K: *Animal physiology: adaptation and environment*, ed 5, Cambridge, UK, 1997, Cambridge University Press.

109. Schönbaum E, Lomax P: Temperature regulation and drugs: an introduction. In Schönbaum E, Lomax P, editors: *Thermoregulation physiology and biochemistry*, New York, 1990, Pergamon.

110. Segal SS, Faulkner JA, White TP: Skeletal muscle fatigue in vitro is temperature dependent, *J Appl Physiol* 61:660, 1986.

111. Sessler DI: Perianesthetic thermoregulation and heat balance in humans, *FASEB J* 7:638, 1993.

112. Sessler DI: Perioperative hypothermia, *N Engl J Med* 336:1730, 1997.

113. Sessler DI: Perioperative thermoregulation and heat balance. In Blatteis CM, editor: *Physiology and pathophysiology of temperature regulation*, Singapore, 1998, World Scientific Publishing.

114. Shanahan TL, Czeisler CA: Light exposure induces equivalent phase shifts of the endogenous circadian rhythms of circulating plasma melatonin and core body temperature in men, *J Clin Endocrinol Metab* 73:227, 1991.

115. Shibasaki M et al: Continuous measurement of tympanic temperature with a new infrared method using an optical fiber, *J Appl Physiol* 85:921, 1998.

116. Simonsen L et al: Thermogenic response to epinephrine in the forearm and abdominal subcutaneous adipose tissue, *Am J Physiol* 263:E850, 1992.

117. Stevens ED: The evolution of endothermy, *J Theor Biol* 38:597, 1973.

118. Stolwijk JAJ, Nadel ER: Thermoregulation during positive and negative work exercise, *Fed Proc* 32:1607, 1973.

119. Takahashi Y et al: Circumventricular organs and fever, *Am J Physiol* 273:R1690, 1997.

120. Tamaki Y, Nakayama T: Effects of air constituents on thermosensitivities of preoptic neurons: hypoxia versus hypercapnia, *Pflügers Arch* 409:1, 1987.

121. Wenger CB et al: Forearm blood flow during body temperature transients produced by leg exercise, *J Appl Physiol* 38:58, 1975.

122. Wood SC: Interactions between hypoxia and hypothermia, *Annu Rev Physiol* 53:71, 1991.

123. Yang Y, Gordon CJ: Regulated hypothermia in the hypothyroid rat induced by administration of propylthiouracil, *Am J Physiol* 272:R1390, 1997.

124. Young CC, Sladen RN: Temperature monitoring, *Int Anesthesiol Clin* 34:149, 1996.

125. Zeisberger E: Biogenic amines and thermoregulatory changes. In Sharma HS, Westman J, editors: *Brain function in hot environment*, New York, 1998, Elsevier Science.

5 Nonfreezing Cold Injuries

Murray P. Hamlet

Nonfreezing cold injuries have a military origin. Although they have probably always occurred in civilians as well, they have not been documented in that population in sufficient numbers or severity to warrant interest. Armies, however, have suffered extensive injuries with significant impact on specific battles and campaigns. Several armies have been decimated by cold, wet conditions. Because of this epidemiology, there is usually a flurry of interest in these injuries immediately after wars. The interest is short-lived, however, probably because little impact has been shown on treatment of the injury. Interest in prevention with new clothing and footwear also flourishes, but it takes another military campaign to prove if the effort was successful. As we become more of an outdoor population, there is a high likelihood that civilians will put themselves in threatening environments more often and for longer times. Two particular groups appear to be producing injuries consistently. One is snowmakers at recreational ski facilities, and the second is rafting crews. The term "river rot" from the rafting community clearly refers to a trench foot injury. This chapter touches on the history, epidemiology, pathophysiology, clinical treatment, and postinjury sequelae of nonfreezing cold injury. Although many references and other sources of information are old, their observations still have significant value in understanding the injuries.

EPIDEMIOLOGY

Production of nonfreezing cold injuries involves having cold, wet extremities for an extended period. Historically, most injuries have been produced at just above the freezing temperature of human tissue. The most challenging condition involves fluctuations of temperatures above and immediately below freezing with wet socks and boots. Standing or sitting for a prolonged period with stagnation of circulation in the extremities and tight, constrictive footwear are major contributing factors. Blunt trauma of marching on cold, wet feet also adds to the severity.

Wetness increases conductive heat loss. Wetness with maceration of skin may contribute to the severity of the injury, but in animal models the injury can be produced with dry, cold air. This probably does not occur in a natural situation. This is because in the military context, the soldier is often unable to do anything to get his or her feet or boots dry because of the combat setting and urgency of the battle. Even if he or she knows what to do, the soldier does not have the time or the ability to attain an appropriate remedy. When the battle is over and the victim has time to warm and dry the feet, they become hot, swollen, and extremely painful. If the extremities are repeatedly exposed to injurious cold, the damage is compounded.

PERNIO

The civilian setting (e.g., rafting, snowmaking, winter hiking) often involves consecutive days of wearing wet boot liners and socks from hiking in wet weather or having wet feet from water immersion in a boat or life raft. Long canoe outings and sea kayaking trips lend themselves to this injury. The duration of exposure is important in determining the potential severity. Between 3 and 6 hours of cold and moisture produce swelling and tenderness with little or no residual consequences. Subcutaneous vesicles may be present, with or without blue discoloration and tenderness. This is termed *chilblain*. Between 6 and 12 hours of exposure produces more lasting swelling with some pain and deep ache. There is often scaling and desquamation but no deep tissue damage. There may be deep tissue sensitivity to pressure and subsequent resistance to wearing boots or shoes for a few days. After 12 hours to 3 days of being cold and wet, there may be deep pain and thin, partial-thickness skin eschars that form on the dorsum of the hands and feet. The eschars will slough without scarring but create persistent pain. This condition is termed *pernio*. The acute nature of the symptomatology is an early warning for the long-term sequelae of pernio. Although healing appears to occur as the edema subsides and the plaques slough, the pain persists and there may be later symptoms of tingling, paresthesia, skin scaling, and edema, even from mild cold exposure. Walking may be difficult, and shoes may cause enough constant pain that the individual has to go shoeless most of the day. This injury is seen in schoolchildren with tight, cold, and wet footwear who repeatedly walk home in slush without caring for their feet. It is seen in mild cold settings, such as logging, snowmaking, and kayaking, where the feet are cold and wet and the acute symptoms do not provoke the individual to protect the feet. In a battle setting, soldiers are often unable to take care of their feet, and their footwear is often poor. Prisoners of war often have pernio or trench foot from forced marches in cold and wet conditions.

One histopathologic study of nine victims of pernio noted a unique lymphocytic vasculitis. Edema of the papillary dermis was a variable feature, as was perivascular lymphocytic infiltration (characteristic of systemic lupus erythematosus, erythema multiforme, or drug eruption). In all likelihood, trench foot and chilblains share a common pathophysiology that includes sympathetic instability and vascular hypersensitivity to cold, with microvascular stasis and thrombosis.

Prevention is paramount for this injury. Awareness of the threat and training on keeping the feet dry, changing socks, massaging feet, and emergency care are essential. Preexposure training and daily foot checks are essential. A few minutes of scrutiny can prevent serious damage and decrease the likelihood of requiring medical assistance. Leaders in summer camps and outdoor training must be constantly aware of foot care.

The treatment for pernio is simply to dry and massage the feet. Active, gentle warming above 30° C (86° F) as for frostbite usually produces significant pain and discomfort. Elevation is helpful to treat edema. Nonsteroidal antiinflammatory medication may be beneficial empirically but has not been studied in a randomized, prospective manner. Pain on warming may not respond to narcotics. Ketorolac tromethamine (Toradol) might be used, but there is no reference for its success.[10] Topical substances do not appear to have any beneficial effects, although an antiinflammatory topical may be tried.

Sequelae of Pernio

Pernio produces long-term sequelae of pain, numbness, and paresthesia even with mild cooling. On occasion, healing is followed by hyperpigmentation. The victim is prone to recurrences on lesser exposure. Pain from pressure may limit the victim to loose-fitting footwear. Some relief can be had by resting feet on a brushlike surface, such as Astroturf. Sandals that support on points or small knobs seem to give relief and promote gradual desensitization to pain and pressure in the feet.

TRENCH FOOT (IMMERSION FOOT)

An excellent historical review of nonfreezing cold injury was offered by T.J.R. Francis in 1984.[5] The term *trench foot* derives from World War I, when troops would stand in water-filled trenches for days and acquire this injury, severely limiting available manpower. There are earlier descriptions of cold, wet injuries. Critchie[3] found references in 1727 describing the injury in shipyard workers and explorers. There is little doubt that Napoleon's surgeon Baron Larrey's description of cold "conjulgation" involved many nonfreezing cold injuries along with true frostbite. In the Crimean War (1845-1855), when British troops were poorly equipped and deployed in winter and were wracked with dysen-

tery, there were 1924 reported injuries. Regimental medical officer B. Hughes first described the three stages of trench foot, the tenets of drying and massaging the feet, and the notion that dry socks and rubber overboots were responsible for a significant decrease in injury. After Smith, Ritchie, and Dawson's experimental work and observation,[12] there were general orders issued to commanders to take steps to prevent the injury. These procedures carried over to the British troops in World War II, where few nonfreezing cold injuries occurred. Unfortunately, the American army suffered 4560 cold injuries in 2½ months in 1943-1944. Significant medical research and description of nonfreezing cold injury was performed by Ungley.[14-16] He first recognized the similarities between trench foot and immersion foot symptoms and pathology from individuals in life rafts immersed in water. These descriptions of the pathophysiology are still the most detailed and useful. Nonfreezing cold injury was rarely reported in the Korean War. Postwar interviews with veterans indicate a high incidence of frostbite and some trench foot. British exposure in the Falklands Campaign defined a significant number of injuries with no amputations, but which required dismissal of many soldiers from military service. The Argentines suffered 274 amputation injuries from trench foot.

When one looks at the circumstances that have produced large numbers of nonfreezing cold injury in military operations, it is easy to transfer them to the civilian wilderness medicine setting. Poorly trained, tired, frightened, and dehydrated soldiers with thin socks and tight-fitting boots who are deployed in a cold and wet environment are unable to maintain foot care because of the battle setting. After several days of exposure, they are able to rest in a warm tent and remove their boots, where they begin to manifest the first stages of trench foot. Civilians in an outdoor setting who are similarly cold, wet, exhausted, and dehydrated are unwilling or unable to take the time and effort to care for themselves. Many are unaware of the threat and simply go to bed with wet feet or continue to put on wet socks and boots day after day. Uninformed outdoorspersons are simply naïve about the role of wet feet in producing trench foot.

The linchpin to disaster in a cold, wet environment is a pair of tight-fitting boots. Wetness increases conductive heat loss caused by the footwear. The cold produces peripheral constriction, and the tight boots add to tissue ischemia. Reduced blood flow from sympathetic nervous system–mediated vasoconstriction along with dehydration leads to sluggish or nonexistent blood flow to the foot. Tissue anoxia leads to cellular compromise and death.

At the cellular level, there appears to be a hierarchy of sensitivity, with neurons, muscle cells, and endothelial cells being the most susceptible. The ischemic injury to different cell types determines eventual outcome. With damage to neurons and their axons, there is paresthesia, pain, and muscle atrophy. With damage to sympathetic nerves, the result is hyperhidrosis and cold sensitivity. With damage to muscle and fat cells, there is atrophy and replacement with fibrous connective tissue, along with cramping and muscle spasms. Bone injury leads to bone infarcts and lysis, effects similar to osteoporosis, and subsequent arthritic changes. If one understands the cellular pathology, it is easy to envision the etiology of postinjury sequelae.

SIGNS AND SYMPTOMS

Trench foot and immersion foot are essentially the same injury. Both are produced by long-term cooling of the extremities. Trench foot occurs from wearing wet boots and socks, whereas immersion foot involves immersion of the feet in water, such as in a life raft or boat. Water temperature associated with trench foot is often 0° to 10° C (32° to 50° F). The pathogenesis of the injuries appears to be the same, but trench foot may include the blunt trauma of marching, which adds to the severity of the injury. Also, immersion foot is generally a single experience, whereas trench foot often involves repeated injury to the feet.

These injuries are vasomotor in the sense that the end result combines with damage to small blood vessels, peripheral nerves, and adjacent dermal organs; sympathetic, motor, and sensory nerves are affected. Symptomatology reflects injury to these nerves and damage to sweat glands, blood vessels, nail beds, muscle, cartilage, and bone.

Prehyperemic Phase

When one observes the limb immediately after exposure, it appears blanched, yellowish-white, and cold to touch. "Cold and numb" are the most common descriptions of the prehyperemic phase. The distal vessels may be pulseless for some time after admission. The victim describes "walking on wooden limbs," "walking on wool," or "walking in someone else's feet." Balance is impaired, and there is a shuffling gait.

Hyperemic Phase

The hyperemic phase lasts 6 to 10 weeks. Shortly after warming, the feet become hot, painful, red, dry, and swollen (Figure 5-1). This often occurs before medical management. Pain can be excruciating and is described as a deep, burning ache with throbbing. Definitive medical care is often sought at this time. Approximately 7 to 10 days later, shooting or stabbing pains occur down the foot, across the arch, out to the toes, and up the limb. Victims cannot tolerate even light pressure on their feet, and the bedsheets must be tented to prevent touching them at night. Nerve damage is evident

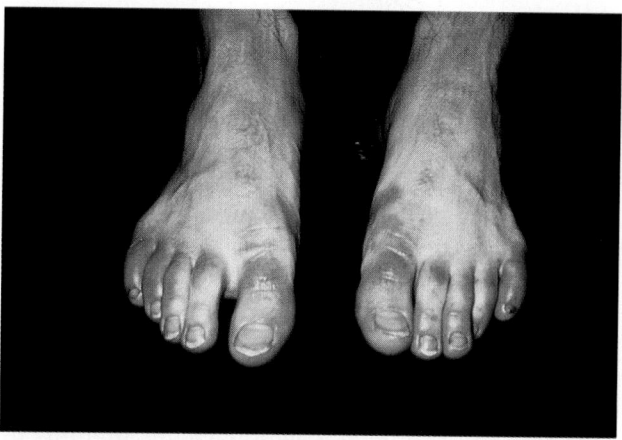

Figure 5-1 Moderate trench foot. No amputation. *(Courtesy M.P. Hamlet.)*

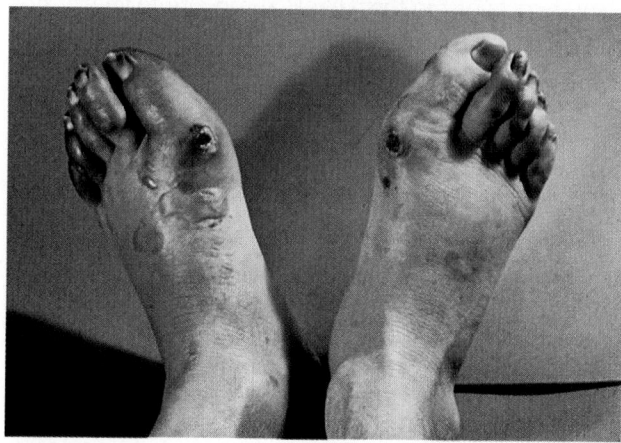

Figure 5-2 Immersion injury from a life raft. Note pressure necrosis from the shoes. This severe injury resulted in the amputation of all toes but the great toe. *(Courtesy M.P. Hamlet.)*

by loss of sensation and motor control, tingling pain, and paresthesias. Paresthesias and alternating pain and numbness increase with warming and dependency of the limb. Throbbing, pulsatile pain may last for weeks. Vibratory sensation is also diminished or lost. Hyperhidrosis occurs from nerve damage and local injury to sweat glands.

Vascular injury is reflected in the reactivity of the vessels. If the limb is elevated, it blanches. When lowered, it becomes blue or deep purple-red. Swelling occurs rapidly when the limb is warmed. Blisters may form with clear fluid or be hemorrhagic, indicating more severe injury.

The skin thins, indurates, and scales. Circular ulcerations may be superficial or deep. Black eschar forms and later sloughs, leaving pink, sensitive skin. Nails slough (Figure 5-2) without pain and continue to do so intermittently for years. Distal gangrene may be dry and mummifying or, more consistently, moist and liquefied. This often requires early surgical debridement.

Muscle is damaged with loss of muscle mass and strength. Electromyography shows slowing, deep tendon reflexes are sluggish or absent, and deep pain often results from muscle activity. A wasting deformity ("hollowing") of the sole of the foot occurs from loss of intrinsic muscles. Bone lesions representing decalcification of phalanges and periarticular lysis and loss of joint integrity occur.

Posthyperemic Phase

Swelling, hyperhidrosis, alternating pain and numbness, Raynaud's phenomenon, and cold sensitivity comprise the postinjury picture. Muscle wasting causes weakness and cramping when the victim attempts to stand. Neurologic damage with loss of proprioception and motor control leads to gait abnormalities that can last a lifetime. Wasting of intrinsic muscles results in claw defects of the toes. Areas that were formerly hot and painful now become cold and cold-sensitive. They show pallor and cyanosis and are slow to rewarm. Affected areas become hyperhidrotic, may become swollen, and may harbor shooting pains, as well as intermittent return of the dull ache.

PATHOGENESIS

Ungley[15] wrote that this injury should be described as a "peripheral vasoneuropathy after chilling," which in consideration leads to a sound understanding of trench foot. Although there has been significant effort to define the pathogenesis, the precise cause remains somewhat elusive. Reviewing past research and pathology information leads to the possibility of trench foot being a reperfusion injury. Green[6] wrote that there was little damage while tissue was cold and that injury occurred upon rewarming. He believed that as tissue warmed, there was a mismatch between the nutrients and oxygen delivered during a state of vasoconstriction and the increased metabolic demands of cells. If the limb was warmed slowly, then there was less symptomatology and less damage. However, Smith, Rickles, and Dawson[12] and Blackwood[1] believed that cold itself damaged different cell types, although they had difficulty differentiating the effects of ischemia from the direct effect of cold on these cells.

Nerve damage was first thought to occur to small A and C fibers because pain was the predominant feature. It was later found that large myelinated fibers were also damaged but not as early. Small peripheral nerve endings are perhaps the most sensitive, but a precise hierarchy of injury has not been defined. Hyaline degeneration, swelling and disruption of neurolemmal sheaths, and precipitation of neural proteins appear in all nerves to some degree, depending on the severity and duration of the insult. Damage to autonomic nerve fibers is extensive and equates with the

symptomatology at different stages. During the hyperemic stage, there is redness, swelling, and pain, along with anhidrosis. This is replaced in the posthyperemic phase with cold sensitivity, hyperhidrosis, and cooling of the limb.[4] Although some regeneration of partially damaged neurons is possible, this ability appears limited, and long-term neurologic symptomatology is common.

Fibrous connective tissue deposits in vessel walls render them less compliant or rigid. Fat cells in muscle appear to be damaged early. Muscle cells show degeneration, swelling, loss of structure, hyaline degeneration, and complete loss of internal material. Muscle cells shrink and become fibrotic and nonfunctional.

Skin atrophy and thinning occur, and dry, scaly patches develop. In abraded areas, such as the bottom of the foot, the skin thickens and cornifies with thick calluses. Skin on the upper part of the foot becomes thin, friable, and very sensitive to pressure. There are collagen deposits around damaged nerve endings, small blood vessels, and damaged sweat glands. Hyperhidrosis may be from damage to autonomic innervation or from the direct effect of cold. Nerve endings in the skin send mixed messages. Pain vs. numbness and hot vs. cold all emanate from skin late in the posthyperemic phase.

Blisters followed by ulceration and subsequent eschar formation indicate local ischemia. Dry, mummifying gangrene may form tight, shieldlike eschars over toes and metatarsal areas. Demarcation may take weeks, but early infection, liquefaction, fever, and elevated muscle enzymes call for surgical intervention.

CLINICAL EVALUATION

Early clinical evaluation does not alter initial management. An accurate history of the duration and severity of cold exposure is the essential starting point to estimate severity of the injury later. Late evaluations of cold sensitivity, thermal threshold analysis,[10] and infrared thermography after mild cold exposure have proven to be most useful in defining severity of injury. They are particularly important in the determination of the degree of disability for compensation or for continued military assignment.

TREATMENT

Drying and slight elevation of the feet with passive rewarming from core heat are indicated. Cool fanning of the feet at 20° C (68° F) may help minimize pain. There is no "silver bullet" for treatment; free radical scavengers and cytokine-blocking agents have the most potential for future investigation. Pain relief is not effective because nonsteroidal antiinflammatory agents and narcotics do not alleviate the different kinds of pain produced.

Oakley[10] described the use of amitriptyline (50 to 150 mg at night) as somewhat beneficial. Patients should not be allowed to traumatize their feet during the hyperemic and early posthyperemic phase. Walking can be so painful that patients will refuse even mild physical therapy. Other medications, such as nifedipine and thymoxamine, were at first thought to offer some relief but have not been proven effective.[10] Later, the feet should be kept warm and dry with thick socks and loose-fitting shoes. Avoidance of cold exposure is essential to prevent painful episodes. The remainder of treatment is symptomatic and often fairly nonproductive.

SEQUELAE OF TRENCH FOOT

Although the acute injury is difficult, long-term sequelae are the real problems with nonfreezing cold injury. Relatively minor injuries often produce clinically significant problems years later. With minor injury, short-term pain and dysfunction can be expected for days to weeks until recovery. There is often persistent mild cold sensitivity, but this is minor and quite tolerable. Years later, paresthesias, Raynaud's syndrome, chronic fungal infections, swelling, and alternating pain and numbness develop. Gait changes from pain avoidance and loss of proprioception include widened stance, shortened stride, and shuffling gait. Hyperhidrosis leads to chronic paronychial fungal infections that are refractory to treatment. Thick, deformed nails require professional podiatry care.

The more severe the acute injury, the quicker and more intense the sequelae. Moderate to severe injury often leads to symptoms early after acute recovery. Scaling, ulceration, and nail loss occur intermittently throughout life with no apparent precipitating events. Injured individuals are extremely cold sensitive, often requiring changes in job or residence. A complete lifestyle change may be required to tolerate symptomatology.

Individuals with severe injuries (e.g., necrosis and amputation) are never symptom free. There is a long healing time for ulcerations and amputation stumps. During this time, severe symptoms often occur proximal to the amputation site. Muscle atrophy that occurs proximal to the injury site often limits joint motion and flexibility. Cramping is common. Deep muscle aching while standing or even sitting for extended periods is also common.

There is a psychologic component to this injury. Because treatment for relief of symptoms is not very productive, patients become frustrated. The changes in lifestyle are significant. Victims may become depressed and home-ridden. Alcohol abuse is not uncommon. Because other vascular and neurologic conditions affect the lower extremities with aging, the combination with cold injury sequelae is often confusing to the examining physician.

CRYOGLOBULINS

Cold-induced precipitation of serum proteins was first reported in a patient with multiple myeloma by Wintrobe and Buell.[18] Subsequently, the term *cryoglobulin* was introduced to denote a group of serum proteins that have the common property of reversibly precipitating or gelling in the cold.[8] The vast majority of cryoglobulins are either intact monoclonal immunoglobulins (IgGs) or immunoglobulin complexes (that is, mixed cryoglobulins) in which one component, usually IgM, is directed against IgG.[7] Symptoms directly attributable to monoclonal cryoglobulins are quite variable and include cold intolerance with typical Raynaud's phenomenon, dependent purpura, cutaneous vasculitis with ulceration, retinal hemorrhages, coagulopathies, and cerebral thrombosis. In many cases, only inexact correlations exist among the concentration of the cryoglobulin, the temperature of cryoformation, and the presence of symptoms.[7] Of clinical relevance is the composition of the cryoprecipitate. Since acral temperatures of 30° C (86° F) are present in the hands and feet,[2] in vivo cryoprecipitation may directly contribute to impaired capillary blood flow in the extremities; this has been demonstrated by biomicroscopy of conjunctival and nail bed capillaries.[11] In patients with monoclonal cryo IgM, the higher intrinsic viscosity of IgM compared with IgG is greatly amplified and attendant symptoms can often be directly related to hyperviscosity.[7]

In a large clinical series, only two thirds of the patients had skin lesions or vasomotor attack at initial examination.[2] Cold sensitivity was apparent in less than half of these patients. Less common early symptoms were renal failure, mucosal bleeding, visual disturbance, and abdominal pain. In cryoglobulinemia without severe symptoms and in the absence of an underlying disease requiring active treatment, the decisions for treatment and type of treatment are difficult. Primary treatment should be directed toward minimizing cold exposure. Cyproheptadine (Periactin) 4 mg three or four times daily for approximately 1 to 2 weeks is useful when urticaria occurs.[17] This is probably due to its antihistamine and antikinin activity. Avoidance of prolonged standing is important in patients to prevent dependent purpura. With severe manifestations, plasmapheresis may be required for emergency treatment.

COLD URTICARIA

Cold urticaria is a fairly common form of physical urticaria.[9] It is characterized by local or generalized wheals, either on continuous cold exposure or on rewarming of sites previously exposed to cold. Local symptoms include redness, itching, wheals, and edema in cold-exposed skin. Systemic symptoms include fa-

tigue, headache, dyspnea, tachycardia, and rare anaphylactic shock. Usually the diagnosis is made by an
ice cube or ice water immersion test, in which a wheal
reaction appears in the exposed skin within 20 minutes.
Primary acquired cold urticaria is the most common
form. It occurs at any age, has an equal male/female
incidence, and tends to be self-limited, although it may
become chronic. Secondary acquired cold urticaria is
associated with an underlying disorder, such as cold
agglutinins or paroxysmal hemoglobinuria. Familial
cold urticaria is rare.

The cause of cold urticaria is unknown. It has been
reported to be mediated by IgE and IgM and to involve
the release of histamine or other inflammatory mediators.[9,17,18] Avoidance of cold is not always effective in
preventing cold urticaria, since the rate of cooling and
not absolute temperature appears to be the principal
stimulus. Desensitization may achieve only short-term
benefit. Cyproheptadine has been the most successful
drug, but doxepin, hydroxyzine, and ketotifen have
also been shown to be effective.[9,13,17,18]

REFERENCES

1. Blackwood W: Injury from exposure to low temperature: pathology, *Br Med J* 4, 1944.
2. Brouet JE et al: Biologic and clinical significance of cryoglobulins: a report of 86 cases, *Am J Med* 57:775, 1974.
3. Critchie M: *Shipwreck survivors: a medical study*, London, 1943, J & A Churchill.
4. Emmelin N, Trendelenburg B: Degeneration activity after parasympa-thetic and sympathetic denervation. In *Reviews of psychology*, Berlin, 1972, Springer-Verlag.
5. Frances TJR: Non-freezing cold injury: a historical review, *J R Naval Med Serv* 70:134, 1984.
6. Green R: Frostbite and kindred ills, *Lancet* 2, 1941.
7. Grey HM, Kohler PF: Cryoimmunoglobulins, *Semin Hematol* 10:87, 1973.
8. Lerner AM, Barnum CP, Watson CJ: Studies of cryoglobulins. 11. The pre-cipitation of protein from serum at 5° C in various disease states, *Am J Med Sci* 214:416, 1947.
9. Neittaanmaki H: Cold urticaria: clinical findings in 200 patients, *J Am Acad Dermatol* 13:636, 1985.
10. Oakley EHN: *Non-freezing cold injury*, Technical Report, Institute of Naval Medicine, UK.
11. Rinfret AP: *Cytobiology in cryogenic technology*, New York, 1962, Wiley.
12. Smith JL, Ritchie J, Dawson J: Clinical and experimental observations on the pathology of trench frostbite, *J Pathol* 20, 1915.
13. St.-Pierre JP, Kobric M, Rackham A: Effect of ketotifen treatment on cold-induced urticaria, *Ann Allergy* 55:840, 1985.
14. Ungley CC: Immersion foot and immersion hand, Bulletin of *War Medicine* 4:61, 1943.
15. Ungley CC, Blackwood W: Peripheral vasoneuropathy after chilling. "Immersion foot and immersion hand," *Lancet* 2:447, 1942.
16. Ungley CC, Channell CD, Richards RL: The immersion foot syndrome, *Br J Surg* 33:17, 1945.
17. Wanderer AA, Ellis ES: Treatment of cold urticaria with cyproheptadine, *J Allergy Clin Immunol* 48:366, 1971.
18. Wintrobe MM, Buell MV: Hyperproteinemia associated with multiple myeloma, *Bull Johns Hopkins Hosp* 52:156, 1933.

SUGGESTED READINGS

Adnot J, Lewis CW: Immersion foot syndromes, *J Assoc Mil Dermatol* 11:87, 1985.

Akers WA: Paddy foot: a warm weather water immersion foot syndrome vari-ant. Part I. the natural disease epidemiology, *Mil Med* 139, 1974.

Akers WA: Paddy foot: a warm weather water immersion foot syndrome vari-ant. Part II: field experiments, correlation, *Mil Med* 139, 1974.

Berson RC, Angelucci RJ: Trenchfoot, *Bulletin of the US Army Medical Department* 77, 1944.

Blackwood W: Studies in the pathology of human immersion foot, *Br J Surg* 31:329, 1944.

Catterall MD: Warm water immersion injuries of the feet—a review, *J R Nav Med Serv* 61, 1975.

Crouch C, Smith WL: Long term sequelae of frostbite, *Pediatr Radiol* 20:365, 1990.

Douglas JS, Eby CS: Silicone for immersion foot prophylaxis: where and how much to use, *Mil Med* 137, 1972.

Endrich B, Hammersen F, Messmer K: Microvascular ultrastructure in non-freezing cold injuries, *Res Exp Med (Berl)* 190:365, 1990.

Frances TJR, Golden FStC: Non-freezing cold injury: the pathogenesis, *J R Nav Med Serv* 71:3, 1985.

Fraser IC, Loftus JA: "Trench foot" caused by the cold, *Br Med J* 14:1, 1979.

Friedman NB: The pathology of trench foot, *Am J Pathol* 21, 1945.

Ganor S: Corticosteroid therapy for pernio, *J Am Acad Dermatol* 8:136, 1983.

Gill KA: Report of a field study on silicone ointments MDX-4-4056 and MDX-4-4078, *Naval Medical Field Research Laboratory Report* 17:16, 1967.

Irvin MS: Nature and mechanism of peripheral nerve damage in and experi-mental model of non-freezing cold injury, *Ann R Coll Surg Engl* 78:372, 1996.

Irwin MS et al: Neuropathy in non-freezing cold injury (trench foot), *J R Soc Med* 90:433, 1997.

Keatinge WR, Harmon MC: Local mechanisms controlling blood vessels. In *Monographs of the physiological society*, No 37, London, 1980, Academic Press.

Kennett RP, Gilliatt RW: Nerve conduction studies in experimental non-freezing cold injury: I. Local nerve cooling, *Muscle Nerve* 14:553, 1991.

Kennett RP, Gilliatt RW: Nerve conduction studies in experimental non-freezing cold injury: II. Generalized nerve cooling by limb immersion, *Muscle Nerve* 14:960, 1991.

Marcus P: "Trench foot" caused by the cold, *Br Med J* 3:1, 1979.

Mills WJ Jr et al: Frostbite: experience with rapid rewarming and ultrasonic therapy, Part II, *Alaska Med* 35:1, 1993.

Montgomery H: Experimental immersion foot: review of the pathophysiology, *Physiol Rev* 34, 1954.

Nukada H, Pollack M, Allpress S: Experimental cold injury to peripheral nerve, *Brain* 104(Pt 4):779, 1981.

Orr KD, Fainer DC: Cold injuries in Korea during the winter of 1950-51, *Medicine* 31, 1952.

Ramstead KD, Hughes RG, Webb AJ: Recent cases of trench foot, *Postgrad Med J* 56, 1980.

Rennie DW, Adams T: Comparative thermo-regulatory response of negroes and white persons to acute cold stress, *J Appl Physiol* 11, 1957.

Rustin MH et al: The treatment of chilblains with nifedipine: the results of a pilot study, a double-blind placebo-controlled randomized study and a long-term open trial, *Br J Dermatol* 20:267, 1989.

Smith JL, Ritchie J, Dawson J: On the pathology of trench foot, *Lancet* 11, 1915.

Spittell JA Jr, Spittel PC: Chronic pernio: another cause of blue toes, *Int Angiol* 11:46, 1992.

Vayssairat M: Chilblains, *J Mal Vasc* 17:229, 1992.

Webster DR, Woolhouse FM, Johnson JL: Immersion foot, *J Bone Joint Surg* 24, 1942.

Whayne TF, DeBakey ME: *Cold injury: ground type*, Washington, DC, 1958, Office of the Surgeon General, Department of the Army.

White AD: Chilblains, *Med J Aust* 154:406, 1991.

White JC, Schoville WB: Trench foot and immersion foot, *N Engl J Med* 232, 1945.

White JC, Warren S: Causes of pain in feet after prolonged immersion in cold water, *War Med* 5, 1944.

Zdeblick TA, Field GA, Shaffer JW: Treatment of experimental frostbite with urokinase, *Am J Hand Surg* 13:948, 1988.

6 Accidental Hypothermia

Daniel F. Danzl

Although used for medical purposes for millennia, cold modalities were not scientifically evaluated until the eighteenth century. The hemostatic, analgesic, and therapeutic effects of cold on various conditions were well known. Biblical references cite truncal rewarming of King David by a damsel; various remedies were mentioned by Hippocrates, Aristotle, and Galen.[214]

The effects of cold on human performance are perhaps best documented in military history. Frosty conditions have decided many battles.[116] Most cold injuries encountered today affect the urban destitute and wilderness and sports enthusiasts, such as skiers, hunters, sailors, climbers, and swimmers.[133,234] The popularity of Arctic and mountain expeditions has increased the number of persons at risk. Among those challenging the environment are climbers of Mt. Everest, Mt. Hood, and Mt. McKinley.[108]

EPIDEMIOLOGY

In most countries, primary hypothermia deaths are considered violent and are classified as accidental, homicidal, or suicidal.[32] Deaths from secondary hypothermia are usually considered natural complications of systemic disorders, including trauma, carcinoma, and sepsis. The true incidence of secondary hypothermia throughout the world is unknown because hypothermic persons found indoors usually have other serious and diverting secondary medical illnesses. In addition, delays are common between hospital admission and death, so secondary hypothermia is significantly underreported. In contrast, death certificate data more accurately quantify primary hypothermia.

Hypothermia occurs in various locations and in all seasons.[180,196,278] In a multicenter North American survey of 428 cases of civilian accidental hypothermia, 69 occurred in Florida.[49] Urban settings account for the majority of cases in most of the industrialized countries.[51,137,257] During 1979-1995, there was an annual average of 723 deaths attributed to hypothermia in the United States. Around half of these fatalities were patients over age 65.[33]

Classifications

Accidental hypothermia is best defined as the unintentional decrease of around 2° C (3.6° F) in the "normal" core temperature of 37.2° to 37.7° C (98.9° to 99.9° F) without disease in the preoptic and anterior hypothalamic nuclei (Table 6-1).[182] Classically, hypothermia is

defined as a core temperature below 35° C (95° F). Hypothermia is both a symptom and a clinical disease entity. When sufficient heat cannot be generated to maintain homeostasis and the core temperature drops below 30° C (86° F), the patient becomes poikilothermic and cools to the ambient temperature.

Among the clinical classifications, the most practical division includes healthy patients with simple environmental exposure (primary), those with specific diseases producing hypothermia (secondary), and those with predisposing conditions. Other divisions reflect the etiology of hypothermia and include immersion vs. nonimmersion and acute vs. chronic heat loss.[183,199]

Various physiologic stressors and other factors can impair thermoregulation. Age extremes, the state of health and nutrition, the type of exposure, and a multitude of intoxicants or medications can jeopardize thermostability by decreasing heat production or increasing heat loss. Physiologic stressors also include dehydration, sleep deprivation, and fatigue. These challenges increase heat loss via evaporation, radiation, conduction, and convection, and compensatory responses often fail.[183] The resulting mortality rates range from the highly suspicious zero to well over 50% in many clinical series, depending largely on the severity of risk factors and on patient selection criteria.[51,196,278]

For safety, experimental investigations of induced hypothermia in human volunteers usually terminate cooling at about 35° C (95° F). Naturally this precludes analysis of some of the more significant pathophysiologic features of moderate or severe hypothermia. Design limitations also occur in studies of anesthetized animals, since the results of these experiments require variable degrees of extrapolation to humans. For example, large differences exist both in the cardiovascular responses to interventions and in the amounts of peripheral musculature that are present, particularly in nonporcine animal models. As a result, clinical treatment recommendations must be predicated on the degree and duration of hypothermia and on the predisposing factors that are subsequently identified.[106]

NORMAL PHYSIOLOGY OF TEMPERATURE REGULATION

Warm-blooded animals maintain a precariously dynamic equilibrium between heat production and heat loss.[135,136] The normal diurnal variation in humans is

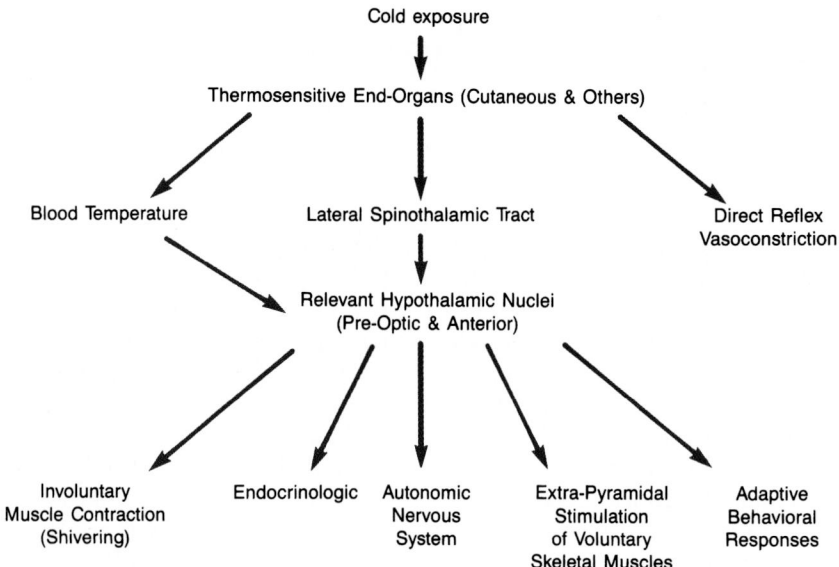

Figure 6-1 Physiology of cold exposure.

TABLE 6-1. Fahrenheit to Centigrade Conversion Scale*

FAHRENHEIT	CENTIGRADE	FAHRENHEIT	CENTIGRADE	FAHRENHEIT	CENTIGRADE
95	**35**	73	22.78	52	11.11
94	34.44	72	22.22	51	10.56
93	33.89	71	21.67	**50**	**10**
92	33.33	70	21.11	49	9.44
91	32.78	69	20.56	48	8.89
90	32.22	**68**	**20**	47	8.33
89	31.67	67	19.44	46	7.78
88	31.11	66	18.89	45	7.22
87	30.56	65	18.33	44	6.67
86	**30**	64	17.78	43	6.11
85	29.44	63	17.22	42	5.56
84	28.89	62	16.67	**41**	**5**
83	28.33	61	16.11	40	4.44
82	27.78	60	15.56	39	3.89
81	27.22	**59**	**15**	38	3.33
80	26.67	58	14.44	37	2.78
79	26.11	57	13.89	36	2.22
78	25.56	56	13.33	35	1.67
77	**25**	55	12.78	34	1.11
76	24.44	54	12.22	33	0.56
75	23.89	53	11.67	**32**	**0**
74	23.33				

*C = (F − 32) × 5/9. Each 5° C = 9° F.

only 1° C (1.8° F). Since physiologic changes occurring in humans are modified by predisposing or contributory factors, the normal responses to severe temperature depression require significant extrapolation.[203]

Basal heat production usually averages 40 to 60 kcal/m² body surface area per hour. It increases with shivering thermogenesis,[194,195] food ingestion, fever, activity, and cold stress. Normal thermoregulation in vertebrates involves transmitting cold sensation to hypothalamic neurons via the lateral spinothalamic tracts and the thalamus (Figure 6-1). The physiologic characteristics of the four zones of hypothermia appear in Table 6-2. A complete discussion of the physiology of cold exposure and thermoregulation is presented in Chapter 4.

TABLE 6-2. Characteristics of the Four Zones of Hypothermia

| STAGE | CORE TEMPERATURE | | CHARACTERISTICS |
	° C	° F	
Mild	37.6	99.6 ± 1	Normal rectal temperature
	37.0	98.6 ± 1	Normal oral temperature
	36.0	96.8	Increase in metabolic rate and blood pressure and preshivering muscle tone
	35.0	95.0	Urine temperature 34.8° C; maximum shivering thermogenesis
	34.0	93.2	Amnesia, dysarthria, and poor judgment develop; maladaptive behavior; normal blood pressure; maximum respiratory stimulation; tachycardia, then progressive bradycardia
	33.30	91.4	Ataxia and apathy develop; linear depression of cerebral metabolism; tachypnea, then progressive decrease in respiratory minute volume; cold diuresis
Moderate	32.0	89.6	Stupor; 25% decrease in oxygen consumption
	31.0	87.8	Extinguished shivering thermogenesis
	30.0	86.0	Atrial fibrillation and other arrhythmias develop; poikilothermia; pupils and cardiac output two thirds of normal; insulin ineffective
	29.0	85.2	Progressive decrease in level of consciousness, pulse, and respiration; pupils dilated; paradoxical undressing
Severe	28.0	82.4	Decreased ventricular fibrillation threshold; 50% decrease in oxygen consumption and pulse; hypoventilation
	27.0	80.6	Loss of reflexes and voluntary motion
	26.0	78.8	Major acid-base disturbances; no reflexes or response to pain
	25.0	77.0	Cerebral blood flow one third of normal; loss of cerebrovascular autoregulation; cardiac output 45% of normal; pulmonary edema may develop
	24.0	75.2	Significant hypotension and bradycardia
	23.0	73.4	No corneal or oculocephalic reflexes; areflexia
	22.0	71.6	Maximum risk of ventricular fibrillation; 75% decrease in oxygen consumption
Profound	20.0	68.0	Lowest resumption of cardiac electromechanical activity; pulse 20% of normal
	19.0	66.2	Electroencephalographic silencing
	18.0	64.4	Asystole
	13.7	56.8	Lowest adult accidental hypothermia survival[91a]
	15.0	59.2	Lowest infant accidental hypothermia survival[208]
	10.0	50.0	92% decrease in oxygen consumption
	9.0	48.2	Lowest therapeutic hypothermia survival[203]

PATHOPHYSIOLOGY

Nervous System

Numbing cold depresses the central nervous system, producing impaired memory and judgment, slurred speech, and decreased consciousness. Temperature-dependent enzyme systems in the brain do not function properly at cold temperatures that are well tolerated by the kidneys.[94] As a result, most patients are comatose below 30° C (86° F), although some remain amazingly alert.

Neurons are initially stimulated by a 1° C (1.8° F) drop in temperature, but the brain does not always cool uniformly during accidental hypothermia. After the initial increase, there is a linear decrease in cerebral metabolism by 6% to 10% per degree Centigrade from 35° C (95° F) to 25° C (77° F). Hypothermia affords cerebral protection because of the diminished cerebral metabolic requirements of oxygen.[86,93]

The electroencephalogram is abnormal below 33.5° C (92.3° F) and becomes silent at 19° to 20° C (66.2° to 68° F).

The triphasic waves commonly noted in hypothermia are also observed in various metabolic, toxic, and diffuse encephalopathies. Visual evoked potentials, another objective measure of cerebral function, become smaller as the mercury drops. After cerebral cortical function becomes impaired, lower brainstem functions are also deranged.

Cerebrovascular autoregulation is protectively intact until the temperature drops below 25° C (77° F). Although vascular resistance is increased, blood flow is disproportionately redistributed to the brain. In canine studies, blood flow in the brain, muscle, kidney, and myocardium recovers quickly to control levels after rewarming. Flow deficits in the pulmonary, digestive, and endocrine systems persist for up to 2 hours after rewarming.[49]

Chilling the peripheral nervous system increases muscle tension and preshivering tone, eventually leading to shivering. Shivering, which is also centrally controlled, is a much more efficient heat producer than voluntary muscle contractions of the extremities.

Cardiovascular System

Many cardiovascular responses caused by or associated with hypothermia are well described but not well understood.[160,161] Cold stress increases the consumption of myocardial oxygen. Autonomic nervous system stimulation causes tachycardia and peripheral vasoconstriction, both of which increase systemic blood pressure and cardiac afterload.

After premonitory tachycardia, decremental bradycardia produces a 50% decrease in heart rate at 28° C (82.4° F). Since this bradycardia is caused by decreased spontaneous depolarization of the pacemaker cells, it is refractory to atropinization. If there is a "relative" tachycardia not consistent with the degree of hypothermia, the clinician should be concerned. Associated conditions include occult trauma with hypovolemia, drug ingestion, and hypoglycemia.

During hypothermic bradycardia, unlike normothermia, systole is prolonged longer than diastole. In addition, the conduction system is much more sensitive to cold than is the myocardium, so the cardiac cycle is lengthened. Cold-induced changes in pH, oxygen, electrolytes, and nutrients also alter electrical conduction.[179]

Hypothermia progressively decreases the mean arterial pressure and cardiac index. Cardiac output drops to about 45% of normal at 25° C (77° F). Systemic arterial resistance, determined by invasive hemodynamic monitoring, is increased. Even after rewarming, cardiovascular function may remain temporarily depressed, with impaired myocardial contractility, metabolism, and peripheral vascular function.[262]

Mild, steady hypothermia in patients with poikilothermic thermoregulatory disorders causes electrocardiographic (ECG) alterations and conduction abnormalities.[181] First the PR, then the QRS, and most characteristically the QTc intervals are prolonged. Clinically invisible increased preshivering muscle tone can obscure the P waves; ST segment and T wave abnormalities are inconsistent.

The J wave (Osborn wave or hypothermic hump; Figure 6-2), first described by Tomaszewski in 1938,[261] occurs at the junction of the QRS complex and ST segment. It is not prognostic but is potentially diagnostic.[210] J waves occur at any temperature below 32.2° C (90° F) and are most frequently seen in leads II and V₆. When the core temperature falls below 25° C (77° F), J waves are found in the precordial leads (especially V₃ or V₄). The size of the J waves also increases with temperature depression but is unrelated to arterial pH. J waves are usually upright in aV_L, aV_F, and the left precordial leads.

J waves may represent hypothermia-induced ion fluxes, resulting in delayed depolarization or early repolarization of the left ventricle, or there may be an unidentified hypothalamic or neurogenic factor. J waves are *not* pathognomonic of hypothermia but also occur with central nervous system lesions, focal cardiac ischemia, and sepsis. They may also be present in young, healthy persons. When pronounced, J waveform abnormalities can simulate a myocardial infarction. Computer software is not widely available that can successfully recognize and suggest the diagnosis of hypothermia.

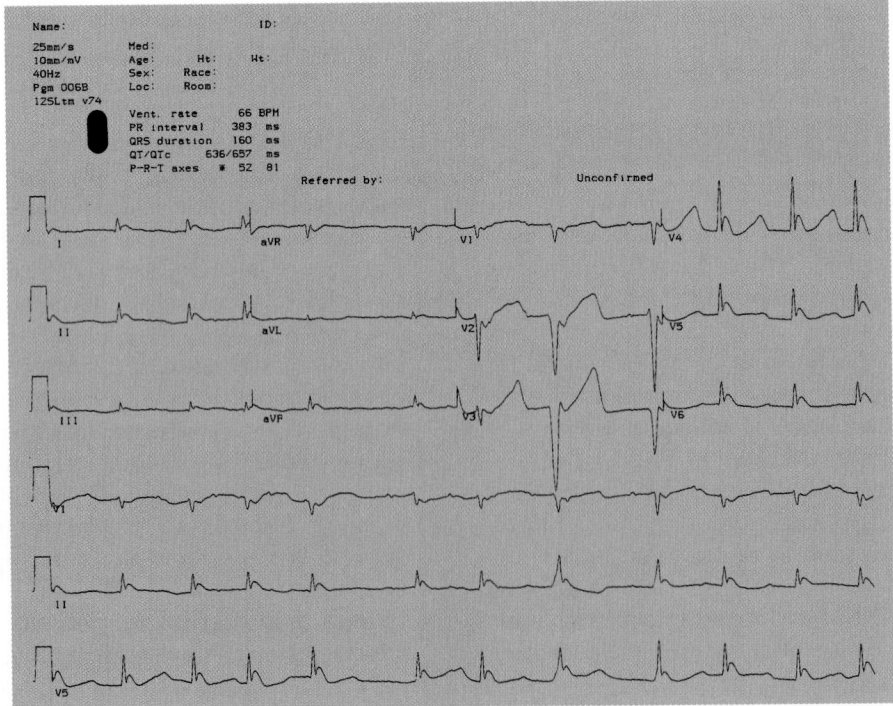

Figure 6-2 The J or Osborn wave of hypothermia.

Such a capability can be important in rural and wilderness settings, since prehospital thrombolytic therapy will expand as the role of the field 12-lead ECG is refined.[46] Thrombolysis is unstudied in hypothermia but would be expected to exacerbate coagulopathies.[95]

Below 32.2° C (90° F), all types of atrial and ventricular arrhythmias are encountered.[64] The His-Purkinje system is more sensitive to cold than is the myocardium. As a result, conduction velocity decreases and electrical signals can disperse. Since conduction time is prolonged more than the absolute refractory period, reentry currents can produce circus rhythms that initiate ventricular fibrillation (VF).

In addition to causing bradycardia, widening the QRS complex, and prolonging the QT interval, hypothermia increases the duration of action potentials (Figure 6-3).[15,16] During rewarming, nonuniform myocardial temperatures can disperse conduction and further increase the action potential duration, another mechanism to develop the unidirectional blocks that facilitate reentrant arrhythmias. At temperatures between 25° and 20° C (77° and 68° F), myocardial conduction time is prolonged further than the absolute refractory period. Another arrhythmogenic mechanism is development of independent electrical foci that precipitate arrhythmias.

Selection of the class III antiarrhythmic drug *d*-sotalol may be problematic.[16] It has temperature-dependent effectiveness and lengthens prolonged action potentials more efficiently at long pacing cycle lengths. Various electrolyte abnormalities can further complicate the situation during hypothermic conditions, since they exacerbate the effects of prolonged action potentials. Most conspicuously, hypothermia-induced cellular calcium loading mimics digitalis toxicity and may predispose to a forme fruste of torsades de pointes.

Hypothermia-induced VF and asystole often occur spontaneously below 25° C (77° F). The VF threshold and the transmembrane resting potential are decreased.

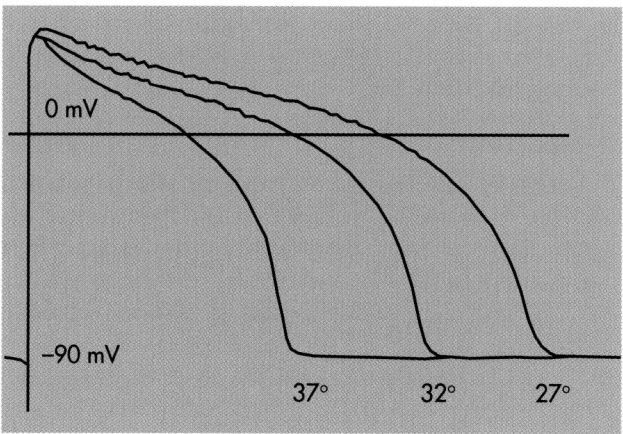

Figure 6-3 Example of the effects of temperature on action potentials in cardiac cells.

Since the heart is cold, the conduction delay is facilitated by the large dispersion of repolarization, and the action potential is prolonged. The increased temporal dispersion of the recovery of excitability is linked to VF. In a way, nature's model of resistance to VF is the heart of hibernating animals during rewarming.[132] Animals with this capacity seem to be protected by a shortened QT duration and a calcium channel handling system that prevents intracellular calcium overload.

Asystole may be the more common on initial examination, and VF may be iatrogenic. Both rhythms may result from hypovolemia, tissue hypoxia, therapeutic manipulations, acid-base fluxes, autonomic dysfunction, and coronary vasoconstriction coupled with increased blood viscosity.[49]

Core Temperature Afterdrop

Core temperature afterdrop refers to the continued decline in a hypothermic patient's temperature after removal from the cold (see also Chapter 8). Contributing to afterdrop is the simple temperature equilibration between the warmer core and the cooler periphery. Circulatory changes account for another set of observations. The countercurrent cooling of blood that perfuses cold extremities results in a core temperature decline until the existing temperature gradient is eliminated. In cold-water immersion, postrescue collapse may also result from abrupt hypotension after loss of the hydrostatic squeeze in the water.

The incidence and magnitude of core temperature afterdrop vary widely in clinical experiments and in surgically induced hypothermia.[88,89,91,106] Hayward[109] measured his own esophageal, rectal, tympanic, and cardiac temperatures (via flotation tip catheter) during rewarming after being cooled in 10° C (50° F) water. On 3 different days, rewarming was achieved via shivering thermogenesis, heated humidified inhalation, and warm bath immersion. Coincident with a 0.3° C (0.5° F) afterdrop during warm bath immersion, Hayward's mean arterial pressure fell 30% and his peripheral vascular resistance fell 50%. These results provide impressive support for the circulatory hypothesis as one of the contributors to afterdrop.

Another study of peripheral blood flow during rewarming from mild hypothermia in humans suggests that minimal skin blood flow changes can lead to afterdrop (Figure 6-4). Harnett, Pruitt, and Sias[106] precipitated the largest core temperature afterdrops when their subjects were rewarmed with plumbed garments and heating pads.

In summary, core temperature afterdrop appears to become most clinically relevant when a large temperature gradient exists between the periphery and the core, particularly in dehydrated, chronically cold patients. Both conductive and convective mechanisms are responsible for afterdrop.[86,89] Stimulating periph-

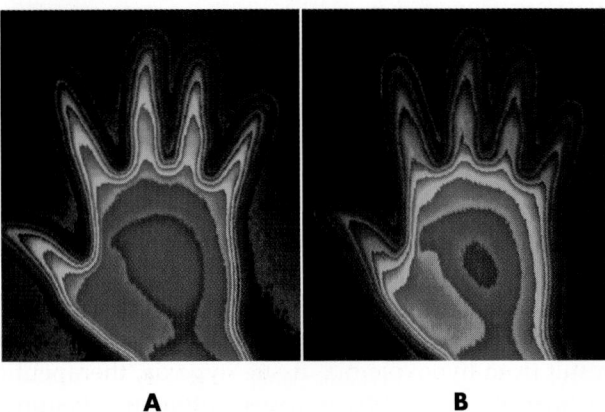

A   **B**

Figure 6-4 Infrared scan of the palmar hand surface. Blue color = 43° C (109.4° F); red color = 68° C (154.4° F). **A,** At room temperature. **B,** After 5 minutes in a cold room, with evidence of vasoconstriction. *(Courtesy Naval Health Research Center, San Diego, Calif.)*

---

eral blood flow can increase afterdrop. Major afterdrops are also observed when frostbitten extremities are thawed before thermal stabilization of the core temperature.

Respiratory System

Any exposure to a big chill initially stimulates respiratory drive, followed by progressive depression of respiratory minute volume as cellular metabolism is depressed. Respiratory rate often falls to 5 to 10/min below 30° C (86° F), and ultimately brainstem neurocontrol of ventilation fails. Carbon dioxide production drops 50% for each 8° C (14° F) fall in temperature. In severe hypothermia, carbon dioxide retention and respiratory acidosis reflect the aberrant responses to normothermic respiratory stimuli.[85]

Other pathophysiologic factors contributing to a ventilation-perfusion mismatch include decreased ciliary motility, increased quantity and viscosity of secretions, hypothermic respiratory distress syndrome, and noncardiogenic pulmonary edema. The thorax loses elasticity while pulmonary compliance drops. The respiratory "bellows" stiffen and fail because the contractile efficiency of the intercostal muscles and diaphragms declines.

Pertinent potentially protective or detrimental factors that affect tissue oxygenation in endothermic humans are listed in Box 6-1.

Renal System

The kidneys respond briskly to hypothermia-induced changes in the vascular tree's capacitance. Peripheral vasoconstriction can result in a relative central hypervolemia, producing diuresis, even with mild dehydration. In addition, renal blood flow is depressed by 50% at 27° to 30° C (80.6° to 86° F), which decreases glomerular filtration rate. Nevertheless, there is an initial large diuresis of this dilute glomerular filtrate, which does not efficiently clear nitrogenous wastes.

The multifactorial etiology of the cold diuresis is still debated.[98,99] Some of the suggested mechanisms include inhibition of antidiuretic hormone (ADH) release and decreased renal tubular function. Neither hydration nor ADH infusions seem to influence the diuretic response, which appears to be an attempt to compensate for initial relative central hypervolemia caused by vasoconstrictive overload of capacitance vessels.

The diuresis may be pressure related caused by impaired autoregulation in the kidney. Cold diuresis has circadian rhythmicity and correlates with periods of shivering. Cold water immersion increases urinary output 3.5 times, and the presence of ethanol impressively doubles that diuresis.[49]

Coagulation

The significant effects of temperature on coagulation continue to be investigated.[249] Coagulopathies often develop in hypothermic patients because the enzymatic nature of the activated clotting factors is depressed by cold.[72,224] In vivo, prolonged clotting is proportional to the number of steps in the cascade. For example, at 29° C (84.2° F) a 50% to 60% increase in the partial thromboplastin time (PTT) would be expected. Kinetic tests of coagulation, however, are normally performed in the laboratory at 37° C (98.6° F). As the blood warms in the machine, the enzymes between each factor in the cascade are activated. The sample of warmed in vitro blood will then clot normally.

The reversible hemostatic defect created by hypothermia may not be reflected by the "normal" prothrombin time (PT) or PTT.[229] This coagulopathy is basically independent of clotting factor levels and cannot be confirmed by laboratory studies performed at 37° C. Treatment is rewarming and not simply administration of clotting factors.[225]

Thrombocytopenia as a cause of bleeding becomes progressively significant in severe hypothermia. Proposed mechanisms include direct bone marrow suppression and splenic or hepatic sequestration. Thromboxane B_2 production by platelets is also temperature dependent, so cooling skin temperature in baboons produces reversible platelet dysfunction. Thrombocytopenia is a common but poorly recognized corollary of hypothermia in the elderly and neonates.

Coagulopathy in trauma patients is attributed to enzyme inhibition, platelet alteration, and fibrinolysis. The critical temperature at which enzyme activity slows significantly is 34° C (93.2° F).[273] In addition, clot strength weakens as a result of platelet malfunction. Fibrinolysis was not significantly affected at any temperature in the range measured (33° to 37° C [91.4° to 98.6° F]) (also see Trauma).

Physiologic hypercoagulability develops during hypothermia, with a sequence similar to that seen in disseminated intravascular coagulation (DIC). This produces a higher incidence of thromboembolism during hypothermia. Causes include thromboplastin release from cold tissue, simple circulatory collapse, and release of catecholamines and steroids. Since fibrin split product levels can be normal, bleeding is not always considered a hematologic manifestation of DIC. One distinctive hypothermic hematologic picture includes thrombocytopenia, sideroblastic anemia, and erythroid hypoplasia.[49]

Whole blood viscosity increases with the hemoconcentration seen after diuresis and the shift of fluid out of vascular compartments. Red blood cells (RBCs) simply stiffen and have diminished cellular deformity when chilled.[217] The elevated viscosity of hypothermia is also exacerbated with cryoglobulinemia. Cryofibrinogen is a cold-precipitated fibrinogen occasionally seen with carcinoma, sepsis, and collagen vascular diseases. Blood viscosity is also increased by the transient increase in platelet and RBC counts seen with mild surface cooling. This could explain the increased mortality from coronary and cerebral thromboses that occur in winter.[183]

PREDISPOSING FACTORS

The factors that predispose to hypothermia can be separated into those that decrease heat production, increase heat loss, or impair thermoregulation.[183] There is significant overlap among these groups (Box 6-2).

Decreased Heat Production

Thermogenesis is decreased at both extremes of age. In the elderly, neuromuscular inefficiency and decreased physical activity impair shivering. Aging progressively diminishes homeostatic and cold adaptive capabilities. Although most elderly persons have normal thermoregulation, they tend to develop conditions that impair heat conservation.

The elderly are physiologically less adept at increasing heat production and the respiratory quotient (the ratio of the volume of carbon dioxide produced to the volume of oxygen consumed per unit of time). Impaired thermal perception, possibly caused by decreased resting peripheral blood flow, leads to poor adaptive behavior. Metabolic studies also demonstrate that in severely hypothermic elderly persons, lipolysis occurs in preference to glucose consumption.[172]

Neonates have a large surface area/mass ratio, a relatively deficient subcutaneous tissue layer, and virtually no behavioral defense mechanisms.[131] Newborn "unadapted" infants attempt to thermoregulate with initial vasoconstriction and acceleration of metabolic rate. In contrast, "adapted" infants who are older than 5 days of age can increase lipolysis immediately and burn oxidative brown adipose tissue.

No cause-effect relationship has been found between hypothermia and the mortality rate of premature infants.[110,237] Although the smaller infants in a neonatal intensive care unit are at the greatest risk of hypothermia, mortality is related to hypothermia only in larger neonates.

Emergency deliveries and resuscitations are responsible for most acute neonatal hypothermia. Other common risk factors are prematurity, low birth weight, inexperienced mother, perinatal morbidity, and low socioeconomic status. In more chronically induced subacute hypothermia, lethargy, a weak cry, and failure to thrive are common.[259]

Many cold infants have "paradoxical rosy cheeks," looking surprisingly healthy. After the first few days of life, hypothermia frequently indicates septicemia and carries a high mortality rate.[44] Low weight and malnutrition are common. Hypothermia in a low-birthweight neonate should suggest the possibility of intracranial hemorrhage; hypothermia is also observed in shaken baby syndrome.

Endocrinologic failure, including hypopituitarism, hypoadrenalism, and myxedema, commonly decreases heat production. Interestingly, congenital adrenal hyperplasia with mineralocorticoid insufficiency is more common in cold climates, possibly an adaptive response to prolonged exposure to cold temperatures, since "normal" cold diuresis is reduced in these patients.

Box 6-2 FACTORS PREDISPOSING TO HYPOTHERMIA

DECREASED HEAT PRODUCTION

Endocrinologic failure

Hypopituitarism
Hypoadrenalism
Hypothyroidism
Lactic acidosis
Diabetic and alcoholic ketoacidosis

Insufficient fuel

Hypoglycemia
Malnutrition
Marasmus
Kwashiorkor
Extreme physical exertion

Neuromuscular physical exertion

Age extremes
Impaired shivering
Inactivity
Lack of adaptation

IMPAIRED THERMOREGULATION

Peripheral failure

Neuropathies
Acute spinal cord transection
Diabetes

Central failure/neurologic

Cardiovascular accident
Central nervous system trauma
Toxicologic
Metabolic
Subarachnoid hemmorrhage
Pharmacologic
Hypothalamic dysfunction
Parkinson's disease
Anorexia nervosa
Cerebellar lesion
Neoplasm
Congenital intracranial anomalies
Multiple sclerosis
Hyperkalemic periodic paralysis

INCREASED HEAT LOSS

Environmental

Immersion
Nonimmersion

Induced vasodilation

Pharmacologic
Toxicologic

Erythrodermas

Burns
Psoriasis
Ichthyosis
Exfoliative dermatitis

Iatrogenic

Emergency childbirth
Cold infusions
Heatstroke treatment

MISCELLANEOUS ASSOCIATED CLINICAL STATES

Multisystem trauma
Recurrent hypothermia
Episodic hypothermia
Shapiro's syndrome
Infections: bacterial, viral, parasitic
Pancreatitis
Carcinomatosis
Cardiopulmonary disease
Vascular insufficiency
Uremia
Paget's disease
Giant cell arteritis
Sarcoidosis
Shaken baby syndrome
Systemic lupus erythematosus
Wernicke-Korsakoff syndrome
Hodgkin's disease
Shock
Sickle-cell anemia
Sudden infant death syndrome

Hypothyroidism is often occult, with no history of cold intolerance, dry skin, lassitude, or arthralgias. The physician should check for a thyroid scar or any history of thyroid hormone replacement. The degree of temperature depression correlates fairly directly with mortality. Eighty percent of patients in myxedema coma, which is several times more common in females, are hypothermic.

The effects of insufficient nutrition extend from hypoglycemia to marasmus to kwashiorkor. Kwashiorkor is less often associated with hypothermia than is marasmus because of the insulating effect of hypoproteinemic edema. Central neuroglycopenia distorts hypothalamic function. Many alcoholic patients with hypothermia are hypoglycemic. Malnutrition decreases insulative subcutaneous fat and directly alters thermoregulation. In 744 elderly women with femoral neck fractures, poor nutrition predisposed to hypothermia and its attendant clumsiness.[11] Partly because of fuel depletion, hypothermia is as great a threat as hyperthermia in marathon races run in cool climates. Among 62 runners, participants slowing from fatigue or injury late in a race were at serious risk of hypothermia.[189]

Increased Heat Loss

Poorly acclimated and insulated individuals often have high diaphoretic, convective, and evaporative heat losses during exposure to cold. Because the skin functions as a radiator, any dermatologic malfunction increases heat loss. Such erythrodermas include psoriasis, exfoliative dermatitis, and toxic epidermal necrolysis.[171] Hypothermia with hypernatremic dehydration is also seen in congenital lamellar ichthyosis.

Burns and inappropriate burn treatment cause excessive heat loss, as do other iatrogenic factors, including massive cold intravenous infusions and overcooling heatstroke victims.[151] When carbon dioxide is used for abdominal insufflation before laparoscopy, warming the gas before administration helps prevent hypothermia. Environmental immersion exposure is discussed in detail in Chapter 8.[87]

Many pharmacologic and toxicologic agents both increase heat loss and impair thermoregulation.[135] The most common is ethanol, which interacts with every thermoregulatory neurotransmitter. Although ingestion of ethanol produces a feeling of warmth and perhaps visible flushing, it is the major cause of urban hypothermia.[51,196] In fatal cases of accidental hypothermia, many victims are under the influence of ethanol. In children with ethanol intoxication, hypothermia is common.

Ethanol is also a poikilothermia-producing agent that directly impairs thermoregulation at high or low temperatures.[1,134] Body temperature is lowered both from cutaneous vasodilation with radiative heat loss and from impaired shivering thermogenesis. Chronic ethanol ingestion damages the mamillary bodies and posterior hypothalamus, which modulates shivering thermogenesis.[218] Ethanol also increases the risk of being exposed to the environment by modifying protective adaptive behavior. The ultimate example is paradoxical undressing, or removal of clothing in response to a cold stress. As an organic solvent, ethanol confers a few theoretically redeeming qualities in freezing cold injuries by lowering the cellular freezing point.[98,99]

The neurophysiologic effects of ethanol are modified by duration and intensity of exercise, food consumption, and applied cold stress.[78] Aging increases sensitivity to the hypothermic actions of ethanol in some primate experiments. Chronic ingestion yields tolerance to its hypothermic effects, and rebound hyperthermia may be seen during withdrawal. Conditions associated with ethanol ingestion that adversely affect heat balance include immobility and hypoglycemia.

Inhibited hepatic gluconeogenesis coexists with malnutrition. Hypothermic alcoholic ketoacidosis is re-

ported.[278] Intravenous thiamine is diagnostic and therapeutic for Wernicke's encephalopathy, another cause of reversible hypothermia. The acute triad of global confusion, ophthalmoplegia, and truncal ataxia is often masked by hypothermia, and temperature depression may persist for weeks.

Impaired Thermoregulation

Various conditions that impair thermoregulation can be considered as having central, peripheral, metabolic, pharmacologic, or toxicologic effects.

Central. Central conditions may directly affect hypothalamic function and mediate vasodilation. Traumatic lesions include skull fractures, especially basilar, and intracerebral hemorrhages, most commonly chronic subdural hematomas. Pathologic lesions include neoplasms, congenital anomalies, and Parkinson's disease. Patients with Parkinson's disease or Alzheimer's disease, because of global neurologic impairment, are particularly at behavioral risk. Finally, cerebellar lesions also impede heat production because of inefficient choreiform shivering.

Hypothermia can occur with Reye's syndrome. In Hodgkin's disease, hypothermia is seen only in previously febrile patients with advanced disease, independent of cell type. This seems to be a disease-associated functional disorder of thermoregulation, similar to that seen in anorexia nervosa. Centrally induced hypothermia is completely antagonized with thyrotropin-releasing hormone.

Peripheral. Peripheral thermoregulation fails after acute spinal cord transection. Victims are functionally poikilothermic as soon as peripheral vasoconstriction is extinguished.[193] Other peripheral impediments to thermostability include neuropathies and diabetes mellitus. Hypothermia is more common in elderly diabetics than in the general population, even after excluding patients with diabetic metabolic emergencies. The common denominator in metabolic derangements may be abnormal plasma osmolality that interferes with hypothalamic function. Similar causes of hypothermia include hypoglycemia, diabetic ketoacidosis, and uremia. Remarkably, the pH was 6.67 in one hypothermic survivor with lactic acidosis and 6.41 in another.[201]

Pharmacologic/Toxicologic. Numerous medications and toxins in therapeutic or toxic doses impair centrally mediated thermoregulation and vasoconstriction.[215,287] Of 103 critically ill patients with overdoses, 27 were hypothermic.[141] The usual offenders are barbiturates, benzodiazepines, phenothiazines, and the tricyclic antidepressants. Reduced core temperature may be a prodrome of lithium poisoning. Organophosphates, narcotics, glutethimide, bromocriptine, erythromycin, clonidine, fluphenazine, bethanechol, atropine, acetaminophen, and carbon monoxide all cause hypothermia.[17] In experimental studies, hypothermia after acute carbon monoxide poisoning is associated with increased mortality.

Recurrent Hypothermia

Recurrent and episodic hypothermia are widely reported. The recurrent variety is more common and is usually secondary to ethanol abuse, with one person having survived 12 episodes. Severe, recurrent presentations are also caused by self-poisoning and anorexia nervosa.[49]

Persons with episodic hypothermia can be divided into two groups, albeit with significant overlap, as follows:

Group 1: Diaphoretic episodes precede the temperature decline, which lasts several hours; includes those with hypothalamic lesions and agenesis of the corpus callosum (Shapiro's syndrome) and persons with spontaneous periodic hyperthermia. Resultant hyperhidrosis and hypothermia are successfully treated with clonidine, a centrally acting α-adrenergic agonist. The hypothermia of corpus callosum agenesis is also seen with hypercalcemia and status epilepticus; since no hypothermia results from experimental sectioning of the corpus callosum, associated lesions, including lipomas, probably cause thermoinstability. Spontaneous periodic hyperthermia may reflect a diencephalic autonomic seizure disorder and can accompany paroxysmal hypertension. Vasomotor and thermoregulatory mechanisms are successfully treated with anticonvulsants. Florid psychiatric symptoms often mask these intermittent hypothermic episodes.

Group 2: Consists of persons who remain cold for days to weeks, rather than hours; these have more seizure disorders, and the central hypothalamic thermostat is set abnormally low.

Patients with intermittent hypothermia usually show some characteristics from both groups.[183] Circadian rhythm disturbances are also seen in persons with neurologic disorders who have chronic hypothermia.

Predisposing Infections/Conditions

Among the infestations and infections that not only elevate but often depress core temperature are septicemia, pneumonia, peritonitis, meningitis, encephalitis, bacterial endocarditis, typhoid, miliary tuberculosis, syphilis, brucellosis, and trypanosomiasis.[168] Other diseases, in addition to cerebrovascular and cardiopulmonary disorders, that produce secondary hypothermia include lupus, carcinomatosis, pancreatitis, and multiple sclerosis. Hypothalamic demyelination may explain the episodic hypothermia observed in some patients with multiple sclerosis.

Hypothermia can also result from low cardiac output after a major myocardial infarction, which can be reversed by intraaortic balloon counterpulsation. Finally, causes include vascular insufficiency, giant cell arteritis, uremia, sickle cell anemia, Paget's disease, sarcoidosis, and sudden infant death syndrome. Magnesium sulfate infusion during preterm labor has produced hypothermia with fetal and maternal bradycardia, and hypothyroidism can be manifested as hypothermia after preeclampsia (see Box 6-2).

Trauma

The relationship of hypothermia to trauma is still being actively investigated.[83] Hypothermia protects the brain from ischemia but can result in arrhythmias, acidosis, and coagulopathies, and it can extract a high metabolic cost during rewarming. Hypothermia hinders the protective physiologic responses to acute trauma and affects the pharmacologic and therapeutic maneuvers necessary to treat the injuries.[11]

There is usually an inverse relationship between the injury severity score and the core temperature of traumatized patients on arrival in the emergency department (ED). This observation does not settle whether hypothermia is just another risk factor for increased mortality or reflects the fact that the most severely injured patients are in hemorrhagic shock.

One study assesses the impact of hypothermia as an independent variable during resuscitation from major trauma.[83] Patients not aggressively rewarmed with continuous arteriovenous rewarming (CAVR) had increased fluid requirements, increased lactate levels, and increased acute mortality.

Of the clinical entities associated with hypothermia, traumatic conditions causing hypotension and hypovolemia most dramatically jeopardize thermostability.[139] Hypothermia is often obscured by obvious hemorrhaging and injuries. Conversely, traumatic neurologic deficits, including paresis and areflexia, can be misattributed to hypothermia. In trauma patients requiring surgery, the mean temperature loss was greater in the ED than in the operating room.[101] Thermal insults are often added during a trauma resuscitation. The patient is completely exposed for examination, and resuscitative procedures cause further heat loss.

In a study stratifying subjects with the anatomic Injury Severity Scale (ISS), hypothermic patients had a higher mortality rate than did similarly injured patients who remained normothermic.[140] Another study did not corroborate this finding,[251] but those investigators stratified using Trauma Revised Injury Severity Scale (TRISS) methodology, which is probably less valid during hypothermia because its physiologic components overestimate injury severity. To illustrate this point, some component of hypotension is normal for a given degree of hypothermia.

Various adverse physiologic events accompany hypothermia with trauma.[190] Decreased skin and core temperatures without compensatory shivering thermogenesis are reported in patients with major trauma as defined by the ISS.

Hypothermia directly causes coagulopathies in trauma patients through at least three avenues (see Coagulopathy).[26] The cascade of enzymatic reactions is impaired and plasma fibrinolytic activity is enhanced, producing a clinical presentation similar to DIC. Also, platelets are poorly functional and become sequestered.

Hypothermia protects only when induced before shock occurs. This reduces adenosine triphosphate (ATP) utilization while ATP stores are still normal, as during elective surgery. ATP stores in traumatized patients are already depleted. Hypothermia worsens the effects of endotoxins on clotting time in vitro and may synergistically exacerbate the coagulopathy seen in trauma.[73] The average temperature of 123 initially normothermic trauma patients in whom lethal coagulopathies developed was 31.2° C (88.2° F).[144] In another study, postinjury life-threatening coagulopathy in the seriously injured who require massive transfusion is predicted by persistent hypothermia and progressive metabolic acidosis.[41]

The appropriate target core temperature for a hypothermic patient with an isolated severe head injury may be 32° to 33° C (89.6° to 91.4° F). This target temperature balances neuroprotection against the adverse hematologic and physiologic consequences of hypothermia.[185,186,285]

PRESENTATION

The patient's history may suggest hypothermia.[26] Diagnosis becomes fairly simple when exposure is obvious, as with avalanche victims. Subtle presentations, however, predominate in urban settings. Victims often complain only of vague symptoms, including hunger, nausea, fatigue, and dizziness. Predisposing underlying illness or ethanol ingestion is also common, as are major trauma, immersion, overdose, cerebrovascular accidents, and psychiatric emergencies (Box 6-3).

During the head, eye, ear, nose, and throat examination, abnormal findings can include decreased corneal reflexes, mydriasis, strabismus, flushing, erythropsia, facial edema, rhinorrhea, and epistaxis. Mild hypothermia usually does not depress pupillary light reflex. Cardiovascular findings after initial tachycardia include bradyarrhythmias and hypotension. Heart sounds may be muffled and distant.

Tachypnea, an early respiratory finding, is usually followed by progressive hypoventilation with bronchorrhea and adventitious sounds. Because the gastrointestinal tract is depressed, abdominal distention or rigidity, ileus, obstipation, and poor rectal tone are often present.

Gastric dilation is common in neonates and myxedematous adults. Genitourinary output ranges from initial polyuria resulting from cold diuresis to anuria. Interestingly, the incidence of testicular torsion reportedly increases because of cremasteric contractions.

Diffuse neurologic abnormalities vary widely. Some persons can still converse at 32° C (89.6° F) and are normoreflexic. The level of consciousness generally declines proportionate to the degree of hypothermia. The presence of ataxia and dysarthria may mimic a cerebrovascular accident. Speed of reasoning and memory registration are also impaired. Amnesia, antinociception, anesthesia, or hypesthesia can develop. Cranial nerve signs are present after bulbar damage from central pontine myelinolysis. These extraocular muscle movement abnormalities, similar to extensor plantar responses, do not directly correlate with the degree of hypothermia.[75]

Hyperreflexia predominates from 35° to 32.2° C (95° to 90° F) and is followed by hyporeflexia. The plantar response remains flexor until 26° C (78.8° F), when areflexia develops. The knee jerk is usually the last reflex to disappear and the first to reappear during rewarming. From 30° to 26° C (86° to 78.8° F), both contraction and relaxation phases of reflexes are prolonged equally. In myxedema, however, the relaxation phase of the ankle reflex is more prolonged than is the contraction phase.[183] Most importantly, spinal cord and other central nervous system lesions may be obscured by depressive neurologic changes that normally accompany hypothermia.[75]

Psychiatric presentations and suicide attempts associated with hypothermia are commonly misdiagnosed initially. Preexisting psychiatric disorders can blossom in the cold, even if they were stabilized in temperate climates. Mental status alterations include anxiety, impaired judgment, perseveration, neurosis, and psychosis. Leaders of expeditions can become moody, apathetic, uncooperative, and risk taking. Elderly patients often withdraw in confusion, become silent, and display lassitude and poor judgment. A peculiar flat affect is common, and psychomotor impairment can resemble an organic brain syndrome.

Early in hypothermia, simply losing effective use of the hands can be devastating. Appropriate behavior adapted to the cold, such as seeking a heat source, is often lacking. An extreme example is paradoxical undressing.[149] The clothing is removed in a preterminal effort to address impending thermoregulatory collapse, and many persons have been mistakenly identified as sexual assault victims. This phenomenon is also seen in hypothermic children.

Musculoskeletal posturing can extend to pseudo–rigor mortis. Preshivering muscle tone is increased before core temperature drops to 35° C (95° F), and muscular rigidity, paravertebral spasm, and even opis-

Box 6-3 SIGNS OF HYPOTHERMIA

HEAD, EYE, EAR, NOSE, THROAT

Mydriasis
Decreased corneal reflexes
Extraocular muscle abnormalities
Erythropsia
Flushing
Facial edema
Epistaxis
Rhinorrhea
Strabismus

CARDIOVASCULAR

Initial tachycardia
Subsequent tachycardia
Arrhythmias
Decreased heart tones
Hepatojugular reflux
Jugular venous distention
Hypotension
Peripheral vasoconstriction

RESPIRATORY

Initial tachypnea
Adventitious sounds
Bronchorrhea
Progressive hypoventilation
Apnea

GASTROINTESTINAL

Ileus
Constipation
Abdominal distention or rigidity
Poor rectal tone
Gastric dilation in neonates or in adults with myxedema
Vomiting

GENITOURINARY

Anuria
Polyuria
Oliguria
Testicular torsion

NEUROLOGIC

Depressed level of consciousness
Ataxia
Dysarthria
Amnesia
Anesthesia

NEUROLOGIC—cont'd

Areflexia
Poor suck reflex
Hypoesthesia
Antinociception
Initial hyperreflexia
Hyporeflexia
Central pontine myelinolysis

PSYCHIATRIC

Impaired judgment
Perseveration
Mood changes
Peculiar "flat" affect
Altered mental status
Paradoxical undressing
Neuroses
Psychoses
Suicide
Organic brain syndrome
Anorexia
Depression
Apathy
Irritability

MUSCULOSKELETAL

Increased muscle tone
Shivering
Rigidity or pseudo–rigor mortis
Paravertebral spasm
Opisthotonos
Compartment syndrome

DERMATOLOGIC

Erythema
Pallor
Cyanosis
Icterus
Scleral edema
Ecchymosis
Edema
Pernio
Frostnip
Frostbite
Panniculitis
Cold urticaria
Necrosis
Gangrene

thotonos may occur. Extremity compartment syndromes often develop because of associated conditions causing prolonged compression and immobility, in addition to compartment hypertension seen during reperfusion of frostbitten extremities.

Dermatologic presentations of hypothermia include erythema, pallor, edema, and scleral edema. Cold urticaria, frostnip, frostbite, and gangrene should also cause the clinician to consider this diagnosis. Pernio is also observed with chronic myelomonocytic leukemia.

LABORATORY EVALUATION

Acid-Base Balance

The strategy for achieving and maintaining acid-base balance in hypothermia differs from that of normothermia.[57,107,126] After initial respiratory alkalosis from hyperventilation when a person first becomes chilled, a common underlying disturbance is mixed acidosis. The respiratory component of the acidosis is caused mainly by direct respiratory depression. In addition, as the temperature decreases, solubility of carbon dioxide in the blood increases. Further contributors to the metabolic component of this acidosis include impaired hepatic metabolism and acid excretion, lactate generation from shivering, and decreased tissue perfusion.[113] Nevertheless, reliable clinical prediction of the acid-base status in accidental hypothermia is not possible. In one series of 135 cases, 30% were acidotic and 25% alkalotic.[196]

Circulatory changes also prevent adequate mobilization and delivery of organic acids to buffer systems. As in normothermia, mixed venous blood may best reflect acid-base status during resuscitation.[255] Despite flow changes in a moderately hypothermic canine model, a significant correlation persists between arterial and mixed venous pH. The arteriovenous change in pH is ±0.03 to 0.04 pH unit. The buffering capacity of cold blood is also markedly impaired. In normothermia, when the $PaCO_2$ increases 10 mm Hg, a decrease in pH of 0.08 unit occurs. At 28° C (82.4° F), the decrease in pH doubles to 0.16.

The optimal strategy to maintain acid-base homeostasis during treatment of accidental hypothermia has changed from earlier days.[230] The accepted earlier assumption was that 7.42 was the ideal "corrected" patient pH at all temperatures and that therapy should be directed at maintenance of the corrected arterial pH at 7.42.[277] A better intracellular pH reference is electrochemical neutrality, at which pH equals pOH. Since the neutral point of water at 37° C (98.6° F) is pH 6.8, Rahn[219] has hypothesized that this normal 0.6 unit pH offset in body fluids should be maintained at all temperatures.[223] Because the neutral pH rises with cooling, so should blood pH (Figure 6-5).

Relative alkalinity of tissues makes physiologic sense. Intracellular electrochemical neutrality ensures optimal function of the enzyme systems and transport proteins at all temperatures and allows excretion of the neutral intracellular waste product urea.[9]

Depressed metabolism and carbon dioxide generation are the physiologic responses to temperature depression, since each temperature has its associated metabolic rate. Ventilation is intrinsically adjusted to maintain a net charge on the defended parameter, the peptide-linked histidine imidazole buffering system.

One homeostatic approach to maintain a steady pH is to keep the bicarbonate content constant. This is

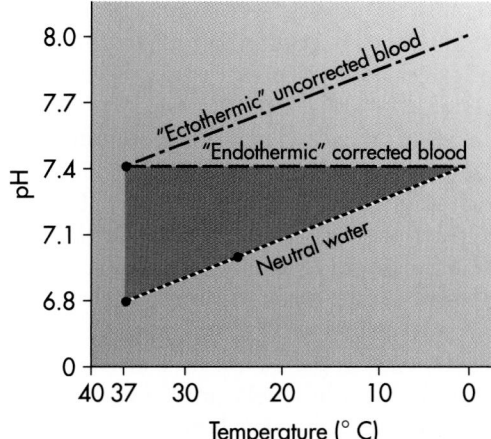

Figure 6-5 Neutrality is the pH of water at any given temperature. At 25° C (77° F) the neutral pH of water is 7.0; at 37° C (98.6° F) it is 6.8. Ectotherm's physiologic 0.6 pH offset from neutral water progressively diminishes if the arterial blood gases are temperature corrected. After the in vitro sample is warmed in the analyzer to 37° C, do not mathematically correct the reported values to reflect the in vivo temperature.

achievable only if the total blood carbon dioxide content does not change. Since carbon dioxide solubility increases with temperature depression, alveolar ventilation must increase to compensate by lowering the $PaCO_2$. The active ectotherms exhibit this respiratory adaptation and do not depress their respiratory minute volume when cold. This response, termed the *ectothermic*, or *alpha-stat, strategy*, allows them to maintain total bicarbonate and carbon dioxide content while increasing pH.[213] Hibernating mammals are far more acidic and use an acid-base strategy that suppresses metabolism, termed the *endothermic*, or *pH stat, strategy*.

In summary, accidental hypothermia in a human should not be considered a protective form of "hibernation." The endothermic strategy using arterial blood gas values that are mathematically "corrected" after the values are determined by the analyzer is dangerous.[13] The ectothermic approach assures adequate alveolar ventilation and acid-base balance at any temperature when the uncorrected pH is 7.4 and the uncorrected $PaCO_2$ is 40 mm Hg.

Hematologic Evaluation

The severity of blood loss is easily underestimated. Hematocrit value increases because of a decline in plasma volume and a 2% increase per 1° C (1.8° F) fall in temperature. In addition, total RBC mass might already be low because of preexisting anemia, malnutrition, leukemia, uremia, or neoplasm.

White blood cell count is frequently normal or low, even if sepsis is present. As a result, systemic leukopenia does not imply absence of infection, especially if the patient is at either age extreme, debilitated, intoxicated, myxedematous, or has secondary hypothermia.[168] Leukocyte count also drops during hypothermia because of direct bone marrow depression and hepatic, splenic, and splanchnic sequestration.

Serum electrolyte levels must be continuously monitored and rechecked during warming. There are no safe predictors of electrolyte values.[49,106] Serum electrolytes fluctuate with temperature, duration of exposure, and rewarming technique selected. Both membrane permeability and sodium-potassium pump efficiency also change with temperature. Isolated temperature depression per se has no consistent effect on sodium and chloride levels until well below 25° C (77° F). Plasma electrolyte levels are also affected by ongoing fluid shifts, prehydration, rehydration, and endocrine or gastrointestinal dysfunction.

Plasma potassium level is independent of temperature. Empirical potassium supplementation during hypothermia often results in normothermic toxicity. From a clinical perspective, hypokalemia occurs as potassium moves into the musculature and not simply out of the body through kaliuresis. The physiologically illogical discrepancy of decreasing potassium level with decreasing pH results from greater intracellular than extracellular pH changes. Hypokalemia is much more common in prolonged or chronically induced hypothermia.

Systemic potassium deficiencies can also be exacerbated by prior diuretic therapy, alcoholism, diabetic ketoacidosis, hypopituitarism, and inappropriate antidiuretic hormone secretion. Hypokalemic digitalis sensitivity can be masked by hypothermia, and gradual correction of persistent and severe hypokalemia during rewarming is necessary for optimal cardiac and gastrointestinal function.

When hyperkalemia is identified, the physician should search for other causes of metabolic acidosis, crush injury or rhabdomyolysis, renal failure, postsubmersion hemolysis, or hypoaldosteronism. Temperature depression can increase hyperkalemic cardiac toxicity. The well-known diagnostic ECG changes are often obscured, and VF can occur with serum potassium levels below 7 mEq/L.

Hypothermia has no consistent effect on magnesium or calcium levels. Severe hypophosphatemia is reported during treatment of profound hypothermia. Although increases in serum enzyme levels are not seen in mild experimental hypothermia, numerous serum enzymes are elevated when diffuse intracellular structural damage occurs in severe accidental hypothermia. Creatine kinase (CK) levels over 200,000 IU are observed, and rhabdomyolysis is often present in these instances.[49]

Inhibition of cellular membrane transport decreases glucose utilization. In addition, insulin release and activity are markedly reduced below 30° C (86° F). Because target cells are insulin resistant, hyperglycemia is commonly seen initially. Markedly elevated glucose levels often correlate with hyperamylasemia and increased cortisol secretion.[278]

Acute hypothermia initially elevates serum glucose level through catecholamine-induced glycogenolysis. However, chronic exposure after exhaustion and glycogen depletion leads to hypoglycemia. The symptoms often resemble those of hypothermia. Cold-induced renal glycosuria is common and does not imply normoglycemia or hyperglycemia. When hypoglycemia and central neuroglycopenia are present, correction improves level of consciousness only to that expected for the current core temperature. Cholesterol and triglyceride levels are also often below normal.

Hyperglycemia that persists during and after rewarming should suggest diabetic ketoacidosis or hemorrhagic pancreatitis. Insulin is ineffective until core temperature is well above 30° to 32° C (86° to 89.6° F) and therefore should be withheld to avoid iatrogenic hypoglycemia after rewarming. Although prior renal disease should be a consideration, blood urea nitrogen (BUN) and creatinine concentrations are often elevated because of decreased nitrogenous waste clearance by cold diuresis. Because of ongoing fluid shifts, BUN is a poor reflector of circulatory volume status.

The relationship between primary accidental hypothermia and hyperamylasemia appears to correlate with the severity of temperature depression, but preexisting or hypothermia-induced pancreatitis is present in up to 50% of patients in some urban series. Since the abdominal examination is frequently unreliable, amylase and lipase levels should be measured, except in minor cases. Ischemic pancreatitis is attributable to microcirculatory collapse in hypothermia. Decreased pancreatic blood flow activates many proteolytic enzymes. The extent of hyperamylasemia can correlate with mortality rates. Hypothermia with hypothalamic astrocytoma and pancreatitis also occurs.[49]

TREATMENT

Prehospital Management

The combination of cold and exhaustion is a common cause of hypothermia in the field.[197] The individual's cold tolerance depends on temperature, wind, clothing worn, and wetness. It does not take an extremely cold temperature to produce hypothermia after energy depletion. As mental function decreases, the victim cannot respond to the rising threat. Judgment is impaired, and the victim seldom takes necessary precautions to prevent further disaster.[21]

Field presentation of victims who are awake covers a wide spectrum. Some persons are obtunded but conscious. The British term for this is the "stumbling slobbers" because of the incoordination. Victims may or may not be shivering and often have a distant gaze and slurred speech.

Comatose victims require careful handling because they are extremely sensitive to VF and asystole. Rough handling causes VF (Figure 6-6). Gurneys should be carried or rolled slowly to avoid jostling, and "code 3 full lights and sirens" transport should be avoided if victims are perfusing adequately.

The initial rescuer and first responder often encounter obstacles to preventing further heat loss.[198] Because cold, stiff, and cyanotic patients with fixed and dilated pupils have been "reanimated," the treatment dictum for prehospital personnel remains, "No one is dead until warm and dead."[6] A succinct summary of prehospital care of the hypothermic patient is rescue, examine, insulate, and transport.

In certain imposing geographic settings, treatment protocols are helpful to standardize treatment while tacitly acknowledging that available health care facilities may offer limited expertise and equipment.[231] Aeromedical transport is often ideal in these circumstances.[282] In difficult environments, proper protocols with rehearsal and critique of mass casualty plans in the cold are far more important than similar adjuncts in flat and consistently sunny terrain.

The history obtained at the scene helps determine optimal treatment. The pertinent past medical history regarding prior cardiopulmonary, endocrinologic, or neurologic conditions is particularly helpful. The circumstances of discovery, duration of exposure, associated injuries or frostbite, and obvious predisposing conditions should be recorded, as should the Glasgow Coma Scale score, although not predictive. No prognostic neurologic scale during hypothermia is valid, but trends are often useful.

Accurate field measurement of core temperature is generally impractical. Low-reading glass oral thermometers that record down to 25° C (77° F) give a rough estimate of the temperature in cooperative persons who are not tachypneic, but these thermometers are often unreliable outdoors in cold ambient conditions. The failure to consider accidental hypothermia in the differential diagnosis can present unforeseen problems.

Prolonged field treatment should be avoided whenever possible, although the rescuer must attempt to prevent further heat loss (Box 6-4). The rescuer should

anticipate the presence of an irritable myocardium, hypovolemia, and a large temperature gradient between the periphery and the core.

Passive external rewarming with dry insulating materials minimizes conductive, convective, evaporative, and radiant heat losses. Remove any wet clothing from awake victims and insulate them with sleeping bags, insulated pads, bubble wrap, blankets, or even newspaper. In a survey of common field rewarming methods used by Mountain Rescue teams, the most common techniques include chemical pads, sleeping bags, and hot water bottles.[104]

If extrication will be delayed, it may be safe to give warm, sweet drinks, warm gelatin (Jell-O), Tang, juice, tea, or cocoa. Avoid heavily caffeinated drinks. Because

Box 6-4 PREPARING HYPOTHERMIC PATIENTS FOR TRANSPORT

1. The patient must be dry. Gently remove of cut off wet clothing and replace it with dry clothing or a dry insulation system. Keep the patient horizontal, and do not allow exertion or massage of the extremities.
2. Stabilize injuries (i.e., the spine; place fractures in the correct anatomic position). Open wounds should be covered before packaging.
3. Initiate intravenous infusions (IVs) if feasible; bags can be placed under the patient's buttocks or in a compressor system. Administer a fluid challenge.
4. Active rewarming should be limited to heated inhalation and truncal heat. Insulate hot water bottles in stockings or mittens and then place them in the patient's axillae and groin.
5. The patient should be wrapped. The wrap starts with a large plastic sheet, on which is placed an insulated sleeping pad. A layer of blankets, a sleeping bag, or bubble wrap insulating material is laid over the sleeping bag; the patient is placed on the insulation; the heating bottles are put in place along with IVs, and the entire package is wrapped layer over layer. The plastic is the final closure. The face should be partially covered, but a tunnel should be created to allow access for breathing and monitoring of the patient.

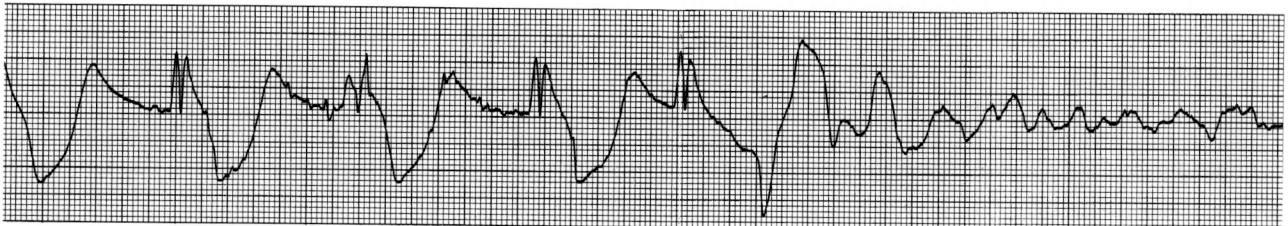

Figure 6-6 In this patient, ventricular fibrillation developed during a code 3 transport by emergency medical services to the emergency department. Note the pronounced J wave after the QRS complex.

a significant diuresis is usually associated with the cooling process, the victim's fluid balance must be assessed. Once mildly hypothermic victims are well hydrated, they can be walked out to safety.

Handle severely hypothermic victims gently, immobilizing them to prevent exertion. Although exercise can rewarm a person more rapidly than shivering, it also markedly increases afterdrop.[88,89] Because of autonomic dysfunction, victims should be kept in a horizontal position whenever possible to minimize orthostatic hypotension. Vigorously massaging cold extremities is also contraindicated, since skin rubbing, like ethanol, suppresses shivering thermogenesis and increases cutaneous vasodilation.

Field management of the comatose victim first involves ventilation to raise oxygen saturation. Mouth-to-mouth or mouth-to-nose rescue breathing is appropriate but may be difficult because of chest stiffness and significant resistance to diaphragmatic motion. Forced ventilation increases oxygenation, which helps stabilize the heart electrically. The single greatest factor in maintaining perfusion is oxygenation provided during severe hypothermia.

During a storm, prolonged field rewarming may be the only viable option until meteorologic conditions become more favorable for land or, preferably, aeromedical evacuation.[282] Many prehospital medications freeze in solution. If this occurs, their pharmacologic activity after thawing is indeterminate (see Appendix at end of this book). When available, consider whether administration of 50% dextrose or naloxone is indicated.

Give an intravenous (IV) fluid challenge with 250 to 500 ml heated (37° to 41° C [98.6° to 105.8° F]) 5% dextrose in normal saline solution. If that is unavailable, any crystalloid infusion with dextrose can be used. Improvisation during transport is often helpful. For example, a plastic IV container can be placed under the patient's back, shoulders, or buttocks to add warmth and infusion pressure. Taping heat-producing packets to IV bags is another option. These heating agents may be chemical packets or phase change crystals, which produce heat for up to several hours. IV fluid compressors are bulb-inflating cuffs that surround IV pouches to maintain flow. The Israeli army has a spring steel compressor system for IV bags.

Peripheral vessels may be difficult to locate, and IV lines are hard to maintain during transport. Ideally, IV fluids should be warmed to body temperature or slightly higher, but total body warming is not accomplished with IV fluids in the field. Using intraosseous infusions may provide a reasonable pathway for fluid replacement in the field when peripheral vessels have collapsed and cannot be entered.

The methods selected to stabilize core temperature should be tailored to the severity of hypothermia and the field circumstances. Gently removing or cutting off wet clothing while the patient remains prone may be the best option to limit heat loss and prevent orthostasis. Passive external rewarming with waterproof insulation suffices for mild chronic hypothermia. In their series of patients requiring cardiopulmonary bypass (CPB), Walpoth[269,270] "maintained" hypothermia during transport. Whether supplemental active field rewarming should be initiated en route to the ED, and in which subsets of patients, is not definitively established. Intentionally maintaining hypothermia during transport seems wise only for patients with an isolated closed head injury.

"Field rewarming" is a misnomer, since adding much heat to a hypothermic patient in the field is extremely difficult.[68] Warmed IV solutions, heated sarongs, or heated humidified oxygen can provide only a small amount of heat input. Hot water bottles or heat packs can be placed in the axillae, in the groin, and around the neck. Casualty evacuation bags are available in many models and designs. Some have more insulation than others, and some have specialized zippers and openings that allow access to the victim during transport. Most bags are windproof and waterproof.

Inhalation therapy is safe for active rewarming of victims with profound hypothermia in the field.[106] It helps prevent respiratory heat loss, which represents an important percentage of heat production when the core temperature is below 32° C (89.6° F). Technical difficulties experienced while using inhalation rewarming devices in volunteers suggest the importance of proper instruction for the rescuer.[253]

The current rewarming device weighs 3 kg, including oxygen tank, and consists of an oxygen cylinder, demand valve, 2-L reservoir bag, soda lime, and pediatric water canister. An in-line thermometer measures mean air temperature at the face mask. In the field, heat and moisture exchangers are practical, light, and inexpensive. They are, however, less efficient than active humidifiers.[173,175]

The Res-Q-Air (CF Electronics, Inc., Commack, N.Y.) is a lightweight, portable first-aid device that delivers heated humidified air or oxygen at temperatures ranging from 42° to 44° C (107.6° to 111.2° F) down to ambient conditions of −20° C (−4° F). This system consists of a heating chamber connected via a corrugated hose to a one-way flow valve and an oronasal mask. The temperature is controlled by a transducer in the one-way flow valve that provides feedback to the electronic control circuits. Supplemental oxygen and bag adaptation are possible.

Although surface rewarming suppresses shivering, it may be the only option when the victim is isolated from medical care. Active external rewarming options include radiant heat, warmed objects placed on the patient, and body-to-body contact.[90] Care must be exercised not to burn victims with hot objects, including commercially produced "hot packs." Total body contact rewarming may carry some risk, [90,106] but logistical impediments limit the use of this method unless extrication will be significantly delayed.

A hydraulic sarong or vest, in which heated water is circulated via hand pump, is also used occasionally.[104] Immersion rewarming is dangerous in the field because monitoring and resuscitation capabilities are limited.

The Norwegian Personal Heater Heat Pac may be a useful device for field transport of hypothermic patients. This device uses a single "D" battery and burns 30 hours on a single charcoal block. It is durable, lightweight (1 kg), efficient, and effective. It circulates hot air within a blanket or sleeping bag and provides a comfortable, warm and dry environment for transporting victims. In a human model with shivering inhibited by meperidine, the rate of rewarming with passive external rewarming over 150 minutes is not improved with inhalation rewarming.[96]

Another option under development is the use of a modified forced-air warming system for field use.[62,63,88] The Portable Rigid Forced-Air Cover is heated with a Bair Hugger 505 Heater/Blower (Augustine Medical, Inc., Eden Prairie, Minn.). It covers the patient's trunk and thighs and can adapt to various transport vehicle power sources.

Prehospital Life Support (Figure 6-7)

A patent airway and the presence of respirations must be established. The victim may appear apneic if respiratory minute ventilation is significantly depressed. A common error in tracheally intubated patients is overzealous assistance of ventilation, which can induce hypocapnic ventricular irritability. The indications for prehospital endotracheal intubation are identical to those under normothermic conditions. Appropriate ventilation with 100% oxygen may protect the heart during extrication and transport. Avoid overinflation of the tracheal cuff with frigid ambient air. As the victim warms, air in the cuff can expand and kink the tube. Careful protection and fixation of the tubing of the cuff port during extremely cold conditions are necessary to prevent breakage and cuff leak.

Palpation of peripheral pulses is often difficult in vasoconstricted and bradycardic patients. Apparent cardiovascular collapse may actually reflect depressed cardiac output just sufficient to meet minimal metabolic demands. The rescuer should auscultate and palpate for at least 1 minute to find pulses. Iatrogenic VF can easily result from unindicated chest compressions.

If a cardiac monitor is available, use maximal amplification to search for QRS complexes. If the victim is in VF, the rescuer should attempt defibrillation initially with 2 watt sec/kg up to 200 watt sec. If the second and

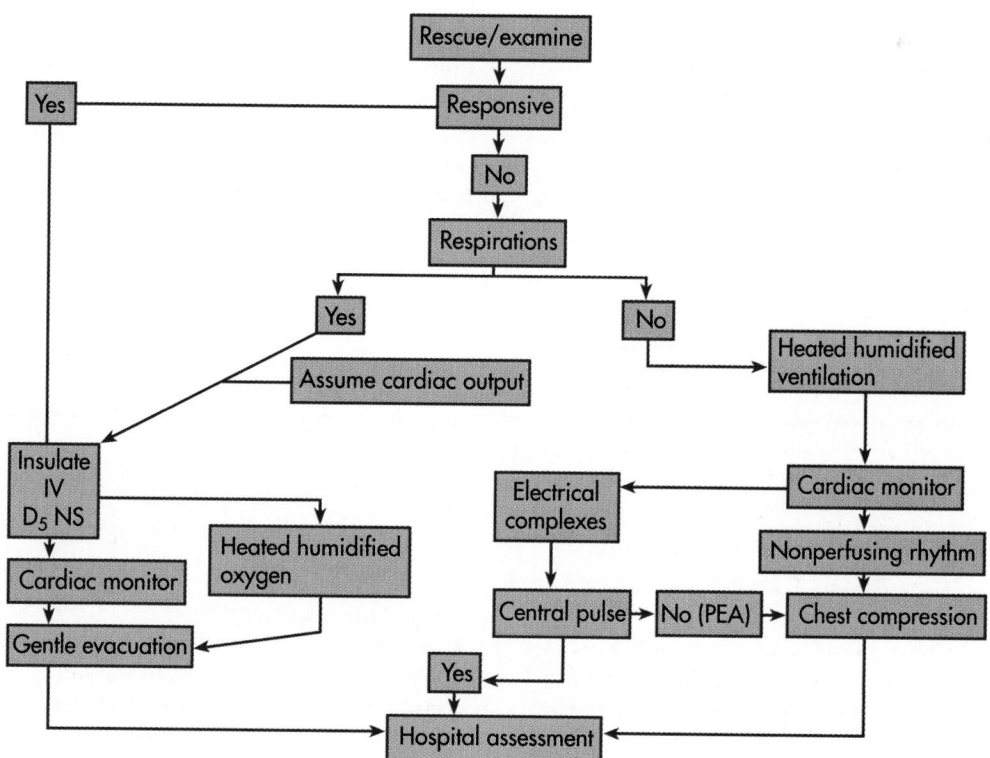

Figure 6-7 Prehospital life support. *PEA*, Pulseless electrical activity.

third attempts at 360 watt sec are unsuccessful, assume that the victim must be rewarmed before further attempts. Do not perform defibrillation if electrical complexes are seen on the monitor. Most monitors and defibrillators have not been tested for operation at temperatures below 15.5° C (59.9° F). Standard monitor leads do not always stick well to cold skin, so benzoin may be useful. If this fails, needle electrodes may be necessary. Another option is to puncture the gel foam conventional monitor pad with a small-gauge injection needle.[274]

Carefully assess unresponsive victims for a central pulse before assuming they have pulseless electrical activity (PEA). The lowest temperature at which mechanical reestablishment of cardiac activity has been successful is 20° C (68° F),[54] and defibrillation attempts rarely succeed below 30° C (86° F). If resuscitation in the field is unsuccessful, rewarming and cardiopulmonary resuscitation (CPR) should be continued during transport to the ED.

Management in the Emergency Department

The history obtained from a hypothermic patient is often unreliable; therefore it is prudent to confirm hypothermia and monitor with continuous core temperature measurements. Diagnostic errors in the ED usually result from incomplete monitoring of vital signs. Doppler ultrasound may be necessary to locate a pulse and should be supported by continuous ECG monitoring. The physician should also address the requirements for resuscitation and initiate advanced life support when necessary (Box 6-5).

Temperature Measurement. Some hospitals lack adequate equipment for accurate core temperature measurement.[204] Rectal measurements are most practical clinically but may not reflect cardiac or brain temperatures.[112] An indwelling thermistor probe placed to a depth of 15 cm is fairly reliable unless adjacent to cold feces. Rectal temperature lags behind core temperature fluctuations and is also affected by lower extremity temperatures[280] (Table 6-3).

Simultaneous esophageal temperature measurements may be helpful when airway protection is provided with endotracheal intubation. Esophageal temperature approximates cardiac temperature. Since the upper third of the esophagus is near the trachea, the probe may read falsely high during heated inhalation therapy. The probe should be placed 24 cm below the larynx. The greatest discordance between rectal and esophageal temperatures is noted during the transition phase between cooling and rewarming. Correct selection, accuracy, and use of devices that measure urine

---

Box 6-5 RESUSCITATION REQUIREMENTS

Thermal stabilization
  Conduction
  Convection
  Radiation
  Evaporation
  Respiration
Maintenance of tissue oxygenation
  Adequate circulation
  Adequate ventilation
Identification of primary vs. secondary hypothermia
Rewarming options
  Passive external rewarming
  Active external rewarming
  Active core rewarming

TABLE 6-3. Core Temperature Measurements

TYPE	ADVANTAGES	CONSIDERATIONS
Rectal	Convenient Continuous monitoring	Insert 15 cm Lags during cooling to rewarming transition Falsely elevated with peritoneal lavage Falsely low if probe in cold feces or with frozen lower extremities
Esophageal	Convenient Continuous monitoring	Insert 24 cm below larynx Tracheal misplacement Aspiration Falsely elevated with heated inhalation
Tympanic	Approximates hypothalamic temperature via internal carotid artery	Probe: tympanic membrane perforation; canal hemorrhage Infrared: unreliable; cerumen effect
Bladder	Convenient Continuous monitoring	Unreliable Falsely elevated with peritoneal lavage Falsely low with cold diuresis

temperature are debated. Crystalloid resuscitation and cold-induced diuresis both produce erratic readings.

Tympanic temperature theoretically approximates hypothalamic temperature and can be accurately measured with thermometers in contact with the tympanic membrane. Since these are impractical except in anesthetized patients, external auditory canal thermometers that measure infrared emission from the tympanic membrane have been developed. These are not actually "tympanic" thermometers, but this term is used extensively.[288]

External auditory canal thermometers are poorly sensitive for fever when used in clinical settings. Tympanic thermometers alone in patients with suspected hypothermia may also be very insensitive. Although bladder temperature measurement devices can be incorporated into the urinary drainage catheter, the readings are frequently unreliable. They will be falsely elevated with peritoneal lavage and, more commonly, low as a result of cold-induced diuresis.

Initial Stabilization. After core temperature measurement, all clothing should be gently removed or cut off with minimal patient manipulation.[212] Immediately insulate the patient with dry blankets. Apply a cardiac monitor, and insert intravenous catheters as needed. Arterial catheter insertion may help in managing selected profoundly hypothermic patients. Pulmonary artery catheters can precipitate cardiac arrhythmias and should be reserved for complex cases. Insertion of pulmonary artery catheters into cold vessels may perforate the pulmonary artery.[39] Do not use central venous catheters in the right atrium, since this could precipitate arrhythmias.[244]

Accuracy of pulse oximetry during conditions of poor perfusion is unclear. In one study of hypothermic patients on CPB, the finger probes were inaccurate.[36] The probe may be fairly reliable if a vasodilating cream is applied first. The value of end-tidal carbon dioxide measurements to assess adequacy of tissue perfusion and tracheal tube placement has been established at normal temperatures. Most of these devices, however, only measure the carbon dioxide content of dehumidified air and thus cannot be used during airway rewarming.

Laboratory evaluations to be considered, except in some cases of mild hypothermia, include blood sugar, arterial blood gases, complete blood cell count, electrolytes, BUN, creatinine, serum calcium, serum magnesium, serum amylase and lipase, PT, PTT, international normalized ratio (INR), platelet count, and fibrinogen level. A toxicologic screen should be considered if the level of consciousness does not correlate with the degree of hypothermia. Selective studies of thyroid function, cardiac isoenzyme levels, and serum cortisol levels are indicated.

The indications for radiography should be liberalized from normothermia. Radiologic evaluation of poorly responsive patients must include cervical and other spine films to detect occult trauma. Chest radiographs may predict collapse during rewarming when cardiomegaly and redistribution of vascularity are already present. Abdominal films should be obtained when the physical examination is unreliable. Bowel sounds are usually diminished or absent in severe hypothermia, and rectus muscle rigidity is frequently present. Pneumoperitoneum, pancreatic calcifications, or hemoperitoneum may be noted. Small bowel dilation is associated with cold-induced mesenteric vascular occlusion, and colonic dilation is often present in conjunction with myxedema coma. The use of focused abdominal sonography may be helpful.

Nasogastric tube insertion should be performed after endotracheal intubation in moderate or severe hypothermia, since gastric dilation and poor gastrointestinal motility are common. Indwelling bladder catheters with urine meters are needed to monitor urine output and the cold diuresis.

FLUID RESUSCITATION

Most fluid shifts are reversed by rewarming, and mild hypothermia usually requires only an IV lifeline. In more severe cases, volume shifts and elevated blood viscosity from hemoconcentration, lowered temperature, increased vascular permeability, and low flow state mandate aggressive fluid resuscitation. The viscosity of blood increases 2% per degree Centigrade drop in temperature; therefore hematocrit values over 50% are commonly seen. Low circulatory plasma volume is often coupled with elevated total plasma volume during rewarming. Hemodilution is usually not a problem, seen only during massive crystalloid resuscitation of actively hemorrhaging patients.[49]

Assume that patients will be significantly dehydrated, with free water depletion elevating serum sodium concentration and osmolality. During the descent into a hypothermic state, normal physiologic cues for thirst become inactive and access to water is often difficult. Since hypothermia results in natriuresis, saline depletion may be present. Further causes of sodium losses include prior diuretic therapy and gastrointestinal losses. Preexisting total body sodium excess is seen with congestive heart failure, cirrhosis, and nephrosis. In these cases serum sodium and osmolality values are often normal. Rarely, serum sodium level is low because of free water excess. Other causes include myxedema, panhypopituitarism, and inappropriate antidiuretic hormone secretion.[49]

Most patients with core temperature below 32.2° C (90° F) should receive an initial fluid challenge with 250 to 500 ml of 5% dextrose in warmed normal saline solution. Theoretically, Ringer's lactate solution should be avoided because a cold liver cannot metabolize lactate. Any potential advantages of colloids over crystalloids remain uncertain. Some clinicians administer colloids to patients who are not responding to crystalloids.

Monitor the victim for standard clinical signs of fluid overload, including rales, jugular venous distention, hepatojugular reflux, and S_3 cardiac gallop. Persistent cardiovascular instability often reflects inadequate intravascular volume. In this case, a properly placed central venous pressure catheter that does not enter and irritate the right atrium has a role. Pulmonary wedge pressure measurements should generally be deferred until after rewarming. The need for RBC transfusions is determined by the corrected hematocrit; blood dilution with warmed infusate does not cause significant hemolysis.

In many cases, rapid volume expansion is critical. Circulatory volume is decreased, and peripheral vascular resistance is increased. In neonates, adequate fluid resuscitation markedly decreases mortality. Adults receiving hemodynamic monitoring have shown improvement of cardiovascular efficiency during crystalloid administration. VF immediately after rescue has been attributed to both core temperature afterdrop and vascular imbalance in patients who are moved from a horizontal supine position.[174] The fluxing relationship between active vascular capacity and circulating fluid volume depends not only on the mechanism of cooling but also on the method of rewarming.

The safety and efficacy of the pneumatic antishock garment in hypothermia are unknown. Application presents several theoretic circulatory and limb hazards. Since the vasculature is already maximally vasoconstricted, provision of more peripheral vascular resistance by the garment will not be significant. Hypothermic patients, particularly those with frostbite, are at high risk for extremity compartment syndromes and rhabdomyolysis. Pneumatic trousers should be considered only to temporarily stabilize coexistent exsanguinating major pelvic fractures.

REWARMING OPTIONS

Passive External Rewarming

Because hypothermia is an extremely heterogenous condition and no controlled studies exist, rigid treatment protocols are not suggested.[231,235,289] A versatile approach to rewarming can be developed after careful consideration of the observations from animal experiments, human experiments on mild hypothermia, and various clinical reports[102] (Box 6-6).

The initial key treatment decision is whether to use active or passive rewarming (Box 6-7). Noninvasive passive external rewarming (PER) is ideal for most previously healthy patients with mild hypothermia. The patient is covered with dry insulating materials in a

---

Box 6-6 REWARMING TECHNIQUES

PASSIVE EXTERNAL

Thermal stabilization

ACTIVE

External

Radiant heat
Hot water bottles
Plumbed garments
Electric heating pads and blankets
Forced circulated hot air
Immersion in warm water
Negative pressure rewarming

Core

Inhalation rewarming
Heated infusions
Gastric and colonic lavage
Mediastinal lavage
Thoracic lavage
Peritoneal lavage
Diathermy
Hemodialysis
Venovenous extracorporeal blood rewarming
Arteriovenous extracorporeal blood rewarming

Box 6-7 INDICATIONS FOR ACTIVE REWARMING

Cardiovascular instability
Moderate or severe hypothermia (<32.2° C [90° F]) (poikilothermia)
Inadequate rate or failure to rewarm
Endocrinologic insufficiency
Traumatic or toxicologic peripheral vasodilation
Secondary hypothermia impairing thermoregulation
Identification of predisposing factors (see Box 6-2)

---

warm environment to minimize the normal mechanisms of heat loss. When the wind is blocked, less heat escapes via radiation, convection, and conduction. Conditions with higher ambient humidities slightly limit respiratory heat loss.

Aluminized body covers significantly reduce heat loss.[69,120] Nevertheless, endogenous thermogenesis must generate an acceptable rate of rewarming for PER to be effective.[205] Humans are functionally poikilothermic below 30° C (86° F), and metabolic heat production is less than 50% of normal below 28° C (82.4° F). Shivering thermogenesis is also extinguished below 32° C (89.6° F). This thermoregulatory neuromuscular re-

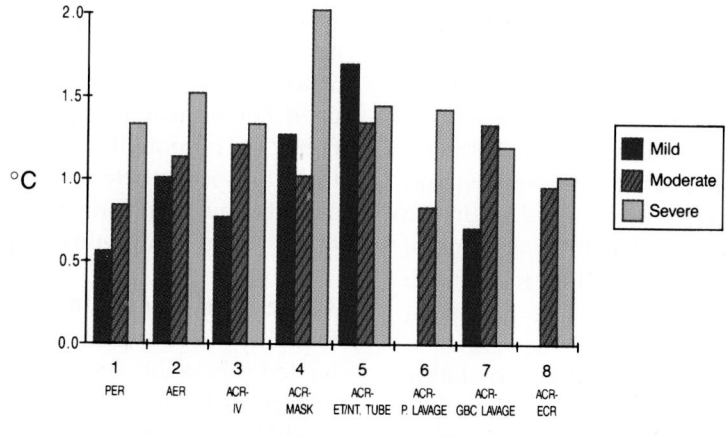

Figure 6-8 First-hour rewarming rates from a large multicenter survey. *ACR*, Active core rewarming; *AER*, active external rewarming; *ET*, endotracheal tube; *GBC*, gastric-bladder-colon lavage; *IV*, intravenous; *NT*, nasotracheal tube; *P*, peritoneal lavage; *PER*, passive external rewarming. (*Data from Danzl DF et al:* Ann Emerg Med *16:1042, 1987.*)

sponse to cold normally increases heat production from 250 to 1000 kcal/hr unless glycogen is depleted during cooling.

Elderly patients in whom mild hypothermia develops gradually are acceptable candidates for PER. Peripheral vasoconstriction is maintained, which minimizes the circulatory component of core temperature afterdrop. When rewarming times are markedly prolonged (over 12 hours), complications tend to increase.

Patients who are centrally hypovolemic, glycogen depleted, and without normal cardiovascular responses should be stabilized and rewarmed at a conservative rate. In a multicenter survey the first (0.75° C ± 1.16), second (1.17° C ± 1.17), and third (1.26° C ± 1.28) hour rewarming rates for the elderly far exceeded 0.5° C per hour with no increase in mortality rate (Figure 6-8).[51]

Active Rewarming

Active rewarming, which is the direct transfer of exogenous heat to a patient, is usually required with temperatures below 32° C (89.6° F).[162] Rapid identification of any impediment to normal thermoregulation, such as cardiovascular instability or endocrinologic insufficiency, is essential.[163,196] Intrinsic thermogenesis may also be insufficient after traumatic spinal cord transection or pharmacologically induced peripheral vasodilation. Some patient populations generally require active rewarming.[154] For example, aggressive rewarming of infants minimizes energy expenditure and decreases mortality.[284] In these circumstances, vigorous monitoring for respiratory, hematologic, metabolic, and infectious complications is essential.

When active rewarming is needed, heat can be delivered externally or to the core. Active external rewarming (AER) techniques deliver heat directly to the skin. Examples include forced air rewarming, immer-

sion, arteriovenous anastomoses rewarming, plumbed garments, hot water bottles, heating pads and blankets, and radiant heat sources.

Active External Rewarming. The interpretation of survival rates with AER is affected by various risk factors and patient selection criteria. In some reports, "active" is an artificial description, since rewarming required more than 24 hours. One author reported a 100% success rate with immersion rewarming.[77]

Some experimental and clinical reports link AER with peripheral vasodilation, hypotension, and core temperature afterdrop, but previously healthy, young, acutely hypothermic victims are usually safe candidates for AER.[25] Heat application confined to the thorax may mitigate many of the physiologic concerns pertaining to the depressed cardiovascular and metabolic systems, which are unable to meet accelerated peripheral demands. Combining truncal AER with active core rewarming may further avert many potential side effects.

Forced Air Rewarming. Forced air warming systems efficiently transfer heat.[7,88,130] The Bair Hugger (Augustine Medical, Inc.) uses hot forced air circulated through a blanket. The air exits apertures on the patient side of the cover, permitting the convective transfer of heat.[191,240] In one study that rewarmed accidental hypothermia victims in the ED, rewarming shock and core temperature afterdrop were not noted[250] with the use of heated inhalation and warmed IV fluids. A group also treated with a convective cover inflated at 43° C (109.4° F) rewarmed 1° C (1.8° F) per hour faster than a group covered with a cotton blanket (1.4° C [2.5° F] per hour).

A study of full-body forced air warming compared a commercially available convective blanket with simple air delivery beneath bed sheets.[148] Directed 38° C (100.4° F) warm air under the sheets warmed standardized thermal bodies containing water very efficiently.

The use of forced air warming systems is most practical in the ED.[153,158,165] Although these devices decrease shivering thermogenesis, afterdrop is minimized and heat transfer can be significant. Thermal injury to poorly perfused, vasoconstricted skin using some of the other external heat application techniques is a hazard in both adults and children.[104,151]

IMMERSION. Immersion in a 40° C (104° F) circulating bath presents difficulties in monitoring, resuscitation, treatment of injuries, and maintenance of extremity vasoconstriction to prevent core temperature afterdrop. "Bobbing" CPR is impossible in the tub. In normothermic men with coronary artery disease, the cardiovascular stress and arrhythmogenic response to immersion in a hot tub are mild, less than those induced by exercise.[2] In contrast, placing the hands and feet in warm water theoretically opens arteriovenous shunts and accelerates rewarming in acute hypothermia. The attraction to Scandinavian palmar heat packs may reflect this physiology.

ARTERIOVENOUS ANASTOMOSES REWARMING. The original description of this noninvasive AER technique was by Vangaard[264] in 1979. Exogenous heat is provided by immersion of the lower parts of the extremities (hands, forearms, feet, calves) in 44° to 45° C (111.2° to 113° F) water. The heat opens arteriovenous anastomoses (AVAs). These organs are 1 mm below the epidermal surface in the digits.[14,61,195] As a result, there is increased flow of warmed venous subcutaneous blood returning directly to the heart. Countercurrent heat loss is minimized because the superficial veins are not close to the arterial tree.

To be efficacious, the cutaneous heat exchange area must include the lower legs and forearms, and the water must be 44° to 45° C. Reported advantages with AVA rewarming include patient comfort and decreased postcooling afterdrop.

A permutation of AVA rewarming is negative pressure rewarming. Under hypothermic conditions, the AVAs remain closed during peripheral vasoconstriction. In combination with localized heat application, application of subatmospheric pressure theoretically distends the venous rate and increases flow through the AVAs.

To initiate negative pressure rewarming, the forearm is inserted through an acrylic tubing sleeve device fitted with a neoprene collar. This allows an airtight seal to form around the forearm. After −40 mm Hg vacuum pressure is created, heat is applied over the dilated AVAs.[247] The thermal load can be provided via an exothermic chemical reaction or via a heated perfusion blanket.

The clinical efficacy and safety of AVA rewarming in accidental hypothermia remains to be determined. Studies concluding that heat exchange is ineffectual used cooler water applied only on the hands and feet.[30,43] The potential for superficial burns of anesthetic, vasoconstricted skin is a consideration. Another caveat is hypotension precipitated in hypovolemic patients who remain semi-upright with this technique.

Active Core Rewarming. Various techniques can effectively deliver heat to the core,[228,239,264] including heated inhalation, heated infusion, diathermy, lavage (gastric, colonic, mediastinal, thoracic, peritoneal), hemodialysis, and venovenous and continuous arteriovenous rewarming. Formal CPB is the definitive core rewarming technique. Average first-hour rewarming rates reported with some of these techniques in one multicenter study are listed in Figure 6-8.

AIRWAY REWARMING. Heated, humidified oxygen inhalation has been studied extensively for both prehospital and ED rewarming.[173] The effectiveness of the respiratory tract as a heat exchanger varies with technique and ambient conditions.[192] Since dry air has low thermal conductivity, complete humidification coupled with inhalant temperature of 40° to 45° C (104° to 113° F) is required.[222] The main benefit of airway rewarming is prevention of respiratory heat loss. Heat yield can represent 10% to 30% of the hypothermic patient's heat production when respiratory minute volume is adequate.[23]

The rate of rewarming is greater using an endotracheal tube (ETT) than by mask. In one series, the reported rewarming rate with 40° C aerosol was 0.74° C (1.33° F) per hour via mask and 1.22° C (2.2° F) per hour via ETT.[196] In the multicenter survey the average first- and second-hour rewarming rates in severe cases were 1.5° to 2° C (2.7° to 3.6° F) per hour. Because of the decremental efficiency at higher temperatures, the rate is slower in mild cases.[51]

Thermal countercurrent exchange in the cerebrovascular bed of humans[56] affects the efficiency and influence of heated mask ventilation during hypothermia. Known as the *rete mirabile*, this system could preferentially rewarm the brainstem. Heated inhalation via face mask continuous positive airway pressure (CPAP) has been successfully used and may correct the ventilation-perfusion mismatch.[31] Heated humidified oxygen via face mask may not be feasible in some patients with coexistent midface trauma.

Heat liberated during airway rewarming is produced mainly from condensation of water vapor. The latent heat of vaporization of water in the lung is slightly lower than 540 kcal/g H_2O. This is multiplied by the liters per minute ventilation to calculate the quantity of heat transfer. When core temperature is 28° C (82.4° F), the rate of rewarming with heated ventilation at 42° C (107.6° F) equals endogenous heat production. Although the effect on overall thermal balance can be minimal, there may be preferential rewarming of thermoregulatory control centers.

Heated humidified inhalation ensures adequate oxygenation, stimulates pulmonary cilia, and reduces the amount and viscosity of cold-induced bronchorrhea. Although preexisting premature ventricular contractions (PVCs) may reappear during rewarming, there is no evidence that inhalation rewarming precipitates new, clinically significant ventricular arrhythmias.[50] Vapor absorption does not increase pulmonary congestion or wash out surfactant. When the pulmonary vasculature is heated, warmed oxygenated blood that returns to the myocardium could attenuate intermittent temperature gradients. The amplitude of shivering is also lowered, an advantage in more severe cases. In theory, this suppression could decrease heat production in mild hypothermia, although experimentally the core temperature continues to rise.[43]

There are numerous oxygenation considerations in hypothermia (see Box 6-1). The "functional" value of hemoglobin at 28° C (82.4° F) has been calculated to be 4.2 g/10 g in patients on CPB.[76] The oxyhemoglobin dissociation curve also shifts to the left (Figure 6-9). This impairs release of oxygen from hemoglobin into the tissues. Although some patients can self-adjust their respiratory minute volume (RMV) for current carbon dioxide production, this may not be possible if there are additional toxins or metabolic depressants.

Most humidifiers are manufactured in accordance with International Standards Organization (ISO) regulations. The humidifier will not exceed 41° C (105.8° F) close to the patient outlet with a 6-foot tubing length.[268] If the decision to alter the equipment is made, carefully monitor the temperature and do not exceed 45° C (113° F). The only report of thermal airway injury was in a patient ventilated via endotracheal tube for 11 hours with 80° C (176° F) inhalant.

Strategies to circumvent the 41° C ceiling include reduction of tubing length, adding additional heat sources, disabling the humidifier safety system, and placing the temperature probe outside the patient circuit.[268] Label all modified equipment to avoid routine use. A volume ventilator with a heated cascade humidifier can also deliver CPAP or positive end-expiratory pressure (PEEP) if needed during rewarming. The airway rewarming rates clinically range from 1° to 2.5° C (1.8° to 4.5° F) per hour.[51]

Heat and moisture exchangers function like artificial nares by trapping exhaled moisture and then returning it. They provide inadequate humidification to treat accidental hypothermia. With prolonged use, ETT occlusion and atelectasis are both problems.[38,97] In the field, heat and moisture exchangers are practical, lightweight, and inexpensive, although less efficient than active humidifiers.[173]

Airway rewarming is indicated in the field when the equipment is available and in the ED when core temperature is lower than 32.2° C (90° F) on arrival. Although airway rewarming provides less heat than other forms of active core warming, it prevents normal respiratory heat and moisture loss and is safe, fairly noninvasive, and practical in all settings.

HEATED INFUSIONS. Cold fluid resuscitation of hypovolemic patients can induce hypothermia. In one series of previously normothermic patients with major abdominal vascular trauma, the average postresuscitation temperature was 31.2° C (88.2° F) in those with refractory coagulopathies.[144] IV fluids are heated to 40° to 42° C (104° to 107.6° F), although some authors suggest higher temperatures may be safe. The amount of heat provided by solutions becomes significant during massive volume resuscitations.[245] One liter of fluid at 42° C provides 14 kcal to a 70-kg patient at 28° C (82.4° F), elevating the core temperature almost 0.33° C (0.6° F).

Microwave heating of IV fluids in flexible plastic bags is a widely available option.[238] The plasticizer in the polyvinyl chloride containers is stable to microwave heating. Thermal packs, jackets, or insulation on IV bags also help preserve heat.[20] Heating times should average 2 minutes at high power for a 1-L bag of crystalloid. The fluid should be thoroughly mixed before administration, since "hot spots" are common in ovens. Fresh frozen plasma can also be thawed in under 5 minutes.

Significant conductive heat loss occurs through IV tubing, so long lengths of IV tubing increase heat loss, especially at slow flow rates.[70] There are various methods to achieve and maintain ideal delivery temperature of IV and lavage fluids in hypothermia but no standardized approach.[105]

Blood preheated to 38° C (100.4° F) in a standard warmer is useful, but clotting and shortened RBC life are hazards with blood-warming packs. Local mi-

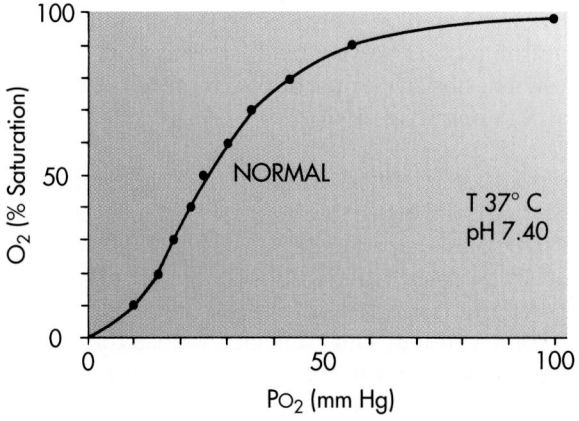

Figure 6-9 Oxyhemoglobin dissociation curve at 37° C (98.6° F). At colder temperatures the curve shifts to the left.

crowave overheating hemolyzes blood. An alternative is to dilute packed RBCs with warm calcium-free crystalloid. The Level 1 Fluid Warmer (Life Systems, Inc., Southfield, Mich.) warms cold crystalloid and blood from 10° C to 35° C (50° F to 95° F) via a heat exchanger at flow rates of up to 500 ml/min.

Rapid administration of fluid into the right atrium at a temperature significantly different from that of circulating blood may produce myocardial thermal gradients.[244] In one study, heated IV fluid, up to 550 ml/min, was administered through the internal jugular vein without complication. In an experimental canine model with adequate cardiac output, central infusion of extremely hot (65° C [149° F]) IV fluids was reported to accelerate rewarming without hemolysis.[74,241]

Using amino acid infusions may accelerate energy metabolism. Fever is common in patients receiving hyperalimentation. In patients recovering from elective surgery, however, amino acids have had no significant thermogenic effect.[117] The results might differ in energy-depleted patients with chronically induced accidental hypothermia.

In summary, intravenous solutions and blood are routinely heated during hypothermia resuscitations. Various blood warmers are available commercially, but countercurrent in-line warmers and rapid warm saline admixture are the most efficient techniques.[128]

HEATED IRRIGATION

Gastrointestinal irrigation. Heat transfer from irrigation fluids is usually limited by the available surface area, so do not use irrigation as the sole rewarming technique. Direct gastrointestinal irrigation is less desirable than irrigation via intragastric or intracolonic balloons because of induced fluid and electrolyte fluxes. Exceeding 200- to 300-ml aliquots may force fluid into the duodenum; therefore frequent fluid removal via gravity drainage minimizes "lost" fluid. A log of input and output is essential. This facilitates estimation of fluid balance during resuscitation and helps determine if irrigation should be abandoned in anticipation of dilutional electrolyte disturbances.

To avoid these limitations, a double-lumen esophageal tube has been investigated, as have other modified Sengstaken tubes.[155] Patients should be tracheally intubated before gastric lavage. Because of the proximity of an irritable heart, overly vigorous placement of a large gastric tube seems ill advised. In the multicenter survey, gastric, bladder, and colon lavage rewarmed severely hypothermic patients at 1° to 1.5° C (1.8° to 2.7° F) for the first hour and 1.5° to 2° C (2.7° to 3.6° F) for the second hour.[51]

Commercially available kits designed for gastric decontamination are convenient (Figure 6-10). The use of a Y connector and clamp simplifies the exchanges. Ideal dwell times for thermal exchange depend on flow rates

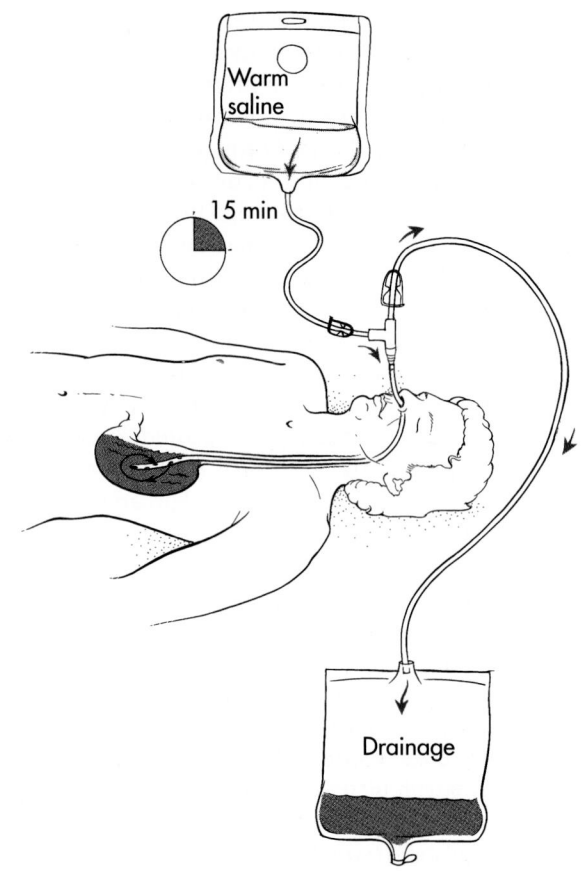

Figure 6-10 Gastric lavage.

and may average several minutes. In direct gastric lavage, warmed electrolyte solutions, such as normal saline or Ringer's lactate, are administered via nasogastric tube.[167] After 15 minutes the solution is aspirated and replaced with warm fluids. Disadvantages include the small surface area available for heat exchange and the large amount of fluid escaping into the duodenum.[28] Regurgitation is common, and the technique must be terminated during CPR. Some authors continue to support the concept of esophageal heat exchange, but clinical success is limited.[157,221,274,275]

Bladder irrigation should be limited to around 200- to 300-ml aliquots to prevent bladder distention. A number of aesthetic obstacles must be overcome to maintain successful colonic irrigation.

Mediastinal irrigation. Mediastinal irrigation and direct myocardial lavage are alternatives in patients lacking spontaneous perfusion. A standard left thoracotomy is performed while CPR is continued. Opening the pericardium is unnecessary unless an effusion or tamponade is present. The physician bathes the heart for several minutes in 1 to 2 L of an isotonic electrolyte solution heated to 40° C (104° F), then performs suction and replacement of warm fluids.[29]

The physician may attempt internal defibrillation after myocardial temperature reaches 26° to 28° C (78.8 to 82.4° F). Unless a perfusing rhythm is achieved, lavage is continued until myocardial temperature exceeds 32° to 33° C (89.6° to 91.4° F). A standard post-thoracotomy tube in the left side of the chest could provide an avenue for continued rewarming via thoracic irrigation.

A median sternotomy also allows ventricular decompression and direct defibrillation.[166] One potential disadvantage of both these techniques is that open cardiac massage of a cold, rigid contracted heart may not generate flow.[3,45] Unless immediate CPB is an option, mediastinal irrigation and direct myocardial lavage are indicated only if cardiac arrest has occurred. In this circumstance, personnel skilled in the technique should also initiate all other available rewarming modalities.

Closed thoracic lavage. Irrigation of the hemithoraces is a valuable rewarming adjunct.[10,29,272] Two large-bore thoracostomy tubes (36 to 40 Fr in adults; 14 to 24 Fr, ages 1 to 3; 20 to 32 Fr, ages 4 to 7) are inserted in one or both of the hemithoraces. One is placed anteriorly in the second to third intercostal space at the midclavicular line, and the other in the posterior axillary line at the fifth to sixth intercostal space. Normal saline heated to 40° to 42° C (104° to 107.6° F) is then infused via a nonrecycled sterile system (Figure 6-11, A). Hypothermic coagulopathies in extreme situations might necessitate the use of cautery at the incision sites.

A high-flow countercurrent fluid infuser (Level 1 Fluid Warmer)[27] heats to 40° C and delivers normal saline in 1-L or preferably 3-L bags into the afferent chest tube.[27,246] I prefer connecting into the Level 1 tubing with standard 3/16-inch-internal-diameter suction connection tubing and a sterilized plastic graduated two-way connector, since this facilitates adaptation to any size chest tube (Figure 6-11, A). The effluent is then collected in a thoracostomy drainage set. The reservoir must be emptied frequently. Alternatively, when a single chest tube is used, 200- to 300-ml aliquots are used for irrigation, and suctioning is achieved through a Y connector. The Y connector is also useful for irrigating both hemithoraces with a single fluid warmer (Figure 6-11, B).

The clinical experience reported with closed thoracic lavage remains limited.[142,281] Fluid has been infused into the anterior higher chest tube (afferent limb) and suctioned or gravity drained out the lower posterior tube (efferent limb) into a water seal chest drain.[103] Infusion inferoposteriorly with suction anteriorly can increase dwell times.[129] The efficiency of thermal transfer varies with flow rates and dwell times. If the patient has been successfully rewarmed, the upper tube should be removed and the lower one left in place to allow residual drainage.

Closed sterile thoracic lavage seems a natural choice in the ED during cardiac arrest resuscitations. In patients who are perfusing, this technique should be considered hazardous unless extracorporeal rewarming capability is immediately available. Many hypothermic trauma patients have been irrigated successfully in the operating room.

The clinically reported rates range from 180 to 550 ml/min. The overall rate of rewarming should easily equal or exceed that achievable with peritoneal lavage and is often 3° to 6° C (5.4° to 10.8° F) per hour. An added benefit is preferential mediastinal rewarming. In addition, closed chest compressions during cardiac arrest can maintain perfusion. Open cardiac massage of a rigid, contracted heart may not be possible in severe cases before bypass, which is a problem with mediastinal irrigation.[3,45,47]

Various complications should be considered. Left-sided thoracostomy tube insertion into patients who are perfusing could easily induce VF. Patients with pleural adhesions have poor infusion rates, and subcutaneous edema may develop. If the fluids are infused under pressure without adequate drainage, intrathoracic hypertension or even a tension hydrothorax could develop and cause the expected adverse cardiovascular effects. Insufficient data are available to assess the effects on pulmonary ventilation and perfusion.

Peritoneal lavage. Heated peritoneal lavage is a technique available in most facilities (Figure 6-12). Heat is conducted intraperitoneally via isotonic dialysate delivered at 40° to 45° C (104° to 113° F).[265] This technique is not a practical option in the field.

Before lavage is initiated, chest and abdominal radiographs should be obtained because subsequent films may reveal subdiaphragmatic air introduced during the procedure. The bladder and stomach must be emptied before insertion of the catheter. The two common techniques for introducing fluid into the peritoneal cavity are the minilaparotomy and the percutaneous puncture.

The "minilap" requires an infraumbilical incision through the linea alba. A supraumbilical approach is necessary if previous surgical scars, a gravid uterus, or pelvic trauma is identified. The peritoneum is punctured under direct visualization and dialysis catheter(s) inserted. A much simpler and more rapid technique is the guidewire, or Seldinger's, variation of the percutaneous puncture. The site is infiltrated if necessary with lidocaine and a small stab incision is made. An 18- to 20-gauge needle penetrates the peritoneum, and a guidewire is introduced. Entry into the peritoneum is usually recognizable by a distinct "pop." A disposable kit is available (Arrow Peritoneal Lavage Kit [AK-0900], Arrow International Inc., Reading, Pa.). The 8-Fr lavage

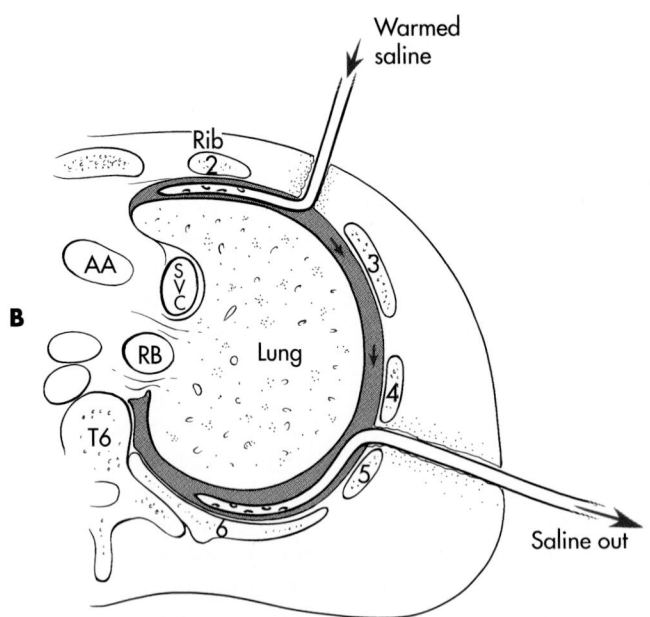

A Fluid warmer

Saline

Heat exchanger

Air eliminator

Midclavicular line

Postaxillary line

Autotransfusion bag

Water seal chest drain

B

Warmed saline

Rib
2

AA

S
V
C

RB

Lung

T6

3

4

5

6

Saline out

Figure 6-11 Thoracic lavage. **A,** Cycle. **B,** Cross section.

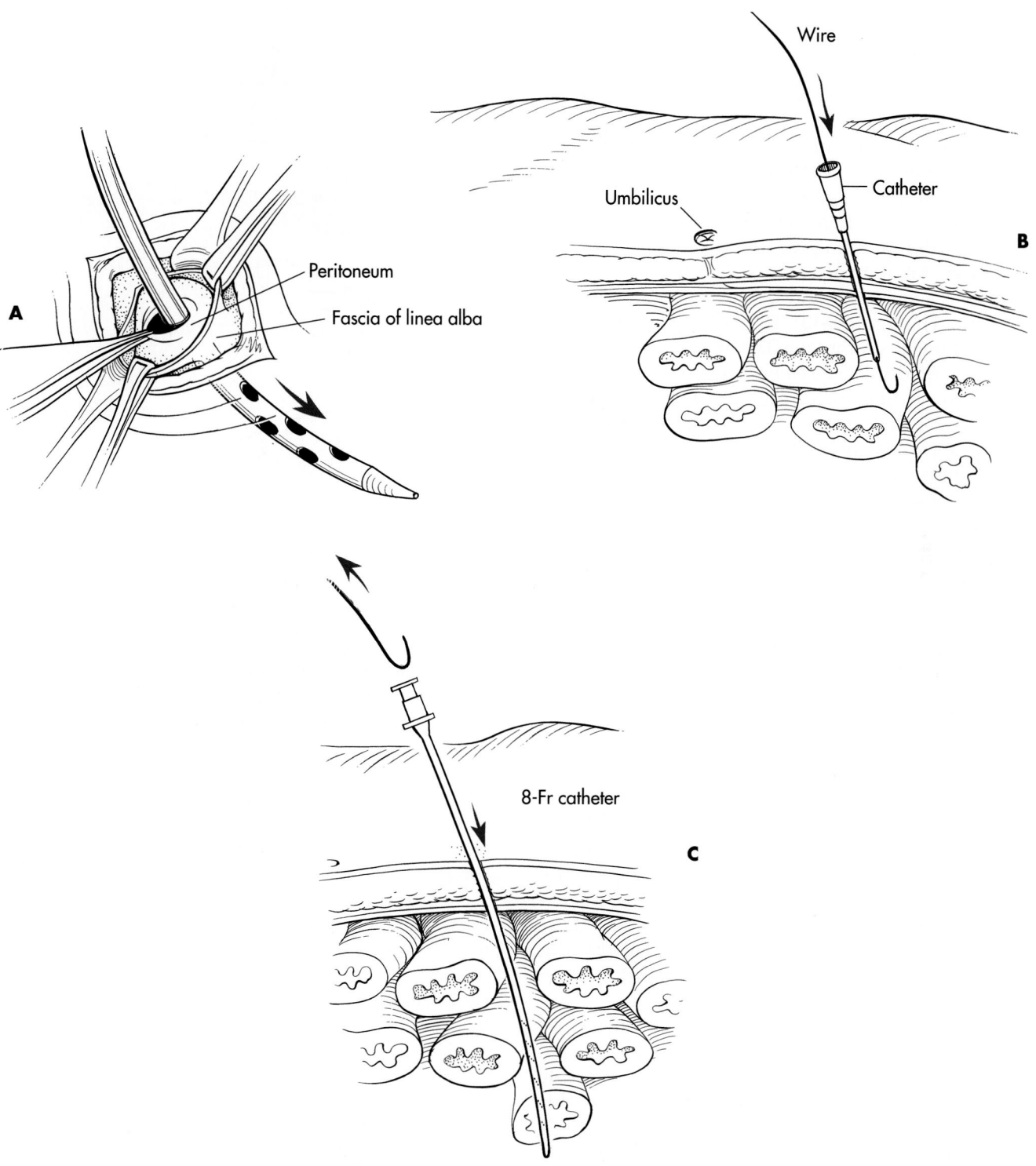

Figure 6-12   Peritoneal lavage. **A,** Minilaparotomy for peritoneal lavage. **B,** The catheter in place with the needle removed and the wire introduced. **C,** An 8-Fr catheter is introduced over the wire, and the wire is then removed.

catheter is inserted over the wire and advanced into one of the pelvic gutters. Double-catheter systems with outflow suction speed rewarming.

Normal saline, lactated Ringer's solution, or standard 1.5% dextrose dialysate solution with optional potassium supplementation can be used.[246] Isotonic dialysate is heated to 40° to 45° C. Up to 2 L is then infused (10 to 20 ml/kg), retained for 20 to 30 minutes, and aspirated. The usual clinical exchange rate is 6 L/hr, which yields rewarming rates of 1° to 3° C (1.8° to 5.4° F) per hour. An alternative for severe cases is a larger catheter, as found in cavity drainage kits (Arrow 14 Fr [AK-01601]) (Figure 6-13). The catheter can be placed with Seldinger's technique. The higher drainage capability markedly increases exchange rates and minimizes dwell times necessary for maximal thermal transfer. The flow rate via gravity through regular tubing is approximately 500 ml/min, which can be tripled under infusion pressure.

A unique advantage of peritoneal dialysis is drug overdose and rhabdomyolysis detoxification when hemodialysis is unavailable. In addition, direct hepatic rewarming reactivates detoxification and conversion enzymes. Peritoneal dialysis worsens preexisting hypokalemia. Vigilant electrolyte monitoring is essential before empirical modification of the dialysate. The presence of adhesions from previous abdominal surgery increases the complication rate and minimizes heat exchange.

Peritoneal dialysis during standard mechanical CPR is as effective as partial cardiac bypass in resuscitating severely hypothermic dogs. Unlike the group of dogs receiving AER, peritoneal lavage rewarming did not require significantly greater quantities of crystalloids and bicarbonate. In another canine study, peritoneal dialysis at a rate of 12 L/hr rewarmed dogs more rapidly than did heated, humidified inhalation.[279] This exchange rate is rarely possible in humans. Bowel infarction may be a concern when using prolonged warm peritoneal dialysis in severe hypothermia with inadequate visceral perfusion during CPR.[12]

Peritoneal lavage is invasive and should not be routinely used in treating stable, mildly hypothermic patients. Extracorporeal rewarming should be available in case of rare major complications, including VF. This technique is indicated in combination with all available rewarming techniques in cardiac arrest patients.

EXTRACORPOREAL BLOOD REWARMING

Cardiopulmonary bypass. Partial or complete CPB should be considered in severely hypothermic patients.[100,227] Favorable considerations include absence of severe head injury or a history of asphyxia. Some centers only initiate CPB if the presenting arterial pH is above 6.5, serum potassium is below 10 mmol/L, and core temperature is above 12° C (53.6° F).[55,119,260,270] A major advantage of CPB is preservation of oxygenated

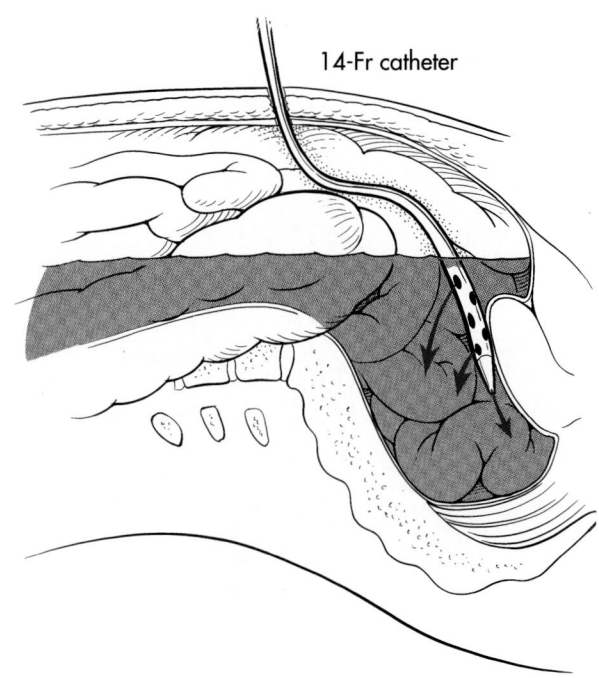

14-Fr catheter

Figure 6-13   Peritoneal lavage. A 14-Fr catheter is of greater caliber and can infuse fluids more rapidly.

flow if mechanical cardiac activity is lost during rewarming.[60,125,127,187] CPB is three to four times faster at rewarming than other active core rewarming (ACR) techniques and reduces the high blood viscosity associated with severe cases. CPB should also be considered when severe cases do not respond to less invasive rewarming techniques, in patients with completely frozen extremities, and when rhabdomyolysis is accompanied by major electrolyte disturbances.[138]

Various extracorporeal rewarming (ECR) techniques can be lifesaving in selected profound cases of hypothermia.[48,108] Althaus[3] describes complete recovery in three severely hypothermic tourists after prolonged periods of cardiac arrest and CPR. In another review of 17 cases, there were 13 survivors.[248] Walpoth[269,270] reports rewarming 32 patients with CPB, of which 15 are long-term survivors. The average age was 25.2 years. Their mean presenting T_{esoph} was 21.8° C (71.2° F), and the mean interval between discovery and CPB was 141 minutes.

The standard femoral-femoral circuit includes arterial and venous catheters, a mechanical pump, a membrane or bubble oxygenator, and a heat exchanger (Figure 6-14). A 16- to 30-Fr venous cannula is inserted via the femoral vein to the right atrium/inferior vena cava junction. The tip of the shorter 16- to 20-Fr arterial cannula is inserted 5 cm or proximal to the aortic bifurcation. Antretter[5] uses 32-Fr venous and 28-Fr arterial cannulas with the open surgical technique, and 21-Fr venous and 19-Fr arterial cannulas if inserted percutaneously. Closed chest compressions can be maintained

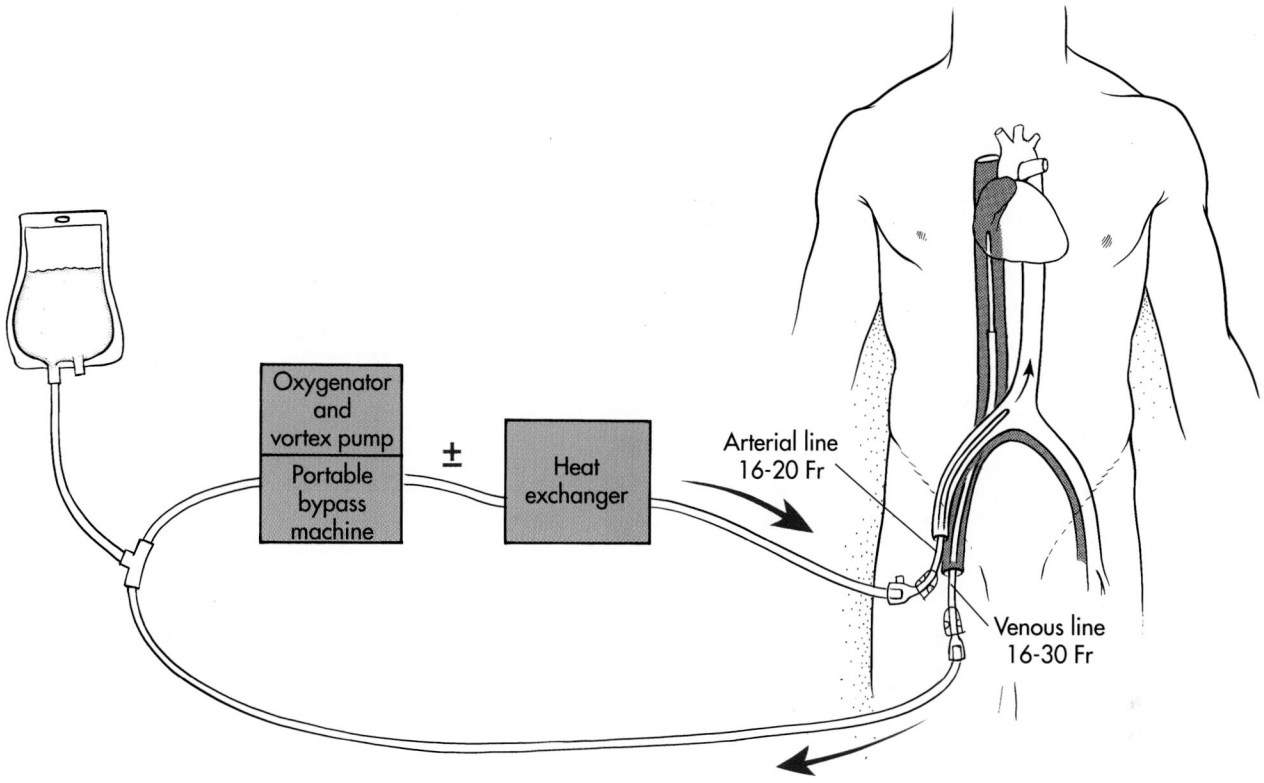

Figure 6-14 Femoral-femoral bypass.

during percutaneous or open surgical technique insertion and may help decompress the dilated nonbeating heart. Transesophageal echocardiography can help evaluate ventricular load and valve function.

Techniques have been developed to decrease the need for IV anticoagulation with heparin, which previously limited clinical applicability.[271] Heparin-coated perfusion equipment was used successfully without systemic heparinization in a patient with hypothermic cardiac arrest (23.3° C [73.9° F]) and intracranial trauma.[266] The use of nonthrombogenic pumps, coupled with enhanced physiologic fibrinolysis seen in the first hour of CPB, also has succeeded experimentally.[58]

Heated, oxygenated blood is returned via the femoral artery. Femoral flow rates of 2 to 3 L/min can elevate core temperature 1° to 2° C (1.8° to 3.6° F) every 3 to 5 minutes. In Splittgerber's review,[248] the mean CPB temperature increase was 9.5° C (17.1° F) per hour. Most pumps can generate full flow rates up to 7 L/min. Long[178] recommends considering the use of vasodilator therapy with IV nitroglycerin to facilitate perfusion. He initiates bypass flow rates at about 2 L/min and gradually increases to 4 to 5 L/min. Vasoactive agents may be needed to maintain the cardiac index at 30 or more and for a (low) systemic vascular resistance of 1000 or less.

The optimal temperature gradient and bypass rewarming rates are unknown. One study of rewarming via CPB in a swine model cooled to 23° C (73.4° F) addresses this concern. An excessive temperature gradient between brain tissue and circulant adversely affected electroencephalography (EEG) regeneration.[226] The other theoretical concern is the possibility of increased bubbling if high perfusate temperature gradients are used. Most current investigators use 5° C (9° F) gradients[18] or 10° C (18° F) gradients.[19] Eventually, neuromonitoring during rewarming will provide some answers. In severe cases, evoked cerebral responses before EEG regeneration could help assess the recovering brain.

Complications with the standard technique include vessel damage, air embolism, hemolysis, DIC, and pulmonary edema (Box 6-8). Endothelial leakage increases compartment pressures and exacerbates frostbite. If adequate flow rates of 3 to 4 L/min (50 to 60 ml/kg/min) cannot be maintained, thoracotomy or a venous catheter with side holes, augmenting intravascular volume, should be considered.

Arteriovenous rewarming. CAVR involves the use of percutaneously inserted femoral arterial and contralateral femoral venous catheters.[80-82,84] This technique requires a blood pressure of at least 60 mm Hg. Seldinger's technique is used to insert 8.5-Fr catheters. Heparin-bonded tubing circuits obviate the need for

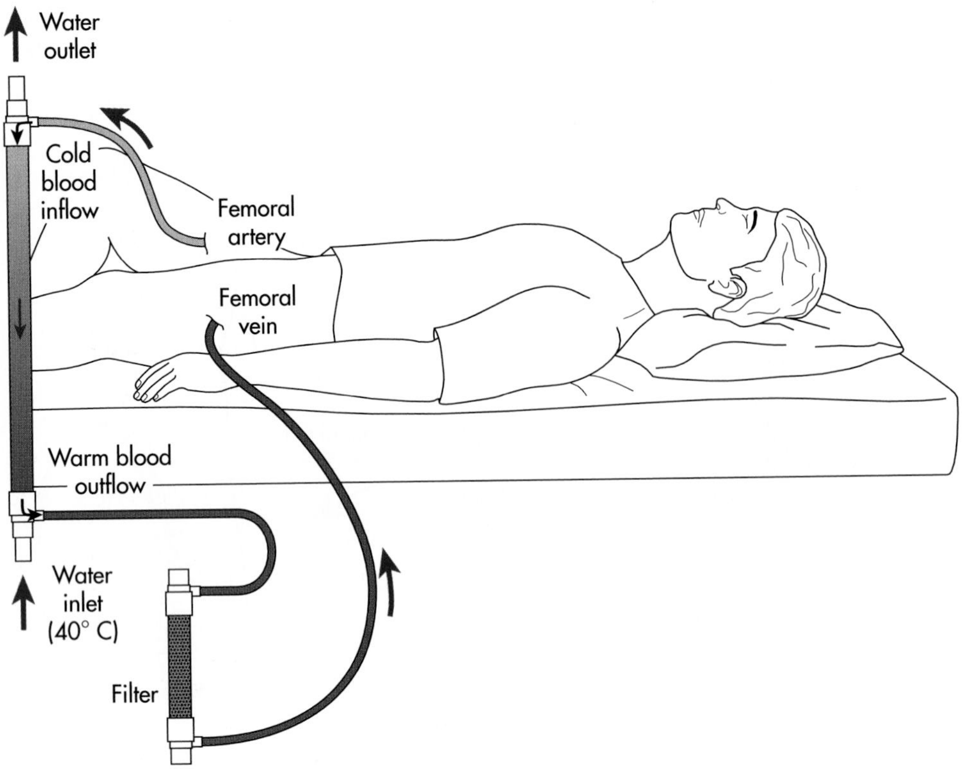

Figure 6-15 CAVR schematic.

Box 6-8   EXTRACORPOREAL REWARMING

COMPLICATIONS

Vascular injury
Air embolism
Pulmonary edema
Coagulopathies (hemolysis, disseminated intravascular coagulation)
Frostbite tissue damage
Extremity compartment syndromes

CONTRAINDICATIONS

CPR is contraindicated (see Box 6-9)
Lack of venous return
Intravascular clots or slush
Complete heparinization would be hazardous*

*Unless with athrombogenic tubing or adequate physiologic fibrinolysis.

---

systemic anticoagulation. CAVR has principally been performed on traumatized patients (Figure 6-15).

The blood pressure of spontaneously perfusing traumatized hypothermic patients creates a functional arteriovenous fistula by diverting part of the cardiac output out the femoral artery through a countercurrent heat exchanger (e.g., Level 1; Flo Temp-IIe). The heated blood is then returned with admixed heated crystalloids via the femoral vein. The additional fluids are titrated and infused by piggyback until hypotension is corrected.

The rate of rewarming exceeds hemodialysis. CAVR does not require the specialized equipment and perfusionist necessary for CPB.[79] The average flow rates are 225 to 375 ml/min, resulting in a rate of rewarming of 3° to 4° C (5.4° to 7.2° F) per hour. Since the catheters are 8.5 Fr, the patient must weigh at least 40 kg. Coagulation begins to appear in the heparinized circuits at around 3 hours.

Venovenous rewarming. In extracorporeal venovenous rewarming, blood is removed, usually from a central venous catheter, heated to 40° C (104° F), and returned via a second central or large peripheral venous catheter. Flow rates of 150 to 400 ml/min have been achieved.[100,111]

The circuit is not complex and is more efficient than many other nonbypass modalities. There is no oxygenator, and since the method does not provide full circulatory support, volume infusion is the only option to augment inadequate cardiac output.

In another variation of the extracorporeal venovenous circuit, blood is removed from the femoral vein, heparinized, and sent through a blood rewarmer via an infusion pump accelerator. It is neutralized with protamine before reinjection into the subclavian or internal jugular vein, which would preferentially rewarm the heart.

Hemodialysis. Standard hemodialysis is widely available, practical, portable, efficient, and should be strongly considered in patients with electrolyte abnormalities, renal failure, or intoxication with a dialyzable substance.[202] Two-way flow catheters allow cannulation of a single vessel.[159] A Drake-Willock single-needle dialysis catheter can be used with a portable hemodialysis machine and external warmer. After central venous cannulation, exchange cycle volumes of 200 to 250 ml/min are possible.

Although heat exchange is less than with standard two-vessel hemodialysis, the ease of percutaneous subclavian vein placement is a major advantage. Hemodialysis via two separate single-lumen catheters placed in the femoral vein can achieve continuous blood flow at 450 to 500 ml/minute.[114,115] In-line hemodialysis also simplifies correction of electrolyte abnormalities. Local vascular complications, including thrombosis of vessels and hemorrhage secondary to anticoagulation, may occur.

With all of these techniques there is no proof that rapid acceleration of the rate of rewarming improves survival rates in perfusing patients. Potential complications of uncontrolled rapid rewarming in severe hypothermia include DIC, pulmonary edema, hemolysis, and acute tubular necrosis.

In hypothermic cardiac arrest, rewarming should be attempted via CPB and hemodialysis when CPR is not contraindicated (Box 6-9), unless frozen intravascular contents prevent flow. Clotted atrial blood or failure to obtain venous return also cause these techniques to fail. If experienced personnel and necessary equipment are unavailable, all other rewarming techniques should be used in combination.[18,282]

DIATHERMY. Diathermy, the transmission of heat by conversion of energy, has been evaluated as a rewarming adjunct in accidental hypothermia.[118,176] Large amounts of heat can be delivered to deep tissues with ultrasonic (0.8 to 1 MHz) and low-frequency (915 to 2450 MHz) microwave radiation. Short-wave (13.56 to 40.68 MHz) modalities are high frequency and do not penetrate deeply. Contraindications include frostbite, burns, significant edema, and all types of metallic implants and pacemakers.

Under ideal conditions in a laboratory study, radiowave frequency (13.56 MHz) electromagnetic re-

---

Box 6-9 CONTRAINDICATIONS TO CARDIOPULMONARY RESUSCITATION IN ACCIDENTAL HYPOTHERMIA

Do-not-resuscitate status is documented and verified.
Obviously lethal injuries are present.
Chest wall depression is impossible.
Any signs of life are present.
Rescuers are endangered by evacuation delays or altered triage conditions.

From Danzl DF et al: *Ann Emerg Med* 16:1042, 1987. Developed in conjunction with the Wilderness Medical Society.

---

gional heating of hypothermic dogs after immersion did not damage tissue at 4 to 6 watts/kg and rapidly elevated the core temperature.[280] Zhong[290] successfully rewarmed 16 piglets with microwave irradiation "until they squealed and suckled." Subsequently, 20 of 28 human infants who were rewarmed with microwave irradiation at 90 to 100 watts survived. The temperature rose an average 1° C (1.8° F) after 6 to 7 minutes, and the average infant required 45 minutes to achieve a rectal temperature of 36° C (96.8° F). In an experimental study of men cooled to 35° C (95° F), warm water immersion rewarming was more rapid than radiowave rewarming with 2.5 watts/kg.[146]

Both ultrasonic and low-frequency microwave diathermy can deliver large quantities of heat below the skin. As dosimetry guidelines are developed, potential complications and ideal application sites for this experimental technique deserve further study in the hospital. In the field setting, potential problems with power supply and electronic and navigational interference have compounded the physiologic problems.

CARDIOPULMONARY RESUSCITATION

Basic and advanced life support recommendations in hypothermia continue to evolve (Figure 6-16).[252] Cardiac output generated with closed chest compressions maintains viability in selected patients with hypothermia.[254] The optimal rate and technique are unknown. Definitive prehospital determination of cardiac activity requires a cardiac monitor, since misdiagnosis of cardiac arrest is a hazard. Peripheral pulses are difficult to palpate when extreme bradycardia is present with peripheral vasoconstriction.

Some authors contend that asystole is a more common presenting rhythm than is VF. In the field, differentiating VF from asystole may be impractical. Possible causes of VF include acid-base fluxes, hypoxia, and coronary vasoconstriction with increased blood viscosity. Chest compressions and various therapeutic interventions are also implicated. The role of acid-

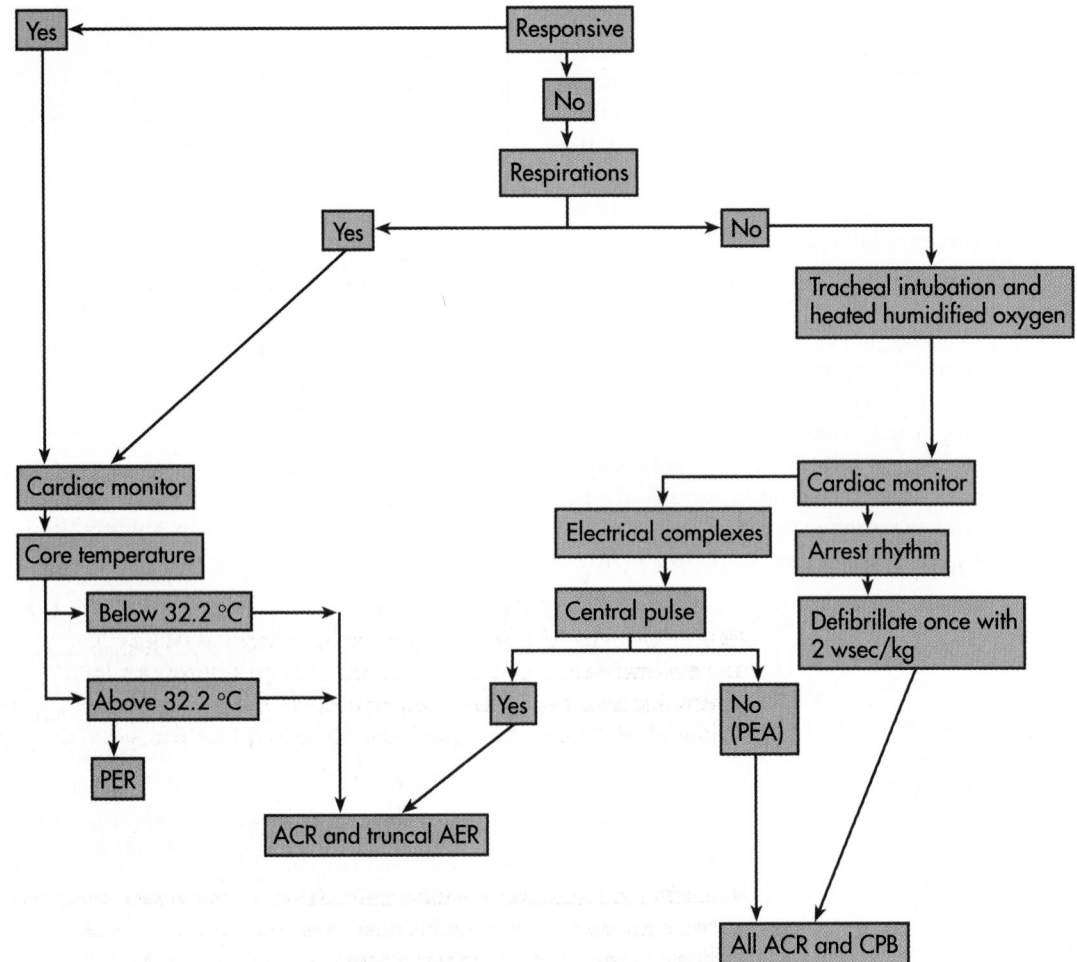

Figure 6-16 Emergency department algorithm. *ACR*, Active core rewarming; *AER*, active external rewarming; *CPB*, cardiopulmonary bypass; *PEA*, pulseless electrical activity; *PER*, passive external rewarming.

base fluxes is not clear. Mild alkalosis appears somewhat protective against VF during controlled, induced hypothermia.[156]

Blood Flow During Chest Compressions

During normothermic conditions, blood flow partially results from phasic alterations in intrathoracic pressure and not just from direct cardiac compression. Niemann[206] demonstrated that antegrade flow occurs without left ventricular compression in a normothermic canine model. Closed chest compressions increase intrathoracic pressure. When thoracic inlet venous valves are competent, the resultant pressure gradient between arterial and venous compartments generates supradiaphragmatic antegrade flow.

Some clinical observations challenge the supremacy of the "cardiac pump" model. This model is predicated on closure of the mitral valve and opening of the aortic valve during chest compression. This allows a forward stroke volume. During release of compression, transmitral flow can fill the left ventricle. Optimal cardiac output is thus generated by achieving the maximal compression rate, which allows maximal left ventricular end diastolic filling. Interestingly, transesophageal echocardiography in a canine model demonstrates mitral valve closure during chest compression except during low-impulse (downstroke momentum) compressions. Compression of a cold, stiff chest wall may be equivalent to low impulse.[45]

In hypothermia the role of a "thoracic pump" with the heart as a passive conduit is an attractive hypothesis. The phasic alterations in intrathoracic pressure generated by compressions are equally applied to all of the cardiac chambers and thoracic vessels. The mitral valve remains open during compression, and blood continues to circulate through the left side of the heart.

Myocardial compliance can be severely reduced in hypothermia. Althaus[3] noted in one of three hypothermia survivors at thoracotomy that "the heart was found to be hard as stone and it is hardly conceivable how effective external cardiac massage could have been." Chest wall elasticity is also decreased with cold, as is pulmonary compliance. Lastly, more force is needed to depress the chest wall sufficiently to generate intrathoracic vascular compartment pressure gradients. Despite these potential physiologic explanations, a large number of neurologically intact survivors remain after prolonged closed chest compressions. The explanation lies in measuring intrathoracic pressures during hypothermic closed chest compressions.

Perfusion enhancement maneuvers remain largely unstudied in hypothermia. Ancillary abdominal binding, as with the abdominal compartment of antishock trousers, might favorably inhibit paradoxical diaphragmatic motion.[45,206] Simultaneous compression and ventilation can increase flow in the heart's left side. Ventilation with the proper carbogen concentration also allows high ventilatory rates while maintaining uncorrected $PaCO_2$ at 40 mm Hg. Placement of a counterpulsation intraaortic balloon is another option. Mechanical thoracic compression devices could be useful during prolonged resuscitations with limited availability of personnel and no bypass capabilities.

During hypothermic cardiac arrest in swine, the cardiac output, cerebral blood flow, and myocardial blood flow averaged 50%, 55%, and 31%, respectively, of those achieved during normothermic closed chest compressions.[184] Blood flow to these areas did not decrease with time, unlike in the normothermic group. No significant difference in flow generated appeared between normothermic and hypothermic swine at 20 minutes. Hypothermic rheologic changes, including increased viscosity, also affect flow. Peripheral vascular resistance is expected to increase during vasoconstriction, but in the swine there was no difference in systemic and organ vascular resistance between normothermic and hypothermic CPR.[184]

In a multicenter survey of 428 cases, 9 of the 27 patients receiving CPR initiated in the field survived, as did 6 of 14 patients with emergency department-initiated CPR.[49] Based on these cases and a literature review, refinements of the American Heart Association's CPR standards in hypothermia have been proposed (see Box 6-9).[67]

Since cardiac output is the product of heart rate and stroke volume, the optimal closed chest compression rate should be the fastest rate allowing optimal ventricular filling. Many patients have recovered neurologically following slow compression rates. One recovered after 220 minutes at half the normal compression rate.[207] The optimal rate probably has a direct linear relationship with the degree of hypothermia.[45]

Tissue decomposition, apparent rigor mortis, dependent lividity, and fixed, dilated pupils are not reliable criteria for withholding CPR. In addition, intermittent flow may provide adequate support during evacuation. Therefore CPR should not be withheld only because continuous chest compressions cannot be ensured.[35] The

lowest temperature documented in an infant survivor of accidental hypothermia is 15.2° C (59.4° F), in an adult is 13.7° C (56.8° F),[91a] and in induced hypothermia is 9° C (48.2° F).[42,54,203,208] One patient recovered after 6½ hours of closed chest compressions.[169] In Saskatchewan in 1994 a 2-year-old child reportedly recovered from a core temperature of 13.9° C (57° F).

Respiratory Considerations

When cardiopulmonary arrest develops during resuscitation, noncardiac causes are often pulmonary emboli or progressive respiratory insufficiency. Provision of adequate oxygen supply is essential during rapid rewarming. For each 1° C (1.8° F) rise in temperature, oxygen consumption increases up to three times[76] (see Box 6-1).

Endotracheal intubation and ventilation decrease atelectasis and ventilation-perfusion mismatch. Complete airway protection averts aspiration, which is otherwise common in depressed airway reflexes, bronchorrhea, and ileus. Carbon dioxide production also drops by half with an 8° C (14.4° F) fall in the temperature. During induced hypothermia, carbogen (1% to 5% carbon dioxide added to oxygen) facilitates acid-base management by allowing adjustment of the fractional inspired CO_2 concentration ($FiCO_2$) while adjusting the ventilation.[188]

Past controversy regarding the hazards of endotracheal intubation reflected coincidental episodes and a miscitation by Fell[71] of a series of hypothermic overdoses by Lee and Ames.[164] Fell stated that "endotracheal intubation was followed by cardiac arrest in a large proportion of cases," whereas Lee and Ames merely cautioned of that possibility. In a multicenter survey, endotracheal intubation was performed on 117 patients by multiple operators in various settings.[51] No induced arrhythmias were recognized, which is consistent with several reports. Danzl and Miller[46,196] also nasotracheally intubated 40 hypothermic patients without incident, and Ledingham and Mone[163] did not note arrhythmias in their series of 44 cases. Potential arrhythmogenic factors include hypoxia, mechanical jostling, and acid-base or electrolyte fluctuations.

The indications for endotracheal intubation in hypothermia are identical to those in normothermia.[48,52,92] It is required unless the patient possesses intact protective airway reflexes. Ciliary activity is depressed in hypothermia, frothy sputum produces chest congestion, and bronchorrhea resembles pulmonary edema. Fiberoptic or blind nasotracheal intubation is preferable to cricothyroidotomy when cold-induced trismus or potential cervical spine trauma is present. Oral rather than nasal intubation is advisable in coagulopathic patients to avoid causing major epistaxis.

As expected, hypothermia prolongs the duration of neuromuscular blockade. With pancuronium the block is prolonged because metabolism into inactive metabolites is markedly decreased. Neuromuscular blockade is also prolonged with vecuronium and atracurium.

RESUSCITATION PHARMACOLOGY

The pharmacologic effects of medications are temperature dependent. The lower the temperature, the greater the degree of protein binding. Enterohepatic circulation and renal excretion are also altered, so abnormal physiologic drug responses should be anticipated. The usual clinical scenario consists of substandard therapeutic activity while the patient is severely hypothermic, progressing to toxicity after rewarming.[193] Medications are not given orally because of decreased gastrointestinal function, and intramuscular medications are avoided because they may be erratically absorbed from vasoconstricted sites.

The pharmacologic manipulation of respiratory drive, pulse, and blood pressure is generally not indicated. When relative tachycardia is not consistent with temperature depression, the possibility of hypovolemia, hypoglycemia, or a toxic ingestion should be considered. Vasopressors are potentially arrhythmogenic, lower VF threshold, and cannot increase peripheral vascular resistance if the vasculature is already maximally constricted.[163] Vasodilators can precipitate core temperature afterdrop.

If intraarterial pressure is not consistent with the degree of hypothermia, judicious use of inotropic agents may be necessary.[211] Dopamine can be a successful adjunctive treatment.[236] Dopamine reverses cardiovascular depression under hypothermic conditions equivalent to up to 5° C (9° F) rewarming. Dopamine decreases systemic vascular resistance at low infusion doses and increases it at high infusion rates.[211]

There is conflicting evidence regarding cardiovascular function after rewarming. In some studies, there was complete reversal of cold-induced changes, whereas in another, the physiologic response to norepinephrine was paradoxical.[276]

Patients with profound hypothermia after ethanol ingestion have been resuscitated with low-dose dopamine support. In frostbite victims, however, the use of catecholamines may jeopardize the extremities.[178] Catecholamines also exacerbate preexistent occult hypokalemia.

The effect of temperature depression on the autonomic nervous system is still being investigated. In primates, cooling produces a biphasic response in plasma catecholamine concentrations. After an initial increase, the autonomic nervous system switches off at 29° C (84.2° F),[34] suggesting that catecholamine support might be useful below that temperature. The initial rise in catecholamine levels could also be caused by acute respiratory acidosis, which stimulates the sympathetic

nervous system.[24] Low-dose dopamine (1 to 5 mg/kg/min) or other catecholamine infusions are generally reserved for severely hypotensive patients who do not respond to crystalloid resuscitation and rewarming.

Thyroid

The most dramatic "Rip Van Winkle" rude awakening from hypothermic myxedema coma was Dr. Richard Asher's patient in the 1950s. He was successfully metabolically aroused from a 7-year 30° C (86° F) slumber. Ironically, so was a quiescent oat cell carcinoma.

Cold induces stimulation of the hypothalamic-pituitary-thyroid axis. Unless myxedema is suspected, empirical therapy is not recommended. A history of neck irradiation, radioactive iodine, Hashimoto's thyroiditis, or surgical treatment of hyperthyroidism should heighten the clinician's suspicion of myxedema. Failure to rewarm despite an appropriate course of therapy is a further clue.[183]

Myxedema coma is usually precipitated in elderly patients with chronic hypothyroidism who are stressed by trauma, infection, anesthesia, or medication ingestion. Typical nonspecific laboratory abnormalities include hyponatremia, anemia, and liver enzyme and lipid elevations. If myxedema coma is suspected, thyroid function studies, including serum thyroxine (T_4) by radioimmunoassay, triiodothyronine (T_3) resin uptake, and thyroid-stimulating hormone, should be obtained and serum cortisol level measured.

Given the appropriate index of suspicion, the physician should administer 250 to 500 μg levothyroxine (T_4) intravenously over several minutes without waiting for confirmatory laboratory results. Daily injections of 100 μg are required for 5 to 7 days. It is appropriate to consider adding at least 100 to 250 mg of hydrocortisone to the first 3 L of intravenous fluid. Absorption of T_4 is erratic if the drug is given orally or intramuscularly. The onset of action of T_3 is more rapid, which jeopardizes cardiovascular stability; therefore T_3 is avoided in acute replacement therapy. The onset of action of T_4 is 6 to 12 hours, evidenced by continuous improvement of the vital signs during rewarming. Up to one half of the T_4 is eventually converted by the peripheral tissues into T_3.[49]

Steroids

Acute cold stress and many coexisting disease processes stimulate cortisol secretion. The free active fraction of cortisol decreases as the temperature drops because of increased protein binding, and cortisol utilization is similarly decreased. The increase in adrenocorticotropic hormone (ACTH) and adrenal steroid secretion may also be a neurogenic or emotional response in the conscious subject to an unpleasant environment. In rodents, inhibition of ACTH secretion during hypothermia is mediated by decreased hypothalamic secretion of arginine vasopressin and oxytocin. This decreases pituitary responsiveness to corticotropin-releasing factor, inhibiting corticotropin release. Thus exogenous arginine vasopressin could prove helpful during rewarming.

Cold exposure also induces adrenal unresponsiveness to ACTH. As a result, false diagnosis of decreased adrenal reserve is possible and does not represent functional adrenal insufficiency, since ACTH levels return to normal after rewarming. Serum cortisol levels are commonly elevated. Secondary adrenal insufficiency resulting from panhypopituitarism may also coexist with myxedema. Empirical administration of steroids is not indicated unless hypoadrenocorticism is suspected based on a previous history of steroid dependence, suggestive physical findings, or an inexplicable failure to rewarm. The use of narcotic antagonists in hypothermia is reported. Naloxone may reduce the severity of hypothermia in drug overdoses and in spinal shock and appears to have activity at the mu receptor sites.[49]

RESUSCITATION COMPLICATIONS

Atrial Arrhythmias

All atrial arrhythmias, including atrial fibrillation, should have a slow ventricular response with the temperature depression. Atrial fibrillation is commonly noted below 32° C (89.6° F) in accidental hypothermia victims.[278] Atrial fibrillation usually converts spontaneously during rewarming, and digitalization is not warranted. Electrophysiologic studies show that the interval prolongation present on His bundle electrocardiography is unresponsive to atropine. Mesenteric embolization is a potential hazard when the rhythm converts back to sinus rhythm.

Hypothermia renders the negative inotropic effects of calcium channel blockers redundant. Although verapamil has been used to resuscitate a profoundly hypothermic patient after near drowning, any additional cerebral protective effects are speculative. In summary, all new atrial arrhythmias usually convert spontaneously during rewarming and should be considered innocent. Attention is directed toward correcting acid-base, fluid, and electrolyte imbalances while avoiding administration of atrial antiarrhythmics.

Ventricular Arrhythmias

Since preexisting chronic ventricular ectopy may be suppressed in a cold heart, the physician noting ectopy during rewarming is placed in a quandary. The history from the hypothermic patient may be unproductive, and the past cardiac history is often unavailable.

Transient ventricular arrhythmias are generally to be ignored. In one study of 22 continuously monitored patients with hypothermia, supraventricular arrhythmias

were common (nine cases) and benign.[220] Ventricular extrasystoles developed in 10 patients, but none experienced ventricular tachycardia (VT) or VF during rewarming. The terminal rhythm in the eight who died while being monitored was asystole and not VF. The energetics of the fibrillating hypothermic ventricle are under investigation because asystole may consume less energy and be more protective.

Pharmacologic options are limited, since hypothermia induces complex physiologic changes that result in abnormal responses.[283] Drug metabolism and excretion are both progressively decreased. In normothermia, class IA ventricular antiarrhythmics have negative inotropic and indirect anticholinergic effects, and moderately decrease conduction velocity (Box 6-10). Procainamide increases the incidence of VF during hypothermia. Quinidine has been useful during induced profound hypothermia, preventing VF during cardiac manipulation at 25° to 30° C (77° to 86° F). No reports detail the effects of disopyramide. In class IB, lidocaine is yet to be proven effective for prophylaxis and is ineffective in facilitating defibrillation. In animal studies, lidocaine and propranolol have

---

Box 6-10   ANTIARRHYTHMIC AGENTS

Class I. Sodium channel blockers
  IA. Conduction and depolarization moderately slowed
    Action potential duration (APD) and repolarization
      prolonged
      Disopyramide
      Procainamide
      Quinidine
  IB. Conduction and depolarization minimally slowed
    APD and repolarization shortened
      Lidocaine
      Mexiletine
      Moricizine
      Phenytoin
      Tocainide
    Conduction and depolarization markedly slowed
      APD and repolarization prolonged
      Encainide
      Flecainide
Class II. β-Adrenergic blockers
Class III. Antifibrillatory properties
  APD prolonged
    Amiodarone
    Bretylium
    d-Sotalol
Class IV. Calcium channel blockers
  Diltiazem
  Verapamil
Unclassified
  Adenosine
  Magnesium sulfate

minimal hemodynamic effects in hypothermia. If normothermic effects persisted during hypothermia, the class IB agents would appear attractive because they minimally slow conduction while shortening the action potential duration (APD).

The class III agent bretylium tosylate, a unique bromobenzyl quaternary ammonium compound, has been extremely effective in several animal studies.[65] This class of agents seems most ideal pharmacologically because it possesses direct antifibrillatory properties. The ability to prolong the action potential duration is temperature dependent. Ideally, a drug would lengthen the APD only in warmer regions to reduce dispersion. (See Box 6-11.)

Bretylium causes chemical sympathectomy and is both an antiarrhythmic and antifibrillatory agent. Bretylium increases the VF threshold, APD, and effective refractory period. Interestingly, at least at normal temperatures, antifibrillatory effects occur more acutely than do antiarrhythmic effects.

In the first study to evaluate the effects of bretylium administered after induction of hypothermia, Murphy[200] noted that only one of 11 dogs given bretylium (mean 40.5 mg/kg) before five invasive maneuvers developed VF. No dog, including control subjects, showed fibrillation during endotracheal intubation. Of note during discussions regarding prophylaxis, three of the 11 dogs converted to VF during the drug infusion. The effect of bretylium on plasma catecholamines and electrically induced arrhythmias has also been studied. Since catecholamine levels increase during cooling, the demonstrated protection appears to result from alteration of electrophysiologic properties of the cardiac tissues.[209] Amiodarone, another class III drug that possesses direct antifibrillatory activity, would be an interesting agent to study during hypothermic conditions. Also of note, magnesium sulfate at a dose of 100 mg/kg IV can spontaneously defibrillate most patients on CPB at 30° C (86° F) with induced hypothermia.

Emergency transvenous intracardiac pacing of bradyarrhythmias is extremely risky with cold hearts because it commonly precipitates VF. New arrhythmias that develop after rewarming may require pacing on rare occasions. Transcutaneous pacing (TCP) with low-resistance electrodes seems far preferable before stabilization. In a canine model, TCP restored and maintained hemodynamic stability and rewarmed hypothermic animals twice as rapidly as it did the controls.[59]

In summary, bretylium is the only agent shown to have antiarrhythmic activity during hypothermic conditions. Two cases of chemical ventricular defibrillation after infusion of bretylium 10 mg/kg in accidental hypothermia are reported.[47,152] Bretylium appears to be the agent of choice for VF in hypothermia. Bretylium prophylaxis is investigational because toxicity, optimal dosage, and particularly the ideal rate of infusion are unknown.

Sepsis

Our knowledge of the pathophysiology of sepsis in hypothermia continues to improve.[37] Classic signs of infection, including erythema and fever, are absent. Rigors and shakes resemble shivering. The initial history, physical, and laboratory data are often unreliable, so repeated evaluations and comprehensive culturing are mandatory in the ED. The 10% subset of patients with sepsis syndrome who manifest a hypothermic response have a significantly increased frequency of shock and death, and this secondary hypothermia does not appear to be protective.

Hypothermia compromises host defenses and results in serious bacterial infections. These significant infections can be accompanied by minimal inflammatory response. Some common etiologic organisms include gram-negative bacteria, gram-positive cocci, oral anaerobes, and Enterobacteriaceae.[168]

The core endotoxin components of gram-negative bacteria normally signal macrophages. At a normal or elevated temperature, active cytokine triggers include tumor necrosis factor, interleukin-1, and interleukin-6. The potential role of antiendotoxin monoclonal antibodies in patients with accidental but not cytokine-induced hypothermia is unresolved. Bone marrow release and circulation of neutrophils are compromised for up to 12 hours. In addition, human and porcine neutrophils are susceptible to hypothermia. In vitro, neutrophil migration and bacterial phagocytosis are reduced at 29° C (84.2° F). Neutrophilic extermination of various bacteria, including *Staphylococcus aureus* and *Streptococcus faecalis*, is also impaired.

Acquired neutrophil dysfunction is also identified. In addition, hypothermia was associated with decreased neutrophil levels in 40 near-drowned children. As a clinical demonstration of the importance of these factors, therapeutic maintenance of hypothermia to control cerebral edema in near drowning has been abandoned because of the substantial incidence of infectious complications.[49]

The reported incidence of infection varies dramatically with the victim's age and the clinical series re-

---

Box 6-11 ANTIARRHYTHMIC CHARACTERISTICS

The ideal ventricular antiarrhythmic would:
1. Cause no further decrease in conduction velocity
2. Shorten action potential duration (APD)
3. Only lengthen the APD in warmer regions of the myocardium to reduce dispersion
4. Possess direct antifibrillatory properties

ported.[168,278] In one group of 51 infants, 27 had sepsis.[44] Although there were no reliable indicators of infection, some suggestive clues were present. Serum glucose and leukocyte abnormalities, anemia, uremia, and bradycardia were often identified. In addition to *Staphylococcus* and *Streptococcus,* the predominant organisms were *Haemophilus* and Enterobacteriaceae.

Lung infections, usually in the right upper lobe, were reported in 80 of 138 hypothermic infants by El-Radhi et al.[66] Evaluation of the gastric aspirate was another diagnostic predictor of sepsis in 36 of 44 infected infants. In several studies, sepsis was found in 8% to 74% of hypothermic infants.[44] In this age group, empirical broad-spectrum antibiotics are warranted.

In adults the incidence of infection ranges from less than 1% to over 40%, depending on patient selection criteria.[51,168,278] In Lewin's series,[168] serious soft tissue or pulmonary infections were present in 24 of 59 patients and in nine the infection was undiagnosed when the patient was admitted from the ED. Occult bacteremia was present in less than 1% of White's series[278] of 102 patients, and results were negative in all of the 46 lumbar punctures. In other studies of hypothermic elderly patients admitted to hospitals, most have had evidence of probable or definite infections.[53]

Invasive hemodynamic monitoring, although risky, may suggest an infection. Before patients are rewarmed, the combination of an elevated cardiac index and decreased systemic vascular resistance should suggest bacteremia. Right heart catheterization is more hazardous in hypothermia than during normothermia.

In summary, unlike children and the elderly, most previously healthy young adults do not need empirical antibiotic prophylaxis. Nevertheless, treatment indications should be liberalized from normothermia. They should include failure to rewarm or any suspicion or evidence of aspiration, myositis, chest x-ray infiltrate, bacteriuria, or persistent altered mental status. In choosing broad-spectrum coverage, the physician should consider altered drug interactions, volumes of distribution, protein binding, hepatic metabolism, and renal excretion. The combination of an aminoglycoside with a broad-spectrum β-lactam antibiotic is often appropriate.

FORENSIC PATHOLOGY

Macromorphologic and micromorphologic lesions are variable and nonspecific in hypothermia, and there is no single pathognomonic finding at autopsy.[170] Establishing hypothermia as the primary cause of death requires an adequate history of exposure and the absence of other lethal findings at necropsy.[4] For example, unnatural deaths in nursing home patients may be significantly underreported for these reasons.[40]

Macroscopic skin changes can suggest the diagnosis. Hyperemia of the dorsa of the hands and knees is commonly found. Nonpathognomonic findings have been identified in the pancreas, lungs, and heart.[116] Pancreatic findings include fat necrosis, aseptic pancreatitis, and hemorrhage. Pulmonary changes consist of intraalveolar, interstitial, and intrabronchial hemorrhages.

An eye that has been directly exposed to the environment could be a chemical indicator of both the environmental and victim temperature at the time of death. Vitreous humor chemistry profiles at autopsy can reveal that glucose concentration and total carbon dioxide content vary inversely with temperature, with values significantly higher in the winter. An elevated vitreous glucose in a nondiabetic victim should suggest hypothermia.

The total urinary catecholamine content, particularly epinephrine, was high in one group of casualties known to be hypothermic. Erosions of the gastric mucosa, termed *Wischnewsky spots,* are also frequently found.[256] In addition, exposure to extreme cold should be suspected when unusual intravascular hemolysis, which is seen after freezing of blood, is observed in a corpse.[150]

PREVENTION

To function optimally "as the water stiffens" requires an understanding of the principles of heat conservation and loss.[143] Well-trained and educated urban adults can participate in prolonged Arctic maneuvers safely.[242,243,258] To maintain core temperature in the narrow band necessary for peak functioning in cold environments, appropriate adaptive behavioral responses are essential.[121] Autonomic and endocrinologic mechanisms are only supplemental.

Studies of human cold adaptation have reached highly variable conclusions. Explanations for these discrepancies include changes in core and shell temperatures and in metabolic rates before and after cold adaptation. Some observations indicate hypothermic insulative isometabolic cold adaptation associated with local cold adaptation of the extremities.[232]

Excellent physical conditioning with adequate rest and nutrition is paramount.[22] Hikers and skiers must be accompanied by a partner and should wear effective thermal insulation. Wet inner garments must be changed promptly. Persons who exert themselves, including long-distance skiers, should switch garments depending on current exertional heat production.[122-124] Since dehydration must be avoided, drinking from a cold stream is preferable to snow ingestion. Significant energy is needed to convert ice at 0° C (32° F) into water at 0° C.

All areas with a large surface area/volume ratio should be well insulated.[286] The uncovered head can lose a large percentage of the body's total heat production. Of note, adrenergic vasoconstriction does not occur effectively in the head and neck region,[99] which is why a nightcap (not originally Kentucky bourbon) is effective when worn to bed. Excellent synthetic insulating materials include Gore-Tex, Thinsulate, and taslanized nylon.

Flectalon, a web of aluminized polyvinyl chloride fibers, is also a good insulating material. In comparing its insulating efficacy with that of other materials, the "critical" temperature was determined. This is defined as the lowest environmental temperature at which the core temperature can be maintained without increased oxygen consumption. Flectalon lowers the critical temperature more than Thinsulate and may prove useful as an insulator to prevent and treat hypothermia.

Under certain circumstances, insidious hypothermia may develop during exposure to cold water because of the effects of increased insulation on compensatory physiologic events.[8,145] The army mnemonic "COLD," in reference to insulation with clothing, is *clean, open* during exercise to avoid sweating, *loose* layers to retain heat, and *dry* to limit conductive heat losses. For a complete discussion of preventive measures, refer to Chapters 9 and 71.

Prevention of urban accidental hypothermia requires continuous public education. For example, the optimal safe indoor temperature recommendation for the elderly has risen to 21.1° C (70° F).[172] Energy assistance and temporary sheltering are effective measures, and selective heating of sleeping quarters and use of electric blankets are economical suggestions. Prewarming bed and bedroom at night may be the best overall advice to the elderly.

OUTCOME

Even during normothermia, there is often no consensus regarding for how long to continue resuscitative efforts. Partially because of the dramatic reports of reanimations, the standard of care has been that "no one is dead until they are warm and dead." In reality, some victims are clearly dead when they are cold and dead, and it would be useful to safely identify them.[6]

Survival is difficult to predict because human physiologic responses to temperature depression vary so widely.[216] The type and severity of the underlying or precipitating disease process are two determinants. Age extremes, although not statistically correlated with survival, are commonly associated with severe illnesses. In a multicenter survey, however, there were no significant age differences in mortality.

Gender, trauma, infection, and toxin ingestions affected survival differently in multiple, uncontrolled clinical studies. There were no clinically significant differences in male vs. female profiles in the multicenter survey.[51] From a large hypothermia database, a hypothermia outcome score has been developed that could enable multiple observers at differing sites to assess treatment modalities and outcome predictors. Prehospital cardiac arrest, low or absent blood pressure, elevated BUN, and the need for either endotracheal or nasogastric intubation in the ED were significant predictors of outcome after multivariant analysis.[52,147,233]

In a multiple regression analysis of 234 cases in Swiss clinics,[177] the biggest negative survival factors were asphyxia, slow rate of cooling, invasive rewarming, asystole, and development of pulmonary edema or adult respiratory distress syndrome. Positive predictors of survival include rapid cooling rate, presence of VF during cardiac arrest, and narcotic or ethanol intoxication. In a study of 29 patients below 30° C (86° F), mode of cooling was the only independent risk factor.[216]

In a study of CPB survivors, 15 of the 32 patients are long-term survivors.[270] Their neuropsychologic functioning after prolonged prehospital circulatory arrest is very encouraging. These patients were not asphyxiated before becoming hypothermic. Vretenar[267] reviewed the literature regarding the outcomes of 68 other patients resuscitated with CPB. The survival rate was 60%, and the coldest survivor was 15° C (59° F).

There is need for a valid triage marker of death, since vital organ damage is difficult to predict. In one retrospective analysis of primarily avalanche burial victims, extreme hyperkalemia was noted on initial examination and resuscitation proved fruitless.[233] In the Mt. Hood tragedy the nonsurvivors also were hyperkalemic (serum potassium greater than 10 mmol/L).[108] In both of these reports, asphyxia and compression injury may have been contributory. Other indicators of a grave prognosis include a core temperature below 12° C (53.6° F), arterial pH below 6.5, or evidence of intravascular thrombosis (direct visualization; fibrinogen below 50 mg %).

REFERENCES

1. Albiin N, Eriksson A: Fatal accidental hypothermia and alcohol, *Alcohol Alcohol* 19:13, 1984.
2. Allison TG et al: Cardiovascular responses to immersion in a hot tub in comparison with exercise in male subjects with coronary artery disease, *Mayo Clin Proc* 68:19, 1993.
3. Althaus U, Aeberhard P, Schupbach P: Management of profound accidental hypothermia with cardiorespiratory arrest, *Ann Surg* 195:492, 1982.
4. Ambach E, Tributsch W, Henn R: Fatal accidents on glaciers: forensic, criminological, and glaciological conclusions, *J Forensic Sci* 36:1469, 1991.
5. Antretter H, Bonatti J, Dapunt OE: Accidental hypothermia, *N Engl J Med* 332:1033, 1995.
6. Auerbach PS: Some people are dead when they're cold and dead, *JAMA* 264:1856, 1990 (editorial).
7. Avidan MS et al: Convection warmers—not just hot air, *Anaesthesia* 52:1073, 1997.
8. Bagian JP, Kaufman JW: Effectiveness of the space shuttle anti-exposure system in a cold water environment, *Aviat Space Environ Med* 61:753, 1990.
9. Baraka AS et al: Effect of alpha-stat versus pH-stat strategy on oxyhemoglobin dissociation and whole body oxygen consumption during hypothermia cardiopulmonary bypass, *Anesth Analg* 74:32, 1992.
10. Barr GL, Halvorsen LO, Donovan J: Correction of hypothermia by continuous pleural perfusion, *Surgery* 103:553, 1988.
11. Bastow MD, Rawlings J, Allison SP: Undernutrition, hypothermia, and injury in elderly women with fractured femur: an injury response to altered metabolism? *Lancet* 1:143, 1983.

12. Baumgartner FJ et al: Cardiopulmonary bypass for resuscitation of patients with accidental hypothermia and cardiac arrest, *Can J Surg* 35:184, 1992.

13. Becker H, Vinten-Johansen JI, Buckberg GD: Myocardial damage caused by keeping pH 7.40 during systemic deep hypothermia, *J Thorac Cardiovasc Surg* 82:810, 1981.

14. Bergersen TK, Eriksen M, Walloe L: Effect of local warming on hand and finger artery blood velocities, *Am J Physiol* 269:R325, 1995.

15. Bjornstad H, Tande PM, Refsum H: Cardiac electrophysiology during hypothermia: implications for medical treatment, *Arctic Med Res* 50:71, 1991.

16. Bjornstad H, Tande PM, Refsum H: Class III antiarrhythmic action of d-sotalol during hypothermia, *Am Heart J* 121:1429, 1991.

17. Block R et al: Does hypothermia protect against the development of hepatitis in paracetamol overdose? *Anaesthesia* 47:789, 1992.

18. Bolgiano E, Sykes L, Barish RA: Accidental hypothermia with cardiac arrest: recovery following rewarming by cardiopulmonary bypass, *J Emerg Med* 10:427, 1992.

19. Bolte RG et al: The use of extracorporeal rewarming in a child submerged for 66 minutes, *JAMA* 260:377, 1988.

20. Bowen DR: Efficiency of the thermal jacket on the delivered temperature of prewarmed crystalloid intravenous fluid, *AANA J* 60:369, 1992.

21. Bowman W: *Outdoor emergency care: comprehensive first aid for non-urban settings,* Lakewood, Colorado, 1988, National Ski Patrol System.

22. Bracker MD: Environmental and thermal injury, *Clin Sports Med* 11:419, 1992.

23. Brandson RD, Chatburn RL: Humidification of inspired gases during mechanical ventilation, *Respir Care* 38:461, 1993 (editorial).

24. Brimioulle S: Sympathetic nervous system activity during hypothermia, *Crit Care Med* 12:924, 1984.

25. Bristow GK, Sessler DI, Giesbrecht GG: Leg temperature and heat content in humans during immersion hypothermia and rewarming, *Aviat Space Environ Med* 65:220, 1994.

26. Britt LD, Dascombe WH, Rodriguez A: New horizons in management of hypothermia and frostbite injury, *Surg Clin North Am* 71:345, 1991.

27. Browne DA, deBoeck R, Morgan M: An evaluation of the Level 1 blood warmer series, *Anaesthesia* 45:960, 1990.

28. Brunette DD et al: Comparison of gastric and closed thoracic cavity lavage in the treatment of severe hypothermia in dogs, *Am J Emerg Med* 16:1222, 1987.

29. Brunette DD et al: Internal cardiac massage and mediastinal irrigation in hypothermic cardiac arrest, *Am J Emerg Med* 10:32, 1992.

30. Cahill CJ, Balmi PJ, Tipton MJ: An evaluation of hand immersion for rewarming individuals cooled by immersion in cold water, *Aviat Space Environ Med* 66:418, 1995.

31. Canivet JL, Larbuisson R, Lamy M: Influence of face mask-CPAP in one case of severe accidental hypothermia, *Acta Anaesthesiol Belg* 40:281, 1989.

32. Cattermole TJ: The epidemiology of cold injury in Antarctica, *Aviat Space Environ Med* 70:135, 1999.

33. CDC: Hypothermia-related deaths—Vermont, October 1994-February 1996, *MMWR* 45:1093, 1996.

34. Chernow B et al: Sympathetic nervous system "switch-off" with severe hypothermia, *Crit Care Med* 11:677, 1983.

35. Chochinov AH et al: Recovery of a 62 year old male from prolonged cold water immersion, *Ann Emerg Med* 31:127, 1998.

36. Clayton DG et al: A comparison of the performance of 20 pulse oximeters under conditions of poor perfusion, *Anaesthesia* 46:3, 1991.

37. Clemmer TP et al: Hypothermia in the sepsis syndrome and clinical outcome. The Methylprednisolone Severe Sepsis Study Group, *Crit Care Med* 20:1395, 1992.

38. Cohen IL et al: Endotracheal tube occlusion associated with the use of heat and moisture exchangers in the intensive care unit, *Crit Care Med* 16:277, 1988.

39. Cohen JA et al: Increased pulmonary artery perforating potential of pulmonary artery catheters during hypothermia, *J Cardiothorac Vasc Anesth* 5:235, 1991.

40. Corey TS, Weakley-Jones B, Nichols GR: Unnatural deaths in nursing home patients, *J Forensic Sci* 37:222, 1992.

41. Cosgriff N et al: Predicting life-threatening coagulopathy in the massively transfused trauma patient: hypothermia and acidoses revisited, *J Trauma* 42:857, 1997.

42. Currie AE: How cold can you get? A case of severe neonatal hypothermia, *J R Soc Med* 87:293, 1994.

43. Daanen HA, Van De Linde FJ: Comparison of four noninvasive rewarming methods for mild hypothermia, *Aviat Space Environ Med* 63:1070, 1992.

44. Dagan R, Gorodischer R: Infections in hypothermic infants younger than 3 months old, *Am J Dis Child* 183:483, 1984.

45. Danzl DF: Blood flow during closed chest compressions in hypothermic humans, *Wilderness Med* 7:12, 1991.

46. Danzl DF, O'Brien DJ: The ECG computer program: mort de froid, *J Wilderness Med* 3:328, 1992.

47. Danzl DF, Pozos RS: Accidental hypothermia, *N Engl J Med* 331:1756, 1994.

48. Danzl DF, Pozos RS: Accidental hypothermia, *N Engl J Med* 332:1033, 1995 (correspondence).

49. Danzl DF, Pozos RS, Hamlet MP: Accidental hypothermia. In Auerbach PS, editor: *Management of wilderness and environmental emergencies,* ed 3, St Louis, 1995, Mosby.

50. Danzl DF, Thomas DM: Nasotracheal intubations in the emergency department, *Crit Care Med* 8:677, 1980.

51. Danzl DF et al: Multicenter hypothermia survey, *Ann Emerg Med* 16:1042, 1987.

52. Danzl DF et al: Hypothermia outcome score: development and implications, *Crit Care Med* 17:227, 1989.

53. Darowski A et al: Hypothermia and infection in elderly patients admitted to hospital, *Age Ageing* 20:100, 1991.

54. DaVee TS, Reineberg EJ: Extreme hypothermia and ventricular fibrillation, *Ann Emerg Med* 9:100, 1980.

55. Deimi R, Hess W: Successful therapy of a cardiac arrest during accidental hypothermia using extracorporeal circulation, *Anaesthesist* 41:93, 1992.

56. Deklunder G et al: Influence of ventilation of the face on thermoregulation in man during hyper- and hypothermia, *Eur J Appl Physiol* 62:342, 1991.

57. Delaney KA et al: Assessment of acid-base disturbances and their physiologic consequences, *Ann Emerg Med* 18:72, 1989.

58. DelRossi AJ et al: Heparinless extracorporeal bypass for treatment of hypothermia, *J Trauma* 30:79, 1990.

59. Dixon RG et al: Transcutaneous pacing in a hypothermic dog model, *Ann Emerg Med* 29:602, 1997.

60. Dobson JAR, Burgess JJ: Resuscitation of severe hypothermia by extracorporeal rewarming in a child, *J Trauma* 40:483, 1996.

61. Ducharme MB et al: Efficacy of forced-air and inhalation rewarming in humans during mild (T_{co}=33.9° C) hypothermia. In Shapiro Y, Moran DS, Epstein Y, et al: *Environmental ergonomics: recent progress and new frontiers,* London, 1996, Freund Publishing Co.

62. Ducharme MG, Tikuisis P: Role of blood as heat source or sink in human limbs during local cooling and heating, *J Appl Physiol* 76:2084, 1994.

63. Ducharme MG et al: Forced-air rewarming in −20° C simulated field conditions, *Ann NY Acad Sci* 813:676, 1997.

64. Duguid H, Simpson RG, Stowers JM: Accidental hypothermia, *Lancet* 2:1213, 1961.

65. Elenbaas RM et al: Bretylium in hypothermia-induced ventricular fibrillation in dogs, *Ann Emerg Med* 13:994, 1984.

66. El-Rahdi AS et al: Infection in neonatal hypothermia, *Arch Dis Child* 58:143, 1983.

67. Emergency cardiac care committee and subcommittees: Guidelines for cardiopulmonary resuscitation and emergency cardiac care. IV. Special resuscitation situations, *JAMA* 268:224, 1992.

68. Ereth MH, Lennon RL, Sessler DL: Limited heat transfer between thermal compartments during rewarming in vasoconstricted patients, *Aviat Space Environ Med* 63:1065, 1992.

69. Erickson RS, Yount ST: Effect of aluminzed covers on body temperature in patients having abdominal surgery, *Heart Lung* 20:255, 1991.

70. Faries G et al: Temperature relationship to distance and flow rate of warmed IV fluids, *Ann Emerg Med* 20:1198, 1991.

71. Fell RH et al: Severe hypothermia as a result of barbiturate overdose complicated by cardiac arrest, *Lancet* 1:392, 1968.

72. Ferrara A et al: Hypothermia and acidosis worsen coagulopathy in the patient requiring massive transfusion, *Am J Surg* 160:515, 1990.

73. Ferraro FJ Jr et al: Cold-induced hypercoagulability in vitro: a trauma connection, *Am Surg* 58:355, 1992.

74. Fildes J, Sheaff C, Barrett J: Very hot intravenous fluid in the treatment of hypothermia, *J Trauma* 35:683, 1993.

75. Fishbeck KH, Simon RP: Neurological manifestations of accidental hypothermia, *Ann Neurol* 10:384, 1981.

76. Fisher A et al: Oxygen availability during hypothermic cardiopulmonary bypass, *Crit Care Med* 5:154, 1977.

77. Frank DH, Robson MC: Accidental hypothermia treated without mortality, *Surg Gynecol Obstet* 151:379, 1980.

78. Gallaher MM et al: Pedestrian and hypothermia deaths among Native Americans in New Mexico; between bar and home, *JAMA* 267:1345, 1992.

79. Garlow L, Kokiko J, Pino-Marina R: Hypothermia in a 62 year old man: use of the continuous arteriovenous rewarming technique, *J Emerg Nurs* 22:477, 1996 (case review).

80. Gentilello LM, Rifley WJ: Continuous arteriovenous rewarming: report of a new technique for treating hypothermia, *J Trauma* 31:1151, 1991.

81. Gentilello LM et al: Continuous arteriovenous rewarming: experimental results and thermodynamic model simulation of treatment for hypothermia, *J Trauma* 30:1436, 1990.

82. Gentilello LM et al: Continuous arteriovenous rewarming: rapid reversal of hypothermia in critically ill patients, *J Trauma* 32:316, 1992.

83. Gentilello LM et al: Is hypothermia in the victim of major trauma protective or harmful? A randomized, prospective study, *Ann Surg* 226:439, 1997.

84. Gentilello LM et al: Continuous arteriovenous rewarming: experimental results and thermodynamic model simulation of treatment for hypothermia, *J Trauma* 30:1436, 1998.

85. Giesbrecht GG: The respiratory system in a cold environment, *Aviat Space Environ Med* 66:890, 1995.

86. Giesbrecht GG, Bristow GK: Decrement in manual arm performance during whole body cooling, *Aviat Space Environ Med* 63:1077, 1992.

87. Giesbrecht GG, Bristow GK: Influence of body composition on rewarming from immersion hypothermia, *Aviat Space Environ Med* 66:1140, 1995.

88. Giesbrecht GG, Bristow GK: Recent advances in hypothermia research, *Ann NY Acad Sci* 813:676, 1997.

89. Giesbrecht GG, Johnston CE, Bristow GK: The convective afterdrop component during hypothermic exercise decreased with delayed exercise onset, *Aviat Space Environ Med* 69:17, 1998.

90. Giesbrecht GG et al: Treatment of mild immersion hypothermia by direct body-to-body contact, *J Appl Physiol* 76:2373, 1994.

91. Giesbrecht GG et al: Inhibition of shivering increases core temperature afterdrop and attenuates rewarming in hypothermic humans, *J Appl Physiol* 83:1630, 1997.

91a. Gilbert M et al: Resuscitation from accidental hypothermia of 13.7° C with circulatory arrest, *Lancet* 355:375, 2000.

92. Gillen JP et al: Ventricular fibrillation during orotracheal intubation of hypothermic dogs, *Ann Emerg Med* 15:412, 1986.

93. Ginsberg MD et al: Temperature modulation of ischemic brain injury—a synthesis of recent advances, *Prog Brain Res* 96:13, 1993.

94. Globus MY et al: Detection of free radical activity during transient global ischemia and recirculation: effects of intraischemic brain temperature modulation, *J Neurochem* 65:1250, 1995.

95. Glusman A, Hasan K, Roguin N: Contraindication to thrombolytic therapy in accidental hypothermia, *Int J Cardiol* 28:269, 1990.

96. Goheen MSL et al: Efficacy of forced-air and inhalation rewarming using a human model for severe hypothermia, *J Appl Physiol* 83:1635, 1997.

97. Goldberg ME et al: Do heated humidifiers and heat and moisture exchangers prevent temperature drop during lower abdominal surgery? *J Clin Anesth* 4:16, 1992.

98. Granberg PO: Alcohol and cold, *Arctic Med Res* 50:43, 1991.

99. Granberg PO: Human physiology under cold exposure, *Arctic Med Res* 50:23, 1991.

100. Gregory JS et al: Comparison of three methods of rewarming from hypothermia: advances of extracorporeal blood rewarming, *J Trauma* 31:1247, 1991.

101. Gregory JS et al: Incidence and timing of hypothermia in trauma patients undergoing operations, *J Trauma* 31:795, 1991.

102. Gregory RT, Doolittle WH: Accidental hypothermia. II. Clinical implications of experimental studies, *Alaska Med* 15:48, 1973.

103. Hall KN, Syverud SA: Closed thoracic cavity lavage in the treatment of severe hypothermia in human beings, *Ann Emerg Med* 19:204, 1990.

104. Hamilton RS, Paton BC: The diagnosis and treatment of hypothermia by mountain rescue teams: a survey, *Wilderness Environ Med* 7:37, 1996.

105. Handrigan MT et al: Factors and methodology in achieving ideal delivery temperatures for intravenous and lavage fluid in hypothermia, *Am J Emerg Med* 15:350, 1997.

106. Harnett RM, Pruitt JR, Sias FR: A review of the literature concerning resuscitation from hypothermia. II. Selected rewarming protocols, *Aviat Space Environ Med* 54:487, 1983.

107. Hauge A, Kofstad J: Acid-base regulation during hypothermia: a brief review, *Arctic Med Res* 54:76, 1995.

108. Hauty MG et al: Prognostic factors in severe accidental hypothermia: experience from the Mt. Hood tragedy, *J Trauma* 27:1107, 1987.

109. Hayward JS, Eckerson JD, Kemna D: Thermal and cardiovascular changes during three methods of resuscitation from mild hypothermia, *Resuscitation* 11:21, 1984.

110. Hazan J, Maag U, Chessex P: Association between hypothermia and mortality rate of premature infants—revisited, *Am J Obstet Gynecol* 164:111, 1991.

111. Heise D, Rathgeber J, Burchardi H: Severe, accidental hypothermia: active rewarming with a simple extracorporeal veno-venous warming-circuit, *Anaesthesist* 45:1093, 1996.

112. Henker RA, Brown SD, Marion DW: Comparison of brain temperature with bladder and rectal temperatures in adults with severe head injury, *Neurosurgery* 42:1071, 1998.

113. Hering JP et al: Influence of pH management on hemodynamics and metabolism in moderate hypothermia, *J Thorac Cardiovasc Surg* 104:1388, 1992.

114. Hernandez E, Praga M, Alcazar JM: Accidental hypothermia, *N Engl J Med* 332:1034, 1995 (letter).

115. Hernandez E et al: Hemodialysis for treatment of accidental hypothermia, *Nephron* 63:214, 1993.

116. Herr RD, White GL Jr: Hypothermia: threat to military operations, *Mil Med* 156:140, 1991.

117. Hersio K et al: Changes in whole body and tissue oxygen consumption during recovery from hypothermia: effect of amino acid infusion, *Crit Care Med* 19:503, 1991.

118. Hesslink RL Jr et al: Radio frequency (13.56 MHz) energy enhances recovery from mild hypothermia, *J Appl Physiol* 67:1208, 1989.

119. Hill JG et al: Emergency applications of cardiopulmonary support: a multi-institutional experience, *Ann Thorac Surg* 54:699, 1992.

120. Hindsholm KB et al: Reflective blankets used for reduction of heat loss during regional anesthesia, *Br J Anaesth* 68:531, 1992.

121. Hodgdon JA et al: Norwegian military field exercises in the Arctic: cognitive and physical performance, *Arctic Med Res* 50:132, 1991.

122. Holmer I: Assessment of cold stress, *Arctic Med Res* 50:83, 1991.

123. Holmer I: Resultant clothing insulation during exercise in the cold, *Artic Med Res* 50:94, 1991.

124. Holmer I: Prediction of responses to cold, *Arctic Med Res* 54:48, 1995.

125. Husby P et al: Deep accidental hypothermia with asystole: a successful treatment with heart-lung machine after prolonged cardiopulmonary resuscitation, *Tidsskr Nor Laegeforen* 111:183, 1991.

126. Imon H et al: Optimal pH and PaCO$_2$ during moderate hypothermia, *Jpn J Anesthesiol* 41:603, 1992.

127. Ireland AJ et al: Back from the dead: extracorporeal rewarming of severe accidental hypothermia victims in accident and emergency, *J Accid Emerg Med* 14:255, 1997.

128. Iserson KV, Huestis DW: Blood warming: current applications and techniques, *Transfusion* 31:558, 1991.

129. Iversen RJ et al: Successful CPR in a severely hypothermic patient using continuous thoracostomy lavage, *Ann Emerg Med* 19:1335, 1990.

130. Iwasaka H et al: Heat conservation during abdominal surgery, *Masui* 41:666, 1992.

131. Iyengar J, Bhakoo ON: Prevention of neonatal hypothermia in Himalayan villages: role of the domiciliary caretaker, *Trop Geogr Med* 43:293, 1991.

132. Johannsson BW: The hibernator heart: nature's model of resistance to ventricular fibrillation, *Arctic Med Res* 50:58, 1991.

133. Johnson DE, Gamble WB: Trauma in the arctic: an incident report, *J Trauma* 31:1340, 1991.

134. Johnston CE et al: Alcohol lowers the vasoconstriction threshold in humans without affecting core cooling rate during mild cold exposure, *Eur J Appl Physiol* 74:293, 1996.

135. Johnston CE et al: Eucapnic hypoxia lowers human cold thermoregulatory response thresholds and accelerates core cooling, *J Appl Physiol* 80:422, 1996.

136. Johnston CE et al: Hypercapnia lowers the shivering threshold and increased core cooling rate in humans, *Aviat Space Environ Med* 67:438, 1996.

137. Jolly BT, Ghezzi KT: Accidental hyothermia, *Emerg Med Clin North Am* 10:311, 1992.

138. Jones AI, Swann IJ: Prolonged resuscitation in accidental hypothermia: use of mechanical cardio-pulmonary resuscitation and partial cardiopulmonary bypass, *Eur J Emerg Med* 1:34, 1994.

139. Jones DR et al: The successful resuscitation of a hypothermic multi-trauma patient, *WV Med J* 87:298, 1991.

140. Jurkovich GJ et al: Hypothermia in trauma victims: an ominous predictor of survival, *J Trauma* 27:1019, 1987.

141. Kallenback J et al: Experience with acute poisoning in an intensive care unit: a review of 103 cases, *S Afr Med J* 59:587, 1981.

142. Kangas E, Niemela H, Kojo N: Treatment of hypothermic circulatory arrest with thoracotomy and pleural lavage, *Ann Chir Gynaecol* 83:258, 1994.

143. Kanzenbach TL, Dexter WW: Cold injuries. Protecting your patients from the dangers of hypothermia and frostbite, *Postgrad Med* 105:72, 1999 (review).

144. Kashuk JL et al: Major abdominal vascular trauma: a unified approach, *J Trauma* 22:672, 1982.

145. Kaufman JW, Bagian JP: Insidious hypothermia during raft use, *Aviat Space Environ Med* 61:569, 1990.

146. Kaufman JW et al: Comparative effectiveness of hypothermia rewarming techniques: radio frequency energy versus warm water, *Resuscitation* 29:203, 1995.

147. Keatinge WR: Hypothermia: dead or alive? *Br Med J* 302:3, 1991 (editorial).

148. Kempen PM: Full body forced air warming: commercial blanket versus air delivery beneath bed sheets, *Can J Anaesth* 43:1168, 1996.

149. Kinzinger R, Risse M, Puschel K: Irrational behavior in exposure to cold: paradoxical undressing in hypothermia, *Arch Kriminol* 187:47, 1991.

150. Kiuchi M, Kimura Y: Unusual intravascular hemolysis in a case of fatal hypothermia, *Am J Forensic Med Pathol* 13:222, 1992.

151. Klinge U et al: Hypothermia and polytrauma: a case report (28° C), *Anasth Intensivther Notfallmed* 25:436, 1990.

152. Kobrin VI: Spontaneous ventricular defibrillation in hypothermia, *Kardiologiia* 31:19, 1991.

153. Koller R, Schnider TW, Neidhart P: Deep accidental hypothermia and cardiac arrest rewarming with forced air, *Acta Anaesthesiol Scand* 41:1359, 1997.

154. Kornberger E, Mair P: Important aspects in the treatment of severe accidental hypothermia, *J Neurosurg Anesthesiol* 8:83, 1996.

155. Kristensen G et al: An oesophageal thermal tube for rewarming in hypothermia, *Acta Anaesthiol Scand* 29:846, 1985.

156. Kroncke GM et al: Ectothermic philosophy of acid-base balance to prevent fibrillation during hypothermia, *Arch Surg* 121:303, 1986.

157. Kulkarni P et al: Clinical evaluation of the oesophageal heat exchanger in the prevention of perioperative hypothermia, *Br J Anaesth* 70:216, 1993.

158. Kurz A et al: Forced-air warming maintains intra-operative normothermia better than circulating-water in infants and children, *Anesth Analg* 77:89, 1993.

159. Laub GW et al: Percutaneous cardiopulmonary bypass for the treatment of hypothermic circulatory collapse, *Ann Thorac Surg* 47:608, 1989.

160. Lauri T: Cardiovascular responses to an acute volume load in deep hypothermia, *Eur Heart J* 17:606, 1996.

161. Lauri T et al: Cardiac function in hypothermia, *Arctic Med Res* 50:63, 1991.

162. Lazar HL: The treatment of hypothermia, *N Engl J Med* 337:1545, 1997.

163. Ledingham IM, Mone JG: Treatment of accidental hypothermia: a prospective clinical study, *Br Med J* 280:1102, 1980.

164. Lee HA, Ames AC: Hemodialysis in severe barbiturate poisoning, *Br Med J* 1:1217, 1965.

165. Lennon RL et al: Evaluation of a forced air system for warming hypothermic postoperative patients, *Anesth Analg* 70:424, 1990.

166. Letsou GV et al: Is cardiopulmonary bypass effective for treatment of hypothermic arrest due to drowning or exposure? *Arch Surg* 127:525, 1992.

167. Levitt MA et al: A comparative rewarming trial of gastric versus peritoneal lavage in a hypothermic model, *Am J Emerg Med* 8:285, 1990.

168. Lewin S, Brettman LR, Holzman RS: Infections in hypothermic patients, *Arch Intern Med* 141:920, 1981.

169. Lexow K: Severe accidental hypothermia: survival after 6 hours 30 minutes of cardiopulmonary resuscitation, *Arctic Med Res* 50:112, 1991.

170. Lifschultz BD, Donoghue ER: Forensic pathology of heat-and cold-related injuries, *Clin Lab Med* 18:77, 1998.

171. Livingstone SD, Nolan RW, Keefe AA: Heat loss caused by cooling the feet, *Aviat Space Environ Med* 66:232, 1995.

172. Lloyd EL: Hypothesis: temperature recommendations for elderly people: are we wrong? *Age Ageing* 19:264, 1990.

173. Lloyd EL: Equipment for airway warming in the treatment of accidental hypothermia, *J Wilderness Med* 2:330, 1991.

174. Lloyd EL: The cause of death after rescue, *Int J Sports Med* Oct 13 (suppl 1):S196, 1992.

175. Lloyd EL: Accidental hypothermia, *Resuscitation* 32:111, 1996.

176. Lloyd JR, Olsen RG: Radio frequency energy for rewarming of cold extremities, *Undersea Biomed Res* 19:199, 1992.

177. Locher T et al: Accidental hypothermia in Switzerland (1980-1987): case reports and prognostic factors, *Schweiz Med Wochenschr* 121:1020, 1991.

178. Long WB: Cardiopulmonary bypass for rewarming profound hypothermia patients: critical decisions in hypothermia, Annual International Forum, Portland, Ore, Feb 28, 1992.

179. Maaravi AY, Weiss AT: The effect of prolonged hypothermia on cardiac function in a young patient with accidental hypothermia, *Chest* 98:1019, 1990.

180. MacDonell JE, Wrenn K: Hypothermia in the summer, *South Med J* 84:804, 1991.

181. MacKenzie MA et al: Effects of steady hypothermia and normothermia on the electrocardiogram in human poikilothermia, *Arctic Med Res* 50:67, 1991.

182. Mackowiak PA, Wasserman SS, Levine MM: A critical appraisal of 98.6° F, the upper limit of the normal body temperature and other legacies of Carl Reinhold August Wunderlich, *JAMA* 268:1578, 1992.

183. Maclean D, Emslie-Smith D: *Accidental hypothermia*, Philadelphia, 1977, JB Lippincott.

184. Maningas PA et al: Regional blood flow during hypothermic arrest, *Ann Emerg Med* 15:390, 1986.

185. Marion DW et al: Resuscitative hypothermia, *Crit Care Med* 24:S81, 1996.

186. Marion DW et al: Treatment of traumatic brain injury with moderate hypothermia, *N Engl J Med* 336:540, 1997.

187. Martens P: Rewarming by extracorporeal circulation, *Intensive Care Med* 16:342, 1990.

188. Matthews AJ, Stead AL, Abbott TR: Acid-base control during hypothermia, *Anaesthesia* 39:649, 1984.

189. Maughan RJ, Leiper JB, Thompson J: Rectal temperature after marathon running, *Br J Sports Med* 19:192, 1985.

190. McCallum AL: Update on trauma care in Canada: trauma and hypothermia, *Can J Surg* 33:457, 1990.

191. McGuire JP, Giesbrecht GG: A comparison of three forced-air patient warming systems, *Anesth Analg* 76:S256, 1993.

192. Mekjavic IB, Eiken O: Inhalation rewarming from hypothermia: an evaluation in minus 20° C simulated field conditions, *Aviat Space Environ Med* 66:424, 1995.

193. Menard MR, Hahn G: Acute and chronic hypothermia in a man with spinal cord injury: environmental and pharmacologic causes, *Arch Phys Med Rehabil* 72:421, 1991.

194. Mercer JB: The shivering response in animal and man, *Arctic Med Res* 50:18, 1991.

195. Mercer JB: Enhancing tolerance to cold exposure—how successful have we been, *Arctic Med Res* 54:70, 1995.

196. Miller JW, Danzl DF, Thomas DM: Urban accidental hypothermia: 135 cases, *Ann Emerg Med* 9:456, 1980.

197. Mills WJ Jr: Field care of the hypothermic patient, *Int J Sports Med* Oct 13(suppl 1):S199, 1992.

198. Mills WJ Jr: Accidental hypothermia: management approach, 1980 (classical article), *Alaska Med* 35:54, 1993.

199. Moss J: Accidental severe hypothermia, *Surg Gynecol Obstet* 162:501, 1986.

200. Murphy K, Nowak RM, Tomlanovich MC: Use of bretylium tosylate as prophylaxis and treatment in hypothermic ventricular fibrillation in the canine model, *Ann Emerg Med* 15:1160, 1986.

201. Murray BJ: Severe lactic acidosis and hypothermia, *West J Med* 134:162, 1981.

202. Murray PT, Fellner SK: Accidental hypothermia, *N Engl J Med* 332:1034, 1995.

203. Niazi SA, Lewis FJ: Profound hypothermia in man: report of a case, *Ann Surg* 147:264, 1958.

204. Nicholson RW, Iserson KV: Core temperature measurement in hypovolemic resuscitation, *Ann Emerg Med* 20:62, 1991.

205. Nielsen HK et al: Hypothermic patients admitted to an intensive care unit: a fifteen year survey, *Dan Med Bull* 39:190, 1992.

206. Niemann JT, Rosborough JP, Petikan P: Hemodynamic determinants of subdiaphragmatic venous return during closed chest CPR in a canine cardiac arrest model, *Ann Emerg Med* 19:1232, 1990.

207. Nordrehaug JE: Sustained ventricular fibrillation in deep accidental hypothermia, *Br Med J* 284:867, 1982.

208. Nozaki R et al: Accidental profound hypothermia, *N Engl J Med* 315:1680, 1986 (letter).

209. Orts A et al: Bretylium tosylate and electrically induced cardiac arrhythmias during hypothermia in dogs, *Am J Emerg Med* 10:311, 1992.

210. Osborn JJ: Experimental hypothermia respiratory and blood pH changes in relation to cardiac function, *Am J Physiol* 175:389, 1953.

211. Oung CM et al: Effects of hypothermia on hemodynamic responses to dopamine and dobutamine, *J Trauma* 33:671, 1992.

212. Parke TR: Resuscitation from hypothermia, *J Accid Emerg Med* 15:69, 1998.

213. Patel RL et al: Alpha-stat acid-base regulation during cardiopulmonary bypass improves neuropsychologic outcome in patients undergoing coronary artery bypass grafting, *J Thor Cardiovasc Surg* 111:1267, 1996.

214. Paton BC: Accidental hypothermia, *Pharmacol Ther* 22:331, 1983.

215. Perry HE et al: Baclofen overdose: drug experimentation in a group of adolescents, *Pediatrics* 101:1045, 1998.

216. Pillgram-Larsen J et al: Accidental hypothermia: risk factors in 29 patients with body temperature of 30° C and below, *Tidsskr Nor Laegeforen* 111:180, 1991.

217. Poulos ND, Mollitt DL: The nature and reversibility of hypothermia-induced alterations of blood viscosity, *J Trauma* 31:996, 1991.

218. Pozos RS, Wittmers LE: *The nature and treatment of hypothermia,* Minneapolis, 1983, University of Minnesota Press.

219. Rahn H: Body temperature and acid-base regulation, *Pneumonologie* 151:87, 1974.

220. Rankin AC, Rae AP: Cardiac arrhythmias during rewarming of patients with accidental hypothermia, *Br Med J* 289:874, 1984.

221. Rasmussen YH, Leikersfeldt G, Dranck NE: Forced-air surface warming versus oesophageal heat exchanger in the prevention of perioperative hypothermia, *Acta Anaesth Scand* 42:348, 1998.

222. Rathgeber J et al: Is reduction of intraoperative heat loss and management of hypothermic patients with anesthetic gas climate control advisable? Heat and humidity exchangers vs. active humidifiers in a functional lung model, *Anaesthesist* 45:807, 1996.

223. Ream AK, Reitz BA, Silverberg G: Temperature correction of $PaCO_2$ and pH in estimating acid-base status: an example of emperor's new clothes? *Anesthesiology* 56:41, 1982.

224. Reed RL et al: Hypothermia and blood coagulation: dissociation between enzyme activity and clotting factor levels, *Circ Shock* 32:141, 1990.

225. Reed RL et al: The disparity between hypothermic coagulopathy and clotting studies, *J Trauma* 33:465, 1992.

226. Rekland T et al: Neuromonitoring in hypothermia and in hypothermic hypoxia, *Arctic Med Res* 50:32, 1991.

227. Roeggla G et al: Immediate use of cardiopulmonary bypass in patients with severe accidental hypothermia in the emergency department, *Eur J Emerg Med* 1:155, 1994.

228. Rogers I: Which rewarming therapy in hypothermia? A review of the randomized trials, *Emerg Med* 9:213, 1997.

229. Rohrer MJ, Natale AM: Effect of hypothermia on the coagulation cascade, *Crit Care Med* 20:1402, 1992.

230. Rosenthal TB: The effect of temperature on the pH of blood and plasma in vitro, *J Biol Chem* 173:25, 1948.

231. Samuelson T: Experience with standardized protocols in hypothermia, boom or bane? The Alaska experience, *Arctic Med Res* 50:28, 1991.

232. Savourey G, Vallerand AL, Bittel JH: General and local cold adaptation after a ski journey in a severe arctic environment, *Eur J Appl Physiol* 64:99, 1992.

233. Schaller MD, Fischer AP, Perret CH: Hyperkalemia: a prognostic factor during acute severe hypothermia, *JAMA* 264:1842, 1990.

234. Schissel DJ, Barney DL, Keller R: Cold weather injuries in an arctic environment, *Mil Med* 163:568, 1998.

235. Schrijver G, van der Maten J: Severe accidental hypothermia: pathophysiology and therapeutic options for hospitals without cardiopulmonary bypass equipment, *Neth J Med* 49:167, 1996.

236. Schroder T et al: Dopamine dependent diastolic dysfunction in moderate hypothermia, *J Cardiovasc Pharm* 23:689, 1994.

237. Schulman H et al: CT findings in neonatal hypothermia, *Pediatr Radiol* 28:414, 1998.

238. Schwaitzberg SD et al: Rapid in-line blood warming using microwave energy: preliminary studies, *J Invest Surg* 4:505, 1991.

239. Segers MJ et al: Three patients with accidental hypothermia: customized rewarming, *Ned Tijdschr Geneeskd* 141:1369, 1997.

240. Sessler DI: Mild perioperative hypothermia, *N Engl J Med* 336:1730, 1997.

241. Sheaff CM et al: Safety of 65° C intravenous fluid for the treatment of hypothermia, *Am J Surg* 172:52, 1996.

242. Shephard RJ: Some consequences of polar stress: data from a transpolar ski-trek, *Arctic Med Res* 50:25, 1991.

243. Shephard RJ: Asphyxial death of a young skier, *J Sports Med Phys Fitness* 36:223, 1996.

244. Shields CP, Sixsmith DM: Treatment of moderate-to-severe hypothermia in an urban setting, *Ann Emerg Med* 19:1093, 1990.

245. Silbergleit R et al: Hypothermia from realistic fluid resuscitation in a model of hemorrhagic shock, *Ann Emerg Med* 31:339, 1998.

246. Sklar DP, Doezema D: Procedures pertaining to hypothermia. In Roberts JR, Hedges JR, editors: *Clinical procedures in emergency medicine,* ed 3, Philadelphia, 1998, WB Saunders.

247. Soreide E et al: A novel technique for treatment of hypothermia: the combined application of negative pressure and heat to specific surface areas, *Proceedings of the 10th Annual Trauma and Critical Care Symposium,* Baltimore, 1997 (abstract).

248. Splittgerber FH et al: partial cardiopulmonary bypass for core rewarming in profound accidental hypothermia, *Am Surg* 52:407, 1986.

249. Staab DB et al: Coagulation defects resulting from ambient temperature-induced hypothermia, *J Trauma* 36:634, 1994.

250. Steele MT et al: Forced air speeds rewarming in accidental hypothermia, *Ann Emerg Med* 27:479, 1996.

251. Steinemann S, Shackford SR, Davis JW: Implications of admission hypothermia in trauma patients, *J Trauma* 30:200, 1990.

252. Steinman AM: Cardiopulmonary resuscitation and hypothermia, *Circulation* 74(suppl IV):29, 1986.

253. Sterba JA: Efficacy and safety of prehospital rewarming techniques to treat accidental hypothermia, *Ann Emerg Med* 20:896, 1991.

254. Stoneham MD, Squires SJ: Prolonged resuscitation in acute deep hypothermia, *Anaesthesia* 47:784, 1992.

255. Swain JA et al: Relationship of cerebral and myocardial intracellular pH to blood pH during hypothermia, *Am J Physiol* 260:1640, 1991.

256. Takada M et al: Wischnevsky's gastric lesions in accidental hypothermia, *Am J Forensic Med Pathol* 12:300, 1991.

257. Tanaka M, Tokudome S: Accidental hypothermia and death from cold in urban areas, *Int J Biometeorol* 34:242, 1991.

258. Taylor MS: Cold weather injuries during peace time military training, *Mil Med* 157:602, 1992.

259. Thompson DA, Anderson N: Successful resuscitation of a severely hypothermic neonate, *Ann Emerg Med* 23:1390, 1994.

260. Tisherman SA et al: Profound hypothermia (less than 10° C) compared with deep hypothermia (15° C) improved neurologic outcome in dogs after two hours' circulatory arrest induced to enable resuscitative surgery, *J Trauma* 31:1051, 1991.

261. Tomaszewski W: Changements electrocardiographiques observes chez un homme mort de froid, *Arch Mal Coeur* 31:525, 1938.

262. Tveita T et al: Hemodynamic and metabolic effects of hypothermia and rewarming, *Arctic Med Res* 50:48, 1991.

263. Tyndal CM Jr et al: Profound accidental hypothermia in the deep South: clinical exposure, *Perfusion* 11:57, 1996.

264. Vangaard L et al: Arteriovenous anastomoses (AVA) rewarming in 45° C water is effective in moderately hypothermic subjects, *FASEB J* 12:A90, 1998.

265. Vella J et al: The rapid reversal of profound hypothermia using peritoneal dialysis, *Ir J Med Sci* 165:113, 1996.

266. von Segesser LK et al: Reduction and elimination of systemic heparinization during cardiopulonary bypass, *J Thorac Cardiovasc Surg* 103:790, 1992.

267. Vretenar DF et al: Cardiopulmonary bypass resuscitation for accidental hypothermia, *Ann Thorac Surg* 58:895, 1994.

268. Wallace W: Does it make sense to heat gases higher than body temperature for the treatment of cold water near-drowning or hypothermia? A point of view paper, *Alaska Med* 39:75, 1997.

269. Walpoth BH et al: Accidental deep hypothermia with cardiopulmonary arrest: extracorporeal blood rewarming in 11 patients, *Eur J Cardiothorac Surg* 4:390, 1990.

270. Walpoth BH et al: Outcome of survivors of accidental deep hypothermia and circulatory arrest treated with extracorporeal blood warming, *N Engl J Med* 337:1500, 1997.

271. Wang LS et al: A reevaluation of heparin requirements for cardiopulmonary bypass, *J Thorac Cardiovasc Surg* 101:153, 1991.

272. Waters DJ et al: Portable cardiopumonary bypass: resuscitation from prolonged ice-water submersion and asystole, *Ann Thorac Surg* 57:1018, 1994.

273. Watts DD et al: Hypothermic coagulopathy in trauma: effect of varying levels of hypothermia on enzyme speed, platelet function and fibrinolytic activity, *J Trauma* 44:846, 1998.

274. Weinberg AD: Hypothermia, *Ann Emerg Med* 22:370, 1993.

275. Weinberg AD: The role of inhalation rewarming in the early management of hypothermia, *Resuscitation* 36:101, 1998.

276. Weiss SJ et al: The physiological response to norepinephrine during hypothermia and rewarming, *Resuscitation* 39:189, 1998.

277. White FN: Reassuring acid-base balance in hypothermia: a comparative point of view, *West J Med* 138:255, 1983.

278. White JD: Hypothermia: the Bellevue experience, *Ann Emerg Med* 11:417, 1982.

279. White JD et al: Controlled comparison of humidified inhalation and peritoneal lavage in rewarming immersion hypothermia, *Am J Emerg Med* 2:210, 1984.

280. White JD et al: Rewarming in accidental hypothermia; radio wave versus inhalation therapy, *Ann Emerg Med* 16:50, 1987.

281. Winegard C: Successful treatment of severe hypothermia and prolonged cardiac arrest with closed thoracic cavity lavage, *J Emerg Med* 15:629, 1997.

282. Wisborg T, Husby P, Engedal H: Anesthesiologist-manned helicopters and regionalized extracorporeal circulation facilities: a unique chance in deep hypothermia, *Arctic Med Res* 50:108, 1991.

283. Wong KC: Physiology and pharmacology of hypothermia, *West J Med* 138:227, 1983.

284. Wyatt JS, Thoresen M: Hypothermia treatment and the newborn, *Pediatrics* 100:1028, 1997.

285. Xiao F, Safar P, Radovsky A: Mild protective and resuscitative hypothermia for asphyxial cardiac arrest in rats, *Am J Emerg Med* 16:17, 1998.

286. Xu X, Werner J: A dynamic model of the human/clothing/environment system, *Appl Human Sci* 16:61, 1997.

287. Young DM: Risk factors for hypothermia in psychiatric patients, *Ann Clin Psychiatry* 8:93, 1996.

288. Zehner WJ, Terndrup TE: Ear temperatures during rewarming from hypothermia, *Ann Emerg Med* 23:901, 1994.

289. Zell SC, Kurtz KJ: Severe exposure hypothermia: a resuscitation protocol, *Ann Emerg Med* 14:339, 1985.

290. Zhong H, Qinyi S, Mingjlang S: Rewarming with microwave irradiation in severe cold injury syndrome, *Chin Med J* 93:19, 1980.

7 Frostbite

Robert L. McCauley, David J. Smith, Martin C. Robson, and John P. Heggers

Cold-induced injuries are almost exclusively a result of humans' inability to properly protect themselves from the environment. Cold injuries may be either systemic or localized, depending on the temperature and length of exposure. Systemic injury is hypothermia (see Chapter 6), whereas localized injury is frostbite. Although much confusion exists in the literature regarding the myriad of clinical terms used to describe localized injury, the correct term is frostbite.

HISTORICAL ASPECTS

Numerous historical accounts discuss armies exposed to cold sustaining large numbers of cold-induced casualties. Although Hippocrates described some of the symptoms and sequelae of frostbite, cold injuries were probably not prevalent in ancient Greece. In 218 BC, Hannibal lost nearly half of his army of 46,000 to cold injuries in only 15 days when they crossed the Pyrenean Alps. In 210 BC, Xenophon described cold injuries suffered by Spartan soldiers during a retreat across the Carduchion mountains after leaving Alexander's armies. In 1778, Dr. James Thatcher wrote that 10% of George Washington's army had been left to perish in the winter cold during his campaign against the British soldiers.[70]

Despite these accounts, it was not until 1805 that the first official report was published on the effect of cold injury.[88] The first authoritative account of mass casualties was the description by Baron de Larrey, surgeon-in-chief of Napoleon's army during the invasion of Russia in the winter of 1812-1813.[34] Larrey wrote, "When some external part of the body is caught by cold, instead of submitting it to heat, which provides gangrene, it is necessary to rub the affected part with substances containing very little calorick—for it is well known that the effect of calorick on an organized part that is almost deprived of life is marked by an acceleration of fermentation and putrefaction."[34]

Larrey introduced the concept of friction massage with ice or snow, the avoidance of heat in thawing, and the idea that cold injuries were similar to burn injuries. These concepts are better understood against the background as viewed by Larrey.[34] Soldiers with cold injuries rapidly rewarmed their extremities over roaring fires of 66° to 77° C (150° to 170° F) after long marches, only to renew the trek and refreeze their extremities the next day. Larrey recognized that warming was good but cautioned against the use of excessive heat and ul-timately recognized the freeze-thaw-freeze cycle. Napoleon left France with 250,000 men and returned 6 months later with only 350 effective soldiers. The remainder were casualties to cold or starvation.[34]

During the Crimean War (1854-1856), 300,000 French troops sustained 5000 cases of frostbite and 1000 deaths. During World War I (1917-1918), World War II (1941-1945), and the Korean conflict (1950-1953), at least 1 million cases of frostbite occurred.[59,60,78,80] In November and December 1942, the Germans performed 15,000 amputations for cold injuries.[78,79] High-altitude frostbite, first described in 1943, was recognized from the treatment of aviators in World War II.[80] The most prevalent form of this injury was seen in B-17 and B-24 crews flying between 25,000 and 35,000 feet in temperatures of −32° to −43° C (−25° to −45° F). When attacked, the only way the waist gunners of the aircraft could operate their machine guns was to open the large waist pots through which the guns were fired. The gunners often took off their bulky mittens and jackets to improve the dexterity they felt was crucial to saving their lives.[80]

Until the 1950s, treatment of cold injuries basically followed Larrey's guidelines. In 1956, experimental laboratory work by Merryman encouraged Hamill, the Public Health Service district medical officer in Tanana, Alaska, to try rapid rewarming at 38° C (100° F) on a patient with frostbite and hypothermia.[9,49] This was the genesis and has become the cornerstone of the method currently used in Alaska and popularized by Mills.[49]

TEMPERATURE HOMEOSTASIS IN HUMANS

No comprehensive statistical data are available on the incidence of frostbite. The Royal College of Physicians in London estimated that 10% of elderly British home dwellers were hypothermic, but no comparable data were available for frostbite.[15] Frostbite is much more prevalent during military campaigns and is a known hazard for mountain climbers and explorers. In the nonadventurer civilian population, Mills collected 500 cases in Alaska by 1963; Cook County Hospital in Chicago recorded 843 cases from 1962-1972; Maria Hospital in Helsinki, Finland, reported 110 cases in 1968; and Detroit Receiving Hospital reported on 154 patients treated from 1982 to 1985.[4,22,32,50]

Physiologically, humans are tropical beings, better suited to losing heat than retaining it. When naked and at rest, a person's neutral environmental temperature is 28° C (82° F); with an environmental drop of only

8° C (14.5° F), the metabolic rate must double to avoid a lowering of body temperature. In comparison, the Arctic fox can maintain a steady thermal state within an external temperature of −40° C (−40° F) and by doubling its metabolic rate could cope with an outside temperature of −120° C (−184° F).

Putting on clothes in response to cold is not a reflex but requires a conscious decision. When the ability to decide or to act is impaired, there is a risk of cold-induced injury.[11] Alcohol has been implicated in many cases of frostbite.[27,28] Alcohol- or drug-intoxicated persons whose consciousness, judgment, or self-protective instincts are depressed often expose themselves to dangerous environmental hazards. Knize[28] noted that alcohol intake or mental instability led directly to cold injury in 50% of their patients. Once the injury had occurred, alcohol intake probably did not significantly alter the course of events. Barillo et al[1] experimentally demonstrated increased mortality and a detrimental effect of ethanol on tissue perfusion associated with severe murine frostbite. Alcohol consumption promotes peripheral vascular dilation and increases heat loss. This may make an exposed part more susceptible to frostbite.

The type and duration of cold contact are the two most important factors in determining the extent of frostbite injury.[80-82] Touching cold wood or fabric is not nearly as dangerous as direct contact with metal, particularly by wet or even damp hands. Air alone is a poor thermal conductor. Cold alone is not nearly as dangerous a freezing factor as a combination of wind and cold.[87] Wind velocity in combination with temperature establishes the windchill index. For example, an ambient temperature of −6.7° C (20° F) with a 45 mph wind has the same cooling effect as −40° C (−40° F) temperature with a 2 mph breeze.[80-82] Thus it is important to think in terms of heat loss, not cold gain. Frostbite occurs when the body is unable to conserve heat or protect against heat loss.

Because many serious cases of frostbite originate at high altitude, it has been assumed that physiologic changes occurring with increased altitude make persons more prone to frostbite. However, present data suggest that reduction in atmospheric pressure has little or no effect on susceptibility to frostbite. Increased red blood cell concentration does not increase blood viscosity, impede capillary circulation, or have any other apparent bearing on cold injury.[80-82] On the other hand, deep, loose snow, which traditionally has been thought to insulate from the cold, may actually contribute to frostbite. Temperature measured beneath deep snow is frequently much lower than that on the surface. Washburn[82] recounts one expedition to Mt. McKinley, Alaska, when members of his party found it extremely difficult to keep their feet warm, despite a clear, sunny, −16° C (3° F) day with little wind. One member inadvertently dropped a thermometer in the snow and noted that it registered −25.6° C (−14° F). Feet must be dressed for the temperature at their level, not for surface temperature protection.[82]

Development of frostbite does not depend simply on ambient temperature and duration of exposure. Along with wind chill, humidity and wetness also predispose to frostbite. Skin wetting adds an increment of heat transfer through evaporation and causes wet skin to cool faster than dry skin.[56] More important, water in the stratum corneum can terminate supercooling by triggering water crystallization not only in this layer but also in the underlying tissue. Skin wetness is therefore conducive to frostbite because it allows crystallization to terminate supercooling after approximately half of the exposure time required by dry skin. This substantiates the clinical observation that "it has been found that supercooling displays itself in greater degree in skin that remains unwashed. Washing the skin encourages freezing, while rubbing the skin with spirit and anointing it with oil discourages it. The capacity to supercool greatly would seem to be connected with relative dryness of the horny layers of the skin. It is well known that Arctic explorers leave their skins unwashed."[36]

The degree of inadequacy of protective clothing varies with conditions and may contribute to insufficient conservation of body heat. Tight-fitting clothing may produce constriction, which hinders blood circulation and lessens the benefit of heat-retaining air insulation. Wet clothing transmits heat from the body into the environment because water is a thermal conductor superior to air by a factor of about 25.[27] Clothing that transmits moisture away from the body may be protective if an outer wind-resistant layer decreases heat loss. However, this wind-resistant layer must retain the same transmission capabilities; otherwise, clothing will still become moist. Clothes that decrease the amount of surface area may decrease frostbite risk. Mittens are more protective than gloves, since gloves have greater surface area and prevent air from circulating between fingers. Eighty percent of total body heat loss can occur through exposed head and neck areas. Poorly fitted boots notoriously generate frostbite injuries.

During World War II and the Korean conflict, clinical studies indicated that cold injuries occurred with higher frequency among soldiers in retreat.[59,60,86] Fatigue and apathy also increase the incidence of cold injury. When warfare is proceeding toward defeat or in conditions of starvation, soldiers often become indifferent to personal hygiene and clothing and the frequency of frostbite increases.[26] Overexertion increases heat loss. A large amount of body heat can be expended by panting, and perspiration further compounds the problem of chilling.[80-82] Both panting and sweating consume energy, which compounds the fatigue factor.

Impaired local circulation is a primary contributor to frostbite. Cigarette smoking causes vasoconstriction, decreased cutaneous blood flow, and tissue loss in random skin flaps.[35] Reus et al[67] documented that smoking induced arteriolar vasoconstriction and decreased blood flow in a nude model. Although red blood cell velocity increased, the net effect was a decrease in blood flow in the cutaneous microcirculation during and immediately after smoking. Curiously, habitual heavy smokers do not appear to be more prone to frostbite. Other drugs known to have vasoactive properties may also predispose to or compound a frostbite injury. Disease states that alter tissue perfusion, such as atherosclerosis or arteritis, predispose to frostbite.

Based on clinical observations, an individual who has experienced prior cold injury is placed in a high-risk category during subsequent cold exposure.[53,86] For undefined reasons, cold injury sensitizes an individual so that subsequent cold exposure, even of a lesser degree, produces more rapid tissue damage.[27] Military studies emphasize that long periods of immobility contribute to the extent of cold injury.[27,28] Motion produces body heat and improves circulation, especially in endangered limbs.

Civilian clinical studies are inadequate for statistical evaluation of factors such as race and previous climatic environmental exposure.[27,44] Military studies suggest that dark-skinned soldiers are more susceptible than whites to cold injury under the same combat conditions.[87] Individuals from warmer climatic regions within the United States tend to be more susceptible.[86] There are no data to suggest influence of age or gender in the incidence of frostbite.

THE SKIN

The skin is an individual's interface with the environment, serving as an organ of protection. It controls the invasion of microorganisms, maintains fluid balance, regulates temperature, protects against injury from radiation and electricity, and provides immunologic surveillance. Each function is specifically related to a cell or area within the skin.[24]

The skin is a highly specialized bilaminate structure resting on a subcutaneous layer of padding. Generally, the skin is about 1 to 2 mm in thickness, but it varies between 0.5 and 6 mm. The highly cellular epidermis and underlying dermis are in contact by multiple interpapillary ridges and grooves. The outermost layer of the epidermis, the stratum corneum, functions for protection. The innermost layer, the stratum germinativum, or basal layer, contains the only proliferating cells within the epidermis. Between these two layers are keratinocytes in various stages of differentiation. Other cells derived from the neural crest (melanocytes) and mesenchyme (Langerhans' cells), as well as cells of unknown etiology (Merkel's cells), migrate into the epidermis and become organized in specific association with certain keratinocytes.

The dermal-epidermal junctions undulate in most areas of the body, increasing surface contact between the two layers to provide resistance to shearing. The dermal-epidermal junction is a complex of structures referred to as the basement membrane zone, which functions as a filter to inhibit or prevent passage of molecules greater than 40 kD.

The dermis, or deeper layer of skin, is 20 to 30 times thicker than the epidermis. It contains nervous, vascular, lymphatic, and supporting structures for the epidermis and harbors the epidermal appendages. Regions of the dermis differ in structural organization and biochemistry, and each responds uniquely to systemic disease, genetic disease, and environmental assault. The papillary dermis and reticular dermis compose the two main dermal zones. The dermis contains fibrous and nonfibrous matrix molecules. Fibrous proteins, primarily collagen, impart bulk, density, and tensile properties to skin but also allow compliance and elasticity. Nonfibrous matrix molecules, glycosaminoglycans and glycoproteins, form ground substance that influences the osmotic properties of skin, permits cellular migration in a more fluid milieu, and serves as an integrative, continuous medium for all of the other structural elements.[23]

The papillary dermis is only slightly thicker than the overlying epidermis. It is separated from the underlying reticular dermis by a horizontal plexus of vessels. This plexus provides the overlying papillary dermis with a rich blood supply. The papillary dermis is more commonly altered in environmentally induced skin lesions (such as actinic damage) than in systemic disease or inherited diseases of connective tissue metabolism.

The majority of dermis is reticular dermis. Epidermal appendages either terminate in the lower levels of the reticular dermis or penetrate even deeper into the subcutaneous tissue. Blood vessels pierce the dermis, yielding branches to hair follicles and sweat glands.

Thermoregulation is one body function in which the stratum corneum is not important. The rate at which heat is lost by radiation is a function of the temperature of the cutaneous surface, which in turn is a function primarily of the rate of blood flow through the skin. Heat is poorly conducted from warmer internal tissue to the cutaneous surface because adipose tissue is a good heat insulator.

Thus cutaneous circulation is key to the genesis of frostbite. Because of its role in thermoregulation, the normal blood flow of skin far exceeds its nutritional obligation. The skin holds a complex system of capillary loops that empty into a large subcapillary venous plexus containing the majority of the cutaneous blood volume. Under normothermic conditions, 80% of an extremity's blood volume is in the skin and muscle veins. Skin blood volume depends in part on the tone in the resistance and capacitance vessels, and tone in turn depends largely on ambient and body temperature. Under basal conditions, a 70-kg human has a total cutaneous blood flow of 200 to 500 ml/min. With external heating to maintain skin temperature at 41° C (105.8° F), this may increase to 7000 to 8000 ml/min, whereas cooling the skin to 14° C (57° F) may diminish it to 20 to 50 ml/min.

Blood flow through apical structures, such as the nose, ears, hands, and feet, varies most markedly because of richly innervated arteriovenous connections. Blood flow to hand skin can be increased from a basal rate of 3 to 10 ml/min/100 g of tissue to a maximum of 180 ml/min/100 g of tissue. This cutaneous vascular tone is controlled by both direct local and reflex effects. Indirect heating (warming a distant part of the body) results in reflex-mediated cutaneous vasodilation, whereas direct warming results in vasodilation dominated by local effects. When both types (central and peripheral) of heating or cooling are present, their effects are additive.

Cutaneous vessels are controlled by sympathetic adrenergic vasoconstrictor fibers. Vascular smooth muscles have both α- and β-receptors, although the significance of the β-receptors is yet to be defined. Vasodilation in the hands and feet is passive, so maximal reflex vasodilation occurs after sympathectomy. After sympathectomy, residual local control of vascular tone persists so that direct heat or cold continues to alter blood flow.

When the hand or foot is cooled to 15° C (59° F), maximal vasoconstriction and minimal blood flow occur. If cooling continues to 10° C (50° F), vasoconstriction is interrupted by periods of vasodilation and an associated increase in blood and heat flow. This cold-induced vasodilation (CIVD), or "hunting response," recurs in 5- to 10-minute cycles to provide some protection from the cold. There is considerable individual variation in the amount of CIVD, which might explain some of the variation in susceptibility to frostbite. Prolonged repeated exposure to cold will increase CIVD and offer some degree of acclimatization. Eskimos, Lapps, and Nordic fishermen have a very strong CIVD response and very short intervals between dilations, which may contribute to maintenance of hand function in the cold environment.[19]

There is little evidence that humans have any significant physiologic adaptation to cold. They remain homeothermic, warm weather, tropical animals who neither tolerate nor adapt well to the cold. They must find a well-defined microclimate to keep skin temperature close to 32.8° C (91° F). Normal skin maturation and tissue function rely on the maintenance of permeability and integrity of all tissue membranes. A steady rate relationship of prostaglandins, particularly prostaglandin E_2 (PGE$_2$; vasodilator) and PGF$_{2\alpha}$ (vasoconstrictor), is crucial for normal skin function. An imbalance may disrupt cell membrane equilibrium. This relationship is controlled through PGE$_2$-9-ketoreductase and nicotinamide adenine dinucleotide phosphate (NADPH). Low con-

centrations of PGE$_2$-9-ketoreductase found in normal skin emphasize an active biologic presence.

FROSTBITE INJURY

The frostbite injury has classically been divided into four pathologic phases[31]:

1. Prefreeze phase. This is secondary to chilling and before ice crystal formation. Changes are caused by vasospasticity and transendothelial plasma leakage. Tissue temperature ranges from 3° to 10°C (37° to 50° F). Cutaneous sensation is generally abolished at 10° C (50° F).
2. Freeze-thaw phase. This is caused by actual ice crystal formation. Tissue temperature drops below the freezing point as the ambient environmental temperature dips below −15° to −6° C (5° to 21° F). Because of the underlying radiation of heat energy, skin must be supercooled to −4° C (24.8° F) to freeze. With no circulation, skin temperature may drop at a rate in excess of 0.5° C (0.9° F) per minute. After it is completely frozen, the tissue rapidly exhibits poikilothermy. The susceptibility of tissue to freezing varies, with endothelium, bone marrow, and nerve tissue more sensitive than muscle, bone, and cartilage.
3. Vascular stasis phase. This involves changes in blood vessels, including spasticity and dilation, and includes plasma leakage, stasis coagulation, and shunting.
4. Late ischemic phase. This is a result of thrombosis and arteriovenous shunting, ischemia, gangrene, and autonomic dysfunction.

Overlap occurs among these phases.[30] The changes during each phase vary with rapidity of freezing and duration and extent of injury. It is therefore conceptually clearer to divide pathologic changes occurring in frostbite into those resulting from direct cellular injury and those from indirect cellular effects. Changes caused by direct injury include the following[89]:

1. Extracellular ice formation
2. Intracellular ice formation
3. Cell dehydration and shrinkage
4. Abnormal intracellular electrolyte concentrations
5. Thermal shock
6. Denaturation of lipid-protein complexes

Cells subjected to a slow rate of cooling (hours) develop ice crystals extracellularly in the cellular interspaces. Rapid cooling (seconds to minutes) produces intracellular ice crystals, which are more lethal to the cell and less favorable for cell survival. In a clinical cold injury, the slower rate of freezing does not produce intracellular crystals[46]; however, the extracellular ice formed is not innocuous. It draws water across the cell membrane, contributing to intracellular dehydration. The theory of cellular dehydration was originally proposed by Moran[57] in 1929 and subsequently supported by Merryman's study of "ice-crystal nucleation."[45,46,47] Cellular dehydration produces modification of protein structure by high electrolyte concentration, alteration of membrane lipids, alteration of cellular pH, and imbalance of chemical activity.[41,42,47] This phenomenon subsequently permits a marked and toxic increase of electrolytes within the cell, leading to partial shrinkage and collapse of its vital cell membrane. These events are incompatible with cell survival.

Not all the water within a cell is freezable. A small amount of unfrozen water, "bound water," constitutes up to 10% of the total water content and is held tightly in the protein complex within the cell. No matter how rapid or marked the cold injury, this bound water remains liquid. At temperatures below $-20°$ C ($-4°$ F), approximately 90% of available water is frozen.[87] Although the theory of ice crystal disruption of cell structure is attractive, it has yet to be conclusively proven.

Thermal shock defines the phenomenon of sudden and profound temperature change in a biologic system.[18] Precipitous chilling has been theorized to be incompatible with life, but the severity of this phenomenon is debatable. Another poorly understood concept is the manner in which subzero temperatures produce denaturation of lipid-protein complexes. One theory hypothesizes detachment of lipids and lipid-protein from cell membranes as a consequence of the solvent action of a toxic electrolyte concentration within a cell.[37,38] There is no direct evidence supporting an alteration of enzyme activity during freezing, but deoxyribonucleic acid (DNA) synthesis is inhibited.[25] On the other hand, there is indirect evidence of ox liver catalase inactivation caused by denaturation and structural alteration of lactic acid dehydrogenase after freezing and thawing.[39,77]

Indirect cellular damage secondary to progressive microvascular insults is more severe than the direct cellular effect. This is supported by the observation that skin tissue subjected to a standard freeze-thaw injury, which consistently produced necrosis in vivo, survived as a full-thickness skin graft when transplanted to an uninjured recipient site.[83] Conversely, uninjured full-thickness skin did not survive when transferred to a recipient area pretreated with the same freezing injury. Thus direct skin injury is reversible. The progressive nature of injury is probably secondary to microvascular changes.

Approximately 60% of skin capillary circulation ceases in the temperature range of $3°$ to $11°$ C ($37.4°$ to $51.8°$ F), whereas 35% and 40% of blood flow ceases in arterioles and venules, respectively.[68] Capillary patency is initially restored in thawed tissue, but blood flow declines 3 to 5 minutes later. Three nearly simultaneous phenomena occur after thawing: momentary and initial vasoconstriction of arterioles and venules, resumption of capillary circulation and blood flow, and showers of emboli coursing through microvessels.[89] Ultimately, there is progressive tissue loss caused by progressive thrombosis and hypoxia. This is similar to tissue loss seen in the distal dying random flap and the no reflow phenomenon. For both of these, in addition to the effect of arachidonic acid metabolites, oxygen free radicals have been shown to be detrimental and contribute to tissue loss. This may be the case in the frostbite injury.[8]

Considerable evidence points to the primary alteration of the cold injury being injury to vascular endothelium.[89] Seventy-two hours after a freeze-thaw injury, there is loss of vascular endothelium in the capillary walls, accompanied by significant fibrin deposition. The endothelium may be totally destroyed, and fibrin may saturate the arteriole walls.[89] Ultrastructural derangement of endothelial cells after the thaw period has been observed by electron microscopy in capillaries of the hamster cheek pouch after subzero temperatures.[65] The endothelial injury was confirmed by demonstrating fluid extravasation from vessels almost immediately after thawing.[89] As in other forms of trauma, vascular endothelial cells swell and protrude inward into the lumen until they lyse.

Venules appear more sensitive to cold injury than are other vascular structures, partly because of lower flow rates. Arterioles, with a rate of flow almost twice that of venules, are less damaged by freezing and develop stasis later than venules. Capillaries manifest the fewest direct effects of cold injury, but their flow is quickly arrested as a result of their position between arterioles and venules. Generalized stasis and cessation of flow are noted at the point of injury within 20 minutes after freeze and thaw. "White thrombi" (blood cells and fibrin) follow platelet thrombi as blood flow progressively slows. Sludging and stasis result in ultimate thrombosis. Microangiography after cold injury shows that, although spasm of the arterioles and venules exists, it is not marked enough to completely account for the decreased flow of progressive microvascular collapse.[2] It has been postulated that defects seen in angiograms are caused by local factors, possibly thrombi. It has also been observed that vascular thrombosis after cold injury advances from the capillary level to that of the large vessels and ultimately results in ischemic death of progressively larger areas.[29,31] Viable dermal cells may be observed histologically in cold-injured tissues for up to 8 days or until occlusion of local vessels occurs. This emphasizes that a major role is played by vascular insufficiency, and that direct injury to cellular structures and mechanisms may be reversible.

Because Cohnheim had shown changes in cold injury to be similar to changes seen in other inflammatory states, Robson and Heggers[69] postulated that progressive ischemia seen in frostbite might be due to the same inflammatory mediators responsible for progressive dermal ischemia in the burn wound. They evaluated blister fluid from victims with hand frostbite, measuring levels of PGE_2, $PGF_{2\alpha}$, and thromboxane B_2 (TxB_2). Levels of the vasoconstricting, platelet-aggregating, and leukocyte-sticking prostanoids ($PGF_{2\alpha}$ and TxA_2) were markedly elevated. The investigators postulated that massive edema after cold injury was due either to leakage of proteins caused by release of these prostanoids or to leukocyte sludging in the capillaries and increased hydrostatic pressure. Recent studies have confirmed the similarity between cold injury and the burn wound.[8]

Severe endothelial damage was observed by researchers studying a minimal cold injury model in the hairless mouse.[5] In addition, the sequence of endothelial damage, vascular dilation, vascular incompetence, and erythrocyte extravasation was confirmed. This led to speculation that arachidonic acid metabolites, which may originate from severely damaged endothelial cells, are important in progressive tissue loss. Significantly absent from in vivo and microscopic observations were vascular spasm, thrombosis, and fibrin deposition, all of which have previously been implicated as pathophysiologic mechanisms. A rabbit ear model demonstrated increased tissue survival after blockade of the arachidonic acid cascade at all levels.[66] The most marked tissue salvage resulted when specific TxA_2 inhibitors were used. This has now been shown to be effective in clinical situations.[22]

Skin Changes in Response to Frostbite

Reports in the 1940s documenting the histopathology of frostbite injury to the skin have been scarce and incomplete. Historically, studies by several investigators have been limited to skin biopsies without documentation of location, exposure time, temperature, or post injury intervals.[72] More recently, experimental studies have been able to document the histopathology of skin changes under controlled conditions.

In 1988, Schoning and Hamlet[74,75] used a Hanford miniature swine model for frostbite injury ($-75°$ C [$-103°$ F] exposure for up to 20 minutes) to note progressive epithelial damage. Early changes included vacuolization of keratinocytes, with loss of intercellular attachments and pyknosis over a period of 1 week or more. This subsequently progressed to advanced cellular degeneration and the formation of microabscesses at the dermoepidermal junction. Later changes include epithelial necrosis and regeneration, both separately or together within the same tissue. Such histopathologic data favor the current standard of conservative management of frostbite injury.

However, Marzella et al[40] used a New Zealand white rabbit ear model of frostbite injury and proposed that the skin necrosis induced by frostbite injury was merely a reflection of damage to the target cell: the endothelial cell. After submersion of a shaved rabbit ear in 60% ethyl alcohol at $-21°$ C ($-5.8°$ F) for 60 seconds, the entire microvasculature demonstrated endothelial dam-

age within 1 hour; erythrocyte extravasation occurred within 6 hours. These early vascular changes in the rabbit ear model are in contradistinction to the timing of vascular changes in the Hanford miniature swine model reported by Schoning et al.[75] These authors performed biopsies on animals exposed to frostbite injury ($-75°$ C for up to 20 minutes) and evaluated the specimens for vascular inflammation, medial degeneration, and thrombosis. The earliest change documented both grossly and microscopically was hyperemia. Within 6 to 24 hours, leukocyte migration and vasculitis were noted. However, the most severe vascular changes of thrombosis and medial degeneration were not documented for 1 to 2 weeks after the injury.

Whether or not the changes in the epidermis are primary or secondary to damage to the underlying endothelial cells, it is clear that these tissues have a potential, although limited, capacity for regeneration. This further supports a conservative approach to the management of frostbite injury.

Clinical Presentation

Classically, frostbite has been described by its clinical presentation. Initially, it is difficult to predict the extent of frostbite damage.[28,52] Mills[51] favors the use of two simple classifications: mild (without tissue loss) and severe (with tissue loss). Historically, frostbite has been divided into "degrees of injury" based on acute physical findings after freezing and rewarming. First-degree injury shows numbness and erythema. There is a white or yellowish, firm plaque in the area of injury. There is no tissue loss, although edema is common. Second-degree injury results in superficial skin vesiculation (Figures 7-1 to 7-3). A clear or milky fluid is present within the blisters, surrounded by erythema and

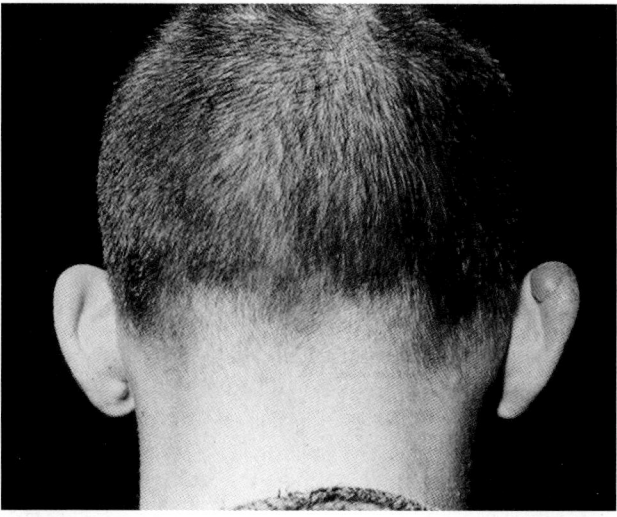

Figure 7-1 Vesiculation of right ear with clear fluid characteristic of second-degree frostbite.

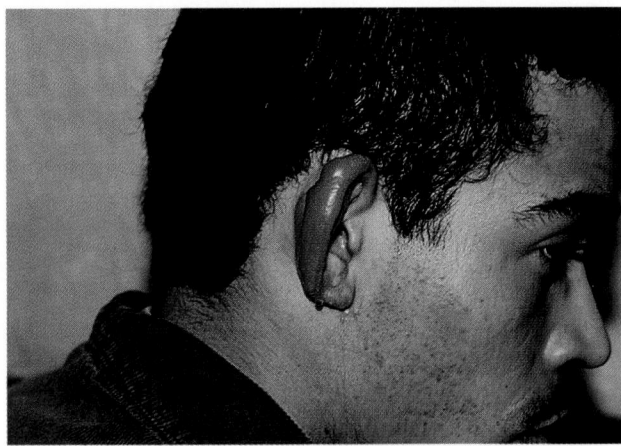

Figure 7-2 Minor first degree frostbite of the ear. Note blister formation on the back of the pinna. One day postthaw. *(Photo by Murray P. Hamlet, DVM.)*

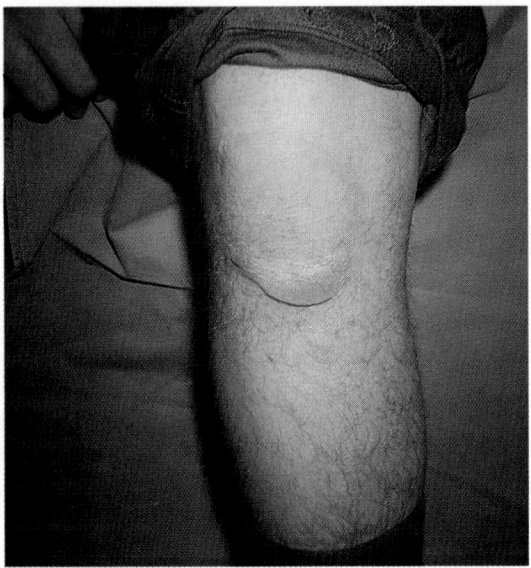

Figure 7-3 First-degree frostbite of the knee from kneeling to change a tire. Twelve hours postthaw. *(Photo by Murray P. Hamlet, DVM.)*

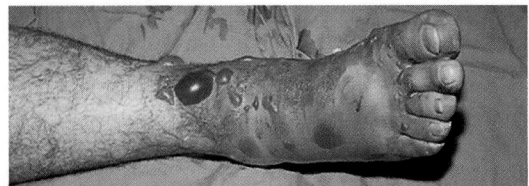

Figure 7-4 Edema and blister formation 24 hours after frostbite injury occurring in an area covered by a tightly fitting boot. *(Courtesy Cameron Bangs, MD.)*

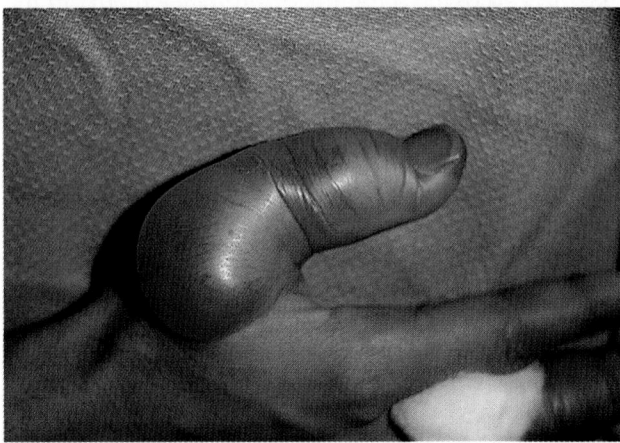

Figure 7-5 Deep second and third degree frostbite with hemorrhagic blebs. One day postthaw. *(Photo by Murray P. Hamlet, DVM.)*

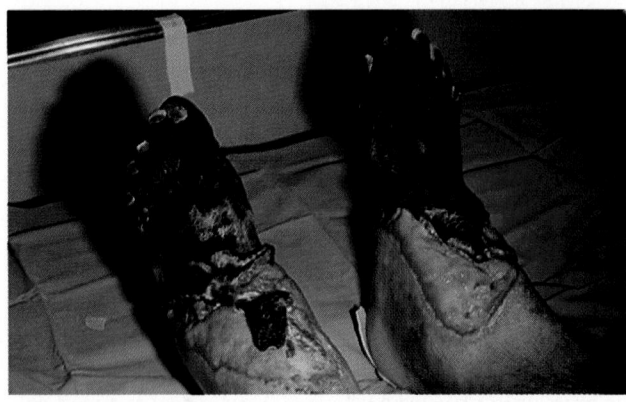

Figure 7-6 Gangrenous necrosis 6 weeks after frostbite injury shown in Figure 7-4. *(Courtesy Cameron Bangs, MD.)*

edema. Third-degree injury shows deeper blisters, characterized by purple, blood-containing fluid (Figures 7-4 and 7-5). This indicates that the injury is into the reticular dermis and beneath the dermal vascular plexus. Fourth-degree injury is completely through the dermis and involves the relatively avascular subcuticular tissues (Figures 7-6 and 7-7). This tends to cause mummification (Figures 7-8 and 7-9), with muscle and bone involvement. Less severe bone injury in children may affect the growth plate and result in developmental digital deformities.[7,10]

Frostbite Symptoms

The severity of frostbite symptoms generally parallels the severity of the injury. In the civilian population, frostbite most frequently occurs on the extremities, with the lower extremity being far more common. It can also appear on the nose or ears and has been reported on the scrotum and penis in joggers.[82]

Mere numbness followed by tingling after rewarming does not constitute bona fide frostbite. Even in its mildest form, true frostbite damages the affected tissue. In most victims the initial clinical observation is coldness of the involved extremity, with numbness present in more than three fourths of victims. This ultimately causes the in-

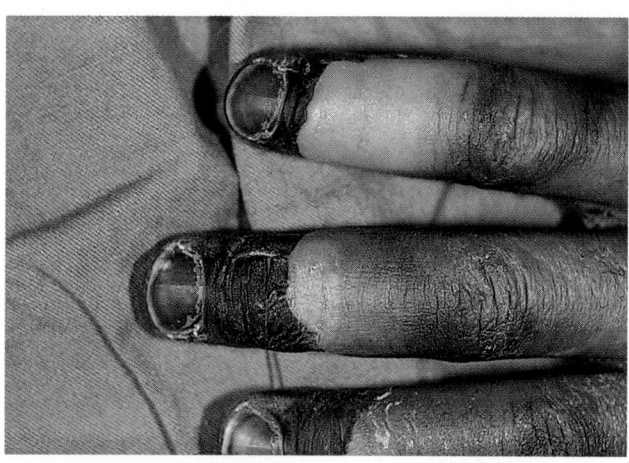

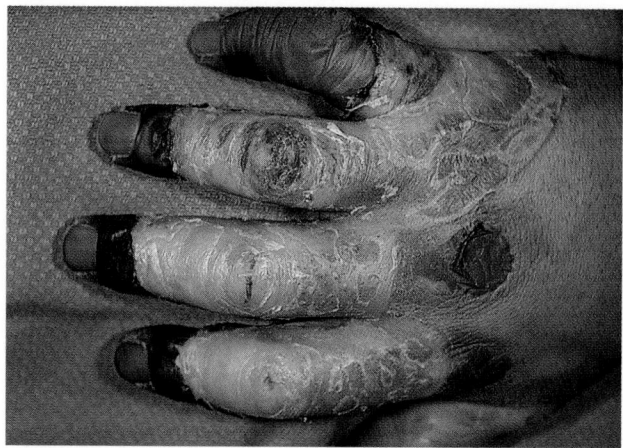

Figure 7-7 Fourth-degree frostbite. Note sharp line of demarcation under eschar, depigmentation of third degree skin proximally and indurated distal fingertips. Fingertips will autoamputate. Four weeks postthaw. *(Photo by Murray P. Hamlet, DVM.)*

Figure 7-9 Fourth-degree frostbite. Fingertips will autoamputate. Note dried or absent bleb surface. Depigmentation and flexure contractures. Five weeks postthaw. *(Photo by Murray P. Hamlet, DVM.)*

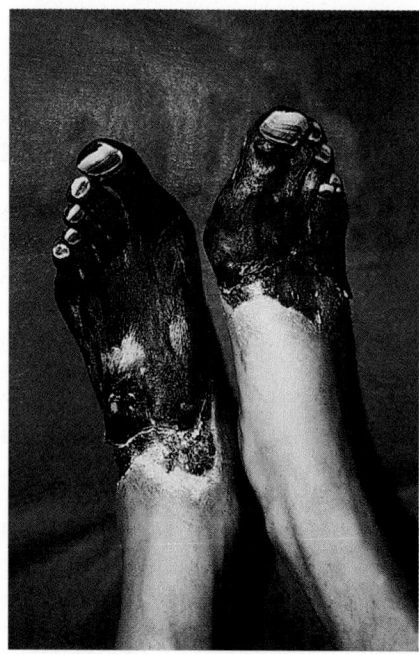

Figure 7-8 Severe fourth-degree frostbite. Note no infection, sharp line of demarcation, and partially removed eschar. Eight weeks postthaw. *(Photo by Murray P. Hamlet, DVM.)*

volved part to feel clumsy or absent and has been attributed to ischemia after intense vasoconstriction. When numbness is initially present, it frequently is followed by extreme pain (76% of victims) during rewarming. Throbbing pain begins 2 to 3 days after rewarming and continues for a variable period, even after the tissue becomes demarcated (22 to 45 days). After about a week, the victim usually notices a residual tingling sensation, probably caused by ischemic neuritis. For this reason, this sensation tends to persist longer than do other symptoms. The severity of the injury usually defines the extent of neu-

ropathologic damage. There may be a great deal of variation in symptoms, with some victims never noticing pain at the onset of the injury. In victims without tissue loss, symptoms usually subside within 1 month, whereas in those with tissue loss, disablement may exceed 6 months. In all cases, symptoms are intensified by a warm environment. Other sensory deficits include spontaneous burning and electric current–like sensations. The burning sensation, which is frequently early in presentation, subsides within 2 to 3 weeks. This sensation is not present in victims with tissue loss. In victims without tissue loss, it may resume on wearing shoes or increasing activity. The electric current–like shock is almost universal (97%) in victims with tissue loss. It usually begins 2 days after injury, lasts for about 6 weeks, and is particularly unpleasant at night. All frostbite victims experience some degree of sensory loss for at least 4 years after injury and perhaps indefinitely.

The clinical appearance of frostbite may be deceiving.[4,59] Only a few victims arrive with tissue still frozen. Originally the extremity appears yellowish white or mottled blue. It may be insensate and may appear frozen solid. Regardless of the depth of the injury, the extremity may have the appearance of being frozen. With rapid rewarming there is almost immediate hyperemia, even with the most severe injury. Sensation returns after thawing and persists until blebs appear. At this point, some effort may be made to assess the severity of the injury. Although "degrees" of injury have been defined, one usually differentiates between superficial (first- or second-degree) and deep (third- or fourth-degree) injuries. Even these distinctions are somewhat artificial, since the initial treatment of frostbite is identical. The degree system may have some importance in retrospective analysis of cases.

After the extremity is rewarmed, edema appears within 3 hours and lasts 5 days or longer, depending

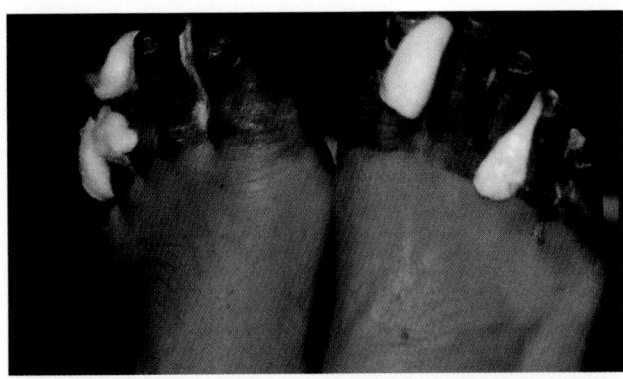

Figure 7-10 Frostbitten toes demarcate three weeks after injury. Note the cotton padding between the toes. Minimal tissue loss occurred. *(Photo by Paul Auerbach, MD.)*

on the severity of the case.[59] Vesicles, or bullae, form 6 to 24 hours after rapid rewarming.[46,60] During the first 9 to 15 days, severely frostbitten skin forms a black, hard, and usually dry eschar whether vesicles are present or not (Figure 7-10).[60] Mummification forms an apparent line of demarcation in 22 to 45 days.[59]

Favorable prognostic signs include sensation to pinprick; normal color; warmth; and large, clear blebs that appear early and tend to extend to tips of the digits. Unfavorable signs include small, dark blebs that appear late and do not extend to the digit tips; the absence of edema; and the presence of cyanosis that does not blanch with pressure.[51]

Techniques that have been used to estimate the extent of injury and to predict ultimate tissue loss include intravenous radioisotope scanning (^{131}I RISA, ^{133}Xe, ^{99m}Tc MDP, ^{99}Tc stannous pyrophosphate), angiography, routine roentgenography, and digital plethysmography. These modalities have also been recommended for estimating the vascular response to vasodilators and identifying tissue boundaries for surgical management. No prognostic technique is absolutely accurate in the immediate postthaw period; a delay of 2 to 3 weeks is necessary to exceed the period of transitory vascular instability.

Ophthalmic Injuries

Ophthalmic injuries, particularly freezing of corneas, occur in individuals who try to force their eyes open in high windchill situations. Snowmobilers and cross-country skiers are particularly susceptible. Blurred vision, photophobia, blepharospasm, tearing, and pain on rewarming suggest such an injury. Rapid rewarming and patching are the only effective treatments. Corticosteroids are contraindicated. Corneal transplantation may be required if keratitis and corneal opacification are irreversible and debilitating. Snowblindness caused by ultraviolet exposure is discussed in Chapter 14.

Management

In 1947, Hurley stated, "Tissue cells can be affected by freezing in three different ways: 1) a certain number of cells are killed; 2) a certain number remain unaffected; and 3) a large number are injured but may recover and survive under the right circumstances."[24] Obviously the major treatment effort must be to salvage as many cells in category 3 as possible.

Frostbite treatment is directed separately at the prethaw and postthaw intervals. If a victim is referred from a nearby location, no attempt at field rewarming may be indicated. Vigorous rubbing is ineffective and potentially harmful. The extremity should not be intentionally rewarmed during transport and should be protected against slow partial rewarming by keeping the victim away from intense campfires and car heaters. All constrictive and wet clothing should be replaced by dry, loose wraps or garments. The extremity is padded and splinted for protection, but no other treatment is initiated. Although there is a correlation between the length of time tissue is frozen and the amount of time required to thaw that tissue, there is no direct correlation between the length of time tissue is frozen and subsequent tissue damage. Therefore rapid transport of frostbite victims (within 2 hours) is appropriate. Otherwise, rapid rewarming should be instituted and the victim transported with protective dressings to prevent refreezing. Blisters should be left intact. Victims with long transport times are at greater risk for recurrent injury. All efforts should prevent subsequent refreezing, since this creates an infinitely worse result than does delayed thawing. A victim who must walk through snow should do so before thawing frostbitten feet. During transport, the extremities should be elevated and tobacco smoking prohibited.[50] Alcohol ingestion is contraindicated.

Once in the emergency department, rapid rewarming should be started immediately. Associated traumatic injuries or medical conditions should be identified. Systemic hypothermia should be corrected to a core temperature of at least 34° C (93° F) before frostbite management is attempted. Fluid resuscitation is usually not a problem with frostbite injuries, although one case of rhabdomyolysis and acute renal failure has been reported.[71]

Treatment is directed at the specific pathophysiologic effects of the frostbite injury, either blocking direct cellular damage or preventing progressive microvascular thrombosis and tissue loss. Direct cellular damage is treated by rapid thawing of all degrees of frostbite with immersion in gently circulating water warmed to between 40° and 42° C (104° and 108° F) (Figure 7-11).[27] Adherence to this narrow temperature range is important, since rewarming at lower temperatures is less beneficial for tissue survival,[16,22] and rewarming at higher temperatures may compound the injury by producing a burn wound.[54] Heated tap water

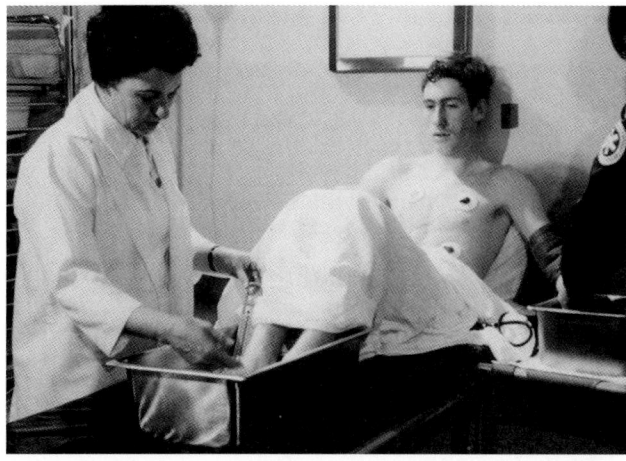

Figure 7-11 Technique to rapidly warm all four extremities simultaneously. The water is 40° to 42° C (104° to 108° F), monitored by a thermometer, and circulated manually. Thawing is usually complete in 30 minutes, when the extremities are pliable and color and sensation have returned.

(50° to 60° C [122° to 140° F]) is too hot and will cause profound discomfort and possible tissue damage. Frozen extremities should be rewarmed until the involved skin becomes pliable and erythematous at the most distal parts of the frostbite injury. This usually takes less than 30 minutes. Active motion during rewarming is helpful, but massage may compound the injury. Extreme pain may be experienced during thawing, and unless otherwise contraindicated, parenteral analgesics are administered. Rapid return of skin warmth and sensation with the presence of an erythematous color is a favorable sign, whereas the persistence of cold, anesthetic, and pale skin is unfavorable.

Rapid rewarming reverses the direct injury of ice crystal formation in the tissue. However, it does not prevent the progressive phase of the injury. McCauley et al[43,44] have designed a protocol based on the pathophysiology of progressive dermal ischemia that has been quite successful in minimizing the production of local and systemic thromboxane by injured tissues (Box 7-1). All but the most minor frostbite cases should be admitted to the hospital. Victims with minor injuries should be admitted if, after rapid rewarming, a warm environment cannot be ensured for the victim. No patient should ever be discharged into subfreezing weather. Even with a warm car waiting, the patient should be allowed to leave only with proper clothing (such as stocking cap, wool mittens, and wool socks). Since the majority of frostbite injuries necessitate admission to the hospital, a discussion of the protocol is warranted. White or clear blisters, which represent more superficial injury, are debrided to prevent further contact of $PGF_{2\alpha}$ or TxA_2 with the damaged underlying tissues. Unlike the clear blisters, hemorrhagic blisters reflect structural damage to the subdermal plexus. It

may be worthwhile to aspirate the thromboxane-containing fluid out of these blisters, but debridement may allow desiccation of the deep dermis and allow conversion of the injury to full thickness. Therefore hemorrhagic blisters are left intact. A specific thromboxane inhibitor is placed on the wounds to prevent further formation of this vasoconstricting mediator (Figure 7-12). Aspirin was originally given systemically to block production of $PGF_{2\alpha}$ and TxA_2. Since the correct dose of aspirin is not known, aspirin has been replaced by ibuprofen.[80] Ibuprofen not only inhibits the arachidonic acid cascade but also has the additional benefit of fibrinolysis. Elevation of the extremity minimizes dependent edema. Since edema inactivates the normal streptococcidioidal properties of the skin, parenteral penicillin is administered during the edema phase of the injury.[11] Antitetanus prophylaxis is given if indicated by the patient's immunization history.[12] Tetanus killed thousands of Napoleon's soldiers in the Russian campaign. There was a report as recently as April 1985 documenting tetanus associated with a frostbite injury. Since frostbite generally involves injuries to the extremities, appropriate physical and occupational therapy should be initiated early. Daily hydrotherapy for active and passive range of motion is extremely valuable in the preservation of function.[14]

Between 1982 and 1985, 56 patients were treated with the previous frostbite protocol and 98 were treated by other "standard" methods. Of the 56 patients treated with the protocol, 18 were admitted with first-degree frostbite, 25 with second-degree frostbite, and 13 with third-degree frostbite. Thirty-two suffered acute frostbite, and 24 had subacute (presenting for treatment more than 24 hours after injury). The mean length of hospital stay for the acute protocol patients was 8.5 days and for the subacute group, 14.9 days. Overall, 67.9% of the protocol group healed without tissue loss, 25% healed with some tissue loss, and 7% required amputation. Of the nonprotocol patients, 11 were admitted with first-degree frostbite, 51 with second-degree frostbite, and 36 with third-degree frostbite. Fifty-six were acute cases, and 42 were subacute. The mean length of hospital stay was 17.5 days for the acute, nonprotocol patients and 19 days for the subacute group. Of this group, 32.7% healed without tissue loss, 34.6% healed with tissue loss, and 32.7% required amputation ($p < .001$; includes all groups of protocol-treated patients). These data indicate therapeutic efficacy of the protocol by virtue of less tissue loss, lower amputation rate, and significantly shorter hospital stay.[22]

Other Therapies

A number of other therapeutic modalities have attempted to prevent progressive thrombosis and tissue loss. Most were proposed before the pathophysiology of the injury was found to be related to inflammatory

---

Box 7-1 PROTOCOL FOR RAPID REWARMING

1. Admit frostbite patients to a specialized unit if possible.
2. Do not discharge or transfer to another facility victims of acute frostbite requiring hospitalization unless it is necessary for specialized care. Transfer arrangements must protect the victim from cold exposure.
3. On admission, rapidly rewarm the affected areas in warm water at 40° to 42° C (104° to 108° F), usually for 15 to 30 minutes or until thawing is complete.
4. Upon completion of rewarming, treat the affected parts as follows:
   a. Debride white blisters and institute topical treatment with aloe vera (Dermaide aloe) every six hours.
   b. Leave hemorrhagic blisters intact and institute topical aloe vera (Dermaide aloe) every six hours.
   c. Elevate the affected part(s) with splinting as indicated.
   d. Administer antitetanus prophylaxis.
   e. For analgesia, administer morphine or meperidine (Demerol) intravenously or intramuscularly as indicated.
   f. Administer ibuprofen 400 mg orally every 12 hours.
   g. Administer penicillin G 500,000 units intravenously every six hours for 48 to 72 hours.
   h. Perform hydrotherapy daily for 30 to 45 minutes at 40° C (104° F). The solution should meet the following specifications:
      (1) Large tank capacity—425 gallons
          Fill level estimate—285 gallons
          Sodium chloride—9.7 kg
          Calcium hypochlorite solution—95 ml
      (2) Medium tank capacity—270 gallons
          Fill level estimate—108 gallons
          Sodium chloride—3.7 kg
          Calcium hypochlorite solution—36 ml
      (3) Small tank capacity—95 gallons
          Fill level estimate—72 gallons
          Sodium chloride—2.5 kg
          Potassium chloride—71 g
          Calcium hypochlorite solution—24 ml
5. For documentation obtain photographs on admission, at 24 hours, and serially every two to three days until discharge.
6. Discharge patients with specific instructions for protection of the injured areas to avoid reinjury and follow up weekly until wounds are stable. If the patient is being discharged with no open lesions, instruct him or her to use wool socks, wear a hat, and use mittens instead of gloves to decrease the loss of heat between the fingers. Explain to patients that they are more susceptible to refreezing, so they should avoid exposure to cold and should wear warm clothing and shoes or boots if going outside is necessary. Give similar instructions to patients who are discharged with open lesions. Also instruct these patients to keep the affected extremity elevated and to take ibuprofen 400 mg orally every 12 hours. Aloe vera should be applied to the involved areas, or scarlet red ointment used if the open areas are small.

---

mediators. These therapeutic attempts deserve comment. It has been observed that cold-injured vessels, shortly after thawing, became dilated and filled with clumps of erythrocytes. These clumps can be easily dislodged by gentle manipulation and do not represent true thrombosis. Although the mechanism that leads to erythrocyte clumping is not completely understood, it may reflect a cold-induced increase in blood viscosity. This suggests that the use of low-molecular-weight dextran may be of benefit in the early treatment of frostbite. Although no controlled clinical trial of low-molecular-weight dextran has been reported, there has been experimental evidence to support its use. Weatherly-White, Sjostrom, and Paton[83] demonstrated that the use of low-molecular-weight dextran, 1 g/kg/day, protected against tissue loss in the rabbit ear model. This led to the suggestion that the use of 1 L of 6% dextran intravenously on the day of injury, followed by 500 ml on each of 5 successive days, might be of benefit.[70] With our present understanding of the etiology of frostbite, there appear to be few instances when it may be used and have demonstrable benefit.

Although true thrombi are not present in dilated, erythrocyte-filled vessels immediately after thawing, they form over the next few days. Heparin has been suggested as a possible treatment for frostbite. Lange and Loewe[33] demonstrated its usefulness in experimental frostbite. Subsequent investigations have been unable to substantiate these findings, and at the present time there is no evidence that heparin alters the natural history of the frostbite.[76]

Intraarterial reserpine has also been shown experimentally to be of use in frostbite. Porter et al[62] reported its clinical use in five patients. Three of the patients were treated within 2 weeks of injury. Angiography of the involved extremities was performed before and after injection (Figure 7-13). Reserpine appeared to be effective in relieving vasospasm. However, treatment did not retard progression of tissue loss. A multiarmed clinical study compared slow rewarming combined with

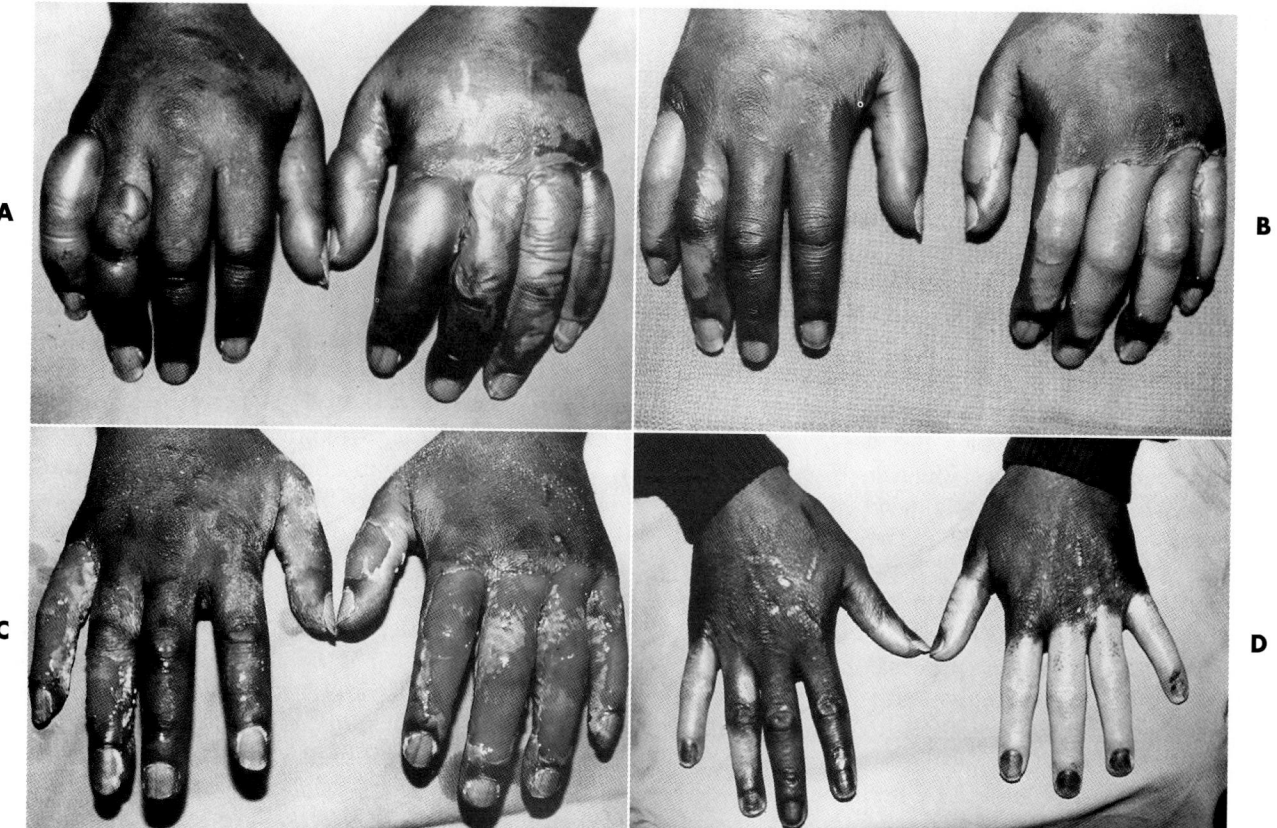

Figure 7-12 **A,** Acute frostbite injury with clear fluid in superficial blisters. **B,** Blisters before treatment but after debridement. **C,** After 48 hours of therapy with topical aloe vera (Dermaide aloe). **D,** Sixteen days after injury.

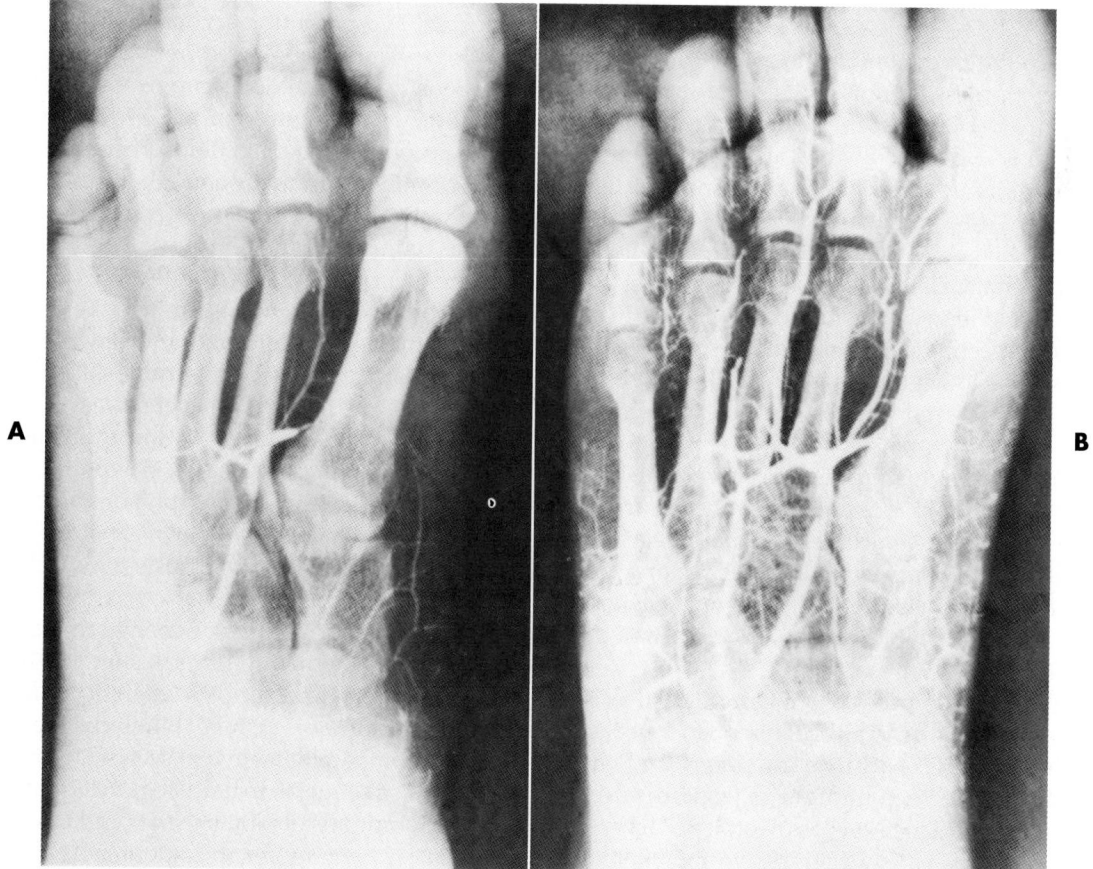

Figure 7-13 Angiograms of the left foot of a 30-year-old man with cold injury. **A,** Initial angiogram. **B,** Angiogram taken 2 days after intraarterial injection of reserpine. (*From Gralino BJ, Porter JM, Rosch J:* Radiology *19:301, 1976.*)

intravenous dextran, intraarterial tolazoline, intraarterial reserpine, and various combinations of these drugs.[79] All of the drug treatments were superior to simple slow rewarming. However, rapid rewarming was as effective as any of the drug treatments. Therefore reserpine might be effective when patients are brought for treatment late and have not been rapidly rewarmed. To date, no anticoagulant or vasodilation treatment has proved useful in controlled clinical trials.

Several reports from Europe and the United States after World War II supported the use of sympathetic block and sympathectomy.[6] However, this remains controversial. If the sympathetic nervous system is involved, it seems reasonable that early sympathectomy would be beneficial. However, experimental evidence indicates that sympathectomy performed within the first few hours of injury increases edema formation and accelerates the pathologic process of tissue destruction.[17,83] On the other hand, sympathectomy performed 24 to 48 hours after thawing seems to hasten resolution of edema and decrease tissue loss.[17] The role of sympathectomy will not become clear until there is a verifiable clinical rating to evaluate results.[13] Similar problems exist in evaluation of the use of hyperbaric oxygen. Although some experimental data support its use, only occasional anecdotal cases are reported.[58] Furthermore, its use is predicated on the original theory of the frostbite injury and not the most recent experimental data.

Early surgical intervention has no role in the acute care of frostbite, unless there is ischemia from a constricting eschar or subeschar infection that cannot be controlled by topical antimicrobials. Decompressing escharotomy incisions are rarely necessary to increase the distal circulation. If such escharotomies are necessary to decompress digits and facilitate joint motion, incisions along the transaxial line are best. It is important that incisions avoid injury to the underlying structures. If uncontrolled infection is present early, escharotomy may be necessary. However, this is rare with the use of penetrating antibacterial agents, such as mafenide acetate.

Surgical intervention is properly reserved for late treatment of frostbite. This is most often necessary if frostbite is very severe or if treatment has been delayed. Normally, aggressive therapeutic measures can prevent progressive injury and gangrene. If gangrene ensues, amputation or debridement with resurfacing may be necessary (Figure 7-14).

This should be accomplished only after the area is well demarcated, which generally requires 3 to 4 weeks. Historically, aggressive early debridement and attempted salvage have been thought to jeopardize recovering tissue and add to tissue loss. Gottlieb, Zachary, and Krizek[18] have taken a more aggressive approach to coverage of severe frostbite injury. Using technetium phosphate and bone scans, they identify nonperfused tissue by the tenth day after injury and surgically remove necrotic tissue. The remaining nonvascularized, nonviable, yet nonnecrotic and noninfected, tissue is salvaged by early coverage with well-vascularized tissue. Theoretically, if nonvascularized tissue has not undergone autolysis and is not infected, it should behave as a composite graft. Preliminary reports are promising.[18]

Late Sequelae

Until 1957, little was recorded about the long-term sequelae of frostbite injuries. Blair, Schatzki, and Orr[3] studied 100 veterans of the Korean conflict 4 years after their injuries. In order of decreasing frequency, the victims reported excessive sweating, pain, coldness, numbness, abnormal skin color, and stiffness of the joints. In addition, the investigators noted frequent asymptomatic abnormalities of the nails, including ridges and inward curving of the edges. In general, the degree of long-term disability was related to the severity of the original injury. Symptoms were worse in cold than in warm weather. This is attributed to the fact that vessels do not react as well to stress.[78] Previously injured blood vessels do not constrict when exposed to cold as effectively as do normal vessels, and they do not dilate as effectively when vasoconstriction is blocked.

Hyperhidrosis is probably both a cause and a result of frostbite. Hyperhidrosis suggests the presence of an abnormal sympathetic nervous response induced by cold injury and is abolished by sympathetic denervation. Sensitivity to cold and predisposition to recurrent cold injury should suggest hyperhidrosis. Blanching and pain on subsequent cold exposure may be a nuisance or may be dramatic enough to suggest a diagnosis of Raynaud's phenomenon. Almost without exception a painful, shiny, cyanotic, and sweaty limb becomes warm, dry, and useful with sympathetic interruption.[74,75] Schoning[73] examined the changes in the sweat glands of Hanford miniature swine after experimental frostbite injury to determine the etiology of hyperhidrosis. She noted that severe sweat gland changes were of two types: degeneration with necrosis and squamous metaplasia. Clearly, if hypohidrosis were a sequela of frostbite injury, morphologically normal and active sweat glands would be an expected finding. We may conclude that hyperhidrosis may lack histologic documentation.

The late abnormalities of change in skin color, including depigmentation of dark skin and appearance resembling erythrocyanosis in light skin, are most likely the result of ischemia.[3] Similarly, the nail abnormality is comparable with that seen with ischemia. Neither of these sequelae usually requires treatment.

Late symptoms of joint stiffness and pain on motion are relatively common and undoubtedly are related to the underlying scars and mechanical problems occa-

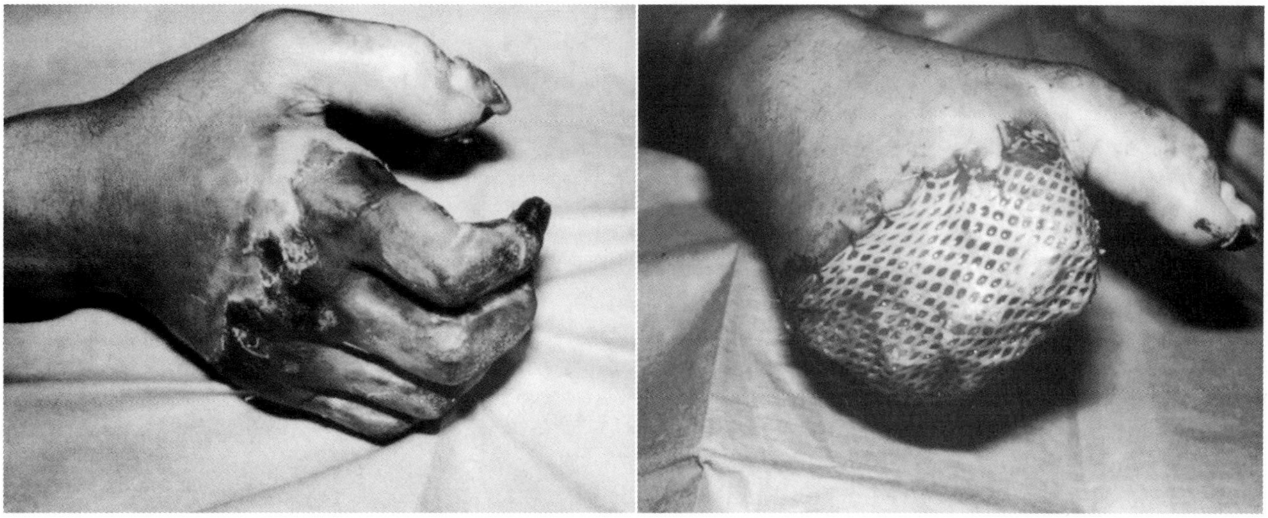

Figure 7-14 **A,** Gangrene from third-degree frostbite. **B,** Treated with partial hand amputation in preparation for toe-to-hand transfer.

sioned by the variety of amputations. "Punched-out" defects in subchondral bone of involved limbs have been noted. These localized areas of bone resorption generally appear within 5 to 10 months after injury and may heal spontaneously. Vascular occlusion is the probable cause of these lesions. Such bone involvement in close proximity to joint surfaces may help explain joint symptoms.

The effects of frostbite on premature closure of epiphyses in the growing hand have recently been reemphasized.[85] The extent of premature closure has been correlated with the severity of the frostbite and noted in partial-thickness injuries. In the digits, premature closure is more frequent from a distal to proximal direction (distal interphalangeal greater than proximal interphalangeal greater than metacarpophalangeal). The thumb has been less often involved. In only 2% of cases does partial epiphyseal closure cause angular deformity.

One of the characteristic features of frostbite is the surprising salvage possible in an apparently badly injured extremity. Amputation should therefore be performed with great conservatism and as late as possible. The line of demarcation may not be decided definitively for weeks or months after injury. As long as secondary sepsis does not intervene, patience often rewards both the patient and surgeon with maximal length of the useful limb. This is particularly true in the upper extremities.

Conditioning and Prevention

Frostbite can usually be prevented by experienced leadership, good physical condition, adequate food, and intelligently used equipment. Probably the two most important basic factors in prevention of frostbite are the heat-producing capacity of the body and the effectiveness of measures to conserve heat once it has been produced. The most fundamental defense against frostbite is a healthy body.

As previously noted, there are no data to support the belief that high altitude increases susceptibility based on changes in blood viscosity. On the other hand, living conditions at high altitude may contribute to increasing danger from frostbite. Cold becomes more intense, as do the violence and severity of storms. Shelter is less appealing and protective. Loss of sleep, inadequate diet, altered digestion, and nervous tension all contribute to a greater degree of fatigue than normally experienced at lower heights. Hypoxia reduces reasoning powers and leads to a tendency to laziness, carelessness, indecision, and lack of normal insight and judgment.[82]

The body requires the same amount of oxygen for various tasks regardless of the attitude. At higher altitudes, however, the body must process more air to gain that same amount of oxygen. Individuals must carefully regulate their activity; otherwise, they will not only exhaust the body but will also cool it. Large quantities of heat can be lost through the lungs by panting and overexertion,[63] which also adds to fatigue.

At higher altitudes, the natural protective mechanism of shivering is impaired and heat production during rest can be significantly reduced. If an individual becomes unable to exercise, the body cannot maintain adequate heat production. The body reduces blood flow to its surface and extremities in an effort to maintain core temperature. In such a situation, no amount of insulation can prevent frostbite and nothing but vigorous warming and administration of oxygen can avert serious results. Since the use of auxiliary oxygen was introduced in mountaineering, frostbite has become less common.

Cold weather increases caloric needs, and variations in diet can have an effect on tolerance.[55] In the cold, cooking, dishwashing, thawing food, and melting water are arduous tasks. Fluid requirements far exceed what is empirically thought to be necessary.

Frostbite is rarely experienced by healthy individuals who are standing still and adequately clothed. It seems to be related almost always to factors such as fatigue, a sudden storm, an accident, or combinations of these. Alcohol intoxication is a frequent forerunner of frostbite. Injury to any part of the body, combined with fear or panic, can allow frostbite in a situation where climatic effects alone would not cause trouble to a seasoned, uninjured person.[82]

Because impaired local circulation is the primary cause of frostbite, anything with even a mildly adverse effect on normal peripheral circulation, such as tobacco or alcohol, should be avoided. Smoking results in varying degrees of diffuse vascular spasm, reducing normal peripheral circulation. Alcohol is not recommended at any time on the trail.[21]

Previous frostbite injury usually results in a prolonged reduction in tolerance to cold by the injured part. Conversely, the concept of physiologic adaptation to cold is extremely controversial. There can be no argument that Eskimos and Tibetans in cold, rugged climates "feel" cold much less than do non-natives. They certainly seem to resist cold more than others and obviously tolerate cold better than those who live in temperate and tropical climates. However, many medical experts allege that this "resistance" is really no more than the result of experience in Arctic survival and day-to-day living. Furthermore, Eskimos, even though they do not feel cold as fast, freeze just as fast and badly as others, given the same actual contact situation. There is increasing evidence that tolerance exists, but even if it is proved, it may be of only academic interest. The basic reason most outdoorspeople are not frostbitten is that they tend to be in good physical condition and know how to act and dress properly.

Many physicians enjoy mountain climbing. Those involved in the Everest exploration wrote about the effects of cold and how to protect against it.[44,82] They suggested that overall physical well-being, good clothing, and intelligent operations in the field were by far the best insurance against frostbite. When a person is exhausted, hungry, ill, injured, or hypoxic, the chances for frostbite injury are increased.[21]

The following measures for frostbite protection are based on Washburn's recommendations[82]:

1. Dress to maintain general body warmth. In cold, windy weather the face, head, and neck must be protected, since enormous amounts of body heat can be lost through these parts.
2. Eat plenty of appetizing food to produce maximum output of body heat. Diet in cold weather at low altitude should tend toward fats, with carbohydrates intermediate and proteins least important. As altitude increases above 3048 m (10,000 feet), carbohydrates become most important and proteins remain least important.
3. Do not climb under extreme weather conditions, particularly at high altitudes on exposed terrain, or get too early a start in cold weather. The configuration of a mountain can help the climber find maximum shelter and solar warmth.
4. Avoid tight, snug-fitted clothing, particularly on the hands and feet. Socks and boots should fit closely, with no points of tightness or pressure. In putting on socks and boots, a person should carefully eliminate all wrinkles in socks. Old matted insoles are to be avoided.
5. Avoid perspiration under conditions of extreme cold; clothing that is adequately ventilated should be worn. If perspiring, remove some clothing or slow down.
6. Keep the feet and hands dry. Even with vapor-barrier boots, socks must not become too wet. All types of boots must be worn with great care during periods of inactivity, especially after exercise has resulted in damp socks or insoles. Wet socks in any type of boot soften the feet and make the skin more tender, greatly lowering resistance to cold and simultaneously increasing the danger of other foot injuries, such as blistering. Extra socks and insoles should always be carried. Light, smooth, dry, clean socks should be worn next to the skin, followed by one or two heavier outer pairs.
7. Wear mittens instead of gloves in extreme cold, except for specialized work, such as photography or surveying, in which great manual dexterity is required for short intervals. In these situations, a mitten should be worn on one hand and a glove temporarily on the other. If bare finger dexterity is required, silk or rayon gloves should be worn, or a metal part that must be touched frequently covered with adhesive tape. The thumbs should be removed and fists held in the palm of mittens occasionally to regain warmth of the entire hand.
8. Be careful while loading cameras, taking pictures, or handling stoves and fuel. The freezing point of gasoline (−57° C [−70° F]) and its rapid rate of evaporation make it very dangerous. Metal objects should never be touched with bare hands in extreme cold or in moderate cold when the hands are moist.
9. Mitten shells and gloves worn in extreme cold should be made of soft, flexible, dry-tanned deer-skin, moose, elk, or caribou hide. Horsehide is less favorable because it dries stiffly after

wetting. Removable mitten inserts or glove linings should be of soft wool.

10. Mittens should be tied together on a string hung around the neck or tied to the ends of parka sleeves. Oiled or greased leather gloves, boots, or clothing should never be used in cold weather operations.

11. Keep toenails and fingernails trimmed.

12. Hands, face, and feet should not be washed too thoroughly or too frequently under rough weather conditions. Tough, weather-beaten face and hands resist frostbite most effectively.

13. Wind and high altitude should always be approached with respect. They can produce dramatic results when combined with cold. Exercise should not be too strenuous in extreme cold, particularly at high altitude, where undue exertion results in panting or very deep breathing. Cold inspired air will chill the whole body and under extreme conditions may damage lung tissue and cause internal hemorrhage.[82]

14. When a person becomes thoroughly chilled, it takes several hours of warmth and rest to return to normal, regardless of superficial feelings of comfort. A person recovering from an emergency cold situation should not venture out again into extreme cold too soon.

15. Avoid tobacco or alcohol at high altitudes and under conditions of frostbite danger.

16. A person who is frostbitten or otherwise injured in the field must remain calm. Panic or fear results in perspiration, which evaporates and causes further chilling.

17. Tetanus immunity should be current.

FROSTNIP

Frostnip is superficial and reversible ice crystal formation associated with intense vasoconstriction. Chilblains result from chronic intermittent exposure to environmental conditions of high humidity and ambient temperature above freezing, without the development of tissue freezing. Frostnip is characterized by discomfort in the involved parts. The symptoms usually resolve spontaneously, and no tissue is lost. There is some question whether this qualifies as cold-induced injury, since neither frozen extracellular water nor progressive tissue loss is routinely demonstrated.

THE FROSTBITE UPDATE

Animal Studies

Recent animal studies by Miller and Koltai[48] and Ozyazgan et al[61] suggest that pentoxifylline with *aloe vera* cream, or defibrotide alone, is beneficial in the treatment of frostbite. Miller and Koltai used the Weatherly-White rabbit model[83] to examine the therapeutic efficacy of pentoxifylline and Dermaide aloe, both alone and in combination.[48] They concluded that, although Dermaide aloe and pentoxifylline were comparable in tissue survival, combining these two therapeutic drugs created a synergistic response when compared with untreated controls (Figure 7-15). All three treated groups were significantly different from the control ($p < .05$). This substantiates earlier animal and human studies conducted by Raine et al,[66] McCauley et al,[43] and Heggers et al,[22] using the thromboxane inhibitor Dermaide aloe.

Ozyazgan et al[61] believed that the events occurring in frostbite were not completely elucidated but suggested that inflammatory mediators, such as PGI_2 and TxA_2, may be the major factors in tissue damage resulting from frostbite coupled with reperfusion injury. Using the Weatherly-White rabbit model for frostbite injury, they established three groups: without freezing, with freezing but no treatment, and with freezing and treated with defibrotide, a polideoxyribonucleotide-naturium-salt that protects endothelium and is also antithrombolytic, anti-polymorphoneutrophilic (PMN), and anti-mast cell (MC). They treated the frostbitten rabbits with defibrotide with a 40mg/kg/day dose twice a day intraperitoneally for 3 days. The frostbitten control received saline, while the nonfrozen control remained untreated.

By measuring PGI_2 and TxA_2 levels and making histologic assessments of PMNs and MCs, it was noted that a significant decrease in these cells did not cause a decrease in tissue survival. It was also noted that PGI_2 was significantly higher than TxA_2 in the treated group when compared with the remaining two groups, which suggests that previous investigators were correct in

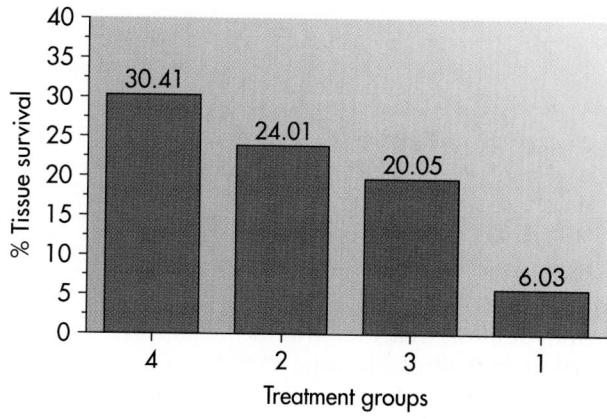

Figure 7-15 Percent tissue survival: Group 4, treatment group with both drugs; Group 2, treatment group with Dermaide aloe alone; Group 3, treatment with pentoxifylline; and Group 1, untreated controls. (*Modified from Miller MB, Koltai PJ: Arch Otolaryngol Head Neck Surg 121:678, 1995*).

TABLE 7-1. Tissue Survival of Patients Treated with Cook County, Illinois, Formula for Frostbite

PATIENT	INJURY	RESULTS
1	Feet bilateral digits 1 week postinjury	Partial amputation proximal interphalangeal joint 2 to 4 digits right; total amputation of digits 1 to 5 left
2	Feet bilateral digits 24 hours postinjury	Partial amputation of the proximal interphalangeal joints 2 to 5 right and 4 to 5 digits left, with total amputation of digits 1 to 3 left; nonambulatory
3	Feet, ankles, legs bilateral 24 hours postinjury	Bilateral open through-the-knee amputation; wheelchair-bound
4	Right foot wet, 6 hours in freezer, 3 days postinjury	Healed with cold sensitivity
5	Feet bilateral 5 hours exposure	Bilateral transmetatarsal amputation; ambulates independently

From Pulla RJ, Pickard LJ, Carnett TS: *J Foot Ankle Surg* 33:53, 1994.
NOTE: All patients were treated with povidone-iodine wet-to-dry dressings.

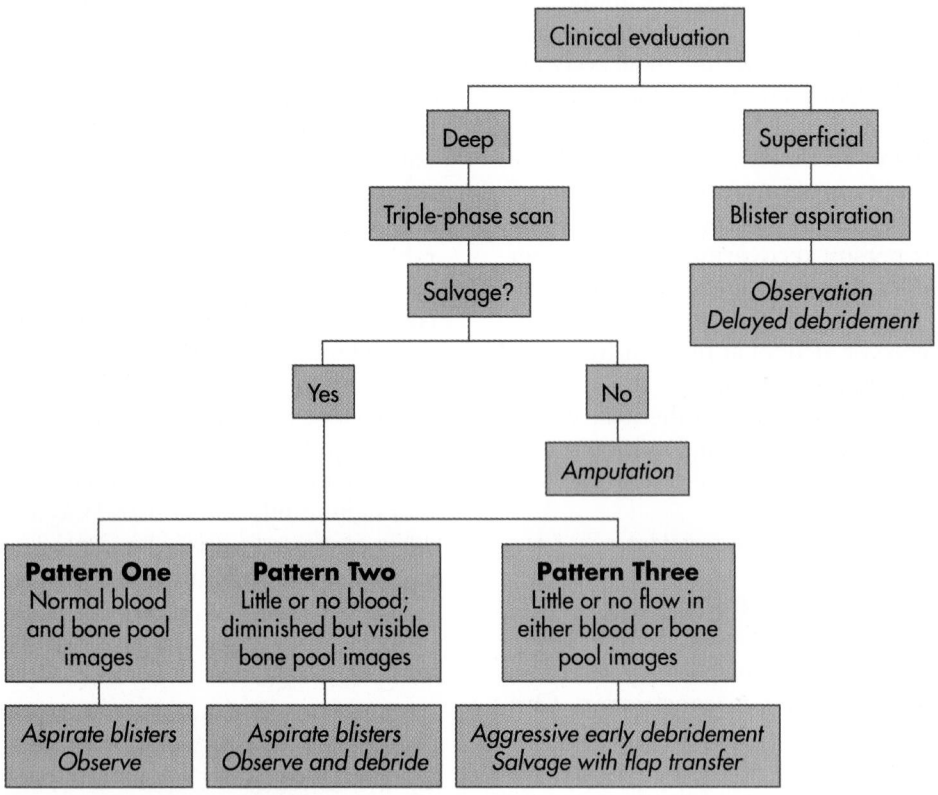

Figure 7-16 Algorithm for treatment of frostbite. Clinical determination of depth forms the first decision tree. Superficial injuries are treated according to standard protocol: aspiration of blisters and delayed debridement. Deep injuries are assessed for suitability of salvage. Salvage attempts follow protocol using triple-phase scanning. Scanning can also be used in the nonsalvage candidate if early debridement is planned. (*Modified from Greenwald D et al:* Plast Reconstr Surg *102:1069, 1998*)

their hypothesis that TxA_2 was the major cause of tissue ischemia in the frostbite injury.[22,43,66]

Human Studies

In recent human frostbite literature, Pulla et al[64] presented five case studies of frostbite injury. Their treatment protocol was based on the McCauley et al[43] frostbite treatment plan (see Box 7-1); however, reserpine and phen-oxybenzamine hydrochloride were used to decrease the incidence of vasospasm. Dermaide aloe and/or silver sulfadiazine were used when available. When rapid rewarming was recommended, a solution of hexachlorophene, povidone iodine, or plain water was used as a wet-to-dry dressing between daily debridements.

Surgical intervention was based on technetium 99m pertechnate scintigraphy, which can assess viable tissue. It was suggested that the scan be performed within 24 to 48 hours after injury and repeated between 7 to 19 days after. Four of the five patients treated required amputation (Table 7-1).

Consequently they reported 80% morbidity compared with the 7% morbidity reported in the study by Heggers et al.[22] Using antivasospasm therapy and povidine-iodine wet-to-dry dressings may have been detrimental. Povidine-iodine is toxic to debrided tissue and might have precipitated further tissue ischemia.

Greenwald et al[20] developed an innovative approach to determining the amount of tissue damage caused by frostbite, thus circumventing the traditional approach of the victim being treated with expectant observation. (With the exception of early blister aspiration, tissues are usually allowed to demarcate before definitive debridement is undertaken.) They used triple-phase bone scanning to define the extent of lethally injured tissues in an endeavor to allow early debridement, wound closure, and aggressive salvage of the extremities with flap reconstruction. Tendon, ligament, bone, and nerve were preserved and covered with vascularized tissue before the first indication of frank necrosis. Postoperative scans revealed revascularization of these tissues. Based on these findings, the authors developed an algorithm for the assessment and treatment of frostbite (Figure 7-16).

ACKNOWLEDGMENTS

The authors are indebted to Ms. Cassie Maness for her care in the preparation of the manuscript. We also compliment Mr. Lewis Milutin, Ms. Tina Garcia, and Ms. Sandra Baxter for their photography and artwork.

REFERENCES

1. Barillo DJ et al: Detrimental effects of ethanol on murine frostbite, *Am Surg* 50:649, 1984.
2. Bellman S, Adams RJ: Vascular reactions after experimental cold injury, *Angiology* 7:339, 1956.
3. Blair JR, Schatzki R, Orr ND: Sequelae to cold injury in one hundred patients: follow-up study four years after occurrence of cold injury, *JAMA* 163:1203, 1957.
4. Boswick JA, Thompson JD, Jonas RA: The epidemiology of cold injuries, *Surg Gynecol Obstet* 149:326, 1979.
5. Bourne MH et al: Analysis of microvascular changes in frostbite injury, *J Surg Res* 40:26, 1986.
6. Bouwman DL et al: Early sympathetic blockade for frostbite: is it of value? *J Trauma* 20:744, 1980.
7. Brown FE, Spiegel PK, Boyle WE Jr: Digital deformity: an effect of frostbite in children, *Pediatrics* 71:955, 1983.
8. Bulkley GB: The role of oxygen free radicals in human disease processes, *Surgery* 94:407, 1983.
9. Campbell R: General outcooling and local frostbite. In *Proceedings of the Symposium on Arctic Biology and Medicine. IV. Frostbite*, Fort Wainwright, Alaska, 1964, Arctic Acromedical Laboratory.
10. Carrera GF et al: Radiographic changes in the hands following childhood frostbite injury, *Skel Radiol* 6:33, 1981.
11. Cold hypersensitivity, *BMJ* 1:643, 1975.
12. Didlake RH, Kukora JS: Tetanus following frostbite injury, *Contemp Orthop* 10:69, 1985.
13. Ducuing J: Les troubles trophiques des produits par de froid sec en pathologic de guerre, *J Chir* 55:385, 1940.
14. Edstrom, LE, Robson, MC, Headley BJ: Evaluation of exercise techniques in the burn patient, *Burns* 4:113, 1977.
15. Fox RH et al: Body temperature in the elderly: a national study of physiological, social and environmental conditions, *BMJ* 1:200,1973.
16. Fuhrman FA, Crissman JM: Studies on gangrene following cold injury. VII. Treatment of cold injury by immediate rapid rewarming, *J Clin Invest* 26:476, 1947.
17. Golding MR et al: Protection from early and late sequelae of frostbite by regional sympathectomy: mechanism of "cold sensitivity" following frostbite, *Surgery* 53:303, 1963.
18. Gottlieb LJ, Zachary LS, Krizek TJ: *Aggressive surgical treatment of frostbite injuries.* Presented at Midwestern Association of Plastic Surgeons meeting, May 1987.
19. Greenfield ADM, Shepherd IT, Whelan RF: Cold vasoconstriction and vasodilatation. *Irish J Med Sci* 309:415, 1951.
20. Greenwald D, Cooper B, Gottlieb L: An algorithm for early treatment of frostbite with limb salvage directed by triple phase scanning, *Plast Reconstr Surg* 102:1069, 1998.
21. Headley BJ, Robson MC, Krizek TJ: Methods of reducing environmental stress for the acute burn patient, *Phys Ther* 55:5, 1975.
22. Heggers JP et al: Experimental and clinical observations on frostbite, *Ann Emerg Med* 16:1056, 1987.
23. Holbrook KA, Byers PH, Pinnell SR: The structure and function of dermal connective tissue in normal individuals and patients with inherited connective tissue disorders, *Scanning Electron Microscopy* 4:1731, 1982.
24. Hurley LA: Angioarchitectural changes associated with rapid rewarming subsequent to freezing injury, *Angiology* 8:19, 1957.
25. Johnson BE, Daniels F Jr: Enzymes studies in experimental cryosurgery of the skin, *Cryobiology* 11:22, 1974.
26. Kinmouth JB, Rob CG, Simeone FB: *The cryopathies in vascular surgery,* London, 1962, E Arnold.
27. Knize DM: *Cold injury in reconstructive plastic surgery: general principles,* vol 1, ed 2, Philadelphia, 1977, WB Saunders.
28. Knize DM et al: Prognostic factors in the management of frostbite, *J Trauma* 9:749, 1969.
29. Kulka JP: Histopathologic studies in frostbitten rabbits. In *Cold injury,* New York, 1956, Josiah Macy, Jr.
30. Kulka JP: Vasomotor microcirculatory insufficiency: observations on nonfreezing cold injury of the mouse ear, *Angiology* 12:491, 1961.
31. Kulka JP: Microcirculatory impairment as a factor in inflammatory tissue damage, *Ann NY Acad Sci* 116:1018, 1964.
32. Kyosola K: clinical experiences in the management of cold injuries: a study of 110 cases, *J Trauma* 14:32, 1974.
33. Lange K, Loewe L: Subcutaneous heparin in the pitkin mastruum for the treatment of experimental human frostbite, *Surg Gynecol Obstel* 82:256, 1946.
34. Larrey DJ: *Memoirs of military surgery,* vol 2, Baltimore, 1814, Joseph Cushing.
35. Lawrence WF et al: The detrimental effect of cigarette smoking on, flap survival: an experimental study in the rat, *Br J Plast Surg* 37:216, 1994.
36. Lewis T: Observations on some normal and injurious effects of cold upon the skin and underlying tissues: III. Frostbite, *BMJ* 2:869, 1941.
37. Lovelock JE: Physical instability in thermal shock in red blood cells, *Nature* 173:659, 1954.
38. Lovelock JE: The denaturation of lipid-protein complexes as a cause of damage by freezing, *Proc R Soc Biol* 147:427, 1957.
39. Marhert CL: Lactate dehydrogenase isozymes: dissociation and recombination of subunits, *Science* 140:1629, 1963.
40. Marzella L et al: Morphologic characterization of acute injury to vascular endothelium of skin after frostbite, *Plast Reconstr Surg* 83:67, 1989.
41. Mazur P: Studies in rapidly frozen suspension of yeast cells by differential thermal analysis and conductometry, *Biophys J* 3:323, 1963.
42. Mazur P: Causes of injury in frozen and thawed cells, *Fed Proc* 24(suppl 14-15):5, 1965.
43. McCauley RL et al: Frostbite injuries: a rational approach based on the pathophysiology, *J Trauma* 23:143, 1983.
44. McCauley RL et al: Frostbite: methods to minimize tissue loss, *Postgrad Med* 88:67, 1990.
45. Merryman HT: Mechanisms of freezing in living cells and tissues, *Science* 124:515, 1956.
46. Merryman HT: The exceeding of a minimum tolerable cell volume in hypertonic suspension as a cause of freezing injury. In *The frozen cell,* London, 1970, Churchill.
47. Miller JW, Danzl DF, Thomas DM: Urban accidental hypothermia: 135 cases, *Ann Emerg Med* 9:456, 1980.
48. Miller MB, Koltai PJ: Treatment of experimental frostbite with pentoxifylline and aloe vera cream, *Arch Otolaryngol Head Neck Surg* 121:678, 1995.

49. Mills W Jr: Summary of treatment of the cold-injured patient, *Alaska Med* 15:56,1973.

50. Mills WJ: Out in the cold, *Emerg Med*, Jan 1976, p 134.

51. Mills WJ Jr: Clinical aspects of frostbite injury. In *Proceedings of the Symposium on Arctic Medicine and Biology. IV. Frostbite.* Fort Wainwright, Alaska, 1964, Arctic Aeromedical Laboratory.

52. Mills WJ Jr: Frostbite, *Alaska Med* 15:27, 1973.

53. Mills WJ, Whaley R: Frostbite: a method of management. In *Proceedings of the Symposium on Arctic Biology and Medicine. IV. Frostbite,* Fort Wainwright, Alaska, 1964, Arctic Aeromedical Laboratory.

54. Mills WJ, Whaley R, Fish W: Frostbite: experience with rapid rewarming and ultrasonic therapy, *Alaska Med* 3:28, 1961.

55. Mitchell HH, Edman M: *Nutrition and climatic stress with particular reference to man,* Springfield, Ill, 1951, Charles C Thomas.

56. Molnar GW et al: Effect of skin wetting on fingercooling and freezing, *J Appl Physiol* 35:205, 1973.

57. Moran T: Critical temperature of freezing living muscle, *Proc R Soc Lond (Biol)* 105:177, 1929.

58. Okuboye JA, Ferguson CC: The use of hyperbaric oxygen in the treatment of experiments frostbite, *Can J Surg* 11:78, 1968.

59. Orr KD, Fainer DC: *Cold injuries in Korea during winter of 1950-1951.* Fort Knox, Ky, 1951, Army Medical Research Laboratory.

60. Orr KD, Fainer DC: Cold injuries in Korea clinic: the winter of 1950-1951. *Medicine* 31:177, 1952.

61. Ozyazgan M et al: Defibrotide activity in experimental frostbite injury, *Br J Plast Surg* 51:450, 1998.

62. Porter JM et al: Intra-arterial sympathetic blockage in the treatment of clinical frostbite, A, *J Surg* 132:625, 1976.

63. Pugh G: Expedition to Cho Oyo, *Geogr J (Lond)* 119:137,1953.

64. Pulla RJ, Pickard LJ, Carnett TS: Frostbite: an overview with case presentations, *J Foot Ankle Surg* 33:53, 1994.

65. Rabb JM et al: Effect of freezing and thawing on the microcirculation and capillary endothelium of the hamster cheek pouch, *Cryobiology* 11:508, 1974.

66. Raine TJ et al: Antiprostaglandins and antithromboxanes for treatment of frostbite, *Surg Forum* 31:557, 1980.

67. Reus WF et al: Acute effects of tobacco smoking on blood flow in the cutaneous micro-circulation, *Br J Plast Surg* 37:213, 1984.

68. Rinfret AP: *Cryobiology in cryogenic technology,* New York, 1962, Wiley.

69. Robson MC, Heggers JP: Evaluation of hand frostbite blister fluid as a clue to pathogenesis, *J Hand Surg* 6:43, 1981.

70. Robson MC, Krizek TJ, Wray RC: Care of the thermally injured patient. In *Management of trauma,* Philadelphia, 1979, WB Saunders.

71. Rosenthall L et al: Frostbite with rhabdomyolysis and renal failure: radionuclide study, *AJR Am J Roentgenol* 137:387, 1981.

72. Schechter DS, Sarot IA: Historical accounts of injuries due to cold, *Surgery* 63:527, 1968.

73. Schoning P: Experimental frostbite in the Hanford miniature swine. Ill. Sweat gland changes, *Int J Exp Pathol* 71:713, 1990.

74. Schoning P, Hamlet MP: Experimental frostbite in Hanford miniature swine. I. Epithelial changes, *Br J Exp Pathol* 70:41, 1989.

75. Schoning P, Hamlet MP: Experimental frostbite in Hanford miniature swine. II. Vascular changes, *Br J Exp Pathol* 70:51, 1989.

76. Schumaker HB et al: Studies in experimental frostbite: the effect of heparin in preventing gangrene, *Surgery* 22:900, 1947.

77. Shikama K. Yamazaki I: Denaturation of catalase by freezing and thawing, *Nature* 190:83, 1961.

78. Simeone FA: Surgical volumes of the history of the United States Army Medical Department in World War 11: cold injury, *Arch Surg* 80:296, 1960.

79. Snider RL, Porter JM: Treatment of experimental frostbite with intra-arterial sympathetic blocking drugs, *Surgery* 77:557, 1975.

80. Vaughn PB: Local cold injury: menace to military operations, a review, *Mil Med* 145:305, 1980.

81. Wanderer AA, Ellis ES: Treatment of cold urticaria with cyproheptadine, *J Allergy Clin lmmunol* 48:366, 1971.

82. Washburn B: Frostbite—what it is—how to prevent it—emergency treatment, *N Engl J Med* 266:974, 1962.

83. Weatherly-White RCA, Sjostrom B, Paton BC: Experimental studies in cold injury, *J Surg Res* 4:17, 1964.

84. Weissman G: Prostaglandins in acute inflammation. In *Current concepts,* Kalamazoo, Mich, 1980, Scope Publications.

85. Weuzl JE, Burke EC, Bianco AJ Jr: Epiphysical destruction from frostbite of the hands, *Am J Dis Child* 114:668, 1967.

86. Whayne TJ, DeBakey MF: *Cold injury, ground type,* Washington, DC, 1958, US Government Printing Office.

87. Wilson O, Goldman RF: Role of air temperature and wind in the time necessary for a finger to freeze, *J Appl Physiol* 29:658, 1970.

88. Zacarian SA: Cryogenics: the cryolesion and the pathogenesis of cryonecrosis. In *Cryosurgery for skin and cutaneous disorders,* St Louis, 1985, Mosby.

89. Zacarian SA, Stone D, Clater H: Effects of cryogenic temperatures in the microcirculation in the golden hamster cheek pouch, *Cryobiology* 7:27, 1970.

90. Zingg W: The management of accidental hypothermia, *Can Med Assoc J* 96:214, 1967.

8 Immersion into Cold Water

Alan M. Steinman and Gordon G. Giesbrecht

Immersion in cold water is a hazard for anyone who participates in recreational, commercial, or military activities in the oceans, lakes, and streams of all but the tropical regions of the world. Recreational aquatic activities include swimming, fishing, sailing, power-boating, ocean kayaking, white-water rafting, canoeing, ocean-surfing, windsurfing, waterskiing, diving, hunting, and the use of personal watercraft. In addition, use of a snowmobile, although not technically a water sport, can involve cold water exposure resulting from accidental entry into lakes and streams.[1] Commercial activities involving water include fishing, shipping, offshore oil drilling, and diving. Military operations over cold water include Coast Guard, Navy, and Marine Corps missions; Army, Air Force, and Marine Corps forces, as well, may encounter cold water exposure during winter operations on land.

The definition of cold water is variable. The temperature of thermally neutral water, in which heat loss balances heat production for a nude subject at rest (i.e., not shivering), is approximately 33° to 35° C (91° to 95° F).[16,17] Hypothermia eventually results from immersion in water below this temperature. For practical purposes, significant risk of immersion hypothermia usually begins in water colder than 25° C (77° F).[104,153,154] Table 8-1 shows the variation of water temperatures throughout the year at various sites in North America,[170] and Figure 8-1 shows typical worldwide sea-surface temperatures for April.[119] Using 25° C as the definition of cold water, the risk of immersion hypothermia in North America is nearly universal during most of the year.

Cold water immersion is associated with two significant medical emergencies: near drowning and hypothermia. This chapter discusses the physiologic responses to and treatment of immersion hypothermia. In addition, this chapter discusses the risk of near drowning with respect to the physiologic consequences of sudden immersion in cold water and the problems of survival in rough seas. Chapter 6 discusses land-based hypothermia, Chapter 56 provides a more complete discussion of drowning, and Chapter 57 discusses diving injuries.

HISTORICAL AND STATISTICAL ASPECTS

The history of human association with the sea and with inland waters provides abundant examples of the effects of accidental cold water immersion. The following case studies demonstrate the scope of the problem:

Perhaps the most famous occurrence was the sinking of the *Titanic* in 1912. After striking an iceberg at approximately 11:40 PM on April 14, the ship sank in calm seas. Water temperature was near 0°C (32° F). Of the 2201 people on board, only 712 were rescued, all from the ship's lifeboats. The remaining 1489 people died in the water, despite the arrival of a rescue vessel within 2 hours. Nearly all of these people were wearing "life preservers," yet the cause of death was officially listed as drowning.[112] More likely the cause of death was immersion hypothermia.[95,102]

In 1963 the cruise ship *Lakonia* caught fire and sank in approximately 18° C (64° F) water off the coast of Madeira in fairly calm seas. Two hundred people abandoned ship into the sea; all wore self-righting life jackets, but 120 died. The cause of death for most victims was hypothermia. Since rescuers reported that small waves washed over the faces of unconscious people, drowning was probably the terminal event.[94]

Numerous examples of maritime occupational accidents exist. In 1982 the offshore mobile oil-drilling platform *Ocean Ranger* collapsed in mountainous seas near Newfoundland, Canada. Water temperature was −1° C (30.2° F). Eighty-four workers were plunged into the water, and despite the presence of a rescue vessel, all died. Immersion hypothermia was a significant factor in these deaths, although the inability of the workers to combat the rough seas and maintain airway freeboard (the distance between the water surface and the mouth) was also a major problem.[106]

Fishing vessel mishaps are a common cause of immersion hypothermia. The following cases illustrate the problems facing the commercial fishing industry:

In 1983 the fishing vessels *Altair* and *Americus* capsized and sank in the Bering Sea in 1° C (33.8° F) water. Fourteen fishermen lost their lives, making it the worst commercial fishing accident in American history. A Coast Guard investigation found vessel over-loading, stability, and crew training and experience as possible factors in the mishaps.[29,171]

In September 1988 the *Cougar,* a Coast Guard–inspected passenger vessel used for fishing, sank with nine persons on board in 13° C (55.4° F) water 45 miles off the Oregon coast. Four occupants died from immersion hypothermia. The five survivors were rescued after spending 17 hours in the sea. Most of the survivors were severely hypothermic, with core temperatures as low as 25° C (77° F). One of the survivors, remarkably, did not require hospitalization; before res-

TABLE 8-1. Mean Water Temperatures (°C) (Temperatures less than 25° C Noted in Bold)

SITE	JAN	FEB	MARCH	APRIL	MAY	JUNE	JULY	AUG	SEPT	OCT	NOV	DEC
Kodiak, AK	**0**	**0**	**2**	**4**	**7**	**9**	**12**	**12**	**10**	**7**	**4**	**2**
Victoria, BC	**7**	**7**	**7**	**9**	**10**	**11**	**11**	**11**	**11**	**10**	**9**	**8**
Astoria, OR	**4**	**5**	**7**	**10**	**13**	**16**	**19**	**19**	**17**	**13**	**9**	**5**
San Francisco, CA	**11**	**11**	**12**	**12**	**12**	**12**	**13**	**13**	**12**	**12**	**11**	**11**
San Diego, CA	**14**	**14**	**15**	**16**	**17**	**18**	**20**	**20**	**20**	**18**	**16**	**15**
Mobile, AL	**10**	**10**	**14**	**21**	**23**	28	29	29	27	**23**	**19**	**14**
Miami, FL	**21**	**21**	**23**	**25**	27	29	30	30	29	27	25	**23**
Norfolk, VA	**17**	**16**	**15**	**18**	**20**	**24**	26	26	25	25	**21**	**19**
Cape May, NJ	**3**	**3**	**5**	**10**	**14**	**19**	**23**	**23**	**21**	**17**	**11**	**6**
Traverse City, MI	**2**	**1**	**1**	**1**	**1**	**3**	**5**	**10**	**10**	**6**	**5**	**4**
Puerto Rico	26	26	26	26	26	27	27	27	28	27	27	26
Honolulu, HI	**24**	**24**	**24**	**24**	25	25	26	26	27	26	25	25

cue, he managed to get out of the water and spend most of the time sitting atop a buoyant life-float.[107]

The best-selling book *The Perfect Storm: A True Story of Men Against the Sea* (made into the feature film *The Perfect Storm*) documents the tragic sinking of the fishing vessel *Andrea Gail* in October 1991. Six fishermen lost their lives in this accident, in which their vessel was caught in an intense Atlantic storm with hurricane-force winds and seas running to 100 feet.[89]

In January 1999 the fishing vessel *Beth Dee Bob,* with a crew of four, sank 13 miles off the New Jersey coast in rough seas. A Coast Guard helicopter responded to the vessel's distress call and arrived on-scene in about an hour. The rescue crew found two empty life rafts and only one crew member alive. He was floating in a life preserver in the 4° C (39.2° F) water while holding onto a strobe light. Unfortunately, he died of hypothermia after transport to a nearby hospital.[171]

In January 1999 the *Kavkaz,* a fishing vessel from Homer, Alaska, capsized in rough seas, trapping two fishermen underneath the boat for 24 hours. Both men wore insulated dry suits (survival suits). However, the zipper on one of the suits was broken, destroying the integrity of the suit and allowing cold water to contact the fisherman's body. He did not survive the ordeal. The other fisherman survived but was moderately hypothermic with a core temperature of 30.5° C (86.9° F).[33]

A 1999 U.S. Coast Guard Fishing Vessel Casualty Task Force Report[171] found that in just 2 months (December 1998–January 1999), 20 commercial fishing vessels were lost at sea. In these mishaps, 21 persons on board died, mainly from exposure to cold water resulting from vessel sinking, capsizing, or the persons falling overboard. From 1994 through January 1999, U.S. Coast Guard statistics show that 396 fishermen lost their lives while fishing. Of these, 298 died from cold water immersion secondary to falling overboard or to the vessel sinking, capsizing, or flooding. In 1998 the death rate for fishermen was 179 per 100,000 workers, a

rate 16 times higher than that for firefighters or for police officers.

Recreational aquatic activities are another major source of immersion incidents. In 1997, Coast Guard statistics show that there were 8047 recreational boating accidents producing 821 deaths, 4555 injuries, and over $29 million in property damage. Over two thirds of these recreational boating fatalities involved exposure of the occupants to water through falling overboard or through vessel capsizing, flooding, swamping, or sinking. Hypothermia or drowning accounted for 74.3% of these fatalities.[172] The following cases illustrate the potential problems with immersion hypothermia in recreational boating and other activities:

In December 1996, three young adults died from hypothermia after their boat sank in 7.3° C (45.1° F) water off East Moriches, New York. The three were experienced boaters and well-versed in cold water survival and safety. Unfortunately, because the weather was unusual for a winter's day in the Northeast (calm winds and seas with an air temperature of 7.3° C), the three left their safety gear and protective clothing at home. When they ended up in the cold seas, their lack of immersion-protective clothing led to death from hypothermia.[8]

In October 1997, three persons died of immersion hypothermia when their 15-foot bass boat was swamped by the wakes of passing boats in Lake Mille Lacs, Minnesota. The four-person crew was forced to spend the night hanging onto their overturned boat in 15.5° C (59.9° F) water. They did not have a radio to call for assistance. Although they were wearing life jackets, they did not have immersion-protective clothing for insulation against hypothermia.[124]

In the winter of 1997-1998, four people died when their snowmobile broke through the thin ice of Lake Scugog, near Toronto, Ontario, Canada. The deaths occurred, ironically, during Snowmobile Safety Week in North America. The Canadian Safety Council reported that in 1997, 101 people were killed in snowmobile

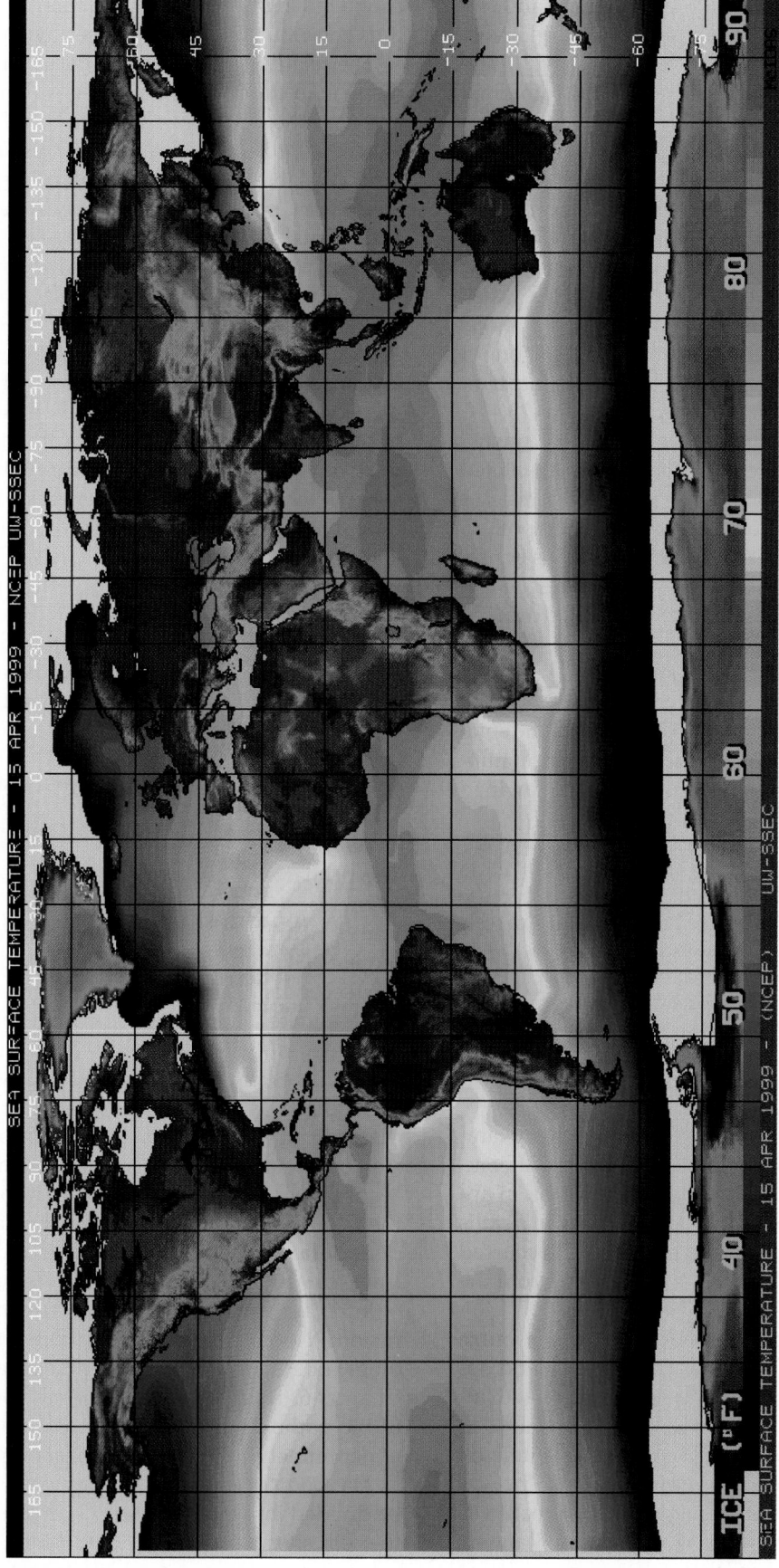

Figure 8-1 Worldwide sea surface temperatures for April 1999. *(From Space Science and Engineering Center, University of Wisconsin, http://www.ssec.wisc.edu/data/sst/latest_sst.gif, 1999. Data provided by National Center for Environmental Prediction.)*

mishaps, the majority of them from drowning and hypothermia after crashing through ice on frozen rivers and lakes.[1]

In the winter of 1988, two men died of hypothermia when their nine-man rowing scull sank in a winter storm on a small lake in western Canada. The nine rowers were immersed in 4° C (39.2° F) water, struggling to hang onto their overturned vessel in 0.6- to 1-m (2- to 3-foot) waves and 30 km/hr winds for over 50 minutes before rescuers could reach them. One man drowned just before rescue; the others were all conscious when pulled from the water. However, during the 13-minute boat transport to shore, three of the thinnest victims lost consciousness and one of these men suffered cardiopulmonary arrest. His core temperature in hospital, 44 minutes after rescue, was 23.4° C (74.1° F); subsequent resuscitation efforts were unsuccessful. The remaining seven survivors were resuscitated from core temperatures as low as 25° C (77° F). This case illustrates the rapidity of onset of immersion hypothermia in lean subjects, and the potentially serious consequences of cardiovascular instability, circum-rescue collapse, and postrescue core temperature afterdrop in immersion hypothermia.[77]

The extensive use of combat ships and aircraft in World War II, particularly in the north Pacific and north Atlantic oceans, provided many examples of accidental immersion in cold water. Molnar reviewed several hundred of these cases.[117] Among them was the following:

"A ship was rammed, and it sank in 3 minutes. Thirty survivors were picked up from rafts after exposure of 1.5 to 4 hours. Some drowned and others died of exposure because the water was 4° C with high seas and a wind velocity of scale 7. Some of the survivors who held on to ropes couldn't let go and rescuers had to cut frozen rope to release them. It appears miraculous how the survivors could have endured such cold water. Most of those who were rescued were in an unconscious state and, when they became conscious complained of numbness of extremities and hands."

The Falklands War in 1982 provided further examples of immersion hypothermia related to naval combat. The Argentine cruiser *General Belgrano* sank in approximately 5° C (41° F) water, resulting in the deaths of many sailors. Some of the deaths from cold occurred even after the sailors had managed to emerge from the water into life rafts.

Maritime military operations are not the only source of hypothermia casualties in the armed forces; land operations, either in combat or in training, also have immersion hypothermia risks. In March 1995, four U.S. Army Rangers died and four others were hospitalized during a training mission in a Florida swamp. The water at the exercise site was deeper and colder than was customary for this exercise. Consequently the Rangers were forced to spend more than 6 hours in cold, wet conditions, much of the time partially immersed in 15° C (59° F) water. Night conditions and difficulties en-

countered in the medical evacuation of the accident victims contributed to the hypothermia deaths.[67]

The relatively high fatality rate from accidental immersion in cold water in various military, commercial, and recreational settings has stimulated technologic advances in protective clothing and rescue devices. Current availability of commonplace items of survival equipment (such as wet suits, dry suits, survival suits, and inflatable life rafts) is primarily a response to the needs of people who work in cold water environments. The value of various types of protective clothing is examined later in this chapter.

In summary, numerous case histories and statistical evidence document the significance of cold water immersion as a cause of the environmental emergencies of drowning and hypothermia. Although drowning is relatively easy to prevent (e.g., through the use of personal flotation devices, water safety training, or restriction of alcohol use), hypothermia is not. Hypothermia is now more widely recognized than in the past, but prevention of immersion hypothermia is still a difficult and often expensive proposition. Therefore, in regions of cold water, which include most of the North American continent, cold water safety, knowledge of cold water risks, and use of appropriate flotation and protective clothing are essential.

PHYSIOLOGIC RESPONSES TO COLD WATER IMMERSION

The primary pathophysiologic effects of hypothermia are decrease in tissue metabolism and gradual inhibition of neural transmission and control. However, in the *initial* stages of cooling of an intact, conscious victim, secondary responses to skin temperature cooling predominate. Sudden immersion in cold water results in immediate decline in skin temperature, which in turn initiates shivering thermogenesis with increases in metabolism (V_{O_2}), ventilation (V_E), heart rate (HR), cardiac output (CO), and mean arterial pressure (MAP). As body temperature declines and shivering ceases, V_{O_2}, HR, MAP, and CO decrease proportionally with the fall in core temperature while hematocrit and total peripheral resistance increase. Renal diuresis and extravascular fluid shifts can lead to a considerable loss of intravascular volume, thus decreasing systemic perfusion. A more detailed description of the pathophysiologic effects of systemic hypothermia is provided in Chapter 6. This section describes the pragmatic effects of the pathophysiologic changes accompanying cold water immersion and their impact on survival.

The body's responses to cold water immersion can be divided into three phases: (1) initial immersion and the cold shock response; (2) short-term immersion and loss of performance; and (3) long-term immersion and the onset of hypothermia. Each phase is accompanied by specific survival hazards for the immersion victim from a variety of pathophysiologic mechanisms. Deaths have occurred in all three phases of the immersion response.

Phase 1: Initial Immersion and the Cold Shock Response

The cold shock response occurs within the first 1 to 4 minutes of cold water immersion and depends on the extent and rate of skin cooling. The responses are generally those affecting the respiratory system and those affecting the heart and the body's metabolism (Figure 8-2).[34,156] Rapid skin cooling initiates an immediate gasp response, the inability to breath-hold, and hyperventilation. The gasp response may cause drowning if the head is submersed during the initial entry into cold water. Subsequent inability to breath-hold may further potentiate drowning in high seas. Finally, hyperventilation causes arterial hypocapnia, which leads to decreased brain blood flow and oxygen supply. This may lead to disorientation, loss of consciousness, and drowning.

Skin cooling also initiates peripheral vasoconstriction, as well as increased CO, HR, and arterial blood pressure. Increased workload on the heart may lead to

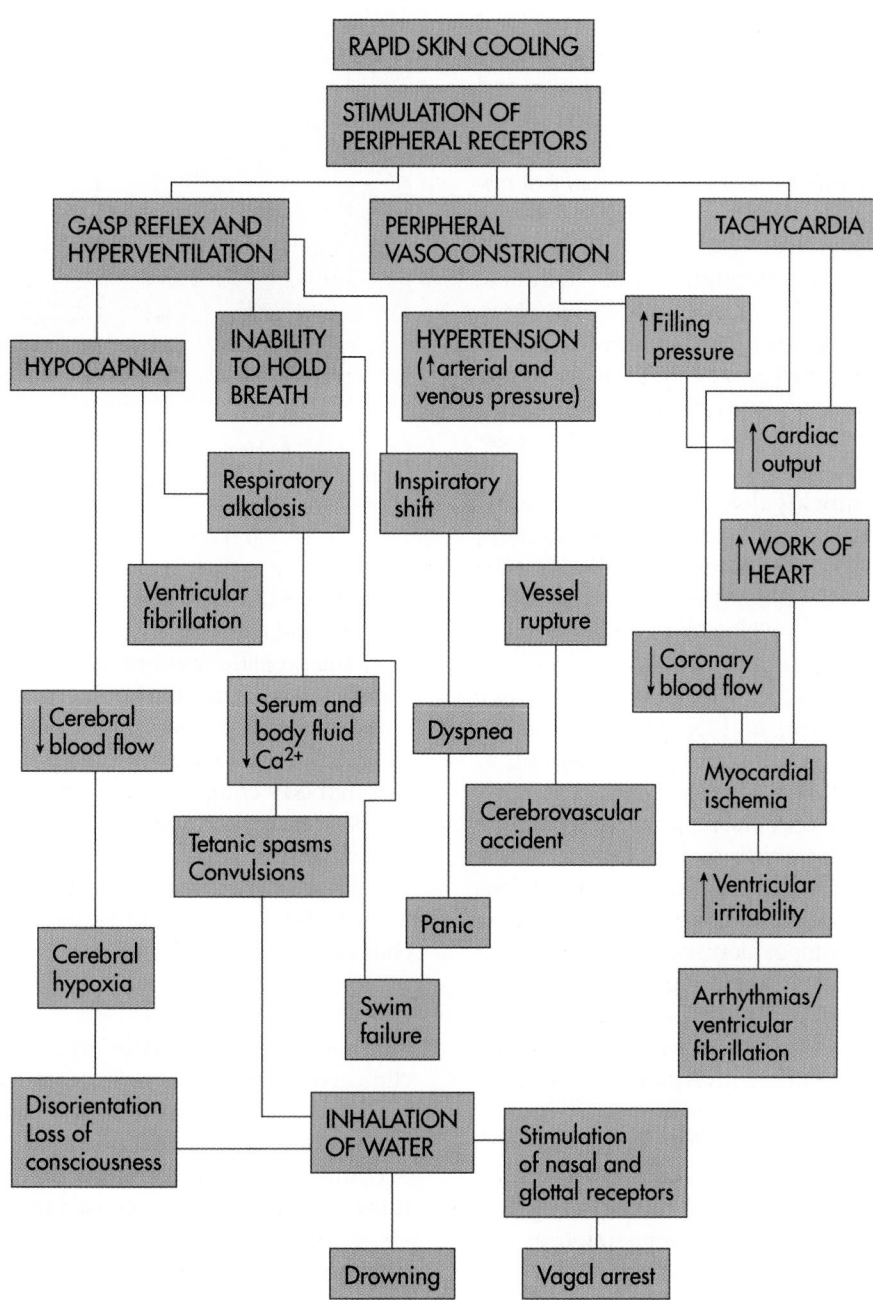

Figure 8-2 Possible cold shock responses. ↑, Increase; ↓, decrease. *(From Edmonds C, Lowry C, Pennefather J: Cold and hypothermia. In* Diving and subaquatic medicine, *Oxford, UK, 1992, Butterworth-Heinemann.)*

myocardial ischemia and arrhythmias, including ventricular fibrillation (VF). Thus sudden death can occur either immediately or within a matter of minutes after immersion (i.e., resulting from syncope or convulsions leading to drowning, vagal arrest of the heart, and VF) in susceptible individuals.[21,42,96,111,158]

Phase 2: Short-Term Immersion and Loss of Performance

For those surviving the cold shock response, significant cooling of peripheral tissues, especially in the extremities, continues, with most of the effect occurring over the first 30 minutes of immersion. This cooling has a direct deleterious effect on neuromuscular activity.[173] This effect is especially significant in the hands, where blood circulation is negligible,[30] leading to finger stiffness, poor coordination of gross and fine motor activity, and loss of power.[38,45,125,126,177] It has been shown that this effect is primarily due to peripheral and not central cooling.[53] Loss of motor control makes it difficult, if not impossible, to execute survival procedures, such as grasping a rescue line or hoist. Thus the ultimate cause of death is drowning, either through a failure to initiate or maintain survival performance (e.g., keeping afloat, swimming, grasping onto a life raft) or excessive inhalation of water under turbulent conditions.

These phenomena have obvious survival implications. It is, of course, advisable to avoid cold water exposure completely. However, if cold water immersion occurs, it is best to quickly determine and execute a plan of action: (1) try to enter the water without submersing the head; (2) escape (i.e., pull oneself out of the water, inflate and board a life raft); (3) minimize exposure (i.e., get as much of one's body as possible out of the water and onto a floating object); (4) ensure flotation if one must remain in the water (i.e., don or inflate a personal flotation device); and (5) call for assistance (i.e., activate signaling devices). It may be difficult to execute these actions while the cold shock responses predominate. However, once the respiratory effects are under control, immediate action should be taken. If self-rescue is not possible, actions to minimize heat loss should be initiated by remaining as still as possible in the heat escape lessening position (HELP), where arms are pressed against the chest and legs are pressed together, or huddling with other survivors (Figure 8-3).[79] Drawstrings should be tightened in clothing to decrease the flow of cold water within clothing layers.

Phase 3: Long-Term Immersion and the Onset of Hypothermia

Most cold water deaths likely result from drowning during the first two phases of cold water immersion, as discussed earlier and during the introduction to this chapter. In general, true hypothermia usually only becomes a significant contributor to death if immersion lasts more

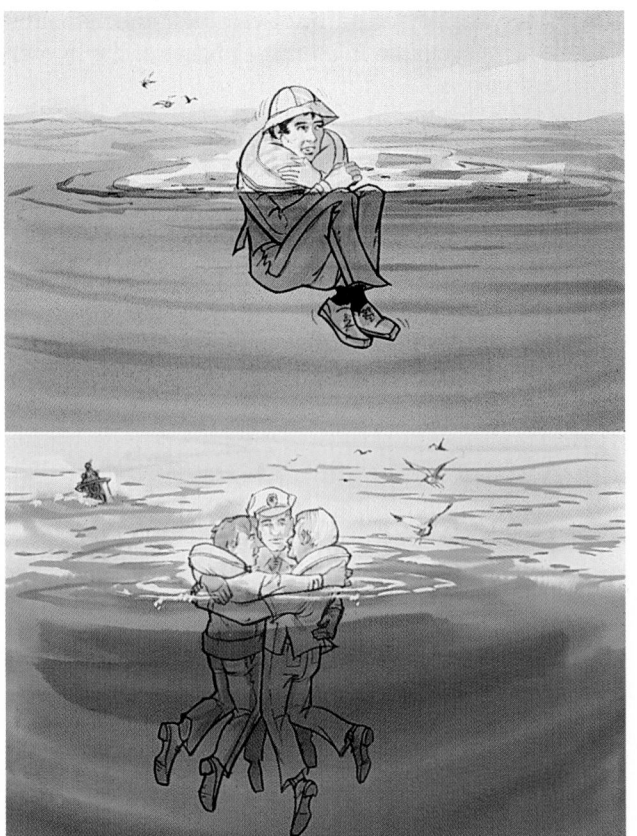

Figure 8-3 **A,** Heat escape lessening posture (HELP) and **B,** huddle techniques for decreasing cooling rates of survivors in cold water. (*From Hayward JS, Eckerson JD, Collis ML: J Appl Physiol 38:1073, 1975.*)

than 30 minutes. The individual who survives the immediate and short-term phases of cold water immersion faces the possible onset of hypothermia because continuous heat loss from the body eventually decreases core temperature (T_c). Many predictive models to determine the T_c response to cooling are based on the relationships among body composition, thermoregulatory response (i.e., shivering thermogenesis), clothing/insulation, water temperature, and sea conditions.[83,154,182,186,190] These variables and their impact on survival time are discussed in more detail in the Cold Water Survival section of this chapter.

Body Core Cooling

Normal body T_c fluctuates around 37° C (98.6° F). The clinical definition of hypothermia is a T_c of 35° C (95° F) or lower; however, any exposure to cold that lowers the temperature below normal levels results in the body becoming hypothermic. Although various temperatures and terms have been used to classify different levels of hypothermia, the following classifications are used here and in Chapter 6. In mild hypothermia (T_c = 32° to 35° C [89.6° to 95° F]), thermoregulatory mechanisms continue to operate fully, but ataxia, dysarthria,

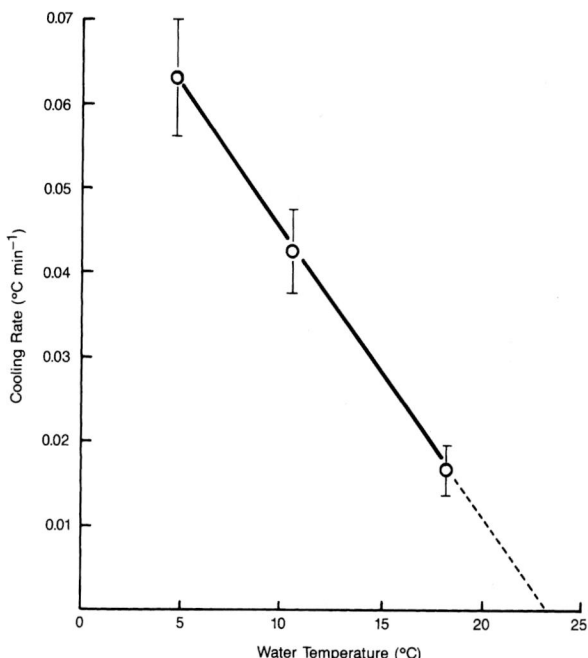

Figure 8-4 The relationship between water temperature and the mean rectal temperature cooling rate in lightly clothed, nonexercising men and women during immersion in seawater. (*From Hayward JS: The physiology of immersion hypothermia. In Pozos RS, Wittmers LE, editors: The nature and treatment of hypothermia, Minneapolis, 1983, University of Minnesota Press.*)

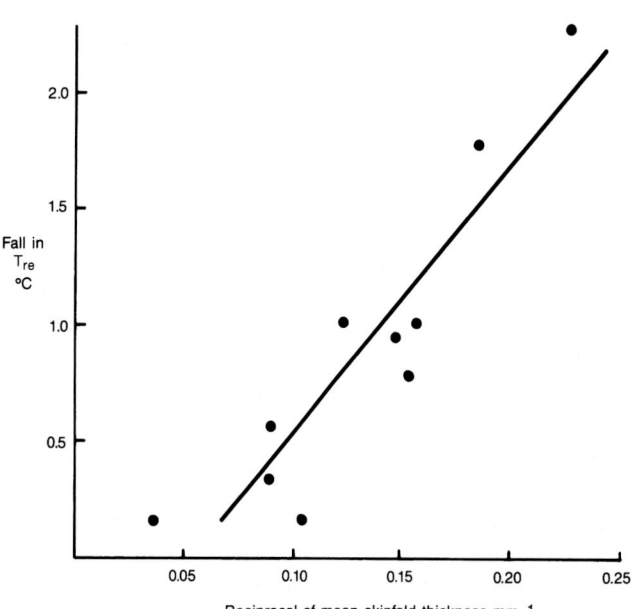

Figure 8-5 The relationship between subcutaneous fat thickness in 10 men and the decline in rectal temperature during 30-minute immersions in stirred water at 15° C (59° F). Skinfold thickness is mean of readings at biceps, abdomen, subscapular, and subcostal sites. T_{re}, rectal temperature. (*From Keatinge WR: Survival in cold water, Oxford, UK, 1969, Blackwell Press.*)

apathy, and even amnesia are likely. In moderate hypothermia (T_c = 28° to 32° C [82.4° to 89.6° F]), effectiveness of the thermoregulatory system (i.e., shivering thermogenesis) diminishes until it fails, there is continued decrease in level of consciousness, and cardiac arrhythmias may also occur. In severe hypothermia (T_c < 28° C), consciousness is lost, shivering is absent, acid-base disturbances develop, and the heart is susceptible to VF or asystole. Death from hypothermia is generally from cardiorespiratory failure.

The rate of body core cooling during cold water immersion depends on the following variables:
1. Water temperature and sea state
2. Clothing
3. Body morphology
4. Amount of the body immersed in water
5. Behavior (e.g., excessive movement) and posture (e.g. HELP, huddle) of the body in the water
6. Shivering thermogenesis
7. Other nonthermal factors

Water Temperature, Sea State, and Clothing Insulation.

These variables are all critically important to intensity of the cold shock response, onset of physical and mental impairment, and rate of core cooling. Figure 8-4 graphically illustrates the inverse linear relationship between water temperature and T_c cooling

rate.[74] Water has a specific heat 4000 times that of air and a thermal conductivity approximately 25 times greater.[118] Immersion in cold water is thus associated with a high rate of heat transfer from skin to water, at least 100 times greater than in air of the same temperature.[118] Sea state and clothing insulation are discussed in more detail in the Cold Water Survival section of this chapter.

Body Morphology (Size and Composition).

Children cool faster than do adults because children have a greater surface area–to–mass ratio. Cooling rate is generally proportional to surface area, whereas the amount of heat that can be lost is proportional to mass. Thus a large surface area–to–mass ratio favors cooling. Similarly, smaller adults generally cool faster than do larger adults, and tall, lanky individuals cool faster than do short, stout individuals. Body composition is also important. Subcutaneous fat is a very efficient insulator against heat loss, and cooling rate is inversely related to skinfold thickness. For example, subjects in the 10th percentile for skinfold thickness wearing light clothing in 5° C (41° F) water have nine times the cooling rate of 90th percentile subjects.[123] Figure 8-5 shows the linear relationship between change in T_c and mean skinfold thickness.[95] Shivering, which is a primary defense against core cooling, also varies with skinfold thickness. At a given skin temperature, the shivering response is less in humans with greater amounts of subcutaneous fat.[99] In moderately cold water temperatures (18° to 26° C [64.4° to 78.8° F]), core cooling has been shown to proceed at the same rate in high- and low-fat individuals because of the greater shivering thermogenesis in the low-fat subjects. However, at colder water temperatures (8° C [46.4° F]), core cooling is attenuated by greater amounts of subcutaneous fat and body mass resulting from increased insulation.[46]

In general, for a survivor immersed in cold water, the core cooling rate is fairly linear once T_c begins to decline. This has been shown to be true for mildly hypothermic experimental subjects. The only data that exist for severely hypothermic humans are those from the infamous Dachau concentration camp atrocities, in which conscious victims, who were cooled to death in ice water, had linear cooling rates.[2] Since these unfortunate victims were emaciated and ill, these data may not apply to healthy cold water immersion subjects.

Amount of Body Immersed. Because of the difference in thermal conductivity between air and water (discussed above), heat loss from body surfaces immersed in cold water is far greater than from body surfaces exposed to cold air, even considering the effect of windchill. Thus immersed victims should attempt to get as much of their bodies out of the water as possible. This issue is discussed in greater detail in the Cold Water Survival section of this chapter.

Behavior and Posture of the Body in Cold Water.
Behavioral variables also affect the core cooling rate. Hayward et al used infrared thermography to demonstrate that, despite marked peripheral vasoconstriction, heat losses are high in the groin, lateral and central thorax, and neck.[78] In the groin and neck, regions with a relatively thin layer of peripheral soft tissue, blood flow through the large, relatively superficial femoral vessels, carotid arteries, and jugular veins potentiates heat flow to the cold water. In the lateral and central thorax, the relative absence of tissue insulation (muscle and subcutaneous fat), combined with high thermal conductivity of rib bone, potentiates heat loss from relatively warm lungs to the cold environment. Furthermore, exercise or excessive movement in the water greatly increases heat loss from active musculature.

The effect of activity on total heat balance depends on the balance among the many factors illustrated in Figure 8-6. In normothermic circumstances, heat produced locally in peripheral muscles is transferred to the core via venous return. In cold water immersion, by contrast, physical activity may actually increase heat loss through increased blood flow to the periphery. This is especially true when immersed victims engage in excessive movement in the water (e.g., swimming or vig-

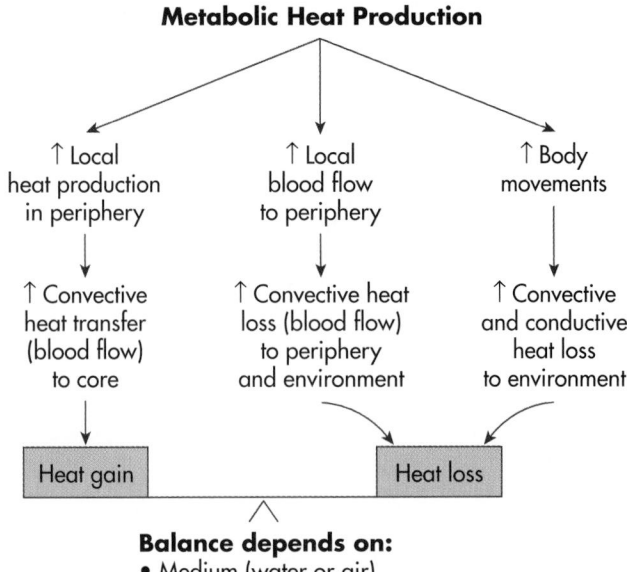

Figure 8-6 Factors influencing total thermal balance during increases in metabolic heat production (e.g., voluntary exercise and involuntary shivering).

orous extremity movements necessary to maintain airway freeboard in rough seas).

Hayward et al[79] demonstrated that minimizing both voluntary activity and the exposure of major heat loss areas of the skin to cold water is the most effective way to minimize the decline in T_c. They showed that treading water and drownproofing significantly increased the cooling rate. In spite of increased metabolic heat production during exercise, increased surface heat loss resulted in faster core cooling during exercise in cold water. They also developed two well-known cold-water survival techniques: HELP and the group huddle (see Figure 8-3). These adaptive behaviors reduce core cooling by 69% and 66% that of control conditions, respectively.[74] In conditions in which the sea is not calm, it may be difficult to perform the group huddle with complete thermal efficiency. However, other advantages of this position include maintenance of group contact and morale. Sagawa et al concluded that the lowest water temperature in which humans could maintain normal T_c by generating body heat through muscular activity is 25° C (77° F), although there may be individual variation in absolute water temperature.[137]

Shivering. Shivering is a thermoregulatory function in which involuntary muscle contraction increases heat production in an effort to prevent or minimize body core cooling. Shivering intensity increases as core and skin temperatures decrease. Generally, shivering inten-

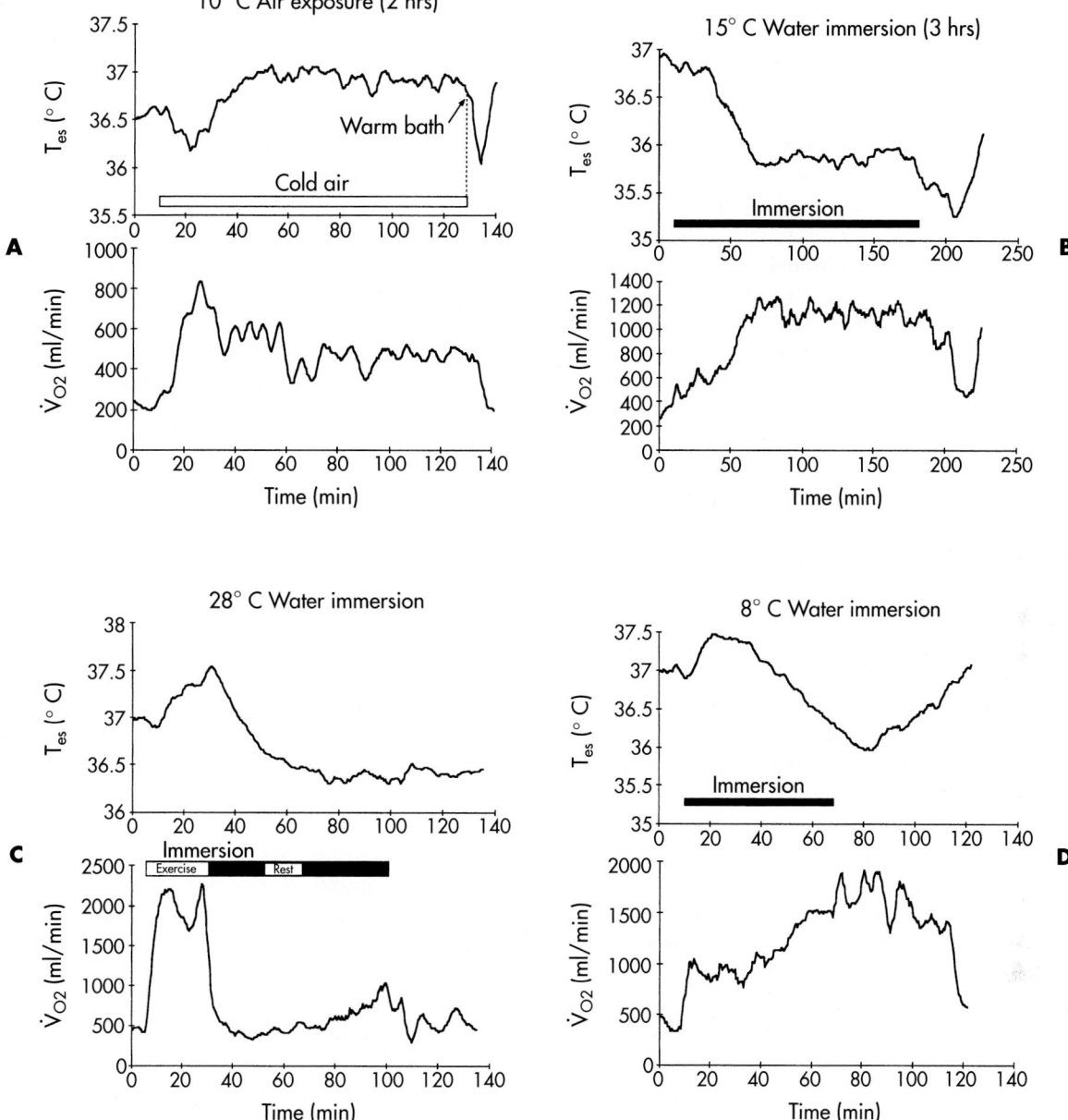

Figure 8-7 Effectiveness of shivering heat production in preventing onset of hypothermia during exposure to **A,** 10° C (50° F) air; **B,** 15° C (59° F) water; **C,** 28° C (82.4° F) water; and **D,** 8° C (46.4° F) water. *Tes,* esophageal temperature.

sity is maximal at T_c = 32° to 33° C (89.6° to 91.4° F) and T_{skin} = ~20° C (68° F); however, shivering heat production is lower, at any given skin temperature, in individuals with higher levels of subcutaneous fat.[99,184]

Thermal balance during shivering depends on the same factors as during voluntary activity (see Figure 8-6). Figure 8-7 illustrates how shivering heat production can maintain T_c in cold air and can arrest the fall in T_c in both warm and cool water. In colder water, the combination of shivering thermogenesis and body insulation (resulting from peripheral vasoconstriction) may result in maintenance of a steady-state T_c, albeit

below normothermic levels. At even lower water temperatures, T_c will continue to decrease, and this decrease will accelerate when shivering thermogenesis eventually stops because of hypothermia-induced thermoregulatory impairment (below ~ T_c = 30° C [86° F]). The power of shivering is especially important in the consideration of the clinical classification of hypothermia and rewarming therapies, since this valuable heat source is an efficient mechanism for rewarming the core during postimmersion recovery and resuscitation. This is discussed in more detail in the Rescue and Management section of this chapter.

Nonthermal Factors. Underwater divers often experience "symptomless," or "undetected," hypothermia. Several factors contribute to increased cooling. First, heat is lost through direct conduction to cold water and through breathing compressed air. Breathing compressed air at depth also alters human thermoregulation. Mekjavic et al studied the effects of hyperbaric nitrogen at 6 atm[110]; these researchers also simulated inert gas or "nitrogen" narcosis with inhalation of 30% nitrous oxide.[129] They demonstrated a decrease in the T_c threshold for shivering and an increase in the rate of core cooling of up to twofold under these conditions. In a separate study, Mekjavic et al demonstrated qualitatively similar effects of insulin-induced hypoglycemia.

Hypercapnia and hypoxia may also be present in various underwater scenarios. Hypercapnia has been shown to lower the shivering threshold[88] and transiently inhibit shivering itself.[103] Both hypercapnia[88] and hypoxia[87] have also been shown to accelerate core cooling.

Alcohol consumption is frequently associated with immersion hypothermia, since ethanol impairment of mental and motor performance is often the cause of accidental immersion. Social drinking can result in carelessness. Intoxicated mariners or others near water often fall from a boat, ship, gangway, wharf, or bridge into the water. Drunken drivers capsize or collide. On the basis of frequency of occurrence alone, the consequences of alcohol ingestion warrant special considerations.

Studies on the effect of moderate doses of ethanol (blood alcohol levels of 50 to 100 mg/dl, the range associated with legal impairment) on cold stress have established the following:

1. Rate of heat loss is not significantly increased. Alcohol has a primary vasodilatory effect under normothermic conditions.[37,84,101] Under hypothermic conditions, where vasoconstriction predominates, alcohol lowers the vasoconstriction threshold during a moderate cold stress of 28° C (82.4° F) water immersion but does not affect the shivering threshold or rate of core cooling.[86]
2. Rate of heat production is slightly decreased. For immersion in water colder than 28° C, a moderate ethanol dose inhibits the metabolic response to cold.[40,108] Shivering thermogenesis is reduced in cold water by approximately 10% to 20%.
3. Cooling rate is not significantly increased.[40,86,108] Because the body's cooling rate in cold water is influenced more by rate of heat loss than by rate of heat production, the slight reduction in shivering thermogenesis induced by moderate ethanol ingestion is outweighed by factors affecting heat loss (e.g., peripheral vasoconstriction and body fat). Since these do not vary with alcohol use when the person is cold stressed, cooling rate does not change.

4. Fatigue potentiates thermoregulatory impairment by alcohol. Exhaustive exercise leading to fatigue (characterized by hypoglycemia and depletion of glycogen reserves), combined with a moderate dose of ethanol, significantly reduces resistance to cold.[70,95] Alcohol inhibits gluconeogenesis[68,90] so that the ability to provide glucose to maintain shivering is reduced. If a person enters cold water in this condition, cooling rate is likely to be greater than in the absence of ethanol.
5. Perception of cold is diminished. Experimental studies of humans in cold water show that moderate alcohol dosage to some extent relieves feelings of intense cold.[40,95] This cognitive alteration may be functionally related to reduced shivering response.
6. Cold-induced diuresis is increased. Alcohol inhibition of antidiuretic hormone augments immersion diuresis.[24] During the first hour of cold water immersion, urine flow rate can be more than six times normal (approximately 8 ml/min). For longer immersions, alcohol potentiates the development of dehydration and hypovolemia.

For most humans, high doses of alcohol (blood levels greater than 200 mg/dl) have an anesthetic effect. Major impairment of mental, motor, and involuntary function (including thermoregulation) occurs. Alcoholics who "pass out" in cold locations ("urban hypothermia") rapidly and passively become hypothermic (see Chapter 6 for a complete discussion of hypothermia).[27,114] When highly intoxicated persons enter cold water (usually by falling in), hypothermia is seldom a problem because such persons usually drown quickly.

Cold Water Submersion

Cold water submersion, or near drowning, is covered in detail in Chapter 55. However, a brief discussion is included here to provide a more complete discussion of cold water immersion. There have been several recent advances in our understanding of why individuals can survive cold water submersion for as long as 66 minutes[9] with full or partial neurologic recovery (cold water near drowning). The most important factor in these unusual cases is the low water temperature and subsequent brain cooling. This principle has been used in clinical practice for years. For example, cardiopulmonary bypass was used to cool neurosurgical patients to a T_c ~9° C (48.2° F) to arrest brain blood flow for at least 55 minutes with full neurologic recovery.[128] The full explanation for these recoveries relates to both (1) the mechanisms for, and amounts of, brain/body cooling that occurs, and (2) the mechanisms for the protective effect of this cooling.

Mechanisms for Brain/Body Cooling

Children have an advantage in cold water submersion incidents because their greater surface area–to–mass ratio allows faster conductive cooling, which provides cerebral protection based on decreased cerebral metabolic requirements of oxygen (CMR_{O2}). The mammalian dive reflex, which initiates intense bradycardia and shunts blood flow to important core organs, such as the heart and brain, has also been implicated. A third factor that has recently been explored is the possibility that cold water ventilation may result in rapid and extensive cooling during submersion (see below).

The effectiveness of the human dive reflex, especially the breath-hold response, is controversial. Nemiroff, who has one of the largest series of successful resuscitations of near-drowning victims, believes that the dive reflex plays an important role, particularly in children and infants, and especially in neonates.[120,121] Hayward et al[82,131] think that the enhanced success in resuscitation associated with cold water near drowning is more due to hypothermia than to the dive reflex.

It is important to note that the protective effect of cooling depends on the T_c at cessation of oxygen delivery and the subsequent rate and extent of the decrease of T_c. Since T_c is likely to be near normal at the onset of an accidental submersion, rapid cooling after onset of ischemia is important for survival. Conduction alone probably cannot account for the rapid decrease in T_c that occurs in cold water submersion incidents. Conn et al[20] studied cold water (4° C [39.2° F]) drowning in shaved, anesthetized dogs. They found that submersed dogs continued to breathe the cold water for an extended period of time. T_c decreased 11° C (19.8° F) in 4 minutes in the completely submersed dogs compared with only 3° C (5.4° F) in the control (immersed with head out) dogs who did not breathe cold water. It is likely that rapid cooling was due to convective heat exchange in the lung compared with only surface conduction in the control dogs. The general conclusion that brain cooling is accelerated considerably by respiration of cold water has been proposed by others[47,61,65] and mathematically predicted by Xu et al.[189] Although breath holding may occur during submersion, a physiologic break point occurs where involuntary breathing movements predominate.[3] This factor, coupled with unconsciousness, could reasonably be expected to result in respiration of water under at least some circumstances. Experimental and anecdotal evidence in humans is rare. However, one helicopter crash survivor reported that, after being trapped underwater for some time, he recalled feeling he was about to die and that he was breathing water in and out just before escaping the cockpit.[12]

Mechanisms for the Protective Effect of Brain Cooling.
Hypothermia provides an advantage during anoxic periods, such as cold water submersion, because of what is known as the "metabolic ice-box." Whole body, or focal, hypothermia has long been used to extend biologic survival time during surgery under isch-

emic conditions. Cerebral protection under hypothermic conditions has commonly been attributed to decreased cerebral metabolic requirements for oxygen according to the Q_{10} principle. Although the Q_{10} of the whole body is about 2, the Q_{10} of the brain increases from ~3 between 27° and 37° C (80.6° and 98.6° F) to 4.8 between 18° and 27° C (64.4° and 80.6° F).[113] Based on these values, if the brain could survive an ischemic insult for 5 minutes at 37° C, cooling to 27° C or to 17° C would provide 15- and 72-minute protection, respectively, based solely on decreased CMR_{O2} (Figure 8-8). Although long survival times at brain temperatures below 20° C (68° F) may be predicted on the basis of increasing Q_{10} and diminishing CMR_{O2}, some additional mechanism(s) may be required to explain intact survival after prolonged submersion in which reported core temperatures are often above 30° C (86° F; these factors are schematically shown in Figure 8-9). Over the past decade, several studies, directed mainly towards protection of the brain during or after cerebral ischemic events, have demonstrated that even moderate brain cooling of 3° to 5° C (5.4° to 9° F) provides substantial cerebral protection from ischemic insult.*

Submersion likely promotes cerebral death as tissue ischemia depletes high-energy phosphates and leads to membrane depolarization. This stimulates release, into the extracellular space, of excitatory neurotransmitters, such as glutamate and dopamine, which mediate postsynaptic depolarization, causing calcium entry into the cell. Calcium influx mediates the production of oxygen and hydroxyl free radicals (which may be involved in reperfusion injury), and release of free fatty acids, re-

---

*References 14, 15, 55, 105, 116, 138, 188.

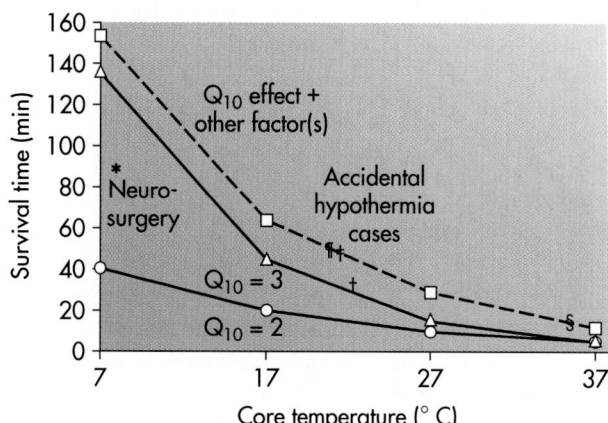

Figure 8-8 Schematic presentation of survival time at different core/brain temperatures. Bottom line, prediction based on a Q_{10} of 2. Middle line, prediction based on the Q_{10} of 3. Top line, prediction based on the Q_{10} effect plus other factors, such as changes in neurotransmitter release (i.e., glutamate and dopamine). Actual survival times are from both neurosurgical and accidental hypothermia cases. Most of these cases fall outside the range predicted based on Q_{10} alone; thus some other factors must also contribute to survival.

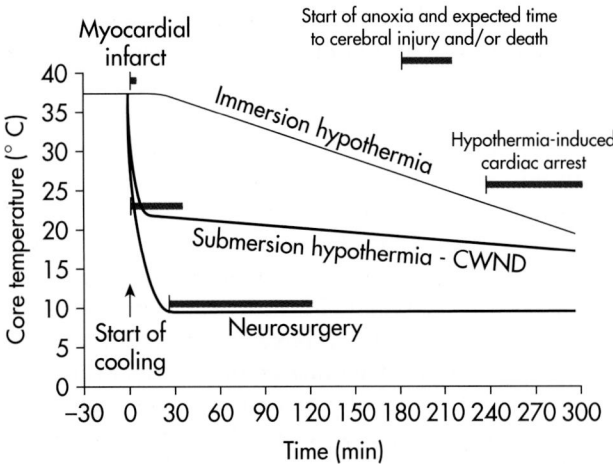

Figure 8-9 Schematic representation of theoretic times to cerebral injury and/or death after sudden onset of anoxia. Examples include anoxia induced by myocardial infarction at normal core temperatures, hypothermia-induced cardiac arrest during immersion hypothermia, ischemia-induced cardiac arrest after cold water near drowning (CWND), and electrically induced arrest after protective cooling for neurosurgery. Note that the times shown are representational; actual survival times may vary.

sulting in eicosanoid synthesis.[167] Various animal studies have shown that cooling the brain by only 3° to 5° C before ischemia delays terminal depolarization and reduces the initial rate of rise of extracellular potassium,[91] results in complete suppression of glutamate release and 60% reduction in the peak release of dopamine,[15] attenuates ischemia-induced damage to endothelial cells,[28] reduces hydroxyl radical production,[57] and improves postischemia glucose utilization.[55] These results relate to mechanisms other than decreased CMR_{O2}, which may explain cerebral protection during cold water near drowning.

In summary, these findings indicate that: (1) if the brain cools even by only 3° to 5° C, it is protected in excess of what would be predicted from decreased CMR_{O2} alone; (2) protection results from additional protective mechanism(s) of cooling related to neurotransmitter release, calcium flux, eicosanoid synthesis, etc.; (3) the mammalian dive reflex may result in some cold-induced circulatory adjustments that favor conservation of oxygen for the heart and brain; and (4) any cold water ventilation may accelerate brain cooling and provide further protection.

Implications for Survival

The paradox of whether core cooling is an advantage or a disadvantage depends on whether there is cessation of oxygen delivery, and if so, the value of T_c when anoxia occurs and how much T_c subsequently declines. These factors are schematically illustrated in Figure 8-9. If oxygen delivery is not compromised (e.g., immersion hypothermia), then core cooling will eventually lead to

death from cardiac arrest. However, if oxygen delivery is compromised (e.g., submersion hypothermia and cold water near drowning), core/brain cooling will prolong survival compared with a condition in which core cooling does not occur (e.g., myocardial infarction). These factors are important in understanding whether children have a survival advantage over adults during cold stress. Because children cool faster, their body size would be an advantage when oxygen supply is compromised during cold water submersion. However, when the oxygen supply is uninterrupted in head-out immersion or in cold air, the small body size becomes a disadvantage because the onset of severe hypothermia will be faster.

Afterdrop and Circum-Rescue Collapse

Anecdotal cases of fatalities among immersion hypothermia victims have been noted in the immediate prerescue and postrescue periods despite the survivors being recovered in an apparently stable and conscious condition. These events are often referred to as cases of "rewarming shock" or "postrescue collapse." Golden et al[64] have noted that deaths can occur either shortly before rescue, during rescue, or after rescue, and they have used the term *circum-rescue collapse* to describe these events. Deaths have occurred within minutes before rescue, while climbing out of the water, while being hoisted to a helicopter, within a few minutes after entering a warm compartment of a rescue vessel, 20 to 90 minutes after rescue, in hospital after transport, and during the 24-hour period postrescue.[59,64,94,109] Three causes of circum-rescue collapse have been proposed: (1) afterdrop—a continued drop in T_c after recovery; (2) collapse of arterial pressure; and (3) factors that potentiate the risk of VF (e.g., hypoxia, acidosis, rapid changes in pH). Each of these causes is discussed below.

Afterdrop is a well-known phenomenon that occurs after removal of a victim from cold water immersion. T_c continues to decline (i.e., afterdrop) in both animate and inanimate objects, even though cold water immersion has ended.* Afterdrop of as much as 5° to 6° C (9° to 10.8° F) has been observed in humans.[6,41,152] This afterdrop was long proposed as the major cause of postrescue death because further cooling of the heart might result in a temperature at which VF or cardiac arrest could occur.[13]

Golden et al[64] discount the importance of this phenomenon and propose collapse of arterial pressure as the cause of death during rescue. They correctly point out that an afterdrop occurring in victims who were hypothermic, yet warm enough to climb on board a ship without assistance, would be unlikely to cause enough myocardial cooling to result in cardiac arrest or VF.

---

*References 2, 13, 18, 54, 63, 133, 139, 179.

Rather, Golden et al propose that removal from cold water results in a precipitous fall in blood pressure, inadequate coronary blood flow, and myocardial ischemia, possibly precipitating VF. This mechanism is likely the main factor in collapse before and during rescue. The fall in blood pressure *before* removal from the water may be due to reduced sympathetic tone or catecholamine secretion when rescue is imminent. Finally, hypotension *during* and shortly *after* rescue may be due to the sudden decrease in hydrostatic pressure on the body (i.e., removal of the "hydrostatic squeeze" of water pressure during immersion), hypovolemia, and/or impaired baroreceptor reflexes. However, this mechanism cannot fully account for all other postrescue deaths occurring 20 minutes to 24 hours postrescue.

The importance of continued myocardial cooling cannot be discounted. Fibrillation of a cold heart can be initiated by mechanical stimuli,[127] hypoxia and acidosis,[122] and by rapid changes in pH.[95] In dogs, myocardial cooling from 30° C to 22° C (86° F to 71.6° F) has been shown to cause a fivefold decrease in the electrical threshold for fibrillation.[23] It is also likely that an increase in the *rate* of myocardial cooling may stimulate fibrillation. Based on the large afterdrop values described above, it is plausible that continued core cooling in significantly hypothermic victims could result in VF, either primarily caused by spontaneous fibrillation of the cold myocardium, or secondarily caused by cold-induced increase in sensitivity to other fibrillation stimuli.

RESCUE AND MANAGEMENT

This section describes prehospital management of hypothermia with specific reference to immersion pathophysiology. Hospital management of both accidental immersion and land-based hypothermia is described in Chapter 6. Prehospital management of hypothermia patients, both in the field and during transportation to a site of definitive medical care, varies with the victim's level of hypothermia, with the rescuer's level of training, with the resuscitative equipment available, with the type of transportation, and with the time required for delivery to definitive care. Medical personnel must exercise good clinical judgment in balancing all these factors to select appropriate therapeutic modalities.

The primary goals in prehospital management of victims of accidental immersion hypothermia are prevention of cardiopulmonary arrest, prevention of continued T_c decline, moderate core rewarming if practicable, and transportation to a site of definitive medical care.[71,148] Aggressive rewarming in the field is usually contraindicated, since the means to either diagnose or manage the many potential complications of severe hypothermia are unavailable in this setting.[115] In unusual circumstances, when transportation to a site of definitive care is impossible, definitive rewarming in the field, using the principles and techniques of management described in the following paragraphs, may be appropriate.

Rescue

Retrieval of a victim from cold water immersion must be performed with caution. Sudden reduction of the "hydrostatic squeeze" applied to tissues below the water's surface may potentiate hypotension, especially orthostatic hypotension.[64] Since a hypothermic patient's normal cardiovascular defenses are impaired, the cold myocardium may be incapable of increasing cardiac output in response to a hypotensive stimulus. Putting a victim into vertical posture may also potentiate hypotension. Hypovolemia, secondary to combined cold- and immersion-induced diuresis, and increased blood viscosity potentiate these effects.[25] Peripheral vascular resistance may also be incapable of increasing, since vasoconstriction is already maximal because of cold stress. The net result of sudden removal of a hypothermic patient from the water is similar to sudden deflation of antishock trousers worn by a patient in hypovolemic shock: abrupt hypotension. This has been demonstrated experimentally in mildly hypothermic human volunteers[60] and has been suspected as a cause of postrescue death in many immersion hypothermia victims.[64,148] Accordingly, rescuers should attempt to maintain hypothermic patients in a horizontal position during retrieval from the water and aboard the rescue vehicle (Figures 8-10 and 8-11).[64,143,148] If rescuers cannot recover the patient horizontally, they should place the victim in a supine posture as quickly as possible after removal from cold water.[148]

The victim's T_c may continue to decline (depending on the quality of insulation provided, the victim's endogenous heat production, active or passive manipulation of extremities, and the site of T_c measurement) even after he or she has been rescued, because of the physiologic processes described earlier for "afterdrop." To diminish this effect, the victim's physical activity must be minimized. Conscious persons should not be required to assist in their own rescue (e.g., by climbing up a scramble net or ship's ladder) or to ambulate once out of the water (as by walking to a waiting ambulance or helicopter).[43,115,148] Physical activity increases afterdrop, presumably by increasing perfusion of cold muscle tissue with relatively warm blood.[11,44,46,48] As this blood is cooled, venous return (the circulatory component to afterdrop) contributes to a decline in myocardial temperature, increasing the risk of VF.[80] Experiments on moderately hypothermic volunteers (esophageal temperature 33° C) demonstrated a threefold greater afterdrop during treadmill walking than while lying still.[10,51] Such exercise-induced enhancement of afterdrop could precipitate postrescue collapse. Throughout the rescue procedures and during subsequent management, hy-

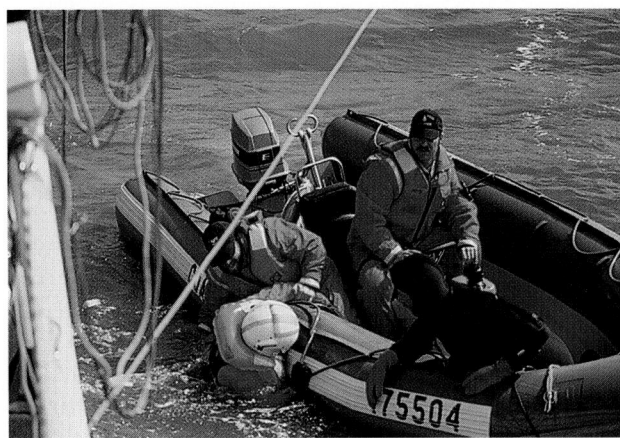

Figure 8-10 U.S. Coast Guard crew keep a hypothermia victim in a horizontal posture during rescue operations.

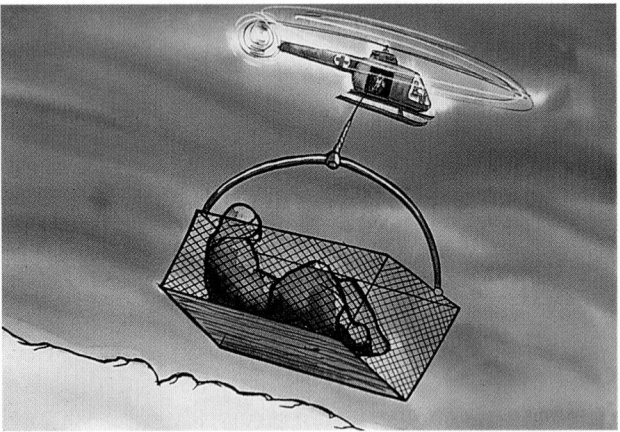

Figure 8-11 Immersion hypothermia victim in a semihorizontal posture during helicopter basket hoist.

pothermic victims must be handled gently.[69,115,143] Excessive mechanical stimulation of the cold myocardium is another suspected cause of deaths after rescue.[102,178]

Examination and Life Support

Since hypothermia affects virtually every physiologic process, rescuers should manage a severely hypothermic patient as they would a victim of multiple trauma.[147,148] Rescuers should not focus solely on T_c to the exclusion of other potentially life-threatening problems. Conversely, when the incident includes cold exposure, care must be taken to not focus solely on trauma injuries. Several victims have died of hypothermia when treatment focused only on non–life-threatening physical injuries. Figure 8-12 shows a recommended algorithm for treatment of hypothermia. In accordance with standard emergency medical procedures, the ABCs (airway, breathing, and circulation) of first aid are essential.[143,148] Rescuers should ensure an open airway and

confirm the presence of adequate ventilation and circulation. If the patient is severely hypothermic, respiration and pulse may be slow, shallow, and difficult to detect.[143,147] Therefore rescuers should take 30 to 45 seconds to assess these vital signs.[143] If neither pulse nor breathing is detectable, rescuers should commence CPR in accordance with normal basic life support protocols.[143,147]

Cardiac rhythm should be carefully monitored, if possible. Percutaneous electrodes may be required to overcome interference from muscle fasciculation or shivering.[143] Endotracheal intubation and the administration of heated, humidified air or oxygen are useful in the management of apnea or hypoventilation and in reducing further respiratory heat loss.[143] Mouth-to-mouth or mouth-to-mask ventilation also provides heated, humidified air. If oxygen is available, it may supplement mouth-to-mouth or mouth-to-mask ventilation. Mouth-to-mouth or mouth-to-mask ventilation has the added advantage of providing a small amount of carbon dioxide to the patient's inspired gases. This may be useful in preventing hypocapnia secondary to relative hyperventilation in a severely hypothermic victim whose metabolic production of CO_2 is diminished.[27] This is important because hypocapnia may decrease the threshold for VF.

Hypothermic patients with *any* detectable pulse or respiration do not require the chest compressions of cardiopulmonary resuscitation (CPR), even though severe bradycardia and bradypnea may be present.[143,147] This differs from normothermic CPR protocols, where chest compressions may be indicated if bradycardia fails to provide sufficient cardiac output or systolic pressure.[143] Since the metabolic requirements of hypothermic patients are reduced, the observed bradycardia and bradypnea may still meet tissue oxygen requirements.[26,43] Inappropriate administration of chest compressions in an attempt to augment cardiac output may precipitate VF from mechanical stimulation of the irritable myocardium.[26]

If a victim of immersion in cold water is found floating face down, near drowning should be suspected and managed accordingly (see Chapter 56). In this case, correction of anoxia is paramount, and consideration of hypothermia is of secondary importance.[121,143] Normal advanced cardiac life support (ACLS) protocols should not routinely be applied to severely hypothermic patients in cardiac arrest, since management beyond basic life support differs from that used in normothermia.[26,143] Defibrillation and pharmacologic interventions are usually ineffective for myocardial temperatures below 30° C (86° F).[7,26,143] Furthermore, repeated defibrillatory shocks may damage the myocardium.[143,147] Defibrillation should be limited to three shocks at 200 joules (J), 300 J, and 360 J, consecutively, in patients colder than 30° C.[143] Administered medications are not only ineffective but may accumulate to toxic levels, since drug metabolism

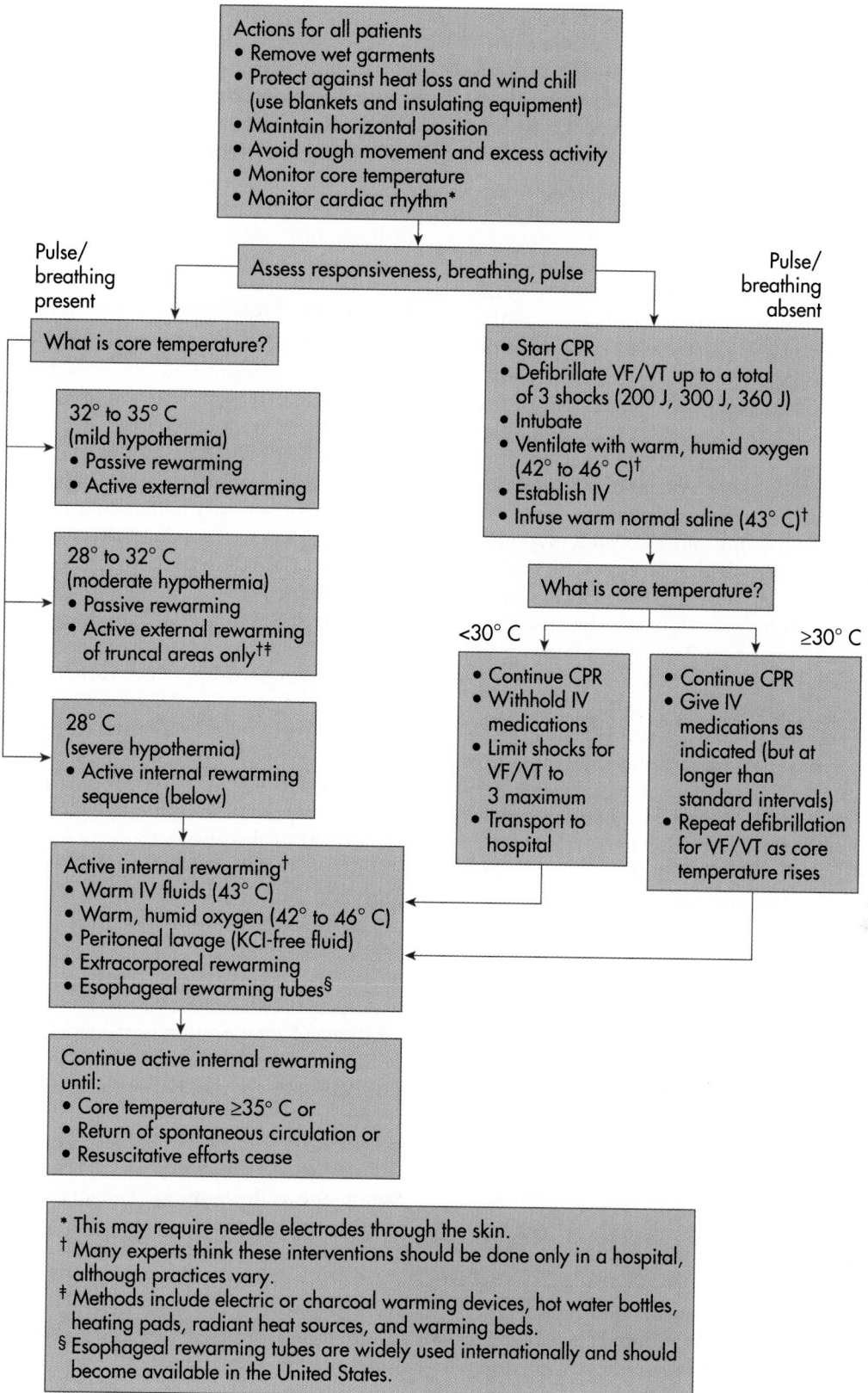

Figure 8-12 Algorithm for treatment of hypothermia. (*Adapted from Standards and guidelines for cardiopulmonary resuscitation and emergency cardiac care, JAMA 268:2172, 1992.*)

by the hypothermic liver and kidneys is reduced.[26,181] For hypothermic patients with a T_c greater than 30° C, normal ACLS protocols may be used.[143] All intravenous (IV) fluids should be warmed before administration. However, it may be necessary to extend the recommended interval for IV medications because of the patient's reduced metabolic rate.

For the unconscious hypothermic patient who is not in cardiopulmonary arrest, endotracheal or nasotracheal intubation should be performed gently. Insertion of pacemaker wires and central venous catheters has been suspected of precipitating VF, but prior ventilation with 100% oxygen has been associated with decreased risk for this complication.[25,27] Rescuers should not withhold intubation, if indicated, for fear of precipitating VF.[143]

If the patient does not require immediate life support intervention, a thorough and systematic examination must be performed as quickly as possible before initiation of hypothermia therapy. Since severely hypothermic patients may have markedly depressed mental status, they may not respond normally to painful stimuli. Victims of immersion hypothermia may have suffered trauma before entering or while in the water. Central nervous system, skeletal, and soft tissue injuries may be overlooked without careful examination.

Attention should be paid to the patient's mental status and other central nervous system signs. Rescuers should evaluate level of consciousness, presence or absence of shivering, and pupillary size and light reflex. Pupils may appear fixed and dilated in an unconscious, severely hypothermic patient, simulating the appearance of death. The diagnosis of death should not be made in a hypothermic patient, particularly in a field setting, unless resuscitation efforts fail after adequate rewarming efforts.

Vital signs should be carefully measured, with particular attention to T_c. A low-reading thermometer (capable of recording down to 20° C [68° F]) is required. Esophageal temperature (at the level of the atria) is the most clinically useful T_c obtainable, since this site most closely parallels cardiac temperature.[51,80] However, most rescue personnel are not equipped to measure esophageal temperature. Rectal temperature is the most easily obtained T_c, yet rescuers often show reluctance to obtain a recording from this site in the field, and incorrect thermometer placement may cause an erroneous reading. If neither esophageal nor rectal temperature is taken, oral or axillary temperature may be of value. Neither of these will be an accurate reflection of T_c in a victim of immersion hypothermia. Facial cooling affects oral temperature, and cold skin temperature affects axillary recordings. However, the victim's true temperature will not be lower than indicated by an oral or axillary recording. Thus rescuers can use even superficial temperatures in a limited way to monitor the patient's status, although this is not ideal.

Hemorrhage should be controlled in the usual manner. However, antishock trousers are normally contraindicated because they are likely to be ineffective in the face of maximal vasoconstriction already present in a severely hypothermic patient.[26] Since hypothermia itself can cause hypotension without massive fluid losses, antishock trousers should be used only if the victim's hypotension is severe and secondary to hemorrhage, or if required for temporary stabilization of major pelvic fractures.[26]

Insulation, Stabilization, and Rewarming

After recovery of the victim from the water, and after management of immediate life-threatening emergencies, the next objectives are prevention of further heat loss and efforts at moderate rewarming (i.e., 1° to 2° C/hr [1.8° to 3.6° F/hr]). Strategies for moderate rewarming in the field vary with equipment available, training of rescue personnel, environmental conditions, and length of time required for transport to a site of definitive care. Maximum insulation of the whole body from any further cooling by the environment is an obvious first requirement. The main goal for rescue personnel is to maintain or improve cardiorespiratory stability and to minimize T_c afterdrop, which can depress cardiac temperature and potentiate VF, as previously discussed. All sources of heat loss (evaporation, conduction, convection, respiration, and radiation) should be controlled. Rescuers should maintain the victim in a horizontal posture to prevent hypotension, as discussed above. Movement of the victim must be kept to a minimum; clothing should be cut away if it is wet. The victim's skin should be dried, and he or she should be protected by dry, insulative clothing and blankets, sleeping bag, or specialized rescue bag. This protection must include the head and neck. Incorporation of a windproof and waterproof layer is of obvious value in preventing convective and evaporative heat loss. This is particularly important for victims requiring helicopter evacuation, since downwash from helicopter rotor blades can reach wind speeds in excess of 160 km/hour (100 mph), thus potentiating significant heat loss from windchill.[148]

Spontaneous Rewarming. Patients who are only mildly hypothermic (exposed to cold water for a relatively short time, fully conscious, and vigorously shivering with a T_c greater than 32° to 33° C [89.6° to 91.4° F]) are usually capable of rewarming themselves without difficulty. Heat production from shivering can reach levels five to six times that of resting metabolic rate.[36] Shivering is thus a highly effective means of rewarming, particularly if rescuers insulate the patient's head and body with vapor barrier garments to minimize evaporative heat loss.[51] Vigorous shivering has been shown to be capable of producing rewarming rates as high as 3° to 4° C/hr (5.4° to 7.2° F).[43,51,52] Victims who are conscious and vigorously shivering are generally not a medical emergency and usually do not require immediate transportation for definitive care. However, rescuers should be aware that prolonged periods of shivering consume the patient's endogenous energy reserves. Thus rescuers should administer oral glucose-containing fluids to conscious persons who have adequate cough and gag reflexes. Attention to energy reserves in unconscious, severely hypothermic victims is also important. Warmed IV glucose solutions are useful in these persons as part of definitive resuscitative and rewarming protocols (see below).[26,143] Alcoholic beverages are contraindicated in all cases.

Inhalation Warming.

Rescuers should attempt to minimize respiratory heat losses. Hypothermic patients lose up to 11 to 13 kcal/hr through the inhalation of relatively cold, dry air and through the exhalation of water-saturated air at near T_c.[185] Administration of heated, humidified air or oxygen at approximately 42° to 46° C (107.6° to 114.8° F) can result in a net positive gain of 17.1 kcal/hr.[185] Although this is a relatively small amount of heat compared with the total kilocalories required to completely rewarm the hypothermic patient, heated and humidified ventilation is of value in insulating the airway from further evaporative heat loss. Some studies have shown, however, that inhalation rewarming reduces metabolic heat production through shivering.[47] In experimental subjects whose shivering was pharmacologically inhibited, inhalation warming did not appear to provide any advantage over spontaneous rewarming.[58] Other suggested benefits of inhalation warming include rehydration, stimulation of mucociliary activity in the respiratory tract, and direct heat transfer from the upper airways to the hypothalamus, brainstem, and other brain structures. Any resultant warming of the respiratory, cardiovascular, or thermoregulatory centers could be of benefit. While research continues on the efficacy of airway rewarming, most hypothermia treatment protocols continue to recommend inhalation warming as an adjunct to overall rewarming strategies.*

Warmed IV Fluids.

Administration of warmed IV fluids is beneficial in reversing hypothermia-induced dehydration and hypovolemia.[26,147] Replacement of fluids before rewarming has been shown in dogs to augment cardiac output.[132] Dextrose 5% in water or normal saline, or normal saline alone, is preferable to lactated Ringer's solution, since a hypothermic liver may be unable to metabolize lactate normally.[148] Administration of 300 to 500 ml should be given fairly rapidly, with the remainder of the liter administered over the next hour.[5] In no case should cold IV fluids be administered. Plastic IV bags can be easily carried inside a rescuer's clothing (preferably next to the skin) to keep the fluids warm and to supply some perfusion pressure.

Body-to-Body Rewarming.

Body-to-body warming of the patient has long been advocated as an acceptable field treatment of the hypothermic patient. Sir John Franklin, in his 1823 text, *Narrative of a Journey to the Shores of the Polar Sea in the Years 1819, 20, 21*, describes this technique for resuscitation of an expedition member recovered from ice water.[39] When wrapped together in a blanket or sleeping bag, a rescuer can donate body heat to a hypothermic patient. Experimental studies on human volunteers, however, have failed to demonstrate a rewarming advantage of this technique in shivering individuals. When subjects were cooled to an average core temperature (T_{es}) of 34.6° C (94.3° F), body-to-body rewarming proved no better than shivering alone.[52] In this study, the heat donated by the "rescuers" was only sufficient to offset the heat lost by inhibition of shivering. Several theoretic arguments mediate against routine use of body-to-body rewarming in shivering victims in the field: (1) the large heat loss of an immersion hypothermic victim (e.g., 300 kcal in cooling an average normothermic adult to a T_c of 33° C [91.4° F]) is unlikely to be reversed by the relatively small amount of heat provided by the donor (e.g., a resting, nonshivering adult produces only about 100 kcal/hr)[52]; (2) rescuers provide a relatively small surface area in direct contact with the hypothermic victim through which to donate heat; (3) peripheral vasoconstriction in the victim will limit heat flow to the core[35]; and (4) external heat from body-to-body contact will inhibit the hypothermic victim's endogenous heat production through shivering.[51] However, in severely hypothermic, nonshivering victims, or in victims whose shivering thermogenesis is inhibited by alcohol, medications, age, etc., body-to-body rewarming may be indicated. Furthermore, body-to-body rewarming may provide important psychologic support to the patient. For these reasons, rescuers should weigh response implications against the advantages and disadvantages of body-to-body rewarming in devising a field rewarming strategy for any particular hypothermic patient.

Heating Pads.

Application of external moderate heat sources to hypothermic patients has been a traditional method of field rewarming. Particularly when applied to the patient's neck, thorax, and groin (areas with high potential for conductive heat transfer),[78] hot water bottles, chemical or charcoal heat packs, heating pads, or other warmed objects have been used in an attempt to stabilize the patient's T_c. Experimental evidence is lacking, however, to demonstrate the efficacy of this treatment modality over spontaneous shivering thermogenesis alone.[19,51,72,151] Only when combined with a source of heated, humidified ventilation has a heating pad been experimentally shown (on mildly hypothermic, shivering volunteers) to be marginally effective in shivering subjects.[130] For more severely hypothermic patients who are not shivering, these types of external

---

*References 25, 26, 43, 143, 148, 180.

heat sources may be indicated in helping stabilize the patient's T_c. Indeed, a recent study has demonstrated that charcoal heating provides a significant rewarming advantage in hypothermic subjects when shivering was pharmacologically inhibited.[85]

Rescuers should be aware of several potential hazards with this rewarming technique. Hypothermic skin is very sensitive to heat and easily injured. All sources of external heat must be separated from direct contact with the victim's skin to prevent severe thermal burns.[147] Third-degree burns have resulted from application of a lukewarm hot-water bottle directly to a hypothermic child's skin.[120] Furthermore, heatpacks that use burning charcoal as a heat source can create a carbon monoxide hazard within an enclosed space.[151]

Arteriovenous Anastomoses Rewarming. This technique relies on the physiologic arteriovenous anastomoses (AVAs) that exist in human digits and on the superficial venous rete in the forearms and lower legs. Warming these areas opens the AVA and increases superficial venous return via the rete. Warmed venous blood thus reaches the core without excessive countercurrent heat loss to cold arteries (i.e., superficial veins are not in close contact with arteries). Because of the pioneering work of Vanggaard and Gjerloff,[175] who proposed AVA rewarming, the Royal Danish Navy has been using this technique since 1970.[174] Recent experimental studies have confirmed the efficacy of this technique.[176] Mildly hypothermic subjects (T_{es} = 34.2° C [93.6° F]) whose hands, forearms, feet, and lower legs were immersed in either 42° C or 45° C (107.6° F or 113° F) water, had a smaller postcooling afterdrop than from shivering alone (0.4° C [0.72° F] compared with 0.6° C [1.08° F]) and a significantly faster rate of rewarming (6.6° C/hr and 9.9° C/hr [11.88° F/hr and 17.82° F]) compared with shivering alone (3.4° C/hr [6.12° F/hr]). Although this technique may be difficult to implement in some field settings, it may be practical in mildly hypothermic victims on rescue vessels or other vehicles where a source of warm water is available. As with heating pads and other sources of external heat, however, rescuers should be concerned about the possibility of thermal burns. In the above study, no burns were observed in the experimental subjects, even when their extremities were immersed in 45° C (113° F) water, although some subjects complained of initial discomfort at this temperature. Rescuers opting to use AVA rewarming should perhaps start with a 42° C (107.6° F) water temperature and gradually raise the temperature to 44° C (111.2° F).[176]

Another concern with AVA rewarming concerns potential cardiovascular instability. Hypotension may occur secondary to increase in peripheral blood flow in a hypovolemic patient. If the victim is required to be in a semiupright posture to receive AVA rewarming, orthostatic hypotension could potentially add to cardiovascular instability. No experimental data support these potential cardiovascular problems, but studies on AVA rewarming have only been performed on mildly hypothermic subjects.[176] Further research is required to evaluate the efficacy and safety of AVA warming on severely hypothermic patients.

Forced Air Warming. Forced air warming (FAW) is a technique derived from a treatment modality used to prevent or reverse hypothermia in surgical patients.[98,140] Convective heat transfer is provided by warm air blown into warming covers over the patient's body. Both experimental and clinical data support the efficacy of this technique on mild to moderate and on severely hypothermic patients. In mildly hypothermic experimental subjects, FAW was associated with a 30% smaller afterdrop than that found with shivering alone. Furthermore, in the initial 35 minutes of rewarming, shivering patients experienced a net heat loss of 30 to 50W, compared to a net heat gain from FAW of 163 to 237W.[50] In moderately to severely hypothermic patients (mean T_{re} = 28.5° C [83.3° F]) treated in an emergency room, FAW (when used in conjunction with warmed IV fluids and inhalation warming) achieved a rewarming rate (2.4° C/hr [4.32° F/hr]) nearly twice that of patients treated only with warmed IV fluids and inhalation warming (1.4° C/hr [2.52° F/hr]).[144]

In another series of experiments using human subjects, a FAW device designed for field use was associated with a significantly higher core rewarming rate (5.8° C/hr [10.44° F/hr]) than that of shivering alone (3.4° C/hr [6.12° F/hr]) but showed no advantage over shivering in decreasing afterdrop.[31] When shivering was inhibited with meperidine in human volunteers,[54] FAW was associated with a 50% decrease in afterdrop and a 600% increase in rewarming rate compared with spontaneous rewarming alone.[58] A different prototype FAW device, using a collapsible rigid patient cover and evaluated experimentally on nonshivering human volunteers, was associated with a smaller afterdrop and faster rewarming rate than spontaneous rewarming alone.[49]

In summary, FAW has shown significant promise as both a field and hospital treatment modality. It is a safe, noninvasive technique that can both decrease afterdrop and increase core warming rate of immersion hypothermia patients. Figure 8-13 schematically illustrates T_c responses to various rewarming methodologies under mild (shivering intact) and severe (shivering absent) hypothermic conditions.

Transportation

Stabilization, insulation, and rewarming of the hypothermic victim should be started during transport to an appropriate medical center for definitive rewarming. If possible, the receiving facility should be selected

Rewarming

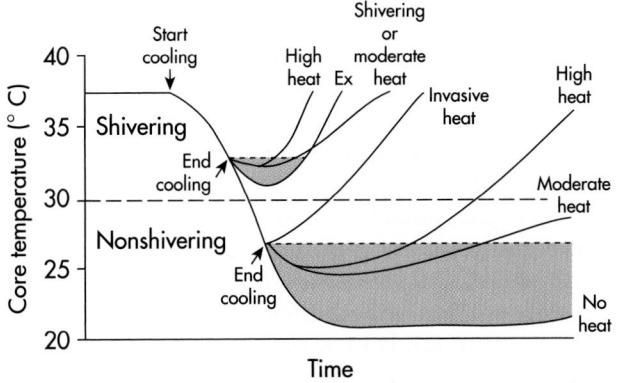

Figure 8-13 Schematic illustration of the effectiveness of various rewarming techniques under shivering and nonshivering hypothermic conditions. Dashed line (at 30° C) indicates approximate core temperature at which shivering is spontaneously abolished. *Ex,* External rewarming.

on the basis of knowledge and experience in managing hypothermic patients. In the same manner that victims of multiple trauma are most appropriately managed in trauma centers, severely hypothermic patients are best managed in hospitals equipped to handle potential complications and to provide core rewarming therapies. For example, a hospital with cardiac bypass rewarming capabilities may be a better choice for managing a severely hypothermic patient than a hospital without such qualifications, even though the former may require a longer transport time.

During transport to a site for definitive medical care, emergency medical personnel should frequently monitor the patient's T_c and other vital signs. In addition, they should attach an electrocardiogram (ECG) monitor; continue administration of warmed IV fluids and heated, humidified air or oxygen; and continue other rewarming efforts discussed above. Rescuers should maintain the hypothermic victim in a supine posture and should restrict the voluntary movements of conscious individuals. At the receiving facility, rescuers should ensure that the patient is carried, and not allowed to walk, to the treatment location.

COLD WATER SURVIVAL

Cold water survival depends on avoidance of drowning and hypothermia and on the many factors related to these risks[145,146,149]:

1. Ability to swim
2. Ability to keep the head out of the water (even without flotation aids)
3. Ability to avoid panic
4. Sea state
5. Availability and type of personal flotation device (PFD)

6. Availability of a life raft
7. Availability of other floating objects to increase buoyancy (such as a capsized boat)
8. Water temperature
9. Physical characteristics of the survivor
10. Type of protective clothing worn against immersion hypothermia and initial immersion cold shock
11. Behavior of the survivor in the water
12. Availability of signaling devices (whistles, flares, strobe lights, radios, and mirrors) and the ability to use these devices
13. Proximity of rescue personnel

Drowning is the most immediate survival problem following water entry. To maintain airway freeboard and to avoid drowning, a survivor must possess the physical skills and psychologic aptitude to combat the effects of wave action.[146,160] Although a PFD assists in maintenance of airway freeboard, waves can still submerge a survivor's head, even in moderately calm seas.[56,145,168] To reduce the risk of drowning in rough seas, a survivor can increase effective airway freeboard by partially exiting the water (e.g., clinging to an overturned vessel or other debris floating in the water) or by climbing totally out of the water into a life raft or onto a capsized vessel. In both these environments, the survivor may still have to cope with the effects of cold wind, spray, and waves.

As previously discussed, sudden immersion in cold water initiates a cardiorespiratory cold shock response that significantly potentiates the risk of drowning. These reflexes and the resulting incapacitation that can accompany them have been suspected as the primary cause of drowning after short-term (<10 minutes) immersion in cold water.[156] Abrupt tachycardia and hypertension induced by sudden immersion in cold water can produce incapacitating cardiac arrhythmias in susceptible individuals and myocardial infarction or cerebrovascular accident in persons with arterial disease or hypertension.[156] In addition, reflex gasp and hyperventilation[156,163] significantly shorten breath-holding duration.[76,82,156] Figure 8-14 illustrates this phenomenon. Loss of breath-holding capacity can have severe consequences for survivors attempting underwater egress from a submerged vehicle, capsized vessel, or aircraft or for survivors simply trying to maintain airway freeboard in a rough sea or white-water river.[82,136,160]

The respiratory difficulties induced by the cold-shock reflexes makes breathing while swimming extremely difficult. Golden and Hardcastle[62] have demonstrated a "swim stroke/respiration asynchrony" leading to water inhalation and swimming failure, and Golden et al[66] have shown that even persons who are considered good swimmers (at least in warm water) can only swim in cold water for a few minutes. Swimming ability and survival time in cold water is further diminished by

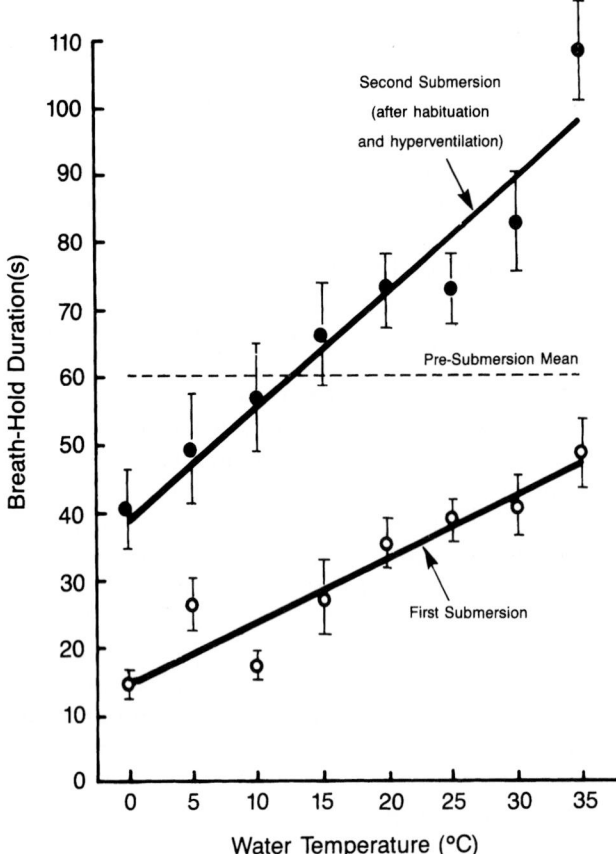

Figure 8-14 Effect of water temperature on maximum breath-hold duration in young, physically fit human subjects (80 men and 80 women). First submersion was sudden after sitting comfortably in air at a mean temperature of 11.3° C (52.34° F). Second submersion followed 2 minutes of acclimatization to the water. The last 10 seconds of the acclimatization was accompanied by 10 seconds of hyperventilation. (*From Hayward JS et al: J Appl Physiol 56:202, 1984.*)

subjective perception of shortness of breath and by panic reactions from unexpected cold water immersion.[156] The work required to swim in cold water is greater than that in warm water because of the former's higher viscosity (e.g., water at 4.7° C [40.5° F] has a viscosity 67% higher than water at 23.7° C [74.7° F]).[97] The increased work of swimming in cold water potentiates the onset of fatigue. The combination of all these factors may incapacitate even physically fit, capable swimmers. Keatinge et al[97] observed sudden incapacitation in two experimental subjects (who were good swimmers) immersed in 4.7° C water. One inhaled water from respiratory difficulty and fatigue after swimming for 7½ minutes and had to be pulled out of the water. The second subject lasted only 1½ minutes before he "floundered and sank without managing to reach the side of the pool, which was about 1 meter from his head, and had to be pulled" out of the water.[97] The observed frequency of such swimming failures and unex-

pected submersions has led the U.S. Coast Guard to coin the term *sudden disappearance syndrome* to describe the phenomenon.[168]

The magnitude of the cold shock response can be attenuated through habituation to cold immersion. Tipton et al demonstrated that habituating subjects to 10° C (50° F) water resulted in 16% reduction in respiratory rate during the first 30 seconds of immersion in 10° C water and 26% reduction in respiratory rate during the 30-second to 180-second interval after immersion in 10° C water. Tidal volume and heart rate response showed similar declines in habituated subjects.[161] Habituation through cold water survival training may thus be an important safety measure for workers in cold water environments.

Protective clothing also diminishes the cold shock response from initial immersion in cold water. Clothing that limits the amount and ingress velocity of water reaching a subject's skin (e.g., well-fitted wet suits and dry suits with adequate seals) significantly decreases the cardiorespiratory reflex responses to sudden immersion.[111,162,164,165] Furthermore, Tipton and Golden demonstrated that subjects wearing a wet suit that protected the torso but left the limbs exposed had a significantly reduced respiratory reflex response but not a reduced heart rate response compared with control subjects with neither torso nor limbs protected. They concluded that the limbs may be more important than the torso in the cardiac response to sudden cold water immersion.[165] Tipton et al[162] also demonstrated that even loose-fitting, poorly insulated clothing can attenuate the magnitude of the cold shock response compared with immersion in swimming trunks only. When volunteers were immersed in 10° C (50° F) water wearing either conventional clothing or conventional clothing plus windproof/showerproof foul-weather clothing, cardiopulmonary and thermal responses were significantly less than those found with swimming trunks alone.

If a victim of cold water immersion can avoid drowning during the initial few minutes after water entry, prevention of hypothermia becomes an important problem. Survival time in cold water, based on the pathophysiologic effects of decreasing T_c, is not a precise calculation. Large individual variations among survivors in body morphology and state of health and fitness, combined with many exogenous variables affecting cooling rate (e.g., clothing, water temperature, sea state, flotation, and behavior), preclude exact predictions of survival time. However, sufficient experimental data and case history findings exist to allow generalizations. At a T_c of 34° C (93.2° F), there is a significant deleterious effect on manual dexterity and "useful function" in cold water.[22,123] If a survivor is trying to combat rough seas, this level of dysfunction may potentiate drowning. At a T_c of 30° C (86° F), unconsciousness is probable.[17,26,149,150,154] Even if a survivor is wearing a self-righting PFD designed to maintain airway freeboard in an unconscious person, drowning is probable at this T_c in all but the calmest seas. At T_c below 25° C (77° F), VF or asystole often occur spontaneously.[26] Of these three core temperatures, 30° C is the most practical for defining the limits of survival in cold water.

For immersion hypothermia, the most important variables affecting cooling rates in cold water are:

1. Water temperature
2. Survivor's height, weight, and percent body fat
3. Type of protective clothing worn by the survivor
4. Sea state
5. Survivor's behavior in the water
6. Amount of the survivor's body immersed in the water
7. Metabolic heat production

The advantage of body fat as an insulator against cold has been discussed previously in the Body Morphology (Size and Composition) section covering pathophysiology and cooling rates. Using an extrapolation of linear cooling rate to 30° C (86° F), Figure 8-15 shows predicted *calm water* survival times of lightly clothed, nonexercising humans in cold water. The graph shows a line for the average expectancy and a broad zone that indicates the large amount of individual variability associated with different body size, build, and degree of fatness. The zone would include approximately 95% of the variation expected for adult and teenage humans under the conditions specified. In the zone where death from hypothermia is highly improbable, cold water still potentiates death from drowning from "cold shock" (as discussed above) in the first few minutes of immersion, especially for those not wearing personal flotation devices. It is important to note that Figure 8-15 discusses only calm water survival times. Since rough water conditions decrease survival times, as discussed below, Figure 8-15 may be useful for estimating *maximum* survival times for an individual immersed in cold water. Search and rescue organizations might find such a maximum survival time helpful, since they often use the longest possible survival time in deciding when to terminate a search effort.

A large number of studies over the past few decades have evaluated the relationship of different types of protective clothing to heat loss and cooling rates.* Nearly all of these studies have been conducted in calm water or in laboratory settings. As illustrated by the cooling rate data in Tables 8-2 and 8-3, such studies have generally shown that in calm water, intact, "dry," insulated garments provide better protection than do "wet" insulated garments, and well-insulated garments

*References 4, 32, 75, 81, 92, 93, 100, 123, 141, 149, 150, 157, 162, 164, 165, 166, 183, 187.

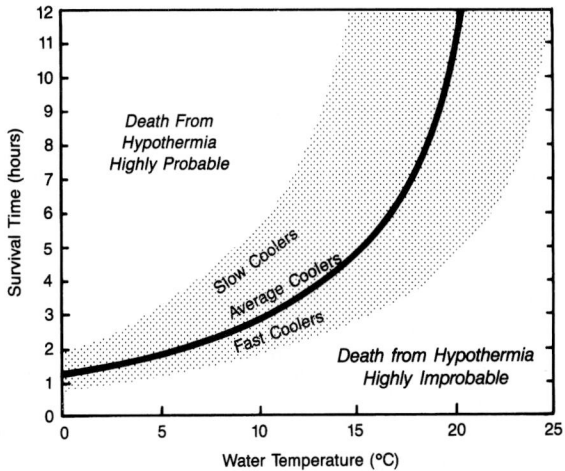

Figure 8-15 Predicted calm water survival time (defined as the time required to cool to 30° C [86° F]) in lightly clothed, nonexercising humans in cold water. The graph shows a line for the average expectancy and a broad zone that indicates the large amount of individual variability associated with different body size, build, fatness, physical fitness, and state of health. The zone would include approximately 95% of the variation expected for adult and teenage humans under the conditions specified. The zone would be shifted downward by physical activity (e.g., swimming) and upward slightly for heavy clothing or protective behaviors (e.g., huddling with other survivors or adopting a fetal position in the water). Specialized insulated protective clothing (e.g., survival suits, wet suits) is capable of increasing survival time from 2 to 10 times (or more) the basic duration shown here. In the zone where death from hypothermia is highly improbable, cold shock on initial immersion can potentiate death from drowning, particularly for those not wearing flotation devices. (*From US Coast Guard:* Addendum to the National Search and Rescue (SAR) Manual, *COMDTINST M16120.5 and COMDTINST M16120.6, 1995.*)

provide significantly better protection than do poorly insulated garments. Figure 8-16 shows various types of cold water protective garments.

Although calm water studies have value in comparing the relative degree of protection afforded by different types of protective clothing, many immersion accidents occur in rough water.[135,159,160] In this environment, a survivor's cooling rate may be affected by swimming to maintain airway freeboard, passive body movements caused by waves, flushing of cold water through "wet" suits, and leakage of cold water into "dry" suits. For example, subjects in a wave tank demonstrate higher energy expenditure and faster cooling rates than do subjects in calm water.[73] Several experimental studies have demonstrated significantly faster cooling rates for human volunteers wearing "wet" protective garments in rough or turbulent water[134,150,187] than for persons in calm water. Even "dry" suits have shown degradation of protection in rough water. In a recent study of dry immersion suits in 16° C water, Ducharme and Brooks[32] found that wave heights up to 70 cm resulted in a 14% decrease in total suit insulation and an

TABLE 8-2. Mean Linear Cooling Rates for Lean Men (Mean Body Fat = 12%) Dressed in Various Types of Garments in 10° C Calm Water

TYPE OF PROTECTIVE CLOTHING	COOLING RATE (° C/HR ± SD)
Control (equivalent to ordinary street clothes)	3.2 ± 1.1
"WET DESIGN"	
Thermal "float coat" (loose-fitted, 5.4-mm closed-cell foam–insulated jacket)	1.6 ± 0.6
Short "wet suit" (custom-fitted, 3.2-mm closed-cell foam covering arms, trunk, and upper thighs)	1.2 ± 0.4
"Insulated coveralls" (loose-fitted, 3.2-mm closed-cell foam covering extremities and trunk)	1 ± 0.4
Full "wet suit" (custom-fitted, 4.8-mm closed-cell foam covering extremities and trunk)	0.7 ± 0.3
"DRY DESIGN"	
"Immersion suit" (loose-fitted, 4.8-mm closed-cell foam with sealed openings)	0.5 ± 0.3

From Steinman AM et al: *Aviat Space Environ Med* 58:550, 1987.

TABLE 8-3. Comparison of Mean Cooling Rates for Thin Men (Mean Body Fat = 9.1%) Wearing Various Types of Protective Clothing in 11.8° C Calm Water

CLOTHING TYPE	MEAN COOLING RATE (° C/HR)	RATIOS TO CONTROL	
		DIRECT	INVERSE
Dry, closed-cell foam insulation (4.8 mm thick)	0.31	0.14	7.35
Wet, closed-cell foam insulation (4.8 mm thick)	0.54	0.23	4.26
Dry, uninsulated (watertight shell over lightweight clothing)	1.07	0.47	2.15
Control (lightweight clothing alone)	2.3	1	1

From Hayward JS et al: Design concepts of survival suits for cold-water immersion and their thermal protection performance, *Proceedings of the 17th Symposium of the SAFE Association*, Van Nuys, Calif, 1980.

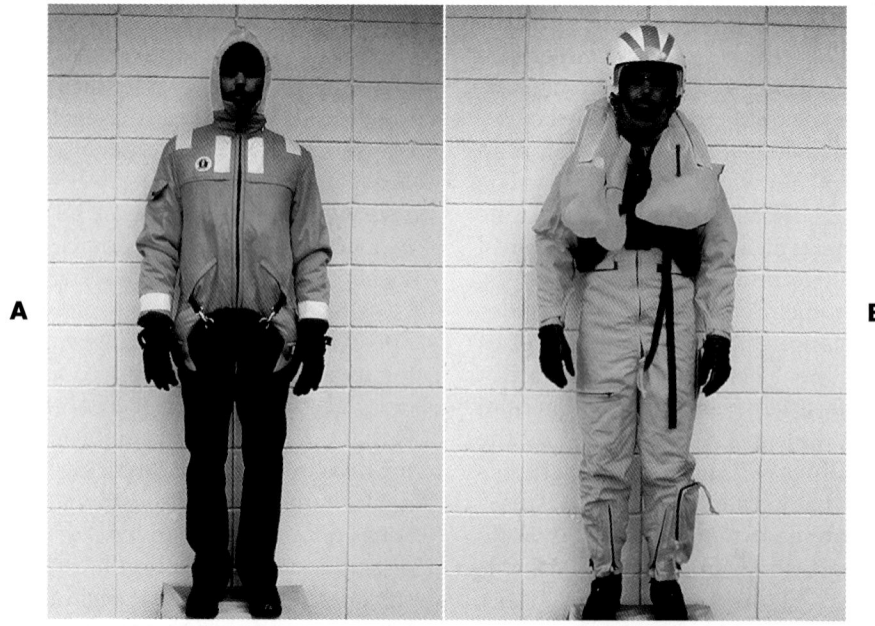

Figure 8-16 Antiexposure garments. **A,** Float coat. **B,** Aviation coveralls with personal flotation device.

Continued

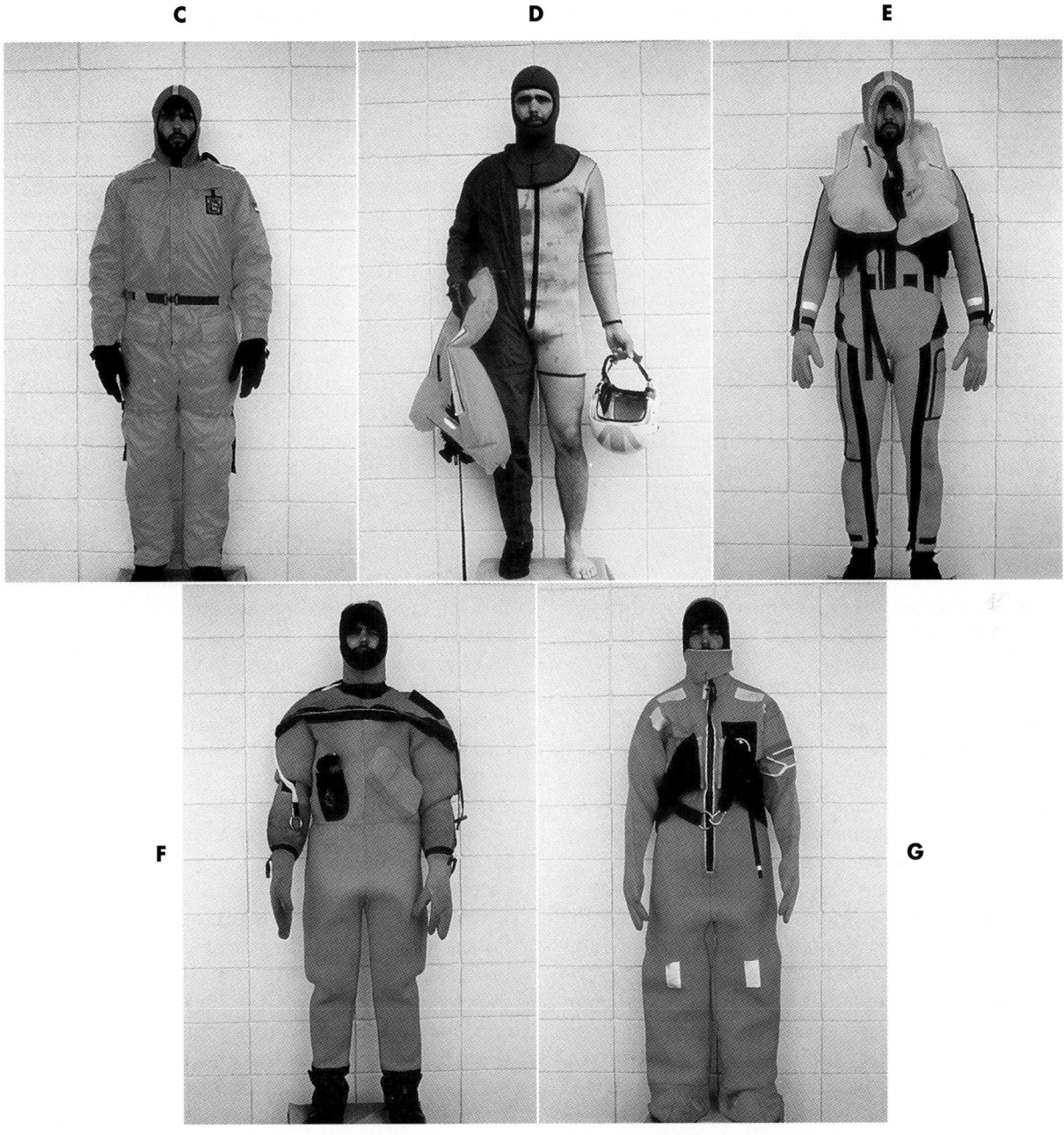

Figure 8-16, cont'd C, Boat crew coveralls or snowmobile suit. **D,** Short wet suit worn as an undergarment. **E,** Full wet suit with personal flotation device. **F,** Insulated dry suit. **G,** Immersion suit. Garments **A** to **C** are loose-fitting, closed-cell foam–insulated wet suits; garments **D** and **E** are tight-fitting closed-cell foam–insulated wet suits; garments **F** and **G** are closed-cell foam–insulated dry suits.

average 45% decrease in thermal resistance at the head and trunk regions of the suits.

Figure 8-17 shows a comparison of cooling rates for lean males dressed in the various types of protective clothing shown in Figure 8-16 in both calm and rough water at approximately 10° C (50° F).[150] The most dramatic differences occurred in the loose-fitted, "wet" protective clothing (such as the float coat and insulated coveralls), where cooling rates nearly doubled in rough

seas over those in calm seas. This was primarily due to flushing of cold water through the garments. However, even the tight-fitted, full "wet" suit allowed a 30% faster cooling rate in rough water over that in calm water. The "dry" suit, which did not leak, showed no significant difference between calm and rough seas.

Estimated survival times in rough seas, based on experimental data, were published for thin men wearing different types of protective clothing in 6° C (42.8° F)

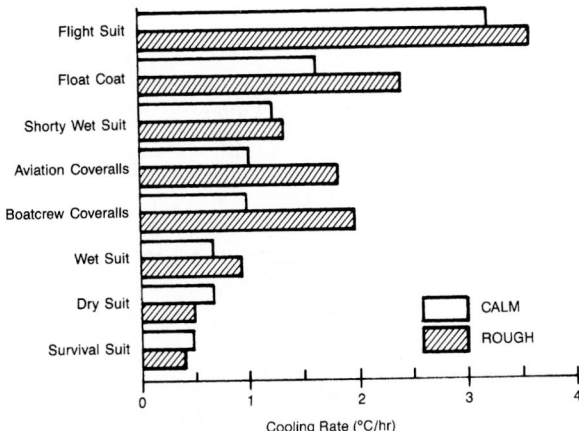

Figure 8-17 A comparison of mean rectal temperature cooling rates in lean male subjects in calm vs. rough seas at 10.7° C (51.26° F). The flight suit, used as a control garment, is equivalent to light clothing. (*From Steinman AM et al:* Aviat Space Environ Med 58:550, 1987.)

water.[149] Table 8-4 shows these times for three different levels of survival. The following assumptions underlie these estimations:

1. Cooling rates are linear.[81,149,150,154]
2. Initial T_c is 37.5° C (99.5° F).
3. Survivors are able to maintain airway freeboard until unconsciousness occurs at a rectal temperature of 30° C (86° F).
4. Self-righting flotation maintains airway freeboard when survivors are unconscious.

In comparing these estimated survival times with those of Figure 8-15 (calm water survival times), the reader must recall that Figure 8-15 concerns only survival to a T_c of 30° C. Furthermore, the zone in the graph must be adjusted downward for rough seas and for survivors wearing only light clothing, and upward for survivors wearing insulated clothing. For 6° C (42.8° F) water, the survival times (to a T_c of 30° C) correlate well between Figure 8-15 and Table 8-4. We must emphasize that the estimates in Table 8-4 pertain to lean individuals with a mean body fat of only 11.1%. Since many populations of adults (such as offshore oil workers) in the 30- to 50-year-old age range average 25% to 30% body fat, the estimates of "time to unconsciousness" and "time to cardiac arrest" must be considered conservative for a broader spectrum of adults.

Survivor location also has a significant effect on T_c cooling rate and survival time. The U.S. Coast Guard and other rescue organizations recommend that a survivor of a maritime accident in cold seas get as much of the body out of the water as possible to minimize cooling rate and maximize survival time.[149,168] This recommendation derives from the higher thermal conductivity of water compared with air at the same temperature.

However, survivors exposed to cold air are still at risk from hypothermia secondary to convective, evaporative, and radiant heat losses. In a rough sea environment, wind increases the magnitude of convective heat loss, and spray and periodic wetting from breaking waves result in conductive heat loss.[153,155] Steinman et al[149] confirmed the above observations. The cooling rates of thin male subjects, wearing different types of protective clothing, were compared for three survival situations:

1. Immersion in 6° C (42.8° F) water with 1.5-m (5-foot) breaking waves
2. Exposure to 7.7° C (45.9° F) air, continuous water spray at 6° C, continuous 28 to 33 km/hr wind, and occasional breaking waves while sitting atop an overturned boat
3. Exposure to 7.7° C air and occasional breaking waves while sitting in an open, one-person life raft

The results of the study are shown in Figure 8-18. For each type of garment worn, cooling rates were considerably faster in the water than atop the boat (despite the effects of wind, spray, and breaking waves) or within the raft.

Survivors should therefore attempt to get as much of their bodies out of the water as possible, even if it means exposure to cold wind and spray. Even rescue and medical personnel who frequently work in wilderness environments poorly understand this recommendation. A widespread misunderstanding of the concept of "windchill" causes many to conclude that survivors have higher heat losses if they are exposed to wind, especially if they are wet, than if they are immersed in water.[149] Windchill (a term originally used by Siple and Passel[142] to describe the increase in heat loss from unprotected skin exposed to wind) is frequently used in the communication media without regard to the difference between exposed and unexposed skin. This misleads many to believe that the windchill temperature applies to both clothed and unclothed areas of the body. Furthermore, common experiences during recreational activities at the beach, lake, or swimming pool, where people subjectively feel colder after leaving the water (because of evaporative heat loss from the skin) than they do while swimming, reinforce the misunderstanding. This has occasionally led survivors to abandon a position of relative safety atop a capsized vessel and reenter the water, usually with tragic results. The sensation of coldness (which is skin dependent) does not reliably convey information about rate of heat loss when two radically different environments such as air and water are compared.

Tikuisis[153,154] recently devised a more sophisticated set of survival time estimates for individuals immersed in cold, rough seas and for survivors partially immersed and/or exposed to cold wind under wet conditions. Us-

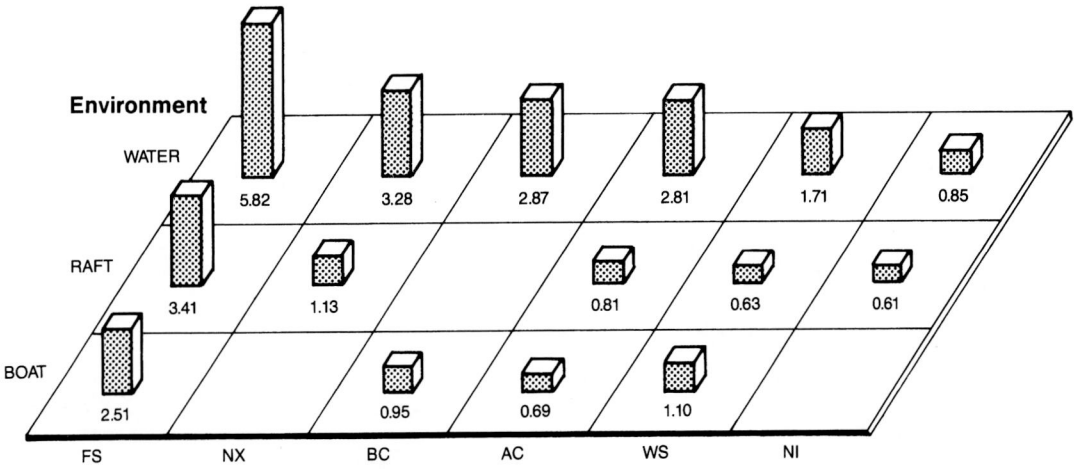

Figure 8-18 Mean linear cooling rates (° C/hr) for lean men in three survival environments: *water* = immersion in 6.1° C (42.98° F) breaking waves; *boat* = 5 minutes immersion in 6.1° C water followed by exposure to 7.7° C (45.86° F) air atop an overturned boat with continuous 28- to 33-km/hr wind, water spray, and occasional breaking waves; *raft* = exposure to 7.7° C air in an open, one-person life raft, preceded by 5-minute immersion in 6.1° C water. *AC,* Air crew coveralls; *BC,* boat crew coveralls; *FS,* flight suit (lightweight clothing); *NI,* intact, non–foam-insulated "dry" coveralls; *NX,* NI with a 5-cm tear in the left shoulder, thus permitting water to leak into the suit and degrade its insulation; *WS,* wet suit. Blank squares indicate combinations of garment and environment that were not tested. *(From Steinman AM, Kubilis P: Survival at sea: the effects of protective clothing and survivor location on core and skin temperature, USCG Rep No. CG-D-26-86, Springfield, 1986, Va, National Technical Information Service.)*

TABLE 8-4. Estimated Survival Times for Lean Subjects (Mean Body Fat = 11.1%) Wearing Various Types of Protective Clothing in Rough Seas

	ESTIMATED SURVIVAL TIME (HR) (95% CONFIDENCE RANGE)		
CLOTHING TYPE	TIME TO INCAPACITY (T = 34° C)	TIME TO UNCONSCIOUSNESS (T = 30° C)	TIME TO CARDIAC ARREST (T = 25° C)
Control (lightweight clothing)	0.4-1.3	0.8-2.6	1.3-4.3
Torn, non–foam-insulated dry coverall (2-inch tear in left shoulder)	0.9-2.7	1.6-5.2	2.5-8.4
Closed-cell foam–insulated, wet coverall (3.2-mm thick insulation in a loose fitted coverall)	1-2.9	1.9-6	3-9.9
Closed-cell foam–insulated, custom-fitted wet suit (4.8-mm thick insulation; tight-fitted)	1.6-4.7	3.1-9.9	4.9-16.2
Intact, non–foam-insulated dry coverall (watertight shell over thick, fiberfill, insulated underwear)	2.9-8.8	5.7-18.2	9.1-30

From Steinman AM, Kubilis P: *Survival at sea: the effects of protective clothing and survivor location on core and skin temperature,* USCG Rep No. CG-D-26-86, Springfield, Va, 1986, National Technical Information Service.

ing computer modeling of human cooling physiology and the experimental data of Steinman et al[149,150] shown above, he developed a series of survival time charts for a range of individual body morphologies while wearing various degrees of protective clothing.[153] Figure 8-19 shows his estimates for lean, average, and fat individuals wearing a loose-fitted, insulated coverall (boat-

crew coverall, snowmobile suit, etc.; see Fig 8-16). Tikuisis defined the lean, average, and fat survivors as having the following morphologic characteristics: height = 1.77 m (5 feet 9½ inches); weight = 66.3, 73.9, and 88.2 kg, respectively, for lean, average, and fat; body fat = 11.2%, 17.7%, and 28.6%, respectively, for lean, average, and fat. Note that the lean definitions fit the experimen-

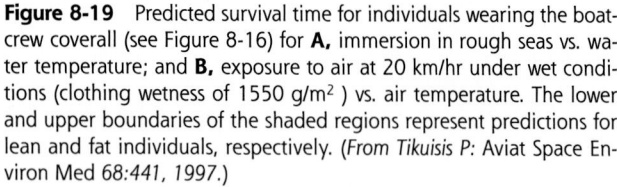

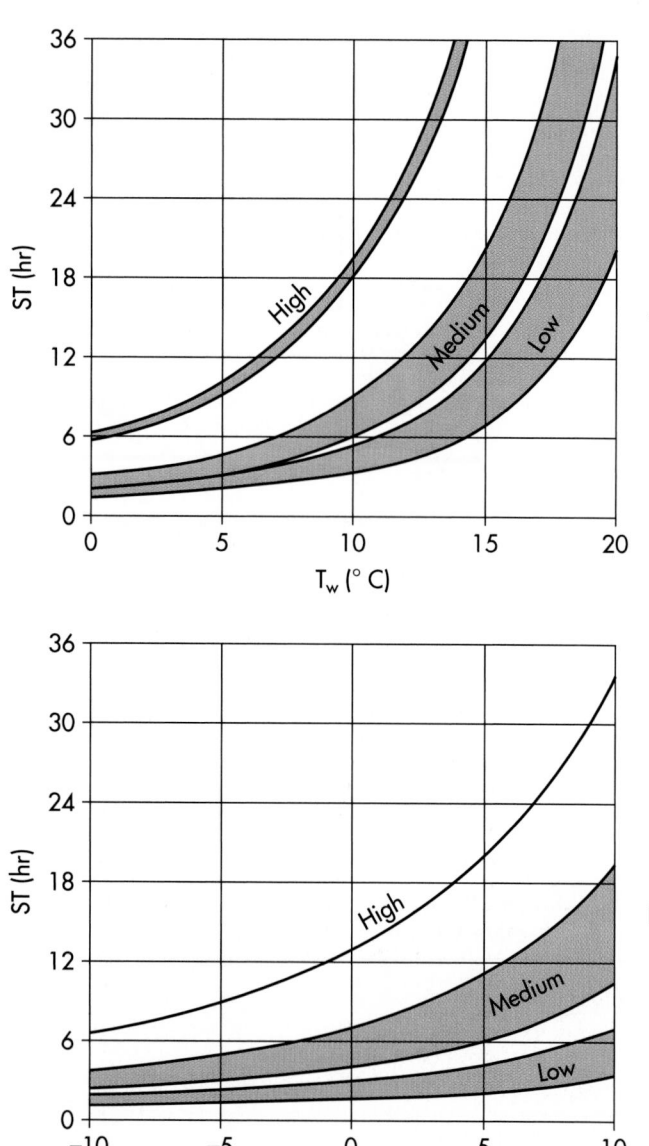

Figure 8-19 Predicted survival time for individuals wearing the boat-crew coverall (see Figure 8-16) for **A,** immersion in rough seas vs. water temperature; and **B,** exposure to air at 20 km/hr under wet conditions (clothing wetness of 1550 g/m²) vs. air temperature. The lower and upper boundaries of the shaded regions represent predictions for lean and fat individuals, respectively. (*From Tikuisis P:* Aviat Space Environ Med *68:441, 1997.*)

Figure 8-20 Prediction of survival time for an average individual under various degrees of clothing protection (See Figure 8-16). **A,** Immersion in rough seas vs. water temperature; *low* = nude, flight suit, float coat, aviation coverall, boat crew coverall, torn coverall; *medium* = short wet suit, full wet suit; and *high* = dry coverall, dry suit. **B,** Exposure to air at 20 km/hr under wet conditions vs. air temperature; *low* = nude, flight suit, aviation coverall; *medium* = float coat, boat crew coverall, short wet suit, full wet suit, dry coverall, torn coverall; and *high* = dry suit. (*From Tikuisis P:* Aviat Space Environ Med *68:441, 1997.*)

tal subjects used by Steinman et al[149] (see Table 8-4). Tikuisis also published a series of survival time charts for the "average" individual (defined above) wearing various types of clothing protection. Figure 8-20 shows his results for low insulation clothing (nude, float coats, average clothing, boatcrew coveralls, leaky "dry" suits), medium insulation clothing (partial or full wet suits), and high insulation clothing (dry, insulated coveralls and survival suits). Both the Canadian and United States Coast Guard in their search and rescue missions are now using these survival charts.

REFERENCES

1. Abocar A: *Canadian snowmobilers falling victim to thin ice,* Reuters, January 23, 1998.
2. Alexander L: *The treatment of shock from prolonged exposure to cold, especially in water.* Combined Intelligence Objectives Subcommittee Item No 24, Office of the Publication Board, Department of Commerce, Washington, DC, 1946.
3. Andersson J, Schagatay E: Effects of lung volume and involuntary breathing movements on the human diving response, *Eur J Appl Physiol* 77:19, 1998.
4. Bagian JP et al: Effectiveness of the space shuttle anti-exposure system in a cold water environment, *Aviat Space Environ Med* 61:753, 1990.

5. Bangs CC: Treating hypothermia. In Wilkerson JA et al, editors: *Hypothermia, frostbite and other cold injuries,* Seattle, 1986, The Mountaineers.
6. Baumgartner FJ et al: Cardiopulmonary bypass for resuscitation of patients with accidental hypothermia and cardiac arrest, *Can J Surg* 35:184, 1992.
7. Bjornstad H, Tande PM, Refsum H: Cardiac electrophysiology during hypothermia: implications for medical treatment, *Arctic Med Res* 50(suppl 6):71, 1991.
8. Bleyer B: On the water; cold water boating can turn deadly, *Newsday,* January 5, 1997.
9. Bolte RG et al: The use of extracorporeal rewarming in a child submerged for 66 minutes, *JAMA* 260:377, 1988.
10. Bristow GK, Giesbrecht GG: Contribution of exercise and shivering to recovery from induced hypothermia (31.2 degrees C.) in one subject, *Aviat Space Environ Med* 59:549, 1988.
11. Bristow GK, Sessler DI, Giesbrecht GG: Leg temperature and heat content in humans during immersion hypothermia and rewarming, *Aviat Space Environ Med* 65:220, 1994.
12. Brooks CJ: Personal communication, 1999.
13. Burton AC: *Man in a cold environment,* London, 1955, Edward Arnold Ltd.
14. Busto R et al: Small differences in intra-ischemic brain temperature critically determine the extent of ischemic neuronal injury, *J Cereb Blood Flow Metab* 7:729, 1987.
15. Busto R et al: Effect of mild hypothermia on ischemia-induced release of neurotransmitters and free fatty acids in rat brain, *Stroke* 20:904, 1989.
16. Carlson LD et al: Immersion in cold water and body tissue insulation, *Aerospace Med* 29:145, 1958.
17. Choi S et al: Thermal balance of man in water: prediction of deep body temperature change, *Appl Human Sci* 15:161, 1996.
18. Collins KJ, Easton JC, Exton-Smith AN: Body temperature afterdrop: a physical or physiological phenomenon? *J Physiol (Lond)* 328:72P, 1982.
19. Collis ML, Steinman AM, Chaney RD: Accidental hypothermia: an experimental study of practical rewarming methods, *Aviat Space Environ Med* 48:625-632, 1977.
20. Conn AW et al: A canine study of cold water drowning in fresh versus salt water, *Crit Care Med* 23:2029, 1995.
21. Cooper KE, Maring S, Riben P: Respiratory and other responses in subjects immersed in cold water, *J Appl Physiol* 40:903, 1976.
22. Cotter JD, Taylor NA: Physiological assessment of the RNZAF constant wear immersion suit: laboratory and field trials, *Aviat Space Environ Med* 66:528, 1995.
23. Covino BG: Pharmacology of local anesthetic agents, *Br J Anaesth* 58:701, 1986.
24. Cupples WA, Fox GR, Hayward JS: Effect of cold water immersion and its combination with alcohol intoxication on urine flow rate of man, *Can J Physiol Pharm* 58:319, 1980.
25. Danzl DF et al: Multicenter hypothermia survey, *Ann Emerg Med* 16:1042, 1987.
26. Danzl DF, Pozos RS, Hamlet MP: Accidental hypothermia. In Auerbach PS, editor: *Wilderness medicine: management of wilderness and environmental emergencies,* ed 3, St Louis, 1995, Mosby.
27. Danzl DF, Pozos RS: Accidental hypothermia, *N Engl J Med* 33:1756, 1994.
28. Dietrich WD et al: The importance of brain temperature in alterations of the blood-brain barrier following cerebral ischemia, *J Neuropathol Exp Neurol* 49:486, 1990.
29. Dillon P: *Lost at sea: an American tragedy,* New York, 1998, The Dial Press.
30. Ducharme MB, Tikuisis P: Role of blood as heat source or sink in human limbs during local cooling and heating, *J Appl Physiol* 76:2084, 1994.
31. Ducharme MB et al: Forced-air rewarming in -20 degrees C. simulated field conditions, *Ann NY Acad Sci* 813:676, 1997.
32. Ducharme MB et al: The effect of wave motion on dry suit insulation and the responses to cold water immersion, *Aviat Space Environ Med* 69:957, 1998.
33. Dzugan J: Alaska Marine Safety Education Association (AMSEA), personal communication, 1999.
34. Edmonds C, Lowry C, Pennefather J: Cold and hypothermia. In *Diving and subaquatic medicine,* Oxford, UK, 1992, Butterworth-Heinemann.
35. Ereth MH, Lennon RL, Sessler DI: Limited heat transfer between thermal compartments during rewarming in vasoconstricted patients, *Aviat Space Environ Med* 63:1065, 1992.
36. Eyolfson D et al: Measurement and prediction of maximal shivering capacity in humans. In Hodgdon J, Heaney JH, Buono MJ, editors: *Environmental Ergonomics VII: International Series on Environmental Ergonomics,* vol 1, San Diego, 1999, NHRC.

37. Fellows IW, MacDonald IA, Bennett T: The influence of environmental temperature upon the thermoregulatory responses to ethanol in man, *Clin Sci* 66:733, 1984.
38. Ferretti G: Cold and muscle performance, *Int J Sports Med* 13:S185, 1992.
39. Forgey WW: *The basic essentials of hypothermia,* Merrillville, Ind, 1991, ICS Books.
40. Fox GR, Hayward JS, Hobson GN: Effect of alcohol on thermal balance of man in cold water, *Can J Physiol Pharmacol* 57:860, 1979.
41. Fox JB et al: A retrospective analysis of air-evacuated hypothermia patients, *Aviat Space Environ Med* 59:1070, 1988.
42. Franks CM et al: The effect of blood alcohol on the initial responses to cold water immersion in humans, *Eur J Appl Physiol* 75:279, 1997.
43. Giesbrecht GG: Cold stress, near drowning and accidental hypothermia: a review, *Aviat Space Environ Med* 71:733, 2000.
44. Giesbrecht GG, Bristow GK: A second postcooling afterdrop: more evidence for a convective mechanism, *J Appl Physiol* 73:1253, 1992.
45. Giesbrecht GG, Bristow GK: Decrement in manual arm performance during whole body cooling, *Aviat Space Environ Med* 63:1077, 1992.
46. Giesbrecht GG, Bristow GK: Influence of body composition on rewarming from immersion hypothermia, *Aviat Space Environ Med* 66:1144, 1995.
47. Giesbrecht GG, Bristow GK: Recent advances in hypothermia research. In Blatteis CM, Blatteis CM, editors: Thermoregulation: Tenth International Symposium on the Pharmacology of Thermoregulation, New York, *Ann NY Acad Sci* 813:663, 1997.
48. Giesbrecht GG, Bristow GK: The convective afterdrop component during hypothermic exercise decreases with delayed exercise onset, *Aviat Space Environ Med* 69:17, 1998.
49. Giesbrecht GG, Pachu P, Xu X: Design and evaluation of a portable rigid forced-air warming cover for prehospital transport of cold patients, *Aviat Space Environ Med* 69:1200, 1998.
50. Giesbrecht GG, Schroeder M, Bristow GK: Treatment of mild immersion hypothermia by forced-air warming, *Aviat Space Environ Med* 65:803, 1994.
51. Giesbrecht GG et al: Effectiveness of three field treatments for induced mild (33.0 degrees C.) hypothermia, *J Appl Physiol* 63:2375, 1987.
52. Giesbrecht GG et al: Treatment of mild immersion hypothermia by direct body-to-body contact, *J Appl Physiol* 76:2373, 1994.
53. Giesbrecht GG et al: Isolated effects of peripheral arm and central body cooling on arm performance, *Aviat Space Environ Med* 66:968, 1995.
54. Giesbrecht GG et al: Inhibition of shivering increases core temperature afterdrop and attenuates rewarming in hypothermic humans, *J Appl Physiol* 83:1630, 1997.
55. Ginsberg MD et al: Temperature modulation of ischemic brain injury—a synthesis of recent advances, *Prog Brain Res* 96:13, 1993.
56. Girton TR, Wehr SE: *An evaluation of the rough-water performance characteristics of personal flotation devices (life-jackets),* USCG Rep No. USCG-M-84-1 (16714), Springfield, Va, 1984, National Technical Information Service.
57. Globus MY et al: Detection of free radical activity during transient global ischemia and recirculation: effects of intra-ischemic brain temperature modulation, *J Neurochem* 65:1250, 1995.
58. Goheen MSL et al: Efficacy of forced-air and inhalation rewarming by using a human model for severe hypothermia, *J Appl Physiol* 83:1635, 1997.
59. Golden FSC: Death after rescue from immersion in cold water, *J R Nav Med Serv* 59:5, 1973.
60. Golden FSC: Problems of immersion, *Br J Hosp Med* 45:371, 1980.
61. Golden FSC: Mechanisms of body cooling in submersed victims, *Resuscitation* 35:107, 1997.
62. Golden FSC, Hardcastle PT: Swimming failure in cold water, *J Physiol (Lond)* 330:60P-61P, 1982.
63. Golden GSC, Hervey GR: The mechanism of the after-drop following immersion hypothermia in pigs, *J Physiol (Lond)* 272:26, 1977.
64. Golden FSC, Hervey GR, Tipton MJ: Circum-rescue collapse: collapse, sometimes fatal, associated with rescue of immersion victims, *J R Nav Med Serv* 77:139, 1991.
65. Golden FSC, Tipton MJ, Scott RC: Immersion, near-drowning and drowning, *Br J Anesth* 79:1, 1997.
66. Golden FSC et al: Hyperventilation and swim failure in man in cold water, *J Physiol (Lond)* 378:94P, 1986.
67. Government Accounting Office: *Army Ranger training: safety improvements need to be institutionalized,* Letter Report GAO/NSIAD-97-29, January 2, 1997.
68. Graham T et al: Effect of alcohol ingestion on man's thermoregulatory responses during cold immersion, *Aviat Space Environ Med* 51:155, 1980.
69. Hackett P et al: *State of Alaska hypothermia and near-drowning guidelines,* Alaska Dept of Health and Human Services, EMS Section, Juneau, Alaska, 1989.

70. Haight JSJ, Keatinge WR: Failure of thermoregulation in the cold during hypoglycemia induced by exercise and ethanol, *J Physiol* 229:87, 1973.

71. Hamilton, RS, Paton BC: The diagnosis and treatment of hypothermia by mountain rescue teams: a survey, *Annual Meeting of Wilderness Medical Society*, 1:28, 1996.

72. Harnett RM et al: Initial treatment of profound accidental hypothermia, *Aviat Space Environ Med* 51:680, 1980.

73. Hayes PA et al: *Reactions to cold water immersion with and without waves*, Farnborough, UK, RAF Institute of Aviation Medicine, RAF IAM Report No 645, 1985.

74. Hayward JS: The physiology of immersion hypothermia. In Pozos RS, Wittmers LE, editors: *The nature and treatment of hypothermia*, Minneapolis, 1983, University of Minnesota Press.

75. Hayward JS: Thermal protection performance of survival suits in ice-water, *Aviat Space Environ Med* 55:212, 1984.

76. Hayward JS: Immersion hypothermia. In Wilkerson JA et al, editors: *Hypothermia, frostbite and other cold injuries*, Seattle, 1986, The Mountaineers.

77. Hayward JS: Personal communication, 1999.

78. Hayward JS, Collis ML, Eckerson JD: Thermographic evaluation of relative heat loss areas of man during cold water immersion, *Aviat Space Environ Med* 44:377, 1977.

79. Hayward JS, Eckerson JD, Collis ML: Effect of behavioral variables on cooling rate of man in cold water, *J Appl Physiol* 38:1073, 1975.

80. Hayward JS, Eckerson JD, Kemma D: Thermal and cardiovascular changes during three methods of resuscitation from mild hypothermia, *Resuscitation* 11:21, 1984.

81. Hayward JS et al: Design concepts of survival suits for cold-water immersion and their thermal protection performance, *Proceedings of the 17th Symposium of the SAFE Association*, Van Nuys, Calif, 1980.

82. Hayward JS et al: Temperature effect on the human dive response in relation to cold-water near-drowning, *J Appl Physiol* 56:202, 1984.

83. Holmer I: Prediction of responses to cold, *Arctic Med Res* 54:48, 1995.

84. Hughes JH, Henry RE, Daly MJ: Influence of ethanol and ambient temperature on skin blood flow, *Ann Emerg Med* 13:597, 1984.

85. Hultzer M et al: Efficacy of torso rewarming using a human model for severe hypothermia, *Proceedings of the World Congress on Wilderness Medicine* 80, 1999 (abstract).

86. Johnston CE et al: Alcohol lowers the vasoconstriction threshold in humans without affecting core cooling rate during mild cold exposure, *Eur J Appl Physiol* 74:293, 1996.

87. Johnston CE et al: Eucapneic hypoxia lowers human cold thermoregulatory response thresholds and accelerates core cooling, *J Appl Physiol* 80:422, 1996.

88. Johnston CE et al: Hypercapnia lowers the shivering threshold and increases core cooling rate in humans, *Aviat Space Environ Med* 67:438, 1996.

89. Junger S: *The Perfect storm: a true story of men against the sea*, New York, 1997, WW Norton & Co.

90. Kalant H, Le AD: Effects of ethanol on thermoregulation, *Pharmacol Ther* 23:313, 1984.

91. Katsura K et al: Changes of labile metabolites during anoxia in moderately hypo- and hyperthermic rats: correlation to membrane fluxes of potassium, *Brain Res* 590:6, 1992.

92. Kaufman JW, Dejneka K: *Cold water evaluation of constant wear anti-exposure suit systems*, Rep No NADC-85092-60, Naval Air Development Center, Warminster, Penn, 1985.

93. Kaufman JW et al: Insidious hypothermia during raft use, *Aviat Space Environ Med* 61:569, 1990.

94. Keatinge WR: Death after shipwreck, *Lancet* 2:1537, 1965.

95. Keatinge WR: *Survival in cold water*, Oxford, UK, 1969, Blackwell Press.

96. Keatinge WR, McIlroy MB, Goldfien A: Cardiovascular responses to ice-cold showers, *J Appl Physiol* 19:1145, 1964.

97. Keatinge WR et al: Sudden failure of swimming in cold water, *Br Med J* 1:480, 1969.

98. Kurz A et al: Forced-air warming maintains intra-operative normothermia better than circulating-water in infants and children, *Anesth Analg* 77:89, 1993.

99. LeBlanc J: Subcutaneous fat and skin temperature, *Can J Biochem Physiol* 32:354, 1954.

100. Light IM et al: Immersion suit insulation: the effect of dampening on survival estimates, *Aviat Space Environ Med* 58:964, 1987.

101. Livingstone SD et al: The effect of alcohol on body heat loss, *Aviat Space Environ Med* 51:961, 1980.

102. Lloyd EL: Accidental hypothermia, *Resuscitation* 32:111, 1996.

103. Lun V et al: Effects of prolonged CO_2 inhalation on shivering thermogenesis during cold-water immersion, *Undersea Hyperb Med* 20:215, 1993.

104. Marino F, Booth J: Whole body cooling by immersion in water at moderate temperatures, *J Sci Med Sport* 1:73, 1998.

105. Marion DW et al: Resuscitative hypothermia, *Crit Care Med* 24:S81, 1996.

106. *Maritime Casualty Report, Mobile Offshore Drilling Unit (MODU) Ocean Ranger: Capsizing and sinking in the Atlantic Ocean on 15 Feb 1982 with loss of life*, USCG 001 HQS 82, Springfield, Va, 1983, National Technical Information Service.

107. Markle RL: *A study of lifesaving systems for small passenger vessels*, US Coast Guard, Commandant (G-MSE-4), March 1991.

108. Martin S, Diewold RJ, Cooper DE: Alcohol, respiratory, skin and body temperature changes during cold water immersion, *J Appl Physiol* 43:322, 1977.

109. McCance RA et al: The hazards to men in ships lost at sea, 1940-44, *Med Res Council Spec Rep Series* 1, 1956.

110. Mekjavic IB et al: Nitrogen narcosis attenuates shivering thermogenesis, *J Appl Physiol* 78:2241, 1995.

111. Mekjavic IB et al: Respiratory drive during sudden cold water immersion, *Respir Physiol* 70:21, 1987.

112. Mersey, Lord (Wreck Commissioner): *Report of a formal investigation into the circumstances attending the foundering on 15th April 1912 of the British Steamship 'Titanic' of Liverpool after striking ice in or near latitude 41 deg 46' N, longitude 50 deg 14' north Atlantic Ocean, whereby loss of life ensued*, London, 1912, His Majesty's Stationery Office.

113. Michenfelder JD, Milde JH: The relationship among canine brain temperature, metabolism, and function during hypothermia, *Anesthesiology* 75:130, 1991.

114. Miller JW, Danzl DF, Thomas DM: Urban accidental hypothermia: 135 cases, *Ann Emerg Med* 9:456, 1980.

115. Mills WJ: Field care of the hypothermic patient, *Int J Sports Med* 13:S199, 1992.

116. Minamisawa H et al: The influence of mild body and brain hypothermia on ischemic brain damage, *J Cereb Blood Flow Metab* 10:365, 1990.

117. Molnar GW: Survival of hypothermia by men immersed in the ocean, *JAMA* 131:1046, 1946.

118. Nadel ER: Energy exchanges in water, *Undersea Biomed Res* 11:149, 1984.

119. National Center for Environmental Prediction, Space Science and Engineering Center, Madison, Wisc, 1999, University of Wisconsin, http://www.ssec.wisc.edu/data/sst/latest_sst.gif.

120. Nemiroff MJ: Personal communication, 1999.

121. Nemiroff MJ: Near-drowning, *Resp Care* 37:600, 1992.

122. Niazi SA, Lewis EJ: Profound hypothermia in the dog, *Surg Gynecol Obstet* 102:98, 1956.

123. Nunneley SA, Wissler EH, Allan JR: Immersion cooling: effect of clothing and skinfold thickness, *Aviat Space Environ Med* 56:1177, 1985.

124. Oakes L: Lone survivor relates ordeal on Mille Lacs, *Minneapolis Star Tribune*, October 7, 1997.

125. Oksa J, Rintamaki H, Makinen T: Cooling alters force-velocity relationship of upper body and arms, *International Conference on Human-Environmental Systems* 587, 1991.

126. Oksa J et al: Gross efficiency of muscular work during step exercise at -15 degrees C and 21 degrees C, *Acta Physiol Scand* 147:235, 1993.

127. Osborne L, Kamal El Din AS, Smith JE: Survival after prolonged cardiac arrest and accidental hypothermia, *Br Med J Clin Res Ed* 289:881, 1984.

128. Parkinson D: Carotid cavernous fistula: direct repair with preservation of the carotid artery, *J Neurosurg* 38:99, 1973.

129. Passias TC, Mekjavic IB, Eiken O: The effect of 30% nitrous oxide on thermoregulatory responses in humans during hypothermia, *Anesthesiology* 76:550, 1992.

130. Pozos RS et al: *Rewarming methodologies in the field*, Naval Health Research Center Rep No NHRC-93-4, Springfield, Va, 1993, National Technical Information Service.

131. Ramey CA, Ramey DN, Hayward JS: The dive response of children in relation to cold water near-drowning, *J Appl Physiol* 63:665, 1987.

132. Roberts DE et al: Fluid replacement during hypothermia, *Aviat Space Environ Med* 56:333, 1985.

133. Romet TT: Mechanism of afterdrop after cold water immersion, *J Appl Physiol* 65:1535, 1988.

134. Romet TT et al: Immersed clo insulation in marine work suits using human and thermal manikin data, *Aviat Space Environ Med* 62:739, 1991.

135. Roythorne C: Cold in North Sea operations. In Adam JA, editor: *Hypothermia ashore and afloat*, Aberdeen, Md, University Press, 1981.

136. Ryack BL, Luria SM, Smith PF: Surviving helicopter crashes at sea: a review of studies of underwater egress from helicopters, *Aviat Space Environ Med* 57:603, 1986.

137. Sagawa S et al: Water temperature and intensity of exercise in maintenance of thermal equilibrium, *J Appl Physiol* 65:2413, 1988.

138. Sano T et al: A comparison of the cerebral protective effects of isoflurane and mild hypothermia in a model of incomplete forebrain ischemia in the rat, *Anesthesiology* 76:221, 1992.

139. Savard GK et al: Peripheral blood flow during rewarming from mild hypothermia in humans, *J Appl Physiol* 58:4, 1985.

140. Sessler DI, Moayeri A: Skin-surface warming: heat flux and central temperature, *Anesthesiology* 73:218, 1990.

141. Shender BS et al: Cold water immersion simulations using the Wissler Texas Thermal Model: validation and sensitivity analysis, *Aviat Space Environ Med* 66:678, 1995.

142. Siple PA, Passel CF: Measurements of dry atmospheric cooling in subfreezing temperatures, *Proc Am Phil Soc* 89:177, 1945.

143. Standards and guidelines for cardiopulmonary resuscitation and emergency cardiac care, *JAMA* 268:2172, 1992.

144. Steele MT et al: Forced air speeds rewarming in accidental hypothermia, *Ann Emerg Med* 27:479, 1996.

145. Steinman AM: A few thoughts on water survival, *On-Scene National Maritime Search & Rescue Review* 2:12, 1984.

146. Steinman AM: A few more thoughts on water survival, *On-Scene National Maritime Search & Rescue Review* 3:14, 1984.

147. Steinman AM: Cardiopulmonary resuscitation and hypothermia, *Circulation* 74:29, 1986.

148. Steinman AM: Prehospital management of hypothermia: rescue, examine, insulate and transport, *J Emerg Med Serv* 1987.

149. Steinman AM, Kubilis P: *Survival at sea: the effects of protective clothing and survivor location on core and skin temperature,* USCG Rep No. CG-D-26-86, Springfield, Va, 1986, National Technical Information Service.

150. Steinman AM et al: Immersion hypothermia: comparative protection of anti-exposure garments in calm vs rough seas, *Aviat Space Environ Med* 58:550, 1987.

151. Sterba JA: Efficacy and safety of prehospital rewarming techniques to treat accidental hypothermia, *Ann Emerg Med* 20:896, 1991.

152. Stoneham MD, Squires SJ: Prolonged resuscitation in acute deep hypothermia, *Anaesthesia* 47:784, 1992.

153. Tikuisis P: Predicting survival time for cold exposure, *Int J Biometeorol* 39:94, 1995.

154. Tikuisis P: Predicting survival time at sea based on observed body cooling rates, *Aviat Space Environ Med* 68:441, 1997.

155. Tikuisis P, Frim J: *Prediction of survival time in cold air,* DCIEM Report No. 94-29, Department of National Defence, North York, Ontario, Canada, 1994.

156. Tipton MJ: The initial responses to cold-water immersion in man, *Clin Sci* 77:581, 1989.

157. Tipton MJ: Laboratory-based evaluation of the protection provided against cold water by two helicopter passenger suits, *J Soc Occup Med* 41:161, 1991.

158. Tipton MJ: The relationship between maximum breath hold time in air and the ventilatory responses to immersion in cold water, *Eur J Appl Physiol* 64:426, 1992.

159. Tipton MJ: The concept of an integrated survival system: for protection against the responses associated with immersion in cold water, *J R Nav Med* 79:11, 1993.

160. Tipton MJ: Debating point—immersion fatalities: hazardous responses and dangerous discrepancies, *J R Nav Med Serv* 81:101, 1995.

161. Tipton MJ, Eglin CM, Golden FSC: Habituation of the initial responses to cold water immersion in humans: a central or peripheral mechanism? *J Physiol (Lond)* 512:621, 1998.

162. Tipton MJ, Stubbs DA, Elliott DH: The effect of clothing on the initial responses to cold water immersion in man, *J R Nav Med Serv* 76:89, 1990.

163. Tipton MJ, Stubbs DA, Elliott DH: Human initial responses to immersion in cold water at three temperatures and after hyperventilation, *J Appl Physiol* 70:317, 1991.

164. Tipton MJ, Vincent MJ: Protection provided against the initial responses to cold immersion by a partial coverage wet suit, *Aviat Space Environ Med* 60:769, 1989.

165. Tipton MJ et al: The influence of regional insulation on the initial responses to cold immersion, *Aviat Space Environ Med* 58:1192, 1988.

166. Tipton MJ et al: The effect of water leakage on the results obtained from human and thermal manikin tests of immersion protective clothing, *Eur J Appl Physiol* 72:394, 1996.

167. Todd MM, Warner DS: A comfortable hypothesis reevaluated: cerebral metabolic depression and brain protection during ischemia, *Anesthesiology* 76:161, 1992.

168. US Coast Guard: *A pocket guide to cold-water survival,* Commandant Instruction M3131.6, Washington, DC, 1991, US Government Printing Office.

169. US Coast Guard: *Addendum to the National Search and Rescue (SAR) Manual,* COMDTINST M16120.5 and COMDTINST M16120.6, 1995.

170. US Coast Guard: *Commandant (G-NRS) data,* 1999.

171. US Coast Guard:*Living to fish, dying to fish: fishing vessel casualty task force report,* March 1999.

172. US Coast Guard: *Recreational boating accident statistics for 1997,* Commandant (G-MSE-4), 1999.

173. Vanggaard L: Physiological reactions to wet-cold, *Aviat Space Environ Med* 46:33, 1975.

174. Vanggaard L: *Laegebog for Sofarende (authorized ship captain's guide),* Copenhagen, 1987, Tellus.

175. Vanggaard L, Gjerloff CC: A new simple technique of rewarming in hypothermia, *Inter Rev Army Navy Air Force Med Serv* 52:427, 1979.

176. Vanggaard L et al: Immersion of distal arms and legs in warm water (AVA Rewarming) effectively rewarms hypothermic humans, *Aviat Space Environ Med* 70:1081, 1999.

177. Vincent MJ, Tipton MJ: The effects of cold immersion and hand protection on grip strength, *Aviat Space Environ Med* 59:738, 1988.

178. Walpoth BH et al: Outcome of survivors of accidental deep hypothermia and circulatory arrest treated with extracorporeal blood warming, *N Engl J Med* 337:1500, 1997.

179. Webb P: Afterdrop of body temperature during rewarming: an alternative explanation, *J Appl Physiol* 60:385, 1986.

180. Weinberg AD: The role of inhalation rewarming in the early management of hypothermia, *Resuscitation* 36:101, 1998.

181. Weinberg AD et al: *Cold weather emergencies: principles of patient management,* Branford, Conn, 1990, American.

182. Werner J, Webb P: A six-cylinder model of human thermoregulation for general use on personal computers, *Ann Physiol Anthrop* 12:123, 1993.

183. White GR et al: Cold water survival suits for aircrew, *Aviat Space Environ Med* 50:1040, 1979.

184. White MD, LeBlanc J: Paradoxical absence of shivering in obese humans, *Thermal Physiol* 1993:143, 1993.

185. Wilkerson J, Zigler S, Wilkerson E: Heat transfer by heated aerosols. In Bangs C, editor: *First Annual International Forum: Critical Decisions in Hypothermia,* Portland, Ore, 1992.

186. Wissler EH: Mathematical simulation of human thermal behavior using whole body models. In Shitzer A, Eberhart RC: *Heat transfer in medicine and biology,* New York, 1985, Plenum Press.

187. Wolff AH et al: Heat exchanges in wet suits, *J Appl Physiol* 58:770, 1985.

188. Xiao F, Safar P, Radovsky A: Mild protective and resuscitative hypothermia for asphyxial cardiac arrest in rats, *Am J Emerg Med* 16:17, 1998.

189. Xu X, Tikuisis P: A mathematical model for human brain cooling during cold water near-drowning, *J Appl Physiol* 86:265, 1999.

190. Xu X, Werner J: A dynamic model of the human/clothing/environment system, *Appl Human Sci* 16:61, 1997.

9 Polar Medicine

Betty Carlisle and Bern Shen

Like much of wilderness medicine, polar medicine's identity derives to a large extent from its setting. "Polar," however, can be defined in several different ways.[33] Geographically, the Arctic and Antarctic circles, at latitudes 66°33' north and south, delimit areas in which the sun does not rise or set on at least 1 day of the year. A more functional definition is the 10° isotherm, which joins those areas in which the average temperature in the warmest month of the year is 10° C (50° F); this correlates roughly with the tree line. Still other definitions or subdivisions are based on the extent of permafrost, tundra, or sea ice.

For medical purposes, the definition of "polar" is more complex. Although climate and geography are clearly important, the salient features of polar medicine are logistic and experiential. Unlike high-altitude medicine or hyperbaric medicine, for example, polar medicine is not unified by an underlying pathophysiology. Although fields such as the former are medicine *because of* the environment's effect on the human organism, polar medicine is largely medical practice *within* the setting.

Medical practice in spite of isolated settings is paradigmatic of wilderness medicine; the patient population is essentially if not literally a small demographic island. A provisional definition of polar medicine, then, could be formulated as "the practice of medicine in isolated settings"; to borrow an anthropologic term describing isolated "island" communities, it could be called Fourth World medicine.[56,120,165]

DISTINCTION BETWEEN ARCTIC AND ANTARCTIC MEDICINE

Although the Polar Regions share the predominant attributes of cold and isolation, they display many important contrasts. The Arctic has been described as a sea nearly surrounded by land, whereas Antarctica is a land and ice mass circumscribed by ocean. The moderating effect of the North Polar waters compared with the elevation (2835 m [9302 feet]) of the South Polar plateau accounts for the roughly 40° C (72° F) differences in wintertime low temperatures. On a plot of temperature vs. humidity, the South Pole is more similar to Mars than to the rest of the earth.

Such environmental contrasts are reflected in population density and diversity of flora and fauna. In contrast to the Arctic's boreal forest, tundra, and growing population of over 2 million, Antarctica is a high, dry, icy desert continent with almost nonexistent flora and fauna, no indigenous population, and transient influxes of a few thousand people each summer and merely a few hundred in winter.

The differences in population patterns mark an important north-south disjunction in polar studies in general,[44] and in polar medicine in particular.[187] There are actually two overlapping but distinct spectra of medical problems—those of indigenous Arctic people and those of visitors to either polar region. As we shall see, many of the medical problems among the Inuit, Sami, Chukchi, Nenet, and other northern groups are those of populations making the often Faustian demographic and cultural transition to a Western industrialized society. Thus medical practice among these groups is similar to that among many other displaced aboriginal populations.

In contrast, medical problems among the usually young and fit scientific, commercial, tourist, or expedition personnel are often related to trauma and the environment and thus fall more appropriately under the purview of travel or expedition medicine. In a sense, the current illnesses and health risks of the indigenous Arctic populations are the result of too much contact with other cultures, whereas those of the sojourners to either polar region are largely the result of too little connection with the culture and medical facilities of home.

The indigenous vs. sojourner or essentially north-south disjunction in polar medicine poses a challenge to a meaningful synthesis. In the spirit of a trend in travel medicine,[72] I recognize that it makes sense to focus not only on the health of elite visitors to remote areas but also on the health problems surrounding and sometimes even caused by them.

A rigorous discussion of health risks, practices, and outcomes ultimately depends on much finer resolution of local climate, culture, and occupational conditions. Even among the remarkably consistent linguistic cultures of the Arctic, there are clearly confounding variables in trying to metaanalyze, for example, health studies among reindeer herders in an isolated Sami village in northern Finland, Inuit apartment block dwellers in Nuuk, Greenland, and Alaskan pipeline workers on the North Slope. Likewise, in the Antarctic there are important differences among the living conditions and health determinants of a marine biologist on the Antarctic Peninsula, a geologist in the Dry Valleys, and a power plant mechanic at the South Pole Station.

IMPORTANCE OF POLAR MEDICINE

Increase in Tourism and Expeditions

The combined geographic polar regions cover about one sixth of the world's surface,[158] and their territory in the imagination has been enlarged by several remarkable expeditions and recent popular magazine articles and books.* Despite, or perhaps because of, the forbidding environment, tourism of various sorts to polar regions is increasing.[13,89,109,177] Junkets "to the North Pole" are popular, despite being costly. Antarctica has become a trendy destination for adventure seekers. Even though no permanent settlement is there, roughly 100,000 tourists a year visit Nordkapp on the tip of Norway.[107] At the other end of the globe, in 1980 it was estimated that 31,000 paying tourists, adventurers, or guests of national scientific expeditions had visited Antarctica.[133] More recently, the number of tourists has increased 33% per year since 1990-1991, when roughly 3200 tourists a year visited "the Ice." In 1998, there were 11,200 tourist visits, not including researchers and support personnel. Even further increases are anticipated in the new millennium.[10] Commercial tourists have even been brought to the South Pole, including one ill-fated sky diving venture with the death of three of the four participants.

Geopolitical Concerns

The interest of governments in polar regions has not lagged behind that of tourists.[57,63,80,176,192] Political and territorial concerns have been important in both polar regions; with increasing exploration of mineral and oil reserves[86] and fishing potential, migrating humans will bring medical problems with them. Although the Antarctic Treaty of 1959 prohibits territorial or commercial claims, a number of nations have made sectoral claims on the continent. Some countries encourage couples to give birth to a child during their tour in Antarctica and thus claim true Antarctic "citizens."[180] Concern about the environmental impact of increasing human activity in polar regions† seems to be tempering the pace of development, but it appears likely that the pool of potential civilian and military patients in polar regions will increase.[170]

Increasing Research Activities

Scientific research has been a part of polar exploration throughout this century.‡ There are scientific and medical journals devoted to the polar regions, and thousands of articles are indexed each year in the Antarctic Bibliography alone.[64] A 45,000-square-foot science facility has been completed at McMurdo,[55] and the re-

placement of the current South Pole Station is expected to be completed by the year 2005.[121] The Australian Stations have completed expansion and updating of research and medical facilities.[94] The Australian program also requires that the physicians undergo rigorous training before deployment.

Here as well, some observers have discerned a north-south split, perceiving research in Antarctica as having more of a political motivation, and that in the Arctic as more practical in orientation.[41] For both scientific and political reasons, an important part of the scientific research in polar regions concerns environmental issues.[30,79] The remoteness of these regions enhances their value as a benchmark for studies of pollution. Studies have revealed several worrisome facts about the contamination of the formerly pristine wilderness, such as the prolonged effective half-life of radioactive fallout deposits[171] and the increased chemical contamination, particularly in animals high on the food chain, with persistent organic compounds (POCs), heavy metals, and other contaminants.[4,30,61,171] As occupational and environmental health issues draw more attention in the next few years, this aspect of polar medicine will assume greater importance.

Interest in Analogies to Space Missions

Several articles and conferences have explored analogies between isolated and confined environments of polar research stations and space stations.* Data from polar (primarily Antarctic) stations tend to be more available and recent than from other space station analogs, such as nuclear submarines.[181] International cooperation in polar health care and human research is coordinated by the Scientific Committee on Antarctic Research (SCAR).[94] It is just a matter of time before long-distance human spaceflight begins, so polar studies may give planners more information of relevance to these future space missions.[117]

BRIEF HISTORY OF HUMAN HABITATION IN POLAR REGIONS

A perspective on the contrasts between Arctic and Antarctic medicine may be sharpened by review of an extremely brief summary of human habitation in the polar areas.

Humans are known to have inhabited Arctic regions for at least 4500 years. Anthropologists have uncovered evidence for several waves of population migration from Siberia through northern Canada to Greenland. Each of these migrations was probably linked to climatic conditions, and each resulted in a distinct set of cultures. The general pattern was of a nomadic life with population

---

*References 9, 84, 90, 101, 109, 127, 130, 158.
†References 13, 60, 103, 113, 116, 177.
‡References 6-8, 44, 155, 157, 178.

*References 59, 76, 94, 118, 162, 182.

densities of approximately 1 person per 400 km²[2,73,164] In more recent times, this long-established and remarkable adaptation to a hostile environment has been disturbed. The pace of cultural change increased dramatically during the second half of the nineteenth century, when the whaling industry moved into Hudson Bay, leading to sustained contact between Europeans and Inuit. In the early part of the twentieth century, religious missions, trading company posts, government stations, and eventually medical clinics and schools began to encourage permanent settlements, roughly quadrupling the population density.[73] This change in population distribution and the contact, and sometimes conflict, between the indigenous and European cultures had medical consequences.

In contrast to the Arctic, the known history of human exploration of the Antarctic is quite recent. Recorded sightings of the continent date only to around 1800, and "winter-over" sojourns did not occur for another century. One can also construct waves of settlement in Antarctica: sealing in the early nineteenth century, whaling in the early twentieth, and scientific since the mid-twentieth.[164] The heroic era of Antarctic exploration occupied the early years of the twentieth century, with exploits such as the highly publicized race for the South Pole between Roald Amundsen and Robert Scott in 1911, and the extraordinary survival of the crew of the 1914 *Endurance* expedition, led by Ernest Shackleton.[84] Perhaps because of these and other dramatic events, and perhaps because of the absence of an indigenous population and the scarcity of easily exploited resources, human activities in the Antarctic have retained a somewhat more expeditionary flavor than in the Arctic. This has helped shape the contrasts in medical practice between North and South Polar Regions.

ARCTIC MEDICAL PROBLEMS

Somatic Health Problems

Effects of Cultural and Demographic Transition.
Medical problems among indigenous populations in the Arctic are characteristic of those of displaced aboriginal people elsewhere in the world. On the one hand, recent episodes, such as the 1987 trichinosis outbreak in Salluit,[96,97] the 1980 rabies outbreak in the Svalbard Islands,[131] and continued problems with diphyllobothriasis[31] and toxoplasmosis,[100] reflect diseases characteristic of nonindustrial lifestyles. On the other hand, increased contact with industrialized cultures has brought problems, as well as benefits. For many years, health care has lagged behind national norms, with infant mortality in the Canadian Arctic greater than 10%, life expectancy in 1970 only 60% of the national average, and widely prevalent tuberculosis, alcoholism, and tobacco use.[105,106,164,185] Despite dedicated individual efforts, catastrophes such as the 1948 outbreaks of influenza originating at Cambridge Bay,[71] the 1949 polio epidemic among Hudson Bay Inuit,[71,108] and widespread tooth decay and even malnutrition with the introduction of new foods[71,72] have demonstrated negative medical consequences of cultural contact.

As indigenous Arctic populations and their environment make the cultural and demographic transition to a Western industrialized way of life, the spectrum of medical problems has shifted. Even isolated mining villages in Greenland no longer exhibit traditional patterns of illness.[51] Changing social patterns have resulted in disturbing trends; more than half the births in Greenland in the 1970s were to unwed mothers,[143] and the prevalence of gonorrhea and syphilis among Greenlanders is one in three,[56] raising concerns about other transmissible diseases, such as viral hepatitis and acquired immunodeficiency syndrome (AIDS).[154]

Environmental and Occupational Health Problems.
A consequence of the transition to industrialized life is a change in environmental health risks.[3] Popular attention has been focused by such recent catastrophes as the Severomorsk submarine base explosion in May 1984 and the *Exxon Valdez* accident in Prince William Sound. The nuclear accident at Chernobyl in May 1986 led to cesium 134 and 137 levels in reindeer meat 50 to 100 times those considered safe, forcing destruction of the Sami reindeer herds. During that same time, lake fishing and berry picking were curtailed because of contamination.[56] Industrial emissions from neighboring regions, including an estimated 100 million tons of sulfur dioxide, have led to the phenomenon of the "Arctic haze," a gradual whitening of the historically deep blue Arctic sky.[56]

Environmental impacts have direct health consequences.[32,120,137] During the last 500 years, industrial pollution has led to a sevenfold increase in lead levels in human tissues in the Arctic.[56] Another survey found blood mercury levels above the normative limit in over 10% of Sami reindeer herders in northern Finland, an index of ocean contamination and concentration of heavy metals in fish.[95] Further contamination of the food chain with long-lasting POCs, including polychlorinated biphenyls (PCBs) and many organic pesticides, is increasingly identified. The long-term consequences of these environmental pollutants on the health of the Arctic dwellers is just recently being studied.[4]

Nontoxicologic factors also make important contributions to Arctic morbidity and mortality. It is striking that Alaska's occupational death rate is five times that of the U.S. national average of 7.6 deaths per 100,000 workers.[142] This reflects in part inherently hazardous working conditions and occupations[17] and possible demographic biases of a young population.[85,147] Other factors, however, may play a role. Recently, aircraft safety has attracted increasing attention.[29,147] Since aircraft are a predominant mode of transportation in polar regions, it is perhaps not surprising that Alaska accounted for almost one fourth of the fatal or serious commuter air crashes in the United States in a recent 5-year review.[142] Nonscheduled or commuter plane (less than 30 seats) flights commonly used in isolated areas may pose a six-fold risk of a fatal crash relative to scheduled airliner flights,[12,183] a figure not surprising given the often extremely challenging flying conditions (Figure 9-1).

Psychosocial Health Problems

With social disruption and increased environmental and occupational health risks, it comes as no surprise that psychologic problems in the Arctic have achieved higher visibility in recent years. For a variety of reasons, stress seems to be higher in winter[58]; seasonal affective disorder (SAD) is discussed below. One survey of over 7000 adults living north of the Arctic Circle found a prevalence of midwinter mental distress of 14% in men and 19% in women[58]; most other studies suggest that this figure may be low. Depression, suicidality, and domestic violence are prominent reasons for visits to the Baffin Consultation Service,[1,191] as well as for consultations in other communities.[38] Studies among scientific staff at research stations are relatively uncommon but show patterns of sleep disturbances, depression, and alcohol use reminiscent of those in Antarctic stations.[27]

The double apparent risk factors of high latitude and being a displaced aboriginal population have made alcohol abuse and concomitant violence a serious problem in the Arctic. In Greenland, one in three Inuit dies a violent death, and roughly 25,000 adults consume 28 million cans of beer a year, one of the highest per capita consumptions of alcohol in the world.[56] Accidents are the leading cause of death in Greenland, and one third of these are estimated to be alcohol related, as are most of the crimes and domestic violence.[143] Similarly, in the Canadian Arctic, alcohol consumption is one and a half times the national average, and Inuit and Indians between 15 and 24 years have a suicide rate six times the national average.[56]

Current and Future Trends

Fortunately, there are encouraging signs related to Arctic health care. The incidence of low birth weight, 5.5% in the central Canadian Arctic, is low compared with many other populations,[40] although it is higher than the non-Arctic dwellers.[4,144] Tuberculosis, which incapacitated up to 20% of the Canadian Inuit by 1950, has been largely brought under control.[73] Perhaps most surprisingly, the age-standardized prevalence of diagnosed diabetes among circumpolar indigenous populations in Russia, Alaska, and Canada is low compared with the U.S. all-race prevalence of 23.5 per 1000, and quite low compared with the presumably genetically similar North American Indian groups.[193]

An important development in recent years has been the institution of trauma registries to track and target significant causes of morbidity and mortality.[47] A recent excerpt from Alaska's trauma registry reports that the leading category of death was firearms related (32%), whereas that of injury was falls (19%).[75] Recent research has increasingly emphasized that injury prevention is not solely a function of safer design of equipment but a complex interplay of environment, activity, and people, notably including personal risk-taking behavior.[81] If current trends toward greater economic independence and education of Arctic peoples continue, such potentially modifiable health behaviors may recede in importance in coming years.

ANTARCTIC MEDICAL PROBLEMS

Medical practice, problems, and their study in the Antarctic are somewhat different from those in the Arctic. After a description of the U.S. medical stations in Antarctica, some highlights of health problems as a spectrum from primarily somatic to primarily psychologic are mentioned.

Medical Stations in Antarctica

The medical facilities in the Antarctic polar regions can be conveniently divided into permanent and expeditionary facilities. As a result of community expectations and the long-term commitment to research in Antarctica, a notable shift has occurred in many of the Antarctic programs, "from an expeditionary, to an operational attitude."[94,145] Although I describe facilities in the United States program, other nations have similar facilities. The United States maintains several small summer camps and three larger year-round stations: McMurdo

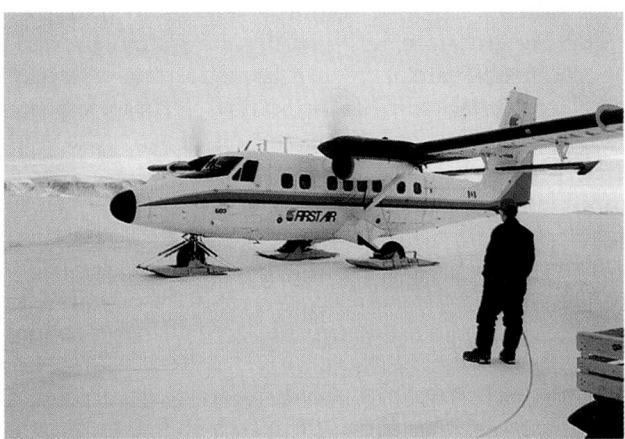

Figure 9-1 Polar air travel is fraught with the ever-present danger of a crash. Sudden and unpredictable weather changes, lack of navigational aids and extreme cold add to the extremely challenging flying conditions. *(Courtesy Stephen Warren.)*

(77°53'S, 166°40'E) on the Ross Ice Shelf, Palmer (64°46'S, 64°03'W) on the Antarctic Peninsula, and Amundsen-Scott (90°S) at the geographic South Pole. There are 40 other stations, mostly coastal, that are maintained by more than a dozen other countries.

McMurdo on Ross Island is the largest settlement and major staging area for U.S. Antarctic activities. The summer population is about 1500 and the winter population is about 200. Monthly mean temperatures vary from −3° C (26.6° F) in summer to −22° C (−7.6° F) in midwinter; cold weather limits aircraft operations and physically isolates McMurdo from late February to late August. The medical facilities consist of a well-equipped infirmary staffed during the summer by two physicians, a nurse practitioner, and several technicians. During the winter, staffing contracts to one physician, a nurse practitioner, and a technician. The vast majority of patient visits are for routine minor medical problems. The rare patient requiring medical evacuation can be flown to Christchurch, New Zealand, during the summer. Unfortunately, the logistically difficult winter evacuation has been required several times. These have primarily been for medical emergencies. The most recent occurred in 1999, when a participant at the South Pole was evacuated in the late spring because of cancer.

Palmer Station on Anvers Island in the Antarctic Peninsula has summer and winter populations of about 44 and 10, respectively. With monthly mean temperatures between −10° C and 2° C (14° F and 35.6° F), it is a popular Antarctic destination for cruise ships. Because of over a thousand visitors a year, there has been active debate regarding the proper role of station personnel in receiving commercial tourists.[145] This issue was highlighted during the 1992 season when a tourist suffered an apparent myocardial infarction and required evacuation. The infirmary has been recently reorganized to facilitate rapid access to emergency medications and equipment.[83]

In contrast to McMurdo and Palmer, Amundsen-Scott South Pole Station at 90°S is at an altitude of 2835 m (9302 feet) on the polar plateau and has monthly mean temperatures of −28° C (−18.4° F) in December and −60° C (−76° F) in July. Its summer and winter populations are roughly 120 and 25, respectively. However, with the recent building of a new station, the population has increased to 250 in summer and 45 in winter. One physician staffs the medical facility. It has a fairly well-stocked pharmacy, dental equipment, x-ray, darkroom, laboratory, bathtub for hypothermia, and a treatment/crash room that can be used for simple operations. In addition, there are two holding beds. Station personnel have undergone training in cardiopulmonary resuscitation and "trauma team" drills[21,35,67,146] (Figure 9-2). There have been recent cases of pulmonary edema and carbon monoxide poisoning, high-altitude

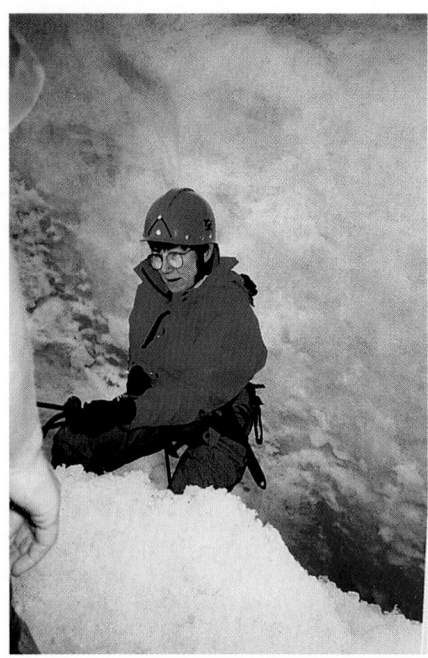

Figure 9-2 Trauma and rescue teams are frequently composed of volunteers and at least one experienced and trained individual. This rescuer is practicing for possible extrication of a victim from a crevasse. *(Courtesy Betty Carlisle, MD.)*

illness, preinfarction syndrome, complex dislocation of a thumb requiring open reduction, and cancer. Fortunately, no deaths have occurred in station personnel since a cervical spine fracture in 1980. However, there were three fatalities in a tragic tourism sky diving event in 1997.

Somatic Health Problems

Many of the primarily somatic health problems in Antarctica have to do with cold, altitude, and trauma and are thoroughly covered in the chapters on those topics. In a midwinter setting where a tossed mug of coffee freezes before the liquid hits the ground, the dangers of frostbite are obvious. Anyone gasping for breath on "Heart Attack Hill" at the South Pole, or losing 5 kg in the first 2 weeks from resting tachycardia and tachypnea, can appreciate the physiologic stresses of rapid ascent to an equivalent of 3200 m (10,499 feet). Likewise, the dangers of ultraviolet exposure at altitude with an ozone hole and snow surface reflectance of 80% to 90% can become painfully evident to the unwary visitor.[148] A few points, however, deserve further mention.

Cold-Related Problems. Cold, of course, is a dominant factor in polar medicine. It can be a source of humor, such as the infamous "300 Degree Club" at the South Pole, for which membership requires sprinting from a 200° F (93.3° C) sauna to the Pole at −100° F (−73.3° C) while somewhat less than completely clothed. Similarly, the quintessential polar first-aid story involves creative solutions to the problem of finding warm fluids,[2] but it would be reckless to forget the ever-present danger of such a hostile environment. Wind chill commonly drops far below $-72°$ C ($-100°$ F). It has been estimated that under the most severe winter conditions, an inactive person in full polar clothing would undergo a life-threatening drop in core temperature to $27°$ C ($80.6°$ F) in only 20 minutes.[46] Airplane refueling crews and others working with liquids at ambient temperatures are constantly reminded that even a small splash can mean instant frostbite.

Rescue and treatment are complicated by the additional need for both victim and rescuer to avoid hypothermia and frostbite.[74] Disorientation and confusion from hypothermia, clumsiness from bulky clothing, and degraded performance characteristics of equipment and intravenous (IV) fluids can complicate otherwise straightforward procedures. A recent case report describes almost immediate freezing of fluid in IV lines and shattering of the plastic IV tubing despite vigorous attempts to warm them.[74] Simple devices commonly used in warmer settings, such as air splints and pneumatic antishock garments, would be similarly unusable. In more sophisticated equipment, batteries would rapidly fail, unwinterized mechanical moving parts would seize, and metal objects would become dangerous sources of frostbite.

Clothing, not normally considered a medical topic, assumes special importance in the polar environment.[65,66,69] Although the clothing used for many polar research programs in the summer seems adequate, a strong argument can be made for specialized winter gear, possibly adapted from the space program, that would allow relatively delicate manipulation of scientific equipment while offering protection from the cold (Figure 9-3). In fact, at temperatures below even that of most military specifications, material properties of equipment, including plastic electrical insulation, create unexpected and novel occupational hazards. Fortunately, the importance of ergonomic issues in the design of machinery and clothing for polar conditions is receiving increased attention.[40,175]

Nutrition Studies. Nutrition has occupied a key niche throughout the history of polar expeditions.[42] Early expeditions in both polar regions provided several examples of nutritional illnesses, including scurvy and possible hypervitaminosis A and lead poisoning.[9,179] More sophisticated nutritional analyses have been possible in recent expeditions,[149,160] and advances continue to be made in development of lightweight but nutritionally dense rations.[39]

During the Canadian-Soviet transpolar ski trek, participants skiing some 20 km/day at a speed of about 3.5 km/hr while carrying 37- to 45-kg packs showed in-

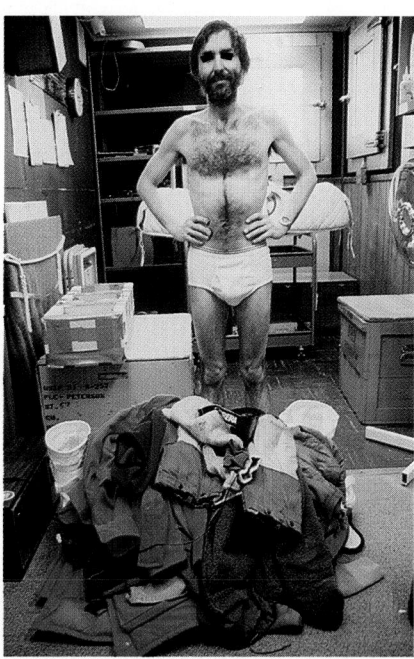

Figure 9-3 Clothing is an important topic in polar medicine. A researcher prepares to go out for extended period in ambient temperature of $-56.7°$ C ($-70°$ F). Total weight of clothes 25 lbs. Notice multiple layers for each area of the body. *(Courtesy Stephen Warren.)*

creased strength, decreased body fat, and increased high-density lipoprotein (HDL) cholesterol. However, a paradoxical drop in aerobic power was noticed, perhaps because of intensive pretraining and conditioning, as well as the increased efficiency of skiing as the trip progressed.[148] Monika Christensen's expedition reported a daily expenditure of roughly 3000 kcal but noted that the men on the expedition consumed up to 6000 kcal/day by the end of the 2½-month trip, possibly related to the drop in temperature from $-5°$ C to $-40°$ C ($23°$ F to $-40°$ F).[25] Although strenuous expedition activities can require caloric intake of up to 7000 kcal/day,[101,161] the applicability of these figures to more sedentary polar sojourners is probably limited.

Infection and Epidemiology. With particular reference to analogs in space colonies, a number of studies have taken advantage of the physical isolation of Antarctic stations as a natural laboratory for infectious disease epidemiology.[28] For example, transmission of *Escherichia coli* has been shown to correlate with population structure.[174] Since microorganisms are thought not to survive the cold long enough to be carried in by winds, midwinter respiratory tract infection outbreaks caused by parainfluenza viruses 1 and 3 and a rhinovirus in the absence of outside contacts have suggested that such organisms could persist in clothing or other fomites.[128] A similar study using swabs of 28 men isolated for a year demonstrated that *Staphylococcus au-*

reus could be temporarily suppressed but not permanently eradicated by antibacterial agents.[82]

Despite a widely reported leukopenia and decrease in cell-mediated immunity during the isolation of overwintering,[184] it is not clear whether persons emerging from Antarctic stations are more susceptible to infection. One study of 125 new and 75 winter-over crew at McMurdo during a 1977 outbreak of adenovirus type 21 showed that during a further 5-week isolation period, 89% of the population were susceptible but only 15% were infected (much less than in usual outbreaks). No significant difference was found between winter-over crew and newcomers.[150]

Circadian Rhythms, Endocrine Studies, and Sleep Research.

Pioneering studies of Natani[111] and Shurley[152] on sleep electroencephalograms at the old South Pole station demonstrated clear patterns of sleep disturbances and "free cycling" of the sleep-activity cycle. Some of these findings have been extended in more recent studies. For example, among four subjects at a small winter-over camp, summer sleep cycles synchronized within the group and with clock time. During 126 days of sunless winter, rhythms free cycled in all four people, and then resynchronized with reappearance of the sun.[78] The degree of synchrony vs. free cycling appears to depend on a number of factors, notably zeitgeber strength, although the number of subjects studied has not been large.[48]

A number of studies have examined the effect of prolonged polar residence on diurnal variations in the level of melatonin. Its important role in free radical scavenging and sleep regulation is beginning to be elucidated.[122] Therapy with full-spectrum bright light (greater than 2500 lux) seems to facilitate daily resetting of the melatonin cycle.[104] Other endocrine fluctuations also appear to be correlated with the length of the day.[173]

Other endocrine studies have examined effects of prolonged residence in polar regions with a longer than diurnal time constant. Twenty-four-hour urinary excretion of catecholamines increases in the cold, but social stresses appear to overwhelm climatic determinants of catecholamine metabolism, correlating with increases in diastolic blood pressure and pulse during the year.[14] A more consistent pattern of decreased free thyroid hormones after several months has been demonstrated by several groups.[54,134] There has even been identified a pattern of increased pituitary release of thyroid-stimulating hormone in response to IV thyrotropin releasing hormone and increased serum clearance of orally administered triiodothyronine (T_3), dubbed the "polar T_3 syndrome,"[135] but the clinical significance of these findings remains unclear.

Environmental Health Issues.

Because of Antarctica's isolation, it seems a particularly disturbing site for litter and pollution. As in the Arctic, events such as the early problems with a nuclear reactor at McMurdo (since removed) and the 1989 oil spill from the *Bahia Paraiso* near Palmer Station,[115] and studies by groups such as Greenpeace, have focused attention on environmental health risks in the Antarctic.[19,113] Environmental inspections at a broad range of Antarctic stations have raised concern about toxic effluents and heavy metal residues,[129] as well as radioisotopes used for research.[145] In an attempt to address these issues, a number of countries have begun to implement more responsible waste management policies.

Occupational Health and Injury Prevention.

Rigorous studies of risk are important for injury prevention.[49] Unfortunately, they are complex and often bedeviled by challenges, including controversial data, multiple variables, imprecise heuristics, and biases. For example, for purposes of occupational epidemiology, it may ultimately prove useful to stratify the Antarctic sojourner population into groups such as sport expeditions, military, commercial, and scientific, but the health behaviors of these groups overlap, and currently few studies have gone beyond aggregate descriptive statistics.

Even from these broad statistics, however, some figures emerge that may be useful cognitive anchors. Forty-five percent of medical cases in the Davis 1982 expedition were related to accidents.[34] A larger study of 1301 injuries among Australian expedition members found that 93% were minor, 3% were major, and 4% were environmental, working out to roughly one injury per person per year.[92] About 7% of the injuries were thought to be alcohol related. There were 16 fatalities from 1947 to 1999, but only one fatality in the past 10 years in the Australian Antarctic Program. Among 3500 scientists and support personnel (2000 person years), there were four medical deaths, two myocardial infarctions, one case of appendicitis, one perforated gastric ulcer, and one cerebral hemorrhage. The remainder of events were accidents involving falls, head injuries, hypothermia, drowning, crush injury, and burns.[98] There have been 57 deaths[93] in the U.S. Antarctic Program since 1946. Relative rankings by cause are aviation 61%, vehicles 11%, ships 7%, recreational 7%, station/industrial 5%, field activities 5%, and other 4%.[102,144,145] Other reports describe overuse, repetitive work syndromes, and noise pollution.[22,68] Often, it is more difficult to adhere to standard occupational safety practices when in a remote location.[146] Environmentally related dermatologic problems may have an incidence of up to 40%.[91,136] A recent report highlights the use of cyanoacrylate glue to hasten healing of disabling fingertip fissures.[11]

Fire Safety.

In the face of extreme cold, it is somewhat counterintuitive that fire has been labeled as "the major concern and principal danger at all Antarctic stations."[45,114] This initially surprising assessment rests on a number of factors. Cold temperatures severely limit the utility of water for fire suppression. Firefighting equipment may become inoperative in extreme cold, and frequent high winds can fan fires. The extremely low absolute humidity in many polar regions results in an even lower relative humidity when outside air is warmed in station dwellings. This in turn leads to an increase in static electricity and dryness of combustibles, already at risk from frequent use of space heaters. Finally, alternative food and shelter are limited or nonexistent.

Elaborate predeployment training, frequent on-site drills, and a keen awareness of potential fire hazards have correlated with a satisfactory fire safety record to date, but this good fortune cannot be taken for granted. At least four major fires have occurred in Antarctica in the last 15 years.[145] Fortunately, only one person died, but there were several injuries, and the Soviet Vostok winter crew had to endure 8 months without a power plant to supply heat.

Tourist Safety. Polar regions are imbued with a sense of the exotic, conjuring up "images of hardship, personal valor, danger, adventure, and of course, the hero."[145] As transportation increasingly opens up previously inaccessible areas, this image attracts growing tourist traffic and, with it, hot debate from both legal and environmental viewpoints.[19]

The essential medicolegal issue is the extent of governmental organizations' responsibility for medical care of participants in nongovernmental activities, whether scientific, political, or commercial.[145] When a tourist group requires aid beyond its own capabilities, whose responsibility is it? To what extent should a research station with limited medical supplies be required to divert some of those supplies to an individual who presumably bears responsibility for planning his or her own medical coverage?

Although the ethical course of action seems clear in the preceding scenarios, there is still uncertainty in our litigious society regarding the relative strengths of the Good Samaritan principle and the doctrine of assumed risk.[62] Perhaps eventually there will be a mandatory rescue insurance policy for tourists similar to the one currently being adopted in Mt.Rainier and Denali National Parks[166] (Figure 9-4).

Air Safety. As in the Arctic, reliance on aircraft for transportation has highlighted the critical importance of air safety. The worst Antarctic air accident was the crash of an Air New Zealand tourist "flightseeing" DC-10 on Mt. Erebus in November 1979. This accident killed all 257 people aboard and effectively ended such flights, which had flown an estimated 11,000 tourists in the previous 2 years.[9] There have been 35 air-related fa-

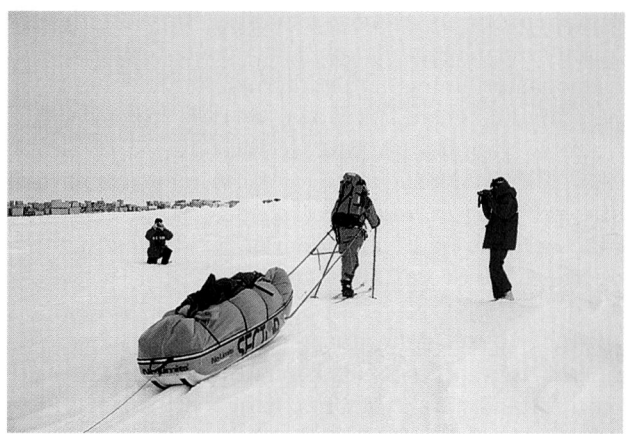

Figure 9-4 Increased numbers of nongovernmental Antarctic expeditions have created increased awareness of the continent, as well as occasional requests for assistance. A lone traveler departs from South Pole in an attempt to do a solo traverse of Antarctica. *(Courtesy Betty Carlisle, MD.)*

talities in the U.S. Antarctic Program since 1946 from crashes related to either fixed-wing or rotor aircraft.[102,145] A ski-equipped LC-130 Hercules crashed at the remote D-59 camp in 1971. Fortunately, none of the 10-crew members aboard were injured, but during a salvage operation in 1987 another LC-130 bringing supplies to D-59 crashed nearby, killing two and injuring nine.

Psychosocial Health Problems

For many polar living arrangements, psychosocial issues may be more important than strictly medical or environmental factors.* Psychiatric problems are mentioned even in reports of early expeditions,[9,168] and almost any participant in expeditions will recognize Thor Heyerdahl's observation[168]:

The most insidious danger on any expedition where men [sic] have to rub shoulders for weeks is a mental sickness that might be called "expedition fever"—a psychological condition which makes even the most peaceful person irritable, angry, furious, absolutely desperate because his perceptive capacity gradually shrinks until he sees only his companions' faults while their good qualities are no longer recorded by his grey matter.

In fact, as Shurley notes, "minor mental troubles are both common and temporary."[151] This is particularly important because there is growing evidence that psychologic and somatic health issues are linked.[81,125] Stress can lead to increased risk of accidents, and conversely, the fear of medical emergencies can lead to increased stress.[162] Confidence in the medical staff and facilities in isolated polar settings is a key factor in countering the concerns arising from isolation. In addi-

*References 27, 37, 52, 136, 148, 159.

tion, appropriate exercise facilities, opportunities for quality mental stimulation, and frequent contact with friends and family via the Internet and telephone can help maintain stability. However, data from the Australian National Antarctic Research Expedition (ANARE) do not suggest a higher incidence of psychiatric problems in Antarctica. In fact, "except for insomnia, which is perhaps endemic, it is lower than expected in the overall population."[94]

Alcohol Abuse. Adjustment to psychosocial stresses in polar communities depends on a complex array of sociocultural factors.[124,163] One coping mechanism is alcohol use. As in many isolated communities at high latitudes, alcohol use can disrupt and lubricate social interactions. At one station, annual per capita absolute alcohol consumption was calculated at 16.9 L.[184] At another, a summer support staff member had to be terminated because of alcohol abuse and two winter-over staff had to be prohibited from purchasing alcohol from the station store; one of these actually required disulfiram to ensure abstinence.

At many Antarctic stations, alcohol is easily available and may be subsidized. In some stations, rations can be excessive or nonexistent. Although relatively few serious incidents involving intoxicated staff have been reported, the potential for serious accidents remains real, particularly during winter when medical evacuation flights are impossible. Recommendations have called for routine monitoring of alcohol levels of anyone involved in an accident[145] or even prohibition of alcohol at Antarctic stations.[37] However, as with prohibition in other countries, this might create more problems than it might solve.

Psychoneuroimmunology. The concept of psychologic or meteorologic modulation of immune function and other physiologic responses is gradually gaining some credence and remains largely unexplored. For example, perhaps an alternative explanation for leukopenia during winters is not absence of antigenic stimulation, as previously thought, but increased stress from interpersonal interactions.[16] In the last few years, SAD has been largely accepted as a useful construct, and it will be intriguing to see if related findings, particularly by ex-Soviet station scientists, on weather-related pathophysiology are confirmed.

Psychologic stress at research stations may arise from several sources.[5,140] One is the environment itself; environmental severity has been found to be an independent predictor of hostility and anxiety after wintering over.[124] Perhaps more important is the perception of the environment. Newcomers to the South Pole station are usually observed wearing a full 12-kg polar outfit at $-20°$ C ($-4°$ F) for several weeks after arrival. By midwinter, the same individuals may eventually

think little of walking from the gym to their rooms dressed only in running shorts and T-shirt at $-60°$ C ($-76°$ F).

Stress can also result from disjunction between a person's original motivation for joining the program and realities of life in the station. Studies suggest that people who go to Antarctic stations to seek thrills or to challenge themselves often have more difficulty sustaining their motivation and performance than those who go to accomplish a scientific mission or even those primarily motivated to earn money. In general, older individuals who are somewhat introverted are able to set work goals and work toward them, and persons who have broadly defined hobby interests seem to cope better with the social isolation and dynamics of wintering over.[37]

Small Group Dynamics. In addition to external climate and internal motivational factors, stress can arise from interpersonal interactions. Although there are many exceptions, participants in the Antarctic program often speak of a tendency for personnel to form cliques or microcultures. People may cluster according to ordinary personal chemistry, along lines of OAE (Old Antarctic Explorer) vs. novice, winter-over vs. summer status, or according to scientific, civilian, or military affiliation.[39] With time, such social clusters can be a source of support or of friction. Nuances of body language and proximity can take on heightened significance,[156] conferring a premium on social adaptability and compatibility. In an attempt to unify the core group, winter-overs participate in a mini Outward Bound type of group bonding experience before deployment.

Social isolation is of course an important factor in polar communities. Although this isolation has been lessened by modern communications and transportation, polar communities resemble in many ways the "asylums" studied by Goffman, "a place of residence and work where a large number of like-situated individuals, cut off from the wider society for an appreciable period of time, together lead an enclosed, formally administered round of life."[50]

A number of studies have drawn parallels between group processes in polar stations and those in other isolated and confined environments, such as submarines or in space.[77,112,118,181] Unfortunately, much of the submarine data are a decade or more old, raising questions of temporal drift and external validity, and the astronaut programs seem to have had little real interest in psychologic issues and so have missed some opportunities for research in this field.[168]

Winter-Over Syndrome. Stressors such as those mentioned previously can result in what has been termed the winter-over syndrome. The historically oft-mentioned "Big Eye" or "20-foot stare in a 10-foot room" seems to be less common now, perhaps because the stations are increasingly comfortable and stimulating environments, but the constellation of depression, hostility, sleep disturbances, and impaired cognition seems to be both common and underreported.[162]

The winter-over syndrome is not a static condition but a time- and individual-dependent process. At the South Pole research station, for example, winter-over staff characteristically report a recognizable pattern of fluctuating activity and mood. There is often a mixture of relief, pride, and fearful anticipation as the last LC-130 flight departs in mid-February, followed by a period of frenetic activity to beat inventory deadlines, file resupply orders, launch projects, and prepare the station for winter. As work and recreation routines develop, mood generally drops with the setting sun and increasing anticipation develops around the upcoming midwinter airdrop of "freshies" (fruits and vegetables), mail, and supplies. However, since the 1995-1996 season, regular airdrops have not been scheduled because of budgetary constraints. A possible benefit of the canceling of the midwinter airdrop may be a less severe August nadir that occurred after the excitement surrounding the airdrop faded. Finally, a rise in mood generally occurs toward the end of the year, although studies at the Australian stations at Mawson and Macquarie Island suggest that the influx of new staff at station opening may actually be associated with increased depression.[184] As usual, the convenience of a descriptive label does not guarantee explanatory or predictive power or validity.

Seasonal Affective Disorder. A probable contributor to and confounder of the winter-over syndrome is the apparently fairly consistent exacerbation of stress and depression under conditions of winter or night. The term *seasonal affective disorder* was first used in 1984 by Rosenthal et al[138,139] to describe the annual recurrence of bipolar affective disorder, hypersomnia, and overeating, which was alleviated by daily exposure to bright (2500 lux) light. Although correlations with melatonin levels have been demonstrated, the detailed pathophysiology of SAD remains an active area of inquiry and may involve retinal signal transduction, as well as timing of light intensity.* Sunlamps have been used informally in some Antarctic stations for years, and full-spectrum lighting has been installed in many public areas since 1987. Given the current indoor lighting and self-selection of winter-overs, SAD may be no more prevalent in Antarctica than at lower latitudes.

Beneficial Effects of Isolation. An interesting point is that isolation may have positive and negative effects.[67]

---

*References 15, 87, 88, 104, 172, 190.

Isolation is not synonymous with loneliness and depression, as Amundsen reported from his sojourn at Framheim.[153] In one study it was found that, except for insomnia, the more severe the environment, the less severe the symptoms of depression, hostility, and anxiety.[126] In fact, a subset of "professional isolates" may actually prefer polar stations to "normal" society.[167]

Reentry. An important issue familiar to many travelers and expedition members is that of reentry or social reintegration on return from a polar sojourn.[140] Although several studies suggest that personality traits are fairly stable during a polar stay, station personnel often require 6 months or more to normalize after returning from Antarctica.[168]

A question that has not been answered fully is whether subtle long-term disabilities might be induced by prolonged isolation at polar stations. Although there have been impressions of cognitive and sensory decrements after wintering over, these have not been confirmed in a number of studies.[168] As for somatic complaints, a study of enlisted Navy personnel who wintered over between 1963 and 1973 found fewer hospitalizations for medical problems on follow-up than among a similar cohort who qualified for wintering over but did not actually go.[6]

Screening and Selection. Based on the preceding findings, several attempts have been made to refine the selection and screening process for successful polar sojourners.[188] These efforts have used a number of methods and instruments to cope with the methodologic constraints common to many studies of complex human systems.[23,53,136,168] Perhaps unsurprisingly, previous successful polar experience seems to be among the best predictors of subsequent high performance. In general, biographic data, peer ratings, psychometric testing, and interviews all seem helpful in selection, although each has weaknesses and inconsistencies.

Early studies led to the tripartite "ability, stability, compatibility" criteria for successful participation in the Antarctic programs.[53] This simple but useful scheme recognizes that technical skill, emotional equilibrium, and interpersonal skills all play important roles in an individual's performance and internal satisfaction. It would be desirable to improve measurement and predictive usefulness of these factors; such studies remain an active frontier for Antarctic research.

OVERVIEW AND FUTURE DEVELOPMENTS

A point made early in this chapter was the challenge inherent in meaningfully synthesizing Arctic and Antarctic medicine. Reflection on some of the issues raised previously suggests several common areas of linkage and directions for future work.

Issues of Methodology and Medical Epistemology

The state of knowledge about the Arctic and the Antarctic is still rudimentary. Studies in polar settings are often handicapped by extremely difficult research conditions and may never achieve the statistical power and validity expected of counterparts in more forgiving climes. Commonly encountered methodologic problems include most notably small sample sizes, unknown effect sizes, measurement of proxy variables, and multiple confounders.

In one study, cold tolerance of five Antarctic divers and five nondivers at the station were compared during the year, using finger immersion tests with measurements of index finger pulp temperature, onset of cold-induced vasodilation, and pain scores.[18] No difference was found between the groups, perhaps, as the authors suggest, because of either whole body cooling or insufficient cold exposure during dives. In another review, it was pointed out that simplifying assumptions of laboratory studies of cold adaptation may overlook the intermittent pattern of chilling and overheating under actual field conditions.[20] In yet another report, cardiac and respiratory functions were measured in Antarctic expedition members during a 3-month summer sojourn, and no persistent changes were noted; the authors suggest that the degree and duration of cold exposure may have been inadequate to produce notable changes.[189]

The preceding examples are offered not to level specific criticism; in fact, the studies were carefully performed and analyzed. As the authors themselves point out, however, inherent difficulties of research under polar conditions weaken the conclusions derived from it. Methodologic issues are perhaps even more complex in studies of social phenomena, such as group dynamics, task performance, or depression. In these situations, it may prove necessary to use multiple triangulating techniques of observational, qualitative, quasiexperimental, and experimental designs.[26,99,168] Given the high cost of supporting studies in a polar setting,[141] a major challenge is to design studies that can uncover meaningful results despite limited resources.

Fourth World Medical Decision Making

Given the relative paucity of rigorous studies on polar medical phenomena, a second challenge is to optimally design polar medical practice. Polar medical lore is replete with stories such as that of the physician of the 6th Soviet Antarctic Expedition who performed an appendectomy on himself[36] or those of retrospectively humorous cold-related injuries.[111] Although the basic principles of emergency medicine, epidemiology, occupational health, psychology, and other disciplines still apply in polar settings,[70] the spectrum of health problems and some important aspects of their management are undoubtedly skewed.[132] As with attempts to improve health care in the so-called developing countries, wholesale transplantation of the U.S. model of medicine may prove inappropriate. As polar medicine continues to evolve,[119] it will need to adapt the Western industrialized model to local conditions.

Fourth World medicine requires distillation of medical practice into a compact yet comprehensive package that will be robust enough to travel well. Novel constraints and the inherently unpredictable nature of a hostile environment further stretch the usual, already tentative rules and thresholds of medical decision making. Perhaps to a greater extent than in most settings, prevention and preparation are paramount in polar medicine. As might be imagined, the risks from even minor mishaps are exacerbated by cold and its effects on both humans and equipment, by altitude and impaired tissue oxygenation and wound healing, and by restricted dexterity and vision from bulky clothing. Isolation from medical facilities exerts a multiplier effect on these risks[147]; a victim extrication and resuscitation that would be routine in most urban or suburban settings presents an overwhelming challenge in polar settings.

With lives at stake, arguments have been made for planning for worst-case scenarios rather than only for likely situations.[145,146] On the other hand, a realistic balance point on the cost/utility curve must be set for each situation based on estimated risks. As polar health care workers have strived to build facilities and offer care of the highest quality, there have even been proposals for such luxuries as anesthesiologist-staffed helicopters and regionalized extracorporeal circulation equipment for rewarming hypothermic patients.[186] Such suggestions, although in line with the polar paradigm of projecting expertise into isolated regions, perhaps overemphasize therapeutic rather than preventive priorities. Given existing fiscal and logistic constraints, preventive measures should take priority over higher-cost options.

A recurrent medical issue in polar stations involves contingency planning and the optimum level of inventory. This question applies equally to drugs, equipment, training, and personnel and is faced immediately by any incoming physician. Given finite (even scarce) resources, space, and resupply, does the physician have enough X on station, has he or she completed enough training to handle Y, is there enough help available to take care of Z? "Just in time" principles of inventory management are not likely to be appropriate. This issue is well illustrated by the recurrent debate over whether to maintain a frozen blood bank at polar stations.[22,67,145,146]

A promising tool for both improved data gathering and medical diagnosis and treatment is informatics. When combined with improved communications systems, the computer offers a flexible and powerful solution to the problems of isolation.[24] Telemedicine embraces a broad range of possible activities. The advantages of rapid access to organized databases and remote consultations for radiology and other specialties via video are promising. Telemedicine is already in place and functioning in some northern Arctic regions. The Australian Antarctic Program has been using it successfully for a number of years.[92] Physiologic, psychologic,[169] and occupational health data[120] can be monitored or retrieved, ultimately linking geography and information flow.

REFERENCES

1. Abbey S et al: Psychiatric consultation in the eastern Canadian Arctic. III. Mental health issues in Inuit women in the eastern Arctic, *Can J Psychiatry* 38:32, 1993.
2. Adler A: Arctic first aid, *N Engl J Med* 326:91, 1992.
3. Akerblom H: Human exposure to environmental hazards in the Arctic, *Arctic Med Res* 52:3, 1993 (editorial).
4. AMAP Assessment Report, delivered at the Ministerial Conference, Alta, Norway, June 1997, http://www.grida.no/amap/assess/soaer-cn.htm#chapter12
5. Anderson C: Polar psychology: coping with it all, *Nature* 350:290, 1991.
6. Anderson C et al: Research in Antarctica: exploring the still unexplored, *Nature* 350:287, 1991.
7. Anderson P: Astrophysics goes south, *Science* 252:1491, 1991.
8. Antarctic wilderness, *Nature* 348:267, 1990.
9. *Antarctica: great stories from the frozen continent*, Sydney, Australia, 1985, Reader's Digest.
10. ASOC Information Paper, delivered at the XXIII ATCM, Lima, Peru, May 1999.
11. Ayton J: Polar hands: spontaneous skin fissures closed with cyanoacrylate (Histoacryl Blue) tissue adhesive in Antarctica, *Arctic Med Res* 52:127, 1993.
12. Baker S et al: Human factors in crashes of commuter airplanes, *Aviat Space Environ Med* 64:63, 1993.
13. Beck P: Regulating one of the last tourism frontiers: Antarctica, *Appl Geogr* 10:343, 1990.
14. Bodey A: *Human acclimatisation to cold in Antarctica, with special reference to the role of catecholamines*, Hobart, Australia, 1988, Australian National Antarctic Research Expedition (ANARE).
15. Bower B: Here comes the sun: scientists shed new light on winter depression, *Science News* 142:62, 1992.
16. Bower B: Marital tiffs spark immune swoon, *Science News* 144:153, 1993.
17. Brattebo G, Wisborg T, Fredriksen K: Crush injuries in Arctic off-shore fisheries: initial treatment to prevent acute renal failure, *Arctic Med Res* 50(suppl 6):104, 1991.
18. Bridgman S: Peripheral cold acclimatization in Antarctic scuba divers, *Aviat Space Environ Med* 62:733, 1991.
19. Broder IE, Keller LR: Fairness of distribution of risks with applications to Antarctica. In Mellers BA, Baron J, editors: *Psychological perspectives on justice*, New York, 1993, Cambridge University Press.
20. Budd G: Ergonomic aspects of cold stress and cold adaptation, *Scand J Work Environ Health* 15(suppl 1):15, 1989.
21. Carlisle E: *South Pole end of season report*, 1992, US Antarctic Program.
22. Carlisle E: *Palmer Station medical turnover report*, 1993, US Antarctic Program.
23. Cazes G et al: The quantitative and qualitative use of the Adaptability Questionnaire (ADQ), *Arctic Med Res* 48:185, 1989.
24. Chiang E, Wiesnet D, Merson R: Satellites: application to the United States Antarctic Program operations and the international potential. In Thomson R, editor: *Space and airborne technology applications to Antarctic operations*, Christchurch, NZ, 1989, Dept of Scientific and Industrial Research.
25. Christensen M: *90° south: final report*, London, 1988, Royal Geographical Society.
26. Cochran W: *Planning and analysis of observational studies*, New York, 1983, John Wiley.
27. Cochrane J, Freeman S: Working in Arctic and subarctic conditions: mental health issues, *Can J Psychiatry* 34:884, 1989.
28. Cosman B, Brandt-Rauf P: Infectious disease in Antarctica and its relation to aerospace medicine: a review, *Aviat Space Environ Med* 58:174, 1987.
29. Cottrell J et al: In-flight medical emergencies: one year of experience with the enhanced medical kit, *JAMA* 262:1653, 1989.
30. Cross M: Antarctica: exploration or exploitation? *New Scientist* 130:29, 1991.
31. Curtis M, Bylund G: Diphyllobothriasis: fish tapeworm disease in the circumpolar north, *Arctic Med Res* 50:18, 1991.
32. Dahlstrom G: Work in the cold: an information and research program in occupational health, *Arctic Med Res* 51(suppl 7):92, 1992.
33. Dawson M: Arctic environments: the physical setting. In Jacobs M, Richardson J, editors: *Arctic life: challenge to survive*, Pittsburgh, 1983, Carnegie Institute.
34. Dick A: *Study of the health and physiological adaptation of an expedition in Antarctica, with special reference to occupational factors*, Hobart, Australia, 1987, Australian National Antarctic Research Expeditions.
35. Dilley D: Personal communication, 1993.
36. Douglas W: Psychological and sociological aspects of manned spaceflight. In *The human experience in Antarctica: applications to life in space*, Sunnyvale, Calif, 1987, National Aeronautics and Space Administration.
37. Draggan S: *Performance in isolated environments*, 1987, Washington, DC, National Science Foundation.
38. Durst D: Conjugal violence: changing attitudes in two northern native communities, *Community Ment Health J* 27:359, 1991.
39. Edwards J, Roberts D: The influence of a calorie supplement on the consumption of the meal, ready-to-eat in a cold environment, *Mil Med* 156:466, 1991.
40. Eisma T: Handling the cold with dexterity, *Occup Health Saf* 60:16, 1991.
41. Elzinga A, Bohlin I: Politics of science in polar regions, *Ambio* 18:71, 1989.
42. Feeney R: Food technology and polar exploration, *Arctic Med Res* 51:35, 1992.
43. Finnemore B: Low birth weight in the central Canadian Arctic, *Arctic Med Res* 51:117, 1992.
44. Fogg G: *A history of Antarctic science*, Cambridge, 1992, Cambridge University Press.
45. Fowler A: Antarctic logistics, *Oceanus* 31:80, 1988.
46. Freitas CD, Symon L: Bioclimatic index of human survival times in the antarctic, *Polar Rec* 23:651, 1987.
47. Frimodt-Moller B, Bay-Nielsen H: Classification of accidents in the Arctic: a suggestion for adaptation of the Nordic classification for accident monitoring, *Arctic Med Res* 51(suppl 7):15, 1992.
48. Gardner P et al: Adaptation of sleep and circadian rhythms to the Antarctic summer: a question of zeitgeber strength, *Aviat Space Environ Med* 62:1019, 1991.
49. Glickman T, Gough M, editors: *Readings in risk*, Washington, DC, 1990, Resources for the Future.
50. Goffman E: *Asylums: essays on the social situation of mental patients and other inmates*, Garden City, NY, 1961, Anchor Books.
51. Gottlieb J: Episodes of illness and medical service in a geographically isolated mine village in Greenland, *Arctic Med Res* 49:128, 1990.
52. Gunderson E: Psychological studies in Antarctica. In Gunderson E, editor: *Human adaptability to Antarctic conditions*, Washington, DC, 1974, American Geophysical Union.
53. Gunderson E, Palinkas L: *Review of psychological studies in the US Antarctic Program*, 1988, US Naval Health Research Center.
54. Hackney A, Hodgdon J: Thyroid hormone changes during military field operations: effects of cold exposure in the Arctic, *Aviat Space Environ Med* 63:606, 1992.
55. Haehnle R: Designing a new science facility for McMurdo Station, *Antarctic J US* 23:4, 1988.
56. Hall S: *The fourth world: the heritage of the Arctic and its destruction*, New York, 1988, Vintage Books.
57. Hamzah B, editor: *Antarctica in international affairs*, Kuala Lumpur, Malaysia, 1987, Institute of Strategic and International Studies.
58. Hansen V, Jacobsen B, Husby R: Mental distress during winter: an epidemiological study of 7759 adults north of the Arctic Circle, *Acta Psychiatr Scand* 84:137, 1991.
59. Harrison A, Clearwater Y, McKay C: The human experience in Antarctica: applications to life in space, *Behav Sci* 34:253, 1989.
60. Hart P: Growth of Antarctic tourism, *Oceanus* 31:93, 1988.
61. Hemmings A, Hay J, Towle S: Environmental science: coming of age in Antarctica. In Hay J, Hemmings A, Thom N, editors: *Antarctica 150: scientific perspectives, policy futures*, Auckland, NZ, 1990, University of Auckland.
62. Herr R: The climb physician: an endangered species? *J Wilderness Med* 1:144, 1990 (editorial).

63. Herr R, Hall H, Haward M, editors: *Antarctica's future: continuity or change?* Hobart, Tasmania, 1990, Australian Institute of International Affairs.

64. Hibben S, editor: *Antarctic bibliography,* Superintendent of Documents No LC33.9, Washington, DC, 1992, Library of Congress.

65. Holmer I: Protective clothing against cold: performance standards as method for preventive measures, *Arctic Med Res* 51(suppl 7):94, 1992.

66. Holmer I, Gavhed D: Resultant clothing insulation during exercise in the cold, *Arctic Med Res* 50(suppl 6):94, 1991.

67. Houseal M: *Medical department of 1991 end-of-season report,* 1991, US Antarctic Program.

68. Houseal M: Lyme disease in the Antarctic, *N Engl J Med* 326:351, 1992.

69. Hubbs K: Antarctic Development Squadron Six (VXE 6) and its role in the test/evaluation of extreme cold weather clothing and equipment. In *US Navy Symposium on Arctic/Cold Weather Operations of Surface Ships,* Washington, DC, 1989, Department of the Navy.

70. Hughes E: Medical problems in the Antarctic, *Med J Aust* 143:95, 1985.

71. Illingworth F: *North of the circle,* New York, 1951, Philosophical Library.

72. International Society of Travel Medicine: *2nd Conference on International Travel Medicine,* Atlanta, 1991.

73. Jacobs M, Richardson JI, editors: *Arctic life: challenge to survive,* Pittsburgh, 1983, Carnegie Institute.

74. Johnson D, Gamble W: Trauma in the Arctic: an incident report, *J Trauma* 31:1340, 1991.

75. Johnson M, Moore M, Kennedy R: Injuries in the Alaskan Arctic, *Arctic Med Res* 51(suppl 7):45, 1992.

76. Johnson R, Kingsley T: Antarctic research and lunar exploration: useful parallels. In *Space 88,* Albuquerque, 1988, American Society of Civil Engineers.

77. Kanas N: Psychological, psychiatric, and interpersonal aspects of long-duration space missions, *J Spacecraft Rockets* 27:457, 1990.

78. Kennaway D, Dorp CV: Free-running rhythms of melatonin, cortisol, electrolytes and sleep in humans in Antarctica, *Am J Physiol* 260:R1137, 1991.

79. Kerr R: Ozone hole: not over the Arctic—for now (news), *Science* 256:734, 1992.

80. Kimball L: *Southern exposure: deciding Antarctica's future,* Washington, DC, 1990, World Resources Institute.

81. Klen T: Accidents in the Arctic: a psychological point of view, *Arctic Med Res* 51(suppl 7):71, 1992.

82. Krikler S: *Staphylococcus aureus* in Antarctica: carriage and attempted eradication, *J Hyg* 97:427, 1986.

83. LaBarre R: *Palmer end-of-season report,* 1992, US Antarctic Program.

84. Lansing A: *Endurance: Shackleton's incredible voyage,* New York, 1986, Carroll & Graf.

85. Leigh J: Estimates of the probability of job-related death in 347 occupations, *J Occup Med* 29:510, 1987.

86. Lemonick M: Antarctica, *Time,* Jan 15, 1990.

87. Lewy A, Sack R: Light therapy and psychiatry, *Proc Soc Exp Biol Med* 183:11, 1986.

88. Lieberman H et al: Possible behavioral consequences of light-induced changes in melatonin availability, *Ann NY Acad Sci* 453:242, 1985.

89. Logan H: Tourism and other activities. In Hay J, Hemmings A, Thom N, editors: *Antarctica 150: scientific perspectives, policy futures,* Auckland, NZ, 1990, University of Auckland.

90. Lopez B: *Arctic dreams: imagination and desire in a northern landscape,* New York, 1986, Scribner.

91. Lugg D: Antarctic epidemiology: a survey of ANARE stations 1947-72. In Edholm O, Gunderson E, editors: *Polar human biology,* London, 1973, Heinemann.

92. Lugg D: ANARE, personal communication, 1999.

93. Lugg D, Gormely P, King H: Accidents on Australian Antarctic expeditions, *Polar Rec* 23:720, 1987.

94. Lugg DJ: Antarctica: Australia's remote medical practice. ///Al/australia polar med.htm

95. Luoma P et al: Blood mercury and serum selenium concentration in reindeer herders in the Arctic area of northern Finland, *Arch Toxicol* 15(suppl):172, 1992.

96. MacLean J et al: Trichinosis in the Canadian Arctic: report of five outbreaks and a new clinical syndrome, *J Infect Dis* 160:513, 1989.

97. MacLean J et al: Epidemiologic and serologic definition of primary and secondary trichinosis in the Arctic, *J Infect Dis* 165:908, 1992.

98. MacMillan HL et al: Aboriginal health, 1996, http://www.cma.ca/cmaj/vol-155/issue-11/1569.htm

99. Marshall C, Rossman G: *Designing qualitative research,* Newbury Park, Calif, 1989, Sage Publications.

100. McDonald J et al: An outbreak of toxoplasmosis in pregnant women in northern Quebec, *J Infect Dis* 161:769, 1990.

101. Mear R, Swan R: *A walk to the Pole: to the heart of Antarctica in the footsteps of Scott,* New York, 1987, Crown Publishers.

102. Mehar H, National Science Foundation: Personal communication, January 1999.

103. Meyer-Rochow V: Observations on an accidental case of raw sewage pollution in Antarctica, *Zentralbl Hyg Umweltmed* 192:554, 1992.

104. Midwinter M, Arendt J: Adaptation of the melatonin rhythm in human subjects following night-shift work in Antarctica, *Neurosci Lett* 122:195, 1991.

105. Millar W: Smokeless tobacco use by youth in the Canadian Arctic, *Arctic Med Res* 49(suppl 2):39, 1990.

106. Millar W: Smoking prevalence in the Canadian Arctic, *Arctic Med Res* 49(suppl 2):23, 1990.

107. Modzelewski M: At the top of Europe, *New York Times,* Aug 29, 1993.

108. Moody J: *Arctic doctor,* New York, 1955, Dodd, Mead.

109. Murphy J: *South to the Pole by ski,* St Paul, Minn, 1990, Marlor Press.

110. Myhre U, Goode P, Miller I: Jogger's phimosis, *Br J Urol* 63:549, 1989.

111. Natani K et al: Long-term changes in sleep patterns in men on the South Polar plateau, *Arch Intern Med* 125:655, 1970.

112. National Aeronautics and Space Administration: *The human experience in Antarctica: applications to life in space,* Sunnyvale, Calif, 1987, National Aeronautics and Space Administration.

113. National Science Foundation: *US Antarctic Program final environmental impact statement,* Washington, DC, 1980, The Foundation.

114. National Science Foundation: *Survival in Antarctica,* Washington, DC, 1984, The Foundation.

115. National Science Foundation: *Antarctic J US* 24(2), 1989.

116. National Science Foundation: *Antarctic research: program announcement and proposal guide,* Washington, DC, 1993, The Foundation.

117. Nicholas J: Small groups in orbit: group interaction and crew performance on space station, *Aviat Space Environ Med* 58:1009, 1987.

118. Nicholas J, Foushee H: Organization, selection, and training of crews for extended spaceflight: findings from analogs and implications, *J Spacecraft Rockets* 27:451, 1990.

119. Norman J: Medical care and human biological research in the British Antarctic Survey Medical Unit, *Arctic Med Res* 48:103, 1989.

120. Norman J, Brebner J: Remote health: occupational health care in the Antarctic, *Occup Health (Lond)* 40:602, 1988.

121. Osgood S, Haehnle R: *Environment one: a master plan study for a new scientific research station at the geographic South Pole.* In International Cold Regions Engineering Specialty Conference, 6th (Feb 26-28), 1991, West Lebanon, NH, American Society of Civil Engineers.

122. Oxidation strongly linked to aging but quenched by ubiquitous hormone, *Science News* 144:109, 1993.

123. Palinkas L: Health and performance of Antarctic winter-over personnel: a follow-up study, *Aviat Space Environ Med* 57:954, 1986.

124. Palinkas L: Sociocultural influences on psychosocial adjustment in Antarctica, *Med Anthropol* 10:235, 1989.

125. Palinkas L: Going to extremes: the cultural context of stress, illness and coping in Antarctica, *Soc Sci Med* 35:651, 1992.

126. Palinkas L, Gunderson E, Burr R: *Psychophysiological correlates of human adaptation in Antarctica.* In International Symposium on Antarctic Research, Tianjin, China, 1989, Ocean Press.

127. Parfit M: *South light: a journey to the last continent,* New York, 1985, Macmillan.

128. Parkinson A, Muchmore H, Scott E: Rhinovirus respiratory tract infections during isolation at South Pole Station, *Antarctic J US* 19:186, 1984.

129. Poorter MD, Schmidt S: Greenpeace environmental and scientific programme in Antarctica. In Hay J, Hemmings A, Thom N, editors: *Antarctica 150: scientific perspectives, policy futures,* Auckland, NZ, 1990, University of Auckland.

130. Porter E: *Antarctica,* New York, 1978, EP Dutton.

131. Prestrud P, Krogsrud J, Gjertz I: The occurrence of rabies in the Svalbard Islands of Norway, *J Wildl Dis* 28:57, 1992.

132. Priddy R: "Acute abdomen" in Antarctica, *Med J Aust* 143:108, 1985.

133. Pyne S: *The ice,* Iowa City, 1986, University of Iowa Press.

134. Reed H et al: Changes in serum triiodothyronine (T_3) kinetics after prolonged Antarctic residence: the polar T_3 syndrome, *J Clin Endocrinol Metab* 70:965, 1990.

135. Reed H et al: Decreased free fraction of thyroid hormones after prolonged Antarctic residence, *J Appl Physiol* 69:1467, 1990.

136. Rivolier J et al, editors: *Man in the Antarctic,* London, 1988, Taylor & Francis.

137. Rodahl K: Working in the cold, *Arctic Med Res* 50(suppl 6):80, 1991.

138. Rosenthal N et al: Seasonal affective disorder, *Arch Gen Psychiatry* 41:72, 1984.

139. Rosenthal N et al: Antidepressant effects of light in seasonal affective disorder, *Am J Psychiatry* 142:163, 1985.

140. Rothblum E: Psychological factors in the Antarctic, *J Psychol* 124:253, 1990 (review).

141. Schneider C: Funding research in Antarctica: a look at NSF support to scientists, *Antarctic J US* 25:1990.

142. Schnitzer P, Bender T: Surveillance of traumatic occupational fatalities in Alaska: implications for prevention, *Public Health Rep* 107:70, 1992.

143. Schuurman H: *Canada's eastern neighbor: a view on change in Greenland*, Ottawa, Ontario, 1976, Ministry of Indian and Northern Affairs.

144. Schweickart R: *Safety in Antarctica: report of the U.S. Antarctic Program Safety Review Panel*, 1988, National Science Foundation doc #88-78.

145. Schweickart R et al: *Safety in Antarctica*, Washington, DC, 1988, National Science Foundation.

146. Shen B: Report to Antarctic safety committee. In Schweickart R et al, editors: *Safety in Antarctica*, Washington, DC, 1988, National Science Foundation.

147. Shen B: Risks of travel in small aircraft: is commuter flying too dangerous? *Travel Med Advisor* 3:14, 1993.

148. Shephard R: Some consequences of polar stress: data from a transpolar ski-trek, *Arctic Med Res* 50:25, 1991.

149. Shephard R: Fat metabolism, exercise and the cold (review), *Can J Sport Sci* 17:83, 1992.

150. Shult P et al: Adenovirus 21 infection in an isolated Antarctic station: transmission of the virus and susceptibility of the population, *Am J Epidemiol* 133:599, 1991.

151. Shurley J: Physiological research at US stations in Antarctica. In Gunderson E, editor: *Human adaptability to Antarctic conditions*, Washington, DC, 1974, American Geophysical Union.

152. Shurley J et al: Sleep and activity patterns at South Pole Station, *Arch Gen Psychiatry* 22:385, 1970.

153. Simpson-Housley P: *Antarctica: exploration, perception and metaphor*, London, 1992, Routledge.

154. Skinhoj P: Epidemiology of viral hepatitis in circumpolar populations, *Arctic Med Res* 50:177, 1991.

155. Smith D: Stargazing at the South Pole, *New Scientist* 130:33, 1991.

156. Sommer R: *Personal space: the behavioral basis of design*, Englewood Cliffs, NJ, 1969, Prentice-Hall.

157. Stix G: Run silent, run (not so) cheap, *Sci Am* 269:26, 1993.

158. Stonehouse B: *North Pole, South Pole: a guide to the ecology and resources of the Arctic and Antarctic*, London, 1990, ION.

159. Strange R, Youngman S: Emotional aspects of wintering over, *Antarctic J US* 6:255, 1971.

160. Strivastava K, Kumar R: Human nutrition in cold and high terrestrial altitudes, *Int J Biometeorol* 36:10, 1992.

161. Stroud M: Nutrition and energy balance on the "footsteps of Scott" expedition 1984-86, *Hum Nutr Appl Nutr* 41A:426, 1987.

162. Stuster J: *Space station habitability recommendations based on a systematic comparative analysis of analogous conditions*, Mountain View, Calif, 1986, National Aeronautics and Space Administration.

163. Suedfeld R, Bernaldez J, Stossel D: The Plar Psychology Project (PPP): a cross-national investigation of polar adaptation, *Arctic Med Res* 48:91, 1989.

164. Sugden D: *Arctic and Antarctic*, Totowa, NJ, 1982, Barnes & Noble.

165. *Symposium on Medical Problems in Sparsely Populated Areas*, Oulu, Finland, 1978, Nordic Council for Arctic Medical Research.

166. Take a risk, pay the price, *New York Times*, Sept 19, 1993.

167. Taylor A: Professional isolates in New Zealand's Antarctic research programme, *Int Rev Appl Psychol* 18:135, 1969.

168. Taylor A: *Antarctic psychology*, Wellington, 1987, DSIR Science Information Publishing Centre.

169. Taylor A: *Collection and transmission of behavioural data by computer and satellite*. In International Symposium on Antarctic Research, Tianjin, China, 1989, Ocean Press.

170. Taylor M: Cold weather injuries during peacetime military training, *Mil Med* 157:602, 1992.

171. Thomas D et al: Arctic terrestrial ecosystem contamination, *Sci Total Environ* 122:135, 1992 (review).

172. Thorington L: Spectral, irradiance, and temporal aspects of natural and artificial light, *Ann NY Acad Sci* 453:28, 1985.

173. Tkachev A, Ramenskaya E, Bojko J: Dynamics of hormone and metabolic state in polar inhabitants depend on daylight duration, *Arctic Med Res* 50(suppl 6):152, 1991.

174. Tzabar Y, Pennington T: The population structure and transmission of *Escherichia coli* in an isolated human community: studies on an Antarctic base, *Epidemiol Infect* 107:537, 1991.

175. Vayrynen S: Ergonomic design of machinery for use in the cold: a review based on the literature and original research, *Arctic Med Res* 51(suppl 7):87, 1992.

176. Vuori H: WHO and Nordic council for Arctic medical research: partners in health, *Arctic Med Res* 50:54, 1991 (editorial).

177. Wace N: Antarctica: a new tourist destination, *Appl Geography* 10:327, 1990.

178. Walton D, editor: *Antarctic science*, Cambridge, 1987, Cambridge University Press.

179. Was the ill-fated Franklin expedition a victim of lead poisoning? *Nutr Rev* 47:322, 1989.

180. Watts A: *International law and the antarctic treaty system*, Hersch Lauterpacht Memorial Lectures, vol 11, Cambridge, 1992, Grotius Publications.

181. Weybrew B: Three decades of nuclear submarine research. In *The human experience in Antarctica: applications to life in space*, Sunnyvale, Calif, 1987, National Aeronautics and Space Administration.

182. Wharton R et al: *Use of analogs to support the Space Exploration Initiative*, Washington, DC, 1990, National Aeronautics and Space Administration and National Science Foundation.

183. Wiant C et al: Work-related aviation fatalities in Colorado 1982-1987, *Aviat Space Environ Med* 62:827, 1991.

184. Williams D: *Health, hormonal and stress-related studies on ANARE*, 1989, Hobart, Australia, Australian National Antarctic Research Expeditions.

185. Wilton P: "TB voyages" into high Arctic gave MDs a look at a culture in transition, *Can Med Assoc J* 148:1608, 1993.

186. Wisbory T, Husby P, Engedal H: Anesthesiologist-manned helicopters and regionalized extracorporeal circulation facilities: a unique chance in deep hypothermia, *Arctic Med Res* 50(suppl 6):108, 1991.

187. World Health Organization: *Health problems of local and migrant populations in Arctic regions*, 1979, The Organization.

188. World Health Organization: *Selection of personnel to work in circumpolar regions*, 1985, The Organization.

189. Xue Q et al: Changes in cardiac and respiratory function of Antarctic research expedition members, *Proc Chin Acad Med Sci* 4:112, 1989.

190. Yerevanian B et al: Effects of bright incandescent light on seasonal and nonseasonal major depressive disorder, *Psychiatry Res* 18:355, 1986.

191. Young L et al: Psychiatric consultation in the eastern Canadian Arctic. II. Referral patterns, diagnoses and treatment, *Can J Psychiatry* 38:28, 1993.

192. Young O: *Arctic in world affairs*, Seattle, 1989, University of Washington.

193. Young T et al: Prevalence of diagnosed diabetes in circumpolar indigenous populations, *Int J Epidemiol* 21:730, 1992.

10 Pathophysiology of Heat-Related Illnesses

Stephen L. Gaffin and Daniel S. Moran

Since the publication of the third edition of this text in 1995, developments in immunology, molecular biology, and systemic and cell physiology have broadened the understanding of heat-related illnesses. A brief outline of a few advances that are opening new avenues of investigation serves as introduction to a more detailed discussion.

Systemic mechanisms underlying heatstroke based on recent studies of induced cellular tolerance to heat,[233] organ blood flow,[205] and hemodynamics in heatstroke[269] are presented. New explanations of the causes and consequences of voluntary dehydration[240] are explored along with the expected impact of water and salt depletion on normal physiology and exercise performance.

The demonstration that strenuous exercise can produce systemic endotoxemia[52,64] and that endotoxins and the cytokine cascade have been implicated in acute heatstroke[56] and in other stressors, such as fear and even depressed mood,[276] may open new avenues of diagnosis and treatment. We present an update to the classic systemic approach to understanding the physiologic dysfunction in heatstroke and, where possible, relate it to emerging shock models involving bacterial toxins and cytokines, such as tumor necrosis factor.

OVERVIEW OF HEAT ILLNESS

A characteristic property of warm-blooded animals is the ability to raise body temperatures greater than ambient temperature (T_{amb}). However, this property is not limited to vertebrates. For instance, eastern tent caterpillars can raise their body temperatures above T_{amb} by 30° C (86° F) or more, using solar radiation.[100] Certain plants even produce heat; a philodendron flower may have a temperature as high as 46° C (115° F) at T_{amb} of 4° C (39.2° F).[450]

Accidental overheating is a danger in all organisms, but sometimes in nature, overheating is intentional and used as a weapon. Hornets occasionally attack the hives of Japanese honeybees. In response, scores of bees crowd closely around the invading hornet to form a "ball of bees" several layers thick. The bees vibrate their muscles rapidly, raising their own core temperature (T_c), which in turn heats the hornet to approximately 43.3° C (110° F). The hornet dies of "heatstroke"; the bees are relatively heat-tolerant and survive.

In humans and probably most animals, hyperthermia is not always painful and may even induce euphoria. It is this lack of a pain warning that is the major facilitator of heat illnesses. As a result, an athlete or soldier may choose to continue performing severe exercise in the heat, even as the risk of heat injury increases.

It is convenient to classify the more familiar heat disorders such as heat syncope, heat exhaustion (including that induced by exertion, and water or salt depletion), heat cramps, and classic and exertional heatstroke (EHS) into separate, well-defined categories. Even so, the symptoms often overlap.

HEAT STRESS AND THERMOREGULATION

Mechanisms of Heat Transfer

The human body obeys the laws of thermodynamics, as heat is transferred from a higher to a lower temperature. Applying these principles, Santee and Gonzalez[433] and Gonzalez[193] provide excellent discourse on characteristics of the thermal environment, the biophysics of heat transfer, the heat balance equation, and clothing considerations. When environmental temperature is higher than skin temperature, the body gains heat; when it is lower, the body loses heat. As a result, elevated environmental temperature adds to the heat burden of the body and interferes with heat dissipation. There are four mechanisms of heat transfer: conduction, convection, radiation, and evaporation. The environmental parameters that determine the potential for heat exchange constitute the thermal environment, which has been defined as "a biophysical aggregate of air temperature, wind speed, relative humidity, and radiation."[492]

Conduction. Conduction is heat exchange between two surfaces in direct contact. Since the areas are usually small (feet in contact with the ground) during the day in most mammals, conduction is generally the least important in quantitative terms, and behavioral thermoregulation generally intervenes (e.g., wearing of insulated boots while walking on hot desert sand). However, lying uninsulated while sleeping on either hot or cold ground can result in significant heat exchange, especially in a person under the influence of vasodilating drugs or alcohol. A person can usually hold the handle of a very hot cooking pot with a dry towel (containing a large number of tiny cells filled with air) without discomfort. However, if the towel is wet (the cells are filled with water), it rapidly heats up because conduction of heat through water is much faster (32 times) than through air. Within a few seconds the pot becomes too hot to hold.

Convection. Convective heat exchange refers to heat transferred from a surface to a gas or fluid, usually air or water. It is a more complex process than conduction because the medium of heat transfer (air or water) is usually moving. The rate of heat exchange by convection depends on many variables, including the density of the fluid (e.g., water vs. air), the temperature gradient, the surface area exposed, and the flow rate of the fluid. Heat loss during cold water immersion is faster than standing nude in air because of the high thermal capacity of water, the greater body surface exposed, and the greater thermal conductivity of water.[400,406] Convective heat exchange varies with velocity of air movement. As T_{amb} rises to approach skin temperature (T_{sk}), heat loss becomes minimal. Once air temperature exceeds mean skin temperature, heat is gained by the body. Loose-fitting clothing maximizes convective and evaporative heat loss. By the same token, body motion alters heat exchange by convection both within (the air pocket between the skin surface and fabric) and on the surface of clothing.

Radiation. Radiation refers to the transfer of heat between the body and its surroundings by electromagnetic waves. All matter absorbs and emits thermal radiation,[471] which is the "radiant energy emitted by a medium that is due solely to the temperature of the medium." Clothing reduces the radiant heat impinging on the skin from industrial sources (e.g., boilers and motors), as well as the solar load in broad daylight. Solar load is a major source of heat gain in hot climates—up to 250 kcal/hr in a seminude man[185] (approximately the same as walking; see later discussion) and 100 kcal/hr in a clothed man. The amount varies with the angle of the sun, season, clouds, and other factors. Concurrently, clothing affects the evaporative process.

Highly pigmented skin is protected from ultraviolet radiation, but it absorbs approximately 20% more heat than does nonpigmented or relatively nonpigmented skin.[274] Increasing blood flow to the skin (BF_{sk}, at $T_{sk} > T_{amb}$) maximizes heat loss from the skin[219,420] by convection and radiation. Although heat is carried by convection and conduction from the body core to the skin, the main role of elevated BF_{sk} in a warm environment is to deliver the heat necessary to vaporize sweat.[189]

Evaporative Cooling. Evaporative, "wet," or insensible heat exchange is usually a one-way heat flow from a body surface to the environment. The heat of vaporization (2.45 J/kg) is "absorbed" slowly with an undetectable change in temperature of the skin or blood. As water is converted from a liquid to a gaseous state in insensible heat exchange, the rate of evaporation of water from the skin, and hence the cooling effect, is proportional to the difference between vapor pressures of water in sweat on the skin surface and that of the surrounding air. A lowered NaCl concentration in sweat increases this difference, hence increasing the rate of evaporation. Since acclimatization leads to lower sweat NaCl concentrations, this increases the sweat evaporation rate.[231]

If the body is unable to maintain thermal equilibrium by radiation, convection, and conduction and core temperature rises, sweating must occur to permit heat loss by vaporization of water.[189] Evaporative heat loss is accompanied by the loss of 580 kcal/L of water evaporated or heat loss of approximately 1 kcal/1.7 ml of sweat vaporized.

Since rates of gastric emptying and delivery of water to the intestines can exceed 1 L/hr, a 1 L/hr sweat rate appears sustainable without significant dehydration if fluid is consumed. Higher sweat rates (e.g., 1500 ml/hr) could theoretically achieve greater rates of heat loss (1500 ml/1.7 ml/kcal = 882 kcal) but are almost never achieved because some of the sweat drips off the skin and thus has no cooling effect. Moreover, these high sweat rates are often at the expense of total body water, since gastric emptying does not keep pace. Knochel[288] has estimated that 650 kcal/hr is a more reasonable figure for an upper limit of heat dissipation.

Certain parts of the body surface are more important than others in providing cooling through sweating. The scalp, face, and upper torso are most important. Only about 25% of total sweat is produced by the lower limbs.[512] Therefore, although wearing a shirt may be critical in the development of heat illness, wearing long or short pants is much less important. The wearing of protective headgear may be most important in the development of heat illness, as shown by a training exercise. In bareheaded persons, the exercise was merely grueling, but 33% of those wearing hats suffered heat illness casualties,[224] as cited in Porter.[397]

The maximum rate of sweat vaporization depends on air dryness and movement. In a hot climate, the limit to heat dissipation is a function of sweat rate and the "atmospheric cooling power," or maximal evaporative cooling capacity of the environment.[190,440] The environment's capacity to vaporize sweat varies primarily with humidity and also with wind velocity. As humidity approaches 100%, evaporative heat loss is minimized. The major effect of wind occurs in humid environments at a velocity between 0.5 and 5 m/sec.[141] Sweat that drips from the body provides no cooling, and sweat evaporated from clothing is considerably less efficient than sweat evaporated directly from skin.[141] Risk of hyperthermia increases with air temperature and humidity. As a result, military trainers and coaches tend to conduct early morning runs to avoid high T_{amb} and the increased incidence of heat illness in humid climates, despite the lower dry bulb temperatures (T_{db}). Sutton[482] pointed out that EHS is reported with increasing frequency during "fun runs" and marathons when the temperature is not particularly hot. This reinforces the simple definition that exertion-induced heatstroke occurs whenever the rate of heat production of an exercising individual exceeds the rate of heat loss, causing body temperature to rise to critical levels.

Heat Stress Indexes. The ability to work in a hot environment is inversely related to the prevailing heat stress level; the higher the heat stress level, the shorter the ability to carry out work and the greater the risk of heat illness. Safety in a hostile environment depends on following strict rules and limitations concerning exposure time and work intensity. The need for a quantitative index that combines environmental heat stress factors to provide a reliable and consistent correlation with the induced physiologic strain was recognized 100 years ago.[203]

In 1905, Haldane suggested the use of wet bulb temperature (T_w) as an index of the severity of a warm environment in Cornish tin mines.[203] T_w is lower than T_{db} because of the cooling effect of evaporation of water from the thermometer, which in turn, varies inversely with relative humidity (RH). However, the relationship between T_w and physiologic strain (rises in T_c, HR, respiratory rate, etc.) was not valid at high-humidity levels and in hot-dry climates.[33] In 1923, Houghten and Yaglou[238] developed the effective temperature (ET) index to define thermal comfort limits. This index was a combination of T_w, T_{amb}, and wind velocity (Va), and produced an equivalent thermal sensation. However, several deficiencies were recognized, including overestimation of the effects of T_{amb} at high temperatures and underestimation of Va in hot-wet climates.[33]

In 1957, Yaglou and Minard[535] suggested the wet bulb globe temperature (WBGT) index, which consisted of combining T_{amb}, T_w, and black globe temperature (T_g) according to unequal weights:

$$\text{For outdoor use: WBGT} = 0.7T_w + 0.2T_g + 0.1T_{amb}$$

$$\text{For indoor use: WBGT} = 0.7T_w + 0.3T_{amb}$$

However, calculation of WBGT involves measuring T_g from a thermometer surrounded by a 6-inch blackened sphere, which is inconvenient and not practical under many circumstances. Nevertheless, the WBGT index is the most widely used index to describe environmental heat stress for outdoor and indoor use and is used for setting limits of U.S. military training exercises in hot

weather.[69,117] It is also used to set limits in industrial plants,[369] by sports associations as guidance to prevent heat injury,[33,337] and by workers in different occupations as a safety index.[83,164,202,463] However, WBGT is limited for two main reasons: (1) it cannot be applied to persons wearing different types of clothing (e.g., protective clothing), and (2) measuring T_g is inconvenient. Wearing protective clothing imposes a higher heat stress equivalent to adding 6° to 11° C (10.8° to 19.8° F) to the WBGT index.[392] As a result, for WBGT to accurately reflect environmental stress, corrections and adjustments must be made for the type of clothing worn and the metabolic rate.[228,271]

Thus attempts were made to develop alternatives to WBGT. In 1971, Botsford[53] suggested the wet globe thermometer (WGT), known also as the Botsball, which combined measuring T_{amb}, T_w, and radiation into a single reading. Unfortunately, the WGT index did not provide adequate precision values for hot climates, and its readings were significantly lower than the WBGT index.[335]

In 1962, Sohar et al[470] suggested the discomfort index (DI), using a combination of T_{amb} and T_w, which has been used extensively in Israel. However, a recently modified DI (MDI) suggested altering constants to the parameters T_{amb} and T_w to achieve a better correlation with the WBGT index.[349] However, uncertainties in the radiation component in any heat stress index would limit its assessment (e.g., solar radiation measurement for the shade vs. open sky). The most widely used WBGT index is computed from three separate environmental measurements, and the equipment to measure this index is cumbersome and more suited to a fixed-site station than a mobile situation. Furthermore, measuring T_g by a black globe thermometer requires about 30 minutes for the instrument to reach equilibrium. Thus the need for a reliable portable field instrument for measurement of this heat stress index in a mobile situation (e.g., training in the field) is essential.

In a Marine training base with 17,000 to 25,000 recruits per year, clinical studies from the 1950s reported a large number of heat casualties occurring upon strenuous physical exercise when the WBGT was higher than 26.7° C (80° F).[344] As a result, new regulations and guidelines were implemented for different heat categories, which reduced the numbers of casualties. However, Kark et al[266] reported 1425 cases of exertional heat illness during the period of 1982-1991 and showed that 25% of the cases occurred between 7:00 to 9:00 AM at WBGT level of 26.7° C. These cases occurred in spite of the preventive measures taken on Parris Island, South Carolina, which involved rescheduling of training and physical activity according to newly categorized WBGT values. In addition, further attention was given to clothing, equipment, workloads, and hydration. Exertional heat illnesses continue to be a common problem during training in a warm environment despite preventive measures taken.[266] The WBGT index provides for measurement of heat load, but its practical application in current army doctrine is limited. If the "weather station" was alongside the trainees at the training site and the environmental measurements were taken continuously and not every hour, this might help in preventing some of the heat casualties.

Work and sports in a hot environment require a fairly accurate measurement of the stress index to prevent heat illnesses and to determine safety behavior patterns (e.g., water consumption rates and work/rest cycles). To implement the current guidelines and limitations for exercise in a hot climate, there is great need for development of an accurate, portable heat stress measurement device. We suggest that current technology, including very small electronic sensors to measure T_{amb} and RH, a miniature display, and a miniature programmable microprocessor for calculating and storing the MDI index, in a wristwatch format are already available to devise a new portable heat stress monitor. Such a tool could help in the decision-making process relating to permissible strain when working in a hostile environment, for use by medical monitors, leaders, or others directly exposed to heat stress. These measures would clearly help prevent heat illnesses and would decrease the dependency on weather station reports.

Temperature Regulation (See Also Chapter 11 and Box 10-1)

To prevent or appropriately manage heat illness, the clinician must understand thermal stress[161] and human thermoregulation.[189,214,480] Temperature regulation refers to both behavioral and autonomic thermoregulatory processes that modify the rates of heat production by shivering and variations in basal metabolism, and heat loss by sweating and peripheral vasomotor tone.[189] These processes act to maintain the temperature of the body within a restricted range with a variable internal or external heat load. The regulated temperature is generally considered that of the "body core," or T_c.

Behavioral Thermoregulation.
Hyperthermia appears to represent a more serious problem than hypothermia, since humans have developed a greater capacity for heat elimination (vasodilation, sweating) than for heat conservation (vasoconstriction).[159,214] To live, work, and reproduce successfully in arid or tropical climates, humans depend not only on physiologic mechanisms to acclimatize to heat but also on behavioral responses to assist temperature regulation. Thus humans possess two control systems (behavioral and physiologic) to regulate body temperature.

Although behavioral responses augmenting shivering seem obvious in a cold environment (e.g., seeking shelter, wearing clothes, and building fires), behavioral factors for thermoregulation in the heat (resting in the heat of the day, seeking shade or water when thirsty)

Box 10-1 COMMONLY HELD FALLACIES REGARDING HEAT ILLNESS*

1. The sine qua non for diagnosis of heatstroke includes hot, dry skin; temperature greater than 42° C; and coma.
2. Unlimited access to fluids allows the exercising individual to maintain adequate hydration despite heat stress.
3. Development of salt depletion heat exhaustion requires 4 to 5 days of exposure to marked heat stress.
4. Consumption of commercially available electrolyte-containing beverages during exercise in the heat tends to return plasma potassium levels to resting values.
5. The primary underlying mechanisms for the development of heat cramps are hypokalemia and hypovolemia.
6. Consumption of excessive volumes of fluid to the point of development of nausea promotes the maximal clearance of free water by the kidneys.
7. When the patient is evaluated in the emergency department, a normal body temperature when combined with normal serum transaminases precludes the diagnosis of heatstroke.
8. The most physiologically appropriate method to achieve rapid reduction in body temperature from hyperthermia is the use of warm air spray.
9. The risk of dilutional hyponatremia should preclude consumption of fluids in the absence of thirst.
10. Endotoxemia is a rare complication of ultramarathon running in the heat.
11. Review of the medical literature reveals that an individual sustaining a single episode of heatstroke remains at increased risk for future heat injury.
12. A high degree of aerobic conditioning, when combined with an appropriate period of heat acclimation, prevents the development of heat illness.
13. Adherence to published guidelines using wet bulb globe temperature to modify physical activity in the heat prevents the development of heat illness.
14. Carpopedal spasm is a relatively rare complication of exercise-induced heat exhaustion.
15. Violent shivering is a common complication in response to whole body cooling of patients with heat exhaustion.

*These fallacies are discussed in greater detail later in the chapter.

---

are also important. Behavioral responses are conscious actions, and therefore the subjective sensations of thermal discomfort inducing the behavior anticipate actual changes in T_c.[102]

Heat Production.
The basal metabolic rate of the average (70 kg) man in a sitting position amounts to approximately 50 to 60 kcal/hr/m[2] of body surface area or 100 kcal/hr.[292] With increased activity, metabolic heat production increases significantly (walking pro-

duces 250 to 300 kcal/hr; walking rapidly with a load, up to 400 to 450 kcal/hr) and may reach 20 times baseline level with strenuous exertion. Depending on the exercise task, usually 70% to 85% of the metabolic rate is released as heat that must be dissipated to maintain thermal balance. If there were no means to dissipate heat, the addition of 70 kcal to a 70-kg person would theoretically be able to increase core temperature approximately 0.8° C (1.4° F), assuming the average specific heat of the human body is 0.8 (kcal/kg/° C). Cellular metabolism increases 13% for each 1° C (1.8° F) rise in temperature until the body approaches heatstroke temperature; at that point, cellular metabolism increases more rapidly. It is 50% above normal at 40.6° C (105.1° F).[71]

Body Temperature Ranges. Normal internal temperatures range from 36° to 38° C (96.8° to 100.4° F), whereas the limits of body temperature for efficient thermoregulation are 35° to 40° C (95° to 104° F).[479] However, during athletic events, T_c increases to 40° to 42° C (104° to 107.6° F).[120,356,532] One marathoner was able to maintain a T_c greater than 41.5° C (106.7° F) for at least 44 minutes during a race.[329] Survival limits of body temperatures are exceptions to these ranges. For example, one heatstroke victim survived a measured T_c of 46.5° C (115.7° F). [466]

Sensing, Relaying, and Central Integration Functions. Physiologic temperature regulation involves detecting changes in body temperature by sensory mechanisms and relaying thermal signals from central and peripheral locations to a central integrative area. This directs effector organs to increase or decrease heat storage appropriately[189] and is mediated by the autonomic nervous system. Sensitive nerve endings within the hypothalamus and near the skin surface of most of the body act as thermoreceptors[224,361] to monitor T_c and T_{sk}.

The primary means of regulating T_c are (1) vasomotor alterations in blood flow and its distribution, (2) shivering, and (3) sweating. The threshold temperatures for sweating, BF_{sk}, and forearm venous volume depend on both T_c and T_{sk}. Heating the skin lowers these threshold temperatures.[94,438,517] At any given T_c heating the skin increases the effector response. Mathematical modeling suggests that T_c is nine times as important as T_{sk} in the reflex control of BF_{sk}.[436] However, the importance of T_{sk} should not be minimized; whereas T_c varies over a narrow range of 7° C (12.6° F), the variation in T_{sk} is threefold to fourfold as great, enabling the system to accommodate to a wide range of environmental temperatures.

During exercise, an increase in T_c elicits an effector response (sweating) with only a minimal change in T_{sk}. The rise in body temperature is proportional to the increased metabolic rate and does not depend on T_{amb}

over a wide range.[368] However, as anyone who has experienced heat exhaustion knows, this relationship does not hold under extremely hot or humid conditions or conditions of maximum effort. This disparity between theory and common experience gave rise to the concept of "prescriptive zone," or a set of conditions in which the magnitude of the core temperature response for everyday work was independent of the environmental temperature.[314]

The preoptic area of the anterior hypothalamus of the brain is generally believed to be the primary site for integration and generation of a "thermal command signal." This area contains many neurons that alter their firing rate in response to warming or cooling.[57] The brain is well perfused relative to its mass and responds rapidly to only a few tenths of 1° C (1.8° F) change in blood temperature.[40,41]

Sweating and skin vasodilation increased linearly above a "set point" temperature of approximately 37° C (98.6° F).[40,41] Local heating accelerates sweating. Thus central and peripheral mechanisms cause sweating when skin temperature is elevated. Local heating may result in a greater release of neurotransmitter for a given sudomotor signal,[137] or heating increases the sensitivity of the gland to a given dose of neurotransmitter.[376] Conversely, lower skin temperatures may inhibit sweating during exercise.[40] Since sweating is not completely abolished by cervical cord transection, spinal centers for temperature regulation appear to contribute.[491]

Set Point Hypothesis. The concept that the central nervous system is a functional interface ("central integrative area") between the thermosensors and thermoregulatory effectors is not accepted by all physiologists.[461] However, it provides a rationale for envisioning a thermostat, or "set point," that shifts all effector thresholds in the same direction.[189] This concept of a central thermostat provides a conceptual framework that fits a variety of situations.

The principal mechanisms involved in temperature regulation during exercise in the heat are venodilation, increased BF_{sk}, and sweating. Dilation of superficial veins increases the efficiency of heat flow from the core to skin and increases the time available for heat transfer between the blood and skin. The cutaneous vasculature is therefore an effector system in thermoregulation because BF_{sk} controls the rate of heat transfer between the body core and surface.[189,420] Unless the rate of heat storage exceeds the capacity of the thermoregulatory system (e.g., a breakdown of heat dissipation mechanisms), effector responses will increase until heat balance is restored.

Vasomotor System. The term vasomotor system refers only to the arterioles that control organ blood flow, vascular resistance, and arterial blood pressure.[420] Since arterioles and the heart together regulate blood pressure, a change in blood pressure is corrected by changes in vascular resistance or cardiac output (CO).[189,215,420] Vasomotor adjustments optimize and regulate the distribution of CO within and between different organ systems. Central thermal receptors alter vasomotor outflow to redirect blood flow to the skin. BF_{sk} in humans exposed to cold can be reduced to 1 ml/100g skin/min and can increase during maximal heat stress to 150 ml/100g skin/min, greater in the extremities than in the trunk.[231]

Blood flow to the skin is under dual vasomotor control. In the cold, adrenergic vasoconstrictor fibers reduce skin blood flow.[160] However, during heat exposure, blood flow increases to the hands, lips, nose, and ears as a result of vasodilation, largely because of the withdrawal of vasoconstrictor tone.[160] Active sympathetic vasodilation over most of the skin area[421] reduces vascular resistance below basal tone. There is a relationship between active sympathetic vasodilation and sweating, perhaps through the release of vasoactive intestinal polypeptide (VIP).[498] The simultaneous release of both transmitters (VIP and acetylcholine) could help explain the apparent relationship between eccrine sweat secretion and cutaneous vasodilation.[320]

Venomotor System. The venomotor system controls the veins; it should be noted, however, that there is a dual venous drainage of the limbs. The deep veins draining mainly from the muscles have relatively poor sympathetic innervation,[510] whereas the superficial veins draining the skin are richly innervated. Although venodilation and increased BF_{sk} enhance heat transfer,[192] they increase the amount of blood pooled in compliant peripheral vessels. As a consequence, filling of these veins reduces central blood volume; at some point, the redistribution of blood could compromise venous return and cardiac filling.[420,421] This system may be altered by fundamental changes in the smooth muscles of the various vessels. Heat increases the speed and extent of contraction of femoral arteries to K^+ and catecholamines (i.e., increases vascular resistance) and may therefore inappropriately slow blood flow to and from the extremities.[382]

CLASSIC HEATSTROKE

The pathologic features of heatstroke are similar irrespective of the cause of the heat illness and are manifested by swelling and degeneration of tissue and cell structures, and widespread microscopic to massive hemorrhages.[456] Most organs are congested, with increased masses and swollen cells. In the gastrointestinal tract, postmortem examination often shows massive ulcerations, hemorrhages, and engorged intestinal vessels.[456] A discussion of the gut is important in any dis-

cussion of heat illness for two reasons: (1) its function determines whether ingested fluid and solutes are delivered to the systemic circulation to correct losses and thereby attenuate hyperthermia, dehydration, and reductions in splanchnic blood flow and gut distress; and (2) heatstroke may result from or be exacerbated by gastrointestinal dysfunction, leading to "leakage" of gut-derived endotoxin into the circulation, endotoxemia, and circulatory collapse. There is an equivalence between the rehydration demand, the capacity of the stomach to deliver water (gastric emptying under optimal conditions can provide 1.8 L/hr) and the intestine to absorb (1.4 to 2.2 L/hr) ingested fluids.

Classic heatstroke occurs when environmental heat stress is maximal.[134,216,476] Populations at risk include the elderly, the poor (who lack adequate air conditioning), those who suffer from malnutrition, and those who have chronic diseases or substance addiction.[216] In classic heatstroke, in contrast to EHS, physical effort is *not* a primary determinant of excessive heat storage and therefore the onset of classic heatstroke is slower. Predisposing factors commonly intervene over days rather than minutes or hours. As a result, there is often ample time for fluid and electrolyte imbalances to develop.

Under some circumstances, passive hyperthermia can develop rapidly in extremely hot environments, such as when infants and small children are left in locked vehicles in the summer heat. This is also true for adults who are passengers in improperly ventilated or non–air-conditioned vehicles. Within minutes under desert conditions, cabins and cargo spaces of vehicles can reach 54° to 60° C (129.2° to 140° F), depending on environmental temperature (T_{amb}) and solar radiation.[242] Similar high temperatures may occur in closed or confined spaces, such as enclosed attics, or in places where there is a high radiant load from machinery or power plants, such as boiler rooms.[292] Individuals who depend on others for fluid intake because of age (the very young or the elderly) or illness are at risk of involuntary dehydration. Infants are more heat labile because of their immature thermoregulatory systems.[442] (See later discussion of thermoregulation in children.)

Epidemiology—Heat Waves

When environmental heat stress is maximal, strenuous exercise is not necessary to produce heat illness.[134,195,216,476] In Peking in 1743, a heat wave reportedly caused 11,000 deaths[456]; 411 cases of severe heatstroke in Nanjing were reported.[326] During the July 1996 Atlanta Olympics there were 1059 heat casualties reported, of which 88.9% were spectators and volunteers.[520] In a separate heat wave,[150] 42 of 44 cases occurred within 8 consecutive days during which the maximum ambient temperature varied from 38.9° to 41.1° C (102° to 106° F). The patients' local environment temperatures were probably much higher, since air conditioning was not widely available at the time.

Only 7 of 44 persons were less than 50 years of age, and the greatest frequency of age distribution was in the range of 60 to 70 years.

In Boulder City, Nevada, July 8 to 18, 1936, T_{amb} reached higher than $38.3°$ C ($100.9°$ F) daily. Forty-four heatstroke victims were admitted to the Boulder City Hospital with progressively increasing daily admission rates during that period.[119] The increasing number of admissions over time suggests that there is a progressive deterioration of the body with prolonged hot weather. This may be related to elevated cytokine levels. In a different heat wave near Dallas, Texas, lasting 26 days, the first case occurred on day 10 of the heat wave and the last case occurred 10 days after the end of the heat wave, with half the cases (14 of 28) occurring over a 3-day period on days 20 to 22. Age was a factor in both heat waves, with 8 of 72 victims above 80 years of age, and a mean age of 59 years in Boulder City and 70.5 years in Dallas. Alcoholism and degenerative diseases were contributing factors in both waves. The victims characteristically had a high rectal temperature (T_{re}) and dry skin, and half of the Boulder City patients and 24 of 28 Dallas patients were comatose. Of the 44 Boulder City patients, 23 showed a fiery red skin rash over the body, particularly over the chest, abdomen, and back.[119] The most common presentation in Dallas patients was that of respiratory alkalosis, often accompanied by metabolic acidosis.[216] All Dallas patients with blood lactate greater than only 3.3 mMol/L (normal range 0.6 to 1.8 mMol/L) suffered a poor outcome, whereas those with initial lactate less than 3 mMol/L did well. That is, what in exercise studies would be only modest elevations in blood lactate become adverse prognostic indicators in classical heatstroke. Furthermore, 9 of 28 classic heatstroke patients arriving with normal serum potassium subsequently became hypokalemic, and all victims were hypokalemic at some point in their course.[216]

A heat wave in Chicago in July 1995 resulted in more than 600 deaths, and more than 3300 emergency department visits and intensive care unit admissions for near-fatal heatstroke. In a group of 58 of these victims with classic heatstroke, 100% experienced multiorgan dysfunction with neurologic impairment, 52% showed moderate to severe renal insufficiency, 45% had disseminated intravascular coagulopathy, and 10% had acute respiratory distress syndrome. Fifty-seven percent of the victims had infections on admission. In-hospital mortality was 21%.[112]

During a July 1988 heat wave in Nanjing, at least 4500 cases of heat illness cases were treated, with 411 of them classified severe.[538] (See Table 10-1 and Box 10-2.) The mean age for males and females was 69.5 and 75.6 years, respectively, and persons over 60 years of age accounted for 77.4% of total deaths. Interestingly, some of these victims showed severe *overhydration*,

TABLE 10-1. Core Temperature of Heatstroke Victims in Nanjing, July 1988

T_c ON ADMISSION (°C)	DEATH RATE (%)	NUMBER OF DEATHS*
<39	11.5	52
39-39.9	13.4	112
40-40.9	31.0	126
41-41.9	40.0	85
>42	83.3	36

Data from Zhi-cheng M, Yi-tang W: *Chinese Med J* 104:256, 1991.
*Overall deaths = 124/411 (30.2%). Victims older than 60 years accounted for 77.4% of all deaths.

Box 10-2 COMPLICATIONS AND SYMPTOMS OF HEATSTROKE VICTIMS IN NANJING, JULY 1988

COMPLICATIONS (%)
Various chronic diseases (24.5)
Hypertension (24.3)
Coronary artery disease (6.1)
Diabetes mellitus (5.8)
Obesity (5.3)
Cardiac insufficiency (4.6)
Cerebral vascular accidents (4.1)
Chronic bronchitis (1.7)
Neoplasm (1.7)

SYMPTOMS (RATE %)
Headache (35.5)
Dizziness (29.2)
Weakness (29.2)
Incontinence (19.2)
Thirst (19)
Numbness of extremities (14.4)
Dysphagia and dysphonia (7.1)
Kinetic imbalance (2.4)
T >40° C (60.1)
Delirium (14.8)
Coma (45.3)
Convulsions (31.6)
Xerosis and hot skin (46.7)
Moist skin (3.2)

Data from Zhi-cheng M, Yi-tang W: *Chinese Med J* 104:256, 1991.

with electrolyte values falling to as low as Na^+ 98, K^+ 2.1, Ca^{2+} 1.52, and Cl^- 97.4 mMol/L.

During 5 heat wave years (1952-1955 and 1966) the average number of heatstroke or heat exhaustion deaths in the United States jumped from 179 to 820 deaths per year.[138,139] In addition, the number of deaths classified as heat-precipitated was more than 8000 during heat wave years. There appears to be a reluctance to certify heatstroke or heat exhaustion as a cause of death, and epidemiologic estimates of the incidence are probably conservative.[456] As an example, heat-related death rates in the Chicago July 1995 heat wave were calculated by two methods: classification of heat-related deaths by the Cook County Medical Examiner's Office (CCMEO) and the excess mortality rates based on total mortality differentials during and before the heat wave. This analysis showed an underestimation of heat-related deaths in areas with high death rates. These results indicate that current practice does not adequately measure actual heat-related deaths. Nevertheless, those numbers may still be practical to use as an indicator to target specific communities for prevention and relief efforts.[455]

Hyperthermia commonly occurs in the presence of numerous and varied host factors.[27,242] These include many that affect thermoregulation through altering heat loss mechanisms (e.g., lack of acclimatization, fatigue, lack of sleep, dehydration, skin disorders), whereas others contribute to heat production (e.g., obesity, lack of physical fitness, dehydration, febrile illness, sustained exercise).

Classic heatstroke tends to be a disease of the elderly, the alcoholic, and the infirm. EHS is different, typically affecting young, healthy, and even euhydrated men and women during exercise, and is a syndrome involving hyperventilation and respiratory alkalosis.[59]

EXERTIONAL HEATSTROKE

Physical training increases heat tolerance, whereas a sedentary lifestyle decreases it. A sedentary lifestyle leads to a loss of muscle protein and strength and gain of fat. As a result, more energy is required to carry out any given physical task per gram of body mass, consequently increasing metabolic heat production. Physical training improves tolerance to heat mainly by improving efficiency of the cardiovascular system, increasing the rate of sweat production, and reducing the threshold T_c at which cooling mechanisms are activated.[16]

Within certain body temperature limits, normal thermoregulatory mechanisms are capable of restoring T_c to 37° C (98.6° F) from either hyperthermia or hypothermia. However, if T_c rises to approximately 42° C (107.6° F), then metabolic pathways may be so altered that inappropriate physiologic responses occur. Vascular collapse, shock, and death can follow unless countermeasures such as cooling and volume therapy are initiated. It is not certain whether there is a single critical intracellular derangement occurring at 42° C that ultimately leads to the activation of many harmful metabolic pathways and heatstroke death, or if several harmful pathways become established independently at about the same time in response to the given T_c.

EHS often affects fit and highly motivated individuals participating in sporting events or undergoing performance tests, such as those for military recruits and firefighter and police officer candidates. There will be increases in exertional heat illness because of the increased numbers of individuals participating in sports[216,288,289] and fitness activities, such as jogging,[212] fun-running,[246,367,408,483] bicycling,[456] and long-distance sporting events.[215,532] For example, an estimated 25 million Americans and 1 million Canadians participate in organized road races annually.[216]

EHS has been reported during every season, even in winter. During a winter night a father totally covered his 9-month-old infant with a blanket and a thick quilt because its crying disturbed his sleep. In the morning the child was found dead with many petechial hemorrhages in the upper chest and thoracic viscera, the blood was concentrated (indicating dehydration), and the bedclothes were extremely wet with sweat. This was listed as an accidental death resulting from exertional self-overheating in bed.[539]

Heat Storage Rate

A temperature of 40.4° C (104.7° F) represents a threshold hyperthermia above which heatstroke mortalities occur in exercised, heat-stressed rats.[244,245] The increase in an individual's heat storage, as shown by a rise in T_c, may be rapid (minutes to hours) and metabolic in origin because of overloaded heat loss mechanisms. For brief periods of intense effort, heat production may exceed 1000 kcal/hr.[390] An Olympic marathoner produced metabolic heat in excess of 1400 kcal/hr.[17] Under conditions that limit heat dissipation, such as high humidity or impermeable clothing, this rate of heat storage would cause body temperature to rise approximate 0.5° C/min (0.9° F/min) and produce heatstroke within 10 to 12 minutes. Even under a moderate workload (300 kcal/hr), a person who cannot sweat effectively and thereby dissipate heat can experience a rise in T_c of 5° C/hr (9° F/hr).[356,390]

Others at increased risk of exertional heat illness because of occupation include miners,[531] heavy industry workers,[123,129] and individuals in the military.[70,322,323,344] The yearly pilgrimage to Mecca has resulted in hundreds of fatalities from heat illness.[277] Wearing impermeable garments during physical activity leads to rapid loss of sweat, overload of heat loss mechanisms, and hyperthermia. These events may occur voluntarily (e.g., dieters, wrestlers) or by occupation (e.g., firefighters, hazardous waste handlers). Some cases of EHS have a genetic component.[381]

Failed thermoregulation can have its origin in the dysfunction of either central (hypothalamic) control or peripheral responses of heat loss mechanisms (sweating and vasodilation). A variety of drugs and toxins can produce hyperthermia and are implicated in some cases of severe heat illness.[4,5]

Individuals at Higher Risk

To preserve body temperature in its optimal range of 36.5° to 38.5° C (97.7° to 101.3° F), and to prevent an increase above 40.5° C (104.9° F), it is essential that the body delicately balance metabolic heat production, dry heat exchange, and evaporative heat dissipation. This requires highly developed and effective mechanisms of thermoregulation and temperature sensation. Heatstroke can be completely prevented by providing proper health education and following some simple regulations.[451,452] Prompt recognition, attention, and treatment usually result in complete recovery from heatstroke.

Preventive measures include acclimation to environmental conditions, adjusting physical efforts to match physical fitness, scheduling training to avoid the warmer hours of the day, establishing regulations to induce proper rehydration, and commanding adequate rest periods during activity. The medical team supervising the event should play a major role in preventing exertional heat illness during strenuous physical activity. It should also have the authority to cancel any strenuous activity whenever weather conditions are adverse. Before exercise, medical personnel must examine and evaluate each subject predisposed to heatstroke and, if necessary, exclude him or her from the activity. These measures were successfully implemented in the Israeli Defense Forces (IDF) and have been in practice there for many years. Recently these criteria also became an official position offered by the American College of Sports Medicine.[8]

Heat-susceptible persons include those who are obese, unfit, dehydrated, unacclimated; (perhaps) those with a previous history of heatstroke; and those who suffer from acute febrile illness, diarrhea, or chronic disturbances of the sweating mechanism. These persons carry risk factors for heat illnesses and should be prevented from participating in strenuous exercise, particularly in hot environments.[142] Prescription drugs or drug abuse are among the acquired factors that underlie heat intolerance and may predispose individuals to excessive heat strain by altering thermoregulatory functions physiologically or behaviorally. Potentially harmful drugs include diuretics, anticholinergics, vasodilators, antihistamines, central nervous system inhibitors, muscle relaxants, tranquilizers and sedatives, β-blockers, amphetamines, and tricyclic antidepressants.[380]

Most EHS victims are highly motivated, young, healthy individuals who exert themselves beyond their physiologic capacity (Box 10-3). In a recent review of 82 cases of EHS in soldiers,[143] it was found that most cases occurred during basic training (57%) and an additional 21% occurred during screening tests for special forces—in which motivation is a key issue. Most of the EHS cases occurred in highly motivated but relatively unfit soldiers. Overmotivated soldiers misinformed the medical team regarding various issues that otherwise would have prevented their participation in the activity and therefore resulted in heatstroke.[451] Shapiro and Moran[451] concluded that in the young, active population, physiologic maladaptation is associated mainly with lack of acclimatization, dehydration, presence of infectious diseases or skin disorders, fatigue, and overweight. Although an internal "alarm system" should warn the human body to cease physical activity, during thermoregulatory maladaptation, it fails in the individual

---

Box 10-3 EXERTIONAL HEATSTROKE IN THE FIELD

The following historical narrative from the middle of the nineteenth century describes vividly the devastating impact of heat and dehydration on a military unit in Texas during the Indian Wars, excerpted from "A Cavalry Detachment Three and a Half days Without Water" by CPT J.H.T. King, Assistant Surgeon, U.S. Army Post Surgeon, Fort Concho, Texas:

. . . The next day found them still marching onwards, and the mid-day tropical heat causing great suffering. The desire for water now became uncontrollable. The most loathsome fluid would now have been accepted to moisten their swollen tongues and supply their inward craving. The salivary and mucous secretions had long been absent, their mouths and throats were so parched that they could not swallow the Government hard bread . . .

Vertigo and dimness of vision affected all; they had difficulty in speaking, voices weak and strange sounding, and they were troubled with deafness, appearing stupid to each other, questions having to be repeated several times before they could be understood; they were also very feeble and had a tottering gait. Many were delirious . . . As the horses gave out they cut them open and drank their blood . . . (which) was thick and coagulated instantly on exposure; nevertheless, at the time it appeared more delicious than anything they had ever tasted.

This horse blood quickly developed into diarrhea, passing though the bowels almost as soon as taken; their own urine which was very scanty and deep colored, they drank thankfully, first sweetening it with sugar. The inclination to urinate was absent and micturition performed with difficulty. A few drank the horses' urine, although at times it was caught in cups and given to the animals themselves. They became oppressed with dyspnea and a feeling of suffocation as though the sides of the trachea were adhering . . . prolonging the intervals between each inspiration as much as possible, . . . their lips . . . were . . . covered with a whitish, dry froth and had a ghostly, pale, lifeless appearance as though they would never be opened again. Their fingers and the palm of their hands looked shriveled and pale; some who had removed their boots suffered from swollen feet and legs.

who is overmotivated and/or under peer pressure. The most common underlying factors for heat sensitivity that may lead to heatstroke are summarized in Box 10-4.

Mechanisms of temperature regulation have close functional relationships with other homeostatic mechanisms, that is, regulation of blood pressure, body fluid volumes, electrolytes, and acid-base balance.[451] When these are intact, the thermoregulatory system has the physiologic potential to cope appropriately with any strain resulting from exercise-induced metabolic heat production. This will protect the body from the hazards involved with excessive heat accumulation and elevated body temperature. The defense from the threatening combination of intense physical effort (high metabolic rate) and low environmental potential to

evaporate sweat (high humidity) is expressed by several body alarms that ultimately should result with cessation of physical activity. The subjective "alarm" may be caused by the thermoregulatory system and expressed by elevated body temperature or by the cardiovascular system and manifested by elevated HR.[451] Heatstroke is a maladaptive state whereby the body temperature exceeds a temperature of 40.5° C (104.9° F) or greater, depending upon the severity of any recent exercise, as a result of the mismatch between heat production and heat dissipation.

Imbalances in fluids and electrolytes are common during hot spells, especially when salt losses in sweat are compounded by loss of appetite. Fluid and electrolyte losses resulting from illness (diarrhea or vomiting) often contribute to heat illness. In some cases, dehydration is the primary cause of death.[456]

Sleep deprivation has an insidious effect. Prolonged sleep deprivation is fatal in animals, leading to immunosuppression and a sepsis-like death. That is, sleep is essential for optimal immune function.[38] During hyperthermia, sleep deprivation increases the T_c threshold for the onset of sweating and, in women, reduces BF_{sk}.[118,303] During moderate-intensity exercise, this delayed sweating onset reduced BF_{sk} in the heat, decreased total body sweat rate, reduced evaporative and dry heat loss, and led to elevated T_c.[435] On the other hand, hyperthermia may disrupt the sleep-state pattern, decreasing the duration of rapid eye movement (REM) episodes, thereby degrading the quality of sleep and imposing a psychologic stress.[175]

Combinations of factors that create a threat may be subtle. The presence of air conditioning in the home, workplace, and transportation may decrease the risk for the development of classic heatstroke. However, by diminishing the state of heat acclimatization and respect for the environment, air conditioning may increase a person's risk for developing EHS. Intense and prolonged exposure during weekends and holidays accounts for many cases of sunburn and heat illness.

Military Training

From 1942 to 1944, there were at least 198 deaths from heat illness during military training in the United States.[440] Gardener et al[177] recently studied exertional heat illnesses in Marine recruits at Parris Island. During 12-week basic training of Marine recruits, the rate of exertional heat illness depended upon fitness. These rates correlated with body mass index (BMI) and time-to-complete a 1½-mile run during the first week of the training. Those recruits with a BMI greater than 22 kg × m^{-2} and a run-time greater than 12 minutes had eight times the risk for developing heat illness than those with lower values.[177] In this study of 217,000 Marine recruits (90% male, 80% age 18-20 years), there were 1454 cases of exertional heat illness, with 89%

Box 10-4   RISK FACTORS FOR EXERTIONAL HEAT ILLNESS

FUNCTIONAL-PHYSIOLOGIC

Dehydration
Poor physical fitness
Lack of acclimatization
Heat illnesses history (controversial)
Obesity
Age
Fatigue
Pregnancy

CONDITIONAL CIRCUMSTANCES

Hot climate
External load
Inadequate rest periods
Impermeable clothing
Insulated materials
Missed meals

CONCURRENT DISEASES AND CONGENITAL ABNORMALITIES

CNS lesions
Sweat gland dysfunction
Infectious diseases
Diabetes mellitus
Skin disorders
Diarrhea

DRUGS

Drug abuse
Medications
Alcohol
Caffeine

PSYCHOLOGIC STRESS

Overmotivation
Peer pressure

men and 11% women,[177] and with a peak rate of 2% of recruits in summer. The frequency of reported cases closely correlated with daily heat load (a combination of T_w, T_{db}, and solar radiation) but did not correlate well with T_{amb}. Most cases occurred between 7:00 and 9:00 AM, during training that would have been restricted at elevated T_{amb} later in the day. During those hours, the rate of heat casualties increased substantially as WBGT increased, beginning at levels as low as 18.3° C (65° F). At WBGT of 23.9° to 26.7° C (75° to 80° F), heat illness rates increased 26-fold (over baseline rates at T_{amb} < 18.3° C [65° F]) and 39-fold for the day before exercise. Exposure to WBGT of greater than 80° F was infrequent (25%) among the early morning cases at the time of illness. However, a fascinating observation was made: on the day before illness, high T_{amb} was common (87%), suggesting a prolonged biochemical/physiologic effect of heat exposure.[266] Regardless of the current temperature, if the day before was cool, the frequency of heat cases was low; if it was hot, the frequency was high. Since the recruits were forced to drink large amounts of water, enough to keep them urinating during the night, elevated rate of heat casualties could not have been related to an accumulated dehydration from the day before. *The presence of a high environmental temperature caused an unspecified physiologic predisposition to heatstroke lasting for at least a day.*

Thus even following widely published guidelines based on WBGT for physical activity does not preclude risks. Perhaps a better index should be developed. High rates of metabolic heat production (e.g., running) combined with conditions that limit evaporative heat loss (e.g., high relative humidity, impermeable garments) appear to present a significant risk regardless of T_{db}. Furthermore, prevention is complicated by the observation that conditions on the prior day contribute to the current risk of heatstroke.

Gender differences were found for the incidence of heat illnesses. Female rates were higher during the early hot season (May) and male rates were higher than those for females in the late hot season (September). Although May was cooler than September, there was a higher overall rate in May, probably reflecting less acclimatization in the spring. Comparing the days of the week, only 1.1% of casualties occurred on Sundays, reflecting decreased physical activity. In another study, obesity increased the risk of heat disorders in soldiers training in a hot and humid environment (Singapore).[89]

In the IDF, 82 cases (of 150 suspected) were positively diagnosed as EHS from 1988 to 1996.[143] More than 50% of these cases occurred during the first 6 months in service, mainly in summer (June-September), but 30% of the cases occurred during the spring, and some cases occurred during the winter season. EHS was not related to time of the day. Many cases occurred during the night

or early morning, even under mild heat load. Interestingly, evaluated by the heat load index,[470] 40% of the cases occurred during very short activities, whereas 60% occurred within the first 2 hours of exercise. The temperature regulation mechanism is efficient and the potential core-to-periphery conductance and sweating rate in the 82 heatstroke victims were higher than needed. Therefore EHS is more likely to occur when there is a severe thermal imbalance as a consequence of disturbance in the homeostatic mechanism aggravated by one or more predisposing factors[451] (see Box 10-4).

Although heatstroke may be due to accident, lack of knowledge, poor judgment, or neglect, it is a preventable illness. Therefore cases of fatal heatstroke should be investigated for criminal intent. For instance, in the IDF, almost all cases of EHS occurred when regulations were not strictly followed.[143] In a most unusual incident, an herbalist was convicted of manslaughter in Australia[338] because he "treated" a young boy by immersing him for 40 minutes in a heap of fermenting horse manure, and the boy died of heatstroke. Educational efforts by both the media and the health care community aimed at parents of small children during heat waves should be made with the same enthusiasm as public service announcements of windchill factors during subzero temperatures. If participants develop heat injuries during sporting events that occur in hot weather outside the heat stress guidelines, coaches and organizers of the event should be held legally responsible. The military has long recognized the preventable nature of heat injuries that result from the intense physical activity in hot weather; a passage in the June 10, 1865 *Lancet* reads: "Commanding Officers of volunteers are very apt to err in this particular; and the spirit of their men is such that they shrink from complaint and persevere in efforts which may easily, under a burning sun, become dangerous to life."

Sports

EHS is a true sports emergency. There are several reports each year of heat illnesses with some fatal results, especially in competitive games. Incidence and mortality statistics for athletes are difficult to ascertain, but some have been reported. Undoubtedly, the incidences of unreported nonfatal heatstrokes are higher. From 1990 to 1995, there were 84 reported deaths resulting from heatstroke in athletes participating in American football.[399] In 1995, five American high school football players were reported to have died of heatstroke.[432] Interior linemen are at higher risk because of the their large muscle bulk. The uniform worn by football players covers almost the entire body and adds to heat load. In a 10-year study, 10% of 136 American high school and college athlete deaths were caused by EHS.[500] In the Falmouth, Massachusetts, road race, there are between 10 and 15 heatstroke victims every year.[432] Cyclists and tennis players, in particular, tend to have great problems with dehydration, the cyclists because their sweat evaporates rapidly as they ride causing them to underestimate their fluid loss.[222] In tennis, the duration of the game varies considerably and drinking is permitted only during changeover. The players' sweating rates can reach 2 L/hr, which presents a practical challenge for adequate fluid volume replacement.[43] In soccer, 4.5% of injuries in 480 games were related to heat illnesses.[279] Marathon runners thermoregulate at elevated core temperature (~40° C [104° F]) during a run, and approximately 0.6% of the runners suffer from heat illnesses.[396]

Training Injuries

Although it is clear that the rate of heat illnesses is greater in summer than in winter, the development of musculoskeletal and other injuries is a less obvious consequence of seasonal variations in climate. During basic military training, the incidence of musculoskeletal injuries severe enough to cause a time loss is higher in summer than in fall.[286] That is, the injury rate increases with temperature and at T_{amb} = 33.3° C (92° F) is 2.6 times as high as that at T_{amb} = 16.7° C (61° F) for men and 1.8 times as high for women. This effect is also seen in elite athletes[296] and in British professional rugby players, with summer seasons showing almost double the injury rate of winter (696.8/1000 hours and 363.6/1000 hours, respectively).[393] In various studies, women had 1.5 to 3 times the injury rate of men.[287] Risk factors for injury are poor physical fitness, cigarette smoking, physical inactivity, longer running distances, and use of old running shoes (those 6 months to 1 year old more than doubled the injury rate).[176] Other risk factors for injury include older age, high-arched feet, and being "knock-kneed."[286]

Heat Strain Indexes

How can one best quantify the dyshomeostasis and body injury, or the inability to maintain T_c at the level prescribed by the thermoregulatory center,[203] resulting from exercise and heat? Heat strain is not simply a matter of T_c alone because heatstroke and other heat illnesses could may occur at T_c less than 41° C (105.8° F). During the last century, environmental parameters and physiologic variables were combined to develop a unified heat strain index. Although more than 20 heat strain indexes have been described, none are accepted as a universal physiologic strain index. The main reasons for their lack of generality are related to the number and complexity of the interactions among recognized determining factors and their limited validity.

The existing indexes can be divided into two main categories: (1) "effective" temperature (ET) scales[238] based on meteorologic parameters only (e.g., ambient temperature, T_w, and T_g) and in which the WBGT index is derived[535]; and (2) "rational" heat scales that include a combination of environmental and physiologic parameters (e.g., radiative and convective heat transfer, evaporative capacity of the environment, and rate of metabolic heat production). ET indexes have been widely applied to both assess and predict heat strain but cannot accurately account for different levels of metabolic rate, and different types of clothing (e.g., encapsulating).[271,392]

In 1937 the operative temperature index was developed,[527] which combined the rates of metabolic heat production (M), heat transfer between the body and the environment (H_{r+c}) and the evaporative capacity of the environment to dissipate heat (E_{max}).[34] Its best known modification is the Heat Strain Index (HSI), which relates total evaporation required (E_{req}, the sum of M and H_{r+c}) to E_{max}. HSI is widely accepted because it combines environmental variables and body activity. However, in certain situations, the heat strain was seriously in error and further modifications have not been fully satisfactory.[34,228] HSIs based on physiologic parameters were also suggested but found unsatisfactory.[304] Collectively, although many HSIs were developed, some simple to apply, others highly complex, all were found to be valid only under certain specific conditions.

Recently, Moran et al[350] introduced a new physiologic strain index (PSI) based upon adding equally-weighted the individual strains of T_{re} and heart rate (HR), which represent the combined strains of thermoregulatory and cardiovascular systems. Each strain system was scaled 0 to 5. Thus the PSI is scaled 0 to 10 and can be calculated continuously on-line or during data analysis. The PSI can be applied at any time whenever T_c and HR are measured, including during rest or recovery periods, unlike some of the other indexes.[350] In a recent series of studies, PSI successfully evaluated the strains generated by different clothing ensembles, climatic conditions, different levels of hydration, and exercise intensity for gender during heat stress, for different age groups during acclimatization, and during acute exercise heat stress.[348,351] Furthermore, this index, when adjusted for animal values, successfully rated and correctly discriminated between trained and acclimated rats exposed to exercise heat stress.[352]

PSI differs from previous indexes. It is easier to interpret and use than other indexes available and includes the ability to assess rest and recovery periods. PSI overcomes the shortcomings of previously described indexes and can be used over a wide range of conditions.

Heat strain is well known to correlate with environmental heat load and metabolic heat production, resulting in higher values of T_{re}, HR, and T_{sk}, and a reduced ability to maintain exercise. Various types of clothing with different degrees of water permeation create microclimates differing from that of the environment and lead to higher strains. The combination of different climates, impermeable garments, and hydration levels during different exercise intensities is a challenge for assessment of the individual physiologic strain. However, in two recent studies when different HSIs were applied to quantify the heat strain, PSI was successful at all levels of heat exposure while the other indexes were limited in their abilities.[350] The applicability of PSI was further successfully shown for various sweat rates and relative exercise intensities in different climates and for exercise heat stress and gender at different combinations of exercise intensity and climate.[348]

Gender

In many experiments, women exposed to acute heat stress and exercise thermoregulated less effectively than did men, resulting in the general conclusion that women are less heat-tolerant than are men.[340,453,459] However, in most studies, women generally had lower cardiorespiratory fitness, higher percentage of body fat, lower body weight, lower body surface area, and higher surface area–to–mass ratio than men.[316,387,391] Those physiologic differences are probably not intrinsically gender-specific but result from inequalities in fitness and acclimatization attributable to differences in lifestyle.[372] When such variables were controlled, most of the physiologic differences were narrowed, although mean sweat rate (msw) still remained lower for women.[10,186,340,533] Stephenson and Kolka[474] suggested that the apparent physiologic differences in msw were based on comparing unmatched genders, mainly aerobically fit men to relatively unfit women. They argued that most of the studies comparing responses of men and women were not controlled for menstrual cycle phase and thus were limited in their conclusions. Furthermore, Sawka et al[437] concluded that when men and women were matched for aerobic fitness, they then had similar heat tolerances and body temperature responses during exercise in the heat. For instance, acclimatized men and women have comparable responses to rest and exercise in a desert environment.[514] However, hormonal fluctuations of estrogen and progesterone concentrations associated with the menstrual cycle may alter women's performance and tolerance to exertional heat stress.[316] In a recent study, Moran et al[351] applied the PSI in three climates to evaluate the strain of men and women who were matched for maximal aerobic power (Ap$\dot{V}O_2$max) and intensity for 60 minutes. All subjects underwent a matrix of nine experimental combinations of three different exercises.[23,260,437] The PSI confirmed previous studies that when men and women were matched for Ap$\dot{V}O_2$max and selected physiologic parameters, there is no difference in strain between the two groups.

For middle-aged women, the effects of hormone replacement therapies on the thermoregulatory system

were studied.[65,66,186,489] The luteal phase, with its increased progesterone-to-estrogen ratio, was associated with an elevated T_c, whereas elevated levels of unopposed estrogen were associated with a lower T_c at rest and during exercise heat stress.[489]

In summary, although mean physiologic responses to exercise heat stress suggest poorer thermoregulation for women, this is not necessarily an intrinsic gender difference but reflects a combination of social factors serving to reduce fitness in women.

Aging

In general, middle-aged and older men and women are less tolerant to heat and exercise, suffering more physiologic strain than younger individuals.[237,505] They developed higher HR, T_{sk}, and T_c and lower msw than younger men and women during exercise heat stress. However, it is uncertain whether this is related to age per se or to other factors, such as disease states, decreased physical activity, and lowered aerobic fitness.[386]

A subgroup of middle-aged men who were "habitually active" displayed the same strains to acute exercise heat tolerance and acclimated to heat at about the same rate and degree as when they were younger.[414] Some studies on aging emphasize the importance of aerobic fitness and physical characteristics, such as body fat and body weight in maintaining work heat tolerance. In one study, old and young men and women were matched for Ap$\dot{V}O_2$max, surface area, and surface area–to–mass ratio but differed in age by 35 years.[272] During 75 minutes of light exercise at 37° C (98.6° F) and 60% RH, all groups showed the same degree of physiologic strain. In 1988, Pandolf et al[388] compared responses to acute heat tolerance between young and middle-aged men who were matched for Ap$\dot{V}O_2$max and morphologic factors. The middle-aged mens' tolerance times were actually half an hour longer than the younger mens' during the first day of acclimation (49° C [120.2° F], 20% RH) and they were also at a thermoregulatory advantage during the few days of heat acclimation, although both groups eventually acclimated to the same absolute degree. However, in these studies the middle-aged men were more chronically active than the younger men before heat acclimation. Under different environmental conditions, such as 30° C (86° F) with 80% RH and 40° C (104° F) with 20% RH, no differences were seen between the two groups.[467] In summary, when properly matched subjects are studied, heat stress of middle-aged men resulted in either the same or reduced physiologic strain as that of younger men.

CELLULAR HEATSTROKE

Whatever physiologic derangements occur in the whole body as a result of overheating, some primary derangements must first occur in individual cells.

Subcellular Disruption

Heating alters subcellular structures in many cell types, including detachment of cortical microfilaments from the plasma membrane,[99,133] collapse of the cytoskeleton, swelling of the mitochondria and the endoplasmic reticulum,[50] and disaggregation of polyribosomes and nucleoli.[80,339] Furthermore, heating increases membrane fluidity, grossly distorting the plasma membranes and forming bulges known as "blebs."[30,113,402] Blebs alter membrane function,[13] increasing membrane permeability[494] with solute leakage.[404,424] Such changes are not necessarily lethal; up to a point, the bleb formation may be adaptive, increasing cell survival.[51,261] Red blood cells undergo rearrangements in their cytoskeleton with heat, but rather than forming blebs, they form spheroids at elevated temperatures.[206] These enlarged spherically shaped cells are much less efficient at gas exchange than are normal red blood cells and probably contribute to reduced Po_2 in the tissues at elevated temperatures. Spheroid formation has been found in athletes during long-distance running and may contribute to their physical collapse during exercise.[206]

Apoptosis

Cells are destroyed within the body by the processes of apoptosis and necrosis. In apoptosis, certain individual cells within the body are genetically programmed to die. In this process, cells are broken into small vesicles containing condensed chromatin surrounded by intact cell membranes and are phagocytosed by neighboring cells. During necrosis, a variety of factors, including inflammation, cause swelling, destruction of the plasma membrane, and spewing of cell contents into the environment.[332] Apoptosis may be induced by a variety of stressors, including hyperthermia, aging, and certain toxins (*Pseudomonas* endotoxin, diphtheria toxin, and ricin).[131] A few minutes' exposure to temperatures of 41.5° to 42° C (106.7° to 107.6° F) triggers apoptosis in both cultured mammalian cells and experimental animals by activating Jun N-terminal kinase (JNK).[101,428] The organs producing the greatest number of apoptotic cells from whole body hyperthermia are the thymus, spleen, lymph nodes, and mucosa of the small intestine. The heat shock protein HSP-70 (see below) prevents this activation and contributes to acquired thermotolerance in mammalian cells.[166]

Ionic Changes

Ions do not readily cross lipid bilayers despite their large concentration gradients across plasma membranes. In general, they require specialized channels or carriers to do so. Membrane channels are proteins that contain hydrophilic "pores" penetrating the lipid bilayer, permitting the diffusion of specific ions down their electrochemical gradients to enter or leave cells.[528] Cotransporters are fundamentally different types of pathways that move ions across the cell membranes up their electrochemical gradients by coupling the translocation of at least two ions (e.g., K^+ and Cl^-) using the energy stored in adenosine triphosphate (ATP)-dependent preformed chemical gradients, such as those of H^+ or Na^+ (rather than the concentration gradients of the transported ions).[528]

Potassium ions enter cells by at least two pumping mechanisms, the membrane Na^+K^+ ATPase pump and the "ouabain-resistant pump."[207,537] K^+ exits cells through several types of membrane channels, including voltage-gated, ATP-gated, arachidonic acid-gated, and "leak" channels.[281,364,473] Although the rate of K^+ transport by each pathway varies with temperature, during heating, the overall resultant flux is a net loss of intracellular K^+ and a primary rise in plasma K^+.[174,168,425,475]

Hyperthermia increases the rate of Na^+ influx, leading to a net rise in intracellular sodium (Nai) that is prolonged and not rapidly reversed by cooling. At a sufficiently high temperature, the Na transport mechanisms become denatured and, because of the increased "leakiness" of the plasma membrane and the transmembrane Na concentration gradient, Nai progressively rises until death.[171] Acidifying cells leads to an explosive influx of Na^+ upon heating. Hyperthermia leads to at least mild cytoplasmic acidification,[523] and therefore the combined stresses of heating and acidification lead to increased intracellular Na^+.

Moderate heat activates a Ca^{2+} ATPase pump to temporarily lower intracellular calcium (Cai). However, severe heating causes a net rise in Ca^{2+} through the activation of at least two transport systems and therefore is expected to alter a number of metabolic pathways.[294] Depending on the temperature, Ca^{2+} enters the cell from the extracellular fluid by means of the "reversed mode" of the plasma membrane Ca^{2+}-ATPase pump and enters the cytoplasm from intracellular Ca^{2+} stores.

Some ionic changes in mammalian cells induced by heating, for example, in Ca^{2+} and Na^+, are mediated by inhibition of the Na-H exchanger, activation of Na^+K^+ ATPase, and changes of membrane conductance for ions.[465] See Gaffin[168] for a review of these mechanisms.

Although heating acts directly on the rates of fundamental cell processes, heat also has indirect effects by causing the release of a variety of hormones. These hormones, singly or in combination, further alter the activities of virtually all the ionic pathways. For instance, catecholamines stimulate the muscle membrane Na^+K^+ ATPase (by approximately 100% in rat soleus), increasing both the intracellular K^+ concentration (Ki)[92] and membrane potential.[67] Epinephrine in the presence of insulin stimulates active Na^+/K^+ transport and hyperpolarizes membrane potential in muscle.[156] This effect may be so powerful that, for a time, it "masks" the primary decrementing effect of the heat-induced hyperkalemia on performance.

In addition to the effect of heat on pathway activities, the rise in activity of the various ion pumps provides more metabolic heat, which, near the limit of sweat secretion, increases body temperature still more.

Increased membrane permeability from hyperthermia leads to rises in circulating enzymes. Creatine kinase is the first enzyme detected at T_c as low as 39.5° C (103.1° F) in monkeys (S. Constable and S.L. Gaffin, unpublished observations), and 42.5° C (108.5° F) in rats, followed by lactate dehydrogenase.[324]

Stress Pathways

Early unicellular forms of life were preyed upon by their neighbors and, over geologic time, they developed an immune system for protection. This is a nonspecific immunity and is basic to all phyla today. The original mechanism destroyed the invader's cytoplasm by active oxygen species, including free radicals, produced by the host. In modern mammalian species, specialized inflammatory cells, such as macrophages and natural killer (NK) cells, are especially enriched in those enzymes and chemical pathways producing the toxic free radicals. They also contain additional pathways that allow these cells to recognize invaders and penetrate tight epithelia so that they may easily reach and destroy them. The immune cells are activated by means of circulating and locally produced cytokines, such as tumor necrosis factor (TNF) and interleukin-1 (IL-1), as part of a stress reaction mediated by the hypothalamus. Thus there exists a common stress reaction in vertebrates that is activated by stresses other than infections, such as hyperthermia, and that activates pathways producing toxic species, which may now be inappropriate and toxic to the organism.[169]

Severe hyperthermia in mammals leads to a common response pathway involving the secretion of corticotrophin releasing factor (CRF, also called corticotropin releasing hormone [CRH]) by parvicellular neurons of the paraventricular nucleus of the hypothalamus,[31,497] activation of the sympathetic nervous

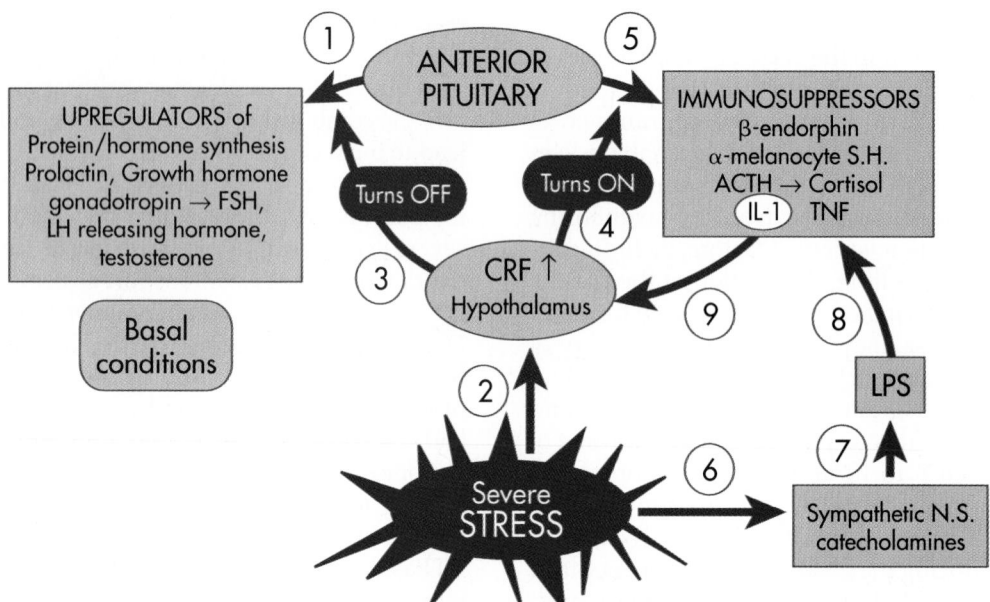

Figure 10-1 Stress and the hypothalamic-pituitary-adrenal axis. Under basal conditions *(1)* the anterior pituitary secretes the immunostimulants prolactin, growth hormone, thyroid-stimulating hormone (TSH), and gonadotropin-releasing hormone, leading to the secretion of luteinizing hormone (LH), follicle-stimulating hormone (FSH), and testosterone. Severe stress *(2)* acts on the paraventricular nucleus in the hypothalamus, producing CRF *(3)*, downregulating the secretion of the immunostimulants and gonadal hormones, and *(4, 5)* upregulating the secretion of the immunosuppressors β-endorphin, α-melanocyte-stimulating hormone, and ACTH, the latter of which upregulates the secretion of the immunosuppressor cortisol. Stress also *(6)* activates the sympathetic nervous system, and catecholamines are secreted. These further downregulate the production of immunostimulants and *(7)* may reduce splanchnic blood flow sufficiently to cause ischemia of the intestinal vascular bed, local damage to the gut wall, and the leakage of lipopolysaccharide (LPS) into the circulation. LPS in turn *(8)* causes the production of the powerful immunosuppressors TNF and IL-1. TNF and IL-1 are also secreted within the hypothalamus in direct response to stress, leading to their participation *(9)* in a positive feedback loop, augmenting the secretion of CRF and resulting in even greater immunosuppression. NOTE: Moderate stress may have the opposite effect and increase the secretion of immunostimulants. *(From Gaffin SL, Hubbar RW:* Wilderness Environ Med *4:312, 1996.)*

system, and secretion of cortisol and catecholamines (Figure 10-1). CRF is directly transported via the hypothalamo-hypophyseal portal system to the anterior pituitary, where it has two important effects: (1) it downregulates eosinophilic cells that secrete the immunostimulants (growth hormone, prolactin, gonadotropin stimulating hormone, luteinizing hormone, and follicular stimulating hormone),[15,127] and (2) it upregulates the pro-opiomelanocortin (POMC) gene in basophilic cells, leading to the secretion of immunosuppressors (β-endorphin, α-melanocyte stimulating hormone, and adrenocorticotropic hormone [ACTH], in turn leading to the secretion of the immunosuppressor cortisol) (see Figure 10-1). A rise in IL-1 is part of a positive feedback loop, causing a further rise in CRF and ACTH.[249,257]

These are not just theoretic predictions based on animal studies. In human subjects, circulating levels of CRF, ACTH, cortisol, and arginine vasopressin (AVP) rose during graded work rates until exhaustion. It appears that high-intensity exercise favors AVP release, whereas prolonged duration favors CRF release.[250]

Energy-Depletion Model

During hyperthermia and continued heat stress, cellular Na^+K^+ ATPase pumps operate at elevated rates, hydrolyzing ATP more rapidly and liberating waste heat into the body faster. If the body cannot dissipate this heat through radiation, conduction, convection, and sweat evaporation, then according to the laws of thermodynamics, T_c must rise further, leading to still greater rates of the Na^+K^+ ATPase pumps-an ominous positive feedback loop. The amount of energy available to a cell is limited. Therefore, at a certain elevated temperature, ATP utilized by the activated Na^+K^+ ATPase pump can no longer be resynthesized sufficiently rapidly to be available for normal cellular processes and the cell becomes "energy-depleted." Experimental support for this concept is the presence of swollen cells (implying a slowing of ion pumps, which affect water transport) and the rapid development of rigor mortis (caused by depletion of ATP) at the end stage of heatstroke pathophysiology. Persons exercising in the heat develop lethal heatstroke at lower T_c than do those at rest. This can be explained by the concept that exercise lowers ATP stores (i.e., creatine phosphate) and therefore less is available for other important cellular processes.[241]

CARDIOVASCULAR STRAIN AND EXERCISE

Severe heat illness involves every system and affects the regulatory (cardiovascular), the integrative (neuroendocrine), and ultimately the basic cellular systems of the body. Probably no greater strain is put on the human body than heavy physical exertion in the heat. This impact of heat stress on the cardiovascular system represents the strain resulting from increased demand for cardiac output to transfer heat and water to the skin for evaporative cooling.

Severe and prolonged exercise leads to changes in body compartments and the cardiovascular system, persisting for hours to days. For instance, a group of men carrying 20-kg backpacks during a 110-km march under warm conditions, eating and drinking ad lib, lost 3.4% of body weight and their plasma volume (PV) fell by 6.1%. However, the next day their PV *dropped still further* to −8.4%, even though they were not exercising. During the following day, PV rose to +3.7% above baseline and remained elevated 4 days after the march.[21]

The hemodynamic displacement of blood to the periphery is aggravated by gravitational displacement of blood volume resulting from upright posture. In an upright human, about 70% of the blood volume is below heart level. Venous pooling of blood in the skin and in the great veins below the level of the heart leads to reduced venous return to the heart and consequent reduced cardiac filling.[421] If active skeletal muscle then vasodilates to supply the increased demands for blood flow in support of muscle metabolism, the competing demands for blood flow between vascular beds translate into a major regulatory problem.[420]

The potential conductance of the vasculature (skin 8 L/min^{-1}, viscera 3 L/min^{-1}, and muscle 65 to 70 L/min^{-1}) is enormous and far exceeds the pumping capacity of the normal human heart (about 22 L/min^{-1}).[255,422] Since the combined blood flow requirements of these vascular beds cannot be met, an inherent competition takes place between the mechanisms that maintain blood pressure and those that maintain blood flow to support metabolism and thermoregulation.[243]

The existence of a variety of types of heat illnesses suggests: (1) the physiologic strain resulting in homeostatic failure produces heat illness; (2) a certain biologic variability is expressed in the response to heat and exercise; (3) hemodynamic stability often takes precedence over thermoregulation; (4) volitional behavior, expressed as exercise performance, is often maintained even as the risk of heat injury increases; and (5) the onset and increase in hyperthermia are not painful.[242] Not surprisingly, the physiologic threat to homeostasis is worsened when accompanied by fluid/electrolyte imbalance.[240,383] Treatment is then directed at the major sources of homeostatic failure: cease the activity, lie down, cool down, and rehydrate. Sometimes the cause of collapse or the other symptoms involved (such as headache, nausea, vomiting, and vertigo) is obvious; sometimes, it is not readily appreciated.

Sweating

Although human eccrine sweat glands generally behave physiologically and pharmacologically as if under parasympathetic or cholinergic control, they also respond to adrenergic stimulation.[434] There are 2 to 3 million sweat glands distributed with decreasing density in the skin of the palms and soles, head, trunk, and extremities, with an average density of about 100 to 200/cm². One g of sweat glands can secrete up to 250 g of sweat per day. Eccrine sweat is always hypotonic, contains variable concentrations of sodium, and is generally 99.5% water by weight.[141] That 0.5% of sweat solids is important, since 1 L of 0.5% sodium chloride contains 5 g of salt, a potential cause of serious salt depletion.

The process of sweat secretion and sweat rate depend on activation of the sweat center in the hypothalamus, which discharges over the cholinergic fibers of the sympathetic nervous system. Rising blood temperatures increase both the number and the rate of sweat glands responding, until the body reaches a thermal equilibrium or the maximum sweat rate occurs.[189] Dehydration and hyperosmolality each leads to reduced sweat rates,[439] with hyperosmolality the more effective (Figure 10-2).

One of the highest sweat rates ever recorded in a human was in a world-class Olympic runner.[17] He pro-duced sweat at a rate of 3.71 L/hr after 19 days of heat acclimation training. Because the maximum rate of gastric emptying is much less than the maximum sweat rate (1.2 vs. 3.7 L/hr), rehydration cannot keep pace with sweat losses under those conditions[18] and an athlete faces significant risk of dehydration despite frequent drinking.[19,20,243] Since rates of gastric emptying can exceed 1 L/hr, as a rule of thumb, a 1 L/hr sweat rate appears sustainable without significant dehydration.

Fluid and Electrolyte Imbalance

Heatstroke Model. Determining the time courses of changes in various physiologic and biochemical parameters caused by heatstroke is difficult or impossible in humans for ethical considerations. Use of rodents precludes the determining of many parameters simultaneously because of lack of blood volume. Miniswine have been used as models because of their considerable physiologic similarities to humans and their practical size. When anesthetized miniswine were passive heated to $T_{amb} = 43°$ C (109.4° F), HR and mean arterial pressure (MAP) rose only slightly until T_c reached 42° C (107.6° F) (Figure 10-3, A). At this T_c, the HR rose to a

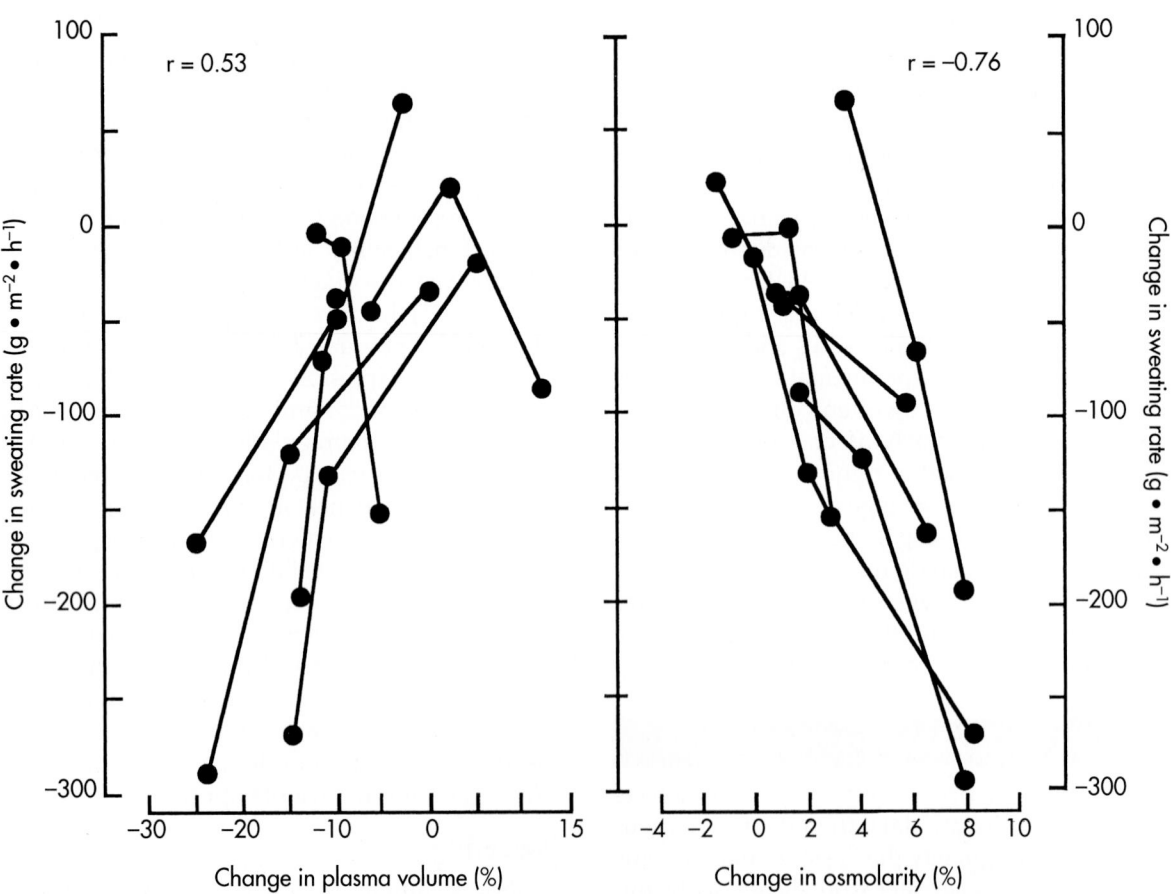

Figure 10-2 Effect of reduced plasma volume or increased osmolarity on sweat rates in six individuals. (*Modified from Sawka MN et al: J Appl Physiol 59:1394, 1985.*)

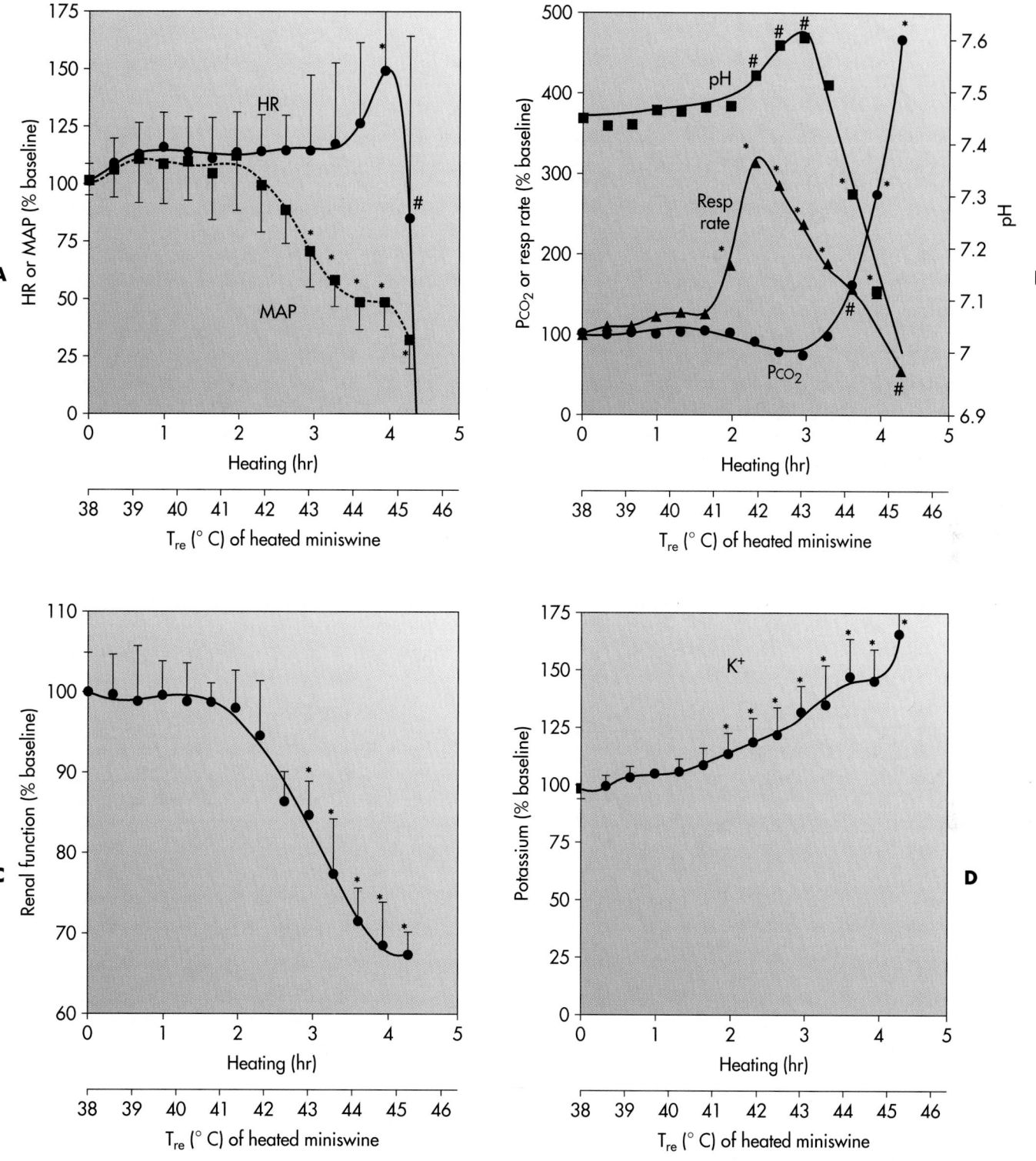

Figure 10-3 **A,** Effect of hyperthermia on mean arterial pressure (MAP) and heart rate (HR) in anesthetized miniswine. After 1-hour baseline, environmental temperature was raised to 42° to 43° C (107.6° to 109.4° F). $*$ = $P < 0.05$ compared with controls; $\#$ = $P < 0.05$ compared with own baseline values. **B,** Effect of hyperthermia on respiratory rate (resp rate), Pco_2, and arterial pH in anesthetized miniswine. Changes from baseline levels. $*$ = $P < 0.05$ compared with controls; $\#$ = $P < 0.05$ compared with own baseline values. **C,** Effect of hyperthermia on renal function. Percent baseline level. $*$ = $P < 0.05$ compared with controls; $\#$ = $P < 0.05$ compared with own baseline values. **D,** Effect of hyperthermia on arterial potassium, calcium, and inorganic phosphate in anesthetized miniswine. $*$ = $P < 0.05$ compared with controls; $\#$ = $P < 0.05$ compared with own baseline values. (*From Gaffin LS et al: J Thermal Biol 23:341, 1998.*)

peak and rapidly fell until death while MAP gradually fell until death but with a shoulder corresponding to the HR peak. The respiratory rate rose, peaking at approximately 42° C, and then continuously fell until death (Figure 10-3, B). Because of the increased ventilation, P_{CO_2} fell until shortly before death, but then rose to very high levels. As ventilation increased, plasma pH rose, but gradually fell as ventilation fell and CO_2 rose. Renal function was stable until 41° to 42° C (105.8° to 107.6° F), the same T_c that reduced MAP (Figure 10-3, C). Serum K^+ continuously rose with T_c (Figure 10-3, D).

A schematic model of normal thermoregulation and pathophysiology of heat stress and heatstroke (based on most of the preceding considerations) is shown in Figure 10-4. Core temperature has been divided into two regions to clarify physiologic mechanisms.

NORMAL THERMOREGULATION. Under a moderate heat load, as skin or core temperature (or both) rises, thermoreceptors (1) increase skin blood flow and (2) cause the secretion of sweat to (3) result in evaporative cooling. To prevent a drop in blood pressure (4), blow flow to the splanchnic regions and to muscle is reduced and (5) stroke volume and then (6) heart rate are increased. Then (7) catecholamines are secreted, followed by corticotropin-releasing factor (CRF), which lead to the secretion of adrenocorticotropic hormone followed by (8) cortisol. Catecholamines (9) cause leukocytosis, while cortisol (10) causes leukopenia, leading to (11) changes in amounts of subsets of leukocytes. If the heart stress is prolonged and severe, the immunosuppression could (12) lead to subsequent increased susceptibility to infections and decremented physical and mental performance. As temperature rises, (13) the respiratory rate increases. As a result of sweating, (14) plasma volume decreases and (15) hematocrit and (16) plasma osmolality rise, leading to (17, 18) the sensation of thirst and ADH release. Reduced plasma volume (14), together with (4) reduced renal blood flow, leads to (19) rises in water-sparing hormones and reduced kidney function.

IMPAIRED HOMEOSTASIS. As temperature continues to rise above approximately 40° C (104° F), direct hyperthermic damage (A1) to cells commences with increases in membrane fluidity and permeability, increases in metabolic rate, including the activity of the Na^+, K^+-ATPase, increases in a variety of metabolites, and decreases in cellular ATP content. At about the same time the reduction in intestinal blood flow (4) becomes more severe, leading (A4) to ischemic injury of the gut wall. This in turns leads to rises in (A5) circulating lipopolysaccharide (LPS) and (A6) cytokines. By activating a blood factor (A7), LPS causes (A8) disseminated intravascular coagulation and a consequent rise in blood viscosity. Thermal injury of endothelia (A3) to-

gether with (A6) cytokines leads to (A9) enhanced metabolism of ω-6 fatty acids, including (A10) the production of thromboxanes and leukotrienes, (A11) oxygen free radicals and further (A12) cellular injury, the probable production of the highly toxic nitric oxide, and (A13) increased vascular permeability. This leads to the loss of fluids into the tissues, and thus (A14) reduced venous return and (A15) consequent reduced central venous pressure. Through Starling's law of the heart (A16), cardiac output begins to fall. This is made more serious (A17) by electrolyte changes in the blood. Eventually (A18) blood pressure falls, leading (A19) to reduced tissue perfusion. In the case of the lung (A20), reduced perfusion leads to (A21) systemic hypoxemia and eventually (A22) ischemia of various tissues and organs and its consequent (A23) contribution to further cellular damage. (A24) Reduced blood flow to the brain (A25), as well as (A26) probable direct thermal denaturation, leads to damage of centrally mediated homeostatic mechanisms, (A27, A28) reduced skin blood flow and drop in cooling rate, and eventually (A29) a fall in respiration. In a separate pathway, cardiac output is also depressed as a result of (A30) a too rapid pulse rate causing (A31) incomplete cardiac filling. Electrolyte derangements are made more severe by (A32) an increased metabolic rate and (A33) reductions of renal blood flow in the kidney.

Hydration. "Water discipline," meaning fluid deprivation, is an attempt to reduce the body's water requirements during activities in the desert or jungle. However, it is an outdated, incorrect, and dangerous concept. Voluntarily or involuntarily withholding water from persons in the heat, in the face of severe thirst, leads to unnecessary deaths and permanent neurologic damage in the survivors of heatstroke.[390a]

If an athlete is hypohydrated when commencing strenuous physical exercise in the heat, he or she will be at a disadvantage compared with a euhydrated person. He overheats earlier, physical and mental performance decrements sooner, and the victim is more susceptible to hemorrhage and trauma. Frequent spitting and withholding water are often done by collegiate wrestlers to qualify for a lower weight class. This behavior must be regarded as a serious risk for developing heat illnesses.

With normal nutrition, ingesting commercial electrolyte/carbohydrate-containing beverages offers no advantage over water in maintaining PV or electrolyte concentration or in improving intestinal absorption. However, under conditions of caloric restriction or repeated days of sustained sweat losses, there might be a benefit to consuming an electrolyte-containing beverage. For athletes, use of glucose polymer solutions may be considered. For the vast majority of individuals, however, the primary advantage of using

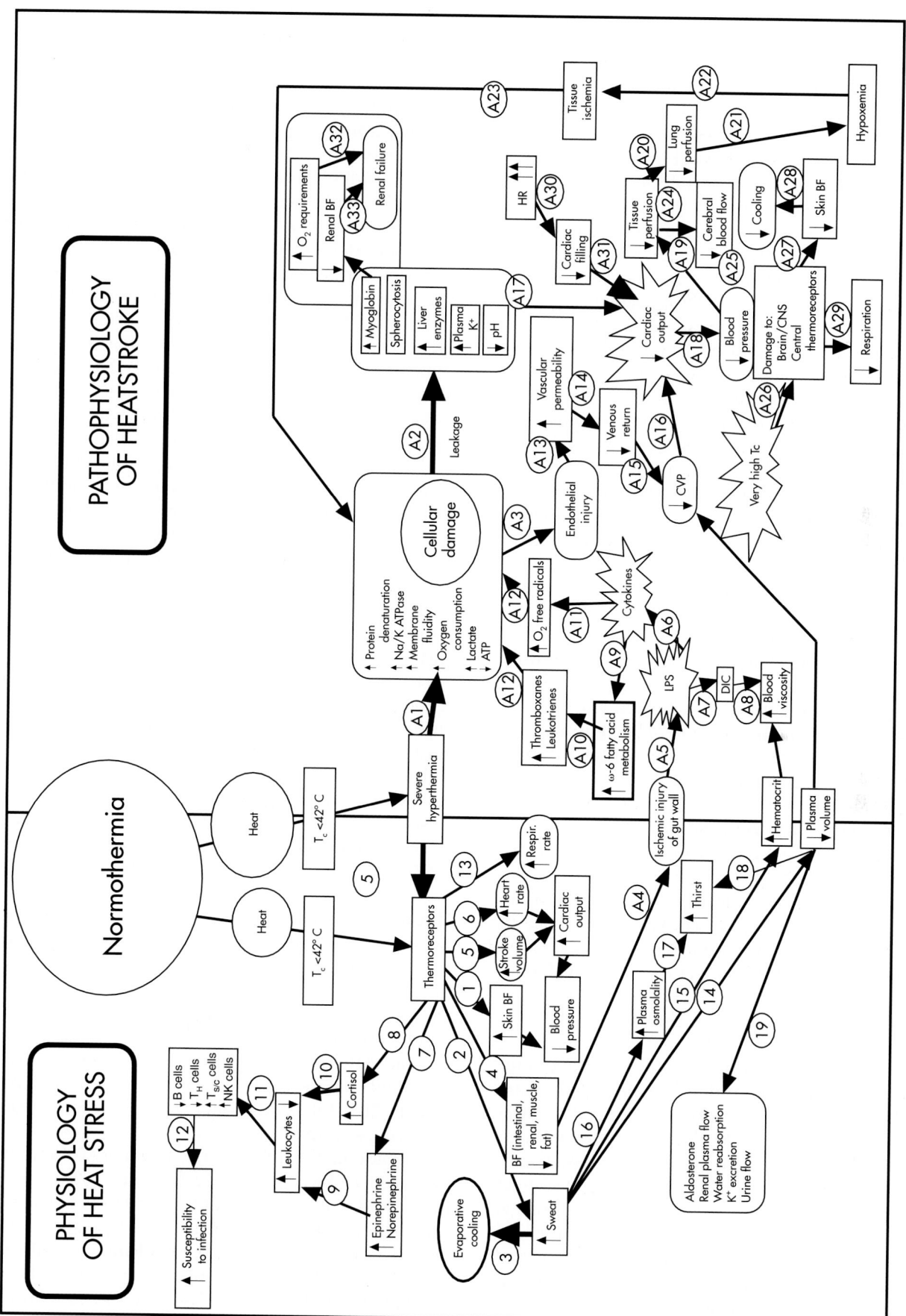

Figure 10-4 Model of the physiology and pathophysiology of heat stress and heatstroke. See text for description. (*From Hubbard RW, Gaffin SL, Squire DL: Heat-related illnesses. In Auerbach PS: Wilderness medicine: management of wilderness and environmental emergencies, ed 3, St Louis, 1995, Mosby.*)

electrolyte- or carbohydrate-containing drinks appears to simply improve taste, thereby enhancing voluntary consumption of fluids. This factor could become important if regulated intake is impossible.

Dehydration, as a dynamic change from euhydration to hypohydration, reduces or compromises the physiologic advantages of physical training or heat acclimation. Involuntary dehydration can produce serious water deficits, such as found in persons cast adrift on tropical seas or stranded in the desert without water. Survival under these conditions requires knowledge of the trade-offs between the benefits of increased physical activity to obtain water and the consequences of increased sweat and dehydration. Adolph et al[1] described both the symptoms and the expected dehydration rates under these circumstances.

The *minimum* unavoidable daily water loss approximates 1.5 L or about 2% of body weight as body water.[330] Although hard work in the heat can elicit this sweat loss in 1 hour (1.5 L/hr), resting in the shade can reduce sweat losses to minimum values (50 to 300 ml/hr at air temperatures from 26.7° to 37.8° C [80° to 100° F]). Assuming that a 12% body weight loss as a water loss produces shock, then survival time could vary between 1 and 5 days. *In the desert, for every 20 miles walked at night, one should carry 1 gallon of water and, during the day, 2 gallons.*[1]

Normal oxidation of carbohydrates produces a small amount of metabolic water that may have survival value. Approximately 500 ml may be produced per day, which represents 30% of the daily obligate water loss at rest. However, as running time in the heat, this represents only about 20 minutes.

Thirst and Voluntary Dehydration. The sensation of thirst does not become prominent until osmotic dehydration exceeds the renal capacity to deal with it physiologically.[240] Therefore inadequate fluid intake also can occur where drinking is possible. That is, the delay in thirst is a manifestation of the body's osmotic control. Although there is wide variation in the individual thirst threshold, it has an average value close to the upper normal value of 295 mOsm/kg H_2O (normal range = 280-295 mOsm/kg H_2O).[328,411,413]

The most potent stimulator of both thirst and antidiuretic hormone (ADH) is dehydration.[12] Within any one individual, the plasma vasopressin response (ADH release) is linearly related to plasma osmolality[413] and therefore to plasma sodium. For example, at an osmolality of 280 mOsm/kg H_2O, ADH release is almost completely inhibited and the osmolality of the urine is minimal (<100 mOsm/kg H_2O). As dehydration occurs, Na rises, causing a rise in plasma ADH concentration (0.5 to 5 pg/ml). ADH causes conservation of water by increasing renal reabsorption of solute-free water.[412] This action increases the concentration of urine (a rise in plasma by 1 mOsm increases urine osmolality by almost 100 mOsm/kg) and decreases its flow. At the thirst threshold of 295 mOsm/kg H_2O, urine flow is reduced tenfold to twentyfold.[328]

In summary, for most people, small osmolality rises resulting from water loss do not normally initiate the sensation of thirst. During work in the heat, *men never voluntarily drink as much water as they lose,* and they usually replace only two thirds of the net water loss.[394] Adolph and co-workers[418] called this phenomenon "voluntary dehydration" and found that it increases with elevated sweat rate induced by higher T_{amb} or work rate, by inadequate time allowed for rehydration, and by greater effort involved in acquiring water. *All persons in the heat should be considered dehydrated* (except immediately after a meal), unless they have recently been forced to drink more water than they desired. Consequently, in the past, heatstroke was almost always accompanied by some degree of dehydration.

However, in the past decade or so, medical authorities have fairly successfully educated athletes to drink adequate amounts of fluids during physical exercise in the heat, even if they are not thirsty. This has led to the routine establishment of water stations along marathon routes for participants to obtain drinks on the run and to drinking "on command" in the military. In a small number of cases, however, too much water was ingested, leading to overhydration, hyponatremia, physical collapse, and even deaths.[178] The administration of intravenous (IV) infusions to all collapsed marathon runners must be recorded, and all subsequent medical teams must be notified about the infusion. Since most collapsed athletes superficially appear similar, Noakes[370] emphasized that there is a significant danger of overhydrating persons who collapsed in the heat. Therefore it is essential to determine the patient's hydration status unless one is certain that the victim has not ingested adequate water.

Chronic Hypohydration. The significant delay between the threshold for ADH release (>280 mOsm) and the thirst threshold (>295 mOsm) is important. It frees the individual from being "forced" to drink immediately in response to changes in osmolality. On the other hand, certain individuals and groups[240] maintain a chronic state of hypohydration just below the thirst threshold (294 mOsm/kg), which represents a deficit of some 2L in total body water (TBW), according to the following example:

It is assumed that the total body water (TBW) in the idealized 70-kg person is 42 L (about 60% of body mass), and that two thirds of this water (28 L) is intracellular and one third is extracellular (3.5 L of plasma and 10.5 L of interstitial fluid). By calculation,[148] the intravascular or PV is equivalent to one twelfth of the total body water (42 L TBW/12 = 3.5 L PV). It is further assumed that there is no salt loss.

Therefore TBW at the thirst threshold, compared with euhydration, is calculated by:

Normal TBW × normal plasma osm =
thirst TBW × thirst plasma osm

$$42 L \times 280 \, mOsm/kg = ? \, L \times 295 \, mOsm/kg$$

$$11{,}760 \, mOsm/295 \, mOsm/kg = 39.9 \, L$$

That is, TBW at the thirst threshold is 39.9 L.

Therefore the actual water loss to reach threshold is 42 L − 39.9 L = 2.1 L, which represents nearly 3% of body weight ([2.1 kg/70 kg] × 100). By exercising in the heat for only about 2 hours, one can incur an additional water loss of 2.1 L (= 4.2 L total), which then results in a water deficit equivalent to 6% of body mass. This 6% TBW deficit decrements performance and increases risk of heat illness. The relationship between hydration state, rise in T_c, and physical performance decrement is best shown in a classic work by Montain et al,[346] who measured performance at three work rates and in three states of hydration. See Figure 10-5.

Primary Water Depletion. Hypohydration caused by primary water depletion and increased fluid losses is characterized by thirst and oliguria and is completely relieved by drinking pure water.[355] Sample calculations based on some commonly accepted estimates highlight the role of reduced water intake vs. missed meals and sweat (water and salt) losses in the dehydration process. In the absence of sweating, a pure water deficit caused by inadequate fluid intake slowly raises plasma Na^+ and can eventually lead to symptoms of circulatory shock. Clinical shock from pure water deficit generally coincides with a sodium concentration above 170 mEq/L (normal range 135-145 mEq/L, mean 140 mEq/L).[148] The water deficit vs. euhydration for an assumed plasma Na^+ = 175 mEq/L can be estimated using the following formula:

$$TBW_{normal} \times Na^+_{normal} = TBW_{dehydrated} \times Na^+_{dehydrated}$$

$$42 \, L \, (see \, above) \times 140 \, mEq/L = ? \, TBW \times 175 \, mEq/L$$

Then TBW for this dehydrated state = 33.6 L. Therefore the water deficit in TBW = 42 L − 33.6 L = 8.4 L.

Thus it is calculated that a loss of 8.4 L of body water or 12% of body mass in a 70-kg person produces shock. At minimal rates of water loss (1.5 to 2.0 L/24 hours), this could be produced in 4 to 5 days.

Therefore, by definition, if a pure water loss occurs (no salt loss), the loss would be apportioned over all the fluid spaces, with two thirds of the loss from the intracellular water (8.4 L × ⅔ = 5.6 L), one third from the extracellular water (8.4 L/3 = 2.8 L), and one twelfth

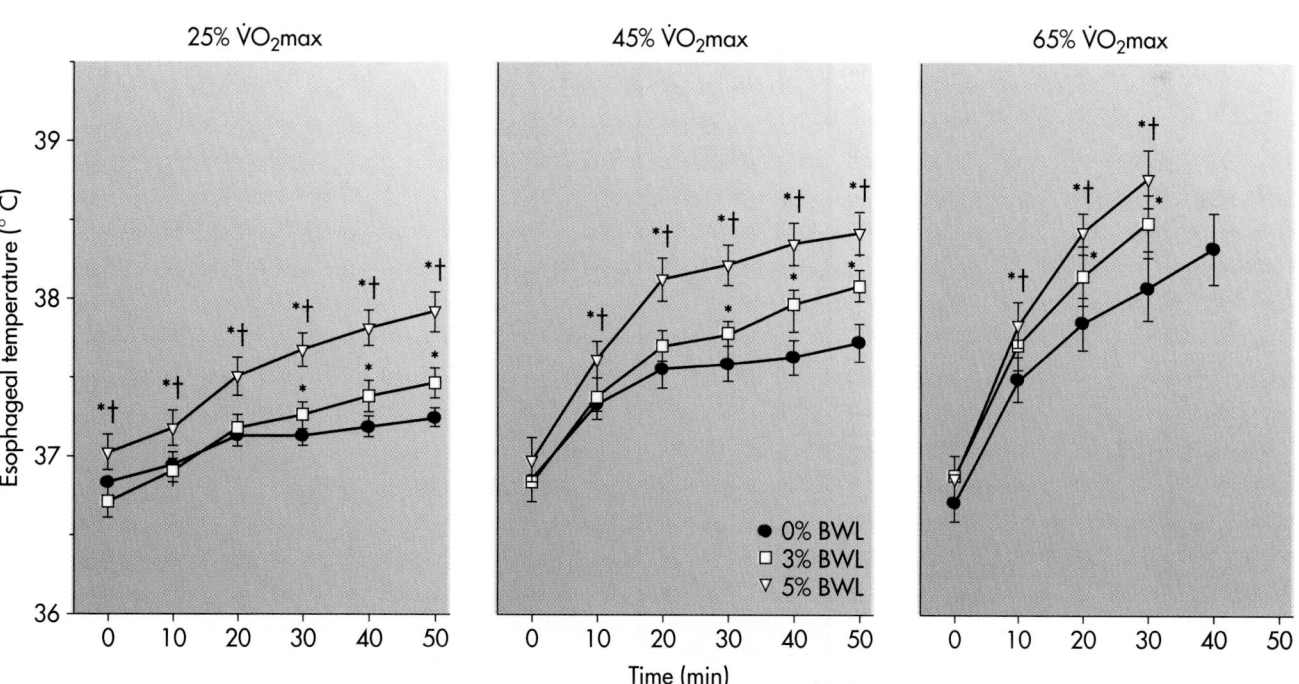

Figure 10-5 Influence of hydration level and exercise intensity on esophageal temperature. *BWL,* Body weight loss; *ApV̇o₂max,* maximal O₂ uptake. (*Data from Montain SJ, Latzka WA, Sawka MN: J Appl Physiol 79:1434, 1995.*)

TABLE 10-2. Effect of Sweat Losses (Salt and Water) on Plasma Volume and Osmolality

Body Weight Loss		Hypotonic Sweat (Percent × 280 mOsm)															
		50%				25%				12.5%				As Pure Water			
		ΔPl Vol		ΔPl Osm		ΔPl Vol		ΔPl Osm		ΔPl Vol		ΔPl Osm		ΔPl Vol		ΔPl Osm	
%	L	ml	%	mOsm	Na	ml	%	mOsm	Na	ml	%	mOsm	Na	ml	%	mOsm	Na
0	0	0	0	280	140	0	0	280	140	0	0	280	140	0	0	280	140
2	1.4	−233	−6.7	285	142	−175	−5	287	144	−146	−4.2	288	142	−117	−3.3	290	145
4	2.8	−467	−13.3	290	145	−350	−10	295	148	−292	−8.3	298	149	−233	−6.7	300	150
6	4.2	−700	−20	296	148	−525	−15	303	152	−437	−12.5	307	154	−350	−10	311	156
8	5.6					−700	−20	312	156	−583	−16.7	318	159	−466	−13.3	323	162
10	7									−729	−20.8	329	164	−583	−16.7	336	168
12	8.4													−700	−20	350	175

from the plasma space (8.4 L/12 = 700 ml). This loss represents approximately 20% of the PV. In practice, usually less than one twelfth of the water loss comes from the plasma space because of its increased plasma protein oncotic pressure.

Sweat Salt Losses. In contrast to the above loss of water only is the situation in which an unacclimatized individual has skipped a prior meal and is losing salt as well as water by producing hypotonic sweat assumed to be 0.41% NaCl = 140 mOsm/Kg = 0.5 × normal plasma osmolality. He is assumed to be euhydrated before commencing exercise in the heat for a 2- to 3-hour period, losing 6% of body mass (4.2 L) as sweat. Since this 4.2 L is at 0.5 × normal osmolality, it is equivalent to a loss of half that volume (2.1 L) of normal saline (280 mOsm/kg) and half (2.1 L) of pure water. That is, the extracellular space (3.5 L [plasma] + 10.5 L [interstitial] = 14 L; the sodium space) would lose 2.1 L of isotonic saline, of which the plasma contributes one fourth (3.5 L/14 L = 1/4). This is equivalent to 525 ml (2.1 L/4) of PV.

In addition, the plasma would contribute one twelfth of the pure water deficit (2.1 L), or 175 ml (2.1 L/12). If these PV losses are added (525 ml + 175 ml = 700 ml), the plasma could lose 20% of its volume ([100 ml/3500 ml] × 100), which is close to the shock threshold (Table 10-2).

This means a 4.2 L loss of sweat has theoretically as much impact on the PV (20%) as *twice* the volume (8.4 L) of pure water loss (20%). In this example, however, inadequate salt and water intake (skipped meals, no drinking) has a role, as does the rapidity of sweat losses (hours vs. days).

ACCLIMATIZATION

Prior heat exposure enhances heat tolerance by expanding circulating PV; increasing the maximum capacity of cutaneous vasodilatation and sweating; and reducing the threshold temperature for increased BF_{sk} and sweating, that is, commencing cooling mechanisms at lower temperatures.[187,516] An acclimatized person shows a lower T_c, T_{sk}, and HR and a higher msw in response to a standard heat stress. A further important benefit of heat acclimation is reduced loss of sodium (both urinary and in sweat) and therefore a reduced likelihood of developing salt-depletion heat illnesses from high sweat losses. When these physiologic adjustments occur in response to heat exposure in a controlled laboratory setting, they are termed *acclimation,* and if induced by the natural environment, *acclimatization.* The physiologic adaptations in the acclimation to heat and to severe physical exercise (training) are very similar; acclimation to one partly but not completely acclimates to the other.

The process of human acclimatization to heat produces both short-term and long-term changes in ther-

moregulatory responses involving sweating, skin circulation, and thermoregulatory set point. For instance, in some studies, short-term heat adapted people sweated more rapidly, whereas those who were long-term adapted sweated more slowly.[231] Other equally impressive changes, but not specifically thermoregulatory, include cardiovascular alterations (HR, stroke volume, and PV) and endocrine adjustments. In the acclimatized state, a given heat and/or exercise load leads to reduced physiologic responses, for example, lowered T_c, lowered HR, elevated cardiovascular reserve, and increased cooling capacity through a reduced threshold for vasodilation.

Importantly, the rates of heat and exercise acclimatization are not uniform within a body but vary from tissue to tissue. As a result, there are periods when compensation processes in different organs are out of phase with one another and the overall effect may be negative.[448] For example, in rats, the immediate heat adaptation response of both the salivary glands and heart is a temporary period of decreased sensitivity of those organs to their respective neurotransmitters, causing a reduced intrinsic secretion of saliva and HR. These intrinsic failures may be "masked" during the acclimation processes by overstimulating those organs through especially high autonomic activities.

Over time, different genes are activated within each organ, leading to the replacement of certain metabolic enzymes with isoforms more appropriate to elevated temperatures. These new isoforms have improved thermostability, altered reaction rates, and specificities, leading to the development of more efficient dynamic processes with reduced heat absorption by the body. In the final adaptive state, these altered enzymes have improved cellular performance, even with normal autonomic activities.[152,235,309]

Depending on a given individual's constitution, state of physical fitness, and thermal history, a specific thermal stress and intensity of exercise will produce some degree of thermal strain. However, each person acclimatizes heat stress in his or her own way, with considerable variation in indexes of heat strain (e.g., weakness, rapid pulse, narrow pulse pressure, flushing of the face and neck, headache, shortness of breath, dizziness, cramps, nausea, and vomiting).[448] Many early studies have been shown to be unreliable because of small sample sizes, incomplete acclimation, or inappropriate measurements. Furthermore, Pandolf[385] has noted that more is known about the time course for the acquisition of acclimation than its decay or loss. Recently, the use of sophisticated molecular biology techniques indicating the participation of heat shock proteins[233] has shed new light on the fundamental processes involved in acclimation.

What is the fundamental event during exercise heat stress that causes the biochemical and physiologic alterations in the body that ultimately result in heat tolerance? At the moment this is unknown. In humans, exercise in the heat causes a rise in aldosterone concentration within a few minutes. An elevated aldosterone concentration increases the number of Na$^+$K$^+$ ATPase pumps on plasma membranes.[162] Simply stimulating rabbit muscle over several days increased the number of Na$^+$K$^+$ pumps on the sarcolemma[197] and exercise training in humans raised the number of Na$^+$K$^+$ ATPase pumps on sarcolemma within 1 week. As a result, severe exercise no longer caused a normal rise in plasma K$^+$, probably because the increased number of Na$^+$K$^+$ pumps attenuated the loss of K$^+$ from working muscle.[197]

Physiologic Changes

One benefit of adaptation is clearly shown by the incidence of heat syncope among persons suddenly exposed to living in a hot environment (Figure 10-6). Syncope, as described below, is caused by reduced cerebral blood flow resulting from a combination of peripheral blood pooling, reduced CO, and orthostatic hypotension. Syncope peaks on the first day of heat exposure and falls to zero by day 5. Although persons can acclimate to hot environments over a period of 1 to 2 weeks, they also deacclimate over approximately the same period of time.

In general, symptoms lessen as acclimation progresses. Nearly complete acclimation to a given level of daily exercise and heat stress can be achieved in 7 to 10 days (Figure 10-7).[385] The physiologic changes produced by heat or physical training include a lowered threshold temperature for the onset of BF$_{sk}$, sweating (see Figure 10-7),[410] increased PV, increased stroke volume, decreased HR, decreased skin temperature, decreased T$_{re}$, and increased Ap$\dot{V}$O$_2$max.[16] Physical training also increases aerobic capacity. Practically, this means that a fit but untrained person who runs a 500-m race and develops a T$_{re}$ of 40° to 43° C (104° to 109.4° F) could, after acclimation, run the same race under the same environmental conditions and have a T$_{re}$ of only 37.5° C (99.5° F).[288]

Although many controversial issues remain, a general rule is that either strenuous interval training or continuous exercise at an intensity greater than 50% Ap$\dot{V}$O$_2$max accounts for about 50% of the improvements found with classic acclimation procedures.[188] This may be important to the individual who wants to

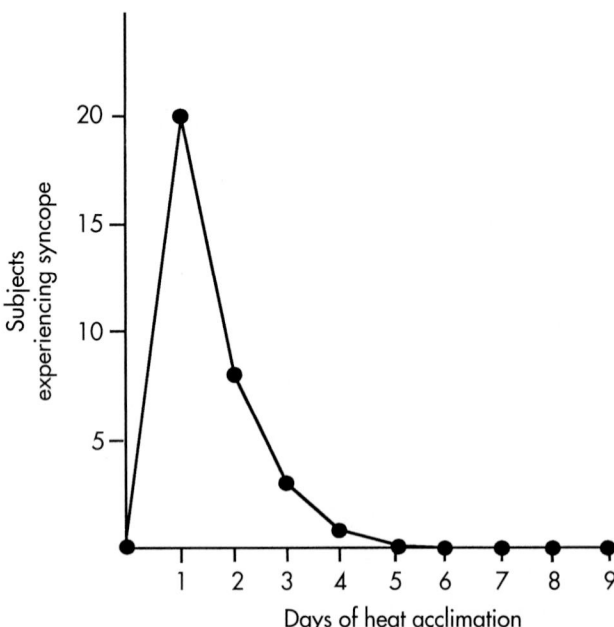

Figure 10-6 Incidence of syncope among 45 subjects living in a hot environment for 24 hours each day and undergoing exercise trials. (*Modified from Bean WB, Eichna LW:* Fed Proc 2:144, 1943, by Hubbard RW, Armstrong LE. In Pandolph KB et al: Human performance: physiology and environmental medicine at terrestrial extremes, *Indianapolis, 1988, Benchmark Press.*)

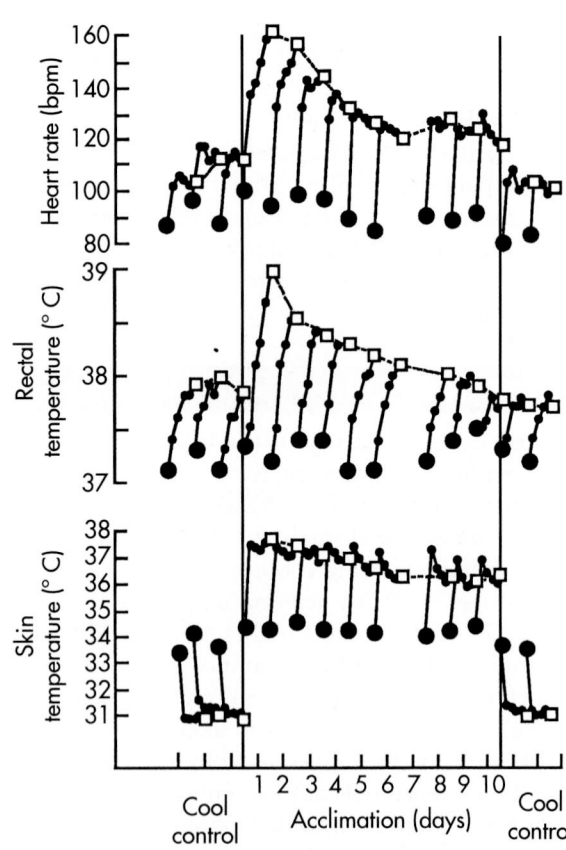

Figure 10-7 Effect of 10 days' acclimation on heart rate and rectal and skin temperatures during a standard exercise (five 10-minute periods of treadmill, separated by 2-minute rests) in dry heat. Large circles show values before start of the first exercise period each day, with small circles showing successive values. Squares show the final values each day. Controls of exercise in cool environment before and after acclimation. (*Modified from Eichna LW et al:* Am J Physiol 163:585, 1950.)

prepare for an acute change in thermal climate but does not have the means to safely elevate his or her core temperature in the heat.

The primary mechanism of the heat acclimation process is to raise internal body temperature sufficiently to induce moderate sweating. This can be achieved with moderate exercise in the heat or by wearing more clothing in a cooler environment. In the unacclimated individual, usually an hour per day of exercise in the heat is sufficient to produce an effect over days of exposure. As a rule, 10 days of successive treadmill walks in dry heat lower final exercise HRs by about 40 beats/min; lower rectal and skin temperatures by 1° and 1.5° C (1.8° and 2.7° F), respectively; and increase sweat production by about 10%.[135] Generally, the degree of acclimation is related to the daily heat stress; that is, daily 100-minute bouts in the heat conferred more acclimation after 9 days than did 50-minute bouts.[315] Most of the improvement in HR occurs in 4 to 5 days, and the improvement is nearly complete after 7 days (see Figure 10-7). As heat acclimation progresses, the onset of thermal sweating occurs at lower core temperatures and the peak sweat rate is higher or even doubled (1.5 to 3 L/hr). Furthermore, the ability to sustain sweating for prolonged periods improves, along with the ability to increase sweating in skin areas that sweated the least before acclimation. Acclimation tends to make the sweating response over different skin areas more uniform.

These effects result, in part, from central mechanisms, as well as from intrinsic fundamental changes in the pharmacologic activity of the sweat glands.[96] Heat acclimation increases the sweat glands' capacity to reabsorb sweat sodium at any given sweat rate.[6] Depending on the state of acclimation, the sodium concentration in sweat varies between approximately 5 and 60 mEq/L (10 to 20 mOsm/kg H_2O) (see Table 10-2) and increases with sweat rate but declines with the state of acclimation. The salt-sparing effect of acclimation seems to depend on the secretion of aldosterone, triggered by the combined effects of sodium depletion and heat stress.[295]

Skin vasodilation, especially in the forearm where it can be measured, occurs at a lower core temperature after acclimation (Figure 10-8). Since these changes parallel the threshold T_c for sweating, they suggest that alterations are occurring in skin blood vessels at the same time as those in skin sweat glands.[161] During acclimatization, despite the vasodilation of skin in the heat, BP is maintained for a long period and without reducing splanchnic blood flow (BF_{spl}). Improved vascular contraction results from improved responsiveness of α adrenoreceptors and decrease in β receptors.

Changes in HR and PV decrease in parallel during the first week of acclimation.[448] The decrease in HR and increase in stroke volume may begin as early as the second day of work in the heat.[534] These changes are

nearly complete by day 5, whereas final rectal temperatures are still declining with subsequent exposures. Many authors have reported that PV increases with the days of heat exposure. However, the mechanisms involved, including salt retention, addition of protein to the vascular space, and fluid shifts between compartments, are unclear.[447] What is interesting, however, is a return of PV to baseline levels after about 2 weeks without apparent thermoregulatory impairment.[29] Horowitz et al[236] have shown that long-term acclimation increased the compliance of rat ventricles in isolated hearts, resulting in a greater diastolic volume at any end-diastolic pressure, hence greater Starling contractility. This promising model has produced recent insights described below.

Climatic Effects

There is a seasonal effect on the threshold temperature (T_{th}) for the onset of sweating; T_{th} is highest in winter and lowest in summer. Therefore, for a given heat stress, BF_{sk} and sweat rate are highest in summer and lowest in winter.[358] Rapid air travel to a desert or jungle climate leads to incomplete acclimatization, or to none at all, and a very much increased rate of heat illnesses. For instance, military personnel have higher heat illness rates in summer than in winter in a number of locations.[63,300] In a 4-year period, there were 10 severe heat casualties among soldiers visiting Cyprus during mili-

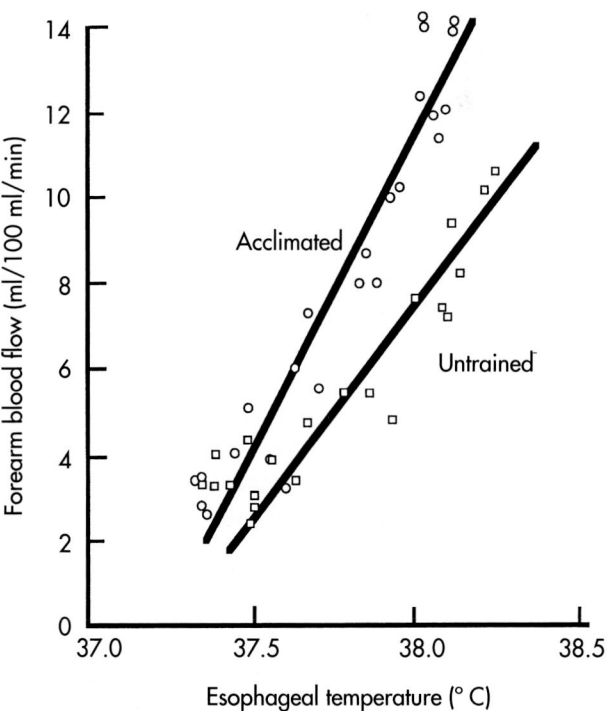

Figure 10-8 Effect of acclimation on forearm blood flow vs. esophageal temperature in one subject. (*Modified from Roberts MF et al: J Appl Physiol 43:133, 1977.*)

tary training, largely because of incomplete acclimatization. The rate was highest during summer months when the WBGT was 26° to 29° C (78.8° to 84.2° F).[63]

The time course of acclimation is similar in hot climates that are equivalent in WBGT. Acclimation to a defined hot environment confers equal acclimation to any other equivalent climate.[200] In groups of unacclimated healthy men subjected to heat for 9 days, those exercising under humid conditions produced better and more complete acclimatization than those exercising under dry conditions at similar WBGTs. Practically, when training at any given T_{amb}, a humid environment—and consequent higher heat load—leads to a more rapid acclimatization than training in a dry environment.[357]

Athletes have thinner skinfold thickness that do nonathletes. This leads to an increased rate of heat loss from the core, across the skin barrier into air by radiation, convection, and conduction. Exercise training improves heat dissipation not only by the reflex physiologic changes previously described but also by causing a reduction in the thickness of subcutaneous fat. Importantly, skinfold thickness is thinner in summer than in winter, thereby improving heat dissipation when it is most needed.[231]

Biochemical Changes

Heat Shock Proteins. The metabolic heat produced by severe exercise can raise the temperature of exercising human muscle to 45° C (113° F), and T_c up to 44° C (111.2° F). These temperatures can damage muscle mitochondria so that they generate O_2^- and H_2O_2, causing oxidative damage in addition to thermal stress.[430]

All cells have the potential of being stressed by heat and other stressors. To survive they have developed the ability to rapidly synthesize specialized proteins known collectively as *heat shock proteins* (HSPs), which protect them against ordinarily lethal conditions. Many cell types are ordinarily destroyed by 5 minutes at $T_{amb} = 49°$ C (120.2° F). However, if they are first heated to 42° C (107.6° F) for 15 minutes, protective HSPs are induced within the cells so that they can survive $T_{amb} = 49°$ C.[427] HSPs refold denatured proteins into their normal conformation and stabilize normal proteins against thermal injury. The binding of HSPs to denatured proteins does not cause immediate global conformational change of the unfolded proteins; rather, HSPs act locally on small regions of exposed hydrophobic amino acids through repeated cycles of binding, folding, and release reactions that are energized by the hydrolysis of ATP.[68] HSPs are produced as a general response to all known stresses, if sufficiently intense, including hypoxia; free radicals; cold, acidic environment; starvation; ionizing radiation; a variety of chemical toxins; and even electromagnetic fields.[68,147,313,271] Furthermore, HSPs may protect parasites against host defenses.[441] Heat shocking a variety of cells and animals increased

HSP content and protected them against not only heat but apoptosis, ischemia/reperfusion injury to the mucosa, and ionizing radiation.[354,378,431,477] Overall, in mammalian tissues, heat shock appears to provide a protective advantage of at least 2° C (3.6° F) against morbidity and mortality caused by high temperatures.[333]

HSPs are induced not only by physical and chemical stresses, including sepsis, cocaine, and tobacco smoke,[45,111,503] but apparently even by psychologic stresses, such as loud noise, isolation in darkness, restraint, water immersion, inescapable irritation, seizures, and sleep deprivation[86,165,218,226,239] Indications of elevated levels of HSP-60 were found in one small study of schizophrenics.[444]

The production of high levels of HSPs is not without cost, otherwise they would be present in cells all the time. HSPs may interfere with the spontaneous folding of new proteins, and the stresses sufficient to induce HSPs redirect cellular machinery to produce HSPs at the expense of producing other proteins. This would be particularly damaging to rapidly growing cells, such as during fetal maturation.[147]

HSPs are grouped into a series of families based upon their molecular masses; for example, the most important HSP-70 family contains several proteins of 68-75 kDa. In each cell, certain HSPs from each family are normally present and increase only moderately following heat, for example, HSP-73, which is sometimes referred to as "constitutive HSP-70." Other HSPs are normally absent from the cell or present in only very low amounts but are rapidly induced by heat ($T_{amb} > 41°$ C [105.8° F]) to become the most common protein in the cell, for example, HSP-72. The widely used, but ambiguous, term *HSP-70* refers to any or all members of the family.

The threshold temperature for the induction of HSPs depends upon the species and cell type but is approximately 4° C (7.2° F) above the normal environmental temperature encountered by the cell. A temperature as low as 5° C (41° F) induces HSPs in Antarctic algae, which normally live at −1° to 1° C (32° to 33.8° F).[502] Most investigators suggest that the threshold in mammalian cells is approximately 41° C (105.8° F), although temperatures as low as 39° C (102.2° F) have been reported.[90]

The rate of heating may also be an important factor in thermal injury, since the production of HSPs and cell survival also depend upon the rate of heating.[46,225] HSP production is also organ-dependent. In heat-shocked rats (42° C [107.6° F]), HSP-72 was produced in the order of liver >> small intestine > kidney, quadriceps > brain.[155] In rat brain, lung, and skin, HSP-70 concentration peaked at 1 hour and returned to baseline at 3 hours poststress. In liver, however, HSP-70 peaked 6 hours poststress.[46] The determination of HSP-72 may be useful as a diagnostic probe of recent heat injury when a rapid assay is developed.[61]

Most studies on HSPs have been carried out in isolated cells and in rodent models. In humans, the threshold T_c and duration for a single heat shock to induce HSPs is not certain. Cells could survive very brief exposures (1 second) to temperatures as high as 60° C (140° F) because they induced HSPs that rendered them thermotolerant.[58] Following a single heat shock in human peripheral blood mononuclear cells, HSP-72 concentration is unchanged for 1 to 2 hours, then rises rapidly to plateau at 4 hours and gradually falls after 12 to 18 hours, but remains above baseline at 24 hours (Gaffin, unpublished observations). Overall, however, upon a single supra-threshold stress, HSPs probably rise within an hour or two of the stress and remain elevated for 12 to 48 hours and possibly for as long as a week.[211] During sport or exercise in summer, however, elevations in T_c would be repeated, and multiple stimuli may have profound effects on the time course of HSP elevation and protection.[233]

This *temporary* thermoprotection by HSPs to heat and exercise is not "acclimatization." Acclimatization is a different process, although it may in part involve HSPs. It develops over a period of several days in response to several periods of moderate heat and may persist for weeks.

In the work of Horowitz et al,[233] acclimatization involves alterations in autonomic, cellular, and molecular responses to heat, varying in their intensities and interrelationships over time. Some studies suggest that increased HSP-72 during rigorous exercise is one of the adaptive mechanisms to cope with increased stress.[234,311] Rats run on a treadmill for 30 minutes per day at 75% Ap$\dot{V}O_2$max showed increases in HSP-72 within 10 weeks.[116] Endurance exercise–trained rats had higher levels of HSP-72, as well as lower levels of lipid peroxidation in their ventricles, and could develop higher systolic pressures.[115,398]

The presence of HSPs is extremely important, since during exercise in moderate and warm temperatures or at rest in tropical or desert heat, T_c may rise to levels that severely decrement performance or may lead to heatstroke, collapse, and even death. A better understanding of the role of HSPs may ultimately lead to methods for faster acclimatization to heat. The ability to produce HSPs may depend upon the diet, since vitamin D–deficient animals showed reduced HSP production.[270]

PROTECTION. HSPs appear to be beneficial to membranes, cells, tissue, and organs. HSP-70 elevated by a variety of stresses (heat shock, brief cyanide, arsenite, peroxide, hypoxia, and toxins) protected cells and their ultrastructure against these or other stressors.[9,49,278,507] HSPs protect against membrane damage caused by toxins (ionomycin) and cytokines.[201,301] Well-healing wounds show high levels of hsp70mRNA, whereas poorly healing wounds have lower levels.[375] Overexpression of HSP-70 in transgenic mice rendered their hearts more resistant to ischemic injury.[327] Those human cell types normally exhibiting great resistance to hypoxia (proximal tubular epithelia) also contain high basal levels of HSP-70.[495] Elevated HSP-72 (by heat shock or arsenite) protected rats against heatstroke morbidity and mortality.[536]

Elevated HSP-72 blunted the liberation of inflammatory mediators (interleukin-6 and thromboxane B_2) in lipopolysaccharide (LPS)-challenged swine and improved the course of hemodynamic variables (decreased peak pulmonary artery pressure and pulmonary vascular resistance index values, increased systemic artery pressure and systemic vascular resistance index values, and favorably altered hypodynamic/hyperdynamic CO).[283] Elevated HSP-70 (by heat shock) protected rat intestine against toxin (ricin)-induced acute intestinal inflammation, with reduced generation of leukotriene B_4 and neutrophilic infiltrate in their ileums.[478] Monocytes and granulocytes constitutively express more HSP-70 and are more heat-resistant than lymphocytes. LPS raises HSP-70 content even more and may be the reason that those cells can survive and function in hostile inflammatory microenvironments.[153]

Not only is raising HSP levels protective against heat, but reducing them is damaging during stress. For example, reducing HSP-72 induction by 40% (by a specific toxin) rendered cardiac myocytes more susceptible to hypoxic injury.[359]

In principle, it may be possible in humans and experimental models to elevate HSPs by one stress (e.g., temporary hypoxia) to render athletes more tolerant to heat, cold, or toxins. This would benefit not only athletes but also soldiers deployed to hot climates and patients soon to undergo surgery.

AGE. In normal adult rats, heat and exercise can each induce HSP-72. However, in aged rats, only exercise could induce HSP-72[299]; that is, aging caused them to lose their ability to induce HSPs by heat. In humans, the elderly have lower levels of HSP-70 in their peripheral blood mononuclear cells (PBMCs) than do the young.[109] This loss of HSP protection may in part account for increased susceptibility of the aged to classical heatstroke, as is seen in heat waves.

RACE. HSP production may be race-related. In one study, heat-induced HSP levels were very intense in cells isolated from native Turkish men living in the hot desert of middle Asia but very weak in Russians living in moderate climatic regions of European Russia. At the same time, those cells isolated from Turkish men better survived heat stress.[253] Not surprisingly, organisms living many generations in hot climates become better adapted to it over time. No systematic study of racial influences on HSPs has been reported.

TRAINING. Long-term exercise training in the heat induced HSPs. In one study of rat brains, HSP-70 content rose only if the exercising rats became hyperthermic, whereas exercise alone did not induce central HSP-70 expression.[506] On the other hand, in spleen cells, peripheral lymphocytes, and soleus muscles, exercise alone induced HSP-60, HSP-70, HSP-90, and HSP-100.[319] In male rowers in training, the HSP-70 content in an active muscle rose each week (181%, 405%, 456%, and 363%) with maximum HSP production at the end of the second training week.[521] In humans walking 30 minutes on a treadmill at their individual anaerobic thresholds, messenger ribonucleic acid (mRNA) for HSP-70 rose but not the HSP-70 protein itself. That is, a single bout of exercise in humans may not be sufficient to induce HSP-70.[401]

Combined stressors may be additive or synergistic in their effect. Exposure of cells to either a moderately elevated temperature or to a low level of ethanol do not induce HSPs. However, when the two stresses were applied at the same time, the cells induced large amounts of HSPs. Thus hyperthermia and ethanol acted synergistically to increase HSP gene expression.[415] Practically, that implies that HSPs may be induced by overlapping periods of exercise, heat, hypoxia, and/or sleep deprivation.

CONSEQUENCES. There is a downside to the production of HSPs during stress injury: the cell ceases or slows production of many other proteins. As a result, in cells at normal temperatures, the synthesis of HSPs (induced by a short heat stress) retards cell growth[146] even as it protects against subsequent heat injury. Not only is growth retarded; heat-shocked immune cells secreted reduced amounts of cytokines in response to LPS.[407] Therefore, persons with elevated HSPs may have reduced or inappropriately altered immune function. Clearly, the potential benefits of deliberately inducing HSPs, with presumed improved resistance to heat, hypoxia, and certain chemicals and toxins, must be weighed against the potentially decremented ability to resist infections. More research in the field is necessary for the required quantitative data.

Thyroid Hormone and Protein Isoforms. Recent studies indicate that thyroid gland function is an important component of heat acclimation. IL-1 reduces the release of thyroid hormone from the thyroid gland.[103,127] Since IL-1 becomes elevated in response to many stresses (see Figure 10-1),[170] its ability to lower thyroid hormone release may be part of the overall protective mechanisms and responses to stress.[267]

Alterations in thyroid hormone concentrations have a number of physiologic and biochemical consequences. Deficiency of thyroid hormone has a negative cardiac chronotropic effect, reducing cardiac contractility and increasing systemic vascular resistance.[62] The basal metabolic rate (BMR) falls with thyroxine deficiency, and since its secretion rate is lower in summer and higher in winter, there is a corresponding seasonal alteration in the BMR and all other processes influenced by thyroxine concentrations.[231] One component of heat acclimatization is a reduction in BMR.[231] Chronic heat stress decreases blood flow to the thyroid[204] and reduces the production rate of thyroid hormone, leading to decreased food intake, growth rate, and oxygen consumption, and lower BMR.[419] The consequences of deficiency in thyroid hormone during acute stress may be fatal. A young woman was discovered unconscious in a sauna and later died with a diagnosis of heatstroke. On autopsy, preexisting Hashimoto's thyroiditis was found.[460]

Muscle contains characteristic isoforms of myosin, each with differing intrinsic metabolic activities, such as the rate of its actin-activated ATPases. Myosin molecules are composed of heavy and light subunits that associate in a specific manner, each of which is specific to muscle type during development and maturation; that is, ventricular myosin of a fetal heart is different from that of an adult heart.[82] In some muscles, acclimation leads to a higher proportion of "slow" myosin ATPase, such as the replacement of myosin heavy chain type IIb (MHCIIb) with type IIx.[124,236] Hearts isolated from heat-acclimated rats became more efficient in terms of amount of oxygen required per unit force time per gram of tissue,[232] due presumably to the presence of altered isoforms of contractile proteins. Between 30 and 90 minutes of daily exercise for 10 weeks reduced the percentage of MHCIIb fibers in rats and increased the slower, but more efficient, MHCIIa fibers in rat hind limb muscle. That is, increasing the training duration increases the fast-to-slow shift in myosin isoforms.[114] Excess thyroid hormone increases the amount of the myosin isozyme V1 with its high rate of ATPase and contractile speed, at the expense of the normal V3 isozyme, leading to greater speed and strength but reduced efficiency. In the case of sweat secretion, upon acclimation, there is intrinsically a greater secretion rate of sweat along the secretory tubules because of isoform alterations.

The administration of thyroid hormone to neonatal rats rapidly replaces fetal cardiac ventricular myosin with its adult isoform. On the other hand, if the synthesis of thyroid hormone is suppressed, then the slower, fetal isoform predominates;[62] that is, thyroid hormone concentration regulates protein isoforms, activities, and therefore the output of metabolic heat.[88]

The speed and extent of contractility of heart muscle depend upon the number of the Ca release channels in the sarcoplasmic reticulum (more channels permit faster Ca^{+2} entry into the cytoplasm and faster contraction), and the rate of Ca uptake by the sarcoplasmic reticulum (SR; faster uptake means faster relaxation). In ventricles, low thyroid hormone levels reduce the number of Ca release channels, which depresses contractility. In the atria, low thyroid hormone also increases the density of muscarinic receptors, rendering them more sensitive to negative chronotropic agents. In summary, low thyroid hormone levels depress cardiac function and render the heart more sensitive to agents that decrease atrial contraction and less sensitive to agents that increase HR and contraction.[14,282,298,416]

Acclimation occurs under conditions of relative or actual hypothyroidism. As a result, the acclimated heart shows altered myosin isoforms and increased phospholamban content but lowered contractile velocity, rate of Ca ATPase Ca uptake by the SR, and relative oxygen consumption. These changes increase overall efficiency of the heart at the expense of contractile velocity.[75,345]

Thyroid hormone increases the number of Na^+K^+ ATPase pumps[91] and decreases the density of voltage-dependent calcium channels on plasma membranes (leading to a reduced intracellular Ca^{2+} content).[149] Thyroid hormone and sustained aldosterone, such as from excess sweat loss and elevated Na, also alter metabolic processes and electrical activity of cells by regulating intracellular Na and K concentrations. In the short term, they increase the number of functional Na^+K^+ ATPase pumps by recruiting preformed but inactive pumps and their subunits to the plasma membrane. In the long term, they induce the synthesis of new pump subunits.[91,144] Therefore the prolonged reduced levels of thyroid hormone seen during acclimatization decrease the number of those pumps, hence reducing metabolic activity.[449]

Almost any traumatic insult to the body alters hormonal levels. It decreases thyroid hormone, gonadotropin, and gonadal steroid concentrations and increases ACTH, cortisol, growth hormone (GH), and prolactin levels[44] (see Figure 10-1). The reduction in thyroid hormone concentration commences within a few hours, may be maximal after 1 to 4 days, and persists for the duration of the illness.[529] Among heatstroke victims, the decreases in serum thyroid hormone correlated with severity of the heatstroke, according to peak T_c.[84] After the patients completely recovered, the thyroid function tests returned to normal. That is, the severity of heatstroke was related to the depression of thyroid function. The hypothyroid state may be protective by preventing undesirable catabolic effects. Therefore replacement therapy is not currently recommended.[84]

In summary, long-term acclimatization to heat and exercise involves changes on a molecular level, including alterations in intracellular HSP concentrations, increased IL-1, reduced thyroid hormone, increased aldosterone, increased number of Na^+K^+ ATPase membrane pumps, alterations in protein isoforms, altogether contributing to the physiologic adaptations in organ function.[232]

IMMUNE SYSTEM

In the processes of digestion and absorption of ingested food, chyme remains in the intestines for hours to days. Although we receive a large share of the nutrients, bacteria present in the gut lumen also absorb nutrients from the chyme and reproduce rapidly, reaching concentrations of 10^9 to 10^{12} organisms/g.[181] Dead gram-negative bacteria slough off into their milieu large amounts of the highly toxic cell wall component (endotoxin), which may reach concentrations of 1 mg/g in feces.

As long as LPS remains within the intestines, it is not harmful. Small amounts that "leak out" into the circulation are rapidly inactivated by several mechanisms: some LPS is phagocytosed by bound Kupffer's cells within the liver reticuloendothelial system (RES), where it is partly detoxified and then bound by hepatocytes for further degrading[493]; some LPS binds to circulating antilipopolysaccharide antibodies[167]; some binds to high-density lipoprotein (HDL)[496]; and some binds to LPS-binding protein (LBP).[530]

However, large amounts of LPS rapidly entering the circulation would overwhelm the protective systems, allowing LPS to express its toxic effects rapidly. At plasma concentrations between approximately 10 and 100 pg/ml, LPS initiates a cascade of molecular events, leading to nausea, vomiting, diarrhea, fever, and headache.[42] Higher concentrations can lead to conditions identical to those of gram-negative bacteremia, including vascular collapse, shock, and death.[76] In fact, at the time of death from gram-negative bacteremia, there may be no live bacteria in the plasma, and the circulating LPS appears to be the immediate cause of septic shock.[519]

Intestinal Ischemia and Lipopolysaccharide Release

During exercise, blood flow to muscle may rise from a resting value of 1 to 2 ml/100 g/min to as high as 300 ml/100 g/min to provide oxygen and nutrients. As T_c rises, blood flow to the skin also rises to provide cooling. This strains the cardiovascular system's ability to maintain blood flow to the heart, brain, and liver.[291,334] It is important that blood flow to the liver be maintained during heavy exercise to remove lactate and other metabolites from the blood and to provide glucose for energy.[291]

To maintain blood pressure under still more intense exercise and thermal stress, blood flow is reduced to the less immediately critical organs, the intestines and kidneys. If splanchnic blood flow drops sufficiently, it causes regions of local ischemia and transitory gut wall damage. If this is prolonged, there may be permanent ischemic injury to the gut wall.[400,403] Furthermore, several transitory bouts of local hypoxia and metabolic stress in splanchnic tissues may generate free radicals, exacerbating ischemic injury.[208] Exercise at 80% Ap$\dot{V}O_2$max for 30 minutes at 22° C (71.6° F) increased the permeability of human intestines to small molecules.[384] Ischemic injury of the intestines causes the diarrhea or water intoxication occasionally encountered during a marathon run as a consequence of the inability to reabsorb water ingested during the race.[291] For example, in one extreme case, Fogoros[158] reported that after winning a marathon in 1979, Derek Clayton stated that "two hours later . . . I was urinating quite large clots of blood, and I was vomiting black mucus and had a lot of black diarrhea." Intense and prolonged running is a common cause of gastrointestinal bleeding; up to 85% of ultramarathoners demonstrate guaiac-positive stools from a 100-km race.[28] The ultimate consequences of reduced gut blood flow—endotoxemia—may be severe.

Because of the high LPS gradient across the gut wall, almost any insult to the integrity of the gut wall leads to a rise in plasma LPS. Hemorrhage to 45 mm Hg reduces splanchnic blood flow and therefore reduces oxygen delivery to the walls of the stomach, small intestine, and sigmoid colon.[347] This has led to local elevations in the permeability barrier of the gut wall and caused endotoxemia.[172] In a swine model, blood flow through the superior mesenteric artery was progressively occluded, leading to progressive tissue hypoxia and a local shift to anaerobic metabolism, producing lactate and a fall in the pH of the gut wall.[154] At about the same time, LPS entered the circulation. This may lead to an ominous positive feedback loop, since infusing LPS causes hypotension, reduced splanchnic blood flow, and an increase in gut permeability so severe that bacteria can be translocated into the circulation.[154,515]

The size of putative "holes" in the gut wall accounting for the rise in LPS permeability depends on the duration of the ischemia. When the superior mesenteric artery of canines was occluded, LPS (molecular or micellar) leaked out into the circulation within 20 minutes, but the appearance in the circulation of whole live bacteria (several orders of magnitude larger) required 6 hours of occlusion.[389] In other species, these times may be much shorter.[110]

In a different model, nonhuman primates breathed a hypoxic gas mixture for an hour.[173] The resultant hypoxemia rapidly initiated a reflex response designed to maintain oxygenation of the heart and brain at the expense of the rest of the body. This reflex caused intestinal blood flow to fall and was so intense that it resulted in transient ischemic injury to the gut wall and translocation of LPS into the circulation within only 5 to 10 minutes of hypoxia. When the immune system was suppressed by radiation, hypoxia caused LPS to rise to higher levels and persist in the blood for a longer period. On the other hand, when the gut flora had been reduced by administration of nonabsorbable antibiotics, there was no detectable translocation of LPS and bacteria by hypoxia.[110,181]

There is a fitness component to alterations in splanchnic blood flow. When experimental animals were heat stressed, the fit ones with their greater cardiovascular capacity maintained BF_{spl} better, had reduced amounts of ischemic damage to the gut wall, and reduced quantities of LPS translocated into the circulation than did sedentary animals.[429] That is, fitness may reduce the LPS load during severe exercise.

Such studies show that the permeability barrier in the gut wall is rapidly damaged by hypotension, reduced blood flow, and hypoxia, thus permitting LPS to enter the portal and systemic circulations at a high rate.

The development of secondary fever and infection with a high death rate is common after the cooling of patients with heatstroke.[458] The susceptibility of such patients to infections[458] may be due to a combination of changes in lymphocyte subpopulations, together with the increase in gut wall permeability to LPS and bacteria caused by hyperthermia and associated hypotension.[110]

Cytokines and Shock

Cytokines are a class of protein cell regulators produced by a wide variety of cell types throughout the body. They control the timing, amplitude, and duration of the immune response.[93] They are relatively low-molecular-weight proteins (<80 kDa), usually act at short range in a paracrine or autocrine manner rather than as circulating hormones,[122] and interact with high-affinity cell surface receptors regulating the transcription of several cellular genes, resulting in changes in cell behavior.[24] The various cytokines are extraordinarily active, have overlapping and important activities and may induce each other so that it is difficult to establish which cytokine has what critical function. The local concentration probably determines which regulatory influence a cytokine has at a particular time. After induction by a single stress, various cytokines may be present for hours to days.

Cytokines are usually grouped into two families, proinflammatory and antiinflammatory. The proinflammatory family cytokines are largely cytotoxic. They destroy invading microorganisms and loosen contacts between adjacent cells in a tissue to increase permeability and permit the entry of macrophages into the tissue. Antiinflammatory cytokines facilitate B-cell activation and production of antibodies.

LPS causes septic shock, but LPS itself is not a contact poison. Rather, LPS present in the bloodstream is first bound by LPB to form a complex, which circulates until it encounters a specific high-affinity LPS receptor, CD-14, on a macrophage.[445] Binding of CD-14 by the LPS-LBP complex initiates a cascade of reactions within the macrophage involving hypersecretion of cytokines. Because of their inappropriate and excessive local concentrations, cytokines become highly toxic. Although the correlation between mortality and plasma concentration of any single cytokine is low in persons with sepsis, mortality correlates closely ($p < .001$) with a "score" consisting of a summation of the concentrations of individual cytokines.[79]

Most of the symptoms of gram-negative bacterial shock can be induced by injection of some of the purified cytokines alone. The first two (and most important) cytokines induced by LPS are TNF and IL-1.[342] TNF administration to humans causes fever, tachycardia, increase in stress hormones, and leukocytosis,[342] with the intensity of symptoms closely correlating with peak concentrations of TNF.

TNF rapidly induces IL-1, which causes fever, sleep, anorexia, and hypotension.[325] IL-1 acts directly on vascular endothelium (which would be an organ the size of the liver if concentrated in one place) to increase local concentrations of nitric oxide and to raise circulating prostaglandin concentrations, ultimately resulting in vasodilation, hypotension, and, possibly, shock.[122] IL-1 may also have a more subtle effect. IL-1 changes the norepinephrine responses of arteries in different vascular beds.[395] It decreases norepinephrine-induced contraction by about 50% in the aorta, carotid, and pulmonary arteries but increases contraction in femoral arteries. By so doing, IL-1 may cause abnormalities in regional blood flow during sepsis.[409] Heatstroke raises circulating catecholamine concentrations, which in the presence of IL-1 may redirect blood flow inappropriately.[3]

In Marine recruits, the frequency of heat illnesses during training increases with the highest temperature on the previous day.[266] That is, high T_{amb} may lead to a prolonged rise in cytokines within the body, which in turn may lower the threshold for developing exertional heat illness (EHI) during exercise the following day. High T_{amb} leads to elevated T_c with apoptosis of "inappropriate" cells, including intestinal mucosal cells, over the next several hours, permitting leakage of toxic bacterial contents from the lumen into the circulation, rendering the person at risk from exercise.

Possible New Therapy. A single injection of IL-1 receptor antagonist (IL-1ra) immediately after the onset of heatstroke in rats blunted the hypotension response to heat; they survived much longer (91 minutes vs. 17 minutes) than did controls.[87] However, with continuous perfusion of IL-ra, the survival time increased to *10 hours* from the onset of heatstroke. Currently, the beneficial effects of IL-1ra have not been proved in humans, and we do not recommend such therapy. However, if clinical trials should prove its effectiveness, then after initiating cooling procedures, volume therapy and transportation to a hospital, administration of IL-1ra may be become part of heatstroke therapy.[87]

Arachidonic Acid, Leukotrienes, and Prostaglandins.
At the biochemical level, binding of IL-1 to its specific membrane receptor activates G protein, which increases intracellular cyclic adenosine monophosphate (cAMP)

concentration, which in turn activates membrane phospholipases. Activation of the phospholipases ultimately leads to cell damage and organism pathophysiology.[81,191] The phospholipases hydrolyze phospholipid esters of fatty acids, which in Western diets are largely the ω-6 fatty acids.[252,305] ω-6 fatty acids are hydrolyzed into the key metabolite, arachidonic acid.

Cells contain two major enzyme classes that can act on arachidonic acid: lipoxygenases and cyclooxygenases. Lipoxygenase acts on arachidonic acid to enter a pathway, forming 5-hydroperoxyeicosatetraenoic acid (5-HPETE) and a series of toxic leukotrienes. Of them, LTB_4, LTC_4, and LTD_4 are the most important. LTB_4 induces inflammation, increases capillary leakage, and causes leukocytes to aggregate. LTC_4 and LTD_4 are the strong bronchoconstrictors involved in asthma.[97,210] Cyclooxygenase converts arachidonic acid into prostaglandin G_2 (PGG_2), which is converted into PGH_2 with the formation of toxic free radicals. PGH_2 is a central metabolite on which a variety of enzymes act to form mainly toxic products, such as thromboxane A_2 (TxA_2) and many different prostaglandins, including the toxic PGD_2. TxA_2 causes platelets to aggregate, is a strong vasoconstrictor, and increases capillary leakage. To a person in shock or with another circulatory disorder, such agents could convert a severe but treatable condition into a lethal one. In summary, eating a normal Western diet results in the presence of large amounts of ω-6 fatty acids in phospholipid cell membranes, predisposing to the formation of arachidonic acid and a large number of its toxic metabolites. For a review of prostaglandin and thromboxane biochemistry, see Oates et al[373,374] and Bottoms and Adams.[54]

However, in fish-enriched diets laden with ω-3 fatty acids, a high proportion of the ω-6 fatty acids in plasma membranes are replaced by the ω-3 fatty acids, phospholipases hydrolyze the phospholipids into eicosapentaenoic acid, and no arachidonic acid is produced. Therefore no strongly toxic thromboxanes, prostaglandins, and leukotrienes are produced. Instead, only slightly toxic leukotriene B_5 is formed.

Dietary fish oil (rich in ω-3 fatty acids) dramatically downregulates key immunoregulatory cytokines involved in an autoimmune disease.[256] Mice fed fish oil for 6 weeks showed reduced fever and weight loss caused by LPS injection and did not have the rise in PGE_2 that normally results from LPS activity. These changes suggest that, indeed, the pathophysiology induced by toxic arachidonic acid metabolites can be reduced or prevented by dietary replacement of ω-6 fatty acids with ω-3 fatty acids.[297] However, there was an exaggerated rise in TNF-α, a toxin in itself, possibly because of the lack of the negative feedback from PGE_2. Therefore, although these studies appear promising, they must be interpreted with extreme caution and are not recommended to guide a prophylaxis for heatstroke. There has not yet appeared a clinical study showing that injection or ingestion of ω-3 fatty acids protects humans against heat illnesses. However, supplementing a normal Western diet with fish oil capsules replaces a significant proportion of ω-6 fatty acids by ω-3 fatty acids in human cell membranes within 6 weeks, and possibly much less.[140]

Fever. Fever, in contrast to exercise hyperthermia, represents a physiologic state in which the "thermostat" has been reset above 37° C (98.6° F) by exogenous pyrogens released by bacteria or viruses[121] or from IL-1,[138,258,353] IL-2, and interferon-α and interferon-β.[48]

Cytokines may be responsible in part for other clinical symptoms of fever, including fatigue, malaise, and edema. α-Melanocyte stimulating hormone inhibits IL-1–induced fever and the acute phase response.[318] Interestingly, neutralizing antibodies to IL-1 and TNF have been found in the sera of both normal and sick individuals and may play a role in their regulation.[485] Current evidence suggests that aspirin-like cyclooxygenase inhibitors interfere with IL-1–induced fever or shock responses by inhibiting prostaglandin synthesis.[379]

Defervation. Circulating LPS reaches the thermoregulatory control center in the anterior hypothalamus, activates cyclooxygenase, and induces prostaglandins.[229,343] LPS also is bound by the liver, where it stimulates the vagus nerve to signal the hypothalamus to produce prostaglandins.[417] At the onset of a fever, a patient often feels "chilled" and shivers to elevate T_c by additional metabolic heat. A new, higher preferred ambient temperature is behaviorally established.[376] The physiologic change is even more important. Once this new set point temperature is established, the thermoregulatory center uses all available thermoregulatory mechanisms to maintain it. As a result, attempts at whole body cooling are met with sensations of extreme discomfort and violent shivering. Thus unsuccessful attempts to cool patients with suspected heat illness that results in chills and violent shivering suggest coexistent infection or disease.

This prostaglandin-mediated pathway may be responsible for fever, for normal circadian temperature variation, for pathologic temperature elevations, and for temperature elevations related to stress.[39,285] Although there may be pyrogens that do not act via prostaglandins,[105,251] treatment, if necessary, should be directed at agents that block the action of the pyrogen at the hypothalamic receptor sites.

The external application of cold to reduce true fever is illogical[481] and often ineffective, even after antipyretic therapy.[25,366] The body defends the higher temperature set point against environmental cooling. Therapy for fever that uses agents to block the causative molecular interaction is the most rational and clinically effective approach. Aspirin and other antipyretic agents, such as acetaminophen, indomethacin, ibuprofen, and other newer nonsteroidal antiinflammatory compounds, are effective and act either directly or indirectly through inhibition of the prostaglandin mechanism.[107]

Fever and Resistance to Infections. In simple heat stress or mild hyperthermia produced by passive heat exposure or an exercise-induced increase in metabolism, body temperature will usually fall spontaneously toward normal levels.[353] The normal febrile response is generally self-limited in both magnitude and duration.[518] Vasopressin[504] and melanotropin[362] appear to act centrally to suppress temperature elevation and may be important in preventing extreme hyperthermia.

Should Antipyretic Therapy Be Routine? High temperatures enhance resistance to viral infections in experimental animals.[37,77,151] For example, replication of deoxyribonucleic acid (DNA) viruses is inhibited by mild hyperthermia,[184,227,321] and measles virus membrane protein is selectively blocked by heating cultures to 39° C (102.2° F).[377] Some host defense functions[423,501] that become more effective at 40° C (104° F) than at 37° C (98.6° F) level off or diminish at 42° or 43° C (107.6° or 109.4° F).[481] Although fever has long been recognized as a manifestation of disease[22] and may be identified as a debilitating problem even in the absence of other signs or symptoms,[513] antipyretic therapy should not be instituted routinely for every febrile episode.[157,196] Furthermore, although administration of aspirin lowers fever by altering the thermoregulatory set point in the hypothalamus, it also leads to a greater rise in T_c in response to a standardized heat stress and therefore is not a universal temperature-lowering agent.[145]

In summary, at T_c up to approximately 40° C (104° F), the febrile process has a role in host defense and routine antipyretic therapy for fever is generally unnecessary and conceivably harmful,[481] especially with a link between aspirin and Reye's syndrome.[481] Instead, treatment should be based on evaluation of relative risks[47,128,284] in the individual case and reassessed if the anticipated benefits are not achieved.[481]

Role of Lipopolysaccharide in Heatstroke Pathophysiology

Heatstroke temperatures greater than 43° C (109.4° F) caused a large increase in permeability of isolated rat intestinal walls to LPS and persisted even after the temperature was reduced to 37° C (98.6° F).[365] This suggests a direct thermal injury of the gut wall. The time course of the movement of LPS through the intestinal wall into the circulation resulting from hypoxia, ischemia, and ionizing radiation was determined in nonhuman primates[363] and compared with hyperthermia ($T_{amb} = 41°$ C [105.8° F], RH = 100%, 3 to 4 hours).[310] As T_c rose, the plasma LPS concentration remained low until 42° to 43° C (107.6° to 109.4° F) (Figure 10-9). At this temperature, there was a sudden rise in LPS concentration, first in the portal vein, and 10 to 15 minutes later in the systemic circulation. This sequence appears to be the main route of LPS: out of the lumen of the intestines, through the portal vein and liver, and into the vena cava as a result of intestinal ischemia and heatstroke.[182]

In a previous study of infection by injecting live gram-negative bacteria, Gaffin and coworkers[519] noted that when the concentration of live gram-negative bacteria or LPS rose, the concentration of measurable circulating LPS-specific antibodies fell because they bound to circulating LPS and were "consumed" and no longer detectable by an immunoassay.[519] It had been expected therefore that in the heatstroke experiments the concentration of "natural" anti-LPS antibodies would also immediately fall at 42° to 43° C (107.6° to 109.4° F). Contrary to expectations, natural anti-LPS began to decline at temperatures as low as 39° to 40° C (102.2° to 104° F) (see Figure 10-9).[182] This suggests that as T_c rose to only 39° to 40° C, LPS actually commenced to leak into the circulation at a slow rate, gradually consuming the anti-LPS antibodies. As T_c continued to rise, at a certain point massive damage to the gut wall occurred, leading to rapid leakage of LPS into the portal vein. Currently it is not clear how much of this damage is caused by reduced oxygen delivery from reduced intestinal blood flow, how much by direct thermal damage of the gut wall, and how much by other causes.

Anti-LPS antibodies were protective against heatstroke in vervet monkeys up to a T_c of 43.5° C (110.3° F),

but no higher.[180] This suggests that LPS-induced toxicity is important in the pathophysiology of heatstroke death only up to 43.5° C (108.5° F). Above this temperature, other mechanisms are more important, such as direct thermal damage to nervous tissue.

LPS had previously been implicated as a factor in heatstroke death by indirect observations. Injection of very low doses of LPS leads to rapid "tolerance" to ordinarily lethal doses of LPS.[126,198] Administration of low doses of LPS protected rats against heatstroke. When the activity of the reticuloendothelial system (the main mechanism for removal of LPS from the circulation) was reduced, the mortality of heatstroke increased.[125] Ryan et al[426] found the inverse effect. Rats were heated to T_c of 42.5° C (108.5° F) and then were passively cooled. The next day they were challenged with a lethal dose of LPS, and the mortality rate dropped from 71% in the control rats to zero in the previously heat-stressed rats.

The importance of LPS in heatstroke death was confirmed in a canine model of heatstroke.[220] T_c was raised to 42.5° C (108.5° F) for 3 hours and then cooled to 38° C (100.4° F). Deaths occurred only if the animals had rises in plasma LPS concentration.

Exertional Heatstroke. Several studies support the idea that the immune system and LPS are involved in the pathophysiology of heatstroke. Leukocytosis is a general response to most forms of stress, including muscular activity,[179] administration of epinephrine or glucocorticoid, and excitement. Prolonged or severe exercise initiates mobilization and activation of neutrophils and causes proteolysis of skeletal muscle and production of acute phase proteins by the liver.[72] Exercise leads to local disruption of tissues and sloughing of tissue fragments that circulate and activate the complement system. This activation primes monocytes for further activation by LPS or by fragments of tissue subsequently damaged.[74]

Severe exercise impaired renal function, causing a 100-fold increase in urinary excretion of proteins so profound that it led to an actual depletion of circulating proteins.[395] Although it is well known that hyperthermia in humans results in a reduction in splanchnic blood flow,[400] only recently has sufficient evidence accumulated to provide a mechanism of how this may contribute to the pathophysiology of heatstroke. To consider the relationship of this evidence to heatstroke it is necessary to consider the contents of the intestinal lumen and the likely results of their leakage into the systemic circulation.

It was first reported that many of the clinical signs in a heatstroke victim, including blood clotting disturbances, were similar to those seen in septic shock cases.[194] LPS activates a blood factor leading to disseminated intravascular coagulation,[336,540] a common com-

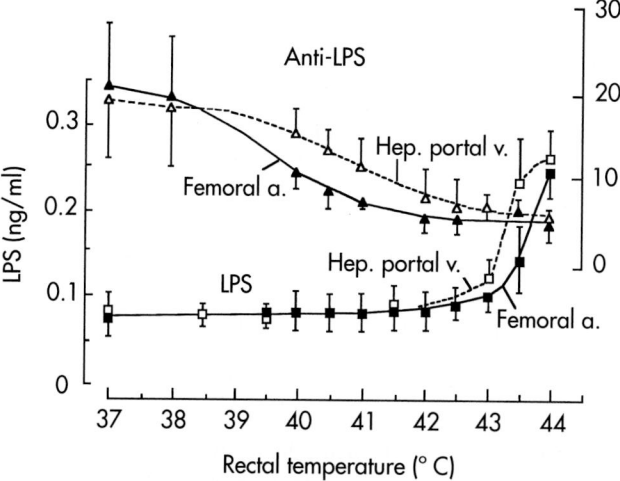

Figure 10-9 Endotoxemia caused by heatstroke in anesthetized nonhuman primates. At T_{re} of 42° to 43° C (107.6° to 109.4° F), plasma lipopolysaccharide (LPS) concentration rose first in the hepatic portal vein and 10 to 15 minutes later in the systemic circulation. However, a decline in "consumed" anti-LPS antibodies occurred at temperatures as low as 39° to 40° C (102.2° to 104° F). (*Modified from Gathiram P et al: Circ Shock 25:223, 1988.*)

plication of septic shock. The authors therefore suggested that LPS participates in the pathophysiology of heatstroke. Similarities between heatstroke and septic shock are described in Box 10-5.

Since core temperatures of long-distance runners may rise above 40° C (104° F), we examined runners who collapsed during an ultramarathon (89.5 km) on a warm day[64] and who reached or were carried into the medical tent at the finish line. Blood samples were taken from 98 patients before therapy. Eighty of 98 had plasma LPS levels raised above normal values, including two in the 1 ng/ml lethal range! It should be noted that the body can tolerate short periods of much higher concentrations, and the lethal concentration usually given as of 1 ng/ml refers to a long-term level, after detoxifying mechanisms come into play.[519] Although hypovolemia and hemoconcentration resulting from sweating may have caused a few "high normals" to cross into the elevated range, this was not the case of the majority. Of those who finished the race, the smaller group with the normal, low LPS levels finished faster. Furthermore, this normal group had higher levels of "natural" anti-LPS in their plasma; that is, the presence of high levels of anti-LPS antibodies correlated with low levels of LPS and better performance. This low LPS and high anti-LPS group also had reduced indexes of

nausea, vomiting, and headache and recovered faster (within 2 hours) than did the larger high LPS and low anti-LPS group (up to 2 days).

In triathlon participants, the concentrations of anti-LPS antibodies fell and LPS rose at the end of the third race.[52] Some athletes had higher levels of "natural" anti-LPS antibodies than did others. When individuals were questioned about their training regimen, it became clear that those who trained the hardest (miles swum, bicycled, and run the 3 weeks before the triathlon) had the highest levels of anti-LPS. It may be that one component of the benefit of physical training is the increase in levels of natural anti-LPS antibodies. We proposed that as a result of severe training, temporary periods of intestinal ischemia occurred, leading to the entry of low to moderate levels of LPS into the circulation, which was enough to stimulate the immune system and induce anti-LPS antibodies. When a marathon was run on a cold day, no elevations in plasma LPS were seen (T. Noakes and S. Gaffin, unpublished observations). At present, it is not clear what combinations of heat load and exertional factors are required to decrease BF_{spl} sufficiently to damage the gut wall for translocation of LPS into the circulation.

Classic Heatstroke. The survival of hospitalized heatstroke patients depends in large part on the rapidity of cooling on entry to a hospital intensive care unit. This time factor may be important because of the time required for the production of cytokines, which is in the range of minutes to hours. Seventeen Hadj patients with classic (nonexertional) heatstroke were admitted to a hospital an average of 2 hours after the onset of heatstroke.[56] Each victim's T_c was greater than 40.1° C (104.2° F). They suffered from delirium, convulsions, and coma. Their plasma LPS concentrations ranged from 8 to 12 ng/ml, that is, extremely high and in the potentially lethal range.[508] Furthermore, their TNF and IL-1 concentrations were also very high. The authors suggested that those cytokines exacerbated the hyperthermia of heatstroke through the induction of prostaglandins.

Nine of eleven heatstroke patients showed a marked leukocytosis resulting from a large increase in the number of T suppressor cytotoxic cells (CD8) and NK cells (CD16/CD56).[55] This leukocytosis increased with increasing T_c. There were also substantial decreases in T helper cells (CD4) and B cells (CD19) as a result of heatstroke. Heatstroke is known to elevate catecholamine levels.[3] Since epinephrine causes leukocytosis with an increase in NK and T suppressor/cytotoxic cells, these authors suggested that heatstroke raised catecholamines, which in turn altered the lymphocyte subpopulations.

On the other hand, hyperthermia causes elevated cortisol[264,265] and cortisol causes lymphocytopenia.[55] In the preceding study, 2 of the 11 heatstroke patients had a decreased number of lymphocytes. To account for the reduction in lymphocytes, the authors suggested that

---

Box 10-5 COMMON FACTORS IN HEAT ILLNESSES AND SEPSIS

CLINICAL

Neurologic symptoms
    Fatigue, weakness, confusion, delirium, stupor, coma, dizziness, paralysis, amnesia
Tachycardia
Nausea, vomiting, diarrhea
Headache
Myalgia
Hypotension
Spasm, rigors
Oliguria, renal failure
Hyperventilation
Organ failure
Shock

LABORATORY

Metabolic acidosis
Hct elevated
Urea elevated
Lactate elevated
Disseminated intravascular coagulation
Cytokines elevated
Hepatic dysfunction
LPS elevated

in those two patients the effects of cortisol, rather than of catecholamines, were dominant. That is, changes in subpopulations of lymphocytes in heatstroke may depend (on an individual basis) on the relative rises in concentration of catecholamines and cortisol, as well as on individual sensitivities to them. However, this is not yet clearly established.

Adaptation and the Immune System. Activity of the immune system through cytokine expression not only alters susceptibility to heat illnesses but determines the winners and losers of athletic competitions or battles as much as skill, strength, and speed. A sick athlete or professional soldier may be defeated by an inferior but healthy opponent. Through appropriate training an athlete may reach his or her peak muscular strength, cardiovascular capacity, coordination, and maximal oxygen consumption. However, at the same time, other environmental, psychologic, or nutritional factors may degrade the immune system, such that he or she becomes more susceptible to an opportunistic infection, very rapidly becomes unfit for competition, and is at risk for heat illnesses.

Mammals possess a programmed universal response to various stressors known as the *general adaptation syndrome.* This includes responses to heat, trauma, hemorrhage, toxins, cold, infections, and nervous irritation.[446] Prolonged heat provokes the general adaptation syndrome, leading to shrinkage of immune tissues and organs with a decrease in immune function.[163] Among various lymphoid subclasses, human NK cells and their precursors are especially sensitive to heat and are completely inactivated by $T_{amb} = 42°$ C (107.6° F) for 60 minutes.[259]

There are relatively few published studies of cytokine secretion following exercise and heat. A new journal, *Exercise Immunology Review,* was established to promote this kind of investigation. Early studies may have been hampered by problems in sampling tissue. Urine samples taken after a race showed large increases in interferon, TNF, IL-1, IL-6, and soluble IL-2r.[472] Failure to detect changes in plasma cytokine concentrations may have been due to rapid renal clearance from the circulation. Rises in IL-1 were observed in human skeletal muscle after muscle-damaging eccentric exercise.[73] Ingestion of vitamin E prevented a rise in IL-1 in vitro from leukocytes obtained from persons subjected to severe exercise.[74] IL-1 causes muscle proteolysis by inducing branched chain keto acid dehydrogenase. This is a rate-limiting enzyme for the oxidation of amino acids in skeletal muscle. As this enzyme increases in concentration, amino acids are progressively oxidized, leading to muscle protein breakdown. Severe exercise suppressed mouse lung macrophages and increased their susceptibility to infections, with greater morbidity and mortality than in moderately exercised mice.[106]

Fourteen consecutive heatstroke patients were found immunosuppressed at admission from depressions in the number of T and T helper cells, CD11a, CD11c, CD44, CD56, and CD54 and rises in T suppressor/cytotoxic T cells. (The many subpopulations of immune cells are usually defined by CD markers.) Cooling led to partial or complete normalization, further derangements, or overcorrection.[209] After a marathon race, leukocyte levels approximately tripled and cortisol concentration rose approximately fivefold.[213] The concentrations of NK cells and B cells fell, although no changes occurred in number of lymphocytes.

Adequate lymphocyte activity is required for normal muscle function. Overtraining may be harmful. A combination of intense physical training and the stress of competition makes some athletes immunosuppressed and more susceptible to infection. One possible mechanism of overtraining muscle injury is that glutamine induces HSPs that protect muscle cells, and overtraining reduces the amount of glutamine available for normal lymphocyte function.[454] There may be a point at which laboratory techniques can quantitatively determine that the disadvantage of immunosuppression is greater than any benefit from exercise training, and that exercise should be curtailed.[213]

HEAT-RELATED ILLNESSES—VARIANTS OF HEATSTROKE

A number of clinical situations arise in which hyperthermia develops that is sufficiently severe (>40° C [104° F]) that it be included as a subgroup of EHS. Neuroleptic seizures and overdose of recreational drugs share with EHS the features of massive muscle contractions (with consequent overuse of high-energy compounds) and rhabdomyolysis.[290] Since the use of recreational drugs is not expected to decline and the number of persons using neuroleptic drugs is probably on the increase, the involvement of heatstroke pathophysiology should be considered in treating those cases. In an unusual situation during mountaineering in summer, two persons died of heatstroke and acute rhabdomyolysis. Both patients had received treatment with antipsychotic drugs, including phenothiazine.[293] In summary, heatstroke in a summertime vacation area might be complicated by the use of therapeutic or recreational drugs.

Malignant Hyperthermia

Malignant hyperthermia is a rare life-threatening disorder involving hypermetabolism, rapid rise in body temperature, and rigidity of skeletal muscle. It is induced by exposure to volatile anesthetics during surgical procedures in affected patients. In about half these patients, mutations were seen in the gene for the Ca^{2+} release channel (RyR).[98,306,511] The anesthetic binds to

RyR and activates the Ca^{++} release channel, causing massive calcium entry into the cytoplasm. This activates contractile proteins, calmodulin, and a variety of calcium-sensitive enzymes, which leads to muscle rigidity, hypercatabolism, fulminating hyperthermia, and metabolic acidosis.[98]

Rhabdomyolysis, hyperkalemia, and myoglobinemia[443] are commonly associated with malignant hyperthermia, with plasma K^+ rising as high as 10 mmol/L.[341] Underlying illnesses in five cases of rhabdomyolysis included heatstroke, high fever, and grand mal seizures with associated hyperthermia. Nevertheless, there were multiple factors responsible for rhabdomyolysis in each case, such as hypokalemia, hypophosphatemia, shock, and arteriosclerosis.[360] A 41-year-old man susceptible to malignant hyperthermia developed an infection and self-medicated with a cold medicine. He presented with high fever, dysarthria, dysphagia, and progressive weakness of his muscles and developed massive rhabdomyolysis with acute renal failure.[268]

Neuroleptic Seizure

The treatment of psychiatric patients with neuroleptic drugs, as well as with antidepressants, antiemetics, and others,[130] may lead to the uncommon but often fatal neuroleptic malignant syndrome, characterized by hyperthermia as high as 42° C (107.6° F),[7] "lead pipe" (skeletal muscle) rigidity, dyspnea, coma, extrapyramidal syndrome, rhabdomyolysis, severe metabolic acidosis, leukocytosis, and elevated creatine phosphokinase.[221,258,488] A number of factors predispose to neuroleptic seizure, including dehydration, exhaustion, aggression, and restraints[254]; high environmental temperature; high doses of neuroleptics; abrupt discontinuation of antiparkinsonism agents; and administration of lithium.[130] Successful treatment of these cases includes immediate withdrawal of the drug, administration of dantrolene, and either oral bromocriptine or the combination of levodopa and carbidopa.[130]

Drug Overdose

Although the toxicity of drug overdose is well recognized, it is not often appreciated that the hyperthermia attained can be in the range reported for heatstroke. Such hyperthermia has been induced with cocaine[120] and amphetamine derivatives, such as 3,4-methylenedioxymethamphetamine (MDMA, "ecstasy") and 3,4-methylenedioxyethamhetamine (MDEA, "Eve").[490] Other components of this syndrome include hyperkalemia, rhabdomyolysis,[462] sympathetic hyperactivity, convulsions, rectorrhagia, psychosis, disseminated intravascular coagulation in the absence of positive blood cultures, and acute renal failure.[223]

Susceptibility to Heatstroke

There may be an inherited susceptibility to EHS. Muscle biopsy specimens taken from two men in military service who had recovered from EHS had abnormal responses to halothane, a well-known cause of malignant hyperthermia.[511] Furthermore, muscles from members of their families had abnormal responses to halothane or ryanodine, a drug that binds to the Ca^{2+} release channels of the sarcoplasmic reticulum.[230] A ryanodine contracture test has been proposed as an in vitro diagnostic test to screen for surgical patients susceptible to malignant hyperthermia.[230] This test might be useful in identifying, retrospectively, a possible subgroup of patients with EHS.

Changes in Cognitive Function

Changes in cognitive function appear to occur before the development of the physical symptoms associated with heat stress.[78] Typically, heat stress causes distortion of the sense of time,[35,36,104] memory impairment,[525] deterioration in attention, and decreased ability to calculate mathematical problems.[85,199,524] Health care personnel should be trained to recognize that confusion, changes in affect, and impaired ability to function in the work environment can be early signs of heat injury under heat stress conditions.[78]

Vasovagal Syncope. Syncope is the cause of about 3% of emergency department visits and 6% of hospital admissions.[183] Vasovagal syncope is responsible for 28% to 38% of syncope patients aged 35 to 39 years.[108,263,331] Benign presyncope or syncope may result from diminished venous return to the heart because of blood pooling in the peripheral circulation. Syncope encompasses psychologic disturbances activating an autonomic vasodilation response; reflex syncope caused by heavy coughing, micturition, and pressure on an irritable carotid sinus; or reduced vasomotor tone caused by hypotensive drugs or alcohol.[132]

Interestingly, the frequency of vasovagal syncope is greater in the young than in the elderly, whereas orthostatic hypotension is more common in older persons.[317] Propranolol does not prevent the vasovagal reaction in response to head-up tilt.[317] Therefore, after the age of 40, presyncope may suggest a more serious condition, such as gastrointestinal bleeding, myocardial or valvular heart disease, or severe anemia. Cardiovascular syncope resulting from arrhythmia carries a 1-year mortality rate of about 30%.[262]

Hyperventilation Dizziness. A slight but prolonged increase in respiratory rate or tidal volume may accompany an increase in anxiety.[132] This can lead to increased blood oxygen content and decreased P_{CO_2}, with accompanying alkalosis. Altogether, these lead to generalized cerebrovascular vasoconstriction with ischemia and dizziness.

Heat-Induced Syncope. The associated clinical syndromes vary in severity depending on the cause of the hyperthermia and therefore so does the duration of central nervous system (CNS) dysfunction. Transient or temporary loss of consciousness associated with a mild form of heat syncope has its origins primarily in the cardiovascular system. It is a consequence of a reduced "effective" blood volume rather than an actual loss of volume.

In an upright and stationary person, blood volume is displaced into the dependent limbs by gravity. If that person is also heat stressed, more blood is displaced into the peripheral circulation to support heat transfer at the body surface. These combined reductions in the effective blood volume can temporarily compromise venous return, CO, and cerebral perfusion. Patients are usually erect at the outset and sometimes report prodromal symptoms of restlessness, nausea, sighing, yawning, and dysphoria.[280] Hypotension results predominantly from vasodilation and bradycardia. This systemic disorder is self-limited because when the person faints and assumes a horizontal position, central blood volume is restored, cardiac filling rises, blood pressure is restored, and the problem remedied.

Fainting is usually brief and responds to horizontal positioning and improved venous return. The patient should be allowed to rest in cooler, shadier surroundings and be offered cool water. The patient should be cautioned against protracted standing in hot environments, advised to flex leg muscles repeatedly while standing to enhance venous return, and warned to assume a sitting or horizontal position at the onset of warning signs or symptoms, such as vertigo, nausea, or weakness. Normally, muscles in the legs act as a "second heart" and in concert with venous valves promote venous return, thereby counteracting orthostatic

pooling and the predisposition to syncope. Consistent with this, nonfainters have higher intramuscular pressure than fainters.

The transient loss of consciousness in syncope has a metabolic basis within ischemic cells of the brain. Despite this, the effects, although startling to onlookers and frightening to the patient, appear readily reversible. There is no risk of direct thermal injury to brain cells complicating the circulatory origin of this sudden decline in effective arterial volume.

The incidence of syncopal attacks falls rapidly with increasing days of work in the heat (see Figure 10-6), suggesting the importance of salt and water retention in preventing this disorder.[242] Thus individuals medicated with diuretics would be at high risk. Furthermore, potassium depletion and hypokalemia may lower blood pressure and blunt cardiovascular responsiveness.[292] In stark contrast to simple syncope is the profound CNS dysfunction dominating the early course of heatstroke. Thus, if a person faints in a setting where hyperthermia is possible and does *not* rapidly return to consciousness, heatstroke should be suspected and body temperature measured.

Exertion-Induced Syncope, Cramps, and Respiratory Alkalosis. During basic military training, a cluster of 17 syncopal episodes was associated with a seldom-described form of heat exhaustion[247] (Table 10-3). In contrast to hypovolemic salt depletion, this heat exhaustion was characterized by hyperventilation, respiratory alkalosis, syncope, and tetany. Most victims also experienced abdominal cramps, yet this was independent of lactic acidosis and hyponatremia. These descriptions were unique in that the heat syncope episodes were not

TABLE 10-3. Clinical Data in 17 Patients with Heat Exhaustion

CASE NO.	AGE	ACTIVITY	SYNCOPE	CRAMPS	T_{re} (° F)	RR	Na$^+$	pH	Pco$_2$
1	19	Marching	Yes	Abd	99.6	24	142	—	—
2	20	Running mile	Yes	Legs/abd	98.4	30	145	—	—
3	20	Rifle range	No	No	99.4	24	143	—	—
4	21	Marching/running	Yes	Hands	100.4	22	162	7.47	34.0
5	21	Marching	No	Severe abd/legs	102.4	35	141	7.50	32.4
6	22	Marching	No	Legs	100.0	22	152	7.70	14.8
7	20	Rifle range	No	Mild	100.0	22	140	—	—
8	20	Marching	Yes	Abd/legs	100.8	30	145	7.52	28.8
9	20	Marching	No	Abd	101.4	24	—	7.69	19.8
10	18	Marching	Yes	Chest	100.8	18	140	7.56	29.4
11	19	Marching	Yes	Tetany	101.5	30	160	7.44	34.2
12	18	Marching	Yes	Severe	100.6	30	130	7.71	17.2
13	20	Marching	No	Mild	98.6	26	141	7.77	15.2
14	19	Marching	Yes	Abd/legs	100.7	30	145	7.76	16.3
15	23	Rifle range	Yes	Abd/legs	101.0	32	148	7.66	19.7
16	18	Marching	Yes	Chest/legs	101.2	28	148	7.78	14.7
17	17	Marching	Yes	Abd	101.6	22	146	7.53	28.4

Abd, Abdomen; *RR*, respiratory rate.

those classically described as the venous pooling or postural hypotension variety.[32,368] The incapacitated trainees arrived at a heat ward within 10 to 30 minutes of the onset of symptoms and blood samples were drawn immediately on admission. They exhibited a moderate to marked respiratory alkalosis, but only two appeared to be severely dehydrated; nearly all (16 of 17 patients) had severe cramps of the abdominal or extremity muscles.

Clinical data recorded on admission are shown in Table 10-3. Almost all the casualties occurred in the afternoon during July 1971 at Fort Polk, Louisiana. All were diagnosed as heat exhaustion resulting from training in the field (12 of 17 while speed marching). Rectal temperatures on admission were elevated, even though most of the victims had been doused with water before evacuation. Serum electrolytes were in the normal range in the majority of the victims. However, hemoconcentration with elevated serum sodium level was observed in four patients. Only 1 of 17 patients had a low serum sodium level and also experienced severe muscle cramps.

The majority of these patients were not water or salt depleted, and 15 of the 16 remaining patients with cramps had normal to elevated serum sodium and chloride levels (not shown). The mean arterial pH for this group of patients was 7.62 ± 0.03 (SEM), and 5 had a pH of 7.67 or greater. Arterial P_{CO_2} was reduced to a mean value of 23.5 ± 2 mm Hg. Thus all patients had moderate to marked respiratory alkalosis, and nine had obvious tetany with carpopedal spasm.[60] The presence of carpopedal spasm and paresthesias in the distal extremities and perioral area helps distinguish this form of cramps from the classic variety.

These data associate exertion-induced heat exhaustion with a form of respiratory alkalosis characterized by syncope, tetany, and muscle cramps and may possibly be the result of "an exaggeration of the normal physiological ventilatory response to thermal extremes."[60] Hyperventilation with its resulting decrease in cerebral blood flow[275,457,509] could account for a significant number of cases of exercise-induced heat syncope. Recumbency, rest, and oral replacement of fluid and electrolyte deficits are usual recommendations. Rebreathing of expired air is directed at alleviating carpopedal spasms but should be done with extreme caution because of its hypoxemic effect.

Classic syncope is usually associated with postural hypotension, whereas heat exhaustion and heat cramps are usually associated with water and electrolyte imbalance. Most literature suggests that unacclimated workers have higher salt losses in the heat than those who are acclimated.[302,308] Thus this series is a good example of the real world with a "mixed bag" of heat illness symptoms. To explain these clinical results, one should recall that acclimated individuals have higher sweat rates (2.5 L/hr

vs. 1.5 L/hr) than do nonacclimated persons but also have increased tolerance to exercise. If both groups voluntarily work at maximum sweat rates for any given task, those who are heat-acclimated could produce higher salt losses, despite their reduced sweat sodium concentrations. Under such a scenario, the acclimated individuals would be predicted to be the more prone to heat cramps.[11] However, Table 10-2 indicates that there are higher salt losses for unacclimated individuals at any given sweat rate or volume of sweat lost. The differential diagnosis of heat cramps should also include exercise-induced peritonitis.[484]

Heat-Induced Tetany

It has long been known that in excessively hot environments, men at rest hyperventilate.[203] Adolph and Fulton[2] described dyspnea and tingling in the hands and feet of men being dehydrated in the heat. In 1941, during a voyage through the intense heat of the Persian Gulf, a ship's engineer was reported experiencing spontaneous hyperventilation and attacks of tetany.[526] He could reproduce these symptoms simply by deliberately overbreathing. This appeared to be the first clinical description of heat-induced hyperventilation tetany.

The exposure of male test subjects to hot, wet conditions led to physiologic changes and onset of symptoms ranging from slight tingling of the feet and hands to more severe carpopedal spasms.[247,248] The frequency and severity of symptoms were apparently not related to the absolute change in the four measured parameters (P_{CO_2}, CO_2, pH, and T_{re}) but rather to the rate of change as depicted in Figure 10-10. There was a direct relationship between the rate of change of the four parameters and the incidence of symptoms. When the subject's tolerance time was short, changes occurred rapidly and the incidence of symptoms was high; conversely, when the tolerance time was long, the same degree of change occurred but the incidence of symptoms was low. It was suggested that rapid changes lead to imbalance between intracellular and extracellular compartments and that this imbalance may be one of the factors inducing symptoms. Again, treatment consists of rest, cooling, and rebreathing expired air.

Heat Cramps

Heat cramps typically occur in conditioned athletes who compete for hours in the sun. They can be prevented by increasing dietary salt and staying hydrated.[136] Heat cramps are brief, intermittent, and often excruciating muscle contractions and are a frequent complication of heat exhaustion and occurred in about 60% of 969 cases of heat exhaustion.[95,308,479] The term "heat cramps" is a misnomer because heat itself does not cause them; rather, they occur in muscles subjected to intense activity and fatigue. The victim with salt de-

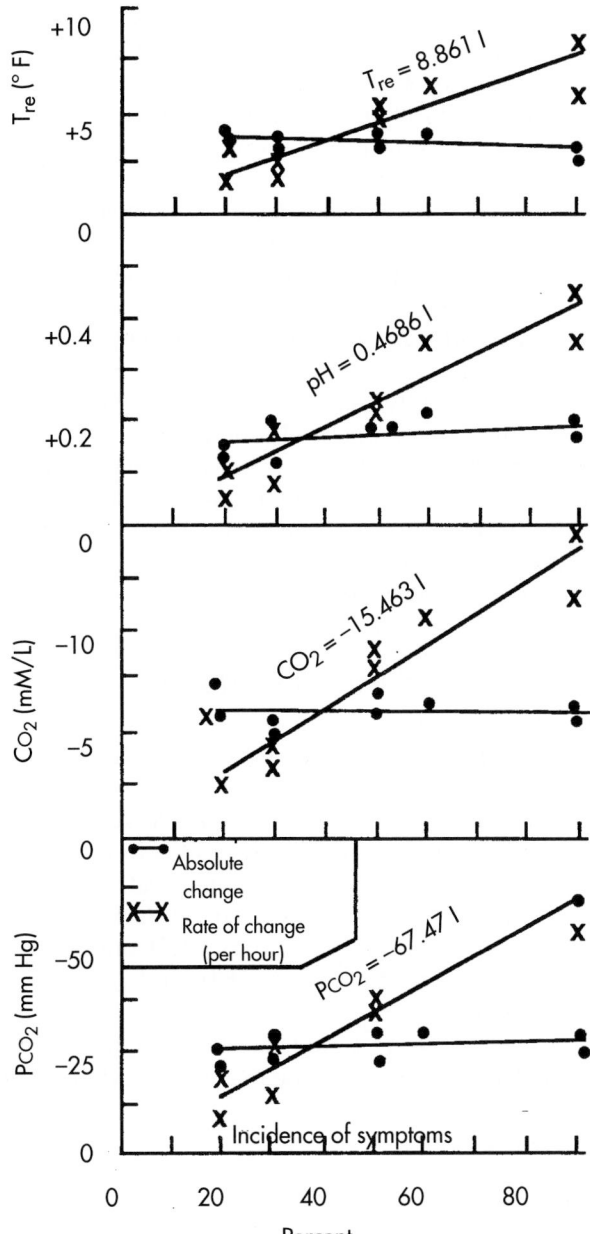

Figure 10-10 Comparison of absolute change and rate of change of P_{CO_2}, CO_2, pH, and T_{re} with incidence of heat-induced tetany. Rate of change values were obtained by dividing the absolute change during exposure by the exposure time in minutes and multiplying by 60. (*From Iampietro PF:* Fed Proc 22:884, 1963.)

pletion at the time of heat exhaustion is obviously ill and has numerous symptoms other than cramps. Furthermore, fatigue, giddiness, nausea, and vomiting are common and may occur before and more prominently than cramps. Sometimes, heat cramps occur as the only complaint with minimal systemic symptoms. Furthermore, there is a difficulty in distinguishing abdominal heat cramps from gastrointestinal upset.

During the 1930s, steel workers, coal miners, sugar cane cutters, and boiler operators were among the most common victims of classic heat cramps.[486,487] Three factors common to most reports are that cramps are preceded by several hours of sustained effort, are accompanied with heavy sweating in hot surroundings, and are combined with the ingestion of large volumes of water. A fourth factor (see later discussion) may be cooling of the muscles. Serum Na^+ levels ranged from 121 to 140 mEq/L (normal 135 to 145 mEq/L).[487] Diagnostic of heat cramps are hyponatremia and hypochloremia that might be due to salt deficit or some degree of water intoxication.[292] If overdrinking causes gastric distention, nausea[405] could trigger vasopressin release and contribute to renal water retention. In an industrial setting, heat cramps occur most commonly late in the day, and after physical activity has ceased; they sometimes occur while a person is showering and occasionally occur in the evening.[308]

Classic heat cramps are distinguished from hyperventilation-induced tetany in that they are limited to contractions of those voluntary skeletal muscle subjected to prior exertion and usually affect only a few muscle bundles at a time. As one bundle relaxes, an adjacent bundle contracts for 1 to 3 minutes. The cramp thus appears to wander over the affected muscle, but the pain can be excruciating in severe cases. Three precipitating conditions (exhaustive work, hemodilution, and cooling the muscle) can each depolarize the muscle cell.[292] This could explain the association of cramps with showering in cool water, since cooling slows sodium transport and depolarizes the cell and may thus reach excitation threshold.[464] The low incidence of heat cramps within the Indian Armed Forces[323] and the fact that Shibolet observed no cases within IDF suggest that heat-acclimated individuals are less likely to experience them. This is consistent with the observation that the incidence was greatest during the first few days of a heat wave.[487]

Heat cramps generally respond rapidly to salt solutions. Mild cases may be treated orally with 0.1% to 0.2% salt solutions (2 to 4 10-grain salt tablets [56 to 112 mEq] or ¼ to ½ teaspoon table salt dissolved in a quart of water). Cooling and flavoring enhance its palatability. Oral salt tablets are gastric irritants and are not recommended. In severe cases, IV isotonic saline (0.9% NaCl) or small amounts of hypertonic saline (3% NaCl) are administered by physicians for rapid relief.

Heat Exhaustion

Classic heat exhaustion is a manifestation of cardiovascular strain resulting from maintaining normothermia. The symptoms of heat exhaustion include various combinations of headache, dizziness, fatigue, hyperirritability, anxiety, piloerection, chills, nausea, vomiting, heat cramps, and heat sensations in the head and upper torso.[16,19,242] Clinical descriptions include tachycardia, hyperventilation, hypotension, and syncope. Although the boundary between heat exhaustion and heatstroke is usually defined as 39.4° to 40° C (102.9° to 104° F), the differential diagnosis is often tenuous[217] or even considered artificial.[456] The victim may collapse with either a normal or an elevated temperature (severe cases around 40° C), usually with profuse sweating. Spontaneous body cooling can occur, which is not prominent in severe heatstroke. The clinical determination of heat exhaustion is primarily a diagnosis of exclusion.

Classic heat exhaustion, like classic heatstroke, tends to develop over several days or longer and presents ample opportunity for the occurrence of electrolyte and water imbalance. The hyponatremia and hypochloremia of patients with either heat cramps or salt depletion heat exhaustion often develop over 3 to 5 days[307] and usually in the unacclimatized individual who has not fully developed his or her salt-conserving mechanisms.[468,469] In salt depletion heat exhaustion, muscle cramps, nausea, and vomiting may be intense, but victims do not feel very thirsty.[242,383] The major route of fluid and electrolyte imbalance (salt depletion, water depletion, water intoxication) involved in a particular heat exhaustion case can be discovered from the events surrounding the collapse and a careful history.[71,292,308,499]

The alternate forms of heat exhaustion are characterized by the type of fluid or electrolyte deficit (primarily pure water or salt deficiency), their underlying causes (prolonged heat exposure vs. intense, short-term exertion), the intensity of the hyperthermia, and the absence or form of CNS disturbance. For example, Table 10-4 is a theoretic demonstration of the impact of body weight loss as either pure water or sweat of varying salt concentrations. If external cooling does not rapidly lower T_c to normal or, conversely, precipitates severe

shivering, intercurrent illness is suspected. Anecdotal experience that in the field suggests that approximately 20% of persons with suspected heat exhaustion have some form of viral or bacterial gastroenteritis. This is especially true if untreated (nonchlorinated) water or ice is available.

At any given loss of body weight (see Table 10-4) the decrement in PV increases with the salt content of sweat. This would be the case for relatively unacclimated individuals. On the other hand, the more dilute the sweat (approaching a pure water deficit) and therefore the greater the rentention of salt the greater the increase in osmolality, plasma, sodium, and thirst. Table 10-4 attempts to compare and contrast the various signs and symptoms of salt and water depletion heat exhaustion with dilutional hyponatremia. It is clear that at some point both syndromes share many symptoms. Vomiting and cramps appear to signal a significant sodium deficit, in addition to some degree of water deficit.

Heat Illness and Coexistent Disease

It has long been known that coexistent illness or infection predisposes an individual to heatstroke.[185] In one study of heat illnesses, 11.2% of patients[522] also had gastrointestinal (choleraic) illness.[522] The reverse is also true: heat waves produce excess deaths from all categories of disease. For example, in one heat wave week in New York in the late summer of 1948, deaths from diseases of the heart and arteries and from diabetes more than doubled (1364 vs. 585), and pneumonia deaths tripled.[139]

Infection predisposes to heat illness and heat stress exacerbates infections, leading to greater morbidity and

TABLE 10-4. Signs and Symptoms of Salt and Water Depletion Heat Exhaustion

SIGNS AND SYMPTOMS	SALT DEPLETION HEAT EXHAUSTION	WATER DEPLETION HEAT EXHAUSTION	DILUTIONAL HYPONATREMIA*
Recent weight gain	No	No	Yes
Thirst	Not prominent	Yes	Sometimes
Muscle cramps	In most cases	No	Sometimes
Nausea	Yes	Yes	Usually
Vomiting	In most cases	No	Usually
Muscle fatigue or weakness	Yes	Yes	No
Loss of skin turgor	Yes	Yes	No
Mental dullness, apathy	Yes	Yes	Yes
Orthostatic rise in pulse rate	Yes	Yes	No
Tachycardia	Yes	Yes	No
Dry mucous membranes	Yes	Yes	No
Increased rectal temperature	Yes	In most cases	No
Urine Na^+/Cl^-	Negligible	Normal	Low
Plasma Na^+/Cl^-	Below average	Above average	Below average

*Data from Armstrong LE et al: *Med Sci Sports Exerc* 25:543, 1993; and Shopes E: *Water intoxication: experience from the Grand Canyon (abstract).* Presented at the 10th Annual Meeting of the Wilderness Medical Society, August 1994, Squaw Valley, Idaho, p 265.

mortality.[312] Relatively few studies have been reported on the susceptibility to infection during heat exposure, or the influence of infection on heat tolerance, and there is a need for further research into the effects of diseases on thermoregulation.[273]

ACKNOWLEDGMENT

This chapter is, in part, a revision of Gaffin SL, Hubbard RW, Squires DL: Heat-related illnesses. In Auerbach P, editor: *Wilderness medicine*, St Louis, 1995, Mosby, pp 167-212, and Dr. Hubbard's original contribution to this chapter is recognized.

The opinions or assertions contained herein are the private views of the authors and should not be construed as official or reflecting the views of the United States Army or Department of Defense. Citations of commercial organizations and trade names in this report do not constitute an official Department of the Army endorsement or approval of the products or services of these organizations. Human subjects participated in these studies after giving their free and informed voluntary consent. Approved for public release; distribution is unlimited.

REFERENCES

1. Adolph EF: *Physiology of man in the desert*, New York, 1947, Interscience.
2. Adolph EF, Fulton WB: The effects of exposure to high temperature upon the circulation in man, *Am J Physiol* 67:573, 1924.
3. Al-Hadramy MS, Ali F: Catecholamines in heat stroke, *Mil Med* 154:263, 1989.
4. Albukrek D: Heat stroke induced cerebellar atrophy: Clinical course CT and MRI findings, *Neuroradiology* 39:195, 1997.
5. Albukrek D, Moran DS, Epstein Y: A depressed workman with heatstroke, *Lancet* 347:1016, 1996.
6. Allan JR, Wilson CG: Influence of acclimatization on sweat sodium concentration, *J Appl Physiol* 38:708, 1971.
7. Allsop P, Twigley AJ: The neuroleptic malignant syndrome. Case report with a review of the literature, *Anaesthesia* 42:49, 1987.
8. American College of Sports Medicine: Position stand on heat and cold illnesses during distance running, *Med Sci Sports Exerc* 28:i, 1996.
9. Amin V et al: The degree of protection provided to neuronal cells by a pre-conditioning stress correlates with the amount of heat shock protein 70 it induces and not with the similarity of the subsequent stress, *Neurosci Lett* 200:80, 1995.
10. Anderson GS, Ward R, Mekjavic IB: Gender differences in physiological reactions to thermal stress, *Eur J Appl Physiol* 71:95, 1995.
11. Anderson RJ et al: Heat injuries: early assessment and management In Wolcott B, Rund DA, editors: *Emergency medicine annual*, vol 1, Norwalk, Conn, 1982, Appleton, Century, Crofts.
12. Andersson B: Regulation of water intake, *Physiol Rev* 58:582, 1978.
13. Anghileri LJ: Role of tumor cell membrane in hyperthermia. In Anghileri LJ, Robert J, editors: *Hyperthermia in cancer treatment*, Boca Raton, Fla, 1986, CRC Press.
14. Arai M et al: Effect of thyroid hormone on the expression of mRNA encoding sarcoplasmic reticulum proteins, *Circ Res* 69:266, 1991.
15. Arkins S, Dantzer R, Kelley KW: Somatolactogens, somatomedins, and immunity, *J Dairy Sci* 76:2437, 1993.
16. Armstrong LE, Pandolf KB: Physical training cardiorespiratory physical fitness and exercise heat tolerance. In Pandolf KB, Sawka MN, Gonzalez RR, editors: *Human performance physiology and environmental medicine at terrestrial extremes*, Indianapolis, 1988, Benchmark Press.
17. Armstrong LE et al: Heat acclimation during summer running in the northeastern United States, *Med Sci Sports Exerc* 19:131, 1986.
18. Armstrong LE et al: Preparing Alberto Salazar for the heat of the 1984 Olympic marathon, *Physician Sportsmed* 14:73, 1986.
19. Armstrong LE et al: Signs and symptoms of heat exhaustion during strenuous exercise, *Ann Sports Med* 3:182, 1987.
20. Armstrong LE et al: Symptomatic hyponatremia during prolonged exercise in heat, *Med Sci Sports Exerc* 25:543, 1993.
21. Ashkenazi I, Epstein Y: Alternations in plasma volume and protein during and after a continuous 110-kilometer march with 20-kilogram backpack load, *Mil Med* 163:687, 1998.
22. Atkins T: Fever-new perspective on an old phenomenon, *N Engl J Med* 308:958, 1983.
23. Avellini BA, Kamon E, Krajewski JT: Physiological responses of physically fit men and women to acclimation to humid heat, *J Appl Physiol* 49:254, 1980.
24. Balkwill F: Cytokines—soluble factors in immune responses, *Curr Opin Immunol* 1:241, 1988.
25. Banet M: Mechanism of action of physical antipyresis in the rat, *J Appl Physiol* 64:1076, 1988.
26. Reference deleted in proofs.
27. Bartley JD: Heat stroke: is total prevention possible?, *Mil Med* 142:528, 1977.
28. Baska RS et al: Gastrointestinal bleeding during an ultramarathon, *Dig Dis Sci* 35:276, 1990.
29. Bass DE, Henschel A: Responses of body fluid compartments to heat and cold, *Physiol Rev* 36:128, 1956.
30. Bass H, Moore JL, Coakley WT: Lethality in mammalian cells due to hyperthermia under oxic and hypoxic conditions, *Int J Radiat Biol* 33:57, 1978.
31. Bateman A et al: The immune-hypothalamic-pituitary-adrenal axis, *Endocr Rev* 10:92, 1989.
32. Bean WB, Eichna LW: Performance in relation to environmental temperature, *Fed Proc* 2:144, 1943.
33. Belding HS: The search for a universal heat stress index. In Hardy JD, Gagge AP, Stolwijk AJ, editors: *Physiological and behavioral temperature regulation*, Springfield, Ill, 1970, Charles C Thomas.
34. Belding HS, Hatch TF: Index for evaluating heat stress in terms of resulting physiological strains, *Heat Pip Air Condit* 27:129, 1955.
35. Bell C, Provins K: Effects of high temperature environmental conditions on human performance, *J Occup Med* 4:202, 1962.
36. Bell C, Provins K: Relations between physiological responses to environmental heat and time judgement, *J Exp Psychol* 66:572, 1963.
37. Bell JF, Moore GJ: Effects of high ambient temperature on various stages of rabies virus infection in mice, *Infect Immun* 10:510, 1974.
38. Benca RM, Quintans J: Sleep and host defenses: a review, *Sleep* 20:1027, 1997.
39. Benedek G et al: Indomethacin is effective against neurogenic hyperthermia following cranial trauma or brain surgery, *Can J Neurol Sci* 14:145, 1987.
40. Benziger TH: On physical heat regulation and the sense of temperature in man, *Proc Natl Acad Sci USA* 45:645, 1959.
41. Benziger TH: The diminution of thermoregulatory sweating during cold-reception at the skin, *Proc Natl Acad Sci USA* 47:730, 1961.
42. Berczi I, Bertok K, Bereznai T: Comparative studies on the toxicity of E. coli lipopolysaccharide endotoxin in various animal species, *Can J Microbiol* 12:1070, 1966.
43. Bergeron MF, Armstrong LE, Maresh CM: Fluid and electrolyte losses during tennis in the heat, *Clin Sports Med* 14:23, 1995.
44. Besedovsky H, Del Rey A: Immune-neuro-endocrine interactions: facts and hypotheses, *Endocr Rev* 17:64, 1996.
45. Blake MJ et al: Neural and endocrine mechanisms of cocaine-induced 70-kDa heat shock protein expression in aorta and adrenal gland, *J Pharmacol Exp Ther* 268:522, 1994.
46. Blake MJ et al: Discordant expression of heat shock protein mRNAs in tissues of heat-stressed rats, *J Biol Chem* 265:15275, 1990.
47. Blatteis CM: Fever: is it beneficial? *Yale J Biol Med* 59:107, 1986.
48. Bocci V: Central nervous system toxicity of interferons and other cytokines, *J Biol Regul Homeost Agents* 2:107, 1988.
49. Borkan SC et al: Heat stress ameliorates ATP depletion-induced sublethal injury in mouse proximal tubule cells, *Am J Physiol* 272:F347, 1997.
50. Borrelli MJ: *The effects of high intensity ultrasound on the ultrastructure of mammalian central nervous tissue*, doctoral thesis, Urbana, Ill, 1984, University of Illinois at Urbana-Champaign.
51. Borrelli MJ, Wong RS, Dewey WC: A direct correlation between hyperthermia induced membrane blebbing and survival in synchronous G1 CHO cells, *J Cell Physiol* 126:181, 1986.
52. Bosenberg AT et al: Strenuous exercise causes systemic endotoxemia, *J Appl Physiol* 65:106, 1988.
53. Botsford JH: Wet globe thermometer for environmental heat measurement, *Am Ind Hyg Assoc J* 32:1, 1971.
54. Bottoms G, Adams R: Involvement of prostaglandins and leukotrienes in the pathogenesis of endotoxemia and sepsis, *J Am Vet Med Assoc* 200:1842, 1992.

55. Bouchama A et al: Distribution of peripheral blood leukocytes in acute heatstroke, *J Appl Physiol* 73:405, 1992.

56. Bouchama A et al: Elevated pyrogenic cytokines in heatstroke, *Chest* 104:1498, 1993.

57. Boulant JA: Hypothalamic control of thermoregulation. In Morgane PJ, Panksepp J, editors: *Handbook of the hypothalamus,* vol 3, New York, 1980, Marcel Dekker.

58. Bowman BJ et al: Survival of human epidermal keratinocytes after short-duration high temperature: synthesis of HSP70 and IL-8, *Am J Physiol* 272:C1988, 1997.

59. Boyd AE, Beller GA: Acid base changes in heat exhaustion during basic training, *Proc Army Sci Conf* 1:114, 1972.

60. Boyd AE, Beller GA: Heat exhaustion and respiratory alkalosis, *Ann Intern Med* 83:835, 1975.

61. Bratton SL, Jardine DS, Mirkes PE: Constitutive synthesis of heat shock protein (72kD) in human peripheral blood mononuclear cells: implications for use as a clinical test of recent thermal stress, *Int J Hyperthermia* 13:157, 1997.

62. Brent GA: The molecular basis of thyroid hormone action, *N Engl J Med* 331:847, 1994.

63. Bricknell MCM: Heat illness in the army in Cyprus, *Occup Med (Oxf)* 46:304, 1996.

64. Brock-Utne JG et al: Endotoxaemia in exhausted runners following a long distance race, *S Afr Med J* 73:533, 1988.

65. Brooks EM, Kenney WL: Chronic hormone replacement therapy does not alter resting or maximal skin blood flow, *J Appl Physiol* 85:502, 1998.

66. Brooks EM et al: Chronic hormone replacement therapy alters thermoregulatory and vasomotor function in postmenopausal women, *J Appl Physiol* 83:477, 1997.

67. Brown GL, Goffart M, Dias MV: The effects of adrenaline and of sympathetic stimulation on the demarcation potential of mammalian skeletal muscle, *J Physiol (Lond)* 111:184, 1950.

68. Bukau B, Horwich AL: The Hsp70 and Hsp60 chaperone machines, *Cell* 92:351, 1998.

69. Burr RE: *Heat illness: a handbook for medical officers,* Technical Report No. T 91-3. Natick, Mass, 1991, US Army Research Institute of Environmental Medicine.

70. Caldwell JA Jr: A brief survey of chemical defense, crew rest and heat stress/physical training issues related to operation Desert Storm, *Mil Med* 157:275, 1992.

71. Callaham ML: *Emergency management of heat illness,* North Chicago, Ill, 1979, Abbott Laboratories.

72. Campbell BG: Cocaine abuse with hyperthermia, seizures and fatal complications, *Med J Aust* 149:387, 1988.

73. Cannon JG et al: Physiological mechanisms contributing to increased interleukin-1 secretion, *J Appl Physiol* 61:1869, 1986.

74. Cannon JG et al: Acute phase response in exercise. II. Associations between vitamin E, cytokines and muscle proteolysis, *Am J Physiol* 260:R1235, 1991.

75. Carafoli E: Intracellular calcium homeostasis, *Annu Rev Biochem* 56:395, 1987.

76. Caridis DT et al: Endotoxaemia in man, *Lancet* 1:1381, 1972.

77. Carmichael LE, Barnes FD, Percy DH: Temperature as a factor in resistance of young puppies to canine herpesvirus, *J Infect Dis* 120:669, 1969.

78. Carter BJ, Cammermeyer M: Emergence of real casualties during simulated chemical warfare training under high heat conditions, *Mil Med* 150:657, 1985.

79. Casey LC, Balk RA, Bone RC: Plasma cytokine and endotoxin levels correlate with survival in patients with the sepsis syndrome, *Ann Intern Med* 119:771, 1993.

80. Cervera J: Effects of thermic shock on HEP2 cells: an ultrastructural and high resolution autoradiographic study, *J Ultrastruct Res* 63:51, 1978.

81. Chang J, Gilman SC, Lewis AE: Interleukin-1 activates phospholipase A2 in rabbit chondrocytes: a possible signal for IL-1 action, *J Immunol* 36:1283, 1986.

82. Chanoine C et al: Myosin structure and thyroidian control of myosin synthesis in urodelan amphibian skeletal muscle, *Int J Dev Biol* 34:163, 1990.

83. Chaurel C et al: Environmental stresses and strains in an extreme situation: the repair of electrometallurgy furnaces, *Int Arch Occup Environ Health* 65:253, 1993.

84. Chen WL et al: Changes in thyroid hormone metabolism in exertional heat stroke with or without acute renal failure, *J Clin Endocrinol Metab* 81:625, 1996.

85. Chiles W: Effects of elevated temperatures on performance of a complex mental task, *Ergonomics* 2:89, 1958.

86. Chin K, Ohi M: New insights into the therapy and pathophysiology of patients with obstructive sleep apnoea syndrome, *Respirology* 3:139, 1998.

87. Chiu WT, Kao TY, Lin MT: Increased survival in experimental rat heatstroke by continuous perfusion of interleukin-1 receptor antagonist, *Neurosci Res* 24:159, 1996.

88. Chizzonite RA, Zak R: Regulation of myosin isoenzyme composition in fetal and neonatal rat ventricle by endogenous thyroid hormones, *J Biol Chem* 259:12628, 1984.

89. Chung NK, Pin CH: Obesity and the occurrence of heat disorders, *Mil Med* 161:739, 1996.

90. Ciavarra RP, Simeone A: T lymphocyte stress response. 1. Induction of heat shock protein synthesis at febrile temperatures is correlated with enhanced resistance to hyperthermic stress but not to heavy metal toxicity or dexamethasone-induced immunosuppression, *Cell Immunol* 129:363, 1990.

91. Clausen T: Regulation of active NaK transport in skeletal muscle, *Physiol Rev* 66:542, 1986.

92. Clausen T, Flatman JA: The effect of catecholamines on NaK transport and membrane potential in rat soleus muscle, *J Physiol (Lond)* 270:383, 1977.

93. Cohen S: Physiologic and pathologic manifestations of lymphokine action, *Hum Pathol* 17:112, 1986.

94. Cohn SM et al: LY171883 preserves mesenteric perfusion in porcine endotoxic shock, *J Surg Res* 49:37, 1990.

95. Collings GH, Shoudy LA, Shaffer FE: The clinical aspects of heat diseases, *Industr Med* 12:728, 1943.

96. Collins KJ, Crockford GW, Weiner JS: The local training effect of secretory activity on the response of eccrine sweat glands, *J Physiol* 184:203, 1966.

97. Cook JA, Tempel GE, Ball HA: Eicosanoids in sepsis and its sequelae. In Halushka PV, Mais DE, editors: *Eicosanoids in the cardiovascular and renal systems,* Lancaster, UK, 1988, MTPP Press Ltd.

98. Cornet C, Moeller R, Laxenaoir MC: Clinical features of malignant hyperthermia crisis, *Ann Fr Anesth Reanim* 8:435, 1989.

99. Coss RA, Dewey WC, Bamburg JR: Effects of hyperthermia (41.5° C) on Chinese hamster ovary cells analyzed in mitosis, *Cancer Res* 39:1911, 1979.

100. Costa JT: Caterpillars as social insects, *American Scientist* 85:150, 1997.

101. Cummings M: Increased c-fos expression associated with hyperthermia-induced apoptosis of a Burkitt lymphoma cell line, *Int J Radiat Biol* 68:687, 1995.

102. Cunningham DJ, Stolwijk JAJ, Wenger CB: Comparative thermoregulatory responses of resting men and women, *J Appl Physiol* 45:908, 1978.

103. Cunningham ET, DeSouza EB: Interleukin 1 receptors in the brain and endocrine tissues, *Immunol Today* 14:171, 1993.

104. Curley MD, Hawkins RN: Cognitive performance during a heat acclimation regimen, *Aviat Space Environ Med* 54:709, 1983.

105. Davatelis G et al: Macrophage inflammatory protein-1: a prostaglandin-independent endogenous pyrogen, *Science* 2432:1066, 1989.

106. Davis JM et al: Exercise, alveolar macrophage function, and susceptibility to respiratory infection, *J Appl Physiol* 83:1461, 1998.

107. Davis MM et al: Accumulation of deuterium oxide in body fluids after ingestion of D_2O-labelled beverages, *J Appl Physiol* 63:2060, 1987.

108. Day SC et al: Evaluation and outcome of emergency room patients with transient loss of consciousness, *Am J Med* 73:15, 1982.

109. Deguchi Y, Negoro S, Kishimoto S: Age-related changes of heat shock protein gene transcription in human peripheral blood mononuclear cells, *Biochem Biophys Res Comm* 157:580, 1988.

110. Deitch EA et al: Effect of hemorrhagic shock on bacterial translocation, intestinal morphology and intestinal permeability in conventional and antibiotic-decontaminated rats, *Crit Care Med* 18:529, 1990.

111. Delogu G et al: Heat shock protein (HSP70) expression in septic patients, *J Crit Care* 12:188, 1997.

112. Dematte JE et al: Near-fatal heat stroke during the 1995 heat wave in Chicago, *Ann Intern Med* 129:173, 1998.

113. Demendoza D, Cronoan JE: Thermal regulation of membrane lipid fluidity in bacteria, *TIBS* 8:49, 1983.

114. Demirel HA et al: Exercise-induced alterations in skeletal muscle myosin heavy chain phenotype: dose-response relationship, *J Appl Physiol* 86:1002, 1999.

115. Demirel HA et al: Exercise training reduces myocardial lipid peroxidation following short-term ischemia-reperfusion, *Med Sci Sports Exerc* 30:1211, 1999.

116. Demirel HA et al: The effects of exercise duration on adrenal HSP72/73 induction in rats, *Acta Physiol Scand* 167:227, 1999.

117. Dep A: *Prevention, treatment and control of heat injury.* Technical Report TB MED 507, NAVMED P-5052-5, AFP 160-1. Washington, DC, 1980, Departments of the Army, Navy, and Air Force.

118. Dewasmes G et al: Regulation of local sweating in sleep-deprived exercising humans, *Eur J Appl Physiol* 66:542, 1993.

119. Dill DB: *The hot life of man and beast,* Springfield, Ill, 1985, Charles C Thomas.

120. Dill DB, Scholt L, MacLean D: Capacity of young males and females for running in desert heat, *Med Sci Sports Exerc* 9:137, 1977.

121. Dinarello CA, Cannon JG, Wolff SM: New concepts on the pathogenesis of fever, *Rev Infect Dis* 10:168, 1988.

122. Dinarello CA, Wolff SM: The role of interleukin-1 in disease, *N Engl J Med* 328:106, 1993.

123. Dinman BD, Horvath SM: Heat disorders in industry: a re-evaluation of diagnostic criteria, *J Occup Med* 26:489, 1984.

124. Dodd SL, Vrabas IS, Stetson DS: Effects of intermittent ischemia on contractile properties and myosin isoforms of skeletal muscle, *Med Sci Sports Exerc* 30:850, 1998.

125. DuBose DA et al: Relationship between rat heat stress mortality and alterations in reticuloendothelial carbon clearance function, *Aviat Space Environ Med* 54:1090, 1983.

126. DuBose DA et al: Role of bacterial endotoxins of intestinal origin in rat heat stress mortality, *J Appl Physiol* 54:31, 1983.

127. Dubuis JM et al: Human recombinant interleukin-1b decreases plasma thyroid hormone and thyroid stimulating hormone levels in rats, *Endocrinology* 123:2175, 1988.

128. Duff GW: Is fever beneficial to the host: a clinical perspective, *Yale J Biol Med* 59:125, 1986.

129. Dukes-Dobos FN: Hazards of heat exposure: a review, *Scand J Work Environ Health* 7:73, 1981.

130. Ebadi M, Pfeiffer RF, Murrin LC: Pathogenesis and treatment of neuroleptic malignant syndrome, *Gen Pharmacol* 21:367, 1990.

131. Editor: Immunotoxin-induced apoptosis. In R&D Systems, editors: *Cytokine bulletin,* Minneapolis, 1999, R&D Systems.

132. Edmeads J: Understanding dizziness: how to decipher this nonspecific symptom, *Postgrad Med* 88:255, 1990.

133. Edwards RHT et al: Effect of temperature on muscle energy metabolism and endurance during successive isometric contractions sustained to fatigue of the quadriceps muscle in men, *J Physiol (Lond)* 220:335, 1972.

134. Eichler A, McFee A, Root H: Heatstroke, *Am J Surg* 118:855, 1969.

135. Eichna LW et al: Thermal regulation during acclimatization in a hot, dry (desert type) environment, *Am J Physiol* 163:585, 1950.

136. Eichner ER: Treatment of suspected heat illness, *Int J Sports Med* 19(suppl 2):S150, 1998.

137. Elizondo R: Local control of eccrine sweat gland function, *Fed Proc* 32:1583, 1973.

138. Ellis FP: Mortality from heat illness and heat-aggravated illness in the United States, *Environ Res* 5:1, 1972.

139. Ellis FP: Heat illness: I. Epidemiology, II. Pathogenesis, III. Acclimatization, *Trans R Soc Trop Med Hyg* 70:402, 1976.

140. Endres S et al: The effect of dietary supplementation with ω-3 polyunsaturated fatty acids on the synthesis of interleukin-1 and tumor necrosis factor by mononuclear cells, *N Engl J Med* 320:265, 1989.

141. Epstein Y, Sohar E: Fluid balance in hot climates: sweating, water intake and prevention of dehydration, *Public Health Rev* 13:115, 1985.

142. Epstein Y, Sohar E, Shapiro Y: Exertional heatstroke: a preventable condition, *Isr J Med Sci* 31:454, 1995.

143. Epstein Y et al: Exertional heat stroke: a case series, *Med Sci Sports Exerc* 31:224, 1999.

144. Ewart HS, Klip A: Hormonal regulation of the Na+K+-ATPase: mechanisms underlying rapid and sustained changes in pump activity, *Am J Physiol* 269:C295, 1995.

145. Fawcett TW, Xu Q, Holbrook NJ: Potentiation of heat stress-induced hsp70 expression in vivo by aspirin, *Cell Stress Chaperones* 2:104, 1997.

146. Feder JH et al: The consequences of expressing hsp70 in *Drosophila* cells at normal temperatures, *Genes Dev* 6:1402, 1992.

147. Feder ME, Hofmann GE: Heat-shock proteins, molecular chaperones, and the stress response: evolutionary and ecological physiology, *Annu Rev Physiol* 61:243, 1999.

148. Feig PU, McCurdy DK: The hypertonic state, *N Engl J Med* 297:1444, 1977.

149. Ferrante J, Triggle DJ: Drug- and disease-induced regulation of voltage-dependent calcium channels, *Pharmacol Rev* 42:29, 1990.

150. Ferris EB et al: Heat stroke: clinical and chemical observations on 44 cases, *J Clin Invest* 17:249, 1938.

151. Feruchi S, Shimizu Y: Effect of ambient temperatures on multiplication of attenuated transmissible gastroenteritis virus in the bodies of newborn piglets, *Infect Immun* 13:990, 1976.

152. Fielding RA et al: Acute phase response in exercise, *Am J Physiol* 265(RICP 34):R166, 1993.

153. Fincato G et al: Expression of a heat-inducible gene of the HSP70 family in human myelomonocytic cells: regulation by bacterial products and cytokines, *Blood* 77:579, 1991.

154. Fink MP et al: Increased intestinal permeability in endotoxic pig, *Arch Surg* 126:211, 1991.

155. Flanagan SW et al: Tissue-specific HSP70 response in animals undergoing heat stress, *Am J Physiol* 268:R28, 1995.

156. Flatman JA, Clausen T: Combined effects of adrenaline and insulin on active electrogenic Na/K transport in rat soleus muscle, *Nature* 281:580, 1979.

157. Fletcher JL, Creten D: Perceptions of fever among adults in a family practice setting, *J Fam Pract* 22:427, 1986.

158. Fogoros RN: Runner's trots, *JAMA* 243:1743, 1980.

159. Fox RH: Heat. In Edholm OG, Bacharach AL, editors: *The physiology of human survival,* London, 1965, Academic Press.

160. Fox RH, Edholm OG: Nervous control of the cutaneous circulation, *Br Med Bull* 19:110, 1963.

161. Fox RH et al: Acclimatization to heat in man by controlled elevation of body temperature, *J Physiol* 166:530, 1963.

162. Francesconi RP et al: Potassium deficiency in rats: effects on acute thermal tolerance, *J Therm Biol* 16:77, 1991.

163. Franci O et al: Influence of thermal and dietary stress on immune response of rabbits, *J Anim Sci* 74:1523, 1998.

164. Froom P et al: Predicting increases in skin temperature using heat stress indices and relative humidity in helicopter pilot, *Isr J Med Sci* 28:608, 1992.

165. Fukudo S et al: Brain-gut induction of heat shock protein (HSP) 70 mRNA by psychophysiological stress in rats, *Brain Res* 757:146, 1997.

166. Gabai VL et al: Hsp70 prevents activation of stress kinases. a novel pathway of cellular thermotolerance, *J Biol Chem* 272:18033, 1997.

167. Gaffin SL: Antibody therapy for shock. In Hardaway RM III, editor: *Shock: the reversible step toward death,* Littleton, Mass, 1988, PSG.

168. Gaffin SL: Simplified calcium transport and storage pathways, *J Therm Biol* 24:251, 1999.

169. Gaffin SL: The immune system and stress. In Pandolf KB, Takeda N, Singal PK, editors: *Adaptation biology and medicine,* vol 2, 1999, New Delhi, Narosa Publishing House.

170. Gaffin SL, Hubbard RW: Experimental approaches to therapy and prophylaxis for heat stress and heatstroke, *Wilderness Environ Med* 4:1, 1996.

171. Gaffin SL, Koratich M, Hubbard RW: The effect of hyperthermia on intracellular sodium concentrations of isolated human cells. In Blatteis CM, editor: *10th International Symposium.* Pharmacology of Thermoregulation, New York, 1996, New York Academy of Sciences.

172. Gaffin SL et al: Protection against hemorrhagic shock in the cat by human plasma containing endotoxin-specific antibody, *J Surg Res* 31:18, 1981.

173. Gaffin SL et al: Hypoxia-induced endotoxemia in primates. Role of the reticuloendothelial system function and anti-lipopolysaccharide plasma, *Aviat Space Environ Med* 57:1044, 1986.

174. Gaffin SL et al: A miniswine model of heatstroke, *J Therm Biol* 23:341, 1998.

175. Galland BC, Bolton DP, Taylor BJ: Apnea and rapid eye movement sleep excess in the piglet during recovery from hyperthermia, *Pediat Res* 34:518, 1993.

176. Gardner JW: *Am J Public Health* 78:1563, 1988.

177. Gardner J et al: Risk factors predicting exertional heat illness in male Marine Corps recruits, *Med Sci Sports Exerc* 28:939, 1996.

178. Garigan T, Ristedt DE: Death from hyponatremia as a result of acute water intoxication in an Army basic trainee, *Mil Med* 164:234, 1999.

179. Garrey W, Bryan W: Variations in white blood cell counts, *Physiol Rev* 15:597, 1935.

180. Gathiram P et al: Anti-LPS improves survival in primates subjected to heat stroke, *Circ Shock* 23:157, 1987.

181. Gathiram P et al: Prevention of endotoxemia by non-absorbable antibiotics in heat stress, *J Clin Pathol* 40:1364, 1987.

182. Gathiram P et al: Portal and systemic arterial plasma lipopolysaccharide concentrations in heat stressed primates, *Circ Shock* 25:223, 1988.

183. Gersh BJ, Hammill SC: Current recommendation for evaluating syncope, *Contemp Intern Med* 80, 1990.

184. Gharpure M: A heat-sensitive cellular function required for the replication of DNA but not RNA viruses, *Virology* 27:308, 1965.

185. Gilat R, Shibolet S, Sohar E: The mechanism of heatstroke, *J Trop Med Hyg* 66:204, 1963.

186. Gilligan DM et al: Acute vascular effects of estrogen in postmenopausal women, *Circulation* 90:786, 1994.

187. Gisolfi CV: Influence of acclimatization and training on heat tolerance and physical endurance. In Hales JRS, Richards DAB, editors: *Heat stress: physical exertion and environment*, Amsterdam, 1987, Elsevier.

188. Gisolfi CV, Cohen JS: Relationships among training, heat acclimation and heat tolerance among men and women: the controversy revisited, *Med Sci Sports Exerc* 11:56, 1979.

189. Gisolfi CV, Wenger CB: Temperature regulation during exercise: old concepts new ideas, *Exerc Sports Sci Rev* 12:339, 1984.

190. Givoni B, Goldman RF: Predicting rectal temperature response to work, environment and clothing, *J Appl Physiol* 32:812, 1973.

191. Godfrey RW, Johnson WJ, Hoffstein ST: Interleukin-1 stimulation of phospholipase in rat synovial fibroblasts. Possible regulation by cyclooxygenase products, *Arthritis Rheum* 31:1421, 1988.

192. Goetz RH: Effect of changes in posture on peripheral circulation, with special reference to skin temperature readings and the plethysmogram, *Circulation* 1:56, 1950.

193. Gonzalez RR: Biophysics of heat transfer and clothing considerations. In Pandolf KB, Sawka MN, Gonzalez RR, editors: *Human performance physiology and environmental medicine at terrestrial extremes*, Indianapolis, 1988, Benchmark Press.

194. Graber CD et al: Fatal heat stroke. Circulating endotoxin and gram-negative sepsis as complications, *JAMA* 216:1195, 1971.

195. Graham BS et al: Nonexertional heatstroke: physiologic management and cooling in 145 patients, *Arch Intern Med* 146:876, 1985.

196. Gray JD, Blaschke TF: Fever: to treat or not to treat, *Rational Drug Ther* 19:1, 1985.

197. Green HJ et al: Altitude acclimatization and energy metabolic adaptations in skeletal muscle during exercise, *J Appl Physiol* 73:2701, 1992.

198. Greisman SE, Hornick RB: Mechanisms of endotoxin tolerance with special reference to man, *J Infect Dis* 128(suppl):S265, 1973.

199. Grether W: Human performance at elevated environmental temperatures, *Aerospace Med* 44:747, 1973.

200. Griefahn B: Acclimation to three different hot climates with equivalent wet bulb globe temperatures, *Ergonomics* 40:223, 1997.

201. Gromkowski SH, Yagi J, Janeway CA Jr: Elevated temperature regulates tumor necrosis factor-mediated immune killing, *Eur J Immunol* 19:1709, 1998.

202. Gun RT, Budd GM: Effects of thermal, personal and behavioral factors on the physiological strain, thermal comfort and productivity of Australian shearers in hot weather, *Ergonomics* 38:1368, 1995.

203. Haldane JS: The influence of high air temperatures, *J Hyg* 55:495, 1905.

204. Hales JRS: Effects of exposure to hot environments on the regional distribution of blood flow and on cardiorespiratory function in sheep, *Pflugers Arch* 344:133, 1973.

205. Hales JRS, Nielson B, Yanase M: Skin blood flow during severe heat stress regional variations & failure to maintain maximal level. In Milton AS, editor: Thermal physiology. In *Proceedings of the IUPS Thermal Commission Symposium*, Aberdeen, Scotland, Aug 1993, International Union of Physiological Science.

206. Hales JRS et al: Lowered skin blood flow and erythrocyte sphering in collapsed fun- runners, *Lancet* 1:1495, 1986.

207. Hall AC, Willis JS: Differential effects of temperature on three components of passive permeability to potassium in rodent red cells, *J Physiol* 348:629, 1984.

208. Hall DM et al: Splanchnic tissues undergo hypoxic stress during whole body hyperthermia, *Am J Physiol* 276:G1195, 1998.

209. Hammami MM et al: Lymphocyte subsets and adhesion molecules expression in heatstroke and heat stress, *J Appl Physiol* 84:1615, 1998.

210. Hammarstrom S et al: Microcirculatory effects of leukotrienes C4 and D4 and E4 in the guinea pig. In Lefer AM, Gee MH, editors: *Progress in clinical and biological research. Leukotrienes in cardiovascular and pulmonary function*, New York, 1985, Alan R Liss.

211. Hang H, Fox MH: Expression of HSP70 induced in CHO cells by 45.0° C hyperthermia is cell cycle associated and DNA synthesis dependent, *Cytometry* 19:119, 1995.

212. Hanson PG, Zimmerman SW: Exertional heatstroke in novice runners, *JAMA* 242:154, 1979.

213. Haq A et al: Changes in peripheral blood lymphocyte subsets associated with marathon running, *Med Sci Sports Exerc* 25:186, 1993.

214. Hardy JD: Physiology of temperature regulation, *Physiol Rev* 41:521, 1961.

215. Harrison MH: Effects of thermal stress and exercise on blood volume in humans, *Physiol Rev* 65:149, 1985.

216. Hart GR et al: Epidemic classical heat stroke: clinical characteristics and course of 28 patients, *Medicine* 61:189, 1982.

217. Hart LE, Sutton JR: Environmental considerations for exercise, *Cardiol Clin* 5:245, 1987.

218. Hashimoto K et al: Behavioral changes and expression of heat shock protein hsp-70 mRNA, brain-derived neurotrophic factor mRNA, and cyclooxygenase-2 mRNA in rat brain following seizures induced by systemic administration of kainic acid., *Brain Res* 804:212, 1998.

219. Havenith G, Middendorp HV: The relative influence of physical fitness acclimatization state anthropometric measures and gender on individual reactions to stress, *Eur J Appl Physiol* 61:419, 1990.

220. Hayano YH: Influence of induced hyperthermia on intestinal blood flow, translocation of endotoxin and other factors in mongrel dogs, *Masui* 40:769, 1993.

221. Heiman-Patterson TD: Neuroleptic malignant syndrome and malignant hyperthermia. Important issues for the medical consultant, *Med Clin North Am* 77:477, 1993.

222. Helzer-Julin M: Sun, heat, and cold injuries in cyclists, *Clin Sports Med* 13:219, 1994.

223. Henry JA, Jeffreys KJ, Dawling S: Toxicity and deaths from 3,4-methylenedioxymethamphetamine ("ecstacy"), *Lancet* 2:384, 1992.

224. Hensel H, Iggo A, Witt I: A quantitative study of sensitive cutaneous thermoreceptors with afferent fibers, *J Physiol* 53:113, 1960.

225. Herman TS et al: Rate of heating as a determinant of hyperthermic cytotoxicity, *Cancer Res* 41:3519, 1981.

226. Hoekstra KA et al: Increased heat shock protein expression after stress in Japanese quail, *Stress* 2:265, 1998.

227. Hoggan MD, Roizman B: The effect of the temperature on inhibition on the formation and release of Herpes simplex virus in infected FL cells, *Virology* 8:508, 1959.

228. Holmer I: Protective clothing and heat stress, *Ergonomics* 39:166, 1995.

229. Holmes SW, Horton EW: The identification of four prostaglandins in dog brain and their regional distribution in the central nervous system, *J Physiol* 195:731, 1968.

230. Hopkins PM, Ellis FR, Halsall PJ: Evidence for related myopathies in exertional heat stroke and malignant hyperthermia, *Lancet* 2:1491, 1991.

231. Hori S: Adaptation to heat, *Jpn J Physiol* 45:921, 1995.

232. Horowitz M: Heat stress and heat acclimation: the cellular response-modifier of autonomic control. In Pleschka K, Gerstberger R, Pierau K, editors: *Integrative and cellular aspects of autonomic functions*, France, 1993, John Libbey Eurotext Ltd.

233. Horowitz M: Do cellular heat acclimatory responses modulate central thermoregulatory activity? *News Physiol Sci* 13:218, 1998.

234. Horowitz M, Maloyan A, Shlaier J: HSP 70 kDa dynamics in animals undergoing heat stress superimposed on heat acclimation, *Ann NY Acad Sci* 813:617, 1997.

235. Horowitz M, Parnes S, Hasin Y: Mechanical and metabolic performance of the rat heart: Effects of combined stress of heat acclimation and swimming training, *Basic Clin Physiol Pharmacol* 4:139, 1993.

236. Horowitz M et al: Heat acclimation: cardiac performance of isolated rat heart, *J Appl Physiol* 60:9, 1986.

237. Horvath SM, Horvath SM: Heat tolerance and aging, *Med Sci Sports* 11:49, 1979.

238. Houghton FC, Yaglou CP: Determining lines of equal comfort, *ASHVE Trans* 29:163, 1923.

239. Hu RQ et al: Neuronal stress and injury in C57/BL mice after systemic kainic acid administration, *Brain Res* 810:229, 1998.

240. Hubbard RW: An introduction: the role of exercise in the etiology of exertional heatstroke, *Med Sci Sports Exerc* 22:2, 1990.

241. Hubbard RW: Heatstroke pathophysiology: the energy depletion model, *Med Sci Sports Exerc* 22:19, 1990.

242. Hubbard RW, Armstrong LE: The heat illnesses: biochemical, ultrastructural, and fluid- electrolyte considerations. In Pandolf KB, Sawka MN, Gonzales RR, editors: *Human performance physiology and environmental medicine at terrestrial extremes*, Indianapolis, 1988, Benchmark Press.

243. Hubbard RW, Armstrong LE: Hyperthermia: new thoughts on an old problem, *Phys Sports Med* 17:97, 1989.

244. Hubbard RW, Bowers WD Jr, Mager M: A study of physiological pathological and biochemical changes in rats with heat and/or work-induced disorders, *Isr J Med Sci* 12:884, 1976.

245. Hubbard RW et al: Rat model of acute heatstroke mortality, *J Appl Physiol* 42:809, 1977.

246. Hughson RL, Sutton JR: Heat stroke in a "run for fun," *Br Med J* 2:1158, 1978.

247. Iampietro PF: Heat-induced tetany, *Fed Proc* 22:884, 1963.

248. Iampietro PF, Mager M, Green EB: Some physiological changes accompanying tetany induced by exposure to hot wet conditions, *J Appl Physiol* 16:409, 1961.

249. Imura H, Fukata J, Mori T: Cytokines and endocrine function: an interaction between the immune and neuroendocrine systems, *Clin Endocrinol (Oxf)* 35:107, 1991.

250. Inder WJ et al: Prolonged exercise increases peripheral plasma ACTH, CRH, and AVP in male athletes, *J Appl Physiol* 85:835, 1998.

251. Iriki M, Riedel W, Simon E: Patterns of differentiation in various sympathetic efferents induced by changes of blood gas composition and by central thermal stimulation in anesthetized rabbits, *Jpn J Physiol* 22:585, 1972.

252. Irvine RF: How is the level of free arachidonic acid controlled in mammalian cells? *Biochem J* 4:3, 1982.

253. Jackson JC et al: Influence of serotonin on the immune response, *Immunology* 54:505, 1985.

254. Jermain DM, Crismon ML: Psychotropic drug-related rhabdomyolysis, *Ann Pharmacother* 26:948, 1992.

255. Johnson JM et al: Regulation of the cutaneous circulation, *Fed Proc* 445:2841, 1986.

256. Jolly CA, Fernandes G: Fish oil and calorie restriction modulates T-cell subset cytokine production in old NZBxNZW F1 female mice, *Proc Congr FASEB*, San Francisco, 1998.

257. Jones TH, Kennedy RL: Cytokines and hypothalamic-pituitary function, *Cytokine* 5:531, 1993.

258. Joshi PT, Capozzoli JA, Coyle JT: Neuroleptic malignant syndrome: life-threatening complication of neuroleptic treatment in adolescents with affective disorder, *Pediatrics* 87:235, 1991.

259. Kalland T, Dahlquist I: Effects of in vitro hyperthermia on human natural killer cells, *Cancer Res* 43:1842, 1998.

260. Kamon E, Kamon E: Sweating efficiency in acclimated men and women exercising in humid and dry heat, *J Appl Physiol* 54:972, 1983.

261. Kapiszewska M, Hoopwood LE: Changes in bleb formation following hyperthermia treatment of CHO cells, *Radiat Res* 105:405, 1986.

262. Kapoor WN, Hammill SC, Gersh BJ: Diagnosis and natural history of syncope and the role of invasive electrophysiologic testing, *Am J Cardiol* 63:730, 1989.

263. Kapoor WN et al: Syncope in the elderly, *Am J Med* 80:419, 1986.

264. Kappel M et al: Effect of in vitro hyperthermia on the proliferative response of blood mononuclear cell subsets, and detection of interleukins 1 and 6, tumor necrosis factor-alpha and interferon-gamma, *Immunology* 3:304, 1991.

265. Kappel M et al: Effects of in vivo hyperthermia on natural killer cell activity, in vitro proliferative responses and blood mononuclear cell subpopulations, *Clin Exp Immunol* 84:175, 1991.

266. Kark JA et al: Exertional heat illness in Marine Corps recruit training, *Aviat Space Environ Med* 67:354, 1996.

267. Karklin A, Driver HS, Buffenstein R: Restricted energy intake affects nocturnal body temperature and sleep patterns, *Am J Clin Nutr* 59:346, 1994.

268. Kasamatsu Y et al: Rhabdomyolysis after infection and taking a cold medicine in a patient who was susceptible to malignant hyperthermia, *Intern Med* 37:169, 1998.

269. Kaufmann SHE: Heat shock proteins and the immune response, *Immunol Today* 11:129, 1990.

270. Kelly DA et al: Effect of vitamin E deprivation and exercise training on induction of HSP70, *J Appl Physiol* 81:2379, 1996.

271. Kenney WL: WBGT adjustments for protective clothing, *Am Ind Hyg Assoc J* 48:A576, 1987.

272. Kenney WL: Control of heat-induced cutaneous vasodilatation in relation to age, *Eur J Appl Physiol* 57:120, 1988.

273. Keren G, Epstein Y, Magazanik A: Temporary heat intolerance in a heatstroke patient, *Aviat Space Environ Med* 52:116, 1981.

274. Kerslake DM: *The stress of hot environments*, New York, 1972, Cambridge University Press.

275. Kety SS, Schmidt CF: The effects of active and passive hyperventilation on cerebral blood flow, oxygen consumption, cardiac output and blood pressure of normal men, *J Clin Invest* 25:107, 1961.

276. Khansari DN, Murgo AJ, Faith RE: Effects of stress on the immune system, *Immunol Today* 11:170, 1990.

277. Khogali M: The Makkah body cooling unit. In Khogali M, Hales JRS, editors: *Heat stroke and temperature regulation*, Sydney, Australia, 1983, Academic Press.

278. Kiang JG, Ding XZ, McClain DE: Overexpression of HSP-70 attenuates in Ca^{2+} and protects human epidermoid A-431 cells after chemical hypoxia. DTIC summary, *Toxicol Appl Pharmacol* 149:185, 1999.

279. Kibler WB: Injuries in adolescent and preadolescent soccer players, *Med Sci Sports Exerc* 25:1330, 1993.

280. Kienzle MG: Syncope: mechanisms and manifestations, *Hosp Pract* 15:73, 1990.

281. Kim D, Clapham DE: Potassium channels in cardiac cells activated by arachidonic acid and phospholipids, *Science* 244:1174, 1989.

282. Kiss E et al: Thyroid hormone-induced alterations in phospholamban protein expression, *Circ Res* 75:245, 1994.

283. Klosterhalfen B et al: The influence of heat shock protein 70 induction on hemodynamic variables in a porcine model of recurrent endotoxemia, *Shock* 7:358, 1997.

284. Kluger MJ: Is fever beneficial? *Yale J Biol Med* 59:89, 1986.

285. Kluger MJ: Further evidence that stress hyperthermia is a fever, *Physiol Behav* 39:763, 1987.

286. Knapik J: Injury control in the US Army, evidence for seasonal variations in injury incidence during basic combat training, *Abstracts from the Fifth Annual Recruit and Trainee Healthcare Symposium*, Beaufort Naval Hospital, Beaufort, SC, April, 1999.

287. Knapik J et al: *Abstracts from the Army Initial Entry Training Injury Prevention PAT AMEDD Center*, Fort Sam Houston, Tex, March 29, 1999.

288. Knochel JP: Environmental heat illness. An eclectic review, *Arch Intern Med* 133:841, 1974.

289. Knochel JP: Dog days and siriasis. How to kill a football player, *J Am Med Assoc* 233:513, 1975.

290. Knochel JP: Heat stroke and related heat stress disorders, *Dis Mon* 35:301, 1989.

291. Knochel JP: Catastrophic medical events with exhaustive exercise: "white collar rhabdomyolysis," *Kidney Int* 38:709, 1990.

292. Knochel JP, Reed G: Disorders of heat regulation. In Kleeman CR, Maxwell MH, Narin RG, editors: *Clinical disorders of fluid and electrolyte metabolism*, New York, 1987, McGraw-Hill.

293. Koizumi T et al: Fatal rhabdomyolysis during mountaineering, *J Sports Med Phys Fitness* 36:72, 1996.

294. Koratich M, Gaffin SL: Mechanisms of calcium transport in human endothelial cells subjected to hyperthermia, *J Therm Biol* 24:245, 1999.

295. Kosunen KJ et al: Plasma renin activity, angiotensin II and aldosterone during intense heat stress, *J Appl Physiol* 41:323, 1976.

296. Koutedakis Y, Sharp NCC: Seasonal variations of injury and overtraining in elite athletes, *Clin J Sport Med* 8:18, 1998.

297. Kozak W et al: Dietary ω-3 fatty acids differentially affect sickness behavior in mice during local and systemic inflammation, *Am J Physiol* 272:R1298, 1997.

298. Kragie L, Kwon YW, Smiehorowski R: Rat cardiac calcium channels and their relationships with β-adrenergic and muscarinic receptors in hypothyroidism, *Endocrine Res* 19:57, 1993.

299. Kregel KC, Moseley PL: Differential effects of exercise and heat stress on liver HSP70 accumulation with aging, *Am J Physiol* 80:547, 1996.

300. Kronfol Z et al: Impaired lymphocyte function in depressive illness, *Life Sci* 33:241, 1983.

301. Kuhlmann MK et al: Heat-preconditioning confers protection from Ca2+-mediated cell toxicity in renal tubular epithelial cells (BSC-1), *Cell Stress Chaperones* 2:175, 1997.

302. Ladell WSS: Disorders due to heat, *Trans R Soc Trop Med Hyg* 51:189, 1957.

303. Landis CA et al: Sleep deprivation alters body temperature dynamics to mild cooling and heating not sweating threshold in women, *Sleep* 21:101, 1998.

304. Lee DHK: Seventy-five years of search for a heat index, *Environ Res* 22:331, 1980.

305. Lee JB, Katayama S: Prostaglandins, thromboxanes, and leukotrienes. In Wilson JD, Foster DW, editors: *Textbook of endocrinology*, Philadelphia, 1985, WB Saunders.

306. Leeb T, Brenig B: Ryanodine receptors and their role in genetic diseases, *Int J Mol Med* 2:293, 1998 (review).

307. Leithead CS, Gunn ER: The aetiology of cane cutter's cramps in British Guiana. In UNESCO, editors: *Environmental physiology and psychology in arid conditions*, Liege, Belgium, 1964, UNESCO.

308. Leithead CS, Lind AR: *Heat stress and heat disorders*, Philadelphia, 1964, FA Davis.

309. Levi E et al: Heat acclimation improves cardiac mechanics and metabolic performance during ischemia and reperfusion, *J Appl Physiol* 75:833, 1993.

310. Levin J, Bang F: Clottable protein in Limulus: its localization and kinetics of coagulation by endotoxin, *Thromb Haemost* 19:186, 1968.

311. Levy E et al: Chronic heat improves mechanical and metabolic response of trained rat heart on ischemia and reperfusion, *Am J Physiol* 272:G2085, 1997.

312. Lewis GBH: Effect of altered environmental temperature on established infection, *Anaesth Int Care* 16:338, 1988.

313. Lin H et al: Electromagnetic field exposure induces rapid, transitory heat shock factor activation in human cells, *J Cell Biochem* 66:482, 1997.

314. Lind AR: A physiological criterion for setting thermal environmental limits for everyday work, *J Appl Physiol* 18:51, 1963.

315. Lind AR, Bass DE: Optimal exposure time for development of acclimatization to heat, *Fed Proc* 22:704, 1963.

316. Lindle RS et al: Age and gender comparisons of muscle strength in 654 women and men aged 20-93 yr, *J Appl Physiol* 83:1581, 1997.

317. Lipsitz LA et al: Reduced susceptibility to syncope during postural tilt in old age: is beta-blockade protective? *Arch Intern Med* 149:2709, 1989.

318. Lipton JM: Neuropeptide alpha-melanocyte-stimulating hormone in control of fever, the acute phase response and inflammation, neuroimmune networks, *Physiol Dis* 243, 1989.

319. Locke M, Noble EG, Atkinson BG: Exercising mammals synthesize stress proteins, *Am J Physiol* 258:C723, 1990.

320. Love AHG, Shanks RG: The relationship between the onset of sweating and vasodilation in the forearm during body heating, *J Physiol* 162:121, 1962.

321. Lwoff A: Factors influencing the evolution of viral diseases at the cellular level and in the organism, *Bacteriol Rev* 23:109, 1959.

322. Malamud N, Haymaker W, Custer RP: Heat stroke: a clinicopathologic study of 125 fatal cases, *Mil Med* 99:397, 1946.

323. Malhotra MS, Ventkataswamy Y: Heat casualties in the Indian Armed Forces, *Ind Med Res* 62:1293, 1974.

324. Manjoo M, Burger FJ, Kielblock AJ: A relationship between heat load and plasma enzyme concentration, *J Therm Biol* 10:221, 1985.

325. Mantovani A, Bussolino F, Dejana E: Cytokine regulation of endothelial cell function, *FASEB J* 6:2591, 1992.

326. Mao ZC, Wang YT: Analysis of 411 cases of severe heat stroke in Nanjing, *Chin Med J* 104:256, 1991.

327. Marber MS et al: Overexpression of the rat inducible 70-kD heat stress protein in a transgenic mouse increases the resistance of the heart to ischemic injury, *J Clin Invest* 95:1446, 1995.

328. Marengo FD, Wang S-Y, Langer GA: The effects of temperature upon calcium exchange in intact cultured cardiac myocytes, *Cell Calcium* 21:263, 1997.

329. Maron MB, Wagner JA, Horvath SM: Thermoregulatory responses during competitive marathon running, *J Appl Physiol* 42:909, 1977.

330. Marriott HL: *Water and salt depletion,* Springfield, Ill, 1950, Charles C Thomas.

331. Martin GJ: Prospective evaluation of syncope, *Ann Emerg Med* 13:499, 1984.

332. Martin SJ: Apoptosis: execution or murder, *Trends Cell Biol* 3:141, 1993.

333. Martinez AA et al: Thermal sensitivity and thermotolerance in normal porcine tissues, *Cancer Res* 43:2072, 1983.

334. Massett MP et al: Vascular reactivity and baroreflex function during hyperthermia in conscious rats, Abstr #5707, *Proc FASEB,* San Francisco, 1998.

335. Matthew WT et al: *Assessment of the reliability of a correction procedure for WGT (Botsball) measurements of heat stress.* Technical Report No T-17-87. Natick, Mass, 1987, US Army Research Institute for Environmental Medicine.

336. McCabe WR: Endotoxin: microbiological, chemical, pathophysiological and clinical correlations. In Weinstein L, Fields BN, editors: *Seminars in infectious diseases,* vol 3, New York, 1980, Thieme-Stratton.

337. McCann DJ, Adams WC: Wet bulb globe temperature index and performance in competitive distance runners, *Med Sci Sports Exerc* 27:955, 1997.

338. McCloskey BP: Manslaughter by heat stroke, *Med J Aust* 2:925, 1976.

339. McCormick W, Penman S: Regulation of protein synthesis in HeLa cells translation at elevated temperatures, *J Mol Biol* 39:315, 1969.

340. McLellan TM: Sex-related differences in thermoregulatory responses while wearing protective clothing, *Eur J Appl Physiol* 78:28, 1998.

341. Mehler J et al: Cardiac arrest during anesthesia induction with halothane and succinylcholine in an infant, *Anaesthetist* 40:497, 1991.

342. Michie HR et al: Detection of circulating tumor necrosis factor after endotoxin administration, *N Engl J Med* 318:1481, 1988.

343. Milton AS, Wendlandt S: Effects on body temperature of prostaglandins of the A, E, and F series on injection into the third ventricle of unanesthetized cats and rabbits, *J Physiol* 218:325, 1971.

344. Minard D, Belding HS, Kingston JR: Prevention of heat casualties, *JAMA* 165:1813, 1957.

345. Mirit E et al: Does low thyroid hormone level switch-on heat acclimation induced changes in cardiac mechanical performance? *Am J Physiol* 276:R550, 1999.

346. Montain SJ et al: Thermal & cardiovascular strain from hypohydration: influence of exercise intensity, *Int J Sports Med* 19:87, 1998.

347. Montgomery A et al: Intramucosal pH measurement with tonometers for detecting gastrointestinal ischemia in porcine hemorrhagic shock, *Circ Shock* 29:319, 1989.

348. Moran DS, Montain SJ, Pandolf KB: Evaluation of different levels of hydration using a new physiological strain index (PSI), *Am J Physiol* 275:R854, 1998.

349. Moran DS, Pandolf KB: Wet Bulb Globe Temperature (WBGT)—to what extent is GT essential? *Aviat Space Environ Med* 70:480, 1999.

350. Moran DS, Shitzer A, Pandolf KB: A physiological strain index to evaluate heat stress, *Am J Physiol* 275(RICP):R129, 1998.

351. Moran DS et al: Can gender differences during exercise-heat stress be assessed by the physiological strain index? *Am J Physiol* 275:R1789, 1999.

352. Moran DS et al: The physiological strain index applied for heat-stressed rats, *J Appl Physiol* 86:895, 1999.

353. Musacchia XJ: Fever and hyperthermia, *Fed Proc* 38:27, 1979.

354. Musch MW et al: Induction of heat shock protein 70 protects intestinal epithelial IEC-18 cells from oxidant and thermal injury, *Am J Physiol* 270:C429, 1996.

355. Nadal JW, Pedersen S, Maddock WG: A comparison between dehydration from salt loss and from water deprivation, *Am J Physiol* 134:691, 1941.

356. Nadel ER et al: Physiological defenses against hyperthermia of exercise, *Ann NY Acad Sci* 301:98, 1977.

357. Nag PK et al: Human work capacity under combined stress of work and heat, *J Hum Ergol (Tokyo)* 25:105, 1996.

358. Nakamura Y, Okamura K: Seasonal variation of sweating responses under identical heat stress, *Appl Human Sci* 17:167, 1998.

359. Nakano M, Mann DL, Knowlton AA: Blocking the endogenous increase in HSP 72 increases susceptibility to hypoxia and reoxygenation in isolated adult feline cardiocytes, *Circulation* 95:1523, 1997.

360. Nakano Y et al: Investigation of etiologies for acute renal failure due to rhabdomyolysis in 5 patients, *Nippon Jinzo Gakkai Shi* 32:1221, 1990.

361. Nakayama T et al: Thermal stimulation and electrical activity of single units of the preoptic region, *Am J Physiol* 204:1122, 1963.

362. Naylor AM, Cooper KE, Veale WL: Vasopressin and fever: evidence supporting the existence of an endogenous antipyretic system in the brain, *Can J Physiol Pharmacol* 65:1333, 1987.

363. Neeman I, Gaffin SL: *A micromethod for the determination of endotoxins.* US Patent No 253,153, pp 1-6 Washington, DC, 1982, US Government Printing Office.

364. Nelson MT et al: Arterial dilations in response to calcitonin gene-related peptide involve activation of K+ channels, *Nature* 344:770, 1990.

365. Neuman F et al: Changes in membrane permeability to endotoxin in heat stroke, *Abstr Isr Soc Int Med* Proc 26, 1978.

366. Newman J: Evaluation of sponging to reduce body temperature in febrile children, *Can Med Assoc J* 132:641, 1985.

367. Nicholson RN, Somerville KW: Heat stroke in a "run for fun," *Br Med J* 1:1525, 1978.

368. Nielsen M: Die Regulation der Korpertemperatur bei Muskelarbeit, *Skand Arch Physiol* 79:193, 1938.

369. NIOSH: *Occupational exposure to hot environments.* Technical Report DHHS 86-113, Washington, DC, 1986, NIOSH.

370. Noakes TD: The hyponatremia of exercise, *Int J Sport Nutr* 2:205, 1992.

371. Nover L: Inducers of HSP synthesis: heat shock and chemical stressors. In Nover L, editor: *Heat shock response,* Boca Raton, Fla, 1991, CRC Press.

372. Nunneley SA: Physiological responses of women to thermal stress: a review, *Med Sci Sports* 10:250, 1978.

373. Oates JA et al: Clinical implications of prostaglandin and thromboxane A_2 formation: part I, *N Engl J Med* 319:689, 1988.

374. Oates JA et al: Clinical implications of prostaglandin and thromboxane A_2 formation: part II, *N Engl J Med* 319:761, 1988.

375. Oberringer M et al: Differential expression of heat shock protein 70 in well healing and chronic human wound tissue, *Biochem Biophys Res Commun* 214:1009, 1995.

376. Ogawa T, Asayama M: Quantitative analysis of the local effect of skin temperature on sweating, *Jpn J Physiol* 36:417, 1986.

377. Ogura H et al: Selective inhibition of translation of the mRNA coding for measles virus membrane protein at elevated temperatures, *J Virol* 61:472, 1987.

378. Ohyama H, Yamada T: Reduction of rat thymocyte interphase death by hyperthermia, *Radiat Res* 82:342, 1980.

379. Okusawa S et al: Interleukin-1 produces a shock-like state in rabbits. Synergism with tumor necrosis factor and the effect of cyclooxygenase inhibition, *J Clin Invest* 81:1162, 1988.

380. Olson KR, Benowitz NL: Experimental and drug-induced hyperthermia, *Emerg Med Clin North Am* 2:459, 1984.

381. Orimo S et al: Two familial cases with exertion-induced heat stroke—relationship to malignant hyperthermia, *Rinsho Shinkeigaku* 32:412, 1992.

382. Padilla J et al: Effects of hyperthermia on contraction and dilatation of rabbit femoral arteries, *J Appl Physiol* 85:2205, 1998.

383. Palmerio C et al: Denervation of the abdominal viscera for the treatment of traumatic shock, *N Engl J Med* 269:709, 1963.

384. Pals KL et al: Effect of running intensity on intestinal permeability, *J Appl Physiol* 82:571, 1997.

385. Pandolf KB: Time course of heat acclimation and its decay, *Int J Sports Med* 19(suppl 2):S157, 1998.

386. Pandolf KB: Aging and human heat tolerance, *Exp Aging Res* 23:69, 1999.

387. Pandolf KB, Sawka MN, Shapiro Y: Factors which alter human physiological responses during exercise-heat acclimation. In Samueloff S, Yousef MK, editors: *Adaptive physiology to stressful environments*, Boca Raton, Fla, 1987, CRC Press.

388. Pandolf KB et al: Thermoregulatory responses of middle-aged and young men during dry-heat acclimation, *J Appl Physiol* 65:65, 1988.

389. Papa M et al: The effect of ischemia of the dog's colon on transmural migration of bacteria and endotoxin, *J Surg Res* 35:264, 1983.

390. Passmore R, Durnin JVGA: Human energy expenditure, *Physiol Rev* 35:801, 1955.

390a. Patton GS Jr: *Notes on tactics and techniques of desert warfare.*

391. Patton JF, Danielis WL: Aerobic power and body fat of men and women during army basic training, *Aviat Space Environ Med* 51:492, 1980.

392. Paull JM, Rosental FS: Heat strain and heat stress for workers wearing protective suits at a hazardous waste site, *Am Ind Hyg Assoc J* 48:458, 1987.

393. Phillips LH, Standen PJ, Batt ME: Effects of seasonal change in rugby league on the incidence of injury, *Br J Sports Med* 32:144, 1998.

394. Pitts GC, Johnson RE, Consolazio FC: Work in the heat as affected by intake of water salt and glucose, *Am J Physiol* 142:253, 1944.

395. Poortmans JR, Jeanloz RW: Urinary excretion of immunoglobulins and their subunits in human subjects before and after exercise, *Med Sci Sports Exerc* 1:57, 1969.

396. Porter AM: Marathon running and adverse weather conditions: a miscellany, *Br J Sports Med* 18:261, 1984.

397. Porter AM: Heat illness and soldiers, *Mil Med* 158:606, 1993.

398. Powers SK et al: Exercise training improves myocardial tolerance to in vivo ischemia-reperfusion in the rat, *Am J Physiol* 275:R1468, 1998.

399. Prentice AT et al: Environment-dependent sports emergencies, *Med Clin North Am* 78:305, 1994.

400. Proppe DW: Alpha adrenergic control of intestinal circulation in heat-stressed baboons, *J Appl Physiol Resp* 48:759, 1980.

401. Puntschart A et al: Hsp70 expression in human skeletal muscle after exercise, *Acta Physiol Scand* 57:411, 1996.

402. Quinn PJ: The fluidity of cell membranes and its regulation, *Prog Biophys Mol Biol* 38:104, 1981.

403. Radigan LR, Robinson S: Effects of environmental heat stress and exercise on renal blood flow and filtration rate, *J Appl Physiol* 2:185, 1949.

404. Reeves RO: Mechanisms of acquired resistance to acute heat shock in cultured mammalian cells, *J Cell Physiol* 79:157, 1972.

405. Reichlin S: Neuroendocrinology. In Wilson JD, Foster DW, editors: *Textbook of endocrinology*, Philadelphia, 1985, WB Saunders.

406. Reuler JB: Hypothermia: pathophysiology, clinical settings, and management, *Ann Intern Med* 89:519, 1978.

407. Ribeiro SP et al: Effects of the stress response in septic rats and LPS-stimulated alveolar macrophages: evidence for TNFα posttranslational regulation, *Am J Respir Crit Care Med* 154:1843, 1996.

408. Richards CRB, Richards DAB: Medical management of fun-runs In Hales JRS, Richards DAB, editors: *Heat stress, physical exertion and environment*, Amsterdam, 1987, Elsevier.

409. Robert R, Chapelain B, Neliat G: Different effects of interleukin-1 on reactivity of arterial vessels isolated from various vascular beds in the rabbit, *Circ Shock* 40:139, 1993.

410. Roberts MF et al: Skin blood flow and sweating changes following exercise, training and heat acclimation, *J Appl Physiol* 43:133, 1977.

411. Robertson GL: The regulation of vasopressin function in health and disease, *Recent Prog Horm Res* 33:333, 1977.

412. Robertson GL, Berl T: Water metabolism. In Brenner BM, Rector FC, editors: *The kidney*, Philadelphia, 1985, WB Saunders.

413. Robertson GL et al: The osmoregulation of vasopressin, *Kidney Int* 10:25, 1976.

414. Robinson S et al: Acclimatization of older men to work in heat, *J Appl Physiol* 20:583, 1965.

415. Rodenhiser DI, Jung JH, Atkinson BG: The synergistic effect of hyperthermia and ethanol on changing gene expression of mouse lymphocytes, *Can J Cytol* 28:1115, 1986.

416. Rohrer DK, Hartong R, Dillmann WH: Influence of thyroid hormone and retinoic acid on slow sarcoplasmic reticulum Ca^{2+} ATPase and myosin heavy chain α gene expression in cardiac myocytes, *J Biol Chem* 266:8638, 1991.

417. Romanovsky AA et al: The vagus nerve in the thermoregulatory response to systemic inflammation, *Am J Physiol* 273:R407, 1997.

418. Rothstein A, Adolph EF, Wills JH: Voluntary dehydration. In Adolph EF, editor: *Physiology of man in the desert*, New York, 1947, Interscience.

419. Rousset B et al: Metabolic alterations induced by chronic heat exposure in the rat: the involvement of thyroid function, *Pflugers Arch* 401:64, 1984.

420. Rowell LB: Human cardiovascular adjustments to exercise and thermal stress, *Physiol Rev* 54:75, 1974.

421. Rowell LB: Cardiovascular aspects of human thermoregulation, *Circ Res* 52:367, 1983.

422. Rowell LB: *Human circulation: regulation during physical stress*, New York, 1986, Oxford University Press.

423. Rozkowski W et al: Effect of hyperthermia on rabbit macrophages, *Immunobiology* 157:122, 1980.

424. Ruifrok ACC, Kanon B, Konings AWT: Correlation between cellular survival and potassium loss in mouse fibroblasts after hyperthermia alone and after a combined treatment with X-rays, *Radiat Res* 101:326, 1985.

425. Ruifrok ACC, Kanon B, Konings AWT: Correlation of colony forming ability of mammalian cells with potassium content after hyperthermia under different experimental conditions, *Radiat Res* 103:452, 1985.

426. Ryan AJ et al: Acute heat stress protects rats against endotoxin shock, *J Appl Physiol* 73:1517, 1992.

427. Sahu SK, Song CW: Thermal sensitivity and kinetics of thermotolerance in bovine aortic endothelial cells in culture, *Int J Hyperthermia* 7:103, 1991.

428. Sakaguchi Y et al: Apoptosis in tumors and normal tissues induced by whole body hyperthermia in rats, *Cancer Res* 55:5459, 1995.

429. Sakurada S, Hales JRS: A role for gastrointestinal endotoxins in the enhancement of heat tolerance by physical fitness, *J Appl Physiol* 84:207, 1998.

430. Salo DC, Donovan CM, Davies KJA: HSP70 and other possible heat shock or oxidative stress proteins are induced in skeletal muscle, heart, and liver during exercise, *Free Radic Biol Med* 11:239, 1991.

431. Samali A, Cotter TG: Heat shock proteins increase resistance to apoptosis, *Exp Cell Res* 223:163, 1996.

432. Sandor RP: Heat illness on-site diagnosis and cooling, *Emergency* 25:35, 1997.

433. Santee WR, Gonzalez RR: Characteristics of the thermal environment. In Pandolf KB, Sawka MN, Gonzalez RR, editors: *Human performance physiology and environmental medicine at terrestrial extremes*, Indianapolis, 1988, Benchmark Press.

434. Sato K: The physiology, pharmacology and biochemistry of the eccrine sweat gland, *Rev Physiol Biochem Pharmacol* 9:51, 1977.

435. Sawka MN, Gonzales RR, Pandolf KB: Effects of sleep deprivation on thermoregulation during exercise, *Am J Physiol* 246:R72, 1984.

436. Sawka MN, Wenger CB: Physiological responses to acute exercise heat stress. In Pandolf KB, Sawka MN, Gonzalez RR, editors: *Human performance physiology and environmental medicine at terrestrial extremes*, Indianapolis, 1988, Benchmark Press.

437. Sawka MN, Wenger CB, Pandolf KB: Thermoregulatory responses to acute exercise-heat stress and heat acclimation. In Fregley MJ, Blatteis CM, editors: *Handbook of physiology: environmental*, Bethesda, Md, 1996, American Physiological Society.

438. Sawka MN et al: Heat exchange during upper and lower-body exercise, *J Appl Physiol* 57:1050, 1984.

439. Sawka MN et al: Thermoregulatory and blood responses during exercise at graded hypohydration levels, *J Appl Physiol* 59:1394, 1985.

440. Schikele E: Environment and fatal heat stroke, *Mil Surg* 98:235, 1947.

441. Schmitz KA et al: Localization of paramyosin, myosin, and a heat shock protein 70 in larval and adult Brugia malayi, *J Parasitol* 82:367, 1996.

442. Schoenfeld Y, Udassin R: Age and sex difference in response to short exposure to extremely dry heat, *J Appl Physiol* 44:1, 1978.

443. Schulte-Sasse U, Eberlein HJ: New findings and experiences in the field of malignant hyperthermia, *Anaesthetist* 35:1, 1986.

444. Schwarz MJ et al: Autoantibodies against 60-kDa heat shock protein in schizophrenia, *Eur Arch Psychiatry Clin Neurosci* 248:282, 1998.

445. Scott RW: Therapeutic applications of neutrophil BPI, *Abstr Adv Diagnosis Prevention & Treatment of Endotoxemia and Sepsis* 3, 1993.

446. Selye H: History of the stress concept. In Goldberger L, Breznitz S, editors: *Handbook of stress,* New York, 1993, The Free Press.

447. Senay LC Jr: Temperature regulation and hypohydration: a singular view, *J Appl Physiol* 47:1, 1979.

448. Senay LC Jr, Mitchell D, Wyndham CH: Acclimatization in a hot, humid environment: body fluid adjustments, *J Appl Physiol* 40:786, 1976.

449. Seppet EK et al: Regulation of cardiac sarcolemmal Ca^{2+} channels and Ca^{2+} transporters by thyroid hormone, *Mol Cell Biochem* 129:145, 1993.

450. Seymour RS: Plants that warm themselves, *Sci Am* 104, 1997.

451. Shapiro Y, Moran DS: Heat stroke: a consequence of mal-adaptation to heat-exercise exposure. In Pandolf KB, Takeda N, Singal PK, editors: *Adaptation biology and medicine: molecular basis,* New Delhi, 1999, Narosa Publishing House.

452. Shapiro Y, Seidman DS: Field and clinical observations of exertional heat stroke patients, *Med Sci Sports Exerc* 22:6, 1990.

453. Shapiro Y et al: Physiological responses of men and women to humid and dry heat, *J Appl Physiol* 49:1, 1980.

454. Sharp NCC, Koutedakis Y: Sport and the overtraining syndrome: immunological aspects, *Br Med Bull* 48:518, 1999.

455. Shen T et al: Toward a broader definition of heat-related death: comparison of mortality estimates from medical examiners' classification with those from total death differentials during the July 1995 heat wave in Chicago, Illinois, *Am J Forensic Med Pathol* 19:113, 1998.

456. Shibolet S, Lancaster MC, Danon Y: Heatstroke: a review, *Aviat Space Environ Med* 47:280, 1976.

457. Shibolet S et al: Fibrinolysis and hemorrhages in fatal heatstroke, *N Engl J Med* 266:169, 1962.

458. Shibolet S et al: Heatstroke: its clinical picture and mechanism in 36 cases, *QJM* 36:525, 1967.

459. Shoenfeld Y et al: Age and sex difference in response to short exposure to extreme dry heat, *J Appl Physiol* 44:1, 1978.

460. Siegler RW: Fatal heatstroke in a young woman with previously undiagnosed Hashimoto's thyroiditis, *J Forensic Sci* 43:1237, 1998.

461. Simon E: Paradigms and concepts in thermal regulation of homeotherms, *NIPS* 2:89, 1987.

462. Singarajah C, Lavies NG: An overdose of ecstasy. A role of dantrolene, *Anaesthesia* 47:686, 1992.

463. Singh AP et al: Environmental impact on crew of armoured vehicles: effects of 24 h combat exercise in hot desert, *Int J Biometeorol* 39:64, 1995.

464. Sjodin RA: *Transport in skeletal muscle,* New York, 1982, John Wiley & Sons.

465. Skrandies S et al: Heat shock- and ethanol-induced ionic changes in C6 rat glioma cells determined by NMR and fluorescence spectroscopy, *Brain Res* 746:220, 1997.

466. Slovis CM, Anderson GF: Survival in a heat stroke victim with a core temperature in excess of 46.5° C, *Ann Emerg Med* 11:269, 1982.

467. Smolander J, Krohonen O, Illmarinen R: Responses of young and older men during prolonged exercise in dry and humid heat, *Eur J Appl Physiol* 61:413, 1990.

468. Sohar E, Adar R: Sodium requirements in Israel under conditions of work in hot climate. In UNESCO, editors: *UNESCO/India Symposium on Environmental Physiology and Psychology,* Lucknow, India, 1962, UNESCO.

469. Sohar E, Kaly J, Adar R: The prevention of voluntary dehydration In UNESCO, editors: *UNESCO/India Symposium on Environmental Physiology and Psychology,* Lucknow, India, 1962, UNESCO.

470. Sohar E, Tennenbaum J, Robinson NA: A comparison of the cumulative Discomfort Index (Cum DI) and the cumulative Effective Temperature (Cum ET) as obtained by meteorological data. In Tromp SW, editors: *Biometeorology,* Oxford, UK, 1962, Pergamon Press.

471. Sparrow EM, Cess RD: *Radiation heat transfer,* Belmont, Calif, 1966, Wadsworth.

472. Sprenger H et al: Enhanced release of cytokines, IL-2r and neopterin after long distance running, *Clin Immunol Immunopathol* 63:188, 1992.

473. Standen NB et al: Hyperpolarizing vasodilators activate ATP-sensitive K+ channels in arterial smooth muscle, *Science* 245:177, 1994.

474. Stephenson LA, Kolka MA: Thermoregulation in women, *Exerc Sport Sci Rev* 21:231, 1993.

475. Stevenson AP et al: Application of compartmental analysis to the determination of ion fluxes in Chinese hamster cells, *J Cell Physiol* 115:75, 1983.

476. Stine RJ: Heat illness, *JACEP* 8:154, 1979.

477. Stojadinovic A et al: Induction of heat-shock protein 72 protects against ischemia/reperfusion in rat small intestine, *Gastroenterology* 109:505, 1995.

478. Stojadinovic A et al: Induction of the heat shock response prevents tissue injury during acute inflammation of the rat ileum, *Crit Care Med* 25:309, 1997.

479. Stolwijk JA: Responses to the thermal environment, *Fed Proc* 36:1655, 1977.

480. Stolwijk JAJ, Hardy JD: Control of body temperature. In Lee DHK, editors: *Handbook of physiology,* Bethesda, Md, 1977, American Physiological Society.

481. Styrt B: Antipyresis and fever, *Arch Intern Med* 150:1589, 1990.

482. Sutton JR: The medical problems of mass participation in athletic competition, *Med J Aust* 2:127, 1972.

483. Sutton JR, Hughson RL: Heatstroke in road races, *Lancet* 1:983, 1979.

484. Sutton JR, Sauder DN: Fever and abdominal pain following exercise, *Med Sci Sports Exerc* 21:S103, 1989.

485. Svenson M et al: IgG autoantibodies against interleukin-1 alpha in sera of normal individuals, *Scand J Immunol* 29:489, 1989.

486. Talbott JH: Heat cramps. In *Medicine,* Baltimore, 1935, Williams & Wilkins.

487. Talbott JH: Heat cramps, *N Engl J Med* 302:777, 1935.

488. Tamion F et al: Malignant neuroleptic syndrome during tiapride treatment, *Clin Exp* 10:461, 1990.

489. Tankersley CG et al: Estrogen replacement in middle aged women: thermoregulatory responses to exercise in the heat, *J Appl Physiol* 73:1238, 1992.

490. Tehan B, Hardern R, Bodenham A: Hyperthermia associated with 3,4-methylenedioxyethamhetamine ("Eve"), *Anaesthesia* 48:507, 1993.

491. Thauer R: Thermosensitivity of the spinal cord. In Hardy JD, Gagge AP, Stiwijk AJA, editors: *Physiological and behavioral temperature regulation,* Springfield, Ill, 1970, Charles C Thomas.

492. Tracey CR, Christian KA: Ecological relations among space, time and thermal niche axes, *Ecology* 67:609, 1986.

493. Treon SP, Thomas P, Broitman SA: Lipopolysaccharide (LPS) processing by Kupffer cells releases a modified LPS with increased hepatocyte binding and decreased tumor necrosis factor alpha stimulatory capacity, *Proc Soc Exp Biol Med* 202:153, 1992.

494. Tsuchido T, Aoki I, Takano M: Interaction of the fluorescent dye 1-N-phenylnapthylamine with Escherichia coli cells during heat stress and recovery from heat stress, *J Gen Microbiol* 135:1941, 1989.

495. Turman MA et al: Characterization of human proximal tubular cells after hypoxic preconditioning: constitutive and hypoxia-induced expression of heat shock proteins HSP70 (A, B, and C), HSC70, and HSP90, *Biochem Mol Med* 60:48, 1997.

496. Ulevitch RJ, Tobias PS: Interactions of bacterial lipopolysaccharides with serum proteins. In Levin J et al, editors: *Bacterial endotoxins: pathophysiological effects, clinical significance and pharmacological control,* New York, 1988, Alan R Liss.

497. Ur E, White PD, Grossman A: Hypothesis: cytokines may be activated to cause depressive illness and chronic fatigue syndrome, *Eur Arch Psychiatry Clin Neurosci* 241:317, 1992.

498. Vaalasti A, Tainio H, Rechardt L: Vasoactive intestinal polypeptide (VIP)-like immunoreactivity in the nerves of human axillary sweat glands, *J Invest Dermatol* 85:246, 1985.

499. Vaamonde CA: Sodium depletion. In Papper S, editors: *Sodium: its biological significance,* Boca Raton, Fla, 1982, CRC Press.

500. Van Camp SP et al: Nontraumatic sports death in high school and college athletes, *Med Sci Sports Exerc* 27:641, 1995.

501. VanOss CJ et al: Effect of temperature on the chemotaxis, phagocytic engulfment, digestion and O_2 consumption of human polymorphonuclear leukocytes, *J Reticuloend Soc* 27:561, 1980.

502. Vayda ME, Yuan ML: The heat shock response of an Antarctic alga is evident at 5 degrees C, *Plant Mol Biol* 24:229, 1994.

503. Vayssier M et al: Tobacco smoke induces both apoptosis and necrosis in mammalian cells: differential effects of HSP70, *Am J Physiol* 275:L771, 1998.

504. Veale WL, Kasting NW, Cooper KE: Arginine vasopressin and endogenous antipyresis: evidence and significance, *Fed Proc* 40:2750, 1981.

505. Wagner JA et al: Heat tolerance and acclimatization to work in the heat in relation to age, *J Appl Physiol* 33:616, 1972.

506. Walters TJ et al: HSP70 expression in the CNS in response to exercise and heat stress in rats, *J Appl Physiol* 84:1269, 1998.

507. Wang YR et al: Heat shock pretreatment prevents hydrogen peroxide injury of pulmonary endothelial cells and macrophages in culture, *Shock* 6:134, 1999.

508. Wardle N: Endotoxin and acute renal failure, *Nephron* 14:321, 1975.

509. Wasserman AJ, Patterson JL: The cerebral vascular response to reduction in arterial carbon dioxide tension, *J Clin Invest* 40:1297, 1961.

510. Webb-Peploe MM, Shepherd JT: Response of large hindlimb veins of the dog to sympathetic nerve stimulation, *Am J Physiol* 215:299, 1968.

511. Wedel DJ: Malignant hyperthermia and neuromuscular disease, *Neuromuscul Disord* 2:157, 1992.

512. Weiner JS: The regional distribution of sweating, *J Physiol (Lond)* 104:32, 1945.

513. Weinstein L: Clinically benign fever of unknown origin: a personal retrospective, *Rev Infect Dis* 7:692, 1985.

514. Wells CL: Responses of physically active and acclimatized men and women to exercise in a desert environment, *Med Sci Sports Exerc* 12:9, 1980.

515. Wells CL et al: Parenteral endotoxin and intestinal function. In Nowotny A, Spitzer JJ, Ziegler EJ, editors: *Cellular and molecular aspects of endotoxin reactions*, New York, 1990, Elsevier.

516. Wenger CB: Human heat acclimatization. In Pandolf KB, Sawka MN, Gonzalez RR, editors: *Human performance physiology and environmental medicine at terrestrial extremes*, Indianapolis, 1988, Benchmark Press.

517. Wenger CB, Roberts MF: Control of forearm venous volume during exercise and body heating, *J Appl Physiol* 48:114, 1980.

518. Werner J: Functional mechanisms of temperature regulation, adaptation, and fever: complementary system theoretical and experimental evidence, *Pharmacol Ther* 37:1, 1988.

519. Wessels BC et al: Plasma endotoxin concentration in healthy primates and during E. coli induced shock, *Crit Care Med* 16:601, 1988.

520. Wetterhall SF et al: Medical care delivery at the 1996 Olympic Games. Centers for disease control and prevention Olympics surveillance unit, *JAMA* 279:1463, 1998.

521. Wichmann MW et al: Melatonin administration following hemorrhagic shock decreases mortality from subsequent septic challenge, *J Surg Res* 65:109, 1996.

522. Willcox WH: The nature prevention and treatment of heat hyperpyrexia, *Br Med J* 1:392, 1920.

523. Willis JS, Ji HL: Explosive increase in Na$^+$ entry to acidified cells at elevated temperature. Evidence for the energy depletion model of heat stroke? *Ann NY Acad Sci* 856:304, 1998.

524. Wing J: Upper thermal tolerance limits for unimpaired mental performance, *Aerospace Med* 36:960, 1965.

525. Wing JF, Touchstone RM: *The effects of high ambient temperature on short-term memory*. Technical Report AMRL-TR-65-103. Aerospace Medical Research Laboratories, Wright-Patterson Air Force Base, Ohio, 1965, Air Force Systems Command.

526. Wingfield A: Hyperventilation tetany in tropical climates, *Br Med J* 1:929, 1941.

527. Winslow CE, Herrington ALP, Gagge AP: Physiological reactions of the human body to varying environmental temperatures, *Am J Physiol* 120:1, 1937.

528. Wolfersberger MG: Uniporters, symporters and antiporters, *J Exp Biol* 196:5, 1994.

529. Woolf PD: Hormonal responses to trauma, *Crit Care Med* 20:216, 1992.

530. Wright SD et al: Lipopolysaccharide (LPS) binding protein opsonizes LPS-bearing particles for recognition by a novel receptor on macrophages, *J Exp Med* 170:1231, 1989.

531. Wyndham CH: Survey of causal factors in heatstroke and their prevention in the gold mining industry, *J S Afr Inst Mining Metallurgy* 1:245, 1966.

532. Wyndham CH: Heat stroke and hyperthermia in marathon runners, *Ann NY Acad Sci* 301:128, 1977.

533. Wyndham CH, Morrison JF, Williams CG: Heat reactions of male and female Caucasians, *J Appl Physiol* 21:357, 1965.

534. Wyndham CH et al: Changes in central circulation and body fluid spaces during acclimatization to heat, *J Appl Physiol* 25:586, 1968.

535. Yaglou CP, Minard D: Control of heat casualties at military training centers, *Arch Ind Health* 16:302, 1957.

536. Yang YL et al: Heat shock protein expression protects against death following exposure to heatstroke in rats, *Neurosci Lett* 7:9, 1998.

537. Zhao MJ, Willis JS: Reduced ion transport in erythrocytes of male Sprague-Dawley rats during starvation, *J Nutr* 118:1120, 1988.

538. Zhi-cheng M, Yi-tang W: Analysis of 411 cases of severe heat stroke in Nanjing, *Chinese Med J* 104:256, 1991.

539. Zhu BL et al: Infant death presumably due to exertional self-overheating in bed: an autopsy case of suspected child abuse, *Nippon Hoigaku Zasshi* 52:153, 1998.

540. Zinner S, McCabe WR: Effects of IgM and IgG antibody in patients with bacteremia due to gram negative bacilli, *J Infect Dis* 133:37, 1976.

11 Clinical Management of Heat-Related Illnesses

Daniel S. Moran and Stephen L. Gaffin

This chapter discusses clinical observations of heatstroke victims, management of heat-related illnesses, and consequences of different levels of hydration on heat illnesses. In heatstroke, the most severe heat illness, early clinical signs are nonspecific. A common picture of heatstroke is sudden collapse of an individual during physical activity carried out in a warm environment. This is usually followed by loss of consciousness with elevated core temperature (T_c) greater than 40° C (104° F), rapid heart rate (HR), tachypnea, hypotension, and, possibly, shock. The severity of heat illness depends on the degree of elevation in T_c and its duration. Therefore, to prevent and minimize complications and save lives, proper management and clinical care are essential.

This chapter focuses on the three different phases of heatstroke (acute, hematologic and enzymatic, and late), problems with recognition of heat illnesses, diagnosis and complications of heatstroke, treatment, and awareness of risk factors. Updated descriptions of issues related to dehydration, hypohydration, hyperhydration, and rehydration are also presented.

CLINICAL AND LABORATORY OBSERVATIONS IN HEATSTROKE

The clinical manifestations of heatstroke vary, depending on whether the victim suffers from classic heatstroke or exertional heatstroke (EHS) (Table 11-1). Some overlap in presentation may occur; treatment with a medication that places an elderly person at risk for classic heatstroke also places an exercising individual at risk for EHS. The clinical picture of heatstroke usually follows a distinct pattern of events in three phases.[76]

Acute Phase

The acute phase is characterized by central nervous system (CNS) disturbances. Since brain function is very sensitive to hyperthermia, this phase presents in all heatstroke patients. Signs of depression of the CNS often appear almost simultaneously in the form of irritability, aggressiveness, stupor, delirium, and coma.[3,37,214] Seizures occur in 60% to 70% of heatstroke cases. After a return to normothermia, the persistence of coma is a poor prognostic sign.[126,214] Other symptoms include fecal incontinence, flaccidity, and hemiplegia. Cerebellar

symptoms, including ataxia and dysarthria, are prominent and may persist.[153,214,242] In over 60% of heatstroke cases, pupils were constricted to pinpoint size.[126,243] Papilledema was found to present in cases of cerebral edema. However, cerebrospinal fluid and pressure were usually within normal values.[3,126,214]

Other common disturbances for the acute phase occur in the gastrointestinal and respiratory systems. Gastrointestinal dysfunction, including diarrhea and vomiting, often occurs. The latter, however, may reflect translocation of toxic gram-negative bacterial lipopolysaccharide (LPS) from the lumen of the intestines because of poor splanchnic perfusion, as well as from CNS impairment.[34,94,214] Hyperventilation and elevation of T_c primarily lead to respiratory alkalosis, which in EHS may be masked by metabolic acidosis as a result of increased glycolysis and the development of hyperlactemia.[39,172] Hypoxemia may be present in cases of respiratory complications.[44,172,222]

Hematologic and Enzymatic Phase

In the hematologic and enzymatic phase of heatstroke, hematologic, enzymatic, and other blood parameters are altered. In humans and experimental animals, hyperthermia results in temporary leukocytosis[107] and changes in lymphocyte subpopulations—both in absolute numbers and in percentages.[1] Leukocytes may range from 20 to 30 $\times 10^3$/mm^{-3} and higher.[21,110] In one study, all fatal cases of exertional heatstroke had disturbances in the blood coagulation system.[215,216] Prothrombin time, partial thromboplastin time and the level of fibrin split products increased with a fall in thrombocytes.[76] Clotting dysfunction peaked 18 to 36 hours after the acute phase of heatstroke, and 2 to 3 days after heatstroke prothrombin levels fell to 17 to 45% of normal. Depending on the severity of heatstroke, thrombocyte values range between 110 $\times$ 10^3/mm^{-3} and zero.[215,216] These clotting disturbances resemble those of gram-negative bacterial sepsis, and it has been suggested that LPS participates in the pathophysiology of heatstroke.[101]

Significant lay interest, scientific research, and commercial product development and marketing have focused on electrolyte abnormalities associated with physical exertion under various conditions. The marked variability in electrolyte content of sweat and intensity

TABLE 11-1. Comparison of Classic and Exertional Heatstroke

	CLASSIC	EXERTIONAL
Age group	Elderly	Men (15-45 yr)
Health status	Chronically ill	Healthy
Concurrent activity	Sedentary	Strenuous exercise
Drug use	Diuretics, antidepressants, antihypertensives, anticholinergics, antipsychotics	Usually none
Sweating	May be absent	Usually present
Lactic acidosis	Usually absent; poor prognosis if present	Common
Hyperkalemia	Usually absent	Often present
Hypocalcemia	Uncommon	Frequent
Hypoglycemia	Uncommon	Common
Creatine phosphokinase/ aldolase	Mildly elevated	Markedly elevated
Rhabdomyolysis	Unusual	Frequently severe
Hyperuricemia	Mild	Severe
Acute renal failure	<5% of patients	25% to 30% of patients
Disseminated intravascular coagulation	Mild	Marked; poor prognosis
Mechanism	Poor dissipation of environmental heat	Excessive endogenous heat production and overwhelming of heat loss mechanisms

Modified from Knochel JP, Reed G: Disorders of heat regulation. In Kleeman CR, Maxwell MH, Narin RG, editors: *Clinical disorders of fluid and electrolyte metabolism*, New York, 1987, McGraw-Hill.

of physical activity, along with ambient temperature (T_{amb}), humidity, and the preexisting state of hydration in the individual, all contribute to the degree of electrolyte abnormalities observed in plasma and sweat.

Plasma Volume Changes. Physical exertion alters plasma volume (PV), depending on several factors: environmental conditions, intensity and duration of exercise, preexisting and coexisting state of hydration, and level of heat acclimatization. In a cool environment, PV is maintained or even increased with exercise. However, in the heat, a few minutes' burst of supramaximal exercise causes a biphasic reduction in PV.[24] During severe exercise, there is rapid efflux of K^+ and metabolites from contracting muscles, causing a local rise in osmotic pressure in the interstitial fluid. As a result, by Starling's law, fluid is initially drawn across capillary walls from the circulation into the extravascular space. This increases the transcapillary osmotic gradient, leading to the observed secondary reduction in PV. The combined processes result in overall sustained reduction of PV by 10% to 15% within 30 seconds.

The volume of sweat lost associated with intense physical activity of 30 minutes or more decreases total body water; if these fluid losses are not replaced, a further reduction in PV results.

Potassium. The literature is contradictory regarding the effect of heat stress on plasma potassium concentration. Generally, most classic heatstroke patients ap-

pear to have normal serum K^+ levels at admission, whereas EHS patients often show hyperkalemia and rhabdomyolysis, but may range from hypokalemia to hyperkalemia.[216]

Mechanisms. Early studies suggested that hypokalemia predisposes to heatstroke[85,119] and the subsequent resultant cellular damage with its elevated K^+ efflux would raise plasma values back to near normal or above.

Only about 2% of total body K^+ is extracellular, and the intracellular environment behaves as a large K^+ reservoir. K^+ passively diffuses out of the cells, down its concentration gradient through K^+ "leak" channels in the plasma membrane. It requires a significant amount of adenosine triphosphate (ATP) to pump it back into the cell. Agents that act on K^+ transport system can cause rapid changes in plasma K^+ concentrations. Elevated extracellular K^+ concentrations depolarize excitable cell membranes. During hyperthermia in several animal models, ranging from crustaceans to miniswine, serum K^+ rose substantially.[14,32,83,130] In some, the higher the K^+, the shorter was the survival time. If the animals had been heat acclimated, the rise in K^+ was blunted.

During prolonged exercise, elevated serum K^+ is usually seen.[204] In some human subjects, serum K^+ levels rose during heat and exercise.[84,183] This would be expected to cause vasodilation of terminal blood vessels within active skeletal muscles. Several days' training lowered this increase in extracellular K^+ for a given workload and improved cardiovascular stability and the ability to dissipate heat. An increase in serum K^+ from exercise may be due in part to the large number of depolarizations of muscle membranes. This elevated K^+ concentration was reduced by insulin injection, but performance was not improved.[147]

In the early stage of heatstroke, victims arriving at a hospital may present with hypokalemia, normokalemia, or hyperkalemia. Rhabdomyolysis, cellular damage, and decreased renal perfusion may in part account for hyperkalemia.*

The loss of K^+ in sweat usually cannot account for hypokalemia in EHS because the normal K^+ of 4 to 5 mmol/L is not significantly affected by prolonged sweating, heat acclimation, or dietary intake of potassium.[52] However, earlier studies suggested that repeated bouts of intense exercise in the heat lead to K^+ deficiency resulting from sweat loss.[135] More recent reports under similar conditions, however, demonstrate normal K^+ levels in plasma and muscles, associated with reduced urinary K^+ excretion. Development of hyperkalemia in heatstroke victims appears be a consequence of increased K^+ permeability, resulting from failure of the Na^+K^+ ATPase pump at the cell membrane level, as described in Chapter 10.

One group concluded that hyperthermia in humans leads first to hypokalemia, probably because of respiratory alkalosis, increased renal secretion, and loss in sweat.[205] This would be followed by metabolic acidosis and hyperkalemia when a potential combination of impaired renal function and general cellular damage develops. Most heatstroke patients admitted during the Hadj exhibited normokalemia or hypokalemia, with concentrations as low as 2 mEq/L or less.[129] Furthermore, once the characteristic hypovolemia had been corrected, serum K^+ fell still further. During exercise in the heat, humans can lose K^+ in an amount of 0.225 mEq/100 g body mass (70% into urine and 30% into saliva).[166] Those differences are not simply a matter of experimental error. Gaffin et al[90] explained these discrepancies in a miniswine model described in Chapter 10.[90]

Sodium. Failure to maintain normal salt intake can suppress triggering of the thirst mechanism, thereby reducing voluntary rehydration. Model experiments indicate that, unlike K^+, intracellular Na^+ content does not change significantly in response to heat treatment until a few minutes before death, at which point there was a small rise.[234,244] However, in some clinical cases serum Na^+ levels were low, reflecting a state of hyperhydration or rhabdomyolysis.[91,106]

The concentration of sodium chloride in sweat may range from 10 to 60 mEq/L, depending on physical activity, heat exposure, the state of heat acclimatization, and the amount of salt ingested.[189] Whereas gender does not affect Na^+ in sweat, children show lower concentrations than adults.[14,66] Values rarely reach 40 mEq/L in prepubertal boys. The average American diet contains about 170 mEq of Na^+ per day, an amount usually adequate to replace all Na^+ lost through sweating by the trained athlete. However, an athlete with an inadequate caloric intake may suffer from dietary salt deficiencies and soldiers in combat usually have insufficient food intake. In such cases, supplementation may be required after moderate sweat losses.

EFFECT OF PHYSICAL ACTIVITY ON SODIUM SWEAT CONCENTRATION. A sudden increase in exercise intensity rapidly increases the electrolyte concentrations of sweat and more slowly increases electrolytes in serum.[29,78,139] The electrolyte concentration of sweat is highest immediately after commencing physical activity and gradually decreases with prolonged exercise, possibly as a passive result of falling body salt content.

Thermal stress alone raises Na^+ and Cl^- concentrations less than those induced by running.[88] In a variety of sports (yachting, rowing, handball, and cycling), initial sweat electrolyte concentrations were dependent on type of sport, duration of performance, and level of training in elite athletes.[29] Cyclists and rowers, whose sports produce high-endurance capability, had significantly lower sweat Na^+ content than did yachtsmen. In addition, participation in an intensive training program led to a further reduction in sweat electrolyte concentration.

The sweat of a trained athlete may show a Na^+ content as low as 17 mmol/L (34 mOsm/kg), a level one third that of a person who is untrained and unacclimated to the heat. Conversely, the untrained, unacclimatized "weekend warrior" or vacationer is at greatest risk for significant Na^+ losses when exercising in the heat (see Table 10-2).

EFFECT OF HEAT EXPOSURE ON RENAL ABSORPTION OF SODIUM. After repeated days of exercise in the heat, there is an increased production of aldosterone with consequent enhanced renal reabsorption of Na^+; thus Na^+ is progressively conserved. After prolonged strenuous exercise and sweating, urinary excretion of Na^+ may almost cease temporarily.[51]

SODIUM DEFICIENCY. In temperate thermal environments, a Na^+ deficit due to exercise is unlikely to be so severe as to require Na^+ supplementation of the normal diet. Similarly, a brief (<2 hours) episode of moderate exercise in the heat rarely causes clinically significant hyponatremia upon voluntary rehydration. However, when sweat loss exceeds 5 L/day, hyponatremia may develop upon rehydration and occur during the initial

---

*References 22, 56, 109, 136, 214, 216.

stage of acclimation to heat, during prolonged and repeated exercise in the heat (training camps), or during ultra-endurance events, such as marathons, 50-mile runs, or triathlons.[170]

In one report, four athletes developed hyponatremia and water intoxication during endurance events lasting more than 7 hours.[177] The cause was thought to be voluntary hyperhydration with hypotonic solutions, combined with moderate losses of Na^+ and Cl^- in sweat. These athletes were slower runners who competed at a lower intensity than did the top finishers.

An interesting case of symptomatic hyponatremia resulting from excessive voluntary intake of water showed paradoxical secretion of antidiuretic hormone (ADH) leading to renal shutdown instead of increased output of urine.[4] Ordinarily, ADH is secreted in response to dehydration but not hyponatremia. However, volume overload of the stomach is known to cause nausea, which is a strong stimulus for production of ADH.

Calcium. In isolated cultured cells, heating may lead to increased permeability of the plasma membrane[234] and an increase (~0.1 μM) in cytoplasmic Ca^{2+} concentration.[85] It is unclear if the rise in Ca^{2+} contributes to the pathophysiology of heatstroke, since elevating the total cell content of Ca^{2+} sixfold had no effects on survivability at 45° C (113° F).[234]

Several studies suggest that hyperthermia leads to a reduction in serum Ca^{2+} as a result of deposition of Ca^{2+} phosphates and Ca^{2+} carbonates in injured skeletal muscles.[205] Other studies, however, indicate that high temperatures may cause acute renal failure or rhabdomyolysis, which in turn releases Ca^{2+} into serum.[134] Moreover, in microswine with heatstroke, we reported a biphasic reduction in Ca^{2+} concentration.[14] At approximately 41° C (105.8° F), Ca^{2+} concentration declined, reaching a minimum at 44° C (111.2° F), and then rapidly rose to near baseline levels. This may account for both the rises and falls in serum Ca^{2+} reported for heatstroke victims.

Fluorescence imaging[138a] and tracer techniques[234] show that heating cultured cells raises cytoplasmic Ca^{2+} concentration.

Magnesium. Concentrations of magnesium in sweat vary from 0.02 to 5 mmol/L and might be expected to cause hypomagnesemia during prolonged exercise in the heat.[47,48,54,231] Significant loss of total body magnesium is prevented, however, because there is a concomitant rapid decrease in renal magnesium excretion.[52,231] Losses during endurance exercise have been estimated to be about 1% of total body magnesium content.[54] Occasionally, an acute fall in serum magnesium occurs following prolonged intense exercise,[25,190] which may be caused by a temporary uptake of Mg^{2+} by erythrocytes,[186] mononuclear cells,[207] and actively contracting muscle,[49] in addition to the losses in sweat.[51] Although some studies suggest that these losses are severe enough to cause symptoms, the consensus is that the development of clinical hypomagnesemia secondary to losses in sweat is unlikely.[146]

Phosphate. Hypophosphatemia is frequently seen in EHS.[31] Heat stress often causes respiratory alkalosis, which increases the rate of cellular uptake of phosphate and reduces its excretion.[168] Other studies suggested that hypophosphatemia was caused by increased renal clearance of phosphorus with a decreased renal threshold, plus contributions from metabolic acidosis and increased uptake of phosphorus by cells.[205] However, hypophosphatemia is not always reported in humans or animal models, and respiratory alkalosis does not always occur at the same time as hypophosphatemia.

Enzymes. One of the prominent and almost pathognomonic characteristics of EHS is the appearance of exceptionally high levels of certain cellular enzymes, implying cell damage or death. Most EHS patients show elevation of serum creatine phosphokinase (CPK) activity and myoglobinuria, suggesting damage of skeletal muscles.[77] CPK activity in the range of 10^3 to 10^4 IU/L was commonly found, with peak values 24 to 48 hours after collapse.[63,206] At T_c of 41.8° to 42.2° C (107.24° to 74.2° F), aspartate aminotransferase (AST) and alanine aminotransferase (ALT) concentrations rose by factors of 25 and 8, respectively, and bilirubin concentration approximately doubled to 1.56 mg/dl.[183]

These rises in enzyme levels are related to tissue damage, which in turn depends upon both T_c and its rate of rise and its duration.[151] CPK, an indicator of skeletal and cardiac muscle damage, was the most sensitive to increases in T_c, followed by lactate dehydrogenase, an index of generalized tissue damage. In microswine with heatstroke, however, we found rises in CPK and lactate dehydrogenase (LDH) only about 20 minutes before death and a rise in AST about an hour before death, but no change in ALT concentration.[90]

In 26 heatstroke victims during the 1994 Hadj, at admission to the heatstroke treatment unit, CPK, AST, ALT, and LDH were elevated in heatstroke victims and remained high after 24 hours. Those who died had higher enzyme levels than the survivors. LDH concentration was useful in distinguishing between those who died and those who had a rapid recovery. The enzymes were better prognostic indicators than T_c, anion gap, and serum K^+.[9]

Glucose. The stress hormones catecholamines and cortisol are secreted during heatstroke, stimulate glycogenolysis, and raise plasma glucose concentrations.[2] Thus classic heatstroke patients are usually hyperglycemic.[31,103] Approximately half of miniswine with heatstroke studied also developed hyperglycemia, but 20 to 30 minutes after a rise in circulating insulin, glucose concentrations sharply declined. In accordance with these observations, patients suffering from heat exhaustion were normoglycemic, but some of those with heatstroke were hypoglycemic.[56]

Late Phase

The late phase of heatstroke is characterized by disturbances in renal and hepatic functions. High bilirubin levels, which may last for several days, reflect both hepatic dysfunction and hemolysis.

Acute renal failure is a common complication of severe cases and occurs in approximately 25% to 30% of EHS patients.[136,150,216] Oliguria and anuria are characteristic features. At this phase, urine has been described as appearing like "machine oil," with a low specific gravity.[182,185,202,216] Usually present in the urine are red and white cells, hyaline and granular casts, and mild to moderate proteinurea.[202] The etiology is of multiple causes,[182] but a major cause is reduced renal blood flow subsequent to heat-induced hypotension, hypohydration, and peripheral vasodilatation. Furthermore, direct thermal injury may also lead to widespread damage of renal tissue.[202] Myoglobinuria and elevated blood viscosity resulting from disseminated intravascular coagulation (DIC) may further contribute to acute oliguric renal failure.[185,202,221,232]

Recovery

CNS dysfunction becomes increasingly severe with prolonged duration of hyperthermia and its associated circulatory failure. Nevertheless, coma persisting for 24 hours, even with subsequent seizures, is usually followed by complete recovery without evidence of mental or neurologic impairment.[3,191] Chronic disability may prevail for several weeks or months in the form of cerebellar deficits, hemiparesis, aphasia, and mental deficiency.[3,136,191] Only in exceptional cases, when coma persists for more than 24 hours, mental and neurologic impairment may become chronic and prevail for some years.[5] However, in one study of classic heatstroke, 78% of patients had minimal to severe neurologic impairment.[63] Shapiro and Moran[206] studied 82 cases of EHS in Israeli soldiers and concluded that associated with each case was at least one factor predisposing to heatstroke (e.g., diarrhea, lack of acclimatization, poor fitness). Correcting those individual risk factors should lead to strategies capable of preventing heatstroke. Indeed, in more than 90% of the victims in whom predisposing background factors were identified and eliminated, and after waiting 6 to 8 weeks to ensure full recovery, the patients were permitted to return to their routine training schedule.

Heat Tolerance Test. In the Israeli Defense Forces, all heatstroke victims must undergo an exercise–heat tolerance test after recovery, in order to rule out any effect of concurrent disease and abnormality in thermoregulation.[75] The patients schedule the test 6 to 8 weeks after the collapse, and before taking the test they are not permitted any activity related to heat stress until they have taken the test. During the test, the individuals wear only shorts and sport shoes. After 10 minutes of rest, they walk on a treadmill at 1.34 m/sec^{-1} at a 2% grade in a hot/dry environment (40° C [104° F], 40% RH) for 120 minutes.[6] Analysis of multiple physiologic variables during the test helps to diagnose any congenital or acquired factors that might compromise body temperature regulation.[75]

CLINICAL MANAGEMENT OF HEAT-RELATED ILLNESS

Heat-Related Illnesses

Classic heatstroke occurs when environmental heat load is very high.[69,109,223] Usually it develops over a few days (e.g., during a heat wave) and affects mainly the elderly, especially those with underlying infection, liver disease, or/and limited access to air conditioning. In classic heatstroke, physical effort is not the primary cause and in most cases is accompanied by dehydration. However, there are many similarities in the pathology of different heat illnesses (classic or EHS, heat exhaustion, etc.), irrespective of the cause of the heat illness (see Chapter 10).

As previously discussed, individuals exercising in the heat develop a spectrum of clinical illnesses ranging from syncope to heatstroke. Further discussion of the clinical management of heat illness focuses on heat exhaustion and heatstroke. The distinction between these two clinical diagnoses is somewhat artificial and may be difficult to establish in the field or at the medical facility.

Exertional Heat Illness. A universal feature of heatstroke is a state of collapse. This puts an abrupt end to the physical effort; activity ceases, body temperature falls, and the victim may spontaneously regain consciousness.

Although strenuous physical exercise (e.g., athletic events, military training, hard labor) in the heat has been notorious in causing heatstroke, it has also occurred at relatively low T_{amb}.[12] In principle, diagnosing exertional heat illness (EHI) is clear: if a previously healthy individual collapses while exercising in a warm environment for more than 1 hour with rectal temperature (T_{re}) greater than 40.5° C (104.9° F), the diagnosis of heatstroke is virtually certain.[44,96,120,144,220] Although EHI might be diagnosed immediately, EHI and its severity can also be diagnosed retrospectively from clinical laboratory data after proper clinical management.[28,65,108,181] Occasionally, T_{re} less than 40° C (104° F) has been seen in cases diagnosed as heatstroke, and later confirmed by blood chemistry.

The presentation of heatstroke is usually acute, with approximately 25% of all casualties exhibiting prodromal symptoms lasting minutes to hours. These include dizziness, weakness, nausea, confusion, disorientation, drowsiness, and irrational behavior. Failure to recognize the first signs of disability, and in some cases an assumption that the subject is malingering, has led to incorrect assessment of true physiologic status. Because of delay in transportation, a heatstroke victim is likely to arrive at the emergency room with T_c lower than that at the site of collapse and partially rehydrated, thus showing only mild CNS disturbances. Therefore a correct diagnosis of heatstroke depends on understanding the entire clinical and pathologic picture (see Chapter 10).

At the time of heatstroke collapse, sweat glands are usually still active and profuse sweating is usually present, in contrast to earlier beliefs about heatstroke.[55,120,144,220] The appearance of dry skin mainly occurs in a very dry climate where sweat evaporates very rapidly or dehydration has become so severe that secretion of sweat is depressed[122]; it is most often seen in classic heatstroke rather than EHS.

It is essential to determine body temperature as soon as possible after collapse, bearing in mind that intense hyperthermia occurs immediately after exercise. Heatstroke has been misdiagnosed from adherence to certain conventional criteria, such as a warm climate, very high body temperature, and lack of sweating. The widely held criterion that T_{re} must be high is incorrect. At the moment of collapse, body temperature probably does exceed a certain critical temperature that usually leads to heatstroke. However, delaying the first measurement of body temperature may provide misleading lower temperatures. In one instance, during transportation between the site of collapse and the hospital emergency room, body temperature dropped from 41.1° C ±0.8 to 37.8° C ±1.2°, a fall of 3.3° C (6.4° F).[226] Furthermore, temperatures may be taken by untrained individuals or measured incorrectly.[121,136,226]

Heat Exhaustion.

Heat exhaustion occurs in individuals who sweat profusely while participating in an endurance event or while engaging in repeated bouts of exercise. This results in significant and unreplaced sweat losses. Prolonged insensible sweat losses, such as occur while sitting in the sun in a moderate breeze, predispose to heat exhaustion if fluid and electrolyte losses are significant.

PROBLEMS WITH RECOGNITION. The early symptoms of heat illnesses are often unrecognized or mistaken for malingering. Failure to attend to these symptoms puts the individual at risk of significant thermal injury. Headache, confusion, drowsiness, and even euphoria may be important warning signals. Individuals who anticipate exposure to hot environmental conditions should be thoroughly versed in the manifestations of heat illness.

The victim of heat exhaustion may arrive at the medical facility with nausea and visual disturbances that mimic the prodrome of a migraine headache. Dizziness or syncope may mistakenly suggest arrhythmia or seizure. Symptoms of chilling, piloerection, sweating, and moderately elevated temperature may suggest an infectious process. Development of altered mental status or ataxia raises the possibility of meningitis, encephalitis, or drug intoxication.

TREATMENT. Treatment is based on symptoms and focuses on both rehydration and reduction in temperature. The victim must immediately cease exercising. Although this appears to be intuitively obvious, some persons develop euphoria and may resist this measure. Furthermore, later return to physical activity on the same day is contraindicated. When possible, the victim should be removed from direct sunlight (which could have a heat load of hundreds of kCal/hr) and restrictive clothing should be loosened. If the victim is unconscious or the T_{re} is greater than 39° C (102.2° F), he or she should be treated as an incipient heatstroke victim and immediately evacuated to a medical facility following the guidelines below.

Body temperature may be lowered by a variety of means. When available, *immersion in ice water facilitates the most rapid drop in body temperature*.[55,89] Alternative measures in the field include sprinkling with water and fanning, or placing ice bags over the superficial great vessels (axillae and groin) and fanning.[46] Periodic toweling of the skin renews the evaporative surface and facilitates evaporative cooling. See Box 11-1.

If the patient is alert, oral rehydration can be instituted with cold water or a fluid replacement beverage; the concentration of carbohydrates in such a beverage should not exceed 6%, otherwise gastric emptying and fluid absorption by the intestines may be delayed. An initial target intake of 1 to 2 L over 2 to 4 hours is reasonable; a greater rate results in limited absorption with inappropriate diuresis. The victim should continue to rest and drink over the next 24 hours. As a general rule, for every pound of weight lost by sweating, one pint (2 cups or 500 ml) of fluid should be consumed. It may require 36 hours to completely restore lost electrolytes and fluid volume to all body compartments via oral intake.

After the acute episode the medical care provider should determine any possible host risk factors for heat illness and review with the victim signs of heat illness and preventive measures.

Heatstroke

Heatstroke is a true medical emergency; before 1950, the mortality rate was 40% to 75%.[13,73] Long-term survival is directly related to rapidly instituting resuscitative measures.

Box 11-1 CURRENT COOLING METHOD FOR EXERTIONAL HEATSTROKE

At the USMC training base at Parris Island, SC, victims of exertional heatstroke are routinely cooled using the following procedures. *NB: These victims are young men and women who are otherwise healthy.* Victims of *classic* heatstroke are usually elderly and with concurrent diseases, and those factors must be taken into consideration.

1. During physical training, the clinic routinely maintains a dedicated room with two bathtubs full of cold water and ice.
2. In the field, the blouse and pants are removed from a collapsed suspected heatstroke patient, leaving on the shorts and T-shirt. Rectal temperature is measured, ice is packed around the groin/axillary areas, and the patient is immediately transported to the clinic on a stretcher. Upon arrival, the stretcher is placed on top of the iced bathtub above the water and ice, with the carrying handles sticking out at both ends.
3. Mental status and other vital signs are assessed and blood drawn for laboratory analyses.
4. One liter of normal saline is administered as a bolus.
5. Sheets are dipped into the tub's icy water and are used to cover and drench the patient. Copious ice is added to the top of the sheet to cool still further, and the skin is massaged to improve skin blood flow. The sheets are frequently rewetted with the icy water.
6. Concurrently, the head is constantly irrigated with more ice water and a fan is directed at the patient.

The victim is not routinely immediately immersed in the ice water in case cardiopulmonary resuscitation becomes necessary. However, if rectal temperature is not lowered sufficiently, then the victim is immersed directly into the ice and water. With this procedure, rectal temperature usually falls to 39.5° C (102.5° F) within 15 to 20 min and the patient is removed from the stretcher, rinsed, and placed on a gurney, and IV fluids and laboratory studies are reviewed.[89]

From Gaffin SL, Gardner J, Flinn S: *Ann Intern Med* 132:678, 2000.

Problems with Recognition. Earlier diagnosis of heatstroke required three signs: severe hyperthermia ($T_c >$ 41° C [105.8° F]), CNS disturbance, and cessation of sweating.[43] This symptom complex represents the extreme or full-blown heatstroke presentation and is now recognized to be *too rigid* and possibly delaying institution of critical interventional measures. We consider each of these criteria in turn.

- The body temperatures reported in heatstroke victims *in the field* may be significantly higher (41.1° C [106.9° F] vs. 37.8° C [100° F]) than those documented in the hospital emergency department.[213] Failure to obtain or record on-site rectal temperatures may hinder prompt diagnosis; similarly, documentation of

only mild elevation in body temperature should *not* preclude the diagnosis of heatstroke.

- The victim's altered mental status may adversely affect the ability of emergency department personnel to obtain a detailed history regarding precipitating events. Lack of such information may also delay diagnosis. Emergency medical transport personnel should attempt to obtain this history before evacuating the victim and communicate the information to the appropriate medical staff.
- Recent investigations have shown that cessation of sweating is a late phenomenon of heatstroke.[187,216] *At the time of collapse, most heatstroke victims continue to sweat profusely.* Failure to consider the diagnosis of heatstroke in a diaphoretic patient could be fatal.
- Unless an alternative cause is obvious, the previously healthy individual who collapses after physical exertion in hot weather should be considered to have EHS.[41,214]

Diagnosis. Shibolet[213] noted that a delay in measurement of T_c or inaccurate methodology in obtaining initial temperature values often led to inappropriately low initial temperature determinations when compared with actual T_c at the time of collapse. Loss of consciousness is an unvarying feature of heatstroke. With cessation of physical activity, the rate of metabolic heat production markedly decreases and T_c will fall if skin temperature (T_{sk}) is greater than T_{amb} and sweating persists. Shapiro and Seidman[210] proposed that the diagnosis of heatstroke should be considered in any person who has lost consciousness during exertion and demonstrates clinical and laboratory signs of heatstroke, even if body temperature was not markedly elevated several hours after collapse. A history of prodromal symptoms as described for heat exhaustion should markedly increase the suspicion for heatstroke.

CNS disturbances (coma, convulsions, confusion, or agitation) accompanying hyperthermia may also be due to CNS infections, sepsis, or other disease processes. Evaluation for these disorders should proceed only after the diagnosis of heatstroke is ruled out. Markedly elevated levels of AST, ALT, and LDH may help in differential diagnosis.[123] However, the clinician should bear in mind that elevation of these enzymes may not occur for 24 to 48 hours after heat injury.[214]

Complications. Observed complications of heatstroke reflect the results of both direct thermal injury and cardiovascular collapse. Autopsy of persons with EHS showed multiple hemorrhages, congestion, and cellular degeneration in most or all of the organs examined.[216] In EHS in particular, rhabdomyolysis is usually present.[137] A brief overview of the specific pathology found should provide a framework for discussion of the therapeutic and supportive management of heatstroke.

CENTRAL NERVOUS SYSTEM. The brain is particularly susceptible to thermal injury. CNS dysfunction is directly related to the duration of hyperthermia and to circulatory failure. The underlying pathology observed on autopsy is brain edema and congestion, with petechial hemorrhage and neuronal degeneration.[150] Cerebrospinal fluid pressure and hematologic features are normal.[214] In Shibolet's study,[213] all patients presented with confusion or agitation or both and 72% had convulsions, but all eventually became comatose. Agitation, delirium, and hallucinations reflect CNS hyperirritability. Pupillary constriction was present in 66% of cases.[127] Seizures occur in approximately 50% of cases.[127] Decerebrate rigidity, oculogyric crisis, and opisthotonos may develop; other findings may include loss of rectal sphincter tone, loss of skeletal muscle tone, and hemiplegia.[214] Cerebellar findings of dysarthria and ataxia are common.

Complete recovery occurs in most cases. However, chronic disability may develop in the form of mental deficiency, dysarthria, ataxia, aphasia, and hemiparesis.

CARDIOVASCULAR SYSTEM. Hypotension does not always occur in heatstroke but is usually present in fatal or severe cases.[216] This hypotension, which may persist even after large volumes of fluid therapy along with vasopressors, is an ominous late feature of heatstroke and may reflect failure of compensatory vasoconstriction of mesenteric blood vessels. As vital organs are hypoperfused, shock develops. Left ventricular subendocardial hemorrhage and focal necrosis of cardiac muscle fibers are commonly found on autopsy.[150,214]

The extreme stress placed on the cardiovascular system of victims with heatstroke results in a universal finding of sinus tachycardia, often with rates exceeding 140 beats/min.[216] Pulse pressure is elevated in the face of low cardiac output (CO) and low diastolic blood pressure.[214] Electrocardiographic findings include ST segment and T wave abnormalities and conduction disturbances.[56] In microswine and monkeys, during heating, HR rose to a plateau shortly after heating and commenced to rise still further at T_c of 41° C (105.8° F), peaking a few minutes before death. Blood pressure was stable or even rose until HR peaked at T_c of 41° C and then declined until death.[90]

PULMONARY SYSTEM. Hyperventilation is a common finding, particularly in EHI. Persistent hyperventilation may lead to respiratory alkalosis and tetany. Coma or seizures may predispose to pulmonary aspiration with consequent lung injury.[214] Pulmonary edema may become severe or fatal; DIC may lead to adult respiratory distress syndrome.[72] Pulmonary infarctions have been found on autopsy.[150]

RENAL SYSTEM. Acute renal failure develops in approximately 25% of heatstroke victims.[133] Hypotension and resultant decreased renal blood flow constitute the primary underlying etiology. As in the CNS, thermal injury may cause direct cellular damage.[202] DIC and myoglobinuria exacerbate the insult to renal tissue. Hematuria, pyuria, proteinuria, and hyaline and granular casts are seen on urinalysis. Eventually, oliguria and anuria may develop.

HEPATIC SYSTEM. Within 12 to 24 hours after heatstroke collapse, elevated AST, ALT, and serum bilirubin levels can be detected.[125] Levels of AST greater than 1000 U/ml are commonly seen in severe heatstroke.[233] Prothrombin level reaches its nadir 48 to 72 hours after heat injury.[201] Cholestasis and hepatocellular necrosis may develop.

GASTROINTESTINAL SYSTEM. Vomiting and diarrhea are common symptoms of heatstroke. Compensatory mesenteric vascular constriction may produce localized areas of gut ischemia and mucosal injury with consequent breakdown of its permeability barrier and translocation of LPS into the circulation.[93] Direct thermal damage to the gut wall may also contribute to gut wall pathophysiology. As previously discussed, the subsequent increase in serum LPS and its role as inducer of potentially damaging cytokines may play a critical part in both the morbidity and potential therapy of heatstroke. In the presence of DIC, hematemesis and melena may develop.[214]

HEMATOLOGIC SYSTEM. White blood cell counts may be elevated to as high as 20,000 to 30,000/ml. Platelet count is depressed, as are levels of clotting factors V and VIII. The commonly seen bleeding diathesis may be manifested as conjunctival hemorrhage, melena, purpura, or hematuria.[214] The primary causes of this coagulopathy are believed to be release of thromboplastic substances secondary to endothelial damage, and endotoxemia resulting in intravascular thrombosis and secondary fibrinolysis.[213] Other contributing factors include direct inactivation of clotting factors by thermal injury, decreased hepatic production of clotting factors, and decreased production of platelets secondary to thermal injury to marrow megakaryocytes. Low levels of fibrinogen and elevated levels of fibrin split products, in the presence of thrombocytopenia, herald the onset of DIC. Clotting abnormalities most often peak 18 to 36 hours after acute heat injury.[213]

ACID-BASE AND ELECTROLYTE ABNORMALITIES. Early in the course of heatstroke, respiratory alkalosis secondary to hyperventilation may be present. As anaerobic or even aerobic glycolysis increases, serum lactate levels rise, generating metabolic acidosis.

Hypernatremia reflects associated dehydration common in heatstroke; however, Na^+ levels may appear normal. In the face of dietary deficiency of Na^+ or profuse sweat losses, initial normonatremia may develop into hyponatremia upon rehydration. Potassium levels may be low or elevated, with hyperkalemia associated with tissue damage and renal compromise. Hypocalcemia, hypomagnesemia, and hypophosphatemia may also occur. Although hypoglycemia may develop in cases of EHS, hyperglycemia secondary to elevated catecholamine release may also be seen.

ON-SITE EMERGENCY MEDICAL TREATMENT

Heatstroke is a medical emergency. Rapid reduction of elevated body temperature is the keystone of management of heatstroke; *duration* of hyperthermia may be the primary determinant of outcome.[133,216] Nevertheless, it is important to follow the ABCs of stabilization while cooling efforts are initiated. See Box 11-2 for basic first aid.

Early diagnosis of heat exhaustion can be vital. Early warning signs include flushed face, hyperventilation, headache, dizziness, nausea, tingling arms, piloerection, chilliness, incoordination, and confusion.[71] Pitfalls in the diagnosis of heat illness include *confusion, preventing self-diagnosis.*[71] Mainstays of therapy include emergency on-site cooling, intravenous (IV) fluids, treating hypoglycemia as needed, IV diazepam for seizures or severe cramping or shivering, and hospitalization if response to therapy is slow or atypical.[71,138]

Cooling should be energetically initiated immediately upon collapse and minimally delayed only for vital resuscitation measures in order to prevent or minimize expected complications. In the field, the sick individual should be placed in the shade and any restrictive clothing removed. The victim's skin should be kept wet by applying large quantities of tap water or water from any source and his or her body constantly fanned. However, it is of utmost importance that these measures do not delay evacuation of the victim to a hospital or the closest medical facility.

In a comatose victim, airway control should be established by insertion of a cuffed endotracheal tube. When available, administration of supplemental oxygen may help meet increased metabolic demands and treat hypoxia commonly associated with aspiration, pulmonary hemorrhage, pulmonary infarction, pneumonitis, or pulmonary edema.[72,150] Positive-pressure ventilation is indicated if hypoxia persists despite supplemental oxygen administration (Figure 11-1).

As discussed previously, resuscitative measures may rapidly lower body temperature. Monitoring and recording rectal temperature on site may be important for the correct diagnosis of heatstroke. Vital signs should be monitored, with attention to blood pressure

---

> **Box 11-2   BASIC FIRST AID FOR HEAT ILLNESSES**
>
> 1. Place the victim in the shade.
> 2. Remove restrictive clothing.
> 3. Apply large amount of water on the victim and keep his or her skin wet.
> 4. Improvise a fan and cool the victim.
> 5. Measure rectal temperature to confirm diagnosis.
> 6. Evacuate to the nearest medical facility.

---

and pulse. Although normotension should not be taken as a reassuring sign, *hypotension should be recognized for the ominous sign it always represents.* If possible, urine and blood samples should be obtained for evaluation before fluid infusion.

Vascular access should be established without delay by insertion of a large-gauge IV catheter. Administration of normal saline or lactated Ringer's solution should be begun. Recommendations regarding the rate of administration of fluids vary. Some authors advise a rate of 1200 ml over 4 hours,[180] but we consider this to be too conservative. Others encourage a 2-L bolus over the first hour and an additional liter of fluid per hour for the next 3 hours.[210] However, vigorous fluid resuscitation may precipitate the development of pulmonary edema, so careful monitoring is indicated. *Ideally, 1 to 2 L of fluid should be administered during the first hour after collapse and additional fluids administered according to the level of hydration.*[76]

Cooling measures should be initiated immediately. However, cooling techniques are ineffective when the victim suffers seizures that increase storage of body heat. Therefore convulsions should be controlled by IV administration of 5 to 10 mg of diazepam, as necessary.

As a result of drastic cooling, skin temperature may decrease enough to cause shivering. IV administration of chlorpromazine (50 mg)[124] or diazepam are effective to suppress shivering and prevent an additional rise in body temperature from metabolic heat production.

Cooling Methods

Much debate exists in the literature regarding the best approach to cooling heatstroke victims.[46,55,102,219,239] Morbidity and mortality are directly related to duration and intensity of elevated T_c. Therefore the rate at which any given method lowers body temperature is extremely important. Another consideration in choosing a cooling modality is the need for access to the victim for continuous monitoring.

Khogali and co-workers[239] developed a body cooling unit designed to maximize evaporative cooling by maintaining cutaneous vasodilation and minimizing

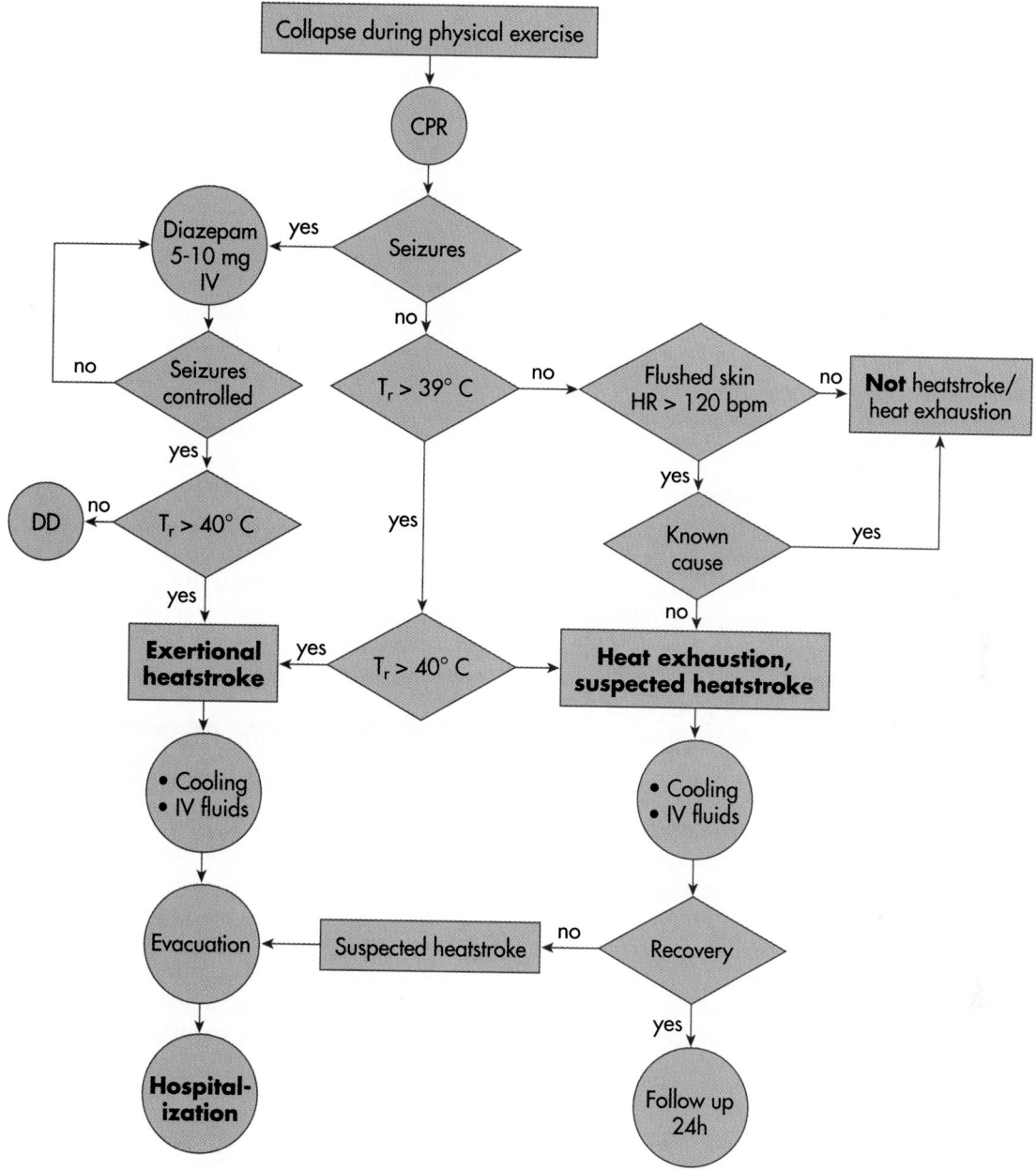

Figure 11-1 Flow chart for on-site emergency medical treatment of exertional heat illnesses. *DD*, Differential diagnosis. (*Modified from Shapiro Y, Seidman DS: Med Sci Sports Exerc 22:6, 1990*).

shivering. The patient is suspended on a net and sprayed from all sides with water at 15° C (59° F). Warm air (45° to 48° C [113° to 118.4° F]) is blown over the victim. Cooling rates of 0.06° C/min (0.11° F/min) have been obtained. Although this method is widely recommended as the treatment of choice, the rate of cooling is actually much less than that accomplished by ice water immersion.

Although not always available, *ice water or cold water immersion is an effective and easily available method of rapidly lowering core body temperature.* However, its use is one of the more hotly debated topics in the heatstroke literature. In most cases, the increased thermal conduc-

tivity of water results in reduction of T_c to less than 39° C (102.2° F) in 10 to 40 minutes.[56] This reflects a mean rate of cooling of 0.13° C/min (0.23° F/min), that is, *twice* the rate of the body cooling unit. Use of cold water rather than ice water resulted in a similar rate of cooling of 0.13° C/min.[180] Cold water immersion is less uncomfortable for the victim than immersion in ice water. In *hundreds* of EHS victims in a military population, there were no fatalities or permanent sequelae after treatment with ice water immersion.[55,56,179] Although other cooling methods reduce the rate of mortality, none has been as successful as ice water–soaked sheets or immersion.[89]

In discussing an alternative cooling method, Khogali[128,239] summarizes the most commonly offered criticisms of ice water immersion:

- Exposure to severely cold temperatures may cause peripheral vasoconstriction with shunting of blood away from the skin, resulting in a paradoxical rise in core temperature.
- Induction of shivering (in response to the cold) may cause additional elevation in temperature.
- Exposure to ice water causes marked patient discomfort.
- Working in ice water is uncomfortable for medical attendants.
- Access to the patient for monitoring of vital signs or administration of cardiopulmonary resuscitation is more difficult.
- There is difficulty maintaining sanitary conditions should vomiting or diarrhea develop.

Although the first two criticisms may appear physiologically appropriate, review of the medical literature fails to provide documentation for a rise in body temperature following ice water immersion or shivering as a problem.[56] In fact, vascular resistance decreased during ice bath cooling and persisted until normothermia.[180] This is an expected observation. The hypothalamic set point for temperature regulation is not raised during heatstroke (unlike during febrile illness), and brain temperature accounts for approximately 90% of the thermoregulatory response, compared with the skin's 10%.[196] The shivering response should only occur if body temperature is allowed to fall below normal. When shivering occurred, chlorpromazine treatment (25 to 50 mg intravenously) was effective.[117] Heatstroke victims rarely require cardiopulmonary resuscitation, so this concern should not preclude the use of ice baths to treat heatstroke. The documented efficacy of ice water immersion in rapidly reducing body temperature, and therefore morbidity and mortality, overrides any consideration of transient personal discomfort for the patient or medical attendants.

If other methods are used initially, any victim whose core temperature does not reach 38.9° C (102.2° F) within 30 minutes after beginning treatment should be placed in a tub containing ice water or on a stretcher above the tub and covered with ice water–drenched sheets and massaged.[89] The tub should be deep enough for submersion of the neck and torso.[188] Rapidly falling core temperature may not be accurately reflected by measured rectal temperature,[44] so with any cooling technique, active cooling should be discontinued when core body temperature falls to 39° C to prevent inducing hypothermia.

In summary, ice water treatment cools EHS patients fastest, can be easily set up with little training, is available in most hospitals without purchasing capital equipment, and may also be used on classic heatstroke victims. However, in treating elderly classic heatstroke patients, a case-by-case judgment call should be made deciding whether the risk of a theoretic, but never-shown, harmful stress by ice water treatment is worth the clear benefit of rapid cooling. Otherwise, cold water or ice water cooling is the method of choice.

Various ancillary modalities have been proposed to facilitate cooling, including administration of cold IV fluids, gastric lavage with cold fluids, and inhaling cooled air. Although these therapies lower body temperature, their effects are minimal compared with ice water immersion. Cooling blankets are ineffective in inducing the rapid lowering of body temperature required in treatment of heatstroke. Use of antipyretics is inappropriate and potentially harmful in heatstroke victims. Aspirin and acetaminophen lower temperature by normalizing the elevated hypothalamic set point caused by pyrogens; in heatstroke, the set point is normal, with temperature elevation reflecting failure of normal cooling mechanisms. Furthermore, acetaminophen may induce additional hepatic damage, and administration of aspirin may aggravate bleeding tendencies. Alcohol sponge baths are inappropriate under any circumstances, since absorption of alcohol may lead to poisoning and coma.

HOSPITAL EMERGENCY MEDICAL TREATMENT

If airway control has not been previously established, a cuffed endotracheal tube should be inserted to protect against aspiration of oral secretions (Figure 11-2). Supplemental oxygen and, when necessary, positive-pressure ventilation should be provided. Temperature should be continually monitored (at 5-minute intervals) by means of an esophageal or rectal probe. Cooling measures should be maintained for T_c greater than 38° C (100.4° F).

IV access should be obtained as quickly as possible. In the emergency room, IV fluid should be administered to EHS victims as a bolus of 1 L. Additional fluid should be based on the clinical situation after laboratory results are obtained to support the circulatory system without risk of inducing pulmonary or cerebral edema. Most heatstroke victims arrive with high cardiac index, low peripheral vascular resistance, and mild right-sided heart failure with elevated central venous pressure. Only moderate fluid replacement is indicated if effective cooling results in vasoconstriction and increased blood pressure. A Swan-Ganz pulmonary artery catheter may be necessary to assess appropriate fluid supplementation. Some victims have low cardiac index, hypotension, and elevated central venous pressure. These persons have been successfully treated with an isoproterenol drip (1 mg/min).[180] Patients with a low cardiac index, low central venous pressure, hypotension, and low pulmonary capillary wedge pressure should receive fluid.

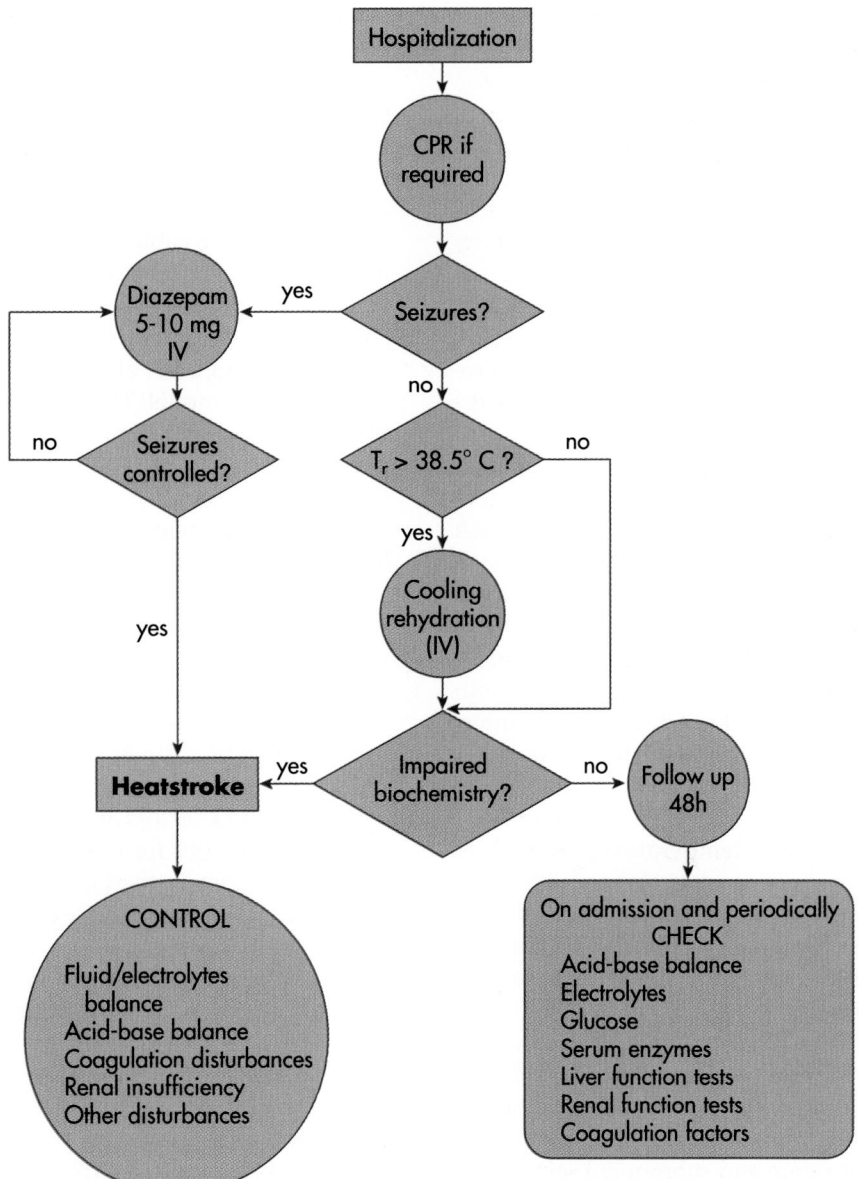

Figure 11-2 Flow chart for hospital medical treatment of exertional heat illnesses. (*Modified from Shapiro Y, Seidman DS:* Med Sci Sports Exerc *22:6, 1990.*)

Cardiac monitoring should be maintained during at least the first 24 hours of hospitalization. Use of norepinephrine and other α-adrenergic drugs should be avoided because they cause vasoconstriction, thereby reducing heat exchange through the skin. Anticholinergic drugs that inhibit sweating, such as atropine, should also be avoided.

As previously discussed, chlorpromazine may be used to treat uncontrollable shivering that might lead to rising body temperature. However, chlorpromazine should be used advisedly because it may cause hypotension or seizures and its anticholinergic effects may interfere with sweating. For these reasons, some physicians prefer to use diazepam to control shivering.

A Foley catheter should be placed to monitor urinary output. Myoglobinuria and hyperuricemia can be prevented by promoting renal blood flow by administering IV mannitol (0.25 mg/kg) or furosemide (1 mg/kg).[210] Early dialysis should be considered if anuria, uremia, or hyperkalemia develops.

Cooling and hydration usually correct any acid-base abnormality; however, serum electrolytes should be monitored and appropriate modifications of IV fluids made. Glucose should be monitored repeatedly because both hypoglycemia and hyperglycemia may occur after heatstroke.[205]

Oral and gastric secretions are evacuated via nasogastric tube connected to continuous low suction. Although antacids and histamine H_2 blockers have been used to prevent gastrointestinal bleeding, no studies to date demonstrate their efficacy in heatstroke victims.

As previously discussed, clotting disturbances peak 18 to 36 hours after onset of heat injury.[214] Coagulation tests (platelet count, prothrombin time, fibrinogen levels, fibrin split products) should be obtained on admission and after 24 hours. DIC may develop 24 to 72 hours after admission and is marked by acute onset of bleeding from venipuncture sites, gingivae, nasal mucosae, lungs, and/or the gastrointestinal tract. DIC is best prevented by rapid cooling of initial hyperthermia and replacement of clotting factors and platelets by transfusion of fresh frozen plasma and platelets.

Acute hepatic dysfunction is exhibited by elevated levels of aminotransferases and bilirubin. The peak levels are seen 36 to 72 hours after collapse. These high levels may last for several days.[76,159,216] Muscle damage is displayed primarily by marked elevation of serum CPK activity levels, which peak 24 to 48 hours after collapse and usually return to normal spontaneously within 5 days. Muscle and liver enzymes and bilirubin values should be carefully followed, but drastic interventions (e.g., liver transplant) are rarely necessary.

Prognosis

Rapid reduction of body temperature, control of seizures, proper rehydration, and prompt evacuation to an emergency medical facility currently result in a 90% survival rate in heatstroke victims, with morbidity directly related to duration of hyperthermia.[209] A poor prognosis is associated with T_c greater than 41° C (105.8° F), prolonged duration of hyperthermia, hyperkalemia, acute renal failure, and elevated serum levels of liver enzymes. Full recovery without evidence of neurologic impairment has been achieved even after coma of 24 hours' duration and subsequent seizures.[216] The persistence of coma after return to normothermia is a poor prognostic sign.[214] In a few victims, some neurologic deficits may persist, but usually for a limited period of 12 to 24 months, and only rarely for a longer period.[5] However, one recent study of classic heatstroke reported that 33% of patients left the hospital with some neurologic impairment.[63]

Dantrolene

Dantrolene has been used very successfully in the treatment of several hypercatabolic syndromes, such as malignant hyperthermia, neuroleptic malignant syndrome, and other conditions characterized by muscular rigidity or spasticity.[224,236] Dantrolene stabilizes the Ca^{2+} release channel in muscle cells, reducing the amount of Ca^{2+} released from the cellular calcium stores. This lowers intracellular Ca^{2+} concentrations, muscle metabolic activity, and muscle tone, and thus heat production.[40,175] In some studies, dantrolene was claimed ef-

fective in treating heatstroke, whereas in others it neither improved the rate of cooling nor improved survival.[38,64,148,228] In six rhabdomyolysis patients, intramuscular Ca^{2+} concentrations were 11 times higher than in controls and dantrolene successfully lowered this elevated Ca^{2+}.[145] Collectively, the limited data available are at best inconsistent. In spite of growing evidence for a possible benefit of dantrolene treatment in heatstroke, justification for its routine use in such cases is not proved, although future clinical trials may change this assessment.[30,112,141,184]

Recently, Moran et al[164] studied dantrolene in a hyperthermic rat model. They found it effective as a prophylactic agent in sedentary animals only. Dantrolene induced more rapid cooling by depressing Ca^{2+} entry into the sarcoplasm. This led to relaxation of peripheral blood vessels with attenuated production of metabolic heat. Dantrolene also may be effective in treating heatstroke by increasing the cooling rate. However, in other animal models, dantrolene was not superior to conventional cooling methods.[245]

Prevention

Prevention of heat illness relies upon awareness of host risk factors, altering behavior and physical activity to match these risk factors and environmental conditions, and a requirement for appropriate hydration during physical exercise in the heat. More aggressive educational activity of the media explaining heat illness and its prevention to the public are to be strongly promoted. Primary care physicians should incorporate this information in the anticipatory guidance of routine health assessment. Despite a wealth of medical literature on heat injury, some athletic coaches continue to use physical or psychologic methods to force athletes to compete or run under intolerably hot conditions. This practice should be viewed as irresponsible, dangerous, and possibly criminally negligent.

AWARENESS OF HOST RISK FACTORS

Risk Factors

Any underlying condition that causes dehydration or increased heat production, or decreased dissipation of heat, interferes with normal thermoregulatory mechanisms and predisposes an individual to heat injury. Older individuals are less heat tolerant than are younger persons to EHI and more susceptible to classic heatstroke because of decreased secretory ability of sweat glands and decreased ability of the cardiovascular system to increase blood flow to the skin (BF_{sk}). When healthy young adults exercise strenuously in the heat, EHS may occur, despite the absence of host risk factors. In particular, persons with type II muscle fiber predominance are more susceptible to EHS because these fibers are "faster" but less efficient than other fiber types.[115] In principle, since women have a thicker subcutaneous fat layer and a T_c 0.4° to 0.5° C (0.7° to 0.9° F) higher during the luteal phase than in the follicular phase, they may be at greater risk for heat injury during the luteal phase, but this has not been documented in controlled studies.[183a,223a]

BMR–to–surface area ratios of children are higher than those of adults. As a result, the child's T_{sk} is higher. Although the secretory rates of sweat glands are lower in children, they have greater numbers of active sweat glands per area of skin than do adults and overall greater sweat rates per unit area.[113] Any reduction in sweat rates would therefore put children especially at risk.

Endocrine abnormalities, such as hyperthyroidism and pheochromocytoma, cause a marked increase in heat production. Acute febrile illness, by virtue of the elevated hypothalamic set point caused by pyrogens, also leads to increased heat production. Muscular activity associated with uncontrolled gross motor seizures or delirium tremens also releases significant metabolic heat.

The primary means of heat dissipation is production and evaporation of sweat. Any condition that reduces this process places the individual at risk for thermal injury. Poor physical conditioning, fatigue, cardiovascular disease, and lack of acclimation all limit the cardiovascular response to heat stress. Obesity places an individual at risk from reduced CO, increased energy cost of moving extra mass, increased thermal insulation, and altered distribution of heat-activated sweat glands.[161] The elderly and the young show decreased efficiency of thermoregulatory functions and increased risk of heat injury.

Several congenital or acquired abnormalities affect sweat production and evaporation. Ectodermal dysplasia is the most common form of congenital anhidrosis. Widespread psoriasis, scleroderma, miliaria rubra ("prickly heat" caused by plugging of the sweat ducts with keratin), or deep burns may also limit sweat production.

Dehydration affects both central thermoregulation and sweating. A mere 2% decrease in body mass through fluid loss produces an increase in HR, increase in T_c, and a decrease in PV. In an otherwise healthy adult, gastrointestinal infection with vomiting and diarrhea may cause sufficient dehydration to place the individual at risk for EHS. Chronic conditions that may contribute to dehydration include diabetes mellitus, diabetes insipidus, eating disorders (especially bulimia), and mental retardation. Alcoholism and illicit drug use are among the 10 major risk factors for heatstroke in the general population.[131] An important effect of alcohol consumption is inhibition of ADH secretion, leading to relative dehydration.

Despite evidence that hypohydration limits physical performance, voluntary dehydration continues to be

routine in certain athletic arenas.[15,36,112,230] Wrestlers, jockeys, boxers, and bodybuilders commonly lose 3% to 5% of their body mass 1 to 2 days before competition. In addition to restricting fluid and food, they also use other pathogenic weight control measures, such as self-induced vomiting, laxatives and diuretics, and exposure to heat (saunas and hot tubs or "sauna suits"). Athletes undergoing rapid dehydration are at risk not only for heat injury but also for other serious medical conditions, such as pulmonary embolism.[60]

Box 11-3 highlights some of the common medications that interfere with thermoregulation. Special attention should be paid to the role of antihistamines in reducing sweating. This class of medications is commonly obtained over the counter, and the general population should be warned of the dangers of exercising in the heat when taking antihistamines.

Although it has been widely believed that sustaining an episode of heatstroke predisposes the individual to future heat injury, this has been refuted in a recent study of heatstroke victims.[16] Ten heatstroke patients were tested for their ability to acclimate to heat; by definition, the ability to acclimate to heat indicates heat tolerance. Nine of these patients demonstrated heat tolerance within 3 months after the heatstroke episode; the remaining patient acclimated to heat a year after his heat injury. In no case was heat intolerance permanent. Although individuals may show transient heat intolerance after thermal injury, evidence for permanent susceptibility to thermal injury is lacking.

Adaptation to Environmental Conditions

Appropriate adaptation to hot environmental conditions encompasses many forms of behavior, including modification of clothing, degree of physical activity, searching for shade, anticipatory enhancement of phys-

---

Box 11-3 DRUGS THAT INTERFERE WITH THERMOREGULATION

DRUGS THAT INCREASE HEAT PRODUCTION
Thyroid hormone
Amphetamines
Tricyclic antidepressants
Lysergic acid diethylamide (LSD)

DRUGS THAT DECREASE THIRST
Haloperidol

DRUGS THAT DECREASE SWEATING
Antihistamines (diphenhydramine)
Anticholinergics
Phenothiazines
Benztropine mesylate

ical conditioning, acclimation to heat stress, and attention to hydration.

Clothing. Different regions of the body are not equivalent in their sweat production.[111] The face and scalp account for 50% of total sweat production, whereas the lower extremities contribute only 25%. When exercising under conditions of high heat load, maximal evaporation of sweat is facilitated by maximum exposure of skin. Clothing should be lightweight and absorbent. Although significant improvement has been made in the fabrication of athletic uniforms, the uniforms and protective gear required by certain branches of the military and public safety officers continue to add to the risk of heat injury. Development of protective clothing that will also permit more effective heat dissipation is indicated.

Activity. Behavioral actions can effectively minimize the occurrence of classic heatstroke. Lack of residential air conditioning places indigent persons at risk during heat waves. By sitting in a cool or tepid bath periodically throughout the day, the individual can decrease the heat stress and thereby prevent heat injury.

Modification of physical activity should not be based solely on any individual parameter of T_{amb}, wet bulb temperature or relative humidity (RH), or solar radiation, since all of these contribute to heat load. The wet bulb globe temperature (WBGT) is an index of heat stress that incorporates all three factors. This value may be calculated (Table 11-2) or obtained directly from portable heat stress monitors that measure all three parameters simultaneously and compute the WBGT. Alternatively, the heat index may be obtained from national weather stations. Current recommendations for prevention of thermal injuries during distance running from the American College of Sports Medicine (ACSM) are based on WBGT.[10] It is stated that "distance races ($\geq$16 km or 10 miles) should not be conducted when the WBGT exceeds 28° C (82.4° F). During periods of the year when the daylight T_{amb} often exceeds 27° C (80° F), distance races should be conducted in the early morning or in the evening to minimize the heat load from T_{amb} and solar radiation."[10] In the British Army, the strenuous Combat Fitness Test (CFT) occasionally leads to heat casualties. To prevent a mean rise in T_c of 0.7° C (1.26° F) and minimize heat illnesses, calculations indicate that CFT should not be undertaken when the end WBGT is expected to be greater than 25° C (77° F).[33]

Table 11-3 presents a suggested modification of sports activity that is also based on the WBGT. Although ACSM guidelines for summer indicate that vigorous physical activity should be scheduled in the mornings or in the evenings, it should be cautioned that *the highest humidity of the day is usually early morning.* Recently, Montain et al[157] updated the replacement guidelines for warm weather training (Table 11-4). It is

TABLE 11-2. Wet Bulb Globe Temperature (WBGT) Heat Index

TEMPERATURE (° F)	EXAMPLE
Wet bulb × 0.7 =	78 × 0.7 = 54.6
Dry bulb × 0.1 =	80 × 0.1 = 8.0
Black globe × 0.2 =	100 × 0.2 = 20.0
HEAT INDEX	82.6

Wet bulb reflects humidity. Dry bulb reflects ambient air temperature. Black globe reflects radiant heat load. Alternative equation: WBGT = (.567) Dry bulb temperature + (393) Environmental water vapor pressure + 3.94.

TABLE 11-3. Modification of Sports Activity Using Wet Bulb Globe Temperature

INDEX (° F)	LIMITATION
<50	Low risk for hyperthermia but possible risk for hypothermia
<65	Low risk for heat illness
65-73	Moderate risk toward end of workout
73-82	Those at high risk for heat injury should not continue to train; practice in shorts and T-shirts during the first week of training
82-84	Care should be taken by all athletes to maintain adequate hydration
85-87.9	Unacclimated persons should stop training; all outdoor drills in heavy uniforms should be canceled
88-89.9	Acclimated athletes should exercise caution and continue workouts only at a reduced intensity; light clothing only
90 or above	Stop all training

important to note that compliance with these recommendations does not remove all risk of heat injury. Developing another index of heat stress that provides a better basis for prevention of EHS is indicated. Recently, a new user-friendly miniaturized (2-inch × 1-inch × 0.5-inch) device based on measuring T_{amb} and RH with microsensors was developed for assessment of heat stress.[162] However, further miniaturization and evaluations of this device are required.

Conditioning. The contribution of cardiovascular conditioning to thermoregulation is discussed in Chapter 10. Ideally, before exercising in the heat, an individual should train under temperate or thermoneutral conditions. For the previously sedentary individual, an exercise regimen incorporating 20 to 30 minutes of aerobic activity 3 to 4 days a week will improve cardiovascular function after 8 weeks.

It is important to remember that even physically active individuals may lack physical conditioning rela-

TABLE 11-4. Fluid Replacement Guidelines for Warm Weather Training (Applies to Average Acclimated Soldier Wearing BDU, Hot Weather)

HEAT CATEGORY	WBGT INDEX (° F)	EASY WORK		MODERATE WORK		HARD WORK	
		WORK/ REST CYCLE	WATER INTAKE (q/hr)	WORK/ REST CYCLE	WATER INTAKE (q/hr)	WORK/ REST CYCLE	WATER INTAKE (q/hr)
1	78-81.9	NL	½	NL	¾	40/20 min	¾
2 (Green)	82-84.9	NL	½	50/10 min	¾	30/30 min	1
3 (Yellow)	85-87.9	NL	¾	40/20 min	¾	30/30 min	1
4 (Red)	88-89.9	NL	¾	30/30 min	¾	20/40 min	1
5 (Black)	>90	50/10 min	1	20/40 min	1	10/50 min	1

From Montain SJ, Latzka WA, Sawka MN: *Mil Med* 164:502, 1999.
BDU, Battle dress uniform; *NL*, no limit to work time per hour.
The work/rest times and fluid replacement volumes will sustain performance and hydration for at least 4 hours of work in the specified heat category. Individual water needs will vary ± ¼ quart/hr.
Rest means minimal physical activity (sitting or standing), accomplished in shade if possible.
CAUTION: Hourly fluid intake should not exceed 1½ quarts.
Daily fluid intake *should not exceed 12 quarts.*
Wearing body armor: add 5° F to WBGT index.
Wearing mission-oriented protective posture (MOPP, chemical protection) overgarment: add 10° F to WBGT index.
EASY WORK: Weapon maintenance; walking hard surface at 2.5 mph, ≤ 30 lb load; manual handling of arms; marksmanship training; drill and ceremony.
MODERATE WORK: Walking loose sand at 2.5 mph, no load; walking hard surface at 3.5 mph, ≤ 40 lb load; calisthenics; patrolling; individual movement techniques, e.g., low crawl, high crawl; defensive position construction; field assaults.
HARD WORK: Walking hard surface at 3.5 mph, ≥ 40 lb load; walking loose sand at 2.5 mph with load.

tive to a particularly stressful competition or activity. Heat illness in runners commonly occurs when novices exceed their training effort during races or when well-trained athletes increase their pace above normal during long-distance events.

Acclimatization. On initial exposure to a hot environment, workouts should be moderate in intensity and duration. A gradual increase in the time and intensity of physical exertion over 8 to 10 days should allow optimal acclimatization[70]; children require 10 to 14 days to achieve a similar response. Acclimation can be induced by simulating hot environmental conditions indoors. If symptoms of heat illness develop during the acclimation period, all physical activity should be stopped and appropriate interventions begun. Acclimation is not facilitated by restricting fluid intake; in fact, conscious attention to fluid intake is required to prevent dehydration. As with physical conditioning, there are limits to the degree of protection that acclimation provides from heat stress. Given a sufficiently hot and humid environment, no one is immune to heat injury.

HYDRATION

Replacement of fluid loss during exercise preserves muscle function. Even after the loss of a large volume of sweat, a well-rehydrated cardiovascular system can maintain CO and blood pressure despite increased BF_{sk}

and continued sweating necessary for optimal temperature regulation.[171]

Throughout this chapter, *euhydration* refers to the idealized "normal" body water content based upon measurements of mass, electrolytes, urine specific gravity, and hematocrit, taken daily for at least 3 days after the first urination of the day and breakfast. *Dehydration* refers to loss of body fluids relative to euhydration, *rehydration* refers to replacement of body fluids, *hypohydration* refers to body fluids debt, and *hyperhydration* refers to excess body fluids.

Dehydration

Under neutral T_{amb}, a person at rest dissipates heat by transitory increases in BF_{sk} to accelerate heat losses by radiation, conduction and convection. When T_{amb} is greater than T_{sk}, exercise generates the need for additional mechanisms to dissipate heat. Evaporation of sweat is the only effective cooling mechanism, but this also causes loss of body fluid. Dripping sweat has no cooling effect and is especially prominent in a hot/wet climate. Under those conditions, the sweat rate ($\dot{m}_{sw}$) will be higher but will not be able to adequately dissipate body heat and lower T_c.[61] Fluid losses through sweating may exceed 2 L/h and up to 15 L/day.[162,196] As a consequence, insufficient drinking for sweat loss may rapidly lead to dehydration, compounding the cardiovascular and metabolic stresses already present.[53]

Blood flow to exercising muscles declines in parallel with dehydration.[97] The combined stresses of dehydra-

TABLE 11-5. Winning and Second-Place Scores in Selected Championship Sports

EVENT	PLACE	ATHLETES	TIME (SEC)	% DIFFERENCE
50 m freestyle—	1	Alexander Popov	22.13	0.59
1996 Olympics	2	Gary Hall	22.26	
200 m freestyle—	1	Danyon Loader	107.6	0.46
1996 Olympics	2	Gustavo Borges	108.1	
400 m freestyle—	1	Danyon Loader	228	0.44
1996 Olympics	2	Paul Palmer	229	
200 m individual medley—	1	Attila Czene	119.9	0.17
1996 Olympics	2	Jani Sievinen	120.1	
400 m individual medley—	1	Tom Dolan	254.9	0.12
1996 Olympics	2	Eric Namesnik	255.2	
Rowing—1996 Olympics	1	Marnie McBean, Kathleen Heddle	416.84	0.36
	2	Mianying Cao, Xiuyun Zhang	418.35	
Men's cycling—	1	Pascal Richard	17,636	0.00
1996 Olympics	2	Rolf Sorensen	17,636	
Four-man bobsled—	1	Czudaj/Voss/Szelig/Lehmann	113.7	0.001
1996 Altenberg World Cup	2	Langen/Kohlert/Ruhr/Hampel	113.83	
Men's Marathon—	1	Abel Anton	7996	0.06
1997 World Championships	2	Martin Fiz	8001	
Men's 5000 m—	1	Daniel Komen	787.4	0.24
1997 World Championships	2	Khalid Boulami	789.3	
Men's discus—	1	Lars Riedel		0.23
1997 World Championships	2	Virgilijus Alekna		
Men's pole vault—	1	Sergei Bubka		0.83
1997 World Championships	2	Maxsim Tarasov		
Men's free rifle—	1	Ennio Falco		0.83
1996 Olympics	2	Miroslaw Rzepkowski		

MEAN DIFFERENCE IN PERFORMANCE BETWEEN WINNING AND LOSING: 0.32%

tion and hyperthermia during exercise in the heat may exceed the body's ability to maintain CO and blood pressure. This renders the dehydrated sportsman less able to cope with hyperthermia.[99]

In a number of studies, 1.9% to 6% dehydration decremented performance in various tasks by 6% to 57% in athletes (Table 11-6).* Among elite athletes, the mean time difference between first and second place in international competitions was 0.32% (range: 0% to 0.83%) (Table 11-5). That is, a small degree of hypohydration may lead to a large decrement in performance among athletes. A dehydrated top-rated athlete can be defeated by a euhydrated but inferior opponent, particularly in endurance events.

Physical and cognitive performance is decremented by 1% dehydration (600 to 800 ml body fluid loss [BFL]), and the decrement becomes more severe with increasing BFL.[100,140] At 7% BFL there is evidence of exhaustion, and collapse is imminent.

Females were thought to be at higher risk for dehydration than males because females have less total body water, comparatively less lean body mass, and proportionately more adipose tissue than do their male

---

*References 59, 95, 104, 192, 200, 225.

counterparts of similar mass.[26] No gender differences were observed in $\dot{m}_{sw}$, but for similar $\dot{m}_{sw}$, females had higher T_{re}, suggesting that females have a less efficient process of evaporating sweat.[211] A larger surface area–to–mass ratio should promote more effective thermoregulation, but nonetheless, if fluid replacement is not sufficient, females may have higher risk for heat illnesses.

How Much to Drink?

The individual should be well hydrated before commencing physical activity in the heat; hypohydration for any reason should preclude physical activity while the individual is heat stressed. The ACSM guidelines recommend that individuals drink 500 ml of fluid about 2 hours before exercise to promote adequate hydration and allow time for excretion of excess water. In general, dehydration can be prevented by replacing body fluid losses through drinking. However, reliance on voluntary fluid intake through the sensation of thirst results in significant dehydration. Ten to 15 minutes before commencing physical activity, 8 oz. (½ cup) of water or appropriate fluid replacement beverage should be ingested. Continued intake of 8 to 12 oz. of fluid every 20 to 30 minutes during exercise should be enforced, or

TABLE 11-6. Decrement in Performance by Dehydration

TASK	DEHYDRATION	PERFORMANCE DECREMENT	REFERENCE
Time to run 1.5, 5, and 10 km	1.9%, 1.6%, 2.1%	3.4%, 7.19%, 6.74%	15
Walk to exhaustion in heat	1.9%, 4.3%	22%, 48%	59
Cycling, CV variables	2.5%-3.2%	23.9%	42
Treadmill during heat at 25%-65% Ap$\dot{V}_{O_2}$max	3%, 5%	0.3° C/3%; 0.7° C/5%; HR 2-18 bpm; CO 0.2-2.3 L/min	159
Submaximal work	3.9%	6.7%	225
Maximal exercise work time	3.8%, 3.6%, 4%	20%, 45%, 57%	192
Submaximal work		T_c: 0.1° C	104
Submaximal work		T_c: 0.5° C	95
Maximal isometric strength, jumping height	3.4%	7.67%-1.9%, 1.51%	235
Isometric and isotonic exercise	3.95%	31%, 29%	230
Maximal exercise work time	4%	12%	200
Various strength, CV measures, wrestlers	4.9%	13.18%, 11.76%, 21.5%, 9.72%, 12.38%	237
Treadmill, wrestlers	4.6%	9.32%, 15.6%	8
Walking, running cross-country	5.7%	21% maximal oxygen uptake	35
Marksmanship	6%	20%	225

Box 11-4   FINDING WATER IN THE DESERT

Persons traveling in hot climates should be prepared for strandings that might lead to death resulting from heat and dehydration. These have included the deaths of large numbers of Egyptian soldiers in the Sinai. The deaths could have been prevented had the soldiers known about subsurface "sweet" water. Another man in the desert who did not drink his car's cooling water also did not lie in the shade below his car and instead wandered off into the desert, where it took a long time to find his body. A woman alone for 2 days in the desert knew enough to stay in the shadow of a cliff. She benefited from the fact that maximal physical activity in the desert may cause a loss of 4 L of water per hour, whereas minimum activity in shade loses approximately 2.5 L per *day.*

1. Sources of water in the desert: Look for green plants.
2. Near the seashore, drinkable water, usually originating from rain, may be found below a sandy/gravel surface, and above any seawater because of its lower density. Particular plants may use this water and show greenery against a gray/brown substrate.
3. Water for drinking may be found at the foot of cliffs that become waterfalls only during a flood. Below these cliffs, pounding water and gravel may have carved a depression in the rocky floor that becomes filled in with gravel saturated with water. At the top of the saturated gravel, evaporation may render the surface dry and hot. However, much of the water often remains in pools or below the soil surface. Green plants often inhabit these areas and are markers for water. Such natural reservoirs retain water for a long time.
4. In wadis, after heavy rain, depressions filled with gravel and rocks become filled with water, with plants surrounding them.

---

urine color should be monitored (when the color becomes darker, it is time to drink more).[17] See Box 11-4.

Sweat rate is a function of individual metabolic rate, clothing, and climatic conditions. During mild work and while wearing cotton clothes, $\dot{m}_{sw}$ ranged between 0.3 and 1.2 L/hr. Performing the same activity but wearing nonpermeable clothing, $\dot{m}_{sw}$ rose to 1 to 2 L/hr. Likewise, during high exercise intensity in a hot climate, an athlete often has $\dot{m}_{sw}$ of 1 to 2.5 L/hr.[195] A high $\dot{m}_{sw}$ of 3.7 L/hr was reported in a marathon runner in the 1984 Olympics.[18] Voluntary matching of fluid consumption to sweat loss is a serious issue because thirst provides a poor index of body water needs.[194] As a result, individuals can dehydrate by 2% to 8% of their body mass during prolonged high sweat rate *even though water may be readily available.*[104] Since about 60% of body mass is water, dehydration of 2% to 8% is equivalent to a loss of 1 to 4 L of body fluids for a person of 75 kg body mass.[194]

The most widely used guideline for fluid replacement was suggested by Shapiro et al.[208] It is based on a mathematical sweat prediction model and is in use by the U.S. Army, as well as by other organizations. Recently, Montain et al[155] adjusted those guidelines for different U.S. Army activities (see Table 11-4).

The color of urine has been suggested as a way to monitor hydration status. This method is based on a color-coding key in which persons pay attention to the color of their urine; darker urine color indicates a higher level of hypohydration. Thus, if urine is strongly yellow-colored, the person is hypohydrated and must drink more water. If urine is clear, he is adequately hydrated. This method is practical for determining moderate degrees of hypohydration and is more sensitive than those based on blood measurements.[20]

The measurements of preexercise and postexercise nude dry weights can also be used as a guide for the need to drink more fluid. For every pound of weight lost during activity, the individual should consume 1 pint (2 cups) of fluid. Fluid loss should be replaced before return to activity in the heat; if a loss greater than 2% of body mass persists, the individual should be withheld from activity. Prehydration slows development of dehydration and temporarily enhances performance.

For assessment of day-to-day hydration status in athletes in the field, Shirreffs and Maughan[217] recently suggested a new method based on a standardized procedure for measuring osmolality of the first urine sample of the day. Urine is collected after wakening and before breakfast to allow day-to-day comparisons of individuals. After analyzing data from 29 athletes, they concluded that their method is reliable for individual hydration status and is a quick and easy method to achieve an approximation of day-to-day hydration status. However, we believe that a better method to evaluate hydration status that is noninvasive, rapidly responsive, and user friendly should be developed.

Advances in biosensor technology and microminiaturization have reduced commercial devices for measuring blood parameters to 2 inches × 6 inches × 1 inch (i-STAT Corporation, Princeton, N.J.), with results as accurate as those obtained from full-sized hospital automated blood chemistry analyzers. The i-STAT analyzer is portable enough to be useful in field scenarios for emergency diagnoses.[138]

The traditional rules of some sports (e.g., field hockey, soccer, tennis, rugby) unintentionally limit opportunities for hydration by failing to provide for time-outs and incorporating brief halftimes. During extremely hot and humid weather, team physicians, trainers, coaches, and officials should work together to incorporate additional breaks (quarters rather than halves) and provide unlimited access to fluids on the sidelines.

Hypohydration

Hypohydration leads to reduced ability to dissipate metabolic heat, rapid elevation in T_c, and more rapid exhaustion. Heat exhaustion occurs at relatively low T_c because blood volume displacement to the skin causes marked cardiovascular strain and instability.[156,199]

The impact of different levels of hypohydration on heat tolerance while wearing clothing was studied under various heat loads.[199,201] Under severe heat stress and wearing impermeable clothing, tolerance time was shortened by hypohydration before commencing the exercise, and the rate of rise in T_c during exercise increased with the degree of hypohydration.[152] The main contributor to excessive rise in T_c was believed to be decreased sweat rate.[104] In warm environments, increased levels of hypohydration result in increased threshold temperature for the onset of sweating and decreased sweat rate at each work rate during exercise.[154]

Hydration status may affect thermoregulatory or cardiovascular responses to exercise via alterations of body fluid volumes or osmolality. Hypovolemia and hyperosmolality, individually or acting synergistically, impair heat loss by elevating threshold T_c for the onset of both peripheral vasodilation and sweating, and possibly by decreasing the gain of these responses.[81,82,174] Hypohydration may also directly impair sweat gland function.[229] Hypohydration of 1.9% (by 24 hours of fluid restriction) increases T_c and serum osmolality during cycling exercise, and decreases blood flow to nonexercising muscles (e.g., forearm) in a normothermic environment.[227] Increasing levels of hypohydration and plasma osmolality, and decreases in PV, cardiac filling, and stroke volume, lead to progressively decremented CO and thermoregulation.[201] During exercise in the heat, each 1% increase in hypohydration levels raised T_c 0.1° to 0.5° C (0.18° to 0.9° F) and increased HR by 4 bpm.[95,104] HR is elevated to compensate for decreased stroke volume presumably caused by reduced central venous pressure and end-diastolic ventricular volume, both consequences of decreased blood volume[98] (see Chapter 10).

When required evaporative heat loss is less than maximal capacity of the environment to support evaporative heat loss ($E_{req} < E_{max}$), then the heat stress is described as "compensable"; if, however, $Er_{eq} > E_{max}$, it is "uncompensable." At an uncompensable heat load, minor levels of hypohydration impair exercise tolerance, even at lower metabolic rates. The impairment becomes evident as the duration of the exercise increases at lower metabolic rates. Hypohydration decreases PV and increases plasma osmolality and inhibits peripheral blood flow and the sweating response, resulting in increased rate of rise in T_c.

The effects of hypohydration on heat strain are well documented. The new physiologic strain index (PSI) showed high correlation between strain and losses of body mass through sweating[160,161,163] (see Chapter 10). However, the effects on skeletal muscle performance and metabolism are less well known.[154,198,199,201] Some studies indicated that hypohydration reduces muscle endurance,[27,77,165] whereas others found no difference.[4,79,114] Recently, Montain et al[157] reported that moderate hypohydration (4% body mass) decreased skeletal muscle performance by 15%. This disagreement with previous studies was explained by inadequate control of prior exercise, heat exposure, and caloric intake in previous studies.[157]

Physiologic Consequences of Hypohydration. Hyperosmolality per se, even without a fall in blood volume, increases the threshold temperatures for onset of skin vasodilation and sweating during exercise in the heat.[57] These effects may be neurally mediated, since preoptic anterior hypothalamic neurons are osmosensitive.[218] Moreover, hypovolemia reduces the rate of sweating during exercise in the heat.[80,201] Decreased PV as a result of lost water and salt, concomitant with increased distribution of blood volume to skin vascular beds, can reduce venous return, central venous pressure, cardiac filling pressure, stroke volume, and CO.[132,173] This would be followed by compensatory increases in HR[158] (Figure 11-3). In addition, increases in plasma hematocrit and viscosity further reduce cardiac filling pressure as a result of increased resistance. In one series of patients with EHS,[213] 35% were hypotensive with systolic blood pressure below 90 torr. Similar findings have been reported for classic heatstroke.[103]

Sinus tachycardia in response to excessive circulatory requirements is consistently present in heatstroke victims.[210] CO and diastolic blood pressure are low, while pulse pressure is high.[214] Depending on the degree of hypoperfusion of vital organs, shock may ensue.[133] Hypohydration compromises thermoregulation,[214] with linear increases in T_c of about 0.15° C (0.27° F) for each 1% decrease in body mass during exercise in the heat.[201] Additionally, hypohydration negates most of the thermoregulatory advantages conferred by high aerobic fitness and heat acclimatization,[35] increasing the risk of heat illness.[214] Sawka et al[199] reported that exhaustion from heat strain occurred at higher T_{re} for euhydrated than for hypohydrated subjects during uncompensable exercise heat stress.

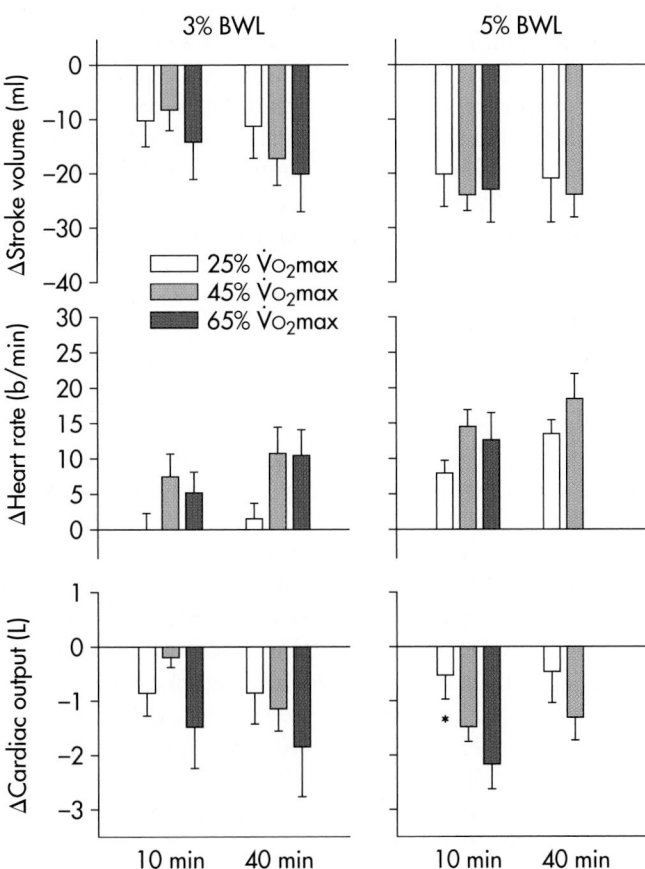

Figure 11-3 Decrements of cardiac performance with 3% and 5% body weight loss. (*From Montain SJ et al:* Int J Sports Med *19:87-91, 1998.*)

Some athletes use diuretics to reduce body weight to compete in a lower weight category. Diuretics increase the rate of urine formation and generally result in loss of solute and volume.[238] Relatively less intracellular water (approximately 65% of total body fluid) is lost after using diuretics because there is no excess of extracellular solute to stimulate redistribution of body water. Unlike either exercise or heat-induced hypohydration, diuretic-induced hypohydration generally results in isoosmotic hypovolemia, since there is a greater ratio of plasma loss to body water loss.[116] Among the common diuretics in use are thiazide, furosemide, and carbonic anhydrase inhibitors.

Hyperhydration

It had been hypothesized that consuming excess water before activity would improve performance during heat stress by expanding blood volume and reducing blood osmolality, thereby reducing cardiovascular and thermal strain during exercise.[86,197] Earlier studies[105,149,167,176] suggested that hyperhydration lowered HR and T_c compared with euhydration. Hyperhydration is usually achieved by drinking water in excess but can also be achieved by ingesting glycerol, since glycerol reduces free water clearance through the kidneys, thereby increasing retention of fluid.[86] In one study, glycerol/water ingestion improved thermoregulation during exercise heat stress.[149] The rise in T_{re} was attenuated by 0.7° C (1.26° F) and the sweat rate was elevated by ~300 to 400 ml/hr above control levels.

More recently, Latzka et al[142,143] studied hyperhydration induced by drinking either water or a water/glycerol mixture during compensable and uncompensable exercise heat stress. Surprisingly, compared with euhydration, hyperhydration did *not* alter T_c, T_{sk}, whole body sweating rate, local sweating rate, sweating threshold temperature, sweating sensitivity, or HR responses. Furthermore, there were no differences in physiologic variables between those achieving hyperhydration with water or by water/glycerol. These data demonstrate that hyperhydration provides no thermoregulatory or cardiovascular advantages over the maintenance of euhydration during compensable or uncompensable exercise heat stress.

Exercise and heat stress each reduce renal blood flow and free water clearance. Therefore the effectiveness of glycerol relative to water as a hyperhydrating agent may be masked. Latzka et al[143] concluded that hyperhydration per se only provides an advantage (over euhydration) in delaying hypohydration during either compensable or uncompensable exercise heat stress. Furthermore, glycerol ingestion caused nausea and headaches on several occasions. The reasons for the conflicting results with previous studies are uncertain but may be due to differences in experimental design. For example, Latzka et al carefully controlled for the initial baseline hydration status for both treatments, whereas earlier studies did not address this important independent variable.

Hyponatremia. Symptomatic hyponatremia is diagnosed when serum Na^+ is less than 130 mEq/L and is generally caused by hypervolemia secondary to drinking large volumes of water or markedly hypoosmotic fluids. This illness has been reported in psychiatric patients and in cases of water overload. However, nonpsychiatric cases are usually associated with enforced water drinking to prevent EHI or with being "too conscientious" in drinking at water stations during a marathon run. There have been several cases of hyponatremia from excessive fluid intake during prolonged exertion in the heat, especially in events such as ultramarathons, triathlons, and recreational hiking, as well as in military training.[23,68,87] Hyponatremia subsequent to water overload is potentially a cause of fatal cerebral and pulmonary edema.[92,178] During the development of hyponatremia, ingested water is absorbed from the gut lumen, diluted blood circulates to the brain, and water enters relatively hypertonic brain tissue by osmosis. Since the brain is enclosed by bone, it cannot swell and intracranial pressure increases. This essentially "squeezes" the cerebrovascular system, reducing intracranial blood flow and occasionally leading to ischemic damage and regulatory collapse. Immediate medical treatment is required.

In the U.S. Army, 125 cases of documented hypoosmolality/hyponatremia were reported over a 7-year epidemiologic study.[67] Many of these cases were associated with excessive water intakes relative to sweat loss, with average serum Na^+ of 121 mEq/L (116 to 133 mEq/L). Such low serum Na^+ values imply that total body water increased by 3 to 5 L.[155] As a result of this report, Montain et al[155] recently revised the U.S. Army fluid replacement guidelines, emphasizing on one hand the need for sufficient fluid replacement during heat stress, while on the other, concern for the danger of overhydration and water intoxication. To achieve an accurate guideline for fluid replacement during heat stress, a two-phase study was carried out by Shapiro et al,[208] who developed a computer model to predict sweating loss ($\dot{m}_{sw}$) during different exercise intensities, followed by validation in a laboratory study. The fluid replacement guidelines presented in Table 11-4 were designed to be a simple and practical tool. These recommendations specify an upper limit for hourly and daily water intake, which safeguards against overdrinking and water intoxication.

TREATMENT OF HYPONATREMIA. It is critical to differentiate between water intoxication and heat exhaustion/ heatstroke because the treatments are very different. In the field, discriminating between hyponatremia and certain heat illnesses may be difficult because of considerable overlap of symptoms.[92] A major difference between water intoxication and heat illnesses would probably be in T_c. In heat illnesses, T_c is generally greater than 39° C (102.2° F), whereas in hyponatremia, T_c is usually normal or close to normal.[23,92] Heat illnesses are treated by cooling and sufficient rehydration, whereas hyponatremia is treated by restricting fluids and gradually correcting Na^+ concentration by infusion of hypertonic NaCl solution. Too rapid a correction of hyponatremia can cause the demyelinating syndrome known as pontine myelinolysis.

Rehydration

Optimal performance is attainable only with sufficient drinking during exercise to minimize dehydration. It is beyond dispute that even low levels of dehydration (1% loss of body mass) impair cardiovascular and thermoregulatory responses and reduce capacity for exercise.[171] Fluid replacement reduces the risk of heat illness and improves exercise performance by preventing or reducing dehydration. Consuming fluids in amounts directly proportional to sweat loss maintains optimal physiologic functions and significantly improves exercise performance, even with exercise lasting 1 hour. However, it is recommended that ingested fluid be cooler than T_{amb} (15° to 25° C [59° to 72° F]) and flavored to enhance palatability and promote fluid replacement.[11]

Once heat injury has progressed to the point of heatstroke, *IV replacement of fluid losses is required. Normal saline solution is the initial IV fluid of choice,* providing excellent expansion of intravascular volume without risking too rapid a correction of undiagnosed hyponatremia. The rate of fluid administration should reflect preexisting or coexisting medical conditions. An initial rate of 1200 ml over 4 hours has been proposed.[180] *Supplemental potassium should be withheld until serum electrolyte levels are known.* This is important because some commercial beverages previously ingested by the victim contain additional K^+. Future choice of fluids should reflect the individual's electrolyte status and cardiac and renal function.

Recommendations for maintaining oral hydration (or, more accurately, minimizing dehydration) are presented in the Prevention section. *The inability to rely on the thirst mechanism to prevent dehydration cannot be overemphasized.* Simple provision of fluids at the sideline during athletic practices and competitions and military training scenarios is not sufficient. Scheduled breaks in activity (every 20 to 30 minutes depending on the degree of heat stress) for required consumption of fluids should become more commonplace.

Rehydration with and without Acclimatization.

Sweating and normal thermoregulation have another impact on the predisposition to clinical states that is widely unappreciated by trainers, coaches, and team physicians. In unacclimatized individuals, sweat salt losses can theoretically produce solute deficits having a profound impact on thirst and therefore on potential rehydration rates.

On average, 60% of body mass is water, so that a 70-kg adult contains 0.6×70 kg = 42 L of total body water (TBW). If he now loses 6% of body mass by hypothetically sweating pure water, then he has lost a volume of 0.06×70 kg = 4.2 L, or (4.2 L/42 L) = 10% of TBW. Thus TBW has been reduced by 4.2 L to 37.8 L.

Since, in this example, all salts are retained within the body, plasma Na^+ rises in proportion to the ratio of euhydrated volume to the new dehydrated volume, $(42 L \div 37.8 L) \times 140$ mEq/L; *Na^+ has risen to 155 mEq/L,* (assuming two osmotically active particles per NaCl molecule) and *310 mOsm/L.*

If, however, that same sweat volume contained NaCl at a concentration of half the normal euhydrated value $(0.5 \times 140$ mEq/L = 70 mEq/L), then there was a sweat loss of 70 mEq/L $\times$ 4.2 L = 294 mEq Na^+, as well as the 4.2 L of water. Since the normal euhydrated plasma Na^+ concentration is 140 mEq/L, crude calculations indicate that the total amount of Na^+ present is 42 L $\times$ 140 mEq/L = 5880 mEq. To calculate the crude final Na^+ concentration, the original total amount of Na^+ must be reduced (5880 − 294 mEq = 5586 mEq) by the 294 mEq lost in sweat, and therefore the *final Na^+ concentration (5586 mEq $\div$ 37.8 L) becomes 148 mEq/L and 296 mOsm/L.* This is high enough to reach the thirst threshold (295 mOsm), so the person feels moderately thirsty and will "desire" to consume only 80 ml of water (vs. 1270 ml; see later discussion) before osmolality is reduced to the thirst threshold. This represents only 1.9% (80 ml/4200 ml $\times$ 100) deficit of the water. Consumption of a solute-rich meal or a fluid-replacement beverage about 2 hours before exercise potentially counteracts the salt loss in sweat of a nonacclimatized individual. This probably also explains, by and large, why water balance is often not fully restored until mealtime in sweating, nonacclimatized individuals.

Another clinically and physiologically relevant aspect of this calculation should be emphasized. It is generally appreciated that fully acclimatized subjects, compared with nonacclimatized ones, sweat sooner (at lower T_c and T_{sk}), with lower sweat salt concentration and in larger volume. That is, acclimated persons sweat more and require larger volumes of replacement fluids than do unacclimatized ones for the same activity.

If this sweat were to contain a Na^+ concentration as low as 0.17% NaCl, the solute loss would be reduced to 235 mOsm, compared with 588 mOsm (see earlier discussion). The dehydrated plasma osmolality would be 305 mOsm/kg, and the thirsty subject would have to consume 1270 ml (a sixteenfold increase) to lower the osmolality to the thirst threshold (30.2% of the water deficit vs. 1.9% above). Although this theoretically important aspect of acclimation on thirst and rehydration volumes has not been experimentally verified, it could significantly improve resistance to heat illness by maintaining more adequate body water stores.

Fluid Replacement Beverages. A more widely investigated and hotly debated topic is appropriate fluid replacement during physical activity in the heat. Confusion has arisen over a need for replacing electrolyte losses, as well as the advantages of carbohydrate supplementation. The benefits of fluid replacement with electrolyte-carbohydrate-containing beverages vs. water was studied in athletes with 1.9% and 3.5% electrolyte losses.[241] No significant difference was found in the maintenance of PV between trials with water and the experimental formulations. During intense exercise lasting longer than 1 hour, the ACSM guidelines for exercise and fluid replacement recommend that carbohydrates be ingested at the rate of 30 to 60 g/hr to maintain oxidation of carbohydrates and delay fatigue.[11]

Early investigators promoted consumption of Na^+-containing fluid to prevent development of hyponatremia during exercise. The rehydration effectiveness of three commercial sports drinks was compared during 4 hours of physical activity.[118] The beverages consisted of prepared solutions containing component individual minerals and glucose. All solutions proved equally effective in maintaining water and electrolyte balance during moderate physical performance. A benefit of ingesting commercial sports drinks appears to be enhanced palatability that increases voluntary fluid consumption, thereby reducing dehydration.[170]

The rate of rehydrating various body compartments depends on the rates of gastric emptying of ingested fluid and the intestinal absorption of water. Gastric emptying is the slower rate-limiting step and depends principally on osmolality and caloric content of the fluid.[74] Which factor predominates depends on physical activity and the temperature and volume of the beverage. Earlier studies suggested that there was a delay in gastric emptying and increased rehydration time when the beverage contained more than 2.5% glucose, sucrose, or fructose. However, more recent studies have reported that there is in fact little or no difference in gastric emptying rates between water and carbohydrate solutions as high as 7%.[62,203] Other investigators have confirmed that under exercise conditions, 5% glucose polymer solutions show a gastric emptying rate similar to water.

A frequent argument for including Na^+ in fluid replacement beverages is to enhance intestinal water absorption, since Na^+ transport is the major determinant of water absorption in the proximal small bowel. Active coupled transport of Na^+ and glucose creates an osmotic gradient that pulls water from the lumen into epithelial cells. However, the rate of intestinal absorption of carbohydrate-electrolyte solutions is equal to, but not faster than, absorption of water.[170,240]

Cold fluids increase the motility of smooth muscles in the gastric wall, thereby speeding gastric emptying more rapidly than do warm drinks. The commonly held belief that consumption of cold water results in stomach cramps has not been confirmed. Such a phenomenon, if it occurs, is more likely related to the volume of the beverage than to its temperature.[50]

Gastric emptying is speeded by stretching the gastric wall. Therefore large volumes of liquid empty from the stomach more rapidly than do small quantities. Athletes, however, are uncomfortable exercising with a nearly full stomach. Indeed, although there may be a benefit to rapid oral rehydration, if the nausea threshold is reached, a secondary increase in ADH secretion may impair the kidneys' ability to excrete excess fluid volume and result in hyponatremia and water intoxication.[19] By drinking smaller volumes (150 to 250 ml) at 15- to 20-minute intervals, athletes can maintain adequate hydration while minimizing gastric distension.

A sports drink should contain 5% to 10% carbohydrate in the form of glucose or sucrose to enhance endurance.[58] However, many athletes suffer cramps, nausea, and diarrhea after drinking a 10% glucose solution. An isocaloric glucose-polymer solution has only one fifth the osmotic pressure. Its lower osmolality allows an increase in the carbohydrate content of a sports drink without risking the gastrointestinal side effects of a high osmolar drink. Several commercial polymer solutions are available.

Carbohydrate feeding during prolonged exercise enhances performance, whether assessed by time to exhaustion or by time to complete a predetermined exercise task.[45,170] Glucose polymer solutions given before and during a soccer game sustained blood glucose concentration and improved performance, although no difference in perceived exertion was found.[212] However, dehydrated soldiers who ingested fluids during exercise in the heat reduced their strain and the intensity of perceived exertion.[169] Whether use of these beverages spares muscle glycogen is a matter of current debate.

A potential problem in using carbohydrate-rich beverages is that they may attract bees and yellow jackets into the vicinity of the athletes, placing them at risk for sting-induced allergic or anaphylactic reactions.

Under normal conditions, use of electrolyte-carbohydrate-containing beverages offers little advantage over water in maintaining PV or electrolyte concentration or in improving intestinal absorption. Consumption of an electrolyte-containing beverage may be indicated under conditions of caloric restriction, prolonged exercise, or repeated days of sustained sweat losses. Drinking carbohydrate solutions during prolonged exercise may enhance performance; athletes who might benefit are those involved in soccer, field hockey, rugby, and tennis. For these athletes, use of glucose polymer solutions may be considered. Under no circumstances should carbohydrate-containing beverages be placed into canteens, since microbial contamination would be unavoidable and subsequent sterilization required.

For the vast majority of individuals, however, the primary advantage of using electrolyte- or carbohydrate-containing drinks appears to enhance voluntary consumption. This factor should not be considered insignificant if regulated intake is impossible.

ACKNOWLEDGMENTS

This chapter is in part a revision of Gaffin SL, Hubbard RW, Squires DL: Heat-related illnesses. In Auerbach P, editor: *Wilderness medicine*, St Louis, 1995, Mosby, pp 167-212. The original contribution by Drs. Hubbard and Squire to this chapter is recognized. We thank Dr. Ralph Francesconi for his helpful suggestions and comments.

The opinions or assertions contained herein are the private views of the authors and should not be construed as official or reflecting the views of the U.S. Army or Department of Defense. Citations of commercial organizations and trade names in this report do not constitute an official Department of the Army endorsement or approval of the products or services of these organizations.

REFERENCES

1. Abderrezak B et al: Distribution of peripheral blood leukocytes in acute heat stroke, *J Appl Physiol* 73:405, 1992.
2. Al-Hadramy MS, Ali F: Catecholamines in heat stroke, *Mil Med* 154:263, 1989.
3. Al-Khawashki MI et al: Clinical presentation of 172 heat stroke cases seen at Mina and Arafat. In Khogali M, Hales JRS, editors: *Heat stroke and temperature regulation*, Sydney, Australia, Academic Press 1983.
4. Albukrek D et al: Heat stroke induced cerebellar atrophy: clinical course, CT and MRI findings, *Neuroradiology* 39:195, 1997.
5. Reference deleted in proofs.
6. Albukrek D et al: Heat intolerance, *Harefuah* 132:563, 1997.
7. Allan JR, Wilson CG: Influence of acclimatization on sweat sodium concentration, *J Appl Physiol* 38:708, 1971.
8. Allen TE, Smith DP, Miller DK: Hemodynamic response to submaximal exercise after dehydration and rehydration in high school wrestlers, *Med Sci Sports Exerc* 9:159, 1977.
9. Alzeer AH et al: Serum enzymes in heat stroke: prognostic implication, *Clin Chem* 43:1182, 1997.
10. American College of Sports Medicine: Position stand on heat and cold illnesses during distance running, *Med Sci Sports Exerc* 28:i, 1996.
11. American College of Sports Medicine: Position stands: exercise and fluid replacement, *Med Sci Sports Exerc* 28:i, 1996.
12. Anderson RJ, Reed G, Knochel JP: Heatstroke, *Adv Intern Med* 1983:835, 1993.
13. Appenzeller O, Atkinson R: *Sports medicine: fitness training injuries*, Baltimore, 1981, Urban & Schwarzenberg.
14. Araki T, Toda Y, Matsushita K: Age differences in sweating during muscular exercise, *Jpn J Phys Fitness Sports Med* 28:239, 1979.
15. Armstrong LE, Costill DL, Fink WJ: Influence of diuretic-induced dehydration on competitive running performance, *Med Sci Sports Exerc* 17:456, 1985.
16. Armstrong LE, Deluca JP, Hubbard RW: Time course of recovery and heat acclimation ability of prior exertional heatstroke patients, *Med Sci Sports Exerc* 22:36, 1990.
17. Armstrong LE, Hubbard RW: Application of a model of exertional heatstroke pathophysiology to cocaine intoxication, *Am J Emerg Med* 8:178, 1990.
18. Armstrong LE et al: Preparing Alberto Salazar for the heat of the 1984 Olympic marathon, *Physician Sportsmed* 14:73, 1986.
19. Armstrong LE et al: Symptomatic hyponatremia during prolonged exercise in heat, *Med Sci Sports Exerc* 25:543, 1993.
20. Armstrong LE et al: Urinary indices of hydration status, *Int J Sports Nutr* 4:265 1994.
21. Assia E, Epstein Y, Shapiro Y: Fatal heat stroke after a short march at night: a case report, *Aviat Space Environ Med* 56:441, 1985.
22. Austin MG, Berry JW: Observation on 100 cases of heatstroke, *JAMA* 161:1525, 1956.
23. Backer HD, Shopes E, Collins SL: Hyponatremia in recreational hikers in Grand Canyon National Park, *J Wilderness Med* 4:391, 1993.
24. Bar-Or O: Children and physical performance in warm and cold environments. In *Advances in pediatric sport sciences*, vol 1, Champaign, Ill, 1984, Human Kinetics.
25. Beller GA, Boyd AE: Heat stroke—a report of 13 consecutive cases without mortality despite severe hyperpyrexia and neurologic dysfunction, *Mil Med* 140:464, 1975.
26. Bergeron MF, Armstrong LE, Maresh CM: Fluid and electrolyte losses during tennis in the heat, *Clin Sports Med* 14:23, 1995.
27. Bijlani RL, Sharma KN: Effect of dehydration and a few regimes of rehydration on human performance, *Indian J Physiol Pharmacol* 24:255, 1980.
28. Birrer RB: Heat stroke: don't wait for the classic signs, *Emerg Med* 9, 1988.
29. Bohmer D: Loss of electrolytes by sweat in sports. In *Sport health and nutrition: the 1984 Olympic Scientific Congress proceedings*, vol 2, Champaign, Ill, 1986, Human Kinetics.
30. Bouchama A, Cafege A, Devol EB: Ineffectiveness of dantrolene sodium in the treatment of heatstroke, *Crit Care Med* 19:176, 1991.
31. Bouchama A et al: Mechanisms of hypophosphatemia in humans with heatstroke, *J Appl Physiol* 71:328, 1991.
32. Bowler K: Heat death and cellular heat injury, *J Therm Biol* 6:171, 1981.
33. Bricknell MCM: Setting heat stress limits for acclimatised soldiers exercising in heat, *J R Army Med Corps* 143:44, 1997.
34. Brock-Utne JG et al: Endotoxemia and long distance races, *S Afr J Sports Med* 1988.
35. Buskirk ER, Iampietro PF, Bass DE: Work performance after dehydration: effects of physical conditioning and heat acclimation, *J Appl Physiol* 12:189, 1958.
36. Caldwell JE: Diuretic therapy and exercise performance, *Sports Med* 4:290, 1987.
37. Carter BJ, Cammermeyer M: A phenomenology of heat injury; the predominance of confusion, *Mil Med* 153:118, 1988.
38. Channa AB et al: Is dantrolene effective in heat stroke patient? *Crit Care Med* 18:290, 1990.
39. Chao NHH: Clinical presentation of heat disorders. In Yeo PPB, Lin NK, editors: *Heat disorders*, Singapore, 1985, Headquarters Medical Services.
40. Chinet A, Giovannini P: Evidence by colorimetry for an activation of sodium-hydrogen exchange of young rat skeletal muscle in hypertonic media, *J Physiol* 415:409, 1989.
41. Choo MHHH: Clinical presentation of heat disorders. In Yeo PPB, Lin MK, editors: *Heat disorders*, Singapore, 1988, Headquarters Medical Services.
42. Claremont AD et al: Heat tolerance following diuretic induced dehydration, *Med Sci Sports Exerc* 8:239, 1976.
43. Clausen T: Regulation of active NaK transport in skeletal muscle, *Physiol Rev* 66:542, 1986.
44. Clowes GHA, O'Donnell TF: Heatstroke, *N Engl J Med* 291:564, 1974.
45. Coggan AR, Coyle EF: Metabolism and performance following carbohydrate ingestion late in exercise, *Med Sci Sports Exerc* 21:59, 1989.
46. Cohen JJ: Apoptosis, *Immunol Today* 14:126, 1993.
47. Consolazio CF, Matoush LO, Nelson RA: Excretion of sodium, potassium, magnesium and iron in human sweat and the relation of each to balance requirements, *J Nutr* 79:407, 1963.
48. Costill DL: Sweating: its composition and effects on body fluid, *Ann NY Acad Sci* 301:160, 1977.
49. Costill DL: Muscle water and electrolytes during acute and repeated bouts of dehydration. In Parizkova V, Rogozkin A, editors: *Nutrition, physical fitness and health*, Baltimore, 1978, University Park Press.
50. Costill DL: Water and electrolyte requirements during exercise, *Clin Sports Med* 3:639, 1984.
51. Costill DL, Branam G, Fink WJ: Exercise induced sodium conservation: changes in plasma renin and aldosterone, *Med Sci Sports Exerc* 8:209, 1976.
52. Costill DL, Cote R, Fink WJ: Muscle water and electrolytes following varied levels of dehydration in man, *J Appl Physiol* 40:6, 1976.
53. Costill DL, Fink WJ: Plasma volume changes following exercise and thermal dehydration, *J Appl Physiol* 37:521, 1974.

54. Costill DL, Miller JM: Nutrition for endurance sport: carbohydrate and fluid balance, *Int J Sports Med* 1:2, 1980.

55. Costrini AM: Emergency treatment of exertional heatstroke and comparison of whole body cooling techniques, *Med Sci Sports Exerc* 22:15, 1990.

56. Costrini AM et al: Cardiovascular and metabolic manifestations of heat stroke and severe heat exhaustion, *Am J Med* 66:296, 1979.

57. Cowles RB, Bogert A: A Preliminary study of thermal requirements of desert reptiles, *Bull Am Museum Nat Hist* 83:265, 1944.

58. Coyle EF, Coggan AR: Effectiveness of carbohydrate feeding in delaying fatigue during prolonged exercise, *Sports Med* 1:458, 1999.

59. Craig FN, Cummings EG: Dehydration and muscular work, *J Appl Physiol* 21:670, 1966.

60. Croyle PH, Place RA, Hilgenberg AD: Massive pulmonary embolism in a high school wrestler, *JAMA* 241:827, 1979.

61. Davies CT, Brotherhood JR, Zeidifard E: Temperature regulation during severe exercise with some observations on effects of skin wetting, *J Appl Physiol* 41:772, 1976.

62. Davis MM et al: Accumulation of deuterium oxide in body fluids after ingestion of D₂O-labelled beverages, *J Appl Physiol* 63:2060, 1987.

63. Dematte JE et al: Near-fatal heat stroke during the 1995 heat wave in Chicago, *Ann Intern Med* 129:173, 1998.

64. Denborough MA: Heatstroke and malignant hyperpyrexia, *Med J Aust* 1:204, 1982.

65. Dickinson JG: Heat-exercise hyperpyrexia, *J R Army Med Corps* 135:27, 1989.

66. Dill DB, Hall FG, Van Beaumont W: Sweat chloride concentration: sweat rate, metabolic rate, skin temperature and age, *J Appl Physiol* 21:99, 1966.

67. Editors: Hyponatremia associated with heat stress and excessive water consumption: outbreak investigation and recommendations, *Med Surveillance Monthly Rep* 3:9, 1997.

68. Editors: *Hyponatremia secondary to overestimation*, Aberdeen Proving Grounds, Md, 1997, US Army Center for Health Promotion and Preventive Medicine.

69. Eichler A, McFee A, Root H: Heatstroke, *Am J Surg* 118:855, 1969.

70. Eichna LW et al: Thermal regulation during acclimatization in a hot, dry (desert type) environment, *Am J Physiol* 163:585, 1950.

71. Eichner ER: Treatment of suspected heat illness, *Int J Sports Med* 19(suppl 2):S150, 1998.

71a. Elias SR, Roberts WO, Thorson DC: Team sports in hot weather: guidelines for modifying youth soccer, *Phys Sportsmed* 19:67, 1991.

72. El-Kassimi FA et al: Adult respiratory distress syndrome and disseminated intravascular coagulation complicating heat stroke, *Chest* 90:571, 1986.

73. Ellis FP: Mortality from heat illness and heat-aggravated illness in the United States, *Environ Res* 5:1, 1972.

74. Endres S et al: The effect of dietary supplementation with ω-3 polyunsaturated fatty acids on the synthesis of interleukin-1 and tumor necrosis factor by mononuclear cells, *N Engl J Med* 320:265, 1989.

75. Epstein Y: Heat intolerance: predisposing factor or residual injury? *Aviat Space Environ Med* 22:29, 1990.

76. Epstein Y, Sohar E, Shapiro Y: Exertional heatstroke: a preventable condition, *Isr J Med Sci* 31:454, 1995.

77. Epstein Y et al: Exertional heat stroke: a case series, *Med Sci Sports Exerc* 31:224, 1999.

78. Felig P, Johnson C, Levitt M: Hypernatremia induced by maximal exercise, *JAMA* 248:1209, 1982.

79. Fogelholm GM et al: Gradual and rapid weight loss: effects on nutrition and performance in male athletes, *Med Sci Sports Exerc* 25:371, 1993.

80. Fortney SM et al: Effect of blood volume on sweating rate and body fluids in exercising humans, *J Appl Physiol* 51:1594, 1981.

81. Fortney SM et al: Effect of hyperosmolality on control of blood flow and sweating, *J Appl Physiol* 57:1688, 1984.

82. Fortney SM et al: Effect of exercise hemoconcentration and hyperosmolality on exercise responses, *J Appl Physiol* 65:519, 1988.

83. Francesconi RP, Mager M: Heat-injured rats: pathochemical indices and survival time, *J Appl Physiol* 45:1, 1978.

84. Francesconi RP, Mager M: Hypo- and hyperglycemia in rats: effects on endurance and heat/exercise injury, *Aviat Space Environ Med* 54:1085, 1983.

85. Francesconi RP et al: Potassium deficiency in rats: Effects on acute thermal tolerance, *J Therm Biol* 16:77, 1991.

86. Freund BJ et al: Glycerol hyperhydration: hormonal, renal, and vascular fluid responses, *J Appl Physiol* 79:2069, 1995.

87. Frizzell RT, Lang GH, Lathan SR: Hyponatremia and ultramarathon running, *JAMA* 255:772, 1999.

88. Fukumoto T, Tanaka T, Fujioka H: Differences in composition of sweat induced by thermal exposure and by running exercise, *Clin Cardiol* 11:707, 1988.

89. Gaffin SL, Gardner J, Flinn S: Current cooling method for exertional heatstroke, *Ann Intern Med* 132:678, 2000.

90. Gaffin SL et al: A miniswine model of heatstroke, *J Therm Biol* 23:341, 1998.

91. Galun E et al: Pathophysiology of exercise-induced hyponatremia and its possible relationship to muscle injury, *Miner Electrolyte Metab* 17:315, 1991.

92. Garigan T, Ristedt DE: Death from hyponatremia as a result of acute water intoxication in an Army basic trainee, *Mil Med* 164:234, 1999.

93. Gathiram P et al: Portal and systemic arterial plasma lipopolysaccharide concentrations in heat stressed primates, *Circ Shock* 25:223, 1988.

94. Gathiram P et al: Changes in plasma lipopolysaccharide concentrations in hepatic portal and systemic arterial blood during intestinal ischemia in primates, *Circ Shock* 27:103, 1989.

95. Gisolfi CV, Copping JR: Thermal effects of prolonged treadmill exercise in the heat, *Med Sci Sports Exerc* 6:108, 1974.

96. Gitin EL, Demos MA: Acute exertional rhabdomyolysis; a syndrome of increasing importance to the military physician, *Mil Med* 139:33, 1974.

97. Gonzalez-Alonso J: Muscle blood flow is reduced with dehydration during prolonged exercise in humans, *J Physiol* 15:895, 1998.

98. Gonzalez-Alonso J et al: Dehydration reduces cardiac output and increases systematic and cutaneous vascular resistance during exercise, *J Appl Physiol* 79:1487, 1995.

99. Gonzalez-Alonso J et al: Dehydration markedly impairs cardiovascular function in hyperthermic endurance athletes during exercise, *J Appl Physiol* 82:1229, 1997.

100. Gopinathan PM, Pichan G, Sharma VM: Role of dehydration in heat stress-induced variations in mental performance, *Arch Environ Health* 43:15, 1998.

101. Graber CD et al: Fatal heat stroke. Circulating endotoxin and gram-negative sepsis as complications, *JAMA* 216:1195, 1971.

102. Graham BS: Features and outcomes of classic heat stroke, *Ann Intern Med* 130:613, 1999.

103. Graham BS et al: Nonexertional heatstroke: physiologic management and cooling in 145 patients, *Arch Intern Med* 146:876, 1985.

104. Greenleaf JE, Castle BW: Exercise temperature regulation in man during hypohydration and hyperhydration, *J Appl Physiol* 39:847, 1971.

105. Grucza R, Szczypaczewwska M, Kozlowski S: Thermoregulation in hyperhydrated men during physical exercise, *Eur J Appl Physiol* 56:603, 1987.

106. Gumaa K et al: The metabolic status of heat stroke patients: the Makkah experience. In Khogali M, Hales JRS, editors: *Heat stroke and temperature regulation*, Sydney, Australia, 1983, Academic Press.

107. Hammarstrom S et al: Microcirculatory effects of leukotrienes C₄ and D₄ and E₄ in the guinea pig. In Lefer AM, Gee MH, editors: *Progress in clinical and biological research: leukotrienes in cardiovascular and pulmonary function*, New York, 1985, Alan R Liss.

108. Hanson G, Zimmerman SW: Exertional heat stroke in novice runners, *JAMA* 242:154, 1979.

109. Hart GR et al: Epidemic classical heat stroke: clinical characteristics and course of 28 patients, *Medicine* 61:189, 1982.

110. Henderson A et al: Heat illness: a report of 45 cases from Hong Kong, *J R Army Med Corps* 132:76, 1986.

111. Herrman F, Prose PH, Sulzberger MB: Studies on sweating. V. Studies of quantity and distribution of thermogenic sweat delivery to the skin, *J Invest Dermatol* 18:71, 1952.

112. Hopkins PM, Ellis FR, Halsall PJ: Evidence for related myopathies in exertional heat stroke and malignant hyperthermia, *Lancet* 2:1491, 1991.

113. Hori S: Adaptation to heat, *Jpn J Physiol* 45:921, 1995.

114. Houston ME et al: The effect of rapid weight loss on physiological functions in wrestlers, *Physician Sportsmed* 9:73, 1981.

115. Hsu YD et al: Blood lactate threshold and type II fibre predominance in patients with exertional heatstroke, *J Neurol Neurosurg Psychiatry* 62:182, 1997.

116. Hubbard RW, Armstrong LE: The heat illnesses: biochemical, ultrastructural, and fluid electrolyte considerations. In Pandolf KB, Sawka MN, Gonzalez RR, editors: *Human performance: physiology and environmental medicine at terrestrial extremes*, Indianapolis, 1988, Benchmark Press.

117. Jesati RM: Management of severe hyperthermia with chlorpromazine and refrigeration, *N Engl J Med* 254:426, 1956.

118. Johnson HL, Nelson RA, Consolazio CF: Effects of electrolyte and nutrient solutions on performance and metabolic balance, *Med Sci Sports Exerc* 20:26, 1988.

119. Kappel M et al: Effects of in vivo hyperthermia on natural killer cell activity, in vitro proliferative responses and blood mononuclear cell subpopulations, *Clin Exp Immunol* 84:175, 1991.

120. Kark JA, Ward F, Gardner J: Prevention of exertional heat illness eliminates unexplained exercise-related death of recruits with sickle cell trait, *Blood* 90(suppl 1):447a, 1997.

121. Kark JA, Gardner J, Ward F: Reducing exercise-related sudden cardiac death rates among recruits by prevention of exertional heat illness, *J Am Coll Cardiol* 31(suppl a):133a, 1998.

122. Kark JA et al: Exertional heat illness in Marine Corps recruit training, *Aviat Space Environ Med* 67:354, 1996.

123. Keren G, Epstein Y, Magazanik A: Temporary heat intolerance in a heatstroke patient, *Aviat Space Environ Med* 52:116, 1981.

124. Keren G, Shonfeld Y, Sohar E: Prevention of damage by sport activity in hot climates, *J Sports Med* 20:452, 1980.

125. Kew MC, Bersohn I, Seftel H: The diagnostic and prognostic significance of the serum enzyme changes in heatstroke, *Trans R Soc Trop Med Hyg* 65:325, 1971.

126. Khogali M: Heat stroke: an overview. In Khogali M, Hales JRS, editors: *Heat stroke and temperature regulation*, Sydney Australia, 1983, Academic Press.

127. Khogali M: Heat stroke and heat exhaustion, *Travel Traffic Med Int* 1:166, 1983.

128. Khogali M: The Makkah body cooling unit. In Khogali M, Hales JRS, editors: *Heat stroke and temperature regulation*, Sydney, Australia, 1983, Academic Press.

129. Khogali M, Mustafa MKY: Clinical management of heat stroke patients. In Hales JRS, Richards D, editors: *Heat stress: physical exertion and environment*, New York, 1987, Elsevier.

130. Khogali M et al: Induced heat stroke: a model in sheep. In Khogali M, Hales JRS, editors: *Heat stroke and temperature regulation*, Sydney, Australia, 1983, Academic Press.

131. Kilbourne EM et al: Risk factors in heatstroke, *JAMA* 247:3332, 1982.

132. Kirsch KA, Vonameln H, Wicke HJ: Fluid control mechanisms after exercise dehydration, *Eur J Appl Physiol* 47:191, 1981.

133. Knochel JP: Environmental heat illness. An eclectic review, *Arch Intern Med* 133:841, 1974.

134. Knochel JP: Dog days and siriasis. How to kill a football player, *JAMA* 233:513, 1975.

135. Knochel JP: Role of glucoregulatory hormones in potassium homeostasis, *Kidney Int* 11:443, 1977.

136. Knochel JP: Heat stroke and related heat stress disorders, *Dis Mon* 35:301, 1989.

137. Knochel JP: Catastrophic medical events with exhaustive exercise: "white collar rhabdomyolysis," *Kidney Int* 38:709, 1990.

138. Kost GJ: Planning and implementing point-of-care testing systems, In Tobin MJ, editor: *Principles and practice of intensive care monitoring*, New York, 1998, McGraw-Hill.

138a. Koratich M, Gaffin SL: Mechanism of calcium transport in human endothelial cells subjected to hyperthermia, *J Therm Biol* 24:245, 1999.

139. Kunstlinger U, Ludwig HG, Stegemann J: Metabolic changes during volleyball matches, *Int J Sports Med* 8:315, 1987.

140. Ladell WS: The effects of water and salt intake upon the performance of men working in hot and humid environments, *J Physiol* 127:11, 1995.

141. Larner AJ: Dantrolene for exertional heat stroke, *Lancet* 339:182, 1991.

142. Latzka WA et al: Hyperhydration: thermoregulatory effects during compensable exercise-heat stress, *J Appl Physiol* 83:860, 1997.

143. Latzka WA et al: Hyperhydration: tolerance and cardiovascular effects during uncompensable exercise-heat stress, *J Appl Physiol* 84:1858, 1999.

144. Leithead CS, Lind AR: *Heat stress and heat disorders*, Philadelphia, 1964, FA Davis.

145. Lopez JR et al: Myoplasmic Ca^{2+} concentration during exertional rhabdomyolysis, *Lancet* 345:424, 1995.

146. Lukaski HC, Bolonchuk WW, Klevay LM: Maximal oxygen consumption as related to magnesium, copper and zinc nutriture, *Am J Clin Nutr* 37:407, 1983.

147. Lundvall J: Tissue hyperosmolality as mediator of vasodilation and transcapillary fluid flux in exercising skeletal muscle, *Acta Physiol Scand* 379(suppl):1, 1972.

148. Lydiatt JS, Hill GE: Treatment of heat stroke with dantrolene, *JAMA* 246:41, 1981.

149. Lyons TP et al: Effects of glycerol-induced hyperhydration prior to exercise in the heat on sweating and T_c, *Med Sci Sports Exerc* 42:477, 1990.

150. Malamud N, Haymaker W, Custer RP: Heat stroke: a clinicopathologic study of 125 fatal cases, *Mil Surg* 99:397, 1946.

151. Manjoo M, Burger FJ, Kielblock AJ: A relationship between heat load and plasma enzyme concentration, *J Therm Biol* 10:221, 1985.

152. McLellan TM et al: Influence of hydration status on rectal temperature response and tolerance during uncompensable heat stress, *Can J Appl Physiol* 24:349, 1999.

153. Mehta AC: Persistent neurological deficits in heat stroke, *Neurology* 20:336, 1970.

154. Montain SJ, Latzka WA, Sawka MN: Control of thermoregulatory sweating is altered by hydration level and exercise intensity, *J Appl Physiol* 79:1434, 1995.

155. Montain SJ, Latzka WA, Sawka MN: Fluid replacement recommendations for training in hot weather, *Mil Med* 164:502, 1999.

156. Montain SJ et al: Physiological tolerance to uncompensable heat stress: effects of exercise intensity, protective clothing and climate, *J Appl Physiol* 77:216, 1994.

157. Montain SJ et al: Hypohydration effects on skeletal muscle performance and metabolism: a ^{31}P-MRS study, *J Appl Physiol* 84:1889, 1998.

158. Montain SJ et al: Thermal & cardiovascular strain from hypohydration: influence of exercise intensity, *Int J Sports Med* 19:87, 1998.

159. Moran DS, Epstein Y, Shapiro Y: Biochemical profile changes during exertional heat stroke. In Hodgdon JA, Heany JH, Buono MJ, editors: *Environmental Ergonomics VIII*, San Diego, 1999.

160. Moran DS et al: Can gender differences during exercise-heat stress be assessed by the physiological strain index? *Am J Physiol* 275:R1789, 1999.

161. Moran DS, Montain SJ, Pandolf KB: Evaluation of different levels of hydration using a new physiological strain index (PSI), *Am J Physiol* 275:R854, 1998.

162. Moran DS, Pandolf KB: Wet Bulb Globe Temperature (WBGT)—to what extent is GT essential? *Aviat Space Environ Med* 70:480, 1999.

163. Moran DS, Shitzer A, Pandolf KB: A physiological strain index to evaluate heat stress, *Am J Physiol* 275(RICP):R129, 1998.

164. Moran DS et al: Dantrolene and recovery from heat stroke, *Aviat Space Environ Med* 70:987, 1999.

165. Moran DS et al: The physiological strain index applied for heat-stressed rats, *J Appl Physiol* 86:895, 1999.

166. Morimoto T: Restitution of body fluid after thermal dehydration. In Hales JRS, Richards D, editors: *Heat stress: physical exertion and environment*, New York, 1987, Elsevier.

167. Moroff SV, Bass DE: Effects of overhydration on man's physiological responses to work in the heat, *J Appl Physiol* 20:267, 1965.

168. Mostellar ME, Tuttle EP: Effects of alkalosis on plasma concentration and urinary excretion of inorganic phosphate in man, *J Clin Invest* 43:138, 1964.

169. Mudambo SMKT, Leese GP, Rennie MJ: Dehydration in soldiers during walking/running exercise in the heat and the effects of fluid ingestion during and after exercise, *Eur J Appl Physiol* 76:517, 1997.

170. Murray R: The effects of consuming carbohydrate-electrolyte beverages on gastric emptying and fluid absorption during and following exercise, *Sports Med* 4:322, 1987.

171. Murray R: Rehydration strategies—balancing substrate, fluid, and electrolyte provision, *Int J Sports Med* 19(suppl 2):S133, 1998.

172. Mustafa MK, Khogali M, Gumaa K: Respiratory pathophysiology in heat stroke. In Khogali M, Hales JRS, editors: *Heat stroke and temperature regulation*, Sydney, Australia, 1983, Academic Press.

173. Nadel ER: Circulatory and thermal regulations during exercise, *Fed Proc* 39:1491, 1980.

174. Nadel ER, Fortney SM, Wenger CB: Effect of hydration on circulatory and thermal regulation, *J Appl Physiol* 49:715, 1980.

175. Nemeth ZH et al: Calcium channel blockers and dantrolene differentially regulate the production of interleukin-12 and interferon-gamma in endotoxemic mice, *Brain Res Bull* 46:257, 1998.

176. Nielsen B et al: Thermoregulation in exercising man during dehydration and hyperhydration with water and saline, *Int J Biometeorol* 15:195, 1971.

177. Noakes TD, Goodwin G, Rayner BL: Water intoxication: a possible complication during endurance exercise, *Med Sci Sports Exerc* 17:370, 1985.

178. Noakes TD et al: The incidence of hyponatremia during prolonged ultraendurance exercise, *Med Sci Sports Exerc* 22:165, 1990.

179. O'Donnell TF: Medical problems of recruit training: a research approach, *US Navy Med* 58:28, 1971.

180. O'Donnell TF, Clowes GHA: The circulatory abnormalities of heatstroke, *N Engl J Med* 287:734, 1972.

181. Parnell CJ, Restall J: Heat stroke: a fatal case, *Arch Emerg Med* 3:111, 1986.

182. Pattison ME et al: Exertional heatstroke and acute renal failure in young women, *Am J Kidney Dis* 11:184, 1983.

183. Pettigrew RT et al: Circulatory and biochemical effects of whole body hyperthermia, *Br J Surg* 61:727, 1974.

183a. Pivarnik JM et al: Menstrual cycle phase affects temperature regulation during endurance exercise, *J Appl Physiol* 72:543, 1992.

184. Portel L et al: Malignant hyperthermia and neuroleptic malignant syndrome in a patient during treatment for acute asthma, *Acta Anaesthesiol Scand* 43:107, 1999.

185. Rajan SF, Robinson GH, Borwer JD: The pathogenesis of acute renal failure in heatstroke, *South Med J* 66:330, 1973.

186. Refsum HE, Meen HD, Stromme SB: Changes in plasma amino acid distribution and urine amino acids excretion during prolonged heavy exercise, *Scand J Clin Lab Invest* 39:407, 1979.

187. Richards D, Richards R, Schofield J: Management of heat exhaustion in Sydney's *The Sun* City-to-Surf fun runners, *Med J Aust* 2:457, 1979.

188. Reference deleted in proofs.

189. Robinson S, Robinson AH: Chemical composition of sweat, *Physiol Rev* 34:202, 1954.

190. Rose LI et al: Serum electrolyte changes after marathon running, *J Appl Physiol* 29:449, 1970.

191. Royburt M et al: Long term psychological and physiological effects of heatstroke, *Physiol Behav* 54:265, 1999.

192. Saltin B: Aerobic and anaerobic work capacity after dehydration, *J Appl Physiol* 19:1114, 1964.

193. Saltin B: Circulatory response to submaximal and maximal exercise after thermal dehydration, *J Appl Physiol* 19:1125, 1964.

194. Sawka MN, Montain SJ, Latzka WA: Body fluid balance during exercise-heat exposure. In Buskirk ER, Puhl SM, editors: *Body fluid balance: exercise and sport,* Boca Raton, 1996, CRC Press.

195. Sawka MN, Pandolf KB: Effects of body water loss on physiological function and exercise performance. In Gisolfi CV, Lamb DR, editors: *Fluid homeostasis during exercise,* Carmel, Calif, 1990, Benchmark Press.

196. Sawka MN, Wenger CB: Physiological responses to acute exercise heat stress In Pandolf KB, Sawka MN, Gonzalez RR, editors: *Human performance physiology and environmental medicine at terrestrial extremes,* Indianapolis, 1988, Benchmark Press.

197. Sawka MN, Wenger CB, Pandolf KB: Thermoregulatory responses to acute exercise-heat stress and heat acclimation. In Fregly MJ, Blatteis CM, editors: *Handbook of physiology: environmental physiology,* Bethesda, Md, 1996, American Physiological Society.

198. Reference deleted in proofs.

199. Sawka MN, Young AJ, Latzka WA: Human tolerance to heat strain during exercise: influence of hydration, *J Appl Physiol* 73:368, 1992.

200. Sawka MN et al: Influence of hydration level and body fluids on exercise performance in the heat, *JAMA* 252:1165, 1984.

201. Sawka MN et al: Thermoregulatory and blood responses during exercise at graded hypohydration levels, *J Appl Physiol* 59:1394, 1985.

202. Schrier RW et al: Renal metabolic and circulatory responses to heat and exercise, *Ann Intern Med* 73:213, 1970.

203. Seiple RS et al: Gastric-emptying characteristics of two glucose polymer-electrolyte solutions, *Med Sci Sports Exerc* 15:366, 1983.

204. Senay LC Jr, Kok R: Effects of training and heat acclimatization on blood plasma contents of exercising men, *J Appl Physiol* 43:591, 1977.

205. Shapiro Y, Cristal N: Hyperthermia and heat stroke: effects on acid-base balance, blood electrolytes and hepato-renal function. In Hales JRS, Richards D, editors: *Heat stress: physical exertion and environment,* New York, 1987, Elsevier.

206. Shapiro Y, Moran DS: Heat stroke: a consequence of mal-adaptation to heat-exercise exposure. In Pandolf KB, Takeda N, Singal PK, editors: *Adaptation biology and medicine: molecular basis,* New Delhi, India, 1999, Narosa Publishing House.

207. Shapiro Y, Moran DS: How significant is magnesium in thermoregulation? *J Basic Clin Physiol Pharmacol* 9:73, 1999.

208. Shapiro Y, Pandolf KB, Goldman RF: Predicting sweat loss responses to exercise, environment and clothing, *Eur J Appl Physiol* 48:83, 1982.

209. Shapiro Y, Rosenthal T, Sohar E: Experimental heatstroke, *Arch Intern Med* 131:688, 1973.

210. Shapiro Y, Seidman DS: Field and clinical observations of exertional heat stroke patients, *Med Sci Sports Exerc* 22:6, 1990.

211. Shapiro Y et al: Physiological responses of men and women to humid and dry heat, *J Appl Physiol* 49:1, 1980.

212. Shephard JR, Leatt P: Carbohydrate and fluid of the soccer player, *Sports Med* 4:164, 1987.

213. Shibolet S: The clinical picture of heat stroke. In *Proceedings of the Tel HaShomer Hospital,* Tel Aviv, Israel, 1962, Tel Aviv University.

214. Shibolet S, Lancaster MC, Danon Y: Heatstroke: a review, *Aviat Space Environ Med* 47:280, 1976.

215. Shibolet S et al: Fibrinolysis and hemorrhages in fatal heatstroke, *N Engl J Med* 266:169, 1962.

216. Shibolet S et al: Heatstroke: its clinical picture and mechanism in 36 cases, *Q J Med* 36:525, 1967.

217. Shirreffs SM, Maughan RJ: Urine osmolality and conductivity as indices of hydration status in athletes in the heat, *Med Sci Sports Exerc* 30:1598, 1998.

218. Silva NL, Boulant JA: Effects of osmotic pressure glucose and temperature on neurons in preoptic tissue slices, *Am J Physiol* 247:R335, 1984.

219. Slovis CM: Features and outcomes of classic heat stroke, *Ann Intern Med* 130:614, 1999.

220. Smith L et al: Unrecognized exertional heat illness as a risk factor for exercise-related sudden cardiac death among young adults, *J Am Coll Cardiol* 29(suppl A):447, 1997.

221. Sohol RS: Heatstroke: an electron microscopic study of endothelial cell damage and disseminated intravascular coagulation, *Arch Intern Med* 122:43, 1968.

222. Sprung CL et al: The metabolic and respiratory alterations of heatstroke, *Arch Intern Med* 140:665, 1980.

223. Stine RJ: Heat illness, *JACEP* 8:154, 1979.

223a. Stephenson LA, Kolka MA: Thermoregulation in women. In Holloszy JO, editor: *Exercise and sport sciences reviews,* Baltimore, 1993, Williams & Wilkins.

224. Strazis KP, Fox AW: Malignant hyperthermia: a review of published cases, *Anesth Analg* 77:297, 1993.

225. Strydom NB et al: Physiological performance of men subjected to different water regimes over a two-day period, *S Afr Med J Suppl S Afr J Lab Clin Med,* p 92, Feb 3, 1968.

226. Sutton JR: Heatstroke from running, *JAMA* 243:1896, 1980.

227. Tankersley CG et al: Hypohydration affects forearm vascular conductance independent of HR during exercise, *J Appl Physiol* 73:1232, 1999.

228. Tayeb OS, Marzouki LN: Effect of dantrolene for treatment on heatstroke in sheep, *Pharm Res* 22:565, 1990.

229. Taylor NAS: Eccrine sweat glands: adaptations to physical training and heat acclimation, *Sports Med* 3:387, 1986.

230. Torranin C, Smith DP, Byrd RJ: The effect of acute thermal dehydration and rapid rehydration on isometric and isotonic endurance, *J Sports Med Phys Fitness* 19:1, 1979.

231. Vernon WB, Wacker WEC: Magnesium metabolism. In *Recent advances in clinical biochemistry,* New York, 1978, Churchill Livingstone.

232. Vertel RM, Knochel JP: Acute renal failure due to heat injury: an analysis of 10 cases associated with a high incidence of myoglobinuria, *Am J Med* 43:435, 1967.

233. Vescia FG, Peck OC: Liver disease from heatstroke, *Gastroenterology* 43:340, 1962.

234. Vidair CA, Dewey WC: Evaluation of a role for intracellular Na^+, K^+ Ca^{2+}, and Mg^{2+} in hyperthermic cell killing, *Radiat Res* 105:187, 1986.

235. Viitasalo JT et al: Effects of rapid weight reduction of force production and vertical jumping height, *Int J Sports Med* 8:281, 1987.

236. Ward A, Chaffman MO, Sorkin EM: Dantrolene: a review of its pharmacodynamic and pharmacokinetic properties and therapeutic use in malignant hyperthermia, the neuroleptic malignant syndrome and an update of its use in muscle spasticity, *Drugs* 32:130, 1986.

237. Webster S, Rutt R, Weltman A: Physiological effects of a weight loss regimen practiced by college wrestlers, *Med Sci Sports Exerc* 22:229, 1990.

238. Weiner IM, Mudge LH: Diuretics and other agents employed in the mobilization of edema fluid. In Gilman A et al, editors: *The pharmacological basis of therapeutics,* New York, 1985, Macmillan.

239. Weiner JS, Khogali M: A physiological body-cooling unit for treatment of heatstroke, *Lancet* 1:507, 1980.

240. Wheeler KB, Banwell JG: Intestinal water and electrolyte flux of glucose-polymer electrolyte solutions, *Med Sci Sports Exerc* 18:436, 1986.

241. White J, Ford MA: The hydration and electrolyte maintenance properties of an experimental sports drink, *Br J Sports Med* 17:51, 1983.

242. Yaqub BA: Neurologic manifestations of heatstroke at the Meccah pilgrimage, *Neurology* 37:1004, 1987.

243. Yaqub BA et al: Heat stroke at the Mekkah pilgrimage: clinical characteristics and course of 30 patients, *Q J Med* 59:523, 1986.

244. Yi PN et al: Hyperthermia-induced intracellular ionic level changes in tumor cells, *Radiat Res* 93:534, 1983.

245. Zuckerman GB et al: Effects of dantrolene on cooling times and cardiovascular parameters in an immature porcine model of heatstroke, *Crit Care Med* 25:135, 1997.

Fire, Burns, and Radiation

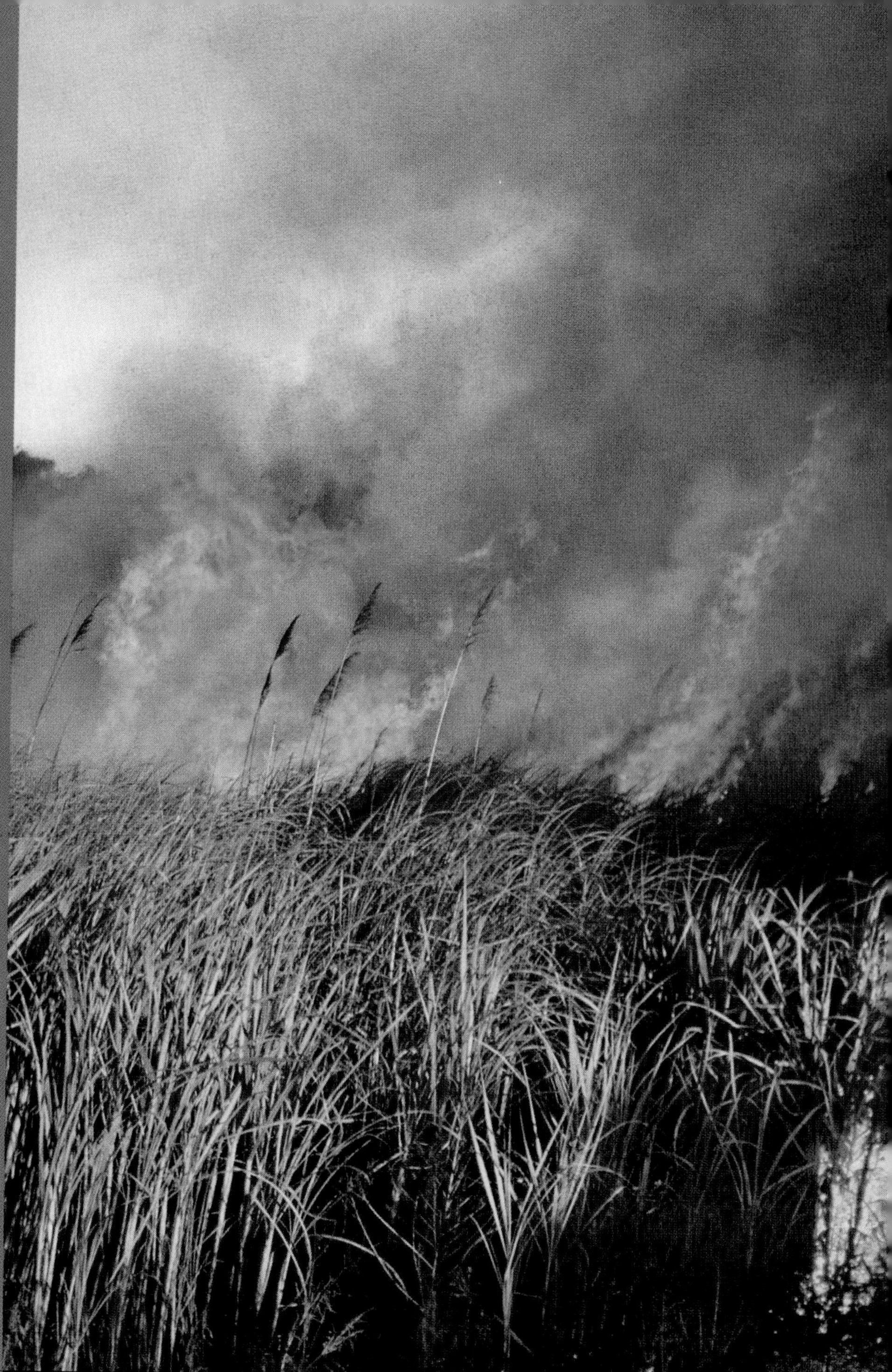

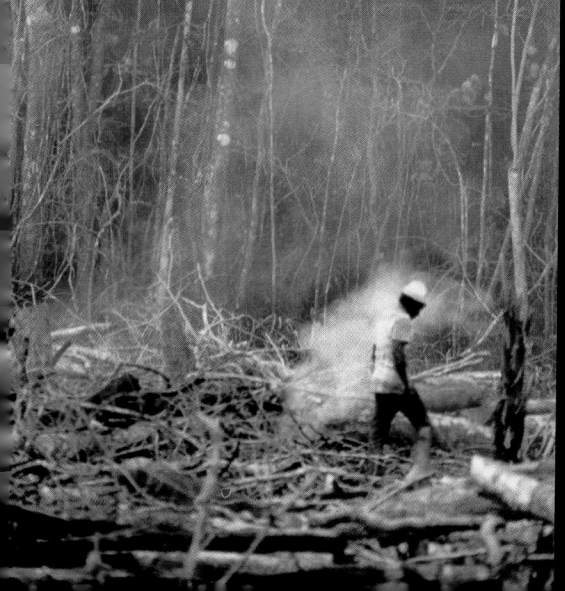

3

12 Wildland Fires: Dangers and Survival

Kathleen Mary Davis and Robert W. Mutch

It is hard to know what to do with all the detail that rises out of fire. It rises out of a fire as thick as smoke and threatens to blot out everything. Some of it is true but doesn't make any difference. Some of it is just plain wrong. And some doesn't even exist, except in your mind, as you slowly discover long afterwards. Some of it, though, is true—and makes all the difference.

Norman Maclean, *Young Men and Fire*, 1992

Describing the 13 fatalities in the Mann Gulch fire near Helena, Montana, in 1949, Norman Maclean wrote, "They were still so young they hadn't learned to count the odds and to sense they might owe the universe a tragedy." The Mann Gulch fire has been called "the race that couldn't be won."[27] Although the crew increased their pace ahead of the fire, the fire accelerated faster than they did until fire and people converged at the end of a race the firefighters could not win. Miraculously, three persons survived the fire. The foreman ignited an escape fire into which he tried to move the crew; two of the smoke jumpers found a route to safety. Many improvements in a person's odds of surviving an encounter with a wildland fire have occurred since 1949. These advances include improved understanding of fire behavior, increased emphasis on fire safety and fire training, and development of personal protective equipment. However, as events such as the Colorado fires of 1994 showed, tragedies continue to occur.

Whether the Mann Gulch fire, the 1871 Peshtigo fire in Wisconsin that killed 1150 people, the Great Idaho fire of 1910 that left 85 dead (Figure 12-1), the 1947 Maine fires that produced 16 victims, or the 1991 Oakland fire that killed 25 people, wildland fires are as much a threat to human life, property, and natural resources on the North American continent as are hurricanes, tornadoes, floods, and earthquakes. This chapter describes the current look of this historical force and discusses new federal fire management policies, the nature and scope of wildland fire hazards, behavior of fires, typical injuries, summary of fatalities (1990-1998), and survival techniques.

WILDLAND FIRE MANAGEMENT AND TECHNOLOGY

Programs for dealing with the overall spectrum of fire are collectively termed *fire management*.[1] They are based on the concept that fire and the complex interrelated factors that influence fire phenomena can and should be managed. The scientifically sound fire management programs that respond to the needs of people and natural environments must also maintain full respect for the power of fire.[1]

Since the early 1900s, federal, state, and local fire protection agencies have routinely extinguished wildland fires to protect watershed, range, and timber values, as well as human lives and property. Fire detection, fire danger rating systems, and fire suppression methods have been developed by fire science laboratories and two equipment development centers maintained by the U.S. Department of Agriculture (USDA) Forest Service. Patrol planes, some with infrared heat scanners, and other aircraft can deliver firefighters, equipment, and fire-retarding chemicals to the most remote fire. These firefighting resources are organized under an Incident Command System that can easily manage simple to complex operational, logistical, planning, and fiscal functions associated with wildfire suppression actions.[3]

Modern fire suppression technology, however, cannot indefinitely reduce the number of hectares burned, as demonstrated by several large fires in recent years: the Greater Yellowstone Area fires in 1988; Mack Lake fire in Michigan in 1980; Foothills fire near Boise, Idaho, in 1992; Silver Complex in Oregon in 1987; and Stanislaus Complex in California in 1989. The hard lesson learned from these fires and others is that wildfires are inevitable. Several factors have coincided to produce massive forest mortality, including drought, epidemic levels of insects and diseases,[21] and unnatural accumulations of fuels as a result of fire exclusion. Many agencies are now using prescribed fire more frequently, deliberately burning under predetermined conditions to reduce accumulations of fuels and to protect human life and property.

Research has indicated that fires are not categorically bad. In fact, many plant communities in North America are highly flammable during certain periods in their life cycles. For example, annual grasses, ponderosa pine, and chaparral plant communities are flammable almost every dry season. Other communities, such as jack pine or lodgepole pine forests, although fire resistant during much of their life cycle, eventually become fire prone when killed by insects, diseases, and other natural causes. The spread of nonnative grasses, such as cheatgrass and red brome, in the arid West has increased the frequency of fires in desert shrublands.

Wildland fires can benefit plant and animal communities. Evolutionary development produces plant species

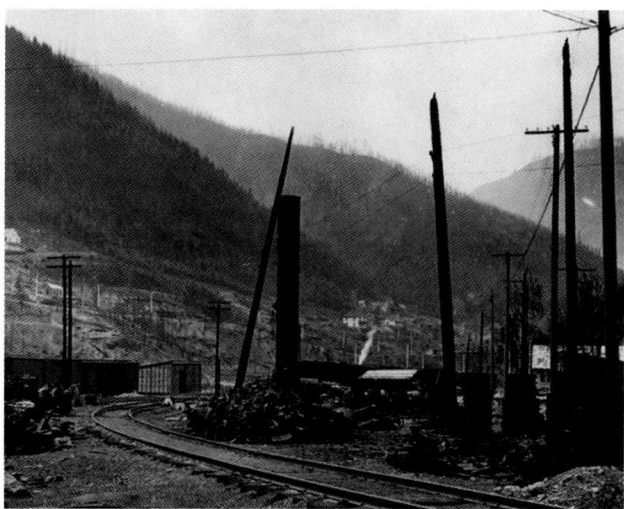

Figure 12-1 Burned ruins of the foundry in Wallace, Idaho, furnish mute testimony to the destructive force of the 1910 fires. The cottage on the terrace was the only one left standing in that part of town. *(Courtesy the USDA Forest Service. Photo by R.H. McKay.)*

well adapted to recurrent fires. Fire tends to recycle ecosystems and maintain diversity.[15] Thus there is growing consensus that fire should be returned to wildland ecosystems where appropriate to perpetuate desirable fire-adapted plant and animal communities and to reduce fuel accumulations.

A landmark report in 1963 to the National Park Service by the Advisory Board on Wildlife Management[14] described how the western slope of the Sierra Nevada had been transformed by fire protection:

When the forty-niners poured over the Sierra Nevada into California, those that kept diaries spoke almost to a man of the wide-spaced columns of mature trees that grew on the lower western slope in gigantic magnificence. Today much of the west slope is a dog-hair thicket of young pines, white fir, incense-cedar, and mature brush—a direct function of overprotection from natural ground fires. Not only is this accumulation of fuel dangerous to the giant sequoias and other mature trees, but the animal life is meager, wildflowers are sparse, and, to some at least, the vegetative tangle is depressing, not uplifting.

The board recommended that the Park Service recognize in management programs the importance of the natural role of fire in shaping plant communities.

Federal Wildland Fire Management Policy

Recent tragedies in the West focused attention on the need to reduce hazardous fuel accumulations. The events of 1994 created a renewed awareness and concern among federal land management agencies about wildfire impacts, leading to a combined review of fire policies and programs. The result was the enactment of a new interagency federal wildland fire management policy, which provided a common approach to wildland fire among federal agencies and called for close cooperation with tribal, state, and other jurisdictions.[37] The principal points of the new federal wildland fire policies are as follows:

1. Firefighter and public safety remains the first priority in wildland fire management. Protection of natural and cultural resources and property is the second priority.
2. Wildland fire, as a critical natural process, must be reintroduced into the ecosystem, accomplished across agency boundaries, and based on the best available science.
3. Where wildland fire cannot be safely reintroduced because of hazardous fuel accumulations, pretreatment must be considered, particularly in the wildland-urban interface.
4. Wildland fire management decisions and resource management decisions are connected and based on approved plans. Agencies must be able to choose from the full spectrum of actions—from prompt suppression to allowing fire to have an ecologic function.
5. All aspects of wildland fire management will involve all partners and have compatible programs, activities, and processes.
6. The role of federal agencies in the wildland-urban interface includes firefighting, hazardous fuel reduction, cooperative prevention and education, and technical assistance. Ultimately, the primary responsibility rests at the state and local levels.
7. Structural fire protection in the wildland-urban interface is the responsibility of tribal, state, and local governments.
8. Federal agencies must better educate internal and external audiences about how and why we use and manage wildland fire.

Prescribed Fire and Fire Use

Prescribed fire, the intentional ignition of grass, shrub, or forest fuels for specific purposes according to predetermined conditions, is a recognized land management practice. The objectives of such burning vary: to reduce fire hazards after logging, expose mineral soil for seedbeds, regulate insects and diseases, perpetuate natural ecosystems, and improve range forage and wildlife habitat. In some areas managed by the National Park Service, USDA Forest Service, and Bureau of Land Management, naturally ignited fires may be allowed to burn according to approved prescriptions; fire management areas have been established in national parks and wildernesses from the Florida Everglades to the Sierra Nevada in California (Figure 12-2). Visitors are increasingly aware that wildland fires can provide an important environment for the enjoyment of park and wilderness experiences.

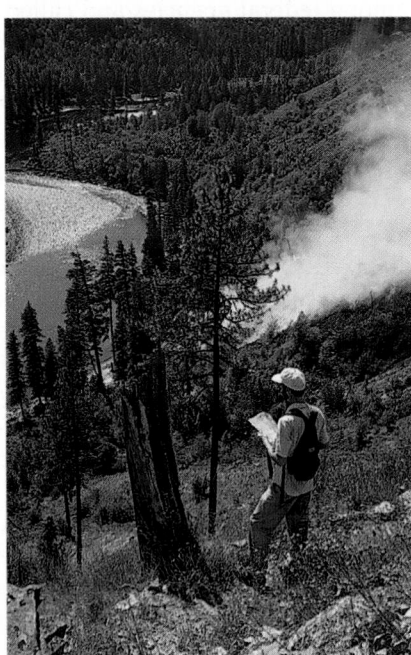

Figure 12-2 Some lightning fires in wildernesses and national parks are now allowed to burn under observation to perpetuate natural ecosystems. *(Courtesy the USDA Forest Service.)*

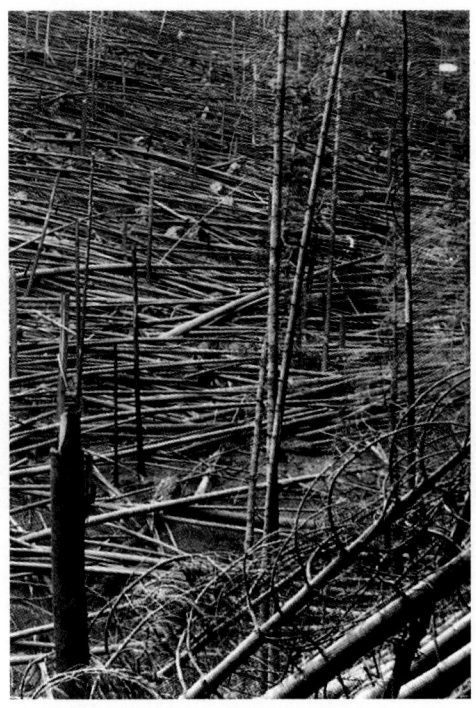

Figure 12-3 These burned-over and wind-thrown trees resulted from the intense behavior of the 1910 forest fire near Falcon, Idaho. *(Courtesy the USDA Forest Service. Photo by J.B. Halm.)*

WILDLAND-URBAN INTERFACE: NEW LOOK OF A HISTORICAL PROBLEM

Just as resource agencies are attempting to provide a more natural role for fire in wildland ecosystems, the general public is increasingly living and seeking recreation in many of these areas. However, past fire exclusion practices have allowed abnormal fuel accumulations, and this fact has combined with the sacrifice of relatively safe perimeter fire suppression strategies in favor of directly protecting people and their possessions.[42] Direct suppression actions *within* the fire's perimeter place firefighters at a greater disadvantage from a safety standpoint. The new interagency policy that emphasizes firefighter and public safety as the first priority will result in less effort to save structures in dangerous situations. What is known of fire behavior and fire survival principles must be readily available to emergency medical personnel, wildland dwellers, and recreationists. In fact, fire protection agencies have been making such information more available to the general public.

Nature of the Problem

Hot, dry, windy conditions annually produce high-intensity fires that threaten or burn homes where wildland and urban areas converge. Can the historical levels of destruction, injury, and fatality be repeated today in the face of modern fire suppression technology? The answer requires an analysis of the conditions that created high-intensity fire behavior in the forests of Idaho and Montana in 1910 (Figure 12-3). The Peshtigo, Michigan, Hinckley, Yacoult, and Maine fires burned hundreds of thousands of hectares and killed more than 2000 people between 1871 and 1947.

On October 8, 1871, the same day that fire wiped out the town of Peshtigo, Wisconsin, the great Chicago fire devastated urban Chicago. Comparative statistics for those two fires highlight the destructive potential of wildland fires. The Peshtigo fire covered 518,016 hectares (1,280,000 acres) and killed 1150 people, whereas 860 hectares (2124 acres) burned and 300 lives were lost as a result of the Chicago fire.[41] The 1910 wildland fires had several common elements: many uncontrolled fires burning at one time; prolonged drought, high temperatures, and moderate to strong winds; and mixed conifer and hardwood fuels with slash from logging and land clearing. These large fires occurred primarily in conifer forests north of the 42nd meridian, or roughly across the northern quarter of the contiguous United States.[2] One of these critical elements that is not as likely to occur today as formerly is the simultaneous presence of many uncontrolled fires. The effectiveness of modern fire suppression organizations reaches the most remote wildland locations. High-velocity winds and more than 1600 individual fires contributed to the spread of the 1910 fires; it is unlikely that a multifire situation of that magnitude would occur today. Prolonged drought, high winds, and flammable fuel types, however, remain significant to the behavior of high-intensity fires.

Some of the fires most potentially damaging to human lives and property occur in areas rich in chaparral shrub fuel in California. Wilson[42] described the severe 1970 fire year in California, in which official estimates showed that 97% of 1260 fires occurring between September 15 and November 15 were held to less than 121 hectares (300 acres). The other 3% of the fires, fueled by a prolonged drought and fanned by strong Santa Ana winds, produced 14 deaths, destroyed 885 homes, and burned more than 242,820 hectares (600,000 acres). Ten years later the situation recurred over 28,330 hectares (70,000 acres) in southern California, resulting in the deaths of 5 persons and loss of more than 400 structures.

More recently, on October 20, 1992, a devastating fire occurred in the hills above Oakland and Berkeley, California. Burning embers carried by high winds from the perimeter of a small fire resulted in a major wildland-urban interface conflagration that killed 25 people, including a police officer and a firefighter, injured 150 others, destroyed nearly 2449 single-family dwellings and 437 apartment and condominium units, burned over 648 hectares (1600 acres), and did an estimated $1.5 billion in damage.[23] The scenario for disaster included a 5-year drought that had dried out overgrown grass, shrubs, and trees, making them readily ignitable. Other factors included untreated wood shingles, unprotected wooden decks that projected out over steep terrain, low relative humidity, high temperatures, and strong winds that averaged 32 km per hour (20 mph) and gusted up to 56 to 80 km per hour (35 to 50 mph). These severe conditions produced a voracious fire that consumed 790 homes in the first hour. Winds lessened to 8 km per hour (5 mph) by the first evening, and firefighters had the situation under control by the fourth day, but not before they had an awful glimpse of what future fires will be.

Wildland fires that threaten human lives and property are not exclusively located in southern California, since the exodus to wildland regions has become a national phenomenon. Fires burned more than 80,940 hectares (200,000 acres) in Maine in October 1947, killing 16 people; another 80,940 hectares (200,000 acres) burned in New Jersey in 1963. On July 16, 1977, the Pattee Canyon fire in Missoula, Montana, destroyed 6 homes and charred 486 hectares (1200 acres) of forests and grasslands in only a few hours.[7] Fires at the wildland-urban interface also have increased internationally. For example, the Ash Wednesday fire disaster in 1983 burned more than 340,000 hectares (840,000 acres) of urban, forested, and pastoral lands in Victoria and South Australia, killing 77

persons, injuring 3500 persons, and destroying 2528 homes.[36] A May 1987 wildfire in northern China added a new perspective regarding the devastating impact wildland fires may have on human lives, property, and natural resources. This fire reportedly burned over 404,700 hectares (1 million acres), killed almost 200 persons, seriously injured another 200, destroyed or damaged 12,000 houses, and forced nearly 60,000 people to evacuate their homes—clearly it was a disaster of major proportions. Protecting lives and property from wildfires at the wildland-urban interface presents one of the greatest challenges faced by wildfire protection agencies.

Large forest fires around the world during the intense El Niño drought conditions of 1997-1998 focused public and media attention once again on the need to evaluate public policies and practices in the forestry and nonforestry sectors that directly or indirectly contribute to the impact of forest fires. The size and damage attributed to these fires was so immense that the *Christian Science Monitor* termed 1998 "the Year the Earth Caught Fire." At times that seemed to be literally true as smoke palls blanketed large regional areas, disrupting air and sea navigation and causing serious public health threats. Seventy people were killed in Mexico alone as a result of the fires, and ecosystems that generally are not subjected to fires, such as the Amazon rain forest and the cloud forest of Chiapas, Mexico, sustained considerable damage. A global fire conference sponsored by the Food and Agricultural Organization of the United Nations (October 1998) brought together specialists from 33 countries to review the serious nature of worldwide fires. Participants at the conference in Rome concluded that governments needed to enact more sustainable land use policies and practices to reduce the impacts of wildfires on people and natural resources. More recently, as of the end of September, 2000, nearly 7 million acres had been scorched by approximately 80,000 fires in the United States.

It is becoming increasingly rare to have a wildland fire situation that does not involve people. However, people are not fully aware of the fire risks and hazards of living and traveling in or near wildlands. *Risk*, in the jargon of the wildland fire specialist, is the probability that a fire will occur. *Hazard* is the likelihood that a fire, once started, will cause unwanted results. Risk deals with causative agents; hazard deals with the fuel complex.[9] The results of two surveys indicated a general feeling of overconfidence by most residents toward the potential danger of forest fire. Eighty percent of Seeley Lake, Montana forest residents who were interviewed thought that the forest fire hazard was low to moderate in their area.[8] Seventy-five percent of Colorado residents interviewed thought that the forest fire hazard was low or moderate in mountain subdivisions of their state.[13] Forest fire hazards in these two areas were much

Box 12-1   RECOMMENDATIONS TO REDUCE LOSS OF LIFE AND PROPERTY IN THE WILDLAND-URBAN INTERFACE

FIRE PROTECTION SERVICES

Remember that firefighter and public safety is the first priority in every fire management activity.

Ensure that all personnel receive regular cross-training in fighting wildfires and structural fires.

In urban departments, in particular, recognize the need to extinguish fires in wildland fuels by using thorough mop-up procedures.

Recognize the need for close coordination of response efforts among neighboring departments or agencies.

Develop specific mutual aid plans for coordinating resources to attack fires in the wildland-urban interface.

Schedule and conduct regular mutual aid training exercises.

Regularly schedule and conduct fire prevention and fire preparedness education programs for the general public and homeowners.

Conduct an assessment of fire risks and prepare a strategic plan to reduce these risks.

Work effectively with lawmakers and other government officials to help prevent unsafe residential and business development.

LEGISLATORS

Examine existing laws, regulations, and standards of other jurisdictions that are applicable for local use in mitigating hazards associated with wildland fires.

Adopt National Fire Protection Association Standard 299 for the Protection of Life and Property from Wildfire. (The purpose of this standard is to provide criteria for fire agencies, land use planners, architects, developers, and local government for fire-safe development in areas that may be threatened by wildfire.)

LEGISLATORS—cont'd

Provide strong building regulations that restrict untreated wood shingle roofs and other practices known to decrease the fire safety of a structure in the wildlands.

PLANNERS AND DEVELOPERS

Create a map of potential problem areas based on fuel type and known fire behavior.

Evaluate all existing or planned housing developments to determine relative wildland fire protection ratings and advise property owners of conditions and responsibilities.

Ensure that all developments have more than one ingress-egress route.

Offer options for fire-safe buildings.

Provide appropriate fuel breaks or green belts in developments.

Ensure that adequate water supplies exist in developments.

Follow specifications in NFPA Standard 299 for the Protection of Life and Property from Wildfire.

PUBLIC AND HOMEOWNERS

Determine the wildfire hazard potential of the immediate area before buying or moving into any home.

Contact federal, state, and local fire services for educational programs and materials regarding fire protection.

Provide a defensible space around structures to help protect them.

Design and build nonflammable homes.

Urge lawmakers to respond with legislative assistance to require appropriate fire safety measures for communities.

---

higher than the public estimates. There is a growing need for the general public, emergency medical personnel, and fire suppression organizations to be well prepared to deal with wildland fire encounters (Box 12-1).

Wildland Lessons

Recommendations to reduce the loss of life and property in the wildland-urban interface will be useless unless they are implemented at the grassroots level by all stakeholders. An excellent example of a community-based program is one implemented at Incline Village and Crystal Bay in the Lake Tahoe basin.[32] The objective of this program is to "reduce the potential for natural resource, property, and human life losses due to wildfire by empowering the communities' residents with the knowledge to address the hazard, providing the resources necessary to correct the problem, and encouraging the

cooperative efforts of appropriate agencies." The three major components of this defensible-space program include neighborhood leader volunteers, a slash removal project, and agency coordination. The key to protecting life and property in the wildland-urban interface is property owners' realization that they have a serious problem and that their actions embody a significant part of the solution. In the Incline Village/Crystal Bay Plan, neighborhood leader volunteers are trained in defensible-space techniques and are expected to teach these techniques to their neighbors and to coordinate neighborhood efforts. Such concerted community action will greatly minimize the threats from Oakland-type "fires of the future."

It is also wise to have sensible land development practices, since tragedies arise not only from ignorance of fuels and fire behavior but also from a greater concern for the esthetics of a homesite than for fire safety. Several aspects of development detract from fire safety in the wildland-urban interface[6,7]:

1. Lack of access to adequate water sources
2. Firewood stacked next to houses
3. Slash (i.e., branches, stumps, logs, and other vegetative residues) piled on homesites or along access roads
4. Structures built on slopes with unenclosed stilt foundations
5. Trees and shrubs growing next to structures, under eaves, and among stilt foundations
6. Roads that are steep, narrow, winding, unmapped, unsigned, unnamed, and bordered by slash or dense vegetation that makes them impossible to drive on during a fire
7. Subdivisions on sites without two or more access roads for simultaneous ingress and egress
8. Roads and bridges without the grade, design, and width to permit simultaneous evacuation by residents and access by firefighters, emergency medical personnel, and equipment
9. Excessive slopes, heavy fuels, structures built in box canyons, and other hazardous situations
10. Lack of fuel breaks around homesites and in subdivisions
11. Living fuels that have not been modified by thinning, landscaping, or other methods to reduce vegetation and litter that contribute to fire intensity
12. Homes constructed with flammable building materials (wooden shakes, shingles)

FIRE BEHAVIOR

Urban and Wildland Fire Threats

Safety precautions for wildland firefighting crews are continually upgraded as new knowledge is gained about fire behavior. Fire sites where people were injured or killed are visited afterward to assess fuel conditions, terrain features, probable wind movements at the time of the fire, and actions of firefighters (Figure 12-4). This information, as well as data about hazards in the wildland-urban interface, is not included in training programs and safety briefings.

In reviewing fire tragedies, a sobering observation is that crew members are almost always experienced and well-equipped firefighters, trained to anticipate "blowup" fire conditions. However, when visibility is lowered to 6 m (20 feet), noise levels preclude voice communication, eyes fill with tears, and wind blows debris in all directions, a person's judgment is badly impaired. Previous training can give way to panic, leading to decisions that result in serious injury or death. This scenario is most evident in urban fires; the pattern of hysteria affecting persons trapped in burn-

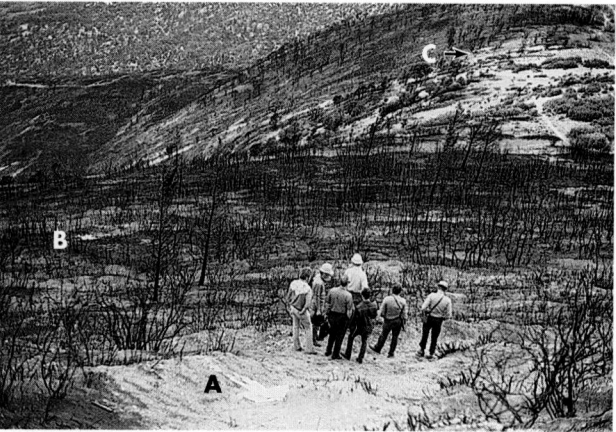

Figure 12-4 In an attempt to avoid the intense heat of this brush fire in southwestern Colorado, four firefighters took refuge in the fireline, in the foreground at point A. Affected by intense convective and radiant heat and dense smoke, one individual ran into the fire and died at point B. Another individual ran approximately 1000 feet down the ridge, where his body was found at point C. The third fatality was a person who remained at point A; he died a short time after this position was overrun by fire. The only survivor also remained in a prone position at point A with his face pressed to the ground. At one point he reached back and threw dirt on his burning pants legs. The survivor sustained severe burns to the back of his legs, buttocks, and arms. The deaths of the other three individuals were attributed to asphyxiation. *(Courtesy the USDA Forest Service.)*

ing buildings is familiar to fire chiefs. The way fire kills in the urban setting can be compared with wildland fires, as shown here[24]:

Heat rises rapidly to upper stories when a fire starts in the basement or on the ground floor. Toxic gases and smoke rise to the ceiling and work their way down to the victim—a vital lesson for families planning protective measures. Smoke poses the double problem of obscuring exit routes and contributing to pulmonary injury and oxygen deprivation.

As the fire consumes oxygen, the ambient oxygen content drops, impairing neuromuscular activity. When the oxygen content drops below 16%, death by asphyxiation will ensue unless the victim is promptly evacuated. Asphyxiation, not fire itself, is the leading cause of fire deaths.

Ambient temperatures may rise extremely rapidly from even small fires. Temperatures of 149° C (300° F) will cause rapid loss of consciousness and, along with toxic gases, will severely damage lung tissues. Warning devices may offer the only possibility for survival due to the rapid onset of debilitating symptoms.

Obvious similarities and differences are seen:
1. Smoke, heat, and gases are not as concentrated in wildland situations as in the confined quarters of urban fires.
2. Flames are not a leading killer in either the urban or wildland situation.
3. Although oxygen levels may be reduced near wildland fires, there is usually sufficient replenishment

of oxygen in the outdoor environment to minimize deprivation. Asphyxiation, however, can also be an important cause of death in wildland fires.

4. Inhalation of superheated gases poses as serious a threat to life in wildland fires as in urban fires.

5. Wildland smoke does not contain toxic compounds produced by combustion of plastics and other household materials, but it does impair visibility, contain carbon monoxide, and have suspended particulates that cause severe physical irritation of the lungs.

6. Automatic early-warning devices and sprinkler systems may protect people from serious injury or death in the urban environment, but in the wildland environment people must rely on their senses, knowledge, and skills to provide early warning of an impending threat to life.

Fire Behavior Knowledge: A Wildland Early-Warning System

The science of fire behavior describes and predicts the performance of wildland fires in terms of rates of spread, intensity levels, ignition probabilities, spotting, and crowning potentials. *Spotting* is a fire spread mechanism resulting from airborne firebrands or embers. *Crowning* is a fire spread mechanism that moves horizontally through the canopies of shrubs or trees. Knowledge of current and predicted weather information and fire danger ratings can be obtained from local wildland fire protection agencies. Experienced firefighters routinely assess the probable behavior of fires using current and expected weather conditions in relation to local fuel and topographic conditions. The emergency medical person, backcountry recreationist, and wildland homeowner must also understand basic fire behavior principles to provide for adequate personal safety. A cardinal rule is to base all actions on current and expected fire behavior. Attention to simple principles, indicators, and rules should enable wildland users to anticipate and avoid fire threats.

Heat, oxygen, and fuel are required in proper combination before ignition and combustion will occur (Figure 12-5).[1] If any one of the three is absent, or if the three elements are out of balance, there will be no fire. Fire control actions are directed at disrupting one or more elements of this basic fire triangle.

Physical Principles of Heat Transfer. Heat energy is transferred by conduction, convection, radiation, and spotting, but generally only the last three processes are significant in a wildland setting. Although conduction through solid objects is important in the burning of logs, this process does not transfer much heat outward from a flaming front.

Convection, or the movement of hot masses of air, accounts for most of the heat transfer outward from the

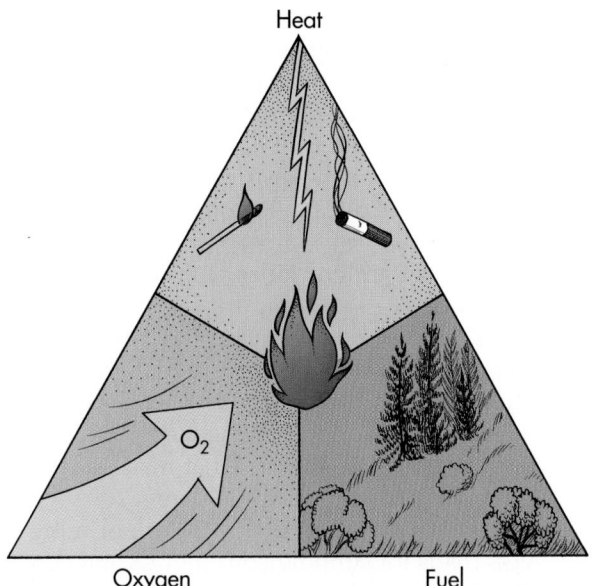

Figure 12-5 Combustion is a process involving the combination of heat, oxygen, and fuel. An understanding of the variation of these three factors is fundamental to an understanding of fire behavior.

fire. Convective currents usually move vertically unless a wind or slope generates lateral movement. Convection preheats fuels upslope and in shrub and tree canopies, which contributes further to a fire's spread and the onset of crown fires.

Via radiation, heat energy is emitted in direct lines of rays; about 25% of combustion energy is transmitted in this manner. The amount of radiant heat transferred decreases inversely with the square of the distance from a point source. More radiant heat is emitted from a line of fire than from a point source. Radiant heat travels in straight lines, does not penetrate solid objects, and is easily reflected. It accounts for most of the preheating of surface fuel ahead of the fire front and poses a direct threat to people who are too close to the fire (Figure 12-6). Many organized fire crew members carry aluminized fire shelters in belt pouches so that they can deploy them quickly when escape is not possible (Figure 12-7). These shelters are used as a last resort to protect from radiant heat.

Spotting is a mass transfer mechanism by which wind currents carry burning or glowing embers beyond the main fire to start new fires (Figure 12-8). In this manner, fire spread may accelerate, unexpected fires occur, and fire intensity and indraft winds may increase.

Factors in Wildland Fire Behavior. A wildland fire behaves according to variations in fuel, weather, and topography. Early warning factors that signal the onset of hotter and faster burning conditions appear in Box 12-2.

When a person encounters a wildland fire, the first

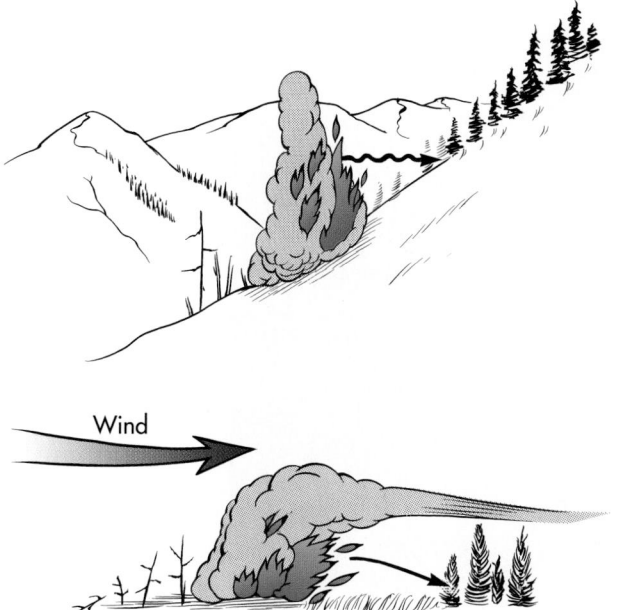

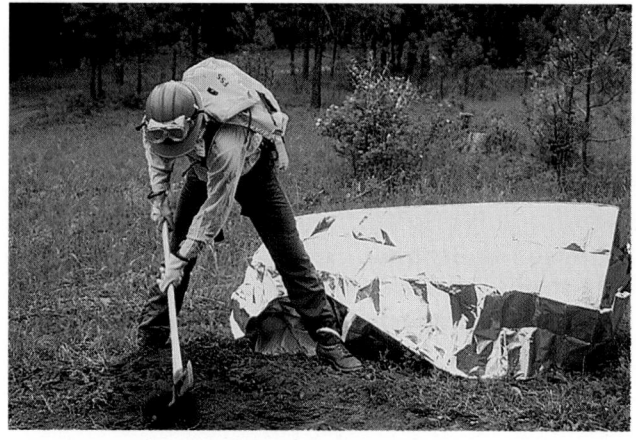

Figure 12-6 Fuels and people upslope or downwind from a fire receive more radiant heat than on the downslope or upwind side.

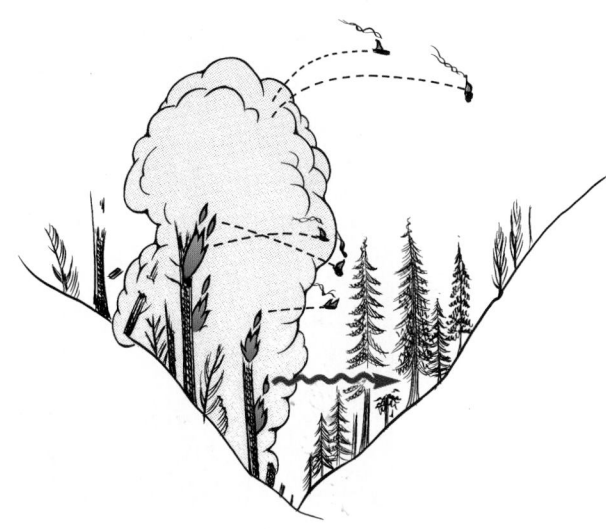

Figure 12-8 Fuels and people on the slope opposite a fire in a narrow canyon are subject to intense heat and spot fires from airborne embers.

Figure 12-7 An aluminized fire shelter, carried in a waist pouch, is deployed by firefighters as a last resort to provide protection from radiant heat and superheated air. *(Courtesy the USDA Forest Service.)*

Box 12-2 EARLY WARNING SIGNALS FOR HOTTER, FASTER BURNING CONDITIONS

FUEL

More fuel; drier fuel; dead fuel; flashy fuel (dead grass, pine needles, and shrubs); aerial fuel (combustible material suspended in crowns of high shrubs and trees, such as branches, needles, lichens, and mosses).

WEATHER

Faster winds; unstable atmosphere (indicators: gusty winds, dust devils, and good visibility); downdraft winds from dry thunderstorms and towering cumulus clouds (erratic and strong winds); higher temperatures, drought conditions, and lower humidities.

TOPOGRAPHY

Steeper slopes; south- and southwest-facing slopes; gaps or saddles; chimneys and narrow canyons (Figure 12-11).

FIRE BEHAVIOR

Rolling and burning pine cones, agaves, logs, hot rocks, and other debris igniting fuel downslope; spot fires that occur ahead of the main fire; individual trees that torch out, or areas of shrubs and trees that burn in a continuous crown fire; fires that smolder over a large area; many fires that start simultaneously; fire whirls that cause spot fires and erratic burning; intense burning with flame lengths greater than 1.2 m (4 feet); dark, massive smoke columns with rolling, boiling vertical development; lateral movement of fire near the base of a steep slope.

---

step should be to review the principles and indicators of fire behavior, sizing up the situation in terms of fuel, weather, topographic factors, and observed fire behavior. After the fire's probable direction and rate of spread are estimated, travel routes that avoid life hazards can be planned (Figure 12-9). The direction of the main body of smoke is often a good indicator of the direction the fire will take.

FUEL. The more fuel that is burning, the hotter the fire will be. Certain types of fuel, such as chaparral, pine, and eucalyptus, burn more intensely because of their fine foliage that contains flammable oils. The size and

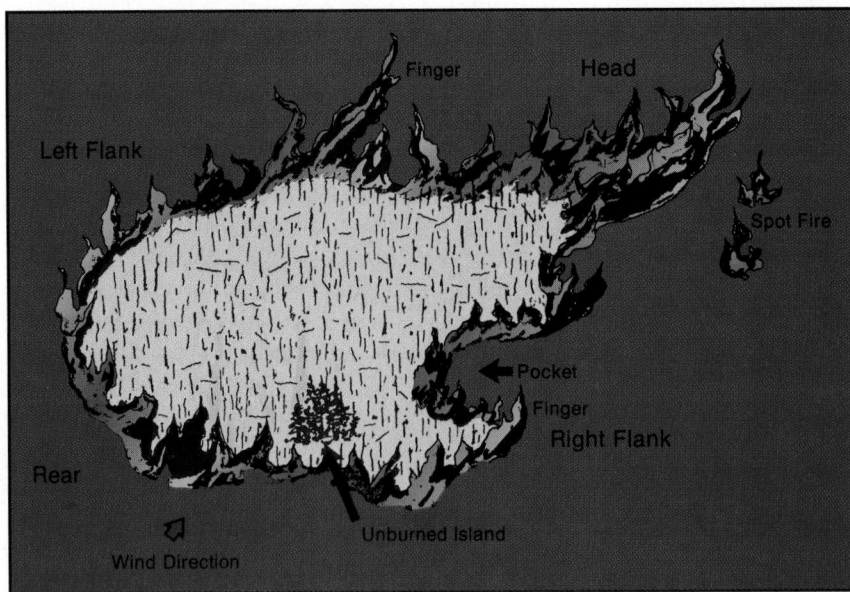

Figure 12-9 The parts of a fire are described in terms of its left flank, right flank, head, and rear. There may also be unburned islands within the fire and spot fires ahead of the fire. The safest travel routes generally involve lateral movement on contours away from the fire's flank or movement toward the rear of the fire. Moving in front of a headfire should be avoided. The burned area inside the fire's perimeter can offer a safe haven, if the flaming perimeter can be safely penetrated by an individual.

arrangement of fuel also influence fire behavior. Small, loosely compacted fuel beds, such as dead grass, long pine needles, and shrubs, burn more rapidly than does tightly compacted fuel. Large fuels burn best when they are arranged so that they are closely spaced, such as logs in a fireplace. Scattered logs with no small or intermediate fuel nearby seldom burn unless they are old and rotten.

WEATHER. The greater the wind, the more rapid the spread of fire. Drier air and higher temperatures cause fuel to dry out more quickly; fire burns more intensely because drying creates more fuel. Prolonged drought makes more fuel available. Fires tend to burn more vigorously when atmospheric conditions are unstable.

The North American continent has been classified into 15 fire climate regions based on geographic and climatic factors (Figure 12-10).[29] Major fire seasons, or periods of peak fire activity, can be used to warn emergency medical personnel and wildland users of the most probable times for life-threatening situations. Although the fire season for the southern Pacific coast is shown as June through September, critical fire weather can occur year round in the most southerly portion. Fire seasons are most active during spring and fall in the Great Plains, Great Lakes, and North Atlantic regions.

TOPOGRAPHY. The steeper the slope, the more rapid the spread of fire. Fire usually burns uphill, especially in

daytime. Changes in topography cause changes in fire behavior (Figure 12-11). On steep terrain, rolling firebrands may cause a fire to spread *downhill*.

Extreme Fire Behavior. Several years of drought combined with a national forest health issue that has produced many dead and dying forests has set the stage for extreme fire behavior conditions that threaten people, property, and natural and cultural resources. Protection from these conditions requires an understanding of the crown fire process. As the name implies, a crown fire is carried through the crowns, or foliage, of a forest or shrubland. Rothermel[26] described the conditions that produce a crown fire:

1. Dry fuels
2. Low humidity and high temperatures
3. Heavy accumulations of dead and downed fuels
4. Small trees in the understory, or "ladder fuels"
5. Steep slope
6. Strong winds
7. Unstable atmosphere
8. Continuous crown layer

The two most prominent behavior patterns of crown fires are wind-driven fires and plume-dominated fires. Each type of crown fire poses a distinct set of threats to people. Fires are seldom uniform and well behaved, so these descriptions of wind-driven and plume-dominated fire behavior may not be readily apparent. The behavior of these types of fires can be expected to

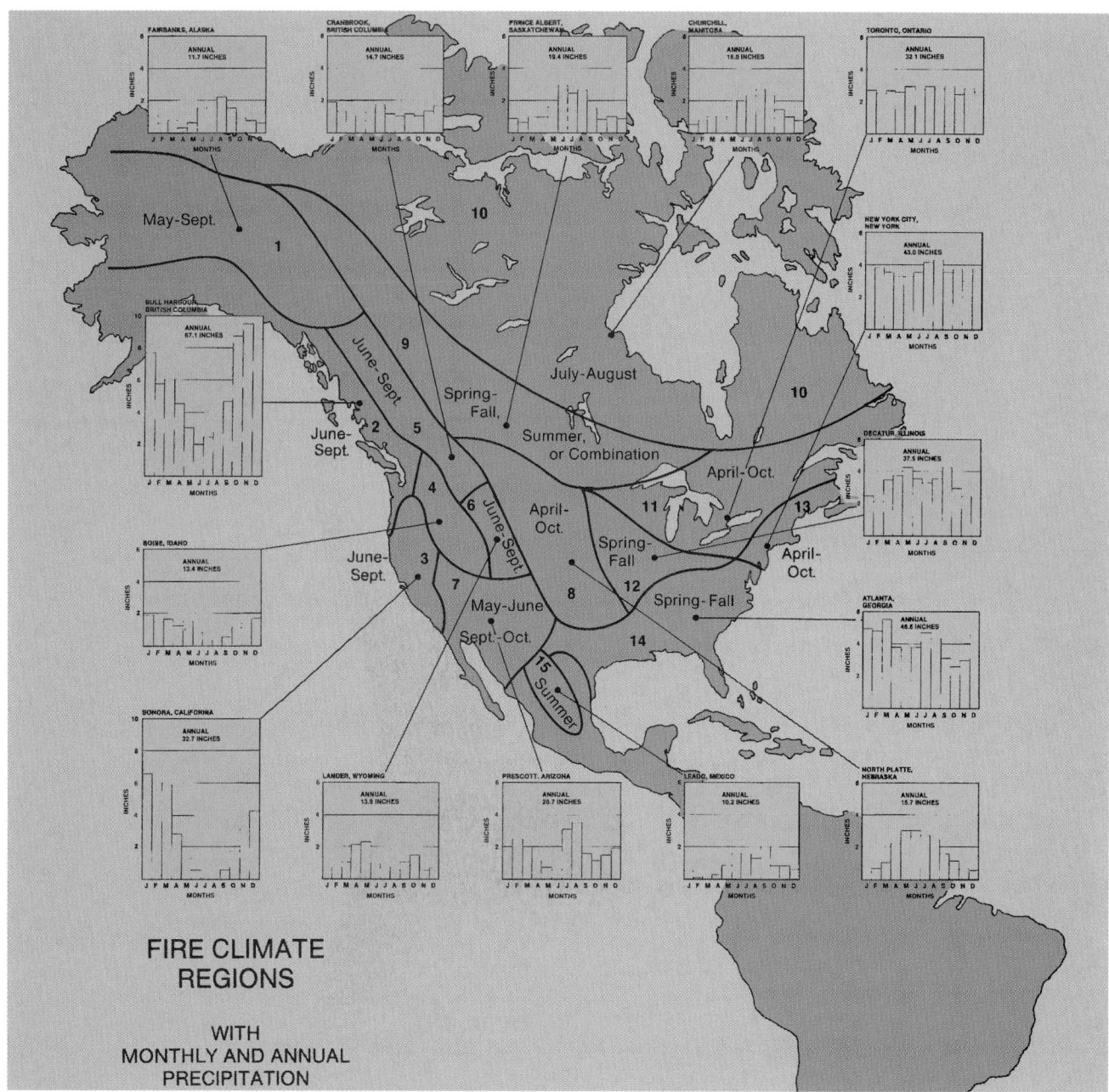

Figure 12-10 Fire climate regions of North America, based on geographic and climatic factors, are as follows: (1) interior Alaska and the Yukon, (2) north Pacific Coast, (3) south Pacific Coast, (4) Great Basin, (5) northern Rocky Mountains, (6) southern Rocky Mountains, (7) Southwest (including adjacent Mexico), (8) Great Plains, (9) central and northwest Canada, (10) sub-Arctic and tundra, (11) Great Lakes, (12) Central States, (13) North Atlantic, (14) Southern States, and (15) Mexican central plateau. The bar graphs show the monthly and annual precipitation for a representative station in each of the fire climate regions. Months on the map indicate fire seasons. (*From Schroeder MJ, Buck CC: Fire weather, Agricultural Handbook 360, 1970, USDA Forest Service.*)

change rapidly as environmental, fuel, and topographic conditions change.[26]

WIND-DRIVEN FIRE. A running crown fire can develop when winds increase with increasing elevation above the ground, driving flames from crown to crown (Figure 12-12). Steep slopes can produce the same effect. Spread rates can vary from 1.6 to 11 km per hour (1 to 7 mph) and possibly faster in mountainous terrain.[26] A running crown fire is accompanied by showers of firebrands downwind, fire whirls, smoke, and the rapid development of a tilted convection column. As long as

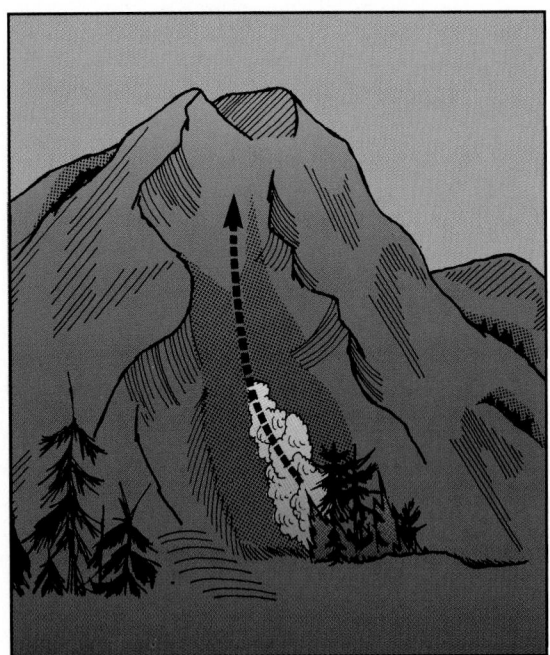 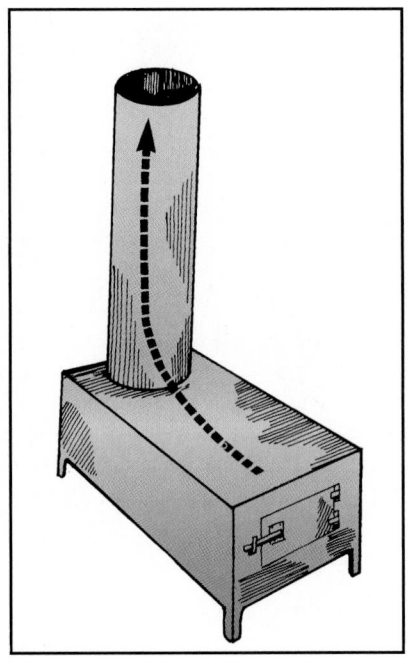

Figure 12-11 Chutes, chimneys, and box canyons created by sharp ridges provide avenues for intense updrafts (like a fire in a stove) and rapid rates of spread. People should avoid being caught above a fire under these topographic conditions.

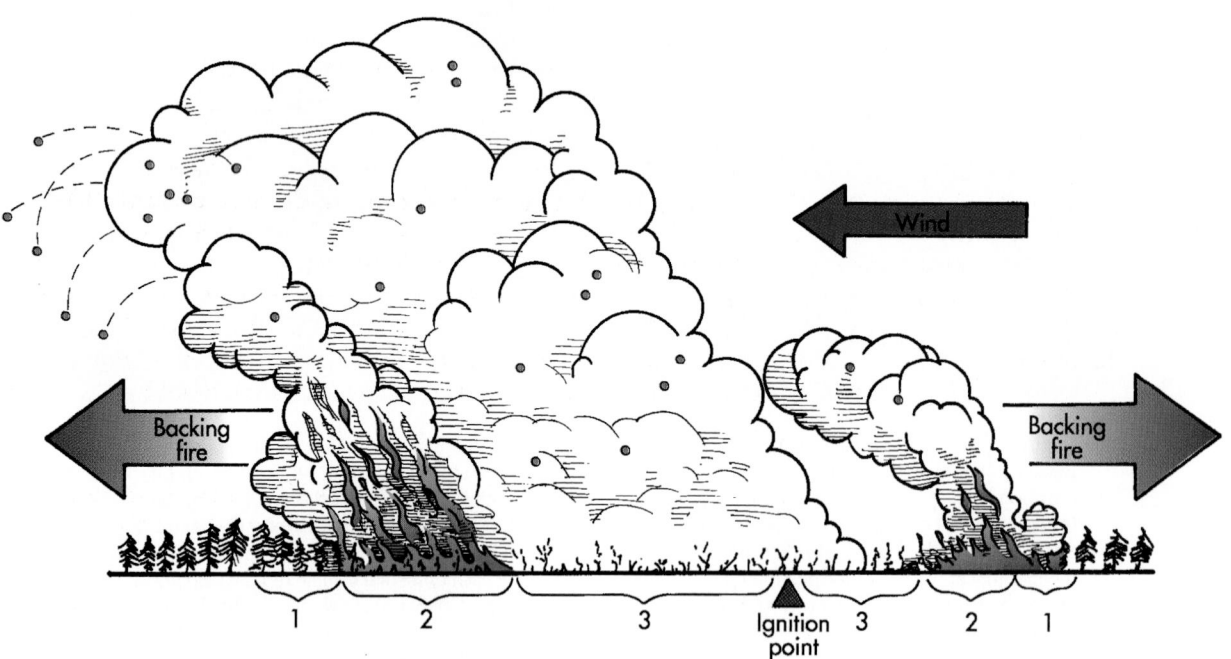

Figure 12-12 Cross-sectional view of a wind-driven crown fire. People are most at risk on the downwind side of a wind-driven fire. This type of fire is caused by winds that increase in velocity with increasing elevation above the ground.

the wind remains fairly constant from one direction, the flanks of the fire can remain relatively safe. The greatest threat is to people who are at the head, or downwind, side of the fire, although long-distance spot fires that ignite from flying embers as far as 1.6 km (1 mile) ahead of the main fire front also pose a risk.

PLUME-DOMINATED FIRE. An alternative form of crown fire develops with relatively low windspeeds or when windspeed decreases with elevation above the ground. This type of crown fire is called a plume-dominated fire because it is characterized by a towering convection column that stands vertically over the fire (Figure 12-13). This type of fire poses a unique threat to people because it can produce spot fires in any direction around its perimeter. It can also spread rapidly as the combustion rate accelerates.

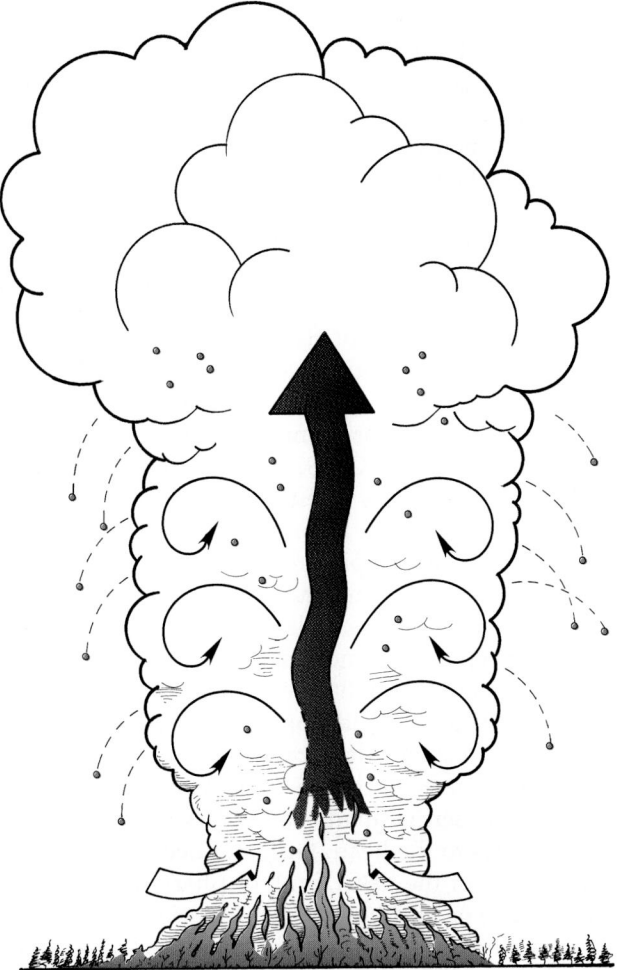

Figure 12-13 Cross-sectional view of a plume-dominated crown fire. People are at risk around the complete perimeter of this type of fire because the fire can spread intensely or spot in any direction. This form of crown fire develops when wind velocities are relatively low or when velocities decrease with elevation above the ground. The convection plume above this type of fire may rise to 7600 to 9100 m (25,000 to 30,000 feet) above the ground.

One form of a plume-dominated fire can be especially dangerous when a downburst of wind blows outward near the ground from the bottom of a convection cell. These winds can be extremely strong[12] and can greatly accelerate a fire. This type of wind occurred during the Dude fire north of Phoenix, Arizona, on June 26, 1990, when six firefighters were killed.

Some indicators help signal the onset of a downburst from a plume-dominated fire. The surest indicator is the occurrence of precipitation of any amount, even a light sprinkle, or the appearance of virga (evaporating rain) below a convective cell.[26] Another indicator is the rapid development of a strong convection column above the fire, or nearby thunder cells. A third and very short warning is the calm that develops when the indraft winds stop before the turnabout and outflow of wind from the cell. This brief period of calm may be accompanied by a humming sound just before the reversing wind flow arrives. If any of these indicators is present, the area should quickly be evacuated. The downburst may also break or uproot trees, creating an additional hazard for people.

FIRE-RELATED INJURIES AND FATALITIES

Most fatalities in wildland fires occur on days of extreme fire danger when people are exposed to abnormally high heat stress caused by weather or proximity to fires. Loss of life is dramatically highlighted under extreme burning conditions; however, many more people are injured than are killed by fires.

One of the worst fire disasters in Australia occurred on February 7, 1967, when 62 persons died in Tasmania.[17] Analysis of location and age of 53 individuals at the time of death is instructive (Tables 12-1 and 12-2). Most people whose bodies were found within or near houses were old, infirm, or physically disabled. More than half of the houses vacated by the 11 people who traveled some distance before being killed were not burned. Most of these victims would probably have

TABLE 12-1. Location of Bodies of 53 Persons Who Died in Tasmanian Fires, February 7, 1967

LOCATION	NUMBER OF DEATHS
Mustering stock	2
Firefighting	11
Traveling in a vehicle	2
Escaping from and found at some distance from houses	11
Within a few meters of houses	10
In houses	17

From McArthur AG, Cheney NP: *Report on southern Tasmania bushfires of 7 February 1967*, Hobart, Australia, 1967, Government Printer.

TABLE 12-2. Age Distribution of 53 Persons Who Died in Tasmanian Fires, February 7, 1967

AGE GROUP	NUMBER IN GROUP	AVERAGE AGE
1-25	1	23
26-50	13	38
51-75	26	64
76-88	13	82

From McArthur AG, Cheney NP: *Report on southern Tasmania bushfires of 7 February 1967*, Hobart, Australia, 1967, Government Printer.

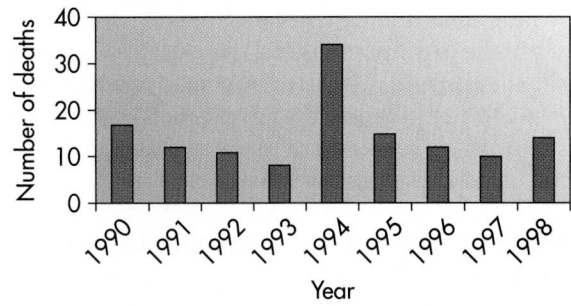

Figure 12-14 The annual death toll for persons who died from all causes while involved in fighting wildland fires from 1990 to 1998 (133 total deaths).

survived if they had remained in their homes. Most of the 11 firefighters who died were inexperienced. Many might have survived if they had observed fire behavior and safety rules.

A review of USDA Forest Service records between 1926 and 1976 shows that 145 men died in 41 fires from fire-induced injuries.[42] Large losses occurred in the Blackwater fire in Wyoming in 1937 (15 deaths), in the Rattlesnake fire in California in 1953 (15 deaths), and in the 1933 Griffth Park fire in southern California (25 fatalities and 128 injuries). Wilson's analysis of people lost to fires in areas protected by other federal, state, county, and private agencies indicated 77 fire-induced fatalities in 26 fires. Wilson[42] identified some common features connecting these fatal fires:

1. Relatively small fires or isolated sectors within larger fires seemed associated with most fatal incidents.
2. Flare-ups of presumed controlled fires were particularly hazardous. Fatalities occurred in the mop-up stage.
3. Unexpected shifts in wind direction or speed occasionally caused flare-ups in deceptively light fuels.
4. Gullies, chimneys, and steep slopes directed fires to run uphill.
5. The violent wind vortices left by helicopters and air tankers may have caused flare-ups in previously controlled areas.

Wilson concluded that the hairline difference between fatal fires and near-fatal fires was determined by the individual's reaction to a suddenly critical situation. Escapes were due to luck, circumstances, advance planning, a person's ability to avoid panic, or a combination of these factors. Frequently, poor visibility and absence of concise fire information threatened survival opportunities by creating confusion and panic.

Nature of Injuries and Fatalies

Fire-related injuries and fatalities are a direct consequence of heat, flames, smoke, critical gas levels, or indirect injuries (Figure 12-14). Injuries and fatalities as-

sociated with wildland fires fall into categories of heat (direct thermal injury, inhalation, and heat stress disorders), flames (direct thermal injury and inhalation), smoke (inhalation and mucous membrane irritation), critical gas levels (oxygen, carbon monoxide, and carbon dioxide), and indirect effects (acute and chronic medical disability and trauma).

Intense fires that produce very high temperatures generally last for only a short time. The duration of intense heat increases with fuel load, being greater in a forest fire where heavy fuels are burning than in a grass or shrub fire. Temperatures near the ground are lower because radiant heat is offset somewhat by inflow of fresh air and the fact that gases of combustion rise and are carried away by convection.[4] Close to the ground, within a few meters of flames reaching up to 11 m (36 feet), air temperatures may be less than 15° C (59° F) above ambient temperature. The breathing of heated air can be tolerated for 30 minutes at 93° C (199° F) and for 3 minutes at 250° C (482° F).[16] Death or severe pulmonary injury occurs when these limits are exceeded. Thermal injuries of the respiratory tract frequently contribute to the clinical picture of smoke inhalation. Persons trapped in a fire may have no choice but to breathe flame or very hot gases. This usually injures the tissues of the upper airway and respiratory tract, most commonly the nose, nasopharynx, mouth, oropharynx, hypopharynx, larynx, and upper trachea. These injuries may result in edema that obstructs the airway and produces asphyxia or that causes tracheitis and mediastinitis.

Signs of thermal injury to the airway include thermal injuries to the head, face, and neck; singed facial hair; burns of the nasal, oral, or pharyngeal mucosa; and stridor or dysphonia.[19,33,45] Associated with a history of exposure to flame and hot gases in a closed space, these clinical findings strongly suggest the presence of a thermal injury to the airway. With the potential for acute airway obstruction, there is obvious urgency in establishing this diagnosis. Most experts who treat thermal injuries of the tracheobronchial tree advocate early visualization of the vocal cords by laryngoscopy and bronchoscopy.[20] Bronchoscopy is a useful predictor of the clinical course and urgency of intensive care unit intervention. In addition, one report shows a significantly greater incidence of pneumonia and late mortality in persons with facial burns than in those without them.[43]

Burns of the lower trachea are rarely reported. In fact, injuries to and beyond the carina are difficult to produce when the trachea is cannulated and hot gases are delivered in the anesthetized dog.[18,44] Air has a very low specific heat and is therefore a poor conductor of thermal energy. In addition, the thermal exchange systems of the upper airway are quite efficient. The hot gas or flame is cooled sufficiently in the upper airway so that it does not burn the bronchi or more distal structures. However, although water or steam in the hot gas mixture is probably rare, it is a far more efficient conductor of heat and permits significant thermal injury to the lower trachea and bronchi.

A delayed onset (2 to 24 hours after smoke inhalation) of pulmonary edema and adult respiratory distress syndrome is widely reported and should be anticipated. Whether this results from direct injury to alveoli, prolonged hypotension, or cerebral hypoxia and cerebral edema is unclear.

Heat stress[30] occurs when air temperature, humidity, radiant heat, and poor air movement combine with strenuous work and insulative clothing to raise body temperature beyond safe limits. Sweating cools the body as moisture evaporates. When water lost through sweating is not replaced, physiologic heat controls can deregulate and body temperature may rise, leading to heat exhaustion or heatstroke (see Chapter 10).

Direct contact with flames causes thermal injury, and death is inevitable with exposure for long periods. Burns may be superficial, partial, or full thickness (see Chapter 13). Immediate death results from hypotension, hyperthermia, respiratory failure, and frank incineration.

The common cause of asphyxia in wildland fire is smoke. Danger increases where smoke accumulates because of poor ventilation, as in caves, box canyons, narrow valleys, and gullies.

Dense, acrid smoke is particularly irritating to the respiratory system and eyes. Excessive coughing induces pharyngitis and vomiting. Keratitis, conjunctivitis, and chemosis may make it impossible to keep the eyes open.

There are concerns about the levels of oxygen, carbon monoxide, and carbon dioxide associated with fire. Critical levels readily occur in a closed space and near burning or smoldering heavy fuels, but the open space of a wildland fire usually contributes to continual mixing of air. Misconceptions about lack of oxygen or excessive carbon monoxide and carbon dioxide in a wildland fire abound in the lay literature.

Flaming combustion can be maintained only at oxy-

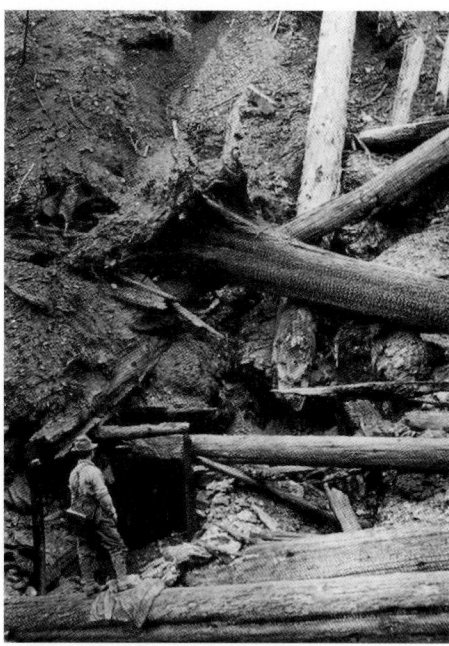

Figure 12-15 Ranger Pulaski led 42 men and 2 horses to this mine tunnel near Placer Creek in northern Idaho to seek refuge from the 1910 fire. One man who failed to get into the tunnel was burned beyond recognition. All the men in the tunnel evidently were unconscious for a period of time. Five men died inside the tunnel, apparently from suffocation. The remainder of the crew was evacuated to the hospital in Wallace, where all recovered. *(Courtesy the USDA Forest Service. Photo by J.B. Halm.)*

gen levels that exceed 12%, a level at which life can also be supported.[4,16] With continued indrafts of air that feed the flames, a fresh source of oxygen is usually present. Even mass fires, in which large tracts of land are burning, rarely reduce oxygen to hazardous levels. Low oxygen levels may occur, however, where there is little air movement, such as in caves (Figure 12-15) or in burned-over land that continues to smoke from smoldering fuels.

Concentrations of carbon monoxide exceeding 800 parts per million (ppm) can cause death within hours. Most fires produce small quantities, but atmospheric concentrations rarely reach lethal levels because of air movement. High concentrations appear to be associated with smoldering combustion of heavy fuels, such as fallen trees or slash piles, and carbon monoxide may also collect in low-lying areas or underground shelters.[5] Outdoors, the danger lies in continual exposure to low concentrations that can increase blood carboxyhemoglobin levels. Prolonged exposure affects the central nervous system, resulting in headache, impaired judgment, progressive lethargy, decreased vision, and other psychomotor deficits.[42]

Carbon monoxide levels of 50 ppm were measured close to a prescribed burn in grass.[8] In another estimate, concentrations of 30 ppm were found roughly 61 m (200 feet) from the fire front. Studies on the 1974 Deadline and Outlaw forest fires in Idaho showed that fire-fighters were exposed to levels above the standards proposed by the National Institute of Occupational Safety and Health (35 ppm over an 8-hour period).[34]

Decreased ambient oxygen may contribute to hypoxia and the overall picture of smoke inhalation (Table 12-3). This mechanism is at least variably operant. When standing gasoline was ignited in a closed bunker, the fire self-extinguished, while the ambient oxygen level remained at 14%, a survivable level.[18] Injecting burning gasoline or napalm into bunkers produced nearly complete and prolonged exhaustion of ambient oxygen. Conflicting data make it difficult to classify definitively situations in which decreased ambient oxygen and subsequent hypoxia of exposed individuals contribute to the clinical picture of smoke inhalation. Studies in which ambient oxygen was measured by scientists did not show significant depletion of the scene of the fire.[11]

Few data are available on levels of carbon dioxide around wildland fires. Although it may be produced in large quantities, it apparently never reaches hazardous concentrations, even in severe fire situations.[4,16]

The quantity of burning fuel and the type of topography affect levels of oxygen and toxic gases. Danger is greater in forest fires where heavy fuels burn over long periods of time than in quick-moving grass and shrub fires. Topography has a major influence; caves, box canyons, narrow canyons, gulches, and other terrain features can trap toxic gases or hinder ventilation, thereby preventing an inflow of fresh air. Although most fatalities result from encounters with smoke, flames, and heat, critical gas levels can induce handicaps sufficient to render the victim more vulnerable to other hazards.

Wildland Fires, Air Toxins, and Human Health

In the United States about 80,000 firefighters are involved with suppression activities on 70,000 wildland fires that burn an average of over 0.8 million hectares (2 million acres) each year. In 1988 over 2 million hectares (5 million acres) of land were burned, with a total combined suppression cost exceeding $600 million. The firefighting effort has another cost that has not been quantified: the effect of smoke on firefighter health and productivity. Over the 4 months of the Greater Yellowstone Area fires, approximately 40% of the 30,000 medical visits made by wildland firefighters were for respiratory problems. More than 600 firefighters required subsequent medical care. In the Happy Camp area during the Klamath fire complex in California in 1987, ambient concentrations of carbon monoxide measured as high as 54 ppm on a volume basis.[36] A better understanding of the effects of wildland fire smoke on people is clearly needed. The combustion products of concern include these classes of materials:

1. Particulate matter
2. Polynuclear aromatic hydrocarbons
3. Carbon monoxide
4. Aldehydes
5. Organic acids
6. Semivolatile and volatile organic compounds
7. Free radicals
8. Ozone
9. Inorganic fraction of particles

Large variances are associated with the development of smoke combustion products and exposure to the materials of concern.[38] Ward et al[39] indicated that the toxicity of the combination of combustion products depends on the relative concentrations of the individual compounds, as well as the overall concentration and length of exposure. Individual toxicities are associated with many of the compounds found in smoke. The combined toxicity of these substances is not known. A detailed set of studies is being carried out to provide answers so that risk management options can be exercised. One of these studies suggested that wildland firefighters experience a small cross-seasonal decline in pulmonary function and an increase in several respiratory symptoms.[28] Eye irritation, nose irritation, and wheezing were associated with recent firefighting.

The strenuous work of fighting or escaping a fire magnifies chronic illnesses, age disabilities, exhaustion, and cardiovascular instability. Common trauma is induced by falling trees or limbs, rolling logs or rocks, vehicular accidents, poor visibility, panic, falling asleep in unburned fuels that later ignite, and leaving the safety of buildings and vehicles. Cuts, scrapes, scratches, lacerations, fractures, and eye injuries (foreign particles, smoke irritation, sharp objects) are other common afflictions. Poison oak, poison ivy, stinging insects, and poisonous snakes are additional sources of trauma during wildland fires. To avoid fire-related injuries and fatalities, a person must keep attuned to mental and

TABLE 12-3. Human Response to Decreased Ambient Oxygen at Sea Level

AMBIENT OXYGEN (%)	HUMAN RESPONSE
20.9	Normal function
16-18	Decreased stamina and capacity for work
12-15	Dyspnea with walking; impaired coordination; variable impaired judgment
10-12	Dyspnea at rest; consciousness preserved; impaired judgment, coordination, and concentration
6-8	Loss of consciousness; death without prompt reversal
<6	Death in 6 to 10 minutes

physical stress levels and be aware of cumulative effects.[30] *Ignorance of this simple principle is disastrous.*

WILDLAND-URBAN INTERFACE FIRE SURVIVAL PRINCIPLES AND TECHNIQUES

History has demonstrated repeatedly that individuals simply were not prepared to make correct choices of survival alternatives under stressful situations. Overconfidence, ignorance, bad habits, lack of preparation, and panic quickly lead to improper and unsafe actions during fire emergencies.[42] "Learning from mistakes" in these settings is not a reasonable education strategy; second chances are frequently unavailable.

The USDA Forest Service organized a task force in 1957 to "study how we might strengthen our ways and means of preventing firefighting fatalities." A major recommendation was to adopt service-wide standard firefighting orders. Ten standard firefighting orders summarize the fundamental principles of safety on the fireline (Box 12-3). Although these were written for firefighters, they apply to all people working, living, or traveling near wildland fires and are adapted here to

---

Box 12-3 TEN STANDARD FIREFIGHTING ORDERS

1. Keep informed of fire weather conditions, changes, and forecasts and how they may affect the area where you are located.
2. Know what the fire is doing at all times through personal observations, communication systems, or scouts.
3. Base all actions on current and expected behavior of the fire.
4. Determine escape routes and plans for everyone at risk and make certain that everyone understands routes and plans.
5. Post lookouts to watch the fire if you think there is any danger of being trapped, of increased fire activity, or of erratic fire behavior.
6. Be alert, keep calm, think clearly, and act decisively to avoid panic reactions.
7. Maintain prompt and clear communication with your group, firefighting forces, and command/communication centers.
8. Give clear, concise instructions and be sure that they are understood.
9. Maintain control of the people in your group at all times.
10. Fight fire aggressively, but provide for safety first. (Nonqualified and improperly equipped persons should fight fire only when it is necessary to assist injured persons.)

---

remind emergency medical personnel, wildland homeowners, and recreationists of safety precautions.

LCES: The Key to Safe Procedures

LCES stands for lookouts, communications, escape routes, and safety zones.[10] These variables are key components in evaluating a fire hazard and determining the best course of action. The wildland fire environment's basic hazards are lightning, volcanoes, fire-weakened trees, rolling rocks and logs, entrapment by running fires, respirable particulates, air toxins, and heat stress. When these hazards exist, there are two options:

1. Do not enter the environment.
2. Adhere to safe procedures according to LCES.

LCES should be viewed from a "systems" point of view, stressing their interdependence. For example, the best safety zone is worthless if the escape route does not offer access at the point of need. People must be familiar with the LCES plan well before it is needed. In addition, the nature of wildland fires dictates that LCES be redefined in pace with changing conditions.

The LCES system is implemented as follows:

1. *Lookouts.* Fixed lookouts or roving lookouts must be where both the hazard and the people can be seen. Lookouts are trained to observe the wildland fire environment and to recognize and anticipate fire behavior changes. When the hazard becomes a danger, the lookout relays this information so people can depart for the safety zone.
2. *Communications.* Communications refers to alerting people to the approaching hazard. Promptness and clarity are essential.
3. *Escape routes.* These paths lead from a currently threatened position to an area free from danger. More than one escape route must be available. Escape routes are probably the most elusive component of LCES, since they change continuously. Timely access to safety zones is the most important component.
4. *Safety zones.* In safety zones those threatened find adequate refuge from danger. The size of the safety zone must provide protection from flames, radiant heat, convective heat, and falling trees and will vary with changes in fuels, topography, wind conditions, and fire intensity.

Eighteen Watch-Out Situations in the Wildland

The following 18 watch-out situations are of particular relevance to emergency medical personnel and wildland users:

1. You are moving downhill toward a fire, but must be aware that fire can move swiftly and suddenly uphill. Constantly observe fire behavior, fuels, and escape routes, assessing the fire's potential to run uphill.

2. You are on a hillside where rolling, burning material can ignite fuel from below. When below a fire, watch for burning materials, especially cones and logs, that can roll downhill and ignite a fire beneath you, trapping you between two coalescing fires.

3. Wind begins to blow, increase, or change direction. Wind strongly influences fire behavior, so be prepared to respond to sudden changes.

4. The weather becomes hotter and drier. Fire activity increases, and its behavior changes more rapidly as ambient temperature rises and relative humidity decreases.

5. Dense vegetation with unburned fuel is between you and the fire. The danger in this situation is that unburned fuels can ignite. If the fire is moving away from you, be alert for wind changes or spot fires that may ignite fuels near you. Do not be overconfident if the area has burned once because it can reignite if sufficient fuel remains.

6. You are in an unburned area near the fire where terrain and cover make travel difficult. The combination of fuel and difficult escape makes this dangerous.

7. Travel or work is in an area you have not seen in daylight. Darkness and unfamiliarity are a dangerous combination.

8. You are unfamiliar with local factors influencing fire behavior. When possible, seek information on what to expect from knowledgeable people, especially those from the area.

9. By necessity, you have to make a frontal assault on a fire with tankers. Any encounter with an active line of fire is dangerous because of proximity to intense heat, smoke, and flames, along with limited escape opportunities.

10. Spot fires occur frequently across the fireline. Generally, increased spotting indicates increased fire activity and intensity. The danger is that of entrapment between coalescing fires.

11. The main fire cannot be seen, and you are not in communication with anyone who can see it. If you do not know the location, size, and behavior of the main fire, planning becomes guesswork, which is an unfavorable response.

12. An unclear assignment or confusing instructions have been received. Make sure that all assignments and instructions are fully understood.

13. You are drowsy and feel like resting or sleeping near the fireline in unburned fuel. This may lead to fire entrapment. *No one should sleep near a wildland fire.* If resting is absolutely necessary, choose a burned area that is safe from rolling material, smoke, reburn, and other dangers or seek a wide area of bare ground or rock.

14. Fire has not been scouted and sized up.

15. Safety zones and escape routes have not been identified.

16. You are uninformed on strategy, tactics, and hazards.

17. No communication link with crew members or supervisor has been established.

18. A line has been constructed without a safe anchor point.

Fifteen Structural Watch-Out Situations for the Wildland-Urban Interface

Because fires occur more often in the wildland-urban interface, these 15 structural watch-out situations have been defined to increase awareness of structural fire dangers[35]:

1. Access is poor (for example, narrow roads, twisting, single lane with inadequate turning).

2. Load limits of local bridges are light or unknown; the bridges are narrow.

3. Winds are strong, and erratic fire behavior is occurring.

4. The area contains garages with closed, locked doors.

5. You have an inadequate water supply to attack the fire.

6. Structure windows are black or smoked over.

7. There are septic tanks and leach lines. (These are found in most rural situations.)

8. A house or structure is burning with puffing rather than steady smoke.

9. Inside and outside construction of structures is wood with shake shingle roofs.

10. Natural fuels occur within 9 m (30 feet) of the structures.

11. Known or suspected panicked persons are in the vicinity.

12. Structure windows are bulging, and the roof has not been vented.

13. Additional fuels can be found in open crawl spaces beneath the structures.

14. Firefighting is taking place in or near chimney or canyon situations.

15. Elevated fuel or propane tanks are present.

Refuge in Vehicles, Buildings, and Fire Shelters

The radiant energy of a fire, although highly intense at a given location, typically lasts for only a short time. Because radiant heat travels in straight lines, does not penetrate solid substances, and is easily reflected, seeking refuge in vehicles, buildings, or fire shelters is often lifesaving.

Vehicles. In the United States, firefighters have survived severe fire storms or the passage of fire fronts by taking refuge in vehicles. The following case histories serve as examples of intense burning situations where lives were saved because people stayed inside vehicles when the fire passed[31]:

In 1958 a veteran Field Section Fire Warden and two young men were fighting forest fires that burned in heavy fuels near the Bass River State Forest in southern New Jersey. A 90 degree wind shift transformed the flank fire into a broad headfire, with advancing flames up to 12 m (40 feet). The men entered their vehicle, a Dodge W300 Power Wagon, which stood in the middle of a sand road 4 m (12 feet) wide. Simultaneously the engine and radio failed.

The Fire Warden repeatedly admonished the crewmen, who wished to flee, to stay in the truck. Subsequently the truck was rocked violently by convection currents and microclimatic changes generated by the flames. The men could neither see nor breathe because of smoke, and the cab began to fill with sparks that ignited the seat. The men stayed with the truck for only 3 or 4 minutes during the passage of the headfire, but they indicated later that the interval involved seemed more like 3 or 4 hours.

At the first opportunity all of them left the vehicle on the upwind side and crouched beside it to escape the searing heat and burning seats. The warden proceeded to burn his hand severely while disposing of a flaming gas can in the truck bed. While the young men escaped virtually unscathed, the older man suffered lung damage and remained on limited duty for 5 years. He has since recovered completely and retired.

In 1976 a firefighter died while fighting a grass fire near Buhler, Kansas, in Reno County. A flashover occurred from a buildup of gases on the lee side of a windbreak. A fire truck was caught in the flashover, and the firefighter working from the back of the vehicle ran and was killed. Although the truck burned, the driver was not seriously hurt.

In a 1962 California Division of Forestry fire in Fresno County, three men, followed by a flank fire that had turned into a headfire, raced back to their truck only a few feet ahead of the flames. The truck would not restart. After the main body of flames passed over the vehicle, the men jumped out in order to breathe, since the truck was burning. Almost completely blinded by smoke and heat, they stumbled headlong into matted fuels, and two received first- and second-degree burns. One man was not burned but had to be treated for smoke inhalation. The truck was a loss.

Sitting in a vehicle during a passing fire front is often perilous, but when a person is trapped, it is almost certain doom to attempt escape by running from the fire. The preceding case histories illustrate a few facts that, if remembered, may prevent panic:

1. The engine may stall and not restart.
2. The vehicle may be rocked by convection currents.
3. Smoke and sparks may enter the cab.
4. The interior, engine, or tires may ignite.
5. Temperatures increase inside the cab because the heat is radiated through the windows.
6. Metal gas tanks and containers rarely explode.
7. If it is necessary to leave the cab after the fire has passed, keep the vehicle between you and the fire.

The type of vehicle determines the amount of protection afforded. Two travelers died in a fire in 1967 in Tasmania, Australia, when they were caught in a canvas-topped vehicle.[16] A later fire in Australia led to further research on various vehicles' protection and the explosiveness of gasoline tanks. In 1969 at Lara, Victoria, Australia, a fast-moving grass fire crossed a four-lane expressway. Several cars stopped in the confusion of smoke and flames. Seventeen people left the safety of their cars and perished. Six people stayed inside their vehicles and survived, even though one car ignited.

Investigations were carried out by the Forest Research Institute (now the Commonwealth Scientific and Industrial Research Organization [CSIRO], Division of Forest Research) in Canberra, Australia, to collect accurate data and dispel the misconceptions that make persons flee a safe refuge if trapped by fire.[4] Cars were placed between two burning piles of logging slash to study a car's ability to shield against radiation. The test was a hotter, longer fire than normally encountered.

Car bodies halved the external radiation transmitted at the peak of the fire, but a person inside would have suffered severe burns to bare skin. Although air temperatures inside the car did not reach hazardous levels until well after the peak radiation had passed, smoke from smoldering plastic and rubber materials would have caused discomfort and made the car uninhabitable. In this study, metal gasoline tanks did not explode, whether intact on cars or separated and placed on a burning pile of slash. Apparently, when tanks are sealed, the space above the liquid contains a mixture too deficient in oxygen vapor to support an explosion.

Cheney[4,5] offered the following advice for survival when in a car and trapped by fire:

1. If smoke obstructs visibility, turn on the headlights and drive to the side of the road away from the leading edge of the fire. Try to select an area of sparse vegetation offering the least combustible material.
2. Attempt to shield your body from radiant heat energy by rolling up the windows and covering up with floor mats or hiding beneath the dashboard. Cover as much skin as possible.
3. Stay in the vehicle as long as possible. Unruptured gas tanks rarely explode, and vehicles usually take several minutes to ignite.
4. Grass fires create about 30 seconds of flame exposure, and chances for survival in a vehicle are good. Forest fires create higher-intensity flames lasting 3 to 4 minutes and lowering chances for survival. Staying in a vehicle improves chances for surviving a forest fire. Remain calm.
5. A strong, acrid smell usually results from burning paint and plastic materials, caused by small quantities of hydrogen chloride released from breakdown of polyvinyl chloride. Hydrogen chloride is water soluble, and discomfort can be relieved by

breathing through a damp cloth. Urine is mostly water and can be used in emergencies.

Buildings. The decision to evacuate a house or remain and defend it is not easy. Fire services generally prefer that residents evacuate the threatened area so that agencies can concentrate on protecting structures. Authorities also agree that evacuation of elderly, very young, infirm, and fearful people is usually a good idea. People should evacuate only if it can be accomplished safely, well in advance of any danger. Several principles should guide the evacuation decision[40]:

1. A fire within sight or smell is a fire that endangers you.
2. More unattended houses burn down.
3. Evacuation when fire is close is too late; evacuation must be done well before danger is apparent.
4. More people are injured and killed in the open than in houses.
5. Learn beforehand about community refuges.
6. Evacuate only to a known safe refuge.

Whether people can find refuge in buildings depends on construction materials and amount of preparation in reducing fuels around the structure. If a home is constructed amid flammable vegetation, plans and procedures to safeguard the home and its occupants are essential. A building usually offers protection while the fire passes even if it ignites later because it shields against radiant heat and smoke. After the fire passes, it may be necessary to exit if the building is burning.

Case histories from Australia demonstrate that homes provide safe havens.[16] In 1967 in Tasmania, 21 people left their houses as fire approached. All died, and some were within a few meters of the buildings. Many houses did not burn and would have been refuges.

When taking refuge in a building, give people useful jobs, such as filling vessels with water, blocking cracks with wet blankets, and tightly closing windows and doors. If possible, assign lookouts to keep watch for spot fires on the outside of the building until the last minute. Before fire approaches the house, take the following precautions[31]:

1. If you plan to stay, evacuate your pets and all family members not essential to protecting the home.
2. Be properly dressed to survive the fire. Cotton fabrics are preferable to synthetics. Wear long pants and boots, and carry for protection a long-sleeved shirt or jacket, gloves, a handkerchief to shield the face, water to wet it, and goggles.
3. Remove combustible items from around the house, including lawn and poolside furniture, umbrellas, and tarp coverings. If they catch fire, the added heat could ignite the house.
4. Close outside attic, eave, and basement vents to eliminate the possibility of sparks blowing into hidden areas within the house. Close window shutters.
5. Place large plastic trash cans or buckets around the outside of the house and fill them with water. Soak burlap sacks, small rugs, and large rags to use in beating out burning embers or small fires. Inside the house, fill bathtubs, sinks, and other containers with water. Toilet tanks and water heaters are an important water reservoir.
6. Place garden hoses so that they will reach any place on the house. Use the spray gun type of nozzle, adjusted to spray.
7. If you have portable gasoline-powered pumps to take water from a swimming pool or tank, make sure they are operating and in place.
8. Place a ladder against the roof of the house opposite the side of the approaching fire. If you have a combustible roof, wet it down or turn on any roof sprinklers. Turn on any special fire sprinklers installed to add protection. Do not waste water. Waste can drain the entire water system quickly.
9. Back your car into the garage and roll up the car windows. Disconnect the automatic garage door opener (in case of power failure, you cannot remove the car). Close all garage doors.
10. Place valuable papers and mementos inside the car in the garage for quick departure, if necessary. In addition, place all pets still with you in the car.
11. Close windows and doors to the house to prevent sparks from blowing inside. Close all doors inside the house to prevent drafts. Open the damper on your fireplace to help stabilize outside-inside pressure, but close the fireplace screen so that sparks will not ignite the room. Turn on a light in each room to make the house more visible in heavy smoke.
12. Turn off pilot lights.
13. If you have time, take down drapes and curtains. Close all venetian blinds or noncombustible window coverings to reduce the amount of heat radiating into the house. This provides added safety in case the windows give way because of heat or wind.
14. As the fire front approaches, go inside the house. Stay calm; you are in control of the situation.
15. After the fire passes, check the roof immediately. Extinguish any sparks or embers. Then check the attic for hidden burning sparks. If you have a fire, enlist your neighbors to help fight it. For several hours after the fire, recheck for smoke and sparks throughout the house.

Fire Shelters. The fire shelter described earlier was developed by the Missoula Technology Development

Center to reduce the number of serious burn injuries and fatalities among firefighters who become trapped while fighting wildland fires. Shelters, designed in the shape of a pup tent, protect the firefighter by reflecting radiant heat. Constructed of an aluminum foil-fiberglass cloth laminate, the shelter reflects approximately 95% of the radiant heat emanating from a fire. The shelter is credited with saving more than 300 lives since its introduction in the 1960s.[25] Why fire shelters work well was demonstrated dramatically on August 29, 1985, when 73 firefighters were forced to take refuge in their shelters for approximately 1½ hours while a severe crown fire burned over them.[22] The incident took place during the Butte fire in the Salmon National Forest in Idaho. Observers described the crown fire that overran the firefighters as a standing wall of flame that reached 61 m (200 feet) above the treetops. Within the shelters, firefighters experienced extreme heat for as long as 10 minutes. Shelters were so hot that they could be handled only with gloves. After leaving the shelters, some firefighters showed symptoms of possible carbon monoxide poisoning, including vomiting, disorientation, and difficulty breathing. Emergency medical technicians administered oxygen to several individuals before evacuation. Five firefighters were hospitalized overnight for heat exhaustion, smoke inhalation, and dehydration. The consensus of those interviewed was that without the shelters, none would have survived.

Entrapment Procedures

Sometimes there may be no chance to escape a fire. When entrapment is imminent, injuries or death may be avoided by following entrapment procedures:

1. Do not panic. Most people are afraid when trapped by fire, so accept this fear as natural, so that clear thinking and intelligent decisions are possible. If fear overwhelms you, judgment is seriously impaired and survival a matter of chance.
2. Do not run blindly or needlessly. Unless a clear path of escape is indicated, do not run. Move downhill and away from the flank of the fire at a 45-degree angle where possible. Conserve your strength.
3. Enter the burned area. Particularly in grass, low shrubs, or other low fuels, do not delay if escape means passing through the flame front into the burned area. Move aggressively and parallel to the advancing fire front. Choose a place on the fire's edge where flames are less than 1 m (3 feet) deep and can be seen through clearly, and where the fuel supply behind the fire has been mostly consumed. Cover exposed skin and take several breaths, then move through the flame front as quickly as possible. If necessary, drop to the ground under the smoke for improved visibility and to obtain fresh air.
4. Burn out. If you are in dead grass or low shrub fuels and the approaching flames are too high to run through, burn out as large an area as possible between you and the fire edge. Step into the burned area and cover as much of your exposed skin as possible. This requires time for fuels to be consumed and may not be effective as a last-ditch effort, nor does this work well in an intense forest fire.
5. Regulate breathing. Avoid inhaling dense smoke. Keep your face near the ground, where there is usually less smoke. Hold a dampened handkerchief over the nose. Match your breathing with the availability of relatively fresh air. If there is a possibility of breathing superheated air, place a dry, not moist, cloth over the mouth. The lungs can withstand dry heat better than moist heat.
6. Protect against radiation. Many victims of forest fires actually die before the flames reach them. Radiated heat quickly causes heatstroke, a state of complete exhaustion. Find shielding to reduce heat rays quickly in an area that will not burn, such as a shallow trench, crevice, large rock, running stream, large pond, vehicle, building, or the shore water of a lake. Do not seek refuge in an elevated water tank. Avoid wells and caves because oxygen may be used up quickly in these restricted places; consider them a last resort. To protect against radiation, cover the head and other exposed skin with clothing or dirt.
7. Lie prone. In a critical situation, lie face down in an area that will not burn. Your chance of survival if the fire overtakes you is greater in this position than standing upright or kneeling.

Arnold "Smoke" Elser, an accomplished Montana outfitter, described how he helped guests avoid entrapment by a forest fire in this personal communication:

The fire began at the bottom of the canyon and proceeded up canyon as fires do. However, the wind currents carried the smoke to the east and not up the drainage to the north; therefore, we received no warning of the fire. The Monture Creek trail goes through some very old mature timber which was not burning as we approached. As my stock, the guests, and I arrived at the fire site and realized that we were in danger, we felt we should fall back and try to flank the fire to the east. Starting back toward this trail, we found a ground fire that made it very hazardous to travel in this direction. Because of my knowledge of the trail and terrain, I knew that our best bet would be to wet down the stock, guests, saddles and outer clothing and try to break through the head of the fire. We successfully did this, receiving only a few minor burns on the horses and the loss of some apparel tied to the backs of the saddles. Some lessons that I learned in this experience were that in handling livestock in a fire situation you must have a very close, firm hand on them. It is also very important that no one panics or shows any excitement, as this alarms the livestock and begins the panic run that is so well known. I found that by talking in very low monotone, keeping the

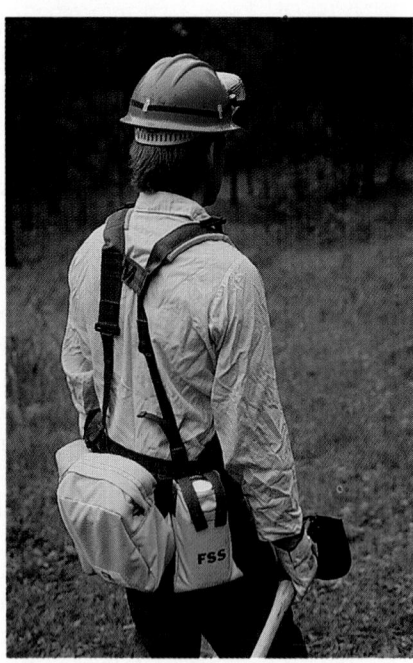

Figure 12-16 Protective clothing for a firefighter includes hard hat and safety goggles, fire-resistant shirt and trousers, leather boots and gloves, and fire shelter carried in a waist pouch. Firefighters also carry canteens to ensure an adequate water supply in a heat-stressed environment. *(Courtesy the USDA Forest Service.)*

pack stock and saddle stock very close together (head to tail), and moving on a good trail, we were able to come through this fire with virtually no harm.

Elser had these additional suggestions for wildland recreationists:

Campers, whether they be livestock oriented, hikers, or boaters, should know where to camp to provide adequate fire barriers around campsites. All campers should consider at least one, and preferably two, safe escape routes and havens (such as rock piles, rivers, and large green meadows) away from heavy fuel areas. Campers should be alert to canyon air current conditions in critical fire seasons. The safety of many recreationists is threatened by nylon and other synthetic fabrics used in the manufacture of most backpacking equipment. These materials melt upon contact with heat. The very nature of good horse packing equipment is a deterrent to fire; canvas mantles that cover the gear and the canvas pack saddles are easily wet down. Leather items such as chaps, good saddle bags, and western hats [that] can shield against heat blasts all provide important protection for the horse user.

Proper Clothing

Clothing protects against radiant heat, embers, and sparks, so it is sensible to dress appropriately (Figure 12-16). Closely woven material is more resistant to radiation and less likely to ignite than is open-weave material. Natural fibers are best. Wool is more flame resis-

tant than cotton, although cotton can be improved by chemical treatment to retard flammability. Synthetic materials are a poor choice because they readily absorb heat, ignite, or melt.

Closely woven materials that provide protection also restrict airflow, so clothes should fit loosely so that they do not interfere with dissipation of body heat. Cotton long johns or undergarments absorb sweat, aid evaporation, and do not melt. Wearing excessive layers of clothing generally contributes to heat stress.

As little skin as possible should be exposed to fire. Long trousers and a long-sleeved shirt should be worn. For maximum protection the shirt should be kept buttoned with sleeves rolled down.

Brightly colored (yellow or orange) coveralls or shirts are worn by organized firefighting crews. These colors improve safety and communications because they are visible in smoke, vegetation, and blackened landscapes.

Other essential apparel includes a safety helmet (hard hat), gloves (leather or natural fiber), leather work boots, woolen or cotton socks, a warm jacket for night wear, goggles, and a handkerchief. Clothing, backpacks, tents, and other camping equipment made of synthetics should be discarded when a person is close to a fire.

Water Intake (see Chapter 11)

Sweating is the primary method for body cooling, although exhaling warm air and inhaling cooler air also decreases body temperature. Because the cooling effect of sweat evaporation is essential for thermoregulation, fluids lost during strenuous work must be replaced. In firefighting, water losses of 0.5 L/hr (1 pint/hr) are common, with losses of up to 2 L/hr (2 quarts/hr) under extreme conditions.[16] Unless water is restored regularly, dehydration may contribute to heat stress disorders, reluctance to work, irritability, poor judgment, and impatience.

Thirst is not a good indicator of water requirements during strenuous work, so additional drinking of small quantities of water at regular intervals is recommended. A useful signal of dehydration is dark, scanty urine.

An excessive amount of electrolytes may be lost through sweating, leading to nausea, vomiting, and muscle cramps. When meals are missed or unseasoned foods are eaten, electrolyte supplements may be needed to replace lost salts. Sweetened drinks should be used as a source of energy if solid food is not available.

Personal Gear

Some rescue and medical missions take a few days. Therefore it is necessary to be prepared for extended periods and changing conditions in the backcountry (Box 12-4).

How to Report a Wildland Fire to Local Fire Protection Authorities

A caller should be prepared to provide the following information when reporting a fire:

1. Name of person giving the report
2. Where the person can be reached immediately
3. Where the person was at the time the fire was discovered
4. Location of the fire; orient the fire to prominent landmarks, such as roads, creeks, and mileposts on highways
5. Description of the fire: color and volume of the smoke, estimated size, and flame characteristics if visible
6. Whether anyone is fighting the fire at the time of the call

Portable Fire Extinguishers

People should know which extinguisher to select for a specific hazard in the home or recreational vehicle and be trained in its use. When a fire is discovered, first

evacuate occupants to safety and promptly report the fire to appropriate authorities. If the fire is small and poses no direct threat, an extinguisher should be used to fight it.

The three major classes of fires are as follows:

Class A fires: Fueled by ordinary combustible materials, such as wood, paper, cloth, upholstery, and many plastics.

Class B fires: Fueled by flammable liquids and gases, such as kitchen greases, paints, oil, and gasoline.

Class C fires: Fueled by live electrical wires or equipment, such as motors, power tools, and appliances.

The right type of extinguisher must be used for each class of fire. Water extinguishers control Class A fires by cooling and soaking burning materials. Carbon dioxide or dry chemical extinguishers are used to control Class B fires by smothering flames. Multipurpose dry chemical or liquefied gas extinguishers control Class A, B, or C fires by a smothering action. Liquefied gas extinguishers also produce a cooling effect. A dry chemical or liquefied gas extinguisher is recommended for recreational vehicles.

Wildfire Fighting Training Course

"Wildfire Fighting," a self-contained 35 mm slide-audiocassette training program produced by the National Fire Protection Association, was designed to help paid and volunteer fire departments, forestry organizations, and individual volunteers prepare for emergencies and carry out effective wildfire fighting operations. It includes useful information on prefire planning, mutual aid, logistic support, safety, fire ground organization, equipment and apparatus, and other topics essential for the safe and successful control of wildfires. The "Wildfire Fighting" program (NFPA Catalog Number SL-104; Harry Abraham, editor) can be ordered from the National Fire Protection Association, Batterymarch Park, Quincy, MA 02269.

"Lessons Learned: Fatality Fire Case Studies" (PMS 490) (1998) uses past fatality fires as a learning tool to help fireline tactical decision-makers avoid similar mistakes. It can be valuable information for emergency response personnel. The course is available from NWCG Publications Management System, National Interagency Fire Center, Attn: Great Basin Cache Supply Office, 3833 S. Development Avenue, Boise, ID 83705, phone 208-387-5104.

CONCLUSIONS

Fire suppression efforts in the late 1800s and early 1900s were largely ineffective because of limited access, absence of trained firefighting organizations, and lack of a fire detection network. During these times, many residents and numerous firefighters died in wildland fires in the United States and Canada. In the recent past, firefighters were more vulnerable to injuries and fatalities from wildland fires than was the general public. Today, with many people living and seeking recreation in wildlands, the odds for serious fire encounters are shifting toward an inexperienced populace. Large property losses and direct injuries are being reported in increasing numbers in the wildland-urban interface. Although wildland fires have not yet posed a serious threat to backcountry recreationists in the United States, the prospect for such confrontations is growing.

Experience with wildland fires allows us to conclude the following:

1. Many indicators point to the fact that increases in investments for only emergency responses to wildfires will result in more damaging and expensive wildfire emergencies in the future. Public policies and public education that link sustainable land use practices with emergency preparedness are likely to be the most successful in the long run.
2. Residential shifts to the wildland-urban interface will increase exposures to life-threatening situations.
3. The expanded use of fire in managing national parks and wildernesses will increase the likelihood that people will encounter fires.
4. The general public tends to underestimate existing fire hazards and is usually not experienced in avoiding fire threats.
5. In some instances, past fire exclusion practices have contributed to the development of more wildland fuel, setting the stage for greater rates of spread and higher intensity levels in some plant communities. The national ecosystem health issue has compounded this problem by producing vast expanses of dead and dying forests, increasing the threat to people from fast-moving, high-intensity fires.
6. Knowledge of fire behavior principles and survival guidelines will prepare people to take appropriate preventive measures in threatening situations.

The general public must share responsibility with suppression organizations to minimize fire hazards created by humans. Care with fire, proper cleanup of debris, fuel reduction efforts on wildland property, fire-safe construction guidelines, and the application of survival skills will minimize fire threats. Such precautions should become as commonplace in the wildland environment as smoke alarms and fire extinguishers have become in the home.

Wildland fire suppression agencies will continue to provide fast, safe, and energetic initial attack responses to protect human life, property, and natural resources. Under conditions of prolonged drought, strong winds, low humidities, and high temperatures, some fires will escape even the best initial attack efforts, directly threatening human life and property. Emergency medical personnel will probably have increasing exposure to wildland fires and will need to know more about fire-related injuries, fire safety, and fire survival.

ACKNOWLEDGMENTS

Line drawings on heat transfer and fire behavior are adapted from J.S. Barrows's *Fire Behavior in Northern Rocky Mountain Forests*. The booklet "Planning for Initial Attack" by the USDA Forest Service was a helpful reference on fire principles.

REFERENCES

1. Barrows JS: The challenges of forest fire management, *Western Wildlands* 1:3, 1974.
2. Brown AA, Davis P: *Forest fire: control and use*, ed 2, New York, 1973, McGraw-Hill.
3. California Department of Forestry: *Field operations guide (ICS-420-1)*, Fire Protection Publications, Oklahoma State University, 1983.
4. Cheney NP: Don't panic—and live, *Nat Dev*, p 1, 1972.
5. Cheney NP: Personal communication, 1981.
6. Colorado State Forest Service: *Wildlife hazards: guidelines for their prevention in subdivisions and developments*, Ft Collins, Colo, 1977, Colorado State University.
7. Fischer WC, Brooks DJ: Safeguarding Montana homes: lessons from the Pattee Canyon Fire, *Western Wildlands* 4:30, 1977.
8. Freedman JD: *A fire and fuel hazard analysis in the Seeley Lake area, Missoula County, Montana*, MA thesis, Missoula, Mont, 1980, University of Montana.
9. Freedman JD, Fischer WC: Forest home fire hazards, *Western Wildlands* 6:23, 1980.
10. Gleason P: LCES: the key to safe procedures, National Fire Protection Association, *Wildfire News and Notes* 5:1, 1991.
11. Gold A, Burgess WA, Clougherty EV: Exposure of firefighters to toxic air contaminants, *Am Ind Hyg Assoc J* 39:534, 1978.
12. Haines D: Downbursts and wildland fires: a dangerous combination, USDA Forest Service, *Fire Management Notes* 49:8, 1988.
13. Hulbert J: Fire problems in rural suburbs, *American Forests* 8:24, 1972.
14. Leopold AS et al: *Wildlife management in the national parks*, Trans American Wildlife and Natural Resources Conference 28:1, 1963.
15. Loucks OL: Evolution of diversity, efficiency, and community stability, *Am Zool* 10:17, 1970.
16. Luke RH, McArthur AG: *Bushfires in Australia*, CSIRO Division of Forest Research, 1978, Australian Government Publishing Service.
17. McArthur AG, Cheney NP: *Report on Southern Tasmanian Bushfires of 7 February 1967*, Hobart, Australia, 1967, Government Printer.
18. Moritz AA et al: The effect of inhaled heat on the air passages and lungs, *Am J Pathol* 21:311, 1945.
19. Moylan JA: Smoke inhalation and burn injury, *Surg Clin North Am* 60:1533, 1980.
20. Moylan JA et al: Early diagnosis of inhalation injury using ^{133}xenon lung scan, *Ann Surg* 176:477, 1973.
21. Mutch RW: *Sustaining forest health to benefit people, property, and natural resources*, In Proceedings of the 1992 Society of American Foresters National Convention.
22. Mutch RW, Rothermel RC: 73 fire fighters survive in shelters, *Fire Command* 53:30, 48, 1986.
23. National Fire Protection Association: *The Oakland/Berkeley Hills fire*, Quincy, Mass, NFPA.
24. Owen HR: *Fire and you*, Garden City, NY, 1977, Doubleday.
25. Putnam T: *Your fire shelter: a facilitator discussion guide*, Missoula Technology and Development Center, 1991, USDA Forest Service.
26. Rothermel RC: *Predicting behavior and size of crown fires in the northern Rocky Mountains*, Research Paper INT-438, 1991, USDA Forest Service.
27. Rothermel RC: *Mann Gulch fire: a race that couldn't be won*, General Technical Report INT-299, 1993, USDA Forest Service.
28. Rothman N et al: Pulmonary function and respiratory symptoms in wildland firefighters, *Occup Med* 33:1163, 1991.
29. Schroeder JJ, Buck CC: Fire weather, *Agr Handbook* 360, 1970, USDA Forest Service.

30. Sharkey BJ: *Heat stress*, Missoula, Mont, 1979, USDA Forest Service, Missoula Equipment Development Center.
31. Smith A et al: Report of U.S.-Canadian task force study of fatal and near-fatal fire accidents, National Wildfire Coordinating Group, 1981 (unpublished report).
32. Smith E, Adams G: *Incline Village/Crystal Bay defensible space handbook*, Reno, Nev, 1991, University of Nevada Reno.
33. Stone JP et al: The transport of hydrogen chloride by soot from burning polyvinyl chloride, *J Fire Flammability* 4:42, 1973.
34. Tietz JG: *Firefighters' exposure to carbon monoxide on the Deadline and Outlaw fires*, Ed T 2424 (Smoke Inhalation Hazards), Missoula, Mont, 1975, USDA Forest Service, Equipment Development Center.
35. Tischendorf JW: Structural watch out situations for the wildland/urban interface. *Wildfire News and Notes* 5(3), National Fire Protection Association.
36. Tokle GO, Marker J: Wildfire strikes home! In Laughlin J, Page C, editors: *Report of the National Wildland/Urban Fire Protection Conference*, 1987.
37. US Department of the Interior and US Department of Agriculture: *Federal wildland fire management policy and program review. Final report.* National Interagency Fire Center, Boise, Idaho, 1995.
38. Ward D: *Air toxics and fireline exposure*, Paper presented at 10th Conference on Fire and Forest Meteorology, Ottawa, Canada, 1989.
39. Ward D et al: The effects of forest fire smoke in firefighters: a comprehensive study plan. A special report for Congressional Committee of Appropriations for Title II–Related Agencies, USDA Forest Service and National Wildfire Coordinating Group, 1989.
40. Webster J: *The complete Australian bushfire book*, Melbourne, Australia, 1986, Thomas Nelson.
41. Wilson CC: Commingling of urban forest fires (a case study of the 1970 California near-disaster), *Fire Res Abs Rev* 13:35, 1971.
42. Wilson CC: Fatal and near-fatal forest fires, the common denominators, *Int Fire Chief* 43:9, 1977.
43. Wroblewski DA, Bower GC: The significance of facial burns in acute smoke inhalation, *Crit Care Med* 7:335, 1979.
44. Zapp JA: Fires, toxicity and plastics. In *Physiological and toxicological products*, 1976, Committee on Fire Research, National Research Council, National Academy of Sciences.
45. Zikria BA et al: Respiratory tract damage in burns: pathophysiology and treatment, *Ann NY Acad Sci* 150:618, 1968.

SUGGESTED READINGS

Barrows JS: *Fire behavior in northern Rocky Mountain forests*, USDA Forest Service, Northern Rocky Mtn For and Range Exp Sta, Station 1951, Paper No 29.
Cohen S, Miller D: *The big burn*, Missoula, Mont, 1978, Pictorial Histories. (The Northwest's forest fire of 1910.)
Cottrell WH: *The book of fire*, Missoula, Mont, 1989, Mountain Press.
Countryman CM: *Carbon monoxide: a firefighting problem*, USDA Forest Service, Pacific SW For and Range Exp Sta, 1971.
Gaylor HP: *Wildfires: prevention and control*, Bowie, Md, 1974, RJ Brady.
Mangan R: Wildland fire fatalities in the United States, Missoula, Montana, USDA Forest Service, Technology and Development Program, 9951-2808-MTDC, 1999.
National Fire Protection Association: *Black Tiger fire case study*, Quincy, Mass, NFPA.
National Fire Protection Association: *Stephan Bridge Road fire case study*, Quincy, Mass, NFPA.
National Fire Protection Association: NFPA 299 *Protection of life and property from wildfire*, Quincy, Mass, 1991, NFPA.
National Wildfire Coordinating Group: Historical wildland firefighter fatalities, 1910-1996. NFES 1849, 1997.
Pringle L: *Natural fire: its ecology in forests*, New York, 1979, William Morrow.
Radtke K: *Living more safely at the chaparral-urban interface*. USDA Forest Service and County of Los Angeles Dept of Forestry and Fire Warden, Pacific Southwest Forest and Range Exp Sta, 1981.
Radtke KWH: *A homeowner's guide to fire and watershed management at the chaparral-urban interface*, County of Los Angeles, Calif, 1982. (Available from Santa Monica Mountains Residents Association, 21656 Las Flores Hts Rd, Malibu, CA 90265; cost $0.50.)
TriData Corporation: Wildland firefighter safety awareness study (Phase III), Arlington, Va, 1998.
US Department of Agriculture, US Department of the Interior, and US Department of Commerce: South Canyon Fire Investigation, 1994, Washington, DC, USDA, USDI, USDC, US Government Printing Office, Region 8.
Webster J: *The complete Australian bushfire book*, 1986, Thomas Nelson.

13 Emergency Care of the Burned Victim

Roberta A. Mann and David Heimbach

EPIDEMIOLOGY

Each year in the United States approximately 2 million individuals are burned seriously enough to seek the care of a physician, and about 70,000 of these require hospitalization. Fortunately, the number of deaths attributable to burns decreased from 12,000 in 1979 to 6000 in 1990. Although treatment facilities would like to take credit for this decrease, the most likely factor responsible is the widespread use of smoke detectors in both public and private dwellings. It has been estimated that more than 90% of burns are preventable and that most are caused by carelessness or ignorance. During the next few years, the biggest contributions in decreasing burn mortality and morbidity may come not from medical scientists but rather from improved engineering design and more successful programs in teaching burn prevention to the public.

Like other forms of trauma, burns frequently affect children and young adults. The hospital expenses and the social costs related to time away from work or school are staggering. Although most burns are limited in extent, a significant burn of the hand or foot may prevent a manual laborer from working for a year or more and in some cases may permanently prevent a return to former activity. The eventual outcome for the burned victim is related to the severity of the injury, individual physical characteristics of the victim, motivation toward rehabilitation, and the quality of treatment of the acute burn.

Most persons with burns who are seen by physicians visit emergency departments, where judgment in triage, care plan for small burns, and initial management for major burns can influence survival of the victim and eventual cosmetic and functional results. Because most victims are young and about one third are children, they will live with the consequences of the acute treatment for an average of 50 years.

The decisions made at the initial contact with the victim require answers to the algorithm shown in Figure 13-1. This chapter describes first responder care for major burns and is organized to guide assessment of burn severity and initial management of the serious burns, as well as to provide an initial treatment plan for minor burns.

PHYSIOLOGY

For burns other than chemical burns, the primary events of injury occur during the time of heat contact.

Coagulation necrosis takes place within cells, and denaturation of collagen occurs in the dermis. Either blood vessels are completely destroyed or the endothelium is damaged severely enough to cause clotting, which leads to ischemic necrosis of remaining viable cells. The burn wound is not static. Surrounding the "zone of coagulation" is a zone of capillary and small vessel stasis. Red cells form into rouleaux, platelet and white cell aggregates form, and the circulation becomes stagnant. Over the next hours or even days the ultimate fate of the burn wound depends on the resolution or progression of this zone of stasis. Cells and tissue stroma release mediators to initiate the inflammatory response. Histamine, serotonin, prostaglandin derivatives, and the complement cascade all have roles. In victims with burns of less than 10% of the total body surface area (TBSA), the actions of these mediators are generally limited to the burn site itself. Capillary permeability increases, neutrophils marginate, and additional inflammatory cells (monocytes, macrophages) are attracted by chemotaxis to the site of injury, initiating the healing process.

As burns approach 20% TBSA, the local response becomes systemic. The capillary leak, permitting loss of fluid and protein from the intravascular compartment into the extravascular compartment, becomes generalized. Cardiac output falls as a result of marked increased peripheral resistance, decreased intravascular fluid volume from the capillary leak, and the accompanying increase in blood viscosity. The decreased blood volume and cardiac output, accompanied by an intense sympathetic response, lead to decreased perfusion to the skin and viscera. Decreased flow to the skin can convert the zone of stasis to one of coagulation, increasing the depth of the burn. The capillary leak and depressed cardiac output lead to depressed central nervous system (CNS) function, and in extreme cases they result in severe cardiac depression with eventual cardiac failure in healthy patients or in myocardial infarction in patients with preexisting coronary artery disease. The first sign of CNS change is restlessness, followed by lethargy and finally coma. Without adequate resuscitation, burns of 30% TBSA frequently lead to acute renal failure, which in a victim with a severe burn almost invariably leads to a fatal outcome.

Cardiovascular changes begin immediately after a burn. The extent of these changes depends primarily on the size of the burn and to a lesser extent on the depth of the burn. Most victims with uncomplicated

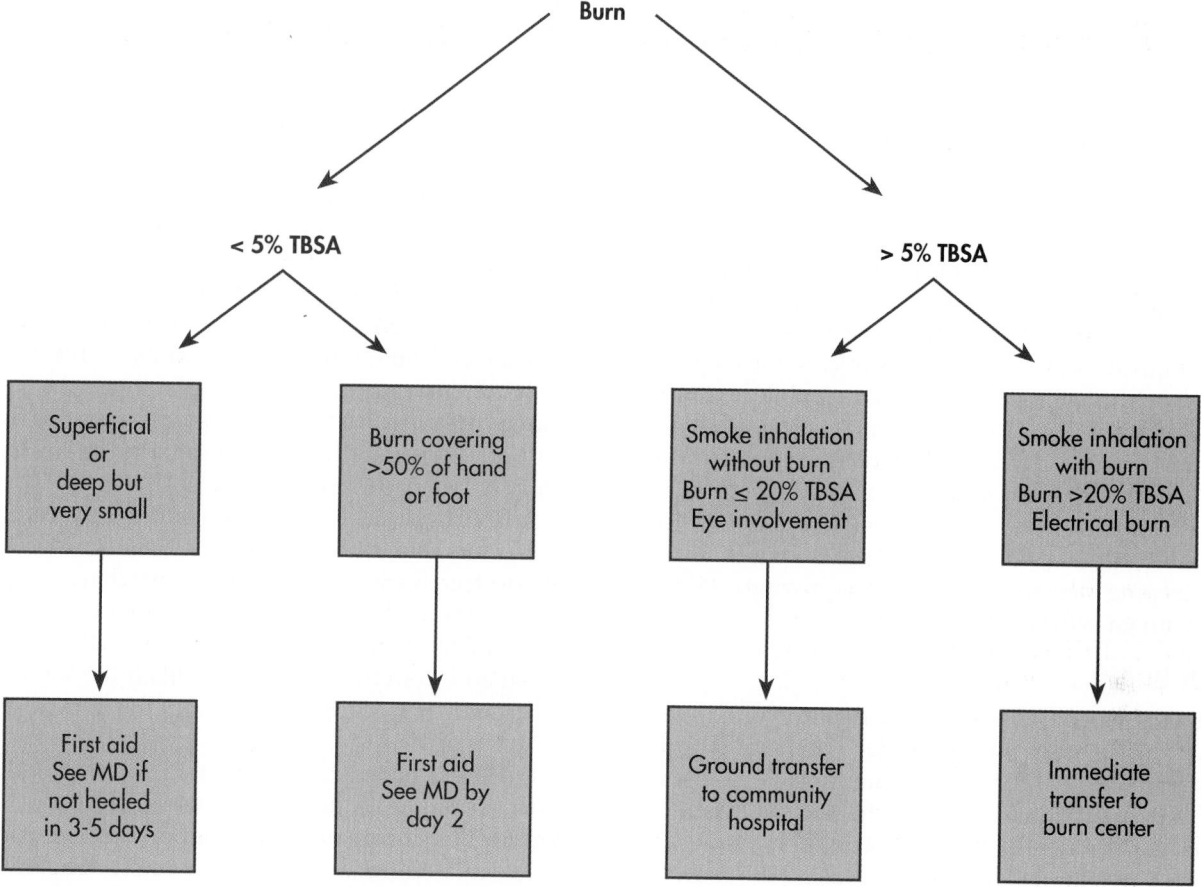

Figure 13-1 Algorithm for decision making at the scene.

burns of less than 15% TBSA can undergo oral fluid resuscitation with some salt-containing solution. As the burn extent passes 20% TBSA, massive shifts of fluid and electrolytes occur from the intravascular into the extravascular (extracellular) space. Reversal of the shifts begins during the second postburn day, but normal extracellular volume is not completely restored until 7 to 10 days after the burn. Unless the intravascular volume is depleted, classic hypovolemic shock occurs. An untreated person will die of cardiovascular collapse; if treatment is poor, irreversible acute tubular necrosis and renal failure will develop.

TYPE OF BURNS

Scald Burns

In civilian practice, scalds, usually resulting from hot water, are the most common cause of burns. Water at 60° C (140° F) creates a deep partial-thickness or full-thickness burn in 3 seconds. At 68.9° C (156° F) the same burn occurs in 1 second. Freshly brewed coffee from an automatic percolator is generally about 82° C (180° F). Boiling water always causes deep burns, and soups and sauces, which are thicker in consistency, remain in con-

tact longer with the skin and often cause deep burns. In general, exposed areas tend to be burned less deeply than areas covered with thin clothing. Clothing retains the heat and keeps the liquid in contact with the skin for a longer time.

Immersion scalds are deep and severe burns.[21,31,97] Although the water may be cooler than with a spill scald, the duration of contact is longer and these burns frequently occur in small children or elderly victims with thin skin. Consequently, many states have passed legislation to set home and public hot water heaters to maximum temperatures well below 60° C (140° F).

Scald burns from grease or hot oil are generally deep partial thickness or full thickness. Cooking oil and grease, when hot enough to use for cooking, may be in the range of 204.4° C (400° F). Tar and asphalt burns are a special kind of scald. The "mother pot" at the back of the roofing truck maintains tar at a temperature of 204.4° to 260° C (400° to 500° F). Burns caused by tar directly from the mother pot are invariably full thickness. By the time the tar is spread on the roof, its temperature has decreased enough that most of the burns are deep partial thickness. Unfortunately, the initial evaluator cannot usually examine these burns because of the adherent tar. The tar should be removed by application of a petroleum-based ointment (such as Vaseline) under a dressing. The dressing may be removed and the ointment reapplied every 2 to 4 hours until the tar has dissolved. Only then can the extent of the injury and the depth of the burn be accurately estimated.[43,96]

Flame Burns

Flame burns are the next most common burn injuries. Although injuries in house fires have decreased with the advent of smoke detectors, a significant number of burn injuries still result from careless smoking, improper use of flammable liquids, automobile accidents, and clothing ignited from stoves or space heaters. Victims whose bedding or clothes have been on fire rarely escape without some full-thickness burns. Outdoor misadventures result from using cooking stoves fueled by white gasoline, taking lanterns into tents, smoking in a sleeping bag, and starting (or improving) charcoal fires with gasoline or kerosene.

Flash Burns

Flash burns are next in frequency. Explosions of natural gas, propane, gasoline, and other flammable liquids cause intense heat for a very brief time. For the most part, unignited clothing protects the skin in flash burns. Flash burns generally have a distribution over all exposed skin, with the deepest areas facing the source of ignition. Flash burns are partial thickness, with the depth dependent on the amount and kind of fuel that explodes. Although such burns generally heat without requiring extensive skin grafts, they may be very large and associated with significant thermal damage to the upper airway.

Contact Burns

Contact burns result from hot metals, plastic, glass, or hot coals. Such burns are usually limited in extent but deep. Victims involved in industrial accidents commonly have both severe contact burns and crush injuries, since these accidents often occur from presses or from hot, heavy objects. With the increased use of wood-burning stoves, an increasing number of toddlers are burned each year. The most common injuries are deep burns on the palms because the child falls with hands outstretched against the stove. Contact burns, especially in unconscious persons or those dealing with molten materials, are frequently fourth degree.[19,56,84] In the wilderness setting the most common contact burn is from hot coals. Intoxicated campers dance around and then into the campfire, architects of "river saunas" mishandle hot rocks, children fall into fires, and beach walkers may sustain deep burns when coals are buried in sand overnight. Even though the injured areas may be small, they can be deep and devastating when the hiker must walk a considerable distance on burned feet.[27]

Electrical Burns

Electrical burns are actually thermal burns from very high–intensity heat. As electricity meets the resistance of body tissues, it is converted to heat in direct proportion to the amperage of the current and the electrical resistance of the body parts through which it passes. The smaller the body part through which the electricity passes, the more intense the heat and the less it is dissipated. Therefore fingers, hands, forearms, feet, and lower legs are frequently totally destroyed, whereas larger-volume areas, such as the trunk, usually dissipate the current enough to prevent extensive damage to the viscera, unless the contact point is on the abdomen or chest. Although cutaneous manifestations may appear limited, massive underlying tissue destruction may be present.[18,36,37,68]

Arc burns occur when current takes the most direct path rather than the one of least resistance. These deep and destructive wounds occur at joints that are in close apposition at the time of injury. Most common are burns of the forearm to the arm when the elbow is flexed and from the arm to the axilla if the shoulder is adducted when current passes from the upper extremity to the trunk.

Electrical burns cause a particular set of other injuries and complications that must be considered during the initial evaluation. As mentioned previously, injuries related to a fall are common. The intense associated muscle contractions may cause fractures of the lumbar vertebrae, humerus, or femur and may dislocate shoulders or hips.

Electrical cardiac damage may have symptoms like those of a myocardial contusion or infarction. Alternatively, the conduction system may be deranged. There can be actual rupture of the heart wall or of a papillary muscle leading to sudden valvular incompetence and refractory cardiac failure. Household current at 110 volts generally either does no damage or induces ventricular fibrillation. Alternating current is more likely to induce fibrillation than is direct current. If no cardiac abnormalities are present when a victim is first seen after shocks of 110 to 220 volts, the likelihood that they will appear later is small.

The nervous system is particularly sensitive to electricity. The most severe brain damage occurs when current passes through the head, but spinal cord damage is possible any time current passes from one side of the body to the other.[47,51] Myelin-producing cells are susceptible. The devastating effects of transverse myelitis may develop days or weeks after injury. Conduction remains normal through existing myelin, but as the old myelin wears out, it is not replaced and conduction stops. Peripheral nerves are commonly damaged and may demonstrate severe permanent functional impairment.[23,34] Every victim with an electrical injury must have a thorough neurologic examination as part of the initial assessment. Myoglobinuria is a frequent accompaniment of severe electrical burns. Disruption of muscle cells releases cell fragments and myoglobin into the circulation to be filtered by the kidney. If untreated, this can lead to permanent renal failure.

Lightning strikes are discussed in Chapter 3. Several recent reviews are available.*

Chemical Burns

Chemical burns, usually caused by strong acids or alkalis, are most often the result of industrial accidents, home use of drain cleaners, assaults, and other improper use of harsh solvents.† In contrast to thermal burns, chemical burns cause progressive damage until the chemicals are inactivated by reaction with the tissue or dilution by flushing with water. Although individual circumstances vary, acid burns may be more self-limiting than are alkali burns. Acid tends to "tan" the skin, creating an impermeable barrier that limits further penetration of the acid. Alkalis combine with cutaneous lipids and saponify the skin until they are neutralized. A full-thickness chemical burn may appear deceptively superficial, appearing as only a mild brownish surface discoloration. The skin may appear intact during the first few days after the burn and then begin to slough spontaneously. Unless the observer can be absolutely certain, chemical burns should be considered deep partial thickness or full thickness until proven otherwise.

CLINICAL PRESENTATION

Cutaneous burns are caused by the application of heat or caustic chemicals to the skin. When heat is applied to the skin, the depth of injury is proportional to the temperature applied, the duration of contact, and the thickness of the skin.

The severity of the burn injury is related to the size of the burn, the depth of the burn, and the part of the body that is burned.

Estimation of Burn Size

Burns are the only quantifiable form of trauma. The single most important feature in predicting mortality, need for specialized care, and the complications expected from the burn is the overall burn size in proportion to the victim's TBSA. Treatment plans, including initial resuscitation and subsequent nutritional requirements, are derived directly from the size of the burn.

A general idea of burn size is provided by the "rule of nines." Each upper extremity accounts for 9% of TBSA, each lower extremity accounts for 18%, the an-

terior and posterior trunk each account for 18%, the head and neck account for 9%, and the perineum accounts for 1% (Figure 13-2). Although the "rule of nines" provides a reasonably accurate estimate of burn size, a number of more precise charts have been developed. A diagram of the burn can be drawn on a chart so that a relatively precise calculation of burned area can be made from the accompanying TBSA estimates given. Children under 4 years of age have much larger heads and smaller thighs in proportion to body size than do adults. In an infant the head accounts for nearly 20% of the TBSA; body proportions do not fully reach adult percentages until adolescence. To further increase accuracy in burn size estimation, especially when burns are in scattered body areas, the observer might calculate the unburned areas on a separate diagram. If the calculations of the unburned areas and the burned areas do not add up to 100%, the observer should begin again with a new diagram to calculate the burned areas. For smaller burns an accurate assessment of burn size can be made by using the victim's hand. The hand amounts to 2.5% TBSA. The dorsal surface accounts for 1%, the palmar surface for 1%, and the vertical surface for 0.5%.

Depth of Burn

An understanding of burn depth requires an understanding of skin anatomy (Figure 13-3). The epidermis, an intensely active layer of epithelial cells under layers of dead keratinized cells, is superficial to the active structural framework of the skin, the dermis. Although metabolically very active, the dermis has no regenerative capacity, and epithelial cells must eventually cover the surface of the dermis before the burn is healed. The skin appendages (hair follicles, sebaceous glands, and sweat glands) all contain an epithelial cell lining, so when the surface epidermis has been killed, epithelial covering must take place from overgrowth of the epithelial cells lining the skin appendages. As these cells reach the surface, they spread laterally to meet their neighbors, creating a new epithelial surface. As the burn extends deeper into the dermis, fewer and fewer appendages remain, and the epithelial remnants must travel farther to produce a new surface covering, sometimes taking many weeks to produce coverage. When the burn extends beyond the deepest layer of the skin appendages, the wound can heal only by epithelial ingrowth from the edges, by wound contraction, or by surgical transplantation of skin from a different site. The thickness of skin varies both with the age and gender of the individual and with the part of the body considered. Although the thickness of the living epidermis is relatively constant, keratinized epidermal cells may reach a height of 5 mm on palms of hands and soles of feet. The thickness of the dermis, on the other hand, may vary from less than 1 mm on eyelids and genitalia

---

*References 24, 25, 28, 29, 57, 68.
†References 26, 38, 62, 64, 76, 79, 86.

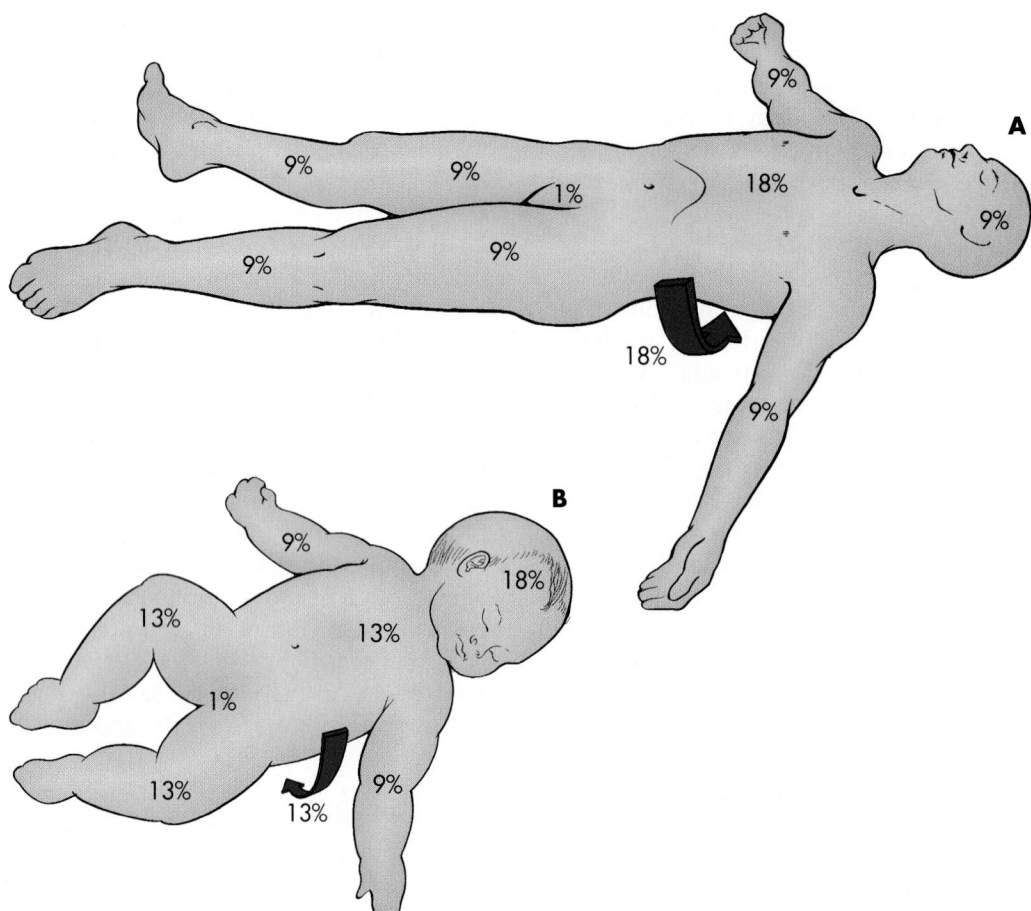

Figure 13-2 Rule of nines used for estimating burned surface area. **A,** Adult. **B,** Infant.

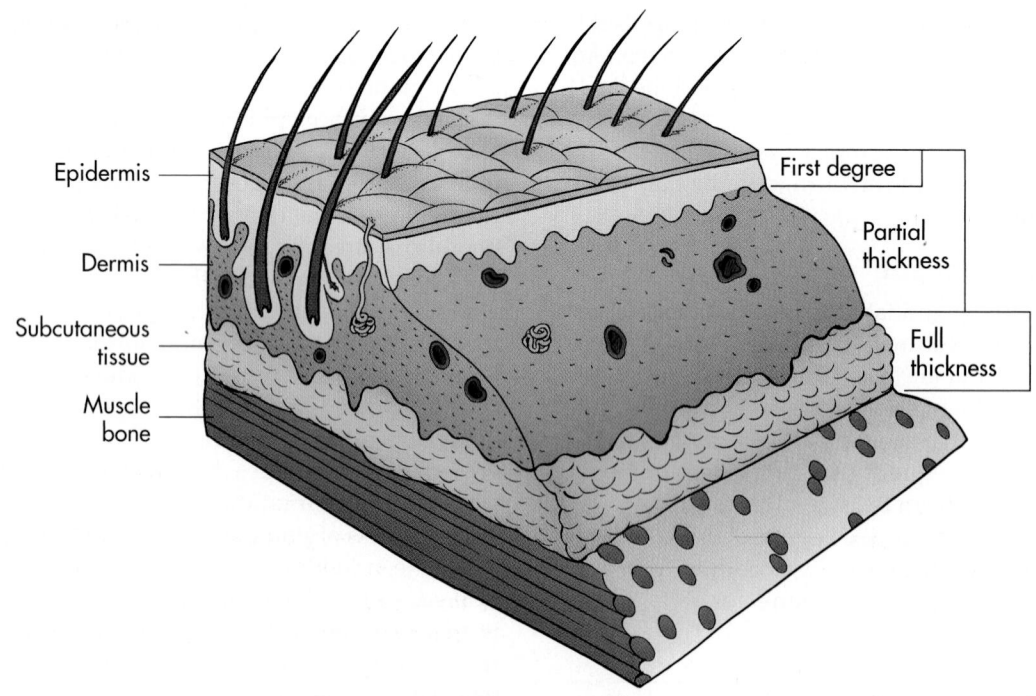

Figure 13-3 Skin anatomy.

to more than 5 mm on the posterior trunk. Although the proportional thickness of skin in each body area is similar in children, infant skin thickness in each specific area may be less than half that of adult skin; the skin does not reach adult thickness until adolescence. Similarly, in patients over 50 years of age, dermal atrophy causes all areas of skin to become quite thin.

Burns are classified by increasing depth as first degree, superficial partial thickness, deep partial thickness, full thickness, and fourth degree.

First-Degree Burns. First-degree burns involve only the epidermis. The prototype is mild sunburn. First-degree burns do not blister. They become erythematous because of dermal vasodilation and are quite painful, both spontaneously and when touched. The erythema and pain subside over 2 to 3 days. By the fourth day the injured epithelium desquamates in the phenomenon of "peeling."

Superficial Partial-Thickness Burns. Superficial partial-thickness burns include the upper layers of dermis and characteristically form blisters with fluid collection at the interface of the epidermis and dermis. Blistering may not occur for some hours after injury. Burns initially thought to be first degree may therefore be diagnosed as superficial partial thickness by day 2. When blisters are removed, the wound is pink and wet and is quite painful as currents of air contact it. The wound is hypersensitive to touch and blanches with pressure, and blood flow to the dermis is increased over that of normal skin. If infection is prevented, superficial partial-thickness burns heal spontaneously within 3 weeks without functional impairment. They rarely cause hypertrophic scarring, but in pigmented individuals the healed burns may never completely match the color of the surrounding normal skin.

Deep Partial-Thickness Burns. Deep partial-thickness burns also blister, but the wound surface is usually a mottled pink and white color immediately after the injury. The victim complains of discomfort rather than pain. When pressure is applied to the burn, capillary refill returns slowly or may be absent. The wound is often less sensitive to touch than is the surrounding normal skin. By the second day the wound may be white and is usually fairly dry. If infection is prevented, such burns heal in 3 to 9 weeks but invariably do so with considerable scar formation. Unless active physical therapy is continued throughout the healing process, joint function may be impaired and hypertrophic scarring, particularly in pigmented individuals and children, becomes inevitable.

Full-Thickness Burns. Full-thickness burns involve all layers of the dermis and can heal only by wound contracture, epithelialization from the wound margin, or skin grafting. Full-thickness burns are classically described as leathery, firm, depressed when compared with the adjoining normal skin, and insensitive to light touch or pinprick. Unfortunately, the difference in depth between a deep partial-thickness burn and a full-thickness burn may be less than 1 mm. Full-thickness burns are easily misdiagnosed as deep partial-thickness burns, since the two types have many of the same clinical findings. For example, they may be mottled in appearance. They rarely blanch with pressure, and they may have a dry, white appearance. The burn may be translucent with clotted vessels visible in the depths. Some full-thickness burns, particularly immersion scalds, have a red appearance and can be confused with superficial partial-thickness burns by the uninitiated. However, these red, full-thickness burns do not blanch with pressure. Full-thickness burns develop a classic burn eschar. An eschar represents the structurally intact but dead and denatured dermis that, over days to weeks, separates spontaneously from the underlying viable tissue.

Fourth-Degree Burns. Fourth-degree burns involve not only all layers of the skin but also subcutaneous fat and deeper structures. These burns almost always have a charred appearance, and frequently only the cause of the burn gives a clue to the amount of underlying tissue destruction.

Although these descriptions appear to separate burns into clearly defined categories, many burns have a mixture of characteristics that give the observer an imprecise diagnostic ability. Considerable research is under way to devise instruments that will more precisely measure the depth of injury. Much of current burn treatment depends on knowledge of the depth of the burn.

TREATMENT

Care at the Scene

Flame Burns. The first responder must remove the injured person from the source of heat. Because of the potential dangers of smoke inhalation in closed areas, the rescuer in a fire must take extreme caution not to become a victim. Persons with burning clothing should be prevented from running and should be made to lie down to keep flames and smoke away from the face. If water is not immediately available, the flames can be smothered with a coat or blanket. If nothing is available, the victim should be rolled slowly on the ground. Once the burning has stopped, the clothes should be removed; some fabrics will continue to smolder and synthetic fabrics may melt, leaving a hot adherent residue on the victim that will continue the burning process.

Scalds and Grease Burns. The victim of a scald or grease burn must be removed from the source of heat.

Any wet clothing or wrap should be removed, since fabric retains moist heat and may continue to burn skin that is in contact with the hot material. Accidents resulting from cooking indoors with grease are particularly hazardous. The startle response to a grease splatter may cause the victim to drop a pan of grease onto the fire, starting a kitchen fire that can rapidly become a dwelling fire.

Airway. Once flames are extinguished, primary attention must be directed to the airway. Any person rescued from a closed space or involved in a smoky fire should be considered at risk for smoke inhalation injury. If compressed oxygen is not available and the victim is coughing independently, he or she should be encouraged to continue to do so. If the victim is unconscious or the airway status is in question, the victim should be placed supine and the airway manipulated manually via the chin lift or jaw thrust maneuver. When possible, 100% oxygen should be administered by tight-fitting mask if smoke inhalation is suspected. If the victim is unconscious and if personnel are trained to insert an endotracheal tube, such a tube should be passed and attached to a source of 100% oxygen. If the airway has to be supported by a tight mask, the rescuers must be aware of the significant danger of aspiration of gastric contents. Air forced into the stomach distends it and causes vomiting. The mask prevents expulsion of the fluid, and the victim rapidly aspirates vomitus into the tracheobronchial tree. No unconscious supine victim should ever be left unattended.

Other Injuries and Transport. Once an airway is secured, the first responder should quickly assess the victim for other injuries and then transport him or her to the nearest hospital.[9,23,68] Victims should be kept flat and warm and should be given nothing by mouth. Aside from establishment of an airway, further resuscitation is unnecessary if the victim will arrive at a hospital within 30 minutes. For transport the victim should be wrapped in a clean, dry sheet and blanket. Sterility is not required.

Cold Application. Smaller burns, particularly scalds, may be treated with immediate application of cool water in hopes of limiting the extent of injury. The application of cold water is controversial, but immediate cooling does decrease the pain, possibly by a decrease in thromboxane production. By the time several minutes have passed, or after arrival in the emergency department, further cooling is not likely to alter the pathologic process. Ice water should not be used except on the smallest burns. Using ice on larger burns can easily induce systemic hypothermia and associated cutaneous vasoconstriction that can extend the thermal damage.

Swelling. During transport, constricting clothing and jewelry should be removed from burned and distal parts, since local swelling begins almost immediately. Constricting objects increase the swelling, and the removal of tight jewelry in the presence of distal edema is time consuming once swelling has occurred.

Electrical Burns. Electrical burns are particularly dangerous, both to the victim and to the rescuer. If the victim remains in contact with the source of electricity, the rescuer must avoid touching the victim until the current can be turned off or the wires cut with properly insulated wire cutters. Once the victim is removed from the source of current, airway, breathing, and circulation must be checked. Ventricular fibrillation or standstill is a common accompaniment to a major transthoracic current; cardiopulmonary resuscitation should be instituted if carotid or femoral pulses are not palpable. If pulses are present but the victim is apneic, mouth-to-mouth resuscitation alone may be lifesaving. Cardiopulmonary resuscitation should continue until a cardiac monitor can be obtained, which will direct treatment with epinephrine for cardiac standstill or defibrillation for ventricular fibrillation. Once an airway is established and pulses return, a careful search must be made for associated life-threatening injuries. Electrocuted victims frequently fall from heights and may have serious head or neck injuries. The intense tetanic muscle contractions associated with electrocution may fracture vertebrae or cause major joint dislocations. Patients with high-voltage electrical injuries should be treated with spinal precautions, and splints if necessary, until fractures can be ruled out.

Chemical Burns. Whenever possible, chemical burns should be thoroughly flushed with copious amounts of water at the scene of the accident. Chemicals will continue to burn until removed; washing for 5 to 10 minutes under a stream of running water may limit the overall severity of the burn. No thought should be given to searching for a specific neutralizing agent. Delay deepens the burn, and neutralizing agents may cause burns themselves; they frequently generate heat while neutralizing the offending agent, adding a thermal burn to the already potentially serious chemical burn.

First Aid at the Scene for Smaller Burns. Not all burns need immediate medical attention. Burns less than 5% TBSA (excluding deep burns of the face, hands, feet, perineum, or circumferential extremity) can be treated successfully in a wilderness setting if adequate first-aid supplies are available and wound care is performed diligently. Except for the very shallow burn that heals within a few days, most burns should be seen by a physician within 3 to 5 days after injury.

Burns should be washed thoroughly with plain soap and water and dried with a clean towel. Any obviously dead skin should be peeled off (which may be painful) or trimmed with sharp manicure scissors (usually painless). Large (greater than 2.5 cm), thin, fluid-filled blisters should be drained and the dead skin trimmed away. Small, thick blisters may be left intact. If any blister begins to leak fluid, it should be drained and trimmed to prevent a potential closed-space infection. Deep burns, as from a flame, are firm and leathery and do not require immediate debridement. A small tube of silver sulfadiazine cream and tubes of antibiotic (such as bacitracin) ointment should be available in the first-aid kit. Either may be used and should be spread lightly over the wound. The wound may then be wrapped in dry, clean gauze, which does not have to be sterile. Simple dressings (one type of topical cream, plain gauze) are sufficient. Some patients prefer nonadherent dressings, such as Telfa, because they are less likely to stick to the wound during dressing changes. The same effect can be achieved by soaking (with water) a plain gauze dressing that appears stuck to the wound, waiting a few minutes, and then removing the dressing with additional water if necessary. Other dressings are available (antibiotic-impregnated silicone gel sheets, calcium aginate). Although patients may prefer one dressing over another for various reasons, no dressing has been shown conclusively to accelerate the healing of burn wounds. The first-aid kit should be stocked with general use supplies; soaps and dressings designed specifically for burns are expensive and unnecessary.

Mobility of the wound area must be actively maintained, and concentrated efforts should be made to avoid dependent positioning, especially when the victim is resting or sleeping. Focal edema in a small burn wound can be painful and alarming and should be prevented with extremity elevation and active range-of-motion exercises several times a day. Wound care should be performed once a day if the dressing remains dry. A wet, sticky dressing needs more frequent wound care. If only the outer dressing is dirty, it be changed as needed. For the quickest healing of superficial burns, daily wound care should remove all exudate and crust, both of which significantly retard wound healing. Items for the first-aid kit include plain (not perfumed) soap, sharp scissors (large and small), a small tube of silver sulfadiazine, tube(s) of bacitracin ointment, cotton gauze, Band-Aids, tape, and acetaminophen.

Emergency Department Care

The primary rule for the emergency physician is to "forget about the burn." Although a burn is usually readily apparent and often a dramatic injury, a careful search for other life-threatening injuries must take priority. Only after an overall assessment of the victim's condition should attention be directed to the specific problem of the burns. Assessment of the non–thermally injured victim is presented in Chapter 18; the following sections consider the specific problems encountered in the victim with burns.

Resuscitation

During the past 30 years more than a dozen resuscitation plans have been suggested. The goal of all resuscitation plans is to complete treatment with a living victim who has normally functioning kidneys and does not have cardiac failure or pulmonary edema. Nearly all of these plans use a combination of colloid and crystalloid solutions, but they vary considerably in the ratio of colloid to crystalloid, the timing of colloid administration, the sodium concentration of crystalloid solution, and to a much lesser extent the total volume of fluid given.* Some require frequent changing of solutions, others require mixing of solutions, and some require careful monitoring of the victim's electrolytes. Intense controversy rages over the "best" resuscitation plan. The controversy, however, need not concern the physician without a special interest in burn physiology. There is general agreement on a few facts. A victim with very large burns will probably need both colloid and crystalloid. Initially, capillaries are permeable to both crystalloid and colloid solutions. The capillary leak to albumin and other large molecules repairs itself between hours 6 and 24.

The choice of formulas for initial resuscitation is probably of relatively little consequence as long as the rate of fluid administration is modified according to the victim's changing requirements as the hours pass. Because of its simplicity, ease of administration, and need for little blood chemistry monitoring, the formula developed by Baxter, known as the Baxter formula, or Parkland formula, has been adopted by most hospitals and has been recommended officially by the American College of Surgeons Committee on Trauma.

According to the Baxter formula, crystalloid is given during the first 24 hours while the capillaries are still permeable to albumin and then colloid is given during the second 24 hours when the capillary leak has presumably sealed. Rapid administration of crystalloid solution results in early expansion of depleted plasma volume, which will return cardiac output toward normal. Once the capillary leak has sealed, colloid (usually in the form of albumin) remains the most effective solution to maintain plasma volume without further increasing edema. The Baxter formula was derived to provide specific replacement of known deficits measured by simultaneous determinations of red blood cell volume, plasma volume, extracellular fluid volume, and cardiac output during burn shock.

---

*References 4, 16, 32, 35, 41, 59, 63, 65.

The first 24-hour and second 24-hour calculations are shown in Box 13-1. The formula calls for the administration of lactated Ringer's solution, 4 ml/kg body weight/percent body surface burned during the first 24 hours after the injury. Half of this fluid should be given in the first 8 hours and the second half during the next 16 hours. Fluid therapy during the second 24 hours consists of the administration of free water in quantity sufficient to maintain a normal serum sodium concentration, as well as plasma (or other colloid) to maintain a normal plasma volume.

The adequacy of resuscitation can best be judged by frequent measurements of vital signs, central venous pressure, and urine output and by observation of general mental and physical responses. Despite myriad new monitoring devices, urine output remains one of the most sensitive and reliable assessments of fluid resuscitation. In the absence of myoglobinuria a urine output of 0.5 ml/kg/hr in adults and 1 ml/kg/hr in children less than 10 kg ensures that renal perfusion is adequate. The victim's sensorium gives an indication of the state of cerebral perfusion and oxygenation. The victim should be alert and cooperative; confusion and combativeness are signs of inadequate resuscitation or warn of other causes of hypoxia.

Victims with burns of less than 50% TBSA can usually be resuscitated with a single large-bore peripheral intravenous (IV) line. Because of the high incidence of septic thrombophlebitis, lower extremities should be avoided as IV portals. Upper extremities are preferable, even if the IV line must pass through burned skin. Victims with burns larger than 50% TBSA or who have associated medical problems, are at the extremes of age, or have concomitant smoke inhalation should have additional central venous pressure monitoring. Because of the extremely unstable state of the circulation in victims with burns over 65%, such victims should be monitored in an intensive care setting where a Swan-Ganz catheter for measuring pulmonary capillary wedge pressure and cardiac output is available.

The presence of myoglobinuria alters the resuscitation plan. Myoglobinuria results from the destruction of muscle cells with release of the red muscle pigment myoglobin. This is most often a problem in victims with associated crush injuries, electrical burns, or extremely deep thermal burns. Characteristic cola-colored urine is an indication to increase the amount of fluid given and to establish a diuresis of 70 to 100 ml urine per hour. An initial bolus of 12.5 g of mannitol with a repeat dose in 15 to 30 minutes should be considered.

Escharotomy

Careful monitoring of the peripheral circulation is required in victims with circumferential full-thickness burns of the extremities. The edema that forms beneath inelastic eschar increases tissue pressure to a point at which it exceeds lymphatic pressure, thereby further increasing edema. When the edema exceeds venous pressure and eventually approaches arterial pressure, it stops all circulation to the extremity distal to the constricted area.

The classic findings of a compartment syndrome, usually considered to be pain, paresthesias, pulselessness, and tense swelling, may or may not be present in the burned extremity. Therefore distal pulses should be carefully monitored with a Doppler ultrasound, and if any of the clinical signs mentioned above occur, or if Doppler signals disappear, an escharotomy should be performed immediately.

Escharotomy is performed as a ward procedure and does not require an anesthetic, since only insensate full-thickness burn is incised. An incision is made through the eschar into subcutaneous tissue, first along the lateral aspect of the extremity and, if symptoms or signs do not improve, along the medial aspect. The incisions need not be as deep as the investing muscle fascia, and bleeding can usually be easily controlled with an electrocautery and the use of topical clotting agents. If arrival to hospital will be within 6 hours, escharotomies should not be done in the field because the victim may bleed to death without proper equipment to control bleeding.

Circumferential full-thickness burns of the trunk in small children occasionally demand an escharotomy to improve pulmonary function. Chest wall escharotomies are made in the anterior axillary line bilaterally, extending from the clavicle to the costal margin. If the

---

Box 13-1 BAXTER (PARKLAND) FORMULA

FIRST 24 HOURS—RINGER'S LACTATE

4 ml/kg/% burn in 24 hours
One half in first 8 hours
One half in second 16 hours

Example: 70-kg man with 50% burn

4 ml × 50% × 70 kg = 14,000 ml in 24 hours
   7000 ml hours 1-8
   3500 ml hours 8-16
   3500 ml hours 17-24

SECOND 24 HOURS—ALBUMIN OR PLASMA AT MAINTENANCE

Maintain normal vital signs
Adequate urine output

Example: 70-kg man with 50% burn

250-500 ml plasma
2000-2500 ml D_5W

abdomen is involved with the burn, the inferior margins of the escharotomy may be connected transversely.

Fasciotomies are rarely needed in victims with thermal burns. However, if distal pulses do not return after medial and lateral escharotomies, fasciotomy should be considered. On the other hand, victims with electrical injuries frequently need fasciotomy. Careful monitoring of all victims with electrical burns and with burns associated with soft tissue trauma or fractures is mandatory. In these circumstances, loss of pulses is a strong indication for urgent fasciotomy under general anesthesia in the operating room.

The need for escharotomy in the burned hand is somewhat controversial. Fingers burned badly enough to require escharotomy are frequently mummified, and the lack of muscles in the fingers puts less tissue at ischemic risk. Escharotomy done in fingers that may not require it runs the risk of exposing the interphalangeal joints, leading to subsequent infection that may ultimately require joint fusion or finger amputation. Both the palmar arch and digital vessels should be monitored with Doppler ultrasound in any significant hand burn. If the signals disappear over the palmar arch or in the digital vessels, consideration should be given to performance of a dorsal interosseous fasciotomy.

Burn Wound Management

The burn wound should be cleansed initially with a surgical detergent. All loose, nonviable skin should be gently trimmed. Debridement should be done gently; small doses of IV narcotic are sufficient analgesia for this procedure. General anesthesia and operating room debridement should be avoided until resuscitation is complete, unless other surgical procedures are necessary.

Once the wound is cleansed, a topical chemotherapeutic agent should be applied. A detailed description of all the agents available is beyond the scope of this chapter, but those most commonly used in the United States and other industrialized countries contain silver sulfadiazine. It comes as a white cream, is soothing to the wound, has a good antimicrobial spectrum, and has almost no systemic absorption or toxicity.[7,40,81,90] The victim should be carefully questioned about allergy to sulfa drugs before their use, however, since allergic reactions are encountered in about 3% of patients. These reactions may be manifested clinically as pain after application rather than the soothing feeling that silver sulfadiazine usually provides. If an allergy is suspected (by history), a small (10 × 10 cm) patch of silver sulfadiazine should be applied as a test. The remainder of the wound can be dressed in bacitracin. If no local reaction occurs after 2 to 4 hours, an allergy is unlikely and silver sulfadiazine is the dressing of choice. If an allergy is confirmed, the victim should be referred to a burn center, where the next choice of topical antimicrobial would probably be silver nitrate solution.

Outpatient Burns

According to guidelines given above, the vast majority of victims with burns do not require hospitalization. In many cases, the burn, if merely kept clean, heals spontaneously in less than 3 weeks with acceptable cosmetic results and no functional impairment. Unfortunately, good results in treating superficial minor burns may entice the unwary physician to treat more complex burns by the same methods. For the victim, the consequences of such a mistake can be the need for subsequent hospitalization, joint dysfunction, and hypertrophic scarring that may be difficult to correct, as well as considerable loss of time from work or school.

First-Degree Burns

Although first-degree burns are very painful, victims rarely seek medical attention unless the area burned is extensive. These victims do not require hospitalization, but control of the pain is extremely important. Aspirin or codeine may be adequate for small injuries, but for large burns, liberal use of a more potent narcotic for 2 to 3 days is indicated.

For topical medication we recommend one of the many proprietary compounds containing extracts of the aloe vera plant in concentrations of at least 60%. Aloe vera has antimicrobial properties and is an effective analgesic.[49,77] Anecdotal evidence suggests that it may decrease subsequent pruritus and peeling.

Burns from ultraviolet rays (sunlight, sunlamp) may initially appear to be only epidermal, but the injury may in fact be a superficial partial-thickness burn with blistering apparent only after 12 to 24 hours. Therefore the victim with such a burn should be cautioned about blisters and should be asked to return if they form, since wound management then becomes more important because of the potential for infection and subsequent scarring.

Superficial Partial-Thickness Burns

Treatment of superficial partial-thickness burns presents little problem. If the wound is kept clean, the victim is kept comfortable, and the joints are kept active, these wounds heal in less than 3 weeks with minimal scarring and no joint impairment.

Initially the wound should be cleansed and debrided as described previously. Small blisters may be left intact. Biochemical analysis of the protein-banding pattern of burn blister fluid, obtained by polyacrylamide gel electrophoresis, has shown it to be similar to that of serum.[93] These authors suggest that the fluid is an exudate mainly from the vascular system, that it provides a good environment for the fibroblasts in the damaged site, and that it facilitates the healing process. Larger blisters are difficult to protect, however, and blister fluid is a rich culture medium for bacteria that live in the skin appendages. Therefore large blisters and small blisters in large burns should usually be totally removed with forceps and scissors. In some instances the blister fluid can be aspirated with a large-bore needle, allowing the blistered epidermis to remain on the wound as a biologic dressing. This dead epidermis, however, is fragile, tends to contract, and rarely stays in place except over small areas.

After debridement these wounds can sometimes be managed with a biologic dressing, such as porcine xenograft.[5,95] Pigskin is available in frozen or lyophilized forms. After a biologic dressing is applied, the burn pain is markedly diminished, and if the xenograft "sticks," no further treatment is necessary except for a periodic wound check. When the burn reepithelizes, the xenograft desiccates and peels away from the new epidermis. Other synthetic dressings, such as those made from plastic film (Op-Site or Epigard) have achieved some popularity.[11,69,88] We find that these dressings adhere poorly (a leaking dressing is not an occlusive one) and provide no advantage. The most commonly used treatment is wound coverage with silver sulfadiazine and application of a light dressing to promote active range of motion. Some very small burns do not require topical agents. For small facial burns, bacitracin ointment may be a better choice than silver sulfadiazine cream because it is less drying.

Pain is managed as for first-degree burns, and the patient usually should return every 2 to 3 days until the wound heals or the patient has demonstrated the ability to manage the wound without supervision.

One home treatment regimen is to have the patient cleanse the wound once daily with tap water and reapply the topical agent and light dressing. During dressing changes, and as often as possible, all involved joints should be put through a full range of motion. The dressing may be unnecessary while the patient is at home, but the patient should dress the wound before leaving the house. This method is highly successful, but it is inconvenient and fairly painful and requires good patient cooperation.

Another treatment regimen advocated by some physicians is a single initial debridement and application of a bulky dressing to be left in place for several days without intermediate cleansing or dressing change. This method reduces pain, but the patient must be careful of the bandage. If the bandage is allowed to become saturated with fluid draining from the wound or to become dirty, it may promote infection.

The "exposure" method has little to recommend it. This method involves leaving the wound open, allowing the wound drainage to desiccate and form a scab. Controlled studies in animals have shown that desiccation and crust formation interfere with wound healing. Our experience has also shown that crusts crack over joints, cause considerable discomfort, and can hide infection.

Deep Partial-Thickness and Full-Thickness Burns

Treatment of deep partial-thickness and full-thickness burns is a matter of grave concern. Full-thickness burns heal only by contraction and epithelialization from the periphery. Epithelium does not begin to migrate until the eschar is removed; the growth rate then is only about 1 mm/day. Thus healing of even a small full-thickness burn may involve many weeks of discomfort and disability.

Deep partial-thickness burns may take 4 to 8 weeks to heal and then leave an unacceptable scar. If a joint is involved, some loss of joint function is the rule. We have adopted a policy of early excision and grafting for such wounds.

Initial outpatient treatment can be followed by elective surgery as soon as it can be scheduled. Small wounds can be treated through day surgery; larger wounds located over dynamically important areas can be closed with only a day or two of hospitalization. The excision and grafting procedures should be done by a surgeon experienced in tangential wound excision.

The advantages of this aggressive approach—a pain-free patient with normal joint function, a better cosmetic result, and a rapid return to work or school—more than compensate for the brief hospitalization and the very small risk associated with minor operation.

Should the excision and grafting plan be unacceptable to the patient or the treating physician, the standard method of daily cleansing and application of sliver sulfadiazine cream is used. Most full-thickness burns need grafting at about 3 to 4 weeks after the injury. Deep dermal burns should be seen by the physician frequently during the healing process; active physical therapy is crucial to ensuring a successful outcome.

REHABILITATION

Physicians who regularly care for people with burn injuries recognize that treatment goals extend far beyond healing of the wounds and survival of the victim. We aim to return victims at least to their preburn functional status physically and to ensure a smooth and timely reentry into family and social situations, including work or school. Awareness that recovery from burn injury often depends on a number of nonphysician health care workers is essential. Depending on the severity of the burn and the associated social situation, participation of nurses, nutritionists, occupational therapists, physical therapists, recreational therapists, social workers, vocational rehabilitation counselors, psychologists, pain management specialists, and clergy is commonly required.

Burn rehabilitation should be initiated by the first physician to see the victim. Once all systemic and wound issues have been addressed, proper positioning of wounded extremities or digits should be assessed by an occupational therapist who has been specially trained in burn management. Splints should be made immediately if deemed appropriate. Range-of-motion exercises should be started on the day of injury, and frequent follow-up by a physical therapist is essential. The best functional outcomes result from meticulous attention to early mobility. Patients almost universally choose not to move a burned body part, and an active ancillary burn staff is essential for satisfactory results. Burn scars require approximately a year to fade, soften, and mature. Physical therapy may be required throughout this time period or longer. Pressure garment therapy may be used in certain cases in an attempt to prevent the development of hypertrophic scars. The interested reader is referred to books dealing with acute burn care, reconstructive plastic surgery, and burn rehabilitation for further discussion.[1,8,14]

INHALATION INJURY

Epidemiology

Of the nearly 500,000 fire victims admitted to hospitals each year, smoke or thermal damage to the respiratory tree may occur in as many as 30%.[71] Carbon monoxide poisoning, smoke poisoning, and thermal injury are three distinctly separate aspects of clinical inhalation injury and are discussed as such. Inhalation injury rarely occurs in an outdoor setting.

Carbon Monoxide Poisoning

PATHOPHYSIOLOGY. Carbon monoxide (CO) is a colorless, odorless, tasteless gas that has an affinity for hemoglobin 200 times greater than that of oxygen. The most simply explained mechanism of action of CO is reversible displacement of oxygen on the hemoglobin molecule. Although worsening hypoxia is important, and the percentage of carboxyhemoglobin in the blood represents in large measure the degree of victim hypoxia, this simple mechanism cannot account for all of the experimental and clinical findings seen with exposure to CO. For example, an experimental group of dogs was exchange-transfused with blood containing 80% carboxyhemoglobin (COHb). They showed no symptoms. In a control group with COHb levels of 80% produced by inhalation of CO, all animals died. Furthermore, the degree of enzyme and muscle impairment may not correlate accurately with the levels of blood COHb.[15,20,30,50]

In vitro, CO combines reversibly with cardiac muscle myoglobin and heme-containing enzymes, such as cytochrome oxidase a$_3$.[15] Despite its intense affinity, it readily dissociates according to the laws of mass action. The half-life of COHb in humans breathing room air is 4 to 5 hours. In humans breathing 100% oxygen, the half-life is reduced to 45 to 60 minutes.[54] In a hyperbaric oxygen chamber at 2 PSI, the half-life is 30 minutes, and at 3 atmospheres in a chamber it is reduced to 15 to 20 minutes.[92]

CLINICAL PRESENTATION. Blood levels of COHb provide a laboratory measure to correlate with associated symptoms of CO poisoning. Levels less than 10% do not cause symptoms, although victims with exercise-induced angina may show decreased exercise tolerance. At levels of 20%, healthy persons complain of headache, nausea, vomiting, and loss of manual dexterity. At 30% they become confused and lethargic and may show depressed ST segments on electrocardiogram. In a fire situation this level may lead to death as the victim loses both the interest and the ability to flee the smoke. At levels between 40% and 60% the victim lapses into coma, and levels much above 60% are usually fatal.

THERAPY. Victims who have not been unconscious and who have a normal neurologic examination on admission almost always recover completely without treatment beyond administration of 100% oxygen. Victims who remain comatose once COHb levels have returned to normal have a poor prognosis, and in our experience they rarely awaken. Although enthusiasts for hyperbaric oxygen treatment (HBOT) consider it a standard of care for CO poisoning,[2,3,52,61] many physicians are skeptical.[78] One controlled study indicated that hyperbaric oxygen made no difference for moderate poisoning, and multiple treatments were no better than a single treatment for victims with severe poisoning.[72] Furthermore, when associated with a major burn, transport to a chamber delays definitive care and is associated with numerous complications, including emesis, seizures, eustachian tube occlusion, aspiration, hypocalcemia, agitation requiring restraints or sedation, arterial hypotension, tension pneumothorax, and cardiac arrhythmia or arrest.[33,87] The issue of whether, and at what time in the progression of CO poisoning, HBOT may be of value will undoubtedly be continued to be studied and debated.

Thermal Airway Injury

PATHOPHYSIOLOGY. The term *pulmonary burn* is a misnomer. True thermal damage to the lower respiratory tract and lung parenchyma is extremely rare unless live steam or exploding gases are inhaled. The air temperature near the ceiling of a burning room may reach 540° C (1000° F) or more, but air has such poor heat-carrying capacity that most of the heat is dissipated in the nasopharynx and upper airway. The heat dissipation in the upper airway, however, may cause significant local thermal injury.

CLINICAL PRESENTATION. Victims who have been in explosions (propane, natural gas, or gasoline) and have burns of the hands, face, and upper torso are particularly at risk for pharyngeal edema.

THERAPY. Maintenance of the airway is the main concern with potential thermal airway injury. Victims injured in explosions should be examined for oropharyngeal erythema and edema. If these are present, the victim should be intubated for 24 to 72 hours until edema subsides. A simple test to determine if intubation should continue is to see if the victim can breathe around the endotracheal tube when the cuff is deflated. If so, the airway edema has probably resolved and extubation should be safe. If doubt exists, extubation should be performed over a fiberoptic bronchoscope or nasogastric tube, which allows easy replacement of the endotracheal tube if necessary. Since this is not a pulmonary parenchymal injury, the purpose of intubation is to protect the airway and not necessarily to assist with ventilation. Ventilator settings should be adjusted accordingly, and vigorous pulmonary toilet should be instituted to prevent the pulmonary problems (atelectasis and pneumonia) commonly seen in intubated victims.

Smoke Poisoning

PATHOPHYSIOLOGY. Some 280 separate toxic products have been identified in wood smoke. Modern petrochemical science has now produced a wealth of plastic materials in homes and automobiles that when burned produce nearly all of these and many other products not yet even characterized.[45,66,85,99] Prominent by-products of incomplete combustion are oxides of sulfur, nitrogen, and many aldehydes. One such aldehyde, acrolein, causes severe pulmonary irritation and edema in concentrations as low as 10 ppm. Although the chemical mechanisms of injury may be different with different toxic products, the overall end organ response is reasonably well defined.* There is an immediate loss of bronchialepithelial cilia and decreased alveolar surfactant. Microatelectasis, and sometimes macroatelectasis, results and is compounded by mucosal edema in small airways. Wheezing and air hunger are common symptoms at this time. After a few hours, tracheal and bronchial epithelia begin to slough and hemorrhagic tracheobronchitis develops. In severe cases interstitial edema becomes prominent, resulting in a typical picture of the adult respiratory distress syndrome (ARDS). Pulmonary alveolar macrophages are poisoned, causing severe impairment of chemotaxis, which undoubtedly contributes to the high incidence of late pneumonia seen in victims with associated cutaneous burns. The activated neutrophils release superoxides and free radicals of oxygen, which together with other inflammatory mediators aggravate alveolar-capillary damage, leading to increased interstitial edema and impaired oxygenation.

CLINICAL PRESENTATION. Any victim who has been indoors in a smoky fire and has a flame burn or was in an enclosed space should be assumed to have smoke poisoning until proven otherwise. The acrid smell of smoke on the victim's clothes should raise suspicion. Rescuers are often the most important historians and should be carefully questioned.

Careful inspection of the mouth and pharynx should be done early. Hoarseness and expiratory wheezes are signs of potentially serious airway edema or smoke poisoning. Copious mucus production and carbonaceous sputum are sure signs, but their absence should not raise false hopes that injury is absent. COHb levels should be obtained; elevated carboxyhemoglobin levels or any clinical symptoms of CO poisoning are presumptive evidence of associated smoke poisoning. In very smoky fires, COHb levels of 40% to 50% may be reached after only 2 to 3 minutes of exposure.[92]

Anyone with suspected smoke poisoning should have a set of arterial blood gases drawn. One of the earliest indicators is an improper ratio (P/F ratio) of the arterial P_{AO_2} to the percent of inspired oxygen (F_{IO_2}). Normally the ratio is 400 to 500, whereas patients with impending pulmonary problems have a ratio of less than 300 (e.g., P_{AO_2} of less than 120 with an F_{IO_2} of 0.40). A ratio of less than 250 is an indication for vigorous pulmonary therapy and not an indication for merely increasing the inspired oxygen concentration.

A number of authorities suggest the routine use of fiberoptic bronchoscopy.[12,55,74,81] It is inexpensive, quickly performed by an experienced clinician, and useful in accurately assessing edema of the upper airway. Aside from the presence of tracheal erythema, however, it does not materially influence the treatment for smoke poisoning. Therefore it should be used only when the diagnosis is in doubt or for experimental studies.

We have correlated by multivariate analysis a constellation of historical items, signs, and symptoms with bronchoscopic findings in 100 consecutive patients with suspected smoke inhalation admitted to the University of Washington Burn Center in Seattle. If the patient had the combination of history of closed space fire, carbonaceous sputum, and a COHb level greater than 10%, there was 96% correlation with positive bronchoscopy. Presence of two of the above features dropped correlation to 70%, and if only one was present, the correlation dropped to 36%. As discussed previously, upper airway edema was best correlated with an explosion (flash burn) that involved both the face and the upper torso. Nearly 50% of such victims had significant upper airway edema and underwent prophylactic airway intubation.

---

*References 10, 17, 39, 42, 53, 54, 75, 83, 98, 99.

THERAPY. There is clear agreement that all victims burned in an enclosed space or having any suggestion of neurologic symptoms should be given 100% oxygen while awaiting measurement of COHb levels. This should be administered through a tight-fitting mask in the field. If the victim demonstrates labored breathing or if a prolonged transport time is anticipated, endotracheal intubation should be performed by trained personnel. One hundred percent oxygen can then be administered by ventilator.

Mucosal burns of the mouth, nasopharynx, and larynx respond with edema formation and may lead to upper airway obstruction at any time during the first 24 hours after the burn. Red or dry mucosa or small mucosal blisters should alert the observer to the possibility of subsequent airway obstruction; they also should raise suspicion that significant smoke inhalation may have occurred. Any victim with burns of the face should have a careful visual inspection of the mouth and pharynx; if abnormalities are found, the larynx should be examined immediately on arrival at the hospital. The presence of significant intraoral and pharyngeal burns is a clear indication for early endotracheal intubation, since the progressive edema may make later emergency intubation extremely hazardous, if not impossible.

The mucosal burns themselves are rarely full thickness and can be successfully managed with good oral hygiene. Once inserted, the endotracheal tube should remain in place for 2 to 5 days until the edema subsides.

Pulmonary functions early in the course of smoke poisoning are variably affected. Typically there are decreased lung volume (functional residual capacity) and vital capacity, evidence of obstructive disease with reduction in flow rates, increased dead space, and rather rapid decrease in compliance. Surprisingly, much of the variability in pulmonary response appears to correlate with the severity of the associated cutaneous burn.[14] Without associated burns the mortality from smoke poisoning is low, the disease rarely progresses to ARDS, and symptomatic treatment usually leads to complete resolution of symptoms in a few days. In the presence of burns, smoke poisoning appears to approximately double the rate of mortality from burns of any size. Pulmonary symptoms (hypoxia, rales, rhonchi, wheezes) are seldom present on admission but may appear 12 to 48 hours after exposure. In general, the earlier the onset of symptoms, the more severe the disease.[91]

No standard treatment has evolved to ensure survival after smoke poisoning; each recommended treatment modality is tempered by opinion and the individual experience of the treating physician. In the presence of increasing laryngeal edema, nasotracheal or orotracheal intubation is indicated. A tracheostomy is never an emergency procedure and certainly should be avoided as initial airway management in victims with burns to the face and neck. A soft-cuffed endotracheal tube should be left in place for 3 to 5 days until the generalized oropharyngeal edema subsides.

Mild cases of smoke poisoning are treated with highly humidified air, vigorous pulmonary toilet, and bronchodilators as needed. Blood gases are drawn at least every 4 hours, and the P/F ratio is calculated. Worsening symptoms, difficulty in handling secretions, and a falling P/F ratio are all indications for intubation and respiratory assistance with a volume ventilator. If oxygenation is impaired (P/F ratio 250 or less), positive end-expiratory pressure (PEEP) or continuous positive airway pressure (CPAP) is initiated and increased by increments of 3 to 5 cm H_2O until no further improvement in the P/F ratio occurs or there is evidence of decreased cardiac output.

The physician must carefully search for other mechanical causes of poor ventilation (e.g., restricted chest wall motion from full-thickness burns, pneumothorax from high ventilator pressures, or mechanical difficulties with the endotracheal tube.)

Prophylactic antibiotics have no value in this chemical pneumonitis, and the subsequent burn management and treatment of eventual bacterial pneumonia can be made more difficult by the development of resistant organisms if antibiotics are used early.

Steroids are commonly used in victims with severe asthma. Clinicians dealing with smoke poisoning often use them for their spasmolytic and antiinflammatory actions. Several authors have studied the use of steroids, but a most convincing study comes from Moylan, who showed in a prospective blinded study of patients with smoke poisoning and associated major burns that the rates of mortality and infectious complications were higher in the steroid-treated patients. In patients with associated burns, Robinson and Seward[76] found that steroids did not alter the hospital course of patients admitted to the hospital after the MGM Grand and Hilton Hotel fires in Las Vegas in 1981.

The decision for hospital admission and the need for specialized care rest on the severity of symptoms from the smoke and the presence and magnitude of associated burns. Any victim who shows symptoms of smoke inhalation and has more than trivial burns should be admitted. If the burns are greater than 15% TBSA, the victim should probably be referred to a special care unit. In the absence of burns, admission depends on the severity of symptoms, presence of preexisting medical problems, and the social circumstances of the victim. Otherwise healthy victims with mild symptoms (only a few expiratory wheezes, minimal sputum production, COHb level less than 10%, and normal blood gas levels) can be watched for an hour or two and then discharged if they have a place to go and someone to stay with them. Victims with preexisting cardiovascular or pulmonary disease should be admitted for observation if they have any symptoms related to the smoke. Victims with moderate symptoms (generalized wheezing, mild hoarseness, moderate sputum production, COHb levels 5% to 10%, and normal blood gas levels) may be admitted for close observation and treated as for asthma. Severe symptoms (air hunger, severe wheezing, and copious [usually carbonaceous] sputum) require immediate intubation and ventilatory support in an intensive care unit setting.

OTHER CONSIDERATIONS

Burns are tetanus-prone wounds. The need for tetanus prophylaxis is determined by the victim's current immunization status. The treating physician should follow the recommendations of the American College of Surgeons.

All victims undergoing IV resuscitation should have an indwelling urinary catheter placed for hourly monitoring of urine output. Arterial lines are useful in victims who need frequent assessment of blood gases or who will need repeated blood sampling. Necessary laboratory work during the resuscitation phase is relatively minimal. Baseline blood chemistries should be drawn. If major operative procedures, such as fasciotomy or multiple escharotomies, are expected, blood should be sent for type and crossmatching for several units of whole blood. Blood gases are mandatory in any victim with a suspected inhalation injury, and arterial pH measurement is useful as an assessment of the overall treatment of shock. If the Baxter formula is used for resuscitation, frequent electrolyte determinations are not necessary because levels will remain in the normal range. By 48 hours, however, careful monitoring of serum sodium and potassium becomes important. High levels of circulating aldosterone result in an increase in renal potassium excretion, and varying degrees of evaporative water loss through eschar dramatically increase the free water requirements of burned victims. Hemoglobin and hematocrit levels are initially high and remain high or normal until the third or fourth postburn day. The blood glucose level commonly is elevated because of the glycogenolytic effect of elevated catecholamines, the gluconeogenic effect of elevated glucocorticoid and glucagon levels, and relative insulin resistance.[44,82,94,100] This well-described "stress diabetes" can become a problem in normal patients if glucose-containing solutions are given during resuscitation and frequently is a serious problem in patients with preexisting diabetes. All diabetic patients require careful monitoring of blood and urine glucose, and most require supplemental insulin during resuscitation.

All medications during the shock phase of burn care should be given intravenously. Subcutaneous and intramuscular injections are unreliably absorbed systemically, and their use should be avoided. Pain control is best managed with small IV doses of morphine given until pain control is adequate without affecting blood pressure.

Before the discovery of penicillin, 30% of burn victims died during the first week after the injury from overwhelming β-hemolytic streptococcal sepsis. The availability of penicillin decreased streptococcal infections but had no influence on mortality or the incidence of bacterial sepsis. Victims then survived the first postburn week only to die of gram-negative penicillin-resistant bacterial sepsis during the second or third week after the burn. The advent of effective topical chemotherapeutic agents applied directly to the burn wounds made possible the control of streptococcal infection, obviating the need for prophylactic penicillin. The use of prophylactic antibiotics in outpatient burns has not been carefully evaluated, so opinion is divided regarding its utility in victims not requiring hospitalization.

Stress ulceration of the stomach and duodenum was once a dread complication, occurring in nearly 30% of victims with burns. Protection of the gastric mucosa by immediate feeding through a small nasogastric tube or, failing that, with instillation of antacids or sucralfate has made stress ulcers rare.[48,61,70,73,89]

Psychosocial care should begin immediately. The victim and family must be comforted, and a realistic outlook regarding the prognosis of the burns should be given, at least to the victim's family. In house fires the victim's loved ones, pets, and many or all possessions may have been destroyed. If the family is not available, some member of the team, usually the social worker, should find out the extent of the damage in hopes of comforting the victim. If the victim is a child and the circumstances suggest that the burn may have been deliberately inflicted or resulted from negligence, physicians in most states are required by law to report their suspicion of child abuse to local authorities.

Burn Severity and Categorization

Severity of injury is proportionate to the size of the total burn, the depth of the burn, the age of the victim, and associated medical problems or injuries. Burns have been classified by the American Burn Association and the American College of Surgeons Committee on Trauma into categories of minor, moderate, and severe.[6] Moderate burns are defined as partial-thickness burns of 15% to 25% of TBSA in adults (10% to 20% in children); full-thickness burns of less than 10% of TBSA; and burns that do not involve the eyes, ears, face, hands, feet, or perineum. Because of the significant cosmetic and functional risk, all but very superficial burns of the face, hands, feet, and perineum should be treated by a physician with a special interest in burn care in a facility that is accustomed to dealing with such problems. Major burns as described previously, most full-thickness burns in infants and elderly victims, and burns combined with diseases or injuries should also be treated in a specialized facility. Moderate burns can be treated in a community hospital by a knowledgeable physician as long as the other members of the health care team have the resources and knowledge to ensure a good result. Newer techniques of early wound closure have made burn care more complex, and an increasing number of victims with small but significant burns are being referred to specialized care facilities to take advantage of these concepts.

The criteria for admission to the hospital of victims with "minor" and "moderate" burns vary according to physician preference, the victim's social circumstances, and the ability to provide close follow-up. In some circumstances, superficial burns as large as 15% can be successfully managed on an outpatient basis. In other circumstances, burns as small as 1% may require admission because of the victim's inability or unwillingness to care for the wound. In general, the threshold for admission of elderly victims and infants should be low. Any victim (child or adult) who the physician suspects of having been abused must be admitted.

Transport and Transfer Protocols

Once an airway is established and resuscitation is under way, burn victims are eminently suitable for transport.[9,22,46] Resuscitation can continue en route, since for the most part patients remain stable for several days. This was well proven during the Vietnam War, when burn victims were transported from Vietnam to Japan and then from Japan to the military burn center in San Antonio, Texas. The transport was generally accomplished during the fist 2 weeks after the burn, with few complications occurring in about 1000 patients transferred.

Hospitals without specialized burn care facilities should decide where they will refer patients and work out transfer agreements and treatment protocols with the chosen burn center well in advance of need. If this is done, definitive care can begin at the initial hospital and continue without interruption during transport and at the burn center. In general, transfer should be from physician to physician, and contact should be established between them as soon as the patient arrives at the initial hospital.

The mode of transport depends on vehicle availability, local terrain, weather, and the distances involved. For distances of less than 50 miles, ground ambulance is usually satisfactory. For distances between 50 and 150 miles, many people prefer helicopter transport. It should be noted, however, that monitoring, airway management, and any changes in therapy are more difficult to achieve in a helicopter. All victims transported by air should have a nasogastric tube inserted and be placed on dependent drainage, since nausea and vomiting usually result during the flight.

Two large-bore IV lines should be functional in case one stops working.

For distances over 150 miles, fixed-wing aircraft are usually satisfactory. Modern air ambulances are completely equipped flying intensive care units, and the personnel are usually well trained for both critical care and the peculiarities of victim care during the flight (see Chapter 27).

The referring physicians must ensure that the victim's condition is suitable for a long transport and prepare the victim for the flight. The victim's airway must be secure. At 9144 m (30,000 feet), planes can be pressurized to an altitude of about 1676 m (5500 feet). Although supplemental oxygen can be given in flight, if the victim's oxygenation is marginal, performing intubation and starting mechanical ventilation before the transport may be preferable. Intubation is difficult en route, so if there is any question of upper airway edema, the victim should be intubated at the referring hospital. Burned victims have difficulty maintaining body temperature, and they should be wrapped warmly before transport. Bulky dressings, a blanket, and a Mylar sheet (usually available from the flight team) can help maintain body temperature. In case the victim has any cardiac irregularities, the plane must be equipped with electronic monitoring capability, since noise and vibrations in flight make clinical monitoring difficult.

Only after all other assessments are complete should attention be directed to the burn itself. If the victim is to be transferred from the initial hospital to a definitive care center during the first postburn day, personnel at the referring hospital can leave the burn wounds alone, merely calculating the size of burn for resuscitation and monitoring pulses distal to circumferential full-thickness burns. The victim can be wrapped in a clean sheet and kept warm until arrival at the definitive care center.

REFERENCES

1. Achauer BM: *Burn reconstruction,* New York, 1991, Thieme Medical.
2. Adir Y, Bentur Y, Melamed Y: Hyperbaric oxygen for neuropsychiatric sequelae of carbon monoxide poisoning, *Harefuah* 122:562, 1992.
3. Adir Y et al: Hyperbaric oxygen treatment for carbon monoxide intoxication acquired in a sealed room during the Persian Gulf war, *Isr J Med Sci* 27:669, 1991.
4. Aharoni A et al: Burn resuscitation with a low-volume plasma regimen: analysis of mortality, *Burns* 15:230, 1989.
5. Alsbjorn BF: Biologic wound coverings in burn treatment, *World J Surg* 16:43, 1992.
6. American Burn Association: Hospital and prehospital resources for optimal care of patients with burn injury: guidelines for development and operation of burn centers, *J Burn Care Rehabil* 11:98, 1990.
7. Aoyama H, Yokoo K, Fujii K: Systemic absorption of sulphadiazine, silver sulphadiazine and sodium sulphadiazine through human burn wounds, *Burns* 16:163, 1990.
8. Artz CP, Moncrief JA, Pruitt BA Jr: *Burns: A team approach,* ed 2, Philadelphia, 1984, WB Saunders.
9. Baac BR et al: Helicopter transport of the patient with acute burns, *J Burn Care Rehabil* 12:229, 1991.
10. Barrow RE et al Cellular sequence of tracheal repair in sheep after smoke inhalation injury, *Lung* 170:331, 1992.

11. Bauman LW et al: Bilaminate synthetic dressing for partial thickness burns: lack of cost reduction for inpatient care, *Am Surg* 57:131, 1991.

12. Bingham HG, Gallagher TJ, Powell MD: Early bronchoscopy as a predictor of ventilatory support for burned patients. *J Trauma* 27:1286, 1987.

13. Blinn DL, Slater H, Goldfarb LW: Inhalation injury with burns: a lethal combination, *J Emerg Med* 6:471, 1988.

14. Boswick JA Jr: *The art and science of burn care,* Rockville, Md, 1987, Aspen.

15. Brown SD, Piantadosi CA: Reversal of carbon monoxide-cytochrome c oxidase binding by hyperbaric oxygen in vivo, *Adv Exp Med Biol* 248:747, 1989.

16. Carvajal HF, Parks DH: Optimal composition of burn resuscitation fluids, *Crit Care Med* 16:695, 1988.

17. Clark CJ et al: Role of pulmonary alveolar macrophage activation in acute lung injury after burns and smoke inhalation, *Lancet* 2:872, 1988.

18. Daniel RK et al: High-voltage electrical injury: acute pathophysiology, *J Hand Surg* 13:44, 1988.

19. Datubo-Brown DD, Gowar JP: Contact burns in children, *Burns* 15:285, 1989.

20. Della-Puppa T et al: Carbon monoxide poisoning and secondary neurologic syndrome: follow-up after hyperbaric oxygen therapy; preliminary results, *Minerva Anesthesiol* 57:972, 1991.

21. Ding YL et al: Extensive scalds following accidental immersion in hot water pools, *Burns Incl Therm Inj* 13:305, 1987.

22. Ellis A, Rylah TA: Transfer of the thermally injured patient, *Br J Hosp Med* 44:206, 1990.

23. Engrav LH et al: Outcome and treatment of electrical injury with immediate median and ulnar nerve palsy at the wrist: a retrospective review and a survey of members of the American Burn Association, *Ann Plastic Surg* 25:166, 1990.

24. Epperly TD, Steward JR: The physical effects of lightning injury, *J Fam Pract* 29:267, 1989.

25. Eriksson A, Ornehult L: Death by lightning, *Am J Forensic Med Pathol* 9:295, 1988.

26. Feldberg L, Regan PJ, Roberts AH: Cement burns and their treatment, *Burns* 18:51, 1992.

27. Field TO Jr, Dominic W, Hansbrough J: Beach-fire burns in San Diego County, *Burns Incl Therm Inj* 13:416, 1987.

28. Fontanarosa PB: Electrical shock and lightning strike, *Ann Emerg Med* 22:378, 1993.

29. Fulde GW, Marsden SJ: Lightning strikes, *Med J Aust* 153:496, 1990.

30. Gorman DF et al: A longitudinal study of 100 consecutive admissions for carbon monoxide poisoning to the Royal Adelaide Hospital, *Anaesth Intens Care* 20:311, 1992.

31. Graitcer PL, Sniezek JE: Hospitalization due to tap water scalds, 1978-1985, *MMWR CDC Surveill Summ* 37:35, 1988.

32. Griswold JA et al: Hypertonic saline resuscitation efficacy in a community-based burn unit, *South Med J* 84:692, 1991.

33. Grube BJ, Marvin JA, Heimbach DM: Therapeutic hyperbaric oxygen: help or hindrance in burn patients with carbon monoxide poisoning? *J Burn Care Rehabil* 9:249, 1988.

34. Grube BJ et al: Neurologic consequences of electrical burns, *J Trauma* 30:254, 1990.

35. Gunn ML et al: Prospective, randomized trial of hypertonic sodium lactate versus lactated Ringer's solution for burn shock resuscitation, *J Trauma* 29:1261, 1989.

36. Haberal M et al: Severe electrical injury, *Burns Incl Therm Inj* 15:60, 1989.

37. Hammond JS, Ward CG: High-voltage electrical injuries: management and outcome of 60 cases, *South Med J* 81:1351, 1988.

38. Herbert K, Lawrence JC: Chemical burns, *Burns* 15:381, 1989.

39. Herndon DN et al: Extravascular lung water changes following smoke inhalation and massive burn injury, *Surgery* 102:341, 1987.

40. Herruzo CR et al: Evaluation of the penetration strength, bactericidal efficacy and spectrum of action of several antimicrobial creams against isolated microorganisms in a burn centre, *Burns* 18:39, 1992.

41. Horton JW, White DJ: Hypertonic saline dextran resuscitation fails to improve cardiac function in neonatal and senescent burned guinea pigs, *J Trauma* 31:1459, 1991.

42. Hubbard GB et al: The morphology of smoke inhalation injury in sheep, *J Trauma* 31:1477, 1991.

43. James NK, Moss AL: Review of burns caused by bitumen and the problems of its removal, *Burns* 16:214, 1990.

44. Jeffries MK, Vance ML: Growth hormone and cortisol secretion in patients with burn injury, *J Burn Care Rehabil* 13:391, 1992.

45. Jones J, McMullen MJ, Dougherty J: Toxic smoke inhalation: cyanide poisoning in fire victims, *Am J Emerg Med* 5:317, 1987.

46. Judkins KC: Aeromedical transfer of burned patients: a review with special reference to European civilian practice, *Burns Incl Therm Inj* 14:171, 1988.

47. Kanitkar S, Roberts AH: Paraplegia in an electrical burn: a case report, *Burns Incl Therm Inj* 14:49, 1988.

48. Kitajima MA et al: Gastric microcirculatory change and development of acute gastric mucosal lesions (stress ulcer), *Acta Physiol Hung* 73:137, 1989.

49. Klein AD, Penneys NS: Aloe vera, *J Am Acad Dermatol* 18:714, 1988.

50. Kodama K et al: A case of "interval" form of acute carbon monoxide poisoning: brain MRI and therapeutic effect of hyperbaric oxygenation, *Rinsho Shinkeigaku* 30:420, 1990.

51. Koller J, Orsagh J: Delayed neurological sequelae of high-tension electrical burns, *Burns* 15:175, 1989.

52. Koren G et al: A multicenter, prospective study of fetal outcome following accidental carbon monoxide poisoning in pregnancy, *Reprod Toxicol* 5:397, 1991.

53. Leduc D et al: Acute and long-term respiratory damage following inhalation of ammonia, *Thorax* 47:755, 1992.

54. Linares HA, Herndon DN, Traber DL: Sequence of morphologic events in experimental smoke inhalation, *J Burn Care Rehabil* 10:27, 1989.

55. Lukånn J, Sånndor L: The importance of fiberbronchoscopy in respiratory burns, *Acta Chir Plast* 32:107, 1990.

56. Lyngdorf P: Occupational burn injuries, *Burns Incl Therm Inj* 13:294, 1987.

57. Massello W III: Lightning deaths, *Med Leg Bull* 37:1, 1988.

58. Mellins RB, Park S: Medical progress: respiratory complications of smoke inhalation in victims of fires, *J Pediatr* 87:1, 1975.

59. Meuli M, Lochbuhler H: Current concepts in pediatric burn care: general management of severe burns, *Eur J Pediatr Surg* 2:195, 1992.

60. Meyer GW, Hart GB, Strauss MD: Hyperbaric oxygen therapy for acute smoke inhalation injuries, *Postgrad Med* 89:221, 1991.

61. Mittal PK et al: Sucralfate therapy for acid-induced upper gastrointestinal tract injury, *Am J Gastroenterol* 84:204, 1989.

62. Moran KD, O'Reilly T, Munster AM: Chemical burns: a ten-year experience, *Am Surg* 53:652, 1987.

63. Morehouse JD et al: Resuscitation of the thermally burned patient, *Crit Care Clin* 8:355, 1992

64. Mozingo DW et al: Chemical burns, *J Trauma* 28:642, 1988.

65. Murison MS, Laitung JK, Pigott RW: Effectiveness of burns resuscitation using two different formulae, *Burns* 17:484, 1991.

66. Narita H et al: Smoke inhalation injury from newer synthetic building materials: a patient who survived 205 days, *Burns Incl Therm Inj* 13:147, 1987.

67. Palmer JH, Sutherland AB: Problems associated with transfer of patients to a regional burn unit, *Injury* 18:250, 1987.

68. Patten BM: Lightning and electrical injuries, *Neurol Clin* 10:1047, 1992.

69. Phillips LG et al: Uses and abuses of a biosynthetic dressing for partial skin thickness burns, *Burns* 15:254, 1989.

70. Prasad JK, Thomson PD, Feller I: Gastrointestinal haemorrhage in burn patients, *Burns Incl Therm Inj* 13:194, 1987.

71. Pruit BA Jr et al: Evaluation and management of patients with inhalation injury, *J Trauma* 30:S63, 1990.

72. Raphael JC et al: Trial of normobaric and hyperbaric oxygen for acute carbon monoxide intoxication (see comments), *Lancet* 2:414, 1989.

73. Rath T, Walzer LR, Meissl G: Preventive measures for stress ulcers in burn patients, *Burns Incl Therm Inj* 14:504, 1988.

74. Richard P et al: Emergency tracheobronchoscopy in children with burns, *Ann Otolaryngol Chir Cervicofac* 107:195, 1990.

75. Riyami BM: Changes in alveolar macrophage, monocyte, and neutrophil cell profiles after smoke inhalation injury, *J Clin Pathol* 43:43, 1990.

76. Robinson MD, Seward PN: Hazardous chemical exposure in children, *Pediatr Emerg Care* 3:179, 1987.

77. Rodriguez M, Cruz NI, Suarez A: Comparative evaluation of aloe vera in the management of burn wounds in guinea pigs, *Plast Reconstr Surg* 81:386, 1988.

78. Roy TM et al: Perceptions and utilization of hyperbaric oxygen therapy for carbon monoxide poisoning in an academic setting, *J Ky Med Assoc* 87:223, 1989.

79. Sawhney CP, Kaushish R: Acid and alkali burns: considerations in management, *Burns* 15:132, 1989.

80. Sawhney CP et al: Long-term experience with 1% topical silver sulphadiazine cream in the management of burn wounds, *Burns* 15:403, 1989.

81. Schneider W et al: Diagnostic and therapeutic possibilities for fibreoptic bronchoscopy in inhalation injury, *Burns Incl Therm Inj* 14:53, 1988.

82. Shangraw RE et al: Differentiation between septic and postburn insulin resistance, *Metabolism* 38:983, 1989.

83. Sharar SR et al: Cardiopulmonary responses after spontaneous inhalation of Douglas fir smoke in goats, *J Trauma* 28:164, 1988.

84. Shugerman R et al: Contact burns of the hand, *Pediatrics* 0:18, 1987.

85. Silverman SH et al: Cyanide toxicity in burned patients, *J Trauma* 28:171, 1988.

86. Singer A et al: Chemical burns: our 10-year experience, *Burns* 18:250, 1992.

87. Sloan EP et al: Complications and protocol considerations in carbon monoxide–poisoned patients who require hyperbaric oxygen therapy: report from a ten-year experience (see comments), *Ann Emerg Med* 18:629, 1989.

88. Smith DJ et al: Biosynthetic compound dressings: management of hand burns, *Burns Incl Therm Inj* 14:405, 1988.

89. Steen J et al: Antacid in the prevention of upper gastrointestinal bleeding in burns, *Acta Chir Scand Suppl* 547:93, 1988.

90. Stern HS: Silver suphadiazine and the healing of partial thickness burns: a prospective clinical trial, *Br J Plast Surg* 42:581, 1989.

91. Stone HH, Martin JD Jr: Pulmonary injury associated with thermal burns, *Surg Gynecol Obstet* 129:1242, 1969.

92. Thom Sr, Keim LW: Carbon monoxide poisoning: a review of epidemiology, pathophysiology, clinical findings, and treatment options including hyperbaric oxygen therapy, *J Toxicol Clin Toxicol* 27:141, 1989.

93. Uchinuma E et al: Biological evaluation of burn blister fluid, *Ann Plast Surg* 20:225, 1988.

94. van Gool JH et al: The relation among stress, adrenalin, interleukin 6 and acute-phase proteins in the rat, *Clin Immunol Immunopathol* 57:200, 1990.

95. Vanstraelen P: Comparison of calcium sodium alginate (Kaltostat) and porcine xenograft (E-Z Derm) in the healing of split-thickness skin graft donor sites, *Burns* 18:145, 1992.

96. Wachtel TL et al: Scalds from molten tar: an industrial hazard, *J Burn Care Rehabil* 9:218, 1988.

97. Walker AR: Fatal tapwater scald burns in the USA, 1979-86, *Burns* 16:49, 1990.

98. Wang CZ et al: Morphologic changes in basal cells during repair of tracheal epithelium, *Am J Pathol* 141:753, 1992.

99. Youn YK, Lalonde C, Demling R: Oxidants and the pathophysiology of burn and smoke inhalation injury, *Free Radic Biol Med* 12:409, 1992.

100. Ziegler MG, Morrissey EC, Marshall LF: Catecholamine and thyroid hormones in traumatic injury, *Crit Care Med* 18:253, 1990.

14 Exposure to Radiation from the Sun

Lee A. Kaplan

Sun exposure, sun damage, and sun protection are increasingly the focus of medical, scientific, and public attention. Adverse effects of sunlight overexposure are well documented,[74,118] but the value and safety of sun-protective strategies are debated. These issues are of particular concern to wilderness enthusiasts who spend considerable time in the sun. Sun protection against acute phototrauma, especially sunburn, is more easily judged than protection against chronic phototrauma—photoaging, cataracts, and photocarcinogenesis. Yet these chronic effects are increasingly relevant to modern societies with demographically aging populations. The economic concerns are huge: billions of dollars are spent annually in the cosmetic and medical industries to repair photodamage, photoaging, and skin cancer. Consumer interest in photoprotection is rapidly expanding. With better sunscreens and, more recently, photoprotective clothing, still more attention and investment will be focused on sun protection.

SOLAR RADIATION

Electromagnetic Spectrum

The sun produces a continuous spectrum of electromagnetic radiation (Figure 14-1). The most energetic rays, those with wavelengths shorter than 10 nm (cosmic rays, gamma rays, x-rays) do not appreciably penetrate to Earth's surface. Phototrauma is primarily due to ultraviolet radiation (UVR). UVR (10 to 400 nm) accounts for about 10% of incident radiation at Earth's surface, visible light (400 to 760 nm) 50%, and infrared (IR; 760 to 1700 nm) 40%.[74]

UVR has four components. Vacuum UVR (10 to 200 nm) is readily absorbed by air and does not penetrate Earth's atmosphere. UVC (200 to 290 nm) is almost entirely absorbed in the stratosphere, 15 to 50 km above Earth's surface, by oxygen and ozone. Man-made sources of UVC—germicidal lamps and arc welding devices—are rarely medically relevant. UVB (290 to 320 nm) is biologically quite active and is principally responsible for tanning, burning, and nonmelanoma skin cancer (NMSC) formation.[74,118] Beneficial effects of UVB include vitamin D production from cutaneous precursors. Approximately 90% of 25-hydroxy vitamin D is formed in this manner.[184] Of the UVR that reaches Earth's surface, UVB accounts for roughly 10%, whereas UVA accounts for 90%, depending on the time of day and season. UVA is typically subdivided into "near" UVA, or UVA II (320 to 340 nm), and "far" UVA, or UVA

I (340 to 400 nm). These subdivisions, although somewhat arbitrary, are based on photobiologic responses. UVA is also biologically active, contributing to tanning, burning, photoaging, and carcinogenesis. UVA penetrates the skin more deeply than does UVB, with less energy lost in the superficial layers of the stratum corneum and epidermis. UVA is the principal trigger for photo-drug reactions. Visible light and IR may cause cutaneous phototrauma, albeit rarely. Solar urticaria has been reported to visible wavelengths. IR alone, and along with UVR, may produce epidermal and dermal alterations.[123]

Environmental Influences on UVR Exposure

UVR intensity is substantially affected by latitude, altitude, season, time of day, surface reflection, atmospheric pollution, and ozone levels. Most UVR reaches Earth in midday; 80% between 9 AM and 3 PM, and 65% between 10 AM and 2 PM.[74] UVB peaks at midday when the sun is at its zenith.[144] UVB is absorbed, reflected, and scattered by the atmosphere; at midday it has less atmosphere to traverse. In early morning and late afternoon, when the sun nears the horizon, UVB decreases considerably. Latitude and season have similar effects; peak UVB exposure is approximately 100 times greater in June than December.[144] For each degree of latitude away from the equator, UVB intensity decreases an average of 3%. UVA varies considerably less than UVB with latitude, time of day, and season, as predicted by Rayleigh's law:

$$\text{Atmospheric light scattering} \propto 1/\lambda^4$$

where λ = wavelength

The shorter the wavelength the greater the atmospheric scattering, so UVB is scattered much more readily than UVA. Additionally, UVA but not UVB is transmitted through window glass, allowing indoor exposure to UVA but not UVB.

UVR may be increased by surface reflection. Water, surprisingly, is a relatively poor reflector. UVR at midday penetrates water up to 60 cm.[144] Reflection from water may increase as the sun nears the horizon, but then there remains little UVB because of atmospheric attenuation. Ice and snow are considerably better reflectors. Clean snow may reflect up to 85% of UVR,[144] accounting for oddly distributed sunburns in spring skiers. Sand, metal, concrete, and other surfaces may reflect UVR to varying degrees.

Clouds may attenuate UVR exposure. Absorption by clouds varies from 10% to 80% but rarely exceeds

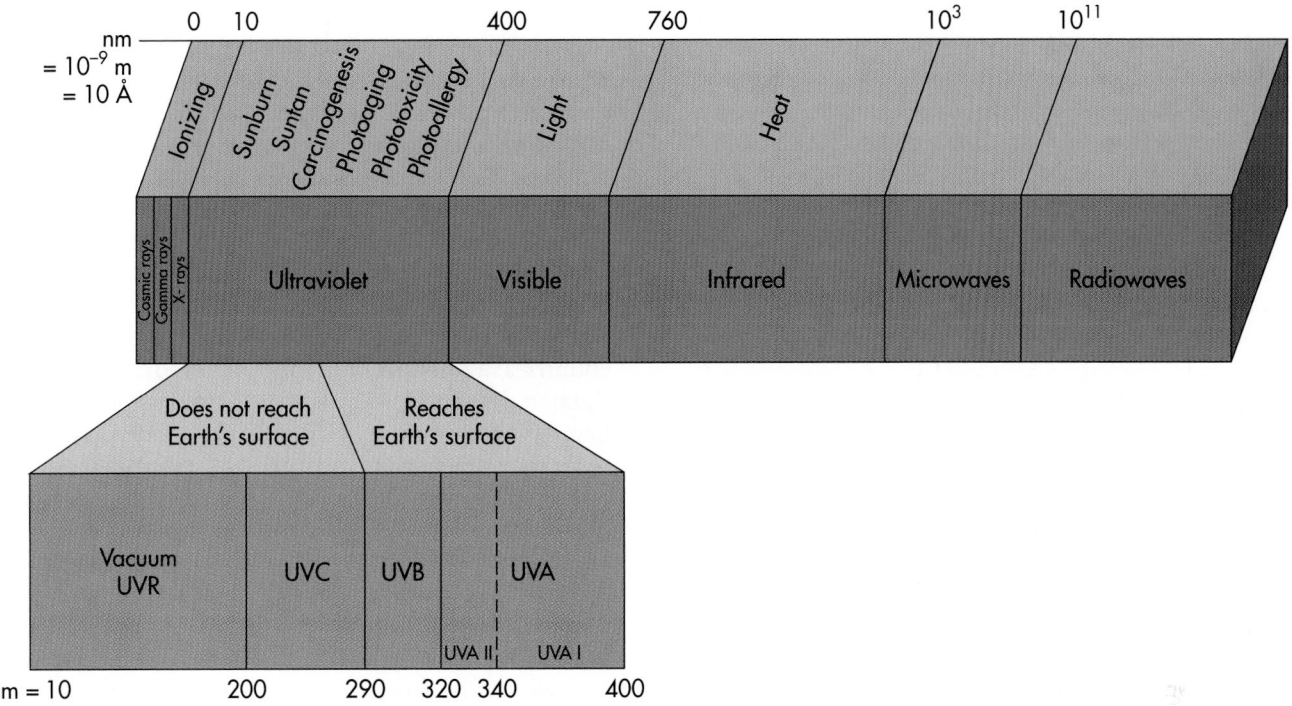

Figure 14-1 Electromagnetic spectrum.

40%.[118] Interestingly, polluted clouds—those containing the greatest concentration of hydrocarbons—are the most effective at absorbing UVR. Clouds are more effective at absorbing heat, in the form of infrared radiation, occasionally seducing hikers and bathers into excessively lengthy midday exposures.

Wind and water augment sunburn. In mice, exposure to wind plus UVR results in more erythema than UVR alone.[177] In humans, wind may reduce heat perception, encouraging longer exposure. Water increases UVR exposure because moist skin reflects less UVR, resulting in greater absorption of UVB. Swimmers and hikers in humid environments may be at risk for increased UVR absorption.[74]

Altitude profoundly influences UVB exposure. Until recently, it was generally accepted that UVB exposure rises 4% for each 305-m (1000-foot) rise above sea level. More recently, however, Rigel et al[190] demonstrated an 8% to 10% increase in UVB for each 305-m rise above sea level. Beginning at the 3353-m (11,000-foot) summit of a ski run in Vail, Colorado, these investigators measured UVB readings every 152 m (500 feet) as they skied down to the base of the run at 2500 m (8200 feet).This study showed that UVB exposure in Vail at 2591 m (8500 feet) is similar to exposure levels in Orlando, Florida, 775 miles further south.

Snow, wind, and altitude may act simultaneously to greatly augment UVB exposure for skiers and climbers. Singh et al[210] reported that 36% (24/67) of climbers de-

veloped significant sunburns during three consecutive expeditions up to 7000 m (23,400 feet) in the western Himalayas, despite the application of sunscreen. These data emphasize the difficulties in providing appropriate UVR protection for high-altitude outdoor enthusiasts.

Ozone Depletion and UVR Exposure

Stratospheric ozone, 15 to 50 km above Earth's surface, provides a thin, fragile shield against UVR. The combination of ozone and oxygen absorbs virtually all of the incident UVC. Ozone attenuates UVB and modestly reduces UVA II but allows transmission of all UVA I.[245] Ozone is continuously created and removed from the stratosphere by natural physicochemical processes that are in turn significantly affected by human-made pollution. Molina and Rowland[164] first suggested that chlorofluorocarbons (CFCs) could cause ozone depletion. CFCs are organic chemicals containing carbon, chlorine, and fluorine, initially developed in the 1970s as refrigerants. Today, CFCs are used in several industrial processes: air conditioning systems, insulation, cleaning solvents, degreasing agents, and metered dose inhalers. Related compounds, halons, contain bromine and also deplete stratospheric ozone. Halons arise from seawater, fire extinguishers, and various industrial processes.[106] CFCs and halons belong to the halocarbon group.

The remarkable stability of CFCs allows them to rise into the stratosphere, where, catalyzed by solar radiation, they release Cl^- and ClO^- that in turn degrade ozone. One prominent chemical pathway by which CFCs deplete ozone is as follows[106]:

$$Cl + O_3 \rightarrow ClO + O_2$$

$$O_3 + UVR \rightarrow O + O_2$$

$$ClO + O \rightarrow Cl + O_2$$

Net reaction: $2O_3 + UVR \rightarrow 3O_2$

Note that Cl^- is preserved in this reaction. The half-life of Cl^- is approximately 75 years,[234] though CFCs may reside in the stratosphere for 50 to 200 years.[106] During that time, each Cl^- molecule may destroy 100,000 molecules of ozone.[234] Over Antarctica, other ozone depletion mechanisms operate: molecular halogens coat the surface of ice clouds, making them even more reactive and able to degrade ozone.[106]

Ozone losses were first reported over Antarctica in 1985[66] by the British Antarctic survey. Ozone showed large declines in the austral springtime (September/October), decreasing a total of 35% during springtimes 1975-1984.[106] Ozone depletion is now documented at all latitudes except the equator. This depletion is uneven, with greater amounts at the poles and less at middle latitudes.[234] Using NASA's Total Ozone Mapping Spectrometer (TOMS) in satellite orbit, ozone depletion has been documented over continental Europe, North and South America, South Africa, New Zealand, and Australia.[136]

Significant increases in UVB have been documented, even in middle latitudes, because of ozone depletion. In Toronto from 1989 to 1993, Kerr and McElroy[121] documented surface UVB increases of 35% per year in winter and 7% per year in summer, corresponding to ozone decreases of 4% per year and 1.8% per year, respectively. Their experimental design allowed the assignment of all of the UVB increase to ozone depletion rather than cloud coverage or pollution. Similar increases in ground level UVB, paralleling decreases in stratospheric ozone, have been documented in Scotland.[168] Typically, in the northern hemisphere's middle latitudes, ozone losses are greater in winter (about 6% per decade) than in summer (3% per decade).[106] Ironically, pollution—smog and particulates—may mitigate UVR increases by absorbing UVB.[234]

The effects of ozone depletion on the biosphere and human skin cancer rates have been estimated. Although estimates vary, generally, for every 1% decrease in ozone, there is a corresponding 2% increase in the incidence of basal cell cancer (BCCa) and a 3% increase in the incidence of squamous cell cancer (SCCa).[50] Melanoma incidence may increase 1%.[234] However, even if UVB triples near the poles, as suggested in worst-case scenarios, polar areas will still receive less UVB than current equatorial levels.[234] Ozone depletion may have its greatest effects on nonhuman biosystems. Plant and plankton yields may be diminished significantly, with uncertain, potentially severe, detriment to terrestrial and marine life.[245]

To prevent ecologic disturbances and restore ozone levels, international agreements have been negotiated. The Vienna Convention in 1985 and the subsequent Montreal Protocol in 1987 were among the first and most notable. The Montreal Protocol, signed by 42 countries, agreed to limit, and then reduce, CFC production, leading to a 50% reduction by 1998.[106] Three later amendments were made to accelerate progress in response to increasing awareness of ozone depletion in middle latitudes. The London Amendment in 1990 required complete phaseout of halocarbon production; and the Copenhagen Amendment in 1992 accelerated the timetable for complete phaseout, stopping production in developed countries by 1996 and undeveloped nations within 10 years. It also extended the protocol to include hydrochlorofluorocarbons. The Vienna Amendment in 1995 revised the phaseout schedule of hydrochlorofluorocarbons.[106, 211]

Although the Montreal Protocol is working—CFC production decreased 75% in the period 1986-1994—its modest limitations would allow continued stratospheric chlorine levels through most of the twenty-first century.[106] In contrast, the stricter limitations of the Copenhagen Amendment will result in ozone levels rising again within the first decade of the twenty-first century.[211] Among the remaining sources of CFC production are metered dose inhalers and cleaning agents for rocket motor manufacturers.[106] American factories may produce 53,500 tons of CFCs annually for export until the year 2005.[20] CFC substitutes are more costly, leading to a black market in CFCs, with an estimated 22,000 tons produced in 1994.[20] A significant portion of this black market is in Freon smuggled to auto air conditioner rechargers. In 1996, an estimated 10,000 tons of CFCs were smuggled into the United States from Mexico and elsewhere.[73] Despite these black market sources, current projections suggest that atmospheric chlorine will begin to fall shortly after 2000. UVB will peak in the first decade of the twenty-first century and then gradually fall by 2050 to levels recorded in the 1950s.

ACUTE EFFECTS OF ULTRAVIOLET RADIATION ON SKIN: SUNBURN AND TANNING

The effects of UVR on skin depend primarily on wavelength, length of exposure, intensity of exposure, repetition of exposure, age at time of exposure, site of exposure, and genetic factors of the individual exposed. To have a biologic effect, UVR must be absorbed. Absorbing molecules are known as *chromophores.* Different chromophores are in the skin for different wavelengths of UVR. Among these are nucleic acids, especially pyrimidine bases, various amino acids in cutaneous proteins, and lipoproteins in cell membranes. These chromophores are at various depths in the skin, accounting in part for the differing photobiologic responses to UVR. As of now, we have only imprecise knowledge of how a given photochemical reaction results in a specific biochemical product, leading to an observable clinical change.

UVC

UVC has no appreciable impact on human health, since it is effectively screened from Earth's surface by stratospheric ozone and oxygen. Even with continued ozone depletion, levels of UVC are not expected to rise. Human-made sources of UVC—germicidal lamps and arc welding devices—have been only rarely associated with cutaneous pathology, as might be predicted, since UVC is effectively absorbed by the stratum corneum, the outermost cutaneous layer.[74]

UVB

UVB acutely induces a cutaneous inflammatory response that is at least partially definable clinically, histologically, and biochemically.[113] Clinically, erythema, or sunburn, is the hallmark of acute overexposure to UVB. The action spectrum for erythema peaks in UVB.[169] Generally, UVB is considered 1000-fold more effective than UVA at inducing erythema. In a human model, 300 nm UVB is 1280-fold more effective at inducing erythema than 360 nm UVA.[246] We usually define erythemogenic doses as multiples of the minimal erythema dose (MED)—the lowest dose to elicit perceptible erythema. In a typical fair-skinned individual, the MED might range from 15 to 70 mJ/cm² for UVB and 20 to 80 J/cm² for UVA.

One MED of UVB for a typical fair-skinned individual would require 20 minutes of midsummer exposure in San Diego, whereas an MED of UVA would require 2 to 3 hours of exposure. In a day's time, a person can receive 15 MEDs of UVB but only 2 to 4 MEDs of UVA.[156] Consequently, although we are exposed to 10-fold to 100-fold more UVA than UVB, more than 90% of sunlight-induced erythema is attributable to UVB. The erythema action spectrum, which peaks in UVB, is remarkably similar to the absorption spectrum of deoxyribonucleic acid (DNA),[169] suggesting that DNA is a principal target chromophore for UVB-induced erythema[247] and pyrimidine dimer formation. Supporting this is the finding that pyrimidine dimer yields correlate with erythema.[98]

Sunburn reflects a local vascular reaction. The causes are multifactorial; DNA damage, prostaglandin activation, cytotoxicity, and other mechanisms are implicated. UVB erythema has its onset 2 to 6 hours after exposure,

peaks at 12 to 36 hours, and fades over 72 to 120 hours.[74,113,118] Acute histologic changes accompanying UVB exposure include edema with vasodilation of upper dermal vasculature[113] and endothelial cell swelling, likely caused by the release of vasoactive mediators.[96] Delayed histologic changes include appearance of sunburn cells in as little as 30 minutes after exposure. These dyskeratotic cells have enlarged nuclei and vacuolated cytoplasm. Initially, sunburn cells are in the lower half of the epidermis but by 24 hours are also in the upper half. These sunburn cells may represent actively cycling, proliferating basal cells that cannot adequately repair UVR-induced DNA lysosomal damage.[46] Beginning 1 hour after exposure, stainable Langerhans' cells are reduced by 25%, and by 72 hours after exposure only 10% remain.[113] In mice exposed to repetitive suberythemogenic doses of UVB, normal numbers of Langerhans' cells return by 8 days after exposure.[113] Vacuolization of melanocytes is seen after 1 hour, returning to normal 4 to 24 hours after exposure.[113] Mast cells decrease in number and granularity within 1 hour, returning to normal in 12 to 72 hours.[113] By 24 to 48 hours after exposure, there is increased melanin synthesis, epidermal proliferation, and thickening of the stratum corneum. Functionally, the epidermal permeability barrier diminishes after UVB exposure because of the altered kinetics of lamellar body–containing cells in the exposed epidermis.[109]

Biochemical changes accompanying sunburn include increased levels of histamine,[113] which return to normal within 74 hours. However, histamine is unlikely to be the sole or even principal mediator of vasodilation and erythema, since antihistamines are ineffective in preventing sunburn. UVR induces increased phospholipase activity, with accompanying increases in prostaglandins. PGD_2, PGE_2, PGF, and 12-hydroxyeicosatetraenoic acid (12-HETE) are increased in suction blister aspirates immediately after UVB, peaking in 18 to 24 hours.[113] Topical and intradermal indomethacin, a prostaglandin inhibitor, blocks UVB-induced erythema for 24 hours after exposure,[212] supporting the thesis that eicosanoids (prostaglandins and leukotrienes) are significant mediators of UVR-induced inflammation.[129] UVB stimulates induction of proinflammatory and mutagenic cytokines tumor necrosis factor-α (TNF-α), interleukin-6 (IL-6), and IL-12.[109] UVR generates free radicals in the skin that likely contribute to the sunburn reaction[152] by causing peroxidative chromosomal, membrane, and protein damage.[14] Topical antioxidants may mitigate sunburn when applied before but not after exposure. Melatonin[14] and vitamin C[48] act protectively by scavenging UVR-generated free radicals; neither absorbs UVR.

UVA

UVA penetrates more deeply into the skin than does UVB. Whereas 95% of incident UVB is reflected or absorbed by the epidermis, nearly 50% of UVA reaches the dermis.[65] UVA contributes modestly to sunburn and may cause clinical erythema. Prolonged daily UVA exposure can approach 125 J/cm^2, significantly exceeding the threshold erythema dose of 20 to 80 J/cm^2.[214] Clinically, UVA erythema has an onset within 4 to 6 hours, peaks in 8 to 12 hours, and fades in 24 to 48 hours.[113,118] Erythema resulting from UVA may have a distinct pathophysiologic mechanism. UVA-induced erythema may be caused by keratinocyte cytotoxicity.[113] Histologically, UVA erythema displays more epidermal spongiosis, fewer sunburn cells, and more dermal changes than does UVB-induced erythema, with a denser, deeper mononuclear cell infiltrate and more vascular damage.[113]

Infrared

IR radiation plays a less well-defined role in photodamage. Near IR preirradiation prevents UVR-induced cytotoxicity,[156] suggesting a possible evolutionary protective mechanism for IR is daily preparation of skin cells to resist UVR-induced damage. However, no data indicate whether IR protects against UVR's mutagenic and carcinogenic effects.

Sunburn Treatment

Sunburn is self-limited, and its treatment is largely symptomatic, involving local skin care, pain control, and antiinflammatory agents (Box 14-1).[13] Cool water soaks or compresses may provide immediate relief, and topical anesthetics are sometimes useful. It is generally preferable to use the nonsensitizing anesthetics menthol, camphor, and pramoxine rather than potentially sensitizing anesthetics containing benzocaine and diphenhy-

---

Box 14-1 SUNBURN TREATMENTS

PAIN CONTROL

ASA
NSAIDs

SKIN CARE

Cool soaks, compresses
Topical anesthetics
  Sarna lotion (menthol + camphor)
  Prax lotion (pramoxine)
  Aveeno Anti-Itch lotion (pramoxine + calamine + camphor)
Moisturizers

STEROIDS

Topical
Systemic

---

dramine. Refrigerating topical anesthetics before application provides added relief. A legion of topical remedies have been suggested anecdotally, including aloe, baking soda, and oatmeal, though controlled studies are lacking. Topical steroids may blanch the reddened skin. Oral nonsteroidal antiinflammatory drugs provide analgesia and may reduce sunburn erythema.[74] Few published studies support the value of systemic steroids, but they enjoy considerable anecdotal support. Sadly, warnings regarding skin cancer are rarely given to sunburned patients seen in the emergency room.[13]

Tanning

Tanning, like sunburning, is caused by UVR. Consequently, persons seeking tan risk sunburn. Tanning is biphasic. After sun exposure, there is immediate pigment darkening (IPD) within minutes, followed by delayed pigment darkening (DPD) in 3 days. IPD is predominantly due to the action of UVA on preformed melanin precursors and occurs in as little as 5 minutes after exposure, peaks in 60 to 90 minutes, and then fades quickly. However, DPD represents new melanin synthesis within melanocytes and the subsequent spread of the richly melanized melanosomes into surrounding keratinocytes. After UVB exposure, DPD is notable by 72 hours, peaks in 5 to 10 days, and slowly fades. DPD is primarily a response to UVB. Most tanning studies have been performed with erythemal doses of UVR. However, multiple suberythemal exposures to UVA are significantly more melanogenic than similarly dosed UVB.[17] The mechanism of DPD is uncertain but is likely multifactorial. UVB stimulates tyrosinase release and arachidonic acid metabolites and releases α-melanocyte-stimulating hormone (α-MSH) from keratinocytes.[5] It also increases the binding affinity of melanocytes for MSH, resulting in increased melanocyte proliferation, melanization, and arborization.[26] UVB increases melanocytes in both exposed and protected human skin,[218] suggesting the possibility of a UVR-stimulated circulating factor that promotes melanocyte proliferation.

CHRONIC PHOTOTRAUMA

Natural Defenses and Skin Type

The absence of erythema does not preclude cutaneous photoreactions. Chronic exposure to UVR is accompanied by insidious cumulative biologic and clinical changes. Although some of these changes are due to broad-band UVR, UVA and UVB often have distinct and different effects on the epidermis, dermis, extracellular matrix, cytokines, and immune response.[236] In response to UVB, the stratum corneum thickens[95] and melanin increases, both protective mechanisms to mitigate further UVB photodamage. The stratum corneum, the outermost layer of skin, is composed of flattened anucleate keratinocytes. It reflects, scatters, or absorbs up to 95% of incident UVB, depending largely on its thickness.[102] With repeated exposure to UVB, the stratum corneum can increase its thickness up to sixfold.[74] As a consequence, the stratum corneum is the main photoprotective factor in Caucasians.[95] Repeated UVA exposures may cause some thickening,[143] but to a much lesser degree. Consequently, UVA tans are not as photoprotective as UVB tans.

Melanin reflects, scatters, and absorbs throughout the UVR spectrum; acts as an antioxidant; and reduces UVR-induced photoproducts.[126] Consequently, constitutive (racial) skin color is a principal determinant of an individual's erythemal response to UVR. Although blacks and whites have similar numbers of melanocytes, these pigment-forming cells are differently melanized and distributed in black and white skin. Increased melanin in blacks can decrease the dermal penetration of UVR up to fivefold[43] and increase the MED up to thirtyfold. In contrast, tanning is much less protective. After an entire summer of tanning, the MED in whites increased only 2.3-fold.[43] Clinically, these racial differences in melanization are reflected in lower rates of burning, photoaging, and skin cancer in blacks.

Susceptibility to photodamage is typically defined by six distinct skin types (Box 14-2). Racial pigmentation alone does not account for differences in skin type. Some redheads tan easily, whereas some blacks burn readily. Reporting errors, typically overstating sun tolerance, are common, further complicating the interpretation of skin types.[185]

Skin type correlates well with MED. Additional factors that influence MED include age and anatomic site. Lower MEDs are recorded in the very young and the very old.[118] Differences in stratum corneum thickness and melanocyte concentration may account for body site–specific differences in MED. For example, the MED of the back is typically less than the MED of the lower leg.

Chronic suberythemal UVA exposures also cause photodamage. Repetitive, low-dose exposures to UVA result in histologic changes,[139,143] including thickened

stratum corneum, granular and stratified cell layers, decreased elastin, vascular dilation, and inflammation.

Aside from stratum corneum thickening and increased pigmentation, intrinsic mechanisms of photoprotection include antioxidants, such as the glutathione peroxidase-reductase system, that mitigate damage from UVR-induced reactive oxygen species. DNA repair enzymes correct most UVR-induced mutations. Carotenoids stabilize biologic membranes from singlet oxygen attack. Urocanic acid absorbs some of the UVR that penetrates the stratum corneum.

Photoaging

Long-term repetitive exposures to sunlight result in photoaging.[69] This process, known as *dermatoheliosis*, is distinctive clinically and histologically from chronologic aging; it is not merely accelerated chronoaging. Photoaged skin is characterized by dryness, roughness, mottling, wrinkling, atrophy, and pebbling and may be studded with precancers (actinic keratoses) or cancers (Figure 14-2). Most of what we consider "old-looking" skin is in fact the result of photoaging and not chronoaging. Although age can be estimated from observing sun-exposed sites, it cannot be estimated from photoprotected sites.[232] The action spectrum for photoaging includes UVB, UVA, and infrared.[143]

Chronically sun-exposed sites have fewer Langerhans' cells. Keratinocytes and fibroblasts from sundamaged skin have diminished lifespans in culture.[90] The most notable histologic change with chronic UVB exposure is deposition of thickened amorphous elastic fibers high in the dermis, demonstrable in photoexposed white skin by age 30. In a transgenic mouse model, UVB but not UVA produces this solar elastosis.[226] Another mouse model suggests that the action spectrum for "photosagging" peaks in UVA at 340 nm,[101] and that this action spectrum is remarkably similar to that for the generation of singlet oxygen by excitation of trans-urocanic acid. These authors conclude that UVA causes photoaging because of its interaction with trans-urocanic acid, releasing reactive oxygen species.

With photoaging, elastin gene expression appears to be activated, although data are conflicting. Tropoelastin and fibrillin synthesis actually diminish with chronic UVB exposure.[235] There is enhanced transcription of other extracellular matrix genes. In particular, photoaged skin demonstrates increased matrix metalloproteinases, potent mediators of connective tissue damage.[69] These arise within hours of UVB exposure, even suberythemal exposure.[68] Interestingly, tretinoin inhibits induction of these UVB-induced proteinases,[68,69] perhaps explaining in part its clinical utility against photoaging.[175,233] Tretinoin also normalizes photoaltered epidermal differentiation and deposits new type I collagen in the upper dermis.[97]

Box 14-2   SKIN TYPES

I: Always burns. Never tans.
II: Often burns. Tans minimally.
III: Sometimes burns. Tans moderately.
IV: Burns minimally. Tans well.
V: Rarely burns. Tans deeply. Moderately pigmented (brown).
VI: Never burns. Deeply pigmented (black).

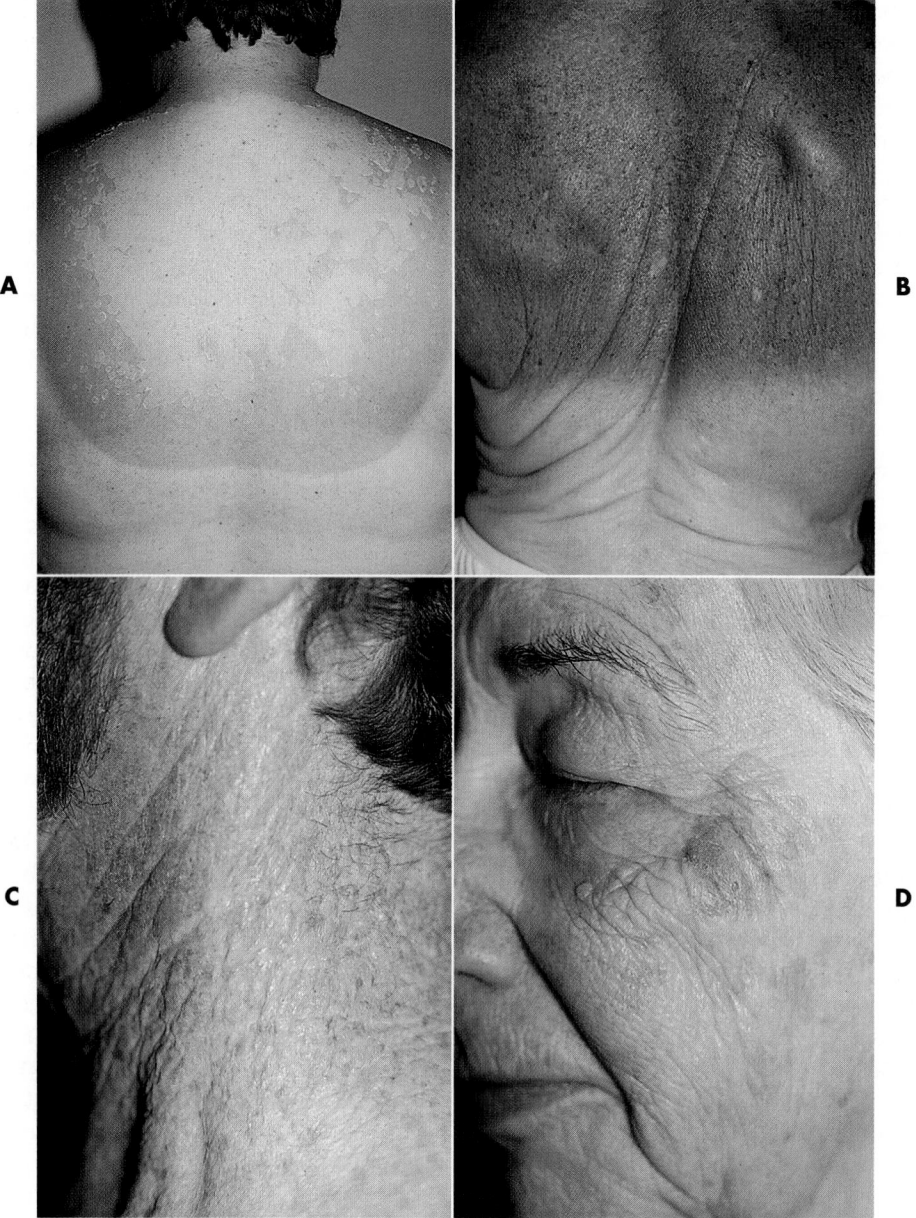

Figure 14-2 Phototrauma. **A,** Tan and peeling after sunburn. **B** to **D,** Dry, mottled, wrinkled, and pebbled skin with photoaging.

Ocular Effects

Acute overexposure to UVB may cause photokeratitis, especially in skiers and climbers ("snowblindness"),[248] whereas chronic exposure to UVR may cause or contribute to pterygia, cataracts, and macular degeneration. A full discussion is presented in Chapter 22.

Sun and Skin Cancer

Skin cancer, the most common of all cancers, is overwhelmingly caused by UVR exposure. In particular, UVR is the principal cause for NMSC—basal and squamous cell cancers. UVR also contributes significantly to melanoma but is not a sine qua non. The incidence of skin cancer is staggering. One in five Americans[190] and two thirds of all Australians[11] born today will develop skin cancer. In addition, the incidences of both NMSC[93] and melanoma continue to increase.[189] Three causative factors seem to predominate:

1. Lifestyle trends, including sun exposure, sunbathing, and tanning bed use
2. Demographic aging of the population
3. Ozone depletion

Since the 1890s, epidemiologic evidence has accumulated linking sun exposure and NMSC in humans. The incidence of skin cancer increases with increasing proximity to the equator.[45] NMSC has a far greater incidence in whites than in blacks and occurs primarily on sun-exposed areas. The risk of NMSC increases with increasing sun exposure, and repeated sunburn is an independent risk factor.[132] Adoption of a sun-protected lifestyle is associated with decreased risk.[108] Patients with xeroderma pigmentosum (XP), with deficient ability to repair UVR-induced DNA damage, have a 1000-fold greater risk of developing NMSC, typically at a very early age.[129]

In the 1920s, laboratory data confirmed that UVR induces and promotes NMSC in mammalian animal models.[118,222] UVC and UVB are effective inducers of SCCa in mice.[113] Although UVB is primarily implicated, UVA augments UVB-induced carcinogenesis,[222] but it is not clearly a carcinogen on its own.

Development of NMSC in humans is related to the time and intensity of exposure. Sun exposure in childhood and adolescence is more predictive of later BCCa.[78] British immigrants to Australia assume the much higher Australian risk of NMSC only if they emigrate before age 18; after 18, immigrants retain the lower British risk.[149] A separate study suggests the risk decreases after age 10.[131] Gallagher et al[78] found that BCCa is associated with sun exposure up to age 19 but not associated with mean annual cumulative summer sun exposure. In this study, risk for BCCa was also associated with fair complexion and freckling. Kricker et al[132] suggest that intermittent, rather than continuous, sun exposure in poor tanners is the most important factor in the development of BCCa.

The relationship of photoexposure and SCCa is distinct and different from that of sun and BCCa. There is significantly increased risk of SCCa with chronic occupational exposure, especially in the 10 years before diagnosis.[79] Although cumulative lifetime photoexposure and SCCa are not associated, risk factors include periodic recreational exposure, pale complexion, and red hair. Persons who develop SCCa seem phenotypically sensitive to UVR with chronic exposure as adults. Household and office exposure to nonsolar UVR does not increase the risk of BCCa and SCCa.[12] In select mouse models, suberythemal UVR causes SCCa.[169] In these models, gradual suberythemal exposures to UVR may be actually more carcinogenic than are erythemal doses.[77] This may be relevant to humans and explain why persons without any prior sunburns may develop SCCa.

Melanoma

Melanoma has a less well-defined relationship to sun exposure. Clearly, however, sun exposure plays a significant role in its development.[4] The ultraviolet action spectrum for melanoma remains uncertain, with different results in different animal models. In *Monodelphis domestica*, a South American marsupial, both UVA and UVB are implicated[54]; in *Xiphophorus* (platyfish and swordtails), UVA, UVB, and visible (blue) light are

causative[54]; and in transgenic mice Tyr-SV40E (C57BL/6 strain), UVB is the etiologic waveband.[122] In humans with XP, the 1000-fold increased incidence of melanoma strongly supports UVB as a causative agent.[130] A unique, recent, and elegant laboratory experiment documented that UVB induces melanocytic hyperplasia, atypia, and melanoma in newborn human foreskin xenografts on RAG-1 (immunodeficient) mice.[5]

Melanoma incidence increases with proximity to the equator in white populations[119] in the United States, Australia, and Scandinavia, as well as in the nonwhite population of India.[135] Intermittent intense exposures pose a high risk for melanoma.[61] Metaanalysis of 15/16 case-controlled studies supports a significantly increased risk of melanoma with a history of sunburn. By contrast, there is only a small increased risk for total exposure and a decreased risk with heavy occupational exposure.[63] Patients with melanoma are twice as likely to relate a history of a prior sunburn and three times as likely to relate a history of multiple prior sunburns, compared with age-matched controls.[63] Persons who tan poorly and burn readily are at higher risk for melanoma.[145] The distribution of melanomas on the trunk (in both genders) and lower legs (in women) is consistent with the hypothesis that intermittent sun exposure is provocative. Note, however, that melanomas also arise in sun-protected sites, especially in nonwhite populations, suggesting an additional cause separate from sun exposure.

A high level of outdoor activity in college is associated with a fourfold risk of later melanoma.[62] Servicemen who served in the Pacific theater during World War II have higher risks of melanoma than those who served in Europe.[34] The incidence of melanoma is increased in indoor workers with higher socioeconomic status, again reflecting the role of intermittent intense sun exposure.[119] Fluorescent light raises some concerns[230] but does not significantly increase melanoma risk, especially when lights have covers or diffusers.[110]

Sunburns in childhood may be particularly relevant to the later development of melanoma. Celtic migrants to Australia arriving before age 10 assume the high melanoma risk of native Australians; migrants older that 15 at arrival have only one-fourth that risk.[200] Europeans who live more than 1 year in a sunny climate have an increased relative risk (RR = 2.7) of melanoma, and the risk increases substantially if they arrive before age 10 (RR = 4.3).[8] However, a recent study suggests that childhood sun exposure contributes a serious risk only if there is subsequent and significant sun exposure as an adult.[9]

This association of increased melanoma risk with youthful sun exposure may be in part attributable to the effect of sun on the development of melanocytic nevi (moles) in children. Several studies confirm that the number of nevi in children increases with increasing acute and chronic sun exposure.[33,81,82,104] In Australia, the number of nevi up to age 12 increases with increasing proximity to the equator.[120] Queensland children have the highest number of nevi in the world, and, not surprisingly, Queensland has the highest incidence of melanoma in the world[104] at 55.8/100,000 for males and 42.9/100,000 for females.[11,23] The number of nevi is a strong predictor of melanoma risk. Melanoma increases with increasing numbers of benign acquired nevi. In a large European case-controlled study, the most important risk factors for melanoma are the number of nevi and number of atypical nevi.[82] Established nevi may develop histologic changes transiently, simulating melanoma after a single UVR exposure,[225] and some recent data suggest that sunburn can induce malignant transformation in benign nevi.[40]

In the United States, melanoma incidence has increased since records were first kept in the 1930s, rising 121% in the 20 years between 1973 and 1994.[99] In 1999, there will have been 44,200 new cases of invasive melanoma.[137] The lifetime risk of melanoma for a child born in the United States today is 1 in 87, and this is anticipated to rise to 1 in 75.[99] Similarly large increases have been noted in Europe, Australia, and even Japan.[119] However, melanoma incidence and death rates show signs of stabilizing and perhaps decreasing for younger cohorts,[92,99,119] likely because of improving sun protective behaviors.

Significant national efforts have been made to educate and protect populations at risk. In Australia, taxes have been removed from sunscreen sales, hats are typically required for children in outdoor sports, and artificial shade is increasingly available in public parks. In addition to improved photoprotection, early detection has been widely promoted. The Skin Cancer Foundation encourages monthly self-examinations, with special attention to pigmented lesions displaying atypical clinical features, the so-called "ABCDs" of melanoma: *A*symmetry, *B*order irregularity, *C*olor variegation, and *D*iameter greater than 6 mm (Figure 14-3). Nevi (moles) with these clinical features, changing nevi, or nevi that bleed should be evaluated by a physician.

Molecular Basis of Photocarcinogenesis

Some photomolecular events are associated with NMSC. UVR causes characteristic photoinsults at sites of adjacent pyrimidines on DNA.[32,166,246] UVR photons are absorbed at the 5-5 double bonds, resulting in cyclobutane dimers if both bonds open and 6-4 (pyrimidine-pyrimidone) photoproducts if a single bond opens.[32] Cyclobutane dimers predominate 3:1, with thymine (T-T) dimers most common.[129]

Suberythemal, as well as erythemal, doses of UVR can induce T-T dimers.[247] Data suggest that cyclobutane dimers and 6-4 photoproducts produce the mutagenic[138] and carcinogenic[129] properties of UVR.

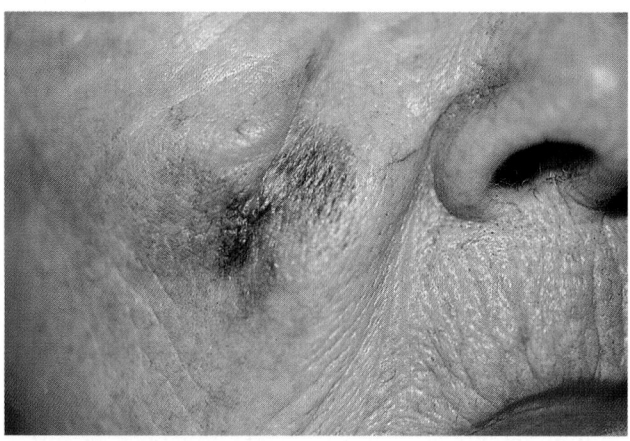

Figure 14-3 Melanoma. Note the asymmetry, border irregularity, color variegation, and diameter greater than 6 mm.

High-performance liquid chromatography can now quantitatively measure UVB photoproducts.[38] Such measurements indicate a thirtyfold interindividual variation in photoproduct yields.[38]

Resultant UVR-induced mutations have a distinctive signature: two thirds display cytosine → thymine (C → T) substitutions at dipyrimidine sites; 10% show CC → TT substitutions.[32] These mutations are relatively unique to UVR damage and allow UVR-induced mutations to be distinguished from chemical mutations.[32]

The most likely target for UVR-induced mutagenic initiation of skin cancer is p53, a tumor suppressor gene.[31,111] Mutations of p53 are the most common genetic alterations yet identified in cancers,[111] found in nearly 50% of all human cancers.[32,129] Approximately 50% of BCCa, 60% of actinic keratoses, and 90% of SCCa contain p53 mutations.[32,250] Although p53 mutations may be found in non–sun-damaged skin with low frequency, 10^{-2} to 10^{-3}, mutations are much more common in sun-exposed sites.[32]

Normal p53 protein is a transcription factor, regulating the cell cycle. DNA damage stimulates p53 protein production, which leads to cell cycle arrest in G1 (a premitotic phase), allowing time for DNA repair.[32] Irreparable damage leads to apoptosis, or programmed cell death. Sunburn cells are examples of apoptotic cells.[250] Cells with mutated p53 are more resistant to apoptosis with subsequent UVR exposures, explaining why p53 inactivation reduces sunburn cells in irradiated mouse skin.[250]

Within the p53 gene there are "hot spots," codons where mutations frequently occur.[32,37] Most p53 mutations result in a single amino acid substitution, typically cytosine to thymine (C → T).[250] Although normal, wild-type p53 has a short half-life and is generally unstable and unstainable, mutated p53 is significantly more stable and consequently stainable by immunohistochemical techniques.[37,190] Both UVA and UVB upregulate p53 expression in human skin.[39] After a single UVR exposure to the forearms, p53 protein expression peaks in 24 hours, returning to baseline after 360 hours.[100]

Mutations in p53 occur as an early, initiating event in photocarcinogenesis.[129] In actinic keratoses, unique p53 mutations are present throughout the lesion,[250] confirming that they occur before, not after, lesion formation. Different actinic keratoses display different p53 mutations, again supporting the role of p53 mutations as initial causative events, followed by clonal expansion of mutated cells to form clinically visible lesions of precancerous actinic keratosis.[250] Altered p53 provides a survival advantage to mutated cells. In response to chronic UVR, neighboring nonmutated cells become apoptotic and die, allowing space for further expansion of the mutated clone with ongoing UVR exposure[32] and ultimately resulting in the development of actinic keratosis or SCCa.

However, p53 mutations alone may be insufficient to produce NMSC. Patients with Li-Fraumeni syndrome, who inherit a mutated form of the p53 gene, have an increased incidence of sarcomas, adenocarcinomas, and melanomas but not NMSC.[129] Consequently, other factors, such as decreased DNA repair and UVR-induced immunosuppression, must play a permissive role. In patients with XP, for example, there are increased numbers of p53 mutations,[32] defective gene repair mechanisms, and greatly increased numbers of NMSC. DNA repair may also be defective in normal, nonsyndromic patients who develop BCCa at an early age[231] and in elderly patients[166] who have a higher incidence of NMSC.

Cutaneous lymphomas may also show a higher frequency of UVR signature p53 mutations.[154] In mycosis fungoides, these mutations are found in the tumor stage but not the plaque stage,[154] suggesting that UVR promotes the clinical progression of this lymphoma. These findings are particularly interesting in view of recent epidemiologic data demonstrating an increased incidence of non-Hodgkin's lymphoma as one moves closer to the equator.[1]

Photoimmunology

UVR produces local and systemic immunosuppression.[172] Locally, UVB depletes Langerhans' cells, which are immunocompetent antigen processing cells, for up to 2 weeks after exposure.[160] In addition, UVB functionally alters Langerhans' cells, diminishing Th1 responses (which promote contact hypersensitivity) while preserving Th2 responses[202] (which suppress contact hypersensitivity), effectively converting the remaining Langerhans' cell from immunogenic to tolerogenic. Antigen-specific suppressor T cells arise, their appearance possibly mediated by UVR-induced synthesis of IL-10 from keratinocytes.[202] As a consequence, contact hypersensitivity and mixed lymphocyte reac-

tions are diminished with UVR exposure. This may explain, at least partially, why UVR-induced skin cancers, which are antigenic, progress into clinical lesions. In mice, this UVR-induced immunosuppression can be transferred with irradiated T lymphocytes.[172] Other proposed mediators of UVR-induced immunosuppression include cis-urocanic acid,[49] TNF-α, prostaglandins,[169] and DNA photoproducts.[161]

Immunoregulatory failure contributes to skin cancer formation.[133] Skin cancer is often more aggressive and occurs at an earlier age in immunosuppressed patients.[64,176] In Australia, 45% of kidney transplant patients develop skin cancer within 11 years and 70% within 20 years.[28] For heart transplant patients in Australia, the incidence of skin cancer is 31% at 5 years and 43% at 10 years, and skin cancer accounts for 27% of patient deaths in this group after the fourth year post-transplant.[176] In these patients, the ratio of SCCa:BCCa is 3:1, precisely opposite the ratio present in non-immunosuppressed patients. These figures are only unusual in that most studies suggest the risk of skin cancer is higher after heart transplant than kidney transplant because of higher doses of immunosuppressive drugs with the former. Chronic sun exposure and fair complexion further increase risks of skin cancer in transplant patients,[176] possibly resulting from overexpression of p53.[88]

PHOTOPROTECTION

Sunscreens

Chemical sunscreens were discovered in 1926. By 1928, the first commercial sunscreen, containing benzyl salicylate and benzyl cinnamate, was marketed in the United States.[74] Subsequent sunscreen evolution was primarily directed toward UVB protection to mitigate the development of sunburn from overexposure to the sun. Paraaminobenzoic acid (PABA) was first advocated as a sunscreen in 1942, patented in 1943, and made commercially available in 1960. By then, national advertisements for sunscreens were blazing the message: tan without burning. Sun protection factor (SPF) 15 formulations only became available around 1980. More recently, as UVA photodamage has been appreciated, UVA sunscreening agents, such as avobenzone, have been introduced. Micronized preparations of titanium dioxide (TiO_2) and zinc oxide (ZnO) have become popular, providing broad-spectrum protection throughout the UVR range. Previously considered "physical" (reflective) as opposed to "chemical" (absorptive) sunscreens, these micronized preparations blur the traditional distinctions. Micronized TiO_2 and ZnO are largely transparent and absorb, reflect, and scatter UVR.[127] Consequently, chemical and physical labels for sunscreens are of diminishing value and perhaps should be dropped.

In the United States, sunscreens are regulated over-the-counter (OTC) products. Until recently, the U.S. Food and Drug Administration (FDA) *Tentative Final Over-the-Counter Drug Products Monograph on Sunscreens,* published in 1993, established the allowable sunscreening agents, testing procedures, and labeling claims for efficacy, water resistance, and safety.[71] This was superceded by the *Final Monograph,* published on May 21, 1999, in the *Federal Register.*[72]

The current FDA-approved sunscreening ingredients are listed in Table 14-1. PABA is an effective UVB absorber but has fallen out of favor. Poorly water soluble, PABA must be formulated in an alcohol vehicle. On the skin, it binds epidermal proteins, enhancing its resistance to water wash-off (substantivity), but provoking contact and photocontact dermatitis in approximately 4% of exposed subjects. Further limiting its acceptability, PABA can permanently stain fabrics a dull yellow color. As a consequence, PABA has been largely replaced by PABA esters—amyldimethyl PABA (padimate A) and octyl dimethyl PABA (padimate O). These absorb well in UVB, are easier to formulate in nonalcoholic vehicles, and are less staining and less allergenic.

TABLE 14-1. Sunscreening Agents Approved in the United States

SUNSCREEN	MAXIMUM %
Aminobenzoic acid	15
Avobenzone	3
Cinoxate	3
Diethanolamine methoxycinnamate*	10
Digalloyl trioleate†	5
Dioxybenzone	3
Ethyl 4- (bis [hydroxypropyl]) aminobenzoate†	5
Glyceryl aminobenzoate†	3
Homosalate	15
Lawsone with dihydroxyacetone*	0.25 with 3
Menthyl anthranilate	5
Octocrylene	10
Octyl methoxycinnamate	7.5
Octyl salicylate	5
Oxybenzone	6
Padimate O	8
Phenylbenzimidazolesulfonic acid	4
Red petrolatum†	100
Titanium dioxide	25
Trolamine salicylate	12
Zinc oxide	25

From Food and Drug Administration: *Final Monograph,* Rockville, Md, May 21, 1999.
*Reserved for inclusion if USP monograph established by May 21, 2001.
†Deleted from FDA *Final Monograph.* To be withdrawn by May 21, 2001.

Cinnamates are the next most potent UVB absorbers. They often replace PABA in "PABA-free" sunscreens, but octyl methoxycinnamate (Parsol MCX) is an order of magnitude less potent than padimate O.[141] Cinnamates are poorly bound to the stratum corneum and may cause contact dermatitis. Cinoxate is the most frequent contact sensitizer, with cross-sensitization to related cinnamates in coca leaves, balsam of Peru, and cinnamon oil.[57]

Salicylates, including homosalate and octyl salicylate, are relatively weak absorbers of UVB and are consequently used in combination with other sunscreening agents. They have the advantage of being nonsensitizing and water insoluble, while helping to solubilize benzophenones in commercial products.[74]

Anthranilates are similarly weak UVB absorbers that also filter UVA. They display peak absorption at 340 nm.[141] Octocrylene is another weak UVB absorber that also absorbs modestly in UVA up to 360 nm. Phenylbenzimidazole sulfonic acid (PBSA) is a unique UVB absorber. Unlike other chemical absorbers, which solubilize in the oil phase of emulsion formulations, PBSA is water soluble. This physiochemical property has resulted in its increasing use in "oil-free" cosmetic sunscreens.[141]

Benzophenones are broader-spectrum sunscreening agents, with good absorption in UVB and UVA up to 360 nm.[141] The three benzophenones available in the U.S. market are oxybenzone, dioxybenzone, and sulisobenzone.

In the United States, dibenzoylmethanes are represented by a single agent—avobenzone (Parsol 1789, butyl methoxydibenzoylmethane). Among the chemical sunscreens, it is the most potent UVA absorber, with little or no absorption in UVB.[141] Its absorption peak at 358 nm falls nearly to zero at 400 nm.[197] Concerns have been raised that photodegradation may limit its effectiveness. Under solar simulated light, avobenzone can be degraded 36% in as little as 15 minutes.[203] However, these data are disputed, and there is debate whether any significant decrease occurs with typical use, especially given the mitigating effect of combined sunscreening agents in commercially available preparations.[203] Additionally, select stabilizing compounds, such as vitamin C, vitamin E, and iron chelators, may retard photodegradation.[155]

Physical sunscreens traditionally refer to opaque agents that primarily reflect, scatter, and, to a lesser extent, absorb UVR. These include calamine, ichthammol, iron oxide, kaolin, red veterinary petroleum, starch, talc, TiO_2, and ZnO. In the wilderness, extemporaneous physical blockers can be made from ashes, mud, and leaves. A sunscreen with a physical filter typically protects throughout the UVR and visible spectra and may even protect against IR-induced erythema.[178] However, classic physical blockers are messy, uncomfortable, and cosmetically undesirable.

In recent years, smaller (micronized or microfine) particle-sized preparations of TiO_2 and ZnO have been made available. Micronized TiO_2 and ZnO have particle size 0.015 to 0.035 μm,[55] making them more soluble in their vehicle base and minimally reflective of visible light. This makes them transparent, or nearly so, in thin coats. ZnO has a lower refractive index than TiO_2 in the visible range, making ZnO less white and more transparent.[163] These micronized preparations significantly absorb UVR, providing broad-spectrum protection from UVB and UVA, blurring the distinction between chemical and physical sunscreens.[55,141,205] TiO_2 and ZnO are sometimes marketed as "chemical-free" sunscreens, clearly a misnomer. Additionally, products containing "physical" sunscreening agents are often marketed as "sunblocks," a misleading term eliminated in the 1999 FDA *Final Monograph*.[72]

Sunscreen Vehicles. Sunscreen vehicles affect efficacy and acceptability. The ideal vehicle spreads easily, maximizes skin adherence, minimizes interaction with the active sunscreening agent, and is noncomedogenic, nonstinging, nonstaining, and inexpensive. In practice, the best vehicle is highly dependent on personal preference. Creams and lotions (emulsions) are most popular. Both are oil-in-water or water-in-oil preparations, although lotions spread more easily. Most sunscreening agents are lipid soluble, accounting for an objectionable, greasy feel. Increasingly popular "dry lotions" minimize the lipid component and often include at least one water-soluble sunscreening agent to reduce oiliness.[141] In contrast, sunscreen oils contain only a lipid phase. Oils spread easily, but thinly, limiting the achievable concentration of active sunscreening agent and thereby limiting protectiveness. In addition, oils are oily and cosmetically less acceptable. Other anhydrous vehicles—ointments and waxes—may be desirable for climbers and winter campers, reducing the risks of chapping and frostbite. Gels are generally nongreasy but tend to wash or sweat off easily. In addition, gels seem to produce more stinging and irritation. Sticks typically incorporate sunscreening agents into wax bases, but application of stick preparations to larger areas is problematic. Aerosols are wasteful, with spray lost to the air, and usually form an uneven film.[141] Increasingly, sunscreens are being incorporated into cosmetics, including foundations, lipsticks, and moisturizers.

Sun Protection Factor. The ability of a sunscreen to protect the skin from UVR-induced erythema is measured by the SPF. The SPF is defined as the ratio of UVR required to produce minimal erythema (1 MED) in sunscreen protected as opposed to unprotected skin.[72,118] It can be represented by the following formula:

$$SPF = \frac{MED \text{ of sunscreen protected skin}}{MED \text{ of unprotected skin}}$$

Testing conditions are standardized by the FDA.[72] The agent to be tested is applied at a standard concentration of 2 mg/cm^2. Testing is performed indoors with a solar simulator on the back between the beltline and scapulae. The SPF is typically determined on a panel of 20 (maximum 25) subjects with skin types I, II, or III. The mean is then determined to be the approved SPF. Using indoor testing with a solar simulator, although more reproducible than outdoor natural sun exposure, may yield a falsely high SPF value. In outdoor testing of more than 30 sunscreens labeled SPF 15, none had SPFs greater than 12.[180] Several factors are responsible: sweating, clothing or towel abrasion, and application variability. In addition, solar simulators generally have reduced outputs of UVA compared with sunlight.[206]

SPF determinations use erythema as their measurable endpoint. Erythema is predominantly a result of UVB, not UVA, exposure. Consequently, SPF is *primarily* a measure of *UVB* protection. The relationship of SPF and UVB absorption is given in Table 14-2.

How high an SPF is necessary? Given that SPF 15 blocks 93% of UVB, some argue that SPF 15 is sufficient[148] and that higher labeling claims are misleading and costly for consumers. However, in several studies, higher SPF sunscreens confer clinical and histologic benefits. In children on Florida beaches, a single application of SPF 25 sunscreen protected just as well as multiple applications for up to 6 hours of exposure.[173] Histologically, an SPF 30 sunscreen provides better protection against sunburn cell formation than does an SPF 15 sunscreen.[116]

Sunscreen Application. Perhaps the most persuasive argument in favor of higher SPF sunscreens derives from variations in application technique. In the real world, sunscreens are applied at much lower concentrations than the 2 mg/cm^2 at which they are tested. Used ad lib, sunscreens are typically applied in concentrations of 0.5 to 1 mg/cm^2.[18,204] The resultant SPF is considerably reduced, typically to about 50% of the labeled SPF for chemical sunscreens.[35] Some suggest the reduction is even greater and that the actual SPF is only 20% to 50% of the labeled value.[219] Physical sunscreens tend to be applied even more thinly, typically

TABLE 14-2. Skin Protection Factor and UVB Absorption

SPF	UVB ABSORPTION (%)
2	50
4	75
8	87.5
15	93.3
30	96.7
50	98

at two thirds the concentration of chemical sunscreens, likely because of their cosmetic visibility.[53] For TiO$_2$ products, application concentrations of 0.65 mg/cm^2 result in SPF values of only 20% to 30% of the intended, labeled value.[219] Not surprisingly, persons who burn more easily tend to apply thicker concentrations of sunscreen.[53] There is no difference in the applied concentrations of higher vs. lower SPF formulations.

Uneven application further reduces sunscreen protection. Using a fluorescent dye, a pattern of spotty use emerges. Individuals typically cover the forehead adequately, but the temples, ears, and posterior neck are often undertreated or missed entirely.[86,142,188] Newly available sunscreens that contain disappearing colorants are popular, allowing visible assurance of complete coverage. Adequate coverage of just the chronically exposed areas (face, ears, and dorsal hands) requires 2 to 3 g,[141] requiring an 8-oz bottle of sunscreen every 80 to 120 days.

Application delay imposes a further decrease in protectiveness. In a study of families on Chicago beaches in summer,[194] sunscreen was applied only after arriving at the beach in 98% of families. The median delay from arrival to application to the last family member was 51 minutes.

Underapplication, uneven application, and delayed application of sunscreens result in unnecessary photoexposure and photodamage. In addition, for hikers, the concomitant use of sunscreen and insect repellent containing diethyltoluamide (DEET) lowers the effective SPF by 34%.[165] Balancing these issues with consumer concerns over SPF inflation, the FDA set a labeling limit of SPF 30+ in the 1999 *Final Monograph*,[72] effective May 21, 2001. This was subsequently extended to December 31, 2002.

UVA Protection Factors. With our increased understanding of UVA-induced photodamage and the recent addition of better UVA blocking agents (avobenzone and micronized TiO$_2$ and ZnO), more attention has been focused on measuring UVA protection. Several measures of UVA protectiveness have been suggested, but none have been widely accepted or used. Among them are the UVA protection factor (APF), analogous to the SPF.[198] The principal drawback to APF determination regards the lengthy exposure times required to induce erythema. A second method, the phototoxic protection factor (PPF), shortens exposure times by sensitizing the skin to UVA with oral or topical psoralens. However, the relevance of PPF data to real-world conditions has been challenged. Other UVA protection factors involve measurement of UVA-induced immediate pigment darkening, suppression of UVA-induced sunburn cell formation in psoralen-treated skin, and UVA-induced photocurrent transmission through various media.[74] In its 1999 *Final Monograph,* the FDA chose not

to impose a specific UVA protection factor but allows a sunscreen to make UVA protection claims as long as it contains an approved UVA sunscreening agent.[72] However, Rosenstein et al[200] found that sunscreens with a labeling claim of UVA protection allow transmission of 6% to 52% of UVA.

Substantivity. The ability of a sunscreen to resist water wash-off is referred to as substantivity. "Water-resistant" sunscreens maintain their SPF after 40 minutes of immersion, "waterproof" sunscreens after 80 minutes. The 1999 FDA *Final Monograph*[72] changes these labels to "water resistant" and "very water resistant," respectively, effective May 21, 2001. Select sunscreening agents, primarily PABA and PABA-esters, are intrinsically substantive resulting from bonding with stratum corneum proteins. Other sunscreens must be incorporated into vehicles that confer substantivity. By applying sunscreen 15 to 30 minutes before water exposure, substantivity can be increased. Reapplication after swimming or sweating helps ensure protection. Numerous high-SPF, waterproof sunscreens are commercially available (Table 14-3).

Conditions for testing substantivity are set by the FDA.[72] Freshwater immersion is required in a pool, whirlpool, or Jacuzzi at 23° to 32° C (73.4° to 89.6° F). This raises some concerns regarding the relevance of substantivity labeling for saltwater ocean enthusiasts, including surfers, sailors, and scuba divers. The MED for skin bathed in salt water is less than the MED for skin bathed in fresh water, and both are lower than the MED of dry skin.[80] Further, cold, churning water; sand abrasion; and toweling may add to sunscreen loss, begging the question of whether waterproof sunscreens are really surfproof. The concerns over saltwater substantivity, amplified by surfer folklore, have led to an almost cultish market of "surfshop" sunscreens, although few published data indicate whether these are more substantive in a saltwater environment.

Sunscreen Prevention of Chronic Photodamage. Sunscreens not only prevent sunburns but also mitigate UVR-induced histologic damage, UVR-induced immunosuppression, photoaging, and photocarcinogenesis. Sunscreens reduce UVR-induced DNA damage,[228] but not entirely.[38] Reductions are seen in pyrimidine photoproducts in humans,[38] as well as in UVR-induced p53 mutations and skin cancer in mice.[3] Sunscreen nearly eliminates the overexpression of p53 in mice after acute[183] and chronic[80] UVR exposure. In humans, an SPF 15 sunscreen reduces p53+ cells by 33% after chronic UVR exposure.[21]

The published effects of sunscreen on immunosuppression are contradictory, largely resulting from the complex relationships of UVR dosing and sensitivity in different experimental models. SPF is not a reliable

TABLE 14-3. Select Sunscreen Products

PRODUCT	SPF	ACTIVE INGREDIENTS	PRODUCT	SPF	ACTIVE INGREDIENTS
HIGH SPF WATERPROOF BROAD-SPECTRUM LOTIONS			**HIGH SPF STICKS**		
Bain de Soleil All Day Waterproof Sunblock	30	B, C, OC, Ti	Bullfrog Stick	18	B, C
Banana Boat Ultra Sunblock	30+	B, C, S	Neutrogena Sunblock Stick	25	B, C, S
BioSun Maximum Sunblock Lotion	45	B, C, OC, S	Shade Stick	30	B, C, S
Coppertone All Day Waterproof Sunblock Lotion	45	B, C, S	**SPECIALTY SUNSCREENS**		
Durascreen Lotion	30	B, C, PBSA, S, Ti	Bullfrog Body Gel	36	B, C, OC
Hawaiian Tropic Super Water-proof Sunblock Lotion	30	C, S, Ti	AloeGator Total Sun Block	40+	B, C, OC, S
Neutrogena Sunblock Lotion	45	B, C, S	Saurus Prosport	44	B, C, OC, S
Ombrelle Sunscreen Lotion	30	A, B, OC, S	Dermatone Sun Protector	23	B, C, PB
PreSun Sensitive Skin Sunscreen	29	B, C, S	**LIP SCREENS**		
Shade UVA Guard	30	A, B, C, S	Banana Boat Aloe Vera Lip Balm	30	B, C, PB, S
Solbar PF Lotion	50	B, C, OC	Chapstick Ultra Lip Protection Sunblock	30	B, C, O, S, Ti
TI Screen Moisturizing Sunscreen Lotion	30	A, B, C, OC, S	Coppertone Lipkote	15	B, C
Vaseline BlockOut Moisturizing Sunblock Lotion	40+	B, C, PB, S, Ti	Neutrogena Lip Moisturizer	15	B, C
Water Babies UVA/UVB Sunblock Lotion	45	B, C, OC, S	Vaseline Lip Therapy	15	B, C
			Water Babies Little Licks Lip Balm	30	B, C, S
HIGH SPF GELS			**"PHYSICAL" SUNSCREENS**		
BioSun Sunblock Gel	30	A, B, C, S	Neutrogena Sensitive Skin Sunblock	17	Ti
PreSun Ultra Clear Gel Sunscreen	30	A, B, C, S	PreSun Block	28	Ti
Shade Sunblock Gel	30	B, C, S	TI-Screen Natural Sunblock lotion	16	ZO
TI-Screen Sports Gel	20	B, C, S			
HIGH SPF SPRAYS			**MOISTURIZERS CONTAINING HIGHER SPF SUNSCREEN**		
Banana Boat Kids Sunblock Spray lotion	25+	B, C, S	Eucerin Facial Moisturizing Lotion	25	C, S, Ti, ZO
Neutrogena Sunblock Spray	20	C, MA, S	Lubriderm Daily UV Lotion	15	B, C, S
Ombrelle Spray Mist	15	A, B, C	Neutrogena Moisture	15	B, C, S
PreSun for Kids Sunscreen Spray	23	B, C, PB, S	Oil of Olay Daily UV Protectant	15	C, PBSA
			Purpose Dual Moisturizer	15	C, MA, Ti

A, Avobenzone; *B*, benzophenones; *C*, cinnamates; *MA*, methyl anthranilate; *OC*, octocrylene; *PB*, PABA or PABA ester; *PBSA*, phenylbenzimidazole sulfonic acid; *S*, salicylates; *Ti*, titanium dioxide; *ZO*, zinc oxide.

measure of a sunscreen's ability to block UVR-induced immunosuppression; two sunscreens with identical SPF values may vary considerably in their immuno-protectant effects.[191] Overall, sunscreens mitigate but do not abrogate UVR-induced immunosuppression. In mice, sunscreens prevent UVR-induced depletion of Langerhans' cells, with higher-SPF sunscreens confer-ring greater protection.[16] However, earlier studies noted little or no beneficial effect from sunscreens.[16] A broad-spectrum SPF 15 sunscreen prevents UVR-in-duced suppression of contact hypersensitivity to dini-trochlorobenzene (DNCB), a potent topical allergen, in humans.[207] In C3H mice transplanted with NMSC, sun-screen blocks UVR-induced immunosuppression, al-lowing tumor rejection, again with increased protection with higher SPF values.[193] However, in susceptible mice injected with melanoma, sunscreens failed to ade-quately suppress UVB enhancement of melanoma growth.[238] This finding was overinterpreted and misin-terpreted to support a peculiar antisunscreen stance. The most appropriate interpretation, however, is that sunscreens by themselves are not sufficient to prevent all of the immunosuppressive sequelae of UVR expo-sure, and that sunscreen should be used as part of a larger sun-protective strategy, including avoidance and clothing protection.

Sunscreens reduce sunburn cell formation and solar elastosis[29] in humans. Histologic changes of photoaging in mice are prevented by pretreatment with SPF 15 sunscreen.[124] In mice exposed to UVB for 10 to 20 weeks, subsequent sunscreen use prevents further photodamage and promotes repair of previous damage, even with continued exposure.[125] Higher-SPF sunscreens provide increasing protection against UVB-induced wrinkling in mice.[25] Similarly, histologic and clinical signs of UVA-induced photoaging are prevented by broad-spectrum sunscreens.[103]

Sunscreen use reduces the formation of precancerous actinic keratoses[170,223] and promotes the resolution of preexisting lesions.[223] In a 2-year trial of sunscreens in humans with actinic keratoses, subjects who benefited most had the greatest number of keratoses at enrollment,[170] underscoring the value of continuing sunscreen use in adults. The daily use of SPF 15 sunscreen in adults reduces the incidence of SCCa but not BCCa.[96a] Stern et al[217] estimated that use of an SPF 15 sunscreen from birth until age 18 would reduce the lifetime risk of NMSC by 78%.

Liquid base makeup, even without sunscreen, provides an SPF of approximately 4 because of pigments in the foundation.[141] For women who use lipstick, the incidence of SCCa is lower than in nonusers or men.[182]

Sunscreens and Melanoma. With melanoma incidence and sunscreen sales both rising over several decades, some have suggested that sunscreens cause melanoma. Garland et al[83,84] have put forth two possible mechanisms:

1. They suggest that sunscreens, by primarily blocking UVB and sunburn, seduce us into longer exposures to UVA in sunlight, and that this increased UVA exposure results in an increased incidence of melanoma.
2. Sunscreens, by blocking UVB, decrease vitamin D levels, which in turn favors melanoma development.

However, most modern sunscreens block substantial amounts of UVA, and recent data suggest that the action spectrum for melanoma in humans is in UVB.[5,122] In addition, vitamin D levels are not diminished in even the most rigorous sunscreen users.[150,213] Consequently, the rises in melanoma incidence and sunscreen use generally reflect increased recreational sun exposure.[169]

Nonetheless, epidemiologic studies have generally failed to demonstrate decreased melanoma incidence with sunscreen use. Paradoxically, several studies have shown an increased risk of melanoma with sunscreen use.[7,54] In 1996, Donawho and Wolf[54] reviewed retrospective studies evaluating melanoma risk in sunscreen users. Only one showed a decreased risk,[110] whereas seven showed an increased risk. A more recent case control study in southern Spain showed a decreased

melanoma risk with sunscreen use.[196] Confounding all of these studies, however, are the following:

1. Persons at highest risk for melanoma (those with fair complexion who burn easily) are precisely the same persons who use sunscreens.
2. Earlier sunscreen products generally had lower SPFs and narrower spectrums.
3. Since sun exposure in childhood appears most provocative for melanoma, surveying adults about sunscreen habits may be irrelevant and misleading.

Sunscreens and Herpes. UVB is a potent stimulus for reactivation of herpes labialis in outdoor enthusiasts. Sunscreen, although ineffective at preventing recurrences in skiers on the slopes,[159] is quite effective in preventing recurrences in the clinical laboratory.[199] Further studies will hopefully resolve this issue.

Sunscreen Side Effects. Sunscreen side effects are generally mild and limited. In a prospective study of 603 subjects who applied SPF 15 sunscreen or vehicle control,[70] 19% in both groups had adverse reactions. Most reactions were irritant in nature, and fewer than 10% were allergic. More than half who developed irritation were atopic. These data support the notion that most contact irritant dermatitis to sunscreens is attributable to excipients. Similarly, allergic reactions to sunscreens are more often due to preservative and fragrances than to active sunscreening agents.[57] As a consequence, and contrary to popular belief, higher-SPF sunscreens are not more irritating than lower-SPF sunscreens.[208]

Nonetheless, most sunscreening agents can cause allergic or photoallergic contact dermatitis.[118] For example, PABA is now rarely used because it sensitizes approximately 4% of exposed subjects. Once sensitized, cross sensitization may occur to thiazides, sulfonamides, benzocaine, and hair dyes containing paraphenylenediamine.[192]

Paradoxically, sunscreens have become the leading cause of photoallergic contact dermatitis.[224] Oxybenzone is the most commonly implicated. In 283 cases of photodermatitis, 35 were photoallergic to oxybenzone and 17 to PABA.[221] In a separate study of 108 patients with photodermatitis, 4 were photoallergic to oxybenzone and 4 to other sunscreening agents.[224]

Stinging or burning without accompanying erythema, scaling, or dermatitis is common, especially in periocular areas and particularly in patients with rosacea, although addition of skin "protectants" (dimethicone or cyclomethicone) to the sunscreen vehicle can mitigate this.[171] Certain vehicles, such as alcoholic gels, may be more stinging. Even when periocular application is avoided, perspiration, water immersion, and rubbing may cause sunscreen to migrate, producing symptoms.

Comedogenicity is primarily related to ingredients in the vehicle base. Certain common excipients (almond oil, cocoa butter, isopropyl myristate, isopropyl palmitate, and olive oil) are possible comedogens.

TiO_2 and ZnO can generate reactive molecular species, called free radicals, with sun exposure.[55] TiO_2 is more photoactive than is ZnO.[163] Electromagnetic radiation with λ less than 412.5 nm has sufficient energy to excite TiO_2 electrons from the valence band to the conduction band.[127] Photoactivated TiO_2 can damage DNA in vitro.[107] In vivo, however, it is unlikely that TiO_2 particles penetrate the stratum corneum to reach underlying epidermal cells containing DNA. Transmission electron microscopy fails to demonstrate TiO_2 penetration of the stratum corneum.[58] Data also demonstrate that ZnO is not absorbed, and Zn levels are unchanged after application.[85] Coating TiO_2 or ZnO with silicone halts the photoproduction of reactive species.[55] Still, some concerns have been raised regarding the use of these agents on broken skin.

Concerns regarding sunscreen-induced vitamin D depletion are generally not warranted. Although regular sunscreen use can decrease cutaneous synthesis of 25-hydroxyvitamin D,[153] sunscreen users nonetheless maintain normal levels of vitamin D. One hundred thirteen subjects using an SPF 17 sunscreen throughout an Australian summer maintained adequate vitamin D levels,[150] and 24 subjects using SPF 15 sunscreen for 2 years maintained normal parathyroid hormone levels and normal bone metabolic markers.[67] Moreover, 8 patients with XP maintained normal vitamin D levels for the 6 years observed, despite rigorous photoprotection with sunscreens, clothing, and sun avoidance.[213] Still, vitamin D supplementation should be considered for elderly patients who may have inadequate vitamin D dietary intake and who are especially at risk for osteopenia and fractures.[94]

Clothing Protection

Clothing is a crucial part of sun protection, providing substantive coverage to broad surface areas. However, clothing varies considerably in its ability to block UVR. Robson and Diffey[195] determined an SPF for 60 different clothing fabrics, ranging from 2 (polyester blouse) to 1000 (cotton twill jean). The single most important factor in determining SPF is the tightness of the weave,[89,144,195] then the actual fabric. An extreme example of this is Lycra, which blocks nearly 100% of UVR when lax and only 2% when maximally stretched.[144] Other determinants include wetness and color. Dry, dark fabrics have a higher SPF than otherwise identical wet, white fabrics.[89] A typical dry, white cotton T-shirt has an SPF of 5 to 9.

Accumulating data show that clothing prevents chronic photodamage. In European children, clothing coverage is associated with fewer nevi.[10] Blue denim reduces UVR-induced p53+ cells twice as effectively as an SPF 15 sunscreen.[21] Denim greatly reduces the formation of skin cancers in patients with XP.[19]

Standardized testing of clothing fabrics has produced a new measure, the ultraviolet protection factor (UPF), analogous to the SPF for sunscreens. A collimated UVR source is passed through flat, tensionless, fabric, with resultant transmission measured by a spectroradiometer or broad-band sensor.[89,195,249] The resultant UPF, however, is generally much lower than actual use values, since natural sunlight is scattered and reflected to a far greater extent than a collimated beam.[187]

In the United States, sun-protective clothing is regulated as a medical device (Figure 14-4). Several manufacturing strategies are used to achieve high SPFs. One approved product, Solumbra, is made of tightly woven nylon with an SPF of 30+. In hairless mice, this fabric is significantly better than cotton in reducing the formation of UVR-induced SCCa.[157] By contrast, Solarknit uses chemically treated cotton and cotton-synthetic blends to achieve an SPF of 30+. Rayosan, a UVR-absorbing agent, bonds to various fabrics, increasing their SPF by up to 300%, and lasts through several washings.[144] A new, unique chemical UVR protectant, Tinosorb FD, may be incorporated into detergents, increasing the SPF of clothing with each wash.

Ladies' hosiery provides a surprisingly low SPF; black hose has an SPF of 1.5 to 3.0 and beige hose has an SPF less than 2.[209] Perhaps this explains in part why skin cancers are more common on the lower legs of women than on those of men.

Hats are also protective, with protection varying as a function of brim diameter and wearing style. Small-brimmed (<2.5 cm) hats adequately protect the forehead and upper nose; medium-brimmed (2.5 to 7.5 cm) and wide-brimmed (>7.5 cm) hats protect increasing proportions of the nose, cheeks, chin, and neck,[52] with large-brimmed hats providing an equivalent SPF of 7 for the nose, 3 for the cheeks, and 2 for the chin. Baseball-style caps are especially useful as a part of an overall sun-protective strategy in children. Using hats to protect the forehead and periocular areas, sunscreen application may be limited to areas below the cheekbones, mitigating the risk of stinging near the eyes.

Glasses, contact lenses, and sunglasses protect the corneas from most UVB and variable amounts of UVA.[201] Surprisingly, price is unrelated to protection.[2] A complete discussion is contained in Chapter 22.

Sun Avoidance

An indoor lifestyle is protective but undesirable for most persons. More practical is the avoidance of excessive midday sun, from 10 AM to 3 PM, significantly reducing UVB exposure.[144] Shade provides variable and often lesser protection than generally assumed. In one study, shade beneath leafy trees provided an SPF less

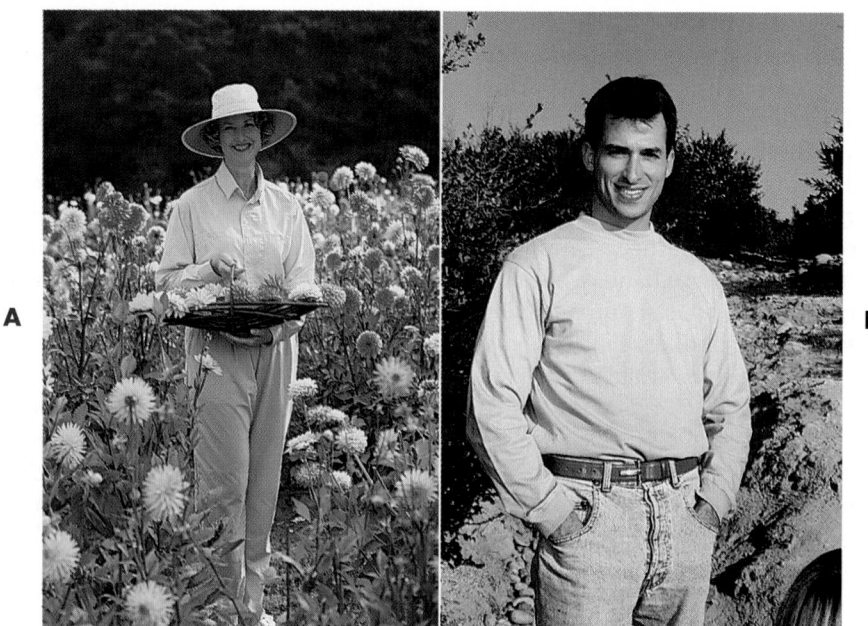

Figure 14-4 Photoprotective clothing. **A,** Solumbra hat, shirt, and pants. **B,** Long-sleeved 100% cotton Solarknit T-shirt. (**A** courtesy Sun Precautions, Inc.; **B** courtesy SunGrubbies.com.)

than 4.[179] Shade cloths allow significantly more UVB exposure than clothing of the same fabrics, largely because of atmospheric scattering and surface reflection.[239]

Automobile windshields typically block UVB and some UVA, whereas side windows block only UVB. This may explain why photodamage is more prominent on the left side of the face in Americans (and on the right side in Australians) who drive a lot.[56] Transparent plastic films, meeting legal requirements in all 50 states, can be applied to block more than 99% of UVR (Llumar UV Shield, CPFilms, Martinsville, Va.).

Sunless Tanning

Bronzers. Most artificial tanners and bronzers contain dihydroxyacetone (DHA, or $C_3H_6O_3$). DHA reacts with amino groups of keratin proteins via the Maillard reaction to form brown pigmented products known as melanoidins.[140] With DHA, bronzing can occur in as little as 1 hour. Often, however, it requires multiple applications to achieve the desired depth of color. Maintaining this bronzed look requires reapplication every few days as the stained stratum corneum is shed from the skin surface. The depth of color is related to the thickness of the stratum corneum and the amount and frequency of application.[141] Frequent cosmetic complaints with DHA include difficulty in obtaining an "even" tan and yellowing of the palms.

DHA + lawsone (a henna dye) is a sunscreening agent. However, DHA alone is an inadequate sunscreen. It absorbs no UVB; rather, DHA absorbs higher-wavelength UVA I and lower-wavelength visible light,[75] making it useful in select photosensitivity disorders, such as porphyrias and polymorphous light eruption. Some commercial bronzing products now contain sunscreen in addition to DHA. However, although the artificial tan in these combination products lasts for days, photoprotection lasts for only hours. Effective May 22, 2000, the FDA *Final Monograph* requires that bronzers without sunscreens display a warning that they do not protect against sunburn.

Certain other products to promote indoor tanning have been used, but few are safe and effective. Tan accelerators, containing melanin precursors such as tyrosine, have no discernible benefit.[114] Sunscreen preparations containing psoralens, most commonly 5-methoxypsoralen (oil of bergamot), are available in Europe. Although these stimulate melanin synthesis, they are tumorigenic in mice.[41] Psoriasis patients treated with psoralen + UVA (PUVA) have a higher incidence of SCCa[215] and, with prolonged use, melanoma.[216] Users of psoralen-containing sunscreen have an increased risk of subsequent melanoma.[7] Oral carotenoids, especially canthaxanthin, have been promoted as tanning pills but are potentially toxic and, consequently, not approved in the United States.

Tanning Salons. Although precise data are lacking, approximately 25 million North Americans, many of them adolescents, use tanning salons each year.[220] In a survey of high school students in St. Paul, Minnesota, 34% admitted to using tanning salons at least four times in the previous year.[174] Until 1980, most sunlamps emitted mostly UVB.[7] Now tanning salons utilize high-output UVA tanning beds and market their services as a way to tan without burning with a subtle but incorrect message that such tans are safe. However, chronic suberythemal UVA contributes to photoaging, immunosuppression, and carcinogenesis. In addition, there is significant variation in the radiation output of tanning beds. In a study of 50 tanning beds in England,[241] UVA outputs varied by a factor of 3 and UVB output varied by a factor of 60. Typically, tanning bed outputs are contaminated with 2% to 10% UVB,[229] more than the average UVB content of natural sunlight. In 38 Scottish tanning units, 10 minutes of exposure yielded the same carcinogenic risk as 30 minutes of peak summer sun at the same latitude.[167]

Tanning bed exposure for 15 to 20 minutes induces DNA damage in fibroblasts.[240] Several case-control studies document a positive association between tanning bed use and the later development of melanoma.[6,230,237] In a Swedish study of 400 patients and 640 controls, persons who used sunbeds or sunlamps before age 30 had a 7.7-fold increased risk of melanoma.[237] In 420 patients from Germany, France, and Belgium, melanoma risks increased 8.97-fold when sunlamps or sunbeds were used for tanning.[6]

Ironically, UVA tans are less effective than natural tans in conferring protection against subsequent sunburn.[117] In addition, maintenance of a yearlong tan provides no protection against subsequent melanoma development.[110] Too often, tanning salons ignore photosensitizing risks in their patrons.[36] Sadly, the damage from tanning salons is insidious. Public awareness and governmental regulation need to be heightened.

Melanin and Thymine Dimers. Cyclobutane T-T dimers, produced by the action of UVR on skin, stimulate melanin synthesis and subsequent pigmentation.[91] Eller et al[60] exposed melanocyte cultures to synthetic T-T dimers and noted twofold to threefold increases in tyrosinase messenger ribonucleic acid (mRNA) and sevenfold increases in melanin production. Topical application to guinea pigs increases pigmentation. This raises the question of whether induction of protective pigmentation in humans might be possible with T-T dimers, whether it is possible to induce a safe tan.

Unique Photoprotectants

Systemic Sunscreens. Safe and effective oral sunscreens remain elusive. Clearly, these would have an advantage in convenience, coverage, and substantivity. Several oral agents have been evaluated, but none has a favorable risk/benefit ratio in normal individuals, although a few are used in patients with photosensitivity disorders. Betacarotene is helpful in erythropoietic protoporphyria, chloroquine in lupus erythematous, and psoralens in polymorphous light eruption.

Antioxidants. UVR exposure results in reactive oxygen species that contribute to DNA damage[181] and the peroxidative destruction of membrane lipids.[113] These effects contribute to DNA structural abnormalities, inflammation, and immune alterations. Protecting the skin from reactive species are various natural antioxidants (vitamins A, C, and E; reduced glutathione; urocanic acid; melanin) and enzymatic systems (catalase, superoxide dismutase).[113] However, chronic exposure to UVR depletes the skin of these antioxidants.[147]

Application of antioxidants before UVR exposure delays skin damage in hairless mice.[24] Select forms of vitamin E, especially tocopherol sorbate, diminish photoinduced free radicals and skin wrinkling in mice.[115] Topical application of vitamins C and E provide protection against the histopathologic changes of photodamage in swine skin.[48] In this animal system, sunscreen plus vitamins C and E provide more protection than sunscreen alone.[48] Although vitamin C does not act as a sunscreen—it does not absorb UVR—it protects against erythema and sunburn cell formation by quenching free radicals that are at least partially causative.[47] Interestingly, the beneficial effect of topical vitamin C in swine skin persists for 72 hours after application, suggesting a potential strategy for longer-term photoprotection.

Topical antioxidants seem more effective than oral antioxidants in preventing photodamage. Orally, 2 g of vitamin C combined with 1000 IU of vitamin E for 8 days increases the MED only modestly.[59] There are some concerns, however, about the routine use of topical antioxidants. For example, vitamin E may provoke contact sensitization and serve as a tumor promoter.[162] Antioxidants might interfere with the normal functioning of p53 protein to produce apoptosis of photodamaged keratinocytes via oxidative enzymes.

Repair Enzyme: T4N5. Recently there has been considerable interest in postexposure therapy for sunburn with topical application of a DNA repair enzyme, T4 endonuclease V (T4N5). Applied in liposomes, it localizes in the epidermis and appendages,[243] enhancing repair of UVR-induced DNA damage in mice and humans.[242] T4N5 prevents UVR-induced immunosuppression[134] and reduces UVR-induced skin cancer in mice.[244] With these qualities, T4N5 may serve in the future as a "morning-after" cream.

PHOTOSENSITIVITY DISORDERS

Endogenous Photosensitivity Disorders

Sun protection is especially important for persons with endogenous photosensitizing disorders, persons who take photosensitizing medications (Box 14-3) and persons exposed to topical photosensitizers (Box 14-4). The most common endogenous photodermatosis is poly-

---

Box 14-3 COMMON ORAL PHOTOSENSITIZING MEDICATIONS

Fluoroquinolones   Sulfonamides
Furosemide   Tetracyclines
Nonsteroidal antiinflammatory drugs   Thiazides
Phenothiazines

Box 14-4 TOPICAL PHOTOTOXINS AND PHOTOALLERGENS

TOPICAL PHOTOTOXIC COMPOUNDS

Dyes

Eosin
Methylene blue

Medications

Phenothiazines
Sulfonamides

Psoralens

Methoxypsoralen
Trimethylpsoralen

Tars

Creosote
Pitch

TOPICAL PHOTOTOXIC PLANTS

Angelica
Carrot
Celery
Cow parsley
Dill
Fennel
Fig
Gas plant
Giant hogweed

TOPICAL PHOTOTOXIC PLANTS—cont'd

Lemon
Lime
Meadow grass
Parsnip
Stinking mayweed
Yarrow

TOPICAL PHOTOALLERGENIC COMPOUNDS

Antiseptics

Chlorhexidine
Hexachlorophene

Fragrances

Methylcoumarin
Musk ambrette

Phenothiazines

Salicylanilides

Sulfonamides

Sunscreens

Benzophenones
Cinnamates
Dibenzoylmethanes
PABA
PABA esters

---

morphous light eruption (PLE), affecting 10% to 14% of whites, predominantly females under age 30. Clinically this presents with pruritus, erythema, macules, papules, or vesicles on sun-exposed skin, arising 1 to 2 days after exposure and resolving spontaneously over the next 7 to 10 days. It is most common with initial sun exposures in spring or early summer; "hardening" of the skin may occur with subsequent exposures. The action spectrum is unclear, although it is most commonly 290 to 365 nm.[74] Sunscreens are only sometimes helpful, although a broad-spectrum sunscreen containing padimate O and avobenzone was quite effective in one study.[76] Sun avoidance and protective clothing are valuable. PUVA, oral antimalarials, and betacarotene have also been used with varying success.

Lupus erythematosus may be exacerbated by sunlight. Although UVB is typically causative, UVA can contribute in some patients. Consequently, broad-spectrum sunscreens, combined with sun avoidance and clothing protection, are most appropriate. A broad-spectrum sunscreen containing padimate O and avobenzone diminished the clinical severity in a 4-week study.[44] Systemic antimalarials may also be used in more serious cases.

Porphyrias are due to inherited abnormalities in heme synthesis. Clinical manifestations vary with the genetic subtype, but photosensitivity is common to this group of disorders. Typically, the action spectrum is in the Soret band, 400 to 410 nm. Consequently, sunscreens other than "physical" blockers are generally inadequate, although topical DHA and oral beta carotene may be useful adjuncts to sun avoidance and protective clothing.

Chronic actinic dermatitis presents as persistent macules and plaques, often infiltrated and lichenified, in chronically sun-exposed sites on older men. These patients may demonstrate dermatitic flares on involved areas with even modest photoexposure to UVR and shorter wavelength visible light. Histologically, the disorder can demonstrate progression from dermatitis to T cell lymphoma. Broad-spectrum sunscreens, sun avoidance, and clothing protection, including brimmed hats, are essential. For advanced cases, therapy with azathioprine, cyclosporine, PUVA, and retinoids has been used.

Persons with persistent light reaction (PLR) display a peculiar and persistent overreaction to sun from a prior topical photoallergy. Musk ambrette, found in many perfumes, has been reported to provoke PLR.[192] UVB is most often causative, although UVA may be involved as well. Broad-spectrum sunscreens, sun avoidance, and clothing protection provide appropriate prophylaxis.

For disorders in which melanocytes are defective or absent, such as albinism and vitiligo, and disorders in which DNA repair mechanisms are deficient, such as xeroderma pigmentosum, the protective triad of sunscreens, sun avoidance, and clothing protection is required.

Phototoxicity

Most oral photodrug eruptions are phototoxic, clinically presenting as exaggerated sunburn on exposed skin. Typically, there are sharp "cutoffs" at the V of the neck and short-sleeve line. Less commonly, there may be photoonycholysis, in which the distal fingernails separate from their underlying beds. Photodrug eruptions are usually triggered by UVA. The most common offending drugs are listed in Box 14-3.

Topical photosensitizers may cause phototoxicity, photoallergy, or both. Phototoxicity results in an exaggerated sunburn, typically followed by postinflammatory pigmentation. Phototoxicity is nonimmunologic. The action spectrum for most topical phototoxic sensitizers is in UVR.

A surprisingly large number of plants contain photosensitizers that can produce phototoxic reactions in exposed human skin (see Box 14-4), resulting in a condition known as phytophotodermatitis. The most common chemical precipitants are furocoumarins, especially psoralens found in limes, lemons, and certain other plants. Phytophotodermatitis is common in farmworkers, bartenders, cannery packers, and vacationers to sunny climates. Oil of bergamot, containing 5-methoxypsoralen, is a frequent cause of phototoxicity in perfumes (berloque dermatitis). Streaks of erythema and subsequent pigmentation on exposed skin

of the face, neck, and wrists typify this eruption. Meadow-grass dermatitis in hikers is another example of phytophotodermatitis. Various common weeds, including meadow parsnip, contain furocoumarins, causing whiplike erythematous streaks and pigment on skin after exposure to sunlight.

Psoralens have been incorporated into sunscreens in Europe to promote tanning, although their use is associated with increasing risks of burns and carcinogenicity.[41] Psoralens, in combination with UVA (PUVA), are used therapeutically for psoriasis and select other dermatoses.

Photoallergy

Although phototoxic reactions may occur in anyone, photoallergic reactions occur only in previously sensitized individuals. Photoallergic reactions are uncommon. They are typically provoked by the interaction of UVA on a topical proallergen, resulting in contact dermatitis within 48 hours. Unlike phototoxic reactions, which are limited to exposed skin, photoallergic reactions can spread to sun-protected adjacent sites. Paradoxically, sunscreens are the current leading cause of photoallergy.[51,112] In the 1970s, a fragrance, 6-methylcoumarin, added to a suntanning product was responsible for a number of cases of photoallergy.[192] In the 1960s, there was a virtual epidemic of photoallergic reactions resulting from antibacterial salicylanilides in soaps.[192] Prevention requires excellent UVA protection, including broad-spectrum sunscreens.

CHANGING ATTITUDES TOWARD PHOTOPROTECTION

In the twentieth century, a tan has become desirable, equated with health, wealth, and stylishness. Characterizing the temper of the times is Coco Chanel's pronouncement in 1929 that "A golden tan is the index of chic." Sadly, this attitude led to dangerous behaviors, resulting in an epidemic of skin cancer.

Several studies document current attitudes toward photoprotection. In a study of Connecticut beachgoers, 70% were there to get or maintain a tan.[252] College students questioned in North Carolina rarely, if ever, used sunscreens.[227] In a U.S. study of 2459 Caucasians, 59% admitted to sunbathing and 25% to sunbathing more than 10 times in the preceding year.[128] Among spring skiers, only two thirds used sunscreens, and, of those, one third were sunburned at the time of the survey.[155] A survey in Leicester, England, found that half of all children sunburn at least once a year.[27] Even patients with sun-related problems often do not adopt adequate sun protection habits. One study documented that patients with dysplastic nevus syndrome, who are at higher risk for melanoma, do not avoid sunburning.[30] Among Israeli patients 1 year after treatment for BCCa, only 49%

wear hats or long sleeves in summer and 62% use less than two bottles of sunscreen per year.[105]

Sunscreen use correlates with knowledge of the harmful effects of sun exposure and understanding of SPF values.[22] In a survey of 1001 adults in the United States, only 42% were aware of the term *melanoma,* and only 34% knew it was some type of skin cancer.[158] Many mistakenly use sunscreens in the belief that sunscreens will promote tanning. Clearly, more education is needed. In Australia, where a significant educational effort is underway, three fourths of adults visiting a family physician report using sunscreens.[151] Increasingly, Australian fashion magazine models are less tan and feature more hats.[42]

Photoprotection education needs to begin in childhood. Up to 80% of lifetime sun exposure occurs by age 18,[217] and childhood exposure may be more significant than lifetime exposure in determining the subsequent risks of BCCa and melanoma. Children who use, or are compelled to use, sunscreens at an early age are more likely to use sunscreens as adolescents.[15] This requires educating parents. Sadly, parents too often ignore, or are ignorant of, photoprotective measures. On beaches in Galveston, Texas, in midday July, only 42 of 82 parents interviewed applied sunscreen to their children.[146] Only a history of prior painful sunburns was correlated with sunscreen use, a finding documented in other studies as well.[251] Hopefully, physicians can alter parental behavior through education, beginning with the first well-baby visit. In the Galveston study, photoprotection was discussed in only 18% of well-baby checkups. Sun avoidance and clothing protection should be advocated for infants under age 6 months, while sunscreen may be added to the photoprotective regimen for older toddlers and children. Consistent use of sun protection in childhood would not only decrease sunburns but would provide lifelong reductions in photoaging and NMSC.[217]

Advertisers and the fashion industry continue to glorify tans with darkly tanned models. Even sunscreen advertisements seem to have a dual and medically incompatible message: tan beautifully while protecting your skin. No wonder the public is confused by oxymoronic enticements to a "healthy tan."[186] Recently, in the United States, there is a glimmer of progress toward photoprotection education in the public media. In a review of models in six popular American fashion magazines, 1983-1993, there is a trend toward lighter tans, more sunscreens, and more sun awareness articles, although men's magazines did not show this trend.[87]

CONCLUSION

Sun exposure is associated with deleterious sequelae, both acute and chronic. Sun protection significantly mitigates these sequelae. Effective sun-protective strategies include sun avoidance, clothing protection, and sunscreens. Sun protection should begin in infancy and continue throughout life; education of parents and children is key to its success. With the introduction of high-SPF, broad-spectrum, waterproof sunscreens and high-SPF clothing fabrics, the office worker and wilderness enthusiast alike can enjoy the outdoors more safely.

REFERENCES

1. Adami J et al: Sunlight and non-Hodgkin's lymphoma: a population-based cohort study in Sweden, *Int J Cancer* 80:641, 1999.
2. Ambach W, Blumthaler M, Grobner J: Sports glasses and ultraviolet protection, *Wilderness Environ Med* 6:29, 1995.
3. Ananthaswamy HN et al: Inhibition of solar simulator-induced p53 mutations and protection against skin cancer development in mice by sunscreens, *J Invest Dermatol* 112:763, 1999.
4. Armstrong BK, Kricker AM: How much melanoma is caused by sun exposure? *Melanoma Res* 3:2, 1995.
5. Atillasoy ES et al: UV induces atypical melanocytic lesions and melanoma in human skin, *Am J Pathol* 152:1179, 1998.
6. Autier P et al: Cutaneous malignant melanoma and exposure to sunlamps or sunbeds: an EORTC multicenter case-control study in Belgium, France, and Germany, *Int J Cancer* 58:809, 1994.
7. Autier P et al: Melanoma and use of sunscreens: an EORTC case-control study in Germany, Belgium and France, *Int J Cancer* 61:749, 1995.
8. Autier P et al: Melanoma risk and residence in sunny area, *Br J Cancer* 76:1521, 1997.
9. Autier P et al: Influence of sun exposures during childhood and during adulthood on melanoma risk, *Int J Cancer* 77:533, 1998.
10. Autier P et al: Sunscreen use, wearing clothes, and number of nevi in 6-to-7-year-old European children, *J Natl Cancer Inst* 90:1873, 1998.
11. Baade PD, Balanda KP, Lowe JB: Changes in skin protection behaviors, attitudes, and sunburn in a population with the highest incidence of skin cancer in the world, *Cancer Detect Prev* 20:566, 1996.
12. Bajdik CD et al: Non-solar radiation and the risk of basal and squamous cell skin cancer, *Br J Cancer* 73:1612, 1996.
13. Baker GE, Driscoll MS, Wagner RF: Emergency department management of sunburn reactions, *Cutis* 61:209, 1998.
14. Bangha, Eisner P, Kistler MS: Suppression of UV-induced erythema by topical treatment with melatonin (N-acetyl-S-methoxytryptamine), *Dermatology* 195:248, 1997.
15. Banks BA et al: Attitudes of teenagers toward sun exposure and sunscreen use, *Pediatrics* 89:40, 1992.
16. Beasley DG et al: Commercial sunscreen lotions prevent ultraviolet radiation-induced depletion of epidermal Langerhans cells in Skh-1 and C3H mice, *Photodermatol Photoimmunol Photomed* 14:90, 1998.
17. Bech-Thomsen N, Ravnborg L, Wulf HC: A quantitative study of the melanogenic effect of multiple suberythemal doses of different ultraviolet radiation sources, *Photodermatol Photoimmunol Photomed* 10:53, 1994.
18. Bech-Thomsen N, Wulf HC: Sunbathers' application of sunscreen is probably inadequate to obtain the sun protection factor assigned to the preparation, *Photodermatol Photoimmunol Photomed* 9:242, 1992-1993.
19. Bech-Thomsen N, Wulf HC, Ullman S: Xeroderma pigmentosum lesions related to UV transmittance by clothes, *J Am Acad Dermatol* 24:365, 1991.
20. Begley S: Holes in the ozone treaty, *Newsweek* p 70, Sept 2, 1995.
21. Berne B, Ponten J, Ponten F: Decreased p53 expression in chronically sun-exposed human skin after topical photoprotection, *Photodermatol Photoimmunol Photomed* 14:148, 1998.
22. Berwick M, Fine JA, Bolognia JL: Sun exposure and sunscreen use following a community skin cancer screening, *Prev Med* 21:302, 1992.
23. Berwick M, Halpern A: Melanoma epidemiology, *Curr Opin Oncol* 9:178, 1997.
24. Bissett DL, Chatterjee R, Hannon DP: Photoprotective effect of superoxide-scavenging antioxidants against ultraviolet radiation-induced chronic skin damage in hairless mouse, *Photodermatol Photoimmunol Photomed* 7:56, 1990.
25. Bissett DL et al: Time-dependent decrease in sunscreen protection against chronic photodamage in UVB-irradiated hairless mouse skin, *J Photochem Photobiol* 9:323, 1991.

26. Bolognia J, Murray M, Pawelek J: UVB-induced melanogenesis may be mediated through the MSH-receptor system. *J Invest Dermatol* 92:651, 1989.

27. Bourke JF, Graham-Brown RAC: Protection of children against sunburn: a survey of parental practice in Leicester, *Br J Dermatol* 133:264, 1995.

28. Bouwes Bavinck JN et al: The risk of skin cancer in renal transplant recipients in Queensland, Australia, *Transplantation* 61:715, 1996.

29. Boyd AS el al: The effects of chronic sunscreen use on the histologic changes of dermatoheliosis, *J Am Acad Dermatol* 33:941, 1995.

30. Brandberg Y et al: Sun-related behaviour in individuals with dysplastic naevus syndrome, *Acta Derm Venereol* 76:381, 1996.

31. Brash DE et al: A role for sunlight in skin cancer: UV-induced p53 mutations in squamous cell carcinoma, *Proc Natl Acad Sci USA* 88:10124, 1991.

32. Brash DE et al: Sunlight and sunburn in human skin cancer: p53, apoptosis, and tumor progression, *J Invest Dermatol Symp Proc* 1:136, 1996.

33. Breitbart M et al: Ultraviolet light exposure, pigmentary traits and the development of melanocytic naevi and cutaneous melanoma, *Acta Derm Venereol* 77:374, 1997.

34. Brown J et al: Malignant melanoma in World War II veterans, *Int J Dermatol* 23:661, 1984.

35. Brown S, Diffey BL: The effect of applied thickness on sunscreen protection: *in vivo* and *in vitro* studies, *Photochem Photobiol* 44:509, 1986.

36. Bruyneel-Rupp F, Dorsey SB, Guin JD: The tanning salon: an area survey of equipment, procedures, practices, *J Am Acad Dermatol* 18:1030, 1988.

37. Buzzell RA: Carcinogenesis of cutaneous malignancies, *Dermatol Surg* 22:209, 1996.

38. Bykov VJ, Marcusson JA, Hemminki K: Ultraviolet B-induced DNA damage in human skin and its modulation by a sunscreen, *Cancer Res* 58:2961, 1998.

39. Campbell C et al: Wavelength specific patterns of p53 induction in human skin following exposure to UV radiation, *Cancer Res* 53:2697, 1993.

40. Carli P et al: Cutaneous melanoma histologically associated with a nevus and melanoma de novo have a different profile of risk: results from a case-control study, *J Am Acad Dermatol* 40:549, 1999.

41. Cartwright LE, Walter JF: Psoralen-containing sunscreen is tumorigenic in hairless mice, *J Am Acad Dermatol* 8:830, 1983.

42. Chapman S, Marks R, King M: Trends in tans and skin protection in Australian fashion magazines, 1982 through 1991, *Am J Public Health* 82:1677, 1992.

43. Cripps D: Natural and artificial photoprotection, *J Invest Dermatol* 76:154, 1981.

44. Cullen JP et al: Safety and efficacy of a broad spectrum sunscreen in patients with discoid or subacute lupus erythematosus, *Cutis* 47:130, 1991.

45. Czarnecki D et al: Squamous cell carcinoma in southern and northern Australia, *Int J Dermatol* 31:492, 1992.

46. Danno K, Takigawa M, Horio T: Relationship of cell cycle to sunburn cell formation, *Photochem Photobiol* 34:203, 1981.

47. Darr D et al: Topical vitamin C protects porcine skin from ultraviolet radiation-induced damage, *Br J Dermatol* 127:247, 1992.

48. Darr D et al: Effectiveness of antioxidants (vitamin C and E) with and without sunscreens as topical photoprotectants, *Acta Derm Venereol* 76:264, 1996.

49. de Fine Olvarius F et al: The sunscreening effect of urocanic acid, *Photodermatol Photoimmunol Photomed* 12:95, 1996.

50. de Gruijl FR, Van Der Leun JC: Estimate of the wavelength dependency of ultraviolet carcinogenesis in humans and its relevance to the risk assessment of a stratospheric ozone depletion, *Health Phys* 67:319, 1994.

51. De Leo V, Suarez S, Maso M: Photoallergic contact dermatitis: results of photopatch testing in New York, 1985-1990, *Arch Dermatol* 128:1513, 1992.

52. Diffey BL, Cheeseman J: Sun protection with hats, *J Dermatol* 127:10, 1992.

53. Diffey BL, Grice J: The influence of sunscreen type on photoprotection, *Br J Dermatol* 137:103, 1997.

54. Donawho C, Wolf P: Sunburn, sunscreen, and melanoma, *Curr Opin Oncol* 8:159, 1996.

55. Draelos ZD: Photoprotection of the skin and hair, *Cosmetic Dermatology* 12:15, 1999.

56. Drivers alert: you may be vulnerable to sun damage, *Sun & Skin News* 16:1, 1999.

57. Dromgoole SH, Maibach HI: Sunscreening agent intolerance: contact and photocontact sensitization and contact urticaria, *J Am Acad Dermatol* 22:1068, 1990.

58. Dussert AS, Gooris E, Hemmerle J: Characterization of the mineral content of a physical sunscreen emulsion and its distribution onto human stratum corneum, *Int J Cosmet Sci* 19:119, 1997.

59. Eberlein-König B, Placzek M, Przybilla B: Protective effect against sunburn of combined systemic ascorbic acid (vitamin C) and d-α-tocopherol (vitamin E), *J Am Acad Dermatol* 38:45, 1998.

60. Eller MS, Yaar M, Gilchrest BA: DNA damage and melanogenesis, *Nature* 372:413, 1994.

61. Elwood JM: Melanoma and sun exposure: contrasts between intermittent and chronic exposure, *World J Surg* 16:157, 1992.

62. Elwood JM: Melanoma and ultraviolet radiation, *Clin Dermatol* 10:41, 1992.

63. Elwood JM, Jopson J: Melanoma and sun exposure: an overview of published studies, *Int J Cancer* 73:198, 1997.

64. Espana A et al: Skin cancer in heart transplant recipients, *J Am Acad Dermatol* 32:458, 1995.

65. Everett MA et al: Penetration of the epidermis by ultraviolet rays, *Photochem Photobiol* 5:533, 1966.

66. Farman JC, Gardiner BG, Shanklin JD: Large losses of total ozone in Antarctica reveal seasonal ClOx/NOx interaction, *Nature* 315:207, 1985.

67. Farrerons J et al: Clinically prescribed sunscreen (sun protective factor 15) does not decrease serum vitamin D concentration sufficiently either to induce changes in parathyroid function or in metabolic markers, *Br J Dermatol* 139:422, 1998.

68. Fisher GJ et al: Molecular basis of sun-induced premature skin aging and retinoid antagonism, *Nature* 379:335, 1996.

69. Fisher GJ et al: Pathophysiology of premature skin aging induced by ultraviolet light, *N Engl J Med* 337:1419, 1997.

70. Foley P et al: The frequency of reactions to sunscreens: results of a longitudinal population-based study on the regular use of sunscreens in Australia, *Br J Dermatol* 128:512, 1993.

71. Food and Drug Administration: Tentative final over-the-counter drug products monograph on sunscreens, *Federal Register* 58:28194, 1993.

72. Food and Drug Administration: Sunscreen drug products for over-the-counter human use final monograph, *Federal Register* 64:27666, 1999.

73. Freon smuggling case just tip of the iceberg? *The San Diego Union Tribune* p A-1, Jan 10, 1997.

74. Friedlander J, Lowe NJ: Exposure to radiation from the sun. In Auerbach PS, editor: *Wilderness medicine: management of wilderness and environmental emergencies*, ed 3, St Louis, 1995, Mosby.

75. Fusaro RM, Johnson JA: Protection against long ultraviolet and/or visible light with topical dihydroxyacetone, *Dermatologica* 150:346, 1975.

76. Fusaro RM, Johnson JA: Topical photoprotection for hereditary polymorphic light eruption of American Indians, *J Am Acad Dermatol* 24:744, 1991.

77. Gallagher CH et al: Ultraviolet carcinogenesis in the hairless mouse skin: influence of the sunscreen 2-ethylbexyl-p-methoxy-cinnamate, *Aust J Exp Biol Med Sci* 62:577, 1984.

78. Gallagher RP et al: Sunlight exposure, pigmentary factors, and risk of nonmelanocytic skin cancer I. Basal cell carcinoma, *Arch Dermatol* 131:157, 1995.

79. Gallagher RP et al: Sunlight exposure, pigmentation factors, and risk of nonmelanocytic skin cancer II. Squamous cell carcinoma, *Arch Dermatol* 131:164, 1995.

80. Gambichler T, Schröpl F: Changes of minimal erythema dose after water and salt water baths, *Photodermatol Photoimmunol Photomed* 14:109, 1998.

81. Garbe C et al: Associated factors in the prevalence of more than 50 common melanocytic nevi, and actinic lentigines: multicenter case-control study of the Central Malignant Melanoma registry of the German Dermatological Society, *J Invest Dermatol* 102:700, 1994.

82. Garbe C et al: Risk factors for developing cutaneous melanoma and criteria for identifying persons at risk: multicenter case-control study of the Central Malignant Melanoma Registry of the German Dermatological Society, *J Invest Dermatol* 102:695, 1994.

83. Garland CF, Garland FC, Gorham ED: Rising trends in melanoma. An hypothesis concerning sunscreen effectiveness, *Ann Epidemiol* 3:103, 1993.

84. Garland FC et al: Occupational sunlight exposure and melanoma in the US Navy, *Arch Environ Health* 45:261, 1990.

85. Gasparro FP, Mitchnick M, Nash JF: A review of sunscreen safety and efficacy, *Photochem Photobiol* 68:243, 1998.

86. Gaughan M, Padilla RS: Use of a topical fluorescent dye to evaluate effectiveness of sunscreen application, *Arch Dermatol* 134:515, 1998.

87. George PM, Kuskowski M, Schmidt C: Trends in photoprotection in American fashion magazines, 1983-1993, *J Am Acad Dermatol* 34:424, 1996.

88. Gibson GE et al: p53 tumor suppressor gene protein expression in premalignant and malignant skin lesions of kidney transplant recipients, *J Am Acad Dermatol* 36:924, 1997.

89. Gies HP et al: Ultraviolet radiation protection factors for clothing, *Health Phys* 67:131, 1994.

90. Gilchrest BA, Murphy G, Soter NA: Effect of chronologic aging and ultraviolet irradiation on Langerhans cells in human epidermis, *J Invest Dermatol* 79:85, 1982.

91. Gilchrest BA et al: Mechanisms of ultraviolet light-induced pigmentation, *Photochem Photobiol* 63:1, 1996.

92. Giles GG et al: Has mortality from melanoma stopped rising in Australia? Analysis of trends between 1931 and 1994, *BMJ* 312:1121, 1996.

93. Gloster HM Jr, Brodland DG: The epidemiology of skin cancer, *Dermatol Surg* 22:217, 1996.

94. Gloth M et al: Vitamin D deficiency in homebound elderly persons, *JAMA* 274:1683, 1995.

95. Gniadecka M et al: Photoprotection in vitiligo and normal skin, *Acta Derm Venereol* 76:429, 1996.

96. Greaves MW, Sondergaard T: Pharmacologic agents released in ultraviolet inflammation studied by continuous skin perfusion, *J Invest Dermatol* 54:365, 1990.

96a. Green A et al: Daily sunscreen application and beta-carotene supplementation in prevention of basal-cell and squamous cell carcinomas of the skin: a randomized controlled trial, *Lancet* 354:723, 1999.

97. Griffiths CE et al: Restoration of collagen formation in photodamaged human skin by tretinoin (retinoic acid), *N Engl J Med* 329:530, 1993.

98. Hacham H, Freeman SE, Gange RW: Do pyrimidine dimer yields correlate with erythema induction in human skin irradiated in situ with ultraviolet light (275-365 nm)? *Photochem Photobiol* 53:559, 1991.

99. Hall HI et al: Update on the incidence and mortality from melanoma in the United States, *J Am Acad Dermatol* 40:35, 1999.

100. Hall PA et al: High levels of p53 protein in UV-irradiated normal human skin, *Oncogene* 8:203, 1993.

101. Hanson KM, Simon JD: Epidermal trans-urocanic acid and the UVA-induced photoaging of the skin, *Proc Natl Acad Sci USA* 95:10576, 1998.

102. Harber LC, DeLeo VA, Prystowsky JH: Intrinsic and extrinsic photoprotection against UVB and UVA radiation. In Lowe NJ, editor: *Physicians guide to sunscreens*, New York, 1991, Marcel Dekker.

103. Harrison JA et al: Sunscreens with low sun protection factor inhibit ultraviolet A and B photoaging in the skin of the hairless albino mouse, *Photodermatol Photoimmunol Photomed* 8:12, 1991.

104. Harrison SL et al: Sun exposure and melanocytic naevi in young Australian children, *Lancet* 344:1529, 1994.

105. Harth Y et al: Sun protection and sunscreens use after surgical treatment of basal cell carcinoma, *Photodermatol Photoimmunol Photomed* 11:140, 1995.

106. Hayman GD: CFCs and the ozone layer, *Br J Clin Pract* 89(suppl):2, 1996.

107. Hidaka H et al: In vitro photochemical damage to DNA, RNA and their bases by an inorganic sunscreen agent on exposure to UVA and UVB radiation, *Photochem Photobiol* 111:205, 1997.

108. Hogan DJ et al: Risk factors for basal cell carcinoma, *Int J Dermatol* 28:591, 1989.

109. Holleran WM et al: Structural and biochemical basis for the UVB-induced alterations in epidermal barrier function, *Photodermatol Photoimmunol Photomed* 13:117, 1997.

110. Holly EA et al: Cutaneous melanoma in women I. Exposure to sunlight, ability to tan, and other risk factors related to ultraviolet light, *Am J Epidemiol* 141:923, 1995.

111. Hollstein M et al: p53 mutations in human cancers, *Science* 253:49, 1991.

112. Hölzle E et al: Photopatch testing: the 5-year experience of the German, Austrian, and Swiss Photopatch Test Group, *J Am Acad Dermatol* 25:59, 1991.

113. Hruza LL, Pentland AP: Mechanisms of UV-induced inflammation, *J Invest Dermatol* 35S, 1993.

114. Jaworsky C, Ratz JL, Dijkstra JW: Efficacy of tan accelerators, *J Am Acad Dermatol* 16:769, 1987.

115. Jurkiewicz BA, Bissett DL, Buettner GR: Effect of topically applied tocopherol on ultraviolet radiation-mediated free radical damage in skin, *J Invest Dermatol* 104:484, 1995.

116. Kaidbey KH: The photoprotective potential of the new superpotent sunscreens, *J Am Acad Dermatol* 22:449, 1990.

117. Kaidbey KH, Kligman AM: Sunburn protection by longwave ultraviolet radiation-induced pigmentation, *Arch Dermatol* 114:46, 1978.

118. Kaplan, LA: Suntan, sunburn, and sun protection, *J Wilderness Med* 3:173, 1992.

119. Katsambas A, Nicolaidou E: Cutaneous malignant melanoma and sun exposure. Recent developments in epidemiology, *Arch Dermatol* 132:444, 1996.

120. Kelly JW et al: Sunlight: a major factor associated with the development of melanocytic nevi in Australian school children, *J Am Acad Dermatol* 30:40, 1994.

121. Kerr JB, McElroy CT: Evidence for large upward trends of ultraviolet-B radiation linked to ozone depletion, *Science* 262:1032, 1993.

122. Klein-Szanto AJP, Silvers WK, Mintz B: Ultraviolet radiation-induced malignant skin melanoma in melanoma-susceptible transgenic mice, *Cancer Res* 54:4569, 1994.

123. Kligman LH: Intensification of ultraviolet-induced dermal damage by infrared radiation, *Arch Dermatol Res* 272:229, 1982.

124. Kligman LH, Akin FJ, Kligman AM: Prevention of ultraviolet damage to the dermis of hairless mice by sunscreens, *J Invest Dermatol* 78:181, 1982.

125. Kligman LH, Akin FJ, Kligman AM: Sunscreens promote repair of ultraviolet radiation-induced dermal damage, *J Invest Dermatol* 81:98, 1983.

126. Kobayashi N et al: Supranuclear melanin caps reduce ultraviolet induced DNA photoproducts in human epidermis, *J Invest Dermatol* 110:806, 1998.

127. Kollias N: The absorption properties of "physical" sunscreens, *Arch Dermatol* 135:209, 1999.

128. Koh HK et al: Sunbathing habits and sunscreen use in 2,459 Caucasian adults: results of a national survey, *Am J Public Health* 87:1214, 1997.

129. Kraemer KH: Sunlight and skin cancer: another link revealed, *Proc Natl Acad Sci USA* 94:11, 1997.

130. Kraemer KH et al: The role of sunlight and DNA repair in melanoma and nonmelanoma skin cancer: the xeroderma pigmentosum paradigm, *Arch Dermatol* 130 1018, 1994.

131. Kricker A et al: A case-control study of non-melanocytic skin cancer and sun exposure in Western Australia, *Cancer Res Clin Oncol* 117(suppl):S75, 1991 (abstract).

132. Kricker A et al: Does intermittent sun exposure cause basal cell carcinoma? A case-control study in Western Australia, *Int J Cancer* 60:489, 1995.

133. Kripke ML, Fisher MS: Immunologic parameters of ultraviolet carcinogenesis, *J Natl Cancer Inst* 57:211, 1976.

134. Kripke ML et al: Pyrimidine dimers in DNA initiate systemic immunosuppression in UV-irradiated mice, *Proc Natl Acad Sci USA* 89:7516, 1992.

135. Krishnamurthey: The geography of non-ocular malignant melanoma in India: its association with latitude, ozone levels, and UV light exposure, *J Cancer* 51:169, 1992.

136. Labin D, Jensen EH: Effects of clouds and stratospheric ozone depletion on ultraviolet radiation trends, *Nature* 377:710, 1995.

137. Landis SH et al: Cancer statistics, *CA Cancer J Clin* 49:8, 1999.

138. Lawrence CW et al: Mutagenesis induced by single UV photoproducts in E. coli and yeast, *Mutat Res* 299:157, 1993.

139. Lavker RM et al: Cumulative effects from repeated exposures to suberythemal doses of UVB and UVA in human skin, *J Am Acad Dermatol* 32:53, 1995.

140. Levy SB: Dihydroxyacetone-containing sunless or self-tanning lotions, *J Am Acad Dermatol* 27:989, 1992.

141. Levy SB, Stanley B: Sunscreens for photoprotection, *Dermatol Ther* 4:59, 1997.

142. Loesch H, Kaplan DL: Pitfalls in sunscreen application. *Arch Dermatol* 130:665, 1994.

143. Lowe NJ et al: Low doses of repetitive ultraviolet A include morphologic changes in human skin, *J Invest Dermatol* 105:739, 1995.

144. Lynde CB, Bergstresser PR: Ultraviolet protection from sun avoidance, *Dermatol Ther* 4:72, 1997.

145. Mackie RM, Aitchison TC: Severe sunburn and subsequent risk of primary cutaneous malignant melanoma in Scotland, *Br J Cancer* 46:955, 1982.

146. Maducdoc LR, Wagner RF, Wagner KD: Parents' use of sunscreen on beach-going children, *Arch Dermatol* 128:68, 1992.

147. Maeda K, Naganuma M, Fukuda M: Effects of chronic exposure to ultraviolet-A including 2% ultraviolet-B on free radical reduction systems in hairless mice, *Photochem Photobiol* 54:737, 1991.

148. Marks R: Summer in Australia: skin cancer and the great SPF debate, *Arch Dermatol* 131:462, 1995.

149. Marks R et al: The role of childhood exposure to sunlight in the development of solar keratoses and non-melanocytic skin cancer, *Med J Aust* 152:62, 1990.

150. Marks R et al: The effect of regular sunscreen use on vitamin D levels in an Australian population, *Arch Dermatol* 131:415, 1995.

151. Martin R: Relationship between risk factors, knowledge and preventing behavior relevant to skin cancer in general practice patients in South Australia, *Br J Gen Pract* 45:365, 1995.

152. Masaki H, Atsumi T, Sakurai H: Detection of hydrogen peroxide and hydroxyl radicals in marine skin fibroblasts under UVB irradiation, *Biochem Biophys Res Commun* 206:474, 1995.

153. Matsuoka LY et al: Chronic sunscreen use decreases circulating concentrations of 25-hydroxyvitamin D: a preliminary study, *Arch Dermatol* 124:1802, 1988.

154. McGregor JM et al: Spectrum of p53 mutations suggests a possible role for ultraviolet radiation in the pathogenesis of advanced cutaneous lymphomas, *J Invest Dermatol* 112:317, 1999.

155. McLean DI, Gallagher R: Sunscreens. Use and misuse, *Dermatol Ther* 16:219, 1998.

156. Menezes S et al: Non-coherent near infrared radiation protects normal human dermal fibroblasts from solar ultraviolet toxicity, *J Invest Dermatol* 111:629, 1998.

157. Menter JP et al: Protection against UV photocarcinogenesis by fabric materials, *J Am Acad Dermatol* 31:711, 1994.

158. Miller DA et al: Melanoma awareness and self-examination practices: results of a United States survey, *J Am Acad Dermatol* 34:962, 1996.

159. Mills J et al: Recurrent herpes labialis in skiers, *Am J Sports Med* 15:76, 1987.

160. Miyagi T, Bhutto AM, Nonaka S: The effects of sunscreens on UVB erythema and Langerhans cell depression, *J Dermatol* 21:645, 1994.

161. Miyauchi-Hashimoto H, Tanaka K, Horio T: Enhanced inflammation and immunosuppression by ultraviolet radiation in xeroderma pigmentosum group A (XPA) model mice, *J Invest Dermatol* 107:343, 1996.

162. Mitchell REJ, McCann R: Vitamin E is a complete tumor promoter in mouse skin, *Carcinogenesis* 14:659, 1993.

163. Mitchnick MA, Fairhurst D, Pinnell SR: Microfine zinc oxide (Z-Cote) is a photostable UVA/UVB sunblock agent, *J Am Acad Dermatol* 40:85, 1999.

164. Molina MJ, Rowland FS: Stratospheric sink for chlorofluoromethanes: chlorine-atom catalyzed destruction of ozone, *Nature* 249:810, 1974.

165. Montemarano AD et al: Insect repellents and the efficacy of sunscreens, *Lancet* 349:1670, 1997.

166. Moriwaki et al: The effect of donor age on the processing of UV-damaged DNA by cultured human cells: reduced DNA repair capacity and increased DNA mutability, *Mutat Res DNA Repair* 364:117, 1996.

167. Moseley H, Davidson M, Ferguson J: A hazard assessment of artificial tanning units, *Photodermatol Photoimmunol Photomed* 14:79, 1998.

168. Moseley H, Mackie RM: Ultraviolet B radiation was increased at ground level in Scotland during a period of ozone depletion, *Br J Dermatol* 137:101, 1997.

169. Naylor MF, Farmer KC: The case for sunscreens. A review of their use in preventing actinic damage and neoplasia, *Arch Dermatol* 133:1146, 1997.

170. Naylor MF et al: High sun protection factor sunscreens in the suppression of actinic neoplasm, *Arch Dermatol* 131:170, 1995.

171. Nichols K, Desai N, Lebwohl MG: Effective sunscreen ingredients and cutaneous irritation in patients with rosacea, *Cutis* 61:344, 1998.

172. Nishigori C et al: The immune system in ultraviolet carcinogenesis, *J Invest Dermatol* 1:143, 1996.

173. Odio MR et al: Comparative efficacy of sunscreen reapplication regimens in children exposed to ambient sunlight, *Photodermatol Photoimmunol Photomed* 10:118, 1994.

174. Oliphant JA, Forster JZ, McBride CM: The use of commercial tanning facilities by suburban Minnesota adolescents, *Am J Pub Health* 84:476, 1994.

175. Olsen EA et al: Tretinoin emollient cream: a new therapy for photodamaged skin, *J Am Acad Dermatol* 26:215, 1992.

176. Ong CS et al: Skin cancer in Australian heart transplant recipients, *J Am Acad Dermatol* 40: 27, 1999.

177. Owens DW et al: Influence of wind on ultraviolet injury, *Arch Dermatol* 109:200, 1974.

178. Pajol JA, Lecha M: Photoprotection in the infrared radiation range, *Photodermatol Photoimmunol Photomed* 9:275, 1992/1993.

179. Parsons PG et al: The shady side of solar protection, *Med J Austr* 168:327, 1998.

180. Pathak MA: Sunscreens: topical and systemic approaches for protection of human skin against harmful effects of solar radiation, *J Am Acad Dermatol* 7:285, 1982.

181. Pence BS, Naylor MF: Effects of single-dose ultraviolet radiation on skin superoxide dismutase, catalase, and xanthine oxidase in hairless mice, *J Invest Dermatol* 95:213, 1990.

182. Pogoda JM, Preston MS: Solar radiation, lip protection, and lip cancer risk in Los Angeles County women, *Cancer Causes Control* 7:458, 1996.

183. Pontén F et al: Ultraviolet light induces expression of p53 and p21 in human skin: effect of sunscreen and constitutive p21 expression in skin appendages, *J Invest Dermatol* 105:402, 1995.

184. Poskitt EM, Cole TJ, Lawson DE: Diet, sunlight and 25-hydroxy-vitamin D in healthy children and adults, *BMJ* 1:221, 1979.

185. Rampen FHJ et al: Unreliability of self-reported burning tendency and tanning ability, *Arch Dermatol* 124:885, 1988.

186. Randle HW: Suntanning differences in perceptions throughout history, *Mayo Clin Proc* 72:461, 1997.

187. Ravishankar J, Diffey B: Laboratory testing of UV transmission through fabrics may underestimate protection, *Photodermatol Photoimmunol Photomed* 13:202, 1997.

188. Rhodes LE, Diffey BL: Quantitative assessment of sunscreen application technique by in vivo fluorescence spectroscopy, *J Soc Cosmet Chem* 47:109, 1996.

189. Rigel D: Malignant melanoma: incidence issues and their effect on diagnosis and treatment in the 1990s, *Mayo Clin Proc* 72:367, 1997.

190. Rigel DS, Rigel EG, Rigel AC: Effects of altitude and latitude on ambient UVB radiation, *J Am Acad Dermatol* 40:114, 1999.

191. Reeve VE et al: Differential protection by two sunscreens from UV radiation-induced immunosuppression, *J Invest Dermatol* 97:624, 1991.

192. Rietschel RL, Fowler JF Jr: Contact photodermatitis. In *Fisher's contact dermatitis*, ed 4, Baltimore, 1995, Williams & Wilkins.

193. Roberts LK, Geasley DG: Sunscreen lotions prevent ultraviolet radiation-induced suppression of antitumor immune response, *Int J Cancer* 71:94, 1997.

194. Robinson JK, Rademaker AW: Sun Protection by families at the beach, *Arch Pediatr Adolesc Med* 152:466, 1998.

195. Robson J, Diffey BL: Textiles and sun protection, *Photodermatol Photoimmunol Photomed* 9:45, 1992.

196. Rodenas JM et al: Sun exposure, pigmentary traits, and risk of cutaneous malignant melanoma: a case-control study in a Mediterranean population, *Cancer Causes Control* 7:275, 1996.

197. Roelandts RJ: Which components in broad spectrum sunscreens are most necessary for adequate UVA protection? *J Am Acad Dermatol* 25:999, 1991.

198. Roelandts RJ, Sohrabrand N, Garmyn M: Evaluating the UVA protection of sunscreens, *J Am Acad Dermatol* 21:56, 1989.

199. Rooney JF et al: Prevention of ultraviolet-light–induced herpes labialis by sunscreen, *Lancet* 338:1419, 1991.

200. Rosenstein BS, Weinstock MA, Habib R: Transmittance spectra and theoretical sun protection factors for a series of sunscreen-containing sun care products, *Photodermatol Photoimmunol Photomed* 15:75, 1999.

201. Rosenthal FS, Bakalian BS, Taylor HR: The effect of prescription eyewear on ocular exposure to ultraviolet radiation, *Am J Public Health* 76:1216, 1986.

202. Saijo S et al: UVB irradiation decreases the magnitude of the Th1 response to hapten but does not increase the Th2 response, *Photodermatol Photoimmunol Photomed* 12:145, 1996.

203. Sayre RM, Dowdy JC: Avobenzone and the photostability of sunscreen products, *Photodermatol Photoimmunol Photomed* 14:38, 1998 (abstract).

204. Sayre RM, Powell J, Rheins LA: Product application technique alters the sun protection factor, *Photodermatol Photoimmunol Photomed* 8:222, 1991.

205. Sayre RM et al: Physical sunscreens, *J Soc Cosmet Chem* 41:103, 1990.

206. Sayre RM et al: Changing the risk spectrum of injury and the performance of sunscreen products throughout the day, *Photodermatol Photoimmunol Photomed* 10:148, 1994.

207. Serre I et al: Immunosuppression induced by acute solar-simulated ultraviolet exposure in humans: prevention by a sunscreen with a sun protection factor of 15 and high UVA protection, *J Am Acad Dermatol* 37:187, 1997.

208. Silber PM et al: Comparative skin irritation of high and low SPF sunscreen products, *J Toxicol Cutan Ocular Toxicol* 9:555, 1989/1990.

209. Sinclair SA, Diffey BL: Sun protection provided by ladies stockings, *Br J Dermatol* 136:239, 1997.

210. Singh KG et al: Incidence of sunburn during mountaineering expedition, *J Sports Med* 26:369, 1986.

211. Slaper H, Velders GJM, Daniel JS: Estimates of ozone depletion and skin cancer incidence to examine the Vienna convention achievements, *Nature* 384:256, 1996.

212. Snyder DS, Eaglstein WH: Topical indomethacin and sunburn, *Br J Dermatol* 90:91, 1974.

213. Sollitto RB, Kraemer KH, DiGiovanna JJ: Normal vitamin D levels can be maintained despite rigorous photoprotection: six years experience with xeroderma pigmentosum, *J Am Acad Dermatol* 37:942, 1997.

214. Stanfield JW et al: Ultraviolet A sunscreen evaluations in normal subjects, *J Am Acad Dermatol* 20:744, 1989.

215. Stern RS, Lunder EJ: Risk of squamous cell carcinoma and methoxsalen (psoralen) and UVA radiation (PUVA): a metaanalysis, *Arch Dermatol* 134:12, 1998.

216. Stern RS, Nichols KT, Vakeva LH: Malignant melanoma in patients treated for psoriasis with methoxsalen (psoralen) and ultraviolet A radiation (PUVA): the PUVA follow-up study, *N Engl J Med* 336:1041, 1997.

217. Stern RS, Weinstein MC, Baker SG: Risk reduction for nonmelanoma skin cancer with childhood sunscreen use, *Arch Dermatol* 122:537, 1986.

218. Stierner V et al: UVB irradiation induces melanocyte increase in both exposed and shielded human skin, *J Invest Dermatol* 92:561, 1989.

219. Stokes R, Diffey B: How well are sunscreen users protected? *Photodermatol Photoimmunol Photomed* 13:186, 1997.

220. Swerdlow AJ, Weinstock MA: Do tanning lamps cause melanoma? An epidemiologic assessment, *J Am Acad Dermatol* 38:89, 1998.

221. Szczcarko C et al: Photocontact allergy to oxybenzone: ten years of experience, *Photodermatol Photoimmunol Photomed* 10:144, 1994

222. Talve L, Stenbeck F, Jansen CT: UVA irradiation increases the incidence of epithelial tumors in UVB-irradiated hairless mice, *Photodermatol Photoimmunol Photomed* 7:109, 1990.

223. Thompson SC, Jolley D, Marks R: Reduction of solar keratoses by regular sunscreen use, *N Engl J Med* 329:1147, 1993.

224. Trevisi P et al: Sunscreen sensitization: a three-year study, *Dermatology* 189:55, 1994.

225. Tronnier M, Wolff H: UV-irradiated melanocytic nevi simulating melanoma in situ, *Am J Dermatopathol* 17:1, 1995.

226. Uitto J et al: Molecular aspects of photoaging, *Eur J Dermatol* 7:210, 1997.

227. Vail-Smith K, Felts WM: Sunbathing: college students' knowledge, attitudes, and perceptions of risks, *J Am Coll Health* 42:21, 1993.

228. Van Praag MCG et al: Determination of the photoprotective efficacy of a topical sunscreen against UVB-induced DNA damage in human epidermis, *J Photochem Photobiol B* 19:129, 1993.

229. Walter SD et al: The association of cutaneous malignant melanoma with the use of sunbeds and sunlamps, *Am J Epidemiol* 131:232, 1990.

230. Walter SD et al: The association of cutaneous malignant melanoma and fluorescent light exposure, *Am J Epidemiol* 135:749, 1992.

231. Wei Q et al: DNA repair and aging in basal cell carcinoma: a molecular epidemiology study, *Proc Natl Acad Sci USA* 90:1614, 1993.

232. Weilepp AE, Kaplan LA, Steinbach JH: Photoassessment of chronologic aging in sun-protected buttock skin, *J Geriatr Dermatol* 4:263, 1996.

233. Weiss JS et al: Topical tretinoin improves photoaged skin: a double-blind vehicle-controlled study, *JAMA* 259:527, 1988.

234. Welch KL: Ozone depletion—is the sky falling? *West J Med* 160:364, 1994.

235. Werth VP et al: Elastic fiber-associated proteins of skin in development and photoaging, *Photochem Photobiol* 63:308, 1996.

236. Werth VP et al: UVB irradiation alters cellular response to cytokines: role in extracellular gene expression, *J Invest Dermatol* 108:290, 1997.

237. Westerdahl J et al: Use of sunbeds or sunlamps and malignant melanoma in southern Sweden, *Am J Epidemiol* 140:691, 1994.

238. Wolf P, Donawho CK, Kripke ML: Effect of sunscreens on UV-radiation-induced enhancement of melanoma growth in mice, *J Natl Cancer Inst* 86:99, 1994.

239. Wong CF: Scattered ultraviolet radiation underneath a shade-cloth, *Photodermatol Photoimmunol Photomed* 10:221, 1994.

240. Woollons et al: Induction of mutagenic DNA damage in human fibroblasts after exposure to artificial tanning lamps, *Br J Dermatol* 137:687, 1997.

241. Wright AL et al: Survey on the variation in ultraviolet outputs from ultraviolet A sunbeds in Bradford, *Photodermatol Photoimmunol Photomed* 12:12, 1996.

242. Yarosh DB, Tsimis J, Yee V: Enhancement of DNA repair of UV damage in mouse and human skin by liposomes containing a DNA repair enzyme, *J Soc Cosmet Chem* 41:85, 1990.

243. Yarosh DB et al: Localization of liposomes containing a DNA repair enzyme in murine skin, *J Invest Dermatol* 103:461, 1994.

244. Yarosh DB et al: Pyrimidine dimer removal enhanced by DNA repair liposomes reduces the incidence of skin cancer in mice, *Cancer Res* 52:4227, 1994.

245. Young AR: The biological effects of ozone depletion, *Br J Clin Prac* 89(suppl):10, 1996.

246. Young AR, Potten CS, Nikaido O: Human melanocytes and keratinocytes exposed to UVB or UVA in vivo show comparable levels of thymine dimers, *J Invest Dermatol* 111:936, 1998.

247. Young AR et al: The similarity of action spectra for thymine dimers in human epidermis and erythema suggests that DNA is the chromophore for erythema, *J Invest Dermatol* 111:982, 1998.

248. Young RW: The family of sunlight related eye diseases, *Optom Vis Sci* 71:125, 1994.

249. Zhang Z et al: Fast measurements of transmission of erythema effective irradiance through clothing fabrics, *Health Phys* 72:2156, 1997.

250. Ziegler A et al: Sunburn and p53 in the onset of skin cancer, *Nature* 372:773, 1994.

251. Zinman R et al: Predictors of sunscreen use in childhood, *Arch Pediatr Adolesc Med* 149:804, 1995.

252. Zitser BS et al: A survey of sunbathing practices on three Connecticut state beaches, *Conn Med* 60:591, 1996.

Injuries and Medical Interventions

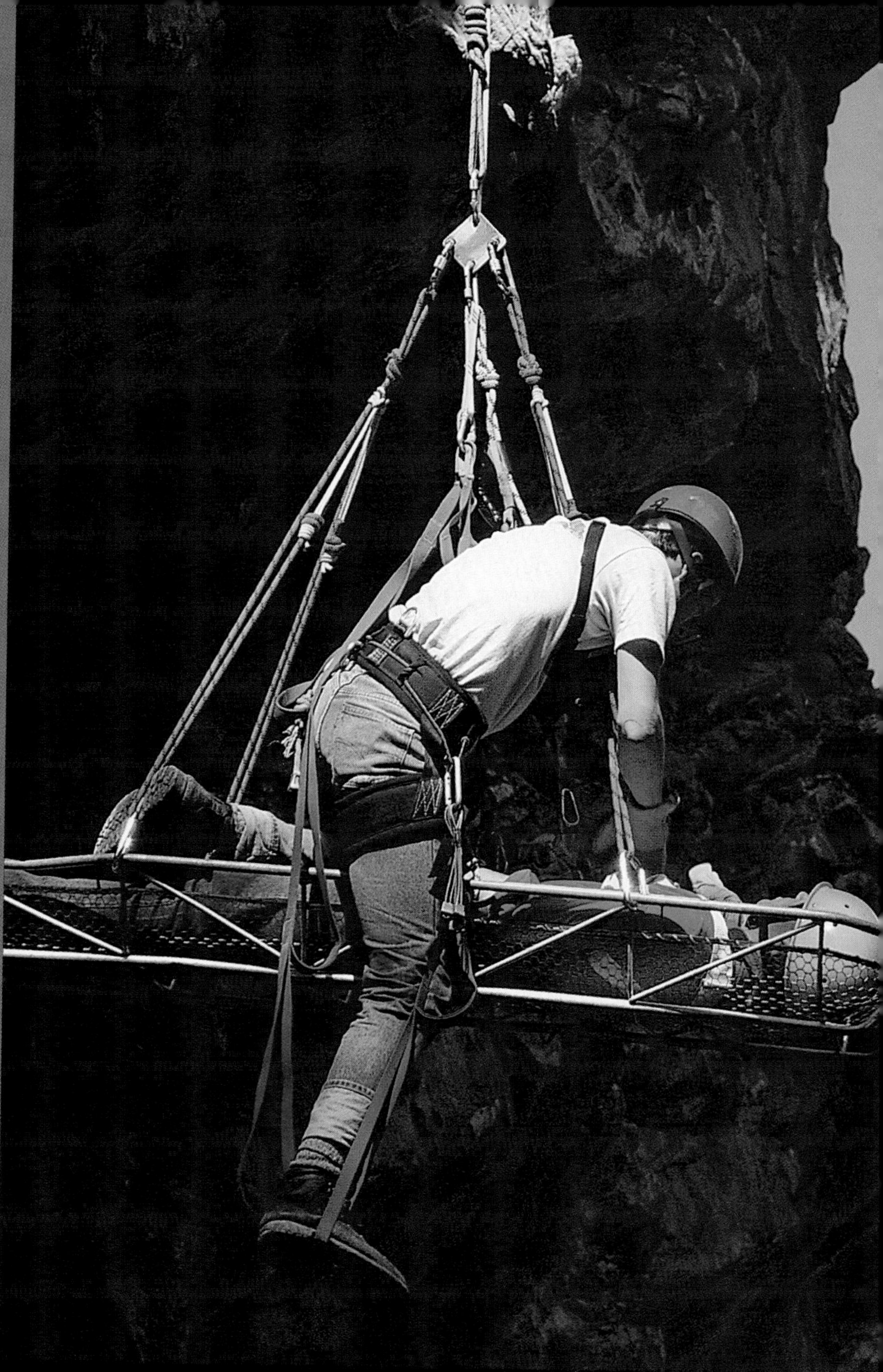

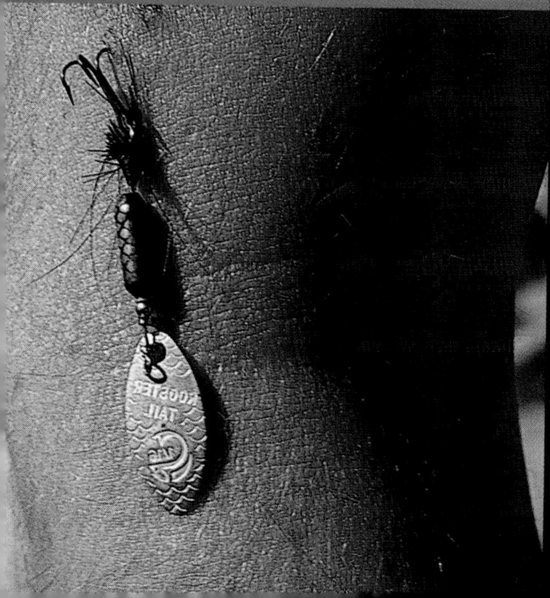

4

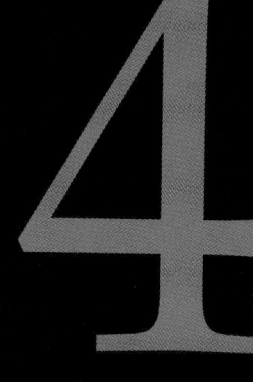

15 Wilderness Injury Prevention

Ariel D. Marks

The feasibility of terrestrial and underwater wilderness exploration and the medical management of related emergencies have changed dramatically as the availability, performance, and distance capabilities of off-road vehicles, watercraft, and vertical-flying, long-range aircraft have allowed access to the most remote and extreme recesses of the planet's environment. Advances in mountain climbing, backpacking, and recreational scuba equipment; affordable cellular telephones; global positioning systems with satellite tracking; computer communications; infrared sensors; radio beacons; and night vision aids have made such exploration safer. Advances in water purification technology, food processing, and preservation techniques extend the potential duration and distance of expeditions. Armed with technologic innovations, novices, children, elders, and persons with disabilities or impaired health now venture into areas once explored only by skilled and experienced wilderness enthusiasts. Accompanying increased access is a rise in the number of associated injuries and fatalities.

CAUSES OF WILDERNESS INJURIES

Contrary to popular belief and media reports, most U.S. wilderness injuries are not due to exotic causes (e.g., wild animal attacks, rock climbing, hang gliding) but occur during common events, such as hiking, swimming, walking, skiing, and driving. Fighting and substance abuse accounted for more than 3 times as many wilderness injuries as did rock climbing,[23] and purely environment-related activity fatalities (e.g., avalanche, shark attack, volcanic fume inhalation) accounted for less than 4% of all deaths.[23] Surprisingly, suicide ranked fourth in a field of 12 activities leading to death.

In one study, researchers found that sprains, strains, and soft tissue injuries accounted for 80% of the injuries; 60% of illnesses were due to nonspecific viral illnesses or diarrhea; and 39% of injuries required evacuation. Researchers concluded that wilderness medical efforts should concentrate on wilderness hygiene and management of musculoskeletal injuries and soft tissue wounds.[14]

MORBIDITY AND MORTALITY STATISTICS

Injury rates in traditional sporting activities are well studied, but wilderness-related injuries are not.[14] In the United States, no general database tracks the incidence of wilderness-related morbidity and mortality. Thus only a sample of the total number of participants and injury rates can be examined. Data reveal that more than 11 million people participated in backpacking or wilderness camping in 1990. The morbidity and mortality figures from eight national parks in California between 1993 and 1995 reported 1708 injuries and 78 fatalities.[23]

There are more than 5 million certified scuba (self-contained underwater breathing apparatus) divers in the United States, with approximately 650,000 annual certifications. The Divers Alert Network (DAN) at Duke University Medical Center, Durham, North Carolina, reported approximately 800 serious diving-related injuries and 80 to 90 diving-related fatalities each year between 1990 and 1993.[10]

From 1990 through 1995 an estimated 32,954 persons were involved in injuries related to personal watercraft. No estimate of total participants has been recorded.[5]

In western Washington, 40 pediatric wilderness-activity related deaths were recorded between 1987 and 1996.[26] Ninety percent of the victims were male, and 83% were age 13 to 19 years. The most common cause of death was by drowning (55%), followed by closed head injury (26%). Injuries or mortalities resulted from lack of preparation, lack of training for wilderness activities, and inadequate basic safety equipment; alcohol use and rescue delays were contributing factors. Of note, the presence of adults did not appear to be significant in reducing the incidence of mortality among the pediatric population.

INJURY PREVENTION IN MEDICAL PRACTICE

Relatively few physicians recognize injury as a disease process with predictable patterns based on patient demographics, geographic locations, and temporal variation. Moreover, most physicians do not yet embrace injury prevention as a realistic dynamic of medical practice. Traditional medical training emphasizes intervention over prevention, and it does not often approach injury as a "preventable disease."

Minimizing the risks of wilderness environments and effectively evaluating and treating illnesses and injuries in remote settings constitute the central mission of wilderness medicine. Because wilderness injuries occur in remote settings, distant from usual sources of medical care, injury control is very important. This chapter distinguishes accidents from injuries, presents the principles of wilderness injury prevention, examines equipment designed to protect or limit injury, lists injury prevention practices in wilderness settings, and identifies vehicular safety strategies.

ACCIDENTS VS. INJURIES

Accidents are defined as unpredictable acts of fate or chance events. *Injuries* are defined as corporeal damages resulting from such events.[28] Injuries are prevented by stopping or reducing the number of accidents causing them. By applying this principle, practitioners of injury prevention estimate that 90% of all injuries are predictable and preventable. For example, by inspecting, testing, and replacing rappelling gear, mountain climbers consciously attempt to prevent accidents related to equipment failure. If equipment-related accidents do occur, mountain climbers then minimize injury by safeguarding their bodies through the use of protective devices, such as helmets, harnesses, and ropes.

Active vs. Passive Injury Prevention Strategies

Injury prevention strategies are either active or passive.[28] Active injury prevention strategies require wilderness enthusiasts to change their behaviors when exposed to risks.[33] For example, wilderness enthusiasts must be convinced that wearing seatbelts reduces the risk of injury when riding in off-road vehicles, then must take the action of buckling up every time they ride.

Passive injury prevention strategies require no action. Rollover bars on off-road vehicles are passive injury prevention devices because, unlike seatbelts, they do not rely on the beliefs or behaviors of passengers. Making off-road vehicles safer by equipping them with rollover bars has done more to decrease injuries from accidents than warnings to wear seatbelts.[29] Another example of passive injury prevention would be to select a campsite well away from steep drops or water hazards to protect children from potential dangers.[17] Passive injury prevention strategies are generally more likely to decrease injury rates than are active injury prevention strategies.[19]

PRINCIPLES OF WILDERNESS INJURY PREVENTION

Planning, preparation, and problem anticipation are the three principles of wilderness injury prevention.

Planning

Careful planning builds the foundation for a safe wilderness outing. This multifaceted task includes thoroughly researching all aspects of the wilderness activity or destination. Today, critical and up-to-date information regarding weather, trail conditions, best times to travel, permit requirements, etc., can be easily and readily obtained. Planning includes developing a comprehensive equipment checklist, a realistic activity timeline, acceptable alternate plans, and emergency procedures. A critical determinant for trip planning is weather, but even the most recent detailed forecast can be wrong, so one must be prepared for unexpected weather.

Planning includes identifying and understanding the potential hazards and risks associated with a wilderness activity or destination. For example, the injury most often associated with kayaking is anterior shoulder dislocation caused by the "high brace" maneuver. Knowing this, kayakers can incorporate shoulder strengthening exercises into fitness regimens and practice "low brace" maneuvers that minimize the risk of shoulder dislocation when paddling in white water.

Planning for health and safety includes establishing limitations that directly minimize any known potentials for harm in specific wilderness activities. High-altitude mountain and rock climbers may plan to limit daily ascent rates not only to allow for acclimatization but also to avoid headaches, fatigue, and dizziness—symptoms of acute mountain sickness.[16]

Preparation

When traveling, many people focus on the logistical aspects of a trip, taking health for granted and assuming standards of health and hygiene similar to those at home. They should be prepared for the worst possible eventuality and expect poor hygiene practices and substandard medical services when traveling to remote locations.

Physical Preparation. Physical preparation includes maintaining excellent fitness and health in anticipation of the added stress of outdoor activities. Because wilderness activities take place in remote settings, distant from usual sources of medical care, a much higher level of medical self-sufficiency is required. Reading a book is a far cry from actually performing these physical functions under duress and challenging environmental conditions, so it is a good idea to rehearse hands-on first-aid procedures.

Mental Preparation. Mental preparation emphasizes being confident about the planned trip. Confidence is based on knowing that you have the skills and experience necessary to handle the situation and not exceeding your limits. Possible evacuation routes and emergency procedures should be established, and you must be aware of each participant's level of comfort with self-treatment and their specific abilities. Determine the location of and distance to known medical care facilities. Notify a friend or neighbor of your departure date, planned length of stay, and anticipated return date and time. Plan your trip, establish priorities, and carry out the plan. Be prepared to take charge in the event of an emergency situation.

Material Preparation. Material preparation involves acquiring proper equipment, testing and organizing equipment, and having backup equipment should something fail. Have sufficient equipment to survive the night under the worst possible environmental conditions for that time of the year.

The wilderness explorer must have all equipment maintained regularly and inspected carefully before a trip. Have emergency bivouac equipment. Carry equipment (in excess of personal needs) that could be given to a person overcome by sudden illness or injury.

If traveling with partners, review what each person is responsible for bringing. Try to "streamline" the equipment so that it does not get caught on things, will be easier to handle, and will be maneuverable when traveling under windy conditions or in water.

Use battery-powered items that require the same size and type of batteries. Keep a gear checklist to avoid forgetting essential items. Depending on your wilderness activity, essential equipment may include an avalanche beacon, compass, duct tape, emergency blankets, emergency bag, extra clothing, extra food, firestarter, first-aid kit, flashlight, ground insulation, knife, maps, matches, sunglasses, sunscreen, shelter (e.g., emergency tube tent), survival whistle, water, water disinfection system, and timepiece. If the risk of human immunodeficiency virus (HIV) or hepatitis B is great, carry a small kit containing sterile needles, syringes, intravenous catheters, and supplies for suturing.

Having adequate light on a trail is essential. Headlamps are particularly useful because they free up the hands.

Problem Anticipation

Discuss and agree on a travel route. Choose a leader, and review each member's capabilities and what equipment and supplies are necessary. Bring adequate protection from environmental and recreational hazards. Be sure to have all the appropriate immunizations. Maintain safe drinking and food hygiene practices. Make sure you have a working knowledge of first aid relevant to the environment at hand.

If using specialized equipment, take a course in its proper use and maintenance. Specialty courses available through retail outlets, clubs, and wilderness organizations prepare and train you for most outdoor activities. For example, a course in avalanche safety will help if you plan to travel through avalanche areas.

INJURY PREVENTION

Scuba Diving and Snorkeling

DAN reported 1132 cases of decompression illness treated in hyperbaric chambers and 104 recreational dive facilities in 1995.[11] Other data collected by DAN reveal approximately 800 serious scuba diving accidents per year and approximately 80 to 90 annual fatalities.[10]

Common causes of injury while diving or snorkeling include drowning, barotrauma, environmental exposure, bites, and stings. Unique to diving are arterial gas embolism, decompression sickness, and nitrogen narcosis.

Preventing drowning includes always wearing a buoyancy control device and a quick-release weight belt, as well as not diving or snorkeling under hazardous weather conditions. Diving with a buddy ensures that you will have someone to assist you if a muscle cramp, exhaustion, entanglement, or other adverse situation occurs. Carrying an underwater knife helps in case of entanglement in monofilament fishing line or seaweed. Carrying a whistle, beacon, or other attention-getting device, such as an "emergency sausage" (a flexible plastic tube 6 feet long that can be filled with air), visible or audible from a great distance provides a help signal if ocean currents carry a person far from the point of entry.

Because of higher conductive heat loss in water, divers and snorkelers should wear insulating wet suits or dry suits. This outerwear also protects against scrapes, bites, and stings. Booties can protect the feet when walking along a rocky beach while carrying heavy scuba gear. When immersed for any length of time, the skin of the hands and feet becomes soft and more prone to injury. Gloves and booties guard these areas from cuts caused by rock or coral.

When in an underwater environment, pay attention to marine life that bites or stings. Avoid aggressive interactions with marine organisms because their aggressive behavior is generally made in self-defense.

Decompression sickness is prevented by following dive table guidelines to limit ongassing of excessive nitrogen. Divers must attend a training course to understand how dive tables operate.

Preventing arterial gas embolism requires that divers breathe continuously when using compressed air. Persons with certain pulmonary contraindications, such as severe asthma, are generally advised not to dive.

Nitrogen narcosis impairs judgment and can result in disorientation and drowning. Usually occurring at depths exceeding 30 m (100 feet) of salt water, nitrogen narcosis is rapidly reversible by swimming into shallower water. To prevent nitrogen narcosis, avoid diving to depths exceeding 100 feet.

The most common site of barotrauma is the tympanic membrane external to the middle ear space, resulting from inadequate equalization of pressure during descent. Preventing barotrauma is achieved by "equalizing" properly.

Injury prevention behaviors for diving include the following:

1. Breathe continuously. Never hold your breath.
2. Clear your ears. Do not dive if your sinuses are congested. Do not dive if you have a medical contraindication to diving.
3. Know how to use and follow the dive tables.

4. Dive with a buddy. Review underwater and top-side communications.
5. Inspect your dive gear regularly.
6. Know your training and physical limitations.
7. Procure air refills from a reputable air station.
8. Get a predive orientation. Learn about the environment and be prepared to abort a dive if conditions are hazardous.
9. Do not use drugs or alcohol before, immediately after, or when diving.
10. Leave your dive plan with a friend or neighbor so that rescue procedures can be initiated if you do not return when expected.

Kayaking, Canoeing, and Rafting

Kayaking, canoeing, and rafting have become the third largest outdoor recreational industry in the United States,[15] with 76 million people participating in these activities. New equipment designs, such as self-bailing inflatable rafts and lightweight, plastic polymer kayaks, have opened up more remote and difficult waterways for exploration and commercial recreation. The American Canoe Association reports approximately 130 white-water fatalities each year, and the most common contributing factor is failure to wear a personal flotation device (PFD).[31]

Exposure to cold water stimulates cardiorespiratory reflexes that make it difficult for submersed swimmers to keep their heads above water.[20] The preferred type of PFD, therefore, when participating in kayaking, canoeing, or rafting, is a vest-type jacket (Coast Guard Type III PFD) that provides heads-up buoyancy. A PFD should fit snugly and not ride up over the head when the user is in the water. Some PFDs include crotch straps as an added safety feature.

PFDs also provide some protection from hypothermia. Closed-cell foam flotation material also protects the thorax from impact injuries during falls on slippery rocks or when swimming rapids. A PFD can also be used as an improvised splint.

Helmets should also be worn by all white-water enthusiasts to protect against head trauma after capsizing. From 10% to 17% of all kayaking accidents involve head injury.[21,32] White-water rafting enthusiasts have used polypropylene helmets similar to those used by bicyclists, having foam liners, nylon chin straps, and drainage holes for head protection. The helmet should have a hard outer shell to protect the skull from impact with sharp rocks. The ears should always be covered and protected. Portholes that allow rapid exit of water from the inside of the helmet should be included so that the helmet does not become waterlogged and add to drag when submerged. The chinstrap should be secure and waterproof so that it does not stretch when wet. These brightly colored, highly visible helmets aid in locating an injured individual in the water.

An athlete is 60 times more likely to sustain a dental injury when not wearing a mouth guard.[25] Mouth guards shield the teeth and protect the lips, cheek, tongue, mandible, neck, temporomandibular joint, and brain.[34] Presently, three types of mouth guards exist—stock, mouth-formed, and custom models—with costs and protective benefits of each increasing, respectively. The American Dental Association currently "recognizes the preventing value of orofacial protectors and endorses the use of orofacial protectors by all participants in recreational sport activity." This endorsement includes recommendations for water sports, such as water skiing, surfing, and water polo.[1,15] In the future, this recommendation should be extended to include high-velocity water sports, such as operating a personal watercraft.

Rope should be readily accessible and secured so that it can be rapidly deployed without entanglement. The type of rope used should not absorb water and should stretch somewhat. Rope can be used to rescue a paddler who has fallen out of a vessel or thrown to a paddler who is pinned or broached.

Injury relating to kayaking, canoeing, and rafting commonly occurs when portaging vessels. If proper lifting techniques are not used, portaging a kayak or canoe can cause back strain. Careful attention to using leg muscles rather than those of the lower back can prevent lower back injury. Injuries resulting from poor conditioning, improper stroke technique, muscle overuse, shoulder dislocation, low back strain, tendonitis in the wrist, extensor tenosynovitis of the forearm, muscle strains, and sprains are relatively common. Prevention and correction involve maintaining physical fitness, engaging in a conditioning program, relaxing the grip on the oar, and taping the wrist in a neutral position. Blisters are also common and can be prevented by wearing properly fitted gloves. Warm-up exercises, including stretching, are beneficial.

All paddlers should watch where they step to avoid ankle sprains and fractures, especially when stepping out of vessels onto wet rocks. "Reef walkers" or neoprene booties with antiskid soles are helpful.

Enthusiasts should also apply sunscreen often, carry a first-aid kit, and avoid drinking river water and eating unrecognizable plants. They should watch the weather and modify activities accordingly. If paddling in cold water, paddlers should dress appropriately, wearing wet suits, gloves, booties, and woolen pullover hats to avoid hypothermia in case of capsizing. They should also avoid ingesting alcohol or illicit drugs, since these intoxicants impair judgment, balance, and heat production. (Alcohol is believed to be a contributing factor in as many as half of all drowning deaths.) Paddlers should apply insect repellent and keep tetanus immunization current.

Backpacking and Hiking

A common injury that occurs during hiking and backpacking is low back pain. It is frequently caused by carrying excessive or poorly distributed loads. Several improvements in backpack design have been developed to prevent low back injury.

The two basic types of backpacks are those with external frames and those with internal frames. The frames are designed to transfer the weight of the backpack from the shoulders and back to the hips and legs. An ideal backpack weight distribution is 20% on the shoulders and 80% on the hips. This distribution lowers the body's center of gravity, making it more stable (Figure 15-1).

Backpacks with External Frames. An external frame pack allows a larger amount of weight to be carried, using a ladderlike frame made of aluminum or plastic. A hip belt and shoulder strap are attached to the frame, usually with clevis pins and split rings. Some backpacks are adjustable to fit the length of the spine. Hikers should look for lumbar padding, a conical hip belt, recurved shoulder pads/straps, and a chest compression strap that improves distribution of weight and increases comfort.

A backpack with an external frame allows air space between the back and the pack, reducing sweating. With an external frame pack, the weight is carried

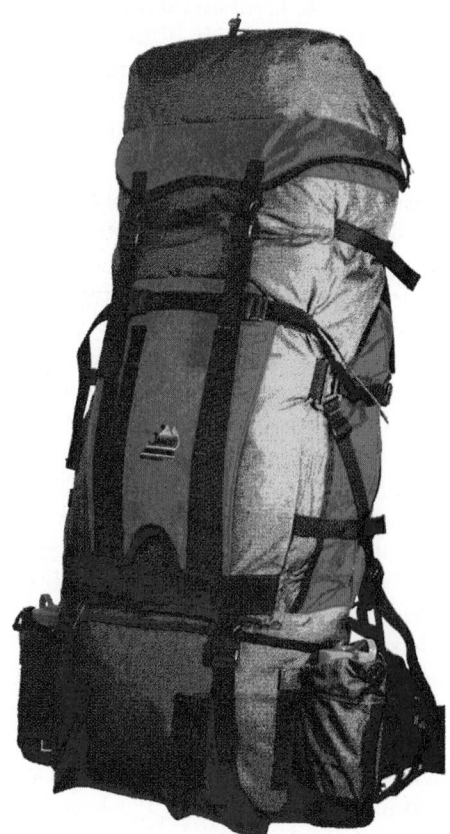

Figure 15-1 To prevent injuries, a backpacker should limit the contents of a backpack to 25% of body weight. *(Courtesy Jandd Mountaineering.)*

higher in the pack, allowing for a more upright posture. However, the pack frequently wobbles side to side during walking.

Backpacks with Internal Frames. The internal frame backpack conforms more to the body, allowing for better balance, and can be worn comfortably for longer periods of time. However, back perspiration can be a problem. Since the bulk of the weight is carried lower, one must bend more, which in turn alters proper posture and can predispose to low back strain. Compression straps can compact the contents of the pack, keeping it more stable.

Backpack Considerations. Backpack size is an important consideration for injury prevention. Hikers need to be sure that all the equipment necessary for the duration of the trip can be carried without putting excessive strain on the shoulders and back muscles. The amount of weight that can be carried in a backpack is determined by the size, body weight, and fitness level of the backpacker. For multiday trips, one should attempt to limit the contents to 25% of body weight. When loading the backpack, 50% of the weight should be in the upper third of the pack. To accomplish this distribution, lighter and bulkier items should be packed in the bottom and heavier items should be packed in the top. The heaviest items should be packed on the top, closest to the frame.

Backpack Lifting. The least injurious method for donning a backpack is to have someone hold and stabilize the pack while the carrier slips his or her arms into the shoulder straps. If a second person is not available, the backpacker can lift and rest the backpack on an object that is waist high and slip into it.

If a backpack must be donned from the ground, it is not recommended that the carrier sit down, slip into the backpack, and stand up. Rather, he or she should lift the backpack onto a bent knee and slide one arm through the shoulder strap. After adjusting the strap so that the backpack rests on the shoulder, the carrier should lean forward and rotate the body slightly, allowing the free arm to slide through the other shoulder strap. While still leaning forward with bent knees, the backpacker adjusts the second strap and hip belt.

To prevent low back strain, a backpacker should use the knees rather than the lower back to bend. Good abdominal muscle tone helps limit back strain.

Backpacks and Children. Backpacks that carry small children can be dangerous. Risks include strangulation if a child becomes entangled in the carrier's harness and head and body injury if a child wiggles out of the harness and falls or is struck by an overhead obstruction, such as a tree branch. Be certain to use a well-structured carrier with a design that restrains the ambitious, mobile child.

Hiking Footwear. Blisters are a common backpacking and hiking injury, but careful selection of shoes and socks limits this problem. The purposes of footwear are protection, cushioning, support, and grip. Selecting, fitting, breaking in, and caring for footwear help them last a long time and maximize comfort. Size footwear in the afternoon, since feet swell during the day. Also, try footwear on both feet before purchase. If one foot is larger than the other, select the size where the larger foot has the best fit.

Size your feet using a Brannock device, which measures not only the length and width of a foot but also the ball-to-heel (arch) length. When selecting footwear, check the length first. If your toes touch the end, leaving no space for the heel, the shoe is too small. When you slide your foot forward into an unlaced shoe or boot, you should be able to insert a finger between the footwear and your heel. If you can't do this, the footwear is too short and will bruise your toes, especially on long downhill walks. When hiking, wear shoes that extend above the ankle to reduce the likelihood of an ankle sprain.

Footwear should fit comfortably with moderate tension on the laces so that they can be tightened or loosened as needed. To avoid blister formation, seams should not rub against any part of the foot. The tongue of the footwear should be aligned and laced properly; otherwise the tongue can slide into a bad position and cause blisters. Ankles should be comfortably supported by stiff heel counters or heel cups and should not slip with toe flexion, causing blisters because of repetitive rubbing. With the foot on the ground, there should be no more than 6 to 12 mm of heel lift.

The soles are protected with layers of cushioning thick enough to prevent bruising but pliable enough to allow natural heel-to-toe flexion. Thick soles insulate against cold and heat. The tread provides grip. Support comes from a fit that stops the foot from slipping inside the shoe but that is not so tight that it prevents the foot from expanding when it swells.

Socks. Many boots feature sock liners or booties made from vapor-permeable membranes, such as Gore-Tex and Sympatex, hung between the lining and outer aspect of the boot. These make boots waterproof when they are new, but most boots leak after a few weeks in wet weather. In addition, lack of breathability means that water vapor cannot penetrate the barrier, resulting in hot, sweaty feet. Socks cushion the feet, preventing abrasion. They also wick away moisture, keeping the feet at the right temperature and humidity. New synthetic materials, such as polypropylene, Capilene, and Thermax, wick away moisture quickly, making them good choices for an inner layer.[13] Pile or fleece socks do not wick away moisture very well.

Wool offers many advantages. It is warm in winter, cool in summer, absorbs and wicks away sweat, and keeps the feet warm when wet. Furthermore, during long trips, it rinses well in cold stream water, can be worn for days at a time without wear, and does not matte down like cotton socks with terry loop liners.

It is worth the time to check socks for loose threads, knots, or harsh stitching that might cause blisters or sore spots. Flat seams at the toes are important. Bulky seams rub and cause blisters. Consider wearing one pair of fairly heavy socks (rag wool) and one pair of light liner socks next to your skin. With one sock, the boot and the outer sock tend to move as a unit. They rub against the heel and the top of the toes at the metatarsal heads. A lightweight liner sock tends to cling to the foot. As the boot moves, the socks rub against each other, not against foot skin.

Foot Hygiene. Keep toenails short and cut them square. Keep feet dry to avoid skin softening. Immediately stop walking and attend to the first sign of a sore or "hotspot" to prevent further injury. Protect any reddened areas with moleskin, tape, or molefoam. Be sure that the covering extends beyond the reddened area.

Avoid getting blisters. Once formed, they must be protected to prevent rupture and infection. If a blister has already formed, relieve external pressure by applying a doughnut-shaped piece of molefoam. A blister should not be unroofed unless absolutely necessary. If this is required, wash the area with soap and water and insert a decontaminated needle ("sterilized" by a flame or with rubbing alcohol) into the edge of the blister. Gently press out the fluid. Apply a sterile dressing. If the blister has already broken, cleanse and cover the area. Topical antiseptic ointment may be beneficial.

Exposure. Overexposure caused by inadequate skin covering results in several problems. An essential area to protect is the head. From preventing heat loss to blocking ultraviolet (UV) exposure, hats are an integral component of the wilderness wardrobe. The uncovered head is a source of considerable heat loss, since it can dissipate up to 70% of total body heat production.[4] Because there is no substantial decrease in blood flow to the head in cold conditions, hats should be worn to stay warm. Hats large enough to cover the ears, face masks, and neck warmers (gaiters) are popular among skiers. The preferred type of hat for wilderness expeditions is the stocking type.

In warm climates, hats with visors and brims provide considerable protection from UV exposure to the face, nose, and ears. Hats also provide some degree of insect protection, especially if sprayed with insect repellent, and reduce radiant heat exposure. They repel light rain, keep leaves and twigs out of the hair, and hold a mosquito net in place. In addition, when worn in the jungle where larger arboreal animals reside, hats can protect the head and hair from airborne droppings. Hats should be lightweight, light colored, and preferably vented. It is helpful to have a retention neck or chin strap for windy days and to have snaps to fasten the brim up when traveling on a trail. Hats do not need to be waterproof. They should be loose fitting.

Eye protection is also essential. Sunglasses provide protection against injury caused by UV exposure, which can contribute to ocular complications, including photokeratitis (snowblindness), cataracts, pterygium, and macular degeneration (Figure 15-2).

The major variables to consider in selecting sunglasses are light transmission, coloration, polarization, and lens construction. Lenses for wilderness exposure should absorb 99% of UV radiation. If used in high solar reflection areas, lenses should also absorb 85% to 95% of visible light.

The preferred lens is made of glass or polycarbonate. Polycarbonate lenses are lightweight, scratch resistant, and shatterproof (a major consideration if impact is possible). Plastic lenses scratch easily and are generally not recommended.

When wearing dark lenses in a bright environment, the pupils dilate and allow more harmful radiation exposure to the retina. Photochromic lenses (those that darken with increasing sun intensity) are potentially dangerous when driving. If fully darkened in bright sunlight, photochromic lenses limit vision considerably when traveling through a tunnel. It is preferable to have a less dark pair of sunglasses for driving. Amber lenses or rose lenses enhance contrast. Polarization is particularly useful in reducing reflective solar glare from water, snow, and ice. UV-absorbing contact lenses do not provide adequate protection from UV radiation and should not be used as substitutes for sunglasses. Sunglasses are still needed to cover the entire eye area, including eyelids.

Choose sunglasses that are close-fitting and have larger lenses, or are of the wraparound variety to prevent UV rays from entering from the side. Children, including infants, should wear sunglasses. Glasses should be secured with some type of strap. Commercial lens "defoggers" are available, although any surfactant, such as soap, rubbed or washed onto lenses will have the desired defogging effect.

In severe blizzard conditions, goggles improve visibility. The goggle's foam mesh vents help reduce fogging. A wide elasticized headband helps keep them in place. For protection from impacts and foreign bodies, safety glasses or goggles should be worn when traveling on bicycles, horses, or any off-road motorized vehicle without a windshield.

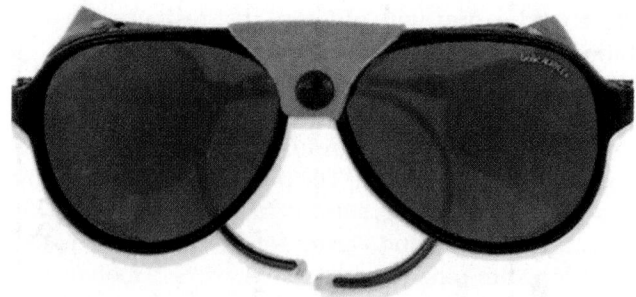

Figure 15-2 Sun protection for the eyes is critical in outdoor activities to prevent premature cataracts, photokeratitis, and other ocular injuries. *(Courtesy Black Diamond Equipment.)*

Hiking Accessories. A useful injury prevention adjunct is a hiking pole or staff to provide stability on rough ground and diminish impact on knees and ankles. A staff can support a good walking rhythm and prevent imbalance when carrying a heavy load. Hiking poles allow for probing and identifying hidden rocks and deep spots and can hold back bushes, barbed wire, stinging plants, and other trail obstructions. They can even be used to fend off aggressive dogs or wildlife.

Using two staffs or poles takes the load off the legs and hips and redistributes part of the weight to the upper body musculature. On a steep area, hiking poles enable tripoding, or having three points of contact with the ground.

Injury Prevention for the Genitourinary Tract. To prevent genitourinary infections during wilderness outings, enthusiasts should maintain superb genital hygiene and assure adequate hydration. To counteract the tendency to bathe less frequently during an extended outing, a shower should be part of the daily schedule (Figure 15-3).

Infections and irritation of the genitourinary tract are more common in women than in men, since the female urethra is shorter, leaving the bladder more predisposed to colonization by bacteria. Infrequent urination and urethral trauma from vigorous activity or bruising from a bike seat, saddle, or climbing harness are common contributing factors to urinary tract infections.

VAGINITIS. Vaginitis can occur with increased stress, sweating, or strenuous and vigorous activities, as well as with changes in the environment, including heat and humidity. To avoid vaginitis, women should keep themselves cool and dry by wearing loose-fitting clothing that maximizes air circulation and minimizes the optimal conditions for bacterial and fungal growth.

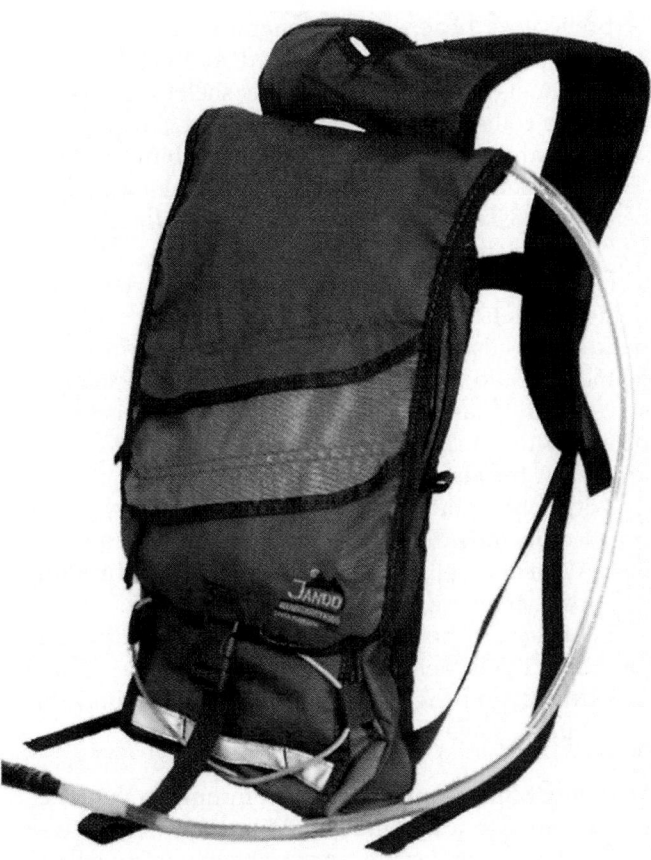

Figure 15-3 Several new and effective methods of transporting water into the wilderness have been developed. A biking hydration system can help prevent urinary tract infection by facilitating the opportunity for adequate hydration. *(Courtesy Jandd Mountaineering.)*

Avoid nylon undergarments because they retain humidity. Cotton underwear is preferable.

SANITARY PROTECTION FOR MENSTRUATION. If menstruating while in the wilderness, women should change their tampons or sanitary napkins just as frequently as at home to avoid infection or toxic shock syndrome. Women who use tampons should make sure their hands are scrupulously clean before insertion. For environmental reasons, tampons with cardboard rather than plastic applicators should be used if wilderness disposal is a possibility.

PERIANAL HYGIENE. Whenever possible, cleanse the anal area with fresh water. If pruritus ani develops, medicated wipes, such as witch hazel tucks or moisture-blocking ointments, have been shown to be beneficial for some individuals. "Porta-showers" or "sunshowers" are particularly helpful to maintain good anal hygiene. Baby wipes are often quite soothing.

For wilderness excursions, biodegradable toilet paper is recommended. Select toilet paper that is dye and perfume free. Use double zip-lock bags for packing to keep the toilet paper dry and clean. Burning toilet paper creates a fire hazard, so, ideally, it should be packed out. If buried, it should be placed 6 inches from the ground surface and at least 60 m (~200 feet) from any natural water supply. Toilet paper decomposes more rapidly if wet and not buried too deeply.

Trail Safety. Finding one's way in the wilderness, sometimes in unfavorable and extreme weather conditions; negotiating cliffs, loose scree, uneven and hazardous terrain, including snow, ice, and mud; and facing other hazards, such as wild animals, can be challenging. Do not assume that because a trail is marked that it is safe, clear, and well maintained. Take a switchback route across slopes when possible. Utilize rest areas.

Balance is key to crossing rough terrain. Watch for unstable rocks and boulders. Keep body weight over feet, with knees bent, and do not lean backward. When traveling along scree, do not have anybody traveling directly below or above you because stones can dislodge and fall. If this occurs, shout a warning, but the person below should not look up. For rock climbers, do not climb what you cannot descend.

At altitude, strong winds can make walking impossible. Be prepared to descend early or take an alternate route if weather worsens. It may be necessary to "sit out" bad weather.

When fording rivers and streams, remember that water is very powerful. The use of safety ropes is recommended.

Hammock Safety. Small, lightweight minihammocks are popular in camping and backpacking. These hammocks have no spreader bars and can be folded easily. The U.S. Consumer Product Safety Commission (CPSC) warns that children can become trapped and strangle on certain minihammocks; two deaths and one nonfatal incident have involved minihammocks or backpacker hammocks. If a hammock is rigged too high off the ground, a child will have difficulty climbing into it and may become trapped or entangled, leading to strangulation. To prevent injuries, install a minihammock near the ground.[9]

Maps. Knowing where you are is a key wilderness skill. Carry maps and know how to read them. Always establish entry, check, and exit points on your maps. Even on marked trails, an inadvertent turn can rapidly create confusion and allow you to become lost.

Two types of maps are available—planimetric (two dimensional) and topographic (three dimensional).

Planimetric maps identify features on the ground. Topographic maps provide information about the shape of the ground itself. Topographic maps use contour lines to identify points of equal elevation. The standard United States Geologic Survey 1:24000 maps have contour intervals of 40 feet. More recent Bureau of Land Management maps use a metric 50-m interval. The closer together the contour lines, the steeper the slope.

Global Positioning Devices (see Chapter 73). The global positioning system (GPS) is a government-operated system consisting of approximately 28 satellites at 12,000 miles altitude. Each satellite orbits the earth twice a day, emitting continuous signals of time and position. By carrying a GPS receiver on the ground, your position can be triangulated.

Line of sight is required between the receiver and satellite. Therefore position determination may be impossible in dense forests, jungles, or below steep cliffs. Furthermore, electronic GPS receivers are sensitive to mishandling, extremes of temperature, and battery failure. They should be an addition to, and not a replacement for, traditional maps and compasses. Natural references, such as sun position, wind, and topography, can provide useful clues to your position.

Cellular Telephones. Cellular telephones can provide ready access to the outside world, as well as an additional form of security when traveling in remote locations. They are sensitive to mishandling and have limited battery life. Since signal transmission relay stations are infrequent in the wilderness, there is a real chance of telephone failure.

If emergency assistance is needed during a wilderness activity, dialing 911 can connect you to a service that will assist with wilderness rescue. Calling the local National Park Service office, a search and rescue organization, or even the local sheriff's office may result in an earlier and more efficient rescue response.

Other Emergency Forms of Communication. The international distress signal (SOS) consists of three short signals, followed by three long signals, and then three short signals, repeated at intervals. This signal can be transmitted with light, sound, or Morse code. Ground-to-air signals can be used with any material visible from the air.

Climbing

Common climbing injuries involve falls, often from great heights. One of the most critical pieces of safety equipment is a helmet, since the head is a major area of potential injury.

Helmet Composition and Fit. The purpose of a helmet is to absorb the energy of an impact, minimizing or preventing head injury. Generally, crushable, expanded polystyrene foam is used for this purpose. Most helmets now have a hard outer shell to protect the head in a collision with a sharp object. It is prudent to wear a hard-shelled helmet when climbing because falling rocks can cause significant damage. It is also beneficial to have a visor attached to the helmet to protect the face and eyes.

Helmets should have a snug, but comfortable, fit. Some helmets have varying thicknesses of internal padding to custom fit the helmet to the user. Ideally, helmets should be lightweight and have a buckle that stays securely fastened. No combination of twisting or pulling should remove the helmet from the head or loosen the buckle on the strap (Figure 15-4).

Additional guidelines for effective helmet wearing practices include the following:
1. Wear the helmet flat atop your head, not tilted back at an angle.
2. Make sure the helmet fits snugly and does not obstruct your field of vision.
3. Make sure the chin strap fits securely and the buckle stays fastened.

Climbing Equipment. To prevent trauma to the torso when climbing, a harness should be worn. Harnesses secure the wearer's center of gravity to a safety line. If footing is lost, free-fall injuries are abated by the harness and safety line. To be effective, a harness must fit securely and be made of strong material with reinforced stitching. It should be inspected regularly for wear.

A useful accessory if climbing at altitude is an "AvaLung." The AvaLung is worn like a life jacket and can help keep a person alive in an avalanche (see Chapter 2). A victim buried in snow can breathe for approx-

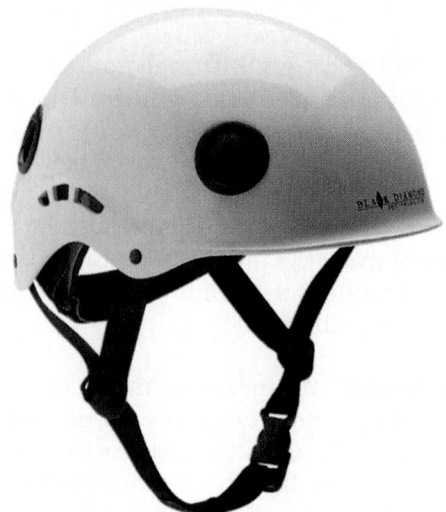

Figure 15-4 Helmets should be worn by all wilderness enthusiasts involved in activities that might result in head injury. *(Courtesy Black Diamond Equipment.)*

imately 10 minutes without and up to 1 hour with the AvaLung vest. The additional time is gained by increasing the surface area for air exchange, using the vest as a "breathing membrane" (Figure 15-5).

Knee guards, elbow guards, and wrist guards are useful protective devices when traveling with heavy packs or on slippery surfaces. Crampons are metal devices that attach to the outside bottom of footwear to provide traction on ice. Although crampons allow the crossing of ice and hard snow without slipping, walking with them involves a change in gait. Because they have sharp metal serrated edges, stress injury to the medial aspect of the knee can occur unless a wider gait is maintained during walking.

Altitude. Along with the limitation of oxygen because of reduced partial pressures, a major consideration at altitude is hypothermia. Hypothermia is prevented through proper exposure protection and common sense. Potential hypothermic situations must be managed before they become serious (see Chapter 6).

Recognize the environmental conditions that lead to hypothermia. Wear appropriate clothing for cold and wet conditions and always wear a hat. Use polypropylene underwear to wick water away from the skin. Wear multiple layers, including but not limited to wool, and a wind and waterproof covering.

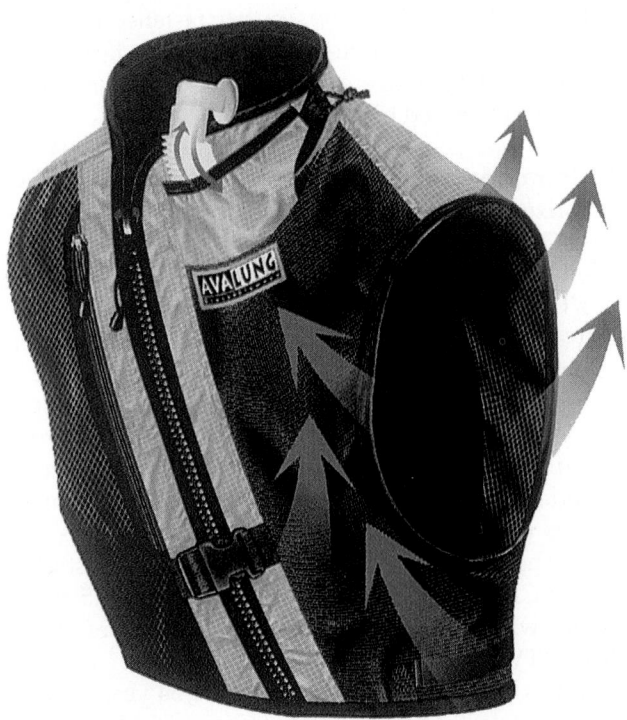

Figure 15-5 The AvaLung is a life jacket worn by avalanche victims. It allows them to breathe while buried.

Physical fitness, continuous exercise, high-calorie food intake, and consumption of hot beverages will prevent the onset of mild hypothermia. Avoid exhaustion, panic, and energy-depleting activities. Carry fire-starting materials and some form of improvisation shelter. Pack a VHF radio and know how to use it. Learn to recognize warning signs of hypothermia.

An ice ax is imperative for traversing snow and ice at altitude. A walking staff or ski pole is entirely inadequate for crossing hard-packed snow or ice. On these surfaces, a slip can quickly become an out-of-control fall. Limiting this fall (self-arrest) involves proper use of an ice ax, which can also be used to cut steps into ice.

Boating (see Chapter 56)

The single most useful injury prevention device for boating is the personal flotation device.[3] A PFD or life jacket should be used when participating in any water-related activity, such as canoeing, kayaking, or jet skiing, but it is not a replacement for knowing how to swim. Brightly colored so that it can be seen at a distance, the PFD is designed to provide the wearer a stable, face-up position in calm water when the head is tilted back. However, most PFDs do not hold up the face of an unconscious wearer, although some newer models assure flotation even with an unconscious user. In rough water, the wearer's face may often be covered by waves, since the PFD is not designed for extended survival in rough water. The styles that ensure face-up flotation and that are designed for the body habitus and the weight of the user are safest.

PFDs require routine minor maintenance. Check the PFD frequently for rips, tears, and holes. Confirm that the seams, fabric, straps, and hardware are in good working order. If caught in riptides, undertows, or strong currents, ride the current out and work your way back to the shore in the area adjacent to the current where the water is calmer.

Personal Watercraft

The use of personal watercraft (PWC), such as jetskis or waverunners, in water recreation has increased rapidly since 1990. Personal watercraft are less than 4 m (13 feet) in length and designed to be operated by persons sitting, standing, or kneeling on the craft, instead of within the confines of the hull.[30] These watercraft allow swifter movement and attain faster speeds in less time than larger, motor-drive boats.

From 1990 through 1995, there were an estimated 33,000 injuries associated with PWC use. Injury rates increased fourfold from an estimated 2860 in 1990 to more than 12,000 in 1995. Injuries and deaths to both the watercraft drivers and bystanders occurred disproportionately among the very young or the intoxicated.[18]

Almost 86% of injured persons were 15 to 44 years of age. The median age was 25 years. Of injured persons, 71% were male. An estimated 7% of the persons injured in the cited report were 14 years old or younger. The rate of injuries related to PWC treated in emergency departments was about 8.5 times higher than the rate of emergency department–treated injuries from motorboats. Kinetic energy is the pathogen of PWC injuries.[29] Increased speed equals increased crash fatality risk and large increases in death tolls.[27]

Given the fast speeds that can be achieved with PWCs, training requirements and enforcement may reduce the number of injuries considerably. Parental or adult supervision is recommended for minor children. Right-of-way guidelines currently in place for boat operators, including maintaining safe distances and reduced speeds, should be extended to PWC users. PWCs should not be used where others are swimming or wading. PWCs offer no protection from impact to the driver or the bystander. No federal laws govern the safe conduct of these vehicles, and many injuries involve swimmers and other unprotected water enthusiasts. The impact of a PWC on a swimmer can be equivalent to a pedestrian being hit by a small truck at high speed.

Hunting (see Chapter 20)

Over 35,000 firearm fatalities have occurred in the United States each year since 1989, and it is estimated that there are three nonfatal firearm injuries for each death associated with a firearm.[2] Hunter safety courses are available in every state and are a prerequisite in most states to obtaining a hunting license. Key recommendations include warning nonhunters of hunting season, limiting hunting to hunting areas, and wearing international orange clothing articles when traveling in areas frequented by hunters. Hunters should always be sure of their target before shooting. A safety harness should be worn when using a tree stand. Care should be taken to use appropriate techniques when cleaning game. Eye protection should always be worn with impact-resistant lenses to prevent injury from ricocheting fragments and shotgun pellets. Ammunition should always be stored separately from guns.

High-frequency hearing loss is common among hunters because of the loud report of the firearm. Earplugs and headsets, although impractical for most hunting situations, can provide good protection for the ears. In most scenarios, a single earplug for the ear closest to the muzzle will protect the ear most likely to be injured.

The greatest potential serious injury from hunting is a gunshot wound. Every effort should be made to ensure that inadvertent misfires do not occur. Most injuries relating to firearms occur during common gun-related activities, such as cleaning and inspection and are therefore self-inflicted. Further studies are needed to evaluate the efficacy of gun safety training courses and to assess the potential role of various gun safety devices, such as trigger locks and loading indicators.

Vehicular Safety

Off-road travel is challenging for both vehicle and driver. Off-road path conditions are usually poor, with deep potholes, large boulders, and mud that limit traction. Because of a lack of clearing and the absence of street lighting, visibility is usually low. There is also the chance of encountering wildlife, which may jump out in front of the vehicle.

Off-road four-wheel-drive vehicles have high centers of gravity to allow for ground clearance so that boulders and rocks do not damage the vehicle's underside. This means that the vehicles are top heavy and prone to tipping, especially when turning corners at high speeds. Care should be taken to travel slowly.

Since most four-wheel-drive vehicles have stiff suspensions (for better maneuverability), always wear a three-point harness and be cognizant of bumping and jarring that can injure the spine. Secure all equipment.

Many off-road vehicles have no air bags or cabs, and many only have lap-belt restraint systems. They often have thin-walled bodies and frames and are not well designed for impact.

Rollover protective structures (ROPS) are essential. These can be enclosed in the cab or unenclosed (resembling one or more exposed rollover bars). ROPS are structural components attached to vehicles designed to protect the operator from being crushed if the vehicle overturns. Although ROPS offer some degree of protection, passengers must be securely fastened with seat belts so they are not ejected from their seats if the vehicle rolls over. Passengers must remain confined within the space protected by the ROPS.

All-terrain vehicles. All-terrain vehicles (ATVs) are motorized recreational cycles with four (and sometimes three) large soft tires. These vehicles are designed for off-the-road use on various terrains.

ATVs have become enormously popular, particularly among the young, with approximately 2.5 million vehicles in use. Although ATVs give the appearance of stability, the three-wheeled design is unstable, especially on hard surfaces. Stability is further compromised by a high center of gravity. The hazard is compounded by the fact that all-terrain vehicles can achieve speeds up to 30 to 50 mph. Moreover, their use by youths has sometimes been promoted.[29] Recent studies by the CPSC showed the risk of injury is 2.5 times higher when children younger than 16 years of age drive ATVs than for drivers 16 to 34 years of age, and 4.5 times higher than for drivers 35 to 54 years of age. Over 2400 deaths associated with three- and four-wheel ATVs occurred from 1982 to 1993.[8]

The majority of injuries associated with ATVs occur when the driver loses control, the vehicle rolls over, the driver is thrown off the vehicle, or the driver collides with a fixed obstacle. Children are often injured when struck by a fence wire or tree branch while traveling at a high speed. In a recent study of three-wheeled ATVs in Alaska,[12] risk factors were found to include intoxication with alcohol, excessive speed, lack of proper protective helmet usage, and rider inexperience.

ATVs should only be used in daylight or driven very slowly at night. These vehicles should never be used on unfamiliar terrain or on public roadways. ATVs should not carry more than one person at a time. Riders should always wear helmets, eye protection, and protective clothing, such as gloves and hand guards.

Drivers should always use the buddy system, driving with other ATVs. In case of injury in a remote area, a buddy ATV can go for help.

In 1982 an estimated 12,000 children 14 years of age and younger suffered motorized minibike- and trail-bike-related injuries.[24]

All-terrain bikes and mountain bikes are a popular form of recreation for wilderness enthusiasts. The rider may be traveling on uneven trails with multiple obstacles, including logs, rocks, and streams. Falls usually cause the rider to lunge forward and sustain concomitant injury to the face and head. Consequently, riders should wear full-face helmets with chin guards to limit maxillofacial injuries. Other forms of injury prevention gear include gloves and hand, elbow, knee, and shin guards. The rider should also wear eye protection if it is not a part of the helmet.

Snowmobiles. In New Hampshire, between January 1989 and February 1992, there were 12 fatal and 165 nonfatal snowmobile injuries.[6] None of the snowmobile drivers who died had taken an off-highway recreational vehicle (OHRV) course. Overall, 76% of the fatal incidents were associated with alcohol use and 67% with excessive speed. Of 165 persons nonfatally injured, 104 (63%) were reported to have been wearing helmets. Helmets were reported to have been worn by 31 (57%) of 54 persons with nonfatal head injuries, compared with four of six persons (67%) with fatal head injuries. In Maine, from fall of 1991 through spring of 1995, 25 (81%) of the 31 who died from snowmobile-related causes were wearing helmets at the time of the incident.[7] The observation that a large percentage of deaths occurred in persons wearing helmets demonstrates that this behavior modification does not ensure survivability. Other contributing factors, such as excessive speed, alcohol, and lack of other corporeal protection, have significant impact on outcome.

In Alaska, between 1993 and 1994, injury, death, and hospitalization rates were greater for snowmobiles than for on-road motor vehicles.[22] A total of 26 snowmobile injury deaths were reported. Seven decedents drowned after breaking through ice, and eight were ejected from vehicles. More than half (58%) of the snowmobile injury deaths involved a natural object, such as a boulder, ravine, or river. Of the 17 decedents for whom blood alcohol concentrations were available, 11 (65%) had blood alcohol concentrations greater than or equal to 100 mg/dl. Thus natural obstacles, excessive speed, and alcohol intoxication contribute to the high risk of injury death associated with snowmobile use.

INTERNET RESOURCES

Look for Internet sources related to wilderness injury prevention online at http://www.WildernessMD.com.

REFERENCES

1. American Dental Association House of Delegates: *Resolution 80H—amendment of policy on orofacial protectors*, Chicago, 1995, the Association.
2. Annest JL et al: National estimates of nonfatal firearm-related injuries: beyond the tip of the iceberg, *JAMA* 273:1749, 1995.
3. Bever D: *A personal focus*, St Louis, 1996, Mosby.
4. Bowman W:. Wilderness survival. In Auerbach PS, Geehr EC, editors: *Management of wilderness and environmental emergencies*, St Louis, 1989, Mosby.
5. Branche CM et al: Personal watercraft-related injuries: a growing public concern, *JAMA* 278:663, 1997.
6. Centers for Disease Control and Prevention: Leads from the morbidity and mortality weekly report, Atlanta, GA: injuries associated with use of snowmobiles—New Hampshire, 1989-1992, *JAMA* 73:448, 1995.
7. Centers for Disease Control and Prevention: Injuries and deaths associated with use snowmobiles—Maine 1991-1996, *JAMA* 277:526, 1997.
8. Children's Safety Network: *ATV safety*, Marshfield, Wisc, 1995, Rural Injury Prevention Resource Center.
9. Consumer Product Safety Commission: Children can get trapped and strangle on some hammocks: safety alert, 1999, http://cpsc.gov/spscpub/pubs/5043.html.
10. Divers Alert Network: *1991 report on diving accidents and fatalities*, Durham, NC, 1993, Duke University Medical Center.
11. Divers Alert Network: *Report on 1995 diving accidents*, Durham, NC, 1997, Duke University Medical Center.
12. Ferguson A: Child accident prevention as a health promotion issue—how extensive is the problem and how far have A & E departments responded to the recommendations made? *Accid Emerg Nurs* 2:193, 1994.
13. Gentile DA, Kennedy BC: Wilderness medicine for children, *Pediatrics* 88:967, 1991.
14. Gentile DA et al: Wilderness injuries and illnesses, *Ann Emerg Med* 21:853, 1992.
15. GMA Research: *National Sporting Goods Association survey*, Bellevue, Wash, 1989.
16. Hackett PH, Roach RC: High-altitude medicine. In Auerbach PS, editor: *Wilderness medicine: management of wilderness and environmental emergencies*, St Louis, 1995, Mosby.
17. Haddon W: Strategy in prevention medicine: passive versus active approaches to reducing human wastage, *J Trauma* 14:353, 1972.
18. Hamman BL et al: Injuries resulting from motorized personal watercraft, *J Pediatr Surg* 38:920, 1993.
19. Karlson T: Injury control and public policy, *Crit Rev Environ Control* 22:195, 1992.
20. Keatings W, Evans M: The respiratory and cardiovascular response to immersion in cold water, *Q J Exp Physiol* 46, 1961.
21. Kizer K: Medical aspects of whitewater kayaking, *Physician Sports Med* 15(128), 1987.
22. Landen M et al: Injuries associated with snowmobiles, *Public Health Rep* 114:48, 1999.

23. Montalvo R et al: Morbidity and mortality in the wilderness, *West J Med* 168:248, 1998.

24. National Information Clearing House: *National electronic injury surveillance data*, Bethesda, Md, 1985, US Consumer Product Safety Commission.

25. National Youth Foundation for the Prevention of Athletic Injury: *Dental injury fact sheet*, Needham, Mass, 1992, the Foundation.

26. Newman LM et al: Pediatric wilderness recreational deaths in western Washington State, *Ann Emerg Med* 32:87, 1998.

27. Nilsson G: *The effect of speed limits on traffic accidents in Sweden*, Linköping, Sweden, 1992, National Road and Traffic Institute.

28. Rivara R et al: Injury prevention. First of two parts (see comments), *N Engl J Med* 337:543, 1997.

29. Robertson L: *Injuries: causes, control strategies, and public policy*, Lexington, Mass, 1983, Lexington Books.

30. US Coast Guard: *Boating statistics 1994*, Washington, DC, 1995, US Department of Transportation.

31. Walbridge C, editor: *River safety report*, Phoenicia, NY, 1992, American Canoe Association.

32. Wallace D: Scary numbers and statistics—results of AWA close calls and serious injuries survey, *AWA J* 3-4:27, 1991.

33. Waller J: *Injury control: a guide to the causes and prevention of trauma*, Lexington, Mass, 1985, Lexington Books.

34. Woodmansey KF: Athletic mouth guards prevent orofacial injuries, *J Am Coll Health* 45:179, 1997.

16 Principles of Pain Management

Bryan L. Frank

Safe and effective pain management in the wilderness is subject to the effects of remote location, extrication considerations, and concomitant illness or injury on physical modalities, anesthetics, analgesics, and other pharmacologic agents. More adventurers with chronic pain syndromes are traveling into remote settings. World travelers are often exposed to various indigenous therapies for conditions, and many of these therapies are increasingly available to American wilderness travelers as "complementary and alternative" medicine. These therapies can be integrated with conventional medical therapies and may be superior to conventional approaches in treating acute or chronic pain in the wilderness.

The old adage "nobody ever died of pain" may be very inappropriate in a wilderness setting. Effective pain management can dramatically enhance a rescue effort and minimize morbidity and mortality. Pain management advances over the last decade that have dramatically altered care in hospitals and clinics also impact care in the wilderness.

PATHOPHYSIOLOGY OF PAIN

Perception of pain is critical for the survival of most organisms. Detection of tissue injury leads to a nociceptive response that initiates protective behavior. The simple response seen with acute injury becomes complex in chronic pain syndromes, where the original insult is long past. Numerous clinical pain entities have been recognized, including acute nociceptive pain (somatic and visceral), postoperative pain (posttraumatic), neuropathic pain, terminal pain, chronic pain, and psychogenic pain. Acute nociceptive pain and chronic pain can generally be managed effectively by the wilderness physician who is informed and prepared.

Acute Nociceptive Pain

Designed to protect us from danger, acute pain is critical to human survival and well-being. In acute trauma, the human peripheral nervous system receptors detect noxious events, peripheral transmission relays information centrally for processing, and the response apparatus is triggered.[51]

Free nerve endings, commonly called *polymodal nociceptors*, respond to mechanical, thermal, and chemical stimuli. These nerve fibers are generally A-delta and unmyelinated C fibers and are most prevalent in the skin. Greater stimuli lead to greater frequency of action potentials. Acting as transducers, these nociceptors transmit their signals to the spinal cord via primary afferent nerve fibers.[52,53]

The peripheral nerve terminals experience a change in milieu after tissue damage and subsequent plasma extravasation resulting from increased capillary permeability. The result is a red flush at the site of trauma secondary to arteriolar dilation, local edema caused by increased capillary permeability, and primary and secondary hyperalgesia. There may also be pain from normally nonnoxious stimuli (allodynia), and an exaggerated response to noxious stimuli (hyperpathia). Tissue substances released in response to injury may magnify the body's nociceptive response. Histamine and serotonin further stimulate free nerve endings and produce vasodilation. Kinins, including bradykinin, are also released and stimulate free nerve endings, as can lipidic acids, cytokines, and various primary afferent peptides (calcitonin gene-related peptide, substance P, and others)[52,53] (Box 16-1).

In the dorsal horn of the spinal cord, connections are made from peripheral nerves to one of five zones, known as laminae I to V. Connections within these laminae differ based on cell type, interneural connections, and histochemistry. Neurochemicals within the dorsal horn include substance P, β-endorphin, enkephalins, dynorphin, serotonin, dopamine, norepinephrine, vasoactive intestinal peptide, γ-aminobutyric acid (GABA), neurotensin, thyrotropin-releasing factor, and oxytocin.[51,53]

Somatic afferent fibers and large-diameter myelinated primary afferent axons, with cell bodies in the dorsal root ganglia, ascend within the spinal cord and terminate in the cuneate and gracile nuclei. Other branches terminate in the anterior horn of the spinal cord. The spinothalamic tracts (neo- and paleo-) ascend the anterolateral pathways after crossing from the contralateral dorsal horn. These fibers then terminate in the thalamic nuclei or with collateral connections in the brainstem and midbrain, where they may modulate sensory transmission.[51]

Descending inhibitory pathways use enkephalins, serotonin, noradrenaline, and probably other neurotransmitters. Central structures include the somatosensory cortex, periventricular gray matter, periaqueductal gray matter, dorsal raphe nuclei, reticular formation, medulla, and nucleus raphe magnus.[51] These mechanisms and others modulate the nociceptive experience.

Box 16-1 NEUROCHEMICALS OF PAIN TRANSMISSION

NEUROPEPTIDES

Adrenocorticotropin
β-Endorphin
Bombesin
Calcitonin gene-related peptide
Cholecystokinin (CCK)
Corticotropin-releasing factor
Dynorphin
Enkephalins (leu-enkephalin, met-enkephalin)
Galanin
Neurotensin
Oxytocin
Somatostatin
Substance P
Substance K
Vasoactive intestinal peptide
Vasopressin

MONOAMINES

Dopamine
Norepinephrine
Serotonin

AMINO ACIDS

Aspartate
GABA
Glycine
Glutamate
Taurine

Chronic Pain

With chronic pain, the sensation of pain no longer warns of trauma and danger. The initial stress response of acute pain is no longer present. Chronic pain is poorly defined through coinvolvement of peripheral and central mechanisms. The pain's duration is not what characterizes pain as "chronic." Rather, it is the prevalence of cognitive-behavioral aspects that supersede nociception. Prolonged pain that is traumatic, postoperative, neuropathic, or terminal is not "chronic" if the pathophysiologic and psychologic characteristics of acute pain are maintained.[51]

Psychologically, the chronic pain patient is commonly depressed. The sufferer may seek secondary gain and demonstrate psychosis, neurosis, or a premorbid personality. Pharmacologic interventions for chronic pain are often more challenging than in acute pain. Antiinflammatory agents, neural blockade, sedative-hypnotics, and narcotics are often ineffective or contraindicated, but antidepressants, cognitive coping strategies, and behavioral modification may be useful.

Recent therapies for chronic pain of use to wilderness travelers include implantable infusion pumps that deliver narcotic and nonnarcotic medications, dorsal column spinal stimulators, and transcutaneous electrical nerve stimulators (TENS).

GOALS OF WILDERNESS PAIN MANAGEMENT

Wilderness pain control may be difficult to achieve because of complex physiologic and environmental challenges. The primary goal should be safety and the secondary goal effective pain relief. However, failure to provide adequate analgesia may place a sick or injured person, as well as the rescue party, at grave risk.

The nature of the injury or illness is assessed and the diagnosis determined while addressing the need for and choice of pain therapy. It is often important to withhold pain therapy until a reasonable diagnosis can be determined, which may be difficult without sophisticated diagnostic equipment. However, history taking and physical examination should lead to an appropriate diagnosis.

Evaluation of the Pain Patient

Through the medical history, the location of the pain, time of onset, precipitating or aggravating factors, frequency and duration, character, severity, and previous treatment are established. Included is past medical and surgical history; menstruation and pregnancy; environmental exposures; dietary intake; medications; and associated symptoms of nausea or vomiting, fever, vertigo, and dyspnea. Many wilderness injuries are reasonably straightforward to diagnose, but pain related to medical illness may be a dilemma. Open-ended questioning may provide greater insight than direct questioning. Changes in cognition may compromise victim evaluation. Pretravel history forms and information or observations of traveling companions may be critical in evaluating a painful condition.

If pressed by critical environmental or patient conditions, the physical examination is performed quickly and systematically, targeted by clues obtained during the history. When possible, a focused examination including a general assessment of contributing factors such as blood pressure and pulse, mental status, cranial nerve function, motor and sensory function, deep tendon reflexes, and strength may provide vital information.[12]

Physical Methods for Treatment of Pain

Wilderness pain management includes simple physical measures, such as applying pressure, cold, heat, or splinting, which are important adjuncts to narcotic analgesics, anesthetics, and other pharmaceutical agents using topical, oral, intranasal, rectal, or parenteral administration (Box 16-2). Additionally, pain

Box 16-2 METHODS OF PAIN MANAGEMENT

PHYSICAL MODALITIES

Compression
Cryoanalgesia
Heat therapy
Splinting
Transcutaneous electric nerve stimulation

PHARMACOLOGIC MODALITIES

Analgesics

Narcotic agonists
Narcotic agonist/antagonists
Nonsteroidal antiinflammatory drugs
Salicylates
ρ-Aminophenols
Dissociative analgesics/anesthetics
Local anesthetics

ADJUNCTIVE PHARMACEUTICALS

Antidepressants
Anticonvulsants
Muscle relaxants
Antihistamines

COMPLEMENTARY AND ALTERNATIVE THERAPIES

Acupuncture
Herbal/botanical remedies
Magnetic therapy

treatment modalities characterized as "complementary and alternative" therapies may provide significant pain relief with less physiologic risks.

Compression Analgesia. Although compression is taught more as a method for establishing hemostasis than for pain management, compression can reduce pain. An injured extremity is wrapped distal to proximal, with a cloth wrap or rubber Esmarch bandage, or a simple constiction band may be placed on the limb proximal to the site of the injury. Resultant anesthesia may occur because of compression of the peripheral nerves.[34] Compression anesthesia may be safe and appropriate in a wilderness setting if other methods or pharmacologic agents are unavailable or contraindicated.

Cryoanalgesia. Hippocrates first recorded the use of ice and snow packs to relieve pain in the fourth century BC. Cryoanalgesia experienced a significant modification by Richardson in 1866 with the introduction of refrigerant ether spray, subsequently replaced by the use of ethyl chloride spray in 1890. Cooper advanced cryoanalgesia in 1961 through the development of the liquid nitrogen probe, which served as prototype for the current generation of nitrous oxide or carbon dioxide cryoanalgesia devices in common use today.[34,41]

Wilderness cryoanalgesia may be applied with ice, snow, or frigid water. Additionally, metal cylinders containing gasoline or ethyl alcohol (freezing point –114.5° C [–174.1° F])[9] remain liquid at temperatures below water's freezing point and may be used to provide a dry cold compress.[49] These containers of subzero temperature liquids may lead to serious frostbite injury. As cold absorbs heat from the adjacent tissues, nerve conduction is reversibly blocked. Conduction ceases in the larger myelinated fibers before the unmyelinated fibers; all nerve conduction ceases at 0° C (32° F). Upon rewarming, nerve conduction resumes, unless the intracellular contents have turned to ice crystals. Extreme cryotherapy leads to wallerian degeneration of axons and myelin sheaths, although the perineurium and epineurium may remain intact and sometimes allow regeneration.[41]

Although a selective cryolesion is the goal of many pain management treatments in chronic pain clinics, this deliberate cell injury is not appropriate in a wilderness setting. Prevention of iatrogenic frostbite and generalized hypothermia while using cold therapy is critical. How long a tissue will tolerate a cold compress before experiencing cellular damage depends on preexistent tissue hypothermia, peripheral vs. central nature of the tissue, and temperature and pressure of the cold compress. Cold water immersion may induce frostbite in persons with snakebite because of venom-compromised tissues. Cold packs are beneficial for marine envenomations[16] (see Chapters 60 and 61). Commercial cold packs typically contain a gel of water and propylene glycol, or other similar antifreeze and heat exchange substances, which may be cooled in cold water or snow.[23] A reasonable guide is to place a dry, thin cotton cloth or foam between the skin and cold metal cylinders, ice, or snow, or cold packs and to remove cold therapy each 15 minutes to assess tissue status.

Heat Therapy. Heat application is not usually recommended for initial (up to 48 hours) pain management of acute trauma because it may lead to increased edema and bleeding. However, heat can be used for pain management in the wilderness. Muscle relaxation, attributed to decreased gamma fiber activity, has been demonstrated after applying heat to the overlying skin. Collagen tissues become more extensible with heat therapy, requiring less force for movement and resulting in less mechanical damage with stretching. These effects may be useful for patients pursuing wilderness travel, especially with chronic pain conditions. Further, heat applied to the skin of the abdomen may markedly reduce gastrointestinal (GI) peristalsis and uterine contractions and thus decrease pain associated with these organs.[46]

Application of heat need not be extreme. Temperatures of 37.8° to 40° C (100° to 104° F) for 10 to 20 minutes generally provide comfort without thermal injury. Heat therapy should be avoided in cognitively impaired patients and for tissue that is anesthetic or ischemic, to prevent further unintended tissue injury. Heat therapy may improve or worsen marine envenomations, or lead to lymphangitis[17] (see Chapters 60 and 61).

Liniments and balms are not true heat transfer agents but consist of multiple botanical or chemical substances that make the tissue feel warm through counterirritant effects and subsequent vasodilation. These substances may help a traveler's soreness and stiffness abate. Common ingredients include menthol, camphor, mustard oil, eucalyptus oil, methyl nicotinate, methyl salicylate, and wormwood oil.[6] These products are generally only recommended on intact skin with a light cloth or plastic covering and should not be placed on mucous membranes; neither should they be used with tight compresses or external heat sources.

Splinting. Splinting allows positioning and immobilization of injured body parts and prevents further damage to soft tissues, blood vessels, nerves, and bones. Preventing bony fragments from damaging surrounding tissue diminishes pain and often facilitates mobilization and extrication of a victim.

Splints (see Chapter 18) should be padded to prevent further surface trauma. They may be accompanied by pressure dressings or cold compresses for additional pain management. Regular reevaluation of tissue circulatory status is critical to prevent damage from swelling, frostbite, or ischemia in immobile, splinted limbs.

Pharmacologic Treatment of Pain
Analgesics (Tables 16-1 and 16-2)

NARCOTIC ANALGESICS. Opium emerged as the first widely used narcotic analgesic by the time of the Renaissance, generally as a powder or sticky gum. It was often combined with alcohol to form laudanum. Prussian pharmacist Frederich Sertürner isolated morphine from opium. Development of the hypodermic needle and syringe by Rynd in Ireland and Pravaz in France greatly enhanced morphine's clinical utility in pain management.[34]

Narcotic agonists affect the opiate receptors in the central nervous system (CNS).[40] Morphine and other opioids are administered orally, intranasally,[43] sublingually, transdermally, subcutaneously, intramuscularly, intravenously, and rectally. Morphine is metabolized primarily in the liver; approximately 10% is excreted through the kidneys. Hepatic and renal damage affects the recipient's response, so that tolerance for a given dose must not be presumed with these conditions.

Morphine is a potent analgesic with sedative and euphoric effects that also depresses the CNS and respiratory drive. Critical patient assessment is always required when using narcotic analgesics to detect respiratory depression and hypotension.

Other narcotic agonists include codeine, which is a "controlled substance" in the United States but available over the counter (OTC) in most other countries, and meperidine, methadone, propoxyphene, and hydromorphone. Newer semisynthetic narcotics that exhibit much shorter durations of action include fentanyl and sufentanil.

Potential adverse side effects may include anaphylaxis, nausea, vomiting, rash, respiratory depression, and hypotension. Narcotic antagonists such as naloxone and other emergency resuscitative medications should be available when using narcotics in the wilderness, just as in the contemporary clinical setting. Do not give potent narcotic analgesics to victims with suspected head injury or neurologic illness.[50]

Naloxone (Narcan) is a narcotic antagonist that may reverse narcotic effects. Doses of 0.2 mg intravenously (IV) or 0.4 mg IV, intramuscularly (IM) or subcutaneously (SC), may be given and repeated each 2 to 5 minutes until CNS, respiratory, or hypotensive narcotic symptoms are reversed, to a maximum dose of 10 mg. Nalmefene is a similar narcotic antagonist with longer duration of action initially given in IV doses of 0.25 mg each 2 to 5 minutes to a total dose of 1 mg (4 doses).[6] Continuous monitoring of blood pressure, mental status, and respiratory status is critical, with possible repeat doses necessary in 1 to 2 hours. Pain may return with aggressive narcotic reversal, and a balance between pain alleviation and physiologic stability is desired. Additionally, narcotic antagonists may lead to acute narcotic withdrawal symptoms in persons with a tolerance to and dependence on narcotics.

Narcotic agonist-antagonist combinations first became popular with pentazocine, which has less addictive potential than pure narcotic agonists. However, these agents may depress the brain and respiration.[35] These may be of special significance in a high-altitude setting where impaired pulmonary and cerebral function may occur. These medications do not provide narcotic agonist effects needed in narcotic-dependent persons, and they may experience withdrawal symptoms without narcotic agonists. Familiar drugs in this class include buprenorphine, butorphanol, and nalbuphine.

NONNARCOTIC ANALGESICS. Nonnarcotic analgesics provide mild to moderate pain relief and are generally safer than narcotics. Acetylsalicylic acid (aspirin) reduces fever, inhibits platelet function, and diminishes inflammation. It has significant GI effects, including gastric irritability, erosion, and bleeding ulcers, and is often better tolerated in an enteric-coated formulation.

TABLE 16-1. Common Oral Analgesics: Dosage Recommendations in 70-kg Adults*

DRUG	DOSAGE (mg)	INTERVAL (hr)	RISKS, PRECAUTIONS
SALICYLATES			
Acetylsalicylic acid (aspirin)	325-650	3-4	GI distress, inhibits platelet function, contraindicated in children with viral illnesses
Diflunisal	300-600	8-12	Similar to aspirin
ρ-AMINOPHENOL			
Acetaminophen	300-650	4-6	Hepatic toxicity in overdose
INDOLES			
Indomethacin	50	4-6	Similar to aspirin
Sulindac	50-75	4-6	Similar to aspirin
Ketorolac	30-60	4-6	Similar to aspirin
PROPIONIC ACIDS			
Fenoprofen	400-600	4-6	Similar to aspirin
Ibuprofen	300-400	4-6	Similar to aspirin
Naproxen	250-500	8-12	Similar to aspirin
COX-2 INHIBITORS			
Rofecoxib	12.5-50	24	GI distress, hypertension
Celecoxib	100-200	12-24	GI distress, skin rash
NARCOTIC AGONISTS			
Codeine	30-60	3-4	Narcotic side effects
Oxycodone	5-10	4-6	Narcotic side effects
Methadone	2.5-10	8	Narcotic side effects
Propoxyphene	32-65	4-8	Narcotic side effects

*Data from Burham T et al, editors: *Drug facts and comparisons,* St Louis, 1999, Facts and Comparisons; and Lubenow TR, McCarthy RJ, Ivankovich AD: Management of acute postoperative pain. In Barash PG, Cullen BF, Stoelting RK, editors: *Clinical anesthesia,* ed 2, Philadelphia, 1993, JB Lippincott.

TABLE 16-2. Common Parenteral Analgesics*

DRUG	DOSAGE (mg)	INTERVAL (hr)	RISKS, PRECAUTIONS
NARCOTIC AGONISTS			
Codeine	15-60 IM	4-6	Narcotic side effects
Hydromorphone	1-4 IM	2-3	Narcotic side effects
Morphine	10-20 IM, 2.5 IV	2-4	Narcotic side effects
Meperidine	50-100 IM, 25-50 IV	2-4	Narcotic side effects
NARCOTIC AGONIST/ANTAGONISTS			
Buprenorphine	0.3-0.6 IM	6-8	May precipitate withdrawal
Butorphanol	2-4 IM	3-4	May precipitate withdrawal
Dezocine	5-20 IM, 5-10 IV	2-4	May precipitate withdrawal
Nalbuphine	10-20 IM, 1-5 IV	3-6	May precipitate withdrawal
NSAID			
Ketorolac	15-30 IM, 2-5 IV	4-6	Similar to aspirin
DISSOCIATIVE ANALGESIC/ANESTHETIC			
Ketamine	50-75 IM, 15-30 IV	2-4	Increased intracranial pressure

*Data from Burham T et al, editors: *Drug facts and comparisons,* St Louis, 1999, Facts and Comparisons; and Lubenow TR, McCarthy RJ, Ivankovich AD: Management of acute postoperative pain. In Barash PG, Cullen BF, Stoelting RK, editors: *Clinical anesthesia,* ed 2, Philadelphia, 1993, JB Lippincott.

Persons with a history of GI ulcers or severe indigestion should avoid aspirin. Dosage should not exceed 650 mg orally every 4 hours. Other salicylate analgesics include diflunisal, choline magnesium trisalicylate, and salsalate. The latter two have minimal GI toxicity and antiplatelet effects. Salicylates are contraindicated in persons with known allergy to the class of drugs and in children under age 15 years with viral respiratory illnesses because their use has been linked to Reye's syndrome.[1]

Acetaminophen is a paraaminophenol that is a mild analgesic and antipyretic.[10] It has no antiplatelet, antiinflammatory, or antiprostaglandin effect and is less likely to cause serious gastric irritation. Dose should not exceed 650 mg every 4 hours. Ingestion of more than 10 g over 24 hours may lead to severe hepatic damage; the drug should be used with extreme caution in anyone with preexisting liver disease. Many OTC medications contain acetaminophen, so these should not be used in combination with pure acetaminophen or in persons with liver disease.

Indomethacin is an indoleacetic acid derivative with analgesic, antipyretic, and antiinflammatory (antiprostaglandin) effects. Both rectal and oral administration lead to rapid absorption. Use reasonable caution in persons with hepatic or renal dysfunction. GI toxicity has been reported with its use, including gastric ulceration and perforation, as well as bone marrow suppression. Other acetic acid derivatives include sulindac, tolmetin, ketorolac, and diclofenac.

Ibuprofen is a nonsteroidal propionic acid derivative antiinflammatory agent with prostaglandin antagonist activities. Its analgesic and antipyretic properties are similar to those of aspirin and acetaminophen, but it may be better for women with dysmenorrhea because its antiprostaglandin effects somewhat relax the uterus. Its antiinflammatory properties may be very useful for arthritis and acute injuries. Like aspirin, ibuprofen can be a gastric irritant and should be avoided in persons with a history of GI ulcer, indigestion, or hiatal hernia. Oral and rectal administration leads to rapid absorption. Ibuprofen has been reported to cause nonspecific fluid retention. Although not studied in wilderness medicine research to this point, its potential to aggravate high-altitude illnesses from acute mountain sickness to high-altitude pulmonary or cerebral edema should be considered. Usual dosage is 400 to 600 mg every 4 to 6 hours. Other propionic acid derivatives include naproxen, fenoprofen, ketoprofen, and flurbiprofen.[10]

The newest class of nonsteroidal antiinflammatory drug (NSAID) medications currently available in the United States is the cyclooxygenase-2 (COX-2) inhibitor group, consisting of rofecoxib and celecoxib. These medications inhibit inflammation and also demonstrate analgesic and antipyretic properties. Mechanism of action is believed to be through inhibition of prostaglandin synthesis via inhibition of COX-2. These medications may be taken orally once per day and are not yet cleared for patients under age 18 years or for patients with advanced renal disease. Elimination is primarily via hepatic metabolism, with little of the drug recovered in the urine. Side effects primarily include GI distress, hypertension, skin rashes, and peripheral edema. The recommended dosage for rofecoxib is 12.5 to 25 mg once daily. Celecoxib may be given either 100 mg bid or 200 mg daily, with no clinical advantage seen with either method of administration.

Local Anesthetics (Table 16-3)

LOCAL ANESTHETIC PHARMACOLOGY. For centuries, coca shrub leaves indigenous to the Andes Mountains were used, creating a mouth-numbing effect. Gaedicke extracted the alkaloid *erythroxylin* in 1855, from which Niemann isolated cocaine in 1860.[8] Carl Koller first reported using ophthalmic cocaine anesthesia in 1884. Subsequent enthusiasm led to the use of cocaine for anesthesia of the nasopharynx and oropharynx for surgery of the ear, nose, and throat. Erdtman of Sweden synthesized lidocaine in 1943.[8]

Local anesthetics block nerve conduction through sodium-blocking properties in free nerve endings, peripheral nerves, spinal roots, and autonomic ganglia. Normally, the cell's sodium-potassium pump constantly pumps sodium out of and potassium into the cell to restore membrane ionic gradients. The anesthetic renders the membrane impermeable to the influx of sodium during depolarization, and the nerve cell thus remains polarized. Anesthetic drug binding occurs within the sodium channel after the drug enters the channel from the intracellular side of the nerve membrane.[11] Variables such as nerve length, rate of nerve impulse transmission, concentration, and volume of local anesthetic will determine the rate of onset and extent of therapeutic effect. Anesthetic potency, as well as

TABLE 16-3. Comparable Anesthetic Doses for Peripheral Blocks and Local Infiltration (No Epinephrine Included)

DRUG	DOSE (mg/kg)
AMIDE ANESTHETICS	
Lidocaine	5
Prilocaine	5
Etidocaine	4
Mepivacaine	5
Bupivacaine	2
ESTER ANESTHETICS	
Procaine	5
Tetracaine	1-2
2-Chloroprocaine	5

onset and duration of action, depends on factors that include lipid solubility, protein binding, and ionization. In general, the "S" stereoisomer has less toxicity and greater duration than the "R" stereoisomer. Anesthetic metabolism and elimination are functions of the specific anesthetic's chemical structure.[11]

Lidocaine was the first of the amino amide class of local anesthetics. It is metabolized by hepatic microsomal enzymes. Since its metabolites do not include paraaminobenzoic acid (PABA), allergic reactions are rare. Procaine is a synthetic amino ester local anesthetic. This class of anesthetic is hydrolyzed by cholinesterase to form paraaminobenzoic acid, which is responsible for allergic reactions seen with ester anesthetics. Because the esters are relatively unstable, they do not tolerate repeated autoclaving for sterilization.[7] Although no specific studies have addressed temperature extremes experienced by supplies in wilderness settings, it is prudent to protect these medications from heat as much as is reasonably possible.

A local anesthetic may provide relief in a topical application before more invasive cleansing and debridement. TAC is a mixture of tetracaine 0.5%, adrenaline 1:2000, and cocaine 11.8% in saline, which may be soaked into a sterile bandage and placed directly over a wound. This combination may provide good analgesia and moderate vasoconstriction.[38] Adverse effects to cocaine absorbed by this method have been reported. The local anesthetic EMLA is a eutectic mixture of 5% lidocaine and prilocaine. After this cream is applied to intact skin under a nonabsorbent dressing for at least 45 minutes, an invasive procedure such as IV needle insertion may be more easily tolerated.

ANESTHETIC TOXICITY. Blood level of anesthetic after tissue injection depends on absorption, dosage, metabolism, and elimination, with increased tissue vascularity and vasoactivity of the anesthetic having great effects. Infiltration into a highly vascular site, such as around an intercostal nerve, leads to more rapid escalation of blood level than does injection into less vascular subcutaneous tissues. Use of an anesthetic/epinephrine mixture leads to slower absorption but must be avoided when injecting distal extremities and digits, where epinephrine-induced vasoconstriction may lead to acute ischemic injury. Because of the possibility of unintentional direct intravascular injection, all local and regional anesthetic infiltrations should be made after negative aspiration for blood and in small aliquots between aspiration attempts.

As anesthetic toxicity levels are approached, common early symptoms include circumoral numbness, tinnitus, and cephalgia. CNS toxicity in the form of seizures occurs at lower anesthetic blood levels than does cardiotoxicity seen as ventricular arrhythmias and cardiovascular collapse. Lidocaine's CNS effects are ac-

tually paradoxical. At blood concentrations of 3 to 5 μg/ml, lidocaine is an anticonvulsant, whereas blood concentrations of 10 to 12 μg/ml are associated with seizures. Generally, cardiotoxicity is achieved at approximately 150% of the blood level concentrations required for anesthetic CNS toxicity. Bupivacaine has demonstrated increased cardiotoxicity out of proportion to its increased potency, relative to lidocaine.[11]

Anesthetic allergy per se is uncommon, with perhaps 99% of all adverse anesthetic reactions actually related to pharmacologic toxicity of the anesthetic or to epinephrine mixed with the agent.[11] Ester anesthetic allergies are related to PABA metabolites; therefore intolerance to PABA-containing sunscreens may indicate allergic tendency to ester anesthetics. Allergies to amide anesthetics in preservative-free vials are rare. There is no known evidence of cross-sensitivity between amide and ester anesthetic classes.

Anesthetic Infiltration Techniques and Nerve Blocks. Soft tissue analgesia is accomplished with local injection of 1% lidocaine. Generally, the maximum injectable dose for lidocaine is 4 mg/kg. Take care to inject from the wound periphery toward the wound's center to decrease the chance of spreading bacteria or foreign matter to adjacent tissue.[38] In larger wounds, injections proceed from an area previously anesthetized to lessen discomfort from subsequent injections.

Local anesthetic injection typically causes temporary pain resulting from the solution's pH. Buffered solutions are available or may be created by adding sodium bicarbonate (1 mEq/ml) to lidocaine or other anesthetic in a 1:10 ratio, bicarbonate to anesthetic. Tolerance to the injection is improved by gentle and slow injection, allowing prudence with the total dose of anesthetic. Adding epinephrine is not generally recommended for soft tissue, although it may provide useful hemostasis, especially in head and scalp lacerations. Avoid using epinephrine on nose tips, ear lobes, distal extremities, and digits to avoid ischemic injury or even subsequent necrosis.

Many central and regional nerve blocks require special training, including a thorough knowledge of anatomy and management of potential complications, but several blocks can be appropriate in a wilderness setting if the physician is cautious and limits the amount of anesthetic injected. Make all infiltrations after aseptic preparation of the skin, whenever possible.

DIGITAL NERVE BLOCKS (Figure 16-1). Anesthesia to the digits is easily accomplished with a low-volume field block to the medial and lateral aspects of the digit at the base of the respective phalanx. Approach the digital nerves from the dorsum of the hand or foot rather than from the palm or sole. The dorsal digital nerves and proper digital nerves course along the medial and lateral aspects of the digits roughly at the 10 and 2 o'clock

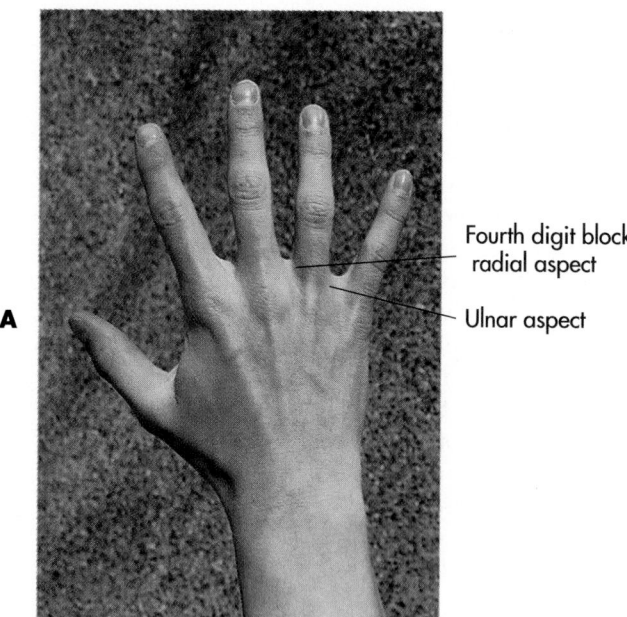

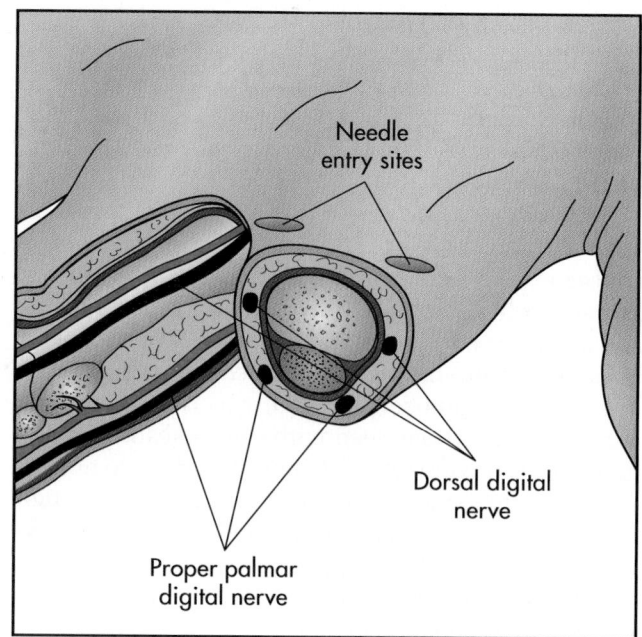

Figure 16-1 A, Site of digital nerve block. **B,** Digital nerve anatomy. *(A courtesy Bryan L. Frank, MD.)*

and 4 and 8 o'clock positions, respectively. From 3 to 5 ml of lidocaine 0.5% to 1.0% injected as a field block with a 25-gauge (or 27-gauge) needle to the medial and lateral aspects of the proximal digit gives a satisfactory digital block. *Do not use an epinephrine-containing anesthetic* because this could lead to circulatory compromise and possible necrosis of the digit.

WRIST BLOCKS (Figure 16-2). The entire hand may be anesthetized by blocking the nerves at the wrist. The radial nerve supplies the cutaneous branches of the dorsum of the hand and thumb, and distally to the distal interphalangeal joints of the index, long, and radial aspect of the ring fingers. Median nerve sensory distribution includes the palmar surface of the hand, the ulnar aspect of the thumb, the palmar aspect of the index finger, and the long and radial portion of the ring finger. The median nerve innervation extends dorsally over the index, long, and ring fingers to the distal interphalangeal joint. The ulnar nerve gives sensation to the palmar and dorsal surfaces of the lateral hand, the fifth finger, and the ulnar half of the ring finger.[5]

Using a 25-gauge needle, inject 2 to 4 ml of lidocaine 1% in the subcutaneous tissue overlying the radial artery. A superficial subcutaneous injection from this point and over the radial styloid anesthetizes cutaneous branches from the proximal forearm and extending into the hand.[42] Block the median nerve with 2 to 4 ml of lidocaine 1% just proximal to the palmar wrist crease between the tendons of the palmaris longus and the flexor carpi radialis muscles. Make the

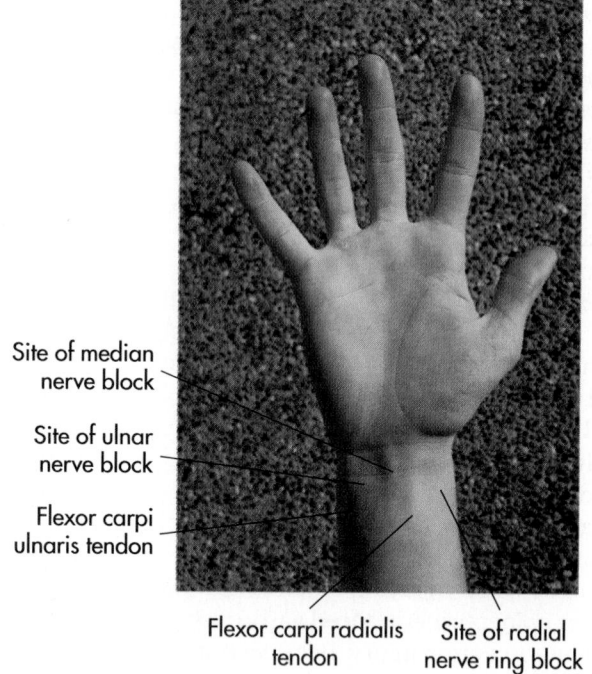

Figure 16-2 Landmarks for wrist block. *(Courtesy Bryan L. Frank, MD.)*

injection deep to the volar fascia. If a paresthesia is elicited (resulting from contact with the nerve), withdraw the needle slightly before injection. Block the ulnar nerve with 2 to 4 ml of lidocaine 1% injected just lateral to the ulnar artery, which is radial to the flexor carpi ulnaris tendon at the level of the ulnar styloid.

ANKLE BLOCKS (Figure 16-3). Anesthesia of the foot is easily accomplished with blocks of the sensory nerves at the ankle. Using a 25-gauge needle, block the deep peroneal nerve, providing sensation between the great and second toes, with 5 ml of lidocaine 1% between the tendons of the tibialis anterior and the extensor hallucis longus at the level of the medial and lateral malleoli. The needle may be passed to the bone just lateral to the dorsalis pedis artery. Inject the superficial peroneal nerve with 5 ml of lidocaine 1% with a superficial ring block between the injection of the deep peroneal nerve and the medial malleolus. This blocks sensation to the medial and dorsal aspects of the foot. Inject the posterior tibial nerve with 5 ml of lidocaine 1% just posterior to the medial malleolus, adjacent to the posterior tibial artery. Paresthesias are sought in these blocks and will increase the likelihood of success.[28] Posterior tibial nerve distribution includes the heel and plantar foot surface. Follow paresthesias by a slight withdrawal of the needle before injection. Block the sural nerve, providing sensation to the posterolateral foot, with a similar volume of lidocaine 1% between the lateral malleolus and Achilles tendon, followed by a subcutaneous infiltration from this site and over the lateral malleolus.[42]

TRIGGER POINT INJECTIONS. Persons who suffer from neck and shoulder or lower back strain may benefit greatly from deactivation of myofascial trigger zones. The pain relief may be profound and enable an adventure to continue without disruption. Travell and Simons have extensively described primary and secondary painful points and their referral patterns. Myofascial pain may be intense and be referred to a large zone of the body.[45] Successful deactivation of trigger zones may be accomplished with either dry needling (acupuncture) or injection of lidocaine 1%. In the absence of anesthetic or acupuncture needles, trigger point deactivation may be accomplished with a 27-gauge needle.

Injection of a trigger zone is typically performed directly into the painful myofascial point and in a four-quadrant zone from the center of the trigger point, advancing 1 to 2 cm into the adjacent tissue at a 45- to 60-degree angle from the skin surface. Muscle twitches, or fasciculations, may accompany the injections though need not be sought. A volume of 1 to 2 ml of lidocaine 1% is usually ample for each trigger zone. There is no benefit to adding corticosteroids to the anesthetic. Using an acupuncture needle (or a 27- or 30-gauge needle) may deactivate the trigger zones nicely using a similar four-quadrant pecking of the myofascial zone, without injection of anesthetic. A 1- to 1½-inch needle may be used to peck briskly several times in each direction, also at a 45- to 60-degree angle from the center of the trigger zone. Depth of insertion is typically 1 to 2 cm. Soiled skin should be prepared similar as for an IM injection.

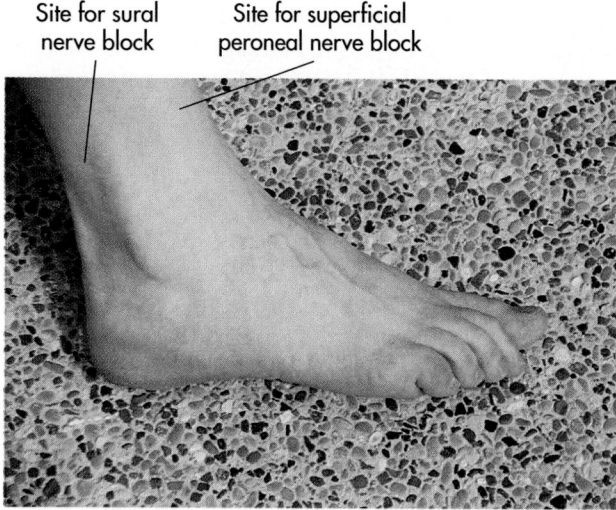

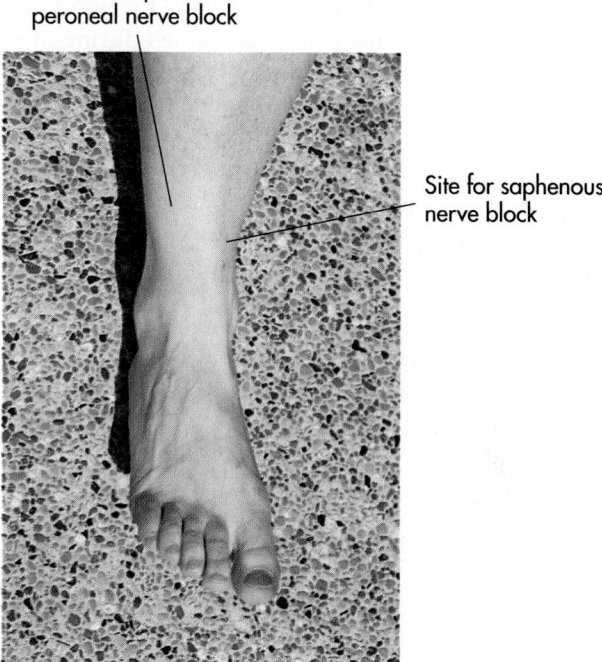

Figure 16-3 Landmarks for ankle block. *(Courtesy Bryan L. Frank, MD.)*

Intravenous Regional Anesthesia or Bier Blocks. The Bier block may provide significant anesthesia to stabilize an arm or leg fracture for a physician unfamiliar with the anatomy and technique of a more sophisticated proximal nerve block. Because a tourniquet is necessary, a Bier block is generally not useful for longer than 60 to 90 minutes.

A vein of the hand or foot on the extremity to be blocked is cannulated with a 20- to 22-gauge IV catheter or butterfly, which is then capped and taped in place. The extremity is then raised above the level of the heart for 1 to 2 minutes to diminish the volume of blood in the distal limb. If tolerated, wrap an Esmarch (rubber) bandage or elastic bandage from the hand or foot toward the proximal arm or leg to exsanguinate the limb. If a compression bandage is not tolerated, elevate the extremity for 5 to 10 minutes or apply an inflatable splint. Apply a tourniquet and hold the pressure at 50 to 100 mm Hg above systolic blood pressure. In the wilderness, a blood pressure cuff is effective, or a strap, rope, or tubing may be used. Place the limb horizontally for the injection, using 25 ml of lidocaine 1% for the upper extremity and 35 ml of lidocaine 1% for the lower extremity. Slowly infuse the anesthetic through the previously inserted intravenous catheter or butterfly at a rate of approximately 0.5 ml per second. Take care to avoid extravasation of the anesthetic into the surrounding tissues.

Anesthesia will ensue over the first 10 to 15 minutes as the lidocaine diffuses from the intravascular space and binds to the soft tissue. Discontinue the injection if the tourniquet pressure is not maintained during injection to prevent anesthetic toxicity from an unrestricted IV bolus injection. The tourniquet should remain inflated for 60 to 90 minutes, when most of the anesthetic should be protein bound in the soft tissues. Then release the tourniquet all at once and the anesthetic effect will diminish within 5 to 10 minutes.

Other Pain Pharmaceuticals

Pharmaceutical agents other than narcotic analgesics and local anesthetics may offer significant relief and prevent or decrease the potential adverse effects of analgesics and anesthetics.

Ketamine. Ketamine is a dissociative anesthetic agent that provides significant analgesia. Its mechanism of action is probably related to its agonist effects on the glutamate receptor of the *N*-methyl-D-aspartate (NMDA) subtype.[53] NMDA may affect central or peripheral neuropathic pain transmission more than nociceptive transmission in tactile or thermal modalities.[3,26] Ketamine is believed to activate μ-opioid receptors responsible for analgesia and δ-opioid receptors for dysphoria.[19] In wilderness settings where respiratory depression may be a significant concern, ketamine may provide significant analgesia and a dissociative state with tolerable respiratory depression and some loss of glossopharyngeal reflexes. Ketamine possesses sympathomimetic activity that may prove useful in injured persons with depressed cardiac function or shock and may also provide bronchodilation for victims with reactive airway disease. It is contraindicated with head injury because it increases intracranial pressure.[25] Intracranial pressure increase results from augmented cerebral blood flow and direct cerebral vasodilatation. Cerebral metabolic oxygen requirements increase as well.[4]

An IV dose of 0.2 to 0.4 mg/kg ketamine provides analgesia and 1 to 2 mg/kg IV or 2 to 4 mg/kg IM leads to profound analgesia and a dissociative state. A quiet and calm setting diminishes unpleasant dissociative experiences for the recipient.

Nonsteroidal Antiinflammatory Drugs. NSAIDs are effective for mild to moderate pain and may provide ample clinical benefit without producing the respiratory depression seen with narcotic analgesics. The mechanism of action is most likely due to inhibition of a prostaglandin-mediated amplification of chemical and mechanical irritant effects on the sensory pathways.[33] NSAIDs undergo rapid absorption after oral or rectal administration, followed by hepatic metabolism and renal excretion of their conjugated metabolites. Injectable forms of various NSAIDs have also been developed in recent years. This nonsteroidal class of medications includes chemically unrelated compounds grouped together by their therapeutic actions, represented by agents such as acetic acid, propionic acid, oxicam, and pyrazolone derivatives.

Adverse effects of NSAIDs include GI distress and bleeding, CNS disturbances (vertigo, drowsiness), and prolonged bleeding from platelet function inhibition. In certain circumstances, NSAID-induced immunosuppression increases a propensity to bacterial infection.

Antidepressants. Wilderness travelers may be taking antidepressant medications for chronic pain or psychoemotional dysfunction. Continuation of these medications is important to avoid intensification of pain or psychoemotional lability. Chronic pain conditions that may benefit from antidepressants include migraine cephalgia, postherpetic neuralgia, and diabetic neuropathy. The tertiary amine tricyclic drugs (e.g., amitriptyline, imipramine, doxepin, and clomipramine) are commonly used for pain problems. Antidepressant medications are presumably effective for treating chronic pain problems by blocking presynaptic reuptake of serotonin and/or norepinephrine by the amine pump.[2] These drugs are rapidly absorbed after oral administration, although this may be decreased by antimuscarinic effects. They are highly protein-bound and have half-lives of 1 to 4 days. They are generally oxidized by the hepatic microsomal system and conjugated with glucuronic acid. Elimination occurs via urine and feces.[24]

Side effects may include dry mouth, urinary retention, constipation, and hyperactivity.[18] Photosensitivity may place wilderness travelers at risk for sunburn, and orthostatic hypotension may lead to falls. Overdoses produce excessive sedation, anticholinergic effects on the cardiac conduction system, significant hypotension, respiratory depression, arrhythmias, and coma.

Anticonvulsants. Of all the drugs classified as anticonvulsants, four are useful as adjuvant medications in pain management: phenytoin, valproic acid, carbamazepine, and clonazepam. Their chemical structures bear little relationship to one another. Serum levels have not been clearly established as useful parameters in pain management. The mechanism of action of each of these drug classes is unique and varies from altering sodium, calcium, and potassium flux, to enhancing GABA activity or binding.[24]

Side effects vary but may include nausea and vomiting and CNS effects, such as drowsiness, ataxia, and confusion. It is important to rule out drug effects as a factor in wilderness-related illnesses. These drugs are not recommended for acute pain management in the wilderness.

Antihistamines. Antihistamines may be useful adjuvants. Specifically, hydroxyzine provides additive analgesic effect in combination with narcotic analgesics while also lending antiemetic and sedative properties. Hydroxyzine may cause ataxia and disinhibition and on rare occasions is associated with convulsions when used in high doses.[24] A dose of 50 to 100 mg IM may improve clinical pain management . Similarly, oral antihistamines, such as diphenhydramine 25 to 50 mg PO, may provide useful adjuvant effects.

Muscle Relaxants. The term *muscle relaxants* refers to a diverse group of drugs with similar clinical effects but different pharmacologic properties. They are not true skeletal muscle relaxants in the sense of blocking neuromuscular transmission but act by depressing reflexes, generally in the CNS. They are indicated for the relief of muscle spasm related to acute, painful, musculoskeletal injuries. Side effects include decreased alertness, motor coordination, and physical dexterity.

Common centrally acting muscle relaxants include carisoprodol (Soma), 350 mg PO tid-qid; metaxalone (Skelaxin), 800 mg PO tid-qid; and methocarbamol (Robaxin), 1.5 g PO qid for the first 48 to 72 hours, then 1 g PO qid. The specific mechanism of action is unknown but appears to be related to centrally acting sedation. Cyclobenzaprine (Flexeril), 10 to 20 mg PO tid, is structurally related to the tricyclic antidepressant medications. Diazepam (Valium), 2 to 10 mg PO, IM, or IV, is a benzodiazepine that induces calm and anxiolysis via effects on the thalamus and hypothalamus.[6]

Transcutaneous Electrical Nerve Stimulation

Shealy and Liss developed the transcutaneous electrical nerve stimulator as a trial for patients considering spinal cord electrical stimulation to relieve chronic pain.[1] TENS units are so commonly used that wilderness physicians will probably encounter persons using these devices. The mechanism of action is believed to involve stimulation of large, myelinated A fibers, which block C fiber pain sensation from reaching the brain.

This process is explained at least in part by the gate control theory of Melzack and Wall.[37] Additionally, Pomeranz and others have shown the neurohumoral effects of electrical stimulation to include endorphins, enkephalins, serotonin, GABA, adrenocorticotropic hormone (ACTH), and other modulators. High-intensity, low-frequency electrical stimulation elicits an endorphinergic response, whereas low-intensity, high-frequency electrical stimulation leads to spinal segmental analgesia, and monoamine-based presynaptic and postsynaptic inhibition of pain signals.[44] Increased plasma and cerebrospinal fluid (CSF) levels of endorphins with high- or low-frequency electrical stimulation are sometimes seen. Conventional TENS units offer stimulation frequencies of 50 to 80 Hz, whereas acupuncture-like TENS devices use stimulation frequencies from less than 10 Hz to greater than 100 Hz.

Wilderness physicians familiar with TENS units may find them useful to treat acute traumatic pain, but more likely, a traveler will have a TENS unit. Most persons have developed personal preferences for TENS unit settings and skin electrode placement. Rigorous physical activity may cause difficulty maintaining electrode placement. Application to clean, dry skin is important. Preparing the skin with topical benzoin may significantly increase the duration of adhesiveness. Because benzoin is an iodine-based topical solution, avoid it in persons with sensitivity or allergy to iodine.

Complementary and Alternative Medicine Therapies

"Complementary and alternative" denote therapies and modalities that may not be supported by Western-designed prospective, randomized studies, that are not commonly taught in U.S. medical colleges, or that are not generally covered by traditional health insurance plans.[14,15,48] Some may contribute significantly to wilderness pain management.

Acupuncture. Acupuncture has developed over 3 to 5 millennia in Asia and has existed over the past several hundred years in the Western world. Conditions in which acupuncture developed are very similar to those found by wilderness travelers. The use of acupuncture by physicians to treat trauma and illness in wilderness settings has been described recently in medical literature.[20,22] Properly administered acupuncture should have a very low risk of morbidity and may be extremely effective in alleviating pain and even restoring function to an injured wilderness traveler (Figures 16-4).

Pomeranz and others have demonstrated endorphin, enkephalin, monamine, and ACTH release with acupuncture stimulation.[44] Other effects, such as the gate theory and altered sympathetic activity,[30] may apply as well. Clinically, improved microvascular circulation may lead to decreases in tissue edema, which in

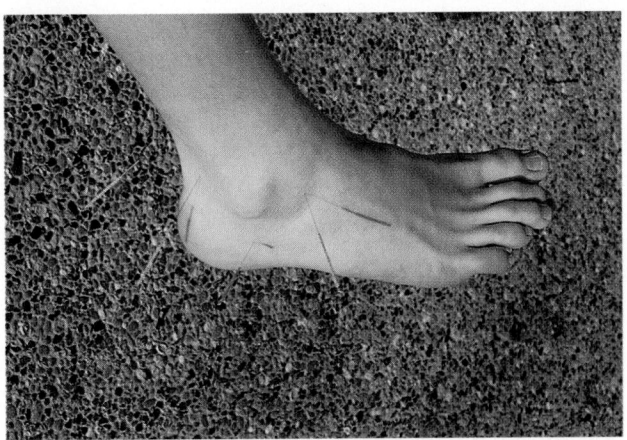

Figure 16-4 Typical acupuncture needle placement for lateral ankle strain. *(Courtesy Bryan L. Frank, MD.)*

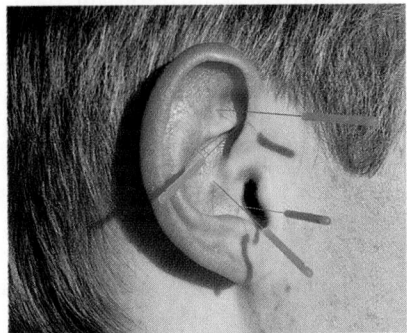

Figure 16-5 Patient with auricular needles in place. *(Courtesy Bryan L. Frank, MD.)*

turn may diminish pain and aid in restoring function. The release of ACTH leads to increased circulating corticosteroids; decreased inflammation may contribute to decreased pain and improved healing.[27]

Contemporary medical acupuncturists are typically trained in a variety of styles or traditions. Many physicians use a combined approach of acupuncture point selections based on neuroanatomy and those believed to have energetic effects in the body. Additionally, acupuncture microsystems are often used, in which the entire body is represented in a small area such as the ear, scalp, or hand. These microsystems are often quite beneficial for acute pain[22] (Figure 16-5).

Sterile acupuncture needles are compact, lightweight, and easy to include in a day pack or first-aid kit. Integration of acupuncture into the biomedical care of wilderness trauma, pain, and illness may dramatically enhance patient comfort and facilitate extrication from a remote setting.

An energetic style of acupuncture that is especially useful for common trauma utilizes the tendinomuscular meridians (TMM) of the acupuncture energetic sub-

systems. The indications for activation of the TMM treatment include acute strains, sprains, abrasions, and hematomas. A needle is placed in the "Ting" point of one to three of the meridians involved in the lesion. This is followed by placing a needle in the "Gathering" point for the meridian(s), then by placement of needles approximately 1 cm around the area of induration, swelling, or bruising. All needles in this treatment are placed to only 2 to 3 mm depth and are left in place for 20 to 45 minutes.

For example, sprained ankles often respond to acupuncture. Commonly, a lateral ankle sprain involves both the gall bladder and bladder TMM zones. The Ting points for these meridians are at GB 44 and BL 67 on the lateral angles of the fourth and fifth toes, respectively. The Gathering point for these meridians is at SI 18, just below the zygoma in line with the lateral canthus. Local needles typically include four to six placed around the swelling or ecchymosis of the ankle sprain. Recovery from the sprain may proceed much more rapidly with this type of acupuncture input than with conventional therapies of rest, ice, compression, and elevation (RICE) alone. Failure to respond with 70% to 85% or greater decrease in pain over 24 to 48 hours may in fact alert the medical acupuncturist that an injury may be more serious than initially appreciated.

Most acupuncture treatment requires substantial training to be responsibly integrated with conventional Western therapies. National and international standards of training have been established for Western-trained physicians who desire to incorporate acupuncture into their traditional medical practices. The American Academy of Medical Acupuncture (AAMA) represents physician acupuncturists whose training meets or exceeds standards established by the World Health Organization, the World Federation of Acupuncture and Moxibustion Societies, and the International Congress of Medical Acupuncture and Related Therapies (ICMART). Physicians interested in learning acupuncture may contact the AAMA at (323) 937-5514 for information on training programs designed specifically for physicians. The National Commission for Certification of Acupuncture and Oriental Medicine provides testing and resources primarily for nonphysician acupuncturists.[21]

Herbal/Botanical Remedies (See Chapter 50). The term *herb* is broadly defined as a nonwoody plant that dies down to the ground after flowering. The term *botanical* is a more general description of flora, although common interpretation includes any plant used for medicinal therapy, nutritional value, food seasoning, or dyeing another substance as an herb.[13] As with acupuncture, the use of botanicals may be encountered in wilderness travels as a part of the indigenous culture and medical care. Botanicals are often prepared as infusions, with the plant's soft portions placed in a pot and covered by boiling water to create a supernatant. Herbal decoctions are traditionally prepared in special earthen crocks, or in containers of stainless steel, ceramic, or enamel by contemporary practitioners, specifically avoiding aluminum and alloy metal pots. The herb is placed in the container and covered with cold water that is then boiled, covered, and simmered. Travelers may encounter an herbal remedy dispensed as a poultice, botanical liniment, ointment, or oil to be applied to the skin. Alternately, many modern herbalists utilize capsule forms of herbs for ease of administration. Combinations of several herbs are often more effective than a single herb, and common formulas have been recorded worldwide for centuries.[29] Appropriate application or prescription of botanical products rarely leads to toxicity or adverse reactions, although such are possible if botanicals are used excessively or carelessly.

Certain botanical products used for pain include morphine, isolated from the opium poppy, and cocaine, from coca leaves (*Erythroxylon coca*). Often used as a seasoning or food, oregano (*Origanum vulgare*) has been beneficial for rheumatic pain.[29] Sunflower (*Helianthus annuus*) is a source of phenylalanine, useful for general pain. Turmeric (*Curcuma longa*) contains curcumin, an antiinflammatory substance beneficial for rheumatoid arthritis, and ginger (*Zingiber officinale*) is beneficial for rheumatoid arthritis, osteoarthritis and fibromyalgia. Clove (*Syzygium aromaticum*) is endorsed by the German botanical resource, Commission E, topically for dental pain. Red peppers (*Capsicum* species) contain substance P–depleting capsaicin and also salicylates. Often taken as an infusion or decoction, kava kava (*Piper methysticum*) contains both dihydrokavain and dihydromethysticin, which have analgesic effectiveness similar to that of aspirin. Evening primrose (*Oenothera biennis*) is a great source of tryptophan and has been demonstrated to relieve pain associated with diabetic neuropathy. Lavender (*Lavandula* species) contains linalool and linalyl aldehyde, which appear to be useful for pain of burns and other injuries in topical and aromatherapy form.[13]

Willow (*Salix* species), used to treat pain since 500 BC, contains salicin and other salicylate compounds. The German Commission E has recognized willow as an effective pain reliever for headaches, arthritis, and many other pains.

Salicylate-containing plants include red peppers, wintergreen, and birch bark. Avoid all botanicals containing salicylates in persons who are sensitive or allergic to aspirin products. Further, children who have viral infections, such as a cold or influenza, should avoid these products because salicylates have been implicated in the development of Reye's syndrome.[13]

Chamomile (*Matricaria chamomilla*) contains chamazulene, which is reportedly beneficial for abdominal pain related to GI spasm or colic; as an antihistaminic, it has mild calming or sedative properties. It is used in Europe to treat leg ulcers and may be beneficial for painful, irritated bites and stings.[13] Plantain major (*Plantago major*) is also commonly used for bites and stings, poison ivy discomfort, and toothache, and has been used traditionally by Native Americans as a wound dressing. Aloe gel (*Aloe vera*) has been used since ancient times to treat burns and sunburn and to promote wound healing.

Especially useful for sprains and strains is the mountain daisy or arnica (*Arnica montana*), which is also endorsed by Commission E. Arnica was in *the U.S. Pharmacopoeia* in the early 1800s to 1960s and has long been used by Native Americans and others for relieving back pain and other myofascial pains and bruising. It is used topically or internally, often in homeopathic form. Comfrey (*Symphytum officinale*) has been used since ancient Greece for skin problems.[13] It contains alloin, which is antiinflammatory, and is endorsed by Commission E to topically treat bruises, dislocations, and sprains. Comfrey has experienced a controversial safety record because oral ingestion of its pyrrolizidine alkaloids has been associated with hepatotoxicity and/or carcinogenicity.[13] For this reason, only topical use of comfrey is recommended.

Magnet Therapy. Magnetic therapy has been described for approximately 4000 years in the Hindu Vedas and the Chinese acupuncture classic, Huang Te Nei Ching. The application of magnetic stones, or *lodestones,* is said in ancient legends of Cleopatra and others to have decreased pain and preserved youth. Early Romans used the discharge of the electric eel to treat arthritis and gout.[31]

Danish physicist Oerstad proved in 1820 that an electric current flowing through a wire had its own magnetic field. Modern medicine's most familiar use of magnetic energy is with magnetic resonance imaging (MRI). There are various theories about the effectiveness of permanent magnets for use in pain and healing. Lawrence[31] reports increased blood circulation and increased macrophage activity and Lednev,[32] Olney et al,[39] and McLean et al[36] have hypothesized effects on peripheral nerves, including blockage or modification of sensory neuron action potentials and enhanced regeneration of peripheral nerves.[47]

Most permanent magnets marketed at this time for management of pain measure approximately 200 to 1200 gauss in strength. At this level, there is little if any risk in trying a magnet for pain reduction, assuming the patient is properly evaluated to provide other appropriate care. Many patients report significant pain reduction within hours, whereas others report relief after wearing the magnets for a week or more. In wilderness travel, it is reasonable to carry a few magnets because they are usually lightweight, compact, and unbreakable. Magnets marketed for pain therapy range in size from a 2-inch circle to 6- by 12-inch rectangular pads. Most are only a few millimeters thick and are often flexible. These are becoming more readily available through multilevel marketing, television "infomercials," health food stores, and the Internet. Some people have experienced pain relief with simple, small magnets used to place notes and photographs on a refrigerator. Placement of the magnet should be directly over the area of pain, and it should be held in place with tape, clothing, or straps.

REFERENCES

1. Abram SE: Electrical stimulation for cancer pain treatment. In Abram SE, Haddox JD, Kettler RE, editors: *The pain clinic manual*, Philadelphia, 1990, JB Lippincott.
2. Abram SE, Haddox JD: Chronic pain management. In Barash PG, Cullen BF, Stoelting RK, editors: *Clinical anesthesia*, ed 2, Philadelphia, 1993, JB Lippincott.
3. Bazal MK, Gordon FJ: Effect of blockade of spinal NMDA receptor on sympathoexcitation and cardiovascular response produced by cerebral ischemia. In Waldman SD, Winnie AP, editors: *Interventional pain management*, Philadelphia, 1996, WB Saunders.
4. Bendo AA et al: Neurophysiology and neuroanesthesia. In Barash PG, Cullen BF, Stoelting RK, editors: *Clinical anesthesia*, ed 2, Philadelphia, 1993, JB Lippincott.
5. Brown DL: *Atlas of regional anesthesia*, Philadelphia, 1992, WB Saunders.
6. Burnham T et al, editors: *Drug facts and comparisons*, St Louis, 1999, Facts and Comparisons.
7. Covino BG: Local anesthetics: update. In Stanley TH, Ashburn MA, Fone PG, editors: *Anesthesiology and pain management*, Dordrecht, Netherlands, 1991, Kluwer Academic.
8. de Jong RH: Local anesthetics in clinical practice. In Waldman SD, Winnie AP, editors: *Interventional pain management*, Philadelphia, 1996, WB Saunders.
9. Dean JA, editor: *Lange's handbook of chemistry*, ed 14, New York, 1992, McGraw-Hill.
10. Denson DD, Katz JA: Nonsteroidal antiinflammatory agents. In Raj PP, editor: *Practical management of pain*, ed 2, St Louis, 1992, Mosby.
11. DiFazio CA, Woods AM: Pharmacology of local anesthetics. In Raj PP, editor: *Practical management of pain*, ed 2, St Louis, 1992, Mosby.
12. Donohoe CD: Evaluation of the patient in pain. In Waldman SD, Winnie AP, editors: *Interventional pain management*, Philadelphia, 1996, WB Saunders.
13. Duke JA: *The green pharmacy: new discoveries in herbal remedies for common diseases and conditions from the nation's foremost authority on healing herbs*, Emmaus, Penn, 1997, Rodale Press
14. Eisenberg DM et al: Unconventional medicine in the United States—prevalence, costs, and patterns of use, *N Engl J Med* 328:246, 1993.
15. Eisenberg DM et al: Trends in alternative medicine use in the United States, 1990-1997: results of a follow-up national survey, *JAMA* 280:1569, 1998.
16. Exton DR, Fenner PJ, Williamson JA: Cold packs: effective topical analgesia in the treatment of painful stings by *Physalia* and other jellyfish, *Med J Aust* 151:625, 1989.
17. Fenner PJ et al: First aid treatment of jellyfish stings in Australia: response to a newly differentiated species, *Med J Aust* 158:498, 1993.
18. Foley KM: The role of adjuvant drugs and aesthetic blocks in the management of patients with cancer and pain. In Stanley TH, Ashburn MA, Fone PG, editors: *Anesthesiology and pain management*, Dordrecht, Netherlands, 1991, Kluwer Academic.
19. Fragen RJ, Avram MJ: Nonopioid intravenous anesthetics. In Barash PG, Cullen BF, Stoelting RK, editors: *Clinical anesthesia*, ed 2, Philadelphia, 1993, JB Lippincott.
20. Frank BL: Medical acupuncture and wilderness medicine: an integrated medical model in third world settings, *Medical Acupuncture* 8:11, 1996.
21. Frank BL: Medical acupuncture: a model of integrated healthcare from alternative to mainstream medicine, *Colorado Medicine* 94: 252, 1997.
22. Frank BL: Medical acupuncture enhances standard wilderness care: a case study from the Inca Trail, Machu Picchu, Peru, *Wilderness Environ Med* 8:161, 1998.
23. Gilman AG et al, editors: *Goodman and Gilman's pharmacologic basis of therapeutics*, ed 8, New York, 1990, Pergamon Press.
24. Haddox JD: Neuropsychiatric drug use in pain management. In Raj PP, editor: *Practical management of pain*, ed 2, St Louis, 1992, Mosby.
25. Hartrick C: Pain due to trauma including sports injuries. In Raj PP, editor: *Practical management of pain*, ed 2, St Louis, 1992, Mosby.
26. Hassenbusch III SJ: Receptors at the spinal cord level: the clinical target. In Waldman SD, Winnie AP, editors: *Interventional pain management*, Philadelphia, 1996, WB Saunders.
27. Helms JM: *Acupuncture energetics: a clinical approach for physicians*, Berkeley, Calif, 1995, Medical Acupuncture Publishers.
28. Katz J, Renck H: *Handbook of thoraco-abdominal nerve block*, Orlando, Fla, 1987, Grune & Stratton.
29. Kenner D, Requena Y: *Botanical medicine: a European professional perspective*, Brookline, Mass, 1996, Paradigm Publications.
30. Knardahl S et al: Sympathetic nerve activity after acupuncture in humans, *Pain* 75:19, 1998.
31. Lawrence R, Rosch P, Plowden J: *Magnet therapy: the pain cure alternative*, Rocklin, Calif, 1998, Prima Publishing.
32. Lednev LL: Possible mechanisms for the influence of weak magnetic fields on biological systems, *Bioelectromagnetics* 12:71, 1991.
33. Lubenow TR, McCarthy RJ, Ivankovich AD: Management of acute postoperative pain. In Barash PG, Cullen BF, Stoelting RK, editors: *Clinical anesthesia*, ed 2, Philadelphia, 1993, JB Lippincott.
34. Madigan SR, Raj PP: History and current status of pain management. In Raj PP, editor: *Practical management of pain*, ed 2, St Louis, 1992, Mosby.
35. Mather LE: Clinical pharmacokinetics of analgesic drugs. In Raj PP, editor: *Practical management of pain*, ed 2, St Louis, 1992, Mosby.
36. McLean MJ et al: Blockage of sensory neuron action potentials by a static magnetic field in the 10 mT range, *Bioelectromagnetics* 16:20, 1995.
37. Melzack R, Wall PD: Pain mechanisms: a new theory, *Science* 150:971, 1965.
38. Morris JA, Swiontkowski MF, Herrmann HJ: Wilderness trauma emergencies. In Auerbach PS, editor: *Wilderness medicine: management of wilderness and environmental emergencies*, ed 3, St Louis, 1995, Mosby.
39. Olney RK et al: A comparison of magnetic and electrical stimulation of peripheral nerves, *Muscle Nerve* 11:21, 1998.
40. Ready LB: Choice of methods for acute pain control. In Stanley TH, Ashburn MA, Fone PG, editors: *Anesthesiology and pain management*, Dordrecht, Netherlands, 1991, Kluwer Academic.
41. Saberski LR: Cryoneurolysis in clinical practice. In Waldman SD, Winnie AP, editors: *Interventional pain management*, Philadelphia, 1996, WB Saunders.
42. Scott DB: *Techniques of regional anesthesia*, Norwalk, Conn, 1989, Appleton & Lange/Mediglobe.
43. Striebel HW et al: Patient-controlled intranasal analgesia (PCINA) for the management of postoperative pain: a pilot study, *J Clin Anesth* 8:4, 1996.
44. Stux G, Pomeranz B: *Basics of acupuncture*, Berlin, 1998, Springer-Verlag.
45. Travell JG, Simons DG: *Myofascial pain and dysfunction: the trigger point manual*, Baltimore, 1992, Williams & Wilkins.
46. Vasudevan S et al: Physical methods of pain management. In Raj PP, editor: *Practical management of pain*, ed 2, St Louis, 1992, Mosby.
47. Weintraub MI: Chronic submaximal magnetic stimulation in peripheral neuropathy: is there a beneficial therapeutic relationship? *Am J Prev Med* 8:12, 1998.
48. Wetzel MS et al: Courses involving complementary and alternative medicine at U.S. medical schools, *JAMA* 280:784, 1998.
49. Wilkerson JA: Cold injuries. In Wilkerson JA: Basic medical care and evacuation. In Wilkerson JA, editor: *Medicine for mountaineering & other wilderness activities*, ed 4, Seattle, 1992, The Mountaineers.
50. Wilkerson JA: Medications. In Wilkerson JA, editor: *Medicine for mountaineering & other wilderness activities*, ed 4, Seattle, 1992, The Mountaineers.
51. Wilson PR, Lamer TJ: Pain mechanisms: anatomy and physiology. In Raj PP, editor: *Practical management of pain*, ed 2, St Louis, 1992, Mosby.
52. Yaksh TL: Neurotransmitter systems involved in nociceptive transmission. In Stanley TH, Ashburn MA, Fone PG, editors: *Anesthesiology and pain management*, Dordrecht, Netherlands, 1991, Kluwer Academic.
53. Yaksh TL: Pharmacology of the pain processing system. In Waldman SD, Winnie AP editors: *Interventional pain management*, Philadelphia, 1996, WB Saunders.

17 Emergency Airway Management

Anne E. Dickison

Emergencies involving the airway are among the most urgent conditions necessitating medical intervention. Airway management in the field is a combination of careful physical and scene assessment, recognition of risk, optimization of airway mechanics, and communication to bring the victim to definitive care.

Because the wilderness ability to provide an artificial airway or to assume control of respirations may be quite limited, optimally the victim can be an active participant in the remote-site rescue effort. The drive to breathe is one of the most powerful brainstem reflexes. Although they may be depressed, the autonomic reflexes to cough, gag, swallow, gasp, flare nostrils, open the vocal cords during inspiration, hyperventilate in response to hypoxemia or head injury, and recruit accessory muscles of respiration are generally preserved until the victim is near death. The wilderness rescuer must avoid any medications or interventions that might impair these reflexes.

Only a small minority of airway emergencies occur instantaneously, such as sudden complete airway obstruction by an aspirated foreign body (Table 17-1) or a crushed larynx from impact with a steering wheel. Certain other rapidly evolving life-threatening emergency situations have major immediate airway considerations, but if the underlying condition can be stabilized or relieved, the need to manage the airway becomes less pressing. Examples in this second category include suffocation, thoracic squeeze, near drowning, intoxication, or any circumstance in which absence of breathing (apnea) can be converted to spontaneous respiratory effort or an obstructed airway can be converted to a patent one.

Airway compromises that are anticipated to worsen with time fall into a third important category. Without timely and anticipatory intervention, an otherwise viable victim might die from a potentially preventable airway death. Examples in this third category include airway injury from inhalation burns; soft tissue trauma to the mouth, tongue, or neck; infections involving the pharyngeal or hypopharyngeal soft tissues; allergic reactions; and angioneurotic edema. Although there could be hours between onset of airway compromise and progression to end-stage respiratory failure, the more compromised and distorted the airway becomes, the greater the skill (and luck) required to effectively intervene. In a multicasualty incident, the victim with airway compromise in evolution would be prioritized as first to be evacuated.

A fourth category of airway emergency involves the need to establish an artificial airway as a mechanism for providing sustained positive-pressure ventilation. The primary problem in this category is not airway anatomy or patency but rather a situation leading to alveolar hypoventilation. Examples of these circumstances include flail chest with pulmonary contusion; spinal cord injury; pulmonary aspiration resulting in noncompliant lungs or presence of particulate or chemical matter needing to be removed; or pulmonary edema from burns, altitude, or near drowning. In a multicasualty incident, this victim would be triaged as less immediate and, in all likelihood, resuscitative measures would not be initiated.

RECOGNITION OF AIRWAY OBSTRUCTION

The usual indicators for initiating cardiopulmonary resuscitation (CPR) are poor color and unresponsiveness to stimulation. Poor color can be anything from pallor, cyanosis, and mottling to perimortem or postmortem livedo reticularis and livor mortis. Although a very important diagnostic sign, the presence of poor color, even overt cyanosis, does not necessarily mean that the victim is compromised because of an airway emergency or that resuscitative measures should include airway intervention. Cyanosis can be present without airway compromise, and significant airway compromise can be present without cyanosis.

Cyanosis in the absence of airway compromise can result from hypothermia, anemia, hypovolemia, insufficient cardiac output, intrapulmonary or intracardiac shunts, or inadequate tissue perfusion. An allergic reaction with airway edema and vasodilation (causing flushed red skin) is one example of an airway emergency in the absence of cyanosis; unconsciousness (with associated upper airway obstruction) resulting from carbon monoxide poisoning is another.

If cyanosis is not a certain indicator of airway compromise, then what is? The two most important aspects of respiratory assessment are (1) the presence or absence of attempts to breathe; and (2) if attempts are being made, an appreciation of the degree of labor and posture adjustment required to support air exchange. The first observation assesses the integrity of the central nervous system, and the second the patency of airway corridors in combination with elasticity of the lungs and strength of the chest wall.

Labored respirations are typified by a rate that is forcefully rapid, irregular, or gasping. Unusual sounds

TABLE 17-1. Causes of Airway Obstruction

CAUSE	INTERVENTION
Aspiration of foreign body	Heimlich maneuver
	Removal by direct visualization and extraction
	Cricothyrotomy
Unconsciousness	Positioning
	Consider airway adjuncts
	Consider cricoid pressure
Apnea	Open airway
	Initiate rescue breathing
	Check for obstruction
	Consider airway adjuncts
Facial or neck trauma	Careful physical examination
	Remove debris in mouth
	Account for teeth
	Assess potential for swelling
	Positioning
	Secretion assistance
Allergic reactions	Remove from source of allergy
	Epinephrine if available
	Consider cool mist
	Consider topical or sprayed vasoconstrictors
	Consider inhaled β-agonists
	Consider airway adjuncts
Seizures	Pad environment
	Consider padded stick between side molars (no fingers)
	If possible, turn on side to facilitate gravity drainage of saliva or vomit

TABLE 17-2. Description of Airway Sounds

SOUND	DESCRIPTION
Stridor	A sharp, high-pitched squeaky sound with vocal quality that emanates from the larynx and is usually more prominent on inspiration than expiration
Wheezing	A sustained whistling sound made by air passing through narrowed airways usually distal to the larynx, and generally more prominent in expiration than inspiration; the pitch is lower than stridor and higher than rhonchi
Rhonchi	Gurgling, congested, low-pitched rattling sounds in the chest caused by secretions in the large and medium-sized airways
Grunting	A staccato glottic noise heard in end-expiration only, with a lower pitch than that of stridor; usually found in association with restrictive lung disease or with thoracic or abdominal pain
Snoring	A characteristic low-pitched, very low-frequency inspiratory noise caused by periodically interrupted airflow through the soft tissues of the pharynx

or noisy respirations could be present. Accessory muscles of the chest wall, shoulders, neck, and abdomen strain with the effort. If respiratory effort causes chest wall retractions, there may be an airway emergency in evolution.

Retractions result from mismatch between chest wall effort (when the rib cage expands) and ease of pulmonary air inflow. Pulmonary air inflow can be impeded by upper airway obstruction or by stiff lungs that do not readily expand. The pattern of retractions and the noises made in breathing can indicate which of these two possibilities is more dominant. The "restrictive" respiratory pattern for *stiff lungs* typically involves intercostal retractions, tachypnea, and the respiratory noises of rales (alveolar fine crackles) and "grunting" (the brief holding of breath at end-inspiration, then letting it go with an expulsive and audible quick exhalation).

In contrast, the "obstructive" respiratory pattern for *upper airway obstruction* exhibits greater use of neck and abdominal accessory muscles; comparatively greater supraclavicular, subcostal, and sternal retractions; and

fewer rales relative to the presence of wheezes, stridor, snoring, gurgles, or other abnormal respiratory noises (Tables 17-2 and 17-3). In the obstructed airway, expiration tends to be slowed or prolonged, and is not expulsive or accompanied by a "grunt," though it may be audibly wheezy.

Partial obstruction can be recognized by decreased volume exchange (decreased air entry by auscultation or decreased chest rise by inspection) or by increased transit time during inhalation or exhalation. In the normal breathing pattern, a pause occurs between exhalation and the next inspiration. During this resting pause, no respiratory muscles contract to move air. The duration of the pause depends on inspiratory time, expiratory time, and how rapidly a person must breathe to meet the body's obligate metabolic requirements to acquire oxygen and get rid of carbon dioxide. No pause between breaths is an ominous sign. This suggests that there exists a significant airway obstruction (prolonging the inspiratory and expiratory times) or that respiratory failure (to meet metabolic demands) is present or impending.

Any emergent respiratory problem could be "mixed" and have contributions from stiff lungs and from upper airway obstruction. Appreciating the relative contributions of obstruction vs. restriction is important for triage and for evaluating options for airway intervention.

TABLE 17-3. Sounds Associated with Airway Obstruction

SITE OF OBSTRUCTION	DISEASE EXAMPLE	SOUND TRANSMISSION
Nose	Upper respiratory infection, broken nose, sinusitis, allergic rhinitis	Dull, less resonant voice; blunting of consonants such as "m"
Nasopharynx	Adenoiditis, injured palate, bulbar palsy	Cannot raise soft palate well, so alteration of vowels, flattening of phonation, "cleft palate" enunciation
Tongue	Macroglossia, swollen tongue, airway burns	Vocal quality unchanged but enunciation is greatly affected, especially with "s," "j," "l," and "w"; snoring may be prominent, especially if the person is asleep or supine
Oropharynx	Tonsillitis, peritonsillar abscess, Ludwig's angina	"Hot potato" phonation; muffling of voice, coarse snoring with sleep
Hypopharynx	Epiglottitis, retropharyngeal abscess, supraglottitis, airway burns	Muffled voice, diminished volume of sound, facial grimacing with effort to speak or swallow, reluctance to vocalize or cry, occasional hoarseness, occasional snoring, rare stridor
Larynx	Croup, laryngomalacia, laryngeal injury/edema, vocal cord dysfunction, broken larynx, airway burns	Stridor common; hoarseness or raspiness on vocalization; wheezing, whistling, or vocal squeak may be present in exhalation; enunciation of consonants not altered, but vowels (especially "e" and "u") may lose their quality and identity
Trachea	Croup, tracheomalacia, airway burns	Hollow, brassy, barking cough that "carries"; wheezing may be prominent; quality of vocalization or resonance may be altered if additional upper airway pathology coincides (e.g., nasal stuffiness, laryngitis)
Large and medium airways	Asthma, aspirated objects, airway burns, near drowning	Wheezing is characteristic; cough often congested, with prominent rhonchi; quality of vocalization or resonance may be altered if additional upper airway pathology coincides (e.g., sinusitis, tonsillar hypertrophy, laryngeal inflammation)

HEAD POSITIONING

The most common causes of upper airway obstruction are a floppy tongue and lax pharyngeal muscles (deep sleep, unconsciousness, muscle weakness, cranial nerve dysfunction), or soft tissue enlargement from infection, edema, or hypertrophy. Because teeth play such an important role in preserving the size and patency of the oropharynx, edentulous persons (the young, elderly, poorly dentitioned, and recently traumatized) are most vulnerable to upper airway obstruction. Upper airway obstruction is almost always improved by optimal head positioning, mouth opening, clearing of nasal passages, and/or tongue manipulation.

Keeping open the mouth of an unconscious person is very important. With the interior of the mouth in view, one can visually gauge the position of the tongue and the presence of vomit, foreign debris, or pooling of secretions, and can hear the quality and regularity of respiratory noises, even at a distance. In the obtunded infant or small child, the site of upper airway obstruction

is usually between the tip of the tongue and the hard palate in the front of the mouth. This is easily overcome by flattening the tongue down to the floor of the mouth using a finger, tongue blade, or other smooth object. In an obtunded adult, the site of upper airway obstruction from the tongue is more posterior, usually between the base of the tongue and the posterior oropharynx (back of the throat) (Figure 17-1). When the tongue is retrodisplaced, it causes the epiglottis to fold over and close off the tracheal introitus, which results in a secondary site of upper airway obstruction. Relief of both of these sources of obstruction will come from lifting the jaw upwards (Figure 17-2), "dislocating" the jaw hinge to simultaneously keep the mouth open and the jaw lifted (Figure 17-3), or by traction on the tongue itself.

The optimal head position for airway alignment and patency varies with age. However, no matter what the person's age, the most desirable posture is maintaining "neutral" (not flexion, not hyperextension) head position with the chin "proudly" jutted forward, nose in the "sniffing" position, mouth open, tongue resting on the

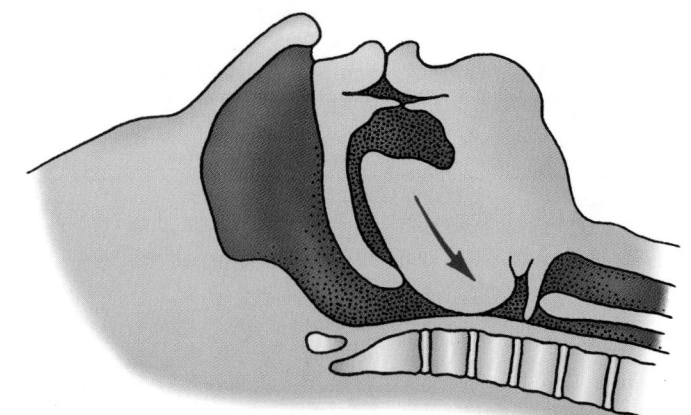

Figure 17-1 Tongue position in the unconscious adult. Note airway obstruction by the base of the tongue against the posterior pharyngeal wall with closure of the epiglottis over the trachea.

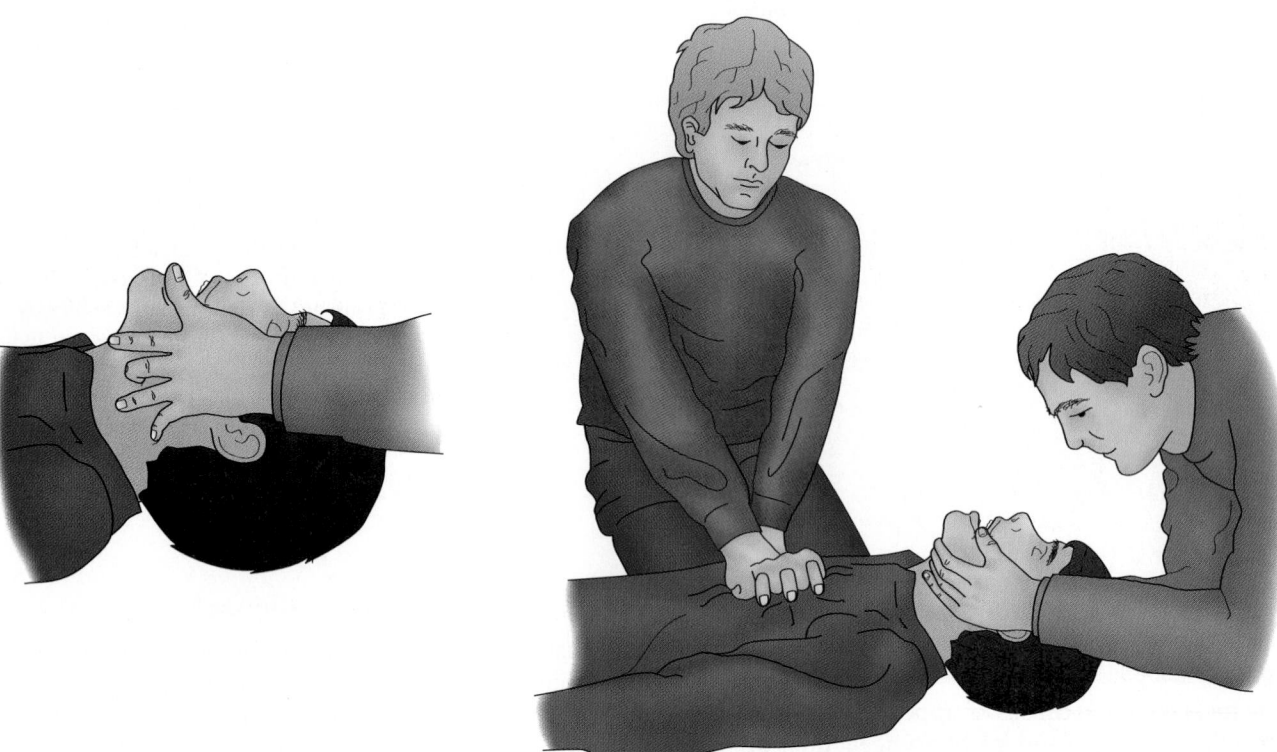

Figure 17-2 Triple maneuver airway support: maintain axial alignment of the cervical spine, lift up on the angle of the mandible, and hold open the mouth. Located midway between the chin and the angle of the mandible, the facial artery pulse may be monitored at the same time.

Figure 17-3 Jaw thrust. *(Courtesy University of Florida College of Medicine, Department of Anesthesiology.)*

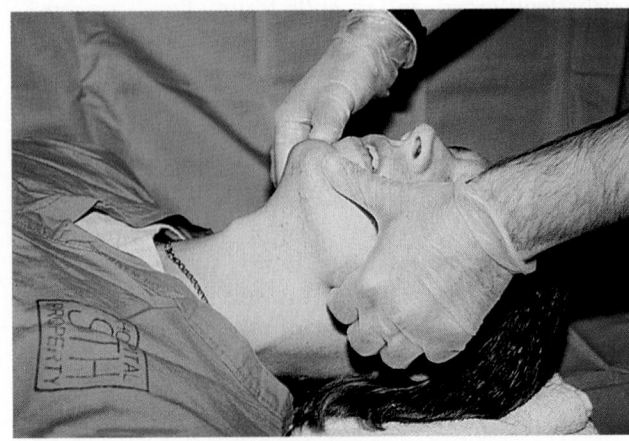

floor of the mouth, and angle of the mandible perpendicular to the ground (Figure 17-4). The least desirable head position in any age group is with the neck flexed and chin pointed towards the chest. Flexion also increases unfavorable stresses on a potentially unstable cervical spine. Extreme hyperextension of the head in any age group stresses ligaments, angulates the airway, and is to be avoided.

Head shape, relative head size, and curvature of the cervical spine change with age, so optimal head positioning and pillow support also change. Because of prominence of the cranial occiput in an infant, the baby's airway is best supported with a shoulder roll or built-up surface for the back. The child does best without a pillow or with a built-up cushion for the back and only a small pad for the occiput. The adult's airway is best supported in the sniffing position with a small pillow under the head, the chin pointed in the air, and a preserved natural lordosis of the cervical spine. Improvisationally, the sniffing position can be achieved with a soda can behind the neck and a folded T-shirt under the head (see Figure 17-4).

If the mechanism of injury or physical examination suggests a possibility for cervical spine injury, efforts to stabilize the neck and head should be undertaken, and the victim should be spared neck flexion, hyperextension, or lateral rotation. Fortunately, the best head position for the airway is also good for the cervical spine. If a cervical spine immobilization method is utilized, the airway should be evaluated for obstruction both before and after application.

BODY POSITIONING

We are accustomed to seeing patients presented to us supine. However, the supine position may be neither desirable nor achievable. Because of gravity, some airways are better maintained in a side-lying or prone position. Nontraditional positioning for stabilization and transport may be necessary because of burns, vomiting, secretion management, or location of impaled objects. Principles of transport for patients in nonsupine positions have to do with preservation of good perfusion and mechanical alignment in all body parts under pressure, maintaining neck straightness, and assuring the ability of the rescuer to monitor airway patency.[1-3,9] In a nonsupine position, the same airway posture is sought: minimal torsion of the cervical spine, neck in a sniffing position, mouth open, and tongue on the floor of the mouth (Figure 17-5).

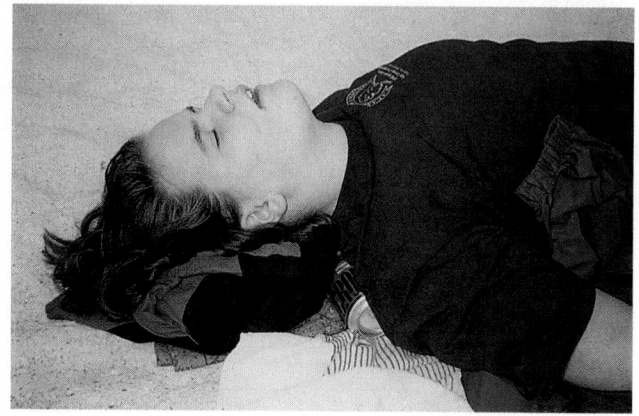

Figure 17-4 Sniffing position of adult attained by using an improvised pillow. The line of the mandible should be perpendicular to the ground. *(Photo from Anne E. Dickison, MD.)*

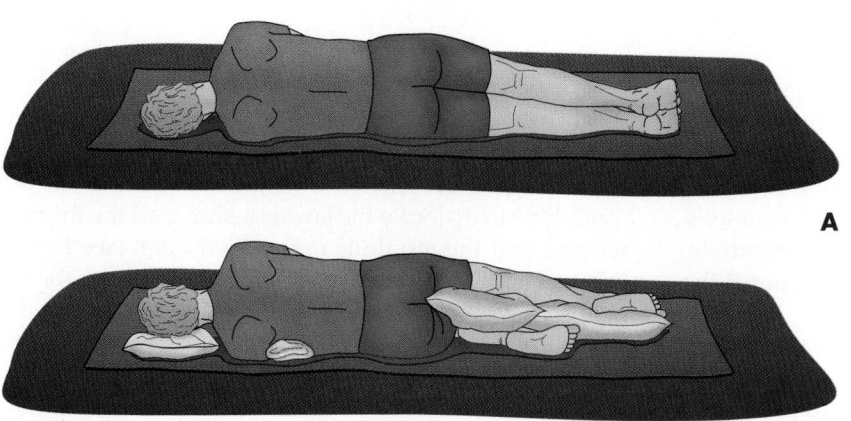

Figure 17-5 A, Patient lying on side with airway/neck in good position and pressure points protected. Flexing the down-side leg stabilizes the torso. The pillow and axillary roll help maintain the spine in good alignment. *Continued*

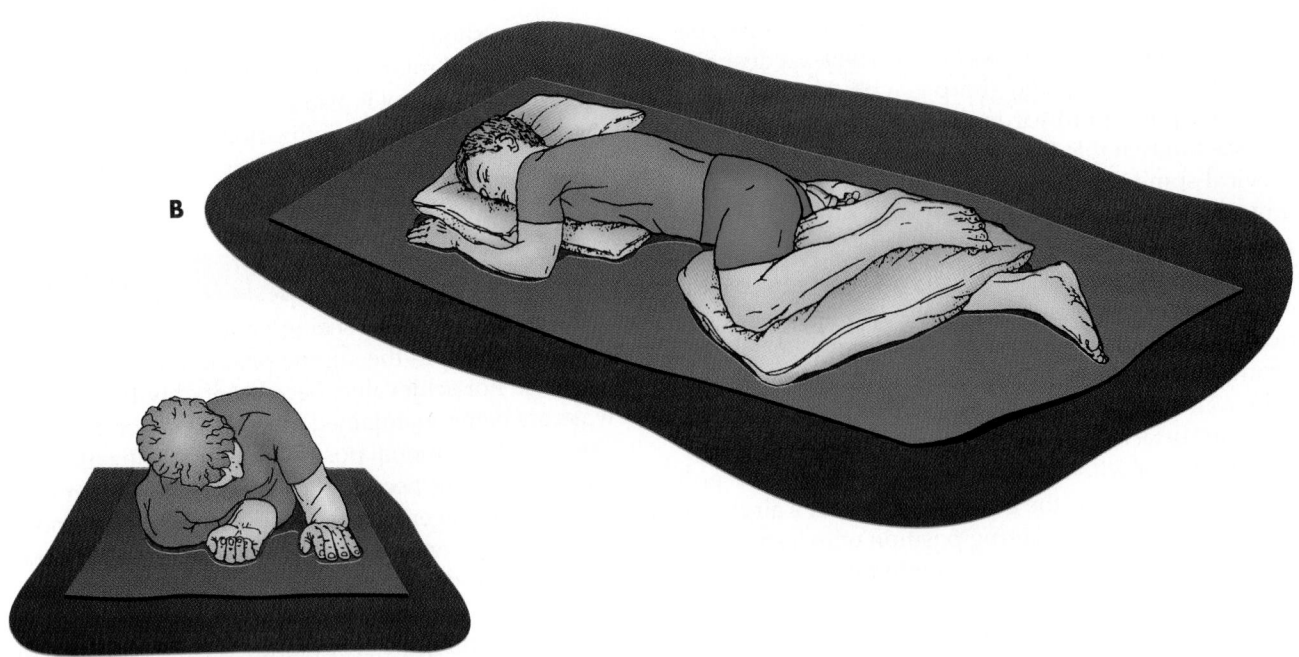

Figure 17-5, cont'd   B, Patient positioned semiprone to facilitate gravity drainage of secretions. A pillow under the head keeps the spine in relative alignment. With no pillow under the head, the width of the shoulder inclines the pharynx downward at a steeper angle.

NONINVASIVE AIRWAY MANEUVERS

If the upper airway is obstructed, there are four basic noninvasive airway opening maneuvers. The most simple is the *head tilt, chin lift.* The heel of one of the rescuer's hands is pressed down on the victim's forehead, and the fingers of the other hand are placed under the chin to lift it up. The intended result is the sniffing position (Figure 17-6). Problems arise if the mouth is closed or soft tissues are infolded because of the chin lift. In addition, downward pressure on the forehead tends to lift the eyebrows and open the eyelids, so measures may need to be taken to protect the eyes.

A second maneuver is the *jaw thrust* (Figure 17-7, *A*). Pressure is applied to the angle of the mandible to dislocate it upwards while forcefully opening the mouth. This is painful, and the conscious or semiconscious victim will object by clamping down or writhing.

A third maneuver is the *internal jaw lift* (Figure 17-7, B). The rescuer's thumb is inserted into the victim's mouth under the tongue, and the mandibular mentum (chin) is lifted, thus stretching out the soft tissues and opening the airway. This is the best maneuver for the unconscious victim with a shattered mandible. The internal jaw lift is dangerous to the rescuer if the victim is semiconscious and can bite.

A fourth noninvasive airway maneuver takes some practice but serves several purposes and is the best one if done correctly. In this two-handed *triple maneuver,* the

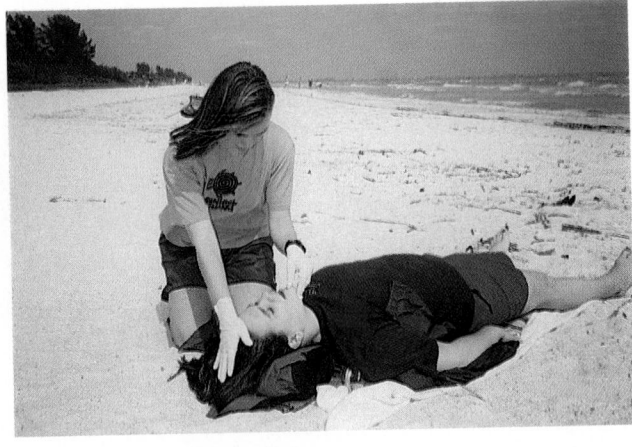

Figure 17-6   Head-tilt, chin-lift maneuver, mouth open. *(Photo from Anne E. Dickison, MD.)*

head is held between two hands to prevent lateral rotation and to maintain neck control. The fourth and fifth fingers are hooked behind the angle of the mandible to dislocate the jaw upwards, and the thumbs ensure that the mouth is maintained open (see Figure 17-2). The third finger may be positioned over the facial artery as it comes around the mandible so that the pulse can be monitored at the same time. For greatest stability, the rescuer's elbows should rest on the same surface upon which the victim is lying.

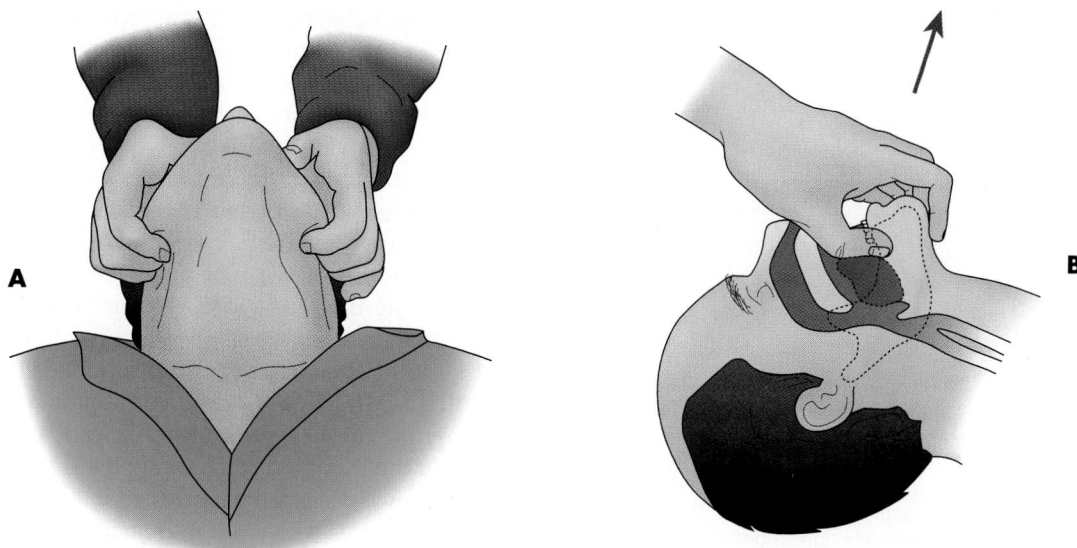

Figure 17-7 **A,** External jaw thrust. **B,** Internal jaw lift.

All noninvasive airway maneuvers except tongue traction and the internal jaw lift can be conjoined with rescue breathing or bag-valve-mask assisted ventilation.

RESCUE BREATHING AND FOREIGN BODY ASPIRATION

The principles of rescue breathing and response to foreign body aspiration are well presented by courses in basic life support (BLS), advanced cardiac life support (ACLS), advanced trauma life support (ATLS), neonatal advanced life support (NALS), and pediatric advanced life support (PALS).

CRICOID PRESSURE

Cricoid pressure, or the Sellick's maneuver, is a noninvasive maneuver intended to protect the airway from potential pulmonary aspiration of gastric contents. This maneuver has become a mainstay of airway management for any victim considered to have a "full stomach" and who is, or is about to become, neurologically depressed and unable to fully protect the airway. Full stomach conditions that place the obtunded victim at risk for passive regurgitation and pulmonary aspiration include obesity, pregnancy, intoxication, ascites, ulcer disease, gastroesophageal reflux, diabetes or other cause of delayed gastric emptying, increased intracranial pressure, bowel obstruction, and any form of major trauma.[1,3,9] In general, infants and children are at greater risk for vomiting and aspiration, since they eat more often, vomit more readily when distressed, have a shorter distance between stomach and mouth, and are at greater risk for abdominal and head trauma (re-

sulting from pediatric body proportions) than are adults. What time a victim last ate a meal is irrelevant to whether or not there is risk for vomiting, but knowing this information may forewarn the rescuer about what sort of stomach contents could appear during rescue and resuscitation.

Cricoid pressure may be applied any time during resuscitation when securing and protecting the airway with an endotracheal tube is not an option, or when intubation attempts have failed and the victim needs positive-pressure ventilation to stay alive. Positive-pressure breaths, whether from rescue breathing or bag-valve-mask resuscitation, follow the path of least resistance. By exerting occlusive pressure on the esophagus, properly applied cricoid pressure directs inflations into the lungs while helping to prevent abdominal distention, compromised diaphragmatic excursion, and increased risk for emesis and gastric rupture.

There are two major concerns about using cricoid pressure on a person with neck trauma. Theoretically, pressure on the anterior side of C6 (opposite the cricoid cartilage) could cause vertebral subluxation if ligaments were disrupted or lax between C5 and C7. Potentially a spinal cord lesion could be caused to progress from partial to complete. No known case of this complication has been reported.[1]

Cricoid pressure should *not* be applied if there is a suspected laryngotracheal injury. Pressure may cause connective tissues "hanging on by a thread" to disrupt completely. Several cases of cricotracheal separation with total loss of airway patency and death have been reported under these circumstances.[1] Laryngeal trauma is suspected when there is bruising over the anterior midneck; when the thyroid cartilage (Adam's apple) is

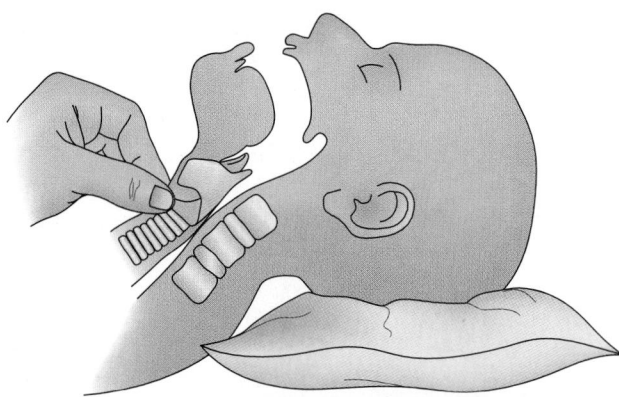

Figure 17-8 Schematic of cricoid pressure (Sellick's maneuver). The cricoid cartilage completely encircles the trachea and has a flat back side which may be pressed against the flat vertebral body across from it, thereby closing shut the esophagus in between. The shape of the cricoid cartilage is similar to that of a signet ring.

riding high, low, or askew; when crepitus is palpable over the larynx; when the victim is unable to vocalize or if the quality of the voice is hoarse and raspy; or when the traumatized person is unable to swallow. To help distinguish between vocal cord dysfunction (from an injured larynx) and other face and neck injuries that might impair speech or interfere with swallowing, the conscious person is asked to hum, and the unconscious victim is observed for alterations in the sound of a cough or moan.

To apply cricoid pressure, the rescuer forms a V between the thumb and index finger. Pressure of 10 to 15 mm Hg is applied, just enough to indent the tissues, but not enough to leave lasting fingernail impressions. Pressing down with the thumb exclusively leads to excessive force and poor control over lateral displacement of the cricoid ring, which in turn cause kinking and occlusion of the subglottic trachea. The V is correctly applied over the cricoid cartilage midneck 1 to 2 cm below the thyroid cartilage (Figure 17-8). A common error is to place the pressure directly on the thyroid cartilage or above the thyroid cartilage at the hyothyroid membrane. Since the soft-sided vocal cords lie just beneath the shield-shaped thyroid cartilage, pressure at this level or above will not preserve patency of the trachea while closing the esophagus. Only the cricoid cartilage completely surrounds the trachea and has a posterior firm flat edge against the esophagus. Pressure applied to any tracheal cartilage other than the cricoid "ring" will not work.

SUCTIONING

In the wilderness, one must remove secretions without the benefit of electricity, customary suction devices, or aesthetic and sterile protective barriers. A number of innovative products are on the market that the prehos-

pital responder, extended care provider, or potential expedition medic might want to consider for the expedition first-aid kit (see Chapter 69).

Gloves and a face barrier (plastic square with a small one-way valve to place over the victim's face) can be tucked into an old 35-mm film container or one of the small pouches marketed specifically for this purpose. Alternatively, a plastic baggie with a slit in it for the mouth and nostrils can be placed over the victim's face for rescue breathing. Debris can be swept from the mouth with a finger wrapped in a T-shirt or other available cloth. The victim can be positioned so that gravity facilitates drainage of blood, vomit, saliva, and mucous; something absorbent or basinlike can be placed at the side of the mouth to catch drained effluvia.

Turkey basters can be included in an expedition first-aid kit not just for secretion management purposes but also for gentle wound irrigation and burn dressing or wet compress moisturizing. The rubber self-inflating bulbs marketed for infant nasal suctioning can also be used to suction out debris from the mouths and noses of adults.

If time permits and the supplies are available, a "mucous trap" suction device can be improvised from a jar with two holes poked in its lid and two tubes or straws duct-taped into the holes. One straw goes to the rescuer, who provides suction, and the other is directed towards whatever has accumulated in the airway. The jar serves to trap the removed secretions so that the rescuer is spared the distasteful experience of suctioning bodily fluids or foreign substances such as mud directly into his or her own mouth.

Secretion removal by gravity or suctioning is key to the management of epistaxis and for maintaining the airway of a victim with mandibular fractures (see Chapter 23).

AIRWAY EQUIPMENT

Stethoscope

A stethoscope is a useful addition to an expedition first-aid kit. However, auscultating breath sounds without a stethoscope is very easy. Either place the ear directly to the chest or isolate and amplify the breath sounds by listening through a hollow object, such as a cup, empty water bottle, or soda can, or through the cardboard center of a roll of toilet paper. The additional merit of a real stethoscope is that it can be disassembled to harvest compliant tubing that might be used improvisationally to substitute for nasopharyngeal airways, cricothyrotomy tubes or stents, straws for suction devices, chest tubes, restraining tethers, lymphatic constriction bands, or other medical devices not on hand.

Masks and One-Way Valves

The purpose of the one-way nonrebreathing flap-valve is to permit air to be pushed into the victim through one aperture while exhaled air (and secretions) are exhausted through a separate route, thus helping minimize exposure to infectious substances.[2] These one-way valves are small, lightweight, and inexpensive and would be easy to tuck into a small container along with gloves and a face barrier.

Face masks differ in shape, type of seal, transparency, and materials used for construction. The mask is composed of three parts: body, seal (or cushion), and universal connector. The mask body is usually domed to allow room for a wide range of chin, mouth, and nose sizes and is usually transparent or semitransparent to facilitate visualization of emesis or blood. The seal is the brim of the mask that comes into contact with the face. The two types of seals are the cushion type (often inflatable) and a soft rubber type that is an extension of the body of the mask molded to fit the contours of the face. The universal connector at the peak of the mask dome provides a 22-mm female adaptor that connects the mask to a one-way valve to go to the rescuer's mouth, the elbow of an Air-Mask-Bag-Unit (AMBU bag), or the breathing circuit of a ventilator.

Noncushioned masks are more difficult to use and demand a greater array of sizes. The cushioned masks are a far better choice for responding to out-of-hospital emergencies. In general, the more generous the cushion, the greater its adaptability to a variety of facial sizes and shapes, and the less practice required to achieve and maintain a good seal between mask and face. On the other hand, the greater the volume of air involved in creating the cushion and the more flexible the materials of the cushion, the more vulnerable the cushion becomes to the effects of altitude and temperature. For a mask intended for use in the wilderness, the feature of a self-sealing nipple to permit adjustment of the volume and pressure of air within the cushion is strongly advised.

For maximum ease of use, a high-volume, low-pressure cushion (the softest, biggest one) should be kept well enough inflated so that there is an air-filled buffer and yet a smooth contact surface between the cushion and the various contours of the face. Despite optimal cushion inflation, however, some facial shapes provide special challenges. For example, a seal may be difficult to achieve on the bushy-bearded individual. If the beard cannot be rapidly modified, the rescuer could consider using petroleum jelly, hand lotion, bag balm, or K-Y jelly to try to slick down the beard and seal over areas where air could leak out. This maneuver has the disadvantage of making the rescuer's hands slick and the cushion of the mask slippery, so both of the rescuer's hands will be needed to maintain the mask fit. The rescuer also runs the risk of greasing up anything else handled during the resuscitation. Alternatively, a large, clear intravenous site dressing (e.g., Tegaderm

10×12 cm, 3M Health Care, St. Paul, Minn.) can be placed over the mouth and beard. The nostrils are left uncovered, and a slit the width of the mouth permits full mouth opening while sealing over the beard and improving the security of a rescuer's grip.[4]

Another challenging facial contour is the prominently chinned, long-faced, and edentulous older individual. With the facial laxity that comes with age and without bordering teeth, the cheeks tend to cave in. Again, a two-handed mask technique is probably necessary. The thumbs press down on either side of the mask, and the fingers pull up on the jaw and bunch up as much of the cheek tissues as possible. A second pair of hands might be needed to bunch up the tissues around the entire lower perimeter of the mask. The stiffer the cushion, the harder it is to make this seal. Another maneuver to consider in this situation is to roll up two gauze or cloth packs to tuck into the mouth and distend the cheeks. The risks of this maneuver are dislodgement and possible aspiration of the packs, and retrograde displacement of the tongue despite a good jaw lift. If there is any choice in the matter, it is almost always easier to mask-ventilate an individual with dentures in place than one with dentures removed, so if intact and secure, dentures should be left in place during field resuscitation.

A third challenging facial contour is that of the average infant, any chubby-cheeked baby-toothed tonsil-abundant young child, or a moon-faced short-necked adult. The key to successful mask ventilation in these situations is to keep the victim's mouth open and the soft tissues from folding in on themselves from gravity and extrinsic compression. One approach is to mask-ventilate over a pacifier, oral airway, nasopharyngeal airway, or improvisational hollow object intended to hold the lips apart, the mouth open, and the tongue pressed down to the floor of the mouth and away from the back of the throat.

Several masks with one-way valves are specifically packaged and marketed for the adventurer or remote-site responder. Carrying cases for traveler's mask-and-valve products can be impact- and puncture-resistant, colorful and readily identifiable, and usable for alternate purposes (e.g., catching water, corraling small objects, or transporting severed digits or avulsed teeth) and can display instructions for CPR or useful illustrations of airway anatomy.

To select the most widely adaptable "first-aid kit" mask-and-valve product, look for the following features: transparent and easily bendable mask body materials that retain little "memory" of residing in their carrying positions and do not become stiff, brittle, or nondeformable in cold temperatures; an inflatable cushion seal that can be adjusted for changes in temperature and altitude; a flexible high-volume low-pressure cushion seal able to conform to many different face sizes and shapes; a mask span that can be used on both small and large victims; tough materials resistant to cracks and punctures; and a compact mask or carrying case that does not take up disproportionate space in the first-aid kit (Figure 17-9).

Oropharyngeal Airway

An oropharyngeal airway (OPA) holds the base of the tongue away from the posterior pharyngeal wall and keeps the mouth open and the lips apart. It may stimulate gagging or induce vomiting and is not well tolerated in the responsive or semiconscious victim. Improper or forceful insertion can cause soft tissue, palatal, or dental injury, as can subjecting the structures of the mouth to prolonged or intense pressures from biting down or holding the OPA in place with tethers.

An OPA should be wide enough to contact two or three teeth on both the maxilla and mandible, and should be rigid enough to withstand compression, yet compressible enough so that the biting teeth do not damage themselves. There are three parts to the OPA: a flanged end that protrudes from the lips and keeps the airway in sight; a flat straight surface that rides between the front teeth, and a semicircular posterior section that follows the curvature of the tongue to its base in the hypopharynx (Figure 17-10, *A*). An air channel in the interior or deep grooves along the sides allow for air passage. These characteristics should be mimicked with any improvisational OPA substitute.

If an oral airway does not conform to the size and shape of the victim's natural airway, upper airway obstruction may worsen. An overly large oral airway will either plug the tracheal introitus with its tip or will press down on and cause the epiglottis to fold over and occlude the glottis. Additionally, glottic stimulation can result in laryngospasm and a complete loss of airway. Too small an oral airway will miss the curvature of the tongue and will press down in the middle of it, worsening occlusion at the base of the tongue or causing the epiglottis to close over the glottis (Figure 17-10, *B*). Furthermore, an overly small oral airway can be swallowed entirely or partially swallowed and left hung up midneck between the larynx and the thoracic inlet.

Recently, Mallinckrodt (St. Louis, Missouri) introduced a cuffed oropharyngeal airway (COPA). The high-volume, low-pressure cuff at the distal end of the OPA is intended to passively lift the epiglottis and position the base of the tongue while it gently occludes the posterior pharynx. The proximal end of the COPA is fitted with a standard 15-mm male connector for easy adaptation to positive pressure ventilation. Insertion of the proper size is critical to successful seating of the cuff. Typically the COPA will be one size larger than a normal OPA. Compared with a standard OPA and the

laryngeal mask airway (LMA), the COPA is more difficult to place correctly and requires a greater number of subsequent airway maneuvers to maintain its luminal patency.[6]

Nasopharyngeal Airway

Compared with the OPA, the nasopharyngeal airway (NPA) is better tolerated in the awake or semiconscious person. Since it does not have to withstand the forces of biting teeth, the NPA can be more flexible and compliant. A flange outside the nostril prevents the NPA from slipping or being swallowed or aspirated. The flange can be improvised with a safety pin through the tube itself (Figure 17-11) or by securely duct-taping a circle of something to the outside of the nostril end of the tube. The gentle curvature of the NPA follows the superior surface of the hard palate, descends through the hidden nasopharynx and down the visible posterior oropharynx, and ends up in the hypopharynx behind the base of the tongue (Figure 17-10, *C*). An endotracheal tube can be shortened and softened in warm water to substitute for a commercial nasal trumpet. Any flexible tube of appropriate diameter and length can be used as an improvisational substitute for the NPA.

The key to successful and atraumatic insertion involves lubrication (saliva works well); an understanding of nasal anatomy; and steady, gentle pressure. If the NPA has a bevel, the flat edge of the bevel is oriented toward the nasal septum. The direction of insertion is straight back toward the occipital prominence of the skull. As the NPA passes through the turbinates, there will be mild resistance, but once the tip has entered the nasopharynx, there will be sensation of a "give." The tube should be visible in the oropharynx as it passes behind the tonsils, and the tip should come to rest behind the base of the tongue but above the vocal cords.

Complications of NPAs include failure to pass through the nose (usually resulting from a deviated septum), epistaxis, accidental avulsion of adenoidal tissue, mucosal tears or avulsion of a turbinate, submucosal tunneling (the tube tunnels out of sight behind the posterior pharyngeal wall), and creation of pressure sores. If the NPA or any nasal tube is left in place for more than several days, impedance to normal drainage may predispose the victim to sinusitis or otitis media.

Other Airway Adjuncts

Other commercial airway adjuncts used in prehospital circumstances include the esophageal-tracheal Combitube, the esophageal obturator airway (EOA), the esophageal–gastric tube airway (EGA), the pharyngotracheal lumen airway (PTLA), and the LMA. Successful insertion of these devices requires formal instruction and practice. Their use in the wilderness setting is

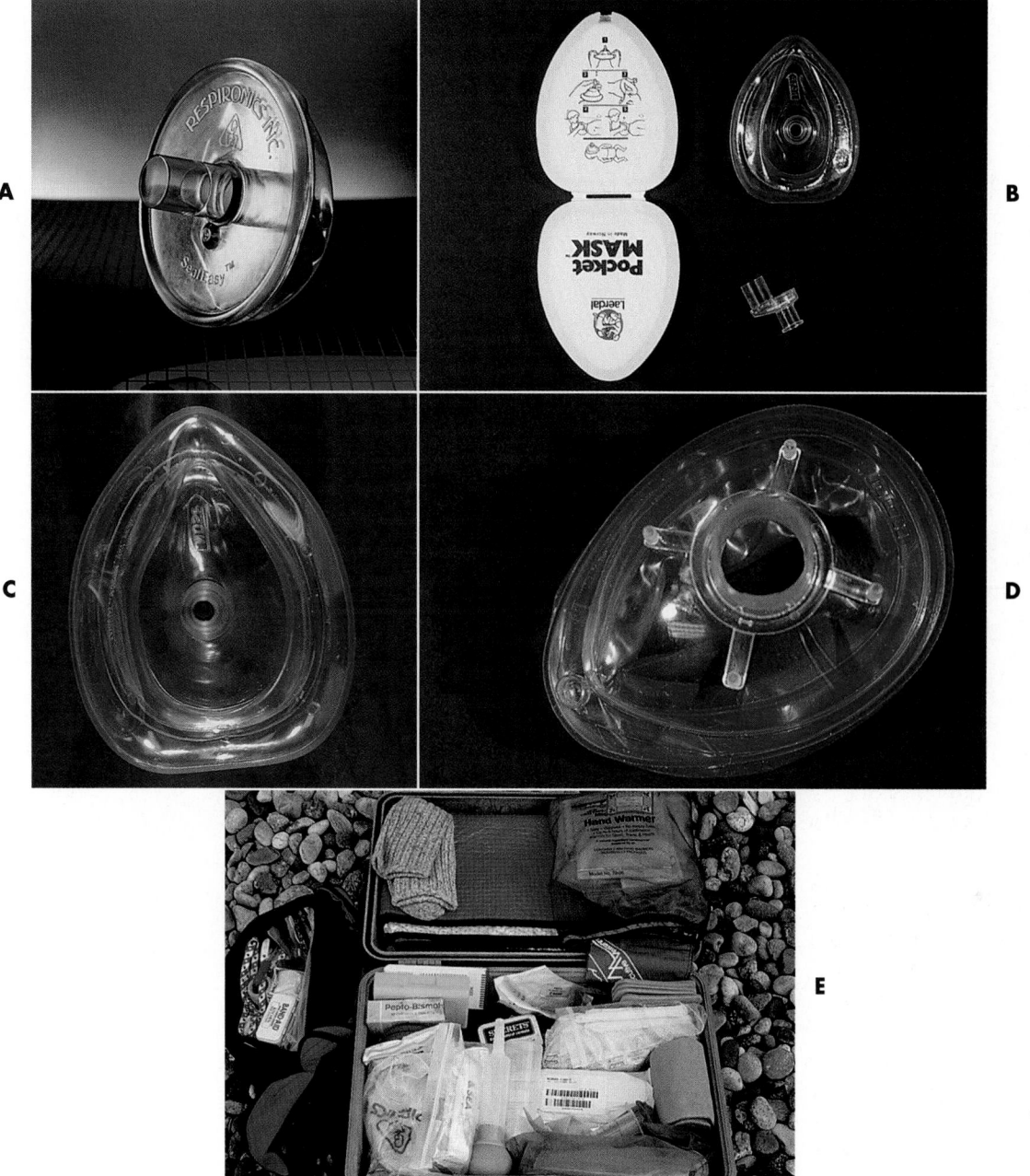

Figure 17-9   A, Respironics SealEasy mask. Note the high-volume, low pressure cushion and the self-sealing nipple for adjusting cushion volume and pressure. **B,** Laerdal pocket mask, one-way valve, and convenient carrying case. **C,** Note the cushion indentations from changes in altitude and temperature. This mask does not have a self-sealing nipple for volume adjustment. **D,** Typical anesthesia mask. Note the tall dome, high-volume low-pressure cushion, needle-less cushion inflation port, and prongs to secure the mask to the head in order to free up the hands of the operator. **E,** First Aid Kit in a Pelican Case. Note the turkey baster for secretion removal and two different types of facial airway masks. In a separate baggie in the upper right under the medication bag are airway adjuncts and potential improvisational airway components. *(**A,** Courtesy Respironics. **B** to **E,** Photos from Anne E. Dickison, MD.)*

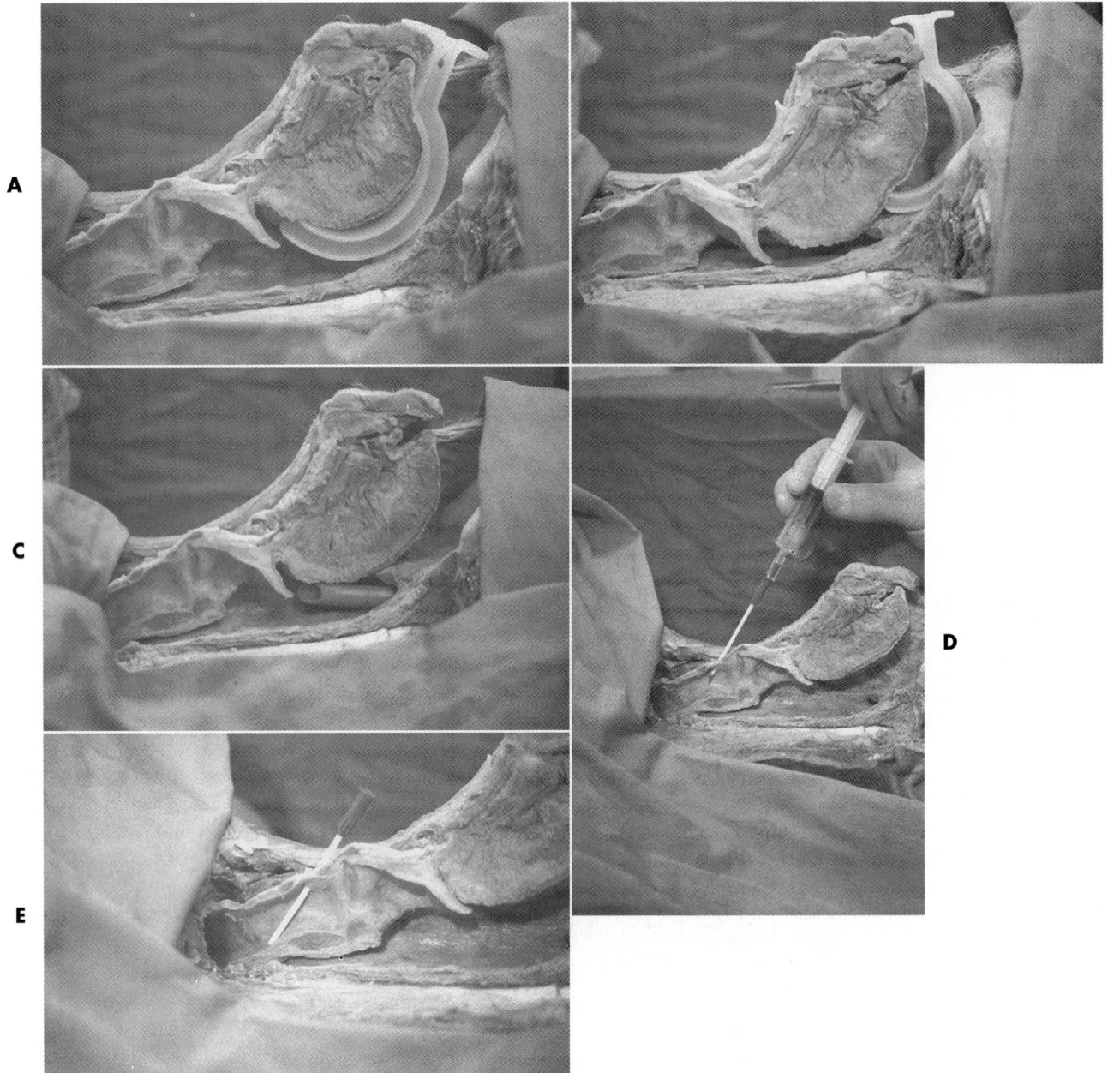

Figure 17-10 **A,** Cadaveric sagittal section demonstrating proper placement of an oropharyngeal airway. The OPA fits to the curvature of the tongue with the flange outside the lips and the tip just above the epiglottis. Note the angle of the epiglottis and its distance from the posterior pharyngeal wall. **B,** Cadaveric sagittal section demonstrating the consequence of using too small an OPA. Note the OPA pushes the tongue towards the back of the throat, which causes obstruction as the epiglottis comes in contact with the posterior pharyngeal wall and folds over the entrance to the trachea. **C,** Cadaveric sagittal section demonstrating proper placement of a nasopharyngeal airway. Note the NPA emerging from the nasopharynx, passing through the posterior oropharynx, and ending with its tip behind the tongue just above the epiglottis. **D,** Cadaveric sagittal section demonstrating the proper location, depth, and angle for insertion of a percutaneous needle cricothyrotomy. **E,** The catheter has been advanced off the needle and the stylet has been withdrawn. The challenge now will be to secure the catheter so that it does not kink or become displaced. *(Courtesy Michael S. Gorback, MD.)*

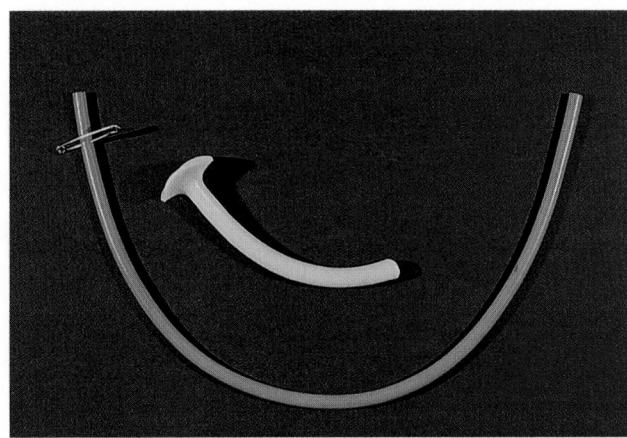

Figure 17-11 Any flexible small tube of sufficient length can be used improvisationally. This tube was marketed as a restraint for sunglasses. Note the use of a safety pin to create a "flange." The other item is a form of nasopharyngeal airway, the "nasal trumpet." *(Photo from Anne E. Dickison, MD.)*

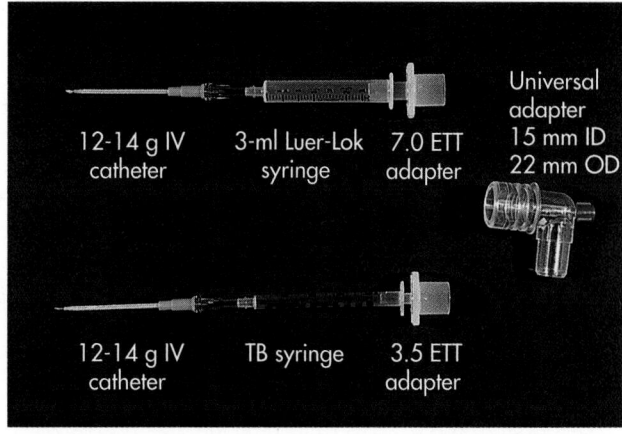

Figure 17-12 Combination of catheter assemblies to allow connection of a needle cricothyrotomy to a 15/22-mm standard adaptor for AMBU ventilation. *(Photo from Anne E. Dickison, MD.)*

appropriately limited to trained and experienced providers.

CRICOTHYROTOMY

If the upper airway is completely obstructed and obstruction cannot be relieved or bypassed, the only way to avoid death is to create an air passage directly into the trachea. The most accessible and least complicated access site is through the cricothyroid membrane. Even in experienced hands, the relatively high complication rates for emergent cricothyrotomies (10% to 40%)[1] are still less than those for tracheostomies. Complications include bleeding, puncture of the posterior trachea and esophagus, creation of a false passage, inability to ventilate, aspiration, subcutaneous and mediastinal emphysema, vocal cord injury, and subsequent tracheal stenosis.

The cricothyrotomy hole may be made percutaneously with a trocar or needle or surgically with a knife blade. When the trachea is successfully entered, a gush of air will exit, often with a cough. If a syringe containing 1 ml of water or lidocaine is attached to the needle used for puncture, bubbles may be seen as the needle tip enters the trachea. Once the cricothyroid membrane is punctured, it is essential to maintain patency of the tract and identify the hole with a tube, stylet, obturator, tweezers, wire, or another temporary place marker. It is very easy to lose the tract and create a false passage while trying to instrument or cannulate the route.

Making a small (1- to 1.5-cm) vertical incision in the skin over the cricothyroid membrane facilitates the ease of the next step, puncture through the lower third of the dime-sized membrane. Vertical skin incisions have advantages over horizontal incisions because vertical in-

cisions tend to be more controlled and better positioned in reference to landmarks. The needle/catheter is advanced in the midline of the neck at a 45-degree angle aiming toward the lower back (Figure 17-10, *D*). Once the needle or introducer aspirates air, the catheter is slid off the stylet and the stylet is withdrawn (Figure 17-10, *E*). Taking care not to kink a flexible catheter at the insertion site, the hub may be secured in place with tape or sutures or may be attached to a Luer-Lok syringe-adaptor mechanism. With anything other than a commercial cricothyrotomy set or endotracheal tube, provision of positive-pressure ventilation requires the creative assembly of an adapter connecting the apparatus in the trachea to the female connector on an AMBU bag. Figure 17-12 shows an example of the step-up series of connections needed for this type of extension.

If the catheter in the trachea is to be replaced by a stiffer or bigger cannula, a guidewire is inserted through the catheter several centimeters down the trachea, the catheter is withdrawn with the guidewire remaining, and a dilator is advanced over the guidewire, then withdrawn. Next, the intended cannula is threaded over the guidewire until it is seated with its flanges flush to the skin. The process of identifying a lumen with an introducer, marking the lumen with a guidewire, dilating the entry site, then placing the final apparatus over the guidewire is called the Seldinger technique, and the procedure of replacing a smaller tube with a larger one is termed a dilational cricothyrotomy.

A temporary cricothyrotomy trocar-and-tube can be fashioned from a tuberculin or 3-ml syringe that has been cut on the diagonal then forcefully inserted through the cricothyroid membrane (Figure 17-13). Since the improvised trocar point of the syringe is sharp and irregular, insertion is apt to be traumatic.

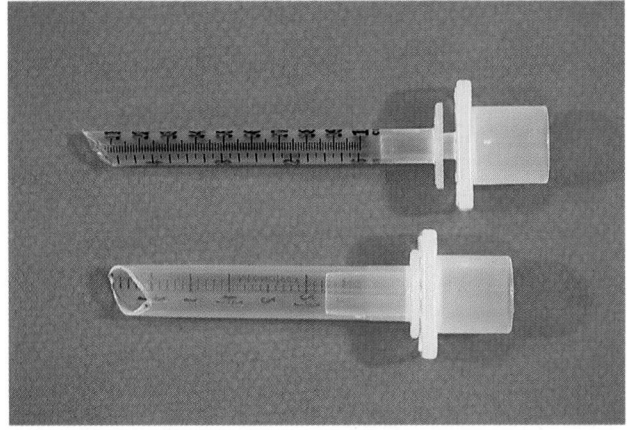

Figure 17-13 A tuberculin or 3-ml syringe can be cut on the diagonal to improvise a combination trocar-cricothyrotomy tube. Caution must be taken with insertion not to traumatize the posterior pharyngeal wall. *(Photo from Anne E. Dickison, MD.)*

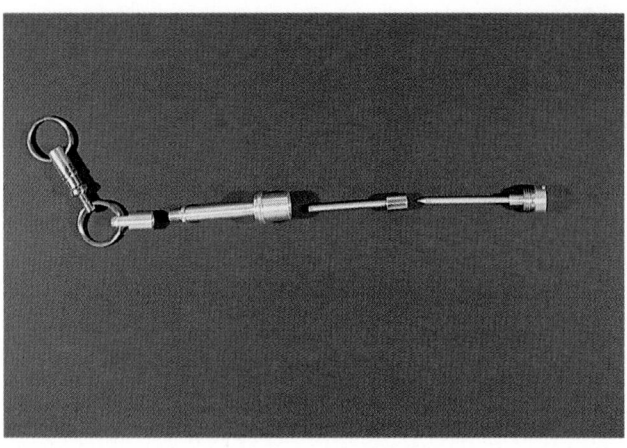

Figure 17-14 Lifestat keychain emergency airway set. *(Photo from Anne E. Dickison, MD.)*

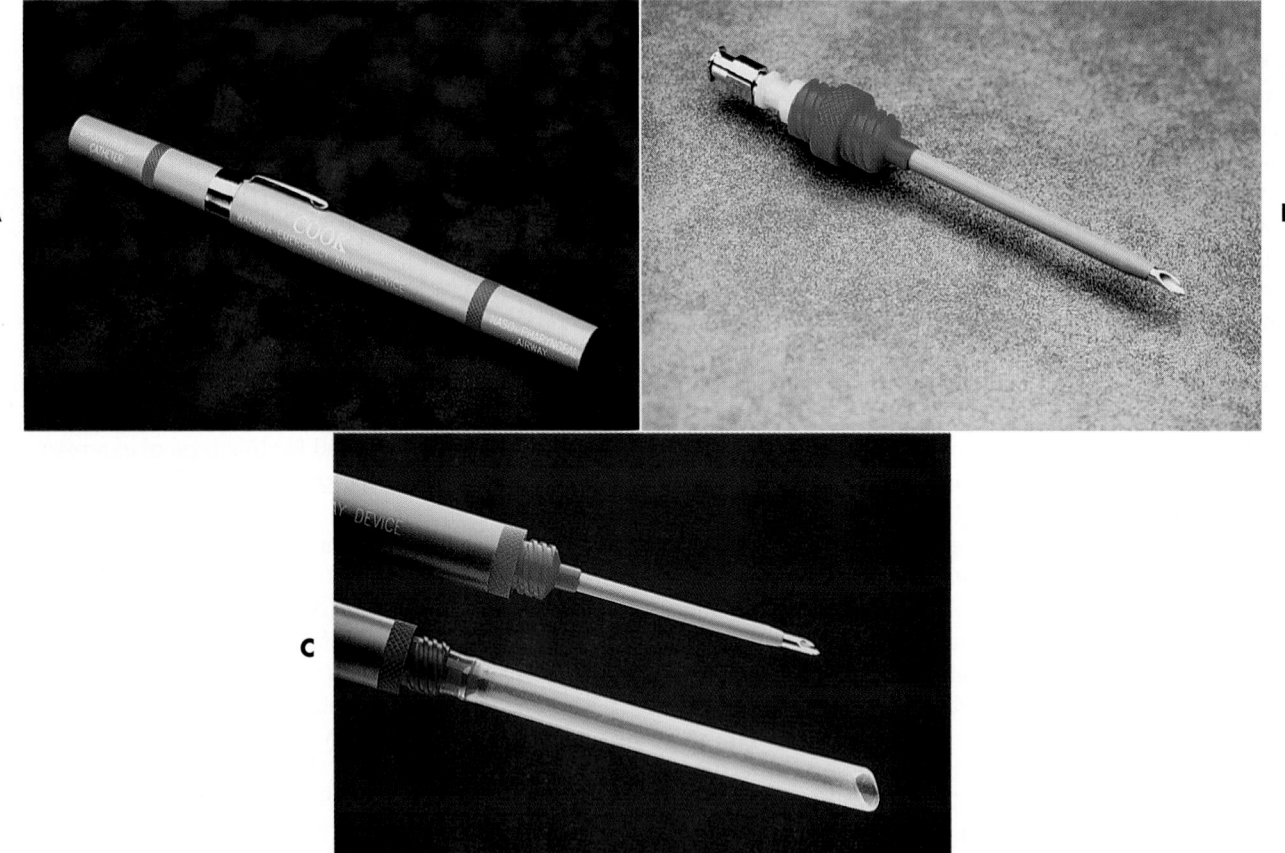

Figure 17-15 **A,** Wadhwa Emergency Airway Device. **B,** Wadhwa transtracheal catheter with removable stylet and Luer-lock connection for jet ventilation. **C,** Internal components of the Wadhwa Emergency Airway Device. Both the transtracheal catheter and the nasopharyngeal airway screw into the case for an extension with a 15-mm adaptor. *(Courtesy Cook, Inc.)*

Care must be taken to not lacerate the posterior tracheal wall or create a tracheoesophageal fistula.

Even with a universal adapter (15/22-mm) connection, without a jet ventilation device or cricothyrotomy tube of the proper diameter, curvature, and length, it is extremely difficult to positive-pressure ventilate a victim through a needle catheter or improvisational substitute. The victim has the best chances at survival if spontaneous respiratory effort can be preserved; it is easier for the victim to draw air in through a critically small opening than it is for a rescuer to generate the pressure needed to force air in through the same aperture. Pressures sufficient to make a chest rise can be generated by a rescuer blowing through the needle catheter, but such efforts rapidly lead to rescuer fatigue. Temporary transtracheal oxygenation and ventilation through a 12- or 14-gauge needle can be provided using a flow rate of 15 L/min or by jet ventilation (40 psi) at a slow intermittent rate of 6 breaths per minute and an inspiratory to expiratory ratio of 1:14.[7] The very long expiratory time is necessary to allow passive expiration through a restrictive channel.

Packaged dilator cricothyrotomy sets, such as those manufactured by Melker, Arndt, and Corke Cranswick, contain a scalpel blade, syringe with an 18-gauge over-the-needle catheter and/or a thin introducer needle, guidewire, an appropriately-sized dilator, and a polyvinyl airway cannula. The Patil set (Cook Critical Care, Bloomington, Ind.), the Portex Minitrach II (Concord/Portex, Keene, N.H.), and the military version of the Melker set are sold without the guidewire and appeal to prehospital providers unfamiliar with the Seldinger technique. Pertrach (Pertrach, Inc., Long Beach, Calif.) is similar in concept except the guidewire and dilator are forged as a single unit so a finder catheter cannot be used, and the introducer must be peeled away. The Nu-Trake device (International Medical Devices, Inc., Northridge, Calif.) is complicated to use, has a rigid airway that risks trauma to the posterior trachea, and is difficult to secure.[8]

In terms of expedition kit portability, three transtracheal puncture emergency airway devices deserve special mention. Lifestat (New Orleans, La.) manufactures a key chain emergency airway set that consists of a sharp-pointed metal trocar introducer that fits through a straight metal cannula that screws into a metal extension with a universal 15-mm male adaptor. Lightweight and less than 3 inches long, the three-component apparatus is attached to a separate and detachable keychain (Figure 17-14). Cook Critical Care offers a 6-Fr reinforced-catheter emergency transtracheal airway catheter (order number C-DTJV-6.0-7.5-BTT) with a molded Luer-Lok connection for jet ventilation or added assembly of a 15-mm adaptor for standard modes of positive-pressure ventilation. Cook Critical

Box 17-1 FUNDAMENTAL GOALS OF AIRWAY MANAGEMENT IN THE FIELD

The fundamental goals of airway management in the field are to
1. Promote conditions supporting airway patency
   Optimal positioning
   Facilitated removal of secretions or debris
   Close observation for emesis, bleeding, seizures, or other intercurrent events leading to obstruction or aspiration
2. Avoid doing or administering anything that could further depress respirations, obstruct airway, or depress respiratory reflexes
3. Assess the potential for worsening
   Plan the evacuation accordingly
   Communicate the situation and concerns to others
   Prepare for escalated intervention

Care also offers the Wadhwa Emergency Airway Device (order number C-WEAD-100). This lightweight, impact-resistant assembly is 7.25 inches long and the diameter of a highlighter pen (Figure 17-15). It disassembles to yield a 12-Fr Teflon-coated cricothyrotomy catheter with removable metal stylet (with a molded plastic Luer-Lok connection for oxygen or jet ventilation), plus a flexible nasopharyngeal airway adhered to a molded plastic flange. Both the cricothyrotomy catheter and the NPA screw into the Wadhwa case to provide a low-resistance extension and a 15-mm (male) connection for standard positive-pressure ventilation equipment.

SUMMARY

The conscious or semiconscious person with an airway emergency instinctively seeks an optimal posture for air exchange (Box 17-1). The unconscious person, unless deeply anesthetized, paralyzed, or profoundly hypoxic, continues effort to breathe until death is very near. If a victim shouts or cries out, the airway is intact and the lungs are filling. If a victim is breathing but obstructed, determination should be made as to why. If a victim is making no respiratory effort at all, a choice must be made about whether or not to initiate CPR.

REFERENCES

1. Benumof JL: *Airway management: principles and practice,* St Louis, 1996, Mosby.
2. Bowman WD: *Outdoor emergency care: comprehensive prehospital care for nonurban settings,* ed 3, Lakewood, Colo, 1998, National Ski Patrol System, Inc.

3. Capan LM, Miller SM, Turndorf H: *Trauma anesthesia and intensive care,* Philadelphia, 1991, JB Lippincott.
4. Dickison AE: *Improvisational airway management,* syllabus of the World Congress on Wilderness Medicine, Whistler, BC, Canada, 1999; Colorado Springs, Colo, Wilderness Medical Society.
5. Gorback MS: *Emergency airway management,* Philadelphia, 1991, BC Decker.
6. Greenberg RS et al: A randomized controlled trial comparing the cuffed oropharyngeal airway and the laryngeal mask airway in spontaneously breathing anesthetized adults, *Anesthesiology* 88:970, 1998.
7. Kirby RR, editor: Critical care, vol 1. In Miller RD, editor: *Atlas of anesthesia,* Philadelphia, 1997, Churchill Livingstone.
8. Melker RJ, Florete OG: Percutaneous dilational cricothyrotomy and tracheostomy. In Benumof JL, editor: *Airway management: principles and practice,* Philadelphia, 1996, Mosby.
9. Miller RD, editor: *Anesthesia,* vol 2, ed 5, Philadelphia, 2000, Churchill Livingstone.
10. Roberts JR, Hedges JR: *Clinical procedures in emergency medicine,* ed 2, Philadelphia, 1991, WB Saunders.

18 Wilderness Trauma and Surgical Emergencies

Eric A. Toschlog and John A. Morris, Jr.

PURPOSE

This chapter is written with the intent to provide physicians and health care practitioners with a concise, pragmatic approach to the management of trauma and surgical emergencies encountered in a wilderness environment. Our focus is directed primarily at the health care professionals responsible for the well-being of expedition members.

Wilderness expedition health care providers will have varied capabilities, experience, and resources, but it is the environment that will most influence patient outcome. Complex interventions in the field are frequently impractical. With ongoing debate concerning issues ranging from the value of field resuscitation for internal hemorrhage to the method (if any) of closure of animal bite wounds, it remains clear that identifying injuries, establishing an airway, and making expedient evacuation plans most strongly influence survival.[22,25,71]

The key to successful management of wilderness emergencies is preparedness. Knowledge of the advanced trauma life support (ATLS) protocols provides a scaffold for preparation for wilderness travel. The simple, concise principles contained in ATLS concepts are well suited to the management of wilderness emergencies, where resources are scant and prompt response is essential to victim survival.

WILDERNESS TRAUMA EMERGENCIES

Overview

Management of wilderness trauma is based on military and civilian prehospital principles, including rapid assessment and diagnosis of injury, treatment, and, if necessary, evacuation. These principles and those promulgated by the Committee on Trauma of the American College of Surgeons (ACS) are formally taught in the ACS ATLS program. Any physician planning to be a medical officer on a wilderness expedition should be familiar with the material taught in the ATLS program. Optimally, the complete ATLS course should be successfully completed before assuming responsibility for the care of participants in a wilderness expedition.[1-3,45]

Background

Trauma remains the leading cause of death in the first four decades of life, and in terms of trauma-related ex-penditures and significant long-term disability, the societal cost is staggering. Epidemiologic data indicate that death from trauma occurs in a trimodal time distribution.[5,95] The first peak occurs within seconds to minutes and represents catastrophic injury. The second peak occurs within minutes to hours after injury. Injuries responsible for the second mortality peak are those associated with significant head injury, pneumothorax, and/or significant blood loss. This distribution emphasizes the concept of the "golden hour," the postinjury time interval when rapid and aggressive intervention may significantly influence mortality.

The medical literature is limited regarding the incidence of injury incurred during wilderness-related activities. It is estimated that greater than 10 million Americans participate in wilderness backpacking and camping activities annually. A study by Gentile et al[33] documented the injury and evacuation patterns recorded by the National Outdoor Leadership School over a 5-year period. Injuries occurred at a rate of 2.3 per 1000 person-days of exposure, with orthopedic and soft tissue injuries most frequent. A recent study by Montalvo et al[61] analyzed case incident report files from eight California National Park Service parks and found an injury incidence of 9.2 nonfatal events per 100,000 visits, with 78 fatalities reported in a 3-year period. Both studies document a low risk of injury but highlight the possible morbidity resulting from wilderness injury and the need for rapid, uniform intervention.

Establishing Priorities

There are three immediate priorities in managing wilderness trauma:

1. Control oneself. It is normal to feel anxious when confronted with an injured victim. However, anxiety must not be transmitted to the victim or other members of the expedition team. One must be in control of oneself to take control of the situation.
2. Control the situation. The first priority in controlling the situation is ensuring the safety of the uninjured members of the party. Expeditious evacuation of a victim requires that all expedition members function at maximal efficiency; even minor injuries to other members in the group can jeopardize physical strength, functional manpower, and the success of the evacuation. Although the physician member of the team may

not be the expedition leader, his or her position is automatically elevated during a medical crisis. However, this does not mean that the physician should dominate the evacuation process. Although the expedition leader must rely on the medical assessment provided by the physician, the leader is best prepared to plan the evacuation.

3. Obtain an overview of the situation. The victim's general condition should be evaluated. Is the victim in immediate distress from a condition that requires relatively simple management, such as airway control? Is the victim in such a precarious environmental situation that he or she needs to be moved before resuscitation? Scene security may be integral to the safety of the injured and caregiver. Is the victim properly protected from the elements, including sun, wind, cold, and water? Hypothermia remains one of the most important contributors to trauma-related coagulopathies.[92]

After the victim has been placed in the most stable and safe environment, the examining physician is ready to implement the ATLS-based five steps of wilderness trauma management:

1. Primary survey
2. Resuscitation
3. Secondary survey
4. Definitive plan
5. Packaging and transfer preparation

The purpose of the primary survey is to identify and begin initial management of life-threatening conditions by assessing the following (called the ABCDE of trauma care):

1. *Airway* maintenance and cervical spine stabilization
2. *Breathing*
3. *Circulation*, with control of significant external hemorrhage
4. *Disability*: Neurologic status
5. *Exposure/Environmental* control: Completely undress the victim with careful attention to the prevention of hypothermia

After the primary survey is performed, resuscitation efforts are initiated. The level of resuscitation depends on the equipment and expertise available. At a minimum, resuscitation consists of control of external hemorrhage. In the emergency department, resuscitation would also include the administration of oxygen and intravenous (IV) fluids.

The third step is the secondary survey, a head-to-toe evaluation of the trauma victim that uses inspection, percussion, and palpation techniques to evaluate each of the body's five regions: head and face, thorax, abdomen, skeleton, and skin. A history should be taken at the same time as performance of the secondary survey. The specifics of the mechanism of injury, if unknown to the physician or caregiver, may be of vital importance. Loss

of consciousness, head injury, the height of a fall, or the species of attacking animal may influence treatment and evacuation plans, as well as contribute to the stability of the scene. The ATLS AMPLE method of rapid history-taking is discussed in further detail in the Secondary Survey section. After this survey, the examining physician should formulate a definitive plan. It is useful to record all observations on paper if the circumstances permit. Such data may prove to be of critical importance to evacuating or hospital personnel.

The first step in formulating a plan is to compile a list of the injuries present. The next step is to determine if any injury warrants evacuation. A determination needs to be made as to the route of evacuation: air, land, or water. Aeromedical evacuation is expensive and, depending on the environment, could pose a risk to both the victim and medical evacuation team. Aeromedical evacuation should be considered only for victims with potentially life- or limb-threatening injuries where the environment allows such a modality.

Packaging the victim for evacuation is the final step. The evacuation effort requires organization, coordination, and great effort on the part of the expedition team. Transfer protocol will be discussed within the respective injury sections.

Fluid Precautions in the Wilderness

A number of life-threatening viruses are transmitted through contact with bodily fluids. The Centers for Disease Control and Prevention (CDC) have established a set of standard precautions to be applied in all cases of contact with human body fluids:

1. Goggles
2. Gloves
3. Fluid-impervious gowns
4. Shoe covers and fluid-impervious leggings
5. Mask
6. Head covering

In the wilderness setting, the materials necessary for standard precautions are rarely available. However, every victim in the wilderness must be assumed to carry a communicable disease. Every effort should be made to approximate universal precautions, particularly covering the hands and eyes.

Primary Survey

Persons injured in the wilderness should be assessed and their treatment priorities established based on their mechanism of injury, the vital signs, and the specific injuries incurred. Logical treatment priorities must be established in a critically injured victim, including the need for evacuation when the primary survey is complete. The victim's vital signs must be assessed quickly and efficiently, with restoration of life-preserving vital functions. This sequence constitutes the ABCDE of trauma care and is designed to identify and treat life-threatening conditions within the "golden hour."

Airway (see Chapter 17). The upper airway should be assessed for patency. This rapid assessment should include inspection for signs of airway obstruction, including foreign bodies and signs of facial or tracheal fractures that may lead to airway obstruction. The chin lift (see Figure 17-6) or jaw thrust (see Figure 17-3) may be helpful in establishing an airway. If the victim is able to speak, the airway is likely not jeopardized, but this is not an absolute and frequent, repeated evaluation is mandatory. Additionally, a Glasgow Coma Scale (GCS) of 8 or less is indicative of the possibility of a precarious airway and requires establishment of a definitive airway.

Specific attention should be directed toward the possibility of cervical spine injury. The victim's head or neck should never be hyperextended, hyperflexed, or rotated to establish or maintain an airway. Approximately 10% of victims with head injuries or facial fractures have a concomitant cervical spine fracture. Such a fracture should be assumed to exist in any person with a significant injury above the level of the clavicle. If a situation requires removal of immobilizing devices, in-line *stabilization*, not *traction*, must be maintained. For a detailed discussion of airway management, please refer to Chapter 17.

Breathing and Ventilation. The victim's chest should be exposed and chest wall movement observed. Because oxygenation and carbon dioxide elimination require adequate function of the diaphragm, chest and abdominal musculature, and ribs, any trauma sustained by these structures may preclude adequate ventilation. Therefore establishment of an airway in the primary survey does not ensure ventilation.

Conditions that can lead to asymmetric chest wall movement include tension pneumothorax, open pneumothorax, and flail chest. Upon auscultation, absent or asymmetric breath sounds may be produced by improper placement of an endotracheal tube, pneumothorax, or hemothorax.

Circulation. Evaluation of circulation is divided into assessment of cardiac output and control of major external hemorrhage. Manometric blood pressure measurement is not easily performed in the field, although it may provide useful data. Important information regarding perfusion and oxygenation can be obtained rapidly by assessing the victim's level of consciousness, taking the victim's pulse, looking at skin color, and assessing capillary refill time.

The pulse should be assessed first. Although the following are only general estimates and carry some inaccuracy, approximations of systolic blood pressure can be used if a palpable pulse is present:
1. Radial artery—80 mm Hg
2. Femoral artery—70 mm Hg
3. Carotid artery—60 mm Hg

When circulating blood volume is reduced, cerebral perfusion pressure may be critically impaired, resulting in altered level of consciousness. Do not assume that altered level of consciousness is attributable to head injury. It must be noted that conscious victims may be in class III shock with impending death.

Skin color and capillary refill allow rapid initial estimation of peripheral perfusion. Pressure applied to the thumbnail or hypothenar eminence causes underlying tissue to blanch. In a normovolemic person, color returns to the nail bed within 2 seconds. In a hypovolemic, poorly oxygenated person, capillary refill requires more than 2 seconds.

If hypovolemia is suspected, on the basis of either absent pulses or prolonged capillary refill, the examiner should immediately assess the neck veins. Distended neck veins, although a nonspecific sign, may suggest tension pneumothorax or pericardial tamponade in the context of hypotension. Flat neck veins suggest hypovolemia and hemorrhagic shock.

Major hemorrhage can occur in five anatomic areas:
1. Chest
2. Abdomen
3. Retroperitoneum
4. Thigh
5. External environment

Exsanguinating external hemorrhage should be identified and controlled during the primary survey. Blood loss should be controlled by direct pressure on the wound. Tourniquets should not be used for control of external bleeding. Proper stabilization of a femur fracture can minimize blood loss into the thigh. In the field, little can be done about significant intrathoracic or intraabdominal hemorrhage.

Disability and Neurologic Assessment. The neurologic assessment of the injury victim conducted during the primary survey should be rapid and efficient. The victim's level of consciousness should be established. In addition, pupillary size and reactivity should be assessed. Level of consciousness should be assessed using the Glasgow Coma Scale (Box 18-1). It is critical that the neurologic assessment be repeated frequently, particularly if evacuation is delayed. Deterioration in mental status portends a poor prognosis, although a variety of conditions other than intracranial injury can affect mental status. Hypoxia, hypovolemia, and hypothermia should be expeditiously corrected.

Exposure and Environmental Control. The victim should be fully undressed and exposed, if possible in a protected environment. Garments and gear should be removed by cutting them away, unless the garments can be dried and are essential for future protection from the environment. Wet clothing must be removed early to prevent hypothermia. It is mandatory to visualize the entire victim to document and assess injury. However, this step of the primary survey should be per-

Box 18-1 GLASGOW COMA SCALE

This scale evaluates the degree of coma by determining the best motor, verbal, and eye opening response to standardized stimuli.

EYE OPENING

Spontaneous	4
To voice	3
To pain	2
None	1

VERBAL RESPONSE

Oriented	5
Confused	4
Inappropriate words	3
Incomprehensible words	2
None	1

MOTOR RESPONSE

Obeys command	6
Localizes pain	5
Withdraw (pain)	4
Flexion (pain)	3
Extension (pain)	2
None	1
TOTAL	

formed with caution. First, it is imperative to cover the victim immediately after removal of clothing. Hypothermia and its effects on mental status, cardiovascular function, and coagulation is one of the most underappreciated entities in the care of the trauma victim. The possibility of hypothermia should be entertained in all environments, since it is most prevalent in trauma victims during warm summer months. Second, clothing and gear should not be pulled from the victim unless complete immobilization of injuries can be achieved. Expedition members may be wearing a variety of gear and clothing, including biking, skiing, or climbing helmets. Helmets should be removed with in-line stabilization of the cervical spine.

Shock

Shock is defined as cellular hypoxia secondary to inadequate circulation of blood. It was defined historically by John Collins Warren as "a momentary pause in the act of death." Nowhere is this adage more applicable than in the wilderness setting. Any physician who cares for trauma victims has witnessed an apparently "stable" victim rapidly deteriorate and die. With only clinical acumen, the wilderness physician must be sufficiently astute to identify the subtle signs of shock.

The treatment of shock is resuscitation, which may be defined as any intervention that restores blood flow and cellular oxygenation. The power of the primary survey lies in the fact that it is essentially a form of resuscitation. Rapid identification of conditions leading to hypoperfusion facilitates their reversal. Although the majority of trauma victims exhibiting signs of shock in the wilderness have sustained acute blood loss, a simple entity such as a pneumothorax may be responsible for shock.

Hemorrhagic shock is classified according to the blood volume that has been lost. A central question in caring for victims of blood loss in the wilderness is the reliability of vital signs in quantifying degree of hemorrhage. Associated with each class of hemorrhage are clinical signs that allow a caregiver to quantify blood loss (Table 18-1). It is evident that assessing blood pressure alone is a poor way to predict impending deterioration. When hypotension can be measured, a normal individual has already lost 30% of his or her blood volume and salvage may be impossible. Resuscitation should be initiated at the first sign of shock, equating to class II hemorrhage, and evacuation planned accordingly.

Vascular Access

Vascular access must be obtained promptly. The standard method of obtaining access is by insertion of two large-bore (16-gauge or larger) catheters, preferably into peripheral veins of the upper extremity. Alternatives include using lower extremity veins and obtaining central venous access. If peripheral access cannot be secured, the femoral vein should be the next site attempted. Advantages of femoral vein access include ease of cannulation relative to jugular and subclavian access and fewer complications.[93]

Depending on expertise, the internal jugular and subclavian veins may be accessed. Despite a higher incidence of complications compared with peripheral access, central access complication rates in trauma centers have been demonstrated to be less than 5% in most studies.[93] If peripheral access is inadequate or unobtainable, it is clear that the next site attempted should be determined by the provider's level of confidence and expertise. Failure to obtain peripheral or central venous access mandates venous cutdown, which is most easily performed at the distal greater saphenous vein (Figure 18-1). Despite fewer complications than central access, cutdowns are more experience-dependent.

Children in the wilderness less than 6 years of age in whom venous access cannot be obtained should undergo intraosseous resuscitation. This is accomplished by introducing a needle through the periosteum of the tibia just inferior to the tibial tuberosity (Figure 18-2). Needles that are 18- to 20-gauge are preferable, but any needle strong enough to penetrate the periosteum without bending can be used.

Of the resuscitative therapies that potentially may be initiated in a well-prepared expedition, volume resus-

TABLE 18-1. Classes of Hemorrhagic Shock

	CLASS I	CLASS II	CLASS III	CLASS IV
Blood loss (ml)	Up to 750	750-1500	1500-2000	>2000
Blood loss (% blood volume)	Up to 15%	15%-30%	30%-40%	>40%
Pulse rate	<100	>100	>120	>140
Blood pressure	Normal	Normal	Decreased	Decreased
Pulse pressure (mm Hg)	Normal or increased	Decreased	Decreased	Decreased
Respiratory rate	14-20	20-30	30-40	>35
Urine output (ml/hr)	>30	20-30	5-15	Negligible
CNS/mental status	Slightly anxious	Mildly anxious	Anxious, confused	Confused, lethargic
Fluid replacement (3 : 1 rule)	Crystalloid	Crystalloid	Crystalloid and blood	Crystalloid and blood

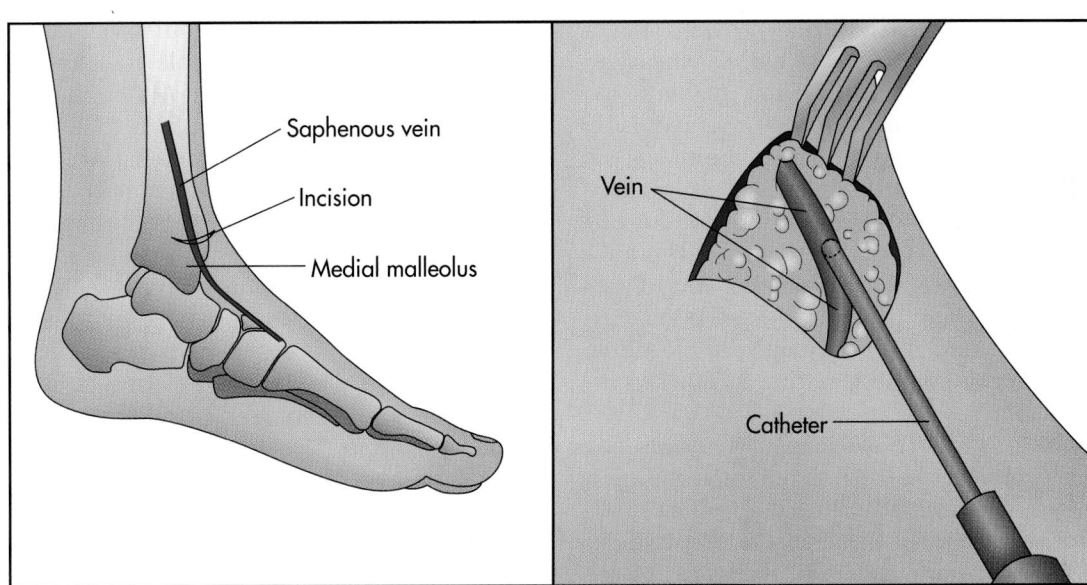

Figure 18-1 Venous cutdown performed at the distal greater saphenous vein.

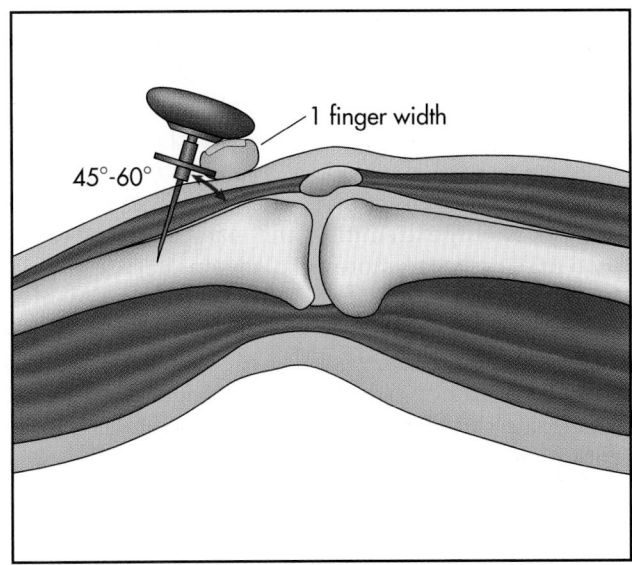

Figure 18-2 Intraosseous resuscitation performed by introducing needle through the periosteum of the tibia joint inferior to the tibial tuberosity.

citation deserves considerable attention. Fluid resuscitation in trauma has been a contentious topic, perhaps overly so, relative to fluid type and amounts used. A number of recent studies focusing on the prehospital administration of fluids in trauma victims not only rehashed the fluid composition debate but also called into question the efficacy of prehospital resuscitation.[71] Although further prospective trials are needed relative to fluid type and prehospital use, an impressive compilation of data has been amassed looking at resuscitative fluids in the trauma victim. Past studies have not only compared colloids with crystalloids[88] but have explored the use of blood and plasma substitutes, and hypertonic saline. An analysis of the details of such studies is beyond the scope of this chapter, but a summary of fluid recommendations is in order.

In small volumes, hypertonic saline has been shown to be an effective resuscitative fluid, and its efficacy in closed head injury is under evaluation. Currently, no improvement in survival has been demonstrated using hypertonic saline compared with crystalloid, and its use has been associated with hypokalemia, pulmonary edema, and dramatic increases in serum sodium and osmolarity.[6] The significance of these reported complications in trained hands is questionable, and hypertonic fluids may have a future role in resuscitation. Further study is warranted in the use of hypertonic saline, but its use in the wilderness setting is not recommended at this time.

Artificial blood products, such as perfluorocarbons and diaspirin cross-linked hemoglobin, have been shown to be efficient resuscitative fluids in animal studies.[20,77,86] However, they are expensive and not yet adequately studied in humans. Additional studies are needed concerning artificial blood products, since no benefit relative to crystalloid has yet been demonstrated in trauma victims. Their relatively experimental nature, cost, and lack of proven superiority over crystalloid preclude use in the wilderness setting at this time.

Based on the current literature, it is clear that both colloids (including hetastarches and albumin) and crystalloids are efficient volume expanders.[79] Certainly, larger volumes of crystalloids than colloids are needed to achieve similar resuscitative endpoints, usually in a ratio of 3 to 1. However, no benefit in survival using colloids has been demonstrated, and recent studies indicate that their use in critically ill patients may increase mortality.[19,68] Additionally, no proven detriment, including increased extravascular lung water, impaired wound healing, or decreased tissue oxygen diffusion, has been proven with the use of large volumes of crystalloids. Crystalloids are safe, nonantigenic, easily stored and transported, effective, and inexpensive. Most experts in trauma care agree that crystalloid is preferable to colloid infusion in the prehospital, early resuscitative phase of trauma care. Accordingly, the re-

suscitative fluid recommended by ATLS protocol is normal saline.

Several animal studies and recent human clinical trials in trauma victims have found that treatment with IV fluids before control of hemorrhage resulted in increased mortality rates.[9,56] Although these data are compelling, they have been accumulated in victims with penetrating injuries and short prehospital times, and the definition of prehospital *resuscitation* within these studies comprised widely varying volumes. Clearly, prehospital resuscitative protocols remain in evolution, and it is likely that current common practices will be altered in the future. However, application of these particular data to the wilderness setting at the current time is dangerous for a number of reasons. First, the leading cause of death in wilderness trauma is head injury. Many multiple trauma victims have a head injury, and it may be impossible to discern whether an intracranial lesion is present. Although under continued study, the current approach to management of head injury is aggressive maintenance of cerebral perfusion pressure to control intracranial pressure. Underresuscitation in the context of an intracranial injury could be catastrophic. Second, the multisystem-injured victim frequently presents with associated orthopedic injuries. A victim with closed extremity fractures with significant contained hemorrhage benefits from fluid resuscitation. Third, a victim with significant external hemorrhage that can be controlled before evacuation benefits from intravascular repletion.

In summary, resuscitation with IV fluids should be initiated in the field, particularly in victims with head injury and unquantified multiple trauma. Victims should have vascular access secured and resuscitative fluids given in the form of normal saline as dictated by severity of injuries and hemodynamics.

Secondary Survey

The secondary survey is an extension of the primary survey and should not be undertaken until the primary survey is complete and the victim has been stabilized. Additionally, resuscitative regimens, if available, should have been initiated. The secondary survey is a head-to-toe assessment of the victim including history and physical examination. The face, neck, chest, abdomen, pelvis, extremities, and skin should be examined in sequence. A more detailed neurologic examination should be completed, including reassessment of the GCS. The neck should be examined independently of the thoracolumbar spinal cord. Examination of the pelvis should not include the traditional "rocking" to determine stability, since this may exacerbate existing comminution.

The detailed secondary survey should not delay evacuation packaging. As in the nonwilderness setting, it is imperative to repeat the primary survey as the victim's condition warrants. Specific examinations will be discussed in the sections covering regional injuries.

History. The victim's history should be assessed during the secondary survey. Knowledge of the mechanism of injury and any comorbid medical conditions or allergies may enhance understanding the victim's physiologic state.

The ATLS "AMPLE" history is a useful and rapid mnemonic for this purpose:

Allergies
Medications currently used
Past medical history/*Pregnancy*
Last meal
Event or *Environment* related to the injury

Adjuncts. Resuscitation should be initiated simultaneous with the primary survey. The degree of resuscitation depends on available resources, experience of the rescuer(s), and environmental conditions. Under optimal circumstances, resuscitation allows oxygenation, fluid administration, and cardiac and vital sign monitoring. As adjuncts to the secondary survey, it also includes placement of urinary and nasogastric (NG) catheters. This degree of resuscitation will be almost universally unavailable in the wilderness setting. Here, resuscitation may be limited to oral administration of warm, high-calorie fluids and maintenance of victim comfort and body temperature.

A nasogastric tube and indwelling urinary (Foley) catheter should be placed if available and appropriate. In a victim with depressed level of consciousness or nausea and vomiting, gastric decompression assists in protection against aspiration—which could prove catastrophic in a remote area. In addition, children can exhibit deterioration in hemodynamics secondary to massive gastric distention. Nasogastric tubes should be placed in persons who are endotracheally intubated in the field. The tube can be aspirated sequentially with a syringe or left open to gravity drainage. If there is suspicion of a facial fracture(s), an NG tube should not be placed through the nares.

A Foley catheter can assist in volume assessment and hemodynamic status determination in a critically injured victim. Hourly urine output typically does not decrease until the onset of class III hemorrhagic shock, with loss of 30% to 40% of blood volume. Contraindications to urinary catheter placement in the field are blood at the urethral meatus, high-riding prostate, scrotal hematoma, and personnel not experienced in placement.

PNEUMATIC ANTISHOCK GARMENT. The pneumatic antishock garment (PASG) is a noninvasive device inflated around the lower extremities and abdomen to augment peripheral vascular resistance and increase blood pressure. It was widely instituted as a treatment for shock in the 1980s, largely based on anecdotal data. Prospective data relevant to penetrating chest and abdominal trauma[42,57] and retrospective data in blunt trauma[7] indicate an increase in mortality with its use. The PASG has theoretical benefits in the stabilization of hemodynamically unstable pelvic fractures, although no scientific evidence exists for this application.[71] Further prospective studies in blunt trauma are needed, and use of the PASG is not indicated in the wilderness setting for blunt trauma at this time.

Injuries to the Head, Face, and Neck. The secondary survey begins with examination of the entire head and scalp for evidence of skull or facial fractures, ocular trauma, lacerations, and contusions. The scalp is thoroughly palpated for tenderness, depressions, and lacerations. The bones of the face—including the zygomatic arch, maxilla, and mandible—are palpated for fractures. Detailed discussion of oral, facial, and eye injuries is presented in Chapters 22 and 23. Elements of the GCS are repeated.

The wilderness eye is discussed in detail in Chapter 22, but general examination principles are as follows. Significant periorbital edema may preclude examination of the globe, and assessment should be carried out rapidly. The globe should be evaluated for visual acuity, pupillary size, conjunctival hemorrhage, lens dislocation, and entrapment. Persons with significant facial trauma have a high incidence of associated ocular or orbital injuries.[75] Recent studies of ocular injuries in trauma victims have emphasized underappreciation of ocular and periocular signs indicative of significant underlying injury by many disciplines involved in the victim's care.[70]

Head Injuries

Background. Approximately 500,000 to 2 million cases of head injury occur in the United States yearly.[34] Of these, approximately 10% die before reaching a hospital.[5] Long-term disability and sequelae associated with head injury are significant, with more than 100,000 persons suffering varying degrees of permanent impairment. Because of the high-risk nature of traumatic brain injury (TBI) and the impact of initial management on disability and survival, clinical management objectives must address both immediate survival and long-term outcome. No standardized management guidelines for head injuries in a wilderness setting have been developed, and a wide range of clinical approaches are used in hospital settings.[34] However, available literature suggests that morbidity and mortality can be reduced by means of a protocol that includes early airway control with optimization of ventilation,[38] prompt cardiopulmonary resuscitation, and rapid evacuation to a trauma care facility.

In the wilderness setting, triage, resuscitation, and initial management of the head-injured victim must focus on maintenance of ATLS protocol, attempts to prevent secondary brain injury, and expeditious evacuation to a neurosurgical center.

First and foremost, secure the airway. Multiple clinical and experimental studies have demonstrated the detrimental effects of hypoxia on the injured brain. A definitive airway should be established if any degree of compromise exists. Because of the high incidence of concomitant cervical spine injuries in this patient population, optimal immobilization is paramount in prevention of further devastating neurologic injury.

The focus must then be directed to prevention of secondary brain injury. The purpose of the wilderness head injury protocol is to allow individuals with widely varying levels of experience and expertise to identify signs of significant head injury, begin proper resuscitation in the context of prevention of secondary brain injury through airway maintenance and hemodynamic support, and evacuate appropriately.

Anatomy. The scalp is comprised of five layers of tissue that cover the calvaria: skin, connective tissue, galea aponeurotica, loose areolar tissue, and periosteum of the skull. The galea is a fibrous tissue layer with important ramifications in closure of scalp wounds, discussed later in this chapter. Loose areolar tissue beneath the galea represents the site of accumulation of blood in scalp hematomas. A rich vascular network located between the dermis and the galea supplies the scalp. When lacerated, these vessels can be a significant source of hemorrhage, which may be of importance if evacuation is impossible or delayed.

The skull is composed of two groups of bones that form the face and cranium. Cranial bones are divided into the calvaria and base. The calvaria is composed of frontal, ethmoid, sphenoid, parietal, and occipital bones. The calvaria is especially thin in the temporal region, whereas the skull base is irregular with outcroppings, such as the anterior temporal fossa.

The covering of the brain within the skull is composed of three membranous layers: a thick and fibrous dura, a thinner arachnoid layer, and the innermost pia. In the wilderness environment, the layers have little clinical relevance, and their distinction—with the exception of defining a closed vs. open injury—bears little significance.

Pathophysiology of Traumatic Brain Injury. TBI can be divided into primary and secondary injury. Primary injury is comprised of the physical or mechanical insult at the moment of impact, and the immediate and permanent damage to brain tissue and cranium. Little can be done in the wilderness setting relative to primary brain injury. Secondary injury is the biochemical and cellular response to initial mechanical trauma and includes physiologic derangements that may exacerbate primary injury. Such physiologic alterations include

hypoxia, hypotension, ischemia, and hypothermia. Elevated intracranial pressure (ICP) may cause and exacerbate secondary brain injury.

Many forms of head injury cause elevated ICP, the duration of which is significantly correlated with poor outcome. Thus elevated ICP is not only is indicative of significant underlying pathology but also contributes negatively to the outcome. The Monro-Kellie doctrine states that the volume of intracranial contents must remain constant. If the normal compensatory response to increased volume, which consists of decreasing venous blood and cerebrospinal fluid (CSF) volume, is overcome, then small increases in volume cause exponential increases in ICP. The volume-pressure curve in Figure 18-3 relates the small but critical time period between decompensation and brainstem herniation. With ICP elevation directly correlating with secondary brain injury, it is evident that the field provider must attempt to keep the head-injured victim in the flat portion of the curve, minimizing ICP.

The most important priority in minimizing secondary brain injury in the field is optimizing cerebral perfusion pressure (CPP). CPP is relates to ICP and mean arterial pressure (MAP) as follows:

$$CPP = MAP - ICP$$

A CPP less than 70 mm Hg after head injury correlates with increased morbidity and mortality.[5,37] Cerebral blood flow (CBF) should be maintained at approximately 50 ml/100 g brain tissue/minute.[54] At 5 ml/100 g/min, irreversible damage and potential cell death occur.[5] Study data have shown a correlation between low CBF and poor outcome.[54] At a MAP between 50 mm Hg and 160 mm Hg, cerebral autoregulation maintains

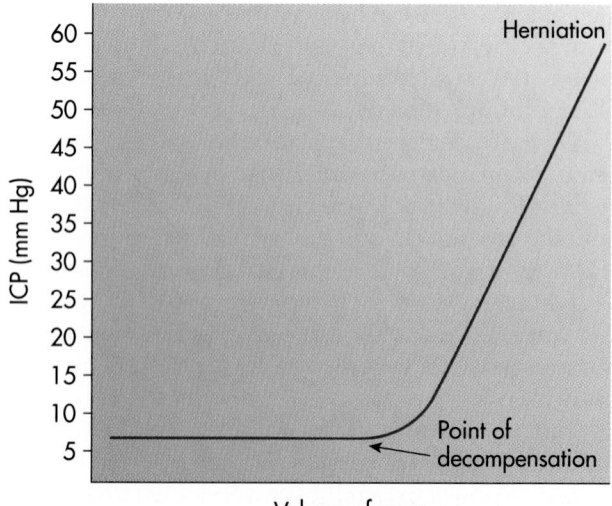

Volume-Pressure Curve

Figure 18-3 Critical time period between decomposition and brainstem herniation after traumatic brain injury.

CBF at relatively constant levels. Not only is autoregulation known to be disturbed in injured regions of the brain but also a precipitous fall in MAP can additionally impair autoregulatory function, decreasing CBF and exacerbating ischemia-induced secondary injury. Intuitively, it can been seen that the field provider has a means to combat rises in ICP simply by optimizing the MAP through aggressive resuscitation.

Diagnosis. There are three useful descriptions of head injury that may be applied to field recognition.

History. The history, including the mechanism and timing, severity, and morphology of the injury, can assist in the decision-making process regarding resuscitation and evacuation.[5] The mechanism may be identified as blunt or penetrating. The anatomic demarcation between blunt and penetrating injury is traditionally defined by the dura mater. Blunt injuries in the wilderness setting most often result from falls. Falling objects and assaults comprise the remainder of the majority of blunt injuries. Penetrating injuries are most commonly gunshot or arrow wounds.

Severity. Severity of injury can be estimated by quantifying the GCS and the pupillary response. The generally accepted definition of coma is a GCS score of less than 8. With regard to the primary survey and the essential component of airway protection, it has been demonstrated that GCS score does not specifically correlate with need to intubate, and the airway may be acceptable below a score of 8. It is important to note the victim's *best* motor response, since it is most predictive of outcome. Any victim with a GCS score less than 15 who has sustained a head injury should be evacuated if possible. A low or declining GCS suggests increased ICP, which demands attention to optimizing MAP and consequently CPP. Abnormal or asymmetric pupillary responses relative to size or responsiveness also suggest intracranial mass lesion and elevated ICP.

Morphology. Injury morphology may be difficult to assess in the wilderness setting and relies on level of suspicion and clinical signs and symptoms. Following attention to the primary survey, including airway and immobilization, the physical examination of the secondary survey is imperative and can provide information as to the existence of TBI.

Injury Classification. Intracranial injuries range from concussion to massive subdural hematoma. Subdural hematomas are more common than are epidural hematomas, comprising 20% to 30% of mass lesions. "Subdurals" result from torn bridging veins between the cerebral cortex and draining venous sinuses. Their prognosis is worse than that of "epidurals," although prompt recognition and drainage improve outcome. Epidermal hematomas are most commonly located in the temporal region and result from injury to the middle meningeal artery, often associated with a fracture. They may present loss of consciousness followed by a lucid interval before rapid deterioration, although this sequence is frequently not observed. Hemorrhagic contusion is also quite frequent, constituting 35% of traumatic injuries; this lesion has the propensity to result in significant increases in ICP. *Diffuse axonal injury* (DAI) is the term used to describe a prolonged posttraumatic coma not resulting from a mass lesion or ischemic insult. Similar to hemorrhagic contusion, DAI may result in elevated ICP.

Physical Examination. The physical examination should be done so that it does not delay evacuation. The GCS should be reassessed. The hallmark of TBI is altered level of consciousness. Physical signs that may denote underlying brain injury include significant scalp lacerations, contusions, scalp hematomas, facial trauma, and signs of skull fracture, including Battle's sign (see below) and periorbital ecchymosis (raccoon eyes). Hemotympanum and bleeding from the ears, or CSF rhinorrhea or otorrhea, also suggest skull fracture and underlying TBI.

The pupillary examination may provide valuable data in the assessment of underlying TBI. Temporal herniation may be heralded by a mild dilation of the pupil and a sluggish response to light. Further dilation of the pupil followed by ptosis, or paresis of the medial rectus or other ocular muscle, may indicate third cranial nerve compression by a mass lesion. Table 18-2 relates pupillary examinations to possible underlying

TABLE 18-2. Interpretation of Pupillary Findings in Head-Injured Victims

PUPIL SIZE	LIGHT RESPONSE	INTERPRETATION
Unilaterally dilated	Sluggish or fixed	Third nerve compression secondary to tentorial herniation
Bilaterally dilated	Sluggish or fixed	Inadequate brain perfusion; bilateral third nerve palsy
Unilaterally dilated or equal	Cross-reactive (Marcus-Gunn)	Optic nerve injury
Bilaterally constricted	Difficult to determine; pontine lesion	Opiates
Bilaterally constricted	Preserved	Injured sympathetic pathway

brain lesions. Most dilated pupils are on the ipsilateral side of the mass lesion. With direct globe injury, traumatic mydriasis may result. Additionally, 5% to 10% of the population has congenital anisocoria. Neither direct trauma nor congenital anisocoria should be assumed in a head-injured victim exhibiting mental status change in the wilderness.

After quantification of GCS score, pupillary examination, and examination of the head and face for signs of external trauma, a concise neurologic examination should be performed. The goal of the field neurologic examination is to identify motor or sensory focal deficits suggestive of intracranial injury. Sensory

deficits follow general dermatome patterns shown in Figure 18-4. Unilateral hemiplegia may signify uncal herniation resulting from mass effect in the contralateral cortex because of compression of the corticospinal tract in the midbrain. Ipsilateral pupillary dilation associated with contralateral hemiplegia is a classic and ominous sign of tentorial herniation. Reflex changes in the absence of altered mental status are not indicative of TBI. With the exception of the performance of gag and corneal reflex evaluations, the brainstem cannot be evaluated in the wilderness environment. The "doll's eyes maneuver" should never be performed without complete radiologic evaluation of the cervical spine. Ice

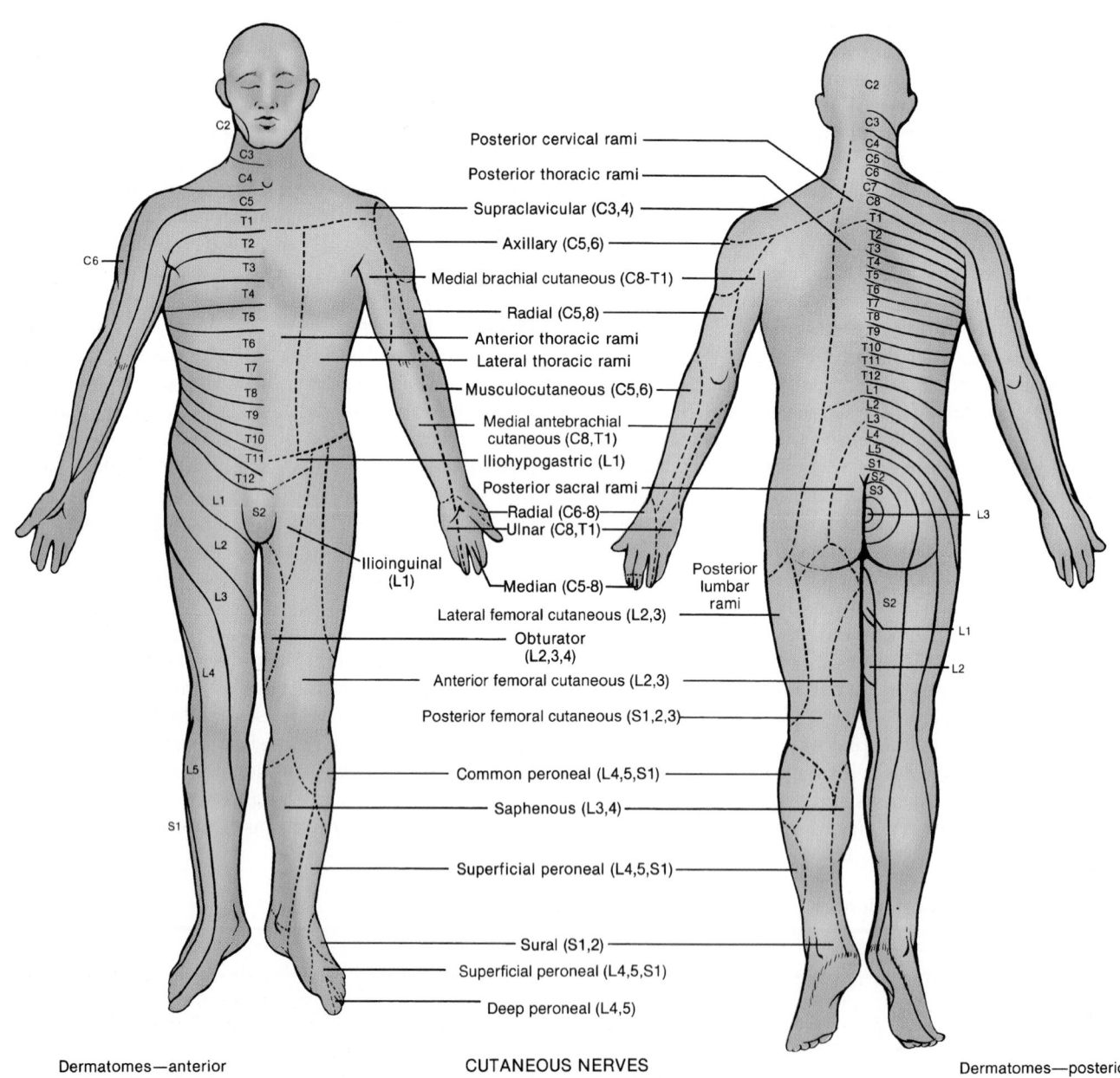

Dermatomes—anterior   **CUTANEOUS NERVES**   Dermatomes—posterio

Figure 18-4 Dermatome pattern, the skin area stimulated by spinal cord elements. Sensory deficits following general dermatome patterns.

water irrigation of the tympanic membrane intended to evoke nystagmus adds nothing to an evacuation decision and should not be performed outdoors.

Resuscitation. Resources and circumstances permitting, resuscitation should be initiated as an adjunct to the primary survey. The primary focus for the head-injured victim, similar to any traumatized victim, is the airway. During the primary survey and performance of the ABCDE sequence, IV access should be established. If IV resuscitation is impossible, it is *not* advisable to administer fluids orally to the victim with head injury because of the likelihood of vomiting, airway compromise, and aspiration.

Individuals sustaining head trauma have a high incidence of concomitant injuries. Up to 32% of persons with severe head injury will have a long bone or pelvic fracture, 20% to 25% a chest injury, and 10% an abdominal injury. A victim who does not have a palpable femoral pulse or manifests other signs of hypotension in the context of suspected head injury must be assumed to have a nonneurogenic etiology of shock. Resuscitation is critical in this setting for multiple reasons. First, management of a head injury should be secondary to other life-threatening injuries, which, if not addressed, may preclude survival. Second, as previously discussed, maintenance of MAP and thus CPP is critical in preventing secondary brain injury.

The type of resuscitative fluid administered is controversial. Previously, recommendations existed warning of the dangers of overhydration in head injury, to the extent of implementing fluid restriction. Fluid restriction has not been shown to reduce ICP or edema formation in the laboratory, and hypotonic solutions do not decrease cortical water content.[87] The need for resuscitation and intravascular volume support is now well established. Possible resuscitative fluids now include primarily isotonic crystalloids, colloids, or hypertonic crystalloids. Hypotonic fluids are not appropriate in TBI because they can cause increased brain water and thus elevated ICP. Recent data from animal studies suggest that colloids offer no advantage over isotonic crystalloids, such as lactated Ringer's solution, in head injury in terms of augmenting CBF or preventing cerebral edema.[98] As previously noted, no clear prospective trial has documented any advantage of colloid over crystalloid administration in the victim with multiple systemic injuries. Evidence is accumulating that hypertonic solutions, particularly hypertonic saline, may be beneficial in TBI.[89,94] However, an advantage has not been demonstrated in trauma victims overall, and expertise is necessary for their use. Thus the recommended resuscitative fluid for the head-injured victim in the wilderness setting is isotonic crystalloid. MAP should be optimized at 90 mm Hg based on cuff pressure or extrapolation from distal pulses.

Further Management. Numerous adjuncts exist in the management of the head-injured victim, few of which are applicable in the wilderness setting. Once the primary and secondary surveys are complete, the airway is secured, resuscitation has been initiated, and spine immobilization has been achieved, the victim should be placed in a 30-degree head-up position. This position assists in control of ICP and thus CPP through augmentation of venous outflow. This maneuver should not be attempted if the spine cannot be adequately immobilized.

If endotracheal intubation is possible, ventilation should be optimized *without* hyperventilating the victim. Hyperventilation has been used aggressively in the past to promote hypocarbia-induced cerebral vasoconstriction, thereby increasing CBF. However, if $PaCO_2$ falls below 25 mm Hg, severe vasoconstriction ensues, effectively reducing CBF and promoting ischemia. Studies have demonstrated worse outcomes in victims with severe head injury who were hyperventilated.[64] Because of the inability to measure or titrate this variable in the wilderness, ventilation should be controlled to approximate normal minute ventilation.

All bleeding from the scalp or face should be controlled with direct pressure. Scalp hematomas, regardless of size, should not be decompressed. Open wounds, particularly skull fractures, should be irrigated and covered with the most sterile dressing available. Fragments of displaced cranium overlying exposed brain tissue should not be replaced. If signs of skull fracture are present, immunization against tetanus and broad-spectrum antibiotic prophylaxis are recommended.

Although diuretics have been widely utilized in the intensive care management of intracranial hypertension, no rationale exists for their use in the field. The wilderness trauma victim may have many injuries that are impossible to diagnose. In this setting, particularly in the presence of hemorrhagic shock, attempts to induce osmotic diuresis to decrease ICP may be life-threatening. Diuretics such as furosemide or mannitol may exacerbate hypotension and alkalosis and induce renal complications in the absence of physiologic monitoring.[4]

Steroids have no role in head injury in the field or intensive care unit. Studies have documented no beneficial impact on ICP or survival. Attempts at brain preservation by slowing metabolic rate and oxygen consumption have no role in the wilderness setting. Barbiturates have been used for elevated ICP refractory to other measures but may induce hypotension, depress myocardial function, and depress the neurologic examination.[4] Compared with minimizing ICP, they offer no proven benefit.[37]

Approximately 15% of persons with severe head injury experience posttraumatic seizures. Phenytoin, if available, can be safely administered in the field, but only after a witnessed seizure. Prophylactic administration has not been shown to decrease long-term seizure activity.

Skull Fracture. Skull fracture in the wilderness mandates evacuation. Therapeutic options in the field are few, with intervention limited to identifying the injury and arranging rapid transport. Skull fractures may be open or closed, linear or stellate, and may occur in the vault or skull base. Basilar skull fractures often manifest signs that aid in the diagnosis, including periorbital ecchymosis (raccoon eyes), retroauricular ecchymosis (Battle's sign), CSF leaks, or eighth cranial nerve palsy. Skull fractures are associated with a high incidence of underlying intracranial injury. In an awake and alert victim with a skull fracture, the chance of brain injury is increased 400-fold.[5]

Skull fractures with depression greater than the thickness of the skull may require elevation. No attempt at elevation should be made in the field. Any exposed brain surface should quickly be covered with the most sterile covering available, preferably moistened with crystalloid solution. Loose bone or brain fragments should not be manipulated. If a broad-spectrum antibiotic is available, it should be administered. After attention to the wound and stabilization of associated injuries, the victim should be rapidly evacuated.

Penetrating Head Injuries. The majority of penetrating head injuries in the wilderness are gunshot wounds, although knives and arrows may penetrate the cranium. Such injuries are usually catastrophic. However, examples of survival exist in small caliber, low-velocity injuries and tangential wounds.[55] As with closed head injury, management priorities consist of maintenance of airway, prevention of secondary brain injury, and rapid evacuation. If the cranium has been violated, the victim should receive antibiotics and tetanus immunization in the same manner as for open skull fracture. Some authors recommend 7 days of anticonvulsant therapy.[55] In the rare instance that the projectile is embedded in the skull, no attempt at removal should be undertaken. If the length of the projectile makes immobilization or transport cumbersome, excess length may be removed, but only if this may be done easily and without displacement of the intracranial segment.

Evacuation. Survival and outcome of head injury in the wilderness correlate directly with the rapidity of evacuation. Certain situations dictate immediate evacuation. Any person with evidence of an open or closed skull fracture should be evacuated. The incidence of TBI associated with skull fractures is variable but significant throughout the literature. Recent data predict that 30% to 90% of persons with raccoon eyes or Battle's sign will have an abnormal computed axial tomography (CAT) scan.[11,18] Similarly, any person who sustains a penetrating injury should be evacuated.

The decision to evacuate victims who have sustained closed head injuries can be simplified by dividing the victims into three groups based on probability of injury.

The high-risk group is composed of persons with GCS score of 13 or less. Focal neurologic signs or evidence of decreasing level of consciousness requires evacuation. The low-risk group includes persons who have suffered a blow to the head but are asymptomatic, did not lose consciousness, and complain only of mild headache or dizziness. Data from recent studies suggest that persons who meet low-risk criteria (including GCS of 15, no loss of consciousness, minimal symptomatology, and unlikely mechanism) have a minimal chance of having significant TBI[11,18] and may be closely observed.

The group for which the evacuation decision is most difficult is the moderate-risk group. These persons have a history of brief loss of consciousness or change in consciousness at the time of injury, or a history of progressive headache, vomiting, or posttraumatic amnesia. If any of these signs is present in the face of concurrent systemic injury, the victim should be evacuated immediately. Studies associating clinical variables and abnormal computed tomography (CT) scans have demonstrated the significance of decreased GCS, symptoms, and loss of consciousness. If these signs are present in isolation and the evacuation can be completed in less than 12 hours, the evacuation should proceed. If the evacuation is impossible or will require longer than 12 hours, the victim should be closely observed for 4 to 6 hours. If the examination improves to normalcy during the observation period, it is reasonable to continue observation.

Neck Injuries

Blunt Neck Injuries. Injuries to the neck may be classified as blunt or penetrating. Significant blunt injuries include cervical spine injuries and laryngotracheal injuries. Seventy-five percent of injuries to the trachea are confined to the cervical region.[69] Fracture of the larynx and disruption of the trachea usually require surgical intervention unavailable in the wilderness. The sooner laryngeal repair is accomplished, the better the outcome with respect to phonation.[21] Victims present with a history of a significant blow to the anterior neck. Physical examination findings include difficulty with phonation, subcutaneous emphysema that may extend as far inferiorly as the abdominal wall, stridor, odynophagia, and, often, acute respiratory distress.

Treatment is focused on establishing and maintaining an airway until evacuation can occur. Frequently, the airway will be in jeopardy, and because of the propensity for injuries of this type to result in significant and progressive edema, endotracheal or nasotracheal intubation is often necessitated. If these options are unavailable, airway maintenance techniques as described in the Primary Survey section should be used. In the event of intubation failure or lack of availability with impending hypoxic death, a surgical cricothyroidotomy may be necessitated. A recent study of prehospital cricothyroidotomy demonstrated that success rates were high regardless of medical specialty as long as previous training had been instituted.[51] For further descriptions of airway management, refer to Chapter 17.

BACKGROUND. Vertebral column injury, with or without neurologic deficits, must be identified in any wilderness multiple trauma victim. Approximately 2.6% of victims of major trauma suffer acute injury of the spinal cord.[16] Fifteen percent of victims sustaining an injury above the clavicles and 5% to 10% of persons with a significant head injury will have a cervical spine injury. Additionally, 55% of spinal injuries occur in the cervical region.[55] In the wilderness setting, fractures or dislocations of the cervical spine are a result of falls from significant heights, or of high-velocity ski or vehicular injuries. Twenty-eight percent of persons with cervical spine fractures have fractures elsewhere in the spine.[10]

ANATOMY. The cervical spine consists of seven vertebrae. The anteriorly placed vertebral bodies form the weight-bearing structure of the column. The bodies are separated by intervertebral disks and held in place anteriorly and posteriorly by longitudinal ligaments. The paraspinal muscles, facet joints, and interspinous ligaments contribute as a whole to the stability of the spine. The cervical spine, based on its anatomy, is more susceptible to injury than are the thoracic and lumbar spine. The cervical canal is wide from the foramen magnum to C2, with only 33% of the canal comprised by the spinal cord itself. The clinically relevant tracts in the spinal cord include the corticospinal tract, the spinothalamic tract, and the posterior columns.

CLASSIFICATION AND RECOGNITION. Fractures of the cervical spine frequently result in neurologic deficit, with total loss of function below the level of injury.[50] Resultant spinal cord injuries should be classified according to level, severity of neurologic deficit, and spinal cord syndrome. Fractures of the C1-C2 complex generally result from axial loading (a C1 ring fracture, or Jefferson's fracture) or an acute flexion injury (a C2 posterior element fracture, or hangman's fracture). Approximately 40% of atlas fractures have an associated fracture of the axis. The atlas fracture, if survived, is rarely

associated with cord injury but is unstable and requires strict immobilization. Generally, a complete neurologic injury at this level is unsurvivable owing to paralysis of respiratory muscle function. One third of victims sustaining an upper cervical spine injury die at the scene. The most common mechanism of injury is flexion, and the most common level of injury at C5-C6.[10]

Fractures and dislocations may result in partial or complete neurologic injury distal to the fracture or in no neurologic injury at all. Partial injuries to the spinal cord result from typical patterns of injury. Because flexion injuries are the most common type of injury to the cervical spine, the anterior cord syndrome (see below) is the most commonly seen serious neurologic picture. A careful neurologic examination in the field to grade motor strength and to document sensory response to light touch and pinprick yields important information that should be documented and reported to the treating physician at the definitive care facility. The presence or absence of the Babinski's reflex should be noted, as well.

When appropriate resources are available, a rectal examination should be performed. Complete lack of tone and failure of the sphincter muscles to contract when pulling on the penis or clitoris (the bulbocavernosus reflex) indicate the presence of spinal cord injury.

When individuals with cervical spine fractures or dislocations are transported, the neck must be stabilized to prevent further injury to the spinal cord or nerve roots at the level of the fracture or dislocation. Approximately 28% of persons with cervical spine fractures have fractures elsewhere in the spine;[10] therefore the entire spine must be protected during transport.

Occasionally, a pure flexion event can result in dislocation of one or both of the posterior facets without fracture or neurologic injury. The victim may complain only of neck pain and limitation of motion. If so, the victim should be transported with the neck rigidly immobilized. With this injury, posterior instability is present (since the interspinous ligament is ruptured), and any further flexion stress could produce a spinal cord injury.

PHYSICAL EXAMINATION. A thorough neurologic examination should be performed. Initial documentation of deficits and frequent repeat examinations are critical to follow-up care. The classification of injury in the field begins with determination of the level of injury. Knowledge of sensory dermatomal and motor myotomal patterns is invaluable (see Figure 18-4). The sensory level is the lowest dermatome with normal sensation and may differ on each side of the body. C1 to C4 are variable in their cutaneous distribution, and assessment should begin at C5. The examiner must not be confused by the occasional innervation of the pectoral skin by C1 to C4, known as the "cervical cape." Light touch and pinprick should be assessed.

Motor function should be assessed by the myotomal distribution listed in Box 18-2. Each muscle should be graded on a six-point scale:

0—Total paralysis
1—Palpable or visible contraction
2—Full range of motion without gravity
3—Full range of motion against gravity
4—Full range of motion with decreased strength
5—Normal strength

Each muscle must be tested bilaterally and documented. The reflexes alluded to in the classification section must be tested, as well as anal sphincter tone.

SYNDROMES. Central cord syndrome is characterized by a disproportionate loss of motor power between the upper and lower extremities, with greater strength retained in the lower extremities. Sensory loss is variable. The mechanism of injury usually involves a forward fall with facial impact and hyperextension of the spine.

Anterior cord syndrome is characterized by paraplegia and loss of pain and temperature sensation. It is the most common presenting syndrome caused by cervical spine injury and carries a poor prognosis.

Brown-Séquard's syndrome results from hemisection of the cord. It consists of ipsilateral motor loss and position sense with contralateral sensory loss two levels below the level of injury. It is usually secondary to penetrating injury.

IMMOBILIZATION. After identification of injury, the caregiver faces a critical decision with important ramifications—whether or not to immobilize.[31] Victims who would as a matter of course be immobilized in an urban setting might not be appropriate candidates for immobilization in the wilderness. The decision to immobilize converts an otherwise ambulatory victim who can actively participate in his or her own evacuation to one requiring more involved evacuation procedures. The subsequent evacuation can be dangerous to the victim and rescuers and demands significant expense and resource utilization.

Risk criteria for cervical spine injury and the need for immobilization have been defined.[40,53] All criteria for the exclusion of immobilization must be satisfied. These include normal mental status without chemical influence; lack of distracting injury; normal neurologic examination; and a reliable neck examination without midline neck pain, deformity, or tenderness. Figure 18-5 presents an evidence-based algorithm for determining need for immobilization. Although the need for immobilization poses hazards for the evacuation process, if criteria are met, immobilization takes precedent over ease of evacuation.[58] A difficult balance must be struck in the wilderness between the likelihood of true injury and the danger to the expedition members and rescuers that may ensue when the victim is immobilized.

If a rigid litter is not available, the victim should be maintained on the flattest surface possible. A rigid cervical collar should be placed. All collars allow some degree of movement, particularly rotation. Soft collars offer the least immobilization.[30] The Philadelphia collar

---

Box 18-2 SENSORY AND MOTOR DEFICIT ASSESSMENT

SENSORY

C5: Area over deltoid
C6: Thumb
C7: Middle finger
C8: Little finger
T4: Nipple
T8: Xiphisternum
T10: Umbilicus
T12: Symphysis
L3: Medial aspect of thigh
L4: Medial aspect of leg
L5: First toe web space
S1: Lateral foot
S4 and S5: Perianal skin

MOTOR

C5: Deltoid
C6: Wrist extensors
C7: Elbow extensors
C8: Finger flexors, middle finger
T1: Small finger abductors
L2: Hip flexors
L3: Knee extensors
L4: Ankle dorsiflexors
L5: Great toe extensors
S1: Plantar flexors

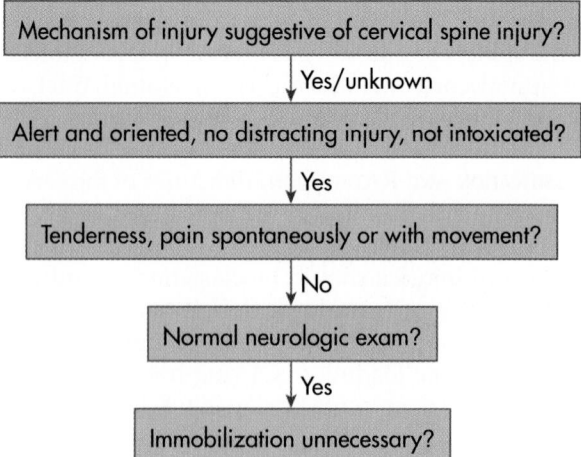

Figure 18-5 Clinical assessment of cervical spine stability. Failure of any criterion suggests need for immobilization.

has been shown to allow 44% of normal rotation and 66% of normal lateral bending.[55] To achieve 95% immobilization, a halo and vest are necessary. Any number of materials may be used to improvise an immobilizing device. Restriction of flexion, extension, and rotation must be achieved to the greatest degree possible. Optimal immobilization consists of a long spine board or litter, rigid collar, bolsters to the sides of the head, and tape or straps restricting movement (Figure 18-6).

TREATMENT. The issue of pharmacotherapy for spinal cord injury is under continuous study. Currently, based on data accumulated by the National Acute Spinal Cord Injury Study Group, documented *blunt* spinal cord injury should be treated with a bolus of 30 mg/kg of methylprednisolone within 8 hours of injury followed by a continuous infusion of 5.4 mg/kg over the next 23 hours.[13] Steroids are not recommended in the field unless a victim clearly manifests a spinal cord injury in the absence of head injury.

Because little definitive treatment for cervical spine injury can be accomplished in the field, survival and outcome depend on speed of transport and maintenance of airway. This is particularly true considering the association of cervical spine injury with head injury and major systemic trauma. Transport all victims with proven or suspected cervical spine injury to a definitive care facility.

Penetrating Neck Injuries. Similar to penetrating head injury, penetrating neck injury is usually due to gun or knife wounds. Most penetrating injuries do not confer bony instability; however, stability should not be assumed. Neurologic deficits, if present, can progress with further movement of an unstable spine. Projectiles should not be removed if embedded in the neck. Penetrating injuries to the neck may not directly injure the spine, but neurologic sequelae may result from blast effect. The same immobilization criteria should be implemented as when dealing with blunt injuries.

Penetrating injuries to the neck are classified according to anatomic zones of injury (Figure 18-7). Zone I injuries extend from the clavicles to the cricoid cartilage. Zone II injuries occur between the cricoid and the angle of the mandible. Zone III injuries occur superior to the angle of the mandible.

Historically, treatment has been based on penetration of the platysma muscle. In the wilderness setting, if the examiner is confident that platysmal penetration has not occurred, the victim may be observed and the wound considered a laceration. Much debate has occurred over management of platysmal penetration within respective topographic zones, with treatment arms consisting of surgical exploration vs. radiographic evaluation. In the wilderness setting, such considerations are not irrelevant. A penetrating injury violating the platysma muscle indicates the possibility of significant neurovascular, esophageal, and/or tracheal injuries, so the victim should be evacuated with close attention to the airway. If hemorrhage uncontrollable by direct pressure is present, careful insertion of a Foley catheter into the wound with balloon inflation may provide temporizing tamponade.[21]

Injuries to the Thorax

Background. The mortality from thoracic trauma is approximately 10%. Approximately 25% of all trauma

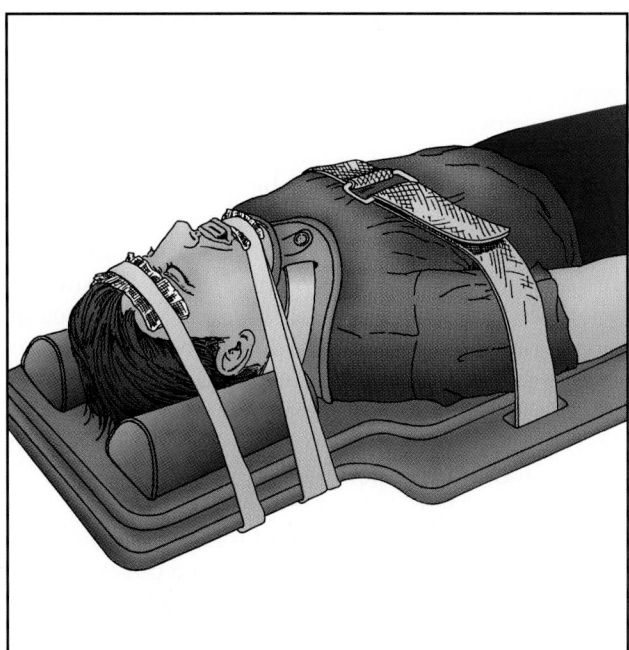

Figure 18-6 Proper spine immobilization.

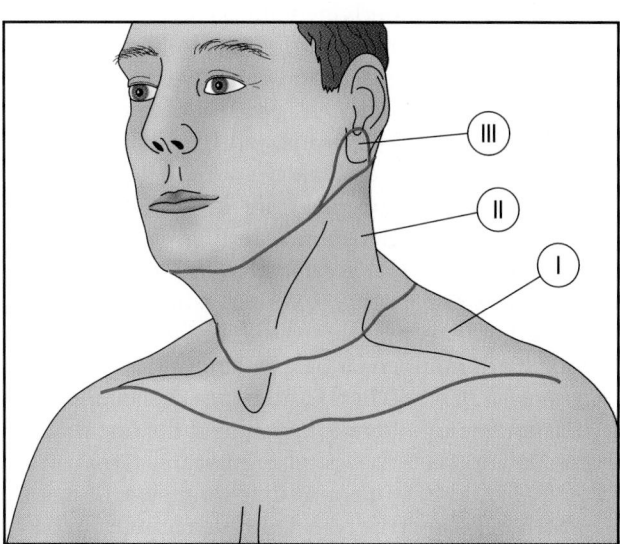

Figure 18-7 Zones in penetrating neck trauma.

deaths in the United States are attributable to chest injury.[5] However, only 15% of persons with major thoracic trauma require thoracotomy. Early intervention can play a critical role in survival, and many deaths are preventable. Prompt identification of life-threatening injuries in the immediate postinjury period may facilitate proper, lifesaving intervention.

In the wilderness environment, blunt thoracic injuries usually result from falls or direct blows to the chest. Penetrating injuries result from gun, knife, or arrow wounds, or from impalement after a fall. Immediate, life-threatening thoracic injuries include airway obstruction, tension pneumothorax, flail chest, and cardiac tamponade. The hallmark of significant thoracic injury is hypoxia, which may sometimes be remedied in the field.

Pathophysiology. Chest injuries often result in hypoxia, hypercarbia, and acidosis. The tissue hypoxia of thoracic trauma can be multifactorial. Inadequate delivery of oxygen can be from hemorrhagic shock, direct lung injury with ventilation-perfusion mismatch (pulmonary contusion, atelectasis, hematoma), and/or changes in normal intrathoracic pressure dynamics (tension or open pneumothorax). Hemodynamic instability and inadequate oxygen delivery may also result from cardiac tamponade or contusion.

Physical Examination. Thorough physical examination begins with visualization and inspection of the chest. Exposure of the chest should be completed in the primary survey. The airway is assessed for patency and air exchange, and the pattern of breathing is noted. In the immediate postinjury period, most trauma victims are tachypneic, partly from pain and anxiety. Dyspnea, cyanosis, the use of accessory muscles of respiration, or intercostal muscular retraction are abnormal and may give clues to the underlying injury.

Chest wall movement during respiration should be symmetric. Paradoxical chest wall movement is associated with flail chest. The chest wall should be inspected for contusions and abrasions, which may herald underlying bony or visceral injury.

Distention of the external veins in a person who has just suffered thoracic trauma and is hypotensive or tachycardic (heart rate greater than 130 beats per minute) suggests impairment of venous return to the heart. This finding may be seen in situations of increased intrathoracic or intrapericardial pressure and is associated with tension pneumothorax and pericardial tamponade. In tension pneumothorax, deviation of the trachea is in a direction opposite the lesion. Significant sternal bruising may herald fracture or cardiac contusion.

The thorax should be palpated systematically for bony tenderness, starting at the distal clavicles and working medially toward the sternum. The sternum is divided into the manubrium, gladiolus (body), and xiphoid cartilage. The manubrium is joined to the gladiolus by fibrocartilage, but mobility at this joint is minimal.

Each rib should be palpated individually. Ribs 1 to 7 are vertebrosternal; their costal cartilages join the sternum. Ribs 8 through 10 are vertebrochondral, with each costal cartilage commonly joining the cartilage of the rib above. Ribs 11 and 12, vertebral ribs, have no attachment to the sternum. Point tenderness over a rib can be associated with contusion or fracture. Displaced fractures can be palpated; occasionally, bone grating can be palpated during respiration.

Subcutaneous emphysema may extend up into the neck and down to the level of the inguinal ligaments. In the trauma situation, subcutaneous emphysema is invariably associated with pneumothorax.

Vocal fremitus describes palpation of vibrations transmitted through the chest wall. During speech, the victim's vocal cords emit vibrations in the bronchial air column that are conducted to the chest wall. Diminished vocal fremitus is associated with pneumothorax or hemothorax. To test for vocal fremitus, the examiner applies the palmar arch of the examining hand against the person's anterior chest wall. The person is asked to repeat "one, two, three" using the same pitch and intensity of voice with each repetition. If the vibrations are not well perceived, the patient is asked to lower the pitch of the voice. The chest should be symmetric, left to right.

Percussion is used to detect changes in the normal density of an organ. Percussion of the chest is performed by placing the examining fingertip on the chest wall and sequentially striking the fingertip with the tip of the finger of the other hand. In the trauma victim, dullness replacing resonance in the lower lung suggests hemothorax. Hyperresonance or tympany replacing resonance occurs only with a large pneumothorax or tension pneumothorax.

If a stethoscope is not available, primitive chest auscultation can be performed using a rolled piece of cardboard or paper. Any cylinder that can transmit sound through a column of air accentuates breath sounds when placed against the chest wall. The absence of sounds normally produced by the tracheobronchial air column indicates blockage in the airways or abnormal filtering of sound by fluid within the pleural cavity. In the trauma victim, this is invariably associated with pneumothorax or hemothorax.

Blunt Chest Trauma. Blunt chest trauma in the wilderness is most often associated with either a direct blow or a deceleration injury. The mechanism usually relates to a fall from variable heights. Compression of the chest wall by moving or falling debris may also contribute to intrathoracic injuries, as may be seen in traumatic asphyxia associated with burial in an avalanche or earthquake.

RIB FRACTURES. Rib fractures range in severity from an isolated nondisplaced single fracture, which causes only minor discomfort, to a major flail segment, which can be associated with an underlying hemopneumothorax and pulmonary contusion. Rib fractures are characterized by painful respiration, most severe on inspiration. Victims often breathe in a characteristically rapid, shallow pattern. Point tenderness is palpated over the fracture, and displacement can occasionally be detected. Rib fractures are detected with a compression test, in which pressure is exerted on the sternum while the victim lies supine. This will elicit pain over the fracture site.

Isolated rib fractures are managed with oral analgesics and rest. Thoracic taping and splinting are not necessary or helpful. Multiple rib fractures are significant because of the potential seriousness of associated injuries and increased pain. However, this pain responds well to an intercostal nerve block. Victims with multiple rib fractures need to be evacuated as conditions permit. After administration of an intercostal block, a person may regain the ability to hike out of the wilderness.

The morbidity of rib fractures relates to decreased inspiratory tidal volume secondary to pain and splinting. In the wilderness setting, management must focus on pain control and pulmonary toilet. If oral analgesia is insufficient to control pain, an intercostal block is ideal. Depending on the anesthetic used, varying lengths of analgesia can be attained, perhaps allowing transient ambulation for evacuation. Deep breathing should be encouraged 10 times hourly to help prevent atelectasis.

COSTOCHONDRAL SEPARATION. It is difficult to distinguish between a rib fracture and costochondral separation. With the latter, pain is more likely to be predominantly anterior over the costochondral junction. Pain increases with inspiration and worsens with direct palpation. Costochondral separation also responds to intercostal nerve block and oral and IV analgesics.

STERNAL FRACTURE. A sternal fracture is usually associated with a direct blow to the anterior chest wall. The injury is characterized by severe, constant chest pain that worsens with direct palpation. Sternal instability is unusual and can be associated with a significant underlying visceral injury, including pulmonary or myocardial contusion. The victim should immediately be evacuated by litter or helicopter.

PNEUMOTHORAX. Simple pneumothorax can occur from an injury that allows air to enter through the thoracic

wall or, more frequently, from an injury to the lung that permits air to escape into the pleural space. Symptoms include tachypnea, dyspnea, resonant hemithorax, absence of breath sounds, and tactile fremitus. A person with chest pain after a blunt blow to the chest, particularly with accompanying rib fracture(s), should be suspected of having a pneumothorax.

Treatment of pneumothorax involves decompression of the pleural space. In the wilderness environment, tube thoracostomy is rarely possible. Fortunately, although victims with isolated pneumothorax may complain of chest pain or dyspnea, they are not completely disabled. With analgesia to control pain, ambulation facilitates evacuation. It may be easier and more prudent to set a slow pace with frequent rest periods than to perform an unnecessary litter evacuation.

If resources and expertise allow placement of a thoracostomy tube, it should be performed only when clinically indicated. Considering possible morbidity in a remote area, prophylactic decompression should never be undertaken. Suspicion of a pneumothorax alone on physical examination does not warrant a catheter or chest tube. When a high index of clinical suspicion is accompanied by incapacitating symptoms, such as shortness of breath, decompression should be considered. The key to saving a victim's life is the understanding that a condition exists that can rapidly progress from a nondisabling condition to a life-threatening condition. Once the diagnosis of pneumothorax is entertained, vigilant observation and a high index of clinical suspicion are necessary in the event of progression to a tension pneumothorax. Symptoms should be closely monitored and frequent repeat examinations should be performed.

TENSION PNEUMOTHORAX. A tension pneumothorax develops when a one-way air leak follows lung rupture or chest wall penetration. Air is forced into the thoracic cavity with no means of escape, and pressure mounts within the hemithorax. With sufficient increases in intrathoracic pressure, the mediastinum is shifted to the contralateral side, which impedes venous return from both the superior and inferior vena cavae. Cardiac output is diminished and the victim soon exhibits signs and symptoms of shock. Victims with tension pneumothorax manifest distended neck veins and tracheal deviation away form the side of the lesion. There is unilateral absence of breath sounds, and the hemithorax is hyperresonant or tympanitic. Respiratory distress, cyanosis, and frank cardiovascular collapse may occur.

Tension pneumothorax is life-threatening and frequently associated with additional serious injuries. It mandates rapid chest decompression, followed by evacuation to a medical facility.

Decompression is performed by inserting a needle or catheter into the chest and converting the tension into an open pneumothorax. Ideally, a 14-gauge catheter is inserted percutaneously over the second rib in the midclavicular or anterior axillary line (Figure 18-8). Once the rib is identified with the tip of the needle, the needle is marched over the anterior superior surface of the rib and inserted through the intercostal muscles and pleura into the thoracic cavity. As the pressure within the hemithorax is released, a distinct rush of air is heard. The plastic catheter is advanced over the tip of the needle, the needle withdrawn, and the catheter left in place to ensure continued decompression. The needle should not be reintroduced into the catheter because it may damage or sever the catheter. Because tension pneumothorax is commonly associated with severe injury, the victim should be evacuated to a medical facility as rapidly as possible. A rubber glove or a finger cot can be attached to the external catheter opening to create a unidirectional flutter valve that allows egress of air from the pleural space.

If resources are limited and treatment is needed, any number of devices can be used to decompress the chest.

A sharp instrument and hollow tube, sterilized as well as possible, are all that is needed. Rapid cleansing of the skin surface is accomplished with antiseptic, alcohol, or water. A Heimlich valve kit is ideal for decompression and represents a valuable addition to the expedition first aid arsenal.

If resources permit placement of a thoracostomy tube, adequate anesthesia and expertise are required. The skin should be sterilized if possible, and local anesthesia should be infiltrated into the skin and periosteum of the rib. Insertion is most effectively accomplished through the fifth intercostal space at the anterior axillary line. A small incision is made and the subcutaneous tissue bluntly separated with a finger or clamp. A blunt instrument, preferably a clamp, is forcefully inserted into the pleural space closely adhering to the superior surface of the rib to avoid the inferiorly located intercostal neurovascular bundle. Having entered the pleural space, a tube (36 F or greater in size) is inserted apically and posteriorly.

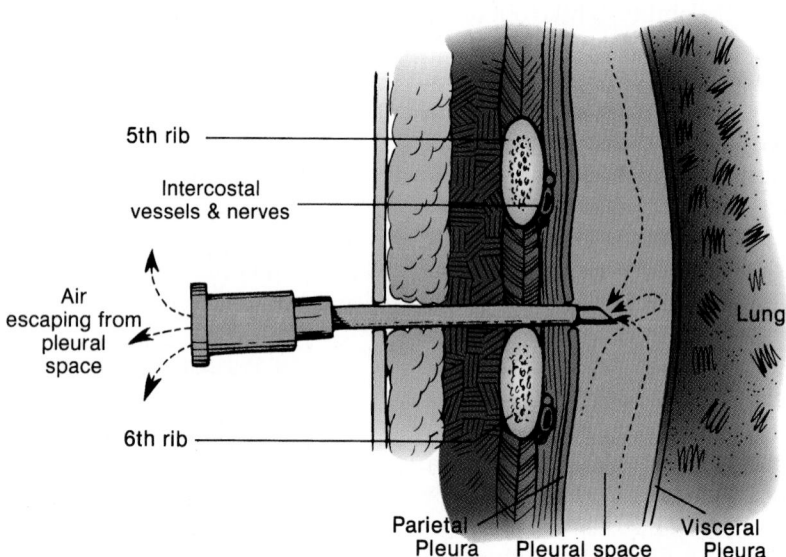

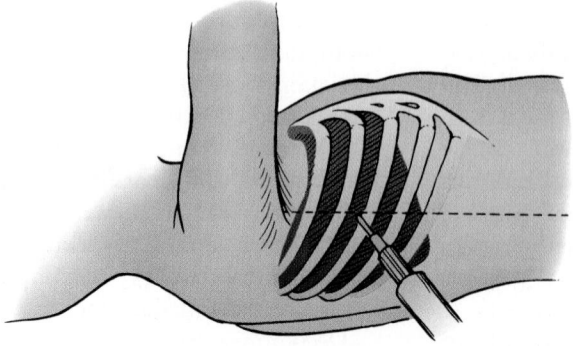

Figure 18-8 Needle decompression of tension pneumothorax. This procedure is performed only for tension pneumothorax in patients with hemodynamic instability.

The tube should then be secured with suture or tape and 10 to 20 cm H_2O suction or underwater seal applied. A tube open to the atmosphere can accomplish decompression. The end of the tube can be covered with a rubber glove, finger cot, or plastic bag; one-way flow evacuating the chest is the goal. It must be emphasized that this procedure is not without morbidity and should only be used by trained personnel under optimal conditions. Antibiotics with gram-positive coverage should be initiated if the pleural space is penetrated with an indwelling catheter or tube.

HEMOTHORAX. Hemothorax is usually associated with multiple rib fractures resulting from a direct blow to the chest. The primary cause of a hemothorax is laceration of the lung, intercostal vessel, or internal mammary artery. The victim complains of chest pain, tenderness associated with rib fractures, inspiratory pain, and dyspnea. Vocal fremitus is absent, percussion may be flat or dull, and breath sounds are diminished or absent.

A chest tube may be placed if proper equipment is available and evacuation may be delayed. Needle aspiration of a hemothorax is unnecessary in the immediate postinjury period and may precipitate a pneumothorax. As in the case of pneumothorax, treatment is strictly based on clinical deterioration. Isolated hemothorax from blunt trauma leading to shock is unusual and commonly associated with other massive injuries.

FLAIL CHEST. When a series of three or more ribs is fractured in both the anterior and posterior plane, a portion of the chest wall may be mechanically unstable. As negative intrathoracic pressure develops during inspiration, the unstable segment paradoxically moves inward and inhibits ventilation. A flail segment indicates a severe direct blow to the chest wall with associated multiple rib fractures and decreased tidal volumes, often with associated underlying pulmonary contusion. The contusion can be expected to progressively impair ventilation and oxygenation over the succeeding 48 hours. Victims will often tolerate a flail segment for the first 24 to 48 hours, after which they require mechanical ventilation.

Any victim with a flail segment should be rapidly evacuated. Because the victim is usually incapable of participating in evacuation, a litter should be prepared or aeromedical evacuation considered. Intercostal nerve block may assist in short-term management of pain and pulmonary toilet. Restrictive (to chest wall expansion during inhalation) external chest wall supports, including taping or extensive stabilization with sandbags, are contraindicated. These measures hinder chest wall movement, decrease vital capacity, and are less effective than intercostal nerve block in pain control. However, focal stabilization or cushioning of the flail segment only to control unnecessary motion and pain may provide minimal relief from the discomfort.

BLUNT CARDIAC INJURIES. Blunt cardiac injuries leading to pericardial tamponade or cardiac contusion are rare. Pericardial tamponade is life-threatening. The pericardial sac is fibrous and expands little. A small amount of intrapericardial blood can severely restrict diastolic function. Blunt injury resulting in tamponade is usually from chamber rupture and rarely survivable, particularly in a remote setting.

The diagnosis of tamponade can be difficult, particularly in the wilderness. Beck's triad, which consists of distended neck veins, hypotension, and muffled heart sounds, is present in less than 33% of cases of tamponade and is particularly difficult to ascertain under nonoptimal conditions. Pulsus paradoxus, an increase in the normal physiologic decrease in blood pressure with inspiration, may be indicative of tamponade. Kussmaul's sign, or a rise in venous pressure with spontaneous inspiration, is possible to assess outdoors.

Once pericardial tamponade is diagnosed, immediate evacuation is required. Treatment consists of median sternotomy in a hospital operating room. The only temporizing measure pending evacuation is pericardiocentesis. This procedure can be lifesaving, particularly if a cardiac injury with a slow leak exists. However, its application in the wilderness setting should occur only if there is a high index of suspicion, coupled with shock and impending death unresponsive to resuscitative efforts. A long (approximately 15 cm) 16- to 18-gauge needle with an overlying catheter is introduced through the skin 1 to 2 cm below and to the left of the xiphoid. The needle is advanced at a 45-degree angle with the tip directed at the tip of the left scapula. When the pericardial sac is entered, aspiration with a syringe follows. The catheter is left in place and secured for possible repeat aspirations as the victim's condition warrants. Immediate evacuation should follow.

Cardiac contusion is a rare, nebulous condition resulting from a severe blow to the precordium. An overlying sternal contusion or fracture may be present. The diagnosis should be suspected in an isolated high-velocity blow to the precordium with unexplained evidence of increased venous pressure and hemodynamic instability. Chest pain is invariably present, usually resulting from musculoskeletal contusion. Morbidity results from ensuing arrhythmias. The diagnosis, if hemodynamically significant, is difficult to distinguish from blunt trauma–induced tamponade. Diagnosis can only be definitively made at autopsy. Electrocardiographic abnormalities after injury have correlated with subsequent arrythmias.[52] In the wilderness setting, any person who is unstable or symptomatic from an arrhythmia should be evacuated. If evacuation is not possible, it is noteworthy that fatal arrhythmia potential decreases significantly after 24 hours.

TRAUMATIC ASPHYXIA. Traumatic asphyxia is a rare syndrome of craniocervical cyanosis, facial edema, petechiae, subconjunctival hemorrhage, and occasional hypoxemia-related neurologic symptoms that results from severe thoracic crush injury. In the wilderness environment, it is associated with land or mudslides, avalanches, or falling debris. Any significant blunt compressive force to the thorax can result in the syndrome. Children are particularly susceptible because of high compliance of the chest wall.[16] Traumatic asphyxia is not a benign condition, as a result of a high incidence of serious associated injuries,[67] and mortality in natural disasters is consequently high.[32] A number of studies have documented the severity of associated injuries, with the syndrome useful as an indicator of potentially lethal injury.[24] As documented in natural disasters, a significant crush injury component may accompany traumatic asphyxia.[32] Crush injuries and rhabdomyolysis are discussed in the Extremity Injury section of this chapter.

The pathophysiology of traumatic asphyxia involves two elements. The crush injury results in acute increases in intrathoracic pressure and thus inferior and superior vena caval pressures. Venous flow is reversed in the veins of the head, which contain no valves. Venous hypertension leads to capillary rupture and the characteristic facial edema and petechiae. Recognition of the physical findings is imperative in diagnosing the syndrome and identifying concomitant injuries (Figure 18-9).

Treatment consists of carefully extracting and, if necessary, immobilizing the victim. Rapid extrication is the single most important factor in improving survival. Establishment and maintenance of an airway is critical because significant facial and laryngeal edema may rapidly develop. Associated injuries should then be addressed in the primary survey. Subsequent care is supportive, consisting of airway control, administration of oxygen, head elevation of 30 degrees, treatment of associated injuries, and possible evacuation.

Mortality is low in civilian environments but higher in wilderness disaster settings. Mortality is due to pulmonary dysfunction and associated injuries. Morbidity is secondary to neurologic damage; however, the majority of neurologic sequelae clear within 24 to 48 hours. If the victim survives, long-term sequelae are rare.

Penetrating Chest Trauma. Penetrating chest trauma above the nipple line is associated with hemopneumothorax and may also be associated with significant visceral injury. A victim with penetrating chest trauma below the nipple line often has intraabdominal penetration in addition to possible thoracic injury. Such a victim requires immediate rapid evacuation.

The open ("sucking") chest wound produces profound intrathoracic physiologic alterations. Normal chest expansion creates negative intrathoracic pressure, which pulls air into the trachea and allows the lungs to expand. When the diaphragm and chest wall relax, positive pressure creates expiration. If the chest wall sustains an injury approximately two-thirds the tracheal diameter, negative intrathoracic pressure for inspiration is lost, the ipsilateral lung collapses, and the loss of negative intrathoracic pressure affects the good lung. Consequently, it is important to rapidly reconstruct chest wall integrity. Initially, this is most easily done by placing a hand over the sucking chest wound. Field treatment includes placing a petrolatum gauze on top of the wound, covering it with a 4 × 4 gauze pad, and taping it on three sides (Figure 18-10). The untaped fourth side serves as a relief mechanism to prevent tension pneumothorax. Persons with sucking chest wounds should be rapidly evacuated to sophisticated medical care.

Injuries to the Abdomen

Intraabdominal injuries in the wilderness setting are unique because they are often difficult to recognize. *However, once recognized or suspected, all intraabdominal injuries require rapid resuscitation and immediate evacua-*

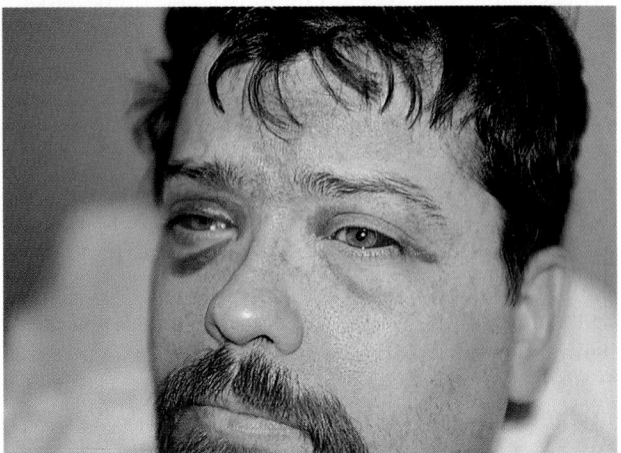

Figure 18-9 Typical clinical facial appearance of traumatic asphyxia.

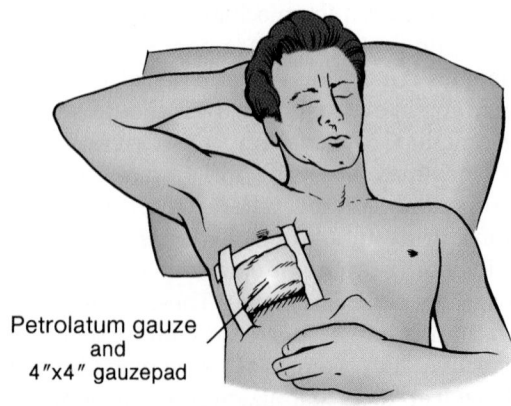

Petrolatum gauze
and
4"x4" gauzepad

Figure 18-10 Treatment of a sucking chest wound. Sealing the wound with a gel defibrillator pad works best because this pad adheres to wet or dry skin. Petrolatum gauze or Saran Wrap also works well. Note that one side is not sealed to allow egress of air.

tion. The abdomen represents the most frequent site of life-threatening hemorrhagic shock; however, in the wilderness setting, few diagnostic and treatment options exist.

Blunt Abdominal Trauma. Blunt intraabdominal injury is commonly associated with falls. Abdominal injuries are often associated with fractures or closed head injuries. Often the decision for evacuation is made on the basis of other injuries; however, the wilderness physician must be attuned to the potential for intraabdominal hemorrhage as an occult injury.

ANATOMY. For descriptive purposes, the abdomen may be divided into thoracic, true, and retroperitoneal compartments. The thoracic abdomen contains the liver, spleen, stomach, and diaphragm. The liver, spleen, and—more rarely—stomach may be injured by direct blows to the ribs or sternum. Twenty percent of persons with multiple left lower rib fractures have a ruptured spleen. A direct blow to the epigastrium may result in increased intraabdominal pressure with subsequent rupture of the liver or diaphragm. The true abdomen contains the small bowel, large bowel, and bladder. Isolated bowel injuries are rare in the wilderness setting. Blunt bladder or rectal injury usually occurs in conjunction with severe pelvic fracture and carries high mortality. The retroperitoneal abdomen contains the kidneys, ureters, pancreas, and great vessels. It is notoriously difficult to evaluate by physical examination. Life-threatening hemorrhage can occur into the true abdomen or the retroperitoneal space.

DIAGNOSIS. Although much progress has been made in the last decade to evaluate for the presence of blunt intraabdominal injury, modalities such as CT, ultrasound, and diagnostic peritoneal lavage are irrelevant in the wilderness setting. The wilderness physician must have a high index of suspicion and perform a superlative history and physical examination.

PHYSICAL EXAMINATION. The physician should look for signs of early shock: tachycardia, tachypnea, delayed capillary refill, weak or thready pulse, and cool or clammy skin. Physical examination of the abdomen begins with visualization and inspection. Contusions and abrasions may be the only harbingers of occult visceral injury. Periumbilical ecchymosis associated with abdominal hemorrhage (Cullen's sign) is virtually never present in a victim with acute abdominal trauma. Abdominal distention secondary to hemorrhage is a very late sign and never present before shock and cardiovascular collapse. Abdominal inspection should survey the flanks, lower chest, and back. Inspection of the back should follow palpation of the spine while the victim is supine. The victim should be very carefully logrolled if there is any suspicion of spinal injury.

Looking for muscle guarding, the examiner gently palpates the abdomen in all four quadrants. *Any* persistent guarding or tenderness after wilderness trauma mandates rapid evacuation. Percussion tenderness is an indicator of peritoneal irritation, also mandating evacuation. The presence or absence of bowel sounds has little prognostic significance. Bowel sounds may be present in the face of significant intraabdominal hemorrhage or, conversely, absent in victims when extraabdominal injuries induce ileus.

Referred pain to the left shoulder (Kerr's sign) strongly suggests the presence of a ruptured spleen. This pain is often exaggerated by placing the victim in Trendelenburg's position, increasing the amount of left upper quadrant blood irritating the diaphragm. Pain from the retroperitoneal abdomen associated with injuries to the kidney or pancreas may be referred to the back. However, referred pain is usually a late finding and not helpful in the evaluation of acute trauma.

Gross hematuria that does not clear immediately or is coupled with an associated injury, such as pelvic fracture or abdominal or back pain, requires immediate evacuation. To minimize blood loss, the victim should be kept stationary and the evacuation team brought as close to the victim as possible.

In a wilderness setting, rectal and vaginal examination adds little to the evacuation decision when evaluating for abdominal trauma. The unstable pelvic fracture associated with rectal and vaginal injuries is usually the determinant for evacuation.

Penetrating Abdominal Trauma. Penetrating intraabdominal injuries may result from gunshot, stab, or arrow wounds. The social context in which these injuries occur (accidental, intentional, or self-inflicted) makes little difference in the wilderness setting. Recrimination, guilt, and blame only interfere with the paramount goal of immediate evacuation.

GUNSHOT WOUNDS. Low-caliber gunshot injuries often present with small entrance and no exit wounds. High-caliber, high-velocity gunshot injuries may have relatively innocuous entrance wounds but may be associated with large, disfiguring exit wounds and extensive internal injuries. No matter what the caliber or trajectory and no matter where the entrance and exit, all gunshot wounds from the nipple line to the inguinal ligament should be presumed to have penetrated the abdominal cavity and created an intraabdominal injury. These injuries mandate immediate surgical intervention. A victim of gunshot wounds to the head, neck, chest, abdomen, or groin should undergo immediate evacuation accompanied by the administration of a single-agent broad-spectrum antibiotic, such as an oral fluoroquinolone (e.g., ciprofloxacin, 750 mg po bid). Gunshot wounds (hunting injuries) are discussed in Chapter 20.

Shotgun Injuries. Shotgun injuries to the torso are managed in the same manner as gunshot wounds. Shotgun injuries have potentially lower incidence of underlying visceral injury than gunshot wounds, but there is often extensive soft tissue damage requiring surgical debridement. The potential exists for delayed development of peritonitis from a single penetrating pellet to the viscera. Consequently, shotgun injuries should also be treated with emergency evacuation and a broad-spectrum antibiotic, as recommended above for gunshot wounds.

Occasionally, a close-range shotgun blast results in a soft tissue defect large enough for the injured bowel to extrude through the wound. The injured bowel should not be placed back into the abdomen. Injured bowel displaced from the abdominal cavity conceptually should be treated as though it were an enterocutaneous fistula. Since evacuation is often delayed in the wilderness, it is better to have fecal contents outside, rather than inside, the peritoneal cavity. The exteriorized bowel should be kept moist and covered at all times. Uncovered bowel outside the peritoneal cavity rapidly desiccates and becomes nonviable, mandating later surgical resection. Exposed bowel should be covered with an abdominal pack or cloth moistened with sterile saline at best, or at worst with potable water. The dressing should be checked and remoistened at least every 2 hours.

Stab Wounds. The penetrating object is usually a knife but may be as varied as a piton, ski pole, or tree limb. Any deep skin laceration from the nipple line to the groin should be considered to have damaged an intraabdominal organ. Whereas the odds of an abdominal gunshot wound injuring a visceral organ exceed 95%, the odds of a stab wound injuring a visceral organ are between 50% and 60%.

In certain urban hospitals, the high incidence of negative surgical explorations for stab wounds had led to a more selective approach toward patients with abdominal stab wounds.[65] This approach uses local wound exploration, diagnostic peritoneal lavage, and frequent physical examination.

Although no data exist addressing the management of stab wounds in the wilderness environment, the following approach is practical and reasonable. If the wound extends into the subcutaneous tissue, the evacuation decision depends on local wound exploration. This procedure is simple to perform, even in the wilderness environment. The skin and subcutaneous tissue are infiltrated with local anesthetic, and the laceration is extended several centimeters to clearly visualize the underlying anterior fascia. It is helpful to use lidocaine (Xylocaine) 1% with epinephrine to minimize slight but annoying bleeding that can impair visualization. The wound should never be probed with any instruments, particularly if overlying the ribs.

Wound exploration is confined to the area from the costal margin to the inguinal ligament. Local wound exploration is contraindicated in wounds that extend above the costal margin, because it is possible for such exploration to communicate with a small pneumothorax, potentially exacerbating respiratory distress.

If thorough exploration of the wound shows no evidence of anterior fascial penetration, and if the victim demonstrates no evidence of peritoneal irritation, the wound can be closed with tape (Steri-Strips) or adhesive bandages, dressed, and the evacuation process delayed. Physical examination should be performed every few hours for the next 24 hours. If no peritoneal signs develop and the victim feels constitutionally strong, a remote expedition may resume with caution and an eye to evacuation should the victim become ill.

In the wilderness environment, it is prudent to have a low threshold for evacuation because of technical difficulties in performing wound exploration—such as insufficient light and inadequate instruments. Persons who have been impaled by long objects, such as tree limbs or ski poles, should have the object left in place, and carefully shortened, if possible, to facilitate transport.

Pelvic Trauma

In the wilderness setting, fractures of the pelvis are generally associated with falls from significant heights, high-velocity ski accidents, or vehicular trauma.

Pelvic fractures can be lethal. With opening of the pelvic ring, there may be hemorrhage from the posterior pelvic venous complex and occasionally branches of the internal iliac artery. For hemodynamically unstable victims with severe pelvic fracture, resuscitative efforts should be instituted. Additionally, simple techniques to reduce any increased pelvic volume through the application of sheets or slings may slow bleeding.

The key factor in initial management of pelvic fractures is identification of posterior injury to the pelvic ring. Posterior ring fractures or dislocations are associated with a greater incidence of significant hemorrhage, neurologic injury, and mortality than are other pelvic fractures. The diagnosis of a posterior ring fracture is based on instability of the pelvis associated with posterior pain, swelling, ecchymosis, and motion. Persons with posterior ring fractures must be immediately evacuated on backboards, with care taken to minimize leg and torso motion.

The flank, scrotum, and perianal area should be inspected for blood at the urethral meatus, swelling or bruising, or a laceration in the perineum, vagina, rectum, or buttocks suggestive of an open pelvic fracture. The pelvis should be examined carefully once, without any aggressive rocking motion. The first indication of mechanical disruption is leg length discrepancy or rotational deformity in the absence of an obvious leg fracture or hip location. For more information on pelvic fracture, see Chapter 21.

Extremity Trauma

The majority of wilderness-related extremity injuries involve fractures and sprains, which are discussed in Chapter 21. This section focuses on the general field management of significant extremity vascular injury, traumatic amputation, and recognition and treatment of rhabdomyolysis.

Vascular Injuries. Injury to the major vessels supplying the limbs can occur with penetrating or blunt trauma. Fractures can produce injury to the vessels by direct laceration (rarely) or by stretching, which produces intimal flaps. Penetrating injuries can be devastating if transection of a vessel occurs. Significant vascular injuries, from both penetrating and blunt causes, can result in multiple vessel injury subtypes, each of which may be limb-threatening. Injury subtypes include laceration, transection, contusion with spasm, thrombosis, or aneurysm formation (true and false), external compression, and arteriovenous fistula. An accurate history, expeditious physical examination, and swift evacuation are the keys to life and limb salvage.

HISTORY. A complete history of the time and mechanism of injury is invaluable in planning further management. Although no absolute ischemia time has been established, a goal of less than 6 hours to reperfusion is prudent.[30] The amount of blood present at the scene should be quantified. A history of bright pulsatile blood that abates is suggestive of arterial injury. Thirty-three percent of victims with arterial injuries have intact distal pulses.

PHYSICAL EXAMINATION. Vascular examination in the field can be highly variable. Hypovolemia, hypothermia, and hostile conditions make an accurate examination challenging. Skin color and extremity warmth should be assessed first. Distal pallor and asymmetric hypothermia are suggestive of a vascular injury. Pulses should be palpated. In the upper extremity, the axillary, brachial, radial, and ulnar arteries should be assessed. In the lower extremity, the femoral, popliteal, posterior tibial, and dorsalis pedis pulses should be assessed. Location and direction of the wound should be determined, hemorrhage quantified, and the presence of hematomas or a palpable thrill noted.

A good neurologic examination that quantifies motor and sensory deficits is critical. Because of the high metabolic demands of peripheral nerves, disruption of oxygen delivery makes neuronal cells highly susceptible to ischemic death. Conversely, skeletal muscle is relatively resistant to ischemia. Loss of sensation or limb paralysis is an alarming sign of impending anoxic necrosis.

TREATMENT OF VASCULAR INJURIES. Significant hemorrhage should be identified and controlled in the primary survey. All hemorrhage should be controlled with direct pressure at the site of injury. Tourniquets should be applied only when direct pressure fails to control bleeding. Tourniquets should be released every 5 to 10 minutes to prevent further ischemia.

Hematomas should never be explored or manually expressed. Attempts to clamp or ligate vessels are not recommended. Frequent repeat neurovascular examinations are mandatory.

Once bleeding is controlled and the wound is covered with a sterile but noncompressive dressing, completion of the primary survey, identification and stabilization of associated injuries, and appropriate resuscitation with normal saline should follow. The extremity should be splinted to prevent further movement. The need for evacuation depends directly on the results of the physical examination. Examination results can be grouped into "hard signs," indicative of ischemia or continued hemorrhage, and "soft signs" that are suggestive but not indicative of ischemia (Boxes 18-3 and 18-4).

All victims with hard signs should be evacuated emergently. Based on current data, an isolated soft sign may warrant observation alone, depending on the remoteness of the expedition and the risks of evacuation. The data for observation of soft signs has emerged from hospital settings and must be applied with great caution in the wilderness. If soft signs are present, clinical suspicion is high, and evacuation can be accomplished

Box 18-3 VASCULAR "HARD SIGNS"

Pulsatile bleeding
Palpable thrill
Audible bruit
Expanding hematoma
Six "P's" of regional ischemia
    Pain
    Pulselessness
    Pallor
    Paralysis
    Paresthesia
    Poikilothermia

Box 18-4 VASCULAR "SOFT SIGNS"

Injury in proximity to major vessel
Diminished but palpable pulses
Isolated peripheral nerve deficit
History of minimal hemorrhage

safely, the victim should be transported and observed in a medical facility.

Traumatic Amputation. In the wilderness environment, amputation victims require immediate evacuation. Hemorrhage is controlled during the primary survey with direct pressure, and resuscitation is instituted. Tourniquets are rarely required. The victim should be kept warm and calm. Reassurance and analgesics should be administered. Amputations should only be completed if minimal tissue bridges exist and it is clear that the neurovascular supply has been interrupted.

Amputation of a mangled extremity, defined as an extremity with high-grade open fracture and soft tissue injury, should not be carried out in the wilderness except in the case of uncontrollable hemorrhage threatening the life of the victim, and then only by experienced surgical personnel. All other severely injured extremities should be wrapped in available sterile materials, splinted, and kept moist.

Amputated extremities should be cooled if possible, optimally in a plastic bag in ice or ice water. Avoid placing the extremity in direct contact with ice. Without cooling, the amputated extremity remains viable for only 4 to 6 hours; with cooling, viability may extend to 18 hours. The amputated extremity should accompany the victim throughout the course of the evacuation.

Crush Injuries and Rhabdomyolysis. Rhabdomyolysis is a potentially fatal syndrome that results from lysis of skeletal muscle cells. In its fulminant form, rhabdomyolysis can affect multiple organ systems. Compartment syndrome, renal failure, and cardiac arrest represent the major complications.

Any condition resulting in significant acute or subacute striated muscle damage can precipitate rhabdomyolysis. Crush injuries of the extremities and pelvis, revascularization of ischemic tissue, ischemic extremities, animal bite and snakebite,[17,23] frostbite, and traumatic asphyxia[32] can all result in rhabdomyolysis in a wilderness setting. Crush injuries are frequently a result of avalanches, falls from heights, or rock slides.

The pathophysiology of rhabdomyolysis remains controversial. The exact mechanism of muscle injury appears not to be simple direct force or isolated ischemia and is probably multifactorial.[32] The common cellular derangement is interference of the normal function of muscle cell membrane sodium-potassium adenosine triphosphatase (ATPase) with intracellular calcium influx and cell death.[74] After cell death, multiple intracellular constituents, including myoglobin, creatine kinase, potassium, calcium, and phosphate, are released into the systemic circulation.

The metabolic derangements of rhabdomyolysis depend directly on the release of intracellular muscle constituents. Myoglobinemia, hypercalcemia, hyperphosphatemia, hyperkalemia, hyperuricemia, metabolic acidosis, coagulation defects, and contracted intravascular volume result.

The clinical presentation of rhabdomyolysis may include muscle weakness, malaise, fever, tachycardia, abdominal pain, nausea and vomiting, or encephalopathy. Symptoms may mimic those of persons with spinal cord injury.[8] The danger of the syndrome lies in the cardiovascular effects of electrolyte disturbances and renal failure[66] secondary to changes in renal perfusion and direct toxicity of myoglobin to tubular cells.

Successful treatment relies on prompt diagnosis based on clinical signs and urinalysis, aggressive hydration, and forced diuresis. Myoglobin turns urine tea-colored, which is an important indicator of significant muscle death and need for aggressive treatment.

Normal saline should be administered intravenously at 1 to 2 L/hr to achieve a urine output of 100 to 300 ml/hr. Victims who are trapped in rubble should have resuscitation initiated before extrication, if possible. The addition of agents to alkalinize the urine and promote diuresis have been shown to improve clearance of myoglobin but not to alter survival. Additionally, diuretics may be detrimental in multisystem trauma victims who are hypovolemic. All victims demonstrating myoglobinuria should be evacuated.

Injuries to the Skin and Wilderness Wound Management

The goals of wilderness wound management are to minimize wound complications and promote healing. Treatment should begin with an approach to the victim as a trauma patient. Within the context of the primary survey, hemorrhage should be controlled. Then, the victim should be examined and the wound inspected. Steps to minimize infection should be undertaken, incorporating anesthesia, assessment of need for tetanus immunization and antibiotics, irrigation, and debridement. After attempts to minimize infection, a definitive plan should be established, including the need for evacuation (Box 18-5).

Box 18-5 GUIDELINES FOR WILDERNESS WOUND MANAGEMENT

1. Identify and stabilize associated traumatic injuries
2. Control hemorrhage
3. Examine wound
4. Minimize infection
   a. Tetanus immunization as indicated
   b. Antibiotics for high-risk wounds
   c. Irrigation
   d. Debridement
5. Implement definitive care

Wound Morphology. Major lacerations are often the most obvious sign of trauma; however, injuries to the integument are rarely life-threatening. Contusions, abrasions, and lacerations should force the examiner to focus on areas of potential occult injury. Contusions often overlie extremity fractures or, when present on the torso, suggest the potential for underlying visceral injury. Extremity lacerations may be associated with fractures or may extend into the joint space.

The four basic types of skin injuries are lacerations, crush injuries, stretch injuries, and puncture wounds. Lacerations rarely require closure in the wilderness environment. Commonly, multiple wound morphologies are present in the same injury, and an array of wound presentations are possible.

Crush injuries may be associated with significant tissue necrosis, impaired healing, increased rates of infection, and underlying muscle damage with subsequent rhabdomyolysis. Fortunately, they are rare in the wilderness.

Stretch injuries produce a split in the skin but, more important, may be associated with underlying nerve or tendon damage.

Puncture wounds often appear innocuous but have a high propensity for infection. Animal bite wounds, discussed in detail in Chapters 41 to 44, can manifest any of these wound morphologies alone or in combination.

Primary Survey. Many skin and soft tissue wounds encountered in the wilderness setting accompany significant injuries. Therefore the wound must never distract the physician from associated life-threatening injuries. The ATLS primary survey should be performed in the usual fashion.

Control of Hemorrhage. The vast majority of bleeding will be controlled with direct pressure, applying the most sterile covering available. Applying pressure over major arterial pressure points is discouraged, as is the use of tourniquets. In the event of bleeding not controlled by direct pressure, tourniquets may be applied with the knowledge that limb sacrifice is possible. If applied, tourniquets should be released every 5 to 10 minutes if possible to transiently restore perfusion and to assess if they are still necessary. Clamping bleeding vessels is not advised, since this may cause unnecessary neurovascular injury.

Physical Examination. Wound inspection and physical examination are critical in any setting. This phase of treatment may need to be abbreviated and should not delay packaging and evacuation. Although it is important to assess the extent of injury, including tissue loss and underlying musculoskeletal and neurovascular injury, aggressive wound exploration may worsen existing injuries.

Detailed knowledge of regional anatomy is useful. The detailed neurovascular examination should be documented before anesthesia and definitive care, including assessment of pulses and regional perfusion. The neurologic examination should quantify sensory and motor function, with particular attention to functional assessment of muscle groups traversing the injured region. Two point discrimination should be assessed in wounds involving the hands or fingers. Wounds over joints and tendons should be put through full range of motion.

Anesthesia. Pain management in the wilderness is discussed in Chapter 16. Administration of anesthesia occurs before mechanical wound cleansing and definitive care. The three methods of anesthetic administration briefly discussed here are topical, local, and regional.

Topical anesthesia was originally introduced for mucosal lacerations but has been shown to be effective for skin wounds. TAC (sterile tetracaine 0.5%, adrenalin 1:2000, and cocaine 11.8% in saline) has been used with success as a topical anesthetic. Complications have included seizure and death.[90] An alternative preparation consisting of lidocaine, adrenalin, and tetracaine (LAT) has been shown to be as effective as TAC without the associated complications.[29] Topical anesthetics may be soaked into a sterile gauze and placed on the wound surface for 7 to 10 minutes. Disadvantages of topical anesthetic include potential for a slightly increased risk of infection and less versatility than locally injected lidocaine.

Local anesthesia is the standard method for achieving soft tissue analgesia. Typically, 1% lidocaine without epinephrine is used. In adults, the maximum injectable dose of lidocaine is 300 to 400 mg subcutaneously. Lidocaine should not be injected directly from within the wound to the periphery because this increases the chance of introducing bacteria deeper into the soft tissue.[60] The injection should proceed from the periphery of the wound, with each successive needle stick entering the skin through a previously anesthetized area.

Local anesthesia can be administered with relatively little discomfort using a 25-gauge needle and a 1-ml tuberculin syringe. Although using a small syringe increases the time to anesthetize a larger wound, this method minimizes both the anesthetic dose and the distortion of soft tissue planes, facilitating tissue repair. Pain associated with administration of local anesthesia is due to the acidity and stretching of nerve endings within the dermis and subcutaneous tissue. Burning sensation associated with lidocaine injection is directly proportional to the rate of administration. Warming the local anesthetic,[44] buffering the solution with sodium bicarbonate to a concentration of 1%, and administering anesthetic slowly in small doses all minimize pain.

Regional anesthesia, defined as sensory nerve blockade proximal to the wound, is an excellent mode of anesthetizing wounds of the upper and lower extremities. Two types are regional nerve block and Bier block. Regional nerve blocks require skill and a detailed knowledge of regional anatomy. They are not suitable for the first-time user in the wilderness environment.

The Bier block is easier to administer and is preferred in the wilderness setting. It involves injection of local anesthetic into a cannulated hand or foot vein, with concurrent control of venous outflow using a tourniquet.

Irrigation. Once the wound is anesthetized, irrigation, debridement, and closure can proceed. Irrigation removes dirt, debris, foreign bodies, and bacteria from the wound. Irrigation has been extensively studied in traumatic wounds and clearly results in a decreased incidence of infection, reducing infection rates as much as twentyfold when proper technique is used.

The type of irrigation fluid and the technique utilized will be resource-dependent in the wilderness setting. The cleanest fluid available should be used. Wilderness fresh water sources that are not grossly contaminated can be boiled or filtered.[31] Any concentration of sterile crystalloid solution can be used, although normal saline remains the most readily available, economical, and cost-effective irrigant. Recent data suggest that tap water may be as effective as normal saline.[62]

The amount of irrigation necessary is difficult to quantify. Some authors use 60 ml of irrigant per centimeter wound length as a guide,[44] but in the wilderness setting where precision is more difficult to attain, irrigation should be continued in amounts and time intervals sufficient to remove visible debris from the wound.

Many bactericidal and bacteriostatic irrigants, including commercial soaps, ethyl alcohol, iodine solutions, and hydrogen peroxide, are available in wilderness first-aid kits. Many of these agents have been shown to result in significant microcellular destruction of tissues[14] and, when used in high concentrations, may impair wound healing. They offer no advantage over copious irrigation with sterile water or crystalloid. Although addition of antibiotics to irrigant solutions is an attractive concept, they are costly, difficult to store, and offer no advantage over irrigation with sterile water alone.

The method of wound irrigation, as well as the pressures used, have been studied extensively. The goals of irrigation are to remove bacteria, assist in the mechanical debridement of necrotic tissue, and remove foreign bodies that can impair subsequent wound healing. Optimal irrigation pressures are 5 to 8 psi, delivered through a syringe with a 16- to 20-gauge needle.

In summary, irrigation consisting of normal saline or sterilized potable water should be delivered in a continuous fashion by the most sterile implement available at a pressure sufficient to dislodge debris but not overtly damage tissue.

Debridement. Like irrigation, debridement has been shown to decrease the incidence of wound infection. Additionally, debridement has the potential to improve long-term cosmesis. Debridement should be carried out sharply. Scrubbing the wound with abrasive materials does not improve infection rates and may cause damage to healthy tissue. Similarly, soaking the wound has never been shown to improve outcome. Hair removal should be undertaken only if it impairs visualization and inspection of the wound,[90] or if tape is to be used as a method of temporary closure.

The goal of debridement in the wilderness should be to remove grossly contaminated or devitalized tissue and to remove foreign bodies and bacteria embedded in such tissue. The extent of tissue removal should be based on the experience and training of the caregiver.

Tetanus Prophylaxis. The spores of *Clostridium tetani* are ubiquitous in the environment, in such places as soil, animal teeth, and saliva. Any animal bite that penetrates the skin can be responsible for a tetanus infection. The majority of cases of tetanus infection in the United States follow failure to attain adequate immunization.[76] This fact accentuates the preventable nature of tetanus infections and the essential role of proper immunization. If available in the wilderness setting, tetanus prophylaxis should be administered as outlined in Table 18-3.

Definitive Care of Lacerations. "Definitive" care may have many definitions, depending on the setting. The planned approach to management of wounds in the wilderness is determined by a combination of morphology of the wound, infection risk factors, available resources, level of expertise, and type of expedition.

Major lacerations or those associated with significant injury should be evacuated. If wound management cannot acceptably minimize infection risk factors, the victim should be evacuated. In general, wounds that can be closed or managed open and that do not impose excessive infection risk factors and do not immobilize the expedition member or group can be treated definitively in the wilderness. The wound must not impair physical ability in a way that the victim risks further injury or jeopardizes group safety.

WOUND CLOSURE. Lacerations can be closed if they are small to intermediate in size; have minimal infection risk factors; are on well-vascularized regions, such the scalp and face; are less than 6 hours old; and have no anatomic contraindications.

TABLE 18-3. Tetanus Prophylaxis

HISTORY OF IMMUNIZATION (DOSES)	CLEAN MINOR WOUNDS		MAJOR DIRTY WOUNDS	
	TOXOID*	TIG†	TOXOID	TIG
Unknown	Yes	No	Yes	Yes
None to one	Yes	No	Yes	Yes
Two	Yes	No	Yes	No (unless wound older than 24 hours)
Three or more				
Last booster within 5 years	No	No	No	No
Last booster within 10 years	No	No	Yes	Yes
Last booster more than 10 years ago	Yes	No	Yes	Yes

*Toxoid: Adult: 0.5 ml dT intramuscularly (IM).
      Child less than 5 years old: 0.5 ml DPT IM.
      Child older than 5 years: 0.5 ml DT IM.
†Tetanus immune globulin (TIG): 250 to 500 units IM in limb contralateral to toxoid.

Closure may be accomplished with suture, staples, tape and similar bandages, or adhesives. Tape, and—less frequently—adhesives, are viable alternatives to sutures. Healing and cosmetic outcome depend directly on dermal apposition, which is the goal of any closure method.

Advantages of sutures include meticulous closure and high wound tensile strength. The primary disadvantage is the skill necessary to place them. The suture selected is dictated by morphology of the wound. To simplify selection in the wilderness environment, absorbable sutures, such as chromic gut and polyglactin (Vicryl), should be used to close deep layers and for subcuticular closures. Nonabsorbable suture, such as nylon (Ethilon) and polypropylene (Prolene), should be used on the skin. Silk is reactive, has poor tensile strength, and should be avoided. *No wound should be sutured by an individual who is inexperienced in basic surgical technique.* Additionally, no wound incurred in the wilderness is truly risk-free regarding infection. In general, the safest management strategy for lacerations in the wilderness setting is open management or closure with nonsuture alternatives.

Surgical staples are easily placed, are nonreactive, have lower infection rates than sutures, and minimize time of closure.[90] They should be avoided on areas of cosmetic importance, such as the face.

Tapes and adhesives offer a preferable alternative to sutures. Tape and adhesive strips (e.g., Steri-Strips) are easily applied and require little technical ability. If a wound is appropriate for closure, tape offers a rapid, safe, painless, and inexpensive alternative to sutures and staples.[27] The only requirement of tape use is conformity to principles of dermal apposition. Disadvantages of tape include need for adhesive solutions, such as benzoin; low tensile strength; and lack of applicability over any region

of tension.[90] A critical limiting factor in wilderness use of tape closure is the need for the wound to remain dry.

Tissue adhesives in wound closure have been studied for 20 years.[26] Recently, use of octylcyanoacrylate and similar synthetic agents have been shown to be equal in strength and cosmesis compared with sutures at 1 year.[78] Advantages of adhesives include ease of application, safety, patient comfort, and low cost.[91] Similar to tape, immediate tensile strength is poor and dehiscence is more likely compared with sutures.[90] If closure is possible and other means are unavailable or impractical, adhesives may be used.

SCALP LACERATIONS. The extent and severity of scalp lacerations are often initially obscured by surrounding hair that is matted with blood. Hydrogen peroxide and water effectively remove blood from hair, although hydrogen peroxide should not be used to irrigate the wound. Interestingly, and most likely owing to the vascularity of the scalp, irrigation did not alter outcome in clean lacerations in one study.[41]

Hair surrounding the laceration is removed only if absolutely necessary to clean the wound using a safety razor. Hair removal should be limited to the immediate area of the laceration, since the surrounding hair can later be twisted into strands and used to approximate the wounds edges if necessary. Once wound margins have been identified, anesthetic should be applied.

The key to examination of the scalp is determining the integrity of the galea. Significant degloving injury or galeal laceration may mandate evacuation. The scalp is highly vascularized. An extensive scalp laceration bleeds freely, and if it follows a fall or direct blow to the head, may be associated with an underlying skull fracture. Superficial scalp lacerations often bleed freely and may require pressure dressings to achieve hemostasis.

Minor scalp lacerations can be effectively treated in the wilderness setting, after following the aforementioned infection-minimizing steps. Of note, debridement of scalp wounds should be kept to a minimum because it may be difficult to mobilize wound edges to cover the resulting soft tissue defect. In addition, cosmesis is not a significant concern on the hair-covered scalp. Acceptable closure of a minor scalp laceration can be performed using strands of hair to approximate wound edges. This method minimizes shaving.

FACIAL LACERATIONS. Facial lacerations are relatively simple to manage because they rarely damage underlying structures and are well vascularized. If suspicion exists regarding damage to cranial nerves or the parotid duct, the wound should be managed in an open fashion. Debridement should be limited to obviously necrotic tissue. Because of vascularity of the face, infection is rare, and most wounds can be closed. For small wounds, tape is a useful closure technique.

TORSO LACERATIONS. Torso lacerations require evaluation for fascial penetration. Anterior fascial penetration in the torso converts the wound from a skin wound to one requiring management of underlying chest or abdominal structures. Tissue debridement may be more aggressive over the torso, since surrounding tissue planes can be mobilized for closure. Adipose tissue should not be approximated with suture, and subdermal dead space should be obliterated with deep, nonadipose approximating sutures.

Hand Injuries. Severe contusions to the hand commonly occur with crush or rope injuries. The hand should be carefully protected if marked swelling and pain with motion are present. If no joint instability or fracture is identified, a bulky hand dressing should be applied with the wrist dorsiflexed 10 degrees, the thumb abducted, and the metacarpophalangeal joints flexed 90 degrees, known as the position of function. Cotton wadding or bandages can be placed in the palm and between the fingers, and an elastic bandage can be used as an overwrap. A volar splint allows this position to be maintained until definitive care is reached.

Lacerations of the finger flexor or extensor tendons occur with accidents involving knives or other sharp objects. A flexor tendon laceration, partial or complete, can be a serious problem if not repaired early. The open wound should be cleansed and loosely taped closed if no infection risk factors are present, and the finger should be splinted in slight flexion at the interphalangeal joints and in 90 degrees of flexion at the metacarpophalangeal joint. To achieve optimal results, this injury should be managed by a hand surgeon within the first 3 to 5 days.

For an extensor tendon, the open wound should be cleansed and taped closed, and a splint should be applied with the metacarpophalangeal joint in slight flexion and the interphalangeal joint extended. The victim should be seen by an orthopedic surgeon within 7 days.

The nerves most commonly injured by laceration include the superficial radial nerve at the wrist, ulnar nerve at the elbow or wrist, and median nerve at the wrist. Digital nerves are commonly lacerated in accidents with knives. In general, the wound should be cleansed and taped loosely and a splint should be applied to the wrist and hand. The victim should see a hand surgeon within 7 days.

Puncture Wounds. Puncture wounds carry significant infection risk where organic contamination is frequent. Significant puncture wounds to the torso should be treated according to the guidelines outlined in the section on penetrating trauma to the chest and abdomen. Puncture wounds to the extremities should be unroofed if they are proximal to the wrist or ankle. The unroofed wound should be irrigated as previously described and then packed open with sterile gauze. Delayed primary closure with tape can occur at 48 to 96 hours. Puncture wounds to the hands and feet should not be explored in the absence of detailed knowledge of anatomy. If this expertise is not available, the wound should be cleaned and the victim started on antibiotics, such as cephalexin (Keflex), 500 mg po q6h.

If the skin is punctured with a fishhook, the skin surrounding the entry point should be cleansed with soap and water. Fishhook removal techniques are discussed in Chapter 20.

Antibiotic Use and Infectious Complications. The use of prophylactic antibiotics for wounds incurred in the wilderness is not recommended. Antibiotic treatment usually begins after the injury has occurred and therefore is never truly "prophylactic." The use of antibiotics in lacerations and bite wounds should be confined to victims with significant infection-risk factors, such as animal bites, heavily contaminated wounds, or comorbid medical conditions. This includes high-risk wounds, such as puncture wounds and those occurring on the hands. Debridement and irrigation are far more important than antibiotics in eliminating infection and remain the mainstay of risk reduction in any wound incurred in the wilderness.

If antibiotics are indicated, selection should be tailored by available resources and coverage of likely contaminating organisms. Many single-agent broad-spectrum oral antibiotics are available. If any sign of infection develops in a wound—closed or open—including pain, discharge, erythema, edema, or fever, antibiotics should be administered. In an infected closed wound, the adhesive or sutures should be removed and the wound irrigated. Wet-to-dry dressings with normal saline should be started and the wound closely observed. Elevation and splinting may assist in relieving pain.

Management of Animal Attacks and Bite Wounds.
See Chapters 41 to 44.

WILDERNESS SURGICAL EMERGENCIES

The Acute Abdomen

In the wilderness, the critical distinction between the surgical and nonsurgical abdomen determines whether the victim should be evacuated. A myriad of nonsurgical conditions mimic a surgical abdomen. It has been extensively reported that the bite of the black widow spider (*Latrodectus mactans*) can induce abdominal pain indistinguishable from a surgical acute abdomen,[49] and mushroom ingestion can cause severe gastroenteritis.[82] Pain, anorexia, nausea, vomiting, and fever are characteristic manifestations of an acute abdominal disorder. Tenderness and guarding are the hallmarks of peritoneal irritation and suggest that surgery is needed.

The approach to someone with abdominal pain begins with a detailed history that includes the person's age, gender, systemic symptoms, and past medical history. This information provides a framework for more detailed questioning about the character of the pain, its mode and time of onset, severity, and precipitating and palliating factors.

In persons 15 to 40 years of age, females are more likely to have abdominal pain, but males have a higher incidence of surgical disease. Common genitourinary causes for abdominal pain in men include epididymitis, renal colic, urinary retention, and testicular torsion. Common causes in women include pelvic inflammatory disease (PID), urinary tract infection, dysmenorrhea, ruptured ovarian cyst, and ectopic pregnancy.

Pain is the hallmark of a surgical abdomen (Table 18-4). It can be characterized by mode and time of onset, severity, localization, and precipitating factors. The onset of abdominal pain can be explosive, rapid, or gradual. The person who is suddenly seized with explosive, agonizing pain is most likely to have rupture of a hollow viscus into the free peritoneal cavity. Colic of

TABLE 18-4. Differential Diagnostic Features of Abdominal Pain

DISEASE	LOCATION OF PAIN AND PRIOR ATTACKS	MODE OF ONSET AND TYPE OF PAIN	ASSOCIATED GASTRO-INTESTINAL SYMPTOMS	PHYSICAL EXAMINATION
Acute appendicitis	Periumbilical or localized generally to right lower abdominal quadrant	Insidious to acute and persistent	Anorexia common; nausea and vomiting in some	Low-grade fever; epigastric tenderness initially; later, right lower quadrant
Intestinal obstruction	Diffuse	Sudden onset; crampy	Vomiting common	Abdominal distention; high-pitched rushes
Perforated duodenal ulcer	Epigastric; history of ulcer in many	Abrupt onset; steady	Anorexia; nausea and vomiting	Epigastric tenderness; involuntary guarding
Diverticulitis	Left lower quadrant; history of previous attacks	Gradual onset; steady or crampy	Diarrhea common	Fever common; mass and tenderness in left lower quadrant
Acute cholecystitis	Epigastric or right upper quadrant; may be referred to right shoulder	Insidious to acute	Anorexia; nausea and vomiting	Right upper quadrant pain
Renal colic	Costovertebral or along course or ureter	Sudden; severe and sharp	Frequently nausea and vomiting	Flank tenderness
Acute pancreatitis	Epigastric penetrating to back	Acute; persistent, dull, severe	Anorexia; nausea and vomiting common	Epigastric tenderness
Acute salpingitis	Bilateral adnexal; later, may be generalized	Gradually becomes worse	Nausea and vomiting may be present	Cervical motion elicits tenderness; mass if tuboovarian abscess is present
Ectopic pregnancy	Unilateral early; may have shoulder pain after rupture	Sudden or intermittently vague to sharp	Frequently none	Adnexal mass; tenderness

renal or biliary origin may also be sudden in onset but seldom causes pain severe enough to prostrate the victim. If someone has rapid onset of pain that quickly worsens, acute pancreatitis, mesenteric thrombosis, or small bowel strangulation should be suspected. The person with gradual onset of pain is likely to have peritoneal inflammation, such as that accompanying appendicitis or diverticulitis.

Severity of the pain may be characterized as excruciating, severe, dull, or colicky. Excruciating pain unresponsive to narcotics suggests an acute vascular lesion, such as rupture of an abdominal aneurysm or intestinal infarction. Both conditions are unusual in the wilderness environment. Severe pain readily controlled by medication is characteristic of peritonitis from a ruptured viscus or acute pancreatitis. Dull, vague, and poorly localized pain suggests an inflammatory process and is a common initial presentation of appendicitis.

Colicky pain characterized as cramps and rushes is suggestive of gastroenteritis. The pain from mechanical small bowel obstruction is also colicky but has a rhythmic pattern, with pain-free intervals alternating with severe colic. The peristaltic rushes associated with gastroenteritis are not necessarily coordinated with colicky pain.

Physical examination of the abdomen is initiated by inspection. Valuable clues to the underlying condition that may be obtained in this manner include stigmata of cirrhosis, distention, hyperperistalsis, or incarcerated herniae. The victim may not be able lie still, which is indicative of renal or biliary colic. Persons lying perfectly still frequently have peritoneal inflammation. Auscultation is helpful if the classic "rushes and tinkles" of small bowel obstruction are present. Palpation in the wilderness setting is most helpful in documenting the presence or absence of peritoneal signs. Shake or percussive tenderness, particularly in the context of fever, nausea, and or vomiting, indicates a need for evacuation. Rectal and vaginal examinations should be performed, if practical.

General Field Treatment Principles. When evaluating someone with a possible emergent surgical condition in the wilderness, correctly identifying the etiology of a given condition is less important than identifying peritoneal inflammation and the need for operation.

When dealing with a surgical abdomen or other condition requiring evacuation, adjuncts to definitive hospital treatment can be initiated in the field.

Dehydration and intravascular volume depletion accompany many surgical conditions, particularly when the disease process has progressed and evacuation is delayed. Initiation of crystalloid resuscitation in the field is intuitively beneficial for persons who have developed or have the potential to develop septic or hypovolemic shock. Dehydration is common in the wilderness, and frank hypovolemia can result from vomiting associated with gastroenteritis, appendicitis, renal colic, and small bowel obstruction. Perforated viscus, pancreatitis, cholecystitis, small bowel obstruction, PID, and necrotizing soft tissue infections all may feature volume depletion. The goal in the wilderness setting is to recognize the signs of hypovolemia and initiate resuscitation to decrease eventual perioperative morbidity.

Nasogastric tube decompression of the stomach can prove beneficial in alleviating emesis secondary to abdominal pain or obstruction. Large-bore catheters are best and can be easily aspirated with a syringe. Placement should be confirmed by aspiration of gastric contents or auscultation of gastric air after insufflation of the stomach.

Foley catheters are becoming increasingly more available in wilderness first-aid kits. Recording urine output provides an effective estimate of intravascular volume status. Foley catheter placement should never hinder the possibility of ambulatory evacuation.

Appendicitis. Acute appendicitis is the most common cause of a surgical abdomen in persons under the age of 30 years. Acute appendicitis is really more than one single disease entity. In terms of physical signs and symptoms, appendicitis proceeds from inflammation to obstruction to ischemia to perforation, all within approximately 36 hours. Symptoms reflect the stage of the disease. Unfortunately, the time frame for the progression of clinical events is highly variable.

Differential diagnosis of appendicitis includes gastroenteritis and mesenteric adenitis, the most common inflammatory disorders in adults. The first symptom of gastroenteritis is typically vomiting, which precedes the onset of pain and is often associated with diarrhea; it is rarely associated with localizing signs or muscular spasm. Bowel sounds are usually hyperactive. A rectal examination rarely shows abnormalities in gastroenteritis but frequently does so in adults with appendicitis.

Mesenteric adenitis is often preceded by an upper respiratory infection and is associated with vague abdominal discomfort that often begins in the right lower quadrant. Abdominal examination reveals only mild right lower quadrant tenderness that is often not well localized.

The incidence of PID in young women with abdominal pain confounds the diagnosis of appendicitis. Some clinicians have documented a relationship between menses and onset of pain. If abdominal pain occurs within 7 days of menses, the incidence of PID is twice that of appendicitis. If onset of pain occurs greater than 8 days from menses, appendicitis is twice as likely as PID. This history with a pelvic examination may enable the examiner to differentiate between the two entities.

Acute appendicitis mandates evacuation because untreated perforation retains significant mortality. Broad-spectrum antibiotics (if IV capability, cefotetan [Cefotan] 2 g IV q12h, or as an alternate, piperacillin/taxobactam [Zosyn] 4.5 g IV q8h; if only oral antibiotic capabilities, a fluoroquinolone, such as ciprofloxacin [Cipro] 750 mg po bid) should be initiated, attempting coverage against gram-negative and anaerobic organisms. Intravenous crystalloid resuscitation should be initiated, particularly if the victim is older or perforation is suspected, and the victim should be placed at bowel rest.

Acute Cholecystitis and Biliary Colic. Biliary colic refers to pain induced by obstruction of the cystic duct, usually by gallstones. The label of this condition as "colic" is a misnomer, since the pain is usually constant. The condition is rarely seen before adulthood and is several times more common in women than in men. A sufferer often relates a past history of gallstones and previous episodes of similar pain, which is described as constant right upper quadrant and/or epigastric pain, radiating to the right scapula and back. Onset ranges from insidious to acute and frequently follows a meal. The episode usually lasts 15 minutes to 1 hour and then abates.[63] If pain is severe, nausea and vomiting may be present (60% to 70%).

Acute cholecystitis is an infection of the gallbladder secondary to cystic duct obstruction, usually from gallstones. In the wilderness setting, it is useful to think of these interrelated conditions as a continuum of one unified disease process. Both biliary colic and cholecystitis present with right upper quadrant pain; however, biliary colic has the potential to be self-limiting and may not require evacuation. Not all persons with biliary colic develop cholecystitis, and signs of infection should be excluded.

Cholecystitis symptoms typically escalate in severity. Pain that persists more than 1 to 2 hours is suspicious for cholecystitis, particularly when accompanied by fever, more significant nausea and vomiting, and right upper quadrant rebound tenderness. Recent studies have shown that fever may be an unreliable predictor of severity of infection.[36] Acute cholecystitis mandates hospitalization, and evacuation plans should be instituted. The disease can progress to gangrenous changes in the gallbladder wall, leading to perforation and death if untreated.

The definitive treatment of cholecystitis is cholecystectomy. In the field, IV antibiotics (ampicillin/sulbactam [Unasyn] 3 g IV q6h or PO alternative ciprofloxacin [Cipro] 750 mg po bid) should be given, directed at common biliary organisms, including *Escherichia coli*, *Klebsiella*, *Bacteroides*, *Enterobacter*, *Streptococcus*, and *Proteus* species. Oral antibiotics with optimal bioavailability should be initiated in the absence of parenteral

forms, ensuring the broadest spectrum of coverage available. As with most abdominal infections, IV hydration should be started in the field. If significant nausea and vomiting are present, nasogastric decompression may improve comfort and prevent aspiration.

Peptic Ulcer Disease. The incidence of peptic ulcer disease (PUD) is decreasing in the United States. With the advent of treatment of *Helicobacter pylori* infections and the variety of acid-reducing agents available, it is less often a disease seen by surgeons. The exception is perforation of gastric or duodenal ulcer, which should be considered in the differential diagnosis of acute abdomen in the wilderness. Victims frequently relate a history of PUD and need for medication. This history, in combination with acute onset of unrelenting epigastric pain radiating to the back, is suspicious for perforation of an ulcer.

The physical examination greatly assists in the differentiation between simple ulcer disease symptoms and perforation. Pain may be severe. Gastric secretions are caustic to the peritoneum, and as a result, the abdomen frequently displays a rigid, boardlike character with associated diffuse peritoneal signs.

History and examination consistent with gastric or duodenal perforation mandates evacuation. Dehydration may be significant. IV resuscitation should be started and the victim placed on bowel rest. Antibiotics are not indicated.

Diverticulitis. Diverticulitis is localized infection of a colonic diverticulum. Impacted material in the diverticulum, usually feces, leads to a localized inflammatory process that can lead to abscess formation and perforation. Diverticulitis presents over a wide range of severity, ranging from mild, localized infection to intraabdominal catastrophe. It is more common in middle age; one third of the population over the age of 45 have diverticula, 20% of which will develop diverticulitis.[86]

Victims often relate a history of previous attacks. Pain is typically described as gradual in onset and localized in the left lower quadrant of the abdomen, although right-sided diverticulitis can occur. Diarrhea and fever are frequently associated complaints. Examination findings range from mild left lower quadrant abdominal tenderness to frank peritonitis, depending on the severity of the underlying infection.

Treatment in the wilderness setting consists of hydration, bowel rest, antibiotics, and evacuation. If evacuation is impossible or significantly delayed, oral broad-spectrum antibiotics may be effective. Mild cases of diverticulitis are frequently treated on an outpatient basis with oral antibiotics,[80] such as broad-spectrum fluoroquinolones, such as cefotetan 2 g IV q12h, or an alternative oral fluoroquinolone such as ciprofloxacin 750 mg po bid. Antibiotic therapy is directed primarily at gram-negative aerobic and anaerobic bacteria, and single-agent therapy covering these organisms has been demonstrated to be as effective as multiple-agent regimens.[48] Because of unpredictability of response to antibiotic treatment, evacuation is indicated.

Mechanical Small Bowel Obstruction. Small bowel obstruction is a true emergency in the wilderness. When the obstruction is complete, expedient surgery is the only treatment. Small bowel obstruction in the United States is almost invariably the result of adhesions from previous laparotomy or incarceration of abdominal hernias, and the history often makes the diagnosis. Victims complain of sudden onset of diffuse, crampy abdominal pain associated with vomiting and obstipation. With progression of the process to strangulation and infarction of bowel, fever and tachycardia develop.

Late physical examination findings reveal a distended, tympanitic abdomen. Although variable, high-pitched tinkling bowel sounds suggest obstruction. A thorough inspection for hernias should be performed.

Progression of examination findings to frank peritonitis is alarming and suggests ischemic bowel. The adage, "Don't let the sun set on a small bowel obstruction," is sound advice in the wilderness setting. All persons suspected of having a small bowel obstruction should be evacuated immediately. In the interim, the stomach should be decompressed with a nasogastric tube to relieve vomiting and abdominal distention, and aggressive IV hydration should be started.

Incarcerated Abdominal Wall Hernias. Abdominal wall hernias are common; groin herniorrhaphy is the most common major general surgical operation performed in the United States.[59] Hernias can become incarcerated or strangulated, which constitutes a surgical emergency. Seventy-five percent of hernias occur in the groin[83]; the majority of incarcerated hernias presenting in the wilderness setting will be inguinal hernias. Other common hernias with the capacity for incarceration are incisional and umbilical hernias.

Many people live with bulging asymptomatic hernias. Others manually reduce symptomatic hernias. New painful hernias or known hernias that can no longer be reduced elicit concern. The pain of inguinal hernias is usually intermittent. A description of constant pain is suspicious for incarceration. Associated symptoms of fever, tachycardia, nausea, and vomiting are indicative of possible incarceration or strangulation.

On physical examination, a mass should be sought along the course of the spermatic cord. Masses may present from the external inguinal ring to the scrotum. The differential diagnosis for painful inguinal or scrotal masses includes lymphadenopathy, testicular torsion, and epididymitis. Associated tenderness of the spermatic cord may be present. A painful mass at the umbilicus or previous incision site, or below the inguinal ring, indicates possible incarcerated umbilical, incisional, or femoral hernia, respectively.

Bowel within an incarcerated hernia sac can become gangrenous in as little as 4 to 5 hours;[59] therefore it is important to attempt to identify time of incarceration. The decision to evacuate is determined by the presence of contraindications to manual reduction (see below), which are essentially physical signs that progression to strangulation may be occurring.

Femoral hernias should not be reduced. The danger is en masse reduction of compromised or gangrenous bowel. Contraindications to reduction include associated signs of toxicity, such as fever, tachycardia, or evidence of bowel obstruction in association with a painful irreducible mass. If the hernia itself is exquisitely tender to palpation and the overlying skin is erythematous and warm, the hernia should not be reduced. Victims with incarcerated hernias with signs of systemic or local toxicity should be evacuated. Similarly, victims with irreducible hernias—which require emergent surgery—should be evacuated.

A newly incarcerated hernia without contraindications to reduction may be reduced by personnel experienced in such techniques. Gentle pressure is exerted on the hernia mass toward the inguinal ring, optimally with the victim flat and hips elevated. Analgesia and sedation may aid in reduction. Gangrenous bowel can rarely be reduced by this method.[90] If successful, the victim should be closely observed for signs of recurrence or abdominal pain.

Urologic Emergencies

Renal colic describes a symptom complex resulting from acute obstruction of the urinary tract secondary to calculus formation. The goal of the wilderness physician is to recognize the symptom complex and institute treatment. After obstruction of the urinary tract, the pain crescendo of renal colic begins in the flank. The pain progresses anteriorly over the abdomen and radiates to the groin and testes in men and the labia in women. Because the autonomic nervous system transmits visceral pain, many abdominal complaints may manifest. Nausea and vomiting are common. With severe colic, the victim writhes in pain and is unable to find a comfortable position.

Physical findings are less revealing than is the review of systems. Tenderness to deep palpation of the region of obstruction or percussion of the flank is present. Diagnosis in the wilderness is assisted by the presence of gross hematuria.

Management is directed primarily at pain control. Although almost universally deployed, forced diuresis may reduce ureteral peristalsis. Thus forced oral fluids or aggressive IV hydration are of questionable benefit.[97] The majority of calculi pass spontaneously in 4 to

6 hours. The goal of management is to control pain until passage of the stone has occurred. A number of pharmacologic approaches may be used. Nonsteroidal antiinflammatory drugs, such as ibuprofen and ketorolac, have been shown to be effective in the management of renal colic.[97] Narcotic analgesics are most effective given parenterally; however, agents such as meperidine, codeine, and hydromorphone (Dilaudid) may be given orally. For symptoms uncontrolled by antiinflammatory agents, narcotics may be added. Antiinflammatory agents and analgesics can be combined. An antiemetic may be added to relieve nausea. When administering pain medication in the field, particular attention should be given to airway maintenance and induced nausea and vomiting.

Any person whose symptom complex cannot be controlled must be evacuated. Additional indications for evacuation include calculus anuria and evidence of obstruction-induced infection.

Urinary Retention. Urinary retention is an unpleasant and painful experience that requires immediate medical, and often surgical, intervention.[12] The etiology of urinary retention ranges from prostatism[46] in men to atonic bladder in women. In general, causes have been broadly divided into four groups: obstructive, neurologic, pharmacologic, and psychogenic.[96] Twenty-five percent of men reaching 80 years of age will experience acute retention,[12] which has been shown to increase prostate surgery perioperative mortality.[73] Acute urinary retention can lead to incapacitating symptoms in the wilderness; prompt recognition and intervention are necessary.

Principal symptoms are bladder distention and pain that may mimic acute abdomen, overflow incontinence, dribbling, and hesitancy. Physical examination findings include prostatic enlargement in men and lower midline abdominal tenderness and distention. If painful distention of the bladder is present, decompression should be undertaken.

Bladder decompression should be initially attempted with a standard Foley catheter. In men with prostatic hypertrophy, passage of the catheter may be challenging, and a large catheter or catheter coudé should be used if a standard Foley catheter cannot be passed. Instrumentation of the urethra with hemostats or dilators is dangerous and should not be attempted in the field.

If multiple attempts are unsuccessful and symptoms are severe, needle decompression is indicated. The skin of the suprapubic region should be anesthetized, if possible. The distended bladder is palpated to guide aspiration. A 22-gauge needle attached to a syringe is introduced through the skin of the lower abdomen two finger breadths above the pubic symphysis and directed at the anus. The needle is advanced with simultaneous aspiration of the syringe until free-flowing urine is visualized. Palpation of the bladder in combination with adherence to this technique should lead to successful decompression.

Complications related to decompression can occur.[81] Drainage of greater than 300 ml/hr can induce mucosal hemorrhage. In addition, 10% of victims develop postobstructive diuresis that may lead to dehydration, in which case crystalloid repletion should be undertaken. Finally, it must be recognized that the situation has been temporized and that retention will recur. Treatment may need to be continued or repeated. Drainage of the bladder acutely relieves symptoms and may allow ambulatory evacuation, but the underlying etiology must be addressed in a medical facility.

The Acute Scrotum. Acute onset of scrotal pain and swelling requires immediate attention. Etiologies are multiple, but incarcerated hernia and testicular torsion are the most clinically significant in the field. Although any one aspect of the history and physical examination may not be diagnostic, when taken as a whole, they frequently suggest the etiology of the scrotal pathology.[47]

Testicular torsion can occur at any age, but it is more likely near puberty. The likelihood of testicular salvage is inversely proportional to elapsed time from torsion; this is a true surgical emergency. Acute onset of severe testicular pain is the hallmark. Mild to moderate pain is more suggestive of a torsed testicular appendage or epididymitis. It has been stated that victims who can ambulate with minimal pain are less likely to have a torsed testicle. In addition, nausea and vomiting may accompany torsion, whereas fever, dysuria, and frequency are associated with epididymitis.

Physical examination reveals a firm-to-hard testis frequently associated with bluish discoloration at the superior pole (blue dot sign).[47] Scrotal skin may be edematous and discolored. Unilateral scrotal swelling without skin changes is more indicative of a hernia or hydrocele. In testicular torsion, the affected testis is often larger than the unaffected side. Testicular torsion can be somewhat differentiated from acute epididymitis by Prehn's sign,[85] which is relief of pain accomplished by elevation of the testicle. Because torsion twists the spermatic cord and elevates the testicle, pain in not relieved by elevation (negative Prehn's sign). Conversely, pain is relieved in epididymitis with elevation (positive Prehn's sign). This maneuver has low sensitivity in distinguishing the two conditions but is helpful in conjunction with other findings.[85]

Treatment consists of surgical detorsion, which should be accomplished within 12 hours of torsion.[47] Manual detorsion is not the treatment of choice; however, remoteness of the wilderness environment may mandate manual attempts. Studies of manual detorsion are scant and the cohorts small.[39]

If manual detorsion is necessitated, the victim should be placed supine. If the left testis is affected, the right hand of the examiner should grip the testis between thumb and forefinger to elevate the testis toward the inguinal ring. A counterclockwise (epididymis turning medially) rotation should be used. If successful, the testis will descend to its normal position and relief will be felt by all. The right testis is grasped with the left hand and rotated counterclockwise.

The surgical treatment of testicular torsion includes pexis of the testis to prevent recurrent torsion. Thus, although detorsion may temporize an acute situation in the field, all victims must be evacuated for proper follow-up.

Prostatitis. Fifty percent of men will experience prostatic symptoms in their adult life.[74] A number of forms of prostatitis have been defined, including viral, bacterial (5%), nonbacterial (65%), and chronic forms, as well as prostatodynia.[76] The acute bacterial form may potentially lead to severe infection.

Bacterial prostatitis is an infection of the prostate caused primarily by gram-negative bacteria, with 80% attributable to *Escherichia coli*. It is an acute, febrile illness characterized by perineal pain radiating to the low back, chills, malaise, and voiding symptoms, such as urgency, frequency, and dysuria. Urinary retention is not uncommon, and cystitis frequently accompanies the infection. On rectal examination, the prostate gland is usually boggy, warm, and tender. Enlargement is variable.

In an ideal situation, treatment is individualized to the cause, which may be difficult to discern in the wilderness. The infection may respond to an oral antibiotic. Ciprofloxacin (750 mg po bid), ampicillin (500 mg po qid), or trimethoprim (80 mg with sulfamethoxazole 400 mg po bid) is an effective regimen. Penetration of prostatic secretions has been shown to be best achieved by trimethoprim/sulfamethoxazole (TMP/SMX). The chosen antibiotic should be administered for 30 days. If retention is present, catheterization or suprapubic aspiration should be undertaken.

Acute bacterial prostatitis can escalate in severity to systemic toxicity. Persons who have evidence of systemic toxicity unresponsive to a trial of oral or parenteral antibiotic therapy should be evacuated.

Urinary Tract Infection

Urinary tract infections (UTIs) are extremely common and include episodes of acute cystitis and pyelonephritis occurring in otherwise healthy individuals. These infections predominate in women; approximately 25% to 35% of women age 20 to 40 report having had a UTI.[43] Conversely, men between the ages of 15 and 50 rarely develop a UTI.

Despite the striking difference in prevalence, symptoms are similar between men and women. The symptoms may represent urethritis, cystitis, or an upper urinary tract infection; the distinction is often difficult. Common symptoms include frequency, urgency, dysuria, suprapubic pain, flank pain, and hematuria. Flank pain with tenderness to percussion suggests pyelonephritis. On urinalysis, pyuria is nearly invariably present and hematuria may assist in the diagnosis. Definitive diagnosis is based on significant bacteriuria. The leukocyte esterase test has a screening sensitivity of 75% to 96% and a specificity of 94% to 98% in detecting greater than 10 leukocytes per high-power field.[43]

Treatment in the wilderness setting for both men and women should be directed at the most common causative agents, although 50% to 70% of cases resolve spontaneously if untreated. Causative bacteria include *Escherichia coli* (70% to 95%); *Staphylococcus* species (5% to 20%); and, less frequently, *Klebsiella*, *Proteus*, and enterococci. Fortunately, oral antibiotics are highly effective. Although resistant *Escherichia coli* strains are being reported, TMP/SMX (Bactrim DS) is an excellent first-line drug. Alternative regimens include nitrofurantoin, a fluoroquinolone, or a third-generation cephalosporin. A 3-day course of therapy has been shown to be more effective than single-dose therapy.[43] For pyelonephritis, similar antibiotics in a 10- to 14-day course is acceptable initial treatment. Evacuation should be reserved for systemic toxicity unresponsive to oral antibiotics.

Gynecologic Emergencies

See Chapter 75.

Skin and Soft Tissue Infections

Poor hygiene, superficial skin wounds, blisters, dermatologically significant plants, and insect bites contribute to disruption of the skin barrier. Most often seen are superficial pyodermas that do not extend beyond the level of the skin. These include erysipelas, impetigo, folliculitis, furunculosis, and carbunculosis. The majority of superficial skin infections are self-limited. However, with less than optimal hygiene and limited resources, skin infections may progress to deep soft tissue infections.

Cellulitis. Cellulitis is acute infection of the skin involving subcutaneous tissue. The superficial form of cellulitis, erysipelas, is identified by well-demarcated, warm, and erythematous plaques with raised borders. The face, scalp, hands, and lower extremities are most often affected. Cellulitis is frequently preceded by a superficial wound.

In the wilderness setting, there are ongoing infection risk factors. Members of expeditions may be physically stressed and nutritionally depleted. High altitude is associated with immunosuppression. *Clostridia* species and other pathogens are ubiquitous in the soil, and proper initial wound care may be suboptimal. Under such conditions, cellulitis can progress to abscess formation and tissue necrosis, leading to septicemia. Wounds that develop erythematous, warm, and boggy margins should be treated with antibiotics and closely observed. The margins of erythema should be marked to gauge progression.

Treatment consists of proper wound hygiene and antibiotic therapy. Local wound measures include elevation, application of moist heat every 4 to 6 hours, and immobilization. Antibiotic therapy is directed at common causative pathogens. Group A streptococci and *Staphylococcus aureus* are most commonly implicated. If complications occur and the cellulitis appears to be progressing, a mixed infection is likely.

Because Gram's stain and culture-directed therapy are not possible, the most broad-spectrum antibiotic available should be administered. Parenteral antibiotics are indicated for serious or mixed infections. Penicillin G (1 to 2 million units every 2 to 3 hours) is recommended, with first-generation cephalosporins as an alternative. Because oral antibiotics may be the only available therapy, they should be initiated early in the field. Suggested agents include erythromycin (for the penicillin-allergic victim); cephalexin; a macrolide, such as clarithromycin; or a fluoroquinolone, such as ciprofloxacin or levofloxacin.

Lymphangitis. Acute lymphangitis is an infectious process involving subcutaneous lymphatic channels. Its recognition in the wilderness setting is important relative to its propensity to follow puncture wounds, hand wounds, infected blisters, and animal bite wounds. Clinical presentation involves linear erythematous streaks that originate in the lymphatic drainage basin of the wound and "point" to the draining nodal group. Causative agents are similar to those common for cellulitis, with the addition of *Pasteurella multocida* from animal bite wounds.

Treatment consists of antibiotics, warm moist soaks every 4 to 6 hours, and immobilization and elevation of the extremity. Optimal treatment consists of parenteral antibiotics, but as with cellulitis, oral agents should be initiated if parenteral drugs are not available. Broad-spectrum agents with good oral bioavailability and gram-positive coverage are recommended.[84]

Abscess Formation. When untreated, many superficial skin infections convert to abscesses. Development of a raised, fluctuant mass with overlying warmth and erythema should raise suspicion that surgical drainage is necessary. Frequently, the lesion will "point" when purulent fluid has amassed below the dermis and rupture is impending. Warm soaks and observation are recommended by some clinicians, particularly if the presence of drainable pus is uncertain. However, the definitive treatment is drainage. Antibiotics are recommended if significant associated cellulitis is present, but penetration may be poor.

Local anesthesia should be administered before incision. The lesion should be incised in line with tissue planes over the point of maximum fluctuance. The value of cruciate incisions over linear incisions is debatable; the important feature is assurance of adequate drainage to prevent recurrence. If drainage is undertaken, the incision must be large enough to adequately drain the cavity. All purulent material should be evacuated and the cavity copiously irrigated with saline or water.

Packing is unnecessary if adequate continued drainage is ensured. The wound should be covered with a sterile dressing, changed 2 to 3 times per day with concurrent irrigation, and closely observed for reaccumulation of purulence.

Necrotizing Infections. Necrotizing skin and soft tissue infections are life-threatening conditions caused by virulent, toxin-producing bacteria. Depth of tissue involvement is variable and may involve skin, fascia, or muscle. The etiology of necrotizing infections is related to breaks in normal cutaneous defenses associated with some form of injury. Although rare, such infections are of importance to the wilderness physician because of the array of documented inciting injuries and the reduction in mortality possible if diagnosis and treatment are rapid.[28] Necrotizing infections have developed after innocuous-appearing injuries, including simple scratches, insect bites, ankle sprains, and sore throats.[35]

The incidence of necrotizing soft tissue infections is unknown, and there is no age or gender predilection. They most commonly occur on the extremities, abdominal wall, and perineum, within 1 week of the inciting event. Common pathogens include streptococcal species, *Staphylococcus*, *Vibrio* species, *Clostridia*, *Pseudomonas*, *Aeromonas*, *Enterobacter*, and fungi. Many infections become polymicrobial.

The clinical manifestations can be subtle. An area of cellulitis is commonly the first indication of infection. Pain is often excruciating, and fever is usually present. The infection then progresses to spreading erythema, induration, blue-black discoloration, and blister formation. Necrosis of skin, subcutaneous fat, muscle, and/or fascia follows, depending on the organism involved. Necrotic tissue exudes a foul-smelling, watery "dishwater" fluid. Subcutaneous emphysema may be present, particularly with clostridial infections, although enteric organisms may also produce air in tissues.

Unfortunately, treatment is limited in the wilderness environment. Debridement of infected tissue should be carried out to the greatest degree humanely possible, but further debridement in a hospital setting is invariably necessary. The extent of debridement necessitated is often striking.

After debridement, parenteral antibiotics are necessary. Vancomycin and gentamicin are appropriate first-line agents. The most broad-spectrum oral antibiotic available should be initiated, and the victim expeditiously evacuated. Time is of the essence because the infection can only be halted by aggressive surgical intervention.

REFERENCES

1. Abraham BR: The impact of advanced trauma life support course on graduates with a non-surgical medical background, *Eur J Emerg Med* 4:11, 1997.
2. Ali J: Effect of Advanced Trauma Life Support program on medical students' performance in simulated trauma patient management, *J Trauma* 44:588, 1998.
3. Ali J: Comparison of performance of interns completing the old (1993) and new (1997) Advanced Trauma Life Support courses, *J Trauma* 46:80, 1999.
4. Allen CH, Ward JD: An evidence-based approach to management of increased intracranial pressure, *Crit Care Clin* 14:485, 1998.
5. American College of Surgeons: *Advanced trauma life support for doctors,* ed 6, Chicago, 1997, American College of Surgeons.
6. Baron BJ, Scalea TM: Acute blood loss, *Emerg Med Clin North Am* 14:35, 1996.
7. Berendt BM, Van Nieuwerburgh P: Survival not improved by MAST use in ITEC trauma registry, *The ITEC Newsletter* 16:6, 1991.
8. Better OS, Stein JH: Early management of shock and prophylaxis of acute renal failure in traumatic rhabdomyolysis, *N Engl J Med* 322:825, 1990.
9. Bickell WH, Wall MJ Jr, Pepe PE: Immediate versus delayed fluid resuscitation for hypotensive patients with penetrating torso injuries, *N Engl J Med* 331:1105, 1994.
10. Bohlman HH, Ducker TB, Lucas JT: *Spine and spinal cord injuries in the spine,* Philadelphia, 1982, WB Saunders.
11. Borczuk P: Predictors of intracranial injury in patients with mild head trauma, *Ann Emerg Med* 25:761, 1995.
12. Boyle P: Some remarks on the epidemiology of urinary retention, *Arch Ital Urol Androl* 70:77, 1998.
13. Bracken MB et al: Administration of methylprednisolone for 24 or 48 hours or tirilazad mesylate for 48 hours in the treatment of acute spinal cord injury, *JAMA* 277:1597, 1997.
14. Branemark P, Ekholm R: Tissue injury caused by wound disinfectants, *J Bone Joint Surg* 49A:48, 1967.
15. Burney RE et al: Incidence, characteristics, and outcome spinal cord injury at trauma centers in North America, *Arch Surg* 128:596, 1993.
16. Campbell-Hewson G, Egleston CV, Cope AR: Traumatic asphyxia in children, *J Accid Emerg Med* 14:47, 1997.
17. Carroll RR, Hall EL, Kitchens CS: Canebrake rattlesnake envenomation, *Ann Emerg Med* 30:45, 1997.
18. Cheung DS, Kharasch M: Evaluation of the patient with closed head trauma: an evidence-based approach, *Emerg Med Clin North Am* 17:9, 1999.
19. Cochrane Injuries Group Albumin Reviewers: Human albumin administration in critically ill patients: systematic review of randomised controlled trials, *BMJ* 317:235, 1998.
20. Deangeles DA et al: Resuscitation from hemorrhagic shock with diaspirin cross-linked hemoglobin, blood, or hetastarch, *J Trauma* 42:406, 1997.
21. Demetriades D et al: Complex problems in penetrating neck trauma, *Surg Clin North Am* 76:661, 1996.
22. Demetriades D et al: Paramedic vs. private transportation of trauma patients: effect on outcome, *Arch Surg* 131:133, 1996.
23. Denis D et al: Rhabdomyolysis in European viper bite, *Acta Paediatr* 87:1013, 1998.
24. Dunne Jr, Shaked G, Golocovsky M: Traumatic asphyxia: an indicator of potentially severe injury in trauma, *Injury* 27:746, 1996.
25. Eckstein M: Outcomes of trauma patients with airway intervention in the prehospital setting, *Ann Emerg Med* 27:123, 1996.
26. Edlich RF: Tissue adhesives—revisited (editorial), *Ann Emerg Med* 31:106, 1998.
27. Edlich RF: Tissue adhesives (comment), *Ann Emerg Med* 32:274, 1998.
28. Elliot DC, Kufera JA, Myers RAM: Necrotizing soft tissue infections: risk factors for mortality and strategies for management, *Ann Surg* 224:672, 1996.
29. Ernst AA et al: LAT (lidocaine-adrenaline-tetracaine) versus TAC (tetracaine-adrenaline-cocaine) for topical anesthesia in face and scalp lacerations, *Am J Emerg Med* 13:151, 1995.
30. Feliciano DV, Moore EE, Mattox KL: *Trauma,* ed 3, Stamford, Conn, 1996, Appleton & Lange.
31. Forgey WW: *Practice guidelines for wilderness emergency care,* ed 1, Old Saybrook, Conn, 1995, Globe Pequot Press.
32. Gans L, Kennedy T: Management of unique clinical entities in disaster medicine, *Emerg Med Clin North Am* 14:301, 1996.
33. Gentile DA et al: Wilderness injuries and illnesses, *Ann Emerg Med* 21:853, 1992.
34. Ghajar J et al: Survey of critical care management of comatose head-injured patients in the United States, *Crit Care Med* 23:560, 1995.
35. Green RJ, Dafoe DC, Raffin TA: Necrotizing fasciitis, *Chest* 110:219, 1996.
36. Gruber PJ et al: Presence of fever and leukocytosis in acute cholecystitis, *Ann Emerg Med* 28:273, 1996.
37. Gruen P, Liu C: Current trends in the management of head injury, *Emerg Med Clin North Am* 16:63, 1998.
38. Hanley DF: Neurologic critical care and the management of severe head injury in the united states, *Crit Care Med* 23:433, 1995.
39. Hawtrey CE: Assessment of acute scrotal symptoms and findings, *Urol Clin North Am* 25:715, 1998.
40. Hoffman JR et al: Low risk criteria for cervical-spine radiography in blunt trauma: a prospective study, *Ann Emerg Med* 21:1454, 1992.
41. Hollander JE et al: Irrigation of facial and scalp lacerations: does it alter outcome? *Ann Emerg Med* 31:73, 1998.
42. Honigman B et al: The role of pneumatic antishock garment in penetrating cardiac wounds, *JAMA* 266:2398, 1991.
43. Hooton TM, Stamm WE: Diagnosis and treatment of uncomplicated urinary tract infection, *Infect Dis Clin North Am* 11:551, 1997.
44. Howell JM, Chisholm CD: Wound care, *Emerg Clin North Am* 15:417, 1997.
45. Jabbour M, Osmond MH, Klassen TP: Life support courses: are they effective? *Ann Emerg Med* 28:691, 1996.
46. Jacobsen SJ et al: Natural history of prostatism: risk factors for acute urinary retention, *J Urol* 158:481, 1997.
47. Kass EJ, Lundak B: The acute scrotum, *Pediatr Clin North Am* 44:1251, 1997.
48. Kellum JM et al: Randomized prospective comparison of cefoxitin and gentamicin/clindamycin in the treatment of acute colon diverticulitis, *Clin Ther* 14:376, 1992.
49. Kemp ED: Bites and stings of the arthropod kind: treating reactions that range from annoying to menacing, *Postgrad Med* 103:96, 1998.
50. Kiwerski JE: Neurologic outcome from conservative treatment of cervical spinal cord injured patients, *Paraplegia* 31:192, 1993.
51. Leibovici D et al: Prehospital cricothyroidotomy by physicians, *Am J Emerg Med* 15:91, 1997.
52. Maenza RL, Seaberg D, DiAmico F: A meta-analysis of blunt cardiac trauma: ending myocardial confusion, *Am J Emerg Med* 14:237, 1996.
53. Mahadevan S et al: Interrater reliability of cervical spine injury criteria in patients with blunt trauma, *Ann Emerg Med* 31:197, 1998.
54. Mansfield RT: Head injuries in children and adults, *Crit Care Clin* 13:611, 1997.
55. Marion DW: Head and spinal cord injuries, *Neurol Clin* 16:485, 1998.
56. Martin RR et al: Prospective evaluation of preoperative fluid resuscitation in hypotensive patients with penetrating truncal injury: a preliminary report, *J Trauma* 33:354, 1992.
57. Mattox KL et al: Prospective MAST study in 911 patients, *J Trauma* 29:1104, 1989.
58. Meldon SW et al: Out-of-hospital cervical spine clearance: agreement between emergency medical technicians and emergency physicians, *J Trauma Inj Infect Crit Care* 45:1058, 1998.
59. Mensching JJ, Musielewicz AJ: Gastrointestinal emergencies, part II: abdominal wall hernias, *Emerg Med Clin North Am* 14:739, 1996.
60. Mills J, Ho MT, Trunkey DD: *Current emergency diagnosis and treatment,* Los Altos, Calif, 1983, Lange.
61. Montalvo R: Morbidity and mortality in the wilderness, *West J Med* 168:248, 1998.
62. Moscati R et al: Comparison of normal saline with tap water for wound irrigation, *Am J Emerg Med* 16:379, 1998.
63. Moscati RM: Gastrointestinal emergencies, part II: cholelithiasis, cholecystitis, and pancreatitis, *Emerg Med Clin North Am* 14:719, 1996.
64. Muizelaar JP, Marmarou A: Adverse effects of prolonged hyperventilation in patient with severe head injury: a randomized clinical trial, *J Neurosurg* 75:731, 1991.
65. Nance FC et al: Surgical judgement is the management of penetrating wounds of the abdomen: experience with 2,212 patients, *Ann Surg* 193:639, 1931.
66. Naqvi R: Acute renal failure due to traumatic rhabdomyolysis, *Ren Fail* 18:677, 1996.

67. Nunn CR et al: Traumatic asphyxia syndrome, *Tenn Med* 90:144, 1997.
68. Offringa M: Excess mortality after human albumin administration in critically ill patients, *BMJ* 317:223, 1998.
69. Pate JW: Tracheobronchial and esophageal injuries, *Surg Clin North Am* 69:11, 1989.
70. Pelletier CR et al: Assessment of ocular trauma associated with head and neck injuries, *J Trauma Inj Infect Crit Care* 44:350, 1998.
71. Pepe PE, Eckstein M: Reappraising the prehospital care of the patient with major trauma, *Emerg Med Clin North Am* 16:2, 1998.
72. Pewett EB, Schaeffer AJ: Urinary tract infection in urology, including acute and chronic prostatitis, *Infect Dis Clin North Am* 11:623, 1997.
73. Pickard R, Emberton M, Neal DE: The management of men with acute urinary retention. national prostatectomy audit group, *Br J Urol* 81:712, 1998.
74. Poels PJE, Gabreels FJM: Rhabdomyolysis: a review of the literature, *Clin Neurol Neurosurg* 95:175, 1993.
75. Poon A et al: Eye injuries in patients with major trauma, *J Trauma Inj Infect Crit Care* 46:494, 1999.
76. Prevots R et al: Tetanus surveillance-United States, 1989-1990, *MMWR CDC Surveill Summ* 41:1, 1992.
77. Przybelski RJ et al: Cross-linked hemoglobin solution as a resuscitative fluid after hemorrhage in the rat, *J Lab Clin Med* 117:143, 1991.
78. Quinn J et al: Tissue adhesives versus suture wound repair at 1 year: randomized clinical trial correlating early, 3-month, and 1-year cosmetic outcome, *Ann Emerg Med* 32:645, 1998.
79. Roberts JS, Bratton SL: Colloid volume expanders: problems, pitfalls and possibilities, *Drugs* 55:621, 1998.
80. Roberts P et al, The Standards Task Force American Society of Colon and Rectal Surgeons: Practice parameters for sigmoid diverticulitis, *Dis Colon Rectum* 38:125, 1995.
81. Rosen P: *Emergency medicine: concepts and clinical practice,* ed 4, St Louis, 1998, Mosby.
82. Roy S, Wiemersheimer P: Non-operative causes of abdominal pain, *Surg Clin North Am* 77:1433, 1998.
83. Sabiston DC Jr: *Sabiston's textbook of surgery,* ed 15, Philadelphia, 1997, WB Saunders.
84. Sadick NS: Current aspects of bacterial infections of the skin, *Derm Clin* 15:341, 1997.
85. Samm BJ, Dmochowski RR: Urologic emergencies: trauma injuries and conditions affecting the penis, scrotum, and testicles, *Postgrad Med* 100:187, 1996.
86. Schultz SC et al: The efficacy of diaspirin crosslinked hemoglobin solution resuscitation in a model of uncontrolled hemorrhage, *J Trauma* 37:408, 1994.
87. Shackford SR, Zhuang J, Schmoker J: Intravenous fluid tonicity: effect on intracranial pressure, cerebral blood flow, and cerebral oxygen delivery in focal brain injury, *J Neurosurg* 76:91, 1992.
88. Shires GT, Barber AE, Illner HP: Current status of resuscitation: solutions including hypertonic saline, *Adv Surg* 28:133, 1995.
89. Simma B et al: A prospective, randomized, and controlled study of fluid management in children with severe head injury: lactated ringer's versus hypertonic saline, *Crit Care Med* 26:1265, 1998.
90. Singer AJ, Hollander JE, Quinn JV: Evaluation and management of traumatic lacerations, *N Engl J Med* 337:1142, 1997.
91. Singer AJ et al: Prospective, randomized, controlled trial of tissue adhesive (2-octylcyanoacrylate) vs. standard wound closure techniques for laceration repair. the octylcyanoacrylate study group, *Acad Emerg Med* 5:94, 1998.
92. Spiess BD: Traumatic coagulopathies, *Anesthesiol Clin North Am* 14:29, 1996.
93. Sweeney MN: Vascular access in trauma: options, risks, benefits, and complications, *Anesthesiol Clin North Am* 17:97, 1999.
94. Taylor G et al: Hypertonic saline improve brain resuscitation in a pediatric model of head injury and hemorrhagic shock, *J Pediatr Surg* 31:65, 1996.
95. Trunkey DD: Trauma, *Sci Am* 249:28, 1983.
96. van der Linden EF, Venema PL: Acute urinary retention in women, *Ned Tijdschr Geneeskd* 142:1603, 1998.
97. Walsh PC: *Campbell's urology,* ed 7, Philadelphia, 1998, WB Saunders.
98. Zhuang J et al: Colloid infusion after brain injury: effect on intracranial pressure, cerebral blood flow, and oxygen delivery, *Crit Care Med* 23:140, 1995.

19 Wilderness Improvisation

Eric A. Weiss and Howard J. Donner

At the heart of wilderness medicine is improvisation, a creative amalgam of formal medical science and commonsense problem solving. Defined as "to fabricate out of what is conveniently at hand," improvisation encompasses many variations, is governed by few absolute rights and wrongs, and is limited more often by imagination than by personnel or equipment.

GENERAL GUIDELINES

When you work with an improvised system, you should test your creation on a noninjured person ("work out the bugs") before applying it to a victim. Include materials that lend themselves to improvisation in the wilderness survival kit to enhance efficiency. Creativity is needed when searching for improvisational materials. The victim's gear can provide needed items (e.g., backpacks can be dismantled to obtain foam pads and straps). When possible, practice constructing improvised systems before they are required in an actual rescue.

IMPROVISED AIRWAY MANAGEMENT

Airway obstruction in the semiconscious or unconscious victim is usually caused by relaxation of the oropharyngeal muscles, which allows the tongue to slide back and obstruct the airway. If only one rescuer is present, maintaining a patent airway with the jaw thrust or chin lift technique precludes further first-aid management. You can improvise a nasal trumpet type

of airway from a Foley catheter, radiator hose, solar shower hose, siphon tubing, or inflation hose from a kayak flotation bag or sport pouch.

Establish a temporary airway by attaching the anterior aspect of the victim's tongue to the lower lip with two safety pins (Figure 19-1). An alternative to puncturing the lower lip is to pass a string through the safety pins and hold traction on the tongue by securing the other end to the victim's shirt button or jacket zipper.

Surgical Airway (Cricothyroidotomy)

Cricothyroidotomy—the establishment of an opening in the cricothyroid membrane—is indicated to relieve life-threatening upper airway obstruction when a victim cannot be ventilated effectively from the mouth or nose, and endotracheal intubation is not feasible. This may occur in a victim with severe laryngeal edema, or with trauma to the face and upper larynx. Cricothyroidotomy may also be useful when the person's upper airway is obstructed by a foreign body that cannot be extracted by a Heimlich maneuver or direct laryngoscopy.

In the wilderness, you can perform cricothyroidotomy by cutting a hole in the thin cricothyroid membrane and then placing a hollow object into the trachea to allow for ventilation (Box 19-1). Locate the cricothyroid membrane by palpating the victim's neck, beginning at the top. The first and largest prominence felt is the thyroid cartilage ("Adam's apple"), whereas the second (below the thyroid cartilage) is the cricoid carti-

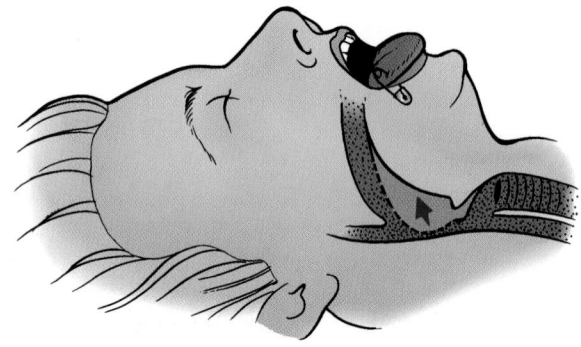
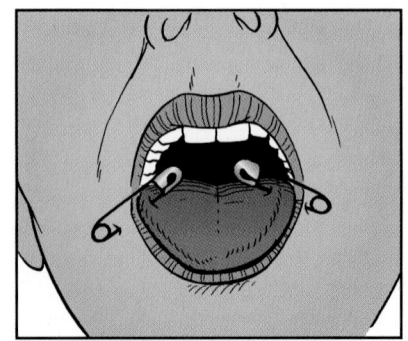

Figure 19-1 Safety pinning tongue to open airway. (*From Auerbach PS, Donner HJ, Weiss EA:* Field guide to wilderness medicine, *St Louis, 1999, Mosby.*)

Box 19-1   IMPROVISED CRICOTHYROIDOTOMY TUBES

1. IV administration set drip chamber: Cut the plastic drip chamber of a macro drip (15 drops/ml) IV administration set at its halfway point with a knife or scissors. Remove the end protector from the piercing spike and insert the spike through the cricothyroid membrane. The plastic drip chamber is nearly the same size as a 15-mm endotracheal tube adapter and fits snugly in the valve fitting of a bag-valve device (Figure 19-2).
2. Syringe barrel: Cut the barrel of a 1- or 3-ml syringe with the plunger removed at a 45-degree angle at its

midpoint to create an improvised cricothyroid airway device. The proximal phalange of the syringe barrel helps secure the device to the neck and prevents it from being aspirated (Figure 19-3).
3. Any small hollow object: Examples include a small flashlight or penlight casing, pen casing, small pill bottle, and large-bore needle or IV catheter. Several commercial devices are small and lightweight enough to be included in the first-aid kit.

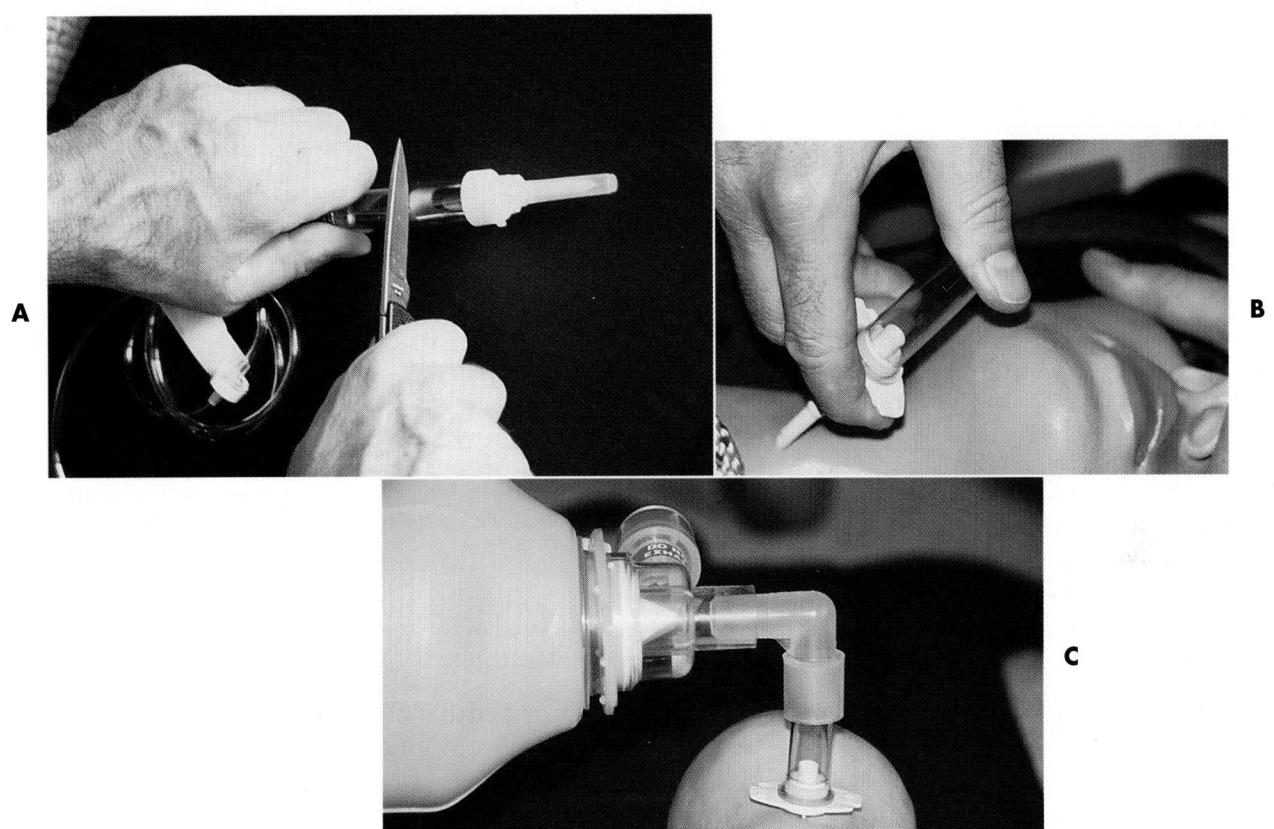

Figure 19-2   A, Cut plastic drip chamber at halfway point. **B,** Insert spike from drip chamber into the cricothyroid membrane. **C,** Bag-valve device will fit over the chamber for ventilation.

lage. The small space between these two, noted by a small depression, is the cricothyroid membrane (Figure 19-4). With the victim lying on his or her back, cleanse the neck around the cricothyroid membrane with an antiseptic if one is readily available. Put on protective gloves. Make a vertical 1-inch incision through the skin with a knife over the membrane (go a little bit above and below the membrane) while using the fingers of

your other hand to pry the skin edges apart. Anticipate bleeding from the wound. After the skin is cut apart, puncture the membrane by stabbing it with your knife or other sharp penetrating object (Figure 19-5, *A*). Stabilize the larynx between the fingers of one hand, and insert the improvised cricothyroidotomy tube through the membrane with your other hand (Figure 19-5, *B*). Secure the object in place with tape.

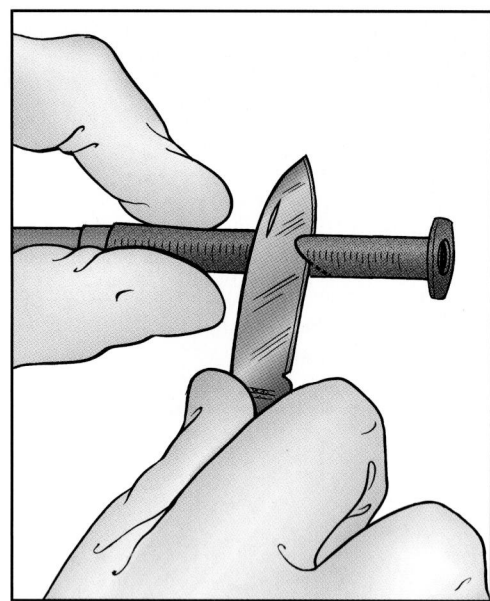

Figure 19-3 Improvised cricothyroid airway device can be created by cutting barrel of syringe at 45-degree angle at its midway point. (*From Auerbach PS, Donner HJ, Weiss EA: Field guide to wilderness medicine, St Louis, 1999, Mosby.*)

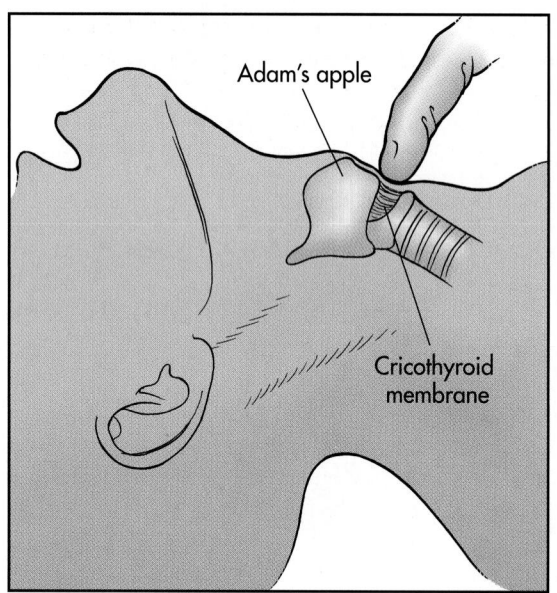

Figure 19-4 Cricothyroid membrane is found in the depression between the Adam's apple (thyroid cartilage) and the cricoid cartilage. (*From Auerbach PS, Donner HJ, Weiss EA: Field guide to wilderness medicine, St Louis, 1999, Mosby.*)

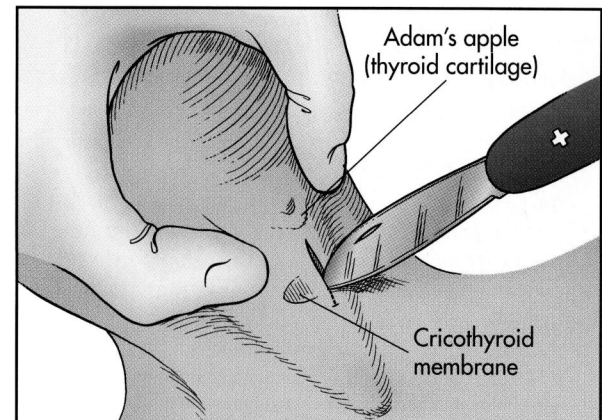

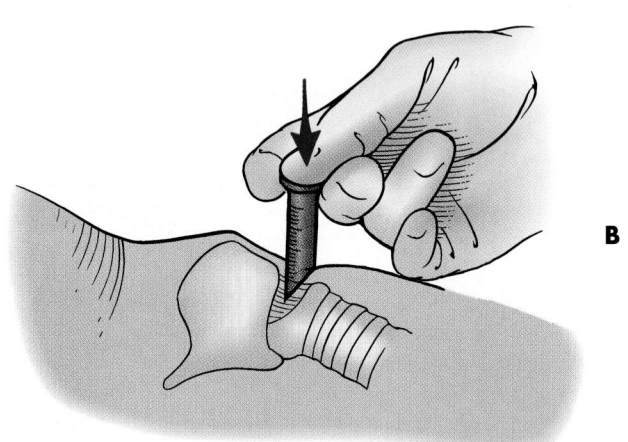

Figure 19-5 Cricothyroidotomy. **A,** Locate cricothyroid membrane and make a vertical 1-inch incision through the skin. **B,** Insert pointed end of improvised cricothyrotomy tube through the membrane. (*From Auerbach PS, Donner HJ, Weiss EA: Field guide to wilderness medicine, St Louis, 1999, Mosby.*)

Complications associated with this procedure include hemorrhage at the insertion site, subcutaneous or mediastinal emphysema resulting from faulty placement of the tube into the subcutaneous tissues rather than into the trachea, and perforation through the pos-terior wall of the trachea with placement of the tube in the esophagus.

Improvised Barrier For Mouth-To-Mouth Rescue Breathing

A glove can be modified and used as a barrier shield for performing rescue breathing. Cut the middle finger of the glove at its halfway point and insert it into the victim's mouth. Stretch the glove across the victim's mouth and nose and blow into the glove as you would to inflate a balloon. After each breath, remove the part of the glove covering the nose to allow the victim to exhale. The slit creates a one-way valve, preventing backflow of the victim's saliva (Figure 19-6).

EAR, NOSE, AND THROAT EMERGENCIES

Epistaxis is a common problem in travelers. The reduced humidity in airplanes, cold climates, and high-altitude environments can produce drying and erosion of the nasal mucosa. Other etiologic factors include fa-

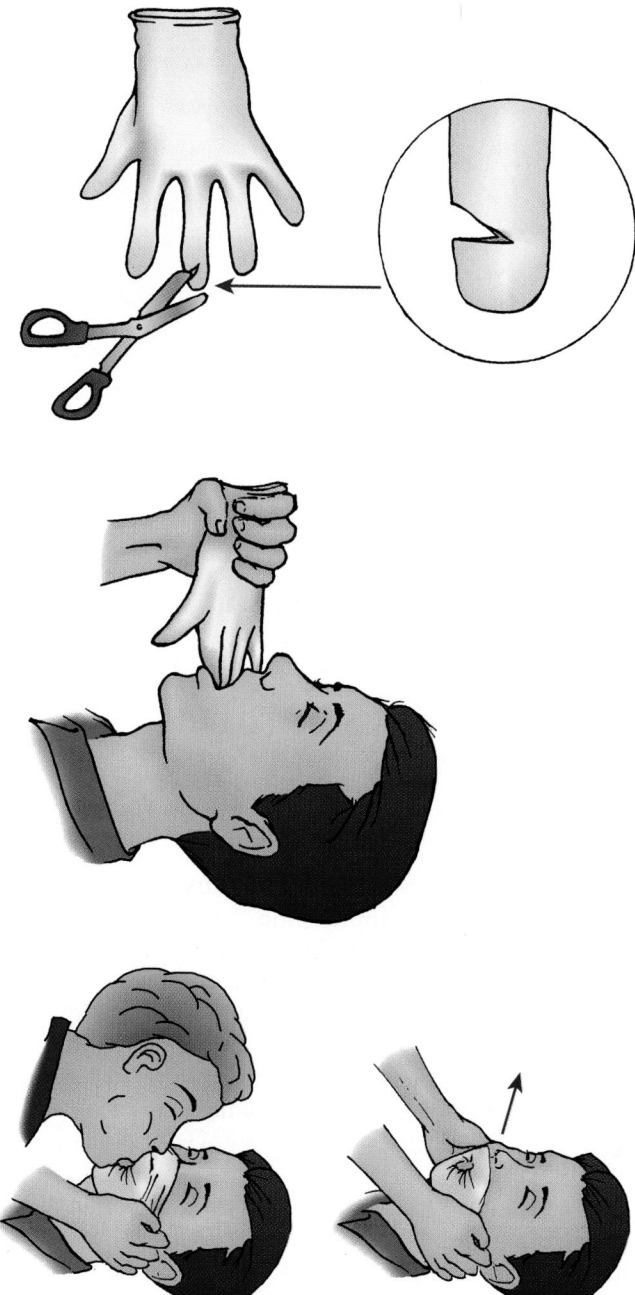

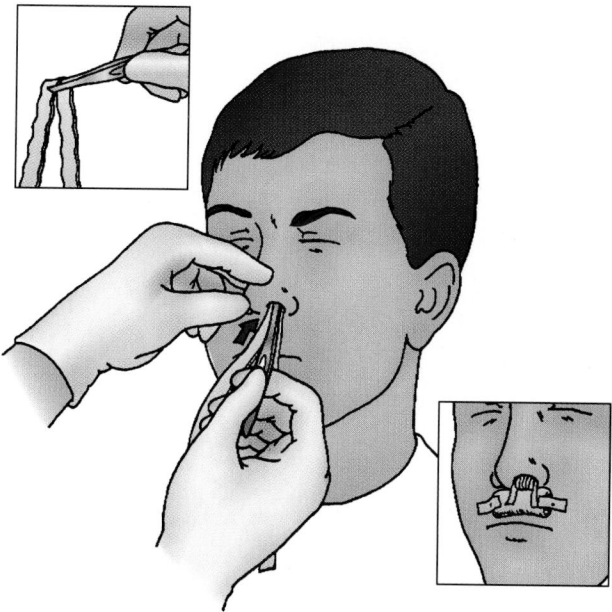

Figure 19-7 Anterior epistaxis from one side of the nasal cavity can be treated using nasal packing soaked in a vasoconstrictor. Vaseline-impregnated gauze or strips of nonadherent dressing can be packed in the nose so that both ends of the gauze remain outside the nasal cavity.

Figure 19-6 Improvised cardiopulmonary resuscitation (CPR) barrier is created using a latex or nitrile glove. Make a slit in the middle finger of the glove.

cial trauma, infections, and inflammatory rhinitis. Although most cases of epistaxis are minor, some present life-threatening emergencies.[32]

Anterior epistaxis from one side of the nasal cavity occurs in 90% of cases.[7] If pinching the nostrils against the septum for a full 10 minutes does not control the bleeding, nasal packing may be needed. Soak a piece of cotton or gauze with a vasoconstrictor, such as oxymetazoline (Afrin) nasal spray, and insert it into the nose, leaving it in place for 5 to 10 minutes. Vaseline-impregnated gauze

or strips of a nonadherent dressing can then be packed into the nose so that both ends of the gauze remain outside the nasal cavity (Figure 19-7). This prevents the victim from inadvertently aspirating the nasal packing.[32]

Complete packing of the nasal cavity of an adult victim requires a minimum of 1 m (3 feet) of packing to fill the nasal cavity and tamponade the bleeding site.[7] Expandable packing material, such as Weimert Epistaxis Packing or the Rhino Rocket, is available commercially. A tampon or balloon tip from a Foley catheter can also be used as improvised packing.[32]

Anterior nasal packing blocks sinus drainage and predisposes to sinusitis. Prophylactic antibiotics are usually recommended until the pack is removed in 48 hours.[32]

If the bleeding site is located posteriorly, use a 14- to 16-Fr Foley catheter with a 30-ml balloon to tamponade the site.[10] Prelubricate the catheter with either Vaseline or a water-based lubricant, then insert it through the nasal cavity into the posterior pharynx. Inflate the balloon with 10 to 15 ml of water and gently withdraw it back into the posterior nasopharynx until resistance is met. Secure the catheter firmly to the victim's forehead with several strips of tape. Pack the anterior nose in front of the catheter balloon as described earlier.

Esophageal foreign bodies may cause significant morbidity. Respiratory compromise caused by tracheal compression or by aspiration of secretions can occur. Mediastinitis, pleural effusion, pneumothorax, and abscess may be seen with perforations of the esophagus

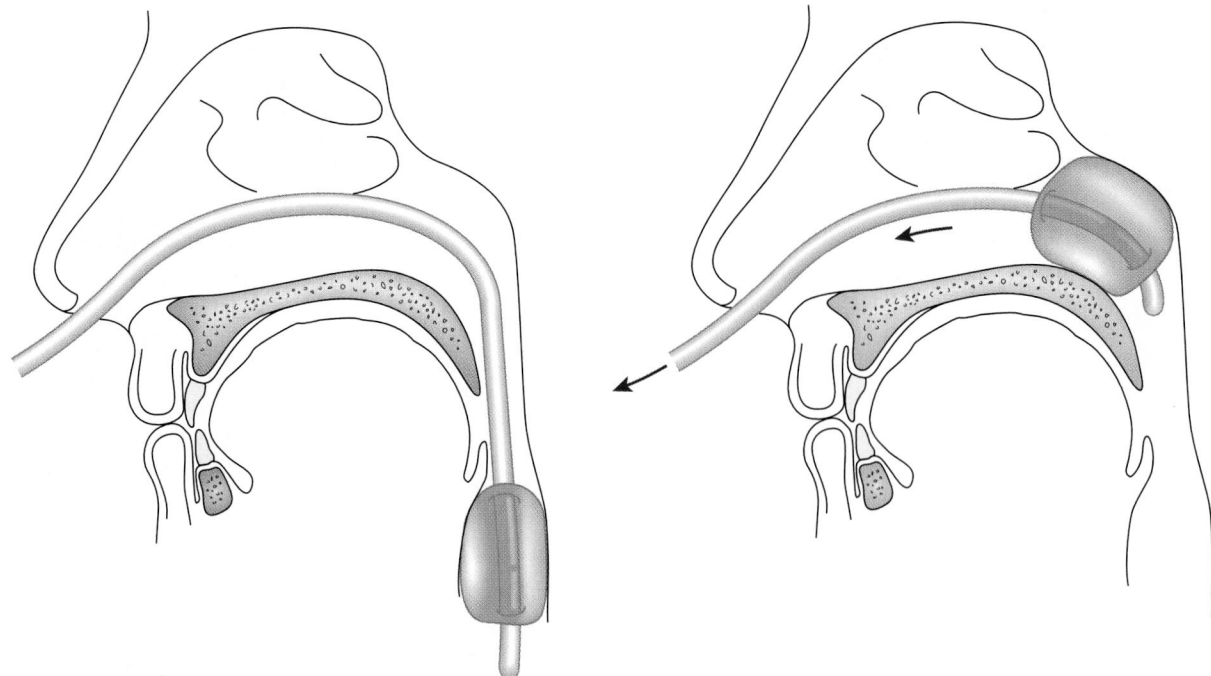

Figure 19-8 Packing the back of the nose. Insert a Foley catheter into the nose and gently pass it back until it enters the back of the throat. After the tip of the catheter is in the victim's throat, carefully inflate the balloon with 10 to 12 ml of air or water from a syringe. Inflation should be done slowly and should be stopped if painful. After the balloon is inflated, gently pull the catheter back out until resistance is met.

from sharp objects or pressure necrosis caused by large objects.[20]

The use of a Foley balloon-tipped catheter can be a safe method for removing blunt esophageal foreign bodies.[4,5,12] Success rates of 98% have been cited.[4] Associated complications include laryngospasm, epistaxis, pain, esophageal perforation, and tracheal aspiration of the dislodged foreign body.[20] Sharp, ragged foreign bodies or an uncooperative victim precludes use of this technique (Figure 19-8).[28]

Lubricate a 12- to 16-Fr Foley catheter and place it orally into the esophagus while the victim is seated. After placing the victim in Trendelenburg's position, pass the catheter beyond the foreign body and inflate the balloon with water. Withdraw the catheter with steady traction until the foreign body can be removed from the hypopharynx or expelled by coughing. Take care to avoid lodging the foreign body in the nasopharynx. Any significant impedance to withdrawal should terminate the attempt.[28] Use of this technique is recommended only in extreme wilderness settings or when endoscopy is not available.

IMPROVISED PLEURAL DECOMPRESSION OF A TENSION PNEUMOTHORAX

Signs and symptoms of a tension pneumothorax include distended neck veins, tracheal deviation away from the side of the pneumothorax, unilateral absent breath sounds, hyperresonant hemithorax to percussion, subcutaneous emphysema, respiratory distress, cyanosis, and cardiovascular collapse. Tension pneumothorax mandates rapid pleural decompression if the victim appears to be dying. Possible complications of pleural decompression include infection; profound bleeding from puncture of the heart, lung, or a major blood vessel; or even laceration of the liver or spleen.

Technique

Swab the entire chest with povidone-iodine or another antiseptic. If sterile gloves are available, put them on after washing your hands. If local anesthesia is available, infiltrate the puncture site down to the rib and over its upper border.

Insert a large-bore intravenous (IV) catheter, needle, or any pointed, sharp object that is available into the chest just above the third rib in the midclavicular line (midway between the top of the shoulder and the nipple in a line with the nipple approximates this location) (Box 19-2). If you hit the rib, move the needle or knife upward slightly until it passes over the top of the rib, thus avoiding the intercostal blood vessels that course along the lower edge of every rib. The chest wall is 1½ to 2½ inches thick, depending on the individual's muscularity and the amount of fat present. A gush of air signals that you have entered the pleural space; do not push the penetrating object further. Releasing the tension converts the tension pneumothorax into an open pneumothorax.

Box 19-2 IMPROVISED PLEURAL DECOMPRESSION DEVICES

1. Large-bore (12- or 14-gauge) IV catheter or needle
2. Endotracheal tube
3. Foley catheter with a rigid support ("stylet"), such as a clothes hanger, placed into the lumen
4. Section of a tent pole
5. Hose from a hydration pouch

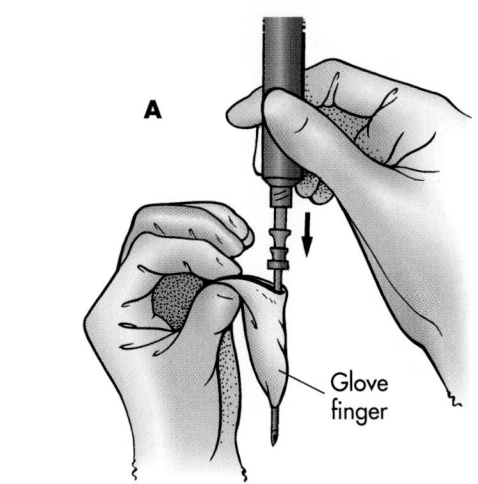

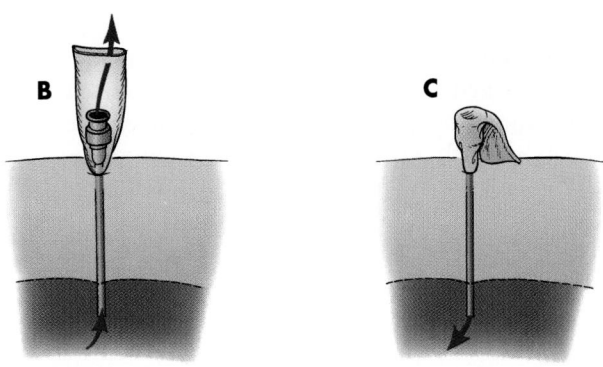

Figure 19-9 A, Finger of glove is attached to needle or catheter to create flutter valve. **B,** Flutter valve allows air to escape. **C,** Flutter valve collapses to prevent air entry. (*From Auerbach PS, Donner HJ, Weiss EA: Field guide to wilderness medicine, St Louis, 1999, Mosby.*)

Leave the needle or catheter in place and place the cut-out finger portion of a rubber glove with a tiny slit cut into the end over the external opening to create a unidirectional flutter valve that allows continuous egress of air from the pleural space (Figure 19-9). To create a one-way flutter valve, cut a finger portion of a latex glove off at the proximal end of the finger and insert the needle or catheter into the open end of the glove finger and through the tip as shown (see Figure

19-9, *A*). The cut-out–finger portion of the glove creates a unidirectional flutter valve that allows egress of air from the pleural space during expiration but collapses to prevent air entry on inspiration (see Figure 19-9, *B* and *C*).

OPEN ("SUCKING") CHEST WOUND

Penetrating trauma to the chest can produce a chest wound that allows air to be sucked into the pleura on inspiration. Place a piece of plastic food wrap, aluminum foil, or one side of a plastic sandwich bag on top of the wound and tape it on three sides. The untaped fourth side serves as a relief valve to prevent formation of a tension pneumothorax.

IMPROVISED SPLINTING AND TRACTION*

Cervical Spine Injuries

Because of its mobility, the cervical spine is the spinal column area most commonly injured in trauma. Any obvious or suspected cervical spine injury demands full spinal immobilization with use of both a rigid or semirigid cervical collar and long board immobilization. Historically, dogma about cervical spine injuries has specified a "splint 'em as they lie" approach. Transporting a victim who is not in anatomic position is arduous in the backcountry. It is uncomfortable for the victim, difficult for the rescuers, and increases the risk of further injury. In general, gentle axial traction back to anatomic position is indicated unless (1) return to anatomic position significantly increase pain or focal neurologic deficit or (2) movement of the head and neck results in any noticeable mechanical resistance.[17]

All cervical spine injuries (or suspected injuries) deserve full long board immobilization. Movement of the pelvis and hips laterally is potentially more dangerous than anterior-posterior movement; therefore it is appropriate during extended transport to allow gentle flexion at the hip with immobilization in that position if the victim is more comfortable. Soft pads behind the knees and the small of the back also add to the victim's comfort during a long transport.[9]

Cervical Collars. Cervical collars are always adjuncts to full spinal immobilization and never used alone. The improvised cervical collar is used in conjunction with manual cervical spine stabilization followed by complete immobilization of the victim on a spine board. A properly applied and fitted collar is a primary defense

---

*Specific aspects of fracture care are covered in detail in other chapters. This chapter focuses on improvised *systems*, not on definitive orthopedic *management*. Improvised systems rarely provide the same degree of protection as commercial systems. Good judgment is needed.

against axial loading of the cervical spine, particularly in an evacuation that involves tilting the victim's body uphill or downhill. Improvised cervical collars have had a bad reputation, and textbooks continue to depict them made from a simple cravat wrapped around the neck. This type of system is no more effective than the soft cervical collars often used by urban plaintiffs trying to impress a jury.

An improvised cervical collar works effectively *only* if it has the following features:

1. It is rigid or semirigid.
2. It fits properly (many improvised designs are too small).
3. It does not choke the victim.
4. It allows the victim's mouth to open if vomiting occurs.

The following are improvisational approaches to cervical collars.

Closed-Cell Foam System. The best closed-cell foam systems incorporate a full-size or three-quarter-length pad folded longitudinally into thirds and applied by being centered over the back of the victim's neck and wrapped forward. The pad is crossed under the chin, contoured underneath opposite axillae, and secured. If the pad is not long enough, you can tape or tie on extensions. This system also works well with blankets, beach towels, or even a rolled plastic tarp. Avoid small flexible cervical collars that do not optimally extend the chin-to-chest distance.

Padded Hip Belt. A padded hip belt or fanny pack removed from a large internal or external frame backpack can sometimes be modified to work perfectly. Wider is usually better. Take up excess circumference by overlapping the belt, and secure the excess material with duct tape (Figure 19-10).

Clothing. Bulky clothing, such as a fiberpile or fleece jacket, can be rolled and then wrapped around the victim's neck to make a cervical collar. The extended sleeves can be used to secure the collar. Prewrapping a wide elasticized (Ace) wrap around the jacket compresses the material to make it more rigid and supportive.

Malleable Aluminum Splint. A well-padded, aluminum splint (e.g., SAM splint) can be adjusted to fit almost any size neck (Figure 19-11).

Improvised Spinal Immobilization. As noted, the improvised cervical collar is only an adjunct to full spinal immobilization. Two immobilization systems are (1) short board immobilization, which is useful for short-duration transport (that is, getting the victim out of immediate danger) or when used in conjunc-

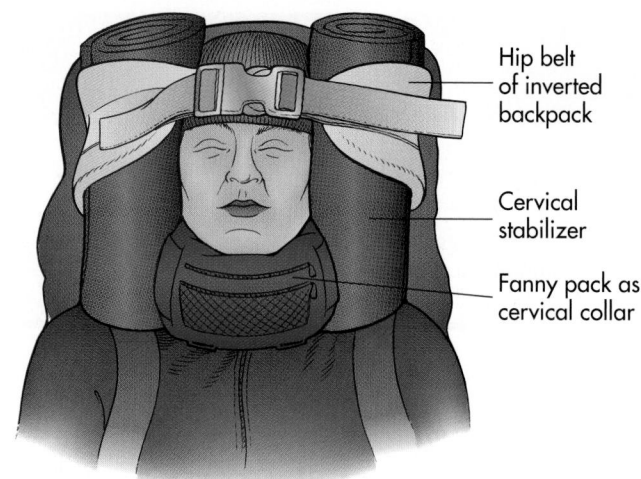

Figure 19-10 Inverted pack used as spine board. (*From Auerbach PS, Donner HJ, Weiss EA:* Field guide to wilderness medicine, *St Louis, 1999, Mosby.*)

tion with a long board; and (2) long board immobilization, used for definitive immobilization during extensive transport.

Use all of these systems in conjunction with a rigid or semirigid cervical collar, as described previously. Improvised lateral "towel rolls" are often added to these systems for additional head and neck support. These rolls can be improvised from small sections of Ensolite. Alternatively, a U-shaped head support or "horse collar" can be made from any rolled garment, blanket, tarp, or tent fly; this is placed over the victim's head in an inverted U and used with the improvised cervical collar and spine board. Hiking socks or stuff bags filled with dirt, sand, or gravel also work well for this purpose. Stuff bags filled with snow for support should *never* be used because the snow can melt during transport and allow excessive head and neck motion. However, snow-filled stuff bags can act as temporary support while more definitive systems are being constructed.

Improvised Short Board Immobilization

Internal frame pack and snow shovel system. Some internal frame backpacks can be easily modified by inserting a snow shovel through the centerline attachment points (the shovel handgrip may need to be removed first). The victim's head is taped to the lightly padded shovel (Figure 19-12); in this context the shovel blade serves as a head bed. This system incorporates the remainder of the pack suspension as designed (that is, shoulder and sternum straps with hip belt) and works well with other long board designs, such as the continuous loop system (see Continuous Loop System section).

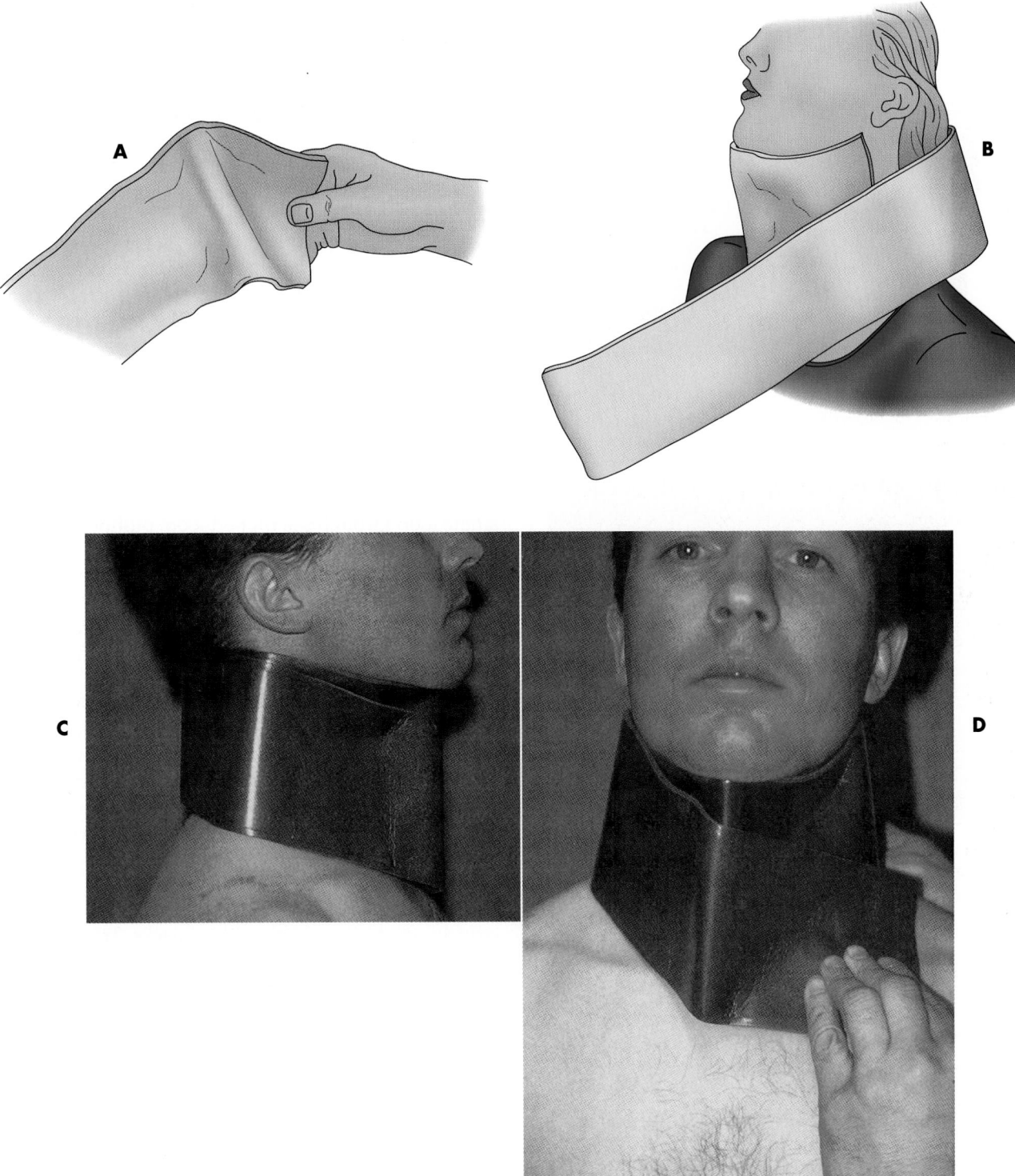

Figure 19-11 Malleable aluminum splint cervical collar. **A,** Place a vertical bend in the malleable aluminum splint approximately 6 inches from one end to form a vertical pillar. Then, add bilateral flares to make the splint comfortable for the victim where it rides against the lower mandible. **B,** Place the anterior pillar securely beneath the victim's chin and wrap the remaining length of the splint around the victim's neck. **C,** Side view of cervical collar fashioned from SAM splint. **D,** Frontal view. The end is angled inferiorly to provide an adequate chin-to-chest distance.

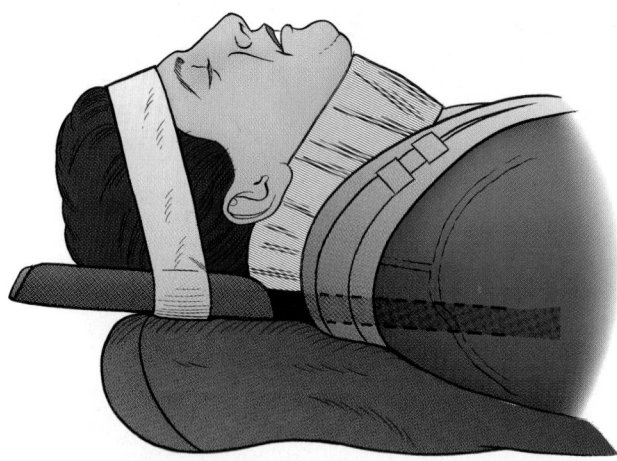

Figure 19-12 Head immobilized on a padded shovel.

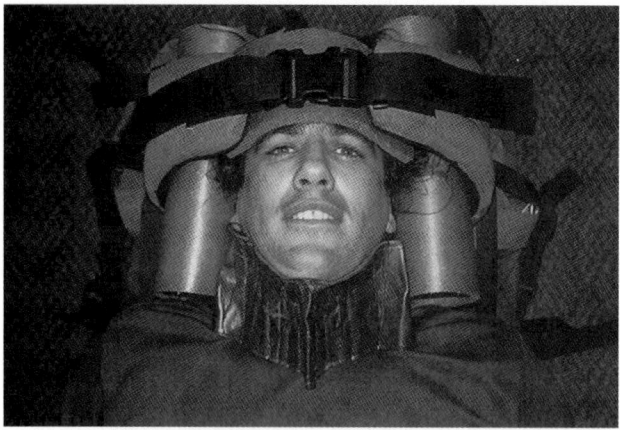

Figure 19-13 Short board using an inverted pack system. The backpack waistbelt can be seen encircling the head.

Inverted pack system. An efficient short board can be made using an inverted internal or external frame backpack. The padded hip belt provides a head bed, and the frame is used as a short board in conjunction with a rigid or semirigid cervical collar (Figure 19-13).

Turn the pack upside down, and lash the victim's shoulders and torso to the pack. Fasten the waist belt around the victim's head, as in the top section of a Kendrick extrication device. The hip belt is typically too large, but you can eliminate excess circumference with bilateral Ensolite rolls. Unlike the snow shovel system, this system requires that the victim be lashed to the splint.

Snowshoe system. A snowshoe can be made into a fairly reliable short spine board (Figure 19-14). Pad the snowshoe and rig it for attachment to the victim as shown.[19]

IMPROVISED LONG BOARD IMMOBILIZATION

Continuous loop system. For the continuous loop system (also known as the daisy chain, cocoon wrap, or mummy litter), the following items are needed:

1. A long climbing or rescue rope
2. A large tarp
3. Sleeping pads (Ensolite or Therm-a-Rest)
4. Stiffeners (such as skis, poles, snowshoes, canoe paddles, or tree branches)

Lay the rope out with even U-shaped loops as shown in Figure 19-15, *A.* The midsection should be slightly wider to conform to the victim's width. Tie a small loop at the foot end of the rope and place a tarp on the laid rope. On top of the tarp, lay foam pads the full length of the system (the pads can be overlapped to add length). Then lay stiffeners on top of the pads in the same axis as the victim (Figure 19-15, *B*). Add multiple foam pads on top of the stiffeners followed optionally with a sleeping bag (Figure 19-15, *C*). Place the victim on the pads. To form the daisy chain, bring a single loop through the pretied loop, pulling loops toward the center, and feeding through the loops brought up from the opposite side. It is important to take up rope slack continuously. When the victim's armpits are reached, bring a loop over each shoulder and tie it off (or clip it off with a carabiner) (Figure 19-15, *D*).

One excellent modification involves adding an inverted internal frame backpack. This can be incorporated with the padding and secured with the head end of the rope. The pack adds rigidity and padding, and the padded hip belt serves as a very efficient head and neck immobilizer (see Figures 19-10 and 19-13).

Backpack frame litters. Functional litters can be constructed from external frame backpacks. Traditionally two frames are used, but three or four frames (as illustrated in Figure 19-16) make for a larger, more stable litter. Cable ties or fiberglass strapping tape simplifies this fabrication. These litters can be reinforced with ice axes or ski poles.

Kayak system. Properly modified, the kayak makes an ideal rigid long board improvised litter. First, remove the seat along with sections of the upper deck if necessary. A serrated river knife (or camp saw) makes this improvisation much easier. Open deck canoes can be used almost as is once the flotation material has been removed.

Canoe system. Many rivers have railroad tracks that run parallel to the river canyon. The tracks can be used to slide a canoe by placing the boat perpendicular to the tracks and pulling on both bow and stern lines.

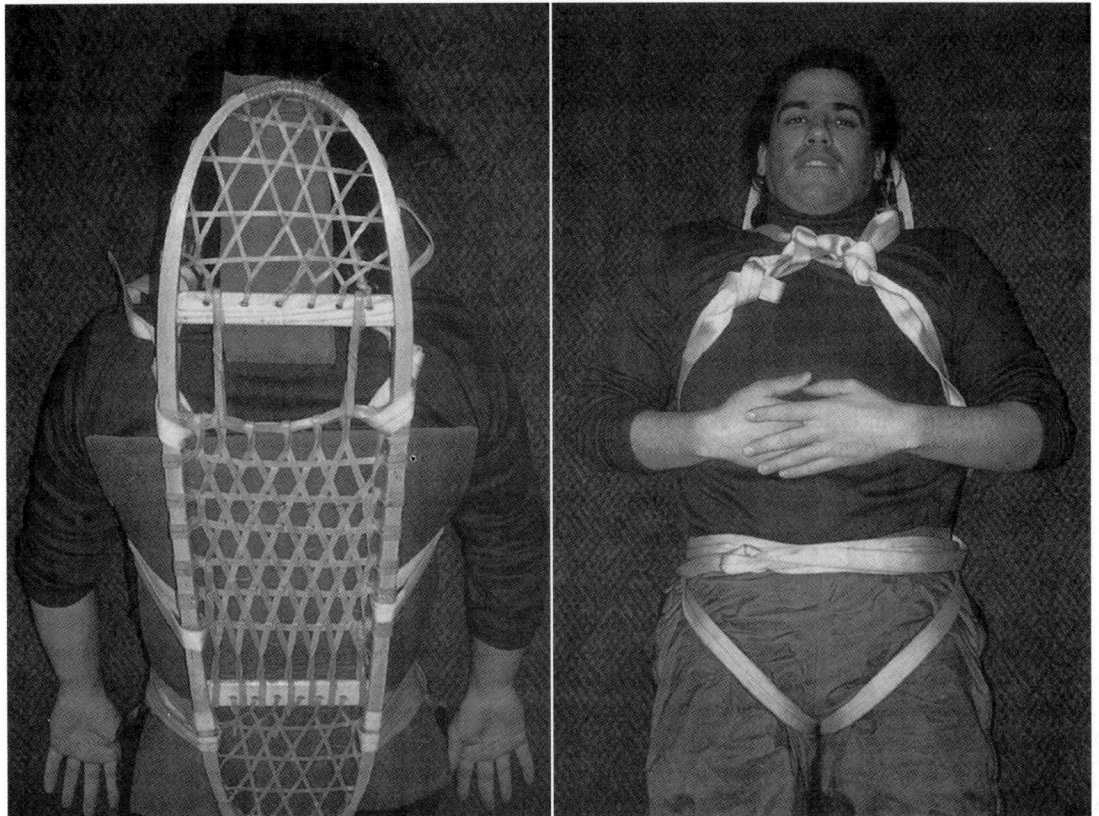

Figure 19-14 Improvised snowshoe short board. A well-padded snowshoe is prerigged with webbing and attached to the victim as shown. This system can also be used in conjunction with long board systems, such as the continuous loop system.

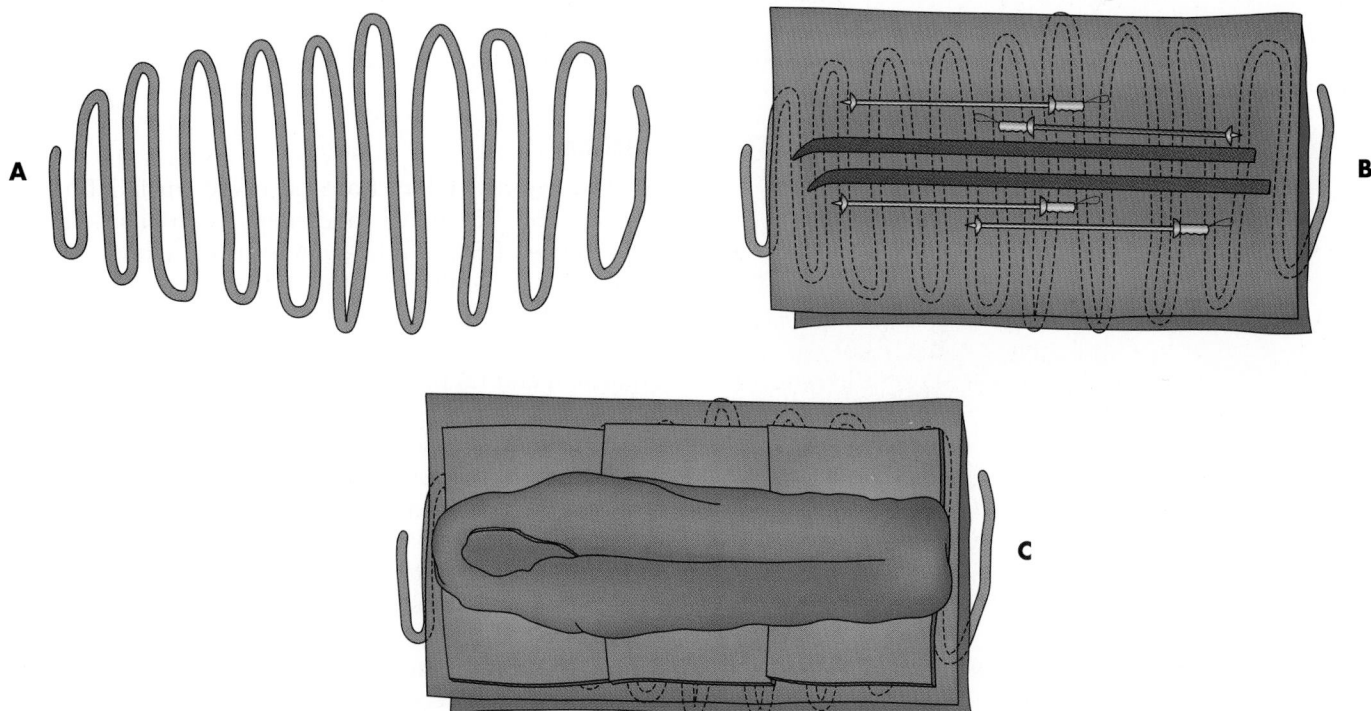

Figure 19-15 Continuous loop, or "mummy," litter made with a climbing rope. **A,** Rope is laid out with even U-shaped loops. **B,** Stiffeners such as skis and poles are placed underneath the victim to add structural rigidity. It is important to pad between the stiffeners and the victim. **C,** A sleeping bag may be used in addition to the foam pads. *Continued*

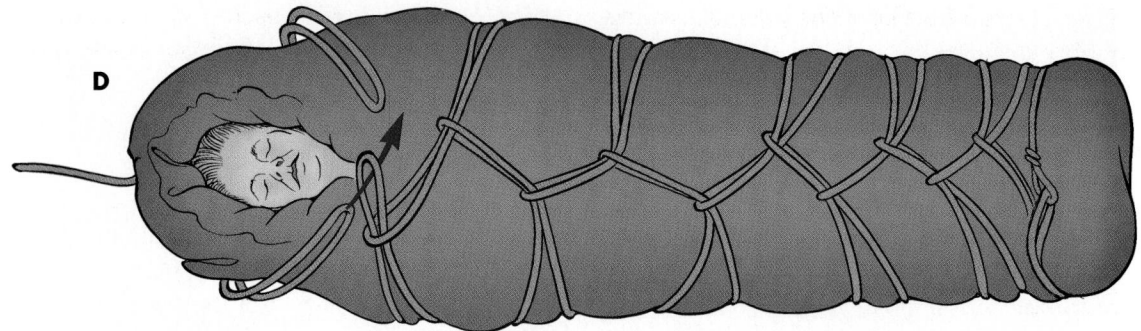

Figure 19-15, cont'd **D,** Loop of rope is brought over each shoulder and tied off (see text).

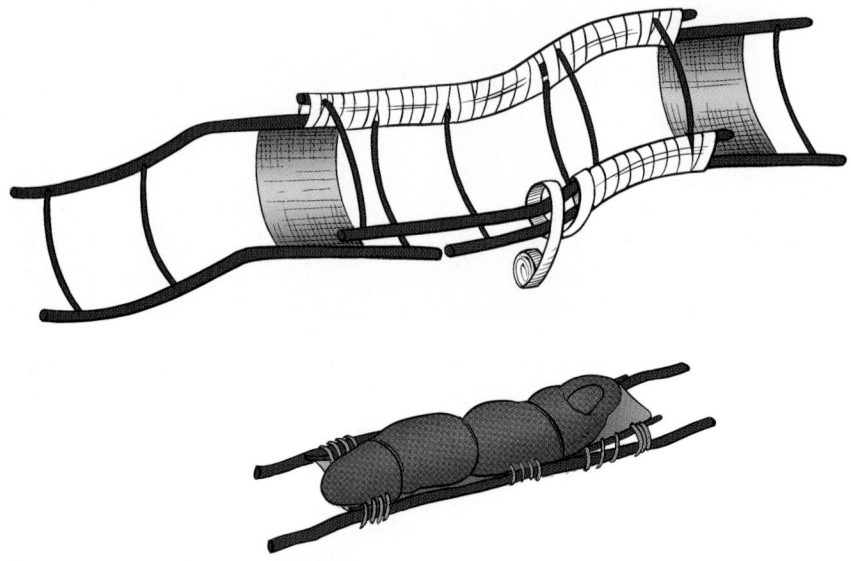

Figure 19-16 Backpack frame litter.

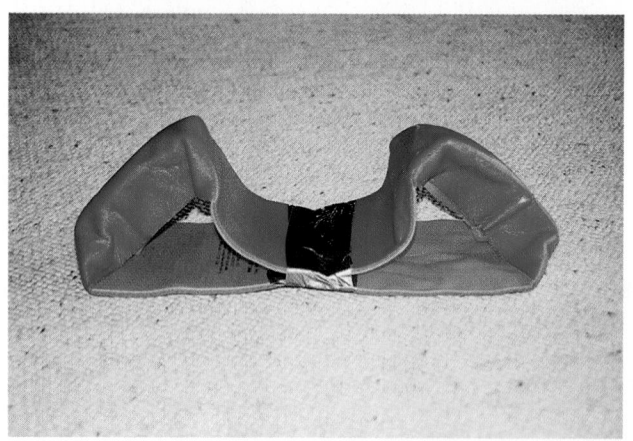

Figure 19-17 Improvised head bed.

Improvised head bed. A malleable aluminum splint can be formed as shown to create a head bed to assist in securing the immobilized head of an injured victim. Tape this head bed to a commercial or improvised backboard (Figure 19-17).

Traction

Why are improvised traction systems so crucial? Traction can be lifesaving in certain situations.[6] The importance of femoral traction in urban emergency medicine is generally accepted. In the backcountry environment, traction is essential for two fundamental reasons: (1) the general inability to provide IV volume expansion and (2) prolonged transport time to definitive care.

The primary purpose of backcountry femoral traction is to *limit blood loss into the thigh*. For a constant surface area, the volume of a sphere is greater than the volume of a cylinder. Pulling (via traction) the thigh compartment back into its natural cylindric shape limits blood loss into the soft tissue. Although the main objective is to control hemorrhage and prevent shock, enhanced comfort for the victim and decreased potential for neurovascular damage are important secondary benefits. Properly applied, improvised femoral traction can save lives in the backcountry, particularly on extended transports where IV fluids are not available.

General Principles of Traction. The potential variety of traction designs is unlimited, but five key design principles should be considered when evaluating any femoral traction system:

1. Does the splint provide inline traction? Or does the splint incorrectly pull the victim's leg off to the side or needlessly plantar flex the ankle?
2. Is the splint comfortable? Be sure to ask the victim.
3. Does the splint compromise neurologic or vascular function? Constantly check distal neurovascular function.
4. Is the splint durable, or will it break when subjected to backcountry stresses? As stated earlier, it might help to try the traction design on an uninjured person and then knock the device around a bit to determine its strength.
5. Is the splint cumbersome? Many reasonable splint designs become so bulky and awkward that litter transport, technical rescue, or helicopter evacuation is impossible. For example, a full-length ski splint is not compatible with evacuation in a small helicopter.

Femoral Traction Systems. Every femoral traction system has six components:

1. Ankle hitch
2. Rigid support that is longer than the leg
3. Traction mechanism
4. Proximal anchor
5. Method for securing the splint to the leg
6. Additional padding

ANKLE HITCH. Various techniques are used to anchor the distal extremity to the splint. Many work well, but some are impossible to recall in an emergency. Choose an easy-to-remember technique and practice it. It is best to leave the shoe on the victim's foot and apply the hitch over it. Cut out the toe section of the shoe to periodically check the circulation.

Single runner system. Loop a long piece of webbing, shoelace, belt, or rope over itself, bringing one end through the middle to create a stirrup. After rotating it away from the person by 180 degrees, slip the hitch over the shoe and ankle.

Double runner system. In this very straightforward technique, lay two short webbing loops ("runners") over and under the ankle as shown (Figure 19-18, *A*). Pass the long loop sides through the short loop on both sides (Figure 19-18, *B*) and adjust as needed (Figure 19-18, *C*). One advantage of this system is that it is infinitely adjustable, enabling the rescuer to center the pull from any direction. As always, proper padding is essential, especially for long transports. The victim's boot can distribute pressure over the foot

and ankle but will obscure visualization and palpation of the foot. A reasonable compromise is to leave the boot on and cut out the toe section for observation.

S-configuration hitch. This type of hitch is preferred if the victim also has a foot or ankle injury because traction is pulled from the victim's calf instead of the ankle. Lay a long piece of webbing or other similar material over the upper part of the ankle (lower calf) in an S-shaped configuration. Wrap both ends of the webbing behind the ankle and up through the loop on the other side. Pull the ends down on either side of the arch of the foot to tighten the hitch and tie an overhand knot (Figure 19-19).

Victim's boot system. Another efficient system uses the victim's own boot as the hitch. Cut two holes into the side walls of the boot just above the midsole and in line with the ankle joint. Thread a piece of nylon webbing or cravat through to complete the ankle hitch (Figure 19-20). Cutting away the toe may be necessary for neurovascular assessment.

Buck's traction. For extended transport, Buck's traction can be improvised using a closed-cell foam pad (Figure 19-21). Wrap the pad around the lower leg as shown and loop a stirrup below the foot from medial calf to lateral calf. Fasten this assembly with a second cravat wrapped circumferentially around the calf over the closed-cell foam (duct tape or nylon webbing can be used instead of cravats). This system greatly increases the surface area over which the stirrup is applied and decreases the potential for neurovascular complications and dermal ischemia. In addition, improvised Buck's traction has been used to manage backcountry hip fractures. However, recent literature indicates that this technique may have little benefit.[1] If Buck's traction is used for a hip injury, use smaller amounts of traction (roughly 5 pounds or less).

RIGID SUPPORT. The rigid support can be fabricated as a unilateral support (similar to the Sager traction splint or Kendrick traction device) or as a bilateral support, such as the Thomas half ring or Hare traction splint. Unilateral supports tend to be easier to apply than bilateral supports. The following are some ideas for rigid support.

Double ski pole or canoe paddle system. This is fashioned like a Thomas half ring, with the interlocked pole straps slipped under the proximal thigh to form the ischial support. Some mountain guides carry a prefabricated drilled ski pole section or aluminum bar that can be used to stabilize the distal end of this system (Figures 19-22).

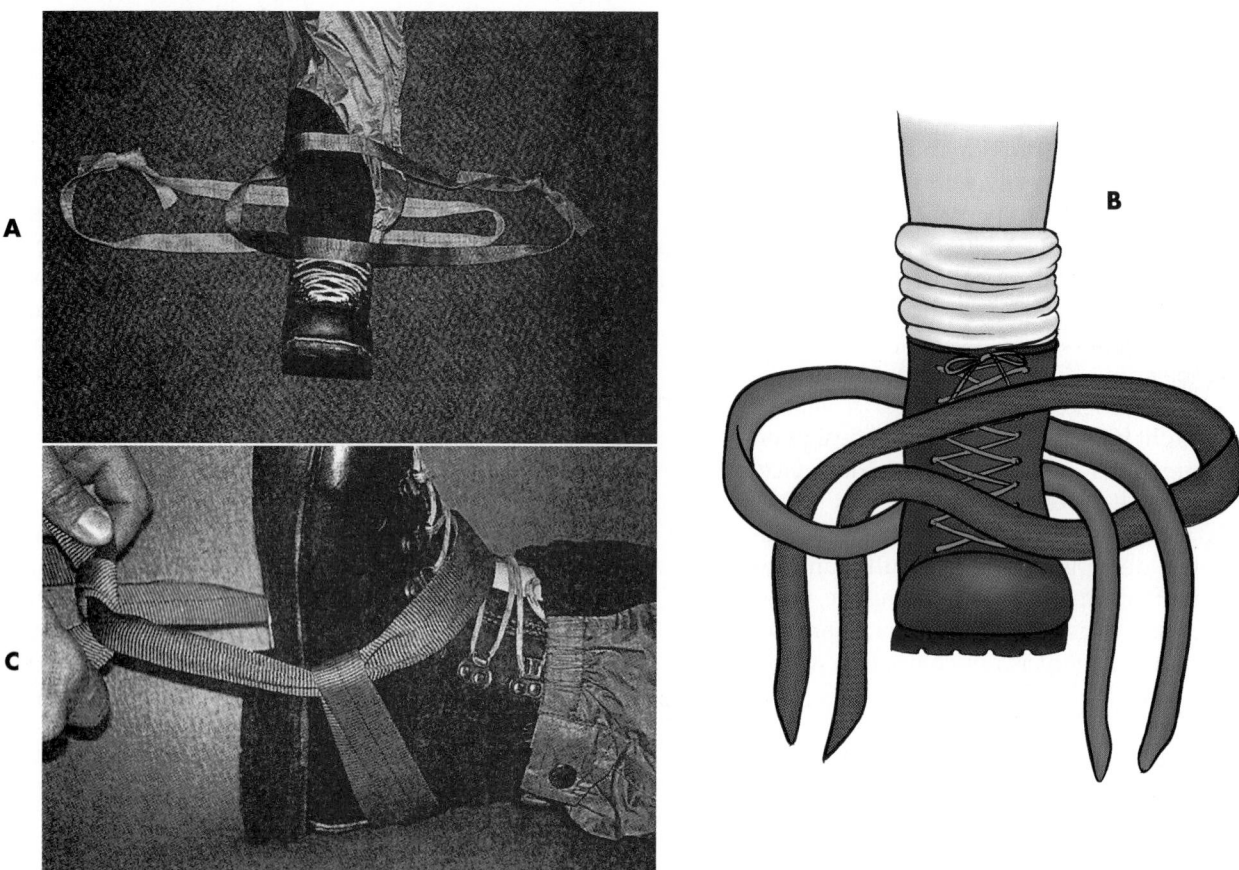

Figure 19-18 Double runner ankle hitch. **A** and **B,** Two webbing loops (runners) are laid over and under the ankle. **C,** Completed double runner ankle hitch. The beauty of this system is its infinite adjustability. The traction can be easily centered from any angle, ensuring in-line traction.

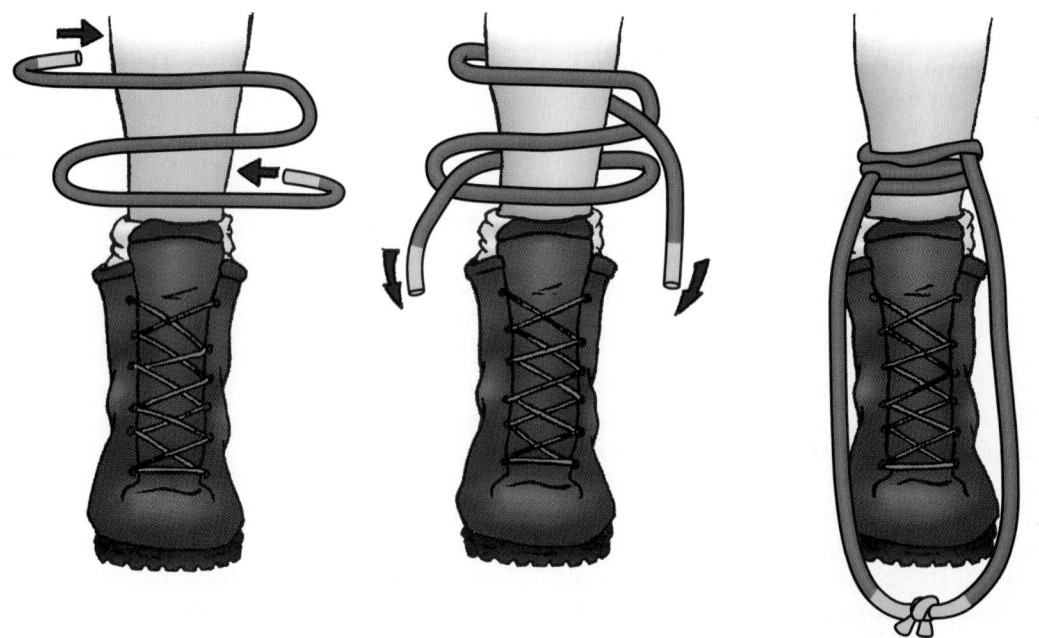

Figure 19-19 S-configuration hitch for traction splinting.

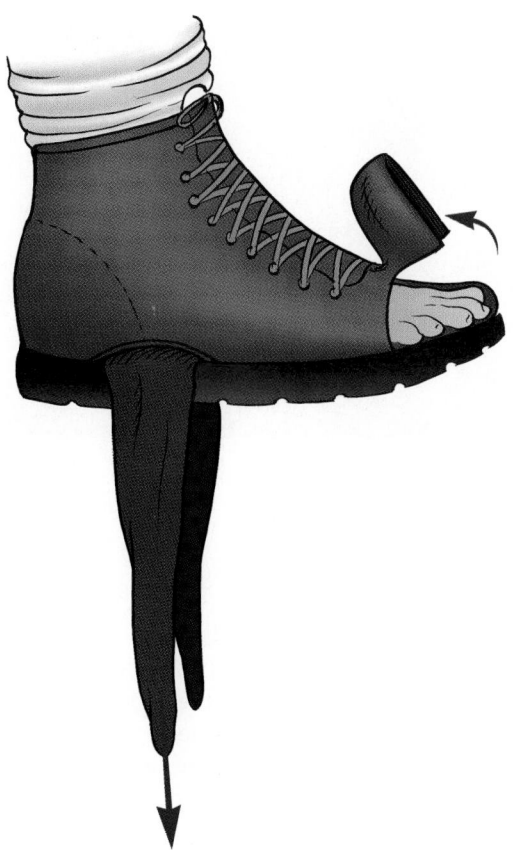

Figure 19-20   Traction using cut boot and cravat.

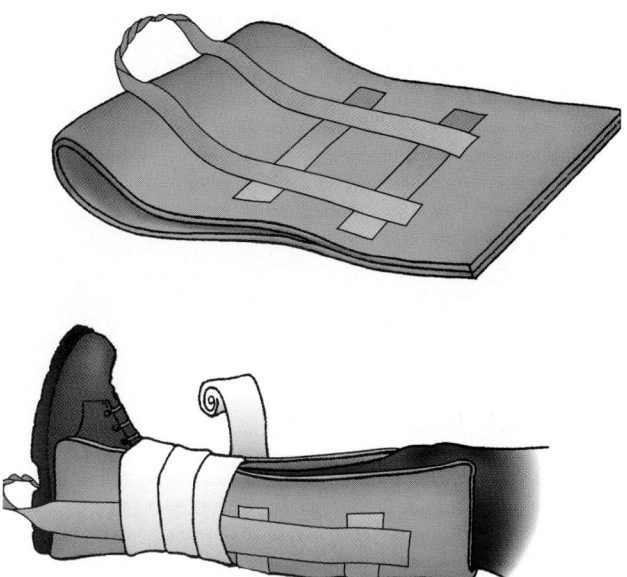

Figure 19-21   Buck's traction. Duct tape stirrups are added to a small foam pad that is wrapped around the leg. The entire unit is wrapped with an Ace bandage. This system helps distribute the force of the traction over a large surface area.

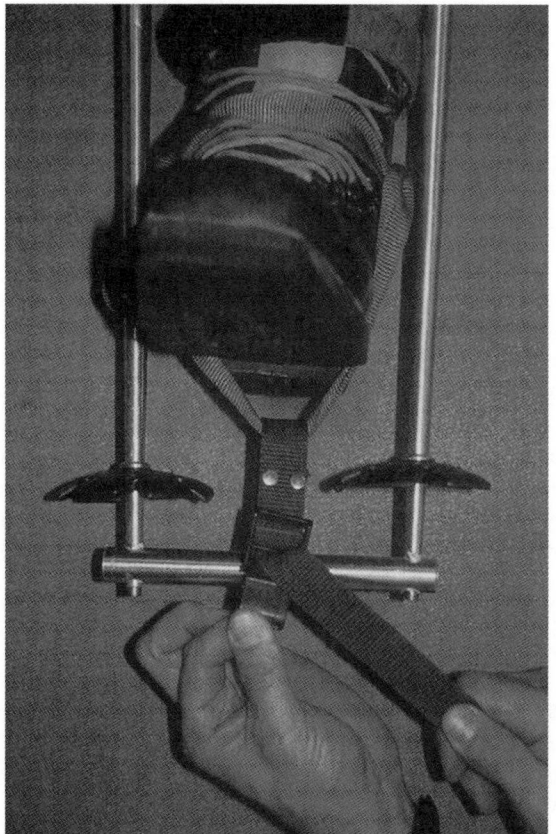

Figure 19-22   Double ski pole system with prefabricated cross-bar and webbing belt traction. A prefabricated drilled ski section is used to attach the ends of two ski poles. Traction is applied with a webbing belt and sliding buckle.

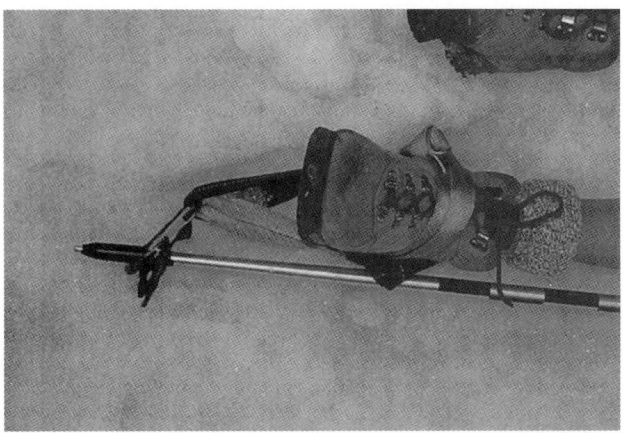

Figure 19-23 Single ski pole system. An adjustable telescoping ski pole is used as the rigid support. A stirrup is attached to a carabiner placed over the end of the pole. Traction is applied by elongating the ski pole while another rescuer provides manual traction on the victim's leg. Additional padding and securing follow (not shown).

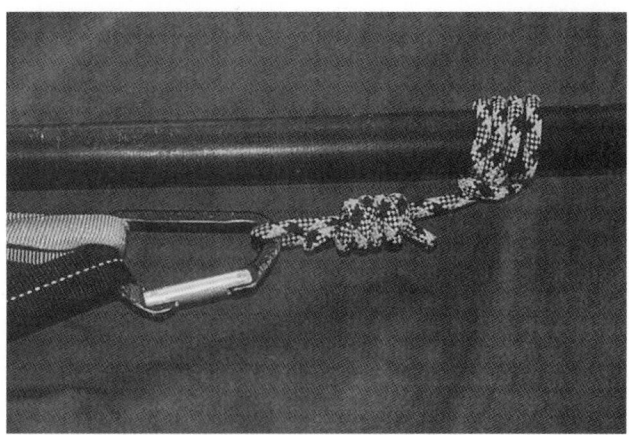

Figure 19-26 Two Prusik wraps are shown. Three or four wraps provide additional friction and security. If the Prusik knot slips, it can be easily taped in place.

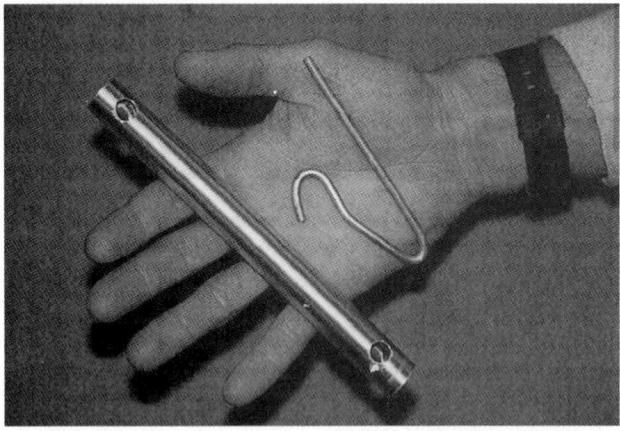

Figure 19-24 Prefabricated drilled tent pole section and bent tent stake. The ski pole section is used to stabilize the end of a double ski pole traction system. This can be improvised on site if necessary. The bent tent stake serves as a distal traction anchor if a tent pole is used as the rigid support.

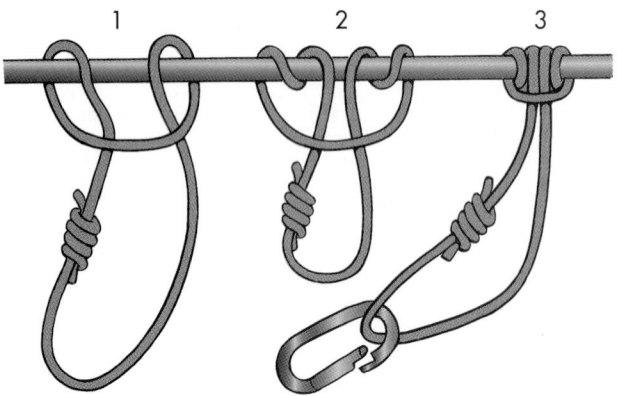

Figure 19-25 A Prusik knot made from a small-diameter cord is used as an adjustable distal traction anchor. Although two wraps are shown in the illustration, an additional wrap adds further security when applied to a smooth surface, such as a kayak paddle.

Single ski pole or canoe-kayak paddle. Use a single ski pole or paddle either between the legs, which is ideal for bilateral femur fractures, or lateral to the injured leg. The ultimate rigid support is an adjustable telescoping ski pole used laterally. Adjust the pole to the appropriate length for each victim, making the splint compact for litter work or helicopter evacuation (Figure 19-23).

Tent poles. This system uses conventional sectioned tent poles. Fit the poles together to create the ideal length rigid support. Because of their flexibility, tent poles must be well secured to the leg to prevent them from flexing out of position. Place a blanket pin or bent tent stake (Figure 19-24) in the end of the pole to provide an anchor for the traction system. Alternately, use a Prusik knot (Figure 19-25) to secure the system to the end of the tent pole (Figure 19-26).

Miscellaneous. Any suitable object, such as a canoe or kayak paddle (see Figure 19-26), two ice axes taped together at the handles, or a straight branch can be used to make a rigid support. Although skis immediately come to mind as suitable rigid components, they are too cumbersome to work effectively. Because of their length, skis may extend far beyond the victim's feet or require placement into the axillae, which is unnecessary and inhibits mobility (e.g., sitting up during transport). Premanufactured canvas pockets, available from the National Ski Patrol System, provide a ski tip and tail attachment grommet for use with the ski system.

TRACTION MECHANISM. The first modern popularized improvised traction mechanism was the Boy Scout–style Spanish windlass. Although these systems work and look good in the movies, they can be awkward to apply

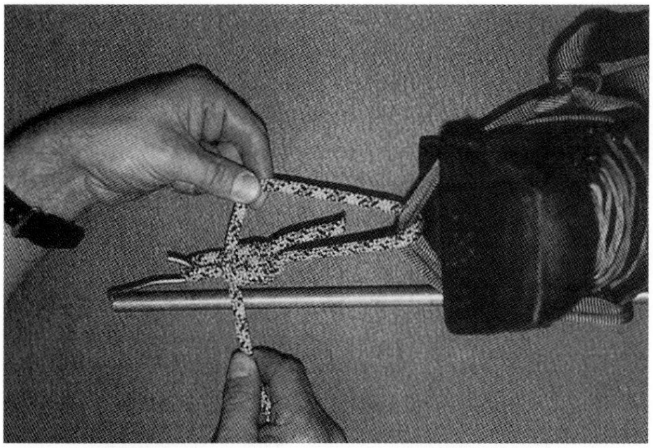

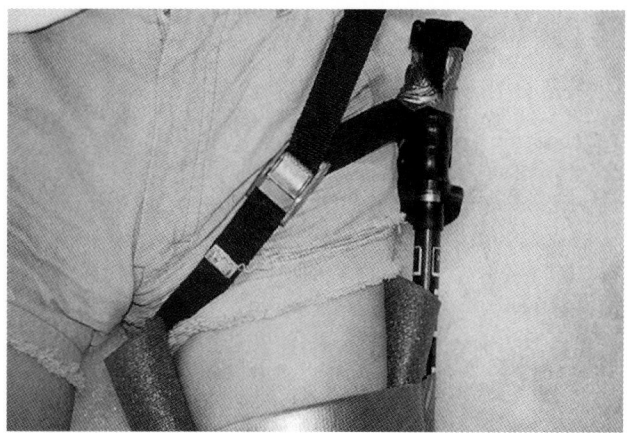

Figure 19-27 Tent pole traction with trucker's hitch. A bent tent stake is placed into the end of the tent pole as the distal traction anchor. A simple trucker's hitch is used to provide traction.

Figure 19-28 Proximal anchor using cam lock belt. The belt is applied as shown. A ski pole is used laterally as the rigid support. Duct tape is useful for securing components. Padding is helpful but is not always necessary if the victim is wearing pants.

and are often not durable. The windlass can unspin if it is inadvertently jarred and can apply rotational forces to the leg.

The amount of traction required is primarily a function of comfort. A general rule is to use 10% of body weight or about 10 to 15 pounds for the average victim. After the traction is applied, always recheck distal neurovascular function (circulation, sensation, movement).

Cam lock or Fastex-like slider. This simple, effective system uses straps that have a Fastex-like slider. Such straps are often used as waist belts or to hold items to packs. Alternately, a cam lock with nylon webbing can be used. Attach the belt to the distal portion of the rigid support and then to the ankle hitch. Traction is easily applied by cinching the nylon webbing (see Figure 19-22).

Trucker's hitch. A windlass can be easily fashioned using small-diameter line (parachute cord) and a standard trucker's hitch for additional mechanical advantage (Figure 19-27).

Prusik knot. Almost any system can be rigged with a Prusik knot (see Figure 19-25). Prusiks are ideal for providing traction from rigid supports with few tie-on points (such as a canoe paddle shaft or a tent pole). The Prusik knot can be used to apply the traction (by sliding the knot distally) or simply as an attachment point for one of the traction mechanisms already mentioned.

Litter traction. If no rigid support is available and a rigid litter such as a Stokes is being used, apply traction from the rigid bar at the foot end of the litter. If this system is used, ensure that the victim is immobilized

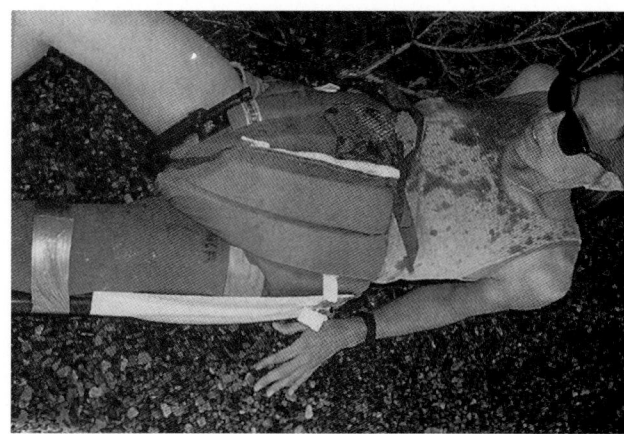

Figure 19-29 Life jacket proximal anchor. An inverted life jacket worn like a diaper forms a well-padded proximal anchor. A kayak paddle is rigged to the life jacket's side adjustment strap.

on the litter with adequate countertraction, such as inguinal straps.

PROXIMAL ANCHOR. The simplest proximal anchor uses a single proximal thigh strap, which can be made from a piece of climbing webbing or a prefabricated strap, belt, or cam lock (Figure 19-28). A cloth cravat can be used in a pinch. On the river a life jacket can be used (Figure 19-29). When climbing, a climbing harness is ideal.

SECURING AND PADDING. Check all potential pressure points to ensure that they are adequately padded. An excellent padding system can be made by first covering the upper and lower leg with a folded length of Ensolite (Figure 19-30). This is preferred over a circum-

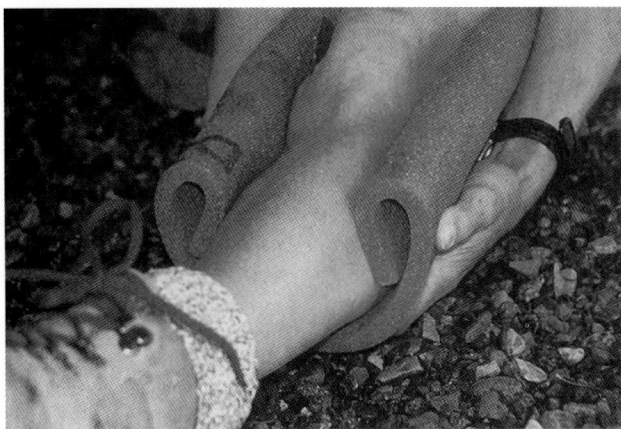

Figure 19-30 Folding Ensolite padding often provides better visualization of the extremity than does a circumferential wrap.

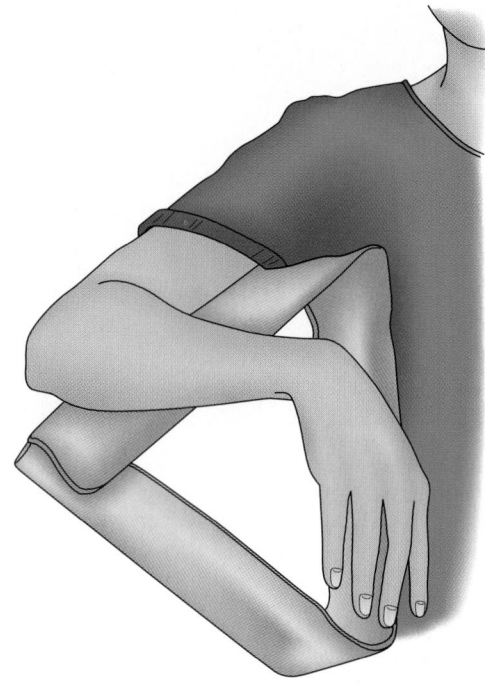

Figure 19-31 Tripod splint for unreduced anterior shoulder dislocation. This splint holds the arm in abduction when adduction is not possible. Additional padding should be added where necessary and the splint secured to the arm with an elastic wrap or other bandaging material.

ferential wrap because the folded system allows you to see the extremity. The victim is more comfortable if femoral traction is applied with the knee in slight flexion (padding placed beneath the knee during transport). Secure the splint firmly to the leg. Almost any straplike object will work, but a 4- to 6-inch Ace bandage wrapped circumferentially provides a comfortable and secure union. Finally, strap or tie the ankles or feet together to give the system additional stability. Tying the ankles together also prevents the injured leg from excess external rotation and jarring during transport.

Extremity Splints

Splint all fractures before the victim is moved unless his or her life is in immediate danger. In general, make sure the splint incorporates the joints above and below the fracture. If possible, the splint should be fashioned on the uninjured extremity and then transferred to the injured one.

On ski trips, skis and poles can be used as improvised splints. On white-water trips, canoe and kayak paddles can be used in a similar manner. Airbags used as flotation for kayaks and canoes can be converted into pneumatic splints for arm and ankle injuries. The mini-cell or ethafoam pillars found in most kayaks can be removed and carved into pieces to provide upper and lower extremity splints. A life jacket can be molded into a cylinder splint for knee immobilization or into a pillow splint for the ankle.

The flexible aluminum stays found in internal frame packs can be molded into upper extremity splints. Other improvised splinting material includes sticks or tree limbs, rolled-up magazines, books or newspapers, ice axes, tent poles, and dirt-filled garbage bags or fanny packs.

Ideally a splint should immobilize the fractured bone in a functional position. In general, "functional position" means that the legs should be straight or slightly bent at the knee, the ankle and elbow bent at 90 degrees, the wrists straight, and the fingers flexed in a curve as if the person were attempting to hold a can of soda or a baseball.

Splints can be secured in place with strips of clothing, belts, pieces of rope or webbing, pack straps, gauze bandages, or elastic bandage wraps.

Padded aluminum can be molded into various configurations to splint extremity injuries (Figures 19-31 to 19-36).

Functional Splints

Although most splints are designed to completely immobilize an injured extremity, in the backcountry a splint may need to allow for a limited range of motion so the victim can facilitate his or her own rescue. Many functional splints can be quickly improvised using nothing more than a closed-cell foam sleeping pad and some tape or elastic wrap. With the advent of inflatable sleeping pads (e.g., Therm-a-Rest), foam pads are not as ubiquitous as they once were in the backcountry. However, many of these splints can be made using a partially inflated Therm-a-Rest. Once applied, these pads can be inflated to provide the necessary support, fit, and comfort (Figure 19-37).

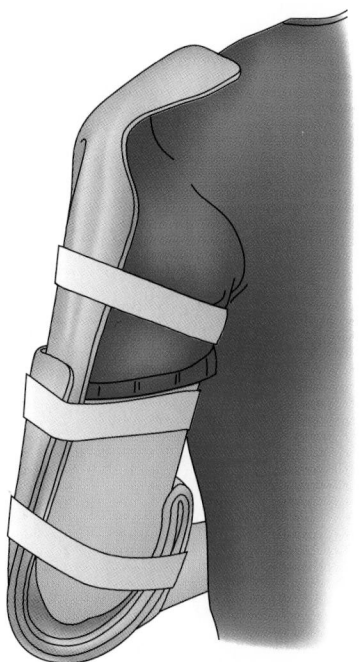

Figure 19-32 Humerus splint. Used in conjunction with a sling and swath, this splint adds extra support and protection for a fractured humerus.

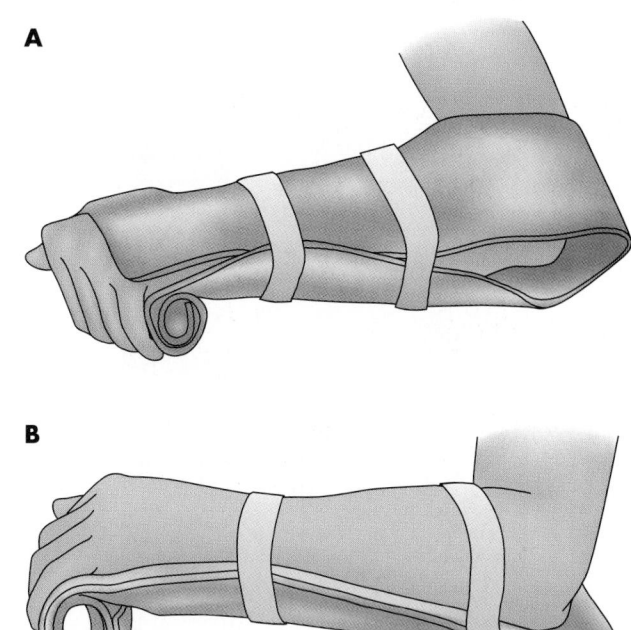

Figure 19-33 Forearm splint. These splints are used for the treatment of wrist or forearm fractures. The sugar-tong splint **(A)** prevents pronation and supination and has the advantage of greater security and protection than the volar splint **(B)** because of its anterior-posterior construction.

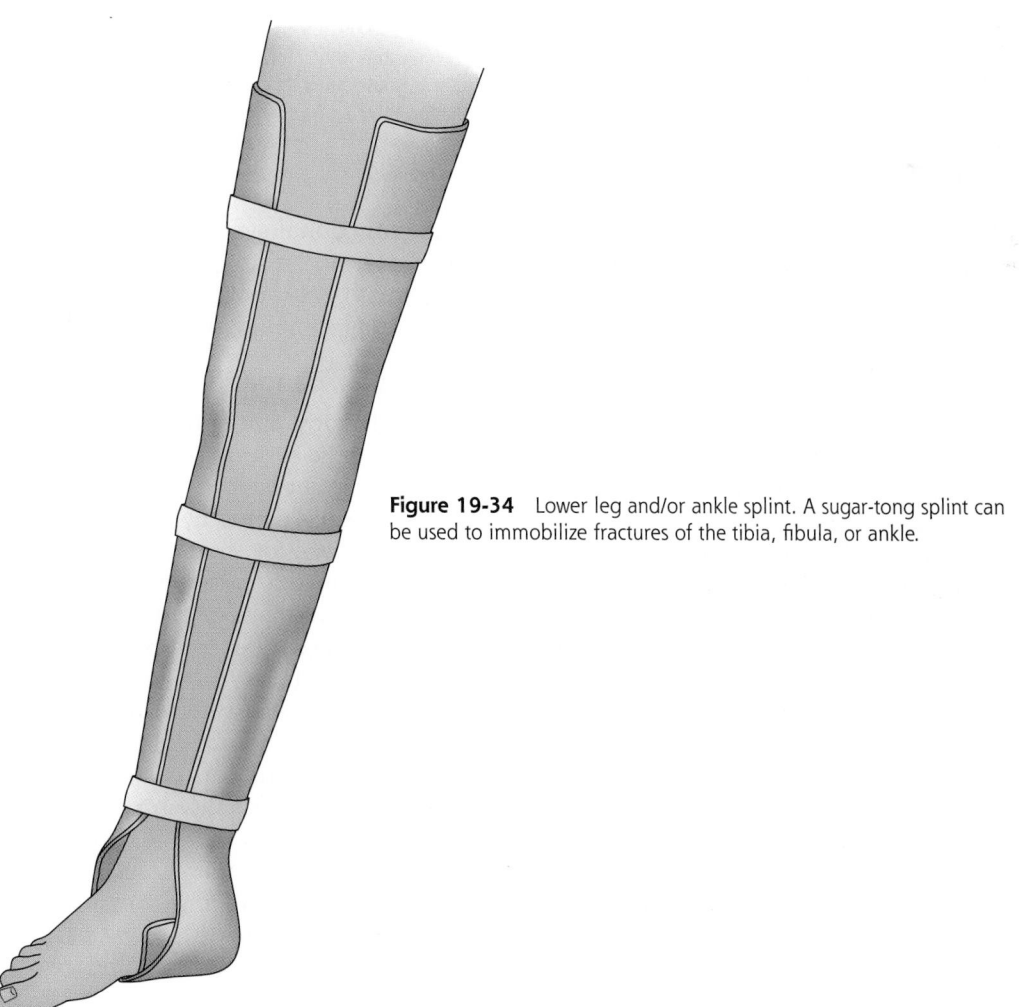

Figure 19-34 Lower leg and/or ankle splint. A sugar-tong splint can be used to immobilize fractures of the tibia, fibula, or ankle.

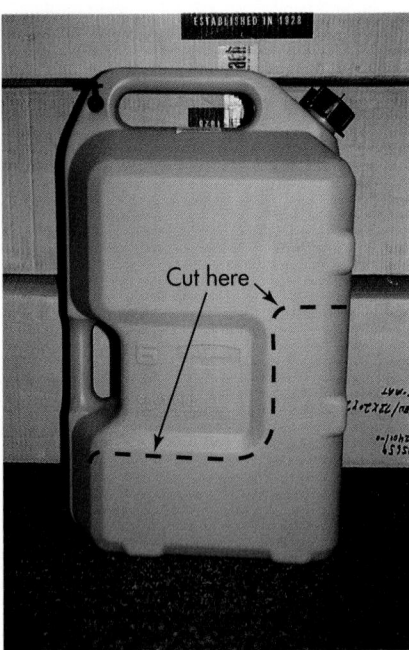

Figure 19-35 Posterior arm splint. This splint is cut from of a 5- to 9-gallon plastic fuel or water can (jerry can). When used with appropriate padding, this forms an excellent splint for injured or fractured elbows.

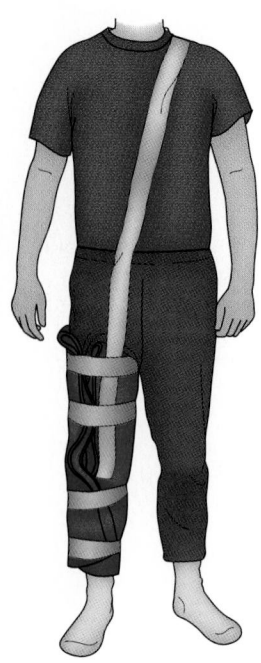

Figure 19-37 Functional knee and lower leg immobilizer. Wrap a sleeping pad around the lower leg from the midthigh to the foot. Fold the pad so that the top of the leg is not included in the splint. This provides better visualization of the extremity and leaves room for swelling. A full-length pad forms a very bulky splint and may need to be trimmed before rolling. Because of the conical shape of the lower extremity and the effects of gravity, foam pad lower extremity splints tend to work their way inferiorly when the victim ambulates. A simple solution is to use "duct tape suspenders" to keep the splint from migrating downward.

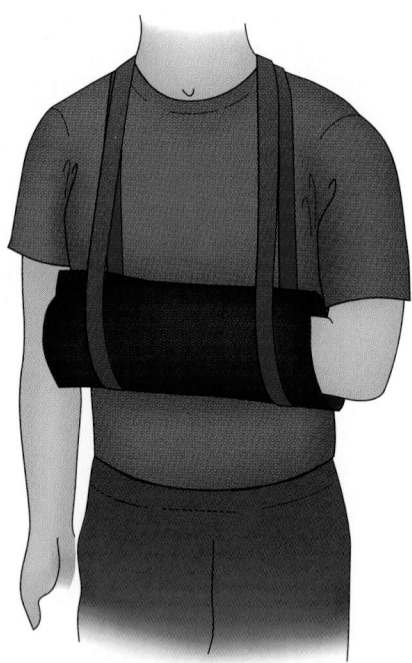

Figure 19-36 Webbing sling. An 8-foot length of 1-inch tubular or flat webbing is used to form a functional arm sling. A Crazy Creek Chair can be used to improvise both upper and lower extremity splints. Its inherent integral strapping system precludes the need for additional straps or tape.

Functional Shoulder Immobilizer (Shoulder Spica Wrap).
After a dislocated shoulder is reduced, standard treatment is to completely immobilize the arm with a sling and swath. This, however, prevents the victim from using the extremity to facilitate evacuation. A more functional system can be made using a 6-inch elastic wrap. This method allows the victim limited function (e.g., ski poling or kayak paddling) while still preventing complete abduction of the arm.

Triangular Bandage
One of the most ubiquitous components of first-aid kits and one of the easiest to replace through improvisation is the triangular bandage. The need to carry this bulky item, which is commonly used to construct a sling and swath bandage for shoulder and arm immobilization, can be eliminated by carrying two or three safety pins. Pinning the shirt sleeve of the injured arm to the chest portion of the shirt effectively immobilizes the extremity against the body (Figure 19-38, *B*).

If the victim is wearing a short-sleeved shirt, the bottom of the shirt can be folded up and over the arm to create a pouch. This can be pinned to the sleeve and chest section of the shirt to secure the arm (Figure 19-38, *A*).

Triangular bandages are also used for securing splints and constructing pressure wraps. Common items, such as socks, shirts, belts, pack straps, webbing, shoe laces, fanny packs, and underwear, can easily be substituted.

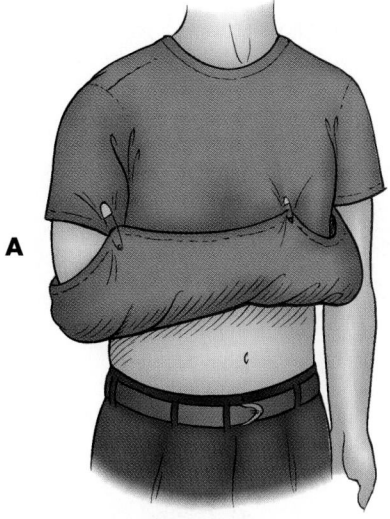

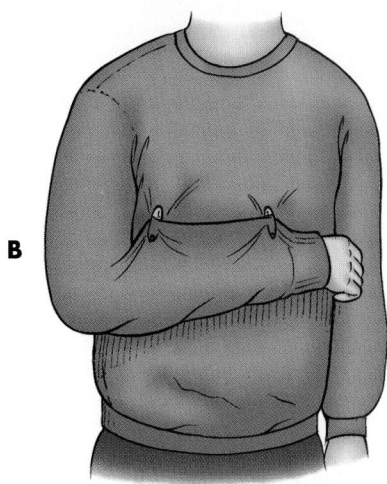

Figure 19-38 Techniques for pinning the arm to the shirt as an improvised sling. **A,** With a short-sleeved shirt the bottom of the shirt is folded up over the injured arm and secured to the sleeve and upper shirt. **B,** With a long-sleeved shirt or jacket the sleeved arm is simply pinned to the chest portion of the garment.

IMPROVISED WOUND MANAGEMENT

The same principles that govern wound management in the emergency department apply in the wilderness. The main problem faced in the wilderness is access to adequate supplies. In deciding to close a wound primarily or pack it open, take into account the mechanism of injury, age of the wound, site of the wound, degree of contamination, and ability to effectively clean the wound.

Wound Irrigation

The primary determinants of infection are bacterial counts and amount of devitalized tissue remaining in the wound.[15] Ridding a wound of bacteria and other particulate matter requires more than soaking and gen-

> **Box 19-3   RECOMMENDED TECHNIQUE FOR WOUND IRRIGATION**
>
> 1. Fill a sandwich or garbage bag with disinfected water.
> 2. Disinfect the water with iodine tablets, iodine solution, or povidone-iodine or by boiling it.
> 3. Normal saline can be made by adding 2 teaspoons of salt (9 g) per liter of water.
> 4. Seal the bag.
> 5. Puncture the bottom of the bag with an 18-gauge needle, safety pin, fork prong, or knife tip.
> 6. Squeeze the top of the bag forcefully while holding it just above the wound, directing the stream into the wound.
> 7. Use caution to ensure that none of the irrigation fluid splashes into your eyes.

tle washing with a disinfectant.[18] Irrigating the wound with a forceful stream is the most effective method of reducing bacterial counts and removing debris and contaminants.[21,27] The cleansing capacity of the stream depends on the hydraulic pressure under which the fluid is delivered.[14,26] Irrigation is best accomplished by attaching an 18- or 19-gauge catheter to a 35-ml syringe or a 22-gauge needle to a 12-ml syringe. This creates hydraulic pressure in the range of 7 to 8 lb/in^2 and 13 lb/in^2, respectively.[14,23,26] The solution is directed into the wound from a distance of 1 to 2 inches at an angle perpendicular to the wound surface and as close to the wound as possible. The amount of irrigation fluid varies with the size and contamination of the wound, but should average no less than 250 ml.[14] Remember, "The solution to pollution is dilution."

Which irrigation solution is best for open wounds? Those who subscribe to the dogma that nothing should enter a wound that could not be instilled safely into the eye believe that normal saline is the best solution.[8,16] In a study of 531 patients with traumatic wounds, there was no significant variation in infection rates among sutured wounds irrigated with normal saline, 1% povidone-iodine, or pluronic F-68 (Shur-Clens).[11]

Tap water was recently found to be as effective for irrigating wounds as sterile saline. In fact, the infection rate was significantly lower after irrigation with tap water, and no infections resulted from the bacteria cultured from the tap water.[2]

Improvised wound irrigation requires only a container that can be punctured to hold the water, such as a sandwich or garbage bag, and a safety pin or 18-gauge needle (Box 19-3).

Wound Closure

Before a wound is closed, remove all foreign material and grossly devitalized tissue. You can accomplish de-

Box 19-4 WOUND TAPING TECHNIQUE

1. Obtain hemostasis and dry the wound edges.
2. Apply benzoin or cyanoacrylate glue to the skin adjacent to the wound. Benzoin should be left to dry until it becomes tacky, but the tape should be applied to the glue while the glue is still wet.
3. Tape should be cut to ¼-inch or ½-inch widths, depending on the size of the laceration, and to a length that allows for 2 to 3 cm of overlap on each side of the wound.
4. Secure one half of the tape to one side of the wound. Oppose the opposite wound edge with a finger while the tape is secured to the other side.
5. Wound tapes should have gaps of 2 to 3 mm between them to allow for serous drainage.
6. Cross-stays of tape can be placed perpendicular over the tape ends to prevent them from peeling off.
7. Additional glue can be applied to the tape edges every 24 hours to reinforce adhesion.

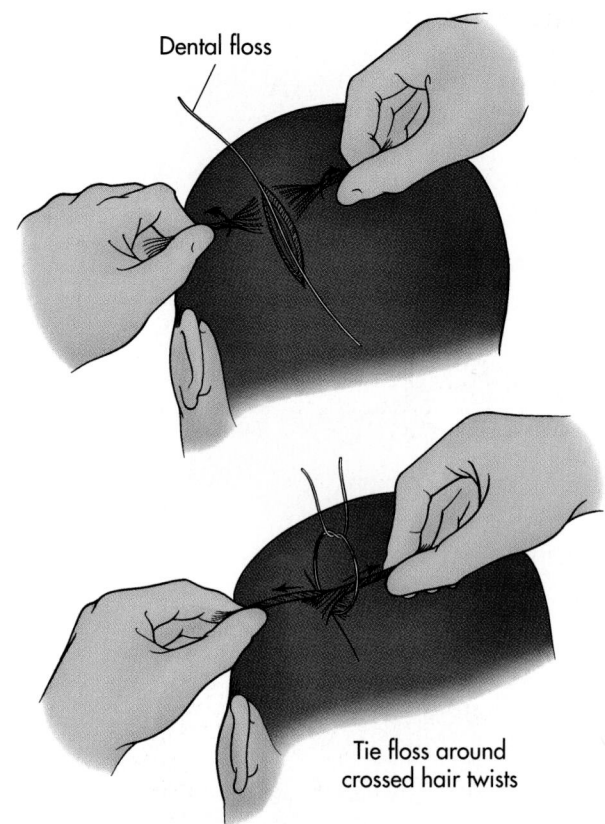

Figure 19-39 Scalp laceration closed using dental floss. (*From Auerbach PS, Donner HJ, Weiss EA:* Field guide to wilderness medicine, *St Louis, 1999, Mosby.*)

bridement using scissors, a knife, or any other sharp object. Close wounds with sutures, staples, tape, pins, or glue. Although suturing is still the most widely used technique, stapling and gluing are ideal methods for closing wounds in the wilderness.

Clinical studies of the use of staples to close traumatic lacerations have found various advantages of stapling over suturing: wound tensile strength is greater, there is less inflammation, the time required for closure is shorter, and fewer instruments are needed.[24] Most important, the cosmetic outcome is not compromised.[13] Staplers are lightweight, presterilized, and easy to use.

Wound Taping. Skin tapes are useful for shallow, nongaping wounds and have several advantages over suturing, including reduced need for anesthesia, ease of application, decreased incidence of wound infection, and availability. Any strong tape can be used to improvise skin tape strips, but duct tape works especially well (Box 19-4). Puncturing holes in the tape before application helps prevent exudate from building up under the tape.

Wipe the skin with a solvent such as acetone first to remove oil and sweat. Then apply benzoin to the skin before the tape to augment adhesion. Wound taping does not work well over joints or on hairy skin surfaces unless the hair is first removed.

Hair-Tying a Scalp Laceration. If you are faced with a bleeding scalp laceration and the injured person has a healthy head of hair, you can tie the wound closed using the victim's own hair and a piece of suture (0-silk

works best), dental floss, sewing thread or thin string. Take the material and lay it on top of and parallel to the wound. Twirl a few strands of hair on each side of the wound and then cross them over the wound in opposite directions so that the force pulls the wound edges together. Have an assistant tie the strands of hair together with the material while you hold the wound closed with the strands of hair. A square knot works best (Figure 19-39). Repeat this technique as many times as necessary, along the length of the wound, to close the laceration.

Gluing. The concept of gluing wounds is not new; the U.S. Army used a quick-sealing glue to treat battlefield wounds in Vietnam, and Histoacryl (butyl-2-cyanoacrylate) tissue adhesive has been used in Europe and Canada for sutureless skin closure for more than a decade.[31]

The U.S. Food and Drug Administration (FDA) has recently approved a topical skin adhesive to repair skin lacerations. Dermabond (2-octyl cyanoacrylate) is packaged in a small single-use applicator and costs about $30 per tube. Tissue glue is ideal for backcountry use because it precludes the need for topical anesthesia, is

Box 19-5   TECHNIQUE FOR GLUING LACERATIONS

1. Irrigate the wound with copious amounts of disinfected water.
2. Control any bleeding with direct pressure. Place a gauze pad moistened with oxymetazoline (Afrin) nasal spray into the wound to help control bleeding.
3. Once hemostasis is obtained, approximate the wound edges using fingers or forceps.
4. Paint the tissue glue over the apposed wound edges using a very light brushing motion of the applicator tip. Avoid excess pressure of the applicator on the tissue because this could separate the skin edges, forcing glue into the wound. Apply multiple thin layers (at least three), allowing the glue to dry between each application (about 2 minutes).
5. Glue can be removed from unwanted surfaces with acetone, or loosened from skin with petrolatum jelly.

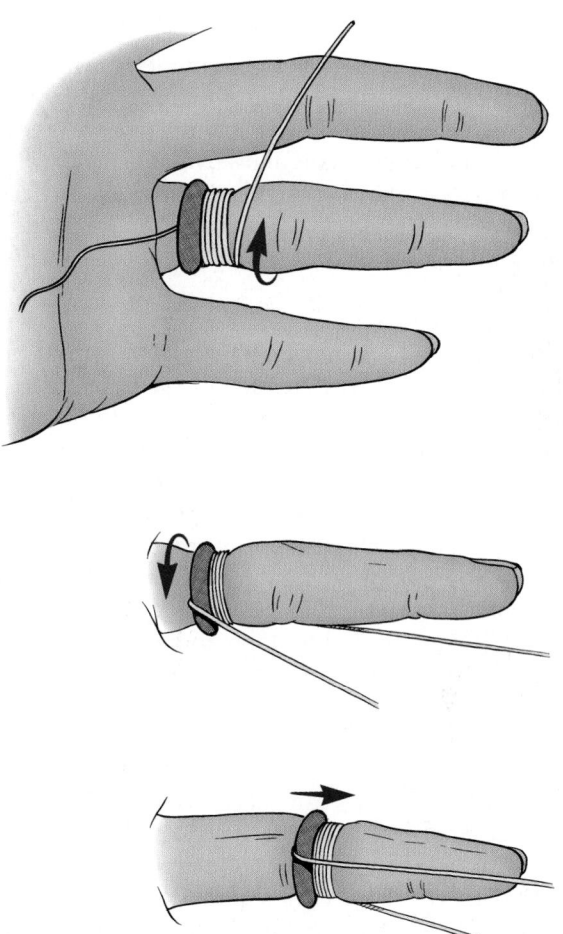

Figure 19-40   String technique for removing a ring from a swollen finger.

easy to use, reduces the risk of needle stick injury, and takes up much less room than a conventional suture kit. When applied to the skin surface, tissue glue provides strong tissue support and peels off in 4 to 5 days without leaving evidence of its presence.[23] It provides a faster and less painful method for closing lacerations than does suturing and has yielded similar cosmetic results in children with facial lacerations (Box 19-5).[22] Tissue glue evokes a mild acute inflammatory reaction with no tissue necrosis.[30]

Dermabond has 4 times the three-dimensional breaking strength of Histoacryl and forms a more flexible bond, thus providing a stronger and longer bond than its European counterpart. Petroleum-based ointments and salves, including antibiotic ointments, should not be used on the wound after gluing, since these substances can weaken the polymerized film and cause wound dehiscence.

Tissue glue has also been used successfully to treat superficial painful fissures of the fingertips ("polar hands"), which commonly occur in cold climates and at high elevations.[3]

RING REMOVAL

Remove rings quickly from injured fingers and after any trauma to the hands. Progressive swelling may cause rings to act as tourniquets. If a ring cannot be removed with soap or lubricating jelly, the string wrap technique can be used. Pass a 20-inch length of fine string, dental floss, umbilical tape, or thick suture between the ring and the finger. Pull the string so that

most of it is on the distal side of the digit and then wrap it around the swollen finger from proximal to distal, beginning next to the ring and continuing past the proximal interphalangeal joint. Place successive loops of the wrap close enough together to prevent any swollen skin from bulging between the strands. Remove the ring by unwinding the proximal end of the string and forcing the ring over the distal string. If the string is not long enough, the technique may require repeated wraps (Figure 19-40).

IMPROVISATIONAL TOOLKIT

Some people, convinced they could whittle a Swan-Ganz catheter from a tree branch, enter the wilderness with nothing more than a Swiss Army knife. However, a little foresight and preparation make improvisation much easier. Efficiency translates into speedy preparation and assembly, which ultimately results in better care. The following section lists items that facilitate improvisation in the field.

Knife

The knife can be a fairly simple model, but it should have an awl for drilling holes into skis, poles, sticks, and so on. The awl on a Swiss Army knife works quite well for this purpose. This allows you to create well-fitted components during improvisation (e.g., a drilled cross-bar attached to ski tips for an improvised rescue toboggan).

Tape

Carry some form of strong, sticky, waterproof tape. (This item *cannot* be improvised.) Use either cloth adhesive tape (already in the medical kit) or duct tape. Duct tape is ideal for almost all tasks, even being useful on skin when needed (e.g., to close wounds, treat blisters, or tape an ankle). Some persons may be sensitive to the adhesive. Fiberglass strapping tape has greater tensile strength and is ideal for joining rigid components, such as taping two ice axes together. However, it is less sticky than duct tape and not as useful for patching torn items. Extra tape can be carried by wrapping lengths of it around pieces of gear.

Plastic Cable Ties

Lightweight cable ties can be used to bind almost anything together (for example, binding pack frames together for improvised litters or ski poles together for improvised carriers). They are also perfect for repairing many items in the backcountry.

Parachute Cord

Parachute cord has hundreds of uses in the backcountry. It can be used for trucker's hitch traction and for tying complex splints together. Parachute cord is light; carry a good supply.

Safety Pins

Safety pins have various uses (Box 19-6).

Wire

Braided picture-hanging wire works well because it is supple and ties like line. Its strength makes it superior for repairing and improvising components under an extreme load, such as fabricating improvised rescue sleds or repairing broken or detached ski bindings.

Bolts and Wing Nuts

Bolts and wing nuts make the job of constructing an improvised rescue sled much easier (see Improvised Rescue Sled or Toboggan section). Bolts are useful only if holes can be created to put them through. Therefore a knife with an awl is needed for drilling holes through skis, poles, and so on.

Prefabricated Cross-Bar

The prefabricated cross-bar can be used for double ski pole traction splint systems. A cross-bar is easily fabri-

Box 19-6   USES OF A SAFETY PIN
Using two safety pins to pin the anterior aspect of the tongue to the lower lip to establish an airway in an unconscious victim whose airway is obstructed
Replacing the lost screw in a pair of eyeglasses to prevent the lens from falling out
Improvising glasses: Draw two circles in a piece of duct tape where your eyes would fit. Use the pin to make holes in the circles, then tape this to your face. The pinholes will partially correct myopic vision and protect the eyes from ultraviolet radiation. Slits can also be used for improvised sunglasses.
Neurosensory skin testing
Puncturing plastic bags for irrigation of wounds
Removing embedded foreign bodies from the skin
Draining an abscess or blister
Relieving a subungual hematoma
As a fishhook
As a finger splint (mallet finger)
As a sewing needle, using dental floss as thread
Holding gaping wounds together
Replacing a broken clothing zipper
Holding gloves or mittens to a coat sleeve
Unclogging jets in a camping stove
Pinning triage notes to multiple victims
Removing a corneal foreign body (with ophthalmic anesthetic)
In a sling and swath for shoulder or arm injuries
To fix a ski binding
To extract the clot from a thrombosed hemorrhoid
To pin a strap or shirt tightly around the chest for rib fracture support
Tick removal

cated from a branch or short section of a ski pole, but carrying a prefabricated device, such as a 6-inch predrilled ski pole section, saves time (see Figure 19-22).

Ensolite (Closed-Cell Foam) Pads

Since the introduction of Therm-a-Rest types of inflatable pads, closed-cell foam has become increasingly scarce; however, closed-cell foam (Ensolite) is still the ultimate padding for almost any improvised splint or rescue device. The uses for closed-cell foam are virtually unlimited. Even die-hard Therm-a-Rest fans should carry a small amount of closed-cell foam, which is lightweight and doubles as a comfortable seat cushion. Furthermore, unlike inflatable pads, Ensolite will not puncture and deflate.

Therm-a-Rest pads also have their place, being useful for padding for long bone splints and immobilizers (e.g., an improvised universal knee immobilizer). An inflatable pad can also be used to cushion pelvic fractures. First, wrap the deflated pad around the pelvis.

Then secure the pad with tape and inflate it, creating an improvised substitute for military antishock trousers (MAST device).

Fluorescent Surveyor's Tape

Surveyor's tape can be used much like Hansel and Gretel's bread crumbs to help relocate a route into or out of a rescue scene. It is also ideal for marking shelters in deep snow and can serve as a wind sock during helicopter operations on improvised landing zones. Surveyor's tape is not biodegradable, so it should always be removed from the site after the rescue is completed.

Space Blanket or Lightweight Tarp

For improvising hasty shelters in times of emergency, some form of tarp is essential. In the snow a slit trench shelter can be built in a matter of minutes using a tarp. Otherwise, the complex and time-consuming construction of improvised structures such as snow caves, igloos, or tree branch shelters might be necessary. Typically, little time or help is available for this task during emergencies. In addition, tarps are essential for "hypothermia wraps" when managing injured persons in cold or wet conditions. The only advantage of a space blanket over other tarps is its small size, which means there is a good chance it was packed for the trip.

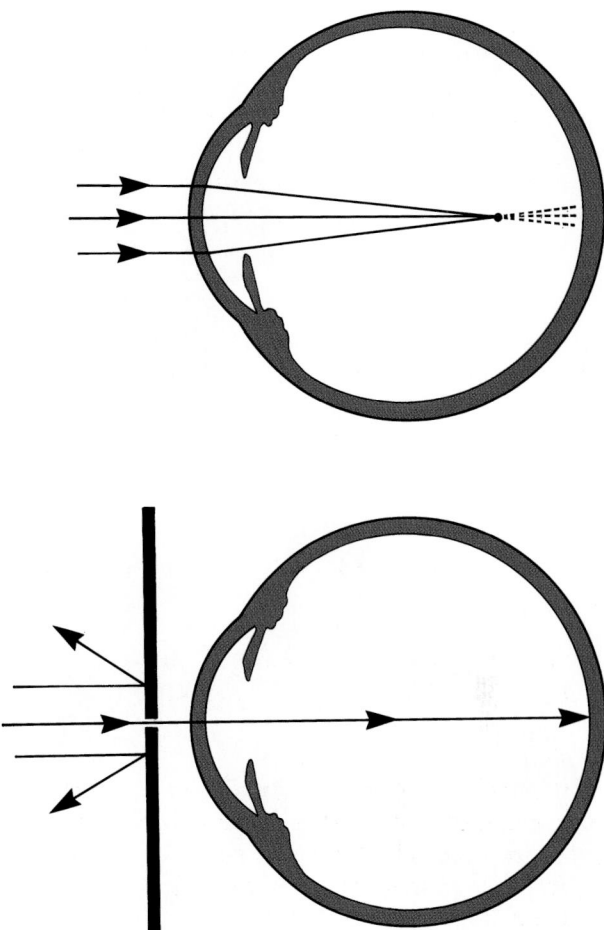

Figure 19-41 Pinhole in cardboard to improve vision in person with myopia.

IMPROVISED EYEGLASSES

Exposure of unprotected eyes to ultraviolet radiation at high altitudes may produce photokeratitis (snow blindness). Symptoms are delayed, and the victim is often unaware that an eye injury is developing. When sunglasses are lost at 4267 m (14,000 feet) in the snow, photokeratitis can develop in 20 minutes. You can improvise sunglasses from duct tape, cardboard, or other light-impermeable material that can be cut. Cardboard glasses with narrow eye slits can be taped over the eyes for protection.

Slits can also be cut into a piece of duct tape that has been folded over on itself with the sticky sides opposing. After a triangular wedge is removed for the nose, apply another piece of tape to secure the glasses to the head.

Pinhole tape glasses can improve vision in a myopic person whose corrective lenses have been lost. With myopia, parallel light rays from distant objects focus in front of the retina. The pinhole directs entering light to the center of the cornea, where refraction (bending of the light) is unnecessary. Light remains in focus regardless of the refractive error of the eye (Figure 19-41). Pinhole glasses decrease both illumination and field of vision, so puncture a piece of duct tape or cardboard repeatedly with a safety pin, needle, fork, or other sharp object until enough light can enter to focus on distant objects. Secure the device to the face.

IMPROVISED TRANSPORT

Carries

Two-Hand Seat.* Two carriers stand side by side. Each carrier grasps the other carrier's wrists with opposite hands (for example, right to left). The victim sits on the rescuers' joined forearms. The carriers each maintain one free hand to place behind the back of the victim for support (support hands can be joined). This system places great stress on the carriers' forearms and wrists.

Four-Hand Seat. Two carriers stand side by side. Each carrier grasps his or her own right forearm with the left hand, palms facing down. Each carrier then grasps the forearm of the other with his or her free hand to form a square "forearm" seat. With the forearm seat, the victim must support himself or herself with a hand around the rescuers' backs.

---

*Both the two-hand seat and the four-hand seat are useful only for very short carries over gentle terrain.

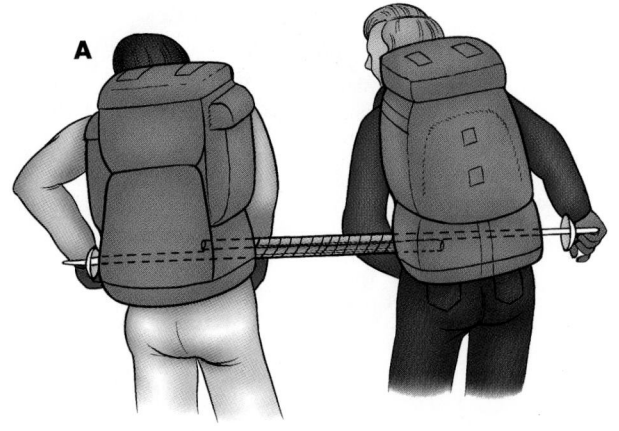

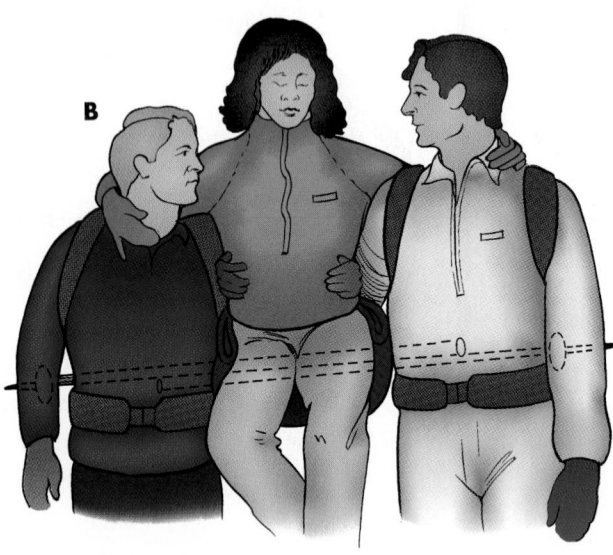

Figure 19-42 Ski pole seat. **A,** Ski poles are anchored by the packs. **B,** The victim is supported by the rescuers.

Ski Pole or Ice Ax Carry. Two carriers with backpacks stand side by side with four ski poles or joined ice ax shafts, resting between them and the base of the pack straps (Figure 19-42). The ski poles or ice ax shafts can be joined with cable ties, adhesive tape, duct tape, wire, or cord. Because the rescuers must walk side by side, this technique requires wide-open, gentle terrain. The victim sits on the padded poles or shaft with his or her arms over the carriers' shoulders.

Split-Coil Seat ("Tragsitz"). The split-coil seat transport uses a coiled climbing rope to join the rescuer and victim together in a piggyback fashion (Figure 19-43). The victim must be able to support himself or herself to avoid falling back, or must be tied in.

Two-Rescuer Split-Coil Seat. The two-rescuer split-coil seat is essentially the same as the split-coil Tragsitz transport, except that two rescuers split the coil over their shoulders. The victim sits on the low point of the

rope between the rescuers (Figure 19-44). Each rescuer maintains a free hand to help support the victim.

Backpack Carry. A large backpack is modified by cutting leg holes at the base. The victim sits in it like a baby carrier. Some large internal frame packs incorporate a sleeping bag compartment in the lower portion of the pack that includes a compression panel. With this style of pack, the victim can sit on the suspended panel and place his or her legs through the unzipped lower section without damaging the pack, or the victim can simply sit on the internal sleeping bag compression panel without the need to cut holes.

Nylon Webbing Carry. Nylon webbing can be used to attach the victim to the rescuer like a backpack (Figure 19-45). At least 4.6 to 6.1 m (15 to 20 feet) of nylon webbing is needed to construct this transport. The center of the webbing is placed behind the victim and brought forward under the armpits. The webbing is then crossed and brought over the rescuer's shoulders, then down around the victim's thighs. The webbing is finally brought forward and tied around the rescuer's waist. Additional padding is needed for this system, especially around the posterior thighs of the victim.

Three-Person Wheelbarrow Carry. This system is extremely efficient and can be used for prolonged periods on relatively rough terrain. The victim places his or her arms over two rescuers' shoulders (the rescuers stand side by side). The victim's legs are then placed over a third rescuer's shoulders. This system equalizes the weight of the victim very efficiently.

Litters (Nonrigid)

Many nonrigid litter systems have been developed over the years. These systems are best suited for transporting non–critically injured victims over moderate terrain. They should *never* be used for trauma victims with potential spine injuries.

Blanket Litter. A simple nonrigid litter can be fabricated from two rigid poles, branches, or skis and a large blanket or tarp. The blanket or tarp is wrapped around the skis or poles as many times as possible and the poles are carried. The blanket or tarp should not be simply draped over the poles. For easier carrying, the poles can be rigged to the base of backpacks. Large external frame packs work best, but internal frame packs can be rigged to do the job. Alternatively, a padded harness to support the litter can be made from a single piece of webbing, in a design similar to a nylon webbing carry.

Tree Pole Litter. The tree pole litter is similar to the blanket litter described previously. In the tree pole lit-

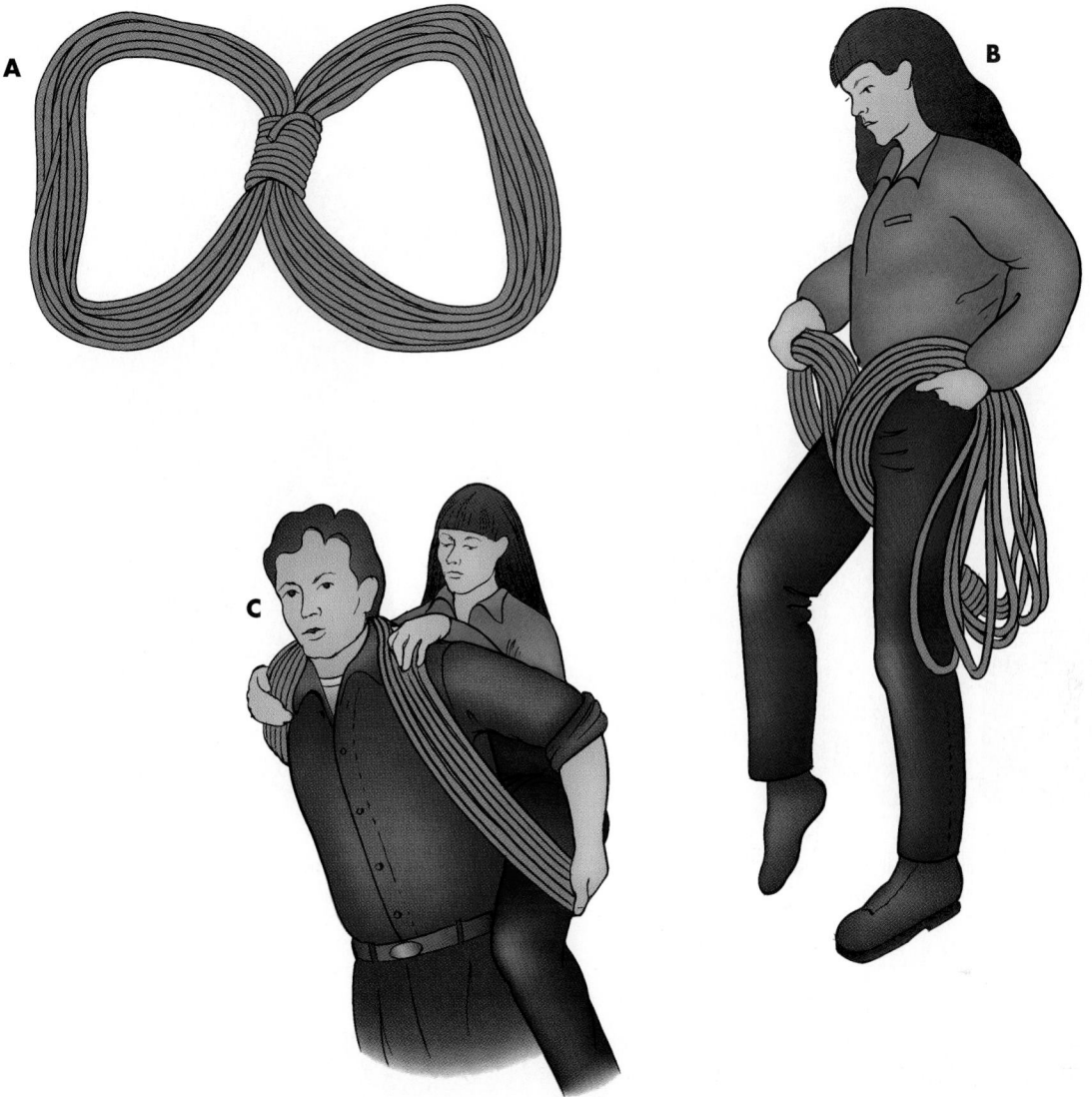

Figure 19-43 Split-coil seat. **A,** Rope coil is split. **B,** Victim climbs through rope. **C,** Rescuer hoists the sitting victim.

ter, instead of a blanket or a tarp, the side poles are laced together with webbing or rope and then padded. Again, the poles may be fitted through pack frames to aid carrying. To give this litter more stability and to add tension to the lacing, the rescuer should fabricate a rectangle with rigid cross-bars at both ends before lacing.

Parka Litter. Two or more parkas can be used to form a litter (Figure 19-46). Skis or branches are slipped through the sleeves of heavy parkas, and the parkas are zipped shut with the sleeves inside. Ski edges should be taped first to prevent them from tearing through the parkas.

Internal Frame Pack Litter. The internal frame pack litter is constructed from two to three full-size internal

frame backpacks, which must have lateral compression straps (day packs are suboptimal). Slide poles or skis through the compression straps; the packs then act as a support surface for the victim.

Life Jacket Litter. Life jackets can be placed over paddles or oars to create a makeshift nonrigid litter.

Rope Litter. On mountaineering trips the classic rope litter can be used, but this system offers little back support and should never be used for victims with suspected spine injuries. The rope is uncoiled and staked onto the ground with 16 180-degree bends (eight on each side of the rope center). The rope bends should approximate the size of the finished litter. The free rope ends are then used to clove hitch off each bend (leaving 2 inches of bend to the outside of each clove hitch). The

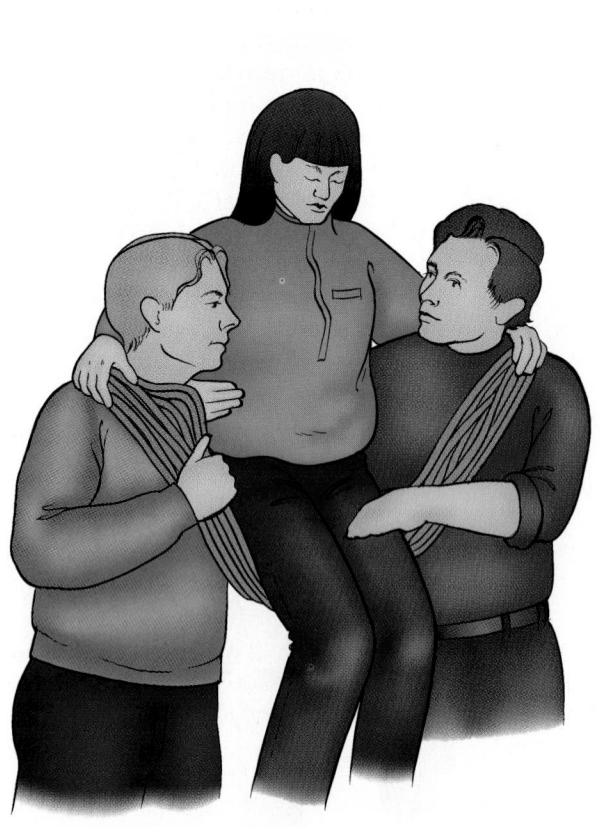

Figure 19-44 Two-rescuer split-coil seat. Balance could be improved by using a longer coil to carry the victim lower.

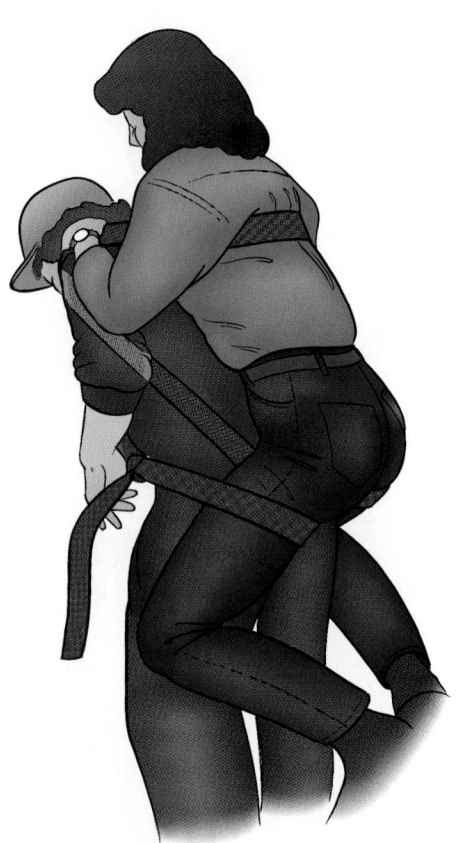

Figure 19-45 Webbing carry. Webbing crisscrosses in front of the victim's chest before passing over the shoulders of the rescuer.

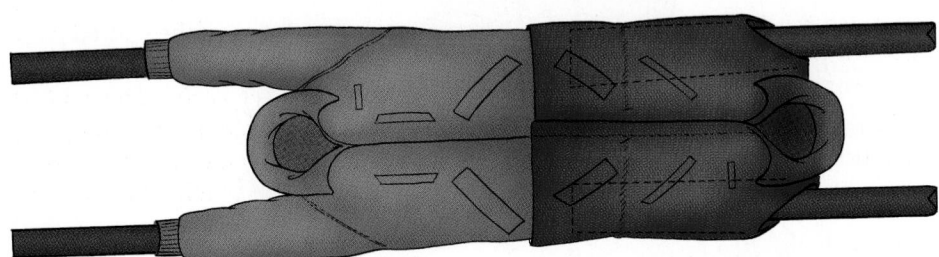

Figure 19-46 Parka litter. On the right the sleeves are zipped inside to reinforce the litter.

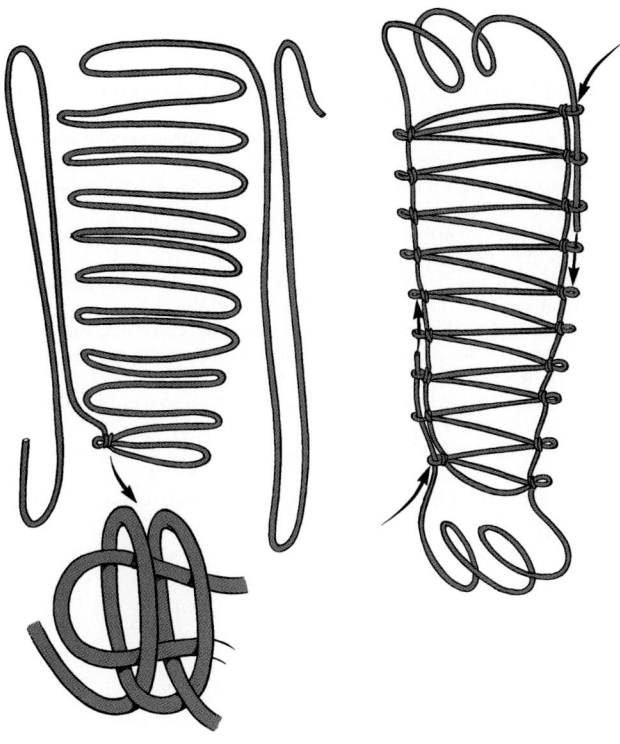

Figure 19-47 Rope litter.

leftover rope is threaded through the loops at the outside of each clove hitch. This gives the rescuers a continuous handhold and protects the bends from slipping through the clove hitches. The rope ends are then tied off (Figure 19-47). The litter is padded with packs, Therm-a-Rest pads, or foam pads. This improvised litter is somewhat ungainly and requires six or more rescuers for an evacuation of any distance. A rope litter can be tied to poles or skis to add lateral stability if needed.

Improvised Rescue Sled or Toboggan

A sled or toboggan can be constructed from one or more pairs of skis and poles that are lashed, wired, or screwed together. Many designs are possible. Improvised rescue sleds may be clumsy and often bog down hopelessly in deep snow. Nonetheless, they can be useful for transporting a victim over short distances (to a more sheltered camp or to a more appropriate landing zone). They have sometimes been used for more extensive transports, but they do not perform as well as commercial rescue sleds.

To build an improvised rescue sled/toboggan, the rescuer needs a pair of skis (preferably the victim's) and two pairs of ski poles; three 2-foot-long sticks (or ski pole sections); 24.4 m (80 feet) of nylon cord; and extra lengths of rope for sled hauling.

The skis are placed 0.6 m (2 feet) apart. The first stick is used as the front cross-bar and is lashed to the

ski tips. Alternately, holes can be drilled into the stick and ski tips with an awl, and bolts can be used to fasten them together. The middle stick is lashed to the bindings. One pair of ski poles is placed over the crossbars (baskets over the ski tips) and lashed down. The second set of poles is lashed to the middle stick with baskets facing back toward the tails. A third rear stick is placed on the tails of the skis and lashed to the poles. The lashings are not wrapped around the skis; the cross-bar simply sits on the tails of the skis under the weight of the victim. Nylon cord is then woven back and forth across the horizontal ski poles. The hauling ropes are passed through the baskets on the front of the sled. The ropes are then brought around the middle cross-bar and back to the front cross-bar. This rigging system reverses the direction of pull on the front cross-bar, making it less likely to slip off the ski tips.[29]

Another sled design incorporates a predrilled snow shovel incorporated into the front of the sled. A rigid backpack frame can also be used to reinforce the sled. This requires drilling holes into the ski tips and carrying a predrilled shovel. This system holds the skis in a wedge position and may offer slightly greater durability.[25]

A FINAL NOTE

Under certain conditions, improvised systems are entirely *suboptimal* and may not meet standard of care criteria. It would, for example, be ill advised to fabricate a litter for transporting a victim with a suspected spine injury when professional rescue is only a few miles away. An improvised litter system might be entirely appropriate, however, if the injured person is 40 miles out and needs transport to a sheltered camp or potential helicopter landing zone. The context of the situation should be considered. At times, persons are obligated to do whatever they can, and a resourceful approach to problem solving combined with a little ingenuity could save a victim's life.

REFERENCES

1. Anderson GH et al: Preoperative skin traction for fractures of the proximal femur, *J Bone Joint Surg* 75B:794, 1993.
2. Angeras MH, Brandberg A: Comparison between sterile saline and tap water for the cleansing of acute traumatic soft tissue wounds, *Eur J Surg* 158:347, 1992.
3. Ayton JM: Polar hands: spontaneous skin fissures closed with histoacryl blue tissue adhesive in Antarctica, *Arctic Med Res* 52:127, 1993.
4. Bancewicz J: Oesophageal bolus extraction by balloon catheter, *BMJ* 1:1142, 1978.
5. Bigler FC: The use of a Foley catheter for removal of blunt foreign objects from the esophagus, *J Thorac Cardiovasc Surg* 51:759, 1966.
6. Borschneck AG: Why traction? *J Emerg Med Serv* 10:44, 1985.
7. Bratton JR: Epistaxis management: conservative and surgical, *J S Carolina Med Assoc* 80:395, 1984.
8. Bryant CA et al: Search for a non-toxic surgical scrub solution for periorbital lacerations, *Ann Emerg Med* 5:317, 1984.
9. Chan D et al: The effect of spinal immobilization on healthy volunteers, *Ann Emerg Med* 23:48, 1994.
10. Cook PR, Renner G, Williams F: A comparison of nasal balloons and posterior gauze packs for posterior epistaxis, *Ear Nose Throat J* 64:446, 1985.

11. Dire D: A comparison of wound irrigation solutions used in the emergency department, *Ann Emerg Med* 19:704, 1990.

12. Dunlap LB: Removal of an esophageal foreign body using a Foley catheter, *Ann Emerg Med* 10:101, 1981.

13. Dunmire SM et al: Staples versus sutures for wounds closure in the pediatric population, *Ann Emerg Med* 18:448, 1989.

14. Edlich RF: Current concepts of emergency wound management, *Emerg Med Rep* 5:22, 1984.

15. Edlich RF et al: Principles of emergency wound management, *Ann Emerg Med* 17:1284, 1988.

16. Edlich RF, Sinkinson CA: Current concepts of emergency wound management. Part II, *Emerg Med Rep* 5:173, 1984.

17. Isaac J, Goth P: *The Outward Bound wilderness first aid handbook,* New York, 1991, Lyons & Burford.

18. Lammers RL et al: Effect of povidone-iodine and saline soaking on bacterial counts in acute, traumatic, contaminated wounds, *Ann Emerg Med* 19:709, 1990.

19. Lyons S, Wilderness Professional Training, Crested Butte, Colo, personal correspondence, 1994.

20. Nandi P, Ong GB: Foreign body in the esophagus: review of 2394 cases, *Br J Surg* 65:5, 1978.

21. Peterson L: Prophylaxis of wound infections, *Arch Surg* 50:177, 1945.

22. Quinn JV et al: A randomized, controlled trial comparing a tissue adhesive with suturing in the repair of pediatric facial lacerations, *Ann Emerg Med* 22:1130, 1993.

23. Rodeheaver GT et al: Wound cleansing by high pressure irrigation, *Surg Gynecol Obstet* 141:357, 1975.

24. Roth JH, Windle BH: Staple versus suture closure of skin incisions in a pig model, *Can J Surg* 31:19, 1988.

25. Schimelpfenig T, Lindsey L: *NOLS wilderness first aid,* Wyoming, 1991, NOLS Publications.

26. Sinkinson CA: Maximizing a wound's potential for healing, *Emerg Med Rep* 10:11, 1989.

27. Stevenson T et al: Cleansing the traumatic wound by high-pressure syringe irrigation, *J Am Coll Emerg Phys* 5:17, 1976.

28. Taylor RB: Esophageal foreign bodies, *Emerg Med Clin North Am* 5:2, 1987.

29. Tilton B: *The basic essentials of rescue from the backcountry,* Merrilville, Ind, 1990, ICS Books.

30. Toriumi DM et al: Histotoxicity of histoacryl when used in a subcutaneous site, *Laryngoscope,* April 1991.

31. Watson DP: Use of cyanoacrylate tissue adhesive for closing facial lacerations in children, *Br Med J* 299:1014, 1989.

32. Yonkers AJ et al: Etiology and management of epistaxis, *Ear Nose Throat J* 60:453, 1981.

20 Hunting and Other Weapons Injuries

Edward J. Otten

*E*ven as Nimrod the mighty hunter before the Lord.

Genesis 10:9

Anthropologists have many theories concerning the origins and importance of hunting in the evolution of the human species. The physical attributes of bipedal locomotion, binocular vision, and an opposable thumb all make humans more efficient hunters. Whether these exist because humans have an innate compulsion to hunt or whether humans are hunters because of these traits is debatable. There is no debate, however, that human social evolution, language, the use of tools, and domestication of animals are directly related to more efficient hunting. In a survival situation, and in some ways with regard to evolution, hunter-gatherer animals have a distinct advantage over strictly vegetarian animals because of the relative food value of meat over plants. Hunters tend to be males. Approximately three fourths of all calories in modern hunter-gatherer groups are derived from plants, and this portion of the food is usually supplied by the women in the group. Even in Eskimo tribes where plants make up little of the diet, the women do most of the fishing while the men hunt.

Hominids were at a disadvantage, even in groups, when hunting large animals or driving off other predators from their kills until they began using stones, long bones, and sticks to enhance their relatively weak teeth and claws. Implements for hunting and skinning animals were the earliest tools found by anthropologists. Human cultural evolution followed closely the technologic changes in weapons, although sports, business, and war had replaced the need for hunting in most cultures even by the time Nimrod walked the earth. Bows and arrows, slings, spear throwers, nets, harpoons, traps, and firearms were designed to extend the reach and increase the lethality of the human hand. Unfortunately, humans discovered that they could kill each other with these weapons. Since the discovery of gunpowder, the development of weapons technology has surpassed all other forms of human endeavor, including medicine and transportation.[6,7]

HUNTING IN THE UNITED STATES

Only a few cultures still depend on hunting as their primary food-gathering method. Examples are the Mbuti tribe, Andaman Islanders, and Eskimos. Many cultures, however, use hunting to supplement agriculture, plant gathering, or raising livestock. Most hunting in the United States is done for sport or pleasure, although in some areas of the country hunting and trapping are still the primary source of income for a few people. The total number of hunters and trappers is unknown. Many participate illegally and are not licensed. Throughout the United States, 30 million hunting licenses were sold in 1988. Although hunting seasons are regulated and relatively short, hunters spent 16 million visitor-days in the national forests.

The North American Association of Hunter Safety Coordinators, a division of the New York State Office of Wildlife Management, reported 860 fatal hunting injuries during the 4-year period 1983-1986, with a total of 6992 injuries from firearms. Interestingly, 34% of the total injuries and 89% of the handgun injuries were self-inflicted. Shotguns accounted for 106 of the fatalities and 906 of the total injuries, whereas rifles accounted for 79 fatalities and 465 injuries. Hunting injuries are only a small portion of the total number of unintentional firearm deaths in the United States. Of 131 firearm deaths in California from 1977 to 1983, only eight were the result of hunting accidents.* Hunting injury data may be inaccurate for a number of reasons. Many minor nonfatal injuries may go unreported, and most states do not differentiate accidental firearm hunting deaths from deaths that occur during any other activity. Also, automobile and all-terrain vehicle accidents that occur while hunting, or gunshot wounds inflicted while "cleaning a gun" at home, could be considered nonhunting injuries.

Types of Injuries Encountered

Most injuries to hunters are the same types of injury seen in backpackers, fishermen, and climbers. Frostbite, sprains, burns, and fractures occur with the same frequency in hunters as in others who visit wilderness areas.

A common type of injury in hunters that is not associated with weapons is the tree stand injury. Tree stands are platforms designed to hold hunters several feet off the ground so that they can more easily kill large game. Whether homemade or of commercial design, the platforms generally are small and attached to the trunks of trees, with some method, usually a ladder or steps, for

---

*References 8, 10, 22, 29, 36, 40.

495

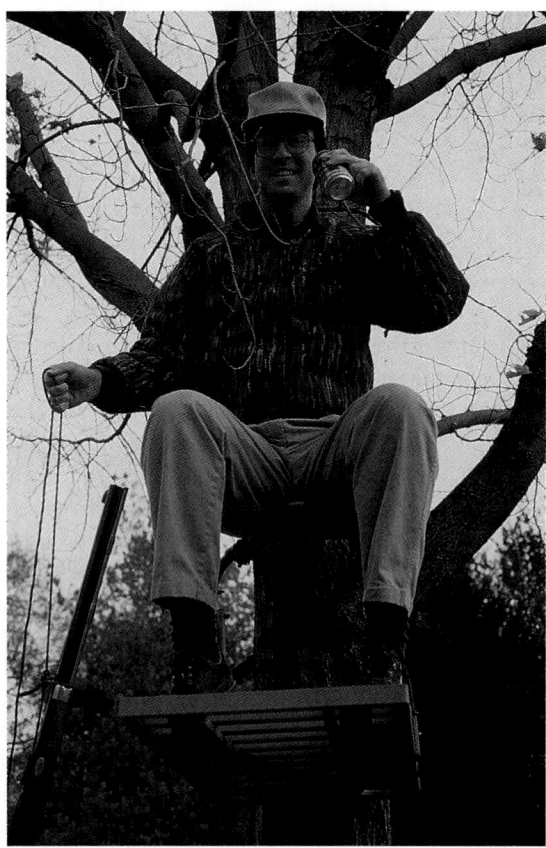

Figure 20-1 The wrong way to use a tree stand. This hunter is not wearing a safety harness, is drinking alcohol, and is pulling his firearm into the tree stand with the muzzle pointing upward.

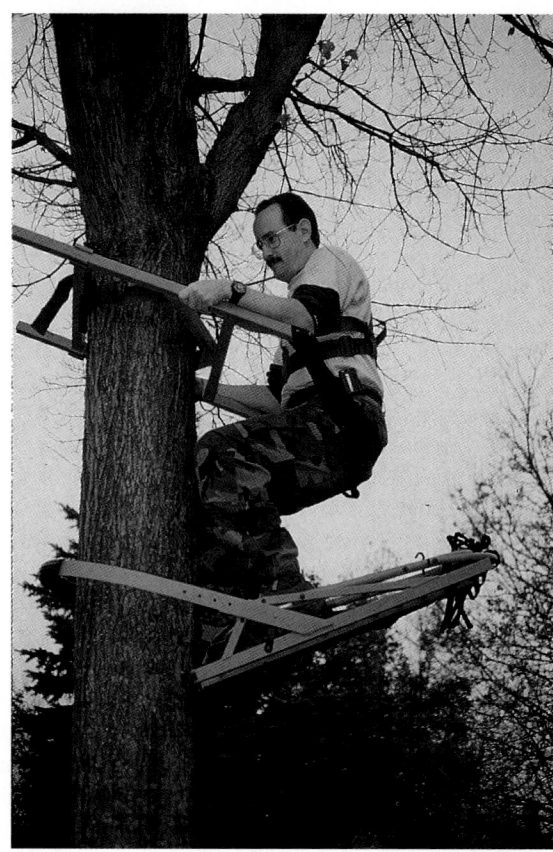

Figure 20-2 A commercially produced tree stand can be used to climb the tree and obviates the need for a ladder or steps, which are the cause of many falls.

climbing the tree (Figures 20-1 and 20-2). Hunters often fall asleep in the platforms and fall off, or fall while climbing up or down trees. At least half of these injuries could be prevented if all hunters wore tree stand safety harnesses. Although most of the injuries are similar to those seen with any type of fall, occasionally a hunter drops a firearm, which discharges, or falls on an arrow or rifle, causing an additional weapons injury (Figure 20-3). Over 10 years, injuries of this type in Georgia accounted for 36% of reported hunting injuries and 20% of hunting fatalities.[35,37]

Injuries that are unique to hunters are those caused by their weapons. Most hunting is done with firearms. Shotguns and rifles are more commonly used, although handguns are increasing in popularity. Other types of weapon include the bow or crossbow and arrow. These are popular because an extended hunting season is allowed in several states if this type of "primitive" weapon is used. The rationale is that these weapons are less dangerous to innocent bystanders at long range compared with rifles and shotguns, and that more skill is needed to hunt with this type of weapon.

Other weapons are used for hunting but are less likely to be encountered. For example, spears, har-

poons, and nets are used by some hunters in the Arctic, Australia, and Africa. Trap injuries may be included in the definition of hunting injuries. Most traps are designed to catch and hold small game. Injuries usually occur when a trapper triggers a spring-loaded trap prematurely. Crush injuries and puncture wounds to the hands are most common. Hikers occasionally tread on unmarked traps, and domestic animals such as dogs are accidentally caught in poachers' traps. Another problem with traps occurs when an animal (wild or domestic) is caught in a trap and attacks the trapper while being released. Many knife lacerations occur when hunters clean game. Lack of familiarity with the process or techniques for field dressing and cleaning game is the likely cause. Failing to wear protective gloves; using the wrong type of knife; working with bloody, slippery material; and having cold hands all contribute to accidents.

Arrow Injuries. Modern arrows are usually made from aluminum, graphite, or fiberglass, although many beginners still use inexpensive wooden arrows. A number of types of arrowhead are in use,

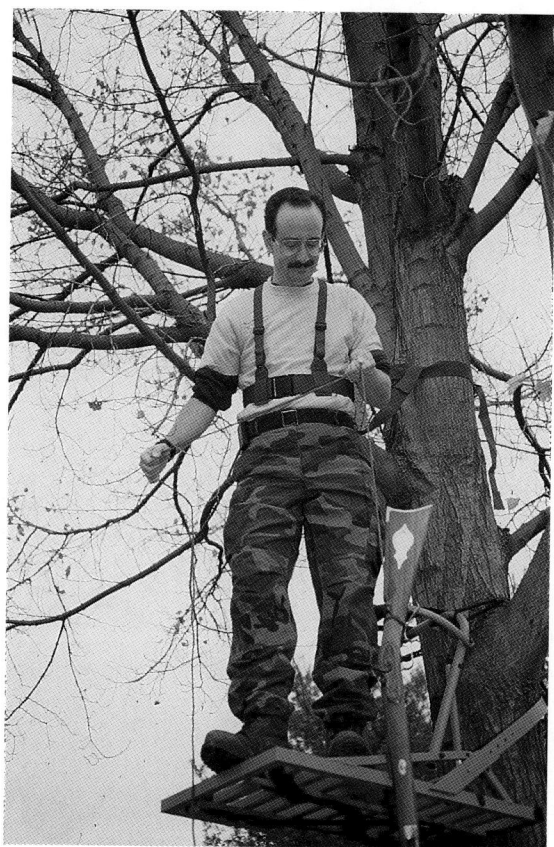

Figure 20-3 The correct way to bring a firearm into the tree stand, with the muzzle pointing down and the hunter wearing a safety harness at all times.

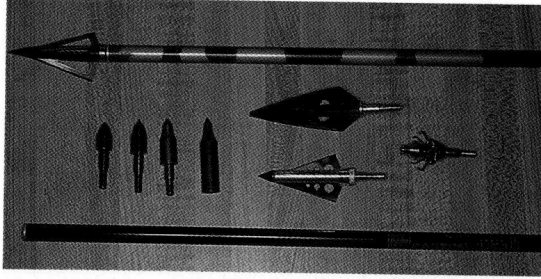

Figure 20-4 Types of arrows. *Top,* Aluminum shaft arrow with hunting broadhead. *Middle (left to right),* Four field points of various weights: two types of broadheads and small game blunt hunting head with spring claws to prevent arrow loss from burrowing into the ground. Bottom, Fiberglass shaft for interchangeable heads.

such as field points and target points, but most injuries are due to broadheads. These come in a variety of sizes and shapes and are designed to inflict injury by lacerating tissue and blood vessels, thereby causing bleeding and shock. Unlike firearms, which are designed to kill quickly by tearing tissue and transferring large amounts of energy, arrows usually kill more slowly with less tissue damage (Figure 20-4).[4,19] Arrows are propelled by a conventional bow, which may be straight, recurved, or compound, or by a crossbow. The force used to propel the arrow is usually measured in "draw weight," which is the number of foot-pounds necessary to draw a 28-inch arrow to its full length. The higher the pound draw, the more powerful the bow and the deeper the penetration the same type of arrow will have. Arrows have a much shorter range than bullets and must be more accurately placed to kill the animal quickly; therefore most shots are taken under 50 m (164 feet). Because brush and tree branches can easily deflect an arrow, most shots are taken with a clear field of view. For these reasons, target identification is usually not a problem and a bow hunter is less likely to shoot another hunter. Most arrow injuries occur when hunters fire illegally at night in heavy brush and are not

sure of their target. Another common injury occurs when a hunter runs after a wounded animal and falls on an arrow that was to be used for a second shot or falls out of a tree stand onto an arrow. A loaded crossbow is similar to a loaded gun. Hunters have been accidentally shot when dropping the weapon or snagging the trigger on a branch or fence. Hunting arrowheads are quite sharp; injuries commonly occur when a hunter is sharpening the blade of the arrow or returning an arrow to the quiver.

Injuries from Firearms. Firearms discharge a projectile by using air, modern fast-burning powders, or old-fashioned black powder. Air guns use a spring or carbon dioxide cartridge to push the projectile from the barrel. Although air guns are quite accurate at short distances, the projectiles cannot usually penetrate skin from distances greater than 100 m (328 feet). Air guns are commonly used by children, who cannot legally obtain or use other types of firearms. Well-meaning parents buy them as toys, erroneously believing them to be safe. The wounds they cause can be lethal, especially from the spring-propelled guns, which can send out lead pellets at sufficiently high velocities to penetrate bone. Black powder weapons use a solid propellant that is ignited with a spark from flint striking steel or a percussion cap. When ignited, the propellant is rapidly converted to a gas that expands and pushes a lead ball out of the barrel of the weapon. These weapons are quite accurate and are used to hunt large game, such as deer and elk. The injuries from black powder weapons are similar to those from modern weapons and are discussed below. The same precautions should be used when hunting with or shooting any type of firearm, whether the propellant is air or gunpowder.[24,28,39]

The powder (propellant) in weapons that use modern gunpowder is encased in a brass or aluminum shell for rifles and handguns and in a plastic or paper shell for shotguns. Shells are open on one end for the actual projectiles to be inserted, and in the case of shotgun shells, plastic or cotton wadding is used to keep the projectiles from moving around inside the shells. The powder is detonated from the opposite end by an explosive primer that is in either the rim of the shell, as with the .22 caliber long rifle cartridge, or the middle of the shell, as with the 12-gauge shotgun shell or 30/30 rifle cartridge. Detonation occurs when the firing pin on the weapon strikes the primer, igniting the powder. Upon detonation the powder produces a rapidly expanding gas that pushes the projectile (and wadding) out of the barrel of the weapon. Not all of the powder is burned, so that in case of close-proximity wounds, powder stippling may appear on clothing or skin. With contact wounds the escaping gases may cause bursting of the skin and a stellate laceration near the point of entrance. The projectile may vary in size and shape from 1 mm in circumference and a few milligrams in weight to 2 cm in circumference and 100 g in weight. The projectiles are usually made of lead or steel and may be covered with a copper jacket. They are usually single when shot from a rifle or pistol and multiple when fired from a shotgun, although some hunters prefer large single (deer slug) rounds fired from shotguns.

Hundreds of types of bullets or rounds are available for firearms. They may be factory loaded or hand loaded, which adds the variables of propellant amount and type. Small arms are classified according to caliber, which is expressed in fractions of an inch; for example, .22 caliber means the diameter of the bullet is 0.22 inch; .45 caliber is 0.45 inch; and so forth. The caliber may be expressed in metric measurement; for example, a 9 mm bullet is 9 mm in diameter, which also happens to be 0.357 inch. This system can be made more complicated when considering the amount of powder used, the year the bullet was adopted, or the name of the person who first introduced the round. Examples of these types are .45/70 (70 grains of powder), .30-06 (adopted in 1906), and .35 Whelen (the man who developed the round). Shotgun terminology is a little less complicated, based on the number of lead balls, the diameter of the barrel, and how many lead balls it takes to make a pound. For example, a 12-gauge shotgun has a barrel that is the same diameter as a lead ball that weighs 1/12 pound, a 20-gauge, 1/20 pound. The higher the gauge, the smaller the barrel and the smaller the round. The only exception is the .410 shotgun, which is caliber .410 or 0.410 inch in diameter. The recent introduction of the term "magnum" refers more to the type and amount of powder than to the size of the bullet used (Figures 20-5 and 20-6).

The type and severity of wounds inflicted by a firearm depend on several factors. The most often quoted factor, but the least important, is the amount of energy the bullet (projectile) has when leaving the firearm. The kinetic energy formula, $KE = \frac{1}{2} MV^2$, can be applied to any moving object or to calculate the

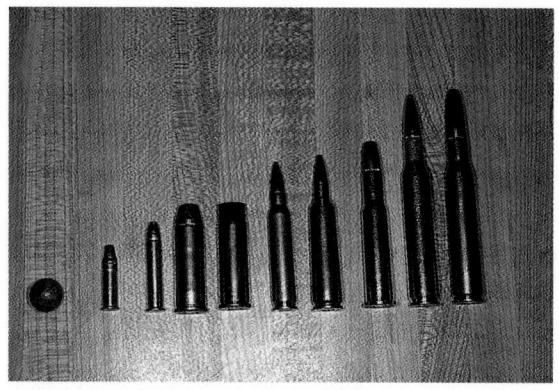

Figure 20-5 Examples of hunting bullets. *Left to right,* .50 caliber black powder lead bullet, .22 caliber lead bullet, .22 caliber long rifle lead bullet, .44 magnum semijacketed hollowpoint bullet, .44 magnum shotshell, .223 caliber (5.56 mm) full metal jacket bullet, .22/250 caliber semijacketed soft point bullet, .30/30 caliber soft point flat nose bullet, .270 caliber pointed soft point bullet, and .30-06 caliber round nose soft point bullet.

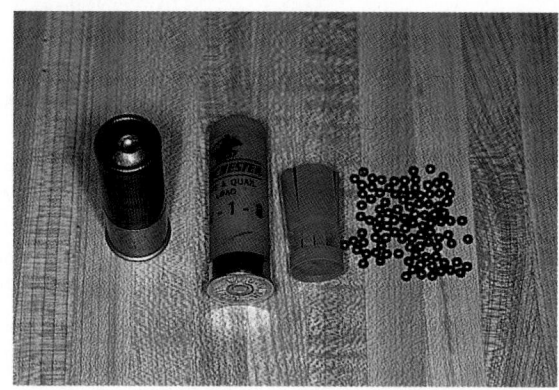

Figure 20-6 Examples of shotgun rounds. *Left to right,* 12-gauge slug round, empty 12-gauge plastic round, plastic 12-gauge wadding, and number six shotgun pellets.

muzzle energy for a particular type of firearm. Energy increases much more as a function of the velocity of the bullet than as a function of the mass. For this reason, most firearms are classified according to muzzle velocity. The higher the velocity of the bullet, the greater the energy and the greater the potential for injury. Firearms with muzzle velocities greater than 2500 feet/sec are considered high velocity, 1500 to 2500 feet/sec medium velocity, and less than 1500 feet/sec low velocity (Table 20-1). Bullets cause damage to tissue by crushing. The energy of a bullet may be transmitted to the tissue in part or in total depending on the surface area the bullet presents to the tissue. Bullets that strike at an angle, yaw, mushroom, or fragment present more surface area than do bullets that stay in one axis and maintain one shape. Hunting bullets are designed to manipulate shape and composition to maximize surface area. By the Geneva Convention, military bullets must have a full metal jacket and be less than .50 caliber. This is de-

TABLE 20-1. Comparison of Bullet Caliber, Weight, Velocity, and Muzzle Energy

CALIBER	WEIGHT (g)	MUZZLE VELOCITY (feet/sec)	MUZZLE ENERGY (foot-pounds)
.22	40	1080	90
.223	55	3250	1280
.44 magnum	180	1600	1045
.30/60	150	2750	2500

signed to minimize surface area. However, most military rounds travel at such high velocities (greater than 2700 feet/sec) that fragmentation reliably occurs even with full metal jackets. Fragmentation may also occur when a bullet strikes bone and sends splinters in several directions. The bone fragments cause injuries within the body similar to those from bullet fragments and may even exit the body to injure bystanders. Another phenomenon is temporary cavitation, which occurs at all velocities to some degree but becomes a factor only at high velocities. A permanent cavity occurs when a bullet or fragment crushes tissue. The bullet also creates a radial dispersion wave as a result of acceleration of tissue away from its path, which creates a temporary cavity. This wave is well tolerated by most elastic tissue, such as muscle, bowel, and lung; however, inelastic tissues, such as liver or brain, do not tolerate it and may be severely damaged by the temporary cavity. In high-velocity bullet wounds the temporary cavity may be several times larger than the permanent cavity. The total effect of high energy, fragmentation, mushrooming, yaw, and temporary cavity formation injures tissue. Although the kinetic energy formula cannot be denied, the other factors are probably more important to injury production. The type of tissue struck is the most important factor. As can be seen from Table 20-1, the .22 caliber long rifle bullet has a low mass and velocity and thus a low muzzle energy, yet more fatalities have occurred from this round than from any other. It is very inexpensive, can be fired from a number of rifles and handguns, is commonly used to hunt game, and is not thought of as particularly dangerous by inexperienced hunters. For these reasons, most people are shot by this round. The bullet is highly lethal when striking the brain, the heart, or a major blood vessel.*

Other rare problems associated with firearms are explosions that occur within the firearm itself. These can cause burns or fragment types of injuries. When firearms are loaded with excessive amounts of powder or the wrong powder is used in reloading bullets, the resultant detonation may cause the frame or cylinder of the firearm to explode. The burning powder or fragments of metal can cause injuries to the shooter. These injuries usually occur to the face and hands; penetrating eye injuries are also common. Obstruction of the barrel of the firearm by snow, mud, or other foreign material may cause a similar explosion.

Trap Injuries. Traps are designed to either kill animals or to capture them alive and uninjured. The latter type poses no risk to humans unless they should happen upon a trap and attempt to free the animal or otherwise approach the trap. The trapped animal will often bite or claw anyone within range. Leg hold traps designed to kill or injure an animal may occasionally cause problems for unwary hikers or campers. These traps have a spring-loaded jaw that closes when triggered by touching a trigger plate usually only involving 1 to 2 pounds of pressure. Most injuries involve the foot, but any area of the body that can fit between the jaws can potentially be injured. The jaws can be released by compressing the spring controlling the jaws (Figure 20-7). Very large traps used to trap poachers or to catch large animals, such as tigers or bears, cannot easily be released without help. These traps may also be attached to large weights, such as logs or concrete blocks, to prevent escape. Fortunately, most of these large traps are now collector's items and not used in the field. Nonconventional traps, such as snares, deadfalls, and pit traps, may rarely be encountered, but the mechanisms and types of injuries are quite variable. Trap guns are illegal in most areas of the world; injuries are similar to gunshot wounds.

Unexploded Ordnance. There are many areas in the world where unexploded ordnance can be found. This may include aerial bombs, rockets, artillery and mortar shells, grenades, and mines. Any area of the planet where a war has been fought in this century has potential for harboring these items. Crews excavating streets in urban areas of England, France, and Germany often uncover unexploded ordnance from World War I or World War II. Many areas of the United States that have been used for bombing or artillery ranges are adjacent to wilderness regions and, although they are usually well marked as impact areas, still pose a risk for the unwary traveler. Many areas of the shallow ocean accessible to scuba divers have sunken munition transports and warships that contain massive amounts of unexploded bombs, shells, and torpedoes. Another problem that has arisen is the use of mines and booby traps to protect marijuana and opium fields and illegal drug laboratories throughout the world.

Currently, unexploded land mines represent a significant health problem in Southeast Asia, the Balkans, Central America, Egypt, Iran, and Afghanistan. The International Red Cross estimates that someone is killed

---

*References 1, 2, 12-16, 27, 34, 38.

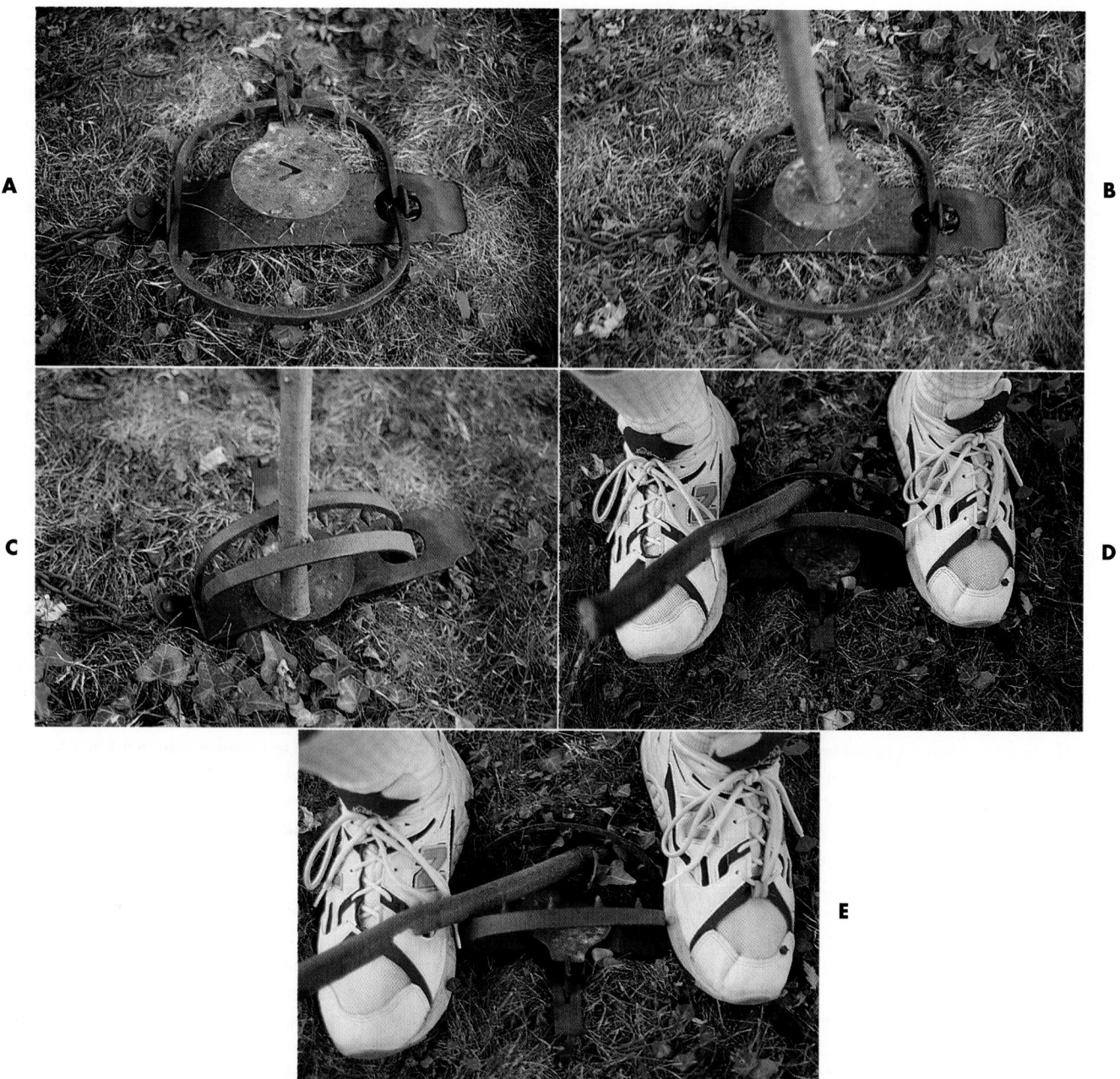

Figure 20-7 **A,** A leghold trap set. **B** and **C,** A leg hold trap sprung. **D** and **E,** How to release a trap that has been sprung by standing on each end of the trap and compressing the spring.

or injured by a land mine every 22 minutes. The average number of mines deployed per square mile in Bosnia is 152, in Iran 142, in Croatia 92, and in Egypt 59. There are a total of 23 million mines in Egypt alone. Land mines may be commercially manufactured or produced locally from available materials (Figure 20-8). Commercial, currently produced United States land mines have a limited active life and self-destruct after their active life has expired. Unfortunately, this is not true of older types of mines or mines produced by other countries. Locally produced mines have no stan-

dard size, shape, or detonation pattern and may be very difficult to detect and defuse. These types of land mines are used extensively in El Salvador, Malaysia, and Guatemala. Land mines have two primary functions, the first of which is to cause casualties; these are so-called antipersonnel mines. These may be blast or fragmentation type; the fragmentation type may be either directional or nondirectional (Figure 20-9). These may cause lethal or nonlethal injuries in several persons. Wounded soldiers require more care than killed soldiers do, and the tactical effect may be the same. The

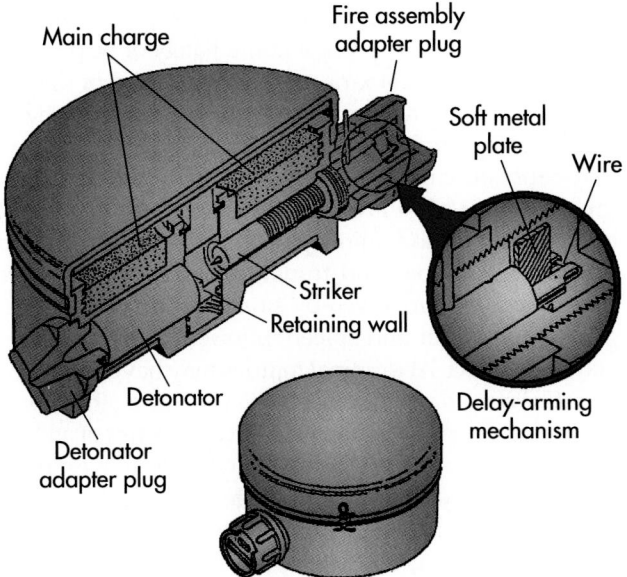

Figure 20-8 An example of an antipersonnel mine manufactured by the Soviet Union.

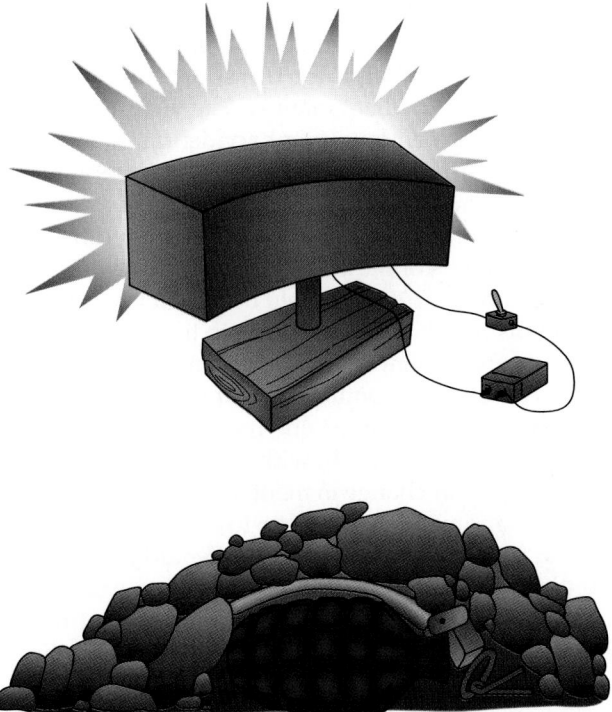

Figure 20-9 *Above,* A directional type mine used against unarmored vehicles or personnel. *Below,* An improvised mine, or booby trap, manufactured from a hand grenade and materials at hand.

second primary function is to destroy vehicles, such as tanks, so these mines are usually much larger. All mines have three basic components: (1) a triggering device, (2) a detonator, and (3) a main explosive charge. The triggering device differs, depending on the type of

mine. Blast mines usually involve pressure types of triggers and occasionally are command detonated, especially for antitank purposes. Many antitank mines will not explode unless a pressure of 300 to 400 pounds is applied. The M14 blast antipersonnel mine needs only 20 to 30 pounds of pressure to trigger the detonation. Fragmentation mines are usually triggered by trip wires or similar "touch" devices. The M18A1 fragmentation mine, or "claymore" mine, is designed to be command detonated by an electronic trigger. Booby traps other than land mines may be mechanical, chemical, or explosive. During the Vietnam War, venomous snakes were used, as well as the notorious sharpened bamboo spikes known as "punji" traps. The distribution of mines usually entails spreading them on the surface of the ground; by air along roads, railways, and defensive positions; or hiding them by burying or camouflage along trails or suspected routes of approach.

Injuries from land mines depend on several factors: type of mine (blast or fragmentation), position on the ground, method of detonation, whether it explodes above the ground, position of the victim, environment, and type of soil. Four general patterns of injuries occur with land mines. Pattern A injuries occur with small blast mines, such as the U.S. M14 and the Chinese Type 72. These injuries usually involve only the leg below the knee. Complete or partial foot amputations are most common, and trunk or head injuries are rare. Pattern B injuries are caused by larger blast mines, such as the Russian PMN. These mines contain 4 to 6 times as much high explosive material, and the cone of explosion is much larger. The injuries seen with this type of land mine usually involve massive soft tissue injuries to both legs below and above the knee and commonly the pelvis, abdomen, and chest. Pattern C injuries are generally caused by Russian PFM-1, or "butterfly," mines. These mines are usually distributed by air, and the wings are designed to help spread the mines. They are triggered by pressure applied to the wings; handling the mine commonly does this. Most of the injuries involve amputation of the hand at the wrist, but often the head, neck, and chest are injured also. Unfortunately, the loss of one or both eyes is not uncommon with this mine. Pattern D injuries are caused by fragmentation mines. These may be bounding mines, such as the U.S. M16 or the Russian OZM, or directional mines, such as the U.S. M18A1 or the Russian MON. They are designed to spread metallic fragments over a wide area at the height of a person's waist. The fragments lose their energy much faster than a bullet projectile but at close range can be devastating. The lethal range is usually 25 to 50 m (82 to 164 feet), with casualties occurring out to 200 m (656 feet). The injuries are quite similar to gunshot wounds and are often multiple. Large, unexploded artillery shells or bombs may cause a combination of blast and fragment injuries but on a larger scale, sometimes involving scores of victims.

The treatment of these injuries can be very complex and involve vascular, orthopedic, soft tissue, abdominal, and craniofacial procedures. The wounds are usually highly contaminated with soil, clothing, and fragments, so massive debridement is necessary. Rarely, unexploded ordnance may be imbedded in soft tissues and body cavities and must be removed in the operating room, possibly endangering the lives of medical personnel. Most victims who survive never completely regain normal function, especially if the initial treatment was delayed or inadequate. Postsurgical infection of mine injuries is common and greatly increases morbidity and mortality. Initial treatment involves airway control, treating tension pneumothorax, and controlling hemorrhage. Tourniquets are often necessary to control the bleeding from amputated limbs. Splinting the injured extremity and covering the wound to prevent further contamination is necessary. Initial debridement must be done carefully; removal of fragments may cause bleeding to recur. Penetrating injuries of the pelvis and abdomen usually require laparotomy, and soft tissue injuries may require multiple reconstructive procedures. Broad-spectrum antibiotics and tetanus prophylaxis are appropriate in all cases and fluid resuscitation usually indicated with extremity injuries.

Blast injuries without fragmentation may cause tympanic membrane rupture, blast lung resulting from alveolar rupture, and intestinal rupture, although the latter is more common with underwater mine explosions. The mechanism is production of an overpressure wave that travels through tissue of various density and causes tear injuries at membrane interfaces. These injuries must be suspected in any victim involved in a blast, whether from a land mine or other explosive device. Scuba divers and swimmers who are involved in underwater explosions may have more serious injuries because of the increased speed of sound in a liquid medium. This can cause more severe tearing of membranes at the fluid-air interface and additional trauma secondary to a "water hammer" effect and spalling. The position of the victim and the number of shock waves caused by reflection of the blast wave off of walls and ground may increase the amount of damage. Victims in contact with solid objects, such as the hull of a ship or vehicle, may have increased injuries because of increased velocity of the blast wave through solids. Burns and translational injuries, whereby the victim is thrown by the blast and has injuries similar to a fall or motor vehicle crash, also occur.

Generally speaking, the closer the victim is to the blast, the greater the injury. The tympanic membrane will rupture at overpressures of 5 psi. This causes acute hearing loss, pain, and tinnitus. Blast lung is caused by the overpressure wave passing through the chest wall and may involve one or both lungs. Chest pain, dyspnea, and hemoptysis may present immediately or be delayed up to 48 hours. Chest x-ray may show patchy or diffuse infiltrates, pneumothorax, subcutaneous air, and/or hemothorax. Implosion of air into the vascular system may cause air embolism and sudden death. Abdominal injuries in air blast are uncommon but in water blast may present as abdominal pain, nausea, vomiting, and tenesmus. Sigmoid and transverse colon injuries are most often seen, followed by small bowel and solid organ (such as liver and spleen) injuries from the "water hammer" effect. Abdominal injuries may have a delayed (up to several days) presentation. The key to therapy is to be suspicious of occult injuries in any victim of a blast, whatever the cause. Most injuries will present within the first hour; however, because injuries may be delayed in presentation, observation and close follow-up are critical. Treatment is generally supportive for ear and lung injuries and operative for abdominal injuries.*

Treatment of Hunting Injuries

The treatment of hunting injuries involves standard principles and priorities of trauma care. Airway, breathing, circulation, bleeding control, immobilization of the spine and fractured extremities, wound care, and stabilization of the victim for transport should be performed in an expedient manner. The victim should always be disarmed to prevent accidental injury to the rescuer or further injury to the victim. Removing the firearm or arrow from the vicinity of patient care is usually sufficient, but ideally the firearm should be made safe by removal of the ammunition and opening of the firing chamber. Arrows should be placed in a quiver, or the points may be wrapped in cloth to prevent injury.

The management of common traumatic injuries and illnesses, such as hypothermia and mountain sickness, is no different except for one important point: *always disarm the victim*. A victim with a charged weapon and a head injury or change in mental status for any reason presents an immediate danger to a well-meaning rescuer. If the person attempting to offer aid to an injured hunter is not familiar with weapons, it is usually best to move the weapon several feet from the victim and point it in a direction where an accidental discharge will do the least harm.

Arrow Injuries. Lacerations from razor-sharp hunting points are not unusual and can be treated like any similar laceration. The wound should be irrigated, any foreign material removed, and the laceration closed primarily. Victims pierced by an arrow should be stabilized, and the arrow should be left in place during transport, if possible. Attempts to remove the arrow by

---

*References 3, 5, 9, 11, 17, 18, 20, 21, 23, 25, 26.

pulling it out or pushing it through the wound may cause significantly more injury and should be avoided. It is acceptable to cut off the shaft of the arrow and leave 3 or 4 inches protruding from the wound to make transport easier if this can be accomplished with a minimum of arrow movement. A large pair of paramedic types of shears can usually cut through an arrow shaft if it is stabilized during cutting. The portion of the arrow that remains in the wound should then be fixed with gauze pads or cloth and tape. A similar approach should be used for spears and knives. The victim should be transferred as quickly as possible to an operating room, where the arrow can be removed under controlled conditions. Radiographs are helpful to identify associated anatomic structures before removal is attempted in the operating room (Figure 20-10).

Gunshot Wounds. Emergency department care of the gunshot wound includes securing the airway, placing two intravenous lines in unaffected extremities, performing cardiac monitoring, and providing oxygen therapy. The patient with a neck wound and expanding hematoma should be endotracheally intubated as soon as possible. If endotracheal intubation is not possible, a needle cricothyrotomy followed by a tube cricothyrotomy should be performed. Relief of tension pneumothorax with a needle or tube thoracostomy or occlusion of a sucking chest wound should be done immediately. Any external bleeding should be controlled by direct pressure. A radiograph should be obtained of the involved area, and where there is a presumed entrance wound without an exit wound, multiple x-ray studies may be needed to find the location of the bullet. On rare occasion, bullets have been observed to embolize from the chest area via the aorta to the lower extremity arteries or to the heart via the vena cava. A type

and crossmatch and basic trauma laboratory tests should be performed. Tetanus toxoid and immunoglobulin should be administered as indicated by the victim's history. Broad-spectrum antibiotics should be administered to cover the wide range of pathogens associated with gunshot wounds, especially with complex wounds to the abdomen and extremities. Victims in shock should be taken to the operating room immediately. If this is not possible, type O-negative or type-specific blood should be transfused. Autotransfusion, when available, can be an ideal way to replace lost blood in the victim in shock. Military antishock trousers or pneumatic antishock garments have not been shown to be beneficial in the treatment of shock secondary to penetrating trauma. Emergency thoracotomy is indicated for victims who have lost vital signs shortly before reaching the emergency department or while in the emergency department. Injuries to the heart or great vessels can be occluded with Foley catheter balloons, pericardial tamponade can be relieved, and the aorta can be cross-clamped. Hypothermia is commonly unrecognized in the trauma victim and may lead to coagulopathy, cardiac arrhythmias, or electrolyte disturbances. Rectal temperatures should be obtained and only warmed fluids and blood given to the victim.

Many myths associated with the management of gunshot wounds should be repudiated. The size or caliber of a bullet cannot easily be determined from the size of the wound; skin is quite elastic and stretches before being torn by a blunt bullet. The path of the bullet cannot be determined by connecting the entrance and exit wounds, since bullets may bounce and only a fragment may exit. The exit wound may be larger or smaller than the entrance wound, and the point of entrance or exit is not easily determined by looking at the wound. Wounds from high-velocity bullets are similar to other types of wounds, and standard rules of debridement should be followed. Wide debridement of normal-appearing tissue is unnecessary and should not be done. In general, victims of gunshot wounds should be evacuated quickly and stabilized if possible. Most victims (80%) of gunshot wounds to the chest who survive the first 30 minutes can be treated with a thoracostomy tube and observation. All gunshot wounds to the abdomen should be explored in the operating room. Radiographs should be used to identify bullets, bullet fragments, and bony injuries. Extremity wounds can be treated conservatively unless signs of vascular injury are present. Experience in combat has shown that vascular injuries do best when identified and treated immediately. Obviously, major bony injuries and nerve injuries eventually need operative therapy, but immediate intervention is rarely necessary. Most important, the underlying injury cannot be determined by examination of the external wound.

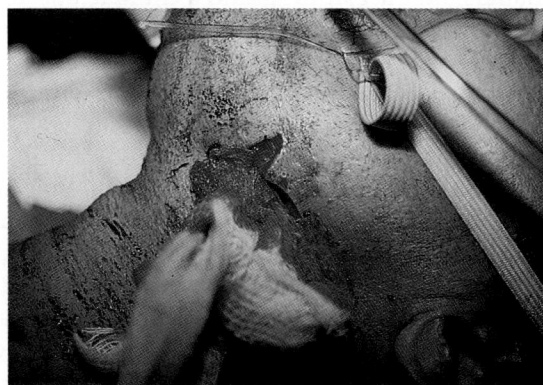

Figure 20-10 Arrow wound to the left side of the neck near the mandible. The shape of the wound resembles the blades of the broadhead as shown in Figure 20-4.

Vascular injuries may not be identified during the initial examination; therefore noninvasive, portable, Doppler ultrasound studies can be extremely valuable in the emergency department. Contrast angiography should be performed on any victim with a suspected vascular injury. The removal of the bullet or bullet fragment is not necessary unless the bullet is intravascular, intraarticular, or in contact with nervous tissue, such as the spinal cord or a peripheral nerve. Bullets found during exploratory laparotomy or wound debridement should be removed, but it is unnecessary to explore soft tissue, such as muscle or fat, solely to remove a bullet. Shotgun pellets that have minimal penetration can be removed from the skin with a forceps. Often the plastic or cloth wadding is found in superficial shotgun wounds and should be removed. Shotgun blasts may produce large soft tissue defects that need extensive debridement and either skin grafting or surgical flap rotation to maximize coverage. Patients with powder burns should have as much of the powder residue removed as possible with a brush under local anesthesia. The powder will tattoo the skin if it is not re-

moved, and the deep burns may need dermabrasion or surgical debridement (Fig. 20-11).[12,27,38]

Retained lead bullets and shotgun pellets for the most part are not hazardous; however, when they are within joint spaces or the gastrointestinal tract, significant amounts of lead can be absorbed and toxicity can occur.[33]

Prevention of Hunting Injuries

Most state fish and wildlife agencies have recognized that hunters are at risk for injuries and have tried to develop programs to minimize morbidity and mortality. National organizations such as the Boy Scouts of America and the National Rifle Association have been teaching firearm and hunting safety for decades. The Hunter Education Association and the North American Association of Hunter Safety Coordinators (NAAHSC) have attempted to identify high-risk groups and situations by collecting data on both fatal and nonfatal hunting-related injuries. NAAHSC-approved Hunter Safety Programs are available in every state, and all states except Alaska, Massachusetts, and South Carolina require the course before issuing a license to hunt. These courses are roughly 12 hours long and cover hunter responsibility, firearms and ammunition, bow hunting, personal safety, game care, and wildlife identification. They stress respect for the wilderness and a rational approach to game management. All hunters, potential hunters, and persons going into hunting areas should take one of these courses. Approximately 650,000 hunters complete a hunter safety course annually. Since the first course given in Kentucky in 1946, more than 18 million hunters have been certified.

Most injuries could probably be prevented by following a few simple rules. Nonhunters should be aware of hunting seasons and designated hunting areas and wear international orange clothing articles while in hunting areas. Hunters should always be sure of their target before shooting, use safety harnesses in tree stands, and use appropriate technique and tools for cleaning game. Tree stands should be well constructed. Hunters should never consume alcohol or mind-altering drugs that might interfere with their judgment. Eye protection in the form of safety glasses should be worn while hunting or target shooting to prevent injuries from ricocheting fragments and shotgun pellets. High-frequency hearing loss is common in hunters because of the loud report of the firearm. Although earplugs and headsets can protect the hunter, they are impractical for most hunting and are used mainly for target shooting. Some hunters use a single ear plug for the ear closest to the muzzle of the firearm. This protects the ear most likely to be injured but still allows the hunter to hear approaching game and other hunters. Bow hunters should always use wrist and finger protection to prevent injuries from the arrow

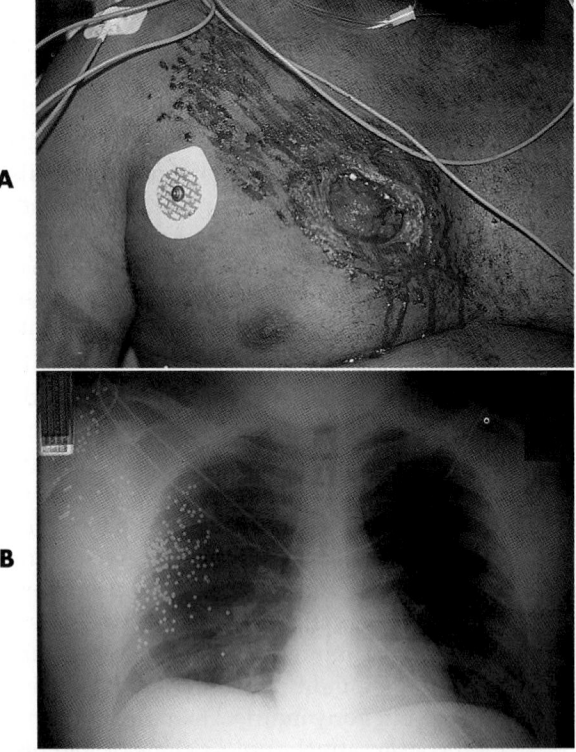

Figure 20-11 **A,** Close-range 12-gauge shotgun wound to the right side of the upper chest. The large central wound was caused by the plastic wadding, and the pellets have struck at an angle toward the shoulder. The patient was turning to the right when shot. The external appearance of the wound indicates a massive injury to the chest. **B,** Chest radiograph of the patient in **A.** No pellets have penetrated the chest, and there was no pneumothorax, pulmonary contusion, or vascular injury. The injury was totally superficial, and the patient was admitted for observation and local wound care.

fletching and the bowstring. All arrows should be carried in a quiver until ready for use. The arrow broadhead should always be pointed away from the hunter. These few steps would probably eliminate most hunting injuries.[30,31]

FISHING INJURIES

Sport fishing is associated with a large number of relatively minor injuries compared with hunting. The usual problems associated with outdoor recreation are common among fishermen: sunburn, frostbite, hypothermia, near drowning, sprains, fractures, motion sickness, and heat illness. Lacerations are relatively more common because of the use of knives to cut bait and fishing lines and to clean fish. These lacerations are often contaminated with a variety of marine and freshwater pathogens that may increase the incidence of wound infection. Thorough debridement of the wound and copious irrigation with sterile saline solution are the best initial methods to prevent infection (see Chapters 60 to 62).

Fishhook Injuries

Fishhooks are designed to penetrate the skin of fish easily and to hold fast while the fish is played and landed. To perform this dual role, they are extremely sharp at the tip, have a barb just proximal to the tip, and are curved so that the more force applied to the hook, the deeper it penetrates. Fishhooks may be single or in clusters of two, three, or four to increase the chance of catching the fish. Some state fishing laws limit the number of hooks allowed on a single line when fishing for certain game fish to make it more sporting. Unfortunately, the increased number of hooks on a lure or line also increases the chance of catching a fisherman. The most common fishhook punctures occur when fish are removed from hooks. The combination of sharp hooks, slippery fish, and an inexperienced fisherman leads to puncture wounds or embedded fishhooks. Many fishermen use commercial fishhook removers or large Kelly forceps to remove hooks. Some fishing guides simply cut the hook with a side-cutting pliers; they believe the remaining segment of hook will eventually oxidize in the victim and disintegrate. Often, fishhooks are stepped on with a bare foot or fishermen catch themselves or another person on the backcast.

Fishhooks can penetrate skin, muscle, and bone. They may pierce the eye or the penis. Care must be taken in removing a fishhook so that further damage to underlying structures is avoided. The first step is to remove the portion of the hook that is embedded from any attached lines, fish, bait, or lure. This is best done with a sharp side-cutting pliers. A bolt cutter may be needed for large, hardened hooks. A number of techniques are used for removing embedded fishhooks, but

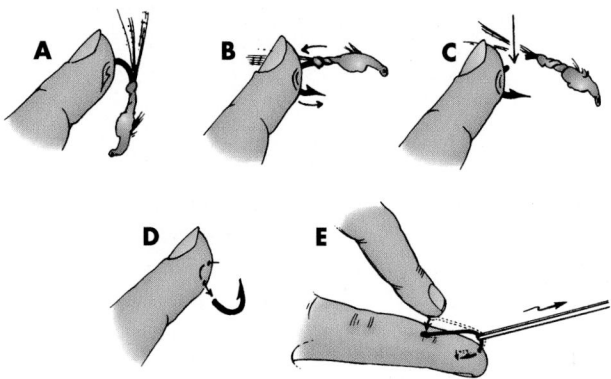

Figure 20-12 **A** to **D,** Removal of a fishhook that has penetrated a fingertip. **E,** "Press-and-yank" method of fishhook removal.

all involve a certain amount of movement of the hook, which causes increased pain. A local anesthetic should be infiltrated around the puncture site to minimize pain and movement of the patient. The first method can be used if the hook is not deeply embedded. Pressure is applied along the curve of the hook while the hook is pulled away from the point. Because the barb is on the inside of the curve of the hook, this enlarges the entrance hole enough to allow the barb and point to pass through. Sometimes a string looped through the curve of the hook facilitates the process. If the hook is deeply embedded, pressure can be applied along the curve of the hook until the point and barb penetrate the skin at another place, and then the barb can be cut off and the remainder of the hook backed out (Figure 20-12). Fishhooks embedded in the eye should be left in place, the eye covered with a metal patch or cup, and the victim referred to an ophthalmologist for further care. Rarely, hooks become embedded in bone or cartilage; this victim must be taken to the operating room to have the hook removed via a surgical incision.

Fishing Spear Injuries

Fishing spears, like fishhooks, are designed to penetrate and hold fish. They may be jabbed or thrown or propelled by rubber straps or carbon dioxide cartridges. The more force used to propel the spear, the deeper penetration into tissue. Although arrows are designed to cause bleeding and bullets to cause crushing, fishing spears are designed to hold the fish until it drowns or is otherwise dispatched. Spears may penetrate the human chest or abdominal cavity, skull, or any other anatomic area. Some bleeding may occur, especially if major blood vessels are struck. The victim should be removed from the water as soon as possible and immediate attention given to airway, breathing, and bleeding control. The spear should be stabilized in place, and the victim immediately transported to a medical facility. Penetrating neck and chest injuries may require endo-

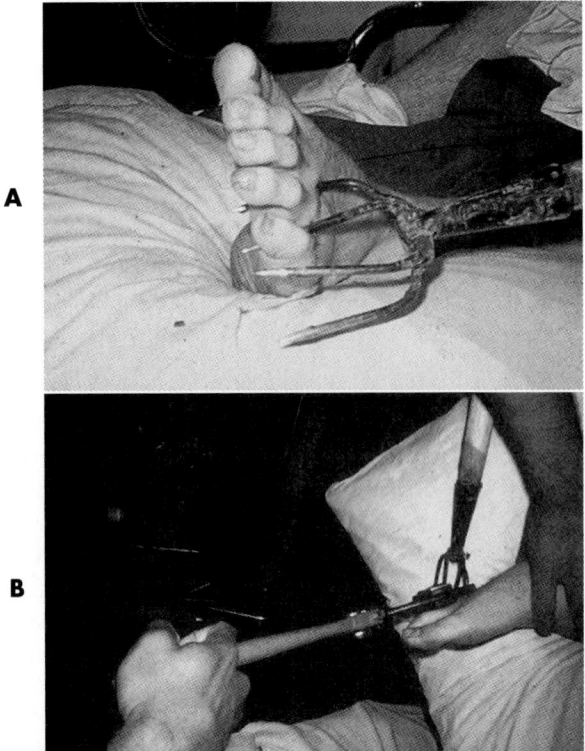

Figure 20-13 **A,** Male patient with a multipronged fishing spear through the foot. He said he saw something move and he speared it. **B,** Same patient with the spear being cut off in the emergency department with a bolt cutter. The patient was taken to the operating room to have the remainder of the spear removed.

tracheal intubation and tube thoracostomy. If a spear is embedded in the cheek and interfering with the victim's airway, cutting it off with a bolt cutter and removing it through the mouth is permitted. Spears in all other locations should be left in place, although they may be cut off to facilitate transportation or improve the victim's comfort (Figure 20-13).

REFERENCES

1. Adams DB: Wound ballistics: a review, *Mil Med* 147:831, 1982.
2. Amato JJ et al: Bone as a secondary missile: an experimental study in the fragmentation of bone by high-velocity missiles, *J Trauma* 29:609, 1989.
3. Argyros GJ: Management of primary blast injury, *Toxicology* 121:105, 1997.
4. Bear F: *Fred Bear's world of archery,* Garden City, NY, 1979, Doubleday.
5. Belvoir Research, Development, and Engineering Center: *Mine/countermine guide for low intensity conflict environment in Central America,* Fort Belvoir, Va, 1989, Countermine Systems Directorate.
6. Blumenschine RJ, Cavallo JA: Scavening and human evolution, *Sci Am* 267:90, 1992.
7. Campbell BG: Hunting and the evolution of society. In *Humankind emerging,* Boston, 1979, Little, Brown.
8. Carter GL: Accidental firearm fatalities and injuries among recreational hunters, *Ann Emerg Med* 18:406, 1989.
9. Cernak I et al: Recognizing, scoring and predicting blast injuries, *World J Surg* 23:44, 1999.
10. Cole TB, Patetta MJ: Hunting firearm injuries, North Carolina, *Am J Public Health* 78:1585, 1988.
11. Department of the Army: *Field manuals FM 20-32 mine/countermine operations and FM 5-34 engineer field data,* Washington DC, 1989, US Government Printing Office.
12. Fackler ML: Wound ballistics: a review of common misconceptions, *JAMA* 259:2730, 1988.
13. Fackler ML, Bellamy RF, Malinowski JA: Wounding mechanism of projectiles striking at more than 1.5 km/sec, *J Trauma* 26:250, 1986.
14. Fackler ML, Ballamy RF, Malinowski JA: The wound profile: illustration of the missile-tissue interaction, *J Trauma* 28:S21, 1988.
15. Fackler ML, Malinowski JA: The wound profile: a visual method for quantifying gunshot wound components, *J Trauma* 25:522, 1985.
16. Fackler ML et al: Bullet fragmentation: a major cause of tissue disruption, *J Trauma* 24:35, 1984.
17. Giannou C: Antipersonnel landmines: facts, fictions, and priorities, *BMJ* 315:1453, 1997.
18. Guy RJ et al: Physiologic response to primary blast, *J Trauma* 45:983, 1998.
19. Hain WH: Fatal arrow wounds, *J Forensic Sci* 34:691, 1988.
20. Jeffrey SJ: Antipersonnel mines: who are the victims? *J Accid Emerg Med* 13:343, 1996.
21. Krug EG et al: Preventing land mine related injury and disability: a public health perspective, *JAMA* 280:465, 1998.
22. Lambrecht CB, Hargarten SW: Hunting-related injuries and deaths in Montana: the scope of the problem and a framework for prevention, *J Wilderness Med* 4:175, 1993.
23. Landmine related injuries, 1993-1996, *MMWR Morb Mortal Wkly Rep* 46:724, 1997.
24. Lawrence HS: Fatal nonpowder firearm wounds: case report and review of the literature, *Pediatrics* 85:177, 1990.
25. Lein B et al: Removal of unexploded ordnance from patients: a 50 year military experience and current recommendations, *Mil Med* 164:163, 1999.
26. Liebovivi D, Ofer NG, Shmuel CS: Eardrum perforation in explosion survivors: is it a marker for pulmonary blast injury? *Ann Emerg Med* 34:168, 1999.
27. Lindsey D: The idolatry of velocity, or lies, damn lies and ballistics, *J Trauma* 20:1068, 1980.
28. Lucas RM, Mitterer D: Pneumatic firearm injuries: trivial trauma or perilous pitfalls? *J Emerg Med* 8:433, 1990.
29. National Safety Council: *Accident facts 1987,* Washington, DC, 1987, The Council.
30. *Ohio hunter safety education student handbook,* Ohio Division of Wildlife, Seattle, 1981, Outdoor Empire.
31. Pryce D: *Safe hunting,* New York, 1974, David McKay.
32. Strada G: The horror of land mines, *Sci Am* p 40, May 1996.
33. Stromberg BV: Symptomatic lead toxicity secondary to retained shotgun pellets, *J Trauma* 30:356, 1990.
34. Sykes LN, Champion HR, Fouty WJ: Dum-dums, hollow-points, and devastators: techniques designed to increase wounding potential of bullets, *J Trauma* 28:618, 1988.
35. Tree stand–related injuries among deer hunters—Georgia, 1979-89, *MMWR Morb Mortal Wkly Rep* 38:697, 1989.
36. US Department of the Interior, Fish and Wildlife Service: *1985 national survey of fishing, hunting and wildlife associated recreation,* Washington, DC, 1988, US Government Printing Office.
37. Urquhart CK et al: Deer stands: a significant cause of injury and mortality, *South Med J* 84:686, 1991.
38. Walker ML, Poindexter JM, Stovall I: Principles of management of shotgun wounds, *Surg Gynecol Obstet* 170:97, 1990.
39. Walsh IR et al: Pediatric gunshot wounds—powder and non-powder weapons, *Pediatr Emerg Care* 4:279, 1988.
40. Wintemute GJ et al: Unintentional firearm deaths in California, *J Trauma* 29:457, 1989.

21 Orthopedics

Thomas J. Ellis and Marc F. Swiontkowski

SKELETAL SYSTEM INJURIES

In the wilderness, initial management of a person with a musculoskeletal injury must consider the cause of the injury; the direction of force in relation to the individual or limb so the victim can be checked for injuries to adjacent bones and joints; the time of the injury, because the length of time to treatment may determine prognosis; and the environment where the accident has occurred, including cold, wind, or heat exposure, especially with open wounds that communicate with fractures.

Once the victim's condition is stabilized, examine the skeletal system closely beginning with the spine, moving to the pelvis, and ending with the extremities.

SPINAL INJURIES

Cervical Spine

In the wilderness, cervical spine fractures or dislocations result from falls off significant heights or high-velocity ski or vehicular injuries. Because head and cervical spine injuries are highly associated, individuals with significant head injuries are considered to have a cervical spine injury, especially if unconscious. Ideally, a person with a suspected cervical spine injury is placed on a backboard, with neck immobilization, and evacuated.

Neurologic deficit often results from cervical spine fracture. Fracture of the C1-2 complex results from axial loading (a C1 ring fracture—Jefferson's fracture) or an acute flexion injury (a C2 posterior element fracture—hangman's fracture). Complete neurologic injury at this level is fatal because of paralysis of the respiratory muscles, so surviving victims generally have partial deficits or are neurologically intact. Axial cervical spine fractures may result from flexion (most common), extension, rotational forces, or a combination of these, and most commonly occur at C5-6.[3]

Fractures and dislocations may result in neurologic insult distal to the bony injury. Because flexion injuries are the most common cervical spine injuries, the neurologic deficit is generally an anterior cord syndrome. The victim suffers complete motor and sensory loss but retains proprioception. The field examination aims to grade motor strength, document sensory response to light touch and pinprick, and note the presence or absence of Babinski's reflex.

When appropriate supplies are available, do a rectal examination. Complete lack of tone and failure of the sphincter muscles to contract when pulling on the penis or clitoris (the bulbocavernosus reflex) indicate spinal cord injury.

When transporting an individual with a cervical spine fracture or dislocation, stabilize the neck to prevent further injury. Because 28% of persons with cervical spine fractures also have other spinal fractures, protect the entire spine.[3] A pure flexion event may dislocate one or both posterior facets, producing neck pain and limitation of motion. Because the interspinous ligament is ruptured, transport this victim with the neck rigidly immobilized to accommodate the posterior instability.

Thoracolumbar Spine

Thoracolumbar spine fractures occur most frequently at the thoracolumbar junction. Because the thoracic spine is well splinted by the thoracic cage, when an axial or flexion load is applied, the ribs diminish forces on the thoracic vertebral bodies and transmit the force to the upper lumbar levels. In the wilderness, falls from significant heights or high-velocity sporting vehicular trauma produce these fractures (Figure 21-1). Thoracolumbar spine fracture is frequently associated with major hindfoot fractures (particularly of the calcaneus). With these mechanisms of injury and unilateral or bilateral calcaneus fracture, assume there is a spine fracture and transport the victim with spine precautions.

Perform a careful neurologic examination as part of the secondary survey, paying close attention to the dermatomal response to light touch and pinprick, motor function, and the presence or absence of cord level reflexes. With significant head injury, assume a spinal injury is present. Logroll the victim, maintaining perfect spinal alignment, and carefully place him or her on a backboard, or use the scoop stretcher (see Chapter 26). Because significant fluctuations in sympathetic tone may occur, monitor blood pressure and body temperature, taking appropriate steps to cool or warm the victim.

PELVIC INJURIES

Pelvic fractures generally occur in a fall from significant height, high-velocity ski accident, or vehicular trauma. The direction of force is directly related to the fracture and influences definitive management.[9,11] Penna and Tile[5,11] divide pelvic fractures into anteroposterior (AP) compression injuries, lateral compression (LC) injuries, and vertical shear (VS) injuries. In

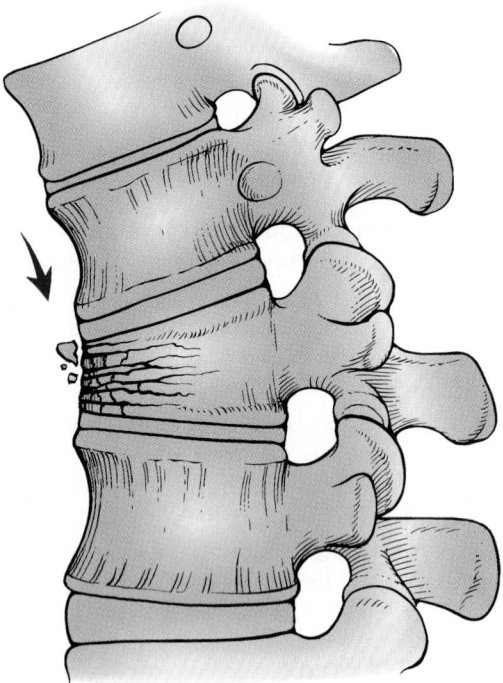

Figure 21-1 Wedge compression fracture from axial or flexion loading at the thoracolumbar junction.

addition, there are simple, nondisplaced inferior or superior ramus fractures and avulsion fractures. On clinical examination, these latter fractures are generally seen as an area of tenderness but no instability.

The key factor in pelvic fracture is identification of posterior injury to the pelvic ring, which is associated with significant hemorrhage, neurologic injury, and mortality. Posterior ring fractures are revealed by instability of the pelvis associated with posterior pain, swelling, ecchymosis, and motion. Immediately evacuate this victim on a backboard, taking care to minimize leg and torso motion. Bleeding associated with a pelvic injury is from cancelleous bone at fracture sites, retroperitoneal lumbar venous plexus injury, or, rarely, pelvic arterial injuries.

LC injuries are usually stable, with impaction of the posterior structures but seldom any complications. AP compression injuries demonstrate anterior instability, palpable ramus fractures, or pubic symphysis gapping. These fractures are often accompanied by bladder, prostatic, or urethral injury. Transport the victim on a backboard with the feet internally rotated to help reduce the anterior pelvic diastasis. With severe injury and hemodynamic instability, medical antishock trousers (MAST) provide stability and decrease intrapelvic blood loss. Keep them inflated until transfer to a definitive care center. If MAST are not available, tie a garment securely around the pelvis. Because vertical shear injuries are both rotationally and vertically unstable, definitive care is directed toward providing posterior stability, as it is

for those few lateral compression injuries with unstable posterior fractures. In an AP injury, symphyseal widening exceeding 2.5 cm indicates injury to the anterior capsular structures of the sacroiliac joint, requiring stabilization with internal or external fixation.

EXTREMITY INJURIES

Physical Examination

Physical examination addresses circulatory, nerve, skeletal, and joint function.

Circulatory Function. Penetrating or blunt trauma can injure the major vessels supplying the limbs. Fractures can produce injury by direct laceration (rarely) or by stretching, which produces intimal flap tears that can occlude distal flow or lead to platelet aggregation and delayed occlusion. Thus circulatory function examination is done before and after the victim's arrival at the definitive care center. Assess the color and warmth of the skin or distal extremity; pallor and asymmetric regional hypothermia may indicate vascular injury. In the upper extremity, palpate the brachial, radial, and ulnar arteries, using hand-held, battery-powered sound Doppler units if available. If blood loss, hypothermia, or obesity makes these pulses difficult to assess, evaluate temperature and color. Any suspected major arterial injury mandates immediate evacuation after appropriate splinting.

Nerve Function. Nerve function may be impossible to assess in an unconscious or uncooperative person. If possible, establish nerve function to the distal extremity after the victim's condition is stabilized. Then compare these initial findings periodically with repeat examinations during transport, noting any deterioration.

Carefully document the results of light touch and pinprick tests. For spinal and pelvic injuries, assess the dermatomal distribution of spinal nerves, and evaluate muscle function by observing active function and grading the strength of each group against resistance.

Skeletal Function. The long bones of the lower extremity serve as the major structural supports for locomotion, whereas those of the upper extremity stabilize the soft tissues, enabling positioning of the hand in space. A visible angular deformity reveals a fracture; palpable crepitus confirms the diagnosis. Perform appropriate splinting after aligning the limb with axial traction. Other than noting the degree and orientation of the limb's position when the victim is found, do not delay aligning and splinting fractures. Distinguishing joint injuries and intraarticular or very proximal or distal fractures must wait for the definitive care facility. Similarly, distinguishing wrist or ankle ligamentous injury from a fracture is not required for initial treatment.

Joint Function. Muscle forces act across joints to improve the position of the lower limbs for ambulation and the hand for handling objects. Each joint has a certain minimum function to allow for stability and a normal range of motion. Making the diagnosis of a joint injury in the field allows appropriate splinting and prevents further damage during transport.

Begin palpation of long bones distally and proceed across all joints. Apply a splint if there is palpable crepitus, swelling, deformity, or a block to motion. If the victim can cooperate, take each joint through an active range of motion to quickly locate the injury. When this is not possible, evaluate passive motion of each joint after palpation for crepitus and swelling.

Reduce any dislocations after completing the neurocirculatory examination. This generally relieves the victim's discomfort considerably. Next, evaluate stability by careful, controlled motion. Joints with associated fractures or interposed soft tissues are frequently unstable after reduction. Take great care in applying splints to prevent redislocation. Report details of the reduction maneuver, including orientation of the pull, amount of force involved, amount of sedation, and residual instability of the joint, to the definitive care physician.

Splinting Techniques (see also Chapter 19)

With suspected cervical or thoracolumbar spine trauma, transport the victim on a hard surface. Backboards or scoop stretchers (see Chapter 26) are most effective, but improvisation with any hard piece of wood, fiberglass, or straight tree limbs lashed together may be needed. If cervical spine injury is suspected, place a roll of clothes or a water bottle as high as the victim's mid face on either side of the head to prevent rotational movement. Apply tape from the supporting stretcher across the objects and the victim's forehead to add stability. Transport victims with a suspected major pelvic injury in similar fashion, stabilizing the lower extremities.

For shoulder fractures or dislocations, use a commercially available sling or improvised triangular bandage to take the weight of the arm off the injured structures. Whenever possible, splint the upper extremity in the position of function. It may be difficult to place an injured elbow in 90 degrees of flexion and neutral pronation-supination.

Securely fix the limb to the splint with tape or elastic bandages. Air splints, when inflated, can adequately splint the upper extremity in this position. These splints are lightweight and compact but should be used with caution under conditions such as heat and rapid increase in altitude in which they might expand and compress the limb. Splints may also be made from plaster or fiberglass, which can be applied over cotton softroll. Lightweight fiberglass splints, such as Orthoglass (Smith and Nephew), are easy to use and effective in

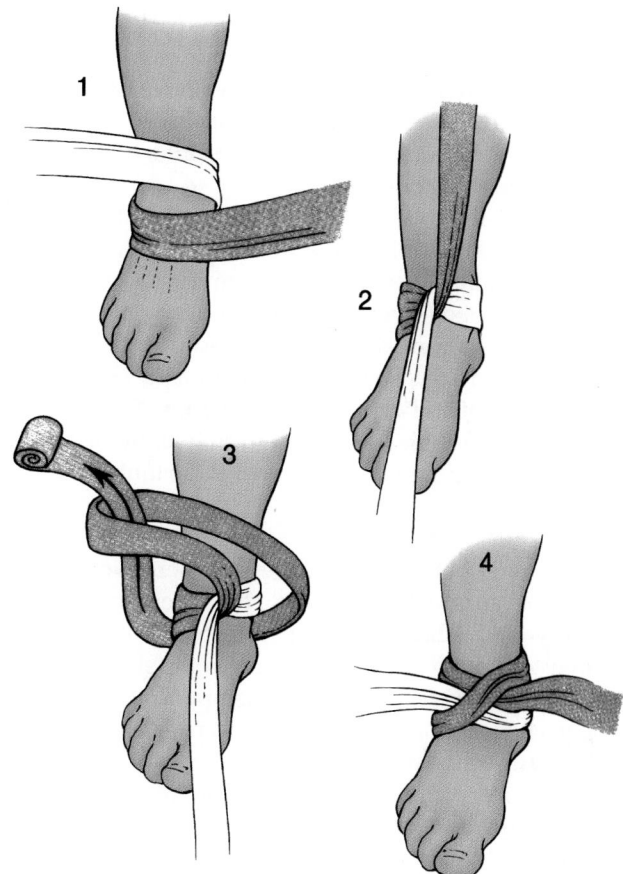

Figure 21-2 Improvisation of an ankle wrap to be used for traction.

the initial management of these injuries. These splints are prepadded and can be applied with either cold or warm water. The warmer the water, the faster the fiberglass sets and the greater the exothermic reaction. Avoid hot water because it may generate an excessively exothermic reaction and possibly burn the skin. Immerse the fiberglass in the water, gently squeeze out the excess, and apply the splint. An elasticized bandage helps hold the splint where desired until the fiberglass is hard. Wooden or metal splints, custom made or improvised, also work.

Splints are used to immobilize the limb securely in functional position until definitive care is reached. Apply hand splints with the metacarpophalangeal (MCP) joints flexed 90 degrees and the interphalangeal (IP) joints extended. This position places the collateral ligaments at maximum length and prevents later joint contracture. Position the lower extremity for transport with the hip and knee extended and the ankle in neutral position. With hip or femur fractures or dislocations, apply traction whenever possible, improvising when necessary (Figure 21-2). Usually, a Thomas splint with a Spanish windlass is available. The ring of the splint rests against the victim's ischium and pubis, and traction is applied through the windlass, stabilizing the joint or fracture fragments. The Kendrick traction device is lightweight and packaged for easy transportation. If commercial splints are unavailable, strap the injured leg to the noninjured leg, placing a tree limb or walking stick between them. If possible, transport the victim on a backboard.

For the lower leg, air splints provide adequate immobilization of tibia-fibula fractures or ankle fractures and dislocations. Splints made from plaster or fiberglass may be applied over cotton padding with elasticized wraps. Custom-made or improvised metal splints can be stabilized with elastic bandages or tape. Hold the ankle in neutral and apply the splint firmly. Transport victims with unstable lower extremity fracture or dislocation in the recumbent position with the limb elevated.

Open Fractures

Recognizing an open fracture is imperative; without prompt surgical treatment, the incidence of osteomyelitis is high. In an open fracture, the fractured bone communicates with a break in the skin. Consider all lacerations near a fracture as open. With subcutaneous bones (tibia), open fractures are easily identified, but with other bones (humerus, femur, pelvis) that have more surrounding soft tissue, identification is more difficult because the fractured bone end usually retracts once it punctures the skin and is then covered by soft tissue. Most open fractures persistently ooze blood from the laceration, which may facilitate diagnosis. Fat globules may be extruding from the wound.

General care of an open fracture outdoors depends on evacuation time. Open fractures require prompt operative irrigation, debridement, and stabilization. If evacuation can be completed within 8 hours, realign the fracture, give a broad-spectrum antibiotic, and splint the extremity. If the fractured ends of the bones are sticking out of the skin, try to realign the fracture and reduce the bone ends under the skin. If bone ends extrude through the skin, cover the exposed bone with a povidone-iodine solution–soaked gauze sponge, splint the extremity, and arrange for prompt evacuation. If evacuation time exceeds 8 hours, attempt irrigations, limited debridement, and stabilization with a splint in the field. Antibiotic options are listed in Box 21-1.

Amputation

In the wilderness, the amputation victim requires immediate evacuation. Control hemorrhage using direct pressure; tourniquets are virtually never indicated. Without cooling, an amputated part remains viable for only 4 to 6 hours; with cooling, viability may be extended to 18 hours. Cleanse the amputated part with saline or water, wrap it in a moistened sterile gauze or towel, place it in a plastic bag, and transport it in an ice-water mixture. Do not use dry ice. Keep the amputated part with the victim throughout evacuation.

Box 21-1 ANTIBIOTIC OPTIONS

INTRAVENOUS

Cefazolin (Ancef) 1 g q8h and gentamicin (5 mg/kg) q24h or ticarcillin (Timentin) 3.1 g q8h

INTRAMUSCULAR

Ceftriaxone (Rocephin) 1 g q24h
Oral ciprofloxacin 750 mg BID and cephalexin (Keflex) 500 mg QID

WATER EXPOSURE

Ciprofloxacin 400 mg IV/750 mg po BID or sulfamethoxazole (Bactrim) DS 1 po BID and cefazolin (Ancef) 1 gm IV q8h/cephalexin (Keflex) 500 mg po q6h

DIRT OR BARNYARD

Add penicillin 20 million units IV qd/500 mg po q6h

PENICILLIN ALLERGIC

Use clindamycin 900 mg IV q8h or 450 mg po q6h in place of penicillins and cephalexin (Keflex)

ALTERNATIVES

Erythromycin 500 mg q6h or amoxicillin 500 mg po q8h

Compartment Syndrome

A compartment syndrome begins when locally increased tissue pressure reduces arterial blood flow to a muscle compartment. When local blood flow is unable to meet metabolic demands of the tissue, ischemia ensues. In the wilderness, compartment syndromes most frequently occur in association with fractures or severe contusions. This syndrome can occur when the victim has been lying for some time across a limb so that the body weight occludes the arterial supply. Elevated local tissue pressure (compartment pressure within 10-20 mm Hg of diastolic arterial blood pressure) can occur with acute hemorrhage or after revascularization of an ischemic extremity. Hypotension can lower the risk of a compartment syndrome.

The lower leg and forearm are the most common sites for a compartment syndrome because of the tight fascia in these regions, but it also occurs in the thigh, hand, foot, and gluteal regions. The conscious victim complains of severe pain out of proportion to the injury. The muscle compartment feels extremely tight, and applied pressure increases the pain. There is decreased sensation to light touch and pinprick stimuli in the areas supplied by the nerves traversing the compartment. Stretching muscles within the compartment produces severe pain. The most reliable signs of a compartment syndrome are pain, tight compartments, hypesthesia, and pain on passive stretch. Pulselessness, pallor, and slow capillary refill may not be observed, even with a severe compartment syndrome.

Emergency evacuation is required. The victim must be definitively treated in the first 6 to 8 hours after onset to optimize return of function to the involved limb. Emergency fasciotomy, the treatment of choice, relieves the pressure. Limited fasciotomies can be performed in the field by an experienced surgeon if evacuation will require more than 8 hours.

RICE Principle

The general principle in the acute management of all extremity injuries is rest, ice, compression, and elevation (RICE). For unstable fractures, immobilization is also indicated. Avoid heat for the first 72 hours after injury. Premade chemical cold packs work well, but cold packs made from ice or snow suffice. If ice is used, mix some water in a bag with the ice to more evenly distribute the cold. Wrap the cold pack to the injured area with an elasticized bandage. Place a thin piece of fabric between the cold pack and the victim's skin to prevent burning of the skin. Apply the ice to the elevated (above the level of the heart) extremity for 30 to 45 minutes every 2 hours, or, if cold packs are unavailable, immerse the extremity intermittently in a cold mountain stream. A compressive dressing also helps decrease swelling, but should not be used if compartment syndrome is possible. In this situation, keep the limb at the level of the heart and avoid compressive dressings.

UPPER EXTREMITY FRACTURES

Clavicle

Fracture of the clavicle usually occurs in the middle or lateral thirds of the bone and is associated with a direct blow or with a fall onto the lateral shoulder. Clavicle fractures are common with snow skiing. The victim complains of shoulder pain, which may be poorly localized. Arm or shoulder motion exacerbates the pain. To localize the problem, gently palpate the clavicle to identify the area of maximum tenderness. The presence of crepitus at the clavicle confirms the diagnosis. Although rare, a clavicle fracture can be associated with a pneumothorax because the cupula of the lung is punctured; therefore auscultate the chest for breath sounds. Shortness of breath and deep pain on inspiration increase suspicion for a pneumothorax. Clavicle fracture may also accompany injury to the brachial plexus and axillary artery or subclavian vessels. Perform a thorough neurocirculatory examination of the affected extremity and examine the skin carefully. Approximately 3% to 5% of clavicle fractures may be open because of the bone's subcutaneous location. Evacuate the victim if there is a significant open wound, suspected pneumothorax, or nerve or vascular injury. Field treatment

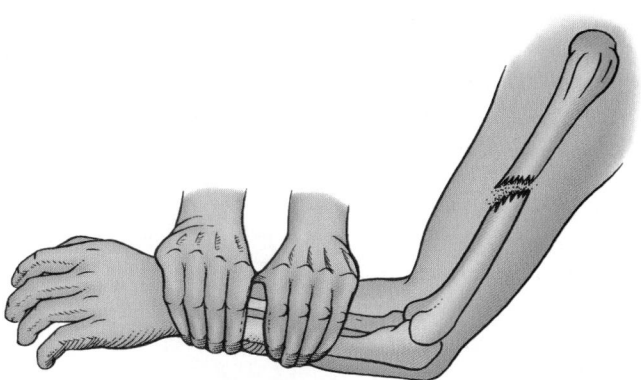

Figure 21-3 To control pain, a fractured humerus should be stabilized manually until a splint can be applied.

for a clavicle fracture consists of a figure-eight bandage or sling and judicious use of analgesics.

Humerus

Fracture of the humeral shaft may result from a direct blow or torsional force on the arm. This fracture frequently occurs with a fall, rope accident, or skiing accident. Fractures of the midshaft and junction of the middle and distal third of the humeral shaft violate the spiral groove path of the radial nerve. If there is arm pain with deformity and crepitus, stabilize the arm, and carefully check the sensory and motor function of the radial nerve as part of the overall neurocirculatory examination (Figure 21-3). Evaluate radial nerve function by checking sensation in the dorsal thumb web space and MCP extension with the proximal and distal IP joints flexed. When fracture of the humeral shaft is suspected, firmly apply an appropriate coaptation splint made of plaster, fiberglass, or wood with an elastic bandage on the medial and lateral sides of the humerus. Use a sling for comfort. Acute reduction of the fracture is not routinely required.

Fracture of the proximal humerus is often difficult to differentiate from shoulder dislocation in the acute phase. The mechanism is frequently a high-velocity fall onto an abducted, externally rotated arm, or a direct blow to the anterior shoulder. The victim complains of severe pain around the shoulder with palpation or any arm motion. Palpable crepitus confirms the diagnosis. This fracture does not routinely require acute reduction; application of an arm sling is appropriate field management.

Fracture-dislocation of the proximal humerus can also occur, with most dislocations being anterior. Anterior or posterior fullness, with crepitus on the injured side compared with the uninjured side, suggests the diagnosis. This is a more severe injury, so perform a very careful neurocirculatory examination. Any significant nerve or vascular injury should prompt evacuation to a definitive care center. If the injury is identified and definitive care

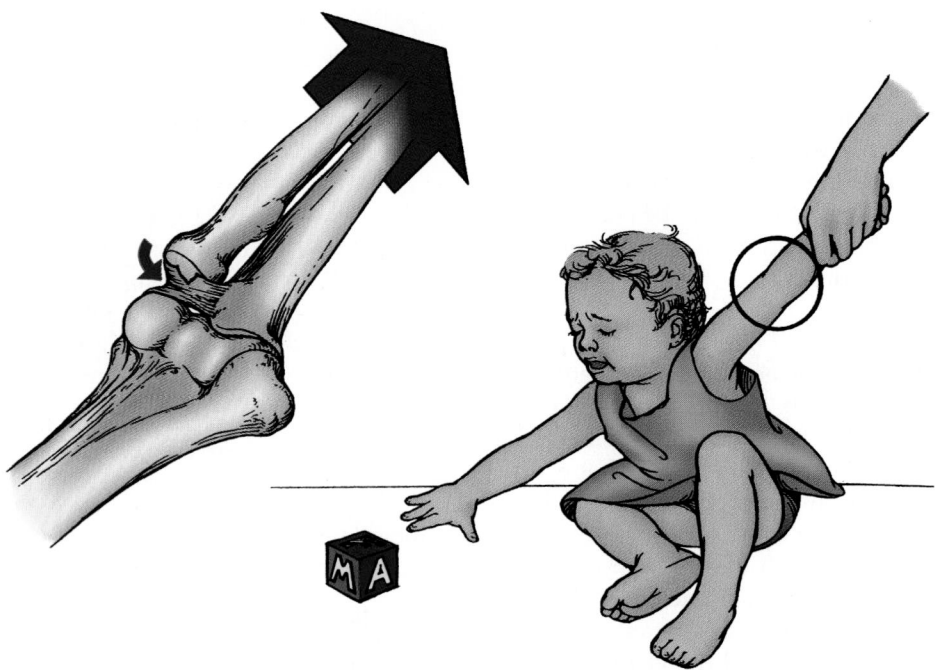

Figure 21-4 Nursemaid's elbow most commonly occurs when a longitudinal pull is applied to the upper extremity. Usually the forearm is pronated. There is a partial tear in the orbicular ligament, allowing it to subluxate into the radiocapitellar joint. (*From Rockwood CA Jr, Willkins KE, King RE, editors:* Fractures in children, *ed 3, Philadelphia, 1991, JB Lippincott.*)

is more than 1 to 2 hours away, attempt reduction. Using available sedation, stabilize the trunk while applying firm longitudinal traction in line with the arm. Have an assistant apply anterior pressure to the humeral head to ease it back into the glenoid joint space. Avoid any maneuver that compresses the brachial plexus (i.e., a foot in the axilla for countertraction).

Fracture of the distal humerus is more frequently extraarticular in children and intraarticular in adults. Children generally sustain supracondylar fractures after falls from heights. Extension-type injuries are much more common than flexion-type, and they most commonly occur in children ages 4 to 8 years. Deformity, swelling, pain, and crepitus are present, and the diagnosis is fairly obvious. Perform a careful neurocirculatory examination, then focus the motor examination on flexion of the thumb and distal IP joint of the index finger, because injury to the anterior interosseus nerve is frequently associated. If the radial pulse is absent, try to flex or extend the elbow while palpating the radial pulse. If the pulse improves, splint the limb in that position for transport. If the pulse does not improve and definitive care is more than 1 hour away, perform a reduction. After available sedation is given, extend the supinated elbow with gentle longitudinal traction. Reduce the fracture by flexing the elbow while maintaining longitudinal traction, then splint the elbow in 90 degrees of flexion. Evacuation should be performed promptly.

For the adult with pain, crepitus, deformity, and swelling after a fall, perform the neurocirculatory examination, then apply a splint with the elbow at 45 or 90 degrees of flexion, depending on the victim's comfort. Do not attempt reduction without radiographic confirmation because crepitus is more often associated with a fracture than with a dislocation. Evacuate the victim promptly if there is an open fracture or neurocirculatory deficit.

Subluxation of the radial head in children (nursemaid's elbow) occurs when a longitudinal pull is applied to the upper extremity (Figure 21-4). The orbicular ligament partially tears, allowing a portion of it to slip over the radial head. An audible snap may be heard at the time of the injury. The initial pain from the injury subsides rapidly, and the child does not seem distressed, but refuses to use the extremity. Any attempt to supinate the forearm brings about a cry of pain and distress. If a definitive care center is nearby, splint the injury and arrange for evacuation. Otherwise, if the history and examination are consistent with the diagnosis, attempt a reduction. First supinate the slightly flexed forearm; if this fails to produce the characteristic snapping sensation of reduction, maximally flex the elbow in supination until the snapping sensation occurs (Figure 21-5). If the reduction is successful, the child is usually content and playing within 5 to 10 minutes, and no immobilization of the joint is indicated. If the reduction is unsuccessful, the child contin-

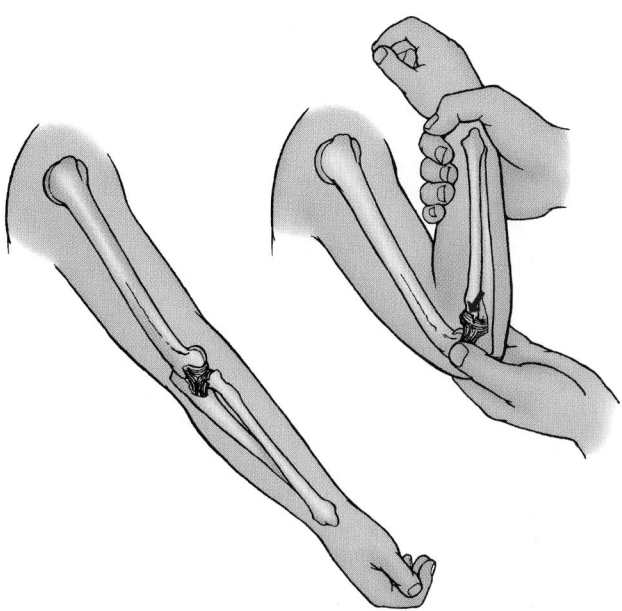

Figure 21-5   Reduction of nursemaid's elbow injury. *Left*, the forearm is supinated. *Right*, the elbow is then hyperflexed. The rescuer's thumb is placed laterally over the radial head to feel the characteristic snapping as the ligament is reduced. (*From Rockwood CA Jr, Willkins KE, King RE, editors: Fractures in children, ed 3, Philadelphia, 1991, JB Lippincott.*)

ues to avoid using the involved arm and should be evacuated for definitive care.

Radius

Radial shaft fracture is commonly associated with a motor vehicle or industrial accident but may occur with a fall involving angular or axial loading of the forearm. A radial shaft fracture may be associated with dislocation of the distal radioulnar joint (Galeazzi's fracture), so examine the wrist for tenderness, swelling, and deformity. The victim generally complains of pain, and deformity and crepitus are noted over the radial shaft after a fall or direct blow, with any arm motion exacerbating the pain. When both the radius and ulna are fractured, forearm instability is marked. Always examine the joint above (elbow) and the joint below (wrist) for tenderness, crepitus, and deformity. Once a fracture of the radius or both bones of the forearm is identified, splint the wrist, forearm, and elbow in the position of function.

Fractures of the radial head generally occur in young to middle-aged adults who fall onto outstretched hands. The victim complains of pain about the elbow, with loss of full extension, and pain at the radial head on the lateral side of the elbow with gentle pressure and rotation of the forearm. Fracture of the radial head frequently produces an elbow hemarthrosis, which is identifiable by fullness posterior to the radial head and anterior to the tip of the olecranon. A fluid wave can be balloted. If equipment is available and you are confident of the di-

agnosis, aspirate the hemarthrosis and instill 5 ml of lidocaine. Gently move the elbow through a range of motion and then place it in a posterior splint in 90 degrees of flexion with the forearm supinated. On a prolonged expedition when definitive care cannot be reached, remove the splint after 5 days and have the victim perform intermittent range of motion exercises (both flexion/extension and pronation/supination), reapplying the splint for comfort. With more comminuted radial head fractures, attempts at motion produce pain and crepitus and motion remains restricted. These injuries require operative treatment. With nondisplaced or minimally displaced radial head fractures, early motion prevents permanent loss of motion, although most individuals lose some extension and pronation/supination. Splint the arm in supination to prevent contracture of the intraosseus ligament and loss of supination.

Fracture of the distal metaphyseal radius is generally associated with a fall onto the outstretched hand of an older osteoporotic individual. In the wilderness, these fractures occur in younger adults with falls from significant heights onto outstretched hands. Intraarticular distal radius fracture often accompanies fracture of the ulnar styloid. Pain, deformity, and crepitus are obvious. Perform a distal neurocirculatory examination, focusing on the sensory function of the median nerve. When there is neurocirculatory compromise, and definitive care is more than 1 to 2 hours away, perform a gentle reduction. Place one hand on the forearm to provide countertraction and the other around the wrist of the involved extremity. Dorsiflex the wrist and apply longitudinal traction as the wrist is returned to a neutral position. Apply a splint that immobilizes the wrist and elbow. Distal radius and ulna fractures occur most commonly in girls ages 11 to 13 years and in boys ages 13 to 15. These fractures are not usually comminuted but can be difficult to reduce (Figure 21-6). In cases involving an open fracture, significant distal neurologic deficit, or abnormal circulatory examination, splinting and evacuation should be prompt. Keep the limb elevated above the heart during transport.

Ulna

Ulna shaft fracture is most often associated with fracture of the radial shaft at the same level. When isolated, it usually occurs as a result of a direct blow, the so-called *nightstick fracture*. Fracture of the ulnar shaft can be associated with dislocation of the radial head (Monteggia's lesion), so assess elbow function carefully. In the wilderness, the most frequent mechanism of injury is bracing a fall or collision with the forearm. Pain, localized swelling, and crepitus are present. Apply a long-arm splint in the position of function. An open fracture is an indication for prompt evacuation.

Fracture of the proximal ulna (olecranon) results from a fall onto the posterior elbow, or avulsion with

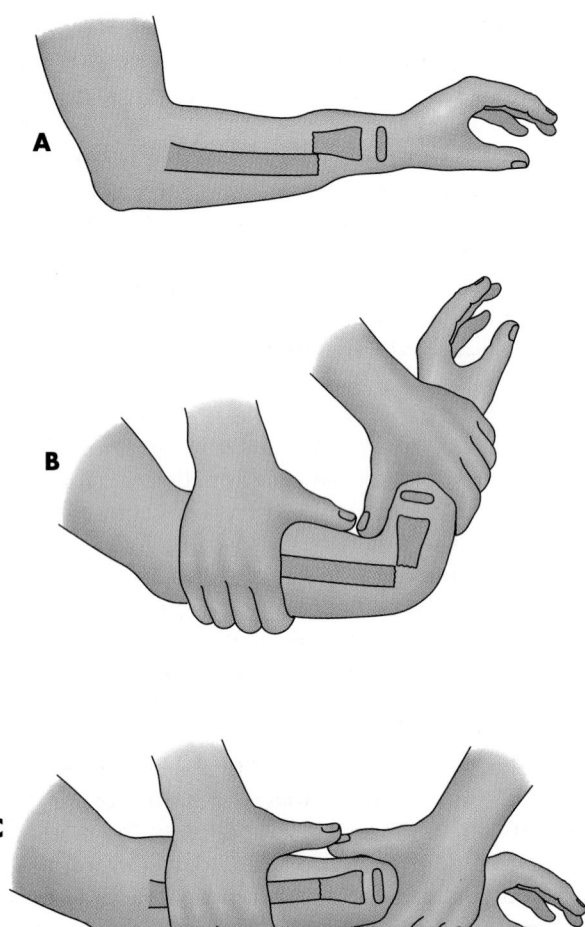

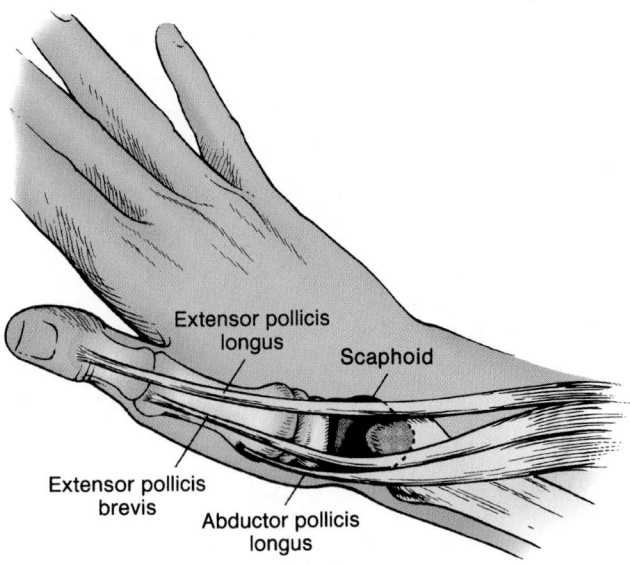

Figure 21-7 The scaphoid (navicular) bone sits in the "anatomic snuffbox" of the radial aspect of the wrist

Figure 21-6 Technique for reduction of a complete fracture of the forearm. **A,** Initial fracture position. **B,** Hyperextend fracture to 100 degrees to disengage the fracture ends. **C,** Push with the thumb on the distal fragment to achieve reduction. (**B** and **C** modified from Levinthal DH: Surg Gynecol Obstet 790, 1933. **A** to **C** from Green N, Swiontkowski MF: Skeletal trauma in children, vol 3, ed 2, Philadelphia, 1998, WB Saunders.)

violent asymmetric contraction of the triceps muscle. The victim may be unable to extend the elbow actively against gravity if the triceps is dissociated from the forearm with a complete olecranon fracture. On initial examination, the victim has pain, significant swelling, and a palpable gap in the olecranon. With severe trauma, olecranon fracture may be associated with an intraarticular fracture of the distal humerus, which can only be diagnosed radiographically. Do a complete distal neurocirculatory examination, examine the shoulder and wrist, then apply a splint in the position of function and comfort. An open fracture, absent pulse, severe swelling, or neurologic deficit should prompt immediate evacuation.

Wrist

Wrist fractures occur with significant rotational forces or high axial loading forces, as occur in falls onto the hand. The victim first complains of pain and later wrist swelling. Hand use or forearm rotation produces significant pain. Many carpal bone fractures are associated with wrist dislocation. Reduction of dislocations is described later.

Carpal bone fractures cannot be diagnosed without radiographs. Scaphoid (navicular) fracture is the most common fracture and is suspected when the patient's area of maximum tenderness is in the "anatomic snuffbox" (Figure 21-7). If appropriate splinting materials are available, apply a thumb spica splint, immobilizing both the radius and the entire thumb. With fracture of the hook of the hamate bone, the victim complains of pain at the base of the hypothenar eminence. This injury occurs when the hand is used to apply significant force to an object with a handle on it, such as an ax or hammer, and great resistance is met. A short-arm splint suffices for this injury, and for other suspected carpal injuries, until definitive treatment is obtained. With open fractures or those accompanied by median nerve dysfunction, promptly evacuate the victim.

Metacarpals

Fracture of the metacarpal base or shaft occurs with crush injuries or with axial loads when rocks or other immovable objects are struck. Fractures at the base of the digit metacarpals are suspected when tenderness, crepitus and, occasionally, deformity are present. Manage these with a short-arm splint.

Fractures of the metacarpal necks also occur by the same mechanism and usually involve the fifth and fourth metacarpals. These fractures occur at the base of the knuckles and can be associated with significant flexion deformity. Up to 40 degrees of flexion in the fifth and fourth digits can be accepted without compromising hand function, so these fractures rarely require reduction. Rotational deformity of the metacarpal is poorly tolerated and should be anticipated with suspected metacarpal fractures. With the MCP and the IP joints flexed 90 degrees, the fingernails should be parallel to one another and perpendicular to the orientation of the palm. The terminal portions of the digit should point to the scaphoid tubercle.

When malalignment or significant shortening with a suspected shaft fracture is noted, reduce the fracture with longitudinal traction on the involved digit. Immobilize a fractured metacarpal shaft or neck by applying an aluminum splint (or stick) to the volar surface and taping the involved digit to the adjacent digit, with the MCP joint at 90 degrees. This is the point of maximum length of the collateral ligaments. Immobilizing the joint in this position prevents contractures that can lead to subsequent loss of motion.

Fracture of the base of the thumb metacarpal often occurs with an axial force directed against a partially flexed thumb metacarpal. If the fracture extends into the joint, it often requires operative fixation. If this fracture is suspected, immobilize the thumb and wrist in a thumb spica splint. An open metacarpal fracture needs cleansing, debridement, and presumptive antibiotic therapy for 48 hours or until definitive care is obtained.

Phalanges

Fractures of the digital phalanges occur with crush injuries or when the digits are caught in ropes or within equipment being used to haul objects. Angular or rotational deformity and crepitus make these fractures obvious. Without radiographs, an intraarticular fracture with subluxation or dislocation is difficult to differentiate from an IP joint dislocation. Angular deformities in these fractures can be reduced using a pencil or thin stick placed in the web space as a fulcrum to assist in reduction. Reduce a fracture of the shaft of a phalanx by applying traction and correcting the deformity. Immobilize the fractures by taping the injured digit to the neighboring uninjured digit or to a volar splint. Cleanse nail-bed fractures or crushes with soap, apply a sterile dressing, and apply a protective volar splint to prevent further injury.

UPPER EXTREMITY DISLOCATIONS AND SPRAINS

Sternoclavicular Joint

Traumatic dislocation of the sternoclavicular joint generally requires tremendous force, either direct or indirect, applied to the shoulder, and consequently it is rare. Anterior dislocation is most common, with the medial head of the clavicle going anterior to the manubrium of the sternum. The victim complains of pain around the sternum and frequently has difficulty taking a deep breath. When the dislocation is posterior, significant pressure may be placed on the esophagus and superior vena cava. The victim may complain of difficulty swallowing and have engorgement of the veins of the face and upper extremities, representing superior vena cava obstruction syndrome. A step-off between the sternum and the medial head of the clavicle (compared with the uninjured side) confirms this diagnosis.

Unreduced anterior dislocation does not produce neurocirculatory compromise and is treated with a sling. It is usually unstable after reduction. Attempt reduction of a posterior dislocation as soon as possible if any neurocirculatory compromise is present. Place the victim supine with a large roll of clothing or other firm object between the scapulae. Apply traction to the arm against countertraction in an abducted and slightly extended position. You may need to manually manipulate the medial end of the clavicle to dislodge the clavicle from behind the manubrium (Figure 21-8). If this fails, apply sharp, firm pressure posteriorly to both shoulders. Repeat this maneuver several times, placing a larger object between the scapulae if reduction attempts are initially unsuccessful. Alternatively, seat the victim and place your knee between the shoulders, then pull back on both shoulders. If the victim remains in extremis, grasp the midshaft clavicle with a towel clip or pliers and forcefully pull it out of the thoracic cavity. Once reduced, the injury is usually stable. This type of dislocation requires evacuation.

Acromioclavicular Joint

The acromioclavicular joint is injured by a blow on top of the shoulder (Figure 21-9). Because using the hand increases pain, place the arm on the affected side in a sling. As long as the individual can tolerate the discomfort associated with such an injury, evacuation is not necessary.

Glenohumeral Joint

The head of the humerus at the shoulder joint is generally dislocated anteriorly and inferiorly. The usual mechanism of injury is a blow to the arm in the abducted and externally rotated position. This frequently occurs in skiing as the individual crosses his or her ski tips or goes forward on a mogul and lands face first with the arms in this position.

Recurrent dislocations and dislocations in younger patients may be easier to reduce than first-time dislocations in older patients. Do a thorough motor, sensory, and circulatory examination of the involved extremity. Carefully assess axillary and musculocutaneous nerves because they are the nerves most commonly injured with an anterior dislocation. Do serial examinations of distal pulses, capillary refill, and forearm compartments.

The preferred method of reduction is linear traction along the axial line of the extremity while stabilizing

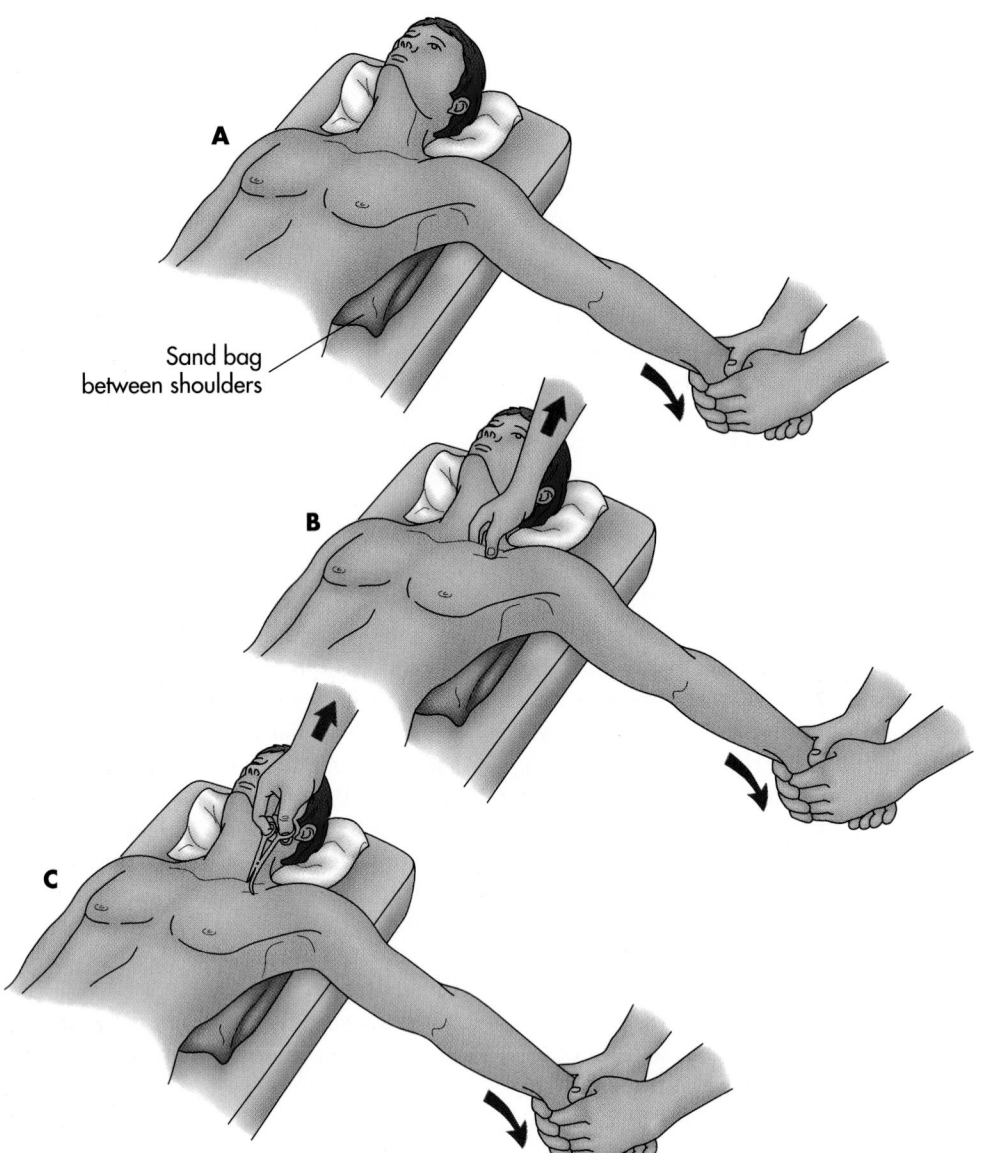

Figure 21-8 Technique for closed reduction of the sternoclavicular joint. **A,** The patient is positioned supine with a sandbag placed between the two shoulders. Traction is then applied to the arm against countertraction in an abducted and slightly extended position. In anterior dislocation, direct pressure over the medial end of the clavicle may reduce the joint. **B,** In posterior dislocation, in addition to the traction it may be necessary to manipulate the medial end of the clavicle with the fingers to dislodge the clavicle from behind the manubrium. **C,** In a stubborn posterior dislocation, it may be necessary to sterilely prepare the medial end of the clavicle and use a towel clip to grasp around the medial clavicle to lift it back into position. *(From Rockwood CA Jr, Green DP, Bucholz RW, editors: Rockwood and Green's fractures in adults, ed 3, Philadelphia, 1991, JB Lippincott.)*

the torso with a blanket or rope (Figure 21-10). Narcotic or benzodiazepine premedication can be extremely helpful, but avoid this in a multiply-injured victim if you are concerned about altering mentation or adversely affecting blood pressure. You may tie a sheet, belt, webbed strapping, or avalanche cord around your waist and the victim's bent forearm, so that you (standing or kneeling) can lean back to apply traction, keep-

ing your hands free to guide the head of the humerus back into position (Figure 21-11). Place padding in the armpit and bend of the elbow to prevent pressure injury to sensitive nerves beneath the skin. In the Milch technique, place the patient prone or sitting upright. Place your right hand in the axilla for a dislocated right shoulder and hold the victim's hand with your left. Gently abduct the victim's arm and apply pressure to

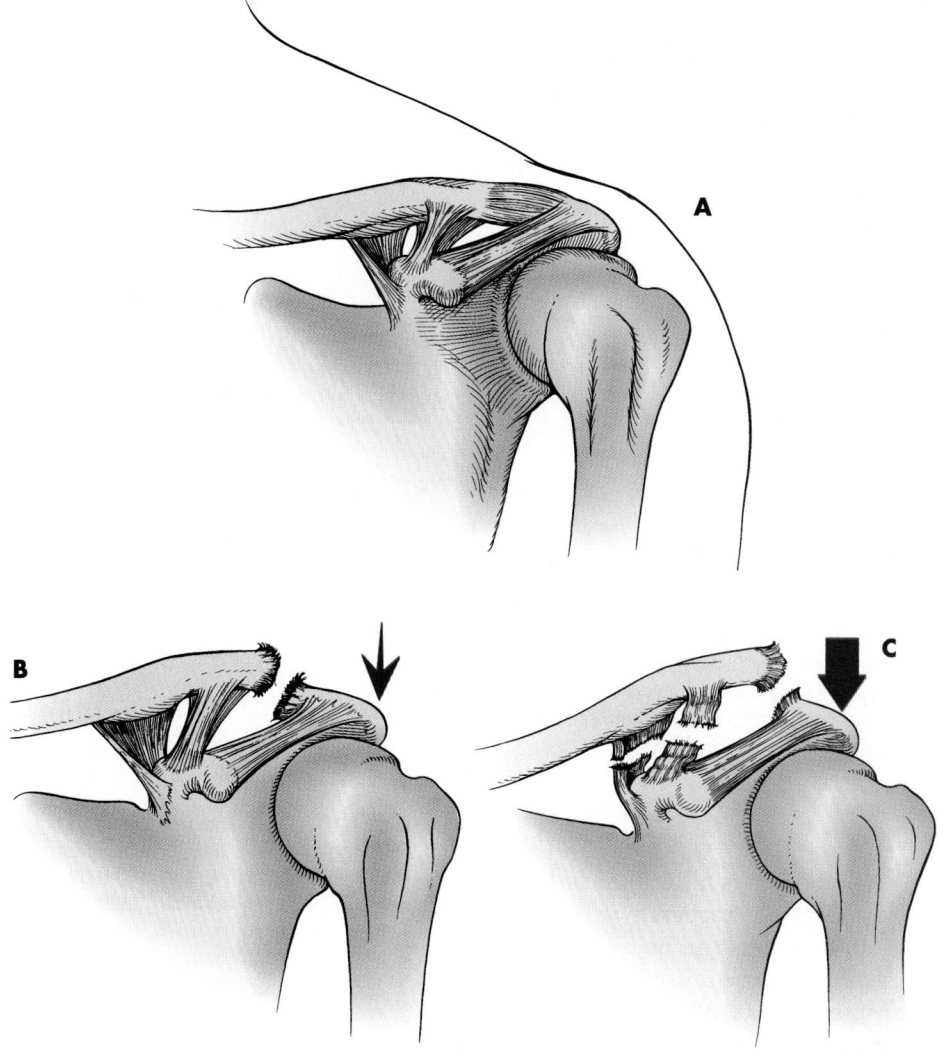

Figure 21-9 Acromioclavicular joint surgery. **A,** Normal anatomy. **B,** Second-degree injury. **C,** Third-degree injury.

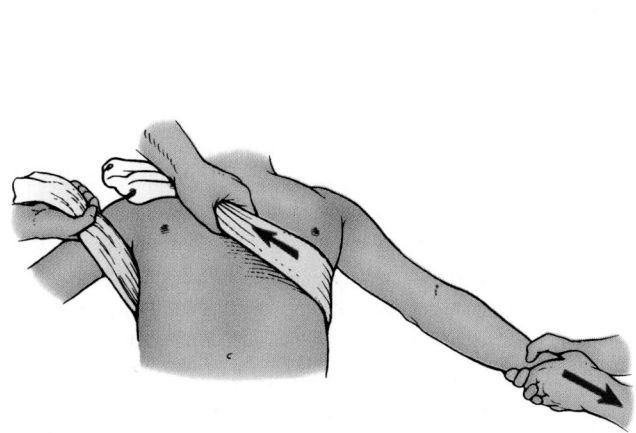

Figure 21-10 Traction and countertraction for dislocated shoulder reduction.

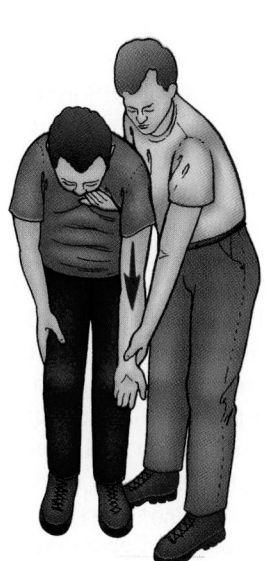

Figure 21-11 Pulling on the hanging arm to relocate a dislocated humerus. (*From Auerbach PS:* Medicine for the outdoors: the essential guide to emergency medical procedures and first aid, *ed 3, New York, 1999, The Lyons Press.*)

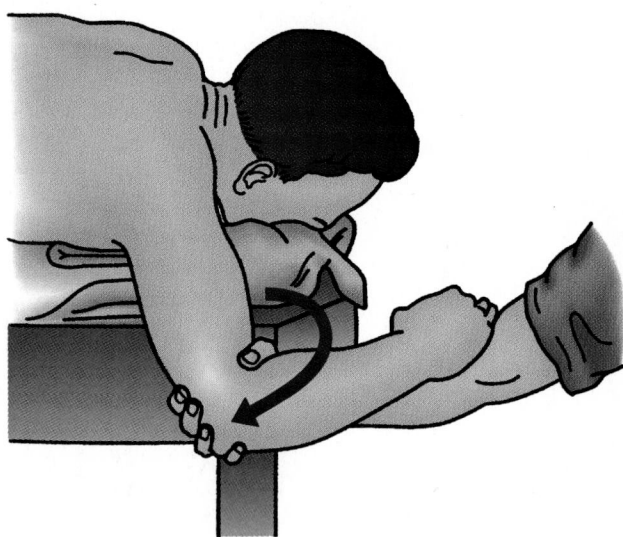

Figure 21-12 Milch technique of closed reduction of anterior gleno-humeral dislocation with the patient prone. The arm can be manipulated in the same manner with the patient supine. (*Redrawn from Lacey T II, Crawford HB: J Bone Joint Surg 34A:108, 1952. In Browner BD et al: Skeletal trauma, vol 2, ed 2, Philadelphia, WB Saunders, 1998.*)

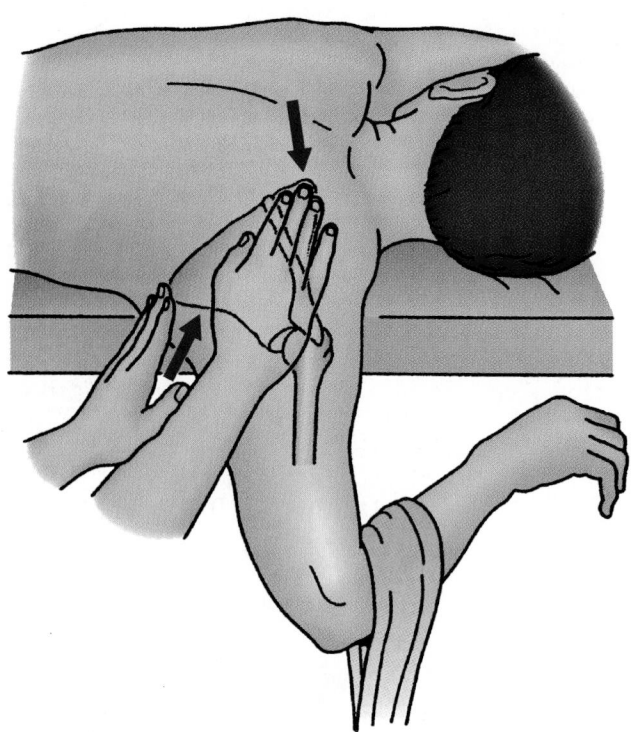

Figure 21-13 Scapular manipulation technique for closed reduction of anterior glenohumeral dislocation. (*Redrawn from Anderson D, Zvirbulis R, Ciullo J: Clin Orthop 164:181, 1982. In Browner BD et al: Skeletal trauma, vol 2, ed 2, Philadelphia, 1998, WB Saunders.*)

the humeral head. When the arm is fully abducted, rotate it externally and apply gentle traction to reduce the humeral head. This slow process can be highly successful in the acute setting because it usually does not require analgesics or muscle relaxants (Figure 21-12).[6] The success of this maneuver decreases as the time after dislocation increases.

Scapular manipulation is also minimally traumatic and highly successful.[2] Place the victim prone and apply 5 to 15 pounds of traction on the arm. Once relaxation is obtained, raise the inferior angle of the scapula and rotate it toward the spine; rotate the superior aspect away from the spine (Figure 21-13). This can also be done with the victim in the standing position (Figure 21-14). If the victim is standing, it may help to pull the arm forward, as well as down. This technique generally requires excellent relaxation, but can be highly successful.

An alternative method is to have the victim lie prone so that the injured arm dangles free. Place a thick pad under the injured shoulder. Attach a 10 to 20 lb (4.5 to 9 kg) weight to the wrist or forearm (do not have the victim attempt to hold the weight) and allow it to exert steady traction on the arm, using gravity to relocate the humeral head (Figure 21-15). A standing victim can bend forward at the waist as you pull steadily downward on the arm to simulate the gravity effect. Use gentle side-to-side motion at the wrist to assist with the reduction (Figure 21-16). Avoid the Hippocratic maneuver (Figure 21-17) of placing a foot in the axilla of the injured limb to achieve countertraction because of increased pressure on the structures within the axillary sheath.

Posterior dislocation of the glenohumeral joint makes up less than 5% of shoulder dislocations. It may occur with adduction and axial loading of the shoulder, a direct blow to the anterior aspect of the shoulder, or as a result of marked internal rotation accompanying a grand mal seizure. Frequently, the dislocation is associated with either a humeral head impaction injury or a glenoid fracture. The victim complains of significant pain and loss of shoulder motion. Generally, external rotation is completely lost. On palpation of the shoulder, you can usually detect posterior fullness not found on the uninjured side. This dislocation can be more difficult to reduce than an anterior dislocation, so excellent analgesia is generally required. Flex the arm forward, rotate it internally, and adduct it to disengage the head from the posterior glenoid rim. Occasionally, lateral traction on the humeral shaft is also required. With longitudinal traction and anterior pressure on the humeral head from behind, reduction is achieved.

If the reduction maneuver is successful, place the arm in a sling until definitive care is reached. If possible, hold a posterior dislocation in neutral or slight external rotation. Because of the significant incidence of fractures with these injuries, radiologic examination is required to make the diagnosis, and evacuation is mandated.

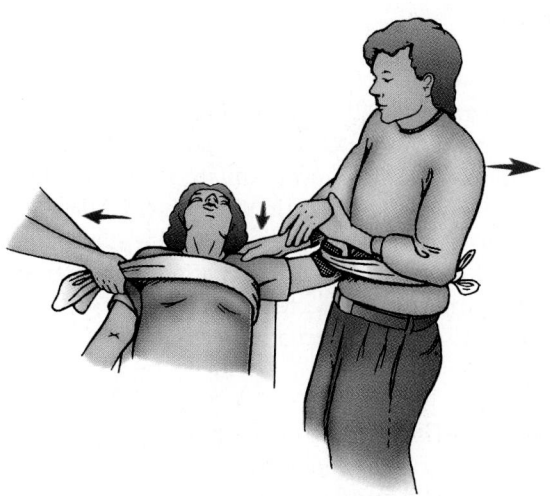

Figure 21-14 Repositioning a dislocated shoulder. Attached to the victim's forearm with a strap, rope, or sheet, the rescuer uses his body weight to apply traction, leaving his hands free to manipulate the victim's arm. A second rescuer applies countertraction, or the victim can be held motionless by fixing the chest sheet to a tree or ground stake. (*From Auerbach PS:* Medicine for the outdoors: the essential guide to emergency medical procedures and first aid, *ed 3, New York, 1999, The Lyons Press.*)

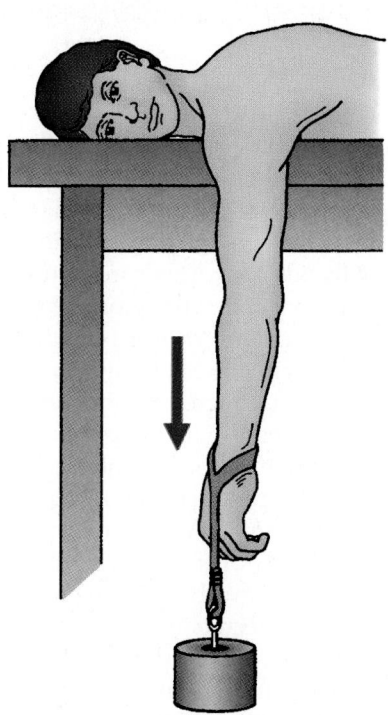

Figure 21-15 Stimson technique. (*Redrawn from Rockwood CA, Green CP, editors:* Fractures in adults, *vol 1, Philadelphia, 1984, JB Lippincott. In Browner BD et al:* Skeletal trauma, *vol 2, ed 2, Philadelphia, 1998, WB Saunders.*)

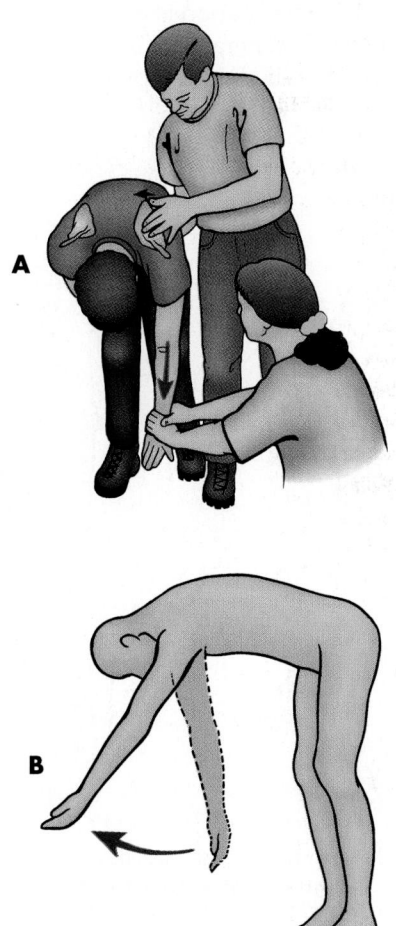

Figure 21-16 A, Pushing the lower edge of the scapula toward the spine while an assistant pulls downward on the hanging arm to assist in the relocation of a dislocated humerus. **B,** The downward pull on the arm may be slightly forward to help put the humerus back in the shoulder socket. (*From Auerbach PS:* Medicine for the outdoors: the essential guide to emergency medical procedures and first aid, *ed 3, New York, 1999, The Lyons Press.*)

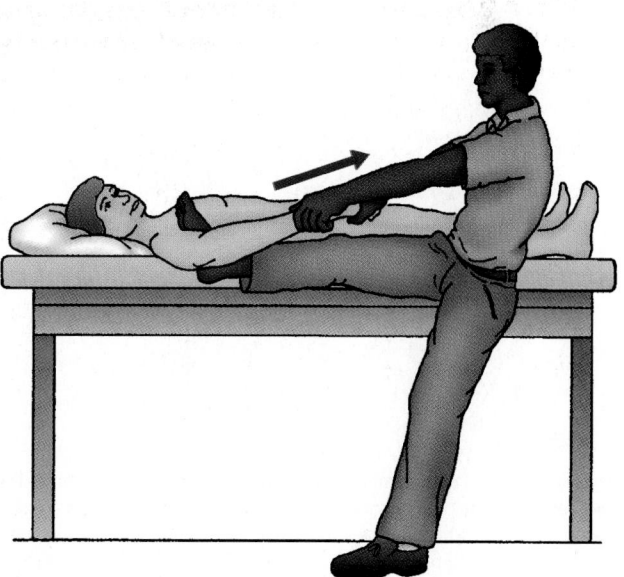

Figure 21-17 Hippocratic technique of closed reduction of anterior glenohumeral dislocation. The foot is placed against the proximal humerus, and longitudinal traction is applied to the upper extremity. (*Redrawn from Rockwood CA, Green CP, editors:* Fractures in adults, *vol 1, Philadelphia, 1984, JB Lippincott. In Browner BD et al:* Skeletal trauma, *vol 2, ed 2, Philadelphia, 1991, WB Saunders.*)

Elbow

Dislocation of the elbow occurs with hyperextension or axial load from a fall onto the outstretched hand. It is generally posterior and lateral. The diagnosis is obvious, with posterior deformity at the elbow and foreshortening of the forearm. After carefully assessing distal sensory, motor, and circulatory status, perform reduction. With countertraction on the upper arm, apply linear traction with the elbow slightly flexed and the forearm in the original degree of pronation and supination. Downward pressure on the proximal forearm to disengage the coronoid from the olecranon fossa may be helpful. Avoid hyperextension. Adequate analgesia can be extremely helpful. An alternative method is to place the patient prone over a log or makeshift platform and apply gentle downward traction on the wrist for a few minutes. As the olecranon begins to slip distally, lift up gently on the arm. No assistant is needed, and if the maneuver is done gently, no anesthesia is required (Figure 21-18). A modification of this maneuver is to hang only the forearm over the platform and apply gentle downward traction via the wrist. Guide the reduction

of the olecranon with the opposite hand (Figure 21-19). Reduction provides nearly complete relief of pain and restoration of normal surface anatomy. Apply a posterior splint with the elbow in 90 degrees of flexion and the forearm in neutral position, using a sling for comfort. If reduction is not successful after three attempts or if a nerve injury is suspected, apply a splint to the arm as it lies and initiate evacuation.

Wrist

Wrist dislocations, which are frequently associated with carpal fractures, are generally produced by a fall onto the outstretched hand. A wrist dislocation may be difficult to differentiate clinically from a fracture of the distal radius. However, in either case, perform a reduction maneuver after careful assessment of distal neurocirculatory function, emphasizing median nerve function. The reduction maneuver is similar to that for a distal radius fracture. Use one hand to stabilize the forearm and the other to grasp the hand. First, dorsiflex the wrist if the dislocation is dorsal (most common) or volarflex it if the dislocation is volar, then apply longitudinal traction. In general, significant dorsiflexion is required to obtain reduction, and premedication can be

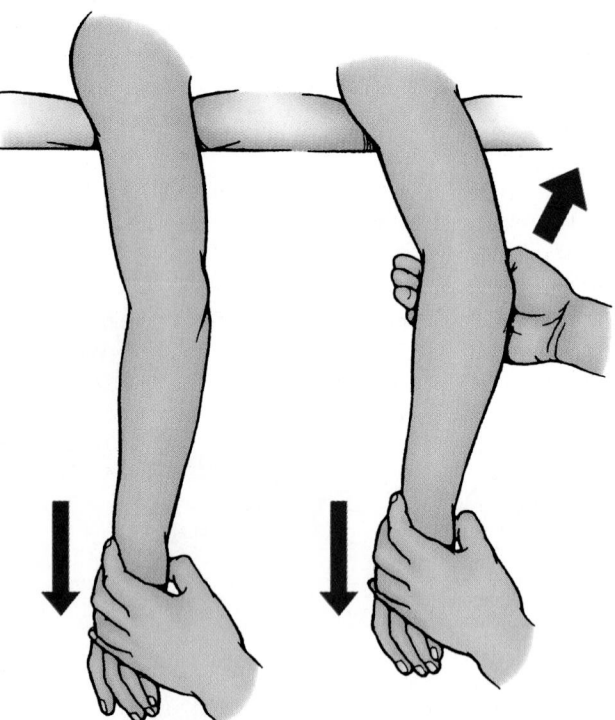

Figure 21-18 Parvin's method of closed reduction of an elbow dislocation. The patient lies prone on a stretcher, and the physician applies gentle downward traction on the wrist for a few minutes. As the olecranon begins to slip distally, the physician lifts up gently on the arm. No assistant is required, and if the maneuver is done gently, no anesthesia is required. (*Redrawn from Parvin RW: Closed reduction of common shoulder and elbow dislocations without anesthesia, Arch Surg 75:972, 1957. In Rockwood CA Jr, Green DP, Bucholz RW, editors: Rockwood and Green's Fractures in adults, ed 3, Philadelphia, 1991, JB Lippincott.*)

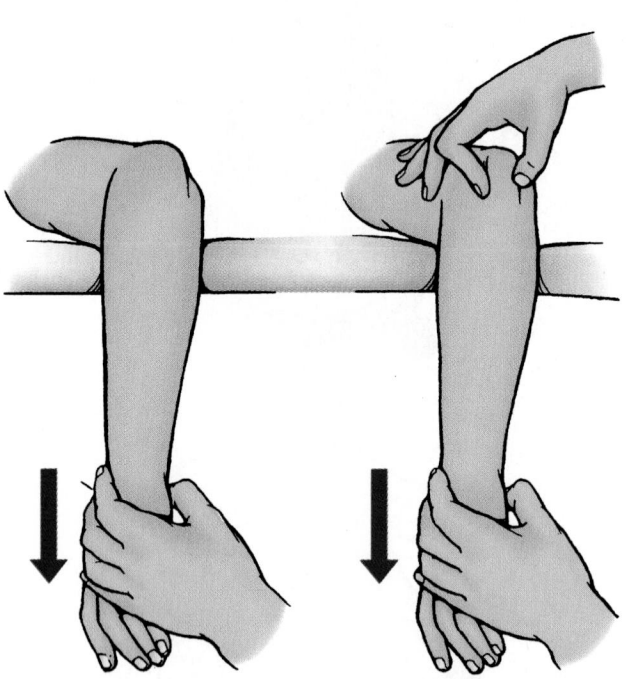

Figure 21-19 In Meyn and Quigley's method of reduction, only the forearm hangs from the side of the stretcher. As gentle downward traction is applied on the wrist, the physician guides reduction of the olecranon with the opposite hand. (*Redrawn from Meyn MA, Quigley TB: Reduction of posterior dislocation of the elbow by traction on the dangling arm, Clin Orthop 103:106, 1974. In Rockwood CA Jr, Green DP, Bucholz RW, editors: Rockwood and Green's Fractures in adults, ed 3, Philadelphia, 1991, JB Lippincott.*)

extremely helpful. If reduction is unsuccessful after three attempts or if there is median nerve dysfunction, initiate evacuation. Apply a short-arm splint if reduction is successful, and elevate the arm above the level of the heart until definitive care is procured. Consider pain and tenderness about the wrist with no significant deformity an intercarpal ligamentous disruption or a carpal fracture and apply a short arm splint.

Metacarpophalangeal Joint

MCP joint dislocation is rare, being produced by a crush injury or when the hand is caught in a rope. This dislocation may be dorsal or volar, with dorsal dislocation being most common. Clinically, the joint is hyperextended and the phalanx shortened. Most dorsal dislocations are easily reduced. First, hyperextend the proximal phalanx 90 degrees on the metacarpal, then push the base of the proximal phalanx into flexion, maintaining contact at all times with the metacarpal head to prevent entrapment of the volar plate in the joint (Figure 21-20). Avoid straight longitudinal traction because it may turn a simple dislocation into a complex dislocation (see below). Flex the wrist and IP joints to relax the flexor tendons, and the joint usually reduces easily with a palpable and audible clunk. Apply a dorsal-volar splint, with the joint held at 90 degrees of flexion. Irreducible or complex dislocations also occur when the volar plate is interposed in the joint. Clinically, the joint is only slightly hyperextended and the volar skin is puckered over the joint. These dislocations are most common in the index, thumb, and little finger. A single attempt at reduction using the technique just described is indicated, but these dislocations usually require open reduction. If reduction of an MCP joint dislocation is unsuccessful, splint the joint in the position of comfort and obtain definitive treatment as soon as possible.

The thumb MCP joint is most commonly injured. Dislocations are reduced as already described. Injury to the ulnar collateral ligament of this joint (skier's or gameskeeper's thumb) results from a valgus stress, as may occur when an individual falls holding an object in the first web space. The victim complains of tenderness over the ulnar aspect of the MCP joint. There may be instability to radial stress with the joint held in 30 degrees of flexion, an indication for surgical repair. In the field, apply a thumb spica splint and seek definitive care within 10 days. If splinting material is not available, tape the thumb until definitive care can be obtained (Figure 21-21).

Proximal Interphalangeal Joint

Proximal interphalangeal (PIP) joint dislocations may be dorsal, volar, or rotatory, with dorsal dislocation by far the most common. Dorsal dislocation occurs with hyperextension, and the volar plate is always ruptured. It can be associated with fracture of the volar lip of the middle phalanx, creating instability after reduction. Perform reduction as described for dorsal MCP dislocation. Avoid straight longitudinal traction to prevent entrapment of the volar plate into the joint. After reduction, tape the finger to an adjacent finger to avoid hyperextension and allow early motion (Figure 21-22). As with MCP dislocation, a complex dislocation can occur, but it is rare. This is difficult to reduce closed and often requires open reduction.

Volar dislocations are rare. For this injury to occur, the central slip must be disrupted, and the potential for a boutonniere deformity is present. Reduce the digit by flexion of the PIP joint, pushing the base of the middle phalanx dorsally. Treat the PIP joint like a rupture of the central slip, with the PIP joint splinted in extension. Leave the distal interphalangeal (DIP) and MCP joints free to allow motion.

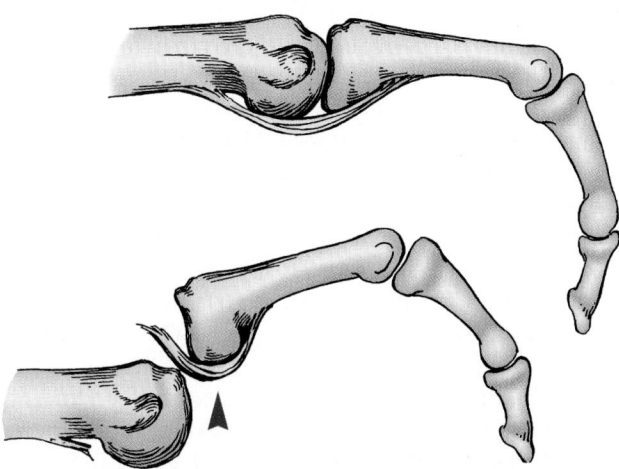

Figure 21-20 The single most important element preventing reduction in a complex MCP dislocation is interposition of the volar plate within the joint space, and it must be extricated surgically. (*From Rockwood CA Jr, Green DP, Bucholz RW, editors: Rockwood and Green's Fractures in adults, ed 3, Philadelphia, 1991, JB Lippincott.*)

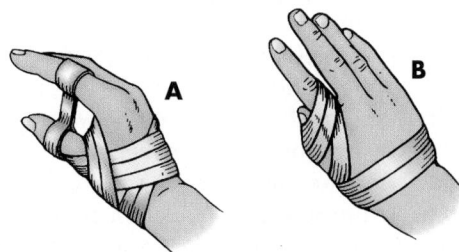

Figure 21-21 Taping the thumb for immobilization. **A,** The buddy-taping method. **B,** A thumb-lock; if possible, padding should be placed between the thumb and forefinger. (*From Auerbach PS: Medicine for the outdoors: the essential guide to emergency medical procedures and first aid, ed 3, New York, 1999, The Lyons Press.*)

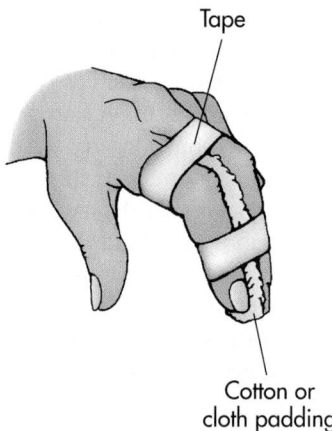

Tape

Cotton or
cloth padding

Figure 21-22 Buddy-taping method to immobilize a finger. (*From Auerbach PS:* Medicine for the outdoors: the essential guide to emergency medical procedures and first aid, *ed 3, New York, 1999, The Lyons Press.*)

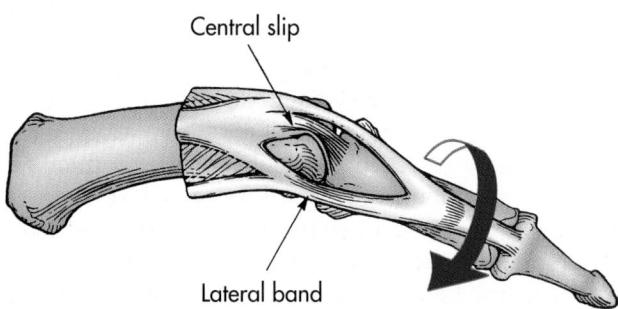

Central slip

Lateral band

Figure 21-23 Rotary subluxation of the PIP joint. The condyle of the head of the proximal phalanx is button-holed between the lateral band and central slip, both of which remain intact. (*From Rockwood CA Jr, Green DP, Bucholz RW, editors:* Rockwood and Green's Fractures in adults, *ed 3, Philadelphia, 1991, JB Lippincott.*)

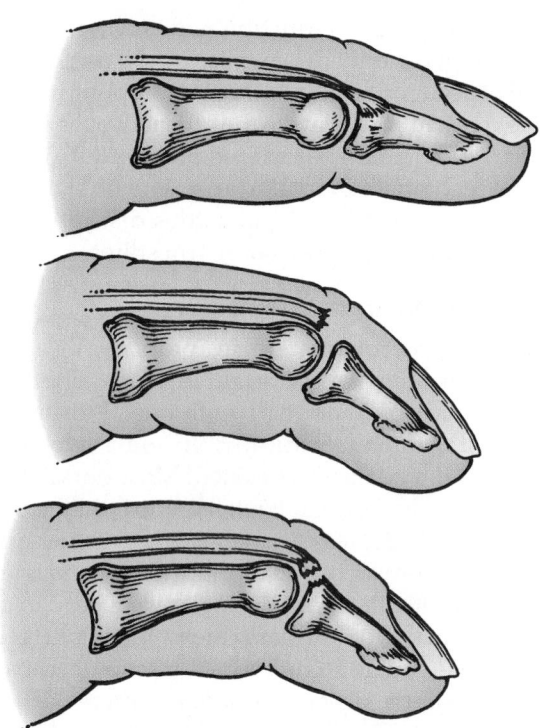

Figure 21-24 The three types of injury that cause a mallet finger of tendon origin. *Top,* The extensor tendon fibers over the distal joint are stretched without complete division of the tendon. Although there is some drop of the distal phalanx, the patient retains weak active extension. *Center,* The extensor tendon is ruptured from its insertion on the distal phalanx. There is usually a 40- to 45-degree flexion deformity, and the patient has loss of active extension at the distal joint. *Bottom,* A small fragment of the distal phalanx is avulsed with the extensor tendon. This injury has the same clinical findings as that shown in the center drawing. (*From Rockwood CA Jr, Green DP, Bucholz RW, editors:* Rockwood and Green's Fractures in adults, *ed 3, Philadelphia, 1991, JB Lippincott.*)

Rotatory subluxation of the PIP joint is also rare (Figure 21-23), occurring after a twisting injury. The condyle of the head of the proximal phalanx is buttonholed between the lateral band and the central slip, both of which remain intact. This injury can be difficult to reduce. With both the MCP and PIP joints flexed, apply gentle traction to the finger. This relaxes the volarly displaced lateral band and allows the band to be disengaged and slip dorsally when a gentle rotary and traction force is applied. You can achieve further relaxation of the lateral band by dorsiflexion of the wrist. After reduction, buddy tape the finger and begin early motion. With any dislocation of the PIP joint, seek definitive care promptly to ensure adequate reduction of the injury.

"Jammed" fingers may be just as debilitating and painful as dislocated digits. With these injuries, stress the involved joint both radially and ulnarly to ensure collateral ligament integrity. If the joint is stable, the finger can be buddy taped to an adjacent digit and immediate care is not indicated. If the finger is unstable, seek definitive care.

Distal Interphalangeal Joint

The DIP joint is less frequently injured than the PIP joint. Pure dislocations are rare and are usually dorsal and associated with an open wound. The reduction maneuver is similar to that used for dorsal PIP joint dislocation, and the injury is stable after reduction. More commonly, a mallet-finger injury occurs when the extensor tendon is taut, as when striking an object with the finger extended. The basic injury is incompetence of the extensor tendon at its insertion into the distal phalanx. The three types of mallet injuries are shown in Figure 21-24. Individuals with this injury lack full extension of the DIP joint when the MCP and PIP joints are kept in extension. Holding these joints in extension isolates the extensor tendon by neutralizing the intrinsic muscles. If an extension lag is noted, splint the joint in slight extension for 6 to 8 weeks, leaving the PIP and DIP joints free (Figure 21-25). Obtain a radiograph within the first 10 days to ensure that the joint is reduced.

Occasionally, the flexor digitorum profundus (FDP) tendon is avulsed from its insertion on the distal pha-

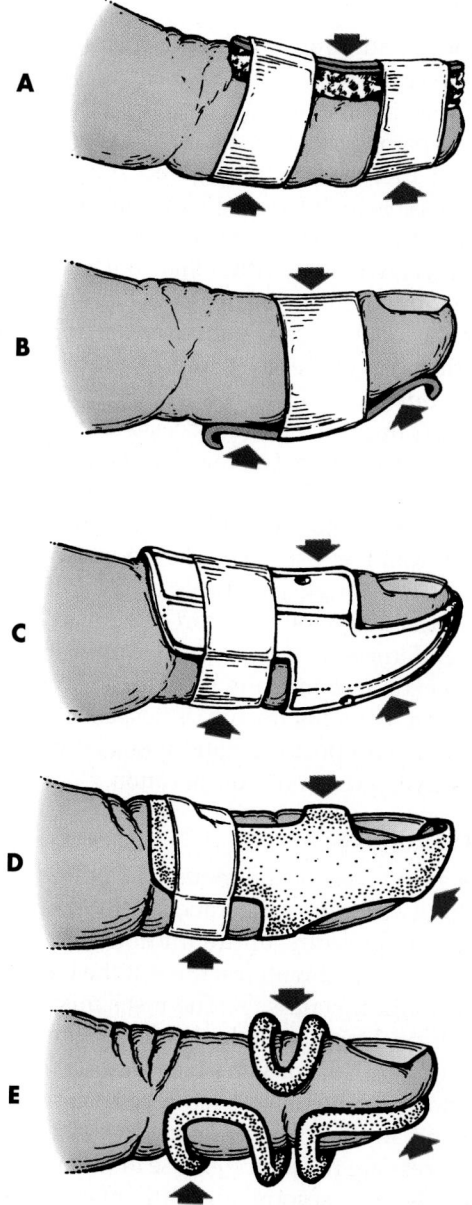

Figure 21-25 Mallet finger can be treated by immobilizing the DIP joint with a dorsal padded aluminum splint **(A)**, a volar unpadded aluminum splint **(B)**, a Stack splint **(C)**, a modified Stack splint **(D)**, or an Abouna splint **(E)**. Note that each of these splints uses a three-point fixation principle. (*From Rockwood CA Jr, Green DP, Bucholz RW, editors: Rockwood and Green's Fractures in adults, ed 3, Philadelphia, 1991, JB Lippincott.*)

lanx. This occurs with forced hyperextension of the DIP joint while the FDP is maximally contracted. The ring finger is most commonly injured. The diagnosis is made by demonstrating inability to flex the DIP joint with the PIP joint held in extension. Pain and local tenderness are more common over the PIP joint, where the retracted end of the tendon usually lies. Splint the digit in flexion, and seek care within 7 days from a surgeon specializing in the upper extremities.

LOWER EXTREMITY INJURIES

Femur and Patella

In general, healthy, active individuals sustain fractures of the proximal femur only in falls from significant heights or from high-velocity injuries sustained during water or snow skiing. These fractures occur in the femoral neck or intertrochanteric region. When the head and spinal cord are uninjured, the victim complains of pain within the proximal thigh. In all but the thinnest individuals, there is little local reaction in terms of swelling or deformity around the hip region to aid in diagnosis. Any movement of the affected limb produces significant pain. In many cases, the affected limb is noticeably shortened and externally rotated. Following a careful sensory, motor, and circulatory examination, realign the limb and apply a Kendrick, Thomas, or REEL splint, if available. An improvised traction splint can be fabricated (see Chapter 19). If none is available, transport the victim on a backboard, with the limbs strapped together or tied to a board with a tree limb placed between them. Fracture of the femoral neck is associated with a significant risk of posttraumatic femoral head necrosis. Without a radiograph, this fracture is impossible to distinguish from an intertrochanteric hip fracture. Because there is evidence that emergency treatment of a fracture of the femoral neck decreases the risk of posttraumatic avascular necrosis,[10] arrange rapid evacuation of any victim in whom this injury is suspected.

Fracture of the femoral shaft occurs by similar mechanisms. Crepitus and maximum deformity are noted in the midportion of the thigh. After neurocirculatory examination, place the limb in traction or protect it as noted previously. Correct any gross deformity of the shaft with gentle traction, and repeat the neurocirculatory examination. This fracture may be an open injury, so split the victim's pants to complete the examination. Discovery of an open wound should prompt rapid evacuation.

Fracture of the distal end of the femur is frequently intraarticular and occurs with high-velocity loading when the knee is flexed. With axial loading on the femur, the patella becomes the driving wedge and the femoral condyles suffer direct impact, producing either a patella fracture or a fracture of the femoral condyles or distal metaphysis. With a patella fracture, the injury may be obvious on deep palpation. This is often an open injury because there is very little soft tissue overlying this sesamoid bone. Instability of the distal femur with crepitus indicates a supracondylar femur fracture, not a patella fracture. The definitive diagnosis is made radiographically. After initial neurocirculatory examination, realign the limb to avoid compression of the popliteal artery and vein. Apply a posterior splint to the realigned limb for transportation. As with all fractures, open wounds in the region of the fracture, or an abnormal nerve or vascular examination should prompt immediate evacuation.

Tibia and Fibula

The tibial plateau is the broad intraarticular surface of the upper tibia that articulates with the distal femur. This area can be fractured with a fall or leap from a height. Frequently, angulatory moments across the knee are associated. A valgus moment produces a fracture of the lateral tibial plateau, whereas a varus moment produces a medial plateau fracture. Pain, swelling, and deformity are obvious on initial examination. With a tibial plateau fracture, significant hemarthrosis develops quickly. Because of anatomic tethering of the popliteal artery by the fascia of the soleus complex, arterial injury may result from this fracture, especially when associated with a knee dislocation. Assess distal pulses and capillary refill at 1-hour intervals, keeping in mind the possibility of a compartment syndrome. After initial examination, carefully realign the limb and apply a posterior splint for transportation.

Tibial shaft fractures are associated with fibular shaft fractures in 90% of cases. These fractures result from high-impact trauma. Before the development of higher, anatomically conforming ski boots, these fractures were the most common ski injuries. The injury was sustained when the body rotated around a fixed foot (occurring with a ski caught against a rock or tree stump), which produced a torsional, spiral fracture of the tibia and fibula.

Tibial shaft fracture is the most common type of open fracture in the wilderness setting. When this injury is suspected, inspect the entire limb for distal sensory, motor, and circulatory function before realignment. Apply a posterior splint for transport. Take great care in serially examining the limb for the possibility of a compartment syndrome because this is the most common anatomic location for this problem.

Ankle

The intraarticular distal tibia, medial malleolus, and distal fibula, or any combination of these, may be involved in an ankle fracture, which is generally produced by large torsional moments about a fixed foot. With the distal tibia, axial loading from a fall or jump may also be involved. Note if there is significant pain and swelling as the shoe is removed. Palpation along the medial and lateral malleoli confirms the clinical suspicion. After the shoe is removed to inspect the skin for open wounds, perform a neurocirculatory examination.

If there is a rotational deformity in the ankle, realign the ankle with gentle traction before applying a posterior splint with the ankle in neutral position. During transport, elevate the limb above the level of the heart.

Tarsal Bones

The calcaneus and talus are usually fractured during falls or jumps from significant heights when the victim lands on his or her feet. With a calcaneus fracture, significant heel pain, deformity, and crepitus are immediately evident after the boot is removed. A talus fracture may be impossible to differentiate from an ankle fracture on clinical grounds. An ankle fracture is tender at the malleolus level, whereas with a talar fracture, the tenderness is located distal to the malleoli. Talus fracture occurs when the foot is forced into maximum dorsiflexion. Knowing the point of the foot's impact with the ground is helpful in differentiating a talus fracture from an ankle fracture. Talus fracture may be associated with subtalar or ankle joint dislocation, but this deformity is more severe. Arrange for emergency evacuation because these injuries are very difficult to reduce closed, and pressure on the skin from the displaced talar body can produce significant skin slough. Fractures of the other tarsal bones are exceedingly rare but can be defined by localizing the tenderness to a specific site. Apply a short-leg splint with extra padding and elevate the limb during transportation. If a talus fracture is suspected, expedite evacuation because posttraumatic avascular necrosis of the talar body is a common complication.

Metatarsal Bones

Fractures at the base of the metatarsals often accompany midfoot dislocation (Lisfranc's dislocation). These injuries occur across the entire midfoot joint and are commonly associated with fractures at the bases of the second and fifth metatarsals. The mechanism usually occurs with axial loading of the foot in maximum plantar flexion as a result of vehicular trauma, most frequently snowmobiling. The victim complains of midfoot pain and swelling; on removing the shoe, crepitus and tenderness are noted at the base of the metatarsals (especially the first, second, and fifth metatarsals) and plantar ecchymosis may be present. Overall foot alignment is maintained, but stressing the midfoot by stabilizing the heel and placing force across the forefoot in the varus and valgus directions reveals instability. Place the foot in a well-padded posterior splint and elevate it whenever possible. Do not allow the victim to ambulate. Swelling associated with this injury can produce a compartment syndrome.

Metatarsal shaft fracture occurs with a crush injury or a fall or jump from moderate height. Midshaft metatarsal fractures also occur as "fatigue," or so-called "march" fractures, which often occur with prolonged hiking or running with poor preconditioning. Pain and localized tenderness are the hallmarks of this diagnosis. The dull pain at the midshaft of a metatarsal (often the second or fifth) may be converted to more severe pain with associated crepitus by a jump from a log or a rock. You can temporarily manage these fractures with a stiff-soled boot or orthotic insert. If there is fracture instability or extreme pain, apply a short-leg splint and allow no further weight bearing.

Phalanx

Toe phalanges are fractured by crush injuries and can be prevented by the use of steel-toed or hard-toed boots. A great-toe phalanx fracture can be a significant problem because force is placed on this digit during the toe-off phase of gait. Manage phalanx fractures by buddy taping the toe to an adjacent uninjured digit with cotton placed between the toes. Displaced intraarticular fracture of the proximal phalanx of the great toe may need operative fixation. Stiff-soled boots minimize discomfort during weight bearing.

LOWER EXTREMITY DISLOCATIONS AND SPRAINS

Hip

Posterior hip dislocation is produced by axial loading of the femur with the hip flexed and adducted.[7] It generally occurs in vehicular trauma but can follow a fall or sledding or skiing accident. With posterior dislocation, the victim complains of severe pain about the hip and the affected limb appears shortened, flexed, internally rotated, and adducted. Any hip motion increases the pain. It is not clinically possible to determine if there is an associated acetabular or femoral neck fracture. With the rare anterior dislocation, the limb is externally rotated and slightly flexed and abducted. This

type of dislocation is generally produced by wide abduction of the hip caused by significant force.

Place the victim in a supine position to do a complete survey of all organ systems. Carefully examine the distal limb for associated fractures, and perform a thorough sensory and motor examination. The peroneal division of the sciatic nerve is most susceptible to injury with a posterior dislocation. Hip dislocations are an orthopedic emergency because time to reduction is directly linked to the incidence of avascular necrosis of the femoral head. Immediate transfer to a definitive care center is desirable because hip radiographs may reveal an associated femoral neck fracture that could become displaced if closed reduction is attempted. However, if it will be more than 6 hours before the victim can be evacuated to a definitive care center, attempt closed reduction. With the Allis technique (Figure 21-26), position the victim supine on the ground or a stretcher. Stand above the victim and pull in-line traction on the extremity while an assistant applies counter traction to the iliac wings. With anterior dislocation, apply traction with the leg slightly abducted and externally rotated and the hip gently extended. Reduce posterior dislocations by flexing the hip 60 to 90 degrees. Internal rotation and adduction of the hip will facilitate the reduction. Successful reduction is usually indicated by an audible "clunk" and restoration of limb alignment. As with any reduction maneuver, adequate analgesia and a slow, progressive increase in traction force are helpful. The Stimson gravity technique (Figure 21-27) may not be as practical in the wilderness. Position the patient prone on a makeshift platform. With a posterior dislo-

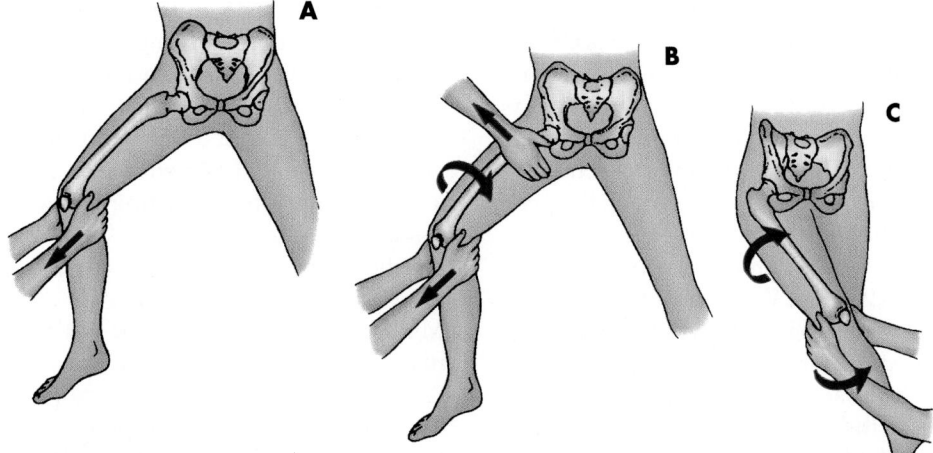

Figure 21-26 The Allis technique for reduction of a hip dislocation. The surgeon's position must provide a mechanical advantage for the application of traction. **A,** Internal and external rotation is gently alternated, perhaps with lateral traction by an assistant on the proximal thigh. **B,** In-line traction with hip flexed. **C,** Adduction is often a helpful adjunct to in-line traction. (**A** to **C,** redrawn from DeLee JC. In Rockwood CA Jr, Green DP: Fractures, vol 2, ed 2, Philadelphia, 1985, JB Lippincott. In Browner BD et al: Skeletal trauma, vol 2, ed 2, Philadelphia, 1998, WB Saunders.)

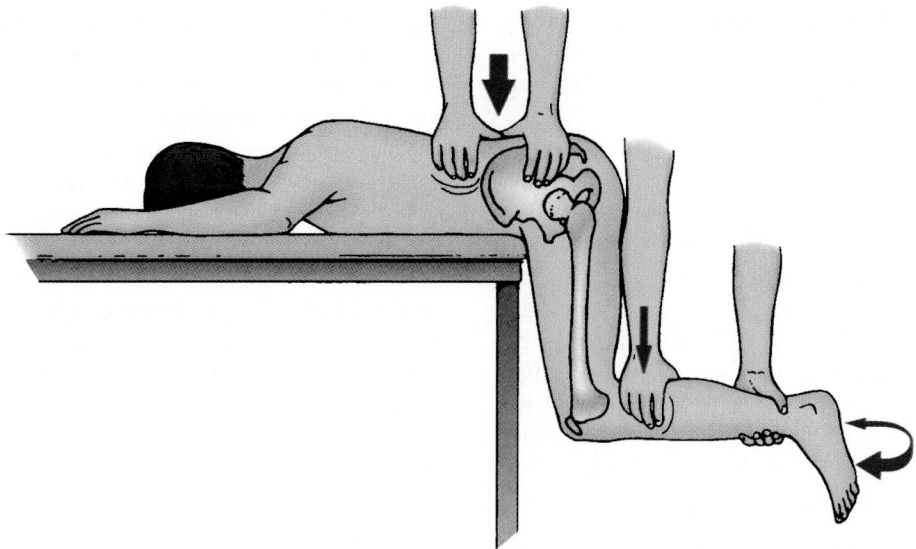

Figure 21-27 The Stimson gravity reduction technique. This method has limited application in patients with multiple injuries. (*Redrawn from DeLee JC. In Rockwood CA Jr, Green DP: Fractures, vol 2, ed 2, Philadelphia, 1985, JB Lippincott, 1985. In Browner BD et al: Skeletal trauma, vol 2, ed 2, Philadelphia, 1991, WB Saunders.*)

cation, the hip and knee are flexed 90 degrees. Apply longitudinal traction in addition to adduction and internal rotation. The reduction maneuver is actually the same for both techniques, with one performed with the victim supine and the other with the victim prone.

Knee

Knee dislocation is obvious because of the amount of deformity. The tibia may be dislocated in five directions: anterior, posterior, lateral, medial, and rotatory. The most common directions are anterior and posterior. This represents a true emergency because 5% to 40% of knee dislocations have associated vascular injuries.[1,3,4,8,12] In a large series, Green and Allen[4] reported an above-knee amputation rate of 86% for vascular injuries associated with knee dislocations that were not repaired within 8 hours of injury. The vascular injury occurs because of tethering of the popliteal vessels along the posterior border of the tibia by the soleus fascia. A knee dislocation is a high-velocity injury usually produced by vehicular trauma or a fall. When this injury is suspected, do a careful screening neurocirculatory examination. Intact distal pulses do not definitively rule out an arterial injury. Intimal flap tears can produce delayed thromboses of the popliteal artery. In addition, injury to the peroneal nerve can occur.

Many knee dislocations spontaneously reduce and may lead the examiner to underestimation of the seriousness of the injury. Instability in extension to either varus or valgus stress indicates disruption of at least one of the cruciate ligaments and should alert you to the potential for a knee dislocation.

After initial examination, reduce the persistent dislocation. Anterior dislocation is reduced with traction on the leg and gentle elevation of the distal femur. Posterior dislocation is reduced with traction in extension and anterior elevation of the tibia. Posterolateral rotatory dislocation can be very difficult to reduce and usually requires open reduction. It occurs when the medial femoral condyle buttonholes through the medial capsule. A transverse furrow on the medial aspect of the knee is pathognomic for this injury. For transport, apply a posterior splint to the limb and move the victim on a backboard. Be vigilant to the possibility of an arterial lesion or emerging compartment syndrome. Emergency evacuation is advised because of the risk of amputation related to vascular injury.

Isolated ligament or meniscal injuries can also occur. Anterior cruciate ligament (ACL) injury happens with a hyperextension or twisting injury to the knee, often associated with an audible "pop" and rapid onset of swelling and pain. On examination, the victim has both a pivot shift and increased laxity on a Lachman's test. Meniscal injuries also occur with a twisting mechanism. These injuries show a slower onset of swelling (24 to 48 hours), with pain to palpation over the joint line. The victims may complain of the knee catching, locking, or giving way, especially with twisting motions. Medial collateral ligament (MCL) injury occurs with a valgus stress to the knee. The victim complains of tenderness along the medial aspect of the proximal tibia and sometimes over the medial femoral condyle. Valgus stress with the knee in 30 degrees of flexion is painful. With a partial or complete tear, laxity will be present. It is difficult to determine if a concomitant meniscal injury is present acutely because both injuries can be painful over the joint line. Instability to valgus stress in full extension indicates injury to the MCL and at least one of the cruciate ligaments. Wrap the knee with an elasticized bandage to contain the swelling, and place in an immobilizer if instability is present. Transport the victim to a definitive care center.

Frequently, the patellofemoral joint is dislocated. Because of the increased femorotibial angle in females, this injury is far more common in women. Generalized ligamentous laxity may predispose to this problem. Dislocation of the kneecap may result from a twisting injury or asymmetric quadriceps contraction during a fall. These mechanisms routinely occur with hiking, climbing, and skiing accidents. The patella winds up lateral to the articular surface of the distal femur. Although neurovascular injuries rarely occur in association with a dislocated patella, conduct a screening examination.

The patella can often be reduced by simply straightening the knee. If this is not successful, apply gentle pressure to the patella to push it back up onto the distal femoral articular groove. Apply a knee splint with the joint in extension; weight bearing is allowed. Keep the knee in extension until definitive care can be obtained. A radiograph is ultimately required to rule out osteochondral fractures, which are frequently associated with this injury.

Ankle

Ankle dislocations are almost always accompanied by fractures of both malleoli. These dislocations generally occur with falls onto uneven surfaces or with twisting injuries of moderate velocity. Carefully examine the area about the ankle for open injuries and conduct a neurocirculatory examination to obtain a baseline status. Then align the ankle joint by grasping the posterior heel, applying traction with the knee bent (to relax the gastrocnemius-soleus complex), and bringing the foot into alignment with the distal tibia. After this maneuver, reexamine the foot, dress any wounds, and apply a posterior splint. During transport, elevate the limb above the level of the heart.

The most common musculoskeletal injury occurring in the wilderness setting is an ankle sprain. Ligament sprain, or tearing of the fibers, is separated into three grades. Grade 1 injury is partial disruption of some of the ligament fibers, represented grossly by mild intersubstance hemorrhage. Grade 2 injury is complete disruption of a portion of the ligament fibers. The main substance of the ligament remains intact, and the injury is characterized by moderate hemorrhage with grossly visible torn ligament fibers. Grade 3 injury is complete disruption of the ligament fibers, which can result in instability of the related joint.

The medial ligament complex consists of the deltoid ligament, which runs from the medial malleolus to the talus (Figure 21-28). The ligament complex on the lateral side is much more complex and consists of three separate ligaments named for their origins and insertions: the calcaneofibular ligament, the anterior talofibular ligament, and the posterior talofibular ligament (see Figure 21-28). The lateral ligament complex is the most frequent site of an inversion injury. When such an injury occurs, remove the shoe and sock and conduct a screening neurocirculatory examination. Palpate each ligament individually for tenderness, and then evaluate the ankle for instability with the anterior drawer test. This test is performed by stabilizing the tibia with one hand and grasping the posterior heel to pull the foot forward with the other hand. If the talus slides forward within the ankle mortis (using the uninjured side as a comparison), the injury represents a grade 3 injury. Place the foot and ankle into a posterior splint or air splint. If possible, keep the victim from bearing weight on the limb. If this examination does not reveal instability and is thus indicative of a grade 1 or 2 sprain, apply an elasticized bandage or ankle taping (see Chapter 19). All injuries should be acutely treated following the RICE principle. Commercially available stirrup air splints also aid in ambulatory management of these injuries.

A more serious ankle sprain is the high ankle sprain, which affects the anterior inferior tibiofibular ligament (portion of the syndesmotic ligament) and occurs in up to 10% of ankle sprains. The victim complains of pain to palpation over the distal tibiofibular joint and also with dorsiflexion and external rotation of the foot relative to the tibia. Compression of the fibula and tibia in the proximal half of the calf produces pain over the syndesmosis. Unlike stable lateral ankle sprains, these injuries take 4 to 6 weeks to resolve. Treat initially with a short leg splint or walking boot. Failure to recognize this injury will produce prolonged disability.

In the field, tape the ankle both to decrease pain and to limit swelling (Figure 21-29; see also Chapter 19). During taping, keep the victim's ankle perpendicular to the tibial shaft. This makes walking easier, because the ankle is not plantar flexed, and it helps prevent development of an Achilles tendon contracture. If available, an Aircast ankle brace provides additional ankle support and can be used with a shoe or boot.

A fracture of the lateral process of the talus may be confused with a lateral ankle sprain, so radiographs are generally needed to rule out this injury. Inversion injuries are also infrequently associated with fractures at the insertion of the peroneus brevis tendon. You can identify this injury by the point tenderness at the base of the fifth metatarsal, but a radiograph is required for definitive diagnosis. Early management is the same as for an ankle sprain.

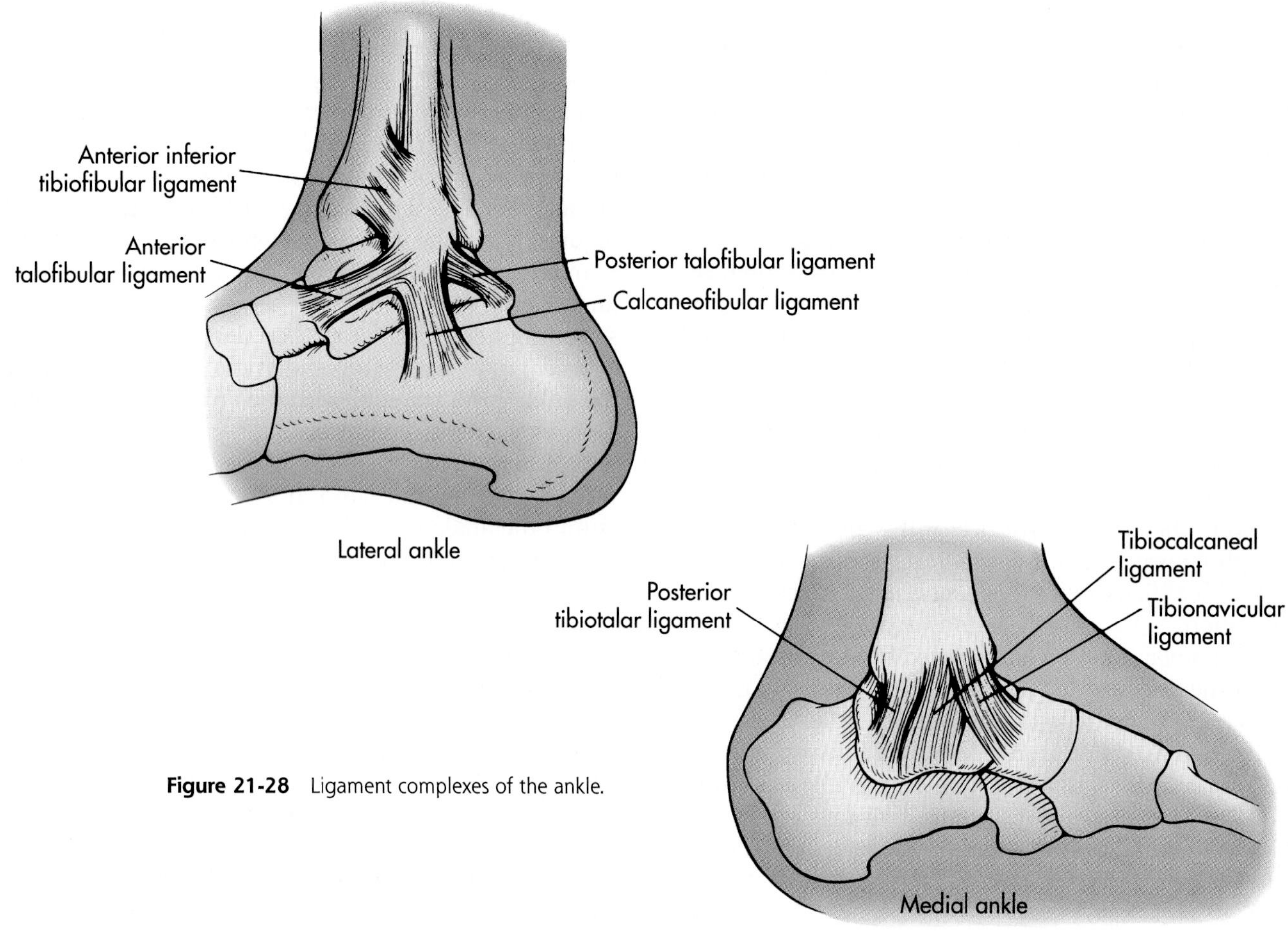

Anterior inferior
tibiofibular ligament

Anterior
talofibular ligament

Posterior talofibular ligament

Calcaneofibular ligament

Lateral ankle

Figure 21-28 Ligament complexes of the ankle.

Posterior
tibiotalar ligament

Tibiocalcaneal
ligament

Tibionavicular
ligament

Medial ankle

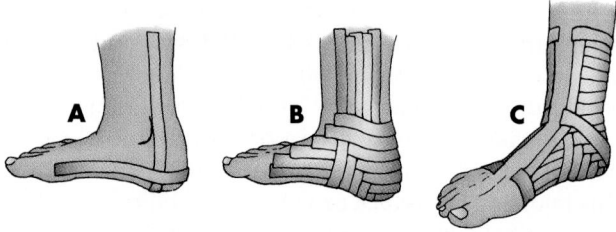

Figure 21-29 Taping a sprained ankle. **A,** Strips of adhesive tape are placed perpendicular to each other to **(B)** lock the ankle with a tight weave. **C,** The tape edges are covered to prevent peeling. (*From Auerbach PS: Medicine for the outdoors: the essential guide to emergency medical procedures and first aid, ed 3, New York, 1999, The Lyons Press.*)

Hindfoot

The subtalar joint may infrequently be dislocated in a significant fall or jump when an individual lands off balance or on an uneven surface. The calcaneus may be dislocated medially or laterally relative to the talus, the latter being slightly more common. Assess the position of the heel relative to the ankle. With either dislocation, attempt a reduction if it will be more than 3 hours until the victim will reach a definitive care center.

Medial dislocation is reduced more easily than is lateral dislocation, in which the posterior tibial tendon frequently becomes displaced onto the lateral neck of the talus, blocking the reduction. The maneuver is the same for both: grasp the heel with the knee flexed (relaxing the gastrocnemius-soleus complex), accentuate the deformity, apply linear traction, and bring the heel over to the ankle joint. This maneuver is generally successful for medial dislocation, but lateral dislocation, especially when associated with open wounds, often requires open treatment. After reduction is attempted, apply a posterior splint and elevate the limb above the heart. Even if the reduction is successful, do not allow the victim to bear weight until definitive care is obtained.

Midfoot

Midfoot fracture dislocation (Lisfranc's injury) is described in the metatarsal fracture section.

Metatarsophalangeal and Interphalangeal Joints

Metatarsophalangeal (MTP) joint dislocations of the toes are relatively uncommon but can occur when a moderate axial force is directed at the great toe. Crush injuries and rock-climbing accidents while the victim is wearing flexible-soled shoes can produce this injury; wearing boots with reinforced toe boxes of adequate depth generally prevents it. Injuries of this type at the great toe may be associated with fractures of the metatarsal or phalanx. The dislocation is generally dorsal. Because these may be open injuries, inspect the foot carefully. Reduce the joint in a manner similar to that used for dorsal PIP joint dislocation of the hand. MTP dislocation of the great toe can occasionally require open reduction if the head of the metatarsal buttonholes through the sesamoid–short flexor complex.

The lesser MTP joints are generally dislocated laterally or medially. The most common mechanism for this injury is striking unshod toes on immovable objects. Relocate the toes by applying linear traction with the victim supine and using the weight of the foot as countertraction. Similar mechanisms produce dislocations of the IP joints, which are also reduced by applying linear traction with gentle manipulation. Once reduced, tape the injured toe to the adjacent toe for 1 to 3 weeks and have the victim wear a protective boot with a stiff sole and deep toe box.

OVERUSE SYNDROMES

Plantar Fasciitis

Plantar fasciitis is inflammation of the fascia (tough connective tissue) on the sole of the foot. An individual with plantar fasciitis complains of insidious onset of pain at the origin of the plantar fascia, which is located at the most anterior aspect of the heel pad. Any activities that stretch the plantar fascia elicit pain. The pain is worse when first getting up in the morning or after resting, and is accentuated when the ankle and great toe are dorsiflexed (i.e., during push-off). Conservative treatment consists of (1) heel cord stretching 20 minutes twice a day, (2) antiinflammatory medications, and (3) wearing an orthotic that cups the heel, has a soft spot under the tender area, and supports the arch. It may take several weeks for symptoms to improve, but conservative therapy is successful in 90% of cases. An ankle-foot splint worn at night may also help because it holds the foot in a neutral position, keeping the plantar fascia slightly stretched. The orthosis also provides significant pain relief if used while walking. In severe cases, taping the arch can provide pain relief (Figure 21-30). A thin layer of benzoin or spray tape adhesive is applied to the bottom of the foot. Fix an anchor strip of ¾-inch adhesive tape in a U shape around the heel from just under the malleoli (prominences of the ankles) up to just behind the level of the "knuckles" of the toes (Figure 21-30, A). Next, lay fairly tight cross-strips of ½-inch tape across the bottom of the foot, with their ends torn to lay on the anchor strip (Figure 21-30, B). This creates a "sling" of tape under

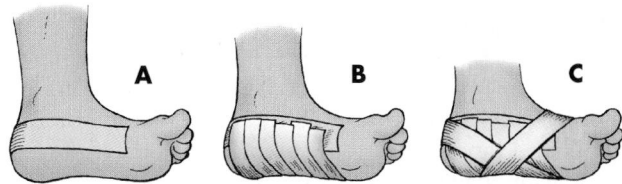

Figure 21-30 Taping for arch support. **A,** Fix an anchor strip under the heel. **B,** Attach strips across the bottom of the foot. **C,** Lock the crosspieces. (*From Auerbach PS: Medicine for the outdoors: the essential guide to emergency medical procedures and first aid, ed 3,* New York, *1999, The Lyons Press.*)

the foot for the support. Finally, apply another U-shaped piece of tape around the heel that crosses under the center of the arch and locks down the crosspieces (Figure 21-30, C).

Carpal Tunnel Syndrome

Carpal tunnel syndrome (CTS) occurs when the median nerve is compressed within the carpal tunnel. The carpal tunnel is located on the palmar side of the wrist and is formed by the transverse carpal ligament volarly and the carpal bones dorsally. The FDP and superficialis tendons to the second through fifth digits, the long thumb flexor, and the median nerve pass through this canal. Individuals complain of pain and paresthesias along the palmar aspect of the radial digits. They also complain of frequently dropping objects. Symptoms are worse at night and aggravated with prolonged wrist extension or flexion. Phalen's sign, which is numbness and tingling in the median nerve distribution after sustained wrist flexion, is suggestive of CTS. Thenar muscle atrophy is only seen in severe cases. Consider other causes, such as more proximal sites of nerve compression (especially the cervical spine), dialysis, pregnancy, or acute and chronic trauma. Treatment consists of wrist splinting in slight extension (especially at night), activity modification, and antiinflammatory medications.

Tibial Fatigue Fractures

Tibial fatigue fractures can also occur in individuals who suddenly increase their activity. Victims complain of pain with weight bearing, swelling, tenderness to palpation, and increased warmth at the fracture site. The most common site in the tibia is the proximal two thirds of the tibial diaphysis. Fracture of the distal third of the fibula can also occur. Treatment consists of activity reduction, protective weight bearing, and avoiding activities that produce pain. Failure to decrease activity level completes fracture of the tibia. As the pain subsides, the activity level can be increased. Two to three months may be required for resolution of symptoms.

EVACUATION DECISION

The issues surrounding the decision to evacuate an orthopedically injured individual vary depending on the goals and support of the expedition. A group of 25 climbers in the Himalayas with physician support and a field hospital at base camp will have very different criteria for evacuating an injured person than will a family of four spending a week hiking in the Rockies. In all cases, party leaders should have a plan for contacting evacuation support teams if a serious injury occurs.

Musculoskeletal injuries that warrant immediate evacuation to a definitive care center are listed in Box 21-2. These include any suspected cervical, thoracic, or lumbar spine injuries. A victim who has a suspected pelvic injury with posterior instability, significant suspected blood loss, or injury to the sacral plexus should receive emergency evacuation on a backboard. Any open fracture requires definitive debridement and care within 8 hours to prevent development of deep infection and should prompt emergency evacuation. Victims with suspected compartment syndromes must be evacuated on an emergency basis. Joint dislocations involving the hip or knee warrant immediate evacuation because of the associated risk of vascular injury or posttraumatic avascular necrosis of the femoral head. Lacerations involving a tendon or nerve warrant urgent evacuation to a center where an upper-extremity surgeon is available. In all but the most serious wilderness expeditions, arrangements should be made to evacuate the victim when the treating individuals are not reasonably sure of the injury with which they are dealing or its appropriate management.

Box 21-2   INDICATIONS FOR EMERGENT EVACUATION

Suspected spine injury
Suspected pelvic injury
Open fracture
Suspected compartment syndrome
Hip or knee dislocation
Vascular compromise to an extremity
Laceration with tendon or nerve injury
Uncertainty of severity of injury

REFERENCES

1. Almekinders LC, Logan TC: Results following treatment of traumatic dislocations of the knee joint, *Clin Orthop* 284:203, 1992.
2. Anderson D, Zvirbulis R, Ciullo J: Scapular manipulation for reduction of anterior shoulder dislocations, *Clin Orthop* 164:181, 1982.
3. Bohlman HH, Ducker TB, Lucas JT: *Spine and spinal cord injuries in the spine,* Philadelphia, 1982, WB Saunders.
4. Green NE, Allen BL: Vascular injuries associated with dislocation of the knee, *J Bone Joint Surg* 59A(2):236, 1977.
5. Penna GF et al: Pelvic disruption: assessment and classification, *Clin Orthop* 157:12, 1980.
6. Russell JA, Holmes EM, Keller DJ et al: Reduction of acute anterior shoulder dislocations using the Milch technique: a study of ski injuries, *J Trauma* 21:802, 1981.
7. Schatzker J, Barrington TW: Fractures of the femoral neck associated with fractures of the same femoral shaft, *Can J Surg* 11:297, 1968.
8. Shelbourne KD et al: Low-velocity knee dislocation, *Orthop Rev* 20(11):995, 1991.
9. Slatis P, Huittinen VM: Double vertical fractures of the pelvis: a report on 163 patients, *Acta Chir Scand* 138:799, 1972.
10. Swiontkowski MF, Winquist RA, Hansen ST: Fractures of the femoral neck in patients between ages twelve and forty-nine years, *J Bone Joint Surg* 66A:837, 1984.
11. Tile M: *Fractures of the pelvis and acetabulum,* Baltimore, 1984, Williams & Wilkins.
12. Varnell RM et al: Arterial injury complication knee disruption, *Am Surg* 5(12):699-704, 1989.

22 The Eye in the Wilderness

Frank K. Butler, Jr.

In the practice of ophthalmology, where the diagnosis often rests primarily on what is seen with a slit lamp, any locale that does not afford ready access to this modality could be considered wilderness. Another aspect of wilderness medicine practice is unfavorable environmental conditions, such as extremes of temperature or exposure to hypoxic or hyperbaric stress. Remote locations often make determining the urgency with which a victim should be referred for specialty care one of the most challenging aspects of treating medical disorders in the wilderness.

This chapter considers several commonly encountered types of eye disorders: periocular trauma; chemical injury to the eye; sudden vision loss in a white, quiet eye; acute orbital and periorbital inflammation; and the acute red eye. A diagnostic and therapeutic approach to these disorders suitable for the wilderness environment is presented. Finally, eye problems that are encountered in diving and altitude exposures are discussed.

PRELIMINARY PLANNING

Pertinent ocular items in a preliminary medical survey include contact lens wear; previous episodes of nontraumatic iritis; previous episodes of herpetic keratitis; and a history of corneal transplantation, retinal detachment, radial keratotomy, or other ocular surgery. A positive response to these questions may alert the health care professional to specific ocular problems that may be encountered on the proposed trip. In addition, a basic wilderness eye kit (described below) should be assembled and taken on the trip.

THE WILDERNESS EYE KIT

Box 22-1 contains the suggested items for a basic wilderness ocular emergency kit. A topical fluoroquinolone, such as ciprofloxacin or ofloxacin, is the antibiotic eye drop of choice. These medications are preferred for treatment of bacterial keratitis in a wilderness setting. Topical tetracaine and fluorescein strips are important for diagnosis. Topical prednisolone is an excellent ocular antiinflammatory medication. The choice of an oral antibiotic is based on the efficacy of the proposed antibiotic in treating preseptal cellulitis, orbital cellulitis, and penetrating trauma to the globe. The fluoroquinolone family of antibiotics offers several good choices for these indications. Trovafloxacin (500 mg tablets) is a systemic fluoroquinolone with excellent coverage against gram-positive, gram-negative, and anaerobic bacteria.[29,80] It also offers the convenience of once-daily dosing, but currently there have been a number of unpublished reports of hepatotoxicity with trovafloxacin that may limit the usefulness of this medication.[57] Levofloxacin (500 mg tablets) is another systemic fluoroquinolone with very good activity against a wide variety of gram-positive and gram-negative organisms but less anaerobic coverage than trovafloxacin.[57] Ciprofloxacin has been shown to have excellent ocular penetration when given orally[40] but is less efficacious against gram-positive organisms than is levofloxacin. Weighing these factors, levofloxacin is my current recommendation for the preferred oral antibiotic. Bacitracin is an antibiotic ointment suitable for use in patching corneal abrasions. Ophthalmic ointments are best applied by using downward pressure on the lower lid to pull it away from the eye and then applying a 1-cm ribbon of ointment to the conjunctiva of the lower lid. When released, the lid returns to its normal position and normal blinking distributes the ointment over the corneal surface. Oral prednisone has three possible treatment uses in the wilderness—refractory iritis, giant cell arteritis, and orbital pseudotumor. Topical scopolamine (0.25%) is used to reduce ciliary muscle spasm, which causes much of the discomfort associated with iritis and corneal abrasion. Scopolamine, however, has the disadvantage of dilating the pupil (making the eye very sensitive to bright light) and preventing accommodation (making reading very difficult) for 5 to 7 days. Artificial tears are used to treat ocular surface drying and to flush conjunctival foreign bodies from the eye. Diclofenac 0.1% drops have been shown to decrease corneal sensitivity, especially when multiple drops are used.[68,78,79] They have been found helpful in reducing the discomfort associated with traumatic corneal abrasion[31] and excimer laser refractive surgery.[20,81,82] In the unlikely event of angle-closure glaucoma in a wilderness setting, 2% pilocarpine may be used. The medications in Box 22-1 are listed in my recommended priority order. In the spirit of making do in the wilderness, all of the disorders mentioned in this chapter can be managed with only the medications mentioned above, but alternative therapies are also discussed.

VISUAL ACUITY MEASUREMENT IN THE WILDERNESS

Evaluation of visual acuity is an essential element of the eye examination. Serial measurements of visual acuity are used to monitor an individual's progress while being treated for an eye disorder. Lack of an eye chart does not preclude the ability to obtain some quantitative measure of visual acuity. A near vision card can be used for this purpose. It should be held the prescribed distance—usually 14 inches—from the eye. If a near card is not available, the ability to read print in a book is a useful alternative measure. If glasses have been lost, use a piece of paper with a pinhole created by the tip of a pen or pencil to help compensate for the lost refractive correction. Remember that individuals 40 years of age and older may need a pinhole or reading correction to help them focus on a near target. Although a marked decrease in visual acuity can be an important warning of a significant ocular disorder, visual acuity cannot always be considered a reliable indicator of the severity of disease. A corneal abrasion victim may initially have worse visual acuity than a person with a retinal detachment or corneal ulcer, despite the fact that the latter two entities are much more serious disorders.

GENERAL THERAPEUTIC APPROACH

The recommendations made in this chapter are not necessarily the preferred management of the disorders mentioned when one is not in the wilderness setting. Of special interest is the recommendation for a nonophthalmologist to use a topical steroid in the management of several of the disorders discussed. The use of topical ocular steroids is generally best undertaken by ophthalmologists for two reasons: first, steroids are usually indicated only for relatively serious ocular disorders, which should be followed by an ophthalmologist when pos-

sible. Second, topical steroid use may result in elevated intraocular pressure, cataracts, and exacerbation of certain eye infections. All of the disorders for which steroids are recommended below should be referred to an ophthalmologist for follow-up as soon as possible upon return from the wilderness. Caution should be exercised in prescribing a topical steroid for longer than 3 days. Although cataracts are typically associated with long-term steroid use, a significant rise in intraocular pressure may occur within just a few days after initiation of topical steroid therapy.[23]

The requirement for expedited evacuation is one of the questions that must be answered when treating an eye disease in the wilderness. In the sections below, the need for evacuation may be considered nonurgent unless an *emergent* (as soon as possible) or *expedited* evacuation (as soon as is deemed reasonable given the resources required to accomplish the evacuation) is specified in the recommendations for treatment.

ACUTE PERIOCULAR INFLAMMATION

Causes of acute periocular inflammation are listed in Box 22-2. Preseptal cellulitis means that the infectious process is confined to the tissues anterior to the orbital septum. Preseptal cellulitis therefore presents as erythema and edema of the eyelids without restricted ocular motility, proptosis, pupillary change, or decrease in visual acuity. However, some of these findings may be difficult to appreciate in the presence of marked lid edema. Historical clues include antecedent periocular trauma or insect bite or sting. In the past, this disorder has been treated very aggressively because of the high incidence of *Haemophilus influenzae* infection, especially in pediatric patients, with subsequent septicemia and meningitis. The advent of *H. influenzae type* B vaccine has changed the microbiology of this disorder and may dictate changes in treatment strategies in the future.[15] Persons who present with this disorder may be treated with levofloxacin 500 mg once a day and should have an expedited evacuation. Alternative antibiotic choices include ciprofloxacin 750 mg twice a day, dicloxacillin 500 mg every 6 hours, or cephalexin 500 mg 4 times a day.

Dacryocystitis (infection of the lacrimal sac) may mimic the findings of preseptal cellulitis, but erythema, edema, and tenderness are localized to the area inferior to the medial aspect of the eye, over the nasolacrimal sac and duct. The presence of this condition generally indicates obstruction in the opening between the lacrimal sac and the nasal cavity. Surgical intervention to restore the patency of this opening is usually undertaken after the acute infection is treated. The most common pathogens in acute dacryocystitis are *Staphylococcus aureus*, *Streptococcus* species, and (in children) *H. influenzae*.[52] Treatment should be initiated with

---

Box 22-2 DIFFERENTIAL DIAGNOSIS OF ACUTE PERIOCULAR INFLAMMATION

Preseptal cellulitis
Orbital cellulitis
Dacryocystitis
Orbital pseudotumor
Insect envenomation

---

levofloxacin 500 mg once a day and warm compresses. Alternative antibiotic choices include ciprofloxacin 750 mg twice a day or amoxicillin/clavulanate 875 mg/125 mg every 8 hours. Worsening of the condition after 24 to 48 hours should be managed with an expedited evacuation.

Periocular insect envenomation is a preseptal cellulitis look-alike. Although secondary infection may follow envenomation, the envenomation itself may produce significant erythema and edema. Diagnostic clues include a history of insect bite or a periocular papular lesion at the site of the envenomation. Ice or cool compresses may be used to treat the envenomation, with levofloxacin 500 mg once a day, dicloxacillin 500 mg every 6 hours, or cephalexin 500 mg 4 times a day added if secondary infection is suspected.

The term *orbital cellulitis* means that the infection has spread to or originated in the tissues posterior to the orbital septum. This may be manifest as diplopia or restriction in ocular motility as the extraocular muscles are affected, proptosis as edema in the orbit pushes the globe forward, decreased vision as the optic nerve is affected, or pupillary change if innervation of the pupil is affected. Fever is suggestive of orbital cellulitis in the differential diagnosis of periocular inflammation. This condition is more commonly associated with sinusitis than with periocular trauma as an antecedent disorder.[42] Most series report a 50% to 75% incidence of sinusitis or other upper respiratory infection in association with orbital cellulitis.[83] The bacteria that most commonly cause orbital cellulitis are *Staphylococcus aureus*, *Streptococcus pyogenes*, and *Streptococcus pneumoniae*.[52] Anaerobes are frequently present in cases of chronic sinusitis and should be suspected in orbital cellulitis associated with long-standing sinus disease.[52] If not treated aggressively, orbital cellulitis may be associated with life-threatening infection of the central nervous system. Before antibiotics became available, approximately 19% of persons with orbital cellulitis died of intracranial complications and 20% of survivors became blind in the involved eye.[52] This disorder requires hospitalization and intravenous antibiotic therapy. Interim therapy should include levofloxacin 500 mg twice a day. Alternative antibiotic choices are ciprofloxacin 750 mg twice a day or amoxicillin/clavulanate 875 mg/

125 mg every 8 hours. A decongestant should be added if sinusitis is present, and emergent evacuation should be undertaken.

Orbital pseudotumor is an inflammatory disease of the orbit that may present very much like orbital cellulitis. The differentiation between these two entities may be difficult.[42] There would typically not be a history of preceding sinusitis. A reasonable approach in the wilderness is to begin therapy with levofloxacin 500 mg twice a day and arrange for emergent evacuation. Prednisone (80 mg a day) should be added if there is no response to antibiotic therapy, there is no fever or sign of central nervous system involvement, and evacuation has not been possible by 24 to 48 hours after presentation. If prednisone therapy is initiated, its efficacy should be evaluated after 48 hours. If there has been a decrease in pain, erythema, edema, or proptosis, therapy should be continued until evacuation is accomplished. If there has been no response after 48 hours, the prednisone may be discontinued without tapering.

PERIOCULAR TRAUMA

Eyelid Laceration

The most important aspect of managing an eyelid laceration is to carefully exclude the presence of penetrating injury to the globe. Clues to the presence of an open globe are noted in that section below.

A lid laceration that is horizontally oriented on the eyelid, does not penetrate the full thickness of the lid, and does not involve the lid margin is relatively easily managed. In the absence of an ability to properly irrigate, disinfect, and suture the laceration, it should be managed by irrigation with the cleanest disinfected water available, application of topical antibiotic drops (ciprofloxacin, ofloxacin, or tobramycin) to the laceration, drying the surrounding skin surface, and then closing the laceration with tape strips. The wound may then be treated with antibiotic ointment (bacitracin or erythromycin) 4 times a day for 3 to 4 days. Alternatively, the laceration may be left open, treated with antibiotic ointment 4 times a day, and repaired 1 or 2 days later.[42] The laceration should be observed frequently while healing. If redness or discharge develops, the victim should be started on levofloxacin 500 mg once daily or dicloxacillin 500 mg every 6 hours, the wound closure tape should be removed from the laceration, and evacuation should be expedited, especially if the response to oral antibiotics is poor.

Complicated lid lacerations, defined as stellate or complex, or involving the lid margin or the canthi (medial or lateral end of the palpebral fissure), are more difficult to manage. These lacerations may result in secondary functional difficulties if ocular lubrication or lacrimal drainage becomes impaired. In addition, cosmesis may be poor if a meticulous repair is not done. These wounds should be managed by irrigation with the cleanest disinfected water available, application of antibiotic ointment, and coverage with a sterile dressing. Evacuation for definitive repair should be expedited.

Instillation of Adhesive Drops into the Eye

Inadvertent instillation of a "superglue" (cyanoacrylate-type adhesive) compound into the eye may bind the lids tightly together. Overnight application of a pressure patch with eye pads presoaked with water has been reported to make manual separation of the lids possible and eliminate the need for general anesthetic and surgical separation of the lids.[58] Ophthalmic ointment inserted through any small opening in the adherent lids has also been reported to facilitate resolution.[48] Once the lids are separated, the eye should be checked for a corneal abrasion.[71]

CHEMICAL INJURY TO THE EYE

The mainstay in the management of any chemical eye injury is immediate and copious irrigation of the ocular surface with water from whatever source is most readily available. In the wilderness, bottled water or intravenous solution is the best option. If neither of those is available, treated (filtered and disinfected) water from a drinking container is the next best option, with untreated water a last resort. Instillation of several drops of tetracaine will make the procedure much less uncomfortable for the victim. Irrigation should be continued for a minimum of 30 minutes.[42] The two most damaging chemicals are strong acids and alkalis.[42] Sulfuric acid from an exploding car battery is a typical acid, whereas cleaning products, such as drain cleaners, are typical alkalis. Caustic alkalis are more likely to damage the eye than acids because of their profound and rapid ocular penetration. Do not attempt to neutralize the corneal surface with acidic or alkaline solutions. Chemicals other than acids and alkalis may be uncomfortable when they are encountered but are less likely to produce significant long-term damage.

After a minimum of 30 minutes of flushing has been completed, the eye should be examined for retained particles. These should be removed with a moistened cotton-tipped applicator.[42] Treatment for an acid- or alkali-induced injury includes ciprofloxacin or ofloxacin drops 4 times a day until fluorescein staining confirms that the corneal epithelial defect that typically accompanies these injuries has resolved. Topical prednisolone 1% should be added if there is significant inflammation. Prednisolone drops should be used every hour while awake for 3 days. Eye pain is managed with scopolamine drops 4 times a day for 3 days and oral pain medications.[69] Evacuation should be expedited if: (1) the cornea is found to be opaque, (2) a large epithelial defect is found on fluorescein staining, or (3) significant

pain persists after 3 days. Another sign of serious injury is blanching of the conjunctiva in the limbal area.[42]

ACUTE LOSS OF VISION IN A WHITE, QUIET EYE

Vision may be variably decreased with many of the disease entities that are noted later in the Acute Red Eye section. This section addresses sudden loss of vision that occurs in a white, quiet eye. A differential diagnosis is provided in Box 22-3. Disorders that cause this symptom are often difficult to diagnose without ophthalmic instruments (none of which are included in the kit shown in Box 22-1). There are few treatments for most of these disorders likely to be effective in a wilderness setting. Although an afferent pupillary defect (Marcus Gunn pupil) may be present, this is a nonspecific finding that would be expected with most of the disorders in Box 22-3, except for vitreous hemorrhage and high-altitude retinal hemorrhage.

An important question that must be asked in the face of acute loss of vision in a white, quiet eye is "Does this person have giant cell arteritis?" Giant cell arteritis (GCA), also called temporal arteritis, can cause devastating anterior ischemic optic neuropathy, often first noted on waking and which usually becomes permanent.[24] Subsequent involvement of the second eye is common if GCA in the first-stricken eye is not promptly treated.[24] Although visual loss has been reported to occur in both eyes simultaneously, there is typically a delay of 1 to 14 days before the second eye is affected.[1] Loss of vision in the second eye can be prevented in most cases by the prompt initiation of high-dose corticosteroid therapy.[1,24,28,55]

Arteritic anterior ischemic optic neuropathy is typically a disease of older individuals, with one large study reporting a mean age of 70 years and the age of the youngest patient as 53 years.[1] Clues to diagnosis are temporal headache, jaw claudication, fever, weight loss, transient visual obscurations, and polymyalgia rheumatica (generalized myalgias).[55] The visual obscurations seen in GCA usually last 2 to 3 minutes.[55] If a person is felt to be

---

Box 22-3   DIFFERENTIAL DIAGNOSIS OF ACUTE LOSS OF VISION IN A WHITE, QUIET EYE

Retinal detachment
Central retinal artery occlusion
Anterior ischemic optic neuropathy
Optic neuritis
Central retinal vein occlusion
Arteritic anterior ischemic optic neuropathy
Vitreous hemorrhage
High-altitude retinal hemorrhage

suffering from GCA, he or she should be started on prednisone 80 mg qd and evacuation expedited.

If one suspects a retinal detachment based on a history of high myopia (extreme nearsightedness), floaters, or photopsias (flashing lights), expedited evacuation should be undertaken because of the need for surgical repair. Loss of central vision caused by a retinal detachment usually means that the macula is involved and that surgical repair is urgent rather than emergent. Ross and Kozy[65] found that a delay to surgery of up to 1 week in macula-off rhegmatogenous retinal detachments did not affect final visual acuity. Expedited evacuation to a facility that has retinal surgery capability will allow for more precise determination of the urgency for surgical repair.

If the victim is at altitude (above approximately 3048 m [10,000 feet]), high-altitude retinal hemorrhage (discussed below) should be suspected and further ascent avoided.[10] Descent of at least 915 m (3000 feet) should be undertaken as soon as feasible.[10]

Another potentially treatable cause of sudden loss of vision in a white, quiet eye is central retinal artery occlusion (CRAO). Previous conventional therapy for CRAO of ocular massage, pentoxifylline, and anterior chamber paracentesis has been reported to be unsuccessful in restoring vision in 40 of 41 patients with CRAO, even though 11 patients presented within 6 hours of visual loss and 17 presented within 12 hours.[66] Primate retinas can tolerate no more than 100 minutes of ischemia caused by a complete blockage of retinal blood flow.[27] However, fluorescein angiography has shown that in humans, CRAO is seldom complete, and that therapy begun up to 6 hours after visual loss may be successful in restoring vision.[66]

Hyperbaric oxygen was reported successful in restoring vision on two separate occasions in one patient with recurrent branch retinal artery occlusions associated with Susac's syndrome.[41] Oxygen is supplied to the retina from both the retinal and choroidal circulations. Under normoxic conditions, approximately 60% of the retina's oxygen is supplied by the choroidal circulation. Under hyperoxic conditions, the choroid is capable of supplying 100% of the oxygen needed by the retina.[41] When retinal arterial flow is interrupted, the retinal tissue undergoes a period of ischemia. Blood flow may be spontaneously reestablished, as frequently happens with arterial obstruction, or ischemia may continue until cell death and necrosis occur.[45] The period of time during which the tissue is ischemic, yet capable of recovery, is called the ischemic penumbra.[45] Hyperbaric oxygen is not always required for a reversal of retinal ischemia. The author has treated a monocular patient who suffered a central retinal artery occlusion in his only seeing eye and presented to the emergency department within an hour of visual loss. The victim's vision improved from 20/400 to 20/25 within minutes on supplemental oxygen by mask. Unfortunately, however, his vision decreased rapidly to 20/400 whenever the supplemental oxygen was removed. The victim was heparinized and maintained on supplemental oxygen for approximately 10 hours, at which time the removal of oxygen no longer caused a decrease in vision. If oxygen is being carried for an extreme altitude summit attempt or for other purposes, a person with sudden painless loss of vision should be given a trial of oxygen administered in as high a concentration as possible to see if this therapy results in visual improvement.

Care should be taken when monocular visual loss occurs. Although central vision may still be normal in the fellow eye, depth perception may be impaired and the victim may therefore be at increased risk of a fall during evacuation.

ACUTE RED EYE

Box 22-4 provides a partial list of disorders that can result in an acute red eye. In the absence of a slit lamp, the diagnosis must rely on the basic techniques of history, penlight inspection, fluorescein staining, response to administration of topical anesthesia, and pupillary status. The discussion of the differential diagnosis of the acute red eye that follows uses these clinical findings to establish the diagnosis. A pictorial representation is shown in Figure 22-1. The term *fluorescein positive* is used to denote an eye with a discrete area of staining noted with cobalt blue light after instillation of fluorescein dye. Some conditions, such as blepharitis, viral keratoconjunctivitis, and ultraviolet (UV) keratitis, may cause a pattern of punctate staining referred to as *superficial punctate keratitis* (SPK).

Traumatic Ocular Disorders

Obvious Open Globe. If there is a history of trauma and penlight inspection of the eye reveals an obvious open

---

Box 22-4   DIFFERENTIAL DIAGNOSIS OF THE ACUTE RED EYE

Obvious open globe	Iritis
Corneal abrasion	Scleritis
Corneal ulcer	Conjunctivitis
Subconjunctival hemorrhage	Blepharitis
Traumatic iritis	Ultraviolet keratitis
Hyphema	Episcleritis
Occult open globe	Conjunctival foreign body
Herpes simplex virus keratitis	Dry eye
Corneal erosion	Contact lens overwear syndrome
Acute angle closure glaucoma	

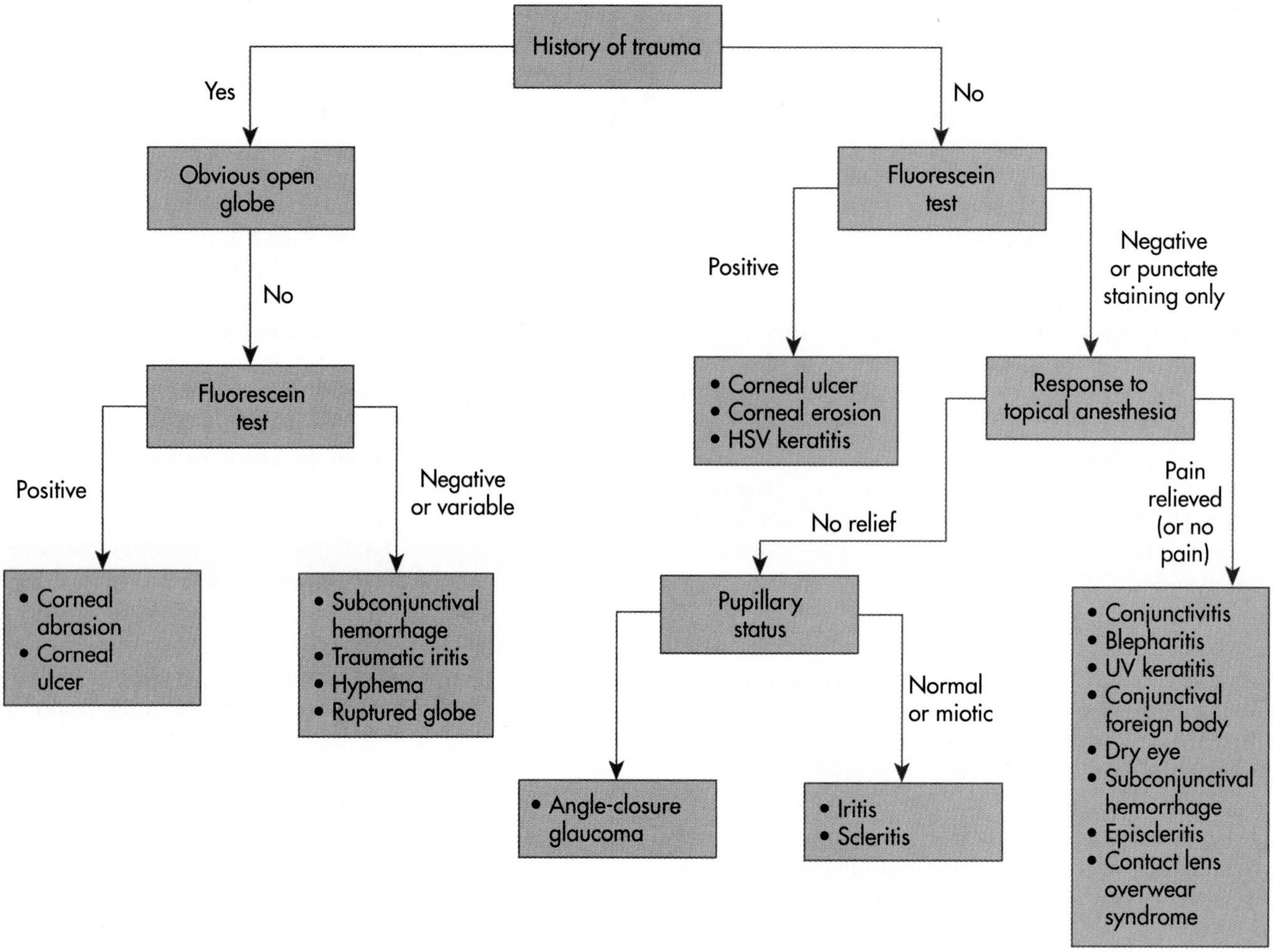

History of trauma

Yes — Obvious open globe

No — Fluorescein test

Obvious open globe → No → Fluorescein test

Fluorescein test:
- Positive → • Corneal abrasion • Corneal ulcer
- Negative or variable → • Subconjunctival hemorrhage • Traumatic iritis • Hyphema • Ruptured globe

Fluorescein test:
- Positive → • Corneal ulcer • Corneal erosion • HSV keratitis
- Negative or punctate staining only → Response to topical anesthesia

No relief → Pupillary status
- → • Angle-closure glaucoma
- Normal or miotic → • Iritis • Scleritis

Pain relieved (or no pain) →
- • Conjunctivitis
- • Blepharitis
- • UV keratitis
- • Conjunctival foreign body
- • Dry eye
- • Subconjunctival hemorrhage
- • Episcleritis
- • Contact lens overwear syndrome

Figure 22-1 Algorithm showing wilderness diagnostic procedure for the acute red eye.

globe (such as the eye in Figure 22-2), the examination should be discontinued and a protective shield placed over the eye. Do not apply a pressure patch or instill any topical medication. There are two primary concerns in the management of this condition. The first is to minimize manipulation or additional trauma to the eye that might raise intraocular pressure and result in expulsion of intraocular contents through the corneal or scleral defect. The second is to prevent development of posttraumatic endophthalmitis, an infection of the aqueous and vitreous humors of the eye. This typically has devastating visual results, with only 30% of victims in one study retaining visual acuity greater than or equal to 20/400.[38] *Staphylococcus epidermidis* is the most common pathogen implicated, but *Bacillus cereus* is a very aggressive pathogen often isolated in this condition.[38] After the shield is placed, the victim should be started on levofloxacin 500 mg twice a day. Trovafloxacin 200 mg once a day is a reasonable alternative choice for prophylaxis because of its very broad antibacterial spectrum[29,80] and good ocular penetration.[50] Ciprofloxacin 750 mg twice a day is a third option. A person with an obvious open globe needs surgical repair as soon as possible and

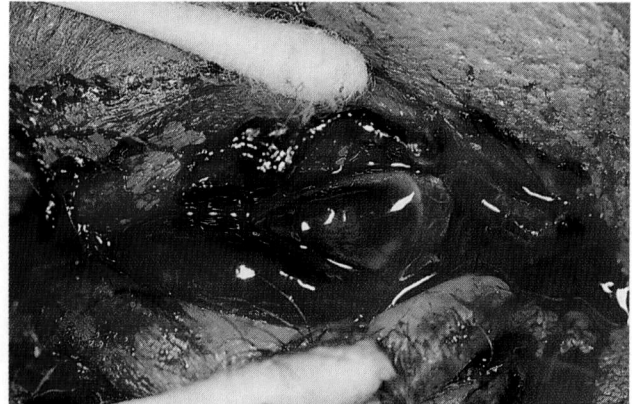

Figure 22-2 Obvious open globe (corneoscleral laceration). *(Courtesy Steve Chalfin, MD.)*

should be evacuated emergently. Because there is a possibility that air may have been introduced into the eye, barometric pressure changes during evacuation should be minimized, if possible. However, this consideration is secondary to the need for expeditious transport to a facility where surgical repair can be performed.

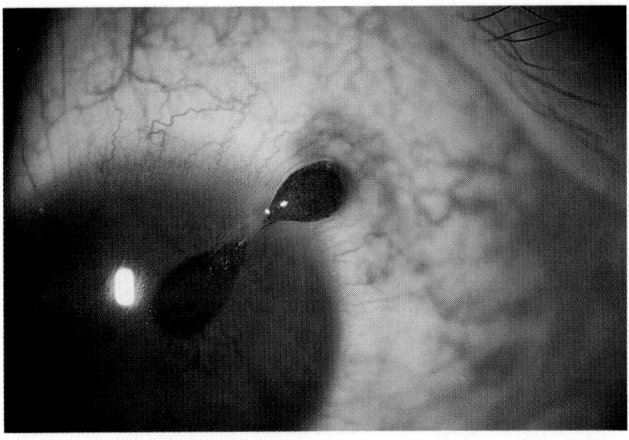

Figure 22-3 Occult open globe with uveal pigment at the limbus and a peaked pupil. *(Courtesy Steve Chalfin, MD.)*

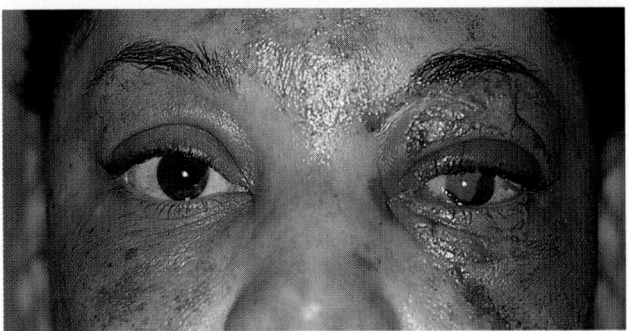

Figure 22-4 Corneal abrasion. *(Courtesy Steve Chalfin, MD.)*

Occult Ruptured Globe. A penetrating injury to the eye or a ruptured globe may not always be obvious. Clues to occult rupture include large subconjunctival hemorrhage with chemosis, dark uveal tissue present at the limbus, distorted pupil (Figure 22-3), fluorescein leak from a linear or punctate corneal epithelial defect, mechanism of injury (hammering metal on metal, impaling injury, etc.), or decrease in vision. If an occult globe rupture is suspected, the victim should be treated as described previously for an obvious open globe. The relatively less severe appearance of the injury does not eliminate the threat of endophthalmitis, so levofloxacin therapy should be initiated.

Corneal Abrasion. A corneal abrasion is disruption of the protective epithelial covering of the cornea (Figure 22-4). This results in intense pain, tearing, light sensitivity (photophobia), and increased susceptibility to infection until the defect has healed (usually in 2 to 3 days). There is typically a history of antecedent trauma or contact lens wear. The sine qua non for this diagnosis is an epithelial defect on fluorescein staining. Standard treatment consists of bacitracin ointment followed by application of a pressure patch, although a recent study has shown that small (less than

10 mm^2), noninfected, and non–contact lens-related abrasions healed significantly faster with less discomfort when they were not patched.[33] In a wilderness setting, the nonpatching option has the additional advantage of not rendering the victim completely monocular and adversely affecting visual field and depth perception. If the nonpatching option is chosen, the victim should be treated with topical fluoroquinolone drops or bacitracin ointment 4 times a day until the corneal epithelium is healed. Diclofenac drops 4 times a day should be helpful in reducing discomfort. Sunglasses help alleviate photophobia. Repeated use of a topical anesthetic for pain control is contraindicated. If the abrasion is contact lens-related, the eye should *not* be patched because of the increased risk of corneal ulcer present with a contact lens-related abrasion[60]; contact lens-related corneal abrasions should be treated with topical fluoroquinolone drops every 2 hours while awake until the epithelial defect has resolved to ensure coverage against *Pseudomonas*. An abrasion associated with vegetable matter should also not be patched.[60] If the abrasion is large or the victim's discomfort severe, scopolamine drops once or twice a day may be added to the antibiotic. (Wait 5 minutes between each drop.) Much of the pain associated with corneal abrasion and ulcer is due to ciliary muscle spasm, which is relieved by scopolamine. The rationale for using scopolamine only with a very painful abrasion in the wilderness is that this medication will cause the pupil to dilate (and the eye to become very sensitive to light) and accommodation to relax (with a resultant decrease in near visual acuity) for approximately 5 to 7 days.

An oral analgesic may be required for pain control. The victim should be monitored daily for development of a corneal ulcer (noted on penlight examination as a white or gray infiltrate on the cornea) and for progress in healing of the epithelium (as measured by resolution of fluorescein staining).

Corneal Ulcer. The term *corneal ulcer*, as used here, denotes acute bacterial, fungal, or protozoal infection of the cornea. Chronic corneal epithelial defects caused by a variety of autoimmune or inflammatory processes are also referred to as corneal ulcers at times, but these disorders are beyond the scope of this chapter. Although a corneal ulcer (Figure 22-5) is an infectious process, it is often preceded by a traumatic corneal abrasion. The other predisposing condition for a corneal ulcer is contact lens wear, which results in microtrauma to the corneal epithelium and may allow bacteria or other microorganisms to infect the cornea. Corneal ulcers are typically significantly painful. A small white or gray infiltrate on the cornea can be appreciated by a careful penlight examination. If not treated aggressively, the small initial lesion may progress to the much larger infiltrate shown in Figure 22-5 with a correspondingly

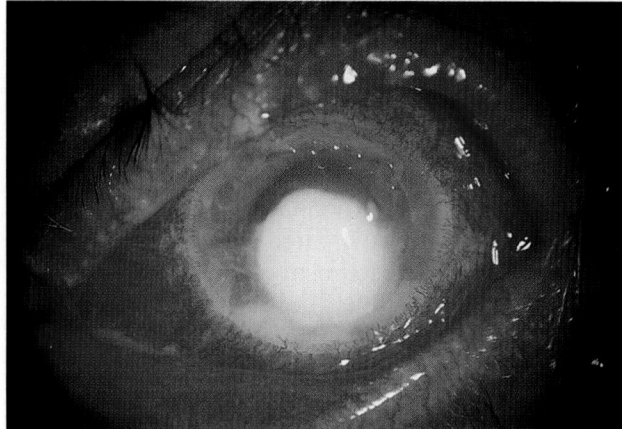

Figure 22-5 Corneal ulcer. *(Courtesy Steve Chalfin, MD.)*

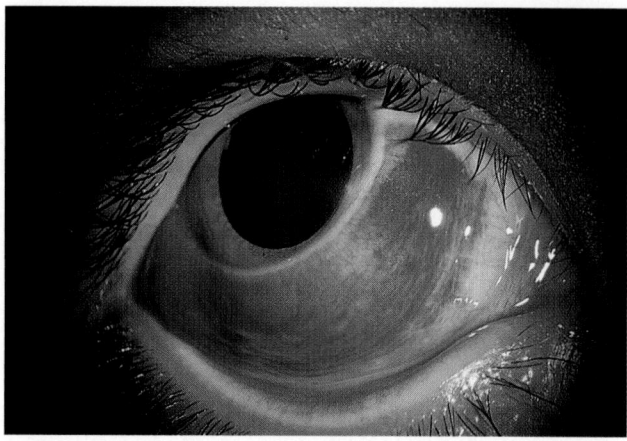

Figure 22-6 Subconjunctival hemorrhage. *(Courtesy Steve Chalfin, MD.)*

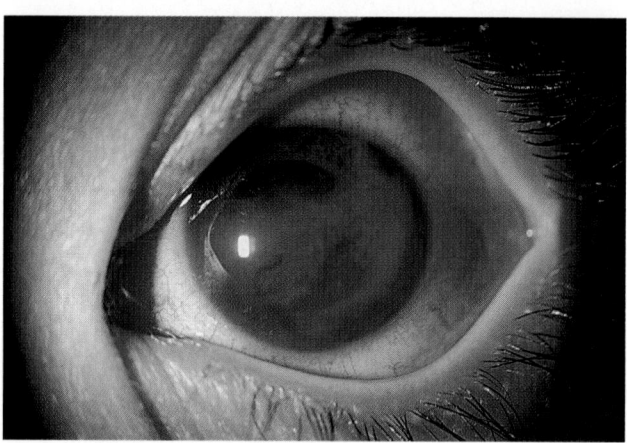

Figure 22-7 Hyphema. *(Courtesy Steve Chalfin, MD.)*

more severe impact on visual acuity. Fluorescein staining reveals an epithelial defect overlying the infiltrate. The associated pain is usually significantly decreased by application of a topical anesthetic, but ciliary spasm may cause pain relief to be incomplete.

An inadequately treated corneal ulcer may result in visual loss from dense corneal scarring or ocular perforation with subsequent endophthalmitis. Management of this disorder in the past included hospital admission for treatment with concentrated and frequently administered aminoglycoside and cephalosporin topical drops. Recently, outpatient therapy with fluoroquinolone eye drops has been shown to be comparable in efficacy with fortified antibiotic preparations.[30,53] Treatment for corneal ulcer, then, should be with ciprofloxacin or ofloxacin, 1 drop every 5 minutes for 3 doses initially, then 1 drop every 15 minutes for 6 hours, then 1 drop every 30 minutes thereafter around the clock.[60] Scopolamine 1 drop 2 to 4 times a day may help relieve discomfort caused by ciliary spasm. Repeated use of topical anesthetics for pain control is contraindicated. Systemic analgesia may be required if pain is severe. Expedited evacuation is recommended.

Traumatic Iritis. Iritis refers to inflammation of the iris or, more accurately, the anterior uveal tract of the eye. It may also be called *anterior uveitis* or *iridocyclitis*. The sine qua non of this condition is inflammatory cells in the anterior chamber of the eye, which must be visualized with a slit lamp. In the wilderness, this diagnosis must be presumptive. Iritis may accompany a corneal abrasion or result from blunt trauma. The diagnosis rests primarily on the presence of significant posttraumatic pain without a corneal abrasion or ulcer noted on fluorescein staining, or on pain that persists after the abrasion is healed. Treatment is with prednisolone 1 drop 4 times a day for 3 days. Scopolamine 1 drop twice a day may be added if pain is severe enough to justify the blurred vision that scopolamine therapy will entail.

Subconjunctival Hemorrhage. Subconjunctival hemorrhage (Figure 22-6) is a bright red area over the sclera of the eye that results from bleeding between the conjunctiva and the sclera. It is easily visible without the use of a slit lamp. This injury is innocuous and resolves over a period of several days to several weeks without treatment. In the presence of antecedent trauma, one should be alert for another, more serious injury. In particular, if hemorrhage results in massive swelling of the conjunctiva (chemosis), an occult globe rupture should be suspected.

Hyphema. The term *hyphema* is defined as blood in the anterior chamber. Although this is usually seen in the setting of acute trauma, it may also be caused by other conditions, such as iris neovascularization. The eye should be examined with the victim sitting upright. If enough blood is present, it collects at the bottom of the anterior chamber and is visible as a layered hyphema (Figure 22-7). This may not be appreciated if the victim is examined while in a supine position or if the amount of blood is very small.

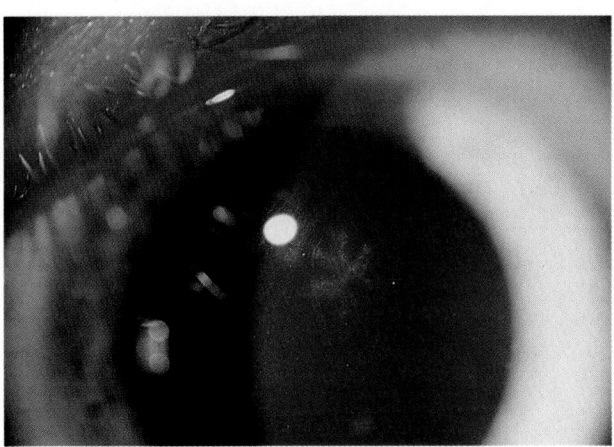

Figure 22-8 Herpes simplex virus keratitis. *(Courtesy Steve Chalfin, MD.)*

Although most hyphemas resolve without sequelae, this disorder may be complicated by an acute rise in intraocular pressure or corneal blood staining. Treatment in the wilderness consists of activity restriction (walking only), prednisolone drops 4 times a day, avoidance of aspirin or nonsteroidal antiinflammatory drugs (NSAIDs), and use of an eye shield until the hyphema has resolved. Diamox 250 mg 4 times a day by mouth should be added if available to treat the potentially increased intraocular pressure. Retinal injury and/or an occult ruptured globe may accompany traumatic hyphema. A hyphema victim requires ophthalmologic evaluation, so expedited evacuation should be undertaken.

Nontraumatic Fluorescein-Positive Acute Red Eye

Herpes Simplex Virus Keratitis. The essential element in this diagnosis is the characteristic dendritic epithelial pattern on fluorescein staining (Figure 22-8). There will often be a history of previous episodes of herpes simplex virus (HSV) keratitis. Treatment is trifluorothymidine 1% drops 9 times a day.[60] Treatment is continued until the corneal staining has resolved, at which time the frequency of dosing is reduced to 4 times a day for 1 week. Trifluorothymidine was not included in the list of eye medications to be taken on the expedition because trifluorothymidine drops require refrigeration. If a significant delay is anticipated before evacuation, HSV keratitis may be treated by using tetracaine 3 to 5 drops given 1 minute apart to anesthetize the cornea and then performing a gentle Q-tip debridement of the epithelial lesion.[60] The resulting epithelial defect should then be treated as described in the Corneal Abrasion section.

Corneal Erosion. A corneal erosion is an epithelial defect caused by nontraumatic disruption of the corneal epithelium. The fluorescein staining pattern seen with corneal erosion may be identical to that seen with corneal abrasion; pain and photophobia are present with both

disorders. The diagnosis is made when the apparent corneal abrasion has no history of trauma to explain its presence. There is often a history of previous similar episodes. The two primary causes for corneal erosion are corneal dystrophies and previous ocular trauma.[55] Recurrent corneal erosions are believed to be caused by a defect in healing between the hemidesmosomes of the corneal epithelium and the underlying basement membrane.[42] At night, the epithelium may become adherent to the closed eyelid during sleep. When the individual awakens and opens his or her eyes, the corneal epithelium is pulled away from the basement membrane by movement of the lid. This accounts for the typical history of acute onset of pain on awakening. Signs and symptoms include pain, tearing, and foreign body sensation.[42]

Treatment of these lesions may be difficult. The cornea should be inspected for a loose sheet of epithelium that remains partially attached to the corneal surface. If this is present, try to debride it with a cotton-tipped applicator after topical anesthesia with tetracaine. The lesion is then managed initially in the same manner as a corneal abrasion. There is a high rate of recurrence if follow-up treatment with 5% sodium chloride ointment each evening or anterior stromal puncture is not undertaken.

Corneal Abrasion and Corneal Ulcer. Both lesions may occur as complications of contact lens wear. Management has been described above. Contact lens-related corneal abrasions have a relatively high incidence of progressing to corneal ulcers.[33] Therefore they should not be patched and should receive topical antibiotic therapy with ciprofloxacin or ofloxacin drops every 2 hours while awake until the epithelial defect has resolved. Contact lens wear *in both eyes* should be discontinued immediately. If an ulcer is related to contaminated lens solutions, infection in the first eye may be followed rapidly by a similar occurrence in the other eye.

Nontraumatic Fluorescein-Negative Acute Red Eye (Pain Not Significantly Improved by Topical Anesthesia)

Acute Angle-Closure Glaucoma. This diagnosis is easily made when the intraocular pressure can be measured with a tonometer. Intraocular pressure is normally between 10 and 21 mm Hg. With acute angle-closure glaucoma, the pressure may increase to 50 or 60 mm Hg or higher. Although handheld tonometers are available, they will not often be present outside of hospitals or clinics. The most important clues to the diagnosis of angle-closure glaucoma in the wilderness setting are the characteristics of the pain and the status of the pupil. Angle-closure glaucoma victims do not have the mild burning or foreign body type of pain typically seen with conjunctivitis, blepharitis, or other external eye diseases. Angle-closure glaucoma produces a pain that is usually deep and severe. Although corneal abrasions and corneal ulcers may also be accompanied by severe pain, the pain in these two disorders is usually significantly relieved by topical anesthetics. This is not true of the pain seen with acute glaucoma, scleritis, or iritis. In these disorders, the pain is rarely if ever significantly relieved by topical anesthetics. In acute angle-closure glaucoma, the pupil is usually found to be mid-dilated (6 to 7 mm) and vision is usually decreased. This disorder generally affects persons over 50 years of age[42] and is more common in persons of Asiatic ethnic origins. There is often a history of previous transient episodes of eye pain. Nausea and vomiting may be present. An eye with acute angle-closure glaucoma is shown in Figure 22-9.

The usual treatment is topical antiocular hypertensive medications and laser iridotomy, which allows the aqueous humor to bypass the pupillary block. This relieves the angle closure with a resultant decrease in intraocular pressure.[42] In the wilderness setting, treatment should be with 2% pilocarpine one drop every 15 minutes for 4 doses,[55] then 4 times a day in *both* eyes, since there is a high rate of subsequent occurrence of angle-closure glaucoma in the fellow eye. Pilocarpine alone may be successful in relieving the angle closure and lowering the pressure, but this is not a reliably effective treatment because ischemia of the pupillary sphincter muscle may prevent pilocarpine from exerting its miotic effect. Diamox 250 mg 4 times a day by mouth should be added if available. Evacuation should be emergent if pain is not relieved, since even 1 day of very high intraocular pressure may result in permanent damage to the optic nerve and loss of vision.

Nontraumatic Iritis. Signs and symptoms of nontraumatic iritis that may be appreciated without a slit lamp include pain, redness, photophobia, limbal flush, and decreased vision.[55] There is often a history of previous episodes. An eye with nontraumatic iritis is shown in Figure 22-10. (The pupil is iatrogenically dilated.) Iritis not associated with corneal trauma is typically more se-

vere than the traumatic variety but may range from mild to very severe and typically is not significantly relieved by topical anesthesia. Fluorescein staining is negative and the pupil is usually miotic, thus helping differentiate iritis from angle-closure glaucoma. Iritis is far more common than angle-closure glaucoma and may be associated with a number of systemic infectious and inflammatory diseases. In the wilderness setting, the emphasis should be on immediate treatment with prednisolone 1% 1 drop every hour while awake. Scopolamine 1 drop 1 to 4 times a day may be added for pain control and to prevent posterior synechiae (pupillary scarring) if inflammation is severe. If pain is not significantly decreased in 24 to 48 hours, oral prednisone 80 mg a day should be added to the treatment regimen and maintained until evacuation. Evacuation should be expedited, since posterior synechiae and elevated intraocular pressure may develop.

Scleritis. It may be difficult to differentiate between nontraumatic iritis and scleritis without a slit lamp, but scleritis is much less common than iritis. The characteristics of the pain are similar, with pain, photophobia, scleral injection, and tearing.[55] Scleritis is often associated with rheumatologic disease and may be either nodular or diffuse.[55] The diffuse form of scleritis is shown in Figure 22-11. The initial treatment of scleritis in the wilderness setting is topical prednisolone drops 1 drop every hour while awake and an NSAID, if available. Prednisone 80 mg a day should be added if there is no improvement in 24 to 48 hours and maintained until an expedited evacuation.

Nontraumatic Fluorescein-Negative Acute Red Eye (No Discomfort or Discomfort Improved by Topical Anesthesia)

Conjunctivitis. One of the most common disorders in this diagnostic category is conjunctivitis. Etiologic agents of infectious conjunctivitis include bacteria,

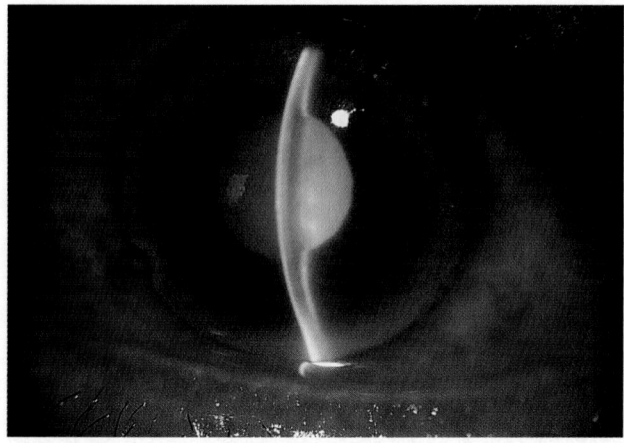

Figure 22-9 Angle-closure glaucoma. *(Courtesy Steve Chalfin, MD.)*

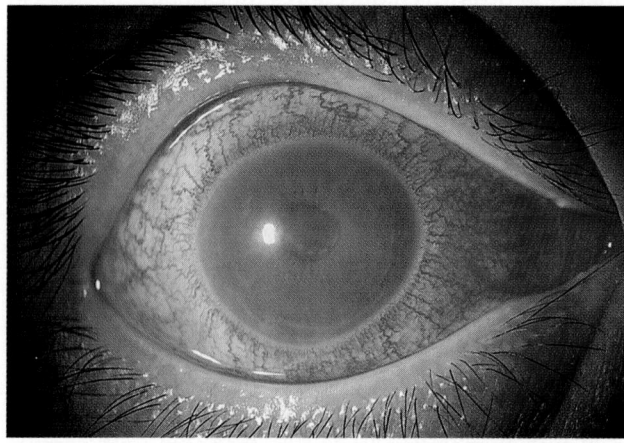

Figure 22-10 Nontraumatic iritis. *(Courtesy Steve Chalfin, MD.)*

viruses, chlamydiae, fungi, and parasites.[42] Acute allergic conjunctivitis may also be encountered, especially in a wilderness setting. The keys to diagnosis are the presence of discharge or tearing, relatively mild burning or foreign-body type discomfort that is relieved by topical anesthesia, and a negative (or SPK) fluorescein staining pattern. The diagnosis of conjunctivitis should be questioned in the absence of discharge or tearing. The primary exception to this statement is allergic conjunctivitis, which may not generate a significant discharge. In this case, bilaterality, significant ocular itching, and a history of ocular or systemic allergies will help make the diagnosis. With infectious conjunctivitis, there are often signs or symptoms of an accompanying upper respiratory infection (URI) or a history of contact with other persons who have recently suffered from conjunctivitis.

Treatment of conjunctivitis in the wilderness setting is with ciprofloxacin or ofloxacin drops (1 drop 4 times a day for 5 days) if there is a yellowish discharge. Tobramycin 0.3% drops or trimethoprim/polymixin B drops are acceptable alternatives.[42] This should be an adequate treatment time if conjunctivitis is bacterial. Symptoms that persist for more than 5 days suggest a viral etiology. These symptoms may take several weeks to clear, just as some viral URIs take several weeks to resolve. If there is only tearing or a watery discharge, suggesting a viral etiology, treatment with artificial tears and cool compresses may be substituted for antibiotic therapy. The victim should be instructed on infection precautions, since viral conjunctivitis can spread rapidly through a group. This is especially true if the discomfort caused by conjunctivitis is severe and accompanied by significant photophobia. These symptoms suggest epidemic keratoconjunctivitis (EKC), which, in addition to having a prolonged course, is very uncomfortable because of the corneal involvement. An eye with EKC is shown in Figure 22-12. Sunglasses should be part of the treatment. Scopolamine 1 drop 2 to 4 times a day may be required to reduce discomfort.

As noted previously, if the predominant ocular symptom is itching, allergic conjunctivitis should be suspected. Allergic conjunctivitis may be treated with cool compresses and/or systemic antihistamines. Severe ocular itching may be treated with a 3-day course of prednisolone, 1 drop 4 times a day.

Hyperacute conjunctivitis with marked lid edema, conjunctival hyperemia, chemosis, and copious purulent discharge should alert the care provider to the possibility of a gonococcal etiology.[42] Gonococcal conjunctivitis may progress to vision-threatening keratitis and should be treated aggressively with levofloxacin 500 mg once a day, ciprofloxacin or ofloxacin drops 4 times a day, and expedited evacuation.

Bacterial and viral conjunctivitis are highly contagious. Individuals with infectious conjunctivitis should be informed of this fact and the importance of infection precautions emphasized.

Blepharitis. Blepharitis is probably the most common external eye disease seen in the general ophthalmologist's office.[16] It is often misdiagnosed as conjunctivitis. Differentiation may often be made by the history. Blepharitis tends to be a bilateral, chronic disease with recurrences and exacerbations. There is chronic flaking and irritation of the skin at the base of the eyelashes that may occasionally be complicated by bacterial superinfection. An eye with blepharitis is shown in Figure 22-13. There may be an association with skin disorders, such as seborrheic dermatitis or acne rosacea.[16] The victim often has a history of chronic ocular itching and burning. Fluctuating vision may be present as well.[16] A history of excessive mucous discharge in the eyes on waking is often present.

Treatment for blepharitis should focus on the lid margins. Bacitracin or erythromycin ophthalmic ointment should be applied thinly to the lid margins at bedtime for 4 weeks. Lid hygiene is directed at reducing the amount of debris on the lid margins and con-

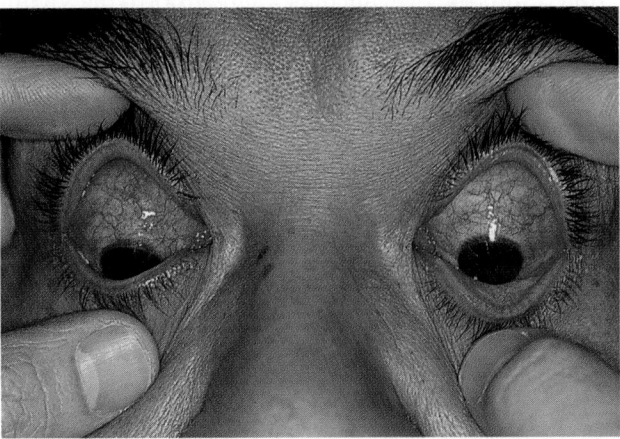

Figure 22-11 Diffuse scleritis. *(Courtesy Steve Chalfin, MD.)*

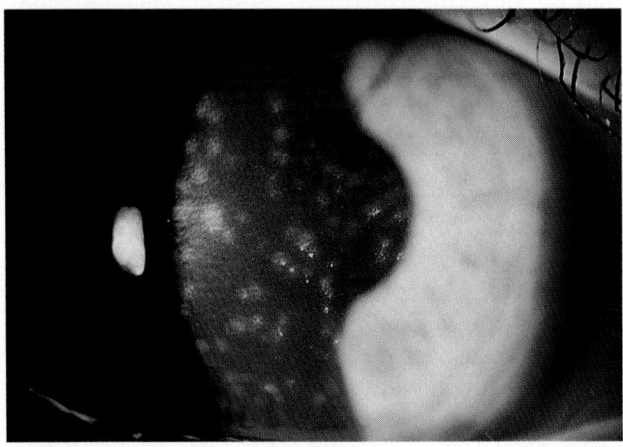

Figure 22-12 Epidemic keratoconjunctivitis (EKC). *(Courtesy Steve Chalfin, MD.)*

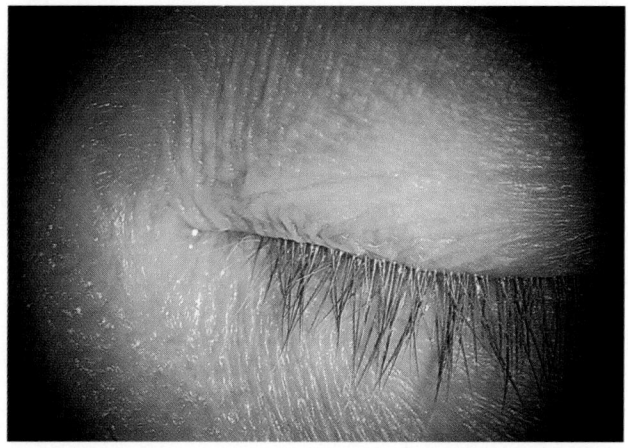

Figure 22-13 Blepharitis. *(Courtesy Steve Chalfin, MD.)*

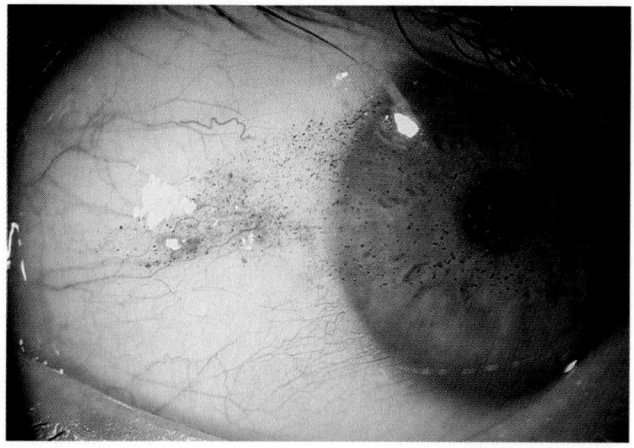

Figure 22-14 Conjunctival foreign body. *(Courtesy Steve Chalfin, MD.)*

sists of warm, moist compresses applied to the eyelids 1 to 4 times a day for 5 to 10 minutes, followed by gently wiping away the moistened lash debris. Artificial tears may relieve the sensation of "dry eye" that often accompanies blepharitis.[16]

Ultraviolet Keratitis. The diagnosis of ultraviolet keratitis is easy to make in the presence of a severely sunburned face and bilateral red, painful eyes. The discomfort typically does not start until 6 to 10 hours after UV exposure and may awaken the victim.[55] Symptoms range from mild irritation and foreign body sensation to severe pain, photophobia, and lid spasm.[55] Fluorescein staining usually reveals a punctate staining pattern.

Treatment consists of bacitracin or erythromycin ophthalmic ointment applied to the eye 4 times a day (an acceptable alternative would be fluoroquinolone drops 4 times a day) and sunglasses. In a severe case, one or both eyes may be patched to aid in pain control, although it may be better to patch only the more severely affected eye so that the victim is not deprived of vision in both eyes.[10] Scopolamine (1 drop twice a day) may be added for pain control. Systemic analgesia may also be required. The victim should be reexamined every day until there is no longer an SPK pattern present on fluorescein staining, at which time antibiotic therapy may be discontinued. The duration of discomfort from UV keratitis is typically 24 to 48 hours.[55]

Conjunctival Foreign Body. The symptom of ocular foreign body sensation does not necessarily mean that a conjunctival or corneal foreign body is present. Although the presence of a conjunctival foreign body may be strongly suspected based on the abrupt onset of discomfort following a gust of wind or other mechanism for depositing foreign material in the eye, definitive diagnosis requires visualization of the offending material, which may sometimes be quite difficult. Figure 22-14 shows an eye with a conjunctival foreign body. The vic-

tim is often able to help with foreign body localization before the instillation of topical anesthetic drops.

Treatment consists of a careful search for the foreign body using adequate lighting. Topical anesthesia makes the victim much more agreeable during the search and removal efforts. A handheld magnifying lens or pair of reading glasses will provide magnification to aid in the visualization of the foreign body. Eyelid eversion with a cotton-tipped applicator helps the examiner identify foreign bodies located on the upper tarsal plate. Once located, the foreign body should be removed with a cotton-tipped applicator after the eye has been anesthetized and the cotton-tipped applicator moistened with tetracaine. The eye is then stained with fluorescein to check for a corneal abrasion. If no foreign body is visualized but the index of suspicion is high, vigorous irrigation with artificial tears or sweeps of the conjunctival fornices with a moistened cotton-tipped applicator after topical anesthesia may be successful in removing the foreign body.

Several types of foreign body merit special mention. If the foreign body identified is one that may have penetrated into the eye, such as a large thorn, the victim should be managed as described in the Obvious Open Globe section. Hot ashes or cinders from a campfire may strike the eye, resulting in both a foreign body and a thermal burn. Immediate instillation of topical anesthesia will provide temporary pain relief to facilitate foreign body removal and will also stop any ongoing thermal injury. After the foreign body has been removed, the corneal abrasion that typically results from a thermal injury to the cornea should be managed as outlined in that section.

Dry Eye. Symptomatic dry eye is commonly encountered in the wilderness, especially in mountainous areas where the air is very dry and significant wind is often present.[10] Dry eye is usually bilateral and may result in secondary tearing.[60] There may be a history of previous episodes of symptomatic dry eye. Individuals with chronic dry eyes are usually middle-aged or older and may have a history of autoimmune disorders. The discomfort is usually relieved by topical anesthesia.

Treatment is with artificial tears used as often as needed to relieve symptoms. Dehydration may contribute to this condition, and adequate fluid intake should be maintained. The use of sunglasses may provide protection from the wind and be of significant benefit in managing this disorder.

Contact Lens Overwear Syndrome. The considerations here are much as described in the Dry Eye section, except that the symptoms are magnified by the presence of contact lenses.

Contact lens rewetting drops and sunglasses are the first line of management. Should these measures be ineffective in relieving symptoms, the contact lenses should be removed. If significant SPK are present on fluorescein staining, ciprofloxacin or ofloxacin drops 4 times a day should be used until the SPK have resolved.[10] Contact lenses should not be replaced in the eye until the eye is symptom-free. An individual who wears contact lenses in the wilderness should *always* carry a pair of glasses that can be used if contact lens problems arise.

Episcleritis. Episcleritis is a benign, self-limited, inflammatory condition of the lining of the eye between the conjunctiva and the sclera.[42] There is usually sectorial redness without discharge (Figure 22-15). There is often a history of previous episodes. Discomfort is typically mild or absent. The presence of severe pain, photophobia, or decrease in vision suggests another cause. Episcleritis is often misdiagnosed as conjunctivitis, but the lack of a discharge and the sectorial redness usually seen in episcleritis will help differentiate between the two disorders.

Episcleritis is usually self-limited and resolves without treatment over 3 to 4 weeks.[42] If symptoms are troublesome, it may be treated with prednisolone drops 4 times a day for 3 to 5 days.

SOLAR RETINOPATHY

The retina is protected from UV radiation damage because this high-energy radiation is absorbed by the cornea and the lens of the eye. However, visible and near-infrared light of sufficient intensity may reach the retina and cause photochemical damage.[42] In the wilderness setting, this would most likely occur as the result of staring at the sun or a solar eclipse. Shortly after such an exposure, the individual may experience blurred or distorted vision, a central scotoma, and/or a headache. Visual acuity is often reduced to the 20/40 to 20/70 range. There is no effective therapy for this injury, but visual acuity may return to normal over a period of several months in mild cases.

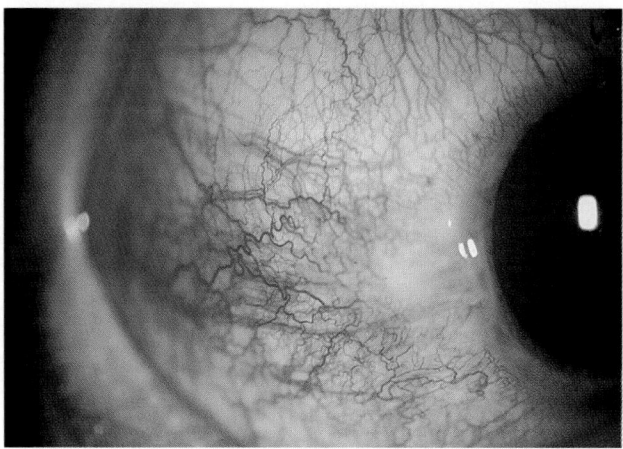

Figure 22-15 Episcleritis. *(Courtesy Steve Chalfin, MD.)*

LOCATING A DISPLACED CONTACT LENS

Soft contact lens wearers may occasionally have one of their lenses become displaced, causing blurred vision and a foreign body sensation. Once the lens is displaced, it may be hard to locate. The conjunctival fornix of the lower lid is easily examined by distracting the lens from the globe with gentle downward finger pressure applied to the lower lid. If the contact lens has been displaced into the superior conjunctival fornix (usually the case), it may be more difficult to locate. If visual inspection with a penlight and a handheld magnifying lens is not successful in finding the lens, gentle digital massage over the closed upper lid directed towards the medial canthus often results in the contact lens emerging at that location. Several minutes of massage may be required. A few drops of artificial tears often facilitates the process. If this maneuver is unproductive, the eye may be anesthetized with a drop of tetracaine, the upper lid distracted from the globe with upward finger pressure, and the fornix swept with a moistened cotton-tipped applicator.

IMPROVISATION (see also Chapter 19)

If you encounter a person with known or suspected globe rupture, it is of paramount importance to ensure that subsequent inadvertent trauma does not cause extrusion of ocular contents. If an eye shield is not available, one may be fashioned with duct or rigger's tape and any available rigid flat or concave object that can be placed over the eye. Examples include small cups or bowls to provide a good standoff distance between the eye and the improvised shield. Improvised wound closure strips can be made by tearing rigger's or duct tape into ¼-inch widths. Spectacles and sunglasses can be improvised by making a pinhole in a piece of paper or cardboard. (Make the pinholes before placing the paper or cardboard in front of the eyes!) Take note of the

TABLE 22-1. Pressures and Equivalent Oxygen Fractions at Altitude

FEET	METERS	ATMOSPHERIC PRESSURE (mm Hg)	EQUIVALENT OXYGEN (%)	PARTIAL PRESSURE OF OXYGEN (mm Hg)
Sea level	Sea level	760	20.9	159
4,000	1,219	656	18.0	137
7,000	2,134	586	16.1	122
10,000	3,048	523	14.4	109
15,000	4,572	429	11.8	89
20,000	6,096	347	9.5	73
25,000	7,620	282	7.8	60
29,028	8,848	253	7.0	53

restriction in peripheral vision caused by using pinhole glasses. If the purpose is to improvise sunglasses rather than to achieve a refractive effect, the pinhole can be larger or fashioned into a horizontal slit to improve peripheral vision. Improvised magnifying glasses for examining the eye or other small areas may be made by simply using a pair of reading or hyperopic glasses. Another refractive improvisation technique involves a handheld magnifying lens. This convex lens with its plus refracting power can be used to provide a variety of hyperopic refractive corrections by moving the lens to various distances in front of the eye.

THE EYE AT ALTITUDE

Ocular disorders associated with altitude exposures have been addressed in a recent review article.[10] The sections from that paper that address ocular disorders likely to be encountered in mountaineering are included below.

Altitude Exposures and Ocular Physiology

A number of significant effects on visual function resulting from the hypoxia of altitude were described by Wilmer and Berens[88] in their classic article. The decrease in ambient pressure at altitude causes a hypobaric hypoxia despite a constant oxygen fraction of 0.21 as noted in Table 22-1. Retinal blood flow has been shown to increase by 128% after 4 days at 5300 m (17,384 feet).[22] This increase in blood flow results in clinically observable changes, such as increase in diameter and tortuosity of retinal vessels and optic disk hyperemia, which are seen in most unacclimatized persons at altitudes above 4573 m (15,000 feet).[22,35,46,59]

Because of its avascularity, the cornea receives most of its oxygen supply from the surrounding atmosphere,[74] so it may suffer hypoxic dysfunction even if the inspired gas mix is not hypoxic, as noted below in the Refractive Changes at Altitude after Refractive Surgery section. This is an important factor when considering topics such as the suitability of contact lenses and refractive surgical procedures for mountaineers and aviators.

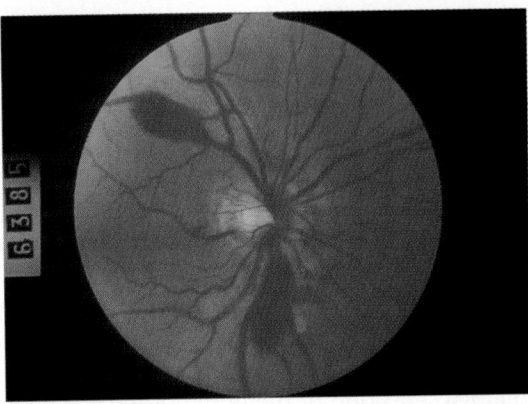

Figure 22-16 High-altitude retinal hemorrhages. *(Courtesy Dr. M. McFadden, UBC, Vancouver, BC, in association with Dr. C. Houston, Burlington, Vt.; Dr. G. Gray, DCIEM, Toronto, Ontario; and Drs. Sutton and P. Powells, McMaster University, Hamilton, Ontario.)*

High-Altitude Retinal Hemorrhage

There are many reports of retinal hemorrhages (Figure 22-16) in mountain climbers.* These have been described as high-altitude retinal hemorrhages (HARH) or as part of the more inclusive term *altitude retinopathy*.[8] A classification for HARH has been developed by Weidman.[85,86] Butler, Harris, and Reynolds[8] reported an incidence of HARH of 29% in climbers on a Mt. Everest expedition at altitudes ranging from 5300 to 8200 m (17,385 to 26,896 feet). McFadden et al[46] found that 56% of their subjects had HARH at an altitude of 5360 m (17,581 feet) and that one had a retinal nerve fiber layer infarct (cotton wool spot) (Figure 22-17). They also reported that exercise at altitude was associated with both an increased incidence of HARH and fluorescein leakage from the retinal vessels. Hackett and Rennie[26] described HARH in 4% of 140 trekkers examined at 4243 m (13,917 feet) at Pheriche in the Himalayas. These authors also found a significant correlation of retinal hemorrhages with symptoms of acute mountain sickness (AMS). Kobrick and Appleton[35] found no reti-

*References 8, 21, 26, 37, 39, 46, 59, 61, 67, 70, 84.

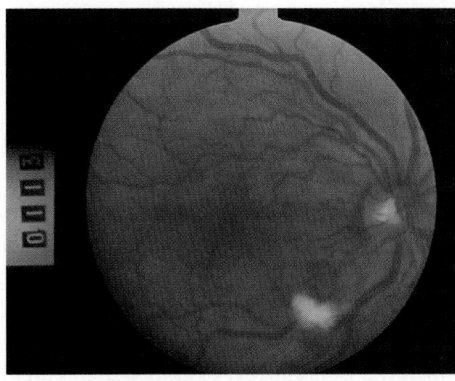

Figure 22-17 Cotton wool spots seen at 5400 m. This occurred in a climber after Valsalva maneuver and represents the most severe form of retinopathy. *(Courtesy Dr. M. McFadden, UBC, Vancouver, BC, in association with Dr. C. Houston, Burlington, Vt.; Dr. G. Gray, DCIEM, Toronto, Ontario; and Drs. Sutton and P. Powells, McMaster University, Hamilton, Ontario.)*

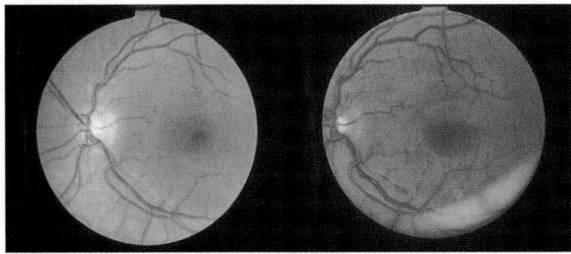

Figure 22-18 The normal fundus as sea level (left). The same fundus at 5400 m (right). Note the vascular engorgement and tortuousness at altitude. *(Courtesy Dr. M. McFadden, UBC, Vancouver, BC, in association with Dr. C. Houston, Burlington, Vt.; Dr. G. Gray, DCIEM, Toronto, Ontario; and Drs. Sutton and P. Powells, McMaster University, Hamilton, Ontario.)*

nal hemorrhages in eight subjects examined after 48 hours at 4573 m (15,000 feet) in a hypobaric chamber, although all subjects displayed the marked vascular engorgement and tortuosity typical of the eye at altitude (Figure 22-18). Differences in the incidence of HARH for exposures at similar altitudes may be due to differences in time at altitude before examination, acclimatization schedule, exercise levels, examination techniques, and the presence of concurrent conditions that may predispose to HARH.

HARH has been reported to be associated with both altitude headache and a history of vascular headache at sea level.[67] Rimsza et al[61] noted that HARH may occur at lower altitudes in individuals with chronic lung disorders that interfere with oxygenation. Their case report described a woman with cystic fibrosis who had climbed as high as 3049 m (10,000 feet) but was at 1677 m (5500 feet) when she noted a sudden decrease in vision associated with preretinal hemorrhage of the right eye. They also noted that the ocular findings of cystic fibrosis are similar to those seen with altitude retinopathy.[61]

Although HARHs are often not associated with acute visual symptoms,[8,59,84,91] they may result in a loss

of visual acuity or paracentral scotomas.[21,39,70,84] Lang and Kuba[39] reported a person who experienced decreased visual acuity and central scotoma from HARH resulting from a 7000-m (22,960-foot) altitude exposure. Permanent deficits in visual function are uncommon but have been reported.[70,84] Shults and Swan[70] reported that four survivors of an ill-fated Aconcagua expedition in Argentina in 1973 were found to have severe HARH after an altitude exposure of 6860 m (22,500 feet). Two of the survivors suffered apparently permanent paracentral scotomas.

No reports were found of a progressive decrease in visual acuity or progressive enlargement of paracentral scotomas as a result of remaining at altitude after the development of HARH.[10] Weidman[84] reported a case in which further ascent after the development of HARH resulted in additional lesions. HARH that results in decreased visual acuity should be a contraindication to further ascent.[10] Butler and Harris[8] recommended that evacuation of individuals with decreases in visual function resulting from HARH (in the absence of high-altitude cerebral edema [HACE] or high-altitude pulmonary edema [HAPE]) be considered nonemergent unless reexamination indicates a progressive deterioration of vision or increasingly severe retinopathy. HARH resolves over a period of 2 to 8 weeks after the altitude exposure is terminated.[84]

Cortical Blindness at High Altitude

Hackett[25] reported six cases of cortical blindness at high altitude. These victims were found to have intact pupillary reflexes. Descent, Gamow (hyperbaric) bag recompression, or supplemental oxygen breathing should be used in persons with neurologic dysfunction at altitude.

Ocular Motility

Kramar[37] reported that convergence insufficiency was found in women with altitude illness. Basnyat[2] noted that lateral gaze palsy and other focal neurologic deficits, often in the absence of other symptoms of AMS or HACE, are seen commonly by physicians in the Himalayan Rescue Association. Rennie and Morrissey[59] reported a person with nystagmus at altitude that was associated with ataxia and intention tremor. Ocular motility abnormalities should be managed in the same way as cortical blindness at high altitude as described in the preceding paragraph.

Contact Lenses in Mountaineering

Contact lenses may be used successfully at high altitude.[11,91] Clarke[11] noted that contact lenses were used successfully by five members of the British Everest Expedition in 1975 up to altitudes as high as 7317 m (24,000 feet). Use of contact lenses at altitude during trekking or mountaineering entails several considerations beyond those encountered in normal use. In general, overnight use of extended-wear contact lenses is not recommended because of the associated increased rate of microbial keratitis. Even soft contact lenses decrease the oxygen available to the cornea. Lid closure during sleep further accentuates corneal hypoxia. Removing contact lenses at night, however, presents logistical problems in the mountaineering setting. Practicing acceptable lens hygiene during an expedition is difficult. The mountaineer who leaves contact lenses in a case filled with liquid solution in the tent outside of his or her sleeping bag at night may awaken to find the solution and lenses frozen solid.

Guidelines for military personnel using contact lenses in austere environments have been developed and apply to the expedition setting[10]:

1. Disposable extended-wear lenses may be left in the eye for up to 1 week. If the wearer is still in the field at the end of this period, the lenses should be removed and discarded. After an overnight period without lenses, new lenses may be inserted, with strict attention to contact lens hygiene.

2. Contact lens wearers should *always* have backup glasses available for use in the wilderness in case a lens is lost or becomes painful.

3. Individuals who wear contact lenses on expeditions should carry both fluoroquinolone eye drops and contact lens rewetting solution. Both types of drops may freeze if not protected from the cold.

4. Contact lens wearers often note that their eyes become dry. This discomfort may be alleviated with contact lens rewetting drops.

5. Contact lens wearers often note increased sensitivity to sunlight. Individuals who wear contact lenses in the field during daylight hours should carry sunglasses.

Continuous wearing of disposable contact lenses for a week, followed by discarding of the lenses and insertion of fresh lenses after an overnight period without a lens, is a controversial approach to contact lens wear in an expedition setting. Whether or not the reduction in lens handling offsets the increased risk of microbial keratitis resulting from overnight wear is not known. The decision to wear contact lenses while mountaineering should be made carefully. Microbial keratitis (corneal ulcers) can pose a significant threat to vision under the best of circumstances. Should this disorder occur with a 7- to 10-day delay to definitive ophthalmologic care, the danger of permanent loss of vision is great. Any eye pain that occurs in contacts lens wearers in the wilderness should be managed as described previously in the Acute Red Eye section. Considering all the potential problems, a good pair of prescription glacier glasses or laser refractive surgery might be a more reasonable alternative than contact lenses as a long-term solution to the refractive needs of mountaineers.

Refractive Changes at Altitude after Refractive Surgery

An acute hyperopic shift in persons who have had radial keratotomy (RK) and then experience an altitude exposure was reported by Snyder in 1988[75] and White and Mader in 1993.[87] This effect has been observed at altitudes as low as 2744 m (9000 feet).[75] A dramatic example of this phenomenon was that experienced by Dr. Beck Weathers in the Everest tragedy of May 1996 in which eight climbers lost their lives. Dr. Weathers had undergone bilateral RK years before the expedition. He noted a decrease in vision, which started early during his ascent.[36] Author Jon Krakauer recalls that ". . . as he was ascending from Camp Three to Camp Four, Beck later confessed to me, 'my vision had gotten so bad that I couldn't see more than a few feet.'"[36] This decrease in vision forced Dr. Weathers to abandon his quest for the summit shortly after leaving Camp Four and nearly resulted in his death. Another report describes two expert climbers who experienced hyperopic shifts of three diopters or more during altitude exposures of 5000 m (16,400 feet) or higher on Mt. McKinley and Mt. Everest.[12]

Mader and White[43] found that the magnitude of the hyperopic shift was 1.03 +/− 0.16 diopters after 24 hours at 3659 m (12,000 feet) and 1.94 +/− 0.26 diopters at 5183 m (17,000 feet). Ng[51] reported no refractive change after 6 hours in post-RK eyes at a simulated altitude of 3659 m, suggesting that the hyperopic shift requires more than 6 hours to develop. Further studies by Mader et al[44] at 4299 m (14,100 feet) on Pike's Peak revealed that: (1) subjects who had undergone RK demonstrated a progressive hyperopic shift associated with flattened keratometry findings during a 72-hour exposure; (2) control eyes and eyes that had undergone laser refractive surgery (photorefractive keratectomy [PRK]) experienced no change in their refractive state; (3) peripheral corneal thickening was seen on pachymetry in all three groups; and (4) refraction, keratometry, and pachymetry all returned to baseline after return to sea level. Winkle[89] demonstrated that exposing post-RK corneas to 100% nitrogen via goggles at one atmosphere for 2 hours caused a significant hyperopic shift of 1.24 diopters and corneal flattening of 1.19 diopters in post-RK eyes. Corneal thickness increased in both post-RK and control eyes but was not associated with a hyperopic shift in control eyes. This is strong evidence that the effect of altitude exposures on post-RK eyes is caused by hypoxia rather than by hypobarism and further illustrates that breathing a normoxic inspired gas mix will not protect against the development of hypoxic corneal changes.

The effect of the post-RK hyperopic shift seen at altitude depends on the postoperative refractive state (undercorrected patients may actually have their vision improve) and the accommodative abilities of the individual.[43] The work of Mader and his colleagues has provided compelling evidence for myopic mountaineers that PRK instead of RK is their refractive surgical procedure of choice. Individuals who have undergone RK and plan to undertake an altitude exposure of 2744 m (9000 feet) or higher while mountaineering should bring multiple spectacles with increasing plus lens power.[43] To my knowledge, a post-RK hyperopic shift has not been reported in airline passengers or flight crew. This may be because the latent period required for this phenomenon to develop exceeds the duration of most commercial flights or because the approximate 8000-foot cabin pressure on most commercial flights does not produce sufficient corneal hypoxia for a hyperopic shift to occur.

Ultraviolet Radiation Damage
(see also Chapter 14)

Ultraviolet radiation is divided into UV-A (320 to 400 nm), UV-B (290 to 320 nm), and UV-C (100 to 290 nm). Almost all UV-C radiation is absorbed by the earth's ozone layer.[54,77] The cornea absorbs all radiation with wavelengths of less than approximately 300 nm, and the lens absorbs almost all of the remaining UV-B radiation that reaches it.[77] UV radiation is increased with high altitude, low latitude, and highly reflective environments.[54] Altitude exposures associated with mountaineering entail exposures to increases in the amount of both incident and reflected UV light.

Acute exposure to high levels of UV radiation may result in UV photokeratitis,[14,77] whereas chronic exposures may be associated with cortical lens opacities,[13] posterior subcapsular lens opacities,[4] pterygia,[3] and squamous cell carcinoma of the conjunctiva.[49]

Diagnosis and management of UV keratitis are discussed previously in this chapter. The best strategy for dealing with UV radiation–induced disorders is prevention. Most experienced mountaineers and trekkers are well aware of the need for sunglasses with high rates of UV absorption. UV attenuation in sunglasses depends on the size, shape, and wearing position, as well as the absorption properties of the optical material used.[63] The use of a brimmed hat is another effective means of decreasing UV exposure to the eye.[54,64] In conjunction with the use of topical sun-blocking agents, a hat may also help prevent a series of cutaneous neoplasms from being a lasting reminder of previous mountaineering expeditions.

Sunglasses Selection in Mountaineering

What type of sunglasses should be worn by individuals on mountaineering expeditions? Absorption of essentially all UV radiation is a key consideration, since radiation in this portion of the electromagnetic spectrum is not visible and serves only to produce adverse effects in the eye. Another critical consideration is the amount of visible light transmitted. Sunglasses that suf-

fice for everyday use may not be adequate for use in the mountains, especially while on snow or glaciers. The comfort zone for luminance is approximately 350 to 2000 candelas/m^2.[77] An outdoor environment consisting of sunlit fields and foliage may have a luminance of 3000 to 7000 candelas/m^2; a bright beach may have a luminance of 6000 to 15,000 candelas/m^2. Standard sunglasses that transmit 15% to 25% of visible light reduce the luminance in these situations to within the comfort range. In contrast, bright sun reflected off snow or clouds may result in luminances of 15,000 to 30,000 candelas/m^2. Sunglasses with visible light transmittance in the 5% to 10% range are needed to reduce luminance to a comfortable range in these circumstances. (The 1986 American National Standards Institute [ANSI] standards for nonprescription sunglasses recommend that tinted lenses with visible light transmittances of less than 8% not be used for driving.[77]) Sideshields or deeply wrapped lens designs should be used.[77] Infrared absorption is important in certain industrial occupations, such as glass, iron, and steelworkers,[77] but is less important in protective eyewear to be used outdoors. Table 22-2 provides desirable characteristics in selecting sunglasses for mountaineering or other environments with high levels of luminance and UV radiation.[10]

Photochromic Lenses

Photochromic lenses change transmittance or color when exposed to light or UV radiation.[77] They are designed to transmit a greater percentage of incident light

TABLE 22-2. Sunglasses Selection Criteria for Mountaineering

SUBJECT	CHARACTERISTICS
UV absorption	99% to 100%
Visible light transmittance	5% to 10%*
Lens material	Polycarbonate or CR-39†
Optical quality	Clear image without distortion‡
Frame design features	Large lenses; side shields or "wraparound" design; fit close to face; good stability on face during movement; lightweight; durable
Color	Gray§

*Glasses with less than 8% transmittance of visible light should not be worn while driving. Sunglasses or any tinted lenses with a visible light transmittance of less than 80% should not be worn while driving at night.[77]

†Glass lenses typically have very good optical clarity and scratch resistance but are heavier and more expensive.

‡Hold the sunglasses at arm's length and move them back and forth. If the objects are distorted or move erratically, the optical quality is probably less than desirable. Also, compare the image quality between several different pairs of sunglasses to get a basis for comparison.

§The use of colored lens tints can alter color perception and possibly compromise the visibility of traffic signals. Neutral gray absorbs light relatively constantly across the visible spectrum and avoids these problems.[77]

when indoors or in conditions of reduced illumination and a reduced amount of light when exposed to higher levels of illumination. This is accomplished in one example of glass lenses by incorporating an inorganic silver halide into the lens. When the lens is exposed to sunlight, this compound decomposes into its component silver and halide ions and the lens turns dark gray.[77] When the lens is removed from sunlight, the process reverses. When selecting photochromic lenses, the adequacy of indoor light transmittance can be judged while trying them on. The outdoor transmittance should be approximately 5% to 10% as noted in Table 22-2 if the glasses are to be used for mountaineering. Most photochromic lenses have outdoor transmittances of approximately 20%, which should suffice for less highly reflective outdoor environments.[77]

Several plastic photochromic lenses are now available. The darkening process in plastic lenses is accomplished by organic light-sensitive compounds that are suspended in a thin layer near the front of the lens. Plastic photochromic lenses generally do not darken well enough to be used as sunglasses in bright environments. In addition, unlike glass photochromic lenses, the photochromic reaction typically used in plastic lenses usually fades in 1 to 2 years.[77]

THE EYE AND DIVING

The ocular aspects of scuba diving and other hyperbaric exposures were reviewed in a 1995 paper.[9] The sections from that paper that address the hyperbaric environment, ocular barotrauma, the ocular manifestations of decompression sickness and arterial gas embolism, ophthalmic considerations in fitness-to-dive evaluations, and the differential diagnosis of decreased vision after diving are included here. An expanded discussion of these items, as well as additional material on diving after eye surgery, the effect of common eye medications on fitness to dive, and the use of hyperbaric oxygen to treat ocular disorders, may be found in the review article.

The Hyperbaric Environment
(see also Chapter 59)

At sea level, the body is exposed to one atmosphere (ATA) of pressure. This magnitude of pressure may also be expressed as 760 mm Hg, 33 feet of sea water (FSW), and 14.7 pounds per square inch (psi).

The normal atmospheric pressure of 1 ATA is often used as a reference point from which other pressures are measured. When one states that the intraocular pressure (IOP) is 15 mm Hg, what is meant is that the IOP is 15 mm Hg more than the surrounding environment. In point of fact, the absolute pressure inside the eye at sea level is 775 (760 + 15) mm Hg. The IOP that is measured with a tonometer is therefore a "gauge" pressure, meaning that the pressure displayed is the actual pressure minus the atmospheric pressure.

Ophthalmic Considerations in the Fitness-to-Dive Evaluation

A diver should have adequate visual acuity to be able to read his or her gauges and function safely underwater. Possession of a driver's license is a convenient indication that a potential diver has sufficient visual acuity to meet this standard.[9] A person who has recently undergone ophthalmic surgery should refrain from diving until the recommended convalescent interval has passed.[9] Individuals who suffer from glaucoma may dive safely unless they have had glaucoma filtering surgery performed.[9] Systemic carbonic anhydrase inhibitors are best avoided in glaucoma patients who wish to dive because of possible confusion between medication-induced paresthesias and decompression sickness.[9] Any individual who is suffering from an acute ocular disorder that causes significant pain, decreased visual acuity, or other disabling symptoms should refrain from diving until these symptoms have resolved.[9]

Underwater Refractive Correction

If contact lenses are to be used for diving, soft contact lenses are preferred.[5,17,32,47] Hard (polymethylmethacrylate) contact lenses have been associated with corneal edema during decompression and after dives.[72,73] These changes are caused by formation of nitrogen bubbles in the precorneal tear film during decompression, which interferes with normal tear film physiology and results in epithelial edema. Bubble formation would be expected to be more common during dives with significant decompression stress.

Although the increased gaseous diffusion properties of rigid gas-permeable contact lenses theoretically decrease the chance of bubble formation in the tear film, use of these lenses while diving has been demonstrated to cause bubble formation under the lens, leading to secondary corneal epithelial disruption.[76] The author has treated one diver with foreign body sensation and blurred visual acuity that occurred during ascent while wearing gas-permeable contact lenses. Symptoms resolved upon removal of the lens at the surface.

Corneal edema was not observed in one series in which soft contact lenses were studied.[73] The most frequent complication of soft contact lens use in diving is loss of the lens.[32,34] The risk of lens loss can be minimized by ensuring a good seal on the face mask and minimizing the amount of water that gets into the air space of the mask. Should the mask become displaced during the dive, narrowing of the palpebral fissures helps decrease the chance of the contact lens floating off the surface of the eye.[32]

A prescription ground face mask is another refractive alternative, as is a face mask with a lens bonded onto the surface of the mask. Masks and lenses may be lost in high swells or rough surf, however, leaving a diver without refractive correction. When contemplating the purchase of an expensive prescription face mask, one needs to be mindful of the corollary of Murphy's law that applies to diving: "Weight belts always fall on the face masks with prescription lenses."

Ocular Barotrauma

The eye is normally filled with noncompressible fluid and solid tissues and is therefore protected from barotrauma. However, once a mask is placed over the face, a different circumstance exists. The face mask is an air-filled space bounded on one side by the eyes and ocular adnexa. As a diver descends, if he or she does not expel gas through the nose into the airspace of the face mask, a relative negative pressure develops in this space. If this negative pressure becomes great enough, the eyes and ocular adnexa are drawn towards the space. Marked lid edema with ecchymosis and subconjunctival hemorrhage may develop as tissues and blood vessels are disrupted by this distention. These signs may be alarming to the diver but typically resolve without sequelae. In a more severe case, such as that which may occur when an unconscious diver sinks a significant distance in the water column, more serious injury, including hyphema, may occur.[19] A diver with face mask barotrauma is shown in Figure 22-19.

Barotrauma is also possible in persons with gas bubbles in the anterior chamber or vitreous cavity. Pressure-induced changes in the volume of this bubble may result in retinal, uveal, or vitreous hemorrhage, as well as partial collapse of the globe. Permanent loss of vision may ensue. One person who attempted to dive while an iatrogenic bubble was present in the vitreous cavity noted the immediate onset of very severe eye pain upon descent and quickly aborted his dive.[56] Persons with in-

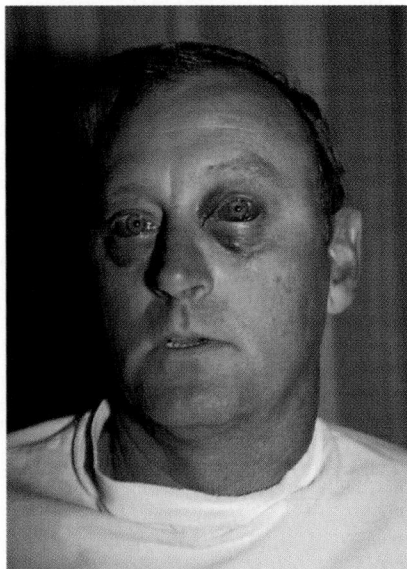

Figure 22-19 Mask squeeze in a diver who descended to 45 FSW without exhaling into his mask. *(Courtesy Kenneth W. Kizer, MD.)*

traocular gas should not be allowed to dive as long as the bubble remains in the eye. The necessity of adding extra gas to the face mask during descent makes it obvious that swim goggles, which cover only the eyes and not the nose, should never be used for diving.

Decompression Sickness

Ocular involvement in decompression sickness (DCS) was first reported by Sir Robert Boyle, who observed gas bubbles in the anterior chamber of the eye of a viper that had been experimentally exposed to increased pressure.[6] Ocular manifestations of DCS are infrequently reported in the ophthalmic literature,[9] but there are a number of reports of ocular involvement with DCS in the diving medical literature.[7,9,18,62] Reported manifestations include nystagmus, diplopia, visual field defects, scotomas, homonymous hemianopias, orbicularis oculi pain, cortical blindness, convergence insufficiency, optic neuropathy, and central retinal artery occlusion.[9] The incidence of visual symptoms in patients with DCS was found to be 7% in one large series.[62]

Fluorescein angiography of divers has documented retinal pigment epithelial abnormalities indistinguishable from those seen in eyes with choroidal ischemia. These changes are attributed to decompression-induced intravascular gaseous microemboli. The incidence of these lesions was related to the duration of diving and a history of DCS. Although no diver was reported to have suffered a loss of visual acuity from these abnormalities, the long-term effects of this phenomenon remain to be studied.[9]

DCS may also result when an individual without a hyperbaric exposure is suddenly exposed to a decrease in pressure. Altitude DCS presenting as optic neuropathy has been reported.[7] The risk of DCS may be increased if an altitude exposure is undertaken after diving without allowing a sufficient time interval for excess nitrogen taken up during the dive to leave the body.[9]

DCS is treated with oxygen breathing and recompression on an emergent basis. Ophthalmologists seldom encounter this disease in an acute setting because most divers know to seek recompression therapy for signs or symptoms of DCS. Since treatment generally results in resolution of all symptoms, most persons with visual symptoms before treatment are asymptomatic after recompression treatment and are therefore not referred to ophthalmologists.[6] Should an ophthalmologist encounter a person with acute ocular disturbances consistent with DCS after a hyperbaric or hypobaric exposure, the victim should be referred emergently to the nearest available recompression chamber and diving medicine specialist, since DCS may worsen rapidly if not treated. Physicians unsure of the location of the nearest diving medicine specialist or recompression chamber can call the Divers Alert Network at Duke University (919-684-8111).

Incomplete response to treatment or recurrence of symptoms after treatment may bring a victim with ocular DCS to the ophthalmologist on a less emergent basis. The victim should be managed in conjunction with a diving medicine specialist. Recompression therapy and hyperbaric oxygen should be administered even when a significant delay has occurred between the onset of symptoms and initial evaluation of the victim, since treatment may be effective despite delays of up to several weeks.[7,9]

Arterial Gas Embolism

Retrochiasmal defects, such as hemianopias or cortical blindness, are found with arterial gas embolism. Central retinal artery occlusion may result from gas emboli in the ophthalmic artery.[9] Management is similar to that for DCS, with emergent recompression and hyperbaric oxygen therapy indicated in all cases.

Differential Diagnosis of Decreased Vision after Diving

DCS and arterial gas embolism should be considered whenever vision is acutely decreased after diving because of the possible emergent need for recompression therapy, especially if any other manifestation of DCS or arterial gas embolism are present. Other disorders may also affect vision after a dive. Corneal edema resulting from the formation of gas bubbles under polymethylmethacrylate and rigid gas-permeable contact lenses may cause decreased vision. A soft contact lens wearer who complains of blurred vision after a dive may have a lost or displaced lens.

Another possible cause of nondysbaric decreased vision after a dive is epithelial keratopathy induced by chemical agents used to reduce face mask fogging. The time-honored application of saliva or toothpaste to the interior surface of the mask reduces but does not eliminate fogging. This led to the development of commercial antifog agents designed to be applied to the inside surface of face masks. These agents may contain volatile compounds potentially toxic to the corneal epithelium, including glycols, alcohols, and phenol derivatives. Exposure to these compounds may result in blurred vision, photophobia, tearing, and blepharospasm that may not develop until several hours after the dive.[90] Slit lamp examination typically reveals diffuse superficial punctate keratopathy. Development of this syndrome commonly results from improper use of the antifog agent, such as overly generous application or failure to rinse the mask before use.

The author has treated several persons with recurrent mild ocular irritation and blurring of vision after dives on which soft contact lenses were worn. The lenses were noted to be tightly adherent to the cornea, probably as a result of a decrease in water content in the lens after contact with hypertonic sea water. Symptoms were relieved with a few drops of isotonic artificial tears.

> **Box 22-5 DIFFERENTIAL DIAGNOSIS OF DECREASED VISION AFTER DIVING**
>
> Decompression sickness
> Arterial gas embolism
> Bubbles under contact lenses
> Displaced contact lens
> Antifog agent keratopathy
> Contact lens adherence syndrome
> Transdermal scopolamine

A diver sometimes uses a transdermal scopolamine patch (placed behind the ear) to prevent motion sickness. This may result in mydriasis, decreased accommodation, and blurred vision in the ipsilateral eye. A differential diagnosis of decreased vision after diving is presented in Box 22-5.

ACKNOWLEDGMENTS

I thank Drs. Steve Chalfin, Dave Harris, and Dave Perlman for their much-appreciated contributions to the preparation of this chapter.

REFERENCES

1. Aiello PD et al: Visual prognosis in giant cell arteritis, *Ophthalmology* 100:550, 1993.
2. Basnyat B: Seizure and hemiparesis at high altitude outside the setting of acute mountain sickness, *Wilderness Environ Med* 8:221, 1997.
3. Bergmanson JP, Soderberg PG: The significance of ultraviolet radiation for eye diseases: a review with comments on the efficacy of UV-blocking contact lenses, *Ophthalmic Physiol Opt* 15:83, 1995.
4. Bochow TW et al: Ultraviolet light exposure and risk of posterior subcapsular cataracts, *Arch Ophthalmol* 107:369, 1989.
5. Davis JC, Bove AA: Medical evaluation for sport diving. In Bove AA, Davis JC, editors: *Diving medicine*, ed 3, Philadelphia, 1997, WB Saunders.
6. Butler FK: Decompression sickness. In Gold DH, Weingeist TA, editors: *The eye in systemic disease*, Philadelphia, 1990, JB Lippincott.
7. Butler FK: Decompression sickness presenting as optic neuropathy, *Aviat Space Environ Med* 62:346, 1991.
8. Butler FK, Harris DJ, Reynolds RD: Altitude retinopathy on Mount Everest 1989, *Ophthalmology* 99:739, 1992.
9. Butler FK: Diving and hyperbaric ophthalmology, *Surv Ophthalmol* 39:347, 1995.
10. Butler FK: The eye at altitude, *Int Ophthalmol Clin* 39:59, 1999.
11. Clarke C: Contact lenses at high altitude: experience on Everest southwest face 1975, *Br J Ophthalmol* 60:479, 1976.
12. Creel DJ, Crandall AS, Swartz M: Hyperopic shift induced by high altitude after radial keratotomy, *J Refract Surg* 13:398, 1997.
13. Cruickshanks KJ, Klein BE, Klein R: Ultraviolet light exposure and lens opacities: the Beaver Dam Eye Study, *Am J Public Health* 82:1658, 1992.
14. Dolin PJ, Johnson GJ: Solar ultraviolet radiation and ocular disease: a review of the epidemiological and experimental evidence, *Ophthalmic Epidemiol* 1:155, 1994.
15. Donahue SP, Schwartz G: Preseptal and orbital cellulitis in childhood: a changing microbiologic spectrum, *Ophthalmology* 105:1902, 1998.
16. Driver PJ, Lemp MA: Meibomian gland dysfunction, *Surv Ophthalmol* 40:343, 1996.
17. Edmonds C, Lowry C, Pennefather J: *Diving and subaquatic medicine*, ed 3, Oxford, UK, 1992, Butterworth-Heinemann.
18. Elliott DH, Moon RE: Manifestations of the decompression disorders. In Bennett PB, Elliott DH, editors: *The physiology and medicine of diving*, ed 4, London, 1993, WB Saunders.
19. Fletcher C: Personal communication.
20. Forster W et al: Topical diclofenac sodium after excimer laser phototherapeutic keratectomy, *J Refract Surg* 13:311, 1997

21. Frayser R et al: Retinal hemorrhages at high altitude, *N Engl J Med* 282:1183, 1970.

22. Frayser R et al: The response of the retinal circulation to altitude, *Arch Intern Med* 127:708, 1971.

23. Friedberg MA, Rapuano CJ: *Office and emergency room diagnosis and treatment of eye disease,* Philadelphia, 1990, JB Lippincott.

24. Ghanchi FD, Dutton GN: Current concepts in giant-cell (temporal) arteritis, *Surv Ophthalmol* 42:99, 1997.

25. Hackett H: Cortical blindness in high altitude climbers and trekkers: a report on six cases (abstract). In Sutton JR, Houston CS, Coates G, editors: *Hypoxia and cold,* New York, 1987, Praeger.

26. Hackett PH, Rennie D: Rales, peripheral edema, retinal hemorrhage, and acute mountain sickness, *Am J Med* 67:214, 1979.

27. Hayreh SS, Kolder HE, Weingeist TA: Central retinal artery occlusion and retinal tolerance time, *Ophthalmology* 87:75, 1980.

28. Hayreh SS, Podhajsky PA, Zimmerman B: Ocular manifestations of giant cell arteritis, *Am J Ophthalmol* 125:509, 1998.

29. Hooper DC: Expanding uses of fluoroquinolones: opportunities and challenges, *Ann Intern Med* 129:908, 1998

30. Hyndiuk RA et al: Comparison of ciprofloxacin ophthalmic solution 0.3% to fortified tobramycin-cefazolin in treating bacterial corneal ulcers, *Ophthalmology* 103:1854, 1996.

31. Jayamanne DG et al: The effectiveness of topical diclofenac in relieving discomfort following traumatic corneal abrasions, *Eye* 11:79, 1997

32. Josephson JE, Caffery BE: Contact lens considerations in surface and subsurface aqueous environments, *Optom Vis Sci* 68:2, 1991.

33. Kaiser PK, the Corneal Abrasion Patching Study Group: A comparison of pressure patching versus no patching for corneal abrasions due to trauma or foreign body removal, *Ophthalmology* 102:1936, 1995.

34. Kinney JS: *Human underwater vision: physiology and physics,* Bethesda, Md, 1985, Undersea and Hyperbaric Society.

35. Kobrick JL, Appleton B: Effect of extended hypoxia on visual performance and retinal vascular state, *J Appl Physiol* 31:357, 1971.

36. Krakauer J: *Into thin air,* New York, 1997, Random House.

37. Kramar PO et al: Ocular functions and incidence of acute mountain sickness in women at altitude, *Aviat Space Environ Med* 54:116, 1983.

38. Kressloff MS, Castellarin AA, Zarbin MA: Endophthalmitis, *Surv Ophthalmol* 43:193, 1998.

39. Lang GE, Kuba GB: High altitude retinopathy, *Am J Ophthalmol* 123:418, 1997.

40. Lesk MR et al: The penetration of oral ciprofloxacin into the aqueous humor, vitreous, and subretinal fluid of humans, *Am J Ophthalmol* 115:623, 1993.

41. Li HK, Bejean BJ, Tang RA: Reversal of visual loss with hyperbaric oxygen treatment in a patient with Susac Syndrome, *Ophthalmology* 103:2091, 1996.

42. MacCumber MW: *Management of ocular injuries and emergencies,* Philadelphia, 1998, Lippincott-Raven.

43. Mader TH, White LJ: Refractive changes at extreme altitude after radial keratotomy, *Am J Ophthalmol* 119:733, 1995.

44. Mader TH et al: Refractive changes during a 72 hour exposure to high altitude after refractive surgery, *Ophthalmology* 103:1188, 1996.

45. Mangat HS: Retinal artery occlusion, *Surv Ophthalmol* 40:145, 1995.

46. McFadden DM et al: High altitude retinopathy, *JAMA* 245:581, 1981.

47. Mebane GY, McIver NK: Fitness to dive. In Bennett PB, Elliott DH, editors: *The physiology and medicine of diving,* ed 4, London, 1993, WB Saunders.

48. Morgan SJ: Use of ophthalmic ointment to separate adhesive, *Arch Ophthalmol* 107:15, 1989.

49. Newton R et al: Effect of ambient solar radiation on incidence of squamous-cell carcinoma of the eye, *Lancet* 347:1450, 1996.

50. Ng EW et al: Treatment of experimental *Staphylococcus epidermidis* endophthalmitis with oral trovafloxacin, *Am J Ophthalmol* 126:278, 1998

51. Ng JD et al: Effects of simulated high altitude on patients who have had radial keratotomy, *Ophthalmology* 103:452, 1996.

52. O'Brien TP, Green WR: Periocular infections. In Mandell GL, Bennett JE, Dolin R, editors: *Principles and practice of infectious diseases,* ed 4, New York, 1995, Churchill Livingstone.

53. Ofloxacin Study Group: Ofloxacin monotherapy for the primary treatment of microbial keratitis, *Ophthalmology* 104:1902, 1997.

54. Olson CM: Increased outdoor recreation, diminished ozone layer pose ultraviolet radiation threat to eye, *JAMA* 261:1102, 1989.

55. Pavan-Langston D: *Manual of ocular diagnosis and therapy,* ed 4, Boston, 1996, Little, Brown.

56. Peterson T: Personal communication.

57. Perlman D: Personal communication.

58. Raynor LA: Treatment for inadvertent cyanoacrylate tarsorrhaphy, *Arch Ophthalmol* 106:1033, 1988.

59. Rennie D, Morrissey J: Retinal changes in Himalayan climbers, *Arch Ophthalmol* 93:395, 1975.

60. Rhee DJ et al: *The Wills eye manual: office and emergency room diagnosis and treatment of eye disease,* New York, 1998, Lippincott-Raven.

61. Rimsza ME, Hernried LS, Kaplan AM: Hemorrhagic retinopathy in a patient with cystic fibrosis, *Pediatrics* 62:336, 1978.

62. Rivera JC: Decompression sickness among divers—an analysis of 935 cases, *Mil Med* 129:314, 1964.

63. Rosenthal FS et al: The effect of sunglasses on ocular exposure to ultraviolet radiation, *Am J Public Health* 78:72, 1988.

64. Rosenthal FS et al: The ocular dose of ultraviolet radiation to outdoor workers, *Invest Ophthalmol Vis Sci* 29:649, 1988.

65. Ross WH, Kozy DW: Visual recovery in macula-off rhegmatogenous retinal detachments, *Ophthalmology* 105:2149, 1998.

66. Schmidt D, Schumacher M, Wahkloo AK: Microcatheter urokinase infusion in central retinal artery occlusion, *Am J Ophthalmol* 113:429, 1992.

67. Schumacher GA, Petajan JH: High altitude stress and retinal hemorrhage: relation to vascular headache mechanisms, *Arch Environ Health* 30:217, 1975.

68. Seitz B et al: Corneal sensitivity and burning sensation. Comparing topical ketorolac and diclofenac, *Arch Ophthalmol* 114:921, 1996

69. Shingleton BJ, Hersh PS, Kenyon KR: *Eye trauma,* St Louis, 1991, Mosby.

70. Shults WT, Swan KC: High altitude retinopathy in mountain climbers, *Arch Ophthalmol* 93:404, 1975.

71. Silverman CM: Corneal abrasion from accidental instillation of cyanoacrylate into the eye, *Arch Ophthalmol* 106:1029, 1988.

72. Simon DR, Bradley ME: Corneal edema in divers wearing hard contact lenses, *Am J Ophthalmol* 85:462, 1978.

73. Simon DR, Bradley ME: Adverse effects of contact lens wear during decompression, *JAMA* 244:1213, 1980.

74. Slamovits TL, editor: *Fundamentals and principles of ophthalmology,* American Academy of Ophthalmology basic and clinical science course, Section 2, p 152, 1993-1994.

75. Snyder RP, Klein P, Solomon J: The possible effect of barometric pressure on the corneas of an RK patient: a case report, *International Contact Lens Clinics* 15:130, 1988.

76. Socks JF, Molinari JF, Rowey JL: Rigid gas permeable contact lenses in hyperbaric environments, *Am J Opt Phys Optics* 65:942, 1988.

77. Stephens GL, Davis JK: Spectacle lenses. In Tasman W, Jaeger EA, editors: *Duane's textbook of clinical ophthalmology,* Philadelphia, 1996, Lippincott-Raven.

78. Sun R, Gimbel HV: Effects of topical ketorolac and diclofenac on normal corneal sensation, *J Refract Surg* 13:158, 1997

79. Szerenyi K et al: Decrease in normal human corneal sensitivity with topical diclofenac sodium, *Am J Ophthalmol* 118:312, 1994

80. Trovafloxacin, *Med Lett Drugs Ther* 40:30, 1998.

81. Tutton MK et al: Efficacy and safety of topical diclofenac in reducing ocular pain after excimer photorefractive keratectomy, *J Cataract Refract Surg* 22:536, 1996

82. Weinstock VM, Weinstock DJ, Weinstock SJ: Diclofenac and ketorolac in the treatment of pain after photorefractive keratectomy, *J Refract Surg* 12:792, 1996

83. Westfall CT, Shore JW, Baker AS: Orbital infections. In Gorbach SL, Bartlett JG, Blacklow NR, editors: *Infectious diseases,* ed 2, Philadelphia, 1998, WB Saunders.

84. Wiedman M: High altitude retinal hemorrhage, *Arch Ophthalmol* 93:410, 1975.

85. Weidman M: High altitude retinal hemorrhages: a classification. In Henkind P, editor: *Acta XXIV International Congress of Ophthalmology,* Philadelphia, 1980, JB Lippincott.

86. Weidman M: Altitude illness. In Gold DH, Weingeist TA, editors: *The eye in systemic disease,* Philadelphia, 1990, JB Lippincott.

87. White LJ, Mader TH: Refractive changes with increasing altitude after radial keratotomy, *Am J Ophthalmol* 115:821, 1993 (letter).

88. Wilmer WH, Berens C: Medical studies in aviation: V. The effect of altitude on ocular functions (1918), *Aviat Space Environ Med* 60:1018, 1989.

89. Winkle KR et al: The etiology of refractive changes at high altitude after radial keratotomy, *Ophthalmology* 105:282, 1996.

90. Wright WL: SCUBA divers' delayed toxic epithelial keratopathy from commercial mask defogging agents, *Am J Ophthalmol* 93:470, 1982.

91. Zafren K, Honigman B: High altitude medicine, *Emerg Med Clin* 15:191, 1997.

23 Dental and Facial Emergencies

Henry J. Herrmann

Acute conditions involving the mouth and related structures can disrupt recreational activities in the outdoors. A simple toothache, although not life threatening, can cause disabling pain. At the other end of the spectrum, odontogenic infections or major facial trauma are associated with high morbidity and mortality. This chapter discusses toothaches, temporomandibular joint (TMJ) disorders, oral infections, maxillofacial trauma, local anesthesia for dental emergencies, the dental first aid kit, and prevention.

MAXILLOFACIAL PAIN

The causes of maxillofacial pain are myriad, and the diagnosis of head and neck syndromes can be exceedingly difficult. Box 23-1 is a partial listing of pain-producing conditions. Fortunately, most of these syndromes are relatively rare. Only the most commonly encountered are covered in this chapter.

Pulpitis

The common toothache is caused by inflammation of the dental pulp. It may be difficult for the victim to identify the offending tooth because the pain often radiates to the eye or ear region, or is referred from one dental arch to the other. The painful tooth is rarely sensitive to percussion or palpation. An obvious cause, such as a large carious lesion, is sometimes found on examination of the mouth, but often all of the teeth appear intact. If the pulpitis is mild, the condition is characterized by pain that is only elicited by hot, cold, or sweets, and disappears within seconds when the stimulus is removed. Moderate pulpitis is characterized by greater discomfort and an increasing interval between removal of the stimulus and resolution of the pain. In its most severe form, pulpitis causes intense, continuous, and debilitating pain.[4,17] Emergency treatment recommendations follow.

Mild Pulpitis (Characterized by Transient Thermal Sensitivity). Examine the mouth visually. Structures will likely appear within normal limits. However, if a defect in a tooth is found, it should be temporarily filled. Reassure the victim that although this condition is annoying, rapid progression is unlikely.

Moderate Pulpitis (Longer Episodes of Pain). Proceed as for mild pulpitis. Treat with a nonnarcotic analgesic (ibuprofen 600 mg PO q6h prn pain).

Severe Pulpitis (Intense, Continuous Pain). The preferred approach to severe pulpitis is pain relief using a local anesthetic, followed by evacuation of the victim. A nerve block with bupivacaine 2% with 1:200,000 epinephrine (Marcaine) can provide up to 8 hours of excellent pain relief without central nervous system (CNS) depression (see section on local anesthesia). Large doses of narcotics should not be used because they are likely to compromise the victim's ability to participate in evacuation. In an extraordinary circumstance, an experienced rescuer could locate the offending tooth, expose the pulp, remove the inflamed pulpal tissue with a barbed broach, and cover the opening with a temporary filling material. Extraction is also an option in a case of severe pulpitis, but is to be discouraged for a number of reasons (see section on exodontia).

Periapical Osteitis

Inflammation of the supporting structures at the root of a tooth is characterized by constant, often throbbing pain. Unlike pulpitis, the affected tooth is easily located. The victim can usually point to the exact source of the pain, or the examiner may gently tap individual teeth, observing for tenderness. The area over the apex of the tooth is usually tender to palpation, but there is no frank swelling. Although trauma to a tooth can result in periapical inflammation, the most common cause is egress of bacteria and breakdown products from the necrotic pulp. Minor swelling around the apex extrudes the tooth slightly, causing increased forces on the tooth during occlusion and thus intensifying the pain. Emergency treatment includes an analgesic (ibuprofen 600 mg PO q6h prn pain) and/or a local anesthetic and a soft diet. Ideally, the contacting areas of the opposing tooth are reduced to relieve occlusal forces. Because this is generally impractical in the field, the victim should be given a strip of leather or something similar to place between the teeth on the nonpainful side. This will keep the offending tooth out of occlusion and reduce the pain.

Cracked Tooth Syndrome

With cracked tooth syndrome (CTS), the victim complains of momentary, sharp pain when chewing certain foods. Often, the victim reports that the tooth feels "weak" or that "it only hurts when I bite on something hard just the right way." These symptoms occur when forces of the proper magnitude and direction open the incomplete fracture within the tooth. Significantly, there is no pain on chewing soft foods. This condition usually progresses slowly. The victim should be advised to avoid chewing on the affected side and to seek definitive dental treatment as soon as possible.

Maxillary Sinusitis

The pain of maxillary sinusitis is generally described as a relatively continuous, throbbing ache that is intensified by postural change. A typical statement is "My tooth really hurt when we were hiking down that hill. I could feel it pound with every step. When we got to camp, I lay down, but it got even worse." The pain may be unilateral or bilateral. It is usually located in the infraorbital region and is often referred to the cheek, frontal region, and the maxillary premolars and molars. A complaint of multiple toothaches in the maxilla, with little or no evidence of carious teeth, should immediately raise suspicion for maxillary sinusitis. In addition to pain, there is tenderness elicited by pressure infraorbitally or over the bony prominence above the first molar. The victim also generally has an elevated temperature and nasal or postnasal discharge. Treatment of maxillary sinusitis includes an analgesic (ibuprofen 600 mg PO q6h prn pain), inhala-

tion of steam, oxymetazoline (Afrin) 0.05% in each nostril, 1 spray bid, to shrink the nasal membranes and improve sinus drainage, and an antibiotic. Appropriate choices include amoxicillin 875 mg with clavulanic acid 125 mg (Augmentin) PO bid for 10 days, or trimethoprim 160 mg with sulfamethoxazole 800 mg (Septra DS) PO bid for 10 days. Azithromycin (Zithromax), 500 mg PO the first day and 250 mg PO for four days, is a convenient alternative.

Temporomandibular Disorders

Considerable disagreement remains concerning the etiology, classification, and treatment of temporomandibular disorders (TMD). The subject is confusing because TMD is actually a cluster of unrelated conditions, multifactorial in origin and with overlapping symptoms, that often respond to a variety of therapies, including placebos.[6] Included under the classification of TMD are two groups of sufferers: those with masticatory muscle involvement (myofascial pain and dysfunction [MPD]) and those with TMJ problems. A brief summary follows.

Myofascial Pain and Dysfunction. Muscle hyperactivity is an important etiologic factor in MPD. In some persons this may result from parafunction (e.g., gum chewing, clenching or grinding the teeth). Occlusal interferences can also cause muscle hyperactivity. This occurs when a lower tooth contacts an upper tooth prematurely during mouth closure and a reflex causes jaw muscle contraction that shifts the mandible in such a way as to avoid the premature contact. Psychologic stress is also an important factor in causing excessive muscle tension.

Participants in wilderness activities are exposed to many of the risk factors for MPD. The high physiologic and psychologic demands of many expeditions lead to considerable stress. Increased jaw function, such as that required to chew granola, jerky, and other dried foods common on wilderness expeditions, is another factor that may precipitate an acute episode of MPD. Symptoms of MPD include pain in the muscles of mastication, which is usually unilateral and increases with chewing, headache, earache, intermittent clicking of the TMJ, limitation of jaw movement, and a change in bite. The victim may have a history of acute onset, or a long saga of exacerbation, remission, and various treatments.

The examiner may find objective signs, such as audible clicking of the TMJ, tenderness of the jaw muscles to palpation, tenderness of the TMJ to palpation, and abnormal jaw movements, such as inability to open the mouth widely, or deviation of the chin to one side on opening. Emergency treatment consists of resting the muscles (e.g., soft diet and control of tooth clenching and grinding habits) and the application of moist heat. Holding a soft material such as a folded gauze between the front teeth often gives immediate relief because it keeps the teeth from touching and allows the muscles to relax. An analgesic (ibuprofen 600 mg PO q6h) should be given on a scheduled basis, rather than as needed, to break the cycle of muscle pain and spasm. A muscle relaxant, such as metaxalone (Skelaxin) 800 mg PO tid or cyclobenzaprine (Flexeril) 10 mg PO tid, or sedative, such as diazepam (Valium) 2 to 10 mg PO tid, may be helpful if primary treatment is ineffective. Muscle relaxants and sedatives, especially in higher doses, can cause significant CNS depression, so they should be used in the lowest effective dosage and only if more conservative therapy has failed.

Mandibular Dislocation. Dislocation of the mandible and inability to close the mouth can result from external trauma or sudden wide opening of the mouth, such as occurs with yawning. The condition may be unilateral or bilateral. If there is a history of trauma, a condylar fracture should be suspected (Figure 23-1). A dislocated mandible is reduced by placing the rescuer's thumbs on the victim's lower molars and moving the mandible down, then posteriorly, and then up. If muscle spasm is severe, sedation might be necessary.[6] After reduction of the mandible, the victim must avoid wide mouth opening. The victim should place one hand under the chin or position the chin against the chest when yawning. It is also helpful to place a bandage around the head and under the chin for several days to limit jaw movement.

Anterior Disc Displacement. Anterior displacement of the TMJ's cartilaginous disc with reduction to a normal position on mouth opening causes clicking in the joint. Generally, this is not associated with pain or severe dysfunction. However, if the disc is displaced and does not

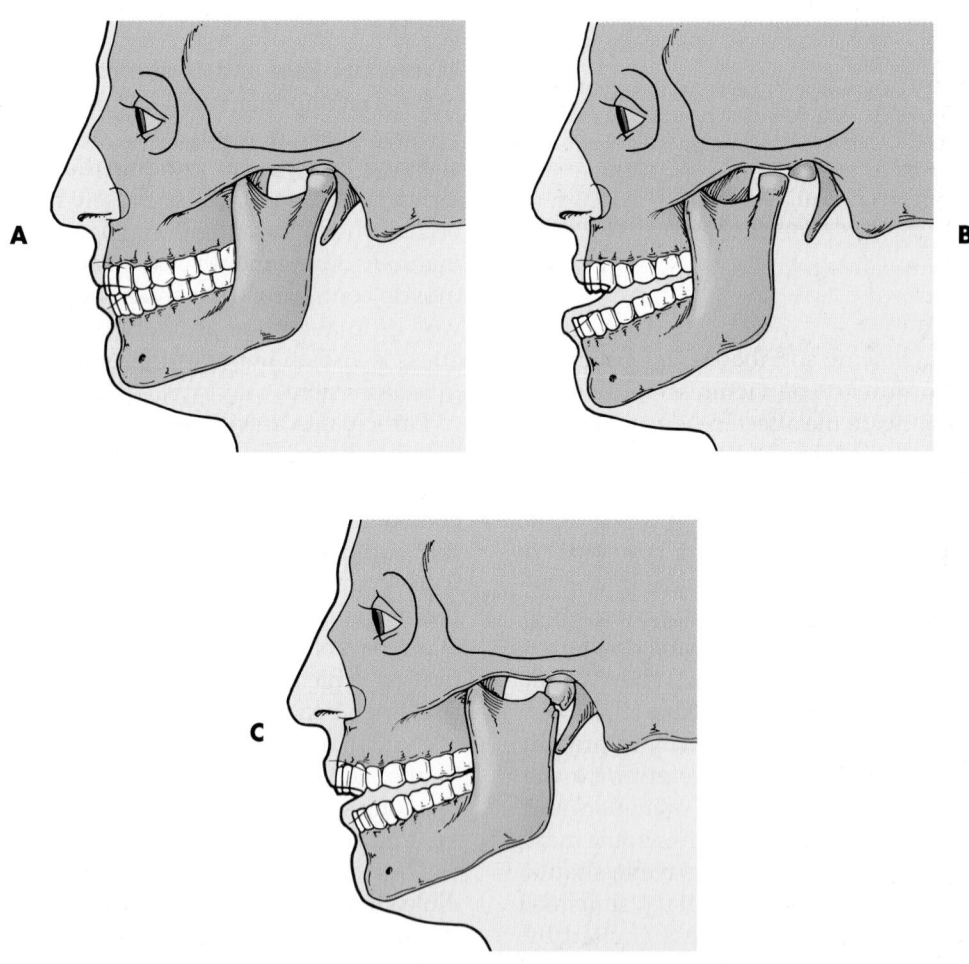

Figure 23-1 Open and closed lock vs. condylar fracture. **A,** The normal temporomandibular joint with cartilaginous disc, shown in blue. **B,** In a mandibular dislocation, the condylar head is anterior to the cartilaginous disc. No teeth are touching. **C,** In a condylar fracture, the joint is positioned normally, but the muscles of mastication have pulled the posterior portion of the mandible upwards, creating premature contact of the posterior teeth.

reduce on mouth opening, the victim may not only have pain, but also limited jaw movement (closed lock). Closed lock can occur suddenly while eating or talking, it may be present on awakening, or it can be associated with trauma. There is joint tenderness, and the chin deviates toward the affected side on attempted mouth opening.[6] Similar restriction of mandibular function may be caused by muscle spasm. However, with myospasm the affected muscles are firm and extremely tender, whereas in closed lock the muscles are usually normal.

The victim can often reduce a closed lock. Have the victim close his or her mouth until the teeth almost touch, then move the mandible as far as possible to the affected side, and finally swing the mouth fully open. If these maneuvers fail after three attempts, consider manual reduction. The rescuer places his thumbs on the victim's lower molars, presses downward, pulls the mandible forward, then gradually moves the mandible up and back.[6] This may require sedation with oral diazepam (Valium) 2 to10 mg.

MAXILLOFACIAL INFECTIONS

Aphthous Ulcers

The etiology of aphthous ulcers is unclear. One opinion is that they represent an autoimmune attack on the oral mucosa, followed by secondary infection. The lesions are round, superficial, and have a red halo. They occur on movable mucosa and can be quite painful. The victim usually gives a history of similar ulcerations. The lesions typically last 10 to 14 days.

Many treatments have been proposed, but none have been found to be predictably effective. The best approach appears to be application of a topical steroid to reduce pain and hasten healing by 3 to 4 days. Mix fluocinonide 0.05% (Lidex) ointment with Orabase and place the mixture gently over each ulcer 6 to 8 times per day, especially after meals and before bedtime. Do not mix the medications until you are ready to apply them, and do not rub the mixture into the lesions. Other options include premixed preparations, such as Kenalog in Orabase, which can be applied to the ulcer 6 to 8 times per day; these preparations are more convenient but deliver only about 10% of the antiinflammatory effect. Dexamethasone (Decadron) elixir (0.5 mg/5 ml, rinse with 5 ml for 2 minutes and expectorate qid) or a systemic steroid (prednisone, 40 mg PO qd for 3 days, then taper) can be used for a very severe case.[20] If these preparations are not available, tincture of benzoin or a topical anesthetic (viscous lidocaine 2%) can be applied to the dried surface of the ulcer before meals and at bedtime to control the pain.

Viral Infections

Herpes labialis (cold sore, fever blister) is the most common oral viral infection. It is characterized by yellow, fluid-filled vesicles that rupture to leave ragged ulcers. Other locations for recurrent herpetic outbreaks include the palate, tongue, and buccal mucosa. The victim can be given acyclovir (Zovirax) 200 mg PO five times daily for 5 days. It is important to begin treatment as soon as the victim becomes aware of a prodromal "tingle" or paresthesia. Use of sun-blocking agents on the lips helps prevent herpes labialis (see Chapter 14).

Primary herpetic gingivostomatitis is characterized by a thin zone of very red, painful gingiva just next to the teeth. Other areas of mucosa, such as the tongue, may also be involved, and close inspection may reveal tiny vesicles or ulcers. Sore throat, lymphadenopathy, and low-grade fever are also present. This and other viral infections of the oral cavity are self-limited. The victim should be reassured that the condition will resolve in about 10 days. Treatment involves the use of an analgesic (ibuprofen 600 mg PO q6h prn pain) and soothing mouth rinses such as warm saline or a mixture of equal amounts of diphenhydramine (Benadryl) elixir 12.5 mg/5ml with kaolin-pectin (Kaopectate) and viscous lidocaine 2% (rinse and expectorate 5 ml q2h).

Yeast Infections

Oral yeast infections occur most commonly in persons who are debilitated, immunocompromised, or taking an antibiotic. Classic oral candidiasis (thrush) is characterized by white patches on the mucosa that can be rubbed off, leaving a red and raw surface. Candidiasis can also present as an erythematous mucosa without any white patches, or as chronic angular cheilitis. Candidiasis is treated with an antimycotic mouth rinse (nystatin oral suspension 100,000 units/ml, rinse with 5 ml for 2 minutes and swallow qid for 10 days) or lozenges (clotrimazole [Mycelex] troche 1 qid, leave in mouth 5 minutes and expectorate remains). In the field, nystatin preparations meant for vaginal treatment can be used (Mycostatin vaginal suppository used as an oral lozenge tid for 10 days).

Bacterial Infections

A bacterial infection in the maxillofacial region can become a serious health threat. In a wilderness setting, it should be treated aggressively. The majority of odontogenic infections are caused by mixed populations of aerobic and anaerobic bacteria. These organisms are almost always present as normal oral flora, but because of a change in the relative numbers of various bacteria or because of a change in the oral environment, an infection can become aggressive.

The behavior of an organism, such as the production of collagenase or hyaluronidase, determines the clinical presentation. Thus an infection may present as a diffuse cellulitis or localize as an abscess. Oral infections generally spread slowly, but rapid spread to a deep facial space can occur. Regional lymphadenopathy is common, whereas severe systemic symptoms are rare. Although bone is often involved, osteomyelitis is uncommon.

Acute Apical Abscess/Cellulitis. An acute apical infection begins with bacteria invading the dental pulp. The infection then spreads to surrounding bone through the apical foramen and then along the path of least resistance. Because the apices of most teeth are located closer to the facial aspect of the jaw, swelling is much more common in the facial soft tissues, as opposed to those on the lingual or palatal side.

The victim presents with pain and swelling, often fluctuant and usually in the buccal vestibule. There is often a history of prior toothache, but at this stage tooth pain is often absent. The offending tooth can be localized by percussion, the site of the swelling, the condition of the teeth, and by using radiographs if available. The affected tooth does not respond at all to hot or cold. The victim may be dehydrated from decreased fluid intake.

The primary treatment for an apical abscess (Figure 23-2). is drainage.[5,7] This can be accomplished with incision, extraction, or endodontic therapy. The treatment chosen depends on the equipment and personnel available, the advisability of retaining the offending tooth, and ultimately, on clinical judgment. An antibiotic is necessary only if complicating factors exist[5,7,17] (Box 23-2). Penicillin (Pen VK 500 mg PO qid) is the most commonly used antibiotic in dental practice,[17] but a cephalosporin, such as cephalexin (Keflex) 500 mg PO qid, typically carried on wilderness expeditions, is acceptable. Combination antibiotic therapy is not indicated except for life-threatening sepsis or when organisms particularly sensitive to combination therapy have been identified. There is some evidence that hesitance to obtain drainage combined with over-reliance on chemotherapy can lead to serious exacerbation of dental infections.[7]

Incision and Drainage. Incision and drainage (I and D) is often the treatment of choice in an emergency situation. An I and D can be performed by someone other than a dentist using commonly available supplies. It is indicated for fluctuant swelling caused by an apical abscess, and it may also be effective for nonfluctuant swelling associated with infection. Infiltration of a local anesthetic helps to reduce the pain of incision. If a local anesthetic is unavailable, adequate anesthesia can often be obtained by applying cold to the area to be incised, using ice, snow, or frigid water. An incision is made down to bone in one swift motion and a knife blade or the beak of a hemostat is used to spread the incision. A T-shaped drain may be improvised from a piece of latex glove (Figure 23-3) and retained without sutures. Hydration, a soft diet, an analgesic (ibuprofen 600 mg PO q6h prn pain), and warm saline rinses are helpful postoperative measures.

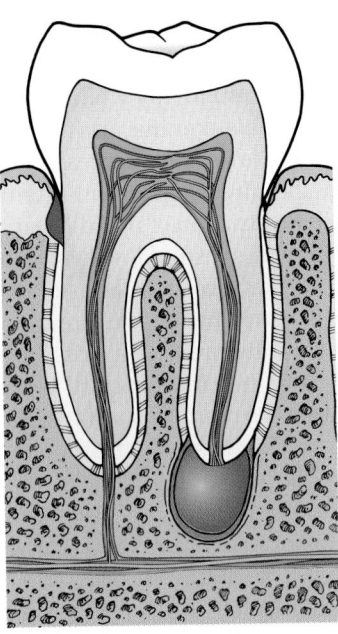

Figure 23-2 The left side of the figure shows a periodontal abscess. A periapical abscess is depicted on the right.

Box 23-2 INDICATIONS FOR ANTIBIOTIC USE IN DENTAL EMERGENCIES

Prophylaxis for persons at risk of bacterial endocarditis
Prophylaxis for persons having prosthetic joint implants within the past 2 years
Local infections
    If the victim is immunocompromised
    If drainage cannot be established
    If there will be a long delay to definitive care
Disseminated infections
    Lymphadenopathy
    Fascial plane involvement
    Systemic symptoms (fever, chills, malaise)
Compound maxillofacial fractures, including all fractures of tooth-supporting bone
Exarticulation (avulsion) of teeth
Soft tissue wounds open for 6 hours or more before closure
Surgical procedures under nonsterile conditions

Deep Fascial Space Infections. An acute apical infection occasionally spreads beyond the local region. The rescuer should be suspicious of any dental infection that causes swelling or tenderness in the floor of the mouth, swelling of the tongue, dysphagia, breathing difficulty, or trismus, or that fails to respond to appropriate therapy. The most commonly involved fascial spaces are the canine, buccal, masticator, and submandibular spaces.

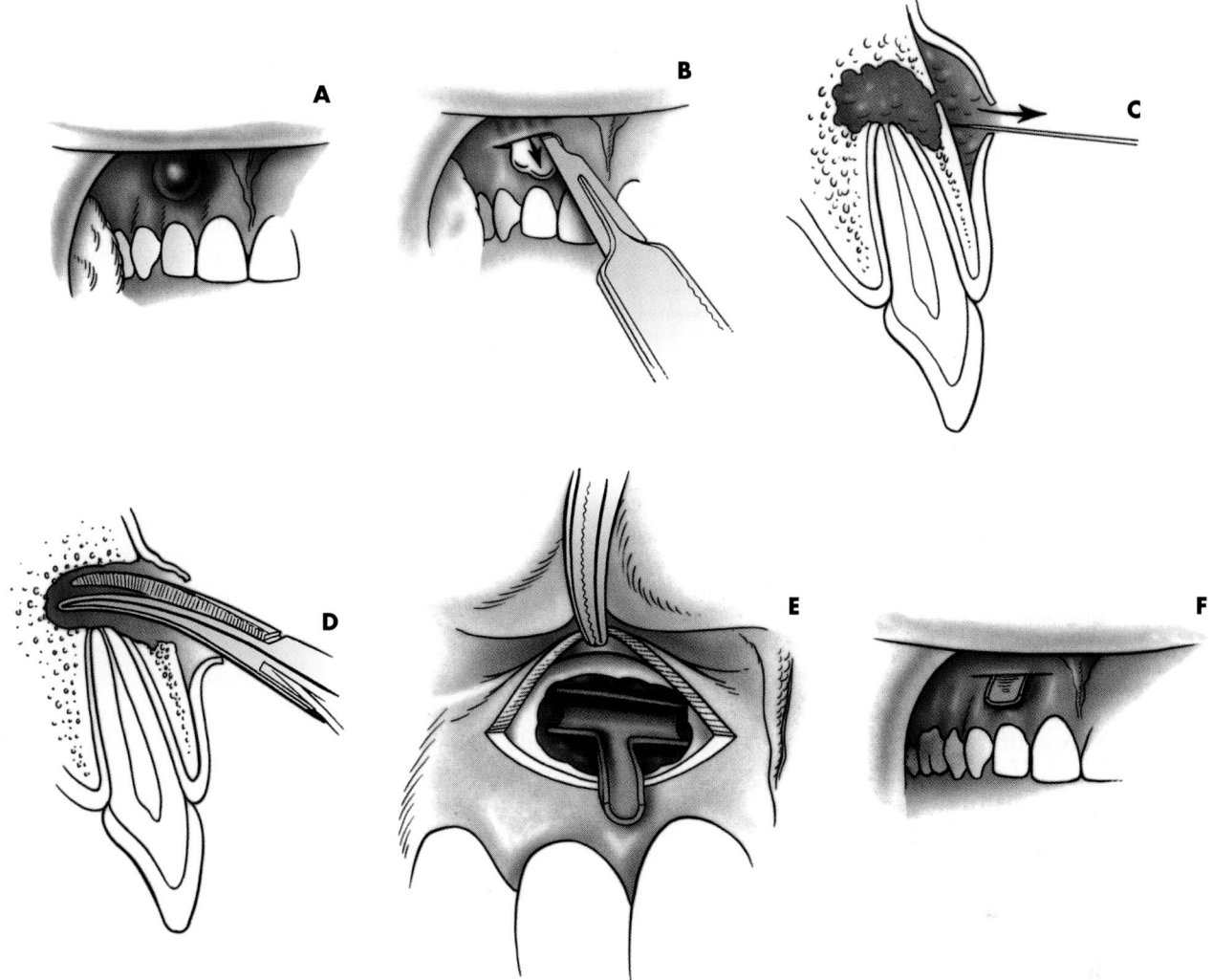

Figure 23-3 Incision and drainage technique. **A,** Fluctuant abscess. **B,** Abscess incised with scalpel. Purulent drainage is removed by suction or caught in gauze sponges. **C,** Cross section showing incision carried to the bone. **D,** The incision is spread with a hemostat. **E,** A "T" drain will often stay in place without sutures. **F,** Drain in place. (*Redrawn from Ingle JI, Beveridge EE:* Endodontics, *ed 2, Philadelphia, 1976, Lea & Febiger.*)

The canine space is located lateral to the nose. Infection originates in the maxillary canine tooth, and swelling causes the eye to close. The infection is drained through an intraoral approach over the root of the canine tooth.

Buccal space infection is characterized by a rounded swelling of the cheek. The offending teeth are the maxillary and mandibular molars. Drainage is obtained extraorally through an incision below the lower border of the mandible that will hide the scar.

The masticator space is divided into the masseteric, pterygoid, superficial temporal, and deep temporal spaces, all of which communicate. The hallmark of involvement is trismus. Swelling may be minimal because of the deep location of the abscess. The masseteric and pterygoid spaces are drained at the angle of the mandible, whereas the temporal space may be drained from an intraoral approach or through an incision just superior to the zygomatic arch.

The mylohyoid muscle divides the floor of the mouth into the sublingual and submandibular spaces. These communicate posteriorly and with their counterparts across the midline. An infection originating in a mandibular tooth can involve these spaces. If only the sublingual space is infected, an intraoral approach is used for drainage, avoiding damage to Wharton's duct. If the submandibular space is involved, an extraoral approach is used. All incisions in the facial area are made parallel to the branches of the facial nerve.[8,16]

Fascial space infections are potentially life threatening. The likelihood of widespread sepsis increases, cavernous sinus venous thrombosis and mediastinitis are possible, and the airway may become compromised.[9] The most feared infection is Ludwig's angina, a bilateral submandibular space infection that elevates the tongue, obstructs breathing, and is associated with high mortality. A mild dental infection can progress to a life-threatening emergency in as little as 48 hours.[7]

Treatment of fascial space infections includes airway management, proper hydration and electrolyte balance, aggressive I and D, intravenous antibiotics, and pain control.[7,9,19] Because these objectives are best met in a controlled environment, any person with a suspected fascial space infection should be evacuated immediately.

Chronic Apical Abscess. The hallmark of chronic apical infection is a draining fistula or "gum boil." Because the bacteria have a route to escape, they do not cause pressure or pain, although the tooth may be mildly sensitive when eating. Such an abscess is not truly an emergency, but if the victim is overly concerned that the condition may worsen before definitive care is provided, an antibiotic can be given.

An infected deciduous tooth also usually presents with a fistula and a mild amount of swelling at most. Happily for the child, pain is rarely present. Emergency care involves an antibiotic, with the dosage adjusted for the child's weight; I and D is performed only if the abscess is not draining. Extract the tooth only if it is very loose and it will be weeks until comprehensive care is available.

Periodontal Abscess. A periodontal abscess is an accumulation of pus between the gingiva and the tooth (see Figure 23-2). Swelling is near the gingival margin rather than in the vestibule, as would be the case with a periapical abscess. The tooth is sensitive to percussion, but responds appropriately to hot and cold. There is always a potential communication between the abscess and the mouth. The passage can be found by probing the gingival margin with a small, blunt instrument, using a local anesthetic if available. Gentle probing will establish drainage; no incision is necessary. Hot saline rinses are prescribed, and a rapid recovery is almost invariable.

Pericoronitis. Pericoronitis is an infection of the gingival flap over a partially erupted tooth. The most common site is the mandibular third molar. Pericoronitis is usually caused by streptococci and seldom produces purulence. The condition may mimic streptococcal pharyngitis or tonsillitis. The primary site of infection is always tender, and trismus is a common sign. Field treatment consists of saline irrigation of the space under the flap using a syringe. Place the victim on hot saline rinses every 2 hours and begin antibiotic therapy.

Acute Necrotizing Ulcerative Gingivitis (ANUG). ANUG, also known as *trench mouth*, is characterized by ulceration and blunting of the interdental papillae. The

gingiva between the teeth appears punched out and is covered by a gray/white pseudomembrane, whereas the surrounding gingival tissue is very red. The victim's primary complaint is pain, but he or she may also report gingival bleeding, a metallic taste, and a foul odor. This infection is caused by fusiform bacteria and spirochetes. It usually occurs in young adults with poor oral hygiene, stress, and suboptimal nutrition (conditions that may be present during difficult wilderness expeditions). The most important treatment is gentle debridement of plaque, calculus, and food from around the teeth. Resolution may require several sessions of careful cleaning 1 to 2 days apart. Each session of debridement will result in some healing, which will allow more aggressive treatment the next time. The victim is also given an antibiotic (metronidazole [Flagyl] 500 mg PO qid) and analgesic (ibuprofen 600 mg PO q6h prn pain) and instructed to keep the area clean with good brushing, flossing, and rinsing (warm saline and/or diluted hydrogen peroxide, if available).[4]

EXODONTIA

A dental extraction is considered definitive treatment and should be attempted in the field only under extraordinary circumstances (Box 23-3). Extraction requires trained personnel, specialized instruments, and profound anesthesia, which may be difficult to obtain. Premedication with a sedative and/or narcotic may be necessary. Intraoperative and postoperative complications are common. Providers of emergency care should focus on treating

---

Box 23-3 FACTORS TO CONSIDER BEFORE EXTRACTION OF TEETH

Desires of the victim
Victim's medical history
Available alternative treatments
Difficulty/desirability of evacuation
Certainty of diagnosis (are you sure you have the correct tooth?)
Possible complications if the tooth is not extracted
Factors relating to the difficulty of the procedure
   Mobility or immobility of the tooth
   Position of the tooth
   Condition of tooth structure above the gingiva
   Patient's mouth-opening ability
   Available supplies and instruments
   Experience of rescuers
Possible complications arising from the extraction
   Fractured root(s)
   Fractured alveolus
   Soft tissue injury
   Root tip lost in the sinus
   Prolonged bleeding
   Localized osteitis (dry socket)

pain and infection with local anesthetics, analgesics (ibuprofen 600 mg PO q6h prn pain or hydrocodone 7.5 mg and acetaminophen 750 mg [Vicodin ES] PO q4 to 6h prn pain), I and D, and/or antibiotics (see section on periapical abscess) as appropriate for each case. Extraction or other definitive care can then be rendered after evacuation, and the tooth can often be saved.

Other factors to consider before exodontia are the degree of mouth opening possible, the relationship of the root to the maxillary sinus, the condition of the clinical crown, the alignment of the tooth in the dental arch, and a history of previous endodontic treatment (after root canal treatment, a tooth is usually very brittle).[14] If, after careful consideration of all factors, extraction is deemed the best course of treatment, proceed as follows.

Review the victim's medical history. In a wilderness setting, it is unlikely you will be faced with a case complicated by medical conditions such as a blood dyscrasia, anticoagulant therapy, or severe cardiovascular dis-ease, but you must be certain before the surgery begins. Persons with most types of heart murmurs or recent prosthetic implants should be premedicated with an antibiotic[10] (Boxes 23-4 and 23-5). Consider the emotional state of the victim and decide if sedation is prudent.

Plan the procedure and gather all necessary equipment. Secure a good light source and a means to keep the field dry—either suction or plenty of gauze. It is important to have the victim's head supported. Therefore it may be best to place the victim in a supine position with the head slightly elevated. Obtain good local anesthesia and test by touching the soft tissues with a sharp instrument. A 4 × 4-inch gauze curtain placed in the rear of the victim's mouth will prevent aspiration of teeth and debris.

Teeth are inflexible and brittle. Heavy forces, especially if applied quickly (high acceleration), break teeth. Bone has more flexibility, the degree of which depends on the individual victim. Judiciously applied, moder-

---

Box 23-4   RECOMMENDATIONS FOR ANTIBIOTIC PROPHYLAXIS BEFORE INTRAORAL PROCEDURES LIKELY TO CAUSE SIGNIFICANT BLEEDING

CONDITIONS FOR WHICH PREMEDICATION IS RECOMMENDED

Prosthetic joint replacement if within 2 years of placement, or if victim has insulin-dependent diabetes, previous prosthetic joint infection, or hemophilia
Prosthetic heart valve replacement
Previous endocarditis
Complex cyanotic congenital heart disease
Surgically constructed systemic pulmonary shunt or conduit
Most congenital cardiac malformations other than those listed below
Acquired valvular dysfunction (e.g., rheumatic heart disease)
Hypertrophic cardiomyopathy
Mitral valve prolapse with valvular regurgitation and/or thickened leaflets

CONDITIONS FOR WHICH PROPHYLAXIS IS NOT RECOMMENDED

Isolated secundum atrial septal defect
Surgical repair of atrial septal defect, ventricular septal defect, or patent ductus
Previous coronary artery bypass graft surgery
Mitral valve prolapse without valvular regurgitation
Physiologic, functional, or innocent heart murmur
Previous rheumatic fever without valvular dysfunction
Cardiac pacemaker or implanted defibrillator
Coronary artery stent

Box 23-5   REGIMENS FOR ANTIBIOTIC PROPHYLAXIS BEFORE INTRAORAL PROCEDURES LIKELY TO CAUSE SIGNIFICANT BLEEDING

STANDARD REGIMEN

Amoxicillin 2 g PO 1 hour before procedure

CHILDREN

Amoxicillin 50 mg/kg PO 1 hour before procedure, not to exceed adult dose

UNABLE TO TAKE ORAL MEDICATIONS

Ampicillin 2 g IM/IV 30 minutes before procedure

PENICILLIN ALLERGY (CHOOSE ONE OF THE FOLLOWING)

Clindamycin 600 mg PO 1 hour before procedure
Clindamycin 600 mg IV 30 min before procedure
Clindamycin 20 mg/kg PO 1 hour before procedure (for children)
Clarithromycin 500 mg PO 1 hour before procedure
Cephalexin 2 g PO 1 hour before procedure

From Dajani AS et al: *JAMA* 277:1794, 1997.

ate forces will slowly expand the bone. The exodontist must be attentive to feedback from the forceps because the bone and tooth will "tell you what they want to do." The tooth will eventually be delivered in the same direction as if it continued to erupt. However, do not attempt to "pull" the tooth in that direction initially. The direction of force needed to loosen a tooth depends on the anatomy of the root. A straight, conical root can be loosened by twisting forces. This technique often works well on the upper front teeth. Sometimes a tooth can be removed by alternating 30 seconds of steady pressure toward the cheek with 30 seconds steady pressure in the opposite direction until the root gradually loosens.[23]

A variety of instruments can be used to apply force to the tooth. Elevators are firmly wedged between tooth and bone in the interproximal area. Avoid putting pressure on the adjacent tooth. Forceps should be applied as far apically as possible. Spend plenty of time working the forceps well under the gingiva. Lower molars are often removed with "cowhorn" forceps, which in addition to applying the usual forces, are designed to apply force to the tooth in a coronal direction simply by squeezing the handles. However, an experienced exodontist using careful technique and a single forceps (number 151 universal forceps) will have success extracting almost any nonimpacted tooth, whereas a reckless operator using dozens of specialized instruments will still have difficulty.[23]

Despite the utmost care, a tooth may break during the extraction procedure. If this occurs, stop and take a minute to reevaluate the situation. The root canals will probably now be exposed. If you are treating a case of infection, perhaps drainage can be obtained through the root canal. If you are treating a case of severe pulpitis, perhaps the pulpal tissue can now be removed. Remember that you are rendering emergency care, and it may not be necessary to remove the remaining root at that time. Some teeth are impossible to remove without sectioning, or they can be removed in only one direction.

Once the tooth has been removed, compress the expanded socket using the thumb and forefinger. If the gingiva is quite loose, placing a suture may help speed healing. Have the victim apply direct pressure to the wound by biting firmly on a gauze pack for 30 minutes while sitting in an upright position. Complete hemostasis may require several hours of steady pressure. Caution the victim to avoid rinsing, spitting, tooth brushing, and smoking for 24 hours. Application of cold and the use of an appropriate analgesic will reduce swelling and pain. Beginning the day after surgery, have the victim rinse with warm saline to cleanse the area.

A common postoperative complication is persistent bleeding several hours after the extraction, accompanied by a poorly organized clot that looks like a piece of raw liver growing out of the socket. Remove the "liver clot" and have the victim apply firm, uninterrupted pressure to the socket by biting on a gauze pack for 20 minutes. If the victim cannot do this, the rescuer will have to apply manual pressure. If bleeding continues after 20 minutes, consider packing the socket (e.g., using Gelfoam, Surgicel, or sterile gauze) and/or suturing. Then resume direct pressure. A dry tea bag used as a compress may provide chemical hemostasis because of the tannic acid.

Another postextraction complication is acute alveolar osteitis, or "dry socket." The victim reports moderate to severe pain, foul odor, and a bad taste, beginning about 3 days after a dental extraction. Examination reveals an empty socket and exposed bone caused by loss of the blood clot, but no suppuration. Treatment consists of gentle irrigation with warm saline followed by packing with a strip of gauze dipped in eugenol. Also administer an oral analgesic. Change the pack every 24 to 48 hours until the symptoms subside, which may take up to 10 days. The victim should avoid alcohol, smoking, and carbonated beverages during treatment.

TRAUMA TO THE FACE AND JAWS

It is essential to quickly evaluate the general condition of an injured victim (see Chapter 18).[13] The primary survey identifies and corrects any inadequacy in respiration or circulation. The mouth and pharynx should be examined for foreign bodies, such as blood clots, tooth or bone fragments, or dentures. If the airway is still obstructed, it may be necessary to perform a chin lift or jaw thrust, or insert an oropharyngeal airway to hold the tongue forward (see Chapter 17). Care should be taken not to hyperextend the neck because of the possibility of a cervical spine fracture. If there is no indication of a neck fracture, sometimes merely placing a victim on his side rather than in a supine position facilitates respiratory exchange. If all of these measures fail, endotracheal intubation or performance of a cricothyroidotomy or, less commonly, a tracheotomy may be necessary. Once a victim's airway is secured and he is hemodynamically stable, perform a secondary survey.

Injuries to the Teeth and Supporting Tissues

Question the victim about the time and nature of the accident, symptoms, loss of consciousness, nausea, vomiting, visual disturbances, and headache. A baseline mental status examination and cranial nerve assessment may be warranted. Clean the face, mouth, head, and neck of blood and debris. This will unmask soft tissue injuries and facilitate diagnosis. Gently reflect the lips with teeth closed to examine soft tissues and occlusion. Carefully examine any lacerations to determine if they penetrate through the lip and/or contain foreign material. Examine all of the teeth for fractures. A blow to the chin or a whiplash injury may produce fractures of the posterior teeth as the mandible is forcibly closed. Examine fractured teeth carefully for pulp exposure. This will require drying the teeth with gauze. Tap each tooth with an instrument handle. Tenderness denotes injury to the periodontal ligament, whereas a high-pitched, metallic sound indicates ankylosis. Test each tooth for abnormal mobility. Electrical pulp vitality testing, dental radiographs, and soft tissue radiographs are obtained if available.[2,11,15]

A classification of traumatic injuries to the teeth and supporting structures is given in Box 23-6. Note that these injuries often occur in combination, with one tooth exhibiting two or more injuries, or several teeth exhibiting various sequelae of trauma. Each injury requires definitive treatment, but proper emergency care will improve the prognosis and make the victim more comfortable. Treatment of most injuries requires, or is at least facilitated by, infiltration of a local anesthetic.[2]

Specific Dental Injuries

CROWN INFRACTION. Blows to the teeth sometimes produce small craze lines in the enamel. These superficial fractures look like tiny surface cracks on an old porcelain dish. Reassure the victim that minimal damage has occurred and treatment is not necessary.

Box 23-6 CLASSIFICATION OF DENTAL TRAUMA

INJURIES TO THE HARD DENTAL TISSUES AND PULP

Crown infraction
Uncomplicated crown fracture
Complicated crown fracture
Uncomplicated crown-root fracture
Complicated crown-root fracture
Root fracture

INJURIES TO THE PERIODONTAL TISSUES

Concussion
Subluxation
Intrusive luxation
Lateral luxation
Extrusive luxation
Exarticulation

INJURIES TO THE SUPPORTING BONE

Comminution of alveolar socket
Fracture of alveolar socket wall
Fracture of alveolar process
Fracture of jaw

INJURIES TO SOFT TISSUES

From Andreasen JO, Andreasen FM: *Textbook and color atlas of traumatic injuries to the teeth,* ed 3, St. Louis, 1994, Mosby.

UNCOMPLICATED CROWN FRACTURE. In an uncomplicated crown fracture, the tooth has been fractured, but no pulp tissue is visible. The tooth may be sensitive to cold, but otherwise all tests are within normal limits. No emergency treatment may be necessary. Irritating sharp edges can be smoothed with a fingernail file. If thermal sensitivity is moderate to severe, a soothing topical antiinflammatory dressing (e.g., Intermediate Restorative Material [IRM], L.D. Caulk Co., Milford, Delaware) can be held in place with aluminum foil or adhesive tape.

UNCOMPLICATED CROWN-ROOT FRACTURE. Diagnosis and treatment of an uncomplicated crown-root fracture is identical to the uncomplicated crown fracture, except that the fracture is nearly vertical, leaving a small, chisel-shaped fragment attached only by the palatal gingiva (Figure 23-4). Removal of this mobile fragment will make the victim much more comfortable.

COMPLICATED CROWN FRACTURE. In a complicated crown fracture, the pulp has been exposed. A small exposure that has not been grossly contaminated is capped with calcium hydroxide (Dycal, L.D. Caulk Co., Milford, Delaware) or IRM. If the exposure is large, or if the pulp tissue has been exposed for more than 24 hours, amputate about 2 mm of tissue with a sharp, sterile instrument. If bleeding continues for more than a few minutes, use a cotton pellet soaked in local anesthetic solution, hydrogen peroxide, or Dycal to obtain hemostasis. Fill the top of the canal with Dycal or IRM and protect the tooth as for a crown fracture (Figure 23-5).

COMPLICATED CROWN-ROOT FRACTURE. In a complicated fracture of the crown and root, the tooth has been fractured obliquely, resulting in a mobile fragment at-

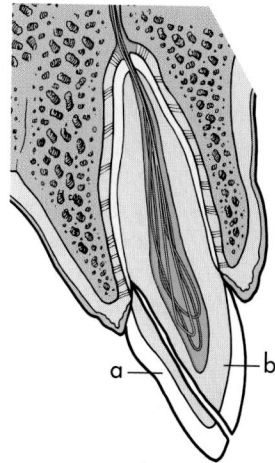

Figure 23-4 Crown-root fracture. The mobile fragment (*a*) should be removed. The larger fragment (*b*) should be left in place.

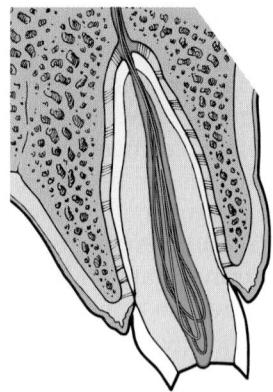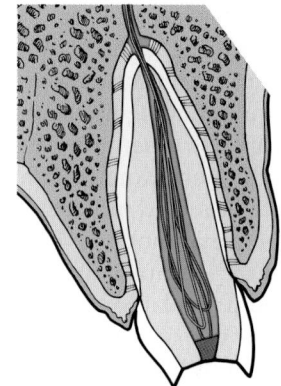

Figure 23-5 Complicated crown fracture. Treatment of a complicated crown fracture.

tached to the palatal gingiva and pulp exposure. First remove the mobile fragment as in a crown-root fracture. Then treat the pulp exposure as in a complicated crown fracture.[2]

ROOT FRACTURE. A root fracture may be difficult to diagnose without radiographs. There will be slight to severe malposition of the crown, but this could be caused by luxation of the entire tooth or a root fracture with luxation of the coronal portion. Reposition the tooth as precisely as possible and splint rigidly (see section on splinting). Hard tissue union of the fragments usually occurs within 3 months. If the coronal portion of the tooth proves impossible to stabilize and definitive treatment is days away, remove the mobile fragment, but do not attempt to extract the apical fragment.[2,15]

CONCUSSION AND SUBLUXATION. Concussion and subluxation injuries to the tooth's supporting structures (i.e., periodontal ligament, bone, and gingiva) cause sensitivity to percussion. The tooth remains in its proper position. However, in subluxation the tooth is abnormally mobile, whereas mobility is normal with concussion. Emergency treatment consists of shortening the opposing tooth so that the victim can occlude comfortably.

INTRUSION. A tooth that has been driven into the bone by a vertical force will demonstrate little mobility and a high-pitched, metallic tone on percussion. Emergency treatment is palliative only. Endodontic treatment (to prevent inflammatory root resorption) and orthodontic extrusion should begin within 2 weeks of injury. Intrusion is associated with a poor long-term prognosis.[2]

EXTRUSION. The extruded tooth is partially displaced from its socket and extremely mobile. Gentle, steady pressure is used to reposition the tooth, allowing time to displace the blood that has collected in the apical region of the socket. After reduction, the tooth is splinted for 2 to 3 weeks. The splint should allow physiologic movement of the injured tooth.

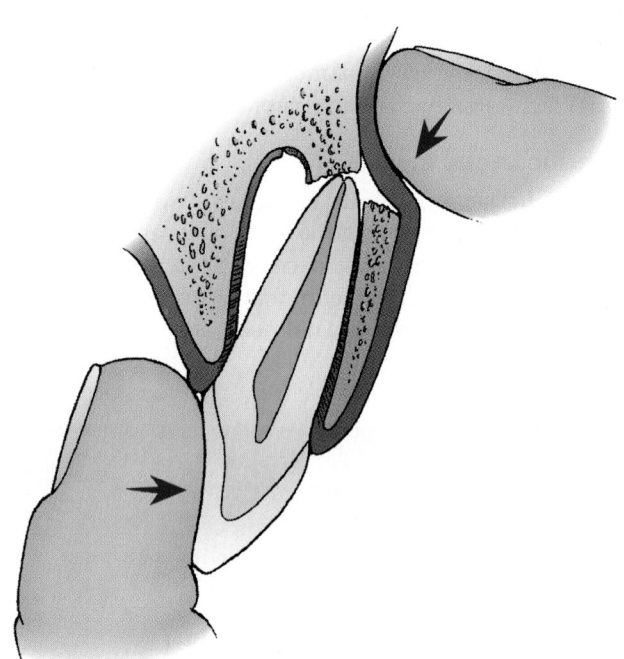

Figure 23-6 Technique used to reduce lateral luxation.

LATERAL LUXATION. In lateral luxation injuries, the tooth is often displaced by a horizontal blow, yet it is not mobile because the apex is locked into its new position in the alveolar bone. A high, metallic tone on percussion is another clue that this has occurred. This injury and its treatment are painful. Figure 23-6 shows how two fingers are used to reduce the tooth. One finger guides the apex down and back while the other repositions the crown.[2] This requires judicious, but sometimes quite firm application of force. The tooth may snap back into position and be quite stable. Splinting is necessary if mobility is present after reduction.

EXARTICULATION. When a tooth is totally avulsed from bone, the prognosis after replantation depends on the health of the periodontal ligament cells, some of which are still attached to the root surface and some of which line the socket wall.[3] To preserve the vitality of these cells, certain guidelines should be observed. Keep the time before replantation to a minimum. Immediate replacement is ideal. If the tooth must be stored, keep it moist. Less than 15 minutes in air is associated with a good prognosis; longer than 2 hours results in a poor prognosis.[3,11] If possible, the tooth should be stored in a Save-A-Tooth container (Smart Practice, Phoenix), which uses a soft mesh to suspend the tooth in Hank's balanced salt solution. Alternative transport mediums are whole milk, saline, the victim's saliva, sports drinks, and water, in that order of preference. The concept is to preserve the health of the periodontal ligament cells in the most isotonic, pH balanced solution at hand. If no container is available, use a plastic bag, plastic wrap, or saturated cloth to keep the tooth from drying. Handle the tooth by the crown only. Never scrub, curette, or use a disinfectant on the root surface; gently rinse with saline to remove debris. When removing clotted blood from the socket, use gentle irrigation and suction, and avoid scraping the socket walls. Ease the tooth back into place with slow, steady pressure. After replantation, nonrigidly splint the tooth for 1 week. Administer an antibiotic for 5 days and give appropriate antitetanus prophylaxis. Endodontic therapy should be instituted within 2 weeks.[3,11,15]

The preferred approach to tooth avulsion or severe luxation is immediate reduction in the field, followed by evacuation for definitive treatment. The next most desirable option is to store the tooth properly and transport victim and tooth for replantation within a few hours of injury. If field conditions prevent either course of action, a delayed replantation procedure is indicated. Store the tooth dry. Three weeks after the injury, the necrotic pulp tissue is removed and the tooth is disinfected, fluoridated, and surgically replanted. The aim of delayed replantation is to produce ankylosis between tooth and bone.[2]

ALVEOLAR SEGMENT FRACTURE. Alveolar segment fracture is characterized by displacement of two or more teeth as a unit. The teeth are not mobile with respect to one another. The apices may be locked into their abnormal position, as in lateral luxation. The segment is repositioned (this may be painful even with local anesthesia), and rigid splinting is placed for 4 to 6 weeks.

Proper Reduction. It is sometimes difficult to know when a displaced tooth has been returned to its proper position. Usually a tooth should be positioned similarly to its contralateral mate. Sometimes asking the victim can help; it may be that one tooth has always been longer than the others, or in a different position. However, occlusion is always the best guide to proper position. If the victim bites and contacts only the injured tooth, further positioning is necessary. In many cases, it is not possible to completely reposition the tooth because of swelling or organized clot formation. There-

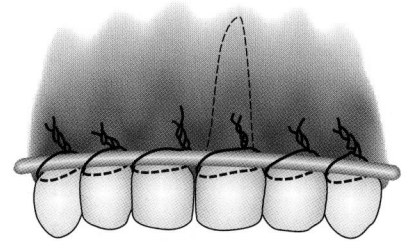

Figure 23-7 Arch bar and wire splint,

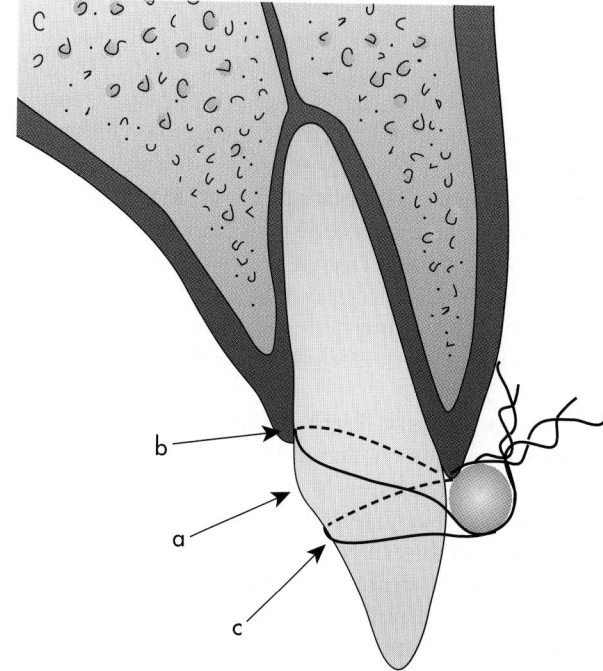

Figure 23-8 Cross sectional view of an arch bar and wire splint. **A,** The widest part of the tooth. **B,** The position of the wire on the stable teeth. **C,** The position of the wire on the mobile tooth or teeth.

fore some adjustment of the opposing tooth (try using an emery board or file from your pocket knife) may be necessary to allow proper occlusion. If the injured tooth receives additional trauma each time the victim bites, it will be uncomfortable, and healing will not occur.

Splinting. When the goal of splinting is to establish a normal, fibrous union between the tooth and the bone, a short-term, nonrigid technique is used. When hard tissue union is desired (e.g., with root fracture or alveolar segment fracture), longer-term rigid splinting is used.[2] Ideally, a single avulsed or loosened tooth is usually bonded to the adjacent tooth or teeth with the acid etch and composite technique.[2,15] For fractures of the jaws or alveolar segments, arch bars and wire splints are often used (Figures 23-7 and 23-8). The rescuer lacking adequate materials must use ingenuity and improvisation to splint teeth. During a very short evacuation, the victim could hold the tooth in approximate position

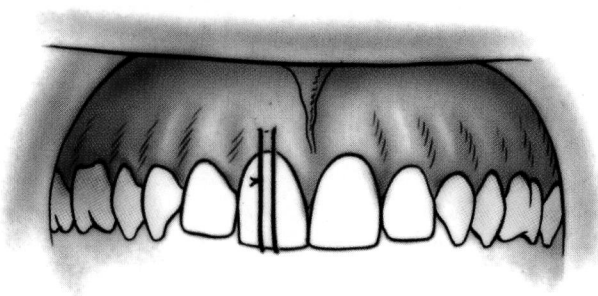

Figure 23-9 Suture used to stabilize a loose or avulsed tooth. The suture also passes through the palatal tissue (hidden from view).

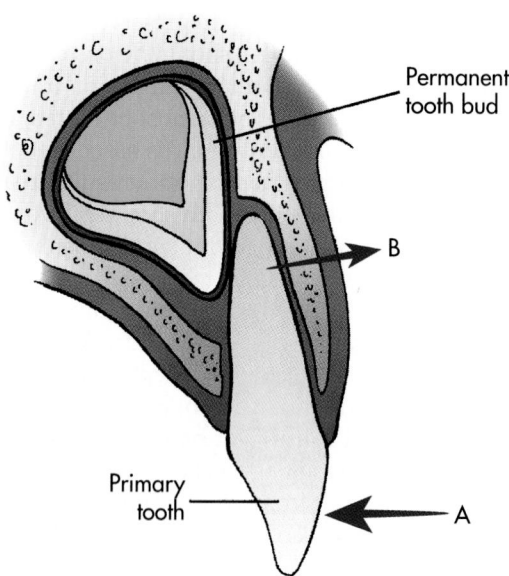

Figure 23-10 When a deciduous tooth is traumatized, the typical direction of force as the child falls forward is shown by arrow *A*, and the apex of the deciduous tooth is levered away from the developing tooth bud, as shown by arrow *B*.

by closing on a gauze pad. Softened wax can be adapted to a loosened tooth and the teeth on either side to lend support. Figure 23-9 shows how a suture can be used to hold a tooth in place for a period of a few days. For a sturdier splint, a crude arch bar can be cut from a SAM splint or made from a paper clip and dead-soft wire obtained from copper wiring or twist ties. Note the proper positioning of the wire on the injured tooth and the anchor teeth (see Figure 23-8).

Injuries to Primary Teeth. Injuries to the deciduous teeth offer unique challenges, not the least of which is behavioral management of a young child. Splinting is very difficult because of the small amount of tooth structure available. In general, heroic efforts should not be made to save primary teeth.[2] Exarticulated deciduous teeth should not be replanted. Severely extruded teeth, infected teeth, or those intruded into the developing permanent tooth should be extracted. Because the permanent tooth follicle lies to the lingual side of the primary tooth root, the typical frontal impact displaces the crown toward the palate, but levers the root apex away from the permanent tooth (Figure 23-10). Most minor subluxations and luxations require only symptomatic treatment. As long as the displaced tooth does not interfere with occlusion, reduction is contraindicated. Spontaneous repositioning often occurs over a period of weeks. Fragments of primary roots need not be extracted because normal resorption will still occur.

Epistaxis

Although most cases of nosebleed are trivial, some can become life threatening as a result of respiratory compromise secondary to aspiration of blood, or extensive blood loss resulting in hypotension. Therefore the condition should never be neglected. The nasal mucosa is laced with numerous superficial blood vessels that serve to warm and humidify inspired air. A particularly rich collection of vessels, and a common site of anterior nosebleed, comprise Kiesselbach's plexus on the nasal septum (Figure 23-11). Spontaneous epistaxis is more common in environments that are cold, dry, dusty, or smoke-filled.

In evaluating a victim with epistaxis, first determine if the bleeding is unilateral or bilateral, and whether it is coming from an anterior or posterior site. A nosebleed usually occurs on one side of the nasal cavity. However, in a victim with profuse bleeding, the blood can pass behind the nasal septum and also appear on the unaffected side. Most victims bleed from an anterior site, which can be visualized on intranasal examination. Posterior epistaxis is usually caused by traumatic injury to the sphenopalatine artery (see Figure 23-11). The bleeding point cannot be seen on intranasal examination.

The first step in treating a person with a nosebleed is to have him sit upright with his head tipped slightly forward so that blood will drip passively out of the nose rather than flow posteriorly into the throat, causing choking and possible aspiration or vomiting of swallowed blood. Ask the victim to blow his or her nose to remove any clots. If suction and a nasal speculum are available, the nasal cavity can then be examined to determine the site of bleeding. When there is minor bleeding from the anterior aspect of the nose, the victim can be instructed to pinch the nostrils together for at least 10 minutes. Hold the soft tissues tightly against the septum. Pinching the bony bridge of the nose will not provide direct pressure on the bleeding vessels.

If nose pinching does not stop the bleeding, apply a topical vasoconstrictor. Choices include cocaine 4%,

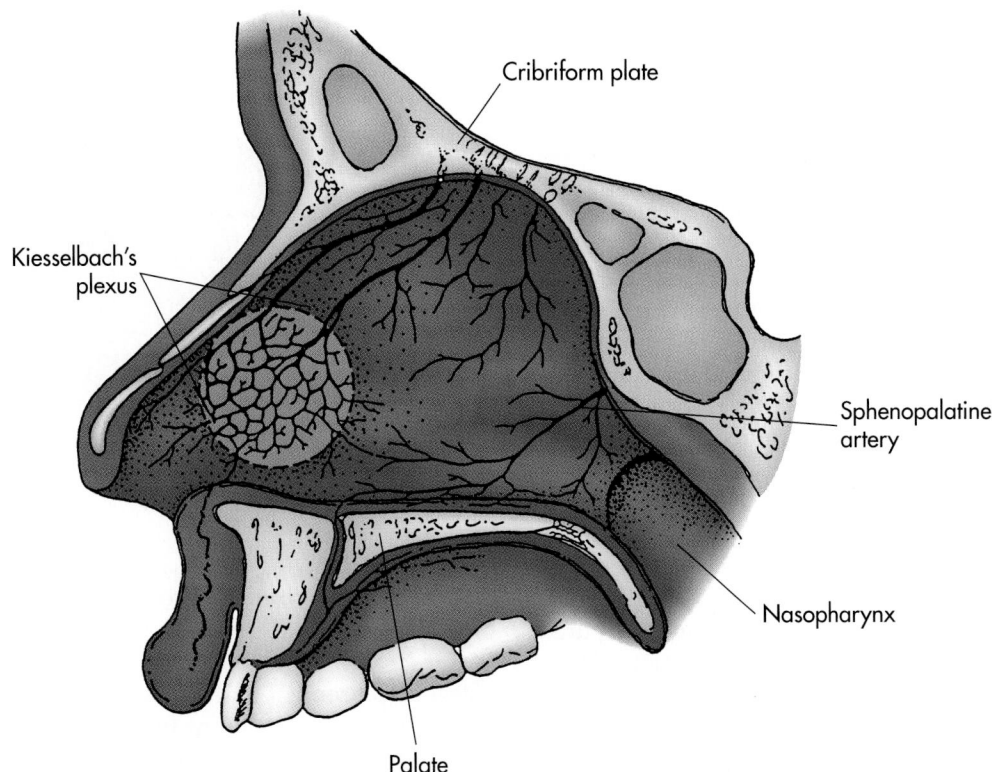

Figure 23-11 Nasal anatomy. Kiesselbach's plexus is the most common site of anterior epistaxis. The sphenopalatine artery is the most common site of posterior epistaxis. Insert tubes and instruments in the direction of the nasopharynx, not the cribriform plate. (*From Fleisher GR, Ludwig S:* Textbook of pediatric emergency medicine, *Philadelphia, 1999, Lippincott Williams & Wilkins.*)

ephedrine 5%, aqueous epinephrine 1:1000, phenylephrine 0.5% (Neo-Synephrine), or oxymetazoline 0.05% (Afrin). Vasoconstrictors can also be found in some local anesthetics, asthma medications, and southwestern desert plants of the genus *Ephedra* (e.g., Mormon Tea, joint-fir, canatilla, tepopote). Vasocontrictors can be applied by drip, spray, on a cotton pledget, or with a cotton-tipped applicator. Objects placed in the nose should have a string attached, or other method of easy removal, and should be aimed posteriorly. Avoid pushing material laterally into the turbinates or superiorly toward the cribriform plate (see Figure 23-11). Leave the vasoconstrictor in place between 10 minutes and 24 hours.

When there is more vigorous anterior nasal bleeding, nose pinching or the topical application of a vasoconstrictor may not be effective. In such an instance, the bleeding site can be injected with 0.5 to 1 ml of lidocaine containing 1:100,000 epinephrine, which will have a tamponading and a vasoconstricting effect. Alternatively, a small piece of oxidized regenerated cellulose (Oxycel or Surgicel), gelatin sponge (Gelfoam), or microfibrillar collagen (Avitene) can be placed directly over the bleeding site. Once the bleeding has stopped, the victim should be instructed not to blow the nose or probe the area for 48 hours. Increasing the humidity of inspired air may help prevent a recurrence of the bleeding. Placing the victim in a tent with several other persons, or with a pot of boiling water, and placing a handkerchief over the victim's nose while outside, will humidify and warm the air before it reaches the nasal mucosa.

If the bleeding cannot be controlled by the previous methods, anterior nasal packing is required. This involves placement of ½-inch strip gauze impregnated with an antibiotic or petroleum jelly into the nasal cavity. The adult victim requires 3 to 4 feet of such gauze to adequately pack the nose and tamponade the bleeding. The gauze is layered in tiers starting on the nasal floor and proceeding to the roof of the nose. Both ends of the gauze are left outside the nose and taped to the face to prevent inadvertent aspiration. Expandable packing (Weimert Epistaxis Packing, Rhino Rocket), with an applicator device for rapid deployment, or a Foley catheter can also be used for anterior nasal tamponade. Because anterior nasal packing blocks sinus drainage and can predispose to sinusitis, the victim should be placed on prophylactic amoxicillin, 875 mg with clavulanic acid 125 mg (Augmentin) PO bid, until the packing is removed in 48 hours.

Because it is not possible to visualize the site of posterior epistaxis, the victim requires a posterior nasal pack or placement of a Foley catheter or nasal balloon.[1] Placing the conventional posterior nasal pack involves first gently inserting a lubricated soft tube into each nostril until the ends can be visualized in the back of the throat, grasped with a hemostat, and brought out through the mouth. Use Foley catheters, nasogastric tubes, chest tubes, or improvised substitutes, such as one of the products used to hold sunglasses in place. A cylindrical pack of 4 × 4-inch gauze pads is prepared and held in shape by tying three silk sutures around it and leaving the ends long. The pack should be the same diameter as a circle made by the victim's thumb and forefinger (the "OK" sign). The two end sutures are attached to the oral ends of the catheters (Figure 23-12). The nasal ends of the catheters are then pulled carefully back out of the nose until the pack is firmly positioned against the posterior aspect of the nasal cavity above the soft palate. The sutures are then detached from the catheters and tied over a bolster placed underneath the nose. The middle suture remains outside of the mouth and is secured externally to be used to remove the pack 48 hours later.

A 14 to 16 French Foley catheter with a 30-ml balloon can also be used as a posterior pack. The lubricated catheter is inserted through the nose into the posterior pharynx, inflated 10 to 15 ml, and then gently pulled back into the nasopharynx and held in position by clamping the external end with a hemostat. Commercially available preshaped nasal balloons can also be used to treat posterior epistaxis.[1] Air is preferred over saline for inflating nasal balloons as a safety precaution in case of breakage.

Nasal Fracture

Because of the prominence of the nose, nasal fracture is the most common facial fracture. It is often accompanied by abrasions, lacerations, and epistaxis. Nasal bleeding should be managed first. Once this bleeding is controlled, any facial wound should be properly cleansed. Local anesthesia may be needed to accomplish removal of foreign material. Plain lidocaine or another local anesthetic without a vasoconstrictor is recommended when injecting the nose. Particulate matter is removed either by irrigation or scrubbing with a sterile brush. This is essential to avoid infection and prevent tattooing.

Abrasions should be covered with an antiseptic or antibiotic ointment (e.g., mupirocin, bacitracin) and washed gently twice daily with a mild soap and warm water to prevent crusting. Small laceration edges can be reapproximated with tape closure. Deeper lacerations require interrupted sutures. Remove sutures in 3 to 5 days, at which time tape strips can be placed if additional stabilization of wound margins is necessary.

Once soft tissue injuries have been managed, the nose should be assessed for possible fracture by observing it for symmetry from the front and from below. If swelling has already occurred, this may be difficult to determine. However, palpation of the bridge may re-

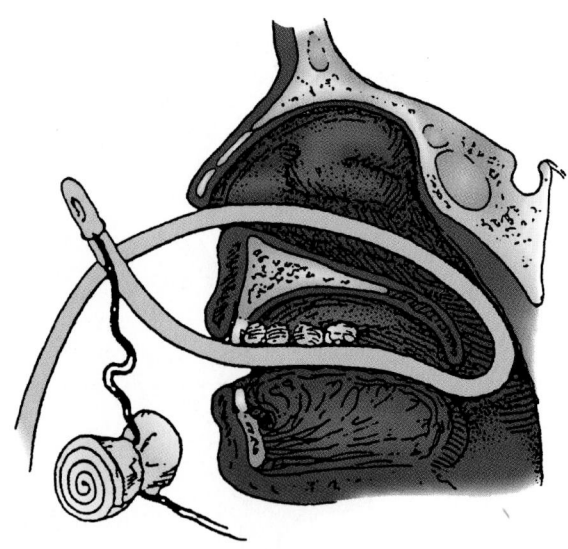

Figure 23-12 Inserting a posterior nasal pack. (*From Fleisher GR, Ludwig S:* Textbook of pediatric emergency medicine, *Philadelphia, 1999, Lippincott Williams & Wilkins.*)

veal displacement that is not visible, and crepitus can sometimes be felt. Point tenderness may also be indicative of a fracture, but it can also be associated with soft tissue injury.

After external examination of the nose, the interior of the nasal cavity should be examined for lacerations and septal hematoma. Remove blood clots with a swab or suction to improve visibility. Small lacerations may not require treatment, but large lacerations should either be closed with resorbable sutures or covered with Oxycel, Gelfoam, Surgicel, or Avitene to control bleeding. Any deviation, bulging, or widening of the nasal septum may be indicative of a hematoma. However, septal deviation may have been present before the injury. To determine if a hematoma is present, the area can be pressed with a cotton-tipped applicator. A hematoma will feel soft, and the area may be temporarily indented by the pressure.

A septal hematoma needs to be drained to prevent pressure necrosis and loss of nasal support or the formation of a septal abscess, which can also produce destruction of the septum. The area is anesthetized by injection of a local anesthetic or the application of a topical anesthetic (benzocaine 20%), and a small incision is made in the most inferior aspect of the hematoma. The nasal passage should then be packed with ½-inch gauze impregnated with petroleum jelly or antiseptic to prevent recurrence of bleeding.

Because most surgeons prefer to treat nasal fracture after the swelling has subsided (5 to 10 days after injury), such an injury does not require immediate treatment.[12] As long as there is no active bleeding, and any abrasions and lacerations have been treated, the victim has at least 3 to 5 days before definitive management is indicated. If the nose appears straight as the swelling subsides, and the victim can breathe easily through both nostrils, there probably was no fracture, or a fracture exists with only minimal displacement and further treatment may not be necessary. In the interim, the nose can be protected from further injury by a splint made by cutting a triangular piece of a SAM splint large enough to fit the contour of the nose. Rest the splint on the adjacent part of the face without placing pressure on the nasal bridge. This shield is held in place by strips of adhesive tape. Nasal packing is not necessary unless it is used to control epistaxis or recurrent septal hematoma. Penicillin VK or amoxicillin 500 mg PO should be administered four times each day for 5 days.

Jaw Fracture

Any person who has suffered a head or facial injury should be examined for a jaw fracture.[13] First, evaluate occlusion by having the victim bite the teeth together. Any deviation of the bite or change in the level of the occlusal plane, especially in the mandible, should raise the suspicion of a fracture. Usually there will also be a tear in the gingival tissues and bleeding and ecchymosis at the site of the discontinuity. A sublingual hematoma is a common sign of a mandibular fracture. In edentulous areas, there will also be a discrepancy in the level of the bone, often accompanied by a disruption in the mucosa.

If no obvious tooth or bone displacement is noted, bimanual examination of the body of the mandible should determine if any abnormal movement can be detected. It is particularly important to evaluate any area of contusion in the soft tissue. In addition to preternatural movement, a grating sound can occasionally be heard when a fracture is present.

The mandibular condyles should be evaluated, especially if the chin has sustained a traumatic blow. A unilateral fracture is suspected when there is a shift of the midline of the mandible to the painful side on mouth opening. A bilateral fracture will often result in an anterior open bite (see Figure 23-1). Normally, the condyles can be palpated by placing a forefinger in front of the external auditory meatus. If the condyle cannot be palpated, or if it does not move significantly when the mouth is opened, a fracture may be present.[13,21]

The maxilla is examined for possible fracture by grasping the anterior segment between the thumb and forefinger and gently rocking the jaw anteroposteriorly and laterally. If a complete (Le Fort I) fracture is present, the entire maxilla will move (Figure 23-13). With a unilateral fracture, only one half of the maxilla will move. If a complete maxillary fracture is detected, the presence of a pyramidal (Le Fort II) fracture extending to the nasal area needs to be considered. The maxilla should again be rocked gently while the bridge of the nose is grasped between the thumb and forefinger of the opposite hand. Any movement of the nasal complex is indicative of a pyramidal fracture. Because this fracture also extends through the infraorbital rim, this

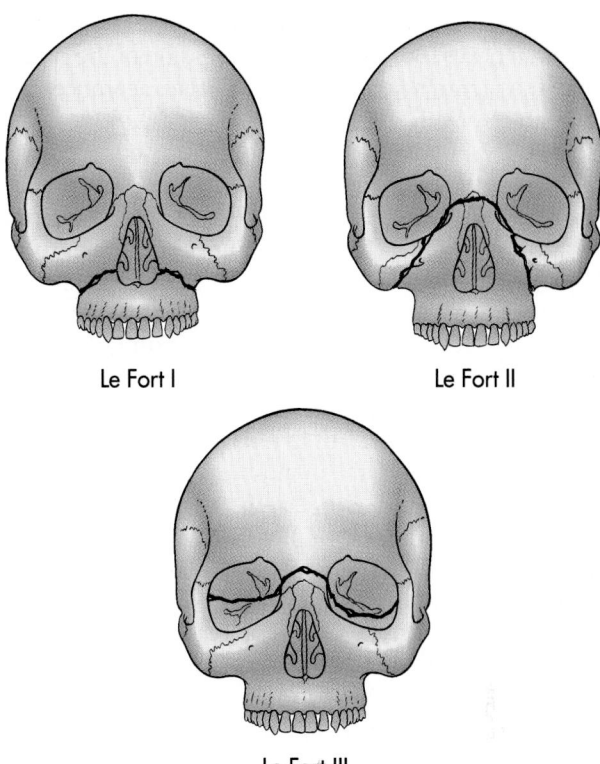

Figure 23-13 Classification of midface fractures. (*Redrawn from* Oral and maxillofacial surgery services in the emergency department, *Rosemont, IL, 1992, American Association of Oral and Maxillofacial Surgeons.*)

area should be palpated for the presence of a step deformity. However, care must be taken not to confuse a fracture with the infraorbital foramen, which can also be felt in this region. If a fracture is present, the victim will feel numbness below the eye and in the upper lip and lateral aspect of the nose. This is caused by injury to the infraorbital nerve.

The third type of midface fracture, the Le Fort III, involves detachment of the midface from the base of the skull. This is a complex injury often accompanied by intracranial trauma. There is generally subconjunctival hemorrhage and bilateral periorbital edema and ecchymosis. Usually the eyelids are swollen shut. Laceration of the meninges causes cerebrospinal fluid (CSF) to leak from the nose. To distinguish CSF from mucus, hold a clean, white handkerchief under the nose for a moment and then allow the material to dry. Mucus will stiffen the fabric, whereas CSF will dry as a double ring without stiffening the fabric. When CSF rhinorrhea is suspected, an antibiotic (penicillin VK 500 mg PO qid) should be administered, but the nose should not be packed.

Fractures of the zygomaticomaxillary complex generally result from a blow to the cheek. The most common findings are subconjunctival hemorrhage and ecchymosis and swelling of the lids. There may be double vision caused by displacement of the globe and/or entrapment of extraocular muscles. As with a Le Fort II fracture, there is numbness in the distribution of the infraorbital nerve. Because of the depression of the cheekbone, the victim's face will have a flat appearance.

Fracture of the zygomatic arch can occur as an isolated injury. Such a fracture results in a depression on the lateral aspect of the face. Because the coronoid process of the mandible is located beneath the zygomatic arch, this type of fracture can also result in inability to fully open the mouth.[13]

The best treatment for a jaw fracture is immediate immobilization. Even if perfect alignment is not achieved, fixation will make the victim more comfortable, reduce bleeding, and avoid further displacement of the fragments. Fractures that pass through the tooth-supporting portion of the mandible may be quickly stabilized with a bridle wire, or more securely held with an arch bar (see Figure 23-7). Fractures in more posterior locations can be temporarily immobilized with a bandage (Figure 23-14), which should pull the mandible in a superior direction. Do not pull the chin posteriorly, because this can displace the fracture and compromise the airway. More rigid fixation can be obtained with intermaxillary wiring, which involves placing arch bars on upper and lower arches, placing the teeth in proper occlusion, and then connecting the upper arch bar to the lower bar with elastics or thin wire.

A posteriorly displaced Le Fort fracture should be disimpacted using forward traction. If the mandible is intact, the maxilla can be held in place by forcing mouth props (commercially available or improvised) between the upper and lower molars. Significant bleeding from the nasal cavities sometimes accompanies midface fractures. However, any tamponade of the nasal cavities will displace the mobile maxilla inferiorly unless it is first stabilized from below with mouth props.

A victim with facial bone fractures should be evacuated to a hospital for definitive treatment. In the interim, an antibiotic (penicillin VK 500 mg PO qid) and pain medication should be given. However, strong narcotics should be avoided if there is an associated head injury to avoid respiratory depression in an already obtunded victim.

Soft Tissue Injuries

Wounds of the oral mucosa and face should be treated after repair of the dental injuries and jaw fractures. Lacerations are likely to be reopened if closed before intraoral manipulations. Soft tissue injuries should be thoroughly irrigated and cleansed of foreign debris to prevent infection and tattooing. Tissue debridement should be very conservative. The excellent blood supply to this region means that wounds can be closed with sutures or other wound closures with little fear of infection if treatment can be accomplished within 6 hours of the injury. Sutures should be removed in 3 to 5 days, after which tape strips can be placed for additional stabi-

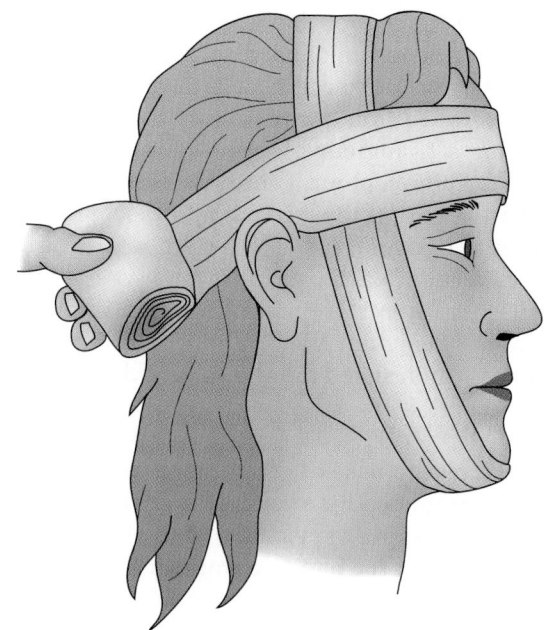

Figure 23-14 A simple bandage can be used to temporarily stabilize a jaw fracture.

lization of the wound margins. Facial abrasions should be gently washed twice daily with mild soap and warm water and then covered with an antiseptic ointment to prevent crusting. Small lacerations of the oral mucosa need not be closed. Use direct pressure for hemostasis.

Through and through lacerations, which are common in the lower lip, are first closed intraorally, after which the remainder of the wound is closed in layers from an extraoral approach. A laceration crossing the vermilion border of the lip requires careful alignment to avoid disfigurement. Deep lacerations of the soft palate will involve the muscles and must be closed in layers. Maintain traction on the tongue while lingual lacerations are sutured. Have an assistant or the victim grasp the tongue with gauze and hold it forward. After any intraoral repair, have the victim avoid rinsing for 24 hours and advise a liquid, nondairy diet. After this period, initiate rinsing four times a day with warm saline, chlorhexidine gluconate 0.12%, or diluted peroxide.

A facial laceration may be complicated by damage to associated structures (Figure 23-15). Injury to the lacrimal drainage system is present if a probe inserted into the punctum at the medial corner of the lid emerges into the laceration. Damage to the parotid duct should be suspected if there is leakage from the wound when Stensen's duct is irrigated with saline. Evidence of facial nerve damage is sought by observing the victim move the eyebrows, eyelids, and mouth. If facial nerve injury occurs behind a vertical line through the lateral canthus of the eye, evacuation for immediate repair is recommended.

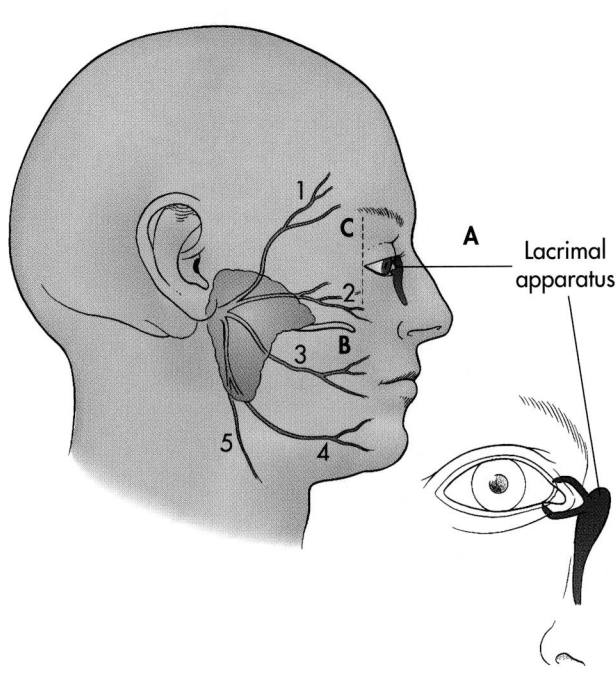

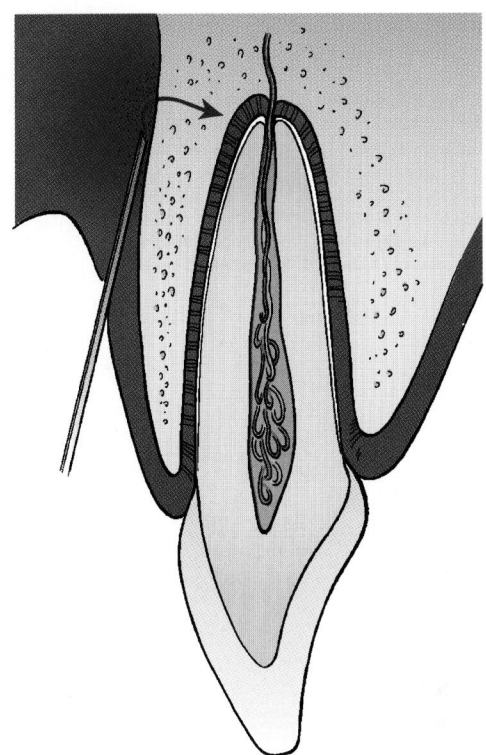

Figure 23-15 Structures that may be injured by facial lacerations. **A,** The lacrimal drainage system. **B,** The parotid duct. **C,** A line drawn through the lateral canthus of the eye. Facial nerve injuries posterior to this line should be repaired as soon as possible. *1-5,* branches of cranial nerve VII. (*Redrawn from* Oral and maxillofacial surgery services in the emergency department, *Rosemont, IL, 1992, American Association of Oral and Maxillofacial Surgeons.*)

Figure 23-16 Technique for infiltration of a local anesthetic.

Orthodontic Emergencies

Orthodontic appliances sometimes cause soft tissue irritation or ulceration. Cover the offending fixture with soft wax. Sometimes a protruding wire can be bent until the sharp portion faces away from the soft tissues. If a bracket or wire becomes excessively loose, it can usually be removed with judicious tinkering. If a wire needs to be cut and small wire cutters are unavailable, try repeatedly bending the appliance until the metal fatigues and breaks.

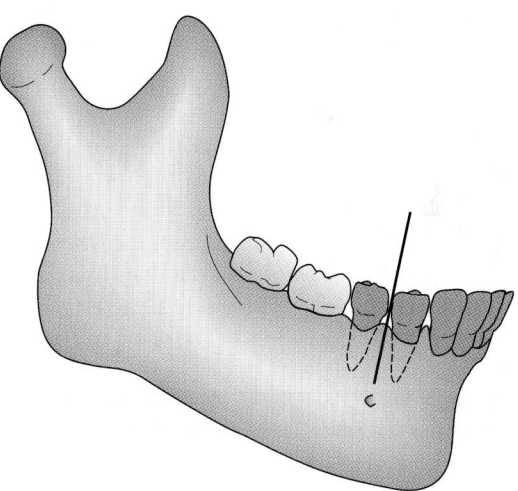

Figure 23-17 Technique for blocking the inferior alveolar nerve near the mental foramen. The shaded teeth will be anesthetized.

LOCAL ANESTHESIA

Local anesthesia is a prerequisite to many emergency dental, oral, and maxillofacial procedures. Anesthesia of any upper tooth and the associated buccal soft tissues can be obtained by infiltration. Approximately 2 ml of a local anesthetic solution is placed as close to the apex of the tooth as possible, just above the periosteum. By holding the syringe parallel to the long axis of the tooth, the needle tip is guided in the proper direction (Figure 23-16). Two percent lidocaine with 1:100,000 epinephrine is commonly used, although 2% bupivacaine with 1:200,000 epinephrine (Marcaine) is useful

for long-term pain relief. Other available local anesthetics can be substituted.

The mental nerve block is a simple method for obtaining anesthesia of the teeth and buccal mucosa from the second premolar forward. Proceed as for the infiltration, except that the target area is the mental foramen, located between the apices of the lower first and second premolars (Figure 23-17). After depositing the solution, gently massage the area for about 30 seconds.

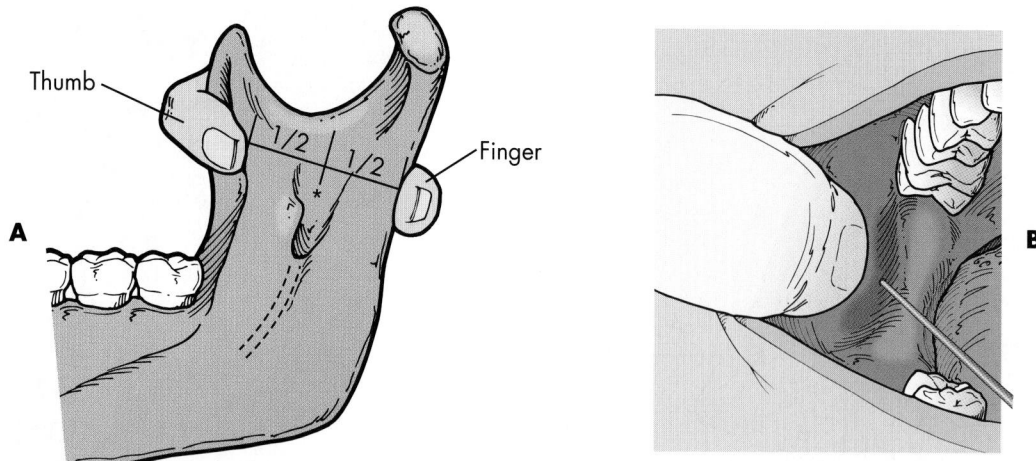

Figure 23-18 When administering the inferior alveolar block, the target area **(A)** lies on the medial surface of the mandibular ramus, halfway between the rescuer's thumb and forefinger. Keep the syringe parallel to the occlusal plane, as shown in **B.**

The inferior alveolar nerve block is more difficult to learn, but it produces anesthesia of all of the lower teeth up to the midline and the buccal soft tissues forward of the mental foramen. The lingual nerve is also blocked by this injection, producing numbness of the anterior two thirds of the tongue and lingual gingiva. Figure 23-18, *A*, shows how the deepest concavity on the anterior border of the mandibular ramus is palpated by the thumb while the deepest concavity on the posterior border is palpated by the index finger. The target area is then halfway between the rescuer's thumb and index finger.[22] In Figure 23-18, *B*, the syringe is kept parallel to the plane of the lower teeth, and the mucosa is punctured just medial to the rescuer's thumbnail. When bone is contacted in the target area, the anesthetic solution is deposited. Experienced dentists miss the target area, and thus fail to produce adequate anesthesia, in about 10% of injections.[22]

DENTAL FIRST-AID KIT

Items necessary to manage dental emergencies can be added to a wilderness first-aid kit without a large sacrifice of space or weight. Cavit (Premier Co., Norristown, Pennsylvania) is temporary filling material that requires no mixing and is easy to use. Squeeze a small amount of the material from the tube and place it in the tooth. Wet a dental packing instrument (or cotton-tip applicator or toothpick) to prevent sticking and pack the Cavit well. Then remove any excess. Have the victim bite to displace material that would interfere with occlusion. The filling material will set in a few minutes after contact with saliva.

Zinc oxide/eugenol cements (Intermediate Restorative Material [IRM], L.D. Caulk Co., Milford, Delaware) consist of a liquid and a powder. Start with two drops of the liquid and begin mixing in the powder. Keep adding powder to make a dough that is as dry as possible. Dip the instruments in some powder to keep the mixture from sticking. Insert and shape the filling material as explained previously. Zinc oxide/eugenol cements have several advantages compared to Cavit. They are significantly stronger and can be mixed to a doughy stage for filling or slightly thinner for use as a cement. Most important is the soothing effect of eugenol on teeth with pulpitis. However, the liquid often leaks from its container, lending a pervasive odor to the backpack and tent; wind tends to blow the powder away; and the material is difficult to mix and is a sticky mess to insert into the tooth.

A more complete kit for extended expeditions should include a number 151 universal extraction forceps and a straight elevator for extracting teeth. A mouth mirror, orthodontic wax, dental floss, dental syringe, 30-gauge needles, and anesthetic cartridges complete the kit. These items fit in a small case and weigh about 14 ounces. A custom dental first aid kit is preferred over commercial dental "travel kits" that contain unnecessary items and lack essential ones.

In an outdoor situation, techniques must often be adapted or improvised depending on the items available. For example, Figure 23-9 shows how a suture can be used to splint an avulsed or extruded tooth. A temporary filling can be fashioned from softened candle wax, an emery board can be used to smooth a sharp tooth, or a pocket knife can be used to perform a drainage procedure.

PREVENTION

The vast majority of dental emergencies can be prevented, beginning with pretrip planning. Before any extended travel in a remote area, each person should have a thorough dental examination, radiographs, periodontal care, and treatment of potentially troublesome teeth. The Peace Corps requires certification that examination and treatment have been performed before assignment to developing countries. The National Science Foundation has similar requirements, and in addition requires impacted and unopposed third molars to be extracted before travel to Antarctica.

Once in the wilderness, minimal precautions can have significant effects. Lip balm with sunscreen can inhibit herpes labialis outbreaks. Routine personal oral hygiene will prevent many odontogenic infections and painful inflammatory conditions. Ideal care should include twice daily tooth brushing and flossing. Toothpaste is not essential, because mechanical removal of plaque and stimulation of the gingiva are the most important aspects of oral care. The fuzzy end of a hickory twig can be used if a toothbrush is not available. In the wilderness, daily oral hygiene not only helps prevent dental emergencies, but it also contributes to an overall sense of well-being and helps buoy morale when, for example, an expedition is tent-bound by bad weather.

Helmets are essential for preventing trauma in rock climbing, white-water kayaking, and mountain biking. It is estimated that custom-made mouth guards prevent over 200,000 injuries every year in interscholastic sports.[18] Their use in backcountry recreation, now almost nonexistent, would probably also be very beneficial in appropriate circumstances.

REFERENCES

1. Abelson TI: Epistaxis. In Paparella MM et al, editors: *Otolaryngology,* ed 3, Philadelphia, 1991, WB Saunders.
2. Andreasen JO, Andreasen FM: *Textbook and color atlas of traumatic injuries to the teeth,* ed 3, St Louis, 1994, Mosby.
3. Andreasen JO et al: Replantation of 400 avulsed permanent incisors: factors related to periodontal ligament healing, *Endo Dent Traumatol* 11:76, 1995.
4. Antonelli JR: Acute dental pain. Part I. Diagnosis and emergency treatment, *Compendium* 11:492, 1990.
5. Baker KA, Fotos PG: The management of odontogenic infections: a rationale for appropriate chemotherapy, *Dent Clin North Am* 38:689, 1994.
6. Blank LW: Clinical guidelines for managing mandibular dysfunction, *Gen Dent* 46:592, 1998.
7. Bridgeman A, Wisenfeld D, Newland S: Major maxillofacial infections: an evaluation of 107 cases, *Aust Dent J* 41:281, 1995.
8. Bridgeman A, Wisenfeld D, Newland S: Anatomical considerations in the diagnosis and management of acute maxillofacial bacterial infections, *Aust Dent J* 41:238, 1996.
9. Chow AW: Life-threatening infections of the head and neck, *Clin Infect Dis* 14:991, 1992.
10. Dajani AS et al: Prevention of bacterial endocarditis: recommendations by the American Heart Association, *JAMA* 277:1794, 1997.
11. Diangelis AJ, Bakland LK: Traumatic dental injuries: current treatment concepts, *JADA* 129:1401, 1998.
12. Doerr TD et al: Nasal fractures. In Cummings CW et al, editors: *Otolaryngology head and neck surgery,* vol 2, St. Louis, 1998, Mosby.
13. Haug RH, Likavec MJ: Evaluation of the craniomaxillofacial trauma patient. In Greenburg AM, editor: *Craniomaxillofacial fractures,* New York, 1993, Springer-Verlag.
14. Hooley JR, Golden DP: Surgical extractions, *Dent Clin North Am* 38:217, 1994.
15. Josell SD: Evaluation, diagnosis, and treatment of the traumatized patient, *Dent Clin North Am* 39:15, 1995.
16. Laskin D: Anatomic considerations in diagnosis and treatment of odontogenic infections, *JADA* 69:308, 1964.
17. Okeson JP, editor: *Orofacial pain: guidelines for assessment, diagnosis, and management,* Carol Stream, IL, 1996, Quintessense Publishing Co.
18. Padilla R, Dorney B, Balidov S: Prevention of oral injuries, *CDAJ* 24:30, 1996.
19. Sands T, Pynn BR, Katsikeris N: Odontogenic infections: microbiology, antibiotics, and management, *Oral Health* 85:11, 1995.
20. Svirsky JA: Recurrent aphthous ulcerations, *Va Dent J* 69:8, 1992.
21. Tiner BD: Facial fractures. In Montgomery MT, Redding SW, editors: *Oral-facial emergencies,* Portland, Ore, 1994, JBK Publishing.
22. Trebus DL, Singh G, Meyer RD: Anatomical basis for inferior alveolar nerve block, *Gen Dent* 46:632, 1998.
23. Zambito RF, Zambito ML: Exodonture: technique and art, *NY State Dent J* 58:33, 1992.

Rescue and
Survival

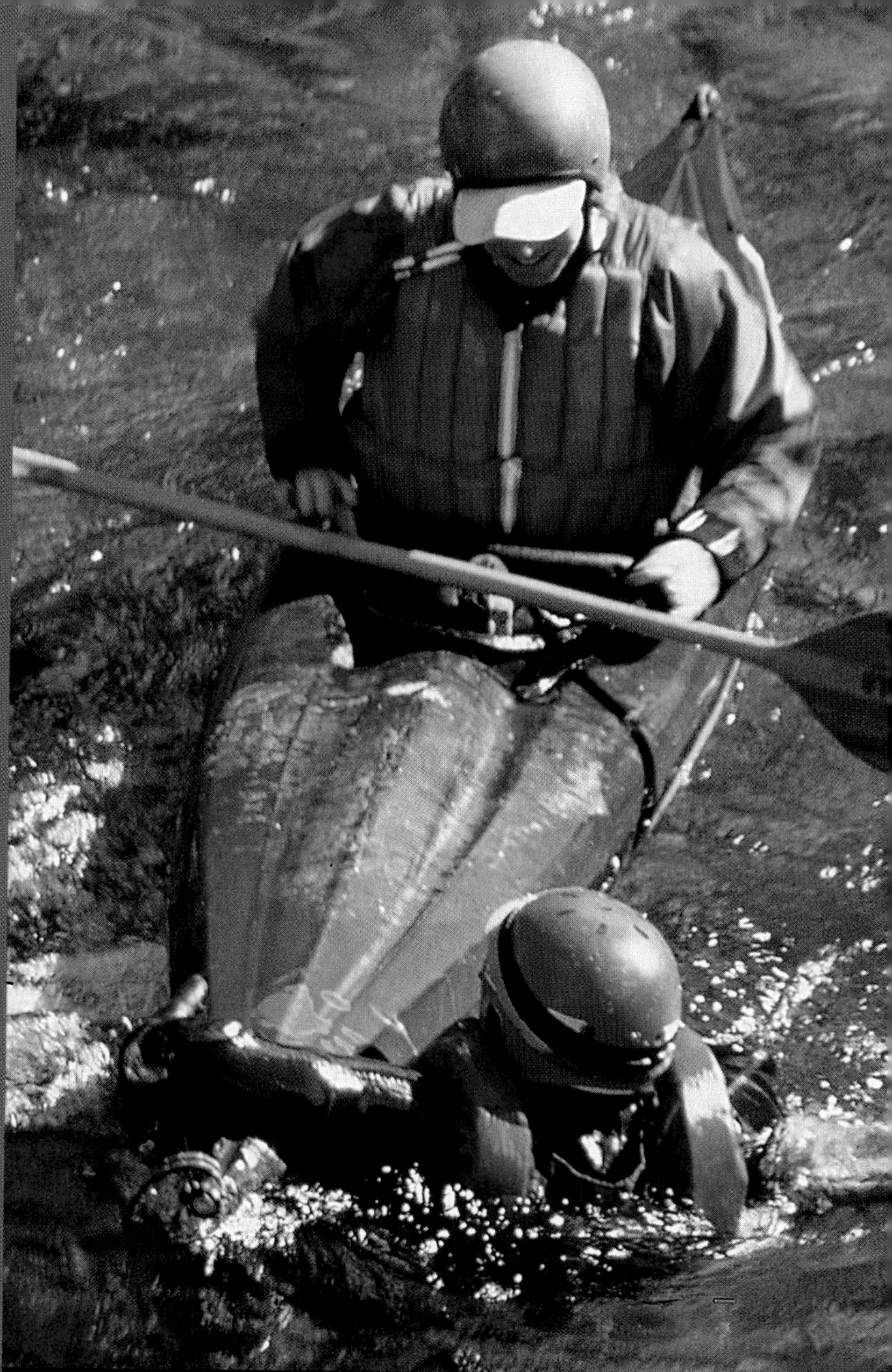

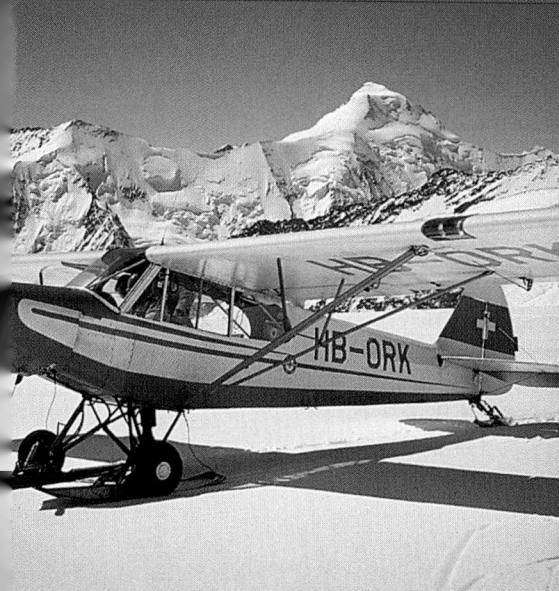

5

24 Wilderness Emergency Medical Services and Response Systems

Franklin R. Hubbell

When an accident or medical crisis occurs in the wilderness or backcountry away from access to immediate assistance, the chain of events set in motion will hopefully lead to a successful rescue. However, how it unfolds varies tremendously, depending on the part of the world in which the critical events occur. Currently, no national or international standard for wilderness emergency medical services (EMS) and response exists. Instead, the configurations of personnel and policies reflect local, national, and international influences. In the United States, wilderness EMS are the most diverse, since they are provided by a wide range of agencies and individuals with a wide variety of training and certification levels, ranging from first aid to paramedic. Canadian wilderness EMS are generally provided through the military, whereas in European wilderness situations, physicians have a prominent role.

The American Alpine Club's Safety Committee gathers, reviews, and analyzes mountaineering accidents that have occurred throughout North America and publishes the annual report *Accidents in North American Mountaineering*. The data collected illustrate both the necessary diversity of wilderness and mountain rescues and current limitations (Box 24-1).

Several states have established (or are in the process of establishing) working protocols for providing care in the wilderness or "extended care" environment. With increased natural and human-made disasters, EMS systems worldwide have suddenly found themselves essentially operating in "wilderness" settings because of prolonged exposure to hostile environments, delayed evacuation and transport times, and lack of medical resources and direction. Prehospital personnel almost always provide care for much longer than the "golden hour" and have been hard pressed to utilize their street-oriented skills in these extended care situations.

Internationally, the Union Internationale des Associations d'Alpinisme (or International Union of Alpine Associations [UIAA]) has established criteria and courses for postgraduate training for physicians in mountain medicine. This allows physicians in the European Union to become certified in wilderness medicine and to practice the relevant skills in an appropriate arena.

The foundation has been set for national standards in providing emergency care and rescue by the adoption and implementation of the Incident Command System (ICS). This system has been used in coordinating forest firefighting tactics in the western United States. It has evolved into a template usable by any agency that may become involved with an emergency effort.

The ICS was developed to coordinate the many departments and individuals responding to large-scale forest fires. Since these fires can involve hundreds of departments with thousands of individuals, a system is needed that establishes a hierarchy of command and a common language of leadership and communication.

The assimilation of ICS into rescue and EMS offers a solution to the single biggest problem facing these services: how to coordinate and interface a variety of teams working on the same rescue effort. When each team follows its own set of operating procedures, standing orders, leadership protocols, terminology, and egos, it often makes it virtually impossible to effectively and safely coordinate a major rescue effort.

The ICS works well, and organizations such as the National Fire Academy and various state EMS offices have tried to adopt and implement it at all levels of emergency response. The ICS is now increasingly the standard for responding to any emergency situation, ranging from a single department answering a call to a minor motor vehicle accident to a complex search and rescue effort involving many agencies and rescue teams. Chapter 25 discusses the basics involved in the ICS. As it becomes widely adopted and used, it will establish a national standard on which can be built national prehospital standards, including wilderness or "extended care" protocols.

Wilderness emergency medicine is a combination of emergency medical training and outdoor wilderness skills. Blending these elements, although essential, is not necessarily natural or easy. The art and science of prehospital emergency medicine began over 30 years ago in the United States and has evolved into a highly regimented and well-defined subspecialty of emergency medicine. We now have first responders, emergency medical technicians (EMTs), and paramedics, and a well-organized EMS system exists nationwide. However, this last statement may be somewhat misleading because each state has an independent EMS system and regulations so that a truly national standard does not yet exist.

The only national prehospital EMS standard that currently exists is via the National Registry of EMTs.

Box 24-1 MOUNTAIN SEARCH AND RESCUE FACTORS IN THE UNITED STATES

1. Search and rescue is the responsibility of national parks, state parks, county sheriffs, or state conservation officers, depending upon the state or park.
2. The vast majority of backcountry and technical rescues are carried out by volunteer rescue groups.
3. Ninety percent of all rescues are carryouts on foot rather than airlifts by helicopter or fixed-wing aircraft.
4. At least 95% of rescues are performed without physicians present, instead using the skills of first responders, emergency medical technicians, and paramedics, who may or may not be trained in wilderness medicine and rescue techniques.
5. Only two of the major climbing areas, Yosemite and Grand Teton National Parks, use helicopters extensively.
6. Only Denali National Park uses fixed-wing aircraft extensively and helicopters occasionally.
7. Only three national parks have rangers who are trained specifically for technical rescue, advanced medical support, and helicopter operations: Yosemite, Grand Teton, and Mt. Rainier National Parks.
8. National and state parks are not mandated with a "duty to rescue." However, virtually all parks provide rescue service. Most parks have a budget for these activities.
9. Many roadside climbing areas and popular backcountry areas are not within the jurisdictions of parks. Technical and backcountry rescues carried out at these locations are often performed by local rescue squads, fire departments, and ambulance units, usually without the benefit of specialized training or technical backcountry skills.

This organization offers individual state EMS systems standardized written and practical examinations for first responders, EMT-basics, intermediates, and paramedics. This guarantees that, regardless of where someone was trained, he or she will be tested using the same standard. According to the Registry, there are approximately 110,000 EMT-basics, 11,000 EMT-intermediates, and 41,000 EMT-paramedics currently certified by their agency. However, since not all states recognize the National Registry certification or participate in this particular standardization, the actual numbers of certified emergency care providers are considerably higher.

Training programs that focus on rapid response, rapid intervention, and rapid transport to advanced care facilities exist nationwide. Prehospital personnel are prepared to work within the framework of the "golden hour," when time is precious and critical actions save lives. This is a nationally accepted urban standard to which all EMS personnel are currently trained. Although this standard is appropriate for evaluating and training urban EMS personnel and response systems, it is often not adequate for rural, wilderness, mountain, or "extended" EMS personnel and response systems. In these situations, patient care is measured in hours and days rather than minutes.

Traditional EMS recognizes rapid notification (the 911 system), dispatch, response, assessment, thorough prehospital care, transport, evaluation, and critical care in a hospital emergency department. Rapidity is the most critical factor that distinguishes urban emergency medical care from wilderness emergency medical care. However, time is not the only difference. Wilderness emergency medicine is governed by a complex set of medical skills and protocols, equipment requirements, and other specialized skills, including different attitudes or psychologic requirements, each of which combine premeditated action with improvisation. A productive mental attitude comes largely from the individual's training, expertise, and experience in the outdoors.

In mountain and wilderness outdoor activities, including mountain and wilderness rescue, haste truly makes waste, which may, in certain circumstances, cost lives. As a result, wilderness and mountain rescue teams must achieve a balance between the urgency of the situation and the necessity for adequate preparation. This is not an easy or natural blend of emotions and skills. On one hand, trained EMS professionals are always primed and ready to go, feel comfortable moving rapidly, act quickly, and think on their feet. On the other hand, skilled outdoorspeople are always eager and willing to travel into the backcountry but understand the necessity of thorough preparedness. This attitude ensures that not only is each team prepared but that each individual is prepared. The team must be organized from a leadership perspective and know where it is headed, what injuries to anticipate, and how weather will affect the rescue. The team counts on each individual member being physically and mentally prepared. This difficult task requires recognition of the differences between short-term and long-term care during a rescue so that a safe and successful extended care rescue can be achieved.

Mountain rescue, wilderness rescue, rural rescue, white-water rescue, expedition medicine, disaster medicine, air-sea rescue, search and rescue, cave rescue, and avalanche rescue are all likely to be extended rescues. Once rescue personnel reach a victim, they will usually be with the person for hours, providing extended emergency care. The terms *extended rescue* and *extended emergency care* refer to rescue efforts that are outside that first golden hour, which has relevance mostly for acute and severe trauma situations.

Many of the recommendations in Box 24-2 need further development and may be considered controversial.

In particular, specialized wilderness medical training with standardized protocols has yet to be developed.

SEQUENCE OF EVENTS IN BACKCOUNTRY RESCUE

The principles and standards of a wilderness or mountain rescue (extended care rescue), including organization, specialized skills and knowledge, and essential components of the team, can best be illustrated by reviewing the sequence of events during a typical backcountry rescue in North America (Box 24-3).

Occurrence of the Critical Event

The critical event occurs when an individual participating in an activity away from immediate help is suddenly stricken by injury or illness. The key factor is immobilization. The fact that the injured or ill person cannot self-evacuate or move to seek shelter or stay warm results in the need for a rescue. Once the victim or others in the party realize this, the need to seek help becomes obvious.

Making the Decision to Get Help

Before anyone leaves to seek assistance, the victim's companions should perform a physical examination, record vital signs, determine the level of consciousness, and provide appropriate emergency care, which may entail moving the victim into protective shelter. Victim information should be summarized in a note that accompanies the individual(s) going for help. A map depicting the victim's exact location and a list of the other party members, noting their level of preparedness to endure the environmental conditions, should be included. The individual(s) going for help should carry appropriate provisions. To prepare information adequately generally takes 30 minutes to 1 hour. However, thorough preparation rarely occurs. Often, someone suddenly yells, "I'll get help" and disappears, running down the trail with sparse vital knowledge.

With the improvements and availability of communications technology, such as cellular phones and global positioning systems, backcountry adventurers may have more rapid access to the EMS system from the mountains. Whether this will increase the number of inappropriate callouts remains to be determined. Recent reports indicate that reliance on fallible technology may be responsible for outdoorspeople using poor judgment in terms of trip planning. Assuming that help is just a phone call away, hikers are taking more risks.

Notifying the Emergency Medical System

Eventually, the messenger notifies someone in authority that an emergency has occurred and help is needed. Usually, the request is made to a central 911 system. If no central service is available, a local dispatch agency is notified. The agency contacts the closest emergency medical service, which can be a rescue squad, ambulance corps, fire department, or first response team.

Activating the Emergency Medical System.

Notification of an emergency usually occurs via pagers worn by individual members. An alert tone is followed by an oral message describing the emergency, its location, and type of response required.

At this point, a wide variety of events can occur, involving agencies within and outside the EMS system. Even in areas of the United States with well-organized extended care rescue teams, the team may be notified last. Ideally, it should be notified immediately, but all too often this is not the case. Instead, local agency responders are notified and rush around trying to determine how quickly they can reach the victim.

Notifying and Mobilizing the Extended Rescue Team.

The first step is to notify team members. In many parts of the United States, organized and coordinated extended rescue teams do not exist, so a "team" is created of relatively untrained volunteers willing to hike in and assist. The task of further organizing and coordinating the rescue effort generally falls on the shoulders of a local rescue squad, fire service, or police department, which may or may not be willing and prepared to manage and execute an extended or technical rescue.

In the parts of the United States where backcountry use is common and backcountry accidents occur regularly, extended care rescue teams have generally evolved from local EMS squads with skilled outdoor enthusiasts. Some teams offering local search and rescue capabilities may be coordinated locally (such as the Appalachian Mountain Club, Stonehearth Open Learning Opportunities [SOLO], and Mountain Rescue Service in the White Mountains of New Hampshire); other teams may be part of a nationwide system responding to incidents throughout the country and be coordinated on a regional or national level (such as the National Cave Rescue Commission). Coordination of extended care rescue teams may also come under the jurisdiction of a law enforcement body, such as state conservation officers (e.g., New Hampshire Fish & Game), sheriff's department (e.g., the Los Angeles County Sheriff in California), or a statewide coordinating system (e.g., the Pennsylvania Search and Rescue Council). Organized teams can be quite sophisticated in their dispatching function so that all members can be notified simultaneously, or they may use a more "low-tech" telephone tree to call out members.

Assembling and Organizing the Rescue Team

Once members are notified, they assemble at a common location (rescue station) to organize the rescue effort. The first task is to define the type of rescue to establish equipment needs. Estimating the time it will take to effect the rescue and assessing the need for other agency involvement and assistance are also primary tasks. The questions to be answered and the variables to be considered may include the following:

1. Time of day: will this be a night rescue?
2. Weather: what are the current weather conditions at the rescue location and what is the forecast?
3. When did the accident occur?
4. What are the supposed injuries?
5. How many victims are there?
6. How many people are in the party?
7. How well prepared are they?
8. Does anyone in the party have medical expertise?
9. Do we know the exact location, or is this a search and rescue?
10. Is a "hasty team" needed? Has it left for the scene yet?
11. Is each of the team members prepared? Does each have personal equipment, a bivouac kit, head lamp, food, and water?
12. Is each member trained and skilled in this particular type of rescue?
13. Who is on the medical team?
14. Who is on the evacuation team?
15. Is the team equipment organized and divided up?
16. How urgent is the situation? Is a helicopter required? Is one available?
17. Are the weather conditions appropriate for an air rescue?
18. Will multiple agencies be involved? If so, are radio frequencies coordinated?

Once the team is assembled and all pertinent issues have been addressed satisfactorily, the team is transported to the trailhead (launch point) to begin the search.

Commonly, a hasty team starts out ahead of the main team. Once the hasty team has enough information to locate the victim, they travel as lightly as possible, with only enough gear to ensure their own safety and to equip them to manage the victim's primary injuries. The goal is to reach the victim as quickly as is reasonably possible and deliver primary care, then apprise the rest of the team of the victim's condition, equipment needs, and environmental concerns.

Locating the Victim

How long it takes to locate the victim varies tremendously, depending on distance, terrain, weather conditions, mode of transportation, and whether the victim's exact location is known. A general rule of thumb for a team responding on foot is that it will take 1 hour for each mile through the backcountry. If a search is involved, all bets are off. A search and rescue effort can involve many agencies, individuals, and days (see Chapter 25).

Providing Appropriate "Extended Emergency Care"

Once the victim is located, appropriate medical care can be provided. The rescue team should ensure its own safety; wet clothes should be replaced with warm, dry clothing, and members should check for emerging problems within their group. While the medical team cares for the victim, the evacuation team secures shelter, prepares warm drinks, establishes and maintains communications, and plans and organizes the evacuation.

Companions with the victim may have been affected by the environment while waiting for the rescue team to arrive and require assistance. They may need to be assessed and treated for hypothermia, frostbite, heatstroke, heat exhaustion, and dehydration.

Regardless of what transpired before the medical team arrived, a complete victim assessment is essential.

Do not assume that all the injuries have been found or that all medical conditions have been managed properly (Box 24-4).

In the extended care environment, the victim must be monitored for *changing* conditions that indicate an underlying problem. Awareness of environmental emergencies is particularly important, with constant care to prevent hypothermia, frostbite, heatstroke, heat exhaustion, and dehydration. To do this, it is necessary to monitor the victim and write a new SOAP note at least every 15 minutes:

Subjective: Is the victim comfortable, too hot, too cold, hungry, thirsty, or in need of urination or defecation?

Objective:

Vital signs—are they stable? Record these.

Victim examination—recheck all dressings, bandages, and splints; are they still controlling bleeding? Are they too tight or too loose? (Swelling limbs can cause bandages or splints to impede circulation, resulting in ischemic injuries or worsening frostbite or snakebite.)

Box 24-4 VICTIM ASSESSMENT

PRIMARY SURVEY: LOCATING AND TREATING LIFE-THREATENING PROBLEMS

A—Airway Management

Is the airway open?
Is the airway going to *stay* open?

B—Breathing

Is air moving in and out?
Is the airway quiet or silent?
Is breathing effortless?
Is the respiratory system intact?
Is breathing adequate to support life?

C—Circulation

Is there a pulse?
Is bleeding well controlled?
Is capillary refill normal (less than 2 sec)?
Is circulation adequate to support life?

D—Disability

Conscious vs. unconscious
Level of consciousness—awake/verbal/painful/unconscious (AVPU) or Glasgow Coma Scale
Cervical spine stabilization

E—Environment

Internal vs. external
Is the victim warm and dry?
Protected from the cold ground
Protected from the elements

SECONDARY SURVEY: WHAT IS WRONG AND HOW SERIOUS IS IT?

Vital signs: Indicate the condition of the victim

RR—respiratory rate and effort
PR—pulse rate and character
BP—blood pressure (systolic/diastolic)
LOC—level of consciousness (AVPU or Glasgow Coma Scale)
TP—tissue perfusion: Skin color, temperature, and moisture
Capillary refill (less than 2 sec)

Victim examination: Head-to-toe examination to locate injuries

AMPLE history:

Allergies
Medicines
Past medical history
Last food/drink
Events leading up

SOAP NOTE: To record and organize victim data

Subjective: Age, gender, mechanism of injury, chief complaint
Objective: Vital signs, victim examination, AMPLE history
Assessment: Problem list
Plan: Plan for each problem

Assessment: Has the initial assessment changed?
Plan: Is the rate of evacuation still the same?

Evacuating the Victim to the Appropriate Facility

While providing emergency care, part of the team is designated as the evacuation team. This group has evaluated the various options for evacuation. To properly evaluate the situation, the first information they need is provided by the medical team leader, since they need to know the status of the victim to establish the pace. If the victim's condition is stable, time is less important; if the victim's condition is critical, time is critical.

The evacuation team must explore different options. If speed is a consideration, weather conditions are reviewed and the availability of a helicopter-assisted rescue is determined. If a helicopter is not an option, the fastest route out is established. If time or speed is not critical, the safest means of evacuation that is easiest on the victim and rescuers is defined. A general rule for the duration of an evacuation is that it will take 1 to 2 hours for every mile to be covered, requiring six well-rested litter bearers for every mile. Thus a 4-mile carryout will require a 24-member litter team and can take 4 to 8 hours to complete. Eventually, the team reaches a trailhead and the victim is transferred to an ambulance for transport to a hospital emergency facility.

Returning to Base

The team returns to base to reorganize equipment in preparation for the next extended rescue, and to debrief. Because people are exhausted and hungry, the debriefing session is often canceled. However, establishing a mechanism to debrief the rescue effort is imperative so that they can learn from the shared experience, discuss victim care, and work through problems. Whenever several different emergency organizations with disparate rescue and emergency personnel combine to perform a complex rescue, there may be tension, bruised egos, and concerns about the medical care provided or evacuation plan used. These problems deserve to be discussed and managed in real time as expediently as possible so that teams will cooperate successfully in the future, improve their performance, and provide the best possible patient care on the next rescue. This process minimizes the burnout syndrome that can occur with volunteer teams.

TEAM ORGANIZATION AND FUNCTION

The organization of an extended care rescue team is based on both training of individuals and type of rescue. The structures of teams can vary from loosely knit groups of friends with no leadership hierarchy to paramilitary organizations with rigid leadership roles.

Team members require personal knowledge, experi-ence, and expertise in the particular aspect of extended care and rescue in which they will participate, as well as knowledge and expertise in the principles of extended emergency care, extended rescue techniques, and technical rescue skills.

Personal Knowledge, Experience, and Expertise

Individuals who want to be part of an extended rescue team need to acquire outdoor skills *before* they become part of a rescue team. Every member must have extensive knowledge of likely environmental emergencies: hypothermia, frostbite, heat syndromes, snakebite, dehydration, lightning strike, and so forth. Each must understand general principles of weather behavior. Rescuers need to be comfortable with route finding, map and compass, personal preparedness, and bivouac and survival skills. The knowledge, skills, and equipment that a skilled outdoorsperson should possess are often referred to as "the ten essentials" (see Box 24-5). The

---

Box 24-5   THE TEN ESSENTIALS

1. *Attitude*
Positive belief that you can make things better
Will to survive
2. *Fuel to burn: food*
   High-carbohydrate foods that require no preparation
   High-carbohydrate foods that can be made into a drink
3. *Quench your thirst: water*
   A minimum of 2 L/day if not active
   Up to 3 L/hr if active
Ability to make more pure disinfected water
4. *Stay warm and dry: clothing*
   Warm clothing that retains heat even if wet
   Waterproof raingear, top and bottom
5. *Get dry: shelter*
Ability to improvise shelter or bivouac
A bivouac ("bivy") kit (see Box 24-6)
6. *Get warm: fire*
   Ability to warm water (stove, candle, fire)
   Ability to build a fire (waterproof matches and tinder)
   Ability to make kindling or tinder (folding knife)
7. *Know where you are going: navigation*
   Map and compass skills and route-finding skills
   Ability to move about at night (headlamp)
8. *Know the environment: weather*
   Basic understanding of weather patterns
   Knowledge of how to react to severe weather, lightning
9. *Getting help: signaling*
   Whistle, preferably plastic
10. *Providing help: first aid kit*
    Basic small personal trauma kit

Box 24-6 BIVOUAC KIT

Two large garbage bags (emergency shelter or raingear)
10 × 10 foot sheet of plastic and 100 feet of parachute
   cord (shelter)
Emergency space blanket (shelter, ground cloth)
Stocking cap (warmth)
Spare socks (warmth and can act as spare mittens)
Metal cup (to warm liquids)
Gelatin (to make a drink)

Two plumber's candles (to warm water or start fire)
Waterproof matches or lighter
Knife
Compass
Whistle
All of these items fit neatly into a small stuff sack that
   is 6 × 6 inches and weighs less than 1 pound when
   filled.

---

same skills, knowledge, and equipment commonly used by the outdoor enthusiast are essential on a mountain rescue.

Extended Rescue Techniques and Skills

Specific skills and techniques applicable to a particular situation include those of search and rescue, vertical and technical rock climbing, and white-water navigation. Snow or winter camping or avalanche rescue may be required, depending on the environment. Extended rescue teams should require their members to have, at a minimum, the working knowledge and equipment in Box 24-7.

Knowledge is acquired over time. Specific medical, rescue, and technical skills are obtained and retained through courses, continuous training, and refresher programs. Appendix A at the conclusion of this chapter provides a list of schools, institutes, and organizations that are involved in mountaineering research, standards development, and training programs.

Wilderness and Mountain Rescue Team Organization

Organization of wilderness and mountain rescue teams is where the greatest diversity exists, since no universal standard has been established. Teams vary from local mountain rescue teams with extreme skills and qualifications for providing mountain rescue care to informal collections of friends without leadership. Other, more "professional," teams are operated under the jurisdiction of law enforcement agencies with paramilitary hierarchy and leadership. This diversity is particularly noticeable in the United States because the vast majority of teams are composed of volunteers who are not reimbursed for their rescue efforts.

In Europe, mountain rescue teams are professional and employ full-time personnel. They charge for rescue efforts, with the fees providing money for personnel, equipment, helicopters, technical gear, and ongoing training. As with any "profession," standards have evolved. As a result, there are more standards in

Europe than in the United States. Still, there is variation from European country to country, especially in leadership and organization.

In many parts of the world, especially remote and wild areas, organized and available rescue teams do not exist. If someone is in need of help, the expedition team necessarily becomes the rescue team.

TRAINING OF WILDERNESS EMERGENCY MEDICAL TECHNICIANS

The best way to develop an appreciation for the vast difference between what is required of the traditional (urban) EMT and what is required of the extended care or wilderness emergency medical technician (WEMT) is to compare their respective course curriculums.

The Department of Transportation (DOT) is responsible for developing and updating the EMT curriculum in the United States. This curriculum is considered the minimum national standard for EMT students to qualify for the National Registry or an individual state practical and written examination. Passage of such an examination enables a student to become certified as a National Registry or state EMT.

A national standard for WEMT curricula does not yet exist. Despite the lack of a DOT-like standard, there are several similar curricula for wilderness emergency care at the EMT level. Based on the recommendations of the Wilderness Medical Society and other groups that address the issues of wilderness prehospital emergency medicine, these curricula adhere to the same principles of long-term patient care, which can be used for comparison with the standard DOT curriculum.

A WEMT course typically contains all of the material in the DOT EMT course curriculum plus what is necessary to acquire the skills attendant to long-term wilderness emergency care. Typical EMT courses are approximately 100 hours with 10 additional hours of emergency department observation time. The WEMT module carries an additional 48 to 80 hours of training.

Box 24-7   KNOWLEDGE, SKILLS, AND EQUIPMENT FOR EXTENDED RESCUE TEAMS

MOUNTAINEERING SKILLS

Understanding fabrics and clothing systems and their seasonal variations (see Chapter 70)
  Fabrics and fibers
  Layering techniques
  Vapor barrier systems
  Waterproof fabrics, raingear systems
  Footgear
Personal protection equipment
  Helmets
  Harnesses
  Gloves
  Goggles, sunglasses
  Hearing protection
Backcountry equipment
  Internal or external frame packs and soft packs
  Shelter (natural and human-made)
  Specialty equipment: snow shoes, crampons, ice axes, stoves, skis
Backcountry travel
  Route finding
  Map and compass: map reading, dead reckoning, types of maps, compass reading, bearings, magnetic vs. true bearing, triangulation, global positioning systems
Survival skills: the ten essentials
  Shelter and warmth; emergency bivouac ("bivy") kits
  Food, water
Understanding how backcountry travel and rescue vary with the seasons
Understanding how backcountry travel and rescue vary with different environments
  Alpine
  Desert
  Forest
  Water (swamp, river, lake, ocean)
  Tropics
  High altitude
Low-impact camping and rescue work
Basics of weather and weather forecasting
  Principles of barometric pressure
  Clouds and their significance in weather forecasting
  Prevailing weather patterns in the rescue area
Personal fitness
  Physical conditioning
  Nutrition and hydration requirements for different activities

MOUNTAIN AND EXTENDED EMERGENCY MEDICAL SKILLS

Emergency medical training should be at a minimal level of first responder or higher (emergency medical technician, paramedic, registered nurse, nurse practitioner, physician's assistant, or physician). Regardless of the level, training must include specific information on wilderness and extended emergency care procedures.

MOUNTAIN AND EXTENDED EMERGENCY MEDICAL SKILLS—cont'd

Topics of extended care training and principles should include the following:
Patient assessment system
Cardiopulmonary resuscitation
Airway management, including endotracheal intubation and needle decompression for tension pneumothorax
Shock and control of bleeding, including the use of intravenous (IV) therapy for fluid resuscitation
Long-term wound care and prevention of infection
Musculoskeletal injury management, including specific information on diagnosis and long-term management of the following:
  Sprains and strains
  Fractures, including how to reduce or realign angulated fractures
  Diagnosis and reduction of dislocations
  Management of compound fractures
  Management of chest injuries, including decompression of a tension pneumothorax with a needle thoracostomy
  Spinal cord injury diagnosis and management
  Head injury, including recognition and management of increasing intracranial pressure
Management of environmental emergencies
  Hypothermia and frostbite, including the use of IV fluids
  Heatstroke and heat exhaustion, including the use of IV fluids
  Dehydration and nutrition, acute and during evacuation
  Lightning injuries
  Animal attacks, insect bites, and reptile and marine envenomations, including anaphylactic reactions and the use of epinephrine and antihistamines
  Contact dermatitis, such as poison ivy, oak, and sumac
  Sunburn and snowblindness
  High-altitude injuries, including acute mountain sickness, pulmonary edema, cerebral edema
  Near drowning
Diagnosis and management of acute medical emergencies
  Chest pain (myocardial infarction, angina, costochondritis)
  Shortness of breath (asthma, anaphylaxis, pneumothorax)
  Seizures and cerebrovascular accidents
  Acute abdomen (peritonitis, constipation, diarrhea)
  Pyelonephritis and septic shock
Victim lifting and handling techniques (body elevation and movement [BEAM], free of any movement [FOAM])
Improvising techniques: "emergency medicine barehanded" (see Chapter 19)
Training in the use of the Incident Command System
Bloodborne pathogens and infectious disease prevention

Continued

Box 24-7 KNOWLEDGE, SKILLS, AND EQUIPMENT FOR EXTENDED RESCUE TEAMS—cont'd

MOUNTAIN AND EXTENDED EMERGENCY MEDICAL SKILLS—cont'd

Monitoring of bodily functions (hunger, thirst, and need to excrete)

General understanding and appreciation for the difference between urban (short-term) and wilderness (long-term) emergency care

MOUNTAIN AND EXTENDED RESCUE SKILLS

Understanding equipment used in wilderness search and rescue operations, including maintenance and care
  Ropes, slings, carabiners, harnesses, helmets
  Litters, litter harnesses, haul systems
  Litter patient packaging equipment
Basic radio communications
  Care and maintenance of communications equipment
  Procedures and protocols
Basic helicopter operations and procedures
  Approach to a helicopter
  Safety considerations
  Landing zones
  Haul techniques
  Interagency relations
Basic understanding of search procedures
Basic understanding of rescue procedures
Basic understanding of Incident Command System and its use in search and rescue management

MOUNTAIN AND EXTENDED RESCUE SKILLS—cont'd

Basic rope handling and knot tying skills
  How to care for and handle ropes
  Rappeling, belaying, and braking techniques
  Knots
    Figure-8
    Figure-8 follow through
    Figure-8 on a bight
    Double figure-8
    Double fisherman's
    Prusik
    Tensionless hitch (round turn and two half hitches)
    Water
    Half hitch and full hitch
    Bowline
    Alpine butterfly
Specific rescue training
  Water search
  White-water
  Avalanche
  Technical or vertical (rock)
  Cave

LEADERSHIP

Leadership and followship training
Ability to use the Incident Command System

A typical WEMT course outline appears in Box 24-8. The topics in boldface are peculiar to a WEMT program, whereas the other topics are those required in a DOT EMT course. Hours per topic illustrate the time required for both EMT and WEMT training. This outline is arranged in the current DOT EMT recommended format, with the WEMT material added on a per topic basis; topics are not necessarily listed in the order that they would be taught for a particular course. An explanation follows of the extended emergency medical care material that WEMTs must learn.

Introduction to Emergency Care

"Wilderness vs. urban emergency care" is an introductory presentation to illustrate the differences between urban ("golden hour") emergency care and extended, or "wilderness," emergency care. For WEMTs, it will in certain instances be necessary to learn two different modalities of therapy, one for short-term (less than 1 hour) care and one for long-term or extended (several hours to days) care.

"Backcountry rescue gear inspection" is a hands-on review of gear for the outdoor practice sessions and backcountry mock rescues. The course staff must in-

spect the participants' boots, clothing, raingear, and rescue equipment to determine their adequacy for the particular environment in which they will be deployed. Inspecting equipment not only ensures the safety of each individual in the course but also teaches a standard for preparedness, awareness, and attention to details that is critical for wilderness travel and emergency care.

"Medical legal issues" is usually offered early in a course so that the participants are aware of the legal concerns surrounding practicing medicine as EMTs and WEMTs. WEMTs need to be aware of protocols existing where they will become licensed.

"The human animal—our natural physiologic limits" is an overview lecture of how humans fit into the natural environment and of their daily nutritional requirements and natural limitations. The WEMT must understand physiologic limits, such as those of endurance, temperature, and altitude, and the consequences when these limits are exceeded.

Patient Assessment Systems

"Patient assessment in the wilderness and practice" takes the newly learned skills of patient assessment and adapts them to the backcountry. The WEMT must be

Box 24-8 EMT AND WEMT COURSE CURRICULA AND HOURS PER TOPIC*

1. Introduction to emergency care
   Wilderness vs. urban emergency care (1 hour)
   Backcountry rescue gear inspection (1 hour)
   Medical legal issues (1 hour)
   Blood-borne pathogens
   Overview of human systems—anatomy and physiology (2 hours)
   The human animal—our natural physiologic limits (2 hours)
2. Patient assessment systems
   Primary survey—ABCs (1 hour)
   Secondary survey (1 hour)
   Patient assessment practice (2 hours)
   Patient assessment in the wilderness and practice (3 hours)
3. Cardiopulmonary resuscitation (8 hours)
   Mannequin practice and certification (8 hours)
   Cardiopulmonary resuscitation (CPR) teaching, practice, and testing to American Heart Association standards
4. Airways, oxygen, and mechanical aids to breathing (3 hours)
   Airways, oxygen, CPR, and mechanical aids to breathing in the wilderness environment—uses and limitations (6 hours)
   Airways: oropharyngeal, nasopharyngeal, esophageal obturator airway, endotracheal intubation
   Oxygen administration
   Suction techniques
5. Bleeding and shock (3 hours)
   Shock, intravenous (IV) fluids, and long-term patient care (4 hours)
   Practice starting IV infusions and fluid administration (4 hours)
   Use of pneumatic antishock garments (PASG) (3 hours)
   Use of PASG in the wilderness (1 hour)
6. Soft tissue injuries (3 hours)
   Long-term wound care (1 hour)
7. Principles of musculoskeletal care
   Fractures of the upper extremities (3 hours)
   Fractures of the pelvis, hip, and lower extremities (3 hours)
   Fracture laboratory—practice in assessment and management (3 hours)
   Musculoskeletal trauma management in the wilderness (3 hours)

8. Injuries of the head, face, eye, neck, and spine (3 hours)
   Practical laboratory: spinal cord injury management (SCIM) (3 hours)
   Head trauma, increasing intracranial pressure (1 hour)
   SCIM: Long-term care and improvising (1 hour)
9. Injuries to the chest, abdomen, and genitalia (3 hours)
   Chest trauma in the wilderness (3 hours)
10. Medical emergencies I (3 hours)
    Poisoning, bites and strings, heart attack, stroke, dyspnea
    Medical emergencies II (3 hours)
    Diabetes, acute abdomen, communicable disease, seizure, substance abuse, and pediatric emergencies
    Medical emergencies in the wilderness (3 hours)
11. Emergency childbirth (3 hours)
12. Burns and hazardous materials (3 hours)
    Long-term care of burns (1 hour)
13. Environmental emergencies (3 hours)
    Hypothermia, frostbite, immersion foot (4 hours)
    Heatstroke, heat exhaustion, dehydration (4 hours)
    Drowning (2 hours)
    High-altitude emergencies (2 hours)
    Barotrauma (2 hours)
    Animals that bite and sting (2 hours)
    Plants—contact dermatitis (2 hours)
    Marine animals that bite and sting (2 hours)
14. Psychologic aspects of emergency care (3 hours)
15. Lifting and moving patients (3 hours)
    Use of Stokes litters and improvising litters (3 hours)
16. Principles of vehicle extrication (4 hours)
    Practice laboratory (3-8 hours)
    Principles of backcountry evacuation (4 hours)
    Search and rescue organization and execution (4 hours)
    Wilderness mock rescue with or without overnight (8-12 hours)
17. Leadership and followship skills
    The Incident Command System
18. Ambulance operations I (3 hours)
    Ambulance operations II (3 hours)
    Helicopter-assisted rescues (3 hours)
19. Review (3-6 hours)
    Testing—written and practical examinations (16-20 hours)
20. Emergency department observation time (10 hours)

*Topics in boldface are peculiar to WEMT programs, whereas the other topics are required topics covered in a DOT EMT course.

knowledgeable and skillful in wilderness patient assessment, a step-by-step approach to the first 5 minutes of scene safety and patient care. The WEMT will develop an awareness of potential life-threatening dangers in the environment, how to ensure personal safety and the safety of others, how to approach a victim safely, how to perform primary and secondary surveys to determine the extent and severity of injuries, and what impact the environment might have on the victim.

Airways, Oxygen, and Mechanical Aids to Breathing

"Airways, oxygen, cardiopulmonary resuscitation, and mechanical aids to breathing in the wilderness environment—uses and limitations" addresses one of the most important lifesaving and life-maintaining skills in emergency medicine: the ability to establish and maintain a patent airway. Unfortunately, most EMTs are not provided with the training and tools they need to properly maintain an open airway in an unconscious victim. Failure to perform endotracheal intubation can be disastrous for such a victim.

Endotracheal intubation is commonly used by EMT-intermediates and paramedics and other advanced life support (ALS) personnel in cardiac arrest settings and for unconscious, unresponsive victims. In the extended care environment, the use of intubation in a cardiac arrest situation is not nearly as common as it is for the normothermic, unconscious, and unresponsive person, who has probably suffered head trauma. In this situation, without intubation, the only way to maintain a patent airway while lifting, moving, and transporting a victim in a litter is to place the victim on his or her side. Gravity pulls the tongue forward and allows secretions to drain from the mouth. Oropharyngeal, nasopharyngeal, and esophageal obturator airways and tongue pin-pull techniques may temporarily keep the tongue from occluding the airway, but they are ineffective in preventing vomitus, blood, or saliva from entering the airway. Also, during evacuation in a Stokes litter, constant monitoring of a victim's airway is virtually impossible, which makes endotracheal intubation of paramount importance. The WEMT should know how to establish and maintain a patent airway, including the use of endotracheal intubation.

"Oxygen administration" presents the use of supplemental oxygen, for which both EMTs and WEMTs follow the same general guidelines. Even though oxygen is important to prehospital care, its use has significant logistic limitations in the backcountry. The WEMT must realize that carrying large quantities of oxygen into the backcountry is impossible. Small D and E cylinders can be carried, but each provides high-flow oxygen for only 20 to 30 minutes. Oxygen is a compressed gas in a tank, so as it expands, it cools dramatically and may contribute to hypothermia. To prevent this, the gas should be preheated by wrapping the oxygen tubing around a chemical heat pack during administration.

"Suction techniques" presents the use of suction devices to clear the airway, which is similar for EMTs and WEMTs. Hand-operated, as distinct from battery-operated, suction devices are usually used in extended care scenarios.

Bleeding and Shock

"Shock, intravenous (IV) fluids, and long-term patient care" and "Practice starting IV infusions and fluid administration" provide information about the care of victims in shock.

In the urban management of shock, the essential component is recognition. Once shock is recognized, the victim can be rapidly transported to an emergency department or intercepted by paramedics for definitive care, namely fluid resuscitation.

In the extended care environment, WEMTs must be able to manage the shock syndrome by providing appropriate definitive care. During extended evacuations, WEMTs should know how to administer IV fluids to stabilize hypovolemia. This includes starting a peripheral IV line, maintaining the catheter placement, using proper fluids, and prewarming the solutions before and during administration.

"Use of pneumatic antishock garments (PASG) in the wilderness" discusses the use of these garments for victims in shock. The practice of treating shock using PASG has largely fallen out of favor. As long as an IV line can be established and maintained, fluid administration is the definitive method for managing shock. The WEMT must be aware that the PASG has other uses. In the extended care situation, use of the PASG may be invaluable in stabilizing a fractured pelvis to control internal blood loss and prevent shock. It may be useful in conjunction with a traction splint for a fractured femur. An added benefit is that the PASG may facilitate a comfortable and well-padded ride for the victim in a Stokes litter. However, WEMTs must recognize the limitations of a PASG. The primary drawback in the backcountry is the potential for cold injury. Once the apparatus is inflated, the decrease in peripheral circulation greatly increases the risk for cold injuries or frostbite to the lower extremities. This can be prevented by properly packing the feet with chemical heat packs and adequately insulating the lower extremities in the litter. Careful monitoring of the lower extremities every 15 minutes is essential.

Soft Tissue Injuries

"Long-term wound care" covers proper wound management once bleeding has been controlled, and further care if more than 12 hours will be required to bring the victim to definitive care. The principles of long-term wound care are to stabilize the wound and prevent and control infection.

To prevent infection, the WEMT must know how to sterilize or disinfect fluid and how to properly debride and rinse out a contaminated wound. Once the wound is cleaned and debrided, the edges can be approximated but not tightly closed, since this may increase the risk of abscess formation and a life-threatening infection. Training in suturing techniques to close wounds is not currently recommended.

Even the most fastidiously cleaned wound can still become infected, particularly in a remote setting, because of constant exposure to microbes. Recognition of wound infections and appropriate management are important. The WEMT must learn to use specific antibiotics in extended care settings of greater than 3 days and for prophylaxis with grossly contaminated wounds and compound fractures. Antibiotic therapy is not controversial, since various safe broad-spectrum antibiotics can cover most wound infections with minimal risk of a severe allergic reaction. In certain circumstances the benefits of antibiotic administration clearly outweigh the risks.

Principles of Musculoskeletal Care

"Musculoskeletal trauma management in the wilderness" presents the treatment of injuries. In an urban setting, the primary concern with fracture and dislocation care is that the injury site be splinted properly to prevent further injury. In the extended care environment, the primary concern is to maintain proper circulation distal to the site of the injury. This may require straightening an angulated fracture or reducing a dislocation.

When an angulated fracture occurs, distal circulation can be impaired, putting the soft tissues at considerable risk for ischemic injury or frostbite. Under normal circumstances, it would take hours for moderate ischemia to cause irreparable soft tissue injury, but in the backcountry, prolonged time under hostile weather conditions frequently occurs, which decreases the amount of heat and oxygen being transferred to the extremity.

Knowing how to properly straighten out an angulated fracture significantly decreases the risk of secondary ischemic injury and frostbite, controls bleeding at the fracture site, and diminishes pain. It is much easier to splint and stabilize a fracture in proper position if it is straight than if it is angulated.

Approximately 3 additional hours of training are needed to teach a WEMT how to straighten an angulated fracture and reduce dislocations. Without an x-ray, it is impossible to see the exact positioning of bone fragments or disarticulated joints, making it difficult to know exactly how to manipulate the bone. The concern is that if a jagged bone end is moved improperly, secondary injury might occur: part of a neurovascular bundle might be severed, a fascial sheath surrounding a muscle might be cut, or the bone ends might erupt through the skin. Fortunately, all of these structures are richly endowed with pain receptors. If the sharp end of a bone fragment begins to impinge, it causes a dramatic increase in pain at the site. A commonly used technique is to straighten the angulated site slowly while maintaining constant gentle traction. With each 1 to 2 cm of movement, the victim is asked if the new position is better or worse (causes less or more pain). If the pain diminishes with movement, the reduction is proceeding properly; if pain increases, all movement is stopped and the extremity is returned to the previous position of improvement. While still under gentle traction, the extremity is repositioned and another attempt at reduction is made.

As long as nothing is forced and movement is achieved slowly under gentle traction, angulated fractures can be easily realigned and dislocations reduced without the need for pain medication or any risk of further injury.

Musculoskeletal injuries in the long-term care setting must be carefully monitored. It is essential to reinspect the injury site at reasonable intervals for circulation, sensation, and motion. Fracture sites swell; as a result, even the best splint can act as an inadvertent tourniquet. Immobilized extremities cool because of lack of activity and impaired circulation, also increasing the risk of ischemic injury or frostbite.

Injuries of the Head, Face, Eye, Neck, and Spine

"Head trauma, increasing intracranial pressure" addresses one of the leading causes of death from backcountry accidents. Many who die of head trauma in the wilderness would have survived in an urban setting because of rapid access to definitive care. The WEMT must be able to recognize a potentially serious head injury long before the victim is at risk of brainstem herniation.

In the extended care environment, there are few situations when the team should hurry. One such situation is the presence of significant head trauma, for which the only appropriate care may be rapid evacuation to a facility where the victim can be put into the hands of a neurosurgeon.

It is important to establish and monitor the level of consciousness. The AVPU (*a*wake, *v*erbal, *p*ain, *u*nresponsive) scale is used. Within the primary survey, an initial evaluation of disability or neurologic status is made. After that, level of consciousness is reevaluated every 15 minutes to observe in particular for any evidence of increasing intracranial pressure.

Injuries to the Chest, Abdomen, and Genitalia

Chest trauma is significant for the WEMT because it can result in a pneumothorax that can evolve into a tension pneumothorax. WEMTs need to be taught how to inspect, palpate, percuss, and auscultate the chest for significant injuries to the respiratory system. It is not difficult to train an individual to detect breath sounds, determine the presence of a pneumothorax, and monitor a pneumothorax for its development into a tension pneumothorax. Unlike increasing intracranial pressure, for which there is little to do but evacuate the victim, a tension pneumothorax can be relieved, increasing the chance of survival. The easiest and most effective technique a WEMT may learn is needle thoracostomy in the fifth intercostal space in the midaxillary line.

Medical Emergencies

Diagnosing medical emergencies in the wilderness requires the WEMTs to be aware of essential signs and symptoms.

Environmental Emergencies

The typical EMT course includes 3 to 6 hours of training in management of environmental emergencies. A WEMT course will have a minimum of 22 hours of additional training in environmental emergencies.

"Hypothermia, frostbite, and immersion foot" covers cold injuries, which are among the most common environmental injuries seen in the backcountry. The WEMT must understand principles of thermoregulation; heat production and heat loss; recognition of hypothermia, frostbite, and immersion foot; and appropriate care.

"Heatstroke, heat exhaustion, and dehydration" provides necessary information about the balance of heat production and heat loss in a hot environment and the fluid requirements necessary to support physiologic cooling. WEMTs need to know how to recognize and provide long-term care for victims of heatstroke, heat exhaustion, and dehydration.

Lifting and Moving Patients

"Use of Stokes litters and improvising litters" discusses the primary device for evacuation from the backcountry. Even when a helicopter is used, the victim is usually "packaged" in a litter before being loaded. WEMTs must know the specific techniques for victim packaging in a litter to protect and support injuries. Use of the proper carrying techniques and methods of belaying a litter up or down a steep slope are critical to the safety of everyone involved.

Ambulance Operations

"Helicopter-assisted rescues" describes the use of helicopters in backcountry rescue efforts and evacuation. WEMT training should address the dangers, hazards, and limitations of helicopters.

APPENDIX

Research, Standards, and Program Resources

The following is a list of organizations and committees dedicated to some aspect of extended medical, rescue, and technical training. Many are also active in mountain, wilderness, marine, or disaster rescue and management efforts.

American Alpine Club
710 Tenth Street, Suite 100
Golden, CO 80401
303-384-0110
Resource: Publishes *The American Alpine Journal* and annual *Accidents in North American Mountaineering*. Has committees dedicated to establishing and promoting standards in safety and education in mountaineering.

American Mountain Guides Association
710 Tenth Street, Suite 101
Golden, CO 80401
Resource: Dedicated to establishing and maintaining standards for mountaineering and professional mountain guides. Publishes quarterly *Mountain Bulletin*.

Appalachian Mountain Club
P.O. Box 298
Gorham, NH 03581
603-466-2727
Resource: Active mountain rescue team that offers a variety of workshops on outdoor skills, environmental issues, and wilderness medical and rescue skills. Publishes quarterly *Appalachia*.

Appalachian Search and Rescue Conference
P.O. Box 440, Newcomb Station
Charlottesville, VA 22904
804-674-2400 (emergencies only)
Resource: Wilderness EMS agency, search and rescue, course and materials development.

Center for Emergency Medicine of Western Pennsylvania
230 McKee Place, Suite 500
Pittsburgh, PA 15213-4904
Resource: Offers various wilderness EMT and wilderness command physician training courses.

International Society for Mountain Medicine
Clinique Generale de Sion
1950 Sion, Switzerland
Resource: An international organization dedicated to research and education in mountaineering. Publishes quarterly *The Newsletter of the ISMM*.

Mountain Rescue Association
5301 D North 33rd Drive
Phoenix, AZ 85017-2802
Resource: National wilderness rescue organization dedicated to the development of standards and certification of mountain rescue teams.

Nantahala Outdoor Center
US 19 West, Box 41
Bryson City, NC 28713
704-488-2175
Resource: Offers a variety of courses on white-water rescue and wilderness medical and rescue training.

National Association for Search and Rescue
4500 Southgate Place Suite 100
Chantilly, VA 20151
703-222-6277
Resource: National information resource for search and rescue, as well as certifications in various search functions. Publishes quarterly journal *Response.*

National Cave Rescue Commission
c/o National Speleological Society
Cave Avenue
Huntsville, AL 35810
205-852-1300
EMERGENCY: *National Rescue Coordination 1-800-851-3051*
Resource: Active national cave rescue team.

National Ski Patrol System, Inc.
Ski Patrol Building, Suite 100
133 South Van Gordon
Lakewood, CO 80228
303-988-1111
Resource: Active rescue teams and ski patrols. Offers an outdoor emergency care course, various ski patrol certifications, avalanche training, and introductory mountaineering training.

Stonehearth Open Learning Opportunities (SOLO) and North American Rescue Institute (NARI)
P.O. Box 3150
Conway, NH 03818
603-447-6711
Resource: An international organization dedicated to developing and offering a variety of courses and certifications in wilderness and marine medicine, rescue, leadership, and outdoor skills. An active mountain rescue team. Publishes bimonthly *Wilderness Medicine Newsletter.*

Union Internationale des Associations d'Alpinisme (UIAA) (International Union of Alpine Associations)
President of the UIAA Medical Commission
Bruno Durrer, MD
Dokterhuus
3822 Lauterbrunnen
Switzerland
Resource: An international organization dedicated to the promotion of standards, safety, awareness, and education in mountaineering worldwide. Produces multiple publications on mountain safety and medicine.

United States Coast Guard Headquarters
2100 Second Street, SW
Washington, DC 20593-0001
202-267-1012 (Boating Operations)
Resource: Active national marine rescue military organization. Source of information and various boating-related certifications.

Wilderness Medical Associates
RFD 2, Box 890
Bryant Pond, ME 04219
207-665-2701, 800-742-2931
Resource: Offers a variety of courses and certifications in wilderness medical and rescue courses.

Wilderness Medical Society
P.O. Box 2463
Indianapolis, IN 46206
317-631-1745
Resource: A physician-based national wilderness medical organization with various committees dedicated to education in wilderness emergency medicine. Particular attention to education for physicians. Publishes quarterly newsletter and *Wilderness and Environmental Medicine* (formerly *Journal of Wilderness Medicine*).

Wilderness Medicine Institute of the National Outdoor Leadership School
300 Tenth Street
P.O. Box 9
Pitkin, CO 81254
303-641-3572
Resource: Offers a variety of courses and certifications in wilderness medicine and rescue.

SUGGESTED READINGS

American Academy of Orthopedic Surgeons: *Emergency care and transportation of the sick and injured,* ed 7, Sudbury, Mass, 1999, Jones & Bartlett.

Auerbach P: *Medicine for the outdoors,* New York, 1999, The Lyons Press.

Bowman W: *Outdoor emergency care,* ed 3, Lakewood, Colo, 1998, National Ski Patrol System.

Forgey W, editor: *Wilderness Medical Society: practice guidelines for wilderness emergency care,* Merrillville, Ind, 1995, ICS Books.

Henry M, Stapleton E: *EMT prehospital care,* ed 2, Philadelphia, 1997, WB Saunders.

Houston C: *Going higher,* ed 4, Seattle, 1998, The Mountaineers Books.

Iverson KV, editor: *Position statements of the Wilderness Medical Society,* Point Reyes Station, Calif, 1989, Wilderness Medical Society.

Lindsay L et al: *Wilderness first responder, wilderness and environmental medicine,* Lawrence, Kan, 1999, Alliance Communications Group

McSwain N et al: *The basic EMT: comprehensive prehospital care,* ed 1, St Louis, 1997, Mosby.

Mistovich J et al: *Prehospital emergency care and crisis intervention,* ed 6, Upper Saddle River, NJ, 2000, Brady.

Schimelpfenig T, Lindsey L: *NOLS wilderness first aid,* Lander, Wyo, 1991, National Outdoor Leadership School.

US Department of Transportation, National Highway Traffic Safety Administration: *Emergency medical technician-basic: national standard curriculum,* ed 4, Washington, DC, 1994, US Government Printing Office.

Wilkerson J, editor: *Medicine for mountaineering,* ed 4, Seattle, 1993, The Mountaineers Books.

Williamson J, editor: *Accidents in North American mountaineering,* Golden, Colo, American Alpine Club, published yearly.

25 Search and Rescue

Donald C. Cooper, Patrick H. LaValla, and Robert C. Stoffel

As ever-increasing numbers of outdoor users turn to the wilderness for recreation, the medical community and search and rescue (SAR) organizations will contend with a growing number of lost, sick, and injured persons. Wilderness search, rescue, and medical intervention are unique in several ways. All aspects of SAR are enormously time consuming. Simply raising the alarm for someone lost or injured in an isolated area may take hours, days, or even weeks. Organizing a response, including obtaining equipment and transportation for responders, requires a variable amount of time, depending on the level of preparedness of the response organization. Finding, gaining access to, stabilizing, and transporting a victim to definitive care can be a lengthy process.

Because it takes many persons to perform a wilderness rescue (six or eight persons are required to carry a litter 1 mile), logistic considerations such as food, shelter, and transportation for responders quickly create their own problems. SAR personnel are subjected to the same risks and environmental stresses that compromise victims. To obviate further tragedy, they must have a heightened awareness of potential danger, adverse conditions, and personal limitations. In addition to basic and advanced life-support training, rescuers must have extensive wilderness experience that combines practicality with creativity and resourcefulness. SAR personnel must have training in survival, improvisation, communications, leadership, navigation (e.g., map, compass, and global positioning system [GPS]), first aid, and specific SAR techniques. Many interventions, such as cardiopulmonary resuscitation, defibrillation, tube thoracostomy, tracheal intubation, and intravenous therapy, are difficult—if not impossible—in the wilderness setting. Examinations may be hampered by the bulky clothing necessary to keep the victim warm and dry. Medications and equipment are subject to rough handling and extremes of temperature, which may render them ineffective, unsterile, or inoperative (see Appendix at end of this book).

Finally, decision making that optimizes patient care while not unduly risking the well-being of SAR personnel requires experienced leadership grounded in both common sense and technical skill. Perhaps the demands of SAR were best summarized by the wise rescuer who said that climbers, divers, hikers, and other outdoor enthusiasts get to choose where they practice their skills, but SAR personnel have no such choice. The situation, usually urgent, dictates where and when rescuers practice their art. The same situation that already compromised at least one person's health or well-being subsequently endangers the SAR participants.

This chapter introduces medical professionals to the unique search, rescue, and medical problems encountered in wilderness, remote (including urban disaster environments), and backcountry situations. The rudiments of SAR coordination, resources, and specialized problems will be discussed. This information will help medical personnel understand how the SAR community works and provide an educational foundation to help prevent situations requiring undue risk, or SAR personnel themselves from having to be rescued.

SEARCH AND RESCUE: AN OVERVIEW

SAR systems provide the response for overdue, lost, injured, or stranded persons, usually in connection with outdoor activities and environments. In the context of SAR, "wilderness" can take on several meanings. For instance, most consider wilderness to be regions that are uninhabited and uncultivated. Personnel may be called out to search a natural area such as a large park or desert, but it is equally likely that a search will be urban, in an area devastated by a natural disaster such as an earthquake or hurricane. Because the majority of the population in the United States resides in urban areas, emergency responders and SAR personnel are far more likely to encounter urban wilderness than a natural one. However, this chapter focuses on the nonurban setting.

Types of SAR emergencies vary nationally, as do the responders. Programs, equipment, and personnel differ geographically in accordance with local needs and available resources. SAR can probably be best defined as "finding and aiding people in distress—relieving pain and suffering."[15] SAR often involves a great many volunteers and entails a multitude of skills. For example, the eruption of Mt. St. Helens, one of the nation's most catastrophic disasters, resulted in the largest peacetime SAR operation in the history of the United States.

SAR operations can benefit comprehensive emergency management, providing a training ground and experience builder for disaster response capability at the most elementary level. The management concepts used in SAR operations establish foundation principles for providing response capability to large-scale emergencies and disasters. Nearly every type of hazard mentioned in comprehensive emergency management plans (local and state disaster coordination plans developed in all states) requires search and rescue.[14] Management of these SAR operations can range from directing the actions of a few responders in a small community hit by a minor earthquake to managing an effort involving thousands of searchers in a large urban calamity. Often, large situations involve several political subdivisions and coordination of air and ground resources. Local governments and other agencies that participate in SAR response must coordinate diverse multiskilled responders. In addition, many agencies that collectively support multiorganizational SAR responses operate under their own specific statutory authority.

SAR operations entail a motivating time factor that focuses on a successful conclusion: finding or rescuing a lost subject before he or she succumbs to the effects of the environment, injuries, or a specific hazard. To be effective, extremely diverse organizations must be drawn together in a life-threatening situation with a commonality of purpose; this is even more true during a community-wide disaster.

Search and Rescue in the United States

National Search and Rescue Plan. SAR involves many agencies and volunteers, and the federal government assumes some responsibilities for overall coordination, especially of federal or military resources requested by local or state agencies.

The U.S. National SAR Plan[20] (*website:* www.uscg. mil/hq/g-o/g-opr/icSAR/nsp.htm) was first published in 1956 and identifies federal responsibilities in search and rescue. It is also the basis for the National Search and Rescue Manual, which discusses SAR organization, resources, methods, and techniques.

The National SAR Plan is implemented and maintained by the National SAR Committee (NSARC), formerly the Interagency Committee on Search and Rescue (ICSAR), which includes representatives from each of the six signatory federal agencies (Departments of Transportation, Defense, Commerce, and the Interior; the National Aeronautics and Space Administration [NASA], and the Federal Communications Commission [FCC]). NSARC reviews SAR matters affecting all agencies, including recommendations by participating agencies for plan revision or amendment, and makes appropriate recommendations. It encourages federal, state, local, and private agencies to develop equipment and procedures that will enhance the national SAR capability and promote coordinated development of all national SAR resources.

There are three geographic regions of jurisdiction identified in the National SAR Plan:

1. *Inland area:* Continental United States, except inland Alaska and waters under jurisdiction of the United States.
2. *Maritime area:* U.S. waters, Hawaii, specific areas off the west coast of Canada (south of Alaska), the

high seas, and those commonwealths, territories, and possessions of the United States lying within the "Maritime area," which has two parts: the Atlantic and the Pacific.
3. *Overseas area:* Overseas unified command areas, inland Alaska, areas not included in Inland or Maritime regions.

A "SAR coordinator" or agency responsible for SAR in the specific region administers each of the areas. The United States Air Force (USAF) is the coordinator for the Inland area, the United States Coast Guard (USCG) is responsible for the Maritime area, and the appropriate overseas unified command (and the Alaskan Air Command) tracks its respective areas in the Overseas area. Each SAR coordinator establishes agreements with military, civilian, state, local, and private agencies to ensure the fullest practical cooperation and utilization in SAR missions. SAR coordinators maintain files of these agreements and lists of the agencies and the locations of their SAR facilities.

Although the federal government provides guidance, national policy protects the desires of state and local agencies to direct and control their own SAR resources. Therefore each state and local government is encouraged to assume SAR responsibility within its geographic boundaries and capabilities. The federal role is to coordinate federal agencies in support of those at the local and state levels to create a cooperative national SAR network.

The USCG and USAF both operate rescue coordination centers (RCCs) in the United States, but each service takes a slightly different approach. The Air Force RCC (AFRCC) coordinates inland SAR activities in the continental United States but does not directly conduct SAR operations. In most situations, the Civil Air Patrol (CAP), state police, or local rescue services carry out the actual SAR operations. In contrast, the USCG not only coordinates but also conducts maritime SAR missions.

U.S. Air Force Rescue Coordination Center. Established in 1947 to meet the growing demand for SAR and its legislated responsibility, the original three AFRCCs have evolved into a single RCC located at Langley Air Force Base in Hampton, Virginia, under the Air Combat Command (ACC). The peacetime mission of the AFRCC is to build a coordinated SAR network, ensuring timely, effective lifesaving operations whenever and wherever needed. As of August 1996, the AFRCC recorded the prosecution of over 58,000 SAR missions, resulting in over 12,800 lives saved.[21]

The AFRCC functions around the clock and is staffed by people trained and experienced in the coordination of SAR operations. The center is equipped with extensive audio and digital communications equipment and maintains a comprehensive resource file listing federal, state, local, and volunteer organizations that conduct or assist SAR efforts in the United States, Canada, and Mexico.

There are four types of authorized AFRCC missions: search, rescue, MEDIVAC, and mercy.

SEARCH. Once a distress situation is determined to exist but a location is unknown, federal SAR forces may be activated to search for, locate, and relieve the distress situation. The object of these searches may take the form of overdue aircraft, emergency locator transmitters (ELTs), hunters, hikers, or children.

RESCUE. A rescue mission entails the use of federal SAR forces to recover persons in distress whose location in a remote area is known, but who need assistance. This may be in the form of transportation to safety or to an adequate medical facility. These requests are normally received by the AFRCC from park-service personnel or the local law-enforcement authority.

MEDIVAC. The transportation by federal assets of persons from one medical facility to another is defined as *aeromedical evacuation,* or MEDIVAC. Requests are normally received from a local hospital when no commercial transportation is available, the person's life is in jeopardy, and time is critical. Each request is evaluated, and the decision to use federal resources is weighted heavily by the attending physician's medical opinions.

MERCY. A mission to transport blood, organs, serum, medical equipment or personnel to relieve a specific time-critical, life-threatening situation is referred to as a *mercy mission.* Requests are normally referred from a local hospital authority or, in come cases, the American Red Cross when commercial transportation is not available.

Although the AFRCC will accept and act on initial notification from any person or agency, it will attempt to determine the urgency and the facts pertaining to the situation before obliging itself. Several aspects of the situation are considered before a mission is opened, including the following:
1. Medical evaluation and urgency
2. State agreement requirements
3. Posse Comitatus Act
4. Conflict of interest with commercial resources
5. Resource availability

The medical condition of the victim or victims is the most important aspect of mission consideration. The AFRCC will only consider a request valid when there is an immediate threat to life, limb, or sight. A mission will only be started to prevent death or the aggravation of a serious injury or illness. The observations and opinions of a physician at the incident site weigh heavily on the decision to open a mission, and a flight surgeon is on call at the AFRCC when a local physician is unavailable.

Each state has an agreement on file in the AFRCC describing the responsible agency and coordinating requirements for the various types of SAR missions. Each request for federal assistance is evaluated to ensure the requirements stipulated in the relevant agreement are met. Title 18 USC 1385 (the Posse Comitatus Act) prohibits military participation in civil law-enforcement activities. Although there are some exceptions to the prohibition, as a general rule, Department of Defense (DOD) forces, including the CAP, will be restricted from participating in searches in which the person being sought is evading searchers, is a fugitive, or when foul play is considered.

On MEDIVAC or mercy missions in which the patient is not eligible for DOD medical benefits, federal assets cannot be used when commercial resources are available. Even when a patient is unable to pay or is destitute, commercial resources will be checked for availability and provided the opportunity to accept the mission before allocating federal resources.

Although any SAR-capable asset belonging to the federal government may be requested, each resource is evaluated for distance from the distress location, special equipment requirements, urgency of the situation, and which resource can best accomplish the mission. Military forces may be called on to assist in civilian SAR missions. However, their participation in these activities must not interfere with their primary military mission.

Once the decision has been made to use federal resources, a mission number is assigned and SAR forces are selected based on the geographic location and mission requirements. The Air Force coordinator will then work closely with the responsible agency in an attempt to provide the resources best suited to accomplish the mission.

The AFRCC can be contacted as follows:

Mailing address: AFRCC, 205 Dodd Blvd., Suite 101C, Langley AFB, VA 23665-2789

For mission use and SAR requests *only:* (800) 851-3051

Administration (Monday-Friday during duty hours): (757) 764-8117

Website: www.acc.af.mil/afrcc

email: afrccrcc@hqaccdo.langley.af.mil

U.S. Coast Guard Rescue Coordination Centers. The USCG is designated as the federal SAR coordinator for the Maritime area, which is divided into two areas: Atlantic and Pacific. These areas are divided into several districts, which are further divided into groups (several per district) and stations. A 24-hour alert status is maintained year round at all levels, and Coast Guard resources can be underway or airborne within minutes of notification of a SAR mission. At its headquarters, each area and district maintains a fully staffed operations center responsible for coordinating operations within that area or district on a 24-hour basis. When coordinating SAR missions, these operations centers are called "rescue coordination centers" (RCCs). Although minor SAR incidents are often resolved at the station or group level, the district or area assumes the duties of the SAR mission coordinator (SMC) in more complex or large-scale missions.

The USCG is arguably involved in more SAR missions than any other organization or agency on the face of the earth. It is also notable that the USCG is a separate federal agency under the Department of Transportation, not the Department of Defense as is the Air Force.

An important global service of the USCG is the Automated Mutual-Assistance Vessel Rescue (AMVER) system. AMVER involves ships, regardless of flag, voluntarily providing information about their capabilities (i.e., medical personnel on board, rescue equipment) and regularly reporting their location to a global computer system that tracks their whereabouts. When a situation arises that requires SAR capabilities, a surface picture (SURPIC) is produced that graphically shows the location of all AMVER participants in the vicinity. The RCC can use this information to select the best one or several ships to respond to the emergency, allowing all others to continue their voyages. Today approximately 12,000 ships from over 140 countries participate in AMVER, representing approximately 40% of the world's merchant fleet. An average of 2700 ships are on the AMVER plot each day, with over 1 million voyages tracked annually. The AMVER system has saved over 1500 lives since 1990.[22]

A "preventive SAR" service provided by the USCG as a direct result of the Titanic disaster is the International Ice Patrol, whose operations are funded by SOLAS (Safety of Life at Sea) Convention signatories. Since 1913, the Ice Patrol has amassed an enviable safety record, with not a single reported loss of life or property caused by collision with an iceberg outside the advertised limits of all known ice in the vicinity of the Grand Banks. However, the potential for a catastrophe still exists, and the Ice Patrol continues its mission using high-tech sensors and computer models.

The USCG also performs or coordinates the medical evacuation of seriously ill or injured persons from vessels at sea if the patient's condition warrants it and USCG assets are within range. For less serious situations, USCG flight surgeons will offer medical advice via radio. On rare occasion, the RCC may coordinate with a U.S. Navy (USN) ship to allow a USCG MEDIVAC helicopter to refuel to extend its range. Also on rare occasion, the RCC may coordinate with the USAF to dispatch pararescue personnel to parachute to the vessel and stabilize the patient. In either case, these actions are taken only in the most serious situations where one or more lives depend on such drastic actions.

If a vessel is reported overdue or unreported (i.e., failed to check in when expected), USCG assets may or may not launch immediately, depending on whether the overdue craft is thought to be in immediate danger. Regardless, an extensive investigative effort will be initiated immediately. During this investigation, a preliminary communications check (PRECOM) and extended communications check (EXCOM) will likely take place. These actually include more than just contacting intended destinations. They also include interviewing persons who may be knowledgeable about the craft and dispatching USCG vehicles and/or small boats to physically check harbors, marinas, launching ramps, and the like. In addition, an urgent all-ships broadcast is initiated requesting information on any recent or future sightings that might be the missing vessel, and EXCOMs are repeated on a regular basis.

If none of these communications and investigation efforts produce positive results (i.e., locating the vessel and/or indications that the persons on board are not in immediate danger), a search will be undertaken. Search planning is conducted by the RCC staff, but additional assets can be requested from other agencies (i.e., USAF and USN) and/or foreign governments in a position to assist. With the assistance of the USCG's Computer Assisted Search Planning (CASP) system, the RCC develops scenarios based on the available information. These scenarios are then weighted according to a subjective estimate of how likely each one is to represent the true situation. The further analysis of available information leads to the development of probability maps (using CASP), after which a search is planned and orders are issued to all participating units. The search continues until either the survivors are found and rescued, or it is deemed that further searching would be fruitless.[6]

Because SAR regions are not construed as boundaries to effective SAR action, and much of the Inland area borders on the Maritime area, coordination between the AFRCC and the USCG RCC is a daily occurrence. Missions that traverse both areas will be coordinated through the AFRCC or the appropriate USCG RCC. It is not unusual for the USCG to call on the AFRCC for a particular resource needed to prosecute a mission in the Maritime area, or conversely, the AFRCC to utilize a USCG resource in the Inland area.

The USCG RCC can be contacted as follows:

Mailing address: USCG Headquarters, Commandant (G-OPR), 2100 Second Street SW, Room 3106, Washington, DC 20593-0001

Phone: (202) 267-1943

Fax: (202) 267-4418

Website (RCC location and contact information): www.uscg.mil/hq/g-o/g-opr/contacts.htm

U.S. Mission Control Center. The U.S. Mission Control Center (USMCC), located in Suitland, Maryland, is the U.S. operational component of a multiagency, multinational program that uses satellites to detect and accurately position emergency beacon signals from aircraft, vessels, and people in distress. This program is called the *SAR Satellite-Aided Tracking (SARSAT)* program, and the USMCC is one of 23 interconnected MCCs around the world that handle data distribution for the system. The National Oceanic and Atmospheric Administration (NOAA) operates Earth-observing satellites that are used to carry, among other things, SARSAT instruments that can detect and relay emergency signals from beacons activated by people in distress. These SARSAT payloads are provided by Canada and France, but Russia operates very similar instruments, known as COSPAS, aboard satellites that are part of a navigation system. The USMCC is administered by the SARSAT Operations Division of NOAA, which also represents U.S. interests in international COSPAS-SARSAT meetings. The USMCC is staffed 24 hours a day, 365 days a year. However, the vast majority of alert data distribution is handled automatically.

Together, the COSPAS-SARSAT system is being used in an international cooperative SAR effort in which the objective is to help save the lives of aviators, mariners, or anyone in distress who activates an emergency beacon. Aircraft carry ELT beacons that are normally triggered by the impact of a crash. Ships carry floating Emergency Position-Indicating Radio Beacons (EPIRBs) that are activated by immersion in water. Both devices can also be activated manually. These devices transmit on a radio frequency of 121.5 Megahertz (MHz) and/or 406.025 MHz. Using Doppler processing techniques, a beacon transmitting on the 121.5-MHz frequency can be located with an accuracy of about 10 to 25 km (5 to 12 miles) and may take as long as several hours to confirm. Alternatively, a beacon alerting on the 406 MHz frequency can be located within an accuracy of about 2 to 5 km (1 to 3 miles) and is usually confirmed in a matter of minutes. In addition, the 406-MHz devices have the capability of transmitting a unique identifier for which the MCCs maintain registration information about the owner of the device if the beacon was previously registered. In the near future, some 406-MHz devices will be coupled with electronic navigational receivers (such as GPS units) and will be able to provide both immediate alerting and accurate position information.

The COSPAS-SARSAT system consists of a network of satellites, ground stations, MCCs, and RCCs. When an emergency beacon is activated, the signal is received by a satellite and relayed to the nearest available ground station. The ground station, called a *Local User Terminal (LUT)*, processes the signal and calculates the position from which it originated. Once calculated, this position is transmitted to an MCC, where it is joined with identification data and other information on that beacon, if such information is available. The MCC then transmits an alert message to the appropriate RCC based on the geographic location of the beacon. If the location of the beacon is in another country's service area, the alert is transmitted to that country's MCC.

Before the inception of COSPAS-SARSAT, monitoring of ELTs depended largely on airborne aircraft or aviation ground facilities. This method provided irregular coverage, particularly in remote regions. Rapid location by satellite significantly reduces SAR time, improves survival chances for accident victims, and reduces exposure of SAR teams to hazardous conditions often encountered during their missions.

Federal Aviation Administration. The Federal Aviation Administration (FAA), through its Air Route Traffic Control Centers (ARTCCs) and Flight Service Stations (FSSs), monitors and flight-follows aircraft filing flight plans in the inland area. In some cases, individual citizens contact an FAA facility when they have knowledge of a probable SAR situation involving aircraft. Therefore the FAA is usually the first agency to alert the AFRCC of a distressed or overdue aircraft. The AFRCC is tied directly into the FAA's computer network, and FAA facilities use this system to alert the AFRCC.

Once the AFRCC is alerted, the FAA and AFRCC work together to determine the urgency of the situation and locate the aircraft. Initially, radio communications are reviewed to determine the last known location of the distressed aircraft. Concurrently, other FAA facilities begin a check of all possible airports where the aircraft might have landed. In the meantime, the AFRCC contacts relatives, friends, and business associates of the pilot or passengers aboard the missing aircraft, with the hope of establishing the whereabouts of the aircraft, or to gather information about the personnel aboard. Through these contacts, the AFRCC determines the pilot's intentions, flying capabilities, emergency equipment aboard, and other pertinent information that would assist if a search becomes necessary. Through experience, the FAA and AFRCC have learned that the majority of alerts for missing aircraft are due to the pilot failing to either close the flight plan or inform some person or agency of his or her intentions. For this reason, only a small percentage of alerts issued by the FAA result in an actual airborne search for a missing aircraft.

All ARTCCs have the capability to recall recorded radar data. The National Track Analysis Program (NTAP) can identify and track targets that are at a sufficient altitude to be tracked by radar regardless of whether they are being controlled by the ARTCC. NTAPs requested by the AFRCC have been proven to be a key ingredient in aircraft searches, providing the route of flight and last radar position.

With the congressional mandate requiring most aircraft to be equipped with an ELT, the FAA works very closely with the USMCC and the AFRCC to readily locate the source of ELT signals. All ELT signals reported to

FAA facilities are immediately forwarded to the AFRCC and jointly investigated as probable distress signals.

Civil Air Patrol. In 1948 the CAP was permanently chartered by the U.S. Congress as the official auxiliary of the USAF. As such, this nonprofit organization of volunteers was charged with three primary missions: the development of aviation through aerospace education, a cadet youth program, and emergency services.

Under their emergency services mission, the CAP provides SAR mission coordinators, search aircraft, ground teams, personnel on alert status, and an extensive communications network to emergency response efforts. Further, they provide services to national relief organizations during a disaster; the transportation of time-sensitive medical materials (e.g., blood and human tissue); and aerial reconnaissance, airborne communications support, and airlift of law-enforcement personnel in the national counter-drug effort. When CAP resources are engaged in a SAR mission, they are reimbursed by the USAF for communications expenses, fuel and oil, and a share of aircraft maintenance expenses. In addition, CAP members are covered by the Federal Worker's Compensation Act in the event of an injury while participating in a SAR mission.

The CAP is the AFRCC's prime air resource for the inland area. The AFRCC maintains an alert roster provided by CAP wings in each of the 48 contiguous states and is the central point of contact for CAP participation in SAR missions. The AFRCC also works closely with CAP national headquarters and directly provides input for CAP training in emergency services.

The CAP can be contacted as follows:
National HQ Civil Air Patrol, 105 South Hansell Street, Bldg. 714, Maxwell AFB, AL 36112-6332
Unit Locator: (800)-FLY-2338
Membership Development: (334) 953-4260
Public Affairs: (334) 953-4287

U.S. Coast Guard Auxiliary. The U.S. Coast Guard Auxiliary is to the USCG as the CAP is to the USAF. The auxiliary is made up of citizens who volunteer their time and boats or aircraft to enhance and maintain the safety of boaters. The passage of the Auxiliary and Reserve Act of 1941 designated that civilian volunteers of the USCG be referred to as *auxiliary.* When America entered World War II, some 50,000 auxiliary members joined the war effort. After the war, their attention returned to recreational boating safety duties in compliance with the auxiliary's four cornerstones: vessel examination, education, operations, and fellowship. Today, as in 1941, auxiliarists are civilian volunteers whose activities are directed by policies established by the commandant of the USCG. Although under the authority of the commandant, the auxiliary is internally autonomous, operating on four organizational levels

(smallest to largest): flotilla, division, district regions, and national.

When auxiliary resources are engaged under USCG "orders," they are reimbursed by the USCG for communications expenses, fuel and oil, and a share of vessel/aircraft maintenance expenses. In addition, auxiliary members are covered by the Federal Worker's Compensation Act in the event of an injury while participating in an authorized mission.

Many members of the auxiliary spend their weekends providing free boating safety courses to the public and free courtesy safety inspections to boaters. However, members also respond to minor SAR incidents, and the local USCG station, group or district RCC coordinates their activities. Some auxiliarists have also become qualified to work in the RCCs or assist regular USCG facilities with regulating and patrolling regattas and other maritime events.[23]

With its 33,000 members, the auxiliary saved nearly 500 lives in 1998 alone, in addition to assisting over 12,000 persons, performing over 139,000 courtesy marine exams, teaching over 6000 public and youth classes, and assisting the USCG in over 50,000 administrative and operational missions.[22]

The USCG auxiliary website URL is: www.cgaux.org/cgauxweb/

Disaster Response in the United States. The Robert T. Stafford Disaster Relief and Emergency Assistance Act (1988) provides the authority for the U.S. federal government to respond to disasters and emergencies to provide assistance to save lives and protect public health, safety, and property. The Federal Response Plan (FRP; available at www.fema.gov/r-n-r/frp/) was designed to address the consequences of any disaster or emergency situation in which there is a need for federal response assistance under authority of this legislation. The purpose of the FRP is to facilitate the delivery of all types of federal response assistance to states to help them deal with the consequences of significant disasters. The FRP outlines the planning assumptions, policies, concept of operations, organizational structures, and specific assignments of responsibility to the departments and agencies in providing federal response assistance to supplement the state and local efforts. It is applicable to natural disasters such as earthquakes, hurricanes, typhoons, tornadoes, and volcanic eruptions; technologic emergencies involving radiologic or hazardous material releases; and other incidents requiring federal assistance under the Stafford Act.[4]

To facilitate federal assistance, the FRP breaks federal response into 12 functions called *emergency support functions* or ESFs. Each ESF is coordinated by a primary federal agency and assisted by multiple support agencies.

FEMA serves as the lead agency for ESF-9 (Urban SAR, or US&R or USAR) and, as such, coordinates the

National Urban SAR Response System. This system is a framework for structuring local emergency services personnel into integrated disaster-response task forces. These task forces, replete with the necessary tools and equipment and requisite skills and techniques, can be deployed by FEMA for the rescue of victims of disaster and structural collapse. Currently, there are 27 FEMA US&R task forces spread throughout the continental United States trained and equipped to handle structural collapse rescue. They encompass local emergency service personnel from 18 states and can be deployed by FEMA to a major area disaster. Two task forces have also responded to several international disasters under the auspices of the U.S. Agency for International Development, Office of Foreign Disaster Assistance.

Each FEMA US&R task force contains 62 specialists, is designed to be self-sufficient for the first 72 hours of operation, and must be able to function for up to 10 days before being replaced. By design, there are two task-force members assigned to each position for the rotation and relief of personnel. This allows for round-the-clock task-force operations. In addition, all task-force members must be sufficiently cross-trained in their SAR skill areas to ensure depth of capability and integrated task-force operations.

After a request for federal assistance from a governor is received and approved by the president, task forces may be activated or placed on alert when a major disaster threatens or strikes a community or region. There are three regions: East, West and Central. Upon activation, alerted task forces start locating personnel and organizing their mobilization. Each task force is tasked with having all its personnel and equipment at the embarkment point within 6 hours of activation (the mobilization window). Depending on the location of the disaster, a task force will respond to the scene either by ground, using its own trucks, or via a military or civilian aircraft. Generally, an operational task force can be heading to its destination in a matter of hours. When the task forces are not on a FEMA-requested response, they function as technical rescue teams in their own communities and, in many cases, provide a regional or state-wide urban SAR capability.

A FEMA US&R task force includes four major functional elements:

1. *Search:* Canine, electronic, and physical capabilities to locate trapped victims.
2. *Rescue:* Evaluate compromised areas, structural stabilization, breaching, site exploration, live-victim retrieval.
3. *Medical:* Minimize health and safety risks, treat both task-force team members and trapped victims, provide critical incident stress debriefing.
4. *Technical:* Provide hazardous materials specialists, structural engineers, heavy rigging, communications specialists, and logistics specialists.

Typically, FEMA US&R task forces conduct the following operations:

- Perform physical SAR operations in damaged or collapsed structures
- Provide emergency medical care to task-force personnel, entrapped victims, and search canines
- Conduct reconnaissance to assess damage and needs and provide feedback to local, state, and federal officials
- Assess and/or shut off utilities to damaged buildings
- Conduct hazardous materials survey or evaluation
- Conduct structural/hazard evaluations of buildings needed for immediate occupancy to support disaster-relief operations
- Stabilize damaged structures, including shoring and cribbing operations

A comprehensive equipment cache totaling 58,000 pounds supports each task force. The cache elements sent to the disaster scene include communications and locating equipment, rope, and materials for rigging, hauling, lifting, and pulling. In addition, devices to facilitate shoring, structural movement sensing, victim extrication, cutting, and drilling are included to address a wide variety of potential SAR challenges.

The medical team includes four medical specialists and two physicians. Many of the medical specialists on US&R teams are both paramedics and firefighters and thus have experience in both rescue and prehospital medical care. Most of the physicians involved in US&R are emergency medicine specialists who have attended additional training in confined-space medicine, crush syndrome, hazardous materials, public health issues relevant to disaster management, and other issues important to the function of a US&R team. The medical team is designed to bring the emergency department to the field and carries all of the advanced life-support equipment available in any advanced life-support (ALS) ambulance.

The State's Role: Coordination and Support. All states have passed legislation that provides for direct support to local government entities during emergencies or life-threatening situations, and most states have a specific agency responsible for overall coordination and support for local SAR problems. This support can take many forms, but most often it is in the area of coordination and "one-stop shopping" for resources. Each state must establish an agency or central location that is familiar with all aspects of emergency management and the resources available to aid in life-threatening situations. Many of these resources belong to the state and can be used to aid local jurisdictions.

A number of states, especially in the Northwest, have designated a state agency to be responsible for directing and coordinating air SAR activities. These state departments, or divisions of aeronautics, develop and maintain aviation SAR response programs with cooperation and support from local and federal agencies. Experience shows that this system usually works better than those in other areas of the country that rely on the federal government to initiate and carry out aircraft SAR activities.

If a local emergency manager, sheriff, or fire chief requests outside assistance in the form of specialized teams, search dogs, air support, or enhanced communications, the state agency for civil defense, emergency services, or emergency management can in most cases locate the nearest resources available and coordinate the response. If any federal resources are needed, such as air support or military personnel, the state agency provides a direct link to that resource. For instance, the AFRCC at Langley Air Force Base in Virginia has working agreements with all states that are updated annually. Technically, the resources of local and state governments must have been exhausted or be unable to perform a task before federal support can be rendered. However, policy provides for immediate aid when time is critical and in life-or-death situations. Much discretion is given to military installation commanders regarding aid to civilian authorities as long as the primary (military) mission of the resource is not impaired. In fact, most commanders appreciate the opportunity to fly actual missions. Access to these resources must be gained through the state and the AFRCC.

Every state's emergency management agency is responsible for providing support, guidance, training, and coordination to local political subdivisions within that state. As such, it produces a vital behind-the-scenes effort to help local jurisdictions prepare for emergencies, including SAR. The state also initiates the laws necessary to enhance effective actions for SAR response. Such legislation often indemnifies volunteer SAR teams, provides their medical coverage and insurance, and in some cases replaces personal property lost during SAR work. Although most volunteers work willingly until the job is done, this recognition and coverage by the state often provide additional incentives for volunteer participation.

Local Response. The official response to the call for a wilderness SAR situation is usually delegated to a political subdivision within the state. The legal responsibility for SAR is generally vested with the county sheriff or chief law-enforcement officer at the local level, but this varies by region and state. In some cases it is the responsibility of state police agencies, and in others it belongs to land management agencies. The SAR response for one jurisdiction may differ greatly from that of another. For instance, many national parks in some areas of the country handle all of their own SAR incidents. Others jointly manage the function, whereas some rely entirely on outside resources. National forest land is managed solely by forest-service personnel, but when it comes to SAR, the forest service usually only supports the functions of the local responders.

In urban and suburban areas, police officers, firefighters, emergency medical technicians, and civil defense emergency organizations maintain some degree of disaster and emergency readiness through daily missions that involve SAR work. Fire departments have historically been responsible for rescue and response to emergencies within certain geographic or political areas, and volunteers augment many departments. Law-enforcement agencies also maintain full-time, efficient response systems designed for their particular SAR requirements. Ambulance and rescue vehicles operated by a variety of private enterprises and volunteer organizations augment existing local government services. Through local emergency response planning and coordination, these services respond to a spectrum of everyday emergencies, including fires, collapsed buildings, hazardous material spills, vehicle extrications, and home medical emergencies.

County sheriffs, reserve law enforcement, volunteer fire departments, and a variety of volunteer and rescue units have been established to address local SAR problems. Delivery of SAR aid to rural and wilderness areas often presents many special logistic problems, which may be compounded by distance, terrain, and weather. The demand for wilderness SAR is often seasonal and unpredictable. Volunteer mountain rescue units, Explorer SAR groups, SAR dog teams, CAP squadrons, motorized units, and many types of volunteer composite teams (i.e., teams that have a variety of capabilities) are usually formed locally in response to the type and nature of recurring SAR problems. Regardless of who does it or what type of SAR emergencies occur, local resources and effort must be developed because they are closest to the problem. State and federal resources are subject to problems with time lag, distance, weather, logistics, and bureaucracy. The same storm or disaster that incapacitates a local area may also prohibit outside (and sometimes inside) emergency response and resupply.

Although official agency responses differ greatly around the country, one major factor remains constant—the dedicated and unfailing willingness of volunteers to respond and work until the job is done. The volunteer effort in SAR nationwide is the backbone of aid to people in distress, as is stated in the rescue service motto: "These Things We Do That Others May Live." The volunteer response has proved crucial to wilderness-type situations. Volunteer organizations, communications, and special skills cannot be replaced by any "official agency" resources.

ORGANIZATION OF A SEARCH AND RESCUE EVENT

SAR requires people who take action and meet objectives to achieve a common goal, often with one or more lives in the balance. For any combination of actions to be effective in a particular situation, the enterprise must be systematically coordinated and organized. All participants must know their responsibilities, what is expected of them, who is in charge, and to whom they answer. If this knowledge is lacking, the effort can quickly become chaotic, ineffective, and, very probably, dangerous. Nowhere are these issues more important than in an emergency situation in which time is of the essence.

Emergency response research is clear and specific. The four operational problems that continue to arise during emergency responses in the United States are ambiguity of authority, inability to communicate between agencies, poor use (or no use) of specialized resources, and unplanned negative interactions with the news media.[14,15] Accordingly, the key elements for success in SAR operations continue to be good coordination of resources (the right people and equipment in the right place at the right time), effective communications, and good management practices with trained leaders.[14]

Incident Command System

The system designed to address the challenges of managing emergency incidents in the United States, including SAR, is called the *Incident Command System (ICS)*. It has been in use in the United States for many years.[17] This function-based system was designed to be adaptable to various types and sizes of incidents in a proactive, rather than a reactive, manner. The system groups similar tasks into five functional areas: command, operations, planning, logistics, and finance/administration. Each of these functions is performed at every incident to one degree or another, and all can easily be expanded as the size and complexity of the situation dictate. This expansion, however, is based on the premise that the span of control (the ratio of the subordinates to each supervisor) should never exceed seven to one and should more commonly be five to one. When this is exceeded, another level is added to the hierarchy to maintain an acceptable span of control (Figure 25-1).

The command section is led by the incident commander and provides overall management of the orga-

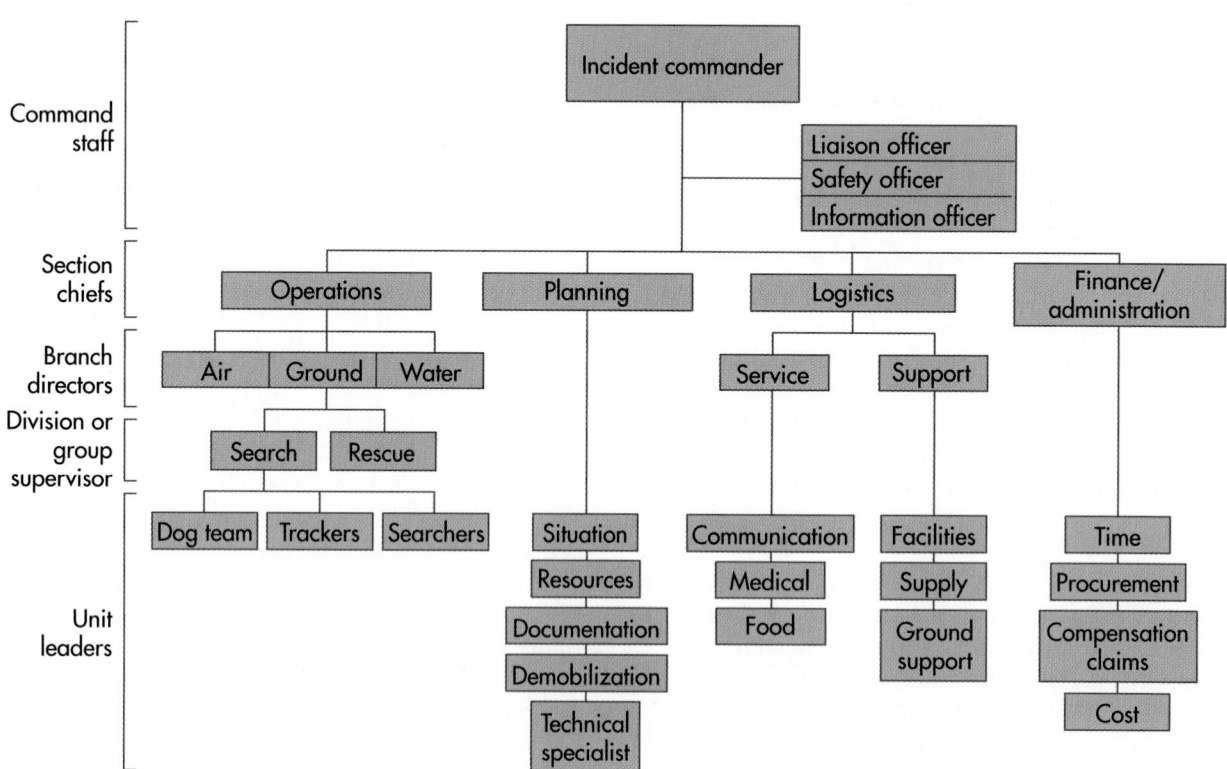

Figure 25-1 Functional hierarchy of the Incident Command System commonly used in SAR in the United States. (*From Cooper DC, LaValla PH, Stoffel RC: SAR fundamentals: basic skills and knowledge to perform search and rescue, ed 3 (rev), Cuyahoga Falls, Ohio, 1996, National Rescue Consultants.*)

nization. Within ICS, the command section is responsible for dealing with other agencies (liaison officer), the news media and other external influences (information officer), and for the overall safety of the operation and its participants (safety officer). If the incident is too small for these functions to be performed by separate individuals, the incident commander performs them.

The operations section is led by the operations section chief, who is responsible for coordinating and performing all tactical operations. This role is commonly performed by the incident commander until the incident becomes large and complex enough that the function must be performed by another individual. When multiple casualties are involved in an incident, their triage, treatment, and transport fall under the purview of the operations section. In such an incident the operations section is divided into functional groups, often including at least triage, treatment, and transport groups. The person in charge of managing and coordinating the efforts of each group is called the *group supervisor*. If the operations section is better divided using geography, a *division* rather than a *group* is formed. For instance, injured persons at an auto accident might be found on two sides of a road. An east division and a west division might be established to deal with the geographic separation of the resources. In a small organization, the supervisor of each division would answer directly to the operations chief.

To respond to specific challenges within an incident, a task force or strike team might be formed. A task force is any combination of single resources assembled for a particular tactical need, with common communications and a leader. For instance, FEMA combines search, rescue, and medical resources to form a US&R Task Force. A strike team, on the other hand, is a combination of a designated number of the same kind and type of resources with common communications and a leader. The number of resources used in the team will be based on what is needed to perform the function. For instance, four three-person hasty search teams may be combined to form a strike team. These two combinations of resources permit the necessary flexibility when allocating resources.

The planning section is led by the planning section chief, who is responsible for collecting, evaluating, and distributing all incident information. As with the other sections, the incident commander performs this function unless the size and complexity of the incident dictate otherwise. In SAR the planning section is particularly important because it evaluates search evidence and determines, based on what has been learned, what future actions should be taken or how current actions should be modified. Because such interpretation and evaluation often require great technical knowledge, personnel such as hazardous materials specialists,

physicians, structural engineers, and other technical specialists may be required to help the planning section develop and revise the incident action plan.

The logistics section is led by the logistics section chief, who is responsible for providing personnel, equipment, and supplies for the entire incident. This awesome task involves ensuring that personnel are available, rested, and fed; that all equipment, including communications equipment, is available and operable; that vehicles are fueled and repaired; and that medical care is provided for all incident personnel. Basically, logistics is charged with seeing that the physical tools required to meet the overall objectives are available, operable, and maintained.

If the size and complexity of the incident prevent the incident commander from monitoring finance and administrative issues, the finance/administration section is led by the finance/administration section chief. This section is responsible for tracking all financial data for the incident, such as personnel hours, resource costs, costs for damage survey, and injury claims and compensation. Because most agencies involved in SAR can handle financial issues on their own, and most incidents are small and of short duration, the incident commander usually performs the functions of this section. Only in the largest or most complex incidents is it necessary for the incident commander to assign an individual or staff to perform finance section duties.

FOUR PHASES OF A SEARCH AND RESCUE EVENT: THE INCIDENT CYCLE

Every SAR event goes through four consecutive phases: locate, access, stabilize, and transport.[2] This sequence, however, could more accurately be described as a continuum that begins with planning or preplanning for the incident. Because planning for the next incident should be affected by what happened during the last, the incident cycle is actually continuous and only pauses between incidents. Once first notice of an incident has been received and the locate phase begins, the goal is to progress through the access, stabilize, and transport phases as quickly, safely, and efficiently as possible. Planning between incidents allows decisions to be made in a calm environment without the urgency that often accompanies a SAR operation. Such plans identify who will be in charge, the organization of the operation, specific procedures, viable alternatives, and other decisions that are best made before an incident occurs (Figure 25-2).

Locate Phase

The first step in addressing any emergency situation is locating the subject or subjects in need of assistance. This may be as simple as asking for an address or as

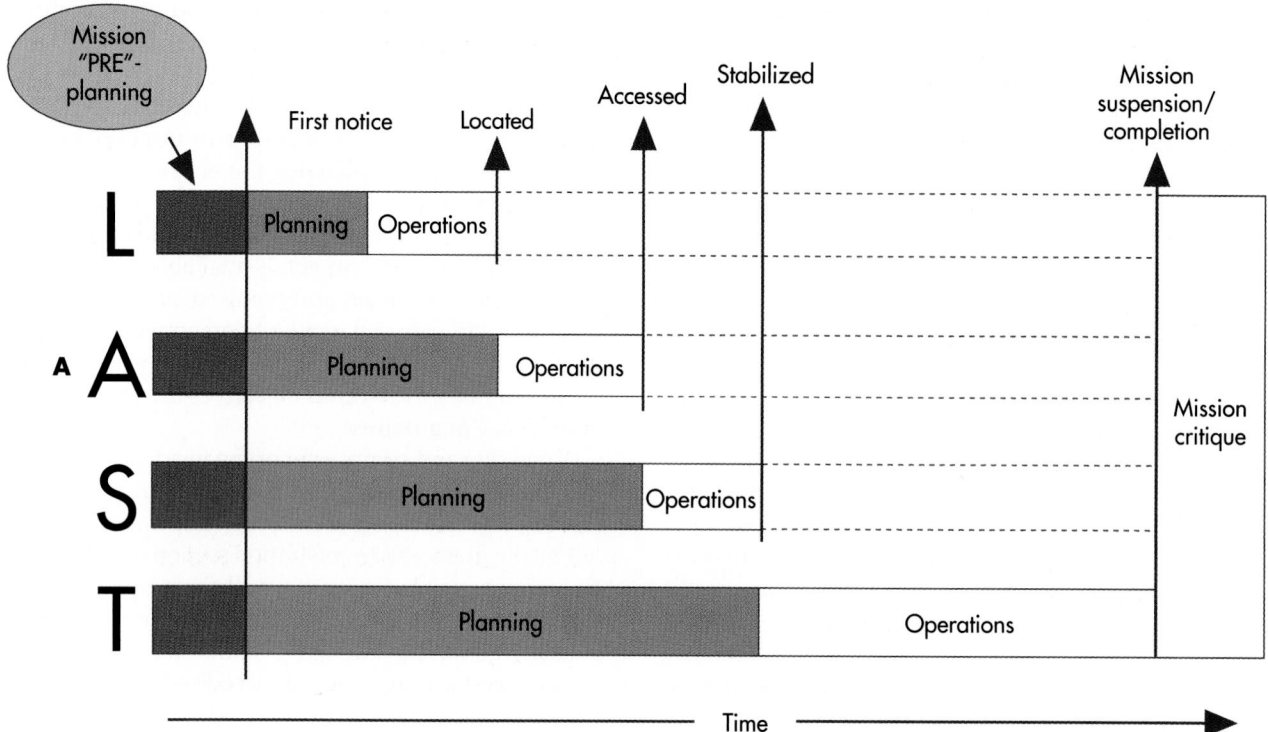

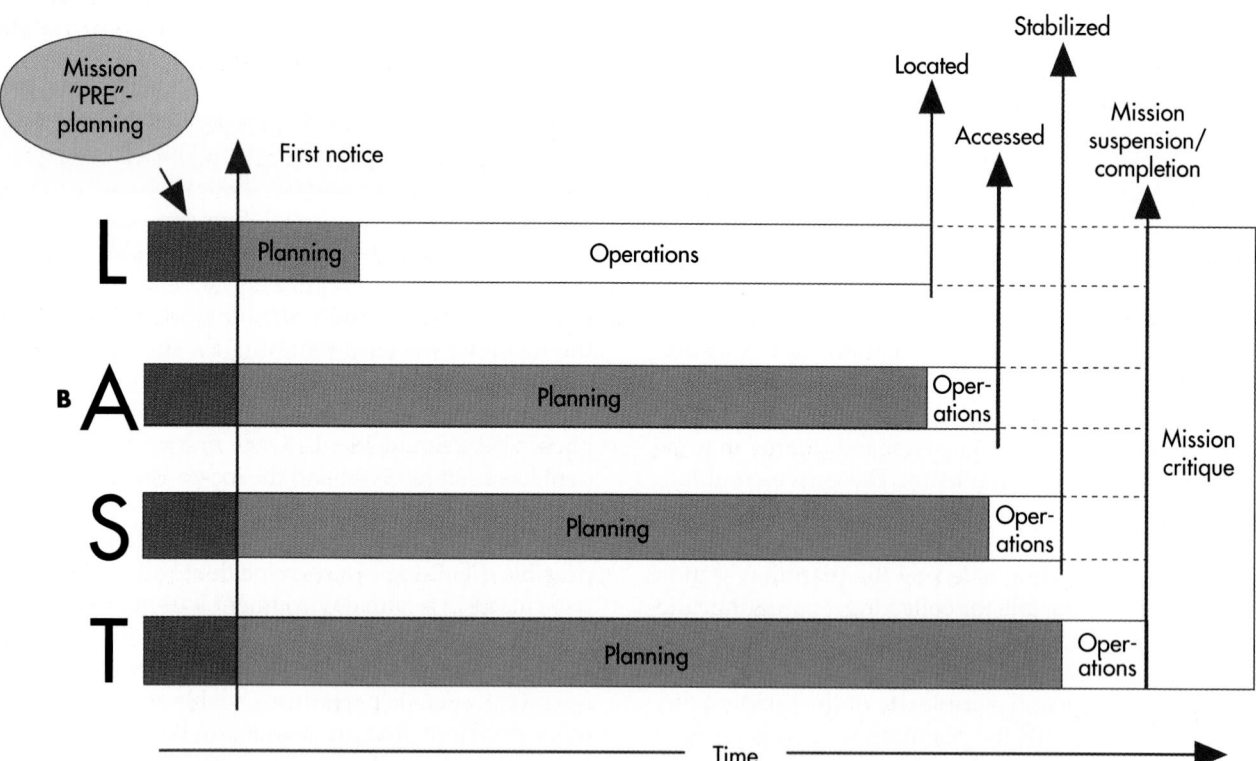

Figure 25-2 The time-specific components of a SAR event vary with the type of incident. Note that all components take place in both incidents but require different amounts of time. **A,** Typical rescue operation. **B,** Typical search operation.

complex as conducting an extended search for a lost person or persons. If the subject is easily found, rescuers can quickly move into the access phase. However, if locating the subject is difficult, this phase may turn into the crux of the SAR problem.

First Notice. The first notice of an incident is often conveyed by relatives who report an injury or missing person, by a witness to an incident, by a government agency reporting distress signals (such as an ELT), by bystanders who perceive a problem, or by a 911 call. Once the initial notice is received, the individual taking the information must know what to do and whom to call next.

Planning Data and Its Uses. Information gathered at the onset of an incident begins an ongoing investigation. It is used to determine the appropriate response and to help predict how the subject or subjects might react to the situation. This information is called *planning data* and includes any information that might affect what should be done to resolve the situation. Examples of planning data include the name of the subject, the situation that caused the problem, the last known location of the subject, the subject's physical and mental condition, the subject's plans (where was he or she going?), what resources are available, weather information (present and predicted), geographic information, and the history of similar incidents in the area. The purpose of collecting all of this information is to help decide what to do next while predicting what the subject might do to help or hinder the situation.

The investigation and gathering of information continue throughout the incident and are used to modify initial plans. As new information is acquired, an action plan is developed and revised until the end of the incident cycle, when planning for the next incident commences.

Once information is gathered, the urgency of the situation is assessed. This assessment ultimately determines the speed, level, and nature of any response and may indicate whether a nonurgent or an emergency response is needed. The specific information used in urgency determination includes the age and condition of the subject, current and predicted weather, and relevant hazards. Figure 25-3 is an Urgency Determination Form, which can be used by SAR managers to determine how urgent their response should be.[15] Urgency also contributes to allowable risks and thus influences searcher safety—a primary consideration for search managers.

Search Tactics. During the initial "locate" phase of the incident, emphasis is on searching for the subject. Exactly how to accomplish this is a priority, especially if

this part of the incident cycle is expected to be a problem. SAR managers first initiate techniques that increase the chances of locating the subject in the shortest time. These techniques are generally termed *tactics* and involve some action performed to find the subject. These actions can be passive (e.g., not requiring actual field searching) or active (requiring deployment of searchers in the field). Examples of passive tactics include confining the search area to limit movement of the subject and others into and out of the area, identifying and protecting the point last seen (PLS) or the last known position (LKP), and attracting the subject, if he or she is expected to be responsive.

Generally, passive techniques are quicker and easier to apply, so they are started first. As the incident progresses, active tactics are initiated. In SAR management, efforts are almost universally made to apply quick response resources in areas likely to offer early success. The best resources are put in the most likely areas as early as possible. In addition, identifying and protecting the PLS or LKP are crucial passive techniques that can mean the difference between success and failure of the entire effort.[15]

Active techniques include sending teams of searchers into an area to search for clues or the subject. They are categorized by level of thoroughness. For instance, a fast, relatively nonthorough search of high-probability areas is called a *type I search* (Table 25-1). *Type II techniques* can be applied when relatively rapid searches of large areas are desired. Thoroughness may increase, but more important, efficiency improves because larger areas can be searched with the same or fewer resources. Thus success is achieved sooner. *Type III techniques* are applied only when the absolute highest level of thoroughness is required. Unfortunately, this is almost always at the expense of time and efficiency. Basically, the greater the thoroughness, the more resource-intensive and time consuming the technique.

Clues and Their Value. Clues are discovered during the investigative and tactical phases of a search. Their importance cannot be overemphasized. They may take the form of physical evidence such as a footprint or discarded item, an account by a witness, or information gleaned from the investigation. Clues serve as the rudder that steers the overall search operation. Relevant clues are the basis for all search strategy and can determine or modify all actions. Their powerful influence should be obvious; this is why searchers are taught to be "clue conscious" and to seek clues, not just subjects. There are many more clues than there are subjects.

People generate clues. A person exudes scent, takes up space, and, when traveling, leaves evidence of passing. This evidence is often discoverable if the appropriate resource is applied in a coordinated, organized

Search Urgency

Remember the lower the number the more urgent the response!!!

Date Completed: _____
Time Completed: _____
Initials: _____

A. SUBJECT PROFILE .... _____

Age
    Very Young 1
    Very Old 1
    Other 2-3
Medical Condition
    Known or suspected injury or illness 1-2
    Healthy 3
    Known fatality 3
Number of Subjects
    One alone 1
    More than one (unless separation suspected) 2-3

B. WEATHER PROFILE .... _____

Existing hazardous weather 1
Predicted hazardous weather (8 hours or less) 1-2
Predicted hazardous weather (more than 8 hours) 2
No hazardous weather predicted 3

C. EQUIPMENT PROFILE .... _____

Inadequate for environment 1
Questionable for environment 1-2
Adequate for environment 3

D. SUBJECT EXPERIENCE PROFILE .... _____

Not experienced, not familiar with the area 1
Not experienced, knows the area 1-2
Experienced, not familiar with the area 2
Experienced, knows the area 3

E. TERRAIN & HAZARDS PROFILE .... _____

Known hazardous terrain or other hazards 1
Few or no hazards 2-3

       TOTAL .... _____

If any of the seven categories above are rated as a one (1), regardless of the total, the search could require an emergency response.

••• THE TOTAL SHOULD RANGE FROM **7** TO **21** WITH **7** BEING THE MOST URGENT. •••

8-11 Emergency Response   *12-16 Measured Response*   *17-21 Evaluate & Investigate*

Figure 25-3 Urgency Determination Form.

TABLE 25-1. Summary of Active Search Tactics

	TYPE I	TYPE II	TYPE III
Criterion	Speed	Efficiency	Thoroughness
Objective	Quickly search high-probability areas and gain information on search area	Rapid search of large areas	Search with absolute highest probability of detection
Definition	Fast initial response of well-trained, self-sufficient, and very mobile searchers, who check areas most likely to produce clues or the subject the soonest	Relatively fast, systematic search of high-probability segments of the search area that produce high results per searcher hour of effort	Slow, highly systematic search using the most thorough techniques to provide the highest possible probability of detection
Considerations	Works best with responsive subject; offers immediate show of effort; helps define search area; clue consciousness is critical; planning is crucial for effective use; often determines where not to search	Often employed after hasty searches, especially if clues were found; best suited to responsive subjects; often effective at finding clues; between-searcher spacing depends on terrain and visibility	Marking search segment is very important; should be used only as a last resort; very destructive of clues; used when other methods of searching are unsuccessful
Techniques	Investigation (personal physical effort); check last known position for clues; follow known route; run trails and ridges; check area perimeter, confine area; check hazards and attractions	Open grid line search with wide between-searcher spacing; compass bearings or specific guides are often used to control search; often applied in a defined area to follow up a discovered clue; no overlap in area coverage; critical separation; sound sweeps	Closed grid or sweep search with small between-searcher spacing; searched areas often overlap adjacent teams for better coverage
Usual team makeup	Two or three very mobile, well-trained, self-sufficient searchers	May include three to seven skilled searchers, but usually just three	Four to seven searchers, including both trained and untrained personnel
Most effective resource	Investigators, trained hasty teams, human trackers, dogs, aircraft, any mobile trained resource	Clue-conscious search teams, human trackers and sign-cutters, dogs, aircraft, trained grid search teams	Trained grid search teams

search effort. Searchers must be sophisticated enough to discover this evidence and interpret its meaning before it is destroyed or decays. Because evidence important to a search effort is often easily destroyed once it is discovered, it is important to protect it from damage until it is completely analyzed.

Search Resources. *Resources* are defined as all personnel and equipment available, or potentially available, for assignment to incident tasks. Specific types of active tactics are categorized by the resource that performs them, such as dog teams, human trackers, ground search teams, and aircraft. Other common resources include management teams (e.g., overhead teams, public information officers), water-trained responders (e.g., river rescue, divers), cold weather responders (e.g., ice climbers, avalanche experts, ski patrollers), specialized vehicle responders (e.g., snowmobiles, four-wheel-drive trucks, all-terrain vehicles, mountain bikes, horses), and technical experts (e.g., communications experts, interviewers,

chemists, rock climbers, physicians, cavers). In addition to these, other less common resources might also be available. These could include attraction devices (such as horns, flags, lights, sirens), mine detectors (military), noise-sensitive equipment (super microphones), infrared devices (forward-looking infrared [FLIR] on aircraft, night-vision equipment, thermal imagers), thermistors, and even witches, seers, prophets, and diviners.

Just about any person or thing imaginable may be available for use in a SAR incident. Their use is limited only by the creativity of those in charge. Here we discuss a few of the most common.

Dogs. Dog teams are a common type of active search resource in the wilderness and are composed of a dog (occasionally more than one) and a human handler. The dog uses scent to search for and follow a subject while the handler interprets signals from the dog and searches visually for evidence. Three common categories are tracking, trailing, and air-scenting dogs.

Tracking dogs follow scent on the ground from a person's footsteps and usually very closely follow the trail where a person traveled, regardless of the wind. Trailing dogs follow scent that has fallen onto the ground from the subject along the route of travel. Unlike the tracking dog, the trailing dog may follow the scent at some distance from the actual tracks of the subject, and may therefore be more affected by wind. Tracking and trailing dogs are most effective when used in areas that have not been contaminated by humans other than the subject. Also, weather and time tend to destroy scent available to these types of dogs, so the earlier they are used in a search, the better their chances of finding something.

Air-scenting dogs work off-lead to follow a subject's scent to its source. Specifically bred and trained air-scenting dogs can even discriminate between individual humans. They may detect scent from articles of clothing and can often follow it to discover a person buried in rubble or snow or even submerged under water. Wind is very important to this type of dog, as are other environmental forces such as sun and rain. But as long as the source exists, an air-scenting dog can usually detect the scent carried in air currents and follow it to the source.

HUMAN TRACKERS. Human trackers use their visual senses to search for evidence left by a person's passing. Human trackers "cut" or look for "sign" or discoverable evidence by examining the area where the subject probably would have passed. This process of looking for the first piece of evidence from which to track is called "sign cutting." Following the subsequent chain or chronology of sign is called "tracking."[3]

In SAR, most trackers use a stride-based approach called the step-by-step method. This simple, methodical approach emphasizes finding every piece of possible evidence left by a subject. However, its most important role is undoubtedly the ability to quickly determine the direction of travel of the subject and thus limit the search area.

Ground Search Teams

Hasty teams. A hasty team is an initial response team of well-trained, self-sufficient, highly mobile searchers whose primary responsibility is to check out the areas most likely to first produce the subject or clues (e.g., trails, roads, road heads, campsites, lakes, clearings, and so on). Their efficiency and usefulness are based on how quickly they can respond and the accuracy of initial information.

Ideally, hasty teams should include two or three individuals who are knowledgeable about tracking. They should be clue oriented, familiar with the local terrain and dangers in the area, and completely self-sufficient. Also necessary are the ability to skillfully interview wit-

nesses and to use navigational skills with pinpoint accuracy. Team members should be trained at least in advanced first aid. Hasty teams usually operate under standard operating procedures so they do not have to wait for specific instructions. They carry all of the equipment they might need to help themselves and the lost subject for at least 24 hours.

Grid teams. Grid searchers use a more systematic approach to searching. They usually examine a well-defined, usually small segment to discover evidence (Figure 25-4). The classic approach to grid searching involves several individuals (almost always too many) standing in a line, shoulder to shoulder, walking through an area in search of either evidence or subjects. The distance between searchers can be varied to change thoroughness and efficiency (wide spacing is less thorough and more efficient). However, such resource-intensive approaches to searching are generally less preferred than those that use fewer personnel in a more efficient manner (such as tracking, dogs, or aircraft). In addition, close-spaced grid searching tends to damage evidence and is generally difficult to coordinate.

Although grid searching may be an acceptable approach in certain limited circumstances, experience has shown that when the subject of a search is a person, searching in this thorough manner should be used only as a last resort. Experiments involving grid searching have suggested that it is better to place searchers farther apart. This is usually a more efficient use of resources.

AIRCRAFT. Aircraft serve the same purpose as grid searchers, only from a greater distance, at a greater speed, over a larger area, and usually with a lower level of thoroughness. Within a search effort, aircraft can serve both as a tactical tool to look for clues and as transportation for personnel and equipment. Both

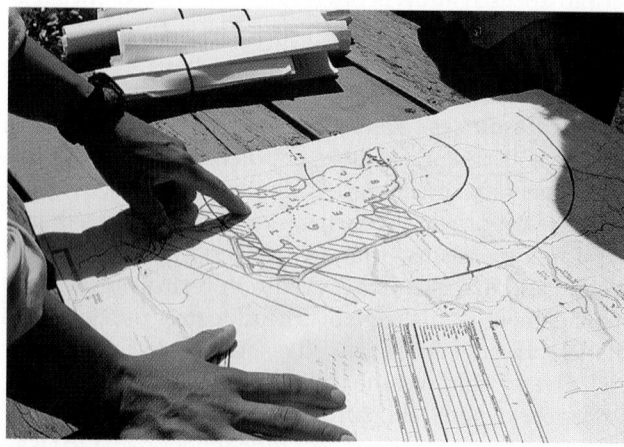

Figure 25-4 Map used to brief ground team. *(Photo courtesy Spectra Communications, Inc.)*

fixed- and rotor-wing aircraft have their place in SAR and, like other resources, have their advantages and limitations. Among the most obvious limitations are the expense and complex use requirements of aircraft. Aircraft not only require specialized personnel and cost a great deal to operate, they also have very strict weather and environmental restrictions. For instance, it would be difficult to search from an aircraft in a snowstorm, and terrain may prevent searching certain areas from the air. However, most of these difficulties can be adequately addressed and minimized in a well-developed preplan.

Search Planning and Management Considerations.

State-of-the-art searching for lost persons has come a long way from the familiar lining up of volunteers shoulder to shoulder and walking in a straight line to search an area. Many new lifesaving concepts have been developed by the national SAR community. By borrowing from psychology, mathematics, and business and analyzing research on past incidents, search management has evolved into a sophisticated science. By studying human behavior, statistics, probabilities, leadership, and management, search managers have been able to improve search effectiveness and efficiency.[15]

Search management is determined by two general considerations: where am I going to look for the lost person? (strategy) and how am I going to find the lost person? (tactics). To be effective, modern searchers follow several basic principles and techniques, including the following:

1. Respond urgently—*a search is an emergency*
2. Confine the search area
3. Search for clues
4. Search at night
5. Search with a plan in an organized manner
6. Grid search (type III) as a last resort

Every day, firefighters, paramedics, police officers, and other emergency responders receive calls to perform their duties, and often they can only guess what they will find once they arrive. In response to this the concept of the "firehouse" response has evolved. This concept calls for emergency responders, much like emergency physicians, to assume the worst until proven otherwise. Thus they respond with "lights and siren" to most calls just in case the situation is serious. Furthermore, they often respond in this way even when the reporting party specifies that the situation is minor, claiming that a certain percentage of individuals reporting incidents are wrong in their assessment. Essentially, the situation is considered an emergency until proven otherwise.

For years, searching has been considered less urgent than other emergencies. While emergency responders were running with lights and sirens to situations reported as "women not feeling well" or "dumpster on fire," reports of a lost child or an overdue hiker were relegated to the "let's wait and see" category. Through years of experience, search managers now know that a search is as much an emergency as any other call for help. Furthermore, if an urgent response is mustered, the situation can be resolved faster, more successfully, and usually with less effort. Thus a search should be considered an emergency that justifies an urgent response, a high priority, a thorough assessment, and immediate action.

Search Theory. The mathematical basis for searching and the study of search theory had its beginnings during World War II in the work of the U.S. Navy's Anti-Submarine Warfare Operations Research Group (AS-WORG) and was originally based on searching for the wakes of warships as seen by aircraft flying over the ocean.[5] The results of this work were collected in a seminal report by B.O. Koopman in 1946,[12] but the report was not declassified and generally available until 1958.[1] In 1980 Koopman developed a somewhat expanded version of this work, which was published in his book *Search and Screening: General Principles with Historical Applications.*[13] Although Koopman's work is clearly aimed at naval interests, the general theory of search he established is applicable to virtually any type of search problem. Since this early work, search theory has undergone continuous research and development by agencies such as the USCG and USN in both the maritime and aeronautical environments, mining and oil businesses in the search for mineral and petroleum deposits, and even archeologists in the search for lost cities, such as Troy.[18]

The fundamental usefulness of search theory lies in its ability to help determine where and how to search. It accomplishes this by (1) quantifying the likelihood of a lost subject being in a particular area, as well as the likelihood of searchers finding the subject; and (2) offering tools with which one can estimate the chances of success of a particular search.

The application of search theory requires the appropriate use of probability theory, a branch of mathematics that is used for estimating the likelihood of uncertain events, in planning a search. The chances that the lost person or clue is in the search area is called *probability of area (POA)*. The probability that a search resource will find the lost person or clue if it indeed is in the area being searched is called *probability of detection (POD)*. The mathematical combination of these two important variables produces a product called *probability of success* (POS = POA × POD). The foremost objective, and major challenge, for search planners is to combine the appropriate search resources (sensors producing POD) with appropriate segments of the search area where the subject is likely to be (POA) to produce the most POS in the least amount of time. On the surface this seems to be a straightforward proposition. However, additional critically important factors, such as resource detection capability, environmental influences, search object characteristics, probability density, probability distribution, coverage and sweep width, conspire to make the most correct search action a complex, unintuitive series of difficult choices.

Although software is available to assist in the mathematical decisions, less than optimum but historically acceptable results have been achieved when a search manager applies the principles of search management as an intuitive combination of hard science and sage experience. In the final analysis, search success is based on more than just science. At its finest, it involves the artistic application of science and a high degree of organizational and management skill sprinkled with intuition and punctuated with a bit of luck.

Lost Subject Behavior. Modern search management is also based on the use of what is called a *complete "subject profile."* Such a profile identifies as much as is known about the missing subject, including general state of health, past experiences, and state of mind, through the use of a form called the *Lost Person Questionnaire.* This information is collected and used by search managers to predict how an individual would react in various situations. Analysis of this information from past incidents and understanding how the involved individuals behaved in given circumstances have offered great insight for search managers.

Although it is not difficult to appreciate the importance of predicting how a subject might react when lost, the scientific approach to the subject began with William G. Syrotuck's seminal paper in 1977, *Analysis of Lost Person Behavior: An Aid to Search Planning.*[19] This paper was based on the premise that individuals will have similar travel habits when compared with others in the same "category." The six categories Syrotuck described include small children (1 to 6 years), children (6 to 12 years), hunters, hikers, elderly (over 65 years), and "miscellaneous adults," such as nature photographers, fruit gatherers, bird watchers, and other outdoor enthusiasts. He also included two "special categories" (mentally retarded persons and despondents) for which he had very little data. In his study, Syrotuck described the behavioral characteristics of a representative member of each category and computed "probability zones" for each based on distances traveled. This distance was measured "as the crow flies," or as a straight-line distance, between the point where the subject was last seen and the location where the subject was eventually found. Realizing that there was likely a substantial difference between how far a lost subject actually traveled and the crow's flight distance, Syrotuck argued that, "it is more important to realize that a known percentage of all lost persons is found within a one- or two-mile radius than it is to know how they got

there." Syrotuck studied 229 cases, most from wooded areas of Washington and New York states, and all involved subjects traveling on foot.[19]

Beyond identifying categories, Syrotuck also documented and described six other factors that may affect the search plan. He suggested that search personnel in possession of the following information could more accurately predict the subject's location:

1. Circumstances under which the person became lost
2. Terrain
3. Personality
4. Weather
5. Physical condition at time of loss
6. Medical problems

He went on to describe how one's general state of health, past experiences, and physical situation (e.g., hot, cold, altitude) contribute to predicting behavior patterns. How one reacts to being lost, he also suggested, can impact the type and quantity of clues (i.e., disrobing, discarding equipment), survivability (i.e., failure to build a fire), detectability (i.e., bright clothing, bad weather), and tendency to follow travel aids such as rivers, roads, and trails. In all, Syrotuck produced the first scientific description of how people might react to being lost, and how searchers could use this information to improve operations.

Following the theme of lost-person behavior and using the crow's-flight distance, Koester and Stooksbury[9] performed a retrospective study of persons who suffered from dementia of Alzheimer's type (DAT) and who became the subjects of organized SAR efforts in Virginia. They studied 82 cases (initially) from the Virginia Department of Emergency Services' (DES) lost subject database and compared the DAT patient's behavior to that of elderly lost subjects that possessed normal cognitive abilities. Their findings were of great interest to search managers in that this was the first time research of this type had been conducted for the inland SAR community. Koester and Stooksbury also described a "subject profile summary" and suggested specific search techniques for lost DAT patients. Notable in their findings were the facts that none of the subjects in the cases they studied yelled for help, and they were usually found 0.5 miles (0.8 km) from the PLS. Since this initial research, Koester[10,11] has continued to analyze the Virginia DES data (Tables 25-2 to 25-4).

Also using the crow's flight distance, Hill[8] described distances traveled and probability zones for lost persons in Nova Scotia. However, Hill found it useful to modify and add to Syrotuck's categories of lost persons. For instance, Hill broke young people into four categories, children 1 to 3 years, children 4 to 6 years, children 7 to 12 years, and youths 13 to 15 years. He described characteristics for fishermen, skiers, and walkaways (i.e., people who walk away from a constant-care situation), and additional characteristics for those who are despondent.

TABLE 25-2. Summary of findings from Koester, 1999[10] and Koester, 2000[11]

	TYPE OF VICTIM				
STATISTIC	ALZHEIMER'S	ELDERLY	DESPONDENTS	RETARDATION	PSYCHOTIC
n	87	33	65	29	25
Age (S.D.)	76 (9.2)	70 (4.3)	37 (15.7)	30 (3.3)	43 (15.9)
Males	67%	67%	76%	60%	63%
Females	33%	33%	24%	40%	37%
Uninjured	51%	48%	34%	85%	72%
Injured	27%	15%	11%	11%	5%
Deceased	22%	37%	55%	4%	22%
Distance from PLS (km)					
Mean	1.0	2.9	2.2	1.4	2.2
S.D.	0.8	0.8	5.3	1.9	3.7
Median	0.8	0.8	0.3	0.8	0.8
Range	0-4.8	0-8.0	0-32.2	7.7	12.9
25%	0.3	0.2	0.2	0.2	0.2
50%	0.8	0.8	0.3	0.8	0.8
75%	1.1	4.0	2.6	1.6	2.0
Max zone	2.4 (94%)	7.7 (95%)	8.0 (96%)	4.0 (95%)	7.7 (92%)

PLS, Point last seen.

TABLE 25-3. Distance Traveled Data, from Koester, 1999[10] and Koester, 2000[11]

DISTANCE FROM THE PLS MILES (km)	TYPE OF SUBJECT			
	ALZHEIMER'S (ADRD)	DESPONDENTS	MENTAL RETARDATION	PSYCHOTICS
n	87	74	29	25
10%	0.1	0	0	0
20%	0.1	0.1	0.1	0.1
30%	0.25	0.1	0.2	0.25
40%	0.3	0.15	0.25	0.3
50%	0.5	0.2	0.5	0.4
60%	0.5	0.25	0.75	0.5
70%	0.7	0.75	1.0	1.0
80%	1.0	1.25	1.7	2.0
90%	1.25	4.0	3.0	4.8
100%	2.0	20	4.8	8.0
Investigative finds	8%*	10%	11%	5%

PLS, Point last seen.
*Investigative finds increase to 25% in urban areas.

TABLE 25-4. Subject Found Location Data, from Koester, 1999[10] and Koester, 2000[11]

	TYPE OF SUBJECT			
	ALZHEIMER'S (ADRD)	DESPONDENTS	MENTAL RETARDATION	PSYCHOTICS
Structure	15%	8%	21%	23%
Yard (open field)	18%	4%	16%	—
Drainage	18%	8%	21%	7%
Woods	7%	33%	16%	30%
Brush/briars	29%	—	11%	7%
Road	7%	—	11%	23%
Powerline/linear	—	13%	5%	—
Other	4%	8% (cliff bottom)	—	—

Taking a slightly different approach, Heth and Cornell[7] published a study of 162 incidents of persons lost in wilderness areas in southwestern Alberta, Canada. They tabulated crow's-flight distance traveled and angular dispersion of travel (the angle from a line that connects the PLS with the intended destination) by different categories of wilderness users. They formed 10 categories of outdoor user (Table 25-5) and included only subjects propelled by muscle (no machinery). Interestingly, Heth and Cornell found a behavioral distinction between "front country" users (i.e., front to parking lots, groomed trails, frequent signage, good and available maps attracted users with a large range of outdoor experience and skill) and "backcountry" users (i.e., remote areas, undeveloped, attracted prepared and experienced users). Not unlike Syrotuck and Hill, Heth and Cornell discovered that, with the exception of despondents, there is a similar distribution of distance traveled by persons lost outdoors. However, they went further and suggested that there might be a linear relationship between certain data sets. For instance, their analysis indicated that hikers travel about 2.3 times farther than campers, and cross-country skiers breaking trail travel about 5.4 times farther than cross-country skiers using groomed trails. The implication is that if archival data are possessed for one category in one region and are compared with categories of lost subjects similar to those described by Heth and Cornell, a scalar parameter could be applied to extrapolate crow's-flight distances for other subject categories. Such a possibility is exciting to search managers who only rarely have access to relevant and reliable archival data.

Search managers have used these behavioral studies, and others, in a number of valuable ways. By direct analysis and limited extrapolation, search managers have been able to find answers to important planning questions that are helpful in determining where and how to search. Such efforts have also taught search managers the importance of collecting behavioral data on lost persons, and the predictive value of such data.

Access Phase

After the subject is located, the search is over. Rescuers must now gain access to the subject to assess and treat injuries, evaluate the situation, and mitigate the problem. Accomplishing these objectives may be as simple as walking into a room with the subject or as complex as reaching an astronaut in space. Regardless, planning for this eventuality should be complete and ready to be carried out at the conclusion of the locate phase.

Once rescuers reach a subject, the situation and scene must be assessed. In emergency services terminology, this is called the *size-up*. The size-up consists of identifying hazards to the subject and rescuers, then developing a strategy to deal with the problems. For instance, a subject might be trapped by a winter storm in a high alpine environment. Safety considerations for rescuers entering such a hostile and dangerous environment would certainly influence further actions and may well take precedence over the entire rescue effort.

Specialized skills may be required for rescuers to safely gain access to the scene. For instance, rescuers may need to rappel to a patient who has fallen onto a ledge in terrain such as the Grand Canyon. Or rescuers may need to climb sheer rock faces to reach an injured mountaineer on Half Dome in Yosemite National Park. These are examples of how complex the access phase of a rescue may be and point to the importance of thorough and proper planning.

If the size-up indicates that the situation or environment is so hazardous that remaining on scene poses an immediate threat to the subject, accelerated rescue techniques may be required. Accelerated rescue techniques are immediate actions required to remove a subject

TABLE 25-5. Formal Estimates of Crow's Flight Distance (in km) Between the PLS and the Point Found for (N) Persons Lost During Different Wilderness Activities

ACTIVITY GROUP	PERCENTILE			
	25	50	75	90
Campers (18)	.722	1.559	3.001	4.931
Cross-country skiers: break trail (5)	4.537	9.795	18.860	30.988
Cross-country skiers: groomed trail (18)	.842	1.819	3.501	5.753
Despondents (6)	.229	.656	1.793	4.664
Hikers (38)	1.691	3.650	7.028	11.548
Hunters (5)	1.222	2.638	5.079	8.345
Mountain bikers (18)	3.759	8.116	15.626	25.675
Scramblers (7)	1.165	2.515	4.843	7.958
Walkaways (14)	.701	2.007	5.486	14.274
Other (13)	1.765	3.812	7.339	12.058

From Heth DC, Cornell EH: *J Environ Psych* Dec 11, 1997.
NOTE: Estimates for despondents and walkaways were based on a different Wakeby distribution than that used to estimate the percentiles of the other user categories.

from a dangerous environment without stabilization. They often entail deviations from local standard operating procedures and protocols. Examples of such situations include poisonous gas environments (e.g., in caves), fires, unstable terrain (such as avalanches and rock slides), adverse weather (hurricanes, thunderstorms, severe snowstorms), or any hostile environment that threatens the subject, rescuers, or both.

Stabilize Phase

The stabilize phase has three primary components: physical, medical, and emotional. Once rescuers have access to the subject, the scene must be quickly evaluated, or sized-up, for immediate physical hazards and threats from the environment or situation. Scene safety is an initial priority in the size-up, and risks to rescuers and the subject must be weighed against the benefits to be gained. An example of physical stabilization would include an occupied automobile teetering on the edge of a cliff. Before the occupant can be medically assessed, the situation (i.e., the automobile) must be stabilized to best protect the rescuers and the patient. Other examples of physical stabilization might include protecting the patient from further injury (e.g., removing them from the hazardous environment, applying a helmet) or removing the hazard (e.g., extinguishing the fire, securing the teetering auto).

Once the physical environment is stabilized and free from immediate hazards, medical management and stabilization commence. This process usually follows accepted procedures, starting with primary and secondary physical examinations and basic and advanced life support. It should include full-body immobilization, usually in a litter; specific site immobilization of fractures and related injuries; treatment of shock and other hemodynamic compromise; and protection from the environment. The goal of medical stabilization is usually to prepare the subject for transportation to a definitive care facility. If medical care is not required, confirming this fact may be all that is required at this stage before moving into the transport phase.

Emotional stabilization is necessary because an anxious victim is a hazard to rescuers and himself or herself. Again, the goal is to best protect both the rescuers and the victim. Simple, calm communication with the victim, slowly describing what happened and what rescuers are doing, is often enough to calm a nervous victim.

Stabilization, like assessment, should continue throughout the transport phase. The overall objective is to prepare the victim for transport to definitive care while maintaining his or her comfort and safety.

Transport Phase

In the fourth phase of SAR, the subject is moved to definitive care. For this to occur, the stabilized subject must be "packaged" so that he or she can be moved safely and efficiently while stabilization and assessment continue. Transportation types range from foot travel, with the subject walking on his or her own, to evacuation by aircraft. The appropriate mode of transportation is determined by weather, type and severity of injuries, overall urgency, terrain, available resources, and other related factors.

Rescue Equipment. Today's rescues occur in many remote and unusual environments and often require extremely technical rescue equipment and skills. Responders trained in the appropriate techniques and technologies should be the only personnel to apply them. Much of the gear and many of the techniques have been derived from those first developed by mountaineers, climbers, cavers, and, more recently, whitewater enthusiasts.

Rescue equipment is generally broken down into three broad categories: personal gear, rescue software, and rescue hardware. Personal equipment includes such items as footwear, gloves, helmets, articles of clothing, eye protection, and other protective apparel. Software is equipment such as rope, webbing, slings, and harnesses that are made of soft, strong synthetic materials specifically designed and manufactured for rescue. Hardware is such equipment as carabiners, cams, friction devices, pulleys, and litters made of steel and alloys specifically designed and manufactured to endure the rigors of rescue.

PERSONAL EQUIPMENT. Rescuers must often wear special equipment to protect them from accidents and hazards. Head, eye, and hand protection is considered mandatory in virtually all rescue environments. Additional personal equipment requirements are dictated by the rescue environment and the specific needs of the situation (Figure 25-5).

Special gear. In addition to the usual challenges of the rescue environment, certain hazards require specialized equipment. Examples of such equipment include fire-resistant clothing worn by structural and wildland firefighters, personal flotation devices (PFDs) used by rescuers in and around water (Figure 25-6), netting used in outdoor settings when insects become a problem, bulletproof garments used by law-enforcement and military rescue personnel, and chemical protective suits worn when exposure to hazardous materials is possible.

No clothing or protective gear meets all of the requirements for involvement in or around a rescue scene. Rescuers study situations so that they understand all hazards before anyone becomes involved. Their conclusions help them identify protective-equipment requirements. Gear that may be necessary for one environment can be dangerous in another. A firefighter's turnout gear may be required in a structure fire but can be deadly in a river rescue situation. Every

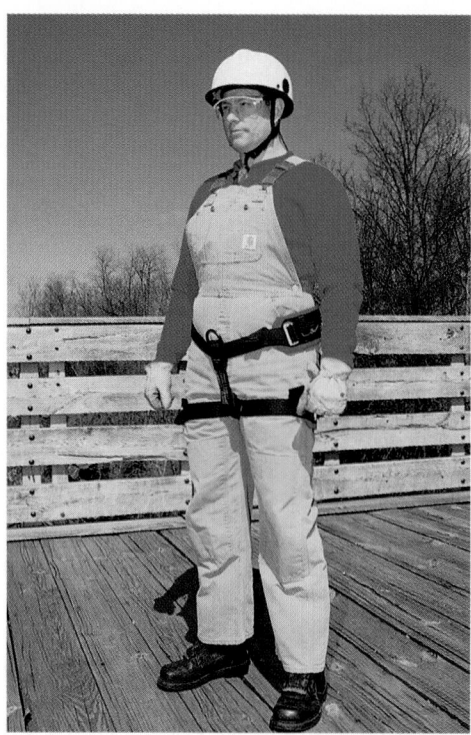

Figure 25-5 Even though the personal equipment necessary is dictated by both the rescue environment and the needs of the specific situation, it includes head, hand, foot, and eye protection as a minimum.

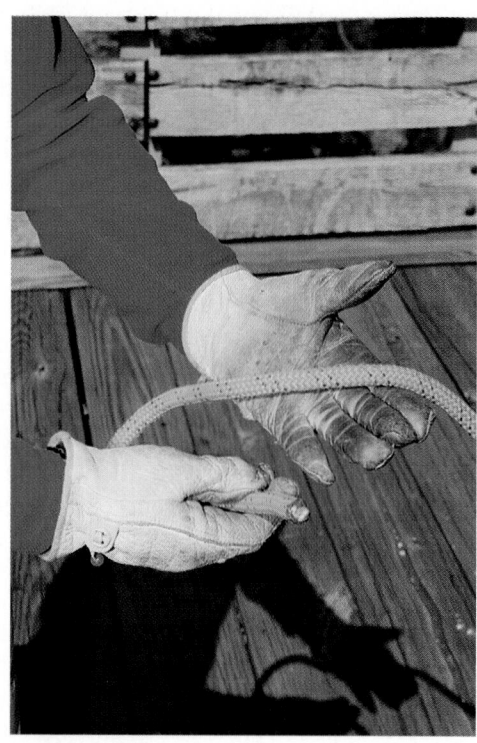

Figure 25-7 Example of ½-inch, nylon, static, kernmantle rope of the type commonly used in rescue. Rescue rope should be checked over its entire length for damage before use.

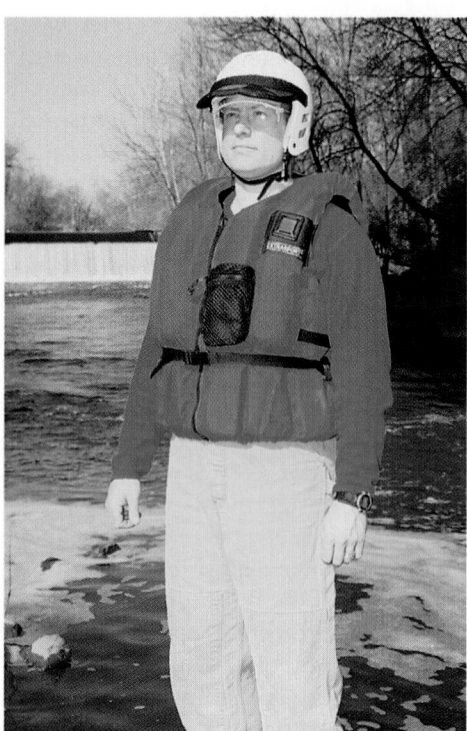

Figure 25-6 Rescuer wearing a personal flotation device (PFD) and helmet often used for rescue in and around moving water.

rescuer is responsible for understanding the rescue environment and how to best prepare for it.

SOFTWARE

Rope. Rope is by far the most versatile piece of rescue equipment and serves as the universal link in most rescue environments. The material from which the rope is made (such as nylon, polyester, or polyolefins) and the design (laid, kernmantle, flat) are important in the consideration of the use for which a rope is intended.

In most rescue environments, nylon is preferred because of its overall strength, resistance to abrasion, and ability to stretch and absorb energy. Natural fiber ropes such as hemp are no longer considered for use in rescue—synthetic materials are far better. Although design and amount of materials used influence strength, new ½-inch diameter nylon rescue rope usually has a tensile strength in excess of 9000 pounds (Figure 25-7).

The most common design of rescue rope is *kernmantle*, a term derived from German, meaning "core in sheath." With this design, a core of material (often parallel fibers) is surrounded by a braided sheath. The sheath protects the inner core, which supplies much of the strength of the overall rope. Other designs such as laid (twisted) and braided are also used in rescue rope.

Kernmantle rope is either "dynamic" or "static." Dynamic kernmantle stretches more than 4% of its length to absorb the impact of a fall, and it is used primarily in lead climbing. Static kernmantle stretches less (no more than 4% of its length); it is used in rescues in which a great deal of stretch would be a nuisance or even dangerous.

Because of the importance of rope in the rescue chain, frequent inspection, care, and maintenance are important. Rope used in rescue is kept clean, inspected often, and protected from sharp edges, high temperatures, sunlight, chemicals, and abrasion. In addition, a detailed history of rescue ropes is kept so that an educated decision can eventually be made regarding each rope's removal from rescue service (see Chapter 72).

Webbing. Flat rope or webbing is another common link in rescue systems. It comes in two common configurations: flat and tubular. Tubular webbing is manufactured as a tube in such a way as to seem flat when in use. In cross section, however, it is obviously tubular and a bit less stiff than true flat webbing. One-inch-diameter tubular webbing can be used in rescues to tie anchor slings and harnesses. It has a tensile strength of approximately 4000 pounds when new.

Flat webbing is flat in cross section. Its strength is directly proportional to the amount of material used in its manufacture. Automobile seat belts are an example of the material used in rescue harnesses, anchor slings, and anywhere strong, flat software is beneficial (Figure 25-8).

Harnesses. Harnesses come in many sizes and shapes; they are used to attach something (usually a rope) to a person's body. They may be "full-body," encompassing the thorax and the pelvis (Figure 25-9); "seat," encompassing only the pelvis (see Figure 25-5); or "chest," encompassing only the thorax. Each type of harness has its use and associated advantages and disadvantages. Classically, the most common harness for climbing has been the seat harness. However, rescue practitioners have been trying to standardize the full-body harness for rescuer use, with the separate seat and chest harnesses having only limited special use by trained individuals.

Webbing can be tied into a large loop (runner) and applied to a person in such a way as to serve as an improvised harness. Although this is not a preferred method of attachment to a rope, it can work if other harnesses are not available.

HARDWARE

Carabiners. Carabiners are large, safety pin–type mechanisms used to connect various elements of a rescue system, such as a rope and anchor. They are occasionally called "biners," "snap links," or "crabs," and consist of a spring-loaded gate that pivots open, a spine that supports most of the load and lies opposite the gate, a latch, and depending on the specific style, a locking mechanism.

Steel and aluminum are the two materials from

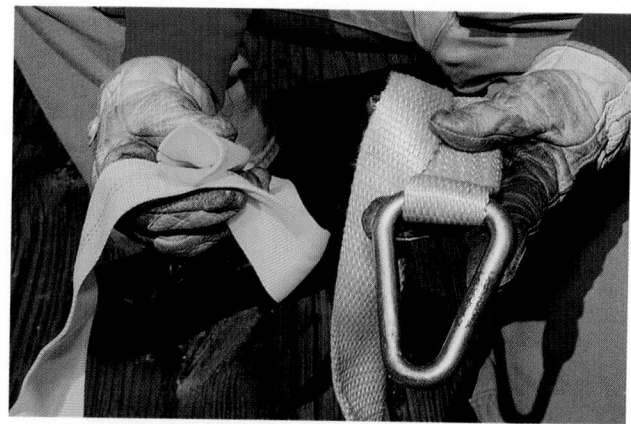

Figure 25-8 *Left,* Tubular webbing with cross section visible. *Right,* Flat webbing used in anchor sling.

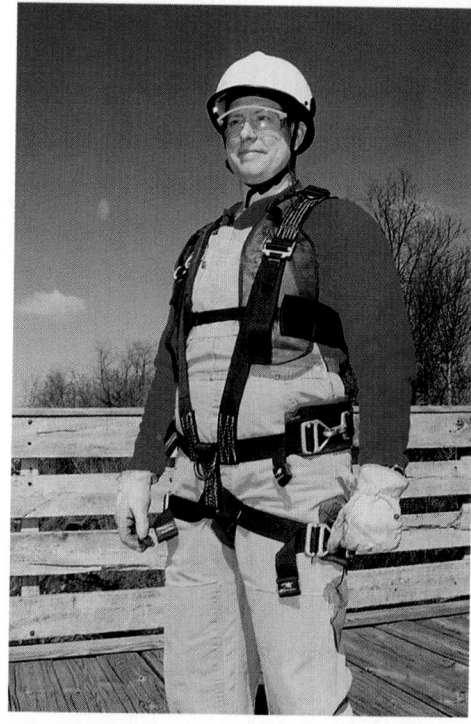

Figure 25-9 Full-body harness. Note that the harness encompasses both the pelvis and the thorax.

which carabiners are most commonly made. Size for size, steel is stronger and heavier, but aluminum is lighter and stronger pound for pound. In rescue, steel is almost always preferred unless weight is a factor, as in remote alpine situations.

Common shapes of carabiners include oval, D, offset D, pear, and large offset D. The design best suited for any situation is dictated by the specific use. No matter what the shape, carabiners used in rescue usually have a mechanism for locking the gate closed so that opening it takes a special effort. This design feature not only

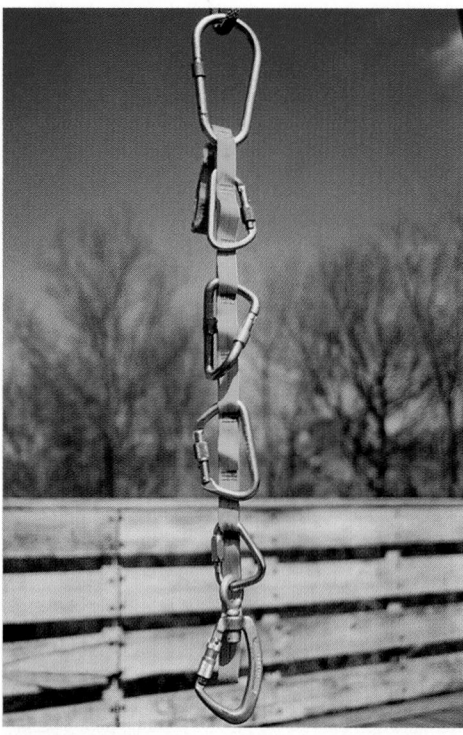

Figure 25-10 Various types of carabiners. *Top to bottom:* (1) RSI Big hook, steel, screw locking hinged gate; (2) alloy, offset D, screw locking hinged gate; (3) RSI Twist Link, steel, screw locking hinged gate; (4) SMC extra large, rescue, steel, screw locking hinged gate; (5) Tri-link, steel, triangular, screw lock; (6) Auto-lock, swivel-mount, steel, quarter twist locking hinged gate (NFPA 1983 certified). Note that locking carabiners should always be locked when in use.

improves the strength of the device, but also reduces the chances that a carabiner will open accidentally at a bad time (Figure 25-10).

Descending/friction devices. Many different descending devices exist today, but they all do primarily the same thing: apply friction to the rope to allow controlled lowering of a person or load. The most common descending devices in rescue are the figure-8 plate and the brake bar rack.

The figure-8 plate gets the name from its general shape. It has two rings of different sizes. The larger ring produces friction on the rope, whereas the smaller ring is used primarily as an attachment for the load (e.g., the rescuer during rappel). Friction is produced by passing a bight of rope through the large ring and around the small ring, then attaching the small ring to either an anchor (for a lowering system) or a rescuer's harness (for a rappel or abseil) with a locking carabiner (Figure 25-11).

The brake bar rack, or simply "the rack," uses either steel or aluminum bars on a steel rack to produce friction on a rope. When the rope is threaded alternately around the bars and the load or rescuer is attached to the "eye" in the rack, friction is applied. The number of bars applied to the rope and the distance between them can be varied to change the friction. This variable friction allows versatility not available with the figure-8 plate; however, the rack takes a bit more training to use safely (Figure 25-12).

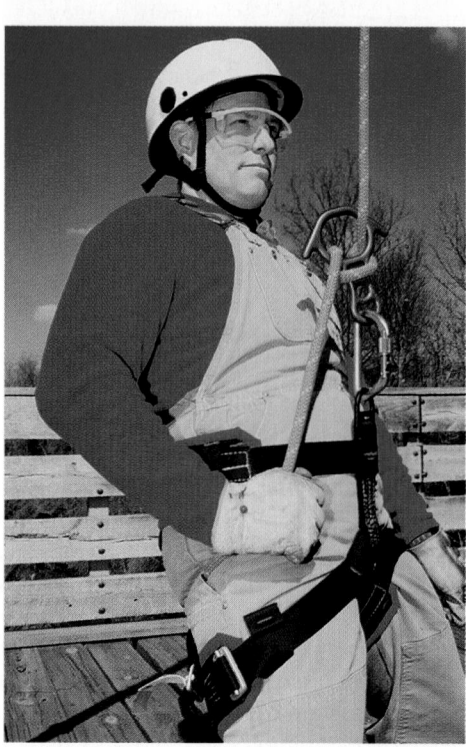

Figure 25-11 Example of figure-8 plate descending device (with "ears") commonly used in rescue.

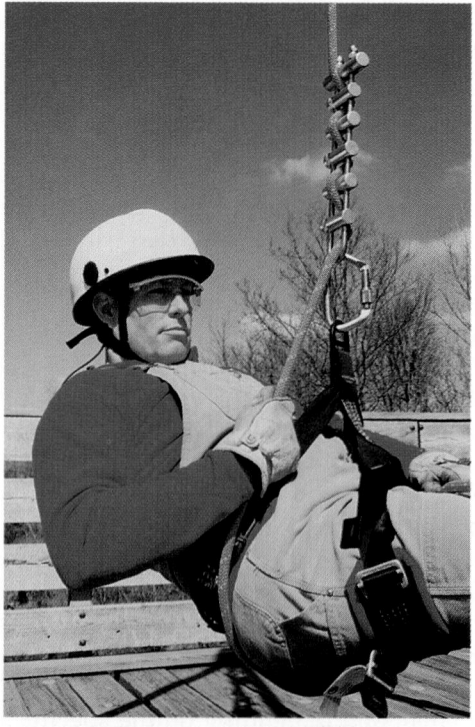

Figure 25-12 RSI Super Rack brake bar rack in use.

Ascenders. Ascenders are devices that grip or hold the rope. They have been adapted from climbing and caving equipment, with which they are used to ascend or climb a fixed rope. In rescue, they are used to climb fixed lines when necessary, but they can also be used in hauling systems to grip the rope. In this way, they hold fast when the rope is pulled in one direction and allow the rope to slide easily when it is pulled in the other direction (Figure 25-13, *A-D*).

When ascenders are used to climb a rope, one is fixed to the rope and supports the load while the other is moved into position ahead. When this action is alternately repeated, a skilled climber can move up a rope with relative speed and ease. Selected rope hitches (e.g., a Prusik hitch) can be used in lieu of an ascender.

Pulleys. Pulleys are simple machines that apply a turning wheel to reduce friction on a rope as it rounds a turn. In rescue, these metal devices serve primarily to change the direction of a rope, such as within a mechanical advantage system. The "sheave" is the wheel or pulley, and there may be more than one. The "side plate" or "cheek" is the side of the device that makes contact with the anchor at the "hook," which is usually the weakest part. The axle or "sheave pin" is what the wheel turns on; it is supported by the side plates. In rescue pulleys the side plates are movable so that the pulley can be attached to a rope anywhere along its length (Figure 25-14).

The larger the diameter of the pulley, the more efficient the device. That is, the bigger the pulley, the more

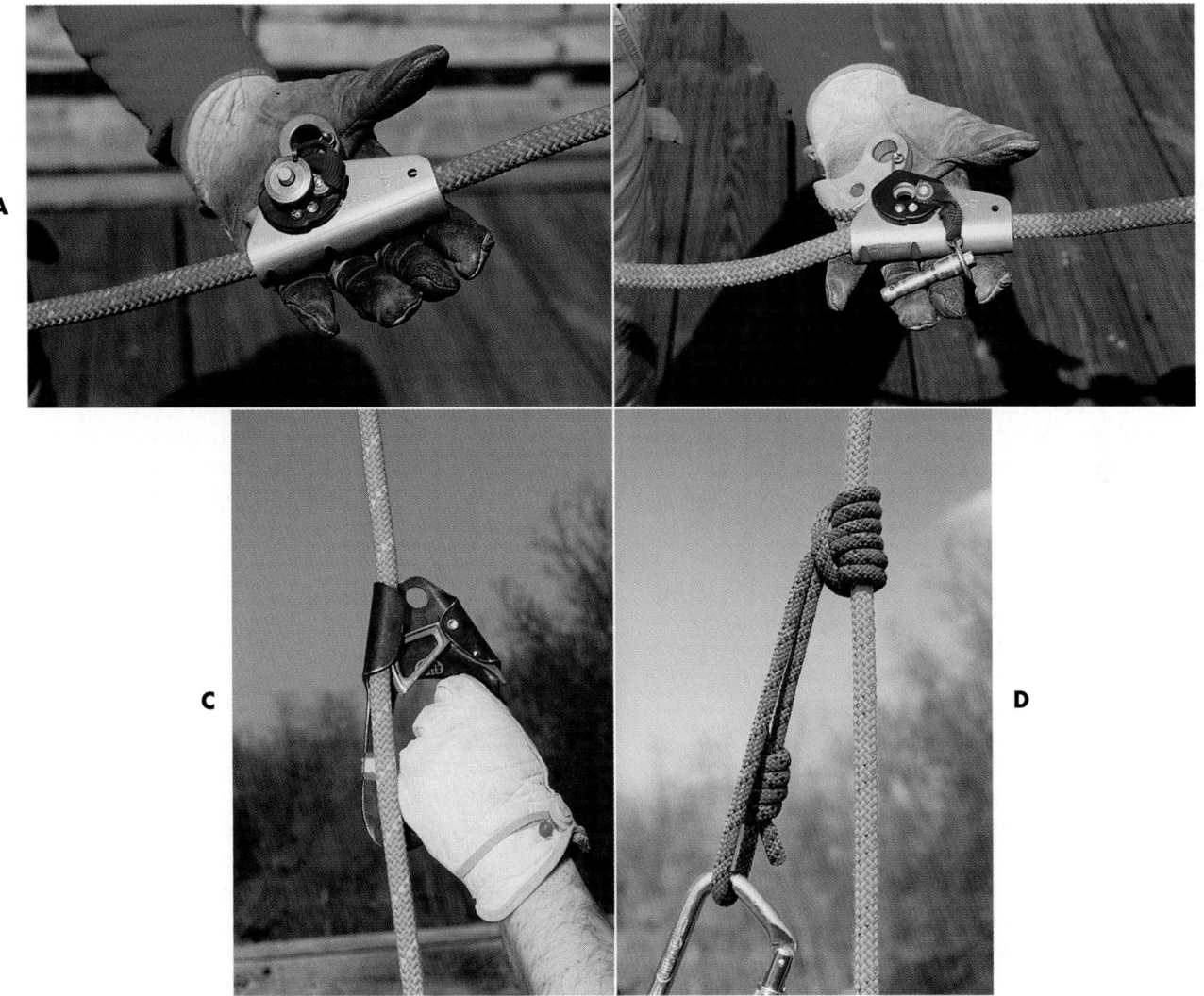

Figure 25-13   A, Gibbs ascender applied to rope. When the eye of the cam is pulled, the cam squeezes the rope and holds fast. When the cam is released, the device can be moved on the rope. **B,** Gibbs ascender dismantled with shell around rope. Note cam *(upper left)* and pin *(bottom)*. **C,** Clog handled ascender. Although used where climbing a fixed rope is required, handled ascenders are rarely used in rescue. **D,** A 3-wrap Prusik hitch can often be used in lieu of a mechanical ascender.

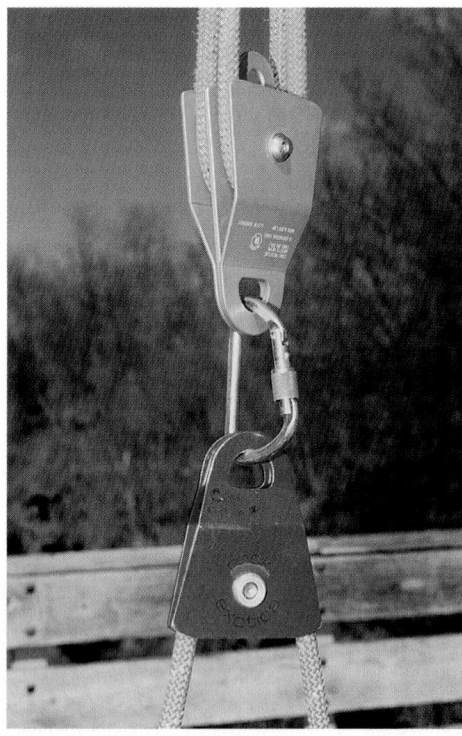

Figure 25-14 Two types of pulleys commonly used for rescue. *Top*, 2-inch double pulley. *Bottom*, 2-inch, "Prusik-minding." Note that rescue pulleys are applied to rope by removing the carabiner and swiveling the side plate to allow the introduction of the rope.

friction (theoretically) is reduced. A rule of thumb often used by rescuers is that a pulley with the largest diameter possible should be used, but never less than four times the diameter of the rope. Therefore, because ½-inch (11 mm) rope is commonly used in rescue, a pulley diameter of at least 2 inches should be used.

A variation of the pulley is the edge roller. This device uses 4- to 6-inch open-face pulleys to both reduce the friction of a rope passing over an edge and reduce damage to the rope by protecting it from excess abrasion. Single units can protect the rope from 90-degree angles, and multiple units tied together can provide protection for complex projections.

Litters. Litters or stretchers are the conveyances in which victims are transported when they cannot travel under their own power. New high-technology materials and designs have greatly improved the choices available. In past years, rescuers were forced to settle for either wooden backboards, old military stretchers, the wire Navy Stokes basket, or the "scoop" stretcher. Today, strong, lightweight synthetic materials and inventive designs have improved the strength, weight, durability, and comfort of litters.

The goals have not changed during the continuing evolution of the perfect wilderness transportation device. Rescuers still want a device that is comfortable for

a person in pain, serves well as a platform for assessment and medical care during transport, allows for full-body immobilization while offering complete security, and protects its occupants from the rescue environment. See Chapter 27 for additional information regarding specific litters, packaging, handling, and evacuation techniques.

ANATOMY OF A SEARCH AND RESCUE INCIDENT

To summarize how all of the previously discussed information fits together, it is convenient to dissect a SAR incident into its component parts and then analyze how all of the parts fit together (Figure 25-15).

From the SAR operative's perspective, an actual callout is merely an interruption of planning for an incident. That is, people involved in SAR are constantly in a state of readiness and prepared to respond. When a situation occurs, this planning stage is suddenly interrupted by the report of an incident or first notice. The individual taking the information is charged with conveying it to the appropriate authority. The authority determines the urgency, continues the investigation process, begins to develop an operational strategy, and generates an incident action plan. At the same time, those in charge begin to muster appropriate resources to carry out the action plan. In SAR, this is termed *resource callout*, or just *callout*.

Once notified of an incident, individual resources are gathered at a collection point and signed in. The sign-in process enhances safety and allows tracking of resources, which helps those in charge determine the quantity and type of resources available. Once signed in, resources are allocated to assignments designed to meet the goals of the action plan within a reasonable time. This physical implementation of plans in the field is called *tactics* and is a direct outgrowth of the incident action plan.

Allocation of resources in the field continues until there is reason to suspend a phase of the operation. If the subject is found, the search is suspended and the access phase can commence. Once rescuers have access to the subject, the focus turns to stabilization and transportation. If at any point the operation cannot be continued (e.g., the subject was never found, access cannot be gained, transportation is impossible), suspension and demobilization may occur without completion of the entire cycle. The decision to discontinue active search efforts is difficult and involves complex management issues, almost always of the no-win variety.

When a situation is resolved, mission suspension and demobilization begin. In larger incidents this may involve structured deactivation of multiple resources, pulling teams out of the field, dismantling facilities, completing documentation, and returning resources to

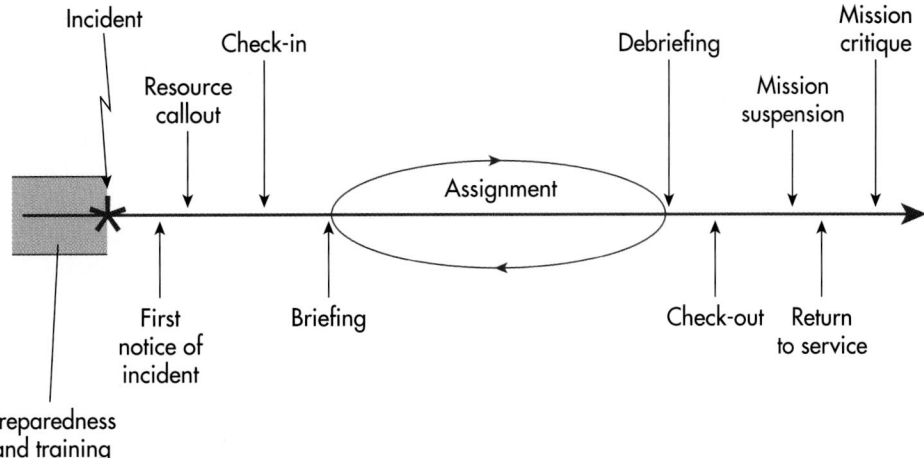

Figure 25-15 Time progression or the "anatomy" of a search from a searcher's (operational) perspective. The process is actually a continuous cycle that pauses in the planning and preparation phase until an incident occurs.

service. Basically, everyone finishes what he or she was doing and gets ready to do it again. All of this takes planning and preparation and should be addressed in the overall preplan long before it is required.

After every incident, participants realize that if they had it all to do again, they would do some things differently. If these thoughts and ideas are not documented, they can be lost, and future responses may be cursed to repeat past mistakes. This is one reason that every incident should contain some type of evaluation of the entire mission, known as the *post-incident critique.* The critique can be formal, involving every participant at a sit-down meeting, or informal, involving just a brief discussion of recent events. The critique documents lessons learned and provides a basis for revising the preplan. Thus the cycle continues, and lessons learned from one mission influence the next.

SEARCH AND RESCUE ENVIRONMENTS WITHIN THE WILDERNESS SETTING[4]

SAR teams throughout the world are frequently called on to solve complex problems in a wide spectrum of environments. Even within the environments addressed in this text, widely diversified subenvironments exist that present unique sets of problems and hazards to SAR personnel. When confronted with the numerous and dangerous environmental conditions found in the wilderness setting, SAR personnel must be prepared to work where others have been unable to cope. A military motto becomes the SAR credo: "Adapt, improvise, overcome."

Some of the specialized subenvironments and their associated conditions within which SAR team members may have to work are listed in Box 25-1.

It is beyond the scope of this text to discuss in detail how SAR personnel adapt to each of these environ-

---

Box 25-1   SEARCH AND RESCUE CONDITIONS

Mountainous terrain
Vertical rock
Vertical ice
Flat ice and ice holes
Snow fields and avalanches
Crevasses
Caves
Mines
Wells
Booby-trapped stills and gardens
Air shafts
Fast water and white-water streams
Coastal white-water surf
Flash floods
Slow-rising floods
High winds and storms
Seas and lakes
Snow and blizzard conditions
Hazardous material dump sites

---

ments, but it is important to note that adaptation and improvisation are required in nearly all wilderness situations. The particular improvisation depends on the situation, as well as the skill and experience of the individuals involved.

Regardless of the type of rescue environment encountered by rescuers, the following general rules should be followed:

1. Use technical personnel for technical rescue.
2. If the subject is dead, evacuate only when there is no risk to team members, or at least when the hazard has been assessed and the risk justified.
3. Stabilize the subject before evacuating; continue stabilization during transport.

4. Find, plan, and use the easiest route for evacuation.
5. If a litter must be carried, appoint someone to serve as route finder, with a radio and markers, to report potential hazards and problems.
6. Litter teams of six to eight persons per team should be used, with three teams minimum. Normally, there should be no more than 20 minutes per shift. Additional personnel may also be required to carry equipment.
7. Use accepted procedures to care for and protect the victim.
8. A radio carrier brings up the rear.
9. If using a helicopter for evacuation, make sure:
   a. That the subject is briefed.
   b. That the subject is protected.
   c. That someone goes with the subject who knows what has been done medically.

Special Environments in Search and Rescue

Specialized SAR environments produce diverse problems and potential complications. Each environment presents its own obstacles to increase the complexity and difficulty of particular rescues.

Technical Rock. Mountaineering, rock climbing, and casual scrambling have created a need for specialized SAR expertise. Individuals and groups involved in rock rescue have refined and developed techniques for most situations. The hallmark of a technical rock rescuer is the ability to improvise and modify tools or techniques to meet any crisis. He or she must be comfortable using climbing gear and being exposed to heights.

Once an individual is located in a rock environment and the situation is surveyed, it is necessary to gain access. Local groups familiar with particular well-known areas will have already solved this problem. The solution will involve either climbing up or dropping down to the victim. Safety for all persons involved is paramount, because an accident during a rescue is almost always catastrophic. Climbing up to the victim requires knowledge of rock-climbing techniques, and proper equipment and familiarity with its use are critical. Local outing clubs or mountaineering stores can be contacted for more detailed assistance. Specialized technical rock rescue teams, such as those sanctioned by the Mountain Rescue Association, routinely practice climbing techniques and solving vertical rescue problems.

Caves and Mines. Standard obstacles in the environment include poor communications, extreme darkness, difficulty in lighting, small and wet spaces, and questionable atmosphere. The various environments included here are collectively termed *confined spaces*.

The levels of moisture in a water, or "live," cave can vary over a considerable range. Some are merely muddy; others have flowing rivers. Caves in the western United States are generally drier than eastern caves; however, humidity, wetness, and cold temperatures create potential for hypothermia in both areas, a fact that is greatly underestimated. Flooding is often a great problem, and many cavers have died because of inattention to the weather on the outside. During heavy rains, the caves become natural drains for streams. Wind and temperature are other underestimated problems associated with cave and mine emergencies. It is not unusual for strong winds to develop along subterranean passages, which intensifies convective air chilling.

Confined passages, low crawls, and squeezes pose unique problems for the rescue of injured cavers. The use of standard items such as litters, backboards, and splints may be impossible in such places. Confined passages with varying, often toxic, constituent gases can lead to difficulties for victims and rescuers alike. Occasionally, a self-contained breathing apparatus or surface-supplied air is required. The potential for toxic gases justifies extensive atmospheric monitoring while operating in the underground environment.

An essential part of any cave or mine rescue operation is thorough orientation to the hazards associated with a particular underground area. This involves pinpointing the locations of pits, waterfalls, siphons, canyons, and other difficult formations that may pose problems in extrication, search, or safety. Many caves have been mapped by the National Speleological Society and the National Park Service.

The real difficulties may begin only after a victim is located. The goal is to move the person rapidly, safely, and comfortably to the surface. Without practice underground, that task will be virtually impossible. Neoprene exposure bags similar to body bags have been used for this purpose and keep the individual dry and protected during what may be a very long and slow evacuation.

Medical care procedures must be performed under dark, cold, and muddy conditions. Experienced cave rescuers agree that repackaging supplies and equipment for underground use is essential. Streamlining kits, packs, and containers is imperative for unobstructed passage through tight spaces in cold, damp conditions.

Team members must carry a minimum of 24 hours of light in a helmet-mounted lamp; two additional sources of light, with spare bulbs and batteries; and waterproof matches and candles. Other equipment needed might include the following:

1. A high-quality helmet with chin strap and headlamp attachment
2. Sturdy, warm clothes and gloves for damp, dirty conditions for up to 24 hours; the material should be wool and the fit should allow good mobility
3. Lug-soled boots that are light and drain water

4. Nonstretch, specialized caving rope that is highly resistant to abrasion
5. Wrap-around-style litter (or even an old conveyor belt) that can aid in dragging an injured person through small passages: a common Stokes litter may not always work well
6. Wet suits for longer missions in extremely wet caves
7. Harnesses and slings resistant to chemicals and water
8. Plastic sheeting to divert water around a victim during evacuation
9. Small portable pumps, a siphon hose, and plastic to divert, dam, or pump water around areas during operations
10. Warm food and drink carried in thermally insulated containers

Essential caving skills include all of the capabilities for rock climbing, including vertical rope technique, ascending, rappeling, belaying, and being comfortable working at the end of a rope. All of these skills must be practiced until they can be done in the cold and wet without the benefit of light. Team practices are conducted both on the surface and underground, with participants being forced to work in mud, suffocatingly tight squeezes, soaking waterfalls, and complete darkness. This may be a difficult evolution for even the most experienced rescuer to endure, but just another "hang in the hole" for a seasoned caver.

White-Water River. There are dozens of potentially dangerous problems in the river SAR (white-water) situation (see Chapter 30). Log and debris piles at various bends in the river can function as "strainers" for the recreational victim, but they may be death traps for the would-be rescuer. The banks of the stream may be deeply undercut, with treacherous overhanging debris and snags that can catch on clothing, equipment, and skin. Combined with muddy and rapidly rising water, these factors render river rescue difficult and unpredictable.

In fast-moving water, the single greatest problem is that responders underestimate the power and threat of moving water. Foolhardy heroics and overenthusiasm frequently lead to further tragedy. Cold-water immersion, coupled with wind and cold temperatures, predisposes everyone to hypothermia. Wet clothing, darkness, and injury add to the insult. The noise of moving water may obviate clear communications, and poor contact between the victim and rescuers or among the rescuers leads to confusion and danger.

All potential responders in this environment must know how to read the water for capsize points and other dangerous phenomena. The hydraulics of low-head dams, collapsed bridges, and other submerged structures can produce a drowning machine for unsuspecting individuals. Rescue team members must know how to protect themselves in fast-moving water at all times. Mandatory in this environment are good judgment, strong swimming ability, knowledge of all types of technical systems and equipment used in climbing, and a thorough understanding of river dynamics and hydraulic influences.

WHITE-WATER AND RIVER RESCUE EQUIPMENT NEEDS. In addition to standard rescue equipment, the following items should be considered when establishing rescue capability in the white-water and river environment:

1. Inflatable rafts or boats (Hard boats may not be as stable and are usually less preferred. Inflatables should be at least 14 to 16 feet long and 6 feet wide, with separate air chambers. The "spider boat," with two pontoons joined together in a catamaran-style craft, makes an excellent, stable rescue platform for moving water.)
2. A line gun or crossbow adaptation that will shoot a line at least 200 feet
3. Power winch or simple "come-along" that can be carried to remote sites
4. Lengthy (150 to 300 feet) durable floating ropes in rope bags
5. Floating throw-rope bags with approximately 60 feet of line
6. A lightweight litter with enough flotation to keep a packaged patient's head out of the water; standard rescue litters often have adaptations for this purpose
7. Fire-hose end caps with air-hose adapters, which allow the fire hose to be inflated with air and used in a shore-based rescue
8. PFDs for every rescuer who will be exposed to the water environment; wet suits and helmets for rescuers who will be directly involved in moving water
9. Dry extra clothing for victims and rescuers
10. Portable "loudhailer" or public address system
11. Portable lighting systems
12. Detailed maps, aerial photographs, or both, of the area, as well as information regarding river hazards during high, medium, and low water levels
13. Dry, buoyant storage bags for sensitive gear
14. Reliable, watertight communications capability for white-water noise and moisture conditions
15. Small surfboardlike Styrofoam boards ("boogie board") for swimming in moving water

White-Water Surf. Like river white water, ocean surf can present some very different problems in rescue because there is no "average" beach. There are recurring rescue situations that pose unique problems in the white-water surf environment.

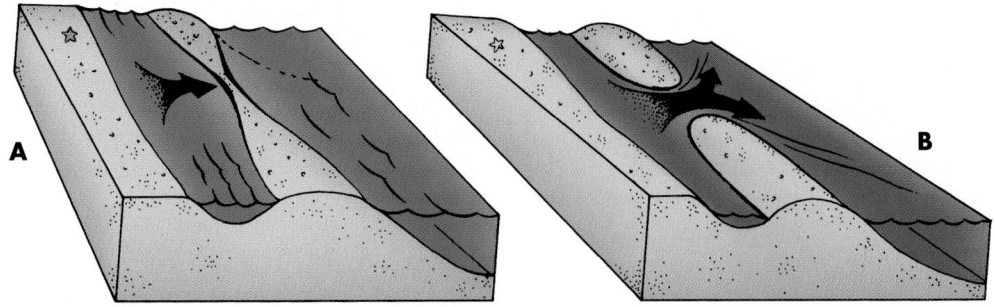

Figure 25-16 Runout. **A,** This phenomenon begins with an offshore sandbar. As waves roll in, the water level builds up behind the bar until a section gives way. **B,** As the sandbar "dam" gives way, the water develops a very rapid current running seaward. The recommended action is to swim across the current until out of the pull.

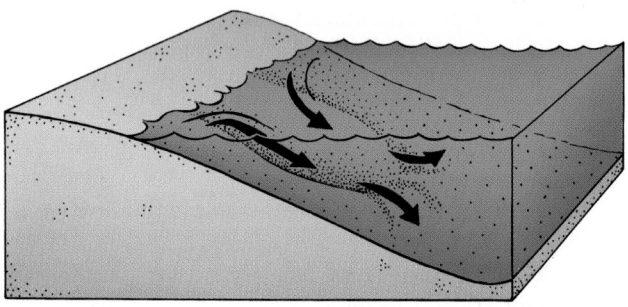

Figure 25-17 Rip. A depression in the beach floor concentrates returning water into a strong current. To escape, a person should ride with the current or swim to the side and out of the pull.

Along with the potential for immersion hypothermia, lacerations and contusions can result from being dashed against barnacle-encrusted rocks in the wild and unpredictable ocean surf. Contact with venomous sea life is always a possibility. However, the greatest threat to ocean beach users is the action of the water itself and the possibility of drowning through inattention or unfamiliarity with ocean surf hazards in the form of runouts, undertows, and rips.

RUNOUT. A runout occurs when an offshore sandbar or ledge is built up over a long period. Millions of tons of water flow over the bar during daily tidal changes. Eventually the water may equal or exceed the level outside the bar. Any weak spot in the bar usually gives way, causing a funnel effect (Figure 25-16). Water rushes toward the bar at a terrific rate, sweeping everything with it. This common phenomenon can be easily spotted from the beach. Usually 15 to 50 yards wide, it is characterized by choppy, jumbled-up, little waves. The water often has a dirty, foamy, or debris-laden surface moving seaward. If a bar is visible offshore, definite breaks can be seen where the water pours through. Surfers often seek runout currents for fast transportation out beyond shoreline waves.

Swimmers caught in a runout have two options. They may swim parallel to the shoreline out of the strip of current, or if the bar is visible (usually characterized by breaking waves), they may relax and let the current complete its runout. About 25 yards beyond the bar the current dissipates. This is an offshore phenomenon—current force increases near the bar but is often negligible near shore.

RIP. A far worse problem close to the beach is a rip, which can knock children and even adults off their feet and carry them to deep water in seconds. Rips are caused by a slight depression on the beach where wave water rushes after breaking on shore. Water rushing to the depression soon becomes an irresistible seaward flow (Figure 25-17). It may be as narrow as 15 yards at its source and usually does not travel as far as a runout. Rips generally dissipate a few yards beyond the breakers. A rip looks like a runout, with a streak of turbulent discolored water or a line of foam leading directly out from shore. A swimmer has the same options as in a runout, either to swim parallel to the beach or to relax and ride the current until it ebbs. A person who swims straight toward the beach will never make it. A beach with several rips moving up and down in unpredictable patterns is very dangerous. An unwary swimmer could panic and drown.

UNDERTOW. On narrow, steep beaches a type of current known as *undertow* can be found. It is caused by gravity acting on water thrown up on the beach by wave action. Water retreating back down the steep shore continues under oncoming waves (Figure 25-18). Undertow is usually of very short duration and is ended by the next breaking wave. Wading near shore on a steep beach, an individual could be pulled under in this current and find himself or herself quickly in deep water. If the person resists the current, the next wave may break directly on the person's back. In some circumstances this could cause traumatic injury, especially to the neck

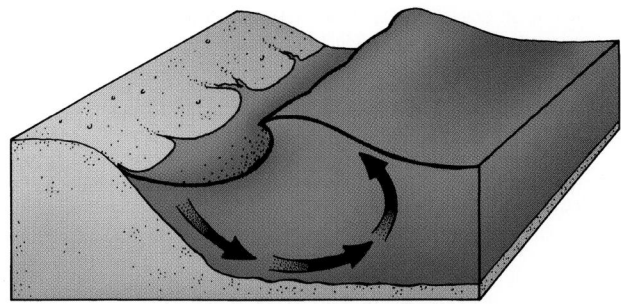

Figure 25-18 Undertow. This hazard develops on a steep beach where the water returns rapidly seaward after being tossed up by the wave action. A person should never fight this action but should relax and rise on the next wave.

and back. A person caught in an undertow should let the current pull until it ceases, then swim to the surface and ride the next wave into shore.

Cold, Snow, and Ice. Perhaps no other type of SAR environment requires a more broadly based foundation of personal and team skills than winter snow and ice. These skills include downhill and cross-country skiing, snowshoeing, technical climbing, winter survival, and a good understanding of snow and ice physics. Unlike rock, snow and ice conditions change on a daily and even minute-to-minute basis. The effects of gravity, wind, temperature, slope, heat exchange, load factors, and avalanche (see Chapter 2) continually impose problems for missions under these conditions. Technical and nontechnical SAR problems in snow and ice environments take longer to address and are more taxing, technical, and complex. Combined with shorter days, extremes of weather, and the ever-present threat of hypothermia and localized cold injuries, technical missions of this type are unacceptable for all but the most experienced SAR personnel.

Versatility and improvisation are essential components of the overall strategy that must be used in snow and ice. Transportation of the victim is often one of the most difficult problems, but it can usually be resolved through detailed preplanning. Innovations such as covering a litter with a canvas cover or improvising an attachment to cross-country skis are clever solutions to common winter problems. Commercial products such as the Hegg Sled and the Sked Litter (see Chapter 26) have streamlined the laborious task of transporting injured people through snow and ice.

MAGNITUDE AND CAUSES OF PROBLEMS IN WILDERNESS SEARCH AND RESCUE

It is impossible to report the exact number of backcountry SAR missions that occur each year in the United States. Some estimates are in excess of 100,000. In the United States, no federal agency is charged with gathering these data. With rare exception, only in the last few years have some states and local jurisdictions begun to collect and analyze SAR mission numbers and related information. Through the efforts of organizations such as the National Association for Search and Rescue, this vital information is now being used as a database to predict victim behavior and to improve the efficiency of SAR management.

Most wilderness accidents are the result of inexperience or lack of preparation, often aggravated by fatigue, lowered body temperature, and other medical management problems, rather than the direct result of natural phenomena such as avalanche or rock fall.

In an effort to save lives through education, the Washington State Department of Emergency Management SAR Division has been recording statistics on SAR missions for over 20 years. The goal of this effort has been to find out what factors in each SAR mission may have caused a problem for the subject. Box 25-2 is an overview of that data, compiled in an attempt to create a preventive SAR subject profile.

In addition to the factors listed in Box 25-2, the data pointed out some extremely interesting characteristics. Using broad-based generalizations, the analysts were able to further describe a potential SAR victim. Although the data were gathered only from the state of Washington, they have application in nearly every state and have to some degree been substantiated by other statistics.

The average SAR victim is a composite outdoorsman (e.g., hunter, fisherman, skier, hiker, climber, boater, photographer). Most do not do any of these activities well and are not members of organized groups that specialize in these pursuits. Most reside in densely populated areas and travel some distance for recreation and outdoor pursuits. They usually travel too fast and too far to acclimatize well to the terrain, altitude, and environmental conditions encountered. Interviews show that they also generally ignore signs of weather change, environmental hazards, body indicators, and written warnings concerning danger or safety. Most wilderness or backcountry emergencies are solved by either the victim or outside help within 72 hours. The decisions and actions taken by the victims during the first 6 hours of the situation (such as emergency shelter, improving clothing, firecraft, signaling) are the most critical and influence the outcome most heavily. Of all precipitating factors, weather contributes the most to misery, carelessness, and the ultimate SAR mission.

REFERENCES

1. Benkoski M, Monticino M, Weisinger J: A survey of the search theory literature, *Naval Research Logistics* 38:469, 1991.
2. Cooper DC, LaValla PH, Stoffel RC: SAR *fundamentals: basic skills and knowledge to perform search and rescue*, ed 3 (rev), Cuyahoga Falls, Ohio, 1996, National Rescue Consultants.
3. Cooper DC, Taylor A: *Fundamentals of mantracking: the step-by-step method*, ed 2, Cuyahoga Falls, Ohio, 1992, National Rescue Consultants.
4. Federal Emergency Management Agency: *The Federal Response Plan*, PL 93-288, as amended, Washington, DC, 1991, Superintendent of Documents.
5. Frost JR: *Search theory enhancement study: prepared for interagency committee on SAR research and development working group*, Fairfax, Va, 1998, Soza and Company, Ltd.
6. Frost JR: Personal communication, March 3, 1999.
7. Heth DC, Cornell EH: Characteristics of travel by persons lost in Albertan wilderness areas, *J Environ Psych* Dec 11, 1997.
8. Hill KA: *Distances traveled and probability zones for lost persons in Nova Scotia*, 1996, unpublished data.
9. Koester RJ, Stooksbury DE: Behavioral profile of possible Alzheimer's disease patients in Virginia SAR incidents, *Wilderness and Environmental Medicine* 6:34-43, 1995.
10. Koester RJ: (1999). *Behavioral and statistical profile of lost mentally retarded and psychotic subjects in Virginia*. Personal communication, July 7, 1999. Based on author's presentation with same title at RESPONSE '99, Annual Conference of the National Association for Search and Rescue, June 1999.
11. Koester RJ: *Behavioral and statistical profiles of lost subjects in Virginia*. Personal communication, June 6, 2000.
12. Koopman BO: *Search and screening* (OEG Report No. 56, The Summary Reports Group of the Columbia University Division of War Research, 1946). Available from the Center for Naval Analyses.
13. Koopman BO: *Search and screening: general principles with historical applications*, New York, 1980, Pergamon Press.
14. LaValla PH, Stoffel RC: *Blueprint for community emergency management: a text for managing emergency operations*, Olympia, Wash, 1991, Emergency Response Institute.
15. LaValla PH et al: *Search is an emergency: a text for managing search operations*, ed 4 (rev), Olympia, Wash, 1998, Emergency Response Institute.
16. Miller AT Jr: Altitude. In Slonin NB, editor: *Environmental physiology*, St Louis, 1974, Mosby.
17. National wildfire coordinating group: *Incident command system, national training curriculum reference text*, NWCG, October, 1994.
18. Soza and Company, Ltd., United States Coast Guard: *The theory of search: a simplified explanation*, (rev), Fairfax, Vir, 1998, the authors.
19. Syrotuck WG: *Analysis of lost person behavior*, Westmoreland, NY, 1977, Arner Publications.
20. US Coast Guard and The Joint Chiefs of Staff: *National search and rescue manual*, vol 1, *National search and rescue system*. Joint Pub 3-50, COMDTINST M16120.5A, Washington, DC, 1991, Superintendent of Documents.
21. United States Air Force: *AFRCC history and mission*, March, 1999, (www.acc.af.mil).
22. United States Coast Guard: U.S. Coast Guard website: www.uscg.mil/hq/g-o/g-opr/, May, 1999.
23. United States Coast Guard Auxiliary: *U.S. coast guard auxiliary history and accomplishments*, website: www.cgaux.org, May, 1999.
24. Worsing RA Jr, editor: *Basic rescue and emergency care*, Park Ridge, Ill, 1990, American Academy of Orthopaedic Surgeons.

26 Litters and Carries

Donald C. Cooper, James Messenger, and Timothy P. Mier

Every search and rescue event goes through a series of four consecutive phases. These phases are illustrated by the acronym LAST (*l*ocate, *a*ccess, *s*tabilize, and *t*ransport). This process ends with the movement of the patient (or patients) from the scene to either a medical facility or an area of comfort and safety (transport)[6] (see Chapter 25).

In the United States the term *stretcher* suggests a flat, unsophisticated frame covered with canvas and used for carrying the sick, injured, and deceased short distances. The term *litter* can mean the same thing but usually suggests an apparatus specifically designed to immobilize and carry a patient longer distances. Over the years the subtle differences in the terms have been lost, and users have gravitated to one or the other. In the United States the term *litter* is used to describe all manner of rescue conveyance. In Great Britain, however, the preference is to use *stretcher* to describe the same devices. In this chapter the two terms are used interchangeably.

SIZE-UP

To select the best method for getting a patient to definitive care, the rescuer must make a realistic assessment of several factors. Scene safety is the initial priority. The necessary evaluation, called the *size-up* (Box 26-1), involves a (usually hasty) determination of whether the victim, rescuer, or both are immediately threatened by either the environment or the situation. Proper immobilization and patient packaging are always preferable, but sometimes the risk of aggravating existing injuries is outweighed by the immediate danger presented by the physical environment. In such a situation the rescuer has little choice but to immediately move the patient to a place of safety before definitive care is provided or packaging is completed.

Evacuation options are limited by three rescuer-related variables: (1) the number of rescuers, (2) their level of fitness, and (3) their technical ability. Carrying a victim, even over level ground, is an arduous task. At an altitude where just walking requires great effort, carrying a victim may be impossible. The specific rescue situation or environment encountered also may present challenges beyond the capability of the available rescuers. Complex rescue scenarios requiring specially trained personnel and special equipment are called *technical rescues* and often involve dangerous environments, such as severe terrain, crevasses, avalanche chutes, caves, or swift water. To avoid becoming victims themselves, rescuers must be realistic when evaluating their ability to perform these types of rescues.

DRAGS AND CARRIES

The most fundamental and expedient method of transporting an ill or injured person is by dragging or carrying them. Although these methods of transportation are far less than ideal and may not meet standard care criteria, the urgency of the situation may outweigh the risks involved. In addition, the process can be physically demanding, and rescuers can quickly become fatigued to the point of hazard. Therefore other options often should be considered before a victim is moved, especially a long distance. A drag or carry may be the best option when a person cannot move under his or her own power, injuries will not be aggravated by the transport, resources and time are limited, the need for immediate transport outweighs the desire to apply standard care criteria, the travel distance is short, or the terrain makes the use of multiple rescuers or bulky equipment impractical.

A "blanket drag" (Figure 26-1, *A*) can be performed on relatively smooth terrain by one or more rescuers rolling the victim onto a blanket, a tarp, or even a large coat and pulling it along the ground. This simple technique is especially effective for rapidly moving a person with a spinal injury to safety because the victim is pulled along the long axis of the body. In extreme circumstances the "fireman's drag" (Figure 26-1, *B*) can be used. In this type of drag the rescuer places the bound wrists of the victim around his or her neck, shoulders, or both and crawls to safety.

A carry should be considered only after it is confirmed that the victim cannot assist rescuers or travel on his or her own. Beyond simply lifting a person over one's shoulder in a "fireman's carry" (Figure 26-2) or acting as a human crutch, a more efficient one-person carry can be accomplished by using equipment, such as webbing, backpacks, coils of rope, or commercial harnesses. Equipment-assisted carries are particularly effective when an injured climber or hiker must be evacuated across a short distance over rough terrain or when a person must be quickly removed from a hazardous environment. In the simplest equipment-assisted carry, 4.5 to 6 m (15 to 20 feet) of webbing is

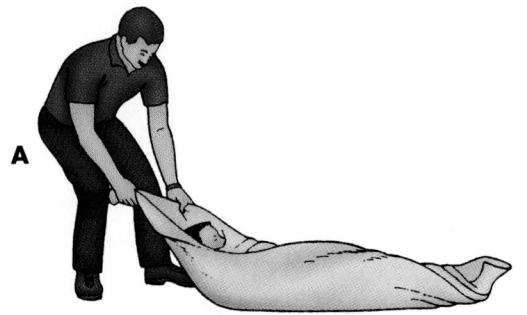

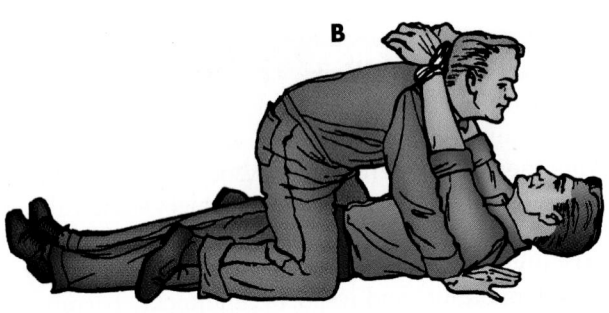

Figure 26-1 A, Blanket drag. **B,** Fireman's drag. Both techniques are intended to be used when expeditious transport over a short distance is required. (*From Auerbach PS: Medicine for the outdoors: the essential guide to emergency medical procedures and first aid, ed 3, New York, 1999, Lyons Press.*)

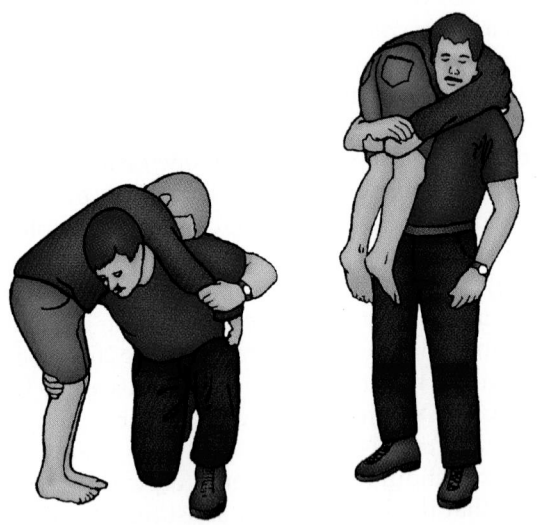

Figure 26-2 Classic fireman's carry: a single rescuer technique for short distance transport only. The rescuer must use his or her legs for lifting. (*From Auerbach PS: Medicine for the outdoors: the essential guide to emergency medical procedures and first aid, ed 3, New York, 1999, Lyons Press.*)

wrapped around the victim, who is "worn" like a backpack by the rescuer (Figure 26-3).

Similarly a backpack or split coil of climbing or rescue rope can be fashioned into a seat around the victim and hoisted by the rescuer. A rescuer can modify a large

---

BOX 26-1 EVACUATION SIZE-UP FACTORS

What are the scope and the magnitude of the overall situation?
Are there immediate life-threatening hazards?
What is the location, and how many victims are there?
What is the patient's condition? Is the subject able to assist rescuers?
  a. No injury (able to walk unassisted)
  b. Slight injury (able to walk unassisted)
  c. Slight injury (assistance required to walk)
  d. Major injury (requires considerable attention and assistance)
  e. Deceased
Is there a need for technical rescue?
Is the scene readily accessible?
What rescue resources (including rescuers and equipment) are available?
How far must the patient (or patients) be transported?
Are ground or air transport assets available?

---

backpack by cutting holes in the bottom for the victim's legs, who then sits in it like a child would sit in an infant carrier (Figures 26-4 and 26-5)

A few commercial harnesses allow a lone rescuer and single patient to be raised or lowered together by a technical rescue system. A Tragsitz is one example (Figure 26-6).

For carrying infants and small children a papoose-style sling works well and can easily be constructed by the rescuer tying a rectangular piece of material around his or her waist and neck to form a pouch. The infant or child is then placed inside the pouch, which can be worn on the front or back of the rescuer's body.

If two rescuers are available, additional and often superior options for carrying a victim become possible. One option consists of two rescuers forming a seat by joining their hands or arms together. The victim sits on the "platform" and holds on to the rescuers for support. It is difficult to cover a long distance or rough terrain when using this technique (Figure 26-7).

A coil of climbing or rescue rope can be used to form a "two-rescuer split coil seat," with each rescuer slipping a side of the rope coil around his or her outside shoulder (Figure 26-8). The patient then sits on the "seat" formed by the rope. A similar approach involves using padded ski poles or stout limbs tied together and supported by backpacks worn by rescuers. The victim sits on the supported poles with his or her arms around the rescuers' shoulders. If the poles are properly padded and securely attached to sturdy rescuers, this technique can be quite comfortable for both rescuer and victim. This approach requires gentle terrain without narrow trails.

Spine injuries generally prohibit the use of drags or carries because the victim cannot be properly immobi-

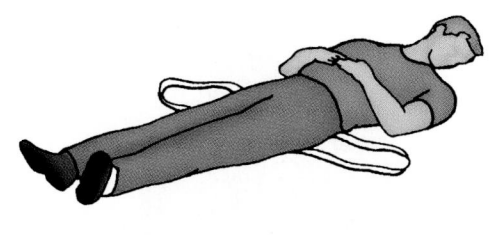
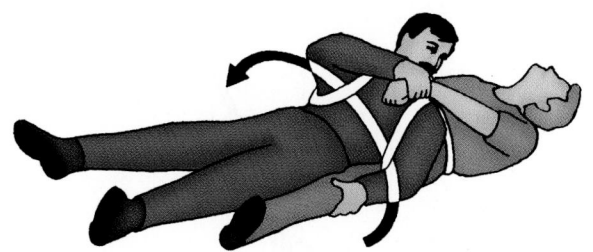

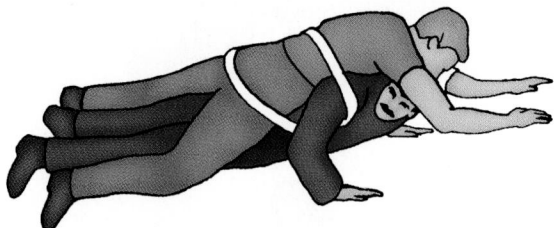
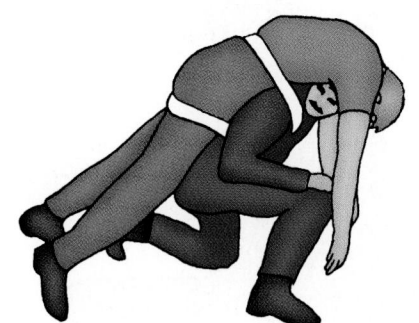

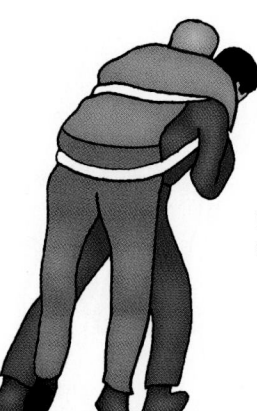

Figure 26-3 Web sling (tied into a loop) used to carry a victim. The rescuer must use his or her legs for lifting

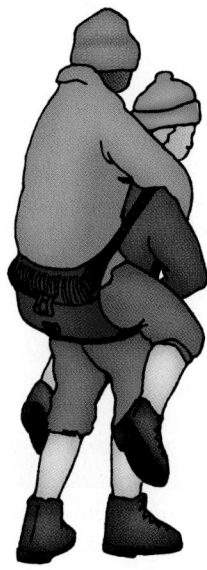

Figure 26-4 Backpack carry.

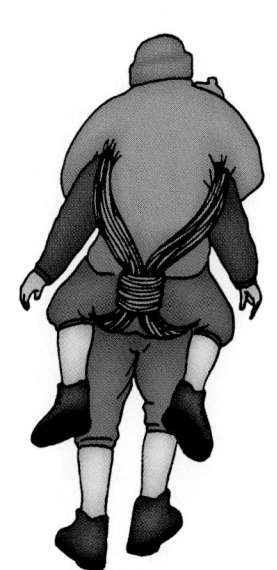
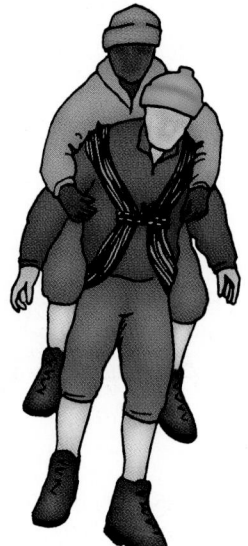

Figure 26-5 Single-rescuer split coil carry. Note that the coil can be tied in front of the rescuer, and the wrists of the victim can be bound and wrapped around the rescuer's neck for more stability.

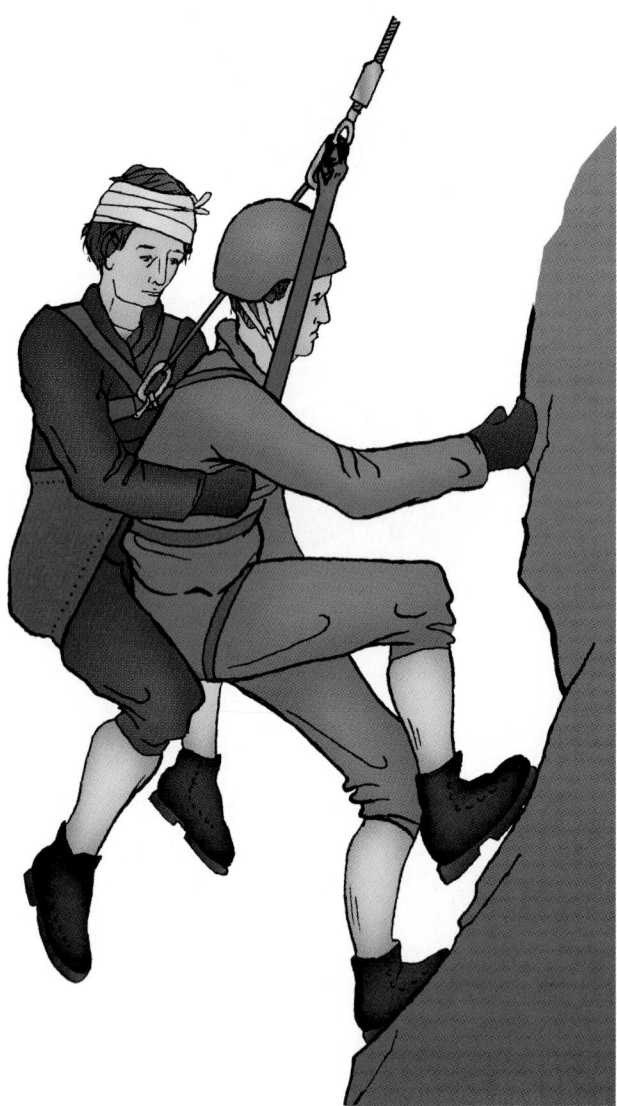

Figure 26-6 Tragsitz harness in use.

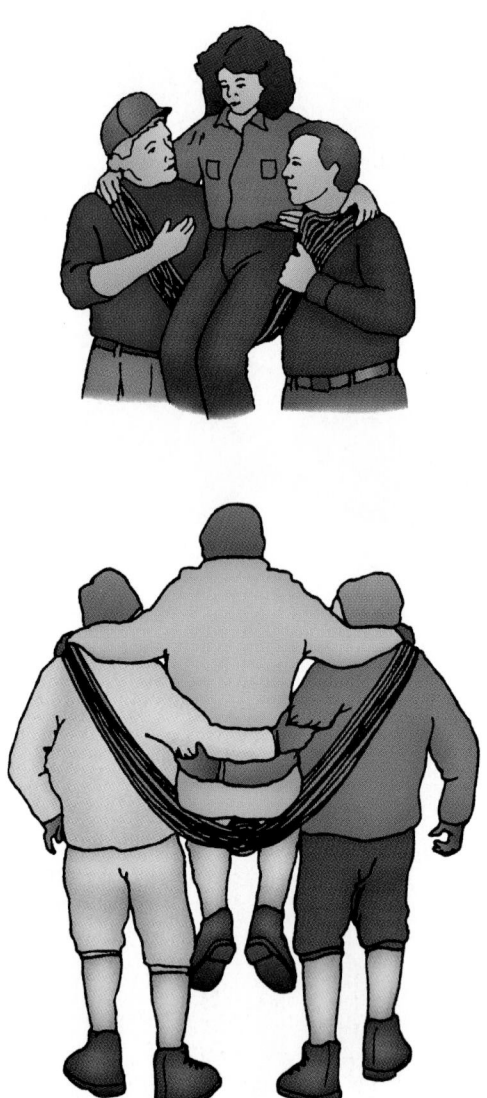

Figure 26-8 Two-rescuer split coil seat.

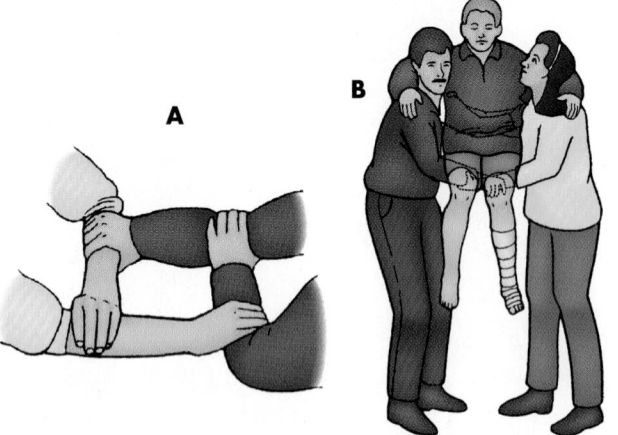

Figure 26-7 A, Four-handed seat used to carry a person. In this technique the upper body is not supported. **B,** Alternative four-handed seat that helps support the victim's back. (*From Auerbach PS:* Medicine for the outdoors: the essential guide to emergency medical procedures and first aid, *ed 3, New York, 1999, Lyons Press.*)

lized, but drags or carries may be acceptable when immediate danger outweighs the risk of aggravating existing injuries. Drags are particularly useful for victims who are unconscious or incapacitated and unable to assist their rescuer (or rescuers) but may be uncomfortable for conscious victims. When a drag is used, padding should be placed beneath the victim, especially when long distances are involved. The high fatigue rate of rescuers makes carries a less attractive option when long distances are involved.

LITTER IMPROVISATION

The simplest improvised litter is made from a heavy plastic tarpaulin, tent material, or large polyethylene bag (Figure 26-9). By wrapping the material around a rock, wadded sock, or glove and securing it with rope

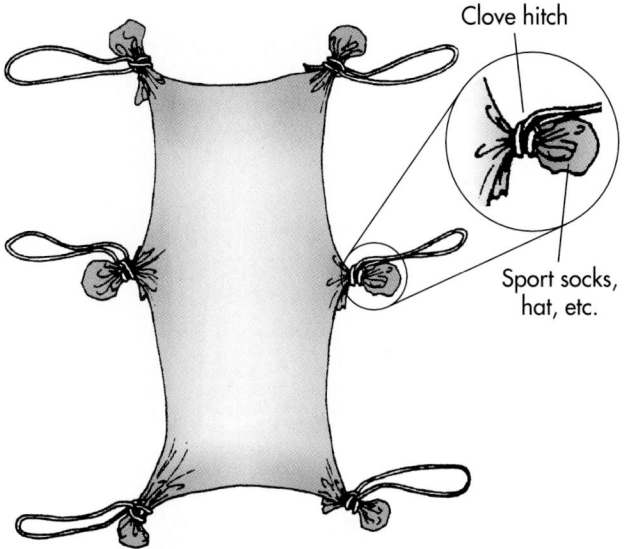

Figure 26-9 Improvised handled soft stretcher.

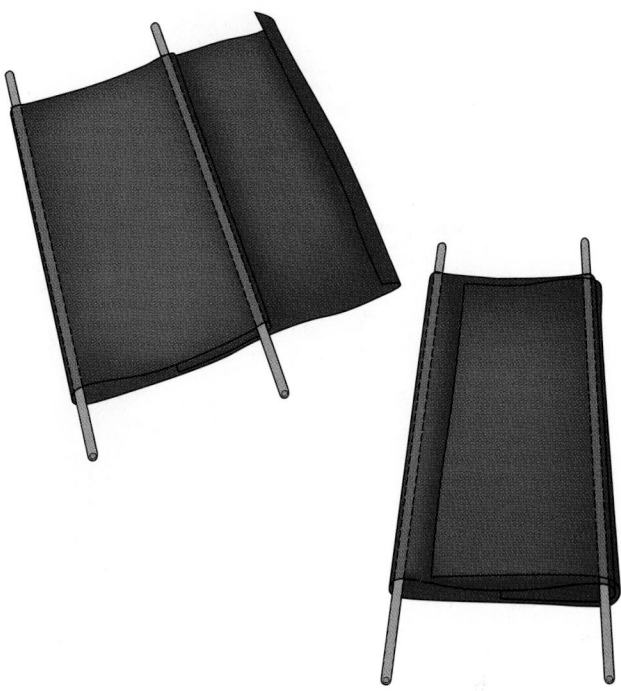

Figure 26-11 Improvising a stretcher from two rigid poles and a blanket or tarp.

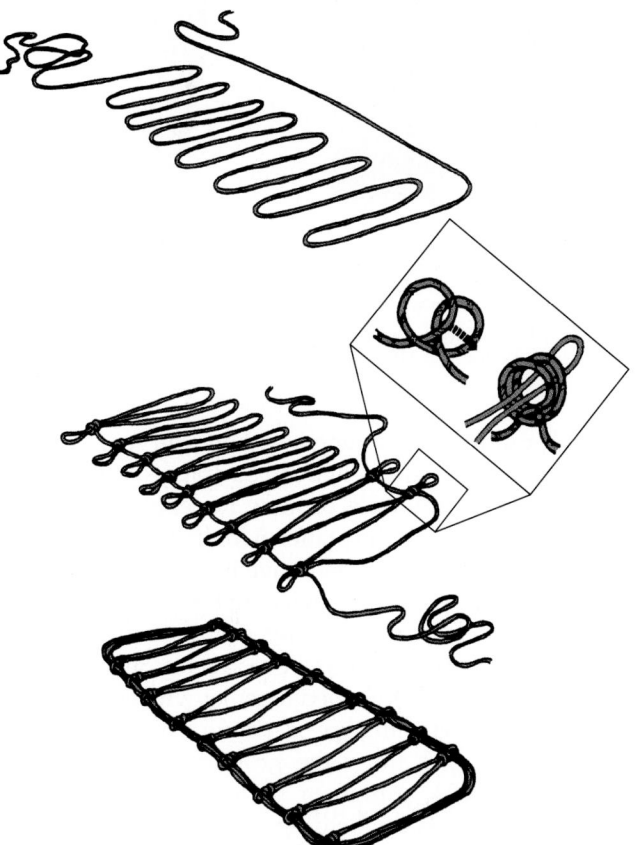

Figure 26-10 Tying an improvised rope (nonrigid) stretcher.

or twine, the rescuer can fashion handles in the corners and sides to facilitate carrying. The beauty of this device is its simplicity, but it can be fragile, so care must be taken not to exceed the capability of the materials used. As an additional precaution, all improvised lit-

ters should be tested with an uninjured person before being loaded with a victim. This type of nonrigid, "soft" litter can be dragged over snow, mud, or flat terrain but should be generously padded, with extra clothing or blankets placed beneath the victim.

A coil of rope also can be fashioned into a litter, called a *rope litter* or *clove hitch stretcher,* but a 46- to 61-m (150- to 200- foot) climbing or rescue rope is required (Figure 26-10). The rescuer constructs the litter by laying out 16 180-degree loops of rope (8 on each side of center) across an area the desired width of the finished litter. The running ends of the rope are used to tie a clove hitch around each of the loops, and then the unused portion of rope can be passed through the loops on the other side and tied off. The litter is then padded with clothing, sleeping pads, and similar material. Lateral stability can be added by tying skis or poles to the finished product. Because of its nonrigid construction, this litter offers little back support and is best suited for victims with injuries that do not require immobilization.

A sturdy blanket or tarp can be used in combination with ski poles or stout tree branches. The blanket or tarp is stretched over the top of two poles, which are held about 1 m (3 feet) apart; tucked around the far pole; and folded back around the other pole. The remaining material lies over the first layer to complete the litter (Figure 26-11). The weight of the victim holds the blanket in place. A similar device can be improvised by passing the poles through the sleeves of two heavy, zipped (closed) parkas.

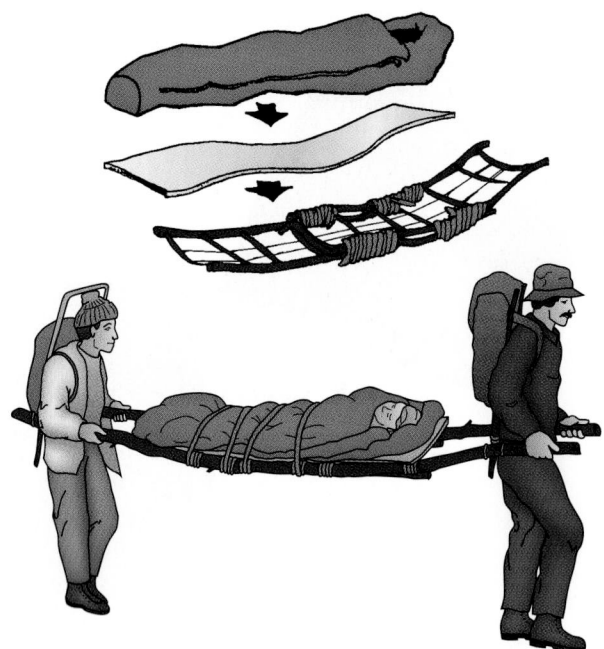

Figure 26-12 Packframe litter. Note that the sapling poles on the litter can be attached to the rescuer's pack frames to help support the victim's weight.

It may be necessary to transport victims with certain injuries (i.e., spine injuries; unstable pelvis, knee, or hip dislocations) on a more rigid litter. Ski poles, stout tree limbs, or pack frames can provide a rigid support framework for such a device. For example, three curved backpack frames can be lashed together to form a platform (Figure 26-12). Ski poles or sturdy branches then can be fastened to the frames for use as carrying handles, and the platform can be padded with ground pads, sleeping bags, or a similar material.

Combining a rope litter with a rigid litter can provide more strength and versatility. The rescuer fashions this type of litter by first building a platform of poles or limbs, using a blanket as in a rigid litter, and placing the victim in a sleeping bag on the platform. The patient and platform are wrapped and secured with a length of rope. Because a mummy sleeping bag is used to encapsulate the victim, this device is sometimes called a *mummy litter*. Although this type of litter offers improved support, strength, and thermal protection, careful thought must be given to the physical and psychological effects such a restrictive enclosure may have on the victim (Figure 26-13).

If long distances must be traveled or if pack animals are available, a litter may be constructed so that it can be dragged or slid along the ground like a sled. One such device is known as a *sledge* (Figure 26-14). This litter is fashioned out of two forked tree limbs, with one side of each fork broken off. The limbs form a pair of sledlike runners that are lashed together with cross members to form a patient platform. The sledge offers a solid platform for victim support and stabilization. If sufficient

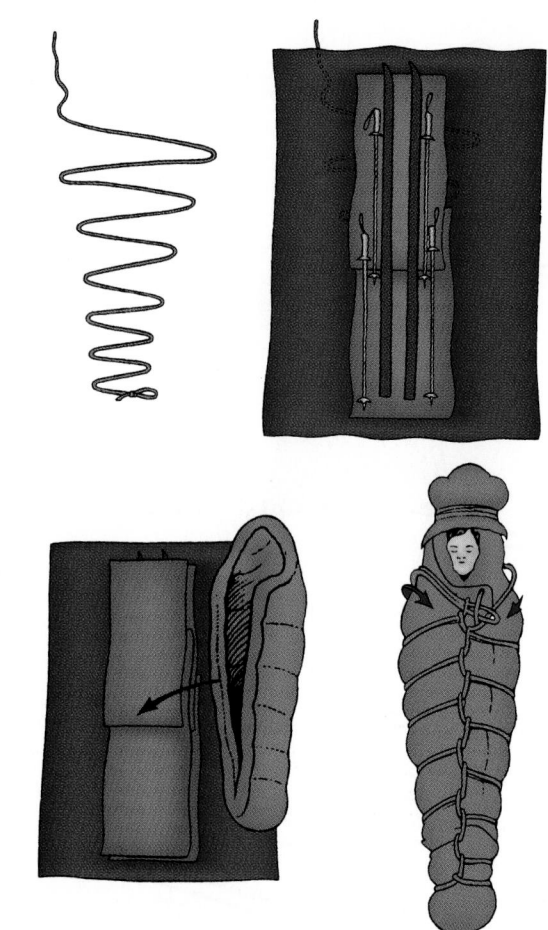

Figure 26-13 Mummy litter. (*From Auerbach PS: Medicine for the outdoors: the essential guide to emergency medical procedures and first aid, ed 3, New York, 1999, Lyons Press.*)

effort is put into fashioning a smooth, curved, leading edge to the runners, a sledge can be dragged easily over smooth ground, mud, ice, or snow. Ropes also can be attached to the front of the platform for hauling and to the rear for use as a brake when traveling downhill.

A travois is a similar device that is less like a sled and more like a travel trailer (without wheels). A travois is a V-shaped platform constructed out of sturdy limbs or poles that are lashed together with cross members or connected with rope or netting. The open end of the V is dragged along the ground, with the apex lashed to a pack animal or pulled by rescuers. Although the travois can be dragged over rough terrain, the less smooth the ground, the more padding and support necessary for comfort and stabilization. A long pole can be passed through the middle of the platform and used for lifting and stabilization by rescuers when rough terrain is encountered.

When victims are transported in improvised litters, especially over rough terrain, they should be kept in a comfortable position, with injured limbs elevated to limit pressure and movement. To splint the chest wall and allow full expansion of the unaffected lung, victims

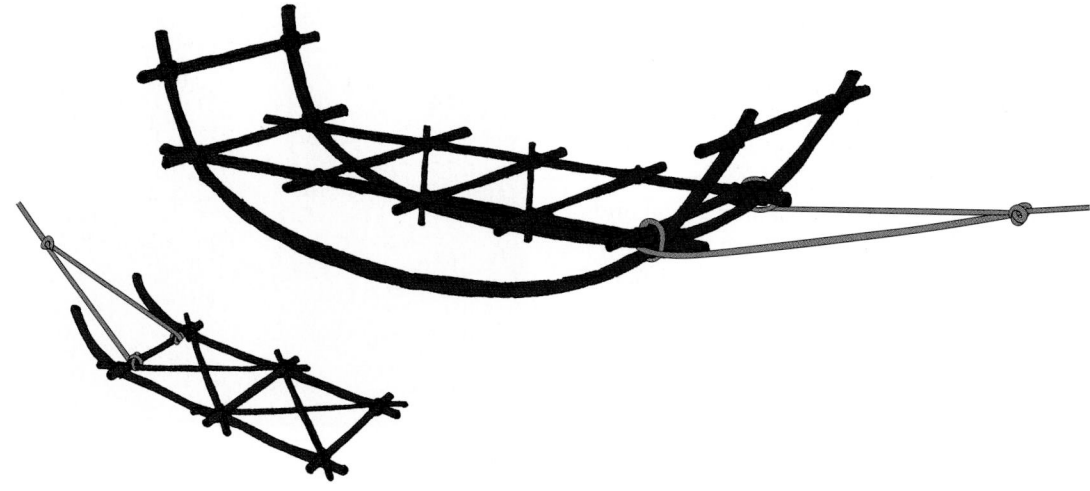

Figure 26-14 A "sledge."

with chest injuries generally should be positioned so that they are lying on the injured side during transport. For a person with a head injury, the head should be elevated slightly, and for persons with dyspnea, pulmonary edema, or myocardial infarction, the upper body should be elevated. Conversely, when the victim is in shock the legs should be elevated and the knees slightly flexed. Whenever possible, unconscious patients with unprotected airways should be positioned so that they are lying on their side during transport to prevent aspiration.[1]

RESCUE LITTERS AND STRETCHERS

The image most often associated with rescue immobilization and transportation devices in the United States is that of a traditional tubular steel and chicken wire–netted basket, which came to be known as the *Stokes basket*. Although this apparatus was and still is ubiquitous, many may recall the Thomas, Duff, Mariner, Brancard Piguillem, Perche Barnarde, Neil Robertson, MacInnes, and Bell stretchers for their evolutionary and robust designs. Today there are a variety of devices that meet the following two primary wilderness medical needs:

1. Immobilization and protection of a victim during transportation
2. Safe, comfortable, and stabilized transportation of a victim to definitive care

DESIRABLE CHARACTERISTICS OF A WILDERNESS STRETCHER

Peter Bell,[2] rescue equipment historian and developer of Bell stretchers, has described several specific characteristics of a high-quality, useful rescue stretcher. Bell claims that "a good stretcher should":

1. Be as strong and robust as possible, with materials compatible with the rescue environment
2. Be as lightweight as possible
3. Have smooth edges that will not snag
4. Be devoid of small spaces that will trap or pinch fingers (rescuers' and patients')
5. Be large enough to provide strength, security, and comfort for the largest of persons when the device is in any position (horizontal, vertical, on its side, upside down, etc.)
6. Prevent worsening of injuries during use
7. Provide security for the victim regardless of his or her condition (e.g., slippery, wet, muddy)
8. Be comforting to the conscious victim
9. Be easy to use in the dark and in temperature extremes (very hot or cold)
10. Protect the victim from the environment (heat, cold, brush, rocks, etc.)
11. Be reliable for many years after many uses in extreme conditions
12. Be easy to carry and use when carrying a heavy, large person
13. Be portable (can be carried in a car, boat, plane, helicopter, etc.)
14. Be impossible to use improperly
15. Be easy to clean and sterilize

STRETCHERS

In the interest of brevity and with some technical latitude, this discussion describes stretchers in four categories: basket-style, flat, wrap-around, and mountain rescue.

Basket-Style Stretchers

The basket-style stretcher derives its name from its shape. The sides curve upward to protect the victim's sides and to prevent the victim from rolling out. Most basket-style stretchers combine a steel frame (solid, tubular, or both) with a shell of either steel wire netting ("chicken wire") or plastic. Many include wooden slats in the bottom to provide additional protection and support.

Most likely, basket-style stretchers initially were adopted by wilderness rescue organizations because they met fundamental needs and were sufficiently robust to endure great abuse in severe terrain. The seminal basket-style stretcher, called the *Stokes*, first appeared in the late 1800s and likely got its name from the fact that it was designed to be used on naval and commercial ships to remove casualties from the "stoke-hold," a room in which the boilers were stoked (Figure 26-15). However, at least one source makes an unsubstantiated claim that the device was invented in 1895 by Charles Stokes.[8] The significant influence of this device is reflected in the fact that the Stokes was the first commercially available basket-style stretcher in the United States.

The original Stokes design included a leg divider meant to separate and support each leg individually. Many came to consider this configuration counterproductive when the use of long (16 × 72 inch) backboards and other spinal, full-body immobilization devices became widespread, especially for early treatment of trauma. Most current designs of the Stokes basket-style stretcher have eliminated the leg divider to allow full immobilization of a patient on a long backboard, which can be inserted into the basket. The Junkin Safety Appliance Company manufactures several Stokes basket-style stretchers, including models that break into two pieces and models with and without wooden slats or leg dividers, that meet the more robust military specifications (MIL-L-37957 and RR-L-1997) (Figure 26-16).

Although the traditional materials and design (i.e., tubular and flat, welded steel with a steel chicken wire covering) are still in use today, basket-style stretchers are more often constructed from tubular stainless steel or aluminum because of the added corrosion resistance, increased strength, and reduced weight. Manufacturers, such as Junkin and Ferno, offer basket-style devices in full-rectangular and tapered-rectangular shapes. Both are also available in break-apart versions for easy carrying. Narrower versions (usually 19 inches wide, instead of 24) are available for use in confined spaces or caves, although cave rescuers rarely prefer any type of chicken wire litter.

Because of the importance of portability in wilderness areas, the break-apart capability is an adaptation to nearly all styles and types of litters. Junkin manufactures a version of the Stokes stretcher completely coated with a plastic material called *Plastisol*, which provides nonsparking, nonconductive, and antistatic properties. Junkin suggests that this coating allows improved purchase (handgrip) on the litter and offers insulation from the temperature of the metal. A collateral benefit of the coating is that it extends the life and integrity of the steel chicken wire netting.

Taking advantage of substantial improvements in polymer research, some manufacturers began produc-

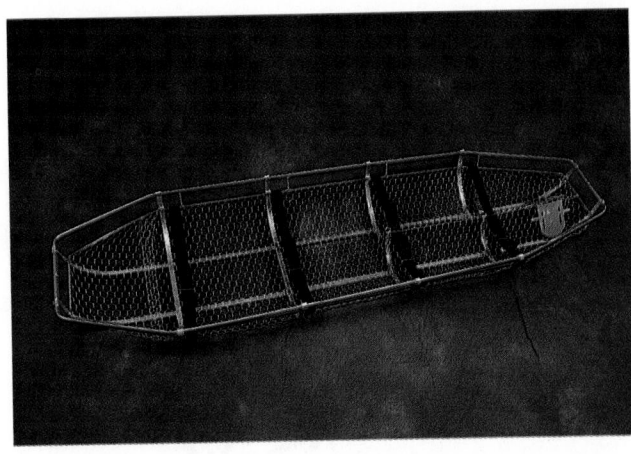

Figure 26-15 Traditional tapered Stokes litter with leg divider. *(Courtesy Junkin Safety Appliance, Inc.)*

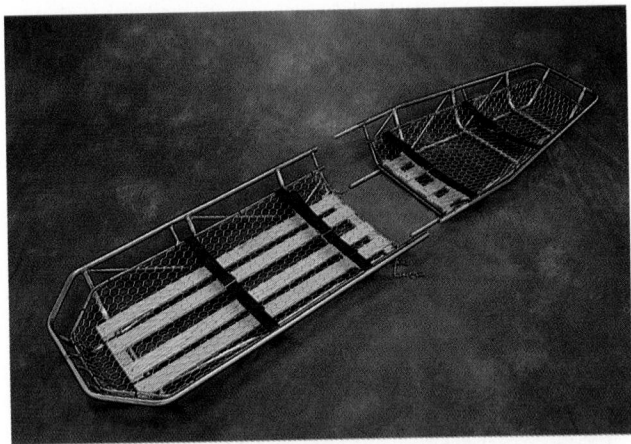

Figure 26-16 Break-apart Stokes litter with wooden slats. Many manufacturers also offer accessory straps or backpack devices that allow the rescuer to carry the litter halves on his or her back. *(Courtesy Junkin Safety Appliance, Inc.)*

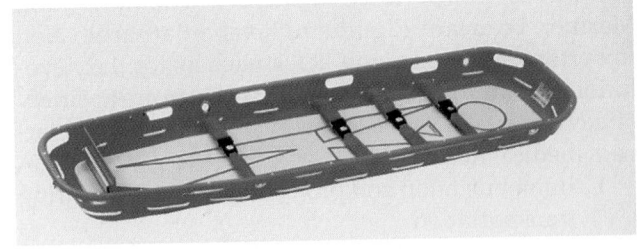

Figure 26-17 Ferno model 71 stretcher. *(Courtesy Ferno.)*

ing a stretcher shell composed of rigid plastic instead of steel mesh. Ferno's model 71 stretcher has an orange plastic shell wrapped around an aluminum frame and secured with aluminum rivets. Brass grommets in the plastic serve as attachment points for a lifting harness (Figure 26-17). At half the weight of a traditional steel Stokes, this device offers protection from snags and obstacle penetration that cannot be provided by the wire netting of the Stokes. In addition, the plastic used is chemical resistant and the molded underside runners make it slide smoothly over flat ground, ice, and snow. Ferno offers a version with tow handles and a chain brake that is designed specifically for ski patrol applications so that a packaged victim can be "skied" down a slope or pulled along a snow-covered trail. The orange Ferno litter has a load limit of 270 kg (600 lb), but its usefulness in a vertical raise configuration depends on the integrity of the aluminum frame and the plastic shell; if one is compromised, both may fail. Because of this limitation and because of the lightweight materials used, bending or twisting the device should be avoided.

International Stretcher Systems also builds a basket-style stretcher with an aluminum frame but uses a different approach for combining the frame with the shell. Their plastic shell is similar to the shell in the Ferno model 71 (high-density polyethylene), but it is placed outside a full aluminum skeleton to facilitate sliding over the ground. Inside the stretcher, a spring-suspended victim "bed" that doubles as the victim retention system has been added to protect the victim from the internal frame members. This bed minimizes transport shock and features built-in shoulder straps, pelvic padding, a head and chin immobilizing harness, foot and ankle straps, and a large "double-security" Velcro body restraint flap that wraps around the victim. The stretcher is lightweight (weighing 10 kg, or 22 lb) and high strength (holding up to 1134 kg, or 2500 lb) (Figure 26-18).

The Junkin model SAF-200-B includes parallel stainless steel top rails. The top tube is larger to allow comfortable hand-gripping and to provide an attachment for lifting bridles, and the smaller solid steel lower rail allows attachment of patient retention straps. The twin rail configuration keeps patient straps and lifting systems from interfering with each other and helps protect the attached materials from abrasion during use. Unlike the International Stretcher Systems device, the stainless steel frame in the Junkin stretcher wraps around the exterior of the basket, which is lined with a smooth-surfaced, permanently padded plastic shell. This design offers comfort for the victim but makes it difficult to slide on the ground because of the external, exposed steel frame members. The unit is heavy (weighing 14.5 kg, or 32 lb) but breaks apart for packing and marries well with a litter wheel to allow easier handling.

Bell Rescue Stretchers offers the Series 2 Ludlow stretcher, which is simply their strongest flat stretcher with deep basket sides added. This strong, stainless steel–framed design has fold-down sides, which simplify access with a backboard. The sides can be completely removed to revert the device back to a flat

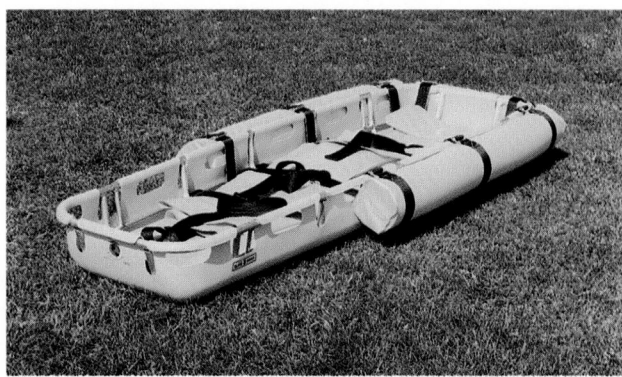

Figure 26-18 International Stretcher Systems' "3-in-1" Basket Litter with flotation added. *(Courtesy International Stretcher Systems.)*

stretcher. Other available variations on this theme from Bell include versions with shorter sides (the Otterburn), an open foot end (the Newark), and a steel plate welded into the bottom of the stretcher to help protect the victim (the Manchester). The Manchester weighs nearly 22.5 kg (50 lb) by itself. The manufacturer claims that the Series 2 models can all accommodate a long spine board and have been "proof tested" to between 500 and 720 kg (1102 and 1587 lb). The "bed" of Bell's Series 2 stretchers is made of 14 polypropylene web straps that cross between the steel frame members. This webbing also passes through two movable stainless steel spinal supports (flat steel frame members that run the length of the caudal two thirds of the litter). Four patient retention straps attached to the outermost rails, a patient shoulder strap, and integral lifting rings are supplied with the device. A slightly smaller, lighter, and less robust version, called the *Bell Emergency Stretcher* (discussed in the next section), also is available.

Flat Stretchers

Flat stretchers are generally flat and have very short or no sides. Restraint straps or built-in tie downs serve as the physical means by which the victim is secured in the litter. Although the specific characteristics of these types of stretchers vary greatly (from extremely lightweight to high strength), generally they are used when specific benefit is derived from their low-profile shape. Although this style of stretcher has been modified to allow dragging or sliding (e.g., mountain rescue stretchers), the primary purpose of the flat design is to reduce weight and profile for carrying or for specific applications, such as loading into an aircraft.

Although a simple, two-pole canvas litter is fine for use over short distances, uncomplicated terrain, or the battlefield (where haste is paramount), the lack of patient protection and immobilization capability limits it usefulness outside of the hospital or battlefield setting. A more modern version of this simple device is made of aluminum, folds for easy storage, and doubles as a long

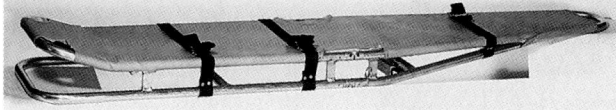

Figure 26-19 The Junkin Air Rescue Stretcher (SAF-350) was designed for use in Bell Jet Ranger helicopters. This lightweight, flat stretcher folds for easy storage but is not designed for long carries. *(Courtesy Junkin Safety Appliance, Inc.)*

backboard. Another version is hinged at one end so that it can be spread along its long axis and slid under a patient on the ground with little movement or rolling. This "scoop" stretcher was commonly used by emergency medical service providers but has been supplanted by the use of long backboards. In the final analysis, both the military and aluminum iterations of the flat stretcher are intended for carrying a person short distances in an environment with few terrain obstacles or where complete security and immobilization are not required.

Several successful varieties of flat stretchers have evolved over the years, including the Brancard Piguillem, the Junkin Air Rescue Stretcher (Figure 26-19), and a few of the Bell stretchers that are categorized as flat for the purposes of this discussion.

The Brancard Piguillem (*Brancard* is French for "stretcher" and *Peguillem* is a proper name) is a flat, old-style stretcher consisting of a canvas patient bed lashed to a steel and aluminum frame (weighing 14 kg, or 30 lb), which folds in half for easy carrying by one person. The design, which has evolved over the years in the European and British mountain rescue communities, includes a patient bed with a permanently attached, integral casualty bag lashed to the frame to protect and secure the victim. Full-length runners raise the stretcher a few inches above obstacles and allow for easy bare-handed gripping. This folding, portable design with integral patient protection made the Brancard Piguillem popular with mountain rescuers and served as the impetus for the evolution of several of the current styles of mountain rescue stretchers.

The Kendall Stretcher, from Bell Rescue Stretchers, has the same features as their Ludlow Stretcher without the basket sides (see the previous section). The Kendall has a stainless steel frame, integral lifting rings, a bed made of polypropylene web straps that cross between the frame members, color-coded patient retention (38-mm web) straps, and a detachable foot loop. The Kendall Stretcher can be used either side up; there is no top or bottom. A slightly less robust version of Bell's flat stretcher is their Basic Emergency Stretcher. This device is smaller and lighter (weighing 5.2 kg, or 11 lb, 8 oz) and works well in commercial and industrial settings where severe terrain is rarely encountered.

Troll Safety and Rescue Equipment produces the Alpine Stretcher, a folding, one-piece, steel-frame

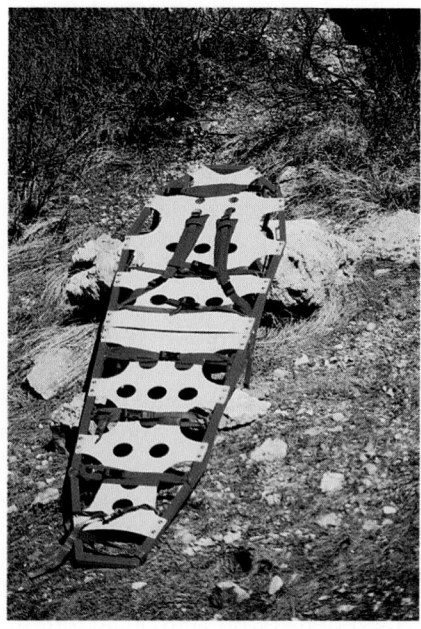

Figure 26-20 The steel-framed Troll Alpine Stretcher has an integral patient retention system and a polyolefin bed. *(Courtesy Troll USA.)*

stretcher that has a short spinal protection strip below a rigid polyolefin bed. It is strong and flat, making it suitable for wilderness and mountain rescues in which vertical evacuation is required. The integral, color-coded full-body harness and folding capability make it easy to transport into the wilderness and securely package a patient (Figure 26-20).

Mountain Rescue Stretchers

Mountain rescue stretchers are essentially stronger, more robust flat litters with runners or skis attached to the bottom for easy movement over rugged terrain. Over the years, engineers and litter designers with mountaineering and rescue backgrounds have adapted rescue litter designs to meet specific practical needs of their environment. The result is the strongest and most robust platform available for patient treatment and transportation, but these benefits come at the cost of weight and size.

The Thomas Stretcher is an early and beautifully simple example of the mountain rescue device. Invented in the U.K. in the 1930s by Eustace Thomas (no relation to Hugh Owen Thomas, who invented the Thomas "half-ring" splint), it consisted of wood (ash) runners, an aluminum frame, a canvas bed, and six or seven patient straps attached to the rails. It also had locking, tubular, retractable handles that stowed in the tubular rails.[5] The Thomas Stretcher is still manufactured, with some modifications, by Bell Rescue Stretchers in the U.K.

In the late 1950s, Donald Duff, a pioneer of mountain rescue in Scotland, designed a stretcher with a steel tubular frame and no handles. Channeled steel runners extended along two thirds of the caudal end of the stretcher. It weighed about 13.5 kg (30 lb) and could be fitted with a wheel and undercarriage for easier movement over rocky terrain. Its profile was low and sleek, and the runners could be detached and the remainder folded in two for backpacking.[4]

Although they have almost completely been replaced by more modern designs, two basket-style mountain rescue stretchers that evolved in Britain and Europe over the first half of this century deserve mention. The Perche Barnarde (*Perche* is French for "perch" or "pole" and *Barnarde* is a proper name) consists of a 2-m (7-foot) square section of steel tube from which a canvas casualty bag is suspended. The tube breaks into three pieces for easy carrying. The bag is attached to the tube at each end. Where the patient's shoulders would fall, a spreader bar is placed to keep the bag open. From each end of the steel tube extend two removable, bicycle-type handlebars fitted with pads so that the handlebars can rest on rescuers' shoulders. Although this device has been used successfully in many difficult mountain evacuations over the years, its limitations regarding patient comfort, protection, and immobilization are obvious.

The Mariner consists of a canvas bed attached to a steel sledlike frame. The bed functionally resembles a reclining chair in that the patient sits flexed at the hips and waist with the lower legs supported by a canvas platform. The frame is rounded from end to end and includes two steel runners to deflect obstacles. Two adjustable handles extend from each end of the frame for carrying. Today, the Mariner is used by several U.K. mountain rescue teams and contributed significantly to the evolution of the mountain rescue stretcher.

The current British standard for mountain rescue stretchers includes two devices that are incredibly strong, durable, and unfortunately heavy. The Mark III Bell Rescue Stretcher (which weighs 24 kg, or 53 lb) and the model 6 MacInnes Rescue Stretcher (which weighs 22 kg, or 48 lb) (Figure 26-21) are intended to survive years of use in extreme mountainous environments. Both have break-apart versions for easy packing into isolated areas, and both incorporate lifting rings, skids, and head guards.

Flexible, Wrap-Around Stretchers

A focus on improving stretchers for particular environments or situations has led to major developments in a number of litter design areas. It is difficult for a single device to excel in every situation because enhancing one capability or characteristic can be detrimental to another. For instance, it can be difficult to achieve a substantial increase in strength while decreasing overall weight. However, new innovative stretcher designs and materials allow structural flexibility to meet specific needs.

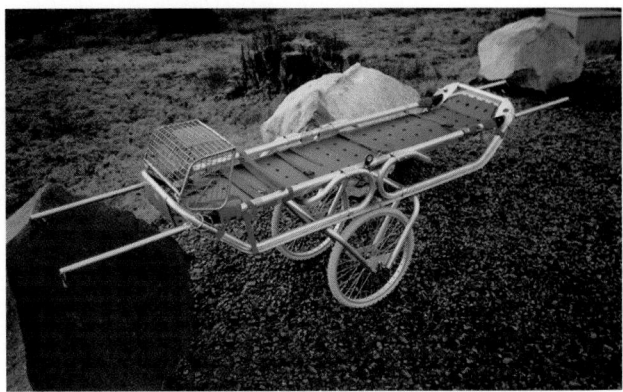

Figure 26-21 MacInnes MK 6 Mountain Rescue Stretcher. Note the extending handles, folding head guard, and optional twin (solid) tires. *(Courtesy MacInnes Rescue Stretchers.)*

Flexible, wrap-around stretchers can be folded, rolled, or otherwise compacted for storage and "wrap around" in that they contain the victim to provide protection, immobilization, and often sufficient support for vertical lifting. The Neil Robertson Stretcher was the impetus for this entire category of device. Adapted from a Japanese design and first produced between 1906 and 1912, this wooden and canvas stretcher was originally made of bamboo and sewn by hand. The "Neil Rob" supplanted the Mansfield military stretcher in the U.K. and was first given the name *Hammock for Hoisting Wounded Men from Stokeholds and for Use in Ships whose Hoists are 2 feet, 6 inches in Diameter.*[3]

The Neil Rob consists of wooden slats covered with semirigid canvas that are sewn the length of the stretcher. These slats wrap around the patient in mummy fashion, with arms in or out, providing protection without bulk. Full-body immobilization, protection, and a small cross section combine to produce a device well suited for use in small spaces or for situations in which the victim must be moved through a small opening.[9]

For situations requiring full-body protection for the victim without complex restraint systems, the Reeves Stretcher (model 321011) and Ferno Flexible Stretcher (model 131 and 137) almost totally encapsulate the patient (Figure 26-22). Although not intended for vertical lifting, both include a durable, vinyl-coated fabric shell that wraps around the sides of the patient and integral wood or synthetic slats that provide longitudinal rigidity. When used in conjunction with a cervical collar and spinal immobilization, these devices provide environmental and mechanical protection while allowing the victim to be carried through narrow passages.

The Reeves Sleeve (model 31220) is a compact immobilizing stretcher suitable for hand-carry situations or vertical environments. The device slides over a full backboard and depends on the backboard or short spinal immobilizer to provide rigidity (Figure 26-23).

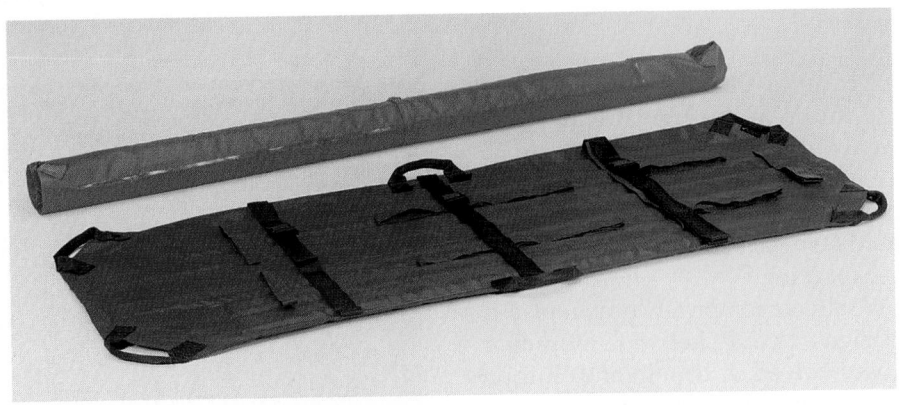

Figure 26-22   Ferno Flexible Stretcher with storage case. *(Courtesy Ferno.)*

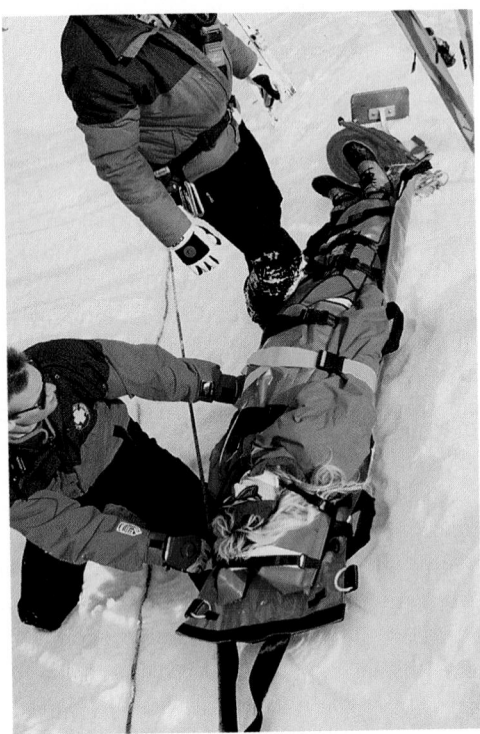

Figure 26-23   Reeves Sleeve in use. *(Courtesy Reeves Manufacturing, Inc.)*

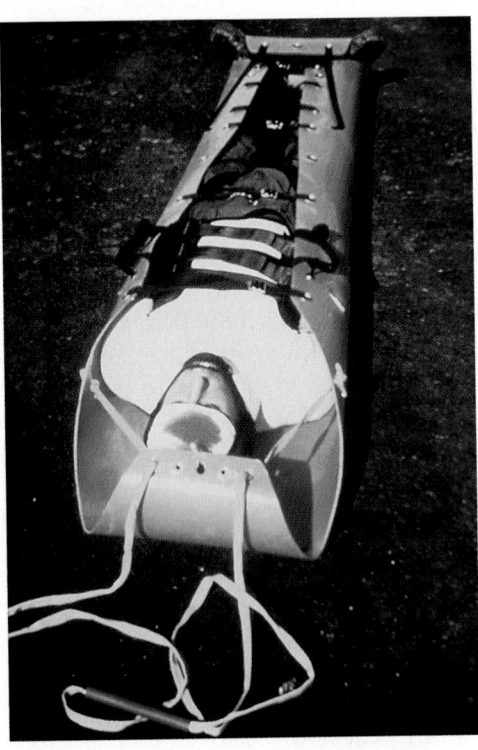

Figure 26-24   SKED Stretcher in use. *(Courtesy Skedco.)*

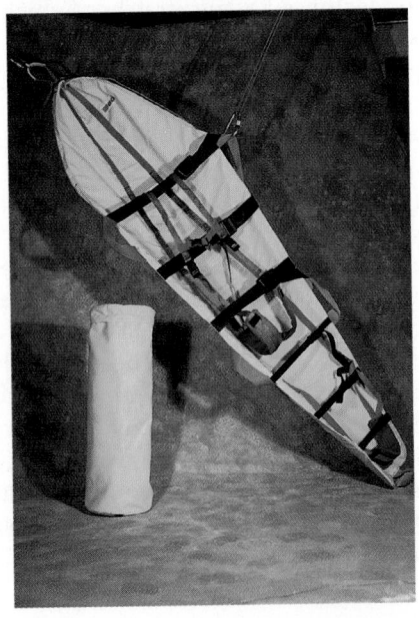

Figure 26-25   Troll Evac II Body Splint and carrying bag. *(Courtesy Troll USA.)*

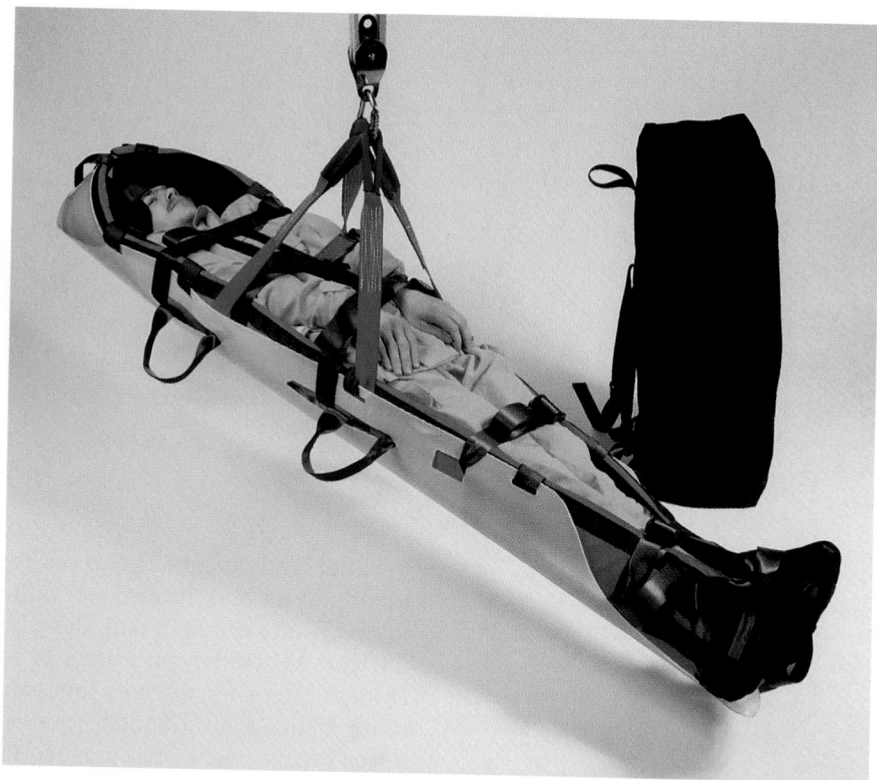

Figure 26-26 The Smith Safety Products (SSP) HD Rescue Stretcher and carrying bag constitute the basic package. When the detachable plastic shell (shown) is added, it becomes the SSP USAR Stretcher. *(Courtesy Smith Safety Products, Inc.)*

Skedco's SKED stretcher provides wrap-around protection similar to the Neil Rob, but a combination of shape and material, rather than integral slats, provides longitudinal rigidity (Figure 26-24). Light and compact when stored in its packable case, the flexible, low-density polyethylene plastic litter wraps around the victim to form a rigid sleeve that is superbly compact for maneuvering in tight quarters. A half-length version is available for moving persons from areas that are too confined for a full-length device when flexing the victim at the hips might facilitate extrication. The hard and smooth plastic material can be easily dragged over a variety of surfaces and offers substantial protection from penetrating obstacles. Though the SKED stretcher provides spinal protection, the manufacturer recommends using an Oregon Spine Splint (Skedco) or similar device when cervical spine immobilization is necessary. External lift slings are included with the SKED to allow vertical or horizontal lifting, and flotation is available for use in a marine environment.

Troll Safety and Rescue Equipment produces the Evac II Body Splint, which is designed for use in confined spaces and for technical rope evacuations (Figure 26-25). A flexible, heavy nylon moisture barrier gives moderate rigidity to the protective nylon covering with sewn-on web handles. The integral body harness eliminates the need for any additional casualty retaining straps, and the lightweight nature of the device allows superior portability in confined areas. However, the substantially tapered shape may make it difficult to package the victim with external splints. The device can be used horizontally, as a transportation device, or vertically, during technical evacuation.

The Ferno Paraguard Rescue Stretcher (model 1411) is based on a narrow patient "bed," which gets its foundation from a stainless steel and aluminum frame. The bed includes color-coded straps and wraps for victim packaging. The stretcher folds in half when not in use. It may be used in vertical environments and includes removable "bicycle-type" handlebars and shoulder harness assist straps that allow two rescuers to carry the stretcher from each end.

Smith Safety Products (SSP) manufactures a wrap-around stretcher system that incorporates many of the features found individually in other products. The SSP HD Rescue Stretcher is based on a wrap-around shell made of multi-ply polyvinyl chloride (PVC) and closed-cell foam encased in a 1000-din Cordura nylon shell (Figure 26-26). According to the manufacturer, this combination forms a comfortable, full-body splint that provides patient protection from temperature extremes. SSP's basic stretcher features built-in patient restraint straps (head, shoulder, and ankle) and a footrest. Their USAR Stretcher package offers, in addition to the basic

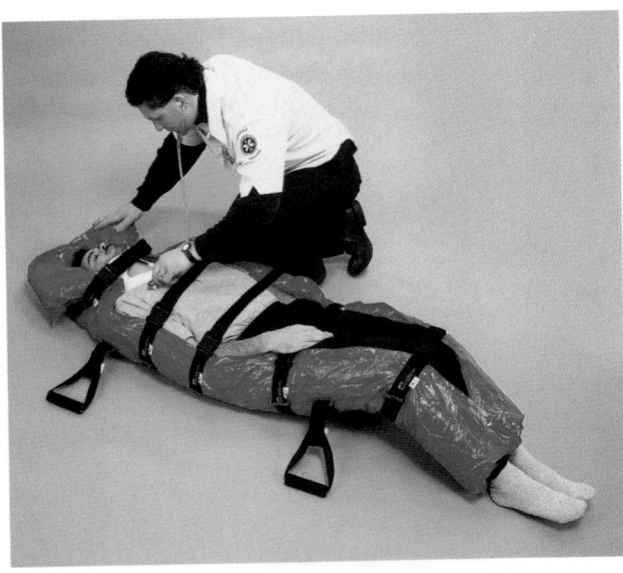

Figure 26-27 The Medical Devices International Immobile-Vac Full Body Mattress is a full-body splint that can be carried or inserted into other litters. *(Courtesy Medical Devices International.)*

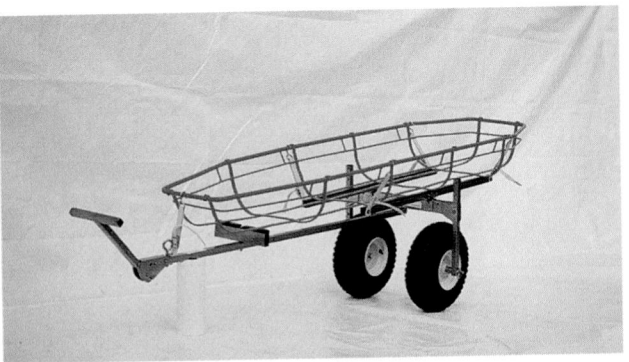

Figure 26-28 The Stokes Chariot from Farrington Chariots. *(Courtesy Farrington Chariots.)*

features, a detachable plastic shell that provides a smooth surface for dragging or sliding and protection from snags or penetration. The USAR Response Set adds a patient bag made of thermal fleece.

Medical Devices International (MDI) makes the Immobile-Vac Full Body Mattress, which is a full-body vacuum splint on which the victim is carried (Figure 26-27). The vinyl-coated, fabric patient bed contains loose polystyrene (Styrofoam) beads similar to those in a beanbag chair. Once the victim is positioned on the mattress, a small hand pump is used to expel air from within it. This process creates a rigid, full-body splint that conforms to the victim's shape. This "cocoon" immobilizes the spinal column and extremities while providing a comfortable platform. The mattress has integrated web carrying straps that can be used to carry the patient directly, or the mattress can be inserted into a basket-style stretcher for added versatility and strength. The use of a basket stretcher will be necessary for high-angle rescue because the MDI device is not designed for vertical rescue by itself.

TRANSPORTATION HARDWARE ACCESSORIES

A number of wheeled devices can be attached to most basket-style stretchers. These devices take the carrying burden off rescuers in nontechnical evacuations and reduce the load on low-angle haul systems. One example is the Russ Anderson Litter Wheel, which incorporates a large, underinflated all-terrain vehicle tire into a lightweight aluminum frame that clamps to the underside of the litter. This single wheel is positioned under the center of gravity, and the rescuers walk alongside the litter to steady and guide it, with the wheel carrying most of the load. When they encounter large obstructions, such as logs or trenches, rescuers simply lift the litter and continue rolling. One advantage of this device is that it reduces the number of rescuers required to move a litter safely over a long distance. When using this device, only two rescuers (one at each end) are required to tend the litter, but more may be used as necessary.

To meet a similar need, the Stokes Chariot (Farrington Chariots) employs a collapsible stainless steel frame with two attached 16-inch (outer diameter) wheels. With no axle between the wheels, the tires can be set to the outside of the frame for greater side-to-side stability or to the inside and under the frame to negotiate narrow trails or doorways. The draw bar end of the "chariot" is set up to receive either the T bar handle, for towing by rescuers on foot, or a hitch adapter, for towing behind motorized vehicles (Figure 26-28). International Stretcher Systems makes a similar device out of aluminum. It also can be folded for storage and employs wheels that can be repositioned on the frame.

Junkin and CMC Rescue market two useful stretcher accessories. The CMC Rescue Stretcher Insert is based on Yosemite Search and Rescue's idea to replace the chicken wire in the Stokes litter with a nylon bed, because chicken wire requires padding to allow even minimal patient comfort. A nylon bed allows for an integrated patient restraint system (harnesses) and greatly improves patient comfort. Junkin's Comfo-Pad takes a slightly different approach to the same problem by supplying padding where it is needed in this type of uncomfortable stretcher.

MacInnes and Bell integrate steel wire head protectors in their mountain rescue stretcher designs. This feature is important where falling rock is a hazard. CMC Rescue markets a similar aftermarket device

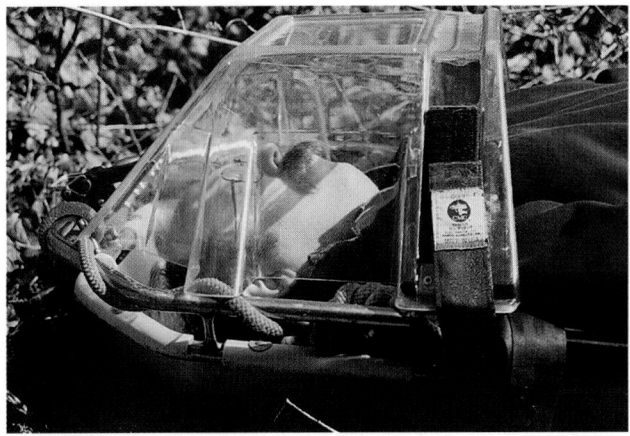

Figure 26-29 The CMC Litter Shield protects the victim from falling debris while allowing access to the head and face.

made of clear polycarbonate under the trademark CMC Rescue Litter Shield (Figure 26-29). It protects the victim's face from falling debris; allows for easy, rapid airway access; and can be moved out of the way because it hinges on the end of the litter. The shield stores compactly in the litter when not in use.

Flotation systems are available for some litters. Ferno and Skedco each offer this option to make their devices safer and more versatile in swift or open water rescue situations.

Most litter manufacturers offer specific devices or methods for carrying their devices into isolated areas. For instance, the SKED, Troll Evac II, and SSP HD Rescue Stretchers can be rolled up and carried in a special backpack by a single rescuer. Other manufacturers sell special backpacks or integral carrying harnesses for carrying half of their break-apart litters because of the greater weight.

Carrying a Loaded Litter

An evacuation is defined as *high angle* or *vertical* when the weight of the stretcher and tenders (stretcher attendants) is primarily supported by a rope and the angle of the rope is 60 degrees or greater.[7] This type of situation is often encountered when a rescue is performed on a cliff or overhang or over the side of a structure and usually requires only one or two tenders. In high-angle rescues, most often the stretcher is used in the horizontal position to allow only one tender and to keep the victim supine and comfortable. However, when the packaged victim and stretcher must be moved through a narrow passage or when falling rock is a danger, the stretcher may be positioned vertically.

In a scree or low-angle evacuation, the slope is not as steep (less than 60 degrees), the tenders support more of the weight of the stretcher, and a rope system is still needed to help move the load. In this type of rescue, more tenders (usually four to six) are required and the rope is attached to the head of the stretcher. The head of the litter is kept uphill during a low-angle rescue.

In a nontechnical evacuation, tenders completely support the weight of the stretcher during a carry out. Generally the terrain dictates the type of evacuation. If the stretcher can be carried without the support of a rope, it is a nontechnical evacuation. If rope is needed to support the load or to move the stretcher, it is either a low- or high-angle evacuation, depending on the angle of the slope.

Carrying a litter in the wilderness is difficult and requires many resources. It takes at least six rescuers to carry a person in a litter a short distance (0.4 km, or ¼ mile, or less) over relatively flat terrain. With six rescuers, four can carry the litter while the other two clear the area in the direction of travel and assist in any difficult spots. However, depending on the terrain and the weight of the victim, all six rescuers may be needed to safely carry the litter any distance. If the travel distance is longer, many more rescuers are required (Figure 26-30).

PATIENT PACKAGING

Patients (victims) on stretchers must be secured, or "packaged," before transport. Packaging consists of stabilization, immobilization, and preparation of a victim for transport. Physically strapping a person into a litter is relatively easy, but making it comfortable and effective in terms of splinting can be a challenge. The needs of a person secured and transported in a litter are great and should not be overlooked or underestimated. The rescuer's goals are as follows:

1. Package the person to avoid causing additional injury.
2. Ensure the victim's comfort and warmth.
3. Immobilize the victim's entire body in such a way as to allow continued assessment during transport.
4. Package the victim neatly so that the litter can be moved easily and safely.
5. Ensure that the victim is safe during transport by securing him or her within the litter and belaying the litter as necessary.

Generally, proper patient packaging must provide for physical protection and psychological comfort. Once packaged in a carrying device, a person feels virtually helpless, so transport preparation must focus on alleviating anxiety and providing rock-solid security. With this in mind, rescuers must provide for the victim's ongoing safety, protection, comfort, medical stabilization, and psychologic support.[6]

Splinting and spinal immobilization are usually acheived by using a full or short backboard. The victim

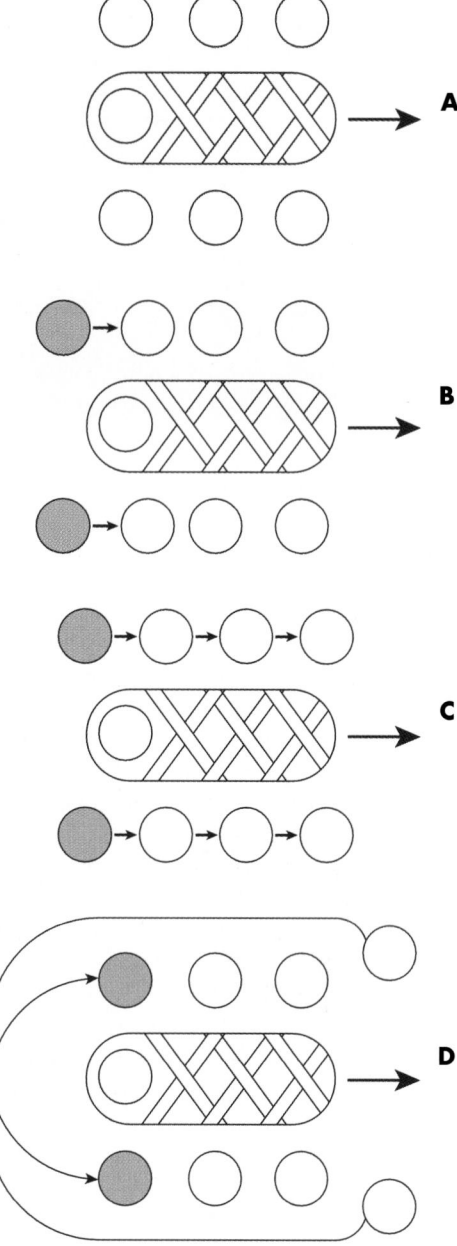

Figure 26-30 Litter-carrying sequence. **A,** Six rescuers are usually required to carry a litter, but rescuers may need relief over long distances (greater than 0.4 km, or ¼ mile). **B,** Relief rescuers can rotate into position while the litter is in motion by approaching from the rear. **C,** As relief rescuers move forward, others progressively move forward. **D,** Eventually the rescuers who are furthest forward can release the litter (peel out) and move to the rear. Rescuers in the rear can rotate sides so that they alternate carrying arms. Carrying straps (webbing) also can be used to distribute the load over the rescuers' shoulders. In most cases the litter is carried feet first, with a medical attendant at the head monitoring airway, breathing, level of consciousness, and so on.

is secured to the board, and then the victim (on the board) is placed into the litter. When the immobilized patient is finally placed into the litter, adequate padding (e.g., blankets, towels, bulky clothing, sleeping bags) placed under and around him or her contributes to comfort and stability. During transport, victims like to have something in their hands to grasp, to have pressure applied to the bottom of their feet by a footplate or webbing, and to be able to see what is happening around them.[6]

Because persons are so vulnerable to falling debris when packaged in a litter, especially in a horizontal high-angle configuration, a cover of some type should always be used to protect the victim (Figure 26-31). A blanket or tarpaulin works well as a cover to protect most of the body, but a helmet and face shield (or goggles) are also recommended to protect the head and face from projectiles. Alternatively a commercially available litter shield can be used and allows easy access to the airway, head, and neck (Figure 26-29). Because the head and neck usually require immobilization, the technique and equipment used to protect them should allow this. Remember also that the conscious victim desires an unobstructed view of his or her surroundings.

Carrying a person in the wilderness often requires that the litter be tilted, angled, placed on end, or even

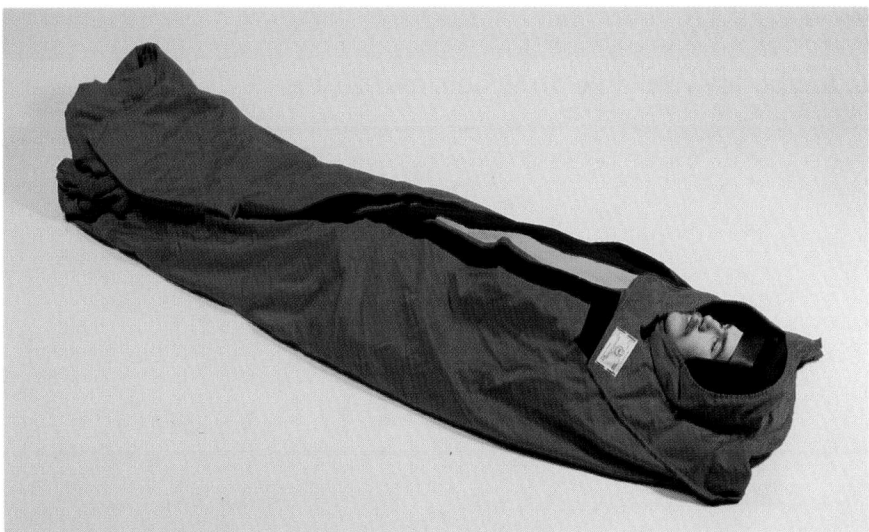

Figure 26-31 Smith Safety Products (SSP) Thermal Fleece Patient Bag (model 323) was designed to provide thermal protection for the SSP HD Rescue Stretcher but also offers limited protection from falling debris. *(Courtesy Smith Safety Products, Inc.)*

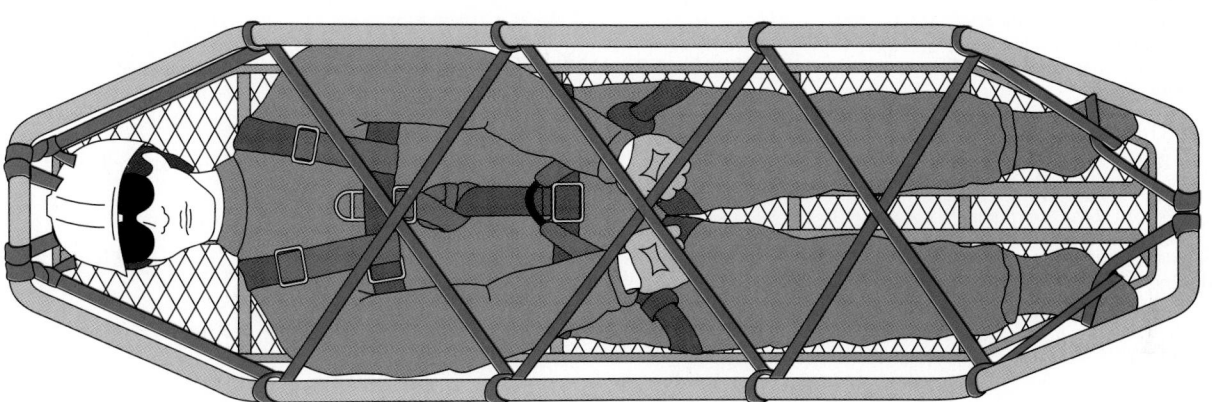

Figure 26-32 One 10-m (30-foot) web or rope can be used to secure a person into a litter.

inverted. In all of these situations the victim must remain effectively immobilized and securely attached to the litter, the immobilizing device within the litter, and any supporting rope. Poor attachment can cause patient shifting, exacerbation of injuries, or even complete failure of the rescue system.

Manufacturers have taken several approaches to securing a person within the litter. Most integrate a retention or harness system directly into the litter. However, a few require external straps to secure the victim to the device. Many users suggest that an independent harness be attached directly to the victim to provide a secondary attachment point in case any link in the attachment chain fails.

When a harness is not available, tubular webbing, strips of sturdy material, or even rope can be used to secure the victim. One approach uses tubular webbing slings in a figure eight at the pelvis and shoulders to prevent the victim from sliding lengthwise in the litter.

A 10-m (30-foot) piece of 5-cm (2-inch) webbing or rescue rope can be used to achieve the same goal (Figure 26-32). The rope or web is laced back and forth between the rails of the litter in a diamond pattern until the victim is entirely covered and secure. Such a technique also easily incorporates a protective cover and support of the victim's feet.

Regardless of the techniques and equipment used, frequently checking vital signs (i.e., distal pulse and capillary refill) during transport can help ensure that any strapping does not obstruct circulation.

APPENDIX

Comparison of Contemporary Available Stretchers and Litters

	APPROX. RETAIL COST (US $)	DIMENSIONS L × W × H	WEIGHT lbs (kg)	FRAME MATERIALS	SHELL MATERIALS
BASKET STRETCHERS					
Bell Series 2—Ludlow	2280	2080 × 585 mm	38.5 (17.5)	Stainless steel	Poly web bed
Ferno Basket Model 71-S	655	85.25 × 24 × 8 inches	26 (11.8)	Tubular aluminum	High-density polyethylene
International Stretcher Systems "3-in-1" Basket Litter[1]	900	81 × 25 × 8 inches	22 (10)	Aluminum schedule 80 pipe, butt welded	Recyclable polyethylene shell; vinyl-coated nylon bed insert
Junkin Basket, break-apart Model SAF-300-B	1000	80.5 × 22.5 × 8 inches	34 (15.4)	Welded steel tube	Steel hexagonal mesh netting
Junkin Plastic Stretcher, break-apart Model SAF-200B	560	84.5 × 24 × 7..5 inches	32 (14.5)	Steel tube	High-density polyethylene
Junkin Confined Space Stokes Model SAF-300CS	240	81.5 × 18.5 × 7.75 inches	23 (10.45)	Welded stainless steel tube	Steel hexagonal mesh netting
FLAT STRETCHERS					
Junkin Air Rescue SAF-350	300	73 × 16 × 7 inches	14 (6.3)	Aluminum tube	Vinyl-covered nylon
Medical Corp Stretcher ex: Junkin SAF-501-NA, Ferno 108	150	87 × 4.5 inches	14 (6.36)	Anodized aluminum side poles with 4 hardwood handles	Vinyl-coated nylon
"Scoop" stretcher ex: Junkin SAF-400, Ferno 65	515	79 × 16.75 × 3 inches	20 (9)	Aluminum tube	Aluminum
Troll Alpine Stretcher	975	78 × 23 × 3.25 inches	25 (11.3)	Square tubular steel (16 g)	Polyolefin bed
MOUNTAIN RESCUE STRETCHERS					
MacInnes Mountain Rescue Stretcher Mark 6	1324	218 × 47 × 26 cm	44 (20)	Stainless steel tube and rod	Aluminum
MacInnes Superlight Stretcher	896	189 × 53 × 31 cm	26.4 (12)	Stainless steel and aluminum tube	Aluminum alloy
Bell Mountain Rescue Stretcher Mark 3	3192	2000 × 578 mm	48.4 (22)	Stainless steel, aluminum, titanium	Stainless steel wire mesh
WRAP-AROUND STRETCHERS					
Ferno Flexible Stretcher Model 137	350	76.5 × 27.25 × 1 inches	19 (8.6)	Oak wooden slats	Vinyl-coated nylon

Y, Yes; *N*, no; *NA*, not applicable; *NN*, not needed; *NR*, not rated; *NP*, not published; 1 = low, unlikely; 10 = high, very likely.
[1]The weight of the ISS basket alone is 22 lbs; complete is 40 lbs (shell = 7 lbs; frame = 22 lbs; bed insert, lifting straps, restraint system, belts, and buckles = 11 lbs).
[2]The welded lift points on the Troll Alpine Stretcher are rated at 6000 lbs each.

RATED STRENGTH (R) OR PROOF LOAD (P)	YES OR NO								RELATIVE SUBJECTIVE INDEX					COMMENTS
	RUNNERS OR SKIDS?	FOLDS, ROLLS OR BREAKS APART FOR CARRYING?	FLOTATION AVAILABLE AS OPTION?	DESIGNED FOR HORIZ. OR VERT. LIFTING?	CAN WHEEL(S) ATTACH?	HOLDS FULL BACKBOARD?	DESIGNED FOR AIR-CRAFT USE?	INTEGRAL PATIENT RESTRAINTS	DURABILITY AND ROBUSTNESS	LIKELY TO SNAG IN USE	LIKELY TO PINCH FINGERS	RESCUER COMFORT (WITHOUT ADJUNCTS)	PATIENT COMFORT (WITHOUT ADJUNCTS)	
500 kg (P)	N	N	Y	Y	Y	Y	N	Y	10	5	4	6	5	Six patient restraint straps; sides fold down
600 lbs (R)	Y	Y	Y	Y	Y	Y	N	Y	7	2	5	5	5	Four-point restraints; integral hand-holds
2500 lbs (P)	Y	N	Y	Y	Y	Y	N	Y	10	2	2	5	8	Adjustable lifting slings, flotation available for head & back (6-inch bats) or as self-righting kit for rough seas
1200 lbs (R)	N	Y	Y	Y	Y	Y	Y	Y	5	8	5	3	8	Four patient restraint straps included
1200 lbs (R)	Y	Y	Y	Y	Y	Y	N	Y	7	4	1	6	5	Four seat-belt type patient restraint straps
1500 lbs (R)	Y	N	Y	Y	Y	Y	N	Y	8	7	1	6	5	Four patient restraint straps; integral upper tube hand holds
400 lbs (R)	N	Y	N	N	Y	Y	Y	Y	5	4	5	3	8	Made to fit inside Bell Jet Ranger helicopter; integral handles with tube frame; three patient restraint straps
500 lbs (R)	Y	Y	N	N	N	Y	N	Y	5	5	5	2	8	Four steel legs act as skids
350 lbs (R)	N	Y	N	N	N	NN	N	Y	8	4	8	3	5	Handles integral with tubular frame; adjustable length for different size patients; three patient restraint straps
6000 lbs (R)[2]	Y	Y	N	Y	Y	Y	N	Y	8	6	4	5	7	According to the mfg., this device spins very little when hoisted under a helicopter
1000+ kg (P)	Y	Y	N	Y	Y	Y	Y	Y	10	6	5	7	8	Four patient restraint straps included; wheel available; pole handles extend from ends; headguard extra
NP	Y	Y	N	Y	Y	Y	Y	Y	9	5	6	7	7	Six patient restraps; helicopter lift cables; side bearer straps; folds into backpack; two folding transverse shafts
1000 kg (P)	Y	Y	Y	Y	Y	Y	N	Y	10	6	7	7	8	Fold down head guard; front/rear folding pole handles; rotation available; full price includes pack frames
350 lbs (R)	N	Y	N	N	Y	Y	N	Y	4	4	1	8	7	Six web handles; provides c-spine immobilization with integrated restraints

Continued

	APPROX. RETAIL COST (US $)	DIMENSIONS L × W × H	WEIGHT LBS (kg)	FRAME MATERIALS	SHELL MATERIALS
WRAP-AROUND STRETCHERS—cont'd					
Ferno Paraguard Model 1411	1828	72 × 11 × 4 inches	36.5 (16.6)	Stainless steel and aluminum alloy slats	NA
Reeves Flexible Stretcher Model 101	215	78 × 28 inches	14 (6.3)	Wooden slats	Vinyl-coated nylon
Reeves Sleeve Model 122	400	73 × 24 inches	14 (6.3)	NA	Vinyl-laminated nylon
MDI Immobile-Vac Full Body Matress Model 81-A5000	445	81 × 36 inches	12 (5.5)	NA	PVC-coated polyesther mesh
SKED	450	84 × 36 inches	18 (8.1)	NA	Low-density easy glide polyethylene
SSP HD Rescue Stretcher[5]	445	77 × 12 inches	8.9 (4)	Polyethylene sheeting	Cordura nylon
Troll Evac II Body Splint	575	79 × 26 inches	12 (5.5)	Polyolefin	Nylon 6.0 finished coated

Y, Yes; *N*, no; *NA*, not applicable; *NN*, not needed; *NR*, not rated; *NP*, not published; 1 = low, unlikely; 10 = high, very likely.
[3]Strength rating is for bridle only.
[4]A KED, Oregon Spine Splint, or similar short spine board device is recommended for spinal immobilization.
[5]Smith Safety Products (SSP) adds an external polyethylene sheet to their "HD" (320) model to upgrade it to the "USAR" (321) model, which is less likely to snag obstacles than is the "HD" model.
[6]The rated strength listed is the tensile strength of the 44-mm flat web handles on the Troll Evac II Body Splint.

REFERENCES

1. Auerbach P: *Medicine for the outdoors: the essential guide to emergency medical procedures and first aid*, ed 3, New York, 1999, Lyons Press.
2. Bell P: *So, what makes a good stretcher?* Bell Rescue Stretchers website, www.rescuestretchers.co.uk/study.html, April, 1999.
3. Bell P: *The Neil Robertson stretcher.* Bell Rescue Stretchers website, www.rescuestretchers.co.uk/nrob.html, May, 1999.
4. Bell P: *Rescue stretchers in the U.K.* Bell Rescue Stretchers website, www.rescuestretchers.co.uk/hist.html, May, 1999.
5. Bell P: *The Thomas stretcher.* Bell Rescue Stretchers website, www.rescuestretchers.co.uk/thomas.html, May, 1999.
6. Cooper DC, LaValla PH, Stoffel RC: *Search and rescue fundamentals: basic skills and knowledge to perform search and rescue*, ed 3 (revised), Cuyahoga Falls, Ohio, 1996, National Rescue Consultants.
7. Frank JA, Smith JB: *CMC rope rescue manual*, ed 2, Santa Barbara, Calif, 1992, CMC Rescue.
8. Hudson S, editor: *Manual of U.S. cave rescue techniques*, ed 2, Huntsville, Ala, 1988, National Speleological Society.
9. U.S. Navy: Rescue and transportation. In *Virtual naval hospital: standard first aid*, www.vhn.org/StandardFirstAid/chapter11.html, May 1999.

RATED STRENGTH (R) OR PROOF LOAD (P)	RUNNERS OR SKIDS?	FOLDS, ROLLS OR BREAKS APART FOR CARRYING?	FLOTATION AVAILABLE AS OPTION?	DESIGNED FOR HORIZ. OR VERT. LIFTING?	CAN WHEEL(S) ATTACH?	HOLDS FULL BACKBOARD?	DESIGNED FOR AIR-CRAFT USE?	INTEGRAL PATIENT RESTRAINTS	DURABILITY AND ROBUSTNESS	LIKELY TO SNAG IN USE	LIKELY TO PINCH FINGERS	RESCUER COMFORT (WITHOUT ADJUNCTS)	PATIENT COMFORT (WITHOUT ADJUNCTS)	COMMENTS
400 lbs (R)	N	Y	N	Y	N	NN	Y	Y	5	5	5	7	6	Detachable end handles; four web handles; shoulder harness attaches to end handles
300 lbs (R)	N	Y	N	N	N	N	N	N	4	4	1	8	7	Rolls lengthwise for carrying; requires external patient restraint straps; web handles
Vertical: 5000 lbs (P) Horiz.: 1250 lbs (P)	N	N	N	Y	N	Y	N	Y	6	5	1	8	5	Requires backboard for rigidity and immobilization; six web handles
NA	N	Y	N	N	N	NN	N	Y	5	5	2	3	9	Two web handles per side with padded tube over web
Horiz.: 10000 lbs (R)[3] Vertical: 5800 lbs (R)[3]	N	Y	Y	Y	N	Y[4]	N	N	5	1	1	5	8	Four nylon web handles (more can be added); weight is with all accessories; suggest adjunct c-spine immobilizer be used
6000 lbs (P)[3]	N	Y	Y	Y	N	NN[4]	N	Y	8	2	1	9	10	Six web handles; wrap around bridle
6000 lbs (R)[6]	N	Y	N	Y	N	NN[4]	N	Y	7	3	2	5	8	This device will work in the horizontal position but is designed to be used in the vertical position

27 Aeromedical Transport

James P. Bagian and Robert C. Allen

Rapid provision of appropriate definitive care to acutely ill and injured patients is a major goal of all emergency medical services (EMS) systems throughout the world. The ability to rapidly transport and initiate treatment of severely ill or traumatized patients is important in decreasing morbidity and mortality. This is particularly germane to wilderness and environmental emergencies, where medical resources are scarce, transport times to definitive care facilities are often prolonged, and terrain and weather conditions are inherently difficult. Aeromedical transport crews can deliver emergency medical care at the scene, and the time to definitive care can be greatly decreased. This maximizes the patient's chance for a successful recovery.

AEROMEDICAL EVOLUTION

Rapid evacuation of trauma victims from an injury scene to the location of definitive care is a modern concept with roots in antiquity. The New Testament documented an early instance of prehospital care and transport: "A certain Samaritan . . . went to him and bound up his wounds, pouring oil and wine, and set him on his own beast and brought him to an inn, and took care of him."[78]

The greatest impetuses to the advancement of emergency care and transportation have been epidemics and wars.[61] Before the classical Greco-Roman period, injured soldiers were often left on the battlefield to die. Later, Homer described the use of chariots to evacuate fallen warriors during the Trojan War.[48] Napoleon's forces devised horse-drawn carriages, or *ambulance volantes,* for the same purpose.[52] The North American Indians devised the *travois,* a litter that could be pulled by a person or animal to transport ill or injured persons.[59] The U.S. Army began a similar practice during the Seminole War of 1835-1842 and used it again in the Civil War. Major Jonathan Letterman established the process of rapidly clearing wounded soldiers to a point behind the battle line where they could be further triaged to an expectant area for persons with mortal wounds, a local treatment area for the "walking wounded," or a hospital if definitive care was feasible. The central concept was efficient access to surgery for the victim of trauma.

These developments were soon followed by the invention of flying machines. In France, Richet had prophesied the potentials of air transport in 1869.[61] This was before the first balloon airlift. The prophesy was validated the following year during the Franco-Prussian War when the first documented aeromedical evacuations took place. During the Prussian siege of Paris, 160 wounded soldiers were evacuated and transported by hot air balloon over enemy lines.[80]

In the United States, air evacuation took place soon after the Wright brothers flew in 1903.[39] Grossman and Rhoades presented their idea of air transport of patients to the War Department in 1910, but the government refused to fund them. It was not until World War I that the U.S. military began to utilize aircraft to carry injured soldiers, and this occurred only rarely. However, the French transported patients as early as 1912 aboard Dorland ARII fighters converted to carry litters, despite the government's objection to the concept of aeromedical transport: "Are there not enough dead in France today without killing the wounded in airplanes?"[39]

The United States began utilizing its first dedicated air ambulances in 1920, using the deHavilland DH-4A, followed by the Cox-Klemin XA-I. World War II saw the widespread application of fixed-wing aircraft for evacuation. More than 1.4 million were transported from front-line hospitals to tertiary care facilities, with only 46 deaths en route.[86] During this time the concept of medical care during transport was implemented. In November 1942 the War Department began to train flight surgeons, flight nurses, and enlisted medical personnel for aeromedical transport.[39] Also during 1942, Igor Sikorsky produced a rotor-wing aircraft, called a "helicopter," which the army configured with external litters. It was used in an air evacuation for the first time in 1944 in Burma.[36]

Helicopters did not enjoy widespread use until more reliable machines became available. The Sikorsky S-51 and later the Bell 47-B were deployed over the rugged terrain and uncertain roads of Korea with great success to provide wide-scale evacuation of wounded soldiers to Mobile Army Surgical Hospital (MASH) units. Although only 11 dedicated "Medevac" helicopters were used, more than 17,700 casualties were evacuated. For the first time, injury victims could travel directly from the point of injury to definitive surgical care.

This set the stage for the Army helicopter evacuation ("Dust Off") operations in Vietnam in 1962. With the

TABLE 27-1. Mortality Rates and Evacuation Times During Major Wars

CONFLICT	EVACUATION TIME (HR)	MORTALITY RATE (%)
World War I	18	18
World War II	4-6	3.3
Korea	2-4	2.4
Vietnam	1-2	1.8

From Stewart RD: *Trauma Q*, May 1985, p 1.

Bell UH-IA Iroquois ("Huey") under the leadership of Major Charles Kelly, the Army's 57th Medical Detachment became known for the courage and hard work of flight crews, who flew despite darkness, adverse weather, and enemy fire. Later, the turbine-powered Bell model UH-1H was used to evacuate up to nine patients at a time by hoist from above a dense jungle canopy. By 1967, about 94,000 injured men had been evacuated.[69]

As air evacuation matured, the time from wound to definitive care declined from 18 hours in World War I to between 1 and 2 hours in Vietnam.[88] Although medical advances have contributed to improved survival, battlefield mortality has steadily declined from 18% in World War I to 1.8% in Vietnam, perhaps more because of rapid aeromedical transport to definitive care (Table 27-1).

Unfortunately, emergency medical care for civilians greatly lagged behind the developments in the military. In the late 1960s, rescue efforts were more organized, skilled, and rapidly performed for a man shot in the Vietnam conflict than for a civilian injured on U.S. highways.[61] Civilian ambulances were said to be no faster than taxis.[77]

Civilian transport began to change dramatically in the United States in 1966 when the National Academy of Sciences–National Research Council put forth the white paper *Accidental Death and Disability. The Neglected Disease of Modern Society* (U.S. Department of Health, Education and Welfare). This document was the impetus for improving EMS systems through the country, and soon the civilian sector began to emulate the military model.

Outside the United States, Germany and Switzerland had developed a network of helicopter and fixed-wing air evacuation and transport services that continue to provide rapid access to care from even the most remote areas.[38] The first U.S. civilian aeromedical program was begun in 1969 as a joint effort between the Maryland State Police and the University of Maryland Center for the Study of Trauma (now the Maryland Institute for Emergency Medical Service Systems). Certain hospitals were designated as trauma centers, and

victims of highway and other trauma were flown by police pilot-paramedic teams in a primary response role at the accident scene. Since 1970 the service has flown more than 199,000 missions.[82]

With the development of faster and more powerful helicopters, reconfiguration of fixed-wing aircraft for aeromedical needs, enhanced knowledge of aeromedical physiology, and experience accumulated through more than 50 years of transport experience, the acceptance, utilization, and success of aeromedical transport are universal. The role of aeromedical transport in the wilderness setting continues to evolve as its importance in providing rapid emergency medical care to sick and injured patients is recognized.

TYPES OF AEROMEDICAL TRANSPORT PROGRAMS

Hospital-Based Programs

The most ubiquitous type of program is hospital based. Helicopter service is often provided in *primary* (to the accident scene) and *secondary* (to the community hospital emergency department) response roles. In addition, many hospitals provide fixed-wing transport in a secondary response role for long-distance transports or when transport by helicopter is impractical.

According to the Association of Air Medical Services, in early 1994 there were more than 175 hospital- or health care provider–affiliated and 20 freestanding rotor-wing transport programs in the United States. These services transported more than 172,000 patients in 1993. Nationally, approximately 70% of all flights are interfacility transports, and 30% are flights from the scene.[63]

In a hospital-based transport program the hospital frequently leases the helicopter from a vendor, who also supplies the pilots, maintenance, and fuel. The hospital has the responsibility for providing the medical crew and determining the configuration of the crew. In addition, the program directors are responsible for medical control and quality improvement.

The hospital may choose to own the aircraft and contract with a vendor for operations or employ its own pilots and mechanics. In most cases the helicopter resides on a helipad atop or near the hospital, and the crew, which may consist of a specially trained flight nurse, flight paramedic, and physician, is quartered in the hospital ready for immediate launch (see Flight Crew).

Non–Hospital-Based Programs

Non–hospital-based service is provided by an entity that may be supported by a consortium of hospitals, or it may be an independent corporation, ambulance service, or aviation fixed-base operator (FBO). The aircraft may be owned or leased by the entity or by an aviation contractor. Although this is not a common model for helicopter services in the United States, many fixed-wing services operate in this manner. A corporate airplane may be provided on demand for use in an air ambulance mode with its interior reconfigured, or a dedicated airplane may be provided with a custom-made air-ambulance interior configuration, usually under a Supplemental Type Certificate (STC).

Public Safety, Police, or State Services

The aircraft (usually a helicopter) may be owned and operated by a governmental agency such as the state highway patrol and operated under part 135 of the Federal Aviation Regulations (FAR). As in the Maryland model, flight personnel typically include police pilots and emergency medical technician-paramedics.

Military Assistance to Safety and Traffic Program

The Military Assistance to Safety and Traffic (MAST) program was established to supplement the civilian EMS systems. Under this program, air medical evacuation services are supplied by active-duty military medical units to the extent that their training budgets allow, provided they can use actual patient transports instead of training exercises. The MAST mission is "secondary"; it is available only when its personnel and equipment are not being used in support of the unit's primary mission. MAST may be requested by the local EMS or disaster management agency. Typical aircraft include the Bell UH-1 and Sikorsky UH-60 (Blackhawk). The medical crew usually consists of medical corpsmen. The MAST program may not compete with similar civilian services.

Other Military Resources

The U.S. Air Force provides aeromedical transport in support of U.S. military disaster conditions. This service can be requested through the Rescue Command Center at Langley Air Force Base in Virginia. Other available resources include the Air National Guard and the U.S. Coast Guard. Many states have organizations (e.g., California Department of Forestry) that may be called on to assist in search and rescue (SAR) operations in preparation for aeromedical transport. Many other countries have analogous units; the Israeli Air Force, for example, operates a squadron that provides civilian and military rescue and evacuation services.

PATIENT MISSION TYPES

Primary Response

In a primary response role the aeromedical transport service responds to an accident scene or field location, usually at the request of police, fire, or local EMS personnel, and serves as the initial and sole mechanism of transport to the hospital. In this instance the aeromed-ical crew may function as "first responders." Helicopters are most suited to a primary response role. The required response times must be short (less than 10 minutes from call to take-off); thus the flight crew must be stationed at or near the launch site 24 hours a day. The service radius ("stage length") is short (typically less than 50 miles), and crews need to be experienced in techniques for landing in proximity to obstacles, under poor conditions, and on uncertain surfaces. In prehospital situations, patients' conditions vary widely, and often, little or no assessment or stabilization is performed before arrival of the flight crew. Medical personnel must possess a high degree of training and experience and should possess at a minimum emergency medical technician (EMT) skills required for patient extrication and stabilization at the scene.

Secondary Response

In the secondary response role a patient has already been transported by other means to a hospital where some degree of stabilization may have occurred. The aeromedical service transports the patient in the early stages of care from the emergency department of a hospital to a facility better equipped to offer definitive care. Response times required for this type of mission must be competitive with one-way ground transport times. Stage lengths are short to intermediate (150 miles). The transport vehicle is typically a helicopter, although in some remote and wilderness areas, fixed-wing services are also suited to this role. Flight crews used in a secondary response vary depending on the needs of the patient (see Medical Mission Types). The responding aeromedical service typically consists of flight nurses, paramedics, and in some cases flight physicians.

Tertiary Response

In a tertiary response an inpatient who requires specialized services unavailable at the current facility or who requests relocation is transported to a new facility. Tertiary transports may involve helicopters or fixed-wing aircraft, depending on the level of urgency, stage length, and the cost of transport. Commercial entities throughout the world specialize in this type of service.

MEDICAL MISSION TYPES

The needs of different patient types may be categorized by medical problem; this in turn dictates the requirements of the aeromedical transport service. In most hospital-based helicopter programs the majority of patients transported are categorized as adult trauma, cardiac, or medical noncardiac. A number of programs offer or specialize in pediatric, neonatal, perinatal, and organ transplant services, for which specialized crews and equipment may be required. In addition, aeromedical transport programs that provide SAR operations require specialized equipment and training.

Trauma Patients

Trauma patients transported in the primary or secondary response modes may account for 20% to 60% of a hospital-based helicopter service's transport activity, depending on the hospital's function and capability as a trauma center and the relationship between the aeromedical service and the community EMS and public safety network. A study of one urban setting noted that 20% of helicopter missions were to injury scenes, which were located at a mean distance of 14.4 miles from the hospital. Of patients transported, 19% had penetrating trauma, and 81% blunt trauma (66% from motor vehicle accidents). The most common organ system injuries involved the head (65%), extremities (39%), chest (31%), and abdomen (27%). The overall mortality of transported patients was 24%. The most common procedures required at the scene were endotracheal (ET) intubation (41%) and cardiopulmonary resuscitation (CPR) (18.7%). The most common life-threatening conditions were cardiac arrest (18.7%), airway obstruction (5.1%), cardiac tamponade (3.2%), and tension pneumothorax (1.7%).[33]

A multicenter study of blunt trauma victims transported by helicopter aeromedical services from both urban and rural environments found a mean trauma score of 13 (of 16), mean age of 29 years, and overall mortality rate of 15%.[8]

These and other studies indicate the need for skilled crews in the transport of trauma patients.[91] Medical personnel must have the ability to assess the patient adequately to detect frequent in-flight complications and to intervene with appropriate procedures, including intravenous (IV) cannulation, ET intubation, CPR, chest decompression, and at times a surgical airway (Box 27-1).

In wilderness areas the flight crew must be skilled at victim extrication and operating in rugged terrain. They must be familiar with standard trauma care and the range of clinical entities most frequently seen in the wilderness setting. In addition, because resources may be limited and backup unavailable, they may be required to function semiautonomously. For this reason, protocols and standing orders are valuable. Most important are training, skill, and judgment.

Patients with Cardiac Disease

Patients with most cardiac disease most often are transported in a secondary or tertiary response role, by either helicopter or fixed-wing aircraft. They typically account for 20% to 50% of an aeromedical service's transport activity. The conditions of these patients are often medically complex. Technologically sophisticated

---

Box 27-1 TRAUMA CARE ABOARD EMERGENCY MEDICAL SERVICES HELICOPTERS

MECHANISM OF INJURY

Motor vehicle accident
Fall
Industrial or agricultural accident
Gunshot or stab wound
Burn
Sporting accident
Drowning
Hypothermia

PROCEDURES PERFORMED BY FLIGHT CREW

Endotracheal intubation
Cardiopulmonary resuscitation
Intravenous lines
Central venous access
Extrication and splinting
Bladder catheterization
Nasogastric tube insertion
Venous cutdown
Tube thoracostomy
Cricothyrotomy
Pericardiocentesis
Antishock garment application

---

treatment modalities may include antiarrhythmics, vasopressors, inotropes, vasodilators, thrombolytic agents, cardiac monitoring, arterial and central venous pressure monitoring, pacemakers, implantable defibrillators, and intraaortic balloon counterpulsation devices.[23,30,37,50] The flight crew must have sophisticated knowledge, expertise, and experience and may include a cardiac critical care nurse and a physician.

Patients with Medical, Noncardiac Conditions

Patients with medical, noncardiac conditions, like those with cardiac disease, are most often transported in the secondary or tertiary response mode by either helicopter or fixed-wing aircraft. This group consists largely of patients with acute neurologic disease or shock or who require assisted ventilation.[41] The spectrum of potential in-flight challenges includes cardiovascular problems, arrhythmias, hypotension, respiratory difficulties requiring acute airway management, seizures, and alterations in level of consciousness. The flight team must be able to manage an airway and operate a ventilator. Additional considerations relate to the cabin environment and need for pressurization if hypoxemia is present, if barotrauma is likely, or if trapped gas exists, as well as the need to predict the requirement for and manage finite oxygen resources in flight.

Pediatric Patients

Pediatric patients may have traumatic or medical conditions.[9,44] In a study of 636 pediatric patients transported by air in the Salt Lake City area, 57.5% were transported by helicopter and 37.5% by fixed-wing aircraft, with a mean stage length of 207 miles (helicopter, 82 miles; fixed-wing, 452 miles). Less than 1% of flights were from the scene. The patient age ranged from 3 weeks to 16 years, with 45% less than 1 year old. Trauma was the most common diagnosis (15.3% head injury, 9.3% multiple injuries), followed by neurologic illness (24.2%), respiratory failure or infection (20.1%), gastrointestinal or genitourinary problems (10.2%), metabolic disease (9.2%), cardiovascular disease (6%), and general pediatric surgical problems (5.7%). The overall mortality was 7%.[60] Many of the considerations for pediatric transport are similar to those for adults, especially with older children. Infants may require an incubator, however, and flight crews must be experienced in caring for infants and children. Specifically, knowledge of pediatric advanced cardiac life support skills, including pediatric drug dosages, airway sizes, and fluid management, is essential.

Perinatal Patients

The need for expedient evaluation, preparation, and transport of the obstetric-gynecologic patient is increasing. Types of problems include ectopic pregnancy, pelvic inflammatory disease, toxic shock syndrome, abnormal fetal presentation, multiple gestation, diabetes in pregnancy, placenta previa, abruptio placentae, disseminated intravascular coagulation, preeclampsia-eclampsia, and preterm labor. The decision to transport patients in advanced preterm labor should be based on such factors as distance between hospitals, time required to cover the distance, personnel available for the transport, gestational age, and speed with which labor has progressed. The flight crew must be knowledgeable about these problems and comfortable with their treatment so as to ensure a favorable outcome for both mother and child.

Neonates

Neonates have unique anatomy and physiology, and the diseases that affect them require specific knowledge and skills by those involved in their transport. Specific issues include newborn assessment, including assignment of an Apgar score, airway clearance, temperature, homeostasis, and familiarity with neonatal resuscitation.[3] Access to references concerning neonatal emergency drug dosages should be available.[2,72]

The ability to perform umbilical vein catheterization is an important skill for any member of the transport team involved in neonatal care. In addition, knowledge of fluid, electrolyte, and glucose requirements is essential.[53] The flight crew involved in the transport of a neonate often includes a neonatal nurse and a neonatologist.

Search and Rescue

Wilderness search and rescue is a unique aspect of aeromedical care and transport that requires significant training and expertise. Most dedicated aeromedical aircraft in the United States are not well suited for SAR operations (see Aircraft for Search and Rescue). Most standard aeromedical crews are not trained in SAR techniques. Many aeromedical helicopters and some fixed-wing aircraft become involved in SAR activities, however, so it is important to be familiar with SAR techniques. In addition, outside the United States, persons providing aeromedical transport are frequently involved in SAR activities (see Chapter 25).

The keys to a successful SAR operation include proper communications, transport, evacuation, and medical treatment, in the setting of favorable weather conditions and topography. The helicopter, equipped with a hoist and winch, is one of the most effective means of providing SAR in the wilderness setting and is essential in mountainous regions. A long delay between the time of the accident and the call for assistance, combined with a serous injury, adversely affects patient outcome.

Helicopters are helpful in various SAR activities, including low-altitude search activity, search area evaluation, and movement of supplies and equipment. They may be the only means of extrication and rescue from the scene. Fixed-wing aircraft are also useful for search and can provide secondary transport, especially when long distances are involved.

The U.S. Air Force routinely uses helicopters and fixed-wing aircraft for long-distance SAR operations. Fixed-wing aircraft often arrive at the scene first and may deploy pararescuemen by parachute. If the rescue site is over water, the aircraft may also deploy an inflatable boat with motor and rescue equipment. The pararescuemen and their survivors are then recovered by surface vessels or by rescue helicopters that have been refueled aerially in order to reach the rescue site (Figure 27-1). This capability permits the rapid deployment of rescuers while allowing the most expeditious recovery of survivors and their delivery to definitive care. Theses services are on alert for all space shuttle launches to provide SAR support in the event of a mishap.

In the United Kingdom the Royal Air Force operates a helicopter SAR service that flew 1490 missions from 1980 to 1989, almost all of which involved vacationers along the coasts or in the mountains.[55] The Danish helicopter rescue service was founded in 1966 and uses a Sikorsky (S-61) helicopter. Since 1973 its crew has included a physician trained in aerospace medicine and helicopter transport. From 1973 to 1989 it flew 5733

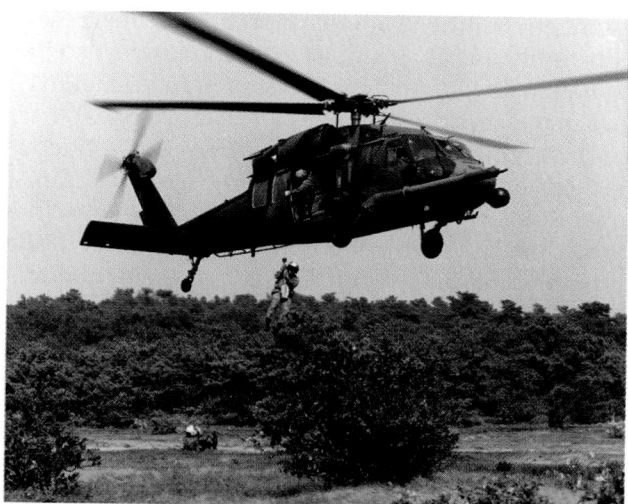

Figure 27-1 MH-60G Pave Hawk hoisting a pararescueman during a search and rescue exercise. A variant of the UH-60 Blackhawk, the Pave Hawk is flown by U.S. Air Force rescue squadrons. Modifications include forward-looking infrared equipment, night-vision-compatible cockpit lighting, terrain and navigation radar, air refueling probe, auxiliary fuel tanks, and hoist. *(Courtesy U.S. Air Force.)*

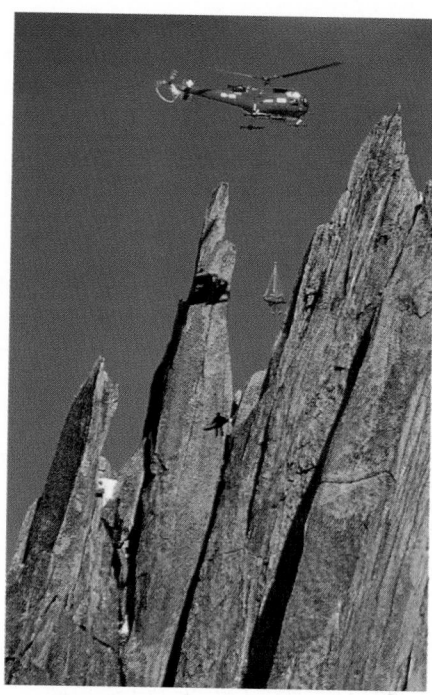

Figure 27-2 Helicopter rescue in extremely difficult terrain. *(Courtesy P. Bärtsch, MD, and the Swiss Alpine Club.)*

missions, 2075 of which involved direct medical intervention. The most frequent problems were abdominal trauma and cardiopulmonary diseases.[95]

In the high Alps, more than 90% of all rescues are performed using helicopters (3000 per year).[4] Of these, 5% are combined rescues; that is, the helicopter carries the rescuers below cloud level, near the site of the accident. Only 5% of mountain rescues are purely ground rescues, mainly necessitated by visibility.[76] Currently a network of SAR systems extends throughout the Alps. In some countries (France, Italy, Germany, Austria, and Spain), air rescues are managed partially or totally by the army or the state. The aircraft most often used for this purpose are the Alouette III, Lama, Ecureil (French), Bolkow 105, 117 (German), Augusta AK 117 (Italian), and Bell (United States). In Switzerland the rescue system in remote terrain is managed by the Swiss Alpine Club and three air rescue companies, Swiss Air Rescue (REGA), Air Glaciers, and Air Zermatt. Switzerland may be unique in that its 18 strategically placed helicopter rescue bases allow an aircraft to reach any accident scene within 15 minutes of take-off. Since the foundation of REGA in 1952, more than 150,000 patients have been transported by either fixed-wing aircraft or helicopter.

Up to 8000 patients (5500 from accident scenes) are transported by helicopter every year. Twenty percent of these rescues require a winch, with one third of all winch operations occurring in accident sites that are difficult to reach.[28] More than 75% of all persons rescued by winch were thought to have injuries requiring physician assistance at the scene. Eighty percent of all

Swiss air rescue missions are physician assisted, and 20% have a paramedic in charge. All the physicians and rescue crews are physically fit and trained in alpine techniques, since two thirds of all rescue missions performed from 1990 to 1993 were in topographically remote and difficult terrain (Figure 27-2).

Difficult helicopter SAR operations are those that involve low visibility, strong winds, night missions, high-angle rescues, and long-line hoist operations (extension of the hoist cable up to 120 m [394 feet]). In addition, in mountainous regions, power cables and transport cables present a considerable risk. In all cases the rescue risks to the flight crew (as well as to the patient) must be weighed against the degree of injury and risk of further morbidity. The U.S. Air Force, Army, Navy, and Coast Guard equip and train groups to operate in these hostile rescue environments. Helicopters are frequently equipped with precision navigation systems and night vision, forward-looking infrared (FLIR), and thermal imaging equipment. The intense training and specialized equipment permit rescue operations under much more demanding conditions than those encountered by civilian services. Of the military services, only the U.S. Coast Guard has a primary mission of civilian SAR; Army, Navy, or Air Force groups may be requested to assist in civilian rescues in areas where they are available.

An increasing number of people participate in alpine sports, including mountain climbing, downhill skiing, mountain biking, and paragliding.[30] A typical representation of the type of mountaineering accidents experienced in the Swiss Alps is shown in Table 27-2. In addition to SAR in mountainous regions, aeromedical rescue presents great challenges to the medical and flight crews involved in rescues from sea and white water, floods, vertical rock faces, and avalanches.

Medical treatment of the survivors should begin immediately at the site of the accident unless weather conditions are deteriorating or the scene is inherently unsafe. If a hoist extraction is needed, the patient with potential multisystem trauma should be evacuated by a rescue net or basket (Stokes) litter with careful spinal immobilization. A tag line attached to the litter prevents spinning during hoist operations. The tag line should be attached with a weak link so that the tag line will break away if the litter becomes uncontrollable. Persons with minimal or isolated injuries may be hoisted by a jungle penetrator (Figure 27-3), rescue basket, or other dedicated hoist device. If a hoist device is not available, the victim may be hoisted by climbing harnesses or rescue belts.[27] The climbing harness or belt should be carefully inspected to make sure that it has not been damaged in the mishap, that it will withstand the strain of the hoist operation, and that it can be safely attached to the hoist cable.

The extent of medical treatment rendered on site before extraction depends on many factors, including the victim's condition, scene safety, medical supplies available, medical skill of the rescuers, weather conditions, aircraft loiter time, and flight time to definitive care.

TABLE 27-2. Mountaineering Accidents in the Swiss Alps, 1992 (N = 1845 Persons)

ACTIVITY	NUMBER OF PATIENTS RESCUED
Delta gliding	18
Paragliding	196
Off-slope skiing	35
Ski touring	238
Mixed climbing	456
Rock climbing	178
Hiking	723

From Dürrer B, Hassler R, Mosimann U: *Mountaineering accidents in the Swiss Alps and rescue activities of the Swiss Alpine Club, 1992.*

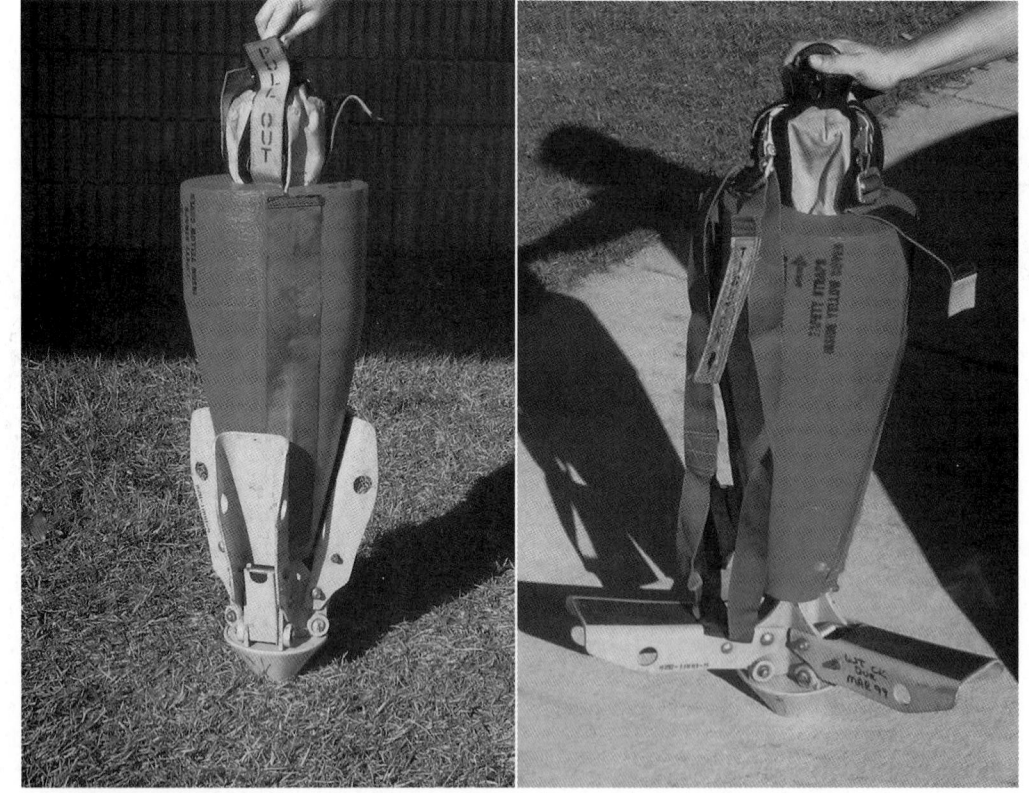

Figure 27-3 **A,** Jungle penetrator used as a hoist device on most military rescue helicopters. The streamlined shape allows it to slip through dense tree canopies to reach the ground. A foam flotation collar can be attached, making the penetrator buoyant. **B,** Jungle penetrator rigged for hoist. The seats are flipped down, and the safety straps are pulled out from their stowed position and passed over the head and under the arms of the victim, who then straddles one of the seat paddles. Although the penetrator has three seats, usually only one or two personnel are hoisted at a time. *(Courtesy Robert C. Allen.)*

Good communication between the flight crew and the rescue team is essential to the decision process. Aeromedical crews involved in mountain rescue need to have a thorough understanding of the unique medical problems frequently found in high-altitude rescue situations.

AEROMEDICAL AIRCRAFT

Many different types of aircraft can be adapted to the air ambulance role. Each type has its strengths and weaknesses. On the other hand, not all aircraft are well suited for SAR in wilderness areas. Matching the physical and flight characteristics of the aircraft to the needs of the mission is vital. In many circumstances, compromises must be made because of aircraft availability. Rescuers must consider the physical characteristics of the aircraft when caring for a victim in flight.

Cabin Space

Cabin space should be considered not only in terms of total interior volume in cubic feet, but also with regard to floor space, headroom, and the ergonomics of cabin layout. Ample headroom should be available for the patient to lie comfortably on a secured stretcher and for access by two crew members to all parts of the body. Specifically, access to the head is needed for intubation, the chest for CPR, and the extremities for monitoring perfusion. Some helicopters, such as the Aerospatiale AStar/TwinStar or the MBB BO-105, provide ample upper body access but only limited lower body access while in flight. The relationship of flight crew members when seated (and secured by seat belts) in proximity to the patient is important. The ideal configuration places one medical crew member at the patient's head for airway management and verbal interaction and one at the patient's side to monitor vital signs and perform necessary non-airway-related procedures. This arrangement is typified by the MBB BK-117 helicopter (Figure 27-4).

Although some rotor-wing aircraft, such as the BK, are theoretically capable of transporting two patients, this greatly increases demands on the flight crew and the aircraft and diminishes access to both patients. Policies and procedures regarding two-patient transport in these aircraft should be carefully considered. In some large helicopters, such as the CH-46, CH-47 or MH-53, there is enough room to work on multiple patients. Even on relatively large (by civilian standards) military helicopters, however, such as the Coast Guard HH-60J Jayhawk (Figure 27-5), space for patient care can be at a premium.

Cabin space can be more generous in fixed-wing aircraft. Cabin-class airplanes, such as the Beech King Air and Piper Cheyenne III, provide an aisle and capability to carry more than one patient and additional crew or family members.

Access for Patient Loading

The cargo door should be wide enough that the patient's stretcher can be maneuvered into the aircraft without undue tilting, and it should be positioned comfortably near stretcher height to obviate the need for strenuous lifting during ground loading. Standard door configurations on many aircraft do not meet these needs. The "clamshell" doors on an MBB BK-117 helicopter and the oversized cargo door on a Gulfstream Commander 1000 work well for patient loading (Figure 27-6).

Useful Load

One of the most important considerations for a given patient transport is the aircraft's useful load. This difference

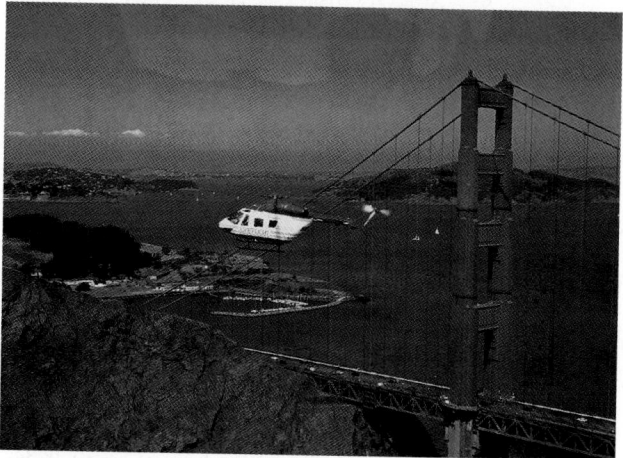

Figure 27-4   Stanford LifeFlight MBB BK-117. *(Courtesy Geralyn Martinez.)*

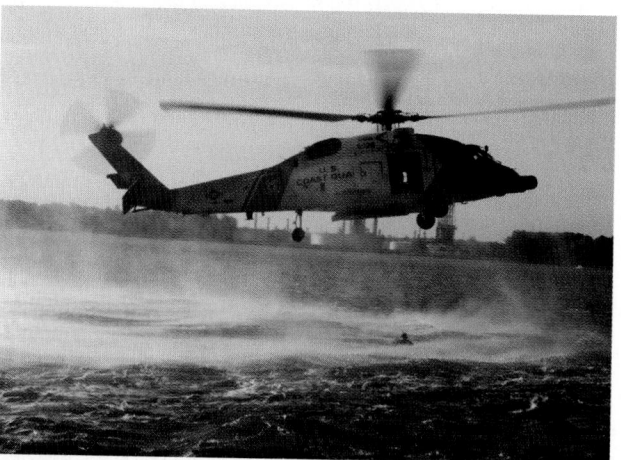

Figure 27-5   U.S. Coast Guard HH-60J Jayhawk helicopter in low hover over water, preparing to lower hoist cable to the rescue swimmer. Note the extensive spray under the aircraft. The Jayhawk, a variant of the UH-60 Blackhawk, is a medium-range helicopter used for search and rescue, drug interdiction, and maritime law enforcement. *(Courtesy US Coast Guard.)*

between the maximum take-off weight and the basic empty weight is a reflection of the load-carrying capability. In most EMS helicopters the useful load ranges between 1500 and 2800 pounds. On-board avionics, medical equipment, fuel, and crew weights must be subtracted from this value to yield the maximum allowable patient weight (Figure 27-7). Fuel weighs 6 pounds per gallon; a twin-engine helicopter may burn 70 gallons per hour (420 pounds per hour), requiring it to carry 600 pounds or more fuel for a 30-minute-radius flight (with 30-minute reserve). Thus it becomes evident that a flight crew of three weighing a total of 500 pounds with a full load of fuel, oxygen, and medical gear may not have the capability to carry even a small patient, especially on a hot day when the helicopter's performance (lift) is reduced. This consideration can become critical on flights from the accident scene, where terrain obstacles may require vertical take-off and climb-out, demanding maximum helicopter performance. Density altitude (a factor of the air temperature and the pressure altitude) is critical in the performance of helicopters in mountain regions. High altitude combined with hot weather can seriously degrade the performance of even the most powerful helicopters.

Weight and Balance

Not only must the weight of the loaded aircraft remain at or below the maximum allowed take-off weight for that aircraft, but the center of gravity (CG) must lie within fore and aft limits established by the manufacturer. Each loading configuration places the CG in a unique position, which must be calculated by the pilot before flight, or the flight characteristics may be adversely affected, compromising safety. This consideration may dictate where certain pieces of medical equipment, such as oxygen bottles, may be placed or where heavier crew members must sit.

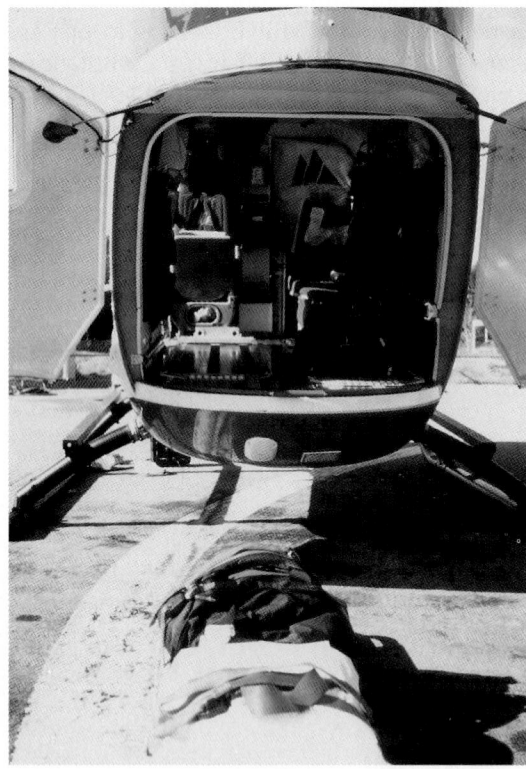

Figure 27-6 MBB BK-117 with rear clamshell doors open. *(Courtesy Susan Lockman, Stanford Lifeflight.)*

Maximum take-off weight[a]	
Less basic empty weight[b]	−
Less fuel on board[c]	−
Less pilot and crew	−
Less medical gear[d]	−
Maximum "patient payload"	=

[a]Maximum take-off weight is certificated for each aircraft type and can be found in the operating manual.

[b]Basic empty weight includes added avionics, permanent equipment, fluids, and unusable fuel. It is different for each aircraft and is recorded in the aircraft's operating manual.

[c]The quantity of fuel on board depends on the mission needs. Divide round-trip distance by cruise speed to yield time en route. Add time for warm-up, climb, approach, and a 30-minute reserve (VFR) to yield total engine time. Multiply total engine time by rate of fuel consumption to yield total fuel consumed. Fuel weight 6 lb/gal.

[d]Medical gear includes carry-on and nonpermanent items.

Figure 27-7 Weight calculation aboard aircraft.

On flights from the accident scene the patient's weight is approximated before departure. With pressure to hasten departure, accurate weight and balance calculations are difficult. Thus the aircraft used must have enough margin in the CG envelope that CG limits are not easily exceeded for the given mission profile.

Cruise Speed

One of the most basic reasons for transporting a patient by air is to take advantage of the greater speed of aircraft compared with ground vehicles. This allows the patient earlier arrival at the destination and minimizes time spent out of the hospital. Not only do aircraft have a speed advantage, but they can travel in a straight line from origin to destination without the curves and deviations present in surface travel. For an aircraft to compete with a ground vehicle in speed in a primary or secondary response mode, it must be at least twice as fast as an ambulance, since the helicopter must fly round trip (outbound to destination and inbound with patient) in the time that the ambulance would travel one way. This is possible with most EMS helicopters, unless (1) the referral location has no suitable landing area (necessitating a time-consuming transit of crew and stretcher to and from the location), (2) ground "packaging" times for the flight crew with the patient are excessive, or (3) an ambulance has a clear, straight highway as a means of alternative transport.

Most EMS helicopters are capable of attaining 120 to 150 mph over the ground, although a headwind or tailwind may hinder or improve these figures (Table 27-3). Piston twin-engine aircraft have a cruise speed range of 220 to 275 mph, turboprop aircraft of 300 to 385 mph, and jets of 400 to 535 mph or more.[22,70]

Range

Aircraft range is limited by the amount of fuel, which is a function of fuel tank capacity and useful load. In most cases a trade-off is made between payload and fuel; the more weight in fuel, the less weight in passengers (or patients). The maximum time aloft can be calculated by dividing usable fuel on board by rate of fuel burn per hour at cruise speed. Multiplying maximum time aloft by cruise speed yields the maximum range. The Federal Aviation Administration (FAA), under FAR part 91.23, requires that a 45-minute fuel reserve remain at the conclusion of all flights conducted under instrument flight rules (IFR), and a 30-minute reserve under visual flight rules (VFR). Most EMS helicopters operate under VFR, whereas most fixed-wing operations are IFR. Because helicopters typically fly to and from a point at which refueling is not available, round-trip fuel must be carried; this effectively limits the customary radius of operation to approximately half the range (less required reserves). Although it is possible to refuel en route to an airport, this adds to the flight time. Therefore helicopters typically operate within a radius of 150 miles or less, unless the transport is one-way outbound or unless refueling at the destination is feasible. Fixed-wing aircraft operate from airport to airport; thus the radius of operation is closer to the maximum range with reserves. Many fixed-wing aircraft are capable of ranges in excess of 1000 miles, with some jets able to travel more than 2000 miles.

Pressurization

The partial pressure of oxygen in the atmosphere declines with increasing altitude so that at 5486 m (18,000 feet) it is one-half that at sea level. Part 91.32 of FAR requires the use of supplemental oxygen for the pilot at flight altitudes above 3810 m (12,500 feet) for longer

TABLE 27-3. Helicopters Frequently Used for Aeromedical Transport

HELICOPTER	CRUISE SPEED (MPH)	ENGINE(S)	SHP	USEFUL LOAD (LB)	SERVICE CEILING (FT)	RANGE (MILES)*
Bell 206L-3	130	SE-T	650	1950	20,000	325
AStar 350D	140	SE-T	615	1868	15,000	379
TwinStar 355F1	147	TE-T	420 each	2391	13,120	368
MBB BO-105 CBS	145	TE-T	420 each	2732	17,000	334
Agusata 109A II	163	TE-T	420 each	2605	15,000	359
Bell 222UT	152	TE-T	684 each	3376	15,800	380
MBB BK-117	160	TE-T	650 each	2645	17,000	368
Sikorsky S-76	167	TE-T	650 each	4700	15,000	550
Dauphin 2	161	TE-T	700 each	4118	15,000	564

Data from Collins RL et al: *Flying 1985 annual & buyer's guide,* New York, 1985, Ziff-Davis; and 1987 hospital aviation directory, *Hosp Aviat* 6(4):8, 1987.
SE-T, Single engine, turbine; *TE-T,* twin engine, turbine; *SHP,* shaft horsepower.
*Range includes fuel for warmup, taxi, climb, and 30-minute reserve.

TABLE 27-4. Fixed-Wing Aircraft Used for Aeromedical Transport

AIRCRAFT	CRUISE SPEED (MPH)	CABIN	ENGINES	USEFUL LOAD (LB)*	SERVICE CELING (FT)	RANGE (MILES)†	TAKE-OFF (FT)‡
Seneca III	221	NP	TE-P	1921	25,000	721	1250
Baron 58TC	277	NP	TE-P	2447	25,000	1150	2700
Cessna 402C	245	NP	TE-P	2774	26,900	1164	2200
Navaho 350	250	NP	TE-P	2533	24,000	1200	2200
Cessna 414	258	P	TE-P	2386	30,800	1300	2600
Cessna 421	277	P	TE-P	2807	30,200	1522	—
Cessna 441	330	P	TE-T	4124	35,000	2195	—
Cheyenne II	293	P	TE-T	4053	31,000	1275	2500
Cheyenne III	347	P	TE-T	4448	35,000	1789	3200
MU-2	317	P	TE-T	3975	27,300	1412	—
King Air F90	309	P	TE-T	4383	31,000	1315	2900
Commader 1000	323	P	TE-T	3965	30,750	2149	
Citation I	410	P	TE-J	5222	41,000	1500	3000
Lear 25D	509	P	TE-J	7150	51,000	1600	4000

Data from Collins RL et al: *Flying 1985 annual & buyers guide,* New York, 1985, Ziff-Davis; 1987 hospital aviation directory, *Hosp Aviat* 6(4):8, 1987; and McNeil EL: *Airborne care of the ill and injured,* New York, 1983, Springer-Verlag.
NP, Nonpressurized; *P,* pressurized; *TE-P,* twin-engine, piston; *TE-T,* twin-engine, turboprop; *TE-J,* twin-engine, turbojet/turbofan.
*Useful load excluding avionics, fuel, passengers.
†Range estimated at cruise speed, less 45-minute reserve.
‡Approximate nonbalance-field take-off length.

than 30 minutes.[31] Above 4267 m (14,000 feet), supplemental oxygen must be used by the pilot and all *minimum required* flight crew at all times. Technically a medical flight crew member is not a *required* minimum crew member for the operation of the aircraft; neither is the copilot of an aircraft operated under FAR part 135 and certified for single-pilot operations (as with most aeromedical aircraft). Thus the medical crew member is not required to wear supplemental oxygen, although doing so would be prudent, especially for smokers. At altitudes greater than 4572 m (15,000 feet), in addition to the above requirements, each occupant must be provided with supplemental oxygen (although there is no legal requirement to use it).

The effects of hypoxia with increases in altitude are more pronounced in patients with lung disease and preexisting hypoxia; this necessitates supplemental oxygen at much lower altitudes. Supplemental oxygen at night will enhance night vision even at altitudes below 3810 m and should be considered for the flight crew, based on operational requirements.

To eliminate the need to provide supplemental oxygen, pressurization is available in many larger, fixed-wing aircraft (Table 27-4). A pressurized aircraft is able to pump air into the cabin to maintain a pressure differential between the cabin and outside air, generally 4 to 8 pounds per square inch (PSI). This allows the cabin atmosphere to be maintained at or below the equivalent of a 2438-m (8000-foot) altitude, despite actual altitudes of 9144 m (30,000 feet) or higher.[62] Pressurization obviates the need for supplemental oxygen for crew members and nonpatient passengers, but passengers with lung disease may still require it. Also, by limiting the drop in cabin pressure that occurs with altitude, changes in trapped gas volumes, such as in ET tube cuffs, air splints, and the gastrointestinal tract, can be decreased or eliminated. Special categories of patients include those with dysbarism. Exposure to increased altitude, with its concomitant decrease in ambient pressure, should be avoided. If possible, sea-level ambient pressure should be maintained when transporting these patients.

On the other hand, helicopters are nonpressurized and generally fly at lower altitudes where altitude-related hypoxia is unlikely. One exception occurs in mountainous regions where altitudes required to rescue victims or cross mountain passes may exceed 3658 m (12,000 feet). Reasons for transporting patients at higher altitudes include terrain avoidance, the need to surmount adverse weather (which usually occurs within 6096 m [20,000 feet] above ground), and greater speed and fuel efficiency at higher altitudes.

Service Ceiling

The service ceiling is the maximum altitude at which an aircraft can still maintain a rate of climb of 30.5 m (100 feet) per minute. This ceiling is important in predicting an aircraft's ability to climb above adverse terrain and weather and in taking advantage of favorable winds aloft to maximize ground speed. In the western

United States, mountainous areas require flight at least 610 m (2000 feet) above the highest terrain along the route of flight, which means a 3658- to 4877-m (12,000- to 16,000-foot) service ceiling. These altitudes restrict most helicopters and require use of supplemental oxygen in nonpressurized airplanes. Flight operations that typically require flight at these altitudes should have access to aircraft with sufficiently high service ceilings and pressurization.

Runway Length

Although not a factor in helicopter operations, runway length restricts certain fixed-wing aircraft from landing. Most airports in rural areas have runway lengths between 610 and 1220 m (2000 and 4000 feet). Higher-performance airplanes usually have progressively longer runway requirements and may be unable to land and take off safely on these strips. Thus, when transport from a rural location with a short runway is requested, it is important to determine the capability of the aircraft being used. Piston twin-engine aircraft can usually operate safely from a 762- to 914-m (2500- to 3000-foot) strip but may have difficulty with 610 m (2000 feet); turboprop airplanes require 762 to 1067 m (2500 to 3500 feet); and jets usually require runway lengths of 1220 m (4000 feet) or more.[62] The take-off roll for airplanes increases with increasing temperature and airport altitude; on a hot day, many airplanes may be incapable of taking off from a short runway if heavily loaded.

In winter conditions, operating on icy runways may pose a safety hazard for braking. Turboprop airplanes and jets have a reverse thrust mode that can slow the aircraft on rollout without braking.

Weather Operations

Adverse weather conditions that may affect a given flight include restrictions in visibility resulting from precipitation, fog, haze, or clouds, as well as airframe icing, turbulence, and wind shear. Flight during instrument meteorologic conditions (IMC) requires adherence to IFR, whereas visual meteorologic conditions (VMC) allow alternative use of VFR. VMC for airplanes are defined as visibility of at least 3 miles and ceiling of at least 305 m (1000 feet) (departing from an airport in controlled airspace).[31] The ability to fly IFR not only improves the likelihood that the mission can be undertaken and completed safely should clouds or adverse weather be present but also enhances the ability of the air traffic control center to follow the flight and properly separate aircraft.

IFR capability has drawbacks. Sophisticated and expensive equipment and training are required. Virtually all fixed-wing aircraft are capable of IFR operations, but most EMS helicopters are not. IFR operations are usually conducted from airport to airport (where an instrument approach is available), but most helicopters travel to and from nonairport points without an instrument approach. The percentage of actual missions canceled or aborted because of IMC is small in most rotor-wing programs. One study determined that inadvertent excursions into IMC occurred about 1.3 times per pilot per year, and the anticipated percentage of operations that would be conducted IFR, if it were available, was 9.4%.[68] For most hospital-based programs the cost of upgrading to a more expensive IFR-equipped helicopter (especially if a copilot is necessary for IFR certification), plus the added expense of maintaining pilot IFR proficiency, would be prohibitive. As a rule, military helicopters fly with a pilot and copilot and are usually capable of flying in IFR conditions, although IMC are far from ideal for SAR operations.

Performance

Closely related to aircraft speed is its ability to climb, expressed in feet per minute (fpm). Known as performance, this ability dictates the type of aircraft used for a given aeromedical transport mission (see Table 27-2). The greater the performance (a complex function of power, weight, wing, propeller, and air density characteristics), the better is the aircraft's ability to outclimb adverse weather or to avoid rising terrain or obstacles. Helicopters are unique in their ability to hover above the ground effect, that is, to climb vertically out of the supporting cushion of air produced by the rotor wash. Helicopters perform better when they have a running start, building up forward speed while still in the cushion of ground effect until translational lift is developed. Translational lift results from the forward to backward flow of air over the rotor blades. A helicopter's ability to climb vertically out of ground effect is limited by horsepower and weight. On a hot day at high altitude, performance may be insufficient to take off vertically.[46] This must be considered when selecting a landing site away from an airport. If a confined space surrounded by obstacles is selected, a vertical take-off may be required.[18]

Fixed-wing aeromedical aircraft are virtually all twin engine not only for enhanced speed, performance, and cabin space but also for the necessary redundancy of systems required for IFR operations under FAR part 135. If one engine fails, a second is available to allow flight to be maintained; however, if failure occurs during take-off, single-engine climb performance may not be adequate to provide lift. This fact may be critical if insufficient altitude has been gained to allow a return to the airport before obstructions are encountered. Therefore single-engine climb performance for various types of aircraft must be considered, especially if operating out of high-altitude airports, in hot weather, or in mountainous regions (see Table 27-4). In general, single-engine climb performance is about 200 to 290 fpm

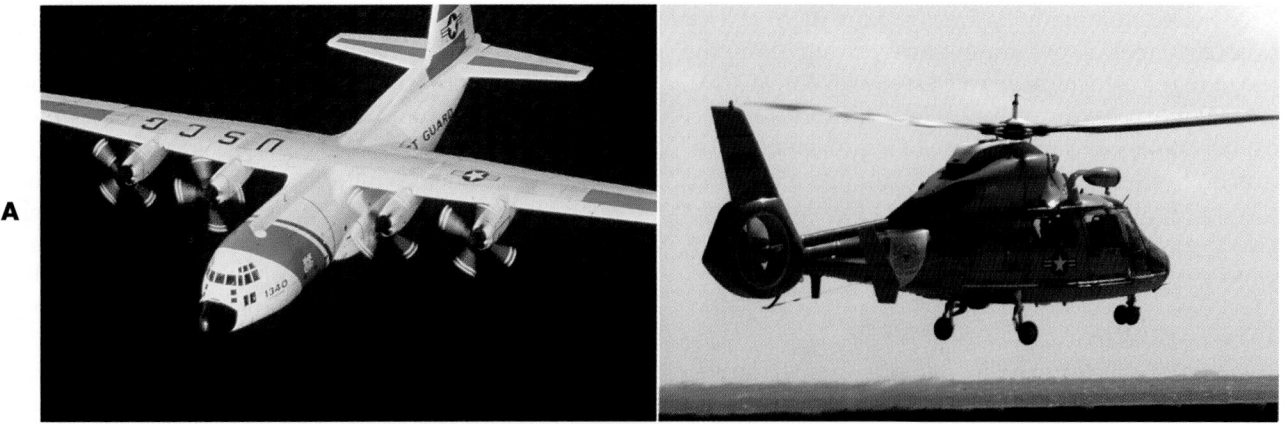

Figure 27-8 **A,** U.S. Coast Guard C-130 Hercules aircraft. This long-range aircraft is used for ice patrol, fisheries management, and search and rescue. **B,** Coast Guard HH-65 Dolphin helicopter. This short-range light-lift helicopter is used for near-shore search and rescue, maritime fisheries enforcement, and law enforcement. *(Courtesy US Coast Guard.)*

in piston twins, 600 to 900 fpm for turboprops, and 1000 to 2000 fpm for jets.[62] The airplane with the best single-engine climb performance will provide the greatest margin of safety, but the cost of equipment, pilot training, and adequate runways will be high.

Aircraft for Search and Rescue

Search and rescue is a special type of aeromedical transport that demands aircraft uniquely suited to this role. The aircraft should have good visibility to the sides and below, the ability to fly slowly and to hover, the ability to land away from an airport, and adequate performance in high-density altitude conditions. In addition, certain extrication situations require the capability to hoist victims from rugged or hostile terrain.

Helicopters are the aircraft of choice for many SAR missions (Figure 27-8). Few hospital-based EMS helicopters are configured for hoist operations, and hospital flight crews are typically not trained in SAR techniques. The SAR mission differs from other types of medical missions in its requirement for low-level flight over potentially hostile terrain, its use of flight crews for visual surveillance for survivors or wreckage, the need for a prolonged hover if hoist operations occur, and the need for flight crew training in wilderness survival principles if a mishap occurs. Experience and training in these activities are essential for safety. In general, military helicopters and their crews are better equipped and trained to carry out SAR operations. For example, U.S. Coast Guard and U.S. Air Force helicopters have radio locating equipment to pinpoint emergency location transponders (ELTs), also known as emergency position-reporting beacons (EPRBs); possess night vision and FLIR cameras to maximize the probability of visually locating a survivor; and have hoists that enable them to extract survivors from areas where landing is not an option.

Flight crews on these missions must be specially trained in the use of rescue equipment and must possess the appropriate medical qualifications and experience to deal properly with atypical EMS situations. U.S. Navy and U.S. Coast Guard rescue swimmers and U.S. Air Force pararescuemen are trained to enter the water or proceed on land to aid in the recovery of survivors. Navy and Coast Guard rescue swimmers receive basic medical training; pararescuemen are trained to the EMT-paramedic level and are given additional training in long-term care of trauma victims.

Special hazards exist in mountainous areas. High-density altitudes may limit an aircraft's performance, but local weather patterns may be erratic. On the leeward side of mountains or ridges, severe downdrafts may prevent a helicopter from hovering out of ground effect. The landing site selected should be free of terrain obstacles and should allow for a long, shallow approach and departure. Open areas away from the leeward side of mountains or ridges are preferable.

SAR aircraft may not routinely carry the same medical equipment (e.g., ventilators, pacemakers, and defibrillators) as the typical EMS helicopter. Therefore care should be taken to verify that the medical equipment carried on a SAR aircraft is adequate for the intended mission (see Chapter 25).

Pilot Requirements

Helicopter EMS are usually VFR operations, and the FAA has established minimum requirements for pilot experience. FAR part 135.243 specifies that the pilot in command of a helicopter carrying passengers for hire must have at least 500 hours of flight time, including at least 100 hours of cross-country time with 25 hours at night. Fixed-wing services are typically IFR operations, and pilots must have at least 1200 hours of flight time, including 500 cross-country, 100 night, and 75 hours of actual or simulated instrument time. They must also be instrument rated and possess a commercial certificate.

Most EMS helicopter pilots have much more experience than the minimum requirements; one survey found 59% had more than 4000 hours and none fewer than 2000 hours.[32] The pilot in command is solely responsible for the safety of all passengers and must decide whether to accept or decline a mission. For this reason the pilot is often not told the nature of the medical mission until a decision to go is made. This decision should be based on the destination, weather conditions, environmental circumstances, and estimated time at the scene, airport, or destination facility. No mention of patient type or severity should be made to the pilot before the launch decision is made so that this decision is objective. The pilot has the final say on all decisions related to safety of flight.

Communications

Helicopter EMS units must have the capability to communicate on very-high-frequency (VHF) airbands assigned for air traffic control, flight service, and local airport Unicom. In addition, the ability to communicate with ground EMS and public safety via VHF and ultrahigh-frequency (UHF) airbands is essential. Air use frequencies are accessible through standard aircraft communications transceivers, but EMS communications require additional radio equipment designed for this purpose. Additional needs include communication with the helicopter's base station, either on a locally assigned public-use frequency or a Federal Communications Commission (FCC)–assigned discrete frequency in the VHF airband. Another means of communication is aircraft 800-MHz radiotelephones that can access the surface telephone network. Communication over airband frequencies requires strict adherence to FAA communications guidelines and a radiotelephone operator permit from the FCC.[26]

Medical Equipment and In-Flight Monitoring

On-board medical supplies and equipment are typically tailored to the needs of a specific transport program and include medications, airway and ventilation supplies, dressings and bandages, IV fluids, immobilization devices, military antishock trousers (MAST), and stretchers.[73] The U.S. Department of Transportation (DOT), in conjunction with the American Medical Association (AMA), has published guidelines for on-board equipment for air ambulance operation (Box 27-2).[92]

Power

Most aircraft systems operate from 14 or 28 volts of direct-current (DC) power supplied by an engine-driven alternator or generator. This is not adequate to operate most medical devices, which require 110 to 120 volts of alternate-current (AC) power. Such devices can-

not be used without an internal battery of sufficient charge to provide power for the duration of the mission, or unless a 110- to 120-volt AC power source is available from a power inverter, which must be installed under an STC. Power inverters are common components of EMS helicopters and dedicated fixed-wing aircraft that have been retrofit with a custom-made air ambulance cabin configuration, but they may not be a standard component in fixed-wing aircraft that support a dual role and use an interchangeable corporate configuration.

Stretcher

The patient stretcher must be secured to the aircraft according to the requirements of FAR part 23.561 or 25.561 for seats: 3.0 g's upward (2.0 g's, part 25), 9.0 g's forward, and 1.5 g's sideways. For helicopters the requirements are 1.5 g's upward, 4.0 g's forward, and 2.0 g's sideways. Special configurations, especially those incorporating oxygen bottles and metal framework, may require an STC. Other guidelines (recommendations only) for stretcher configurations are for clear view and access to the patients with at least 30 inches of headroom and at least 12 inches of aisle beside the head. The stretcher should be at least 19 inches wide by 73 inches long.[92] If the patient is positioned with head forward, the acceleration that occurs during take-off of a fixed-wing aircraft may cause venous pooling in the lower extremities and transient hypotension. To prevent this, the patient can be positioned with feet forward.

Climate Control

The aircraft must be capable of maintaining a comfortable interior environment; about 24° C (75° F) is recommended. During summer months the extensive glass area on a helicopter can produce a greenhouse effect, which may necessitate air conditioning for the comfort of both crew and patient.

Lighting

Lighting should be available to enable the crew to attend to the patient' s needs but not interfere with cockpit operations. Curtains or other physical barriers may satisfy this need.

Suction

Suction is a requirement for ambulance operations in most states and should be available at all times during aeromedical transport. Integral suction as a custom retrofit system or a portable battery-powered device can be used.

Oxygen

In general, enough oxygen should be provided for the flight, plus a 45-minute reserve (IFR; 30 minutes VFR).

Box 27-2 U.S. DEPARTMENT OF TRANSPORTATION–AMERICAN MEDICAL ASSOCIATION GUIDELINES FOR ON-BOARD MEDICAL EQUIPMENT FOR AEROMEDICAL TRANSPORT

BASIC MEDICAL EQUIPMENT RECOMMENDED FOR EACH FLIGHT

1/patient	Litter or stretcher with approved restraints
2/patient	Sheets
2/patient	Blankets
1/patient	Pillow with cover impervious to moisture
1/patient	Pillowcase
1 set	Spare sheets and pillowcase (if weight and space allow)
1 unit	Medical oxygen with manual control; adjustable flowmeter with gauge (0 to 15 L/min); attachment for humidification (NOTE: The oxygen unit must be attached to the aircraft in an approved manner. The amount of oxygen to be carried is determined by multiplying the prescribed flow rate times the length of time the patient must be on oxygen and adding a 45-minute reserve. The minimum amount of oxygen carried should be enough to supply one patient for 1 hour at 10 L/min. It may be necessary to carry a portable oxygen unit if oxygen is not available for patient transfer at some point in the flight.)
2 each	Oxygen masks in adult, child, and infant sizes
6	Connecting tubes
1	Oxygen key
1 unit	Portable suction with connecting tubes
2 each	Suction catheters (various sizes)
2	Tonsil suction tips
1 unit	Squeeze bag-valve-mask unit capable of receiving oxygen through an inlet, and delivering 80% to 100% oxygen through the mask; with masks in adult, child, and infant sizes (bags in adult and small child/infant sizes)
1 unit	Oxygen-powered, manually triggered breathing device (100-L/min flow rate)
1	Blood pressure cuff, sphygmomanometer
1	Stethoscope (NOTE: To record blood pressure readings, a Doppler or electronic stethoscope may be required if noise or vibration levels are high. An electronic unit must not cause electromagnetic interference on aircraft equipment.)
2 each	Oropharyngeal airways in adult, child, and infant sizes
1	Emesis basin
1	Urinal or bedpan or both
1/patient	Sound suppressors
1	Pneumatic antishock trousers with pressure relief valve
2	Cervical collars
2	20-gallon trash bags

BASIC MEDICAL EQUIPMENT RECOMMENDED FOR EACH FLIGHT—cont'd

1 box	Zipper-lock plastic bags or similar product
1	Flashlight, 2 D batteries or equivalent with spare batteries and bulb
2	Locking hooks (or other positive locking device for intravenous fluid containers)
1 qt	Drinking water
12	Paper cups

DRESSINGS AND SUPPLIES KIT, DESIGNED TO BE CARRIED ON EACH FLIGHT

4	Cardboard or air splints or equivalent in arm and leg sizes
12	Tongue depressors
2	Mouth gags or padded tongue depressors
1	Bandage scissors
4	Tourniquets
1 each	Rolls of adhesive tape, ½, 1, 2, 3 inch
1 each	Rolls of paper tape, various sizes
4	Kling bandages or equivalent
1	3-inch elastic bandage
1	4-inch elastic bandage
4	Kerlix rolls or equivalent
2 pairs	Sterile gloves
3	Petrolatum gauze
1 box	Adhesive bandages
6	Disposable surgical face masks
2 each	Syringes, 3, 5, and 10 ml (TB and insulin)
3 each	Needles, 18, 20, and 22 gauge
3 each	Needles, 19, 21 gauge, scalp/vein
2	Surgical dressings
24	Sterile gauze pads
6	Nonsterile gauze pads
2	Triangle bandages
2	Wrist restraints
2	Eye covers
1 roll	Aluminum foil, sterilized and wrapped
1	Large safety pin
2	Clinical thermometers
4	Airsick bags
12	Waterless towelettes
1 box	Tissues

MEDICATION AND INTRAVENOUS KIT, DESIGNED TO BE CARRIED ON EACH FLIGHT

2	Epinephrine HCl, 1:1000, 1 ml, prefilled syringe
2	Epinephrine HCl, 1:10,000, 10 ml, prefilled syringe with intracardiac needle
2	Aminophylline inj., 500 mg in 2-ml ampules
4	Atropine sulfate, 0.5 mg in 5-ml prefilled syringe

Modified from US Department of Transportation, National Highway Traffic Safety Administration; American Medical Association Commission on Emergency Medical Services: *Air ambulance guidelines*, Washington, DC, 1981, The Department. *Inj.*, Intramuscular injection; *Fr*, French; *ECG*, electrocardiogram.

Box 27-2   U.S. DEPARTMENT OF TRANSPORTATION–AMERICAN MEDICAL ASSOCIATION GUIDELINES FOR ON-BOARD MEDICAL EQUIPMENT FOR AEROMEDICAL TRANSPORT—cont'd

MEDICATION AND INTRAVENOUS KIT, DESIGNED TO BE CARRIED ON EACH FLIGHT—cont'd

2	Diphenhydramine HCl, 50 mg/ml, 1-ml prefilled syringe
2	Dextrose, 25 g/50 ml, prefilled syringe
2	Intravenous injection sets with microdripper
2	Lidocaine HCl, 2 g/10 ml, prefilled syringe
3	Lidocaine HCl, 20 mg/ml, 5-ml prefilled syringe
6	Naloxone HCl, 0.4 mg/ml, 1-ml ampules
1	Nitroglycerin, 0.4 mg, sublingual tablets, 100
2	Digoxin inj., 0.5 mg/2 ml, ampules
4	Furosemide, 10 mg/ml, 2-ml ampules
2	Chlorpromazine HCl, 25 mg/ml, 1-ml ampules
6	Sodium bicarbonate inj., 3.75 mg/50 ml, prefilled syringe
2	Morphine sulfate, 15 mg/ml, prefilled syringe
1	Hydrocortisone sodium succinate, 100 mg/vial
1	Methylprednisolone sodium succinate, 1000 mg/vial
1	Plasma protein fraction, 250 ml with infusion set
2	Sterile water for injection, 20 ml
3	Diazepam, 5 mg/ml, 2-ml prefilled syringe
6	Alcohol swabs
1	Phenylephrine HCl, 0.25%, nasal spray
2	Ammonia inhalant solution, 0.5-ml ampule
2	Isoproterenol HCl, 1:5000, 1-ml ampules
1	Tourniquet
1	0.9% sodium chloride inj., 500-ml bag
1	0.9% sodium chloride inj., 250-ml bag
1	Lactated Ringer's inj., 250-ml bag
1	Lactated Ringer's inj., 500-ml bag
2	Lactated Ringer's inj., 1000-ml bag
3	Needles, 15 gauge, 1½ inch
1	Dextrose, 5% in water, 250 ml
1	Dextrose, 5% in water, 500 ml
1	Dextrose, 5% in normal saline, 250 ml
1	Dextrose, 5% in normal saline, 500 ml
1	Pressure pack or infusion pump
1 each	Drip tubing, regular and pediatric
2	Armboards
6	Alcohol wipes
1	Clean hemostat
1 each	Sterile hemostat, curved and straight
1	Nasogastric tube, 14 gauge
2	Sterile normal saline for injection, 20 ml
2 pair	Sterile gloves
1	Knife handle
1	Subclavian set
1	No. 15 blade
1	Intravenous infusion cuff
1 each	Rolls of tape, 1 and 2 inch

AIRWAY MANAGEMENT KIT, DESIGNED TO BE CARRIED ON EACH FLIGHT

1	Laryngoscope with curved and straight blades in various sizes; spare batteries and bulb
As required	Adapters for attaching endotracheal tubes to oxygen, etc.
1	Rubber-shod forceps
1	Magill forceps
1	Esophageal obturator airway with gastric suction capability
1	McSwain dart or Heimlich valve
1	Syringe, 60 ml
1	Needle, 14 gauge
1	Syringe, 10 ml
1 each	Rolls of adhesive tape, 1 and 2 inch
1	Viscous lidocaine HCl, 2%
1 tube	Surgical lubricant

BURN KIT, TO BE CARRIED WHEN REQUIRED

3	Normal saline, 1 ml in plastic container
1	Sterile burn sheet, 57 × 80 inch
5 packs	Xeroform gauze, 5 × 9 inch
1	Irrigating syringe, 50 ml
2 pairs	Sterile gloves
4	Kerlix rolls
2 packs	Fluffy gauze

POISON DRUG OVERDOSE KIT, TO BE CARRIED WHEN REQUIRED

1	Irrigation tray
1	Surgical stomach tube for lavage
1 each	Specimen bottles for urine, gastric, and miscellaneous
2 each	Stomach tubes, 14, 16, and 18 Fr
1	Rubber stomach tube, no. 20
1 tube	Lubricant
1 box	Glucagon, 1 unit
2	Ipecac Syrup, 30 ml
1	Physostigmine salicylate, 1 mg/ml, 2-ml ampules
1	Pralidoxime chloride, 1-g kit
1	Activated charcoal, 10 g

OBSTETRIC KIT, TO BE CARRIED WHEN REQUIRED

1	Disposable obstetric pack with sheets, cord clamps, DeLee suction, plastic bag, silver swaddler, sterile gloves
2	Oxytocin, 10 units/ml, 1-ml ampule
1	Episiotomy scissors
1	Ring forceps

Continued

Box 27-2   U.S. DEPARTMENT OF TRANSPORTATION–AMERICAN MEDICAL ASSOCIATION GUIDELINES FOR ON-BOARD MEDICAL EQUIPMENT FOR AEROMEDICAL TRANSPORT—cont'd

PEDIATRIC KIT, TO BE CARRIED WHEN REQUIRED AND ALWAYS WITH OBSTETRIC KIT

1	Pediatric laryngoscope handle with blades
1 each	Pediatric endotracheal tubes with stylette, 2.5, 3, 3.5, and 4 Fr
1	Pediatric Magill forceps
2	Bulb syringes
2	DeLee suction
2	Pediatric drip intravenous tubing
1 each	Feeding tubes, 3.5, 5, and 8 Fr
1	Pediatric blood pressure cuff, sphygmomanometer

ADDITIONAL EQUIPMENT FOR TRAUMA PATIENTS, TO BE CARRIED WHEN REQUIRED

1	Scoop stretcher
1	Long backboard
1	Foley catheter set
1	Femur traction splint
1	Suture kit

ADDITIONAL EQUIPMENT FOR CARDIAC PATIENT, TO BE CARRIED WHEN REQUIRED

1 unit	Cardiac monitor with strip chart recorder
1 each	Spare ECG electrode for each lead
1	Spare roll of ECG recording paper
1 unit	Defibrillator with four pads and conductive gel (defibrillator may come as a unit with the cardiac monitor)
1	Rubber mat or other means of electrically isolating the patient from the aircraft
1	Cardiac board

ADDITIONAL EQUIPMENT FOR SPECIFIC PATIENTS, TO BE CARRIED WHEN REQUIRED

1 unit	Respirator capable of continous ventilation, with ventilator, tubing, exhaled volume measuring device, set of tracheostomy endotracheal adaptors
1 unit	Incubator, with all equipment suitable for neonatal care

---

In addition, oxygen should be carried to allow for ground handling time at either end. The amount of oxygen required can be obtained by multiplying the desired flow rate in liters per minute (L/min) by the total duration of transport and patient loading and unloading. Table 27-5 lists the capacities of various types of oxygen tanks and their respective weights. Some portable ventilators have a gas-driven logic circuit that requires additional air or oxygen. Electrically powered ventilators have a lower requirement for oxygen but carry the additional need for a power inverter. Most patients are transported with oxygen supplied by nasal cannulae (1 to 6 L/min). A single E-sized oxygen cylinder is adequate for short flights, although backup cylinders are usually carried. Patients intubated and maintained on 100% oxygen, as well as those ventilated on long flights, will exceed the capacity of an E cylinder quickly; several E cylinders or an H cylinder will be required.

Ventilators

On short flights, most patients can be bag ventilated manually, with the addition of a positive end-expiratory pressure (PEEP) valve as needed. Manual ventilation has drawbacks. Minute ventilation can rarely be precisely controlled, leading either to respiratory acidosis or more often to alkalosis. The patient's tidal volume limits may be exceeded, with resultant pulmonary barotrauma. More important, the medical attendant will be completely occupied with ventilation and is

TABLE 27-5. Oxygen Tank Specifications

CYLINDER SIZE	WEIGHT (lb)	CAPACITY* (L)	ENDURANCE† (HR) AT 2 L/min	ENDURANCE† (HR) AT 10 L/min
D	11	356	2	1
G	32	1200	10	2
Q	70	2320	19.3	3.8
H and Q	150	6900	57.5	11.5

From National EMS Pilot's Association: *Hosp Aviat* 5(6):17, 1986.
*At 21° C (70° F), 14.7 PSI. Capacity varies with ambient conditions.
†Estimated endurance; actual values may vary.

thus unavailable to perform other tasks. This takes on added importance if complex infusions are being administered or in-flight complications occur. The likelihood that manual ventilation will be unsatisfactory increases with the duration of transport, medical complexity of the patient, and severity of underlying lung disease.

Compact ventilators are available for use in the aeromedical transport environment.[12] The simplest are pressure ventilators with a timing valve mechanism that will deliver a predicted minute ventilation at a given rate and tidal volume adjustable to patient size. These require that the patient have normal airway compliance. If airway resistance increases, smaller tidal volumes will result, and tidal volumes usually cannot be varied independently from rate. Volume-cycled ventilators are superior and available in configurations in which tidal volume and rate can be varied independently. Oxygen bottles, a 50-PSI regulator, high-pressure gas lines, a patient breathing circuit, and source of humidification need to be present.

As mentioned, ET tube cuffs need to be appropriately monitored during flight to prevent overinflation resulting from decreased ambient pressure.

Infusion Devices

Several methods of IV infusion delivery are available in the aeromedical setting: gravity-feed microdrip or macrodrip tubing with the drip rate manually adjusted, gravity-feed automatic infusion regulators with a closed-loop drip-monitoring feedback mechanism controlling drip rate, and infusion pumps. If a pump is used over moderate or long transport distances, the internal battery power may be inadequate, necessitating an external source of power, usually an AC power inverter. With infusions that must be carefully maintained, an infusion pump is preferable. With frequent patient movement and manipulation, tubing can bend and kink, altering resistance to fluid flow. Air trapped in tubing (or in glass IV bottles) can expand with changes in altitude and increase or decrease the infusion pressure. Thus a reliable servocontrolled infusion system provides a margin of safety.

Monitor-Defibrillator

Combination monitor-defibrillators operate from internal batteries when 110 to 120 volts AC is not available. Other monitors capable of pressure monitoring from arterial lines or pulmonary artery catheters may be used, but these may have limited usefulness on flights of short duration, during which vibration and motion (turbulence) can introduce artifact and erroneous readings, as may occur aboard a helicopter. These devices may find a greater role with dedicated fixed-wing aircraft that frequently transport critically ill patients over long distances. Noninvasive blood pressure measurement is reasonably accurate in most patients, although these devices may have insufficient sensitivity.[57]

Potential hazards of defibrillation while airborne remain a concern, although trials support its safety.[23,43] Caution is still advised, and care should be taken to ensure that crew and aircraft systems are isolated from potential electrical contact (see Common Aeromedical Transport Problems). The pilot should be notified before defibrillation. It is unlikely that defibrillation will cause a problem with the aircraft, but if in a critical phase of flight (e.g., take-off, landing), the pilot may delay the shock until the critical phase of flight is accomplished.

Oximetry

Pulse oximetry is often indicated for optimal patient care. Pulse oximeters use a colorimetric method, with placement of a soft probe over a fingertip, in a thin skinfold such as an earlobe, or against the conjunctiva.[1,84] They may be extremely useful in aeromedical transport, during which other methods to detect changes in respiratory status are difficult.

Mechanical Resuscitators

Cardiac arrest resuscitation while airborne in a small cabin is difficult and physically demanding. In most instances a standard medical crew of two will be completely occupied in performing chest compressions and ensuring ventilation. Additional tasks may be impossible. Therefore a mechanical resuscitator may be used to prevent fatigue and free crew members for other tasks.[67] Mechanical resuscitators are gas-powered devices capable of providing ventilation and chest compressions automatically. Some models provide only chest compressions.

FLIGHT CREW

Crew Configuration

One of the continuing controversies in aeromedical transport involves crew composition (Table 27-6). The ideal crew composition varies considerably with the mission profile. When the aircraft is involved in a primary response to the accident scene, inclusion of an EMT may be beneficial. The transport of patients whose illness or injuries are complex or whose clinical conditions are extremely unstable may benefit from the presence of a physician. All aeromedical transport programs include one or more of the following providers in the transport medical crew.

Emergency Medical Technician–Paramedic

EMTs are increasingly a part of the aeromedical flight team. In 1993, 71% of rotor-wing transport programs reported using an EMT-paramedic (EMT-P) as a member of the flight team, vs. 44% in 1988.[15] Paramedics vary in their level of training depending on the state in which they work but usually follow DOT guidelines, which include three levels of certification. EMT-basic provides basic ambulance, rescue, and first-aid skills. EMT-intermediate may include IV and intubation skills. The EMT-paramedic level involves such skills as intubation, IV techniques, medication administration, defibrillation, and arrhythmia recognition and treatment. For an aeromedical flight team member, additional training relating to the aeromedical environment is desirable.[81,92]

EMTs can be of particular value in operations that necessitate frequent interaction with ground EMS. In some regions, helicopter EMS service is integrated into the regional primary response network so that they arrive at the accident scene before ground units, and flight team members experienced in scene assessment and victim extrication are essential.

TABLE 27-6. Medical Attendants in Aeromedical Transport, 1988-1993

	PERCENTAGES				
	1988	1990	1991	1992	1993
HELICOPTER					
Medical crew					
One attendant	8	3	3	2	2
Two attendants	92	97	97	98	98
Crew configuration					
RN/paramedic	44	54	53	57	71
RN/RN	15	11	11	19	21
RN/physician	10	12	11	10	3
RN/other	17	15	20	7	2
Other	14	8	5	7	3
Regular-duty shift length					
8 hours	2	2	4	6	3
12 hours	62	68	70	82	63
24 hours	18	16	15	11	10
12 and 24 hours	9	9	5	0	19
Other	9	5	6	1	5
FIXED-WING AIRCRAFT					
Medical crew					
One attendant	17	17	10	4	5
Two attendants	83	83	90	96	95
Crew configuration					
RN/paramedic	41	38	36	54	59
RN/RN	17	15	25	18	24
RN/physician	5	3	2	0	6
RN/other	22	35	32	18	9
Other	15	9	5	10	2
Regular-duty shift length					
8 hours	—	3	2	2	8
12 hours	46	43	50	47	46
24 hours	14	14	14	19	8
Other	40	40	34	32	38

From Cady G: *Air Med J* 12:308, 1993.
RN, Registered nurse.

Flight Nurse

At least one flight nurse is part of almost all aeromedical transport programs; in 1993, 21% of rotor-wing programs reported using two flight nurses as the sole team members.[15] Critical care or emergency nursing experience is usually a prerequisite, with additional training that includes patient assessment, advanced cardiac life support (ACLS), a trauma life support course, prehospital care skills, certain procedures such as ET intubation, advanced IV cannulation techniques, and in some cases, needle thoracotomy, venous cutdown, cricothyrotomy, and other specialized patient care activities. The flight nurse often is also a certified EMT.

Flight Physician

The experience and training of physicians involved in aeromedical transport depend on their role. Those who function as the on-line medical control physician communicate via radio or 800-MHz radiotelephone with the flight crew, monitors care, and gives necessary orders. In the United States, physicians fly as a component of the flight team in a minority of aeromedical transport programs; in 1993, only 3% of all rotor-wing transport programs reported the routine use of a physician, vs. 10% in 1988.[15] In helicopter EMS operations an emergency physician or trauma surgeon may be appropriate, whereas with fixed-wing transport of intensive care unit (ICU) patients an intensivist may be of value.

Physicians functioning in this role must have a current level of skill and expertise sufficient to address a wide range of clinical problems. They must also possess additional training relative to the airborne environment, including flight physiology, aircraft operations, and prehospital care (Box 27-3). Most important, they must function in this role with sufficient frequency so as to maintain their skills and remain safe and comfortable within the aeromedical setting. In doing so, they become an asset to the flight team rather than a distraction or liability.

Studies during the late 1980s and early 1990s attempted to determine whether a physician crew member has an effect on the outcome of patients transported by helicopter.* Some studies concluded that a physician crew member had a positive impact on patient outcome, whereas others found no difference in outcome between similar cohorts of patients transported by flight crews with two nurses or a nurse and a paramedic. The cost of using a physician crew member is substantially higher than that of a nurse-nurse or nurse-paramedic crew configuration. Some argue that this higher cost would be offset by the decrease in hospital stay or lost person-years that would occur if a physician were a standard member of the flight crew. With advanced training in critical procedures and treatment protocols combined with on-line medical direction, a nonphysician flight crew usually functions as well as a crew that includes a physician. No objective evidence supports the benefit of a physician as a standard flight crew member.

Crew Member Stress

By its nature, aeromedical transport involves moving a gravely ill patient into an adverse environment with

---

*References 5, 6, 14, 40, 42, 75, 83, 85.

Box 27-3 SPECIALIZED TRAINING FOR AEROMEDICAL TRANSPORT

Aviation physiology
Atmospheric pressure changes with altitude
Gas expansion with altitude
Changes in partial pressure of oxygen with altitude
Effects of motion and acceleration
Effects of noise and vibration
Changes in temperature and humidity
Aircraft safety
Aircraft systems and equipment operations
In-flight emergency procedures
Survival techniques
Patient extrication and immobilization
Patient loading and handling aboard an aircraft
Patient care techniques in the aeromedical environment
Respiratory support and ventilation aboard the aircraft
Pertinent Federal Aviation Administration regulations
  and procedures
Familiarity with the local EMS system
Radio communications skills and techniques

Hazardous materials response procedures
Record keeping and documentation in aeromedical
  transport
Preflight, in-flight, and postflight procedures
Clinical procedures
Cardiopulmonary resuscitation aboard the aircraft
Defibrillation aboard the aircraft
Intravenous cannulation
Endotracheal intubation
Tube thoracostomy
Needle thoracotomy
Cricothyrotomy
Central vein catheterization
Pericardiocentesis
Nasogastric tube insertion
Bladder catheterization
Antishock trouser application
Interosseous line placement
Umbilical vein catheterization

limited resources. Under these conditions a medical crew of only two or three persons must perform complex tasks, solve difficult problems, and make life-or-death decisions. They must perform in a physically confining space that may be uncomfortable, and they must do so under time pressure and with little or no physical assistance. In some cases, rescuers' lives may be at risk. This scenario occurs in few other arenas of civilian medical care.

"Stress" describes an array of adverse physiologic and psychologic reactions that occur when a person perceives a threat to existence. Although stress may not diminish performance, it may be responsible for errors, faulty judgment, and uneven manual skill performance. It may also affect the physical and psychologic health and satisfaction of the flight crew member.[16]

When measured during patient flights, the level of anxiety among aeromedical crew members was significantly higher than during a baseline period on the ground.[87] Factors that correlate with high in-flight anxiety levels include adverse weather conditions (e.g., low ceilings, high winds), severity of the patient's medical condition, complexity of illness or injuries, and the crew member's fatigue.

Efforts should be made to minimize stress among crew members. This includes frequent and adequate training; continuing education and feedback; adequate medical backup, including on-line medical direction, written protocols, and treatment guidelines that can aid in difficult decisions; a supportive rather than an intimidating or critical quality assurance program; ade-

quate rest; and safe weather minimums. Both routine mission debriefing and critical incident stress debriefing (CISD) should be an integral part of all transport programs.[64,65]

FLIGHT PHYSIOLOGY

Aeromedical care is different from ground-based care not only because of special equipment and the space-limited environment, but also because of the hostile physical milieu.

Hypoxia and Altitude

The earth is blanketed by a sea of air. The troposphere lies in the first 9144 to 18,288 m (30,000 to 60,000 feet) and contains atmospheric moisture. Vertical convection currents, as well as a temperature decline with increasing altitude at a lapse rate of 2° C per 305 m (3.6° F per 1000 feet), occur here. Virtually all atmospheric weather occurs in this layer. Above this level lies the stratosphere, extending from 18,288 to 30,480 m (60,000 to 100,000 feet), where temperature remains relatively constant and no moisture or vertical convection currents exist.

Air exerts pressure on everything it contacts in an amount equal to the weight of the column of air above the point of reference. At sea level the atmospheric pressure is 14.7 PSI or 760 mm Hg. As the person ascends, a progressively smaller air mass remains to exert weight, and the pressure diminishes. At 5486 m (18,000 feet) the atmospheric pressure is one half of that at sea level, and at 8534 m (28,000 feet) it is one third as great

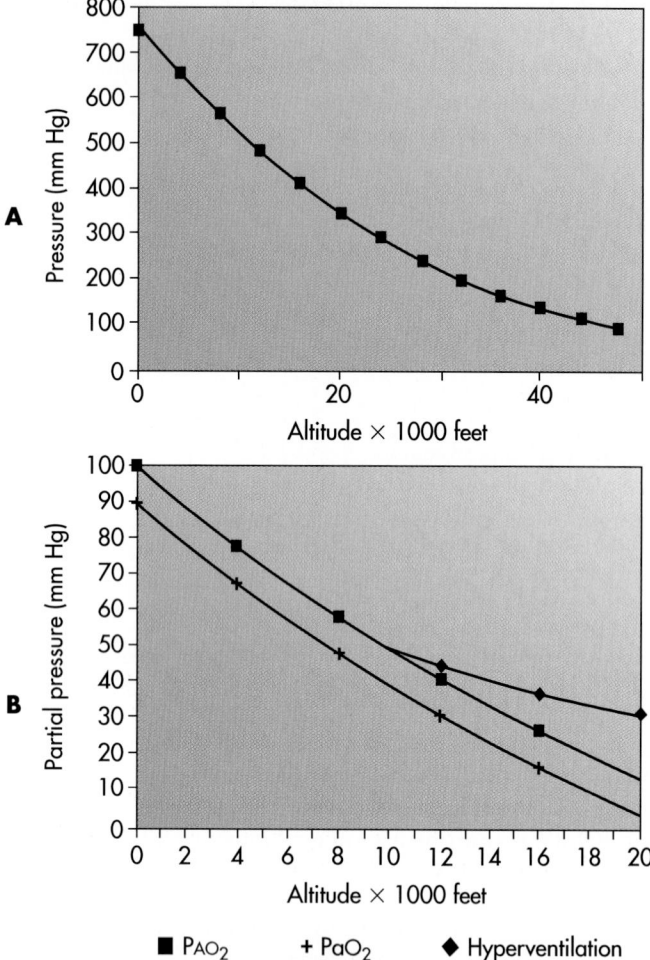

Figure 27-9 **A,** Atmospheric pressure vs. altitude. **B,** Alveolar (P_{AO_2}) and arterial (P_{aO_2}) oxygen tensions vs. altitude.

TABLE 27-7. Composition of Air

GAS	PERCENT
Nitrogen	78.09
Oxygen	20.95
Carbon dioxide	0.03
Other gases	0.07
Water vapor	1-5 at sea level

From Del Vecchio RJ: *Physiologic aspects of flight,* Oakdale, NY, 1977, Dowling College Press.

(Figure 27-9). Similarly, under the weight of air, individual molecules tend to compact, so the density of air is also greatest at the surface and diminishes with increasing altitude.

These phenomena underlie most of the important physiologic consequences of flight. Air is composed of several gases, of which oxygen makes up approximately 21%, an amount that is relatively constant despite increasing altitude (Table 27-7).[25,73] Henry's law

states that the quantity of gas that goes into solution depends on the partial pressure of that gas (and its solubility characteristics) as exerted at the air-water interface. The partial pressure of oxygen in alveolar air (P_{AO_2}) is determined by multiplying the fractional composition of oxygen in inspired air (F_{IO_2}) by the atmospheric pressure (barometric pressure, P_B) after the opposing vapor pressure of water (P_W, 47 mm Hg) has been subtracted. This is the basis of the alveolar air equation, as follows:

$$P_{AO_2} = F_{IO_2} \times (P_B - P_W) - P_{CO_2}/R$$

where P_{CO_2} is the arterial carbon dioxide tension and R is the respiratory quotient (approximately 0.8). Arterial oxygen tension (P_{aO_2}) in normal individuals is within 10 to 15 mm Hg of the P_{AO_2}. With lung disease characterized by ventilation-perfusion mismatch, intrapulmonic shunting, or severe diffusion defects, the alveolar-arterial (A-a) oxygen gradient is much larger, and higher amounts of inspired oxygen are required to produce sufficient oxygenation of arterial blood. The atmospheric P_{O_2}, P_{AO_2}, and the P_{aO_2} all decline with altitude (Figure 27-9). To some extent, P_{aO_2} can be maintained through hyperventilation as P_{CO_2} is reduced, but eventually P_{aO_2} will decline below 60% and hemoglobin will begin to desaturate greatly.

It is important during aeromedical transport to maintain hemoglobin saturation at or above 90%. Knowledge of the patient's preflight P_{aO_2} will enable a calculation of the patient's A-a oxygen gradient, which can then be subtracted from the P_{AO_2} calculated for the anticipated en route altitude (or cabin altitude in a pressurized craft) to yield the expected en route P_{AO_2}. Nomograms can be devised for this purpose (Figure 27-10). If the en route expected P_{aO_2} is unacceptably low, supplemental oxygen is required. The F_{IO_2} required to maintain the P_{AO_2} at a given level can be calculated from the alveolar air equation as follows:

$$F_{IO_2} = (P_{AO_2} + P_{CO_2}/R)/(P_B - P_W)$$

Or, if $P_{CO_2} = 40$, $R = 0.8$, and $P_W = 47$ mm Hg, then:

$$F_{IO_2} = (P_{AO_2} + 50)/(P_B - 47)$$

This allows P_{AO_2} to be determined by adding the P_{aO_2} desired (the minimum acceptable is 60 mm Hg) to the known A-a oxygen gradient (calculated from the preflight blood gas). P_B can be estimated over the first 15,000 feet (4572 m) of ambient or cabin altitude as follows:

$$P_B = 760 - (23 \times Alt)$$

where Alt is the altitude above sea level in thousands of feet. Transport cabin environments rarely ex-

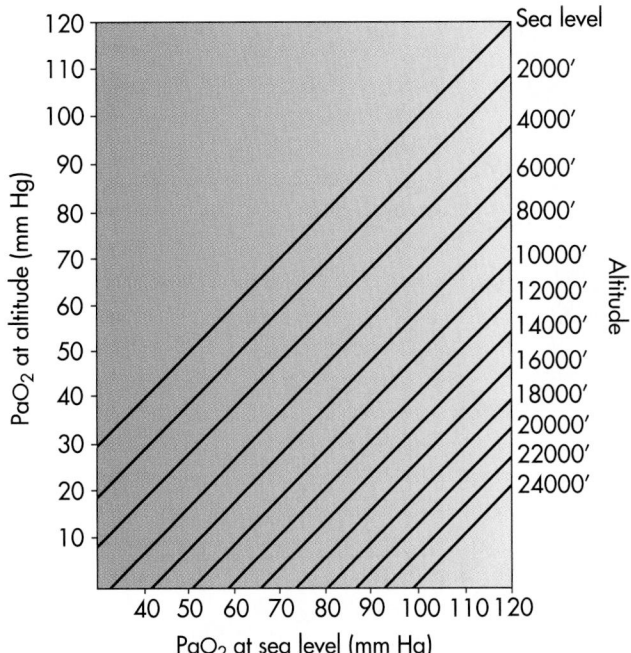

Figure 27-10 Arterial oxygen tension (Pao$_2$) at altitude vs. Pao$_2$ at sea level. Locate the sea-level Pao$_2$ on the *x* axis and intersect with the cruise altitude (on the diagonal). Read across to find the Pao$_2$ at altitude (*y* axis).

TABLE 27-8. Clinical Manifestations of Trapped Gas Expansion

TRAPPED GAS LOCATION	CLINICAL MANIFESTATIONS
Intestinal lumen	Abdominal pain, distention
Pleural space	Pneumothorax, tension pneumothorax
Subcutaneous	Subcutaneous emphysema
Paranasal sinuses	Facial pain
Middle ear	Ear pain
Dental root	Tooth pain
Blood	Air embolism, decompression sickness
Air splints, antishock trousers	Compartment syndrome, ischemia
IV bottle and tubing	Fow rate increase
Blood pressure cuff	Tourniquet effect
Endotracheal tube cuff	Air leak, hypoventilation

ceed these altitudes, since pressurized craft are usually capable of maintaining cabin pressure equal to 8000 feet (2438 m) or below at normal cruising altitudes. Nonpressurized craft must provide supplemental oxygen above 15,000 feet. Even a modest increase in FiO$_2$ is usually enough to maintain oxygenation under these circumstances, unless a severe A-a oxygen gradient exists, in which case the addition PEEP may be necessary. The previous equation would predict that a PaO$_2$ of 80 mm Hg at sea level on 40% oxygen would require that an FiO$_2$ of 50% at 8000 feet be maintained. An oximeter can simplify monitoring of oxygenation; as altitude increases, a fall in oxygen saturation can be treated with increases in FiO$_2$.

Effects of Pressure Changes

Trapped Gas. Boyle's law states that the volume of a gas varies inversely with pressure. This means that trapped gases expand as an aircraft ascends to higher altitude (and lower pressure) and contract as it descends. The volume change can be determined from the following equation:

$$P_1 \times V_1 = P_2 \times V_2$$

Clinically, this is manifested by such alterations as expansion or contraction of air splints or MAST pants, changes in ET tube cuff size, expansion of bowel gas in cases of intestinal obstruction or ileus, expansion of pneumothorax air space, and expansion of air trapped in IV lines (or glass IV bottles) (Table 27-8). Certain precautions must be taken, such as the use of plastic IV bags and frequent monitoring of pressure cuffs.

Dysbarism. Decompression sickness occurs mainly in scuba divers that ascend too soon after a dive. Too rapid a decrease in ambient pressure allows nitrogen bubbles to form in the microcirculation, which may lead to ischemia and tissue damage (see Chapter 57). Care must be taken in the transport of an ill or injured diver to allow a surface interval of at least 12 hours before transport. An alternative is to attain at least a level D (PADI) dive stage, with a cabin altitude not to exceed 2438 m (8000 feet). If an individual must be transported abruptly after submersion, the transport must be conducted at the lowest possible safe altitude in a pressurized aircraft, to reduce the risk of decompression illness.

Motion and Acceleration

Aircraft not only move through space in a rectilinear fashion, which cannot be detected by human senses in the absence of visual cues, but also rotate about three axes: longitudinal (roll), vertical (yaw), and horizontal (pitch) (Figure 27-11). Motions about these axes are sensed by the semicircular canals located in the inner ear. Sensations from these organs are useful as an adjunct to visual cues. However, they may quickly lead to spatial disorientation, a phenomenon often experienced by individuals traveling in a turbulent environment without a visual frame of reference. For example, when an aircraft enters a bank to the right, the sensation may be initially correctly interpreted. However, after rollout of the stationary bank to a neutral position, a sensation of

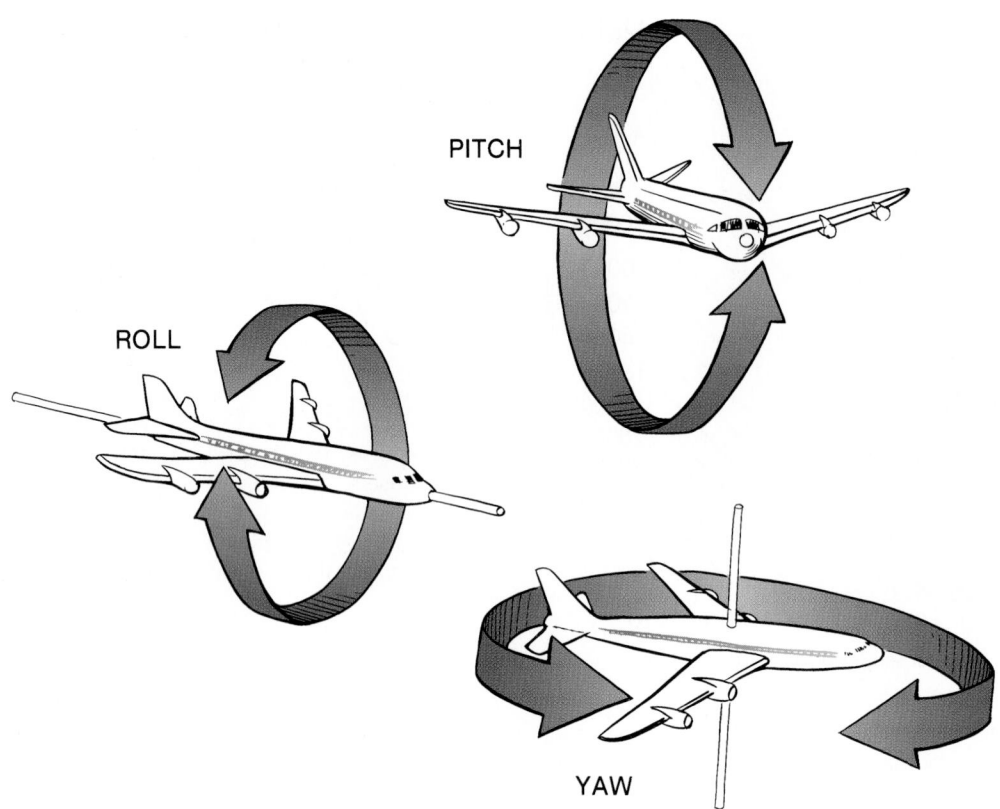

PITCH

ROLL

YAW

Figure 27-11 Axes of movement in aviation.

rolling into a left bank may be sensed. If uncorrected, apprehension may follow. The best remedy for this effect is to maintain a visual reference to the correct position.

Vestibular stimuli, especially in turbulence with limited or no visual frame of reference, may result in motion sickness, manifested most often as nausea or vomiting. Affecting both patients and flight crews, motion sickness can be counteracted with antiemetics such as antihistamines (e.g., dimenhydrinate, 50 mg orally) or phenothiazines (e.g., prochlorperazine, 10 mg orally); however, these may produce sedation and are potentially hazardous in flight. Transdermal scopolamine patches applied behind the ear have been used as effective prophylaxis for nausea and vomiting during flight.

Noise and Vibration

Noise and vibration are components of all aircraft environments, especially helicopters. The most obvious impact of noise is on communications within the cabin, particularly with the patient, who is least likely to have a headset and access to the aircraft's intercom. In addition, the patient's breath sounds are difficult if not impossible to hear, and thus other means to identify changes in respiratory status, such as pulse oximetry, must be employed.

Headsets are essential for effective communication among flight crew members aboard a helicopter, although they are usually unnecessary aboard larger fixed-wing aircraft. Noise may lead to permanent defects in auditory acuity if exposure is prolonged or recurrent. Veteran pilots demonstrate 10- to 20-dB reductions in high-frequency auditory acuity. Noise and vibration may also lead to stress and fatigue.

COMMON AEROMEDICAL TRANSPORT PROBLEMS

Pretransport Preparation

Once the decision is made to transport a patient by air and the appropriate aeromedical service is contacted, preparations must be made to ensure patient safety and comfort and to aid the flight crew in patient care. A study of the causes of ground delays in a rural interhospital helicopter transport program found that on arrival of the flight team, 31% of patients required minor interventions (insertion of IV line or nasogastric tube, blood transfusion, bladder catheterization, MAST application) before take-off, and 33% required major interventions (ET intubation, tube thoracostomy, central venous access).[54] When no intervention was required, the mean ground time was 31.2 minutes, compared

Box 27-4 PRETRANSPORT PREPARATIONS

SCENE RESPONSE

Airway secured
Stabilization on a rigid spine board with cervical immobilization device, neck rolls, and tape
Two large-bore intravenous lines
Antishock garment applied
Landing zone selected and secured

INTERHOSPITAL TRANSPORT

Airway secured
Stabilization on a rigid spine board with cervical immobilization device, neck rolls, and tape
Two large-bore intravenous lines
Tube thoracostomy for pneumo/hemothorax
Bladder catheterization (if not contraindicated)
Nasogastric catheterization (if not contraindicated)
Lactated Ringer's solution hanging
Typed and cross-matched blood if available
Extremity fractures splinted (traction splinting for femur fractures)
Copies of all available emergency department records and laboratory results, including a description of the mechanism of injury

with 57.4 minutes when one or more major interventions were required.

To minimize delays, pretransport preparations should be made for victims of acute trauma (Box 27-4).

Patient Comfort

Motion, vibration, noise, temperature variations, dry air, changes in atmospheric pressure, confinement to a limited position or backboard, and fear of flying may cause patient discomfort.

Patient Movement

Patient handling and movement can contribute to morbidity and mortality in unstable patients.[93] All transported patients should be adequately secured to the stretcher with safety straps to prevent sudden shifting of position or movement of a secured fracture. During transport from the ground to the aircraft cabin, attempts should be made to limit sudden pitching of the stretcher. DOT guidelines recommend design of cabin access such that no more than 30 degrees of roll and 45 degrees of pitch may occur to the patient-occupied stretcher during loading.[62] The stretcher, in turn, should be adequately attached to the floor.

Motion sickness in the patient may be treated with an antiemetic such as promethazine (25 mg orally, intravenously, or intramuscularly) or prochlorperazine (5 to 10 mg orally, intravenously, or intramuscularly).

Scopolamine disks are useful for prolonged flight and do not require parenteral or oral administration, although their antiemetic effects are not always uniform and may not occur until 4 to 6 hours after application. They may be best used to decrease motion sickness in the flight crew.

Noise

Noise can be avoided with hearing protectors, which are devices similar to headphones but without internal speakers. Inexpensive hearing protectors are available as deformable foam ear plugs. In some cases, headphones may be used in an awake patient if the crew wants the patient to communicate on the intercom system.

Eye Protection

When a patient is loaded on or off a helicopter with the rotors turning, the patient's eyes must be protected. Serious eye injuries can result from debris blown into the air. Lightweight sky diver goggles ("boogie goggles") are effective and inexpensive. The eyes must be protected even if the patient is unconscious. Taping temporary patches over the eyes is also effective.

Respiratory Distress

Patients with respiratory disease or distress should have immediately treatable conditions addressed before take-off. ET intubation is essential if airway patency is threatened or if adequate oxygenation cannot be maintained with supplemental oxygen. It is better to err on the side of caution when making a decision about a patient's airway. During flight it is easier to treat restlessness in an intubated patient than airway obstruction or apnea in a nonintubated patient.

Nearly all patients should receive supplemental oxygen. FiO_2 should be increased with increasing cabin altitude to maintain a stable Po_2 (Figure 27-12). When oxygen saturation monitoring is unavailable and pretransport arterial oxygen content unknown, 100% oxygen may be administered throughout the flight to ensure adequate oxygenation. Patients with chronic lung disease who are prone to hypercapnia may have a deterioration in condition if the hypoxic drive is eliminated. In these patients the least oxygen necessary to maintain saturation above 90% is advisable; this amount may be estimated in advance or calculated from the alveolar air equation. Close in-flight monitoring is essential. Finally, altitude changes may affect ET cuff volume, so cuff pressure must be checked frequently.

Cardiopulmonary Resuscitation and Cardiac Defibrillation

CPR in an aircraft is difficult. The rescuers must perform several tasks simultaneously while ventilating the lungs or compressing the chest, all in a physically confining space. The crew must be familiar with modifica-

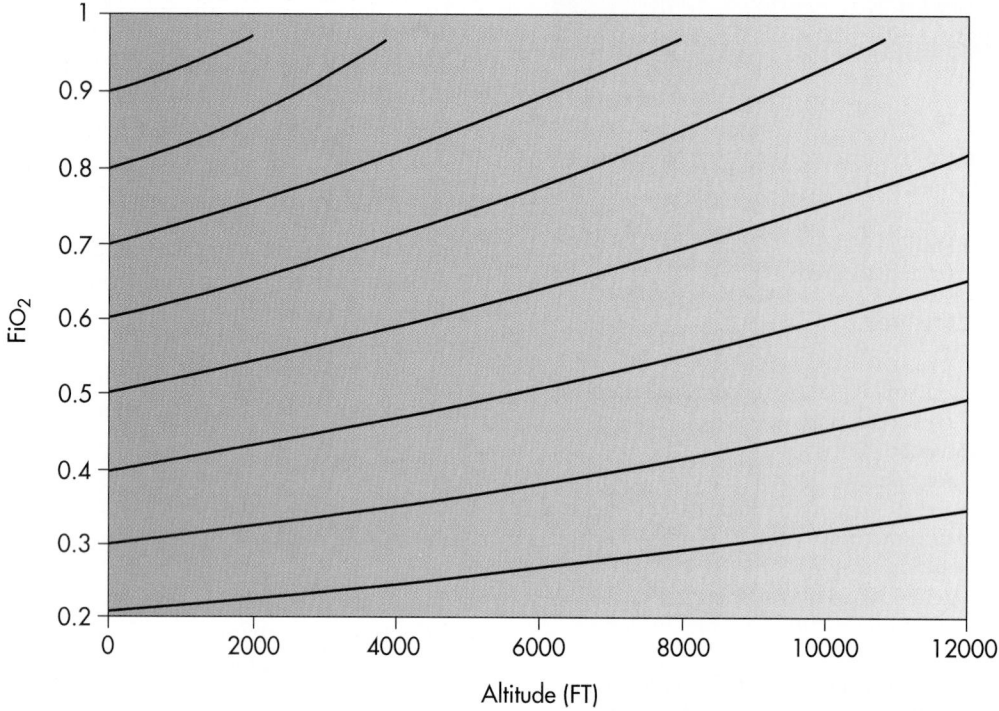

P_B	Altitude					FiO_2				
		0	0.21	0.30	0.40	0.50	0.60	0.70	0.80	0.90	1.00
760	2000	0.23	0.32	0.43	0.54	0.65	0.76	0.86	0.97	PP
707	4000	0.25	0.35	0.47	0.59	0.70	0.82	0.94	PP	PP
656	6000	0.27	0.38	0.51	0.63	0.76	0.89	PP	PP	PP
609	8000	0.29	0.41	0.55	0.69	0.83	0.97	PP	PP	PP
564	10000	0.31	0.45	0.60	0.75	0.90	PP	PP	PP	PP
523	12000	0.34	0.49	0.65	0.82	0.98	PP	PP	PP	PP
483	A-a:	15	79	150	222	293	364	435	507	578

Calculated from the alveolar air equation under standard temperature and pressure conditions. *PP,* Positive pressure required; P_B, barometric pressure (mm Hg); *Alt,* altitude (feet); *A-a,* alveolar–arterial oxygen gradient (mm Hg).
X axis: en route altitude
Y axis: FiO_2 required to maintain PO_2 = 90 mm Hg
To calculate the FiO_2 necessary to maintain PO_2 = 90 mmHg at a specific altitude, choose the value on the Y axis closest to that necessary to maintain PO_2 = 90 mmHg at sea level (altitude = 0 ft) and follow the corresponding line across to the new altitude (X axis). The proper FiO_2 is the Y value corresponding to the new X value.

Figure 27-12 Fraction of inspired oxygen required to maintain oxygen tension at 90 mm Hg (varying with altitude).

tions in technique.[45] As previously mentioned, there should be no concern with airborne defibrillation if all electronic navigational equipment on the aircraft has a common ground, as mandated by the FAA standards. Despite cramped quarters and sensitive electrical equipment, defibrillation can be safely performed in all types of aircraft currently used for emergency transport utilizing standard precautions routinely used during defibrillation on the ground.[23,94] In the interest of safety, however, it is best to notify the pilot before performing defibrillation.

Patient Combativeness

Patients may be combative to the point that they pose a threat to the safety of the flight and crew. An uncontrollable patient may cause sudden shifts in aircraft balance or may strike a crew member or important flight instruments or equipment. Such patients should be properly restrained in advance. If sedation is necessary, a careful neurologic examination documented beforehand is essential. Useful agents include diazepam (5 to 20 mg intravenously) or shorter-acting agents, such as midazolam (2 to 10 mg intravenously or intramuscularly.) Paralyzing agents, such as pancuronium, vecuronium, and succinylcholine, have the advantage of not altering the sensorium, but they require airway control with ET intubation.[90] In addition, it is necessary to sedate a patient who is paralyzed to facilitate intubation and transport.

Endotracheal Intubation

ET intubation may be difficult to perform while airborne, especially in a confining cabin, and should be done before departure if possible. This is especially true in trauma victims with head injuries and in burn victims who have carbonaceous sputum or hoarseness. Special techniques are available to supplement standard methods of intubation, including a lighted stylet, ET tubes with controllable tips, and digital intubation. Sedation or pharmacologic paralysis may be necessary. Of 106 aeromedical transport programs in the United States that reported using neuromuscular blocking agents, 39 use them to facilitate intubations, and 67 use them once a patient is intubated to manage combativeness and ensure airway patency.[79] Induction of paralysis before intubation in the aeromedical setting is controversial. One study reported a 96.6% success rate using succinylcholine to facilitate intubation, with 3.4% of patients requiring an emergency surgical airway.[66] Besides the need for surgical airway if intubation is unsuccessful, concerns exist about cervical spine manipulation during intubation in the paralyzed patient, unrecognized esophageal intubation in a nonbreathing patient, and the relative contraindications to the use of succinylcholine in certain patients. As shorter-acting nondepolarizing paralytic agents (e.g., mivacurium) are developed, this adjunct to airway and combativeness control in the aeromedical setting will be studied further.[51]

In some flight programs, nonphysician crew members are taught to perform emergency cricothyrotomy. Although occasionally lifesaving, this procedure is often difficult to perform and should be undertaken only as a final method to secure an emergency airway.

Thrombolysis

The air transport of patients with acute myocardial infarction often involves thrombolytic therapy. Because bleeding is a major adverse effect of thrombolytic agents, one study investigated whether air transport resulted in a higher incidence of bleeding complications compared with a similar cohort of patients given thrombolytic drugs who were transported by ground ambulance. The study concluded that helicopter transport of patients with acute myocardial infarction after initiation of thrombolysis is comparatively safe and without a clinically significant increase in bleeding complications.[34]

Flight Safety

Because aeromedical transport involves medical care delivered in a hostile environment, the patient and crew are at risk of injury or death in the event of a mishap. Flight crew training must emphasize safety. The pilot is ultimately responsible for the safety of the aircraft's occupants and is trained not only to operate the aircraft skillfully and safely, but also to provide necessary safety instructions and guidance to crew members and passengers. Safely practices vary depending on the type of aircraft but include common guidelines.

Approaching the Aircraft. Helicopters with turning rotor blades must be approached only from the front and sides and only while under pilot observation (Figure 27-13). The tail rotor must be given wide berth, especially on helicopters with rear doors. It is advisable to station a crew member in a safe position to direct approaching individuals away from the tail rotor. Shutting down the helicopter's engines completely, when the situation allows, is prudent before patient loading and unloading. Approaching in a crouched position minimizes the risk of contact with the rotor blades should a sudden gust of wind or movement of the aircraft cause them to dip. Loose clothing and debris should be secured (Box 27-5).

Fixed-wing aircraft should be approached with similar precautions regarding propellers. This is especially important in aircraft with access doors in front of the wing and engine nacelles. Engine shutdown on the side of entry enhances safety of loading and unloading.

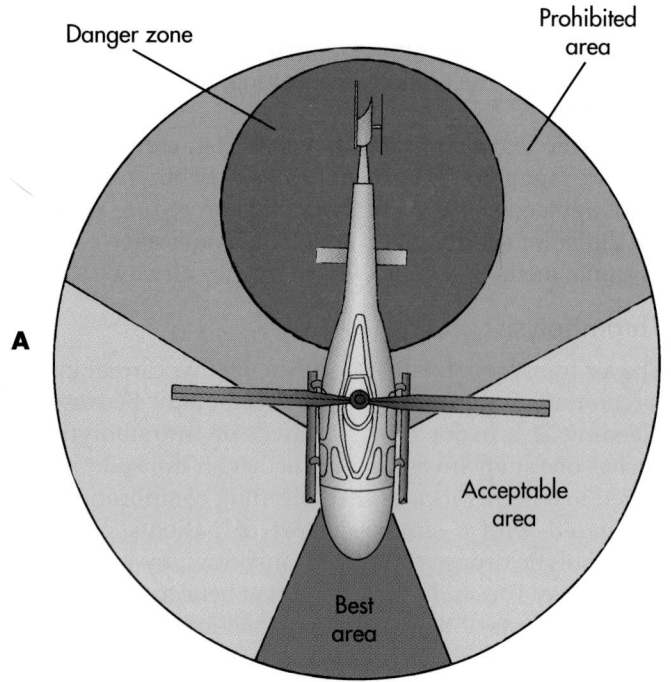

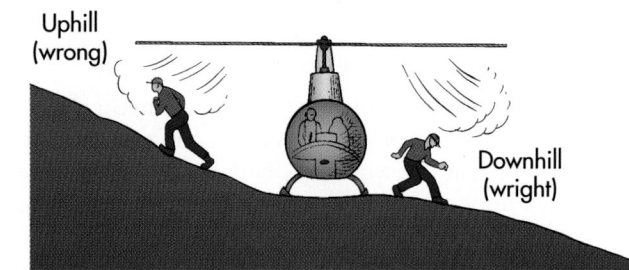

Figure 27-13 Helicopter safety. **A,** Safe approach zones. **B,** The proper way to approach or depart a helicopter.

Box 27-5 HELICOPTER SAFETY

DO:

Approach and depart downhill.
Use crouched position.
Approach after visual contact and approval from pilot.
Await direction of flight crew.
Approach from the front or the sides.
Secure area first of people and then of loose debris.

DON'T:

Approach or depart uphill.
Use tall intravenous poles or other objects.
Use loose sheets or clothing.
Smoke tobacco within 50 feet.
Run near the aircraft.
Drive a vehicle within 30 feet.
Shine headlights or flashlights toward the aircraft.

be required to operate in flight or in an emergency. This includes all aircraft doors, fire extinguisher, communications equipment, oxygen equipment, and electrical outlets. In addition, the crew must be familiar with emergency shutdown procedures. Finally, before take-off, door security must be confirmed by a crew member familiar with the operation of the door.

In-Flight Obstacle Reporting. An extra pair of eyes can be invaluable to a pilot in a busy airspace or on a scene approach complicated by trees and electrical or phone wires. Primarily important in VFR conditions, assistance with obstacle identification can enhance the safety of the mission; however, flight should not occur under conditions in which obstacle reporting by a crew member is essential to safety, since the person must then divide attention between patient care and obstacle reporting.

Ground Coordination and Control. Enthusiastic rescue personnel or curious onlookers may approach the aircraft in a hazardous manner. Flight crew members must be able to communicate with ground units during the landing phase to ensure adequate scene preparation; they may be required to perform crowd control while on the ground. This requires directing individuals away from the rotor blades, propellers, or other hazardous equipment at the scene. If loading or unloading the patient while the rotors or propellers are still turning ("hot loading" or "hot off-loading") is necessary, special precautions must be undertaken for ground crews, the flight crew, and the patient.

Safety Belt Use. The use of safety belts (preferably with shoulder harnesses, especially in helicopters) is an important safety measure. Certain patient care activities (e.g., ET intubation, CPR), however, may be impossible to perform with safety belts secured. The design and selection of aircraft and interior configurations should allow maximal access to the patient with the crew members properly restrained. Throughout the flight the crew members and patient should remain restrained as much as possible in smooth air and at all times in rough air. Movement inside the cabin affects aircraft balance. An aircraft loaded near its aft CG limit may exceed its limits if a crew member moves to a new position within the cabin. Changes in position should be preceded by consultation with the pilot. Light aircraft are sensitive to turbulent air, and appropriate precautions must be taken to avoid being injured from sudden motion.

Proper Use of Aircraft Equipment. Crew members must be familiar with all aircraft equipment they may

Emergency Procedures. All crew members should memorize and routinely practice emergency procedures.

These procedures should address in-flight fires, electrical failures, loss of pressurization, engine failure, emergency landing with and without power, precautionary landing away from an airport, and other in-flight emergencies.

Survival. An emergency or precautionary landing away from an airport necessitates survival before rescue arrives. Under adverse environmental conditions and with injured victims, survival may depend on specific actions by the crew. The crew should be proficient in emergency egress from the aircraft, including escape after crashes and water landings, especially in helicopters. After water landings, helicopters usually roll inverted and sink rapidly. Helicopter "dunker" training is required for all military helicopter crews. The crews are strapped into a simulated helicopter fuselage and lowered rapidly into a pool, simulating a semicontrolled water landing. The fuselage then rolls inverted and the crew must open emergency exits and egress the simulator. This type of training has been shown to save lives in helicopter water crashes. All crew members should be trained in the use of emergency signaling devices, such as ELTs, flares, signal fires, and ground emergency signals. Survival skills should be taught to all crew members, including advanced first aid, building emergency shelters, fire starting, and obtaining water and food from the environment.

Aeromedical Accidents. Attention continues to focus on EMS helicopter accidents. Statistics from 1986 estimated a rotor-wing accident rate of 17.65 with 5.88 fatalities per 100,000 transports.[35] Aviation accident rates are typically reported in relation to flight hours. EMS fatalities therefore amounted to 6.0 per 100,000 flight hours, compared with 3.3 for the helicopter industry in general. The EMS rate subsequently declined, however, with 3.0 accidents per 100,000 transports reported in 1991 (Figure 27-14).[74,88]

From 64% to 84% of EMS accidents result from pilot error, approximately 23% from mechanical causes, and 3% from unknown causes.[19] Of accidents caused by pilot error, adverse weather was a contributing factor in 67% (Table 27-9).[17] In all, two thirds of fatal weather-related accidents occur at night, and 86% of all fatal accidents occur at night or in marginal weather conditions (Table 27-10).[20] Only 35% to 40% of all EMS helicopter flights occur at night. The most common phase of flight for weather-related accidents was en route (86%), with 14% occurring on departure and none on approach (Table 27-11).

Only 5% of fatal EMS helicopter accidents occur in flights to or from the scene, although such flights account for 24% of EMS helicopter missions.[21] When scene-related accidents occur, they result in fatalities 9% and injuries 35% of the time, suggesting a low-energy impact vs. an en route crash. Causal factors related to scene accidents include wire and obstacle strikes (70%),

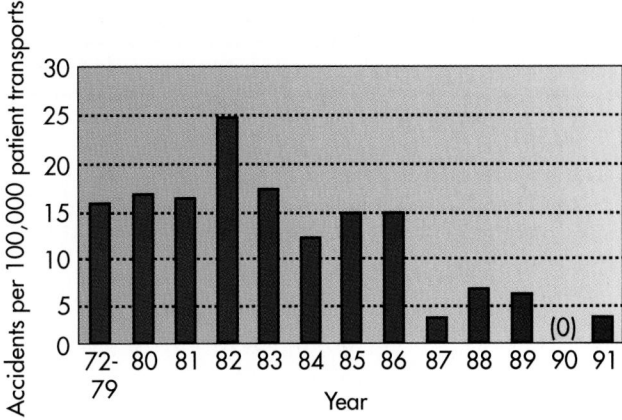

Figure 27-14 Aeromedical helicopter accident rate, 1972 to 1991. (*From Preston N:* J Air Med Transport *11:14, 1992.*)

TABLE 27-9. Major and Primary Causes and Severity of Aeromedical Accidents, 1972 to 1989

	PERCENTAGES		
	1972-1985	1987-1988	1989
MAJOR CAUSES			
Weather	30	30	17
Engine failure	18	9	0
Obstacle strike	18	10	33
Control loss	9	20	17
Other	25	40	33
PRIMARY CAUSE			
Pilot error	64	60	83
Mechanical failure	30	30	0
Unknown	6	10	17
ACCIDENT SEVERITY			
Fatal	36	50	67
Injury	28	30	17
Damage only	36	20	17

From Collett HM: J Air Med Transport 9(2):12, 1990.

TABLE 27-10. Effect of Weather on Accident Seriousness

SEVERITY OF ACCIDENT	WEATHER RELATED	PERCENTAGE
Fatal	14/21	67
Injury	3/17	18
Damage only	1/32	3

From Collett HM: Hosp Aviat 5(11):15, 1986.

TABLE 27-11. Environment of Fatal Accidents

VISIBILITY	ACCIDENTS	PERCENT
Day visual meteorologic conditions	3	14
Night visual meteorologic conditions	4	19
Day marginal	4	19
Night marginal	10	48
TOTAL	21	100

From Collett HM: *Hosp Aviat* 5(11):15, 1986.

loss of control (18%), and mechanical failure (12%). The landing phase is involved in scene-related accidents in 41% of cases, whereas the take-off phase is involved in 59%. Because 40% of scene-related accidents occur at night and approximately 40% of helicopter EMS flights occur at night, scene accidents do not appear more hazardous at night than in the day. Single-engine helicopters have more often been involved in engine failure accidents (77%) than have twin-engine craft (the two types are approximately equal in number in the EMS industry).

Recommendations for enhancing safety include instituting stringent guidelines to limit flights at night or in adverse weather, increasing pilot proficiency training, and reducing pilot fatigue and workload factors. Decisions on the appropriateness of air transport regarding utilization and weather should be based on general protocols that are not subject to the emotional turmoil of a medical crisis.[10] The trend in the industry has been toward twin-engine helicopters for an increased margin of safety from engine failure accidents.

In addition, for dedicated EMS helicopter flights, a statistically strong relationship exists between the ability to fly under IFR and a lower accident rate.[56] The Association of Air Medical Services considered the question of whether all helicopters should be required to have IFR capability when it published its voluntary standards for rotor- and fixed-wing aircraft. This was not mandated because of the tremendous expense and because many programs were unlikely to comply.[58]

Ground to Air Signaling. It is best to have radio communication between the ground party and the helicopter crew. This may not be possible, however, and hand signals may be needed to communicate. Standard hand signals are used by military rescue personnel for communication between a deployed rescue swimmer and the helicopter (Table 27-12). These same signals can be used while on land. To acknowledge the signals, the hoist operator gives a thumbs up or the pilot flashes the rotating beacon.

TABLE 27-12. Swimmer to Helicopter and Ground to Air Signals

INTENTION	ACTION
Deploy medical kit	Arms above head, wrists crossed
Situation OK	Thumbs up
Lower rescue cable with rescue device attached	Arm extended over head, fist clenched
Lower rescue cable without rescue device attached	Climbing-rope motion with hands
Helicopter move in/out	Wave in/out with both hands
Cease operations	Slashing motion across throat
Deploy litter	Hands cupped, then arms outstretched
Personnel secured, raise cable	Vigorously shake hoist cable or thumb up; vigorous up motion with arm
Team recall	Circle arm over head with fingers skyward

Landing Zone Operations. The ideal helicopter landing zone is a wide, flat, clear area with no obstacles in the approach or departure end. Vertical landings and take-offs can be done, but it is safer for the helicopter to make a gradual descent while flying forward. Higher altitudes and higher temperatures require larger landing zones. The center of the landing zone can be marked with V, with the apex pointing into the prevailing wind. Any obstacles can be marked with brightly colored, properly secured clothing.

The size of the landing zone depends on the weather conditions, type of helicopter involved, altitude, temperature, and types of obstacles in the area. Small helicopters such as the Jet Ranger can usually land safely in a 60 × 60–foot landing zone. Larger helicopters such as the Bell 412 require a 120 × 120–foot zone.[95] Large military helicopters may require even greater landing zones. In general, pilots prefer the largest, flattest piece of ground they can find. The condition of the ground (e.g., loose snow, dust, gravel) should be communicated to the pilot before the final approach. Before the helicopter lands, all loose clothing and equipment should be secured. During approach, no personnel or vehicles should move on or near the landing zone.

Once the helicopter is on the ground, it must be approached only from the front and side, and then only while under direct observation of the pilot. The aft portion of the aircraft and areas around the tail rotor must be avoided at all times. Some helicopters (e.g., BK-117) have rear doors for loading and unloading patients, and ground personnel should wait for directions from the crew before approaching the rear area.

If the ground is uneven or slopes, all personnel should approach and depart from the helicopter on the downslope side. It is safest to load the patient into the helicopter with the engines off and the rotors stopped ("cold load"). If the patient must be loaded with the engines on and blades turning ("hot load"), eye and ear protection should be worn by all personnel approaching the helicopter, including the patient. A safety person should be assigned to prevent anyone from inadvertently walking toward the tail rotor.

Once the patient is loaded, all personnel should leave the landing zone, take cover, and stay in place until the helicopter has departed. It is best to be off to the side, not directly in the take-off path.

Hoist Operations. If the helicopter is not able to land and has a rescue hoist installed, hoist operations may be the only means of evacuating the patient. In most circumstances a helicopter crew member rides the hoist down to the site to rig the survivor into the rescue device and to oversee the hoist operation, using the following guidelines:

Do not touch the hoist, rescue device, or cable until after it has touched the ground (or water). Helicopters can build up a very powerful static electricity charge that will be grounded through whatever the hoist touches first. This has been known to knock rescuers and survivors off their feet.

Once the rescue device and cable have touched the ground, put the patient into the rescue device, taking care to keep the hoist cable clear of all personnel. Do not allow the hoist cable to loop around any personnel or around the rescue device, since serious injury is possible when the cable slack is taken up.

Make sure that the patient is properly secured in the rescue device, with all safety straps tightened.

When the patient is secured, move away from the rescue device and signal "up cable."

If the rescue device is a basket (Stokes) litter, use a tag line with a properly installed weak link to prevent the litter from spinning during the hoist.

Night Operations. Night helicopter rescue operations are considerably more dangerous than daylight operations. In most cases it is best to delay helicopter insertion or extraction operations until daylight. If this is not possible, however, night missions can be done safely with careful planning and coordination between the helicopter and ground party. The same rules of daylight helicopter operations apply to night operations, but with extra care taken to ensure that all personnel understand their roles.

In night operations it is virtually mandatory to have radio communications between the ground and the helicopter. "No-comm" night operations should only be attempted by personnel specially trained and experienced in these techniques. The landing zone should be clearly marked and the pilot allowed to make the approach. All personnel should stay clear of the landing zone until the pilot has made a safe landing.

Personnel approaching the landing zone should have a small light or reflective material attached to their outer clothing so they can be clearly seen. The minimum number of people should approach the helicopter, and a safety observer is mandatory to keep the ground team together and clear of the tail rotor and rotor blades.

The landing zone should be as large as possible, preferably at least 50% larger than a daylight landing zone. Any obstacles should be clearly marked with light-colored streamers, small lights, or even light-colored clothing. The landing zone can be illuminated with flashlights at the corners, with another flashlight at the center point. These flashlights should be pointed at the ground, not into the air; flashlights pointed at the helicopter during landing and take-off may distract or momentarily blind the crew. If flashlights are not available, small fires can be used to illuminate the edges of the landing zone, although the helicopter can scatter burning embers for many meters.

If crew members are using night vision equipment, lights must never be flashed at the helicopter. Even the amount of white light from a small flashlight may be sufficient to overload the night vision equipment, functionally blinding the crew.

Dispatch and Communications. The dispatch center is the focal point for communications during aeromedical transport operations. Dispatchers receive incoming requests for service; obtain necessary information relative to the launch decision: coordinate the interaction between essential parties; "scramble" the flight crew; assemble and maintain necessary information regarding destination, weather, local telephone numbers, and frequencies; follow the progress of the flight; input data into the system database; and communicate with ground EMS units and hospitals. Communication may occur through a combination of methods: land telephone lines into a dispatch switchboard, hospital-EMS net transceiver, discrete frequency transceiver (communications with aircraft), or walkie-talkie radios. Familiarity with the EMS system and EMS communications is essential for successful dispatch.

Flight following is an important part of aeromedical safety and involves tracking the position of the aircraft during a mission by plotting the location according to reports from the pilot at 10- to 15 minute intervals. If an accident or in-flight emergency occurs, the dispatcher is soon aware and can initiate SAR to a precise location, which enhances the chances of survival.

APPROPRIATE USE OF AEROMEDICAL SERVICES

Aeromedical transport combines skilled treatment and stabilization capability with rapid access to definitive care, but not without risk, and at high cost ($1 to $2 million per year for a program, or about $2000 per transported patient, which is approximately 400% higher than ground transport).[13] However, the comparative risk of aeromedical transport must be placed in perspective against the risk of patient death from nonreferral or from less timely ground transport with limited medical capability en route.

Although not proved, advanced provider skill levels during prehospital care are considered beneficial, especially in severely ill or injured patients.[49] In rural and wilderness environments, advanced life support (ALS) services may be made more readily available by EMS helicopters. This is especially true in areas that are difficult or impossible to reach by ground.

The speed of access to definitive care is another consideration in choosing the mode of transport. In isolated rural or wilderness locations, a helicopter may be the only means of expedient access. Prolonged victim extrication allows time for a helicopter to arrive at the scene, decreasing total transport time and thereby increasing the advantage of helicopter transport.

Patient comfort also must be considered, especially on long transports over rough roads. Although a helicopter moves in three dimensions, fore and aft acceleration is usually steady, without the starting and stopping motions present during ground transport. However, helicopters typically travel within 914 m (3000 feet) of the ground's surface and are more subject to turbulence than are high-flying fixed-wing aircraft.

Whether aeromedical transport reduces mortality when compared with ground transport has not been determined definitively. An uncontrolled national multicenter study of trauma patients transported by helicopter showed a 21% reduction in mortality from that expected based on predictions from the Trauma Score–Injury Severity Score (TRISS) methodology and national normative trauma outcome data.[8]

A similar study using the TRISS methodology compared actual mortality with helicopter vs. ground transport and showed a 52% reduction from expected mortality when patients were transported by air, vs. no reduction in expected mortality when transport occurred by ground.[7] Another study using TRISS methodology found a benefit of aeromedical transport only in patients with severe trauma (a probability of survival less than 90%).[11]

In 1990 the Association of Air Medical Services (AAMS) issued a position paper on the appropriate use of emergency air medical services. In 1992 these recommendations were accepted by the California Medicaid provider as reasonable criteria for the use of air medical transport. In a review of 558 consecutive patient transports, 98% had met at least one of the AAMS criteria.[71]

The risk of aeromedical transport can be placed in perspective if the overall risk of death using ground transport, estimated from the trauma score, is compared with the risk when patients are transported by air. Assuming a reduction in risk of between 21% and 52% when transport is by air, the additional risk of death from crashes (6 per 100,000 transports, or 0.006 per transport) is negligible in comparison to the benefits. This is probably true, however, only for patients with moderate to severe, but nonmortal, injuries (i.e., trauma scores between 5 and 14). Those having minor injuries, with near 100% likelihood of survival, are unlikely to gain additional benefit; those having mortal injuries, with little hope of survival, are unlikely to be saved by any means attempted or employed.

The decision to transport a patient by air requires judgment and a realistic appraisal of the risks. A patient should be transported by air only if he or she is so ill that transport is necessary; if ground transport is unavailable, delayed, or unable to reach the patient; or if aeromedical transport would reduce the risk of death by permitting more rapid access to definitive care, providing greater medical skill en route, or both.

SUMMARY

It has been estimated that since aircraft took to the sky to assist in the emergency transport of sick and injured patients, more than 1 million have been transported over 100 million miles. With a conservative estimate of mortality reduction of even 10%, close to 100,000 patients may owe their lives to the speed and skill provided by aeromedical transport teams.[47]

DISCLAIMER

The opinions expressed in this chapter are those of the authors and do not necessarily represent the opinion or endorsement of the Department of Veterans Affairs, the Department of Defense, or the United States Air Force.

REFERENCES

1. Abraham E, Lee G, Morgan MT: Conjunctival oxygen tension monitoring during helicopter transport of critically ill patients, *Ann Emerg Med* 15:782, 1986.
2. American Academy of Pediatrics: Emergency drug dosages for infants and children and naloxone use in newborns: clarification, *Pediatrics* 83:803, 1989.
3. Apgar V: A proposal for new method of evaluation of the newborn infant, *Anesth Analg* 32:260, 1953.

4. Bagnoud B et al: *Mountain rescue today: colour atlas of mountain medicine,* London, 1991, Wolfe.

5. Baxt WG: Is there a role for flight physicians on EMS rotorcraft? *Trauma Q* 39, May 1985.

6. Baxt WG, Moody P: The impact of a rotocraft aeromedical emergency care service on trauma mortality, *JAMA* 249:3047, 1983.

7. Baxt WG, Moody P: The impact of a physician as part of the aeromedical prehospital team in patients with blunt trauma, *JAMA* 257:3246, 1987.

8. Baxt WG et al: Hospital-based rotocraft aeromedical emergency care services and trauma mortality: a multicenter study, *Ann Emerg Med* 14:859, 1985.

9. Black RE et al: Air transport of pediatric emergency cases, *N Engl J Med* 207:1465, 1982.

10. Blue B: Aeromedical transport, *J Fam Pract* 36:269, 1993.

11. Boyd CR, Corse KM, Campbell RC: Emergency interhospital transport of the major trauma patient: air versus ground, *J Trauma* 29:789, 1989.

12. Branson RD et al: Utilization of mechanical ventilators in hospital based air ambulance programs, *Hosp Aviat* 5:6, 1986.

13. Burney RE, Fischer RP: Ground versus air transport of trauma victims: medical and logistical considerations, *Ann Emerg Med* 15:1491, 1986.

14. Burney RE et al: Comparison of aeromedical crew performance by patient severity and outcome, *Ann Emerg Med* 21:375, 1992.

15. Cady G: 1993 program survey, *Air Med J,* September 1993.

16. Cauthorne CV, Fedorowicz RJ: Sociological impacts of work/rest schedules on pilots, and their perceptions of performance, *Hosp Aviat* 5:14, 1986.

17. Collett HM: Scene-related accidents, *Hosp Aviat* 5:17, 1986.

18. Collett HM: Weather-related accidents, *Hosp Aviat* 5:15, 1986.

19. Collett HM: Mechanical failure accidents, *Hosp Aviat* 6:11, 1987.

20. Collett HM: Year in review, *Hosp Aviat* 1:3, 1987.

21. Collett HM: 1989 accident review, *J Air Med Transport* 9:12, 1990.

22. Collins RL et al: *Flying 1985 annual & buyers guide,* New York, 1985, Ziff-Davis.

23. Dedrick D et al: Airborne defibrillation study, Washington, DC, 1986, Seventh Annual ASHBEAMS Scientific Assembly (abstract).

24. Defibrillation safety in emergency helicopter transport, *Ann Emerg Med* 18:69, 1989.

25. Del Vecchio RJ: *Physiologic aspects of flight,* Oakdale, NY, 1977, Dowling College Press.

26. Dispatch and communications, *Hosp Aviat* 6:5, 1987.

27. Dürrer B: Practical problems of fixation and evacuation in mountain rescue. In *Proceedings of the International Congress of Mountain Medicine,* Crans, Mont, 1991.

28. Dürrer B: REGA winch rescues,1983 and 1984. In *Proceedings of the International Aeromedical Evacuation Congress,* Zurich, 1985, p 108.

29. Dürrer B, Hassler R, Mosimann U: *Mountaineering accidents in the Swiss Alps and rescue activities of the Swiss Alpine Club, 1992.*

30. Ehrenwerth J, Sonja S, Hackel A: Transport of critically ill adults, *Crit Care Med* 14:543, 1986.

31. Federal Aviation Administration, Department of Transportation: *Federal aviation regulations.* In FAR-AIM 1986, Seattle, 1986, ASA.

32. Fifth annual aircrew survey, *Hosp Aviat* 5:19, 1986.

33. Fischer RP et al: Urban helicopter response to the scene of injury, *J Trauma* 24:946, 1984.

34. Fromom RE et al: Bleeding complications following initiation of thrombolytic therapy for acute myocardial infarction: a comparison of helicopter-transported and nontransported patients, *Ann Emerg Med* 20:1991.

35. Golby SB: Critical care, *AOPA Pilot* 30:39, 1987.

36. Golby SB: Dust off, *AOPA Pilot* 30:46, 1987.

37. Gore JM et al: Evaluation of an emergency cardiac transport system, *Ann Emeg Med* 12:675, 1983.

38. Green B: The aeromedical programs of West Germany, *Hosp Aviat* 6:6, 1987.

39. Guiford FR, Soboroff BJ: Air evacuation, *J Aviat Med* 18:601, 1947.

40. Hamman BL et al: Helicopter transport of trauma victims: does a physician make a difference? *J Trauma* 31:490, 1991.

41. Harless KW et al: Civilian ground and air transport of adults with acute respiratory failure, *JAMA* 240:361, 1978.

42. Harris BH: Performance of aeromedical crew members: training or experience? *Am J Emerg Med* 4:409, 1986.

43. Harris BH: Defibrillation in helicopters, *Ann Emerg Med* 12:517, 1983.

44. Harris BH, Orr RE, Boles ET: Aeromedical transportation for infants and children, *J Pediatr Surg* 10:719, 1975.

45. Hensleigh C, Yelser F: Helicopter megacode, *J Aeromed Health Care* 18, 1984.

46. High altitude operations, *Hosp Aviat,* June 1984, p 4.

47. Hoffman L: Worth their weight in gold, *EMN,* January 1992.

48. Homer: *The Iliad,* Middlesex, England, 1982, Penguin Books (translated by EV Rieu).

49. Jacobs LM et al: Prehospital advanced life support: benefits in trauma, *J Trauma* 24:8, 1984.

50. Kaplan L, Walsh D, Burney RE: Emergency aeromedical transport of patients with acute myocardial infarction, *Ann Emerg Med* 16:55, 1987.

51. Kern L, Komon H: An evaluation of mivacurium chloride: can it be effective in the prehospital setting? *Air Med J* 12:1993 (abstract).

52. Larrey JD: *Memorires de chirurgie militaire et campagnes,* Paris, 1812, J Smith.

53. Lee G: *Flight nursing. principles and practice,* St Louis, 1991, Mosby.

54. Leicht MJ et al: Rural interhospital helicopter transport of motor vehicle trauma victims: causes for delays and recommendations, *Ann Emerg Med* 15:450, 1986.

55. Liskiewicz WJ: An evaluation of the Royal Air Force helicopter search and rescue services in Britain with reference to Royal Air Force Valley, 1980-1989, *J R Soc Med* 85:727, 1992.

56. Low R et al: Factors associated with accidents involving EMS helicopters, *Air Med J* 9:35, 1993.

57. Low RB, Martin D: Accuracy of blood pressure measurements made aboard helicopters, *Ann Emerg Med* 16:510, 1987.

58. Lumpe D: Association of air medical services publishes new voluntary standards, *JEMS* 10:28, 1992.

59. MacDonald RC. Banks JG, Ledingham I: Transportation of the injured, *Injury* 12:225, 1979.

60. Mayer TA, Walker ML: Severity of illness and injury in pediatric air transport, *Ann Emerg Med* 13:108, 1984.

61. McKenny S: Aeromedical evolution, *AMJ,* May-June 1986, p 22.

62. McNeil EL: *Airborne care of the ill and injured,* New York, 1983, Springer-Verlag.

63. Merrill N, Executive Director, Association of Air Medical Services: Personal communication, 1993.

64. Mitchell JT: Stress: the history, status and future of critical incident stress debriefings, *JEMS* 11:47, 1988.

65. Mitchell JT: Stress: development and functions of a critical incident stress debriefing team, *JEMS* 12:43, 1988.

66. Murphy-Macabobby M et al: Neuromuscular blockade in aeromedical airway management, *Ann Emerg Med* 21:1992.

67. National Conference on Cardiopulmonary Resuscitation and Emergency Cardiac Care: Standards and guidelines for cardiopulmonary resuscitation (CPR) and emergency cardiac care (ECC), *JAMA* 255:2905, 1986.

68. National EMS Pilot's Association: Single pilot IFR survey, *Hosp Aviat* 5:17, 1986.

69. Neel S: Army aeromedical evacuation procedures in Vietnam, *JAMA* 204:309, 1968.

70. 1987 hospital aviation directory, *Hosp Aviat* 6:8, 1987.

71. O'Malley R, Watson-Hopkins M: Monitoring the appropriateness of air medical transports, *Air Med J* 9:332, 1993.

72. *Pediatric drug chart,* ed 3, Oregon, 1993, InforMed.

73. Poulton TJ, Kisicki PA: Physiologic monitoring during civilian air medical transport, *Aviat Space Environ Med* 58:367, 1987.

74. Preston N: 1991 air medical accident rates, *J Air Med Transport* 11:14, 1992.

75. Rhee KJ et al: Is the flight physician needed for helicopter emergency medical services? *Ann Emerg Med* 15:174, 1986.

76. Rohrer W et al: *Swiss air rescue medical statistics, 1990/1991.*

77. Rosen P et al: Prehospital care: an integrated concept of emergency medicine, *Top Emerg Med* 1:19, 1980.

78. Sandmel S, editor: *The New English Bible,* Luke 10:33-35.

79. Sayre MR, Weisgerber I: The use of neuromuscular blocking agents by air medical services, *J Air Med Transport,* January 1992.

80. Secretary of the Air Force: *Aeromedical evacuation,* Background Information Rep No 68-3, 1968, US Air Force Office of Information.

81. Shea D: The role of nurses and paramedics on EMS rotorcraft, *Trauma Q,* May 1985, p 33.

82. Shields G: Personal communication, 1993, Maryland State Police.

83. Shufflebarger C, Townsend R: Letter to the editor, *JAMA* 258:2378, 1987.

84. Shufflebarger C et al: Transconjunctival oxygen monitoring as a predictor of hypoxemia during helicopter transport, *Am J Emerg Med* 4:501, 1986.

85. Snow N, Hull C, Severns, J: Physician presence on a helicopter emergency medical service: necessary or desirable? *Aviat Space Environ Med* 57:1176, 1986.

86. Sredl DM: *Airborne patient care management: a multidisciplinary approach,* St Louis, 1983, Medical Research Associates.

87. Stanley L, Saunders CE: Stress in aeromedical transport crews: objective measurement in-flight and associated factors, Milwaukee, 1987, Eighth Annual ASHBEAMS/NFNA Conference (abstract).

88. Steinbrunn RN: Preventing and controlling inadvertent IFR, *Air Med J* 9:315, 1993.

89. Stewart RD: Prehospital care of trauma, *Trauma Q,* May 1985, p 1.

90. Syverud SA et al: Prehospital use of neuromuscular blocking agents in a helicopter ambulance program, *Ann Emerg Med* 16:500, 1987.

91. Thomas F, Clemmer TP, Orme JF: A survey of advanced life support procedures being performed by physicians and nurses used on hospital aeromedical evacuation services, *Aviat Space Environ Med* 56:1213, 1985.

92. US Department of Transportation, National Highway Traffic Safety Administration; American Medical Association Commission on Emergency Medical Services: *Air ambulance guidelines,* Washington, DC, 1981, DOT.

93. Waddell G et al: Effects of ambulance transport in critically ill patients, *Br Med J* 1:386, 1975.

94. Waggoner RR et al: Airborne defibrillation . . . the sequel, *J Air Med Transport,* February 1991.

95. Wegman F et al: Sixteen years with the Danish search and rescue helicopter service, *Aviat Space Environ Med* 61:436, 1990.

96. Whitman J: *Preparing a landing zone,* NEMSPA, September 1991.

28 Wilderness Survival

Warren D. Bowman

This chapter examines the human body's requirements for homeostasis and how they can be satisfied in a wilderness environment where little oxygen, food, or water may be available and where extremes of heat or cold may exist. The requirements are similar whether the individual becomes lost with few resources during a simple day hike or whether injury occurs or severe environmental conditions develop during a well-planned wilderness expedition. Although improvisation and living off the land are mentioned, *anticipation, prevention,* and especially *preplanning* are much more important and form the core of this discussion. As an example taken from Antarctic exploration, Roald Amundsen's style of thorough preparation and the use of well-tested equipment should be emulated rather than Robert Scott's intuitive and untested approach.[12]

The outcome of an encounter with severe environmental stress varies with the type, magnitude, and duration of the stress and with the stressed subject's resources. These resources include the state of acclimatization; physical integrity, particularly conditioning and the presence of illness or injury; experience; equipment and the ability to improvise intelligently; and such intangibles as "backcountry common sense" and the will to survive. The recommendations in this chapter are based on personal experience, the opinions of survival experts, research, and analysis of actual survival situations. General principles are emphasized, but "tricks of the trade" may hold the key to life or death. Unfortunately, most of the lay literature emphasizes tales of misfortune, hazardous adventures, and mindless bravado in the face of unnecessary hardships brought on by errors of the participants, while great deeds go unrecorded or forgotten because the experience and competence of the adventurers kept catastrophic, "newsworthy" experiences to a minimum. In the words of Corneille, "To vanquish without risk is to triumph without glory."[6]

Increased leisure time and growing interest in outdoor activities place more people into settings where survival situations may develop. The cross-country skier, winter mountaineer, and winter camper may be exposed to extremes of cold and storms. The expeditionary mountaineer may explore regions where winter exists year-round and where ambient oxygen is low. The desert traveler may be exposed to extremes of heat and the tropical traveler to extremes of both heat and humidity. Passengers in aircraft, seacraft, or land vehicles may be stranded in almost any type of environment. A common thread in the development of life- or limb-threatening emergencies is the insistence on traveling during storms and other stressful environmental conditions, when more prudent persons would stay put in a comfortable bivouac. Excuses for this include reaching a predetermined but not essential goal on time so that others will not worry. Physicians who participate in wilderness recreation or treat adventurers need to be aware of the physiologic and psychologic impacts of environmental stress and how related deleterious effects can be prevented and treated.

The knowledgeable traveler should plan for unexpected situations using preventive aspects of survival. This includes being familiar with weather forecasts, strategizing worst-case scenarios, carrying emergency items, avoiding solo travel in isolated areas, and leaving notice of the projected route and expected time of return. With good planning, deteriorating weather or an injury-forced bivouac becomes more of an inconvenience than a life-threatening ordeal. However, chance plays a part in survival. Serious but unforeseen hazards can occur, or environmental stresses can be so severe that survival is impossible regardless of preparations. Anyone who ventures into wilderness must accept the possibility, however remote, of death or serious injury.

For survival the body requires a constant supply of oxygen, a core temperature regulated within relatively narrow limits (about 24° to 42° C [75° to 107° F]), water, food, and self-confidence, faith, and will to live. For comfort and optimum performance, body temperature must be close to normal, and the body must be rested, well nourished, in top physical condition, and free from disease and injury. The most immediate of these requirements are maintenance of body integrity (through accident prevention) and regulation of body temperature. Dehydration, starvation, and exhaustion make temperature maintenance more difficult and interfere with the rational thought and agility required to prevent accidents. Insufficient oxygen becomes a contributing factor at extreme altitude or in such mishaps as suffocation caused by avalanche burial or carbon monoxide (CO) poisoning from cooking in an unventilated shelter. Abundant food and water are of little value to a hypothermic person with insufficient clothing and shelter or to the victim of heatstroke, even though lack of food and water eventually weaken and kill an otherwise healthy individual. Lack of self-confidence, faith, and the will to live may cause an attitude of panic and defeatism that prevents a person from taking timely survival actions, such as conserving energy, preparing shelter, or lighting a fire. Poor physical conditioning or the presence of illness or injury may interfere with the body's ability to produce heat by shivering or to lose heat by sweating and increasing skin perfusion, which can hamper wood gathering, shelter building, and other necessary actions.[4]

The most important organ for survival is the *human brain*, since voluntary actions such as preparedness, regulation of energy expenditure, adjustment of clothing, and seeking shelter are more important than involuntary mechanisms of adaptation to environmental stress.

OXYGEN

As a human ascends from sea level, the body is subjected to increasing cold, decreasing oxygen, increasing solar radiation, and decreasing atmospheric pressure. For every 305 m (1000 feet) of altitude gain, the ambient temperature drops by about 2.2° C (4° F), the barometric pressure drops by about 20 mm Hg (0.1 mb/m), and the amount of ultraviolet (UV) radiation increases by about 5%. The percentage of oxygen in the atmosphere remains constant, but the partial pressure of oxygen diminishes with altitude so that at 3077 m (10,000 feet) it is only two-thirds that at sea level and at 5488 m (18,000 feet) only half.[3]

During acute exposure to high altitude the effects of hypoxia initially can cause fatigue, weakness, headache, anorexia, nausea, vomiting, dyspnea on exertion, insomnia, and Cheyne-Stokes respirations (see Chapter 1). These symptoms are probably present to some degree in everyone who goes rapidly from sea level to 2462 m (8000 feet) or above. The clinical effects of hypoxia are often difficult to distinguish from those of cold, high winds, dehydration, and exhaustion. Serious degrees of acute mountain sickness (AMS) are unusual below 3692 to 4308 m (12,000 to 14,000 feet) but have been reported in trekkers as low as 2308 m (7500 feet). In Yellowstone National Park, mild AMS is not infrequently seen in visitors at just over 1829 m (6000 feet). At any height, oxygen in ambient air may be prevented from reaching the cellular level because of interruption of normal transport pathways, generally by illness or injury. Examples of this in the wilderness include the following[4]:

1. Insufficient oxygen in inspired air in avalanche burial, near drowning, or living in a poorly ventilated snow cave
2. Upper airway obstruction from a facial injury, blockage by the tongue in an unresponsive patient, or aspiration of foreign material
3. Interference with proper lung function caused by pneumonia, pulmonary edema, pulmonary hemorrhage, pulmonary contusion, atelectasis, hemothorax, pneumothorax, or chest wall injury
4. Circulatory insufficiency caused by myocardial infarction, pericardial tamponade, shock, or pulmonary embolism
5. Interference with ventilatory control after injury to the respiratory center or hyperviscosity-induced cerebral infarction
6. Interference with the oxygen-carrying capacity of the blood from anemia or CO poisoning

The emergency and definitive treatments of such conditions follow standard techniques detailed elsewhere in this book and include the administration of oxygen, if available. CO poisoning is probably a greater hazard than is generally appreciated. Many famous polar explorers, including Byrd, Andree, and Stefannson, were killed by or had narrow escapes from the effects of stoves operated in tightly enclosed living areas.[20]

REGULATION OF BODY TEMPERATURE

Humans are called *homeotherms* because as warm-blooded animals they maintain a body temperature that varies within very narrow limits despite changes in environmental temperature. In *poikilotherms*, or cold-blooded animals, body temperature varies with that of the environment. Homeothermy is necessary to support the enzyme systems of the human body, which function best at 37° to 37.5° C (98.6° to 100° F). The human body can be viewed as a heat-generating and heat-dissipating machine where internal temperature is the net result of opposing mechanisms that tend to increase or decrease body heat production, increase or decrease body heat loss, and increase or decrease addition of heat from the outside. Through these mechanisms the internal body temperature usually can be regulated successfully despite ambient temperatures that vary more than 55° C (100° F) from the coldest to the hottest seasons in temperate climates.

Basal body heat production occurs at about 50 kcal/m²/hr. This can be increased by muscular activity (involuntary [shivering] and voluntary), eating, inflammation and infection (fever), and in response to cold exposure. Shivering can increase heat production up to 5 times the basal rate and vigorous exercise up to 10 times. Cold exposure increases hunger, the secretion of epinephrine, norepinephrine, and thyroxine, and semiconscious activity such as foot stamping and dancing in place. Eating provides not only needed calories but also the temporary increase in basal metabolic rate that occurs during digestion alone (specific dynamic action, or SDA). The SDA of protein is five to seven times higher than that of fat and carbohydrate and lasts longer. However, the onset of the SDA is much faster with carbohydrate than with protein or fat. Therefore the person who is cold inside a sleeping bag at bedtime should eat carbohydrate, and to stay warm all night, protein.

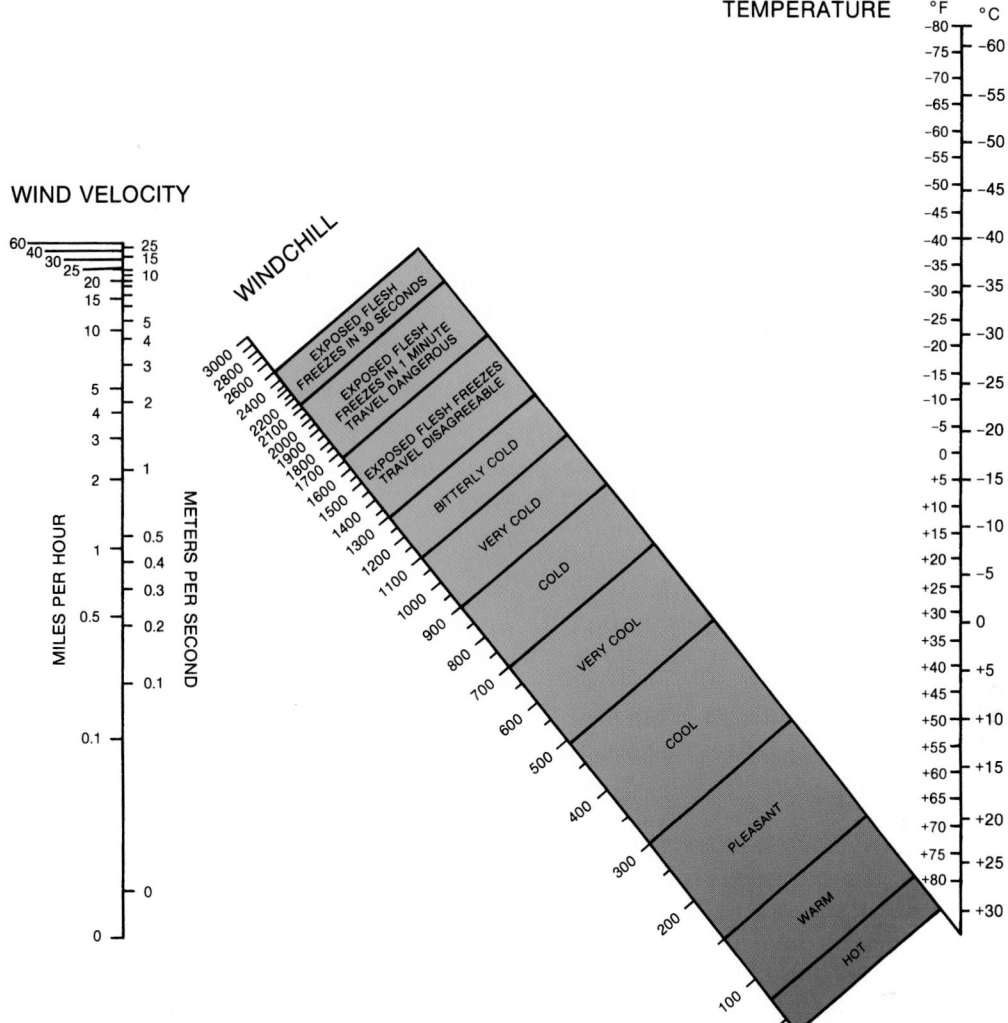

Figure 28-1 Line chart showing windchill and state of comfort under varying conditions of temperature and wind velocity. The numbers along the left margin of the diagonal center block refer to the windchill factor, that is, that rate of cooling in kilocalories per square meter per hour of an unclad, inactive body exposed to specific temperatures and wind velocities. Windchill factors above 1400 are most hazardous.

In hot weather, body heat production can be decreased by slowing muscular activity and avoiding foods with a high SDA.

In cold weather, heat can be added to the body by close exposure to a fire or other heat source, such as sunlight, and by ingesting hot food and drink. In hot weather, external heat addition can be decreased by staying in the shade, wearing clothing that blocks the sun's rays, and avoiding hot objects and hot food and drink.

The body loses heat to the environment by conduction, convection, evaporation, radiation, and respiration. It may gain heat from the environment by the same mechanisms (except for evaporation). The relative importance of these mechanisms depends on temperature, humidity, wind velocity, cloud cover, insulation, contact with hot or cold objects, sweating, and muscular exercise. With a resting body in still air at 21° C (70° F), radiation, conduction, and convection ac-

count for 70% of total heat loss, evaporation for 27%, and urination, defecation, and respiration for only 3%. During work, however, evaporation may account for up to 85% of heat loss.[4]

It is useful to think of the body as composed of a core (heart, lungs, liver, adrenal glands, central nervous system, and other vital organs) and a shell (skin, muscles, and extremities). Most of the adjustments in response to cold or heat exposure occur in the shell. They are designed to maintain a relatively constant core temperature; in below-freezing weather, these adjustments may predispose parts of the shell to frostbite and other types of localized cold injury.

The importance of avoiding travel and seeking shelter during storms and extreme cold cannot be overemphasized. The additive chilling effect of wind when added to cold is impressive. Windchill charts (Figure 28-1) show the relationship between actual temperature,

TABLE 28-1. Fiber Characteristics of Natural and Synthetic Fibers

FABRIC	SPECIFIC GRAVITY* (RATIO TO WATER)	THERMAL CONDUCTANCE† (cal/m²)	EVAPORATIVE ABILITY‡	WICKING ABILITY	MOISTURE REGAIN§
Wool	1.32	2.1	Low	Moderate	17
Cotton	1.54	6.1	Low	High	7.9
Nylon	1.14	2.4	High	Low	4
Polyester	1.38	2.4	High	Low	1
Acrylic	1.15	2.4	High	High	1
Polypropylene	0.91	1.2	High	High	5

Modified from Davis AK: *Nordic skiing—a scientific approach*, Minneapolis, 1980, University of Minnesota.
*The lower the specific gravity, the better the insulating ability.
†The lower the thermal conductance, the slower the flow of heat from the body.
‡The higher the evaporative ability, the shorter the amount of time a fiber will be wet, that is, in a reduced insulative state.
§Moisture regain is the amount of moisture a fiber can absorb before feeling wet.

wind velocity, and "effective" temperature at the body surface. "Windchill" refers to the *rate* of cooling; the actual temperature reached is no lower than it would be if wind were absent (unless evaporation of liquid is occurring from the body surface). The increase in heat loss as the wind rises is not linear; rather, it is roughly proportional to the *square root* of the wind speed.

At moderate ambient temperatures the body's core temperature is kept stable by constant small adjustments in metabolic rate, muscular activity, sweating, and skin circulation. When the body is chilled, automatic and semiautomatic mechanisms increase internal heat production by slightly increasing the metabolic rate, by shivering, and by semiconscious activities (e.g., foot stamping) and reduce heat loss by diminishing sweat production and shell circulation. The person has a strong urge to curl up in a ball, thereby reducing the body's surface area. At the same time the brain tells the body to decrease heat loss by adding insulation and wind protection, to seek shelter, and to increase heat gain by increasing muscular activity, building a fire, seeking sunlight, and eating.[4]

When the body overheats, these actions are reversed. The body increases heat loss by increasing circulation to the skin and extremities and increasing sweating. These mechanisms require more water, which stimulates the thirst response. Heat production is decreased because of a feeling of sluggishness and languor, leading to a reduction in physical activity and in the amount of heat produced by muscles. The brain tells the body to decrease heat gain and increase heat loss by providing shelter from the sun, removing clothing, and fanning oneself.

COLD WEATHER SURVIVAL

Body temperature in a cold environment is maintained by decreasing heat loss, increasing internal body heat production, and adding heat from the outside. The most efficient of these methods is conservation of body heat by decreasing heat loss, generally by using clothing and shelter.

Decreasing Heat Loss

Heat loss from conduction and convection can be prevented by interposing substances of low thermal conductivity, such as clothing made of good insulating materials, between the body and outside air. Clothing creates a microclimate of warmed, still air next to the skin surface. Clothing's value depends on how well it traps air, the thickness of the air layer, and whether these qualities are reduced by wetting (Table 28-1). Traditional insulating materials are wool, down, foam, and older synthetics such as Orlon, Dacron, and polyester. Wool retains warmth when wet because of moderately low wicking action and a unique ability to suspend water vapor within its fibers without affecting its low thermal conductance. It can absorb a considerable amount of water without feeling wet but is heavier than synthetics, itchy, and more difficult to dry. Its toughness and durability, however, make it a good choice for garments subject to hard wear, such as trousers, mittens, and socks. Cotton, particularly denim and corduroy, is a poor insulator. It dries slowly because of low evaporative ability; high thermal conductance is further increased by wetting. Cotton has no place in the backcountry in cold weather.

Orlon, acrylic, and polyester were developed to duplicate the properties of wool without wool's higher cost. They traditionally have been used in hats, sweaters, and long underwear. They are almost as warm and not as itchy as wool, and they evaporate moisture better. A number of newer fabrics are woven from fibers that have lower thermal conductance, greater insulating ability, and better wicking action than traditional fibers. Examples include polypropylene and treated polyesters, such as Capilene, Thermax, and Thermastat. Polyester is also made into pile and fleece, which are light, dry easily, trap air well, and stay warm when wet because the fibers do not absorb water. Examples are Polartec, Borglite, Polarplus, and Synchilla. Fibers used as fillers in quilted garments include hollow synthetic fibers designed on the principle of reindeer hair, such as Hollofil II and Quallofil. Microfibers that provide good insulating ability with less bulk include Thinsulate, Thermoloft, and Thermolite. One of the newest microfibers, Microloft, is supposed to be warmer than down at the same weight. New synthetics come on the market frequently—consult trade journals and "gear" issues of outdoor magazines.

The "layer principle" of clothing is effective in preventing overheating and chilling. Multiple layers of clothing provide multiple layers of microclimate. Layers are added as necessary to prevent chilling or subtracted to prevent excessive perspiration. Since water conducts heat 25 to 32 times faster than air at the same temperature, clothing wetted by perspiration or water may cause rapid heat loss from conduction and evaporation. The need to add or subtract layers should be anticipated before chilling or heavy perspiring occur.

Clothing should be easily adjustable, sweaters should be of the zipper or cardigan type, and outer layers should be cut full enough to allow expansion of inner layers to their full thicknesses. Zippers in the axillary and lateral thigh areas are useful for ventilation.

Loss of heat from convection can be prevented by wearing windproof outer garments of nylon, tightly woven cotton-nylon blends, or water-resistant laminates such as Gore-Tex. Typical examples include a parka with hood and a pair of windproof pants (regular or bib style) or ski warm-up pants.

The loss of heat from infrared radiation can also be prevented by insulation, emphasizing proper covering for body parts with a large surface area/volume ratio. The uncovered head can dissipate up to 70% of total body heat production at an ambient temperature of $-16°$ C ($5°$ F), partly because the body does not reduce blood supply to the head and neck as it does to the extremities in cold weather. High heat loss through radiation during cold nights can be decreased by sleeping in a tent or under a tarp instead of in the open. Coverage for the head, ears, hands, and feet should not restrict circulation. Developed initially for skiers, the "neck warmer," or "neck gaiter," can be pulled up over the back of the head to form a hood or up over the lower face to form a mask.

Heat loss from the respiratory tract can be diminished by avoiding overexertion and overheating with excessively heavy breathing. When it is extremely cold, inspired air can be warmed by pulling the parka hood out in front of the face to form a "frost tunnel."

Heat loss from conduction occurs by direct contact with a colder object. Sitting on a pack, foam pad, log, or other object of lower heat conductivity is preferable to sitting in the snow or on a cold rock. At low temperatures, bare skin freezes to metal. This can be avoided by wearing light gloves when handling metal objects. Gasoline or other liquids with freezing points lower than that of water can cause frostbite if accidentally poured on the skin at low temperatures. During bivouacs in snow shelters, contact with the snow can be avoided by using a foam pad or improvising a mattress of evergreen boughs, grass, or dry leaves. In cold or windy weather an injured person needs windproof insulating material under as well as over and around the body.

Heat loss from conduction and evaporation can be lessened by avoiding wetting and by changing to dry clothes or drying out quickly when wet. Ideally, outer clothing should be windproof, should not collect snow, and should shed water but not be waterproof, since waterproof garments prevent evaporation of sweat. Newer fabrics, such as Gore-Tex, are suited for this and for outermost layers.

Dressing for Cold Weather

Anyone who ventures outdoors in cold weather should have enough clothing, either on the body or in the backpack, for the most extreme environmental conditions likely to be experienced.

First Layer

LONG UNDERWEAR. Wool is still an excellent choice for long underwear but is expensive and may be difficult to find. Merino wool is less itchy. Polypropylene, acrylic, and the newer polyesters may be preferable because of their lower cost, good insulating ability, and good evaporative ability (see Table 28-1). Again, fabrics containing cotton should be avoided. Synthetics tend to retain body odor more than wool after washing.

SOCKS. One or two pairs of moderate to heavy wool or wool/nylon blend socks are excellent, preferably with an additional pair of light polypropylene socks worn underneath next to the skin. At least one spare pair of the wool socks should be carried.

THIN GLOVES (GLOVE LINERS). Light polypropylene, wool, silk, or fingerless wool or pile gloves are useful for moderately cold conditions or when finger dexterity is required, as in adjusting ski bindings. Polyester/Lycra gloves provide a tighter but more stretchable fit to enhance fine finger movements.

Second Layer

SHIRT. Shirts should be made of light, soft wool or a suitable synthetic such as acrylic and should have long sleeves. Large breast pockets with buttons or Velcro are handy to carry items such as sunglasses and a compass. Shirts should open completely in front or at least have a half-zipper. A turtleneck feature protects the neck, as do neck warmers and mufflers, which can be pulled up to protect the lower face.

PANTS. Wool or pile pants are best and should have pockets that are easily accessible for hand warming. Pile pants should have reinforcements at the knees and buttocks and a zipper or Velcro fly for males. Full or partial lateral leg zippers are convenient.

FOOT GEAR. The type of boot chosen depends on the type of activity and the expected environmental temperatures. For moderate temperatures, sturdy leather climbing boots made of full-thickness leather, 6 to 8 inches in height with rubber lug soles and roomy enough to accommodate the desired numbers of socks, are ideal. Boots made of leather and fabric such as Gore-Tex are lighter and suited for trail hiking but are not as durable for rough terrain.

Boots must be long enough so that the toes do not strike the front of the boot during downhill walking. They should be laced firmly enough that the heel does not move up and down, but not so tightly that circulation is restricted and the toes cannot be wiggled easily.

For colder temperatures, double boots are preferable. These can be all-leather boots or can have outer shells of plastic or nylon with inner boots of felt or foam. All-leather versions are becoming difficult to obtain. The Canadian type of shoe-pak (e.g., Sorel) with a removable inner felt liner is a good choice for light snowshoeing and other nontechnical outdoor activities in the cold. Special double ski boots are available for ski touring, Telemark skiing, and ski mountaineering, depending on whether three-pin or mountaineering ski bindings are used.

HAT. Hats should be of the stocking variety, made of wool, pile, Orlon, polypropylene, or wool-polypropylene, and large enough to cover the ears. A small bill feature is desirable to shade the eyes. "Bomber" caps with bills and pull-down earflaps and "Andean" caps with ear coverings are popular. Some arrangement should be provided to protect the face from cold wind, as with a balaclava configuration or a separate face mask. A useful combination is a ski hat with a neck warmer that can be pulled up to cover most of the lower face.

Third Layer

PARKA. The parka can be a standard ski or mountain parka filled with down, Dacron, Quallofil, Thinsulate, or other lofting material. A more versatile combina-

tion is two separate garments: a pile jacket plus a Gore-Tex shell. For snow camping a pile jacket with a thin outer layer of nylon (three-season, squall, or warm-up jacket) may be preferred because, unlike an uncovered pile jacket, it does not collect snow when worn without the shell. The shell should have a hood with a drawstring, a two-way zipper with an overlying weather flap closed with snaps or Velcro, a cloth flap to protect the chin from the metal zipper pull, armpit and/or lateral chest zippers for ventilation, and at least four outer pockets plus one or two inside pockets to contain frequently needed items (e.g., gloves, compass, map, sunglasses, neck warmer). Outer pockets should be located where they can be reached while wearing a backpack with a fastened waist belt. The shell should be fingertip length unless bibs are worn.

Pockets with horizontal openings may close with Velcro, but those with vertical openings should close with zippers. Because the parka is anchored by the shoulders, when using one hand it is generally easier to pull a vertical zipper down than up. In some brands of parkas, vertical zippers are pulled *down* to close the pockets; in other brands they are pulled *up*. I prefer the *down* type because the danger of losing pocket contents from difficulty closing a zipper is worse than any delay from difficulty opening a zipper.

For ventilation, there should be zippered openings at the armpits. These should be large enough so the parka can be converted into a vestlike garment during warm conditions by inserting the wearer's arms through the openings and tucking the sleeves inside the parka. Since these zippers usually perform more easily when pulled from the distal to the proximal direction, this direction should close them, since increasing wind protection is usually more urgent than decreasing it (freezing is more dangerous than sweating).

WIND PANTS. These should be light and water repellent; Gore-Tex is a good choice. Long, zippered side openings are useful to permit donning pants without removing boots, as well as for ventilation and access to inner pants pockets.

HAND GEAR. One of the more serious and still unsolved cold weather problems is how to keep fingers warm while leaving them unhampered enough to do work. Mittens are warmer than gloves since fingers that touch each other warm each other, but even thin mittens do not allow delicate finger movements. An important part of the cold finger solution is to prevent core cooling and compensatory extremity vasoconstriction by addressing core temperature stabilization through exercise, eating, and wearing enough layers on the trunk.

A common strategy is to wear a pair of thin gloves of polypropylene, silk, thin wool, or polyester-Lycra inside a wool or pile mitten covered with a windproof and water-resistant glove shell. For delicate finger work, the gloved hand is removed from the mitten, the work done as fast as possible, and the hand returned to the mitten. However, since insulating materials insulate in both directions, when inside a warm mitten, cold fingers wearing gloves will not rewarm as fast as cold, bare fingers. Therefore another solution is to use bare fingers, which will perform faster than gloved fingers, returning them to warm mittens periodically until the task is done. This is not practical, however, when working with metal in very cold weather. Another approach is to keep a pair of gloves warm in a pocket and put them on after removing the hands from mittens. Polyester-Lycra gloves are easier to don than many other types of thin gloves.

Excellent three-layer mitten sets include windproof shells with leather palms and two sets of removable pile mittens, at least one of which is fastened with Velcro. Another good system is a thin glove liner inside a heavy wool (Dachstein, ragg, or wool-polypropylene) mitten inside a Gore-Tex shell. An option that gives more finger dexterity in moderately cold conditions is a polypropylene glove liner inside a fingerless wool glove inside a shell. However, more layers result in more difficulty working with the hands. Shells should have easily accessible "nose warmers" of pile or mouton on the backs, should be long enough to cover the wrists, and should have palms of soft leather or sticky fabric for securely holding ice axes and ski poles.

GAITERS AND OVERBOOTS. Gaiters, which are long nylon tubes that cover the lower leg and upper part of the boot, are designed to keep snow, sand, and gravel out of boots and socks. They extend upward to just below the knee, open at the side or in front with a zipper or Velcro, and have a strap that fits under the boot sole to keep them snug on the boots and a drawstring at the top to hold them up. Gaiters with a front opening closed by a wide Velcro strap are easiest to don and doff. Shorter versions that extend to just above the ankle are adequate for summer mountaineering and may be preferable for cross-country skiers who need access for tightening boot buckles before descents.

High-altitude mountaineering requires special insulated overboots or lined gaiters.

Fourth Layer. The previous three layers are usually worn on the body. A fourth layer should be easily available in the pack. This should include quilted or pile pants and jacket (or vest).

RAIN GEAR. In moderate climates or in spring conditions when rain and wet snow may be encountered, outer garments of Gore-Tex or similar material should be used. For maritime climates and during seasons of heavy rain, it may be better to have two separate sets of outer garments: a light, thin, windproof nylon jacket and pants and a waterproof (coated nylon) jacket and pants.

Vapor Barrier Systems. Waterproof garments and sleeping bag liners close to the skin can prevent saturation of outer clothing and sleeping bags with sweat and the resulting reduction in insulating value. Sweating is reduced, and body water requirements are decreased. Vapor barriers seem to work better in very cold weather than at moderate temperatures. A light garment of polypropylene or similar material should be worn next to the skin, with the waterproof garment over this. Persons with hyperhidrosis and those who dislike clammy skin may object to a vapor barrier system.

Shelter

Everyone who spends time in the wilderness should practice the construction of several types of emergency survival shelters. The function of a shelter is to provide an extension of the microclimate of still, warm air furnished by clothing and to contain heat generated by the body, a fire, or other heat source. A properly designed shelter should permit easy and rapid construction with simple tools and should give good protection from wind, rain, and snowfall. The type and size of shelter depend on the presence or absence of snow and its depth, on natural features of the landscape, and on whether firewood or a stove and fuel are available. If external heat cannot be provided, a shelter must be small and windproof to preserve body heat.

Small trees, branches, thick grass, leaf piles, small caves, and snow holes under downed trees or dense evergreens can be used. If possible, a shelter should be constructed in the timber to provide protection from the wind and access to firewood. Generally, shelters partway up the side of a ridge are warmer than those in a valley, since cold air tends to collect in valleys and basins during the night. Exposed, windy ridges above the timberline are cold. Areas exposed to flooding (drainages, dry river beds), rockfalls, or avalanches and under dead trees or limbs should be avoided. If open water is available, the camp may be located nearby, although in nonsurvival conditions, camps should be at least 200 feet from bodies of water. To avoid drifting snow, tents and shelters should be located with the entrance at right angles to the prevailing winds.

TABLE 28-2. Thermal Conductivity of Various Substances

SUBSTANCE	CONDUCTIVITY*	TEMPERATURE MEASURED (° C)
Air	0.006	0
Down	0.01	20
Polyester (hollow)	0.016	
Polyester (solid)	0.019	
Snow (old)	0.115	0
Cork	0.128	30
Sawdust	0.14	30
Wool felt	0.149	40
Cardboard	0.5	20
Wood	0.8	20
Dry sand	0.93	20
Water	1.4	12
Brick	1.5	20
Concrete	2.2	20
Ice	5.7	0

*Conductivity is the quantity of heat in gram calories transmitted per second through a plate of material 1 cm thick and 1 cm² in area when the temperature difference between the sides of the plate is 1° C.

Snow is a good insulator (Table 28-2). Its heat conductivity is $\frac{1}{10,000}$ that of copper and somewhat better than wool felt, so snow shelters may be warmer than other types of constructed shelters as long as the inhabitants remain dry. Contact with the snow or cold ground is avoided by using a foam pad, dry leaves, grass, or (in survival conditions only) a bed of evergreen boughs.

Natural Shelters. Caves and alcoves under overhangs are good shelters and can be improved by building wind walls with rocks, snow blocks, or brush. A fire should be built in such a way that heat reflects onto the occupant. The fire should be 5 to 6 feet from the back of the shelter, with a reflector wall of logs or stones on the opposite side of the fire; the occupant should sit between the fire and the back of the shelter (Figure 28-2).

In deep snow, large fallen logs and bent-over evergreens frequently have hollows under them that can be used as small caves. Cone-shaped depressions around the trunks of evergreens ("tree wells") can be improved by digging them out and roofing them over with evergreen branches or a tarp. A fire built to one side of such a shelter will reflect its heat off the snow toward the occupant. Ventilation must be adequate,

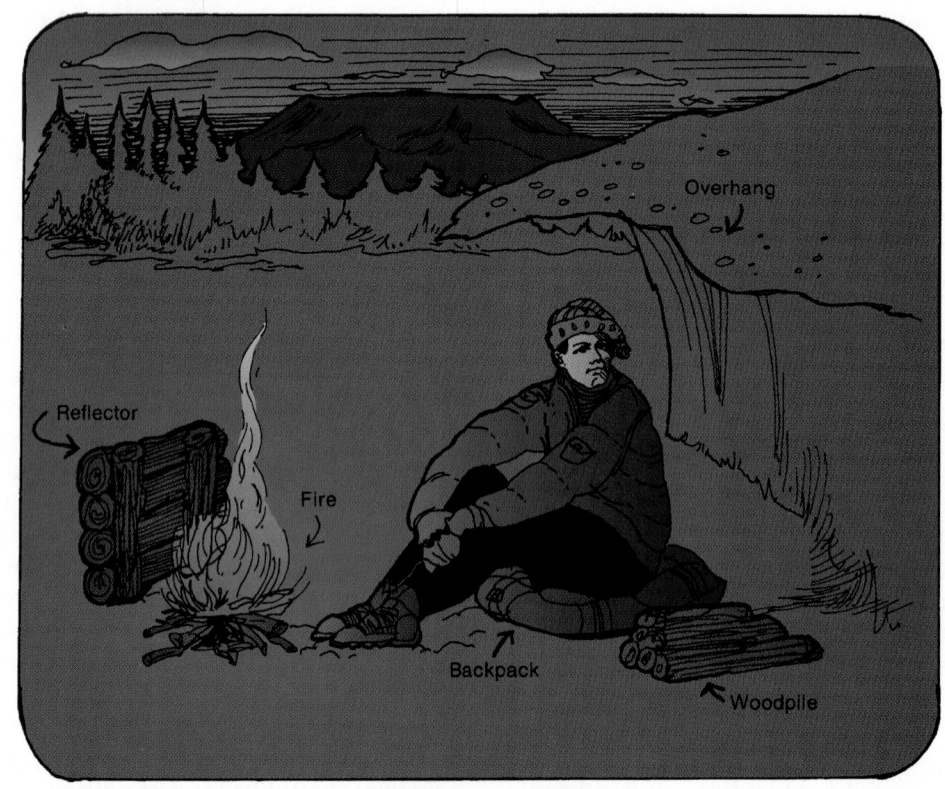

Figure 28-2 Natural shelter.

and the fire should not be positioned under snow-laden branches.

Constructed Shelters. When no snow is available, shelters can be built of small trees, branches, brush, and boughs. A tarp can be rigged into a lean-to shelter. In cold weather the most satisfactory form is a lean-to with two sides closed with brush, a fire at the open front, and a wall of logs or stones on the far side of the fire to reflect heat into the lean-to's interior (Figure 28-3). Walls or roofs of brush, branches, or broad leaves should be thatched (i.e., each layer should overlap the one below it).

Snow Shelters. If snow shelters become too warm, the walls will be wet and the roof will drip. A useful rule of thumb is that persons inside a snow shelter should be able to see their breath at all times.[24]

Snow Trenches. A snow trench is the easiest and quickest survival snow shelter and the one least likely to make the diggers wet. It can be dug in most areas that are flat or on slight to moderate inclines as long as the snow is 3 feet or deeper or can be piled to that depth. A 4 × 6–foot trench can be dug in 20 minutes, one end roofed over with a tarp or boughs, and a fire built at the opposite end (Figure 28-4).

If a large tarp and a stove are available, a trench can be dug that is as comfortable as a snow cave and will hold two or three people. The object is to keep the maximal amount of snow around and over the trench. The trench is dug as narrow as possible at the surface while still providing sufficient room to shovel; a suitable size for the top is 4 feet wide and 8 feet long. It is undercut at the back and sides so that the bottom is 6 to 7 feet wide and 9 to 10 feet long (Figure 28-5). A narrow en-

trance helps contain heat and can be closed with a small plastic sheet or a pack. Four or more skis or small tree trunks are laid from side to side over the top of the trench, with ski poles or branches interwoven at right angles. A tarp is then laid on top of these and snow piled around its edges to hold it down. In very cold weather the entire tarp can be covered by a layer of snow; at least 8 inches is needed for proper insulation. When the entrance is closed, a small stove and the occupants' body heat will raise the interior temperature to −4° to −1° C (25° to 30° F). Higher temperatures should be avoided so that clothing and bedding will not become wet from melting snow.

Above the timberline in deep, wind-packed snow, a similar trench can be roofed with snow blocks that are laid horizontally, set as an A-frame, or laid on skis (Figure 28-6). Chinks between the blocks are caulked with snow.

Snow Caves. Although a small snow cave large enough for one person can be dug with a ski or cooking pot, it is much better to have a shovel. Two shovels are best: a medium-sized general-purpose aluminum scoop

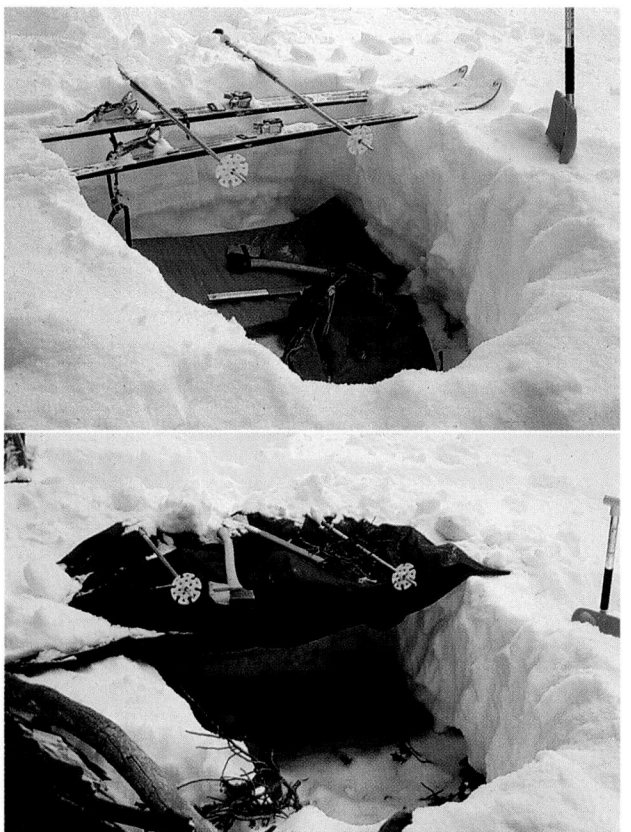

A

B

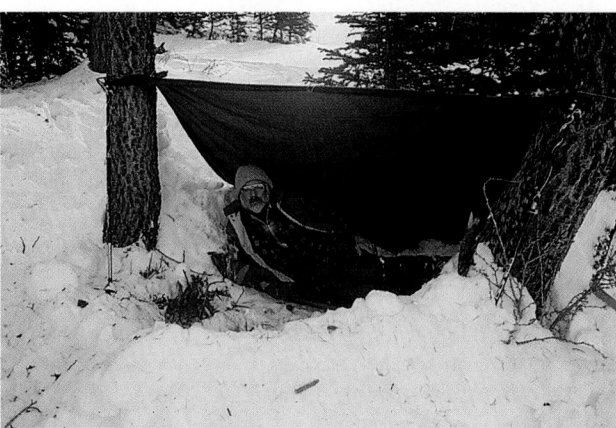

Figure 28-3 Lean-to shelter. Sides should be closed with brush or snow and a fire built in front.

Figure 28-4 Emergency snow trench. **A,** Pit is dug and overlaid with skis and poles. **B,** Tarp is placed over the skis and secured with snow and heavy objects.

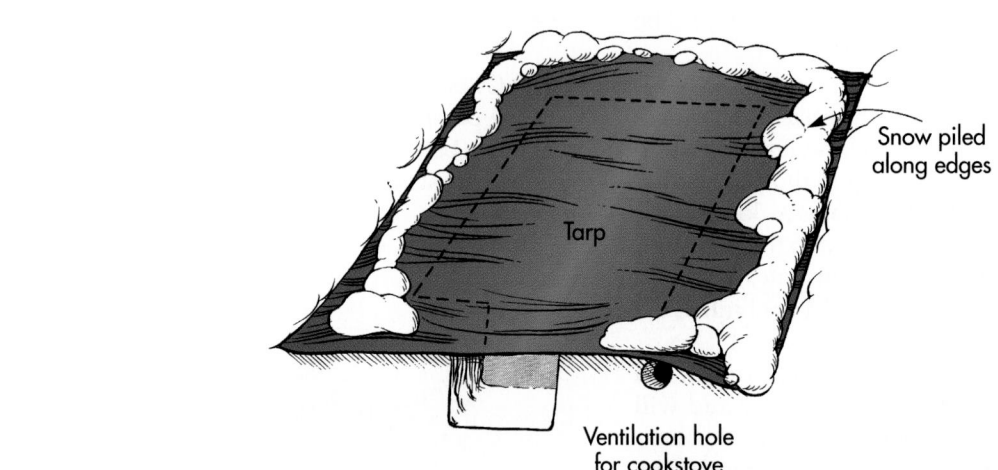

Sides and ends undercut

Narrow entrance

A

Ski poles

Skis

Snow piled along edges

Tarp

Ventilation hole for cookstove

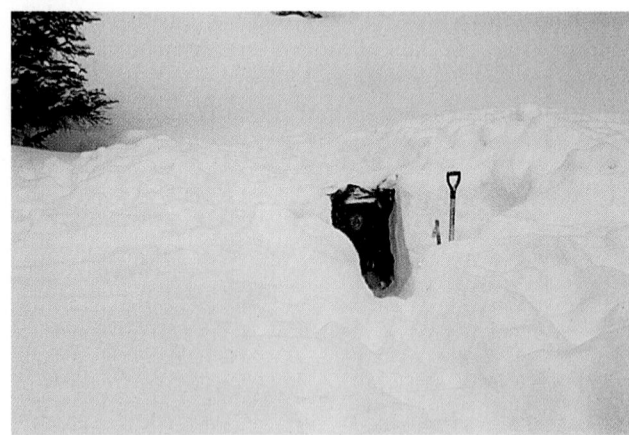

B

Figure 28-5   A, Three-person snow trench. **B,** Completed trench the morning after a heavy snowfall.

shovel and a small, straight shovel (French type) to use while excavating the interior of the cave. The site is a large snow drift such as found on the lee side of a small hill. Areas in avalanche zones are avoided (see Chapter 2). The entrance is dug just large enough to crawl through and is angled upward toward the sleeping chamber (Figure 28-7, *A*), which should be large enough for a stove and two occupants lying side by side. After the entrance is dug with the scoop shovel,

the digger crawls inside, lies supine, and uses the straight shovel to excavate the chamber until room is sufficient to move around and use the larger scoop shovel. A ventilation hole as large as a ski pole basket is cut in the roof over the cooking area. A cave large enough for two persons takes several hours to dig. Pine branches or other natural material are used to cover the floor if a sleeping pad is not available. Since the diggers tend to become wet, water-resistant or waterproof jack-

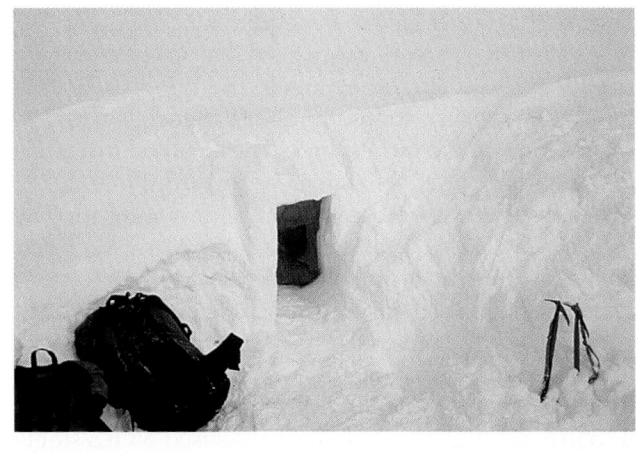

Figure 28-6 A, Above-timberline snow trench. **B,** Completed snow trench the morning after a heavy snowfall.

ets and pants should be worn. A faster method is to excavate a large entrance so there is more room to dig, then partly fill in the entrance hole with snow blocks cut with a shovel or snow saw (Figure 28-7, *B* and *C*).

SNOW DOMES. When the ground is flat or the snow cover is shallow, snow can be piled into a large dome 6 to 7 feet high and left to harden for a few hours (Figure 28-8). A low entrance is dug on one side, and from

there the interior is carved out to make a dome-shaped room large enough to sleep three people. A ventilation hole is cut in the roof over the stove.

IGLOOS. Igloos are the most comfortable arctic shelters but require time, experience, and some engineering skill. They are not recommended for the novice but may be worth the effort if the party will be stranded for any length of time. Igloos require one or ideally two

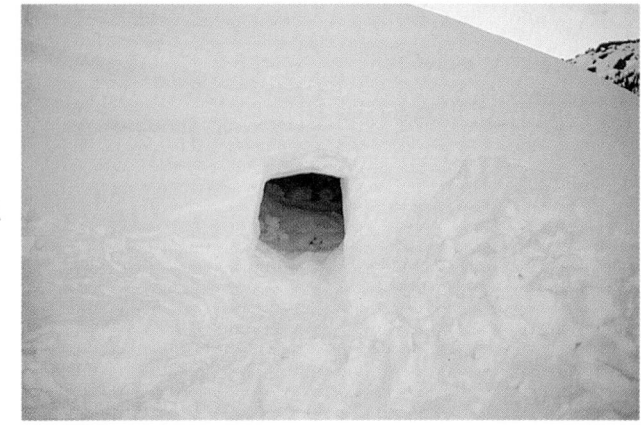

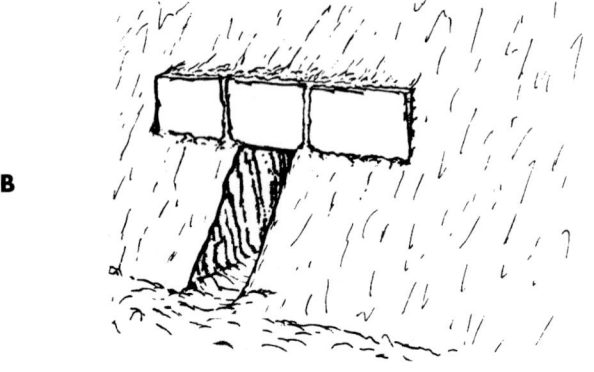

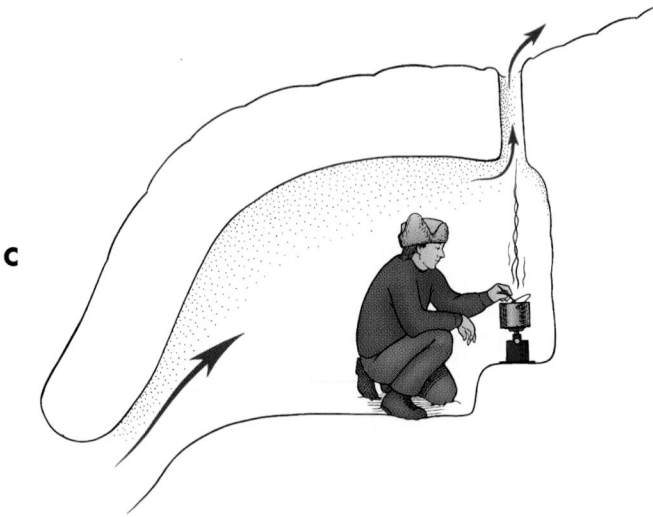

Figure 28-7 **A,** Snow cave entrance. **B,** Snow cave partly closed with snow blocks. **C,** Interior of snow cave.

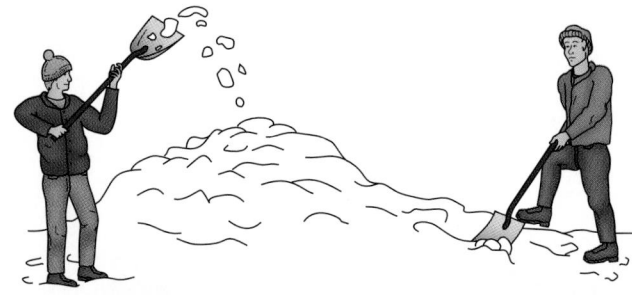

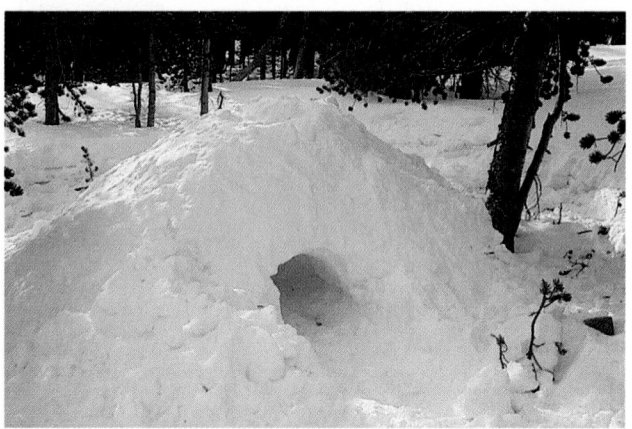

Figure 28-8 **A,** Preparing a snow dome. **B,** Completed snow done.

snow saws and snow of the proper consistency. Wind-blown snow in a treeless area is best; otherwise a large area of snow can be stamped well and left to harden over several hours. To mark the diameter of the igloo, a ski pole is held by the handle and the body turned so that the pole basket makes a large circle. This will outline the

base of an igloo suitable for three people. Cutting some of the snow blocks from inside this circle will lower the floor so that fewer blocks are required for the dome.

At least two persons are needed, one to cut and carry the blocks and the other inside the igloo to lay the blocks. The blocks should be about 18 inches wide, 30 inches long, and 8 inches thick. They are laid in a circle leaning in about 20 to 30 degrees toward the center of the igloo, with the sides trimmed for a snug fit. The tops of the first few blocks in the first circle are beveled so that a continuous line of blocks is laid, with the first few blocks of each succeeding circle cocked upward (Figure 28-9). A common error is not to lean the blocks inward enough, resulting in an open tower instead of a dome. Gaps are caulked with snow. The dome should be 5 to 6 feet high inside and can be closed with a single capstone of snow. The entrance is dug as a tunnel under rather than through the edge of the igloo, preventing warm air from escaping.

Tents and Bivouac Sacs. Tents are generally comfortable and dry but in very cold weather are not as warm as snow shelters. They are preferable to snow shelters at mild temperatures, during damp snow conditions at temperatures above freezing, or when the snow cover is minimal. Bivouac sacs are carried by climbers on

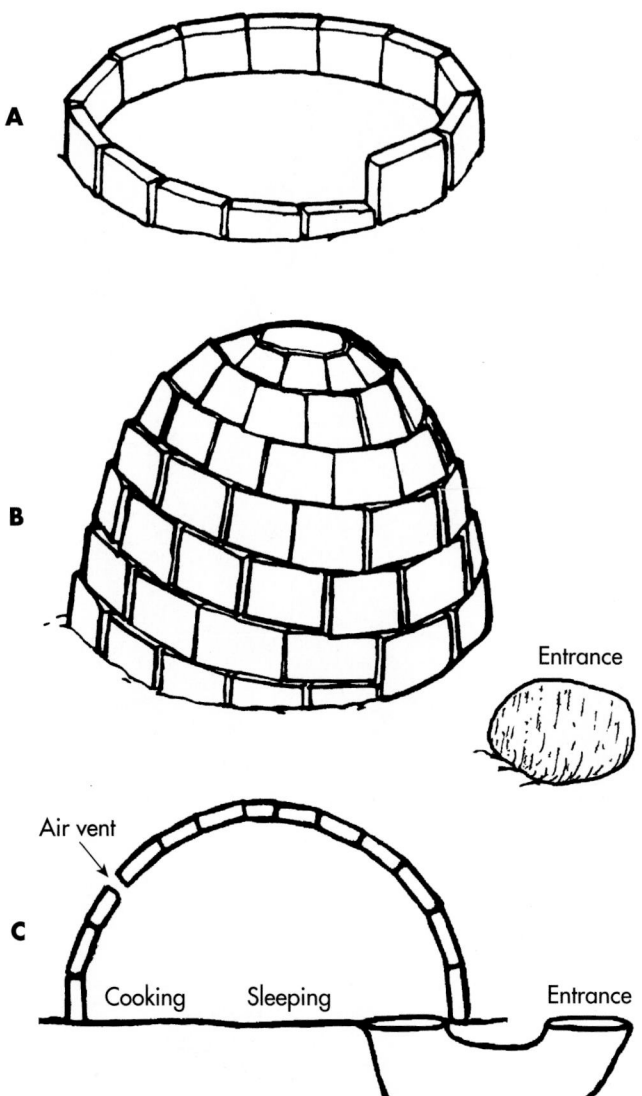

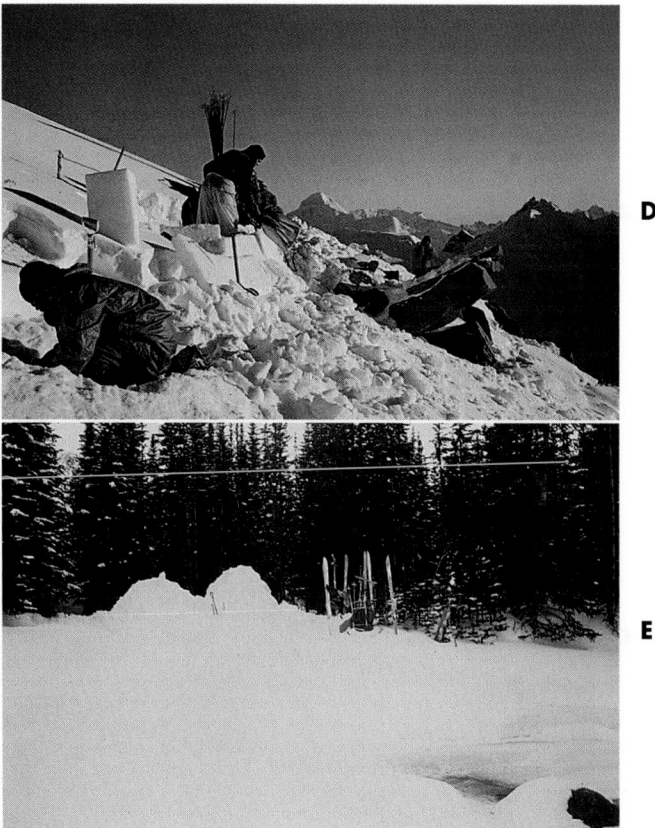

Figure 28-9 **A** to **C,** Stages of igloo construction. **D,** Building an igloo, southeast ridge of Mt. Foraker. **E,** Double igloo for a party of five.

long alpine-style climbs or for emergencies. They are usually made of Gore-Tex or waterproof fabric and hold one or two persons. Many modern packs have extensions, so when used with a cagoule or anorak (roomy, knee-length, hooded pullover garment), they form an acceptable bivouac sac.

Increasing Internal Body Heat Production

Internal body heat production can be increased voluntarily by raising the level of muscular activity and by eating. To obtain maximal heat production from exercise, the body should be well fed and in peak physical condition. This is particularly important for persons with sedentary jobs who participate in vigorous outdoor sports and for rescue personnel who may be subject to severe, unplanned, and prolonged physical stress. A suitable physical conditioning program should develop both aerobic and motor fitness. The

goal of aerobic exercise is efficient extraction of oxygen from alveolar air. This is best developed by rhythmic endurance exercises such as running, cross-country skiing, cycling, swimming, and using exercise bicycles and Nordic skiing simulators. The most effective activities are those that exercise lower and upper extremities simultaneously. Exercise should be vigorous enough to produce a heart rate of 75% of the age-related maximum (0.75 × [220 minus the participant's age]) for at least 15 minutes 4 days a week. Motor fitness, which includes strength, power, balance, agility, and flexibility, is developed by vigorous competitive team sports, selected calisthenics, and weight-lifting exercises.

Providing External Heat: Fire Building

The ability to build a fire under adverse conditions is an essential skill that should be practiced by persons

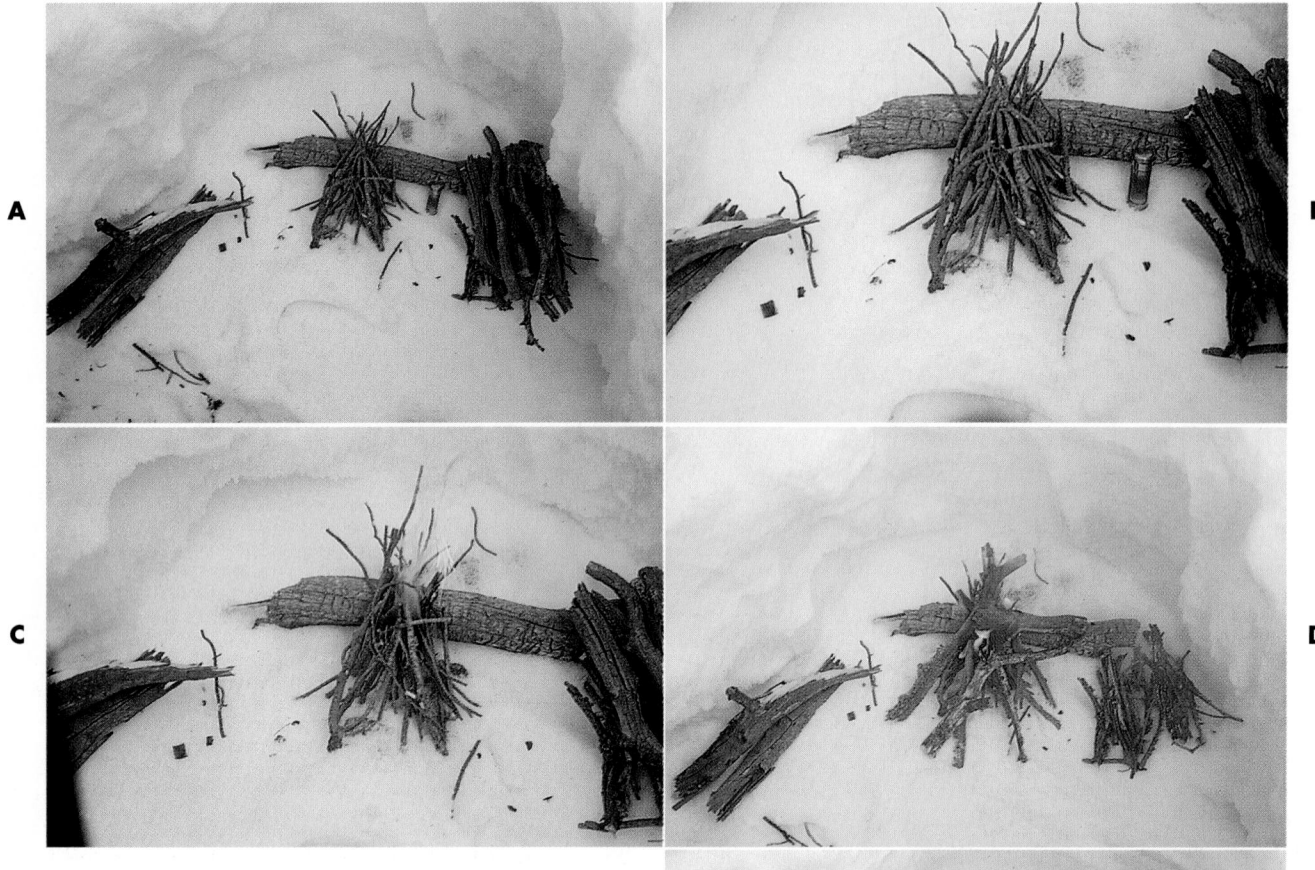

Figure 28-10 Stages of building a fire. **A,** Select a spot out of the wind. Start by placing tinder, such as small, dry evergreen twigs, in a lean-to fashion against a larger branch. **B,** Add a layer of kindling (larger dry branches and split sticks) over the tinder, being sure that air can reach each piece. **C,** Insert a lighted match, candle, or cigarette lighter into the base of the lean-to. **D** and **E,** Add larger pieces of kindling and fuel (large sticks and pieces of split wood) as the fire catches well. Keep the fire small so that you can get close to it.

who engage in outdoor activities (Figure 28-10). Necessary equipment includes a sturdy knife, a candle, and waterproof matches. In addition, a tube of chemical fire starter (available in most outdoor stores) is highly recommended, especially for wet climates.

To burn, a fire needs air, but not too much air. The fire site should be out of the wind behind a rock or log or in a snow pit. If the fire is built on bare ground, all flammable material such as moss and grass should be cleaned off by scraping the ground surface down to mineral soil over an area at least 3 feet in diameter. If snow is too deep to be removed down to bare ground, the fire should be built on a platform of green logs.

Building a fire requires three types of combustible material: tinder, kindling, and fuel. *Tinder* is any type of finely divided, high flammable material. It must be dry. Examples include grass and leaves, inner bark of birch trees, shavings from dry sticks, cotton balls, small sticks, and fine grades of steel wool. The most readily available natural material is the small dry twigs found on the lower, dead branches of evergreens. If the outer wood of small branches is wet, it can be shaved off, or the branches can be split lengthwise into several thinner lengths with a sturdy knife to expose the dry core. The tinder is arranged in lean-to form by placing it against a larger branch, smallest sticks on the bottom and larger ones on top, separated just enough so that air can reach each piece. To conserve matches, one match should be used to light a candle or segment of fire starter, which in turn lights the tinder. The flame should be placed under the middle of the lean-to of tinder so that lower, smaller pieces will set fire to higher, larger pieces.

Kindling is larger material, usually larger pieces of dead branches and large branches that have been split lengthwise with a knife. Once the tinder is burning well, these larger pieces of dry wood are added.

Fuel is the largest material, usually branches and sections of dead tree trunks several inches or more in diameter. These should be split if an ax is available. Standing dead wood is preferable to wood lying on the ground, and wood that has lost its bark to wood with bark, because both will be drier and less rotten than their alternatives. Fuel is added after the kindling is burning well.

Several times more fuel than the predicted need should be collected. When dead branches are gathered, only those that snap loudly when broken off should be selected. If no ax or saw is available, the fire can be built next to a large, downed log, which may catch and burn for several days. Long, dead sections of trees can be shortened by laying them across a fire so that when they burn through, two shorter sections result. Fires generally should be kept small, both to conserve wood and to allow them to be approached more closely. The wood supply should be protected from rain and snow.

A fire can be started without matches by using an automobile cigarette lighter or batteries and steel wood. A "wire" can be made by twisting and pulling out a fine-grade (e.g., 4-0) steel wool. This will catch fire if the ends are touched to the positive and negative terminals of two fresh C or D batteries in tandem. A fire starter can be made by stripping the insulation from the middle of a wire and wrapping the bare portion 7 to 10 times around a dry stick. If the two ends of the wire are touched to the terminals of an automobile battery, the wire will become red hot and the stick will ignite (the wire should be long enough that the flame is not close to the battery, where it could ignite hydrogen gas produced by the battery).

When scraped hard with a file or knife blade, commercial "metal matches" made of magnesium will produce showers of sparks that will ignite tinder such as fine steel wool, cotton, or small dry shavings.

Food*

For optimum performance, the human body requires a daily supply of calories, carbohydrate, protein, fat, minerals, and vitamins. Carbohydrates supply calories and are essential for replacement of muscle glycogen. If diet is inadequate, body carbohydrate and fat stores and finally tissue protein will be depleted to provide calories for heat and energy. Carbohydrate in the form of liver and muscle glycogen is used up first, then fat is used at a steady rate until gone. Protein is used rapidly at first, then more slowly, and finally rapidly again just before death.[9]

A moderately active 70-kg (154-pound) male normally requires the food equivalent of 2800 kcal/day, but if exercising in cold weather, he may require more than twice this amount. Protein intake should be at least 65 g/day, and carbohydrates should make up 60% to 70% of the diet.

Although most persons in a survival situation worry more about food than anything else, food is usually less important than shelter or water because a person can survive for weeks without food, even in cold weather. Enough water must be available, however, and energy expenditure must be kept to a minimum. Most wilderness parties carry adequate supplies of food; problems arise if food is exhausted, lost, or contaminated. Bare ridges, high mountains above timberline, and dense evergreen forests are difficult places to find wild food, even in summer. Success is more likely on river and stream banks, on lake shores, in margins of forests, and in natural clearings. Since in most cases the amount of wild food found by an untrained individual will not provide enough calories to replenish the energy expended in searching for it, it is important *always to carry extra food for emergencies.*

The following general rules about wilderness edibles have many exceptions, so no unfamiliar wild food should be eaten except in extreme circumstances (see Chapters 48 and 49):

1. All wild foods except fruits and berries should be cooked. This will make them more palatable, more digestible, and safer to eat.
2. Persons who spend time outdoors should know the edible plants and animals of familiar areas. Similar species are often found in similar though unfamiliar areas.
3. Plants to avoid include mushrooms and other fungi, buttercups, plants with umbrella-shaped flowers, wild beans and peas, all unknown berries except blue and black ones, all bulbs except those with an onion odor, and all plants with milky or colored sap or shiny leaves. Compound berries (e.g., raspberries, blackberries, thimbleberries, salmonberries) are safe to eat.
4. No one should eat large quantities of a strange plant food without first tasting it.
   a. Touch the plant's sap or juice to the inner forearm or tip of the tongue.
   b. If no ill effects occur, boil plant parts in two 5-minute changes of water. Place 1 teaspoon of the resulting material in the mouth for 5 minutes, and chew but do not swallow it. If a

*References 2, 7, 16, 17, 19, 22, 23, 26.

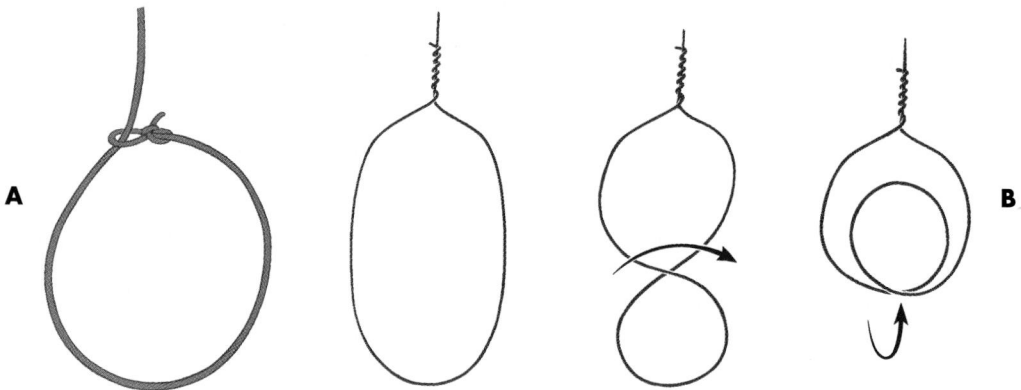

Figure 28-11 Snare loop. **A,** Simple snare loop. **B,** Locking device for a wire snare loop.

burning, nauseating, or bitter taste results, immediately spit if out. If no unpleasant effect occurs, swallow it and wait 8 hours.

c. If no ill effects (e.g., nausea, cramps, or diarrhea) occur after 8 hours, eat 2 tablespoons and wait an additional 8 hours.

d. If no ill effects occur at the end of this period, consider the plant edible.

5. All land mammals, birds, and birds' eggs can be eaten. The entire carcass, both fat and lean, should be eaten, except for canine, seal, and polar bear livers. Crustaceans below the high-tide mark, mollusks, insects, reptiles, and some amphibians can be eaten. Salamanders and frogs should be skinned; toads should be avoided altogether. Fish, crustaceans, and mollusks should be eaten promptly because they spoil quickly. Fish and meat can be preserved by drying. Black mussels, mollusks with cone-shaped shells, Pacific reef fish, "puffers," fish eggs or entrails, and any fish that looks "ugly" should be avoided (see Chapter 54). Any fish with an unpleasant odor, pale slimy gills, flabby skin, flesh that remains pitted when pressed on, or sunken eyes should be avoided, as well as all aquatic life during a red tide.

6. Edible parts of wild plants may include roots, leaves (especially young leaves), stems (usually require peeling), shoots, buds, grass seeds, inner bark (aspen, cottonwood, birch, willow, lodgepole pine, Scotch pine), nuts, and berries (except as noted in 3).

Animal Food. Mammals and birds can be trapped, snared, or shot. Some, such as spruce hens and porcupines, can be clubbed. Fish can be hooked, speared, or trapped. To secure this type of food, however, the hunter must locate the prey. On land this is done by searching for signs such as trails, droppings, burrows, dens, and bedding areas. Carnivore dung usually contains hair and bone; herbivore dung has indigestible plant parts. Trails lead to feeding and watering places. Successful hunting requires patience, skill at stalking, and knowledge of animal behavior. The best times to hunt are at dawn and dusk as animals are moving to or from their bedding areas.

Small animals can be snared or trapped. Snares should be baited or located on a game trail at a place where the animal has no choice but to enter the snare. This can be a naturally narrow or a prepared area. The mouths of dens and burrows are good places to set snares. Gloves should be worn during snare construction to minimize human scent. Snare loops can be made from any type of bare wire or improvised from strips of green bark, cord, shoelaces, or clothing strips. Light, strong wire such as 28-gauge piano wire is best. A small loop is tied at one end of the wire, and the main loop is made by feeding the other end through the small loop (Figure 28-11, A). The main loop is adjusted to catch the animal around the neck and to fit the expected size of the prey (e.g., three fingers in width for squirrels, fist sized for rabbits). Snares using loops are effective because the animal almost always lunges forward, tightening the loop around its neck. A locking device should be included to prevent the wire loop from loosening after the animal is trapped (Figure 28-11, B). Snares should be set at midday when animals are bedded down. The trapper approaches the area at a 90-degree angle to the trail, sets the snare, and backs away, keeping downwind from the animal's expected location and not walking on the game trail. Natural surroundings should be disturbed as little as possible. Snares and traps should be checked twice daily. In general, one animal is caught for every 15 snares set.

Many different types of traps have been invented; most include a trigger arrangement that is baited or located so that it releases when disturbed by the animal's movement. Trigger release allows a counterweight to pin the animal or a bent sapling to straighten and hoist it off the ground (Figure 28-12).

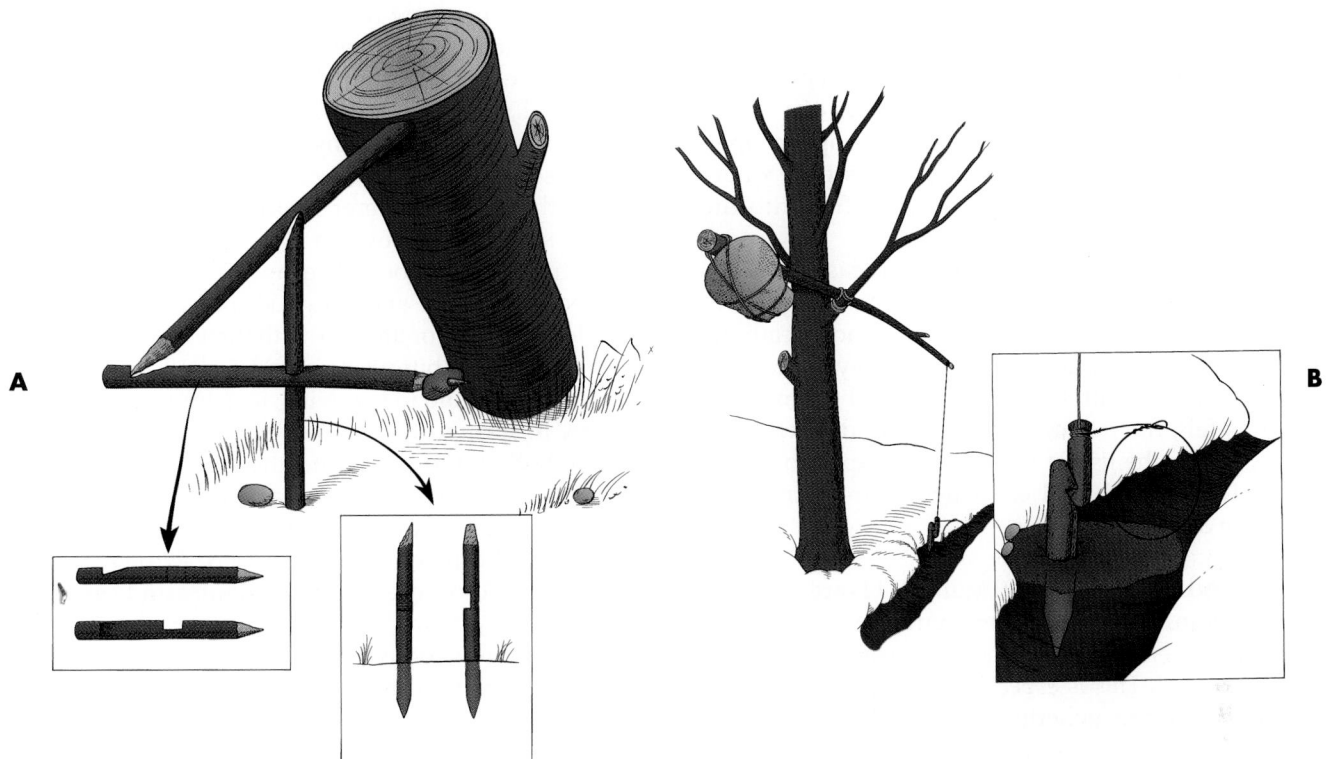

Figure 28-12 **A,** Figure-4 deadfall. **B,** Twitch-up snare.

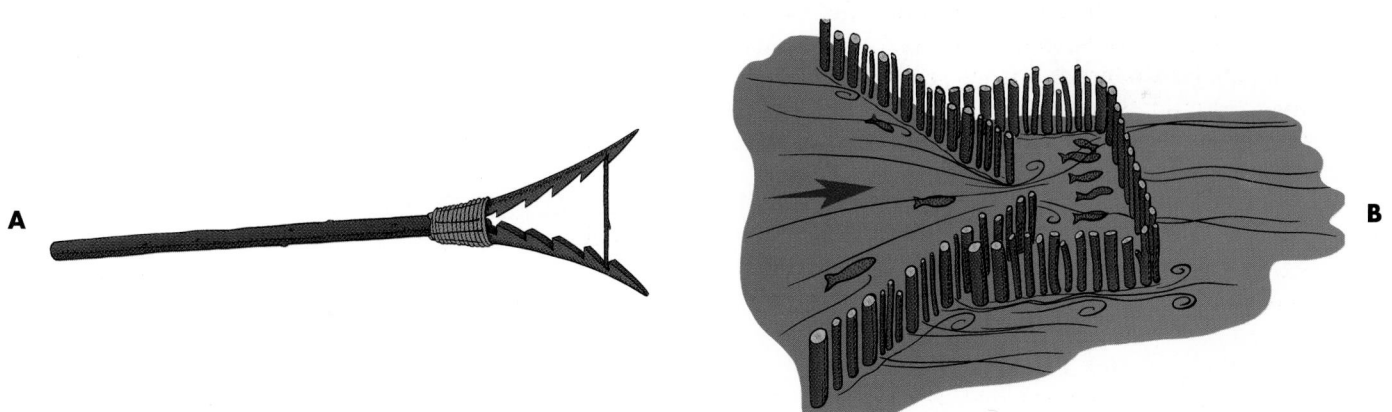

Figure 28-13 **A,** Split-shaft fish spear. **B,** Fish trap.

Birds can be caught with snares or baited fishhooks.

Fish can be taken with hook and line, traps, and spears. Emergency survival kits should contain several hooks and a long length of line. Insects, smaller fish, worms, shellfish, or meat can be used as bait, or lures can be improvised from pieces of brightly colored cloth, feathers, or bits of shiny metal. In open streams the best places to fish are pools below falls and behind rocks. Locating fish is more difficult in the winter, when they retreat into the deep parts of lakes. Holes can be cut in

the ice of frozen lakes. The best time to fish is early morning or dusk. An effective fish spear is the split-shaft type (Figure 28-13, *A*), which has two toothed jaws held apart by an easily dislodged trigger. A spear works best if it is used to pin a fish against the bottom or bank so the fish can be grasped with the hands before it works loose.

In streams, fish traps can be made by using rocks or vertical willow branches to build an enclosure with a funnel-shaped opening, the narrow end extends well into the enclosure (Figure 28-13, *B*). The trap should be located so that the water current drives fish into the wide end of the funnel. Another type of trap can be made by tying the neck and sleeves of a T-shirt closed, placing the shirt with the tail propped open in the water at the downstream end of a pool where fish have been seen, and chasing the fish into the shirt.

Another way to catch large fish (at least 10 inches long) is by "tickling."[17,23] This involves crawling slowly upstream along a stream bank, feeling underneath the bank and under nearby logs for fish. They are usually found lying still with their heads pointed upstream. If a fish is felt, the person moves the hand slowly forward, grasps the fish at the gills, and flips it onto the bank. Tickling fish and constructing and using fish traps are difficult in winter.

Plant Food. Edible plants (Figure 28-14) are common in mountain meadows and even in forests, although considerable energy may be needed to dig up or gather plant material. This is especially true during the winter months, when gathering roots and berries may re-

quire removing snow from large areas and digging in frozen ground. Tender new needles of pines and other conifers are edible, although not very tasty. Pine nuts are found in pine cones, which can be picked from trees. All pine nuts are edible and high in caloric value but are so small in some species that it is impractical to gather them. The gatherer should look for unopened cones, scorch them over a fire, and split them by pounding with a rock. The nuts are removed and roasted. Acorns are another good source of food; they should be boiled for an hour with three changes of water to remove the bitter tannic acid. Cattails and arrowheads can be found in low-lying, marshy areas and lake shores. In spring the sheathed top spike of the cattail can be boiled and eaten and the sprouts eaten raw. Pollen from the blooming flower spike can be used as flour. Although fibrous, the roots contain much starchy material and can be boiled or roasted. Arrowhead tubers are boiled or roasted for 30 minutes and eaten after peeling.

Dandelions, woolly louseworts, wild onions, elk thistle, and bistort can sometimes be found under the snow in mountain meadows. The roots of all these

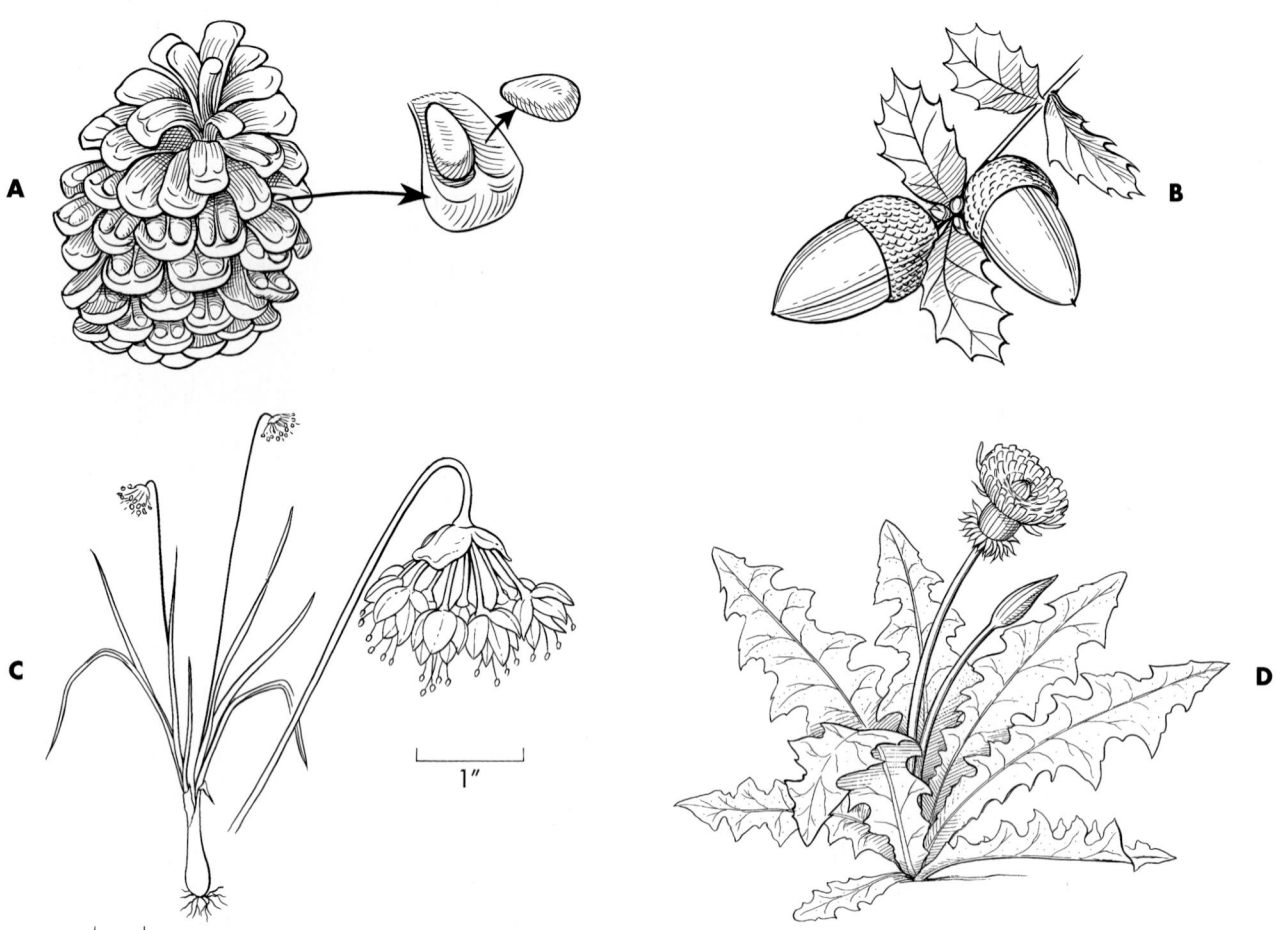

Figure 28-14 Edible wild plants. **A,** Pine cone. **B,** Acorns. **C,** Wild onion. **D,** Dandelion.

plants are edible and nourishing but should be boiled. Many bulbs are poisonous, however, and only those with an onion odor should be eaten. The young leaves and shoots of ferns can be boiled and eaten, and the leaves of mountain sorrel can be eaten raw. Wild rose hips are edible. Elk thistle stems are edible if peeled and boiled. Young dandelion roots and leaves can be eaten; older ones should be boiled in several changes of water to remove the bitter taste. The inner bark of aspen, cot-

tonwood, birch, willow, lodgepole pine, and Scotch pine is edible.

Berries, such as huckleberries, raspberries, crowberries, cranberries, bearberries (Kinnikinnick), salmonberries, and thimbleberries can sometimes be found under or over the snow and are edible (Figure 28-15).

Certain types of lichen can be eaten. Iceland moss should be boiled for an hour, reindeer moss boiled or roasted, and rock tripe dried and then boiled.

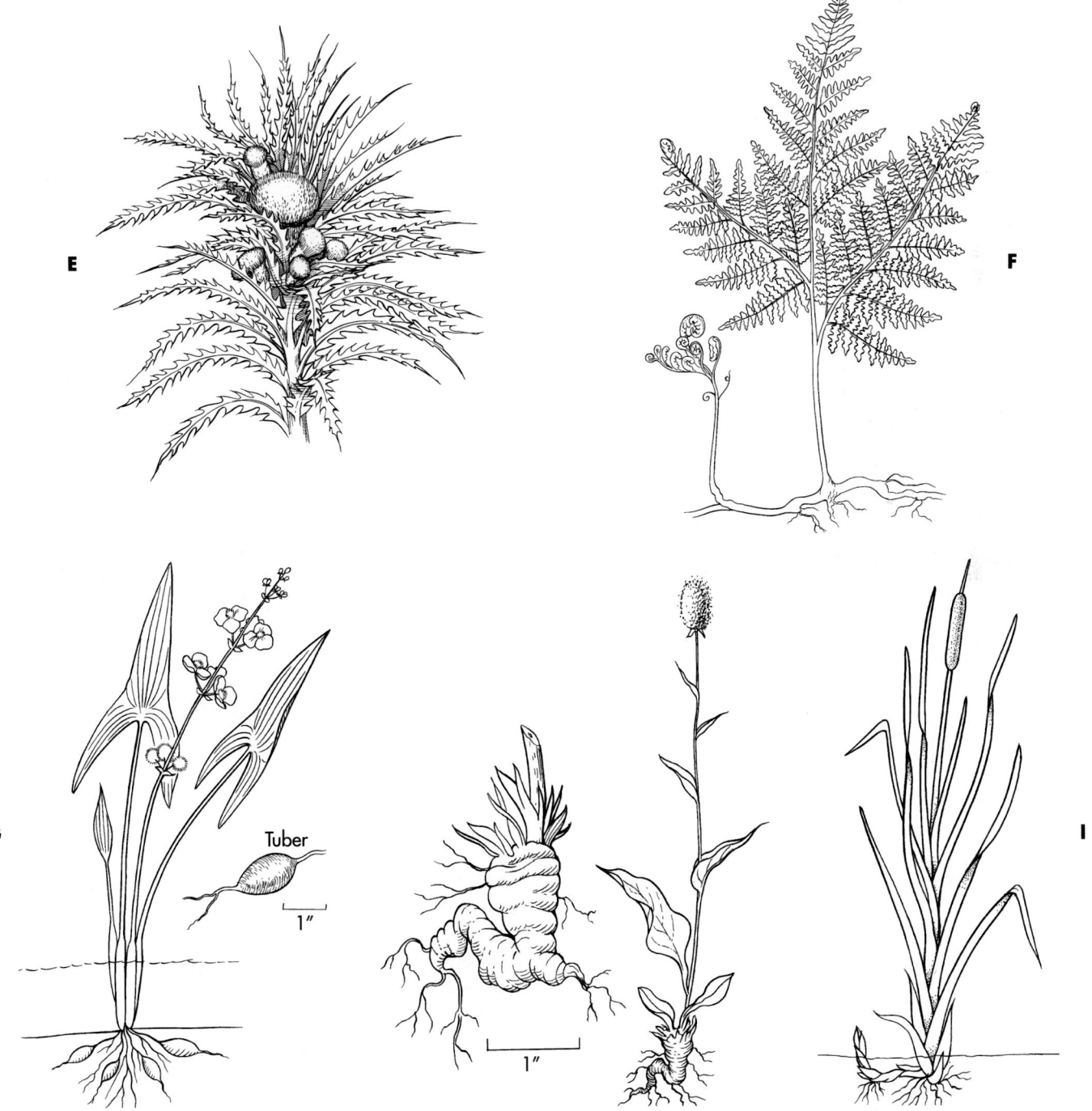

Figure 28-14, cont'd **E,** Elk thistle. **F,** Fern. **G,** Arrowhead. **H,** Bistort. **I,** Cattail.

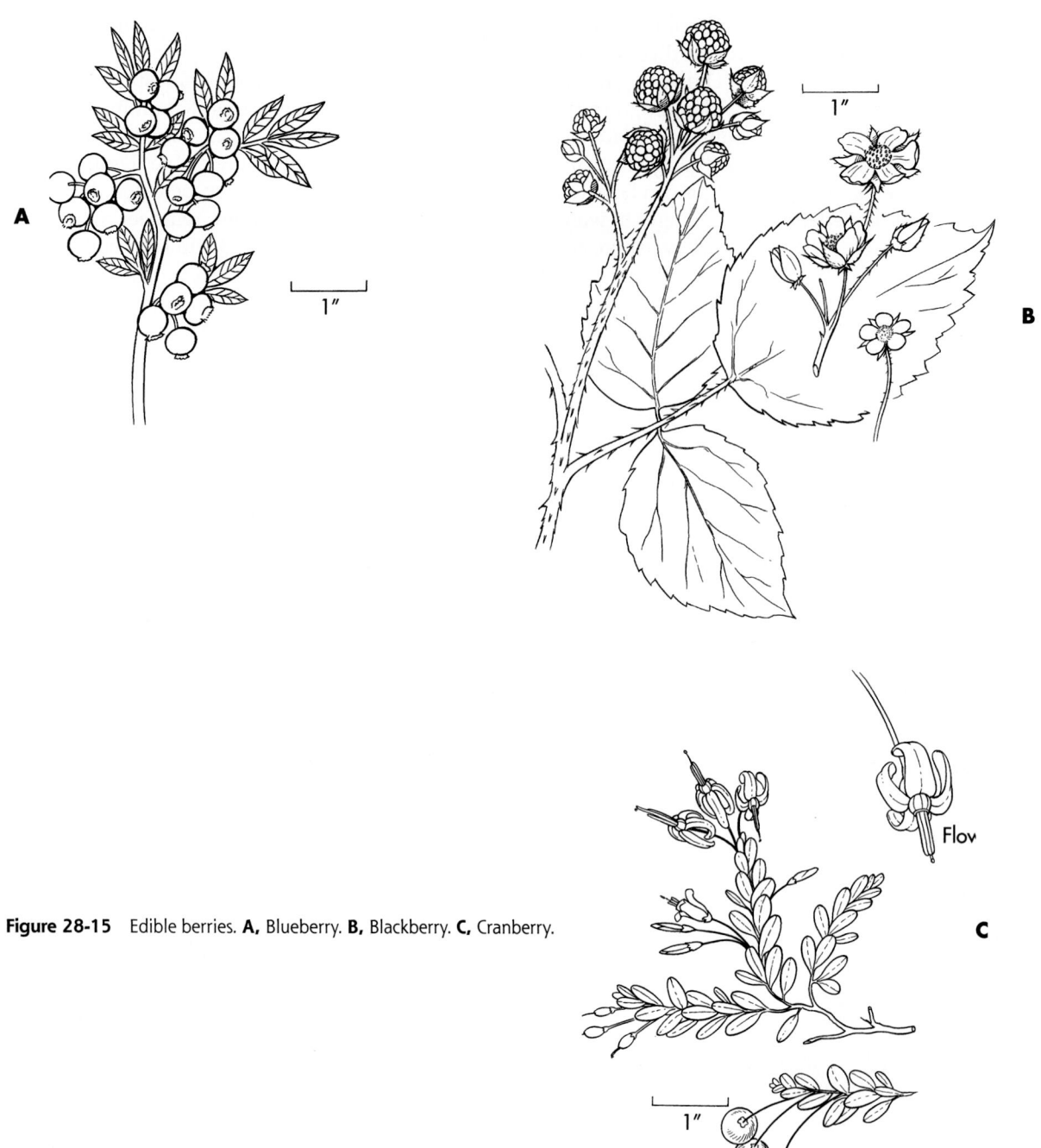

Figure 28-15 Edible berries. **A,** Blueberry. **B,** Blackberry. **C,** Cranberry.

Cooking. As noted, all wild foods except fruits and berries should be cooked. Cooked food is usually more appetizing, easier to chew, more digestible, and safer because cooking destroys microorganisms. Hot food also helps maintain morale.

A large metal container, preferably a pot with a bale (see Appendix A), is indispensable to heat water and other liquids. Since cooking over a fire will cover the outside with soot, a stuff sack is useful to store the pot. Since it can tip over easily, the pot should not be placed directly on burning wood but on two firm rocks or green logs with fire in between. Rocks from a stream or dry wash should not be placed near a fire, since steam from internal moisture can cause an explosion. A pot can also be hung over the fire on a sturdy green stick, one end of which is supported by a forked stick driven into the ground and the other end anchored by rocks.

Most types of wild food can be cooked successfully by boiling, and the cooking water retains the food's fat and natural juices. This water should be consumed as well.

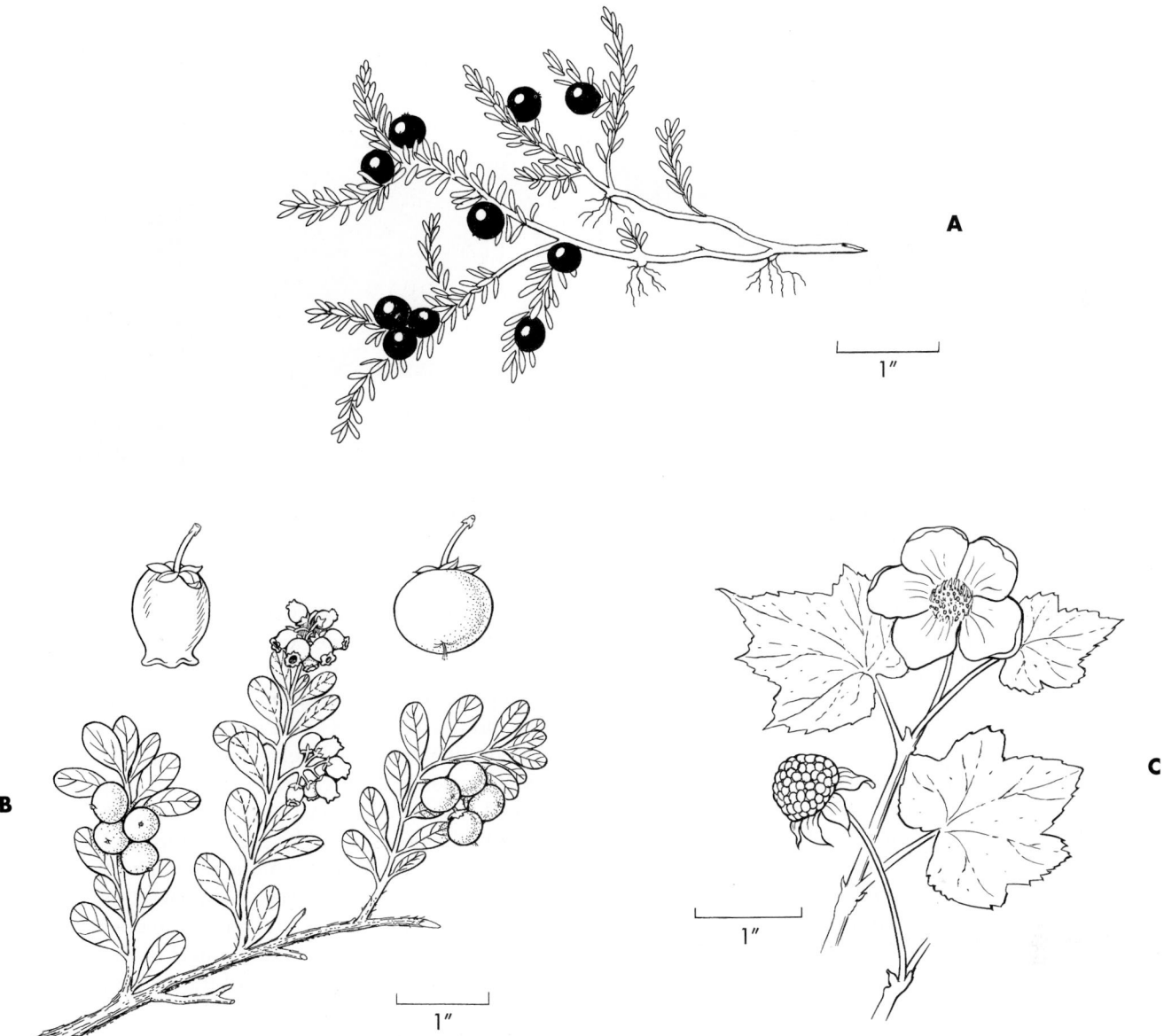

Figure 28-15, cont'd **D,** Crowberry. **E,** Bearberry. **F,** Salmonberry.

Meat and fish can be roasted on a spit made from a green tree branch or can be fastened to a flat rock or the flat surface of a split log tipped on edge to face the fire.

Water

Water constitutes about 60% of the body weight of an average young adult male; the value for a female is slightly lower. The percentage of water tends to decrease with age. In a sedentary adult, normal daily water loss includes about 1400 ml of urine, 800 ml through the skin and lungs, and 100 ml in the stool, for a total of 2300 ml daily. Since about 800 ml of water per day is contained in food and 300 ml produced by metabolism, a minimum daily intake of 1200 ml is necessary in a temperate climate at sea level to avoid dehydration.[9] In a hot dry climate, at high altitude, or with exertion, insensible losses and sweating increase considerably, so fluid intake should be increased proportionally. Monitoring urine output determines whether intake is adequate; 1 to 1.5 L of light-colored urine should be excreted per day. Adding fruit flavors and making hot drinks improve the palatability of water. Electrolyte drinks and salt tablets are generally unnecessary in cold weather, since the electrolytes lost in sweat are easily replaced by a normal diet. When water supplies are limited, overexertion is avoided and sweat "rationed."

Almost all surface water should be considered contaminated by animal or human wastes, with the possible exception of small streams descending from

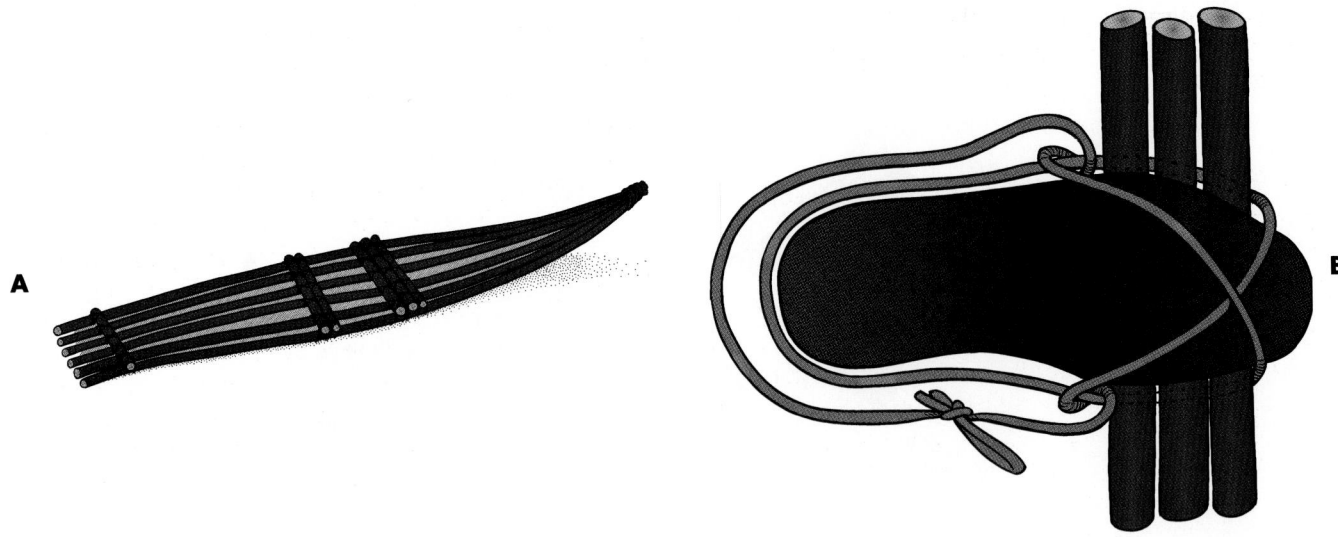

Figure 28-16 **A,** Emergency snowshoe. **B,** Detail of snowshoe binding.

untracked snowfields or high, uninhabited areas. At altitudes below 5488 m (18,000 feet), simply bringing water to a boil will kill *Giardia* cysts and most harmful bacteria and viruses. Water can also be disinfected by filtration or addition of chemicals (see Chapter 51).

At subfreezing temperatures and in locations above the snow line where liquid water is difficult to find, snow or ice must be melted to obtain water. This requires a metal pot (which should be included in every survival kit), fire-starting equipment, and wood for fuel. The time and effort required and decreased thirst in cold weather favor development of dehydration under survival conditions.

Whenever open water is encountered, individuals should drink their fill of disinfected water, then top off all canteens. Each evening, enough snow is melted to provide water for supper plus a full canteen, which is placed in the bottom of the sleeping bag to keep it from freezing and is ready for use during the night or for making breakfast in the morning. Before leaving camp in the morning, melted snow provides everyone with at least a full canteen for the day. Melting ice or hard snow is more efficient than melting light, powdery snow. To avoid scorching the pot, the snow is melted slowly, or water is heated in the bottom of the pot before adding snow. On warmer sunny days, snow can be spread on a dark plastic sheet to melt.

Emergency Snow Travel

Travel in deep snow is almost impossible without skis or snowshoes. Even though travel may be unwise for other reasons, wilderness foot travelers in both subarctic and temperate latitudes should know how to im-

provise snowshoes from natural materials in case they are stranded by a late- or early-season snowstorm. Emergency snowshoes (Figure 28-16, *A*) can be made from poles that are 6 feet long, ¾ to 1 inch thick at the base, and ¼ inch thick at the tip, and sticks ¾ inch thick and 10 inches long.[2] Twelve long poles and 12 short sticks are needed. For each snowshoe, six long poles are placed side by side on the ground, and the middle point of the poles is marked. One short stick is lashed crosswise to the tail (base) of the poles, and three short sticks are lashed side by side just forward of the midpoint of the poles where the toe of the boot will rest. Two sticks are lashed where the heel of the boot will strike the snowshoe. The tips of the six poles are tied together. Each binding (Figure 28-16, *B*) is made of a continuous length (about 6 feet) of nylon cord, preferably braided, since it will eventually fray. The midpoint of the cord is positioned at the back of the boot above the bulge of the heel. Each end of the cord is run under the three side-by-side short sticks at the side of the boot, then up and across the boot toe so that it crosses the other end on top of the toe, forming an X. Then each end is looped around the cord running along the opposite side of the boot, and the ends are brought around the back of the boot heel. The cord is pulled tight around the boot, and the ends are tied together at the lateral side of the heel.

On walking the tip of the snowshoe should rise, the boot heel should rise, and the boot sole should remain on the snowshoe.

Snow travelers should avoid stepping close to trees (because of funnel-shaped "tree wells" around tree trunks), large rocks (because of weak snow or moats around them), and overhanging stream banks. The person who falls into a stream or lake should roll repeatedly in powdery snow to wick the water from clothing, brushing the snow off each time. A fire completes the drying process.[2]

Stalled or Wrecked Vehicles

Persons stranded in automobiles or downed airplanes can survive using the equipment in the vehicles. Survivors should *stay with the vehicle* rather than go for help, since a vehicle is much more visible to rescuers than is a person. Floor mats and upholstery can be used for insulation, but it is much better to have a vehicle survival kit containing extra clothing and blankets (see Appendix D).

Automobiles.[25] In cold weather, drivers should keep their vehicles in the best possible mechanical condition, using winter-grade oil, the proper amount of radiator antifreeze, deicer fluid for the fuel tank, and windshield antifreeze for the cleaning fluid. Windshield wiper blades that are becoming worn should be replaced. A combination snow brush and ice scraper should be available, and a can of deicer is useful on frozen door locks and wiper blades. Snow tires, preferably studded (illegal in some states), are desirable, but chains should be carried as well. All-wheel drive or four-wheel drive is optimal, and front-wheel drive superior to rear-wheel drive. The battery should be kept charged, the exhaust system free of leaks, and the gas tank full (drive on the upper half of your tank). A cell phone or citizen's band radio is useful. The marooned driver should tie a brightly colored piece of cloth to the antenna and at night should leave the inside dome light on to be seen by snowplow drivers and rescuers (headlights use too much current). If necessary for heat, the motor and heater can be run for 2 minutes each hour (after checking to see if the exhaust pipe is free of snow). To avoid CO poisoning, a downwind window is cracked 1 to 2 inches. Reusable CO detectors are available and can be carried in the survival kit. One or two large candles should be carried to provide heat and light if the gasoline supply runs out. Two candles can raise the interior temperature well above freezing.

Airplanes. Airplane fuselages are poorly insulated. Unless a stove is available, survivors are usually better off constructing a shelter than can be heated with a fire (as described earlier), outside but near the aircraft. Batteries and cigarette lighters can be used as fire starters. Oil and gasoline can be used as fuel if poured over a container full of dirt or sand.

HOT WEATHER SURVIVAL

Environmental conditions predisposing to serious heat stress can be found in most temperate zone regions during the summer months and in the tropics year-round. The amount of heat stress is proportional to both temperature and relative humidity; thus a tropical jungle environment with a relatively lower temperature and higher humidity can be as dangerous as a drier desert environment with a relatively higher temperature. Serious heat illness occurs when endogenous heat production plus exogenous heat gain forces the core temperature to dangerous levels (more than 40° to 46° C [104° to 105° F]) despite the body's cooling mechanisms. These mechanisms include involuntary cutaneous vasodilation, sweating, and voluntary mechanisms, such as seeking shelter from the sun, avoiding excess insulation and heat-producing physical activity, and replacing lost fluids and electrolytes (see Chapter 10).

The body adapts better to heat and altitude than to cold. It acclimatizes to heat by increasing the blood volume, dilating skin blood vessels, and improving cardiac efficiency so as to carry more heat from the body core to the shell. The process of acclimatization takes about 10 days, during which the subject starts to perspire at a lower temperature, the volume of perspiration increases, and the perspiration contains fewer electrolytes.

The following discussion emphasizes survival in a desert environment (see also Chapter 29).

Practical Methods for Adjusting to Hot Weather[4]

Heat loss by conduction, convection, and radiation can be increased by exposing the maximum amount of skin to the circulating air. This should be done only when in the shade; when in the sun, skin should be completely protected by clothing. Wearing clothing when exposed to hot sun also reduces water loss by reducing sweating. Because heat loss and sweating may be impaired by sunscreens, a good compromise is to cover the face and hands with a sunscreen having a high sun protection factor (SPF) number and to wear a long-sleeved shirt and long trousers of tightly woven, loose-fitting, light-colored (preferably white) cotton. Avoid T-shirts, which have an SPF of only 5 to 9. Special clothing with an SPF of 30 or greater is available (e.g., Solumbra). If desired, ventilation holes can be cut at the axillae and groin. Hydration is maintained by drinking adequate fluids, some of which can contain electrolyte supplements. Optimal hydration maintains blood volume and shell circulation and supports the sweating mechanism. Enough water *must* be carried or be available in the field. Water bottles should be wrapped with clothing to insulate them and buried in the backpack.

The layer principle of clothing is recommended in the desert as well as in cold weather. Layers can be taken off during the heat of the day and added at night when the dry desert air cools rapidly. Since high winds and sandstorms occur frequently in desert areas, a wind-resistant parka and pants are desirable; since rains occasionally occur as well, the garments should also be water repellent.

Because of its high thermal conductivity, poor insulating ability, and good wicking ability, cotton—which is avoided in cold weather—is the fabric of choice for hot weather clothing. Clothing should be loose to promote air circulation.

Before exposure to prolonged or strenuous hot weather exertion, individuals should allow time for acclimatization.

Heat gain from the environment can be minimized by using clothing to protect the head and body from the direct rays of the sun. A hat with a wide brim or a Foreign Legion–style cap with a neck protector and ventilation holes in the crown is recommended. A neck protector can be improvised from a large bandana by placing it on the head with the point just above the forehead, bringing the two tails around in front of the ears, tying them under the chin, and then replacing the hat.

Travelers should seek shelter during the hottest part of the day. Caves and overhangs can be used, but gulleys and other dry watercourses should be avoided because of the danger of flash floods. A sun shelter can be made by suspending a tarp from brush or cacti or by laying the tarp on a framework of poles. Travelers who become stranded in a vehicle should lie *under* it. Because desert air is much cooler a foot above or a few inches below the ground surface, the desert traveler should lie on a platform or in a scooped-out depression rather than directly on the ground.

Direct contact with the hot ground and other hot objects, particularly hot metal, should be avoided. Sturdy hiking or climbing boots should be worn to protect the feet, not only from the hot ground but also from sharp rocks, the spines of cacti, and snakes. Gaiters should be worn or improvised from strips of cloth to keep sand and insects out of boots and socks. The hands should be protected with leather gloves. Rest periods should be taken in the shade rather than in the direct sun. High-quality sunglasses should be used to protect the eyes; if necessary, sunglasses can be improvised from a piece of cardboard or wood with a narrow slit cut for each eye.

Body heat production can be minimized by avoiding muscular exertion during periods of high heat and humidity. Persons should travel only early in the morning, late in the evening, or at night.

Desert Survival*

About 20% of the earth's land surface is made up of desert. Desert areas average less than 25.4 cm (10 inches) of rainfall annually. Deserts range from barren sand or gravel plains without a living plant for a hundred miles to areas of grass and thorny bushes than can support camels and goats. Despite lack of moisture, many plants and animals have adapted to the hot, arid environment and are able to thrive in many deserts.

Deserts heat up rapidly during the day, but because of low humidity and the low specific heat of the ground, they cool rapidly at night. Daily temperature ranges may be as great as 55° C (100° F).[26] These temperature changes produce alternate expansion and contraction of rocks, causing them to break up into smaller and smaller fragments and eventually to form gravel or sand. Lack of rainfall reduces the eroding effect of water, so wind and wind-borne sand are the most important agents of erosion. When the rare rains occur, water tends to run off rather than sink into the ground, and flash floods may occur; dry watercourses (arroyos, wadis, dry washes) are familiar features. Sudden weather changes are common; desert travelers in the fall, winter, and spring should be prepared for cold as well as hot weather. Dust storms and strong solar glare can be hazardous.

Southerly deserts may be hot year-round, whereas northern ones may have four recognizable seasons. Desert temperatures as hot as 134.4° F in the Sahara at Azizia and 134° F in Death Valley, California, have been recorded.[16] At such temperatures, the ground can become so hot that feet may be burned through shoes, and serious burns can result from touching exposed metal.

Desert plants have developed special characteristics that enable them to conserve water and survive long periods of drought. Some have extensive root systems that quickly absorb rainfall moisture, and others have exceptionally long roots that reach down to the water table. Many plants are dormant during the hottest season; others have thick external coverings that resist evaporative losses. Some are able to store water during wet seasons to allow survival through dry periods. Desert animals forage and hunt during the cool of the evening and night, resting in cool places during the day.

Food. Natural food is difficult to obtain in true deserts but is less important than water. A survivor can live several weeks without food if water is available. More natural food is available in the deserts of the American Southwest than in Old World deserts, such as the Sahara and Gobi (Figure 28-17).

No plant with milky juice should be eaten. All cactus fruits are edible, and the leaves of flat-leafed cacti (e.g., prickly pear) can be peeled and eaten, preferably after boiling. Wild cherries, wild celery, wild currants, wild onions, acacia beans, and piñon nuts are found in some areas. Grass seeds and the soft part of grass stalks are edible. Kangaroo rats, jerboas, rabbits, prairie dogs, lizards, tortoises, snakes, and insects, particularly lo-

---

*References 2, 9, 16, 19, 22, 23.

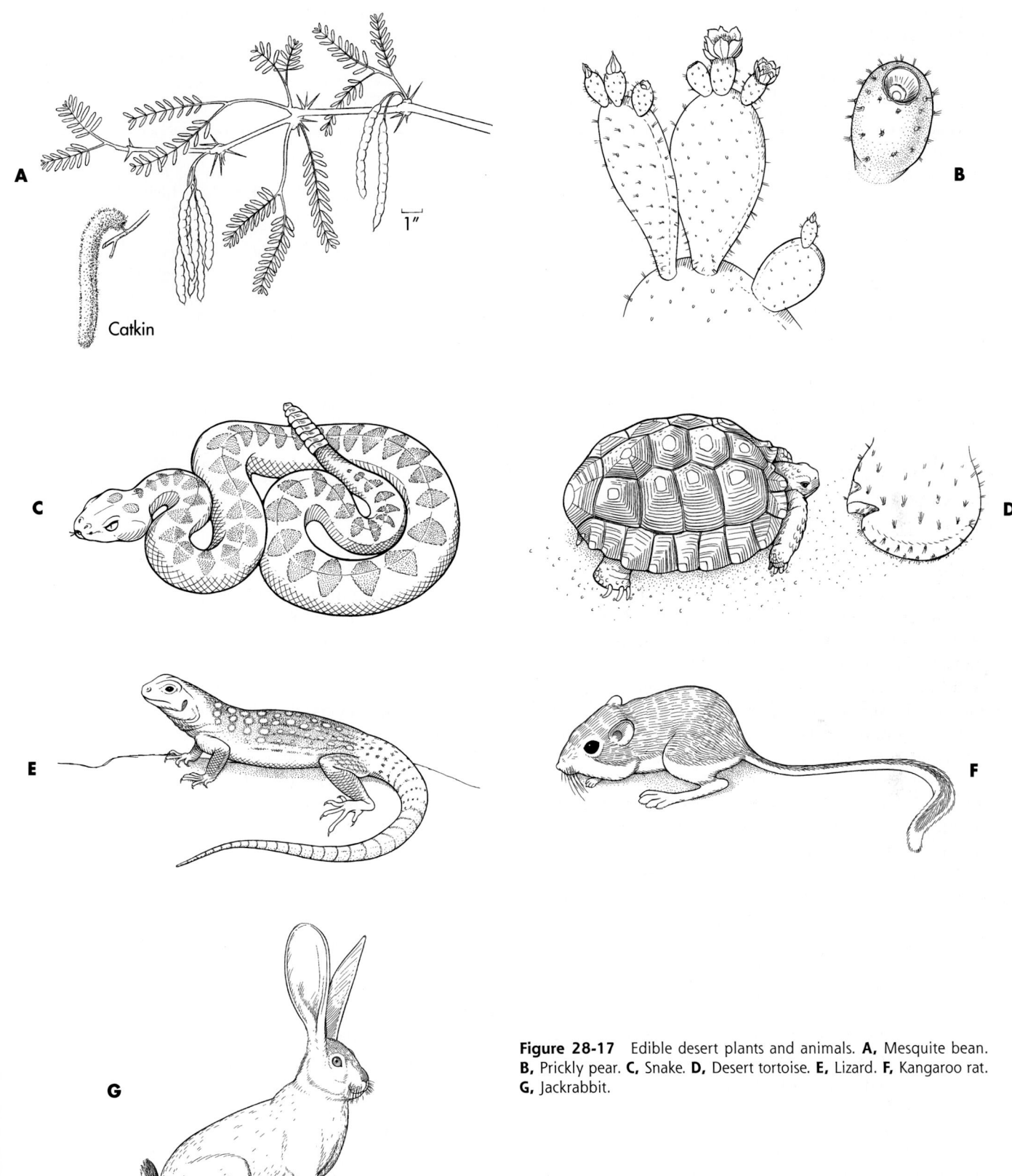

Catkin

Figure 28-17 Edible desert plants and animals. **A,** Mesquite bean. **B,** Prickly pear. **C,** Snake. **D,** Desert tortoise. **E,** Lizard. **F,** Kangaroo rat. **G,** Jackrabbit.

TABLE 28-3. Expected Days of Survival at Various Environmental Temperatures and with Varying Amounts of Available Water

	MAXIMUM DAILY TEMPERATURE IN SHADE (° F)	AVAILABLE WATER PER PERSON (U.S. QUARTS)					
		0	1	2	4	10	20
No walking	120	2	2	2	2.5	3	4.5
	110	3	3	3.5	4	5	7
	100	5	5.5	6	7	9.5	13.5
	90	7	8	9	10.5	15	23
	80	9	10	11	13	19	29
	70	10	11	12	14	20.5	32
	60	10	11	12	14	21	32
	50	10	11	12	14.5	21	32
Walking at night and resting thereafter	120	1	2	2	2.5	3	
	110	2	2	2.5	3	3.5	
	100	3	3.5	3.5	4.5	5.5	
	90	5	5.5	5.5	6.5	8	
	80	7	7.5	8	9.5	11.5	
	70	7.5	8	9	10.5	13.5	
	60	8	8.5	9	11	14	
	50	8	8.5	9	11	14	

From Adolph et al: *Physiology of man*, New York, 1947, Interscience.

custs, are all edible. Small mammals and birds can be trapped or snared as described previously. If firearms are available, larger animals such as antelope, deer, foxes, and badgers can be procured and leftover meat dried in the sun.[16,22,23] If water is limited, however, it is wise to base the diet on carbohydrate rather than protein, since more water is required to excrete the waste products of protein in the urine.

Water. There is no substitute for water in the desert, although a person can prolong life in a survival situation by decreasing water loss. Waterholes and oases are rare in deserts. They occasionally may be located by watching the behavior of animals and birds, which travel toward water at dawn and dusk. Animal trails tend to lead to water and may be joined by other trails and become wider as they approach it. Birds may circle before landing at a waterhole, especially in the morning. A pool of water with no animal tracks or droppings may be poisonous. Muddy and dirty water should be filtered through cloth, and all water should be treated chemically or by filtration or boiling before drinking (see Chapter 51). Persons should not drink urine or water from a vehicle radiator (which contains glycols). Table 28-3 shows the expected days of survival in the desert in relation to the amount of water available.

A useful device for producing potable water is a solar still (Figure 28-18). The materials needed include a 6 × 6–foot piece of sturdy, clear plastic sheeting (preferably reinforced with duct tape in the center), a shovel, a 6- to 8-foot piece of surgical tubing, a 1-quart plastic bowl, duct tape, and a knife. A cone-shaped hole about 3½ feet in diameter and 18 to 20 inches deep should be dug in a low area where water would stand the longest after a rain. With the surgical tubing taped securely to its bottom, the bowl is placed in the center of the hole. The plastic sheet is positioned loosely on top of the hole and weighted with a fist-sized rock in the center so that it sags into a cone whose apex is just above the bowl. Crushed desert vegetation is placed inside the hole to provide additional moisture, preferably barrel and saguaro cactus parts. Unknown or possibly poisonous plants are avoided. Dirt and rocks are piled around the rim on top of the plastic sheet to seal the edges of the hole. Urine can be placed inside the hole in an open container. Contaminated surface water can also be purified inside a solar still, but water from a vehicle radiator should not be used because the glycols will distill along with the water.

The still is not opened once it starts operating. It will produce 1 pint to 1 quart of water per 24 hours without added urine or vegetation and up to 4 quarts with it. The surgical tubing is used to suck water from the bowl periodically as it collects.

If vegetation is plentiful, another type of solar still can be made from a large, clear plastic bag.[21] On a slope, a hole several feet in diameter is dug with a craterlike rim surrounded by a moat that drains downhill into a small hole. The bag is centered on the large hole with its edges over the moat and its mouth downhill at the small hole. An upright stick is placed

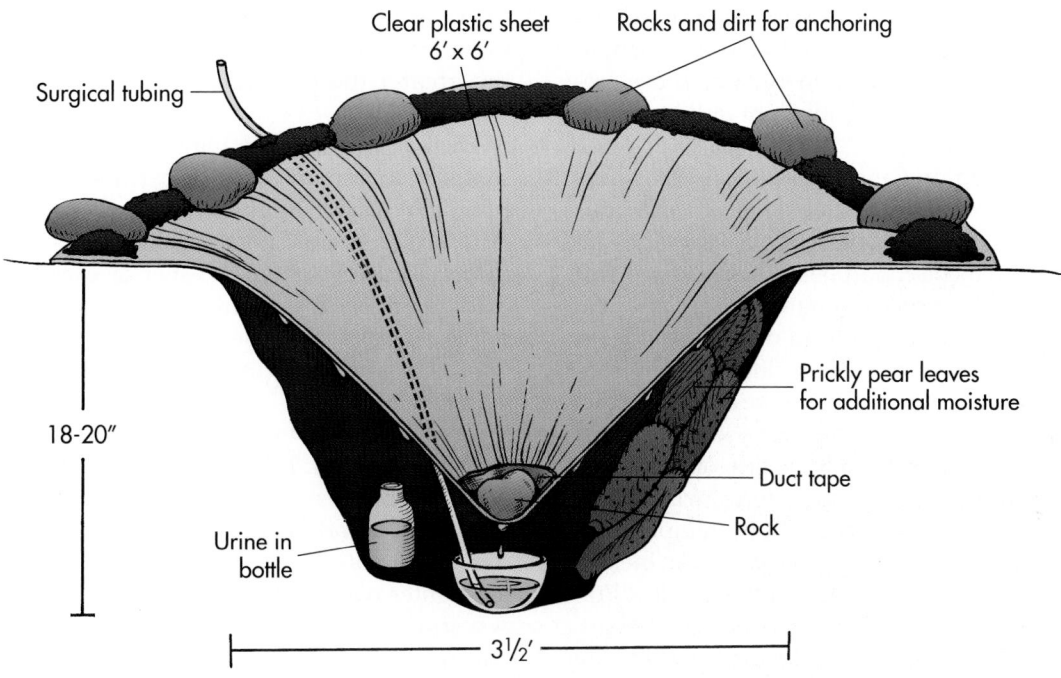

Surgical tubing

Clear plastic sheet
6' x 6'

Rocks and dirt for anchoring

18-20"

Prickly pear leaves
for additional moisture

Duct tape

Rock

Urine in
bottle

3½'

Figure 28-18 Solar still.

inside the bag in the middle and clean rocks along the crater rim inside the bag to keep the bag anchored and ballooned out. Duct tape reinforces the bag where the stick tents it. After the bag is filled with vegetation, its mouth is tied shut. The vegetation should not touch the sides of the bag or spill into the part of the bag that is over the moat. The warmth of the sun causes water to evaporate from the vegetation and condense on the inside of the bag, run down into the part of the bag that is over the moat, run downhill toward the mouth of the bag, and collect in the part of the bag's neck that is in the small hole. Survivors open the mouth of the bag and pour out the water as needed.

NAVIGATION

Even if in a familiar area, backcountry travelers should always to carry a compass, map, and altimeter. Prior training and experience in map reading and compass use are necessary.[13] The best type of compass for the layperson is the Swedish Silva compass, designed to be used in the sport of orienteering. The compass is always followed even if at odds with "gut feelings" about direction. Topographic maps are available at most outdoor stores in both the 7.5- and 15-minute series.

Global positioning system (GPS) units are small, electronic devices that can plot a traveler's position by receiving signals from satellites. Although very useful, especially in poor visibility, they are expensive and bat-tery dependent, require at least three satellites in the unobstructed sky above, and need experience to translate their output into a position on a map.[5] The back-country traveler should be expert with map and compass before considering a GPS unit.

Travelers who lose or forget their compass should still be able to find directions (see Chapter 73). At night, north can be found by identifying the Big Dipper (Northern Hemisphere only) and following the "pointers" (farthest stars on the bowl of the dipper) to the North Star (Polaris), the most distal star in the handle of the Little Dipper, which is located about halfway between the Big Dipper and the W-shaped constellation Cassiopeia. On a sunny day a nondigital watch set to standard time can be used to find direction. When the hour hand is pointed toward the sun, south will be one-half of the shorter of the two distances between the hour hand and 12 o'clock.

WEATHER FORECASTING[5,11,15,18,27]

Travelers entering the backcountry must check expected weather conditions. Modern weather forecasting, because of radar, satellite technology, and other advanced techniques, is accurate but not infallible. Local and national radio and television networks broadcast local and regional reports hourly. The Weather Channel has multiday forecasts and is also available on the Internet at www.weather.com. The best source of up-to-date local weather information is the National Weather Service, which broadcasts

24 hours a day at frequencies from 162.400 to 162.550 MHz on very-high frequency (VHF) FM. Multichannel radios with a weather band receive these frequencies, and inexpensive, lightweight radios receive only these frequencies.

When evaluating avalanche conditions, travelers must know the weather conditions over the previous few days as well. The U.S. Forest Service provides information on avalanche conditions in many mountainous areas, especially in western states (see Chapter 2).

Since weather information from outside sources is usually impossible to access in a wilderness environment, the wilderness traveler should be able to predict weather to some extent. This requires a knowledge of both local weather patterns and basic meteorology, particularly the significance of cloud patterns, wind directions, barometric pressure changes, and temperature changes. Backcountry weather forecasting is an inexact science, however. In Michael Hodgson's words, "Predictions relative to weather are only educated guesses, never statements of fact. Always be prepared for the worst."[11]

The major factors that influence weather are solar radiation, the components of the atmosphere (especially water vapor), topography, physical properties of large water bodies and land masses, and the effects of the earth's daily and yearly rotation on the amount of solar radiation that reaches each part of the earth.

The earth's atmosphere is constantly in motion. The primary motion is basically circular, involving vertical upward motion as air is heated at the equator, then horizontal motion of this warm air toward the poles where it cools, descends, and moves back toward the equator to replace heated, upward-moving air. If the earth did not rotate, this circular motion would be in a north-south direction. The earth's rotation, however, causes the direction of movement to be deflected to the right (in the Northern Hemisphere), so the movement becomes more west to east (Coriolis effect) in the temperate zone (area between Tropic of Cancer and Arctic Circle). Because the earth's surface is covered unevenly by land masses, water bodies, and polar ice, and because these regions are heated irregularly as the earth rotates on its axis, systems of moving cold and warm air masses are formed. Cold, moist air masses tend to form over cold (polar) seas and warm, moist air masses over warm seas. Cold, dry air masses tend to form over cold (polar) land and warm, dry air masses over warm land. The polar regions have large, stable areas of cold, high-pressure air (polar highs), and the equatorial regions (between 10 degrees south and north of the equator) have a large area of stable, warm, moist, and low-pressure air (doldrums).

Atmospheric pressure in air masses depends on their temperature: higher in cold air masses and lower in warm air masses. Winds are caused by air moving from a high-pressure to a low-pressure area; the greater the pressure difference, the higher the wind speed.

Each air mass, which may cover hundreds to thousands of square miles of the earth's surface, is nearly homogenous for temperature and humidity. In the northern temperate zone, air masses generally move from west to east; in North America, exceptions include cold, relatively dry air masses that move south from northern Canada in the winter and warm, moist air masses that move north from the Gulf of Mexico in the summer.

Cold air masses move faster than warm air masses (25 to 35 mph vs. 10 to 20 mph). The boundaries between air masses are called *fronts*. Frontal air is generally unstable and frequently an area of violent weather. A cold front is an area where heavy, cold air is displacing lighter warm air, frequently by coursing under it. A warm front is an area where lighter, warm air is replacing a retreating mass of heavier, cold air.

Warm, low-pressure air masses are called *lows,* or *cyclones;* cold, high-pressure ones are called *highs,* or *anticyclones.* Since air flows from areas of high pressure to areas of low pressure, lows are characterized by winds blowing from their edges toward their centers and highs by winds blowing from their centers toward their edges. The Coriolis effect causes winds in the Northern Hemisphere to move in a clockwise direction from the center to the periphery in a high and in a counterclockwise direction from the periphery to the center in a low. Understanding these principles can help the traveler interpret shifting wind directions as highs and lows pass.

Weather within an air mass is controlled by its moisture content, the relationship between land surface and air mass temperatures, and terrain features such as up or down slopes. Precipitation can occur in either a high or a low but is more common in a low. The amount of moisture in a mass of air can be described as the air's *relative humidity,* or the amount of water vapor in the air compared with the amount it could hold at its current temperature without condensation occurring. Warm air can hold more water vapor than can cold air. The term *dew point* refers to the temperature at which the relative humidity becomes 100% and the water vapor in air starts to condense. Since the temperature drops about 2.2° C (4° F) for every 305 m (1000 feet) of ascent (1.6° C [3° F] if moist, 3° C [5.5° F] if dry), rising air cools and descending air warms. Water vapor in rising air will condense when the air cools to its dew point, producing fog, clouds, and precipitation.

The wilderness traveler should be able to identify the different types of clouds and know their significance. Clouds are divided into four types based on

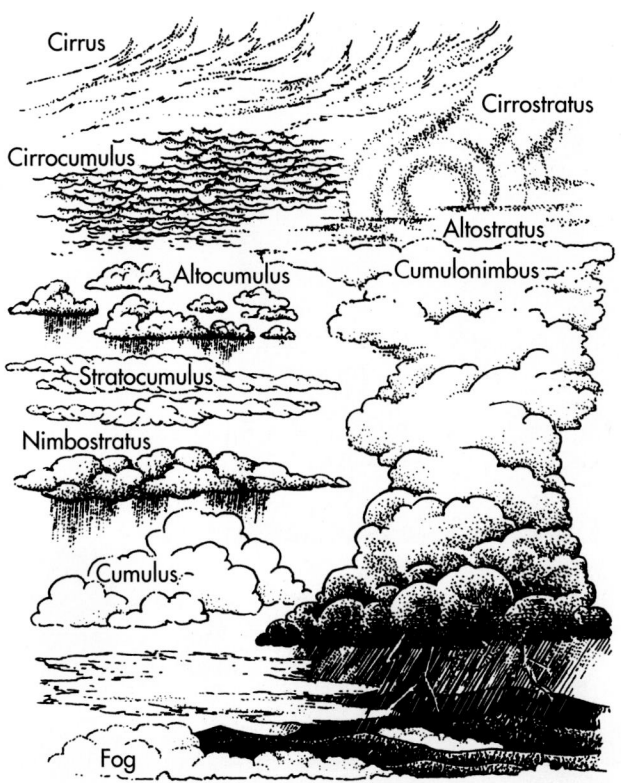

Figure 28-19 Different types of clouds. (*Modified from Woodmencey J: Reading weather, Helena, Mont, 1998, Falcon.*)

level, form, and association with precipitation (Figures 28-19 and 20). The highest clouds are *cirrus* clouds, which develop above 6000 m (20,000 feet). These ice-crystal clouds frequently appear thin, veil-like, and delicate. The feathery ones are called "mare's tails." The sun shines brightly through cirrus clouds. Middle-level clouds (2000 to 6000 m [6500 to 20,000 feet]) have the prefix *alto-* (e.g., altocumulus). Low-level clouds (2000 m or below) have the prefix *strato-* or suffix *–stratus* (e.g., stratocumulus, nimbostratus). These terms are also used to indicate clouds in sheets or layers at high altitudes (e.g., altostratus, cirrostratus).

Clouds of high vertical development (500 to 18,200 m [1600 to 60,000 feet]) are the larger types of cumulus clouds frequently associated with heavy precipitation. Developing ones that ascend to 9100 m (30,000 feet) are called cumulus congestus with billowing tops resembling cauliflowers. The largest ones rise to 18,200 m (60,000 feet) or above, are called cumulonimbus, and have anvil-shaped tops. Both types have darkening bases. Because of these clouds' height, precipitation falls long distances through supercooled water droplets. Depending on conditions, hail, soft hail (graupel), or huge snowflakes may result.

The prefix *nimbo-* or suffix *-nimbus* indicates that a cloud is associated with precipitation. The term *cumu-*

lus refers to any clouds that present as large or small groups of separate fluffy masses (e.g., cirrocumulus, altocumulus, cumulus fractus, depending on their altitude). Cumulus humilis refers to the middle-level, white, cottony clouds with white bases seen in fair weather.

In the inland parts of North America, the worse winter weather (blizzards) is associated with moving masses of warm air (lows) and the worst summer weather (severe thunderstorms) with rising masses of warm air and moving masses of cold air (highs).

There are two types of thunderstorms, both associated with cumulonimbus clouds (thunderheads). *Frontal* thunderstorms result when an arriving cold front slides under a warm air mass. *Air mass* thunderstorms consist of two subtypes. *Orographic* thunderstorms result when moist air is forced up over a mountain range, causing thunderstorms on the windward side. *Convective* thunderstorms result from rising vertical currents of air caused by heating of ground or water by solar radiation. These are the typical afternoon or early-evening thunderstorms, which may be accompanied by tornadoes when severe.

An advancing warm front bringing precipitation has a predictable series of lowering, darkening cloud formations: scattered cirrus, sheets of cirrostratus, sheets of altostratus, then nimbostratus. Precipitation can begin with the appearance of either altostratus or nimbostratus clouds. The combination of cirrus clouds followed by cirrostratus and altostratus clouds usually predicts precipitation within 24 to 48 hours. Cumulus congestus and especially cumulonimbus clouds indicate thunderstorms.

The wilderness traveler can anticipate weather to a limited extent by using a thermometer and altimeter (or barometer), noting the wind direction, and identifying clouds. Some digital watches have altimeter and barometer features. Both measure air pressure, but the altimeter registers higher as altitude increases (pressure drops) and the barometer registers higher as pressure rises. While traveling in mountains, barometer and altimeter readings will change as altitude changes, regardless of a low or high pressure area. In the evening, however, the movable arrow on an anaeroid altimeter can be set or the altitude (or barometric pressure) recorded. The next morning the evening reading is compared with the morning reading. Most severe winter storms are accompanied by an altimeter rise of 150 to 240 m (500 to 800 feet). A rapid altimeter rise (barometer drop) may signify high winds or a short severe storm and a slow steady altimeter rise (barometer drop) a long storm. A rapid altimeter drop (barometer rise) may also mean high winds.

Measuring and recording the air temperature several times daily (remembering that normal temperature drops with increased altitude) can confirm an advanc-

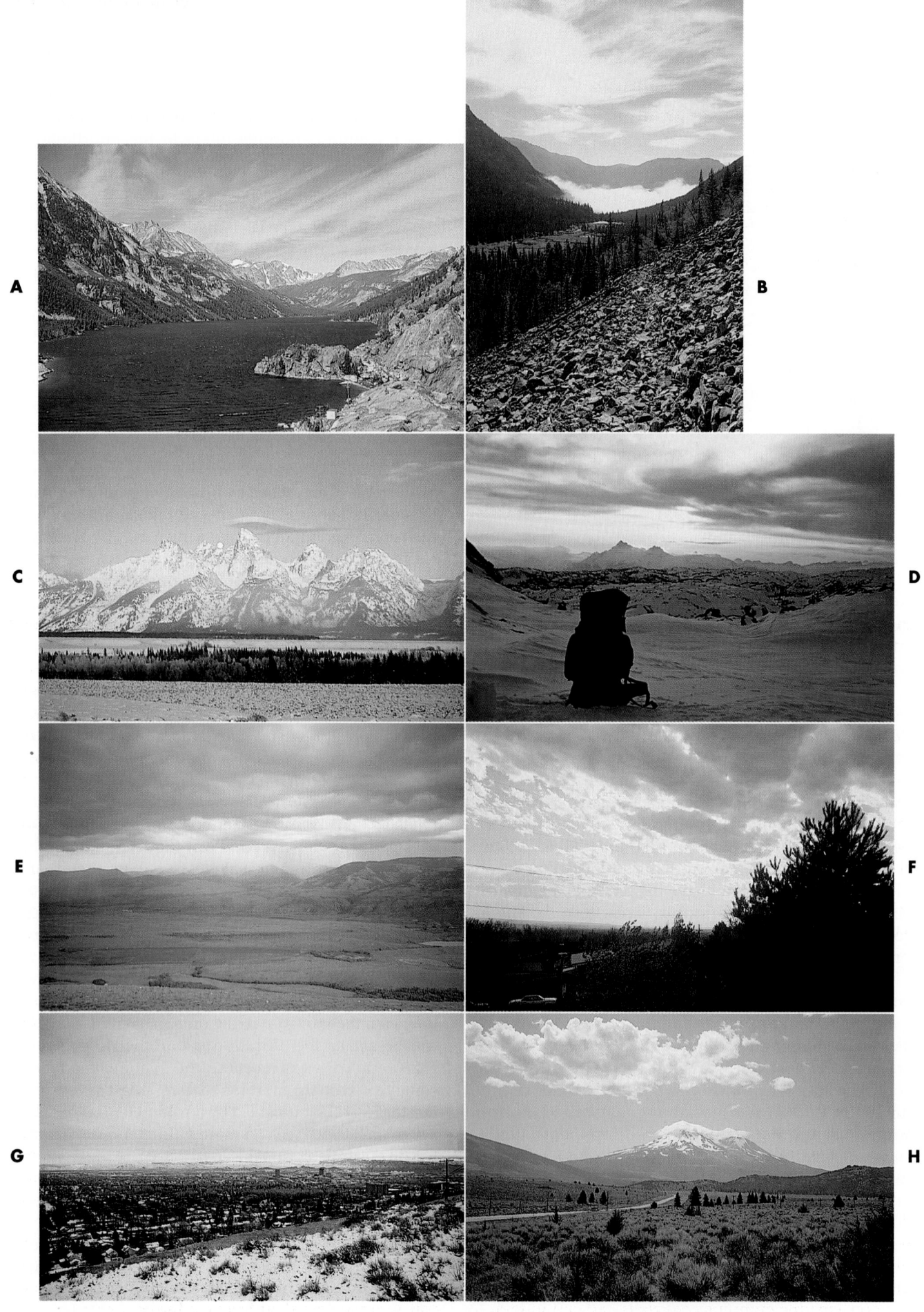

Figure 28-20 **A** and **B,** Cirrus. **C,** Altocumulus lenticularis. **D** and **E,** Altostratus. **F,** Altocumulus. **G,** Nimbostratus. **H,** Cumulus humilis.

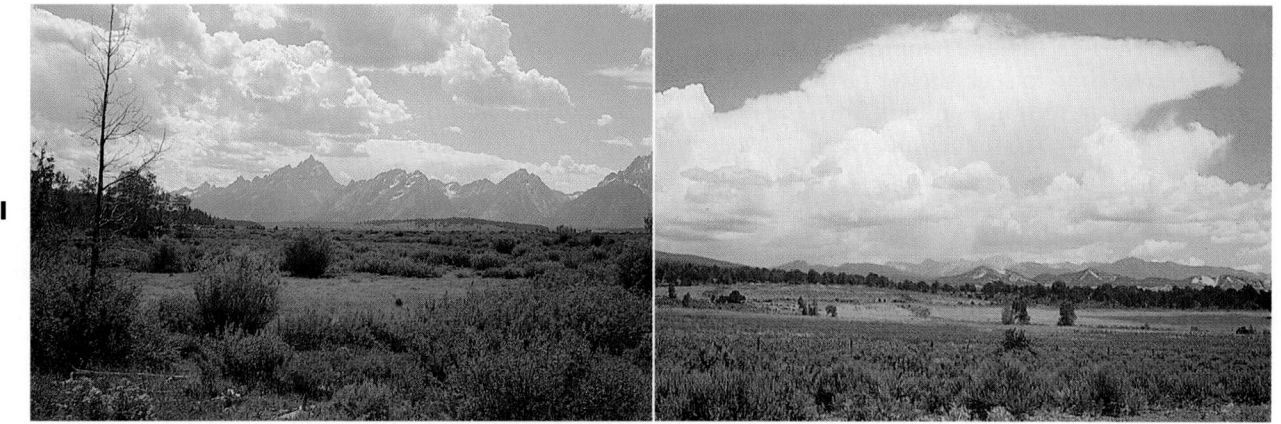

Figure 28-20, cont'd I, Cumulus congestus. **J,** Cumulonimbus.

ing low or high when coordinated with other observations. If a low is moving directly toward you, the wind will shift so that it is blowing from the southeast or south (Northern Hemisphere). If the wind comes from the southwest or west, the low is passing north of you; if from the northeast or east, it is passing south of you. An easy way to check this is to stand with your back to the wind. The low-pressure area will be in front of you and to your left.[5] As a front passes, the wind will gradually shift 180 degrees.

The shores of large bodies of water have characteristic wind patterns because of the difference in warming and cooling rates of water and land. As the land warms, breezes begin to blow from water to shore in the morning. As the land cools, breezes begin to blow from land to water in the evening. Since cloud patterns are always changing, they must be observed at regular intervals throughout each day in order to develop the ability to predict their meanings with any confidence.

Mountain Weather

Mountain weather is more unpredictable than weather in lower, flatter country. Winds frequently blow up and down mountain valleys regardless of their orientation because of the funnel effect of the valley and temperature differentials caused by solar radiation. The funnel effect may also cause heavy snowfalls at passes or the higher ends of valleys.

On a sunny day the sun warms mountaintops and high slopes first, the warm air rises, and winds blow up the slope. In the evening, the tops and high slopes cool first, the cool air descends, and winds blow down the slope. Glaciers and large snowfields produce significant cool, down-slope winds. Except on the clearest days, mountaintops may have clouds over them or nearby because of up-slope winds that carry moist air high enough to reach its dew point. In the summer, mountains warm up during the morning and early afternoon, creating cumulus congestus and cumulonim-

bus clouds that produce thunderstorms, lightning, and hail. Therefore the standard recommendation for summer climbers is to arise early and reach the summit before noon.

Lightning usually precedes rain in a thunderstorm and can strike up to 5 miles away from the storm. Distance is estimated by counting the seconds between the lightning flash and the first noise of thunder; 5 seconds equals 1 mile (see Chapter 3).

Precipitation is frequently heavy on the windward side of large mountain ranges; the leeward sides are usually much drier and in low areas may be desert. Stationary lens-shaped clouds (altocumulus lenticularis) are frequently seen near mountaintops in windy weather and signify high winds at the summits. High winds also produce long snow plumes from summits and ridges. The summit wind speed will be about twice the valley wind speed.[27]

Winds blowing at right angles to a mountain range tend to concentrate at any gaps or passes in the range, creating high winds due to the Venturi effect. Warm winds on down slopes in the winter (Chinook or foehn winds) are produced when cool, dense air blowing over mountaintops loses its moisture as precipitation on the windward side; the drier air then warms rapidly as it descends on the lee side. These warm winds can melt snow rapidly.

Weather is more stable at certain times of the year than others, but the times vary by geographic area. For example, in the northern Rocky Mountains the best times to hike or climb in the summer are the last week of July, all of August, and the first week in September. The best time to ski, tour, or climb in the winter is February. In Alaska the best climbing weather in winter is during February and in spring and summer from April through June. In the Himalaya and Karakorum Mountains, the best climbing weather is immediately before and after the summer monsoon (a seasonal, northward flow of warm, moist air from the Indian Ocean).

The principal value of understanding weather signs is in predicting severe, life-threatening storms and providing adequate time to seek shelter or the option to stay put rather than try for a summit. Travel in severe weather, especially above timberline, should never be undertaken casually.

Summary of Backcountry Weather Forecasting

1. Blue sky, a few cirrus or cumulus humilis clouds, cold temperatures, low to medium winds, and a steady or dropping altimeter are predictors of good weather.
2. A lowering cloud pattern (cirrus followed by cirrostratus, altostratus, and nimbostratus), rising temperatures, wind freshening and shifting to blow from the southeast or south, and an altimeter rise of 152 to 244 m (500 to 800 feet) indicate a possibly severe winter storm.
3. Building cumulus congestus clouds changing to cumulonimbus clouds indicate probable thunderstorms and possible hail. A thunderstorm is frequently heralded by a rush of cold air (cold front).
4. Signs that a severe winter storm is abating include clouds thinning, cloud bases rising, temperature falling, altimeter dropping, and winds shifting to blow from the north or northwest.

SANITATION

Adherence to proper habits of cleanliness and sanitation is as important in the wilderness as at home.[4] The hands are washed with biodegradable soap after urinating and defecating, before cooking and eating, and before dressing open wounds. If soap is unavailable, snow or the cleanest available plain water is used. Dishes and pots are washed with hot water, avoiding soap. Waste water is scattered over a wide area and never dumped into a body of water. Bathing and washing clothes should be done at least 60 m (200 feet) from bodies of water, using water in a container. Gloves, preferably rubber (impermeable) ones, are worn when handling moist animal or human tissues.

Campers should dig and defecate in a "cathole" at least 8 inches deep, 6 inches wide, downhill, and at least 60 m from camp, water sources, or snow to be melted for water, covering feces completely with dirt. No camp should be within 60 m of a lake or stream, which is 70 to 80 normal steps for most adults.

Travelers should urinate on rocks or dirt, not on green plants. When sleeping in a tent or snow shelter, a 500-ml wide-mouth polyethylene bottle can be used as a urinal to avoid going outside, especially at night. Special funnels to use with the bottle are available for women.

PSYCHOLOGIC ASPECTS OF SURVIVAL

Dealing with the psychologic aspects of survival is as important as confronting physical and environmental factors. As mentioned previously, the dangerous mindset that keeps a person continuing on a hazardous course, such as completing a climb or reaching a distant campsite despite conditions that would make a more prudent person bivouac or turn back,[8] is a recurring scenerio. In a survival emergency, a person with adequate oxygen, a stable body temperature, shelter, water, and food may still die if unable to withstand the psychologic stress. Conversely, persons have survived amazing hardships with little more than a strong determination to live. Individual reactions, however, cannot be predicted in advance. Groups faced with unexpected emergencies testify that courage and leadership appear in unexpected places.

If persons possess the necessary skills and have at least a minimum of survival equipment (see appendixes to this chapter), the odds are strongly in their favor. Medical personnel have the advantage of being trained to suppress panic. Fear and surrender are normal reactions that must be opposed by whatever psychologic tools are available. In some cases, religious faith or the desire to rejoin loved ones have been credited with survival.

Anxieties that paralyze action include fear (of the unknown, being alone, wild animals, darkness, weakness, personal failure, discomfort, suffering, and death) and panic. Panic, the uncontrolled urge to run away from the situation, interferes with good judgment, resulting in inappropriate actions, such as abandoning weaker companions, dividing the party, and discarding vital survival equipment. Useless flight saps available energy, leads to exhaustion, and hastens death.

Other psychologic reactions include apathy and the normal desires to be comfortable and to avoid pain.[23] Apathy is giving up, a state of indifference, mental numbness, surrender, and unwillingness to perform necessary tasks. The person shows resignation, quietness, lack of communication, loss of appetite, fatigue, drowsiness, and withdrawal. Apathy in one's self is overcome by faith in abilities and equipment and belief in survival and the possibility of rescue. Apathy in others is combated by communicating plans and positive feelings about resources and outcomes to them, and including all group members in planning and survival activities.

Comfort is not essential to survival. Severe discomfort from injuries, illnesses, thirst, hunger, excessive heat or cold, sleep deprivation, and/or exhaustion is inevitable in a survival situation and must be tolerated in order to live. There are many accounts of adventurers who have survived many days with severe injuries such as open fractures because of the will to live, or who have dragged themselves for miles despite multiple injuries to find help.

Providing an ill or injured party member with psychologic support is important. This includes appearing calm, unhurried, and deliberate yourself while trying to encourage optimism, patience, and cooperation. A person with a minor injury or illness should be encouraged to self-evacuate, accompanied by at least one healthy party member. When a person with a severe injury or illness needs to be evacuated, the party must decide whether to use the resources at hand or to send for help. The decision will depend on the weather, party size, training, available equipment, distance, type of terrain involved, type of injury or illness, victim's condition, and availability of local search and rescue groups, helicopters, and other assistance. Unless the weather is excellent, the party strong and well equipped, the route short and easy, and the victim comfortable and stable, the best course of action generally is to make a comfortable camp and send the strongest party members for help. A written note should include each victim's name, gender, age, type of injury or illness, current condition, and emergency care; the party's resources and location (preferably map coordinates); and names, addresses, and telephone numbers of relatives. The victim who must be left alone should have an adequate supply of food, fuel, and water.

As soon as you realize that you are lost, stop, sit down in a sheltered place, calmly go over the situation, and make an inventory of your survival equipment and other resources. If it is cold or becoming dark, start a fire and eat if you have food. Take out your map or draw a sketch of your route and location based on natural features. Unless you know your location and can reach safety before dark, prepare a camp and wait until morning. Do not allow yourself to be influenced by a desire to keep others from worrying or the need to be at work or keep an appointment. Your life is more important than anyone else's peace of mind.[10]

If you are alone and unquestionably lost, and especially if injured, you must decide whether to wait for rescue or attempt to walk out under your own power. Almost always, it is better to use the time to prepare a snug shelter and conserve strength if rescue is possible. If you decide to leave, mark the site with a cairn or bright-colored material such as surveyor's tape, leave a note at the site with information about your condition, equipment, and direction of travel, and then mark your trail. These actions will aid rescuers and enable you to return to the site if necessary. Travel should never be attempted in severe weather, desert daytime heat, or deep snow without snowshoes or skis. If no chance of rescue exists, prepare as best possible, wait for good weather, and then travel in the most logical direction.

SIGNALING

Besides radios, cell phones, and other electronic equipment, signaling devices are either auditory or visual. Three of anything is a universal distress signal: three whistle blasts, three shots, three fires, or three columns of smoke. The most effective auditory device is a whistle. Blowing a whistle is less tiring than shouting, and the distinctive sound can be heard farther than a human voice. An effective visual ground-to-air signal device is a glass signal mirror, which can be seen up to 10 miles away but requires sunlight. Smoke is easily seen by day and a fire or flashlight by night. On a cloudy day, black smoke is more visible than white; the reverse is true on a sunny day.

Black smoke can be produced by burning parts of a vehicle, such as rubber or oil, and white smoke by adding green leaves or a small amount of water to the fire.

Ground signals (e.g., SOS, HELP) should be as large as possible—at least 3 feet wide and 18 feet long—and should contain straight lines and square corners, which are not found in nature. They can be tramped out in dirt or on grass or can be made from brush or logs. In snow the depressions can be filled with vegetation to increase contrast.

Many pilots do not know the traditional 18 international ground-to-air emergency signals, which have been replaced with the following five simple signals adopted by the International Convention on Civil Aviation[23]:

V   I require assistance
X   I require medical assistance
N   No
Y   Yes
→   Am proceeding in this direction

Air-to-ground signals include the following:

Message received and understood: rock plane from side to side.

Message received but not understood: make a complete right-hand circle.

When using cell phones, radios, and other electronic devices, persons should move out of valleys and gulleys to higher elevations if possible. Operational pay phones in campgrounds closed for the season or other facilities can be used to call for help. Most will allow 911 or another emergency number to be dialed without payment, but carrying the right change and memorizing your telephone credit card number are recommended.

PROTECTION FROM WILD ANIMALS

Although persons in a survival situation often worry about wild animal attacks, these are rare. Many wild animals flee when confronted with a shouting, moving human. Exceptions include polar bears, grizzly bears, moose, bison, cougars, jaguars, wild pigs, elephants, lions, tigers, water buffalo, leopards, wolverines, females with young (e.g., bears, moose, elk, deer), rabid mammals, and feral dogs and cats (see Chapters 41 to 43). Polar bears, some grizzly and black bears, the great cats, and crocodiles may hunt humans as food. Venomous snakes, insects, arachnids (e.g., scorpions and ticks), and marine animals are also a concern (see Chapters 33 to 39 and 60 to 62).

The only effective weapon against large mammals and reptiles is a high-powered rifle, although pepper spray may discourage an attacking bear. Improvised weapons such as a spear tipped with a hunting knife, are useless.

Food should not be kept in a shelter or backpack during the night. All food should be placed in a nylon bag and hung between two trees on a high line. Above the timberline, small rodents such as mice may gnaw holes in expensive tents to reach food inside, so all food should be bagged and hung on a line between two high boulders.

In desert and other snake or scorpion country, travelers should avoid walking barefoot, especially at night, and should not place hands, feet, or other body parts in uninspected places. Desert campers should carry tents with floors and tightly zipped doors. Those sleeping outside should shake out clothing, footgear, and bedding before using them.

In warm weather, insect repellent should be carried and used liberally.

HOW TO PREPARE FOR A POSSIBLE SURVIVAL SITUATION

Basic survival equipment and skills for those interested in wilderness travel should include the following:
1. Practice physical conditioning and healthful habits. Avoid alcohol, tobacco, and "recreational" drugs.
2. Develop the ability to swim well.
3. Learn how to use a map and compass and find directions without a compass.
4. Be able to build a fire under adverse conditions.
5. Have a working knowledge of local weather patterns and be able to use an altimeter, thermometer, cloud forms, and wind directions to predict storms. Avoid exposure to meteorologic hazards, such as blizzards and lightning strikes.
6. Be familiar with the special medical problems of the type of wilderness involved. For example, for cold weather and high-altitude travel, be familiar with the prevention, diagnosis, and treatment of hypothermia, frostbite, and altitude illnesses. Travel in the desert and tropics requires familiarity with tropical infections, snakebites, tropical skin diseases, and heat illness. Understand basic principles of prehospi-

tal emergency care and the improvisation of splints and bandages.
7. Carry a survival kit containing equipment appropriate for the topography, climate, and season (see appendices to this chapter).
8. Be able to construct appropriate types of survival shelters.
9. Acquire a working knowledge of the characteristics of natural hazards and how to predict and avoid them. These include forest fire, lightning strike, avalanche, rockfall, cornice fall, flash flood, white water, deadfall, storms of various kinds, and the hazardous animals and plants of the area of travel.
10. Read and analyze accounts of survival experiences (see Suggested Readings).[1,12,14]
11. Be aware of the psychologic aspects of a survival situation and of errors in judgment that can lead to a survival emergency.
12. Know the edible plants and animals of the area of projected travel, as well as the poisonous or venomous species. Basic hunting, trapping, and fishing skills are valuable.
13. Never travel alone. Always let responsible persons know your destination and expected time of return, and do not fail to notify these persons of your return to avoid unnecessary rescue attempts. After you leave, avoid changing destination and time plans except in unusual circumstances. Failure to follow these guidelines has led to many unsuccessful searches.

APPENDIX A

Everyone should develop the habit of carrying at least a Swiss Army knife and matches in a waterproof container when away from paved roads.

Sample Basic Wilderness Survival Kit

This kit is carried in a small backpack, with a capacity of 3200 to 4000 cubic inches.

Shelter-building equipment:
Plastic or nylon tarp (not a "space blanket")
1/8 inch braided nylon cord, 50 to 100 feet
Folding saw

Fire-building equipment:
Waterproof matches
Candle
Fire starter (substitute: camera film)
Sharp, sturdy hunting knife (e.g., folding Buck knife with 4-inch blade)

Signaling equipment:
Pencil and small notebook
Whistle
Card with ground-to-air signals

Two sets of correct change for pay phone
Signal mirror, preferably glass with sighting device
Flashlight (or preferably headlamp), with spare batteries and bulb

Other:
Compass
Map
Nondigital watch
Metal pot with bale and sack to store it
Metal cup with handle
Spoon
Toilet paper
Sunburn cream
Lip balm with high SPF number
Spare socks (used as spare mittens in emergency)
Emergency food
First-aid kit
Sunglasses
Canteen (full)
Water disinfection equipment: chemicals or filter
Insect repellent (in season)

Repair kit, adapted to type of travel (e.g., ski, snowshoe, kayak):
Leatherman type of tool (or Swiss Army knife) small pliers with wire-cutting feature, small crescent wrench
Small screwdriver with multiple tips
Picture wire
Fiberglass tape
Duct tape
Steel wool for shimming
Assorted nuts, bolts, and screws

Additional considerations:
Altimeter
Thermometer (plastic alcohol type clipped to loop on outside of pack)
Spare eyeglasses
Swiss Army knife with scissors
Fishhooks and line
No. 28 piano wire for snares
Cellular telephone (if service available)
GPS locator
.22-caliber rifle and ammunition
Surveyor's tape
Cigarette lighter

APPENDIX B

Sample Winter Survival Kit

Basic survival items from Appendix A

Spare clothing for severe weather: at least four layers total, including spare mittens
Snow shovel: small grain-scoop type with detachable handle

Optional items:
Piece of Ensolite or Therm-a-Rest mattress
Sleeping bag
Gore-Tex bivouac sac
Stove and fuel
Light ax
Snow saw

APPENDIX C

Sample Desert Survival Kit

Basic survival items from Appendix A

Fold-up steel shovel with short handle

Items for construction of four solar stills:
Four sheets of clear plastic, 6 × 6 feet, reinforced in center by cross of duct tape
Four pieces of surgical tubing, 6 to 8 feet long
Four 1-quart plastic bowls
5-gallon water jug, full
1-liter wide-mouth bottle for use as urinal
Spare sunglasses
Heavy leather gloves
Citizen's band radio
Light rifle or target pistol with ammunition

APPENDIX D

Vehicle Cold Weather Survival Kit[25]

Sleeping bag or two blankets for each occupant
Extra winter clothing, including boots, for each occupant
Emergency food
Waterproof matches
Long-burning candles, at least two
First-aid kit
Spare doses of personal medications, if any
Swiss Army knife
Three coffee cans with lids, for toilet
Toilet paper
Citizen's band radio or cell phone
Flashlight with extra batteries and bulb
Battery booster cables
Extra quart of oil (place some in hubcap and burn for emergency smoke signal)
Tire chains
Snow shovel
Tow chain, at least 20 feet long
Small sack of sand
Two plastic water jugs, full
Tool kit
Gas line deicer
Flagging, such as surveyor's tape (tie to top of radio antenna for signal)

Signal flares

Long rope (e.g., clothesline) to act as safety rope if you leave car in blizzard

Carbon monoxide detector

Ax

Folding saw

Full tank of gas

APPENDIX E

Minimal Equipment for Survival First-Aid Kit (see Chapter 69)

Cravats, at least two

Rubber gloves

Roll of 3-inch Kling (self-adhering roller bandage)

Roll of 2-inch adhesive tape (waterproof preferred)

2-inch rubberized bandage (Ace or Coban)

Small prepackaged bandage strips

Nonadhering sterile gauze pads

Sterile compresses

20-ml syringe and needle or splash shield for irrigating wounds

Steel sewing needle (can be part of sewing kit)

Single-edged razor blade

Thermometer (low readings for cold environments)

Nonprescription analgesic of choice (e.g., acetaminophen, ibuprofen)

Prescription analgesic of choice (e.g., APAP with codeine, 30 mg; APAP with propoxyphene, 100 mg)

Diphenhydramine, 25- or 50-mg capsules

Small bottle or package of swabs of povidone-iodine solution 10%

Duct tape, fiberglass strapping tape (for improvising litters and splints; carried in repair kit); other splinting materials can usually be improvised using ski poles, ice axes, hammers, branches, and parts of backpacks or vehicles

Splinter forceps

Persons who are taking regular medications, such as asthmatics and diabetics, should carry emergency supplies of their medicines in addition to regular supplies; anyone who has had an anaphylactic reaction should carry an emergency epinephrine kit (EpiPen or Ana-Kit)

Physicians may take additional items, such as injectable epinephrine, an injectable narcotic, and skin glue

Other considerations (for longer trips):

Drug for nausea and vomiting (e.g., prochlorperazine or promethazine suppositories)

Drug for diarrhea (e.g., loperamide)

All-purpose antibiotic (e.g., ciprofloxacin)

Topical ophthalmic ointment (e.g., gentamicin)

REFERENCES

1. *Accidents in North American mountaineering*, Golden, Colo, American Alpine Club, and Banff, Alpine Club of Canada (published yearly).
2. *Aircrew survival*, Washington, DC, 1996, Department of the Air Force, US Government Printing Office.
3. Bowman WD: *Winter first aid manual*, ed 4, Denver, 1984, National Ski Patrol System.
4. Bowman WD: *Outdoor emergency care*, ed 3, Denver, 1998, National Ski Patrol System.
5. Clark R et al: *Mountain travel and rescue, a manual for basic and advanced mountaineering courses*, Denver, 1995, National Ski Patrol System.
6. Corneille P: *Le Cid*, Act II, Scene 2, 1636.
7. Craighead FC Jr, Craighead JJ (revised by Smith RE, Jarvis DS): *How to survive on land and sea*, ed 4, Annapolis, Md, 1984, US Naval Institute.
8. Fear G: *Surviving the unexpected wilderness emergency*, Tacoma, Wash, 1979, Survival Education Association.
9. Guyton AC, Hall JE: *Textbook of medical physiology*, ed 9, Philadelphia, 1996, WB Saunders.
10. Harris B: *A handbook for wilderness survival*, New York, 1996, Evans.
11. Hodgson M: *The basic essentials of weather forecasting*, Merrillville, Ind, 1992, ICS Books.
12. Huntford R: *The last place on earth*, New York, 1986, Atheneum.
13. Kjellstrom B: *Be expert with map and compass*, New York, 1994, MacMillan.
14. Logan N, Atkins D: *The snowy torrents: avalanche accidents in the United States 1980-1986*, Denver, 1996, Colorado Geological Survey.
15. Ludlum DM: *The Audubon Society field guide to North American weather*, New York, 1991, Alfred A. Knopf.
16. Nesbitt PH, Pond AW, Allen WH: *The survival book*, New York, 1959, Funk & Wagnalls.
17. Patterson CE: *Surviving in the wilds*, Toronto, 1979, Personal Library Publishers.
18. Reifsnyder W: *Weathering the wilderness, the Sierra Club guide to practical meteorology*, San Francisco, 1980, Sierra Club Books.
19. Shanks B: *Wilderness survival*, New York, 1987, Universe Books.
20. Stefansson V: *Unsolved mysteries of the Arctic*, New York, 1938, Macmillan.
21. Stoffel R, Lavalla R: *Survival sense for pilots and passengers*, Olympia, Wash, 1980, Emergency Response Institute.
22. *Survival*, Field Manual 21-76, Washington, DC, 1986, Department of the Army, US Government Printing Office.
23. *Survival training*, Washington, DC, 1985, Department of the Air Force, US Government Printing Office.
24. Wilkinson E: *Snow caves for fun and survival*, ed 2, Boulder, Colo, 1992, Johnson.
25. *Winter wheeling in Wyoming*, Cheyenne, 1998, Wyoming Department of Transportation.
26. Wiseman J: *The SAS survival handbook*, London, 1996, HarperCollins.
27. Woodmencey J: *Reading weather*, Helena, Mont, 1998, Falcon.

SUGGESTED READINGS

Auerbach PS: *Medicine for the outdoors*, ed 3, New York, 1999, The Lyons Press.

Clifford H: *The falling season*, New York, 1995, HarperCollins.

Kochanski M: *Bushcraft: outdoor skills and wilderness survival*, Vancouver, 1987, Lone Pine.

Krakauer J: *Into thin air*, New York, 1997, Villard.

Lansing A: *Endurance*, New York, 1976, Avon.

MacInnes H: *The price of adventure: mountain rescue stories from four continents*, Seattle, 1978, The Mountaineers.

MacInnes H: *High drama: mountain rescue stories from four continents*, Seattle, 1980, The Mountaineers.

Olson LD: *Outdoor survival skills*, ed 6, Chicago, 1997, Chicago Review Press.

Parr P: *Mountain high mountain rescue*, Golden, Colo, 1987, Fulcrum.

Randall G: *Cold comfort: keeping warm in the outdoors*, New York, 1987, Lyons Books.

Riles MJ: *Don't get snowed: a guide to mountain travel*, Matteson, Ill, 1977, Greatlakes Living Press.

Rutstrum C: *Paradise below zero*, New York, 1974, Collier Books.

Simpson J: *Touching the void*, New York, 1988, HarperCollins.

Waterman J: *Surviving Denali: a study of accidents on Mount McKinley, 1910-1982*, New York, 1983, American Alpine Club.

Waterman J: *Surviving Denali: a study of accidents on Mount McKinley 1903-1990*, ed 2, New York, 1991, AAC Press.

Whittlesey LH: *Death in Yellowstone: accidents and foolhardiness in the first national park*, Boulder, Colo., 1995, Rinehart.

Wilkinson E: *Snow caves for fun and survival*, Denver, 1986, Windsong Press.

29 Jungle Travel and Survival

John B. Walden

Persons who venture into the tropical rainforest step into an exotic and mysterious environment that can be unforgiving. Preparedness makes the difference between misery and pleasure.

TROPICAL ENVIRONMENT

In these forests lies a virtually limitless supply of excitement, joy and wonder to be encountered in new illuminations on the constructs and workings of life on earth.[23]

Tropical rainforests, located between the Tropic of Cancer (23°27' N latitude) and the Tropic of Capricorn (23°27' S latitude), are regions with at least 4 inches of precipitation per month and a mean annual monthly temperature exceeding 24° C (75° F) without any occurrence of frost.[10] Facts and figures fail to capture the essence of tropical rainforests and their extraordinary biologic diversity. Seen from the air, the forest stretches from horizon to horizon in a vast green carpet. In season the crowns of trees in full blossom dot the landscape with vivid splashes of red, orange, and yellow. Sizable streams may be hidden beneath the emerald canopy. Rivers, usually muddy yellow or black, snake through the forest; early-morning or late-afternoon sun transforms these braided rivers into glistening, mirror-like strands of liquid silver.

Observed from the forest floor, the jungle is entrancing. In virgin, deep forest, all is muted and shadowy save for random shafts of light that stream down to spotlight labyrinths of oddly shaped branches and spectacularly colored flowers. Shrubs and herbaceous plants are scarce in forest away from the flood plain, so it is relatively easy to walk undisturbed. The dimness is occasionally disrupted by areas bathed in bright light from larger holes in the canopy caused by a recently fallen tree, sandy beach, or cutting and burning by humans. It is in these sunlit areas that the traveler encounters the lush and nearly impenetrable wall of foliage portrayed in adventure films. The tidy "textbook" division of vegetation into distinct tiers is somewhat arbitrary and not easily confirmed, even by experts.[27]

In addition to upland *terra firme* forests, lowland forests remain submerged for several months each year. Such forests, or *várzeas*, make up only a small percentage of forested land but are infinitely more fertile than their nonflooding and nutrient-poor counterparts.

Despite environmental differences within the jungle, the basics of travel remain the same.

TRIP PREPARATION

Reading

National Geographic[3] and Wilson[35,36] provide an excellent introduction to people, places, and biodiversity issues. *The Emerald Realm*[10] is a superb overview of the world's tropical forests. The references at the end of this chapter offer insights into the complex inner workings of the moist tropical forest.[1,26,27] The books by Kritcher[20] and Forsyth et al[14] are especially helpful.

Trips into the rainforest should be scheduled for the dry season, because trails are more serviceable for trekking at that time. Information on weather patterns can be obtained from agencies of national governments, anthropologists, missionaries, and the excellent series *World Survey of Climatology*.[31]

Attitude

In selecting participants, experienced expedition leaders look for a sense of humor; the ability to see the bright side in difficult times may be an asset more valuable than physical conditioning. Houston[18] and others have discussed the role of humor as a predictor of success. Erb[11,12] noted that successful or failed participation in wilderness ventures also is a significant predictor.

A number of expedition leaders privately note that two individuals who have a sexual relationship often form a team within a team, to the detriment of the expedition as a whole.

Conditioning

Indigenous peoples in jungle regions are almost always slender. After trekking with large numbers of non-indigenous men and women in equatorial regions, I have observed that overweight or powerfully built individuals, particularly men, seem to fare the worst, especially with heat-related illness. Achieving an ideal weight is beneficial on the trail.

Although being in good shape is sensible, a person need not be an elite athlete to trek through the jungle and enjoy the experience. Good leg strength, acquired by training with stair-climbing exercise machines, offers appropriate preparation.

To keep up with native porters and guides, the prospective expedition member should practice hiking at a fast pace. Once in the jungle, travelers should imitate the energy-saving, fluid rhythm of local inhabitants.

Because trekkers frequently encounter single-log bridges, a well-developed sense of balance is desirable. Walking on the rails of train tracks or on curbs may help in preparation. To adapt to the specific situations, trekkers should go to the woodlands and practice walking on logs. Head stability is important. Equilibrium can be enhanced by avoiding brisk head movements and by employing the "gaze-anchoring" technique of tightrope walkers. The person fixes the gaze on a spot near the end of the log and does not stare down at the spot just ahead of the feet.[2,6] Special cleats (Covell) should be considered for crossing log bridges that are high off the ground, long, and slippery. The cleats can be snapped on quickly before crossing a log bridge and promptly snapped off at the other end.

IMMUNIZATIONS

Travelers to rainforest regions should protect against the following diseases by vaccination or with prophylactic medications:

1. Diphtheria, tetanus
2. Hepatitis A, hepatitis B
3. Measles, mumps, rubella
4. Polio
5. Rabies
6. Typhoid
7. Yellow fever (in certain regions of tropical Africa and South America)
8. Malaria

Malaria is prevalent throughout the tropics. Before travel to malarious areas, appropriate prophylaxis is needed. Updated information on the risk of malaria in various regions may be obtained through the International Travelers' Hot Line service at the Centers for Disease Control and Prevention (877-FYI-TRIP, www.cdc.gov). *The Medical Letter on Drugs and Therapeutics* issue on parasitic diseases, published every 2 years, is an excellent source for current recommendations on preventing and treating malaria (see Chapter 66).

Persons traveling into remote regions of Amazonia where Indian groups live in isolation should receive yearly influenza vaccinations to reduce the likelihood of inadvertently transmitting disease to these high-risk native inhabitants. Protection against meningococcal disease should be considered where circumstances warrant.

Medical Kit

The Wilderness Medical Society points out that it is inappropriate to pack medications and equipment when no team member has the knowledge or experience to use them safely.[19] The following items for a basic medical kit (Box 29-1) are adequate for personal use in the rainforest setting (see Chapter 69):

Box 29-1 MEDICAL KIT FOR JUNGLE TRAVEL

Bismuth subsalicylate tablets (48)
Diphenhydramine hydrochloride 25- or 50-mg capsules (15)
Ciprofloxacin hydrochloride 500-mg tablets (20)
Clotrimazole and betamethasone dipropionate cream (60 g)
Epinephrine autoinjector (2)
Ibuprofen 200- or 600-mg tablets (30)
Ketorolac 60-mg single-dose syringe (2)
Lidocaine hydrochloride carpules (3)
Metronidazole 250-mg tablets (21)
Mupirocin ointment 2% (30 g)
Permethrin 5% cream (60 g)
Permethrin 1% shampoo (2 oz)
SAM splint (1)
Sulfacetamide sodium ophthalmic solution 10% (15 ml)
Sunscreen (4 oz) (2)
Tramadol hydrochloride 50-mg tablets (20)

---

1. Bismuth subsalicylate (Pepto-Bismol tablets) is an effective over-the-counter preparation for preventing and treating common traveler's diarrhea. It also is useful for heartburn and indigestion. Pepto-Bismol tends to turn the tongue and stools black.
2. Diphenhydramine hydrochloride (Benadryl, 50-mg capsules) is safe and effective as an antihistamine, for motion sickness, and as a nighttime sleep aid.
3. Ciprofloxacin hydrochloride (Cipro, 500-mg tablets) is highly active against the important bacterial causes of enteritis, including *Escherichia coli*, *Vibrio cholerae*, *Salmonella*, *Shigella*, *Campylobacter jejuni*, *Aeromonas*, and *Yersinia enterocolitica*.
4. Clotrimazole and betamethasone dipropionate (Lotrisone) cream has antifungal properties and a steroid for rashes.
5. Epinephrine autoinjector (EpiPen/EpiPen Jr.) provides for emergency treatment of severe allergic reactions to insect stings, foods, or drugs.
6. Ibuprofen (600-mg tablets) is a good choice for mild to moderate pain from such problems as menstrual cramps, rheumatoid arthritis, and osteoarthritis. It also lowers elevated body temperature caused by common infectious diseases.
7. Ketorolac (Toradol, 60-mg for injection) provides good short-term relief for moderate to severe pain. It is preferred over narcotics only because it is less likely to cause problems with customs officers and police.
8. Lidocaine hydrochloride may be required as a local anesthetic agent for relief of the excruciat-

---

Box 29-2 GEAR FOR JUNGLE TRAVEL

Trail shoes (1 pair)
Camp boots (1 pair)
Covell cleats
Socks (3 pairs)
Hat (1)
Pullover garment (1)
Shirts
   Long sleeved (2)
   Short sleeved (2)
Pants (2 pairs)
Undergarments
   Underpants (3)
   Sports bra (2)
Poncho (1)
Flannel sheet
Hammock or Therm-a-Rest
Mosquito net
Backpack for porter
Personal backpack
Antifogging solution for eyeglasses
Batteries
Binoculars
Camera equipment and film
Campsuds
Candles
Cup/plate

Ear plugs
Fishing supplies
Garbage bags
   30-gallon size (4)
   13-gallon size (4)
Headlamp
Inflatable cushion
Insect repellent
Laminated map(s)
Machete
Waterproof matches/cigarette lighter
Pen
Toilet paper
Leatherman pocket survival tool
Poly bottles (2)
Razor/battery-operated shaver
Spoon
Sport sponge
Sunglasses
Umbrella
Whistle
Zipper-lock bags
   Gallon size (5)
   Quart size (5)
   Pint size (5)

---

ing pain resulting from stingray envenomation and conga ant or caterpillar stings. It should be infiltrated into and around the wound area using a dental aspirating syringe and 25-gauge needle. Lidocaine carpules (used by dentists) are protected and easy to carry and use in the rainforest.[16]

9. Metronidazole (250-mg tablets) is excellent for treating giardiasis, acute amebic dysentery, and *Trichomonas* vaginitis.

10. Mupirocin (Bactroban) ointment 2% should be immediately applied to burns, abrasions, lacerations, and ruptured blisters, which can rapidly become infected in the tropics.

11. Permethrin 5% cream and 1% shampoo should be applied before returning home by travelers who have been in close contact with heavily infested tribal peoples. Many natives, especially in the tropics of Central and South American, are infested with scabies and head lice.

12. The SAM splint is lightweight, waterproof, reusable, and not affected by temperature extremes.

13. Sulfacetamide sodium (Sodium Sulamyd) ophthalmic solution 10% is excellent for treating conjunctivitis, corneal ulcers, or other superficial ocular infections.

14. Sunscreen is essential in open areas such as rivers or jungle clearings. Sunscreens designated "waterproof" retain their full sun protection factor (SPF) rating for longer periods during sweating or water immersion than do products designated "water resistant." Opaque formulations are excellent for the nose, lips, and ears. Visitors to the tropics should wear lightweight, long-sleeved shirts and a wide-brimmed hat when exposed to the sun for prolonged periods (see Chapter 14).

15. Tramadol hydrochloride (Ultram, 50 mg tablets) is used for moderate to severe pain.

Common sense dictates supplementary items. Women on long trips might add miconazole vaginal suppositories to treat yeast infections; older men might take a 16 French catheter and sterile lubricating jelly for dealing with problems from prostatic hypertrophy. The fingers may swell rapidly during vigorous activity in the rainforest. To eliminate the possible need for emergency removal, all rings should be removed before jungle trekking.

Gear

The goal is to travel as light as possible. The more stuff that is packed, the greater is the likelihood of breakdowns, complications, and misery. The items mentioned have withstood the test of time over years of long-distance tropical trekking (Box 29-2).

Gear must hold up under difficult jungle travel conditions that include heat, wetness, and mud. No line of advertised gear is ideally suited for the traveler in the tropics. In the United States, L.L. Bean, Inc. (www.llbean.com) and Recreational Equipment, Inc. (REI) (www.rei.com) are good sources for equipment that is usually satisfactory for the tropics (see Chapter 69).

Footwear. Since feet absorb more punishment than any other part of the body, suitable footwear is the most important item of gear. This is one area where a person absolutely must not carry inferior equipment. If the feet cannot go, nothing can go.

Military-style "jungle boots" are unsuitable for serious, long-distance trekking. After an hour of hard walking through streams and muddy trails, blisters will form on every surface of the foot and the skin will peel off in sheets, bringing a jungle trip to a premature end. Furthermore, safely crossing log bridges and mossy, slime-covered river rocks is almost impossible in these boots.

Two pair of shoes are needed: one suitable for the wet, slippery conditions imposed by the trail and another that meets the need for dryness and comfort in camp.

TRAIL SHOES. The following features are desirable in trail shoes:
1. Uppers that hit just above or just below the ankles. Some people choose a high-cut design, reasoning that the extra height gives some added snake protection.
2. Extra protection over the big toe. Rubber or leather toecaps prevent the big toe from being severely battered and bruised.
3. Moderately deep-tread outsoles. Traction on rugged and muddy terrain is important. Running shoes with hard, "high-impact" soles should not be worn because they become slippery on wet logs or river rocks.
4. Quick drying time. Uppers of Cordura nylon and split leather, in addition to resisting abrasion and being aerated, dry rapidly in the sun. Even though hiking shoes usually become soaked within minutes on the trail, it is a psychologic boost to start each day with dry shoes. Since jungle travelers can be in waist-high water while on the trail, waterproof shoes with Gore-Tex liners are not essential.
5. Snagproof design. Shoes or boots with "quick-lace" steel hooks should be avoided; vines and weeds become tangled around the metal hooks, causing the wearer to stumble and pulling the laces untied. Shoelaces should always be double knotted.
6. Light weight
7. Well broken in

CAMP BOOTS. Footwear needs are different in camp where the trekker wants dry feet. Shoes, although excellent for the trail, are not suited for camp. A boot that comes to midcalf keeps mud off the feet and pants. Rubber remains an excellent material for keeping water away from the feet. Rubber lug soles provide traction. When rubber-soled boots are worn, however, extreme caution is needed when crossing bridges and walking on rocks. Camp boots should be light weight, since they must be carried in a pack on the trail. Discount stores usually carry lightweight, lug-soled rubber boots that meet the criteria for jungle camp boots.

OTHER OPTIONS. The lightweight, comfortable, mesh/neoprene fabric "water" shoes popular for beach and sailboarding activities may have a place on river trips when substantial time will be spent in dugout canoes or rubber rafts.

Thongs and open-toe sandals are fine for most towns and cities in the tropics, but in certain jungle regions such as the Amazon Basin, exposed feet invite hordes of biting insects.

The jungle traveler must never go barefoot. Plant spines and glass can puncture the feet, and larvae of ubiquitous parasites such as hookworm and Strongyloides can enter through the skin. The burrowing jigger flea, *Tunga penetrans*, is a serious pest and can be avoided by wearing shoes.

Socks. Cotton or thin synthetic socks should be worn in the jungle to decrease the risk of blisters from wet trail shoes, to reduce insect bites (particularly from no-see-ums), and to lessen the risk of lacerations from sawgrass.

Clothing. In many countries military green or camouflage-style clothing is strictly contraindicated. This is particularly true in military dictatorships or in remote border regions. To be mistaken for a guerilla or foreign infiltrator by the military, police, or security (undercover) forces can lead to harassment, detention, or worse.

HAT. For protection from radiant heat and objects falling in the forest, the traveler should wear a lightweight, light-colored hat that has a medium or wide brim. It need not be waterproof but should be made of material that can be wadded up. A useful feature is a fastener on each side to snap the brim up for traveling on the trail. A pith helmet, widely regarded as affectatious, is fine for open savanna and river trips, but on the trail, branches make it impractical.

PULLOVER. Drenching rain may leave a person feeling chilled and uncomfortable, particularly when traveling mainly by canoe or raft. Chilling generally is not a problem when hiking on the trail so long as the person keeps moving. A Dacron polyester fleece pullover such as L.L. Bean's Polarlite Pullover, REI's Polarlite Sweater, or a Patagonia pullover will keep a person warm. Wet garments should be wrung out so that they continue to offer thermal protection. Professional white-water boatmen working in tropical regions generally pack a polyester outerwear garment.

SHIRTS. Two light-colored, ultralightweight, long-sleeved cotton shirts should be taken. At the end of the day, the trail shirt should be washed and rinsed so that it will be ready, although perhaps still damp, the next morning. The second shirt can be used in camp or as a spare for the trail. Expensive synthetic shirts guaranteed to wick away moisture are poor jungle trail shirts, and make the person sweaty and sticky.

In camp, if no-see-ums and mosquitoes are few, a lightweight, short-sleeved cotton shirt is practical. Two should be packed. A four-pocket style called the *guayabera*, favored by men throughout Latin America and the Caribbean, is ideal. La Casa de Las Guayaberas (Naroca Plaza, 5840 SW 8th St., Miami, FL 33144; 305-266-9683; fax 305-267-1687) has an exceptional selection of short- and long-sleeved guayaberas; be sure to specify 100% cotton.

PANTS. Two pairs of ultralightweight, light-colored cotton pants are needed. One pair is worn on the trail during the entire trip. Trail pants should be washed often. The other pair is worn around camp and in towns along the way. Jeans become waterlogged as soon as they become wet and are totally unsuitable for tropical trekking. Although synthetic shirts are unsuitable, nylon Supplex pants can substitute for cotton on the trail. Mangrove Sanded Supplex pants (Sportif, 800-776-7843) hold up well, are quick drying, have a built-in mesh brief, and meet criteria for comfort on the trail. Pants with zip-off legs to create instant shorts should be avoided.

UNDERGARMENTS. Underpants and sport bras should be made of cotton.

PONCHO. An ultrathin waterproof poncho is useful on rafting or canoe trips and in villages but is worthless on the trail.

Bedding

FLANNEL SHEET. Tropical rainforests become uncomfortably cold between midnight and sunrise. A cotton sheet does not provide enough warmth, a blanket is too heavy, and a summer-weight sleeping bag retains too much body heat. A flannel sheet sewn together like a mummy bag (40 × 90 inches), but without a taper, provides suitable warmth either in a hammock or on a pad.

Many inhabitants of the tropical forests sleep with their feet near a fire that is tended throughout the night. They have learned that the chill of damp, cool jungle nights can be lessened as long as the feet stay warm. Also, disposable "warm packs" can be wrapped within a sock.

HAMMOCK. Soft cloth hammocks are too bulky and heavy for trips and begin to smell after a few days. Fishnet cotton hammocks tend to fall apart within hours or days. The so-called camping tent-hammocks or military tent-hammocks are usually bulky, heavy, impossible to sling properly, extremely uncomfortable, hot, unstable, and *never* able to keep the rain out in a heavy tropical downpour.

The nylon Double Hammock sold by Wal-Mart (Model EZ-190 by E-Z Sales Manufacturing, 1432 West 166 St., Gardena, CA 90247) has proved nearly ideal for jungle travel. It is compact, lightweight, durable, and reasonably comfortable. It cannot rot or absorb odors. For easier handling, the ski rope tie-end lines that are sold with the Double Hammock should be replaced with 3/8-inch double-braided rope.

THERM-A-REST. The Therm-a-Rest foam pad is the choice of expedition organizers throughout the world. It combines the insulating qualities of foam and the cushioning of an air mattress, rolls up to a compact size, and inflates on its own when the valve is opened.

The traveler who will be sleeping on a pad should pack a 1½ × 2½–yard plastic ground sheet. The sheet should not be placed directly on the jungle floor, where stinging insects and snakes abound. It should be used only in a hut or on an elevated platform. The ground sheet may also be beneficial for temporary rain protection and for keeping bow spray off a person or gear during water travel.

MOSQUITO NETTING. A mosquito net designed for use with a hammock is basically a rectangular box that is open at the bottom with sleeves at each end panel for the passage of the ropes by which the hammock is slung. Such nets are difficult to find outside the tropics. Fortunately, a serviceable mosquito net can easily be made from "no-see-um netting" (available by request from REI).

Backpacks. A sturdy, well-designed backpack should be used to carry gear. Reflective material should be sewn onto the back of each backpack. Iron Horse Safety Specialists (800-323-5889, fax 214-340-7775, e-mail ihss1@aol.com) sells red-orange reflective material for daytime visibility and reflective silver for nighttime reflectivity. On serious jungle treks, porters are present. This frees expedition members to carry much lighter loads.

BACKPACK FOR PORTER. An internal-frame backpack of 3000 to 4000 cubic inch capacity is a good size. It should have external pockets for quick access to liter-sized water bottles.

Indigenous peoples are accustomed to carrying packs and hauling loads with a strap, known as a *tumpline,* slung over the forehead or chest. Many natives, including Amazonian Indians, dislike using the shoulder straps that come as standard equipment on backpacks. Given enough straps, almost any native porter can quickly rig a satisfactory tumpline on a backpack.

PERSONAL PACK. A daypack of 1200 to 2000 cubic inch capacity is useful for carrying a camera, snack food, and other gear that must be kept handy. A waterproof liner will keep perspiration from wicking into the bag and wetting everything inside. The pack should have two outside pockets for quick access to liter-sized water bottles.

PACK FOR RIVER TRIPS. A durable, waterproof "dry" bag, used by river runners, is worth considering, especially if the trip will involve spending days or weeks at a time in dugout canoes or rubber rafts. Most of these packs, however, cannot stand up to the demands of long-distance overland trekking. The straps tend to be uncomfortable and frequently rip out on the trail.

Other Useful Items

ANTIFOGGING SOLUTION FOR EYEGLASSES. Antifog solution, available from dive shops, reduces humidity-induced fogging of glasses.

BATTERIES. Alkaline batteries should be brought from home. Batteries sold in Third World nations do not last long and often leak.

BINOCULARS. The traveler who is an avid bird watcher or enjoys watching butterflies or seeking out orchids high on distant limbs will want to pack a pair of binoculars that are lightweight, compact, shockproof, and waterproof or water resistant.

CAMERA EQUIPMENT. Older-style cameras with mechanical shutters are reliable in regions of high humidity. Film with an ISO of 200 is ideal for use in the low-light conditions of the jungle and much preferred over slower film.

CAMERA CASE OR BAG. Hard-bodied Pelican cases are waterproof and virtually indestructible. The silver-gray color cuts down on heat absorption and is preferred in hot climates. The cases are ideal for rafting or canoe trips but bulky for trekking. On the trail, waterproof "dry" bags protect equipment.

CAMP SOAP. A biodegradable soap should be used. The soap Campsuds works in hot, cold, fresh, or salt water and cleans dishes, clothing, hair, and skin.

CANDLES. Electricity tends to fail at unpredictable times in small towns and even in cities in Third World countries. Travelers should carry dripless candles, but spring-loaded candle lanterns should be avoided.

CUP AND PLATE. A large Lexan polycarbonate cup is unbreakable, does not retain taste or odor, and serves the role of cup, bowl, and plate. Travelers who want an actual plate should buy one made of indestructible Melamine.

EAR PLUGS. Travel in the tropics often involves flying in incredibly loud helicopters, cargo planes, or short takeoff and landing (STOL) aircraft. Sponge ear plugs that roll up and fit in the ear canal offer inexpensive, effective protection against hearing damage.

FISHING SUPPLIES. For additional "food insurance" the jungle traveler should carry 75 feet of 20-pound-test fishing line, a 12-inch steel leader with swivel, and a few hooks. Breakdown travel rods and spincast reels should be considered for sport fishing or adding fresh meat to the daily provisions. Throughout the tropics, most species of fish find Rat-L-Trap lures, particularly the chrome and blue combination, irresistible.

GARBAGE BAGS. Four 30-gallon capacity and four 13-gallon capacity large plastic garbage bags can hold clothes, bedding, and other items that must stay absolutely dry and can keep dirty boots isolated from clean items in the backpack.

HEADLAMP. Battery-operated headlamps offer hands-free convenience at night for reading or going to the latrine. They should shine at least 10 hours on a set of batteries.

INFLATABLE CUSHION OR PILLOW. A small, durable, cloth-covered inflatable cushion is recommended for sitting in a dugout canoe or aluminum boat.

INSECT REPELLENT. To repel mosquitoes, flies, ticks, chiggers, fleas, and gnats (but not no-see-ums), insect repellent should contain 15% to 30% diethyl-toluamide (DEET). Formulations should not contain higher than 30% DEET, often called "jungle juice." These may pose health hazards (see Chapter 32).

Technique is critical when applying insect repellent. Before dressing, the person should spray the ankles, lower legs, and waist. After the socks are put on, a band should be sprayed around the top; a band should also be sprayed around both pant legs to midcalf. A light spray to the shirt, front and back, may also help. The hands should be sprayed, rubbed vigorously, and run through the hair. Some repellent should be dabbed on the face, neck, and ears, carefully avoiding the eyes; contact lens wearers should be especially vigilant when applying insect repellent.

No-see-ums, which are tiny gnats that abound throughout the tropics of the Americas, are the most common source of insect annoyance in many regions. They are active at sunset and attack humans emerging from jungle streams. No-see-ums cannot bite through even the thinnest cloth and are usually inhibited by Skin So Soft (SSS, Avon). (SSS is not effective against ticks, fleas, flies, and chiggers and offers little protection against mosquitoes.) SSS should be applied liberally and often to the wrists, knuckles, bare ankles, face, ears, and scalp. Men with full beards seem to be especially troubled by tiny gnats and may benefit by applying small amounts of SSS to the beard area.

LAMINATED MAP. Accurate maps exist for most regions on earth. From the best map available, travelers should laminate photocopied portions that are relevant to a particular itinerary (see Rescue Strategies).

MACHETE. A machete is the single essential tool for jungle survival and for the many tasks in camp and on the trail that require steel with a sharp edge. It is hazardous to use a machete in the rain or when cutting wet grass, however, since the weapon may fly out of the hand. Also, when cutting brush, the person often encounters sawgrass. The resulting skin lacerations, which are not noticed at the first because sawgrass is razor sharp, may take a week or two to heal. Because of the risks involved, an experienced individual should be in charge of transporting and using the machete.

MATCHES OR CIGARETTE LIGHTER. Waterproof, windproof Hurricane Matches light when damp and stay lit for several seconds even in the strongest wind. Many jungle travelers prefer a butane cigarette lighter.

ORGANIZER BAGS. See-through organizer bags help reduce clutter and minimize the risk of misplacing small items.

PEN. The Fisher Space Pen (Fisher Pressurized Pen, 711 Yucca St., Boulder City, NV 89005) writes upside down without pumping, under water and over grease, and in hot and cold temperature extremes. It has an estimated shelf life of over 100 years.

POCKET TOOL. A favorite pocket tool for the outdoors enthusiast is the Swiss Army knife. The Leatherman Super Tool is recommended for jungle travel and survival and features needle-nosed pliers and 12 locking implements.

POLY BOTTLES. Essential gear includes two quart- or liter-sized wide-mouth water bottles made of high-density polyethylene or Lexan polycarbonate. A 2-ounce, heavy-duty poly bottle comes in handy for carrying a salt and pepper mixture to add flavor to boiled plantains and yucca.

RAZOR OR BATTERY-OPERATED SHAVER. Both men and women should carry lightweight disposable razors. Most men find that lightweight, AA battery–operated shavers give two shaves a day for up to 2 weeks before requiring a change of batteries.

SPOON. Knife-spoon-fork sets are unnecessary. With a knife blade, a good tablespoon made of either Lexan polycarbonate or stainless steel is sufficient for eating.

SPORT SPONGE. A camp towel, made of microporous material, is lightweight, compact, and superabsorbent; it replaces the cotton towel. With the Cascade Designs Pack Towel or similar brand, the body and even hair can be dried much more quickly than with a traditional towel.

SUNGLASSES. Sunglasses should be polarized with full ultraviolet light protection. Many travelers prefer sunglasses with red-tinted lenses. Because red is the complement of green, these lenses make the jungle foliage stand out intensely and sharply, with enhanced contrast and depth of field. Retainers hold eyeglasses securely during vigorous activity.

TOILET PAPER. American toilet paper is much softer than that purchased in Third World countries. The traveler should never wipe with jungle leaves.

UMBRELLA. A collapsible umbrella is useful in tropical cities and in remote villages when walking from hut to hut. It also offers excellent protection from the sun on canoe or raft trips. The umbrella should be reflective silver, not heat-absorbing black.

WHISTLE. A high-quality plastic whistle can be used to signal in case someone strays off the path.

ZIPPER-LOCK BAGS. Heavy-duty zipper-lock freezer bags are excellent for organizing medicines, toiletries, and other small objects. Bring five each of the gallon, quart, and pint sizes.

COPING WITH THE JUNGLE ENVIRONMENT

A visit to the rainforests of the New World tropics can be either a sublime experience or a hellish ordeal.[14]

Wetness

The superhumid lowland rainforest receives up to 400 inches of rain a year; in contrast, Indiana averages about 40 inches. In the higher elevation cloud forest, dense cloud cover throughout the year is accompanied by constant mist or drizzle. In such heat and high humidity, people become mentally fatigued as a result of being constantly wet. Fortunately, travelers can use basic strategies for coping with the physical and psychologic burden of wetness. Wetness is as much a state of mind as a physical condition.

Dryness while trekking or working during the day is not a requisite for physical or mental health. Wetness does not equate with illness, significant discomfort, or dampened spirits. People can tolerate being wet throughout much of the day if they know that they have a dry change of clothes to wear in camp and that they will be dry at night. In addition to the psychologic benefits, being dry at night means that maceration is less likely to develop in intertriginous areas.

Bedding and clothing can be protected from moisture by careful wrapping in plastic garbage bags. Despite all efforts, however, certain "dry" items eventually become damp or accidentally soaked. Wet articles should be spread out on shrubs and bushes. They will dry within 2 hours in full sun. Myiasis caused by the tumbu fly, *Cordylobia anthropophaga*, of sub-Saharan Africa can be avoided by hanging clothing to dry in bright sunlight, never on the ground. Clothing dried over a wood fire absorbs odors that do not wash out.

Health Issues

Health Risks. The subject of the tropics causes many people to think about tropical diseases such as filariasis and animals such as the candirú (see later discussion). Malaria, hepatitis, and motor vehicle accidents are the three leading health problems in most tropical regions. Tropical travelers who venture off the path may be exposed to bodily harm and serious diseases, such as leishmaniasis, onchocerciasis, and Chagas' disease. Bouts of diarrhea or other annoyances will likely occur, regardless of the extent of precautions taken, but death is unlikely.

Duration of Travel and Emotional Response. Cashel et al[5] examined the mood pattern of participants on a wilderness course and noted a high level of confusion, fatigue, anger, depression and tension on day 4. After 2 to 3 weeks of travel in remote areas, the general health of expedition participants deteriorates as a result of insect bites, falls, and noxious plants. Inexperienced trekkers may quickly tire of unfamiliar food and miss usual comforts. Experienced leaders therefore prefer to limit expeditions to 3 weeks.

Preventing Heat-Related Illness. The following guidelines may help prevent heat-related illness (see Chapters 10 and 11).

1. Before undertaking long-distance trekking in the tropics, acclimatize by spending at least 5 days in a hot, humid environment and engaging in moderate daily exercise. This acclimatization will be lost within a week if not maintained.[15]
2. Avoid alcohol and certain drugs. Medications such as β-blockers, anticholinergics, and diuretics increase the likelihood of heat-related illness and should be avoided if possible.
3. Wear ultralightweight, light-colored, and loose-fitting cotton clothing and a wide-brimmed hat.
4. Whenever possible, have a native porter carry all gear.
5. Maintain adequate hydration. Before setting off on the trail, drink a liter of disinfected water. A half hour later, drink a second liter. One hour after the second liter, drink a third, then consume approximately 1 L every 2 to 4 hours while on the trail.

Heat cramps, often severe, tend to occur when large amounts of water are ingested without adequate salt replacement. Oral rehydration salts (ORS), in premeasured packets added to a liter of disinfected water, provide an ideal balance for replacing lost electrolytes. Trekkers should drink at least 1 L of water containing ORS before setting out on the trail and a second liter after especially strenuous days. ORS packets are distributed by the World Health Organization and UNICEF but are difficult to obtain commercially overseas. In the United States, oral rehydration therapy packets may be obtained from Cera Products (888-237-2598) and Jianas Brothers (816-241-2880).

Sport beverages, such as Gatorade, help maintain adequate electrolyte balance but not as well as ORS. Salt tablets are not recommended because they are gastric irritants and may even delay acclimatization because of aldosterone suppression.[15]

Unexpected Isolation

Various factors contribute to unexpected isolation in the jungle, such as inclement weather, mechanical problems, or political turmoil that shuts down public transportation. Many people respond with anger and irritability, which can be devastating to group dynamics. Travelers should accept the situation and use the additional time to appreciate the tropical forest, take photographs, or read paperback books.

It helps to shift out of gear mentally and allow the intellectual machinery to idle. Nearly everyone has the experience of driving for hours and arriving at a destination with virtually no recollection of the trip. The same can be accomplished in the village setting, lying around on a hammock. The hours and days pass surprisingly quickly, akin to cruising in a sailboat with no engine. The person learns patience and develops an appreciation that the rhythms of nature are not governed by the ticking of a clock. Unexpected isolation allows many visitors to experience the biospheric cadence.

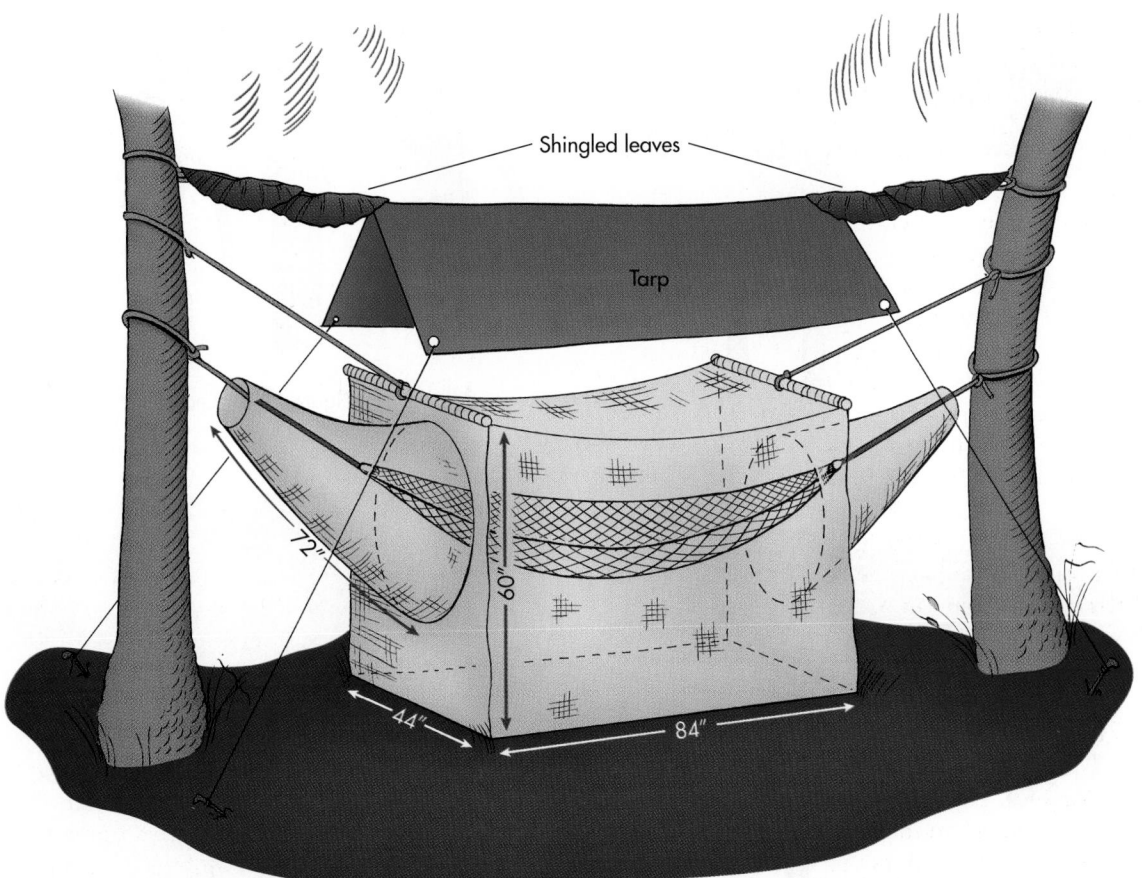

Figure 29-1 Construction of mosquito netting for use with a hammock: sleeve hole = 88 inches in circumference; small hole = 18 inches in circumference; smallest holes (for supporting sticks) = 4 inches in circumference.

Camp Life

Shelter. Natives rarely spend the night in makeshift shelters, and it is usually best to use existing dwellings for a hammock or sleeping pad. Common courtesy governs their placement or sleeping pad inside the hut of a native. Travelers should ask about taboo spots before bedding down.

When huts are not available for use, a tarpaulin provides satisfactory shelter from the rain. Rip-stop polyethylene tarps (8 × 10 feet) are lightweight and waterproof. Coated nylon tarps are also acceptable but must be sealed with a product such as Seam Grip.

Figure 29-1 illustrates a typical method of erecting a tarp. First, a thick line is run between two trees 7 to 8 feet off the ground and cinched tight. The long axis of the tarp is centered over the rope, and a rope attached to the middle grommet on each end is tied to the tree. The corner grommets are tied to available trees, bushes, or strong clumps of grass; a tie-down in the middle on each side is also helpful. The sides of the roof should be made high enough to enter and exit conveniently but not so high that driving rain can come in at an angle.

Once the tarp is up, the hammock ropes are run through the sleeves of the mosquito net. Then the hammock is slung. It should be suspended high enough that it will not sag to the ground during the night as it naturally gives under an adult's weight. Next, the mosquito net is suspended. The ropes running from tree to tarp, from tree to mosquito net, and from tree to hammock should be sprayed with DEET-containing insect repellent to keep ants and other pests from using the ropes as trails. Finally, a few broad leaves (banana leaves or heliconia) folded at the spine are draped over the bare rope extending from the tree to the tarp to keep rain from running down the tarp and hammock ropes.

Knowledge of two knots is needed for slinging a hammock. These knots always hold and always come undone quickly without jamming. The *half hitch* is used to tie the hammock to a horizontal beam, as follows (Figure 29-2):

1. Pass the working end of the rope around the object to which it is to be secured.
2. Pass the working end of the rope around again without crossing over itself.

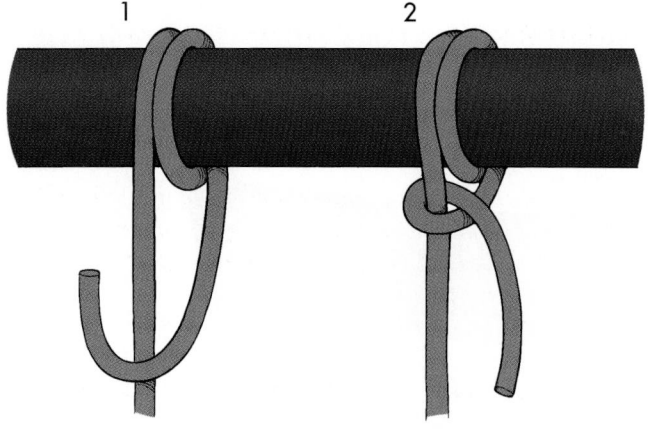

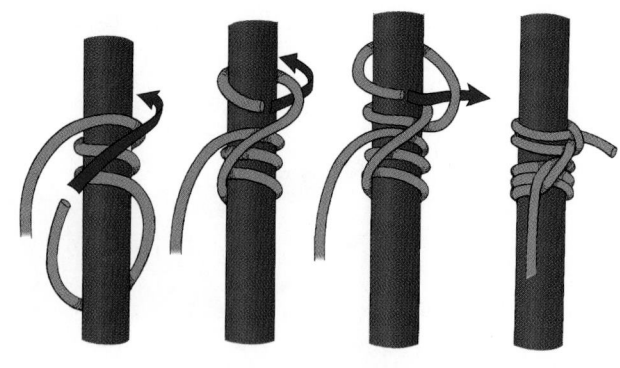

Figure 29-3   Camel hitch.

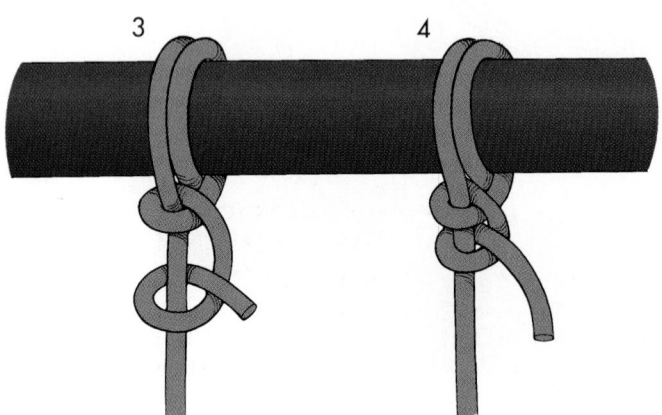

Figure 29-2   Half hitch knot.

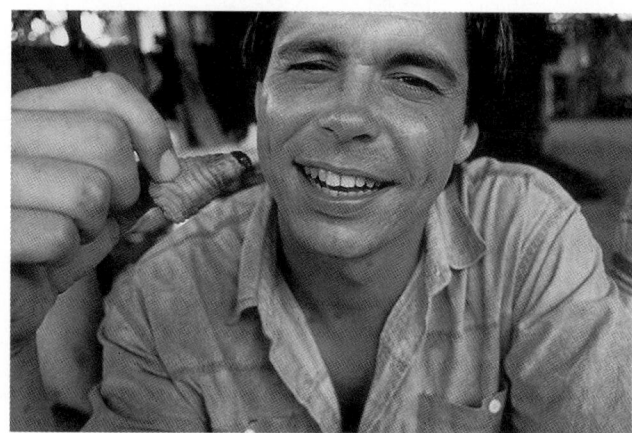

Figure 29-4   The palm grub is a favorite delicacy.

3. Bring the end over and around the standing part and through the loop that has just been created. You have just made a half hitch.
4. Make a second half hitch below the first half hitch.
5. Pull tight.

The *camel hitch* is used to tie the hammock to a vertical post secure, as follows (Figure 29-3):

1. Make three turns around the vertical pole.
2. Bring the working end up and over the turns.
3. Make a turn at the top and pass the end back under itself.
4. Make a second turn at the top and pass the end back under itself.

Weather conditions can change in minutes, and travelers must be prepared with adequate shelter. The use of a tent as shelter in the tropical rainforest is not recommended.

Food. Solitary travelers or small groups usually do not need to pack large amounts of food. Edibles are always available in areas inhabited by friendly natives. As a general rule, food is safe to eat if it is peeled, cooked, or boiled.

Travelers in the tropics must be open to eating local food. Most creatures are edible, such as boiled caiman (alligator), cooked capybara (a 50-kg rodent), or roasted palm grubs (larvae of *Rhynchophorus*). Raw palm grubs, up to 5 inches long, are tasty and a favorite of Amazonian Indians (Figure 29-4). They are eaten by slashing open the thin integument with the thumbnail, extracting and discarding the intestinal tract, placing the opened skin to the mouth, and sucking out the turgid contents.

In addition to palm grubs, more than 20 species of edible insects, including ants and termites, are collected year-round by the people of Amazonia.[9] Large hairy spiders 10 inches in diameter, *Theraphosa leblondi,* are often roasted on an open fire. After the barbed hairs are singed off, the spider is placed in the embers; it has a shrimplike taste.

Indians of the Americas have perfected the art of smoking fish and meat so that they remain safe to eat for long periods. It is common to see huge hunks of tapir meat or slabs of 100-pound catfish resting on racks, coal black from the smoking process.

The tropics have an abundance of flora as food. The yard-long heart of palm is cool and delicious when eaten in its raw state or may be included in a soup spiced with tropical herbs. Familiar tropical fruits include papaya, mango, pineapple, and passion fruit (*Passiflora*). Many New World fruits have no name in English and generally have not found their way into the world market, such as chirimoya, guanabana, pitahayas, naranjilla, uchuva, tamarillo, zapote, sapotilla, and badea.[22,25,34] The boiled fruit of the peach palm, *Bactries gasipaes,* is nutritious and flavorful.

The banana and its cousin, the plantain, provide a large percentage of the total caloric intake of natives in the American and African tropics. Curiously, in many native villages it is difficult to find the sweet, finger-length bananas and the common yellow bananas exported from tropical countries. The green plantain features prominently in the daily fare of inhabitants of the tropics. The plantain has little taste and is exceptionally dry.

Yucca (manioc or cassava), *Manihot esculenta,* is a staple source of carbohydrate nutrition throughout the Americas and much of tropical Africa. The two kinds of yucca, "sweet" and "bitter," are the same species but differ in their distribution and amount of a poisonous constituent, a cyanogenic glycoside, in the root.[30] Sweet and bitter yucca cannot be easily distinguished; one must know which variety was planted. Sweet yucca, common in the eastern lowlands of the Andean countries of Colombia, Ecuador, and Peru, is eaten after the bark containing the toxic substance is peeled off and the root boiled. In bitter yucca the poison is more concentrated and distributed throughout the root, so it must be extracted before consumption. Amerindians use an apparatus called the *tipití* to express the poisonous juice from the peeled and grated flour of manioc roots.

Travelers in a large group should carry dried, packaged foods, since the host village might not be able to provide sufficient foodstuffs or travelers might pass through isolated and uninhabited regions. Packaged foods should also be carried by travelers in regions where natives are unfriendly.

Dried instant food only needs water to make a meal. A few selections should be tried before a large supply for field use is ordered. It is not necessary to add hot water to all packaged foods; adding disinfected, ambient-temperature water produces acceptable results for most foods. Drawbacks to prepackaged foods include expense, space, and disposing of the empty foil packages.

I carry the following supplemental food items for 2- to 3-week treks into remote but inhabited jungle regions: one 2-ounce heavy-duty poly bottle filled with salt and pepper mixed half and half, a few pounds of rice, a tin of long-keeping butter (or oil) for cooking the rice, a few tins of tuna or sardines packed in tropical hot sauce, and several Power-Gel energy packets for trail snacks. Hard caramels can be given to porters after long or difficult passages.

Potable Water.   Potable Aqua (tetraglycine hydroperiodide 16.7%) tablets are recommended for disinfecting water because they are easy to use and have proved effective in killing bacteria, viruses, and most parasite cysts (see Chapter 51). Water filters are not recommended for purifying jungle water; they clog with silt and must be cleaned frequently. If a water filter is used, it should be fitted with a good pre-filter to catch the excess silt.

Jungle Hazards

The following hazards are common in the wilderness jungle setting or thought to be common. Other chapters provide additional insights and viewpoints, particularly with respect to treatment.

Arthropods

ANTS.   The conga ant, *Paraponera clavata,* 1 to 1½ inches long, is the terror of the American tropics. The bite of these large black ants can produce intense pain and fever for up to 24 hours, which provides the Spanish name *veinte-cuatro* (twenty-four). Fortunately, they are conspicuous because their large, shiny black bodies tend to stand out against foliage. Special caution is needed when ducking under or climbing over trees, where ants are often found. A conga bite requires strong pain medication and perhaps the injection of lidocaine at the bite site.

Travelers should avoid touching trees and bushes. Many plants in the tropics provide a home and food for ants, which provide aggressive defense of the plants.

Fire ants are common throughout the tropics and subtropics. Their bite causes discomfort but not excruciating pain. Characteristic pustular lesions in crops often result from fire ant stings.

CHIGGERS.   Chiggers, a form of mite, are a problem throughout equatorial regions. Whereas temperate-climate chiggers may cause mild discomfort for a few days, the tropical chigger sets up an inflammatory and allergic reaction that often persists for weeks.

In the South American tropics, chiggers are found in grassy fields, such as jungle airstrips and yards around mission compounds. Walking through chigger-infested areas without protection could leave a person covered with chigger bites. After a few days the victim begins to itch mildly. As the days pass, the itching intensifies, seems to come in waves, and may change its focus.

Prevention is the best treatment. Areas known to be infested with chiggers should be avoided when possible. Spraying shoes or boots and lower pant legs with repellent containing DEET is highly effective. Pretreatment of clothing with permethrin has been recommended. Travelers in the American tropics should *never* walk through grassy areas in shorts.

JIGGER FLEA. *Tunga penetrans,* the jigger flea or chigoe, originally found in South and Central America, has now spread to East and West Africa and India. The fertilized female flea enters the feet through cracks in the soles, between the toes, and around the toenails. The female swells to the size of a pea and may be readily identified as a white papule with a central pit, through which the female extrudes excrement and eggs. When eggs are ripe for release, intense itching causes scratching that helps release large numbers of flea eggs. Incomplete removal of the jigger frequently results in complications caused by secondary infection. A simple extraction technique virtually eliminates complications. Open the skin over the nest of eggs with a surgical blade. Fold back the flaps, remove the easily identified egg sac, and with tweezers, remove the head of the female flea, which can be seen once the egg sac has been removed. Wash the area with hydrogen peroxide.[16]

MYIASIS. Myiasis (skin infestation by fly larvae) is common in many regions of sub-Saharan Africa (the tumbu fly, *Cordylobia anthropophaga*) and Central and South America (the human botfly, *Dermatobia hominis*). The victim finds an itchy swelling that slowly enlarges into a lesion with a single breathing pore from which bubbles clear or slightly bloody drainage. Later, movement is felt under the skin as the developing larva wriggles around.

Removing the larvae before they emerge on their own is generally advised. Surgical excision, however, should be undertaken with caution because accidental rupture of the larval tegument can lead to secondary infections. Various methods to close off the breathing pore so the larva will emerge on its own include application of bacon fat, meat, chewing gum, or petroleum jelly.

SCORPIONS AND SPIDERS. Stinging scorpions and venomous spiders are common throughout the tropics and provide another reason to exercise caution before sitting down or placing a hand on logs, bushes, or the ground.

VENOMOUS MOTHS, BUTTERFLIES, AND CATERPILLARS. The larvae and adults of a number of moths (genus *Hylesia*) and butterflies bear venomous hairs that may cause skin eruptions. A rash may result from direct contact with the adults or larvae or by windblown hairs. Direct contact with certain Amazonian caterpillars can cause disabling pain.

In the Amazon tropics, noxious smoke from burning garbage (e.g., plastic wrappers) may cause tree-dwelling caterpillars to loosen their hold on overhead branches and rain down on unwary campers.

Treatment of lepidoptera envenomation may require injection of lidocaine at the site of intense pain and administration of analgesics, antihistamines, and corticosteroids (Chapters 36 and 37). Moth hairs may be removed with sticky lint removers used for clothing.

WASP AND BEE STINGS. Sudden, intense pain from the sting of certain species of tropical wasps and bees can be so severe that it knocks the victim to the ground as though hit with an electric shock. Perfumes and brightly colored or flower-patterned clothing should be avoided.[19] Bird watchers should not venture too close to the hanging nests of yellow-rumped caciques and oropendolas, because wasps are invariably associated with these nests.

Fish

STINGRAY. The stingray, a flattened, cartilaginous cousin of the shark, may be encountered buried just beneath the surface of the bottom ooze in tropical rivers and streams throughout the Amazon Basin, Africa, and Indo-China. Rays inflict injury by lashing upward with the caudal appendage, driving one or more retroserrated venomous spines deep into the victim's foot, ankle, or lower leg. This produces agonizing pain, often accompanied by headache, vomiting, and shortness of breath. After the initial phase of envenomation, tissue necrosis may develop. Wearing shoes or boots when wading in water does not always prevent a stingray from jabbing its barb into the foot or leg. Prevention lies in shuffling the feet along the bottom so that the ray will have enough warning to glide away safely (see Chapter 60).

ELECTRIC EEL. The so-called electric eel (actually an eel-shaped fish) is encountered from Guatemala to the La Plata River in South America and is especially common in the Amazon region. A person can drown after being stunned by a jolt from this fish.

Electric eels are said to prefer deep water. Inhabitants of regions heavily infested with eels report a slight tingling sensation when one is close. No practical way exists to prevent these shocks.

CANDIRÚ. The candirú is a toothpick-sized parasitic catfish that inhabits Amazonian waters and may invade the urethra of urinating humans. Orifice penetration by the wily candirú can be prevented by wearing a tight bathing suit and not urinating underwater. Native methods of dislodging these fish from the urethra include drinking a tea made from the green fruit of the jugua tree, *Genipa americana* L. Vitamin C (2 to 5g) may serve the same purpose[4] (see Chapter 62).

PIRANHA. Although no human deaths have been documented, piranha have nipped off the fingertips of canoeists dangling their hands in the water.

Mammals

BATS. Vampire bats are found throughout Mexico, Central America, and South America, especially in areas that have large cattle ranches. Sleeping humans are unaware of the presence of a feeding bat; the phlebotomy is painless. Both vampire and fruit bats carry rabies. Sleeping under mosquito netting prevents bat bites. The risk of rabies can be reduced by prophylactic human diploid cell rabies vaccine.

DOGS. Most native groups keep dogs for hunting. Populations with a history of recent tribal warfare often keep packs of dogs close by as an early warning system. These semiwild dogs should be treated with caution; threatening them may cause immediate attack, since they are not easily intimidated. When approaching huts or villages, the traveler should allow porters to deal with the dogs first.

Dogs intent on biting often adopt particular behavior patterns. The dog protecting its territory crouches low, straightens its back and tail, emits a deep guttural growl, and stares fixedly at a specific part of the person's anatomy. Such behavior indicates imminent attack and a sharp blow to the nose may be necessary. Freezing in place may prevent an attack, and direct eye contact should be avoided.

JAGUARS. Jaguar attacks are rare. Recommendations are based on advice for avoiding a cougar attack. Increase your apparent size by raising your arms above the head and waving an object such as a backpack or stick, or opening a jacket. Yell, shout, whistle, or speak loudly and forcefully in a low, deep tone of voice. Back away slowly; do not turn your back and run.[8]

Reptiles

SNAKES. Snakebites are rare; 450,000 hours of field work at sites in Costa Rican rainforests were documented without a single snakebite.[7]

Most poisonous snakes tend to blend into their surroundings, and nonnatives rarely see them. The most effective protection is putting a jungle-reared guide in front on the trail. Natives almost always spot a poisonous snake and can quickly dispatch it.

Snakes are often encountered along the shoreline of rivers and small streams. Particular caution is needed when hiking in such areas or when disembarking from a canoe or rubber raft. In the forest the hiker should always step onto a log and then step away from it. The log should *not* be straddled; snakes often are encountered where the log makes contact with the jungle floor. Since many venomous snakes in the tropics are heat seeking and hunt at night, caution is needed.

Anacondas (water boas) feature in the folklore of all native cultures in the regions of Amazonia where these enormous snakes (up to 30 feet long) live. These non-poisonous snakes kill by looping coils around prey and then tightening the coils, suffocating the victim. Anecdotal reports of anacondas attacking and swallowing humans, particularly children and women bathing at the edge of jungle streams, are unconfirmed.

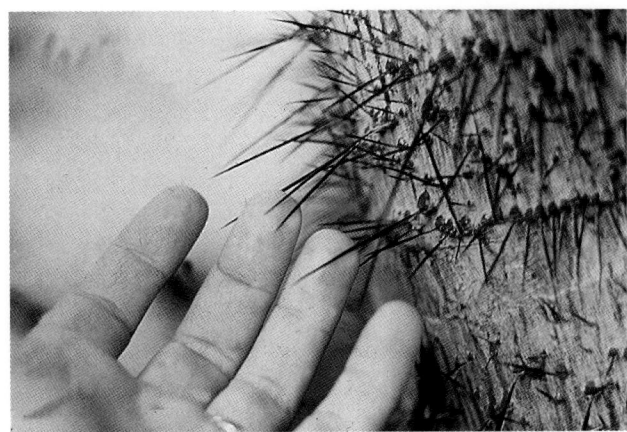

Figure 29-5 Needle-sharp spines ring the peach palm.

ALLIGATORS AND CROCODILES. Although they appear torpid lying in the sun, alligators and crocodiles can move amazingly fast. Humans cannot outswim or outrun a charging crocodile.

Bites should be treated with thorough cleaning of the wound, surgical debridement if necessary, tetanus prophylaxis, and an appropriate antibiotic. A study of the oral flora of 10 alligators captured in Louisiana revealed various aerobic and anaerobic organisms responsive to trimethoprim-sulfamethoxazole.[13]

Plants

ARMED OR SPINE-BEARING PLANTS. Spine-bearing trees abound in forested areas of the tropics. The peach palm (*Bactris gasipaes*), a tall, slender palm whose heart and fruit mesocarp are prized by natives, is found from Nicaragua to Bolivia. The trunk of this tree is ringed with needle-sharp spines (Figure 29-5). Peach palms often grow alongside trails. Contact with this palm can result in penetration of spines deep into the flesh. Spines that enter a joint space may require surgical extraction. Secondary infection and inflammation often occur.

HALLUCINOGENIC PLANTS. Jungle-dwelling tribes throughout Central and South America use hallucinogenic plants. Powerful drugs, such as ayahuasca (*Banisteriopsis*), *Brugmansia*, the virola snuffs, and yopo (*A. peregrina*), are used by shamans seeking the truth.[28,29,30] These powerful intoxicants should be avoided.

SAWGRASS. In many regions of the tropics, sawgrass is an ever-present nuisance. This scalpel-like blades of this

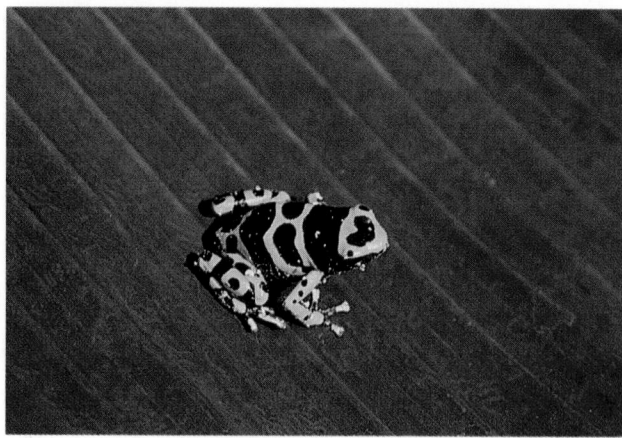

Figure 29-6 Poison-dart frog.

grass can slice into exposed skin. Even when treated with antibiotic ointment, the lacerations often take 1 to 2 weeks to heal. Hikers should avoid sawgrass; special care is needed when working with a machete.

Miscellaneous Hazards

POISON-DART FROGS. Poison-dart frogs, tiny, brilliantly colored species in the genus *Dendrobates,* may be encountered in Central America and Northern South America (Figure 29-6). *Phyllobates terribilis* secretes a toxin from its skin so powerful that a lethal dose could be absorbed if enough secretion entered an open wound. It is wise to avoid all contact with brilliantly colored frogs, caterpillars, and snakes.

FALLING TREES. Tropical trees do not have deep roots and often fall in relatively modest winds. In many regions of the world, risk of snakebite is significantly lower than the risk of injury or death from falling trees. In the forest, hammocks should be slung away from large trees. Travelers setting up camp should always look up at the branches of any trees near camp; although the base of the tree may appear sound, higher areas may be rotted.

FORDING RIVERS. The hiker should never attempt to cross a fast-flowing or deep river with a pack on his back. Regaining footing in a rapidly moving current can be difficult. Unless experienced in crossing such streams, the traveler should take the hand of a native guide or porter.

LOG BRIDGES. On frequently used trails, natives generally place a single log across creeks, ravines, and swampy areas. These log bridges may be up to 20 feet high and 75 feet long. Good balance is essential. Because a backpack impairs balance, a porter should carry it across.

MERCURY CONTAMINATION. Travelers to the Amazon Basin should be aware of the serious, widespread contamination of waterways by mercury that gold miners (*garimpeiros*) use to process their ore. Although most manufacturers of portable water treatment and filtration systems do not specifically claim to remove mercury, any activated carbon system should reduce the risk. The manufacturers of SafeWater Anywhere, (www.safewateranywhere.com), a 1-L squeeze-bottle filter, cite 99.25% mercury removal. Travelers should exercise caution in choosing rivulets as a source of potable water in areas where mercury contamination is known or suspected.

RISING RIVERS. Streams, particularly narrow ones bounded by vertical banks, can rise 20 feet in a few hours as a result of intense rains. Camp should not be set up on an island or beach in a small canyon during the rainy season. A cloudburst in the headwaters can send a wall of water rushing downstream, even though it may be a clear, moonlit night at the campsite.

Traveling with Children in the Tropics

The following guidelines should be considered when trekking with children in the tropical forest:

1. Do not attempt a daylong hike. Unlike indigenous children, others cannot hike all day in the humid tropical forest. Preadolescents should hike only 1 to 2 hours; for children aged 12 to 16 can hike 2 to 3 hours. Do not subject a child to jungle trail conditions unless the child has had extensive experience hiking in temperate climates.
2. Do not attempt difficult or dangerous trails.
3. Avoid trekking during the rainy season.
4. Keep the child well hydrated.
5. Provide proper footwear (running or hiking sneaker-type shoes or boots with an adequate tread). Avoid leather boots.
6. Keep the child ahead of you and behind a native guide. Children should not be out of sight on the trail.
7. When wading across rivers, have an adult native guide hold the child's hand.
8. *Always* have children wear a properly sized life vest while rafting, taking canoe trips, or crossing deep, swift, or wide rivers.
9. Do not allow a child to carry any equipment in a daypack other than 2-L bottles of drinking water.
10. Ensure that routine vaccinations are up to date. Special vaccinations, such as yellow fever and typhoid should be considered for certain jungle areas. Hepatitis A vaccine is recommended. Antimalarials are indicated.

Any child who plans to visit the tropics should be a strong swimmer. Many natives begin swimming in infancy and are accustomed to deep or rapidly flowing water that would be extremely hazardous to visiting children. Swimming holes are often located in the swift-flowing outer loop of jungle rivers, where depths may reach 6 feet or more within a yard of the shoreline.

SURVIVAL

Every year, inexperienced people enter the jungle and become lost. After a person ventures only a mere few yards into the forest, especially jungle that has been cleared and is now a tangle of secondary growth, everything begins to look the same. *To avoid becoming lost, travelers should always have an experienced guide when traversing unfamiliar territory.*

Tribal peoples of the world's tropical forests have an uncanny ability to find their way and arrive at the desired destination, even after days of travel. They can always find food and water and, if necessary, rapidly construct a shelter or a weapon.

Occasionally, travelers are left behind on the trail by indigenous guides. Unintentional desertion occurs when trekkers hire natives who have had no experience with neophytes. Realizing that their charges cannot keep up on the trail, the guides run ahead and sit down to rest, not knowing that others cannot navigate the trail alone. Travelers who want to avoid being left behind on the trail should hire a guide who is experienced in traveling with nonnatives. Suitable guides and porters can usually be identified with the help of a village leader, local school teacher, village health worker, missionary, or anthropologist.

Rescue Strategies

For individuals in a jungle survival situation, lifesaving items include a large-scale map, a global positioning system (GPS) unit, some form of electronic voice communication, and a machete. Topographic maps are available from numerous international and national mapping agencies. Satellite images with extraordinary resolution are available from Space Imaging (1-800-232-9037) or the U.S. Geological Survey (Eros Data Center 47914, 252 ND St., Sioux Falls, SD 57198-0001; 1-800-252-4547; edcwww.cr.usgs.gov).

Small, lightweight GPS units display precise latitude, longitude, and altitude. Such information is extremely useful for navigation and for communicating one's location to rescue aircraft. Newer units quickly lock onto satellites and are more likely to work under the jungle canopy.

Canoeists, rafters, or trekkers contemplating an expedition into largely uninhabited and unexplored regions should consider buying a compact emergency position-indicating radio beacon (EPIRB). The 406 MHz EPIRB units offer a reliable method of alerting various rescue services via a global satellite system. These units should be activated only in a true emergency when lives are at risk.

Hand-held satellite phones are available for worldwide communication. Although currently expensive to purchase and operate, their potential to provide rescuers with precise GPS location makes these lightweight phones worthy of serious consideration for inclusion for wilderness travel.

Lightweight, hand-held, very-high-frequency (VHF) aircraft transceivers are excellent for emergency communications. Visitors to remote areas should know the radio frequencies used by rescue aircraft. VHF transceivers are line-of-sight instruments, so they are most useful when aircraft are overhead without objects, such as trees or mountains, between the hand-held unit and the aircraft. In many regions of the world the Mission Aviation Fellowship (MAF) provides air service to remote airstrips in small villages. If assistance is needed, a hand-held radio transmitter can be used to call an MAF short take-off and landing (STOL) aircraft.

Bush pilots appreciate having information on the condition of seldom-used airstrips. A crude but acceptable device can be constructed to measure airstrip hardness (Figure 29-7). Cut a pole exactly 2 inches in diameter and approximately 6 feet long. Starting exactly 6 inches from one end, taper that end to a point. Lash a cross-member on the pole, and have a person weighing approximately 170 pounds stand with assistance on the cross-member. Make a map of the strip, noting the depth to which the pointed end of the pole sinks into the earth at several dozen sites. Communicate this information to the pilot by radio. If the pole goes in only 2 inches in most areas, the strip is considered ideal; 2 to 4 inches is marginal; penetration beyond 4 inches indicates that the airstrip is unsuitable for landing and take-off.

If rescue is not feasible, the traveler should continually move downstream at a fast pace. Inhabited areas usually have a trail running alongside a stream. The trail may veer away from the stream where natives have cut a path to connect two villages. Marking the trail every 10 yards with a machete makes it easier to return to the starting point. To avoid confusion, the traveler should mark trees only on one side of the trail.

Where human paths are in frequent use, identifying a trail is fairly easy. Seldom-used trails or any trail traversed during times of optimal plant growth may be extremely difficult for the nonnative to identify and follow. Even under adverse circumstances, however, there are clues to trail identification. Paradoxically, concentrating only on the actual foot path will almost certainly cause you to lose sight of the trail. Think of the jungle trail not as a track on the ground but as the intestinal lumen of "some gigantic leafy creature,"[17] with vertical margins, often an overhead horizontal boundary, and sometimes a visible path beneath the

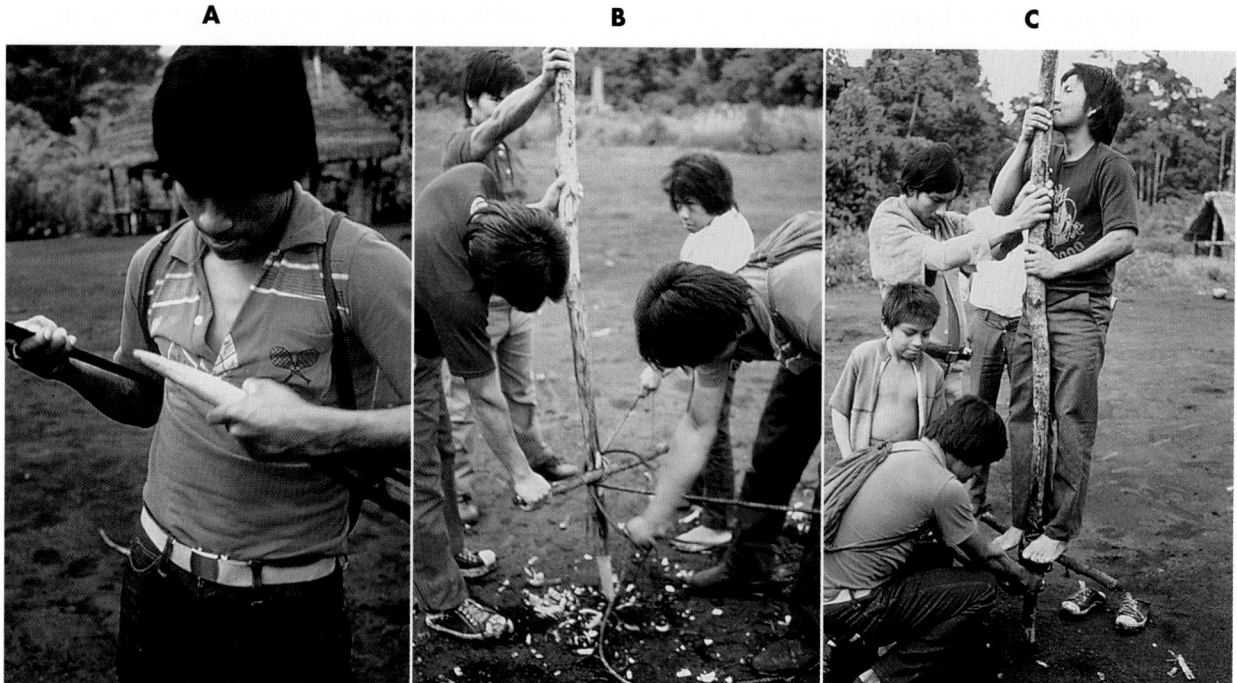

Figure 29-7 **A,** Young man sharpening a stick to a point. **B,** Lashing a cross-member to a pole. **C,** Standing on the pole to take measurements of the depth of penetration into the airstrip.

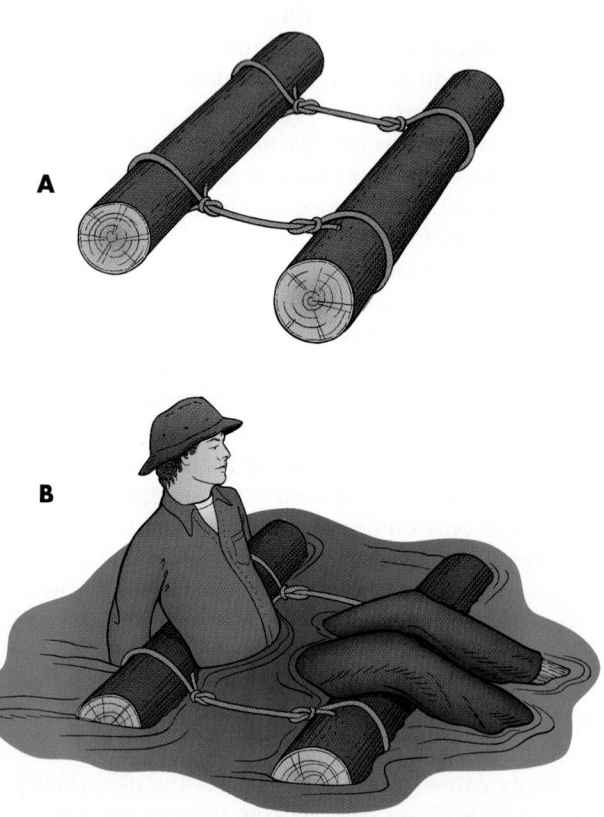

Figure 29-8 Log flotation device. **A,** Two lightweight logs are tied together. **B,** Device in action.

feet. Diagonally sliced saplings or neatly severed branches indicate someone has used a machete. There is a particular reflectivity off the ground where humans have trod; this reflectivity is the best way to follow a trail at night. These trail-finding clues are often so subtle that you may *sense* the trail rather than *see* it. Game trails meander and are narrower than human trails.

In the jungle setting, navigation with a compass for a distance of more than 200 yards is fraught with hazard. Travelers should not attempt to cut overland if lost, inexperienced, or on their own unless a significant landmark is visible or sounds of humans or domesticated animals, indicating a settlement, are clearly heard.

A raft may be constructed by lashing logs together with rope or tough, pliable jungle vines. Balsa trees (*Ochroma pyramidale*), encountered throughout much of Amazonia, make the best rafts. Balsa is often found growing alongside rivers and has the following characteristics: tall, columnar trunk with branches and leaves bunched at the top, which gives the tree a "skinny" look; beige or gray-beige trunk; bark that is smooth but tends to flake, giving it a mottled appearance; and broadly heart-shaped, more or less three-lobed leaves. The key feature of balsa wood is its remarkably light weight. Bamboo also can be used to construct a first-class raft.

A log flotation device may be constructed by tying together two balsa logs or other lightweight wood placed 2 feet apart (Figure 29-8).[32]

A "brush" raft may be made by placing buoyant vegetation within clothing or a poncho. Dry leaf litter ("duff") or plants such as water hyacinth may be used.[32]

Food

Food is readily available in inhabited regions. Even abandoned villages yield enough fruit and vegetables on which to survive. Throughout the tropical world, bananas and the large plantain "cooking banana" are ubiquitous. Root crops such as taro, yams, and yucca should be sought. Yucca roots should be shredded or pounded and then boiled to release their toxic compounds. As an extra precaution, the wet pulp should be flattened into a "pancake" and cooked on a grate to eliminate any remaining volatile hydrogen cyanide gas.

All land crabs, mammals, birds, freshwater fish, turtles, snakes, and lizards are edible but should be cooked first to eliminate parasites. It is virtually impossible to kill game without firearms. In inexperienced hands, traps and snares are not effective. Much better results are obtained from fishing (see Chapter 28).

Water

Water may be made safe by boiling or using chemical disinfectants, such as Potable Aqua tablets. Drinkable water may be found in lianas, often called "water vines," throughout jungle regions. Vines that contain water are fairly easy to identify because they tend to resemble the "grapevines" of North American forests and have rough, scaly bark. These vines may be several inches thick and contain surprising amounts of clear water. Vines that do not contain drinkable water tend to have smoother bark and, when cut, exude sticky, milky liquid. Travelers should *not* drink from vines that contain milky, latex-like sap; this substance is poisonous. Maximal amounts of water are collected from water-bearing vines if the first cut is high on the vine and the second cut is lower on the vine near the ground. When the water stops flowing from the cut section, cutting approximately 6 inches from the opposite end will start the flow again.

Water may be trapped within sections of certain types of green bamboo. Bamboo that contains water makes a sloshing sound when shaken. Water also may be obtained from green bamboo stalks by bending a stalk over, tying it down, and cutting off the top. Water dripping from the severed tip can be collected in a container during the night (Figure 29-9).[32]

Large amounts of water can be found in the voluminous natural cisterns formed by the cuplike interiors of epiphytes (air plants), such as bromeliads. The water should be strained through a cloth.[32]

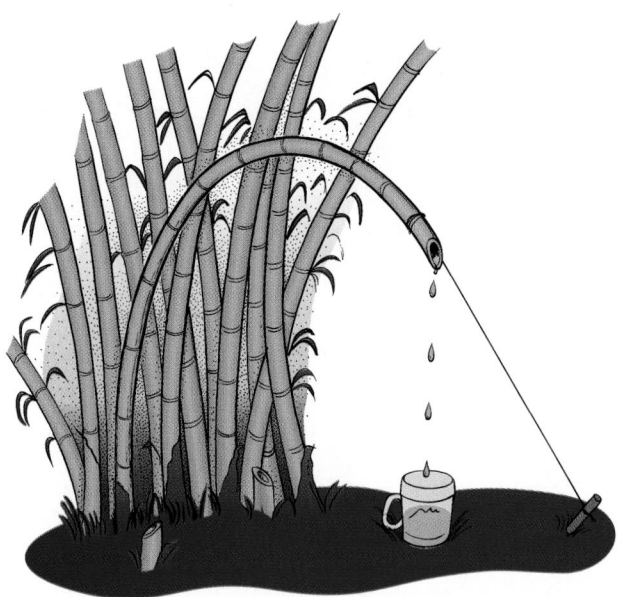

Figure 29-9   Bamboo can be a source of water.

Water may be collected from a banana or plantain plant by cutting the plant approximately 1 foot above the ground and scooping out the center of the stump into a bowl shape. The hollow thus formed fills immediately with water. The first two fillings have a bitter taste and should be dipped out. The third and subsequent fillings are drinkable. A banana plant can furnish water in this fashion for several days (Figure 29-10).[32]

In coastal regions, unripe (green) coconuts provide adequate supplies of refreshing milk. The milk of mature coconuts has a laxative effect and should be avoided.

Shelter

Abandoned, temporary shelters previously constructed by natives on hunting expeditions seem to attract particularly aggressive, large biting spiders and stinging ants. Also, venomous snakes may be attracted to rodents residing in these abandoned shelters. It is often preferable to take the extra time to set up a new camp than to risk encountering venomous insects, arachnids, and snakes.

In an emergency a proper shelter can be constructed using only plant materials. Figure 29-11 illustrates the basics of constructing a sleeping platform and lean-to. A shingled covering can be made quickly and easily from long, broad banana or heliconia leaves. Tropical palms provide a more substantial roof but require more time and skill in construction. After selecting a suitable ground-hugging species or chopping down a slender tall palm (palm trees with spines often provide the best fronds), each frond is separated into halves by grasp-

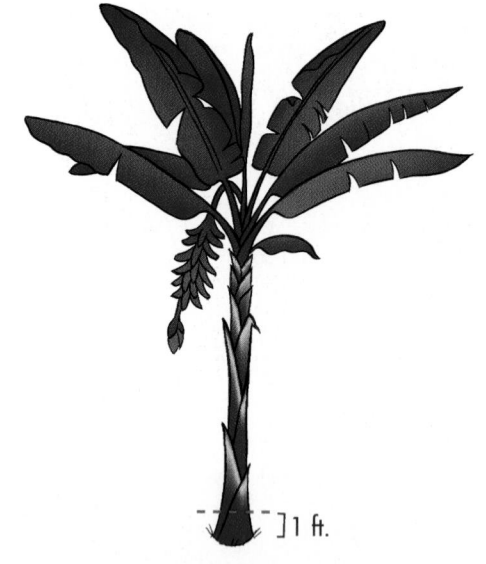

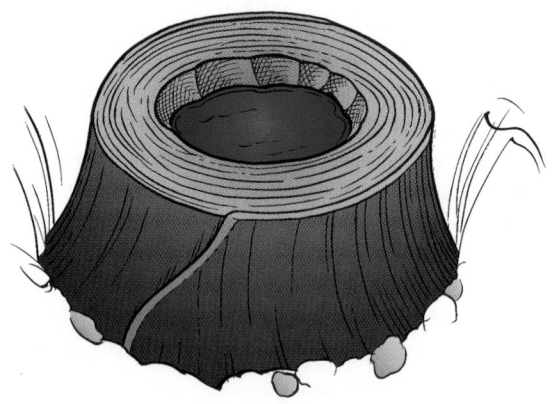

Figure 29-10 Water collected from a banana plant.

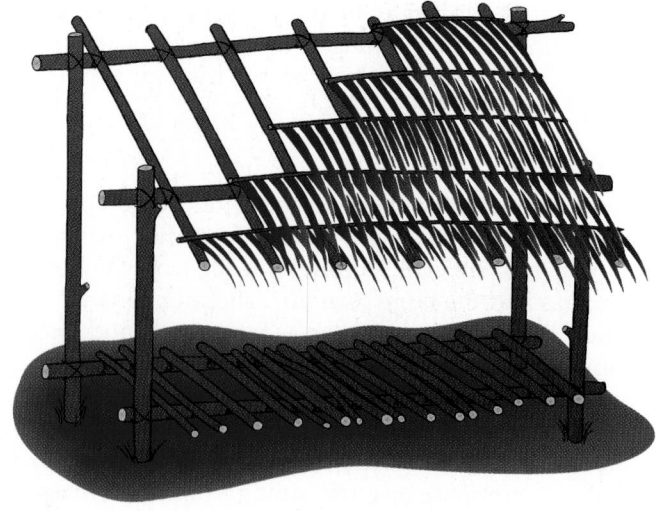

Figure 29-11 Sleeping platform.

ing it at the distal end, separating the leaves as though parting hair down the middle, and splitting the frond in two with a quick jerk (Figure 29-12). The halves should be overlapped like shingles and secured to the roof framework.

It is much easier to construct an adequate shelter using a tarpaulin (see Camp Life).

Psychology of Survival

Travelers reared on movies and novels depicting the horrors of the Amazon may have irrational fears of being lost or stranded in the jungle. Visible daytime threats worsen with the onset of darkness, when perception becomes distorted. Travelers incapacitated by fear may throw away survival items or may flee from rescuers.

Strategies that can increase travelers' confidence in survival include the following:

1. Previous jungle experience. It is helpful to be-gin tropical excursions in the structured setting of small-group travel. Ecotours, particularly in Costa Rica and Ecuador, offer a combination of rainforest trekking and cross-cultural experience.

2. Survival manuals. Military experts and others provide insights from decades of experience.[32,33]

3. Information on the tropical rainforest. Familiarity with exotic plants and animals lessens the likelihood of fear while increasing awareness of potential utility in a survival situation. The anthropological literature is replete with first-person accounts by anthropologists who have lived under trying circumstances with minimally contacted tribal populations throughout the tropics.

4. Classic accounts of adventure and survival. The Adventure Library (800-754-8229) offers an excellent series of survival epics.[21]

5. Courses in wilderness-oriented skills. The National Outdoor Leadership School (NOLS, 307-332-5300, www.nols.edu) teaches wilderness-oriented skills and leadership in a core curriculum stressing safety and judgment, leadership and team work, outdoor skills, and environmental studies.

6. Traveling with a machete, the one indispensable tool. A map, compass and a GPS unit are other recommended items.

7. Taking stock. The traveler facing a wilderness crisis assess a situation analytically and rationally before planning the course of action. *Having survival skills is important; having the will to survive is essential.*[33]

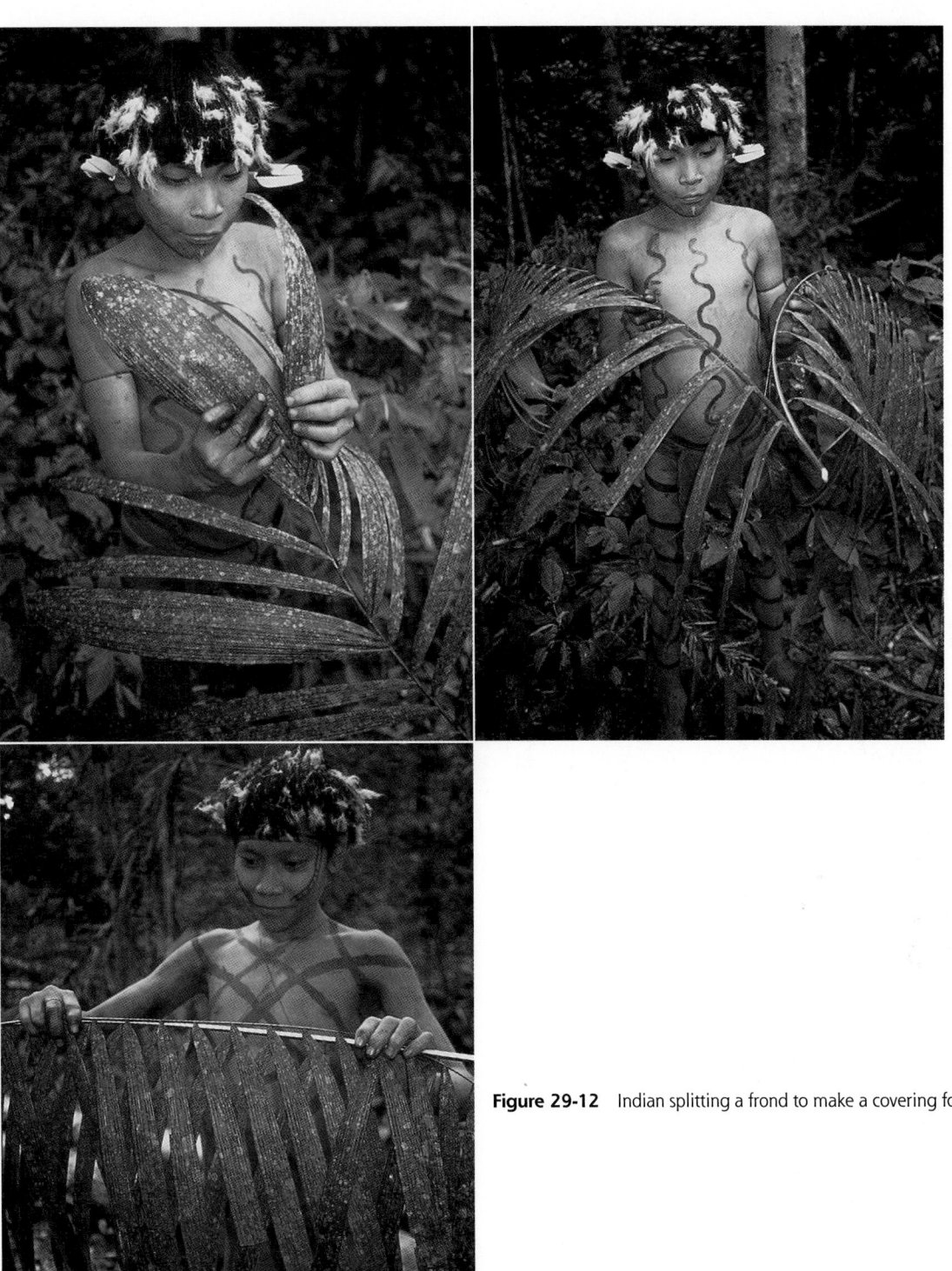

Figure 29-12   Indian splitting a frond to make a covering for a lean-to.

REFERENCES

1. Balick MJ, Cox PA: *Plants, people, and culture: the science of ethnobotany,* New York, 1996, Scientific American Library.
2. Berthoz A, Pozzo T: Head and body coordination during locomotion and complex movements. In Swinnen SP et al, editors: *Interlimb coordination: neural dynamical and cognitive constraints,* New York, 1994, Academic Press.
3. Biodiversity: the fragile web, *Natl Geogr* 195, 1999.
4. Breault JL: Candiru: Amazonian parasitic catfish, *J Wilderness Med* 2:312, 1991.
5. Cashel CM, Layne SWL, Montgomery D: Emotional response patterns of participants during a wilderness experience, *Wilderness Environ Med* 1:9, 1996.
6. Clement G, Pozzo T, Berthoz A: Contribution of eye position to control of the upside-down standing posture, *Exp Brain Res* 73:569, 1988.
7. Colwell RK: A bite to remember, *Nat Hist* 94:2, 1985.
8. Conrad L: Cougar attack: case report of a fatality, *J Wilderness Med* 3:387, 1992.
9. Dufour DL: Insects as food, *Am Anthropologist* 89:383, 1987.
10. *The emerald realm: earth's precious rainforests,* Washington, DC, 1995, National Geographic Society.
11. Erb BD: Predicting success in wilderness ventures, *Wilderness Med Lett* 7:8, 1990.
12. Erb BD: *Medical selection of participants in wilderness ventures.* Presented at the Second World Congress on Wilderness Medicine, Aspen, 1995.
13. Flandry F et al: Initial antibiotic therapy for alligator bites, *South Med J* 82:262, 1989.
14. Forsyth A, Miyata K, Landry S: *Tropical nature,* New York, 1995, Touchstone.
15. Goodman P, Kurtz KJ, Carmichael J: Medical recommendations for wilderness travel, *Postgrad Med* 77:173, 1985.
16. Guderian R: Personal communication.
17. Hansen E: *Stranger in the Forest,* Boston, 1988, Houghton Mifflin.
18. Houston CS: Who will you take on a high mountain expedition? *Wilderness Med Lett* 7:11, 1990.
19. Iserson KV, editor: *Position statements,* Point Reyes Station, Calif, 1989, Wilderness Medical Society.
20. Kritcher J: *A neotropical companion,* Princeton, NJ, 1997, Princeton University Press.
21. Lansing A: *Endurance,* New York, 1994, Adventure Library.
22. *Lost crops of the Incas,* Washington, DC, 1989, National Academy Press.
23. Lovejoy TE: Foreword. In Forsyth A, Miyata K, Landry S: *Tropical nature,* New York, 1995, Touchstone.
24. O'Hanlon R: *In trouble again,* New York, 1990, Vintage Books.
25. Olaya Cl: *Frutas de America,* Bogota, Colombia, 1991, Editorial Norma.
26. Perry DR: The canopy of the tropical rainforest, *Sci Am* 251:138, 1984.
27. Richards P, Baillie I, Walsh R: *The tropical rainforest,* Cambridge, UK, 1996, Cambridge University Press.
28. Schultes RE: *Where the gods reign,* Oracle, Ariz, 1988, Synergetic Press.
29. Schultes RE, Hofmann A: *Plants of the gods,* New York, 1979, McGraw-Hill.
30. Schultes RE, Raffauf RF: *The healing forest,* Portland, Ore, 1990, Dioscorides Press.
31. Schwerdtfeger W, editor: *World survey of climatology,* 16 vols, New York, 1969-1986, Elsevier Scientific.
32. *Survival: AFPAM 36-2246,* Washington, DC, 1996. Department of the Air Force.
33. *Survival: FM 21-76,* Washington, DC, 1992. Department of the Army.
34. Weatherford J: *Indian givers,* New York, 1988, Crown.
35. Wilson EO: Threats to biodiversity, *Sci Am* 261:108, 1989.
36. Wilson EO: *The diversity of life,* New York, 1993, Norton.

30 White-Water Medicine and Rescue

Eric A. Weiss

> *Rivers have what man most respects and longs for in his own life and thought—a capacity for renewal and replenishment, continual energy, creativity, cleansing.*
>
> John M. Kauffman, *Flow East*

Rafting, canoeing, and kayaking have become the third largest outdoor recreation industry in the United States.[34] Over 19 million people canoe and kayak each year, and more than 57 million enjoy rafting.[6] Combined participation in river sports is growing at a rate of 15% annually.[35,43] Kayaks and rafts are also used by law enforcement officers, park rangers, and game wardens to patrol and manage their territories.[29] New equipment designs have opened up more difficult rivers for exploration and commercial recreation.

It is not surprising that the number of river-related accidents and deaths has also increased dramatically. The American Canoe Association reports that approximately 130 white-water fatalities occur each year.[43] This chapter examines the unique and dynamic hazards associated with rivers and white-water paddling. Safety equipment, accident prevention, common injuries, environmental hazards, medical management, and swift water rescue are also reviewed.

HISTORICAL PERSPECTIVE

White-water boating as a recreational activity began in the United States in earnest during the late nineteenth century when adventurers attempted to emulate Major Wesley Powell's Colorado River expedition by rowing boats down many of the West's large rivers.[24] These heavy wooden boats were replaced by inflatable rafts after World War II, when surplus neoprene assault boats and life rafts became available for civilian use.[3] In 1966, fewer than 500 people boated the Colorado River through the Grand Canyon in an entire year. Recently, the figure exceeded 500 per day.[24]

Rafting did not become popular in the eastern United States until the early 1960s. In 1968, commercially guided raft trips were offered for the first time on the New River in West Virginia.[45] The Chattooga River in Georgia attracted many rafters after the movie *Deliverance* was filmed there in 1971. The Youghiogheny River in Pennsylvania and the South Fork of the American River in northern California have become the two most heavily rafted rivers in the country.

Technologic advances have revolutionized river running. Electronically welded plastic has largely replaced rubber as the primary material used in raft construction, making the vessels lighter, stronger, and easier to repair. Self-bailing rafts, introduced in 1983, are now ubiquitous and provide greater maneuverability, allowing rafters to run rivers previously considered too difficult and dangerous. Unfortunately, greater mobility has been paralleled by an increase in the number of accidents occurring far from medical care.

A major innovation in kayaking was the development of the plastic kayak, first manufactured in 1972 by the Holloform Company (Figure 30-1).[45] Kayaks had been previously constructed from resinous materials, such as fiberglass and Kevlar, which were more fragile and less likely to "broach," or wrap around rocks. Paddlers were reluctant to run steep, rocky rivers for fear of breaking their boats. Most recreational white-water kayaks are now made of molded polyethylene plastic, which does not break apart and has the potential to fold when broached or pinned, trapping the paddler. Kayakers with "indestructible" boats are pushing the limits of navigable rivers. Even Niagara Falls has been successfully run by a kayaker!

The enormous popularity of rafting and kayaking has led to exponential growth of professional guide services. In 1990, 35 million people were taken down U.S. rivers by commercial companies.[43] Faced with increased competition, guide services have been leading inexperienced clients with little formal training and few practical skills into difficult and dangerous rivers (Figure 30-2). In the summer of 1988, five U.S. executives died after their raft flipped on the Chilco River in British Columbia. One of the survivors was reported to have said, "We looked at white water as sort of a roller coaster ride."[41]

MORBIDITY AND MORTALITY

There is a paucity of data that document the relative risk of white-water–related activities. In Colorado, fewer people die while engaged in rafting, canoeing, and kayaking than in climbing, bicycling, and skiing. Figures compiled by the Colorado Department of Public Health and Environment showed that 69 people died in climbing or hiking accidents, 36 while bicycling and 32 while snow skiing during a 3-year period ending in 1995. Rafting, canoeing, and kayaking incidents, by comparison, resulted in 19 fatalities (Table 30-1).

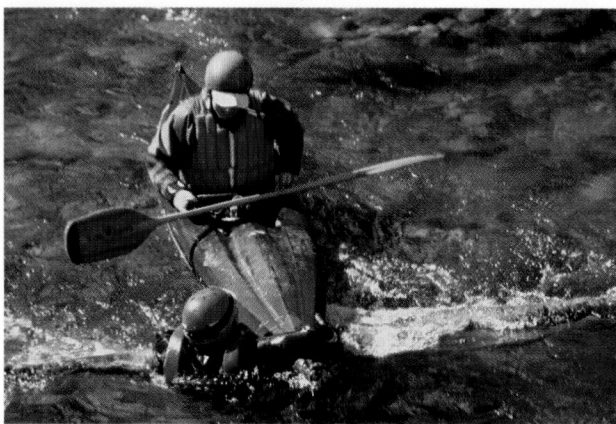

Figure 30-1 River rescue. The plastic kayak has revolutionized white-water sports. *(Courtesy Paul Auerbach, MD.)*

TABLE 30-1. Recreational Fatalities in Colorado, 1993-1995 (252 deaths were the result of recreational activities)

ACTIVITY	RANK	FATALITIES
Climbing/hiking	1	69
Bicycling	2	36
Snow skiing	3	32
Swimming	4	25
Canoeing/kayaking/rafting	5	19
Horseback riding	6	18
Boating/water skiing	7	13
Fishing	8	11
Hunting	9	6

Data from Colorado Department of Public Health and Environment.

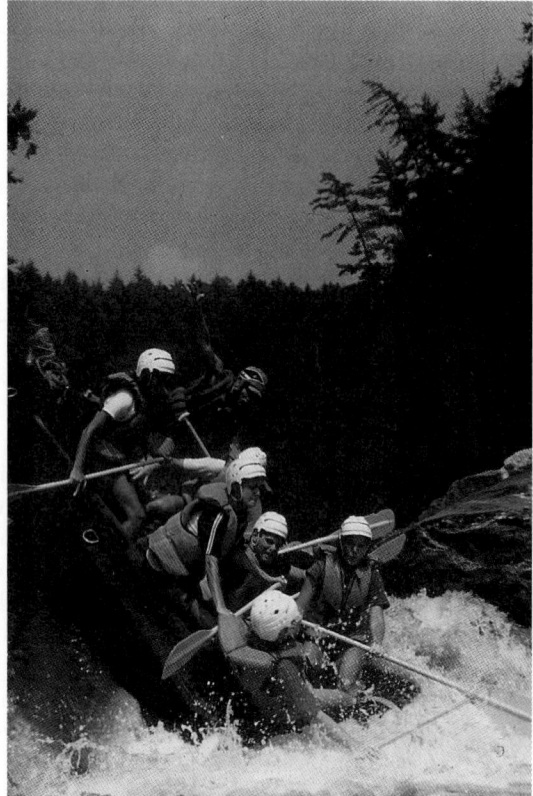

Figure 30-2 Class V commercial rafting on the Chattooga River, Georgia. *(Courtesy Robert Harrison, Whetstone Photography.)*

A retrospective analysis of injury reports submitted by commercial rafting outfitters to the West Virginia Division of Natural Resources from 1995-1997 revealed a total of 200 injuries with a resulting overall injury incidence rate of 0.263 per 1000 rafters. The average age of injured persons was 33.14 years, 53.3% were male, and 59.8% had previous rafting experience.[47]

The body parts most frequently injured during rafting mishaps are the face (33.3%), including the eye (12.1%), mouth (6.6%), other facial parts (5.1%), nose (4.5%), and teeth (4.0%), followed by the knee (15.3%), arm/wrist/hand (11.6%), and other parts of the leg, hip, or foot (10.5%). The most common injury types are lacerations (32.5%), sprains/strains (23.2%), fractures (14.9%), contusions/bruises (9.8%), and dislocations (8.2%). Most injuries occur in the raft as a result of collisions among passengers, being struck by a paddle or other equipment, or entanglement of extremities in parts of the raft.[47] Because most injuries occur in the raft and involve the face, accident-preventive measures include attaching face protection to paddling helmets and carrying fewer passengers per raft.

EQUIPMENT

The dynamic and unpredictable nature of rivers can turn any mishap into a tragedy. For this reason, the initial mission of white-water medicine is to emphasize safety and accident prevention.

According to the U.S. Coast Guard's boating accident statistics, the most common factor contributing to white-water–related deaths is failure to wear a personal flotation device (PFD, or life jacket).[43] Exposure to cold river water can stimulate respiratory and cardiovascular reflexes, making it difficult for a swimmer to keep his or her head above water (maintain freeboard) (see Chapter 8).[25] The Coast Guard is charged with regulating and testing life jackets and classifies PFDs into five types. Of these, only two types are commonly used in white-water sports.

The type III PFD, a vest-type jacket favored by most paddlers, permits greater mobility and comfort. The Coast Guard requires that type III PFDs have a minimum of 15½ pounds of flotation (lift). Because most adults effectively weigh between 10 and 12 pounds in the water, this allows at least 3½ pounds of effective required buoyancy.

Type V PFDs are used by commercial outfitters because they provide greater flotation and are constructed asymmetrically with over half of the jacket's flotation distributed in the front. This is supposed to turn an unconscious wearer face up. Although this may be true in calm water, it does not work reliably in swift water.

A PFD should fit snugly and not ride up over the head when a person is in the water. Because even a well-fitting life jacket can be pulled off by turbulent water, some manufacturers now include crotch straps as an added safety feature. Testifying before a congressional subcommittee, the president of the National Transportation Safety Association cited the Chilco River accident to support his contention that crotch straps be made mandatory on all white water–use life jackets. Several survivors reported that their life jackets rode up over their heads and did not keep their faces above water.

Life jackets with built-in rescue harnesses, pioneered by the Europeans, are now widely available in the United States. A typical harness system uses seatbelt webbing threaded through a metal retainer, then run into a plastic cam-lock buckle with a toggle. The toggle allows the user to find the buckle in white water. To release the system, the user pulls the toggle, opening the buckle and allowing the webbing to slip through the retainer and release. A D-ring mounted on the back of the jacket provides a point for clipping in a rope (Figure 30-3). This quick-release belt allows the wearer to attempt a strong swimmer rescue but also to get free of the tethering line quickly in an emergency.

Beyond flotation, life jackets have other benefits that make them highly useful in wilderness settings. Their insulating properties help prevent hypothermia. The closed-cell foam flotation material acts as thoracic padding during falls on slippery rocks or when swimming rapids after exiting the craft. Life jackets also make excellent improvised splints; they can be fashioned into cervical collars, cylindrical knee braces (Figure 30-4), or padded ankle stirrups.

The American Whitewater Affiliation (AWA) safety code recommends the use of helmets at all times in kayaks and canoes, and in rafts and other craft when attempting rapids of class IV or greater difficulty. Surveys have shown that head trauma after capsizing comprises 10% to 17% of all kayaking accidents.[29,44]

Another vital piece of safety equipment is a rope, which should be readily accessible and secured in a manner that facilitates rapid deployment and prevents entanglement. Throw ropes for river use should float, have a certain amount of dynamic stretch, and not absorb water. Self-contained throw bags have virtually replaced

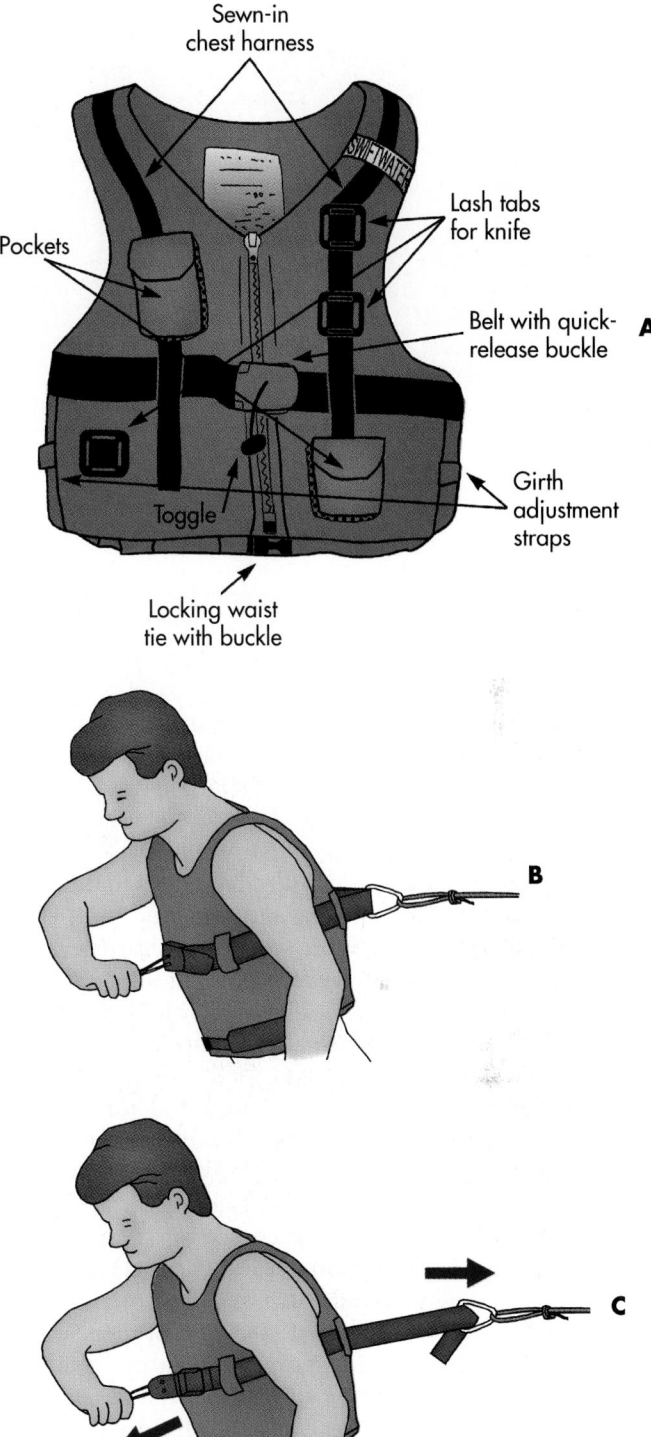

Figure 30-3 A, Life jacket with built-in rescue harness. **B** and **C,** A quick-release buckle allows the wearer to release the tether when necessary. It is essential for swiftwater use.

coiled ropes for river use and generally hold about 50 to 75 feet of ⅜-inch polypropylene rope inside a nylon stuff sack. Newer styles can be attached to life jackets for rapid access. They can also be thrown to rescuers by a paddler who is pinned or broached. Commercial outfitters and

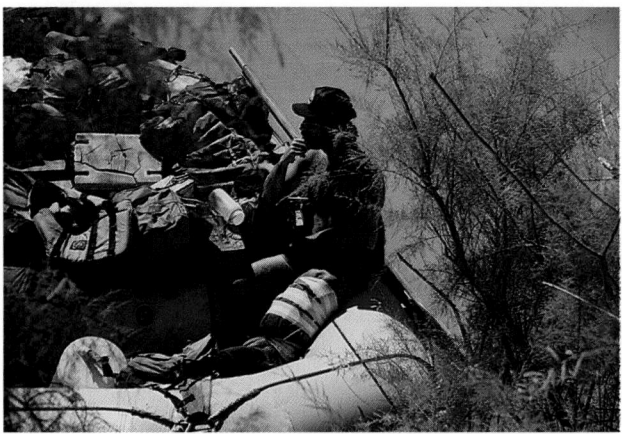

Figure 30-4 A paddler wearing a type III life jacket around his knee as an improvised knee immobilizer to help stabilize a sprained knee.

large groups of rafters should carry at least one 300-foot-long static rope to be used for Telfar lowers, Tyroleans, and other rescue situations where mechanical advantages are used.

Knives should be readily accessible. Fixed blades are preferable to folding ones unless the folded blade can be opened easily with one hand. Double-edged blades can cut in two directions and thus require minimal handling in precarious situations. Some modern knives designed for kayakers feature serrated edges that can cut through plastic boats during entrapment.

Whistles should be worn so paddlers can alert others that an accident has occurred. Paddlers are often spread out over the course of a rapid, and yelling over the roar of the water is usually a frustrating and fruitless endeavor.

Placing adequate barriers between the human body and the environment is of paramount importance in aquatic sports. Functional, insulated clothing should be considered a mandatory safety item to prevent hypothermia. Cotton is a poor choice for river wear; it loses all of its insulating properties when wet and dries slowly. Newer synthetics such as polypropylene and polyester pile absorb no more than 1% of their weight in water and maintain thermal insulating qualities when wet.[27] When combined with a nylon or Gore-Tex paddling jacket, a synthetic underlayer provides effective protection from cold and wind.

Wet suits, previously considered to be optimal garments for paddlers in extreme conditions, are stiff and somewhat constricting.[1] The dry suit, with tight-fitting latex seals at the wrist, ankle, and neck, is the new "gold standard" for cold water boating. By sealing water out and preventing evaporative heat loss, the dry suit can keep a paddler warm even during winter conditions.[17]

Overheating is occasionally a problem with dry suits. Recently a dry suit contributed to profound and unexpected hyperthermia in a kayaker who had suffered a submersion injury in cold water.[4]

RIVER HAZARDS

The International Scale of River Difficulty grades rivers and rapids into classes I to VI. An American version of this rating has been adopted by the AWA for most U.S. rivers (Box 30-1).[42] Some western rivers use the Grand Canyon System, which rates rapids on a scale from 1 to 10. Neither scale is a truly objective standard; individual and regional variations are common, and the margin of difficulty for a particular rapid may differ significantly for kayaks and rafts. Unfortunately, important safety parameters, such as water temperature, remoteness, and evacuation potential, are not taken into consideration.

The difficulty of a river generally increases with the volume of flow and the average gradient. The volume of water in a river is usually expressed as a measure of cubic feet per second (cfs). It is the amount of water moving past a certain point during a given period of time. The volume of a river can be determined by multiplying the width by the depth times the speed of the current. As the water level rises, its speed and power increase exponentially, raising the difficulty of most rapids.[3] Occasionally, however, a rapid becomes easier as the added water submerges hazardous obstacles. Gradient is the amount of drop between two points and is expressed as feet per mile. The steeper the gradient, the faster the water moves.

Not all water flows downstream. The most common upstream flow is an eddy, which is created when water flows around an obstacle. The water piles up higher than the river level on the upstream side of the obstacle, while the water on the downstream side is lower. Water flows around the obstacle then back toward it to fill in the low spot. The line between the upstream and downstream current is the eddy line. Eddies are one of the most important features of the river for boat maneuvering and rescue. Exiting the main current by pulling into an eddy allows the paddler to stop the descent and safely scout the next rapid. It also provides a location for a paddler to set up rescue for his or her companion upstream.

Hydraulics, also known as holes, reversals, rollers, suck-holes, and pour-overs, are the most common hazards in rivers. A hydraulic is created when water flows over an obstacle, causing a depression that produces a relative vacuum within which the downstream water recirculates (Figure 30-5). The water below a hydraulic is typically very aerated and presents a white, foamy appearance. Rafts and kayaks can be turned upside down by the force of a hydraulic, and if the reversal currents are strong enough, crafts and people can become trapped in the recirculating flow. When proceeding into a rapid that contains a hazardous hydraulic,

Box 30-1 AMERICAN VERSION OF THE INTERNATIONAL SCALE OF RIVER DIFFICULTY

CLASS I: EASY

Fast-moving water with riffles and small waves. Few obstructions, all obvious and easily avoided with little training. Risk to swimmers is slight; self-rescue is easy.

CLASS II: NOVICE

Straightforward rapids with wide, clear channels that are evident without scouting. Occasional maneuvering may be required, but rocks and medium-sized waves are easily avoided by trained paddlers. Swimmers are seldom injured, and group assistance, although helpful, is seldom needed.

CLASS III: INTERMEDIATE

Rapids with moderate, irregular waves that may be difficult to avoid and can swamp an open canoe. Complex maneuvers in fast current and good boat control in tight passages or around ledges are often required; large waves or strainers may be present but are easily avoided. Strong eddies and powerful current effects can be found, particularly on large-volume rivers. Scouting is advisable for inexperienced parties. Injuries while swimming are rare; self-rescue is usually easy, but group assistance may be required to avoid long swims.

CLASS IV: ADVANCED

Intense and powerful but predictable rapids requiring precise boat handling in turbulent water. The advanced river may feature large, unavoidable waves and holes or constricted passages that demand fast maneuvers under pressure. A fast, reliable eddy turn may be needed to

CLASS IV: ADVANCED—cont'd

initiate maneuvers, scout rapids, or rest. Rapids may require "must" moves above dangerous hazards. Scouting is necessary the first time down. Risk of injury to swimmers is moderate to high, and water conditions may make self-rescue difficult. Group assistance for rescue is often essential but requires practiced skills. A strong Eskimo roll is highly recommended.

CLASS V: EXPERT

Extremely long, obstructed, or violent rapids that expose a paddler to above-average danger. Drops may contain large, unavoidable waves and holes or steep, congested chutes with complex, demanding routes. Rapids may continue for long distances between pools, demanding a high level of fitness. Eddies may be small, turbulent, or difficult to reach. At the high end of the scale, several of these factors may be combined. Scouting is mandatory but often difficult. Swims are dangerous and rescue is difficult, even for experts. A very reliable Eskimo roll, proper equipment, extensive experience, and practiced rescue skills are essential for survival.

CLASS VI: EXTREME

Class VI runs exemplify the extremes of difficulty, unpredictability, and danger. The consequences of errors are very severe, and rescue may be impossible. For teams of experts only, at favorable water levels, after close inspection and taking all precautions. This class does not represent drops believed to be unrunnable but may include rapids that are only occasionally run.

From *Safety code of the American Whitewater Affiliation,* Phoenicia, NY, 1989, American Whitewater Affiliation.

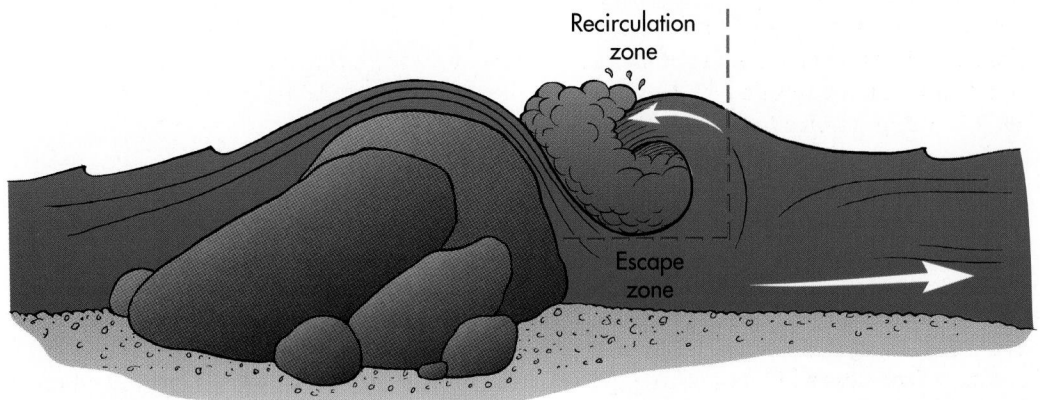

Figure 30-5 Recirculating currents created by a hydraulic. Water and "swimmers" are released downstream beneath the surface.

one of the group should preset a rope below the hole to facilitate rescue.

Hydraulics release water downstream from beneath the surface. This may be the only avenue of escape for a swimmer. Escape from a strong hydraulic may re-

quire a person to stay submerged and to resist the urge to return immediately to the surface. Surfacing too early can result in recirculation. Fortunately, most hydraulics eventually release people regardless of what action they take.

Novice paddlers often misjudge the force of hydraulics. It is not the height of the drop that generates the recirculating power but rather the shape and angle of the obstruction, combined with water volume and adjacent eddy currents. A "smiling" hydraulic has its outer edges curving downstream, so that the recirculating water feeds out into the main current and is thus easier to escape. In a "frowning" hydraulic, the outer edges curve back upstream into the center of the hydraulic, making escape much more difficult.

Low-head dams or weirs form massive hydraulics with enormous recirculating potential. Unlike natural hydraulics, these human-made structures form hydraulics all the way across the river, leaving no escape routes. In the Binghamton Dam disaster of 1975, a 13½-foot Boston whaler with a 20-horsepower engine was pulled into a hydraulic while attempting a rescue, resulting in the deaths of three firefighters.[39]

Undercut rocks are boulders or ledges that have been eroded just beneath the water surface. These usually occur on geologically older rivers. They can be difficult to recognize and pose significant risks for entrapment and drowning, even in class II rapids.

The potential for entrapment can also occur when swimmers attempt to stand up and walk in swift-moving currents. A foot can become wedged in an undercut rock or between rocks beneath the surface, causing the victim to lose his or her balance and fall face down into the river (Figure 30-6, *A*). With the foot entrapped, the victim cannot regain an upright or even face-up position. This type of mishap has caused drownings in water less than 3 feet deep.

A swimmer in a rapid should assume a supine position, with feet at the surface and pointed downstream to serve as shock absorbers. This position minimizes the potential for both foot entrapment and head and neck trauma (Figure 30-6, *B*).

Strainers are obstacles, such as fallen trees, bridge debris, or driftwood lodged between rocks or jutting out from the shore, that allow water to pass through (sieve effect) while trapping the swimmer or boater. Flooded rivers, a favorite of expert boaters, often develop many new strainers as riverbank debris is washed into the flow. In the summer of 1987, five paddlers drowned when their raft struck a large strainer on Canada's Ellaho River.[41]

Negotiating a strainer requires special tactics. The safest option for the swimmer is to swim aggressively into the strainer head first rather than feet first, and then attempt to climb over the debris (Figure 30-7, *A*). Approaching a strainer feet first may lead to underwater entrapment (Figure 30-7, *B*).

Human-made hazards can also pose a threat to river runners. Bridge pilings, submerged automobiles, dams, and low-hanging power lines can pin or injure boaters.

A broach occurs when a boat wraps sideways around an obstacle or when both bow and stern become stuck on separate obstacles simultaneously. Common obsta-

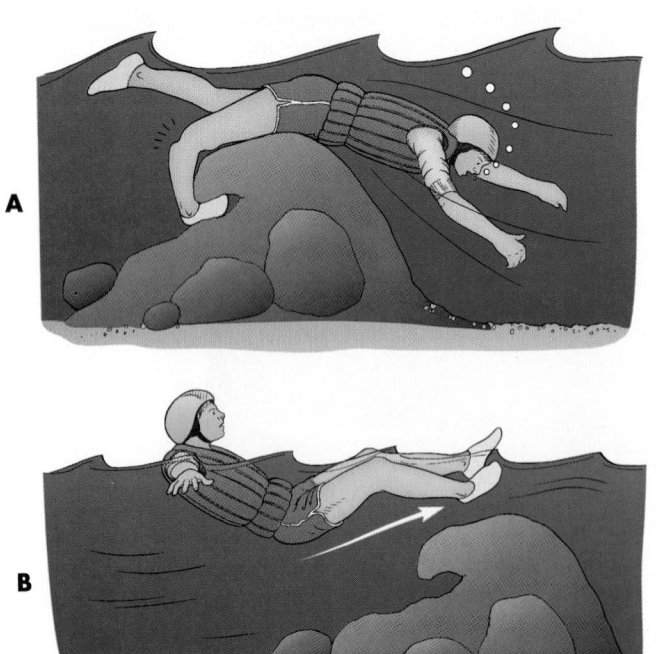
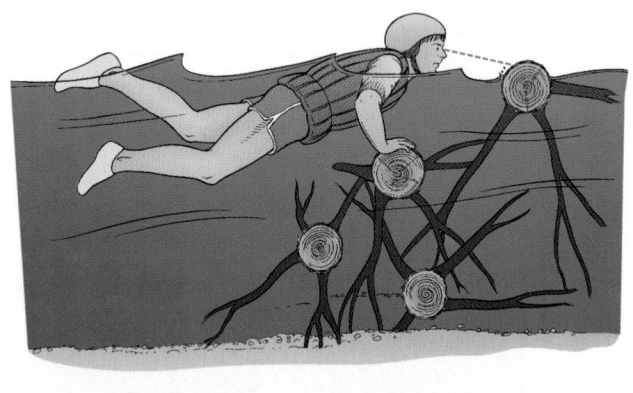
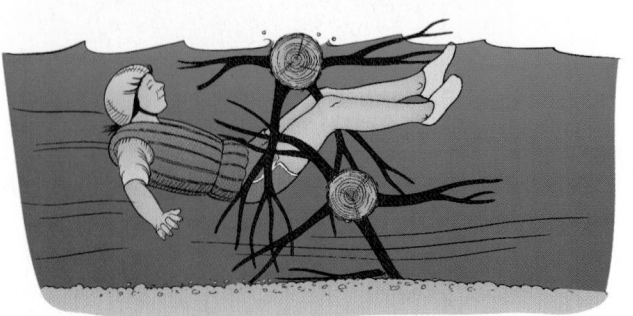

Figure 30-6 **A,** Attempting to stand up in shallow water can produce foot entrapment in an undercut rock. **B,** Proper way to swim while in a rapid.

Figure 30-7 **A,** Proper approach to a strainer. **B,** Incorrect approach to a strainer.

cles include boulders, trees, bridge pilings, and ledges protruding from canyon walls. Drowning can occur if the paddler leans upstream away from the obstacle and flips upside down while still broached or if the boat collapses and entraps the victim (Figure 30-8).

A vertical pin happens when a kayaker plunges over a drop and the end of the boat becomes trapped between rocks beneath the surface. The force of the water can fold a plastic kayak over on itself, trapping the occupant upside down beneath the surface (Figure 30-9).

A survey of 365 members of the AWA revealed that 33% of serious kayaking incidents and 41% of open canoeing mishaps involved either pinning or broaching (Table 30-2).[44] In a separate survey of 500 paddlers between 1989 and 1993, 42% of kayaking fatalities resulted from vertical pins, broaches, or entrapments in strainers.

Kayak construction can have important safety implications in both broach and pin situations. The force of the current against the deck of the boat or back of the paddler can make it impossible for the victim to extract his or her legs and escape. Boat makers have developed kayaks with larger cockpits that make it easier to raise the knees out and escape the craft. Transverse bulk-

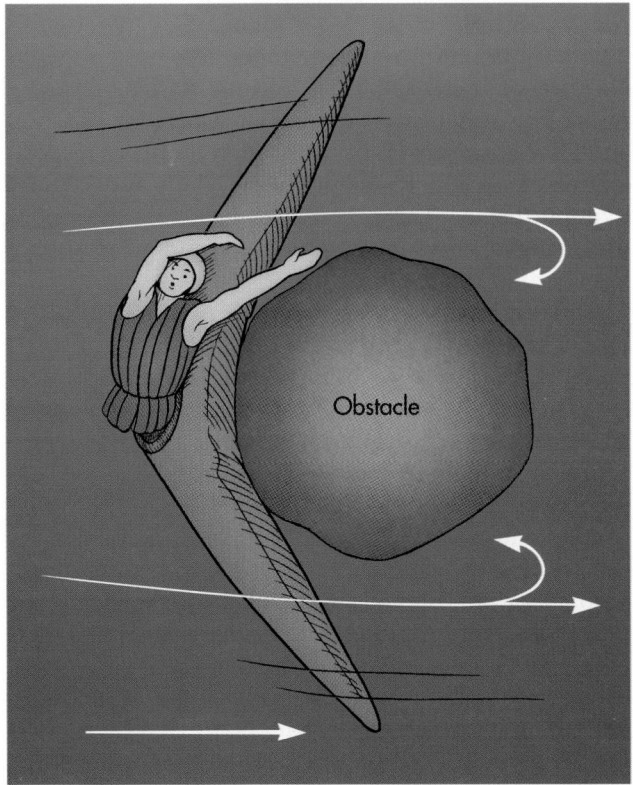

Figure 30-8 Broach.

TABLE 30-2. Serious White-Water–Related Incidents

INCIDENT	NUMBER	PERCENTAGE OF ACCIDENTS
Vertical pin entrapment	18	8
Broach entrapment	46	21
Rock sieve entrapment	16	7
Undercut rock entrapment	23	10
Recirculation in hydraulic	47	21
Long swim	42	19

From Wallace D: *AWA J* 3:27, 1991.

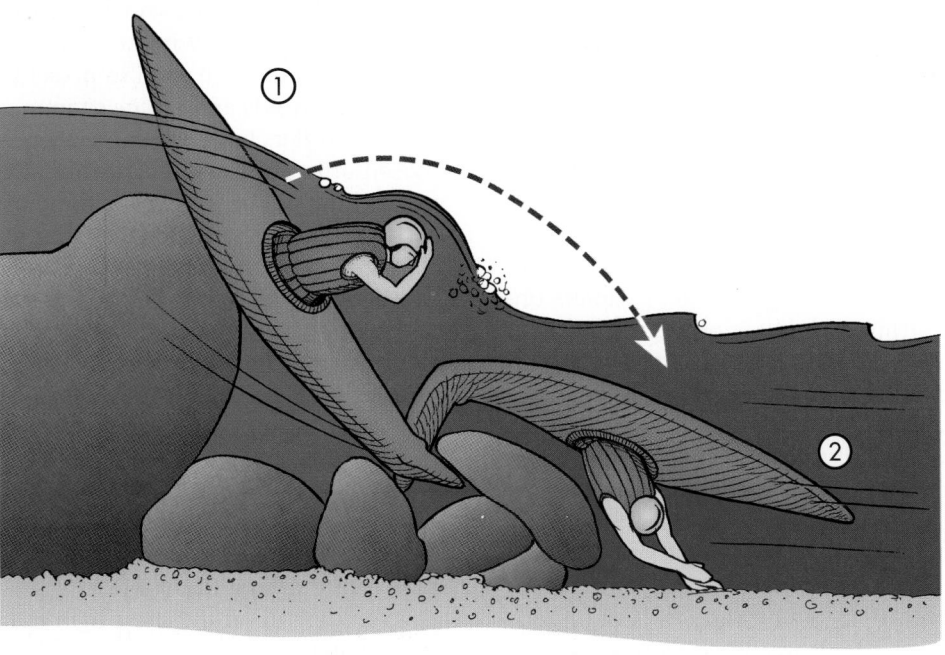

Figure 30-9 *1*, Vertical pin. *2*, Pitchpole pin.

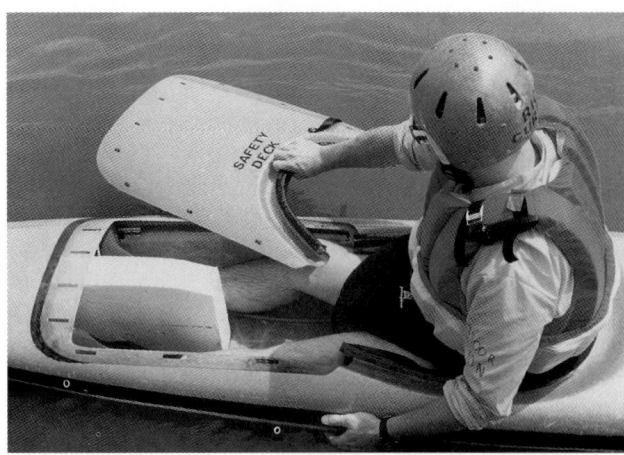

Figure 30-10 Safety Deck system, which offers an emergency exit for a kayaker in distress.

head-type foot braces have replaced pedal-type braces to prevent the kayaker from being shoved forward in the boat. This feature ensures the escape potential offered by larger cockpits. One of the compromises of the larger cockpit, however, is that the sprayskirt is more likely to come off in turbulent water.

Another safety feature, the Safety Deck System (Outdoor Safety Systems, Princeton, NJ), uses a manually releasable foredeck section that can be jettisoned by the paddler for emergency exit (Figure 30-10). During normal use, this deckplate is securely fastened to the boat and does not alter its shape or performance. The Safety Deck System has been tested extensively with positive results, but unfortunately its cost has precluded commercial development.

SUBMERSION ACCIDENTS

Almost all fatalities on rivers result from submersion. Each year the River Safety Task Force of the American Canoe Association compiles accounts of drownings and other accidents. Every 3 years it publishes the *River Safety Report,* which chronicles and analyzes these accidents.[39-41,43]

Most submersion fatalities occur after paddlers unexpectedly swim from their boats or become trapped in them underwater. The exact cause of drowning often remains unclear and is inexplicably blamed on immersion hypothermia. Although hypothermia induces impaired judgment and coordination and may be an important contributing factor, immersion hypothermia is probably never the sole cause of death.[46] Studies by Hayward and others have shown that seminude subjects are able to maintain normal core temperatures for 15 to 20 minutes in 10° C (50° F) water.[19,20] Continuous immersion for up to 1 hour would be required to produce profound hypothermia.[20]

Cold water immersion precipitates drowning by three other mechanisms. Sudden cold water immersion produces profound cardiovascular and respiratory responses. Reflex sympathetic output can markedly increase blood pressure and heart rate, resulting in lethal arrhythmias.[16,25,26]

An immediate and involuntary gasp occurs after cold water immersion. This is followed by hyperventilation.[8] Pulmonary ventilation increases up to fivefold because of increased tidal volume and respiratory rate.[38] The initial gasp can result in aspiration of water and laryngospasm. Hyperventilation produces respiratory alkalosis with resultant muscle tetany and cerebral hypoperfusion.[8] This response can increase the risk of drowning in a person struggling to maintain an airway freeboard in rough water.

The respiratory stimulation produced by cold water immersion significantly decreases breath-holding duration.[21] This fact has enormous implications for kayakers who must hold their breath while attempting to roll up a boat after flipping upside down. This probably accounts for the unexplained swims by expert kayakers who sometimes fail to right themselves after flipping in cold water.

Peripheral cold water–induced vasoconstriction exacerbates rapid cooling of muscles and nerves in the extremities, resulting in loss of strength and coordination.[38] The ability to swim, maintain freeboard, avoid obstacles, and climb from the river may be greatly impaired.[28] Even when the air temperature is warm, paddlers running cold water rivers should wear sufficiently insulated clothing.

The combination of hyperventilation and muscle dysfunction can be lethal for a swimmer in rough water. A PFD helps but does not prevent even small waves from submerging a swimmer's head.[15] These dangers make imperative the need to preset safety systems in significant rapids and rescue swimmers first. Unfortunately, paddlers have drowned when their companions chased after equipment, assuming that the swimmer could climb out of the river without assistance.[40,42]

Safety kayaks with enhanced buoyancy are recommended on commercial raft trips, since they provide additional flotation for clients who fall overboard.

Although some maintain that the respiratory and cardiovascular reflexes can be abolished by repeated exposure of the face to cold water, there are currently no scientific data to support this theory of acclimatization.

TRAUMA

A survey of commercial raft clients revealed that the most common significant injury was a sprained or fractured ankle.[45] Ironically, these injuries usually occur out of the water when persons walk on loose, wet, and slippery rocks during scouting and portaging or when entering or leaving the river. Ankle and other lower extremity injuries also occur on the river when rafters are tossed onto each other in rapids.

Kayakers are prone to ankle injuries from forced dorsiflexion or inversion when the bow of the boat hits an obstruction. The feet are held against the narrow horizontal braces while the heels are pushed underneath, or the entire ankle is inverted. European- and some American-designed kayaks with bulkhead foot braces have reduced this problem.

Management of foot and ankle injuries should begin with ice, elevation, and compression to reduce swelling. Cold river water is usually substituted for ice. Compression wrapping is important after icing to prevent swelling from reflex vasodilation. Splinting is important to reduce pain and edema and to limit exacerbation of the injury during evacuation. Pneumatic splints, still carried by many raft companies, provide adequate support and compression but are prone to overinflation when heated by the sun. Zippers often malfunction when they rust or jam with sand. Neurovascular integrity must be checked frequently with an air splint. Ankle splints can be improvised from life jackets, kayak float bags, articles of clothing, or a SAM splint.

Strains are common in white-water sports. Researchers at Dalhousie University in Halifax, Nova Scotia, analyzed dynamic electromyographic potentials of the various muscle groups used in kayaking and then correlated them with videotaped sequences.[32] Muscles used most often in kayaking that are prone to strain injury are shoulder extensors (latissimus dorsi, teres major, pectoralis major), medial scapula rotators (rhomboideus major and minor, pectoralis minor), lateral scapula rotators (pectoralis minor, serratus anterior), shoulder flexors and horizontal adductors (anterior deltoideus, pectoralis major, coracobrachialis), elbow extensors (triceps), and spine erector muscles. Any training program for kayakers needs to emphasize conditioning of these muscle groups.

Back strain afflicts rafters, kayakers, and canoers. Rafters are prone to back injuries while portaging, pushing stuck rafts off rocks, and carrying the crafts to and from the river. Raft guides are notorious for suffering back strain when pulling capsized customers, who often weigh more than they do, back into the rafts. Kayakers and canoers injure their backs lifting water-laden boats and loading their crafts onto automobile roofs. Sitting for prolonged periods with legs extended and minimal back support leads to muscle fatigue in kayakers, compounding the potential for injury.

Repetitive dorsiflexion of the wrist required to operate an offset (feathered) kayak paddle produces tendinitis and synovitis.[31] A paddle constructed with a 75- to 80-degree offset instead of the traditional 90 degrees can reduce wrist stress. Aspirin or nonsteroidal

TABLE 30-3. Common White-Water–Related Injuries, 1980-1991 (N = 85)

INJURY TYPE	NUMBER	PERCENTAGE OF INJURIES
Shoulder dislocation	14	16.5
Near drowning	11	12.9
Fractures	15	17.6
Head and neck	6	7
Hypothermia	4	4.7
Leg injuries	11	12.9
Lacerations	9	10.5
Fatalities	7	8.2

From Wallace D: *AWA J* 3:27, 1991.

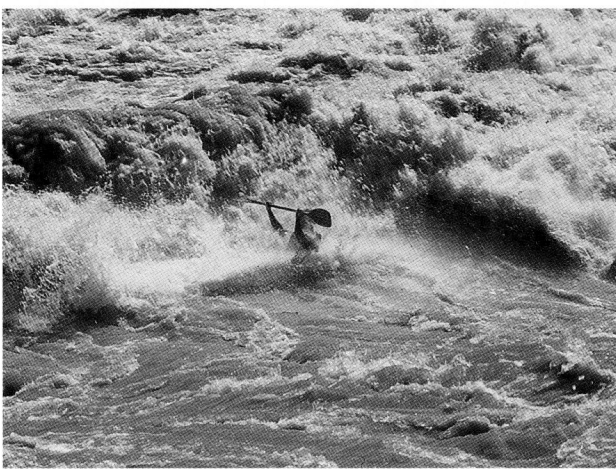

Figure 30-11   High brace maneuver.

antiinflammatory agents ingested 30 minutes before paddling, combined with ice application afterward, may be beneficial. Wrist supports provide limited relief.

The injury most often associated with kayaking is anterior shoulder dislocation. Various surveys have placed its incidence in kayakers at 10% to 16%, making it the second most common white-water–related injury (Table 30-3).[5,30,44,45] The maneuver most notorious for precipitating this injury is the high brace. Often used while supporting the kayaker in a hydraulic, surfing on a wave, or rolling the kayak upright after a flip, the high brace entails abduction of the humerus, with external rotation of the glenohumeral joint (Figure 30-11). If the arm becomes extended behind the midline plane of the body by the force of the current, the triad of abduction, external rotation, and extension of the shoulder can stretch or rupture the glenoid labrum and capsule, resulting in anterior subluxation or dislocation.[37] The paddle acts as a lever to increase the force on the glenohumeral joint.

To minimize the risk of shoulder dislocation, the preferred method of bracing is the "low brace," in which the arm is held in internal rotation and close to the body (adduction). Although initially awkward for the novice paddler, this bracing maneuver is inherently stronger and more versatile because it allows backpaddling out of a hydraulic. Exercises that strengthen the rotator cuff and deltoideus, triceps, and pectoralis muscles reinforce the glenohumeral joint.

The paddler with a dislocation is usually aware that something has gone wrong and holds the extremity away from the body, unable to bring the arm across the chest.[37] The shoulder may appear square because of anterior, medial, and inferior displacement of the humeral head into a subcoracoid position.

Although on-scene reduction of shoulder dislocations is controversial, immediate relief of pain, curtailment of ongoing injury, and subsequent ability to function more actively in evacuation are strong reasons to do it. Several techniques have been advocated for reduction.[36] The key element is rapid initiation, since the longer a shoulder remains dislocated, the more difficult the eventual reduction becomes. Relocation is often delayed because river corridors rarely afford rapid access to a flat and comfortable area upon which to place a victim in the supine or prone position, a requirement for most techniques.

For river and other wilderness settings, reduction is facilitated by using a technique in which the victim is standing or sitting (Figure 30-12). As soon as the diagnosis is made, the victim bends forward at the waist while the rescuer supports the chest with one hand. With the other hand, the rescuer grabs the victim's wrist and applies steady downward traction and external rotation. While maintaining traction, the rescuer can slowly flex the shoulder by moving it in a cephalad direction until reduction is obtained. If two rescuers are available, one should support the victim at the chest while the other pulls countertraction and flexion at the arm. Scapular manipulation by adducting the inferior tip using thumb pressure and stabilizing the superior aspect of the scapula with the cephalad hand may augment reduction (Figure 30-13).[33,36]

Shoulder reduction can also be done while the victim is sitting. Grab the victim's forearm close to his or her elbow with both hands and, with the elbow bent at 90 degrees, pull steady downward traction on the arm. After about a minute of sustained traction, slowly raise the entire arm upward until reduction is complete. Gingerly rotating the forearm outward while pulling traction may facilitate reduction. If a second rescuer is present, scapular manipulation can be performed simultaneously as described above.

Another relocation technique uses the victim's life jacket to allow one rescuer to apply both controlled traction and countertraction.[11] This technique requires that the victim be supine, with room for the rescuer to sit adjacent to the dislocated shoulder. The rescuer then slides his or her foot and leg through the life jacket's arm opening, under the neck, and out through the jacket's head opening. The rescuer's leg functions as a head rest, while the foot braced against the opposite shoulder strap of the life jacket provides countertraction. Holding the forearm of the affected side with the elbow bent at 90 degrees, the rescuer slowly leans back to apply traction while the leg exerts countertraction. The life jacket allows countertraction force to be distributed across the victim's

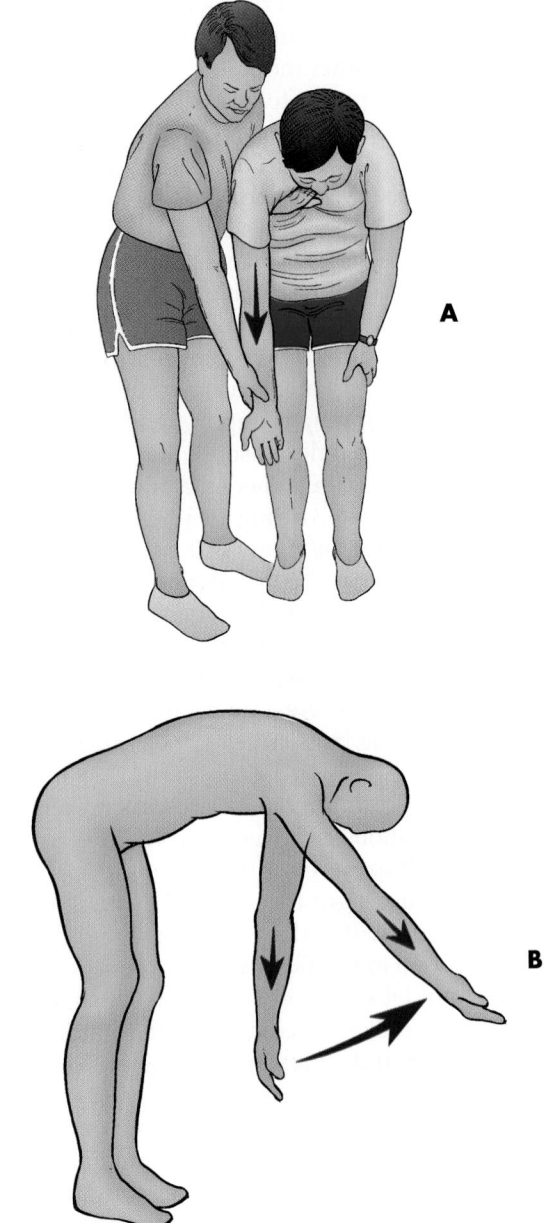

Figure 30-12 Weiss technique for shoulder relocation with the victim standing. **A,** The rescuer supports the victim's chest with one hand and pulls down and forward **(B)** with the other hand.

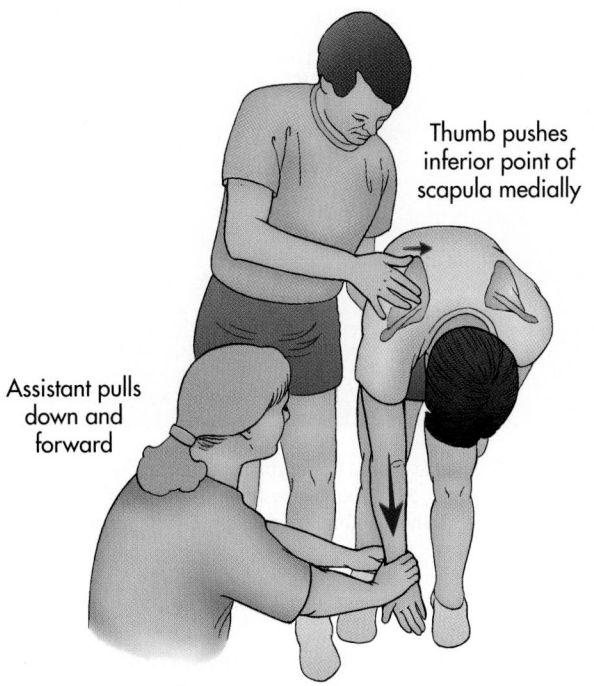

Figure 30-13   If two rescuers are available, scapular rotation to assist shoulder relocation can be performed while the second rescuer pulls the arm down and forward. The inferior top of the scapula is pushed medially.

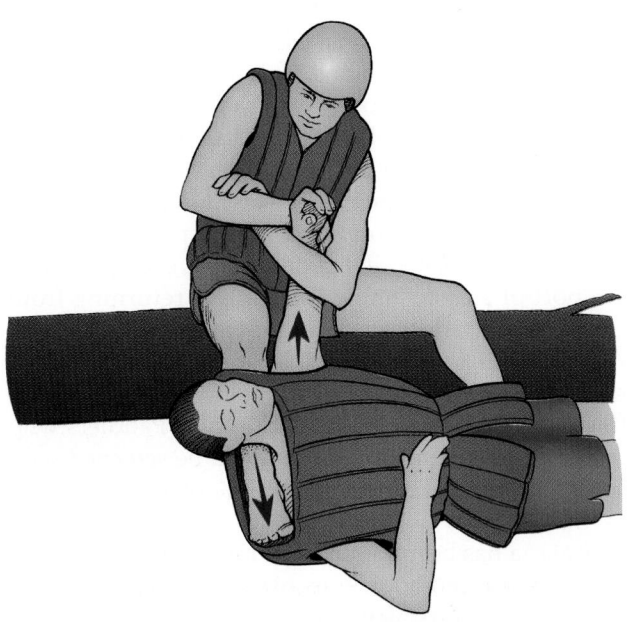

Figure 30-14   Using a life jacket to assist in countertraction for shoulder relocation.

chest. External and internal rotation can be applied to the humerus during traction to facilitate reduction (Figure 30-14).

One should always monitor circulation and motor-sensory function to the wrist and hand before and after attempting a shoulder reduction. To prevent a recurrent

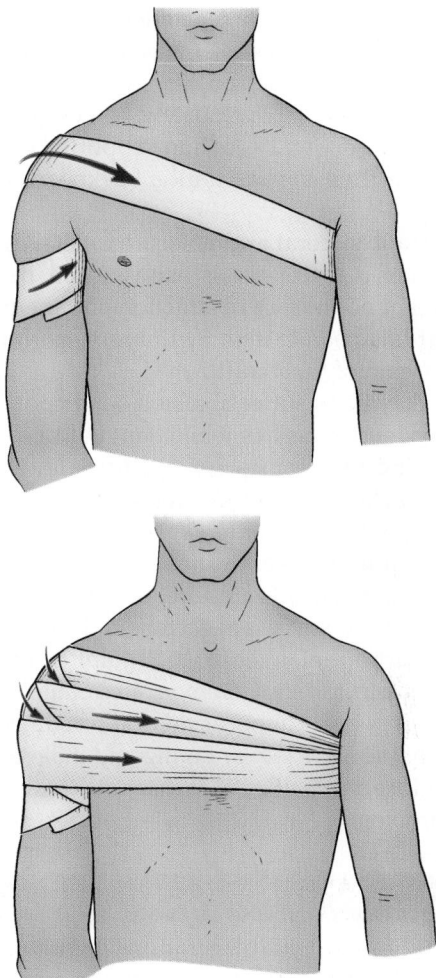

Figure 30-15   Shoulder harness for support after shoulder dislocation.

dislocation, the kayaker's arm should be splinted across the chest with a sling or swath or by safety pinning the sleeve of the arm across the chest. If circumstances preclude exiting the river without further kayaking, the shoulder can be partially stabilized by wrapping an elastic or neoprene wrap around the torso and involved arm to limit abduction and external rotation (Figure 30-15).

Head, facial, and dental trauma are more common in kayakers and decked canoeists than in rafters because of the potential for flipping upside down while still in the craft. Minor abrasions, lacerations, and contusions are common; serious head injury with loss of consciousness is rare. Head and facial trauma can be minimized by wearing a protective helmet and tucking forward, instead of leaning backward, while rolling.

Spine fractures have been reported in kayakers and canoers.[40-41,43] Cervical spine injuries have occurred in kayakers in conjunction with head trauma sustained after flipping upside down. Vertical compression fractures of the thoracolumbar spine have occurred from axial loading when a kayaker landed flat after paddling over a waterfall. One kayaker was rendered paraplegic after landing on his back on rocks while attempting to negotiate a waterfall.[43] Fortunately, his companions recognized the injury and kept him supported on minicell blocks from their kayaks until a backboard could be obtained.

Significant visceral and musculoskeletal injury can occur when a swimmer is sandwiched between a downstream boulder or obstruction and the upstream craft that has been exited. Swimmers should always stay upstream of their craft.

Many kayakers suffer abrasions and contusions to the fingers and knuckles while hanging upside down after flipping. Oar frames, oars, paddles, and the metal ammunition boxes used to keep supplies dry can all inflict injury when rafts are capsized or paddlers are tossed about in turbulent water.

Blisters on the hands are a frequently reported problem in paddling surveys.[45] Kayakers develop them at the metacarpophalangeal (MCP) joint of the thumb along the ulnar aspect. Common sites of blister formation in rafters and canoeists are the proximal palmar surfaces of the MCP joints. Taping and moleskin application reduce the incidence of this potentially incapacitating problem.

INFECTIONS

Blisters, abrasions, and lacerations are always at increased risk for infection in an aquatic environment. Maceration from prolonged immersion in water and exposure to atypical pathogens are contributing factors.

An outbreak of *Staphylococcus aureus* skin infections among raft guides in Georgia and South Carolina nearly led to the demise of two rafting companies.[10] Sharp grommets on the thwarts of the rafts had caused repeated lower extremity abrasions. The causative organism was cultured from rafts up to 48 hours after use. Daily raft disinfection enabled the companies to remain in operation.

Otitis externa (swimmer's ear) is a common problem among paddlers. Water exposure to the ear canal macerates the epithelium and elevates the normally acidic pH of the canal, predisposing the ear to infection.[12] The bacteria most commonly cultured are *Pseudomonas aeruginosa, Proteus vulgaris,* and *Staphylococcus* species.[12,23] Antibiotic eardrops with or without hydrocortisone are widely available and very useful. Irrigation of the canal with commercially available solutions containing acetic acid and alcohol helps prevent infection by lowering the pH and drying the canal.[23] The drops should be applied after each outing (see Chapter 63).

Recent publicity given to water contamination by *Giardia lamblia* has been reinforced by statistics from the Centers for Disease Control and Prevention, which re-

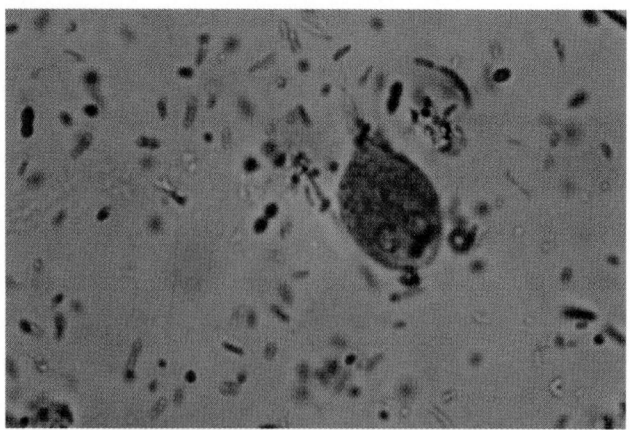

Figure 30-16 *Giardia lamblia* trophozoite seen by methylene blue wet mount staining under oil (1000×). The finding of cysts or trophozoites in a patient with diarrhea is sufficient to make a tentative diagnosis of giardiasis.

port *Giardia* organisms to be the most common pathogenic intestinal parasite in the United States (see Chapters 51 and 52). *Giardia* cysts abound in mountain streams and rivers once considered to be sources of pristine water (Figure 30-16). They persist in very cold water and have no detectable taste or smell. Rivers are contaminated by animals that defecate in or near the water. Studies by the Wild Animal Disease Center at Colorado State University, Ft. Collins, Colorado, have identified more than 30 animal species as *Giardia* carriers.

Paddlers who travel to foreign countries should seek information on local endemic diseases and relevant prophylactic measures. White-water rafting and kayaking in Third World countries subject paddlers to unusual aquatic-related infections. This is exemplified by a report of schistosomiasis in rafters returning from Ethiopia.[22] Schistosomiasis is endemic in large areas of Africa, South America, and the Caribbean and is transmitted to humans who swim or come into contact with fresh water containing the larval stage. Paddlers who return from endemic regions should be screened with serologic testing, since up to 50% of infections are asymptomatic.[31]

Malaria has been reported in rafters returning from New Guinea, and both leptospirosis and hepatitis have stricken kayakers venturing to Costa Rica.[2] In the United States, pulmonary blastomycosis was reported among canoeists in Wisconsin.[7]

ENVIRONMENTAL HAZARDS

Although hypothermia is rarely the cause of death among white-water paddlers, hypothermia-induced impairment of judgment and coordination is a significant contributing factor in many fatalities and accidents.[18,28,39-41] The paddling season usually begins in early spring when air temperatures are cool and snow melt–swollen rivers run extremely cold. Paddlers with rusty skills are more prone to frequent swims and the effects of cold water immersion. Many rivers, especially in the western United States, are controlled by dams that release water from far beneath the surface and thus remain cold year round. Placing adequate barriers between the human body and the environment and carrying adequate food and waterproof matches are of paramount importance.

Another common environmental affliction suffered by paddlers is rhus dermatitis from poison oak or poison ivy. Most cases occur during spring paddling when the vines are potent but the characteristic leaves have not yet appeared. Barrier creams such as StokoGard Outdoor Cream and Tecnu Ivy Shield can be used by individuals highly sensitive to the plants. After plant contact occurs, the oil may be removed from the skin by washing within 30 minutes.[13] A commercial product, Tecnu Oak and Ivy Cleanser, can remove oil from the skin for up to 8 hours after exposure. Any solvent may help remove some of the urushiol oil from the skin. Gasoline, paint thinner, acetone, and rubbing alcohol have all been reported to be effective. Unfortunately, these products can also be irritating to the skin

Treatment of rhus dermatitis consists of oral antihistamines and systemic corticosteroids. A 2-week course is needed to prevent recurrence of the rash (see Chapter 47).[13]

Sunburn and the effects of chronic exposure to solar radiation are compounded by water's ability to reflect up to 100% of ultraviolet radiation (UVR), depending on the time of day. Sand can reflect up to 17% of harmful UVR. Most rivers are situated in mountains, where UVR increases 4% to 5% with each additional 305 m (1000 feet) of altitude.[9] Sunscreens must be applied frequently because they are prone to wash off in the water. Zinc oxide and other barrier creams are more resistant to water and are preferable on areas of intense exposure, such as the nose and lips. Paddlers with fair skin should consider using gloves to protect the hands from UVR exposure.

Eye protection from UVR is often overlooked or avoided by paddlers because sunglasses frequently fog while on the river. Application of Dawn dishwashing soap to the lenses prevents fogging for up to 30 minutes. Polarizing lenses reduce glare off the water, but the polarizing feature does not in and of itself filter UVR and infrared radiation.

Venomous snakes, especially pit vipers, along with scorpions, spiders, and fire ants, are frequently encountered by river enthusiasts and should be considered potential hazards. Paddlers should know appropriate first-aid measures for envenomations.

Paddlers commonly consume wild foliage, which may produce severe illness. In one published report, six rafters were poisoned and one of them died after eating water hemlock, *Cicuta douglaslii*.[31]

SWIFT WATER RESCUE

Time is the most important factor in river rescue and often precludes the use of technical rope-based systems. Experience and an understanding of river dynamics are essential.

The most common rescue scenario involves a swimmer who has exited the craft. The victim may be moving downstream at 5 to 10 miles per hour in the middle of a large river. Since the dynamic nature of swift water does not often allow time for a shore-based rescue system to be established, many white-water rescues are made from a raft, canoe, or kayak. Rafts should stay close together in rapids to render mutual aid. Throw bags can be used directly from the raft to rescue swimmers, or the victim may often be reached with an outstretched arm and a paddle. A swimmer should be pulled back into the raft by grabbing the shoulder straps on his or her life jacket and then leaning backward into the raft to pull the person in. The swimmer can assist by pulling up on the frame, D-ring, or hand line as he or she is being pulled in.

Kayaks can be used to rescue swimmers in midcurrent. The kayak is also an excellent platform to provide additional flotation for a swimmer who is trying to maintain freeboard in rough water. The most common method of rescuing swimmers with kayaks is to have them grab the bow or stern "grab loop" of the boat and then tow them to safety. The loop is usually sized so that it is easy to grab yet will not admit an adult-sized hand. The swimmer can also grab onto the back of the cockpit rim and pull his or her torso onto the back deck. This gets the swimmer out of the cold water and reduces the likelihood of injury from rocks.

Boogie Boards originally developed for use in the ocean surf have been modified for rescue use on rivers. Rescue Boards are larger and come with two sets of handles—one for the rescuer and one for the victim. The boards add a substantial amount of flotation to a rescue swimmer and, when used with swim fins, can provide a maneuverable platform for reaching and picking up a victim.

The latest craft to be adapted to swift-water rescue is the personal watercraft, or Jet Ski. Introduced in 1987, these machines have become increasingly popular with professional rescue agencies. Since they lack an exposed propeller, personal watercraft are safe for swimmers and can negotiate shallow rivers. They can be maneuvered upstream in rapids, and turn within a short radius. Newer versions, adapted for rescue, can tow a backboard or litter device behind them and are quite stable.

Rescue from entrapment requires a higher level of skill and often presents greater potential risk to the

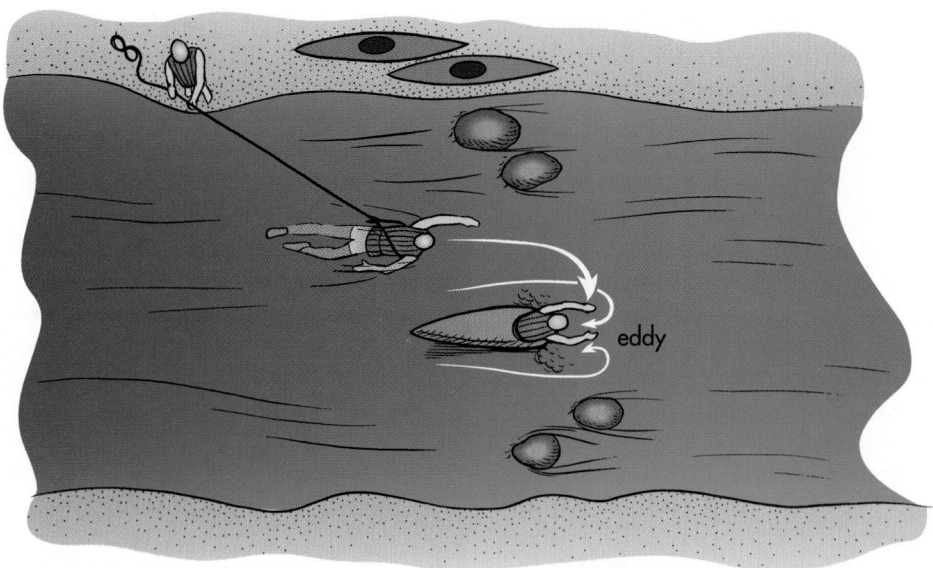

Figure 30-17 Strong swimmer rescue.

rescuer. The method used depends on whether the victim can maintain adequate freeboard. If the entrapment site is accessible, direct contact with the victim is quickest and most effective. A rescuer may wade to the entrapment site or reach it by boat if there is a stable site to exit the craft. When wading, the rescuer should use a paddle for support. Start by facing upstream, with legs slightly wider than shoulder width. Reach out, turn the paddle blade parallel to the current, and plunge it into the water. Just before the blade hits bottom, turn it sideways to the current. The force of the onrushing water will pin it to the bottom. The paddle and your two legs form a tripod, which is more stable than your legs alone. Move slowly across the current, facing upstream, moving only one of these three points at a time. The river downstream should be scouted for hazards before entering and, if possible, a rope thrower should be stationed downstream in the event the rescuer loses footing.

A strong swimmer rescue is the next quickest method but entails significant risk to the rescuer (Figure 30-17). The rescuer is tethered to a rope that provides added stability against the force of the current. If a quick-release harness is not available, a loose loop of rope can be passed under the rescuer's armpits.

A tag line rescue should be considered if the victim cannot be reached directly. A tag line is a rope stretched across the river downstream that is then brought upstream to the victim (Figure 30-18). Getting the line across the river sometimes constitutes an insurmountable obstacle. If the river is narrow, it may be possible to throw the line across. Otherwise, it can be ferried across by a boat or team of swimmers. During a ferry, as much of the rope as possible should be kept out of the water to avoid drag.

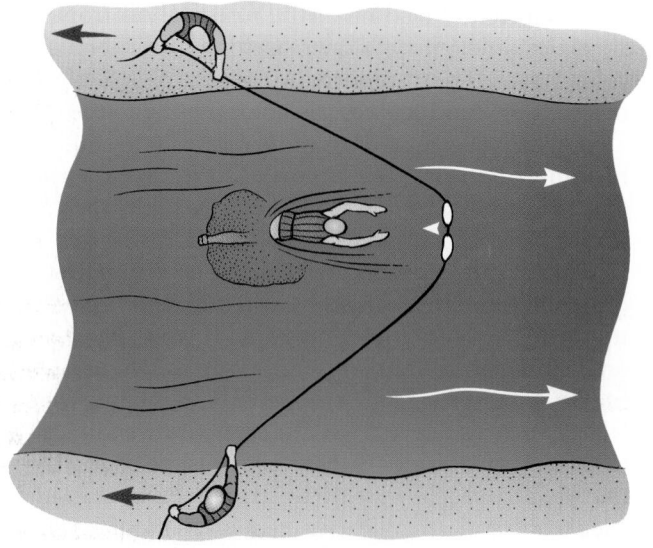

Figure 30-18 Tag line.

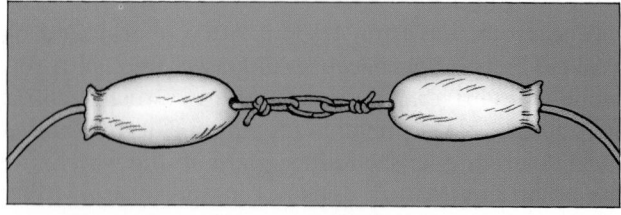

Figure 30-19 Two throw bags connected with a carabiner to make a tag line.

There are two types of tag lines (Figure 30-19). A floating tag line has a life jacket or some other flotation device attached to the middle to keep the rope on the surface, which helps support the victim. A snag tag is a weighted line submerged and walked upstream to

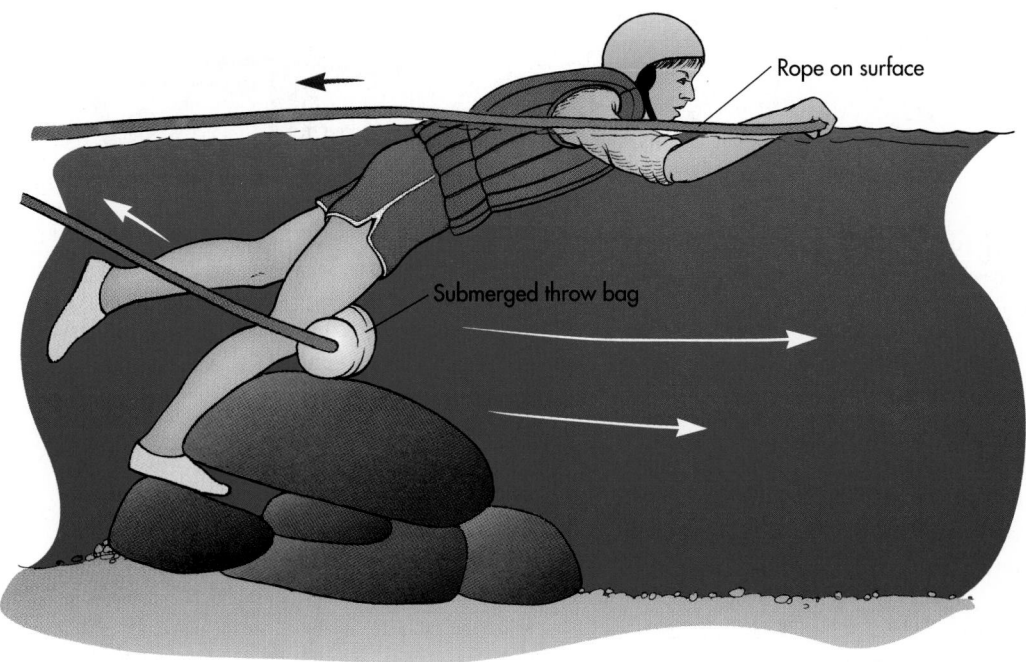

Figure 30-20 Submerged snag tag.

snare a foot or other body part that has been trapped under the surface. A snag tag can be made by joining together two throw bags filled with rocks (Figure 30-20).

APPENDIX A

White-Water First-Aid Kits

The following variables should be considered when designing a white-water first-aid kit: remoteness and accessibility of the river, Third World travel conditions, the number of people the kit will need to support, pre-existing medical conditions; and space and weight restrictions. When assembling a kit, the following components are generally recommended for rafting and kayaking:

Rafting Kit

Waterproof dry bag or Pelican box
Cardiopulmonary resuscitation mouth shield (CPR-Microshield)
Hypothermia/hyperthermia thermometer
Bandage scissors
Fine-point tweezers or forceps
Temporary dental filling (Cavit)
Glutose paste
Irrigation syringe with 18-gauge catheter
Povidone-iodine solution
3M surgical stapler (1 stapler holds 25 staples)
Dermabond tissue glue
Wound closure strips (Steri-Strips)
Tincture of benzoin
Polysporin ointment
Moleskin

Latex or non-latex (hypoallergenic) gloves
Antiseptic towelettes
Safety pins
Waterproof matches
Accident report form and pencil
Large garbage bag
4 × 4-inch sterile dressings
8 × 10-inch trauma pad or Bloodstopper dressing
Eye pads
Nonadherent dressing (Xeroform or Aquaphor)
Triangular bandage
3-inch conforming gauze bandage
3-inch elastic bandage with Velcro closure
1-inch × 10-yard surgical tape
Duct tape (can be wrapped around the paddle shaft)
Strip and knuckle bandages
Cotton-tipped applicators
Aloe vera gel
Diphenhydramine capsules
Cortisone cream
Acetaminophen tablets
Ibuprofen tablets
Eardrops
    Prophylactic eardrops (mixture of rubbing alcohol
        and white vinegar)
    Treatment eardrops (Cortisporin Otic Suspension)
Epinephrine injectable or EpiPen
Prochlorperazine suppository
Diazepam or midazolam
Oxycodone
Oxymetazoline (Afrin) nasal spray
Antibiotics (trimethoprim/sulfamethoxazole, cipro-
    floxacin, cephalexin)

Sunscreen (sun protection factor [SPF] 15 or higher)
Insect repellent
Iodine tablets
Tampons
Tea bags

Kayaking Kit

Waterproof dry bag or small Pelican box
Cardiopulmonary resuscitation mouth shield
Hypothermia/hyperthermia thermometer
Scissors
Fine-point tweezers or forceps
Small surgical stapler (3M) or Dermabond Glue
Wound closure strips
Tincture of benzoin
Polysporin ointment
Latex or non-latex (hypoallergenic) gloves
Antiseptic towelettes
Safety pins
Waterproof matches
Accident report form and pencil
3 × 3-inch sterile dressings
Nonadherent dressings
2-inch conforming gauze bandage
Duct tape
Strip and knuckle bandages
Cotton-tipped applicators
Diphenhydramine
Acetaminophen
Ibuprofen
Prophylactic eardrops
Epinephrine
Prochlorperazine suppository
Diazepam or midazolam
Oxycodone
Sunscreen
Insect repellent
Iodine tablets

APPENDIX B

Universal River Signals

Stop: Potential hazard ahead. Wait for "all clear" signal before proceeding. Form a horizontal bar with your outstretched arms. Those seeing the signal should pass it back to others in the party. (Figure 30-21.)

Help/Emergency: Assist the signaler as quickly as possible. Give three long blasts on a whistle while waving a paddle over your head. (Figure 30-22.)

All Clear: Come ahead (in the absence of other directions, proceed down the center). Form a vertical bar with your paddle or one arm held high above your head. Paddle blade should be turned flat for maximum visibility. To signal direction or a preferred course through a rapid around an obstruction, lower the previously vertical "all clear" by 45 degrees to-

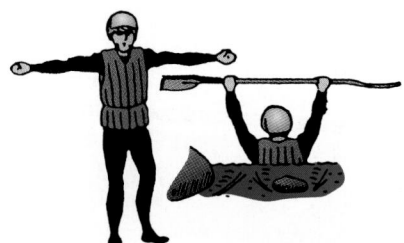

Figure 30-21   Stop signal.

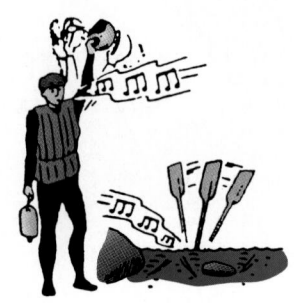

Figure 30-22   Help/emergency signal.

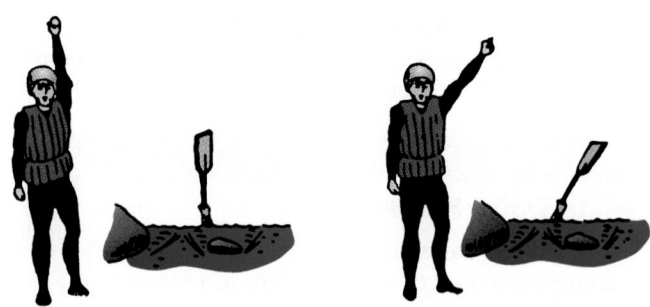

Figure 30-23   All clear signal.

ward the side of the river with the preferred route. Never point toward the obstacle you wish to avoid. (Figure 30-23.)

APPENDIX C

Organizations

American Canoe Association (ACA)
7432 Alban Station Boulevard
Suite B-226
Springfield, VA 22150-2311

American Whitewater Affiliation (AWA)
P.O. Box 85
Phoenicia, NY 12464

Chinook Medical Gear
P.O. Box 1736
Edwards Business Center B11
Edwards, CO 81632

Rescue 3
P.O. Box 4686
Sonora, CA 95370

Safety Deck System
Outdoor Safety Systems
140 Quaker Road
Princeton, NJ 08540

National Organization for River Sports
Box 6847
Colorado Springs, CO 80904

REFERENCES

1. Allan JR, Elliot DH, Hayes PA: The thermal performance of partial coverage wet suits, *Aviat Space Environ Med* 57:1056, 1986.
2. Backer H: Malaria in returned travelers, *Wilderness Med* 4:11, 1987.
3. Bechdel L, Ray S: *River rescue,* Boston, 1989, Appalachian Mountain Club Books.
4. Brody AJ, Mitchell C, Springer M: Submersion injury complicated by hyperthermia in a kayaker wearing a dry suit, *J Wilderness Med* 4:198, 1993.
5. Burrell CL, Burrell R: Injuries in whitewater paddling, *Physician Sports Med* 10:119, 1982.
6. *Canoe Magazine,* Canoe America Associates, Kirkland, Wash, Dec 1993.
7. Centers for Disease Control: Blastomycosis in canoeists—Wisconsin, *MMWR* 29:450, 1979.
8. Cooper KE, Martins S, Riben P: Respiratory and other responses of subjects immersed in cold water, *J Appl Physiol* 40:903, 1976.
9. Daniels F: Physical factors in sun exposure, *Arch Dermatol* 85:98, 1962.
10. Decker MD et al: An outbreak of staphylococcal skin infections among river rafting guides, *Am J Epidemiol* 124:969, 1986.
11. Dutkly P: A simple method of treating shoulder dislocations for the whitewater enthusiast, *Wilderness Med* 5:9, 1988.
12. Ellison RT III, Zimner SH: Infectious disease emergencies. In Kravis TC et al, editors: *Emergency medicine: a comprehensive review,* ed 3, New York 1993, Raven Press.
13. Epstein WL: Plant-induced dermatitis, *Ann Emerg Med* 16:950, 1987.
14. Fraser RE: Paddling precautions advised, *Physician Sports Med* 10:16, 1982.
15. Girten TR, Wehr SE: An evaluation of the high-water performance characteristics of personal flotation devices, *USCG Report,* USCG-M-84-1 (167/4), Springfield, Va, 1984, National Technical Information Service.
16. Golden FS, Golden C: Problems of immersion, *Br J Hosp Med* 45:371, 1980.
17. Goldman RF et al: Wet versus dry suit approaches to water immersion protective clothing, *Aviat Space Environ Med* 37:485, 1966.
18. Harwett RM, Bijlani MG: The involvement of cold water in recreational boating fatalities. I, *Accid Anal Prevent* 14:147, 1982.
19. Hayward JS: The physiology of immersion hypothermia. In Pozos RS, Wittmers LE, editors: *The nature and treatment of hypothermia,* Minneapolis, 1983, University of Minnesota Press.
20. Hayward JS, Eckerson JD: Physiological responses and survival time prediction for humans in ice water, *Aviat Space Environ Med* 55:206, 1984.
21. Hayward JS et al: Temperature effect on the human dive response in relation to coldwater near drowning, *J Appl Physiol* 56:202, 1984.
22. Istre GR et al: Acute schistosomiasis among Americans rafting the Omo River, Ethiopia, *JAMA* 251:508, 1984.
23. Jenkins BH: Treatment of otitis externa and swimmer's ear, *JAMA* 175:402, 1961.
24. Jennings AK: *Whitewater, wildwater,* Royal Oak Press, 1981, West Virginia.
25. Keatinge WR, Evans M: The respiratory and cardiovascular response to immersion in coldwater, *Q J Exp Physiol* 46:83, 1961.
26. Keatinge WR, Hayward MG: Sudden death in coldwater and ventricular arrhythmia, *J Forensic Sci* 16:459, 1981.
27. Keatinge WR et al: The effects of work and clothing on the maintenance of the body temperature in water, *Q J Exp Physiol* 46:69, 1961.
28. Keatinge WR et al: Sudden failure of swimming in coldwater, *BMJ* 1:480, 1969.
29. Kizer KW: Medical aspects of whitewater kayaking, *Physician Sports Med* 15:128, 1987.
30. Kizer KW: Medical problems in whitewater sports, *Clin Sports Med* 6:663, 1987.
31. Kizer KW: Whitewater medicine, *Emerg Med Clin North Am* 29:91, 1987.
32. Mayer PJ: Helping your patients avert canoe and kayak injuries, *J Musculoskel Med* 4:31, 1987.
33. McNamara RM: Reduction of anterior shoulder dislocations by scapular manipulation, *Ann Emerg Med* 21:1140, 1993.
34. *National Sporting Goods Association survey,* Bellevue, Wash, 1989, GMA Research.
35. *Participation in sports activities by selected characteristics: 1990,* Mount Prospect, Ill, 1990, National Sporting Goods Association.
36. Reibel GD, McCabe J: Anterior shoulder dislocation: a review of reduction techniques, *Am J Emerg Med* 9:180, 1991.
37. Serra JB: Management of trauma in the wilderness environment, *Emerg Med Clin North Am* 2:3, 1984.
38. Steinman AM, Hayward JS: Coldwater immersion. In Auerbach PS, Geehr EC, editors: *Management of wilderness and environmental emergencies,* St Louis, 1989, Mosby.
39. Walbridge CW, editor: *Best of the river safety task force newsletter, 1976-1982,* Lorton, Va, 1983, American Canoe Association.
40. Walbridge CW, editor: *River safety report, 1982-1985,* Lorton, Va, 1986, American Canoe Association.
41. Walbridge CW, editor: *River safety report, 1986-1988,* Lorton, Va, 1989, American Canoe Association.
42. Walbridge CW, editor: *Safety code of the American Whitewater Affiliation,* Phoenicia, NY, 1989, American Whitewater Affiliation.
43. Walbridge CW, editor: *River safety report, 1989-1991,* Lorton, Va, 1992, American Canoe Association.
44. Wallace D: Scary numbers and statistics—results of AWA close calls and serious injuries survey, *AWA J* 3-4:27, 1991.
45. Weiss EA: Whitewater medicine, *J Wilderness Med* 2:245, 1991.
46. Whisman SA, Hollenhorst SJ: Injuries in commercial whitewater rafting, *Clin J Sport Med* 9:18, 1999.
47. Wilkerson JA, Bangs CC, Haward JS: *Hypothermia, frostbite and other cold injuries,* Seattle, 1986, The Mountaineers.

31 Cave Rescue

Steve Hudson and Loui H. Clem

A cave can be one of the most hostile environments a rescuer can enter. Not only must a cave rescuer be adept at managing the unique challenges of functioning in the cave environment, he or she must also manage a unique set of rescue problems relating to rescuer safety, equipment, logistics, access and extrication, and mission support. A cave rescue should never be undertaken without qualified cave rescuers on scene. In addition, the incident commander must be familiar with or seek the advice of someone who is familiar with the unique challenges of the cave environment.

The time to learn about caving is not as a medic on a cave rescue. If there is any chance that you will encounter a cave rescue as part of your profession or avocation, time spent familiarizing yourself with caves and caving techniques may be lifesaving.

ENVIRONMENT

Any natural opening in the earth large enough to enter is considered a cave. Human-made mines and tunnels are not caves. Although these often seem similar to caves, their entry often requires special skills and equipment different from those for caves. Caves take many forms, including sinkholes, cracks, sumps, siphons, springs, pits, and caverns. Caves are formidable places, dark and dangerous. Running, seeping, or standing water originally formed most caves, so water is a major part of many cave environments. As caves become less active hydrologically, they may dry up. Some caves are so dry that dust induces respiratory problems in visitors.

Temperature extremes are likely. Caves tend to be at the mean ground temperature of the area. For the most part, U.S. continental caves run from cool to cold. Very warm climates sport warm caves, whereas alpine mountain caves measure close to freezing temperatures and may even contain ice. Tropical and desert caves can be so hot that cavers must wear lightweight garments to explore, but more common is the problem of hypothermia from sitting around underground waiting for the next assignment or struggling in cold and wet passages. It is not uncommon to be supine or prone in 4-inch deep, 13° C (55° F) water with one's back pressed against cold rock, facing a stiff breeze.

Caves can be fragile, often heavily decorated with mineral formations that have formed over thousands of years. Cavers try to protect these formations whenever possible by avoiding walking on or touching delicate areas or otherwise altering the cave. Even the natural oils rubbed off of human hands can alter growth of an active formation. The caver's motto, "leave nothing but footprints, take nothing but pictures, and kill nothing but time," extends to rescue operations. Everything brought in must be packed out at the end of the operation. An abandoned flashlight battery can leach its chemicals and poison the cave-adapted life-forms found in a cave passage.

PERSONAL SAFETY

Whether entering a cave for exploration or for rescue purposes, personal gear requirements are tailored to caving. Clothing should be appropriate to the environment. Caves can be wet, dry, dusty, cold, warm, or a combination of these. Wind can exist in passages because of temperature and pressure differentials between the cave and the outside air, and chill factor becomes a significant consideration. Undergarments should provide the necessary thermal layers, while outerwear provides a protective barrier against the elements.

A mountaineering type of helmet, with a nonelastic "three point" chin strap that keeps it planted properly on the head, is a must. The helmet protects against impact with the hard and often sharp rock of cave ceilings and walls in tight or low passages and offers rockfall protection. It is also a convenient mounting platform for the required light source.

It takes only one episode of trying to navigate in the complete darkness underground to understand why no fewer than three light sources should be carried by each person in a cave. Rescuers underground without functioning lights become other subjects to be rescued. Electric lights are preferred, but carbide lamps may also be used. At least two of these lights should be helmet mountable for hands-free operation, each with sufficient "burn time" capacity or spare batteries to travel in and out of the cave. If carbide lamps are used, care should be taken when working close to victims because it is easy in tight spots to forget that the light on your head is an open flame that can quickly burn anything with which it comes in contact. For this reason, most cave rescuers prefer electric lights.

Many cavers find gloves useful for both thermal insulation and protection against sharp rocks and sticky mud. If the cave has vertical components, leather-palmed gloves are necessary for rope work.

Cave mud is slippery and adheres to everything. It makes walking and scrambling through a cave dangerous. Lug sole boots provide the best traction, and stiff leather uppers help protect feet against sharp rocks. For small passages or "crawlways," a set of durable kneepads is a wise adjunct.

As in any remote environment, the caver should be self-sufficient and able to care for at least himself for an extended period. This requires replacement batteries or carbide, fresh water for drinking, food for energy, a basic first-aid kit, and extra insulation, such as extra thermal layers and a hat that can be worn under the helmet. Cavers often store a folded trash bag in the suspension of their helmets, to be used as an emergency shelter from wind and water, among other possibilities. An additional challenge for the extended cave visit is the requirement to pack out whatever is packed in, including human waste. Strong, leak-proof plastic containers are useful for that purpose.

Use a small, durable pack to carry extra gear. Carry what is needed and no more. Keep in mind that the pack will be alternately carried, pulled, pushed, and dragged through cave passages of different sizes, so things such as straps and external attachments will become an impediment to maneuverability.

Not all caves have vertical drops, but for those that do—or when in doubt—carry a lightweight seat and chest harness, rack or figure-8 descender, and an ascending system. One or two 20-foot sections of 1-inch tubular webbing come in handy for an extra step-up or to construct a quick belay or hand line.

EQUIPMENT

The amount of equipment used during a cave rescue is prodigious. Each person entering the cave must have at least the minimum complement of personal gear. Ropes and hardware are utilized nearly as quickly as they can be produced; items that are difficult to find, such as hard-wired field-phones or cave radio systems, become necessities.

Ropes used underground are usually of the static kernmantle variety. The tougher the sheath, the better the rope. Adequate carabiners, anchor materials, and other hardware should be available for rigging. If multiple locations must be rigged for raising, lowering, or traversing, the best possible scenario is to have enough gear to rig each site individually. Having to derig a system, sort the gear, carry it past the proceeding litter, and rerig another system can be time consuming and a recipe for disaster. Even a small cave might require multiple sites rigged for safe patient extrication. Pre-bagged packages of gear for specific common rigging tasks are often useful. Include anchor webbing, ample carabiners, pulleys, prussiks, belay devices, lowering devices, and rope grabs as required to set up one site per bag.

Although most cave evacuations require litter transport, evaluate the situation carefully to determine whether a litter is really necessary. A properly stabilized "walking wounded" caver can be helped out of a cave in short time and with little manpower. Put that same person into a litter, and the number of rescuers and hours to the hospital goes up exponentially! If litter transport is deemed necessary, the next difficult decision is which litter (or litters) to use. On any given evacuation, this selection requires a fine balance of requirements. Maneuvering a bulky litter through narrow cave passages can be a challenging proposition. In larger caves, or where a vertical raise is required, basket litters are the best choice. Plastic-bottomed versions are preferable over steel and mesh versions, allowing the option of dragging the litter where necessary. In tighter caves, drag-sheet types of litters, such as the wrap-around Sked, provide low-profile advantages but are less comfortable and protective for the victim. Occasionally, a cave is so restrictive that even the length of such a litter is problematic, and a short board, such as a KED or OSS, is the only alternative. It is not unheard of to begin the carry in a tight section of a cave using a OSS, add a Sked once the passage opens up a bit, drop the Sked into a full basket litter for ease of carrying in a large walking passage, then drop all the way back to the OSS to negotiate a tight entrance passage.

When choosing a litter and victim packaging, take comfort into account. Although rescuers are working up a sweat, the victim lying in the litter can be extremely cold. Thermal layers are a necessity and include a sleeping bag, vapor barrier, and moisture barrier to keep the victim dry. The victim should have adequate head and face protection and, if the environment will become vertical at any point, a harness. Anticipate transport time; evacuation can take days, so extra warmth and padding may be needed.

A reasonable first-aid kit should contain writing materials for recording victim condition, basic medications, airway management tools, bandages, cervical collars, and splints. Sealing each item in plastic helps keep out cave grit, and the entire kit can be packaged in a large-mouth bottle or other watertight, durable container.

Because of extended times involved in reporting caving accidents and responding to and accessing injured cavers, most victims are either very stable or dead. The upshot is that advanced life support (ALS) skills and equipment are generally not required. Dragging a defibrillator into the cave with your first-aid kit is for the most part unjustified. This is fortunate, since the effect of cave mud and water would render all but the sturdiest military models ineffective. Newer semi-automatic defibrillators may fare better.

The cave environment is no more friendly to even simple interventions such as intravenous (IV) infusions. In most cases, hanging a gravity-operated IV is not an option, so positive pressure infusion methods must be used. Further, consideration must be given to methods for keeping the insertion point clean, and care taken not to interrupt flow while negotiating tight passageways.

LOGISTICS

Logistics of an underground rescue are complicated at best and a nightmare if not managed well. Lack of easy communication, limited access, extended time, and difficulty in obtaining rest for teams all contribute to complexity.

Communication is essential to keep rescuers from becoming lost, to issue instructions, and to distribute nutrition. Various hard-wired field-phone systems are available for use in cave rescue, but generally only well-established teams have access to these. A relatively new development is the availability of special low-frequency cave radios that can transmit voice through dense rock and soil. Without such systems, message runners are indispensable. A group of swift, agile, safe, and well-trained cavers—and a method for keeping them rested and nourished—is invaluable.

A team of rescuers sent into a known location can take hours or most of a day to reach the victim. It is logistically impractical for these rescuers to carry sleeping bags and food to allow rest and recovery before starting their work assignment. Keeping rescuers rested, fed, watered, and warm many hours away through a challenging cave rescue requires an incident management team that can predict the needs of the underground workers hours before they themselves realize the need.

Whether or not a communication system is available, establishment of a control point at or near the cave entrance(s) is critical. Entrance control should be established as soon as rescuers arrive at the cave. All personnel and equipment entering or leaving the cave should be recorded into a log kept by entrance control. This log becomes invaluable hours later to determine when teams should be replaced, if someone is still in the cave, and who carried in what piece of missing vital gear.

The Incident Command System (see Chapter 24), or a modified version of it, provides the best framework for managing cave rescue personnel, by performing required functions while maintaining a reasonable span of control. Generally, the functions required on a cave rescue are similar to those required on any other rescue, although the specific means of accomplishing the functions will vary.

There should always be one person in command of an operation. This is the foundation of creating accountability and organization, which are the keys to efficiency and safety. The incident commander assesses the incident, activates resources, determines the strategy, and approves the plan for the operation. Other functions vital to success are planning, operations, logistics, and finance. The incident commander may have one or more people to assist, or he or she may be responsible for several of these functions. Someone must plan strategies, supervise the operation, take care of the physical needs of the rescuers and the required equipment, and track the resources used.

CAVE ACCESS

Gaining access to the caver victim is a matter of overcoming an array of obstructions inherent in the cave. Merely to move a few hundred feet through a cave might require rappelling, crawling on one's belly, and squeezing through cracks in the rocks while dragging equipment, climbing over large rocks, swimming, and slithering through mud.

The total darkness of a cave is confining to some, and even this simple matter can quickly become a major obstacle. Noncaver responders may have psychologic inhibitions, such as fear of the dark or confined spaces. In no case should a rescuer ever be pushed beyond his or her comfort level in accessing a victim. Claustrophobia can cause panic and severe dysfunctional behavior.

Other factors inherent to the cave include temperature variables, wetness, and restrictive cave passages. Certain large or weak personnel and/or bulky and heavy equipment might be physically incapable of getting through these tight spaces.

If the cave rescue requires raising or lowering a victim, or traversing the victim over horizontal rope lines, persons skilled in cave rigging should be responsible for building the systems. Rigging in caves is an art because of anchoring difficulties, directional changes, tight squeezes, and minimal working surface. Details on cave rigging and professional training can be acquired through the National Cave Rescue Commission, a nonprofit organization that teaches courses in cave rescue techniques and management.

Many vertical drops in caves are overhung at the top, preventing the caver access to a wall while descending and ascending the rope. In cases where the roped drop has the rope running against a wall, it can be advantageous to place anchors at points throughout the length of the drop. This "rebelay" method allows multiple people to ascend/descend simultaneously, lessens rope wear points, and provides the added safety of having a shorter rope length to protect for each anchor. Practice at crossing rebelays is essential before attempting to enter a cave thus rigged. The caver must be able to essentially transfer from one free-hanging rope to another while hanging in midair. This is easy to do with the correct equipment setup and practice but not so easy when the technique is tried for the first time underground on the way to a medical emergency.

Usually, single rope techniques are used, especially where a free-hanging drop is involved. This means that just one rope is put over the side for the rescuer to ascend or descend. The use of an additional belay line not only requires additional personnel but might prove more hazardous if the two lines become entangled.

In the United States, the most common cave ascending systems are the Mitchell system and various renditions of the ropewalker system. These are both efficient means of ascending and can easily be mastered with practice. The frog system, popular in other countries, requires more climbing effort but is easier to use when ascending past rebelays in the system. It is imperative that an ascending system be fitted to the user. Some rigs work better for tall, lean frames, and others work best for heavier body types. All rescue personnel entering a vertical cave should have their own personally fitted rope climbing system and must have practiced climbing in that system in a safe practice area.

Large holes or boulder slopes inside the cave may best be negotiated by using a highline traverse. Highlines often require great amounts of time to set up properly but can shave away hours of litter movement time by passing above difficult cave terrain that otherwise would present many challenges for a litter carried by hand. Use of a highline is most practical when it is known in advance that there will be sufficient time for rigging. The decision to take the time to rig a traverse should be made based on these three factors: the time it will take to move the victim to the obstacle you want to be traversed, the time necessary to rig the highline, and the time that will be saved by using the highline to move the victim over the obstacle.

HAZARDOUS ATMOSPHERES

One often-overlooked hazard to cavers is the ambient atmosphere. Most caves in the United States breathe naturally either from changes in barometric pressure or from the chimney effect of multiple entrances. Some caves have small rooms that have so little airflow that a few cavers can quickly consume most of the oxygen. Buildup of gases CO, CO_2, methane, and/or hydrogen sulfide is not uncommon in caves. Instances of gasoline seeping into caves from underground storage tanks have been recorded. If poor air quality is suspected, use of an air monitoring device is essential. It is possible to enter a cave containing high levels of unhealthy gases, but only with appropriate caution. In such cases, it is advisable to solicit participation of the local hazardous materials emergency response team.

With the assistance of a hazardous materials or confined space rescue team, "bad air" in caves can be mit-

igated in several ways. One way is to release compressed air into the cave, forcing good air in and bad air out. Success of this method is limited, and because of the massive amounts of air in a cave, this method is slow at best. If this method is used, entrants should carry an air monitor, since "pockets" of bad air may remain trapped in parts of the cave. Another option is to release oxygen into the cave. Although this can speed the air exchange process somewhat, it has its own disadvantages. In addition to being difficult to accomplish, it is possible to elevate the oxygen level in the cave to that of deleterious combustion. Exhaust fans offer a reasonable method, although care must be taken to prevent generator exhaust from entering the cave.

If necessary, rescuers can be equipped for entry with surface-supplied air with bail-out bottles, self-contained breathing apparatus, or rebreathers. Each of these has advantages and disadvantages, but all are difficult to manage in the cave environment and thus should be avoided if possible. Pre-event training and practice in the safe use of any of this equipment is imperative before entering an atmosphere that is hazardous for breathing.

Other airborne hazards, such as histoplasmosis and rabies, are not detectable by air monitor. If these hazards are suspected, no rescuer should enter the environment without an appropriate filter mask and other personal protective equipment.

Water and caves are usually closely associated. Created by water, caves are a natural deposit for overflow or drainage from a variety of sources. Many caves can flood with little or no warning, and a recreational caver or rescuer caught in a flooding cave is in mortal danger.

Flooding is usually associated with heavy rains, which can cause diffuse seepage over a large area of the cave or a high flow into sinkholes. Occasionally, sinking streams can carry floodwater. In some parts of the world, entire rivers disappear underground, flow through caves, and resurface miles away. A flood crest from many miles upstream can pass through these caves without warning.

Flood-prone caves are generally identifiable by their makeup. Cave walls coated with thick mud can be an indication that flooding is not unusual in that section of the cave, and extra caution is warranted. Bedrock cave walls with gravel deposits at key points in the cave, and debris lodged in the ceiling can also be warning signs.

Becoming trapped in a flooding cave is not desirable, but it is survivable. If possible, find a high point in a wide passage, downstream of any major constriction, and wait out the flood. It is also possible, with enough advance warning, to remove a sediment dam downstream that may otherwise cause water to back up into your "safety zone." It is seldom wise to attempt to swim, either upstream or down.

For a rescuer called to assist cavers trapped in a flooded cave, entering the torrent is not wise. If the location of the trapped victims is known, it may be possible to use (or make) another entrance from which to evacuate them.

If entry through the main entrance is necessary, it is imperative that the water level be controlled before entry. Methods of accomplishing this goal vary depending on the situation. Often, it may be enough to simply wait out the flood and let the water level subside naturally. If the water level is still on the rise, however, or if the source remains constant, additional measures may be warranted. Keep in mind that water is a powerful force, and any plan should be engineered by professionals.

One of the simplest diversion methods is to broaden the flood crest so that less of it flows into the cave. Water can be diverted using sandbags, hay bales, or dirt or by digging channels. If this is not possible or feasible, one may be able to lower the water level by digging through debris downstream, thereby expediting the exit. Pumping is also an option, although the hazards inherent in this method should be evaluated closely beforehand.

Entering a flooded cave with scuba equipment is a dangerous, last-resort method that should only be attempted by certified cave divers. A scuba entry may be justified if cavers are known to have been entrapped for an extended period of time, if there is a known medical emergency, or if the cave is completely flooded. In these cases, it may be advisable for certified cave divers to enter and assess the condition of entrapped persons, transport survival supplies, or provide medical assistance. Only in the most dire circumstance is it justified to attempt to transport a victim through a flooded passage.

At a minimum, a scuba entry requires two to three divers, as well as a backup diver. Diving is gear intensive and requires an air compressor, extra tanks, 110-volt electricity to charge dive lights, underwater communications equipment, waterproof bags, full face masks for subjects, water rescue suits, underwater strobe lights, transport cases, and surface personnel to assist with transporting equipment.

VICTIM CARE

As with many remote accidents, the time it takes to report, respond to, and access a caving accident usually means that the victim, if alive, is relatively stable. Although this generalization has exceptions, the treatment issues faced by most rescuers are related to extended transportation times.

Data obtained in *American Caving Accidents* indicate that the leading cause of caving injury is falls, and that hypothermia, fractures, and head injuries top the list of complaints. Unfortunately, spinal injury is invariably present, and this can compound the transportation challenge. The approach to medical care should be similar to any other medical situation, with one notable difference: the victim has suffered an acute injury but will be confined for transport for an extended period. Care, then, will be a combination of acute emergency responses adapted for a victim who is, for all practical purposes, bedridden.

Once the victim has been stabilized and packaged, the assessment process should continue throughout the evacuation. It is best if one medical person can stay with and monitor the victim throughout the evacuation.

Hypovolemia is a common complaint, so establishing an IV early in the intervention can be useful. Take measures to ensure that rescuers will be able to maintain IV access and manage the supplies throughout the evacuation, and infuse only fluids not contraindicated by head or other injury. If the victim is alert and oriented, fluid administration will increase the need to urinate, so take this into consideration. As best as possible, maintain communication with the victim, encouraging him or her to flex muscles to maintain good circulation. Allow the victim to assist in care as much as possible.

Availability of ALS and drug therapy is useful on extended transports, so it is helpful to have strong rapport with the local medical authorities should complex treatment become necessary.

CONCLUSION

Never underestimate a cave rescue. Caves are unique environments, and entry should not be attempted without appropriate technical training and preparation.

The advantage to any rescue group of establishing a good working relationship with local cavers cannot be overemphasized. These are the persons with knowledge of the caves; with the training, equipment, and experience to handle the obstacles and the environment; and who already feel at ease underground. They could prove to be your most valuable resource for a successful cave rescue. Many cavers have taken extensive training in cave rescue techniques and are members of organized cave and cliff rescue teams. The first step to finding cavers is to contact a local chapter, or "grotto," of the National Speleological Society, the largest cave exploration, education and science-oriented organization in the United States. Contact them at:

National Speleological Society
2813 Cave Avenue
Huntsville, AL 35810
nss@caves.org
http://www.caves.org/

Given the unique underground environmental and topographic conditions, nothing can replace formal training in cave rescue techniques and specific cave rescue problems and solutions. Persons interested in enhancing their training should get in touch with the National Cave Rescue Commission (NCRC). The NCRC conducts week-long cave rescue seminars and weekend orientations across the United States. Contact them at the address above as the National Cave Rescue Commission of the National Speleological Society or at:

http://www.caves.org/io/ncrc/

SUGGESTED READINGS

Hudson S, editor: *Manual of U.S. cave rescue techniques,* ed 2, Huntsville, Ala, 1988, National Speleological Society.

Putnam W, editor: *American caving accidents,* published annually, Huntsville, Ala, National Speleological Society.

Insects, Animals, and Zoonoses

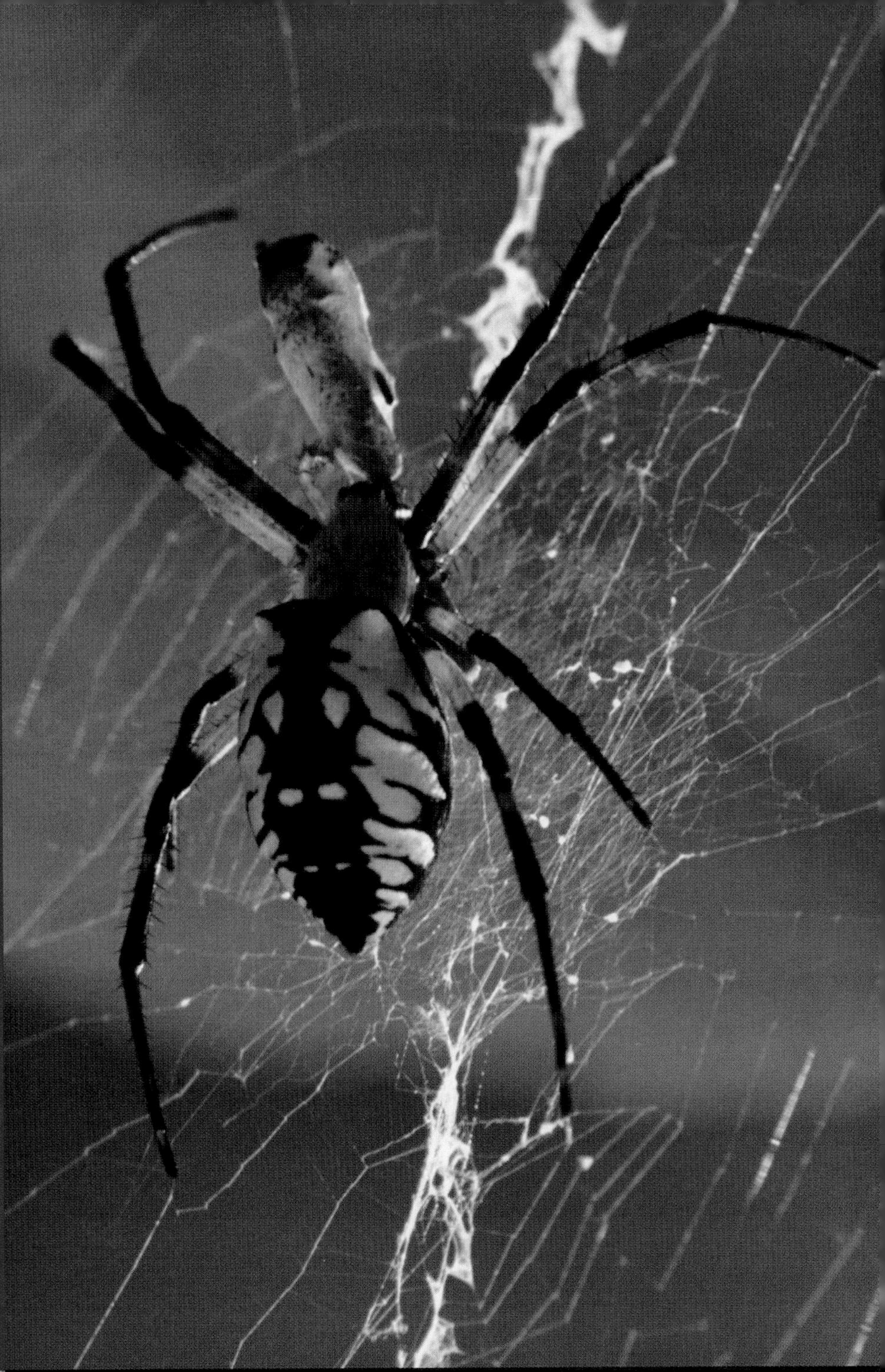

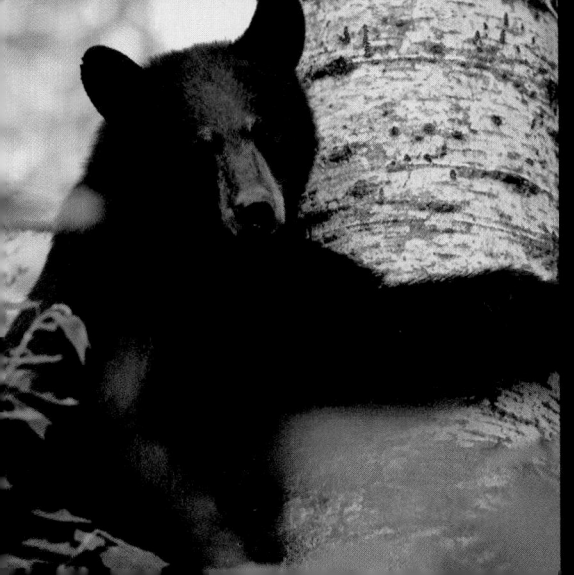

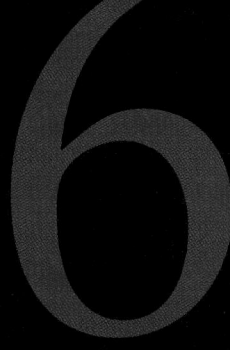

6

32 Protection from Blood-Feeding Arthropods

Mark S. Fradin

BLOOD-FEEDING ARTHROPODS

Of all the hazards, large and small, that may befall the outdoor enthusiast, perhaps the most vexatious comes from the smallest perils—blood-feeding arthropods. Mosquitoes, flies, fleas, mites, midges, chiggers, and ticks all readily bite humans. The resulting bites may, at best, result only in minor annoyance; at worst, arthropod bites may transmit to humans multiple bacterial, viral, protozoan, parasitic, and rickettsial infections (Box 32-1). Mosquito-transmitted diseases alone will be responsible for the deaths of one out of every 17 people currently alive.[108] This chapter reviews the arthropod species that bite humans and discusses various options for personal protection against nefarious insects.

Mosquitoes (Family Culicidae)

Mosquitoes are responsible for more insect bites than any other blood-sucking organism. Mosquitoes are found all over the world, except in Antarctica. These two-winged insects belong to the order Diptera. There are 170 species of mosquitoes in North America and more than 3000 species worldwide. Anopheline, or malaria-transmitting, mosquitoes can be distinguished by their resting position on the skin, characteristically appearing with the bodies raised high, almost as if standing on their heads. Most other species, in contrast, rest with their bodies parallel to the skin surface (Figure 32-1, *A*).

Mosquitoes vector more diseases to humans than do any other blood-feeding arthropod. Mosquitoes transmit malaria to 300 to 500 million people each year, resulting in as many as 3 million deaths per year.[99] They vector multiple arboviruses to humans, including several forms of encephalitis, epidemic polyarthritis, yellow fever, and dengue fever (see Chapter 66). Mosquitoes also transmit the larval form of the nematode that causes lymphatic filariasis.

Only female mosquitoes bite, requiring a blood-protein meal for egg production. Male mosquitoes feed solely on plant juices and flower nectar. Mosquitoes feed every 3 to 4 days, consuming up to their own weight in blood with each feeding. Certain species of mosquitoes prefer to feed at twilight or nighttime; others (such as the aggressive Asian tiger mosquito, *Aedes albopictus*) bite mostly during the day. Some mosquito species are zoophilic (preferring to feed on animals, including birds, reptiles, mammals, and amphibians), whereas others are anthropophilic (preferring human blood). Members of the genera *Anopheles*, *Culex*, and *Aedes* are the most common biters of humans. In some mosquitoes, seasonal switching of hosts provides a mechanism for transmitting disease from animal to human.

Mosquitoes rely on visual, thermal, and olfactory stimuli to help them locate a blood meal.[5,6,12,18,38,49] For mosquitoes that feed during the daytime, host movement and dark-colored clothing may initiate orientation towards an individual. Visual stimuli appear to be important for in-flight orientation, particularly over long ranges, whereas olfactory stimuli become more important as a mosquito nears its host. Carbon dioxide and lactic acid are the best-studied attractants. Carbon dioxide serves as a long-range attractant, luring mosquitoes at distances of up to 36 m (118 feet).[36,37,102] At close range, skin warmth and moisture serve as attractants.[5,12] Volatile compounds, derived from sebum, eccrine and apocrine sweat, and/or the cutaneous microflora bacterial action on these secretions, may also act as chemoattractants.[55,69,95] Floral fragrances found in perfumes, lotions, soaps, and hair-care products can also lure mosquitoes.[30]

There can be significant variability in the attractiveness of different individuals to the same or different species of mosquitoes.[15,50] Men tend to be bitten more readily than women, and adults are more likely to be bitten than children.[50,73] Heavyset people are more likely to attract mosquitoes, perhaps because of their greater relative heat or carbon dioxide output.[83]

During the day, mosquitoes tend to rest in cool, dark areas, such as on dense vegetation, or in hollow logs, tree stumps, animal burrows, and caves. To complete their life cycle, mosquitoes also require standing water, which may be found in tree holes, woodland pools, marshes, or puddles. To minimize the chances of being bitten by mosquitoes, campsites should ideally be situated as far away from these sites as possible.

Blackflies (Family Simuliidae)

At 2 to 5 mm in length, blackflies[3,8,21,39,48] (Figure 32-1, *B*) are smaller than mosquitoes. They have short antennae, stout humpbacked bodies, and broad wings. Blackflies are found worldwide. The adults are most prevalent in late spring and early summer and are most likely encountered near fast-running, clear rivers or streams, which they require to complete their life cycle. Unlike most mosquitoes, blackflies tend to bite during the day-time. They primarily use visual cues to locate a host. Dark moving objects are particularly attractive, but car-bon dioxide and body warmth also serve as attractants. Only the female bites, taking up to 5 minutes to feed. Blackflies may be present in swarms, inflicting numer-ous bites on their victims.

Blackflies are attracted to the eyes, nostrils, and ears

Box 32-1   DISEASES TRANSMITTED TO HUMANS BY BITING ARTHROPODS

MOSQUITOES

Eastern equine encephalitis*
Western equine encephalitis*
St. Louis encephalitis*
La Crosse encephalitis*
Japanese encephalitis
Venezuelan equine encephalitis
Malaria
Yellow fever
Dengue fever
Bancroftian filariasis
Epidemic polyarthritis (Ross River virus)
Chikungunya fever
Rift Valley fever

TICKS

Lyme disease*
Rocky Mountain spotted fever*
Colorado tick fever*
Relapsing fever*
Ehrlichiosis*
Babesiosis*
Tularemia*
Tick paralysis*
Tick typhus

FLIES

Tularemia*
Leishmaniasis*
African trypanosomiasis (sleeping sickness)
Onchocerciasis
Bartonellosis
Loa loa

CHIGGER MITES

Scrub typhus (tsutsugamushi fever)
Rickettsial pox*

FLEAS

Plague*
Murine (endemic) typhus

LICE

Epidemic typhus
Relapsing fever

KISSING BUGS

American trypanosomiasis (Chagas' disease)

*May be found in the United States.

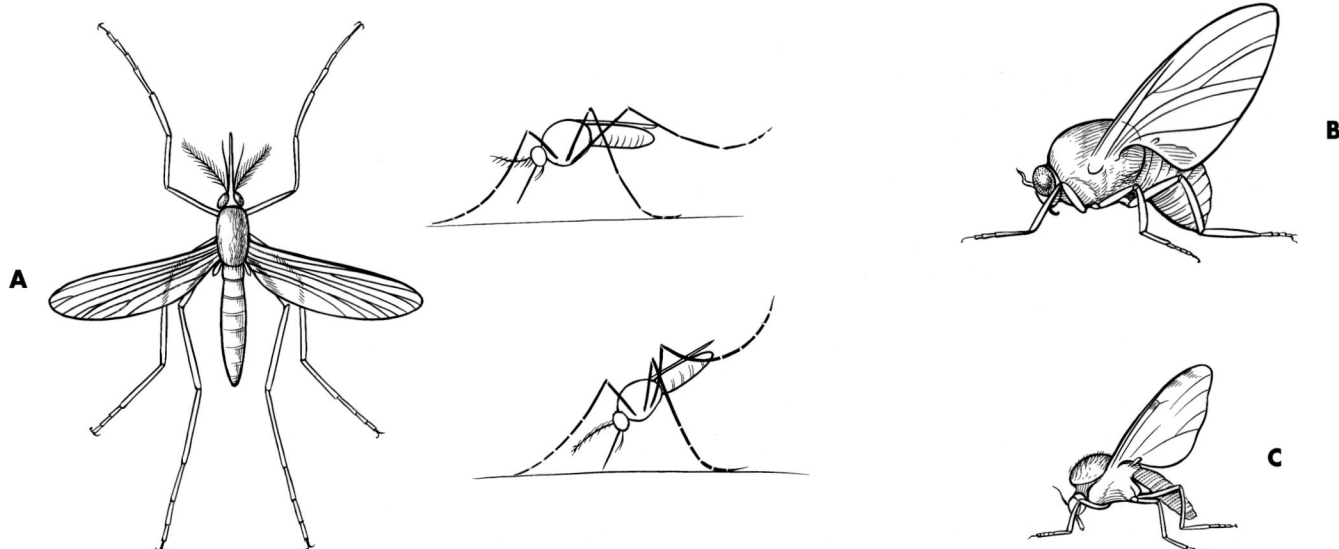

Figure 32-1 Blood-feeding arthropods. **A,** Mosquito: Culex and Anopheles. **B,** Blackfly. **C,** Biting midge.
Continued

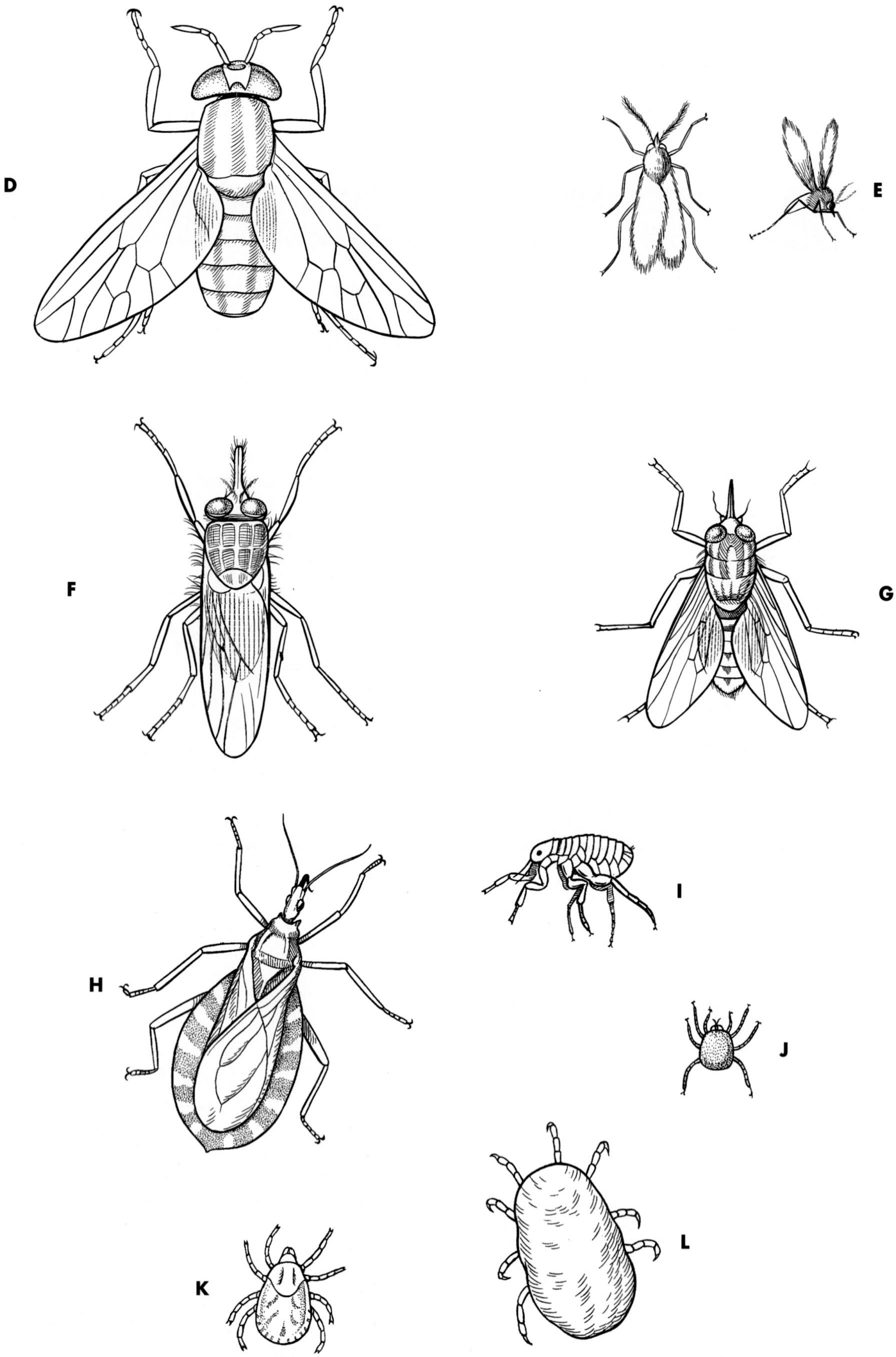

Figure 32-1—cont'd Blood-feeding arthropods. **D,** Tabanid fly. **E,** Sand fly. **F,** Tsetse fly. **G,** Stable fly. **H,** Kissing bug. **I,** Flea. **J,** Chigger mite. **K,** Hard tick. **L,** Soft tick.

of their hosts. They often crawl under clothing or into the hair to feed. The insect's mouthparts are used to tear the skin surface, producing a pool of blood from which the fly feeds. Blood loss from the bite site often persists after the blackfly has departed. The resulting intensely pruritic, painful, and edematous papules are typically slow to heal. Rare systemic reactions, including fever, urticaria, anaphylaxis, and even death, have been reported after blackfly bites. Although these flies are not known to transmit disease to humans in North America, in the tropics, blackflies are vectors of the parasite *Onchocerca volvulus,* which causes river blindness.

Midges (Family Ceratopogonidae)

Also known as *no-see-ums, sand gnats, sand fleas,* and *flying teeth,* biting midges[3,8,21,39,48] are small (less than 2 mm), slender flies with narrow wings (Figure 32-1, *C*). Their small size makes them difficult to see, and they can pass readily through common window screens. Biting midges may be found worldwide. They breed most commonly in salt marshes but may also be found in freshwater wetlands. Despite their inconspicuous size, female midges are aggressive biters, frequently attacking in swarms and inflicting multiple painful and pruritic bites within minutes. Midges often crawl into the hair before biting. Depending on the species, midges may bite during the day or at nighttime. Their activity is greatest during calm weather, declining as wind speed increases. Biting midges are not known to transmit disease in North America.

Tabanids (Family Tabanidae)

The family Tabanidae (Figure 32-1, *D*) includes horseflies, deerflies, greenheads, and yellow flies.[3,8,21,39,48] These insects are relatively large (10 to 20 mm) robust fliers, with numerous species worldwide. Tabanids breed in aquatic or semiaquatic environments, with a life cycle of over a year. They are able to fly for miles and rely primarily on vision to locate a host by movement. These flies are most active on warm, overcast days. Only the females bite, using scissorlike mouthparts to create within the skin a bleeding slash, which is slow to heal. Despite their size, these flies usually bite painlessly, but the resulting reaction can include intense itching, secondary infection, and, rarely, systemic reactions, such as urticaria or anaphylaxis. Since the adult fly usually only lives about a month, and only one generation emerges per year, the potential season for being bitten is fortunately relatively short. In the United States, deerflies have been shown to be capable of transmitting tularemia to humans; in Africa, the deerfly may vector the filarial parasitic worm, *Loa loa.*

Sand Flies (Family Psychodidae)

Sand flies[3,8,21,25,39,48] are tiny (2 to 3 mm), hairy, and long-legged flies, with multisegmented antennae and a char-

acteristic V-shape to the wings when at rest (Figure 32-1, *E*). Only female sand flies are blood-feeders, feeding mostly during calm, windless nights, and resting during the day in animal burrows, tree holes, or caves. Most sand fly bites tend to occur on the face and neck.

In tropical and subtropical climates, sand flies have been shown to vector multiple cutaneous, mucocutaneous, and systemic diseases, including bartonellosis and three forms of leishmaniasis. The only sand fly–transmitted disease in the United States has been cutaneous leishmaniasis, reported in Texas.

Tsetse Flies (Family Glossinidae)

Tsetse flies[3,8,21,39,48] are found only in tropical Africa. They are 7 to 14 mm long, yellowish-brown, with wings that fold over their backs, giving them the appearance of honeybees at rest (Figure 32-1, *F*). Both genders bite, feeding in daytime on a wide variety of mammals, including humans. Tsetse flies seem to rely primarily on vision and movement to identify their hosts. Their bites may cause petechiae or pruritic wheals. Tsetse flies vector African trypanosomiasis (sleeping sickness).

Stable Flies (Family Muscidae)

Stable flies[39,48] resemble common houseflies and are most often encountered in coastal areas. Unlike a housefly, which rests with its body parallel to the surface, a stable fly rests with its head held higher than its posterior (Figure 32-1, *G*). Both male and female stable flies are vicious daytime biters, requiring a blood meal every 48 hours to survive. If disturbed, they will attempt to feed multiple times, preferring to bite the lower extremities. Horses and cattle are the preferred hosts, but hungry stable flies will readily bite humans. These flies have knifelike mouthparts that they use to puncture flesh before pumping up the blood. Stable flies breed in decaying vegetation and in herbivore manure and are frequently found congregated on sunny walls. Stable fly bites are generally self-limited. They are not known to transmit disease to humans.

Kissing Bugs (Family Reduviidae)

Kissing bugs[3,8,21,26,39,48] (assassin bugs) are large (10 to 30 mm in length) insects with cone-shaped heads, overlapping wings, and an alternating pattern of orange and dark brown stripes on the lateral abdomen (Figure 32-1, *H*). Kissing bugs get their name from a tendency to bite around the human mouth, but they may also bite other parts of the body. Both male and female reduviids bite, requiring a blood meal to mature through five nymphal growth stages. Reduviids are nocturnal feeders, attracted to their hosts by warmth, carbon dioxide, and odor. During the day, they rest in trees or indoors in crevices of house walls and ceilings. Kissing bug bites are initially painless, but frequent exposure to the bites can produce erythema, edema, and pruritus at the bite sites. More importantly, kissing bugs are the vector for *Trypanosoma cruzi,* the causative agent of Chagas' disease, which has been reported in Central and South America, as well as in the southwestern United States.

Fleas (Family Pulicidae)

Adult fleas[3,8,21,39,48] are small (2 to 6 mm), wingless insects, with three pairs of powerful legs that enable them to jump distances of up to 30 cm (Figure 32-1, *I*). Hungry fleas of both genders feed on the nearest warm-blooded animal, without clear host preference. Fleas usually move around, probing and biting several times, resulting in grouped lesions of pruritic papules. Fleas are capable of transmitting sylvatic plague and murine typhus.

Chigger Mites (Family Trombiculidae)

Trombiculid mites[3,8,21,39,48] (Figure 32-1, *J*) may be found worldwide. Commonly known as *chiggers, red-bugs,* or *harvest mites,* these reddish-yellow insects are readily encountered in damp, grassy, and wooded areas, especially along the margins of forests, where they may number in the thousands. Only the tiny (less than 0.2 mm) larval stages are parasitic, feeding on mammals, birds, reptiles, and amphibians. Chiggers are most active in the summer and early autumn. They usually infest humans by crawling up the shoes and legs, preferring to attach to skin at areas where the clothing fits tightly, such as at the top of socks or around the elastic edges of underwear. Chiggers do not burrow into the skin or actively suck blood. Rather, they pierce skin with their mouthparts and secrete a proteolytic salivary fluid that dissolves host tissue, which they, in turn, suck up. If undisturbed, chiggers may feed for several days before dropping off. In humans, this rarely occurs because the larvae usually cause enough irritation that they are dislodged by scratching. The host response to chigger bites is brisk, often leading to intensely pruritic, bright red 1- to 2-cm nodules. In Asia, chiggers may serve as vectors of scrub typhus. Rickettsial pox is also transmitted by a mite bite.

Ticks (Families Ixodidae and Argasidae)
(See Chapter 33)

Ticks[3,8,21,39,48,105] are classified as hard ticks (family Ixodidae) and soft ticks (family Argasidae) (Figure 32-1, *K* and *L*). Hard ticks are so named because of the presence of a sclerotized plate, or scutum, that covers part of the body. Both types of ticks may be found worldwide, but hard ticks are more commonly encountered in North America. Hard ticks are usually found in weedy or shrubbed areas, along trails, and at forest boundaries, where mammalian hosts, such as deer, are plentiful. Soft ticks are more resistant to desiccation than are hard ticks. Soft ticks thrive in hot and dry climates and are commonly found in animal burrows or caves.

Both genders are bloodsuckers. Soft ticks are nocturnal and feed rapidly, in just a few minutes. Hard ticks most commonly feed during the day and may feed on a single host for days. Ticks are unable to fly or jump. Hard ticks climb vegetation and "quest," waiting passively for hours or days, forelegs outstretched, until they detect the vibration or carbon dioxide plume of a passing host. When they encounter fur or skin, they climb onto the host and then crawl around in search of an appropriate location on which to attach and feed. The attachment bite is usually painless.

People in suspected tick habitats should check clothing frequently for the presence of ticks. If multiple ticks are seen on clothing, they are most easily removed by trapping them on a piece of cellophane tape, or by rolling a sticky tape-type lint remover across them; hundreds of small ticks can be easily removed by this method.

Attached ticks are more difficult to remove. Tick mouthparts are barbed, and some species of tick also secrete a cement that firmly anchors the tick into the skin. Erythema, pruritus, and edema are commonly seen at the site of a tick bite. Improper partial removal of the mouthparts may initiate a long-lasting foreign body reaction, leading to secondarily infected lesions that are slow to heal, or granuloma formation that may persist for months. (For a discussion of the best method for tick removal, see Chapter 33.)

After the tick is removed, the bite site should be cleansed with soap and water, or an antiseptic, and hands should be washed. It may be prudent to save the tick, in case later identification becomes necessary. Prompt removal of attached ticks will greatly reduce the likelihood of disease transmission. Laboratory studies of attachment times for *Borrelia burgdorferi* (Lyme disease)–infected ticks showed that transmission of the spirochete rarely occurred if the tick was attached for less than 48 hours.[79-82,104,105]

In the United States, soft ticks of the genus *Ornithodoros* are capable of transmitting to humans the *Borrelia* spirochete that causes relapsing fever. Three genera of the hard ticks Ixodidae transmit disease to man: *Ixodes* (which vectors Lyme disease, babesiosis, and tick paralysis), *Dermacentor* (vectors tularemia, Rocky Mountain spotted fever, ehrlichiosis, Colorado tick fever, and tick paralysis), and *Amblyomma* (vectors tularemia, ehrlichiosis, and tick paralysis).[71,105] Larval, nymph, and adult ticks may all transmit disease during feeding. Transovarial transmission also enables female ticks to directly infect their offspring.

Box 32-2 MANUFACTURERS OF PROTECTIVE CLOTHING, PROTECTIVE SHELTERS, AND INSECT NETS

PROTECTIVE CLOTHING (includes hooded jackets, pants, headnets, ankle guards, gaiters, and mittens)

Bug Baffler, Inc.
P.O. Box 444
Goffstown, NH 03045
(888) 774-7391

Insect Out
P.O. Box 49643
Colorado Springs, CO 80919
(888) 488-0285

BugOut Outdoor Wear, Inc.
P.O. Box 185
Centerville, IA 52544
(515) 437-1936

Skeeta
P.O. Box 72103
Fairbanks, AK 99707
(907) 479-9389

The Original Bug Shirt Company
908 Niagara Falls Blvd., #467
North Tonawanda, NY 14120
(800) 998-9096

PROTECTIVE CLOTHING—cont'd

Shannon Outdoor's Bug Tamer
1210-A Peachtree Street
Louisville, GA 30434
(800) 852-8058

PROTECTIVE SHELTERS AND INSECT NETS

Long Road Travel Supplies
111 Avenida Drive
Berkeley, CA 94708
(800) 359-6040

Wisconsin Pharmacal Co.
1 Repel Road
Jackson, WI 53037
(800) 558-6614

Travel Medicine, Inc.
369 Pleasant Street
Northampton, MA 01060
(800) 872-8633

PERSONAL PROTECTION

Personal protection against insect bites may be achieved in three ways: avoiding infested habitats, using protective clothing and/or shelters, and applying insect repellents.

Habitat Avoidance

Avoiding infested habitats reduces the risk of being bitten. Mosquitoes and other nocturnal bloodsuckers are particularly active at dusk, making this a good time to be indoors. To avoid the usual resting places of biting arthropods, campgrounds should ideally be situated in areas that are high, dry, and open, as free from vegetation as possible. Attempts should be made to avoid unnecessary use of lights, which attract multiple insects.

Physical Protection

Physical barriers can be extremely effective in preventing insect bites, by blocking arthropods' access to the skin. Long-sleeved shirts, socks, long pants, and a hat will protect all but the face, neck, and hands. Tucking pants into the socks or boots makes it much more difficult for ticks or chigger mites to gain access to the skin. Light-colored clothing is preferable, since it makes it easier to spot ticks and is less attractive to mosquitoes and biting flies. Ticks will find it more difficult to cling

to smooth, closely-woven fabrics (e.g., nylon).[98] Loose-fitting clothing, made out of tightly woven fabric, with a tucked-in T-shirt undergarment is particularly effective at reducing bites on the upper body. A light-colored, full-brimmed hat will protect the head and neck. Deerflies tend to land on the hat instead of the head, and blackflies and biting midges are less likely to crawl to the shaded skin beneath a hat brim.

Mesh garments or garments made of tightly woven material are available to protect against insect bites. Head nets, hooded jackets, pants, and mittens are available from a number of manufacturers in a wide range of sizes and styles (Box 32-2). Mesh garments are usually made of either polyester or nylon and, depending on the manufacturer, are available in either white or dark colors. With a mesh size of less than 0.3 mm, many of these garments are woven tightly enough to exclude even biting midges and ticks. As with any clothing, bending or crouching may still pull the garments close enough to the skin surface to enable insects to bite through. One manufacturer (Shannon Outdoors, Louisville, Ga.) addresses this potential problem with a double-layered mesh that reportedly prevents mosquito penetration. Although mesh garments are effective barriers against insects, some people may find them uncomfortable during vigorous activity or in hot weather.

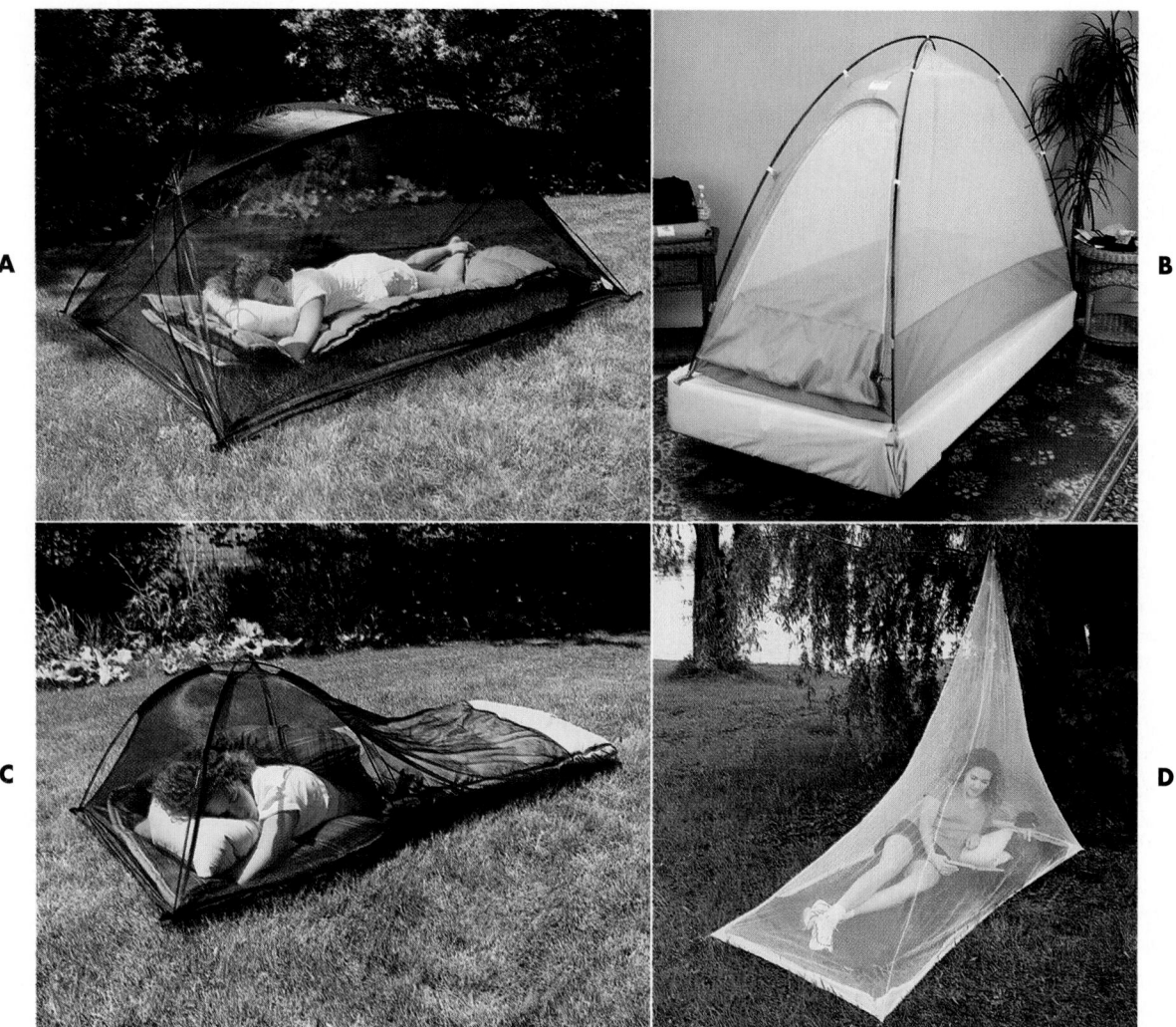

Figure 32-2 **A** to **C,** Protective shelters. **D,** Bed nets. *(**A, C,** and **D** courtesy Wisconsin Pharmacal Co.; **B** courtesy Long Road Travel Supplies.)*

Lightweight insect nets and mesh shelters are available to protect travelers sleeping indoors or in the wilderness (Figure 32-2). The effectiveness of insect nets or shelters may be enhanced by lightly spraying them with a permethrin-based contact insecticide, which provides weeks of efficacy after a single application.

Repellents

For many people, applying an insect repellent may be the most effective and easiest way to prevent arthropod bites. The quest to develop the "perfect" insect repellent has been an ongoing scientific goal for years and has yet to be achieved. The ideal agent would repel multiple species of biting arthropods, remain effective for at least 8 hours, cause no irritation to skin or mucous membranes, possess no systemic toxicity, be resistant to abrasion and wash-off, and be greaseless and odorless. No presently available insect repellent meets all of these criteria. Efforts to find such a compound have been hampered by the multiplicity of variables that affect the inherent repellency of any chemical. Repellents do not all share a single mode of action, and different species of insects may react differently to the same repellent.[88]

To be effective as an insect repellent, a chemical must be volatile enough to maintain an effective repellent vapor concentration at the skin surface but not evaporate so rapidly that it quickly loses its effectiveness. Multiple factors play a role in effectiveness, including concentration, frequency and uniformity of application, the user's activity level and overall attractiveness to bloodsucking arthropods, and the number and species of the organisms trying to bite. The effectiveness of any repellent is reduced by abrasion from clothing; evaporation and absorption from the skin surface; wash-off from sweat, rain, or water; and a windy environment.[34,50,51,67,68,86] Each 10° C (18° F) increase in ambient temperature can lead to as much as 50% reduction in protection time.[51] Presently available insect repellents

TABLE 32-1. DEET-Containing Insect Repellents

MANUFACTURER/ DISTRIBUTOR	PRODUCT NAME	FORM(S)	% DEET
Sawyer Products Tampa, Fla. (800) 940-4464	DEET Plus	Lotion and pump spray	17.5
	Sawyer Gold	Pump spray	17.5
	Sawyer Controlled Release	Lotion	20
	Sawyer Gold	Lotion	30
	Sawyer Gold	Spray aerosol	38
	Maxi-DEET	Pump spray	100
S.C. Johnson Wax Racine, Wisc. (800) 558-5566	OFF! Skintastic Unscented	Pump spray	5
	OFF! Skintastic Unscented	Pump spray	7
	OFF! Skintastic Unscented	Lotion	7.5
	OFF! Skintastic with Sunscreen (SPF 30)	Lotion	10
	OFF! Unscented	Aerosol spray	15
	Deep Woods OFF! with Sunscreen (SPF 15)	Lotion	20
	Deep Woods OFF! Unscented	Aerosol spray	25
	Deep Woods OFF! for Sportsmen	Aerosol spray	30
	Deep Woods OFF! for Sportsmen	Pump spray	100
Tender Corporation Littleton, NH (800) 258-4696	Ben's Backyard	Lotion and pump spray	24
	Ben's Wilderness	Aerosol	27
	Ben's Max 100	Lotion and pump spray	100
Travel Medicine, Inc. Northampton, Mass. (800) 872-8633	Ultrathon	Cream	35
United Industries Corp. St. Louis, Mo. (800) 767-9927	Cutter Just For Kids	Pump spray	7
	Cutter Skinsations with Sunscreen (SPF 15)	Lotion	7
	Cutter Skinsations	Aerosol and pump spray	7
	Cutter Skinsations	Gel; towelettes	7
	Cutter Unscented	Aerosol spray	10
	Cutter Backwoods Unscented	Aerosol and pump spray	23
	Cutter Outdoorsman Unscented	Aerosol; lotion; solid stick	30
Wisconsin Pharmacal Co. Jackson, Wisc. (800) 558-6614	Repel Insect Repellent	Gel	7
	Repel Family Formula	Pump spray	18
	Repel Sportsmen Formula	Pump spray	18
	Repel Sportsmen Formula	Lotion	20
	Repel Family Formula	Aerosol	23
	Repel Sportsmen Formula	Aerosol	29
	Repel Classic Sportsmen Formula	Aerosol	40
	Repel 100	Pump spray	100

NOTE: Some manufacturers give only the concentration of the *m*-isomer; others list total concentrations of all DEET isomers. Technical grade 100% DEET is 95% *m*-isomer and 5% other isomers.

do not "cloak" the user in a chemical veil of protection; any untreated exposed skin can be readily bitten by hungry arthropods.[67]

CHEMICAL DEET. *N,N*-diethyl-3-methylbenzamide (previously called *N,N*-diethyl-*m*-toluamide), or DEET, remains the gold standard of presently available insect repellents. DEET has been registered for use by the general public since 1957. It is a broad-spectrum repellent, effective against many species of crawling and flying insects, including mosquitoes, biting flies, midges, chiggers, fleas, and ticks. The United States Environmental Protection Agency (EPA) estimates that about 30% of the U.S. population uses a DEET-based product every year; worldwide use exceeds 200 million people annu-

ally.[112,114] Decades of empirical testing of more than 20,000 other compounds has not led to the release of a superior repellent.[17,47,53,84,91,111]

DEET may be applied directly to skin, clothing, mesh insect nets or shelters, window screens, tents, or sleeping bags. Care should be taken to avoid inadvertent contact with plastics (such as wrist watch crystals and glasses frames), rayon, spandex, leather, or painted and varnished surfaces, since DEET may damage these. DEET does not damage natural fibers, such as wool and cotton.

In the United States, DEET is sold in concentrations from 5% to 100% in multiple formulations, including lotions, solutions, gels, sprays, and impregnated towelettes and wristbands (Table 32-1). As a general rule, higher concentrations of DEET will provide longer-lasting protection. For most uses, however, there is no need to use the highest concentrations of DEET. Products with 10% to 35% DEET provide adequate protection under most conditions. In fact, most manufacturers, responding to consumer demand, have recently begun to offer a greater variety of low-concentration DEET products. The American Academy of Pediatrics currently recommends that DEET-containing repellents used on children contain no more than 10% DEET.[35,100] Persons adverse to applying DEET directly to their skin may get long-lasting repellency by applying DEET only to their clothing. DEET-treated garments, stored in a plastic bag between wearings, maintain their repellency for several weeks.[15]

Products with a DEET concentration over 35% are probably best reserved for circumstances in which the wearer will be in an environment with a very high density of insects (e.g., a rain forest), where there is a high risk of disease transmission from insect bites, or under circumstances in which there may be rapid loss of repellent from the skin surface, such as under conditions of high temperature and humidity or rain. Under these circumstances, reapplication of the repellent will likely be necessary to maintain its effectiveness.

Two companies (3M, Minneapolis, Minn., and Sawyer Products, Tampa, Fla.) manufacturer extended-release formulations of DEET that make it possible to deliver long-lasting protection without relying on high concentrations of DEET. 3M's product, Ultrathon, was developed for the U.S. military and is currently exclusively sold to the public through Travel Medicine, Inc. (Northampton, Mass.; 800-872-8633). This acrylate polymer DEET formulation, when tested under multiple different environmental/climatic field conditions, was as effective as 75% DEET, providing up to 12 hours of greater than 95% protection against mosquito bites.[2,41,54,72,94,96] Sawyer Products' controlled-release 20% DEET lotion traps the chemical in a protein particle that slowly releases it to the skin surface, providing repellency equivalent to a standard 50% DEET preparation, lasting about 5 hours.[28] Preliminary data suggest that about 50% less of this encapsulated DEET is absorbed when compared with a 20% ethanol-based preparation of DEET.[27]

Given its use by millions of people worldwide for 40 years, DEET continues to show a remarkable safety profile. In 1980, as part of the EPA Registration Standard for DEET,[112] over 30 additional animal studies were conducted to assess acute, chronic, and subchronic toxicity; mutagenicity; oncogenicity; and developmental, reproductive, and neurologic toxicity. The results of these studies neither led to any product changes to comply with current EPA safety standards nor indicated any new toxicities under normal usage. The EPA's Reregistration Eligibility Decision (RED),[114]

released in 1998, confirmed that the Agency believes that "normal use of DEET does not present a health concern to the general U.S. population."

Case reports of potential DEET toxicity exist in the medical literature and are fully reviewed by Fradin.[32] Fewer than 40 cases of significant toxicity from DEET exposure have been documented in the medical literature over the last four decades; over three quarters of these resolved without sequelae. Many of these cases involved long-term, excessive, or inappropriate use of DEET repellents; the details of exposure were frequently poorly documented, making causal relationships difficult to establish. These cases have not shown a correlation between concentration of the DEET product used and the risk of toxicity.

The reports of DEET toxicity that raise the greatest concern involve 14 cases of encephalopathy, 13 in children under age 8 years old.[20,24,32,44,45,64,75,76,120] Three of these children died, one of whom had ornithine carbamoyl transferase deficiency, which might have predisposed her to DEET-induced toxicity.[44,45] The other children recovered without sequelae. The EPA's analysis of these cases concluded that they "do not support a direct link between exposure to DEET and seizure incidence."[114] Animal studies in rats and mice show that DEET is not a selective neurotoxin.[75,89,112] Even if a link between DEET use and seizures does exist, the observed risk, based on DEET usage patterns, would be less than one per 100 million users.[114]

The EPA has issued guidelines to ensure safe use of DEET-based repellents.[114] Careful product choice (most often of a DEET concentration of 35% or less), judicious use, and common-sense application will greatly reduce the possibility of toxicity. Conservative use of low-concentration DEET products is most appropriate when applying repellents to children. Guidelines for properly applying insect repellents are given in Box 32-3.

Questions regarding the safety of DEET may be addressed to the EPA-sponsored National Pesticide Telecommunications Network, available each day from 6:30 AM to 4:30 PM Pacific Standard Time at (800) 858-7378 or via their website at http://ace.orst.edu/info/nptn/.

SKIN-SO-SOFT PRODUCTS. Skin-So-Soft Bath Oil (Avon, New York, N.Y.) received considerable media attention several years ago when it was reported by some consumers to be effective as a mosquito repellent. When tested under laboratory conditions against *Aedes aegypti* mosquitoes, Skin-So-Soft Bath Oil's effective half-life was found to be 0.51 hours.[87] In one study against *Aedes albopictus*, Skin-So-Soft Oil provided 0.64 hours of protection from bites and was 10 times *less* effective than 12.5% DEET.[96] Skin-So-Soft Oil has been found to be somewhat effective against biting midges, but this effect is felt to be a result of its trapping the insects in an

Box 32-3 GUIDELINES FOR SAFE AND EFFECTIVE USE OF INSECT REPELLENTS

For casual use, choose a repellent with 10% to 35% DEET. Repellents with 10% DEET or less are most appropriate for use on children.

Use just enough repellent to lightly cover the exposed skin; do not saturate the skin.

Repellents should be applied only to exposed skin and/or clothing. Do not use under clothing.

To apply to the face, dispense into palms, rub hands together, and then apply thin layer to face.

Young children should not apply repellents themselves.

Avoid contact with eyes and mouth. Do not apply to children's hands to prevent possible subsequent contact with mucous membranes.

After applying, wipe repellent from the palmar surfaces to prevent inadvertent contact with eyes, mouth, and genitals.

Never use repellents over cuts; wounds; or inflamed, irritated, or eczematous skin.

Do not inhale aerosol formulations or get them in eyes. Do not apply when near food.

Frequent reapplication is rarely necessary, unless the repellent seems to have lost its effectiveness. Reapplication may be necessary in very hot, wet environments because of rapid loss of repellent from the skin surface.

Once inside, wash off treated areas with soap and water. Washing the repellent from the skin surface is particularly important under circumstances in which a repellent is likely to be applied for several consecutive days.

If you suspect you are having a reaction to an insect repellent, discontinue its use, wash the treated skin, and consult a physician.

Adapted from United States Environmental Protection Agency, Office of Pesticide Programs, Prevention, Pesticides and Toxic Substances Division: *Reregistration Eligibility Decision (RED): DEET* (EPA-738-F-95-010), Washington, DC, 1998, EPA.

oily film on the skin surface.[66] It has been proposed that the limited mosquito repellent effect of Skin-So-Soft Oil could be due to its fragrance or to the presence of diisopropyl adipate and benzophenone in the formulation, both of which have some repellent activity.[10,53]

Avon Products, Inc. makes no claims about its bath oil being an effective repellent. They currently manufacturer Skin-So-Soft Bug Guard, which contains 0.10% oil of citronella as the active ingredient. In July 1999, Avon introduced a new chemical-based insect repellent to the U.S. market, IR3535, or ethyl-3-(N-butylacetamido) propionate, which can be found in Skin-So-Soft Bug Guard Plus. The limited data presently available to the public on this repellent show that, although it is more effective than most botanical-based repellents, it does not match the overall efficacy of DEET.[22]

Botanical Repellents. Thousands of plants have been tested as sources of insect repellents. Although none of the plant-derived chemicals tested to date demonstrate the broad effectiveness and duration of DEET, a few show repellent activity. Plants with essential oils that have been reported to possess repellent activity include citronella, cedar, verbena, pennyroyal, geranium, lavender, pine, cajeput, cinnamon, rosemary, basil, thyme, allspice, garlic, and peppermint.[7,16,23,40,53,85] Unlike DEET-based repellents, botanical repellents have been relatively poorly studied. When tested, most of these essential oils tended to show short-lasting protection, lasting minutes to 2 hours. A summary of readily-available plant-derived insect repellents is shown in Table 32-2.

CITRONELLA. Oil of citronella was initially registered as an insect repellent by the EPA in 1948. It is the most common active ingredient found in "natural" or "herbal" insect repellents presently marketed in the United States. Originally extracted from the grass plant *Cymbopogon nardus*, oil of citronella has a lemony scent.

Conflicting data exist on the efficacy of citronella-based products, varying greatly depending on the study methodology, location, and species of biting insect tested. One citronella-based repellent was found to provide no repellency when tested in the laboratory against *Aedes aegypti* mosquitoes.[10] However, a field study of the same product showed an average of 88% repellency over a 2-hour exposure. The product's effectiveness was greatest within the first 40 minutes after application and then decreased with time over the remainder of the test period.[107] All Terrain Co. (Encinitas, Calif.; 800-246-7328) produces a citronella-based lotion in which the essential oil has been encapsulated into a beeswax matrix, which slowly releases it to the skin surface, prolonging its efficacy. In laboratory testing against *Aedes aegypti*, this product provided complete protection for the first 2 hours, and 77% protection 4 hours after application.[43]

In general, studies show that citronella-based repellents are less effective than DEET repellents. Citronella provides a shorter protection time, which may be partially overcome by frequent reapplication of the repellent. In 1997, after analyzing available data on the repellent effect of citronella, the EPA concluded that citronella-based insect repellents must contain the following statement on their labels: "For maximum repellent effectiveness of this product, repeat applications at one hour intervals."[113]

Citronella candles have been promoted as an effective way to repel mosquitoes from one's local environment. One study compared the efficacy of commercially available 3% citronella candles, 5% citronella incense, and plain candles to prevent bites by *Aedes* species mosquitoes under field conditions.[62] Subjects

TABLE 32-2. Botanical Insect Repellents

MANUFACTURER	PRODUCT NAME	FORM(S)	ACTIVE INGREDIENT
Avon Corp. New York, NY (800) 367-2866	Skin-So-Soft: Moisturizing Suncare Plus SPF 15 and 30	Lotion	Citronella oil 0.05%
	Bug Guard ± SPF 15	Pump spray	Citronella oil 0.1%
	Bug Guard Moisturizing	Lotion and towelettes	Citronella oil 0.1%
Verdant Brands, Inc. Bloomington, Ind. (800) 643-8457	Blocker	Lotion, oil, and pump spray	Soybean oil 2%
Quantum, Inc. Eugene, Ore. (800) 448-1448	Buzz Away Buzz Away, SPF 15	Towelette and pump spray Lotion	Citronella oil 5%; oils of cedarwood, peppermint, eucalyptus, lemongrass
Tender Corp. Littleton, NH (800) 258-4696	Natrapel	Lotion and pump spray	Citronella 10%
All Terrain Co. Encinitas, Calif. (800) 246-7328	Herbal Armor Herbal Armor SPF 15 Herbal Armor	Lotion Lotion Pump spray	Citronella oil 12%, pep- permint oil 2.5%, cedar oil 2%, lemongrass oil 1%, geranium oil 0.05%, in a slow-release encapsu- lated formula
Green Ban Norway, Iowa (319) 446-7495	Green Ban For People: Regular	Oil	Citronella oil 5%, pepper- mint oil 1%
	Double Strength	Oil	Citronella oil 10%, pepper- mint oil 2%

near the citronella candles had 42% fewer bites than controls who had no protection (a statistically significant difference). However, burning ordinary candles reduced the number of bites by 23%. There was no difference in efficacy between citronella incense and plain candles. The ability of plain candles to decrease biting may be due to their serving as a "decoy" source of warmth, moisture, and carbon dioxide.

The citrosa plant (*Pelargonium citrosum* "Van Leenii") has been marketed as being able to repel mosquitoes through the continuous release of citronella oils. Unfortunately, when tested, these plants offer no protection against bites.[11,70]

BLOCKER. Blocker is a "natural" repellent that was released to the U.S. market in 1997. Blocker combines soybean oil, geranium oil, and coconut oil in a formulation that has been available in Europe for several years.[115] Studies conducted at the University of Guelph, Guelph, Ontario, Canada, showed that this product was capable of providing over 97% protection against *Aedes* species mosquitoes under field conditions, even after 3½ hours of application. During the same time period, a 6.65% DEET-based spray afforded 86% protection, whereas Avon's Skin-So-Soft citronella-based repellent gave only 40% protection.[59] A second study showed that Blocker provided a mean of 200 ± 30 (SD)

minutes of complete protection from mosquito bites.[60] Blocker also provided about 10 hours of protection against biting blackflies; in the same test, 20% DEET only gave 6½ hours of complete protection.[61]

EUCALYPTUS. A derivative (*p*-menthane-3,8-diol, or PMD) isolated from oil of the lemon eucalyptus plant has shown promise as an effective "natural" repellent.[16] This repellent has been very popular in China for years and is currently available in Europe under the brand name Mosi-guard. In field tests against anopheline mosquitoes, PMD showed repellency comparable with 50% DEET.[109] PMD required more frequent reapplication than DEET to maintain its potency but was significantly more effective than 50% citronella oil.[13,110] Release of PMD-based repellents awaits final EPA approval in the United States.

Efficacy of DEET vs. Botanical Repellents. Limited data are available from studies that directly compare plant-derived repellents with DEET-based products. Available data proving the efficacy of "natural" repellents are often sparse, and there is no uniformly accepted standard for testing these products. As a result, different studies often yield varied results, depending on how and where the tests were conducted. In general, when compared with "natural" products, DEET-based repel-

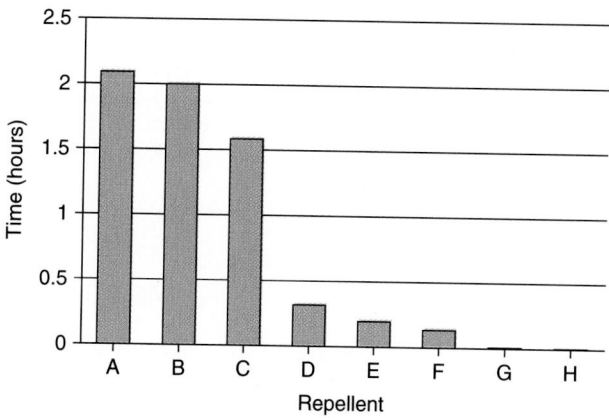

Figure 32-3 Average protection times—DEET vs. botanical repellents. *A,* DEET 6.65%; *B,* DEET 4.75%, *C,* soybean oil 2%, geranium oil, coconut oil; *D,* citronella oil 0.1%; *E,* citronella oil 5%, cedarwood oil, eucalyptus oil, peppermint oil; *F;* prickly pear extract 40%; *G,* citronella oil 0.05%; *H,* DEET 9.5%, impregnated into a wristband.

lents demonstrate longer-lasting effectiveness. In a laboratory study against *Aedes aegypti* mosquitoes, two commercially available "natural" repellents containing citronella (and other plant-derived essential oils) demonstrated no repellent effect, even when applied at twice the concentration that would typically be expected to be used.[10] In the same study, DEET-based repellents (at various concentrations) provided at least 2 hours of protection.[10] Another study comparing "natural" repellents with low-strength DEET products, conducted under carefully controlled laboratory conditions with caged mosquitoes, demonstrated a dramatic difference in effectiveness between several currently marketed insect repellents. Low-concentration DEET lotions (under 7%) consistently proved to be more effective than any of the tested "natural" repellents in their ability to prevent mosquito bites[19] (Figure 32-3).

Alternative Repellents. There has always been great interest in finding an oral insect repellent. Oral repellents would be convenient and would eliminate the need to apply creams to the skin or put on protective clothing. Unfortunately, no effective oral repellent has been discovered. For decades, lay literature has made the claim that Vitamin B_1 (thiamine) works as a systemic mosquito repellent. When subjected to scientific scrutiny, however, thiamine has unanimously been found not to have a repellent effect on mosquitoes.[52,117] The U.S. Food and Drug Administration (FDA), prompted by misleading consumer advertising, issued the following statement in 1983: "There is a lack of adequate data to establish the effectiveness of thiamine or any other ingredient for OTC (over the counter) internal use as an insect repellent. Labeling claims for OTC orally administered insect repellent drug products are either false, misleading, or unsupported by scientific data."[29] Tests of over 100 ingested drugs, including

other vitamins, failed to reveal any that worked well against mosquitoes.[106] Ingested garlic has also never proven to be an effective deterrent.

Insecticides

Permethrin. Pyrethrum is a powerful, rapidly acting insecticide, originally derived from the crushed dried flowers of the daisy *Chrysanthemum cinerariifolium.*[9] Permethrin is a human-made synthetic pyrethroid. It does not repel insects but instead works as a contact insecticide, causing nervous system toxicity, leading to death, or "knockdown," of the insect. The chemical is effective against mosquitoes, flies, ticks, fleas, lice, and chiggers. Permethrin has low mammalian toxicity, is poorly absorbed by the skin, and is rapidly metabolized by skin and blood esterases.[46,119]

Permethrin should be applied directly to clothing or to other fabrics (tent walls[90] or mosquito nets[63]) and not to skin. Permethrins are nonstaining, nearly odorless, resistant to degradation by heat or sun, and will maintain their effectiveness for at least 2 weeks, through several launderings.[92,97]

The combination of permethrin-treated clothing and skin application of a DEET-based repellent creates a formidable barrier against biting insects.[42,54,101] In an Alaskan field trial against mosquitoes, subjects wearing permethrin-treated uniforms and a polymer-based 35% DEET product had greater than 99.9% protection (1 bite/hr) over 8 hours; unprotected subjects were bitten an average of 1188 bites/hr.[58]

Permethrin-sprayed clothing also proved very effective against ticks. One hundred percent of *Dermacentor occidentalis* ticks (which carry Rocky Mountain spotted fever) died within 3 hours of touching permethrin-treated cloth.[56] Permethrin-sprayed pants and jackets also provided 100% protection from all three life stages of *Ixodes dammini* ticks, the vector of Lyme disease.[98] In contrast, DEET alone (applied to the skin) provided 85% repellency at the time of application; this protection deteriorated to 55% repellency at 6 hours, when tested against the Lone Star tick *Amblyomma americanum.*[103] *Ixodes scapularis* ticks, which may transmit Lyme disease, also seem to be less sensitive to the repellent effect of DEET.[93]

Permethrin-based insecticides available in the United States are listed in Table 32-3. To apply to clothing, spray each side of the fabric (outdoors) for 30 to 45 seconds, just enough to moisten it. Allow the fabric to dry for 2 to 4 hours before wearing it. Permethrin solution is also available for soak-treating large items, such as mesh bed nets.

Reducing Local Mosquito Populations

Consumers may still find advertisements for small ultrasonic electronic devices that are meant to be carried on the body and claim to repulse mosquitoes by emit-

TABLE 32-3. Permethrin Insecticides

MANUFACTURER	PRODUCT NAME	FORM(S)	ACTIVE INGREDIENT
Coulston Products Easton, Penn. (610) 253-0167	Duranon Perma-Kill	Aerosol and pump sprays Liquid concentrate	Permethrin 0.5% Permethrin 13.3%
Sawyer Products Tampa, Fla. (800) 940-4464	Permethrin Tick Repellent	Aerosol and pump sprays	Permethrin 0.5%
United Industries Corp. St. Louis, Mo. (800) 767-9927	Cutter Outdoorsman Gear Guard	Aerosol spray	Permethrin 0.5%
Wisconsin Pharmacal Co. Jackson, Wisc. (800) 558-6614	Repel Permanone	Aerosol spray	Permethrin 0.5%

ting "repellent" sounds, such as that of a dragonfly (claimed to be the "natural enemy" of the mosquito), male mosquito, or bat. Multiple studies, conducted both in the field and laboratory, show that these devices do not work.[4,14,31,57] Likewise, mass-marketed backyard bug "zappers," which use ultraviolet light to lure and electrocute insects, are also ineffective: mosquitoes continue to be more attracted to humans than to the devices.[74] One backyard study showed that of the insects killed by these devices, only 0.13% were female (biting) mosquitoes.[33] An estimated 71 to 350 billion beneficial insects may be killed annually in the United States by these devices.[33] Newer technologies, utilizing more specific bait, such as a warm, moist plume of carbon dioxide, as well as other known chemical attractants, may prove to be more successful in luring and selectively killing biting insects. Pyrethrin-containing "yard foggers" set off before an outdoor event can temporarily reduce the number of biting arthropods in a local environment. These products should be applied before any food is brought outside and should be kept away from animals or fish ponds. Burning coils that contain natural pyrethrins or synthetic pyrethroids (such as d-allethrin or d-transallethrin) can also temporarily reduce local populations of biting insects.[65,118] Some concerns have been raised about the long-term cumulative safety of using these coils in an indoor environment.[1,78]

Wood smoke from campfires can also reduce the likelihood of being bitten by mosquitoes. The smoke's ability to repel insects may vary depending on the type of wood or vegetation burned.[77,116]

Integrated Approach to Personal Protection

An integrated approach to personal protection is the most effective way to prevent arthropod bites, regardless of where one is in the world and which species of insects may be attacking. Maximum protection is best achieved through avoiding infested habitats and using protective clothing, topical insect repellents, and per-

methrin-treated garments. When appropriate, mesh bed nets or tents should be used to prevent nocturnal insect bites.

DEET-containing insect repellents are the most effective products currently on the market, providing broad-spectrum, long-lasting repellency against multiple arthropod species. Insect repellents alone, however, should not be relied on to provide complete protection. Mosquitoes, for example, can find and bite any untreated skin and may even bite through thin clothing. Deerflies, biting midges, and some blackflies prefer to bite around the head and will readily crawl into the hair to bite where there is no protection. Wearing protective clothing, including a hat, will reduce the chances of being bitten. Treating one's clothes and hat with permethrin will maximize their effectiveness, by causing "knockdown" of any insect that crawls or lands on the treated clothing. To prevent chiggers or ticks from crawling up the legs, pants should also be tucked into the boots or stockings.

The U.S. military relies on this integrated approach to protect troops deployed in areas where arthropods constitute either a significant nuisance or medical risk. The Department of Defense's Insect Repellent System consists of DEET applied to exposed areas of skin, and permethrin-treated uniforms, worn with the pant legs tucked into boots, and the undershirt tucked into the pant's waistband. This system has been proven to dramatically reduce the likelihood of being bitten by insects.

Persons traveling to parts of the world where insect-borne disease is a potential threat will be best able to protect themselves if they learn about indigenous insects. Protective clothing, mesh insect tents or bedding, insect repellent, and permethrin spray should be carried. Travelers would be wise to check the most current Centers for Disease Control and Prevention (CDC) recommendations about traveling to countries where immunizations (e.g., against yellow fever) or antibiotic prophylaxis (e.g., against malaria) should be undertaken before departure. The CDC maintains these recommendations on its website at www.cdc.gov/travel/index.htm, or by telephone at (888) 232-3228. An excellent summary of information on issues relating to travel health can also be found at www.tripprep.com. This website culls its information daily from the CDC, the *Morbidity and Mortality Weekly Report,* the World Health Organization, and the U.S. State Department.

REFERENCES

1. Achmadi UF, Pauluhn J: Household insecticides: evaluation and assessment of inhalation toxicity: a workshop summary, *Exp Toxicol Pathol* 50:67, 1998.
2. Annis B: Comparison of the effectiveness of two formulations of deet against *Anopheles flavirostris, J Am Mosq Control Assoc* 6:430, 1990.
3. Beaty BJ, Marquardt WC, editors: *The biology of disease vectors,* Niwot, Colo,1996, University Press of Colorado.
4. Belton P: An acoustic evaluation of electronic mosquito repellers, *Mosq News* 41:751, 1981.
5. Bock GR, Cardew G, editors: *Olfaction in mosquito-host interactions,* New York, 1996, John Wiley & Sons.
6. Bowen MF: The sensory physiology of host-seeking behavior in mosquitoes, *Annu Rev Entomol* 36:139, 1991.
7. Brown M, Hebert AA: Insect repellents: an overview, *J Am Acad Dermatol* 36:243, 1997.
8. Busvine JR: *Disease transmission by insects,* New York, 1993, Springer-Verlag.
9. Casida JE, Quistad GB: *Pyrethrum flowers: production, chemistry, toxicology and uses,* Oxford, UK, 1995, Oxford University Press.
10. Chou JT, Rossignol PA, Ayres JW: Evaluation of commercial insect repellents on human skin against *Aedes aegypti* (Diptera: Culicidae), *J Med Entomol* 34:624, 1997.
11. Cilek JE, Schreiber ET: Failure of the "Mosquito Plant," *Pelargonium x Citrosum* 'Van Leenii,' to repel adult *Aedes albopictus* and *Culex quinquefasciatus* in Florida, *J Am Mosq Control Assoc* 10:473, 1994.
12. Clements AN: *The physiology of mosquitoes,* Oxford, UK, 1963, Pergamon Press.
13. Collins DA, Brady JN, Curtis CF: Assessment of the efficacy of quwenling as a mosquito repellent, *Phytotherapy Research* 7:17, 1993.
14. Curtis CF: High frequency radio keeps mosquitoes at bay, *Lancet* 352:992, 1998.
15. Curtis CF et al: The relative efficacy of repellents against mosquito vectors of disease, *Med Vet Entomol* 1:109, 1987.
16. Curtis CF et al: Natural and synthetic repellents. In Curtis CF, editor: *Appropriate technology in vector control,* Boca Raton, Fla, 1990, CRC Press.
17. Davis EE: Insect repellents: concepts of their mode of action relative to potential sensory mechanisms in mosquitoes (Diptera: Culicidae), *J Med Entomol* 22:237, 1985.
18. Davis EE, Bowen MF: Sensory physiological basis for attraction in mosquitoes, *J Am Mosq Control Assoc* 10:316, 1994.
19. Day JF: Personal communication, April 16, 1999, unpublished report, *Efficacy of natural vs. DEET-based repellents,* Florida Medical Entomology Laboratory.
20. deGarbino JP, Laborde A: Toxicity of an insect repellent: *N,N*-diethyltoluamide, *Vet Hum Toxicol* 25:422, 1983.
21. Despommier DD, Gwadz RW, Hotez PJ: *Parasitic diseases,* ed. 3, New York, 1995, Springer-Verlag.
22. Dickens T: Personal communication, September 5, 1999, unpublished report, *Efficacy data on E. Merck 3535, 1976-1979,* USDA Laboratory, Florida.
23. Duke J: USDA Agricultural Research Service Phytochemical and Ethnobotanical Databases, http://www.ars-grin.gov/duke/.
24. Edwards DL, Johnson E: Insect repellent induced toxic encephalopathy in a child, *Clin Pharmacol* 6:496, 1987.
25. Elston DM: What's eating you? Sand flies (Diptera: Psychodidae, Phlebotominae: Lutzomyia, Phlebotomus), *Cutis* 62:164, 1998.
26. Elston DM, Stockwell S: What's eating you? Triatome reduviids, *Cutis* 63:63, 1999.
27. Feller L: Personal communication, May 25, 1999, unpublished report, *Absorption rate of microencapsulated DEET,* Coulston Products.
28. Feller L: Personal communication, July 20, 1999, unpublished report, *Insect repellent test report,* Nomad Traveller's Store.
29. Food and Drug Administration: Drug products containing active ingredients offered over-the-counter (OTC) for oral use as insect repellents, *Fed Red* 48:26987, 1983.
30. Foster WA, Hancock RG: Nectar-related olfactory and visual attractants for mosquitoes, *J Am Mosq Control Assoc* 10:288, 1994.
31. Foster WA, Lutes KI: Tests of ultrasonic emissions on mosquito attraction to hosts in a flight chamber, *J Am Mosq Control Assoc* 1:199, 1985.
32. Fradin MS: Mosquitoes and mosquito repellents: a clinician's guide, *Ann Intern Med* 128:931, 1998.
33. Frick TB, Tallamy DW: Density and diversity of non-target insects killed by suburban electric insect traps, *Ent News* 2:77, 1996.
34. Gabel ML, Spencer TS, Akers WA: Evaporation rates and protection times of mosquito repellents, *Mosq News* 36:141, 1976.
35. Garrettson LK: Commentary—DEET: Caution for children still needed, *J Toxicol Clin Toxicol* 35:443, 1997.
36. Gillies MT: The role of carbon dioxide in host-finding by mosquitoes (Diptera: Culicidae): a review, *Bull Entomol Res* 70:525, 1980.
37. Gillies MT, Wilkes TJ: The range of attraction of animal baits and carbon dioxide for mosquitoes. Studies in a freshwater area of West Africa, *Bull Entomol Res* 61:389, 1972.
38. Gjullin CM: Effect of clothing color on the rate of attack of *Aedes* mosquitoes, *J Econ Entomol* 40:326, 1947.
39. Goddard J: *Physician's guide to arthropods of medical importance,* ed 2, Boca Raton, Fla, 1996, CRC Press.
40. Grainger J, Moore C: *Natural insect repellents for pets, people and plants,* Austin, Tex, 1991, The Herb Bar.
41. Gupta RK, Rutledge LC: Laboratory evaluation of controlled-release repellent formulations on human volunteers under three climatic regimens, *J Am Mosq Control Assoc* 5:52, 1989.
42. Gupta RK et al: Effectiveness of controlled-release personal-use arthropod repellents and permethrin-impregnated clothing in the field, *J Am Mosq Control Assoc* 3:556, 1987.
43. Heal JD, Surgeoner GA: Laboratory evaluation of the efficacy of All Terrain, an essential oil-based product, to repel *Aedes aegypti* mosquitoes, Department of Environmental Biology, University of Guelph, Guelph, Ontario, Canada, 1998.
44. Heick HM et al: Insect repellent, *N,N*-diethyl-toluamide, effect on ammonia metabolism, *Pediatrics* 82:373, 1988.
45. Heick HM et al: Reye-like syndrome associated with use of insect repellent in a presumed heterozygote for ornithine carbamoyl transferase deficiency, *J Pediatr* 97:471, 1980.
46. Insect repellents, *Med Lett Drugs Ther* 31:45, 1989.
47. Jacobson M, editor: *Glossary of plant-derived insect deterrents,* Boca Raton, Fla, 1990, CRC Press.
48. Kettle DS, editor: *Medical and veterinary entomology,* New York, 1982, John Wiley & Sons.
49. Keystone JS: Of bites and body odour, *Lancet* 347:1423, 1996.
50. Khan AA: Mosquito attractants and repellents. In Shorey HH, McKelvey JJ, editors: *Chemical control of insect behavior,* New York, 1977, John Wiley & Sons.
51. Khan AA, Maibach HI, Skidmore DL: A study of insect repellents: effect of temperature on protection time, *J Econ Entomol* 66:437, 1972.
52. Khan AA et al: Vitamin B₁ is not a systemic mosquito repellent in man, *Trans St John's Hosp Dermatol Soc* 55:99, 1969.
53. King WV: Chemicals evaluated as insecticides and repellents at Orlando, Fla. *USDA Agric Handb* 69:1, 1954.
54. Kline DL, Schreck CE: Personal protection afforded by controlled-release topical repellents and permethrin-treated clothing against natural populations of *Aedes taeniorhynchus, J Am Mosq Control Assoc* 5:77, 1989.
55. Knols BG, de Jong R, Takken W: Trapping system for testing olfactory responses of the malarial mosquito *Anopheles gambia* in a wind tunnel, *Med Vet Entomol* 8:386, 1994.
56. Lane RS, Anderson JR: Efficacy of permethrin as a repellent and toxicant for personal protection against the pacific coast tick and the pajaroello tick (Acari: Ixodidae and Argasidae), *J Med Entomol* 21:692, 1984.
57. Lewis DJ, Fairchild WL, Leprince DJ: Evaluation of an electronic mosquito repeller, *Can Entomol* 114:699, 1982.
58. Lillie TH, Schreck CE, Rahe AJ: Effectiveness of personal protection against mosquitoes in Alaska, *J Med Entomol* 25:475, 1988.
59. Lindsay RL, Heal JD, Surgeoner GA: *Comparative evaluation of the efficacy of Bite Blocker, Off! Skintastic, and Avon Skin-So-Soft to protect against* Aedes *species mosquitoes in Ontario,* Guelph, Ontario, Canada, 1996, Department of Environmental Biology, University of Guelph. Sponsored by Chemfree Environment, Inc.

60. Lindsay RL, Heal JD, Surgeoner GA: *Evaluation of Bite Blocker as a repellent against spring* Aedes spp. *mosquitoes,* Guelph, Ontario, Canada, 1996, Department of Environmental Biology, University of Guelph. Sponsored by Chemfree Environment, Inc.

61. Lindsay RL, Surgeoner GA, Heal JD: *Comparative evaluation of the efficacy of Bite Blocker and 20% DEET to repel black flies in Ontario, Canada,* Guelph, Ontario, Canada, 1996, Department of Environmental Biology, University of Guelph. Sponsored by Chemfree Environment, Inc.

62. Lindsay RL et al: Evaluation of the efficacy of 3% citronella candles and 5% citronella incense for protection against field populations of Aedes mosquitoes, *J Am Mosq Control Assoc* 12:293, 1996.

63. Lines JD, Myamba J, Curtis CF: Experimental hut trials of permethrin-impregnated mosquito nets and eave curtains against malaria vectors in Tanzania, *Med Vet Entomol* 1:37, 1987.

64. Lipscomb JW, Kramer JE, Leikin JB: Seizure following brief exposure to the insect repellent N,N-diethyl-m-toluamide, *Ann Emerg Med* 21:315, 1992.

65. Lukwa N, Chandiwana SK: Efficacy of mosquito coils containing 0.3% and 0.4% pyrethrins against *An. gambiae sensu lata* mosquitoes, *Cent Afr J Med* 44:104, 1998.

66. Magnon GJ et al: Repellency of two DEET formulations and Avon Skin-So-Soft against biting midges (Diptera: Ceratopogonidae) in Honduras, *J Am Mosq Control Assoc* 7:80, 1991.

67. Maibach HI, Khan AA, Akers WA: Use of insect repellents for maximum efficacy, *Arch Dermatol* 109:32, 1974.

68. Maibach HI et al: Insects. Topical insect repellents, *Clin Pharmacol Ther* 16:970, 1974.

69. Maibach HI et al: Factors that attract and repel mosquitoes in human skin, *JAMA* 196:263, 1966.

70. Matsuda BM et al: Essential oil analysis and field evaluation of the citrosa plant *"Pelargonium citrosum"* as a repellent against populations of Aedes mosquitoes, *J Am Mosq Control Assoc* 12:69, 1996.

71. McHugh CP: Arthropods: vectors of disease agents, *Lab Med* 25:429, 1994.

72. Mehr ZA et al: Laboratory evaluation of controlled-release insect repellent formulations, *J Am Mosq Control Assoc* 1:143, 1985.

73. Muirhead-Thomson RC: The distribution of anopheline mosquito bites among different age groups, *Br Med J* 1:1114, 1951.

74. Nasci RS, Harris CW, Porter CK: Failure of an insect electrocuting device to reduce mosquito biting, *Mosq News* 43:180, 1983.

75. Osimitz TG, Grothaus RH: The present safety assessment of deet, *J Am Mosq Control Assoc* 11:274, 1995.

76. Osimitz TG, Murphy JV: Neurological effects associated with use of the insect repellent N,N-diethyl-m-toluamide (DEET), *J Toxicol Clin Toxicol* 35:435, 1997.

77. Paru R et al: Relative repellency of woodsmoke and topical applications of plant products against mosquitoes, *P N G Med J* 38:215, 1995.

78. Pauluhn J: Hazard identification and risk assessment of pyrethroids in the indoor environment, *Toxicol Lett* 107:193, 1999.

79. Piesman J: Dynamics of Borrelia burgdorferi transmission by nymphal *Ixodes dammini* ticks, *J Infect Dis* 167:1082, 1993.

80. Piesman J: Dispersal of the Lyme disease spirochete *Borrelia burgdorferi* to salivary glands of feeding nymphal *Ixodes scapularis* (Acari: Ixodidae), *J Med Entomol* 32:519, 1995.

81. Piesman J et al: Duration of tick attachment and *Borrelia burgdorferi* transmission, *J Clin Microbiol* 25:557, 1987.

82. Piesman J et al: Duration of adult female *Ixodes dammini* attachment and transmission of *Borrelia burgdorferi,* with description of a needle aspiration isolation method, *J Infect Dis* 163:895, 1991.

83. Port GR, Boreham PFL: The relationship of host size to feeding by mosquitoes of the *Anopheles gambiae* Giles complex (Diptera: Culicidae), *Bull Entomol Res* 70:133, 1980.

84. Quarles W: Lighted and baited mosquito traps, *Common Sense Pest Control* 12:5, 1996.

85. Quarles W: Botanical mosquito repellents, *Common Sense Pest Control* 12:12, 1996.

86. Rueda LM, Rutledge LC, Gupta RK: Effect of skin abrasions on the efficacy of the repellent DEET against *Aedes aegypti, J Am Mosq Control Assoc* 14:178, 1998.

87. Rutledge LC: Some corrections to the record on insect repellents and attractants, *J Am Mosq Control Assoc* 4:414, 1988.

88. Rutledge LC et al: Comparative sensitivity of representative mosquitoes (Diptera: Culicidae) to repellents, *J Med Entomol* 20:506, 1983.

89. Schoenig GP et al: Absorption, distribution, metabolism, and excretion of N,N-diethyl-m-toluamide in the rat, *Drug Metab Dispos* 24:156, 1996.

90. Schreck CE: Permethrin and dimethyl phthalate as tent fabric treatments against *Aedes aegypti, J Am Mosq Control Assoc* 7:533, 1991.

91. Schreck CE: Protection from blood-feeding arthropods. In Auerbach P, editor: *Wilderness medicine,* ed 3, St Louis, 1995, Mosby.

92. Schreck CE et al: Wear and aging tests with permethrin-treated cotton-polyester fabric, *J Econ Entomol* 73:451, 1980.

93. Schreck CE, Fish D, McGovern TP: Activity of repellents applied to skin for protection against *Amblyomma americanum* and *Ixodes scapularis* ticks (Acari: Ixodidae), *J Am Mosq Control Assoc* 11:136, 1995.

94. Schreck CE, Kline DL: Repellency of two controlled-release formulations of deet against *Anopheles quadrimaculatus and Aedes taeniorhynchus* mosquitoes, *J Am Mosq Control Assoc* 5:91, 1989.

95. Schreck CE, Kline DL, Carlson DA: Mosquito attraction to substances from the skin of different humans, *J Am Mosq Control Assoc* 6:406, 1990.

96. Schreck CE, McGovern TP: Repellents and other personal protection strategies against *Aedes albopictus, J Am Mosq Control Assoc* 5:247, 1989.

97. Schreck CE, Posey K, Smith D: Durability of permethrin as a potential clothing treatment to protect against blood-feeding arthropods, *J Econ Entomol* 71:397, 1978.

98. Schreck CE, Snoddy EL, Spielman A: Pressurized sprays of permethrin or deet on military clothing for personal protection against *Ixodes dammini* (Acari: Ixodidae), *J Med Entomol* 23:396, 1986.

99. Shell ER: Resurgence of a deadly disease, *Atlantic Monthly* 280:45, 1997.

100. Shelov SP, editor: *Caring for your baby and young child: birth to age 5,* New York, 1991, Bantam Books.

101. Sholdt LL et al: Field bioassays of permethrin-treated uniforms and a new extended duration repellent against mosquitoes in Pakistan, *J Am Mosq Control Assoc* 4:233, 1988.

102. Snow WF: The effect of a reduction in expired carbon dioxide on the attractiveness of human subjects to mosquitoes, *Bull Entomol Res* 60:43, 1970.

103. Solberg VB et al: Field evaluation of deet and a piperidine repellent (A13-37220) against *Amblyomma americanum* (Acari: Ixodidae), *J Med Entomol* 32:870, 1995.

104. Sood SK et al: Duration of tick attachment as a predictor of the risk of Lyme disease in an area in which Lyme disease is endemic, *J Infect Dis* 175:996, 1997.

105. Spach DH et al: Tick-borne diseases in the United States, *N Engl J Med* 329:936, 1993.

106. Strauss WG, Maibach HI, Khan AA: Drugs and disease as mosquito repellents in man, *Am J Trop Med Hyg* 17:461, 1968.

107. Surgeoner GA: *Efficacy of Buzz Away Oil against spring Aedes spp. mosquitoes,* Guelph, Ontario, Canada, 1995, Department of Environmental Biology, University of Guelph. Sponsored by Quantum, Inc.

108. Taubes G: A mosquito bites back, *The New York Times Magazine,* pp 40-46, August 24, 1997.

109. Trigg JK: Evaluation of a eucalyptus-based repellent against *Anopheles* spp. in Tanzania, *J Am Mosq Control Assoc* 12:243, 1996.

110. Trigg JK, Hill N: Laboratory evaluation of a eucalyptus-based repellent against four biting arthropods, *Phytotherapy Research* 10:313, 1996.

111. United States Department of Agriculture: Materials evaluated as insecticides, repellents, and chemosterilants at Orlando and Gainesville, Fla., 1952-1964, *USDA Agric Handb* 340:1, 1967.

112. United States Environmental Protection Agency, Offices of Pesticides and Toxic Substances, Special Pesticide Review Division: N,N-diethyl-m-toluamide (Deet) pesticide registration standard (EPA-540/RS-81-004), Washington, DC, 1980, the Agency.

113. United States Environmental Protection Agency, Office of Pesticide Programs, Prevention, Pesticides and Toxic Substances Division: *Reregistration eligibility decision (RED) for oil of citronella* (EPA-738-F-97-002) Washington, DC, 1997, the Agency.

114. United States Environmental Protection Agency, Office of Pesticide Programs, Prevention, Pesticides and Toxic Substances Division: *Reregistration Eligibility Decision (RED): DEET* (EPA-738-F-95-010), Washington, DC, 1998, the Agency.

115. *University of California at Berkeley Wellness Letter: Finally, a safer insect repellent* 13:2, 1997.

116. Vernede R, van Meer M, Alpers MP: Smoke as a form of personal protection against mosquitoes, a study in Papua New Guinea, *Southeast Asian J Trop Med Public Health* 25:771, 1994.

117. Wilson CW, Mathieson DR, Jachowski LA: Ingested thiamine chloride as a mosquito repellent, *Science* 100:147, 1944.

118. Yap HH et al: Field efficacy of mosquito coil formulations containing d-allethrin and d-transallethrin against indoor mosquitos especially *Cules quinquefasciatus* Say, *Southeast Asian J Trop Med Public Health* 21:558, 1990.

119. Young D, Evans S: Safety and efficacy of DEET and permethrin in the prevention of arthropod attack, *Mil Med* 5:324, 1998.

120. Zadikoff CM: Toxic encephalopathy associated with use of insect repellent, *J Pediatr* 95:140, 1979.

33 Tick-Borne Diseases

Douglas A. Gentile and Jason E. Lang

Ticks are familiar pests to those who frequent wilderness or rural areas. They inhabit forests, marshes, deserts, steppes, mountains, and high meadows and have few natural enemies. Most feed on an extremely wide range of hosts, including humans. Ticks are most noted for their high nuisance potential, but they are also efficient vectors for a large number of zoonoses. In fact, ticks transmit a greater variety of infectious agents than any other group of arthropods and run a close second to mosquitoes as vectors of human disease worldwide.[142] In the United States, ticks outrank even mosquitoes as vectors, and tick-borne illnesses constitute an important infectious disease problem, particularly in wilderness and other outdoor recreational areas.

Ticks belong to the class Arachnida, which also includes spiders and scorpions, and they are closely related to mites. Taxonomists divide ticks into two major families: Ixodidae (hard ticks) and Argasidae (soft ticks). Argasid ticks are covered with a leathery integument, and the capitulum (head) is subterminal and not visible from above. Ixodid ticks possess a hard, shield-like scutum, which covers the entire dorsal surface in males but only the anteromedial portion in females (Figure 33-1). The head of ixodid ticks is anterior and visible from above.

Hard ticks have three feeding stages: larva, nymph, and adult. If molting through all stages occurs on the same host, the tick is referred to as a one-host tick. Most Ixodidae are three-host ticks, with each stage feeding on a different host. Hard ticks feed on mammals, reptiles, and birds, and virtually all feed slowly over the course of days. Most take a single adult blood meal, and engorgement with blood is a prerequisite to egg laying. Females may ingest more than 50 times their body weight in blood and other fluids. Ixodid ticks transmit all the major tick-borne diseases in North America, with the exception of relapsing fever.

A typical ixodid life cycle is illustrated by *Dermacentor andersoni*, a major vector for Rocky Mountain spotted fever. The tick hatches as a six-legged larva and actively attaches to a small mammal, often a rodent. After feeding for 3 to 5 days, it drops off and molts to the eight-legged nymph. The nymph hibernates in soil, becoming active again in the spring. After feeding for 4 to 9 days on a larger animal, it again drops off and undergoes a second molt to the adult stage. The mature tick attaches to a third host, on which mating may occur. As with many ticks, *D. andersoni* is capable of surviving for extended periods (more than a year in adults) without a blood meal.

Whereas ixodid ticks are wide ranging, most argasids are nidicolous, or nest loving. Nymph and adult Argasidae generally inhabit the host lair, hiding in cracks and crevices when not feeding. They usually have several nymphal stages (instars), with each stage taking a blood meal. Adults may take several blood meals, feeding rapidly over hours when the host returns.

Although some ticks are host specific, most are opportunists feeding on a variety of hosts. Appendages on the capitulum, the chelicerae, function as piercing and tearing structures, enabling the entire capitulum to be inserted into the host's integument (Figure 33-2). Retrose teeth on the chelicerae help anchor the tick to the host; many ixodid species also secrete a cementlike substance that seals the wound and further secures the attached tick. Salivary glands secrete an anticoagulant, allowing the tick to ingest the host's blood easily.

Tick Envenomation

Ticks cause human disease either by transmitting microorganisms or by secreting toxins or venoms. The nature of most tick toxins is poorly understood. Many appear to be secreted by the tick salivary glands. Some stimulate potent host immune responses; others appear to have direct tissue toxicity. Clinical effects range from localized reactions to anaphylaxis, paralysis, and death.[16]

Local reactions vary from formation of a small pruritic nodule to development of extensive areas of ulceration, erythema, and induration. Lesions may be accompanied by fever, chills, and malaise unrelated to infection. The severity of the reaction varies with both host susceptibility and tick species. A granuloma histologically resembling a lymphoma may develop at the site of a tick bite as long as 6 weeks after the tick is removed.[124] The lesion is believed to be caused by a salivary toxin. Treatment is surgical excision.

Pajaroello Tick Bites

According to local folklore of southern California and Mexico, the bite of the pajaroello tick *Ornithodoros coriaceus* is more feared than the bite of a rattlesnake. In fact, pajaroello bites usually result in a 10 to 30 mm erythematous papule with minimal associated pain and itching. The papule gradually resolves over 3 to 4

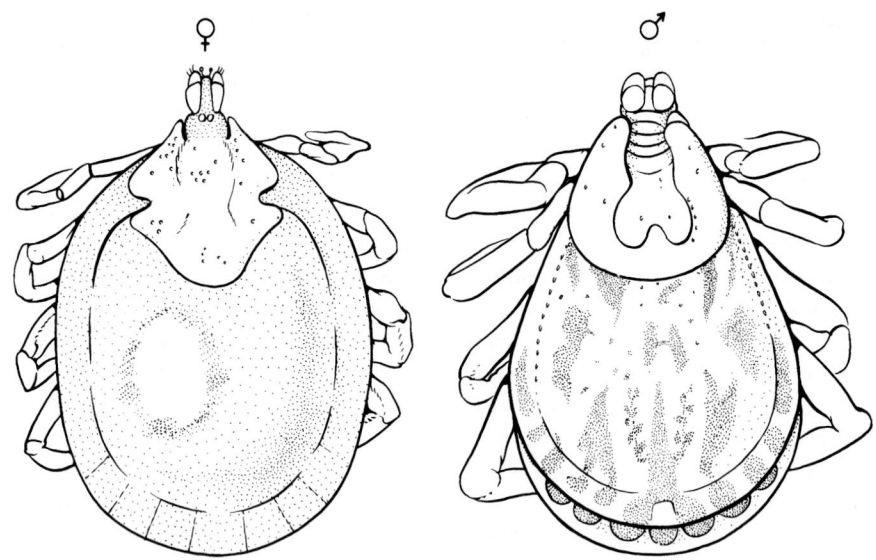

Figure 33-1 Female and male *Dermacentor andersoni*, the tick that causes Rocky Mountain spotted fever.

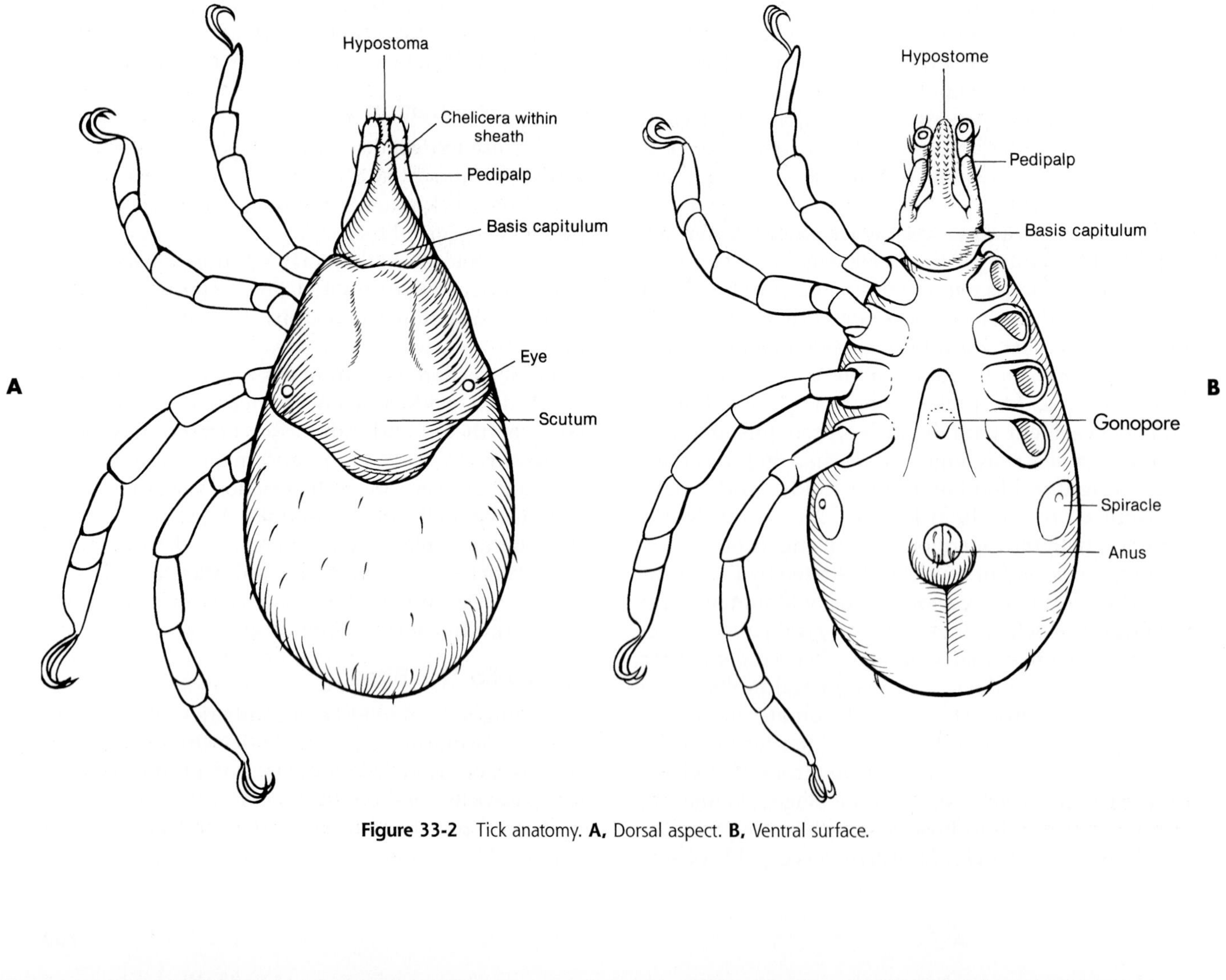

Figure 33-2 Tick anatomy. **A,** Dorsal aspect. **B,** Ventral surface.

weeks. Severe local and systemic reactions have been reported but are rare and probably occur in persons sensitized by previous bites. Local erythema, pain, and edema develop rapidly, followed by tissue necrosis and ulceration. Fever, chills, rigors, and hypotension occur rarely. Severe reactions are probably caused by sensitization to a salivary toxin.[94,114]

Treatment of pajaroello bites includes wound disinfection and administration of tetanus toxoid. The rare severe allergic reaction may require epinephrine, antihistamines, and corticosteroids. When tissue necrosis occurs, excision and primary closure should be considered.

TICK PARALYSIS

As early as 1912, Todd[336] recognized that paralysis occurred in humans and animals after the bite of certain tick species. Tick paralysis has been observed only sporadically in humans since that time but has occasionally constituted a serious veterinary problem.[230] Also known as *tick toxicosis*, tick paralysis is an acute, ascending, flaccid motor paralysis that can appear similar to Guillan-Barré syndrome, botulism, and myasthenia gravis. Although uncommon, familiarity with the clinical features of the disease is important, since prompt diagnosis and removal of the tick are curative.

Tick paralysis has been reported worldwide, but most human cases occur in North America and Australia.[292,360] Forty-three species of ticks, both Ixodidae (hard ticks) and Argasidae (soft ticks), have been reported to cause tick paralysis.[55] Human cases in North America are usually caused by *D. andersoni* or less often *D. variabilis*, although *Amblyomma americanum* (Figure 33-3), *A. maculatum*, and *Ixodes scapularis* have also been implicated.[131] The Pacific Northwest and Rocky Mountain areas account for most cases. In Australia, *Ixodes holocyclus* is primarily associated with the disease, although *I. cornuatus* has been implicated.[132,135]

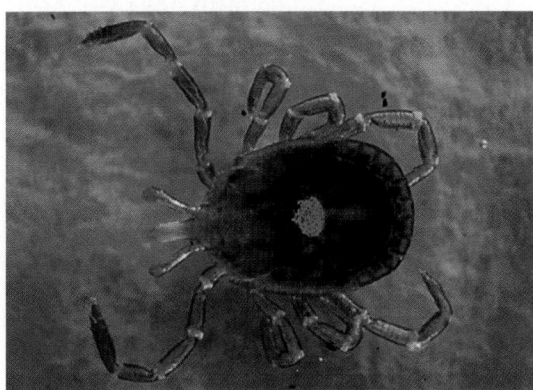

Figure 33-3   Lone star tick *(Amblyomma americanum),* implicated in cases of tick paralysis in North America. *(Courtesy Sherman Minton, MD.)*

Tick paralysis occurs during the spring and summer months (April to June) when nymphs and mature wood ticks are feeding. Children are affected more often than adults, with most cases reported among girls less than 10 years of age. Girls are affected twice as often as boys, probably because ticks on the female scalp are hidden in longer hair.[1] Men account for most of the adult cases, presumably because of increased occupational and recreational exposure to tick habitats.

Tick paralysis in humans develops 5 to 6 days after an adult female tick attaches, usually to the head or neck (male ticks do not cause paralysis). Initially the victim may be restless and irritable and may complain of paresthesias in the hands and feet. Over the ensuing 24 to 48 hours, an ascending, symmetric, and flaccid paralysis develops with loss of deep tendon reflexes. Weakness usually is initially greater in the lower extremities; within 1 to 2 days, severe generalized weakness may develop, accompanied by bulbar and respiratory paralysis. Some victims develop cerebellar dysfunction with incoordination and ataxia.[1,130] Facial paralysis as an isolated finding has occurred in patients with ticks embedded behind the ear.[226] In uncomplicated cases, fever and chills are absent, and the white blood cell (WBC) count and cerebrospinal fluid (CSF) analyses remain normal.

Resolution of paralysis on tick removal establishes the diagnosis. Laboratory aids to diagnosis are not available. In North America, recovery is rapid after removal of the tick, with most victims showing improvement within hours and complete resolution within several days. Undiagnosed, however, tick paralysis may be fatal; mortality in children was 12% in a large Canadian series.[271]

Case reports of Australian tick paralysis suggest that it may be more severe than its North American counterpart. Victims often appear more acutely ill. Paralysis may continue to progress for 48 hours after tick removal, and recovery may be prolonged.[16,17,226] A recent report of six cases in children in Australia however, found little difference in the course between Australian and North American patients.[132]

A neurotoxic venom secreted from the tick salivary glands during a blood meal causes the paralysis. The venom's mechanism of action appears to produce a conduction block in the peripheral branches of motor neurons, diminishing acetylcholine release at the neuromuscular junction.[130,215] Electrophysiologic measurements in humans consistently demonstrate slower motor conduction and reduction in muscle action potential amplitude.[81,212,330] Additionally, the neurotoxin may increase the stimulatory current potential necessary to elicit a response at the motor end plate.[165] A central effect of the toxin has been postulated to explain the cerebellar dysfunction observed in some patients.

After removal of the tick, treatment is supportive. Tick antivenom from hyperimmunized dogs has been developed for Australian tick paralysis and may be beneficial in victims with severe disease, although they have a high incidence of acute allergy and serum sickness.[132,226] The most important aspect of treatment is to consider tick paralysis in any victim with ascending paralysis, then search for and remove the concealed tick.

TICKS AS VECTORS

Ticks transmit a wide variety of infectious agents, all of which cause zoonoses. Ticks may act either as amplifiers or as reservoirs for a given agent.[143] In the agent-tick *amplifier system* the reservoir for the agent is a vertebrate. An immature tick ingests the microorganism while feeding on an infected vertebrate or while feeding concurrently on a vertebrate host with an infected tick. The pathogen replicates in the tick and is passed transstadially, from larval to nymphal to adult stage. The maturing tick transmits the agent to other vertebrate hosts when it feeds. A key epidemiologic feature of this system, transstadial survival of microorganisms, is common in argasid and ixodid ticks but rare in hematophagous insects. This important difference primarily results from the relatively insignificant anatomic changes that occur in the tick during molting.[143]

In the agent-tick *reservoir system*, the microorganism is passed transovarially from one generation of ticks to the next. The agent replicates within the tick and depends solely on the tick population for survival. The agent may also replicate within the vertebrate host of the tick, allowing amplification of the cycle, thereby increasing the density and prevalence of the microorganism.

Table 33-1 lists the major tick-borne diseases in the United States, where Lyme disease, babesiosis, and ehrlichiosis have only recently been recognized. Lyme disease and babesiosis constitute important infectious disease problems in endemic areas, and Lyme disease is now the most common tick-borne illness in the United States and throughout the world. Tularemia and Rocky Mountain spotted fever are observed throughout the United States and continue to produce significant morbidity and mortality. Tick-borne relapsing fever and Colorado tick fever occur in the western states and are particularly likely to affect campers, hikers, hunters, and others who frequent wilderness areas.

Borrelia Infections

Borreliae are bacteria belonging to the order Spirochaetales, which also includes the treponemes and leptospires. *Borrelia* species can be stained with aniline dyes, including routine blood stains such as Wright and Giemsa; this feature allows easy differentiation from the other two genera.[288] Borreliae are helical, actively motile spirochetes, usually 10 to 20 μm long, with three to 10 spirals.[102] Strains cannot be differentiated on the basis of morphology but are classified according to specificity of the tick-spirochete relationship, the range of animals susceptible to infection, and cross-immunity.[19]

TABLE 33-1. Major Tick-Borne Diseases in the United States

DISEASE	ORGANISM	MAJOR VECTORS	GEOGRAPHIC DISTRIBUTION
Lyme disease	*Borrelia burgdorferi*	*Ixodes scapularis,* *I. pacificus*	Coastal mid-Atlantic, northern West Coast, Wisconsin, Minnesota
Rocky Mountain spotted fever	*Rickettsia rickettsii*	*Dermacentor andersoni,* *D. variabilis*	South-central states, coastal southern states
Relapsing fever	*Borrelia hermsii,* *B. turicatae, B. parkeri*	*Ornithodoros hermsi,* *O. turicata, O. parkeri*	Worldwide, most often rural western states
Colorado tick fever	*Orbivirus*	*D. andersoni*	Rocky Mountain states, California, Oregon
Ehrlichiosis	*Ehrlichia chaffeensis*	*Ixodes scapularis?*	Coastal mid-Atlantic states, northern West Coast, Wisconsin, Minnesota
		Amblyomma americanum?	South-central states, coastal southern states
Babesiosis	*Babesia microti*	*Ixodes scapularis*	Coastal southern New England and mid-Atlantic states
Tularemia	*Francisella tularensis*	*A. americanum*	South-central states, Montana, South Dakota

Human *Borrelia* infections occur worldwide, with the possible exception of parts of the southwestern Pacific.[102] All are transmitted by hematophagous arthropods. *Borrelia recurrentis* causes an epidemic form of relapsing fever that is transmitted by the human body louse *Pediculus humanus*. A group of closely related *Borrelia* species causes tick-borne or endemic relapsing fever. A third borrelial disease was recognized in 1982 with the identification of *B. burgdorferi* as the etiologic agent of Lyme disease.

Lyme Disease. An epidemic form of oligoarticular arthritis, originally diagnosed as juvenile rheumatoid arthritis, was recognized in 1975 in the area around Lyme, Connecticut.[308] Subsequent clinical observations revealed a complex, multisystem disorder with dermatologic, cardiac, and neurologic complications. The new disorder was termed Lyme disease.

The rural setting in which most cases occurred, the close geographic and seasonal clustering of cases, and the clinical response to penicillin suggested an arthropod-borne infection. The presence of a distinctive erythematous skin lesion, erythema migrans, preceding the arthritis pointed to a tick vector.[300] Erythema migrans had been observed in Europe since 1910, where it was associated with the bite of the sheep tick *Ixodes ricinus*.[5]

Epidemiologic evidence implicated the deer tick *Ixodes scapularis (dammini)* as the likely vector of Lyme disease. In 1982, Burgdorfer and associates[44] isolated a treponeme-like spirochete, *Borrelia burgdorferi,* from the midgut of *I. scapularis* ticks collected from a known endemic focus of Lyme disease.[28] Subsequently, sera from nine patients clinically diagnosed with Lyme disease yielded high antibody titers to the spirochetes by indirect immunofluorescence.[2] Isolation of *B. burgdorferi* from the blood, CSF, and skin lesions of affected patients finally confirmed the spirochetal etiology of Lyme disease.[26,29,311]

EPIDEMIOLOGY. Lyme disease accounts for more than 90% of all reported vector-borne illnesses in the United States. In 1996 a record 16,461 cases were reported from 45 states, resulting in an overall national incidence of 6.2 per 100,000 population, with 91% of cases in eight states[59] (Box 33-1).

Nantucket County, Massachusetts, reported the highest county-specific incidence nationally with 1247.5 cases per 100,000. The highest proportion of cases occurred in the age groups 0 to 14 years (3784, or 23%) and 40 to 79 (7694, or 47%), with males making up 53% of the gender-reported cases. About 80% of cases occur from May to August, with peak incidence in July.

A cross-sectional survey of 1200 physicians in Maryland revealed that Lyme disease may be greatly underreported, with less than 10% of cases meeting the Centers for Disease Control and Prevention (CDC) diagnostic criteria.[51,66] CDC criteria for Lyme disease include presence of an erythema migrans rash 5 cm or greater in diameter or laboratory confirmation of infection with evidence of at least one manifestation of musculoskeletal, neurologic, or cardiovascular disease. Campbell and associates[51] also found several fold underreporting using a nine-component deterministic model.

The principal vectors of Lyme disease are several closely related ticks of the genus *Ixodes*. The deer tick *I. scapularis (dammini)* is the best documented vector; its geographic distribution correlates with endemic foci of Lyme disease in the northeastern and Midwestern United States.[272,312,351] The range of *I. scapularis* extends from the northeastern United States to the southeastern states. The northern form of *I. scapularis* was originally thought to be a separate species and was named *Ixodes dammini*. Subsequent studies demonstrated mating compatibility and genetic similarity, however, and the two forms are now considered to be the same species.[19] The southern form of *I. scapularis* appears to be responsible for Lyme disease cases in the southeastern United States.[43,232]

Northern *I. scapularis* larvae, abundant in late summer and fall, and nymphs, numerous in spring and summer, are aggressive and parasitize a number of vertebrate species.[43] The preferred host is the deer mouse *Peromyscus leucopus*, which serves as an important reservoir for *B. burgdorferi*.[33,289,297] Transovarial transmission in ticks occurs but appears to be unusual.[40] Adult *I. scapularis* ticks, abundant in spring and fall, have a narrow host range, feeding primarily on deer, which are key hosts in the life cycle of the tick (Figure 33-4). The high incidence of Lyme disease in the northeastern United States has been linked to increases in the deer population.[316,363] In some focal endemic areas, up to 60% of *I. scapularis* ticks are infected with *B. burgdorferi*, and tick populations may be high, even on well-kept lawns.[95]

A third endemic focus in the United States has been identified on the West Coast (California and Oregon),

Box 33-1 INCIDENCE OF LYME DISEASE, 1996 (RATE PER 100,000 POPULATION)	
Connecticut	94.8
Rhode Island	53.9
New York	29.2
New Jersey	27.4
Delaware	23.9
Pennsylvania	23.3
Maryland	8.8
Wisconsin	7.7

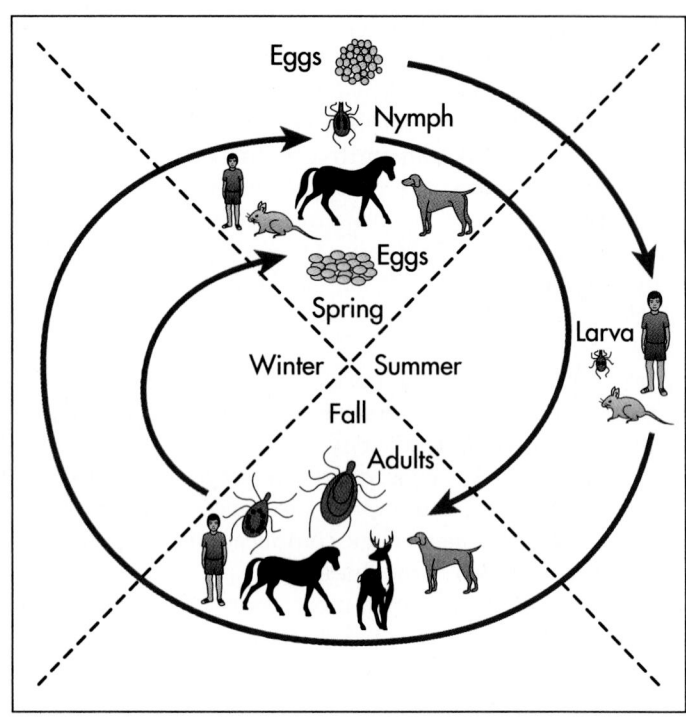

Figure 33-4 Life cycle of *Ixodes scapularis*. The cycle of ixodid ticks typically spans 2 years and includes three blood meals in the spring. The adult female tick releases her eggs, which hatch as six-legged larvae; during the summer, the larvae take a blood meal that lasts approximately 2 days. Larval ticks then enter a dormant phase with cooler fall weather. The ticks then molt in the spring, entering the second phase of their life cycle as eight-legged nymphal ticks. In the late spring or summer, nymphal ticks take a blood meal that typically lasts for 2 to 3 days. The nymphal ticks then molt as eight-legged adults in the fall. The adults mate on white-tailed deer; after mating the male dies, but the female takes one more blood meal before she lays her eggs and dies. *(Modified from Habicht et al: Sci Am 257:78, 1987.)*

where the vector is the western black-legged tick *Ixodes pacificus*, another member of the *I. ricinus* complex. The zoonotic transmission cycle for *I. pacificus* differs from *I. scapularis*, as evidenced by only 1.5% of *I. pacificus* surveyed in northern California and southwestern Oregon being infected with *B. burgdorferi*, a fraction too small to maintain an animal reservoir.[45] In addition, the major hosts for immature *I. pacificus* are species of lizards, which are not competent hosts for *B. burgdorferi*.[175] Instead, the enzootic cycle is maintained by a second tick, *Ixodes neotomae*, which does not bite humans.[18] Up to 15% of *I. neotomae* ticks are infected with *B. burgdorferi*, which is enough to maintain endemic disease. The primary host for *I. neotomae* is *Neotoma fuscipes*, the dusky-footed wood rat, which is a competent reservoir for *B. burgdorferi*.[37] Larval *I. pacificus* ticks feed on a variety of vertebrates and become infected when they feed on *N. fuscipes*. Transmission to humans may then occur from an infected nymph or adult.

Cases of Lyme disease in states outside the range of *I. scapularis* and *I. pacificus* suggest that additional vectors are involved. Ticks from five genera (*Amblyomma, Dermacentor, Haemaphysalis, Ixodes, Rhipicephalus*) and other arthropods, such as mosquitoes, horseflies, and deerflies, are naturally infected with *B. burgdorferi*, but only members of the *I. ricinus* complex appear to be competent vectors for the disease.[172,186,214,232] Investigators have found an uncultivable spirochete in *Amblyomma americanum* ticks, leading to speculation that a related borrelial species is causing a Lyme disease–like

illnesses in the southeastern and south-central United States.

Lyme disease or similar syndromes also occur in Europe, Asia, and Australia. Garin and Bujadoux[116] in France recognized as early as 1922 that neurologic abnormalities occasionally followed erythema migrans. This symptom complex has been described variously as Bannwarth's syndrome, tick-borne meningopolyneuritis, and meningopolyneuritis. The neurologic features include intense radicular pains, chronic lymphocytic meningitis, and peripheral nervous system involvement, particularly facial palsies. The full description of Lyme disease in the United States has led to the recognition of other erythema migrans–associated manifestations (arthritis and cardiac symptoms) in Europe.[121,261,353] Patients with these European diseases (arthritis, carditis, meningoradiculitis) demonstrate increased antibody titers against *B. burgdorferi*.[156,269,321]

The established vector for European erythema migrans, *I. ricinus*, is closely related to the common vectors for Lyme disease in the United States, *I. scapularis* and *I. pacificus*, and the major reservoirs in Europe are species of rodents.[197] Areas of central Europe recently reported that more than 40% of *I. ricinus* ticks are infected by *B. burgdorferi*.[323] *B. burgdorferi* isolated from *I. ricinus* shows minor differences from U.S. strains in morphology, outer surface proteins, plasmids, and deoxyribonucleic acid (DNA) homology.[2,260,298] As a result, *B. burgdorferi* is now di-

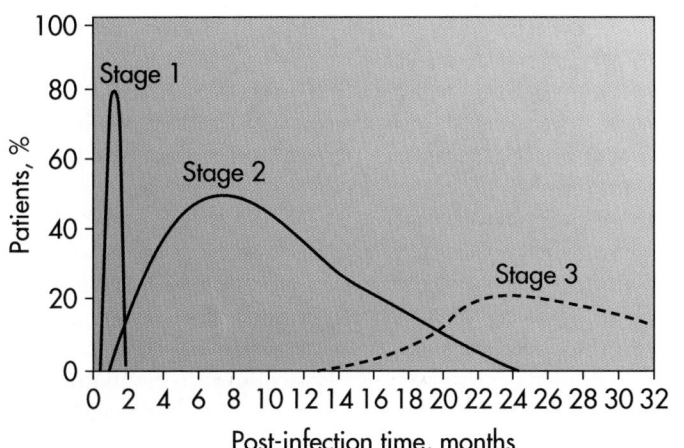

Figure 33-5 Time course and frequency of symptoms. Approximately 50% of victims report recent tick bite. The initial stage I symptoms occur in approximately 70% to 80% of infected individuals. Weeks after the initial tick bite the skin, nervous system, and joints are most often affected as the spirochete spreads hematogenously. Stage II symptoms typically begin 4 to 10 weeks after the initial infection and occur in approximately 50% of untreated patients. Stage III typically starts much later, often 1½ to 2 years and rarely more than 5 years after initial infection. *(Modified from Schmid GP: Rev Infect Dis 11(suppl 6):51460, 1989.)*

vided into three strains: *B. burgdorferi sensu stricto, Borrelia afzelli,* and *B. garinii.*[323] North American isolates are limited to *B. burgdorferi sensu stricto,* but all three strains are found in Europe. These strain variations likely account for differences in clinical manifestations and serologic response between North American and European cases.

Lyme disease cases have also been reported from China, Japan, and Russia, where the principal vector is *Ixodes persulcatus,* and from Australia in the Hunter Valley[320] and along the New South Wales coast.[198] No ticks of the *I. ricinus* complex have been found in Australia, suggesting that other vectors are likely to be identified.

Spirochetal development in most ticks is limited to the midgut, but the organisms disseminate during feeding and appear in saliva, providing the likely mechanism for disease transmission.[33,253] This phenomenon also explains the relationship between duration of tick feeding and *B. burgdorferi* transmission. In one study, nymphal *I. scapularis* transmitted *B. burgdorferi* to one of 14 rodents exposed for 24 hours, five of 14 rodents exposed for 48 hours, and 13 of 14 rodents exposed for 72 hours.[233] A study of persons with tick bites investigated disease progression, as diagnosed by development of erythema migrans, seroconversion on enzyme immunoassay (EIA) and immunoblot, or both. Using the established scutal index to determine length of tick engorgement, investigators found that female and nymph ticks attached for greater than 72 hours were much more likely to induce Lyme disease than ticks attached less than 72 hours.[287]

Although all three stages of the tick may bite humans, the nymph is primarily responsible for transmission of Lyme disease.[312] The small size of nymphs accounts for only 30% of patients with Lyme disease recalling a tick bite.

Box 33-2 LYME DISEASE: STAGE I

Incubation: 7-10 days (range, 3-32 days)
Duration: 28 days (range, 1-14 months)

SYMPTOMS (INCIDENCE)

Erythema migrans (60%-89%)
Mild lymphadenopathy (23%)
Low-grade fever (19%-39%)
Mild fatigue and malaise (54%)
Neck stiffness (35%)
Mild arthralgia and myalgia (44%)

CLINICAL MANIFESTATIONS. Lyme disease is multisystemic and multiphasic. It can be divided into three stages based on chronologic relation to the original tick bite, with different clinical manifestations at each stage (Figure 33-5). The disorder usually begins as a localized infection with erythema migrans and associated symptoms (stage I; Box 33-2).[120,218] Within days to weeks, spirochetes may disseminate through blood or lymph, and neurologic, cardiac, or joint abnormalities may develop (stage II). Finally, chronic, persistent infection (stage III) of the joints, nervous system, skin, or eyes may occur months to years after the onset of Lyme disease. Clinical expression, however, may vary greatly. Incomplete disease presentations occur, and virtually any clinical feature may be present in isolation or recur at intervals, complicating clinical diagnosis.

Although the exact roles of the infecting spirochete, spirochetal antigens, and host immune responses are unclear, tissue invasion and persistence of infection probably cause many later manifestations of Lyme disease. This concept is supported by the isolation of

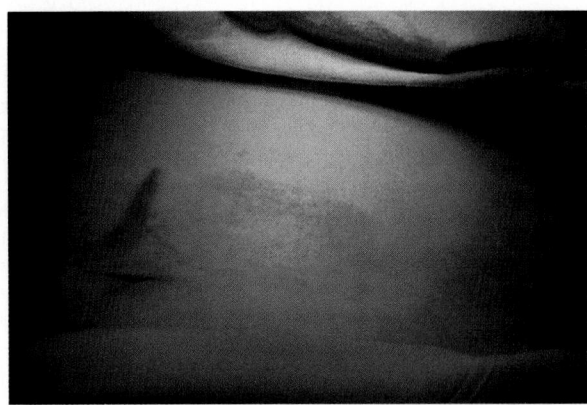

Figure 33-6 Erythema migrans rash of Lyme disease in a pregnant female. *(Paul Auerbach, MD.)*

B. burgdorferi from blood, skin lesions (erythema migrans), and CSF.[28,311] The organism has also been identified in the eye,[314] myocardium,[190] and synovium.[285] Patients at all stages of disease respond to appropriate antimicrobial therapy, and early treatment generally leads to an excellent long-term prognosis.

Stage I: early localized. Erythema migrans is the most characteristic clinical manifestation of Lyme disease (Figure 33-6). An average of 7 to 10 days (range, 3 to 32 days) after inoculation from a tick bite, *B. burgdorferi* spreads locally in the skin, producing an expanding, annular, and erythematous lesion. Initially a central red macule or papule forms at the site. As the lesion expands, partial central clearing may be seen, particularly in larger lesions, whereas the outer borders remain bright red. The borders are usually flat but may be raised and indurated. The center of some early lesions becomes intensely red and indurated or may even become vesicular or necrotic. In some cases, multiple red rings form within the outside margin, or the central area turns blue before clearing. The lesion often reaches a diameter of 15 cm (range, 3 to 68 cm), increasing in size as much as 1 centimeter per day. Erythema migrans may appear anywhere on the body. In cases with a single erythema migrans lesion, the most common sites include the head and neck region (26%), extremities (25%), back (24%), abdomen (9%), axilla (8%), groin (5%), and chest (3%).[120] Erythema migrans is usually warm to the touch and often described by the patient as burning, but occasionally as itching or painful.

Constitutional symptoms may accompany erythema migrans but are usually mild and consist of regional lymphadenopathy, fever, and malaise. Fever is usually low grade but can reach 40° C (104° F) and is more common in children than adults. Lymphadenopathy is typically localized, related to the erythema migrans lesion, but can be generalized.

Erythema migrans fades after an average of 3 to 4 weeks (range, 1 to 14 weeks) without treatment; with antibiotics the lesion resolves after several days. Recurrent lesions may develop 1 to 14 months after the initial lesion in victims who do not receive antibiotic therapy, appearing as erythema migrans, secondary lesions, or both. Rarely, evanescent small red circles and blotches may develop. Patients treated with appropriate antibiotics rarely have recurrent skin lesions.[310]

Retrospective reviews typically note erythema migrans in 60% to 80% of patients with Lyme disease, but a prospective longitudinal cohort study of more than 200 children and an adult prospective population-based study reported erythema migrans in almost 90% of patients.[52,120,295]

It is important to differentiate erythema migrans from local tick bite reactions, insect and spider bites, tinea, cellulitis, and plant dermatitis. Unfortunately, only a minority of victims recall a tick bite. Annular erythematous lesions occurring hours after a tick bite represent hypersensitivity reactions, not erythema migrans. In addition, a rash that resolves in 48 hours is unlikely to be Lyme disease. Biopsy of erythema migrans shows dermal and epidermal involvement at the center, but only dermal changes in the periphery, which are findings suggestive of an arthropod bite.[310]

Although erythema migrans is highly suggestive of Lyme disease, it is not pathognomonic. A study of rashes in the southern United States that clinically resembled erythema migrans found little association serologically or microbiologically with *Borrelia burgdorferi* infection. Many of these rashes were associated with bites from the *Amblyomma americanum* tick, which have recently been found to be infected by *Borrelia lonestarii sp nov.* Currently, no known association exists among *A. americanum, B. lonestarii,* and a Lyme disease–like illness.[50]

Stage II: early disseminated. Within days or weeks after infection, the *B. burgdorferi* may spread from the skin to other organs through the blood or lymph. During this stage, spirochetes can be recovered from the blood. *B. burgdorferi* probably spreads initially to all organs, but like its spirochetal cousin *Treponema pallidum* (syphilis), it appears to sequester in certain niches.[298]

During the hematogenous spread of early disseminated disease, the most common manifestation seen is multiple erythema migrans. These annular secondary skin lesions develop in 20% to 50% of patients in the United States. The secondary lesions are generally smaller, migrate less, and lack indurated centers. They may be located anywhere except the palms

migrans, although patients may present with stage III disease as the initial manifestation of Lyme disease. The skin, joints, and nervous system are most often affected.

Chronic arthralgias and oligoarthritis develop in about 50% of untreated patients.[306] In about 10% of adult patients with arthritis the knees or other large joints become chronically involved, as seen radiographically. Juxtaarticular osteoporosis, cartilage loss, cortical or marginal bone erosions, and joint effusions may be seen. Features of degenerative arthritis, cartilage loss, subarticular sclerosis, and osteophytosis are found less often.[175] Patients usually do not have continual joint inflammation for more than several years, and recurrences tend to become progressively milder.[303] Rheumatoid and antinuclear antibodies are generally absent,[307] although the incidence of B cell alloantigens DR2 and DR4 appears to be increased in patients with chronic Lyme arthritis.[301] The chronic form is unusual in children.[119]

Patients with Lyme disease may develop persistent nervous system involvement months to years after becoming infected. Several distinct but often overlapping syndromes have been described. The best established syndrome is a severe, progressive encephalomyelitis characterized clinically by spastic paraparesis, cerebellar ataxia, cognitive impairment, bladder dysfunction, transverse myelitis, hemiparesis, and cranial neuropathy, particularly of the seventh and eighth cranial nerves.[3] CSF examination typically shows a lymphocytic pleocytosis and intrathecal production of anti–*B. burgdorferi* antibody. Magnetic resonance imaging of the brain may show abnormalities of the white matter. Among seropositive persons, boys seem to develop neurologic symptoms more than girls.

Chronic involvement of the peripheral nervous system also occurs in Lyme disease. Patients may have painless distal paresthesias or painful radiculopathy. The distal paresthesias are generally intermittent, are often symmetric, and involve the legs more frequently than the upper extremities. Radicular pain is more frequently asymmetric and may involve the cervical, thoracic, or lumbosacral segments, often in combination. The pain is typically spinal with radiation into the affected limbs or trunk.[179] Nerve conduction and electromyographic studies suggest a mild axonal polyneuropathy with reductions in motor or sensory nerve conduction velocities and denervation of spinal and limb muscles.[180] The underlying pathophysiologic mechanism appears to be mononeuritis multiplex.[105]

Rarely, patients with neuroborreliosis may have strokes, seizures, or severe dementia.[97] Several syndromes have also been described in which the association with infection by *B. burgdorferi* is less certain. Some patients with serologic evidence of infection develop mild encephalopathy with memory difficulties, depression, mood swings, language disturbances, and fatigue. These patients may or may not have increased intrathecal production of antibodies to *B. burgdorferi*, although some do show improvement with antibiotic treatment.[179] The syndromes termed postborreliosis disorders are more problematic. After treatment for Lyme disease, many patients note persistent fatigue, sleep disorders, depression, or cognitive difficulties. The cause is unknown, and patients do not respond to antibiotics.[105]

Acrodermatitis chronica atrophicans is the best example of prolonged latency followed by persistent infection in Lyme disease. Observed primarily in Europe where the causative organism is *B. afzelli*, the dermatitis may develop years after the onset of illness.[216,298] It begins with an inflammatory phase with bluish red discoloration, often at the site of a previous erythema migrans lesion, preferentially involving the extensor surfaces of the extremities. The inflammatory phase may persist for years or decades, with gradual conversion to atrophy of the skin.[11] After initial hyperpigmentation, hypopigmentation develops, and eventually the skin becomes frail. One third of patients have an associated (usually sensory) polyneuropathy.

Other, unusual late manifestations of Lyme disease include recurrent hepatitis, myositis, eosinophilic lymphadenitis, and ARDS. Several patients with a history of Lyme disease developed a keratitis similar to syphilitic keratitis years after their initial infection.[298] Late Lyme disease occurs infrequently in children.[370]

The roles of persistent infection with *B. burgdorferi* immune mechanisms in late Lyme disease remain unclear. PCR studies show *B. burgdorferi* in joint fluid and CSF of untreated patients with late Lyme disease. After antibiotic therapy, PCR studies may be negative, although inflammation persists within involved joints, especially in patients with HLA-DR4 B-cell alloantigens. [221] Immune mechanisms may also play a role in chronic neurologic disease.

LYME DISEASE DURING PREGNANCY. Lyme disease during pregnancy historically has been of considerable concern because other spirochetes, the treponemes, cause significant congenital infection. The risk of fetal and postnatal complications of Lyme disease during pregnancy require further study, but human transplacental transmission of *B. burgdorferi* has been documented.[184,193,268,354] In each case the infant was either stillborn or died shortly after birth; one mother had been treated with oral penicillin for Lyme disease early in pregnancy.[354] However, fetal infection appears to be rare. In a report of 19 pregnancies complicated by Lyme disease, five had an adverse outcome, although several were minor with no permanent sequelae, and no two outcomes were the same. *B. burgdorferi* infection was not documented in any fetus or neonate, and disease exposure earlier in pregnancy was not associated with increased adverse outcome.[193] Serologic surveys in endemic areas also suggest a low but real risk of fetal transmission. One survey of 2014 pregnant women in Westchester County, New York, showed 0.7% seropositivity, with no significant difference in obstetric outcomes between seropositive and seronegative mothers.[327] In a second report comparing serologic status, 8% of neonates from endemic areas were seropositive for *B. burgdorferi* from cord blood sampling, compared with only 0.8% in infants from nonendemic regions. All neonates with positive serology showed an immunoglobulin (IgG) response, but none had elevated *B. burgdorferi* IgM antibodies. Neonates from the endemic region had fewer malformations but a significantly increased rate of cardiac malformations compared with the non-endemic group.[361]

Despite the increase in Lyme disease, the risk of adverse outcome during pregnancy remains low. No clear association exists between Lyme disease and congenital anomalies, and no distinct pattern of teratogenicity has been identified. The risk of transplacental transmission appears minimal, and currently, no published data support a congenital Lyme disease syndrome.

Despite the relatively low risk, women who acquire Lyme disease during pregnancy should be treated promptly with antibiotics. A 1996 prospective study of 58 pregnant women with erythema migrans given oral or intravenous (IV) penicillin or ceftriaxone reported only seven adverse outcomes, unrelated and none clearly associated with Lyme disease.[188] Although no randomized trials have compared oral with parenteral therapy during pregnancy, the American College of Obstetrics and Gynecology (ACOG) recommends oral penicillin or amoxicillin for three weeks in patients with early localized disease or those with recent deer tick bites. For patients with severe acute disease, neurologic sequelae, or chronic disseminated disease, the ACOG recommends IV therapy with penicillin.[8] Others also recommend IV penicillin, 20 million units/day in divided doses for 10 to 14 days.[354] In patients allergic to penicillin, erythromycin (500 mg four times daily) is an alternative. Ceftriaxone has also been recommended.[216] Pregnant or lactating women should not receive tetracyclines.

DIAGNOSIS. The diagnosis of early Lyme disease is best made using careful consideration of clinical and epidemiologic data. According to the CDC surveillance criteria, the clinical diagnosis includes exposure to an endemic region by a patient presenting with erythema migrans and accompanying generalized symptoms. Diagnosis with early disease does not require laboratory confirmation. However, incomplete cases without erythema migrans may prove difficult to diagnose, presenting as a viral-like illness.[99] Arthritis or neurologic involvement may develop months after the cutaneous eruption, which the patient may not remember. Most patients do not recall a tick bite. The confirmation of late disease requires clinical evidence of disseminated disease plus laboratory evidence of infection.

Routine laboratory studies add little to the early diagnosis of Lyme disease and should not be used as a screening tool in healthy persons. Most patients have a mildly elevated erythrocyte sedimentation rate (ESR), gamma-glutamyltransferase (GGT), aspartate transaminase (AST, SGOT), and alanine transaminase (ALT, SGPT), and decreased absolute WBC count. Some patients have mild anemia. Immunoglobulins A and G are usually normal, whereas IgM may be elevated, especially in severe and neurologic or arthritic disease.

Positive culture for *B. burgdorferi* is the best laboratory evidence of causality but is difficult to obtain. Skin culture may be useful in patients in whom primary erythema migrans lesions are suspected. Saline lavage–needle aspiration and 2-mm punch biopsy of the leading edge of a suspected erythema migrans lesion obtain spirochetes in 29% and 60% of samples, respectively.[371] In specialized laboratories, the success rate of skin biopsy may be as high as 80%.[29] Biopsy from other areas is typically unsuccessful.

Other tests to detect *B. burgdorferi* infection lack sensitivity or are primarily research tools. Direct visualization techniques have yields too low to be clinically useful and are difficult to distinguish from elastin tissue fibers, procollagen fibers, and other artifacts.[279] Urine antigen testing lacks sensitivity. PCR technology amplifies genomic and nongenomic gene sequences of *B. burgdorferi* from tissue samples and can be used as a surrogate to culture. DNA sequences can be detected in blood, urine, CSF, skin, and synovial fluid of patients with Lyme disease. PCR testing is promising but is not standardized and has large interlaboratory variability. Accordingly, routine use of PCR is not currently recommended for the diagnosis of Lyme disease. This leaves detecting indirect evidence of infection—antibodies to *B. burgdorferi*—as the only practical laboratory aid to diagnosis.

Unfortunately, antibody response to *B. burgdorferi* develops slowly. Serologic studies are usually negative in the first 3 to 6 weeks of illness, particularly in patients with limited manifestations. However, patients with complicated Lyme disease (neurologic, cardiac, or joint involvement) or those in remission typically have elevated specific antibody titers.[206,279] IgM antibody titers generally peak between the third and sixth weeks after the onset of illness; IgG antibody titers rise slowly and are highest weeks to months later when arthritis is present. Early treatment with antibiotics may blunt or completely suppress antibody formation. Both IgM and IgG antibodies may persist for months or years after clinical resolution, even after treatment with appropriate antibiotics.[98] Also, patients with early disseminated

Lyme disease (carditis, meningitis, neuropathy) may be seronegative.

Current methods for detecting antibodies to *B. burgdorferi* include indirect immunofluorescent assay (IFA), enzyme-linked immunosorbent assay (ELISA), and Western blot or immunoblot. In most laboratories, ELISA appears to be the test of choice for evaluation of suspected Lyme disease (89% sensitivity, 72% specificity), although IFA can be comparable when performed by experienced technicians.[125,340] Western blot is often used as the second test in a two-test protocol to increase the specificity of serologic testing by demonstrating the presence of antibodies to epitopes that are unique to *B. burgdorferi*.[85] Western blot's particular usefulness lies in identifying false-positive results. Because a positive ELISA result is usually statistically defined as a value two standard deviations above the mean, approximately 5% of the normal population will have a "false-positive" result. Consequently, according to the CDC national consensus panel, positive results from serologic testing are significant only if both ELISA and Western blot are positive. False-positive results are also common in patients with other treponemal diseases (syphilis, yaws, and pinta), leptospirosis, relapsing fever, viral infections (varicella), and autoimmune diseases such as systemic lupus erythematosus (SLE).[206] Patients with Lyme disease, however, do not have positive Venereal Disease Research Laboratories (VDRL) tests. In addition, antibodies directed toward oral flora may cross-react, causing false-positive results.[206,252]

The importance of appreciating the limitations of serologic testing cannot be overstated. Considerable caution must be exercised in interpreting test results. In one study, only 23% of patients referred to the Lyme Disease Clinic at New England Medical Center had active Lyme disease, and a majority of those without Lyme disease had been treated inappropriately with antibiotics.[304] In this study, the most common reason for lack of response to antibiotics was misdiagnosis. The limitations of laboratory testing in Lyme disease include lack of sensitivity and specificity of serologic tests and considerable interlaboratory and intralaboratory variability in test results.[274] The persistence of antibodies in patients with past or asymptomatic infection with *B. burgdorferi* also complicates serologic testing. If another illness develops, as occurred in 20% of patients referred to the New England Medical Center clinic, it may be incorrectly attributed to Lyme disease. This is particularly problematic in patients with nonspecific symptoms of chronic fatigue or fibromyalgia, in whom the predictive value of a positive ELISA is low.

The overdiagnosis of Lyme disease has significant health system and patient care implications. In a study of 209 individuals referred to a university-based Lyme disease clinic with a diagnosis of the disease, only 21% met criteria for active Lyme disease, 60% had no evidence of current or previous infection, and 19% had evidence of previous but not active disease. The 79% of patients without active Lyme disease displayed significant anxiety and stress related to their diagnosis of Lyme disease, used considerable health care resources, and had frequent adverse antibiotic reactions.[249]

Diagnosis of Lyme disease requires careful consideration of epidemiologic and clinical information, supplemented by serologic testing when appropriate. For greatest cost-effectiveness, testing by serologic means should be guided by a patient's pretest likelihood of disease, taking into account exposure history, endemicity, and clinical signs and symptoms. Only 1.2% of tick bites in endemic regions result in erythema migrans.[340] For patients in nonendemic areas and with nonspecific symptoms, the pretest probability of Lyme disease is low, and these patients should not be referred for laboratory testing. Likewise, even patients from endemic areas who only present with nonspecific symptoms (e.g., fatigue, headache, myalgias, arthralgias, palpitations) have a low pretest probability and should not be referred for serologic testing. Serologic testing is most useful in patients with an intermediate pretest probability of having Lyme disease (20% to 80%). Serologic testing should be done in a reference laboratory and confirmed with a Western blot.

In patients from endemic areas who have erythema migrans, serologic tests are not indicated because the pretest probability of Lyme disease is very high; a negative serologic test is likely to be a false negative. Many patients with localized Lyme disease have not developed antibodies at the time of testing, especially if drawn within 2 weeks of symptom onset. These patients should be assumed to have Lyme disease, whether or not serologic tests are positive, and treated empirically. Convalescent titers are not helpful, since early antibiotic treatment may prevent seroconversion. Uncertainty about a lesion being erythema migrans demands careful observation. A lesion that resolves in 1 to 2 days, that does not expand centrifugally, or that is less than 5 cm in diameter is unlikely to be erythema migrans.[118] If Lyme probability appears intermediate after considering the factors of exposure, tick history, and clinical manifestations, the two-step ELISA and Western blot testing is recommended.

Most patients with symptoms of early disseminated or late Lyme disease have positive serologic tests. If clinical and epidemiologic data strongly support the diagnosis of Lyme disease, however, antibiotic treatment is appropriate even with negative findings, since some patients will not have seroconverted. Although patients with symptoms of central nervous system (CNS) involvement often undergo CSF testing for *B. burgdorferi* antibodies, this is not always necessary.[118] The CDC surveillance criteria require diagnostic levels of IgM or IgG antibodies to *B. burgdorferi* in serum or CSF.

Because almost all neuroborreliosis patients have positive serum serologies, CSF testing is not required to diagnose Lyme disease. As noted, a positive test does not establish the diagnosis of Lyme disease but merely indicates that infection has likely occurred in the past. Because immunoglobulins can persist in the serum for years after clinical improvement, serology testing has no role in measuring treatment response. The sensitivity and specificity of T-cell recognition of *B. burgdorferi* antigens are controversial.[298,340]

In patients with isolated nonspecific symptoms such as chronic fatigue, transient musculoskeletal pain, or difficulty concentrating, Lyme serologic tests should not be performed. These symptoms are rarely if ever the sole manifestation of Lyme disease. The pretest probability of Lyme disease in this situation is so low that a positive test is likely to be a false positive.

TREATMENT. Most manifestations of Lyme disease will resolve without treatment; however, appropriate antibiotic therapy hastens resolution in all stages of disease and prevents later complications.[264,312] *B. burgdorferi* is highly sensitive to tetracycline, aminopenicillins, ceftriaxone, and imipenem, both in vitro and in vivo.[151-153] Alternative antimicrobials include penicillin (unlike *Treponema pallidum*, however, *B. burgdorferi* is only moderately susceptible), oxacillin, chloramphenicol, macrolides, and several newer oral cephalosporins. Both cefixime and cefuroxime appear to have equal efficacy to standard therapy.[6,153] Cefuroxime axetil and possibly azithromycin have been found comparable with doxycycline in a clinical trial in patients with early Lyme disease.[183,217,299] Erythromycin also has good in vitro activity but is not as effective as amoxicillin or doxycycline in vivo. Aminoglycosides, sulfa drugs, first-generation cephalosporins, quinolones, and rifampin have little activity against *B. burgdorferi*. Table 33-2 outlines the current approach to antimicrobial therapy in Lyme disease.

In stage I Lyme disease, amoxicillin and doxycycline are the drugs of choice. Amoxicillin is safe in pediatric and pregnant patients. The recommended duration of therapy is at least 14 days and up to 4 weeks if symptoms persist or recur. Because *B. burgdorferi* is very slow growing, prolonged antibiotic exposure may be necessary to kill the organism.[6] Also, some treatment failures have occurred with shorter courses of therapy, so many clinicians recommend at least 21 days of therapy. Choosing an antimicrobial agent for early Lyme disease also depends on attainable CSF levels, since *B. burgdorferi* can invade the CNS early in the course of infection, even in the absence of specific neurologic symptoms.[182] Although some clinicians have used probenecid to increase serum levels of amoxicillin, probenecid may block the entry of beta-lactam antibiotics into brain parenchyma and thus should not be routinely admin-

istered.[368] Oral penicillin and erythromycin are not recommended because they are less effective at preventing late complications (myocarditis, arthritis, meningoencephalitis) than amoxicillin and doxycycline.[310]

Within the first 24 hours of therapy, 15% of patients develop a Jarisch-Herxheimer reaction (JHR), with worsening fever, rash, malaise, and arthralgias.[216,217,312] Treatment for JHR is symptomatic with nonsteroidal antiinflammatory drugs (NSAIDs), and symptoms rarely continue beyond 24 hours from the time of antibiotic administration. Antimicrobials should not be discontinued.

Treatment of early disseminated Lyme disease should be based on the severity of disease. Patients with mild disease, such as facial nerve palsy with normal CSF, first-degree heart block with a PR interval less than 0.30 second, multiple erythema migrans lesions, or early arthritis, can be treated with any of the oral regimens for 3 weeks. In a trial of patients with early disseminated borreliosis without meningitis, a 21-day course of oral doxycycline was equal in efficacy to 14 days of parenteral ceftriaxone.[75]

Patients with severe disease (evidence of meningoencephalitis or more severe heart block) should be treated with parenteral antibiotics. IV penicillin (meningitis dosage), ceftriaxone (2 g every 24 hours for 2 to 4 weeks), and cefotaxime are all effective in treating CNS involvement (meningitis, cranial neuritis, or radiculoneuritis) in Lyme disease.[8,230,303] Ceftriaxone was more effective in some studies than penicillin, and the once-daily dose schedule makes outpatient treatment feasible.[73,74] Meningitic symptoms usually resolve with therapy in 1 week, although complete recovery of motor deficits may require 7 to 8 weeks.[306]

No controlled studies have compared oral vs. parenteral therapy for Lyme carditis, and cardiac manifestations of Lyme disease usually resolve within 1 to 2 weeks, even without antibiotic treatment.[8] However, *B. burgdorferi* can directly invade the myocardium and produce a cardiomyopathy.[294] Other manifestations of disseminated infection also occur in patients with cardiac involvement.[239] For these reasons, patients with evidence of cardiac involvement more severe than a first-degree heart block should be treated with IV antibiotics for at least 2 weeks. Such patients should also be admitted for telemetry and possible temporary pacemaker placement if complete heart block develops.

Optimal therapy for Lyme arthritis remains controversial. Several oral and parenteral regimens have been used successfully. A reasonable approach for patients without evidence of neurologic involvement is to use an oral regimen initially.[308] Four to eight weeks of oral antimicrobial therapy is recommended for acute, intermittent, or chronic arthritis. Generally these patients do well, but treatment failures occur.[69] If an adequate clin-

TABLE 33-2. Antimicrobial Recommendations for Lyme Disease

DRUG	DOSE	DURATION
EARLY LOCALIZED DISEASE		
Adults		
Tetracycline	250 mg po qid	14-28 days
Doxycycline	100 mg po bid	14-28 days
Amoxicillin	500 mg po tid	14-28 days
Cefuroxime	500 mg po tid	14-28 days
Children		
Amoxicillin	50 mg/kg/day po tid	14-28 days
Doxycycline (over 8 yr)	100 mg po bid	14-28 days
Erythromycin	30-50 mg/kg/day po qid	14-28 days
Tetracycline (over 8 yr)	250 mg po qid	14-28 days
Cefuroxime axetil	30-40 mg/kg/day po bid	14-28 days
EARLY DISSEMINATED AND LATE DISEASES*		
LATE DISSEMINATED NEUROLOGIC DISEASE†		
Adults		
Ceftriaxone	2 g/day IV qd	14-28 days
Cefotaxime	2 g/day IV q8h	14-28 days
Penicillin G	20 million IU/day IV q4h	14-28 days
Children		
Ceftriaxone	75-100 mg/kg/day IV qd	14-28 days (max, 2 g/day)
Cefotaxime	90-180 mg/kg/day IV q8h	14-28 days
Penicillin G	300,000 U/kg/day IV q4h	14-28 days (max, 20 million U/day)
LATE DISSEMINATED ARTHRITIS		
Adults		
Amoxicillin	500 mg po qid	28 days
Doxycycline	100 mg po bid	28 days
Ceftriaxone	75-100 mg/kg/day IV qd	14 days
Children		
Amoxicillin	50 mg/kg/day po tid	28 days
Ceftriaxone	2 g/day IV qd	14 days
DISSEMINATED DISEASE AND CARDITIS		
Adults		
Doxycycline	100 mg po bid	21-28 days‡
Amoxicillin	500 mg po q8h	21-28 days‡
Ceftriaxone	2 g/day IV qd	14-28 days§
Children		
Ceftriaxone	75-100 mg/kg IV/IM qd	14-21 days (max, 2 g/day)
Penicillin G	300,000 U/kg/day IV q4h	14-21 days (max, 20 million U/day)

po, Orally; *IV*, intravenously; *IM*, intramuscularly; *bid*, twice a day; *tid*, three times a day; *qid*, four times a day; *qd*, every day; *q4h* or, *q8h*, every 4 or 8 hours.
*For multiple erythema migrans, use treatment for early localized disease for at least 21 days.
For isolated facial palsy, use treatment for early localized disease for at least 21 to 28 days.
†Neurologic involvement limited to an isolated facial palsy should be treated as early disease.
‡For mild cardiac involvement, i.e., first degree atrioventricular block with PR interval less than 0.30 second.
§For second- or third-degree heart block, although no evidence indicates that intravenous is better than oral regimens.

ical response is not obtained, a parenteral regimen can be tried. Clinicians should keep in mind, however, that the response to antibiotics may not occur for 3 months or longer after completion of therapy.[239] Treatment can be augmented with NSAIDs.[216]

In chronic infection (stage III) the outcome after antibiotic treatment is usually favorable, but incomplete resolution is common.[179] In cases of chronic neuroborreliosis, treatment should consist of at least 28 days of IV antibiotics.[74,181] Some experts now advise continuation of treatment for an additional month for late Lyme disease manifestations that do not completely respond to an initial 4-week regimen. In 23 patients with late disease, ceftriaxone had better efficacy than IV penicillin.[74] One case report suggests β-lactam resistance as a possible cause for suboptimal resolution of disease with penicillin treatment.[117]

ASYMPTOMATIC TICK BITES. Patients with asymptomatic tick bites frequently present for care. In one survey, physicians in Maryland reported seeing 11 times as many patients seeking help after "tick bites" than true diagnosed cases of Lyme disease.[66] Three randomized, placebo-controlled studies have addressed antibiotic prophylaxis for tick bites.[7,65,277] Patients in the placebo groups developed Lyme disease or seroconversion 1% to 3.4% of the time, despite 15% to 30% of ticks being infected. No patients in the treatment groups developed Lyme disease. A meta-analysis of the three studies concluded that there was no significant difference between the groups and that routine prophylaxis of tick bites is not warranted, even in endemic areas.[352]

Many physicians do not adhere to this recommendation. Maryland physicians ordered serologic testing in two thirds of patients with asymptomatic tick bite and treated more than half with prophylactic antibiotics.[109] The major area of concern appears to be patients with tick bites who become infected but do not develop erythema migrans (when the disease is easily treated) then develop the late and more serious manifestations of Lyme disease. However, the risk of serious late sequelae in untreated patients with a tick bite is extremely low. First, less than 5 % of those bitten by the *I. scapularis* tick in endemic areas become infected. Second, most patients with an identified tick bite remove the tick before it has been attached for the 36 to 48 hours required to transmit an infectious inoculum of *B. burgdorferi*. Finally, 80% to 90% of the few patients who do become infected will develop erythema migrans, which is easily treated.

Physicians should weigh a number of factors related to the likelihood of disease acquisition in deciding whether to treat asymptomatic tick bites with antibiotics. Those factors include species and stage of the offending tick, duration of attachment, geography, and patient factors such as pregnancy. If a decision is made to treat, the literature supports using a 10-day course of amoxicillin or doxycycline.

VACCINE. The high incidence of Lyme disease and the potential for long-term morbidity have led investigators to focus increasing effort on developing an effective vaccine. Two large trials of vaccines against the outer surface protein A (Osp A) of *B. burgdorferi* have been completed. Efficacy was 49% to 68% after the second dose, increasing to 76% to 92% after three doses.[279,317] Both vaccines were administered in three doses at 0, 1, and 12 months. The vaccines appear to work by neutralizing spirochetes in the midgut of the biting tick during engorgement but before transmission of the organism.[115,281] One of the vaccines, LymeRix, has received Food and Drug Administration (FDA) approval. The vaccine is recommended for individuals 15 to 65 years of age living in highly endemic areas or those in intermediate areas with extensive work outside in forested, grassy areas.

The Osp A vaccine caused few complications in either trial or in earlier safety trials; the most common side effects were localized pain and tenderness.[160] However, these first generation vaccines are not without problems. Because the vaccines are not 100% effective, vaccinated patients can still contract Lyme disease. In recent trials, antibody levels appear to decrease rapidly after vaccination, suggesting the need for boosters to maintain immunity.[115] Follow-up studies are required to determine long-range efficacy beyond 20 months, and new vaccine schedules must be devised with the goal of achieving full immunization within one Lyme disease season. The current vaccines are not approved for children under age 15, despite children representing almost one fourth of Lyme disease cases.[194] In addition, because antibodies to *B. burgdorferi* proteins react in vitro with cardiac and skeletal muscle proteins, neuronal tissue, hepatocytes, and synovial cells, the FDA advisory committee has urged caution in using the Osp A vaccine in persons with arthritis. Finally, the Osp A vaccines result in a positive ELISA result but a negative Western blot.[369] This may lead to confusion if clinicians follow the recommended two-step testing protocol.

Inactivated whole-cell vaccines are effective in laboratory animals and are available for use in dogs. Delays in use of whole-cell vaccines for humans stem from concern that molecular mimicry of whole-cell proteins may lead to immune cross-reactivity and chronic inflammatory conditions.

Relapsing Fever. Relapsing fever is an acute borrelial disease characterized by recurrent paroxysms of fever separated by afebrile periods. It occurs in both endemic and epidemic forms (Table 33-3). The endemic or sporadic form occurs worldwide and is caused by a group of closely related Borrelia species. Argasid ticks belonging to the genus Ornithodoros and wild rodents both serve as reservoir hosts, but the tick serves as the main vector.[338] The epidemic form of relapsing fever is transmitted by the human body louse; it has not been reported in the United States in recent years.

The *Ornithodoros* ticks that transmit tick-borne relapsing fever (TBRF) act as both vectors and reservoirs for *Borrelia* organisms. Transovarial transmission allows all developmental stages to be potentially infective. The

TABLE 33-3. Tick-Borne Relapsing Fever Borreliae

ARTHROPOD VECTOR	*BORRELIA* SPECIES	GEOGRAPHIC DISTRIBUTION
Ornithodoros hermsii	*B. hermsii*	Western United States and Canada
O. turicata	*B. turicatae*	Southwestern United States and Mexico
O. parkeri	*B. parkeri*	Western United States and Mexico
O. moubata	*B. duttonii*	Tropical Africa
O. tholozani	*B. persica*	Central Asia, Middle East, Greece
O. tartakovskyi	*B. latyschevi*	Iran, Central Asia
O. erraticus	*B. crocidurae*	Russia, Middle East, East Africa, Turkey
O. graingeri	*B. graingeri*	Kenya
O. talaje	*B. mozzottii*	Mexico, Central America
O. rudis	*B. venezuelensis*	Central and South America
O. asperus	*B. caucasica*	Iraq, Russia
O. marocianus	*B. hispanica*	Northern Africa, southern Europe

ticks generally feed at night and attach themselves to the host for a short time, usually less than 1 hour. The bite is seldom painful and frequently goes unrecognized. The ticks are extremely resilient and may survive for years between feedings.

Ticks ingest *Borrelia* organisms while feeding on an infected vertebrate, most often a rodent. Borreliae enter the tick hemocele and then spread to other tick tissues, including the salivary glands, coxal organs, and reproductive organs. The coxal organs in argasid ticks are specialized tissues for excretion of excess fluids and solutes accumulated during feeding. In some *Ornithodoros* species, the coxal fluid is released near the mouthparts during feeding, allowing transmission of spirochetes to vertebrate hosts. Transmission may also occur through saliva or regurgitated gut contents.[19] Borreliae remain infective within ticks for many months.[288]

A high degree of specificity exists between the major strains of relapsing fever *Borrelia* and associated tick vectors. For instance, the three *Borrelia* species found in the United States—*B. hermsii*, *B. turicatae*, and *B. parkeri*—show complete specificity for their respective vectors, which are *O. hermsi*, *O. turicata*, and *O. parkeri*. *B. hermsii* can be transmitted only by *O. hermsi*, not by *O. turicata* or *O. parkeri*. This specificity is used extensively in classification of *Borrelia* species.[76]

EPIDEMIOLOGY. *Ornithodoros* ticks generally inhabit rodent burrows and nests, cracks and crevices in human and animal habitats, caves, and similar locations. Habits and patterns of infection vary between tick species. In parts of Africa, ticks live in the dust and cracks of earthen-floored huts, and sporadic cases are seen throughout the year. In the Middle East, Mexico, and southwestern United States, ticks live in the guano of cave floors, and human infection is often associated with visiting or camping in caves.

The majority of cases of TBRF in the United States are attributed to *B. hermsii*. Its vector, *O. hermsii,* inhabits the coniferous forest biome of the western United States and Canada, where it lives in remains of dead trees and burrows inhabited by mice, rats, and chipmunks. Ticks are carried by rodents into poorly maintained cabins and huts; lodging in such shelters by hikers and hunters is a major factor in acquiring relapsing fever.[104,144] Occasional cases are also caused by *O. turicata* (transmitting *B. turicatae*) in Texas (associated with travel into caves) and adjacent areas of the Southwest; *O. parkeri* (transmitting *B. parkeri*) rarely bites humans.[143]

TBRF is found throughout most of the world, although endemic areas include Colorado,[90,144] California,[90] the Pacific Northwest,[104] southern British Columbia, plateau regions of Central and South America, central Asia, Mediterranean countries, and most of Africa. In California, where reporting of relapsing fever is encouraged, two to 12 cases are reported per year.[90] Large outbreaks have been reported from Spokane County, Washington,[333] Colorado,[338] and the north rim area of the Grand Canyon.[53] Between 1985 and 1996, the 285 cases of TBRF reported in the United States occurred in California, Colorado, Idaho, Texas, Washington, Arizona, New Mexico, Nevada, Oregon, Utah, and Wyoming.[338] TBRF is more common in men, presumably because of increased exposure to tick vectors, and occurs primarily during summer months. TBRF is rarely fatal in adults, but in infants less than 1 year of age, case fatality rates may be 20% or higher.[176,288]

CLINICAL MANIFESTATIONS. The characteristic clinical feature of TBRF is abrupt onset of fever lasting about 3 days (range, 12 hours to 17 days), an afebrile period of variable duration, and then relapse with return of fever and other clinical manifestations. The initial febrile period terminates with rapid defervescence or a "crisis," accompanied by drenching sweats and intense thirst. Febrile periods in TBRF are associated with bacteremia. Resolution of fever occurs when the host develops an adequate antibody response to the spirochete. During afebrile periods the spirochete remains "hidden" in organ tissue and undergoes antigenic conversion to a new serotype. Relapse occurs when the new serotype causes bacteremia.

After being bitten by an infected tick, victims may develop a pruritic eschar at the site of the tick bite, but the lesion is usually absent by the onset of clinical symptoms. After an incubation period of approximately 7 days, victims develop fever, frequently accompanied by shaking chills, severe headache, myalgias, arthralgias, upper abdominal pain, photophobia, cough, nausea, and vomiting. The temperature is usually greater than 39° C (102.2° F), and patients may manifest extreme muscular weakness and lethargy. Splenomegaly develops in approximately 40% and hepatomegaly in 18% of TBRF patients. From 10% to 40% have neurologic involvement, approaching the incidence seen in Lyme disease. The most common neurologic complications are meningismus and facial nerve palsy.[48] Facial palsy, when present, typically occurs after the second febrile episode and usually resolves within 2 to 9 weeks with or without treatment. Other reported neurologic complications include neuropsychiatric disturbances, encephalitis, peripheral neuropathy, myelitis, and pathologic reflexes. Iritis or iridocyclitis occurs in up to 15% of untreated cases, typically occurring later in the fever course. Formation of adhesions between the iris and anterior lens capsule frequently leads to visual defects. A rash, ranging from a macular eruption to petechiae and erythema multiforme, develops in 25% to 30% of patients.[288]

Mortality rates have been as high as 40% in some epidemics of louse-borne relapsing fever,[280] but TBRF is generally self-limited, although clinical features may be severe and prolonged. Neurologic complications generally resolve spontaneously, but severe depression may persist for months. Hemorrhagic complications, pneumonia, ARDS, hepatosplenomegaly, petechiae, or myocarditis may develop rarely.[77,104,357]

Relapsing fever in pregnancy results in a high incidence of spontaneous abortion,[288] premature birth, and perinatal morbidity.[156] Fetal death is probably caused by direct placental invasion by spirochetes, resulting in thrombocytopenia and retroplacental hemorrhage.[297] Prior studies have linked pregnancy with a more serious maternal disease course.[132,205,206] A more recent case-control study, however, found no significant difference in pregnant women's mortality or complications.[155] Infection in the neonatal period usually occurs by placental transmission and presents as overwhelming sepsis with very high mortality.[372]

ANTIGENIC VARIATION. The phenomenon of relapse in TBRF is caused by the ability of borreliae to undergo antigenic variation in an infected host. The organisms are capable of spontaneous conversion to many serotypes. Clinically, defervescence occurs when the dominant serotype is eradicated by interaction with host antibody. Spirochetemia probably persists at undetectable levels during the afebrile period and consists of mixed serotypes. Relapse occurs when a variant population reaches detectable levels. Antigenic variation is under complex genetic control and does not appear to require contact of the organism with host antibody.[17,322]

DIAGNOSIS. The clinical diagnosis of TBRF requires thorough knowledge of the epidemiology of the disease and a high index of suspicion. TBRF is uncommon and occurs only sporadically. A history of recent exposure to old cabins, caves, or any rodent-friendly environment suggests the diagnosis. Routine laboratory tests are of little value. The WBC count is usually normal but may be increased or decreased. A left shift is often present. Thrombocytopenia is common but nonspecific. The CSF is often abnormal, with a lymphocytic pleocytosis (typically 10 to 2000 cells/mm³), usually with a normal glucose and elevated protein. A false-positive serologic test for syphilis (Wassermann) occurs in about 5% of cases.[288]

The diagnosis of relapsing fever is confirmed by demonstrating spirochetes on peripheral blood smears. A routine peripheral blood smear (Wright-Giemsa stain) from a febrile patient is initially positive in 70% of cases.[288] The diagnostic yield can be increased by examining thick smears and by staining with acridine orange using fluorescence microscopy.[275] Inoculating laboratory animals (rats, mice) with blood and examining blood smears from the animals will also increase the diagnostic yield. The visual yield of spirochetes in peripheral blood smears diminishes with each successive febrile sampling. *B. hermsii* can be cultured in BSK-II medium, with the yield increasing in acutely febrile patients. Serologic tests are difficult to perform and are not yet practical utility.[338] TBRF is probably underrecognized and underreported and has been misdiagnosed as Lyme disease.[88]

TREATMENT. Tetracycline and erythromycin are both effective in treating relapsing fever. A single oral dose of 500 mg of either drug is effective in louse-borne relapsing fever.[47] However, a 7- to 10-day course (500 mg orally four times a day) is generally recommended in tick-borne disease.[143,288] For children less than 9 years of age, erythromycin is recommended (30-50 mg/kg/day in four divided doses), with the first dose given intravenously. The borreliae are also sensitive to penicillin and chloramphenicol, but treatment failures have been reported with penicillin.[47] Animal studies have shown that early treatment with a β-lactam antibiotic within 24 hours of onset of spirochetemia decreases CNS involvement.[48]

TABLE 33-4. Human Rickettsial Diseases

DISEASE	ORGANISM	ARTHROPOD VECTOR	GEOGRAPHIC DISTRIBUTION
TYPHUS GROUP			
Murine typhus	*Rickettsia mooseri (typhi)*	Flea	Worldwide
Epidemic typhus	*R. prowazekii*	Body louse	Worldwide
Scrub typhus	*R. tsutsugamushi*	Chigger	Asia, Australia
SPOTTED FEVER GROUP			
Rocky Mountain spotted fever	*R. rickettsii*	Ticks	Western Hemisphere
Eastern spotted fevers	*R. conorii*	Ticks	Eastern Hemisphere
	R. sibirica		
	R. australis		
Rickettsial pox	*R. akari*	Mites	United States, Russia
Q fever	*Coxiella burnetii*	Ticks	Worldwide
Trench fever	*Rochalimaea quintana*	Body louse	Africa, Mexico
Ehrlichia	*E. sennetsu*	Ticks	Japan
	E. canis		Worldwide

JHR often occurs after the first dose of antibiotics. In one series, 54% of patients developed a JHR.[88] It is often severe and may be fatal. The reaction begins with a rise in body temperature and exacerbation of existing signs and symptoms; vasodilation and a fall in blood pressure follow. This complex reaction is mediated in part by products of mononuclear leukocytes. The leukocytes are stimulated by increased contact with antibiotic-altered spirochetes. Neither endotoxin nor complement appears to be necessary in the pathogenesis of JHR.[46] JHR typically occurs within a few hours of initial antibiotic dosing and cannot be prevented by prior steroid treatment.

Waiting to begin treatment until the patient is afebrile does not prevent JHR.[144] Pretreatment with acetaminophen and hydrocortisone results in only a mild reduction of hypotension and does not prevent rigors.[47] Patients who are receiving the initial dose of antibiotics for relapsing fever should receive an IV infusion of isotonic saline in anticipation of a possible JHR. This is generally sufficient to counteract the hypotension. Lower initial doses of tetracycline or erythromycin may reduce the frequency of JHR.[144]

Tick-Borne Rickettsial Diseases

Bacteria of the family Rickettsiaceae are small, fastidious intracellular parasites with gram-negative bacterium-like cell walls, typical prokaryotic DNA arrangement, and considerable independent metabolic activity. The six major antigenic groups cause a variety of human diseases worldwide (Table 33-4). Three are potentially transmissible to humans by ticks: spotted fever group (SFG) diseases, Q fever, and *Ehrlichia* infections. Organisms from the genus *Rickettsia* cause the various spotted fevers. *Coxiella burnetii* is the etiologic agent of Q fever. *Ehrlichia* are intraleukocytic Rickettsiaceae that infect humans and a variety of wild and domestic animals.

Spotted Fever Group Diseases. *Rickettsia* of the SFG share intracellular growth characteristics and a group-specific antigen. They are distributed worldwide and, with the exception of *Rickettsia akari* (rickettsial pox), are transmitted by the bite of ixodid ticks (Table 33-5). Ticks serve as the natural hosts, reservoirs, and vectors for the rickettsiae.[200] The organisms replicate freely within the tick host and are passed transovarially and transstadially. Amplification of the cycle occurs when uninfected ticks feed on an infected vertebrate host or concurrently with an infected tick.

In most natural vertebrate hosts the SFG rickettsiae induce an inapparent infection with transient rickettsemia. Human infection occurs through accidental intrusion into the natural cycle of infection or when ticks are transferred into human environments. Humans are incidental and "dead-end" hosts not involved in sustaining the life cycle of the organism.

PATHOGENESIS. The tick-borne SFG diseases share a similar pathogenesis. The usual route of infection is by direct inoculation through the skin through the bite of a tick vector. Infection may also develop after contamination of broken skin with infected tick parts or feces, after blood transfusion from an infected donor,[356] or through aerosol transmission among laboratory personnel working with pathogenic rickettsiae.[224]

Local proliferation of rickettsiae probably occurs at the site of the tick bite, and a primary lesion or eschar frequently develops. Regional lymphadenitis may de-

TABLE 33-5. Spotted Fever Group Diseases

DISEASE	ETIOLOGIC AGENT	MAJOR VECTOR	GEOGRAPHIC DISTRIBUTION	PRIMARY LESION	USUAL SEVERITY
Rocky Mountain spotted fever	*Rickettsia rickettsii*	*Dermacentor andersoni, D. variabilis*	Western Hemisphere	None	Moderate- severe
North Asian tick typhus	*R. sibirica*	*Dermacentor, Haemaphysalis*	Europe to Russian Far East	Often present	Mild
Mediterranean spotted fever	*R. conorii*	*Rhipicephalus sanguineus, Haemaphysalis*	Mediterranean littoral, South Africa, Kenya, India	Often present	Moderate
Queensland tick typhus	*R. australis*	*Ixodes holocyclus*	Australia	Often present	Mild

velop in the distribution of the eschar, suggesting early lymphatic spread. Rickettsemia is typically present at the onset of clinical illness and persists throughout the febrile period.[364]

The SFG diseases are characterized by disseminated vasculitic lesions.[347] The rickettsiae invade, proliferate within, and ultimately destroy capillary and precapillary endothelial cells. In Rocky Mountain spotted fever (RMSF) the organisms spread into larger arterioles and arteries and invade medial smooth muscle cells. Medial necrosis and destruction of the vascular wall may follow. At sites of endothelial cell damage, a perivascular inflammatory response ensues, and platelet and fibrin thrombi tend to form and occlude the vessel lumen. In severe cases, vascular thrombi lead to necrosis of peripheral parts, including fingers, toes, the external ear, and scrotum. Antibodies develop 5 to 7 days after the onset of illness but do not appear to play a significant role in the pathogenesis of the vasculitis.[366] Immunity develops with clinical recovery, tends to be long lasting, and appears to involve both antibody- and cell-mediated mechanisms.

CLINICAL MANIFESTATIONS AND DIAGNOSIS. The SFG diseases display similar clinical manifestations, including fever, chills, headache, and myalgias. Three to 5 days after the onset of illness a characteristic maculopapular rash develops on the ankles, feet, wrists, and hands, then spreads centripetally to involve the entire body, including the palms and soles. With the exception of RMSF, the SFG diseases are generally mild, self-limited illnesses, with deaths seen primarily in elderly or debilitated patients. Untreated RMSF, however, may be severe, with a mortality rate approaching 30%.[40]

Early diagnosis and treatment virtually eliminate mortality and reduce morbidity in SFG diseases. At the onset of illness, however, signs and symptoms are frequently nonspecific, leading to diagnostic confusion with viral or other infectious diseases.[158] Rash, the most

characteristic feature of the illness, may develop late or, rarely, not at all. Identification of the eschar is helpful, but its presence is variable, and it is always absent in RMSF. Only 60% to 70% of patients recall a tick bite. Laboratory data (e.g., hyponatremia, thrombocytopenia) may provide clues to the diagnosis but are nonspecific. Serologic evidence of infection develops late in the illness. Early diagnosis therefore is based primarily on clinical evidence and relies on the ability to correlate clinical signs and symptoms with epidemiologic features.

Rickettsial infection is confirmed by identification of rickettsiae in tissues (not widely available), by isolation of rickettsiae from infected blood or tissues (difficult and hazardous to laboratory personnel), or by demonstration of antibody rise in paired sera. The widely used Weil-Felix test is based on the unique sharing of polysaccharide antigens between certain *Proteus* strains (OX-19, OX-2) and the SFG rickettsiae. This agglutination test lacks both sensitivity and specificity, however, and should be abandoned if other serologic methods are available. Newer and more sensitive serologic methods include complement fixation, microimmunofluorescence, IFA tests, microagglutination, indirect hemagglutination, and ELISA.[63,157,231]

TREATMENT. Early treatment of the spotted fevers is the most important factor in speeding convalescence and reducing mortality. Antibiotic therapy begun early in the course results in rapid resolution of clinical abnormalities. Tetracycline and chloramphenicol are both very effective, although neither drug is rickettsicidal. The antibiotics inhibit the rickettsiae until an adequate immune response by the patient eradicates the infection. Tetracycline is given orally at a dosage of 25 to 50 mg/kg/day in four divided doses (2 g/day in adults); the dose of chloramphenicol is 50 and 75 mg/kg/day for adults and children, respectively. Appropriate IV doses of both drugs may be substituted. Penicillins, streptomycin, and sulfonamides are ineffective. Treatment should be continued until the patient is afebrile for 48 hours, or for a minimum of 5 to 7 days. Relapses are uncommon but may be treated with the same drug when they occur.[366]

ROCKY MOUNTAIN SPOTTED FEVER

Epidemiology. RMSF is the most common fatal tick-borne disease in the United States.[67] It was first recognized in the northwestern United States in the latter part of the eighteenth century and may have been prevalent even earlier in Native Americans of that region. It has since been identified throughout the Western Hemisphere. Human infections have been reported from all 48 contiguous states except Maine. The disease is also seen in Canada, Mexico, and parts of Central and South America.

A major shift in the demographics of RMSF occurred during the twentieth century. Before 1930 most cases were reported from the Rocky Mountains region of the western United States; in recent years more than 90% of cases have been reported from southern and eastern states. Reported cases in the mountain states have actually decreased more than tenfold, with only 2% of cases between 1981 and 1991 occurring in the Rocky Mountain States.[199] "Rocky Mountain" spotted fever has thus become somewhat of a misnomer.

In the early 1970s a marked increase in the reported cases of RMSF was seen in the United States, reaching a peak in 1981 of 1192 cases, for an incidence rate of 0.51 cases per 100,000 population. Reported cases have gradually declined since that time, more recently ranging from 600 to 1200 cases reported each year.[60] Most of this decline has occurred in the South Atlantic states, although they still account for a majority of the cases reported each year. States with the most cases in 1991, for example, were North Carolina (159 cases), Oklahoma (71), Tennessee (58), and Georgia (41).[58]

The changes in the incidence and endemicity of RMSF have been attributed to cyclic changes in tick populations, changes in the virulence of infecting rickettsiae, and the process of suburbanization.[27,137,199] A convincing explanation, however, is still lacking.

RMSF is caused by the gram-negative intracellular bacterium *Rickettsia rickettsii*. The epidemiology of RMSF is determined by the seasonal and geographic distribution of *R. rickettsii*–infected ticks. Many species of ixodid ticks have been implicated as vectors of the disease,[40,173,199] but the most important species in the United States are *Dermacentor variabilis*, the American dog tick, and *Dermacentor andersoni*, the wood tick. Ticks of the *Dermacentor* genus are quite hearty, often living up to 5 years and displaying resilience to desiccation, cold, and starvation. Ticks transmitting RMSF outside the United States include *Rhipicephalus sanguineus* in Mexico and *Amblyomma cajennense* in Central and South America.

D. andersoni is the principal acarine host of *R. rickettsii* in the western United States and Canada. It feeds on virtually any available warm-blooded animal. *D. variabilis* is the primary host in the eastern United States and Canada. The domestic dog is the major host of adult *D. variabilis*, but the tick will feed on a variety of large and medium-sized animals. Nymphal and larval *D. variabilis* feed on various mice, voles, and rabbits. Serosurveys have indicated that a broad range of vertebrate hosts are infected with *R. rickettsii*, although not all sustain rickettsemia of sufficient magnitude to transmit the infection to feeding ticks. *R. rickettsii* occurrence in the United States does not depend on the presence of any given order of mammal.[199]

Domestic dogs become infected with *R. rickettsii* and may become acutely ill with fever and rash. Dogs probably do not play an important role in the amplification cycle of RMSF but may be important in transporting infected ticks close to humans.[128] Several studies have shown an association between domestic dogs and RMSF.[41,128,196] An infected tick may detach from a dog and complete its engorgement on a human, thereby transmitting *R. rickettsii*. Alternatively, infection through abraded skin or conjunctivae may occur during manual deticking of dogs.[349]

Transmission by a tick vector delimits the clinical epidemiology of RMSF. It is a seasonal disease occurring when ticks are active; 95% of U.S. cases occur between April 1 and September 30, with most in May, June, and July. Exposure to wooded areas or areas of high grass increase the risk of disease. In southern states the season is longer with more winter cases, although sporadic cases can occur even in cold climates. RMSF also tends to be focally endemic, with a high proportion of cases occurring in small, circumscribed areas. This may be the clinical expression of "islands" of infected ticks.[196] It is more common in males (60%) and young people (50% less than 20 years of age), who are more likely to be exposed to tick habitats.[332,334] The demographic group with the highest incidence of RMSF is 5- to 9-year-old children in the mid-Atlantic and southern United States.[60,70]

Other factors influencing human transmission include the duration of tick attachment and the prevalence of *R. rickettsii* in ticks. Transmission from the tick salivary glands may occur in as short as 6 to 10 hours of tick attachment, although some cases require more than 24 hours. Only a small percentage of ticks, even in highly endemic areas, are infected by Rickettsia. The chance of exposure to *R. rickettsii* from a tick bite ranges from 1 in 2123 in North Carolina to less than 1 in 1500 in Ohio.

Clinical manifestations. RMSF ranges from mild, even subclinical illness to fulminant disease, with vascular collapse and death occurring within 3 to 6 days of on-

TABLE 33-6. Clinical Findings in Rocky Mountain Spotted Fever

CLINICAL FINDING	PERCENT OF CASES
Fever	99
Headache	80-90
Any rash	85-90
Myalgias	70-85
Petechial rash	45-60
Nausea and vomiting	56-60
Abdominal pain	34-50
Conjunctivitis	30
Stupor	21-37
Diarrhea	19-20
Edema	18
Meningismus	17-18
Splenomegaly	14-29
Hepatomegaly	12-15
Pneumonitis	13-17
Coma	10
Jaundice	8-9
Seizures	8

set. Clinical manifestations reflect the pathogenesis of the infecting rickettsia. Infection typically is through the skin, with spread occurring primarily by blood and lymphatic channels. The rickettsial species attaches to and invades vascular endothelial and smooth muscle cells using surface exposed protein and rickettsial phospholipase. The rickettsial species multiply intracellularly, becoming cytopathic. Vascular injury often ensues, with activation of clotting factors, extravasation of intravascular fluid, and impaired perfusion. Vascular permeability is elevated, with resultant edema, hypovolemia, and hypoalbuminemia. The incubation period ranges from 2 to 14 days (7-day mean onset); severe disease is associated with a shorter incubation period. Typically the victim has sudden onset of fever and chills, with or without headache, and myalgias. The classic triad of fever, rash, and history of tick exposure is present in only 3% to 18% of persons at the initial physician visit.[162] The fever is usually high, greater than 39° C (102.2° F) in two-thirds of patients in the first 3 days of illness, and myalgias and headache may be severe. The most characteristic feature, the rash, usually develops 2 to 5 days after the onset of illness. Other signs and symptoms, including abdominal pain, vomiting, diarrhea, confusion, conjunctivitis, and peripheral edema, are common (Table 33-6). A history of tick exposure is present in 85% of confirmed cases.[334]

The rash in RMSF results from injury to dermal capillaries and small blood vessels. It typically develops first on the wrists, hands, ankles, and feet 2 to 3 days after disease onset. The rash then spreads rapidly and centripetally to cover most of the body, including the palms, soles, and face. Initially the lesions are pink macules, 2 to 5 mm in diameter, that readily blanch with pressure. After 2 to 3 days the lesions become fixed, darker red, papular, and finally petechial. The hemorrhagic lesions may coalesce to form large areas of ecchymoses. Necrosis may develop, especially in areas supplied by terminal arteries, such as fingers, toes, nose, ears, and genitalia. Involvement of the scrotum or vulva is a diagnostic clue.[83]

In its classic form, the rash occurring during the summer months in an endemic area is almost pathognomonic for RMSF. Unfortunately, it is often absent on initial patient presentation, making diagnosis more difficult. The rash is delayed in approximately 10% of patients,[138] with younger patients generally displaying the rash earlier in the disease course. In an additional 10% to 15% of laboratory-confirmed cases of RMSF, no rash is noted ("spotless" fever).[107,137,139] In other patients the rash is evanescent, occurring only with fever spikes. One report indicates a possible actinic nature to the RMSF rash, worsening in sun-exposed areas.[20]

Neurologic involvement in RMSF ranges from mild headache to serious focal or generalized disorders of cerebral function. Headache is very common. Meningismus occasionally develops but does not correlate well with CSF findings, which may be normal or may show modest protein elevation and pleocytosis of both lymphocytes and polymorphonuclear cells (usually 8 to 35 cells/mm³). Cerebral vasculitis may manifest with focal neurologic deficits, which are quite variable but usually transient. Seizures may develop during the acute phase of the illness but rarely persist.[125] Lethargy and confusion are common and may progress to stupor or profound coma. Generalized cerebral dysfunction may be secondary to vasculitic lesions, especially in the reticular network of the brainstem, or to toxicity from severe rickettsial infection (fever, hypotension, hyponatremia, and thrombocytopenia with intracranial hemorrhage). Children with RMSF who develop coma have an increased risk of subsequent behavioral disturbances and learning disabilities. One case report describes Guillain-Barré syndrome as a complication of acute RMSF.[22,129,207,338]

Myocarditis is frequently found at necropsy in fatal RMSF; however, the clinical significance of the cardiac involvement is unclear. Pathologic study shows a patchy, interstitial, mononuclear infiltrate that appears to coincide with the distribution of rickettsiae in myocardial capillaries, venules, and arterioles.[348] Abnormal left ventricular function can frequently be demonstrated echocardiographically in hospitalized patients.[103,191] Overt clinical manifestations of left ventricular dysfunction are uncommon, however, and hypotension and pulmonary edema are generally attributable to noncardiogenic causes. Cardiac enlargement rarely may be seen on chest radiographs.[177,192] ECG abnormalities include nonspecific ST-T changes, conduction abnormalities (primarily first-degree atrioventricular block), and arrhythmias (paroxysmal atrial tachycardia, nodal tachycardia, and atrial fibrillation).[192] Most patients have complete resolution of cardiac abnormalities with clinical improvement, but persistent echocardiographic abnormalities have been noted.[191]

Infection of the pulmonary microcirculation by *R. rickettsii* results in interstitial pneumonitis and increased pulmonary vascular permeability. Although pulmonary involvement is not usually a prominent aspect of RMSF, a significant number of patients complain of cough, chest pain, dyspnea, or coryza.[49] Patchy infiltrates may occasionally be seen on chest radiographs, and noncardiogenic pulmonary edema may develop in severe cases, with potential progression to ARDS.[82,177,262]

Gastrointestinal symptoms are common in RMSF and are prominent complaints in some patients. At autopsy, rickettsial vascular lesions are found throughout the gastrointestinal tract and pancreas, although actual necrosis appears to be a rare event.[240] Occasionally, RMSF presents as an acute abdomen, suggesting appendicitis or cholecystitis.[350]

In the kidneys a focal perivascular interstitial nephritis is concentrated near the corticomedullary junction. Clinically, however, significant renal involvement is usually caused by prerenal azotemia or acute tubular necrosis after a hypotensive episode.[329] Monarticular arthritis in the acute phase of RMSF has been reported.[329]

The major complications of RMSF result from direct vasculitic injury. In late stages of the disease, diffuse vasculitic lesions cause increased systemic capillary permeability, leading to hypovolemia and vascular collapse. Disseminated intravascular coagulation (DIC), acute renal failure, metabolic acidosis, and cardiorespiratory dysfunction may ensue and often presage death. Endothelial leukocyte adhesion molecules and cytokines are thought to play an important role in the pathogenesis of fulminant RMSF. Long-term sequelae include paraparesis; hearing loss; peripheral neuropathy; bladder and bowel incontinence; cerebellar, vestibular, and motor dysfunction; language disorders; and disability from limb amputation.

When death results, it typically occurs after delayed treatment and 8 to 15 days following symptom onset. The exception is with fulminant RMSF, in which death occurs in less than 5 days, with hemolysis the most likely pathogenic cause. Risk factors associated with mortality include elevated serum creatinine, increased AST, increased bilirubin, hyponatremia, thrombocytopenia, and advanced age.[64]

Diagnosis. Before antimicrobials were available, RMSF was frequently a fatal disease. Even with effective antibiotic agents the mortality rate remains approximately 5%.[106,138] Patients older than 30 years, males, and nonwhites are at higher risk.[106,137,138] Elderly patients appear more likely to have a severe course of illness and to have

---

> **Box 33-3** LABORATORY FEATURES OF ROCKY MOUNTAIN SPOTTED FEVER
>
> Normal leukocyte count
> Left shift, toxic granulations, Döhle's bodies
> Thrombocytopenia
> Hyponatremia
> Cerebrospinal fluid pleocytosis
> Increased serum transaminase levels
> Increased serum creatinine levels

---

atypical features, including delayed or absent rash.[139,213] In susceptible individuals, such as those with glucose-6-phosphate dehydrogenase (G6PD) deficiency, RMSF may be fulminant and rapidly fatal.[346]

The most significant factor in deaths from RMSF is a delay in diagnosis and in starting appropriate antibiotic therapy. Before antibiotics the mortality rate (1939 to 1945) was 23%, compared with 5.2% between 1981 and 1992. Patients who receive antibiotic treatment after 5 days of illness may die from advanced disease. Unfortunately, early diagnosis in RMSF is often difficult. The classic triad of rash, fever, and tick bite is actually rare during the first 3 days of illness,[139] and confirmatory laboratory evidence is usually lacking early in the disease. Factors leading to a delay in diagnosis include absence or late appearance of the rash, lack of a history of tick bite or tick exposure, and nonspecific or unexpected initial symptoms leading to an incorrect initial diagnosis.

RMSF rarely is diagnosed by culture results, making historic data and clinical findings imperative. RMSF should be suspected and antibiotic treatment strongly considered in any patient who resides in or has recently visited an endemic area during the summer months and who has fever, headache, and myalgias even in the absence of a rash. Symptoms referable to the pulmonary, gastrointestinal, and central nervous systems often occur in RMSF and should not delay diagnosis.

The differential diagnosis of RMSF is extensive and includes meningococcemia, thrombotic thrombocytopenic purpura, immune complex vasculitis, ehrlichiosis, mononucleosis, measles, enteroviral infections, leptospirosis, and murine typhus. Meningococcemia may be impossible to differentiate initially, but chloramphenicol is effective therapy for both diseases. The rash of atypical measles may mimic that of RMSF.[220] Gastrointestinal infection, respiratory infection (pneumonia, bronchitis), acute abdomen, and meningitis/encephalomyelitis are often misdiagnosed.

Routine laboratory values are nonspecific and provide limited clues to diagnosis, especially early in the course of illness, when serum antibodies are rarely detectable (Box 33-3). Thrombocytopenia has been reported in more than 50% of patients in some series,[346]

Box 33-4 LABORATORY DIAGNOSTIC TESTING FOR ROCKY MOUNTAIN SPOTTED FEVER

SEROLOGIC DIAGNOSIS

Latex agglutination assay
Indirect immunofluorescence assay

SKIN BIOPSY–RELATED DIAGNOSIS

Polymerase chain reaction
Direct immunofluorescence antibody staining
Immunoperoxidase staining

---

although the actual incidence may be closer to 35%.[137,139] Hyponatremia is also common and is probably a result of antidiuretic hormone (ADH) secretion in response to intravascular volume depletion.[98] Other laboratory abnormalities include anemia, azotemia, hypoalbuminemia, CSF pleocytosis with monocytic predominance, increased creatine kinase, and elevated bilirubin and AST/ALT levels. Peripheral WBC count is usually normal.

Laboratory confirmation of RMSF has generally relied on serologic techniques detecting antibody increases in paired sera (Box 33-4). Even with the most sensitive tests, antibody rises are not seen until 5 to 10 days after the onset of symptoms, negating serologies at initial presentation. Early antibiotic therapy may delay titers even longer.[231] Serologic diagnosis requires a fourfold increase in titer between acute and convalescent sera, which does not typically occur until 6 to 10 days after symptom onset.[342] The Weil-Felix test is neither sensitive nor specific for RMSF and should not be used if other tests are available. The complement fixation test is widely available but also lacks sensitivity.[231] False-positive results can occur during pregnancy with latex agglutination assays.[355] The most sensitive and specific serologic tests currently in use appear to be the IFA and indirect hemagglutination tests.[157]

The most promising method for early laboratory diagnosis of RMSF is immunofluorescent identification of *R. rickettsii* in biopsy specimens of the skin rash. Rickettsiae have been identified as early as the fourth day of illness with this method.[367] Sensitivity is 70% to 90%, with a specificity of 100%.[237] Serologic confirmation of RMSF requires a fourfold rise in antibody titers by indirect immunofluorescence or a single titer greater than 64.

Treatment. Mortality is largely eliminated in RMSF by early treatment with tetracycline or chloramphenicol. Patients treated within 4 days of symptom onset are three times less likely to die than those treated later.[70] Treatment should continue for at least 5 to 7 days or until the patient is afebrile for more than 2 days. IV therapy is required only if the patient cannot tolerate oral intake. Treatment with doxycycline may be preferable to chloramphenicol because tetracyclines may be associated with a higher survival rate.[334] Although tetracycline can cause teeth staining in children, the risk is related to cumulative dose. A single course of therapy for RMSF is unlikely to stain teeth. Potential complications of chloramphenicol include bone marrow suppression, aplastic anemia, and gray syndrome. Rickettsiae are sensitive to fluoroquinolones, which remain a potential option even if human data are lacking. Mediterranean spotted fever (*R. coronii*) has been successfully treated with fluoroquinolones.[24] In dogs, tetracycline, chloramphenicol, and enrofloxacin all appear to have equal efficacy in treating RMSF.[35]

In severe cases, supportive therapy is also essential to a favorable outcome. Fluid replacement is critical in the hypotensive patient but must be monitored closely because of the risk of fluid extravasation through damaged vessels. Measurement of pulmonary capillary wedge pressures with a Swan-Ganz catheter may be necessary, especially if pulmonary edema develops. Use of corticosteroids has not been adequately evaluated but may be beneficial in patients with widespread vasculitis or encephalitis.[201,366]

Prophylactic antibiotics after a tick bite are not recommended because of the low incidence of infection and risk of adverse reactions. Routinely testing ticks for rickettsial antigen is not beneficial.[263] Although none currently exists, promising vaccines are in development.

EASTERN SPOTTED FEVER. Three other SFG diseases are transmitted to humans by tick bite: Mediterranean spotted fever (MSF), North Asian tick typhus, and Queensland tick typhus. The three diseases closely resemble one another and have many similarities to RMSF. Generally, the course of illness in all three is milder than in RMSF, although complications and death may occur in susceptible patients. The diseases are characterized by abrupt onset of fever, headache, and malaise after a short incubation period (5 to 7 days). Unlike in RMSF, a primary lesion (eschar, tache noire) is often present at the site of the tick bite and may be associated with regional lymphadenitis. The lesion is classically a small ulcer, 2 to 5 mm in diameter, with a black center and red areola. A rash that varies from maculopapular to petechial usually develops 3 to 5 days after the onset of illness. Untreated, the fever and other symptoms resolve after several days to 2 weeks. Treatment with tetracycline or chloramphenicol significantly shortens the course of illness and, if instituted early, prevents complications.

MSF is caused by *Rickettsia conorii* and has been described under various names, often reflecting its geographic occurrence: Marseilles fever, South African tick bite fever, Kenya tick bite fever, India tick typhus, and boutonneuse fever. As the names indicate, MSF is endemic in areas bordering the Mediterranean Sea, as well as parts of Africa and India. The major vector of MSF in the Mediterranean countries is the dog tick *Rhipicephalus sanguineus*. Several tick species have been implicated as vectors in other areas: *Haemaphysalis leachi* (Kenya, South Africa), *Rhipicephalus simus*, *Dermacentor reticulatus*, and *Ixodes hexagonus*.[101] All stages of *R. sanguineus* occasionally attach to humans, and dogs may be important in transporting the ticks close to humans.[339]

As with other SFG diseases, MSF occurs during the warm weather months. Seasonal occurrence, geographic location, and the presence of a tache noire (noted in 50% to 75% of cases) are the most helpful criteria for early diagnosis.[211,244] Although the disease is usually mild in children and young adults, a malignant form resembling severe RMSF has been described.[243,345]

The elderly, alcoholics, and patients with G6PD deficiency appear particularly at risk.[147,153] The diagnosis can be confirmed by specific serologic testing or by immunofluorescent demonstration of *R. conorii* in cutaneous lesions.[242]

North Asian tick typhus or Siberian tick typhus is endemic throughout Siberia, from European Russia to the Soviet Far East. It is seen primarily in agricultural areas and is closely associated with steppe landscapes.[41] The causative organism, *Rickettsia siberica*, is transmitted to humans by several species of *Dermacentor* and *Haemaphysalis* ticks. In the natural cycle, adult ticks feed on large wild and domestic animals, especially cattle and dogs. As for other SFG rickettsiae, humans are accidental and dead-end hosts.

Queensland tick typhus is caused by *Rickettsia australis*. It is endemic to southern and northern Queensland, and the major vector is the scrub tick, *Ixodes holocyclus*.[41] Both Queensland tick typhus and North Asian tick typhus are benign illnesses of mild to moderate severity with typical rickettsial manifestations: fever, headache, variable appearance of an eschar at the site of the tick bite, and a rash.

SFG rickettsiosis also occurs in Japan, where the causative agent appears to be a distinct serotype of SFG rickettsiae.[331]

Q FEVER. Q fever is a worldwide zoonosis affecting both wild and domestic animals. It was first described in 1937 as an occupational disease of abattoir workers and dairy farmers in Australia.[78] Aerosol spread of *Coxiella burnetii*, the causative organism, is the usual mode of transmission to humans. Sexual transmission has been implicated but not proved.[171] Although ticks may become infected with *C. burnetii* after feeding on an infected vertebrate, tick-borne transmission to humans appears to be very rare.

Fewer than 10 cases of Q fever per year are reported in the United States. Serosurveys have shown widespread prevalence, suggesting frequent asymptomatic infection or underdiagnosis and underreporting.[134,280] The most common clinical presentation of Q fever is an influenza-like illness with fever, headache, myalgias, and pneumonitis. Abnormal liver function tests, jaundice, and hepatomegaly may be seen. Glomerulonephritis has been reported with both acute Q fever and endocarditis-associated chronic infection.[166] *C. burnetii* infection during pregnancy, although not known to be teratogenic, can create placental insufficiency resulting in premature delivery or even intrauterine death.[113,241] A severe case of acute cerebellitis with tonsillar herniation was recently reported.[265] In most victims the illness resolves spontaneously within 2 to 4 weeks of onset, with treatment hastening the resolution.

Q fever may also be a chronic infection, with or without a history of an acute episode. Granulomatous hepatitis and culture-negative endocarditis are the chronic forms of the disease. Endocarditis, fatal in 25% to 60% of patients, can affect native and prosthetic valves (underlying valvular disease is almost invariably present), although it has a predilection for the aortic valve.[123] Infections of aneurysms and vascular prostheses have also been described.[110] A post–Q fever syndrome involving fatigue, myalgia, arthralgia, night sweats, sleep disturbances, and mood alterations has been described and may occur in 20% to 42% of proven cases.[14,228]

Diagnosis of Q fever depends primarily on serologic testing. Two specific complement-fixing antibodies (phase 1 and phase 2) develop after infection with *C. burnetii*. In patients with acute Q fever, phase 2 antibody is usually detectable by the second week of illness; phase 1 is not detectable. The finding of phase 1 antibody indicates chronic infection. IgA subclasses (IgA1 seen in acute and chronic disease, IgA2 seen only in chronic disease) may also help detect chronic vs. acute infection. Only patients with endocarditis were found to have IgA2 antibodies to phase II antigens.[49]

For the acute phase, tetracycline 500 mg orally four times a day will hasten resolution. Treatment of chronic Q fever is not always successful. Patients probably need to be treated with tetracycline for at least 12 months.[7] Some recommend adding another drug, such as lincomycin or cotrimoxazole, but with unproven efficacy.[112,341] Patients with endocarditis typically receive treatment with tetracycline and quinolone for at least 4 years, although new research supports shortened treatment with doxycycline and hydroxychloroquine.[245] A vaccine has been used to prevent infection in high-risk abattoir workers. Prevention through avoidance of potentially infectious animal tissues, especially raw milk and products of conception, should be followed.

TABLE 33-7. Human Forms of Ehrlichiosis

	GRANULOCYTIC	MONOCYTIC
Infecting organism	*Ehrlichia equi-* like agent	*Ehrlichia chaffeensis*
Tick vector	*Ixodes scapularis*	*Amblyomma americanum, Dermacentor variabilis*
Geographic distribution	Northeast, Midwest	South-central states, Southeast

EHRLICHIA INFECTIONS. *Ehrlichia* is a genus in the Rickettsiaceae family. Ehrlichiae are pleomorphic, gram-negative, obligatory intracellular pathogens that cause disease in humans and animals throughout the world. Their life cycle takes place primarily within the cytoplasm of circulating WBCs or platelets. Ehrlichiae can be divided into at least three genogroups based on 16S ribosomal ribonucleic acid (rRNA) gene sequences, but they are clinically classified more often by target cell specificity.

Two forms of ehrlichiosis occur in humans: human monocytic ehrlichiosis (HME) and human granulocytic ehrlichiosis (HGE) (Table 33-7). HME is caused by the *Ehrlichia chaffeensis,* which attacks mononuclear phagocytes. The Lone Star tick (*Amblyomma americanum*) is the primary vector of *E. chaffeensis,* and HME occurs predominantly in the south-central and eastern United States. Serologically and morphologically, *E. chaffeensis* appears to be closely related to *Ehrlichia canis,* which causes an illness in dogs.[185] HGE is caused by an agent similar to *Ehrlichia equi,* infects neutrophils, and is likely transmitted by *Ixodes scapularis* and *Dermacentor variabilis* ticks.[87,222] HGE occurs primarily in the upper Midwestern and northeastern United States. The agent causing HGE is closely related serologically, morphologically, and by genomic sequencing to both *Ehrlichia phagocytophila* and *E. equi,* which are pathogenic to dogs, horses, sheep, goats, and deer.

HME has been reported in more than 30 states since 1986. Most cases occur in the south-central and southern Atlantic states (Oklahoma, Missouri, Virginia, Georgia), principally in areas where RMSF also occurs.[199] In one study, 68% of HME patients reported a tick bite, and 83% reported tick exposure in the 7 to 21 days before disease onset.[108] A recent analysis of ticks in northern California found that more than 13% of *Ixodes* ticks and 20% of *D. variabilis* ticks were infected with *E. chaffeensis.*[167] Most HGE cases occur in Minnesota and Wisconsin, with fewer cases in the southern New England states. Among HGE patients, 6% report tick bites, and almost all report exposure to ticks before

illness. The reservoir hosts for *E. equi*–like agents are thought to be wild rodents, deer, and sheep.[15] In field studies a high proportion of *I. scapularis* in endemic areas are infected with the ehrlichiosis-causing agent.[266] Although most cases of ehrlichiosis are sporadic, reports exist of Army reservist and retirement community outbreaks.[229,293] Patients with ehrlichiosis tend to be older than patients with RMSF, with a slight male predominance. More than 70% of cases occur between May and July.

Human ehrlichiosis has a broad clinical spectrum ranging from subclinical infection to a mild viral-like illness to a life-threatening disease. Because of the shared tick vector and increased seroprevalence of HGE in patients with Lyme disease, confusion surrounds the clinicopathologic spectrum of the disease. As with *Borrelia* and *Babesia* organisms, the vector tick must remain attached for more than 36 hours for effective transmission of *Ehrlichia* organisms. After an average incubation period of 7 days (range, 1 to 21 days), high fever, headache, chills or rigors, malaise, myalgia, and anorexia typically develop. Leukopenia, thrombocytopenia, and elevated liver enzymes may also be present. A rash, usually macular or papular but occasionally petechial or erythematous, develops in 20% to 40% of patients a median of 8 days after the onset of illness.[149] The rash appears to be more common in children than adults and involves the palms or soles in fewer than 10% of cases.[21]

Severe and even fatal complications develop in some patients, usually in elderly or immunocompromised patients or in settings of delayed diagnosis or treatment.[87] Respiratory complications may be relatively common; cough, pulmonary infiltrates, dyspnea, and respiratory failure have all been reported. Other serious complications include encephalopathy, meningoencephalitis, shock, opportunistic infections, gastrointestinal hemorrhage, and renal failure. Immunocompromised patients are a high risk for death. In HME, bone marrow and hepatic granulomas and multiorgan perivascular lymphohistiocytic infiltrates have been observed. In HGE, *Ehrlichia*-mediated defects in host defense and immune suppression have resulted in opportunistic fungal and viral infections.[344]

The most common CNS manifestation that predicts CSF abnormality is altered mental status. In one study of 15 patients with altered sensorium who underwent CSF testing, eight had abnormalities, including elevated lymphocytes (up to 1000 cells/μl) and protein in the CSF. In a review of 21 additional cases with CNS manifestations, 13 of 21 patients had abnormal CSF findings. Fourteen patients underwent brain computed tomography, revealing no abnormalities. Four of the 21 patients with CNS symptoms died.[246]

HGE is clinically similar to HME, although only 8% of HGE patients develop rash.[86] Elevated serum creatinine and transaminases, along with thrombocytopenia, occur in most patients. These abnormalities are usually mild and of short duration.[93]

As with RMSF, the diagnosis of ehrlichiosis depends on clinical findings. Serologic tests can be used to confirm the diagnosis. Indirect IFA testing against *E. chaffeensis* is now available from the CDC, and Western blot can be used to confirm seropositive specimens.[187] Antibody levels rise rapidly during the first 3 weeks and peak after approximately 6 weeks.

Controlled trials of antibiotic therapy have not been conducted for ehrlichiosis, although tetracycline (or doxycycline) appears to be effective. In vitro studies show antibiotic susceptibility to rifampin, quinolones, and doxycycline.[164] Chloramphenicol has been used to treat ehrlichiosis, but treatment failures have been reported, and *E. chaffeensis* is resistant to chloramphenicol in vitro.[36] Rifampin is bactericidal against *E. chaffeensis* in vitro, however clinical experience is limited. Recently, a pregnant HGE patient was treated successfully with rifampin.[39] Currently, tetracycline (doxycycline) should be considered the drug of choice for ehrlichiosis. The optimal dosage and duration of treatment need more investigation, but current recommendations are for oral or IV doxycycline (100 mg twice daily for adults, 3 mg/kg/day in two divided doses for children) for a minimum of 5 to 7 days. Dosing should be minimized as much as possible with children to prevent staining teeth. Because ehrlichiosis is potentially life threatening (2% mortality rate for HME, 7% to 10% for HGE), empiric treatment should be instituted before laboratory confirmation.[343]

Tick-Borne Viral Diseases

Ticks transmit a wide variety of viruses to humans. As with other tick-borne diseases, the viral illnesses are zoonotic. Ticks ingest the organisms while feeding on a viremic host; the virus replicates within the tick and is passed transstadially. Transovarial transmission has been documented for tick-borne encephalitis virus and Crimean-Congo hemorrhagic fever virus; the role of transovarial passage in maintaining these viruses in nature is unknown.[143] Amplification occurs when the infected tick feeds on an uninfected vertebrate. Humans usually are accidentally infected after intrusion into the natural tick-vertebrate cycle.

Tick-borne viruses cause clinical syndromes in humans that can be classified into four broad groups: influenza-like febrile illness with malaise, headache, myalgias, and arthralgias; febrile illness with hemorrhagic complications; febrile illness associated with meningoencephalitis; and subclinical or very mild illness. A specific virus may produce any or all of these syndromes depending on the virulence of the organism, host susceptibility, and the stage of the illness. For example, Colorado tick fever (CTF) virus usually causes an influenza-like febrile illness, but in susceptible hosts it may produce meningoencephalitis or rarely a hemorrhagic diathesis.

Diagnosis of tick-borne viral diseases requires clinical acumen and interpretation of epidemiologic and clinical information. Isolation of the virus, usually by intracerebral inoculation in suckling mice, or demonstration of a rise in antibody titers in the victim confirms the diagnosis. As with most viral diseases, treatment is primarily supportive.

Only CTF occurs with any frequency in the United States. Table 33-8 lists other tick-borne viruses.

Colorado Tick Fever. Colorado tick fever (CTF) is an acute self-limited febrile illness caused by a small, 12-segmented RNA virus of the family Reoviridae and genus Coltivirus. The Salmon River virus, a related but antigenically distinct virus isolated from a patient with likely CTF, is a new putative coltivirus. The distribution of CTF includes the western United States and Canada, specifically the Rocky Mountains, Black Hills, Sierra Nevadas, and coastal range of California, corresponding largely to the range of the Rocky Mountain wood tick, *Dermacentor andersoni.* Distribution exists at altitudes of 1219 to 2048 m (4000 to 10,000 feet), typically among pine-juniper-sagebrush vegetation. The natural reservoir normally depends on the small mammal–tick cycle but also involves small mammals in California outside the known range of *D. andersoni,* suggesting that other tick species are capable of transmitting the virus.[174]

CTF virus is maintained in its natural cycle by transmission between ticks and rodents.[202] Larval stages of *D. andersoni* ingest the virus while feeding on a viremic rodent host and pass it transstadially from larva to nymph to adult. Hibernating nymphs and adults carry the virus through the winter. Infected ticks emerge in the spring and feed on susceptible animals, renewing the cycle. Nymphal and adult ticks may also acquire the virus by feeding on viremic hosts. The virus does not appear to cause disease in its natural hosts; humans are incidental and dead-end hosts, usually infected by adult ticks. Transmission occurs between March and September with a peak between April and June. Risk factors include exposure to outdoor vegetation and often involve camping, hiking, and fishing. Ticks may be carried home on clothing or equipment, leading to infection.

CTF is usually a benign, self-limited febrile illness that is difficult to distinguish from many other agents, especially *Rickettsia rickettsii.* More than 200 cases of CTF are reported annually in the United States, but the actual incidence is probably much higher; many cases are not brought to medical attention or are diagnosed simply as a viral illness. It is a seasonal disease occurring from late March to early October, with a peak incidence

TABLE 33-8. Tick-Borne Viral Diseases

VIRUS	TAXONOMIC GROUP	MAJOR VECTOR	ANIMAL HOSTS	GEOGRAPHIC DISTRIBUTION	HUMAN ILLNESS	FREQUENCY OF RECOGNIZED DISEASE	RISK FACTORS
Colorado tick fever	Reoviridae, genus *Orbivirus*	*Dermacentor andersoni*	Rodents, other small mammals	Mountain highland areas of western United States and Canada	Biphasic FI, ME especially in children, in prolonged viremia	Sporadic, common in endemic areas	Occupational and recreational pursuits in mountain areas
Kemerovo	Reoviridae, genus *Orbivirus*	*Ixodes ricinus, I. persulcatus*	Domestic and wild mammals, birds	Siberia, Czech and Slovak Republics	Mild FI, occasional ME, not fatal	Sporadic, rare	Occupational and recreational pursuits in forested areas
TICK-BORNE ENCEPHALITIS COMPLEX							
Powassan encephalitis	Togaviridae, genus *Flavivirus* ⟶	*I. marxi, I. cookei*	Small mammals	Northern United States, Canada	FI, ME: possible sequelae and death especially in children	Sporadic, rare	Rural areas, pets?
Louping ill		*I. ricinus*	Goats, sheep, cattle, small mammals	Central and eastern Europe	Biphasic ME	Sporadic, common in endemic areas	Agricultural and forestry workers, drinking goat's milk
Russian spring-summer encephalitis		*I. ricinus, I. persulcatus*	Goats, sheep, cattle, small mammals	Siberia	Biphasic ME, possibly severe, with 20% mortality	Sporadic, common in endemic areas	Agricultural and forestry workers
Kyasanur Forest disease		*Haemaphysalis spinigera*	Monkeys, small mammals	Southern India	FI, ME, possible hemorrhagic complications	Sporadic, epidemics occur	Residence in or travel to endemic areas
Omsk hemorrhagic fever		*Dermacentor pictus?*	Muskrats	Western Siberia	FI, hemorrhagic complications	Rare	Direct contact with muskrats
Crimean-Congo hemorrhagic fever	Bunyaviridae, genus *Nairovirus*	*Hyalomma marginatum, H. anatolicum,* others	Domestic and wild mammals	Southern Russia, Middle East, India, Pakistan, central Africa	FI, petechial-ecchymotic rash, hemorrhage, 3%–30% mortality	Sporadic, epidemics occur	Agricultural workers
Dugbe	Bunyaviridae, genus *Nairovirus*	Ixodid species	Cattle	Nigeria, Central African Republic	Acute FI	Rare, primarily children	Herding or caring for livestock
Bhanja	Probably Bunyaviridae	Ixodid species	Domestic and wild mammals	Yugoslavia, Italy, Kenya, Nigeria, India	FI, ME	Rare	Agricultural workers
Thogoto	Possibly Orthomyxoviridae	Ixodid species	Ruminants	Egypt, Kenya, Nigeria	FI, ME, optic neuritis	Rare	Herding or caring for livestock
Quaranfil	Unclassified	*Argas arboreus*	Pigeons, wild birds	Africa, Iran, Afghanistan	FI	Rare	Residence in endemic areas

FI, Febrile illness; ME, meningoencephalitis.

in May and June. All age groups are susceptible to CTF, but it occurs most often in young men, reflecting their greater recreational and occupational activities in outdoor mountain areas. A history of tick exposure can be obtained in approximately 90% of patients with CTF; the usual time between the tick bite and the onset of symptoms is 3 to 6 days (range, 0 to 14 days).[127,291]

CTF usually begins with the abrupt onset of fever. Most victims experience severe headaches, myalgias, and lethargy; complaints of photophobia, ocular pain, anorexia, nausea and vomiting, and abdominal pain are common. A macular or maculopapular rash is reported in 5% to 12% of patients but is not a prominent feature. The most characteristic feature of the illness is a biphasic or "saddle-backed" temperature pattern. Victims initially experience 2 to 3 days of fever, followed by a 1- to 2-day remission and then an additional 2 to 3 days of fever. This pattern is helpful when present but cannot confirm the diagnosis, since it is observed in only about 50% of patients.[127,291]

CTF is usually mild, but severe complications can occur, particularly in children under age 10. Meningoencephalitis has been described in several children.[54,84,282,291] Two children developed a hemorrhagic diathesis and died.[127] Other unusual complications associated with CTF include pericarditis,[1,141] myocarditis,[92] hepatitis,[178] epididymoorchitis,[128] and pneumonitis.[127] Information on CTF contracted during pregnancy is inconclusive, but of five cases reported, one terminated in a spontaneous abortion and in another a liveborn infant had multiple congenital anomalies.[210] CTF virus is teratogenic in mice.[136]

Nearly half the patients with CTF require 3 weeks or longer to recover fully from the illness. The most common persistent symptoms are malaise and weakness. Prolonged symptoms occur most frequently in patients over age 30.[127] Treatment of CTF is supportive; infection generally confers lifelong immunity.

CTF virus circulates free in the plasma and bone marrow of infected patients until the end of the first week of illness, when it is neutralized by antibodies. In the bone marrow the virus infects erythrocyte precursors and persists within mature erythrocytes, where it is protected from antibodies. This allows viremia to persist for a prolonged period, even when clinical recovery is complete. Infective virus can be recovered from the blood for a month or longer in nearly 50% of patients.[127] Persistent viremia in blood donors poses a risk to recipients of blood transfusions; transfusion-acquired infection has been reported.[58]

Other hemopoietic cells may also be affected in CTF. Leukopenia involving both granulocytes and lymphocytes is common and may be helpful diagnostically, although one third of patients have normal WBC counts.[130] Thrombocytopenia may also develop; anemia associated with the virus is rare.

Traditionally, serologic analysis provided little firm evidence of CTF infection during the acute phase because of the delay in appearance of various antibodies. Recently, diagnosis during the acute phase using reverse-transcriptase PCR has been reported, making this method a promising tool for early detection and treatment.[13,149] Isolation of CTF virus from blood or CSF by inoculating suckling mice or cell cultures confirms the diagnosis and has been reported as the most reliable technique.[38] A fluorescent conjugate prepared against CTF viral antigen can be used to stain erythrocyte smears, but the test lacks sensitivity.[127] Serologic tests (neutralizing antibody, complement fixation, IFA) are available, but titers rise slowly, and these are traditionally not diagnostic during the clinical illness. Improvements in early serologic testing are ongoing, with recent reports of IgM detection against synthetic viral peptides and Western blot analysis, facilitating easier diagnosis during the acute phase of illness.

Babesiosis

Babesia species, as with malarial organisms, are pleomorphic intraerythrocytic protozoan parasites. More than 70 distinct species have been described from various vertebrate hosts.[254] Some of the most important species include *B. bigemina, B. bovis,* and *B. divergens* (all in cattle); *B. caballi* and *B. equi* (horses); *B. canis* (dogs); and *B. microti* (rodents). Babesiae are transmitted to vertebrates primarily through the bite of ixodid ticks.

Epidemiology. Babesiosis has long been recognized as an important veterinary disease, receiving biblical reference as the "divine murrain" infecting the cattle of the pharaoh Ramses II (Exodus 9:3). Various epidemics of cattle fever have been documented throughout history.[34] Human disease was originally reported in 1957 in a splenectomized man in Yugoslavia.[283] Five cases of human infection with bovine *Babesia (B. bovis, B. divergens)* were reported from Europe between 1957 and 1976; two cases of babesiosis of unknown species were reported from California in 1968 and 1981; a human case of *B. gibsoni* infection was reported in California in 1993; and a single *B. caucasia* infection was reported from Russia in 1978.[148,254,255] These cases were widely separated geographically, and all occurred in splenectomized individuals.

Since 1970 the incidence of human babesiosis has accelerated, primarily because of an outbreak of *B. microti* infections in the northeastern United States. The first case was recognized in a patient with an intact spleen in 1969 on Nantucket Island, Massachusetts.[358] Since then, more than 450 confirmed cases have occurred in the United States.[71,203] *B. microti* is endemic to the coastal regions of southern New England, where the principal vector is the northern deer tick *Ixodes scapularis.*

Most cases are contracted on Cape Cod and the off-shore islands of Massachusetts (Nantucket, Martha's Vineyard), New York (Shelter Island, Long Island), and Rhode Island (Block Island).[71] Cases have also been reported from Wisconsin and Minnesota, a known focus of *I. scapularis*.[319] The high incidence of *B. microti* infection is caused by its ability to produce disease in individuals with intact spleens. A new strain of *B. microti* called WA-1, thought to be spread by *Ixodes pacificus*, has been isolated from an immunocompetent patient with an intact spleen in Washington State.[238]

The ecology of *B. microti* parallels that of *Borrelia burgdorferi*, the agent of Lyme disease. The major vector in both diseases is *I. scapularis*. White-footed mice (*Peromyscus leucopus*) constitute the major reservoir for *B. microti*. Larval or nymphal ticks ingest the parasite during a blood meal from an infected rodent. Babesiae replicate within the tick and are passed transstadially. Amplification of the cycle occurs when the infected tick transmits the organism to a vertebrate host during the next blood meal. White-tailed deer (*Odocoileus virginianus*) are the principal hosts for adult ticks; larvae and nymphs feed on deer, mice, and other small mammals.[290]

Human babesiosis occurs when humans accidentally intrude on the natural cycle and are bitten by an infected tick. As in other tick-borne diseases, the peak incidence is during the warm weather months from May to September, when ticks are actively feeding. The majority of infections with *B. microti* are asymptomatic. Recent serologic testing shows that although seroconvergence has increased greatly over the past 30 years, it stabilized in the 1990s.

An epidemiologic survey of 136 cases in New York showed that the most important risk factors for severe babesial disease are advanced age, asplenia, and immunodeficiency. Babesial infection appears to be as prevalent in children as in adults, however, the intensity of disease greatly increases over age 40. In one study, 23% of patients with babesiosis had concurrent Lyme disease infection.[203] Case reports have also shown multiple coinfection involving borreliosis, ehrlichiosis, and babesiosis,[209] with more severe symptoms in coinfected individuals compared to single organism infection.[169]

Prolonged, subclinical infection creates the potential for transmission of *B. microti* through blood donation. More than 26 cases of babesiosis acquired by transfusion have been reported.[79,173,189,284,365] Seroprevalence surveys in endemic regions show donor exposure rates of 3% or greater.[80] Currently, control of transfusion-related infection is limited to identifying donors at high risk of exposure (from endemic regions, history of tick bites, seasonal exposure to tick-favorable landscapes). This strategy may become less effective as tick-endemic areas expand. Transfusion

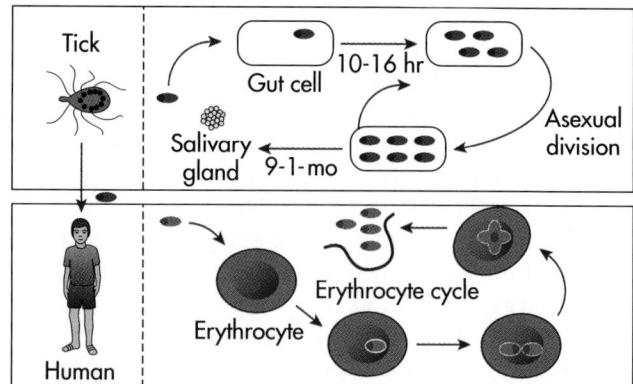

Figure 33-7 *Babesia* life cycle. Within a tick, *Babesia* parasites infect gut cells, undergo asexual division, and eventually migrate to the salivary glands. The organism is introduced into a human when the infected tick takes in a blood meal. Transmission usually involves the nymphal tick, but the duration of attachment required for transmission of *Babesia* species is not known. *Babesia* species can be transmitted to humans concomitantly with *Borrelia burgdorferi*. (*Modified from Boustani MR, Gelfand JA: Clin Infect Dis 22:612, 1996.*)

has also reportedly transmitted new species of *Babesia*, causing significant disease in immunocompetent individuals.[141]

Pathogenesis. Babesiae are transmitted from wild and domestic animal reservoirs to humans by *Ixodes* ticks. The life cycle of *I. scapularis*, the tick responsible for transmission of *B. microti* to humans from rodents, spans 2 years, beginning in the spring with the hatching of the larval form. In the late spring and summer months the larvae feed on a variety of hosts and acquire babesial infection. Typically, larvae become infected from their preferred host, *leucopus*. Ingested Babesiae reach the gut of the feeding tick, where they reproduce sexually. The newly formed zygote eventually spreads throughout the body of the tick. After reaching the salivary glands, the babesial sporoblasts remain dormant until the next spring when the tick larva molts to a nymph. The nymph then seeks a blood meal, infecting a new host (rodents or humans). In endemic areas, as many as 60% of white-footed mice are infected by late summer. The nymph *I. scapularis* is the primary vector of human babesiosis, but adult ticks can also transmit the disease.

After inoculation by a tick bite, *Babesia* sporozoites rapidly invade erythrocytes, where they differentiate into merozoites. Great pleomorphism is displayed,[214] but ring-shaped and ameboid trophozoites are the predominant form. Multiplication occurs by asexual asynchronous budding. After the parasite multiplies, the infected erythrocyte ruptures, freeing the organisms to invade other red blood cells (RBCs); severe hemolytic anemia may ensue (Figure 33-7).

Infection with *B. microti* reduces the malleability of erythrocytes, causing microvascular stasis and decreased RBC life span. Electron microscopy has shown extensive RBC wall damage, including protrusions, perforations, and extrusions in the cell membrane. Asplenia or steroid therapy can worsen the disease and prolong parasitemia. An intact spleen preferentially destroys infected RBCs because of their decreased malleability.

Prolonged parasitemia is common in babesiosis.[257] *B. microti* may persist for as long as 4 months in an otherwise healthy patient.[358] Parasitemia may remain after clinical recovery or may develop in asymptomatic individuals.

An intact spleen is important in resistance to *Babesia* organisms. Although the presence of a spleen is not protective against *B. microti,* the disease is often more severe in splenectomized patients. Age is also an important factor in susceptibility to babesiosis. Children and young adults usually have subclinical or mild, self-limited infections, whereas older adults are more likely to have severe, clinically apparent disease.[25,258] Chronic medical disorders may be an additional risk factor for severe babesiosis.[26]

Clinical Manifestations. Acute *B. microti* infection is characterized by the gradual onset of malaise, anorexia, and fatigue, followed within several days to a week by fever, sweats, and myalgias. Other, less common symptoms include headache, nausea and vomiting, depression, abdominal pain, and dark urine. In a review of 17 patients with babesiosis, 52.9% presented with temperature greater than 38.3° C (101° F), and four of the nine had morning fever spikes; eight had relative bradycardia.[161]

Incubation is 1 to 4 weeks after a tick bite or 6 to 9 weeks after transmission by blood transfusion. Most victims do not recall a tick bite, and rash is not a feature of the illness. If rash resembling erythema migrans appears, Lyme disease coinfection should be considered. Physical examination is usually normal, except for fever (steady or intermittent) and mild splenomegaly in some patients. Petechiae and ecchymosis may rarely occur. Laboratory evaluation reveals a mild to moderate hemolytic anemia; normal to slightly reduced WBC counts; and in some patients, mild to moderate thrombocytopenia. Serum lactate dehydrogenase (LDH) and bilirubin levels are mildly elevated in most patients, reflecting the hemolytic anemia.[126,257] AST and ASL may be elevated, and urine may show proteinuria and hemoglobinuria. In one series, 13 of 17 patients (76.5%) had lymphopenia, and five (29.4%) had rouleau formation in the peripheral blood smear.[161]

A review of 139 hospitalized patients with babesiosis in New York from 1982 to 1993 looked at common signs and symptoms and the prognostic factors associated with poor outcome.[359] Of the 139 patients, 9 (6.5%) died, 35 (25.2%) were admitted to the intensive care unit, and 35 (25.2%) required more than 14 days of hospitalization. In these patients with severe disease the mean age was 62.5 years, and 62% were male. The most common symptoms were fatigue, malaise, weakness (91%); fever (91%); shaking chills (77%); and diaphoresis (69%). Prognostic indicators for severe outcome included high alkaline phosphatase, male gender, and elevated WBC count. Only 12% of patients with severe disease had a history of splenectomy, and only 2% had received a prior blood transfusion.

Although most patients with normal splenic function recover without specific therapy, prolonged fatigue and malaise are common.[257] Splenectomized persons generally have more severe clinical disease with higher levels of parasitemia and more severe hemolytic anemia.[258] Elderly persons, immunocompromised patients, and those with human immunodeficiency virus (HIV) also are at higher risk for severe infection. Pulmonary edema has been reported.[34] Typically, the level of parasitemia ranges from 1% to 10%.

In Europe, babesiosis results from infection with *B. divergens* or *B. bovis* and has been reported only in splenectomized patients. The illness is characterized by high fever, chills, headache, and severe hemolytic anemia, often resulting in hemoglobinuria, jaundice, and renal insufficiency. Major findings on physical examination include fever, hepatomegaly, jaundice, and hypotension. More than half of the reported cases have been fatal.[255]

Only one case of human babesiosis during pregnancy has been reported to date.[247] The patient recovered without specific therapy, and the neonate did not develop babesiosis. Cases of intrauterine infection in animals, however, have been reported.

Diagnosis. Babesiosis should be considered in any person with an unexplained febrile illness who has lived in or traveled to an endemic region in the midsummer months, especially with a history of a tick bite or tick exposure. The diagnosis of babesiosis can be confirmed by identifying the intraerythrocytic parasites on Giemsa-stained blood smears. Persons with intact spleens usually have low levels of parasitemia (less than 5% parasites), and examination of repeated smears may be necessary.[126,257] The predominant forms of *B. microti* closely resemble the small rings of *Plasmodium* species. A later tetrad form may be seen and is positive morphologic evidence of babesiosis. Differentiating *Babesia* from *Plasmodium* may be difficult but is

---

Box 33-5 LABORATORY DIAGNOSIS OF BABESIOSIS

Peripheral blood smear (Wright or Giemsa staining)
   showing intraerythrocytic *Babesia*
Polymerase chain reaction
Indirect immunofluorescent assay
Intraperitoneal inoculation of splenectomized hamsters

---

possible by noting the absence of pigment deposits in erythrocytes parasitized with the older stages of *Plasmodium* species (Box 33-5).

When organisms cannot be detected on blood smears, the diagnosis can made by intraperitoneal inoculation of the patient's blood into splenectomized hamsters. Serologic studies may also be helpful in confirming the diagnosis[259] but are performed in only a few laboratories. A titer greater than 1:64 on IFA testing is considered consistent with seropositivity, and a titer greater than 1:256 is diagnostic of acute infection. No test for circulating *Babesia* antigen is available. PCR testing for *Babesia* can be as sensitive and specific as standard testing and may be reproducible enough for routine use in diagnosis of acute babesiosis.[168]

Treatment and Prevention. Chemotherapy for *B. microti* infection consists of a combination of clindamycin and quinine and should reserved for patients with severe disease or those with asplenia, immunosuppression, or elderly status.[72] The clindamycin dose for adults is 1.2 g intravenously twice daily or 600 mg orally three times daily for 7 days. Children should receive three oral doses of clindamycin for 7 days (20 to 40 mg/kg/day). The quinine dose for adults is 650 mg orally three times daily and for children is 25 mg/kg/day in three divided doses, each for 7 days. Parasites are eradicated from the blood with this therapy, although treatment failures have been reported.[278,284] Recently, azithromycin was used as a successful alternative to clindamycin in one treatment failure.[278] In seriously ill patients with high levels of parasitemia, exchange transfusion may also produce rapid clinical improvement.[147,328]

Patients with mild clinical disease typically recover without specific anti-*Babesia* chemotherapy, although few patients have been followed longitudinally. A recent prospective study showed that parasitemia lasted for a mean of 82 days in 24 asymptomatic subjects not treated with the standard regimen.[170] Even those receiving clindamycin and quinine had delayed resolution of parasitemia, however, and 9 of 22 subjects had significant side effects from standard therapy. Exchange transfusion with clindamycin/quinine therapy has proved to be effective in three cases of *B. divergens* infection.[34]

Avoidance of ticks is the only currently effective method of preventing babesiosis. Splenectomized patients should probably be advised to avoid visiting areas endemic for babesiosis.

TICK-BITE PREVENTION AND PROPHYLAXIS

Prevention of tick-borne diseases is directed toward preventing tick bites. Avoidance of areas (nearby water supply, dense ground cover) supporting the reservoir species, often the white-footed mouse in the northeastern United States, will decrease tick exposure.[273] Protective clothing (long pants cinched at the ankles or tucked into boots or socks) should be worn when in tick-infested areas. Spraying clothes with an insect repellent may provide an additional barrier against ticks. Most repellents contain diethyltoluamide (DEET), which repels ticks but does not kill them. Permanone is an aerosol spray tick repellent for use on clothing. Its active ingredient, permethrin, kills ticks on contact. Field tests have shown Permanone to be 90% to 100% effective in preventing tick bites. Permethrins have very low toxicity in mammals.

Close inspection of all parts of the body at least twice daily should be done when traveling in tick-infested areas. Adult ixodid ticks are generally on the body for 1 or 2 hours before attaching. Even after a tick attaches, disease transmission may be prevented by prompt removal. Proper removal of the tick is important, since infection may be acquired by careless handling of infected ticks, even without a bite. The tick should be grasped as close to the skin surface as possible with blunt curved forceps, tweezers, or protected fingers. The tick should be pulled out with steady pressure, taking care not to crush or squeeze the body, since expressed fluid may contain infective agents. After the tick is removed, the bite site should be disinfected. Traditional methods of tick removal, such as applying fingernail polish, isopropyl alcohol, or a hot match head, do not effect tick detachment and may induce the tick to salivate or regurgitate into the wound.[219] V-shaped devices are available that slide between the tick and the skin so that the tick can be lifted from its attachment.

In general, prophylactic antibiotics are not recommended for tick bites. Clinical trials of antibiotic prophylaxis for RMSF and Lyme disease demonstrate that the risk of infection in a patient who seeks medical treatment for a tick bite is very low. In most areas of the United States the chances are small that a tick harbors an infectious agent. Even if the tick is infected, the agent probably will not be transmitted if the tick is found and removed promptly. Together, these facts suggest that the risk/benefit ratio of an adverse reaction to the antibiotic vs. disease prevention will be high.

REFERENCES

1. Abbott KH: Tick paralysis: a review, *Proc Mayo Clin* 18:39, 1943.
2. Ackermann R et al: *Ixodes ricinus* spirochete and European erythema chronicum migrans disease, *Yale J Biol Med* 57:573, 1984.
3. Ackermann R et al: Chronic neurologic manifestations of erythema migrans borreliosis, *Ann NY Acad Sci* 539:16, 1988.
4. Ackley A, Lupovici M: Lyme-disease meningitis treated with tetracycline, *Ann Intern Med* 105:630, 1986.
5. Afzelius A: Erythema chronicum migrans, *Acta Derm Venereol* 2:120, 1921.
6. Agger WA, Callister SM, Jobe DA: In vitro susceptibilities of *Borrelia burgdorferi* to five oral cephalosporins and ceftriaxone, *Antimicrob Agents Chemother* 36:1788, 1992.
7. Agre F, Schwartz R: The value of early treatment of deer tick bites for the prevention of Lyme disease, *Am J Dis Child* 147:945, 1993.
8. American College of Obstetrics and Gynecology committee opinion: Lyme disease during pregnancy, *Int J Gynaecol Obstet* 39:59, 1992.
9. Anderson BE et al: *Ehrlichia chaffeensis,* a new species associated with human ehrlichiosis, *J Clin Microbiol* 29:2838, 1991.
10. Anderson BE et al: Detection of the etiologic agent of human ehrlichiosis by polymerase chain reaction, *J Clin Microbiol* 30:775, 1992.
11. Asbrink E, Hovmark A: Lyme borreliosis: aspects of tick-borne *Borrelia burgdorferi* infection from a dermatologic viewpoint, *Semin Dermatol* 9:277, 1990.
12. Atlas E et al: Lyme myositis: muscle invasion by *Borrelia burgdorferi, Ann Intern Med* 108:245, 1988.
13. Attoui H et al: Serologic and molecular diagnosis of Colorado tick fever viral infections, *Am J Trop Med Hyg* 59:763, 1998.
14. Ayres JG et al: Post-infection fatigue syndrome following Q fever, *QJM* 91:105, 1998.
15. Bakken JS et al: Human granulocytic ehrlichiosis in the upper Midwest: a new species emerging? *JAMA* 272:212, 1994.
16. Banfield JF: Tick bites in man, *Med J Aust* 2:600, 1966.
17. Barbour AG: Molecular biology of antigenic variation in Lyme borreliosis and relapsing fever: a comparative analysis, *Scand J Infect Dis Suppl* 77:88, 1991.
18. Barbour AG, Fish D: The biological and social phenomenon of Lyme disease, *Science* 260:1610, 1993.
19. Barbour AG, Hayes SF: Biology of *Borrelia* species, *Microbiol Rev* 50:381, 1986.
20. Barson WJ: Probable actinic Rocky Mountain spotted fever, *Pediatr Infect Dis J* 17:850, 1998.
21. Barton LL, Rathore MH, Dawson JE: Infection with *Ehrlichia* in childhood, *J Pediatr* 120:998, 1992.
22. Bell WE, Lascare AD: Rocky Mountain spotted fever, *Neurology* 20:841, 1970.
23. Belman AL et al: Neurologic manifestations in children with North American Lyme disease, *Neurology* 43:2609, 1993.
24. Beltran RR et al: Evaluation of ciprofloxacin and doxycycline in the treatment of Mediterranean spotted fever, *Eur J Clin Microbiol Infect Dis* 11:427, 1992.
25. Benach JL, Habicht GS: Clinical characteristics of human babesiosis, *J Infect Dis* 144:481, 1981.
26. Benach JL, Habicht GS, Hamburger MI: Immunoresponsiveness in acute babesiosis in humans, *J Infect Dis* 146:369, 1982.
27. Benach JL et al: Changing patterns in the incidence of Rocky Mountain spotted fever on Long Island (1971-1976), *Am J Epidemiol* 106:380, 1977.
28. Benach JL et al: Spirochetes isolated from the blood of two patients with Lyme disease, *N Engl J Med* 308:740, 1983.
29. Berger BW, Clemmensen OJ, Ackerman AB: Lyme disease is a spirochetosis: a review of the disease and evidence for its cause, *Am J Dermatopathol* 5:111, 1983.
30. Berger BW et al: Cultivation of Borrelia burgdorferi from erythema migrans lesions and perilesional skin, *J Clin Microbiol* 30: 359, 1992.
31. Bingham et al: Neurologic manifestations in children with Lyme disease, *Pediatrics* 96:1053, 1995.
32. Bloom BJ et al: Neurocognitive abnormalities in children after manifestations of Lyme disease, *Pediatr Infect Dis J* 17:189, 1998.
33. Bosler EM et al: Natural distribution of the *Ixodes dammini* spirochete, *Science* 220:321, 1983.
34. Boustani MR, Gelfand JA: Babesiosis, *Clin Infect Dis* 22: 611, 1996.
35. Breitschwerdt EB et al: Efficacy of chloramphenicol, enrofloxacin, and tetracycline for treatment of experimental Rocky Mountain spotted fever in dogs, *Antimicrob Agents Chemother* 35:2375, 1991.
36. Brouqui P, Raoult D: In vitro antibiotic susceptibility of the newly recognized agent of ehrlichiosis in humans, *Ehrlichia chaffeensis, Antimicrob Agents Chemother* 36:2799, 1992.
37. Brown RN, Lane RS: Lyme disease in California: a novel enzootic transmission cycle of *Borrelia burgdorferi, Science* 256:1439, 1992.
38. Brown SE, Knudson DL: Coltivirus infections. In Porterfield JS, editor: *Exotic viral infections,* London, 1995, Chapman and Hall.
39. Buitrago MI et al: Human granulocytic ehrlichiosis during pregnancy treated successfully with rifampin, *Clin Infect Dis* 27:213, 1998.
40. Burgdorfer W: A review of Rocky Mountain spotted fever (tick-borne typhus), its agent, and its tick vectors in the United States, *J Med Entomol* 12:269, 1975.
41. Burgdorfer W: The spotted fever group diseases. In Steele JH, editor: *CRC handbook series in zoonoses, section A: bacterial, rickettsial, and mycotic diseases,* vol II, Boca Raton, Fla, 1980, CRC Press.
42. Burgdorfer W: Discovery of the Lyme disease spirochete and its relation to tick vectors, *Yale J Biol Med* 57:515, 1984.
43. Burgdorfer W, Gage K: Susceptibility of the black-legged tick, Ixodes scapularis, to the Lyme disease spirochete, *Borrelia burgdorferi, Zbl Bakt Hyg* 263:15, 1986.
44. Burgdorfer W et al: Lyme disease—a tick-borne spirochetosis? *Science* 216:1317, 1982.
45. Burgdorfer W et al: The western black-legged tick, *Ixodes pacificus:* a vector of *Borrelia burgdorferi, Am J Trop Med Hyg* 34:925, 1985.
46. Butler T: Relapsing fever: new lessons about antibiotic action, *Ann Intern Med* 102:397, 1985.
47. Butler T, Jones PK, Wallace CK: *Borrelia recurrentis* infection: single-dose regimens and management of the Jarisch-Herxheimer reaction, *J Infect Dis* 137:573, 1978.
48. Cadavid D, Barbour AG: Neuroborreliosis during relapsing fever: review of the clinical manifestations, pathology, and treatment of infections in humans and experimental animals, *Clin Infect Dis* 26:151, 1998.
49. Camacho MT et al: Distribution of IgA subclass response to *Coxiella burnetii* in patients with acute and chronic Q fever, *Clin Immunol Immunopathol* 88:80, 1998.
50. Campbell GL et al: Epidemiologic and diagnostic studies of patients with suspected early Lyme disease, Missouri, 1990-1993, *J Infect Dis* 182: 470, 1995.
51. Campbell GL et al: Estimation of the incidence of Lyme disease, *Am J Epidemiol* 148, 1018, 1998.
52. Carter ML et al: Epidemiology of Lyme disease in the Lyme, Connecticut area. In *Program and abstracts of the 7th International Congress on Lyme Borreliosis,* San Francisco, June, 1996.
53. Centers for Disease Control: Relapsing fever, *MMWR* 22:242, 1973.
54. Centers for Disease Control: Transmission of Colorado tick fever virus by blood transfusion, *MMWR* 24:422, 1975.
55. Centers for Disease Control: Tick paralysis—Wisconsin, *MMWR* 30:217, 1981.
56. Centers for Disease Control: Update: Lyme disease and cases occurring during pregnancy—United States, *MMWR* 34:376, 1985.
57. Centers for Disease Control: Rocky Mountain spotted fever—United States, 1985, *MMWR* 35:247, 1986.
58. Centers for Disease Control: Summaries of notifiable diseases in the United States, *MMWR* 40:1, 1991.
59. Centers for Disease Control: Lyme disease, 1991-1992, *MMWR* 42:345, 1993.
60. Centers for Disease Control and Prevention:. Summary of notifiable diseases, United States, 1996, *MMWR* 45:3, 1996.
61. Centers for Disease Control and Prevention: Lyme disease - United States, 1996, *MMWR* 46:531, 1997.
62. Clark JR et al: Facial paralysis in Lyme disease, *Laryngoscope* 95:1341, 1985.
63. Clements ML et al: Serodiagnosis of Rocky Mountain spotted fever: comparison of IgM and IgG enzyme-linked immunosorbent assays and indirect fluorescent antibody test, *J Infect Dis* 148:876, 1983.
64. Conlon PJ et al: Predictors of prognosis and risk factors of acute renal failure in patients with Rocky Mountain spotted fever, *Am J Med* 101:621, 1996.
65. Costello CM et al: A prospective study of tick bites in an endemic area for Lyme disease, *Conn Med* 53:338, 1989.
66. Coyle BS et al: The public health impact of Lyme disease in Maryland, *J Infect Dis* 173: 1260, 1996.
67. Coyle PK: Neurologic Lyme disease, *Semin Neurol* 12:200, 1992.
68. Cromley EK et al.: Residential setting as a risk factor for Lyme disease in a hyperendemic region, *Am J of Epidemiol* 147:472, 1998.

69. Culp RW et al: Lyme arthritis in children, *J Bone Joint Surg* 69A:96, 1987.

70. Dalton MJ et al: National surveillance for Rocky Mountain spotted fever, 1981-1992: epidemiologic summary and evaluation of risk factors for fatal outcome, *Am J Trop Med Hyg* 52:404, 1995.

71. Dammin GJ et al: The rising incidence of clinical *Babesia* microti infection, *Hum Pathol* 12:398, 1981.

72. Dammin GJ et al: Clindamycin and quinine treatment for *Babesia microti* infections, *MMWR* 32:65, 1983.

73. Dattwyler RJ et al: Ceftriaxone as effective therapy in refractory Lyme disease, *J Infect Dis* 155:1322, 1987.

74. Dattwyler RJ et al: Treatment of late Lyme borreliosis—randomized comparison of ceftriaxone and penicillin, *Lancet* 1:1191, 1988.

75. Dattwyler RJ et al: Ceftriaxone compared with doxycycline for the treatment of acute disseminated Lyme disease, *N Engl J Med* 337:289-363, 1997.

76. Davis GE: The relapsing fevers: tick-spirochete specificity studies, *Exp Parasitol* 1:406, 1952.

77. Davis RD, Burke JP, Wright LJ: Relapsing fever associated with ARDS in a parturient woman, *Chest* 102:630, 1992.

78. Derrick EH: Q fever, a new fever entity: clinical features, diagnosis and laboratory investigation, *Med J Aust* 2:281, 1937.

79. Dobroszycki J et al: A cluster of transfusion-associated babesiosis cases traced to a single asymptomatic donor, *JAMA* 281:927, 1999.

80. Dodd RY: Transmission of parasites by blood transfusion, *Vox Sanguinis* 74 (suppl 2):161, 1998.

81. Donat JR, Donat JF: Tick paralysis with persistent weakness and electromyographic abnormalities, *Arch Neurol* 38:59, 1981.

82. Donohue JF: Lower respiratory tract involvement in Rocky Mountain spotted fever, *Arch Intern Med* 140:223, 1980.

83. Drage LA: Life-threatening rashes: dermatologic signs of four infectious diseases, *Mayo Clin Proc* 74:68, 1999.

84. Draughn DE, Sieber OF, Umlauf HJ: Colorado tick fever encephalitis, *Clin Pediatr* 4:626, 1965.

85. Dressler F et al: Western blotting in the serodiagnosis of Lyme disease, *J Infect Dis* 167:392, 1993.

86. Dumler JS, Bakken JS: Ehrlichial diseases of humans: emerging tick-borne infections, *Clin Infect Dis* 20, 1102, 1995.

87. Dumler JS, Bakken JS: Human ehrlichiosis: newly recognized infections transmitted by ticks, *Annu Re Med* 49:201, 1998.

88. Dworkin MS et al: Tick-borne relapsing fever in the northwestern United States and southwestern Canada, *Clin Infect Dis* 26:122, 1997.

89. Eckman MH et al: Cost effectiveness of oral as compared with intravenous antibiotic therapy for patients with early Lyme disease or Lyme arthritis, *N Engl J Med* 337:357, 1997.

90. Edell TA et al: Tick-borne relapsing fever in Colorado—historical review and report of cases, *JAMA* 241:2279, 1979.

91. Editorial: Chronic Q fever, *J Infect* 8:1, 1984.

92. Emmons RW, Schade HI: Colorado tick fever simulating acute myocardial infarction, *JAMA* 222:87, 1972.

93. Eng TR et al: Epidemiologic, clinical, and laboratory findings of human ehrlichioses in the United States, 1988, *JAMA* 264:2251, 1990.

94. Failing RM, Lyon CB, McKittrick JE: The pajaroello tick bite—the frightening folklore and the mild disease, *Calif Med* 116:16, 1972.

95. Falco RC, Fish D: Prevalence of *Ixodes dammini* near the home of Lyme disease patients in Westchester County, New York, *Am J Epidemiol* 127:826, 1988.

96. Falco RC, Fish D, Piesman J: Duration of tick bites in a Lyme disease–endemic area, *Am J Epidemiol* 143:187, 1996.

97. Fallon BA et al: The underdiagnosis of neuropsychiatric Lyme disease in children and adults, *Psychiatr Clin North Am* 21:693, 1998.

98. Feder HM et al: Persistence of serum antibodies to *Borrelia burgdorferi* in patients treated for Lyme disease, *Clin Infect Dis* 15:788, 1992.

99. Feder HM et al: Early Lyme disease: a flu-like illness without erythema migrans, *Pediatrics* 91:456, 1993.

100. Feder HM et al: Pitfalls in the diagnosis and treatment of Lyme disease in children, *JAMA* 274: 66, 1995.

101. Feldman-Muhsam B: Ixodid tick attacks on man in Israel: medical implications, *Isr J Med Sci* 22:19, 1986.

102. Felsenfeld O: Borreliae, human relapsing fever, and parasite-vector-host relationships, *Bacteriol Rev* 29:46, 1965.

103. Feltes TF et al: M-mode echocardiographic abnormalities in Rocky Mountain spotted fever, *South Med J* 77:1130, 1984.

104. Fihn S, Larson EB: Tick-borne relapsing fever in the Pacific Northwest: an under-diagnosed illness? *West J Med* 133:203, 1980.

105. Finkel MJ, Halperin JJ: Nervous system Lyme borreliosis—revisited, *Arch Neurol* 49:102, 1992.

106. Fishbein DB et al: Surveillance of Rocky Mountain spotted fever in the United States, 1981-1983, *J Infect Dis* 150:609, 1984.

107. Fishbein DB et al: Unexplained febrile illnesses after exposure to ticks: infection with an *Ehrlichia? JAMA* 257:3100, 1987.

108. Fishbein DB et al: Human ehrlichiosis in the United States, 1985 to 1990, *Ann Intern Med* 120:736, 1994.

109. Fix AD, Strickland GT, Grant J: Tick bites and Lyme disease in an endemic setting: problematic use of serologic testing and prophylactic antibiotic therapy, *JAMA* 279:206, 1998.

110. Fornier PE et al: Coxiella burnetii infection of aneurysms or vascular grafts: report of seven cases and review, *Clin Infect Dis* 26:116, 1998.

111. Francioli PB et al: Response of babesiosis to pentamidine therapy, *Ann Intern Med* 94:326, 1981.

112. Freeman R, Hodson ME: Q fever endocarditis treated with trimethoprim and sulphamethoxazole, *Br Med J* 1:419, 1972.

113. Friedland JS et al: Q fever and intrauterine death, *Lancet* 343:288, 1994.

114. Furman DP, Loomis EC: The ticks of California, *Bull Calif Insect Survey* 25:13, 1984.

115. Gardner P: Lyme disease vaccines, *Ann Intern Med* 129:583, 1998.

116. Garin C, Bujadoux: Paralysie par les tiques, *J Med Lyon* 3:765, 1922.

117. Gasser RNA.: Treatment of Lyme Borreliosis with cefoperazone and sulbactam, *Lancet* 345:8949, 1995.

118. Gerber MA, Shapiro ED: Diagnosis of Lyme disease in children, *J Pediatr* 121:157, 1992.

119. Gerber MA, Zemel LS, Shapiro ED: Lyme arthritis in children: clinical epidemiology and long-term outcomes, *Pediatrics* 102:905, 1998.

120. Gerber MA et al: Lyme disease in children in southeastern Connecticut, *N Engl J Med* 335:1270, 1996.

121. Gerster JC et al: Lyme arthritis appearing outside the United States: a case report from Switzerland, *Br Med J* 283:951, 1981.

122. Goellner MH et al: Hepatitis due to recurrent Lyme disease, *Ann Intern Med* 108:707, 1988.

123. Goffin Y et al: Chronic Q fever, *Lancet* 1:1421, 1981.

124. Goldman L, Johnson P, Ramsey J: The insect bite reaction, *J Invest Dermatol* 18:403, 1984.

125. Golightly MG: Laboratory considerations in the diagnosis and management of Lyme borreliosis, *Clin Pathol* 99:168, 1992.

126. Gombert ME et al: Human babesiosis—clinical and therapeutic considerations, *JAMA* 248:3005, 1982.

127. Goodpasture HC et al: Colorado tick fever: clinical, epidemiologic, and laboratory aspects of 228 cases in Colorado in 1973-1974, *Ann Intern Med* 88:303, 1978.

128. Gordon JC et al: Epidemiology of Rocky Mountain spotted fever in Ohio, 1981: serologic evaluation of canines and rickettsial isolation from ticks associated with human case exposure sites, *Am J Trop Med Hyg* 33:1026, 1984.

129. Gorman RJ, Saxon S, Snead OC: Neurologic sequelae of Rocky Mountain spotted fever, *Pediatrics* 67:354, 1981.

130. Gorman RJ, Snead C: Tick paralysis in three children—the diversity of neurologic presentations, *Clin Pediatr* 17:249, 1978.

131. Goubau PF: Relapsing fevers. a review, *Ann Soc Belg Med Trop* 64:335, 1984.

132. Grattan-Smith PJ et al: Clinical and neurophysiological features of tick paralysis, *Brain* 120:1975, 1997.

133. Gresikova M, Beran GW: Tick-borne encephalitis. In Steele JH, editor: *CRC handbook series of zoonoses, section B: viral zoonoses,* vol I, Boca Raton, Fla, 1981, CRC Press.

134. Guo HR et al: Prevalence of Coxiella burnetii infections among North Dakota sheep producers, *J Occup Environ Med* 40:999, 1998.

135. Haas E et al: Tick paralysis—Washington, 1995, *MMWR* 45:325, 1996.

136. Harris RE, Morahan P, Coleman P: Teratogenic effects of Colorado tick fever virus in mice, *J Infect Dis* 131:397, 1975.

137. Hattwick MAW, O'Brien RJ, Hanson BF: Rocky Mountain spotted fever: epidemiology of an increasing problem, *Ann Intern Med* 84:732, 1976.

138. Hattwick MAW et al: Fatal Rocky Mountain spotted fever, *JAMA* 240:1499, 1978.

139. Helmick CG, Bernard KW, D'Angelo LJ: Rocky Mountain spotted fever: clinical, laboratory, and epidemiological features of 262 cases, *J Infect Dis* 150:480, 1984.

140. Herwaldt BL et al: Transfusion-transmitted babesiosis in Washington state: first reported case caused by a WA1-type parasite, *J Infect Dis* 175:1259, 1997.

141. Hierholzer WJ, Barry DW: Colorado tick fever pericarditis, *JAMA* 217:825, 1971 (letter).

142. Hoogstaal H: Tick-borne Crimean-Congo hemorrhagic fever. In Steele JH, editor: *CRC handbook series in zoonoses, section B: viral zoonoses,* vol I, Boca Raton, Fla, 1981, CRC Press.

143. Hoogstaal H: Argasid and nuttalliellid ticks as parasites and vectors, *Adv Parasitol* 24:135, 1985.

144. Horton JM, Blaser MJ: The spectrum of relapsing fever in the Rocky Mountains, *Arch Intern Med* 145:871, 1985.

145. Indudharan R et al: Intra-aural tick causing facial palsy, *Lancet* 348:613, 1996.

146. Jacobs JC, Stevens M, Duray PH: Lyme disease simulating septic arthritis, *JAMA* 256:1138, 1986.

147. Jacoby GA et al: Treatment of transfusion-transmitted babesiosis by exchange transfusion, *N Engl J Med* 303:1098, 1980.

148. Jerant AF, Arline AD: Babesiosis in California, *West J Med* 158:622, 1993.

149. Johnson AJ, Karabatsos N, Lanciotti RS: Detection of Colorado tick fever virus by using reverse transcriptase PCR and application of the technique in laboratory diagnosis, *J Clin Microbiol* 35:1203, 1997.

150. Johnson JE, Kadull PJ: Rocky Mountain spotted fever acquired in the laboratory, *N Engl J Med* 277:842, 1967.

151. Johnson RC, Kodner C, Russel M: In vitro and in vivo susceptibility of the Lyme disease spirochete, *Borrelia burgdorferi* to four antimicrobial agents, *Antimicrob Agents Chemother* 31:164, 1987.

152. Johnson RC et al: Susceptibility of the Lyme disease spirochete to seven antimicrobial agents, *Yale J Biol Med* 57:549, 1984.

153. Johnson RC et al: Comparative in vitro and in vivo susceptibilities of the Lyme disease spirochete *Borrelia burgdorferi* to cefuroxime and other antimicrobial agents, *Antimicrob Agents Chemother* 34:2133-2136, 1990.

154. Johnson WD: *Borrelia* species (relapsing fever). In Mandell GL, Bennett JE, Dolin R, editors: *Mandell, Douglas and Bennett's principles and practice of infectious diseases*, ed 4, New York, 1995, Churchill Livingstone.

155. Jongen VHWM et al: Tick-borne relapsing fever and pregnancy outcome in rural Tanzania, *Acta Obstet Gynecol Scand* 76: 834, 1997.

156. Kahan A et al: Meningoradiculitis associated with infections by *Borrelia burgdorferi*, *Lancet* 1:148, 1985.

157. Kaplan JE, Schonberger LB: The sensitivity of various serologic tests in the diagnosis of Rocky Mountain spotted fever, *Am J Trop Med Hyg* 35:840, 1986.

158. Kaplowitz LG, Fischer JJ, Sparling PF: Rocky Mountain spotted fever: a clinical dilemma. In Remington JS, Swartz MN, editors: *Current clinical topics in infectious diseases*, vol 2, New York, 1981, McGraw-Hill.

159. Kaplowitz LG, Robertson GL: Hyponatremia in Rocky Mountain spotted fever: role of antidiuretic hormone, *Ann Intern Med* 98:334, 1983.

160. Keller D et al: Safety and immunogenicity of a recombinant outer surface protein A Lyme vaccine, *JAMA* 271:1764, 1994.

161. Kim N, Rosenbaum GS, Cunha BA: Relative bradycardia and lymphopenia in patients with babesiosis, *Clin Infect Dis* 26:1218, 1998.

162. Kirkland KB, Wilkinson WE, Sexton DJ.: Therapeutic delay and mortality in Rocky Mountain spotted fever, *Clin Infect Dis* 20:1118-21, 1995.

163. Kirsch M et al: Fatal adult respiratory distress syndrome in a patient with Lyme disease, *JAMA* 259:2737, 1988.

164. Klein MB et al: Antibiotic susceptibility of the newly cultivated agent of human granulocytic ehrlichiosis: promising activity of quinolones and rifamycins, *Antimicrob Agents Chemother* 41:76, 1997.

165. Kocan AA: Tick paralysis, *J Am Vet Med Assoc* 192:1498, 1988.

166. Korman TM et al: Acute glomerulonephritis associated with acute Q fever: a case report and review of the renal complications of *Coxiella burnetii* infection, *Clin Infect Dis* 26:359, 1998.

167. Kramer VL et al: Detection of the agents of human ehrlichioses in ixodid ticks from California, *Am J Trop Med Hyg* 60:62, 1999.

168. Krause PJ et al: Comparison of PCR with blood smear and inoculation of small animals for diagnosis of *Babesia microti* parasitemia, *J Clin Microbiol* 34:2791, 1996.

169. Krause PJ et al: Concurrent Lyme disease and babesiosis: evidence for increased severity and duration of illness, *JAMA* 275:1657, 1996.

170. Krause PJ et al: Persistent parasitemia after acute babesiosis: *N Engl J Med* 339:160, 1998.

171. Kruszewska D et al: Possible sexual transmission of Q fever among humans, *Clin Infect Dis* 22:1087, 1996.

172. Lane RS, Peisman J, Burgdorfer W: Lyme borreliosis: relation of its causative agent to its vectors and hosts in North America and Europe, *Annu Rev Entomol* 36:587, 1991.

173. Lane RS et al: Ecology of tick-borne agents in California. I. Spotted fever group rickettsiae, *Am J Trop Med Hyg* 30:239, 1981.

174. Lane RS et al: Survey for evidence of Colorado tick fever virus outside of the known endemic area in California, *Am J Trop Med Hyg* 31:837, 1982.

175. Lawson JP, Steere AC: Lyme arthritis: radiologic findings, *Radiology* 154:37, 1985.

176. Le CT: Tick-borne relapsing fever in children, *Pediatrics* 66:963, 1980.

177. Lees RF et al: Radiographic findings in Rocky Mountain spotted fever, *Radiology* 129:17, 1978.

178. Loge RV: Acute hepatitis associated with Colorado tick fever, *West J Med* 142:91, 1985.

179. Logigian EL, Kaplan RF, Steere AC: Chronic neurologic manifestations of Lyme disease, *N Engl J Med* 323:1438, 1990.

180. Logigian EL, Steere AC: Clinical and electrophysiologic findings in chronic neuropathy of Lyme disease, *Neurology* 42:303, 1992.

181. Logigian EL et al: Evaluation of IV ceftriaxone in the treatment of chronic Lyme borreliosis. Presented at the Seventh International Congress on Lyme borreliosis, San Francisco, June, 1996.

182. Luft BJ et al: Invasion of the central nervous system by *Borrelia burgdorferi* in acute disseminated infection, *JAMA* 267:1364, 1992.

183. Lugar SW et al: Comparison of cefuroxime axetil and doxycycline in treatment of patients with early Lyme disease associated with erythema migrans, *Antimicrob Agents Chemother* 39:661, 1995.

184. MacDonald AB, Benach JL, Burgdorfer W: Stillbirth following maternal Lyme disease, *NY State J Med* 87:615, 1987.

185. Maeda K et al: Human infection with *Ehrlichia canis*, a leukocytic rickettsia, *N Engl J Med* 316:853, 1987.

186. Magnarelli L, Anderson JF: Ticks and biting insects infected with the etiologic agent of Lyme disease, *Borrelia burgdorferi*, *J Clin Microbiol* 26:1482, 1988.

187. Magnarelli LA et al: Human exposure to a granulocytic *Ehrlichia* and other tick-borne agents in Connecticut, *J Clin Microbiol* 36:2823, 1998.

188. Maraspin V et al: Treatment of erythema migrans in pregnancy, *Clin Infect Dis* 22:788, 1996.

189. Marcus LC et al: A case report of transfusion-induced babesiosis, *JAMA* 248:465, 1982.

190. Marcus LC et al: Fatal pancarditis in a patient with coexistent Lyme disease and babesiosis: demonstration of spirochetes in the myocardium, *Ann Intern Med* 103:374, 1985.

191. Marin-Garcia J, Barrett FF: Myocardial function in Rocky Mountain spotted fever: echocardiographic assessment, *Am J Cardiol* 51:341, 1983.

192. Marin-Garcia J, Gooch WM, Coury DL: Cardiac manifestations of Rocky Mountain spotted fever, *Pediatrics* 67:358, 1981.

193. Markowitz LE et al: Lyme disease during pregnancy, *JAMA* 255:3394, 1986.

194. Marwick C: Guarded endorsement for Lyme disease vaccine, *JAMA* 279:1937, 1998.

195. Marx RS et al: Rocky Mountain spotted fever—serological evidence of previous subclinical infection in children, *Am J Dis Child* 136:16, 1982.

196. Massachusetts Department of Public Health: On the alert for Rocky Mountain spotted fever, *N Engl J Med* 292:1127, 1975.

197. Matuschka F et al: Capacity of European animals as reservoir hosts for the Lyme disease spirochete, *J Infect Dis* 165:479, 1992.

198. McCrossin I: Lyme disease on the NSW south coast, *Med J Aust* 144:139, 1986.

199. McDade JE: Ehrlichiosis—a disease of animals and humans, *J Infect Dis* 161:609, 1990.

200. McDade JE, Newhouse VF: Natural history of *Rickettsia rickettsii*, *Annu Rev Microbiol* 40:287, 1986.

201. McHugh TP, Ruderman AE, Gibbons TE: Rocky Mountain spotted fever, *Ann Emerg Med* 13:1132, 1984.

202. McLean RG et al: The ecology of Colorado tick fever in Rocky Mountain National Park in 1974, *Am J Trop Med Hyg* 30:483, 1980.

203. Meldrum SC et al: Human babesiosis in New York State: an epidemiological description of 136 cases, *Clin Infect Dis* 15:1019, 1992.

204. Melkert PWJ: Relapsing fever in pregnancy: analysis of high-risk factors, *Br J Obstet Gynaecol* 95:1070, 1988.

205. Melkert PWJ: Mortality in high risk patients with tick-borne relapsing fever analysed by the Borrelia index, *East Afr Med J* 68:875, 1991.

206. Mertz LE et al: Ticks, spirochetes, and new diagnostic tests for Lyme disease, *Mayo Clin Proc* 60:402, 1985.

207. Miller JQ, Price TR: The nervous system in Rocky Mountain spotted fever, *Neurology* 22:561, 1972.

208. Misao T, Kobayashi Y: Studies on infectious mononucleosis (glandular fever). I. Isolation of etiologic agent from blood, bone marrow, and lymph node of a patient with infectious mononucleosis by using mice, *Kyushu J Med Sci* 6:145, 1955.

209. Mitchell PD, Reed KD, Hofkes JM: Immunoserologic evidence of coinfection with *Borrelia burgdorferi*, *Babesia microti*, and human granulocytic *Erlichia* species in resident of Wisconsin and Minnesota, *J Clin Microbiol* 34:724, 1996.

210. Monath TP: Orbivirus (Colorado tick fever). In Mandell GL, Douglas RG, Bennett JE, editors: *Principles and practice of infectious diseases*, New York, 1985, Wiley.

211. Moraga FA et al: Boutonneuse fever, *Arch Dis Child* 57:149, 1982.

212. Morris HH: Tick paralysis: electrophysiologic measurements, *South Med J* 70:121, 1977.

213. Morrison RE et al: Rocky Mountain spotted fever in the elderly, *J Am Geriatr Soc* 39:205, 1991.

214. Mukolwe SW et al: Attempted transmission of *Borrelia burgdorferi* (Spirochaetales: Spirochaetaceae) (JDI strain) by *Ixodes scapularis* (Acari: Ixodidae), *Dermacentor variabilis*, and *Amblyomma americanum*, *J Med Entomol* 29:673, 1992.

215. Murnaghan MF: Site and mechanism of tick paralysis, *Science* 131:418, 1960.

216. Nadelman RB, Wormser GP: Lyme borreliosis, *Lancet* 352:557, 1998.

217. Nadelman RB et al: Comparison of cefuroxime axetil and doxycycline in the treatment of early Lyme disease, *Ann Intern Med* 117:273, 1992.

218. Nadelman RB et al: The clinical spectrum of early Lyme borreliosis in patients with culture-confirmed erythema migrans, *Am J Med* 100:502, 1996.

219. Needham GR: Evaluation of five popular methods for tick removal, *Pediatrics* 75:997, 1985.

220. Nieburg PI, D'Angelo LJ, Herrmann KL: Measles in patients suspected of having Rocky Mountain spotted fever, *JAMA* 244:808, 1980.

221. Nocton JJ et al: Detection of Borrelia burgdorferi by polymerase chain reaction in synovial fluid from patients with Lyme arthritis, *N Engl J Med* 330: 229, 1994.

222. Ogden NH et al: Granulocytic ehrlichiosis: an emerging or rediscovered tick-borne disease? *J Med Microbiol* 47:475, 1998.

223. Olson LJ, Okafar ED, Clements IP: Cardiac involvement in Lyme disease: manifestations and management, *Mayo Clin Proc* 61:745, 1986.

224. Oster CN et al: Laboratory-acquired Rocky Mountain spotted fever—the hazard of aerosol transmission, *N Engl J Med* 297:859, 1977.

225. Pachner AR, Steere AC: The triad of neurologic manifestations of Lyme disease: meningitis, cranial neuritis, and radiculoneuritis, *Neurology* 35:57, 1985.

226. Pearn J: Neuromuscular paralysis caused by tick envenomation, *J Neurol Sci* 34:37, 1977.

227. Peltomaa M et al: Paediatric facial paralysis caused by Lyme borreliosis: a prospective and retrospective analysis, *Scand J Infect Dis* 30:269, 1998.

228. Penttila IA et al: Cytokine dysregulation in the post–Q–fever fatigue syndrome, *QJM* 91:549, 1998.

229. Petersen LR et al: An outbreak of ehrlichiosis in members of an Army reserve unit exposed to ticks, *J Infect Dis* 159:562, 1989.

230. Pfister HW et al: Randomized comparison of ceftriaxone and cefotaxime in Lyme neuroborreliosis, *J Infect Dis* 163:311, 1991.

231. Philip RN et al: A comparison of serologic methods for diagnosis of Rocky Mountain spotted fever, *Am J Epidemiol* 105:56, 1977.

232. Piesman J, Sinsky RJ: Ability of *Ixodes scapularis*, *Dermacentor variabilis*, and *Amblyomma americanum* to acquire, maintain, and transmit Lyme disease spirochetes, *J Med Entomol* 25:336, 1988.

233. Piesman J et al: Duration of tick attachment and *Borrelia burgdorferi* transmission, *J Clin Microbiol* 25:557, 1987.

234. Piras MA et al: Glucose-6-phosphate dehydrogenase deficiency in male patients with Mediterranean spotted fever in Sardinia, *J Infect Dis* 148:607, 1983.

235. Pohl-Koppe A et al: *Borrelia* lymphocytoma in childhood, *Pediatr Infect Dis J*, 17:423, 1998.

236. Poulsen LW, Iversen G: Relapsing fever: differential diagnosis to malaria, *Scand J Infect Dis* 28:419, 1996.

237. Procop GW et al: Immunoperoxidase and immunofluorescent staining of *Rickettsia rickettsii* in skin biopsies: a comparative study, *Arch Pathol Lab Med* 121:894, 1997.

238. Quick RE et al: Babesiosis in Washington State: a new species of *Babesia?* *Ann Intern Med* 119:284, 1993.

239. Rahn DW, Malawista SE: Lyme disease: recommendations for diagnosis and treatment, *Ann Intern Med* 114:472, 1991.

240. Randall MB, Walker DH: Rocky Mountain spotted fever: gastrointestinal and pancreatic lesions and rickettsial infection, *Arch Pathol Lab Med* 108:963, 1984.

241. Raoult D, Stein A: Q fever during pregnancy: a risk for women, fetuses, and obstetricians, *N Engl J Med* 330:371, 1994.

242. Raoult D et al: Laboratory diagnosis of Mediterranean spotted fever by immunofluorescent demonstration of *Rickettsia conorii* in cutaneous lesions, *J Infect Dis* 150:145, 1984.

243. Raoult D et al: Incidence, clinical observations and risk factors in the severe form of Mediterranean spotted fever among patients admitted to hospital in Marseilles, 1983-1984, *J Infect* 12:111, 1986.

244. Raoult D et al: Mediterranean spotted fever: clinical, laboratory and epidemiological features of 199 cases, *Am J Trop Med Hyg* 35:845, 1986.

245. Raoult D et al: Treatment of Q fever endocarditis: comparison of 2 regimens containing doxycycline and ofloxacin or hydroxychloroquine, *Arch Intern Med* 159:167, 1999.

246. Ratnasamy N et al: Central nervous system manifestations of human ehrlichiosis, *Clin Infect Dis* 23:314, 1996.

247. Raucher HS, Jaffin H, Glass JL: Babesiosis in pregnancy, *Obstet Gynecol* 63:7S, 1984.

248. Raucher HS, et al: Pseudotumor cerebri and Lyme disease: a new association, *J Pediatr* 107:931, 1985.

249. Reid MC et al: The consequences of overdiagnosing and overtreatment of Lyme disease: an observational study, *Ann Intern Med* 128:354, 1998.

250. Reik L, Burgdorfer W, Donaldson JO: Neurologic abnormalities in Lyme disease without erythema chronicum migrans, *Am J Med* 81:73, 1986.

251. Reik L et al: Neurologic abnormalities of Lyme disease, *Medicine* 58:281, 1979.

252. Report of the Committee on Infectious Diseases. In 1997 red book, ed 24, American 1997, Academy of Pediatrics.

253. Ribeiro JMC et al: Dissemination and salivary delivery of Lyme disease spirochetes in vector ticks, *J Med Entomol* 24:201, 1987.

254. Ristic M, Healy GR: Babesiosis. In Steele JH, editor: *CRC handbook series in zoonoses, section C: parasitic zoonoses*, vol I, Boca Raton, Fla, 1981, CRC Press.

255. Rosner F et al: Babesiosis in splenectomized adults—review of 22 reported cases, *Am J Med* 76:696, 1984.

256. Rubin DA et al: Prospective evaluation of heart block complicating early Lyme disease, *Pace* 15:252, 1992.

257. Ruebush TK et al: Human babesiosis on Nantucket Island—clinical features, *Ann Intern Med* 86:6, 1977.

258. Ruebush TK et al: Human babesiosis on Nantucket Island—evidence for self-limited and subclinical infections, *N Engl J Med* 297:825, 1977.

259. Ruebush TK et al: Development and persistence of antibody in persons infected with *Babesia microti*, *Am J Trop Med Hyg* 30:291, 1981.

260. Ryberg B: Bannwarth's syndrome (lymphocytic meningoradiculitis) in Sweden, *Yale J Biol Med* 57:499, 1984.

261. Ryberg B et al: Antibodies to Lyme-disease spirochaete in European lymphocytic meningoradiculitis (Bannwarth's syndrome), *Lancet* 2:519, 1983.

262. Sacks HS, Lyons RW, Lahiri B: Adult respiratory distress syndrome in Rocky Mountain spotted fever, *Annu Rev Respir Dis* 123:547, 1981.

263. Sacks JJ, Pinner TAF, Parker RL: Tick testing as a method of controlling Rocky Mountain spotted fever, *Am J Public Health* 73:903, 1983.

264. Salazar JC, Gerber MA, Goff CW: Long-term outcome of Lyme disease in children given early treatment, *J Pediatr* 122:591, 1993.

265. Sawaishi Y et al: Acute cerebellitis caused by Coxiella burnetii, *Ann Neurol* 45:124, 1999.

266. Schauber EM et al: Coinfection of blacklegged ticks (Acari: Ixodidae) in Dutchess County, New York, with the agents of Lyme disease and human granulocytic ehrlichiosis, *J Med Entomol* 35: 901, 1998.

267. Schechter SL: Lyme disease associated with optic neuropathy, *Am J Med* 81:143, 1986.

268. Schlesinger PA et al: Maternal-fetal transmission of the Lyme disease spirochete, *Borrelia burgdorferi*, *Ann Intern Med* 103:67, 1985.

269. Schmedding E et al: Lymphocytic meningoradiculitis (Garin-Bujadoux Bannwarth): from syndrome to disease? *Eur J Pediatr* 144:497, 1986.

270. Schmid GP et al: Surveillance of Lyme disease in the United States, 1982, *J Infect Dis* 151:1144, 1985.

271. Schmitt N, Bowmer EJ, Gregson JD: Tick paralysis in British Columbia, *Can Med Assoc J* 100:417, 1969.

272. Schrock CG: Lyme disease: additional evidence of widespread distribution, *Am J Med* 72:700, 1982.

273. Schutzer SE, Brown T, Holland BK: Reduction of Lyme disease exposure by recognition and avoidance of high-risk areas, *Lancet* 349:9066, 1997.

274. Schwartz BS et al: Antibody testing in Lyme disease—a comparison of results in four laboratories, *JAMA* 262:3431, 1989.

275. Sciotto CG et al: Rapid identification of *Borrelia* in blood and tissue with acridine orange, *Lab Invest* 46:74, 1982.

276. Shapiro ED: Lyme disease, *Pediatr Rev* 19:147, 1998.

277. Shapiro ED et al: A controlled trial of antimicrobial prophylaxis for Lyme disease after deer-tick bites, *N Engl J Med* 327:1769, 1992.

278. Shih CM, Wang CC: Ability of azithromycin in combination with quinine for the elimination of babesial infection in humans, *Am J Trop Med Hyg* 59:4:509, 1998.

279. Shrestha M, Grodzicki RL, Steere AC: Diagnosing early Lyme disease, *Am J Med* 78:235, 1985.

280. Sienko DG et al: Q fever: a call to heighten our index of suspicion, *Arch Intern Med* 148:609, 1988.

281. Sigal LH et al: A vaccine consisting of recombinant Borrelia burgdorferi outer-surface protein A to prevent Lyme disease, *N Engl J Med* 339:216, 1998.

282. Silver HK, Meiklehogn G, Kempe CH: Colorado tick fever, *Am J Dis Child* 101:56, 1961.

283. Skrabalo Z, Deanovi Z: Piroplasmosis in man: report on a case, *Doc Med Geogr Trop* 9:11, 1957.

284. Smith RP et al: Transfusion-acquired babesiosis and failure of antibiotic treatment, *JAMA* 256:2726, 1986.

285. Snydman DR et al: *Borrelia burgdorferi* in joint fluid in chronic Lyme arthritis, *Ann Intern Med* 104:798, 1986.

286. Sonnesyn SW et al: A prospective study of the seroprevalence of *Borrelia burgdorferi* infection in patients with severe heart failure, *Am J Cardiol* 76:97, 1995.

287. Sood SK et al: Duration of tick attachment as a predictor of the risk of Lyme disease in an area in which Lyme disease is endemic, *J Infect Dis* 175:996, 1997.

288. Southern PA, Sanford JP: Relapsing fever—a clinical and microbiological review, *Medicine* 48:129, 1969.

289. Spielman A, Levine JF, Wilson MI: Vectorial capacity of North American *Ixodes* ticks, *Yale J Biol Med* 57:507, 1984.

290. Spielman A et al: Human babesiosis on Nantucket Island, USA: description of the vector, *Ixodes (Ixodes) dammini*, n. sp. (Acarina: Ixodidae), *J Med Entomol* 15:218, 1979.

291. Spruance SL, Bailey A: Colorado tick fever—a review of 115 laboratory confirmed cases, *Arch Intern Med* 131:288, 1973.

292. Stanbury JB, Huyck JH: Tick paralysis: a critical review, *Medicine* 24:219, 1945.

293. Standaert SM et al: A hyperendemic focus of human ehrlichiosis at a golf-oriented retirement community, *N Engl J Med* 333:420, 1995.

294. Stanek G et al: Isolation of *Borrelia burgdorferi* from the myocardium of a patient with long-standing cardiomyopathy, *N Engl J Med* 322:249, 1990.

295. State of Connecticut Department of Public Health: Lyme disease—Connecticut, 1994, *Conn Epidemiol* 15:13, 1996.

296. Steenbarger JR: Congenital tick-borne relapsing fever: report of a case with first documentation of transplacental transmission, *Birth Defects* 18:39, 1982.

297. Steere AC: Conference summary, *Yale J Biol Med* 57:711, 1984.

298. Steere AC: Lyme disease, *N Engl J Med* 321:586, 1989.

299. Steere AC: Effectiveness of early Lyme disease treatment, *Am J Med* 94:553, 1993 (letter).

300. Steere AC, Broderick TF, Malawista SE: Erythema chronicum migrans and Lyme arthritis: epidemiologic evidence for a tick vector, *Am J Epidemiol* 108:312, 1978.

301. Steere AC, Malawista SE: Cases of Lyme disease in the United States: locations correlated with distribution of *Ixodes dammini*, *Ann Intern Med* 91:730, 1979.

302. Steere AC, Pachner AR, Malawista SE: Neurologic abnormalities of Lyme disease: successful treatment with high-dose intravenous penicillin, *Ann Intern Med* 99:767, 1983.

303. Steere AC, Schoen RT, Taylor E: The clinical evolution of Lyme arthritis, *Ann Intern Med* 107:725, 1987.

304. Steere AC et al: Erythema chronicum migrans and Lyme arthritis—the enlarging clinical spectrum, *Ann Intern Med* 86:685, 1977.

305. Steere AC et al: Lyme arthritis—an epidemic of oligoarticular arthritis in children and adults in three Connecticut communities, *Arthritis Rheum* 20:7, 1977.

306. Steere AC et al: Chronic Lyme arthritis—clinical and immunogenetic differentiation from rheumatoid arthritis, *Ann Intern Med* 90:896, 1979.

307. Steere AC et al: Antibiotic therapy in Lyme disease, *Ann Intern Med* 93:1, 1980.

308. Steere AC et al: Lyme disease: cardiac abnormalities of Lyme disease, *Ann Intern Med* 93:8, 1980.

309. Steere AC et al: The early clinical manifestations of Lyme disease, *Ann Intern Med* 99:76, 1983.

310. Steere AC et al: The spirochetal etiology of Lyme disease, *N Engl J Med* 308:733, 1983.

311. Steere AC et al: Treatment of the early manifestations of Lyme disease, *Ann Intern Med* 99:22, 1983.

312. Steere AC et al: Successful parenteral penicillin therapy of established Lyme arthritis, *N Engl J Med* 312:869, 1985.

313. Steere AC et al: Unilateral blindness caused by infection with the Lyme disease spirochete, *Borrelia burgdorferi*, *Ann Intern Med* 103:382, 1985.

314. Steere AC, Dwyer E, Winchester R: Association of chronic Lyme arthritis with the HLA-DR4 and HLA-DR2 alleles, *N Engl J Med* 323:219, 1990.

315. Steere AC et al: Longitudinal assessment of the clinical and epidemiological features of Lyme disease in a defined population, *J Infect Dis* 154:295, 1986.

316. Steere AC et al: The overdiagnosis of Lyme disease, *JAMA* 269:1812, 1993.

317. Steere AC et al: Vaccination against Lyme disease with recombinant *Borrelia burdorferi* outer-surface lipoprotein A with adjuvant, *N Engl J Med* 339:209, 1998.

318. Steigbigel RT, Benach JL: Immunization against Lyme disease—an important first step, *N Engl J Med* 339:263, 1998.

319. Steketee RW et al: Babesiosis in Wisconsin—a new focus of disease transmission, *JAMA* 253:2675, 1985.

320. Stewart A et al: Lyme arthritis in the Hunter Valley, *Med J Aust* 1:139, 1982.

321. Stiernstedt GT et al: Chronic meningitis and Lyme disease in Sweden, *Yale J Biol Med* 57:491, 1984.

322. Stoenner HG, Dodd Y, Larsen C: Antigenic variation of *Borrelia hermsii*, *J Exp Med* 156:1297, 1982.

323. Strle F, Stantic-Pavlinic M: Lyme disease in Europe, *N Engl J Med* 334:803, 1996.

324. Strle F et al: Comparison of culture-confirmed erythema migrans in Europe and the United States (unpublished).

325. Strle F et al: Solitary borrelial lymphocytoma: report of 36 cases, *Infection* 20:201, 1992.

326. Strle F et al: Treatment of borrelial lymphocytoma, *Infection* 24:80, 1996.

327. Strobino B et al: Lyme disease and pregnancy outcome: a prospective study of 2 thousand prenatal patients, *Am J Obstet Gynecol* 169:367, 1993.

328. Sun T et al: Morphologic and clinical observations in human infection with *Babesia microti*, *J Infect Dis* 148:239, 1983.

329. Sundy JS et al: Rocky Mountain spotted fever presenting with acute monarticular arthritis, *Arthritis Rheum* 39:175, 1996.

330. Swift TR, Ignacio OJ: Tick paralysis: electrophysiologic studies, *Neurology* 25:1130, 1975.

331. Takanori O, Tange Y, Kobayashi Y: Causative agent of spotted fever group rickettsiosis in Japan, *Infect Immun* 58:887, 1990.

332. Tanaka R: Rocky Mountain spotted fever—United States, 1986, *JAMA* 258:25, 1987.

333. Thompson RS et al: Outbreak of tick-borne relapsing fever in Spokane County, Washington, *JAMA* 210:1045, 1969.

334. Thorner AR, Walker DH, Petri WA: Rocky Mountain spotted fever, *Clin Infect Dis* 27:1353, 1998.

335. Tibballs J, Cooper SJ: Paralysis with *Ixodes cornuatus* envenomation, *Med J Aust* 145:37, 1986.

336. Todd JL: Tick bite in British Columbia, *Can Med Assoc J* 2:1118, 1912.

337. Toerner JG et al: Guillain-Barré syndrome associated with Rocky Mountain spotted fever: Case report and review, *Clin Infect Dis* 22:1090, 1996.

338. Trevejo RT et al: An interstate outbreak of tick-bourne relapsing fever among vacationers at a Rocky Mountain cabin, *Am J Trop Med Hyg* 58:743, 1998.

339. Tringali G et al: Epidemiology of boutonneuse fever in western Sicily—distribution and prevalence of spotted fever group rickettsial infection in dog ticks (*Rhipicephalus sanguineus*), *Am J Epidemiol* 123:721, 1986.

340. Tugwell et al: Laboratory evaluation in the diagnosis of Lyme disease—clinical guideline, part 2, *Ann Intern Med* 127:1109, 1997.

341. Turck WPG et al: Chronic Q fever, *QJM* 45:193, 1976.

342. Walker DH: Rocky Mountain spotted fever: a seasonal alert, *Clin Infect Dis* 20:1111, 1995.

343. Walker DH: Tick-transmitted infectious diseases in the United States, *Annu Rev Public Health* 19:237, 1998.

344. Walker DH, Dumler JS: Human monocytic and granulocytic ehrlichiosis. Discovery and diagnosis of emerging tick-borne infections and the critical role of the pathologist, *Arch Path & Lab Med* 121:785, 1997.

345. Walker DH, Gear JHS: Correlation of the distribution of *Rickettsia conorii*, microscopic lesions, and clinical features in South African tick bite fever, *Am J Trop Med Hyg* 34:361, 1985.

346. Walker DH, Hawkins HK, Hudson P: Fulminant Rocky Mountain spotted fever—its pathologic characteristics associated with glucose-6-phosphate dehydrogenase deficiency, *Arch Pathol Lab Med* 107:121, 1983.

347. Walker DH, Mattern WD: Rickettsial vasculitis, *Am Heart J* 100:896, 1980.

348. Walker DH, Paletta CE, Cain BG: Pathogenesis of myocarditis in Rocky Mountain spotted fever, *Arch Pathol Lab Med* 104:171, 1980.

349. Walker DH, Raoult D: Rickettsia rickettsii and other spotted fever group rickettsiae (Rocky Mountain spotted fever and other spotted fevers). In Mandell GL, Bennett JE, Dolin R, editors. *Mandell, Douglas and Bennett's principles and practice of infectious diseases*, ed 4, New York, 1995 Churchill Livingstone.

350. Walker DH et al: Rocky Mountain spotted fever mimicking acute cholecystitis, *Arch Intern Med* 145:2194, 1985.

351. Wallis RC et al: Erythema chronicum migrans and Lyme arthritis: field study of ticks, *Am J Epidemiol* 108:322, 1978.

352. Warshafsky S et al: Efficacy of antibiotic prophylaxis for prevention of Lyme disease: a meta-analysis, *J Gen Intern Med* 11:329, 1996.

353. Weber K, Puzik A, Becker T: Erythema-migrans krankheit: Beitrag zur klinik und besiehung zur Lyme-krankheit, *Dtsch Med Wochenschr* 108:1182, 1983.

354. Weber K et al: *Borrelia burgdorferi* in a newborn despite oral penicillin for Lyme borreliosis during pregnancy, *Pediatr Infect Dis* 7:286, 1988.

355. Welch KJ, Rumley RL, Levine JA: False-positive results in serologic tests for Rocky Mountain spotted fever during pregnancy, *South J Med* 84:307, 1991.

356. Wells GM et al: Rocky Mountain spotted fever caused by blood transfusion, *JAMA* 239:2763, 1978.

357. Wengrower D et al: Myocarditis in tick-borne relapsing fever, *J Infect Dis* 149:1033, 1982.

358. Western KA et al: Babesiosis in a Massachusetts resident, *N Engl J Med* 282:854, 1970.

359. White DJ et al: Human babesiosis in New York State: review of 139 hospitalized cases and analysis of prognostic factors, *Arch Intern Med* 158:2149, 1998.

360. Wilkinson PR: Tick paralysis. In Steele JH, editor: *CRC handbook series in zoonoses, section C: parasitic zoonoses*, vol III, Boca Raton, Fla, 1981, CRC Press.

361. Williams C et al: Maternal Lyme disease and congenital malformations: a cord blood serosurvey in endemic and control areas, *Pediatr Perinat Epidemiol* 9:320, 1995.

362. Williamson PK, Calabro JJ: Lyme disease—a review of the literature, *Semin Arthritis Rheum* 13:229, 1984.

363. Wilson ML, Adler GH, Spielman A: Correlation between abundance of deer and that of the deer tick *Ixodes dammini*, *Ann Entomol Soc Am* 78:172, 1985.

364. Wisseman CL: Rickettsial diseases. In Wyngaarden JB, Smith LH, editors: *Cecil textbook of medicine*, Philadelphia, 1985, Saunders.

365. Wittner M et al: Successful chemotherapy of transfusion babesiosis, *Ann Intern Med* 96:601, 1982.

366. Woodward TE: Rocky Mountain spotted fever: epidemiological and early clinical signs are keys to treatment and reduced mortality, *J Infect Dis* 150:465, 1984.

367. Woodward TE et al: Prompt confirmation of Rocky Mountain spotted fever: identification of rickettsiae in skin tissues, *J Infect Dis* 134:297, 1976.

368. Wormser GP: Treatment and prevention of Lyme disease, with emphasis on antimicrobial therapy for neuroborreliosis and vaccination, *Semin Neurol* 17:45, 1997.

369. Wormser GP: Vaccination as a modality to prevent Lyme disease: a status report, *Infect Dis Clin North Am* 13:1, 1999.

370. Wormser GP et al: Lyme disease in children, *N Engl J Med* 336:1107, 1997 (letter).

371. Wormser GP et al: Use of a novel technique of cutaneous lavage for diagnosis of Lyme disease associated with erythema migrans, *JAMA* 268: 1311, 1992.

372. Yagupsky P, Moses S: Neonatal *Borrelia* species infection (relapsing fever), *Am J Dis Child* 139:74, 1985.

34 Spider Bites

Leslie V. Boyer, Jude T. McNally, and Greta J. Binford

INTRODUCTION TO SPIDERS

The spiders number approximately 34,000 described species and are found in all habitats except for the open sea.[37,59,206] They are carnivorous predators with important ecologic roles in most terrestrial ecosystems. Many are capable of wind-borne dispersal (ballooning), which has led to colonization of even the most isolated land masses on earth.

As with ticks, mites, scorpions, and other arachnids, spiders have a body consisting of an abdomen and an unsegmented cephalothorax (prosoma) with chelicerate jaws, pedipalps, and four pairs of legs (Figure 34-1). They are distinct from other arachnids in having loss of abdominal segmentation, and male pedipalpal tarsi are modified as secondary genitalia.[253] In addition, spiders have venom that is produced in a gland in the anterior prosoma and delivered through a cheliceral fang. On the abdomen, they have silk-producing glands and a set of spinnerets.

The primary function of venom in spiders is prey capture or, rarely, defense. Venoms are complex mixtures of neurotoxic and proteolytic peptides, proteins, and biogenic amines.[1,15,102,185,253] Most of these toxins are target specific, acting selectively on arthropods, vertebrates, or other groups, including some with mammalian-specific activity.[1,120,202] Venom composition varies widely across spider species, and variation may exist within species between sexes and among geographically isolated populations.[184] Venom potency also varies within individuals both seasonally and developmentally. Despite this tremendous venom diversity, only a few dozen spider species are considered harmful to people because (1) most others have an insufficient quantity of venom, (2) the toxins do not affect mammals, or (3) the fangs cannot penetrate human skin. In a few species, although laboratory evidence suggests potential mammalian toxicity, human envenomations have not been reported, perhaps because of the rarity of encounters between spiders and humans in some habitats. Table 34-1 lists an assortment of spider families, including those with species that have been reported to bite humans.

All spiders are carnivorous and have the challenge of capturing live prey. Prey capture is a multistep process in which spiders must find prey, ensnare it, immobilize it, and digest it externally before the liquefied meal can be consumed. This process and the role of venom are very diverse. The neurotoxins in spider venom are primarily used for prey immobilization. Venoms of a few spiders are known to have some proteolytic components that likely begin the process of external digestion. The bulk of digestion, however, results from digestive enzymes that are ejected from the mouth, a distinctly separate opening from the venom duct (Figure 34-2). Occasionally, spider digestate may infect wounds created by spider bites, which affects the clinical appearance, although no direct evidence substantiates this suspicion.

In addition to venom, some theraphosids (tarantulas) produce urticating hairs that irritate skin or mucous membranes of animals or humans. Exposure may result from direct contact with the spider or its web or from proximity to airborne hairs launched by an aggravated individual.

GENERAL ASSESSMENT AND TREATMENT OF SPIDER BITES

Awareness of the differential diagnosis is crucial for management of any patient presenting for evaluation of "spider bite," because the offending creature is rarely observed and identified. In general, it is outside of normal biologic activity for spiders to bite humans, except in defense. A defensive bite risks the spider's life and tends to occur only when its life is threatened by being crushed. Thus true spider bites are much less common than insect bites or cutaneous infections. Furthermore, no pathognomonic clinical signs prove the diagnosis without retrieval and identification of a spider that was seen actually biting.[236] Diagnosis of arachnidism without direct evidence can lead to inappropriate treatment and the lack of consideration of more severe underlying medical issues.[145,148,151,228] Therefore the medical history, physical examination, and laboratory evaluation must often consider an alternative etiology. Treatment plans should include careful follow-up and patient counseling to take into consideration any uncertainties in the final diagnosis.

The differential diagnosis of a local lesion may include fungal, bacterial, and viral infection, especially herpes simplex and zoster; the vesiculobullous diseases; arthropod-borne infectious diseases (e.g., Lyme disease); other bites and stings; foreign body reactions; and systemic conditions that predispose to focal skin

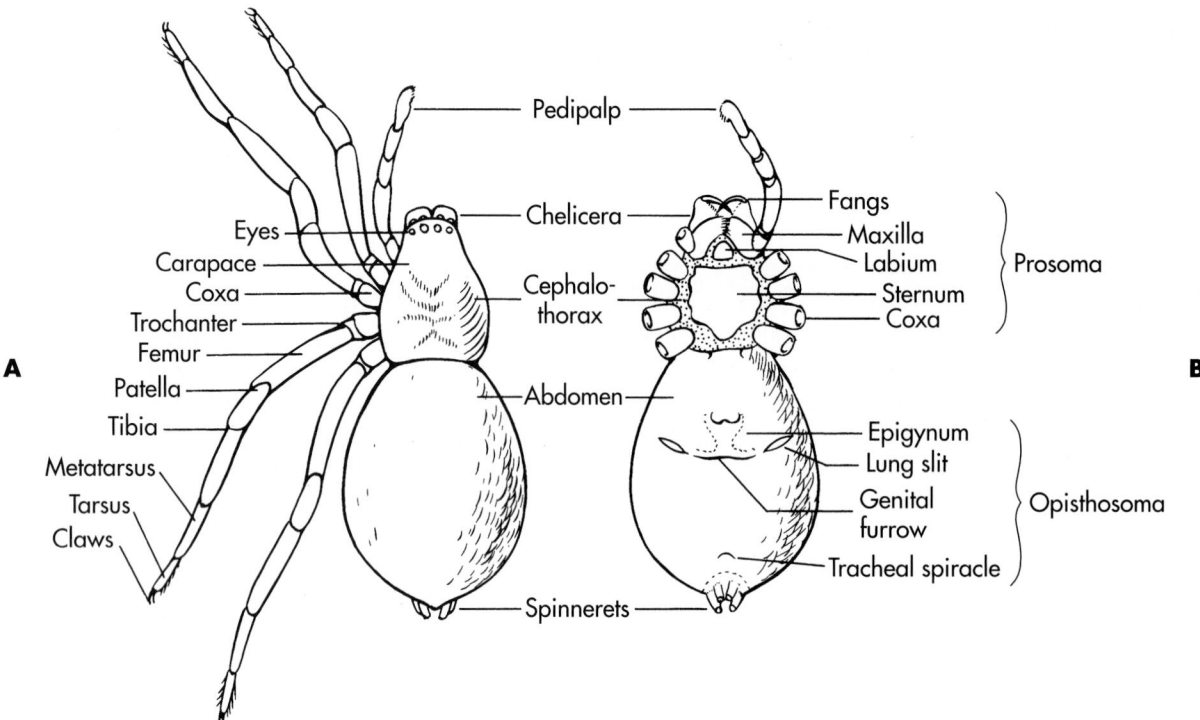

Figure 34-1 External anatomy of an araneomorph spider. **A,** Dorsal. **B,** Ventral (legs omitted).

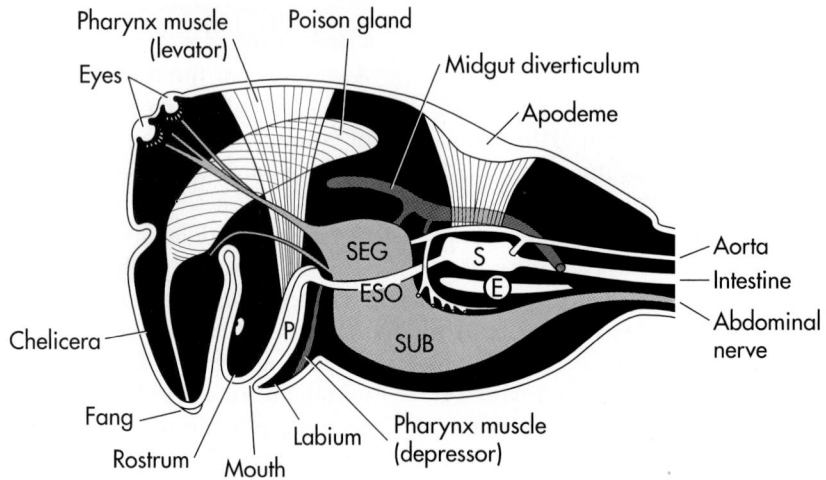

Figure 34-2 Longitudinal section of the prosoma. *E,* Endosternite; *Eso,* esophagus; *P,* pharynx; *SEG,* supraesophageal ganglion; *S,* sucking stomach; *SUB,* subesophageal ganglion. (*Modified from Foelix RF: Biology of spiders, ed 2, Oxford, UK, 1996, Oxford University Press.*)

TABLE 34-1. SPIDERS OF CLINICAL INTEREST

SCIENTIFIC NAME (NUMBER OF GENERA AND SPECIES): COMMON NAME	GEOGRAPHIC RANGE	CLINICAL REMARKS	TAXONOMIC REFERENCES	CLINICAL REFERENCES
Phylum Arthropoda, Class Arachnida, Order Aranea (3 Suborders, 105 families, 3067 genera, approx. 34,000 species): Spiders	Worldwide		59, 208	
Suborder Mesothelae (1 family, 2 genera, 40 species)	Asia (part)	No species believed clinically relevant	209, 212	
Suborder Mygalomorphae (15 families, 260 genera, 2200 species): Mygales	Worldwide		218	
Theraphosidae (86 genera, 800 species): tarantulas and baboon spiders	Worldwide		218	299
Aphonopelma (Rheochostica): tarantula	New World	Minor local reaction; urticating hairs	213, 218	
Rheochostica henzi (previously *Dugesiella henzi*): tarantula	New World		218	
Mygalarachne (previously *Sericopelma*)		Minor local reaction	218	
Pterinochilus: tarantula	Africa	Minor local reaction	218	
Pamphobaetus: tarantula	Brazil	Minor local reaction	218	
Avicularia: tarantula	New World	Minor local reaction	218	
Lasiodora: tarantula	Brazil	Minor local reaction	218	
Grammostola cala: Chilean rose tarantula	New World	Minor local reaction; urticating hairs	218	36, 61
Acanthoscurria: tarantula	New World	Minor local reaction; urticating hairs	218	
Euathlus (previously *Brachypelma*): tarantula	New World	Minor local reaction; urticating hairs	218, 248	
Harpactirella lightfooti: baboon spider or bobbejaan-spinnekop	Africa		218	42, 122, 195
Poecilothuria: tarantula	Australia	Minor local reaction	218	
Selenocosmia	East Indies, India, Australia		218	
Phormictopus	South America, Caribbean		218	
Lampropelma: tarantula	Asia, India	Minor local reaction	218	
Haplopelma minax: Thailand black tarantula	Asia, India	Urticating hairs	218	36
Hexathelidae (11 genera, 74 species): funnel-web mygalomorphs			218	
Atrax	Eastern Australia		115, 218	
Atrax robustus: Sydney funnel-web spider	Eastern Australia	Local pain; severe neurotoxicity	115, 218	90, 91, 126, 262, 263, 271, 303, 305
Hadronyche (Atrax)	Eastern Australia		115, 218	
H. formidabilis: northern funnel-web spider	Eastern Australia	Local pain; severe neurotoxicity	115, 218	11, 118
H. versutus: Australian Blue Mountains funnel-web spider	Eastern Australia	Local pain; severe neurotoxicity	115, 218	11
H. infensus	Eastern Australia	Local pain; severe neurotoxicity	115, 218	11, 299
H. cereberus	Southeastern Australia	Local pain; severe neurotoxicity	115, 218	

Continued

TABLE 34-1. SPIDERS OF CLINICAL INTEREST—cont'd

SCIENTIFIC NAME (NUMBER OF GENERA AND SPECIES): COMMON NAME	GEOGRAPHIC RANGE	CLINICAL REMARKS	TAXONOMIC REFERENCES	CLINICAL REFERENCES
Dipluridae (17 genera, 157 species): funnel-web mygalomorphs	Worldwide		218	
Trechona venosa	South America	Mammalian toxin; no human reports	218	170
Idiopidae (18 genera, 267 species): front-eyed trapdoor spiders	Pantropical, India		218	299
Aganippe subtristis	Australia	Minor local reaction	218	
Arabantis	Australia		218	
Mysgolas (previously *Dyarcyops, Hermea*)	Australia, New Zealand	Minor local reaction	218	
Ctenizidae (10 genera, 116 species): trapdoor spiders	Worldwide, except South America		67, 218	
Bothriocyrtum	North America		218	
Ummidia	North, Central America		218	
Actinopididae (3 genera, 41 species): trapdoor spiders	Australia, Central and South America		218	
Missulena bradleyi: mouse spider	Australia	Mammalian toxin; one case of systemic effects	218	267
Suborder Araneomorphae (90 families, 2700 genera, 32,000 species): true spiders				
Filistatidae (12 genera, 87 species) *Filistata*	Worldwide		156	
Sicariidae (2 genera, 129 species): recluse, brown, or fiddle spiders	Worldwide		156, 210	
Loxosceles : recluse, brown, or fiddle spiders	New World, Mediterranean, Africa		105	10, 20
L. reclusa: brown recluse spider	North America (central, southeast)	Local necrosis; systemic syndrome	105	111, 214, 292
L. arizonica: Arizona brown spider	North America (southwest)	Local necrosis; systemic syndrome	105	
L. rufescens	Worldwide		105, 156	
L. intermedia	Brazil		40	
L. gaucho	Brazil		40	
L. spinulosa	South Africa			
L. laeta: corner spider or spider behind the pictures	South America, Australia, Finland	Painful local lesion; systemic syndrome	105, 156	10
L. parrami	South Africa		193	
Sicarius: six-eyed crab spiders	Neotropics, South Africa	Local necrosis; DIC	196-198	
Dysderidae (20 genera, 371 species): giant-fanged, six-eyed spiders	Worldwide		68	
Dysdera	Worldwide		68	
Desidae (28 genera, 200 species): long-jawed intertidal spiders	Worldwide		230	
Badumna insignis: black house spider	Australia, New Guinea	Local pain, rarely necrosis	117	172, 298, 300
Zodariidae (350 species): hunting spiders	Worldwide			
Supunna picta	Australia	Minor local reaction		38
Tetragnathidae (50 genera, 900 species): long-jawed orb-weaving spiders	Worldwide		166	

TABLE 34-1. SPIDERS OF CLINICAL INTEREST—cont'd

SCIENTIFIC NAME (NUMBER OF GENERA AND SPECIES): COMMON NAME	GEOGRAPHIC RANGE	CLINICAL REMARKS	TAXONOMIC REFERENCES	CLINICAL REFERENCES
Nephila: golden-silk spiders	Pantropical		163	
Argyronetidae (1 genus, 1 species): water spiders	Europe		230	
Argyrontea aquatica	Europe		230	
Gnaphosidae (111 genera, 2156 species): ground and mouse spiders	Worldwide		209	
Herpyllus ecclesiasticus: parson spider	North America	Minor local reaction; brief systemic effects	127	173
Drassodes	Worldwide		207	
Lamponidae (1 genus, 50 species): white-tailed spiders	Australia, Tasmania, New Zealand		209	
Lampona cylindrata: white-tailed spiders	Australia, New Zealand	Minor local reaction; rarely necrotic	209	114, 300
Miturgidae (23 genera): forest floor and cave spiders	Worldwide			
Miturga	Australia, New Zealand			
Heteropodidae (82 genera, 850 species): giant crab, huntsman, and large, wandering crab spiders			92	
Palystes natalius: lizard-eating spider	South Africa	Minor local reaction	64	195, 200
Heteropoda	Worldwide			
Isopeda	Australia, New Guinea, East Indies	Minor local reaction		298
Olios	America, Australia	Local pain, brief nausea	232	298
Delena cancerides: social huntsman spider	Australia	Minor local reaction		
Oxyopidae (9 genera, 400 species): lynx spiders	Worldwide		76	
Peucetia viridans: Green lynx spider	North and Central America, West Indies	Minor local reaction	39	123
Salticidae (475 genera, 4500 species): jumping spiders	Worldwide		80, 216	299
Breda jovialis	Australia	Minor local reaction		
Phidippus	New World	Local pain, minor ulceration		234
Holoplatys	Australia	Minor local reaction, itch, headache		299
Mopsus	Australia			
Thiodina	America			
Opisthoncus	Australia	Minor local reaction	308	299
Thomisidae (160 genera, 1960 species): crab spiders	Worldwide		74, 246	
Misumenoides	Americas		246	
Ctenidae (37 genera, 472 species): wandering spiders	Worldwide			
Phoneutria: armed spiders	South America			
P. nigriventer: Brazilian armed spider	Brazil, Paraguay	Local pain; systemic neurotoxin	82	122, 170
Elassoctenus harpax	Australia			
Cupiennius	South and Central America, West Indies		175	

Continued

TABLE 34-1. SPIDERS OF CLINICAL INTEREST—cont'd

SCIENTIFIC NAME (NUMBER OF GENERA AND SPECIES): COMMON NAME	GEOGRAPHIC RANGE	CLINICAL REMARKS	TAXONOMIC REFERENCES	CLINICAL REFERENCES
Lycosidae (76 genera, 2196 species): wolf spiders	Worldwide		76, 313	
Lycosa: wolf spiders	Worldwide	Local pain		47, 226
L. raptoria	South America	Local pain		
L. tarentula: "tarantula"	Palearctic	Subject of folklore	313	
L. godeffroyi	Australia	Local pain		
L. erythrognatha				
Clubionidae (25 genera, 590 species): sac, running spiders, and two-clawed hunting spiders	Worldwide		75	
Cheiracanthium: sac and running spiders	Worldwide			
C. mildei	Holarctic		75	
C. punctorium	Europe	Minor local reaction; fever	258	32, 180, 181
C. japonicum	Japan, China	Minor local reaction; brief systemic illness	312	203
C. longimanus	Australia	Minor local reaction; brief systemic illness		32
C. lawrencei	Africa	Local necrosis; systemic syndrome		196, 197
C. mordax	Australia	Minor local reaction, brief systemic illness		32
C. inclusum	America	Local pain, nausea	75	32
Corinnidae (51 genera, 659 species): sac spiders	Worldwide		211, 311	
Trachelas		Minor local reaction	211	205, 281
Supunna picta	Queensland	Minor local reaction	65	
Tengellidae (5 genera, 18 species): running spiders	New World			
Liocranoides	Appalachia, California			
Agelenidae (41 genera, 600 species): grass and funnel-web spiders	Worldwide		230	
Tegenaria agrestis: hobo or northwestern brown spider	Europe, America (Pacific Northwest)	Local necrosis; systemic syndrome	231	2, 285, 289
Agelenopsis aperta: grass spider or funnel-web spider	Southwest United States, Mexico		53	290
Zoridae (12 genera)				
Diallomus	Australia			
Superfamily Orbicularia (13 families, 10,300 species)				
Theridiidae (62 genera, 2000 species) comb-footed spiders	Worldwide		311	
Latrodectus: widow spiders	Worldwide	Local pain; systemic neurotoxicity	158, 164	300
L. mactans: black widow spider	North America		164, 168	82
L. mactans hasselti: redbacked spider	Australia		278	97, 140, 272
L. hesperus: black widow spider	North America			56
L. tredecimguttatus	Mediterranean		168	179
L. pallidus	Libya to Russia		168	
L. indistinctus: black button spider	Africa			188
L. geometricus: brown button spider	Worldwide		168	188
Steatoda	Worldwide		159	
S. paykulliana: false black widow spider	Europe, Mediterranean		167	

TABLE 34-1. SPIDERS OF CLINICAL INTEREST—cont'd

SCIENTIFIC NAME (NUMBER OF GENERA AND SPECIES): COMMON NAME	GEOGRAPHIC RANGE	CLINICAL REMARKS	TAXONOMIC REFERENCES	CLINICAL REFERENCES
S. nobilis	England	Local pain; mild systemic effects		294
S. foravae: false button spider	Southern Africa	Minor local reaction		190
Achaeranea tepidariorum	Worldwide	Trivial local reaction	160	
Araneidae (155 genera, 2600 species): orb-weaving spiders	Worldwide			
Argiope: argiopes	Worldwide			110
A. argentata	America	Local pain; vesicle	165	
A. trifasciata	Worldwide		165	
Araneus: cross, garden, and shamrock spiders	Worldwide		161, 162	
Eriophora biapicata	Australia	Minor local reaction		
Neoscona: orb-weaving spiders	Worldwide		30	
Phonognatha graeffei	Australia	Trivial local reaction		

DIC, Disseminated intravascular coagulation.

lesions (e.g., diabetes mellitus, leukemia, lupus erythematosus). "First-aid" interventions by the patient may mask an otherwise benign process by superimposition of trauma, burns, or chemical irritation. Systemic signs and symptoms may require differentiation from the effects of snake or scorpion neurotoxin, pesticide toxicity, sepsis, meningitis, hemolytic anemia, or acute abdomen, depending on the circumstances.

The medical history should include details of the bite circumstances, to demonstrate consistency with expected spider habitat and behavior. This includes location indoors or outside, time of day or night, and human activity at the time of injury. The victim should attempt to recall the appearance of the involved arthropod; if it was believed killed through garments or bedclothes, an attempt should be made to retrieve its remains. Crushed spider parts can be examined and identified by arachnologists or entomologists at many universities and museums. Until identified, spiders may be preserved in 70% to 80% ethanol. The evolution of subsequent wound and systemic symptoms should be noted, along with modifiers, including home treatment and underlying health of the patient. If the local geography lacks species consistent with the suspected pathophysiology, the recent travel history of household contacts should be considered.

Physical examination includes particular attention to the bite site, as well as general assessment for systemic effects. Local findings of importance include anatomic location (spiders are more likely to bite defensively at sites where clothing binds tightly; thin skin is more readily envenomed than callous skin) and number of separate lesions (multiple bites suggest parasitic insect bite rather than spider bite). Central punctae, vesicles, or erosions should be noted, as well as the pattern of peripheral changes, including erythema, pallor, hemorrhage, induration, tenderness or anesthesia, and local lymphatic involvement. Systemic findings, depending on the species involved, may include changes in vital signs, diaphoresis, generalized rash, facial edema, gastrointestinal distress, muscle fasciculations, spasm or tenderness, or altered mental status.

The laboratory evaluation for envenomation is usually simple, seldom requiring more than complete blood count and urinalysis. Assessment for other elements of the differential diagnosis, however, may be much more elaborate. Depending on circumstances, this may include viral, bacterial, or fungal culture; Lyme disease titer; radiography of the abdomen or of the injured part; stool test for occult blood; electrocardiogram; or skin biopsy.

General supportive measures are the mainstay of therapy for most spider bites. These include basic local hygiene, tetanus prophylaxis, analgesics, hydration, and surgical follow-up if indicated for debridement and management of extensive necrotic lesions. Corticosteroids are of unproven benefit and are generally not indicated. Antibiotics, although not of value for simple venom injury, are prescribed when bacterial cellulitis cannot be eliminated from the differential diagnosis. Specific measures, including antivenom, for treatment of envenomation by particular spider species are discussed later in this chapter.

GUIDE TO SPIDER DIVERSITY AND IDENTIFICATION

This chapter provides more information on spider diversity than most reviews in order to (1) inform the reader of the immense diversity of spiders that are

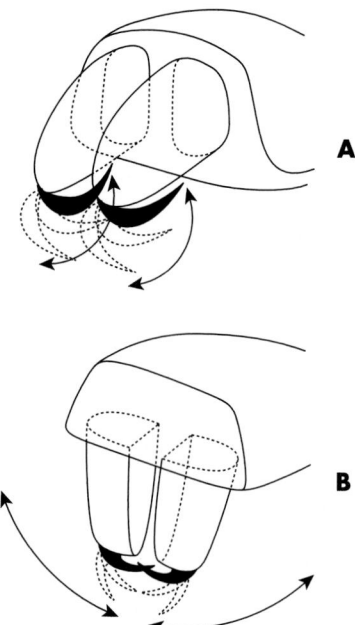

medically insignificant and thus emphasize the rarity of spiders known to cause medical problems; (2) emphasize the need for accurate species identification, particularly in reporting of cases for publication or teaching; and (3) facilitate accurate identification of spiders that are caught in the act of biting by directing professionals to proper identification keys. Table 34-1 includes species worldwide that are currently known or suspected to be medically noteworthy, even minimally, either through the effect of bites or urticating hairs. Geographic range and the most recent systematic work on each group are included. Box 34-1 lists genera of serious medical significance for each continent. For effective communication, groups of spiders must be recognized by the same name worldwide. This chapter uses the current official nomenclature.

Of the three spider suborders, two contain clinically significant species: Mygalomorphae and Araneomorphae. Mygalomorphs include the baboon spiders or tarantulas, trapdoor spiders, purse-web spiders, mygalomorph funnel-web spiders, and several other groups that lack common names. Most spiders are araneomorphs, including jumping spiders, orb-weaving spiders, widow spiders, and wolf spiders (see Table 34-1). The most conspicuous characteristics that distinguish these groups are the orientation of the chelicerae (jaws) and the number of book lungs. Spider fangs are located on the chelicerae, which open sideways in the Araneomorphae and move diagonally in the Mygalomorphae, requiring the latter to rear back for a downward, snakelike strike (Figures 34-3 and 34-4). Mygalomorphae have two pairs of book lungs, whereas most Araneomorphae have only one pair. Lung slits, which open into the book lungs, are easily visible in a ventral view of the anterior abdomen (see Figure 34-1). Characteristics that distinguish families, genera, and species include eye number

Figure 34-3 Movement of the chelicerae in mygalomorphs **(A)** and araneomorphs **(B)**. *(Modified from Foelix RF: Biology of spiders, ed 2, Oxford, UK, 1996, Oxford University Press.)*

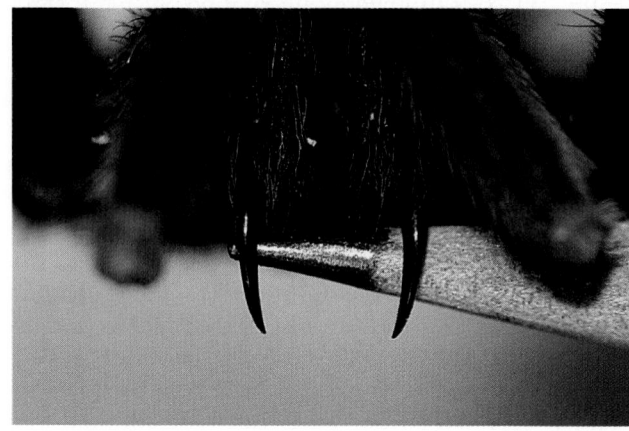

Figure 34-4 Fangs of mature male tarantula (*Aphonopelma* species). *(Courtesy Michael Cardwell & Associates, 1992.)*

and pattern, numbers of tarsal claws, and details of genitalic structure.

Although many spider species are geographically localized (e.g., *Atrax robustus* in Australia, *Phoneutria nigriventer* in Brazil), some, such as the black widow (*Latrodectus mactans*), are found worldwide (see Table 34-1). Others, such as members of the *Loxosceles* genus, are widely distributed in more than one continent, and still others, such as *Tegenaria agrestis*, appear to have naturalized in specific geographic regions distant from their point of ecological origin. Because of the resulting worldwide species diversity and overlap, the remainder of this chapter is structured according to spider taxonomy rather than isolated species or geographic location.

SUBORDER MYGALOMORPHAE

Mygalomorphs make up less than 10% of all spider species. They are found worldwide, with greatest abundance and diversity in tropical regions. Tarantulas (Theraphosidae) are the most famous mygalomorphs and include the largest spiders known, reaching up to 10 cm in body length. Most mygalomorphs are smaller, some less than 1 mm in adult body length. Most live multiple years (some up to 20), and females continue to molt after reaching adulthood. They have diverse habits but typically live in silk-lined burrows or silken tubes. For the purpose of prey capture, mygalomorph silk is only slightly sticky relative to araneomorph silk and is generally used to trigger the presence of prey rather than to ensnare them. Once prey are detected, spiders run out of their retreat, seize prey in their jaws, and return to the retreat to feed. Individuals wander when dispersing, and males leave their retreats in search of females during mating season.

Family Theraphosidae: Tarantulas and Baboon Spiders

Theraphosidae is the largest mygalomorph family with respect to both numbers of species and sizes of the largest individuals (Figure 34-5). Approximately 800 described species are found on all continents, with greatest abundance and diversity in tropical regions. They mature in 3 to 9 years and can live for 15 to 20 years. Individuals live in burrows, with trip-line threads extending from the entrance. These are sometimes located in abandoned rodent burrows or hollow trees. Theraphosids have dense tufts of specialized hairs on their tarsi (feet) that enable them to climb on smooth surfaces and may aid in prey capture. They have two tarsal claws, eight closely grouped eyes, and two pairs of spinnerets. Tarantulas may live for 1 to 25 years. As a group, they are found mainly in tropical and subtropical areas.

Confusingly, "tarantula" was first applied to *Lycosa tarentula,* a species of European spider actually belonging to the wolf spider family, or Lycosidae, which are properly classified within the suborder Araneomorphae, described later in this chapter. In the United States the term *tarantula* usually refers only to the large spiders of the family Theraphosidae, suborder Mygalomorphae.

Grammostola mollicoma is the largest tarantula known, with a body length of 7 to 10 cm and leg spread of 21 to 27 cm.[42,104] *Harpactirella lightfooti,* the baboon spider or bobbejaan-spinnekop, is a mygalomorph spider found in South Africa. Body length is 3 cm; the cephalothorax is brown with a yellowish border.

Venom. Few tarantula venoms have been studied systematically. In the United States, *Rheochostica henzi* and

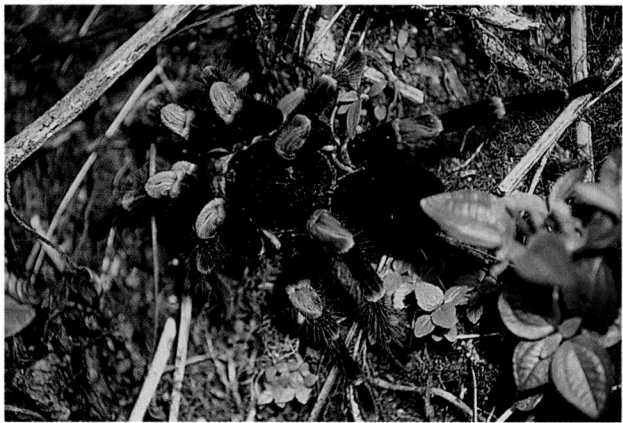

Figure 34-5 *Theraphosidae. (Courtesy Gita Bodner.)*

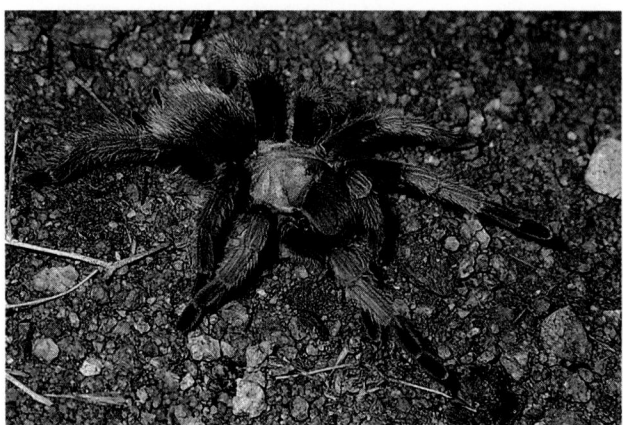

Figure 34-6 Mature female *Aphonopelma iodium. (Courtesy Michael Cardwell & Associates, 1997.)*

members of the genus *Aphonopelma* (Figure 34-6) have venom containing hyaluronidase, nucleotides, and polyamines.[46,54,155,239,240] Polyamines are thought to act as neurotransmitters and increase venom effectiveness, particularly with respect to paralysis of insect prey.[253] Hyaluronidase is postulated to be a spreading factor, and the nucleotide adenosine triphosphate (ATP) potentiates the major effects of the venom on mice. Both venoms cause rapid, irreversible necrosis of skeletal muscle when injected intraperitoneally into mice.[204] *Dugesiella (Rheochostica)* venom was found to have a necrotoxin with several similarities to sea snake venoms.[155] In comparison, the venom of *Scodra griseipes,* an African tarantula, includes higher-molecular-weight (greater than 25,000 daltons) proteins and enzymes plus lower-weight polypeptides (4000 to 9000 daltons); the second group is believed to contain polypeptide neurotoxins.[52] *S. griseipes* venom toxins have a mammalian effect, but this species is not known to be clinically relevant. Recent work suggests that venom chemotaxonomy may be a useful method of nondestructive species recognition, at least within the *Brachypelma* genus.[84]

Urticating Hairs. Several genera of tarantulas, including *Haplopelma*, *Lasiodora*, *Grammostola*, *Acanthoscurria*, and *Brachypelma*, possess urticating hairs irritative to skin and mucous membranes. These genera are located throughout the western hemisphere, with many species indigenous to the United States. When one of these spiders is threatened, it rubs its hind legs across the dorsal surface of its abdomen and flicks thousands of hairs toward the aggressor. These barbed hairs can penetrate human skin, causing edematous, pruritic papules. The itching may persist for weeks. There are four morphologic types of urticating hairs. Tarantulas within the United States possess only type I hairs, which do not penetrate the skin as deeply as type III hairs. Type II hairs are incorporated into the silk web retreat and not thrown off by the spider. Type III hairs can penetrate up to 2 mm into human skin; this is the type of hair most likely to cause inflammation. They are typically found on Mexican, Caribbean, and Central and South American species. Type IV hairs, which belong to the South American spider *Grammostola*, are able to cause inflammation of the respiratory tract in small mammals. Rats and mice have been reported to die of asphyxia within 2 hours after exposure to the hairs.[61,299]

Clinical Presentation. Despite the presence in venom of components toxic to rodent nerves and skeletal muscle, most tarantula bites result in only mild to moderate local symptoms in humans. A few can cause more severe pain and swelling, numbness, or lymphangitis. Species of tarantula implicated as causes of human envenomation include those in genera *Mygalarachne* (formerly *Sericopelma*) of Panama, *Pterinochilus* of Africa, *Aphonopelma* of Mexico and the United States, *Pamphobaeteus* of South America, *Euathlus* of Costa Rica, *Theraphosa* of French Guyana, *Grammostola* of Colombia, *Poecilothuria* of India, *Lampropelma* of Thailand, *Lasiodora* of Brazil, and *Avicularia* of Central America and southwestern United States. Envenomation usually involves immediate pain at the bite site, occasionally followed by some redness and swelling and usually without necrosis or serious sequelae.*

Although no fatalities have been reported, localized pain followed by emesis, weakness, and collapse has been noted after envenomation by *Harpactirella lightfooti*, the baboon spider of South Africa.[42,122,195]

Urticating hairs may cause intense inflammation, which may remain pruritic for weeks. Individuals who handle tarantulas may unwittingly transfer urticating hairs from hand to eye, causing keratoconjunctivitis or ophthalmia nodosa. Keratoconjunctivitis has been de-

scribed after handling of a Thailand black tarantula, *Haplopelma minax*. Fine intracorneal hairs were noted at examination, and inflammation settled quickly with topical corticosteroid treatment; at 36-month follow-up the eye was normal.[36]

More severe ophthalmic complications occurred in two cases after handling of Chilean rose tarantulas, *Grammostola cala*. In these victims, initial findings were similar, with intracorneal hairs and keratoconjunctivitis, but progressive panuveitis followed, with corneal granulomas, iritis, cataract, vitritis, and chorioretinitis apparently related to migration of hairs through the media of the eye. The differences in outcome with exposure to the two species may result from differences in hair morphology, which may also explain differences in other reports of ophthalmic injury from tarantula or caterpillar hair exposure.[36] Similar cases of ophthalmia nodosa have been described.[25,154]

Treatment. Theraphosid bite management is symptomatic. Elevation and immobilization of the extremity and oral analgesics may help reduce pain. All bites should receive local wound care and appropriate tetanus prophylaxis.

Urticating hairs can be removed from skin with repeated application and removal of sticky tape, followed by copious irrigation if necessary; exposed eyes should be irrigated primarily. Topical or systemic corticosteroids and oral antihistamines may also be useful for urticating hair reactions.

Family Hexathelidae: Funnel-Web Mygalomorphs

The family Hexathelidae includes 11 genera and approximately 74 species, which are currently known from the Old World and Chile.[218] The funnel webs that typify members of this group are silk-lined tubular retreats that extend into a protected space, such as a burrow in the ground or a hole in a tree. Sheets of silk radiate from the retreat and signal the presence of prey. These webs superficially resemble webs of araneomorph spiders in the family Agelenidae. Distinguishing characteristics of the spiders include a shiny carapace; long, spiny sensory hairs on the legs; and paired claws lacking claw tufts on the tips of the feet, with teeth lining the medial claw.

Clinically significant hexathelid spiders are species of *Atrax* (Figure 34-7) and *Hadronyche*. Technically, taxonomists now consider *Atrax* and *Hadronyche* species as members of only one genus.[218] To avoid confusion in the literature, species names still use either *Atrax* or *Hadronyche*, depending on their original names. We discuss these species as a cohesive taxonomic group. Among these, the species *Atrax robustus* is best known and most carefully studied. *Atrax* and *Hadronyche* species, all of which are believed to be dangerous, have

---

*References 42, 46, 54, 66, 104, 150, 239.

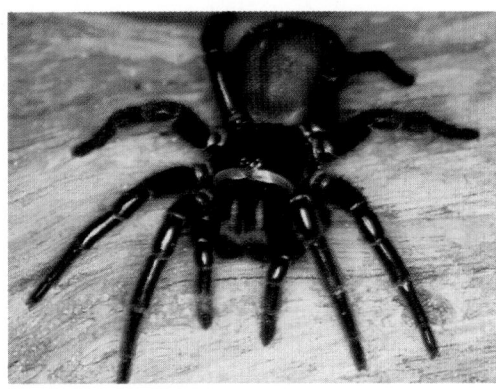

Figure 34-7 Funnel-web spider (*Atrax* species) wearing a wedding ring. *(Courtesy Sherman Minton, MD.)*

been described in southern and southeastern Australia, Tasmania, Papua New Guinea, and the Solomon Islands. As a group, they prefer cool, moist coastal and mountainous regions.[116,118,249]

Genus Atrax/Hadronyche

BIOLOGY. Funnel-web spiders have a glossy ebony cephalothorax and velvety black abdomen. The abdominal undersurface may have brushes of red hair. The fangs reach 4 to 5 mm in length and are capable of penetrating a fingernail or a chicken's skull, sometimes making removal of the spider difficult. Females are somewhat larger than males, with a body length of 4 cm. Mature males are more delicate, with a tibial spur on the second pair of legs and pointed pedipalps.[137,242]

Atrax robustus, the Sydney funnel-web spider, is limited to a 160 km range around the center of Sydney, Australia. The spider creates a tubular or funnel-shaped, silk-lined shallow burrow under rocks, logs, fences, stumps, or thick vegetation or around foundations of houses. Colonies of up to 150 spiders have been found. Females rarely roam far from their webs; males live a vagrant life after reaching maturity. Wandering males may enter houses or other areas of human habitation, especially during the summer months after a heavy rain. Its aggressive behavior and potent venom make the male Sydney funnel-web arachnid one of the most dangerous spiders in the world. It is responsible for all known fatal *Atrax* envenomations.*

Hadronyche formidabilis, the northern funnel-web spider, is found in the central coastal region of New South Wales and the adjacent Blue Mountains. Its tree-dwelling habit was once thought to be unique, but it is now known that other species also live in trees. The webs may be camouflaged in rough-barked trees, such as melaleuca (paper bark), banksia, and eucalyptus.[118]

*References 58, 98, 118, 242, 275, 301.

VENOM. Although many species have venom with significant in vitro toxicity, few have been implicated in human illness. The best described of these is *A. robustus. Atrax* venom causes widespread release of neurotransmitters.[79,118,125,256,263] This may occur by a direct action of the venom on nerve membranes, producing spontaneous action potentials and consequently provoking a global outpouring of transmitters that accounts for the neuromotor and autonomic stimulation seen clinically.

Early efforts to purify the active component of *Atrax* venom resulted in reports of neurotoxins of various molecular weights purified from venom preparations in separate experiments.[261] These were termed *Atraxotoxin* (10,000 to 25,000 daltons, from milked venom),[118] *robustoxin* (4887 daltons, also from milked venom),[250] and *atraxin* (9800 daltons, from ground venom glands).[119] The relationships among these toxins are not clear, but atraxotoxin or atraxin may be a precursor of robustoxin. In addition to these components, *Atrax* venom contains various lower-molecular-weight compounds, including citric acid, lactic acid, phosphoric acid, glycerol, urea, glucose, gamma-aminolevulinic acid, glycine, spermidine, spermine, tyramine, octopamine, and 5-methoxytryptamine.[78]

The best characterized of the toxins is robustoxin, whose 42–amino acid sequence was determined in 1985.[250] It is the sole lethal toxin that can be isolated by cation-exchange chromatography, and its effects in monkeys duplicate the effects of crude venom preparations. A 5 mg/kg intravenous (IV) dose of robustoxin to monkeys causes dyspnea, blood pressure fluctuations culminating in severe hypotension, lacrimation, salivation, skeletal muscle fasciculation, and death within 3 to 4 hours of administration.[191]

Isolated human intercostal muscles were studied to determine the etiology of muscle fasciculations. Muscles treated with *A. robustus* venom developed marked contractions, which were abolished by *d*-tubocurarine.[48] Muscles treated with venom for more than an hour stopped contracting and could be stimulated only by increasing the stimulus duration. *A. robustus* venom has been shown to lack anticholinesterase activity.[260] Contractions are not a direct venom action on the muscle fiber, so acetylcholine appears to have been released from the presynaptic terminals.[96] Muscle fasciculations are apparently caused by abnormal repetitive firing of motor neurons. It was hypothesized that the venom changes the membrane's electric field, activating sodium channels without altering the transmembrane potential or damaging the neuronal membrane ultrastructurally.[79,118,256]

Hypertension in *Atrax* toxicity may have several causes. Morgans and Carroll[186,187] demonstrated direct alpha-adrenergic stimulation with vasoconstriction of isolated arterial preparations exposed to *A. robustus* venom. In rabbit atria an initial decrease followed by an increase in cardiac inotropy and chronotropy may result from vagal acetylcholine and myocardial norepinephrine releases, respectively.[49] The combination of myocardial responses and peripheral vasoconstriction may explain the hypertensive response.

Animal species vary in susceptibility to *Atrax* venom. Rabbits given 15 mg of crude venom intravenously and cane toads given 12 mg of female *Atrax* venom show no effects after envenomation. Primates, including humans, are among the most susceptible species. Newborn mice, also highly susceptible, have been used as an in vivo biologic assay for venom toxicity.[118,265] Sutherland[267] found that a lethal dose of venom from a male *A. robustus* could be neutralized in newborn mice by nonimmune sera from rabbits and other nonprimate vertebrates. Scheumack and coworkers[251] later demonstrated that the active fraction of nonimmune rabbit sera contained immunoglobulins G and M (IgG, IgM).

In addition, venom potency varies with time of year, recent feeding history, maturation and gender of the individual spider.[12] Between 1956 and 1963, Wiener demonstrated significant differences in the venom of male and female *Atrax* spiders. Males had an average venom yield of 1.01 mg, less than the 1.84 average from females. On the other hand, guinea pig lethality was much greater after a bite by a male (75% to 90%) than by a female spider (20%). Weiner concluded that significant qualitative difference exists between the venoms of males and females.

Monkeys, which have a pattern of envenomation similar to that in humans, provide a model in which Sutherland[265,271] has described a biphasic clinical syndrome. Phase I begins minutes after venom injection, with local piloerection and muscle fasciculation. This extends proximally, becoming generalized over the next 10 to 20 minutes. After another 5 minutes, severe hypertension, tachycardia, hyperthermia, and coma with increased intracranial pressure may occur, followed by diaphoresis, salivation, lacrimation, diarrhea, sporadic apnea, borborygmi, and grotesque muscle writhing. Death may result from asphyxia caused by laryngeal spasm, combined with copious respiratory secretions, apnea, or pulmonary edema. Laboratory evaluation reveals metabolic acidosis and elevated plasma creatine phosphokinase. Phase II begins 1 to 2 hours after envenomation, as the phase I symptoms subside. The victim may return to consciousness and appear to recover. In severe cases, hypotension gradually worsens over 1 to 2 hours, with periods of apnea. Pulmonary edema and death may occur despite ventilatory support.

CLINICAL PRESENTATION. Up to 90% of *Atrax* bites may not result in significant envenomation.[299] Intense pain at the bite site may result from direct trauma as well as the venom's effect, but the bite does not provoke cutaneous necrosis. Wiener[303] studied the cutaneous effects of the venom on himself by injecting 0.5 mg intradermally. Local pain and a wheal surrounded by erythema lasted for 30 minutes, followed by localized sweating and piloerection. No systemic effects occurred.

The earliest systemic signs and symptoms may include perioral tingling, nausea and vomiting, diaphoresis, salivation, lacrimation, and dyspnea. Pulmonary edema follows, along with a generalized central and peripheral neurologic syndrome that includes muscle fasciculations, tremor, spasms, weakness, and impaired consciousness. Death may occur secondary to pulmonary failure, hypotension, or cardiac arrest.[262,299]

Thirteen fatalities from *A. robustus* envenomation were recorded between 1927 and 1984. Children are particularly susceptible; those under 12 years may die within 4 hours of the bite.[91,126,268] Before the development of specific antivenom in 1980, severe envenomations resulted in a minimum 8-hour critical period, followed by a 9- to 21-day hospital course.[90,268,271]

No fatalities caused by *H. formidabilis* have been recorded, although, several severe envenomations have occurred.[118] Venoms of *A. robustus*, *A. versutus*, *A. infensus*, and *A. formidabilis* appear to have comparable vertebrate toxicity in vitro.[11]

TREATMENT. Immediate treatment after a bite is modeled after that for Australian snakebite and consists of four steps: (1) wrap the length of the bitten extremity with an elastic bandage, (2) splint to immobilize the extremity, (3) immobilize the victim, and (4) transport to the nearest hospital with the bandage in place.[201,269] A human case report has illustrated the utility of this method, with occurrence, disappearance, recurrence, and reresolution of symptoms coinciding with compression wrap removal and replacement in a man bitten by a male *A. robustus*.[112] An experimental model in *Macaca fascicularis* monkeys has supported efficacy of the pressure immobilization technique.[264,265,273]

Specific antivenom has been the mainstay of treatment for *Atrax* envenomation since 1981. The antivenom is a purified IgG product developed by Sutherland and associates[266,274] at the Commonwealth Serum Laboratories by immunizing rabbits with a combination of male *Atrax* venom and Freund's adjuvant. The antivenom was demonstrated to neutralize *Atrax* venom in vitro and to reverse symptoms in monkeys before its introduction for human use. To date, it has been used with good effect in more than 40 humans bitten by *Atrax* and *Hadronyche* species.[71,271]

If a tourniquet or bandage is in place when the victim presents for hospital care, it should be removed in an intensive care setting, with careful observation for development or progression of symptoms. If systemic signs or symptoms occur, victims are usually treated with antivenom administration. Two ampules of antivenom (100 mg of purified IgG per ampule) are administered intravenously every 15 minutes until symptoms improve. Dosing is the same for children as for adults, and total doses of 2 to 8 ampules have been reported. During a 10-year period, antivenom was given to at least 40 persons, with no adverse effects or deaths reported.[271]

In addition to antivenom administration, management is symptomatic and supportive. Oxygen, mechanical ventilation, and IV fluid support may be indicated in severe cases. Atropine (0.6 mg) may be used to lessen salivation and bronchorrhea. β-Blockers may be indicated for severe hypertension and tachycardia.

Other than antivenom, no consistently effective agent has been found to enhance survival after *Atrax* envenomation. Diazepam, atropine, and furosemide have been found to increase survival in monkeys, but this may not be the case in humans.[89,118]

Scheumack and colleagues[252] developed a toxoid from robustoxin by polymerization with glutaraldehyde. Immunization with the toxoid conferred protection against the lethal effects of 50 mg/kg *Atrax* venom in monkeys for at least 26 weeks after toxoid injection.

Family Dipluridae: Funnel-Web Mygalomorphs

Members of the family Dipluridae are found on all continents and are concentrated in tropical areas. Individuals build funnel webs similar to those of Hexathelidae. Diplurids are distinct from hexathelids in having posterior lateral spinnerets that are very long and widely separated. Most are 5 to 25 mm in length.

Genus Trechona

BIOLOGY. *Trechona venosa* is a large South American funnel-web tarantula with neurotoxic venom potentially dangerous to humans.[42,104,122] As with all *Trechona* species, *T. venosa* is sedentary, living in holes or on plants in tropical forests along the Atlantic coast. The spider may be black or gray-brown with yellow stripes on the abdomen. Mature body length may be 3 to 4.5 cm, with 6- to 7-cm legs and 3- to 4-mm fangs. *T. venosa* is not found in Chile, but in this region it has been confused, particularly in venom studies, with a spider in the family Nemesiidae, *Acanthogonatus subcalpeianus*, which it resembles.[218]

VENOM. The venom of *T. venosa* is extremely toxic to rats, with an apparent action similar to that of *Phoneutria* species.[170]

CLINICAL PRESENTATION. No cases of human envenomation have been reported, although it is pre-

sumed that symptomatic envenomation by *T. venosa* is possible.

TREATMENT. Treatment is symptomatic and supportive.

SUBORDER ARANEOMORPHAE

Enormous diversity is found within the group Araneomorphae, which contains 32,000 of the 34,000 currently described spider species.[59] Araneomorphs, or true spiders, are found throughout the world in all terrestrial (and a few aquatic) habitats. They show tremendous variability in size, appearance, and habit; however, no araneomorphs are as large as the largest tarantulas. Characteristics that distinguish araneomorphs include features of the spinnerets that enable them to produce extremely sticky silk. Also, all but a few groups have only one pair of book lungs. Most have eight eyes, but eye number varies from two to eight. Prey capture tactics usually determine where a spider will be found and are generally consistent within particular groups. Thus these tactics often provide conspicuous clues that help identify spiders.

Family Sicariidae: Recluse Spiders

Sicariidae includes two genera, *Loxosceles* and *Sicarius*, both of which are clinically important. The family falls within a larger group of families (Scytodoids) that all have only six eyes. In these two genera the eyes are in dyad pairs. The chelicerae are fused at the base, and the labium is fused to the sternum. Males have more slender abdomens and more prominent pedipalps than females. Previously, *Loxosceles* was placed in its own family, Loxoscelidae, but this was recently synonymized with Sicariidae.[210]

Genus Loxosceles: Brown Spiders

BIOLOGY. *Loxosceles*, commonly known as brown or fiddle spiders, build small, irregular, and sticky webs in small areas, such as under rocks or wood or in human-made habitats. The genus contains more than 100 species, with centers of diversity in central America and Africa.[20,77,174,238,244] These spiders are 8 to 15 mm in adult body length, are light to dark brown, and have a dark, violin-shaped spot centered anterodorsally, such that the neck of the fiddle extends backward across the cephalothorax. The shape and darkness of the fiddle, relative lengths of the first two pairs of legs, and genitalia characteristics are features that help distinguish species[43,133,244] (Figure 34-8).

From the South American *L. laeta* to the South African *L. spinulosa*, these small arachnids have been associated with human pathologic conditions. Several species have been associated with necrotic arachnidism in the United States: *L. reclusa* (the true brown recluse

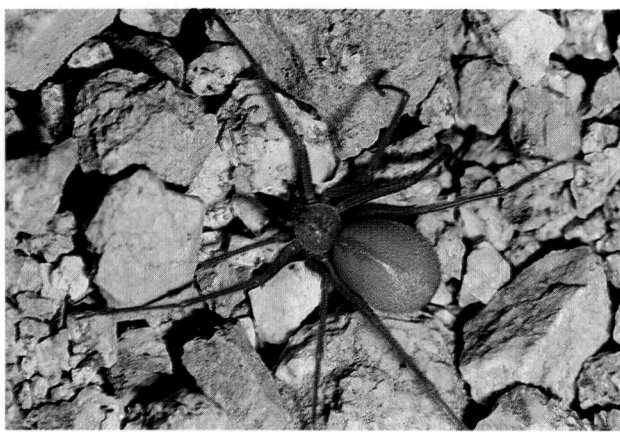

Figure 34-8 Adult female desert violin spider *(Loxosceles deserta)*. *(Courtesy Michael Cardwell & Associates, 1994.)*

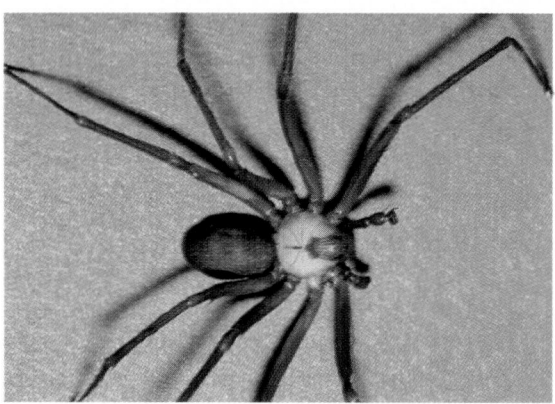

Figure 34-9 Brown recluse spider *(Loxosceles reclusa)*. *(Courtesy Indiana University Medical Center.)*

spider, Figure 34-9), *L. rufescens, L. arizonica,* and *L. laeta.* These spiders are native to all the southernmost states. In the Mississippi River valley, their territory extends as far north as southern Wisconsin. Species native to one region or habitat may adapt successfully to new locations after transport by humans.[197,293]

Brown spiders regularly roam in search of new web sites, and males wander in search of females. They are most active at night from spring through fall, emerging from woodpiles and rats' nests to hunt insects and other spiders. South African savanna species have been observed under stones and logs and in the tunnels of old termite nests; spelean species are found naturally in caves, but have also appeared in homes and export warehouses.[194,196,199] Brown spiders may infest homes, generally preferring warm, undisturbed environments such as vacant buildings and storage sheds. In Chile the tendency to inhabit human dwellings has earned *L. laeta* the names *araña de los rincones* (corner spider) and *araña de detrás de los cuadros* (spider behind the pictures).[245] Molts, or shed exoskeletons, may mark in-

fested areas; the web may be limited to a small, flocculent structure alongside the egg sac. Females may live 1 to 3 years and longer in captivity.[104,134] Naturally unaggressive toward humans, brown spiders are not prone to bite unless threatened or trapped against the skin. Bites typically follow retrieval of old bed sheets or jackets from storage.

VENOM. Fractionated *Loxosceles* venom contains at least eight or nine major protein bands and three or four minor bands identifiable by gel electrophoresis.[223] Hyaluronidase was first identified as a component by Wright and associates.[310] Hyaluronidase probably plays a facilitating role in lesion development, encouraging the spread of other venom components; however, it is not itself a cytotoxin. Hydrolytic enzyme activities include esterase,[310] alkaline phosphatase,[128] lipase,[142] and 5'-ribonucleotide phosphorylase,[103] but none of these alone appears to explain cytotoxicity.

Sphingomyelinase D, a protein fraction of 32,000 dalton, appears to be the most important dermonecrotic factor in *L. reclusa* venom. This component is present in *L. intermedia* spiderlings starting with the third instar, with increasing activity throughout development until adulthood.[108] Injection of the purified fraction produces characteristic lesions in rabbits.[152,280] A protein of similar molecular weight to sphingomyelinase D has been shown to have dermonecrotic activity in the venom of *L. gaucho* of Brazil,[21] and considerable homology has been noted among proteins derived from *L. intermedia, L. laeta, L. gaucho,* and *L. reclusa.*[22] Sphingomyelinase D is postulated to operate by a variety of mechanisms, including cell membrane binding and polymorphonuclear leukocyte neutrophil (PMN) chemotaxis.[100,222,254] Lesions are inhibited in rabbits by pretreatment with nitrogen mustard to deplete PMNs. Histologic studies suggest similarities between venom-induced lesions and those seen with the Arthus and Shwartzmann phenomena.[254]

Some vertebrate species, such as rats and fish, are essentially unaffected by *Loxosceles* venom; others, such as rabbits, mice, and dogs, are highly susceptible to its effects.[243] Injected into humans, the venom is a hemolysin and cytotoxin, with enzymatic activities that may cause dermonecrosis and hemolysis. Pathogenesis of the human lesion is not well understood but depends on the functions of complement and PMNs.[17,244]

Venom from *L. reclusa* has a direct hemolytic effect on human erythrocytes; this process depends on the presence of serum components that include C-reactive protein and calcium.[135,280] Platelet aggregation also is calcium dependent and is induced in vitro with sphingomyelinase D; this process may activate the prostaglandin cascade. Platelet aggregation appears to depend on serum amyloid protein, a serum glycoprotein of previously unknown significance.[99,225,280]

Because *Loxosceles* venom provokes an immune response in experimental animals, efforts to develop diagnostic tests are based on antigen or antibody detection in human blood. In 1973, Berger and associates[29] reported an in vitro lymphocyte transformation assay for *L. reclusa* venom, which turned positive in the lymphocytes of exposed individuals within 4 to 6 weeks of initial exposure. This test may help to document prior exposure but not to diagnose envenomation at the time of the initial bite. Barrett and co-workers[23] reported a passive hemagglutination inhibition test using rabbit antibody and human erythrocytes incubated in vitro with venom from *L. reclusa.*[23] Cardoso and associates, observing that efforts to detect antigen in human serum may fail because of insufficient antigenemia, have demonstrated the presence of *L. gaucho* venom in biopsy homogenate using enzyme-linked immunosorbent assay (ELISA). Barbaro and colleagues[21] demonstrated circulating IgG against *L. gaucho* venom in 4 of 20 patients, detectable between 9 and 120 days after the bite.

Some of the variability in clinical presentation among victims of *Loxosceles* envenomation may be caused by differences in the venom of males and females. Female *L. intermedia* spiders produce a greater amount of more potent venom than males.[63]

CLINICAL PRESENTATION. *Necrotic arachnidism,* or *loxoscelism* in the case of bite by spiders of the genus *Loxosceles,* refers to the clinical syndrome that follows envenomation by a variety of spiders, for which *L. reclusa,* the brown recluse spider, is the prototype. The bites of these spiders often result in serious cutaneous injuries, with subsequent necrosis and tissue loss. Less often, severe systemic reactions may occur with hemolysis, coagulopathy, renal failure, and even death.[292]

Reports of severe reaction to spider bites possibly attributable to brown spiders date to 1872, in a report of a 45-year-old Texas woman with a febrile illness accompanying a large necrotic lesion of her thigh.[50] In 1896, death from renal failure accompanying another bite in Texas was reported.[214] Spider bite was reported as a cause of blackwater fever (massive hemoglobinuria) in Tennessee in 1940.[111] The first documented case of loxoscelism (from *L. rufescens*) was reported by Schmaus[247] in Kansas in 1929. *L. laeta* was identified as the cause of similar lesions in South America in 1937, and *L. reclusa* was the cause of necrotic arachnidism in the Midwestern United States by 1958.[9,10] Since then, numerous cases of cutaneous and more severe reactions have been attributed to spiders of the genus *Loxosceles.*

The clinical spectrum of loxoscelism ranges from mild and transient skin irritation to severe local necrosis accompanied by dramatic hematologic and renal injury. Isolated cutaneous lesions are the most com-

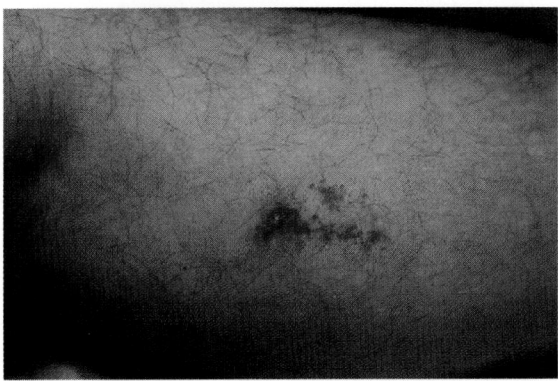

Figure 34-10 Brown recluse spider bite after 6 hours, with central hemorrhagic vesicle and gravitational spread of venom. *(Courtesy Paul Auerbach, MD, and Riley Rees, MD.)*

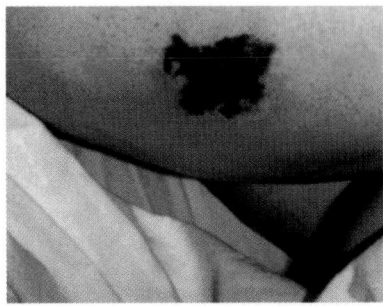

Figure 34-11 Brown recluse spider bite after 24 hours, with central ischemia and rapidly advancing cellulitis. *(Courtesy Paul Auerbach, MD.)*

mon presentation, and most bites may resolve spontaneously without the need for medical intervention.[28,29] Many authors distinguish between simple local presentation and more severe systemic, or viscerocutaneous, loxoscelism.

Local symptoms usually begin at the moment of the bite, with a sharp stinging sensation, although a victim may be unaware of having been bitten. Frequently the bite site corresponds to a portal of entry or a region of constriction of clothing, such as cuff, collar, waistband, or groin. The stinging usually subsides over 6 to 8 hours and is replaced by aching and pruritus as the lesion becomes ischemic from local vasospasm. The site then becomes edematous, with an erythematous halo surrounding an irregular violaceous center of "incipient necrosis" (actually hemorrhage and thrombosis).[44,280] A white ring of vasospasm and ischemia may be discernible between the central lesion and the halo. Often the erythematous margin spreads irregularly in a gravitationally influenced pattern that leaves the original center eccentrically placed near the top of the lesion (Figures 34-10 to 34-12). In more severe cases, serous or hemorrhagic bullae may arise at the center within 24 to 72 hours, and an eschar forms beneath. After 2 to 5 weeks this eschar sloughs, leaving an ulcer of

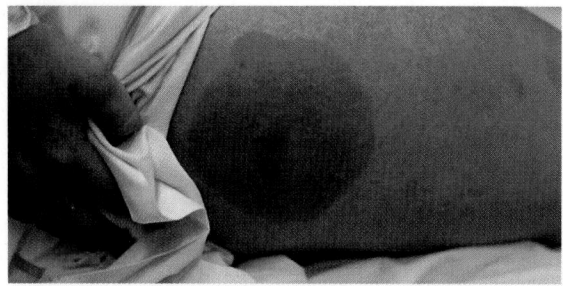

Figure 34-12 Brown recluse spider bite after 48 hours, with incipient central necrosis.

variable size and depth through skin and adipose tissue, but sparing muscle.[130] Lesions involving adipose tissue may be extensive, perhaps from lipolytic action of the venom.[142] The ulcer may persist for many months, leaving a deep scar.[3,235,295] Local sequelae depend on the anatomic location. Persistent segmental cutaneous anesthesia has been attributed to nerve injury after a recluse bite on the side of the neck.[121] Epiglottic and periepiglottic swelling severe enough to require endotracheal intubation has been reported in a recluse bite involving a child's ear.[129]

The bite of the somewhat larger South American spider *L. laeta* is reported to cause intense pain and extensive edema, with proportionately less necrosis than that caused by *L. reclusa*. The edema is notoriously prominent with facial bites and resolves over 2 to 4 weeks.[244]

Systemic involvement is less common but may occur in combination with cutaneous injury from any *Loxosceles* species; it occurs more frequently in children but may be seen in adults.[215,277] Systemic reaction may develop in cases with minor-appearing local findings, making diagnosis difficult.[280] When systemic involvement occurs, hemolytic anemia with hemoglobinuria is often the prominent feature, usually beginning within 24 hours of envenomation and resolving within 1 week.[81] During this time, measured hemoglobin may drop markedly, accompanied by jaundice and hemoglobinuria. The anemia is usually Coombs' test negative, but two cases of Coombs'-positive anemia have been reported.[292] Fever, chills, maculopapular rash, weakness, leukocytosis, arthralgias, nausea, vomiting, thrombocytopenia, disseminated intravascular coagulation (DIC), hemoglobinuria, proteinuria, renal failure, and even death have been reported.[33,70,106,192,292]

The diagnosis of loxoscelism is based on spider observation and identification, typical history, and local and systemic signs. The differential diagnosis of the local injury includes bacterial and mycobacterial infection, herpes simplex, decubitus ulcer, burn, embolism, thrombosis, direct trauma, vasculitis, Lyme disease, and pyoderma gangrenosum.[5,145,217,219,270]

A series of five proved or suspected *L. reclusa* bites to women in the second and third trimesters of pregnancy has been reported. Despite significant local injuries, rash, and microhematuria, no fetal injury was noted.[4]

TREATMENT. Treatment of loxoscelism depends on its severity. Cutaneous loxoscelism can usually be managed on an outpatient basis. Most mild cutaneous envenomations respond to application of local cold compresses,[147] elevation of the affected extremity, and loose immobilization of the part. Tetanus prophylaxis should be provided where indicated. Necrotic lesions may need debridement after erythema has subsided to define the margins of the central eschar. This usually involves significant debridement 1 or 2 weeks after the bite, with close follow-up for several weeks. In severe cases this can be followed with skin grafting or plastic surgery when the wound is stable. Severe necrotic or infected lesions may lead to hospitalization.

Recently the use of dapsone has gained popularity for prevention of lesion progression in potentially necrotic wounds seen within 48 to 72 hours of a bite.[95,101] Dapsone is a leukocyte inhibitor that in theory can minimize the local inflammatory component of cutaneous loxoscelism, thereby preventing or lessening subsequent skin necrosis. In 1983, King and Rees[146] reported the use of dapsone for envenomation in a human bitten by *L. reclusa*, based on a successful trial of dapsone pretreatment in guinea pigs injected with recluse venom. Since that time, no prospective, controlled human trial has proved dapsone efficacy, but a variety of case reports and series have supported its use in the treatment of potentially necrotic wounds treated in the first days after envenomation.[3,26,129,171,296] Typical dosage recommendations are for 50 to 100 mg orally, twice daily. Risks of dapsone therapy include hypersensitivity,[306] methemoglobinemia, and hemolysis in the presence of glucose-6-phosphate dehydrogenase (G6PD) deficiency.

Patients with systemic symptoms should be considered for admission when they have evidence of coagulopathy, hemolysis and hemoglobinuria, or rapid progression of other systemic signs. Care is mainly supportive, usually involving wound care, fluid management, presumptive treatment for bacterial superinfection, and occasionally, blood transfusion. Rarely, hemodialysis has been required for oliguric renal failure.[109] Discharge is appropriate when renal and hematologic status is stable.

For patients with significant local or systemic signs or symptoms, laboratory evaluation should include peripheral blood cell count, basic coagulation screening, and urinalysis. Liver and renal function tests are indicated in severe poisonings. When use of dapsone is considered, a screening test for G6PD deficiency may be indicated. The frequency of follow-up testing depends on the course and severity of envenomation.

Hospitalized patients may need close follow-up of anemia and renal function over several days.

Corticosteroids have been injected either at the wound site or systemically,* but this remains of questionable benefit.[27,221] Antihistamines may help control itching but do not change the lesion.[157] Some advocate early surgical excision of the wound site,[8,16,87,132] but others have demonstrated that outcomes are better with early medical management in human patients,[69,223] as well as in experimental animals.[221] Hyperbaric oxygen (HBO) treatment has been tried empirically in uncontrolled human trials, with reports of good outcome.[276] Comparison of HBO with no treatment in rabbits showed enhanced recovery at 24 days at the histologic level, but with no apparent clinical difference between the two groups.[259]

Loxosceles-specific antivenom has been tried in both the United States and South America. In the early 1980s, Rees and colleagues[221] reported a protective effect of treatment with antivenom in rabbits before or up to 12 hours after envenomation. Small-vessel occlusion, leukocyte infiltration, and necrosis occurred but were diminished in antivenom recipients. Pretreatment in a separate study abolished symptoms of systemic loxoscelism.[220] In one study, 17 patients were separated randomly into dapsone, antivenom, and combination therapy groups; all patients received erythromycin. Individual results suggested that the antivenom was efficacious when given early, but the overall trial was inconclusive, indicating the need for further study.[224] Gomez and colleagues[107a] have studied the intradermal use of an anti-*Loxosceles* Fab-fragment in a rabbit model, suggesting therapeutic efficacy when the antivenom is injected up to 4 hours following envenomation. Currently, no *Loxosceles* antivenom is commercially available in the United States.

In South America an antivenom to *L. laeta* was developed in 1954 by Vellard using immune serum of the donkey. Furlanetto developed *L. laeta* antivenom using immune serum of horses. Reports of the efficacy of systemically administered *L. laeta* antivenom are mixed.[244] An ELISA assay, developed for the detection of circulating venom antigen, has the potential to develop into a tool for clinicians and epidemiologists.[55]

Genus Sicarius: Six-Eyed Crab Spiders

BIOLOGY. About 25 *Sicarius* species are known. Their range is limited to dry regions of South America and South Africa. Individuals live under stones or are sand dwellers. Some hide under sand and emerge to capture passing insects. Their bodies are flattened, and their legs are laterigrade, meaning the tips point anteriorly as in a crab. Adult body size ranges from 12 to 22 mm.

VENOM. The effects of venom of the South African crab spider *Sicarius testaceus* in a rabbit model demonstrated tissue necrosis and increased vascular permeability in the vicinity of the envenomation, as well as a dramatic decrease in platelet count. It is not clear whether this pattern is the same in humans.[283]

CLINICAL PRESENTATION. *Sicarius* species are occasionally implicated in human bites in South Africa. They tend to bite only when provoked and are rarely implicated in human poisonings, despite fairly high toxicity of the venom in laboratory animals. Envenomation reportedly can cause edema, erythema, and necrosis, occasionally associated with DIC.[196-198]

TREATMENT. Treatment of *Sicarius* envenomation is symptomatic and supportive.

Family Desidae: Long-Jawed Intertidal Spiders

Desidae has about 200 species that are distributed worldwide. Their chelicerae are often extended forward and have humps close to the prosomal attachment. Species range in body length from 4.5 to 12 mm. Most spiders in this family build small, irregular webs under rocks or logs. Some desids are closely associated with marine habitats, living in the intertidal zone. These spiders feed on marine animals and at high tide retreat into empty snail shells and worm tubes and seal off the entrance with silk. Others are found only on the water surface.

Genus Badumna: Black House Spider

BIOLOGY. *Badumna insignis* (*Ixeuticus robustus*), or the black window spider, is a common Australian spider associated with a few human bite reports. This species is a nocturnal forager that builds tangled webs with silk retreats in and around human habitations.[299]

VENOM. Venom gland extract from *B. insignis* is reported to cause increased vascular permeability, as well as dose-dependent decreases in arterial pressure in rats, apparently from the presence of a serotonin-like substance in the venom.[149] Venom gland extract does not cause necrosis in cultured human or mouse skin.[14]

CLINICAL PRESENTATION. In one report, *B. insignis* caused local pain, itching, and swelling followed by regional lymph node tenderness and discoloration of the area around the bite. Over 2 weeks the lesion resolved, with some tissue necrosis and sloughing centrally.[172] In a series of five *B. insignis* bites, local lesions were painful but transient and unaccompanied by necrosis.[300] Systemic symptoms have rarely been reported, including nausea, vomiting, abdominal pain, pruritus, and painful knees.[299]

---

*References 28, 72, 73, 136, 139, 176, 214.

TREATMENT. Treatment of *Badumna* envenomation is symptomatic and supportive.

Family Zodariidae: Hunting Spiders

Zodariids are a diverse group of hunting spiders. The estimated 350 species have a worldwide distribution but are primarily found in the tropics and subtropics. They are medium sized (3 to 15 mm), with the anterior spinnerets usually longer than the posterior structures. They hide under stones or burrow in pebbles or sand. Very few reports of documented human envenomation exist, although *Supunna picta*, a common leaf litter–dwelling spider of Australia, reportedly caused a transient erythematous rash and slight itch in a woman bitten at home. The lesion resolved uneventfully.[38]

Family Gnaphosidae: Ground Spiders and Mouse Spiders

Gnaphosids are common and found worldwide, with the highest densities in temperate areas. They are small to medium sized (2 to 14 mm) and usually dark in color (black, gray, or reddish brown). They have long, slightly flattened abdomens, and two of their spinnerets are conspicuous and cylindrical. Gnaphosids are nocturnal hunters, mostly on the ground, and during the day they retreat under rocks and stones or other tight quarters.

Herpyllus ecclesiasticus, the parson spider, is distributed widely throughout the United States under rocks and rubbish and in houses. One case report of a bite by a *H. ecclesiasticus* described pruritus, arthralgia, malaise, and nausea beginning 1 hour after the bite. There was no necrosis.[173,309] Treatment of bites is symptomatic and supportive.

Family Lamponidae: White-Tailed Spiders

Until recently the genus *Lampona* was placed in the family Gnaphosidae. The group was changed to family status because members do not share many of the characteristics that define Gnaphosidae.[209] Specialists believe that many undescribed genera in Australia belong to this group.

Genus Lampona

BIOLOGY. *Lampona cylindrata* is a hunting spider with a distinctive cylindrical shape and white spot at the tip of the abdomen. They are often found indoors in Australia and New Zealand.[299] Individuals are wandering foragers that enter webs of other spiders and prey on them.

VENOM. The venom of *L. cylindrata* appears to increase vascular permeability in rats, perhaps from the release of endogenous bradykinin and prostaglandins.[149] Venom contains histamine and noradrenaline, both more highly concentrated in the venom of male spiders.[217a]

CLINICAL PRESENTATION. *L. cylindrata* was identified as the spider involved in a series of eight cases in Australia. Symptoms included a mild stinging sensation followed by 1 to 10 days of itching, redness, and swelling. In one case a small blister was present for a few hours; no necrosis was reported. The authors suspected that most *L. cylindrata* bites may be benign, despite earlier reports of ulceration after suspected *L. cylindrata* envenomations.[300] Gray[114] reported a case of more significant illness, with nausea, lethargy, and a small zone of necrosis after a known white-tailed spider bite. Although the vast majority of cases are relatively benign, significant skin necrosis occasionally may result from envenomation.[299]

TREATMENT. Treatment of *Lampona* envenomation is symptomatic and supportive.

Family Heteropodidae: Crab Spiders and Hunting Spiders

Biology. Heteropodids, the "giant crab spiders," are distributed worldwide and are mostly tropical. They are large (10 to 40 mm) and resemble crabs, with the tips of all legs angling forward. They have flattened bodies and are capable of moving sideways. They have eight eyes in two straight rows. They are wandering hunters and typically nocturnal. In many places, they are welcome cohabitants with humans because they eat cockroaches.

Palystes natalius, the lizard-eating spider, is one of the largest true spiders in South Africa. It has a brownish gray body with bright yellow and black striped legs. The female is larger than the male, with body length up to 4 cm.

Venom. Venom from the Australian heteropodid *Isopeda montana* has direct beta-adrenoreceptor action, and *Delena cancerides*, the social huntsman spider, appears to have both alpha- and beta-adrenoreceptor activity, although neither of these has been involved in recognized human envenomation. Both have been shown to increase vascular permeability in rats.[131]

Clinical Presentation. Only localized burning accompanied by slight swelling was noted after a female *P. natalius* bite to the left wrist.[195,200] An *Olios calligaster* bite was followed by mild local symptoms, transient nausea, and faintness. Six bites by *Isopeda* species, predominantly *I. pessleri,* resulted in minimal local symptoms only.[300]

Treatment. Treatment of heteropodid bites is symptomatic and supportive.

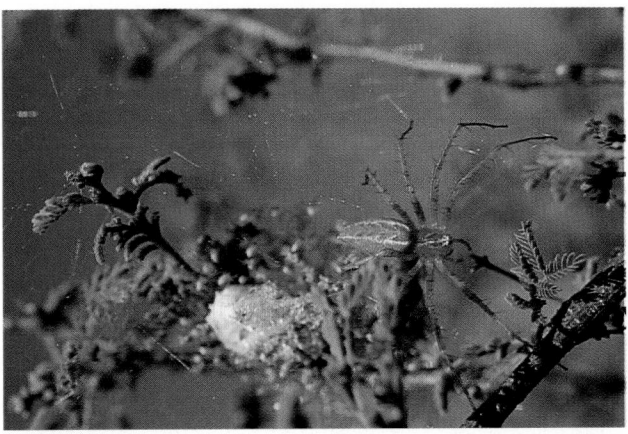

Figure 34-13 Green lynx spider *(Peucetia viridans)*. *(Courtesy Gita Bodner.)*

Family Oxyopidae: Lynx Spiders

Lynx spiders are found worldwide, with the greatest abundance in the tropics. They are small to medium sized (4 to 18 mm) and have a distinctive eye pattern, with six eyes in a hexagon and two smaller eyes below. Their abdomens are pointed posteriorly. They have long leg spines (macrosetae) that help detect motion through vibrations in the air. They are diurnal hunters with good vision and actively search for prey. Most are found on vegetation, and some are arboreal.

Genus Peucetia

BIOLOGY. *Peucetia viridans*, the green lynx spider of the United States and Mexico, is a diurnal hunting spider. *P. viridans* is translucent green, with red eyes and joints[123] (Figure 34-13).

VENOM. Whole venom of *P. viridans* causes total and reversible block of non–*N*-methyl-D-aspartate receptor-mediated transmission in chick central nervous system.[138]

CLINICAL PRESENTATION. The bite results in a burning sensation, pruritus, erythema, and induration.

TREATMENT. Treatment of *Peucetia* bites is symptomatic and supportive.

Family Salticidae: Jumping Spiders

Salticidae is the largest family of spiders, with more than 5000 currently described species and many more yet to be described. They are distributed worldwide, with the highest densities in the tropics. Some have called them the "butterflies of the spider world" because most are brightly colored and some have iridescent scales. Some species mimic ants, beetles, pseu-

doscorpions, and bird droppings. Jumping spiders have excellent eyesight, with large, posteromedian eyes. They visually search for prey, then stalk and ambush with catlike movements. Males are often more brightly colored than females and perform elaborate courtship dances. They are always active during the day and are small, most less than 15 mm.

Bites from spiders of the genus *Phidippus,* such as the jumping spider of the United States, can cause pain, erythema, pruritus, and sometimes minor ulceration. The swelling usually subsides within 2 days.[234] In Australia, local pain has been reported with the bite of spiders from genera *Mopsus, Breda, Opisthoncus* and *Holoplatys*. One patient bitten by a *Holoplatys* reported headache and vomiting.[299]

Family Ctenidae: Wandering Spiders

Ctenidae are mostly found in subtropical and tropical areas. They can be large spiders ranging from 4 to 40 mm. They hunt on the ground or on vegetation. They resemble and are closely related to wolf spiders but are distinguished by their eye arrangement (three rows: two eyes, then four, then two, the last two being the largest). They sometimes travel as stowaways on bananas.

Genus Phoneutria: Banana Spiders (Armed Spiders)

BIOLOGY. The *Phoneutria* spiders of South America are large, nocturnal creatures notorious for their aggressive behavior and painful bite. The best known representative of the genus is *Phoneutria nigriventer*. It is known in Brazil as *aranha armadeira,* meaning "spider that assumes an armed display," because of its characteristic defensive-aggressive display.[242] *P. nigriventer* is the largest, most aggressive true spider found in South America, with an average body length of 35 mm, leg length of 45 to 60 mm, and fangs 4 to 5 mm in length for females. Males are slightly smaller.[241] The body is gray to brown gray with white marks forming a longitudinal band on the dorsal abdomen. A distinguishing characteristic is the red-brown brush of hairs around the chelicerae. *P. nigriventer* is mainly found in southern Brazil, Argentina, and Uruguay. Other species have been found in Bolivia and Colombia. The spiders do not construct a web, since they are nocturnal hunters, often traveling several hundred meters in search of prey. They may enter houses during this time, hiding in clothes in the light of day. According to Bucherl, 600 to 800 spider bites occur each year around the city of São Paulo alone.[41]

VENOM. *Phoneutria* venom is a complex mixture of histamine, serotonin, glutamic acid, aspartic acid, lysine, hyaluronidase, and other polypeptides. Histamine, serotonin, and incompletely characterized kallikrein-kinin activating fractions contribute to local tissue swelling from the increased vascular permeability that may occur with envenomation.[6,177] In addition, the venom contains at least six neurotoxic polypeptides, with molecular weights between 3500 and 8500.[62]

The neurotoxic components include sodium channel poisons that appear to potentiate action potentials along axons, provoking erratic or rapid uncontrolled muscle twitches in invertebrates[83] as well as vertebrates.[7,169] Microscopically, there is acute transient swelling of axons, particularly at the nodes of Ranvier, in a pattern similar to that caused by the venoms of scorpions *Centruroides exilicauda* and *Leiurus quinquestriatus*. The axons recover within a few hours of exposure, but return of nodal width to normal takes several days.[169]

The effects of the venom have been studied in mice, rats, guinea pigs, rabbits, pigeons, and dogs. The venom has little or no effect on frogs and snakes, and it has four times greater toxicity in dogs than in mice. Rats and rabbits are very resistant to the venom's effects, but rabbit vascular smooth muscle contractions appear to be stimulated by a venom protein that acts independently of voltage-dependent sodium and calcium channels.[178] Dogs developed intense pain, manifested by yelping, followed by sneezing, lacrimation, mydriasis, hypersalivation, erection, ejaculation, and death after 200 mg/kg of venom was injected subcutaneously.[242] This is well within the dose that a single spider may inject. Electric stimulation yields an average of 1.6 to 3.2 mg of venom per spider.[41]

CLINICAL PRESENTATION. *P. nigriventer* venom acts on both the peripheral and the central nervous systems.[122] Although the majority of cases are clinically insignificant,[170] humans bitten by *P. nigriventer* may develop severe local pain that radiates up the extremity into the trunk, followed within 10 to 20 minutes by tachycardia, hypertension, hypothermia, profuse diaphoresis, salivation, vertigo, visual disturbances, nausea and vomiting, priapism, and occasionally death in 2 to 6 hours. Respiratory paralysis is generally the cause of death. Severe envenomation is more common among young children. Fatalities may occur in the debilitated or the young, but most people recover in 24 to 48 hours. Workers who handle bananas are frequently bitten because the spider hides in bunches of bananas. Bites have been reported in Switzerland and Argentina in produce workers inadvertently encountering these traveling spiders.[122,241,242]

TREATMENT. In most cases, symptomatic care is all that is necessary. Local pain control may be achieved by infiltration of local anesthetic near the bite site; this reportedly suffices for 95% of cases treated at the Hospital Vital Brasil.[170]

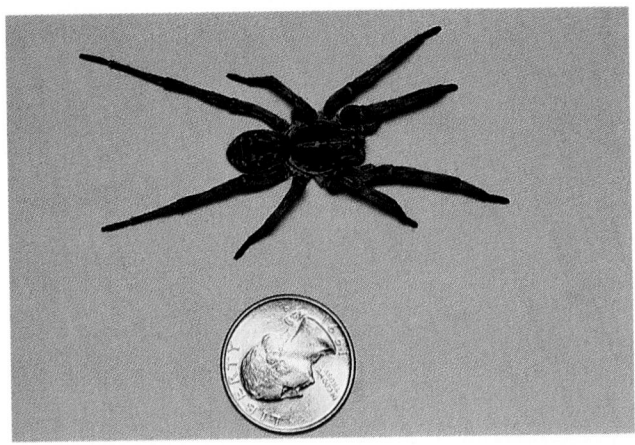

Figure 34-14 Wolf spider (*Lycosa* species). *(Courtesy Arizona Poison & Drug Information Center, 1996.)*

For more severe cases, a polyvalent antivenom (sero antiaracidico polivalente, Instituto Butantan) active against *Phoneutria* species is available in Brazil. Skin testing and antihistamine prophylaxis are recommended before its use. One to five ampules of antivenom are injected intramuscularly and/or intravenously, and clinical response is judged by the relief of pain or resolution of priapism. Opiates may potentiate the venom's effects on respiration and are generally not recommended in cases of systemic envenomation.[122,241,242]

Family Lycosidae: Wolf Spiders

Lycosidae are among the most common spiders. They are diverse, with more than 3000 species distributed worldwide. They are found from beaches to grassy fields and pastures. The Greek name *lycosa* (wolf) comes from the former belief that they hunted in packs.[60,309] They range in size from 3 to 25 mm. Most species wander in active pursuit of prey, generally during the day. A few make deep burrows, and some even cover their burrows with doors. Most live on the ground, but some climb in vegetation. They have good vision, with conspicuously large, posteromedian eyes. Their eyes are arranged in three rows (four eyes, then two, then two). To attract mates, males wave their legs and sometimes stridulate to make sound. The female carries the egg sac attached to her spinnerets. When the young hatch, they climb on their mother's abdomen for transport. They have three claws on their tarsi.

Genus Lycosa: Wolf Spiders

BIOLOGY. *Lycosa* is a large and widespread genus of wolf spiders (Figure 34-14). It includes various middle-sized to large spiders with mildly cytotoxic venom capable of provoking transient inflammation in humans. The most famous wolf spider species is *Lycosa tarentula*, to which "tarantula" was first applied. Its bite was once believed to cause "tarantism," a syndrome of stupor, the desire to dance, and sometimes death, but this historic syndrome is now attributed to *Latrodectus tridecimguttatus* (neither a wolf spider nor a tarantula), and the wolf spider bite is now known to cause little more than stinging pain. The South American *Lycosa raptoria* has been reputed to be more dangerous than other wolf spiders, provoking necrosis at the site of envenomation. It now appears that this was also based on a misunderstanding. Necrotic arachnidism in South America is now attributed mainly to *Loxosceles* species.

VENOM. Lycosid venom is thought to be primarily cytotoxic, without hemolytic or anticoagulant activity.[309] Although scientific reports of necrosis are lacking after envenomation by the Australian wolf spider *L. godeffroyi*, media reports suggest that bites may lead to necrosis. Atkinson and Wright[13] have demonstrated that the raw venom of *L. godeffroyi* causes a strong inflammatory response and cutaneous necrosis when injected into mice. They further hypothesized that this action may result from contamination of the venom with digestive juices, since electrically collected raw venom caused necrosis, whereas venom gland extract did not.[14]

CLINICAL PRESENTATION. A series of 515 cases of confirmed *Lycosa* bites in Brazil showed that most occur between the hours of 6 AM and 6 PM, at a fairly consistent rate year-round. The most common bite sites were feet (40%) and hands (39%). The most common signs and symptoms were all local, with pain in 83%, swelling in 19%, and erythema in 14%. No local necrosis was described.[226]

In the United States five cases of Lycosidae bites have been documented. One resulted in skin necrosis at the bite site, probably from the combined results of envenomation and infection.[47]

TREATMENT. Although South American antivenom active against *Lycosa* venom was available in the past, it was used in only one case of 515 reviewed by Ribeiro and associates.[226] Since 1985 the polyvalent Butantan Institute spider antivenom has not included the antilycosid fraction.[170] Most *Lycosa* cases can be managed with tetanus immunization and ice or oral analgesics; occasionally, local anesthetic block has been used for pain management.[226]

Family Clubionidae: Sac Spiders and Two-Clawed Hunting Spiders

Clubionids are common and distributed worldwide with the highest diversity of species in the neotropics. They are small to medium sized (2 to 15 mm) and are usually light brown to yellowish in color. They hunt nocturnally and make resting tubes in rolled

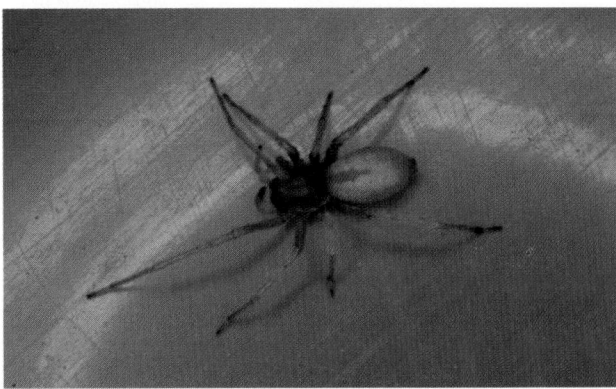

Figure 34-15 *Cheiracanthium inclusum. (Courtesy Sherman Minton, MD.)*

leaves or under rocks or stones, where they retreat during the day.

Genus Cheiracanthium: Running Spiders and Sac Spiders

BIOLOGY. The genus *Cheiracanthium* as a whole has no distinctive marks or patterns.[110,309] Members may be pale yellow, brown, green, or olive. The dorsal abdomen may have a median longitudinal stripe. Body size ranges from 7 to 15 mm, with a total diameter of 3 cm, including long, slender legs.

In the United States, *C. inclusum* is the only indigenous species (Figure 34-15). *C. diversum* is widely found in the Pacific islands. It was transported into Hawaii from Australia approximately 50 years ago. *C. mildei* was introduced from Europe and is now found from New England to Alabama to Utah. It is a common biting spider in Boston; it is most abundant in autumn, when most bites occur.[257]

The South African sac spider *C. lawrencei* is a common nocturnal house spider that forages at night and may become trapped in bedding.[196] During the day these spiders hide in the concavities of leaves, curtains, or windowsills, encased in a silk sac. They are fast moving and aggressive when threatened.[198]

VENOM. Research on *Cheiracanthium* venom is limited. About 75% of guinea pigs bitten by *C. mildei* for the first time developed a wheal within 5 minutes, with 60% developing an eschar within 1 day.[257] Fractionation of dissected venom gland extracts from *C. japonicum* resulted in five fractions with lethal activity in mice. These were considered neurotoxic based on symptoms of dyspnea, flaccid paralysis, and death after intraperitoneal injection.[203]

CLINICAL PRESENTATION. Spiders belonging to the genus *Cheiracanthium* have a documented history of human envenomation since the eighteenth century. Species are known for their tenacious, painful bite. A pruritic, erythematous wheal appears within 30 minutes. Nausea, abdominal cramps, headache, and local necrosis have been reported.

In 1901, Kobert described local swelling, erythema, pain, and fever after the author's third *C. punctorium* envenomation.[32] Maretic[180,181] described local redness, pain, and edema but no necrosis after *C. punctorium* envenomation. In another case, *C. inclusum* caused local pain that radiated from the forearm bite site up the arm, associated with nausea. No other signs developed.[32]

The Australian species *C. mordax* and *C. longimanus* caused local swelling, erythema, and pain associated with malaise, headache, dizziness, and nausea. Symptoms receded within 36 hours after treatment with antihistamines and local anesthetics.[32] Ori[203] found similar signs and symptoms after envenomation by *C. japonicum*.

In South Africa, most *C. lawrencei* bites occur at night during sleep.[196] Paired bite marks 6 mm apart are evident within the first few hours. Local edema and erythema may be slight. By the third day the marks may become necrotic, with more edema, erythema, and pain; headache and fever may accompany this stage. The small ulcer begins to heal 7 to 10 days after the bite.[197]

TREATMENT. The lesion usually heals without problems, provided secondary infections are avoided. Treatment is supportive, consisting of cool compresses, elevation, immobilization, analgesics, and tetanus prophylaxis.

Family Corinnidae: Sac Spiders

Corinnids are ground-dwelling spiders primarily found in tropical regions. They were previously placed in the family Clubionidae and have similar habits. Spiders of the *Trachelas* genus are often encountered in houses in late summer and fall. *T. volutus* and several other *Trachelas* species reportedly cause mild local reactions without necrosis. Bites are painful initially and may swell. No systemic effects have been reported.[205,281] Treatment is symptomatic and supportive.

Family Agelenidae: Hobo, Grass, and Funnel-Web Spiders

The 600 species of Agelenidae are mainly found in temperate regions of the Northern Hemisphere. They are medium-sized spiders, ranging from 8 to 15 mm in body length. Individuals build sheet webs that lead to a long funnel, which the spider uses as a retreat. When prey contacts the web, the spider runs out, bites it, and carries it back into the funnel. The large and conspicuous webs of these spiders often are long lasting, with spiders adding silk to make the sheet larger as the individual grows. Males may be found searching for females.

Genus Tegenaria: Hobo Spiders

BIOLOGY. *Tegenaria agrestis* is commonly called the hobo spider or Northwestern brown spider. It is a 10- to 15-mm, light-brown spider with a yellowish green tint and chevrons on the dorsal abdomen. Individuals typically build funnel webs in disturbed habitats such as abandoned woodlots or along railroad tracks, with a hidden retreat beneath wood, rocks, or debris and silk extending beyond the cover. Spiders mature to adulthood in midsummer and mate and lay eggs in July through September. Adult males live for 1 year, then senesce and die at the end of the mating season. Adult females live for 2 years, so adults are present throughout the year.

T. agrestis spiders are common and widespread natives of Europe and western central Asia.[124] This species was probably introduced in a seaport near Seattle in the early 1900s and was first formally identified in the 1930s.[85,86] It has since expanded its range to British Columbia, Alaska, Oregon, Idaho, Montana, and Utah.[18,227,297] By the 1960s, individuals were often collected in and around human habitations in the Pacific Northwest.

VENOM. The venom of *T. agrestis* has become of interest in the last 15 years because of reports suggesting that their bites result in necrotic lesions. *T. agrestis* venom chemistry is not well characterized, and no necrotoxic component has been identified. Johnson and colleagues[141] identified potent insect-specific neurotoxic peptides and mammalian-specific peptides (5000 and 9000 daltons) that were lethal to mice at high dosage.

Experimental envenomation of rabbits by live male spiders has resulted in extensive cutaneous injury and clear evidence of systemic poisoning. Local erythema appeared and faded within the first day; discolored patches were visible by day 4 and sloughed by day 6. Autopsy revealed petechial hemorrhages on the surfaces of the lungs, liver, and kidneys.[285]

Since the early 1980s medically significant bites in the Pacific Northwest have been attributed to *T. agrestis*.[2,286,288,289] In Europe, no medical problems have been associated with bites from these spiders.[32,42,57] Venom chemistry of American spiders is not different from venoms of English spiders, so the cause of the alleged difference in medical significance is currently under investigation.[35] Bites of males from the Pacific Northwest have more severe necrotic effects on mammalian tissues than bites from females.[285] Necrotic lesions have been attributed to this species all during the year, with a trend toward increased severity in the winter months.[289]

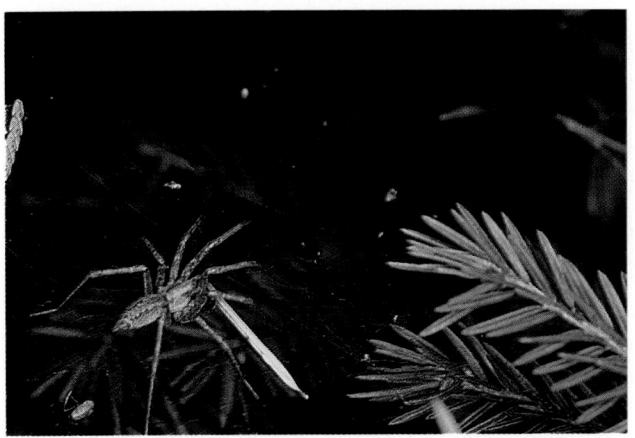

Figure 34-16 *Agelenopsis aperta. (Courtesy Eileen Hebets.)*

CLINICAL PRESENTATION. *T. agrestis* has been implicated in several cases of necrotic arachnidism similar to that seen in *Loxosceles* envenomation. Systemic effects reported include headache, visual disturbances, hallucinations, weakness, and lethargy. Hemorrhagic complications have been reported in experimental animals.

In general, direct observations are scarce of *T. agrestis* biting people, who then develop necrotic lesions.[2] According to Vest,[285,289] who studied 22 cases of "highly probable" *T. agrestis* envenomation, the local lesion followed a pattern reminiscent of loxoscelism. The initial lesion appeared as a small reddened induration, often surrounded by a large zone of erythema. Vesicles occurred within 36 hours, then burst; marked necrosis developed in 50% of cases. The most common symptoms included headache, weakness, and lethargy.[287]

TREATMENT. No studies have investigated treatment for envenomation by *Tegenaria* species. As with mild cases of loxoscelism, patients should be treated supportively, with tetanus prophylaxis, careful wound debridement as needed, and observation.

Genus Agelenopsis: Grass Spiders and Funnel-Web Spiders

BIOLOGY. *Agelenopsis aperta* is common in and restricted to the deserts of the southwestern United States, ranging from California to East Texas (Figure 34-16). They build large, conspicuous sheet webs, with retreats under rocks and logs or in tufts of grass. Adults are 13 mm in body length.

VENOM. The venom of this species is among the best known of all spiders in terms of biochemical composition and neurophysiologic activity of the individual components. Its clinical relevance in humans, however, has only recently been recognized.

Nineteen toxins have been characterized in *A. aperta* venom, with three distinct classes that act synergistically to subdue insect prey rapidly and irreversibly.[202] The μ-agatoxins modify sodium channel kinetics, increasing neurotransmitter release generally; the ω-agatoxins block presynaptic, voltage-sensitive calcium channels; and the α-agatoxins are a family of low-molecular-weight acylpolyamines that block glutamate-sensitive receptor channels in insect muscle. The coexistence of toxins with different mechanisms of neurotoxicity appears to confer a synergistic action to the overall venom effect in insect prey. The ω-agatoxins range in target specificity from invertebrates to mammals.[284]

CLINICAL PRESENTATION. Two cases of envenomation by *A. aperta* have been reported in southern California. A 9-year-old boy developed a tender but nonnecrotic bite site, followed by a 2-day systemic syndrome that included headache, nausea, disorientation, pallor, and unsteady gait. A 54-year-old man developed a painful, indurated lesion that persisted for a week; he had no systemic symptoms.[290]

TREATMENT. Treatment of *Agelenopsis* envenomation is symptomatic and supportive.

Family Theridiidae: Comb-Footed Spiders

The family Theridiidae, sometimes called cobweb or comb-footed spiders, is speciose, diverse, and distributed worldwide. The spiders are small to medium sized (1 to 14 mm, usually less than 8 mm) and often have globose abdomens. They make irregular, tangly webs in which the spider hangs upside down. The silk is very sticky, easily entangling prey. Spiders throw silk over ensnared prey using a tiny comb at the end of the fourth leg. They then envenom prey and suck them dry through a small hole in the exoskeleton, since they have no cheliceral teeth for chewing.

Genus Latrodectus: Widow Spiders

BIOLOGY. Latrodectus (Latin for "robber-biter") species are among the largest theridiids. Females are 12 to 16 mm in body length. Males are much smaller, with longer legs relative to their body size. Individuals build typical theridiid cobwebs with very strong strands of silk. Arthropods are the most common prey, but widows also kill and consume vertebrates (e.g., small lizards and snakes). The folkloric belief that widow females kill and consume their mates does happen, although not as a rule.

The 8- to 10-mm female black widow is shiny black with a characteristic red hourglass marking on the ventral abdomen. Species are distinguished based on hourglass shape and dorsal color patterns. Males are lighter in color, with white and gray markings and a faint

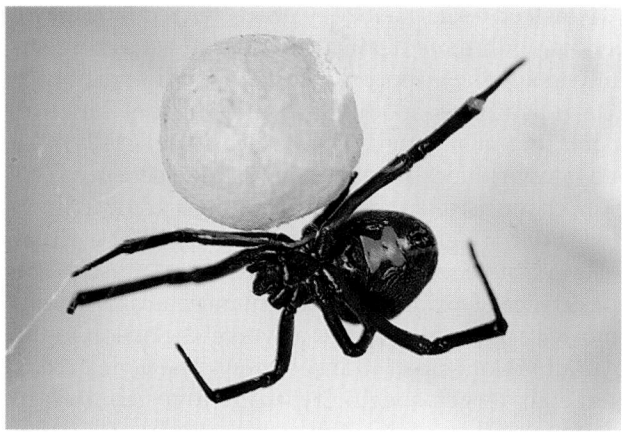

Figure 34-17 Adult female *Latrodectus mactans* with fresh egg case. *(Courtesy Michael Cardwell & Associates, 1999.)*

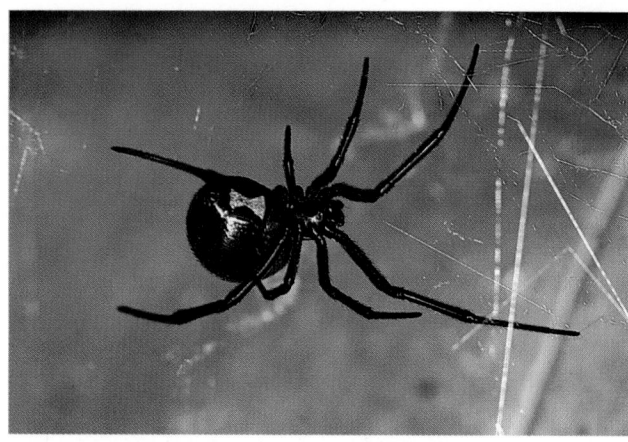

Figure 34-19 Mature female western black widow *(Latrodectus hesperus). (Courtesy Michael Cardwell & Associates, 1993.)*

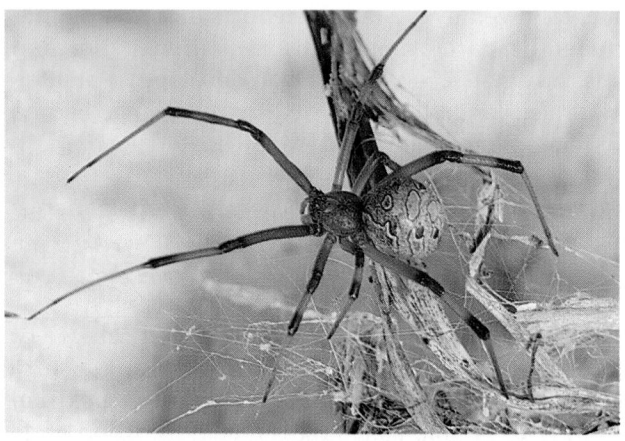

Figure 34-18 Mature female brown widow spider *(Latrodectus geometricus). (Courtesy Michael Cardwell & Associates, 1999.)*

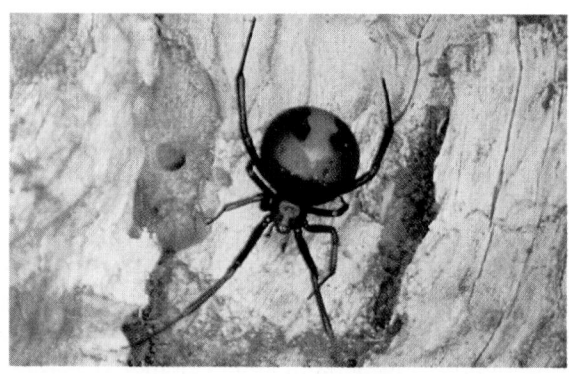

Figure 34-20 Red-backed spider *(Latrodectus mactans hasselti). (Courtesy Sherman Minton, MD.)*

hourglass. This feature becomes more prominent with maturity. The female spins an irregular web in sheltered corners of fields, gardens, and vineyards and under stones, logs, and vegetation. Uncommon in occupied dwellings, the spiders may be plentiful in barns, garages, trash heaps, and outbuildings. A few *Latrodectus* species (e.g., *L. variolus*) are arboreal. The web's tattered "cobweb" appearance may belie an ongoing state of occupation, particularly during the daytime, when the spider is out of sight. The female seldom ventures far from the web, in which she suspends an ovoid or tear-shaped, whitish egg case.

Latrodectus spiders are worldwide in distribution, most plentiful in temperate and subtropical regions, and most abundant during summer.[32] *Latrodectus mactans mactans,* the black widow, is cosmopolitan and occurs in every state except Alaska (Figure 34-17). In North America, species include *L. geometricus* (the brown widow, Figure 34-18), *L. bishopi* (the red-legged widow), *L. variolus,* and *L. hesperus* (Figure 34-19). Species known to envenom humans are endemic to Australia (*L. m. hasselti,* Figure 34-20) and to Europe and South America *(L. tredecimguttatus).* Related species are found in Asia and the Middle East (*L. pallidus*) and in Africa (*L. indistinctus*).

The species *L. tredecimguttatus* is most important in the Mediterranean region, the Middle East, and parts of Russia, where it is sometimes referred to as *L. lugubris.* It may have red or orange spots or may be pure black and is known as *kara kurt* (Russian for black wolf). *L. indistinctus,* the black button spider of South Africa, has a narrow or broken red dorsal band or may be black. The red-backed spider *(L. m. hasselti)* is medically important in Australia, New Zealand, and southern Asia. It has a dorsal red band similar to that of *L. indistinctus,* and the female also has a ventral red hourglass reminiscent of *L. m. mactans. L. geometricus* is brown with black, red, and yellow markings and is common in southern Africa and warmer parts of the Americas.

Widow spiders tend to bite defensively when accidentally crushed. In the Mediterranean basin, southern Russia, and South Africa, bites are associated with grain harvesting and threshing and with grape picking. In the United States, most bites occur in rural and suburban areas of southern and western states, with no special age, gender, or occupational predilection. In regions where outdoor privies are in common use, human envenomations are likely to involve the buttocks or genital area.[34,107,180,307] Outbreaks of latrodectism may occur locally in epidemic fashion, lasting several years, and depend on changes in spider predator and parasite balance and on occupational variations in human-spider contact. Apparent outbreaks may also result from sudden increases in publicity and reporting.[31,143]

VENOM. Unlike many other arthropod venoms, that of the widow spiders appears to lack locally active toxins capable of provoking inflammation. The venom contains several toxic components, including a potent mammalian neurotoxin, α-latrotoxin, which induces neurotransmitter release from nerve terminals.

In 1964, Frontali and Grasso[93] demonstrated three electrophoretically and toxicologically distinct fractions of *Latrodectus* venom. In 1976, Frontali and associates[94] further purified and defined these fractions, encountering one major constituent (the B5 fraction, later renamed α-latrotoxin) with significant toxicity in mice and frogs (other fractions have effects more specific to insect physiology). Alpha-latrotoxin, a protein mix with an average molecular weight of 130,000, caused profound depletion of presynaptic vesicles with swelling of the presynaptic terminal at frog neuromuscular junctions; complete blockade of neuromuscular transmission followed within 1 hour. The toxin binds irreversibly with the lipid bilayer of the cell membrane, producing cation-selective channels and interfering with endocytosis of vesicle membranes.[51,88] The mechanism of action is not fully understood, but multivalent cations, including calcium, may enter the presynaptic nerve terminal through these channels, interfering with calcium-dependent intracellular processes.[113,185] These effects appear to be specific to presynaptic nerves but independent of the transmitter involved. Acetylcholine, noradrenaline, dopamine, glutamate, and enkephalin systems are all susceptible to the toxin.[229]

Grishin[120] has described the venom of *L. tredecimguttatus*, which has a family of seven protein toxins of high molecular weight. These all cause massive neurotransmitter release from presynaptic endings. They differ from each other in the specificity of the target animal. Alpha-latrotoxin acts selectively on vertebrate nerve endings; five latroinsectotoxins act on insects, and one toxin is specific for crustaceans. These large molecules have several functional domains responsible for ionophoric and secretogenic actions. Amino acid sequence analysis of precursor toxins reveals high levels of sequence identity between the different latrotoxins. It also reveals a series of ankyrin-like repeats that might be the structural basis of the interactions between the toxins and the membranes.[120] *L. indistinctus* and *L. geometricus* also contain α-latrotoxin, the former with a greater venom yield per spider.[189]

CLINICAL PRESENTATION. Latrodectism, the syndrome often resulting from *Latrodectus* envenomation, is best known for widespread, sustained muscle spasm rather than for local tissue injury. Although long-term outcomes are usually excellent, victims may have significant hypertension, autonomic and central nervous system dysfunction, and abdominal pain severe enough to be mistaken for acute abdomen.

The initial bite may be sharply painful, but many bites are not recognized initially, so diagnosis is often presumptive and based on local and systemic signs. Local reaction is typically trivial, with only a tiny papule or punctum visible on examination. The surrounding skin may be slightly erythematous and indurated. In most cases, symptoms do not progress beyond this point. In one Australian series, 76% of victims presenting to a hospital for care had local symptoms only.[140]

In some cases, however, neuromuscular symptoms can become dramatic within 30 to 60 minutes as involuntary spasm and rigidity affect the large muscle groups of the abdomen, limbs, and lower back. Rhabdomyolysis has rarely been reported.[97] A predominantly abdominal presentation may closely mimic an acute abdomen. Associated signs include fasciculations, weakness, ptosis, priapism, thready pulse, fever, salivation, diaphoresis, vomiting, and bronchorrhea. Pulmonary edema has been described in Europe[183] and South Africa.[153,291] Respiratory muscle weakness combined with pain may lead to respiratory arrest. Hypertension with or without seizures may complicate management in elderly or previously hypertensive individuals. Isolated (normotensive) seizures do not appear to be a feature of latrodectism. Intractable crying may be the predominant feature in neonates.[45] Pregnancy may be complicated by uterine contractions and premature delivery.[20,133,182,231,237] A characteristic pattern of facial swelling, known as *Latrodectus* facies, may occur hours after the bite and is sometimes mistaken for an allergy to drugs used in treatment. The usual course of an envenomation is to achieve complete recovery after a few days, although pain may last a week or more.

The clinical picture of *Latrodectus* poisoning is similar around the world. In the 1980s in California the most common site of envenomation referred to a toxicology service was the lower extremity (48%), followed by upper extremity (28%), trunk (18%), and head or neck (5%). The most common systemic symptom was abdominal or back pain (58%), followed by extremity pain (38%), hypertension (29%), and diaphoresis (22%).[56] In Australia a 1961 survey showed 37% of victims were bitten on the upper extremities, 27% on the lower extremity, 22% on the buttock or penis, 17% on the trunk, and 4% on the head or neck.[304] A 1978 report showed a decline in incidence of genital and buttock involvement (9.7%), perhaps related to a decrease in the use of outdoor lavatories.[275] Australian envenomations showed a similar pattern of pain and diaphoresis, with more prominent local inflammation and lymphadenopathy and less hypertension than reported in the United States. In South Africa, envenomation by *L. geometricus* results primarily in local pain, whereas *L. indistinctus* provokes a syndrome of generalized pain, diaphoresis, and muscle rigidity similar to that seen in the United States.[188] Victims bitten by *L. tredecimguttatus* may have spasm of facial muscles, swollen eyelids, lacrimation, and photophobia, more often resulting in recognized *Latrodectus* facies. A rash may appear 2 to 11 days after envenomation.[179]

TREATMENT. Although the worst pain usually occurs during the first 8 to 12 hours after a bite, symptoms may remain severe for several days. All symptomatic children, pregnant women, and patients with a history of hypertension should be admitted to the hospital. Discharge is usually possible within 1 to 3 days, when hypertension and muscle spasm have subsided. A patient with a satisfactory response to antivenom may be sent home after several hours' observation.

Care of the local site includes routine cleansing, intermittent application of ice, and tetanus prophylaxis. Severe pain and muscle spasm usually respond to IV narcotics or benzodiazepines. Careful observation of respiratory status is vital when either or both of these are used. Calcium gluconate infusion, advocated in the past, has proved only minimally useful and is no longer recommended. Hypertension may be treated with an infusion of sodium nitroprusside or nifedipine if the patient does not respond to pain control with narcotics or antivenom.

Antivenom active against *Latrodectus* venom is available in the United States from Merck and Co.; in Australia from Commonwealth Serum Laboratories; and in South Africa from the South African Institute of Medical Research. Standards for *Latrodectus* antivenom use vary around the world, as do guidelines for its administration.[56,188,271] In general, antivenom should be used in cases involving respiratory arrest, seizures, uncontrolled hypertension, or pregnancy.[238] In less severe settings, its value must be weighed against the risks of acute hypersensitivity and delayed serum sickness. In Australia, 0.5% to 1% of cases result in anaphylaxis, and some patients develop serum sickness.[275] Death from anaphylaxis has been reported in the United States.[56] The usual therapeutic antivenom dose is one to three vials or ampules. Efficacy of antivenom is reported as satisfactory in 94% of patients in Australia,[298] with anecdotal reports of efficacy even weeks to months after envenomation.[19]

Laboratory evaluation may include complete blood cell count, electrolytes, blood glucose, and urinalysis. Common findings include leukocytosis and albuminuria. In victims with severe muscle spasm, creatine phosphokinase levels may be elevated. Abdominal films and stool examination for occult blood, both of which should be normal after widow spider envenomation, may help with the differential diagnosis of abdominal pain. A pregnancy test should be done if indicated. No specific antigen or antibody detection technique is currently available for clinical diagnosis.

Genus Steatoda: False Black Widow Spiders

BIOLOGY. *Steatoda* species are found worldwide. They are 3 to 8 mm in body length, smaller than *Lactrodectus*, and typically are dark brown, often with white markings on the abdomen. They build tangly cobwebs and sit in crevices under stones, in tree bark, or in cracks of buildings near the web. *Steatoda paykulliana* of Europe, *S. foravae* of southern Africa, and *S. grossa* of the United States bear an external resemblance to members of the *Latrodectus* genus and therefore are referred to as false widow or button spiders.

VENOM. The crude venom of *S. foravae* contains a major polypeptide of the same molecular weight as α-latrotoxin and can elicit a comparable neurotransmitter release syndrome in mice. The median lethal dose, however, is significantly higher, and the relative potency in mice is 10 to 20 times less than for *L. indistinctus*.[190]

CLINICAL PRESENTATION. In humans, *S. nobilis* of southern England has caused brief local pain and slight swelling, followed by local sweating and piloerection, facial flushing, and feverishness.[294] One report of *S. foravae* bite in southern Africa showed minimal local inflammatory response without systemic toxicity.[190] In one Australian report a 2-year-old child bitten by a juvenile *Steatoda* (species unknown) developed lethargy, irritability, diaphoresis, and hypertension 22 hours after the bite. He improved gradually after administration of two ampules of red-backed spider (*Latrodectus*) antivenom.[255]

TREATMENT. In general, care is symptomatic and supportive. Similarities between the neurotoxins in

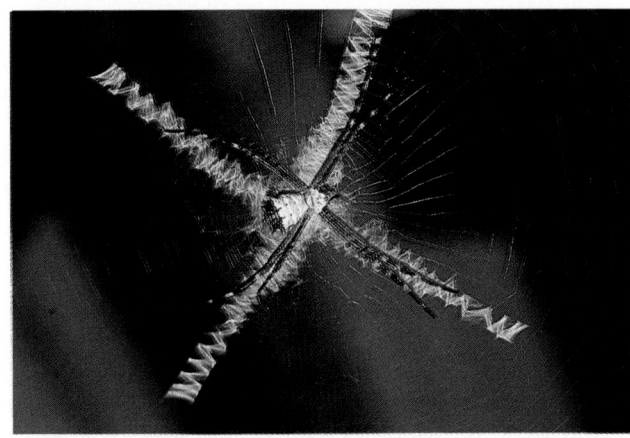

Figure 34-21 Orb weaver *(Argiope species). (Courtesy Eileen Hebets.)*

Steatoda and *Latrodectus* venoms, however, suggest the use of *Latrodectus* antivenom in severely symptomatic cases.

Family Araneidae: Orb-Weaving Spiders

Members of the family Araneidae are familiar to most people because they are common and build conspicuous, mainly circular, two-dimensional orb webs in open places. This is an abundant family, with 4000 species described and distributed worldwide. Species range in adult body size from 2 to 28 mm and often have extreme size dimorphism, with males much smaller than females. They are extremely diverse in size, shape, web design, and prey capture tactics. They can be brightly colored, with typically ovoid abdomens and large chelicerae with several teeth. Although diverse and abundant, they are of minimal clinical concern.

The venoms of many araneid spiders are known to have polyamine neurotoxins that postsynaptically block glutamate receptors in vertebrates.[144] These are currently known from species of *Nephila, Argiope, Araneus,* and *Neoscona.*

Genus Argiope: Argiopes

BIOLOGY. *Argiope aurantia,* known as the golden orb weaver or black and yellow garden spider, is common in California, Oregon, and the eastern United States (Figure 34-21). Other *Argiope* species are found throughout the United States, the Orient, and Australia.[104] It is a large, brightly colored spider with a large, symmetric orb web and a leg spread of up to 7.5 cm.

VENOM. Although *Argiope* venom appears to be cytotoxic in vivo, research indicates the venom has neurotoxic effects in vitro. Venom gland extracts from *Argiope trifasciata* are postsynaptic blockers of neuromuscular transmission at locust glutamate receptors.[282]

CLINICAL PRESENTATION. Bites may cause local pain and erythema. Bites by *Argiope argentata* reportedly cause local pain, erythema, and vesicle formation, which resolve within 24 hours except for the bite marks.[110,309]

TREATMENT. Treatment is symptomatic and supportive.

REFERENCES

1. Adams ME, Olivera BM: Neurotoxins: overview of an emerging research technology, *Trends Neurosci* 17:151, 1994.
2. Akre RD, Myhre: Biology and medical importance of the aggressive house spider, *Tegenaria agrestis,* in the Pacific northwest (Arachnida: Araneae: Agelenidae), *Melanderia* 47:1, 1991.
3. Alario A et al: Cutaneous necrosis following a spider bite: a case report and review, *Pediatrics* 79:618, 1987.
4. Anderson PC: Loxoscelism threatening pregnancy: five cases, *Am J Obstet Gynecol* 165:1454, 1991.
5. Anderson PC: Spider bites in the United States, *Dermatol Clin* 15:307;1997.
6. Antunes E et al: *Phoneutria nigriventer* (armed spider) venom induces increased vascular permeability in rat and rabbit skin in vivo, *Toxicon* 30:1011, 1992.
7. Araújo DAM et al: Effects of a toxic fraction, PhTx$_2$, from the spider *Phoneutria nigriventer* on the sodium current, *Arch Pharmacol* 347:205, 1993.
8. Arnold RE: Brown recluse spider bites: five cases with a review of the literature, *JACEP* 5:262, 1976.
9. Atkins JA, Wingo CW, Sodeman WA: Probable cause of necrotic spider bite in the Midwest, *Science* 126:73, 1957.
10. Atkins JA et al: Necrotic arachnidism, *Am J Trop Med Hyg* 7:165, 1958.
11. Atkinson RK: Comparison of the neurotoxic activitiy of the venom of several species of funnel web spiders *(Atrax),* *AJEBAK* 59:307, 1981.
12. Atkinson RK, Walker P: The effects of season of collection, feeding, maturation and gender on the potency of funnel-web spider *(Atrax infensus)* venom, *Aust J Exp Biol Med Sci* 63:555, 1985.
13. Atkinson RK, Wright LG: A study of the necrotic actions of the venom of the wolf spider, *Lycosa godeffroyi,* on mouse skin, *Comp Biochem Physiol* 95C:319, 1990.
14. Atkinson RK, Wright LG: Studies of the necrotic actions of the venoms of several Australian spiders, *Comp Biochem Physiol* 98C:441, 1991.
15. Atkinson RK, Wright LG: The modes of action of spider toxins on insects and mammals, *Comp Biochem Physiol* 102C:339, 1992.
16. Auer AI, Hershey FB: Surgery for necrotic bites of the brown spider, *Arch Surg* 108:612, 1974.
17. Babcock JL et al: Systemic effect in mice of venom apparatus extract and toxin from the brown recluse spider *(Loxosceles reclusa), Toxicon* 19:463, 1981.
18. Baird CR, Akre RD: Range extension of the aggressive house spider *Tegenaria agrestis* into southern Idaho, Utah, and Montana during 1992 and 1993, *Proc Wash St Ent Soc* 55:996, 1993.
19. Banham NDG, Jelinek GA, Finch PM: Late treatment with antivenom in prolonged red-back spider envenomation, *Med J Aust* 161:379, 1994.
20. Banner W: Bites and stings in the pediatric patient, *Curr Probl Pediatr* 8:69, 1988.
21. Barbaro KC et al: Dermonecrotic and lethal components of *Loxosceles gaucho* spider venom, *Toxicon* 30:331, 1992.
22. Barbaro KC et al: Compared chemical properties of dermonecrotic and lethal toxins from spiders of the genus *Loxosceles* (Araneae), *J Protein Chem* 15:337, 1996.
23. Barrett SM et al: Passive hemagglutination inhibition test for diagnosis of brown recluse spider bite envenomation. Poster presentation at the Society for Academic Emergency Medicine, San Diego, 1989.
24. Reference deleted in proofs.
25. Belyea DA, Tuman DC, Ward TP, Babonis TR. The red eye revisited: ophthalmia nodosa due to tarantula hairs. *South Med J* 91:565, 1998.
26. Benavides MI, Moncada X: Tratamiento de loxocelismo cutaneo con dapsona, *Rev Med Chile* 118:1247, 1990.
27. Berger RS: A critical look at therapy for the brown recluse spider bite, *Arch Dermatol* 107:298, 1973.

28. Berger RS: The unremarkable brown recluse spider bite, *JAMA* 225:109, 1973.

29. Berger RS, Millikan LE, Conway F: An in vitro test for *Loxosceles reclusa* spider bite, *Toxicon* 11:465, 1973.

30. Berman JD, Levi HW: The orb-weaver genus *Neoscona* in North America (Araneae: Araneidae), *Bull Comp Zool* 141:465, 1971.

31. Bettini S, Brignoli PM: Review of the spider families, with notes on the lesser known poisonous forms. In Bettini S, editor: *Arthropod venoms, handbook of experimental pharmacology*, vol 48, Berlin, 1978, Springer-Verlag.

32. Bettini S: Epidemiology of latrodectism, *Toxicon* 2:93, 1964.

33. Bey TA, et al: *Loxosceles arizonica* bite associated with shock, *Ann Emerg Med* 30:701; 1997.

34. Binder LS: Acute arthropod envenomation: incidence, clinical features and management, *Med Toxicol Adverse Drug Exp* 4:163, 1989.

35. Binford GJ: An analysis of geographic and intersexual chemical variation in venoms of the spider *Tegenaria agrestis* (Agelenidae), *Toxicon* (in press).

36. Blaikie AJ, Ellis J, Sanders R, MacEwen CJ: Eye disease associated with handling pet tarantulas: three case reports, *BMJ* 314:1524, 1997.

37. Bond JE, Opell BD: Testing adaptive radiation and key innovation hypotheses in spiders, *Evolution* 52:403, 1998.

38. Boyle CF: Spider bite by a female *Supunna picta*, *Med J Aust* 153:239, 1990.

39. Brady AR: The lynx spiders north of Mexico (Araneae: Oxyopidae), *Bull Mus Comp Zool* 131:432, 1964.

40. Bucherl W: *Loxosceles* e loxoscelismo na America do Sul. V. As especies sul-Americanas do genero *Loxosceles* Heinecken e Lowe 1832, *Mem Inst Butantan* 31:15, 1964.

41. Bucherl W: Biology and venoms of the most important South American spiders of the genera *Phoneutria*, *Loxosceles*, *Lycosa*, and *Latrodectus*, *Am Zool* 9:157, 1969.

42. Bucherl W: Spiders. In Bucherl W, Buckley EE, editors: *Venomous animals and their venoms*, New York, 1971, Academic Press.

43. Butz WC: Envenomation by the brown recluse spider (Aranae, Scytodidae) and related species: a public health problem in the United States, *Clin Toxicol* 4:515, 1971.

44. Butz WC, Stacy LD, Heryford NN: Arachnidism in rabbits: necrotic lesions due to the brown recluse spider, *Arch Pathol* 91:97, 1971.

45. Byrne GC, Pemberton PJ: Red-back spider *(Latrodectus mactans hasselti)* envenomation in a neonate, *Med J Aust* 2:665, 1983.

46. Cabbiness SG et al: Polyamines in some tarantula venoms, *Toxicon* 18:681, 1980.

47. Campbell DS, Rees RS, King LE: Wolf spider bites, *Cutis* 39:113, 1987.

48. Carroll PR, Morgans D: The effect of the venom of the Sydney funnel web spider *(Atrax robustus)* on isolated human intercostal muscles, *Toxicon* 14:487, 1976.

49. Carroll PR, Morgans D: Responses of the rabbit atria to the venom of the Sydney funnel-web spider *(Atrax robustus)*, *Toxicon* 16:489, 1978.

50. Caveness WA: Insect bite, complicated with fever, *Nash J Med Surg* 10:333, 1872.

51. Ceccarelli B et al: Freeze-fracture studies of frog neuromuscular junctions during intense release of neurotransmitter. I. Effects of black widow spider venom and Ca^{2+}-free solutions on the structure of the active zone, *J Cell Biol* 81:163, 1979.

52. Celerier M-L, Paris C, Lange C: Venom of an aggressive African Theraphosidae *(Scodra griseipes)*: milking the venom, a study of its toxicity and its characterization, *Toxicon* 31:577, 1993.

53. Chamberlin RV, Ivie W: North American Agelenidae of the genera *Agelenopsis*, *Calilena*, *Ritalena* and *Tortolena*, *Ann Entomol Soc Amer* 34:585, 1941.

54. Chan TK et al: Adenosine triphosphate in tarantula spider venoms and its synergistic effect with the venom toxin, *Toxicon* 13:61, 1975.

55. Chávez-Olórtegui C et al: ELISA for the detection of venom antigens in experimental and clinical envenoming by *Loxoscele intermedia* spiders, *Toxicon* 36:563, 1998.

56. Clark RF et al: Clinical presentation and treatment of black widow spider envenomation: a review of 163 cases, *Ann Emerg Med* 21:782, 1992.

57. Cloudsley-Thompson JL: Spiders and scorpions (Araneae and Scorpiones). In Lane RT, Crosskey RW, editors: *Medical insects and arachnids*, London, 1993, Chapman and Hall.

58. Clyne D: *A guide to Australian spiders*, Australia, 1969, Nelson.

59. Coddington JA, Levi HW: Systematics and evolution of spiders (Araneae), *Annu Rev Col Syst* 22:565, 1991.

60. Comstock JH: *The spider book*, New York, 1912, Doubleday.

61. Cooke JAL, Miller FJ, Grover RW: Urticaria caused by tarantula hairs, *Am J Trop Med Hyg* 22:130, 1973.

62. Cordeiro MN et al: Purification and amino acid sequences of six TX3 type neurotoxins from the venom of the Brazilian "armed" spider *Phoneutria nigriventer* (Keys), *Toxicon* 31:35, 1993.

63. Cristina de Oliveira K et al: Sex-linked variation of *Loxosceles intermedia* spider venoms, *Toxicon* 37:217, 1999.

64. Croeser PMC: A revision of the African huntsman spider genus *Palystes* L. Koch, 1875 (Araneae: Heteropodidae), *Ann Natal Mus* 37:1, 1996.

65. Davies VT: Araneomorphae (in part), *Zool Cat Aust* 3:49, 1985.

66. De Haro L, Jouglard J: The dangers of pet tarantulas: experience of the Marseilles Poison Centre, *Clin Toxicol* 36:51, 1998.

67. Decae AE: Systematics of the trapdoor spider genus *Cyrtocarenum* Ausserer, 1871 (Araneae; Ctenizidae). *Bull Br Arachnol Soc* 10:161, 1996.

68. Deeleman-Reinhold CL, Deeleman PR: Revision des Dysderinae (Araneae, Dysderidae), les especes Méditerranéennes occidentales exceptees, *Tijdschr Entomol* 131:141, 1988.

69. DeLozier JB et al: Brown recluse spider bites of the upper extremity, *South Med J* 81:181, 1988.

70. Denny WF, Dillaha CJ, Morgan PN: Hemotoxic effect of *Loxosceles reclusa* venom: in vivo and in vitro studies, *J Lab Clin Med* 64:291, 1964.

71. Dieckman J, et al: Efficacy of funnel web spider antivenom in human envenomation by Hadronyche species, *Med J Aust* 151:706, 1989.

72. Dillaha CJ et al: The gangrenous bite of the brown spider in Arkansas, *J Ark Med Soc* 60:91, 1963.

73. Dillaha CJ et al: North American loxoscelism—necrotic bite of the brown recluse spider, *JAMA* 188:153, 1964.

74. Dondale CD, Redner JH: *The insects and arachnids of Canada*. Part 5. The crab spiders of Canada and Alaska, Araneae: Philodromidae and Thomisidae, 1975, Research Branch, Agriculture Canada. 1663:1, 1975.

75. Dondale CD, Redner JH: The insects and arachnids of Canada. Part 9. The sac spiders of Canada and Alaska, Araneae: Clubionidae and Anyphaenidae. Research Branch, *Agriculture Canada*. 1724:1, 1982.

76. Dondale CD, Redner JH: *The insects and arachnids of Canada* Part 17. The wolf spiders, nursery-web spiders, and lynx spiders of Canada and Alaska (Araneae: Lycosidae, Pisauridae, and Oxyopidae), 1990, Canada Department of Agriculture.

77. Duffey PH, Limbacher HP: Brown spider bites in Arizona, *Ariz Med* 28:89, 1971.

78. Duffield PH, Duffield AM, Carroll PR, Morgans D: Analysis of the venom of the Sydney funnel-web spider, *Atrax robustus*, using gas chromatography mass spectrometry, *Biomed Mass Spectrom* 6:105, 1979.

79. Duncan AW, Tibballs J, Sutherland SK: Effects of Sydney funnel-web spider envenomation in monkeys, and their clinical implications, *Med J Aust* 2:429, 1980.

80. Edwards GB, Hill DE: Representatives of the North American salticid fauna. *Peckhamia* 1:110-117, 1978.

81. Eichner ER: Spider bite hemolytic anemia: positive Coombs' test, erythrophagocytosis, and leukoerythroblastic smear, *Am J Clin Pathol* 81:683, 1984.

82. Eickstedt VRD von: Estudo sistemático de *Phoneutria nigriventer* (Keyserling, 1891) e *Phoneutria keyserlingi* (Pickard-Cambridge, 1897) (Araneae; Labidognatha; Ctenidae), *Mem Inst Butantan* 42/43:95, 1981.

83. Entwistle ID et al: Isolation of a pure toxic polypeptide from the venom of the spider *Phoneutria nigriventer* and its neurophysiological activity on an insect femur preparation, *Toxicon* 20:1059, 1982.

84. Escoubas P, Celerier M-L, Nakajima T: High-performance liquid chromatography matrix-assisted laser desorption/ionization time-of-flight mass spectrometry peptide fingerprinting of tarantula venoms in the genus *Brachypelma*: chemotaxonomic and biochemical applications, *Rapid Commun Mass Spectrom* 11:1891, 1997.

85. Exline: *Tegenaria agrestis* (Walckenare), a European agelenid spider introduced into Washington State, *Ann Entomol Soci Am* 44:308, 1951.

86. Exline: New and little known species of *Tegenaria* (Araneidae: Agelenidae), *Psyche* 43:21, 1936.

87. Fardon DW et al: The treatment of brown spider bite, *Plast Reconst Surg* 40:482, 1967.

88. Finkelstein A, Rubin LL, Tzeng MC: Black widow spider venom: effect of purified toxin on lipid bilayer membranes, *Science* 193:1009, 1976.

89. Fisher M, Carr GA: *Atrax robustus* envenomation, *Med J Aust* 2:643, 1972.

90. Fisher M et al: *Atrax robustus* envenomation, *Anaesth Intensive Care* 8:410, 1980.

91. Fisher M et al: Funnel-web spider *(Atrax robustus)* antivenom, *Med J Aust* 2:525, 1981.

92. Fox I: The nearctic spiders of the family Heteropodidae, *J Wash Acad Sci* 27:461, 1937.

93. Frontali N, Grasso A: Separation of three toxicologically different protein components from venom of the spider *Latrodectus tredecimguttatus*, *Arch Biochem Biophys* 106:213, 1964.

94. Frontali N et al: Purification from black widow spider venom of a protein factor causing the depletion of synaptic vesicles at neuromuscular junctions, *J Cell Biol* 68:462, 1976.

95. Futrell JM: Loxoscelism, *Am Med J Sci* 304:261, 1992.

96. Gage PW, Spence I: The origin of the muscle fasciculation caused by funnel-web spider venom, *AJEBAK* 55:453, 1977.

97. Gala S, Katelaris CH: Rhabdomyolysis due to redback spider envenomation, *Med J Aust* 157:66, 1992.

98. Garnet JR, editor: *Venomous Australian animals dangerous to man*, Melbourne, 1968, Commonwealth Serum Laboratory.

99. Gates CA, Rees RS: Serum amyloid P component: its role in platelet activation stimulated by sphingomyelinase D purified from venom of the brown recluse spider *(Loxosceles reclusa)*, *Toxicon* 28:1303, 1990.

100. Gebel HM, Campbell BJ, Barrett JT: Chemotactic activity of venom from the brown recluse spider *(Loxosceles reclusa)*, *Toxicon* 17:55, 1979.

101. Gendron BP: *Loxosceles reclusa* envenomation, *Am J Emerg Med* 8:51, 1990.

102. Geren CR, Odell GV. *The biochemistry of spider venoms*, Marcel Dekker, Inc., New York, 1984, Dekker.

103. Geren CR et al: Isolation and characterization of toxins from brown recluse spider venom *(Loxosceles reclusa)*, *Arch Biochem Biophys* 174:90, 1976.

104. Gertsch WJ: *American spiders*, ed 2, New York, 1979, Van Nostrand Reinhold.

105. Gertsch WJ, Ennik F: The spider genus *Loxosceles* in North America, Central America, and the West Indies (Araneae, Loxoscelidae), *Bull Am Mus Nat Hist* 175:264, 1983.

106. Ginsburg CM, Weinberg AG: Hemolytic anemia and multiorgan failure associated with localized cutaneous lesion, *J Pediatr* 112:496, 1988.

107. Ginsburg HM: Black widow spider bite, *Calif West Med* 46:381, 1937.

107a. Gomez HF et al: Intradermal anti-*Loxosceles* Fab fragments attenuate dermonecrotic arachnidism, *Acad Emerg Med* 6:1195, 1999.

108. Gonçalves de Andrade RM et al: Ontogenetic development of *Loxosceles intermedia* spider venom, *Toxicon* 37:627, 1999.

109. Gonzalez C et al: Insuficiencia renal aguda en loxocelismo cutaneo-visceral: 11 casos, *Rev Med Chile* 114:1155, 1986.

110. Gorham JR, Rheney TB: Envenomation by the spiders *Cheiracanthium inclusum* and *Argiope aurantia*: observations on arachnidism in the United States, *JAMA* 296:158, 1968.

111. Gotten HB, MacGowan JJ: Blackwater fever (hemoglobinuria) caused by spider bite, *JAMA* 114:1547, 1940.

112. Grant SJB, Loxton EH: Effectiveness of a compression bandage and antivenene for Sydney funnel-web spider envenomation, *Med J Aust* 156:510, 1992.

113. Grasso A, Mastrogiacomo A: Alpha-latrotoxin: preparation and effects on calcium fluxes, *FEMS Microbiol Immunol* 105:131, 1992.

114. Gray M: A significant illness that was produced by the white-tailed spider, *Lampona cylindrata*, *Med J Aust* 151:114, 1989.

115. Gray MR: Aspects of the systematics of the Australian funnel-web spiders (Araneae: Hexathelidae: Atracinae) based upon the morphology and electrophoretic data. *In* Austin AD, Heather NW editors: *Australian arachnology*, 1988, Australian Entomological Society.

116. Gray MR: Getting to know funnel-webs, *Aust Nat Hist* 20:256, 1981.

117. Gray MR: The taxonomy of the semi-communal spiders commonly referred to the species *Ixerticus candidus* (L. Koch) with notes on the genera *Phryganoporus*, *Ixeuticus* and *Badumna* (Araneae, Amaurobioidea), *Proc Linn Soc NSW* 106:247, 1983.

118. Gray MR, Sutherland SK: Venoms of the Dipluridae. In Bettini S, editor: *Arthropod venoms, handbook of experimental pharmacology*, vol 48, Berlin, 1978, Springer-Verlag.

119. Gregson RP, Spence I: Isolation and characterization of a protein neurotoxin from the venom glands of the funnel-web spider *(Atrax robustus)*, *Comp Biochem Physiol* 74:125, 1983.

120. Grishin EV: Black widow spider toxins: the present and the future, *Toxicon* 36:1693, 1998.

121. Gross AS et al: Persistent segmental cutaneous anesthesia after a brown recluse bite, *South Med J* 83:1321, 1990.

122. Habermehl GG: *Venomous animals and their toxins*, Berlin, 1981, Springer-Verlag.

123. Hall RE, Madon MB: Envenomation by the green lynx spider, *Peucetia viridans* (Hentz, 1932), in Orange County, California, *Toxicon* 11:197, 1973.

124. Hänngi A, Stöckli E, Nentwig W: Habitats of Central European spiders: characterization of the habitats of the most abundant spider species of Central Europe and associated species, *Misc Faun Helv* 4, 1995.

125. Harriss JB: Toxic constituents of animal venoms and poisons. 2. Spiders, scorpions, marine animals, nonvenomous animals, reactions to antivenoms, *Adverse Drug React Acute Poisoning Rev* 1:143, 1982.

126. Hartman LJ, Sutherland SK: Funnel-web spider *(Atrax robustus)* antivenom in the treatment of human envenomation, *Med J Aust* 141:796, 1984.

127. Heiss JS, Allen RT: The Gnaphosidae of Arkansas, *Bull Ark Agric Exp Stn* 885:1, 1986.

128. Heitz JR, Norment BR: Characteristics of an alkaline phosphatase activity in brown recluse venom, *Toxicon* 12:181, 1974.

129. Herman TE, McAlister WH: Epiglottic enlargement: two unusual causes, *Pediatr Radiol* 21:139, 1991.

130. Hershey FB, Aulenbacher CE: Surgical treatment of brown spider bites, *Ann Surg* 170:300, 1969.

131. Hodgson WC. Pharmacological action of Australian animal venoms, *Clin Exp Pharmacol Phys* 24:10, 1997.

132. Hollabaugh RS, Fernandes ET: Management of the brown recluse spider bite, *J Pediatr Surg* 24:126, 1989.

133. Horen WP: Arachnidism in the United States, *JAMA* 185:839, 1963.

134. Horner NV, Steward KW: Life history of the brown spider, *Loxosceles reclusa*, *Tex J Sci* 19:333, 1967.

135. Hufford DC, Morgan PH: C-reactive protein as a mediator in the lysis of human erythrocytes sensitized by brown recluse spider venom, *Proc Soc Exp Biol Med* 167:493, 1981.

136. Ingber A *et al*: Morbidity of brown recluse spider bites: clinical picture, treatment and prognosis, *Acta Derm Venereol (Stockh)* 71:337, 1991.

137. Ingram WW, Musgrave A: Spider bite (arachnidism): a survey of its occurrence in Australia with case histories, *Med J Aust* 2:10, 1933.

138. Jackson H, Urnes MR, Gray WR, Parks TN: Spider venoms block synaptic transmission mediated by non-*N*-methyl-*D*-aspartate receptors in the avian cochlear nucleus, *Soc Neurosci Abstr* 1:107, 1985.

139. Jansen GT et al: The brown recluse spider bite: controlled evaluation of treatment using the white rabbit as an animal model, *South Med J* 64:1194, 1971.

140. Jelinek GA, Banham NDG, Dunjey SJ. Red-back spider-bites at Fremantle Hospital, 1982-1987, *Med J Aust* 150:693, 1989.

141. Johnson JH et al: Novel insecticidal peptides from *Tegenaria agrestis* spider venom may have a direct effect on the insect central nervous system, *Arch Insect Biochem Physiol* 38:19, 1998.

142. Jong Y-S, Norment BR, Heitz JR: Separation and characterization of venom components in *Loxosceles reclusa*. III. Hydrolytic enzyme activity, *Toxicon* 17:539, 1979.

143. Kaston BJ: Is the black widow spider invading New England? *Science* 119, 1954.

144. Kawai N. Neuroactive toxins of spider venoms, *Toxin Rev* 10:131, 1991.

145. Kemp DR: Inappropriate diagnosis of necrotizing arachnidism: watch out, Miss Muffet, but don't get paranoid, *Med J Aust* 152:669, 1990.

146. King LE, Rees RS: Dapsone treatment of a brown recluse bite, *JAMA* 250:648, 1983.

147. King LE, Rees RS: Brown recluse spider bites: stay cool, *JAMA* 254:2895, 1986.

148. Koh WL: When to worry about spider bites: inaccurate diagnosis can have serious, even fatal, consequences. *Postgrad Med* 103:235, 1998.

149. Korszniak NV, Story DF: Preliminary studies on the inflammatory actions of the venoms of some Australian spiders. *Natural Toxins* 3:21, 1995.

150. Kunkel DB: Arthropod envenomations, *Emerg Med Clin North Am* 2:579, 1984.

151. Kunkel DB: The myth of the brown recluse spider, *Emerg Med* 17:124, 1985.

152. Kurpiewski G et al: Platelet aggregation and sphingomyelinase D activity of purified toxin from the venom of *Loxosceles reclusa*, *Biochem Biophys Acta* 678:467, 1981.

153. LaGrange MAC: Pulmonary oedema from a widow spider bite, *S Afr Med J* 77:110, 1990 (letter).

154. Lasudry JGH, Brightbill FS: Ophthalmia nodosa caused by tarantula hairs, *J Pediatr Ophthalmol Strabismus* 34:197, 1997.

155. Lee CK et al: The purification and characterization of a necrotoxin from tarantula, *Arch Biochem Biophys* 164:341, 1974.

156. Lehtinen PT: Evolution of the Scytodoidae. In *Proceedings of the Ninth International Congress Arachnology,* Panama 1983.

157. Lessenden CM Jr, Zimmer LK: Brown spider bites: a survey of the current problem, *J Kans Med Soc* 61:379, 1960.

158. Levi HW: The spider genus *Latrodectus* (Araneae, Theridiidae), *Trans Am Microscopical Soc,* 78:7, 1959.

159. Levi HW: The spider genera *Steatoda* and *Enoplognatha* in America (Araneae: Theridiidae), *Psyche* 69:11, 1962.

160. Levi HW: American Spiders of the genus *Achaearanea* and the new genus *Echinotheridion* (Araneae: Theridiidae). *Bull Mus Comp Zool* 129:187, 1963.

161. Levi HW: The diadematus group of the orb-weaver genus Araneus north of Mexico (Araneae: Araneidae), *Bull Mus Comp Zool* 141:131, 1971.

162. Levi HW: Small orb-weavers of the genus *Araneus* north of Mexico (Araneae: Araneidae), *Bull Mus Comp Zool* 145:473, 1973.

163. Levi HW: The American orb-weaver genera *Dolichognatha* and *Tetragnatha* north of Mexico (Araneae: Araneidae, Tetragnathinae), *Bull Mus Comp Zool* 149:271, 1981.

164. Levi HW: On the value of genitalic structures and colouration in separating species of widow spiders (*Latrodectus* sp.) (Arachnida: Araneae: Theridiidae), *Vehr Naturwiss Ver Hamburg* 26:195, 1983.

165. Levi HW: The orb-weaver genera *Argiope, Gea,* and *Neogea* from the western Pacific region (Araneae: Araneidae, Argiopinae), *Bull Mus Comp Zool* 150:247, 1983.

166. Levi HW: The neotropical orb-weaver genera *Chrysometa* and *Homalometa* (Araneae: Tetragnathidae), *Bull Mus Comp Zool* 151:91, 1986.

167. Levy G, Amitai P: The cobweb spider genus *Steatoda* (Araneae, Theridiidae) of Israel and Sinai. *Zool Scr* 11:13, 1982.

168. Levy G, Amitai P: Revision of the widow-spider genus *Latrodectus* (Araneae: Theridiidae) in Israel. *Zool J Linnean Soc* 71:39, 1983.

169. Love S, Cruz-Hölfling MA: Acute swelling of nodes of Ranvier caused by venoms which slow inactivation of sodium channels, *Neuropathol (Berl)* 70:1, 1986.

170. Lucas S. Spiders in Brazil, *Toxicon* 26:759, 1988.

171. Mack RB: The bite of the spider woman, *NC Med J* 53:200, 1992.

172. Macmillan DL: Envenomation by a window spider, *Med J Aust* 150:163, 1989.

173. Majeski JA, Durst GG: Bite by the spider *Herpyllus ecclesiasticus* in South Carolina, *Toxicon* 13:377, 1975.

174. Majeski JA, Durst GG: Necrotic arachnidism, *South Med J* 69:887, 1976.

175. Malli H, Vapenik Z, Nentwig W: Ontogenetic changes in the toxicity of the venom of the spider *Cupiennius salei* (Araneae, Ctenidae) *Zool Jb Physiol* 97:113, 1993.

176. Mara JE, Myers BS: Brown spider bites: treatment with hydrocortisone, *Rocky Mt Med J* 74:257, 1977.

177. Maragoni RA et al: Activation by *Phoneutria nigriventer* (armed spider) venom of tissue kallikrein-kininogen-kinin system in rabbit skin in vivo, *Br J Pharmacol* 109:539, 1993.

178. Maragoni S et al: Biochemical characterization of a vascular smooth muscle contracting polypeptide purified from *Phoneutria nigriventer* (armed spider) venom, *Toxicon* 31:377, 1993.

179. Maran B: Pathologic reactions associated with bite of *Latrodectus tredecimguttatus*, *Arch Pathol* 59:727, 1955.

180. Maretic Z: Epidemiology of envenomation, symptomatology, pathology and treatment. In Bettini S: *Arthropod venoms* New York, 1978, Springer-Verlag.

181. Maretic Z: Some clinical and epidemiological problems of venom poisoning today, *Toxicon* 20:345, 1982.

182. Maretic Z: Latrodectism: variations in clinical manifestations provoked by *Latrodectus* species of spiders, *Toxicon* 21(4):457, 1983.

183. Maretic Z, Lebez D: *Araneism with special reference to Europe,* Belgrade, 1979, Nolit.

184. McCrone, JD: Spider venoms: biochemical aspects, *Am Zool* 9:153, 1969.

185. Misler S, Falke L: Dependence on multivalent cations of quantal release of transmitter induced by black widow spider venom, *Am J Physiol* 253:C469, 1987.

186. Morgans D, Carroll PR: A direct acting adrenergic component of the venom of the Sydney funnel-web spider, *Atrax robustus*, *Toxicon* 14:185, 1976.

187. Morgans D, Carroll PR: The responses of the isolated human temporal artery to the venom of the Sydney funnel-web spider (*Atrax robustus*), *Toxicon* 15:277, 1977.

188. Müller GJ: Black and brown spider bites in South Africa, *S Afr Med J* 83:399, 1993.

189. Müller GJ et al: The relative toxicity and polypeptide composition of the venom of two Southern African widow spider species: *Latrodectus indistinctus* and *Latrodectus geometricus*, *S Afr J Sci* 85:44, 1989.

190. Müller GJ et al: Comparison of the toxicity, neurotransmitter releasing potency and polypeptide composition of the venoms from *Steatoda foravae*, *Latrodectus indistinctus* and *L. geometricus* (Araneae: Theridiidae). *Suid-Afrikaanse Tydskrif Wetenskap* 88:113, 1992.

191. Mylecharane EJ et al: Actions of robustoxin, a neurotoxic polypeptide from the venom of the male funnel-web spider (*Atrax robustus*), in anaesthetized monkeys, *Toxicon* 27:481, 1989.

192. Nance WE: Hemolytic anemia of necrotic arachnidism, *Am J Med* 31:801, 1961.

193. Newlands G: A new violin spider from Johannesburg with notes on its medical and epidemiological importance, *Z Angew Zool* 68:357, 1981.

194. Newlands G: A revision of the spider genus *Loxosceles* Heinecken & Lowe, 1835 (Araneae: Scytodidae) in southern Africa with notes on the natural history and morphology, *J Ent Soc S Afr* 38:141, 1975.

195. Newlands G: Review of the medically important spiders in southern Africa, *S Afr Med J* 49:823, 1975.

196. Newlands G, Atkinson P: Behavioural and epidemiological considerations pertaining to necrotic araneism in southern Africa, *S Afr Med J* 77:92, 1990.

197. Newlands G, Atkinson P: A key for the clinical diagnosis of araneism in Africa south of the equator, *S Afr Med J* 77:96, 1990.

198. Newlands G, Atkinson P: Review of southern African spiders of medical importance, with notes on the signs and symptoms of envenomation, *SAMT* 73:235, 1988.

199. Newlands G, Isaacson C, Martindale C: Loxoscelism in the Transvaal, South Africa, *Trans R Soc Trop Med Hyg* 76(5), 1982.

200. Newlands G, Martindale CB: Wandering spider bite—much ado about nothing, *S Afr Med J* 60:142, 1981.

201. Noel V: Funnel-web antivenom, *Med J Aust* 142:328, 1985.

202. Olivera BM, Miljanich GP, Ramachandran J, Adams M: Calcium channel diversity and neurotransmitter release: the w-conotoxins and the w-agatoxins, *Annu Rev Biochem* 63:823, 1994.

203. Ori M: Envenomation of *Cheiracanthium japonicum* and the properties of the spider venom, *Jpn J Med Sci Biol* 31:200, 1978.

204. Ownby CL, Odell GV: Pathogenesis of skeletal muscle necrosis induced by tarantula venom, *Exp Mol Pathol* 38:283, 1983.

205. Pase HA, Jennings DT: Bite by the spider *Trachelas volutus* Gertsch (Araneae, Clubionidae), *Toxicon* 16:96, 1978.

206. Peters W: *Zoology of the arthropods: a colour atlas of arthropods in clinical medicine,* London, 1992, Wolfe.

207. Platnick NI: A revision of the spider genera *Drassodes* and *Tivodrassus* (Araneae: Gnaphosidae), *Am Mus Novit* 2593, 1976.

208. Platnick NI: *Advances in spider taxonomy, 1981-1987,* Manchester, UK, 1987, Manchester University Press.

209. Platnick NI: Spinneret morphology and phylogeny of the ground spiders (Araneae, Gnaphosidae), *Am Mus Novit* 3016, 1990.

210. Platnick NI, Coddington JA, Forster RR, Griswold CE: Spinneret morphology and the phylogeny of haplogyne spiders (Araneae, Araneomorphae), *Am Mus Novit* 3016, 1991.

211. Platnick NI, Ewing C: A revision of the Tracheline spiders (Araneae, Corinnidae) of southern South America, *Am Mus Novit* 3128, 1995.

212. Platnick NI, Sedgwick WC: A revision of the spider genus *Liphistius* (Araneae, Mesothelae), *Am Mus Novit* 2781, 1984.

213. Prentice TR: Theraphosidae of the Mojave Desert west and north of the Colorado River (Araneae, Mygalomorphae, Theraphosidae), *J Arachnol* 25:137, 1997.

214. Presley TE: A case of spider bite, *Memphis Med Monthly* 16:520, 1896.

215. Prince GE: Arachnidism in children, *J Pediatr* 49:101, 1956.

216. Proszynski J: *Catalogue of Salticidae (Araneae): synthesis of quotations on the world literature since 1940, with basic taxonomic data since 1758,* Aaktad Zoologii WSRP, 1990.

217. Rand RP et al: Pyoderma gangrenosum and progressive cutaneous ulceration, *Ann Plast Surg* 20:280, 1988.

217a. Rash LD, King RG, Hodgson WC: Sex differences in the pharmacologic activity of venoms from the white-tailed spider (*Lampona cylindrata*), *Toxicon* 38:1111, 2000.

218. Raven RJ: The spider infraorder Mygalomorphae (Araneae): cladistics and systematics, *Bull Am Mus Nat Hist* 182:1, 1985.

219. Rees RS, Fields JP, King LE Jr: Do brown recluse spider bites induce pyoderma gangrenosum? *South Med J* 78:283, 1985.

220. Rees RS, O'Leary JP, King LE: The pathogenesis of systemic loxoscelism following brown recluse spider bites, *J Surg Res* 35:1, 1983.

221. Rees R et al: Management of the brown recluse spider bite, *Plast Reconstr Surg* 68:768, 1981.

222. Rees RS et al: Interaction of brown recluse spider venom on cell membranes: the inciting mechanism? *J Invest Dermatol* 83:270, 1984.

223. Rees RS et al: Brown recluse spider bites: a comparison of early surgical excision versus dapsone and delayed surgical excision, *Ann Surg* 202:659, 1985.

224. Rees R et al: The diagnosis and treatment of brown recluse spider bites, *Ann Emerg Med* 16:9, 1987.

225. Rees RS et al: Plasma components are required for platelet activation by the toxin of *Loxosceles reclusa*, *Toxicon* 26:1035, 1988.

226. Ribeiro LA et al: Wolf spider bites in São Paulo, Brazil: a clinical and epidemiological study of 515 cases, *Toxicon* 28:715, 1990.

227. Roe AH: The aggressive house spider (hobo spider), *Entomol Extension Utah State University* 86:1, 1993.

228. Rosenstein ED, Kramer N: Lyme disease misdiagnosed as brown recluse spider bite, *Ann Intern Med* 107:782, 1987.

229. Rosenthal L, Meldolesi: Alpha-latrotoxin and related toxins, *Pharmacol Ther* 42:114, 1989.

230. Roth VD: Descriptions of the spider families Desidae and Argyronetidae, *Am Mus Novit*, 2292, 1967.

231. Roth VD: The spider genus *Tegenaria* in the western hemisphere, *Am Mus Novit*, 2323, 1968.

232. Roth VD: American Agelenidae and some misidentified spiders (Clubionidae, Oonopidae and Sparassidae) of E. Simon in the Museum National d'Histoire Naturelle, *Bull Mus Nat Hist Paris* 10:25, 1988.

233. Roth VD, Brame PL: Nearctic genera of the spider family Agelenidae (Arachnida, Araneida), *Am Mus Novit*, 2505, 1972.

234. Russell FE: Bite of the spider *Phidippus formossus*: case history, *Toxicon* 8:193, 1970.

235. Russell FE: Venomous arthropods. In Schachner LA, Hansen R, editors: *Pediatric dermatology*, New York, 1988, Churchill Livingstone.

236. Russell FE, Gertsch WJ: Letter to the editor, *Toxicon* 21:337, 1983.

237. Russell FE, Marcus P, Streng JA: Black widow spider envenomation during pregnancy: report of a case, *Toxicon* 7:188, 1979.

238. Russell FE, Waldron WG, Madon MB: Bites by the brown spiders *Loxosceles unicolor* and *Loxosceles arizonica* in California and Arizona, *Toxicon* 7:109, 1969.

239. Schanbacher FL et al: Composition and properties of tarantula, *Dugesiella hentzi* (Girard) venom, *Toxicon* 11:21, 1973.

240. Schanbacher FL et al: Purification and characterization of tarantula, *Dugesiella hentzi* (Girard) venom hyaluronidase, *Comp Biochem Physiol* 44:389, 1973.

241. Schenberg S, Lima FA: *Phoneutria nigriventer* venom-pharmacology and biochemistry of its components. In Bucherl W, Buckley EE, editors: *Venomous animals and their venoms*, vol 3, New York, 1971, Academic Press.

242. Schenberg S, Pereira Lima FA: Venoms of Ctendiae. In Bettini S, editor: *Arthropod venoms, handbook of experimental pharmacology*, vol 48, Berlin, 1978, Springer-Verlag.

243. Schenone H, Letonja T, Knierim F: Algunos datos sobre el aparato venenoso de *Loxosceles laeta* y toxicidad de su veneno sobre diversas especies animales, *Bol Chile Parasit* 30:37, 1975.

244. Schenone H, Suarez G: Venoms of scytodidae: genus *Loxosceles*. In Bettini S: *Arthropod venoms, handbook of experimental pharmacology*, vol 48, Berlin, 1978, Springer-Verlag.

245. Schenone H et al: Prevalence of *Loxosceles laeta* in houses in central Chile, *Am J Trop Med Hyg* 19:564, 1970.

246. Schick RX: The crab spiders of California (Araneae: Thomisidae), *Bull Am Mus Nat Hist* 129:10180, 1965.

247. Schmaus LF: Case of arachnidism (spider bite), *JAMA* 92:1265, 1929.

248. Schmidt G: *Brachypelma* Simon 1890 or *Euathlus* Ausserer 1875? (Araneida: heraphosidae), *Arachnides* 23:4, 1994 (French).

249. Sheumack DD et al: A comparative study of properties and toxic constituents of funnel-web spider (*Atrax*) venoms, *Comp Biochem Physiol* 78:55, 1984.

250. Sheumack DD et al: Complete amino acid sequence of a new type of lethal neurotoxin from the venom of the funnel-web spider, *Atrax robustus*, *FEBS Lett* 181:154, 1985.

251. Sheumack DD et al: An endogenous antitoxin to the lethal venom of the funnel web spider *Atrax robustus* in rabbit sera, *Comp Biochem Physiol* 99C:157, 1991.

252. Sheumack DD et al: Protection of monkeys against the lethal effects of male funnel-web spider (*Atrax robustus*) venom by immunization with a toxoid, *Toxicon* 29:603, 1991.

253. Shultz S: The chemistry of spider toxins and spider silk, *Angew Chem Int Ed Engl* 36:314, 1997.

254. Smith CW, Micks DW: The role of polymorphonuclear leukocytes in the lesion caused by the venom of the brown spider, *Loxosceles reclusa*, *Lab Invest* 22:90, 1976.

255. South M, Wirth P, Winkel KD: Redback spider antivenom used to treat envenomation by a juvenile *Steatoda* spider, *Med J Aust* 169:642, 1998.

256. Spence I, Adams DJ, Gage PW: Funnel web spider venom produces spontaneous action potentials in nerve, *Life Sci* 20:243, 1977.

257. Spielman A, Levi HW: Probable envenomation by *Cheiracanthium mildei*: a spider found in houses, *Am J Trop Med Hyg* 19:729, 1970.

258. Sterghiu C: Family Clubionidae. In *Fauna Republicii Socialiste România: Arachnida*, Bucharest, 1985, Academia Republicii Socialiste România.

259. Strain GM et al: Hyperbaric oxygen effects on brown recluse spider (*Loxosceles reclusa*) envenomation in rabbits, *Toxicon* 29:989, 1991.

260. Sutherland SK: The Sydney funnel-web spider (*Atrax robustus*). 1. A review of published studies on the crude venom, *Med J Aust* 2:528, 1972.

261. Sutherland SK: The Sydney funnel-web spider (*Atrax robustus*). 2. Fractionation of the female venom into five distinct components, *Med J Aust* 2:643, 1972.

262. Sutherland SK: The Sydney funnel-web spider (*Atrax robustus*). 3. A review of some clinical records of human envenomation, *Med J Aust* 2:643, 1972.

263. Sutherland SK: Venomous Australian creatures: the action of their toxins and the care of the envenomated patient, *Anaesth Intensive Care* 2:316, 1974.

264. Sutherland SK: The management of bites by the Sydney funnel-web spider, *Atrax robustus*, *Med J Aust* 1:148, 1978.

265. Sutherland SK: *Australian animal toxins*, Melbourne, 1980, Oxford University Press.

266. Sutherland SK: Antivenom to the venom of the male Sydney funnel-web spider *Atrax robustus*: preliminary report, *Med J Aust* 2:437, 1980.

267. Sutherland SK: Primum non nocere and the Sydney funnel-web spider, *Med J Aust* 2:105, 1978.

268. Sutherland SK: *Venomous creatures of Australia: a field guide with notes on first aid*, London, 1981, Oxford University Press.

269. Sutherland SK: Sydney funnel web spider bite, *Aust Fam Physician* 14:316, 1985.

270. Sutherland SK: Inappropriate diagnosis of necrotising arachnidism, *Med J Aust* 153:499, 1990 (letter).

271. Sutherland SK: Treatment of arachnid poisoning in Australia, *Aust Fam Phys* 19:47, 1990.

272. Sutherland SK: Antivenom use in Australia. *Med J Aust* 157:734, 1992.

273. Sutherland SK, Duncan AW, Tibballs J: Local inactivation of funnel-web spider (*Atrax robustus*) venom by first-aid measures: potentially lifesaving part of treatment, *Med J Aust* 2:435, 1980.

274. Sutherland SK, Tibballs J, Duncan AW: Funnel-web spider (*Atrax robustus*) antivenom. 1. Preparation and laboratory testing, *Med J Aust* 2:522, 1981.

275. Sutherland SK, Trinca JC: Survey of 2144 cases of red-back spider bites, *Med J Aust* 2:620, 1978.

276. Svendsen FJ: Treatment of clinically diagnosed brown recluse spider bites with hyperbaric oxygen: a clinical observation, *J Ark Med Soc* 83:199, 1986.

277. Taylor EH, Denny WF: Hemolysis, renal failure and death, presumed secondary to the bite of brown recluse spider, *South Med J* 59:1209, 1966.

278. Temoingt M: Certain biomorphological characters of *Latrodectus hasselti* (Thorell, 1870) (Araneae, Theridiidae), *Arachnides* 31:18, 1996 (French).

279. Torda TA, Loong E, Greaves T: Severe lung oedema and fatal consumptive coagulopathy after funnel-web bite, *Med J Aust* 2:147, 1980.

280. Truett AP III, King LE: Sphingomyelinase D: a pathogenic agent produced by bacteria and arthropods, *Adv Lipid Res* 26:275, 1993.

281. Uetz GW: Envenomation by the spider *Trachelas tranquillas* (Hentz), *J Med Entomol* 10:227, 1973.

282. Usherwood PNR, Duce IR, Boden P: Slowly reversible block of glutamate receptor channels by venoms of the spider, *Argiope trifasciata* and *Araneus gemma*, *J Physiol (Paris)* 79:241, 1984.

283. Van Aswegen G et al: Venom of a six-eyed crab spider, *Sicarius testaceus* (Purcell, 1908), causes necrotic and haemorrhagic lesions in the rabbit, *Toxicon* 35:1149, 1997.

284. Venema VJ et al: Antagonism of synaptosomal calcium channels by subtypes of omega-agatoxins, *J Biol Chem* 267:2610, 1992.

285. Vest DK: Emergent patterns in the occurrence and severity of probable hobo spider (*Tegenaria agrestis*) envenomation in humans, *Toxicon* 27:84, 1989.

286. Vest DK: Envenomation by *Tegenaria agrestis* (Walckenaer) spiders in rabbits, *Toxicon* 25:221, 1987.

287. Vest DK: Necrotic arachnidism—Pacific Northwest, 1988-1996, *JAMA* 275:1870, 1996.

288. Vest DK: Necrotic arachnidism in the northwest United States and its probable relationship to *Tegenaria agrestis* (Walckenaer) spiders, *Toxicon* 25:175, 1987.

289. Vest DK: Protracted reactions following probable hobo spider *(Tegenaria agrestis)* envenomation, *Am Arachnol* 48:10, 1993.

290. Vetter RS: Envenomation by a spider, *Agelenopsis aperta* (Family: Agelenidae), previously considered harmless, *Ann Emerg Med* 32:739, 1998.

291. Visser LH, Khusi SN: Pulmonary oedema from a widow spider bite, *S Afr Med J* 75:338, 1989.

292. Vorse H et al: Disseminated intravascular coagulopathy following fatal brown spider bite (necrotic arachnidism), *J Pediatr* 80:1035, 1972.

293. Waldron WG, Madon MB, Suddarth T: Observations on the occurrence and ecology of *Loxosceles laeta* (Araneae: Scytodidae) in Los Angeles County, California, *California Vector Views* 22:29, 1975.

294. Warrell DA et al: Neurotoxic envenoming by an immigrant spider *(Steatoda nobilis)* in southern England, *Toxicon* 29:1263, 1991.

295. Wasserman GS, Anderson PC: Loxoscelism and necrotic arachnidism, *J Toxicol Clin Toxicol* 21:451, 1983.

296. Wesley RE et al: Dapsone in the treatment of presumed brown recluse spider bite of the eyelid, *Ophthalmic Surg* 16:116, 1985.

297. West R, Dondale CD, Ring RA: A revised checklist of the spiders (araneae) of British Columbia. *J Ent Soc Brit Columbia* 81:80, 1984.

298. White J. Envenoming and antivenom use in Australia, *Toxicon* 36:1483, 1998.

299. White J, Cardoso JL, Fan HW. Clinical Toxicology of Spider Bites. In Meier J, White J, editors: *Handbook of clinical toxicology of animal venoms and poisons,* New York, 1995, CRC Press.

300. White J, Hirst D, Hender E: 36 cases of bites by spiders, including the white-tailed spider, *Lampona cylindrata, Med J Aust* 150:401, 1989.

301. Wiener S: The Sydney funnel-web spider *(Atrax robustus).* I. Collection of venom and its toxicity in animals, *Med J Aust* 2:377, 1957.

302. Wiener S: The Sydney funnel-web spider *(Atrax robustus).* II. Venom yield and other characteristics of spider in captivity, *Med J Aust* 2:269, 1959.

303. Wiener S: Observations on the venom of the Sydney funnel-web spider *(Atrax robustus), Med J Aust* 2:293, 1961.

304. Wiener S: Red back spider bite in Australia: an analysis of 167 cases, *Med J Aust* 6:44, 1961.

305. Wiener S: Primum non nocere and the Sydney funnel-web spider, *Med J Aust* 2:104, 1978.

306. Wille RC, Morrow JD: Case report: dapsone hypersensitivity syndrome associated with treatment of the bite of a brown recluse spider, *Am Med J Sci* 296:270, 1988.

307. Wilson H: Acute abdominal symptoms in arachnidism, *Surgery* 13:924, 1943.

308. Wolff RJ: A revision of the jumping spiders of the genus *Thiodina* (Araneae: Salticidae) of North America, Doctoral Dissertation, University of Wisconsin-Milwaukee, 1985.

309. Wong RC, Hughes SE, Voorhees JJ: Spider bites, *Arch Dermatol* 123:98, 1987.

310. Wright RP et al: Hyaluronidase and esterase activities of the venom of the poisonous brown recluse spider, *Arch Biochem Biophys* 149:415, 1973.

311. Wunderlich J: *Spinnenfauna gestern and haute: Fossile Spinnen in Bernstein and ihre heute lebenden Verwandten,* Weisbaden, 1986, Wuelle & Meyer.

312. Yaginuma T: *Spiders of Japan in color,* Osaka, 1986, Hoikusha.

313. Zyuzin AA: Generic and subfamilial criteria in the systematics of the spider family Lycosidae (Aranei), with the description of a new genus and two new subfamilies, *Trudy Zool Inst Leningr* 139:40, 1985.

35 Scorpion Envenomation

Jeffrey R. Suchard and David A. Connor

INTRODUCTION

Scorpion envenomation can result in distinct clinical syndromes. Most scorpion species' stings cause only local pain and inflammation that respond well to minimal supportive therapy and wound care. These scorpions pose no significant management issues and, with few exceptions, are not discussed here in further detail. The truly dangerous scorpions of the world, typified by *Tityus* species in the Caribbean region and in South America, *Androctonus* species and *Buthus occitanus* in North Africa, *Leiurus quinquestriatus* in the Near East, and *Mesobuthus tamulus* in India, cause an "autonomic storm" with prominent cardiopulmonary effects. A third clinical syndrome occurs from stings of *Centruroides* species in the southwestern United States and Mexico and from *Parabuthus* species in southern Africa. These produce prominent neurologic effects associated with excess cholinergic tone. Children are typically more severely affected than adults and often require prompt medical management to avoid morbidity and mortality. The ideal treatment of scorpion envenomation remains controversial, primarily because controlled clinical trials are lacking. Although anecdotal experience and comparisons of historic cohorts demonstrate a benefit from aggressive symptomatic and supportive care, the proper use of antivenins has not been fully resolved.

TAXONOMY AND ANATOMY

Scorpions are grouped in the phylum Arthropoda (Figure 35-1). Scorpions have a crablike or lobsterlike body shape with seven sets of paired appendages (Figure 35-2): the chelicerae, the pedipalps (claws), four sets of legs, and the pectines (a pair of comblike structures on the ventral surface). The segmented tail curves upward dorsally, ending in a terminal bulbous segment called the *telson,* which contains paired venom glands and the stinger (Figure 35-3). The presence and size of a subacular tooth, a small tubercle near the base of the stinger, vary among species and stage of maturity. In the United States, a subacular tooth on a small, slender scorpion usually indicates *Centruroides exilicauda (C. sculpturatus)* (Figure 35-4).[40,129] Many scorpion specimens reveal a broken stinger that does not penetrate human skin well.[132]

Scorpions grasp prey in their pedipalps and then rapidly thrust the tail overhead to sting. The chelicerae tear the food apart. Scorpions feed primarily on ground-dwelling arthropods and small lizards. The scorpion consumes only the juices and liquefied tissues of its prey, discarding the solid parts. Scorpions envenom by stinging; although stings may be reported as bites,[12,45,124] true scorpion bites have not been documented and would be inconsequential if they did occur.

A characteristic physical property of scorpions is that they fluoresce when illuminated by ultraviolet light, as from a "black light" or a medical Wood's lamp (Figure 35-5). This property is used in collecting scorpions for breeding or venom harvesting and in providing pest control. The fluorescent pigment in scorpion cuticle is probably riboflavin.[97]

Scorpions can sting multiple times; however, it appears that the first sting depletes or nearly depletes the telson of venom. A case series of three pairs of scorpion sting victims from India found that consecutive stings by *Mesobuthus tamulus* caused severe cardiovascular manifestations in the first victim but not in the second.[14] We have observed a similar difference in the severity of neurologic manifestations from consecutive *Centruroides exilicauda* stings in Arizona.

GEOGRAPHIC DISTRIBUTION

Scorpions are widely distributed in regions within 50 degrees north and 50 degrees south of the equator[85] and are found on all continents[116] except Antarctica. Scorpions are characteristic of desert areas, semiarid grasslands, and the tropics but may also be found in temperate and subtropical regions.[73,85,97,116] An estimated 5000 deaths from scorpion stings occur annually worldwide,[62] making scorpions second only to snakes as sources of fatal envenomation.[148]

Estimates vary regarding the number of scorpion species. In 1985, Herschkovich et al[84] reported the existence of 500 scorpion species divided into six families. Russell[129] reported 500 to 800 species, others reported 650,[28,36,150] and Neale[116] estimated at least 700 species. More recent reports estimate 1000 species,[62,132] and in 1998, Hutt and Houghton[85] reported 1400 scorpion species divided into nine families (Figure 35-6). The Buthidae is the largest and the most dangerous family and, with few exceptions, contains the only species ca-

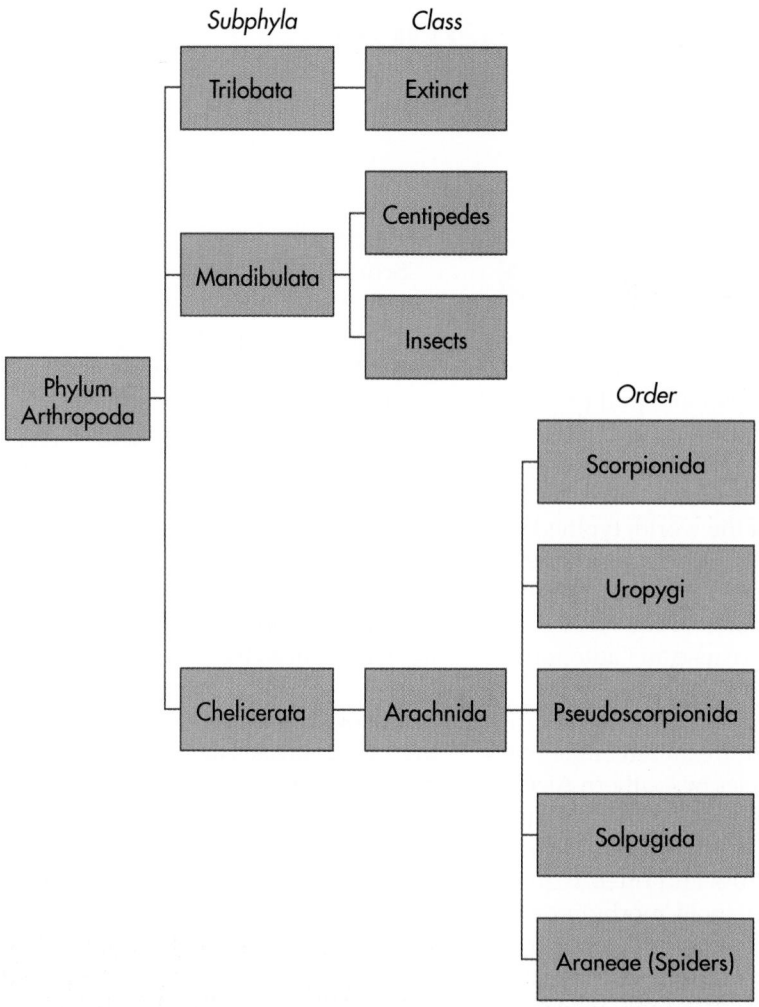

Figure 35-1 Organization of the phylum Arthropoda, showing the relationship of scorpions to spiders and more distantly related insects.

pable of producing clinically significant envenomations, through their neurotoxic venoms.[73,85,132] At least 30 species can inflict potentially fatal stings.[62] All genera commonly recognized as dangerous are buthid scorpions: *Centruroides* and *Tityus* in the Western Hemisphere, and *Androctonus, Buthus, Mesobuthus, Leiurus,* and *Parabuthus* in the Eastern Hemisphere.

VENOM

Scorpion venoms are complex mixtures containing mucopolysaccharides, hyaluronidase, phospholipase, acetylcholinesterase, serotonin, histamine, protease inhibitors, histamine releasers, and neurotoxins.[41,132] Neurotoxins are pharmacologically the most important venom constituents.[132] *Centruroides exilicauda* venom glands contain two types of columnar cells, one secreting mucus and another producing neurotoxins. This species' venom has no enzyme that causes tissue de-

struction, however, so local effects are minimal or absent.[40] The neurotoxins are single-chain, basic polypeptides of 60 to 70 amino acids, reticulated by four disulfide bridges. Each scorpion species' venom contains several neurotoxins, but they all share a similar structure and homologous sequences.[68,132] In neuronal membranes, these toxins cause two effects with regard to fast sodium channels involved in action potential transmission: (1) incomplete inactivation of sodium channels during depolarization, resulting in a widening of the action potential, and (2) a slowly developing, inward sodium current after repolarization, leading to membrane hyperexcitability. The net result is repetitive firing of axons,[40] enhancing release of neurotransmitters (acetylcholine, norepinephrine, dopamine, glutamate, aspartate, γ-aminobutyric acid [GABA]) at synapses and at neuromuscular junctions.[53,59,128,146] This is clinically demonstrated as excessive neuromuscular activity and autonomic dysfunction. Some scorpion

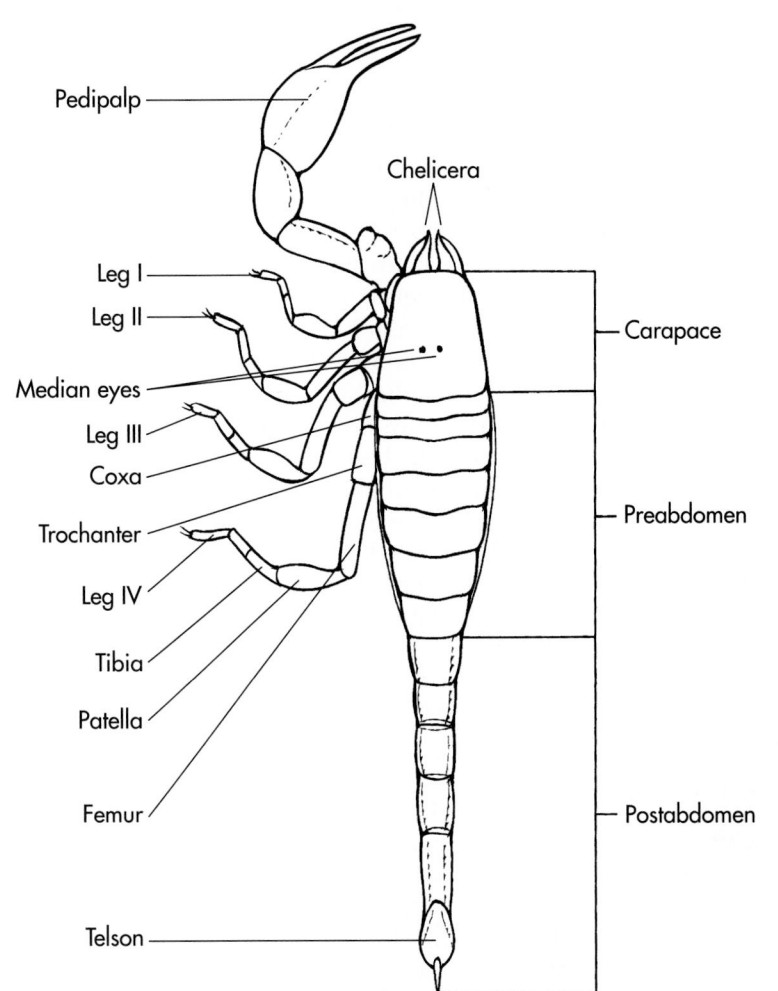

Figure 35-2 Anatomy of a scorpion. *(Redrawn from Keegan HL:* Scorpions of medical importance, *Oxford, Miss, 1980, University Press of Mississippi).*

Pedipalp

Chelicera

Leg I

Leg II

Median eyes

Leg III

Coxa

Trochanter

Leg IV

Tibia

Patella

Femur

Telson

Carapace

Preabdomen

Postabdomen

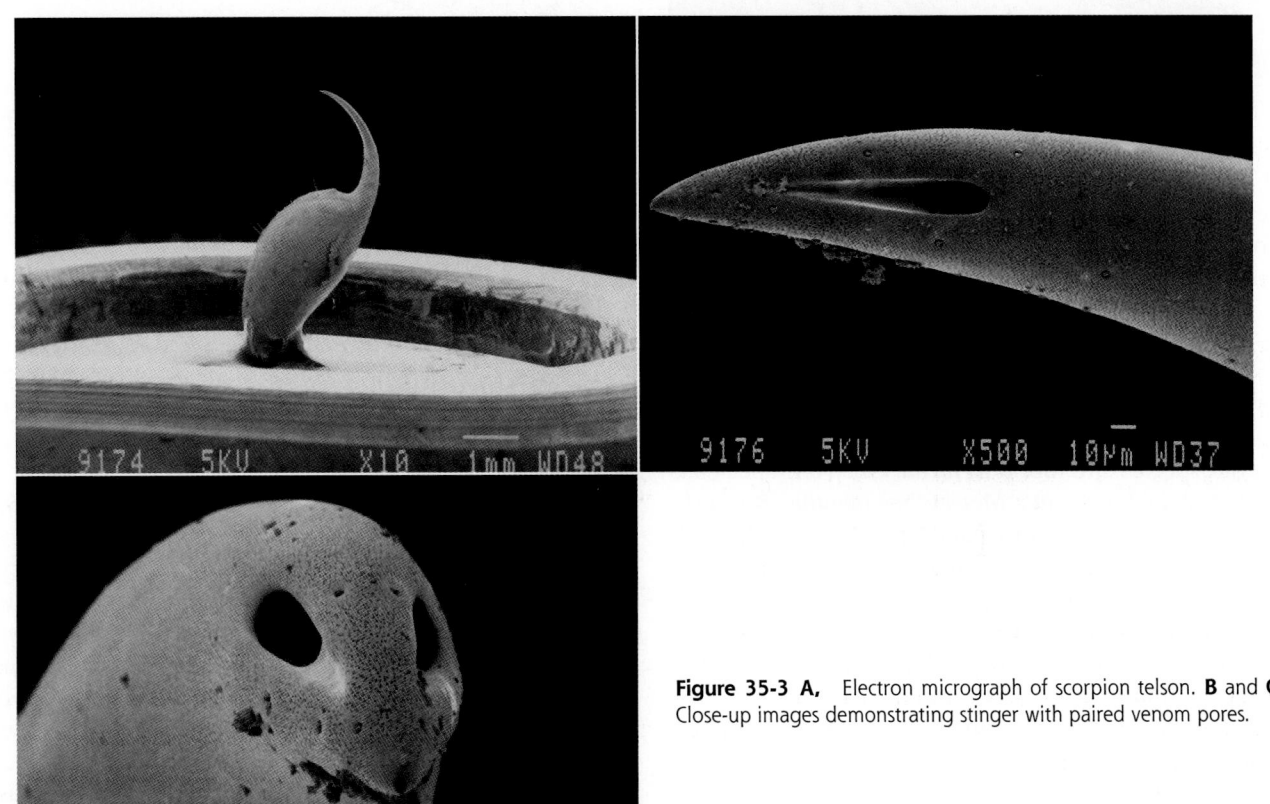

Figure 35-3 A, Electron micrograph of scorpion telson. **B** and **C,** Close-up images demonstrating stinger with paired venom pores.

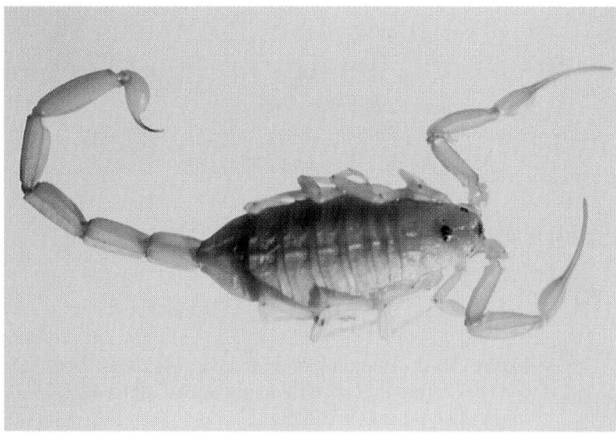

Figure 35-4 *Centruroides exilicauda (C. sculpturatus),* the bark scorpion of Arizona.

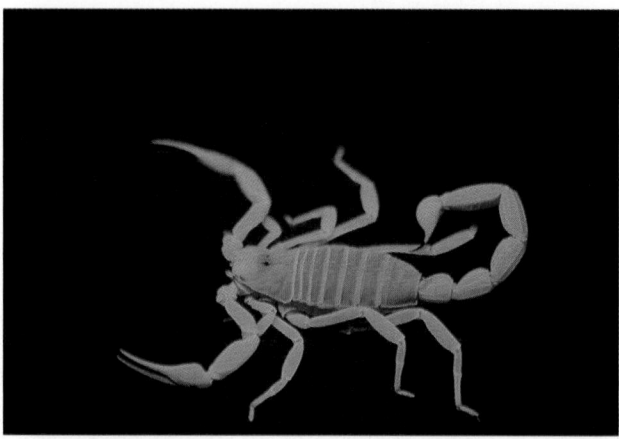

Figure 35-5 Scorpions fluoresce in ultraviolet light.

neurotoxins also have effects on calcium-activated potassium channels,[63,127] chloride channels,[44] and L-type calcium channels.[9]

REGIONAL EPIDEMIOLOGY

India

Between 86 and 99 scorpion species, with at least 45 buthid species, are found in India. Only one species is regarded as dangerous: *Mesobuthus tamulus,* formerly known as *Buthus tamulus,* called the red scorpion.[43,111] *Heterometrus* (formerly *Palamnaeus) gravimanus,* the black scorpion, is a larger species that does not cause systemic toxicity.[15,148] *Heterometrus bengalensis* is common in eastern India.[94] *M. tamulus* is a particular problem in southern coastal India. Stings predominantly occur in April, May, and June at night among young farmers wearing minimal clothing.[15,22] In many cases, stings occur at the tip of an extremity, with the only symptom being pain, which can be controlled with local anesthetic injections.[22,42] Systemic toxicity occurs

from release of catecholamines, with major morbidity and mortality resulting from cardiopulmonary toxicity.* The 30% fatality rates reported in the 1960s and 1970s are now 2% to 3% with treatment using vasodilators and calcium channel blockers.[17,19] An 11.8% mortality rate, however, was found among 152 children admitted in Calcutta from 1985 to 1989, although treatment details were not reported.[28]

Mesobuthus tamulus antivenin is produced for research purposes only. It is not commercially available and would not likely be available in the predominantly rural environment where most stings occur. Bawaskar and Bawaskar[13-22] have developed treatment protocols recognizing the limited medical resources available for the majority of victims, including the potential risks of transporting unstable patients. They recommend oral prazosin and nifedipine for victims with adrenergic toxicity and intravenous (IV) nitroprusside for severe pulmonary edema.

Iran

Radmanesh[121,122] has reported on scorpion envenomation in Khuzestan, a hot and humid province in southwest Iran. A specialized scorpion sting department was established in the provincial capital to study and treat this public health concern, since fatalities occur, especially among children in rural areas during the hot seasons. Over 6 months, 3217 patients were referred to the scorpion sting department, with 200 admitted and the remainder treated as outpatients. Three scorpion species were responsible for almost all cases: *Androctonus crassicauda* (41%) and *Mesobuthus eupeus* (45%) of the Buthidae and *Hemiscorpion lepturus* (13%) of the Scorpionidae.[121] Systemic envenomations by *A. crassicauda,* the Khuzestan black scorpion, resulted in prominent cholinergic signs, such as exocrine gland hypersecretion, urinary frequency and incontinence, and increased gastrointestinal (GI) motility. Adrenergic effects also occurred with lesser frequencies. Neurologic toxicity manifested as delirium, confusion, coma, restlessness, convulsions, localized muscle spasm near the sting site, opisthotonus, and paralysis. A polyvalent scorpion antivenin was ineffective in this series of *A. crassicauda* envenomations.[121]

Hemiscorpion lepturus was responsible for 10% to 15% of stings during the hot season but caused almost all reported stings during winter. This scorpion has a cytotoxic venom, unlike the buthid neurotoxins. Most victims develop a 3- to 4-mm dark-blue macule surrounded by a 1- to 2-cm red halo within the first hour. The skin lesion may enlarge, become indurated and inflamed, and eventually necrose and slough. Serious skin lesions are associated with hemolysis and renal failure. Central nervous system (CNS) and cardiovas-

*References 13, 15, 19, 22, 28, 42.

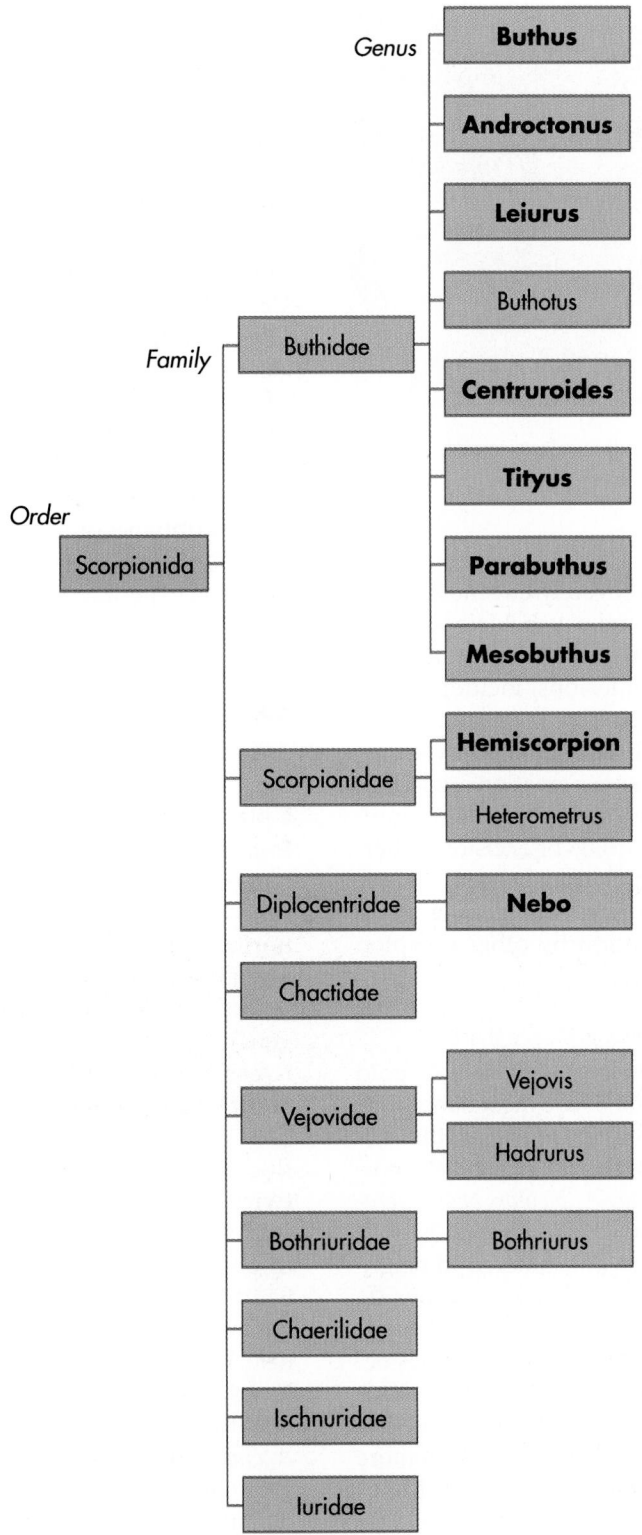

Figure 35-6   Families of the Scorpionida order. Buthidae family contributes the largest number of medically significant genera, as indicated by bold type.

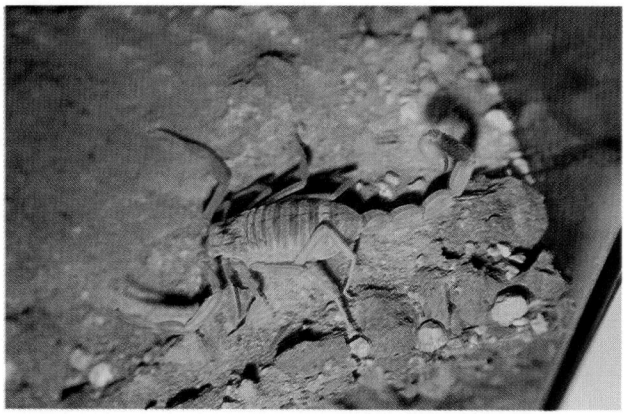

Figure 35-7 *Leiurus quinquestriatus,* the yellow scorpion of North Africa and the Middle East. *(Courtesy R. David Gaban.)*

cular toxicity may be seen in severely envenomed patients. Ankylosis of the joints and psychologic sequelae have also been reported. Local authorities recommend surgical intervention for skin lesions, including prophylactic excision of the sting site, as well as supportive care for hemolysis and renal failure, No antivenin is available.[122] Fatal *H. lepturus* envenomation associated with renal failure has also been reported in Pakistan.[115] No prospective or controlled trials of excisional therapy for *H. lepturus* envenomation have been published, and routine or prophylactic surgical intervention is not recommended for envenomation by other scorpion species.

Israel

Leiurus quinquestriatus, known as the five-keeled gold scorpion or the yellow scorpion, is the most dangerous species found in Israel[31,55,84,127] (Figure 35-7). Other native species include *Buthotus judaicus* (the black scorpion), *Androctonus crassicauda, A. bicolor, Nebo hierochonticus, Scorpio maurus,* and *Orthochirus innesi.*[30,31,55,138] More than 90% of all scorpions encountered in neighboring Jordan are either yellow or black scorpions *(L. quinquestriatus or B. judaicus),*[55] with the yellow being most common.[84] In the Negev desert, 95% of cases occur during the warmer months of April through October. Bedouin children are stung about 6 times more frequently than Jewish children, probably because of more time outdoors and lack of protective footwear. Males are affected 2.3 times more often than females, related to differences in gender roles, such as boys herding sheep or goats.[84] The reported mortality rate in children was 18% among Palestinians living on the West Bank in 1965, 3.7% among children in the Jerusalem area in 1991,[55] and 1.2% among children in the Negev area in 1985.[84]

The *L. quinquestriatus* sting initially produces intense local pain, erythema, and edema, which can be fol-

lowed by an outpouring of catecholamines and acetylcholine from nerve endings. Clinical signs of sympathetic overload predominate, with severe hypertension, tachyarrhythmias, and pulmonary edema.[1,73,74,81,123] Parasympathomimetic action of the venom may also cause bradyarrhythmias or atrioventricular block, usually preceding the sympathetic overload. Cardiomyopathy and myocardial damage with electrocardiographic (ECG) and serum marker (creatine kinase [CK], CK-MB, troponin) changes have been reported.[55,73,131,136] Other common findings from severe stings include agitation, convulsions, encephalopathy, hypersalivation, diaphoresis, priapism, and pancreatitis.[2,133,134] Treatment recommendations differ, but all emphasize aggressive symptomatic and supportive care for severely envenomed patients. However, some authors propose the routine use of antivenin,[55] whereas others argue that serotherapy does not significantly alter outcome based on experimental pharmacokinetic data.[73-75,81] Antivenin also had no demonstrable effect in one clinical series of Israeli patients.[135]

Saudi Arabia

At least 14 species of scorpions are found in Saudi Arabia; the two most common are *Androctonus crassicauda,* a black or dark-brown scorpion, and *Leiurus quinquestriatus,* a yellow scorpion associated with more stings.[7,57,90,99,116] Scorpion envenomation is responsible for 3% to 4% of all pediatric hospital admissions in northwestern Saudi Arabia from May to August, with few admitted in other seasons.[56,57] The incidence of "scorpion sting syndrome" is 1.3 cases per 1000 emergency department patients; 76% of cases occurred between May and October, and 73% of stings occurred at night between 6 PM and 6 AM.[116] Many victims are children playing barefooted outdoors or persons tending flocks of goats or sheep. Males are affected at least twice as often as females.[7,56,116] Mortality rates range from 2% to 5%.[7,56] Antivenin is recommended and routinely administered for scorpion envenomation in Saudi Arabia.[7,56,57,90]

L. quinquestriatus envenomations are reviewed earlier. *A. crassicauda* stings are similar to those of the yellow scorpion, causing hypertension and CNS manifestations, but differ in other ways.[90] The pain from *A. crassicauda* sting has been reported as particularly severe. Generalized erythema was noted in 20% to 25% of children less than 5 years of age; this is not usually seen with other scorpion stings. The cause of this erythema is not clear, especially since elevated catecholamine levels after scorpion envenomation appear to be protective against allergic reaction. Cholinergic effects are seen less often with *A. crassicauda* stings.

Scorpion envenomation became an issue to U.S. soldiers deployed during the Gulf War.[70] *L. quinquestriatus* and *A. crassicauda* were implicated in 57 scor-

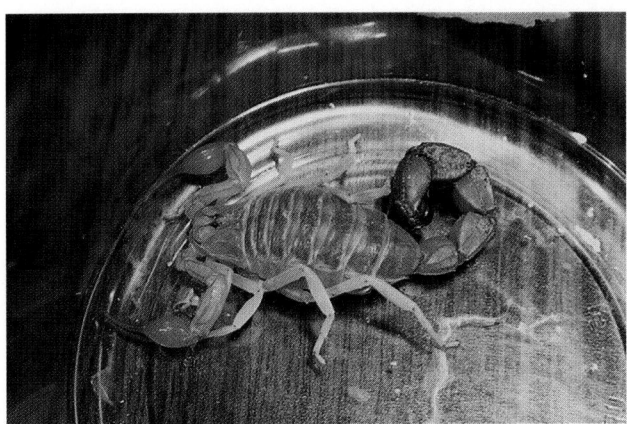

Figure 35-8 *Androctonus australis,* responsible for most severe scorpion envenomations in North Africa. *(Courtesy R. David Gaban.)*

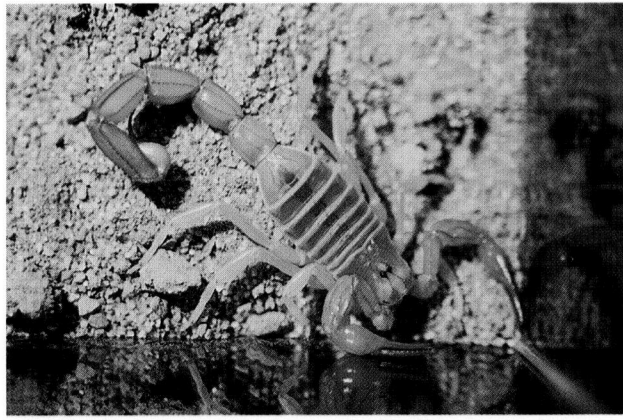

Figure 35-9 *Androctonus amoreuxi,* demonstrating the thin claws and thick tail characteristic of dangerous scorpion species. *(Courtesy R. David Gaban.)*

pion stings over 4 months among 7000 troops of an armored cavalry division stationed in eastern Saudi Arabia. All patients with adequate data for further study recovered fully, usually with only supportive care in the field, probably reflecting that all were healthy adults. No antivenin was available. Typical signs and symptoms included local pain, tachycardia, hypertension, sweating, apprehension, headache, epigastric pain, nausea, restlessness, and local muscle cramping and paresthesias in lower extremity stings. Presumably, victims with only local pain failed to present to battalion aid stations, resulting in an apparently high incidence of systemic effects. Only two persons had significant presentations or subsequent complications. One victim had a clinical picture consistent with anaphylaxis and required intubation for respiratory support. The other victim developed a cutaneous ulcer that healed in 3 weeks with oral antibiotic therapy.[70]

North Africa

Scorpions are a common problem throughout North Africa. Hundreds of scorpion sting deaths occur annually in Algeria.[101] Libya reported 900 stings with seven fatalities per 100,000 population in 1979.[85] Most of the published North African scorpion research is from Tunisia, where 10 scorpion species are found, five of which are responsible for almost all stings.[69] Most stings are caused by *Androctonus australis garzonii, Androctonus aeneas aeneas,* and *Buthus occitanus tunetanus.* *A. australis,* known as the yellow scorpion, accounts for most severe envenomations (Figure 35-8). *A. aeneas* is a dangerous black scorpion found only in the southern part of Tunisia. The next most common species are *Scorpio maurus tunetanus* and *Euscorpius carpathicus sicanus,* another black scorpion found only in the north; both are relatively harmless and have thin tails and thick claws. The more dangerous Tunisian scorpi-

ons have long, thin claws and a thick tail[69,96] (Figure 35-9). Stings occur most often outdoors (92%) on the victim's extremities (95%) during the summer months.[96] Eighty percent of all reported stings occur from July to September, with half of these in August.[69]

Between 30,000 and 45,000 scorpion stings are reported annually, correlating to an incidence of 4.5 to 20 stings per thousand inhabitants, depending on the location. About 2.5% of stings (900 to 1100 per year) result in systemic manifestations requiring hospital admission. The mortality rate ranges from 0.25% to 0.4%, which is about 10% of victims with systemic envenomations, or 35 to 105 deaths per year.[3,69,96-98] Two thirds of reported stings affect adults and older adolescents, but nearly all fatalities occur in younger children; the mortality rate for children is about 1%.[69,96]

The effects of Tunisian scorpion stings have been classified into four stages[69] and three grades[98] based on clinical severity. The first three stages or grades are essentially identical, and the fourth stage is the most severe form of grade III envenomation. The stages or grades do not necessarily reflect the natural time course of envenomation and are designated to aid risk evaluation and to direct treatment.

Grade I envenomations have only local symptoms at the sting site. The most common complaint is intense burning pain. Paresthesias occur in 92% of victims. Mild systemic symptoms, such as irritability and restlessness, occur in 8% to 12% of victims. Local tissue alterations are rare. Grade I cases constitute 90% to 95% of all scorpion stings, and symptoms typically resolve in 3 to 8 hours.

Grade II envenomations have local symptoms as in grade I, sometimes with local edema, associated with moderate systemic symptoms. Irritability (52%), restlessness (48%), tachycardia (34%), and moderate hyperthermia (27%) are characteristic features. Signs of excess cholinergic tone (e.g., diaphoresis, hypersaliva-

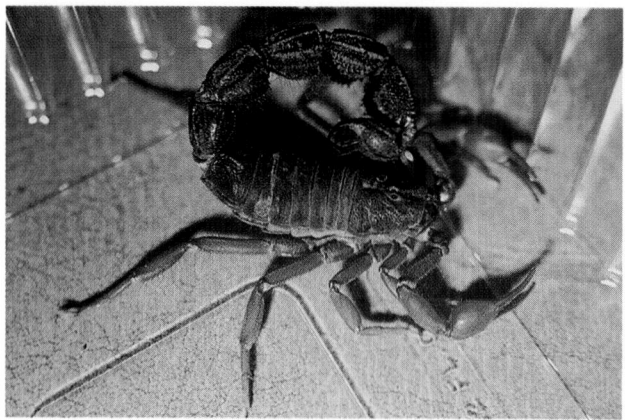

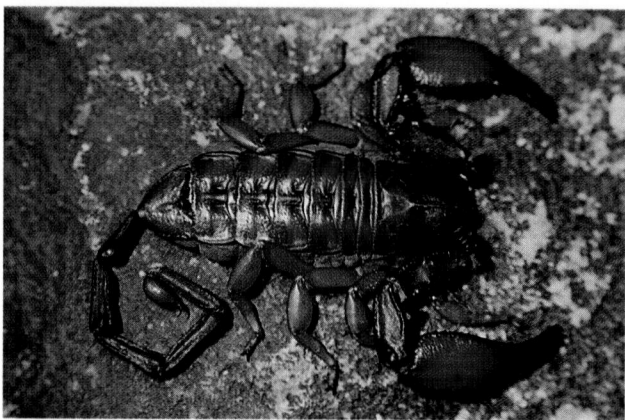

Figure 35-10 *Parabuthus transvaalicus,* a dangerous scorpion of southern Africa. *(Courtesy R. David Gaban.)*

Figure 35-11 *Hadogenes troglodytes,* an impressive-looking yet relatively harmless scorpion of southern Africa, has large claws and a thin tail. *(Courtesy R. David Gaban.)*

tion, rhinorrhea, vomiting, diarrhea) are often found, as well as occasional dyspnea, gastric distention, and priapism. From 5% to 10% of stings present with grade II symptoms. The prognosis is favorable with return to baseline in 3 days, although 1% to 3% of patients initially classified as grade II progress to grade III.

Grade III envenomations involve serious systemic complications, including cardiocirculatory shock, respiratory failure, pulmonary edema, hyperthermia, seizures, priapism, and coma. If the grading system is divided into four stages, the stage III victims have depressed level of consciousness, arterial hypertension, and tachycardia, usually occurring within 2 to 4 hours after the sting. ECG changes consistent with ischemia, respiratory failure, hyperglycemia, and an elevated white blood cell count are also seen. Stage IV signifies worsening neurotoxicity, heralded by profuse vomiting and associated with cardiovascular collapse, pulmonary edema, hyperthermia, seizures, and coma. Even patients with stage III envenomations have a favorable prognosis with appropriate care. Patients who recover will regain consciousness in several hours, and the ECG abnormalities will resolve in 2 to 4 days. All fatalities progress through stage IV, although recovery from stage IV can occur.[69]

South Africa

The majority of scorpion stings in South Africa, Zimbabwe, and neighboring countries do not cause systemic effects, although fatalities occasionally occur.[25,26,100] Scorpions found in southern Africa include the frequently dangerous Buthidae with thin pincers and thick tails (Figure 35-10) and the relatively harmless Scorpionidae, Bothriuridae, and Ischnuridae with thick pincers and thin tails[26,100,110] (Figure 35-11). *Parabuthus* species cause neuromuscular toxicity without the autonomic storm seen from the dangerous scorpions of northern Africa, the Mideast, and India.[25,26,110]

At least 20 *Parabuthus* species are distributed throughout South Africa, Namibia, Botswana, Zimbabwe, and southern Mozambique.[110] Three other species can produce systemic effects but are not considered potentially fatal: *Parabuthus mossambicensis, Uroleptes planimanus,* and *Opistophthalmus glabrifrons.*[24,25] Certain *Parabuthus* scorpions with large venom vesicles are capable of spraying venom when alarmed.[110]

Stings typically occur in the early evening during the warmer months of October through April, with peak incidence in January and February.[25,26,110] Four children died in a series of 42 serious scorpion envenomations from South Africa.[110] No fatalities were noted among 244 patients (17 with severe systemic symptoms) in Zimbabwe.[26] In another study, however, five deaths occurred among 455 patients, with the fatalities in children less than 10 years old or adults over 55.[25] The overall case fatality rate from *Parabuthus* species ranges from 0.3% to 3%.[25,26]

Serious scorpion envenomation in southern Africa closely resembles that seen in the American Southwest from *Centruroides exilicauda.*[25,26,110] Immediate pain, local paresthesias, and hyperesthesia typically occur. Mild cases (60% of stings) are associated with only localized symptoms, moderate cases with three or fewer systemic features, and severe cases (10% to 30%) with more than three systemic signs or symptoms. The pain and paresthesias may generalize, sometimes within minutes in children and usually within 4 to 12 hours in adults. Of victims with severe envenomations, 75% have difficulty swallowing, myoclonic jerks, tongue fasciculations, hypersalivation, and profuse sweating; 50% have bilateral ptosis, slight local swelling, and difficulty urinating (33% with a palpably distended bladder). Children are typically affected more severely and are more likely to exhibit uncontrollable jerking, writhing, and thrashing movements characteristic of neurotoxic scorpion envenomation. Respiratory failure is the most common proximate cause of death.

In untreated cases, urinary retention, ptosis, and sweating resolve in 2 days and dysphagia and hypersalivation in 4 days. After 1 week, 10% of victims still have muscle tremors and tongue fasciculations, and more than half still have localized pain at the sting site. Traditional herbal remedies are frequently used but have no apparent beneficial effect. In fact, rubbing the sting site, as commonly practiced with such herbal remedies, more than doubles the chance of developing a severe envenomation. Antivenin against *Parabuthus transvaalicus* is available commercially and recommended for victims with serious envenomations (see Figure 35-10).

Brazil

About 10,000 cases of scorpion envenomation are reported annually in Brazil,[109] with 80% occurring in southeastern regions.[117] Half the reported stings occur in the state of Minas Gerais,[109] although scorpions are also problematic in São Paulo and Bahia.[33] Most stings occur from December through February.[35,61] *Tityus serrulatus* is the most prevalent species in Brazil and accounts for most fatal stings.[39,109] *Tityus bahiensis* is the next most common species,[117] although severe envenomations are much more likely from *T. serrulatus.*[33] Equine antivenin for either *T. serrulatus* or both *T. serrulatus* and *T. bahiensis* is able to neutralize venom from all Brazilian scorpions studied.[117] Children are much more likely to have severe reactions.[61] In Minas Gerais, children less than 14 years of age accounted for 27% of scorpion envenomation admissions but for all cases of significant morbidity and mortality; 16% were treated in an intensive care unit (ICU) setting. Mortality was 3.5% in 1938[35] but with current treatment now ranges from 1% to 1.1% in children and is 0.28% overall.[61,109,126] Antivenin from a few manufacturers is available in Brazil and routinely used in severe envenomations.[33,35,61,126]

Trinidad

Tityus trinitatis accounts for almost 90% of the scorpion population on Trinidad. Fatalities are rare but occur more often in children. Stings are more frequent in summer months.[11] Systemic effects of serious *T. trinitatis* envenomations include tachypnea, restlessness, vomiting, hypersalivation, cerebral edema, pulmonary edema, hypovolemic shock, seizures, and myocarditis.[41] The most striking clinical observation is the high incidence (up to 80%) of acute pancreatitis; scorpion stings are the most common cause of acute pancreatitis in Trinidad.[11,65]

Venezuela

Tityus discrepans is the most common scorpion in Venezuela.[50,54] The states of Monagas and Sucre in east-

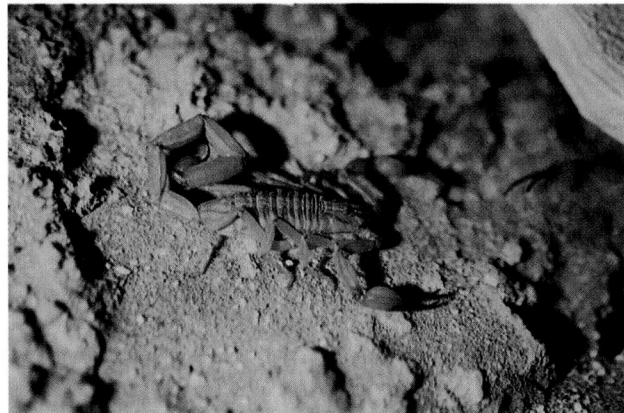

Figure 35-12 *Centruroides limpidus,* one of several closely related, dangerous Mexican scorpions. *(Courtesy R. David Gaban.)*

ern Venezuela are particularly endemic for scorpions.[50] A case series of 64 patients from the state of Merida in southwestern Venezuela classified scorpion envenomations by clinical criteria.[107] Whereas 27 patients had only local manifestations, the remainder had systemic effects of envenomation: 21 primarily had GI complaints, nine had neurologic symptoms and hypertension, and seven had severe envenomations with cardiac arrhythmias, pulmonary edema (five patients), and fatal cardiogenic shock (two patients). These last seven patients all received antivenin produced in Caracas. The survivors received antivenin within 5 hours, whereas the children who died received antivenin later than 5 hours after envenomation.[107]

Mexico

An estimated 200,000 scorpion stings occur annually in Mexico.[46] Of at least 134 native species, eight members of the *Centruroides* family are recognized as significantly dangerous (Figure 35-12): *C. elegans, C. infamatus infamatus, C. limpidus limpidus, C. limpidus tecomanus, C. noxius, C. pallidiceps, C. sculpturatus (exilicauda),* and *C. suffusus suffusus.*[46] *C. noxius* has the most potent venom,[34,102] but *C. suffusus* is usually cited as the most dangerous Mexican scorpion.[132,150] *Centruroides* scorpions are relatively small and described as yellow, tan, or brown in color. Clavigero recognized as early as 1780 that "the venom of the small and yellow scorpions is more active than that of the big grey ones."[108] The 11 Mexican states on the Pacific coast are particularly endemic places for scorpions, with Colima, Nayarit, Guerrero, and Morelos having the highest mortality rates from scorpion envenomation.[46,108] In the 1940s, 7.4 to 8.9 scorpion sting deaths occurred per 100,000 population. This rate decreased to 3.4 to 4.7 per 100,000 in 1957-1958. The great majority occurred in very young children. Approximately 10 times more deaths occurred from scorpions as from all reported snakebites. Most fatal cases occur in the summer months from April through July.[108] In the 1980s, 272 to 401 scorpion fatalities per year occurred nationwide, with respiratory failure as the proximate cause of death; this figure probably underestimates the true total by a factor of 2 to 3.[46]

The following list of signs and symptoms has been reported with Mexican scorpion stings, although not all effects are necessarily seen in the same victim, and no apparent sequence of effects has been observed: hyperexcitability, restlessness, hyperthermia, tachypnea, dyspnea, tachycardia or bradycardia, diaphoresis, nausea, vomiting, gastric distention, diarrhea, lacrimation, nystagmus, mydriasis, photophobia, excessive salivation, nasal secretion, dysphagia with foreign body sensation, dysphonia, cough, bronchorrhea, pulmonary edema, arterial hypertension or hypotension, heart failure, shock, convulsions, ataxia, fasciculations, and coma.[46] Many of these effects appear to be caused by autonomic nervous system dysfunction, which can be seen from either neurotoxic or cardiotoxic scorpions. Unpublished verbal reports by physicians who have treated victims of scorpion envenomation in Mexico suggest that the clinical presentation is virtually identical to that caused by *Centruroides exilicauda* in the United States. The higher mortality from Mexican vs. American scorpion stings most likely results from differences in the human and scorpion population densities, in the ease of access to medical care (e.g., monitoring equipment, ICUs, and antivenin), and perhaps also to cultural differences in housing and protective clothing that promote human-scorpion interactions in Mexico.

Currently, a polyvalent antivenin protective against all native *Centruroides* species is produced by injecting horses with a mixture of macerated venom glands from the most important species (*C. noxius, C. l. limpidus, C. l. tecomanus,* and *C. suffusus*). Antivenin is recommended and often used in patients with systemic symptoms.[46]

United States

About 40 species of scorpions are found in the United States.[36] Only *Centruroides exilicauda* causes a significant number of systemic reactions and is known to be potentially fatal.[23,36,40,129,141] Approximately 30 *Centruroides* species are found distributed throughout the New World,[129] several of which are of medical importance and are mostly found in Mexico.

Centruroides exilicauda (the currently preferred taxonomic designation) is also known as *C. sculpturatus,* or the bark scorpion, because of its preference to reside in or near trees. These scorpions also often hide under wood (old stumps, lumber piles, firewood, loose bark on fallen trees), in ground debris, or in crevices during the daytime. This is troublesome to humans, since the scorpions may hide in shoes, blankets, or clothing left on the floor during daylight hours, as well as under

common ground cover and tents. *C. exilicauda* is found statewide in Arizona and also in some areas of Texas, New Mexico, northern Mexico, small areas of California, and near Lake Mead, Nevada.[40] The bark scorpion is relatively small, measuring up to 5 cm in length. Specimens are variously described as being a uniform yellow, brown, or tan; stripes are uncommon. The pincers (pedipalps) and tail are thin, giving the scorpion a streamlined appearance, in contrast to several of the larger but less dangerous scorpions with thick claws and tails. The presence of a subacular tooth, a tubercle at the base of the stinger, is distinctive to *C. exilicauda* and is helpful in differentiating this neurotoxic scorpion from other species.[40,141]

The bark scorpion presents a significant public health problem in Arizona. About 10% of all calls received by the Samaritan Regional Poison Center in Phoenix are related to scorpion stings, the vast majority of which are known or highly suspected to have been caused by *C. exilicauda;* 6064 such calls were received in 1997, the most recent year with complete data available. The Arizona Poison and Drug Information Center in Tucson reported 2678 scorpion stings the same year. *C. exilicauda* was at one time the number-one killer among Arizona's venomous animals. From 1931 to 1940, more than 40 deaths were attributed to envenomation by this scorpion, mostly in young children and infants. The fatality rate fell dramatically between 1940 to 1970, probably because of improved pest control measures and advances in medical technology and supportive care. In 1972 these scorpion stings were still considered generally fatal to infants less than 1 year of age without treatment, extremely dangerous to older children, and occasionally fatal to adults with hypertension.[141] However, no death has been reported from scorpion envenomation in Arizona since 1968.[23] Because death can apparently be prevented with currently available supportive care, prior fatalities were probably caused by loss of upper airway and respiratory muscle control with the potential for aspiration, exacerbated by metabolic acidosis, hyperthermia, and rhabdomyolysis from excessive muscular activity.[40]

Centruroides vittatus, the common striped scorpion, accounts for the most reported envenomations in the United States after *C. exilicauda. C. vittatus* has a black intraocular triangle and black stripes on the thorax. A review of 558 *C. vittatus* stings reported to Texas poison centers in 1997 found that 96% produced local symptoms of pain, bleeding, burning sensations, erythema, edema, hives, local paresthesias, and pruritus; systemic reactions occurred in 20% of victims.[142] The most common systemic features were paresthesias of the face, tongue, and perioral region, followed by dysgeusia, chills, sweating, dysphagia, fasciculations, nausea, and vomiting. *C. vittatus* is found primarily in the Southwest and Texas but also extends into southern Indiana and Illinois.[145]

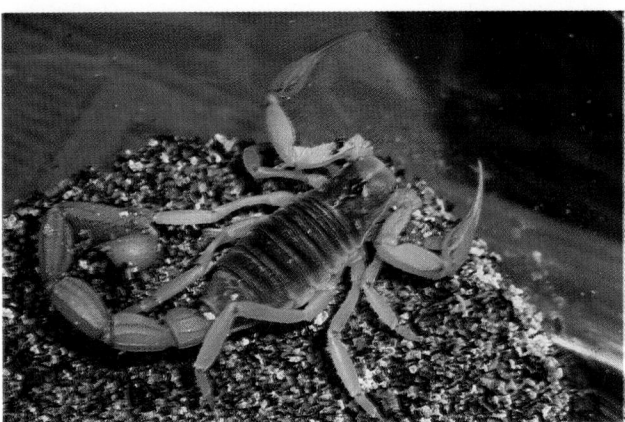

Figure 35-13 *Hadrurus arizonensis*, a "giant hairy scorpion" of the American Southwest. *(Courtesy R. David Gaban.)*

Hadrurus species are the longest and most heavily bodied scorpions native to North America and are known as "giant hairy scorpions" because of their size and conspicuous bristles (Figure 35-13). They are native to Arizona, California, and parts of Utah, Nevada, Idaho, and Mexico. *Vejovis* species have a wide distribution from southern Canada, south through Wyoming, Colorado, and Texas, and west to California. Hypersalivation after *Vejovis* envenomation has been reported. *Uroctonus* species are found in mountain habitats from southern California to Oregon.[129] *Isometrus maculatus* is the only scorpion found in Hawaii[106] but is also found in southern Florida and California.[36] Envenomations cause mild systemic effects (myalgia and nausea), but no fatalities have been reported.[106] *Diplocentrus* species have been found in Florida, Texas, and California.[36] The Midwest and New England are not natural scorpion habitats, although three envenomations in Michigan were caused by scorpions unintentionally transported with personal belongings or with produce, two by *Centruroides hentzi* from Florida, and one by *C. exilicauda* from Arizona.[145] The Samaritan Regional Poison Center in Phoenix has also been consulted regarding stings from bark scorpion stowaways in the mail or personal belongings to Minnesota and Germany, respectively.

Centruroides exilicauda Envenomation. Stings from *C. sculpturatus* often produce significant neuromuscular effects without severe cardiopulmonary toxicity. Curry et al[40] reviewed clinical findings after *C. exilicauda* envenomation and proposed four clinical grades of envenomation to direct treatment (Box 35-1). Grade I envenomation is characterized by local pain and paresthesias at the sting site. Usually, no local inflammation occurs, and the puncture wound is too small to be observed. If no scorpion was seen, the diagnosis may require historical or epidemiologic clues or other physical signs. The "tap test" has been recommended empirically in order to confirm a bark scorpion sting. With the patient looking away or otherwise distracted, gently tapping the sting site will greatly exacerbate the pain, a sign that does not occur with other envenomations.[40,141]

Victims with grade II envenomations have local symptoms plus pain and paresthesias remote from the sting site. The more distant symptoms often radiate proximally up the affected extremity but may occur in even more remote sites (e.g., contralateral limbs) or as generalized paresthesias. Victims may complain of a "thick tongue" and "trouble swallowing" in the absence of objective motor abnormalities. Children and adults frequently rub their nose, eyes, and ears, and infants may present with unexplained crying.[40]

Cranial nerve or somatic skeletal neuromuscular dysfunction is found in grade III envenomations. Cranial nerve dysfunction can be demonstrated as blurred vision, abnormal eye movements, slurred speech, tongue fasciculations, and hypersalivation. The combination of bulbar neuromuscular dysfunction and increased oral secretions may cause problems with airway maintenance. Abnormal eye movements most often are involuntary, conjugate, slow, and roving. Chaotic multidirectional conjugate saccades resembling opsoclonus and unsustained primary positional nystagmus may also be seen.[38] Many patients with abnormal eye movements prefer keeping their eyes closed. Somatic skeletal neuromuscular dysfunction can cause restlessness, fasciculations, alternating opisthotonos and emprosthotonos, and shaking and jerking of the extremities that can be mistaken for a

---

Box 35-2 CENTRUROIDES EXILICAUDA ENVENOMATION, AS REPORTED BY AN INTENSIVE CARE SPECIALIST

Arriving home in the early evening, I decided to go for a run. My running shoes were in the kitchen area, where I had left them the day before. As usual, I would wear my shoes without socks. As I put my left foot into the shoe, I felt an intense burning pain on the dorsum of my first toe. I pulled my foot out of the shoe and along with it came a 1½- to 2-inch, clear-brown scorpion.

Having no idea what to do for a scorpion envenomation, I called the poison control center. I was informed that the systemic toxicity was usually mild for someone my age, and that if the pain was too severe, I should come in and be evaluated. As the minutes went by, I began to salivate and feel perioral paresthesias. As I walked, the paresthesias became more generalized, with a very noticeable paravertebral tingling with each step. After a few more minutes, I decided to call the poison control center to ask for advice. After dialing the number, I was unable to speak clearly because of severe dysarthria and excess salivation. The toe pain seemed to abate as other neurologic symptoms developed.

Since I was unable to talk on the phone, and no neighbors were home to drive me to the hospital, I decided to drive myself. The normal 10-minute drive took

45 minutes. I had coordination difficulties with the gas pedal, clutch, and gear shifting. It was also nighttime, and I could not process the multiple visual inputs of car lights, street lights, and road lines in a way that would allow me to drive more than 5 to 10 miles per hour. I not only had to stop frequently and close my eyes for a few seconds but also had difficulty keeping the car in my driving lane.

After arriving at the emergency department, I was ataxic, dysarthric, and drooling and had difficulty giving the admitting nurse a proper history. I'm certain that I was thought to be either mentally retarded or intoxicated. Examination by the ED physician revealed many abnormal cerebellar findings, continued salivation, inability to swallow liquids, continued symptomatic paresthesias, but no objective motor or sensory deficits. There were no physical signs of envenomation [at the sting site], but tapping the toe produced worsening pain. As my story became clearer to the ED physician, antivenom was ordered and administered. Within 20 minutes of finishing the infusion, all neurologic signs and symptoms were gone, except for toe pain.

Personal account of Dr. Thomas Bajo, Phoenix, Arizona.

---

seizure. The abnormal skeletal muscle activity appears more undulating and writhing, however, than the tonic-clonic movements of generalized seizures. Also, unlike with seizures, the victim often remains awake and alert the entire time.

Grade IV envenomation is characterized by both cranial nerve dysfunction and somatic skeletal neuromuscular dysfunction. On close examination, victims with skeletal muscle hyperactivity (at least grade III) usually also have cranial nerve dysfunction, meeting criteria for grade IV. In the most severe cases, stridor and wheezing occur, suggesting foreign body aspiration or reactive airways disease. Hyperthermia up to 40° C (104° F) probably results from excess motor activity. Respiratory failure, pulmonary edema, metabolic acidosis, sterile cerebrospinal fluid pleocytosis, rhabdomyolysis, coagulopathy, pancreatitis, and multisystem organ failure have also been reported in a few severely ill children.[23] After envenomation, symptoms may begin immediately and progress to maximum severity within 5 hours. Infants can reach grade IV in 15 to 30 minutes.[40] The symptoms abate at a rate that depends on age of the victim and grade of envenomation. Symptomatic improvement occurs within 9 to 30 hours without antivenin therapy.[32,38,40,141] Pain and

paresthesias are exceptions and have been known to persist for days to 2 weeks.

Although adults appear to be envenomed more often, children are more likely to develop severe illness requiring intensive supportive care.[40] A review of 673 patients found that 67.8% of stings occurred in adults older than 20, with 14.9% in children younger than 11. Many more unreported envenomations probably occur in adults, placing the relative incidence for children even lower. Of the patients, 621 (92.3%) had symptoms of either grade I or II envenomations or were asymptomatic and thus required no specific therapy. Younger patients had a higher percentage of the more severe envenomations; 25.9% of children less than 6 years of age had grade III or IV envenomations, or 34% if asymptomatic patients (most likely never stung) are excluded. Only 6.1% of adults had grade III or IV envenomations.[40]

Medically reliable descriptions of the victim's perspective of neurotoxic scorpion envenomation are rare, mostly because of the young age of those most severely affected (Box 35-2).

Other Countries

In Spain from 1974 to 1978, 100 scorpion stings were reported, with most occurring in hot weather and 50%

from *Buthus* species.[67] The poison control center in Marseilles, France, reported 976 scorpion stings from 1973 to 1994.[45] Local signs and symptoms predominated; only a few developed systemic toxicity (nausea, vomiting, tachycardia), and none developed neurotoxicity. Recommended treatment consists of administering analgesics and addressing tetanus immunization status, since hospitalization and antivenin are not necessary.

Scorpions are also found throughout the eastern and tropical regions of Asia. Envenomation by *Buthus martensii* is a common medical problem in China.[147] This scorpion is also used in traditional Chinese medicine for its reputed effects of reversing circulatory failure. The black (Asian forest) scorpion *Heterometrus longimanus* is found in Indonesia, Malaysia, and the Philippines.[83]

Australia is home to approximately 30 scorpion species.[140] *Urodachus yaschenkoi* stings reportedly can disable a young healthy victim for up to 24 hours, with prostration, pyrexia, and sweating. No neurotoxins were found in *U. novahollandiae*, the only Australian species that has had its venom studied.[140]

CLINICAL MANIFESTATIONS

Cardiovascular

Detailed descriptions of myocardial damage and other cardiovascular manifestations from the scorpions of Israel, India, Trinidad, Tunisia, and Brazil have been reported since the 1960s.[73] The overall incidence of heart failure or pulmonary edema is 7% to 32%, with shock reported in 7% to 38% and sudden cardiac death in 7% of victims.

The cardiovascular effects of scorpion envenomation are complex and varied. Stimulation of the sympathetic and parasympathetic branches of the autonomic nervous system results in different clinical presentations that may change with time. Distinct syndromes may dominate the clinical picture in severe scorpion stings. Hypertension or hypotension can occur with or without pulmonary edema, and rhythm disturbances may consist of sinus bradycardia or tachycardia, premature depolarizations, supraventricular tachycardia, atrioventricular block, and ventricular tachycardia.[60,74] A recent Indian study postulated that the cardiovascular effects follow a predictable pattern.[94] Stage I consists of vasoconstriction and hypertension. Stage II is characterized by left ventricular failure manifested as hypotension, with or without pulmonary edema depending on the patient's volume status. Stage III combines both left and right ventricular dysfunction, resulting in cardiogenic shock. A similar progression from a hyperdynamic and hypertensive phase to a hypokinetic, hypotensive phase with left ventricular dysfunction is also reported from Tunisia.[120] Transient parasympa-

thetic effects may occur initially, resulting in bradycardia and hypotension, and are followed by sustained adrenergic hyperactivity.[17]

Sinus tachycardia and hypertension are related to venom-induced catecholamine and angiotensin release.[17,41,76,94,99] Significant hypertension may be seen in up to 77% of patients with systemic envenomation, although a 17.5% to 30% incidence of hypertension is more common.[73] A loud protosystolic gallop, systolic parasternal lift, and transient apical murmur of papillary muscle dysfunction are associated with systemic hypertension.[17,73]

Myocarditis, with ECG changes and biochemical evidence of cardiac injury, is often reported. This myocardial damage is most likely caused by massive catecholamine discharge and sympathetic overstimulation, although direct venom cardiotoxicity has not yet been ruled out.* Many ECG changes consistent with myocardial ischemia and myocarditis have been found in persons stung by scorpions, including Q waves, ST-segment elevation or depression, peaked or inverted T waves, U waves, prolonged QTc intervals, and atrioventricular and bundle branch blocks.[15,35,73,131] Most ECG abnormalities are transient, lasting only as long as the most severe clinical effects. Prolonged QTc intervals last for 48 to 72 hours, however, and T-wave inversions have persisted for 4 to 6 weeks.[14] Echocardiography has demonstrated left ventricular systolic dysfunction, which usually resolves by the next day.[99] Concurrent right ventricular dysfunction supports primary global scorpionic myocarditis rather than secondary myocardial ischemia from systemic hypertension.[120]

Elevated serum levels of CK and CK-MB have been found in about one half of persons with systemic envenomation. Only about one half of those with elevated CK-MB levels also have ECG changes consistent with myocardial injury.[138] Concurrent CK, CK-MB, and troponin-I elevations have also been reported in a victim with transient bradycardia and second-degree (Mobitz type I) atrioventricular block.[131] Histologic examinations of cardiac tissue in fatal human cases have shown a mixed picture of toxic myocarditis and myocytolysis, with interstitial edema and hemorrhage, inflammatory cell infiltrates, focal necrotic foci, and fatty droplet deposition.[41,73]

Respiratory Effects

Respiratory failure after scorpion envenomation has been attributed to direct CNS depression, hypertensive encephalopathy, upper airway obstruction, bronchospasm, impaired surfactant synthesis, and pulmonary edema (PE).[111,134,139] PE is the most severe respiratory feature in severe scorpion envenomation, occurring in 7% to 35% of victims and accounting for

---

*References 17, 41, 61, 73, 120, 136.

about 25% of scorpion-related deaths.[1,2,123] The etiology and pathogenesis of PE from scorpion stings are not clear, and both cardiogenic and noncardiogenic factors have been implicated. Left ventricular systolic dysfunction may cause PE through venom-induced myocarditis and acutely increased afterload.[2,4,72,123] Increased pulmonary capillary wedge pressures,[2] abnormal radionuclide scans,[123] and left ventricular dysfunction demonstrated by Doppler echocardiographic studies[1] support a cardiac origin of PE.

Noncardiogenic causes for PE are less well documented but include shock, primary venom-induced lung injury, oxygen toxicity,[72] and the presence of various inflammatory mediators (interleukins, kinins, platelet activating factor).[4] Histologic and biochemical evidence of increased alveolocapillary membrane permeability has been demonstrated in animal studies and in a fatal human case of *Tityus serrulatus* envenomation.[5] Rabbit studies with *Tityus discrepans* venom found abundant intravascular microthrombi in lungs with PE, and heparin prevented the development of PE.[54] Such findings are atypical of noncardiogenic pulmonary edema, or adult respiratory distress syndrome (ARDS), and the researchers therefore suggest that scorpion venom respiratory distress syndrome (SVRDS) be recognized as a distinct clinical entity.

Neurologic Effects

Centruroides exilicauda (sculpturatus) stings produce significant neuromuscular effects, manifested by pain and paresthesias in lower grades of envenomation and by cranial nerve and somatic skeletal neuromuscular dysfunction in higher grades. These effects are caused by repetitive firing of neurons from venom-induced incomplete sodium channel inactivation.[40] Other scorpions may cause similar neurologic findings as part of their clinical picture. *Centruroides vittatus* causes neurotoxic symptoms in about 20% of victims.[142] Both local and diffuse paresthesias have been reported with *Leiurus quinquestriatus* stings.[31] *Tityus serrulatus* has caused unilateral facial paresthesias and fasciculations in the facial nerve distribution.[119]

Neurologic signs are fairly common among patients with severe envenomations from scorpions categorized here as cardiotoxic. For purposes of discussion, scorpions may be divided into neurotoxic and cardiotoxic categories. In reality, all the scorpions that produce systemic effects are primarily neurotoxic. However, the neurotoxic effects from some species can induce massive release of endogenous catecholamines, causing prominent cardiopulmonary effects. Neurologic signs reported with cardiotoxic scorpions include paresthesias, tremors, shivering, agitation, hyperirritability, apprehension, restlessness, myoclonus, oculogyric crisis (opsoclonus?), convulsions, confusion, delirium, hy-

poreflexia, and coma.* In fatal human cases a preterminal encephalopathic phase is typical.[93]

Intracranial pathology has been noted in several case reports of scorpion envenomation. *Mesobuthus tamulus* and *Heterometrus swannerdani* in India have been implicated in causing hemorrhagic strokes. In two cases, acute arterial hypertension may have ruptured intracranial blood vessels in the basal ganglia,[62,124] although *Heterometrus* species do not cause systemic toxicity related to a catecholamine surge as does *M. tamulus*.[15,148] A third case suggests that frontoparietal hemorrhage results from venom-induced vasculitis.[12] Two earlier cases of hemiplegia associated with scorpion stings in India were believed to result from cerebral thrombosis.[12] A 3-year-old boy stung by *Nebo hierochonticus* developed diffuse intracranial hemorrhages with cortical blindness and deafness, most likely related to disseminated intravascular coagulation (DIC).[8] A 13-year-old Israeli boy stung by *L. quinquestriatus* developed mutism and buccofacial apraxia with bilateral infarcts of the frontal opercular regions,[71] probably related to an episode of cardiogenic shock from ventricular tachycardia.

Many persons with systemic scorpion envenomation exhibit anxiety and agitation, consistent with CNS excitation. Animal experiments have shown that intracerebroventricularly administered *M. tamulus* venom produces similar effects as yohimbine, a known anxiogenic agent.[27] Although in fatal cases of *L. quinquestriatus* envenomation, CNS manifestations always precede terminal hypotension and cardiac arrest, the venom crosses the blood-brain barrier poorly if at all,[88,93,125] so any encephalopathy would be secondary to peripheral effects. Others suggest that CNS manifestations of scorpion stings are caused by hypertensive encephalopathy or excessive levels of circulating catecholamines,[133,134] not a direct venom effect. Hypoxia and pain may also contribute to agitation.

Pancreatitis

Scorpionic pancreatitis was reported by Waterman in 1938 from *Tityus trinitatis* stings and was found in 80% of patients studied by Bartholomew in 1970.[11] Most of these patients had epigastric abdominal pain radiating to the back starting within 5 hours of the sting and resolving within 24 hours. Some patients with hyperamylasemia (38%) did not complain of abdominal pain, suggesting that the true incidence of pancreatitis may be significantly higher. Scorpion stings are the most common cause of acute pancreatitis in Trinidad.[11] Acute pancreatitis is the most common form of the disease, but edematous, hemorrhagic, and chronic relapsing pancreatitis may also occur.[65] Transient pancreatitis has also been reported from *C. exilicauda*[23] and in 93% of

---

*References 22, 33, 35, 55, 81, 98, 116, 122, 134.

children envenomed by *L. quinquestriatus.*[137] The systemic severity of the envenomation or amount of abdominal pain does not appear to correlate with degree of elevation in serum amylase.[11,137] Scorpion venom is known to be a potent secretagogue, stimulating exocrine secretion of the stomach,[144] salivary glands,[40] and pancreas. Enhanced release of proteolytic enzymes, accompanied by spasm of the sphincter of Oddi,[65] is hypothesized to cause acute scorpionic pancreatitis.

Other Gastrointestinal Effects

Nausea, vomiting, gastric distention, abdominal cramping, and occasional diarrhea are reported in victims with severe systemic symptoms.[46,84,99,110] In Tunisia the onset of vomiting heralded worsening neurotoxicity and marked progression from stage III to stage IV envenomation.[69] Gastric distention associated with agitation and depressed level of consciousness place scorpion sting victims at increased risk for pulmonary aspiration of gastric contents. *T. serrulatus* venom increases the volume, acid output, and pepsin output of gastric juice in rats, probably mediated by release of acetylcholine and histamine. Serum gastrin levels are also elevated.[144] Pig studies with *L. quinquestriatus* venom found that despite an increase in oxygen transport and consumption, oxygen utilization in the GI tract was impaired.[139] Such impairment in oxygen utilization may occur in other tissues as well, contributing to metabolic acidosis in severe envenomations.

Endocrine and Other Humoral Effects

Scorpion envenomation has long been known to cause an "autonomic storm" with increased release of endogenous catecholamines, contributing to hypertension, tachycardia, and potentially fatal cardiopulmonary dysfunction. Envenomed patients with abnormal ECG tracings excrete elevated levels of free epinephrine, norepinephrine, and vanillylmandelic acid.[78] Elevated circulating catecholamine levels have also been reported.[5] Release of catecholamines may be caused by direct stimulation of postganglionic sympathetic neurons and the adrenal glands. Hypertension may also be caused by activation of the renin-angiotensin endocrine axis. Elevated levels of renin and aldosterone were found in victims stung by *L. quinquestriatus.*[80]

Stings often induce hyperglycemia related to suppression of insulin secretion,[39,111] in contrast to the enhanced secretion of the exocrine pancreas. Murthy and Hase[111] propose that this results in a syndrome of fuel-energy deficits related to inability to utilize existing metabolic substrates, exacerbating the cardiopulmonary insult. Insulin therapy has been found to reverse ECG changes, reduce angiotensin levels and circulating free fatty acids in experimental animals, and reverse hemodynamic changes and pulmonary edema

in children stung by scorpions.[111,113] *M. tamulus* venom lowers thyroxine and triiodothyronine levels in experimental myocarditis.[112]

Kinins and other inflammatory mediators may play a role in the cardiovascular toxicity. *T. serrulatus* and *C. exilicauda* venoms potentiate the action of bradykinin by inhibiting angiotensin converting enzyme (ACE).[104] Animal experiments show reversal of venom-induced cardiovascular effects with aprotinin,[11,58,93] a kallikrein-kinin inhibitor, and icatibant,[58] a bradykinin antagonist, and augmentation of adverse effects with captopril,[10] an ACE inhibitor.

Serum interleukin-6 (IL-6) levels were greatly elevated in 8 of 10 Israeli children, gradually decreasing toward normal over 24 hours.[138] High levels of circulating IL-1, IL-3, IL-6, IL-10, and granulocyte-macrophage colony-stimulating factor (GM-CSF) have also been found in a severely envenomed Brazilian patient.[4]

Genitourinary Effects

Priapism is frequently reported among male patients with systemic envenomation. Priapism results from enhanced parasympathetic tone and is often associated with vomiting and profuse sweating.[15,16] The incidence of priapism ranges from 4% to 10%[3,7,121] up to 78% to 96%.[84,135] In India, priapism, vomiting, and diaphoresis are considered premonitory diagnostic signs of severe *M. tamulus* envenomation. Priapism is reduced or absent within 6 hours of the sting even in severe cases, and the degree of priapism does not appear to correlate with the severity of envenomation.[15] In Tunisia, however, the incidence of priapism positively correlated with degree of severity.[98]

Urinary retention is found in 33% of victims with systemic envenomation in southern Africa.[25,26,110] This finding, however, is not consistent with increased cholinergic tone, which should produce increased urination, as seen in other series.[7] A dorsal nerve block with 1% lidocaine was successful in treating severe local pain from a *T. serrulatus* sting to the penis.[118]

Hematologic Effects

Scorpion venoms are not generally noted to produce coagulopathies or other significant hematologic effects, although DIC has been reported.[7,103] The occasional "defibrination syndrome" is seen more often in children, probably related to a higher relative dose, and can be experimentally reproduced in dogs. Platelet aggregation can be induced by catecholamines alone, and may therefore be an indirect effect of scorpion venom. Increased osmotic fragility of red blood cells has been demonstrated in some experimental models.[128]

The only scorpion routinely implicated in dangerous hematologic effects is *Hemiscorpion lepturus*, which can cause severe hemolysis and consequent renal failure.[115,122]

Case reports from Saudi Arabia associate severe *Nebo hierochonticus* stings with DIC and intracranial hemorrhage.[7,8] Neither species is from the Buthidae family.

Immunologic Effects

Scorpion toxins are antigenic and therefore capable of eliciting an immune response on reexposure. Positive skin prick and intradermal skin tests and radioallergosorbent assays have been found with the venom from *C. vittatus*[47] and *Androctonus australis hector*[101] in previously envenomed patients. Envenomation by *C. exilicauda* has produced an anaphylactic reaction, with urticaria, wheezing, and facial angioedema but without systemic neurotoxic findings, in an otherwise healthy adult patient previously stung by a scorpion.[149]

Treatment with animal-derived antivenins places a person at risk for both immediate and delayed immunologic reactions. Since the treatment for hypersensitivity reactions includes epinephrine, and because many persons envenomed by cardiotoxic scorpions have elevated circulating catecholamines, such persons should be less likely to have anaphylactic reactions to antivenin. Brazilian patients stung by *T. serrulatus* were separated into groups with or without adrenergic manifestations. Both groups received antivenin.[6] The group with adrenergic toxicity developed significantly less signs and symptoms of early anaphylaxis (8% vs. 42.9%).

Miscellaneous Systemic Effects

Leukocytosis with white blood cell counts as high as $44,000/mm^3$ is common in persons with severe scorpion envenomation.[33,35,94] Mild to moderate hypokalemia was found in 13 of 17 patients with severe *Tityus* envenomations in Brazil[33] and eight patients with *M. tamulus* stings in India,[94] although elevated potassium and lowered sodium levels were found previously.[150] The same venom-induced metabolic changes that inhibit insulin release favor glycogenolysis and lipolysis, leading to elevated circulating levels of free fatty acids.[111,112]

DIFFERENTIAL DIAGNOSIS

Bites or stings from other arthropods should be considered in the differential diagnosis of scorpion envenomation. Pain at the site of *Centruroides exilicauda* sting may be similar to that from a black widow spider (*Latrodectus* species). However, severely ill victims of scorpion envenomation appear unable to lie still, whereas those with black widow spider bites can maintain a position for short periods before moving again to find a comfortable position. Black widow bite may produce hypertension, tachycardia, sweating, and other signs of adrenergic excess but does not produce the abnormal eye movements, fasciculations, and paresthesias found with scorpion sting or induce a positive tap test. Widow spider bites frequently produce a characteristic halo lesion at the site, whereas no lesion is usually visible after *C. exilicauda* sting. Many other arthropods can produce a small puncture wound accompanied by local tissue inflammation. This may be difficult to differentiate clinically from stings by scorpion species in the absence of cardiovascular or neurologic toxicity or without tentative visual identification of the arthropod involved.

The tachycardia, respiratory distress, excessive secretions, and occasional wheezing that occur from *C. exilicauda* sting may be mistaken for asthma, airway obstruction with a foreign body, or poisoning with a cholinergic agent, such as an organophosphate insecticide. In the absence of the history of a scorpion sting, other disorders to be considered include CNS infection, tetanus, dystonic reaction, seizure, and intoxication with an anticholinergic, a sympathomimetic, phencyclidine, nicotine, or strychnine. Autonomic storm from a cardiotoxic scorpion sting may be confused with pheochromocytoma or a monoamine oxidase inhibitor–tyramine reaction. A victim of severe scorpion envenomation presenting late in the course may appear to have cardiac failure or sepsis.

Toxicity from an illegal sympathomimetic is sometimes mistaken for envenomation by *C. exilicauda*. Young children from endemic areas presenting with unusual neurologic symptoms, such as agitation, choreiform or repetitive motion of the trunk and extremities, and abnormal eye movements, may be assumed to have been envenomed even without history of a sting or scorpion.[114] Occasionally the caregivers are aware of this potential for misdiagnosis and claim that their child was stung when they know or suspect that the child ingested methamphetamine. A case series of 18 inadvertent methamphetamine poisonings among children in central Arizona included three victims initially misdiagnosed with a scorpion sting and inappropriately treated with antivenin; one patient had an anaphylactic reaction.[95]

TREATMENT

Ismail et al[93] summarized the current understanding of treating scorpion stings when noting, "It is strange that despite the long experience with scorpion envenomation, most of the treatment protocols advocated are based on isolated clinical observations, are sometimes controversial, and not instituted on rigid or strictly controlled animal or clinical studies. . . . Even in serotherapy, there are no quantitative studies regarding antivenom dosage, routes of administration, time-effectiveness relationship and titre of the antivenom used."

Some treatment recommendations can be eliminated. A so-called lytic cocktail was once considered essential in treating *Mesobuthus tamulus* stings in India.[42] This mixture of pethidine (meperidine), chlorpromazine, and promethazine (equivalent to the DPT cocktail for pediatric sedation, which has fallen into disfavor in the United States) was claimed to induce "artificial hibernation" and improve outcome. Morbidity and mortality statistics, however, have not shown a difference between cohorts historically treated with the lytic cocktail and those not treated. Furthermore, any effect of such treatment would be sedation, which would increase the risk of airway difficulties. Some traditional herbal therapies involve rubbing the area near the sting site, which doubles the chance of developing a severe envenomation.[25,26] Purported herbal therapies for scorpion stings have not been adequately tested and are probably of no benefit.[85] Other therapies no longer recommended include electric shock, barium, iodine, physostigmine, and snake or spider antivenin.[129]

Although much controversy surrounds the proper treatment of scorpion envenomation, some consensus exists. Most victims, even those stung by potentially dangerous scorpions, demonstrate only local signs and symptoms and require only symptomatic outpatient treatment. It is prudent to observe such persons for several hours after the sting to ensure that progression to severe envenomation does not occur. For localized pain, many authorities recommend local anesthesia with lidocaine, bupivacaine, or dehydroemetine by infiltration or nerve block, such as a digital block for fingers or toes.* In southern Africa, Berman[25,26] has reported successful treatment of poorly localized pain radiating up an extremity with an intracutaneous sterile water injection (ISWI), usually also with a local anesthetic infiltrated at the sting site. ISWI is performed by injecting small amounts (about 0.1 ml) of sterile water intradermally into points of maximal pain, producing up to 10 wheals. Pain relief is said to occur within 1 to 5 minutes, but pain may return in 4 to 12 hours and can be persistent. ISWI therapy cannot be generally recommended because it has not been tested in prospective or controlled trials or with scorpion stings elsewhere in the world. Scorpion stings are traumatic puncture wounds, and victims should be given appropriate wound care and tetanus prophylaxis if indicated.

Victims with significant systemic scorpion envenomations should receive supportive and symptomatic care in a monitored hospital setting.[33,56,61,77,81] Many require admission to an ICU, although treatment should begin in the emergency department or outlying facility if available. Airway control must be addressed and continuous cardiovascular and respiratory monitoring instituted. Fluid resuscitation may be indicated secondary to fluid losses from vomiting, sweating, and increased insensible losses from hyperthermia. Both hyperthermia and hypothermia have been reported from scorpion stings, and both appear to worsen toxicity.[92] Hyperthermia usually resolves with standard acetaminophen doses, and hypothermia resolves with warm blankets.

Pharmacologic Therapy

Many drugs have been recommended in the treatment of scorpion envenomations, but few have been rigorously tested. Recommendations for atropine vary. Many victims exhibit signs of excess cholinergic tone, such as bradycardia, vomiting, sweating, and hypersalivation. If venom induces prominent adrenergic effects, the rescuer should not administer atropine.[18,61,81] Parasympathetic venom effects are usually transient and not life threatening, although atropine may be indicated for severe bradycardia. Also, in subsequent phases with more prominent adrenergic toxicity, atropine could worsen tachycardia and hypertension, leading to more severe cardiovascular effects. Atropine may be safe, however, for cholinergic effects from scorpions that do not cause prominent cardiotoxicity. Published cases from southern Africa[25] and anecdotal experience from Arizona suggest that atropine can reverse hypersalivation that interferes with airway control, which may obviate the need for intubation and decrease the risk of aspiration, although caution is still advised.[110] Protocols for the use of atropine and its optimal dosage have not been prospectively determined.

The only therapy to date subjected to prospective, randomized, placebo-controlled human study has been antiinflammatory corticosteroids,[3] which showed no benefit. Treatment with corticosteroids has been regularly recommended and is still common in many countries. In Tunisia, 600 consecutive patients received either 50 mg/kg of hydrocortisone hemisuccinate or a placebo. No differences between the two groups were found in clinical severity (baseline and 4 hours after treatment), mortality, need for artificial ventilation, or duration of hospitalization.[3] Glucocorticoids and antihistamines are not recommended unless administered as treatment for allergic manifestations (e.g., anaphylaxis to antivenin).[26,110]

Vasodilator therapy has received much attention. Since excessive adrenergic tone appears to cause the most significant morbidity, vasodilators should block or reverse severe cardiopulmonary effects from scorpion envenomation. Prazosin is a selective α_1-adrenergic blocker, which is also thought to reverse the inhibition of insulin.[20,21] In India an initial dose of 0.5 mg by mouth for adults and 0.25 mg for children is given to relieve hypertension and pulmonary edema. Repeat doses are given in 4 hours, then every 6 hours as needed for up to 24 hours. Sodium nitroprusside is

---

*References 22, 25, 26, 35, 86, 118.

used in cases of life-threatening pulmonary edema.[22] Nifedipine, 5 to 10 mg "sublingually" by puncturing and swallowing the gelatin capsule, is also used in India along with the initial dose of prazosin. When this protocol was compared with "conventional treatment" (digoxin, furosemide, hydrocortisone, antihistamines, and atropine), the cohort treated with prazosin had significantly reduced morbidity and shortened recovery time.[21,75] In Israel, hypertension from scorpion sting unresponsive to analgesics and sedatives has been treated with IV hydralazine or sublingual nifedipine, which are believed to reverse hypertensive encephalopathy.[133] A potential benefit of vasodilators over antivenin is the rapidity of onset.[75] Captopril has also been used to treat hypertension[94] but theoretically could worsen PE.[10,22,88]

Insulin infusion has been used in India.[111,113] Since scorpion venoms inhibit insulin secretion, this treatment may help reverse the consequent metabolic derangements. "Standard therapy" to which insulin infusions were added consisted of furosemide for elevated central venous pressures or PE, crystalloid for low central venous pressures, and hydrocortisone and dopamine for hypotension. Insulin was given in a glucose solution with 0.3 units regular insulin per gram of glucose, at a rate of 0.1 g glucose per kilogram body weight per hour. Six patients treated with insulin showed improvement in PE and hemodynamics, although furosemide and hydrocortisone appeared to offer little benefit.[111]

Digoxin, diuretics, steroids, antihistamines, dopamine, dobutamine, and β-adrenergic blockers have been used but are not generally recommended. Dantrolene, aminophylline, quinine, and aspirin are potential therapeutic adjuvants in scorpion envenomation.[22,82]

Antivenin

Treatment recommendations seriously diverge regarding antivenin. (We use the term *antivenin* instead of *antivenom*, though either term is acceptable.) Most medical researchers believe that antivenin plays a crucial role in the treatment of seriously envenomed patients.* Proponents believe that (1) antivenin is the only specific therapy available against the primary physiologic insult and (2) it greatly improves outcome. Any previous disappointing experience with antivenin, they argue, probably results from inadequate dosing.[87,88] Researchers from Israel and India do not recommend antivenin.[16,81,135] Opponents believe that (1) morbidity and mortality are not caused by the venom but by autopharmacologic agent release, which should not be reversed by antivenin therapy; (2) pharmacokinetic data do not support a role for antivenin; (3) antivenin has

not improved outcome in Israeli studies; and (4) antivenin is often unavailable and would be prohibitively expensive in India, so other options must be chosen. Some suggest that commercial production of scorpion antivenin is needed in India.[148] Treatment without antivenin consists of managing serious cardiopulmonary and neurologic effects with pharmacologic agents and supportive care. Even when antivenin is administered by its proponents, adjunctive therapies to treat cardiac failure, PE, and other physiologic treatments are also used.

A major issue in the debate regarding the utility of antivenin is the pharmacokinetics of scorpion venom. Detectable circulating levels of venom support the use of antivenin to neutralize the toxins. *Tityus serrulatus* venom injected subcutaneously in rodents rapidly distributes to various tissues, with peak serum levels in 30 to 60 minutes.[125,130] After 2 hours the venom decreased rapidly and was no longer detectable after 8 hours.[125] IV serotherapy therefore should be initiated as soon as possible, since it would become less effective when administered many hours after envenomation.[125]

Ismail et al[88,90] reported that scorpion venoms in animal experiments were rapidly absorbed and distributed to tissues but had more prolonged elimination phases. Scorpion venom has a half-life of 4.2 to 24 hours.[88] The authors concluded that although antivenin would theoretically be most efficacious if given immediately after envenomation, it is still indicated after a delay of several hours or more.[99,130] Interestingly, Gueron et al[73,81] reviewed these data and concluded instead that serotherapy would be ineffective and recommended against it. They suggested that the most severe cardiopulmonary effects would be present early and would not be reversed by antivenin given later. The clinical effects of scorpion envenomation are related to tissue concentrations of *Androctonus amoreuxi* venom in experimental animals,[89] although the slower distribution of antivenin to tissues suggests that it may be less effective when given after a significant delay. A series of 56 victims stung by *T. serrulatus* in Brazil correlated clinical severity to plasma venom concentrations.[48] IV antivenin lowers circulating levels of venom and presumably the clinical severity of envenomation; however, the effectiveness of antivenin on venom bound to other tissues has not been well defined. The role of serotherapy depends on the time to administration, becoming less effective with increasing delay.[96,107] Since scorpion venom acts indirectly through the release of autopharmacologic substances, treatment with specific blockers may be more effective than antivenin in persons with delayed presentation.[89]

Antivenin research is ongoing and may produce improved products in the future. Maximum neutralizing capacity of antivenin is obtained when soluble venom is used as the antigen rather than telson macerates and

---

*References 2, 32, 35, 40, 49, 60, 86, 110.

TABLE 35-1. Scorpion Antivenins

ORGANIZATION	PHONE NUMBER*	SPECIES COVERED
Institut Pasteur, Algiers, Algeria	[213] 2653497	*Androctonus australis hector, Leiurus quinquestriatus, Buthus occitanus*
Institut Pasteur, Casablanca, Morocco	[212] 2275778, [212] 2275206	*Androctonus mauretanicus, B. occitanus, Scorpio maurus*
Institut Pasteur, Tunis, Tunisia	[216] 283022-4, Telex: 14391 PATSU	*A. australis, B. occitanus, Androctonus aeneas, L. quinquestriatus*
The South African Institute for Medical Research, Johannesburg, South Africa	[27] 725-0511, Telex: 4-22211	*Parabuthus transvaalicus,* other *Parabuthus* species
Laboratorios BIOCLON S.A., Mexico City, Mexico (formerly MYN, Zapata, and Grupo Pharma)	[52] 592-87-70, [52] 561-12-11, [52] 592-88-93	*Centruroides* species
Gerencia General de Biologicos y Reactivos, Health Ministry, Mexico City, Mexico		*Centruroides* species
Instituto Butantan, São Paulo, Brazil	[55] 813 7222, [55] 815 1505, Telex: 11-83325-BUTA BR	*Tityus serrulatus, T. bahiensis*
Fundacao Ezequiel Dias, Belo Horizonte, Brazil		Fab$_2$ fragment for *Tityus* species
Refik Saydam Central, Ankara, Turkey		*Androctonus crassicauda, L. quinquestriatus, A. australis, B. occitanus*
Twyford Pharmaceuticals GmbH, Ludwigshafen am Rhein, Germany	[49] (0621) 589-2688, [49] (0621) 589-2896, Telex: 464823	*A. australis, B. occitanus, L. quinquestriatus,* other *Androctonus* and *Buthus* species
Institut d'Etat des Serums et Vaccins, Tehran, Iran	[98] 02221-2005	*A. crassicauda, Buthotus salcyi, Mesobuthus eupeus, Odontobuthus doriae, S. maurus*
Central Research Institute, Kasauli, India (research only)	[91] C.R.I. 22	*Mesobuthus tamulus, Palamnaeus* species, *Heterometrus* species (possibly)
Lister Institute of Preventive Medicine, Elstree, Herts, United Kingdom (not in production)	[44] 081-954-6297	*A. australis, B. occitanus, L. quinquestriatus, A. crassicauda*

*Country code in brackets.

purified toxins.[34] Antibodies have been produced against nontoxic analogs of some scorpion neurotoxins,[52] nontoxic proteins found in scorpion venom,[37,109] and neurotoxin amino acid sequences that are highly conserved among many species.[51] Fab antibody fragments have also been produced against scorpion venoms.[61,102] These fragments induce a lower incidence of hypersensitivity reactions[61] and possess pharmacokinetic characteristics that make them more suitable than whole immunoglobulin G (IgG) antibodies.[91]

Table 35-1 lists scorpion antivenins currently available worldwide.[8,46,126,143]

Centruroides exilicauda Envenomation

Based on the experience of our medical toxicology group in Phoenix, Arizona since the mid-1970s and that of others treating *Centruroides exilicauda* envenomation, we favor the use of antivenin in severe envenomation. We routinely recommend and use antivenin in patients with respiratory compromise, as often seen

in grade III or IV envenomation. Antivenin does not take precedence, however, over appropriate airway protection measures, including endotracheal intubation when indicated. Also, the presence of grade III or IV symptomatology is not an absolute indication for antivenin, and we have seen several victims (usually older children or adults) who met criteria for higher grades of envenomation but were alert with no respiratory distress. In several cases, atropine was the initial treatment given to some very young victims with hypersalivation significant enough to impact respiratory status. No significant adverse cardiovascular effects were noted, and atropine appeared to improve airway maintenance. No prospective studies of atropine in *C. exilicauda* envenomation have been published, so we cannot make a recommendation for or against its routine use.

No widely recognized standard of care exists in the treatment of *C. exilicauda* envenomation in the United States. Some physicians in the Phoenix area routinely treat severely envenomed victims with only supportive and symptomatic care, usually in an ICU. The Arizona Poison and Drug Information Center based in Tucson also generally recommends supportive care without antivenin. For many years the recommended therapy for the neuromuscular hyperactivity seen in severe envenomations was large doses of barbiturates.[141] We believe that sedation with barbiturates, benzodiazepines, or other drugs in a person already with tenuous airway control unduly increases the risk for aspiration and respiratory failure; therefore these drugs should not be given unless the physician is prepared to intubate emergently and artificially ventilate the patient.

A recent case series of patients treated with continuous IV infusions of midazolam was reported by physicians from Tucson, Arizona.[66] Among 33 patients treated in the ICU, the mean infusion time was 9.5 hours and the mean ICU stay was 15 hours, with 85% of patients discharged directly to their homes. Four patients with hypoxia responded to supplemental oxygen. The researchers concluded that continuous midazolam infusions were safe and effective. The neuromuscular hyperactivity of *C. exilicauda* envenomations, however, is not a centrally mediated phenomenon. CNS depressants may decrease motor agitation but only indirectly, whereas antivenin directly treats the underlying cause. Regardless of the method, excessive motor activity should be controlled to avoid potential complications of hyperthermia, rhabdomyolysis, and metabolic acidosis. Antivenin typically works quickly, obviating the need for additional pharmacologic sedation to control hyperactivity. We administer parenteral analgesics for pain and benzodiazepines for agitation to patients not treated with antivenin in the ICU.

The primary concern about using the currently available antivenin is hypersensitivity reactions. Both immediate (type I, or anaphylactic) and delayed (type III, or serum sickness) hypersensitivity reactions may occur. In 1999, Bond[32] reported no anaphylactic reactions to antivenin in 12 patients; 58% developed a delayed rash or serum sickness that resolved with oral antihistamines and corticosteroids. In 1994, Gateau et al[64] reported 145 cases of severe *C. exilicauda* envenomations treated with antivenin, with immediate hypersensitivity reactions in 8% generally characterized as mild; no follow-up for incidence of serum sickness was conducted. In 1999, LoVecchio et al[105] reported a prospective study of 116 patients treated with antivenin. Three patients (2.6%) who developed a rash during the antivenin infusion were treated with hydroxyzine, methylprednisolone, and epinephrine, and the infusions were completed at slower rates. An asthmatic patient who developed wheezing responded to treatment with an epinephrine infusion and an inhaled β-agonist, and was admitted for observation. Nine other patients were admitted for oversedation from medications re-

---

Box 35-3 RISKS AND BENEFITS OF CENTRUROIDES EXILICAUDA ANTIVENIN

SUPPORTIVE AND SYMPTOMATIC CARE
Risks

Typically requires admission to intensive care unit
Symptoms may take many hours to days to resolve
Potential overutilization of limited medical resources
Increased hospitalization costs
Potential for oversedation
Aspiration
Hypoxia
Prolonged artificial ventilation

Benefits

Avoids risks of anaphylaxis and serum sickness

USING ANTIVENIN
Risks

Anaphylaxis: immediate hypersensitivity reaction
Cardiopulmonary monitoring recommended
Serum sickness: delayed hypersensitivity reaction

Benefits

Shorter hospital stay with discharge home likely within a few hours
Rapid symptomatic improvement
Avoids risks of oversedation

---

ceived before antivenin, to rule out aspiration, or for social reasons and all were discharged within 24 hours. During a 3-week follow-up period, 60 of the 99 patients (61%) developed serum sickness that responded to oral corticosteroids and antihistamines; mean duration of symptoms was 2.8 days with medication.

Intravenous antivenin results in rapid reversal of neurologic, respiratory, and cardiovascular toxicity in persons envenomed by *C. exilicauda*. Symptoms completely resolved within 1 to 3 hours in one study[32]; 71% of patients in another study had resolution within 30 minutes.[64] Bond[32] summarized the potential benefits of antivenin administration as decreased time to resolution of symptoms, cost savings in the emergency department (vs. about $1000/day in ICU charges), and the avoidance of sedation, paralysis, and intubation risks.[32] We believe that the data support the safe use of IV antivenin for high-grade scorpion neurotoxicity, and that serious adverse effects are both uncommon and treatable (Box 35-3). Other reasonable and informed physicians have concluded that since fatalities should not occur with appropriate supportive care, patients should not be subjected to any risk of antivenin anaphylaxis.

In the United States, the only currently available scorpion antivenin is produced by the Antivenom Production Laboratory at Arizona State University.[32,40,64]

This antivenin has been produced since 1965 by lyophilizing micron-filtered serum obtained from goats hypersensitized to *C. exilicauda* venom. It is also cross-reactive against at least two Mexican *Centruroides* species, *C. limpidus* and *C. elegans*.[29] Antivenin is produced in batches every 2 to 3 years and is supplied without charge to regional hospitals by Arizona State University. Because of the limited geographic area of its use, the antivenin has not been submitted for U.S. Food and Drug Administration approval, but it is used within the state by special action of the Arizona Board of Pharmacy. Some interest has been expressed by pharmaceutical companies regarding *C. exilicauda* antivenin, but no commercial preparation is currently available.

Recommendations and Procedure. Any of the following relative contraindications (roughly in decreasing order of importance) should suggest withholding animal-derived antivenin in favor of symptomatic and supportive care only: (1) prior administration of antivenin derived from the same species; (2) current β-adrenergic blocker use; (3) history of asthma or atopy; (4) current ACE inhibitor use; and (5) history of allergy to the animal species from which the antivenin is derived, allergy to that animal's milk, or prior extensive exposure to the animal, especially its blood.

The patient is placed on continuous ECG and pulse oximetry monitors. IV access is obtained, preferably with at least two IV lines. Equipment and medications for treating anaphylaxis and respiratory arrest are available. Specifically, we prepare an epinephrine drip, 1 mg in 250 ml of 5% dextrose in water (D5W) or normal saline (NS) on a primed IV line with a pump; IV methylprednisolone and hydroxyzine or diphenhydramine in the room are also made available. The lyophilized antivenin is reconstituted with as much sterile NS or D5W as fills the vial (about 10 ml), with gentle rocking to avoid foaming. The antivenin is then withdrawn from the vial and dissolved in 50 ml of crystalloid (60 ml total) and placed on an IV pump. A skin test is then performed. Up to 0.02 ml of a 1:10 dilution of reconstituted antivenin is injected intradermally with a 27- or 30-gauge needle, the site marked with a pen, and the patient observed for at least 10 minutes for development of a wheal, rash, wheezing, or hemodynamic signs of anaphylaxis. The patient with a reaction is treated appropriately with the medications available. For *C. exilicauda* envenomation, a positive skin test contraindicates further antivenin therapy, and the patient is admitted for supportive care. Skin testing, however, does not always predict adverse reactions. One study showed a 96% sensitivity for mild immediate hypersensitivity reactions but only a 68% specificity.[64]

The antivenin is initially administered at a very slow rate (5 ml/hr), which is doubled every 2 to 3 minutes as long as the patient tolerates the infusion (i.e., develops no signs of anaphylaxis), up to 150 ml/hr. Infusion of one vial by this method takes approximately 30 minutes, and most patients require only one vial of antivenin. The patient is observed for at least 1 hour after the initial antivenin infusion is complete before proceeding with additional antivenin, since most symptoms will resolve in this period. If the symptoms have resolved or regressed to a grade I or grade II envenomation and no complications (e.g., aspiration) are suspected, the patient is discharged.

Since most patients treated with antivenin will develop a delayed hypersensitivity reaction, the patient and caregivers are informed about signs and symptoms of serum sickness before discharge. An urticarial rash developing within a few days to weeks is the most common sign, although malaise, myalgias, and arthralgias also may occur. More serious problems are rare. We recommend discharging the patient with prescriptions for antihistamines (hydroxyzine or diphenhydramine) and a tapering dose of corticosteroids to be started if serum sickness develops. Any persons treated with antivenin must be warned that they are allergic to serum products from the animal species used. Repeated use of antivenin for subsequent envenomations is relatively contraindicated but can be undertaken with extreme caution if necessary.

Consultation with toxicologists experienced in treating *C. exilicauda* envenomations can be obtained by calling the Samaritan Regional Poison Center at (602) 253-3334 or the Arizona Poison and Drug Information Center at (520) 626-6016.

PREVENTION

Many scorpion stings result from human practices that place persons at risk. Residences with small cracks and crevices offer many hiding places, increasing the risk of human-scorpion interactions. In several countries, playing or working outdoors with inadequate protective clothing, especially in the early evening during warm months, is associated with most scorpion stings. In scorpion-infested areas, clothing, shoes, packages, and camping gear should be shaken out and checked for scorpions. Footwear is recommended. Unnecessary ground cover and debris should be removed to reduce potential nesting places.

Certain insecticides, including organophosphates, pyrethrins, and several chlorinated hydrocarbons, are known to kill scorpions. Home spraying is often ineffective because the insecticide does not come in contact with the scorpion. Spraying insecticides around the home can work indirectly by killing other insects in the area and reducing the scorpions' food supply.

REFERENCES

1. Abroug F et al: Assessment of left ventricular function in severe scorpion envenomation: combined hemodynamic and echo-Doppler study, *Intensive Care Med* 21:629, 1995.
2. Abroug F et al: Cardiac dysfunction and pulmonary edema following scorpion envenomation, *Chest* 100:105, 1991.
3. Abroug F et al: High-dose hydrocortisone hemisuccinate in scorpion envenomation, *Ann Emerg Med* 30:23, 1997.
4. Amaral CFS et al: Scorpion sting-induced pulmonary edema: evidence of increased alveolocapillary membrane permeability, *Toxicon* 32:999, 1994.
5. Amaral CFS et al: Children with adrenergic manifestations of envenomation after *Tityus serrulatus* scorpion sting are protected from early anaphylactic antivenom reaction, *Toxicon* 32:211, 1994.
6. Amaral CFS, Rezende NA: Both cardiogenic and non-cardiogenic factors are involved in the pathogenesis of pulmonary oedema after scorpion envenoming, *Toxicon* 35:997, 1997.
7. Annobil SH: Scorpion stings in children in the Asir Province of Saudi Arabia, *J Wilderness Med* 4:241, 1993.
8. Annobil SH, Omojola W, Vijayakumar E: Intracranial haemorrhages after *Nebo hierochonticus* scorpion sting, *Ann Trop Pediatr* 11:377, 1991.
9. Arie-Saadia G et al: Effect of *Leiurus quinquestriatus hebreus* venom on calcium and deoxyglucose uptake in cultured cardiac cells, *Toxicon* 34:435, 1996.
10. Bagchi S, Deshpande SB: Indian red scorpion (*Buthus tamulus*) venom-induced augmentation of cardiac reflexes is mediated through the mechanisms involving kinins in urethane anaesthetized rats, *Toxicon* 36:309, 1998.
11. Bartholomew C: Acute scorpion pancreatitis in Trinidad, *BMJ* 1:666,1970.
12. Barthwal SP et al: Myocarditis and hemiplegia from scorpion bite: a case report, *Indian J Med Sci* 51:115, 1997.
13. Bawaskar HS, Bawaskar PH: Cardiovascular manifestations of severe scorpion sting in India (review of 34 children), *Ann Trop Pediatr* 11:381, 1991.
14. Bawaskar HS, Bawaskar PH: Consecutive stings by red scorpions evoke severe cardiovascular manifestations in the first, but not in the second, victim: a clinical observation, *J Trop Med Hyg* 94:231, 1991.
15. Bawaskar HS, Bawaskar PH: Scorpion sting: a review of 121 cases, *J Wilderness Med* 2:164, 1991.
16. Bawaskar HS, Bawaskar PH: Treatment of cardiovascular manifestations of human scorpion envenoming: is serotherapy essential? *J Trop Med Hyg* 94:156, 1991.
17. Bawaskar HS, Bawaskar PH: Management of the cardiovascular manifestations of poisoning by the Indian red scorpion (*Mesobuthus tamulus*), *Br Heart J* 68:478, 1992.
18. Bawaskar HS, Bawaskar PH: Role of atropine in management of cardiovascular manifestations of scorpion envenoming in humans, *J Trop Med Hyg* 95:30, 1992.
19. Bawaskar HS, Bawaskar PH: Treatment of envenoming by *Mesobuthus tamulus* (Indian red scorpion), *Trans Roy Soc Trop Med Hyg* 86:459, 1992.
20. Bawaskar HS, Bawaskar PH: Vasodilators: scorpion envenoming and the heart (an Indian experience), *Toxicon* 32:1031, 1994.
21. Bawaskar HS, Bawaskar PH: Severe envenoming by the Indian red scorpion *Mesobuthus tamulus*: the use of prazosin therapy, *Q J Med* 89:701, 1996.
22. Bawaskar HS, Bawaskar PH: Scorpion envenoming and the cardiovascular system, *Trop Doct* 27:6, 1997.
23. Berg RA, Tarantino MD: Envenomation by the scorpion *Centruroides exilicauda* (*C. sculpturatus*): severe and unusual manifestations, *Pediatrics* 87:930, 1991.
24. Bergman NJ: *Opistophthalmus glabrifrons* scorpion envenomation, *S Afr Med J* 86:981, 1996.
25. Bergman NJ: Clinical description of *Parabuthus transvaalicus* scorpionism in Zimbabwe, *Toxicon* 35:759, 1997.
26. Bergman NJ: Scorpion sting in Zimbabwe, *S Afr Med J* 87:163, 1997.
27. Bhattacharya SK: Anxiogenic activity of centrally administered scorpion (*Mesobuthus tamulus*) venom in rats, *Toxicon* 33:1491, 1995.
28. Bhattacharya B et al: A retrospective study on scorpion sting in a pediatric age group in a hospital in Calcutta, *Indian J Med Sci* 46:205, 1992.
29. Bloom M: Personal communication, 1999.
30. Blum A, Lubezki A, Sclarovsky S: Black scorpion envenomation: two cases and review of the literature, *Clin Cardiol* 15:377, 1992.
31. Bogomolski-Yahalom V, Amitai Y, Stalnikowicz R: Paresthesia in envenomation by the scorpion *Leiurus quinquestriatus*, *J Toxicol Clin Toxicol* 33:79, 1995.
32. Bond GR: Antivenin administration for *Centruroides* scorpion sting: risks and benefits, *Ann Emerg Med* 21:788, 1992.
33. Bucaretchi F et al: A comparative study of severe scorpion envenomation in children caused by *Tityus bahiensis* and *Tityus serrulatus*, *Rev Inst Med Trop Sao Paulo* 37:331, 1995.
34. Calderon-Aranda ES, Hozbor D, Possani LD: Neutralizing capacity of murine sera induced by different antigens of scorpion venom, *Toxicon* 31:327, 1993.
35. Campos JA et al: Signs, symptoms and treatment of severe scorpion poisoning in children. In Eaker D, Wadstrom T, editors: *Natural toxins*, Oxford, UK, 1980, Pergamon Press.
36. Carbonaro PA, Janniger CK, Schwartz RA: Scorpion sting reactions, *Cutis* 57:139, 1996.
37. Chavez-Olortegui C et al: Neutralizing capacity of antibodies elicited by a non-toxic protein purified from the venom of the scorpion *Tityus serrulatus*, *Toxicon* 35:213, 1997.
38. Clark RF et al: Abnormal eye movements encountered following severe envenomation by *Centruroides sculpturatus*, *Neurology* 41:604, 1991.
39. Correa MM et al: Biochemical and histopathological alterations induced in rats by *Tityus serrulatus* scorpion venom and its major neurotoxin tityustoxin-1, *Toxicon* 35:1053, 1997.
40. Curry SC et al: Envenomation by the scorpion *Centruroides sculpturatus*, *J Toxicol Clin Toxicol* 21:417, 1983-1984.
41. Daisley H, Alexander D, Pitt-Miller P: Acute myocarditis following *Tityus trinitatis* envenoming: morphological and pathophysiological characteristics, *Toxicon* 37:159, 1999.
42. Das S et al: Cardiac involvement and scorpion envenomation in children, *J Trop Pediatr* 41:338, 1995.
43. Das S et al: Scorpion envenomation in children in southern India, *J Trop Med Hyg* 98:306, 1995.
44. DeBin JA, Strichartz GR: Chloride channel inhibition by the venom of the scorpion *Leiurus quinquestriatus*, *Toxicon* 29:1403, 1991.
45. De Haro L, Jouglard J, David JM: Scorpion bites in southern France: experience at the poison-control centre of Marseilles, *Presse Med* 25:600, 1996.
46. Dehesa-Davila M, Possani LD: Scorpionism and serotherapy in Mexico, *Toxicon* 32:1015, 1994.
47. Demain JG, Goetz DW: Immediate, late, and delayed skin test responses to Centruroides vittatus scorpion venom, *J Allergy Clin Immunol* 95:135, 1995.
48. De Rezende NA, Chavez-Olortegui C, Amaral CFS: Is the severity of *Tityus serrulatus* scorpion envenoming related to plasma venom concentrations? *Toxicon* 34:820, 1996.
49. De Rezende NA et al: Efficacy of antivenom therapy for neutralizing circulating venom antigens in patients stung by *Tityus serrulatus* scorpions, *Am J Trop Med Hyg* 52:277, 1995.
50. De Sousa L et al: Scorpion sting epidemiology in Montes municipality of the state of Sucre, Venezuela: geographic distribution, *Rev Inst Med Trop Sao Paulo* 38:147, 1996.
51. Devaux C, Fourquet P, Granier C: A conserved sequence region of scorpion toxins rendered immunogenic induces broadly cross-reactive, neutralizing antibodies, *Eur J Biochem* 242:727, 1996.
52. Devaux C et al: Monoclonal antibodies neutralizing the toxin II from *Androctonus australis hector* scorpion venom: usefulness of a synthetic, non-toxic analog, *FEBS Lett* 412:456, 1997.
53. Dorce VAC, Sandoval MRL: Effects of *Tityus serrulatus* crude venom on the GABA-ergic and dopaminergic systems of the rat brain, *Toxicon* 32:1641, 1994.
54. D'Suze G et al: *Tityus discrepans* venom produces a respiratory distress syndrome in rabbits through an indirect mechanism, *Toxicon* 37:173, 1999.
55. Dudin AA et al: Scorpion sting in children in the Jerusalem area: a review of 54 cases, *Ann Trop Pediatr* 11:217, 1991.
56. El-Amin EO: Issues in management of scorpion sting in children, *Toxicon* 30:111, 1992.
57. El-Amin EO et al: Scorpion sting: a management problem, *Ann Trop Pediatr* 11:143, 1991.
58. Fatani AJ, Furman BL, Zeitlin IJ: The involvement of plasma kinins in the cardiovascular effects of *Leiurus quinquestriatus* scorpion venom in anaesthetised rabbits, *Toxicon* 36:523, 1998.
59. Fletcher PL et al: Action of new world scorpion venom and its neurotoxins in secretion, *Toxicon* 34:1399, 1996.
60. Freire-Maia L, Campos JA: Response to the letter to the editor by Gueron and Ovsyshcher on the treatment of the cardiovascular manifestations of scorpion envenomation, *Toxicon* 25:125, 1987.
61. Freire-Maia L, Campos JA, Amaral CFS: Approaches to the treatment of scorpion envenoming, *Toxicon* 32:1009, 1994.
62. Gambir IS, Singh DS, Pattnaik DN: Stroke in a young woman, *Postgrad Med J* 74:555, 1998.

63. Garcia ML, Hanner M, Kaczorowski G: Scorpion toxins: tools for studying K+ channels, *Toxicon* 36:1641, 1998.

64. Gateau T, Bloom M, Clark R: Response to specific *Centruroides sculpturatus* antivenom in 151 cases of scorpion stings, *J Toxicol Clin Toxicol* 32:165, 1994.

65. George Angus LD et al: Chronic relapsing pancreatitis from a scorpion sting in Trinidad, *Ann Trop Pediatr* 15:285, 1995.

66. Gibly R et al: Continuous intravenous midazolam infusions for *Centruroides exilicauda* envenomations, *Ann Emerg Med* 34:620, 1999.

67. Gonzalez D: Epidemiological and clinical aspects of certain venomous animals of Spain, *Toxicon* 20:925, 1982.

68. Gordon D et al: Functional anatomy of scorpion toxins affecting sodium channels, *J Toxicol Toxin Rev* 17:131, 1998.

69. Goyffon M, Vachon M, Broglio N: Epidemiological and clinical characteristics of the scorpion envenomation in Tunisia, *Toxicon* 20:337, 1982.

70. Groshong TD: Scorpion envenomation in eastern Saudi Arabia, *Ann Emerg Med* 22:1431, 1993.

71. Grosswasser Z, Grosswasswer-Reider I, Korn C: Biopercular lesions and acquired mutism in a young patient, *Brain Injury* 5:331, 1991.

72. Gueron M, Ilia R: Non-cardiogenic pulmonary oedema after scorpion envenomation: a true entity? *Toxicon* 34:393, 1996.

73. Gueron M, Ilia R, Sofer S: The cardiovascular system after scorpion envenomation. A review, *J Toxicol Clin Toxicol* 30:245, 1992.

74. Gueron M, Ovsyshcher I: What is the treatment for the cardiovascular manifestations of scorpion envenomation? *Toxicon* 25:121, 1987.

75. Gueron M, Sofer S: Vasodilators and calcium blocking agents as treatment of cardiovascular manifestations of human scorpion envenomation, *Toxicon* 28:127, 1990.

76. Gueron M, Sofer S: Scorpion envenomation and the heart, *J Wilderness Med* 2:175, 1991.

77. Gueron M, Sofer S: The role of the intensivist in the treatment of the cardiovascular manifestations of scorpion envenomation, *Toxicon* 32:1027, 1994.

78. Gueron M, Weizman S: Catecholamine excretion in scorpion sting, *Isr J Med Sci* 5:855, 1969.

79. Gueron M, Yarom R: Cardiovascular manifestations of severe scorpion sting: clinicopathologic correlations, *Chest* 57:156, 1970.

80. Gueron M et al: Renin and aldosterone levels and hypertension following envenomation in humans by the yellow scorpion *Leiurus quinquestriatus*, *Toxicon* 30:765, 1992.

81. Gueron M et al: The management of scorpion envenomation 1993, *Toxicon* 31:1071, 1993.

82. Guieu R et al: Use of dantrolene in experimental scorpion envenomation by *Androctonus australis hector*, *Arch Toxicol* 69:575, 1995.

83. Gwee MCE et al: The black scorpion *Heterometrus longimanus*: pharmacological and biochemical investigation of the venom, *Toxicon* 31:1305, 1993.

84. Herschkovich Y et al: Criteria map audit of scorpion envenomation in the Negev, Israel, *Toxicon* 23:845, 1985.

85. Hutt MJ, Houghton PJ: A survey from the literature of plants used to treat scorpion stings, *J Ethnopharmacol* 60:97, 1998.

86. Ismail M: Serotherapy of the scorpion envenoming syndrome is irrationally convicted without trial, *Toxicon* 31:1077, 1993.

87. Ismail M: The treatment of the scorpion envenoming syndrome: the Saudi experience with serotherapy, *Toxicon* 32:1019, 1994.

88. Ismail M: The scorpion envenoming syndrome, *Toxicon* 33:825, 1995.

89. Ismail M, Abd-Elsalam MA: Are the toxicological effects of scorpion envenomation related to tissue venom concentration? *Toxicon* 26:233, 1988.

90. Ismail M, Abd-Elsalam MA, Al-Ahaidib MS: *Androctonus crassicauda* (Oliver), a dangerous and unduly neglected scorpion. I. Pharmacological and clinical studies, *Toxicon* 32:1599, 1994.

91. Ismail M, Abd-Elsalam MA, Al-Ahaidib MS: Pharmacokinetics of 125I-labelled *Walterinnesia aigyptia* venom and its specific antivenins: flash absorption and distribution of the venom and its toxin versus slow absorption and distribution of IgG, F(ab')₂ and F(ab) of the antivenin, *Toxicon* 36:93, 1998.

92. Ismail M, Abd-Elsalam MA, Morad AM: Do changes in body temperature following envenomation by the scorpion *Leiurus quinquestriatus* influence the course of toxicity? *Toxicon* 28:1265, 1990.

93. Ismail M, Fatani JY, Dabees TT: Experimental treatment protocols for scorpion envenomation: a review of common therapies and an effect of kallikrein-kinin inhibitors, *Toxicon* 30:1257, 1992.

94. Karnad DR: Haemodynamic patterns in patients with scorpion envenomation, *Heart* 79:485, 1998.

95. Kolecki P: Inadvertent methamphetamine poisoning in pediatric patients, *Pediatr Emerg Care* 14:385, 1998.

96. Krifi MN, El Ayeb M, Dellagi K: New procedures and parameters for better evaluation of *Androctonus australis garzonii* (Aag) and *Buthus occitanus tunetanus* (Bot) scorpion envenomations and specific serotherapy treatment, *Toxicon* 34:257, 1996.

97. Krifi MN et al: Improvement and standardization of antivenoms sera, *Archs Inst Pasteur Tunis* 69:253, 1992.

98. Krifi MN et al: Development of an ELISA for the detection of scorpion venoms in sera of humans envenomed by *Androctonus australis garzonii* (Aag) and *Buthus occitanus tunetanus* (Bot): correlation with clinical severity of envenoming in Tunisia, *Toxicon* 36:887, 1998.

99. Kumar EB et al: Scorpion venom cardiomyopathy, *Am Heart J* 123:725, 1992.

100. Lee NC: Scorpion stings, *S Afr Med J* 79:120, 1991.

101. Leynadier F et al: Allergic reactions to North African scorpion venom evaluated by skin test and specific IgE, *J Allergy Clin Immunol* 99:851, 1997.

102. Licea AF, Becerril B, Possani LD: Fab fragments of the monoclonal antibody BCF2 are capable of neutralizing the whole soluble venom from the scorpion *Centruroides noxius* Hoffmann, *Toxicon* 34:843, 1996.

103. Longenecker GL, Longenecker BE: *Centruroides sculpturatus* venom and platelet reactivity: possible role in scorpion venom-induced defibrination syndrome, *Toxicon* 19:153, 1981.

104. Longenecker GL et al: Inhibition of the angiotensin converting enzyme by venom of the scorpion *Centruroides sculpturatus*, *Toxicon* 18:667, 1980.

105. LoVecchio F et al: Incidence of immediate and delayed hypersensitivity to *Centruroides* antivenin, *Ann Emerg Med* 34:615, 1999.

106. Martin CM: Scorpions and centipedes of the Hawaiian islands: their medical significance, *Hawaii Med J* 30:95, 1971.

107. Mazzei de Davila C et al: Scorpion envenomation in Merida, Venezuela, *Toxicon* 35:1459, 1997.

108. Mazzotti L, Bravo-Becherelle MA: Scorpionism in the Mexican Republic. In Keegan H, MacFarlane W, editors: *Venomous and poisonous animals and noxious plants of the Pacific region*, New York, 1963, Pergamon Press.

109. Moreira-Ferreira AMB et al: In vivo protection against *Tityus serrulatus* scorpion toxins by immunization of mice with a non-toxic protein, *Toxicon* 36:333, 1998.

110. Muller GJ: Scorpionism in South Africa, *S Afr Med J* 83:405, 1993.

111. Murthy KRK, Hase NK: Scorpion envenoming and the role of insulin, *Toxicon* 32:1041, 1994.

112. Murthy KRK, Zare MA: Effect of Indian red scorpion (*Mesobuthus tamulus concanesis*, Pocock) venom on thyroxine and triiodothyronine in experimental acute myocarditis and its reversal by species specific antivenom, *Indian J Exp Biol* 3 6:16, 1998.

113. Murthy KRK et al: Insulin reverses haemodynamic changes and pulmonary oedema in children stung by the Indian red scorpion *Mesobuthus tamulus concanesis*, Pocock, *Ann Trop Med Parasitol* 85:651, 1991.

114. Nagorka AR, Bergeson PS: Infant methamphetamine toxicity posing as scorpion envenomation, *Pediatr Emerg Care* 14:350, 1998.

115. Naqvi R et al: Acute renal failure developing after a scorpion sting, *Br J Urol* 82:295, 1998.

116. Neale JR: Scorpion sting syndrome in eastern Riyadh, *Ann Saudi Med* 10:383, 1990.

117. Nishikawa AK et al: Antigenic cross-reactivity among the venoms from several species of Brazilian scorpions, *Toxicon* 32:989, 1994.

118. Nishioka SDA, Silveira PVP, Pereira CAD: Scorpion sting on the penis, *J Urol* 150:1501, 1993.

119. Nishioka SDA et al: Scorpion sting with cranial nerve involvement, *Toxicon* 30:685, 1992.

120. Nouira S et al: Right ventricular dysfunction following severe scorpion envenomation, *Chest* 108:682, 1995.

121. Radmanesh M: *Androctonus crassicauda* sting and its clinical study in Iran, *J Trop Med Hyg* 93:323, 1990.

122. Radmanesh M: Clinical study of *Hemiscorpion lepturus* in Iran, *J Trop Med Hyg* 93:327, 1990.

123. Rahav G, Weiss AT: Scorpion sting-induced pulmonary edema: scintigraphic evidence of cardiac dysfunction, *Chest* 97:1478, 1990.

124. Rai M et al: Intracerebral hemorrhage following scorpion bite, *Neurology* 40:1801, 1990.

125. Revelo MP et al: Body distribution of *Tityus serrulatus* scorpion venom in mice and effects of scorpion antivenom, *Toxicon* 34:1119, 1996.

126. Rezende NA, Amaral CFS, Freire-Maia L: Immunotherapy for scorpion envenoming in Brazil, *Toxicon* 36:1507, 1998.

127. Rogers DF: Scorpion venoms: taking the sting out of lung disease, *Thorax* 51:546, 1996.

128. Rowan EG et al: The effects of Indian red scorpion *Buthus tamulus* venom *in vivo* and *in vitro, Toxicon* 30:1157, 1992.

129. Russell FE: Venomous arthropods, *Vet Hum Toxicol* 33:505, 1991.

130. Santana GC et al: Pharmacokinetics of *Tityus serrulatus* scorpion venom determined by enzyme-linked immunosorbent assay in the rat, *Toxicon* 34:1063, 1996.

131. Shapira MY, Haviv YS, Sviri S: Second degree atrio-ventricular block and cardiotoxicity secondary to envenomation by the scorpion *Leiurus quinquestriatus* ('yellow scorpion')—an indication for serotherapy? *Hum Exp Toxicol* 17:541, 1998.

132. Sofer S: Scorpion envenomation, *Intensive Care Med* 21:626, 1995.

133. Sofer S, Gueron M: Vasodilators and hypertensive encephalopathy following scorpion envenomation in children, *Chest* 97:118, 1990.

134. Sofer S, Gueron M: Respiratory failure in children following envenomation by the scorpion *Leiurus quinquestriatus:* hemodynamic and neurological aspects, *Toxicon* 26:931, 1998.

135. Sofer S, Shahak E, Gueron M: Scorpion envenomation and antivenom therapy, *J Pediatr* 124:973, 1994.

136. Sofer S et al: Myocardial injury without heart failure following envenomation by the scorpion *Leiurus quinquestriatus* in children, *Toxicon* 29:382, 1991.

137. Sofer S et al: Acute pancreatitis in children following envenomation by the yellow scorpion *Leiurus quinquestriatus, Toxicon* 29:125, 1991.

138. Sofer S et al: Interieukin-6 release following scorpion sting in children, *Toxicon* 34:389, 1996.

139. Sofer S et al: Scorpion venom leads to gastrointestinal ischemia despite increased oxygen delivery in pigs, *Crit Care Med* 25:834, 1997.

140. Southcott RV: Some harmful Australian arthropods, *Med J Aust* 145:590, 1986.

141. Stahnke HL: Arizona's lethal scorpion, *Ariz Med* 29:490, 1972.

142. Stipetic ME et al: A prospective analysis of 558 common striped scorpion (*Centruroides vittatus*) envenomations in Texas during 1997, *J Toxicol Clin Toxicol* 36:461, 1998 (abstract).

143. Theakston RDG, Warrell DA: Antivenoms: a list of hyperimmune sera currently available for the treatment of envenoming by bites and stings, *Toxicon* 29:1419, 1991.

144. Toppa NH et al: Effect of *Tityus serrulatus* scorpion toxin on serum gastrin levels in anaesthetized rat, *Toxicon* 36:1833, 1998.

145. Trestrail JH: Scorpion envenomation in Michigan: three cases of toxic encounters with poisonous stow-aways, *Vet Hum Toxicol* 23:8, 1981.

146. Vatanpour H, Rowan EG, Harvey AL: Effects of scorpion (*Buthus tamulus*) venom on neuromuscular transmission in vitro, *Toxicon* 31:1373, 1993.

147. Wang R et al: Cardiovascular effects of *Buthus martensii* (Karsch) scorpion venom, *Toxicon* 32:191, 1994.

148. Warrell DA: Prazosin: scorpion envenoming and the cardiovascular system, *Trop Doct* 27:1, 1997.

149. Welch S, Thomas R: Anaphylaxis from a *Centruroides sculpturatus* envenomation, *J Toxicol Clin Toxicol* 36:461, 1998 (abstract).

150. Yarom R: Scorpion venom: a tutorial review of its effects in men and experimental animals, *J Toxicol Clin Toxicol* 3:561, 1970.

36 North American Arthropod Envenomation and Parasitism

Sherman A. Minton,† H. Bernard Bechtel, and Timothy B. Erickson

The phylum Arthropoda contains about four fifths of the known animals of the world, and insects are the largest group of arthropods. Insects are an important part of the biota of all terrestrial and freshwater environments that support life; only in marine environments are they relatively unimportant. More species of insects exist than of any other form of multicellular life, and they may well exceed all other land animals in biomass. Insects can use most animal and plant substances as food, and their feeding plays a vital role in recycling organic compounds. They compete with other organisms for the world's food supplies but are themselves a major food source for many forms of life. They are essential for the pollination of many plants. Insect life cycles are diverse and often complex, involving developmental and sexual stages that are widely different in morphology and ways of life. Although sexual reproduction is the rule, parthenogenesis (unisexual reproduction) and pedogenesis occur. Some groups, such as ants, bees, and termites, have developed a high degree of social organization. During at least part of its life cycle, an insect's body is divided into three distinct regions (head, thorax, and abdomen), with three pairs of legs attached to the thorax. Except for a few primitive or parasitic groups, most adult insects have wings.

The greatest direct medical importance of insects is associated with their feeding on human blood and tissue fluids. In doing so, they often inject salivary secretions. This is a highly effective method of transmitting pathogenic microorganisms; moreover, the secretions are often allergenic and sometimes toxic. Other insects may carry human pathogens passively on their feet or mouthparts or in their digestive tracts.

Venoms have evolved in several insect groups, and venomous insects may attack humans, sometimes with lethal results. Skin, hair, and secretions of insects may be irritant or allergenic, producing cutaneous and respiratory syndromes. Finally, insects can be highly annoying.

HYMENOPTERA (BEES, WASPS, AND ANTS)

By far the most important venomous insects are members of the order Hymenoptera, including bees,

wasps, and ants (Figure 36-1). They vary in size from minute to large (up to 60 mm in body length). The abdomen and thorax are connected by a slender pedicle that may be quite long in certain wasps and ants. Bees and most wasps are winged as adults; ants are wingless, except for sexually mature adults during part of the life cycle. Mouthparts are adapted for chewing but in some species are modified for sucking. The life cycle includes egg, larva, and pupa stages before emergence of adults. Immature stages may be protected and provided with food by the adult. Both animal and plant foods are used. Many species are parasitic on other arthropods. All ants and many species of bees and wasps are social insects. Colonies range in size from a few dozen individuals to many thousands. In cold climates, most individuals die in autumn, leaving the fertilized females to winter over and found new colonies in the spring.

Bees

The honeybee (*Apis mellifera*) is one of the few domesticated insects and is maintained in hives in many countries (Figure 36-2). Numerous geographic races of the honeybee exist; the Italian bee (*A. m. ligustica*), a common domestic strain of Europe, is also widely distributed in the United States. Feral honeybee colonies usually nest in hollow trees or crevices in rocks but may nest in the walls of occupied buildings.

An event of considerable health and economic significance in the Americas was the introduction of an African race of the honeybee (*A. m. scutellata*, also referred to as *A. m. adansoni*). This race was introduced from Africa into Brazil because it was thought to be a more efficient honey producer in the tropics. It is characterized by large populations (one queen may lay tens of thousands of eggs), frequent swarming (6 to 12 swarms a year), nonstop flights of at least 20 km, and a tendency toward mass attacks on humans after minimal provocation. As a result, these Africanized honeybees, also known as "killer bees," are much more aggressive than typical Hymenoptera. They attack in swarms of hundreds and chase their victims much greater distances from the hive than does any other species.[54,57]

The first escapes from hives occurred in the state of São Paulo in 1957, and the "Brazilian killer bees,"

---

†Deceased.

863

or "Africanized bees," have spread widely. These bees are actually hybrids between A. *scutellata* and European honeybee races. Cold climate seems to have stopped their southern spread in Argentina, but they have moved steadily northward at 200 to 300 miles per year and in October 1990 reached the southern border of the United States. By mid-1991, 103 swarms had been captured in southern Texas. Populations are established in Arizona, New Mexico, and California.[108] Future populations may eventually be distrib-

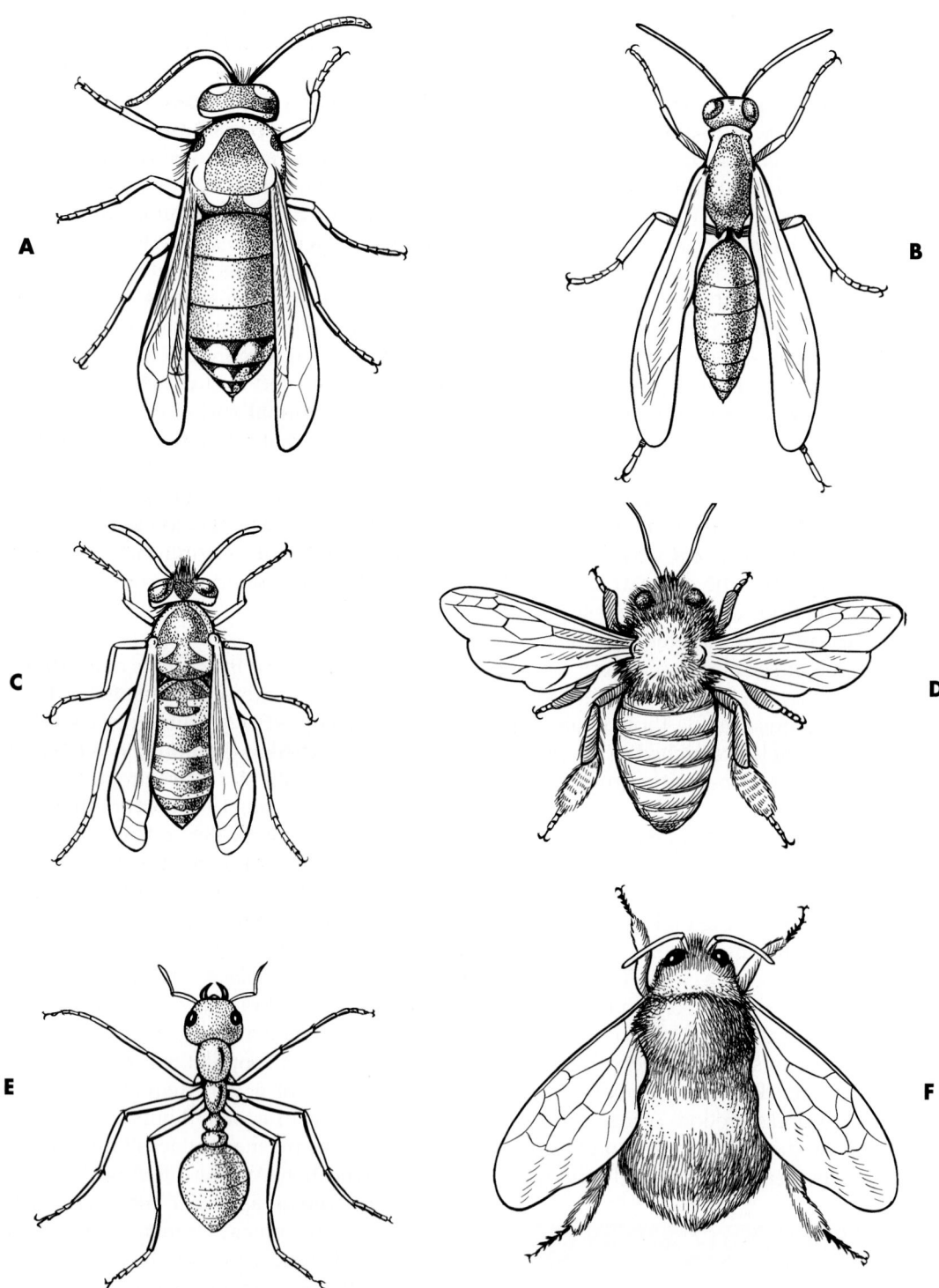

Figure 36-1 Representative venomous Hymenoptera: **A,** hornet *(Vespula maculatal)*; **B,** wasp *(Chlorion ichneumerea)*; **C,** yellowjacket *(Vespula maculiforma)*; **D,** honeybee *(Apis mellifera)*; **E,** fire ant *(Solenopsis invicta)*; **F,** bumblebee *(Bombus species)*.

uted as far east as North Carolina.[133] At least four human deaths have occurred from multiple stings. Unless the bees acquire greater resistance to winter conditions, their range will be confined to the southern third of the United States and may also be restricted by scarcity of suitable flowers in the arid Southwest. The greatest impact of Africanized bees in the United States will probably be economic, related to decreased honey production and less effective pollination of crops. The bees also present a threat to human health. Africanized bee colonies are extremely sensitive to disturbance, respond faster in greater numbers, and are up to 10 times more active in stinging than European bees. The quantity of venom per sting is slightly less in African bees, however, with no significant biochemical or allergenic difference between the venoms.[75,83,110] About 50 simultaneous stings can cause systemic envenomation, and an estimated 500 are necessary to cause death by direct toxicity.[53]

About 350 fatal attacks have been documented worldwide, of which at least 70 occurred in Venezuela during 1977 and 1978. More than 300 bee

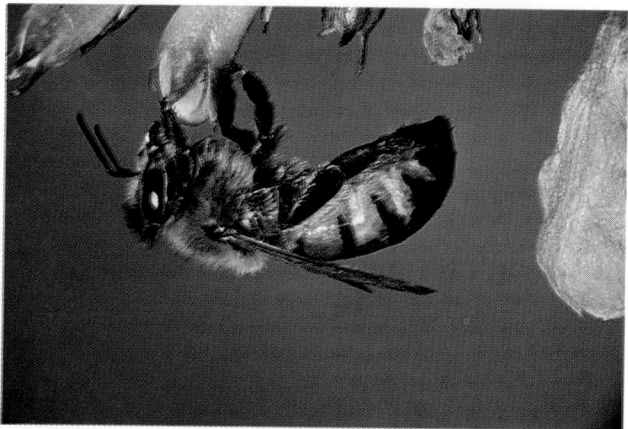

Figure 36-2 Worker honeybee.

attacks occurred in Mexico between 1987 and 1992, with 49 fatalities.[82] A more recent account puts the fatalities at 190, with future estimates of 60 deaths per year.[108] Since Mexico and the southern United States have many feral and domestic honeybee populations, researchers thought that the aggressiveness of the African bees could be dampened by hybridization. Large numbers of male European bees were released to facilitate this, and African queens were replaced by European stock when possible. Recent studies indicate, however, that European bee populations are becoming rapidly Africanized with little reciprocal gene flow, as African females take over European hives.[43,117,134]

Bumblebees (*Bombus* and related genera) are a largely holarctic group often found in quite cold environments. Small colonies usually nest just under the surface of the ground, often in mammal burrows. Some species are aggressive if disturbed, although most have mild dispositions.

Sweat bees (family Halictidae) are small bees of cosmopolitan distribution. They are attracted to sweaty skin and ingest perspiration. They nest in burrows, often in clay banks. Females sting if squeezed or trapped under clothing. The sting is not very painful, but anaphylactic reactions have been reported. The allergens are immunologically unrelated to those in other bee and wasp venoms.[86]

Wasps

Social wasps occur throughout most of the world but are recognized as a medical problem chiefly in the United States and Europe. They often establish colonies close to human dwellings. Yellowjackets (*Vespula* species) may be more important than honeybees as a cause of human stings in the northeastern United States (Figure 36-3). They make underground nests in rotted-out tree stumps, cavities under stones, and mammal burrows. They are strongly attracted to garbage. Paper

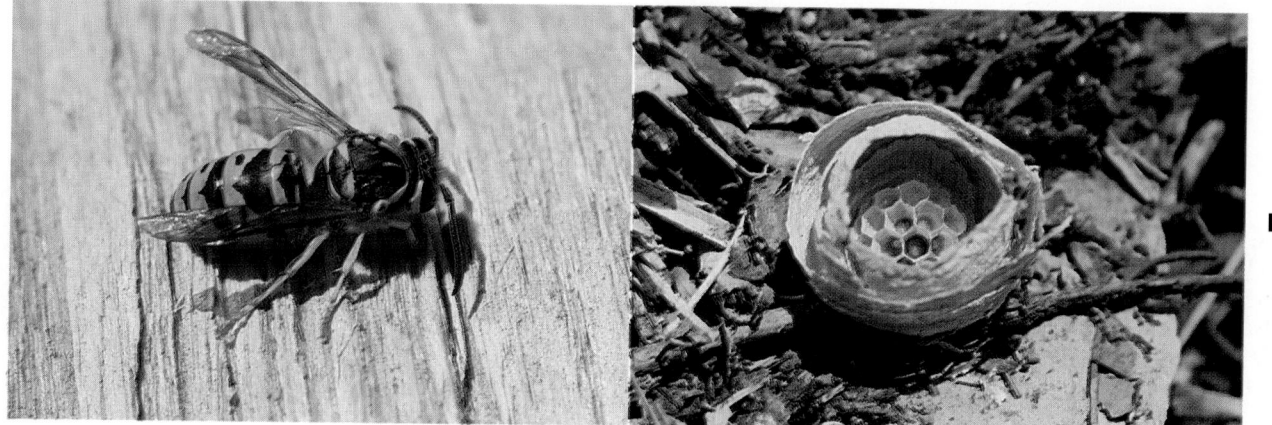

Figure 36-3 **A,** Yellowjacket *(Vespula maculiforma).* **B,** Early nest of yellowjacket.

wasps *(Polistes)* suspend their nests in shaded places, often in shrubbery near houses or below eaves, gutters, or window frames (Figure 36-4). Old World hornets *(Vespa* species) and white-faced hornets *(Dolchiovespula maculata)* create large paper nests that may be plastered to buildings but more typically are hung from tree branches (Figure 36-5).

Solitary wasps are predators, feeding largely on other insects and spiders. Adults often carry the prey alive and paralyzed to the nest as food for the larvae. Some wasps excavate burrows, whereas others make mud nests that may be plastered on shaded walls of buildings or under bridges. Although many nests may be grouped together, the adult wasps have no social organization and make little effort to defend them. The cicada killers *(Specius speciosus)* and tarantula hawks *(Pepsis* species) are among the largest North American wasps. Velvet ants (family Mutillidae) are actually wingless wasp females that are nest parasites of other Hymenoptera (Figure 36-6). They occur in deserts and other dry and open habitat and can inflict a painful sting.

Ants

Ants are social insects, worldwide in distribution over a wide range of habitats. Many ants sting, and others have repugnant secretions. The ant species of greatest medical significance in the United States is the imported fire ant *Solenopsis invicta* (see Figure 36-1, *E*). It apparently was introduced from South America into Mobile, Alabama, in 1939 and has subsequently spread throughout the southern states from southeastern Virginia to central Texas and Oklahoma, largely eliminating another introduced fire ant *(S. richteri)* and two native species. Mound nests are usually found in open grass settings, often in urban areas (Figure 36-7). Other states at risk of harboring fire ants include Arizona, California, New Mexico, Oregon, and Washington.[54] As many as 600 mounds per acre have been reported.

Worker colonies may reach a maximum size of 500,000 ants in 2 years and rapidly give rise to satellite colonies.[118] *S. invicta* is an extremely irritable insect.

Harvester ants *(Pogonomyrmex)* of the southwestern United States and Mexico are of some medical impor-

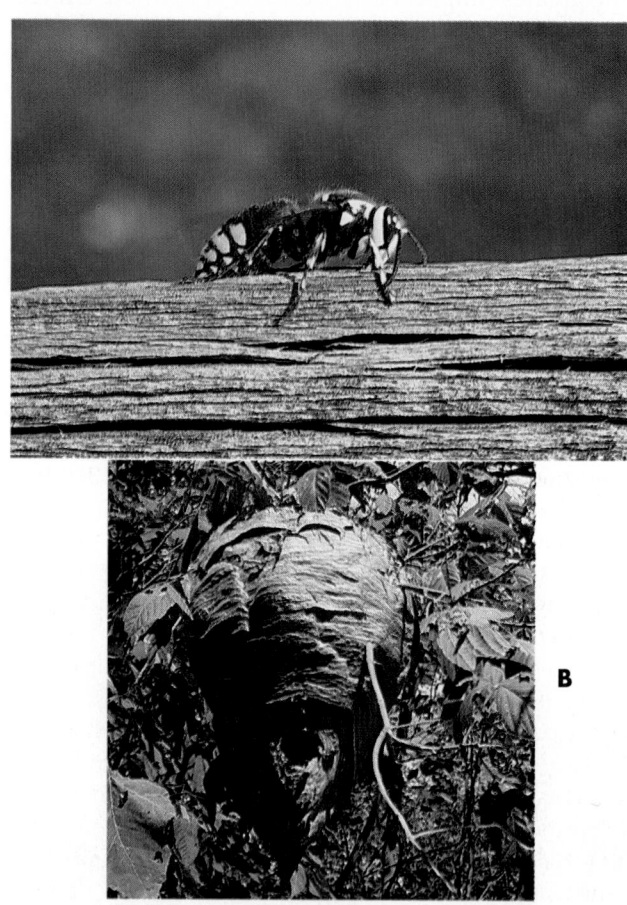

Figure 36-5 **A,** White-faced hornet, *Dolchiovespula maculata,* largest of the common social wasps in the United States. **B,** Typical nest of white-faced hornet.

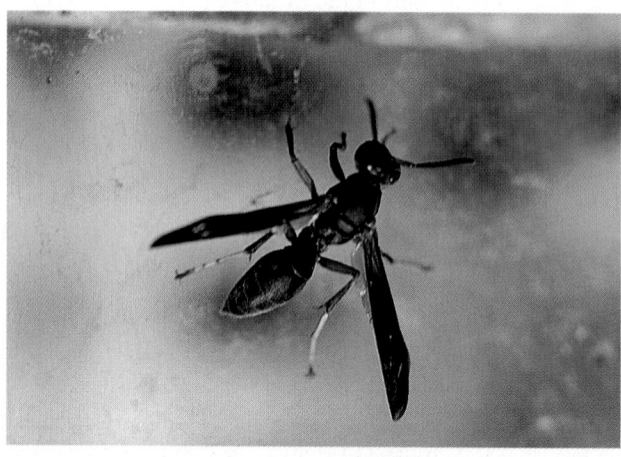

Figure 36-4 Paper *(Polistes)* wasp.

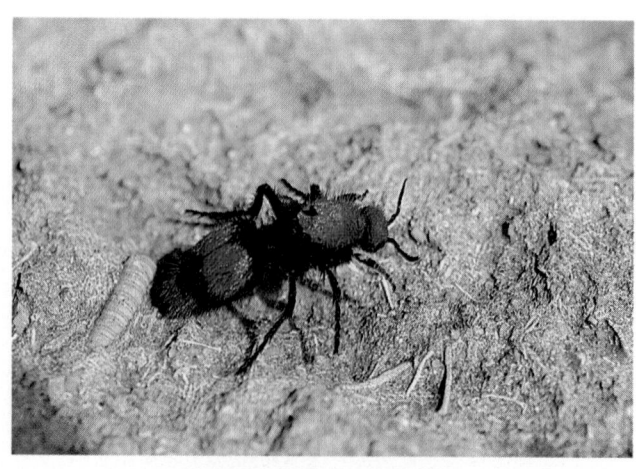

Figure 36-6 Velvet ant.

tance. Entrances to the underground nests are usually surrounded by clear zones and sometimes by rings of soil. Some species react aggressively to disturbance of the nest. The stings are painful and may be accompanied by systemic symptoms; anaphylaxis has been reported.

Stinging Patterns

Multiple stings often result from disturbance of a nest, as the first insects encountered release alarm pheromones that incite aggressive behavior in other members of the colony. With large species such as the white-faced hornet, 40 to 50 stings may create a life-threatening injury.[132] The lethal dose of honeybee venom has been estimated at 500 to 1400 stings.[114] In the United States and other Western nations the incidence of serious insect stings is higher in adults than in children and higher in males than in females. Most persons are stung while engaged in outdoor work or recreation. Beekeeping is a high-risk occupation; however, many beekeepers develop considerable immunity as a result of frequent stings. Other relatively high-risk occupations are farmer, house painter, carpenter, highway worker, and bulldozer operator. Fire ants may invade houses during periods of heavy rain and in hot, dry weather as they seek food and water.[23] Wasps and bees sometimes are swept into the interior of a moving automobile, exposing the occupants to risk of both a sting and a highway accident. Many foods, particularly meats, ripe fruit, or fruit syrups, attract yellowjackets; they often swarm around picnic areas and recycling bins. Syrups, flowers, sweat, and some perfumes attract bees. In such aggregations the insects are not particularly aggressive but may become trapped in clothing or hair. In temperate zones, the incidence of hymenopteran stings is highest in late summer and early fall, when insect populations are highest.[7]

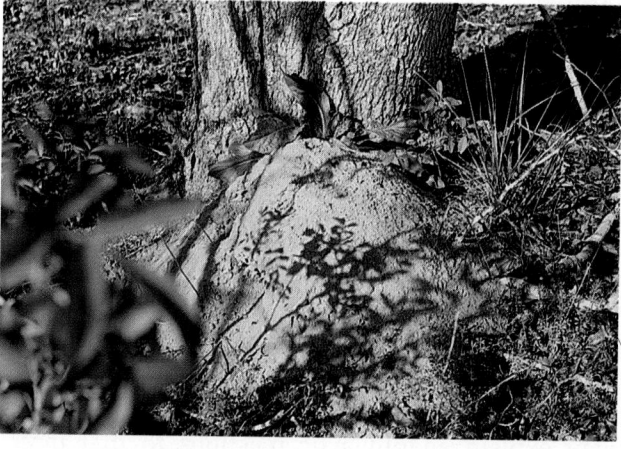

Figure 36-7 Fire ant mound.

Venom and Venom Apparatus

Venom is present in many hymenopteran species and is used for both defense and subjugation of prey. The venom apparatus is located at the posterior end of the abdomen and consists of venom glands, a reservoir, and structures for piercing the integument and injecting venom. Venoms of most medically important Hymenoptera are mixtures of protein or polypeptide toxins, enzymes, and pharmacologically active low-molecular-weight compounds such as histamine, serotonin, acetylcholine, and dopamine. Melittin, a strongly basic peptide, is the principal component of honeybee venom. It damages cell membranes through detergent-like action, with liberation of potassium and biogenic amines. Peptides with similar activity occur in bumblebee venom. Histamine release by bee venom appears to be largely mediated by mast cell degranulating (MCD) peptide. A third peptide, apamin, is a neurotoxin that acts principally on the spinal cord. Adolapin, a recently described bee venom peptide, has antiinflammatory activity, which may explain the effectiveness of bee venom in treating some forms of arthritis. The chief enzymes of bee venom are phospholipase A and hyaluronidase. The former is believed to be one of the major venom allergens and, with melittin, to account for much of the acute lethality. Histamine makes up about 3% of the dry weight of bee venom. The intravenous (IV) median lethal dose (LD_{50}) of honeybee venom for mice is 6 mg/kg. An average sting injects about 50 µl of venom containing approximately 0.05 mg of solids.

Intense pain after stings by hornets and other social wasps is largely caused by serotonin and acetylcholine, which constitute 1% to 5% of dry venom weight. Wasp kinins (peptides) contribute to pain production and have strong, brief hypotensive effects. Mastoparans are similar in action to MCD peptide but are weaker. Phospholipase A, phospholipase B, and hyaluronidase are present in relatively large amounts. Unidentified proteins, some of which appear to be major allergens, are also present. A lethal protein in *Vespa basalis* venom releases serotonin from tissue cells and has hemolytic and phospholipase A activity.[47] The IV LD_{50} of different hornet venoms for mice ranges from 1.6 to 4.1 mg/kg.

Less is known of venoms of solitary wasps. The venom of *Sceliphoron caementarium*, a mud dauber, is comparatively low in protein and contains no acetylcholine, histamine, serotonin, or kinins but contains several unidentified low-molecular-weight compounds. Its proteins are immunologically different from those of honeybee, yellowjacket, and paper wasp venoms. Philanthotoxin (molecular weight 435) from venom of the beewolf (*Philanthus triangulum*) acts at the insect's myoneural junction and has potential value as an insecticide.

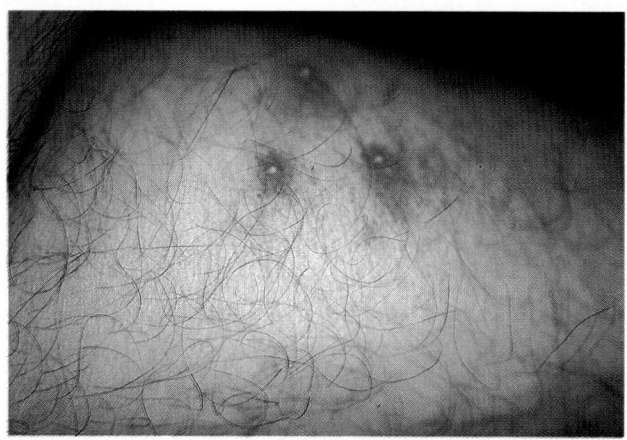

Figure 36-8 Fire ant lesions.

Ant venoms show great variation. Those of more primitive ants (subfamilies Ponerinae, Myrmicinae, and Dorylinae) resemble venoms of social wasps, containing kininlike peptides, enzymes, and unidentified proteins. In more highly evolved ants (subfamilies Dolichoderinae, and Formicinae) a variety of low-molecular-weight compounds (terpenes, ketones, and organic acids) make up the bulk of the secretion, which may be sprayed rather than injected. Venoms of fire ants (*Solenopsis* species) are composed largely of piperidine alkaloids, which cause histamine release and necrosis in human skin. Proteins make up only 0.1% of dry weight of fire ant venoms but are highly allergenic.[35] Hyaluronidase and phospholipase activities have been demonstrated.

Clinical Aspects

Hymenoptera stings are most often inflicted on the head and neck, followed by the foot, leg, hand, and arm. Stings in the mouth, pharynx, and esophagus may occur when bees or yellowjackets in soft drink or beer containers are accidentally ingested.[113] A single wasp, bee, or ant sting in a unsensitized individual usually causes instant pain, followed by a wheal and flare reaction, with variable edema. Fire ants typically grasp the skin with their mouthparts and inflict multiple stings. These produce vesicles that subsequently become sterile pustules (Figure 36-8). Multiple Hymenoptera stings may cause vomiting, diarrhea, generalized edema, dyspnea, hypotension, tachycardia, and collapse. Widespread necrosis of skeletal muscle with hyperkalemia, acute tubular necrosis with renal failure, hepatorenal syndrome with hemolysis, acute pancreatitis, and disseminated intravascular coagulation have been reported after multiple stings.[19,34,59,132] Myocardial infarction, atrial fibrillation, and cerebral infarction in previously healthy individuals may follow multiple hymenopteran stings.[63,99,130]

Large local reactions spreading more than 15 cm beyond the sting site and persisting more than 24 hours are relatively common. They represent a cell-mediated (type IV) immunologic reaction, although more than half these patients also have immunoglobulin E (IgE) antibody against venom or show a positive skin test. Later stings in these individuals usually result in another large local reaction; systemic reactions are rare.[136]

Allergy is the most serious aspect of hymenopteran stings. Anaphylaxis and related syndromes from this source are relatively common outdoor emergencies. An estimated 0.4% of the U.S. population shows some clinical degree of allergy to insect venoms, and 40 to 50 deaths are reported annually.[95] Fatal anaphylaxis due to fire ant stings has also been reported.[90] Asymptomatic sensitization, as shown by positive venom skin test, was observed in 15% of 269 randomly selected subjects with no history of allergic sting reaction.[41] Sensitization is transient but may persist for years. These individuals are at higher risk of systemic allergic reactions than those with negative skin tests.[40]

Sudden death from insect sting may not always be recognized. Of 142 sera obtained after sudden, unexpected death, 23% contained elevated levels of IgE to at least one insect venom. In contrast, 6% of sera from 92 blood donors contained comparable IgE levels. In eight fatal cases of Hymenoptera sting anaphylaxis, IgE to the putative venom source was elevated in all, although levels were not higher than those of some healthy individuals in the same population.[112] Anti–fire ant IgE and elevated serum tryptase were detected in a case of fatal fire ant sting.[81] Elevated levels of venom-specific IgE were detected in two fatal cases of wasp sting.[124]

Wasp and bee venoms contain 9 to 13 antigens, some of which are potent allergens. Available evidence indicates little cross-sensitization between honeybee and wasp venoms. About 50% cross-sensitization occurs between *Polistes* and other social wasp venoms, and nearly 100% between yellowjacket and hornet venoms. Positive radioallergosorbent test (RAST) reactions to imported fire ant venom were seen in 51% of patients allergic to bee and wasp venoms but without exposure to fire ants. The allergen appears to be identical to antigen 5 of wasp venoms.[48]

Examination of sera of hypersensitive individuals for IgE and IgG antibodies against purified venom proteins indicates that phospholipase A, hyaluronidase, and acid phosphatase are important in honeybee venom, whereas phospholipase A, antigen 5, and hyaluronidase are important in wasp venoms. Antigen 5, a nontoxic protein of unknown activity, is reported to have sequence similarity to mammalian testis, human brain tumor, and certain plant leaf proteins. This may explain anaphylactic reactions to first insect stings.[58,131] Despite the small amount of protein in fire ant venoms, about 12% of persons treated for fire ant stings show systemic allergic reactions, and 32 anaphylactic deaths have been confirmed. Four antigens in *Solenopsis invicta* venom have been reported to be allergenic.[12]

Allergic sting reactions occur remote from the sting site and include flushing, pruritus, hives, and angioedema. In life-threatening reactions, marked respiratory distress with airway edema, hypotension, loss of consciousness, and cardiac arrhythmias may be seen. At least half the severe reactions occur within 10 minutes after a sting, and virtually all occur within 5 hours. Most fatalities occur within 1 hour. The interval between the first known sting and the reaction-producing sting is usually less than 3 years but may be as long as 48 years. In a group of 3236 Hymenoptera-allergic individuals, 61.5% were males and 32.3% had a history of atopy. The mean age was 30.5 years. No correlation existed between systemic reactions and number of stings in the past or number of stings per incident and severity of a systemic reaction.[67] In a series of 138 adults with a history of insect sting anaphylactic reactions, 99 had no anaphylactic reactions to later stings, 17 had more severe reactions, and 22 had mild to moderate reactions.[127] In another series of 90 adults with previous anaphylactic reactions, 60 had similar reactions when restung, and 23 had more severe reactions.[94] In children 10 years and younger, life-threatening reactions occur less often than in adults, and repeated sting episodes usually are not increasingly severe. However, 17% of children with a history of systemic bee or wasp sting reactions developed a systemic reaction after a sting challenge test, as did 5% of children who sustained a sting in the field.[44]

Fatalities that occur within the first hour after a sting result from airway obstruction, hypotension, or both. In 69% of fatal cases, obstruction of the respiratory tree by edema or secretions was the principal finding at autopsy; in 12%, vascular pathology was the principal finding; and 7% of the victims had primary central nervous system involvement such as petechial hemorrhages, infarction, and cerebral edema.[4] Hemostatic defects, including reduction of all clotting factors and release of a thrombin inhibitor, may be seen with insect sting anaphylaxis. Severe fetal brain damage, presumably associated with hypoxia, has been reported. Delayed (3 to 14 days) atypical reactions after hymenopteran stings include serum sickness and Arthus reaction, which are caused by systemic and local effects of antigen-antibody complexes; nephrotic syndrome; thrombocytopenic purpura; grand mal and focal motor seizures; transient cerebral ischemic attacks; Guillain-Barré syndrome; and progressive demyelinating neurologic disease. Most appear to be immunologically mediated. In one series, elevated IgE to bee or yellowjacket venom was observed in 6 of 13 such patients.[64,74]

Identification of the individual with potentially dangerous allergy to hymenopteran sting is not always possible. Skin testing with hymenopteran venoms is the most sensitive method; RAST for IgE antibody to venoms is less sensitive.[59] A small but significant number of individuals with no history of sting reactions have IgE antibody specific for hymenopteran venoms; prevalence of this antibody is higher in summer.[139] These methods do not identify all at risk, and antibody levels do not correlate with severity of sting reactions. In a significant number of individuals, particularly children, clinical sensitivity disappears and IgE levels fall virtually to zero 3 to 18 months after a reaction-producing sting. In about 40% of cases, sensitivity may disappear within 3 years.[62] Venom antibody (both IgE and IgG) may be found in healthy individuals (40% of beekeepers, 12% of blood donors) with no history of systemic reaction to insect stings.

Treatment and Prevention

Treatment of anaphylaxis is conventional. Aqueous epinephrine 1:1000 should be administered subcutaneously at the first indication of serious hypersensitivity. The dose for adults is 0.3 to 0.5 ml and for children under age 12 is 0.01 ml/kg, not to exceed 0.3 ml. When symptoms are predominantly respiratory, epinephrine by inhalation (10 to 20 puffs for an adult; 2 to 4 puffs per 10-kg body weight for a child) may provide more rapid relief.[79] In the presence of profound hypotension, 2 to 5 ml of 1:10,000 epinephrine solution may be given by slow IV push, or an infusion may be initiated by mixing 1 mg in 250 ml and infusing at a rate of 0.25 to 1 ml/min. Selective inhaled (nebulized) β_2-adrenergic agents, such as albuterol, can also be effective in relieving bronchospasm at doses of 2.5 mg/3 ml of a 0.08% solution. Aminophylline, 5 mg/kg as a loading dose followed by 0.9 mg/kg/hr as an infusion, may relieve bronchospasm not relieved by epinephrine or albuterol.

In the presence of hypotension, IV crystalloid solutions should be infused; pressor agents such as dopamine may be required. The military antishock trousers (MAST) garment may be helpful if rapid correction of decreased lower extremity peripheral resistance is desired. Oxygen, intubation, and mechanical ventilation may be needed to correct airway obstruction. Antihistamines and corticosteroids are also indicated in acute anaphylactic reactions, although the time of onset with corticosteroids is delayed. Propranolol is contraindicated because of the β-adrenergic blockade effect on the bronchioles. Persons taking β-adrenergic blockers may respond poorly to epinephrine. Those with insect sting anaphylaxis require close observation, preferably in the hospital, for about 24 hours.[79]

For mild hymenopteran stings, ice packs often provide relief. Honeybees frequently and yellowjackets occasionally leave a stinger in the wound. Although recommendations were that stingers should be scraped or brushed off with a sharp edge and not removed with forceps, which might squeeze the attached venom sac and worsen the injury, recent literature has refuted this.[129] Advice to victims on the immediate treatment of bee stings now emphasizes rapid removal by whatever method.[129] Wheal size and degree of envenomation increased as the time from stinging to stinger removal increased, even for a few seconds. The response was the same whether stings were scraped or pinched off after 2 seconds. Home remedies, such as baking soda paste or meat tenderizer applied locally to stings, are of dubious value, although the latter is often regarded as effective. Topical anesthetics in commercial "sting sticks" are also of little value. Local application of antihistamine lotions or creams such as tripelennamine may be helpful. An oral antihistamine such as diphenhydramine, 25 to 50 mg for adults and 1 mg/kg for children, every 6 hours is often effective. No therapy is effective against local effects of fire ant stings, although oral antihistamines and corticosteroids may provide some relief in severe cases. Since infection is common, topical antimicrobials (e.g., mupirocin) and prophylactic oral antibiotics are recommended. Breaking fire ant blisters should be avoided.[18,22]

Corticosteroids such as methylprednisolone, 24 mg/day initial dose tapered off over 4 to 5 days, often help resolve extensive local reactions to bee and wasp stings. This may be combined with cold packs and oral antihistamines.

Envenomation from multiple hymenopteran stings may require more aggressive therapy. IV calcium gluconate (5 to 10 ml of 10% solution) with a parenteral antihistamine and corticosteroid may be helpful in relieving pain, swelling, nausea, and vomiting. Development of a hyperimmune bee venom antiserum is under investigation.[109] Hypovolemic shock is managed conventionally. Plasmapheresis was used successfully to treat a person who sustained about 2000 honeybee stings.[25] Patients should be observed for 12 to 24 hours for coagulopathy and evidence of renal and neurologic damage. Urine output is monitored and urine tested for hemoglobin and myoglobin. Serum potassium, creatine kinase, and lactate dehydrogenase levels should be monitored. Oliguria with myoglobinuria, azotemia, and hyperkalemia are indications that hemodialysis may become necessary.

Immunotherapy. Desensitization with purified venoms produces an excellent blocking antibody response and prevents anaphylaxis in more than 95% of patients. A protective antiidiotypic antibody to honeybee venom has been identified.[56] Venoms for desensitization generally available in the United States are honeybee, yellowjacket, wasp (*Polistes*), and mixed vespid. A whole body extract of fire ant containing at least three venom

antigens is also available. No firm guidelines are available for selecting patients to receive immunotherapy. Skin test results and IgE levels in RAST tests are not reliable. Any adult with a history of systemic allergic reactions should be considered for immunotherapy. Persons receiving β-adrenergic blockers should be shifted to other appropriate medications if possible. Children under 16 with only cutaneous or mild systemic allergic reactions and persons with a history of only large local reactions do not need immunotherapy.[126] Evaluation of anaphylactic risk is recommended in children using wasp venom extract challenges.[107]

Regimens for desensitization attempt to achieve tolerance to venom doses of about 100 μg. A maintenance level of immunity requires about 95 days to achieve. Rapid programs requiring 3 to 7 days for initial immunization appear to be effective.[5,27] Some programs make use of both active and passive immunotherapy.[78] In a series of 1410 patients, 12% had systemic reactions during treatment; no fatalities were reported.[66,68] Experience of 26 women with 43 pregnancies does not suggest significant increased risk from venom immunotherapy during pregnancy.[111] Maintenance doses are required at intervals after basic immunization. Neither skin testing nor determination of IgG and IgE antibody levels against venom will reliably indicate success of immunization, although the majority of persons will be protected by a specific IgG antibody level of 400 RAST units/ml of serum.[125] Actual sting challenge is the most reliable test for determining immunotherapy candidates and desensitization[128] but is not widely used in the United States. It must be done in the hospital with careful monitoring and consideration of economic, ethical, and safety factors.[103] If the skin test is negative after 3 years of immunotherapy, patients may be placed on immunologic surveillance. Few patients require more than 5 years of immunotherapy.[95] For unknown reasons, desensitization to wasp venoms is achieved more quickly than to honeybee venom.[8]

Antivenom Therapy. Recently a group in the United Kingdom developed an ovine Fab-based antivenin as a potential treatment for mass bee stings. Sera from sheep immunized against the venom of *Apris mellifera scutellata* contained high levels of specific antibodies, as demonstrated by enzyme-linked immunosorbent assay (ELISA) and chromatography. Although effective experimentally in a mouse model, no human administration of the antivenin has been documented.[53]

Preparedness and Preventive Measures. Persons with a history of allergic reactions to insect stings (including large local reactions) should carry an emergency kit containing epinephrine and should wear medical identification tags. Kits should be available in work or recreation areas where the risk of insect sting is

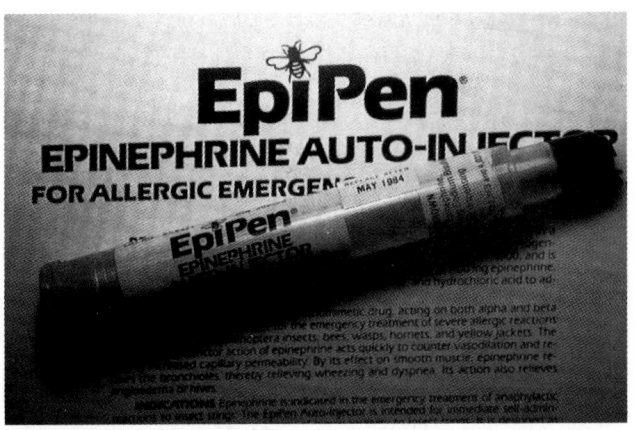

Figure 36-9 EpiPen preloaded delivery system for injection of aqueous epinephrine.

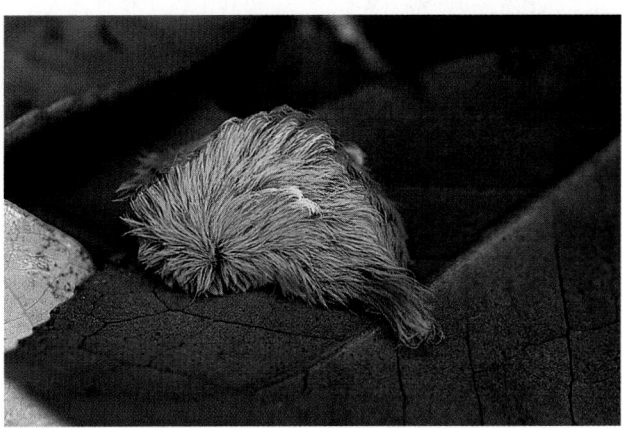

Figure 36-10 Puss caterpillar, *Megalopyge opercularis.*

high. Two kits widely available in the United States are EpiPen (Figure 36-9) and Ana-Kit. EpiPen and EpiPen Jr. are autoinjectors that deliver 0.3 mg or 0.15 mg of epinephrine, respectively. They are quick and easy to use; however, patients should be cautioned against injecting the material into fingers or buttocks or directly over veins. Ana-Kit contains two doses of 0.3 mg of epinephrine in a single conventional syringe, plus chewable antihistamine tablets and a tourniquet. It is more versatile but requires more instruction for the user.

Frequent cleaning of garbage cans and disposal of decaying fruit will make premises less attractive to bees and wasps. Hymenopterans are highly susceptible to many insecticides, and their control around dwellings and other inhabited buildings is rarely difficult. Spraying the nests after dark is safer. Many hymenopterans are economically valuable as pollinators of plants or predators on other insects, so their control on a wide scale is rarely desirable. The fire ant in the southern United States has been the target of massive but marginally effective control campaigns that adversely affected local ecosystems. A new approach uses grain baits containing synthetic insect growth hormones that are carried into the nests, where they disrupt ant caste differentiation and inhibit egg production. Arrays of thousands of hormone-baited traps placed in selected areas of Mexico, however, failed to stop the northward spread of Africanized bees.

LEPIDOPTERA

Venomous Species and Venoms

Insects of the order Lepidoptera typically cause human envenomation, but effects generally are less serious than with hymenopterans. Injury usually follows contact with caterpillars, occurring less frequently with the cocoon or adult stage. The larval lepidopteran (caterpillar) is usually free living, is moderately active, and

feeds on plants, although a few are parasites of insect nests or eat food of animal origin. The pupal stage may be free or encased in a silk cocoon. Wintering over in cold climates is usually in the pupal stage. Adults (butterflies and moths) have wings with microscopic chitinous scales. They primarily feed on nectar and other plant juices, but some eat semiliquid mammalian feces and urine. The adult provides no care or protection of immature stages. No social organization exists, although larvae and adults of some species assemble in large aggregations.

Venomous species occur in about 16 families of Lepidoptera, with no general rules for recognition. Many venomous caterpillars are broad, flat, and sluggish. Some have the dorsal surface densely covered with long hairs. Others are spiny and may have bright, conspicuous colors and markings. Some are highly camouflaged.

Venoms in Lepidoptera are purely defensive. The venom apparatus consists of spines that are simple or branched and frequently barbed. They may be scattered widely over the surface of the insect or arranged in clumps and often are intermixed with nonveniferous hairs or spines. In the most venomous caterpillars the spines are hollow and brittle with venom glands at the bases. Muscles surrounding the glands may help in expelling venom. In other Lepidoptera the spines are solid and function primarily as mechanical irritants or contain surface toxicants. Little is known of the chemistry of caterpillar venoms. Some are heat labile and contain proteins. Histamine and serotonin have been found in caterpillar venoms but are not common. Hairs of the brown-tailed moth (*Euproctis chrysorrhea*) contain enzymes with esterase and phospholipase activity.

Probably the most important venomous caterpillar in the United States is the puss caterpillar (Figure 36-10) or woolly slug (*Megalopyge opercularis*), which occurs in the southern states west through most of Texas and north to Maryland and Missouri. This hairy, flat, and ovoid caterpillar reaches a length of 30 to 35 mm and feeds on shade trees, including elm, oak, and sycamore. Some years it may be plentiful enough to be a nuisance. In southeast Texas in 1958, 2130 persons were treated for stings, with eight hospitalized. A related species, the flannel moth caterpillar *(M. crispata),* occurs in the eastern states north to New England. Its sting is less severe than that of *M. opercularis.* The large, spiny caterpillar of the io moth *(Automeris io)* is pale green with red and white lateral stripes (Figure 36-11). It is widely distributed in the eastern United States but rarely plentiful. The saddleback caterpillar *(Sibine stimula)* and oak slug *(Euclea delphinii)* are flat and almost rectangular; both can deliver a painful injury. The gypsy moth *(Lymantria dispar)* feeds on a variety of plants and has caused thousands of cases of dermatitis in the northeastern United States. Other common nettling caterpillars are *E. chrysorrhea,* which also occurs in Europe, and the tussock or toothbrush caterpillar *(Hemerocampa leucostigma),* with its conspicuous red head and four tufts of bristles. Another tussock caterpillar, *Oryia pseudotsuga,* causes numerous cases of dermatitis and conjunctivitis among lumberworkers and foresters in the northwestern states.

Stinging Patterns

Caterpillar envenomation usually occurs when living insects are touched as they cling to vegetation or drop onto bare skin. Persons cutting branches, picking fruit, or climbing trees are likely to be stung. However, the largest outbreaks have been associated with spines detached from live or dead caterpillars and cocoons. These may be airborne or deposited on bedding or laundry hung outdoors. In temperate regions, caterpillar stings are most common from August to early November. Heavy caterpillar infestations seem to occur during exceptionally favorable weather and with decreases in populations of parasites and predators that serve as natural controls.

Clinical Aspects

Two general syndromes are associated with lepidopteran envenomations. In the case of caterpillars with hollow spines and basal venom glands (e.g., *Automeris, Megalopyge,* and *Dirphia*), direct contact with the live insect causes instant nettling pain, followed by redness and swelling (Figure 36-12). Puss caterpillar stings show a characteristic gridiron pattern of hemorrhagic pinpoint papules. In typical cases, no systemic manifestations occur, and symptoms usually subside within 24 hours. However, pain may be intense with central radiation, accompanied by urticaria, nausea, headache, fever, vomiting, and lymphadenopathy. Hypotension, shock, dyspnea, abdominal tenderness, and convulsions have been reported with puss caterpillar stings.[37,49]

The second syndrome is associated with caterpillars with a less highly developed venom apparatus (e.g., *Lymantria, Euproctis, Thaumetopoea*). Contact with the living insect is not necessary; detached spines are often involved. Little or no immediate discomfort is experienced. An itching, erythematous, papular, or urticarial rash develops within a few hours to 2 days and persists for up to a week. Rarely the lesions may be bullous. Conjunctivitis, upper respiratory tract irritation, and rare asthmalike symptoms may be seen with or without dermatitis. Ophthalmia serious enough to require enucleation may be caused by detached spines lodged in the eye. Acute anaphylactic reactions have not been reported to follow lepidopteran stings. Patch testing has demonstrated both immediate and delayed hypersensitivity.

Treatment and Prevention

Treatment of lepidopteran envenomations is symptomatic. Prompt application and stripping of adhesive tape or a commercial facial peel at the site of the sting may remove many spines and serve as a diagnostic

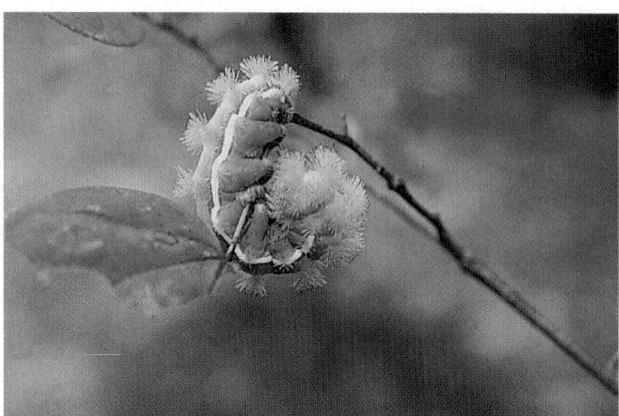

Figure 36-11 Caterpillar of the io moth, *Automeris io.* Widespread in the eastern United States, this species can inflict a painful sting.

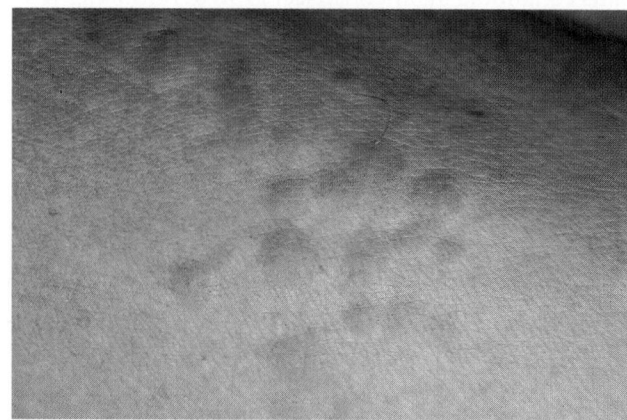

Figure 36-12 Nettle rash from unidentified caterpillar.

procedure, since the spines can be identified by microscopy. Patients with local symptoms usually obtain relief from group I corticosteroid creams and ointments. Over-the-counter preparations containing corticosteroids and antihistamines are not significantly better than simpler preparations such as calamine lotion with phenol. Oral antihistamines such as fexofenadine (60 mg 2 times a day) or antiinflammatory drugs such as tolmetin sodium (400 mg three times a day) are often effective in more severe cases. Occasionally, codeine (30 to 50 mg), meperidine (50 mg), or oxymorphone (1.5 mg) in combination with an antiemetic may be needed to control pain and vomiting. IV calcium gluconate has been used successfully in severe puss caterpillar envenomation.[84,89]

Trees on which caterpillars feed may be sprayed with appropriate insecticides to control species such as the puss caterpillar. Near Shanghai, where chemical insecticides would have been harmful to silkworm culture, *Euproctis* caterpillars were controlled by spraying with an insect virus. Screens on windows and doors protect against moths with toxic spines.

HEMIPTERA (SUCKING BUGS)

The Hemiptera comprise a large order of insects characterized by sucking mouthparts, generally in the form of a beak, and a life cycle with no well-demarcated larval and pupal stages but a gradual transition from the hatchling nymph to adult. Most hemipterans are winged as adults, with the anterior wings generally divided into a chitinized and membranous section. Most feed on plant juices, but several families are predators, and two feed on the blood of humans and other vertebrates.

The assassin bugs (family Reduviidae) are generally recognizable by the long and narrow head, a stout and three-jointed beak, long antennae, and typical hemipteran wings (Figure 36-13). Most are of a dark color; a few are brightly marked or have a checkerboard pattern along the posterior edge of the abdomen. Some species attach fragments of their prey, sand grains, or other debris to their backs. Reduviidae occur on all continents. They have a variety of habitats and are often nocturnal.

The triatomids (e.g., kissing bugs, flying bedbugs, Mexican bedbugs, *barberos*) are a subfamily of the Reduviidae adapted for feeding on blood. They feed on a wide range of mammals and often live in the nests or burrows of their hosts. Armadilloes, dogs, opossums, and pack rats are common hosts in the southern United States and Mexico. Some triatomids adapt readily to life in human dwellings, particularly those of adobe construction. Triatomids are primarily a neotropical group, with species ranging northward in the United States to Utah and southern Indiana. *Triatoma protracta* and *T. sanguisuga* are among the better-known species. The family Cimicidae, or bedbugs, are flat, ovoid, and reddish brown insects whose wings are reduced to a pair of functionless pads. Lack of large terminal claws distinguishes them from lice. Bedbugs are cosmopolitan in distribution. Two species, *Cimex lectularius* and *C. hemipterus*, feed primarily on humans and live in dwellings, where they hide in bedding, under wallpaper, behind baseboards, and in window frames. Homes of poorer persons are more likely to be heavily infested, but the insects may be carried into well-kept residences, hospitals, and hotels. Other species of *Cimex*, normally parasitic on bats and swallows, occasionally attack humans.

Venomous aquatic Hemiptera include the giant water bugs (family Belostomatidae) (Figure 36-14), back swimmers (family Notonectidae), and water scorpions (family Nepidae). Water bugs are distinguished from aquatic beetles by their beak and hemipteran wings; back swimmers have greatly elongated hind legs; and

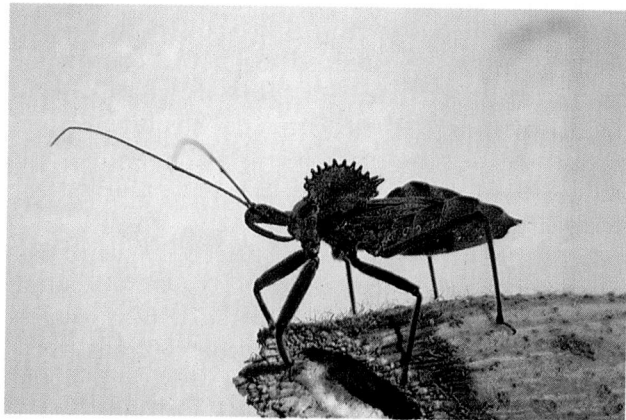

Figure 36-13 Wheel bug, *Arilus cristatus*, a large assassin bug common in the eastern United States.

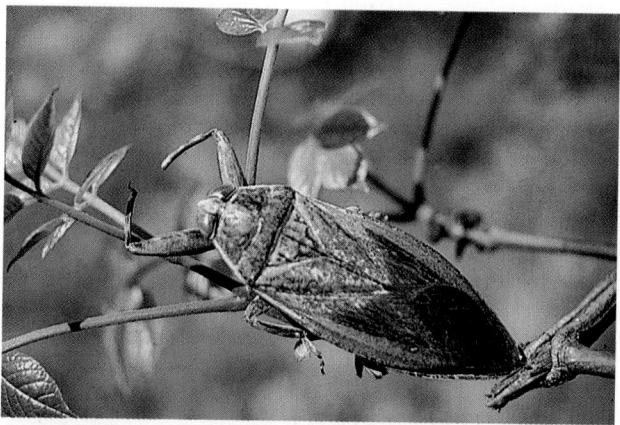

Figure 36-14 Giant water bug, *Benacus griseus*, a large insect common in aquatic habitats in the eastern United States.

water scorpions have a slender body with long, terminal breathing tubes. These insects are widely distributed in freshwater habitats.

The hemipteran venom apparatus consists of two or three pairs of glands in the thorax. Secretions are ejected through half of a double tube formed by the interlocking of the elongated maxillae and mandibles, which have distal tips modified for piercing. Few hemipteran venoms have been studied. Venoms of two reduviids, *Platymeris rhadamanthus* of Africa and *Holotrichus innesi* of the Middle East, contain several enzymes and nonenzymatic proteins.[28,138] Sialase, an enzyme unusual in invertebrates, is found in *Triatoma* venom; it has anticoagulant activity.[1] Venom serves primarily for subjugation and probably digestion of prey, but the insects may defend themselves by biting. Salivary secretions of blood-sucking hemipterans also contain potent allergens.

Clinical Aspects

Triatomids usually bite at night on exposed parts of the body. Feeding may last from 3 to 30 minutes. Bites are painless. On initial exposure there is usually no reaction. Repeated bites are followed by reddish, itching papules that may persist for up to a week. Bites are often grouped in a cluster or line (Figure 36-15) and may be accompanied by giant urticarial wheals, lymphadenopathy, hemorrhagic bullae, fever, and lymphocytosis. Systemic anaphylactoid reactions with respiratory or gastrointestinal manifestations may occur.[50,71] Entomologists and small children are most frequently bitten by assassin bugs, since handling induces the insect to bite. Bites of several U.S. species, such as the wheel bug (*Arilus cristatus*), black corsair (*Melanolestes picipes*), and masked bedbug hunter (*Reduvius personatus*), are described as painful as the sting of a hornet and accompanied by local swelling lasting several hours. Bedbug bites usually raise a pruritic wheal with central hemorrhagic punctum, followed by a reddish

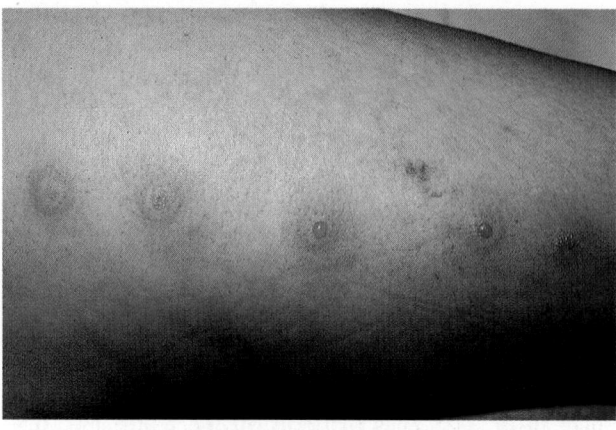

Figure 36-15 Triatomid feeding pattern.

papule that persists for several days. Bullae, generalized urticaria, arthralgia, asthma, and anaphylactic shock are rare sequelae of bedbug bites. Bites by aquatic Hemiptera are similar to those of assassin bugs, but few cases have been described in detail.

Treatment and Prevention

Treatment is symptomatic and not particularly effective. Various antipruritic preparations are helpful in mild cases. Topical or intralesional steroids have generally been disappointing. Immobilization, elevation, and local heat are helpful in severe limb bites. Desensitization with triatomid salivary gland extract has been effective in a small series of patients with history of life-threatening anaphylactic reactions.[101] Triatomids and bedbugs are more difficult to eradicate with insecticides than are many household insects. Benzene hexachloride has been effective against triatomids in Latin America.

BEETLES AND OTHER INSECTS

Beetles (order Coleoptera) are the largest group of insects, with at least 250,000 species. The prothorax of beetles is generally very distinct, whereas the two posterior thoracic segments are more or less fused to the abdomen. In most beetles the anterior wings are heavily chitinized, acting as covers for the posterior membranous wings used in flight. Mouthparts are of the chewing type. The life cycle involves larval and pupal stages before emergence of the adult. Many beetles feed on plants throughout their life cycle, many are predators or scavengers, and a few are parasitic. No beetles have a bite or sting venomous to humans, but several families have toxic secretions that may be deposited on the skin. The blister beetles (family Meloidae) are a cosmopolitan group with numerous representatives in deserts and semiarid regions. A species may suddenly appear by the thousands, especially after rains, persist for a few days, and be replaced by another. The majority are of medium size (about 15 mm) and have soft, leathery forewings (elytra). Some are brilliantly colored. They are plentiful on vegetation, and some species are attracted to lights. A low-molecular-weight toxin, cantharidin, is present in the hemolymph and most of the insect's tissues. It is exuded from multiple sites if the beetle is gently pressed or otherwise disturbed.

In the eastern United States, blister beetle dermatitis is usually caused by *Epicauta* species, which occur on many garden plants. Contact with the beetle is painless and seldom remembered by the victim. Blisters appear 2 to 5 hours after contact and may be single or multiple, usually 5 to 50 mm in diameter and thin walled. Unless broken and rubbed, they are not painful. Cantharidin nephritis has been reported after unusually heavy vesication but more frequently is the result of using a cantharidin preparation as an aphrodisiac.

Darkling ground beetles are moderately large, dark, and heavily chitinized insects that assume a characteristic posture with head down and tail up when disturbed. They are found worldwide in arid regions, where they live under stones and other cover and crawl about at night. Most species can spray irritant secretions, mostly benzoquinones, from the tip of the abdomen to a distance of 30 to 40 cm. These secretions are generally harmless to humans, but blistering of the skin has been reported, and eye injury is possible.

No special treatment for beetle vesication is available. The injuries are best treated as superficial chemical burns. Local preparations containing corticosteroids or antihistamines are not particularly effective.

Other types of insect envenomation are sporadic. Many insects that normally feed on plant juices occasionally inflict annoying bites. This behavior may be initiated by dehydration of the insect or by unknown factors. Small predatory insects, such as lacewing larvae, anthocorids, and *Sclerodermus* species, occasionally attack humans instead of their normal arthropod prey. Thrips may bite and produce itching macules.[80] A small hemipteran, *Leptodemus minutus*, caused numerous cases of dermatitis in Kuwait.[105] The stick insect, *Anisomorpha buprestoides*, a common species in Florida and adjacent states, ejects a noxious fluid from its thoracic region that deters birds and other predators. According to regional folklore, this fluid can be directed toward human eyes with painful consequences. Recently, an outbreak of a blistering disease was reported in a military unit training in the Arizona desert during an unusual heavy rainfall and flooding. Staphylinid (rove) beetles (genus *Paederus*, family Stapylinidae) were collected at the site. These beetles have been responsible for vesicular dermatitis in other parts of the world but were never reported in the United States before this series.[17]

DIPTERA (TWO-WINGED FLIES)

Insects of the order Diptera are characterized by one pair of wings. The second pair is usually modified to form a pair of drumsticklike structures known as halteres. A typical life cycle consists of eggs, limbless larvae, pupae, and winged adults, but numerous variations exist. Mouthparts are of the sucking type. Females of many species, although free living, take blood or other tissue fluids from vertebrates, injecting salivary secretions that are not intrinsically toxic but are potent sensitizing agents for most humans. Larvae of some Diptera are human parasites. Other adult Diptera feed indiscriminately on feces and human foodstuffs. These habits make them by far the most important arthropod vectors of human disease (Table 36-1).

Most of these insects are cosmopolitan in distribution, except tsetse flies, which are restricted to Africa, and tropical and subtropical sand flies. Some species of mosquitoes and blackflies are adapted to cold temperate, sub-Arctic, and alpine environments, where their numbers may make areas uninhabitable during peak activity. Other mosquitoes and biting midges are equally abundant and annoying in some coastal areas and on islands.

Mosquitoes are characterized by a fringe of setae along the posterior margin of the wings and delicate scales along the wing veins. Only the female feeds on blood. Her prominent beak contains a kit of piercing and sucking tools. Most mosquitoes have body lengths of 3 to 4 mm, but some large species may be about twice this size (see Table 36-1). The estimated 3000 species of mosquitoes are cosmopolitan in distribution.

Carbon dioxide, body heat, and sweat gland secretions, especially apocrine, are attractants for mosquitoes; certain skin lipids are repellent.[55] Children under 1 year of age rarely show a skin reaction to mosquito bites, but by age 5 nearly all are reactors. Both immediate and delayed types of hypersensitivity are induced. Typically, immediate pruritic wheals are followed by red, swollen, and pruritic lesions in 12 to 24 hours. These lesions are associated with both IgE and IgG antibody complexes and a lymphocyte response.[87,96]

All the classic types of immunologic injury have been reported after mosquito bites, including injury from circulating immune complexes, asthma, and Arthus reaction.[38,46,120] Seasonal bullous eruptions in a coastal area of Britain were ascribed to *Aedes detritus*. Most of those affected were women with varicose veins or deep venous thromboses. Intense skin reactions accompanied by fever, lymphadenopathy, and hepatosplenomegaly have been described and are associated with infiltration of skin lesions by natural killer lymphocytes.[123] Nodular skin lesions lasting up to a month have been reported after mosquito bites in patients with acquired immunodeficiency syndrome (AIDS) receiving zidovudine.[26] Papulovesicular lesions with eosinophil infiltration were reported following insect (including mosquito) bites in patients with lymphocytic leukemia.[21] Among 21 Japanese patients with severe local and constitutional reactions to mosquito bites, seven died of malignant histiocytosis before age 28. Nine others retained hypersensitivity; three lost it.[46]

Treatment of mosquito bites consists of local application of antipruritic lotions or creams. Antihistamines relieve the itching of early lesions but have no effect on later ones.[97] Group I corticosteroid creams and ointments may be helpful. Desensitization with insect whole body extract is difficult but occasionally successful.[72] Prolonged heavy exposure to mosquito bites

TABLE 36-1. Major Groups of Biting Dipterans

INSECT	RECOGNITION FEATURES OF ADULT	LARVAL AND PUPAL STAGES
Mosquitoes (Culicidae, subfamily Culicinae)	Prominent proboscis; wings with scales; palps of female much shorter than proboscis; usually rests with body parallel to substrate	Aquatic in great variety of habitats; both larval and pupal stages motile
Mosquitoes (subfamily Anophelinae)	Prominent proboscis; wings with scales and often with dark mottling; palps of females about as long as proboscis; usually rests with head down and body held at an angle to substrate	Same as above
Blackflies, buffalo gnats (family Simuliidae)	Stout; humpbacked; short antennae; wings broad with most of veins faint; body length >2.5 mm	Sessile in flowing water; usually attached to rocks and logs, sometimes to crustaceans
Sand flies (family Psychodidae)	Small (usually >2 mm body length); hairy; wings with straight, prominent veins	In damp crevices, animal burrows, leaf litter
Biting midges, sand flies, no-see-ums (family Ceratopogonidae)	Small (>2 mm body length); wings often mottled; most of wing veins faint	In mud, wet sand, rotting vegetation, larvae very motile
Horseflies, deerflies (family Tabanidae)	Large (5-25 mm body length) with large eyes; usually brilliantly colored; body stout; wings with prominent veins	In mud or shallow water
Stable flies (family Muscidae)	Similar to housefly in size and general appearance; sharp-pointed proboscis projects downward and backward	In decaying vegetable matter or urine-soaked straw
Tsetse flies (family Glossinidae)	Large (6-14 mm); proboscis projects forward; wings fold scissorlike over back	Larvae complete most of development in female; pupate in soil a few hours after birth
Snipe flies (family Rhagionidae)	Long legs; relatively slender body; large eyes; wings with prominent veins	Aquatic, in moist soil or rotten wood

causes some individuals to lose sensitivity, occasionally in less than 1 year. Delayed hypersensitivity is lost more readily than immediate hypersensitivity; with decreases in both IgE and IgG[88] (see Chapter 32).

Biting Midges (Culicoides)

Biting midges are very small flies that have a bite out of proportion to their size. Only females feed on blood. The wormlike aquatic larvae usually develop in water-saturated soil; mangrove swamps are a common habitat. Larvae of some species use axils of banana and similar plants. The genus is cosmopolitan but presents the greatest problem in subtropical and tropical coastal regions. Activity is often seasonal. The flies bite most intensely in still air and reduced light.

Bites are immediately painful and result in raised, red, and pruritic lesions that persist from a few hours to a week or more. Some victims develop vesicles, pustules, and superficial ulcers, particularly if bitten by the genus *Leptoconops*. Hypersensitivity is involved, although some persons seem to develop intense reactions on first exposure to the insects.

Treatment of bites is symptomatic and similar to that for mosquito bites. Artificial hyposensitization has not been successful; however, spontaneous de-

crease in skin reactivity may occur in some individuals (see Chapter 32).

Blackflies (Simuliidae)

Blackflies are small stocky flies that have a characteristic humpbacked appearance. Adults prefer open and sunny areas and are good fliers. Not all species are anthropophilic. The sessile larvae and pupae are found in flowing water, from large rivers to small brooks. Blackflies are cosmopolitan, but their abundance and medical significance vary widely. They range well into the Arctic and constitute a major problem for both humans and domestic animals in parts of Europe, Canada, and the northern United States. In the tropics they tend to be more localized, often remaining close to streams.

Blackfly bites are more common on the upper half of the body. They snip the skin and suck the pooled blood, leaving relatively large punctures that may bleed, a symptom rarely seen with bites of other small flies. The local pain, swelling, and redness that follow blackfly bites are unusually intense and persistent. Vesicles and weeping, crusted lesions may last for weeks. Systemic symptoms such as malaise, fever, and leukocytosis may occur. Enlarged indurated lymphatics, particularly in the posterior cervical region, are common in Canadian children living where blackflies are abundant. Hemorrhagic symptoms have been reported in Brazil. Generalized urticaria, bleeding, angioedema, cough, wheezing, toxemia, and even death may occur.[51,60,135]

No specific treatment for blackfly bites is available. Hyposensitization has been attempted with little success. Neither repellents nor ordinary clothes provide satisfactory protection against blackflies when they are present in large numbers. Avoidance of heavily infested areas during fly season is often the most practical solution. Control measures have not proved highly effective (see Chapter 32).

Horseflies and Deerflies (Tabanidae)

Horseflies and deerflies are medium to large (10 to 25 mm body length) stocky flies whose large eyes often are brightly colored. They are strong fliers and prefer open and sunny habitats. The tabanids attack a variety of large mammals, including humans. The predacious maggotlike larvae live in water-soaked soil or shallow water. Bites from these large flies, predominantly the deerfly (*Chrysops* species), are painful and may cause both external and subcutaneous bleeding. An itching wheal up to 1 inch in diameter develops but usually does not last long. In some victims, severe and prolonged swelling of the face or an extremity develops. About 30 cases of systemic anaphylactoid reactions have been reported. One man with a history of systemic reactions to wasp stings had a similar reaction to a horsefly bite.[36,45]

As with other fly bites, treatment is symptomatic. Hyposensitization has been attempted in a few cases, apparently with some success (see Chapter 32).

Other Biting Diptera

Snipe flies (Rhagionidae) primarily prey on insects, but some species, such as *Symphoromyia*, feed on the blood of mammals. Their habits and life history are similar to those of tabanids. Reactions to snipe fly bites range from pain to anaphylaxis. A person who reacts severely may be bedridden for days.

The stable fly (*Stomoxys calcitrans*) is related to the housefly, which it closely resembles. It is plentiful throughout most of the United States, particularly in agricultural districts. Eggs are deposited in piles of decaying vegetation, where the larvae develop. Thunderstorms seem to stimulate fly activity, which accounts for the widespread belief that houseflies bite just before a storm. Bites cause a sharp, stinging sensation, but dermal lesions are uncommon. Itching is brief.

Louse flies (Hippoboscidae) are peculiar Diptera that may lack wings entirely or have them for only part of their adult life. The wingless forms are flat, leathery insects that resemble lice or ticks. They are ectoparasites of birds and mammals. Larvae are carried in the uterus until development is almost complete; the pupal stage

may be spent in the soil or on the host. The sheep ked (*Melophagus ovinus*) is a common species in the United States and sometimes bites sheep shearers and handlers. The related deer ked (*Lipoptena cervi*) is a seasonal pest in wooded sections of northern Europe, causing hundreds of cases of dermatitis annually. The pigeon fly (*Pseudolynchia canariensis*) is an avian parasite that sometimes infests buildings and bites the occupants.

Lesions from hippoboscid bites appear 1 to 24 hours after the bites as reddish itching papules that may persist for up to 3 months. Topical corticosteroids may afford symptomatic relief and hasten resolution of the lesions. Repellents are reported to be ineffective against these insects (see Chapter 32).

Myiasis

The term *myiasis* for parasitism by fly larvae was introduced into the medical literature in 1840, although the condition has been observed since antiquity. More than a hundred species of Diptera have been reported to cause human myiasis.[77] Some are obligate parasites for which humans are one of several hosts; some are opportunistic invaders that find parasitism an alternative to feeding on decaying tissue or its products. Nevertheless, humans are not a particularly good host for most species of fly larvae, and many infections terminate prematurely. Sensitization of host tissues to fly larvae does not occur as readily as with many other arthropod and helminth parasites.

Myiasis may be classified by clinical manifestations or etiologic agents; neither method is totally satisfactory. This chapter discusses only dermal and wound myiasis. Myiasis primarily involving the gastrointestinal tract, urinary tract, eye, and nasopharynx is not covered.

Furuncular Myiasis. In furuncular myiasis the fly larva penetrates the skin but remains sedentary, producing a boil-like lesion that usually has a central opening. Here the larva completes its development but typically emerges to pupate outside the host. As a human problem, this form of myiasis is largely confined to the tropics, although imported cases are being recognized in increasing numbers in other regions of the world (see Chapter 37).

Autochthonous furuncular myiasis may occur in the United States, usually in children. Most cases are caused by larvae of botflies of the genus *Cuterebra*, whose normal hosts are small rodents and rabbits. The fly eggs are attached to low vegetation and hatch on contact with skin of the host. Adult human skin seems impervious to them, but that of children may be penetrated. There is usually a history of outdoor play in weeds or grass or with a pet rabbit, but in one case, eggs apparently were deposited directly on the skin.[39] Lesions typically develop on the head, neck, or chest in

1 or 2 weeks. Once recognized, the larvae can often be removed by simple pressure.[91,116] The syndrome may also be caused by larvae of *Wohlfahrtia vigil*, a large fly native to Canada and the northern United States. Its normal hosts are newborn mammals, particularly mink, dog, and fox. The fly deposits larvae on the skin, which penetrates in about an hour. Human infections are typically in infants under 9 months, and the furuncular lesions are usually on the face. Fever, irritability, and loss of appetite are common. Larvae can usually be expressed from the lesion; surgery rarely is necessary. Netting over the crib or pram when outdoors usually affords protection.

Migratory Myiasis. One type of migratory myiasis is caused by flies of the genus *Hypoderma*. Adult flies are large and hairy, resembling bumblebees. Normal hosts for the parasitic larvae are cattle, deer, and horses. The flies attach their eggs to hairs. Hatchling larvae penetrate the skin and wander extensively through the subcutaneous tissues, eventually locating under the skin of the back, where they produce furuncular lesions. The condition has veterinary importance. Humans are abnormal hosts in which the parasite is unable to complete its development. Human infections usually occur in rural areas where cattle and horses are raised and are more common in winter. Larvae migrate rapidly (as much as 1 cm/hr) and erratically through subcutaneous tissues, producing intermittent, painful swellings over months. The person often senses larval movement. Larvae respond negatively to gravity, so the last lesions are usually on the head or shoulders. Eosinophilia (up to 35% eosinophils on white blood cell differential) and angioedema may be seen. Larvae may emerge spontaneously from furuncles or may die in the tissues. In rare cases, larvae invaded the pharyngeal region, orbit, and spinal canal.

Another form of migratory myiasis is caused by larvae of *Gastrophilus*, which normally are gastrointestinal or nasal parasites of horses (Figure 36-16). In human infections, which are reported more frequently from Europe than from the United States, the young larvae burrow in the skin, producing narrow, tortuous, reddish, and linear lesions with intense itching. Lesions usually advance 1.5 cm/day, but more rapid progress has been reported. Death of the larvae terminates the infection in 1 or 2 weeks without sequelae. This infection is clinically similar to creeping eruption, an invasion of the skin by larvae of the hookworms *Ancylostoma braziliense* and *A. caninum*. The helminthic parasitosis occurs more often in warm, moist regions, including the southern United States, and is associated with dogs and cats. The myiasis is seen more frequently in cooler regions and is associated with horses. Definitive diagnosis can be made only by removal of the parasite from its burrow and microscopic examination.

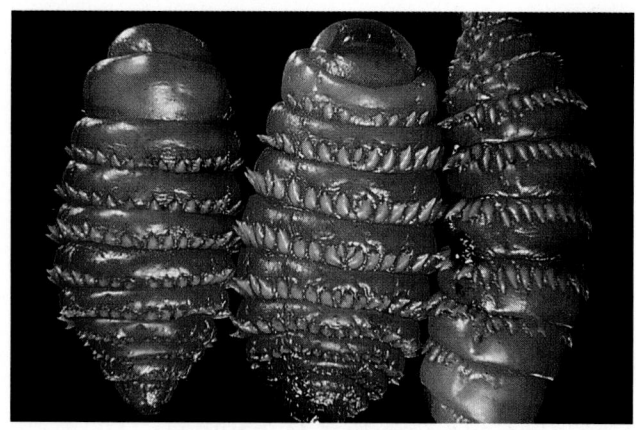

Figure 36-16 Larvae of the botfly *Gastrophilus haemorrhoidalis* from a horse's stomach.

Removal of the larvae by surgery or expression is the usual treatment for migratory myiasis, although local freezing of cutaneous burrows is sometimes successful. Ivermictin given to a patient with *Hypoderma* myiasis resulted in expulsion of the larva.[52] The most effective prevention is control of the infections in domestic animals.

Wound Myiasis. Opportunistic invasion of wounds by fly larvae is often seen during war and natural disasters, when injured persons are exposed to flies and medical facilities are inadequate to cope with the emergency. Wound myiasis may also be seen sporadically in nursing homes and hospitals and often is not reported for cultural and medicolegal reasons.[10] Six of 14 cases in one series were acquired in the hospital. Eleven patients were over 63 years of age, and nearly all had underlying problems, such as diabetes or peripheral vascular disease. Most of the infected lesions were on the feet or ankles.[69] In another series of 16 cases, most victims were debilitated and over age 65. Males were affected more often than females. Seven species of flies were involved.[75] Fifty *Lucilia* larvae were removed from the nose, mouth, paranasal sinuses, and enucleated eye socket of a hospitalized patient left in a room with an open window.[20] The most common fly species involved are *Lucilia* (green-bottle flies), *Calliphora* species (bluebottle flies), *Phorima regina* (black blowfly), *Sarcophaga haemorrhoidalis* (flesh fly), and *Musca domestica* (housefly). The flies, whose larvae normally feed on decaying animal tissues, often deposit eggs or larvae in wounds or around body orifices if a malodorous discharge is present. The larvae feed on necrotic tissue, and damage to healthy tissues and secondary infection are uncommon. They actually may debride wounds, and "maggot therapy" with aseptically bred larvae was briefly used in the 1930s. Recently, laboratory-bred fly larvae have been used to debride venous stasis ulcers and other superficial necrotic areas when antibiotic therapy and surgical debridement were unsuccessful.[115,119] Maggots serendipitously present have been used to debride lesions,[92] but this can be risky.[76] Diagnosis is usually obvious on inspection of the wound. Species identification often requires the larvae to reach maturity. If this is not feasible, examination of the spiracular plates on the last segment of the larva and the chitinized oral structures usually permits adequate identification. Irrigation of the wound and mechanical removal of larvae are generally sufficient for treatment.

LICE (ORDER ANOPLURA)

Species, Life Cycle, and Distribution

Lice are small wingless insects that are ectoparasites of mammals. They are mostly host specific, and two species are human parasites: *Pthirus pubis* (pubic louse) and *Pediculus humanus*, with two varieties, *P. h. capitis* (head louse) and *P. h. corporis* (body louse). They are obligatory parasites, subsisting on blood from the host, and have mouthparts modified for piercing and sucking. The mouthparts are drawn into the head of the louse when not in use.

The adult head louse is about 2 to 4 mm long with an elongated body that is flattened dorsoventrally (Figure 36-17). The head is only slightly narrower than the thorax. The three pairs of legs are about equal in length and possess delicate hooks at the distal extremities. The entire life is spent on the host's body. The eggs (nits) are deposited on hair shafts, generally one nit to a shaft. The nits hatch in about 1 week, and the freshly hatched larvae, which must feed within 24 hours of hatching or die, mature in about 15 to 16 days. The adult female lives for approximately 1 month and may deposit more than 100 eggs during her reproductive life. Body lice are slightly larger than head lice but are similar in appearance with a similar life cycle, although the nits are deposited on fibers of clothing. Head lice and body lice interbreed.

Adult pubic lice are about 1 to 2 mm long, the head is much smaller than the thorax, and the broadly oval body is flattened dorsoventrally (Figure 36-18). The anterior legs are much shorter than the second and third pairs, and the insect resembles a miniature crab. Nits are deposited on hair shafts, often several per shaft, and the egg-to-egg life cycle is approximately 1 month.

Lice are found wherever people are found. Able to exist only briefly away from the human body, lice are spread by close personal contact and by sharing of clothing and bedding. The various species not only have a particular host but often prefer a particular part of the host's body, so generalizing about transmission of the three varieties that parasitize humans is impossible. During biting and feeding, secretions from the louse cause a small red macule. Severe pruritus and marked

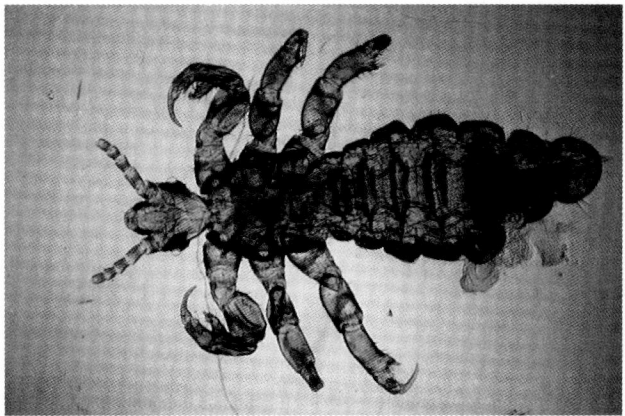

Figure 36-17 Male of the human head louse, *Pediculus humanus capitis.*

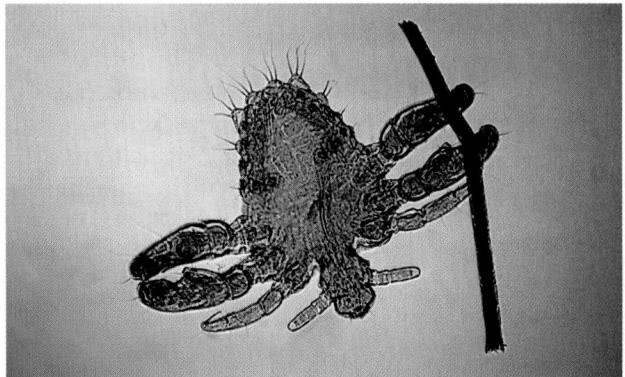

Figure 36-18 Pubic or crab louse, *Phthirus pubis,* grasping a hair.

inflammatory responses to bites are caused by the sensitization that occurs after repeated exposure to bites. Thus a victim may have lice for weeks before pruritus becomes marked. Not all people are equally attractive to lice, possibly because of differences in odor and chemical composition of sweat. Lice are medically important as vectors of systemic illnesses, as well as for dermatitis and discomfort.

Clinical Aspects

The head louse localizes on the scalp and rarely on other hairy areas of the body. Children are most frequently affected, but adults, particularly women, may also be affected. Lice are particularly common in young girls, possibly because of their long hair. Infestation is uncommon in blacks, at least in the United States, probably because the shaft of African hair has an oval cross section that makes it difficult for the louse to grip while depositing eggs. However, pediculosis capitis is found in Africa, where the indigenous head louse is adapted to grip the oval hair shafts. Since nits initially attach to the hair shaft close to the skin and are carried higher as the hair grows, the presence of nits near the tips indicates a longstanding infestation.

Itching is the principal symptom, and physical findings vary with duration and extent of the infestation, cleanliness, excoriations, and degree of secondary infection. Diagnosis is established by identifying nits and lice. It is not always easy to find lice, especially in early and mild cases, when they may be few in number. Lice are very active, but nits are always present and easy to identify. Nits are whitish ovals, about 0.5 mm long, and attached firmly to one side of the hair. Flakes of dandruff, which resemble nits superficially, are not attached to the hair shafts. Occipital and posterior cervical adenopathy is common and may be present even in less severe cases. A pruritic scalp accompanied by adenopathy should prompt a thorough search for lice and nits. In severe cases, oozing and crusting may be present, sometimes with matting of the hair, and lice may be numerous.

The body louse lives chiefly in the seams of clothing and is rarely seen on the skin. These lice leave clothing to feed on the skin or remain attached to the clothing while feeding, and thus they are most abundant where clothing abuts the skin (e.g., beltline). The bite results in a small red macule with a characteristic central hemorrhagic punctum. Excoriations, crusts, eczematization, and other secondary lesions generally obscure the primary lesions by the time the victim seeks medical attention. Shoulders, trunk, and buttocks are favorite sites for bites, and parallel scratch marks on the shoulders are a common finding. The diagnosis is confirmed by identifying parasites or nits from the clothing. Bands of trousers, side seams, and underarm seams are sites of preference. Untreated cases may persist indefinitely, and massive infestations are sometimes seen in vagabonds who have no ready access to frequent laundering or change of clothing or who cannot bathe regularly.

Pediculosis pubis is usually acquired during sexual activity, although it may result from unchanged bedding or nonsexual activity, either from lice that live briefly away from the human body or from egg-infested pubic hairs that are shed. The lice localize principally in the pubic hair, but they are found occasionally in eyebrows, eyelashes, and axillary hairs. Adult pubic lice are not active and hug the skin at the base of the hair shafts, with their heads buried in the follicular orifice. They are not easy to find, but one or more can usually be found if suspicion of the diagnosis is strong enough to prompt a thorough search. A loupe is helpful. Nits are more easily found. Primary bite lesions are almost never seen, but the intense pruritus and pubic scratching are pathognomonic. The secondary infection, crusting, oozing, excoriations, and eczematization that often accompany head and body lice are rarely seen with pubic lice. Peculiar steel-gray macules (maculae caeruleae) may appear in association with some cases of pubic lice. These lesions do not appear until the infestation has been present for several weeks and are most common on the trunk and thighs.

Treatment and Prevention

Treatment of all types of lice strives to eradicate lice and nits and prevent reinfestation. Head lice may be treated with one application of 1% permethrin cream rinse (Nix). Hair should be washed, rinsed, and dried, and the rinse is applied for 10 minutes before being washed off. A fine-toothed comb may be used to remove nits after rinsing. Failure to remove all the nits is a frequent cause of treatment failure. If lice or nits are found after 7 days, retreatment is indicated. Family members and contacts should be treated simultaneously. Hats and scarfs should be machine washed with hot cycle and bed clothing dry-cleaned. Other pediculicides are available if the lice are resistant. Two products, RID (Pfizer, New York, N.Y.) and Triple X (Young's Drug Product, Weatherfield, Conn.) contain 0.3% pyrethrins and 3.0% piperonyl butoxide. One application of either preparation usually eradicates both lice and nits. A few persons may require another application 7 days after the initial treatment.[6] Lindane 1% (hexachlorocyclohexane, Kwell) may be used on persons who fail to respond or who are intolerant of permethrin. Kwell is the medication used most often in the United States for treatment of louse infestations. Lindane penetrates human skin and has potential for central nervous system toxicity. It is contraindicated in neonates and must be used according to strict guidelines in children, pregnant women, and nursing mothers. Alternative treatments contain pyrethrums and piperonyl butoxide as active ingredients. Ivermectin, a macrocyclic lactone antibiotic highly effective against filarial worms and *Strongyloides*, has recently been demonstrated to be effective against lice both topically and orally, but it is not approved for this use at present.[11]

Body lice may be treated with the same medications, but parasites and nits are not generally found on the skin. Eradication of these from the clothing is the primary objective. Treatment includes bathing, laundering all clothing, and changing to fresh clothes free of lice and nits. Dry cleaning eradicates lice and nits, as does ordinary laundering at hot settings. Malathion preparations and γ-benzene hexachloride formulations may be used for mass delousing.

Pubic lice may be treated with the same medications used for head lice. Treatment consists of permethrin 1% cream rinse applied for 10 minutes or lindane 1% shampoo applied for 5 minutes and rinsed. Sexual partners should also be treated.[32] Crotamiton lotion rubbed into the affected area daily for several weeks to destroy hatching ova may also be used. Eyelash infestations may be managed with physostigmine ophthalmic ointment using a cotton-tipped applicator. Machine washing and drying of sheets and clothing at hot settings will kill lice and nits.

FLEAS (ORDER SIPHONAPTERA)

Species, Life Cycle, and Distribution

Fleas are small ectoparasites of mammals and birds. The wingless body, which is covered by a hard shiny integument, is compressed laterally, enabling the fleas to scurry easily among the hairs and feathers of the hosts. They are active insects with legs adapted for jumping, capable of prodigious leaps. Adult fleas subsist on blood. Some species must obtain blood from one particular host, others are less host specific, and all have mouthparts adapted for piercing and sucking. The eggs are laid on or near the host and drop to the ground as the host moves about or shakes. They hatch into small wormlike larvae that feed on droppings from adult fleas, flakes of dried blood from the host, and other organic matter. The life cycle varies among species and may vary considerably within the same species, since each developmental stage is influenced by prevailing temperature and humidity. The customary larval stage of 9 to 15 days may be prolonged for months by adverse conditions, and the pupal stage varies from a week to nearly a year. Individual adult fleas may live for years when circumstances are favorable and can live for months without feeding.

Fleas exist universally, although the distribution of various species is restricted by climate and host. They are of medical importance because of the discomfort resulting from their bites, as a cause of papular urticaria, and as vectors of disease. They are more active in warm weather and cause more problems in warmer climates with a longer breeding season, such as the southwestern United States. They are a particular nuisance in California. High standards of sanitation and personal hygiene in developed countries have discouraged the human flea, *Pulex irritans,* while the same popularity of household pets has been conducive to the proliferation of dog and cat fleas, *Ctenocephalides canis* and *C. felis.* The incidence of other species in mammals and birds remains high. Since dog, cat, and many other fleas are only partially host specific, the fleas associated with many mammals and birds cause disease in humans. Most current flea bite problems are caused by animal fleas. Hungry fleas are more often attracted to people from an area frequented by an animal than from the animal itself. If the family dog is absent, hordes of hungry fleas may persist for months. Consequently, anyone with pet cats or dogs or near domesticated animals is more likely to be bitten, but outbreaks in the absence of pets are common. One epidemic of flea bites among children in a day nursery was traced to dog fleas in a deserted fox nesting area beneath the building.[102] Another outbreak among poultry workers was caused by an infestation of hen fleas, *Ceratophyllus gallinae.*[122] Fleas from flying squirrels also have been documented as the source of bites.

Clinical Aspects

The appearance of flea bites is not diagnostic, and the clinical features depend on degree of sensitivity. A bite produces a small, central hemorrhagic punctum surrounded by erythema and urticaria. A small wheal at the bite site may be nonallergic because of primary urticogenic substances in the flea saliva, but increasingly severe reactions are caused by sensitization to substances in the saliva. Bullae or even ulceration may result from flea bites in highly sensitive individuals. Flea bites are intensely pruritic, and scratching often results in crusting and impetiginization. Fleas have a habit of sampling several adjacent areas while feeding, and bites characteristically appear in irregular groups. Feet, ankles, and legs, as well as the hips and shoulder areas, where clothing fits snugly, are favorite targets. Although an individual lesion produced by a flea bite is not diagnostic, the typical clinical picture of grouped multiple bites is generally sufficient to establish a diagnosis, which is usually confirmed by locating and identifying fleas.

Treatment and Prevention

Ordinary flea bites require symptomatic treatment directed at relief of pruritus and prevention of secondary infection. Corticosteroid creams or calamine lotion with phenol, systemic antihistamines, and antibiotics are helpful when indicated, but the management of flea bites consists largely of prevention. The animals that host the fleas must be treated, as well as such places as chicken coops, rat nests, sleeping sites for dogs and cats, and often dwellings where pets live. Many effective insecticides are available. Typically, *N,N*-diethyl-meta-toluamide (DEET), pyrethrins, piperonyl butoxide, and *d*-trans allethrin are ingredients in sprays and foggers. An insect spray containing permethrin may be effective. Spraying or dusting must eradicate not only adult fleas but also the many larvae and pupae in grass, carpet, floorboards, furniture, and beds. Lindane, carbaryl, and malathion are the active ingredients in many sprays and dusts, and the services of professional exterminators may be necessary.

Veterinary prescriptions are available for control of fleas on dogs and cats. Preparations containing 9.1% imidacloprid (Advantage, Bayer) eliminate or reduce fleas on dogs when applied to the skin; 98% to 100% of fleas are killed within 12 hours of application, and reinfesting fleas are killed for 4 weeks after a single application. An oral preparation used for both dogs and cats contains lufenuron, an inhibitor of insect development. Lufenuron does not kill adult fleas but rather controls flea populations by interrupting the life cycle at the egg stage.

MITES (CLASS ARACHNIDA, ORDER ACARINA)

Species, Life Cycle, and Distribution

Mites make up the largest group in the class Arachnida. Most are small arthropods, and many are barely visible. Mites have two body regions, a small cephalothorax and a larger, unsegmented abdomen. The cephalothorax and abdomen are broadly joined, giving most mites an oblong to globular appearance. Newly hatched larvae have three pairs of legs, and larvae acquire a fourth pair after the first molt. Mites are highly diverse. Some are parasitic, with both vertebrates and invertebrates serving as hosts; some are scavengers, some feed on plants, and many are free living and predaceous. Although most species are oviparous, some are ovoviviparous, and a few are viviparous. They occur worldwide and frequently in great numbers. Mites have been associated with disease transmission, allergies, and dermatologic manifestations. Of the approximately 35,000 species, about 50 are known to cause human skin lesions, and most of the cutaneous lesions are caused by mites feeding or burrowing in the skin. Since children and adults of all races are susceptible to these ubiquitous arthropods, they are responsible for considerable morbidity. The mites of medical importance are some of the sarcoptic mites, some of the trombiculid mites, a number of other acariform mites that infest organic substances such as grains and produce, and the gamasid mites that are vectors of several rickettsial and viral diseases. Dermatologic manifestations of mite bites may be seasonal, as with the trombiculids; individual cases or outbreaks of varying magnitude may be related to contact with mites that infest animals or various foods. Epidemics may occur, as is presently the case with scabies.

Scabies

Life Cycle. The human scabies mite is *Sarcoptes scabiei* var. *hominis,* an obligate human parasite that completes its entire life cycle in and on the epidermis of humans. Unless treated, scabies can persist indefinitely. The adult female is responsible for the symptoms accompanying the infestation. After impregnation, she burrows into the epidermis and remains in the burrow for a life span of about 1 month. She slowly extends the burrow, feeding during travel, during which time several eggs are deposited daily. The ovoid female mite is approximately 0.3 to 0.4 mm long. Numerous transverse corrugations and dorsal spinous processes are adaptations to prevent backward movement in the burrow. The males are much smaller than females, spend more time on the surface, and have a brief life, dying shortly after copulation. The mite is passed in the vast majority of cases by intimate contact, but adult human scabies mites can survive off the host for 24 to 36 hours at room conditions and still remain infestive.[2] Thus scabies can be acquired from infested bedding, furniture, and clothing. Outbreaks not related to sexual activity occur frequently among nursing home patients and personnel; epidemics in schools for small children are also common. Scabies became uncommon after World War II (during the war it was a common problem), but the disease has increased in frequency since 1964 to epidemic proportions worldwide.[85]

Clinical Aspects. Severe nocturnal pruritus is the hallmark of scabies. Itching also may be provoked by any sudden warming of the body and generally does not involve the face. A warm bath or radiant heat may cause a paroxysm of itching. Since the pruritus is caused by sensitization, 4 to 6 weeks may elapse between infestation and the onset of severe pruritus. Reinfestation is common, since eradicating the disease from all contacts simultaneously is often difficult, and reinfestation after cure results in prompt recurrence of symptoms. Cutaneous manifestations are varied. The primary lesion is the epidermal burrow, a tiny linear or serpentine track, rarely longer than 5 to 10 mm. The female mite may burrow anywhere on the body, but sites of predilection include the interdigital spaces, palms, flexor surfaces of the wrists, elbows, feet and ankles, beltline, anterior axillary folds, lower buttocks, and penis and scrotum. The distribution of burrows in infants may be atypical, with burrows frequently found in the scalp and on the soles. In the present epidemic, involving many people with excellent hygiene, cutaneous changes may be almost absent and burrows difficult to find. On the other hand, after the disease has been present for some time, eczematization, lichenification, impetiginization, myriad nonspecific papules and excoriations, and even urticaria may be present. The burrows are often the least conspicuous of various skin changes. The clinical picture varies with differences in personal hygiene, topical treatments used before diagnosis, and individual scratch threshold.

Diagnosis is based on the combination of nocturnal pruritus and cutaneous findings and is confirmed by microscopic examination of burrow contents. The burrow and contents may be collected for examination by scraping with a scalpel blade or by pinching the skin to elevate it and shaving off a superficial layer. Burrows are often inflamed and no longer typical after the disease has been present for some time. The most productive sites to find burrows for examination are finger webs, sides of fingers, wrists, and elbows. Ectoparasites, ova, egg castings, feces, or pieces of mites are diagnostic.

Norwegian scabies is a term describing a particularly severe form of scabies occasionally seen in senile and mentally impaired patients, those with debilitating illnesses, and immunosuppressed patients. Extensive crusting occurs, particularly of the hands and feet. Erythema and scaling may develop, and patients are literally "crawling with mites." This form of scabies is highly contagious resulting from the incredible number of mites on the patient and in the immediate vicinity.[13,61]

Nodular scabies is another troublesome clinical variation. Persistent pruritic nodules develop, particularly on the male genitalia or in the groin, but usually on some covered body part. Nodules may be the only finding and may persist for months after adequate antiscabetic therapy.

Treatment and Prevention. A number of topical treatments are available. In most cases a single overnight application of 5% permethrin cream (Elimite) is curative. Permethrin has the advantages of low mammalian toxicity and high cure rate.[121] Even after adequate therapy, symptoms may persist more than a month until the mite and mite products are shed with the epidermis. The chemical must be applied even beneath the fingernails, since ova and live mites are frequently lodged there as a result of frenzied scratching. If the itching has not abated in several weeks, the patient should be reexamined for treatment failure or reinfestation. Permethrin may be used for retreatment, or alternative scabicides may be considered. Lindane lotion is highly effective but has the potential for central nervous system toxicity, and percutaneous absorption may occur. It is contraindicated in infants and pregnant women and persons known to be allergic to hexachlorocyclohexane. Sulfur in petrolatum (5% to 10%) or another suitable vehicle applied for three consecutive nights is a suitable alternative. Crotamiton 10% cream or lotion applied for two consecutive nights is also used. In the treatment of Norwegian scabies, salicylic acid ointment may be needed to soften scales and permit penetration of the scabicide. Nodular scabies can be a perplexing therapeutic problem and may necessitate intralesional injections of corticosteroids in addition to adequate antiscabetic therapy. Application of crude coal tar to the nodules has been recommended.

Contacts must be treated simultaneously. Clothing and linens should be laundered the morning after treatment to kill mites that may have strayed from the skin. When many members of a household are infested, live mites may be on the furniture; γ-benzene hexachloride sprays are available.

Control of scabies outbreaks in nursing homes and similar epidemic situations can be almost insurmountable because of the number of patients and contacts that must be treated simultaneously. An uncured case of Norwegian scabies as the focus of an epidemic may be surrounded by millions of mites. Ivermectin is an effective antiscabetic when taken orally. A single dose of 250 μg/kg cured 10 of 11 patients with Norwegian scabies and all in a group of otherwise healthy persons with scabies; however,[73] it is presently approved in humans for strongyloidiasis and onchocerciasis.

Zoonotic Scabies. Other burrowing mites similar to the human scabies mite infest animals such as swine, cattle, horses, mules, sheep, dogs, and wild animals. They are relatively host specific but under conditions of close contact may cause self-limited dermatitis in humans. Because of humans' close association with dogs, the most common animal scabies is canine, caused by *Sarcoptes scabiei* var. *canis*. Studies indicate that the dog scabies mites are able to survive for at least 96 hours on human skin, even burrowing and laying eggs, but whether a perpetual life cycle can be established is not yet determined.[29] Infested dogs have reddish papules, scaling, crusting, and evidence of scratching. Humans develop itchy papules, often with some urtication, and scratching may give rise to varying degrees of secondary infection. The initial lesions are most often on areas of skin that come in contact with dogs: forearms, chest, anterior abdomen, and anterior thighs. Outbreaks are frequently traced to a kennel or litter of puppies. In one case, 15 patients developed an itchy dermatitis from five puppies in a single litter.[16] Human infestation with dog scabies mites subsides spontaneously when contact with dogs is discontinued or when the dogs are cured. The dogs must be treated with scabicides and the human victims with symptomatic therapy for pruritus. Cats, also closely associated with humans, have been known to harbor mites that can infest humans. *Notoedres cati* infestation is seen more often in Czechoslovakia and Japan than is dog sarcoptic scabies.[14]

Trombiculid Mites

Mites of the family Trombiculidae are distributed worldwide. In the United States the most important species is *Eutrombicula alfreddugesi* (red bug, chigger, harvest mite). Another species, *E. batatas,* is also indigenous to parts of the United States. Adults are free living and predaceous on small arthropods and their eggs, but the larvae are ectoparasites of vertebrates. Wild and domestic mammals, as well as reptiles, serve as hosts. The larval bite causes human dermatitis. Adult mites lay their eggs among vegetation, and newly hatched larvae crawl up on the vegetation, waiting to attach themselves to a passing host. They attach themselves to the skin with hooked mouthparts and feed on blood, falling off when full. However, humans are not good hosts, and larvae usually do not stay long. Severity of the response depends on the species of trombiculid, the irritating qualities of the mites' saliva, and the host's allergic response. The typical bite is a maddeningly pruritic, hemorrhagic punctum that usually becomes surrounded by intense erythema within 24 hours. Bites may number in the hundreds and can be associated with an allergic reaction. Hypersensitivity causes blisters and weeping of clear fluid with crusting. The surrounding area may be purplish in color, with severe swelling, particularly of the feet and ankles (Figure 36-19). The lesions regress in 1 to 2 weeks, but pruritus is persistent and often paroxysmal during this time, with secondary infection in excoriated skin.

Treatment is symptomatic and consists of topical antipruritic agents, corticosteroids, systemic antihistamines, and occasionally, pulse therapy with systemic corticosteroids. Superpotent topical corticosteroid creams and ointments, such as 0.05% clobetasol, applied sparingly to individual bites several times daily, are effective but must be used properly. Prolonged application can result in atrophy, and absorption can be significant if excessive body surface is treated. Phenol 1% in calamine often is effective. As in all self-limited conditions with no satisfactory cure, home remedies abound, such as meat tenderizer rubbed into the moistened skin. Application of clear nail polish to the individual lesions is a popular home remedy, even though no evidence suggests that this is effective.

Preventive measures consist of avoidance and insect repellents used on skin and clothing. Clothing pretreated with permethrin has resulted in 74.2% increase in protection compared with unprotected controls.[9] Other repellents suggested for treating clothing are ethylhexandiol, DEET, and flowers of sulfur. The symptoms are allergic, and permanent residents in infested areas may develop tolerance to repeated bites.

Miscellaneous Mites

Parasitiformes. This group contains gamasid mites that are parasites of birds, mammals, snakes, insects, and rarely, humans. In addition to being vectors of disease, gamasid mites are responsible for some cases of dermatitis. The chicken mite, *Dermanyssus gallinae*, is responsible for most of the dermatitis caused by this group. This pest of poultry is widespread and is associated with both domestic and wild birds. Poultry workers are common targets, but other persons may be infested from insidious sources, such as a pet canary or bird nest near an intake for ventilation or air conditioning. The clinical picture is nonspecific, but the diagnosis may be made by identifying the mite. Treatment consists of symptomatic therapy and eradication of the mite source.

The tropical rat mite *Ornithonyssus bacoti* has also been reported to cause dermatitis, from such diverse sources as a rat nest in the attic or a colony of laboratory mice.[15,33] Snake mites have been implicated as a

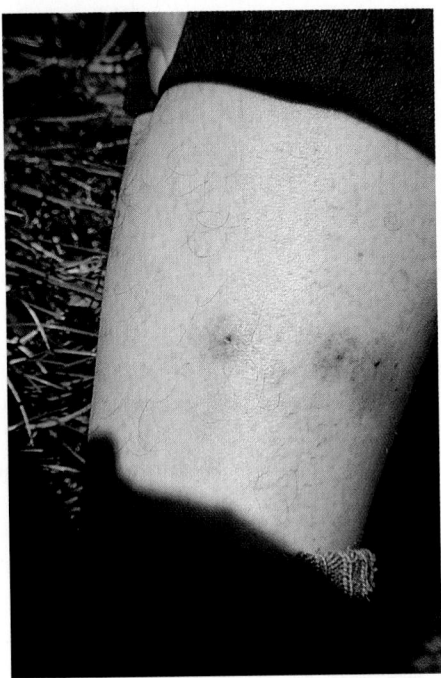

Figure 36-19 Chigger bites.

cause of dermatitis. Four members of one family developed a vesicobullous eruption from *Ophionyssus natricis* harbored by a pet python.[106]

Acariniformes. This huge group includes mites that infest foods, feathers, and furs. Individual infestations and larger outbreaks are common, with increased exposure by occupation, resulting in such terms as *grocer's itch*, *miller's itch*, and *copra itch*. Dogs, cats, and rabbits are primary hosts for mites of the genus *Cheyletiella*, and domestic pets are increasingly the source of mite dermatitis. Pet house cats are often involved.[100]

Mites of the genus *Dermatophagoides* are said to be the principal inhaled allergen of house dust. *D. scheremetewskyi* is an unusual mite that has been found in kapok and feather pillows, in a sparrow's nest, in monkey food, and on rats and other animals. This mite has been reported as the cause of feather pillow dermatitis.[3]

The most common type of dermatitis in this group is grain itch caused by *Pyemotes ventricosus*. This tiny mite parasitizes various insects often found in and around grain and straw. It attacks humans when a large mite population has no ready access to normal hosts. Grain itch implies an occupational bias, but outbreaks not involving farmers or rural workers have been described. During a widespread epidemic of *Pyemotes* infestation of farm workers in the midwestern United States in 1950 to 1951, straw used at the Indiana State Fair was infested. During a 2-year period, 642 visitors were treated for grain itch at a dispensary maintained on the fairgrounds, and about 1100 animal attendants and fair workers were treated over the same period at a separate facility. The reservoir of infestation by *Pyemotes* may be quite obscure. Several cases have been reported associated with the common furniture beetle *Anobium punctatum* in the floor joists of a house.[31] Therapy is symptomatic. Large-scale eradication measures may require services of professional exterminators.

DELUSIONS OF PARASITOSIS

Patients with delusions of parasitosis are convinced, against all evidence to the contrary, that parasites infest their skin and often their homes and clothing. No single cause is known for this condition, although some cases may be associated with proven parasitic infestation. The idea may also be suggested by infestations of relatives or acquaintances. Patients over 50 years are most often female; patients under 50 are equally male and female. Most cases of delusions of parasitosis commence with pruritus, which may be accompanied by crawling, creeping, stinging, and burning sensations. The initial reaction is to scratch, replaced soon by digging to remove the "parasites." Self-mutilation and suicidal behavior may develop. Generally the first contact with a physician is to bring in evidence of the "infestation." Evidence typically consists of scales, lint, crusts, hairs, dust, and small pieces of skin, carefully collected and stored in a small box or folded in facial tissue. Medical attention is often sought not to relieve the symptoms but to eradicate the parasites. Patients may take the evidence to a professional entomologist for identification and may employ professional exterminators for repeated fumigation. Patients may be so convincing that household members or acquaintances come to share the delusion.[24,30]

Many patients with parasitophobia know that their fear is groundless but are still unable to overcome it. Other patients with delusions of parasitosis are convinced that they have an infestation and regard as incompetent the physician who makes the correct diagnosis of no infestation. A complete examination of the patient and the evidence is essential, and investigation of the home or workplace may be indicated. Other medical conditions that may produce cutaneous sensations include liver and renal disease, alcoholism and toxic states, diabetes mellitus, cardiovascular disease, lymphoma, anemia, sideropenia, vitamin B_{12} deficiency, pellagra, peripheral neuritis, dermatitis herpetiformis, drug reactions, and environmental irritants (e.g., arthropods, fiberglass).[70,137]

Psychiatric intervention is often unsatisfactory to both patient and physician. Convinced that the physician is wrong, patients often seek repeated opinions and finally become despondent. Pimozide, a neuroleptic medication used to treat other monosymptomatic hypochondriacal psychoses, has been found useful in treating this condition.[81,93,98] In one group of 14 patients treated with pimozide and followed for an average of 34 months, seven had complete remissions, three had relapses that responded to treatment with pimozide, and four were treatment failures.[65]

IN MEMORIAM

It is with great sadness that we observe the passing of Sherman Minton, MD, who was an outstanding teacher, scientist, and friend. His contributions to this book and the entire wilderness medicine community were extensive and generous, and we will always be in his debt.

Paul Auerbach, MD

REFERENCES

1. Amino R et al: Identification and characterization of a sialase released by the salivary gland of the hematophagous insect *Triatoma infestans, J Biol Chem* 273:24575, 1998.
2. Arlian LG et al: Survival and infestivity of *Sarcoptes scabei* var. *canis* and var. *hominis, J Am Acad Dermatol* 11:210, 1984.
3. Aylesworth R, Baldridge D: Feather pillow dermatitis caused by an unusual mite *Dermatophagoides scheremetewskyi, J Am Acad Dermatol* 13:680, 1985.
4. Barnard JH: Studies of 400 Hymenoptera sting deaths in the United States, *J Allergy Clin Immunol* 52:259, 1973.
5. Bernstein JA et al: Rapid venom immunotherapy is safe for routine use in the treatment of patients with Hymenoptera sting anaphylaxis, *Ann Allergy* 73:423, 1995.
6. Billstein SA, Mattaliano VJ: The "nuisance" sexually transmitted diseases: molluscum contagiosum, scabies and crab lice, *Med Clin North Am* 74:1487, 1990.
7. Bischof RO: Seasonal incidence of insect stings: autumn yellow jacket delirium, *J Fam Pract* 43:271, 1996.
8. Bousquet J et al: Evolution of sensitivity to Hymenoptera venom in 200 allergic patients followed for up to 3 years, *J Allergy Clin Immunol* 84:944, 1989.
9. Breeden GC: Permethrin as a clothing treatment for personal protection against chigger mites, *Am J Trop Med Hyg* 31:589, 1982.
10. Burgess I, Davies EA: Cutaneous myiasis caused by the housefly, *Musca domestica, Br J Dermatol* 123:377, 1991.
11. Burkhart KM, Burkhart CN, Burkhart CG: Update on therapy: ivermectin is available for use in lice, *Infect Med* 14:689, 1997.
12. Butcher BT, Reed MA: Crossed immunoelectrophoretic studies of whole body extracts and venom from the imported fire ant *Solenopsis invicta, J Allergy Clin Immunol* 81:33, 1988.
13. Carslaw RW et al: Mites in the environment of cases of Norwegian scabies, *Br J Dermatol* 92:333, 1975.
14. Chakrabarti A: Human notoderic scabies from contact with cats infested with *Notoedres cati, Int J Dermatol* 25:646, 1986.
15. Charlesworth EN, Clegern RW: Tropical rat mite dermatitis, *Arch Dermatol* 113:937, 1977.
16. Charlesworth EN, Johnson JL: An epidemic of canine scabies in man, *Arch Dermatol* 110:572, 1974.
17. Claborn DM et al: Staphylinid (rove) beetle dermatitis outbreak in the American Southwest, *Mil Med* 164:209, 1999.
18. Cohen PR: Imported fire ant stings: clinical manifestations and treatment, *Pediatr Dermatol* 9:44, 1992.
19. Daisley H: Acute hemorrhagic pancreatitis following multiple stings by Africanized bees in Trinidad, *Trans R Soc Trop Med Hyg* 92:71, 1998.
20. Daniel M, Sramove H, Zalabska E: *Lucilia sericata* causing hospital-acquired myiasis of a traumatic wound, *J Hosp Infect* 28:149, 1994.
21. Davis MDP et al: Exaggerated arthropod-bite lesions in patients with chronic lymphatic leukemia, *J Am Acad Dermatol* 39:27, 1998.
22. De Shazo RD, Butcher BT, Banks WA: Reactions to stings of the imported fire ant, *N Engl J Med* 323:462, 1990.
23. De Shazo RD, Williams DF: Multiple fire ant stings indoors, *South Med J* 88:712, 1995.

24. Dewhurst K, Todd J: The psychosis of association—folie a deux, *J Nerv Ment Dis* 124:451, 1956.

25. Diaz-Sanchez DL, Lipshitz A, Ignocio-Ibarra G: Survival after massive Africanized honeybee stings, *Arch Intern Med* 158:925, 1998.

26. Diven DG, Newton RC, Ramsey KM: Heightened cutaneous reaction to mosquito bites in patients with acquired immune deficiency syndrome receiving zidovudine, *Arch Intern Med* 148:2296, 1988.

27. Duplantier JE et al: Successful rush immunotherapy for anaphylaxis to imported fire ants, *J Allergy Clin Immunol* 101:855, 1998.

28. Edwards JS: The action and composition of the saliva of the assassin bug *Platymeris rhadamanthus* Gaerst (Hemiptera Reduviidae), *J Exp Biol* 38:61, 1961.

29. Estes SA, Kummel B, Arlain L: Experimental canine scabies in humans, *J Am Acad Dermatol* 9:397, 1983.

30. Evans P, Merskey H: Shared beliefs of dermal parasitosis: folie partagee, *Br J Med Psychol* 45:19, 1972.

31. Fine R, Scott HG: Straw itch mite dermatitis caused by *Pyemotes ventricosus*, *J Med Assoc Ga* 52:162, 1963.

32. Forsman KE: Pediculosis and scabies, *Postgrad Med* 98:89, 1995.

33. Fox JG: Outbreak of tropical rat mite dermatitis in laboratory personnel, *Arch Dermatol* 118:676, 1982.

34. Franca FOS et al: Severe and fatal mass attacks by killer bees (Africanized honeybees *Apis mellifera scutata*) in Brazil: clinicopathological studies with measurement of serum venom concentrations, *Q J Med* 87:269, 1994.

35. Freeman TM: Hymenoptera sensitivity in an imported fire ant endemic area, *Ann Allergy Asthma Immunol* 78:369, 1997

36. Freye HB, Litwin E: Coexistent anaphylaxis to Diptera and Hymenoptera, *Ann Allergy Asthma Immunol* 76:270, 1996.

37. Gardner TL, Elston DM: Painful papulovesicles produced by the puss caterpillar, *Cutis* 60:125, 1997.

38. Gluck JC, Pacin MP: Asthma from mosquito bite; a case report, *Ann Allergy* 56:492, 1986.

39. Goddard J: Human infestation with rodent botfly larvae: a new route of entry, *South Med J* 90:254, 1997.

40. Golden DBK et al: Epidemiology of insect venom sensitivity, *JAMA* 262:240, 1989.

41. Golden DBK et al: Natural history of Hymenoptera sensitivity in adults, *J Allergy Clin Immunol* 100:760, 1997.

42. Hall HG: Parental analysis of introgressive hybridization between African and European honeybees using nuclear DNA, *Genetics* 125:611, 1990.

43. Hall HG, Smith DR: Distinguishing African and European honeybee matrilines using amplified mitochondrial DNA, *Proc Natl Acad Sci USA* 88:4548, 1991.

44. Hauk PK, Friedl K, Kaufmehl K: Subsequent insect stings in children with hypersensitivity to Hymenoptera, *J Pediatr* 126:185, 1993

45. Hemmer W, Focke M, Vieluf D: Anaphylaxis induced by horsefly bites. Identification of a 69kd IgE-binding salivary gland protein from *Chrysops* spp by Western blot, *J Allergy Clin Immunol* 101:134, 1998.

46. Hidano KA, Kawakami M, Yago A: Hypersensitivity to mosquito bite and malignant histiocytosis, *Jpn J Exp Med* 52:303, 1982.

47. Ho CL, Hwang LL: Local edema induced by the black-bellied hornet (*Vespa basalis*) venom and its components, *Toxicon* 29:1033, 1991.

48. Hoffman DR: Allergens in Hymenoptera venom XIV: the amino acid sequences of imported fire ant venom allergens, *J Allergy Clin Immunol* 91:71, 1993.

49. Holland DL, Adams DP: Puss caterpillar envenomation: a report form North Carolina, *Wilderness Environ Med* 9:213, 1998

50. Hunt GR: Uncommon insect bites: the reduviid bite, *Tex Med* 73:45, 1977.

51. Irskip HL et al: A survey of the prevalence of biting by the Blanford fly during 1993, *Br J Dermatol* 134:696, 1996.

52. Jelenek T et al: Cutaneous myiasis: review of 13 cases in travelers returning from tropical countries, *Int J Dermatol* 34:624, 1995.

53. Jones RL et al: A novel Fab-based antivenom for the treatment of mass bee attacks, *Am J Trop Med Hyg* 61:361, 1999.

54. Kemp ED: Bites and stings of the arthropod kind, *Postgrad Med* 103:88, 1998.

55. Keystone JS: Of bites and body odour, *Lancet* 347:1423, 1996.

56. Khan RH, Szewcauk MR, Day JH: Bee venom anti-idiotypic antibody is associated with protection in beekeepers and bee-sting sensitive patients receiving immunotherapy against allergic reactions, *J Allergy Clin Immunol* 88:199, 1991.

57. Kim KT: Update on the status of Africanized honeybees in the Western states, *West J Med* 170:220, 1999.

58. King TP: Immunochemical studies of stinging insect venom allergens, *Toxicon* 34:1455, 1996.

59. Kolecki P: Delayed toxic reaction following massive bee envenomation, *Ann Emerg Med* 33:114, 1999.

60. Lacey LA: Anthropophilic blackflies (Diptera: Simuliidae) in Amazon National Park and their effects on man, *Bull Pan Am Health Org* 15:26, 1981.

61. Lang E, Humphries DW, Jaqua-Stewart MJ: Crusted scabies: a case report and review of the literature, *SD J Med* 42:15, 1989.

62. Lantner R, Reisman RE: Clinical and immunologic features and subsequent course of patients with severe insect-sting anaphylaxis, *J Allergy Clin Immunol* 84:900, 1989.

63. Law DA et al: Arterial flutter and fibrillation following bee stings, *Am J Cardiol* 80:1255, 1997.

64. Lazoglu AH et al: Serum sickness reaction following multiple insect stings, *Ann Allergy Asthma Immunol* 75:522, 1995.

65. Lindskov R, Baadsgard O: Delusions of infestation treated with pimozide: a follow-up study, *Acta Derm Venereol* 65:267, 1985.

66. Lockey RF: Immunotherapy for allergy to insect stings, *N Engl J Med* 323:1627, 1990.

67. Lockey RF et al: The Hymenoptera Venom Study I, 1979-1982: demographics and history—sting data, *J Allergy Clin Immunol* 82:370, 1988.

68. Lockey RF et al: The Hymenoptera Venom Study III: safety of venom immunotherapy, *J Allergy Clin Immunol* 86:775, 1990.

69. Lukin LG: Human cutaneous myiasis in Brisbane: a prospective study, *Med J Aust* 150:237, 1989.

70. Lyell A: Delusions of parasitosis, *J Am Acad Dermatol* 8:895, 1983.

71. Lynch PJ, Pinnas JL: "Kissing bug" bites, *Cutis* 22:585, 1978

72. McCormack DR et al: Mosquito bite anaphylaxis: immunotherapy with whole body extracts, *Ann Allergy Asthma Immunol* 74:39, 1995.

73. Meinking TL et al: The treatment of scabies with ivermectin, *N Engl J Med* 333:26, 1995.

74. Meszaros I: Transient cerebral ischemia attack caused by Hymenoptera stings, *Eur Neurol* 25:248, 1986.

75. Mielke U: Nosocomial myiasis, *J Hosp Infect* 37:1, 1997.

76. Miller KB, Hribar LJ, Sanders LJ: Human myiasis caused by *Phormia regina* in Pennsylvania, *J Am Podiatr Med Assoc* 80:600, 1990.

77. Millikan LE: Myiasis, *Clin Dermatol* 17:191, 1999.

78. Muller UR et al: Combined active and passive immunotherapy in honeybee sting allergy, *J Allergy Clin Immunol* 78:115, 1986.

79. Muller UR et al: Emergency treatment of allergic reactions to Hymenoptera stings, *Clin Exp Allergy* 21:281, 1991.

80. Mumcouglu KY, Volman Y: Thrips stings in Israel, a case report, *Isr J Med Sci* 24:715, 1988.

81. Munro A: Monosymptomatic hypochondriacal psychosis manifesting as delusions of parasitosis: a description of 4 cases successfully treated with pimozide, *Arch Dermatol* 114:940, 1978.

82. Munroz-Arizpe RL et al: Insufiencia renal aguda por picadura de abejas africanizadas, *Bol Med Hosp Infant Mex* 49:388, 1992.

83. Nelson DR et al: Biochemical and immunochemical comparison of Africanized and European honeybee venoms, *J Allergy Clin Immunol* 85:80, 1990.

84. Neustater BR, Stollman NH, Manten HD: Sting of the puss caterpillar: an unusual cause of abdominal pain, *South Med J* 89:826, 1996.

85. Orkin M, Maibach HI: Current concepts in parasitology: this scabies pandemic, *N Engl J Med* 298:496, 1978.

86. Pence RL et al: Evaluation of severe reactions to sweat bee stings, *Ann Allergy* 66:399, 1991.

87. Peng Z, Simons FER: A prospective study of naturally acquired sensitization and subsequent desensitization to mosquito bites and subsequent antibody responses, *J Allergy Clin Immunol* 101:284, 1998.

88. Peng Z, Yang M, Simons FER: Immunologic mechanisms in mosquito allergy: correlation of skin reactions with specific IgE and IgG antibodies and lymphocyte response to mosquito antigens, *Ann Allergy Asthma Immunol* 77: 238, 1996.

89. Pinson RT, Morgan JA: Envenomation by the puss caterpillar, *Ann Emerg Med* 20:562, 1991.

90. Prahlow JA, Barnard JJ: Fatal anaphylaxis due to fire ant stings, *Am J Forensic Med Pathol* 19:137, 1998.

91. Rao R, Nosanchuk JS, Mackenzie R: Cutaneous myiasis acquired in New York State, *Pediatrics* 99:601, 1997.

92. Reames MK, Christensen C, Luce EA: The use of maggots in wound debridement, *Ann Plast Surg* 21:388, 1988.

93. Reilly TM: Pimozide in monosymptomatic psychosis, *Lancet* 1:1385, 1975.

94. Reisman RE: Natural history of insect sting allergy: relationship of severity of symptoms of initial sting anaphylaxis to re-sting reactions, *J Allergy Clin Immunol* 90:335, 1992

95. Reisman RE: Stinging insect allergy, *Med Clin North Am* 76:883, 1992.

96. Reunala T et al: Cutaneous reactivity to mosquito bites: effect of cetirizine and development of anti-mosquito antibodies, *Clin Exp Allergy* 2:617, 1991.

97. Reunala T et al: Effects of ebastine on mosquito bites, *Arch Derm Venereol* 77:31, 1997.

98. Riding J, Munro A: Pimozide in the treatment of monosymptomatic hypochondrical psychosis, *Acta Psychiatr Scand* 52:23, 1975.

99. Riggs JE et al: Acute and delayed cerebral infarction after wasp sting anaphylaxis, *Clin Neuropharmacol* 17:384, 1994.

100. Rivers JK, Martin J, Pukay B: Walking dandruff and *Cheyletiella* dermatitis, *J Am Acad Dermatol* 15:1130, 1986.

101. Rohr AS, Marshall NA, Saxon A: Successful immunotherapy for *Triatoma protracta* induced anaphylaxis, *J Allergy Clin Immunol* 73:369, 1984.

102. Rothenborg HW: Of fleas and foxes, *Arch Dermatol* 111:1215, 1975.

103. Rueff F et al: The sting challenge test in Hymenoptera allergy, *Allergy* 51:216, 1996.

104. Sadick N et al: Unusual features of scabies complicating human T-lymphotropic virus type III infection, *J Am Acad Dermatol* 15:482, 1986.

105. Salim MM et al: Insect bite lesions in Kuwait possibly due to *Leptodemus minutus*, *Int J Dermatol* 29:507, 1990

106. Schultz H: Human infestation by *Ophionyssus natricis* snake mite, *Br J Dermatol* 93:695, 1975.

107. Schultze-Werninghaus C: Evaluation of the risk of anaphylactic reactions by wasp venom-extract challenges in children, *Pediatr Allergy Immunol* 10:133, 1999.

108. Schumacher MJ: Significance of Africanized bees for public health, *Arch Intern Med* 155:2038, 1995.

109. Schumacher MJ, Egen NB, Tanner D: Neutralization of bee venom lethality by immune serum antibodies, *Am J Trop Med Hyg* 55:197, 1996.

110. Schumacher MJ, Schmidt JO, Egen NB: Quantity, analysis, and lethality of European and Africanized honey bee venoms, *Am J Trop Med Hyg* 43:79, 1990.

111. Schwartz HJ, Golden DB, Lockey RF: Venom immunotherapy in the Hymenoptera-allergic pregnant patient, *J Allergy Clin Immunol* 85:709, 1990.

112. Schwartz HJ et al: Hymenoptera venom-specific IgE antibodies in postmortem sera from victims of sudden and unexpected death, *Clin Allergy* 18:461, 1988.

113. Shah D, Tsang TK: Bee sting dysphagia, *Ann Intern Med* 129:253, 1998 (letter).

114. Sherman RA: What physicians should know about Africanized honeybees, *West J Med* 163:541, 1995.

115. Sherman RA, My-Tien J, Sullivan R: Maggot therapy for venous stasis ulcers, *Arch Dermatol* 132:254, 1996.

116. Shorter N et al: Furuncular cuterbrid myiasis, *J Pediatr Surg* 32:1511, 1997.

117. Smith DR, Taylor OR, Brown WM: Neotropical Africanized honey bees have African mitochondrial DNA, *Nature* 339:213, 1989.

118. Stafford CT: Hypersensitivity to fire ant venom, *Ann Allergy Asthma Immunol* 77:87, 1996.

119. Stoddard SR et al: Maggot debridement therapy: an alternative therapy for nonhealing ulcers, *J Am Podiatr Med Assoc* 85:218, 1995.

120. Suzuki S et al: A case of mosquito allergy, *Acta Allergol* 2:245, 1976

121. Taplin D et al: Permethrin 5% dermal cream: a new treatment for scabies, *J Am Acad Dermatol* 15:995, 1986.

122. Titchener RW: Infestation of broiler breeder houses with hen fleas, *Parasitology* 79:xiii, 1979.

123. Tokura Y et al: Severe hypersensitivity to mosquito bites associated with natural killer cell lymphocytosis, *Arch Dermatol* 126:362, 1990

124. Trubner K et al: Drei Todesfalle nach Wespenstichen, *Rechtsmed* 1:153, 1991.

125. Urbanek R et al: Venom-specific IgE and IgG antibodies as a measure of the degree of protection in insect-sting sensitive patients, *Clin Allergy* 13:229, 1983.

126. Valentine MD et al: The value of immunotherapy with venom in children with allergy to insect stings, *N Engl J Med* 323:1601, 1990

127. Van der Linden PWG et al: Anaphylactic shock after insect-sting challenge in 138 persons with a previous insect-sting reaction, *Arch Intern Med* 118:161, 1993.

128. Van Hallern HK, Van der Linden PWG, Burgers PW: Hymenoptera sting challenge of 348 patients: relation to subsequent field stings, *J Allergy Clin Immunol* 97:1058, 1997.

129. Visscher PK, Vetter RS, Camazine S: Removing bee stings, *Lancet* 348:301, 1996.

130. Wagdi P et al: Acute myocardial infarction after wasp stings in a patient with normal coronary arteries, *Am Heart J* 128: 820, 1994.

131. Warpinski JR, Bush RK: Stinging insect allergy, *J Wilderness Med* 1:249, 1990.

132. Watemberg M et al: Fatal multiple organ failure following massive hornet stings, *J Toxicol Clin Toxicol* 33:471, 1995.

133. Winston ML: Killer bees: the Africanized honey bee in the Americas, Cambridge, Mass, 1992, Harvard University Press.

134. Winston ML: The Africanized killer bee: biology and public health, *Q J Med* 87:263, 1994.

135. Wirtz RA: Allergic and toxic reactions to non-stinging arthropods, *Annu Rev Entomol* 29:47, 1984.

136. Wright DN, Lockey RF: Local reactions to stinging insects (Hymenoptera), *Allergy Proc* 11:23, 1990.

137. Wykoff RF: Delusions of parasitosis: a review, *Rev Infect Dis* 9:433, 1987.

138. Zerachia T, Bergmann F, Shulov A: Pharmacological activities of the predacious bug *Holotrichus innesi, Toxicon* 10:537, 1972.

139. Zora JA, Swanson MC, Yuninger JW: A study of the prevalence and clinical significance of venom-specific IgE, *J Allergy Clin Immunol* 81:77, 1988.

37 Non–North American Arthropod Envenomation and Parasitism

Sherman A. Minton,† H. Bernard Bechtel, and Timothy B. Erickson

HYMENOPTERA (BEES, WASPS, AND ANTS)

Hymenoptera insects are worldwide in distribution and often consistute a major part of a region's insect fauna. Honeybees are exploited for their honey throughout the world; even the aggressive *Apis mellifera scutellata* is used for honey production in Africa. Honeybees in southern Asia attach huge nests to limbs of forest trees. The giant bee, *Apis dorsata,* of southeast Asia has a reputation for savagery, and deaths from multiple stings have occurred. Yellowjackets and hornets are common in Europe and the Middle East and have similar medical importance as in the United States. Two species, *Vespula orientalis* and *V. vulgaris,* have recently been introduced into Australia, where they have become a significant problem.[30] Paper wasps of the genus *Polistes* are plentiful in tropical America and Australia. Another Australian paper wasp, *Ropalidia revolutionalis,* constructs nests that resemble belts of bullets and hangs them from shrubs and fences. Fire wasps *(Polybia)* are found from Mexico to northern South America. The common species are black with yellow markings. They construct globular, cylindric, or cone-shaped paper nests up to 70 cm long that are usually hung from trees and sometimes under bridges. They may defend these nests with great vigor.

Ants have numerous stinging species in the tropics. Although native to South America, fire ants do not seem to be a major medical problem there, perhaps because of native competitors, predators, and parasites. Two fire ant species are important in areas outside the United States. *Solenopsis geminata* has been introduced into Okinawa and Guam and is widespread in Central America, Mexico, and some Caribbean islands. *S. xyloni* is common in Mexico and also occurs in California and Texas. *S. invicta* has been introduced into Puerto Rico. Amino acid sequences of all fire ant venoms are very similar.[23] Presumably, all fire ant stings are similar and can be managed medically in the same manner.

The samsum ant, *Pachycondyla sennaarensis,* is an ecologic counterpart of the fire ant widely distributed in the African tropics and Arabian peninsula. It nests in the ground but does not make a conspicuous mound. In the United Arab Emirates it is plentiful in urban areas and the cause of many stings.[13] Australian bull ants are large insects (about 20 mm) with prominent jaws (Figure 37-1). They are ground dwelling and common in suburban areas in southeastern Australia. Many neotropical stinging ants live in trees. The giant black ants (16 to 22 mm) of the genus *Paraponera* are found from Nicaragua to the Amazon basin. Although they nest in the ground, workers forage in trees from almost ground level to high in the forest canopy. They are most active at night. The green tree ant of northeastern Australia makes a leaf nest in trees. It has no true sting but ejects formic acid into wounds made by its jaws.

Clinical Aspects

No unique features distinguish Hymenoptera envenomations in other parts of the world from those in North America. Venoms of the various groups show little geographic variation. This is also true of groups at risk, with the possible exception of a few honey-gathering Asian tribes. The incidence of Hymenoptera sting allergy may be slightly higher in western Europe than in the United States, and fatal allergic reactions may be slightly more common.[8] Systemic anaphylactic reactions to stings of Australian bull ants and samsum ants are increasing, with reports of a few fatalities. Patients with history of systemic reactions to samsum ant stings have immunoglobulin E (IgE) and positive skin test reactions to fire ant venom.[13] *Paraponera* ant stings are intensely painful for several hours and may be accompanied by fever and lymphadenitis.

LEPIDOPTERA

The Lepidoptera show high diversity in the tropics with correspondingly greater medical importance, particularly in Latin America. Caterpillars of the genus *Lonomia* native to northern South America can inflict life-threatening stings (Figure 37-2). These caterpillars are 50 to 70 mm long and have numerous branched dorsal spines. They live in primary tropical forests in groups of up to about 50 individuals. Disturbance of their habitat has resulted in an increasing number of envenomations. Venom of *Lonomia* is a protein that activates prothrombin and is stimulated by factor V and calcium ions.[21] Stings cause intense pain but not much local reaction. Signs of coagulopathy, such as ecchy-

---

†Deceased.

888

moses, bleeding gums, hematuria, and melana, may develop in a few hours or be delayed a week or more. Fibrinogen, factor V, factor XII, and plasminogen are decreased; fibrin degradation products are increased; and platelets usually are normal. Acute renal failure, cerebral hemorrhage, and pulmonary hemorrhage may occur. Coagulopathy lasts 2 to 5 weeks.

In one series of 33 cases, four were fatal.[1,6,16] Treatment with prednisone, plasma, and whole blood is ineffective. An antivenom has been developed, and a preliminary report indicates possible clinical effectiveness.[11,12]

Neotropical caterpillars of the genera *Dirphia, Megalopyge,* and *Automeris* are large, stout, spiny, and sometimes covered with hair. Most are forest species but can adapt to areas of cultivation. Agricultural workers are most often stung; the incidence of stings is higher in the rainy season. Intense, centrally radiating pain with local edema and erythema is typical; lymphadenopathy is often seen. Systemic symptoms include nausea, headache, malaise, chills, and fever. Hypotension, shock, and convulsions have been reported. An *Automeris* caterpillar bite reported from French Guyana produced syncopal pain and edematous infiltration of the thigh lasting several days.[10] Symptoms usually subside within 24 hours. Treatment is symptomatic. Oral antihistamines are often effective if given within about

an hour after the sting. Codeine or meperidine is occasionally needed to control pain.

A chronic granuloma of the hands of Brazilian rubber tappers known as *pararama* results from contact with caterpillars of *Premolis semirufa.* Permanent disability may result.[39]

Moths of the genus *Hylesia* occur from southern Mexico to Argentina. The caterpillars have venomous spines, but the greatest problem is created by the moths, which have a coating of spines on their abdomen. The spines or setae are hollow and pointed, contain a toxin of unknown nature, and are freely shed into the air. The moths are attracted to lights in enormous numbers, and their airborne spines can cause great discomfort. Their activity has created serious problems at airports, shipping docks, and tourist resorts. Within a few minutes to a few hours after contact with the spines, victims develop a pruritic, erythematous rash that progresses to urticaria and excoriation. Any portion of exposed skin may be involved, but palms and soles are often spared. Irritation of eyes and mucous membranes is unusual. Symptoms subside in about a week if there is no further exposure. Topical and systemic treatments have had little success.[14]

In Korea, outbreaks of dermatitis, presumably caused by setae of the yellow moth *Euproctis flava,* are well known. In the summer of 1980, hundreds of U.S. soldiers were affected.[3] The caterpillars feed on hardwood trees; great numbers of moths appear in summer and are attracted to lights. Dermatitis usually involves direct contact with moths or their cocoons or with clothing contaminated with setae. The lesions are similar to those described for *Hylesia* and are equally refractory to treatment. Other outbreaks of dermatitis ascribed to *Euproctis* moths and caterpillars have been reported in Japan and China. One outbreak in Shanghai in 1972 affected about 500,000 individuals. Cases of *Euproctis* dermatitis and ophthalmia have also been re-

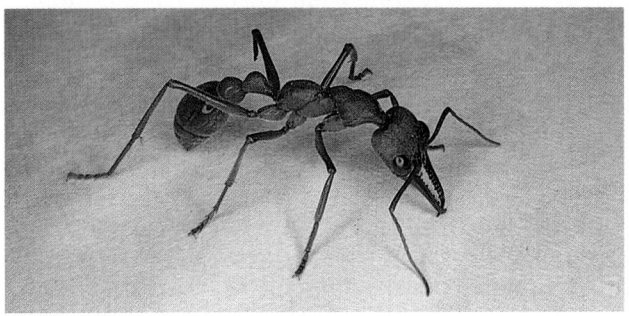

Figure 37-1 Red bull ant.

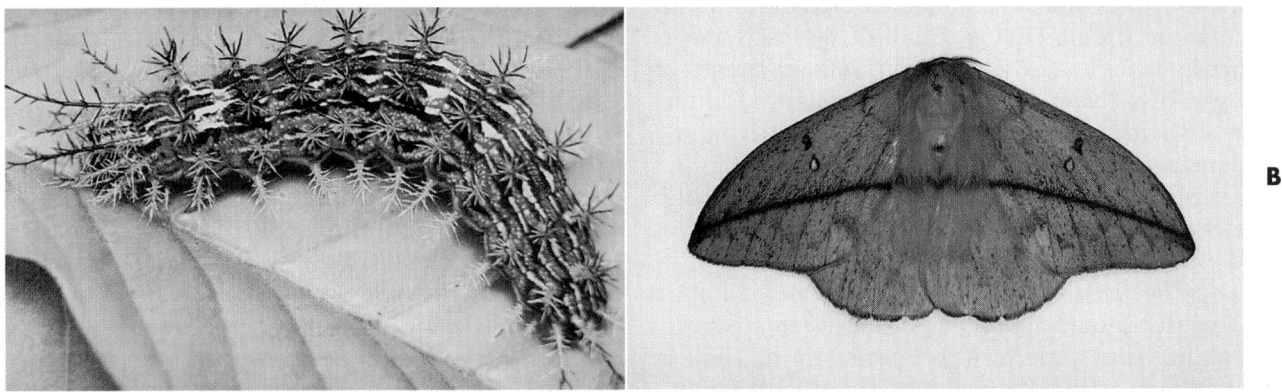

Figure 37-2 **A,** Caterpillar of *Lonomia achelous,* which can inflict injuries characterized by potentially fatal coagulopathy. **B,** Moth of *L. achelous,* which has no venomous spines.

ported in Australia and Great Britain. Sensitization with elevated IgE levels may occur.[39,44]

In the Mediterranean region and Middle East the pine processionary caterpillar, *Thaumetopoea pityocampa*, is plentiful and makes silk nests in trees. Its setae cause a maculopapular rash occasionally accompanied by urticaria, bronchitis, and conjunctivitis. Outbreaks typically occur when groups of tourists and military personnel camp in pine groves. The rash usually results from contact with detached setae rather than with caterpillars. The adult moth stage apparently does not have irritating spines.

Moths of the genus *Calyptera* native to Southeast Asia have a serrate proboscis and feed on mammalian blood, including that of humans. Tropical species of several moth genera feed on human ocular secretions. Their medical importance is unknown.

BEETLES AND OTHER INSECTS

Small rove beetles of the genus *Paederus* are troublesome in many tropical and subtropical regions. The whiplash beetle or Finch Hatton bug *(Paederus australis)* caused evacuation of an entire aboriginal community in northern Australia,[46] and a large suburban hospital in Sri Lanka had 108 cases of painful dermatitis among members of its staff on night duty.[27] Staphylinid (rove) beetle dermatitis epidemics have been reported in Nigeria in 1990, Egypt in 1994, and Kenya in 1998 after sudden floods.[9]

These beetles are slender with elongate abdomens and very short rectangular elytra. They frequent damp habitats and may be plentiful in irrigated crop fields. They usually fly after dark in hot, humid weather and are attracted to lights. Their vesicant secretion is an alkaloid present in greatest concentration in hemolymph; it is usually deposited on human skin when the beetles are pressed or crushed but may occasionally be spontaneously secreted. There is no immediate reaction to the secretion, but after 12 to 24 hours, painful erythematous lesions develop and soon become vesicular. The vesicles last 3 to 7 days and are followed by crusting and pigmentation. Conjunctivitis results if the secretion is rubbed into the eyes. This condition is known in parts of the world as "Nairobi eye" or "Christmas eye."[9] Some persons with extensive skin involvement may show generalized symptoms. Treatment is symptomatic and not very effective. Prompt soap and water washing after insect contact is recommended. Screening of sleeping and working quarters is the best prevention.

Lady beetles (ladybugs, family Coccinellidae) are widely distributed and highly beneficial as predators on aphids and scale insects. Species in the eastern United States often overwinter in houses and do no harm. However, an Australian lady beetle, *Diomus notescens*, is reported to bite, causing papules with small necrotic centers.[40] Two cases of human ear inva-

sion by a predaceous beetle, *Crasydactylus punctatus*, or the carabid beetle, have been reported from Oman. One victim had a severe otologic injury caused by biting and chewing on the external auditory canal and tympanic membrane.[4]

DIPTERA (TWO-WINGED FLIES)

Most dipterans are cosmopolitan in distribution. However, two groups of biting flies and several species involved in human myiasis are largely confined to the tropics and are discussed here (see Table 36-1).

Sand flies (*Phlebotomus* and related genera) are very small biting flies quite distinct from *Culicoides* and its relatives. They are widely distributed in tropical and subtropical regions. They live in damp, shaded places such as mammal burrows, rock crevices, and cracks in walls of houses and other structures. Favorite habitats in Central America are *gambas*, deep clefts between the buttresses of large forest trees. Larval and pupal stages are found in moist detritus in holes and crevices. The adults usually emerge at night when air is still and temperatures are above 13° C (56° F). They are poor fliers. Sand flies are vectors of leishmaniasis and of *Bartonella bacilliformis* in Peru. Sand fly populations can be controlled with pyrethroid insecticide sprayed into the mounds and burrows. Spraying of a 100-m-wide barrier zone around a campsite can reduce sand fly numbers for an extended period.[17]

Tsetse flies (*Glossina* species) are of great importance as vectors of human and animal trypanosomiasis in sub-Saharan Africa. Although not closely related to deerflies and other tabanids, they are similar in appearance and habits (see Chapter 36). Their life history is peculiar in that a single large larva develops in the uterus of the female and is expelled shortly before pupation, which takes place in the soil. Tsetse fly bites produce comparatively little local reaction other than brief pain and itching.

Myiasis

Furuncular Myiasis. This type of myiasis is caused by flies whose larvae penetrate human skin and develop in that location, producing boil-like lesions with an external opening. Formerly, this condition was encountered almost exclusively in the tropics, but with the growing popularity of ecotourism and other travel to unconventional destinations, cases are being seen in many other parts of the world. A German travel clinic reported 13 cases in travelers returning from tropical countries during a 3-year period.[25]

The classic agent of furuncular myiasis is the so-called human botfly, *Dermatobia hominis* (Figure 37-3). Actually, humans are only one of many mammals that serve as suitable hosts for the obligately parasitic larvae of this fly. It is widely distributed in the American tropics and is an important parasite of domestic cattle in many places. Human infection seems to be most prevalent in Central America and northern South America. Adult flies resemble a bumblebee (body length about 15 mm). The do not feed and are infrequently seen. The life cycle of this fly is unique in that the female attaches her eggs to the body of another arthropod for transfer to the host. Large mosquitoes of the genus *Psorphora* are often used (8% were found bearing *Dermatobia* eggs in one study), but about 40 species of insects and ticks have been reported to be egg carriers. When the carrier alights on a mammal, the eggs hatch immediately, and the larvae enter the skin through the bite of the carrier or some other small trauma. Small larvae are fusiform and later become pyriform to ovoid as they reach full development at

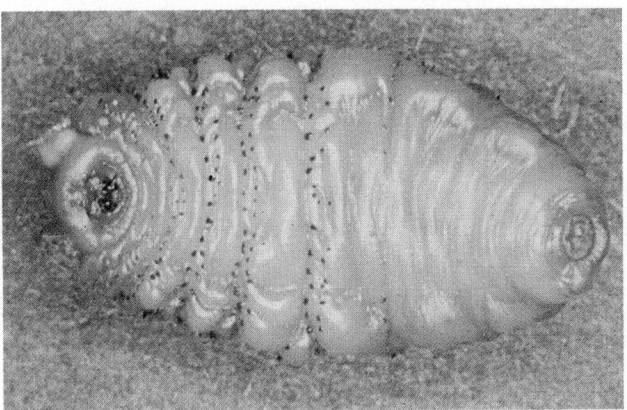

Figure 37-3   Dermatobia larva.

lengths of 15 to 20 mm. They are encircled by several rings of spines. The larval stage lasts 6 to 7 weeks, after which the larva emerges from the skin and drops to the ground, where pupation occurs.

Infection is fairly common among rural people of Central America. Cases in returned tourists and visitors from Latin America have been diagnosed in many parts of the United States. Six cases occurred in one group of tourists visiting archaeologic sites in Guatemala.[15,26,28,37,45] Lesions may be on any part of the body exposed to insect bites and may be single or multiple. An initial pruritic papule becomes a furuncle, with a characteristic opening from which serosanguineous fluid exudes. Pain often accompanies movements of the older larvae, but the lesion is not particularly tender to palpation. Lymphadenopathy, fever, and secondary infection are rare.

This form of myiasis should be suspected in patients with furuncular lesions and history of residence or travel in endemic areas. It must be differentiated from leishmaniasis and onchocerciasis, which have a different prognosis and treatment. The sensation of movement within the lesion, accompanied by pain but little tenderness or inflammation, suggests myiasis. The tip of the larva may protrude from the central opening, or bubbles produced by its respiration may be seen. Often, simple pressure will extrude the organism, particularly if it is small.[36] Occlusion of the breathing hole may cause the larva to emerge sufficiently for it to be grasped and withdrawn. An effective folk remedy is binding a piece of fat, such as bacon, over the opening (Figure 37-4).[5] This often causes the larva to leave its

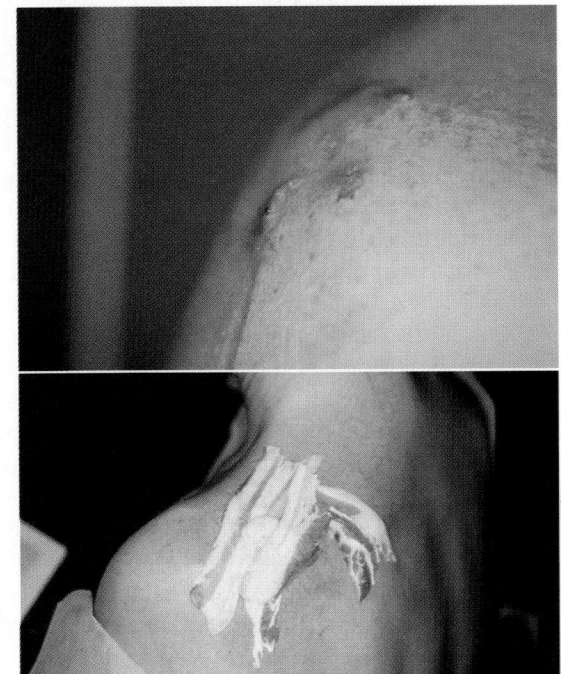

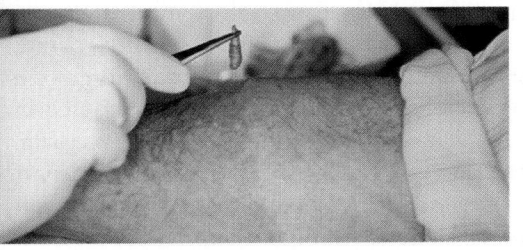

Figure 37-4   A, Lateral view of three lesions cased by infestation with *D. hominis* larvae. The nodules were initially assumed to be furunculosis. A central breathing aperture is present in each nodule. Serosanguineous fluid is draining from two of the nodules. Larval spiracles are visible emerging from the uppermost nodule. **B,** The fatty portion of multiple strips of raw bacon were placed over the larval apertures to obstruct the air supply and encourage the larvae's egress from the skin. **C,** After approximately 2 hours of treatment with bacon therapy, the *D. hominis* larvae have emerged far enough from the subcutaneous tissues to be grasped with forceps. The larva is removed intact. (*From Felsenstein D et al: JAMA 270:2087, 1993.*)

burrow. Another technique is injection of about 2 ml of a local anesthetic into the base of the lesion, thus extruding the larva by fluid pressure.

If these methods are unsuccessful, surgical excision under local anesthesia is indicated. Whatever method is used, care should be taken not to break or rupture the larva. This may cause a strong inflammatory reaction, often followed by secondary infection. Repeated infections tend to confer some immunity that may abort larval development. Screens, protective clothing, and use of insect repellents are helpful in preventing infestation.

Furuncular myiasis in tropical Africa is caused by the tumbu fly, *Cordylobia anthrophophaga*. The larval stage of this fly is an obligate parasite of many mammals, of which rats and dogs are most important epidemiologically. The adult is about the size of a housefly, but stockier. It prefers shade and is most active in early morning and afternoon. Females lay eggs on dry sandy soil or on clothing. They are attracted by the odor of urine. The eggs hatch in 1 to 3 days, and hatchling larvae can survive up to 2 weeks waiting for contact with skin of a suitable host. They can penetrate unbroken skin. They become fusiform to ovoid and reach a length of 13 to 15 mm. The larval stage is completed in 9 to 14 days.

Human infections occur in most nations of sub-Saharan Africa. Transmission increases during the rainy season. Among indigenous peoples, infection is most frequent in children; adults evidently acquire some immunity. Infections among Americans and Europeans visiting Africa are reported regularly.[24,25,43] Lesions may be on any part of the body but are more common on the legs and buttocks. The furuncles are discrete, elevated, and nontender and have a central opening. The number of lesions, up to about 50, is greater than with *Dermatobia*. Infections in children have been mistaken for chickenpox,[35] but the course of the infection is much shorter. An exceptionally heavy infection (about 150 larvae) was caused by *Cordylobia rodhaini*, normally a parasite of forest mammals. It was accompanied by lymphadenopathy, leukocytosis, and elevated IgA. Clothing left to dry on the ground was the presumed source of the parasites.[38] Principles of diagnosis and treatment are much the same as for *Dermatobia*. Avoidance of skin contact with potentially contaminated soil and ironing of clothing and bedding after open-air drying are preventive measures that often are difficult to achieve.

Hematophagous Myiasis. The sole cause of hematophagous myiasis is the Congo floor maggot, *Auchmeromyia luteola*. It is dark, distinctly segmented, ovoid, 15 to 18 mm long, and assumes the larval stage of a moderate-size yellowish fly. It is widely distributed in sub-Saharan Africa and is essentially a human parasite. It is unique among parasitic fly larvae in living apart from its host in the earthen floor of native dwellings. It seeks persons lying or sitting on the floor or on mats

and feeds intermittently on blood, usually at night. The bites are trivial but may interfere with sleep. Sensitization appears to be uncommon.

Wound Myiasis. About 85% to 90% of cases are caused by larvae of flies of the family Calliphoridae, which includes both obligate parasites and opportunists. The most dangerous type of myiasis may be caused by larvae of the screw-worm flies *Callitroga (Cochliomyia) americana (hominivorax)* in the Americas and *Chrysomyia bessiana* in Asia and Africa. The adults are rather stocky flies, 8 to 12 mm in body length, and metallic blue-green to purplish black.

The parasitic larvae are pinkish, fusiform, and strongly segmented, providing the common name. Length at maturity is 12 to 15 mm. They are obligate parasites whose chief hosts are cattle, sheep, and goats. They are a major cause of economic loss among livestock. Enzootic areas are mostly in the tropics and subtropics; in the past, summer infections have occurred as far north as Colorado and Nebraska. Female flies deposit eggs near any break in the skin or around the nose, mouth, or ears if a discharge is present. Larvae invade healthy tissue, often causing considerable damage. The larval stage lasts 4 to 8 days, and the entire cycle is 15 to 20 days in enzootic areas. Screw-worm has been eradicated in the southern United States and some other areas primarily through the release of large numbers of laboratory-bred male flies sterilized by gamma irradiation. Females mate only once, so mating with a sterile male nullifies the female's reproductive effort, greatly reducing the population.

Flies may be dispersed by prevailing winds. Infection is often acquired while resting outside during the day or may result from trauma.[32] Lesions may appear on any exposed part of the body. Those on the scalp may be associated with pediculosis capitis. Typical dermal lesions are ulcers or sinuses that may contain up to 200 larvae. These are surrounded by a zone of induration. Pain is variable. Secondary bacterial infection is common. Tissue destruction may be extensive and mortality is associated with nasopharyngeal invasion.

Topical application of 5% chloroform in olive oil followed by irrigation and manual removal of larvae is often sufficient in dermal infections. Deeper nasopharyngeal and orbital infections require surgery. Antimicrobial therapy as dictated by culture and sensitivity tests, is often necessary. The most effective prevention is elimination of the disease in domestic animals.

BURROWING FLEA

Flea infestations tend to be similar clinically and associated with the distribution of animal hosts. However, one flea, *Tunga penetrans,* is responsible for a distinctive infestation known as tungiasis. The flea has a number of common names: burrowing flea, chigo, sand flea, and jigger. Infestation is common in Central and South America and in Africa, where the burrowing flea is widely distributed, but more cases are seen in the United States as increasing numbers of tourists visit exotic places. One woman resident of New York City developed lesions of tungiasis on her toes after visiting several countries in East Africa, where she frequently wore sandals in rural areas.[47] The primary lesions of tungiasis are produced by the female flea. As soon as it is impregnated, it burrows into the skin until only the posterior end protrudes. Sucking blood, the insect becomes as large as a small pea and deposits eggs that fall to the ground. Lodged in the skin, the gestating female produces a firm itchy nodule, with the posterior end of the flea visible as a dark plug or spot in the center of each nodule. Lesions occur most often on the feet, buttocks, or perineum of persons who wear no shoes or frequently squat, since the burrowing flea is not a good jumper and abounds in the dusty soil surrounding human habitations. If the infestation is extensive, numerous papules may aggregate into plaques with a honeycomb appearance. Secondary infection around each flea is inevitable, resulting in suppuration, ulceration, and rarely gangrene. The lesions become painful or even crippling, and severe infections may lead to death. If the burrowing flea is not removed, the pustule ruptures, leaving an ulcer. Wearing shoes will prevent most cases of tungiasis.

Cases should be treated promptly. One method is curettage of each nodule under local anesthesia, with concomitant use of systemic antibiotics to prevent secondary infection. Ether pledgets applied to the skin will kill the fleas before curettage is begun. Where burrowing fleas are endemic, eradication is important. Floors must be swept free of dust, and insecticides may be sprayed or dusted.

CENTIPEDES AND MILLIPEDES

Centipedes are elongate, flattened arthropods with one pair of legs for each of the typical body segments, which may number from 15 to more than 100. The first segment bears a pair of curved hollow fangs with venom glands at the bases. The last segment bears a pair of filamentous to forcepslike caudal appendages not associated with the venom apparatus. The largest species reach lengths of about 30 cm (12 inches). Most centipedes live in crevices or beneath objects on the ground. Some are burrowers, and others are climbers. Many are nocturnal. *Scutigera coleoptrata*, with body length of 25 mm and long thin legs, is a common house arthropod in much of the United States. *Lithobius* is a cosmopolitan ground-dwelling genus. A species common in eastern U.S. gardens is orange and 30 to 50 mm long. Centipedes prey chiefly on invertebrates, but larger species occasionally eat small vertebrates. Female centipedes of some species curl around their egg clusters and newly hatched young and may actively defend them.

Centipedes use venom primarily to kill prey and only secondarily for defense. Venom may also have a digestive function. Enzymes, including acid and alkaline phosphatase and amino acid naphthylamidase, lipoproteins, histamine, and serotonin, are variably present.[33] Venom of *Scolopendra subspinipes* produces hypotension followed by hypertension. The major lethal toxin is an acidic protein with molecular weight of 60,000 daltons. It produces vasoconstriction, increased capillary permeability, and cardiac arrest.[19,20]

As with spiders, any centipede whose fangs can penetrate human skin can cause local envenomation. Centipede bites are typically pointed in shape, a feature that can help differentiate a bite from a large centipede from a snake.[18] Contrary to popular folklore, centipedes do not inject venom with their feet or caudal appendages. The jaws inject a neurotoxic venom through venom ducts. Centipede bites have been reported from numerous tropical and subtropical regions, but never as a serious medical problem. Most bites have been ascribed to species of *Scolopendra*, which has a wide distribution with several species in the southern United States (Figure 37-5). Fatalities are almost unknown; however, a death in the United

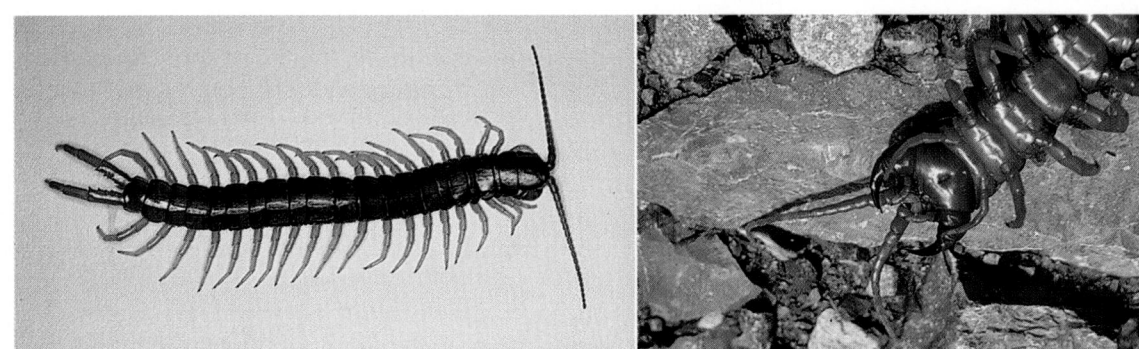

Figure 37-5 A, Centipede, *Scolopendra armidale.* **B,** Centipede fangs.

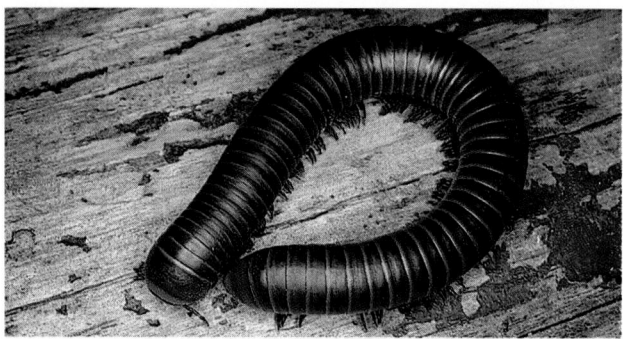

Figure 37-6 *Spirobolus* millipede.

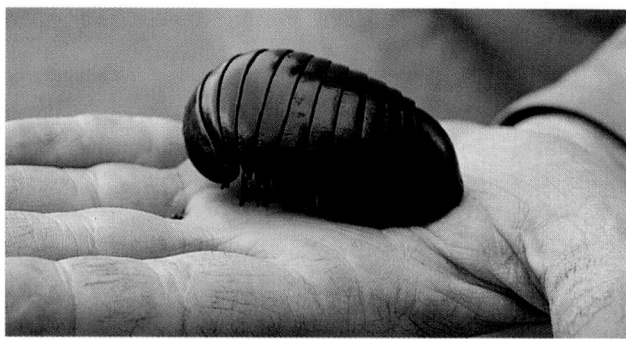

Figure 37-7 Giant Madagascar millipede.

States was recently mentioned, but with no locality or details.[29]

Burning pain, local swelling, erythema, lymphangitis, and lymphadenopathy are common manifestations of a centipede bite. Swelling and tenderness may persist for as long as 3 weeks or may disappear and recur. Superficial necrosis may occur at the site of fang punctures. Few bites with serious systemic reactions have been reported in detail. In one case ascribed to *Scolopendra heros* in the southwestern United States, a woman had massive edema of the leg, necrosis of the peroneal muscles, loss of motor function in the foot, myoglobinuria, and azotemia.[31] An Israeli patient bitten on the neck complained of inability to turn her head, probably because of muscle spasm.[34] Other cases have been characterized by dizziness, nausea, collapse, and pyrexia.[7] An infant that ingested a centipede identified as *Scutigera morpha* developed hypotonia, vomiting, and lethargy, presumably from being bitten in the mouth or pharynx. The child recovered spontaneously after about 48 hours.[2]

Although some centipede bites may be excruciatingly painful, they are not fatal and seldom require more than supportive care. Treatment of centipede envenomation is symptomatic. Infiltration of the bitten area with lidocaine or another anesthetic promptly relieves pain. Antihistamines and steroids have been suggested for more severe reactions. Tetanus prophylaxis is advisable.

Millipedes differ from centipedes in having two pairs of legs per body segment and in lacking apparatus for injecting venom. Several large species of the genus *Spirobolus* are common in the southern United States (Figure 37-6). Some species are broad and short and roll into a ball when disturbed (Figure 37-7). Millipedes are generally ground dwelling and secretive. Occasionally, they aggregate in enormous numbers. They generally feed on decaying vegetation.

Millipedes are exceptionally well endowed with defensive chemical secretions that include hydrogen cyanide, organic acids, phenol, cresols, benzoquinones, and hydroquinones. These effectively deter most predators. Some large species can eject secretions for distances up to 80 cm (32 inches).

Human injury from millipede secretions has been reported from a number of tropical regions. The most common injury is dermatitis that begins with a brown-stained area, which burns and may blister and exfoliate. Millipede secretion in the eye causes immediate pain, lacrimation, and blepharospasm. This may be followed by chemosis, periorbital edema, and corneal ulceration. Blindness has been reported.[22,41] Individuals exposed to large millipede aggregations may complain of nausea and irritation of the nose and eyes. No specific treatment is available. Prompt irrigation with water or saline should be followed by analgesics, antimicrobials, and other measures appropriate for superficial chemical burns. Ophthalmologic evaluation is mandatory for eye injuries.

GENERAL TREATMENT OF INSECT BITES

Oral antihistamines can be effective in reducing the symptoms of insect bites. Cetirizine was given prophylactically in a double-blind, placebo-controlled, 2-week crossover trial to 18 individuals who had previously experienced dramatic cutaneous reactions to mosquito bites.[42] Subjects given the active drug had a 40% decrease in both the size of the wheal response at 15 minutes and the size of bite papule at 24 hours. The mean pruritus score, measured at 15 minutes and 1, 12, and 24 hours after being bitten, was 67% less than that of the untreated controls. These studies have not been done with astemizole, loratadine, or fexofenadine. In highly sensitized individuals, prophylactic treatment with nonsedating antihistamines may safely reduce the cutaneous reactions to insect bites.

A 3.6% ammonium solution (After Bite), relieves the type I hypersensitivity symptoms associated with mosquito bites. In a double-blind, placebo-controlled laboratory trial, 64% of mosquito-bitten subjects experienced complete relief of symptoms after a single application of the ammonium solution, and the remaining 36% had partial relief lasting 15 to 90 minutes.

No subjects treated with placebo reported complete symptom relief.[48]

PROTECTION AND PREVENTION

An integrated approach to personal protection is the most effective way to prevent arthropod bites, regardless of location and species. Insect repellents containing diethyltoluamide (DEET) are the most effective products currently on the market, providing broad-spectrum repellency lasting several hours. Topical insect repellents alone do not provide complete protection. Mosquitoes, for example, can find and bite any untreated skin and may even bite through thin clothing. Deerflies, biting midges, and some blackflies prefer to bite around the head and will crawl into the hair to bite unprotected areas. Wearing protective clothing, including a hat, reduces the chances of being bitten. Treating clothes and hats with permethrin maximizes protection by repelling any insect that crawls or lands on the treated clothing. To prevent chiggers or ticks from crawling up the legs, pants should be tucked into boots or stockings.

Persons traveling to a part of the world where insect-borne disease is a potential threat should be certain to learn about indigenous insects and the diseases they might transmit. Protective clothing, mesh insect tents or bedding, insect repellent, and permethrin spray should be carried.

REFERENCES

1. Arocha-Pinango CL et al: Six new cases of a caterpillar-induced bleeding syndrome, *Thromb Haemost* 67:402, 1992.
2. Barnett PL: Centipede ingestion by a six-month-old infant: toxic side effects, *Pediatr Emerg Care* 7:229230, 1991.
3. Berger TG: Korean yellow moth dermatitis: report of an epidemic, *J Assoc Mil Dermatol* 12:31, 1986.
4. Bhargava D, Victor R: Carabid beetle invasion of the ear in Oman, *Wilderness Environ Med* 10:157, 1999.
5. Brewer TF, Wilson ME, Gonzalez E: Bacon therapy and furuncular myiasis, *JAMA* 270:2087, 1993.
6. Burdmann EA et al: Severe acute renal failure induced by the venom of *Lonomia* caterpillars, *Clin Nephrol* 46:337, 1996.
7. Burnett JW, Calton GJ, Morgan RJ: Centipedes, *Cutis* 37:241, 1986.
8. Charpin D et al: Epidemiology of Hymenoptera allergy, *Clin Exp Allergy* 24:1010, 1994.
9. Claborn DM et al: Staphylinid (rove) beetle outbreak in the American Southwest, *Mil Med* 164 3:209, 1999.
10. Couppie P et al: Venomous caterpillars in French Guyana: 5 cases, *Ann Dermatol Venereol* 125:489, 1998.
11. Dalla Costa LR et al: Efficacy of *Lonomia* antivenom in the treatment of patients with hemorrhagic disorders caused by caterpillars in Brazil, *Toxicon* 37:312, 1999.
12. Dias da Silva W et al: Development of an antivenom against toxins of *Lonomia obliqua* caterpillars, *Toxicon* 34:1045, 1996.
13. Dib G et al: Systemic reactions to the Samsum ant: an IgE mediated hypersensitivity, *J Allergy Clin Immunol* 96:465, 1995.
14. Dinehart SM et al: Caripito itch: dermatitis from contact with *Hylesia* moths, *J Am Acad Dermatol* 13:743, 1985.
15. Dondero TL et al: Cutaneous myiasis in visitors to Central America, *South Med J* 72:1508, 1979.
16. Duarte A, Duarte G, Barrios E: Acute renal failure in accidents caused by caterpillars (*Lonomia obliqua*), *Toxicon* 31:124, 1993.
17. Elston DM: What's eating you? Sand Flies, *Cutis* 62:164, 1988.
18. Elston DM: What's eating you? Centipedes (Chilopoda), *Cutis* 64:83, 1999.
19. Gomes A et al: Pharmacodynamics of venom of the centipede *Scolopendra subspinipes dehaani*, *Indian J Exp Biol* 20:615, 1982.
20. Gomes A et al: Isolation, purification, and pharmacodynamics of a toxin from the venom of the centipede *Scolopendra subspinipes dehaani*, *Indian J Exp Biol* 21:203, 1983.
21. Guerrero B, Arocha-Pinango CL: Activation of human prothrombin by the venom of *Lonomia achelous* caterpillars, *Thromb Res* 66:169, 1992.
22. Haneveld GT: Eye lesions caused by the exudate of tropical millipedes. I. Report of a case, *Trop Geo Med* 10:165, 1958.
23. Hoffman DR: Reactions to less common fire ants, *J Allergy Clin Immunol* 100:679, 1997.
24. Jacobs P, Orrey O: Microabscesses in the swimming trunk area, *S Afr Med J* 87:1559, 1997.
25. Jelenek T et al: Cutaneous myiasis: review of 13 cases in travelers returning from tropical countries, *Int J Dermatol* 34:624, 1995.
26. Johnston M, Dickinson G: An unexpected surprise in a common boil, *J Emerg Med* 14:779, 1996.
27. Komaladasa SD, Perera WDH, Weeratunga L: An outbreak of *Paederus* dermatitis in a suburban hospital in Sri Lanka, *Int J Dermatol* 36:34, 1997.
28. Kpea N, Zywoanski C: "Flies in the flesh": a case report and review of cutaneous myiasis, *Cutis* 55: 47, 1995.
29. Langley RL, Marrow WE: Deaths resulting from animal attacks in the United States, *Wilderness Environ Med* 8:8, 1997.
30. Levick N, Winkle KD, Smith G: European wasps an emerging hazard in Australia, *Med J Aust* 167:650, 1997.
31. Logan JL, Ogden DA: Rhabdomyolysis and acute renal failure following the bite of the giant desert centipede *Scolopendra heros*, *West J Med* 142:549, 1985.
32. Mehr Z, Powers NR, Konkol KA: Myiasis in a wounded soldier returning from Panama, *J Med Entomol* 28:553, 1991.
33. Mohamed AH et al: Proteins, lipids, lipoproteins and some enzymes characteristic of the venom extract from the centipede *Scolopendra morsitans*, *Toxicon* 21:371, 1983.
34. Mumcuoglu KY, Liebovici V: Centipede (*Scolopendra*) bite: case report, *Isr J Med Sci* 25:47, 1989.
35. Nunn P: Tangling with tumbu larvae, *Lancet* 343:646, 1994.
36. Olulmide YM: Cutaneous myiasis—a simple and effective technique for extraction of *Dermatobia hominis* larvae, *Int J Dermatol* 33:148, 1994.
37. Pallali L et al: Case report: myiasis—the botfly boil, *Am J Med Sci* 303:245, 1992.
38. Pampiglione S, Schiavon S, Fioravanti ML: Extensive furuncular myiasis due to *Cordylobia rodhaini* larvae, *Br J Dermatol* 126:418, 1992.
39. Peters W: *A colour atlas of arthropods in clinical medicine*, London, 1992, Wolfe.
40. Poskitt L, Duffill MB: Sleeping with a ladybird: suspected bites from *Diomus notescens*, *NZ Med J* 105:132, 1992.
41. Radford AJ: Millipede burns in man, *Trop Geo Med* 27:279, 1975.
42. Reunala Tet al.: Treatment of mosquito bites with cetirizine, *Clin Exp Allergy* 23:72, 1993.
43. Schorr WF: Tumbu-fly myiasis in Marshfield, Wisconsin, *Arch Dermatol* 93:61, 1967.
44. Southcott R: Moths and butterflies. In Covacevich J, Davie P, Pearn J, editors: *Toxic plants and animals: a guide for Australia*, Brisbane, 1987, Queensland Museum.
45. Sweis IE, Griffith BH, Pensler JM: Souvenirs from Belize: the botfly and the screw worm fly, *Plast Reconstr Surg* 99:868, 1997.
46. Todd RE, Guthridge SL, Montgomery BL: Evacuation of an aboriginal community in response to an outbreak of blistering dermatitis induced by a beetle (*Paedreus australis*), *Med J Aust* 164:238, 1996.
47. Zalar GL, Walther RR: Infestation by *Tunga penetrans*, *Arch Dermatol* 116:80, 1980.
48. Zhai H, Packman EW, Maibach HI: Effectiveness of ammonium solution in relieving type I mosquito bite symptoms: a double-blind, placebo-controlled study, *Acta Derm Venereol (Stockh)* 78:297, 1998.

38 North American Venomous Reptile Bites

Robert L. Norris, Jr. and Sean P. Bush

INTRODUCTION

North America is unique in that it is home not only to venomous snakes, but also to the world's only known venomous lizards. Fortunately, bites by venomous reptiles in North America are relatively uncommon, although precise statistics are not available. The only systematic attempt to evaluate the incidence of venomous snakebite in the United States was done in the late 1960s by Dr. Henry Parrish. He estimated that there were approximately 7000 bites by venomous snakes, of which approximately 15 ended in death.[106] The incidence of venomous snakebite may have changed significantly since Parrish's study, but given that snakebite is not a reportable "disease," no mechanism exists for obtaining reliable data. The incidence of snakebite in Canada is lower than that in the United States because fewer snakes species are found farther north up the continent. In Mexico, however, snakebite takes on increasing medical importance because this country has more venomous snake species than any other nation in the New World.[16] As many as 150 deaths may be caused by snakebite in Mexico each year.[46]

Establishing credible estimates of the incidence of venomous lizard bites is even more difficult than for snakes. The vast majority of victims are bitten while intentionally interacting with the lizard, and since these creatures are legally protected, many bites are probably never reported.

Many physicians called on to render acute care to snakebite victims have had limited experience with the potentially complex syndromes of snake venom poisoning. In addition, convincing research sponsors to fund needed studies evaluating prehospital care techniques, hospital management principles, and antivenom development is difficult when the targeted population size is only a few thousand individuals.

Snake venoms are highly complex mixtures of enzymes, low-molecular-weight polypeptides, glycoproteins, minerals, and other unidentified substances. Venoms vary among species, within a single species depending on its geographic distribution, and even within an individual snake depending on factors such as age, diet, and health.[118] The effects of a particular venom may be different depending on the species of prey or research animal that has been poisoned. Such variables make it difficult to conduct meaningful research into snakebite management techniques.

Table 38-1 lists the species of venomous reptiles found in North America.[16,46,52,74,115] The medically important North American venomous snakes all fall into the families Viperidae (subfamily Crotalinae, the crotalines or pit vipers) and Elapidae (elapids, the coral snakes). Although there are reports of human envenoming by a handful of species of Colubridae—the family of snakes traditionally regarded as harmless—the cases from North America have all been relatively minor and non–life threatening (see Chapter 39).

Pit vipers are widely dispersed throughout most of North America below southern Canada (south of 55 degrees north latitude).[96] In the United States, for example, all 48 contiguous states except Maine have at least one pit viper species.[107] Being poikilothermic and relying on environmental heat energy to support locomotion, feeding, digestion, and reproduction, snakes tend to increase in numbers of species as one moves southward toward the equator. At least 34 species of pit vipers are found in North America, with many more subspecies. Pit vipers can be further divided into rattlesnakes (genera *Crotalus* and *Sistrurus*, approximately 30 species); copperheads, cottonmouth water moccasins, and cantils (genus *Agkistrodon*, three North American species and a number of subspecies); and lance-heads (genus *Bothrops*, with one species in eastern Mexico, *B. asper*).[46]

Rattlesnakes are the most widespread of pit vipers, found throughout most of North America (Figures 38-1 to 38-9). Copperheads (*Agkistrodon contortrix*) are found in the central and southeastern United States and westward into the Big Bend region of Texas (Figure 38-10). Cottonmouth water moccasins (*Agkistrodon piscivorus*) are found in the southeast from Virginia to Florida and extend westward into central Texas (Figure 38-11). In Mexico the copperhead and cottonmouth are replaced by the cantil, *Agkistrodon bilineatus* (Figure 38-12).[52] The pit vipers of North America come in a wide range of sizes. Among the smaller rattlesnakes are the sidewinders (*Crotalus cerastes*), ridge-nosed rattlesnakes (*C. willardi*), and

TABLE 38-1. Venomous Reptiles of North America

GENUS	SPECIES/ SUBSPECIES	COMMON NAME	PRESENT (✓) IN		
			CANADA	U.S.	MEXICO
Crotalus		**Rattlesnakes**			
	adamanteus	Eastern diamondback rattlesnake	—	✓	—
	atrox	Western diamondback rattlesnake	—	✓	✓
	basiliscus	Mexican West Coast rattlesnake	—	—	✓
	catalinensis	Santa Catalina Island rattlesnake	—	—	✓
	cerastes	Sidewinder	—	✓	✓
	durissus	Neotropical rattlesnake	—	—	✓
	enyo	Lower California rattlesnake	—	—	✓
	exsul	Cedros Island diamond rattlesnake	—	—	✓
	horridus	Timber/canebrake rattlesnake	✓	✓	—
	intermedius	Small-headed rattlesnake	—	—	✓
	lannomi	Autland rattlesnake	—	—	✓
	lepidus	Rock rattlesnake	—	✓	✓
	mitchelli	Speckled rattlesnake	—	✓	✓
	mitchelli stephensi	Panamint rattlesnake	—	✓	—
	molossus	Black-tailed rattlesnake	—	✓	✓
	polystictus	Lance-headed rattlesnake	—	—	✓
	pricei	Twin-spotted rattlesnake	—	✓	✓
	pusillus	Tancitaran dusky rattlesnake	—	—	✓
	ruber	Red diamond rattlesnake	—	✓	✓
	scutulatus	Mojave rattlesnake	—	✓	✓
	stejnegeri	Long-tailed rattlesnake	—	—	✓
	tigris	Tiger rattlesnake	—	✓	✓
	tortugensis	Tortuga Island diamond rattlesnake	—	—	✓
	transversus	Cross-banded mountain rattlesnake	—	—	✓
	triseriatus	Dusky rattlesnake	—	—	✓
	unicolor	Aruba Island rattlesnake	—	—	✓
	viridis abyssus	Grand Canyon rattlesnake	—	✓	—
	viridis caliginis	Coronado Island rattlesnake	—	—	✓
	viridis cerberus	Arizona black rattlesnake	—	✓	—
	viridis concolor	Midget faded rattlesnake	—	✓	—
	viridis helleri	Southern Pacific rattlesnake	—	✓	✓
	viridis lutosus	Great Basin rattlesnake	—	✓	—
	viridis nuntius	Hopi rattlesnake	—	✓	—
	viridis oreganus	Northern Pacific rattlesnake	✓	✓	—
	viridis viridis	Prairie rattlesnake	✓	✓	✓
	willardi	Ridge-nosed rattlesnake	—	✓	✓
Sistrurus		**Rattlesnakes**			
	catenatus	Massasauga	✓	✓	✓
	miliarius	Pygmy rattlesnake	—	✓	—
	ravus	Mexican pygmy rattlesnake	—	—	✓
Agkistrodon		**Copperheads, water moccasins, cantil**			
	bilineatus	Cantil	—	—	✓
	contortrix	Copperhead	—	✓	✓
	piscivorus	Cottonmouth water moccasin	—	✓	—
Bothrops		**Lancehead vipers**			
	asper	Terciopelo, cuatro narices	—	—	✓
Micruroides		**Coral snakes**			
	euryxanthus	Sonoran (Arizona) coral snake	—	✓	✓

Continued

TABLE 38-1. Venomous Reptiles of North America—cont'd

GENUS	SPECIES/ SUBSPECIES	COMMON NAME	PRESENT (✓) IN		
			CANADA	U.S.	MEXICO
Micrurus		**Coral snakes**			
	bernadi	Saddled coral snake	—	—	✓
	bogerti	Bogert's coral snake	—	—	✓
	browni	Brown's coral snake	—	—	✓
	diastema	Variable coral snake	—	—	✓
	distans	Clear-banded coral snake	—	—	✓
	elegans	Elegant coral snake	—	—	✓
	ephippifer	Double black coral snake	—	—	✓
	fulvius	North American coral snake	—	✓	✓
	laticollaris	Double collar coral snake	—	—	✓
	latifasciatus	Long-banded coral snake	—	—	✓
	limbatus	Tuxtlan coral snake	—	—	✓
	nebularius	Neblina coral snake	—	—	✓
	nigrocinctus	Black-banded coral snake	—	—	✓
	proximans	Nayarit coral snake	—	—	✓
Heloderma		**Venomous lizards**			
	suspectum	Gila monster	—	✓	✓
	horridum	Mexican beaded lizard	—	—	✓

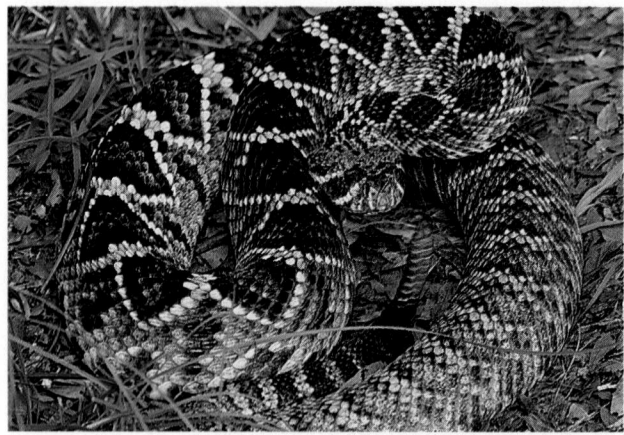

Figure 38-1 Eastern diamondback rattlesnake *(Crotalus adamanteus)* is the largest pit viper of the United States and can attain lengths of 2 m. *(Courtesy Michael Cardwell/Extreme Wildlife Photography.)*

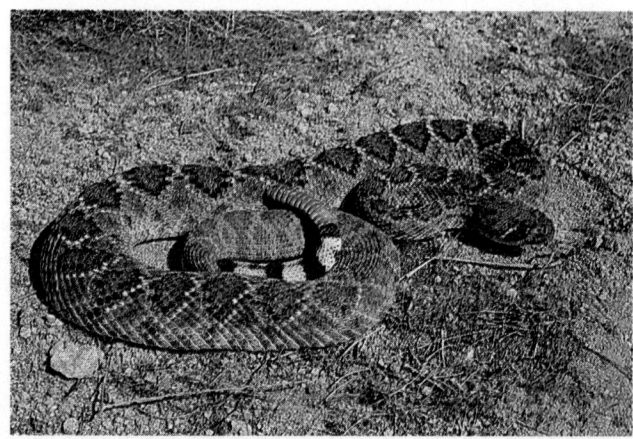

Figure 38-2 Western diamondback rattlesnake *(Crotalus atrox)* causes many serious bites in the U.S. Southwest. *(Courtesy Michael Cardwell/Extreme Wildlife Photography.)*

pygmy rattlesnakes *(Sistrurus miliarius)*, whose adult sizes are routinely less than 65 cm.[74] At the other extreme, the eastern diamondback rattlesnake *(Crotalus adamanteus)* can exceed 2 m.[74]

Outside of North America the family Elapidae contains a number of extremely dangerous species, such as cobras (genus *Naja)*, mambas (genus *Dendroaspis)*, and all the potentially lethal snakes of Australia (e.g., *Oxyuranus, Notechis, Pseudonaja)* (see Chapter 39). The

elapids of North America are all coral snakes and belong to one of two genera, *Micrurus* and *Micruroides* (Figures 38-13 to 38-15). These colorful reptiles are found in Arizona (Sonoran coral snake, *Micruroides euryxanthus)*, the southeastern United States (eastern coral snake, *Micrurus fulvius fulvius)*, and Texas (Texas coral snake, *Micrurus fulvius tenere)*. Mexico has 15 species of coral snake, including *M. euryxanthus* and 14 *Micrurus* species. Because of the inoffensive habits of

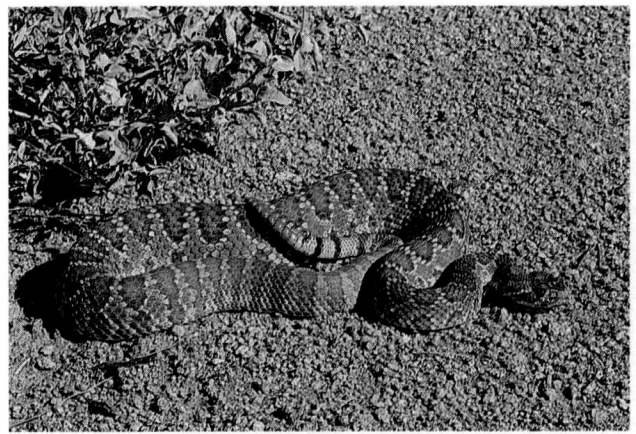

Figure 38-3 Mojave rattlesnake *(Crotalus scutulatus)* has two geographic populations in terms of venom composition, one with predominantly neurotoxic effects and one with more local sequelae. *(Courtesy Michael Cardwell/Extreme Wildlife Photography.)*

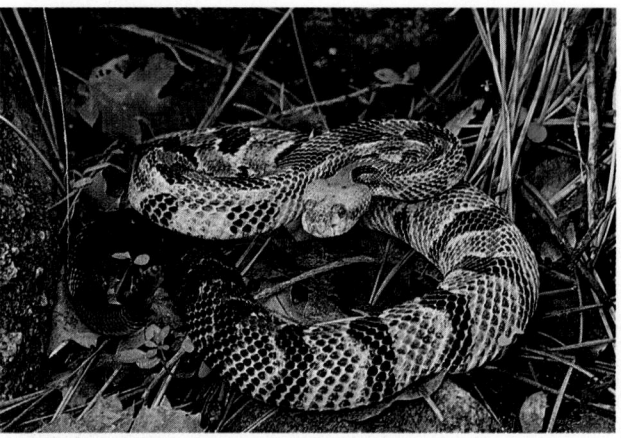

Figure 38-4 Timber rattlesnake *(Crotalus horridus)* is a large, dangerous snake of the eastern United States. *(Courtesy Michael Cardwell/Extreme Wildlife Photography.)*

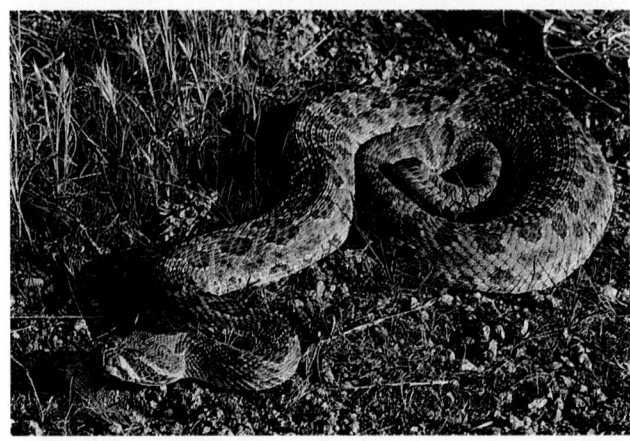

Figure 38-5 Prairie rattlesnake *(Crotalus viridis viridis)* is a widely distributed species of the western United States. *(Courtesy Michael Cardwell/Extreme Wildlife Photography.)*

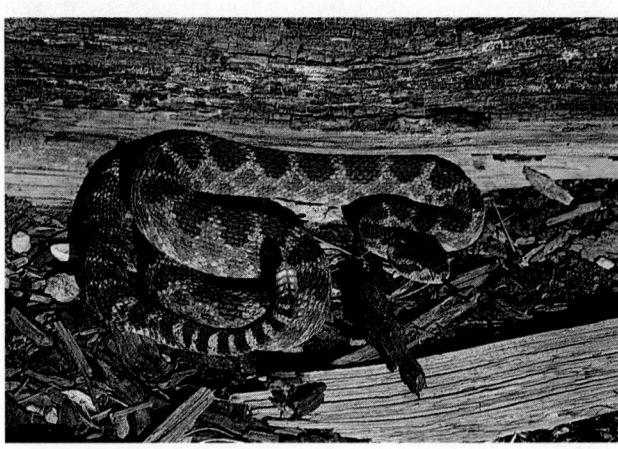

Figure 38-6 Northern Pacific rattlesnake *(Crotalus viridis oreganus)* is a moderate-sized but very toxic snake of the Pacific Northwest. *(Courtesy Michael Cardwell/Extreme Wildlife Photography.)*

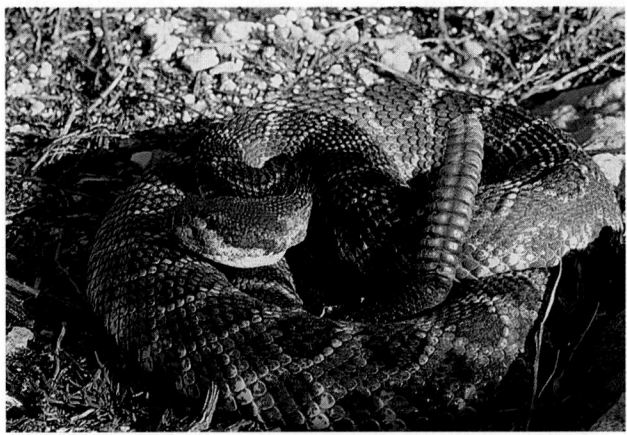

Figure 38-7 Southern Pacific rattlesnake *(Crotalus viridis helleri)* is one of nine subspecies of western rattlesnakes (C. *viridis* subsp.). *(Courtesy Michael Cardwell/Extreme Wildlife Photography.)*

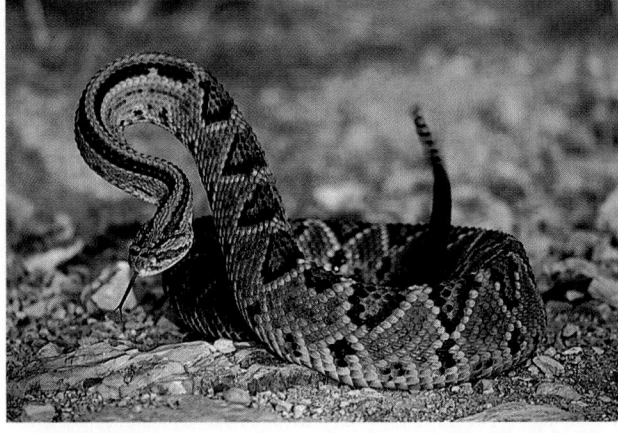

Figure 38-8 Tropical rattlesnake *(Crotalus durissus durissus)* is one of the large, dangerous subspecies of C. *durissus* distributed from southern Mexico through South America. *(Courtesy Michael Cardwell/Extreme Wildlife Photography.)*

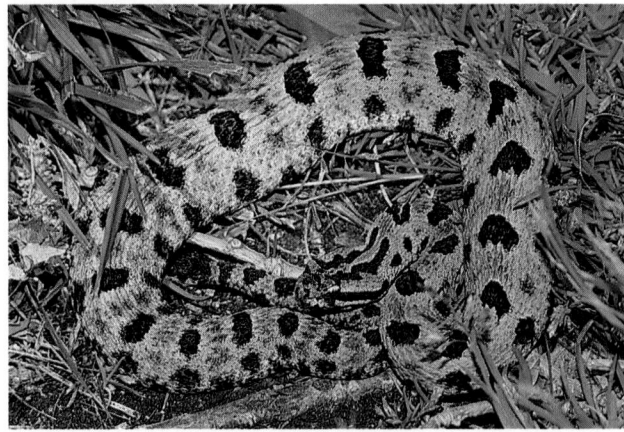

Figure 38-9 Western pygmy rattlesnake *(Sistrurus miliarius streckeri)* is one of the smaller rattlesnake species of North America. *(Courtesy Michael Cardwell/Extreme Wildlife Photography.)*

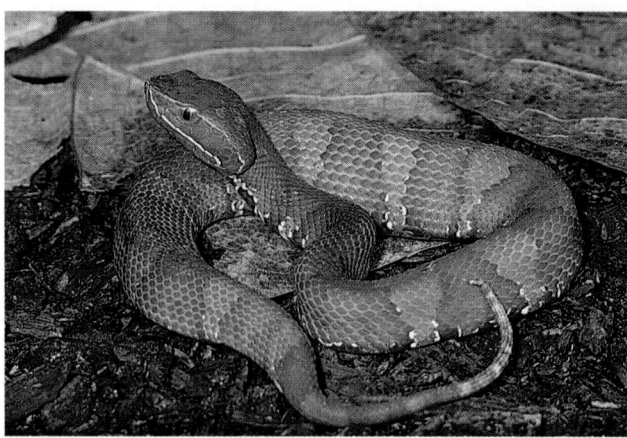

Figure 38-12 Cantil *(Agkistrodon bilineatus)* is a close relative of the copperheads *(A. contortrix)* and cottonmouths *(A. piscivorus)* of the United States. This pit viper is found in Mexico and Central America. *(Courtesy Michael Cardwell and William W. Lamar.)*

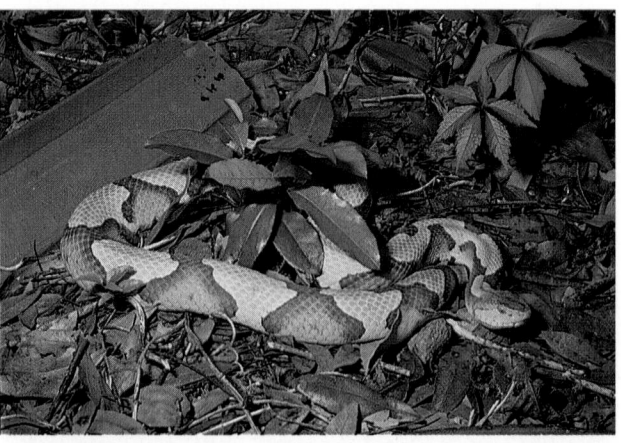

Figure 38-10 Southern copperhead *(Agkistrodon contortrix contortrix)* has markings that make it almost invisible when lying in leaf litter. *(Courtesy Michael Cardwell and Carl Barden Venom Laboratory.)*

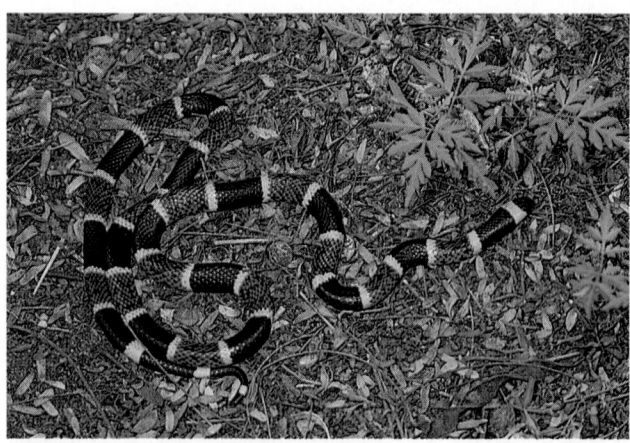

Figure 38-13 Texas coral snake *(Micrurus fulvius tenere)* has a highly potent venom but is secretive, and bites are uncommon. *(Courtesy Michael Cardwell and the Gladys Porter Zoo.)*

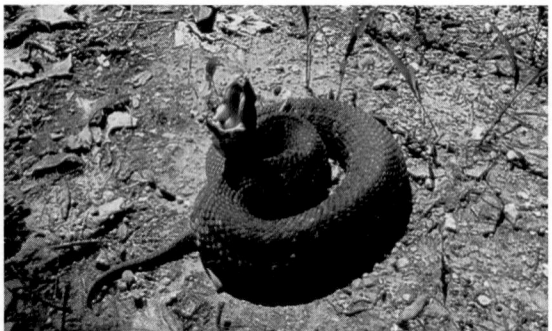

Figure 38-11 Cottonmouth water moccasin *(Agkistrodon piscivorus)* exhibiting its threat display. This snake is found most often around standing water sources in the southeastern United States. *(Courtesy Sherman Minton, MD.)*

these fossorial (burrowing) snakes and their less efficient venom delivery device (see later discussion), bites are very uncommon. Although Parrish and Khan[109] estimated that fewer than 20 coral snake bites occurred in the United States each year, the 1998 report of the American Association of Poison Control Centers (AAPCC) Toxic Exposure Surveillance System listed 61 cases.[90]

The only two known species of venomous lizards in the world are found in North America and belong to the genus *Heloderma.* The Gila monster *(Heloderma suspectum,* with two subspecies) is found in the southwestern United States (Arizona, western New Mexico, southeastern California, southern tip of Nevada, extreme southwestern Utah) and northwestern Mexico (Figure 38-16).[133] The range of the Mexican beaded lizard *(Heloderma horridum,* with three subspecies) is below that of the Gila monster, south to Guatemala

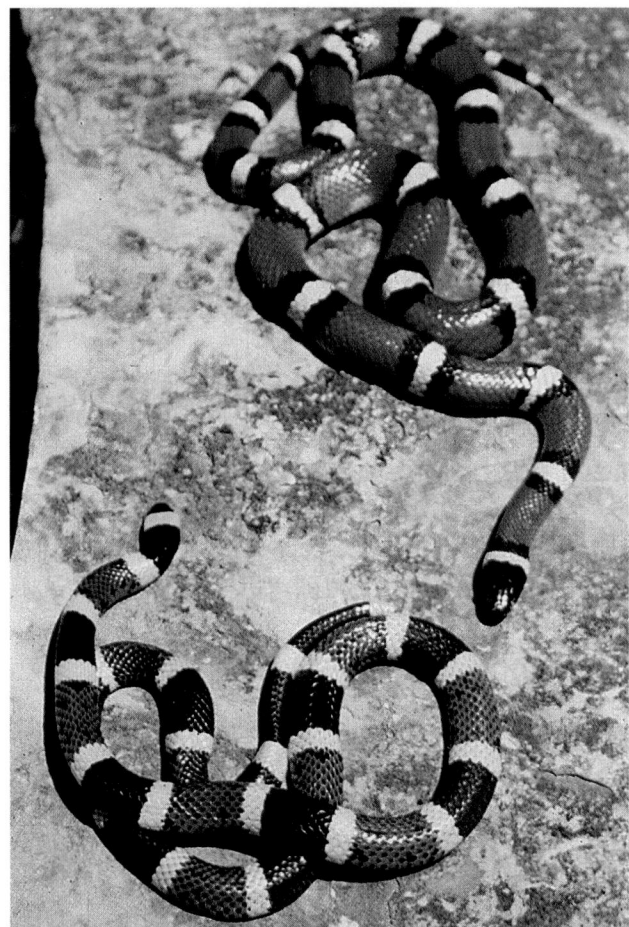

Figure 38-14 Comparison of Texas coral snake *(Micrurus fulvius tenere)* with harmless Mexican milk snake *(Lampropeltis triangulum annulata)*. Coral snake *(bottom)* has contiguous red and yellow bands, whereas the milk snake has its red and yellow bands separated by black. *(Courtesy Charles Alfaro.)*

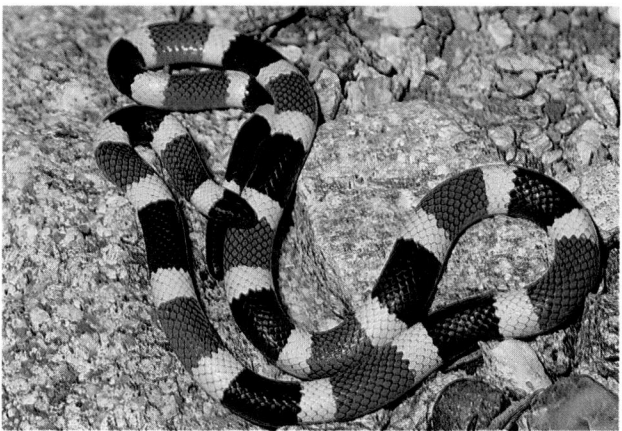

Figure 38-15 Sonoran coral snake *(Micruroides euryxanthus)* is also known as the Arizona coral snake. No documented fatality has followed a bite by this species. *(Courtesy Michael Cardwell and Jude McNally.)*

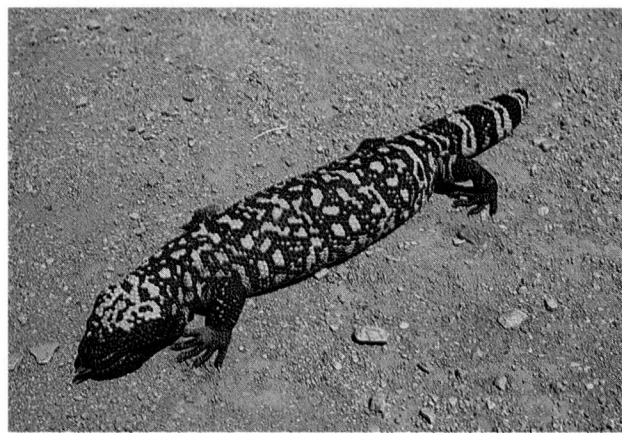

Figure 38-16 Gila monster *(Heloderma suspectum)* is one of only two known venomous lizards and the only species found in the United States. *(Courtesy Michael Cardwell/Extreme Wildlife Photography.)*

(Figure 38-17).[124] The helodermatids are discussed in more detail later in this chapter.

VENOMOUS SNAKES

Anatomy

Pit Vipers. The term *pit viper* comes from the presence of paired, highly sensitive, thermoreceptor organs (pits) present on the forward portion of these snakes' heads (Figure 38-18). These structures, also known as foveal organs, serve the snake in locating prey, aiming strikes, and adjusting venom dose (Figure 38-19). The foveal organs can detect temperature changes of as little as 0.003° C (0.0054° F).[96] A neurologic feedback loop between the foveal organs and the venom delivery apparatus may allow the snake to adjust the volume of venom it injects into a potential meal or a perceived threat.[149]

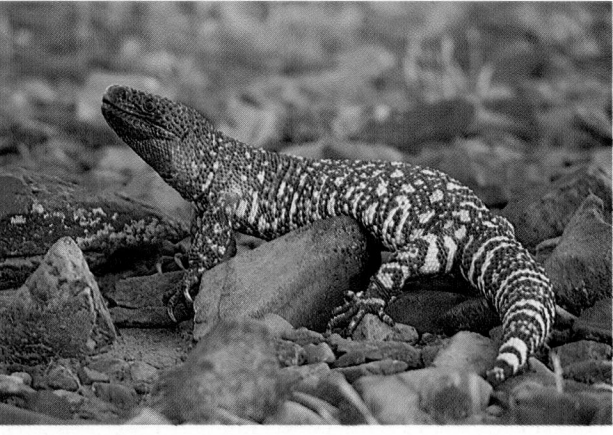

Figure 38-17 Mexican beaded lizard *(Heloderma horridum)* is located south of the Gila monster's range in Mexico. *(Courtesy Michael Cardwell/Extreme Wildlife Photography.)*

The anatomy of the venom delivery system of crotalines is the most sophisticated of all snakes (Figure 38-20). Bilateral glands located at the sides of the head, above and behind the eyes, produce and store the venom. These glands are connected through ducts to more anterior accessory glands that probably serve to activate or potentiate the venom.[118] From here the venom is passed forward through other ducts into the proximal portion of the hollow fangs with which the snake pierces its victim in a stabbing motion. These fangs, found on the anterior surfaces of the maxillary bones, are large (up to 20 mm in large rattlesnakes[74]) and highly mobile. At rest the snake folds the fangs against the roof of its mouth. For the strike, the fangs are brought into an upright position, perpendicular to the maxilla. The snake has voluntary control over its fangs and can open the mouth without raising the fangs or can raise each fang individually. The fangs are relatively brittle and fracture or become dull with time and use. Replacement fangs at varying stages of development behind the functional set move forward on the maxillary bone when needed (Figure 38-21). The speed of a pit viper's strike has been clocked at 8 feet per second; the snake can reach distances of approximately one half of its body length.[149] Table 38-2 lists venom yields for various North American pit vipers.

The fastest crotaline can crawl at a maximum speed of approximately 3 miles per hour, which equates to an average adult walking pace.[149] Pit vipers do not chase people. Accounts suggesting otherwise can be explained by snakes' poor eyesight; when threatened, they may retreat in the direction of people.

The characteristic forked tongue of the snake is an olfactory tool and possesses none of the offensive "stinging" function ascribed to in folklore. The snake extends its tongue to detect chemical odors in its environment. The tongue is then retracted and its tips placed into the paired Jacobson's organs, lined with olfactory epithelium, in the roof of its mouth. This sen-

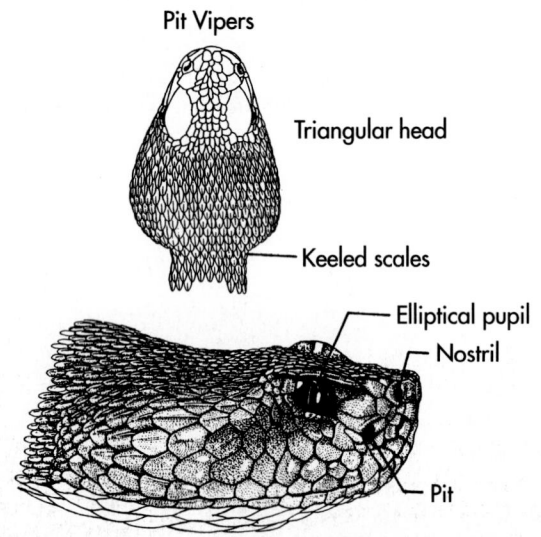

Figure 38-18 Pit viper's head. Note the elliptic pupil and the heat-sensing pit for which these reptiles are named. Viewed from above, the head has a distinctly triangular shape. Many nonvenomous snakes also possess triangular-shaped heads, however, this is not a reliable means of differentiation. *(Marlin Sawyer, 1994.)*

Pit Vipers

Triangular head

Keeled scales

Elliptical pupil

Nostril

Pit

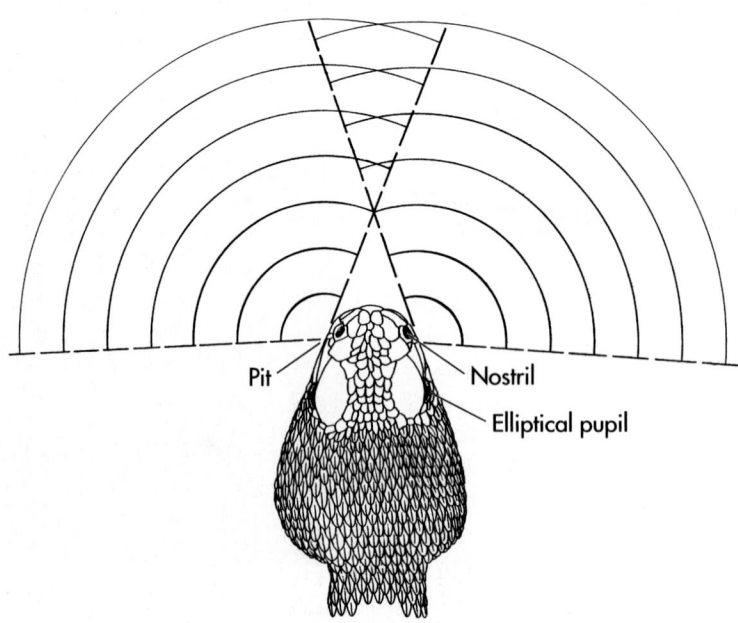

Pit

Nostril

Elliptical pupil

Figure 38-19 Paired heat-sensing pits of the pit vipers used to help the snake locate its prey, direct its strike, and probably determine the volume of venom to be expended. *(Marlin Sawyer, 1994.)*

sory system is highly sensitive, allowing the snake to identify potential mates, locate food, and track down a prey item that has been struck and released.

Pit vipers have elliptic, or catlike, pupils, whereas most North American harmless snakes have round

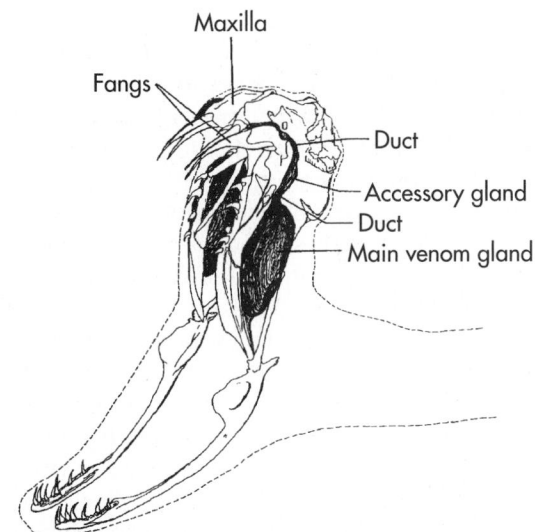

Figure 38-20 Venom delivery apparatus of a pit viper. Venom is produced in large venom glands just posterior to the eyes and is passed through a duct system into the hollow, anterior fangs when the snake bites. *(Marlin Sawyer, 1994.)*

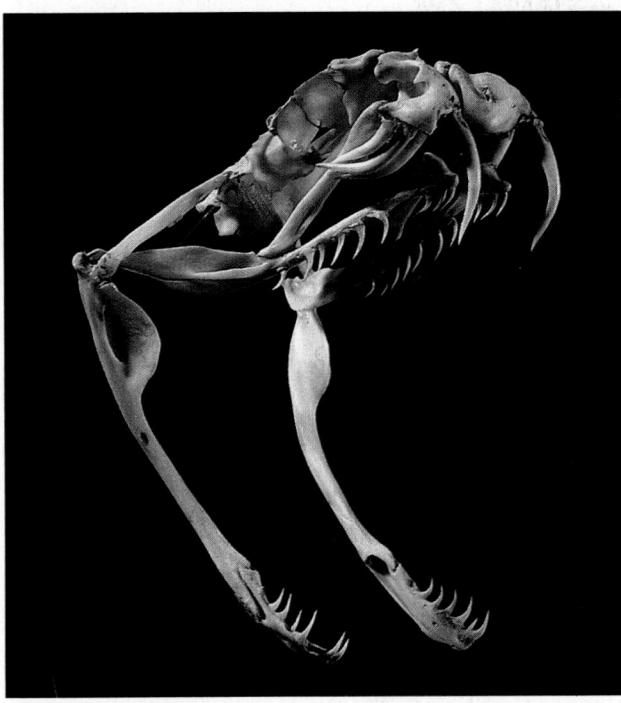

Figure 38-21 Rattlesnake skull. Replacement fangs are behind the primary, functional fangs. The smaller teeth of the palatine, pterygoid, and mandibular bones are used for gripping food. *(Courtesy Michael Cardwell/Extreme Wildlife Photography.)*

pupils. A few essentially harmless, rear-fanged colubrids, such as the night snake *(Hypsiglena torquata)* and lyre snake *(Trimorphodon biscutatus)*, also possess elliptic pupils but lack facial pits. Although these species possess a special venom gland (Duvernoy's gland) in the rear of the mouth, they are innocuous creatures. They are reluctant to bite humans, and their salivary toxins cause few signs or symptoms, other than slight swelling, bruising, and pain. This contrasts with the truly dangerous rear-fanged colubrids of other parts of the world (see Chapter 39). The two species of boas in North America, the rosy boa *(Lichanura trivirgata)* and rubber boa *(Charina bottae)*, also possess elliptic pupils, but their body form (more cigar shaped and lacking the broad, triangular head of a pit viper) and skin patterns are very different from any pit viper.

The caudal rattle of the rattlesnake is composed of loosely interlocked plates of keratin that emit a buzzing sound when the snake rapidly vibrates its tail. This characteristic sound serves as a warning to a perceived threat. A new segment to the rattle is added each time

TABLE 38-2. Venom Yields of Some Medically Important Snakes of North America

SPECIES	MAXIMUM VENOM YIELD (mg DRY WEIGHT)	REFERENCE
Crotalus adamanteus	848	74
Crotalus atrox	1145	74
Crotalus cerastes	63	74
Crotalus durissus	514 (average)	74
Crotalus horridus horridus	160 (average)	97
Crotalus horridus atricaudatus	229	74
Crotalus molossus	540	74
Crotalus scutulatus	141	74
Crotalus viridis helleri	390	74
Crotalus viridis oreganus	289	74
Crotalus viridis viridis	162	74
Sistrurus catenatus	33	41
Sistrurus miliarius	18 (average)	74
Agkistrodon contortrix	45	107
Agkistrodon piscivorus	150	107
Micruroides euryxanthus	6	115
Micrurus fulvius	38	115
Micrurus nigrocinctus	20	115

the snake sheds its skin, which can be from one to several times each year, depending on its age, health, and feeding success. Newborn rattlesnakes have a single button present at birth. Not until after their first shed do they possess a true rattle that can create a sound. Rattles may be broken off during the snake's life and cannot be used reliably to determine age. Although rattlesnakes are quick to sound out a warning when threatened, it is a misconception that they will always do so before striking in defense.

Another distinct anatomic feature of pit vipers is the scale pattern on the underside of the tail, the subcaudal scales. The junction of the snake's body and its tail can be easily ascertained by viewing its ventral side. At this location is a large scale (sometimes divided) known as the anal plate. Just distal to this in pit vipers is a sequence of single scales that entirely cross the ventral surface. In nonvenomous snakes and in coral snakes the subcaudal scales are paired (i.e., each covers approximately half the width of the tail) (Figure 38-23). This feature becomes clinically useful when a snake-

bite victim brings in the body of a decapitated snake for identification and when the skin pattern is unfamiliar to the physician. There are very few exceptions to this anatomic rule. The harmless long-nose snake (*Rhinocheilus lecontei*) and the rosy boas (*L. trivirgata*) and rubber boas (*C. bottae*) possess single subcaudal scales.

Coral Snakes. Coral snakes are identified primarily by color pattern. U.S. coral snakes are banded in a red-yellow-black-yellow-red pattern (see Figure 38-13), and the bands completely encircle the snake's body. The contiguity of the red and yellow bands distinguishes U.S. coral snakes from a number of harmless mimics (e.g., several king snakes and milk snakes, genus *Lampropeltis*), which generally have red and yellow bands separated by black bands. This can best be remembered by recalling the phrase "red on yellow, kill a fellow; red on black, venom lack" or by considering that the red and yellow lights on a traffic signal are the warning lights. Contiguous red and yellow bands on a North American snake warn of its venomous potential. Exceptions to this rule are found south of Mexico city, including some routinely bicolor (red and black) specimens.[98] Although one harmless U.S. colubrid has a contiguous red and yellow banding pattern (the shovel-nosed snake, *Chionactis* species), this is an inoffensive reptile, and its bands do not completely encircle its body. In exceptionally rare cases, coral snakes can be all black (melanistic) or albino.[94]

The coral snake venom apparatus is much less complex than that of the pit vipers. The paired venom glands connect through ducts to slightly enlarged, hollow, maxillary fangs that are fixed in an upright position in the forward portion of the jaw (Figure 38-22). In

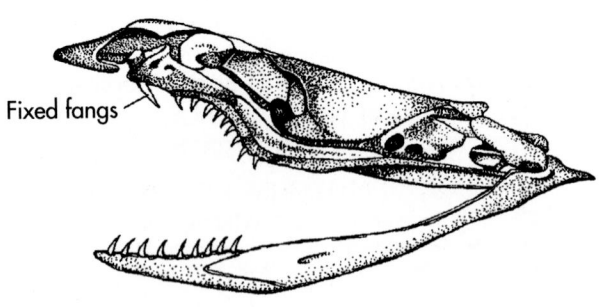

Figure 38-22 Coral snake's skull. Note the slightly enlarged anterior fang that is fixed in its upright position. *(Marlin Sawyer, 1994.)*

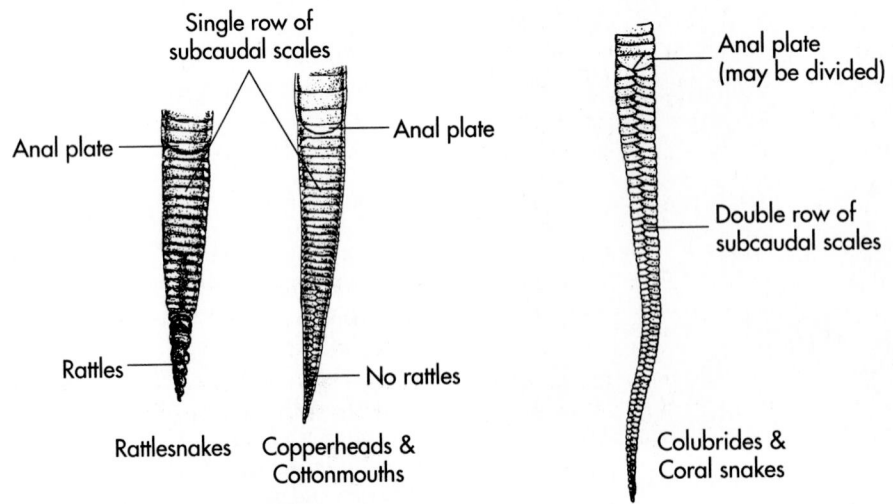

Figure 38-23 Subcaudal scale pattern of pit viper vs. a harmless snake. Pit viper (here, a rattlesnake) has a single scale that spans the ventral side of its tail, just distal to the anal plate, whereas harmless colubrid snake has a double row of scales. Coral snakes also possess a double row of subcaudal scales. *(Marlin Sawyer, 1994.)*

order for the coral snake to inflict a potentially serious bite, it must chew on the victim to inject a sufficient volume of venom through its relatively small fangs. These animals are not capable of striking out with the stabbing motion of the crotalines. In the vast majority of coral snakebite cases, the victim was handling the creature when bitten.

Venoms

Crotaline venoms contain proteins and peptides capable of damaging vascular endothelial cells, leading to increased permeability to plasma and erythrocytes. This results in translocation of fluids, which may progress to hypotension and shock.[148] Specific enzymes common to pit viper venom include proteolytic enzymes, hyaluronidase, thrombinlike enzymes, phospholipase A_2, L-amino acid oxidase, collagenase, RNase, DNase, and arginine ester hydrolase. Proteolytic enzymes damage muscle and subcutaneous tissue and are responsible for necrosis. Hyaluronidase decreases the viscosity of connective tissue, allowing venom to spread. Thrombinlike enzymes act by cleaving either fibrinopeptide A or fibrinopeptide B from fibrinogen without activating factor XIII. This results in formation of an abnormal, unstable fibrin clot, which is readily lysed by both endogenous plasmin and proteolytic enzymes in the venom.[118] This leads to hypofibrinogenemia and increased fibrin degradation products. Phospholipase A_2, common to all pit viper venoms, causes muscle necrosis by damaging cell membranes, which allows calcium influx and release of creatine and creatine kinase (CK). In addition, phospholipase A_2 increases permeability of red blood cell (RBC) membranes, leading to ab-normal RBC morphology and potential hemolysis. Lysolecithin, a by-product of the enzymatic action of phospholipase A_2, damages mast cell membranes and results in histamine release.[21]

Pit viper venom has both offensive (i.e., food gathering) and defensive functions. In predatory strikes the venom immobilizes the prey, facilitates its retrieval by altering its scent, and accelerates digestion.[19,60,62] Defensive strikes are meant to deter predators and tormentors. The amount of venom injected differs from bite to bite. Factors such as prey size and species, duration of fang contact, and time elapsed since last meal influence the amount of venom released.[60,62] Rattlesnakes have been shown to inject significantly more venom into large mice than into small mice.[60] The mass of venom expended probably differs between predatory and defensive bites. In preliminary comparisons, venom expenditure by North American pit vipers appears greater in defensive bites than in predatory bites.[62] In one comparison the northern Pacific rattlesnake (*Crotalus viridis oreganus*) expended almost 4 times more venom when biting a hand model (defensive) than a mouse (predatory).[60,62] The most important

factor influencing potential venom delivery is the size of the snake.[62] A direct relationship has been demonstrated between snake length and mass of venom expended in both predatory and defensive bites.[58,62]

A popular belief is that juvenile rattlesnakes are more dangerous than adult snakes because their venom is more toxic and they are unable to control the volume they release. The venom of some juvenile rattlesnakes may be slightly more toxic, but larger rattlesnakes are capable of delivering much greater amounts of venom in a bite. Juvenile prairie rattlesnakes (*Crotalus viridis viridis*) have venom that is 2 to 3 times more toxic than that of adults.[33] Large adult snakes, however, deliver an average of 17 times more venom than do juveniles.[58] The ability to control venom expenditure has been demonstrated in juvenile rattlesnakes. In a series of first exposures to different-sized prey, "naïve" juvenile rattlesnakes injected similar quantities of venom into all size classes. However, in the second series of exposures, "experienced" snakes injected significantly more venom into larger prey.[59] The clinical relevance of this is uncertain. In many species, venom composition appears to change as the snake ages. Phospholipase A_2 activity decreases with age, probably accounting for some decrease in toxicity. Proteolytic activity, however, increases with age, possibly to aid digestion of larger prey eaten by older, larger snakes.[58] Coagulopathic effects can be different between juvenile and adult western diamondback rattlesnakes (*Crotalus atrox*), partly due to greater amounts of thrombinlike enzymes in younger snakes.[113]

Venom characteristics may vary with geographic origin of the snake.[44] Certain populations of the Mojave rattlesnake (*Crotalus scutulatus scutulatus*) cause human neurotoxicity with severe envenomation while causing minimal local tissue destruction and no hemorrhagic effects.[24,69] Neurotoxic findings may include respiratory difficulty, generalized weakness, and cranial nerve palsies.[24] The venoms of these snakes possess a presynaptic neurotoxin, Mojave toxin, and are classified as venom A populations. Venom B populations lack Mojave toxin and are less toxic. Bites by venom B snakes result in consequences more typical of most rattlesnake venom poisoning: soft tissue swelling, necrosis, and coagulopathy. Venom A populations range from California, across western Arizona, Nevada, Utah, New Mexico, and Texas. Venom B populations are found in more eastern parts of Arizona. A zone of intergradation between venom A and venom B populations occurs along a line between Phoenix and Tucson.[53,147] Toxins with structure and physiologic effects similar to those of Mojave toxin have been isolated from venoms of other species of rattlesnakes, including prairie rattlesnakes (*Crotalus viridis viridis*), midget faded rattlesnakes (*C. v. concolor*), tropical rattlesnakes (*C. durissus*), canebrake rattlesnakes (*C. horridus*), and tiger rattlesnakes (*C.*

tigris).[42,43,61,144] Geographic differences occur in the venoms of other snakes as well. Canebrake rattlesnakes *(C. horridus)* from Florida, Georgia, and South Carolina possess more neurotoxic and myotoxic "canebrake toxin" than do specimens from Alabama, Mississippi, Tennessee, and North Carolina.[43] Differences in concentration of this toxin correlate with variable clinical effects seen after bites by this species from different geographic regions.[17]

Neurotoxicity has been clinically associated with severe myotoxicity in many cases.[13,17,27,69] Severe rhabdomyolysis and myoglobinuric renal failure have been reported after Mojave rattlesnake envenomation and are thought to be related to Mojave toxin.[69] The association between neurotoxicity and myotoxicity has been confirmed in laboratory animals.[3] *C. horridus* specimens possessing significant amounts of the neurotoxin (canebrake toxin) produce a rise in serum CK levels as a biochemical signature of significant venom poisoning. The rise in CK appears to parallel the severity of poisoning by these snakes.[17] Autopsy findings have demonstrated that myonecrosis in this setting is systemic and not focused at the bite site.[17,73] Concomitant rises in MB fractions of creatine kinase can occur in the absence of any clinical evidence of cardiac damage. In one such case, troponin-T was measured as negative despite abnormal total CK and CK-MB.[17] Lesser CK elevations (usually less than 500 U/L) may be seen with other rattlesnake bites, such as that of the eastern diamondback *(Crotalus adamanteus)*. In these cases the elevations appear to more closely parallel local effects.[17]

Mojave toxin is thought to inhibit acetylcholine release at the presynaptic terminal of the neuromuscular junction.[24] *Myokymia,* or muscle fasciculation, is often considered a manifestation of neurotoxicity. This phenomenon, however, occurs through a different mechanism than Mojave toxin–induced neurotoxicity. Muscle fasciculations are believed to be caused by the interaction of certain venom components with calcium or calcium binding sites on the nerve membrane.[24] Fasciculations may occur after envenomation by various species of rattlesnakes, including northern and southern Pacific rattlesnakes *(C. viridis oreganus* and *C. v. helleri,* respectively), eastern diamondback rattlesnakes *(C. adamanteus),* western diamondback rattlesnakes *(C. atrox),* Mojave rattlesnakes *(C. scutulatus),* and timber rattlesnakes *(C. horridus).*[6,24,141]

Coral snake venoms have received less research attention; they are also less complex than pit viper venoms. *Micrurus* and *Micruroides* venoms have minimal proteolytic activity but contain the spreading enzyme hyaluronidase and some phospholipase A_2.[124] The primary lethal component is a low-molecular-weight, postsynaptic neurotoxin that blocks acetylcholine binding sites at the neuromuscular junction.[18,139] In addition, the venom contains at least one myotoxic component that may clinically produce a rise in CK levels.[51]

What coral snake venom lacks in complexity, it makes up in potency. Among U.S. snakes, *Micrurus* and *Micruroides* venom potency, as determined by median lethal dose (LD_{50}) values in mice, are surpassed only by that of the Mojave rattlesnake *(Crotalus scutulatus).*[118] It is estimated that a full-grown coral snake carries enough venom in its delivery apparatus to kill four to five adult humans.[34] It is indeed fortunate that these toxic reptiles are shy, inoffensive, and possess a less effective venom delivery device than the pit vipers.

Clinical Presentation

Pit Vipers. The clinical presentation of pit viper venom poisoning is quite variable, depending on the circumstances of the bite. Important factors include the species, size and health of the snake, age and health of the victim, circumstances that led up to the bite, number of bites and their anatomic locations, and quality of the care rendered to the person, both in the field and in the hospital. Although statistics vary, most accidental bites occur to the lower extremities.[106] The next most common anatomic site is the upper extremity. Many of these bites occur while the victim is intentionally interacting with the snake (e.g., tormenting the animal, trying to catch it, or working with a captive specimen). Less often, bites occur to the head, neck, or trunk. Most bites occur around dawn or dusk, during warmer months, when snakes and people are more active outdoors.[106] A young, intoxicated male bitten on the hand while intentionally interacting with a snake is the most common clinical profile in the United States.

About 75% to 80% of pit viper bites result in envenoming. Approximately one in every four to five bites is "dry," meaning no venom has been injected.[108,118] The snake may voluntarily choose to save its venom for its next meal rather than waste it on a large human. Alternatively, the feedback mechanism may "short-circuit" between the pit organs and the venom apparatus, so that when faced with a huge, heat-radiating mass (a human), the system fails and no venom is expelled. Other possible causes of dry bites include glancing blows that fail to penetrate the skin and an exhausted venom supply. Approximately 35% of cases are mild envenomations, 25% moderate, and 10% to 15% severe.[108] Given their less efficient venom delivery system, coral snakes only effectively envenom approximately 40% of the time.[118]

The clinical findings found in crotaline venom poisoning can be divided into local and systemic signs and symptoms (Table 38-3). After most pit viper bites, severe burning pain at the site begins within minutes. Soft tissue swelling then progresses outward to a variable extent from the bite site. Over hours a bitten extremity can swell all the way to the trunk. Blood may

TABLE 38-3. Signs and Symptoms of Rattlesnake Bites

SIGN OR SYMPTOM	FREQUENCY*
Fang marks	100/100
Swelling and edema	74/100
Pain	65/100
Ecchymosis	51/100
Vesiculations	40/100
Change in pulse rate	60/100
Weakness	72/100
Sweating, chills	64/100
Numbness or tingling of tongue and mouth, scalp, or feet	63/100
Faintness or dizziness	57/100
Nausea, vomiting, or both	48/100
Blood pressure changes	46/100
Change in body temperature	31/100
Swelling regional lymph nodes	40/100
Fasciculations	41/100
Increased blood clotting time	39/100
Sphering of red blood cells	18/100
Tingling or numbness of affected part	42/100
Necrosis	27/100
Respiratory rate changes	40/100
Decreased hemoglobin	37/100
Abnormal electrocardiogram	26/100
Cyanosis	16/100
Hematemesis, hematuria, or melena	15/100
Glycosuria	20/100
Proteinuria	16/100
Unconsciousness	12/100
Thirst	34/100
Increased salivation	20/100
Swollen eyelids	2/100
Retinal hemorrhage	2/100
Blurring of vision	12/100
Convulsions	1/100
Muscle contractions	6/100
Increased blood platelets	16/100
Decreased blood platelets	42/100

Modified from Russell FE: *Snake venom poisoning*, New York, 1983, Scholium International.

*Number of times the symptom or sign was observed per total number of patients.

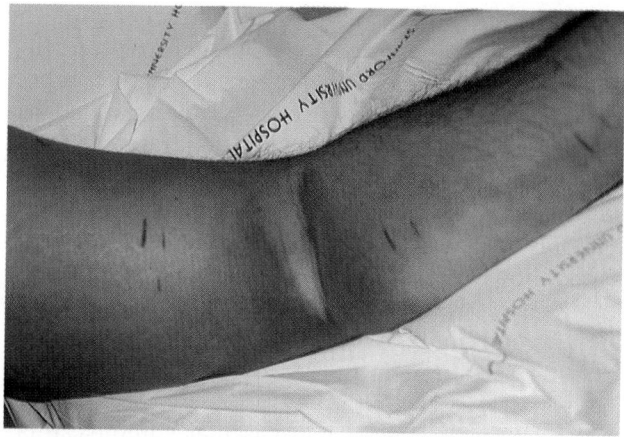

Figure 38-24 Mottled rock rattlesnake *(Crotalus lepidus lepidus)* bite in a young man at 24 hours. Note the exudation of red cells into the soft tissues remote from the bite site. The man was bitten on his left thumb. *(Robert Norris, MD.)*

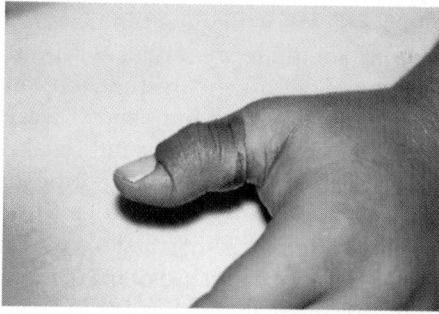

Figure 38-25 Hemorrhagic bleb at the site of a western diamond-back rattlesnake *(Crotalus atrox)* bite at 24 hours. *(Robert Norris, MD.)*

persistently ooze from fang marks, marking the presence of anticoagulant substances in the venom. Ecchymosis is common, both locally and at more remote sites, as the vasculature becomes leaky and RBCs escape into the soft tissues (Figures 38-24 and 38-25). Fang marks are usually evident as small puncture wounds, but the precise bite pattern can be misleading.[100] Most nonvenomous snakebites result in multiple rows of tiny puncture wounds (from the maxillary, palatine, pterygoid, and mandibular teeth), which usually coagulate quickly. Pit vipers also possess palatine, pterygoid, and mandibular teeth, which can result in more than the classic paired puncture marks. Also, a snake may make contact only with a single fang. Thus the associated signs and symptoms should be considered more than the bite pattern in determining whether a bite was inflicted by a pit viper or another snake. Some rattlesnake bites result in little or no local pain despite envenoming; the best example is the Mojave rattlesnake *(Crotalus scutulatus)*. Specimens containing significant amounts of Mojave toxin in their venom tend to cause few local findings. This can lead the treating physician to misjudge the severity of envenoming.[149]

Systemic findings after pit viper bites can be extremely variable because any organ system can be affected. Nausea with or without vomiting is common and may occur early in serious bites. The victim may complain of an overall sense of weakness. An odd sense of taste, such as a rubbery, minty or metallic taste, may be present.[118] Occasionally the victim complains of a numb sensation of the mouth or tongue. The vital signs may be abnormal. The respiratory and heart rates may be increased. The victim may experience respiratory distress due to neurotoxic components of the venom, especially after bites by venom A–producing Mojave rattlesnakes *(C. scutulatus).*[118] Another important cause of respiratory distress is pulmonary edema from pulmonary artery congestion and translocation of intravascular fluid into alveoli. This can be compounded by myocardial depressant factors in some venoms.[118] The victim's blood pressure may be elevated; however, hypotension, which may progress to frank shock, is more common in severe cases. In the first several hours, hypotension is usually caused by pooling of volume in the pulmonary and splanchnic beds. Later, as swelling progresses and fluids exude into remote soft tissues, intravascular volume can become significantly depleted. A rare cause of early shock is an anaphylactic reaction to the venom.[14,29]

Musculoskeletal and neurologic abnormalities can be present. As mentioned, a number of rattlesnake venoms possess a component that can result in local or systemic muscle fasciculations as a sign of significant envenoming. These fasciculations can persist for many hours despite adequate treatment with antivenom. Other findings of neurologic dysfunction can include paresthesias, numbness, and frank motor weakness, especially after bites by some Mojave rattlesnakes *(C. scutulatus)* and eastern diamondback rattlesnakes *(C. adamanteus).*

Although uncommon, hemorrhage can occur at multiple anatomic locations because of the complex procoagulant and anticoagulant fractions of some venoms.[118] Bleeding can occur in the gingival membranes, renal system (microscopic or frank hematuria), gastrointestinal tract (hemoccult-positive stools or frank blood per rectum), pulmonary tree (hemoptysis) or central nervous system.

Laboratory evaluation of a victim of significant pit viper bite may reveal significant abnormalities. The white blood cell count may be elevated. The hematocrit may be elevated from hemoconcentration or may be depressed secondary to bleeding or hemolysis. Serum chemistries may be abnormal. Blood sugar may be elevated. Muscle damage can result in elevated serum potassium and CK levels. Renal dysfunction may result from hypotension, myoglobin and hemoglobin deposition, and direct venom effects.[22] Hepatic dysfunction with elevations of serum transaminases may be seen.[93] Coagulation studies may reveal significant abnormalities. Prothrombin time (PT) and partial thromboplastin time (PTT) can be prolonged. Fibrinogen levels may be depressed, along with an elevation of fibrin degradation products and *d*-dimers.[4] Major abnormalities may be seen in serum coagulation studies in the absence of any clinically significant bleeding (i.e., more serious than gingival oozing or microscopic hematuria).[9] This is particularly relevant in determining when to use blood products in treating these victims. Recurrent co-

agulopathic parameters may persist or recur for as long as 2 weeks after envenomation.[24]

Urinalysis should be obtained to identify hematuria. Proteinuria and glycosuria may also be seen.[123] Each time the victim voids, the urine should be evaluated with bedside testing strips for the presence of blood.

If venom poisoning seems severe or if the victim has significant underlying medical problems (e.g., cardiovascular or respiratory disease), an electrocardiogram (ECG), arterial blood gases (ABGs), and chest radiograph should be obtained. The ECG may reveal evidence of myocardial ischemia. ABGs give important information regarding adequacy of tissue perfusion and respiratory status. Pulmonary vascular congestion or frank pulmonary edema may be seen on the radiograph.

Coral Snakes. The findings of significant coral snake envenoming reflect the predominant neurotoxic effects of these venoms. The victim may have some early, mild, transient pain.[117] Local swelling is uncommon. Fang marks may be difficult to see and should be carefully sought.[102] Systemic signs and symptoms may be delayed as long as 12 or 13 hours after significant bites and can then progress rapidly.[73] The earliest findings may be nausea and vomiting, followed by headache, abdominal pain, diaphoresis and pallor.[32] Victims may complain of paresthesias or numbness or may have altered mental status, such as drowsiness or euphoria.[94] The victim may develop cranial nerve dysfunction (e.g., ptosis, difficulty speaking, difficulty swallowing), followed by peripheral motor nerve dysfunction.[94] In severe cases, respiratory insufficiency and aspiration are significant risks.[73] Cardiovascular insufficiency may also be seen.[123] Unlike many crotaline envenomations, coagulopathy is not a feature of coral snake venom poisoning.

Laboratory studies are of little value in the evaluation of a victim of coral snake bite. Occasionally, a rise in serum CK and myoglobinuria occur, reflecting myotoxicity.[73] ABGs may be useful in evaluating the victim's respiratory status if endotracheal intubation is considered. A chest radiograph is indicated in the setting of apparent cardiac dysfunction or following intubation.

Management
Prehospital Care
PIT VIPERS. Recommendations for first-aid and prehospital treatment of pit viper venom poisoning are often based on speculation and anecdotal experience. Much of the literature is contradictory. In one large retrospective series, first-aid treatment had no relationship to ultimate envenomation severity.[148] Some first-aid measures recommended in the past cause more injury than the snakebite itself, and delays in care have been shown

to increase morbidity and mortality.[29,54] It is inappropriate to use any technique that could potentially injure the patient or impede immediate travel to the nearest facility where antivenom can be administered. General support of the airway, breathing and circulation should be provided based on the capabilities at hand. Oxygen, cardiac monitoring, and intravenous (IV) fluids should be used in the field when available. Although it may be necessary for the victim to hike out from the scene of the incident, activity should be minimized as much as possible. Alternative methods (e.g., helicopter or boat) of extracting the victim from a wilderness setting can be used when available and when conditions such as weather and terrain allow. Jewelry and tight-fitting clothing are removed from the involved extremity in anticipation of swelling. The border of advancing edema is marked with a pen every 15 minutes so that emergency personnel can estimate severity of poisoning by following the rate of progression.

A negative pressure venom extraction device, The Extractor (Sawyer Products, Safety Harbor, Fla.) has been advocated by the Wilderness Medical Society as a temporizing or adjuvant measure before antivenom is available.[35,45] This device, applied directly over fang marks, delivers approximately one atmosphere of negative pressure and requires no skin incisions.[53] To retrieve venom, the device needs to be applied as soon after the bite as possible, probably within 3 minutes.[7] Some recommend that suction continue for 30 to 60 minutes.[2] As blood, tissue fluid, and possibly venom fill the transparent suction cup, the vacuum is lost. The cup is emptied as needed and reapplied as the victim is transported to the hospital. Two small studies suggest some venom retrieval with this device.[7,8] Two patients envenomed by *C. atrox* were treated within 1 minute with an Extractor.[8] The device was applied to each victim a total of 5 times and was left on each time until the suction cup filled. An average of 27.5 μg of venom per milliliter of serosanguineous fluid was removed during the initial suction period, decreasing to 4.4 μg/ml by the end of the fifth application. This is much less than 1 mg of total venom retrieved and probably was not significant because the average venom yield for *C. atrox* is approximately 250 mg.[74] Tissue effects and outcome were not described. In a rabbit study, an estimated 34% of artificially injected, radiolabeled rattlesnake venom was retrieved using the Extractor.[7] The effects on local tissue were not described.

Some suggest the Extractor may exacerbate tissue damage.[38] A study evaluating use of the device in pigs injected with rattlesnake venom demonstrated no difference in swelling between the Extractor group and controls.[11] A circular lesion corresponding to the size of the suction cup, however, developed in some animals and progressed to necrosis. This may have been caused by venom sequestration at the site of envenomation or suction-induced tissue ischemia. Use of the device clinically in humans has been documented in a few anecdotal case reports in nonmedical literature.[55] Its effect on outcome in these cases is difficult to determine, but in two of five cases a dark hemorrhagic bleb conforming precisely to the size of the suction cup formed over the fang puncture sites.

Further research is needed to define the risks and benefits of mechanical suction in crotaline venom poisoning. Other devices producing lesser degrees of suction, such as kits with small, rubber suction cups, are of no benefit. Mouth suction is contraindicated because of the potential for contaminating the wound with oral flora.

Incising the bite site across fang marks is not recommended. This creates additional injury and has never been shown to be effective. Because viperid fangs are curved, incisions may miss the track along which venom is actually injected. Incisions made by laypersons can cause serious injury to underlying blood vessels, nerves, or tendons. In the face of venom-induced coagulopathy, bleeding from such incisions can be severe.[53] Furthermore, the lack of sterile conditions in a field setting increases the risk of infection.

Venom sequestration techniques, such as proper application of a lymphatic/superficial venous constriction band or pressure immobilization, inhibit the systemic spread of venom.[10,135] In a porcine model, lymphatic constriction bands decreased systemic venom absorption without increasing local tissue swelling.[10] It is not clear, however, whether such measures improve outcome after pit viper envenomation. Some argue that restricting spread of potentially necrotizing venom to local tissues may intensify injury.[56] Since local sequelae are the predominant complications after pit viper venom poisoning in North America, and since permanent systemic injury and death are extremely rare, such attempts to limit venom to the bite site may be ill advised.[29] Also, proper placement of a constriction band can be difficult for a lay provider. The band is applied several inches proximal to the bite site and just tight enough (at a pressure of approximately 20 mm Hg) to occlude lymphatic and superficial venous flow while sparing arterial and deep venous perfusion.[10] Appropriate tightness, however, is difficult to gauge. If applied more loosely, the band would be ineffective. If placed too tightly or with ongoing swelling, the band could become an arterial tourniquet.[10,56] Tourniquets have worsened injury when used for snakebite and are contraindicated.[53] Use of a constriction band for a pit viper bite should be based on the situation. If the victim has been bitten by a potentially lethal snake, such as a large rattlesnake (greater than three feet), and is more than 60 minutes from medical care, a constriction band may reduce the chances of a poor systemic outcome, although local necrosis could worsen. More research is also needed on constriction bands.

Pressure immobilization has been used effectively in Australia for field management of elapid snakebites (see Chapter 39).[136] The technique involves wrapping the entire extremity, starting at the bite site, with an elastic or compressive bandage and immobilizing it with a splint. Although one small study suggests this technique is effective in experimental eastern diamondback rattlesnake (*C. adamanteus)* venom poisoning,[135] the concerns about severely restricting venom movement at the site and worsening local necrosis again apply. Patients bitten by pit vipers often complain of severe pain and do not tolerate pressure immobilization well.[56]

The Venom Ex device (Arachnodata, Frauentalweg 97, CH-8045 Zurich) combines a constriction band, incision, and suction.[55] The device consists of six parallel cutting blades (5 mm wide and adjustable to 5 mm in length), a buckled tourniquet (used as a constriction band), and a spring-loaded syringe (20 ml) for suction. The concept is to apply the constriction band, inflict multiple incisions into the bite site, and apply suction to the bleeding wounds. No evidence indicates that this device is beneficial in crotaline bites, and because it uses controversial interventions with potential risks, it is not recommended.

Simple immobilization of the extremity with a splint has not been studied but is unlikely to cause any direct harm. The optimal position for the splinted extremity is not known. The bitten appendage should probably be maintained at heart level, if possible, to balance systemic spread of venom against extremity swelling.

All field management recommendations are based primarily on theory and speculation, with very little science available on which to make an informed decision. This area is open for future research. Until more definitive data are available, the following principles can be used as guidelines. The victim should be calmed, reassured, and transported as expeditiously as possible to the hospital. A splint can be applied en route if materials are immediately available, and the extremity should be kept at heart level unless the victim is required to walk. These measures suffice as adequate prehospital care for the vast majority of cases of pit viper bites in the United States. Decisions regarding the use of a mechanical suction device (e.g., Extractor), a constriction band, or pressure immobilization must take into consideration the risk of worsening local tissue damage.

For the victim of a pit viper bite who is many hours or days from medical care, the best course of action is even less clear and highly dependent on the situation. First-aid measures (reassurance, splint, maintenance of extremity at heart level) should be applied. If present, a companion may hike out for help, if conditions allow

for prompt return of a rescue team. At times, if sufficient rescuers are available, the victim can be carried out. The victim who must hike out should use a makeshift crutch (for a lower extremity bite), should rest frequently, and should maximize oral intake of fluids unless vomiting becomes pronounced.

Electrotherapy was proposed in the late 1980s for first-aid treatment of snakebites and subsequently was popularized by the lay press.[55,63] Guderian et al[49] described 34 indigenous people bitten by unidentified snakes in Ecuador who were treated with electric shocks. Four or five direct-current (DC) shocks (20 to 25 kV, less than 1 mA) were applied to each bite site. Shocks were given every 5 to 10 seconds and lasted 1 to 2 seconds each. The victims apparently developed no local or systemic effects of envenomation, and the authors concluded that treatment was effective. Early proponents recommended application of high-voltage, low-amperage, DC shocks to the bite site using a source such as an outboard motor or lawn mower engine.[48] A "stun gun," typically designed for self-defense, was even modified by one company and marketed for snakebite treatment.[55] This marketing was prohibited by the U.S. Food and Drug Administration (FDA) in 1990 because of total lack of testing or evidence of efficacy. Critics of the Ecuadorian observations suggest many reasons for Guderian's findings. Many of the bites may have been delivered by nonvenomous species, which closely resemble dangerous reptiles in this part of the world, and many indigenous peoples consider all snakes dangerous. The victims who made it to the missionary hospital from the Ecuadorian jungles may have been a self-selected population with less severe bites that would have done well without any treatment.[55,125] In subsequent controlled animal studies, electric shock showed no efficacy in reducing morbidity or mortality after rattlesnake poisoning in mice, rats, or rabbits.[67,70,132] In humans, application of electric shock for snakebite has been associated with acute myocardial infarction and increased local tissue damage secondary to electrical burns.[28,119] Because of its lack of efficacy and inherent risks, electric shock should not be used in the treatment of snakebites.

Local application of ice to the bite wound as a first-aid measure has not been adequately studied as to its benefits or risks. This should not be confused with "cryotherapy," or packing the injured limb in ice for extended periods. This form of treatment was popularized in the 1950s and 1960s. The results of cryotherapy were a significant increase in tissue loss and amputation rate after pit viper bites, and it has now been completely abandoned.[116] Whether brief (e.g., less than 1 hour) application of ice is beneficial (by reducing venom activity or decreasing pain) or harmful (by worsening local ischemia and resulting necrosis) is unknown. The American Red Cross recommends that no cooling measures should be applied in the field management of venomous snakebite.[141]

Indigenous peoples in many parts of the world have long used plants in the treatment of snakebite, either topically or systemically, but little formal research has been done in this area. No current data support the use of any plants in the management of North American snakebite.[66]

Other first-aid measures lacking therapeutic value or potentially more harmful than the snakebite itself include scarification of the bite wound, ingestion of alcohol, use of stimulants, and various folk remedies such as application of ammonia, silver nitrate, oil, potassium permanganate, or saliva. Similarly ineffective is the application of poultices made from various parts of the offending reptile (or other creatures), such as the snake's crushed head, bile, or fat.[118]

Antivenom use in the field can be recommended only when a qualified physician is on scene and when all equipment and drugs are available to manage a potential anaphylactic/anaphylactoid reaction to the serum (including definitive airway management equipment). Newer, potentially safer antivenoms produced using Fab technology (see later discussion) may prove to be safe enough for field use, although monetary costs could be prohibitive.[31]

Attempts to secure or kill the snake are not recommended because of the risk of additional bites to the victim or rescuer and because precious time can be wasted. Currently the same treatment principles and antivenoms apply for all pit viper bites in North America, so absolute identification of the snake is not necessary. Focus is on "treating the bite, not the snake." Serious morbidity and even death have been reported after envenomation by decapitated rattlesnake heads.[17,73,134] In addition, an apparently dead snake or a decapitated snake head can have a bite reflex for up to 1 hour after death. Therefore emergency personnel and hospital care providers should exercise extreme care if handling any specimens accompanying the victim.

CORAL SNAKES. After a bite by a potential coral snake, the animal's skin color pattern should be noted if possible. Because of the potential delay in onset of signs and symptoms after coral snake envenoming and because the recommendation is to administer antivenom to such victims even in the absence of clinical findings, distinguishing between a coral snake and a harmless mimic becomes important. If the snake can be safely captured and contained, this can be helpful if done quickly.

Although research into field management measures for coral snake envenoming is minimal, the Australian pressure immobilization technique would probably be useful. Being elapids, coral snakes are related to the venomous snakes in Australia for which this technique

has been shown to be highly effective in limiting venom absorption (see Chapter 39).

Hospital Care (Box 38-1)

PIT VIPERS. As in all emergent medical care, initial attention must be focused on the victim's airway, breathing, and circulation. Most victims should receive supplemental oxygen until it is clear that they are stable. Pulse oximetry and cardiac monitoring should be instituted and two large-bore IV lines established. The initial management of hypotension or shock should include vigorous fluid resuscitation with crystalloids (normal saline or Ringer's lactate). If organ perfusion remains inadequate after vigorous fluid infusion (e.g., 2 L of crystalloid in an adult, 20 to 40 ml/kg in a child), a trial infusion of albumin should be started. Evidence supports the utility of adding albumin early in this setting because of the rapid onset of increased vascular permeability after significant pit viper envenomation.[126] Vasopressors should be used to treat venom-induced shock only as a last resort, after adequate volume infusion and initiation of antivenom therapy. Prolonged, inadequately treated hypotension has been strongly implicated in fatal cases of venom poisoning.[29,56]

Antivenom is the definitive treatment for serious pit viper envenomation. Antivenin (Crotalidae) Polyvalent (Wyeth-Ayerst Laboratories, Philadelphia, Pa.) has been the only commercially available antivenom in the United States for crotaline envenomation since 1954. Antivenin (Crotalidae) Polyvalent is derived from the serum of horses immunized to the venom of two North American and two South American pit vipers: the eastern diamondback rattlesnake (*C. adamanteus*), western diamondback rattlesnake (*C. atrox*), South American rattlesnake (*C. durissus terrificus*), and fer-de-lance (*Bothrops atrox*). This antivenom can be used for bites by any North American pit viper, as well as all the Central and South American crotalines and some Asian pit vipers. The degree of protection, however, varies according to the species involved. Since this product is manufactured using only four different snake venoms, its ability to protect against crotalines with significantly different venoms (e.g., the Mojave rattlesnake, *C. scutulatus*) is lessened.

As a heterologous serum product, Antivenin (Crotalidae) Polyvalent carries some significant risks in its use. Early, acute reactions to antivenom can be either anaphylactic (type I, IgE mediated) or anaphylactoid (due to direct complement activation).[148] These immediate reactions are clinically indistinguishable and may manifest with urticaria, pruritus, flushing, facial edema, vomiting, diarrhea, crampy abdominal pain, bronchospasm, laryngeal edema, and hypotension. Approximately 20% of patients who receive the Wyeth product can be expected to have an early reaction, and

---

Box 38-1   MANAGEMENT PRINCIPLES IN TREATING A VICTIM OF POTENTIAL PIT VIPER BITE IN NORTH AMERICA

Determine: was the snake venomous?

Determine: is there evidence that venom poisoning has occurred?

Assess and support: airway, breathing, and circulation.

Establish two large-bore intravenous lines for crystalloid infusion.

Obtain appropriate laboratory studies.

Measure the bitten limb's circumference at two or more sites every 15 minutes.

If systemic signs or symptoms or laboratory abnormalities are present, obtain and reconstitute an appropriate antivenom.

Obtain informed consent for antivenom infusion if possible.

Have epinephrine (appropriate subcutaneous dose) drawn up at the victim's bedside for possible acute reaction to antivenom.

Perform skin testing for possible allergy to antivenom if indicated.

If the skin test is negative or if antivenom is to be given without skin testing, pretreat with H$_1$- and H$_2$-blocking antihistamines.

Expand the victim's intravascular volume with crystalloid fluids unless contraindicated.

Dilute the vials of antivenom to be given in crystalloid (1 L for adult, 20-40 ml/kg for child).

Begin antivenom by slow intravenous infusion.

Gradually increase the rate of infusion in the absence of an acute reaction.

If a reaction occurs, stop the antivenom and treat as necessary.

Consider the need for further antivenom:

Further antivenom to be withheld: provide conservative care only.

Further antivenom to be given: dilute the antiserum further; administer intravenous steroids; restart the antivenom at a slower rate.

If reaction continues in the face of severe poisoning:

Admit to the intensive care unit (ICU).

Institute maximal monitoring as needed.

Consult an expert in snake envenomation.

Titrate epinephrine drip against the reaction.

Provide wound care.

Determine management approach:

Apparent dry bite: admit to hospital or observe for a minimum of 8 hours.

Any degree of envenomation: admit to hospital.

Severe venom poisoning: admit to ICU.

---

about half of these are serious.[28,71] Deaths from allergic reactions to antivenom (airway obstruction, cardiovascular collapse) are rare.[71,120] Risk factors for allergy to antivenom (e.g., previous exposure to equine serum, history of allergy to horses) should be considered when deciding on a course of therapy.

Another, more common reaction to Antivenin (Crotalidae) Polyvalent is serum sickness (type III, IgM- and IgG-mediated hypersensitivity reaction), characterized by rash, fever, chills, arthralgias, lymphadenopathy, and malaise. In severe cases, there may be renal or peripheral nerve involvement. Serum sickness may occur in as many as 50% to 75% of patients 3 days to 3 weeks after antivenom administration.[71,149] The likelihood of serum sickness increases with total antivenom dosage and it usually occurs when eight or more vials of Antivenin (Crotalidae) Polyvalent are given.[71]

The risks of adverse reactions to antivenom must be weighed against the potential benefit of improved mortality and morbidity from its administration. Informed consent should be obtained whenever possible.

Severity grading and dosage of antivenom. Deciding when to use antivenom in a case of pit viper venom poisoning can be difficult. The risks of adverse reactions to the antivenom must be weighed against the benefits of reducing venom toxicity. Antivenom should certainly be given when evidence indicates serious envenoma-

tion (e.g., cardiovascular insufficiency, respiratory difficulty) or imminent risk of an acute complication (e.g., life-threatening bleeding, tissue necrosis, compartment syndrome, rhabdomyolysis). Snake venom poisoning is a dynamic process. Initiation of antivenom or administration of additional vials is indicated in the victim with a worsening clinical course (Figure 38-26).

Antivenom therapy is predicated on imparting passive immunity to the victim against circulating snake venom antigens. Once these deleterious antigens bind to their target tissues, antivenom is unable to pull them off or reverse their effects. Therefore, to be most effective, antivenom should be given as soon as possible after the bite, preferably within 4 to 6 hours.[75] Antivenom may be useful, however, in patients with significant coagulopathy or acute renal failure for days after envenomation.[121] Venom antigens have been detected as late as 13 days after venomous snakebite.[39] The clinical implications of prolonged, recurrent, isolated, and mild coagulopathy and the utility of late antivenom administration remain unresolved. No clear endpoints for antivenom's therapeutic window have been established.

Decisions about initial dosing of antivenom in cases of venomous snakebite are based on the apparent or predicted severity of poisoning. The grading scale described in Table 38-4 can be very useful to physicians in determining the severity of North American pit viper bites, but it should not be applied to bites by non-

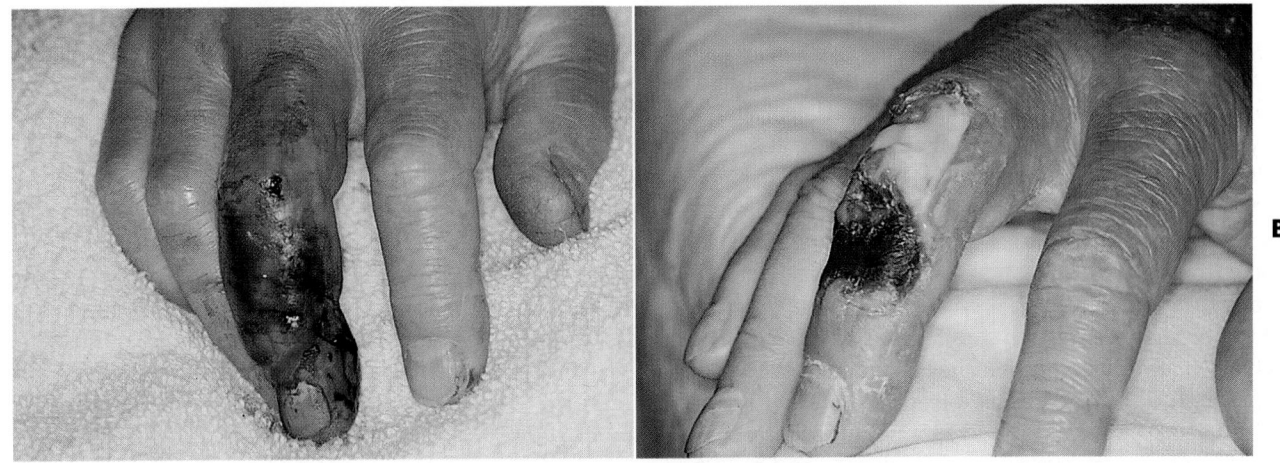

Figure 38-26   A, Soft tissue swelling, hemorrhagic blebs, and early necrosis after red diamond rattlesnake *(Crotalus ruber)* bite to the long finger (day 2). Victim received 10 vials of antivenom 6 hours after the bite and 10 more vials for severe thrombocytopenia on day 2. **B,** Seven weeks later. Note the degree of necrosis. *(Sean Bush, MD.)*

TABLE 38-4. Clinical Severity Grading Scale for Pit Viper Bites in North America

SEVERITY	LOCAL FINDINGS		SYSTEMIC SIGNS AND SYMPTOMS		LABORATORY STUDIES
Nonenvenomation (dry bite)	Puncture wounds only	*and*	None	*and*	Normal
Minimal envenomation	Puncture wounds Swelling limited to bite site Bloody ooze from bite site Local ecchymosis Local pain (may be severe)	*and*	None	*and*	Normal
Moderate envenomation	As for minimal, but swelling may involve entire extremity Severe pain	*and*	Mild (e.g., nausea, vomiting, general weakness, mildly abnormal vital signs)	*or*	Mildly abnormal (e.g., slightly decreased platelet count or fibrinogen; presence of fibrin degradation products; slightly increased PT/PTT; hemoconcentration)
Severe envenomation	May be severe (e.g., severe soft tissue swelling and pain) May be less severe than expected (especially if deep or intravenous deposition of venom)	*and*	Very abnormal vital signs Shock Respiratory distress Significant clinical bleeding	*or*	Profoundly abnormal (e.g., coagulopathy; hemolysis/severe anemia; renal dysfunction)

crotaline species. A more detailed snakebite severity score was developed as a research tool, but is not intended for clinical use.[30]

The grade of envenomation at any given time is determined by whichever parameter (local effects, systemic effects, or laboratory abnormalities) is most severely affected. In nonenvenomations, or "dry bites," fang marks are present but there are no other clinical signs or symptoms and no laboratory abnormalities. The victim has only superficial punctures that require standard wound care, including tetanus prophylaxis as necessary.

Minimal envenomation results in effects confined to the immediate area around the bite site (pain, swelling, erythema, ecchymosis). Systemic effects are absent and laboratory values normal.

In a moderate envenomation, local effects progress beyond the immediate bite area but involve less than the entire body part (arm or leg). Local effects are generally quantified in relation to the extent of involvement of the bitten extremity. Systemic effects begin to appear when venom poisoning reaches moderate severity and may include paresthesias, strange taste sensations, numbness of the mouth and tongue, muscle fasciculations (myokymia), generalized weakness, and mild hypotension. Along with systemic signs and symptoms, laboratory abnormalities occur. Coagulation times (e.g., PT, PTT, international normalized ratio) may be elevated, platelets may drop to less than $90,000/mm^3$, fibrinogen may fall below 90 mg/dl, and CK levels may exceed 500 to 1000 U/L. Although evidence is limited that antivenom corrects venom-induced thrombocytopenia, rhabdomyolysis, or myokymia,[4,24] these abnormalities serve as markers of systemic injury and the need for antivenom therapy.

With severe venom poisoning, local effects may rapidly involve the entire body part and may become limb threatening. Systemic manifestations may include shock, clinically significant hemorrhaging (e.g., hematemesis), respiratory difficulty, and multifactorial renal failure. Severe muscle fasciculations may contribute to respiratory difficulty. Profound laboratory abnormalities, such as thrombocytopenia less than $20,000/mm^3$, coagulopathic parameters associated with potentially life-threatening bleeding, or rhabdomyolysis/myoglobinuric renal failure, also indicated severe envenomation.

Antivenom dosing is directed by clinical severity of venom poisoning. No antiserum is necessary in dry bites, and it is questionable whether the risks associated with the use of Antivenin (Crotalidae) Polyvalent ever justify its use in mild venom poisoning. Some authors recommend a starting dose of 5 vials in mild cases.[118] For moderate poisoning the initial dose should be 10 vials, and for a severe case, 15 to 20 vials. If symptoms, signs, or laboratory parameters continue to deteriorate after the initial dose of antivenom, further dosing in 5- to 10-vial increments every 30 minutes to 2 hours is indicated. A typical total dose of Antivenin (Crotalidae) Polyvalent for a serious rattlesnake envenomation is approximately 20 to 40 vials.

Although few studies have compared children with adults in terms of the effects of crotaline venom poisoning, higher doses of antivenom should be used in pediatric victims.* Children may receive a higher dose of

venom per kilogram of body weight, which may predispose them to greater toxicity. With adequate antivenom administration, however, children do not appear any more susceptible to systemic venom effects than adults.[29]

Special bite situations. Systemic findings may be delayed after bites by venom A–producing Mojave rattlesnakes *(C. scutulatus),* with deceptively minimal local tissue effects. This can lead to underestimation of severity based on the grading scale in Table 38-4. Therefore, in geographic areas where this variant is found, some recommend that antivenom be started empirically for known Mojave bites, regardless of the initial apparent severity of the bite.[12,148] Antivenin (Crotalidae) Polyvalent provides relatively poor coverage for *C. scutulatus* venom, which supports this recommendation.[122] To compensate for reduced overall efficacy in these cases, Wyeth's Antivenin (Crotalidae) Polyvalent is usually given early and in larger doses than for most other rattlesnake bites.

Copperheads *(Agkistrodon contortrix)* and cottonmouths *(A. piscivorus)* generally cause less severe clinical effects that do most rattlesnakes. Many *Agkistrodon* envenomations can be treated without Antivenin (Crotalidae) Polyvalent.[30,146] Severe envenomation, however, regardless of the crotaline species involved, requires antivenom therapy.

Antivenom administration. Reconstituting lyophilized Antivenin (Crotalidae) Polyvalent can be an onerous task. Each vial must be dissolved in 10 ml of diluent. Although the antivenom comes with a vial of 10 ml of sterile water for this purpose, any typical diluent (e.g., sterile water, normal saline) can be used. Using warm diluent helps facilitate reconstitution. Gentle agitation of each vial for several minutes is required to redissolve the proteins. Care must be taken to not denature the antiserum with overzealous shaking. It may take as long as 30 minutes to fully reconstitute the antivenom, so this process should be started as soon as the need for antiserum has been identified.

Wyeth recommends a skin test for possible allergy to equine-derived products before administration of Antivenin (Crotalidae) Polyvalent. This involves intradermal injection of 0.02 to 0.03 ml of a 1:10 dilution of normal horse serum into an unbitten extremity (e.g., volar forearm). A small vial of normal horse serum is packaged along with the lyophilized antivenom and diluent. A positive test is manifested by a wheal and flare reaction within 5 to 30 minutes. Skin testing, however, is very unreliable. As many as 10% to 28% of persons with a negative skin test still manifest an acute reaction to antivenom, and up to 30% with a positive skin test have no reaction if antivenom is still given.[71,130] Furthermore, people can develop an acute reaction or delayed serum sickness to the skin test alone.[130] Since the test takes up to 30 minutes to be called negative, it is reasonable to forego

---

*References 1, 14, 26, 29, 142, 148.

testing in a patient with clear indications for antivenom treatment. If antivenom might be withheld with a positive skin test (e.g., non–life-threatening, moderate envenomation), testing can be considered. In these cases, using actual reconstituted antivenom (further diluted to 1:10 or 1:100) rather than normal horse serum may increase the predictive value of the test. Along with the serum skin test, a similar volume of normal saline should be injected intradermally in the opposite arm as a negative control. Skin testing may be useful in predicting immediate hypersensitivity but has no value in predicting eventual serum sickness. Furthermore, skin testing can sensitize individuals to antivenom, making use of this product even more risky in the event of a future venomous snakebite. Skin testing is *not* recommended when antivenom is either not indicated (dry bite) or clearly indicated (severe bite). Antivenom is still indicated for severe venom poisoning, even with a positive skin test. In this case, management should proceed as for the victim with severe poisoning who reacted adversely to the antivenom during its infusion (see later discussion).

Any time antivenom is given, an acute adverse reaction should be anticipated and preparations made to manage a life-threatening situation. Airway equipment must be immediately available and two functional IV lines secured.

Before beginning antivenom infusion (but after interpreting any administered skin test), the patient may be premedicated with appropriate doses of antihistamines. Both an H_1 blocker (e.g., diphenhydramine, 1 mg/kg) and an H_2 blocker (e.g., cimetidine, 5 mg/kg up to 300 mg) can be given intravenously to prevent or mitigate any acute reaction. Expanding the victim's intravascular volume with an appropriate bolus of crystalloid (e.g., 1 to 2 L in an adult, 20 to 40 ml/kg in a child) may also prevent or blunt such a reaction.[1]

If the risk of allergy is high (e.g., past history of known allergy to horses or horse serum products), a prophylactic dose of epinephrine can be considered as well. Epinephrine has been shown to reduce the incidence of acute reactions to antivenom. Subcutaneous administration of 0.25 ml of epinephrine (1:1000 aqueous) reduced acute adverse reactions from 43% to 11% in one randomized, controlled, prospective series of 105 patients.[111] No patients pretreated with epinephrine had severe reactions to antivenom, whereas 8% of patients who did not receive epinephrine had reactions. Epinephrine must be used with caution in persons at risk for ischemic heart disease or stroke. If coagulopathy is present, prophylactic epinephrine should be avoided because of the risk of elevating blood pressure and causing intracranial bleeding.[145] The very short half-life of epinephrine would certainly limit any potential benefits from its prophylactic use.

Routine premedication with corticosteroids is not common practice in the United States; it is more common in Australia. Since the beneficial effects of steroids in limiting allergic phenomena would not be present for 4 to 6 hours, and since steroids may worsen local effects of venom poisoning by North American pit vipers,[128] steroids are generally not given unless an acute reaction has occurred.

Once the vials of antivenom are dissolved, each should be further diluted before administration. Many early reactions to antivenom are related to the concentration of the product that is given intravenously[1]; therefore Antivenin (Crotalidae) Polyvalent should be given in a relatively dilute form. For adults without preexisting cardiac insufficiency the initial total dose can be placed into a liter of normal saline or Ringer's lactate. For children, the total starting dose should be placed into a volume equivalent to 20 to 40 ml of crystalloid fluid/kg up to 1 L.

The infusion should be started at a slow rate (e.g., 1 ml/min) for the first 10 to 20 minutes, with the attending physician monitoring for signs of acute reaction. If no adverse reaction occurs, the rate is increased to complete the infusion over 1 to 2 hours; children should receive approximately 10 to 20 ml/kg/hr.

If an acute reaction develops, the antivenom infusion should be stopped immediately and the response treated. This may require administration of epinephrine, further antihistamines (both H_1 and H_2 blockers), and steroids. Appropriate ventilatory and circulatory support should be instituted as needed. Once these interventions have stopped the reaction, the physician must determine if antivenom therapy is still indicated. In most cases, antivenom infusion can be restarted, but after further dilution of the antiserum (twofold if the patient's cardiovascular reserve will tolerate the increased volume) and at a slower rate. If the reaction was serious or persists after restarting the antivenom, and if the venom poisoning is life threatening, the patient should be placed in an intensive care setting with maximal cardiovascular monitoring. Invasive monitoring (e.g., arterial line access) is helpful as long as no coagulopathy would make such line placement risky. An epinephrine IV infusion should be established (starting at 0.1 µg/kg/min) and titrated to hold the anaphylactic reaction at bay as further antivenom is infused. Generally, enough antivenom can be administered using this technique to benefit the patient's outcome.[13,91] Careful reevaluation of the need for antivenom should be made before embarking on this hazardous approach. It is advisable to consult with a specialist who manages difficult envenomations.

New antivenoms. Much work has been done worldwide to develop new, more effective, and safer antivenoms for snakebite therapy. For North American pit vipers, a new product may be more potent and less allergenic than Antivenin (Crotalidae) Polyvalent.[25,31]

This antivenom (CroFab, Protherics, London) is derived from four groups of sheep, each immunized to the venom of one of four species of crotaline: eastern diamondback rattlesnake (*Crotalus adamanteus*), western diamondback rattlesnake (*C. atrox*), venom A–producing Mojave rattlesnake (*C. scutulatus scutulatus*), and eastern cottonmouth water moccasin (*Agkistrodon piscivorus piscivorus*). These four genetically dissimilar snakes were chosen to optimize the degree of cross-protection against venoms of all clinically important North American pit vipers.[25]

The ovine IgG molecules from each resulting monospecific antiserum are papain digested into Fc and Fab fragments. The immunogenic Fc portion is precipitated and discarded. The protective Fab portions are isolated by affinity chromatography to the venom against which they are active. These Fab fragments are subsequently desorbed and combined in equal parts to yield a polyspecific, crotaline, Fab antivenom.[25,31] This antivenom should cause fewer allergic reactions than Antivenin (Crotalidae) Polyvalent. Ovine IgG is not glycosylated, unlike equine IgG(T), and therefore is less immunogenic. In addition, Fab fragments, with their single binding site, are incapable of cross-linking immune complexes and stimulating the cascade of mediator release that results in anaphylaxis.[72] Immunologic response is less likely because the immunogenic Fc portion is eliminated and the molecule is smaller.[129] Also, this ovine Fab for injection, with its smaller molecular size, is more rapidly cleared by the kidneys; thus it may prevent serum sickness by reducing immune complex deposition in tissues. A smaller molecule may also allow improved tissue penetration and better access to available venom.[65]

In animal models CroFab has been shown to be 3 to 10 times more potent than Antivenin (Crotalidae) Polyvalent in protecting mice against lethal effects of venom from various North American pit vipers.[25,95] In clinical trials the initial dosage of CroFab ranged from 4 to 12 vials, with repeated doses of 2 to 6 vials given for recurrence or progression of swelling or systemic effects.[24,31,127] Venom effects may recur after initial treatment because Fab fragments are cleared before all venom antigens are neutralized.[127]

In the first 42 patients treated with CroFab, there were 7 early serum reactions (5 with "urticaria," 1 "cough," and 1 "allergic reaction" manifested by urticaria, dyspnea, and wheezing).[104a] There were also 5 late serum reactions (2 with "rash," 1 with "pruritus," 1 with "urticaria," and 1 "serum sickness" manifested by severe rash and pruritus.)[104a]

CroFab received FDA approval in October 2000. Per the manufacturer, it is indicated for mild and moderate North American pit viper venom poisoning.[104a] Almost certainly, the product will be effective in severe cases, as well. The precise degrees of cross protection, however,

for crotaline species other than those used in its manufacture remains to be determined. It is intended for IV administration. No skin test is recommended. No premedication is mentioned in the package insert, but appropriate medications (epinephrine and antihistamines) should be immediately available if a reaction occurs.[104a] The starting dose for CroFab is 4 to 6 reconstituted vials, further diluted to 250 ml of normal saline.[104a] Similar to Antivenin (Crotalidae) Polyvalent administration, CroFab should be started slowly for the first several minutes while observing the patient closely for any signs of adverse reaction. If all goes well, the rate is increased to get the initial dose administered in 1 hour. The victim should then be observed over the course of an additional hour for evidence that control of abnormalities has been achieved. If there is evidence of progression of local findings or if coagulation studies and systemic signs and symptoms fail to return to normal, 4 to 6 additional vials should be given until such stabilization occurs. Then 2 vials should be given every 6 hours for up to 18 hours (3 doses). Further dosage requirements after that time period have not been determined. There is evidence that patients with significant coagulopathies during the initial phase of their poisoning may have recurrence of these findings during the first 2 weeks after the bite.[104a] The clinical significance of these findings and the need for additional antivenom remains to be determined. Certainly, patients should be warned of this potential recurrence of coagulopathy and the need to return if there is any evidence of bleeding and to avoid elective surgical procedures during this time period.

Monitoring therapy. Antivenom administration should continue until the patient is stabilized. This may include reduced swelling, subjective systemic improvement, and stabilization or normalization of vital signs and laboratory values. Muscle fasciculations should not be used as a guide for continued administration of Wyeth's Antivenin (Crotalidae) Polyvalent, since they may be refractory to this therapy. Preliminary reports, however, suggest that myokymia improves with administration of the new Fab antivenom.[24] Neurotoxicity has been documented to improve with antivenom administration, even with delayed administration.[13,24]

The efficacy of antivenom in treating venom-induced coagulopathy and thrombocytopenia is not established. Although Antivenin (Crotalidae) Polyvalent binds to venom antigens responsible for these effects, abnormalities in hemostatic parameters may persist or recur.[4,127] In several reports, venom-induced thrombocytopenia improved after antivenom infusion.[9,57,114] Other reports contradict these findings.[112,138] In a series of patients envenomed by timber rattlesnakes (*Crotalus horridus*), PT and PTT, but not thrombocytopenia, normalized after antivenom therapy.[4] In another series, rattlesnake venom–induced thrombocytopenia usually improved after antivenom infusion, although the degree of improvement was small, frequently incomplete, and did not appear to be related to the total dose of antivenom given.[15] Seifert et al[127] reported investigational use of Fab antivenom (CroFab) in a thrombocytopenic victim of western diamondback rattlesnake (*Crotalus atrox*) venom poisoning. Although the platelet counts rebounded from 12,000/mm³ to 227,000/mm³ within 1 hour, recurrent thrombocytopenia was documented from day 5 through day 10, possibly because of more rapid clearance of Fab fragments than venom antigens.

Blood products. In the rare situation of significant clinical hemorrhage after pit viper venom poisoning (e.g., gastrointestinal bleeding, central nervous system hemorrhage), transfusion of blood products, including platelets, plasma or packed RBCs, may be necessary. Antivenom should always be started before factor replacement to avoid adding further fuel to an ongoing consumptive coagulopathy. Packed RBCs should be considered for acute, severe anemia (e.g., hemoglobin less than 7 g/dl). Solvent/detergent-treated plasma or fresh-frozen plasma may be needed to replace depleted coagulation factors if bleeding is significant, and cryoprecipitate may be added as needed for fibrinogen levels less than 100 mg/dl.[9] Regardless of the presence or absence of bleeding, platelet transfusion should be considered for a count of less than 20,000/mm³. Any improvement in platelet count after transfusion, however, may be temporary.[4,138] Patients with dangerously low platelet counts should be placed on bed rest to lower the risk of bleeding until counts rebound.

Analgesia and wound care. Pain control can be a significant issue after pit viper venom poisoning. Analgesia is best obtained using appropriate, titrated doses of opiates (e.g., IV morphine sulfate, 2 to 10 mg in adults and 0.1 mg/kg in children; repeated as needed if vital signs allow). Aspirin and nonsteroidal antiinflammatory drugs should be avoided because they may exacerbate coagulopathies.

Wound care for pit viper venom poisoning follows standard principles. Tetanus immunization (diphtheria-tetanus toxoid, 0.5 ml intramuscularly) is recommended if the patient's immunization is not up-to-date. Any wounds should be cleaned and the extremity placed in a well-padded splint with additional padding between the digits. The extremity is then elevated above the heart to reduce swelling. Antivenom, if indicated, should be started before elevating the limb.

Although snakes' mouths are colonized with several potentially pathogenic organisms, such as *Pseudomonas aeruginosa*, *Staphylococcus epidermidis*, Enterobacteriaceae species, and *Clostridium* species, wound infections from bites are uncommon, and prophylactic antibiotics are unnecessary in most cases.[23,143] Pit viper

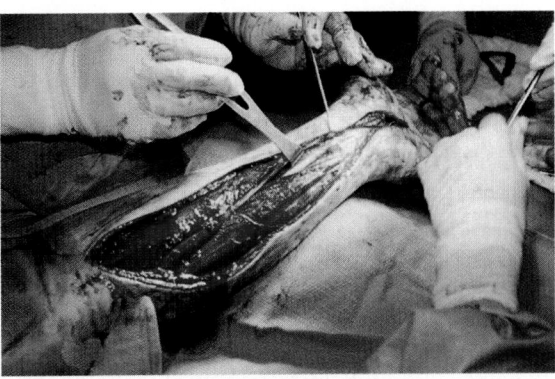

Figure 38-27 Rarely indicated fasciotomy in a victim of severe rattlesnake bite *(Crotalus viridis helleri)*. Compartment pressures were greater than 60 mm Hg despite aggressive antivenom therapy. *(Robert Norris, MD.)*

venom has antibacterial activity, which may account in part for the low incidence of wound infections.[137] If misdirected first-aid efforts included incisions into the bite wound or mouth suction, an appropriate broad-spectrum antibiotic (e.g., amoxicillin/clavulanate) should be considered. If secondary infection occurs, appropriate aerobic and anaerobic wound cultures (and possibly blood cultures, depending on the clinical situation) should be obtained. Empiric therapy should then be started (e.g., ciprofloxacin, 500 mg orally twice a day in adults). If anaerobes are suspected, metronidazole or clindamycin in appropriate doses can be added. Children and pregnant women can be treated with an initial dose of ceftriaxone (50 mg/kg up to 1 g IV or IM) followed by oral amoxicillin/clavulanate (40 mg/kg divided 3 times a day). Daily wound monitoring will guide decisions regarding repeat doses of ceftriaxone until culture and sensitivity results are available. Abscesses should be drained as usual. An infected snakebite should prompt further examination of the wounds for potential retained teeth or fangs. Radiographs may be helpful but are not particularly sensitive.

Compartment syndrome is a rare occurrence after venomous snakebite.[36,101] The diagnosis can be difficult because an envenomed arm or leg is often very swollen, discolored, tender, and painful on attempted range of motion of the digits. These findings may closely mimic a compartment syndrome. To differentiate the subcutaneous swelling from intramuscular swelling, it is relatively simple to measure intracompartmental pressures using a wick catheter or digital readout device. If compartmental pressures exceed 30 to 40 mm Hg, antivenom should be started or continued while the extremity is elevated above heart level. The hemodynamically stable patient should receive IV mannitol (1 to 2 g/kg) over 30 minutes. These measures may reduce the pressures to safe levels.[20] If the pressures fail to decrease within 60 minutes, a fasciotomy is needed (Figure 38-27). A surgical consultant (hand, orthopedic, or general) should be involved if compartment syndrome is a possibility. Prophylactic fasciotomy, however, is not recommended. In animal studies, prophylactic fasciotomy did not reduce the amount of muscle necrosis when rattlesnake venom was injected intramuscularly.[37] Muscle necrosis after pit viper envenomation is primarily caused by direct myotoxic venom effects rather than any increase in intracompartmental pressure. Although the fangs of many pit vipers are long enough to penetrate muscle compartments, most crotaline bites result in subcutaneous deposition of venom.[118]

Management approach. Disposition decisions for patients bitten by pit vipers are generally straightforward. Admission to an intensive care unit (ICU) is prudent for victims with severe envenomations or with progressive clinical findings and need for further antivenom administration. Persons bitten in the head, neck, or trunk should be monitored in an ICU because of the greater risks associated with these bites. Patients who develop a serious adverse reaction to antivenom, such as anaphylaxis, should also be admitted to the ICU. Victims who require a higher level of care than available at the treating institution should be transferred to an appropriate facility. After antivenom infusion and clinical stabilization, victims of moderately severe poisoning can be admitted to a basic floor.

Admission to the hospital should be strongly considered for all persons with apparent envenomation. In one series, more than half of persons with minimal or no signs of envenomation at presentation subsequently developed significant envenomation with moderate to severe swelling, elevated PT, or thrombocytopenia.[68] About 25% of these persons deteriorated more than 8 hours after envenomation. Even with apparent resolution of swelling, victims may later develop severe toxicity.[50] Because onset and progression of signs and symptoms after a pit viper bite vary greatly, all potential victims should be closely watched in the emergency department for a minimum of 8 hours if not admitted. Because of the delayed onset of findings with some Mojave rattlesnake bites, all persons with suspected *Crotalus scutulatus* bites should be admitted to the hospital for 24 hours of observation. Admission is also highly recommended for children with potentially venomous snakebites.

Discharge is considered after 8 hours of observation for victims who apparently sustained a dry bite. These victims have no symptoms or signs other than puncture wounds. All laboratory studies and vital signs must be normal. On discharge, patients should be instructed to return for onset of swelling, increased pain, bleeding, blood in the urine, severe headache, difficulty breathing, rash, joint pain, swollen lymph nodes, fever, or signs of wound infection. The victim should be scheduled for a follow-up reexamination in 24 to 48 hours and should be accompanied and assisted by another if needed.

At time of hospital discharge, patients who received antivenom should be reminded about the possibility of developing serum sickness and that they need prompt medical attention if they develop fever, arthralgias, myalgias, urticaria or other findings consistent with a type III reaction within the first few weeks after treatment. Serum sickness is usually benign and self-limited. Most patients can be adequately treated as outpatients with steroids (e.g., oral prednisone, 1 to 2 mg/kg/day) and antihistamines (e.g., oral diphenhydramine, 25 to 50 mg 4 times a day in adults and 5 mg/kg/day in divided doses for children). Steroids should be continued until signs and symptoms of serum sickness resolve, then tapered over 1 to 2 weeks. In patients more severely affected, treatment can begin in the hospital with IV steroids in equivalent doses.

Discharge instructions to patients should also include information on ways to prevent venomous snakebite. More than half of bites occur during intentional interaction with the reptiles.[99] These usually involve attempts to handle, harass, capture, or kill the snake. The bite may be inflicted by a specimen in captivity. Avoiding intentional interaction with venomous snakes can prevent most injuries. Wearing shoes and long pants can prevent some strikes. In areas where snakes are common, young children should be closely supervised and older children educated to avoid snakes. Animal control services should be called to remove snakes found close to human habitation. If a snake is encountered in the wilderness, people should carefully move a safe distance away from the snake.

Assistance with managing a victim of snakebite can be obtained from regional poison control centers, including the University of Arizona Poison and Drug Information Center (520-626-6016), Rocky Mountain Poison Control (303-739-1123), and San Diego Regional Poison Control (accessed via a central number for California poison control centers, 800-411-8080). The *Antivenom Index,* published by the American Zoo and Aquarium Association (8403 Colesville Rd., Suite 710, Silver Springs, MD 20910; 301-562-0777) and the AAPCC list U.S. antivenom sources.

CORAL SNAKES. Hospital management of coral snake bite victims can be challenging. The first priority in the stable victim is to determine that a coral snake was actually the culprit; photographs of coral snakes and nonvenomous mimics indigenous to the area can be useful. If a coral snake is identified and appears to have inflicted an effective bite, management should proceed in anticipation of a significant envenoming, even if systemic abnormalities are currently absent. Evidence supports this approach because the progression of neurotoxicity can be extremely difficult to halt once it begins, even with antivenom administration.[117]

The patient should receive cardiac and pulse oximetry monitoring, and an IV line should be established. A history and careful physical examination should be performed; local findings are minimal, and fang marks can be difficult to see. The victim typically has little or no swelling and variable local pain. The victim should be carefully assessed for any neurologic abnormalities. Evidence of respiratory dysfunction or difficulty with secretions demands aggressive airway management. Early endotracheal intubation should be considered in such cases to prevent aspiration and its complications.

Laboratory studies have little benefit except for ABGs if respiratory insufficiency is suspected. Bedside pulmonary function testing may be of some benefit in monitoring the patient's status.

If a coral snake inflicted an effective bite, preparation for antivenom administration should begin, even in the absence of systemic signs or symptoms.[73] Several antivenoms are produced for coral snakes of the Western Hemisphere. The antivenom currently available in the United States is manufactured by Wyeth-Ayerst (Antivenin [*Micrurus fulvius*]) using eastern coral snake (*M. fulvius*) venom. It is effective against bites by the eastern (*M. f. fulvius*) and Texas (*M. f. tenere*) coral snakes. It has no proven benefit against Sonoran coral snake (*Micruroides euryxanthus*) venom. No antivenom is currently produced for this species, but it is a small, inoffensive creature, and no deaths have been reported after its bite. Treatment of patients bitten by the Sonoran coral snake is entirely supportive. There is little information regarding efficacy of Antivenin (*Micrurus fulvius*) for other *Micrurus* species of North America. If a significant bite has occurred by a Mexican *Micrurus*, its use is probably warranted.

Preparation for antivenom administration is similar to that for pit vipers. Informed consent is obtained if possible. Skin testing for potential allergy to horse serums is inaccurate and of little benefit in making therapeutic decisions. The victim's intravascular volume should be expanded with prudent crystalloid infusion and the patient premedicated with intravenous antihistamines (both H_1 and H_2 blockers). The starting dose for the antivenom is three to six vials, diluted in 500 to 1000 ml of crystalloid (in 20 ml/kg for pediatric patients).[149] IV infusion is begun at a slow rate, with the physician and epinephrine at the bedside, to ensure no adverse response occurs (anaphylactic or anaphylactoid reaction). The rate is then increased to administer the entire dose over approximately 2 hours.

If a reaction occurs, the antivenom infusion should be temporarily halted and the patient treated as necessary (e.g., epinephrine, further antihistamines, steroids). Once the reaction is treated, the antivenom

can usually be restarted at a slower rate after further dilution of the dose. If a severe reaction occurs, a difficult decision must be made: whether to continue antivenom administration efforts, as outlined for pit viper antivenom reactions, or to treat the patient conservatively (endotracheal intubation as needed and respiratory support). Respiratory paralysis after severe bites can be prolonged and may require days to weeks of mechanical ventilation.[73]

All victims of potential coral snake bite should be admitted to an ICU for close monitoring even if a dry bite is suspected. If signs of neurotoxicity progress after initial antivenom infusion, three to five more vials should be administered; rarely are more than 10 vials required.[104]

Snakebites in Pregnancy

As with all disease states that can occur in pregnant women, the management approach that optimizes fetal outcome is the one that best supports the mother. Fortunately, snake bites are rare in pregnant women in North America. The potential effects of snake venom on the fetus have not been well studied, although fetal malformation has been described.[92] Preterm labor and abruptio placentae have also been reported after pit viper envenomation.[103,150] The anticoagulant and proteolytic actions in most crotaline venoms probably are responsible for disrupting integrity of the placental attachment to the uterus. To inhibit these systemic venom effects, antivenom administration is important, even though antivenom carries an FDA "Category C" designation for safety in pregnancy (i.e., "uncertain safety—animal studies show an adverse effect, no human studies"). Informed consent may be even more important to obtain, if possible, in this situation. Standard doses of antivenom should be used, although the severity rating should be liberally upgraded in pregnant patients.

If an acute allergic reaction develops during antivenom administration, antivenom should be temporarily stopped. Epinephrine should be avoided because of its adverse effects on uterine blood flow. Instead, ephedrine should be given at a dose of 25 to 50 mg by slow IV push.[105] This dose can be repeated every 30 minutes as needed. Other drugs (e.g., antihistamines, steroids) should be given as for the nonpregnant patient. Antivenom administration can usually be restarted in a more dilute concentration and at a slower rate. Additional consultation is advisable.

Other management principles for snake-bitten pregnant women include early obstetric consultation, fetal monitoring, and early ultrasonography for fetal/placental assessment.

Morbidity and Mortality

Pit Vipers. Reliable estimates of morbidity and mortality from snakebite in the United States are not avail-

TABLE 38-5. Snake-Related Deaths Reported to American Association of Poison Control Centers, 1983-1998

YEAR	DEATHS	TOTAL BITES REPORTED*	SPECIFICS
1983	1	717	*Rattlesnake*
1984	1	1347	*Rattlesnake*
1985	0	1676	
1986	0	2416	
1987	1	2701	*Rattlesnake*
1988	0	3076	
1989	1	3851	*Prairie rattlesnake:* 27 year-old male was bitten on two fingertips by 2-foot-long prairie rattlesnake *(Crotalus viridis viridis).* He arrived in ED 15 minutes later. Swelling rapidly progressed to upper arm over next 2½ hours. He skin-tested positive to antivenom but was pretreated with diphenhydramine, epinephrine, and methylprednisolone; 5 vials of antivenom in 250 ml D5W started. After 20 minutes, with 60% of antivenom given, he developed anaphylaxis. He was given IV epinephrine, and cricothyroidotomy was performed because he could not be intubated secondary to laryngospasm. He arrested. Autopsy revealed bronchospasm but no swelling of the upper airway.
1990	0	4461	
1991	1	5255	*Unidentified rattlesnake:* 52-year-old male was bitten on thumb by an unidentified rattlesnake in central Oregon at high altitude. In ED 20 minutes later, he complained of circumoral numbness, tingling, and flushing. Vitals were BP 140/94, pulse 92, and respiration 16. Thumb had "two entrance wounds and minimal swelling." No skin test was performed. He was given 6 ml of a solution of 5 vials of antivenom in 500 ml D5W when he became diaphoretic and dyspneic with increased pulmonary secretions. He became near syncopal. Antivenom was discontinued, and he was intubated and given epinephrine and steroids. He became hypotensive and developed asystole within 15 minutes. Studies showed acidosis, hemoconcentration, and mild coagulopathy. Autopsy revealed extensive coronary artery disease.
1992	2	1055	*Northern Pacific rattlesnake:* 20-year-old male was handling snake when it bit him on the lips. He collapsed, began vomiting, and then was driven 3 miles to hospital. Forty minutes later he was intubated, but arrested during procedure. He was resuscitated with epinephrine, atropine, and 5 vials of antivenom for 30 minutes before recovering a sinus rhythm and BP of 100/60. He developed profound coagulopathy and was given 30 vials of antivenom. He was later determined to be brain dead. Autopsy showed brain edema and herniation. Blood alcohol level was 207 mg/dl. *Black Indian cobra:* 25-year-old male snake expert was bitten on the toe by gravid pet black Indian cobra. He died within minutes. Autopsy revealed bloody pulmonary exudate, cerebral edema, and fine petechial rash.
1993	0	5653	
1994	2	6317	*"Presumptive . . . Mohave [sic] Green rattlesnake":* 40-year-old male was bitten while working in bushes. He collapsed 20 minutes later. In ED 4½ hours later, he was comatose and in atrial fibrillation with labile blood pressure. He was intubated for poor respiratory effort. Fasciculations and metabolic acidosis were noted. Two small puncture wounds 1 cm apart were then noted on the forearm and lower leg. The presumptive diagnosis of *Crotalus scutulatus scutulatus* bite was made and antivenom administered. He was cardioverted to normal sinus rhythm and dopamine was started, but he remained hypotensive. He developed disseminated intravascular coagulation and died on hospital day 8. *Rattlesnake:* 34-year-old male "snake handler" was bitten on the hand when he picked up a rattlesnake on the road. He collapsed 10 minutes after being bitten, and his family began CPR. Medics arrived 30 minutes later, and he was in full arrest. He was intubated, given IV fluids, dopamine, antivenom, and hydrocortisone. He died within 3 hours. Autopsy revealed hemorrhage in the myocardium, alveoli, pancreas, and kidney. Although the airway was patent, he had laryngeal edema, pulmonary edema, and evidence of aspiration. His right coronary artery was 75% stenotic. Blood alcohol level was 118 mg/dl.

TABLE 38-5. Snake-Related Deaths Reported to American Association of Poison Control Centers, 1983-1998—cont'd

YEAR	DEATHS	TOTAL BITES REPORTED*	SPECIFICS
1995	2	7100	*Canebrake rattlesnake:* 35-year-old male was bitten near radial artery while playing with *Crotalus horridus.* He was asystolic when medics arrived 30 minutes later. At autopsy, no necrosis was noted. Blood alcohol level was 250 mg/dl. *Reptile other/unknown*
1996	0	7494	
1997	2	7045	*Rattlesnake:* 4-year-old male bitten on the thigh was treated with 5 vials of antivenom and transferred. He was intubated en route, subsequently developing massive swelling. He arrested, was resuscitated, and given additional antivenom, then arrested again in PICU 7 hours after envenomation. *Poisonous exotic snake*
1998	0	7194	
TOTAL	13	67,358	2 deaths appeared to be caused by anaphylaxis to antivenom. All were male. Ages: 4, 20, 25, 27, 35, 40, 52. 10 rattlesnakes, 2 exotics, 1 unknown. 2 autopsies revealed coronary artery disease. 3 victims were intoxicated with alcohol. Bites: 1 facial, 4 upper extremity, 2 lower extremity, 1 both. Time to death varied from minutes to 8 days.

ED, Emergency department; *D5W,* 5% dextrose in water; *BP,* blood pressure; *CPR,* cardiopulmonary resuscitation; *PICU,* pediatric intensive care unit.
*Includes all bites by reptiles (including exotics, nonpoisonous, and unknowns).

able, but mortality is extremely rare. Extensive work by Parrish in the late 1950s revealed an estimated 7000 venomous snakebites per year with approximately 15 deaths.[106] No one to date has repeated Parrish's systematic evaluation of the problem. The best current information comes from the AAPCC. In 1997, about 7000 reptile bites were reported to regional centers in the AAPCC.[89] Only 10 deaths from endemic venomous snakes were reported to the AAPCC between 1983 and 1998 (Table 38-5).[76-90,140]

When the offending reptile was identified, almost all were rattlesnakes. These numbers are underestimates and can be used only as a rough gauge of incidence and mortality. Not all venomous snakebites, even fatal ones, are reported to the AAPCC. The 1998 statistics, for example, reveal that no fatal snakebite cases were reported to the AAPCC Toxic Exposure Surveillance System.[90] Snakebite is not classified as a reportable disease, and no reliable government statistics exist.

Mortality from snakebite depends on treatment. Before the introduction of Wyeth's Antivenin (Crotalidae) Polyvalent in 1954, mortality rates were estimated as high as 5% to 25%.[108] After this time, mortality rates in patients treated without antivenom declined to approximately 2.6%, largely because of improvements in other aspects of care (e.g., ICU, fluid resuscitation). Antivenom, however, further reduces the mortality rate to 0.28%, a statistically and clinically significant tenfold reduction.[108] This difference should be even more sig-

nificant when newer, safer, and more effective antivenoms become available.

Other than death, permanent systemic morbidity after pit viper envenomation is rare.[29] Local sequelae are more common. The reported incidence of permanent local morbidity is less than 10%, although this does not include complications that may follow surgical interventions.[46] Most patients recover fully after rattlesnake envenomation in the United States, but the incidence of local complications is probably underestimated. Unless careful follow-up is done, including range of motion and sensory testing, permanent disabilities that impact lifestyle and occupation can be missed.[128]

Although not clearly substantiated, children are probably more susceptible to systemic morbidity and mortality from snakebites.[1,26,142] Better pediatric supportive care and improved understanding of how antivenom should be administered have blurred any distinction between pediatric and adult prognosis.[29] Elderly patients appear to have a higher case-fatality rate, probably related to comorbid conditions.[29]

Morbidity and mortality from snakebites also result from efforts to treat the victim. Significant wound complications can follow ill-advised incisions in and around the bite site and application of mouth suction.[40,149] Serious burns and systemic complications, such as myocardial infarction, can follow application of electric shocks to the wound.[28,119] Tourniquets or ice may increase the risk of tissue damage. Equine antivenoms can precipitate early anaphylactic or anaphylactoid reactions and delayed serum sickness (see earlier discussion).

Coral Snakes. Although no deaths have been reported from coral snake bites in the United States since Antivenin *(Micrurus fulvius)* was introduced,[118] the mortality rate if bites were untreated is estimated at approximately 10%.[109] Prolonged muscle weakness is common after severe envenoming, and victims with respiratory compromise may require mechanical ventilation for many days. There are no reports of permanent sequelae in patients who survive coral snake envenomation.

VENOMOUS LIZARDS

Anatomy

The two venomous lizards of the world are impressive creatures about which much misinformation has been spread for centuries. They have been thought to possess supernatural features such as poisonous breath, a stinging tail and the ability to spit their venom.[118] The Gila monster *(Heloderma suspectum)* reaches a maximum length of approximately 50 cm, whereas the beaded lizard *(Heloderma horridum)* is larger, reaching almost a meter. They are both heavily built and possess massive muscles of mastication with powerful biting capacity. The venom delivery apparatus consists of a pair of anterior, multilobed, interior labial glands that open through a series of ducts into the labial mucosa. Their teeth are lancet shaped, grooved, and loosely attached to the jaws. When the reptile becomes agitated, it salivates heavily, producing a flow of venom into the labial mucosa. It bites with a powerful, chewing motion, instilling venom into the wounds by capillary action along the grooves of the teeth. Teeth may be left in the wounds, especially if the lizard must be forcefully removed from the victim (Figure 38-28). The tenacious creature may still be attached when help arrives. Effective envenomation occurs in only about 70% of bites.[5]

Venom

Gila monster and beaded lizard venoms are similar in composition and are as potent as some rattlesnake venoms.[131] They possess enzymatic components, including hyaluronidase (spreading factor), protease, phospholipase A_2, and kallikrein-like substances, and nonenzymatic substances such as serotonin. Venom kallikreins stimulate the release of vasoactive kinins, such as bradykinin, which are largely responsible for occasional hypotension seen after helodermatid bites.[133]

Clinical Presentation

The vast majority of victims bitten by a lizard are attempting to catch or handle the reptile; accidental bites

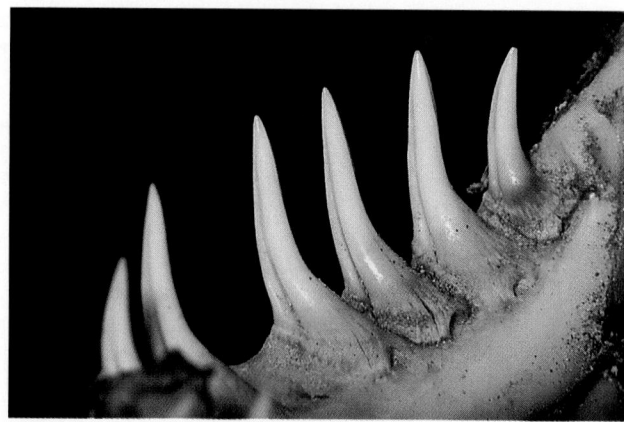

Figure 38-28 Teeth of the helodermatid lizards are grooved to aid instillation of venom during a bite. These teeth are loosely adherent and may become dislodged in the bite wound. *(Courtesy Michael Cardwell/Extreme Wildlife Photography.)*

are rare. Most bites involve captive animals, and many are not reported.

Significant bleeding often occurs from punctured and torn tissues. Throbbing or burning pain may radiate proximally along the bitten extremity. Local edema may be progressive. Victims may complain of generalized weakness, nausea and vomiting, difficulty breathing, profuse sweating, dizziness, and paresthesias.[64,118,133]

On examination the victim may be tachycardic, hypotensive (related to kinin release), and diaphoretic.[64] The wounds generally reveal significant local tissue trauma with variable bleeding. The site may be cyanotic or ecchymotic with local vasospasm.[118] Regional lymphadenopathy may be present on arrival to medical care or appear later.[5]

Management

Prehospital Care. Data are minimal regarding prehospital care of venomous lizard bites. In some cases the first priority is to detach the lizard from the victim. The lizard can be placed under running hot water, or the jaws can be pried apart using a stick or metal instrument.[133] Care must be taken not to injure the victim further and to avoid a second bite, perhaps to the rescuer.

Once freed from the lizard, the victim should be placed at rest and the bite site rinsed and cleaned as much as possible. Any bleeding should be stopped with direct pressure. No evidence supports the use of suction devices, ligatures, or pressure immobilization. Some advocate local ice to reduce pain,[131] but signs of vasoconstriction must be monitored to prevent later tissue loss.[118] A dressing to stop bleeding and a splint to limit movement may be beneficial. Transport to a medical facility should be carried out as expeditiously as possible. Incisions and electrotherapy should be strictly avoided.

Hospital Care. Assuming the lizard has been detached before arrival at the hospital, the victim's airway, breathing and circulation are assessed. Vital signs should be obtained while the patient is being placed on oxygen and cardiac/pulse oximetry monitoring. At least one large-bore IV line should be established with either normal saline or Ringer's lactate. If the victim is hypotensive or tachycardic, a second line should be placed. The victim with hypotension should receive an infusion of physiologic saline (1 to 2 L for an adult, 20 to 40 ml/kg for a child). Hypotension rarely persists after volume resuscitation. If necessary, vasopressors can be added after the victim's intravascular volume has been repleted.[133]

Laboratory studies include complete blood count, serum electrolytes, renal function studies, and coagulation studies. Total WBC may be elevated, and in severe cases, platelets may be decreased.[118] Although lizard venoms do not appear to possess anticoagulant fractions, coagulopathy of unclear mechanism has been reported after severe bites.[5] Hemostatic abnormalities in these victims may not result from the venom but rather from endothelial damage.[133] Urinalysis is useful to assess for microscopic hematuria or renal casts.

These bites can cause transient electrocardiogram (ECG) abnormalities, such as T-wave anomalies and conduction delays.[5,64] Myocardial infarction has been reported after Gila monster bites.[5] An ECG is recommended if the victim shows any sign or symptom of venom poisoning.

Once the victim's overall status is stabilized, attention focuses on wound care. A soft tissue radiograph of the bite site may identify retained lizard teeth but does not replace careful exploration of the wounds.[64] After an assessment of functional status, the wound can be anesthetized using a local or regional block. The bite site should then be carefully explored for damage to underlying vital structures and for retained teeth. Thorough cleansing and irrigation should follow exploration. The wounds are dressed and splinted with generous padding. The extremity is then elevated to reduce swelling and discomfort. Opiates may be necessary in the management of pain during the victim's initial evaluation and for any pain not controlled by local or regional anesthesia. The victim's tetanus immunization status should be updated. Prophylactic antibiotics are not required.[133] Daily wound care should include cleansing with soap and water, followed by hydrogen peroxide, application of a topical antiseptic, and redressing. After the first 24 hours a course of physical therapy can be helpful in more rapidly returning the patient to full function.

If the bite appears to be dry (i.e., victim relatively asymptomatic, vital signs/studies/ECG normal), the victim can be discharged home after approximately 6 hours of observation in the emergency department. This assumes the victim has proper resources for care at home and can return if status deteriorates. Proper wound care instructions should be given and the patient scheduled for reevaluation in approximately 24 to 48 hours. An oral opiate analgesic may be prescribed. Evidence of envenoming (i.e., signs or symptoms besides simple wounds; test or ECG abnormalities) or pain that is difficult to control requires admission. Systemic findings (e.g., chest pain, ECG changes, hypotension, coagulopathy) require monitoring for at least 24 hours.[133]

Morbidity and Mortality

No fatalities from helodermatid bites have been documented in the last 50 years,[95] but a bite might be fatal if a large helodermatid hangs on to the victim for minutes. Such a bite to a child or ill adult is especially dangerous.

Although pain may be prolonged for several hours or even days after these bites, necrosis is rare.[95,118] Wound infections are uncommon. If infection occurs, cultures should be obtained and the victim started on broad-spectrum antibiotic coverage for both gram-positive cocci and gram-negative rods. Culture and sensitivity results should guide further treatment.

ALLERGY TO REPTILE VENOMS

Snake and lizard venoms are highly immunogenic substances, and occasionally, a bitten victim presents with an acute, anaphylactic reaction.[47,110] The risk of such reactions increases in victims previously bitten by venomous reptiles or who work with snake or lizard venoms (e.g., in a venom production or research facility). The presentation can be typical for anaphylaxis, with bronchospasm, hypotension, and urticaria, but differentiating an acute allergic reaction to venom from direct venom toxicity can be difficult. If the precise etiology for hypotension or respiratory distress is unclear, treatment can be rendered for anaphylaxis while antivenom preparation (in the case of snakebite) and supportive care proceed.

BITES BY EXOTIC SNAKES IN THE UNITED STATES

With the growing popularity of herpetoculture in the United States, bites by captive venomous reptiles have increased. Many involve species indigenous to North America, but an increasing number are caused by exotic species. Russell[120] estimated that exotic venomous snakes were responsible for 30 bites in 1984. In 1998, however, 100 such cases were reported to the AAPCC Toxic Exposure Surveillance System.[90] An emergency physician anywhere in North America may see a victim who has been bitten by a king cobra, black mamba, or other exotic species. Management principles in these cases are similar to those outlined earlier (see also Chapter 39).

REFERENCES

1. Banner W: Bites and stings in the pediatric patient, *Curr Probl Pediatr* 1:8, 1988.
2. Blackman J: Viewpoints: response, *J Wilderness Med* 5:216, 1994.
3. Bober MA, Ownby C: Use of affinity-purified antibodies to measure the in vivo disappearance of antibodies to myotoxin a, *Toxicon* 26:301, 1988.
4. Bond GR, Burkhart KK: Thrombocytopenia following timber rattlesnake envenomation, *Ann Emerg Med* 30:40, 1997.
5. Bou-Abboud CF, Kardassakis DG: Acute myocardial infarction following a Gila monster (*Heloderma suspectum cinctum*) bite, *West J Med* 148:577, 1988.
6. Brick JR et al: Timber rattlesnake-induced myokymia: evidence for peripheral nerve origin, *Neurology* 37:1545, 1978.
7. Bronstein AC, Russell FE, Sullivan JB: Negative pressure suction in the field treatment of rattlesnake bite victims, *Vet Hum Toxicol* 28:485, 1986 (abstract).
8. Bronstein AC et al: Negative pressure suction in the field treatment of rattlesnake bite, *Vet Hum Toxicol* 28:297, 1985 (abstract).
9. Burgess JL, Dart RC: Snake venom coagulopathy: use and abuse of blood products in the treatment of pit viper envenomation, *Ann Emerg Med* 10:795, 1991.
10. Burgess JL et al: Effects of constriction bands on rattlesnake venom absorption: a pharmacokinetic study, *Ann Emerg Med* 21:1086, 1992.
11. Bush SP et al: Effects of a negative pressure venom extraction device (Extractor) on local tissue injury after artificial rattlesnake envenomation in a porcine model, *Wilderness Environ Med* 11:180, 2000.
12. Bush SP, Cardwell MD: Mojave rattlesnake (*Crotalus scutulatus scutulatus*) identification, *Wilderness Environ Med* 10:6, 1999.
13. Bush SP, Jansen PW: Severe rattlesnake envenomation with anaphylaxis and rhabdomyolysis, *Ann Emerg Med* 25:845, 1995.
14. Bush SP, Thomas TL, Chin ES: Envenomations in children, *Pediatr Emerg Med Rep* 2:1, 1997.
15. Bush SP, Wu VH, Corbett SW: Rattlesnake venom-induced thrombocytopenia response to Antivenin (Crotalidae) Polyvalent, *Acad Emerg Med* 6:393, 1999 (abstract).
16. Campbell JA, Lamar WW: *The venomous reptiles of Latin America,* Ithaca, NY, 1989, Comstock.
17. Carroll RR, Hall EL, Kitchens CS: Canebrake rattlesnake envenomation, *Ann Emerg Med* 30:45, 1997.
18. Chang CC: The action of snake venoms on nerve and muscle. In Lee CY, editor: *Snake venoms,* New York, 1979, Springer-Verlag.
19. Chiszar D et al: Searching behaviors by rattlesnakes following predatory strikes. In Campbell JA, Brodie ED, editors: *Biology of the pitvipers,* Tyler, Tex, 1992, Selva.
20. Christopher DG, Rodning CB: Crotalidae envenomation, *South Med J* 79:159, 1986.
21. Christy NP: Poisoning by venomous animals, *Am J Med* 42:107, 1967.
22. Chugh KS, Sakhuja V: Renal disease caused by snake venom. In Tu AT, editor: *Handbook of natural toxins: reptile venoms and toxins,* New York, 1991, Marcel Dekker.
23. Clark RF, Selden BS, Furbee B: The incidence of wound infection following crotalid envenomation, *J Emerg Med* 11:583, 1993.
24. Clark RF et al: Successful treatment of crotalid-induced neurotoxicity with a new polyspecific crotalid Fab antivenom, *Ann Emerg Med* 30:54, 1997.
25. Consroe P et al: Comparison of a new ovine antigen binding fragment (Fab) antivenin for United States crotalidae with the commercial antivenin for protection against venom-induced lethality in mice, *Am J Trop Med Hyg* 53:507, 1995.
26. Cruz NS, Alvarez RG: Rattlesnake bite complications in 19 children, *Pediatr Emerg Care* 10:30, 1994.
27. Cupo P, Azevedo-Marques MM, Hering SE: Clinical and laboratory features of South American rattlesnake (*Crotalus durissus terrificus*) envenomation in children, *Trans R Soc Trop Hyg* 82:924, 1988.
28. Dart RC, Gustafson RA: Failure of electric shock treatment for rattlesnake envenomation, *Ann Emerg Med* 20:659, 1991.
29. Dart RC et al: The sequelae of pit viper poisoning in the United States. In Campbell JA, Brodie ED, editors: *Biology of the pitvipers,* Tyler, Tex, 1992, Selva.
30. Dart RC et al: Validation of a severity score for the assessment of crotalid snakebite, *Ann Emerg Med* 27:321, 1996.
31. Dart RC et al: Affinity-purified, mixed monospecific crotalid antivenom ovine Fab for the treatment of crotalid venom poisoning, *Ann Emerg Med* 30:33, 1997.
32. Davidson TM, Eisner J: United States coral snakes, *Wilderness Environ Med* 1:38, 1996.

33. Fiero MK et al: Comparative study of juvenile and adult prairie rattlesnake (*Crotalus viridis viridis*) venoms, *Toxicon* 10: 81, 1972.
34. Fix JD: Venom yield of the North American coral snake and its clinical significance, *South Med J* 73:737, 1980.
35. Forgey WW: More on snake-venom and insect-venom extractors, *N Engl J Med* 328:516, 1993 (letter).
36. Garfin SR: Rattlesnake bites: current hospital therapy, *West J Med* 137:411, 1982.
37. Garfin SR et al: Rattlesnake bites and surgical decompression: results using a laboratory model, *Toxicon* 22:177, 1984.
38. Gellert GA: Snake-venom and insect-venom extractors: an unproved therapy, *N Engl J Med* 327:1322, 1992 (letter).
39. Gillissen A et al: Neurotoxicity, haemostatic disturbances and haemolytic anemia after a bite by a Tunisian saw-scaled or carpet viper (*Echis 'pyramidum'-complex*): failure of antivenom treatment, *Toxicon* 32:937, 1994.
40. Glass TG: Early debridement in pit viper bites, *JAMA* 235:2513, 1976.
41. Glenn JL, Straight RC: The rattlesnakes and their venom yield and lethal toxicity. In Tu AT, editor: *Rattlesnake venoms: their actions and treatment,* New York, 1982, Marcel Dekker.
42. Glenn JL, Straight RC: Venom characteristics as an indicator of hybridization between *Crotalus viridis viridis* and *Crotalus scutalatus scutulatus* in New Mexico, *Toxicon* 28:857, 1990.
43. Glenn JL, Straight RC, Wolt TB: Regional variation in the presence of canebrake toxin in *Crotalus horridus* venom, *Comp Biochem Physiol* 107C:337, 1994.
44. Glenn JL et al: Geographical variation in *Crotalus scutulatus scutulatus* (Mojave rattlesnake) venom properties, *Toxicon* 21:119, 1983.
45. Gold BS: Snake venom extractors: a valuable first aid tool, *Vet Hum Toxicol* 35:255, 1993 (letter).
46. Gomez HF, Dart RC: Clinical toxicology of snakebite in North America. In Meier J, White J, editors: *Handbook of clinical toxicology of animal venoms and poisons,* Boca Raton, Fla, 1995, CRC Press.
47. Gonzalez D: Snakebite problems in Europe. In Tu AT, editor: *Reptile venoms and toxins,* vol 5, New York, 1991, Marcel Dekker.
48. Guderian RH: High-voltage shock treatment for snakebite, *Postgrad Med* 82:250, 1987.
49. Guderian RH, MacKenzie CD, Williams JF: High voltage shock treatment for snakebite, *Lancet* 2:229, 1986 (letter).
50. Guisto JA: Severe toxicity from crotalid envenomation after early resolution of symptoms, *Ann Emerg Med* 26:387, 1995.
51. Guitierrez JM et al: Local effects induced by coral snake venoms: evidence of myonecrosis after experimental inoculations of venoms from five species, *Toxicon* 21:777, 1983.
52. Harding KA, Welch KRG: *Venomous snakes of the world.* Oxford, UK, 1980, Pergamon Press.
53. Hardy DL: A review of first aid measures for pit viper bite in North America with an appraisal of Extractor suction and stun gun electroshock. In Campbell JA, Brodie ED, editors: *Biology of the pitvipers,* Tyler, Tex, 1992, Selva.
54. Hardy DL: Envenomation by the Mojave rattlesnake *Crotalus scutalatus scutulatus* in southern Arizona, U.S.A., *Toxicon* 21:111, 1983.
55. Hardy DL: Fatal rattlesnake envenomation in Arizona: 1969-1984, *Clin Toxicol* 24:1, 1986.
56. Hardy DL, Bush SP: Pressure/immobilization as first aid for venomous snakebite in the United States, *Herpetol Rev* 29:204, 1998.
57. Hardy DL, Jeter M, Corrigan JJ: Envenomation by the northern blacktail rattlesnake (*Crotalus molossus molossus*): report of two cases and the in vitro effects of the venom on fibrinolysis and platelet aggregation, *Toxicon* 2:487, 1982.
58. Hayes WK: Ontogeny of striking, prey-handling and envenomation behavior of prairie rattlesnakes, *Crotalus v. viridis,* Toxicon 29:867, 1991.
59. Hayes WK: Venom metering by juvenile prairie rattlesnakes, *Crotalus v. viridis:* effects of prey size and experience, *Anim Behav* 50:33, 1995.
60. Hayes WK, Lavin-Murcio P, Kardong KV: Northern Pacific rattlesnakes (*Crotalus viridis oreganus*) meter venom when feeding on prey of different sizes, *Copeia* 2:337,1995.
61. Hendon RA, Bieber AL: Presynaptic toxins from rattlesnake venoms. In Tu AT, editor: *Rattlesnake venoms: their actions and treatment,* New York, 1982, Marcel Dekker.
62. Herbert SS: Factors influencing venom expenditure during defensive bites by cottonmouths (*Agkistrodon piscivorus*) and rattlesnakes (*Crotalus viridis, C. atrox*), unpublished Master of Science thesis, Loma Linda University, 1998.
63. Herzberg R: Shocks for snakebites, *Outdoor life* June 1987, p 55.

64. Hooker KR, Caravati EM: Gila monster envenomation, *Ann Emerg Med* 24:731, 1994.
65. Horowitz RS, Dart RC: Antivenins and immunobiologicals: immunotherapeutics of envenomation. In Auerbach PS, editor: *Wilderness medicine: management of wilderness and environmental emergencies,* ed 3, St Louis, 1995, Mosby.
66. Houghton PJ: Treatment of snakebites with plants, *J Wilderness Med* 5:451, 1994 (letter).
67. Howe NR, Meisenheimer JL: Electric shock does not save snakebitten rats, *Ann Emerg Med* 17:254, 1988.
68. Hurlbut KM, et al: Reliability of clinical presentation for predicting significant pit viper envenomation, *Ann Emerg Med* 17:438, 1988 (abstract).
69. Jansen PW, Perkin RM, Van Stralen D: Mojave rattlesnake envenomation: prolonged neurotoxicity and rhabdomyolysis, *Ann Emerg Med* 21:322, 1992.
70. Johnson EK, Kardong KV, Mackessy SP: Electric shocks are ineffective in treatment of lethal effects of rattlesnake envenomation in mice, *Toxicon* 25:1347, 1987.
71. Jurkovich GJ et al: Complications of Crotalidae antivenin therapy, *J Trauma* 28:1032, 1988.
72. Karlson-Stiber C et al: First clinical experience with specific sheep Fab fragments in snake bite: report of a multicentre study of *Vipera berus* envenoming, *J Intern Med* 241:53, 1997.
73. Kitchens CS, Van Mierop LHS: Envenomation by the eastern coral snake (*Micrurus fulvius fulvius*): a study of 39 victims, *JAMA* 258:1615, 1987.
74. Klauber LM: *Rattlesnakes: their habits, life histories, and influence on mankind,* ed 2, Berkeley, Calif, 1997, University of California Press.
75. Kunkel DB et al: Reptile envenomations, *J Toxicol Clin Toxicol* 21:503, 1983-1984.
76. Litovitz TL et al: 1984 annual report of the American Association of Poison Control Centers National Data Collection System, *Am J Emerg Med* 3:423, 1985.
77. Litovitz TL et al: 1985 annual report of the American Association of Poison Control Centers National Data Collection System, *Am J Emerg Med* 4:427, 1986.
78. Litovitz TL et al: 1986 annual report of the American Association of Poison Control Centers National Data Collection System, *Am J Emerg Med* 5:405, 1987.
79. Litovitz TL et al: 1987 annual report of the American Association of Poison Control Centers National Data Collection System, *Am J Emerg Med* 6:479, 1988.
80. Litovitz TL et al: 1988 annual report of the American Association of Poison Control Centers National Data Collection System, *Am J Emerg Med* 7:495, 1989.
81. Litovitz et al: 1989 annual report of the American Association of Poison Control Centers National Data Collection System, *Am J Emerg Med* 8:394, 1990.
82. Litovitz TL et al: 1990 annual report of the American Association of Poison Control Centers National Data Collection System, *Am J Emerg Med* 9:461, 1991.
83. Litovitz TL et al: 1991 annual report of the American Association of Poison Control Centers National Data Collection System, *Am J Emerg Med* 10:452, 1992.
84. Litovitz TL et al: 1992 annual report of the American Association of Poison Control Centers Toxic Exposure Surveillance System, *Am J Emerg Med* 11:494, 1993.
85. Litovitz TL et al: 1993 annual report of the American Association of Poison Control Centers Toxic Exposure Surveillance System, *Am J Emerg Med* 12:546, 1994.
86. Litovitz TL et al: 1994 annual report of the American Association of Poison Control Centers Toxic Exposure Surveillance System, *Am J Emerg Med* 13:551, 1995.
87. Litovitz TL et al: 1995 annual report of the American Association of Poison Control Centers Toxic Exposure Surveillance System, *Am J Emerg Med* 14:487, 1996.
88. Litovitz TL et al: 1996 annual report of the American Association of Poison Control Centers Toxic Exposure Surveillance System, *Am J Emerg Med* 15:447, 1997.
89. Litovitz TL et al: 1997 annual report of the American Association of Poison Control Centers Toxic Exposure Surveillance System, *Am J Emerg Med* 16:475, 1998.
90. Litovitz TL et al: 1998 annual report of the American Association of Poison Control Centers Toxic Exposure Surveillance System, *Am J Emerg Med* 17:435, 1999.
91. Loprinzi CL et al: Snake antivenin administration in a patient allergic to horse serum, *South Med J* 76:501, 1983.
92. Malz S: Snakebite in pregnancy, *J Obstet Gynaecol Br Commonw* 74:935, 1967.
93. McCollough NC, Gennaro JF: Evaluation of venomous snake bite in the southern United States from parallel clinical and laboratory investigations: development of treatment, *J Fla Med Assoc* 49:959, 1963.
94. McCollough NC, Gennaro JF: Treatment of venomous snakebite in the United States, *Clin Toxicol* 3:483, 1970.
95. Mebs D: Clinical toxicology of Helodermatidae lizard bites. In Meier J, White J, editors: *Handbook of clinical toxicology of animal venoms and poisons,* Boca Raton, Fla, 1995, CRC Press.
96. Meier J, Stocker KF: Biology and distribution of venomous snakes of medical importance and the composition of snake venoms. In Meier J, White J, editors: *Handbook of clinical toxicology of animal venoms and poisons,* Boca Raton, Fla, 1995, CRC Press.
97. Minton SA: Variation in venom samples from copperheads (*Agkistrodon contortrix mokeson*) and timber rattlesnakes (*Crotalus horridus horridus*), *Copeia* 4:212, 1953.
98. Minton SA: Identification of poisonous snakes. In Minton SA, editor: *Snake venoms and envenomation,* New York, 1971, Marcel Dekker.
99. Morandi N, Williams J: Snakebite injuries: contributing factors and intentionality of exposure, *Wilderness Environ Med* 8:152, 1997.
100. Norris RL: Fang marks and the diagnosis of venomous snakebite, *Wilderness Environ Med* 6:159, 1995.
101. Norris RL: Envenomations. In Irwin RS, Cerra FB, Rippe JM, editors: *Intensive care medicine,* Philadelphia, 1999, Lippincott-Raven.
102. Norris RL, Dart RC: Apparent coral snake envenomation in a patient without fang marks, *Am J Emerg Med* 7:402, 1989.
103. Osman OH, Gumaa KA: Pharmacological studies of snake (*Bitis arietans*) venom, *Toxicon* 12:569, 1974.
104. Otten EJ: Antivenin therapy in the emergency department, *Am J Emerg Med* 1:83, 1983.
104a. Package insert. CroFab, London, 2000, Protherics, Inc; http://www.protherics.com/CroFab_Package_Insert.pdf.
105. Pantanowitz L, Guidozzi F: Management of snake and spider bite in pregnancy, *Obstet Gynecol Surg* 51:615, 1996.
106. Parrish HM: Incidence of treated snakebites in the United States, *Public Health Rep* 81:269, 1966.
107. Parrish HM: *Poisonous snakebites in the United States,* New York, 1980, Vantage Press.
108. Parrish HM, Goldner JC, Silberg SL: Poisonous snakebites causing no venenation, *Postgrad Med* 39:265, 1966.
109. Parrish HM, Khan MS: Bites by coral snakes: report of 11 representative cases, *Am J Med Sci* 253:561, 1967.
110. Piacentine J, Curry SC, Ryan PJ: Life-threatening anaphylaxis following Gila monster bite, *Ann Emerg Med* 15:959, 1986.
111. Premawardhena AP et al: Low dose subcutaneous adrenaline to prevent acute adverse reactions to antivenom serum in people bitten by snakes: randomised, placebo controlled trial, *Br Med J* 318:1041, 1999.
112. Rao RB, Palmer MB, Touger M: Thrombocytopenia after rattlesnake envenomation, *Ann Emerg Med* 31:139, 1998 (letter).
113. Reid HA: Bites by foreign venomous snakes in Britain, *BMJ* 1:1598, 1978.
114. Riffer E, Curry SC, Gerkin R: Successful treatment with antivenin of marked thrombocytopenia without significant coagulopathy following rattlesnake bite, *Ann Emerg Med* 16:1297, 1987.
115. Roze JA: *Coral snakes of the Americas: biology, identification, and venoms,* Melbourne, Fla, 1996, Krieger.
116. Russell FE: Clinical aspects of snake venom poisoning in North America, *Toxicon* 7:33, 1969.
117. Russell FE: Snake venom poisoning in the United States, *Ann Rev Med* 31:247, 1980.
118. Russell FE: *Snake venom poisoning,* New York, 1983, Scholium International.
119. Russell FE: A letter on electroshock for snakebite, *Vet Hum Toxicol* 29:320, 1987 (letter).
120. Russell FE: AIDS, cancer, and snakebite—what do these three have in common? *West J Med* 148:84, 1988.
121. Russell FE, Banner W: Snake venom poisoning. In Rakel RE, editor: *Conn's current therapy,* Philadelphia, 1988, WB Saunders.
122. Russell FE, Lauritzen L: Antivenins, *Trans R Soc Trop Med Hyg* 60:797, 1966.
123. Russell FE et al: Snake venom poisoning in the United States: experiences with 550 cases, *JAMA* 233:341, 1975.
124. Russell FE et al: Snakes and snakebite in Central America, *Toxicon* 35:1469, 1997.

125. Ryan AJ: Don't use electric shock for snakebite, *Postgrad Med* 82:42, 1987 (letter).

126. Schaeffer RC et al: The effects of colloidal and crystalloidal fluids on rattlesnake venom shock in the rat, *J Pharmacol Exp Ther* 206:687, 1978.

127. Seifert SA et al: Relationship of venom effects to venom antigen and antivenom serum concentrations in a patient with *Crotalus atrox* envenomation treated with a Fab antivenom, *Ann Emerg Med* 30:49, 1997.

128. Simon TL, Grace TG: Envenomation coagulopathy in wounds from pit vipers, *N Engl J Med* 305:443, 1981.

129. Smith DC et al: An affinity purified ovine antivenom for the treatment of *Vipera berus* envenoming, *Toxicon* 30:865, 1992.

130. Spaite D, Dart R, Sullivan JB: Skin testing in cases of possible crotalid envenomation, *Ann Emerg Med* 17:105, 1988 (letter).

131. Stahnke HL, Heffron WA, Lewis DL: Bite of the Gila monster, *Rocky Mtn Med J* 67:25, 1970.

132. Stoud C et al: Effect of electric shock therapy on local tissue reaction to poisonous snake venom injection in rabbits, *Ann Emerg Med* 18:447, 1989 (abstract).

133. Strimple PD et al: Report on envenomation by a Gila monster (*Heloderma suspectum*) with a discussion of venom apparatus, clinical findings and treatment, *Wilderness Environ Med* 8:111, 1997.

134. Suchard JR, LoVecchio F: Envenomations by rattlesnakes thought to be dead, *N Engl J Med* 340:1929, 1999 (letter).

135. Sutherland SK, Coulter AR: Early management of bites by the eastern diamondback rattlesnake (*Crotalus adamanteus*): studies in monkeys (*Macaca fascicularis*), *Am J Trop Med Hyg* 30:497, 1981.

136. Sutherland SK, Coulter AR, Harris RD: Rationalisation of first-aid measures for elapid snakebite, *Lancet* 1:183, 1979.

137. Talan DA: Antibacterial activity of crotalid venoms against oral snake flora and other clinical bacteria, *J Infect Dis* 164:195, 1991.

138. Tallon RW et al: Correspondence, *N Engl J Med* 305:1347, 1981.

139. Van Mierop LHS: Poisonous snakebite: a review—snakes and their venom, *J Fla Med Assoc* 63:191, 1976.

140. Veltri JC, Litovitz TL: 1983 annual report of the American Association of Poison Control Centers National Data Collection System, *Am J Emerg Med* 2:420, 1984.

141. Watt CH: Treatment of poisonous snakebite with emphasis on digit dermotomy, *South Med J* 78:694, 1985.

142. Weber RA, White RR: Crotalidae envenomation in children, *Ann Plast Surg* 31:141, 1993.

143. Weed HG: Nonvenomous snakebite in Massachusetts: prophylactic antibiotics are unnecessary, *Ann Emerg Med* 22:220, 1993.

144. Weinstein SA, Minton SA, Wilde CE: The distribution among ophidian venoms of a toxin isolated from the venom of the Mojave rattlesnake (*Crotalus scutalatus scutulatus*), *Toxicon* 23:825, 1985.

145. White J: Snakebite: an Australian perspective, *J Wilderness Med* 2:219, 1991.

146. Whitley RE: Conservative treatment of copperhead snakebites without antivenin, *J Trauma* 41:219, 1996.

147. Wilkinson JA et al: Distribution and genetic variations in venom A and B populations of the Mojave rattlesnake (*Crotalus scutulatus scutulatus*) in Arizona, *Herpetologica* 47:54, 1991.

148. Wingert WA, Chan L: Rattlesnake bites in southern California and rationale for recommended treatment, *West J Med* 148:37, 1988.

149. Wingert WA, Wainschel J: Diagnosis and management of envenomation by poisonous snakes, *South Med J* 68:1015, 1975.

150. Zugaib M et al: Abruptio placentae following snakebite, *Am J Obstet Gynecol* 151:754, 1985.

39 Non–North American Venomous Reptile Bites

Robert L. Norris, Jr. and Sherman A. Minton†

Snake envenomation is a significant cause of morbidity and mortality in some parts of the world. The only attempt to survey snakebite as a global problem was undertaken in 1954 under the auspices of the World Health Organization.[72] The estimate was an annual incidence of 300,000 bites with 30,000 to 40,000 deaths. Due to methodologic problems, the estimate of incidence was probably much too low. In more recent estimates, as many as 2.5 million envenomations and 125,000 deaths may occur each year.[10] Although reporting from many parts of the world is inadequate, the highest incidence of snakebite occurs in regions where dense human populations coexist with a dense population of venomous snakes, people are engaged in agriculture by nonmechanized methods, and most people reside in small villages. Geographically, these regions include Southeast Asia, sub-Saharan Africa, and tropical America.

The epidemiologic patterns of snakebite in the United States and Europe have changed since 1950. Before that time the bites largely involved persons engaged in agriculture or living in rural environments, although the number was far fewer than those reported from tropical regions. Over the past 40 to 50 years the number of bites from handling captive snakes in a hazardous fashion has increased. In Minton's series of consultations in the United States from 1977 to 1995, 54 of 160 venomous snakebite cases involved nonnative snakes, and 53 of these were by animals in captivity.[48] In addition, 25 of the 106 bites inflicted by native snakes involved captive animals. The popularity of snake keeping as a hobby is increasing. Although most snakes kept in captivity are not dangerous, some people acquire venomous species. In rare cases, venomous snakes may be incorrectly identified and sold as innocuous species. Many snakes in the "pet" trade are not native to the nations where they are sold. Boa constrictors and ball pythons are harmless exotic snakes popular in the United States, whereas the nonvenomous North American king snakes (*Lampropeltis* spp.) and rat snakes (*Elaphe* spp.) are popular in Europe. Venomous species also appear in the international trade. Cobras, large African vipers of the genus *Bitis*, and green arboreal vipers (*Trimeresurus* spp.) from Southeast Asia are among the species commonly sold in the United States, whereas rattlesnakes are prized by collectors in Europe. An informal survey in southern California indicated that nearly 2000 venomous snakes were kept by herpetologists and snake collectors in that area in the early 1960s.[60] Before 1960, bites by nonnative venomous snakes in the United States made up approximately 4% of total bites, largely confined to workers in research laboratories, zoos, and other public displays. In 1972, however, 15% of 410 hospital-treated snakebites were inflicted by nonnative species.[30] An emergency department physician in an urban hospital in the eastern or midwestern United States is almost as likely to be confronted with a bite of an exotic venomous snake as with that of a species native to North America.

Snakebite is a minor hazard for tourists engaged in sightseeing or recreation unless they deliberately capture or handle local reptiles. The risk for those involved in engineering projects, exploration, military operations, scientific fieldwork, and humanitarian activities in regions where venomous snakes are common is somewhat higher but still small. Hardy[26] reported three bites by the large pit viper *Bothrops asper* during 1.5 million person-hours in the field at four operations in Belize, Costa Rica, and Guatemala.

SNAKES OF MEDICAL IMPORTANCE

Snakes are a distinctive and specialized group of reptiles represented by about 2700 species. However, their classification at the family level and beyond has always presented problems to taxonomists. Recent taxonomic changes involving medically important species include redivision of the pit viper genera *Agkistrodon* (North America and Asia), *Bothrops* (tropical America), and *Trimeresurus* (southern Asia) and recognition that some wide-ranging species, such as the Asian cobra (*Naja naja*) and saw-scaled viper (*Echis carinatus*), are actually groups of several similar species.[18,95] Table 39-1 summarizes the major snake families. All species in the families Viperidae, Elapidae, Hydrophiidae, and Atractaspididae, plus an unknown but significant number in the family Colubridae, are venomous. Box 39-1 lists the most medically important venomous species for certain areas of the world.

---

†Deceased.

TABLE 39-1. Major Snake Families

GROUP	DISTRIBUTION	REMARKS
Blind snakes Families: Typhlopidae and Leptotyphlopidae	Tropical and warm temperate zones	Very small, wormlike snakes; none venomous
Boas and pythons Family: Boidae	Mostly tropical and warm temperate zones; pythons in Old World only	Includes both large and small species; none venomous
"Typical" snakes Family: Colubridae	Almost worldwide except for Arctic, Antarctic, southern Australia, and certain islands	Large and extremely varied family; many species with venom glands and posterior maxillary fangs, but few capable of causing clinically significant envenomation
Burrowing asps Family: Atractaspididae	Africa, limited areas of Middle East	About 15 species, all venomous; rather small burrowers; large maxillary fangs used singly with backward stabbing motion
Cobras, mambas, coral snakes, kraits, and others Family: Elapidae	Tropical and warm temperate zones	About 180 species, all venomous; fangs at anterior end of maxillae
Sea snakes Family: Hydrophiidae	Mostly Southeast Asian and Australian coastal waters	About 50 species, all venomous; fangs similar to those of Elapidae
Pit vipers Family: Viperidae Subfamily: Crotalinae	The Americas and much of Asia	About 120 species, all venomous; highly movable fangs on much reduced maxillae; heat-sensing pits between eyes and nostrils
Old World vipers Family: Viperidae Subfamily: Viperinae	Africa, Europe, and Asia	About 40 species, all venomous; fangs like those of pit vipers; no heat-sensing pits

---

Box 39-1 MOST IMPORTANT SPECIES OF VENOMOUS SNAKES IN VARIOUS REGIONS OF THE WORLD

UNITED STATES AND CANADA

Diamondback rattlesnakes (*Crotalus adamanteus, C. atrox*)
Timber rattlesnake (*C. horridus*)
Prairie rattlesnake (*C. viridis viridis*)
Pacific rattlesnake (*C. viridis oreganus* and *C. v. helleri*)
Pigmy rattlesnake (*Sistrurus miliarius*)
Copperhead (*Agkistrodon contortrix*)
Cottonmouth (*Agkistrodon piscivorus*)

MEXICO, CENTRAL AMERICA, WEST INDIES

Western diamondback rattlesnake (*Crotalus atrox*)
Mexican west coast rattlesnake (*C. basiliscus*)
Tropical rattlesnake (*C. durissus*), several subspecies
Cantil (*Agkistrodon bilineatus*)
Terciopelo, barba amarilla (*Bothrops asper*)
Fer-de-lance (*Bothrops lanceolatus, B. caribbaeus*)
Lora, green palm viper (*Bothriechis lateralis*)
Eyelash viper (*Bothriechis schlegelii*)
Hognose viper (*Porthidium nasutum*)
Central American coral snake (*Micrurus nigrocinctus*)

NORTHERN SOUTH AMERICA (TO ABOUT 15° S)

Tropical rattlesnake (*Crotalus durissus*), several subspecies
Terciopelo, mapana, vibora equis (*Bothrops asper, B. atrox*)
Neuwied's lancehead (*Bothrops neuwiedi*)
Amazonian tree viper (*Bothriopsis bilineata*)
Hog-nose vipers (*Porthidium nasutum, P. lansbergii*)

Bushmaster (*Lachesis muta*)
Amazonian coral snake (*Micrurus spixii*)
Red-tail coral snake (*M. mipartitus*)

SOUTHERN SOUTH AMERICA

Brazilian rattlesnake (*Crotalus durissus terrificus*)
Jararaca (*Bothrops jararaca*)
Jararacussu (*B. jararacussu*)
Neuwied's lancehead (*B. neuwiedi*)
Urutu (*B. alternatus*)
Southern coral snake (*Micrurus frontalis*)

EUROPE

European viper (*Vipera berus*)
Asp viper (*V. aspis*)
Nose-horned viper (*V. ammodytes*)

NEAR AND MIDDLE EAST

Levantine viper (*Macrovipera [Vipera] lebetina*)
Palestine viper (*V. palaestinae*)
Saw-scaled vipers (*Echis carinatus, E. coloratus*)
Desert horned viper (*Cerastes cerastes*)

INDIAN SUBCONTINENT AND SRI LANKA

Russell's viper (*Daboia russellii*)
Saw-scaled viper (*Echis carinatus*)
Hump-nose viper (*Hypnale hypnale*)

Continued

Box 39-1 cont'd   MOST IMPORTANT SPECIES OF VENOMOUS SNAKES IN VARIOUS REGIONS OF THE WORLD

INDIAN SUBCONTINENT AND SRI LANKA—cont'd

Indian krait *(Bungarus caeruleus)*
Asian cobras *(Naja naja, N. kaouthia)*
Sea snakes, especially beaked sea snake *(Enhydrina schistosa)*, important in some coastal areas

SOUTHEAST ASIA INCLUDING PHILIPPINES AND MOST OF INDONESIA

Russell's viper *(Daboia russellii)*
Malayan pit viper *(Calloselasma rhodostoma)*
White-lipped tree viper *(Trimeresurus albolabris)*
Wagler's pit viper, temple viper *(T. wagleri)*
Mangrove viper *(T. purpureomaculatus)*
Malayan krait *(Bungarus candidus)*
Asian cobras (chiefly *Naja atra, N. kaouthia, N. philippiensis, N. sputatrix, N. sumatrana)*
King cobra *(Ophiophagus hannah)*
Beaked sea snake *(Enhydrina schistosa)*
Annulated sea snake *(Hydrophis cyanocinctus)*
Hardwicke's sea snake *(Lapemis curtus hardwickii)*

FAR EAST (EASTERN CHINA, TAIWAN, KOREA, JAPAN)

Mamushi *(Agkistrodon blomhoffii, A. halys, A. intermedius)*
Hundred-pace snake *(Deinagkistrodon acutus)*
Okinawa habu *(Trimeresurus flavoviridis)*
Chinese habu *(T. mucrosquamatus)*
Chinese green tree viper *(T. stejnegeri)*
Many-banded krait *(Bungarus multicinctus)*
Chinese cobra *(Naja atra)*
Annulated sea snake *(Hydrophis cyanocinctus)*

NORTHERN AUSTRALIA, NEW GUINEA AND ASSOCIATED ISLANDS

Death adders *(Acanthophis antarcticus, A. praelongus)*
Taipan *(Oxyuranus scutellatus)*
Mulga snake, king brown snake *(Pseudechis australis)*
Papuan black snake *(Pseudechis papuanus)*

Brown snakes *(Pseudonaja textilis, P. nuchalis)*
Ikaheka snake *(Micropechis ikaheka)*
Sea snakes, particularly *Astrotia stokesi, Aipysurus laevis, Lapemis curtus*

SOUTHERN AUSTRALIA AND TASMANIA

Tiger snakes *(Notechis scutatus, N. ater)*
Copperhead *(Austrelaps superbus)*
Death adder *(Acanthophis antarcticus)*
Mulga snake, king brown snake *(Pseudechis australis)*
Red-bellied black snake *(Pseudechis porphyriacus)*
Brown snakes *(Pseudonaja)*, several species

NORTH AFRICA TO SOUTHERN EDGE OF SAHARA

Desert horned viper *(Cerastes cerastes)*
Saw-scaled vipers *(Echis pyramidum, E. ocellatus)*
North African rock viper *(Vipera mauritanica)*
Puff adder *(Bitis arietans)*
Egyptian cobra *(Naja haje)*
Red spitting cobra *(Naja pallida)*
Burrowing asp *(Atractaspis microlepidota)*

CENTRAL AND SOUTHERN AFRICA

Saw-scaled vipers *(Echis pyramidum, E. ocellatus)*
Puff adder *(Bitis arietans)*
Rhinoceros viper *(B. nasicornis)*
Gaboon viper *(B. gabonica)*
Green tree viper *(Atheris squamiger)*
Night adders *(Causus rhombeatus, C. maculatus)*
Spitting cobras *(Naja mossambica, N. nigricollis)*
Egyptian cobra *(N. haje)*
Cape cobra *(N. nivea)*
Ringhals *(Hemachatus haemachatus)*
Black mamba *(Dendroaspis polylepis)*
Green mambas *(D. angusticeps, D. viridis)*
Burrowing asps *(Atractaspis)*, several species
Boomslang *(Dispholidus typus)*

Cobras

Strictly speaking, cobras are snakes of the genus *Naja* (Figures 39-1 to 39-3), but the term is often applied to other snakes of cobralike habitus, particularly the king cobra *(Ophiophagus hannah)* (Figure 39-4), ringhals *(Haemachatus)* (Figure 39-5), water cobras *(Boulengerina)*, and tree cobras *(Pseudohaje)*. Spreading the neck to form a hood is common to all, although this behavior is seen in numerous other snakes of several families, including some nonvenomous species. Nearly all cobras are large snakes, 1.2 to 2.5 m in total length, with the king cobra occasionally reaching 5 m. Cobras of the genus *Naja* occur throughout Africa and tropical and subtropical Asia, except in deserts. They live in a wide variety of habitats and adapt well to agricultural and

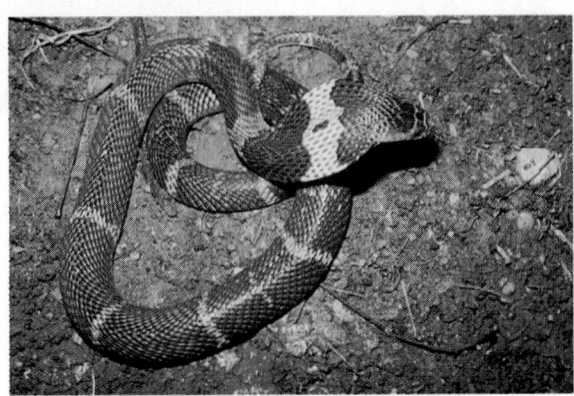

Figure 39-1   Chinese cobra *(Naja atra)*. Cobras are among the world's most venomous snakes, dangerous by virtue of potent venom and distribution in densely populated regions. *(Sherman Minton, MD.)*

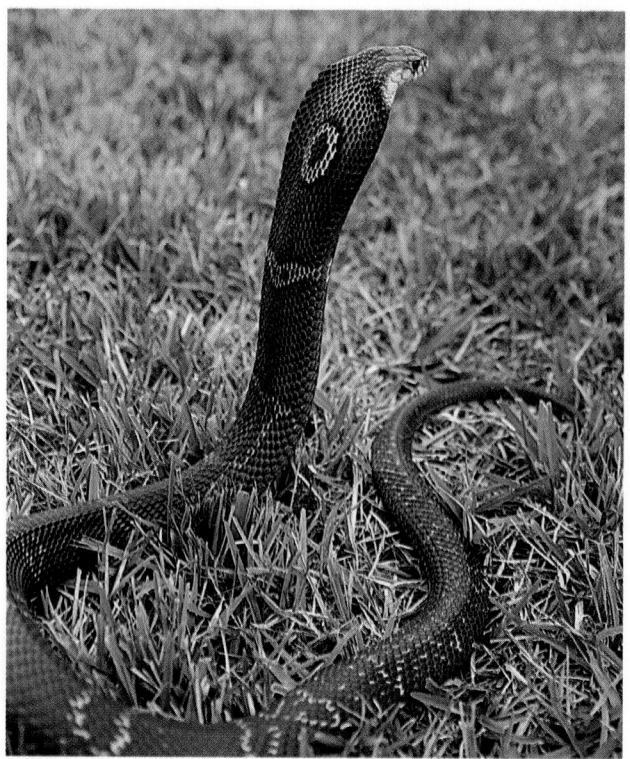

Figure 39-2 The monocellate cobra *(Naja kaouthia)* is one of many cobra species whose venom is known to cause significant local necrosis. *(Courtesy Michael Cardwell and Carl Barden Venom Laboratory.)*

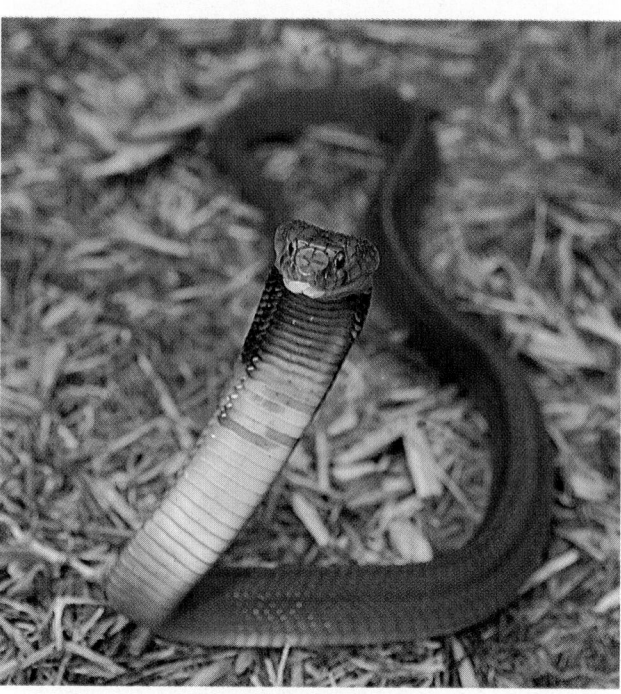

Figure 39-3 The African red spitting cobra *(Naja pallida)* is capable of spraying its venom with great accuracy for distances up to 3 m. *(Courtesy Michael Cardwell and Carl Barden Venom Laboratory.)*

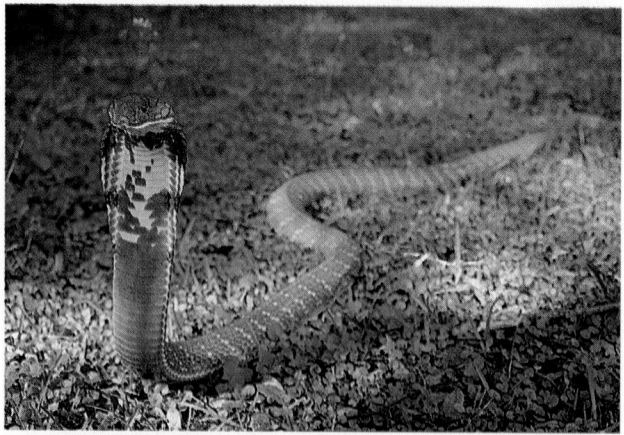

Figure 39-4 The king cobra *(Ophiophagus hannah)* is the largest of the venomous snakes, can reach lengths of up to 5 m, and is widely distributed in Asia. *(Courtesy Michael Cardwell and Carl Barden Venom Laboratory.)*

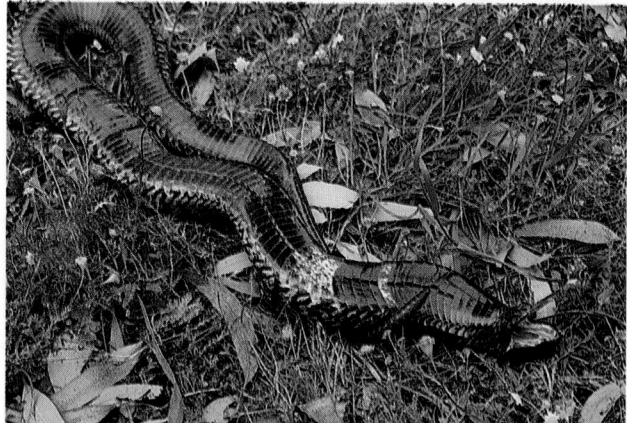

Figure 39-5 Cobralike ringhals *(Hemachatus haemachatus)* of Africa spreads a hood when threatened and can also spit venom. Some specimens feign death, as shown here, causing bites in unsuspecting keepers. *(Michael Cardwell and Cape Town Snake Park.)*

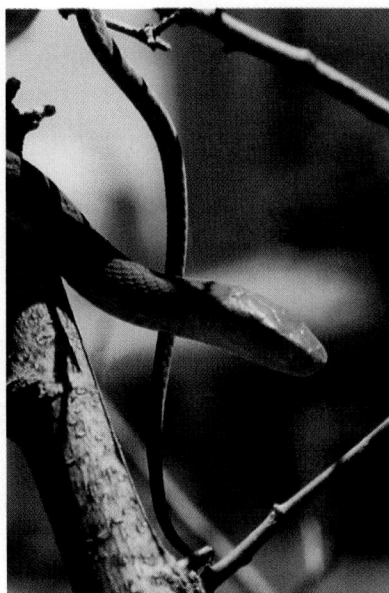

Figure 39-6 Green mamba *(Dendroaspis angusticeps)*. These large, slender arboreal African snakes are quick, alert, and often dangerous. *(Sherman Minton, MD.)*

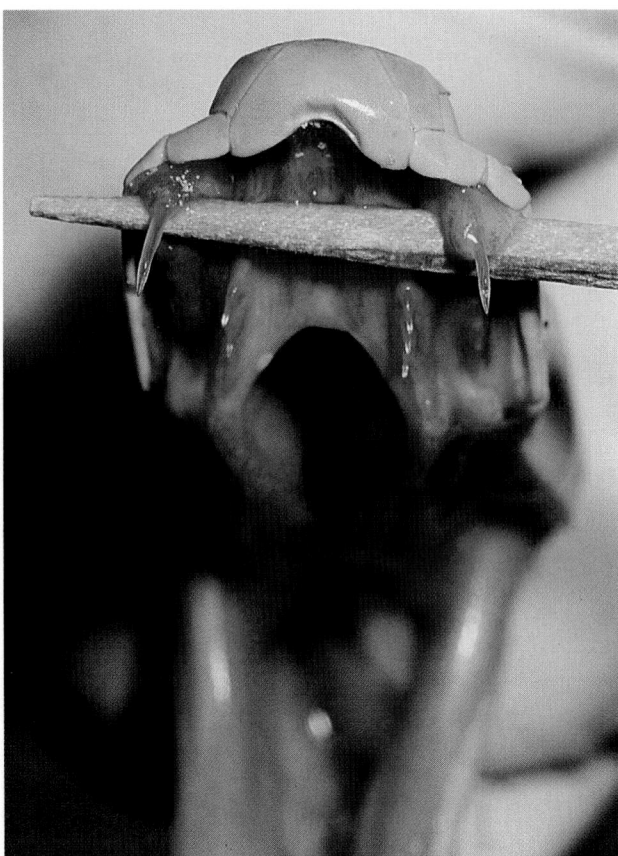

Figure 39-7 Relatively large anterior fangs of green mamba *(Dendroaspis angusticeps)*. Elapids tend to have smaller fangs than do most viperids, but some, as shown here, can be quite large. *(Courtesy Michael Cardwell and Carl Barden Venom Laboratory.)*

suburban situations. The king cobra is restricted to forest areas in southeastern Asia; the ringhals, water cobras, and tree cobras inhabit sub-Saharan Africa. The African spitting cobras, *Naja nigricollis, N. mossambica, N. katiensis, N. pallida,* and *Hemachatus,* have fangs modified for ejecting jets of venom anteriorly and upward for distances up to 3 m with remarkable accuracy. This habit is rarely seen in Southeast Asian cobras.

Mambas

Mambas are slender elapid snakes constituting the genus *Dendroaspis* (Figures 39-6 and 39-7). They are usually 1.5 to 2.2 m long, although the black mamba *(D. polylepis)* may reach 4 m. The four species inhabit most of tropical Africa. Mambas are at least partially arboreal, alert and active, and aggressive under some circumstances.

Kraits

There are about a dozen species of south Asian elapids of the genus *Bungarus* (Figure 39-8). Their average lengths are 1 to 1.2 m, with two species reaching 2 m. Kraits have short fangs and highly toxic venom, are nocturnal, and are often found close to human dwellings. Bites are uncommon, but the case fatality rate is high.

Coral Snakes

All medically important species of coral snakes are in the genus *Micrurus,* which includes about 50 species dis-

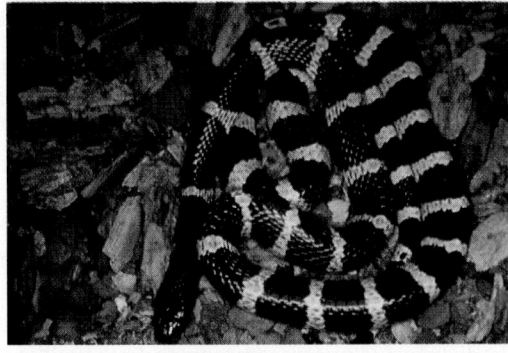

Figure 39-8 Many-banded krait *(Bungarus multicinctus)*. Kraits are widely distributed in southern Asia and have highly lethal neurotoxic venoms. They are nocturnal and rarely aggressive. *(Sherman Minton, MD.)*

tributed from the southern United States to central Argentina (Figure 39-9). Nearly all are in the 0.6 to 1.2 m size range. Most have tricolor patterns of red, yellow, and black. A few species are bicolor. The rules and mnemonics for distinguishing coral snakes from their

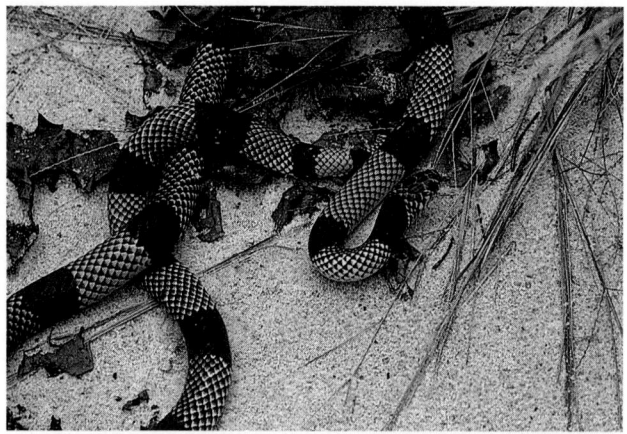

Figure 39-9 Amazonian coral snake *(Micrurus spixii)*. This South American species demonstrates how color patterns can be misleading in identification of coral snakes outside the United States. its red and yellow bands are separated by black rather than being contiguous. *(Courtesy Michael Cardwell and Extreme Wildlife Photography.)*

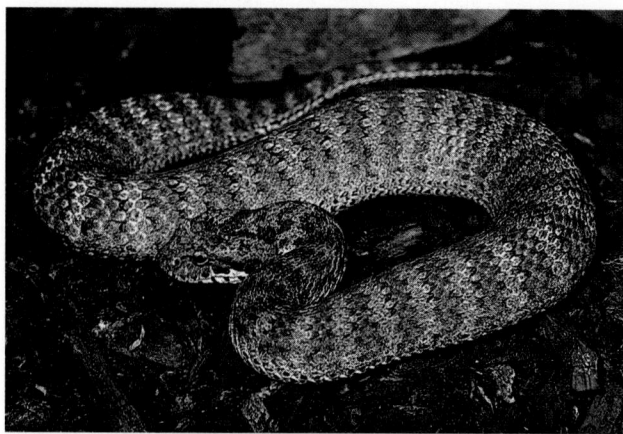

Figure 39-11 Death adder *(Acanthophis antarcticus)*. This viperlike Australian snake is actually an elapid with highly neurotoxic venom. *(Courtesy Michael Cardwell and William W. Lamar.)*

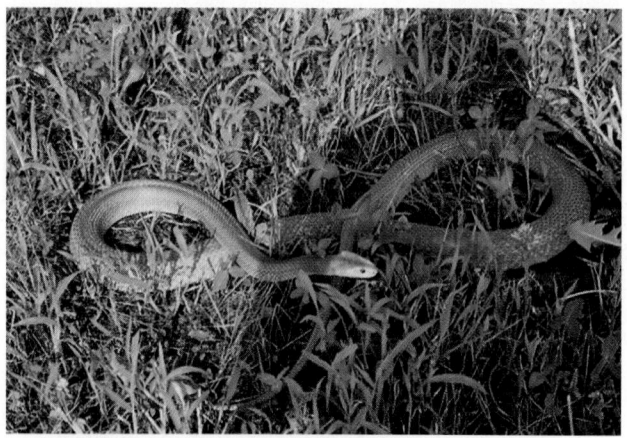

Figure 39-10 Coastal taipan *(Oxyuranus scutellatus)* Australia's largest venomous snake can reach a length of 3 m and can be aggressive. Its range is largely in semitropical Queensland. *(Sherman Minton, MD.)*

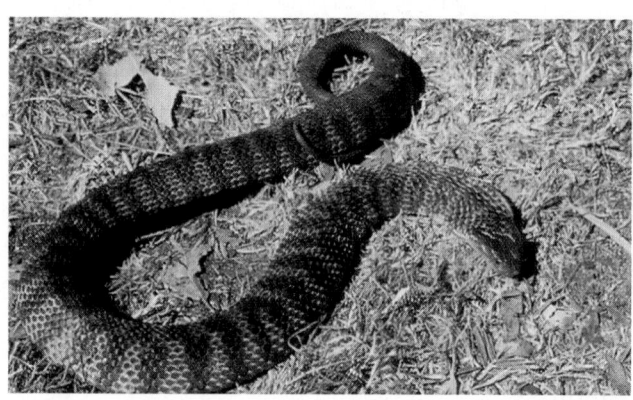

Figure 39-12 Tiger snake *(Notechis scutatus)*. This highly venomous elapid snake is found in the densely populated eastern part of Australia. *(Sherman Minton, MD.)*

mimics become progressively less reliable from central Mexico southward (see Chapter 38). Coral snakes are secretive and not often encountered. The dozen or more species of oriental coral snakes *(Calliophis, Maticora)* are widely distributed but uncommon and not well studied.

Australian Elapids

Elapids are the dominant snakes of Australia, New Guinea, and proximity islands north to the Solomons. The 85 or more species are closely related and part of one evolutionary radiation, which also includes the sea snakes. The diverse elapids range from small (40 to 60 cm), inoffensive burrowers to the potentially aggressive coastal taipan *(Oxyuranus scutellatus)*, which may reach a length of 3.3 m (Figure 39-10). Death adders *(Acanthophis)* are viperlike in appearance, with wide heads

and thick bodies (Figure 39-11). Other dangerous species are tiger snakes *(Notechis)*, which may be plentiful in well-populated eastern coastal districts of Australia (Figure 39-12); brown snakes *(Pseudonaja)*, which are quick and may be dangerous if cornered; and large snakes of the genus *Pseudechis*, including the red-bellied black snake *(P. porphyriacus)* and the king brown snake *(P. australis)*. Venoms of most of these snakes are highly toxic.

Sea Snakes

The 50 or more species of sea snakes inhabit tropical and subtropical sections of the western Pacific and Indian Oceans over the continental shelves, but the pelagic sea snake *(Pelamis platurus)* also occurs on the western coasts of America from Baja California to Ecuador and is occasionally found in Hawaiian waters

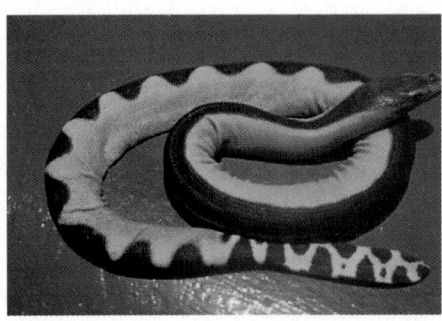

Figure 39-13 Pelagic sea snake *(Pelamis platurus)* is the most widely distributed sea snake and the only species found in American waters. *(Sherman Minton, MD.)*

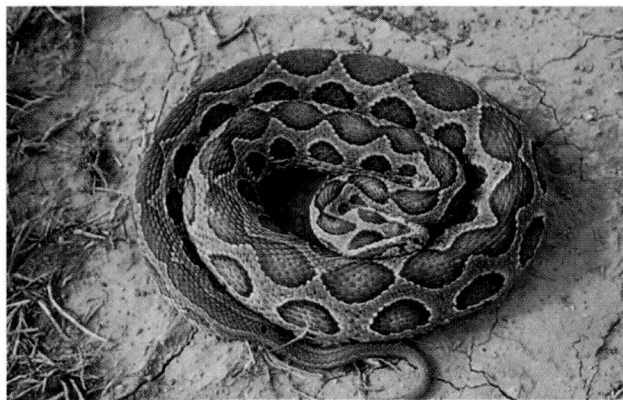

Figure 39-15 Russell's viper *(Daboia russellii).* Plentiful in agricultural regions of southern Asia, these large vipers are a leading cause of fatal snakebites. *(Sherman Minton, MD.)*

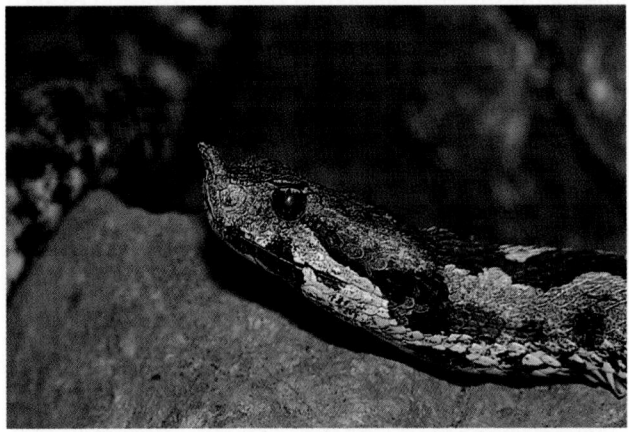

Figure 39-14 Nose-horned viper *(Vipera ammodytes)* is an important cause of snakebites in Europe, but cases are rarely fatal. *(Courtesy Michael Cardwell/Extreme Wildlife Photography.)*

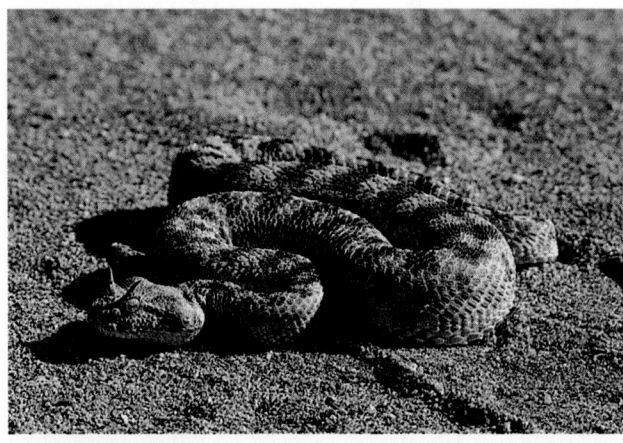

Figure 39-16 Desert horned viper *(Cerastes cerastes).* These relatively small Egyptian vipers are highly adapted to their desert environment. Bites are rarely fatal. *(Courtesy Michael Cardwell and The Living Desert.)*

(Figure 39-13). Similarity in plasma and venom proteins indicates that sea snakes are closely related to Australian terrestrial elapids (see Chapter 61).

Eurasian Vipers

The genus *Vipera* includes approximately a dozen species. Dangerous, large species include the Levantine viper *(V. lebetina),* found from North Africa to Pakistan, and the Palestine viper *(V. palaestinae),* which is native to the Middle East. The European viper *(V. berus)* has one of the most extensive ranges of any land snake and is found from the British Isles to Korea and the eastern limits of Russia. *V. berus* is relatively small (60 to 75 cm). Other species important in Europe are the asp viper *(V. aspis),* Iberian viper *(V. latasti),* and nose-horned viper *(V. ammodytes)* (Figure 39-14). These cause numerous bites, but the case fatality rate is low. The Russell's viper *(Daboia* [formerly *Vipera*] *russellii)* is found from

Pakistan to Taiwan and is one of the world's most dangerous snakes, having a highly lethal venom (Figure 39-15). It adapts well to agricultural environments.

Desert Vipers

The saw-scaled vipers *(Echis)* may cause more fatalities than any other snakes in the world.[83] These snakes live in arid and semiarid regions from India through the Middle East to west Africa; however, they often thrive on cultivated land. Their name comes from the saw-toothed ridges on the lateral scales that are rubbed together to produce a warning sound. These small snakes are rarely more than 60 cm in length but are highly irritable and quick to strike. The venoms cause severe coagulopathy. *Cerastes* has two species in North Africa and the Middle East, including the horned viper of Egypt (Figure 39-16). These snakes are highly adapted to desert conditions. They are relatively small, and their

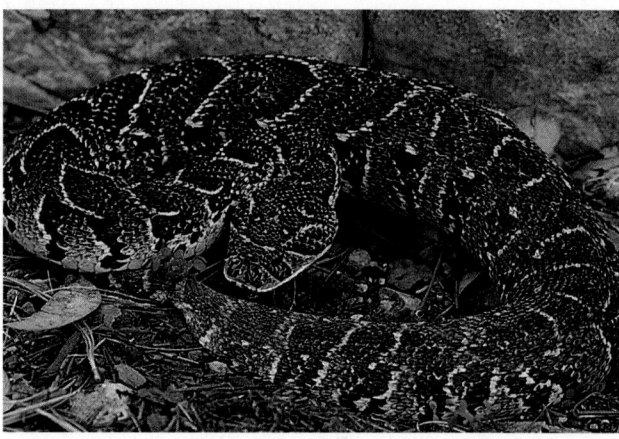

Figure 39-17 Puff adder *(Bitis arietans)*. This large African viper is widely distributed and extremely dangerous. As shown here, its color pattern allows it to blend into background leaf clutter. *(Courtesy Michael Cardwell/Extreme Wildlife Photography.)*

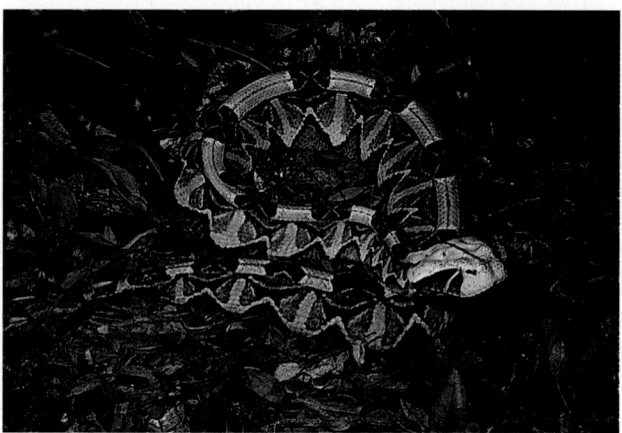

Figure 39-18 Gaboon viper *(Bitis gabonica)*. This impressive African viper possesses the longest fangs of any venomous snake, up to 5 cm. It can deliver massive quantities of hightly toxic venom. *(Courtesy Michael Cardwell and Carl Barden Venom Laboratory.)*

bites are rarely fatal. Two other species in this group are the Persian horned viper *(Pseudocerastes persicus)* and the leaf-nosed viper *(Eristicophis macmahoni)*, both occurring in the Middle East and Pakistan. They are uncommon and of little medical importance.

African Vipers

The genus *Bitis* has 12 species and occurs throughout Africa, exclusive of the northern deserts. The wide-ranging puff adder *(B. arietans)* also occurs in western Saudi Arabia (Figure 39-17). All are stout-bodied, wide-headed snakes. They vary in size from *B. peringueyi* (rarely exceeds 30 cm) to the Gabon viper *(B. gabonica)* (Figure 39-18), which may reach a length of 2 m and a weight of about 10 kg. Habitat ranges from desert to rainforest. The puff adder is a major cause of snakebites in most parts of Africa where it is found. It prefers grassland and often

lives near villages. *Atheris* is an arboreal African viper genus with eight species. They are usually 50 to 65 cm long, and some have a bizarre appearance that makes them popular with zoos and hobbyists; bites are infrequent. Night adders of the genus *Causus* are widespread in Africa south of the Sahara. They are usually 50 to 70 cm long and may be plentiful around fields and villages. Bites are numerous, but fatalities are almost unknown.

Agkistrodon Complex Pit Vipers

The 15 species in the *Agkistrodon* pit viper group are found from the eastern United States to Central America and throughout most of Asia. They are characterized by large shields on the crown of the head, a presumably primitive condition in viperid snakes. American copperheads *(A. contortrix)* and cottonmouths *(A. piscivorus)* are discussed in Chapter 38. The closely related cantil *(A. bilineatus)* is native to Mexico and Central America. The mamushi *(A. blomhoffii)* of Japan, Korea, and eastern China, Siberian pit viper *(A. halys)* of Asian Russia and Mongolia; and central Asian pit viper *(A. intermedius)*, found from Iran to Korea, are all common snakes, usually 60 to 80 cm long and of moderate build. They are the only venomous snakes in much of central and northeastern Asia and account for many snakebites. The case fatality rate is low. The Malayan pit viper *(Calloselasma rhodostoma)* is a distinctive species of Southeast Asia that inhabits forests at low elevation and is particularly common on rubber plantations. It is a major cause of snakebites. The hundred-pace snake *(Deinagkistrodon acutus)* is a large (1.2 to 1.5 m) snake with a strongly upturned snout. It is native to forests in south China and Taiwan and is dangerous but uncommon.

Asian Lance-Head Pit Vipers

The genus *Trimeresurus* is now subdivided by many herpetologists. It includes approximately 40 species. They are distributed from southern India to Indonesia, the Philippines, and the southern islands of Japan (Figure 39-19). The most dangerous species are large (up to 2.3 m), slender snakes with very wide heads. They are often called "habu," a Japanese name. They are mostly terrestrial and may have large populations in sugar cane fields and other areas of cultivation. The Okinawa habu *(T. flavoviridis)* accounts for a high incidence of snakebites on the southern Ryukyu Islands.[63] The Chinese habu *(T. mucrosquamatus)* has a wide range in Southeast Asia and is another plentiful and dangerous species. Arboreal species are often predominantly green, 60 to 100 cm long, and are found throughout the range of the group. *T. albolabris*, the white-lipped bamboo viper, is the most widely distributed member of this group. These vipers cause many snakebites, but fatalities are rare. A third group *(Ovophis* to some) includes five species of stout, short vipers found in mountainous terrain. They seem to be of little medical importance. Wagler's pit viper is a widely

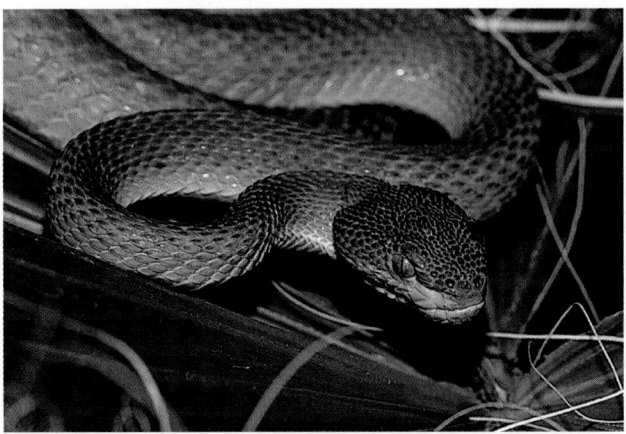

Figure 39-19 Chinese green tree viper *(Trimeresurus stejnegeri)* is found in southern and eastern Asia. *(Courtesy Michael Cardwell/Extreme Wildlife Photography.)*

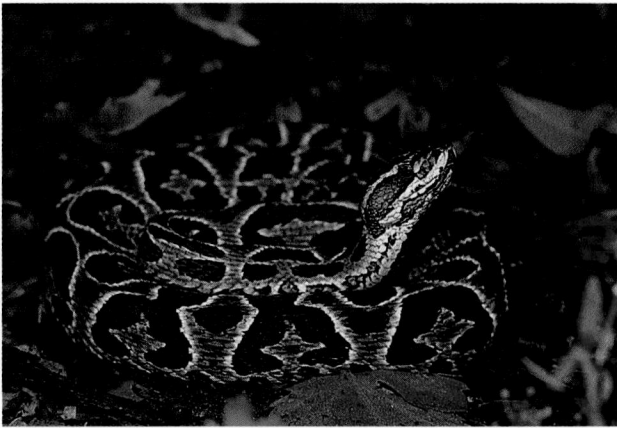

Figure 39-21 Urutu *(Bothrops alternatus).* This large, dangerous South American pit viper is responsible for many severe bites in its distribution. *(Courtesy Michael Cardwell/Extreme Wildlife Photography.)*

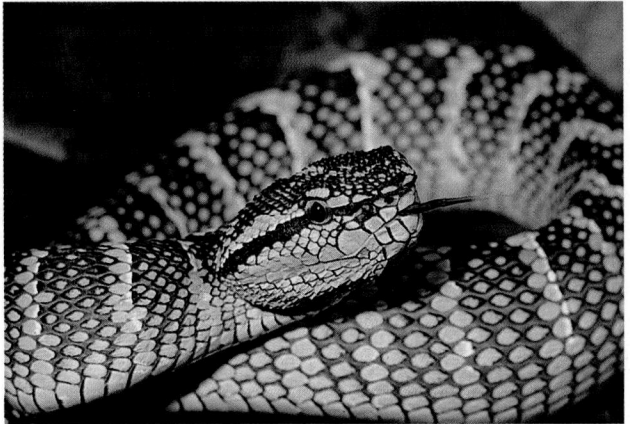

Figure 39-20 Wagler's pit viper, temple viper *(Tropidolaemus wagleri).* This Asian pit viper is popular with amateur snake keepers. *(Courtesy Michael Cardwell and William W. Lamar.)*

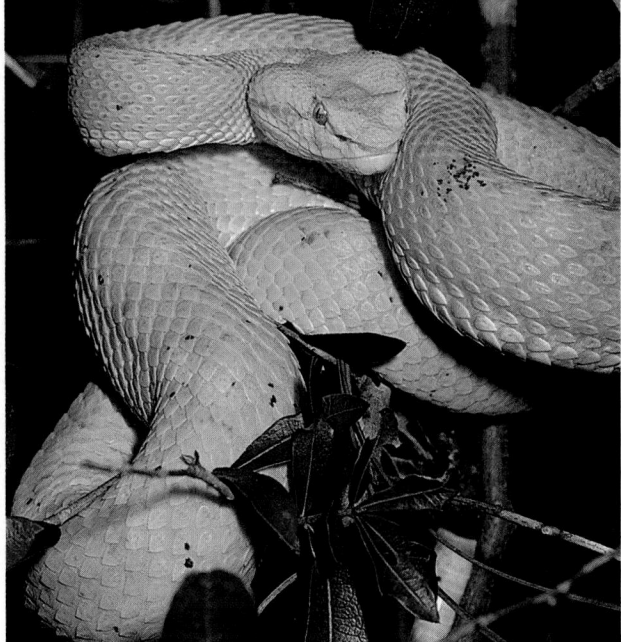

Figure 39-22 Eyelash viper *(Bothriechis schlegelii)* is found in southern Mexico, Central America, and northern South America and is popular with amateur snake keepers. *(Courtesy Michael Cardwell and Carl Barden Venom Laboratory.)*

distributed arboreal species usually assigned to the genus *Tropidolaemus* (Figure 39-20). Its venom contains a peculiar heat-stable toxin, but its bites do not seem to differ from those of arboreal *Trimeresurus.*

Neotropical Pit Vipers

Most of these snakes were formerly assigned to the genus *Bothrops,* which ranges from eastern Mexico to southern Argentina and a few islands of the West Indies (Figure 39-21). The genus contains approximately 30 species, most of which are of medical importance. These are medium to long snakes (0.7 to 2.5 m) of moderate to heavy build with distinctly triangular heads. Habitat ranges from semiarid grasslands to rainforests; several species adapt well to banana and sugar cane plantations. Among the more dangerous species are *B. atrox, B. asper, B. jararaca,* and *B. lanceolatus.* They have many Spanish and Portuguese names, but the name

"fer-de-lance" is often used for these snakes in English language publications. Species of *Bothrops* account for most of the serious snakebites in Latin America. Fifteen arboreal species formerly in *Bothrops* are now in the genera *Bothriopsis* and *Bothriechis.* They are slender snakes with large heads and are 50 to 100 cm in length. Most have green in their pattern. The eyelash viper *(Bothriechis schlegelii)* is a well-known example that accounts for about 20% of venomous snakebites in Costa Rica (Figure 39-22). Fatalities are rare. Fourteen other

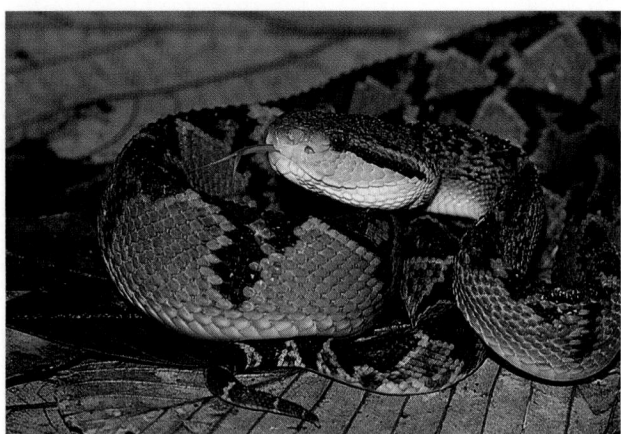

Figure 39-23   Bushmaster *(Lachesis muta)* is the largest pit viper, up to 3.6 m and is found in southern Central America and northern South America. *(Courtesy Michael Cardwell/Extreme Wildlife Photography.)*

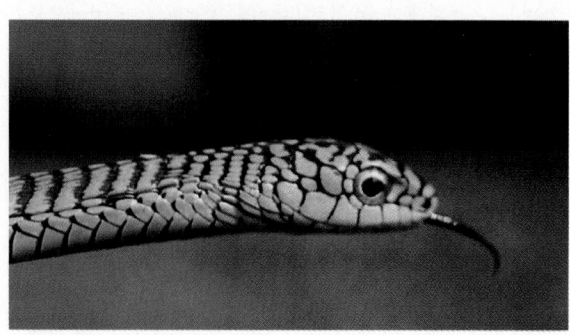

Figure 39-24   Boomslang *(Dispholidus typus)* is the most dangerous of the rearfanged colubrid snakes. This arboreal snake is widely distributed in Africa. *(Sherman Minton, MD.)*

former *Bothrops* species constitute the genus *Porthidium,* which has been further subdivided by some authorities. These are small to moderate-sized snakes (45 to 100 cm) with heavy bodies and wide heads. They are found from eastern Mexico to northern South America, usually in forests and often in highlands. They are terrestrial. Bites are common but fatalities rare. The bushmaster *(Lachesis muta)* is the largest pit viper, usually 1.5 to 2.5 m long but occasionally reaching 3.6 m (Figure 39-23). It has extraordinarily rough scales in the middorsal region and a distinct tail spine. It is found in lowland forests from southern Nicaragua to eastern Brazil and is uncommon. Bushmaster bites are rare, but the case fatality rate is high.

Rattlesnakes

The 31 species of rattlesnakes occur from southern Canada to Uruguay and eastern Argentina, although only two species occur south of the isthmus of Tehuantepec in Mexico. All except one insular species in Baja California can be identified by the presence of a rattle (see Chapter 38).

Burrowing Asps

The 15 species of the genus *Atractaspis* were formerly considered vipers because they have viperlike fangs; however, they have several unique features that justify their recognition as a separate family (Atractaspididae). They are small (50 to 80 cm), moderately slender with small heads, and uniformly black or brown. They are found throughout most of sub-Saharan Africa and in some areas of the Middle East. They frequent habitats ranging from forest to semidesert and are burrowers that may emerge at night and after rains. Bites are fairly common in some parts of Africa, but fatalities are infrequent.

Colubrid Snakes

The colubrids are a large, taxonomically varied family of snakes that lack anterior fangs and the primitive features (e.g., labial heat-sensing pits, pelvic spurs, and so on) associated with boas and some other snakes. Some herpetologists partition this family, but little agreement exists on recognized divisions. In most parts of the world, colubrids make up the majority of snake species, absent only from the Arctic and Antarctic, southern Australia, and some islands. Many species have grooved fangs in the rear of the upper jaw, and others have enlarged but ungrooved rear teeth. Although the vast majority of these species are harmless, more than 50 species of colubrid snakes in 30 genera have caused human envenoming. Most cases are mild because the venom-injecting apparatus is inefficient and the quantity of venom small; however, serious and fatal envenomations have occurred.[47] Most colubrid bites involve the handling of snakes believed to be harmless. The more important species include the boomslang *(Dispholidus typus)* (Figure 39-24), twig snakes *(Thelotornis* spp.), Japanese garter snake *(Rhabdophis tigrinus),* and brown tree snake *(Boiga irregularis).*

VENOM APPARATUS

The venom apparatus of snakes functions mainly to immobilize and kill prey, although it may also be an important means of defense. Dentition is modified in all venomous snakes, although some colubrids have only an enlarged pair of posterior maxillary teeth. The most highly modified dentition is that of vipers, in which a single, large, tubular or deeply grooved fang is attached to a greatly reduced maxillary bone. These fangs have a wide range of rocking movement. Burrowing asps *(Atractaspis* spp.) have large, viperlike fangs used one at a time with a backward stabbing motion as the lower jaw is shifted to the opposite side. They can bite with the mouth virtually closed. Fangs of elapid snakes are short, tubular or grooved, and attached to the anterior end of a longer maxillary bone that may bear additional teeth and has a limited degree of rocking movement. Fangs of sea snakes are even shorter; the maxillary bone is long and usually bears additional teeth. The enlarged teeth or grooved fangs of colubrids are at the rear of the maxillary bone and are typically preceded by additional teeth.

Snake venoms are produced in a pair of glands usually located between the eye and the angle of the mouth. In one genus of oriental elapids (*Maticora*), two species of burrowing asps (*Atractaspis*), and two species of night adders (*Causus*), however, the glands are tubular and extend well back into the body. Histologic and histochemical studies show secretory cells of various types in all snake venom glands.[3,36] Space for venom storage in the lumen of the gland is greatest in viperids and some elapids (e.g., cobras), less in other elapids and sea snakes, and minimal in colubrids. Musculature for emptying the glands is best developed in viperids, moderately effective in elapids and sea snakes, and relatively ineffective in colubrids. This is reflected in quantities of venon injected in natural bites and amounts that can be obtained by extraction.

SNAKE VENOMS

The biochemistry and pharmacology of snake venoms are well studied. The venoms are colorless to amber liquids with solid content that is mostly protein. Pharmacologically active substances include enzymes, polypeptide toxins, glycoproteins, nucleotides, small peptides, and biogenic amines. Many of the enzymes and toxins are very stable. Dried snake venoms can retain lethality and some enzyme activity after three decades of storage.

The postsynaptic neurotoxins, found in most elapid and sea snake venoms, are probably the best understood snake venom toxins. They bind to the nicotinic acetylcholine receptors competitively with acetylcholine and produce a nondepolarizing neuromuscular blockade. The short toxins have 60 to 62 amino acids and four disulfide bridges; the long toxins have 71 to 74 amino acids and five disulfide bridges.

Presynaptic neurotoxins inhibit release of acetylcholine at the neuromuscular junction. Toxins in this group have phospholipase A_2 activity, occur in a variety of elapid and viper venoms, and are similar to myotoxins in some sea snake venoms. The phospholipases of this group have 110 to 125 amino acids and six or seven disulfide bonds. Their neurotoxicity and myotoxicity are not related to hydrolytic activity.

With the exception of sea snake venom, nearly all snake venoms affect blood coagulation, although not always to a clinically significant degree. Thrombinlike activity that converts fibrinogen to fibrin is characteristic of pit viper venoms; the fibrin is abnormal and easily lysed. Enzymes responsible for this activity have been isolated from a number of venoms, including the Malayan pit viper (*Calloselasma rhodostoma*), eastern diamondback rattlesnake (*Crotalus adamanteus*), hundredpace snake (*Deinagkistrodon acutus*), Gaboon viper (*Bitis gabonica*), and jararaca (*Bothrops jararaca*). In sublethal doses these enzymes produce nonclotting blood and do not cause platelet aggregation. Prothrombin activation with formation of thrombin is seen particularly with venoms of the Russell's viper (*Daboia russellii*) and sawscaled vipers (*Echis* spp.), from which the enzymes responsible have been isolated. Prothrombin activation is also seen with venoms of several Australian elapids, some pit vipers, and dangerous colubrids. Some venoms have more than one type of anticoagulant activity.

Hemorrhage and necrosis are often seen with snakebites, particularly those inflicted by vipers. Although attributed to proteolytic enzymes, several hemorrhagic factors have little or no proteolytic activity.[55] Their main mode of action is disruption of the vascular basement membrane.

Extensive myonecrosis is often seen with bites by sea snakes, some Australian elapids, and some pit vipers. Myotoxins have been isolated from several venoms. Most myotoxins show phospholipase A_2 activity, which is more pronounced in those derived from elapids.

The so-called cardiotoxin first described from cobra venom and subsequently found in venoms of some other related snakes is a strongly basic polypeptide whose main action is to produce irreversible depolarization of cell membranes. A specific cardiotoxin with quite different structure and action is found in venoms of some burrowing asps (*Atractaspis* spp.). Its action is directly on the heart, producing coronary vasoconstriction and atrioventricular block.[43,90]

Hyaluronidase is found in most reptilian venoms and facilitates absorption and spread of other venom components. Other enzymes, such as phosphodiesterase, L-amino acid oxidase, 5′ nucleotidase, and acetylcholinesterase, are present in many snake venoms, but their roles in envenomation are poorly understood. Most of the clinical effects of envenomation result from several venom components acting in concert, and venom effects may be compounded by endogenous release of autopharmacologic compounds such as histamine and bradykinin.

SIGNS AND SYMPTOMS OF SNAKE VENOM POISONING

The complexity and diversity of snake venoms are reflected in the wide array of signs and symptoms that can occur after envenomation. The precise clinical pic-

Box 39-2   SIGNS AND SYMPTOMS AFTER SNAKE VENOM POISONING

ELAPIDS (COBRAS, MAMBAS, KRAITS, AUSTRALIAN VENOMOUS SNAKES, CORAL SNAKES)
Local

Findings may be absent or minimal
Significant pain occurs with some species
Regional lymphadenopathy
Necrosis occurs with some species

Systemic

Neurotoxicity (cranial nerve dysfunction, altered mental status, peripheral weakness and paralysis, respiratory failure)
Cardiovascular failure
Coagulopathy
Myonecrosis
Renal failure

SEA SNAKES
Local

Trivial
Fang marks may be difficult to identify

Systemic

Neurotoxicity (cranial nerve dysfunction, peripheral weakness and paralysis, respiratory failure)
Myotoxicity with resulting muscle pain and tenderness, myoglobinemia, myoglobinuria, and hyperkalemia (may precipitate cardiac dysrhythmias and renal failure)

VIPERS AND PIT VIPERS
Local

Pain
Soft tissue swelling
Regional lymphadenopathy
Ecchymosis, bloody exudate from fang marks

Early absence of local findings does not rule out significant envenomation
Local necrosis may be significant

SYSTEMIC

Any organ system may be involved
Cardiovascular toxicity (hypotension, pulmonary edema)
Neurotoxicity (cranial nerve dysfunction, peripheral weakness) with some species
Hemorrhagic diathesis
Renal failure

BURROWING ASPS
Local

Single fang puncture
Pain
Some swelling
Occasional local necrosis

Systemic

Nausea, vomiting
Diaphoresis
Fever
Occasional respiratory distress, cardiac dysrhythmias (atrioventricular block)
Rare fatalities

COLUBRIDS (REAR-FANGED)
Local

Mild to moderate local swelling, pain, and ecchymosis
Bloody exudate from fang marks

Systemic

Nausea, vomiting
Coagulopathy and associated complications
Renal dysfunction

---

ture and degree of severity of any specific venomous snakebite depend on many factors, including the species of snake and its age, size, health, and geographic origin; anatomic location of the bite; size and health of the victim; and therapeutic interventions. The treating physician must anticipate multisystem dysfunction in any victim of snake venom poisoning and must remain vigilant for any constellation of signs, symptoms, and laboratory findings, regardless of the species of snake implicated (Box 39-2).

Elapids

Local findings after most elapid envenomations are unimpressive compared with those seen after typical viperid venom poisoning (Figure 39-25). In many cases it may be difficult to find distinct fang marks.[69,93] The degree of pain varies depending on the species in-

volved. Often, local pain is a minor complaint, but it may be significant after bites by certain cobra species, such as the king cobra (*Ophiophagus hannah*) (see Figure 39-4).[22] Regional lymphadenopathy may be present. Although significant, local soft tissue swelling is uncommon after most elapid envenomations.[11] Some species, such as the African spitting cobras (*Naja mossambica, N. nigricollis*)[76] and some Asiatic cobras (*Naja* spp.),[58,67,75] may produce early edema as an indication of envenomation. Swelling can progress with time to involve the entire bitten extremity. With some of these species, local tissue necrosis may be profound (Figure 39-26).[59,75,85] Some Australian elapids, such as the taipan (*Oxyuranus* spp.) and tiger snake (*Notechis* spp.), also can induce myonecrosis and coagulopathy.[16,59,93] Renal failure has been reported as a complication of envenomation by some elapids.[12,28,59]

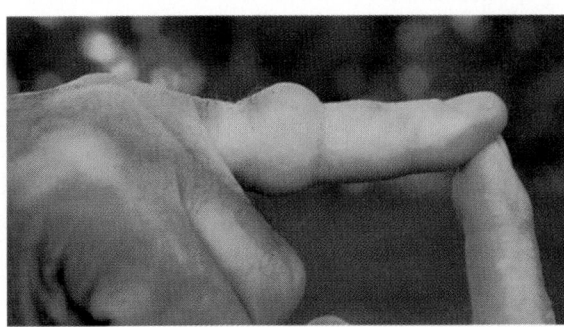

Figure 39-25 Bite of a small Australian elapid snake *(Hemiaspis signata)* resulting in localized swelling with some discoloration but no systemic symptoms. *(Sherman Minton, MD.)*

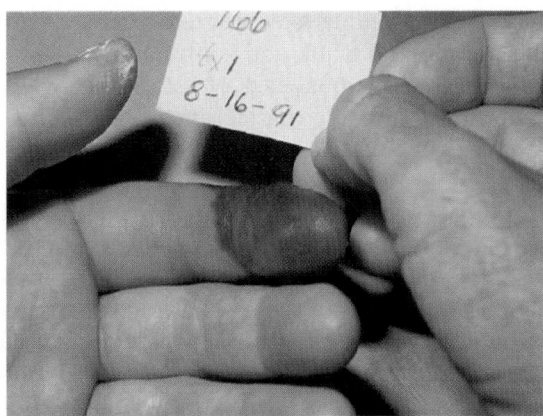

Figure 39-26 Sharply demarcated necrosis, sometimes extensive, often follows bites by both African and Asian cobras. *(Sherman Minton, MD.)*

Neurotoxicity is seen after most elapid envenomations. The time of onset of neuropathic signs and symptoms after envenomation is quite variable. It is usually most rapid after serious cobra and mamba bites and most delayed after some coral snake envenomations. In certain situations the onset may be delayed for 10 hours or more.[59] The earliest systemic manifestations of envenomation by most elapids are signs of cranial nerve dysfunction, especially ptosis, but also difficulty swallowing, dysphonia, and blurred vision.[75] Paresthesias, muscle fasciculations, peripheral weakness, and paralysis, including that of respiratory muscles, may soon follow. Mental status (drowsiness, hallucinations) may be altered.[75] Associated systemic symptoms include hypersalivation and diaphoresis.[11,56] In cases of severe envenomation, cardiovascular depression may result in hypotension and pulmonary edema.[59,91]

Eye exposure to venom from any of the spitting cobras or ringhals results in immediate burning pain and tearing. Significant systemic absorption does not occur, but corneal ulceration, uveitis, and permanent blindness can follow untreated cases.[59,84] Bites by spitting cobras often manifest violent local reactions with hemorrhage and necrosis, but rarely neurotoxicity.

Sea Snakes

Local findings at the bite site after sea snake envenomation are usually trivial. In serious cases, systemic symptoms usually appear within 2 hours.[78] The bite site may show several tiny puncture wounds from the fangs and other teeth, but local pain and soft tissue swelling are negligible (Figure 39-27). Fang marks may be difficult to see.[79]

Sea snake venoms demonstrate significant neurotoxicity in animal studies and in human envenomations.[12,59,79] Neurologic dysfunction is manifested by hypersalivation, dysphagia, dysarthria, muscle spasm, and paralysis. Victims remain conscious if hypoxia is

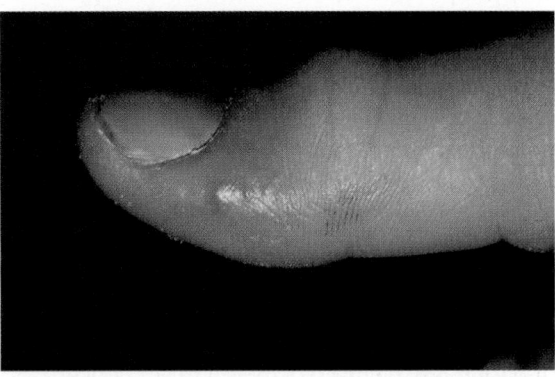

Figure 39-27 Bite of a Southeast Asian water snake *(Enhydrina plumbea)*, generally considered to be nonvenomous. Swelling and ecchymosis were still present after 24 hours. *(Sherman Minton, MD.)*

prevented.[79] Envenomation is also characterized by trismus and diffuse myopathic findings.[56,59] The myotoxic components of sea snake venoms may cause significant outpouring of potassium and myoglobin from injured muscle. Hyperkalemia may precipitate cardiac dysrhythmias, and myoglobinuria can lead to acute renal failure.[5] Untreated sea snake envenomation may result in muscle pain and weakness that persists for months.[59] Death after sea snake envenomation may result from respiratory failure caused by paralysis of the diaphragm, hyperkalemic cardiac arrest, or acute renal failure[79] (see Chapter 61).

Vipers and Pit Vipers (Viperids)

The effects of envenomation by Eurasian and African vipers and Asian and neotropical pit vipers are similar to those seen after bites by the pit vipers of North America (Chapter 38). Severe pain, local soft tissue swelling, subcutaneous ecchymosis, and bloody exudation from the fang marks usually begin within minutes. Regional lymphadenopathy may be present within 30 to 60 minutes, and soft tissue swelling may progress extensively over several hours. The trunk and contralateral extremity may become edematous. Lack of soft tissue swelling, however, does not rule out significant poisoning by some species or after deep intramuscular or intravascular envenoming. After 12 to 24 hours, serum-filled vesicles and hemorrhagic bullae may appear, and ecchymoses may spread throughout the involved extremity.[12]

Systemic envenomation may result in blurred vision, altered taste, weakness, dizziness, diaphoresis, nausea, vomiting, diarrhea, fever, headache, abdominal pain, and bleeding at various anatomic sites.[46,56,59] Hypotension and shock may occur over a variable time course. Early hypotension is caused primarily by pooling of blood in the pulmonary and splanchnic vasculatures. After several hours, transudation of fluid into the bitten extremity and peritoneal cavity, hemolysis, and systemic bleeding may play a role.

Coagulopathy is a characteristic finding after systemic venom poisoning by saw-scaled vipers (*Echis* spp.).[46,57,59] It is also seen after bites by some populations of *Daboia russellii* and many neotropical and Asian pit vipers.[53] Victims can bleed at multiple sites, including the bite wound, soft tissues, gastrointestinal tract, respiratory tract, brain, eyes, and kidneys. The venoms of some populations of *D. russellii* can also cause massive intravascular coagulation and hemolysis.[31,53]

Neurologic findings after pit viper venom poisoning in North America are uncommon (with the notable exception of the Mojave rattlesnake [*Crotalus scutulatus*]; see Chapter 38). Neurotoxicity is a major concern, however, after bites by the South American rattlesnake (*Crotalus durissus terrificus*)[61] and vipers in the Eastern Hemisphere, including the Berg adder (*Bitis atropos*),[84] Palestine viper (*Vipera palaestinae*),[81] and some populations of Russell's viper (*D. russellii*).[82] Signs and symptoms include cranial nerve dysfunction, muscle paralysis, and respiratory failure.[29,52]

Victims may have an altered sensorium (from lethargy to coma) as a result of hypotension, hypoxia, intracranial bleeding, and possibly direct venom effects. Seizures may occur but are uncommon and probably secondary to cerebral hypoxia.

Renal failure may complicate viperid envenoming, as with North American pit vipers or Australian elapids. Etiologic factors include myoglobinuria, hemoglobinuria, hypotension, and direct venom nephrotoxicity. This is especially common after bites from the Russell's viper and saw-scaled viper (*Echis carinatus*).[12,57,59] Onset may be delayed for several days, and any complaints of costovertebral angle pain should arouse suspicion of impending renal failure.[53]

Local bite site necrosis and myonecrosis may be severe after viperid envenomation and may necessitate surgical intervention (amputations, grafting procedures).[46] Although most viperid bites result in venom deposition into subcutaneous tissues, subfascial injection is possible. In these rare cases, direct myotoxicity can produce muscle necrosis. If muscle swelling is significant, a compartment syndrome may develop. The signs and symptoms of compartment syndrome are closely mimicked by the findings after a typical subcutaneous envenomation (swelling, discoloration or cyanosis, pain on palpation, paresthesias). The diagnosis of a compartment syndrome can be confirmed by documenting elevated intracompartmental pressures. This has significant treatment implications, as discussed later.

Burrowing Asps

Envenomation by any of the burrowing asps (*Atractaspis* spp.) may result in severe symptoms, although fatalities have thus far been reported from only *A. microlepidota* and *A. irregularis*.[14,15] Persons bitten by these snakes may have severe local pain followed by numbness, soft tissue swelling, lymphadenopathy, vomiting, diaphoresis, and fever.[15,84] Systemic coagulopathies may occur.[15,24] Local vesicles can be seen at the bite site, and local tissue necrosis occurs rarely.[8,15,84] The cause of death after experimental *Atractaspis* envenomation has been attributed to venom-induced coronary vasospasm.[39]

Colubrids (Dispholidus, Thelotornis, Rhabdophis)

Envenomation by some rear-fanged colubrids may have severe consequences. Fatalities have been reported after bites by the boomslang (*Dispholidus typus*), the bird or twig snake (*Thelotornis kirtlandii*), and the Japanese garter snake or yamakagashi (*Rhabdophis tigrinus*).[38,49,51] Life-threatening envenomation has also occurred after bites by the red-necked keelback (*R. subminiatus*).[6,20,41] Signs and symptoms of envenomation by these snakes include mild soft tissue swelling and, in severe cases, coagulopathy, similar to that seen with viperid venom poisoning.[47,89] Associated findings may include variable local pain, headache, nausea, vomiting, ecchymoses, jaundice, and abdominal pain.[47] Renal dysfunction has been reported after *D. typus*, *T. kirtlandii*, and *R. tigrinus* envenomations.[38,42,51,66] Onset of signs of serious envenomation may be delayed by many hours and possibly even days.[11,21]

MANAGEMENT

Prehospital Care

Prehospital management of a bite by any potentially venomous snake involves placing the victim at rest, offering reassurance, and providing expeditious transport to the nearest facility equipped to handle such an emergency (Figure 39-28). First-aid measures should not cause further harm and should not delay medical care.

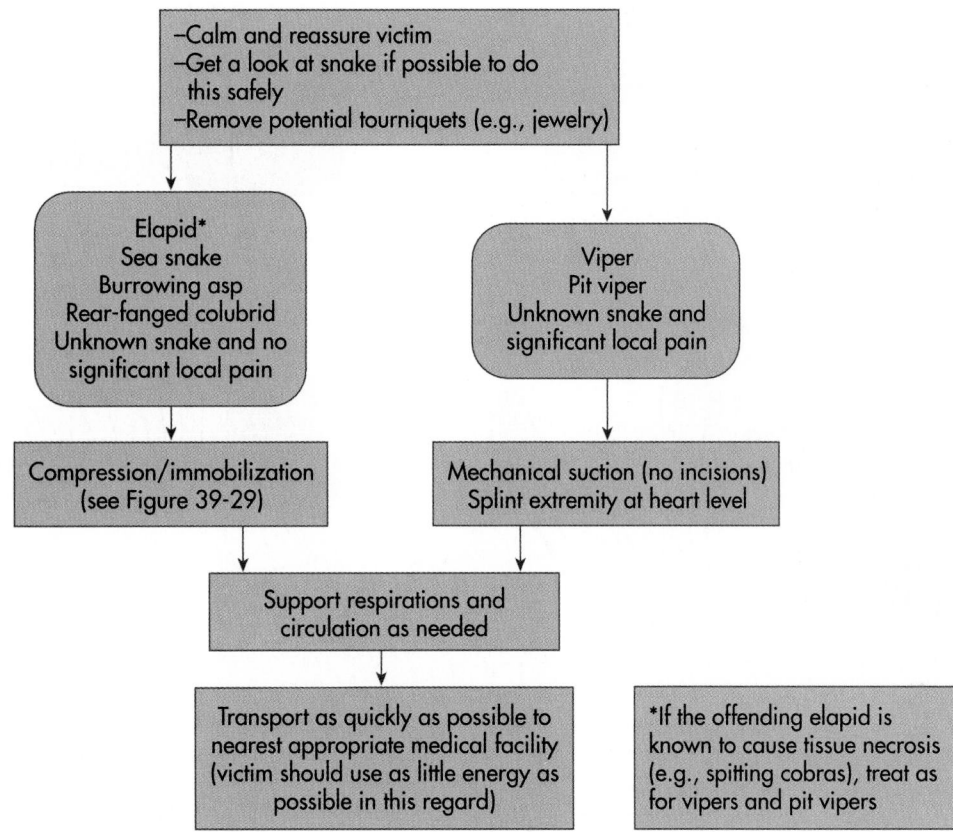

Figure 39-28 First-aid measures for venomous snakebites.

A proven technique of limiting systemic distribution of venom after most elapid and sea snake bites is the Australian pressure immobilization technique (Figure 39-29). This involves immediately wrapping the entire bitten extremity with a crepe bandage, elastic bandage, or article of clothing as tightly as for an acute sprain. This is followed by splinting with any available object.[19,26,71,78] The splinted extremity should be maintained at approximately heart level if possible.

The use of pressure immobilization in cases of bites by snakes capable of causing significant local necrosis (e.g., most viperids, certain cobra species) is controversial.[19] A laboratory study found that pressure immobilization limits pit viper (eastern diamondback rattlesnake, *Crotalus adamanteus*) venom dispersal from the bite site without worsening necrosis.[70] However, localizing a necrotizing venom in the region of the bite site may exacerbate tissue loss.[69,80] Clinical experience with pressure immobilization in human victims of viperid envenomation is limited; the rescuer must weigh the risks against potential benefits. If the offending reptile is a small, innocuous species and transport time to medical care will be short, it may be best to avoid pressure immobilization. If a large or particularly virulent snake is involved and the bite may be life threatening, immobilization may be indicated, especially if in evac-

uation to medical care will be delayed. More definitive recommendations on the use of pressure immobilization in viperid envenoming must await further research and clinical reports.

Respiratory and cardiovascular status should be supported to the extent possible under field conditions. If the time to reach medical care is prolonged and nausea and vomiting are not present, the victim should be encouraged to drink frequent, small volumes of clear, nonalcoholic liquids to support intravascular volume.

Other first-aid measures occasionally recommended for snakebites lack sufficient laboratory or clinical evidence to prove their effectiveness. Using any sharp instrument to incise fang marks in the field does more harm than good by exacerbating local bleeding (especially in the face of coagulopathy), introducing bacteria into the wound under nonsterile conditions, and further devascularizing the wound when perfusion may already be impaired. Applying mechanical suction to the wound using a device such as the Extractor (Sawyer Products, Safety Harbor, Fla; Figure 39-30) without incising the bite may remove a small percentage of venom from the site.[4,5] Further description of the Extractor, including controversies regarding its use, is found in Chapter 38. Measures such as local cooling, electric shock, and the application of topical agents should be avoided because they lack ef-

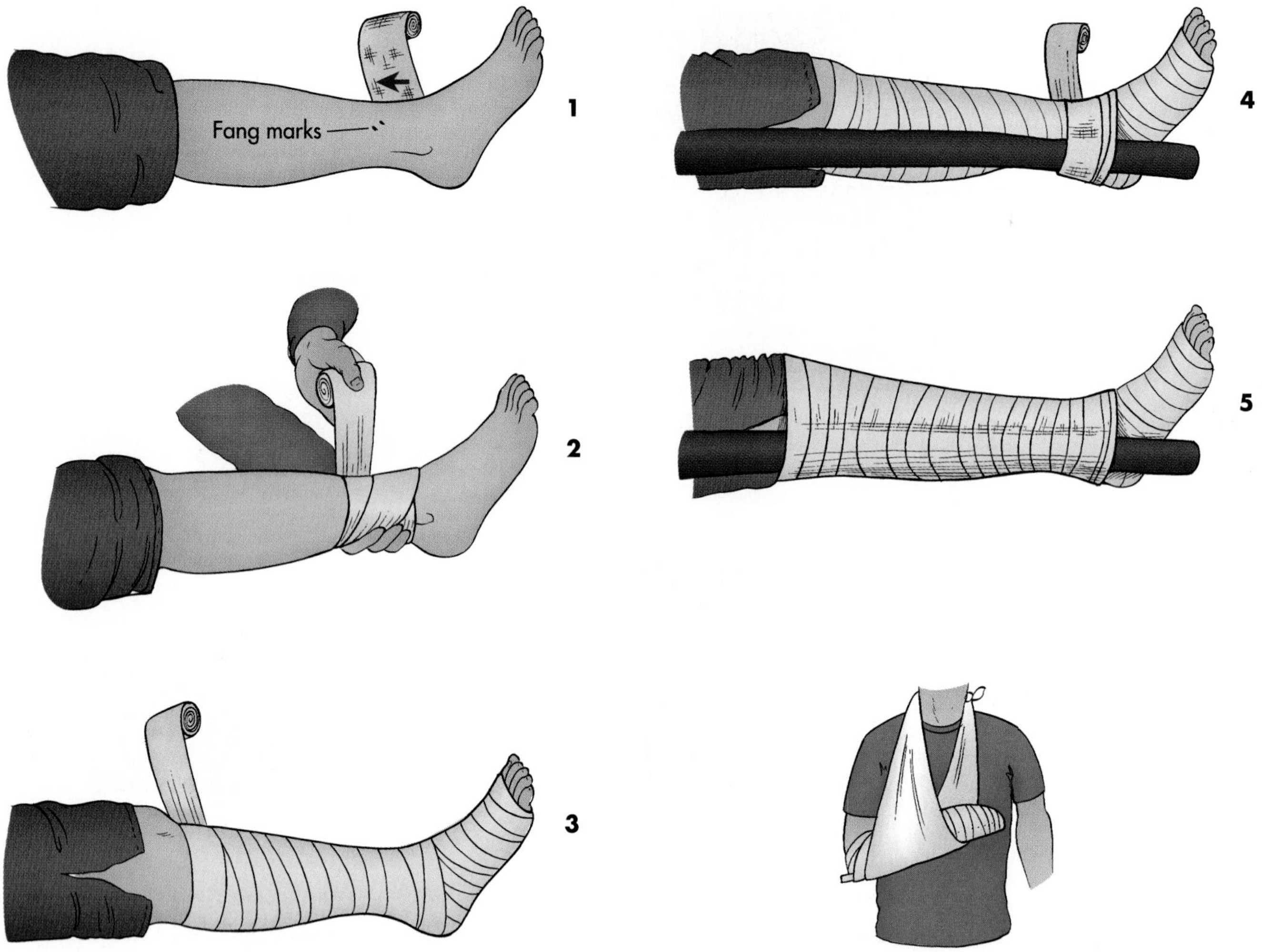

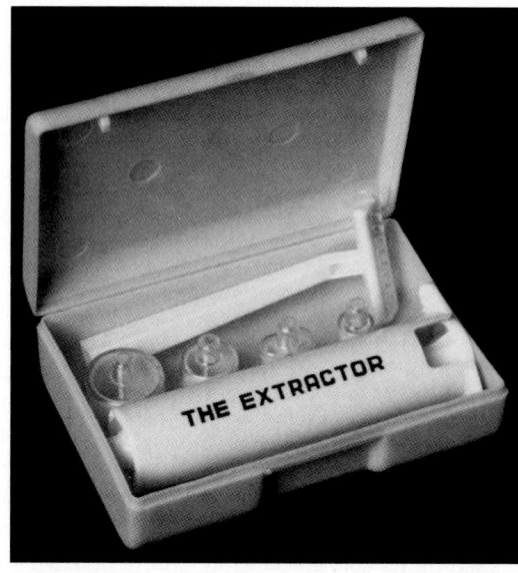

1

2

3

4

5

Figure 39-29 Australian compression and immobilization technique has proved effective in the management of elapid and sea snake envenomations. Its efficacy in viper bites has yet to be evaluated clinically.

Figure 39-30 The Extractor device. The efficacy of this device for applying mechanical suction to snakebites in the field continues to be studied.

ficacy and may actually worsen local tissue damage or the overall clinical outcome. Cold application may drive deleterious venom components deeper into tissues[60] (see Chapter 38).

Evacuating a snakebite victim from a remote field situation can be problematic.[44] The key principles are applying potentially effective first-aid measures (reassurance, splinting, with or without mechanical suction or pressure immobilization), transporting the victim to medical care as soon as possible, and limiting the victim's physical activity to minimize cardiac output and systemic circulation of venom. If the victim is alone and unlikely to be found for several hours, he or she should attempt to hike out, pausing for frequent rest stops and maintaining oral intake of fluids. If a lower extremity is involved, a crutch can be improvised to assist ambulation. If a single companion is present and prompt transportation to medical care is unavailable, first-aid measures should be applied and the victim placed at rest. If unconscious, the victim should be placed in a *recovery position* (left lateral decubitus position with the head downhill and the left

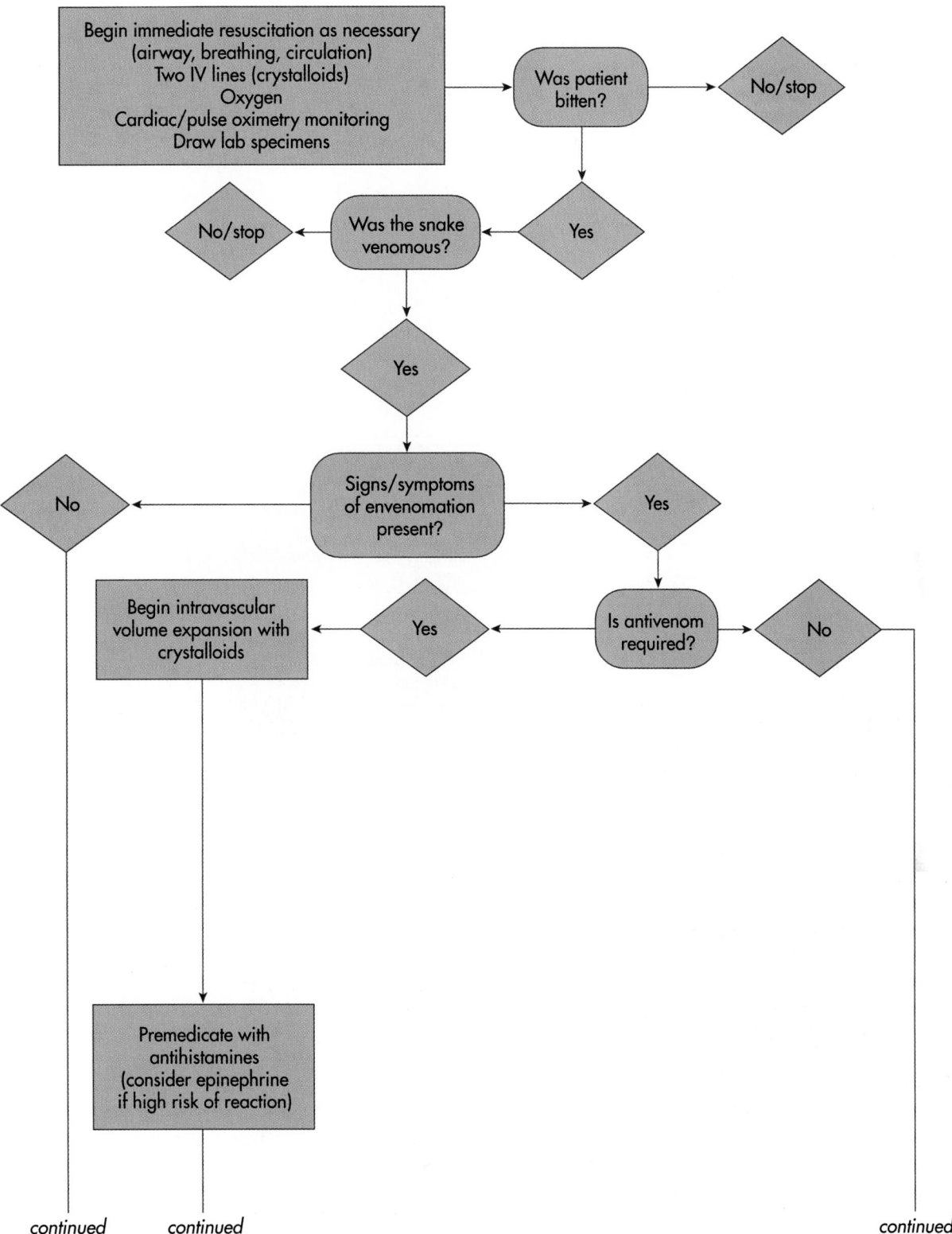

Figure 39-31 Guidelines for the hospital management of venomous snakebite.

knee bent) to keep the airway open and decrease the risk of aspiration. The companion can then hike out in search of help. Any plan to carry the victim out must taken into account the local terrain, weather conditions, and overall distance (see Chapters 25 to 27).

Hospital Care

Initial hospital management of a victim of snake venom poisoning should involve assessment of respiratory and cardiovascular status (Figure 39-31). A patient with significant respiratory distress or in extremis should be

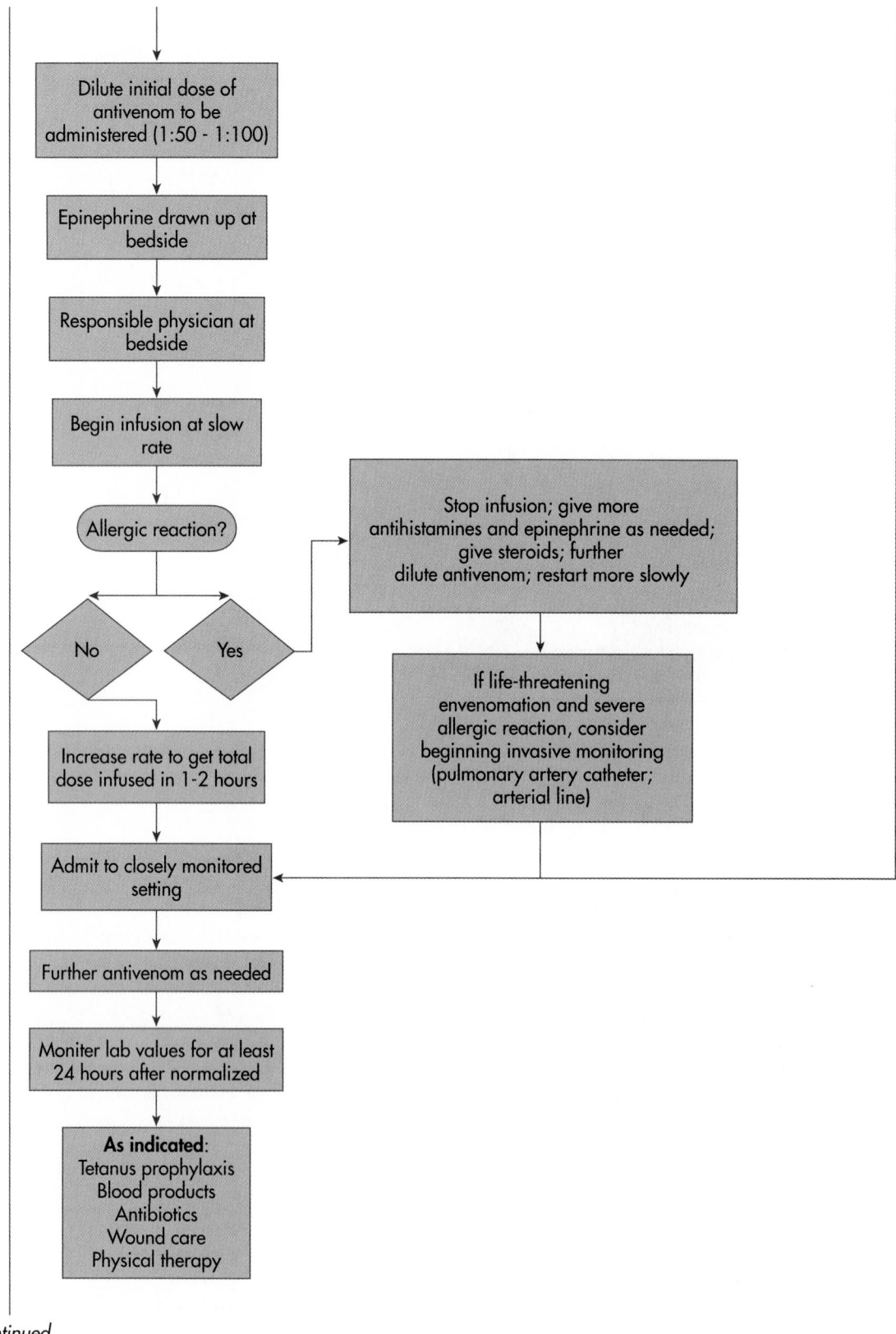

Dilute initial dose of antivenom to be administered (1:50 - 1:100)

Epinephrine drawn up at bedside

Responsible physician at bedside

Begin infusion at slow rate

Allergic reaction?

No

Yes

Stop infusion; give more antihistamines and epinephrine as needed; give steroids; further dilute antivenom; restart more slowly

If life-threatening envenomation and severe allergic reaction, consider beginning invasive monitoring (pulmonary artery catheter; arterial line)

Increase rate to get total dose infused in 1-2 hours

Admit to closely monitored setting

Further antivenom as needed

Moniter lab values for at least 24 hours after normalized

As indicated:
Tetanus prophylaxis
Blood products
Antibiotics
Wound care
Physical therapy

continued

Figure 39-31, cont'd

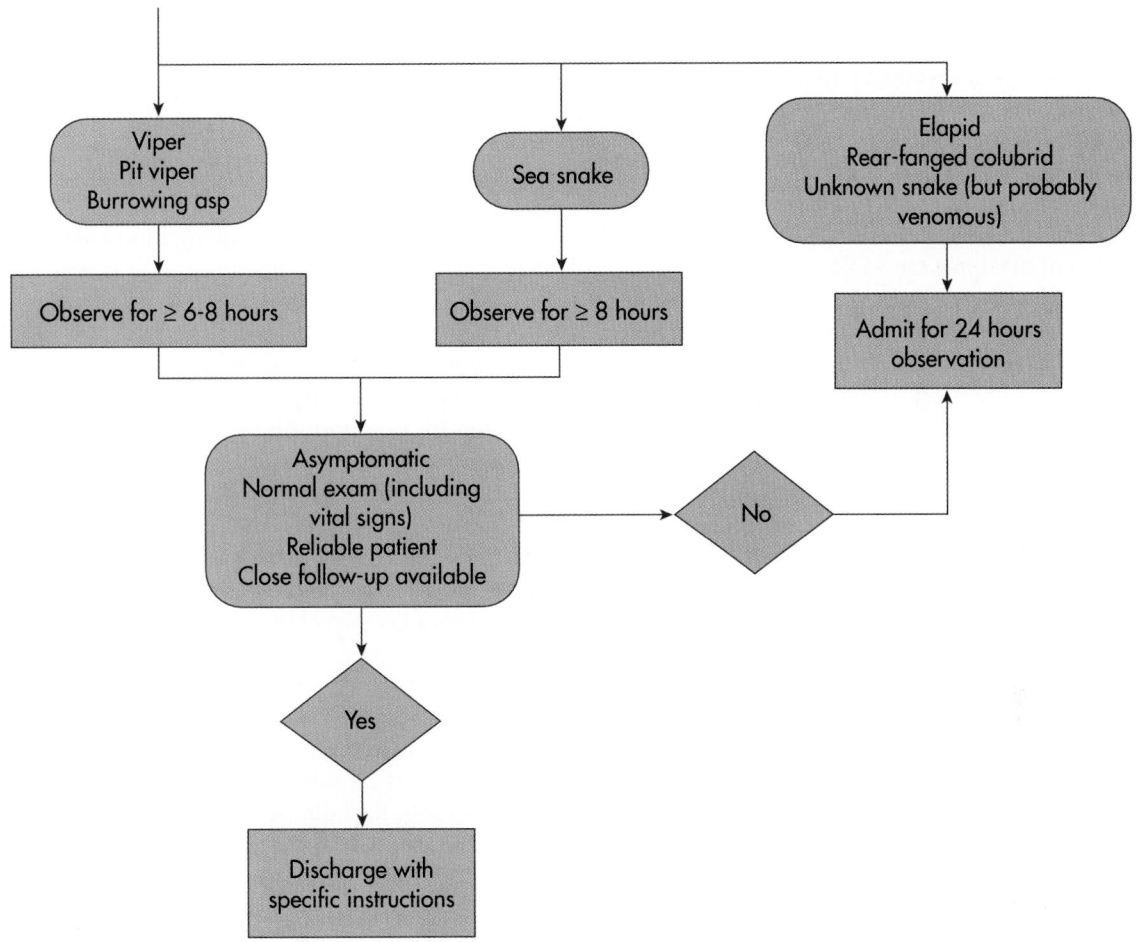

Figure 39-31, cont'd

promptly intubated to support ventilation and prevent aspiration.

Oxygen should be administered to all victims while rapid assessment takes place. Cardiac and pulse oximetry monitoring should be started. If intubation is required, the treating physician should choose the most familiar method. Nasotracheal intubation may be considered, but epistaxis is a risk in victims with coagulopathy. Rapid sequence intubation (RSI) uses sedative-hypnotics and paralytic agents to facilitate oral intubation and is safe and effective. The depolarizing neuromuscular agent succinylcholine should be avoided in RSI of a victim with potential hyperkalemia (e.g., sea snake bite). A nondepolarizing agent, such as vecuronium or rocuronium, can be substituted.

Hypotension is treated initially with intravenous (IV) fluids. Crystalloid, such as Ringer's lactate or normal saline, should be started through at least two large-bore IV lines. Having two lines also allows simultaneous administration of fluids, drugs, and antivenom when indicated. If hypotension persists after the rapid infusion of approximately 2 L of crystalloid in an adult

or 20 to 40 ml/kg in a child, then 5% albumin should be added. Animal research has demonstrated an improvement in physiologic parameters and survival with the use of albumin compared with crystalloids and dextran.[64] Vasopressors should be used only after intravascular volume has been restored. The inappropriate use of vasopressors when volume is required leads to prolonged hypotension, multiple organ failure, and preventable deaths.[25]

If a victim reports being bitten by a snake but appears well, providers must first determine whether the snake is venomous. Identifying the venomous species indigenous to an area is important. Hospital emergency wards should maintain color photographs of the local snake species to aid in identification. The keeper of an exotic snake involved in a bite probably knows its identity, although an amateur hobbiest may know the snake only by its common name. Common names are extremely variable and often applied to a number of unrelated species of snakes. Assistance in definitive identification may be obtained from a local zoo, university, or museum with a herpetologist on staff.

If the snake has been identified as venomous and the victim remains asymptomatic, a careful search for puncture wounds should be made. With bites by sea snakes and smaller venomous snakes, such as coral snakes, identifying fang marks can be difficult.[54,79]

Many bites by venomous snakes occur without injection of venom. These dry bites occur in 20% to 30% of viper bites and 50% to 70% of elapid bites.[37,68] The incidence of dry bites reaches approximately 75% with sea snakes[37] and is even higher with rear-fanged colubrids.[47] A careful history regarding current symptoms and a rapid physical examination looking for abnormalities should be performed. Careful evaluation and monitoring of the victim's vital signs are important. If a pressure immobilization device has been applied in the field and the patient is asymptomatic, it should be removed (after IV access has been secured and appropriate antivenom has been located) to assess the bitten extremity. If obvious signs of envenomation develop, the device should be immediately reapplied and left in place until antivenom administration has begun. If a totally occlusive vascular tourniquet has been applied in the field, a looser constriction band (only tight enough to impede superficial venous and lymphatic return) should be applied more proximally and IV access secured. The arterial tourniquet can then be removed while closely observing the victim for possible deterioration as stagnant, acidotic blood (with or without venom) is released to the central circulation. If signs of significant envenomation are present on arrival, appropriate antivenom administration should begin before removal of any pressure immobilization device or constriction band. Tourniquets are best replaced by constriction bands as soon as possible, however, to avoid adding ischemic insult to venom-induced tissue damage.

Snake venom detection kits are available in Australia and in other regions to help detect the presence of venom in a bitten individual and identify the offending indigenous species.[59,73] This technique, which is both sensitive and specific, uses an enzyme-linked immunosorbent assay (ELISA) to identify venom in tissue fluid taken from the bite site or in the victim's urine. The test is less reliable using blood samples.[93]

The severity of envenomation is assessed. If the victim shows signs of cardiovascular collapse or respiratory distress, prompt action is needed, including antivenom administration. If the patient appears stable, however, the approach is more complicated. Snake venom poisoning is a dynamic process, so a patient who looks well may suddenly develop respiratory distress and hypotension. The physician must anticipate multisystem involvement after snake venom poisoning and be prepared for deterioration in the victim's clinical status. Furthermore, with some snake species, many hours may pass before significant signs or symptoms appear.

The history and physical examination help determine severity. The bitten extremity should be marked at two proximal locations and the circumferences at these sites monitored every 15 minutes for progressive swelling. Rapidly progressive edema indicates a worsening clinical situation. Lack of swelling, however, does not rule out significant venom poisoning.

Laboratory evaluations are also important in judging severity (Box 39-3). A complete blood cell count may reveal a drop in hematocrit with significant bleeding or hemolysis or evidence of hemoconcentration as intravascular fluids leak into soft tissues. Leukocytosis is common, and platelet count may reflect consumptive coagulopathy. The peripheral blood smear may reveal microangiopathic hemolysis. A sample for blood typ-

---

Box 39-3 DIAGNOSTIC STUDIES IN EVALUATION OF VENOMOUS SNAKEBITE VICTIMS

BLOOD AND SERUM

Type and cross-match
Complete blood cell count
Peripheral smear
Coagulation studies (fibrinogen, fibrin degradation products, D-dimer, partial thromboplastin time, prothrombin time)
Electrolytes, glucose, creatinine, blood urea nitrogen, liver enzymes, bilirubin
Arterial blood gases
Myoglobin, creatine kinase

URINE

Bedside tests (glucose, blood, myoglobin [on each voided specimen])
Urinalysis

STOOL

Test for blood

RADIOGRAPHS

Chest (if over 40 years old, history of underlying cardiopulmonary disease, or severe envenomation)
Bite site soft tissue films (if retained fangs possible; poor sensitivity)
Computed tomography of the brain (if presentation suggests intracranial hemorrhage)

ELECTROCARDIOGRAM

If patient is over 40 years old, has a history of underlying cardiopulmonary disease, or has a severe envenomation

ing and screening should be obtained as soon as possible, since both venom toxins and antivenom may later interfere with this procedure. Blood coagulation studies (prothrombin time, partial thromboplastin time, fibrinogen level, fibrin degradation products) can aid in gauging severity in species known to induce coagulopathy. Urine samples should be checked at the bedside with reagent strips for the presence of blood. If positive, formal urinalysis and measurement of urine myoglobin should be performed as well. Stool should be tested for gross or occult blood. Baseline electrolyte and renal function studies are important when hyperkalemia and renal failure are potential complications. Liver function parameters help assess hepatic toxicity. Creatine kinase level, as a marker for myotoxicity, may help determine the presence of envenomation. If elevated, cardiac markers should also be checked to rule out myocardial involvement. If systemic poisoning is evident, an electrocardiogram and chest radiograph should also be obtained. Arterial blood gases should be measured and followed if there is evidence of respiratory involvement or circulatory embarrassment. Signs or symptoms of intracranial bleeding should prompt computed tomographic scanning.

The key principles of treating significant snake venom poisoning are sound supportive care of the victim's physiologic status and the use of appropriate antivenom when available. Antivenoms are available for the vast majority of the world's medically important venomous snakes. Although most antivenoms are still of equine origin, an increasing number of countries are putting ovine Fab or Fab$_2$ antivenoms into clinical use. These antivenoms appear to have an increased safety profile in regard to allergic phenomena and may be more effective than their equine predecessors (see Chapters 38 and 40).[18,33]

Currently, no specific antivenom exists for *Atractaspis* species, and the majority of these bites follow a benign clinical course.[76] Likewise, no antivenoms for colubrid envenomations are widely available, although antivenoms against *Dispholidus typus* and *Rhabdophis tigrinus* venoms are produced in South Africa and Japan, respectively. Management of envenomation by burrowing asps and colubrids relies almost entirely on sound supportive care. The bitten extremity should be splinted and elevated. Mild analgesics may be required in some cases, and antibiotics are indicated if secondary infection occurs. If a coagulopathy develops, careful assessment of the coagulation status of the patient is vital. Fresh-frozen plasma may replace depleted coagulation factors,[51,62] and blood products may be needed to counter a declining hematocrit. However, adding fuel to an ongoing consumptive coagulopathy may exacerbate intravascular clotting.[42] IV steroids (hydrocortisone, 15 mg/kg/day) and aminocaproic acid (70 mg/kg initially, then 15 mg/kg/day) have been bene-

ficial in some cases.[40] The use of heparin for intravascular coagulation has also been recommended but is controversial.[38,66] These modalities have no effect on any direct venom toxicity to the vasculature or internal organs.[51]

For an antivenom to be effective in snake venom poisoning, it must contain antibodies to the specific deleterious antigens present in the offending snake's venom. In regions where more than one antivenom is available to treat bites by various indigenous snakes, identifying the specific snake takes on added importance. In Australia, where multiple monospecific antivenoms are available, this task is aided by ELISA kits. In regions where the only antivenom available is a polyvalent product, identifying the specific snake is less critical as long as all medically important indigenous species are covered by the antivenom. In some situations, antivenom produced for a snake in a particular region may be largely ineffective in treating bites by the same species found in a different region because of significant differences in venom composition. Important examples include the carpet viper *(Echis carinatus)* and Russell's viper *(Daboia russellii)*. Bites by these species should be treated with antivenoms produced using snakes from the same geographic region as the responsible animal.[34]

Using an antivenom developed for unrelated species is generally of no benefit unless cross-protection has been previously demonstrated. Significant risk surrounds use of a heterologous antivenom, however, since all commercially available products carry some variable risks of allergic phenomena (see Chapter 40). In some instances, however, heterologous antivenoms have demonstrated significant cross-protection.[45] An excellent example of this is the efficacy of Commonwealth Serum Laboratory's tiger snake *(Notechis)* antivenom against sea snake venoms.[2,65,78] This should be considered the second-line agent to be used if specific sea snake antivenom is not available.[79] Further research and clinical experience will clarify the antigenic relationships between venoms of seemingly unrelated snake taxa, increasing the list of cross-protective antivenoms.

If there is a choice between a polyvalent antivenom developed to counter the effects of venom poisoning by several snake species found in a geographic area and a monovalent serum specific for one species of snake, the monovalent product should be used if the snake has been definitively identified. It will provide more specific protection with a smaller burden of extraneous, allergenic proteins ineffective against the offending snake's venom. Recommendations regarding antivenom choices can be obtained from experts in snake envenomation or from the *Antivenom Index*.[1,2] This resource contains a list of medically important snakes of the world (scientific and common names), recommended antivenoms for these species, a list of antivenom inventories maintained by participating institutions in the United States, and a list of manufacturers of antivenoms around the world.

Assistance in locating stocks of antivenom within the United States can be obtained by using the *Antivenom Index* or consulting the University of Arizona Poison and Drug Information Center (602-626-6016). Assistance in obtaining an appropriate, exotic antivenom may be obtained from law enforcement agencies or the military.

Once the decision has been made to administer antivenom and an appropriate agent has been obtained, preparations for administration should begin promptly. The patient's intravascular volume should be expanded using crystalloid infusion unless there is a contraindication (e.g., a history of congestive heart failure). Volume expansion may blunt a hypotensive response as a result of direct complement activation by antivenom proteins. An appropriate dose of 1:1000 aqueous epinephrine (0.01 ml/kg, up to 0.5 ml total) should be drawn up in a syringe and placed at the patient's bedside so that it is immediately available for subcutaneous or intramuscular injection if an allergic reaction occurs to the antivenom.

Although most antivenom manufacturers suggest an intradermal test for possible allergy to their product before infusion begins, these tests are extremely nonspecific and unreliable; a significant number of false positives and false negatives occur.[32,88] Furthermore, a positive skin test does not contraindicate the use of antivenom if a significant threat to life or limb exists. If indicated, antivenom should be administered without first performing any test for sensitivity. The treating physician should be at the patient's bedside during the initiation of the infusion in order to intervene immediately if a reaction occurs (see Chapter 40).

The antivenom package insert should be consulted in determining an appropriate starting dose. Antivenom can generally be withheld in an apparently dry bite or minor envenomation while the victim is closely observed for any development or progression of signs or symptoms. For a few species of snakes, antivenom should be administered after *any* bite by an identified specimen regardless of whether symptoms or signs are present. Examples include bites by kraits (*Bungarus* spp.) or large (greater than 50 cm in length) coral snakes (*Micrurus* spp.). Once symptoms begin in these scenarios, they may be difficult to stop even with antivenom.

The potency of different antivenoms is variable, and it is difficult to make general recommendations regarding dosages. For many antivenoms, 20 to 50 ml (further diluted as above) is a reasonable starting dose in treating moderately severe poisoning. In a severe envenomation, especially with evidence of neurotoxicity, 100

to 150 ml is more appropriate.[59] If signs and symptoms or laboratory abnormalities continue to progress after the initial dose is given, more antivenom should be administered. Children should receive the same starting doses as adults or even higher, since children receive larger doses of venom in proportion to their body surface area and intravascular volume.[50,59] In the future, antivenom dosing may be guided by ELISA techniques that quantitate circulating venom.[9]

Before antivenom infusion the patient should be premedicated with IV antihistamines. Fifty to 100 mg of diphenhydramine (1 to 2 mg/kg in children) and 300 mg of cimetidine (5 to 10 mg/kg in children) or equivalent agents can be given. Where antivenom is clearly needed and risk of anaphylaxis is increased (e.g., history of allergy to horses, prior reaction to antivenom), premedicating the patient with a small dose of subcutaneous 1:1000 epinephrine (0.3 ml in adults, 0.01 ml/kg in children) can be considered if there are no contraindications (e.g., coronary artery disease, severe hypertension).

The total antivenom dose to be administered should be added to a bag of diluent (5% dextrose in water or crystalloid) at a dilution of 1:50 to 1:100. The infusion should be begun intravenously at a very slow rate (a few milliliters per minute) with the physician in attendance. If no reaction occurs after a few minutes, the rate can be progressively increased so that the total dose is administered in approximately 1 to 2 hours. If the patient is in extremis, however, the infusion should be more rapid. Antivenom should not be administered by local or intramuscular injection, because it is less effective by these routes, and if a reaction occurs, the drug cannot be discontinued.[11]

If an early reaction occurs, the antivenom should be temporarily halted and the reaction treated (see Chapter 38). The infusion can then usually be restarted at a slower rate. Further diluting the antivenom may also be helpful.

Patients who receive equine antivenom are at risk for immune complex–mediated delayed serum sickness, usually 1 to 2 weeks after administration. This risk increases in direct proportion to the total dose of antivenom administered.

Victims definitely envenomed, particularly those requiring antivenom, should be admitted for close cardiopulmonary monitoring for a minumum of 24 hours and until overall stability is achieved. Any abnormal laboratory values should be remeasured frequently for at least 24 to 48 hours or until normalized. Delayed coagulopathy after antivenom treatment may result from delayed release of venom from depot sites such as skin blisters.[59]

Persons who remain asymptomatic after being bitten by venomous snakes create challenging disposition decisions. If a viperid snake is implicated in such a bite, it is usually safe to discharge the victim after 6 hours of close observation, provided the clinical picture remains normal. For sea snakes, 8 hours is reasonable; for elapids, 24 hours is safer.[11,79] Suspected boomslang (*Dispholidus typus*), bird snake, or twig snake (*Thelotornis* spp.) bites should be observed in the hospital for 24 hours. If coagulation studies remain normal at that time, the patient can be discharged.

If discharged, the person should be instructed about bed rest for 24 hours, increased fluid intake, and monitoring for symptoms, such as increased pain, swelling, dizziness, shortness of breath, numbness, and weakness. Follow-up within 24 hours should be arranged for reevaluation.

With evidence of clinically significant bleeding in the patient with a coagulopathy, administration of appropriate blood products should be considered. Antivenom should be started if possible before blood products are given to stop the continued activation and depletion of coagulation factors. Many viperid bites have laboratory evidence of coagulopathy *without* significant clinical hemorrhage.[46,57] Such cases can be treated with antivenom, bed rest, and close observation while withholding blood products.

Other treatment modalities for snake venom poisoning have demonstrated variable anecdotal benefit, but they do not replace proper conservative care and appropriate antivenom use. Edrophonium and neostigmine, for example, can temporarily reverse neuromuscular blockade after cobra envenomation.[59,75,87] These agents must be used cautiously because either may stimulate cholingeric crisis. Edrophonium combined with atropine might be effective in reversing respiratory muscle weakness in a victim of cobra or krait bite when antivenom is not immediately available. Attempts to temporize in a patient with impending respiratory failure can result in aspiration.[35] It is best to proceed with prompt endotracheal intubation before frank respiratory failure occurs.

Ethylenediaminetetraacetic acid (EDTA) has been touted as an inhibitor of snake venom proteases,[46,60] but its clinical efficacy has not been demonstrated. In fact, increased mortality occurred in animal models when EDTA was given intravenously to treat pit viper venom poisoning.[60]

Other modalities recommended in the past without evidence to support routine use include topical agents (e.g., potassium permanganate) to "deactivate" venom; routine fasciotomy of the bitten extremity (see following discussion); immediate exploration, debridement, or excision of the bite site; administration of heparin to counter disseminated intravascular coagulation; and high-dose steroids. Renal failure can best be prevented by aggressively treating hypotension, maintaining adequate urine output, and using antivenom appropriately. Myoglobinuria should be treated in standard fashion with sodium bicarbonate, mannitol, or loop diuretics. If renal failure develops, care should be directed at maintaining proper electrolyte balance. Peritoneal dialysis or hemodialysis is often required in such cases. Hemodialysis has been anecdotally reported to improve peripheral muscle weakness in victims of severe sea snake envenomation with acute renal failure, probably by reversing hyperkalemic and uremic effects on venom-damaged muscle fibers.[65] Dialysis does not remove circulating venom components, however, and the indications for dialysis are the same as for any other cause of acute renal failure.

Wound care of the bitten extremity should be provided (see Chapter 38). Although controversial, broad-spectrum antibiotics may be used prophylactically for a few days in victims with significant potential for necrosis in an attempt to limit secondary infection. Although the incidence of such infection is low,[13] the risks increase after misdirected attempts to incise or open the bite site under field conditions.[94] Early physical therapy aimed at returning the bitten extremity to its maximal level of function is important, especially in patients with significant soft tissue swelling or necrosis.

If concerned about compartment syndrome, the physician should measure intracompartmental pressures using an appropriate device. Sustained pressures greater than 30 to 40 mm Hg in a normotensive patient may exceed capillary perfusion pressure in the muscles. Ischemia may result if the situation is not addressed, usually by means of a fasciotomy. The pressure at which ischemia ensues is even lower in hypotensive snakebite victims, and the threshold for performing a fasciotomy may need to be lowered in this setting. The overall incidence of compartment syndromes after venomous snakebite, however, is low.[17,23,86] Prophylactic fasciotomies in patients without objectively documented elevated intracompartmental pressures are inappropriate.

The management of a victim with ocular exposure to spitting cobra venom begins with immediate and copious irrigation of the eyes with any readily available, nonirritating fluid.[59,84] Prompt treatment may help prevent local complications. Close ophthalmologic follow-up is important to rule out corneal ulceration or uveitis.

ACTIVE IMMUNIZATION

Rituals and techniques for immunization against snake venom have been practiced for centuries in various parts of the world.[49] More recently, modern immunologic methods have been used. Beginning in 1965, 43,446 individuals in the Ryukyu Islands of Japan, an area of high snakebite incidence, were immunized with habu (*Trimeresurus flavoviridis*) venom toxoid. Follow-up after about 5 years indicated equivocal results, and no further large-scale trials were undertaken, but experimental work continues. Individuals have also been immunized against other snake venoms.[63,77]

MORTALITY

Although mortality rates vary greatly throughout the world, more than 95% of deaths from snakebites occur in underdeveloped countries with inadequate or remote medical resources.[9] The causes of death in fatal cases of elapid envenomation are respiratory paralysis, coagulopathy, renal failure, and cardiac failure.[11,60,92] In viperid-related fatalities the cause is usually protracted hypovolemic shock.[11] This is often related to inadequate fluid resuscitation, inappropriate use of vasopressors, or inadequate or delayed use of antivenom. Sea snake fatalities are related to respiratory failure, cardiac arrhythmias, or renal failure.[7,59,79] The average time to death after envenomation is 5 hours in elapid bites, 2 to 3 days in viperid bites, and 12 to 24 hours in sea snake bites.[58]

REFERENCES

1. American Zoo and Aquarium Association, American Association of Poison Control Centers: *Antivenom index*, Silver Springs, Md, 1999.
2. Baxter EH, Gallichio HA: Cross-neutralization by tiger snake (*Notechis scutatus*) antivenine and sea snake (*Enhydrina schistosa*) antivenine against several sea snake venoms, *Toxicon* 12:273, 1974.
3. Bdolah A: The venom glands of snakes and venom secretion. In Lee CY, editor: *Snake venoms*, Berlin, 1979, Springer-Verlag.
4. Bronstein AC, Russell FE, Sullivan JB: Negative pressure suction in the field treatment of rattlesnake bite victims, *Vet Hum Toxicol* 28:485, 1986 (abstract).
5. Bronstein AC et al: Negative pressure suction in field treatment of rattlesnake bite, *Vet Hum Toxicol* 28:297, 1985 (abstract).
6. Cable D et al: Prolonged defibrillation after a bite from a "nonvenomous" snake, *JAMA* 251:925, 1984.
7. Carey JE, Wright EA: The site of action of the venom of the sea snake *Enhydrina schistosa*, *Trans R Soc Trop Med Hyg* 55:153, 1961.
8. Chajek T et al: Anaphylactoid reaction and tissue damage following bite by *Atractaspis engaddensis*, *Trans R Soc Trop Med Hyg* 68:333, 1974.
9. Chippaux JP: Production and use of snake antivenin. Vol 5 in Tu AT, editor: *Handbook of natural toxins: reptile venoms and toxins*, New York, 1991, Marcel Dekker.
10. Chippaux JP: Snake-bites: appraisal of the global situation, *Bull WHO* 76:515, 1998.
11. Christensen PA: The treatment of snakebite, *S Afr Med J* 43:1253, 1969.
12. Chugh KS, Sakhuja V: Renal disease caused by snake venom. Vol 5 in Tu AT, editor: *Handbook of natural toxins: reptile venoms and toxins*, New York, 1991, Marcel Dekker.
13. Clark RF, Selden BS, Furbee B: The incidence of wound infection following crotalid envenomation, *J Emerg Med* 11:583, 1993.
14. Corkill NL, Ionides CJP, Pitman CRS: Biting and poisoning by the mole vipers of the genus *Atractaspis*, *Trans R Soc Trop Med Hyg* 53:95, 1959.
15. Corkill NL, Kirk R: Poisoning by the Sudan mole viper *Atractaspis microlepidota* Gunther, *Trans R Soc Trop Med Hyg* 48:376, 1954.
16. Currie B, Theakston D, Warrell D: Envenoming from the Papuan taipan (*Oxyuranus scutellatus canni*), *Toxicon* 30:501, 1992.
17. Curry SC et al: Noninvasive vascular studies in management of rattlesnake envenomations to extremities, *Ann Emerg Med* 14:1081, 1985.
18. Dart RC et al: Affinity-purified, mixed monoclonal specific crotalid antivenom ovine Fab for the treatment of crotalid venom poisoning, *Ann Emerg Med* 30:33, 1997.
19. Davidson TM, Schafer SF, Moseman J: Central and South American pit vipers, *J Wilderness Med* 4:416, 1993.
20. Ferlan I et al: Preliminary studies on the venom of the colubrid snake *Rhabdophis subminiatus* (red-necked keelback), *Toxicon* 21:570, 1983.
21. Fitzsimons DC, Smith HM: Another rear-fanged South African snake lethal to humans, *Herpetologica* 14:198, 1958.
22. Ganthavorn S: A case of king cobra bite, *Toxicon* 9:293, 1971.
23. Garfin SR: Rattlesnake bites: current hospital therapy, *West J Med* 137:411, 1982.
24. Gunders AE, Walter HJ, Etzel E: Case of snake-bite by *Atractaspis corpulenta*, *Trans R Soc Trop Med Hyg* 54:279, 1960.
25. Hardy DL: Fatal rattlesnake envenomation in Arizona: 1969-1984, *Clin Toxicol* 24:1, 1986.
26. Hardy DL: *Bothrops asper* (Viperidae) snakebite and field researchers in Middle America, *Biotropica* 26:198, 1994.
27. Hardy DL, Bush SP: Pressure/immobilization as first aid for venomous snakebite in the United States, *Herpetol Rev* 29:204, 1998.
28. Hood VL, Johnson JR: Acute failure with myoglobinuria following tiger snake bite, *Aust NZ J Med* 4:415, 1974.
29. Hurwitz BJ, Hull PR: Berg adder bite, *S Afr Med J* 45:969, 1971.
30. Jenkins M, Russell FE: Physical therapy for snake venom poisoning, *Phys Ther* 54:1298, 1974.
31. Jeyarajah R: Russell's viper bite in Sri Lanka: a study of 22 cases, *Am J Trop Med Hyg* 33:506, 1984.
32. Jurkovich GJ et al: Complications of Crotalidae antivenin therapy, *J Trauma* 28:1032, 1988.
33. Karlson-Stiber C et al: First clinical experience with specific sheep Fab fragments in snake bite: report of a multicentre study of *Vipera berus* envenoming, *J Intern Med* 241:53, 1997.
34. Kemparaju K, Prasad BN, Gowda VT: Purification of a basic phospholipase A$_2$ from Indian saw-scaled viper (*Echis carinatus*) venom: characterization of antigenic, catalytic and pharmacological properties, *Toxicon* 32:1187, 1994.
35. Kitchens CS, Van Mierop LHS: Envenomation by the eastern coral snake (*Micrurus fulvius fulvius*): a study of 39 victims, *JAMA* 258:1615, 1987.
36. Kochva E: The origin of snakes and evolution of the venom apparatus, *Toxicon* 25:65, 1987.
37. Kunkel DB et al: Reptile envenomations, *J Toxicol Clin Toxicol* 21:503, 1983-84.
38. Lakier JB, Fritz VU: Consumptive coagulopathy caused by a boomslang bite, *S Afr Med J* 43:1052, 1969.
39. Lee S et al: Coronary vasospasm as the primary cause of death due to the venom of the burrowing asp, *Atractaspis engaddensis*, *Toxicon* 24:285, 1986.
40. Mandell F et al: Major coagulopathy and "nonpoisonous" snake bites, *Pediatrics* 65:314, 1980.
41. Mather HM, Mayne S, McMonagle TM: Severe envenomation from "harmless" pet snake, *Br Med J* 1(6123):1324, 1978.
42. Mebs D et al: A fatal case of snake bite due to *Thelotornis kirtlandii*. In Rosenberg P, editor: *Toxins: animal, plant and microbial*, Oxford, 1978, Pergamon Press.
43. Meier J, Stocker KF: Biology and distribution of venomous snakes of medical importance and the composition of snake venoms. In Meier J, White J, editors: *Handbook of clinical toxicology of animal venoms and poisons*, Boca Raton, Fla, 1995, CRC Press.
44. Mellor NH, Arvin JC: A bushmaster bite during a birding expedition in lowland southeastern Peru, *Wild Environmental Med* 7(3):236, 1996.
45. Minton SA: Paraspecific protection by elapid and sea snake antivenins, *Toxicon* 5:47, 1967.
46. Minton SA: *Venom diseases*, Springfield, Ill, 1974, Charles C Thomas.
47. Minton SA: Venomous bites by nonvenomous snakes: an annotated bibliography of colubrid envenomation, *J Wilderness Med* 1:119, 1990.
48. Minton SA: Bites by non-native venomous snakes in the United States, *Wilderness Environ Med* 7:297, 1996.
49. Minton SA, Minton MR: *Venomous reptiles*, New York, 1980, Scribners.
50. Mitrakul C et al: Clinical features of neurotoxic snake bite and response to antivenom in 47 children, *Am J Trop Med Hyg* 33:1258, 1984.
51. Mittleman MB, Goris RC: Death caused by the bite of the Japanese colubrid snake *Rhabdophis tigrinus* (Boie) (Reptilia, Serpentes, Colubridae), *J Herpetol* 12:109, 1978.
52. Montgomery J: Two cases of ophthalmoplegia due to Berg adder bite, *Cent Afr J Med* 5:173, 1959.
53. Myint-Lwin et al: Bites by Russell's viper (*Vipera russelli siamensis*) in Burma: haemostatic, vascular, and renal disturbances and response to treatment, *Lancet* 2:1259, 1985.
54. Norris RL, Dart RC: Apparent coral snake envenomation in a patient without fang marks, *Am J Emerg Med* 7:402, 1989.
55. Ohsaka A: Hemorrhagic, necrotizing, and edema-forming effects of snake venoms. In Lee CY, editor: *Snake venoms*, Berlin, 1979, Springer-Verlag.
56. Parrish HM: *Poisonous snakebites in the United States*, New York, 1980, Vantage Press.

57. Prentice CRM: Acquired coagulation disorders, *Clin Haematol* 14:413, 1985.

58. Reid HA, Lim KJ: Sea-snake bite: a survey of fishing villages in northwest Malaya, *Br Med J* 2:1266, 1957.

59. Reid HA, Theakston RDG: The management of snake bite, *Bull WHO* 61:885, 1983.

60. Russell FE: *Snake venom poisoning*, New York, 1983, Scholium International.

61. Russell FE et al: Snakes and snakebite in Central America, *Toxicon* 35:1469, 1997.

62. Saddler M, Paul B: Vine snake envenomation, *Cent Afr J Med* 34:31, 1988.

63. Sawai Y: Vaccination against snake bite poisoning. In Lee CY, editor: *Snake venoms*, Berlin, 1979, Springer-Verlag.

64. Schaeffer RC et al: The effects of colloidal and crystalloidal fluids on rattlesnake venom shock in the rat, *J Pharmacol Exp Ther* 206:687, 1978.

65. Sitprija V, Sribhibhadh R, Benyajati C: Haemodialysis in poisoning by sea-snake venom, *Br Med J* 3:218, 1971.

66. Spies SK, Malherbe LF: Boomslangbyt met afibriongnemie, *S Afr Med J* 36:834, 1962.

67. Stueven H et al: Cobra envenomation: an uncommon emergency, *Ann Emerg Med* 12:636, 1983.

68. Sutherland SK: Mr Ram Chandra and snakebite, *Med J Aust* 1:457, 1979.

69. Sutherland SK: Pressure immobilization for snakebite in southern Africa remains

70. Sutherland SK, Coulter AR: Early management of bites by the eastern diamondback rattlesnake (*Crotalus adamanteus*): studies in monkeys (*Macaca fascicularis*), *Am J Trop Med Hyg* 30:497, 1981.

71. Sutherland SK, King K: *Management of snake-bite injuries*, Hurstville, 1991, Royal Flying Doctor Service of Australia, speculative. South African Med J 85:1039, 1995.

72. Swaroop S, Grab B: Snakebite mortality in the world, *Bull WHO* 10:35, 1954.

73. Theakston RDG: The application of immunoassay techniques, including enzyme-linked immunosorbent assay (ELISA), to snake venom research, *Toxicon* 21:341, 1983.

74. Theakston RDG, Warrell DA: Antivenoms: a list of hyperimmune sera currently available for the treatment of envenoming by bites and stings, *Toxicon* 29:1419, 1991.

75. Tiger ME, Brecher E, Bevan D: Cobra bite in Philadelphia, *Penn Med* 87:53, 1975.

76. Tilbury CR, Branch WR: Observations on the bite of the southern burrowing asp (*Atractaspis bibronii*) in Natal, *S Afr Med J* 75:327, 1989.

77. Toriba M, Sawai Y: Venomous snakes of medical importance in Japan. In Gopalakrishnakone P, Chou LM, editors: *Snakes of medical importance: Asia-Pacific region*, Singapore, 1990, Venom and Toxin Research Group, University of Singapore.

78. Tu A, Fulde G: Sea snake bites, *Clin Dermatol* 5:118, 1987.

79. Tu AT: Biotoxicology of sea snake venoms, *Ann Emerg Med* 16:1023, 1987.

80. Tun-Pe et al: Local compression pads as a first-aid measure for victims of bites by Russell's viper (*Daboia russellii siamensis*) in Myanmar, *Trans R Soc Trop Med Hyg* 89:293, 1995.

81. Van Mierop LHS: Poisonous snakebite: a review—snakes and their venom, *J Fla Med Assoc* 63:191, 1976.

82. Warrell DA: Tropical snake bite: clinical studies in Southeast Asia. Vol 1 in Harris JB, editor: *Natural toxins: animal, plant, microbial*, Oxford, 1986, Clarendon Press.

83. Warrell DA, Arnett C: The importance of bites by saw-scaled or carpet vipers (*Echis carinatus*): epidemiological studies in Nigeria and a review of world literature, *Acta Trop* 33:307, 1976.

84. Warrell DA, Ormerod LD, Davidson NM: Bites by the night adder (*Causus maculatus*) and burrowing vipers (genus *Atractaspis*) in Nigeria, *Am J Trop Med Hyg* 25:517, 1976.

85. Warrell DA et al: Necrosis, haemorrhage and complement depletion following bites by the spitting cobra (*Naja nigricollis*), *Q J Med* 45:1, 1976.

86. Watt CH: Treatment of poisonous snakebite with emphasis on digit dermotomy, *South Med J* 78:694, 1985.

87. Watt G et al: Positive response to edrophonium in patients with neurotoxic envenoming by cobras (*Naja naja philippinensis*): a placebo-controlled study, *N Engl J Med* 315:1444, 1986.

88. Weber RA, White RR: Crotalidae envenomation in children, *Hematol Oncol Clin North Am* 31:141, 1993.

89. Weinstein SA, Kardong KV: Properties of Duvernoy's secretions from opisthoglyphous and aglyphous colubrid snakes, *Toxicon* 32:1161, 1994.

90. Weiser E et al: Cardiotoxic effects of the venom of the burrowing asp, *Atractaspis engaddensis* (Atractaspididae, Ophidia), *Toxicon* 22:767, 1984.

91. Wetzel WW, Christy NP: A king cobra bite in New York City, *Toxicon* 27:393, 1989.

92. White J: Elapid snakes: venom toxicity and actions; aspects of envenomation; management of bites. In Covacevish J, Davis P, Pearn J, editors: *Toxic plants and animals: a guide for Australia*, Brisbane, 1987, Queensland Museum.

93. White J: Snakebite: an Australian perspective, *J Wilderness Med* 2:219, 1991.

94. Wingert WA, Chan L: Rattlesnake bites in southern California and rationale for recommended treatment, *West J Med* 148:37, 1988.

95. Wuster W, Golay P, Warrell DA: Synopsis of recent developments in venomous snake systematics, *Toxicon* 35:319, 1997.

40 Antivenins and Immunobiologicals: Immunotherapeutics of Envenomation

Rivka S. Horowitz and Richard C. Dart

The ideal therapeutic agent effectively treats or prevents a specific medical condition and is free of adverse effects. Commercially available antivenins (antivenoms) are not ideal. The vast majority of antivenins are equine derived and thus possess the potential adverse immunologic effects inherent in the administration of foreign proteins. Although antivenin lowers the morbidity and mortality associated with envenomation, it may have life-threatening side effects. As a result, many physicians are reluctant to administer antivenin even to patients who have a clear indication for its use.

Worldwide, more than 60 commercial laboratories produce almost 200 different antivenin preparations for the treatment of snake, arachnid, fish, and coelenterate envenomations. Theakston and Warrell[48] compiled a list of hyperimmune sera available for the treatment of venom poisoning.

The available crotalid antivenin in the United States is effective against all indigenous North American pit vipers. However, zoos and amateur snake enthusiasts are likely to house non-indigenous, exotic snakes for which the anticrotalid antivenin would be useless. Physicians must expeditiously exploit all available resources to identify and acquire the appropriate antivenins for unusual envenomations. One such resource, the *Antivenin Index*, is compiled by the American Association of Zoological Parks and Aquariums and the American Association of Poison Control Centers (AAPCC). The *Index* lists the location of foreign antivenins stocked by zoos in the United States. Guidance for use of these antivenins and general snakebite management may be obtained through an AAPCC-certified poison center.

PRINCIPLES OF ANTIVENIN THERAPY

Historical Perspective

Immunotherapy against snake venom dates to 1887 with the first report of successful immunization in birds. Sewall[39] reported that pigeons injected with increasing but sublethal doses of *Sistrurus catenatus catenatus* (Eastern massasauga) venom became resistant to venom inoculations seven times the lethal dose. Seven years later, contemporaneous experiments by Calmette[8] and Phisalix and Bertrand[33] demonstrated that immunization with cobra *(Naja naja)* and European viper *(Vipera berus)* venoms, respectfully, protected animals against inoculation with these venoms.

Within a decade of Sewall's landmark experiment, Calmette[9] produced the first therapeutic antivenin derived from immunizing horses with cobra venom. Although Calmette overestimated the effectiveness of his antivenin, erroneously believing that it would protect against all neurotoxic venoms,[8] he recognized an important principle of immunotherapy still operative today: interspecies cross-reactivity.

Another pioneer in the study and production of antivenin, Vital Brazil, further demonstrated both specificity and cross-reactivity through the production of numerous monospecific and polyspecific antivenins. A *monospecific* antivenin is derived from immunizing animals with the venom of a single species, whereas *polyspecific* antivenin is produced either by inoculating animals with the venom of more than one species or by pooling different monospecific antivenins into a final product. Brazil recognized the need for polyspecific antivenins, since snakebite victims were often unable to differentiate among the variety of poisonous snakes indigenous to an area.[14]

To ensure an adequate supply of venom for his research, Brazil organized a unique exchange network throughout the countryside of São Paulo, Brazil. He convinced government and railroad officials to allow free passage for snakes shipped to his institute and sent devices for snake capture and crates for transport to anyone requesting them. For every snake shipped to him, Brazil would send a vial of serum (antivenin); for every six snakes sent, he would provide a needle and syringe for administering the serum.[14] After more than a decade of operating his exchange, Brazil claimed a significant decrease in mortality from snakebites.[5,14]

Neutralizing Antibody

The foundation of antivenin therapy is the antigen-antibody interaction. The component of antivenin responsible for its therapeutic activity is the immunoglobulin G (IgG) antibody molecule. This neutralizing antibody inactivates the antigen by specific, noncovalent, antigen-antibody binding. Thus a neutralizing antibody to phospholipase A_2, a common constituent of snake venoms, prevents or attenuates the neurotoxic or myotoxic activity associated with this venom component.

Understanding the structure of IgG helps to explain both the mechanism of action and the adverse reactions of antivenins. An IgG molecule weighs approximately 150,000 daltons and is composed of two functional parts: the antigen-binding site, consisting of two Fab portions, and the effector site, or Fc region (Figure 40-1). Specific binding of the antigen to the Fab sites neutralizes further activity of the antigen. The Fc region of IgG is responsible for binding and activating immune system cells (e.g., phagocytes, macrophages, mast cells) and triggering a host of immunologic responses. These reactions, which include degranulation of mast cells and activation of the complement cascade, are partly responsible for the immediate, life-threatening allergic reactions to antivenin.

The large size of the IgG antibody has important implications for the immunogenicity, distribution, and elimination of these neutralizing antibodies. Large-molecular-weight entities in general (IgG and other large antivenin components) are more likely to trigger immunologic reactions than smaller ones.[49] The ideal neutralizing antibody would be expected to have a large volume of distribution, implying more extensive tissue penetration and access to venom components. The large size of IgG, however, confines it primarily to the intravascular space and may limit more extensive distribution into tissue compartments. Theoretically, this may limit the effectiveness of IgG in binding antigen within tissue compartments.

The large molecules that make up most antivenin proteins have long elimination half-lives, and may predispose recipients to further immunologic complications. Large antivenin proteins exceed the threshold for filtration and excretion by the kidneys and therefore are eliminated primarily by the reticuloendothelial system (RES), a much slower process than renal elimination. Theoretically, the longer it takes to clear foreign proteins from the body, the more time they will be available to form immune complexes with the patient's endogenous antibodies. These complexes, composed of infused antivenin proteins and the patient's own IgG molecules, may precipitate in susceptible tissue, resulting in clinical disease such as serum sickness.

Enzymatic cleavage of IgG with pepsin and papain produces smaller substituent Fab$_2$ and Fab fragments that are capable of neutralizing venom components. Snake antivenin composed of Fab or Fab$_2$ fragments avoids many of the serious adverse effects of IgG antivenin and thus represents a significant advance in treatment of envenomation (Figures 40-2 and 40-3) (see later discussion).

Modern Production of Antivenin

Antivenin (Crotalidae) Polyvalent, the IgG crotalid antivenin manufactured by Wyeth, has been the mainstay of therapy for crotalid envenomation despite its numerous potential deleterious effects. Efforts to maximize the neutralizing potential of antivenin while minimizing its immunogenicity have become the principal goal of modern antivenin production. Despite major advances in our understanding of the biology of antivenin production, the commercial manufacture of antivenin relies on the same principles of host animal immunization with snake venom described more than a century ago.

All antivenins follow a two-step production process. First, a neutralizing antibody is produced by immunization of a host animal with sublethal doses of venom. This antibody is one of many proteins present in the resulting immune serum preparation. Step two involves purification of antivenin with reduction in the fraction of nonneutralizing proteins. The preparation is then concentrated and packaged in its final lyophilized or liquid form.

Antivenin (Crotalidae) Polyvalent Wyeth. In 2000 the ovine-derived antigen-binding fragment (Fab) anticrotalid antivenin became available for clinical use. Before this, the only available antivenin in the United States against pit viper envenomation was Antivenin (Crotalidae) Polyvalent Wyeth. Manufacture of that antivenin has changed little since its introduction in 1954. In this process, horses are immunized with increasing doses of venom from four crotalid species: *Crotalus adamanteus* (eastern diamondback), *C. atrox* (western dia-

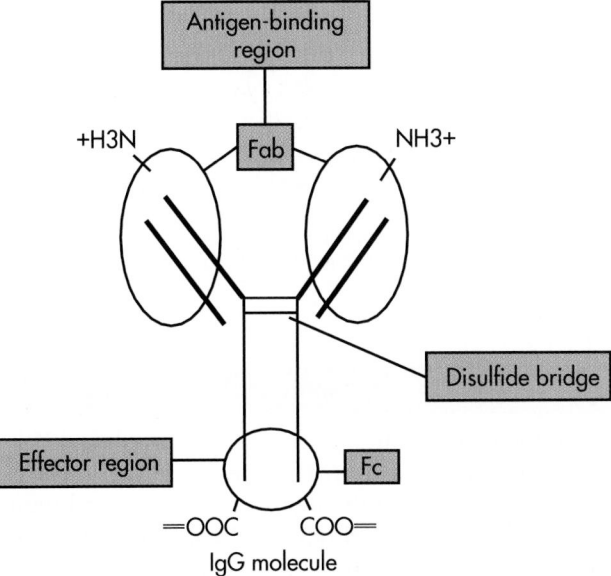

Figure 40-1 Schematic diagram of an IgG molecule. The antigen-binding region (Fab portion) is present at the amino-terminal end. The effector region (Fc portion) interacts with the immune system cells and resides at the carboxyl end of IgG. Note the disulfide bridge.

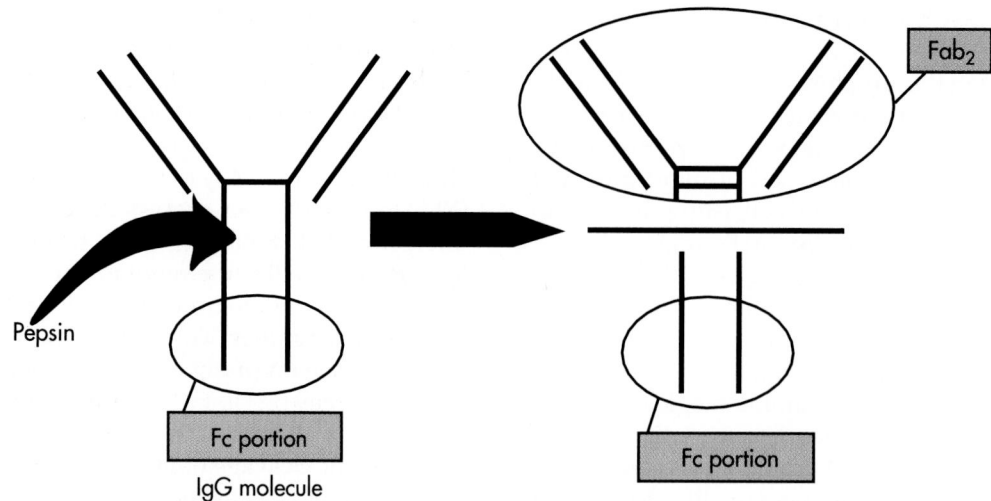

Figure 40-2 Proteolytic cleavage of IgG results in predictable substituent fractions. Pepsin digestion produces Fc and Fab₂ fractions. Fab₂ consists of two Fab portions connected by a disulfide bridge. Molecular weight of Fab₂ is 100,000 daltons.

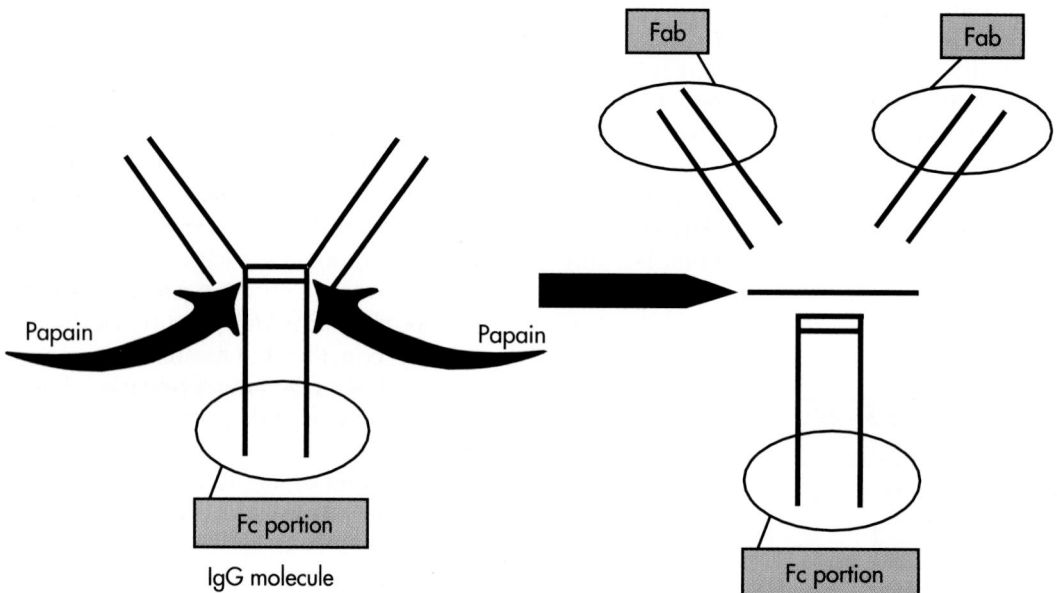

Figure 40-3 Proteolytic cleavage of IgG results in predictable substituent fractions. Papain digestion of IgG yields the Fc and two Fab segments for each IgG molecule. Molecular weight of Fab is 50,000 daltons.

mondback), *C. durissus terrificus* (South American or tropical rattlesnake), and *Bothrops atrox* (fer-de-lance), plus adjuvant for immune system stimulation. The resultant hyperimmune serum is subjected to an ammonium sulfate precipitation, which removes a variety of plasma proteins. Unfortunately, a fraction of neutralizing antibody is also lost in this process, resulting in diminished potency. The product is then precipitated, filtered, resuspended, and lyophilized. The final concentrated antivenin contains 1.5 to 2 g of horse protein, only 15% to 25% of which is IgG.[43]

ADVERSE EFFECTS

Incomplete purification of Antivenin (Crotalidae) Polyvalent Wyeth results in the presence of significant amounts of nonneutralizing proteins, such as albumin, α- and β-globulins, and IgM. Sullivan[43] has quantified the relative contributions of nonneutralizing proteins to the final antivenin product (Box 40-1). The heterologous nature of this antivenin enhances immunogenicity and is responsible for life-threatening anaphylactic and anaphylactoid reactions and the

---

Box 40-1 QUANTITATION OF PROTEINS IN SAMPLES OF WYETH ANTIVENIN	
IgG	2900 mg/ml
IgM	75 mg/ml
Total protein	9.4 g/dl
Albumin	0.28 g/dl
α_1-Globulin	0.74 g/dl
α_2-Globulin	3.50 g/dl
β-Globulin	2.76 g/dl
γ-Globulin	2.12 g/dl

---

more common, but self-limiting, serum sickness (see later discussion). In addition, since the purification process results in denaturation of a portion of the protective IgG fraction,[43] multiple vials of antivenin must be administered for adequate reversal of venom poisoning.

Despite these impurities and being prepared from only four species, the Wyeth antivenin preparation is effective against all crotalids native to North, Central, and South America. This cross-reactivity enables a single preparation of antivenin to be effective against any clinically significant pit viper envenomation.

Anaphylactic and Anaphylactoid Reactions

The spectrum of human immunologic responses to antivenin is well documented. Introduction of heterologous protein may induce type I hypersensitivity (anaphylactic) reactions. This syndrome results from IgE-mediated degranulation of mast cells and release of vasoactive mediators, including histamine, leukotriene, platelet activating factor, adenosine, and neutrophilic and eosinophilic chemotactic factors.[26] These substances induce vasodilation and increased capillary permeability resulting in hemodynamic instability and hypotension. Bronchospasm, laryngospasm, and death can result without airway management and pharmacologic intervention.

Anaphylactoid reactions are clinically indistinguishable from anaphylaxis but are not IgE mediated. In this syndrome, mast cell degranulation is postulated to result from direct interaction of nonneutralizing antivenin protein or the Fc segment of the IgG molecule itself with mast cell membranes. This is often associated with activation of the complement cascade.[45] In addition, large nonneutralizing proteins present in antivenin, as well as aggregates of IgG itself,[3,13,19] may directly activate the complement system, resulting in release of vasoactive mediators. The subsequent hypotension, bronchospasm, and airway compromise require rapid, appropriate interventions. These life-threatening sequelae may occur whether antivenin is administered as the skin test or in the full antivenin dose.

Management of allergic reactions should include epinephrine (intravenous bolus or infusion), antihistamines (both H_1 and H_2 blockers), and aggressive airway support if necessary (Table 40-1).

Allergic Reactions

Patients with significant envenomation and a history of allergy to equine-derived antivenin or to horse serum present a difficult challenge. The decision to treat with Antivenin (Crotalidae) Polyvalent Wyeth must be based on strong clinical and laboratory indications and requires careful but rapid risk-benefit analysis. A patient with a history of allergy to antivenin who requires antivenin because of life- or limb-threatening symptoms may be successfully supported with epinephrine, antihistamines, and airway management. Patients who have experienced life-threatening allergic reactions to antivenin may not necessarily have recurrent reactions when rechallenged. Nevertheless, it is prudent to pretreat such patients with epinephrine and antihistamines (diphenhydramine and cimetidine) before antivenin administration (see Table 40-1).

Serum Sickness

In addition to the acute effects associated with antivenin administration, a delayed type III hypersensitivity reaction is well described. This entity, known as serum sickness, is common,[12,46] particularly in persons receiving more than seven or eight vials of antivenin.[17,50]

The syndrome of serum sickness was originally described in 1905 by two pediatricians, von Pirquet and Schick, who noted that children receiving equine-derived streptococcal antitoxin sometimes developed fever, lymphadenopathy, and rash.[29] They first used the term *serum sickness* to describe this constellation of symptoms resulting from the administration of heterologous serum. Modern definitions of this syndrome have varied little from the original description. Serum sickness is a spectrum of disease, typically characterized by fever, malaise, urticaria, lymphadenopathy, arthralgias, and less commonly, glomerulonephritis and neuritis. The onset of symptoms usually occurs within 1 to 2 weeks after exposure to foreign antigens, in this case, heterologous protein in antivenin.

The pathophysiology of serum sickness results from nonspecific deposition of immune complexes (antigen-IgG) in susceptible tissue. Under nonpathologic conditions, these complexes are cleared by the RES without sequelae. With abnormal vascular permeability and slight antigen excess, however, precipitation of immune complexes occurs. In addition, immune complex deposition tends to occur in tissues where the vasculature has a filtering function.[6] These complexes diffuse between endothelial cells and deposit along the basement membrane.[27] The interaction of immune com-

TABLE 40-1. Treatment Recommendations for Antivenin-Induced Anaphylaxis or Anaphylactoid Reaction

| | EPINEPHRINE | | ANTIHISTAMINES | |
	INFUSION	BOLUS	DIPHENHYDRAMINE	CIMETIDINE
Adult	1-4 μg/min IV	0.5-1 ml of 1:10,000 solution IV	50 mg IV stat, 50 mg IV q6h, prn	300 mg IV stat, then 300 mg IV q6h, prn
Child	0.01-1 μg/kg/min IV	0.01 mg/kg of 1:10,000 solution IV	1 mg/kg IV stat, then 1 mg/kg IV q6h, prn	5-10 mg/kg IV stat, then 5-10 mg/kg IV q6h, prn

IV, Intravenously; *stat,* immediately; *q6h,* every 6 hours; *prn,* as needed.

plexes trapped in the vascular wall with vasoactive mediators results in complement activation, further release of vasoactive mediators, and exacerbation of the inflammatory process. This process characteristically occurs in skin, synovial joints, and the glomerular apparatus, resulting in the clinical manifestations of serum sickness.[10,26,52]

Treatment of Serum Sickness

A large percentage of patients receiving more than seven or eight vials of the standard, equine-derived anticrotalid antivenin develop serum sickness.[17,50] The spectrum of illness in this syndrome is highly variable and may range from mild urticaria, malaise, and low-grade fever to debilitating arthralgias and myalgias. Fortunately, although well described, glomerulonephritis and neuritis are rare complications. The variability of the syndrome requires that treatment be tailored to individual clinical needs.

Patients with serum sickness should receive antihistamines such as diphenhydramine or hydroxyzine and, except in the mildest cases, a 7- to 10-day course of high-dose steroids. Clinical illness typically resolves within 1 to 2 weeks.

SPECIFIC ANTIVENINS

This section covers general aspects of antivenin therapy following envenomation by the black widow spider, coral snake, and pit vipers. Specific indications for each antivenin are covered in their respective chapters (see Chapters 34, 38, and 39), as are specialized or experimental antivenins directed against the venoms of such creatures as scorpions (see Chapter 35) and stonefish, box-jellyfish, and sea snakes (see Chapters 61 and 62).

Arachnid Antivenin: Black Widow Spider

The only nonsnake antivenin approved by the FDA for use in the United States is indicated for envenomation by the black widow spider *Latrodectus mactans* (see Chapter 34). Antivenin *(Latrodectus mactans)* MSD is derived from hyperimmunizing horses with *Latrodectus* venom and is effective in counteracting the pain associated with severe envenomations. A similar antivenin

frequently used in Australia is associated with a low but measurable incidence of anaphylaxis and serum sickness.[47]

Fortunately, the venom from the black widow spider rarely results in life-threatening manifestations. Patients can usually be managed effectively with adequate doses of narcotic analgesics and benzodiazepines. In certain conditions, however, *Latrodectus* antivenin may be indicated. In general, patients with underlying medical problems, such as coronary artery disease or chronic obstructive pulmonary disease, whose pain may trigger secondary ischemic events, and those who may not be able to tolerate large doses of narcotics or benzodiazepines may be appropriate candidates for antivenin. Pregnancy and extremes of age have often been cited as indications for antivenin.[28,38] Patients with severe pain who do not respond to narcotics and benzodiazepines, however, will obtain prompt relief with intravenous (IV) administration of one vial of *Latrodectus* antivenin.[28]

Snake Envenomation

In contrast to black widow spider bites, venomous snakebites do not allow withholding antivenin when signs of envenomation are present (see Chapters 38 and 39). No effective alternative therapy exists for clinically significant snake envenomations other than antivenin.[37] The FDA-approved new, safer anticrotalid antivenin (CroTAb) is available for clinical use. Before this, only equine-derived Antivenin (Crotalidae) Polyvalent Wyeth was available for the treatment of crotalid envenomation from indigenous snakebites in the United States.

Coral Snakes (Elapidae). The AAPCC reported 61 coral snake bites (family Elapidae) in 1998.[22] An effective antivenin is available only for the Eastern *(Micrurus fulvius fulvius)* and Texas *(M. fulvius tenere)* coral snakes. Envenomation by these two species is associated with more serious systemic findings than typically occurs with their Arizona (Sonoran, *Micruroides euryxanthus)* counterpart.[20,36] Signs of local envenomation are minimal, with neurotoxicity in the form of bulbar and respiratory paralysis developing up to 12 hours after the bite.

Immunotherapy for *M. fulvius* envenomation requires IV administration of four to six vials of Antivenin *(Micrurus fulvius)* Equine Origin.[35] Additional vials may be necessary as clinically warranted.[20] Antivenin should be given to patients who have been bitten by an Eastern coral snake that has "chewed" on the affected part and who have evidence of fang penetration through the skin.[20]

Early antivenin treatment is recommended, since cranial nerve dysfunction and respiratory paralysis from Eastern coral snake envenomation may be easier to prevent than to reverse.[20] Once venom components are bound to neuronal target tissue, they may not be readily removed by antivenin, or the end-organ toxicity may not be readily reversible. Thus early administration of antivenin, preferably within 8 hours of the bite, has been advocated.[20] As with any equine-derived product, skin testing is mandatory, and preparations for treatment of anaphylaxis must be in place. Skin testing may be omitted if the patient is hemodynamically unstable as a result of envenomation.

Pit Vipers (Crotalidae). A sheep-derived Fab antivenin, Affinity Purified, Mixed Monospecific Crotalid Antivenom, Ovine Fab for Injection (CroTAb), approved in 2000, represents a major advance in the immunotherapeutics of snake envenomation. Indications for the use of anticrotalid antivenin include signs and symptoms of progressive envenomation, as manifested by increasing local or systemic effects, or laboratory abnormalities consistent with envenomation (see Chapter 38).

Antivenin (Crotalidae) Polyvalent Wyeth. A careful history must be elicited from all envenomed patients. This should include allergy to horse dander, history of atopic reactions, and previous allergy or exposure to horse serum. Patients with positive histories may be at greater risk for allergic reactions to antivenin.

Once the decision to administer antivenin has been made, a skin test determines horse serum sensitivity. Skin testing may be omitted for patients in extremis from snake envenomation, since immediate treatment may be lifesaving. Skin testing should never be done unless a decision to administer antivenin has been made, since life-threatening allergic reactions may occur from skin testing alone. The patient must be in an emergency department or other intensive care setting, with adequate IV access and resuscitation equipment at hand. The attendant staff must be prepared to treat acute anaphylaxis whenever skin testing is performed or antivenin is infused.

PROTOCOL FOR SKIN TEST. The manufacturer recommends the following protocol for skin testing[34]:

1. From 0.02 to 0.03 ml of a 1:10 dilution of antivenin or 0.02 to 0.03 ml of horse serum (provided in the kit as prediluted 1:10 solution) is injected intradermally.
2. A similar control dose of normal saline is injected at a distant site for comparison.
3. Patients with a history of sensitivity to horse serum who require antivenin therapy should be skin tested using a dilution of 1:100 of antivenin or normal horse serum.
4. A positive skin test is usually manifest within 5 to 30 minutes and is characterized by a wheal or without erythema.

A significant percentage of both false-positive and false-negative skin tests occurs. Therefore a negative skin test does not rule out the potential for anaphylaxis associated with the administration of antivenin. Equally important, a positive skin test does not contraindicate the use of antivenin if the patient's life or limb is threatened.[25,34,37] The purpose of a skin test is to identify a patient with obvious severe hypersensitivity so that the health care team can be prepared to manage an allergic reaction.

ADMINISTRATION. In general, the initial dose of this antivenin is 10 vials, although the clinical severity of the bite may necessitate higher initial doses. Eastern diamondback rattlesnake *(C. adamanteus)* envenomations, for example, are typically more severe and may require an initial dose of 10 to 20 vials of antivenin.

Although seemingly a minor detail, dissolving the lyophilized antivenin is yet another challenge in managing the envenomed victim. Provided with each antivenin kit, 10 ml of diluent (bacteriostatic water for injection, USP) is added to the lyophilized antivenin. Gentle swirling and rotating of the vials are mandatory to avoid inactivating the neutralizing component, IgG. Vigorous handling or shaking while solubilizing the antivenin may result in partial denaturation of IgG. Dissolving lyophylized antivenin takes 20 to 30 minutes per vial, so enlisting the help of staff will result in more rapid completion of the process.

Once in solution, the vials of antivenin are diluted in 250 to 500 ml of 5% dextrose in water or normal saline. The initial rate of infusion should be slow, with frequent clinical assessment for evidence of an allergic reaction. If well tolerated, the remainder of the infusion should be administered over 1 hour.

The initial rate of antivenin infusion in patients with positive skin tests should be even slower than for patients with negative skin tests. We support pretreatment of these patients with epinephrine and antihistamines,[31] but this is not universally recommended. If no allergic reaction occurs, the residual infusion may proceed over the next 1 to 2 hours.

If anaphylaxis develops during administration of antivenin, the infusion is stopped, and aggressive airway management and pharmacologic intervention are initiated. Patients should receive epinephrine and antihistamines (both H_1 and H_2 blockers) (see Table 40-1). Persistent life-threatening, systemic signs of venom poisoning may necessitate restarting the antivenin infusion. Under these conditions the antivenin should be further diluted and given at a slower rate than the initial infusion. The patient should be pretreated with antihistamines and epinephrine, and when required, epinephrine should be simultaneously infused at a second IV site (see Chapter 38).

Antigen-Binding Fragment. A major advance in immunotherapy for envenomation involves the use of specific Fab to neutralize venom (see Figure 40-3). Theoretically, use of these smaller antibody fragments has advantages. The ideal immunotherapeutic agent should have: (1) high specificity and affinity for the antigen, (2) rapid and extensive tissue distribution so that it will reach and bind the antigen in a timely fashion, (3) low antigenicity, and (4) rapid clearance from the body.[43] Based on clinical and experimental data, Fab appears to satisfy these criteria.

ADVANTAGES OF FAB VS. IMMUNOGLOBULIN G. Both animal and human experiments, especially with digoxin intoxication, support the efficacy of purified Fab and its superiority to whole IgG. Extensive experience with the digoxin antidote Digibind demonstrates that ovine-derived digoxin-specific Fab fulfills the criteria for an effective immunotherapeutic agent and is superior to whole IgG antibodies.[7,23,41]

In baboon and rabbit models, distribution and elimination half-lives for digoxin-specific Fab were significantly shorter (0.28 to 0.32 and 9 to 13 hours, respectively) than those of the digoxin-specific IgG molecules (4 and 61 hours).[41] In addition, the volume of distribution for digoxin-specific Fab is significantly greater than that of the whole IgG antibody, reflecting its more extensive tissue distribution. In this model, therefore, Fab was more rapidly and extensively distributed to tissue sites than IgG.[41]

Similar kinetic analysis in the dog model of digoxin poisoning revealed significantly shorter distribution half-lives with Fab than with the whole IgG antibody (0.54 hour vs. 2.28 hours). This correlated with shorter mean time to reversal of digoxin-induced cardiotoxicity in the Fab-treated group (36 minutes vs. 85 minutes in the IgG group).[23]

Besides its proven efficacy,[1,40,53] ovine-derived Fab has not caused anaphylaxis or serum sickness despite its extensive use in clinical practice. Digoxin-specific Fab (Digibind) is safe, effective therapy for the rapid reversal of digoxin-induced cardiotoxicity.

ADVANTAGES AND DISADVANTAGES OF FAB ANTIVENIN. Clinical manifestations of crotalid envenomation using polyspecific anticrotalid Fab can be successfully reversed based on (1) the effectiveness of digoxin-specific Fab immunotherapy, (2) the successful clinical trials using Fab antivenin directed against *V. berus*,[18] and (3) the protection against venom-induced lethality in mice after the administration of specific Fab.[44]

Although successful treatment of digoxin toxicity with Digibind is similar to the use of purified Fab fragment antivenin for snake envenomation, important differences include the following:

1. Unlike digoxin, snake venom is a heterogenous mixture of antigens varying greatly in size and structure. The antigenicity of each venom component may vary greatly depending on its physical characteristics.
2. Unlike snake venom, digoxin does not cause permanent cellular damage to target cells. Thus, once digoxin is released from target tissue and bound to Digibind, the cellular toxicity is reversed. The same may not be true of toxic effects of venom.
3. The relatively small size of the digoxin (781 daltons)–Fab (50,000 daltons) complex permits it to be renally excreted. In addition, evidence supports endogenous renal catabolism of such small complexes.[2,21,42,51]

Venom is a complex mixture of proteins, glycoproteins, and peptides, with molecular weights ranging from several thousand to greater than 100,000 daltons.[37] Although Fab complexed to small-molecular-weight venom components may be cleared renally, most of venom proteins have molecular weights greater than 20,000 daltons and are too large to be filtered and excreted by the kidney when complexed to Fab. This may result in significantly longer elimination half-lives of venom-Fab complexes. Theoretically, this may allow sufficient time for dissociation of the venom-Fab complex, resulting in the release of active venom components.

ADMINISTRATION. The new CroTAb antivenom is an affinity-purified, lyophilized preparation of ovine Fab obtained from healthy sheep, each immunized with one of the following North American crotalid snake venoms: *C. atrox* (Western diamondback rattlesnake), *C. adamanteus* (Eastern diamondback rattlesnake), *C. scutulatus scutulatus* (Mojave rattlesnake), and *Agkistrodon piscivorus piscivorus* (cottonmouth or water moccasin). The final product is prepared by isolating the immunoglobulin from the ovine serum, digesting it with papain, and isolating the venom-specific Fab fragments on affinity columns. This procedure produces four different monospecific antivenoms, which are then mixed in equal proportions to prepare the final antivenom.

In mouse lethality studies, CroTAb averaged 5.3 times more potent than Antivenin (Crotalidae) Polyvalent Wyeth in neutralizing the venoms of 10 clinically important North American crotalid snakes.[11] In two prospective, open-labeled, multicenter trials, 42 patients ages 10 and or older had minimal or moderate North American crotalid envenomation (excluding copperhead bites) within 6 hours before admission and showed evidence of worsening in the emergency department. Rapid onset of action was noted in both trials, with reversal of progressive swelling, neurologic, and gastrointestinal symptoms, and prolonged prothrombin time (PT) during the initial CroTAb infusion.

The short half-life of Fab compared with IgG resulted in recurrent signs of envenomation. Therefore a novel dosing schedule for CroTAb is recommended. Four to twelve vials of CroTAb are infused to achieve initial control of the envenomation syndrome, followed by two vials every 6 hours for three additional doses (18 hours), particularly in patients with severe coagulopathy.

COMPLICATIONS. As with all products containing animal proteins, CroTAb causes adverse reactions in about 20% of all reactions during infusion. Nearly all effects were mild. The most severe reaction was bronchospasm, which responded promptly to therapy. No cases of anaphylaxis have been reported. The serum sickness rate is approximately 6%, much lower than with nonpurified serum products, which typically produce serum sickness in 70% to 80% of patients.

Monoclonal Antibodies

Advances in molecular biology have made the use of monoclonal antibodies commonplace in research.[15] A monoclonal antibody is a single, unique molecule produced in large quantity by a clone of cultured B cells. Reports describe the production of monoclonal antibodies directed against specific venom components and activities. For example, monoclonal antibodies with antithrombin-like,[30] antihemorrhagic,[16,32] antimyotoxic,[24] and other activities have been purified. Preincubation of several classes of antiphospholipase A_2 monoclonal antibodies in mice neutralized the myotoxic activity typically seen with *Bothrops asper* (fer-de-lance) envenomation.[24] Monoclonal antibody–based enzyme-linked immunosorbent assays can be used to measure the concentration of venom components and may be more accurate and sensitive than other bioassays.[4] This technique also has diagnostic potential because it can be used to detect unique venom components after envenomation.[30]

Despite these advances, use of monoclonal antibodies for venom poisoning has significant theoretic problems. Traditionally, an effective antivenin has a broad spectrum of activity and can counteract a wide array of clinical sequelae. Because of the complex and heterogenous nature of venoms with their innumer-

able antigenic sites, such antivenin would require pooling of many different monoclonal antibodies. A major advantage of a polyclonal antivenin is its ability to neutralize the effects of venoms of related species within the same genus or family. The very specificity that enables monoclonal antibodies to target unique antigenic determinants might render this approach impractical as an isolated therapeutic modality against envenomation.[25]

Nevertheless, with continued isolation of monoclonal antibodies capable of neutralizing specific clinical effects of envenomation, such as myotoxic effects[24] and thrombinlike activity,[30] "libraries" of monoclonal antibodies may target and counteract predominant signs and symptoms of envenomation. Adjunctive immunotherapy with monoclonal antibodies and a broad-spectrum antivenin may provide the exquisite sensitivity against specific adverse reactions typically absent in standard antivenin.

After a slow start, advances in molecular biology are finally being applied to envenomation therapeutics. We can anticipate a multitude of novel immunotherapeutic modalities in the future.

REFERENCES

1. Antman EM et al: Treatment of 150 cases of life-threatening digitalis intoxication with digoxin-specific Fab antibody fragments: final report of a multicenter study, *Circulation* 81:1744, 1990.
2. Arend WP, Silverblatt JF: Serum disappearance and catabolism of homologous immunoglobulin fragments in rats, *Clin Exp Immunol* 22:502, 1975.
3. Barandun S et al: *Clinical applications of immunoglobulin (gamma globulin): a review of current findings*, Basel, Switzerland, 1982, Sandoz Products.
4. Bignami GS et al: Monoclonal antibody–based enzyme-linked immunoassays for the measurement of palytoxin in biological samples, *Toxicon* 30:687, 1992.
5. Brazil V: *Le defense contre l'ophidisme*, ed 2, São Paulo, 1914, Pocai & Weiss.
6. Buhner D, Grant JA: Serum sickness, *Dermatol Clin* 3:107, 1985.
7. Butler VP Jr et al: Effects of sheep digoxin-specific antibodies and their Fab fragments on digoxin pharmacokinetics in dogs, *J Clin Invest* 59:35, 1977.
8. Calmette A: L'immunisation artificielle des animaux contre le venin des serpents et al therapeutic experimental de morsures venimeuses, *CR Soc Biol* 46:120, 1894.
9. Calmette A: *Le venin de serpants: physiologie de l'envenomation; traitment des morsures venimeuses par le serum des animaux vaccines*, Paris, 1896, Societe de Editions Scientifiques.
10. Cochrane CG, Koffler D: Immune complex disease in experimental animals and man, *Adv Immunol* 16:185, 1973.
11. Consroe P et al: Comparison of a new ovine antigen binding fragment (Fab) antivenin for United States Crotalidae with the commercial antivenin for protection against venom-induced lethality in mice, *Am J Trop Med Hyg* 53:507, 1995.
12. Corrigan P, Russell FE, Wainschel J: Clinical reactions to antivenin, *Toxicon* 1(suppl):457, 1978.
13. Day NK, Good RA, Wahn V: Adverse reactions in selected patients following intravenous infusions of gamma globulin, *Am J Med* 76(suppl 3A):25, 1984.
14. Hawgood BJ: Review article: pioneers of anti-venomous serotherapy: Dr. Vital Brazil (1865-1950), *Toxicon* 30:573, 1992.
15. Henry R, Begent J, Pedley RB: Monoclonal antibody administration: current clinical pharmacokinetic status and future trends, *Clin Pharmacokinet* 23:85, 1992.
16. Iddon D, Hommel M, Theakston RDG: Characterization of a monoclonal antibody capable of neutralizing the haemorrhagic activity of the West African Echis carinatus (carpet viper) venom, *Toxicon* 26:169, 1988.
17. Jurkovich GJ et al: Complications of Crotalidae antivenin therapy, *J Trauma* 28:1032, 1988.

18. Karlson-Stiber C et al: First clinical experiences with specific sheep Fab fragments in snake bite: report of a multicentre study of *Vipera berus* envenoming, *J Intern Med* 241:53, 1997.

19. Kirkpatrick CH: Allergic histories and reaction of patients treated with digoxin immune Fab (ovine) antibody, *Am J Emerg Med* 9 (suppl 1):7, 1991.

20. Kitchens C, Van Mierop L: Envenomation by the eastern coral snake *(Micrurus fulvius fulvius):* a study of 39 victims, *JAMA* 258:1615, 1987.

21. Lathem W et al: The demonstration and localization of renal tubular reabsorption of hemoglobin by stop flow analysis, *J Clin Invest* 39:840, 1960.

22. Litovitz TL et al: 1998 annual report of the American Association of Poison Control Centers, *Am J Emerg Med* 17:435, 1999.

23. Lloyd BL, Smith TW: Contrasting rates of reversal of digoxin toxicity by digoxin-specific IgG and Fab fragments, *Circulation* 58:280, 1978.

24. Lomonte B et al: Neutralization of myotoxic phospholipases A2 from the venom of the snake *Bothrops asper* by monoclonal antibodies, *Toxicon* 30:239, 1992.

25. Malasit P et al: Prediction, prevention and mechanism of early (anaphylactic) antivenom reactions in victims of snake bites, *Br Med J* 292:17, 1986.

26. Melvold R: Review of immunology. In Patterson R et al, editors: *Allergic diseases: diagnosis and management,* ed 4, Philadelphia, 1993, Lippincott.

27. Michael AF Jr et al: Acute poststreptococcal glomerulonephritis, *J Clin Invest* 45:237, 1966.

28. Moss H, Binder L: A retrospective review of black widow spider envenomation, *Ann Emerg Med* 16:188, 1987.

29. Mygind N: *Essential allergy,* Oxford, 1986, Blackwell.

30. Nakamura M, Kinjoh K, Kosugi T: Production of a monoclonal antibody against the thrombin-like enzyme, habutobin, from *Trimeresurus flavoviridis* venom, *Toxicon* 30:1177, 1992.

31. Otten EJ, McKimm D: Venomous snakebite in a patient allergic to horse serum, *Ann Emerg Med* 12:624, 1983.

32. Perez JC, Garcia VE, Huang SY: Production of a monoclonal antibody against hemorrhagic activity of *Crotalus atrox* (Western diamondback rattlesnake) venom, *Toxicon* 22:967, 1984.

33. Phisalix C, Bertrand G: Sur le proriete antitoxique du sang des animaux vaccines contre le venin des vipere, *CR Soc Biol* 46:111, 1894.

34. Product information, Antivenin (Crotalidae) Polyvalent, Wyeth.

35. Product information, Antivenin *(Micrurus fulvius)* Equine Origin, Wyeth.

36. Russell FE: Bites by the Sonoran coral snake, *Micruroides euryxanthus, Toxicon* 5:39, 1967.

37. Russell FE: *Snake venom poisoning,* ed 2, New York, 1983, Scholium International.

38. Russell FE, Marcus P, Streng JA: Black widow spider envenomation during pregnancy, *Toxicon* 17:188, 1979.

39. Sewall H: Experiments on the preventive inoculation of rattlesnake venom, *J Physiol Lond* 8:203, 1887.

40. Smith TW: Review of clinical experience with digoxin immune Fab (ovine), *Am J Emerg Med* 9(suppl 1):1, 1991.

41. Smith TW et al: Immunogenicity and kinetics of distribution and elimination of sheep digoxin-specific IgG and Fab fragments in the rabbit and baboon, *Clin Exp Immunol* 36:384, 1979.

42. Spiegelberg HL, Weigle WO: The catabolism of homologous and heterologous 7S gamma globulin fragments, *J Exp Med* 121:323, 1965.

43. Sullivan JB: Past, present, and future immunotherapy of snake venom poisoning, *Ann Emerg Med* 16:938, 1987.

44. Sullivan JB et al: Protection against *Crotalus* venom lethality by monovalent, polyclonal F(ab) fragments: in search of a better snake trap, *Vet Hum Toxicol* 26:400, 1984.

45. Sutherland SK: Serum reactions: an analysis of commercial antivenoms and the possible role of anticomplementary activity in de-novo reactions to antivenoms and antitoxins, *Med J Aust* 1:613, 1977.

46. Sutherland SK, Lovering KE: Antivenoms: use and adverse reactions over a 12-month period in Australia and Papua New Guinea, *Med J Aust* 2:671, 1979.

47. Sutherland SK, Trinca JC: Survey of 2144 cases of red-back spider bites, *Med J Aust* 2:620, 1978.

48. Theakston RDG, Warrell DA: Antivenoms: a list of hyperimmune sera currently available for the treatment of envenoming by bites and stings, *Toxicon* 29:1419, 1991.

49. Wingert WA: Editorial: treatment of Crotalid envenomation: conservative vs. anticipatory, *J Wilderness Med* 3:113, 1992.

50. Wingert WA, Chan L: Rattlesnake bites in southern California and rationale for recommended treatment, *West J Med* 148:37, 1988.

51. Wochner RD, Strober W, Waldmann TA: The role of the kidney in the catabolism of Bence Jones proteins and immunoglobulin fragments, *J Exp Med* 126:207, 1967.

52. Wolff SM: The vasculitic syndromes. In Wyngaarden JB, Smith LH Jr, Bennett JC, editors: *Cecil textbook of medicine,* ed 19, Philadelphia, 1992, Saunders.

53. Woolf AD et al: Results of multicenter studies of digoxin-specific antibody fragments in managing digitalis intoxication in the pediatric population, *Am J Emerg Med* 9:16, 1991.

41 Bites and Injuries Inflicted by Domestic Animals

Sean Keogh and Michael L. Callaham

Domestic animal bites are common, and their incidence is rising.[15,120,148] Wild animal attacks are often more spectacular, but in the developed world, injuries from domestic animals have a much greater health and economic impact. Humans are not a natural prey of any animal, and most attacks are caused by fear of humans (real or perceived), territoriality, protective instinct, or accident. Occasionally a bite may result from disease (e.g., rabies) or rogue behavior. Injuries range from minimal to fatal, are regularly contaminated with a wide array of pathogens, and may spread systemic disease.

EPIDEMIOLOGY OF BITES AND INJURIES

The 1998 National Pet Owner Survey estimated that more than 39 million households own at least one dog and that 32 million households own at least one cat.[4] The great majority of bites (about 80% to 90%) are inflicted by dogs.[92] Domestic cats account for about 5% to 15%, although some studies report a figure as high as 25%.[92,133,214]

An estimated 1.8% of Americans are bitten by a dog every year, resulting in 4.5 million bite wounds. More than 750,000 of these bite victims seek medical attention.[118,173] From 15 to 30 bites per 10,000 population occur per year, based on patient visits to the emergency department (ED).[120,199] In a survey of 274 million ED visits in the United States between 1992 and 1994, more than 333,000 new dog bite injuries were seen, a rate of 12.9 per 10,000 persons. These injuries produced 0.4% of all ED visits in the United States. Bites to children were common, with boys aged 5 to 9 years having the highest incidence rate at 60.7 per 10,000 persons, which is 3.6% of all injury-related ED visits in this group.[210] These figures represent only bite victims who sought medical attention; one analysis of dog bite incidence in Pittsburgh showed that 790 bites were reported but that an estimated 1388 were unreported, an annual incidence of 58.9 per 10,000 population.[33] Urban areas have a higher reported rate of biting, and some studies suggest that dog bite incidence correlates inversely with socioeconomic status.[184,199]

The victim of a bite is often a pet owner or a member of the owner's family, and injury is frequently sustained while playing with the animal.[38] Surveys of schoolchildren have shown that 55% of boys and almost 40% of girls have been bitten, with 17% requiring medical attention.[12] Childhood bites can produce significant psychologic morbidity.[179] In Thailand, where Buddhist cultural beliefs encourage feeding and protection of stray animals, most dog bites are inflicted by strays and are unprovoked.[14]

The annual incidence of cat bites is about 400,000 in the United States,[5,76,92] which is probably an underestimate. Biting cats are typically stray females, and most human victims are also female.

Human bites on other humans are more common in urban areas, with a reported incidence of 3.6% to 23% of all bites.[27,29,129] One district in Brooklyn, New York, has reported a rate as high as 60.9 bites per 100,000 population.[129] In contrast, human bites in rural communities are less common, with one study reporting that 0.03% of all bites are caused by humans.[177] Children are frequently both the inflicters and the recipients of bite wounds. In a study of day-care centers, 46% of children were bitten by another child over a 1-year period.[73]

About 30 million Americans ride horses, 50,000 of whom are treated for horse-related injury in an ED annually, principally because the rider is unrestrained and can fall off while travelling at speeds up to 40 mph. Horses can kick with a force of up to 1 ton[115] and frequently bite. A 2-year review of animal bites in Oslo revealed that 2% of 1051 recorded bites were caused by horses; 53% of these horse bite victims were children.[43]

The American Ferret Association estimates 6 to 8 million domesticated ferrets reside in the United States. The risk of attack by a ferret is greatest in infants and small children. Bite statistics are scarce, but in Arizona, 11 ferret bites were reported over 11 months, with the ferret population estimated at 4000, about a 0.3% reported bite to ferret population ratio. During the same period, 2265 dog bites occurred, with the dog population estimated at 100,000, for a bite ratio of 2.2%.[180]

Certain occupations carry a greater risk for animal bite; U.S. letter carriers reported 2851 dog bites in 1995,[35] and 64% of veterinarians have sustained a major animal-related injury in their careers.[119] Incidence of biting species varies with exposure. Among veterinarians, most injuries are inflicted by cattle, followed by dogs and then horses.

Box 41-1   ADVICE TO AVOID BEING ATTACKED AND BITTEN BY COMMON PETS*

DOGS

Do not leave a young child alone with a dog.

Never approach or try to pet an unfamiliar dog, especially if it is tied up or confined.

Always ask owners if you can pet their dog.

Do not lean over a dog or pet it directly on the head; do not kiss a dog.

Avoid quick, sudden movements that may startle a dog.

Never pet or step over a sleeping dog.

Never try to take a bone or toy from a dog (other than your own).

Know the appearance of an angry dog: barking, growling, snarling with teeth showing, ears laid flat, legs stiff, tail up, and hair on back standing up.

Never step between two fighting dogs; if you need to separate them, use a bucket of water or a hose.

Do not approach a female dog that is nursing her pups.

Teach injury prevention advice to children from an early age.

CATS

Be aware that some cats do not like prolonged petting.

Know warning signs of an impending bite: twitching of the tail, restlessness, and "intention" bites (i.e., cat moves to bite but does not bite).

FERRETS

Do not sell or adopt a ferret that is known to bite.

Do not push your fingers through the wires of a ferret cage.

Reach for a ferret from the side, palm upward, rather than from above.

Do not handle food and then handle young ferrets without washing your hands first.

Do not poke a ferret or pull on its tail or ears.

Never leave a ferret alone with a child or infant.

If a ferret bites and locks on very tightly, pour cold and fast-running water over its face.

*Prevention of bites and injuries from other animals is addressed in the appropriate sections.

BITE AND INJURY AVOIDANCE

Domestic animals of any kind rarely attack unless provoked, although unrestrained dogs are exceptions.[156] Physical attack is often a last resort, but an animal will often fight if it perceives that it is trapped. Reducing the risk of injury is often based on common sense and knowledge of animal behavior. For example, horses kick backward and with both rear feet, whereas cattle kick forward with only one foot. How humans react during a confrontation with an animal is also important. Nonpredator species such as cattle and deer are very susceptible to human intimidation, whereas a direct stare to a dog is seen as a challenge.

Specific recommendations can reduce the chance of being attacked and bitten by a domestic animal (Box 41-1). Dogs are guided by memory and instinct; fear and self-preservation are very strong instincts, so any perceived threat can lead to an attack. Territoriality is still ingrained in domestic dogs, even if humans provide for them. Protection of food can cause aggression, even in a docile dog. Any threat to a dog's mate, offspring, or owner may result in an attack. Personality changes may lead to aggression; causes include illness (e.g., distemper) or physiological factors (e.g., female in heat).[211] Specific actions can be taken when threatened or under attack by a dog (Box 41-2).

FIELD CARE

Local wound treatment should be initiated at the scene of the bite. This is often more important in determining

---

Box 41-2   SUGGESTED ACTION IF YOU ARE UNDER THREAT OR ATTACKED BY A DOG

Stand totally still, and let the dog come to you.

Stand passively, rather than in an aggressive or submissive pose.

Do not pat the dog.

Keep your eye on the dog, but do not stare at it.

To reprimand the dog, say "no" in a harsh voice; do not attempt to hit the dog.

Do not make any threatening or provocative movement.

Do not fight back, especially against a "fighting" dog.

Do not let the dog get behind you; keep turning to face it.

If you are knocked down, feign death and curl up into a ball until the dog loses interest.

If the dog punches you with its nose, ignore it.

If a dog puts one of your legs in its mouth without tearing the flesh, waiting for a reaction, stay still if you can.

If attacked by more than one dog, try and stand with your back to a wall or car.

Modified from Wilson S: *Bite busters: how to deal with dog attacks,* New York, 1997, Simon & Schuster.

---

the course of healing than any later therapy. When skin is unbroken, but tissue contusion is present, treatment should include prompt and liberal application of ice or other cold packs during the first 24 hours. In wounds producing a penetrating injury, pressure usually controls bleeding; the use of pressure point occlusion or proximal tourniquets should be avoided unless blood loss is extreme and cannot otherwise be controlled. If

Box 41-3   HUMAN AND DOMESTIC ANIMAL BITE RISK FACTORS

HIGH RISK

Location

Hand, wrist, or foot
Scalp or face in infants (risk of cranial perforation)
Over a major joint (risk of perforation)
Through-and-through bite of cheek

Type of wound

Puncture (impossible to irrigate)
Tissue crushing that cannot be debrided (typical of herbivore)
Carnivore bite over vital structure (artery, nerve, joint)

Biting species

Human (hand wound)
Cat (hand and lower extremity wounds)
Pig

Patient factors

Older than 50 years of age
Asplenia

Patient factors—cont'd

Chronic alcoholic
Altered immune status (chemotherapy, AIDS, immune defect)
Diabetes
Peripheral vascular insufficiency
Chronic corticosteroid therapy
Prosthetic or diseased cardiac valve (consider systemic prophylaxis)
Prosthetic or seriously diseased joint (consider systemic prophylaxis)

LOW RISK

Face, scalp, ears, or mouth
Self-bite of buccal mucosa (not through-and-through)
Large clean lacerations that can be thoroughly cleansed
Partial-thickness lacerations and abrasions

---

the victim is more than an hour from treatment, the wounds should be cleansed promptly after resuscitation. Early cleansing reduces the chance of bacterial infection and is extremely effective in killing rabies and other viruses. Tap or drinking water is safe to use. Ordinary hand soap adds some bactericidal, virucidal, and cleansing properties; at least a pint of soapy water should be used. The wound should be thoroughly irrigated and then gently debrided of dirt and foreign objects by swabbing with a soft, clean cloth or sterile gauze. This is particularly important if the biting animal might be rabid, since simple irrigation without actual swabbing of the wound edges may not remove rabies virus. If possible, irrigation should be with a syringe under pressure.

After thorough cleansing, the wound should be covered with sterile dressings or a clean, dry cloth. Wounds of the hands or feet require immobilization. If the wound is high risk (Box 41-3), antibiotics should be started if available, preferably within an hour of wounding. In severe cases, antibiotics are worthwhile even if administered many hours later.

EVALUATION OF INJURIES

Many domestic animals are large, heavy and strong. All victims of animal attacks should be evaluated using advanced trauma life support (ATLS) guidelines, except for the most minor and isolated bite injuries. Severe blunt trauma and life threatening injuries may initially be less obvious than a bite wound. Even apparently minor wounds ultimately require meticulous exploration, because injuries that appear superficial may overlie fractures or lacerated tendons, vessels, and nerves, or may penetrate into joint spaces.[69]

With large herbivores, most of the bite injury may consist of severe contusion without skin disruption.[130,205] Broken skin may result in local wound infection and the transmission of systemic disease. Infection can be caused by organisms carried in the animal's saliva or nasal secretions, by skin microbial flora carried into the wound, or by environmental organisms that enter the wound during or after the attack. Fortunately, most wounds do not become infected, particularly after adequate wound care. The need for tetanus prophylaxis should be assessed and rabies immunoglobulin and vaccine given if required.

Few tests are routinely indicated in the evaluation of most animal bite injuries. Radiographs are useful to exclude fractures, foreign bodies (e.g., teeth), air in the joint after a deep bite wound to the hand, and osteomyelitis in older bite wounds. Films should be taken after any fight-bite injury (e.g., clenched fist) and also after any cranial or facial bite in an infant or small child to exclude bony penetration of the skull or facial fracture.[208] In the first few hours after a bite, white blood cell count or wound culture is not helpful.

DEFINITIVE WOUND CARE

The same principles of irrigation and cleansing used in the prehospital environment apply in the hospital.

Although tap water[9] and normal saline are acceptable wound irrigants,[6] 1% povidone iodine solution should also be used if rabies transmission is a possibility, as it is virucidal.[181,187] Although 1% benzalkonium has been shown experimentally to kill the rabies virus, no data support its use in humans.[48] Besides gauze, a finely porous sponge may be used to cleanse the wound.[36,51,121] Irrigation is best performed with a 19-gauge needle or plastic intravenous (IV) catheter on a 35-ml syringe.[30] Puncture wounds tend to have a higher infection rate because irrigation is difficult, but it can be attempted if the wound is large enough to be held open. Irrigation does not remove dead or devitalized tissue common in bites, so thorough debridement may be required.

Fleisher[69] advises that wounds should be treated and left open initially if they (1) are punctures rather than lacerations, (2) are not potentially disfiguring, and (3) involve the limbs, particularly the hand or foot. Delayed repair is advised if wounds are older than 6 to 12 hours (bites to the arms and legs) or 12 to 24 hours (facial bites). In contrast, many surgeons now advocate primary closure for dog bite wounds of the face, even when several days old.[105] One study from Ghana, where a delay of several days before hospital presentation after injury is common, indicated that immediate closure of human bite injuries to the face is safe. In 90% of cases, wound healing was complete at suture removal, even though some of the wounds sutured were up to 4 days old.[53]

Bites of the hand are common and at high risk for infections and impaired healing. Although dog bites to other areas of the body have wound infection rates of 5% to 10%,[209] dog bite wounds of the hand have infection rates of up to 30%.[26,30,171] Treatment of hand bites should be aggressive, with irrigation, debridement, and antibiotic prophylaxis. The wounds are usually left open, although some authors recommend closing nonpuncture hand wounds.[209] If a dog bite wound to the hand or foot is closed primarily, the part should be immobilized in a bulky dressing and elevated. If infection is present, admission and antibiotics are indicated, with surgical drainage if required. If admission is not possible or practical, the wound should be rechecked daily until signs of infection are no longer present. If there is no evidence of infection, 5 days of splinting and oral antibiotics should be adequate.

WOUND INFECTIONS

Tetanus Prophylaxis

Clostridium tetani is an anaerobic gram-positive rod; its spores are found in the saliva and on teeth of animals and can survive in soil for years. Bite wounds often contain devitalized and crushed tissue, as well as puncture sites. These injuries are particularly suited to the release of the exotoxin *tetanospasmin,* which causes clin-

ical tetanus. The number of cases of human tetanus after bite wounds is small but is double that of bite-related human rabies.[194] Therefore a thorough immunization history is vital for appropriate immunoprophylaxis[161] (see Chapter 66).

Risk Factors for Wound Infection

Risk factors for wound infection after a bite are summarized in Box 41-3.[30,49]

Indications for Cultures

Cultures of fresh bite wound surfaces have no value in the prediction of subsequent infection. Many of the pathogens causing infection take several days to grow and may be very fastidious or difficult to identify, particularly by routine diagnostic laboratory methods. The choice of empiric therapy for infected wounds can occasionally be guided by organisms identified on Gram's stain, but therapeutic decisions are usually made before culture results are known.

Once infection is established, wound culture is indicated if prophylaxis or empiric therapy has failed; if the patient has systemic illness with signs such as pyrexia, rigors, or hypotension (in this case, blood cultures are mandatory); or if the wound or patient is at high risk. Cultures should be both aerobic and anaerobic. Gram's stain of pus may be helpful in determining predominant pathogens. The laboratory must be informed that prolonged cultures of up to 14 days may be necessary, depending on the organism sought. Using specific media for fastidious organisms, such as *Brucella*-supplemented agar to culture *Porphyromonas*, may also increase the isolation rate.[76] This is also important if *Pasteurella* or *Capnocytophaga canimorsus* infection is suspected. Isolates of coliforms should not be dismissed as contaminants and must be identified with antibiotic sensitivities. Reference laboratories, such as those of state health departments or at the Centers for Disease Control and Prevention (CDC) in Atlanta, are more likely to isolate unusual pathogens from bite wound cultures than are local laboratories.[198]

Prophylactic Antibiotics

Surgical wound care rather than antibiotic treatment is the most important factor in decreasing wound infection,[136] but whether to administer "prophylactic" antibiotics after bite wounds remains controversial. Some authors still recommend antibiotic prophylaxis for all dog bites.[134,164,172] Prospective, blinded clinical trials of dog bite wounds suggest that although persons treated with antibiotics may have lower infection rates, this is not statistically significant.[28] Such results have been extrapolated to the bite wounds of other animals. Unfortunately, many trials lacked standardization of wound care, antibiotic choice and dose, and evidence of compliance.

In 1994, Cummings[42] performed a meta-analysis of eight randomized trials to determine whether prophylactic oral antibiotics prevent infection in persons with dog bite wounds. The relative risk for infection in persons given antibiotics was 0.56. This means that 14 persons need to be treated to prevent one infection. This conclusion is skewed, however, because one study had an atypically high infection rate of 60%. If this study is excluded, the benefit of prophylaxis in low-risk wounds is even less convincing. Antibiotic therapy is not cost-effective in low-risk dog bites and should be reserved for wounds at high risk for infection.[28,50] (see Box 41-3). A small controlled trial of antibiotic prophylaxis in cat bites showed a decrease in wound infection in persons given prophylaxis.[60] Deep cat bites are prone to infection and mandate prophylaxis, whereas superficial injuries in low-risk areas do not require it.

The bite victim needing prophylactic antibiotic treatment should be identified early in a wilderness setting or during triage on entry to the ED. After a few hours, bacteria bind to proteins and become encapsulated in a blood and fibrin coagulum that protects them to some extent from antibiotics.[59,207] If infection risk is very high, parenteral antibiotics may be warranted,[207] but in most cases a 3- to 5-day oral regimen is sufficient.

Previous recommendations for choice of antibiotic often assumed that *Pasteurella*, although common in cat bites, was a rare isolate in wounds resulting from dog bites. Recent work by Talan et al[198] suggests that this may not be true. Although 42% of dog bite wounds harbored *Pasteurella stomatis, P. canis,* and *P. dagmatis,*[71] 12% of wounds grew the more virulent *P. multocida.*[198] When infection presents less than 8 hours after injury, *Pasteurella* is probably the infecting organism. Empiric therapy for dog and cat bites should cover at least *Pasteurella, Streptococcus, Staphylococcus,* and anaerobes (see Box 41-5). *Pasteurella* isolates appear susceptible to amoxicillin–clavulanate, ampicillin, penicillin, second- and third-generation cephalosporins, doxycycline, trimethoprim/sulfamethoxazole, fluoroquinolones, azithromycin, and clarithromycin, although the latter two are somewhat less effective.[75-78,80,82-85] Common antibiotics often used for soft tissue wound infections, such as antistaphylococcal penicillins and first-generation cephalosporins, are less active in vitro against *Pasteurella.* Erythromycin, often chosen for the penicillin-allergic patient, is a poor choice for *Pasteurella;* serious clinical failures are well documented.[81,123] *Pasteurella* is resistant to clindamycin.[75]

Amoxicillin-clavulanate is recommended as a first-line agent for cat, dog, human, and most other bite wounds. It is β-lactamase stable and therefore covers all *Bacteroides, Staphylococcus,* and *Streptococcus* species as well as most gram-negative bacteria. It shows activity against all 173 aerobic and anaerobic isolates tested from one series of animal bites.[78] Other options are a second-generation cephalosporin with anaerobic activity (e.g., cefoxitin) or combination therapy with either a penicillin and a first-generation cephalosporin, or clindamycin and a fluoroquinolone (e.g., ciprofloxacin).[198] Azithromycin, which is superior to clarithromycin for treating *Pasteurella,* and the new ketolide antibiotics, such as HMR 3004,[76,85] show in vitro promise, although this may not translate into in vivo success.

For the penicillin-allergic nonpregnant woman, clindamycin and ciprofloxacin are effective in high-risk wounds. For a pregnant woman whose only history of penicillin allergy is a rash, cefoxitin can be given because the chance of cross-sensitivity is low. In the penicillin-allergic pregnant woman the choice is a more difficult. Because neither azithromycin nor clarithromycin is approved for use in pregnancy, erythromycin may need to be prescribed. Because of its limited effectiveness against *Pasteurella,* careful observation of the patient is warranted. Tetracyclines should not be prescribed in pregnancy; ciprofloxacin and tetracycline should not be prescribed for young children (Tables 41-1 and 41-2).

Follow-Up and Indications for Admission

Follow-up of animal bites depends on risk factors (see Box 41-3) and the victim's response to treatment. With a superficial abrasion, infection is unlikely, so a return visit is usually not needed. With a typical, low-risk bite wound, one follow-up visit (in 2 days, to assess any infection) is sufficient. If the patient is well and no sutures have been placed, this visit may not be necessary.

Infected wounds need close follow-up. In a wound that is at high risk for infection, the initial follow-up should be the next day. If an infected wound fails to respond to 5 days of initial antibiotic treatment, a wound culture is usually advised, although switching to a broader spectrum antibiotic may be considered.

Rarely, the victim requires hospitalization (Box 41-4). Response to initial or secondary therapy (particularly in a high-risk patient), age, general health, previous medical history, and social circumstance can influence this decision.

Box 41-4 INDICATIONS FOR CONSIDERATION OF HOSPITAL ADMISSION

Hand bite
Involvement of bone, joint, or tendon
Deep space infection or tenosynovitis
Septicemia from animal bite
Severe wound infection causing systemic toxicity in immunocompetent patient
Cellulitis or local infection in severely immunocompromised patient (diabetes, AIDS, chronic alcoholism, asplenia)*
Cranial injury in an infant
Major trauma inflicted by a large animal

*Possible indication, depending on patient circumstances.

TABLE 41-1. Antibiotic Sensitivities of Common Wound Isolates

ANTIBIOTIC	Pasteurella spp.	BACTEROIDES SP. ANIMAL ORIGIN	BACTEROIDES SP. HUMAN ORIGIN	Fusobacterium	Eikenella	Capnocytophaga	Streptococcus pyogenes	Staphylococcus aureus
Penicillin or ampicillin	+++	+++	+	+++	++	+++	+++	±
Amoxycillin plus clavulanate	+++	+++	+++	+++	++	+++	+++	+++
Erythromycin	–	+	+	–	+	++	++	++
Cephalexin	–	–	–	–	–	+	++	++
Tetracycline*	+++	++	++	+	+	+	++	+
Cefoxitin	++	++	++†	+	++	++	++	++
Clindamycin	–	+	+	++	–	++	+++	+++
Trimethoprim/ sulfamethoxazole	+	–	–	–	–	++	++	++
Imipenem	+++	+++	+++	+++	+++	+++	+++	+++
Piperacillin plus tazobactam	+++	+++	+++	+++	+++	+++	+++	+++
Ciprofloxacin*	+++	–	–	–	±	+++	±	+
Oxacillin	–	–	–	–	–	±	–	+++

+++, Very sensitive; ++, moderately sensitive; +, some sensitivity; ±, predominantly insensitive; −, insensitive.
*Tetracycline should not be prescribed for pregnant women. Ciprofloxacin and tetracycline should not be prescribed for young children.
†*Bacteroides fragilis* may be resistant to cefoxitin.

TABLE 41-2. Suggested Initial Antibiotic Prophylaxis for Domestic Animal and Human Bites

PROPHYLAXIS	ADULT	CHILD
Standard	Amoxicillin-clavulanate	Amoxicillin-clavulanate
If penicillin allergic	Clindamycin plus ciprofloxacin Azithromycin Tetracycline	Azithromycin Tetracycline if child is older
If pregnant	Amoxicillin-clavulanate	—
If pregnant and rash only with penicillin	Cefoxitin*	—
If pregnant and penicillin allergic	Erythromycin†	—

*Chance of cross-sensitivity with penicillin is low.
†Erythromycin has poor activity against *Pasteurella* species, so close clinical observation is necessary.
In the case of pig bite, ciprofloxacin, when not contraindicated, should be added to amoxicillin-clavulanate.

Treatment

If inoculated in sufficiently large numbers, aerobic and anaerobic bacteria can cause localized cellulitis and abscess formation, which are the most common forms of infection. Wound infection may progress to sepsis.

Treatment of wound infection from animal bites is the same as that for other traumatic wounds: elevation and immobilization of the affected part, removal of sutures or staples, and antibiotic therapy. Empiric initial antibiotic therapy is the same as that for prophylaxis (see Table 41-2), except with severe cellulitis or sepsis (see later discussion).

Transmission of Systemic Infection

Approximately 150 systemic diseases of mammals can be transmitted in some manner to humans, but relatively few are transmitted through a bite or scratch. These include rabies, cat scratch, cowpox, tularemia, leptospirosis, infection with *Sporothrix schenckii*, and brucellosis. House cats are an increasing source of human plague in the U.S. Southwest. Since the onset of the human immunodeficiency virus (HIV) epidemic, *Rochalimaea* infection (bacillary angiomatosis) has also become more prominent and is closely associated with exposure to cats.

Sepsis Secondary to Bite Wounds

Although theoretic risks with any animal bite pathogen, bacteremia and sepsis have been reported with only a limited number of organisms. *Capnocytophaga canimorsus*, formerly CDC alphanumeric strain DF-2, is a fastidious, slender, tapering, and gram-negative rod. This facultative aerobe grows poorly in most standard media, making identification difficult. Growth of *C. canimorsus* from blood often takes a week, making Gram's stain of the blood buffy coat taken on admission a useful diagnostic test.[117] Most infections occur after dog bites. Some cases have occurred after nonbite exposure to dogs or no animal exposure.[6] About 80% of persons who become seriously ill with this infection are immunocompromised, particularly because of splenectomy, hematologic malignancy, or cirrhosis. A minor bite in a previously healthy person can also result in catastrophic infection.*

Clinical manifestations include cellulitis, endocarditis, meningitis, pneumonitis, Waterhouse-Friderichsen syndrome, renal failure, shock, and death. Purpuric lesions are seen in one third of cases and may progress to symmetric peripheral gangrene and amputation. Malar purpura is characteristic. In some cases, cutaneous gangrene develops at the bite site, a finding classic to this species of bacteria.

When the diagnosis is known, optimal treatment is with penicillin or a cephalosporin. *C. canimorsus* is susceptible to cefuroxime, ampicillin, erythromycin, and vancomycin. Ciprofloxacin has been used with success.[140] Unlike most gram-negative bacilli, *C. canimorsus* is resistant to aminoglycosides, often used in empiric treatment of sepsis. If *C. canimorsus* infection is suspected, the laboratory should be alerted, and additional blood cultures should be sent to reference laboratories (e.g., the CDC) for identification.

Pasteurella multocida can also produce bacteremia.[143] Usually the source is a cat bite, but dog bites also contribute. Most persons who develop bacteremia, as with those dying of *Capnocytophaga* infection, have cirrhosis, HIV infection, malignancy, or other immunosuppression. The mortality rate can be as high as 36%. Some victims may have been healthy, and even a seemingly trivial bite may produce life-threatening sepsis.[109]

Several options exist for empiric IV antibiotic therapy in severe cellulitis and sepsis (Box 41-5). Clin-

---

*References: 49, 96, 100, 134, 147, 170, 172.

Box 41-5 SUGGESTED EMPIRIC ANTIBIOTIC THERAPY FOR SEVERE CELLULITIS AND SEPSIS FROM BITES

Ciprofloxacin plus clindamycin*
Cefoxitin
Ceftriaxone
Imipenem-cilastatin

*May be given orally in the field or on discharge from hospital.

---

damycin plus ciprofloxacin is an appropriate combination; clindamycin inhibits toxin production in streptococcal infection and covers *Staphylococcus aureus* and anaerobes, and ciprofloxacin has good gram-negative coverage, including *Pasteurella* and *C. canimorsus*. Both drugs can also be given orally, either in the field or as continuation therapy on discharge from hospital.

DOG BITES

Dogs are the only species whose bites have been well studied in large numbers. Most factors contributing to dog bites are related to the owner's level of responsibility.[174]

Although domesticated for at least 12,000 years, dogs retain many of their wild instincts, such as territoriality in a guard dog. Although many people keep dogs to repel burglars, a burglar is a fatal dog attack victim in only 1 of 177 attacks. A fatal dog attack victim is a child in 7 of 10 cases.[35]

Besides the physical and emotional trauma of a dog attack, the financial impact is huge. Recent estimates put the total annual U.S. national cost of ED services for new dog bite–related injuries at more than $102 million.[210] When combined with charges for physician services and subsequent postdischarge care, direct medical care charges for dog bites rise to an estimated $165 million.[165]

Dogs under 1 year of age are responsible for the highest incidence of bites.[215] The incidence of biting increases substantially during the warm summer months. Most bites occur between 1 and 9 PM, probably because more people are on the street.[95] Many bites are inflicted on children coming home from school or playing outdoors. The increased susceptibility of children results from their smaller size, relative inability to defend themselves, interest in animals, and unintentional abuse of animals. Biting dogs (not necessarily those causing fatal wounds) are more likely to be certain breeds, particularly German shepherd, pit bull, and chow chow in the United States.[9,74,90] In a United Kingdom survey of patients receiving plastic surgery for bite wounds, the most common biting dogs were Staffordshire bull terriers, followed by Jack Russell terriers, medium-sized mongrels, and German shepherds.[182]

Pit bulls have become popular in recent years and are often bred for aggressive behavior. Fatal attacks from pit bulls have increased dramatically.[175] Many towns and counties are passing legislation limiting or outlawing ownership of pit bulls, and owners may be charged with manslaughter after fatalities.[39]

Wound Pathophysiology

Although most wounds are minor, the jaws of adult dogs can bite with a force of up to 450 pounds per square inch, enough to puncture light sheet metal.[72] Wounds may comprise a mixture of biting, clawing, and crushing forces. These give a characteristic pattern of lacerations and punctures and may result in avulsion of soft tissues. A dog's bite can break human long bones.[46,48] Treatment may naturally focus on the crushing component of the wound, but the penetrating component may cause the most morbidity.[200] The dog may move and shake its head during the attack, further tearing tissue.[114] Some owners replace their dogs' natural teeth with metal ones to increase their wounding capabilities. Snorting, grunting, or wound manipulation by the biting animal may force air into the tissues.[72] Besides infective organisms, foreign debris and even teeth may be deposited. In a severe attack the dog may eat tissue and blood or scavenge on an unconscious or intoxicated victim.[91,160]

Wound Location

Hand, arm, and lower extremity bites are reported most often in the adult population, with children primarily receiving head and neck wounds.[49] Injuries are typically centered around the nose, lips, and cheeks, and a bite can fracture the victim's maxilla.[70] In one large study the leading sites for wounds in victims of all ages were the face, neck, and head (29%), followed by the upper and then lower limbs.[210] In children up to age 9 years, 73% of injuries were to the face, neck, and head.[210] In Germany, 8500 dog bite injuries to the face are reported each year, and more than 50% of victims are infants or children.[178]

Microbiology of Dog and Cat Wounds

A comprehensive study that evaluated 50 patients with dog bites and 57 patients with cat bites identified a median of five bacterial isolates per culture (Box 41-6).[198] *Pasteurella* species were the most common pathogens in bites of both dogs (50%) and cats (75%), in contrast to many previous studies, where *Pasteurella* was rarely isolated from dog bite wounds.[28] The association of *Pasteurella* with infections of rapid onset was confirmed. In other studies, *Pasteurella multocida* subspecies *multocida*

and *septica* were the most common isolates in cat bite wounds and *P. canis* in dog bites.[16,62,98] *Streptococcus, Staphylococcus, Moraxella, Corynebacterium,* and *Neisseria* were the next most frequent aerobic isolates. *Eikenella corrodens,* usually associated with human bite infections, was found in only one cat and one dog bite wound.[198] *Capnocytophaga* species and *Weeksella zoohelcum,* both of which can cause invasive sepsis, were uncommon in this study and may be opportunistic pathogens. *Fusobacterium, Bacteroides, Porphyromonas,* and *Prevotella* were common anaerobic isolates.

Wound Infection in Dog Bites

Typical nonbite lacerations in an adult ED population have an infection rate of 5% to 15%.[51,89] The rate is lower in the pediatric population.[10] This rate is similar to that of typical outpatient-treated dog bite wounds, when managed properly with irrigation and debridement. Dog bites of the head and neck, all sutured and none treated with antibiotics, have an infection rate as low as 1.4%.[93] Bites of the face and ears, although often requiring extensive plastic surgery, also heal well when treated aggressively and with antibiotics, as do dog bites of the genitalia.[54,195,213] Therefore, dog bite wounds that are not high risk are probably no more infection prone than nonbite, accidental cutaneous lacerations.

Antibiotic therapy for infected dog bite wounds is initially the same as for prophylaxis, unless prophylaxis failed (see Table 41-2).

Law Enforcement Dog Bite Wounds

Law enforcement dogs are usually trained to bite and hold onto a victim until commanded to release. This is not the normal pattern for an attacking dog. The bite-and-hold technique results in deep puncture wounds, severe crush injuries, and large tissue avulsions. Attention should focus on the greater risk for deep nerve, vessel, and musculoskeletal injury.[158] Over 3 years in 486 patients evaluated on a jail ward for police dog bites, 7.2% required angiography of an extremity, and 21% of these had arterial injury.[188] A change in policy, from a bite-and-hold to a find-and-bark technique has been evaluated in Los Angeles. This resulted in a decrease in bites, injuries, and complications and a reduction in hospital admissions from 52% to 33.8% after police dog bite injuries.[102]

Fatal Attacks by Dogs

A dog bite–related fatality can be defined as death caused by acute trauma from a dog attack, often from an exsanguinating neck wound.[72] Fatal attacks by dogs in the United States cause many more deaths than rabies. A vicious attack cannot be predicted from a dog's prior behavior, since most offending dogs revert to normal, friendly behavior after the episode. A review be-

Box 41-6   BACTERIA ISOLATED FROM DOG AND CAT BITES

AEROBES

Pasteurella multocida
Other *Pasteurella* spp.
Streptococcus mitis
Streptococcus mutans
Streptococcus pyogenes
Streptococcus sanguis II
Streptococcus intermedius
β-Hemolytic streptococci, group G
β-Hemolytic streptococci, group F
Other *Streptococcus* spp.
Staphylococcus aureus
Staphylococcus epidermidis
Staphylococcus warneri
Staphylococcus intermedius
Other *Staphylococcus* spp.
Neisseria weaverii
Neisseria subflav
Other *Neisseria* spp.
Corynebacterium minutissimum
Other *Corynebacterium* spp.
Moraxella (Branhamella)
EF-4b
Enterococcus faecalis
Enterococcus avium
Other *Enterococcus* spp.
Bacillus
Pseudomonas aeruginosa
Other *Pseudomonas* spp.
Actinomyces
Brevibacterium
EF-4a
Weeksella zoohelcum
Other *Weeksella* spp.

AEROBES—cont'd

Klebsiella
Lactobacillus
Citrobacter
Flavobacterium
Micrococcus
Proteus mirabilis
Stenotrophomonas maltophilia
Capnocytophaga
Eikenella corrodens
Flavimonas oryzihabitans
Acinetobacter
Actinobacillus
Alcaligenes
Enterobacter cloacae
Erysipelothrix rhusiopathiae
Reimerella anatipestifer
Rothia dentocariosa
Aeromonas hydrophilia
Pantoea agglomerans
Rhodococcus
Streptomyces

ANAEROBES

Fusobacterium
Bacteroides fragilis
Other *Bacteroides* spp.
Porphyromonas
Prevotella
Propionibacterium
Peptostreptococcus
Eubacterium
Clostridium sordellii
Veillonella

Data from Talan DA et al: *N Engl J Med* 340:85, 1999.

tween 1979 and 1988 identified 157 fatalities, a rate of 6.7 deaths per 100 million population per year. Seventy percent of these were in children younger than 10 years.[175] For infants less than 1 year the annual death rate was 68 per 100 million, with half occurring while the infant was sleeping in a crib. Only a minority of fatal attacks were caused by stray dogs. Most victims died at the scene of the attack. Fatal attacks from pit bulls increased from 20% to 62%. German shepherds, huskies, malamutes, and wolf hybrids were the next most common fatal attackers. A review of fatal dog attacks in the US from 1989 to 1994 revealed 109 episodes.[174] Fifty-seven percent of the victims were children under 10 years. The rate of death for neonates was twice that for adults. Most attacks involved an unrestrained dog on the owner's property. Pit bulls were in-

volved in 24 deaths, rottweilers in 16, and German shepherds in 10.

In the most recent American review on dog bite fatalities, covering 1995 to 1996, dogs killed at least 25 people, although this is probably a marked underestimate because of death certificate unavailability.[32] Eighty percent of these deaths involved children, continuing a worrisome trend. Three were neonates less than 30 days old. The rottweiler was the most common breed involved. Sixty-four percent involved more than one dog. Pack behavior increases the likelihood that social facilitation and pack instinct will prolong the attack.[18] A report from southern Ireland notes that many dogs are very timid when alone, but when exposed to a pack environment, their behavior deteriorates dramatically. Of the seven pack attacks in the Irish report, five were by greyhounds.[114] Packs of aggressive dogs should be avoided and aggressive pack behavior toward humans punished by the owner.[18]

Dogs represent a significant potential cause of death for infants and small children. A dog may accept an immobile baby but may have an unpredictable predatory response when the child starts crawling. Severe dog attacks on children occur most frequently in those under 5 years old.[21] Children and severely disabled persons should never be left alone with a dog, regardless of its reputation and prior behavior. Certain breeds (e.g., pit bulls) account for a disproportionate number of cases and should be considered for more effective supervision and controls.

Prevention of Dog Bites

Risk factors for increased biting propensity include male gender and unneutered status. Many dogs that seriously wound or kill humans have long histories of aggressive behavior. Strategies that reduce biting risk include education of owners and the public, selection of dogs, training, care, and socialization.[74] Other strategies, such as the compulsory trimming of canine teeth of sled dogs in Greenland, are also useful.[88]

Laws regarding dangerous dogs should be enforced, although these are not a panacea. In 1991 the Dangerous Dogs Act was quickly enacted in the United Kingdom in response to violent attacks by American pit bull terriers and specified tight restrictions. Any offense meant the dog was euthanized and the owner prosecuted. Unfortunately, difficulties in clearly identifying pit bull terriers in the absence of clear breed standards led to confusion, and the act has received much criticism.[52] It has not yet been shown to decrease injuries by so-called dangerous breeds.[113]

Animal control programs should be introduced and supported. Animal control associations, veterinary societies, and the Humane Society offer such courses.[215] Training in bite avoidance and canine behavior is recommended; for example a dog wagging its tail still may attack. This training should be offered to persons at greatest risk, such as animal control officers and postal workers; children might also benefit.[184] Dog bites should be reported as required by local or state ordinances.

DOMESTIC CAT BITES

Domestic cats are becoming an increasing problem in the United States as the population of strays has exploded, with some estimates at 90 million.[192] This is important because of the opportunity for exposure to wild vectors of rabies. Cats now account for 50% of animal control calls, which has led to proposals for leash and licensing laws for cats. Little information for cat bites by breed is available.

Women, particularly those aged 30 to 40 years, are more likely than men to be bitten by a cat, and 63% of bites are on a hand or finger, usually the right (dominant) hand.[133,198,214] Twenty-three percent of wounds are to the shoulder, arm, or forearm.[198] Seventy percent of wounds are scratches, and 27% are punctures of the skin.[214]

Cats have a weaker biting force than dogs, but possess sharp, slender teeth, often producing deep puncture wounds.[48] Cat bites are notorious for their high infection rate, with 15% to 80% becoming infected.[47,198] Cat bites result in a higher incidence of osteomyelitis and septic arthritis than dog bites.[75] Cat bites frequently possess two risk factors for infection: location on the hand and increased depth of puncture. Other risk factors associated with wound infections include an older victim, longer delay until ED treatment, wound inflicted by a pet rather than a stray, wound care at home, and a more severe wound.[47] Wound infections are more likely to develop in patients with lower extremity wounds who did not receive prophylactic oral antibiotics and in those with puncture wounds without benefit of prophylactic oral antibiotics. Scratches very seldom become infected.[47]

Because the hand and lower extremities are common sites of injury and wounds are deep and penetrating, most cat bites are considered high risk. Such wounds should prompt administration of prophylactic antibiotics (see Table 41-2). Superficial cat bites and scratches elsewhere on the body are not high risk and should receive standard wound care without antibiotic coverage. Bacteria from cat bites and scratches can seed in distant arthritic and prosthetic joints and cause *Pasteurella* septic arthritis, endocarditis, and even mycotic thoracic aortic aneurysm[7,86,99] (see Table 41-2 and Box 41-6).

HUMAN BITES

Human bites are common, particularly in urban areas. They were previously thought to be associated with a higher incidence of infection than other animal bites, but this may not be true. A study of 434 human bites found an infection rate of only 17.7% compared with 13.4% in 803 lacerations in the same patient group.[125] Others have cited a 10% infection rate for human bite wounds.[24] The important high-risk exception is human bites to the hand, especially if treatment is delayed. Unfortunately, bites of the hand often present several days after injury.

Most human bites occur during fights. A wound sustained when human teeth actually bite a part of the human anatomy is termed an *occlusional bite*; in forensic cases this is most common on the hands and arms of men and the breasts and genitalia of women.[75,92] Bites may occasionally be self-inflicted as a result of psychiatric or organic illness.[166,201]

Human bite wounds in developing countries pose special problems. Presentation may be significantly delayed,[127,135,145] and victims may have advanced infections. Many bites are inflicted by women on other women, and many are bites of the face, particularly the lip.[34,53,145] These wounds are intended to be disfiguring and can carry significant social stigma, further delaying treatment. Initial treatment in developing countries may be inappropriate, such as treating fresh bites with very hot water.[127] In the Micronesian Islands the tip of the nose may be bitten off adulterous wives to provoke shame.[20,124] This form of punishment was known under ancient Roman law and Indian custom, and the art of nasal reconstruction originated in India as early as 1000 BC.[151] Traumatic love bites to the neck are well documented, as are bites to the face, breasts and penis during sexual activity.[65,212]

Microbiology

At least 42 different species of bacteria have been identified in human saliva,[128] and 190 species have been found when gingivitis or periodontitis is present (Box 41-7).[137,138] Anaerobes include *Bacteroides fragilis*, *Prevotella*, *Porphyromonas*, *Peptostreptococcus*, *Fusobacterium*, *Veillonella*, and *Clostridium* species. Anaerobes are found in more than 50% of human bite wounds[75] and frequently produce β-lactamase, unlike those from an-

imal bites. Studies show that 41% to 45% of *B. fragilis* infections from human bite wounds are resistant to penicillin.[22,81] Common pathogenic aerobes include β-hemolytic streptococci, *Staphylococcus aureus*, and *Haemophilus* species.[75,92] *Eikenella corrodens*, a fastidious, slow-growing, and gram-negative anaerobic rod, is found on 8.2% of human tooth scrapings and in 0.6% of salivary samples.[167] *E. corrodens* is frequently implicated in fight-bite injury infections and has been found in 10% to 29% of human bite wounds[92] (see Table 41-2).

Human Bites and Systemic Disease

Transmission of actinomycosis has been reported after a human bite,[139] as has syphilis, herpes, hepatitis C, hepatitis B, and tuberculosis.[45,66-68,110,193] Tetanus from a human bite has been documented.[1,144] Herpetic whitlow (infection of the distal phalanx) from herpes simplex virus is a well-known occupational hazard of nurses, physicians, dentists, and oral hygienists.[107] Toxic shock has been reported after a clenched-fist injury.[126]

Human bites had not been thought to pose a significant risk of HIV.[169] HIV is usually not present in the saliva of infected patients, and when present, the titer of virus is very low. Recent data suggest that a slight risk does exist, however, and a human bite is thought to have been the mode of HIV transmission in at least two cases.

Box 41-7 BACTERIA ISOLATED FROM HUMAN BITES

AEROBES

Acinetobacter
Branhamella (Moraxella) catarrhalis
Corynebacterium
Eikenella corrodens
Enterobacter cloacae
Other *Enterobacter* spp.
Escherichia coli
Haemophilus aphrophilus
Haemophilus influenzae
Haemophilus parainfluenzae
Klebsiella pneumoniae
Micrococcus
Moraxella
Neisseria gonorrhoeae
Other *Neisseria* spp.
Nocardia
Proteus mirabilis
Pseudomonas aeruginosa
Other *Pseudomonas* spp.
Serratia marcescens
Staphylococcus aureus
Staphylococcus epidermidis

AEROBES—cont'd

Staphylococcus intermedius
Staphylococcus saprophyticus
α-Hemolytic streptococci
β-Hemolytic streptococci
γ-Hemolytic streptococci

ANAEROBES

Acidaminococcus
Actinomyces
Arachnia propionica
Bacteroides fragilis
Clostridium
Eubacterium
Fusobacterium nucleatum
Peptostreptococcus anaerobius
Peptostreptococcus prevotti
Other *Peptostreptococcus* spp.
Prevotella
Propionibacterium acnes
Other *Propionibacterium* spp.
Veillonella

Modified from Griego RD, Rosen T, Orengo IF, Wolf JE: *J Am Acad Dermatol* 33:1019, 1995.

In one report from Slovenia, a man was bitten while trying to control the airway of a person with acquired immunodeficiency syndrome (AIDS) who had bitten his own tongue during a seizure.[206] The second occurred after a lip bite in a male from a female prostitute.[112]

When bitten by a person who is infected with or at high risk for HIV, the victim should receive unusually vigorous and thorough wound irrigation with a virucidal agent such as 1% povidone-iodine. A baseline HIV blood test and follow-up test in 6 months should be considered.

Human Bites of the Hand

The two forms of bite injury to the hand are the simple, direct occlusional bite to a finger and the fight-bite, or clenched-fist, injury. Osteomyelitis may occur after either injury.[87,204]

The fight-bite injury is more common and at higher risk for infection. Presentation is frequently delayed.[204] From 60% to 80% of fight-bite injuries occur in males, most in the dominant fist after striking an opponent's tooth.[135] In this position the extensor tendon and its underlying bursa are pulled distally over the metacarpophalangeal (MCP) joint. The result is a deep laceration that can disrupt superficial and deep fasciae, the extensor tendon and its bursa, and the joint capsule. When the fingers are extended, the skin and tendon retract proximally, sealing off the contaminated wound.

Any penetrating injury in the vicinity of the MCP joint should be considered a human fight-bite wound until proved otherwise. Radiographs should be requested, and up to 70% of patients may have positive findings[56] (Figure 41-1). Films should be obtained in a

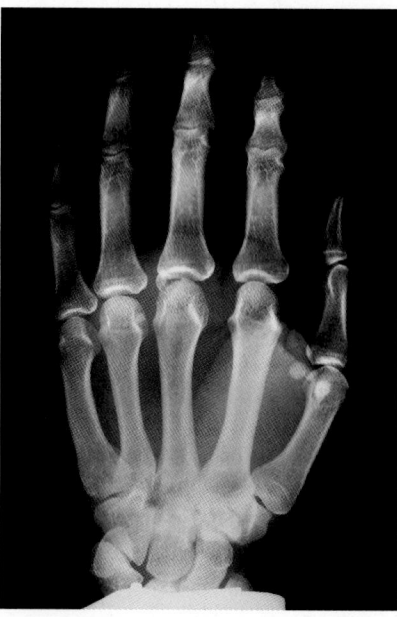

Figure 41-1 Intraarticular fracture of the third metacarpal resulting from a human fight-bite injury.

lateral or steep oblique attitude, since this is the best view for initial soft tissue swelling.[168] The ideal view is the skyline view of the metacarpal head, taken with the x-ray beam in the same plane as the proximal phalanx, with the MCP joint fully flexed.[64]

Treatment of clenched-fist injuries should be rapid and aggressive. Significant injuries should be explored and debrided, preferably in the operating room.[11,204] In the wilderness setting the wounds should be thoroughly irrigated and not sutured. These wounds are at high risk for infection, and antibiotics should be prescribed as soon as possible. Oral antibiotic therapy should result in a very low infection rate.[216] Although evidence is contradictory, few indications exist for primary repair of any type of hand bite. The affected extremity should be immobilized and elevated.

A person with established infection is usually hospitalized and treated with IV antibiotics, although closely supervised outpatient oral therapy is an alternative in the compliant patient after wound cleansing and debridement.[56,191] An appropriate initial antibiotic choice for both prophylaxis and treatment of a clenched-fist injury is amoxicillin-clavulanate.

Human Bites to the Face and Cheek

Facial wounds are at low risk for infection, and a large series of sutured facial human bites treated in a plastic surgery clinic had an infection rate of only 2.5%.[57] Treatment includes aggressive debridement, irrigation, and suturing. Cosmetic considerations are important. Antibiotics are indicated for the same risk factors as in animal bites (see Box 41-3).

Self-inflicted bite wounds of the oral or buccal mucosa have not been well studied. Accidental bites of the mouth and lips have low infection rates, possibly because of protective effects from saliva and resistance of mucosal tissues to the victim's own flora. However, a case of *Haemophilus aphrophilus* vertebral osteomyelitis secondary to an accidental lip laceration was reported in a healthy 36-year-old male despite prophylactic antibiotics.[97]

The literature suggests that oral-cutaneous (through-and-through) wounds are high risk and may benefit from penicillin prophylaxis.[3,155,190] Lacerations that involve only the buccal mucosa, particularly those that do not need suturing, do not require prophylaxis.

Human Bite Forensics

Bite mark evidence has become accepted as a powerful tool in the investigation of crime.[202] Human bite marks are found most often in cases of murder, rape, child abuse, or altercation.[106] The examining physician should document the appearance of the bite carefully, including its shape, color, and size. Determining the age of the bite can be difficult but is often a critical legal issue. The healing dynamics of these bite wounds is poorly understood,[44] and accurate description is better than unsupported speculation. The physician must determine if a criminal act may have occurred; if so, the wound should be photographed. Salivary deoxyribonucleic acid (DNA) can be recovered from bite marks on human skin.[197] Physical comparison of a suspect's teeth to a bite mark injury using hollow-volume comparison overlays is a common forensic odontology technique.[196] Since most physicians are not familiar with these procedures, consultation with a forensic pathologist or dentist is recommended and may be arranged through the local law enforcement agency.

FERRET BITES

Egyptians kept ferrets long before the cat.[154] The two species of ferret in the United States are the common ferret *Mustela putorius furo,* sold as a domestic pet, and the wild black-footed ferret *Mustela nigripes,* which is an endangered species. The pet ferret was domesticated from the wild European polecat and was first introduced into the United States in about 1875.[131] Ferrets are kept in increasing numbers as domestic pets, especially by urban apartment dwellers.

Because of its speed, an attacking ferret can easily run over the shoulders and head of an adult human and inflict multiple bites without stopping.[40] Ferrets were bred to hunt and kill small game and rodents in their burrows and are particularly attracted to suckling animals, possibly because of the scent of milk. Along with a mouth containing 34 teeth, sharp claws are found on all four feet.[8] Severe injuries caused by ferrets are not common. When they occur, an infant is often the victim and typically is sleeping or in a crib. The face, ears, and nose may be mutilated.[154] Scratches, lacerations, and puncture wounds are seen, and the ferret may chew on a victim (e.g., a baby's ear). The neck is also a common target.

In a comprehensive review of 452 ferret attacks over 10 years, virtually all the unprovoked attacks were on the faces of unattended infants.[40] Most victims were less than 3 years of age and were attacked while sleeping or lying down. Several injuries were severe, and one child died. Bites were usually multiple, and sometimes the ferret's jaws had to be pried open or the ferret had to be killed to secure release.[154]

Ferrets are unusually adept at escaping from cages and enclosures, guaranteeing that they will occasionally be loose unsupervised in the house and also that they can escape to the wild, where they will be exposed to endemic rabies. In one study, 4% of biting ferrets were positive for rabies virus.[40] At the University of Georgia, 50 ferrets were inoculated with rabies virus; no animal with virus in the central nervous system showed any evidence of viral shedding in saliva, and only one had rabies in their salivary glands.[55] Ferrets

are now classified in the same category as cats and dogs regarding rabies pathogenesis and viral shedding patterns, rather than as wild terrestrial carnivores. They may be confined and observed for 10 days rather than being routinely euthanized after biting.[103] An effective rabies vaccine for ferrets (IMRAB-3) has been available since 1990.

Little is known of infection rates or bacteriology in ferret-inflicted wounds although unusual species such as *Mycobacterium bovis* have been observed.[108] Initial treatment should be as for dog bites.

BITES AND INJURIES FROM DOMESTIC HERBIVORES

Horses and Donkeys

The horse is inclined to both bite and kick, but most horse-related injuries follow a fall during riding activities. More accidents occur per hour horse riding than motorcycling.[37] Young females are most often injured by falls,[23] and head injuries cause the majority of deaths.[94] When a half-ton horse lands on top of a rider after a fall, pelvic ring injuries and knee ligament injuries are a particular risk.[58] Appropriate helmets and footwear help to reduce the severity of injury.[37]

Horse bites are common but not severe injuries. The occlusal surfaces of both lower and upper incisors are flattened. Most male horses possess canines, however, that may be used to grab onto a mare's neck during mounting. A penetrating wound to the chest after a horse bite in a child has been described.[104] The soft tissue contusions inflicted by a horse can be severe, but in a series of 24 horse bites, 21 healed uneventfully.[58] Bites can produce significant injury, including muscle rupture and fat necrosis, with no external wound. Ultrasound may be useful in the diagnosis of such injuries.[205] Horses also have a propensity for biting human nipples, which are at the same height as a horse's mouth.

Horse kicks from the rear legs can be extremely powerful, causing severe blunt trauma, including cardiac rupture.[19] Kicks have also resulted in massive pulmonary embolism.[159]

Donkeys also bite. One rural worker was bitten twice the same year by the same donkey. The bites were on different forearms, and both resulted in multiple fractures.[189] Death has been reported from fat embolism caused by fractures after a donkey bite.[17]

Cattle and Sheep

Cattle and sheep are usually docile but can inflict a variety of injuries. Serious bites are infrequent, since these animals possess neither upper incisors nor canines. A cow typically weighs 1400 pounds, and a bull can exceed 3000 pounds. Accidental treading on the human victim or butting can cause major crush injuries and fractures. Rams have killed farmers by repeated blunt trauma.[146] Farm animals in Wisconsin kill about six people a year.[25] One hospital in rural Wisconsin treated an average of 22 persons a year for horse and cattle injuries, most of them inflicted by a kick or other assault. Domestic cattle and horses are fairly frequently infected with rabies, but because veterinary workers are immunized against the virus, these animals seldom account for human infection.

Cattle horn injuries (or gorings) present typical and unique damage patterns. The horns are used in an inward hooking motion to butt and fling the victim, or the horn tip can be used for goring. Goring injuries seen in bullfighting typically involve the perineum and thigh; they tend to be deep and sometimes fatal. Scrotal skin avulsion is common in bullfight gorings.[183] By contrast, bull horn injuries from domestic cattle involve a sweeping arc at the level of the bull's head, which is at the level of the human abdomen. The semicircular motion of the horn often produces a relatively superficial laceration, leaving deeper structures of the abdomen intact. In one series of 29 cases in which the peritoneum was breached, usually producing prolapse of bowel or omentum, 27 laparotomies demonstrated no additional injuries. In only a few cases was the bowel itself damaged.[183] The wound infection rate in this series was high (54%), probably because of delayed treatment. Gorings to the eye have also been described; in one case a metal horn cover complete with decorative ribbons was impacted in the orbit.[186]

Farmers or veterinarians examining a sick animal should always have a second person present to assist and warn them.[31] Bulls should be approached only with a protective device (e.g., a heavy stick) and a preplanned exit. A ring in the bull's nose gives a victim something to hang onto besides the horns and a way to yank the bull's nose up, which may stop the attack. Dehorning the bull will not eliminate the potential for crushing. If struck by a bull or cow, the victim should not attempt to stand, since this will provoke being thrown to the ground again, and should try to crawl to safety. Children must be educated about the risks of large animals and kept away from them whenever possible.

Camels

In regions where camels are used for domestic or agricultural purposes, bite injuries are quite common.[176] Although herbivores and usually docile, camels are much more likely to bite in the winter rutting season, and bite fatalities have been reported. Camels have 34 teeth, including large backward-inclined upper canines, or tushes. The lower tushes are placed relatively forward, and the resultant mouth grip is very effective. Jerking movements of the head result in severe tissue damage and sometimes limb avulsion. This whipping motion can also break the victim's neck. The forearm is often injured, and bites to the face are well documented.[150,185] Virtually all bites are single.[176] Injury or death can also occur if the camel presses the victim to the ground and crushes, after gripping the person in its jaws.

Domestic Deer

The most common domesticated deer are the reindeer and the more recently domesticated red and fallow deer. Female deer bite other deer when fighting. Males bite when testosterone levels are low, because at these times antlers are soft, pain sensitive, and cannot be used as weapons. Foreleg kicks are more common, since the deer stands on its back legs. Domestic deer only bite humans when threatened. Since they have a dental pad instead of upper incisors, bites are rarely serious and are usually directed at an arm and the back, which are normally well covered by clothing. These bites are usually single nips.

Microbiology of Herbivore Bites

Little is known about wound infection from herbivore-inflicted injuries. Infection after camel bites is common, up to 86%,[176] although this series did not specify time from injury to treatment. Species of *Actinobacillus lignieresii* and *A. suis*, as well as *Pasteurella multocida*, have been isolated from infected horse and sheep bites.[13,157] All are common organisms in the mouths of herbivores. *Actinobacillus* and *Pasteurella* are closely related genera, distinguished chiefly by biochemical tests. Most domestic herbivores carry *Pasteurella*, and most are given frequent and regular doses of different antibiotics, especially in their feed, leading to antibiotic resistance of bite wound organisms.[162] *Pasteurella caballi* has been isolated from a horse bite wound.[63] *Staphylococcus hyicus* subspecies *hyicus*, a well-known cause of disease in many animals, has been reported as a human wound pathogen after a donkey bite.[153] One child developed *Acinetobacter anitratus* osteomyelitis after a pet hamster bite to his finger.[132]

Bites from horses, donkeys, cattle, sheep, camels, deer, and most other herbivores are treated with the same antibiotics as bites from dogs, cats, and humans (see Table 41-2 and Box 41-5).

INJURY FROM DOMESTIC SWINE

Bites from domestic swine are fairly rare, although pigs have bitten 12% of veterinarians.[119] When they do attack, domestic swine can be aggressive and inflict deep goring or bite injuries, often on the posterior thigh as the pig approaches from behind.[11,149] Goring wounds may be deep, even while deceptively small on the surface.[203]

Among veterinarians, pigs have a reputation of inflicting bites at high risk for infection. Thorough wound exploration and debridement are essential. The usual wide range of bacterial pathogens is reported, including *Pasteurella aerogenes, Bacteroides, Proteus,* and hemolytic streptococci, including *Streptococcus milleri.*[11,122] *Actinobacillus suis* has also been reported.[61] Like many domestic animals, pigs often carry *Pasteurella multocida.* Unusual gram-negative bacteria, such as *Flavobacterium* group IIb, have been isolated, as has *Mycoplasma.*[79,141] Both these organisms are resistant to amoxicillin-clavulanate, so the addition of ciprofloxacin is recommended as prophylaxis for a serious pig bite wound.[141,142]

INJURY FROM BIRDS

Birds may be kept as domestic pets or on farms. They can inflict serious injuries. Attacks on joggers by non-domesticated birds may also occur. European buzzards, red-tailed hawks, and starlings are known to be aggressive on occasion. On farms, rooster attacks, often by male fowl defending their territory, are well documented. Children, especially infants, are particularly vulnerable to attack. Rooster injuries have included serious clawing to the face and a fractured skull.[163] A 2-year-old child sustained a ruptured globe from a rooster attack in a petting zoo.[116] In one report a rooster spur was retained in a wound, resulting in chronic infection.[41] Septic arthritis was reported in a child after a bite from a domestic fowl.[101]

The ostrich is responsible for one to two deaths a year, mostly in Africa, where it is raised commercially. Most of the fatal attacks are kicks to the head and abdomen. The ostrich can kick only forward; a sharp toenail flicks out like a switchblade and can penetrate the abdomen. Since an ostrich can easily outrun a human, the only protection is to lie prone to protect against disembowelment and to cover the neck to protect against pecks. Eventually, the ostrich loses interest and allows the victim to escape.

MEDICOLEGAL IMPLICATIONS

In certain locations and circumstances, animal bites must be reported to public health authorities. Reporting suspected exposure to rabies is mandatory in most regions. If the offending animal is a pet, the victim may seek compensation from the owner, and that the health care provider may be summoned and the medical record reviewed in court. Injuries and their circumstances should be documented as fully as possible, with line drawings or photographs added to the medical record whenever possible. Hand wounds are particularly prone to infection and can lead to permanent, litigation-prone complications. A legible, precise, and complete medical record is the best protection for the health care provider.

Human bites are often inflicted in assaults or fights and may be a marker for child, spousal, or elder abuse.

All these conditions must be reported to law enforcement agents in most jurisdictions. Subsequent criminal investigation may depend heavily on the initial medical record, which must be extensive and complete. Human bites of the hand have a propensity for infection and complications. In addition to providing and documenting thorough and appropriate care of the wounds, the physician should warn the victim of possible complications despite current care.

ACKNOWLEDGMENT

I thank Dr. Marina Morgan for her microbiologic advice and review of this chapter.

REFERENCES

1. Agrawal K et al: Tetanus caused by human bite of the finger, *Ann Plast Surg* 34:201, 1995.
2. Alberio L, Lammle B: Images in clinical medicine. *Capnocytophaga canimorsus* sepsis, *N Engl J Med* 339:1827, 1998.
3. Altieri M, Brasch L, Getson P: Antibiotic prophylaxis in intraoral wounds, *Am J Emerg Med* 4:507, 1986; 5:176, 1987 (erratum).
4. American Pet Products Manufacturers Association: 1998 National Pet Owner Survey.
5. Anderson CR: Animal bites: guidelines to current management, *Postgrad Med* 92:134, 1992.
6. Angeras MH et al: Comparison between sterile saline and tap water for the cleaning of acute traumatic soft tissue wounds, *Eur J Surg* 158:347, 1992.
7. Antuna SA et al: Late infection after total knee arthroplasty caused by *Pasteurella multocida, Acta Orthop Belg* 63:310, 1997.
8. Applegate JA, Walhout MF: Childhood risks from the ferret, *J Emerg Med* 16:425, 1998.
9. Avner JR, Baker MD: Dog bites in urban children, *Pediatrics* 88:55, 1991.
10. Baker MD, Lanuti M: The management and outcome of lacerations in urban children, *Ann Emerg Med* 19:1001, 1990.
11. Barnham M: Pig bite injuries and infection: report of seven human cases, *Epidemiol Infect* 101:641, 1988.
12. Barnham M: Once bitten twice shy: the microbiology of bites, *Rev Med Mirobiol* 2:31, 1991.
13. Benaoudia F, Escande F, Simonet M: Infection due to *Actinobacillus lignieresii* after a horse bite, *Eur J Clin Microbiol Infect Dis* 13:439, 1994 (letter).
14. Bhanganada K et al: Dog-bite injuries at a Bangkok teaching hospital, *Acta Trop* 55:249, 1993.
15. Bhargava A et al: Profile and characteristics of animals bites in India, *J Assoc Physicians India* 44:37, 1996.
16. Biberstein EL et al: Distribution of indole-producing urease-negative pasteurellas in animals, *J Vet Diagn Invest* 3:319, 1991.
17. Bloch B: Fatal fat embolism following severe donkey bites, *J Forensic Sci Soc* 16:231, 1976.
18. Borchelt PL et al: Attacks by packs of dogs involving predation on human beings, *Publi Health Rep* 98:57, 1983.
19. Brathwaite CE et al: Blunt traumatic cardiac rupture: a 5-year experience, *Ann Surg* 212:701, 1990.
20. Brewis A: *Lives on the line: women and ecology on a Pacific atoll,* Fort Worth, Tex, 1996, Harcourt Brace.
21. Brogan TV et al: Severe dog bites in children, *Pediatrics* 96:947, 1995.
22. Brook I: Microbiology of human and animal bite wounds in children, *Pediatric Infect Dis* J 6:29, 1987.
23. Buckley SM, Chalmers DJ, Langley JD: Injuries due to falls from horses, *Aust J Public Health* 17:269, 1993.
24. Bunzli WF et al: Current management of human bites, *Pharmacotherapy* 18:227, 1998.
25. Busch HMJ et al: Blunt bovine and equine trauma, *J Trauma* 26:559, 1986.
26. Callaham M: Prophylactic antibiotics in common dog bite wounds: a controlled study, *Ann Emerg Med* 9:410, 1980.
27. Callaham M: Controversies in antibiotic choices for bite wounds, *Ann Emerg Med* 17:1321, 1988.
28. Callaham M: Prophylactic antibiotics in dog bite wounds: nipping at the heels of progress, *Ann Emerg Med* 23:577, 1994 (editorial).

29. Callaham M: Human and animal bites, *Top Emerg Med* 4:1, 1999.

30. Callaham ML: Treatment of common dog bites: infection risk factors, *JACEP* 7:83, 1978.

31. Casey GM et al: Farm worker injuries associated with bulls, New York State 1991-1996, *AAOHN J* 45:393, 1997.

32. Centers for Disease Control and Prevention: Dog-bite-related fatalities—United States, 1995-1996, *JAMA* 278:278, 1997.

33. Chang YF et al: Dog bite incidence in the city of Pittsburgh: a capture-recapture approach, *Am J Public Health* 87:1703, 1997.

34. Chidzonga MM: Human bites of the face: a review of 22 cases, *S Afr Med J* 88:150, 1998.

35. Children primary focus of National Dog Bite Prevention Week, *Postal News* 51, 1996.

36. Chisholm CD: Wound evaluation and cleansing, *Emerg Med Clin North Am* 10:665, 1992.

37. Chitnavis JP et al: Accidents with horses: what has changed in 20 years? *Injury* 27:103, 1996.

38. Chomel BB, Trotignon J: Epidemiologic surveys of dog and cat bites in the Lyon area, France, *Eur J Epidemiol* 8:619, 1992.

39. Clark MA et al: Fatal and near-fatal animal bite injuries, *J Forensic Sci* 36:1256, 1991.

40. Constantine D, Kizer K: *Pet European ferrets: a hazard to public health, small livestock, and wildlife,* Sacramento, Calif, 1988, Department of Health Services.

41. Cooler JO et al: Retained spur following a rooster attack, *Pediatrics* 90:106, 1992.

42. Cummings P: Antibiotics to prevent infection in patients with dog bite wounds: a meta-analysis of randomized trials, *Ann Emerg Med* 23:535, 1994.

43. Dahl E: Animal bites at the casualty department of the Oslo City Council, *Tidsskr Nor Laegeforen* 118:2614, 1998

44. Dailey JC, Bowers CM: Aging of bitemarks: a literature review, *J Forensic Sci* 42:792, 1997.

45. del Rosario NC, Blair E, Rickman L: A herpetic hickey, *N Engl J Med* 317:54, 1987 (letter).

46. Dimant A et al: [Treatment of open fractures due to dog bite], *Harefuah* 132:461, 1997.

47. Dire DJ: Cat bite wounds: risk factors for infection, *Ann Emerg Med* 20:973, 1991 (erratum 21:1008, 1992).

48. Dire DJ: Emergency management of dog and cat bite wounds, *Emerg Med Clin North Am* 10:719, 1992.

49. Dire DJ, Hogan DE, Riggs MW: A prospective evaluation of risk factors for infections from dog-bite wounds, *Acad Emerg Med* 1:258, 1994.

50. Dire DJ, Hogan DE, Walker JS: Prophylactic oral antibiotics for low-risk dog bite wounds, *Pediatr Emerg Care* 8:194, 1992.

51. Dire DJ, Welsh AP: A comparison of wound irrigation solutions used in the emergency department, *Ann Emerg Med* 19:704, 1990.

52. A dog's dinner of a law, *Vet Rec* 573, 1995.

53. Donkor P, Bankas DO: A study of primary closure of human bite injuries to the face, *J Oral Maxillofac Surg* 55:479, 1997.

54. Donovan JF, Kaplan WE: The therapy of genital trauma by dog bite, *J Urol* 141:1163, 1989.

55. Dreesen D: 4th Symposium on Biosafety, Atlanta, 1996.

56. Dreyfuss UY, Singer M: Human bites of the hand: a study of one hundred six patients, *J Hand Surg* 10A:884, 1985.

57. Earley MJ, Bardsley AF: Human bites: a review, *Br J Plast Surg* 37:458, 1984.

58. Edixhoven P, Sinha SC, Dandy DJ: Horse injuries, *Injury* 12:279, 1981.

59. Edlich RF, Smith QT, Edgerton MT: Resistance of the surgical wound to antimicrobial prophylaxis and its mechanisms of development, *Am J Surg* 126:583, 1973.

60. Elenbaas RM: Evaluation of prophylactic oxacillin in cat bite wounds. *Ann Emerg Med* 13:155, 1984.

61. Escande F et al: *Actinobacillus suis* infection after a pig bite, *Lancet* 348:888, 1996 (letter).

62. Escande F, Lion C: Epidemiology of human infections by *Pasteurella* and related groups in France, *Int J Med Microbiol Virol Parasitol Infect Dis* 279:131, 1993.

63. Escande F, Vallee E, Aubart F: *Pasteurella caballi* infection following a horse bite, *Zentralbl Bakteriol* 285:440, 1997.

64. Eyres KS, Allen TR: Skyline view of the metacarpal head in the assessment of human fight-bite injuries, *J Hand Surg* 18B:43, 1993.

65. Fallouji MA: Traumatic love bites, *Br J Surg* 77:100, 1990.

66. Fenton PA: Hepatitis B virus transmission via bite, *Lancet* 338:1466, 1991.

67. Figueiredo JF et al: Transmission of hepatitis C virus but not human immunodeficiency virus type 1 by a human bite, *Clin Infect Dis* 19:546, 1994 (letter).

68. Fiumara NJ, Exner JH: Primary syphilis following a human bite, *Sex Transm Dis* 8:21, 1981.

69. Fleisher GR: The management of bite wounds, *N Engl J Med* 340:138, 1999 (editorial).

70. Fourie L, Cartilidge D: Fracture of the maxilla following dog bite to the face, *Injury* 26:61, 1995.

71. Ganiere JP et al: Characterization of *Pasteurella* from gingival scrapings of dogs and cats, *Comp Immunol Microbiol Infect Dis* 16:77, 1993.

72. Garcia VF: Animal bites and *Pasturella* infections, *Pediatr Rev* 18:127, 1997.

73. Garrard J, Leland N, Smith DK: Epidemiology of human bites to children in a day-care center, *Am J Dis Child* 142:643, 1988.

74. Gershman KA, Sacks JJ, Wright JC: Which dogs bite? A case-control study of risk factors, *Pediatrics* 93:913, 1994.

75. Goldstein EJ: Bite wounds and infection, *Clin Infect Dis* 14:633, 1992.

76. Goldstein EJ: New horizons in the bacteriology, antimicrobial susceptibility and therapy of animal bite wounds, *J Med Microbiol* 47:95, 1998 (editorial).

77. Goldstein EJ, Citron DM: Comparative activities of cefuroxime, amoxicillin-clavulanic acid, ciprofloxacin, enoxacin, and ofloxacin against aerobic and anaerobic bacteria isolated from bite wounds, *Antimicrob Agents Chemother* 32:1143, 1988.

78. Goldstein EJ, Citron DM: Comparative susceptibilities of 173 aerobic and anaerobic bite wound isolates to sparfloxacin, temafloxacin, clarithromycin, and older agents, *Antimicrob Agents Chemother* 37:1150, 1993.

79. Goldstein EJ, Citron DM, Merkin TE, Pickett MJ: Recovery of an unusual Flavobacterium group IIb-like isolate from a hand infection following pig bite, *J Clin Microbiol* 28:1079, 1990.

80. Goldstein EJ, Citron DM, Richwald GA: Lack of in vitro efficacy of oral forms of certain cephalosporins, erythromycin, and oxacillin against *Pasteurella multocida*, *Antimicrob Agents Chemother* 32:213, 1988.

81. Goldstein EJ, Citron DM, Vagvolgyi AE, Finegold SM: Susceptibility of bite wound bacteria to seven oral antimicrobial agents, including RU-985, a new erythromycin: considerations in choosing empiric therapy, *Antimicrob Agents Chemother* 29:556, 1986.

82. Goldstein EJ, Nesbit CA, Citron DM: Comparative in vitro activities of azithromycin, Bay y 3118, levofloxacin, sparfloxacin, and 11 other oral antimicrobial agents against 194 aerobic and anaerobic bite wound isolates, *Antimicrob Agents Chemother* 39:1097, 1995.

83. Goldstein EJ et al: Activities of HMR 3004 (RU 64004) and HMR 3647 (RU 66647) compared to those of erythromycin, azithromycin, clarithromycin, roxithromycin, and eight other antimicrobial agents against unusual aerobic and anaerobic human and animal bite pathogens isolated from skin and soft tissue infections in humans, *Antimicrob Agents Chemother* 42:1127, 1998.

84. Goldstein EJ et al: In vitro activity of Bay 12-8039, a new 8-methoxyquinolone, compared to the activities of 11 other oral antimicrobial agents against 390 aerobic and anaerobic bacteria isolated from human and animal bite wound skin and soft tissue infections in humans, *Antimicrob Agents Chemother* 41:1552, 1997.

85. Goldstein EJ et al: Trovafloxacin compared with levofloxacin, ofloxacin, ciprofloxacin, azithromycin and clarithromycin against unusual aerobic and anaerobic human and animal bite-wound pathogens, *J Antimicrob Chemother* 41:391, 1998.

86. Goldstein RW, Goodhart GL, Moore JE: *Pasteurella multocida* infection after animal bites, *N Engl J Med* 315:460, 1986 (letter).

87. Gonzales MH: Osteomyelitis of the hand after a human bite, *J Hand Surg* 18A:520, 1993.

88. Gottlieb JO, Misfeldt JC: [Dog bites in the sledge-dog districts of Greenland], *Ugeskr Laeger* 154:2824, 1992.

89. Gravett A et al: A trial of povidone-iodine in the prevention of infection in sutured lacerations, *Ann Emerg Med* 16:167, 1987.

90. Greenhalgh C, Cockington RA, Raftos J: An epidemiological survey of dog bites presenting to the emergency department of a children's hospital, *J Paediatr Child Health* 27:171, 1991.

91. Grellner W, Meyer E, Fechner G: [Simulation of attempted homicide by dog bite in unconscious state], *Arch Kriminol* 201:165, 1998.

92. Griego RD et al: Dog, cat, and human bites: a review, *J Am Acad Dermatol* 33:1019, 1995.

93. Guy RJ, Zook EG: Successful treatment of acute head and neck dog bite wounds without antibiotics, *Ann Plast Surg* 17:45, 1986.

94. Hamilton MG, Tranmer BI: Nervous system injuries in horseback-riding accidents, *J Trauma* 34:227, 1993.

95. Harris D, Imperato PJ, Oken B: Dog bites—an unrecognized epidemic, *Bull N Y Acad Med* 50:981, 1974.

96. Hermann CK et al: [Bacterial infections as complications of dog bites], *Ugeskr Laeger* 160:4860, 1998.

97. Ho JL et al: Hemophilus aprophilus osteomyelitis, *Am J Med* 76:159, 1984.

98. Holst E et al: Characterization and distribution of Pasteurella species recovered from infected humans, *J Clin Microbiol* 30:2984, 1992.

99. Hombal SM, Dincsoy HP: *Pasteurella multocida* endocarditis, *Am J Clin Pathol* 98:565, 1992.

100. Hovenga S et al: Dog-bite induced sepsis: a report of four cases, *Intensive Care Med* 23:1179, 1997.

101. Huang CM et al: Septic arthritis following a chicken bite, *Clin Rheumatol* 17:540, 1998.

102. Hutson HR et al: Law enforcement K-9 dog bites: injuries, complications, and trends, *Ann Emerg Med* 29:637, 1997.

103. Imported dog and cat rabies—New Hampshire, California, *MMWR* 37:559, 1988.

104. Inci I et al: Penetrating chest injuries in children: a review of 94 cases, *J Pediatr Surg* 31:673, 1996.

105. Javaid M, Feldberg L, Gipson M: Primary repair of dog bites to the face: 40 cases, *J R Soc Med* 91:414, 1998.

106. Jessee SA: Recognition of bite marks in child abuse cases, *Pediatr Dent* 16:336, 1994.

107. Jones JG: Herpetic whitlow: an infectious occupational hazard, *J Occup Med* 27:725, 1985.

108. Jones JW et al: Recurrent *Mycobacterium bovis* infection following a ferret bite, *J Infect* 26:225, 1993 (letter).

109. Jones N, Khoosal M: Infected dog and cat bites, *N Engl J Med* 340:1841, 1999 (letter).

110. Kanda T: Induction of asymptomatic HBeAg carrier state in a patient with Down's syndrome following a human bite, *J Med* 25:383, 1994.

111. Kelly IP et al: The management of human bite injuries of the hand, *Injury* 27:481, 1996.

112. Khajotia RR, Lee E: Transmission of human immunodeficiency virus through saliva after a lip bite, *Arch Intern Med* 157:1901, 1997 (letter).

113. Klaassen B, Buckley JR, Esmail A: Does the Dangerous Dogs Act protect against animal attacks? A prospective study of mammalian bites in the accident and emergency department, *Injury* 27:89, 1996.

114. Kneafsey B, Condon KC: Severe dog-bite injuries, introducing the concept of pack attack: a literature review and seven case reports, *Injury* 26:37, 1995.

115. Kriss TC, Kriss VM: Equine-related neurosurgical trauma: a prospective series of 30 patients, *J Trauma* 43:97, 1997.

116. Kronwith SD, Hankin DE, Lipkin PH: Ocular injury from a rooster attack, *Clin Pediatr (Phila)* 35:219, 1996.

117. Kullberg BJ, Westendorp RG, Meinders AE: Purpura fulminans and symmetrical peripheral gangrene caused by *Capnocytophaga canimorsus* (formerly DF-2) septicemia—a complication of dog bite, *Medicine (Baltimore)* 70:287, 1991.

118. Lackmann GM et al: Surgical treatment of facial dog bite injuries in children, *J Craniomaxillofac Surg* 20:81, 1992.

119. Landercasper J et al: Trauma and the veterinarian, *J Trauma* 28:1255, 1988.

120. Langley J: The incidence of dog bites in New Zealand, *NZ Med J* 105:33, 1992.

121. Leibman JB: Proper cleansing of dog bite wounds, *Ann Emerg Med* 24:992, 1994 (letter).

122. Lester A et al: Phenotypical characters and ribotyping of *Pasteurella aerogenes* from different sources, *Int J Med Microbiol Virol Parasitol Infect Dis* 279:75, 1993.

123. Levin JM, Talan DA: Erythromycin failure with subsequent *Pasteurella multocida* meningitis and septic arthritis in a cat-bite victim, *Ann Emerg Med* 19:1458, 1990.

124. Lewis DE: Tungaru conjugal jealousy and sexual mutilation, *Pacific Studies* 13:115, 1990.

125. Lindsey D et al: Natural course of the human bite wound: incidence of infection and complications in 434 bites and 803 lacerations in the same group of patients, *J Trauma* 27:45, 1987.

126. Long WT et al: Toxic shock syndrome after a human bite to the hand, *J Hand Surg* 13A:957, 1988.

127. Loro A, Franceschi F: Human bites and finger infections: a survey at Dodoma Regional Hospital, Tanzania, *Trop Doct* 22:24, 1992.

128. Mann RJ, Hoffeld TA, Farmer CB: Human bites of the hand: twenty years of experience, *J Hand Surg* 2A:97, 1977.

129. Marr JS, Beck AM, Lugo JAJ: An epidemiologic study of the human bite, *Public Health Rep* 94:514, 1979.

130. Marrie TJ et al: Extensive gas in tissues of the forearm after horsebite, *South Med J* 72:1473, 1979.

131. Marshall KR: Ferrets as pets, *J Am Vet Med Assoc* 193:160, 1988 (letter).

132. Martin RW, Martin DL, Levy CS: Acinetobacter osteomyelitis from a hamster bite, *Pediatric Infect Dis J* 7:364, 1988.

133. Matter HC, Sentinella A: The epidemiology of bite and scratch injuries by vertebrate animals in Switzerland, *Eur J Epidemiol* 14:483, 1998.

134. Mellor DJ et al: Man's best friend: life threatening sepsis after minor dog bite, *BMJ* 314:129, 1997.

135. Mennen U, Howells CJ: Human fight-bite injuries of the hand. A study of 100 cases within 18 months, *J Hand Surg* 16B:431, 1991.

136. Moore F: "I've just been bitten by a dog," *BMJ* 314:88, 1997 (editorial).

137. Moore WE et al: Bacteriology of experimental gingivitis in young adult humans, *Infect Immun* 38:651, 1982.

138. Moore WE et al: Bacteriology of severe periodontitis in young adult humans, *Infect Immun* 38:1137, 1982.

139. Morgan MG, Mardel SN: Clenched fist actinomycosis in a penicillin-allergic female, *J Infect* 26:222, 1993 (letter).

140. Morgan MS: Purpura fulminans following a dog bite, *Postgrad Med J* 70:596, 1994 (letter).

141. Morgan MS: Treatment of pig bites, *Lancet* 348:1246, 1996 (letter).

142. Morgan MS: Prophylaxis should be considered even for trivial animal bites, *BMJ* 314:1413, 1997 (letter).

143. Morris JT, McAllister CK: Bacteremia due to *Pasteurella multocida, South Med J* 85:442, 1992.

144. Muguti GI, Dixon MS: Tetanus following human bite, *Br J Plast Surg* 45:614, 1992.

145. Muguti GI, Zvomuya-Ncube M, Bvuma ET: Experience with human bites in Zimbabwe, *Cent Afr J Med* 37:294, 1991.

146. Murray LA, Sivaloganathan S: Rambutt—the killer sheep, *Med Sci Law* 27:95, 1987.

147. Ndon JA: Capnocytophaga canimorsus septicemia caused by a dog bite in a hairy cell leukemia patient, *J Clin Microbiol* 30:211, 1992.

148. Ndon JA, Jach GJ, Wehrenberg WB: Incidence of dog bites in Milwaukee, Wis, *Wis Med J* 95:237, 1996.

149. Nishioka SA, Handa ST, Nunes RS: Pig bite in Brazil: a case series from a teaching hospital, *Rev Soc Bras Med Trop* 27:15, 1994.

150. Ogunbodede EO, Arotiba JT: Camel bite injuries of the orofacial region: report of a case, *J Oral Maxillofac Surg* 55:1174, 1997.

151. Okimura JT, Norton SA: Jealousy and mutilation: nose-biting as retribution for adultery, *Lancet* 352:2010, 1998.

152. Orton DW, Fulcher WH: *Pasteurella multocida*: bilateral septic knee joint prostheses from a distant cat bite, *Ann Emerg Med* 13:1065, 1984.

153. Osterlund A, Nordlund E: Wound infection caused by *Staphylococcus hyicus* subspecies *hyicus* after a donkey bite, *Scand J Infect Dis* 29:95, 1997.

154. Paisley JW, Lauer BA: Severe facial injuries to infants due to unprovoked attacks by pet ferrets, *JAMA* 259:2005, 1988.

155. Paterson JA, Cardo VAJ, Stratigos GT: An examination of antibiotic prophylaxis in oral and maxillofacial surgery, *J Oral Surg* 28:753, 1970.

156. Patrick GR, O'Rourke KM: Dog and cat bites: epidemiologic analyses suggest different prevention strategies, *Publi Health Rep* 113:252, 1998.

157. Peel MM et al: *Actinobacillus* spp. and related bacteria in infected wounds of humans bitten by horses and sheep, *J Clin Microbiol* 29:2535, 1991.

158. Pineda GV et al: Managing law enforcement (K-9) dog bites in the emergency department, *Acad Emerg Med* 3:352, 1996.

159. Politi A, Galli M, Ferrari G: [Massive pulmonary embolism after blunt chest trauma: considerations on pathogenesis and therapy], *G Ital Cardiol* 28:567, 1998.

160. Pollak S, Nadjem H, Faller-Marquardt M: [Agonal dog bite injuries], *Beitr Gerichtl Med* 50:351, 1992.

161. Porter JD et al: Lack of early antitoxin response to tetanus booster, *Vaccine* 10:334, 1992.

162. Post KW, Cole NA, Raleigh RH: In vitro antimicrobial susceptibility of *Pasteurella haemolytica* and *Pasteurella multocida* recovered from cattle with bovine respiratory disease complex, *J Vet Diagn Invest* 3:124, 1991.

163. Preiser G, Lavell TE: Rooster attacks on children, *Pediatrics* 79:426, 1987.

164. Presutti RJ: Bite wounds. Early treatment and prophylaxis against infectious complications, *Postgrad Med* 101:243, 1997.

165. Quinlan KP, Sacks JJ: Hospitalizations for dog bite injuries, *JAMA* 281:232, 1999 (letter).

166. Rashid N, Yusuf H: Oral self-mutilation by a 17-month-old child with Lesch-Nyhan syndrome, *Int J Paediatr Dent* 7:115, 1997.

167. Rayan GM et al: *Eikenella corrodens* in human mouth flora, *J Hand Surg* 13A:953, 1988.

168. Resnick D et al: Osteomyelitis and septic arthritis of the hand following human bites, *Skeletal Radiol* 14:263, 1985.

169. Richman KM, Rickman LS: The potential for transmission of human immunodeficiency virus through human bites, *J Acquir Immune Defic Syndr* 6:402, 1993.

170. Roblot P et al: Septicemia due to *Capnocytophaga canimorsus* after a dog bite in a cirrhotic patient, *Eur J Clin Microbiol Infect Dis* 12:302, 1993 (letter).

171. Rodeheaver GT et al: Pluronic F-68: a promising new skin wound cleanser, *Ann Emerg Med* 9:572, 1980.

172. Saab M et al: Fatal septicaemia in a previously healthy man following a dog bite, *Int J Clin Pract* 52:205, 1998.

173. Sacks JJ, Kresnow M, Houston B: Dog bites: how big a problem? *Inj Prev* 2:52, 1996.

174. Sacks JJ et al: Fatal dog attacks, 1989-1994, *Pediatrics* 97:891, 1996.

175. Sacks JJ, Sattin RW, Bonzo SE: Dog bite–related fatalities from 1979 through 1988, *JAMA* 262:1489, 1989.

176. Saxena PS et al: Camel bite injuries, *J Indian Med Assoc* 79:65, 1982.

177. Scarcella JV: Management of bites: early definitive repair of bite wounds, *Ohio State Med J* 65:25, 1969.

178. Scheithauer MO, Rettinger G: [Bite injuries in the head and neck area], *HNO* 45:891, 1997.

179. Schmitt RL: Injuries from dog bites, *JAMA* 279:1174, 1998 (letter).

180. Searcy RL: Biting the hand that feeds us, *Community Animal Control* 6:14, 1987.

181. Sebben JE: Surgical antiseptics. *J Am Acad Dermatol* 9:759, 1983.

182. Shewell PC, Nancarrow JD: Dogs that bite, *BMJ* 303:1512, 1991.

183. Shukla HS, Mittal DK, Naithani YP: Bull horn injury: a clinical study, *Injury* 9:164, 1977.

184. Sinclair CL, Zhou C: Descriptive epidemiology of animal bites in Indiana, 1990-92—a rationale for intervention, *Public Health Rep* 110:64, 1995.

185. Singh A et al: Multiple fractures following camel bite of the face (a case report), *Acta Chir Plast* 36:85, 1994.

186. Singh RI, Thomas R, Alexander TA: An unusual case of bull gore injury, *Aust NZ J Ophthalmol* 14:377, 1986.

187. Smith JS et al: Unexplained rabies in three immigrants in the United States: a virologic investigation, *N Engl J Med* 324:205, 1991.

188. Snyder KB, Pentecost MJ: Clinical and angiographic findings in extremity arterial injuries secondary to dog bites, *Ann Emerg Med* 19:983, 1990.

189. Stavrev V: A case of open multiple fractures of both forearms caused by a donkey bite, *Folia Med (Plovdiv)* 40:77, 1998.

190. Steele MT et al: Prophylactic penicillin for intraoral wounds, *Ann Emerg Med* 18:847, 1989.

191. Stevenson J, Anderson IW: Hand infections: an audit of 160 infections treated in an accident and emergency department, *J Hand Surg* 18B:115, 1993.

192. Stipp D: Tabbies terrorize our towns, landing cats in the doghouse, *Wall Street Journal*, 1993.

193. Stornello C: Transmission of hepatitis B via human bite, *Lancet* 338:1024, 1991 (letter).

194. Strassburg MA et al: Animal bites: patterns of treatment, *Ann Emerg Med* 10:193, 1981.

195. Stucker FJ et al: Management of animal and human bites in the head and neck, *Arch Otolaryngol Head Neck Surg* 116:789, 1990.

196. Sweet D, Bowers CM: Accuracy of bite mark overlays: a comparison of five common methods to produce exemplars from a suspect's dentition, *J Forensic Sci* 43:362, 1998.

197. Sweet D et al: An improved method to recover saliva from human skin: the double swab technique, *J Forensic Sci* 42:320, 1997.

198. Talan DA et al: Bacteriologic analysis of infected dog and cat bites: Emergency Medicine Animal Bite Infection Study Group, *N Engl J Med* 340:85, 1999.

199. Thomas HF, Voss S: A survey of dog bites in Salisbury, *J R Soc Health* 111:224, 1991.

200. Tuggle DW, Taylor DV, Stevens RJ: Dog bites in children, *J Pediatr Surg* 28:912, 1993.

201. Uchigasaki S, Takahashi H, Suzuki T: Self-inflicted bite injuries associated with intracerebral haemorrhages, *Med Sci Law* 38:179, 1998.

202. Vale GL: Dentistry, bite marks and the investigation of crime, *J Calif Dent Assoc* 24:29, 1996.

203. Van DRS, Van DRJ: Swine bites of the hand, *J Hand Surg* 16A:136, 1991.

204. Van der Werken C: [Clenched fist injuries from teeth: not to be disregarded], *Ned Tijdschr Geneeskd* 142:1297, 1998.

205. Vidal S, Barcala L, Tovar A: Horse bite injury, *Eur J Dermatol* 8:437, 1998.

206. Vidmar L et al: Transmission of HIV-1 by human bite, *Lancet* 347:1762, 1996 (letter).

207. Waldvogel FA et al: Perioperative antibiotic prophylaxis of wound and foreign body infections: microbial factors affecting efficacy, *Rev Infect Dis* 13(suppl 10):S782, 1991.

208. Watson DW: Severe head injury from dog bites, *Ann Emerg Med* 9:28, 1980.

209. Weber EJ, Callaham M: Animal bites and rabies. In Rosen P et al, editors: *Emergency medicine: concepts and clinical practice,* ed 4, St Louis, 1998, Mosby.

210. Weiss HB, Friedman DI, Coben JH: Incidence of dog bite injuries treated in emergency departments, *JAMA* 279:51, 1998.

211. Wilson S: *Bite busters: how to deal with dog attacks,* New York, 1997, Simon & Schuster.

212. Wolf JSJ, Gomez R, McAninch JW: Human bites to the penis, *J Urol* 147:1265, 1992.

213. Wolf JSJ et al: Dog bites to the male genitalia: characteristics, management and comparison with human bites, *J Urol* 149:286, 1993.

214. Wright JC: Reported cat bites in Dallas: characteristics of the cats, the victims, and the attack events, *Public Health Rep* 105:420, 1990.

215. Wright JC: Canine aggression toward people. bite scenarios and prevention, *Vet Clin North Am Small Anim Pract* 21:299, 1991.

216. Zubowicz VN, Gravier M: Management of early human bites of the hand: a prospective randomized study, *Plast Reconstr Surg* 88:111, 1991.

42 Bites and Injuries Inflicted by Wild Animals

Luanne Freer

Wild animal bites are distinct from the other assorted injuries suffered by humans. Tearing, cutting, and crushing injuries are sometimes combined with blunt trauma caused by falls. Animal bites may cause local infection, but this complication is hardly unique. Many offending bacteria reside in numerous environmental sources. However, few traumatic lacerations are as regularly contaminated with as broad a variety of pathogens as are animal bites.

Other special features are as follows:

1. Many victims have been terrorized by an attacking animal.
2. Animals can transmit various systemic diseases, many of which induce substantial morbidity and mortality; detailed discussion of zoonoses is found in Chapter 44.
3. In contrast to the extensive scientific literature on traumatic injuries that do not involve bites, the literature on animal bites, especially wild animal bites, is largely unscientific and often simply anecdotal. As a result, rational treatment decisions are often made without a completely satisfactory scientific basis.
4. Many decisions involved in the treatment of wild animal attack victims are based on experience with domestic animal attacks, namely dog and cat bites.
5. Perhaps most importantly, animal attack injuries are usually preventable. When experience allows humans to understand typical behavior for a species, they can take proper precautions in the vicinity of a potentially dangerous animal.

This chapter interprets the present state of knowledge to make logical, specific recommendations for all of these features.

INCIDENCE OF BITES

Neither the annual number of bites nor the base population at risk can be reliably estimated, especially when the human population is only those exposed to a wild animal or in a wilderness setting. The world supports approximately 4600 species of mammals, 10,000 species of birds, and 6000 species of reptiles,[90] but the actual number of wild animals in the world is estimated to be in the billions. Many people who suffer relatively minor injuries from wild animals do not seek medical attention unless infection or some other complication occurs, or they fear exposure to rabies. If the injury is minor, patients will continue to be treated, released, and unrecorded.

Few studies have examined the incidence of wild animal bites (Table 42-1). In Sweden, three of 1000 inhabitants were injured by animals each year.[19] Domestic animals accounted for over 90% of the total, moose accounted for 6% (almost all involved in auto accidents), and all other animals totaled 4%. However, bites were not examined separately, and many injuries occurred during accidents caused by animals. Some officials estimate there are two bites for every one reported, but a survey of children 4 to 18 years old estimated an incidence of more than 36 times the reported bite rate. Such figures are most likely based on domestic bites, although this was not specifically stated.[14,15]

No reported statistics exist on the typical wild animal attack victim. If all animal bites (including domestic) are considered, two U.S. state health departments report animal bites most often occurring in male children age 5 to 9 years,[120,122] but over 90% of animal attacks in these states are caused by domestic animals so this group is probably not representative of a *wild* animal attack. In undeveloped countries, many persons are exposed every day to bites from species considered "exotic" in the developed world.

Persons in certain occupations in developed countries, such as veterinary and animal control workers and laboratory workers, are at greatest risk of wild animal bite. A British survey reported a 70% incidence of animal-handling injuries during a typical veterinarian career; the rate was 42% in veterinary technical staff.[32] The U.S. Bureau of Labor Statistics reported that in 1 year, less than 0.3% of all occupational injury fatalities were caused by mammals.[130] In one study of 102 animal control officers, the overall bite rate was 2/57 per working day, 175 to 500 times the estimated rate in the general population (this study did not differentiate between wild and domestic animal bites).[14] It is difficult to make conclusions about the financial sequelae of *wild* animal bites because the incidence is substantially lower than with domestic animal bites.

In every statistical series of bites, small numbers of exotic animals, such as ocelots, jaguars, lions, leopards,

TABLE 42-1. Incidence (Percent) of Bites by Species in the United States

SPECIES	REFERENCE				
	A	B	C	D	E
Dog	89	91.6	78		75
Cat	4.6	4.5	16		20
Rodent	2.2	3	<1	65	2.5
Monkey	0.1*	0.2	2.2	15	0.2
Skunk		0.02	0.02	0.1	
Lagomorph	0.2	0.5			1
Large mammal	0.03†	0.01‡	1.2	3§	0.5
Reptile	0.1				
Bat		0.004	0.3	6	0.7
Raccoon		0.08	1	3‖	0.5

A, Marr J, Beck A, Lugo J: An epidemiologic study of the human bite, *Public Health Rep* 94:514, 1979.
B, Scarcella J: Management of bites, *Ohio State Med J* 65:25, 1969.
C, Sinclair CL, Zhou C: Descriptive epidemiology of animal bites in Indiana, 1990-1992—a rationale for intervention, *Public Health Rep* 110:64, 1995.
D, Kizer K: Epidemiologic and clinical aspects of animal bite injuries, *JACEP* 8:134, 1979.
E, Spence G: A review of animal bites in Delaware—1989 to 1990, *Del Med J* 62:1425, 1990.
*Includes 21 monkeys, 4 raccoons, 3 ferrets, 1 weasel, 1 coatimundi, 1 skunk, and 1 goat.
†Includes three lions, one ocelot, one leopard, one polar bear, and one anteater.
‡Includes one goat, one ocelot, one jaguar, and one groundhog, which inflicted a bite on Groundhog Day.
§One coyote.
‖One kinkajou.

polar bears, wolves, anteaters, and weasels, are represented. Bites from these animals occur from exposure to wild and zoo animals, and from the increasing popularity of wild animals as pets, which are usually kept illegally and without adequate understanding and training regarding animal care and behavior.

Several thousand people per year are killed by mammalian bites, with most of the deaths inflicted by man-eating lions and tigers in Africa and Asia (Table 42-2). The World Health Organization (WHO) estimates that roughly 60,000 people per year are killed by snakes and that additional millions are killed by insect-borne diseases.[143] An estimated 200 Americans are killed by animals each year; 131 of these die in traffic accidents involving deer.[62] Bees kill approximately 43 persons, dogs 14, and rattlesnakes 10. Wild animals, such as bears and cougars, kill fewer people than do goats, rats, jellyfish, and a captive elephant. Over 3 million people visit the wilderness in Yellowstone National Park every year; the incidence of serious injury by a wild animal at the park is less than the chance of being struck by lightning.[61]

CIRCUMSTANCES AND PREVENTION OF ANIMAL BITES

Animal Behavior

Prevention of animal bites requires a thorough knowledge of the behavior, personalities, and patterns of various species of animals. A person wishing to avoid the bite of a particular species will often be able to gain expertise about that species' behavior only from those

who work with it regularly. Detailed information on animal behavior and the attack patterns of animals is also available on Internet websites listed in Box 42-1.

Basic Principles For Avoiding Animal Bites

Animals rarely attack people without provocation. Exceptions are large carnivores, which may be relatively unafraid of humans, and creatures clinically infected with rabies. However, carnivores do not commonly hunt humans as preferred prey. The animal's perception of provocation may differ from that of the human. Patterns of behavior and attack differ by species.

People often capture or restrain wild animals, creating stress that may induce even the most benign ani-

TABLE 42-2. Human Deaths from Animal Attacks

SPECIES	ANNUAL ESTIMATED DEATHS	ANNUAL ESTIMATED ATTACKS	PREDOMINANT AREA	COMMENTS
Humans	200,000		Worldwide	Individual murders only; excludes 1 million/yr by war in recent decades
Humans	34,000	3 million	United States only	Deaths by firearm, both intentional and accidental; attacks include all assaults
Snake	60,000		Worldwide	
Crocodile	1000		Africa	Man eating predominantly
Alligator	<1	7	Florida only	Human encroachment on alligator habitat
Tiger	600-800		India	Frequently man eaters
Lion	300-500		Africa	Frequently man eaters
Leopard	400		Africa, India	Frequently man eaters
Elephant	200-500		Central Africa, India	Occasionally rogue man killers; incidence increasing because of environmental pressures
Hippopotamus	200-300		Africa	Unpredictable; bites and trampling common
African buffalo	20-100		Africa	Only if cornered or wounded
American bison	<1	3-5	United States only	Usually only when approached at close range
Moose	1-2	20	Sweden only	Almost always involves vehicle collision with animal
Hyena	10-50	Hundreds	Africa	Frequently bites off face of sleeping victim
Wolf	20-50	200-500	Eurasia (none in North America)	Hundreds per year in previous centuries
Domestic dog	10-20	1,500,000	United States only	
Gorilla	0	2-3	Africa	Only if cornered; injuries usually not severe
Baboon	0	1-2	South Africa	Usually pets
Ostrich	1-2		South Africa	Disembowelment, kick to head, stomping
Emu	None reported	1-2	Worldwide	Usually on farms
Black rhinoceros	<1		Africa	Easily provoked

mal to turn on its captor. Allegedly tame animals are very likely to struggle. Even shy animals that are being captured for treatment of an injury may attempt self-defense and can inflict a life-threatening injury such as goring. Therefore all situations of animal restraint and capture are considered high risk, and careful study of the species' behavior, the individual animal, and the physical environment and resources should precede actual attempts at restraint.

Because people seem drawn to raising wild animals as pets,[84] a large and lucrative market exists, particularly in the United States. No matter how they are raised, these animals remain wild and will never be as predictable, trustworthy, and nonaggressive as animals that have been domesticated for centuries. Often own-ers demonstrate a lack of common sense, as in the case of a pet Bengal tiger that attacked and killed its trainer, then 6 weeks later did the same to its owner.[9,39] Many of these mistakes probably stem from a lack of firsthand experience with wild animals.

Most wild species have a strong sense of territoriality. Individuals, pairs, or larger groups establish a territory that ranges from square feet to square miles and aggressively prevent any intrusion into that territory, particularly by members of their own species. During mating season, this drive may stimulate even small animals to threaten or attack humans, particularly in protection of the nest and young. A Malayan tapir bit off the arm of a zookeeper who came between the usually docile animal and its calf.[66]

A major principle of animal behavior is that physical attack is often the animal's last resort. Animals generally give ample warning of their intentions. Spectacular contests that occur in the wild are governed by elaborate rituals and rules that encourage a nonviolent solution, so that the victor may successfully defend its territory and itself with little or no injury. Humans can often avoid attack and injury by successfully interpreting visual, auditory, and olfactory warning signs. If a human slowly and carefully backs off without making sudden or threatening gestures, usually no harm will be done. The ideal reaction may depend on the species. For example, mountain lions have been turned from a full charge by an angry human who acted aggressively or fought back.[16] Given a choice of victims, such a predator prefers the fleeing, panicky victim who demonstrates expected flight rather than unexpected behavior. Nonpredatory species, such as deer, are extremely susceptible to human intimidation, whereas a canine can be provoked to attack by a direct stare, which is regarded as a challenge.

If capture of an animal is essential, detailed preparation should be undertaken. For small animals, using nets or heavy cloth and wearing extremely heavy gloves and other protective clothing are advisable. Desperate animals can bite with tremendous force; large carnivores can easily amputate a gloved digit. A wolf can tear apart a stainless steel bowl with its teeth, and a hyena can bite through a 2-inch plank.[27] Four men are needed to subdue an adult chimpanzee; an orangutan can maintain a one-fingered grip that an adult human cannot break. Larger animals generally require a team approach by animal control specialists with equipment such as nets, barriers, cages, and immobilizing drugs. Ideal immobilization techniques for various species are detailed in veterinary texts.[49]

PREHOSPITAL CONSIDERATIONS

Attacks by domestic and farm animals are fairly predictable and preventable, unlike attacks in the wilderness. In Africa, life-threatening attacks by large animals, such as water buffalo, lions, tigers, and elephants, are common. Attacks by larger animals can result in major blunt or penetrating trauma, with possible major arterial blood loss, airway damage, broken ribs, pneumothoraces, and intraperitoneal bleeding. The victim's condition and the availability of rapid evacuation determine the extent of treatment in the field. Often medical personnel or supplies are not available and the victim must be moved to a hospital or clinic as soon as possible.

Many, if not most, of the complications and serious infections from animal bites are caused by inadequate first aid and significant delays to medical care. Local wound treatment should be initiated at the scene of the bite (Box 42-2) and can determine the course of healing more than any other therapy. Simple first aid measures must be initiated immediately unless definitive or better treatment is available within a short time. Pressure on the wound or pressure points controls most bleeding; avoid tourniquets unless blood loss cannot be controlled otherwise. If the victim is more than 1 hour from a treatment facility, cleanse the wounds at the scene as soon as resuscitation efforts are complete. Early cleansing reduces the chance of bacterial infection and is ex-

---

Box 42-2 SUMMARY OF ANIMAL-BITE WOUND TREATMENT

MANDATORY FOR ALL WOUNDS

1. Evaluate for potential blunt trauma and injury to deeper and vital structures by penetrating teeth, claws, or horns.
2. Ensure appropriate tetanus immunization.
3. Irrigate wound with copious volume (minimum 100 to 300 ml) of normal saline or 5% povidone-iodine solution.
4. Debride obviously crushed and devitalized tissue.
5. If the animal is suspected to be rabid (atypical behavior, high-risk species), do the following:
   a. Infiltrate wound edges with 1% procaine hydrochloride.
   b. Swab wound surface vigorously with cotton swabs and 1% benzalkonium chloride (Zephiran) solution or other soap.
   c. Rinse wound with normal saline.
   d. Assess need for rabies immune globulin and vaccine.

6. Assess risk factors to decide on further (selective) treatment (see Box 42-3).
7. Do not culture fresh wounds.
8. Do not give prophylactic antibiotics for routine low-risk bite wounds.

SELECTIVE TREATMENT (WOUNDS SELECTED BY RISK FACTORS)

1. Suture, staple, or adhesive strip closure of all skin wounds in the usual fashion unless wounds are high risk (e.g., hand wounds, high-risk species, immunosuppressed patient).
2. Culture infected wounds only if they fail to respond to initial antibiotic therapy, they are very high risk (see Box 42-3), or there is evidence of systemic sepsis.
3. Consider delayed primary closure of high-risk wounds and administration of prophylactic antibiotics to victims with high-risk wounds.

tremely effective in killing rabies and other viruses. Potable water, preferably boiled or treated with germicidal agents, is adequate for wound irrigation. Ordinary hand soap adds some bactericidal, virucidal, and cleansing properties. If a 1% povidone-iodine (Betadine) solution is available, it should be used as an irrigant. Thoroughly irrigate the wound with at least a pint of soapy water and then gently debride it of dirt and foreign objects by swabbing with a soft, clean cloth or sterile gauze. Irrigation with a syringe is much better, but syringes are seldom available (see Chapter 18).

After cleansing, cover the wound with sterile dressings or a clean, dry cloth. Wounds of the hands or feet require immobilization. If the wounds are at high risk for infection, treatment is hours away, and an antibiotic such as amoxicillin-clavulanate, azithromycin, or ciprofloxacin is available, it is reasonable to start immediate treatment with an oral dose[48,57]; to be most effective in preventing subsequent wound infection, this should be given within 1 hour of wounding. However, with a severe wound, it is worthwhile to provide the antibiotic even many hours later. If antibiotics are not available, the wound is infection prone, and medical care is hours or days away, a simple remedy such as filling the wound with honey may be an effective antibacterial strategy.[106]

When definitive medical care cannot be obtained for a day or more, cleanse and irrigate the wound thoroughly. For some wounds, attempting closure is reasonable. Further discussion of bandaging and wound-repair techniques may be found in Chapters 16, 18, and 19.

In addition to treating the bite victim, try to capture the offending animal for examination, if this can be done without risk of further injury. Unusual behavior, such as unprovoked attack by a wild animal in broad daylight or a complete absence of fear of humans, should raise the suspicion of rabies. Live capture is optimal, but freshly killed animals are usually satisfactory for examination for fluorescent rabies antibody (FRA). Avoid damaging the animal's head and brain, because brain tissue is needed for analysis. Availability of the animal can eliminate the need for costly and uncomfortable rabies prophylaxis. If more than 1 hour will elapse before the animal can be transported to a hospital or public health department, refrigerate the body. Do not use preservatives. Rabies is discussed in Chapter 44.

Examination of the animal is not useful for most other diseases and will not help predict local wound infections. Therefore use good judgment in deciding how much time and energy to expend on capture.

EVALUATION AND TREATMENT OF INJURIES

Evaluate all victims of animal bites for blunt trauma and internal injuries, which may be less obvious than the bite wound (see Box 42-2). Many animals are large, strong, and heavy, and victims should be treated like any other victim of blunt or penetrating trauma. Internal organ damage, deep arterial and nerve damage, and penetration of joints are all possible. Particularly in children, animal bites can penetrate vital structures such as joints or the cranium[20,82]; radiographs are needed whenever these injuries are suspected. A complete head-to-toe evaluation for trauma is advised in all but the most trivial and isolated bite injuries. Few laboratory tests are of use in evaluating animal-bite injuries. Unless hematocrit is being assessed for evidence of blood loss from occult trauma, the complete blood cell (CBC) count is not useful because it is a nonspecific and unreliable gauge of infection. Definitive trauma evaluation and treatment are discussed in detail in Chapter 18. Routine wound cultures obtained at the time of initial wounding do not reliably predict whether infection will develop, or, if it does, the causative pathogens.[48]

The principles of wound care for injuries caused by inanimate objects apply to bite wounds as well. Many bite injuries are simple contusions that do not break the skin. The infection potential of these injuries is low; superficial wound cleansing and symptomatic treatment of pain and swelling suffice. Treatment should include prompt and liberal application of ice or other cold packs during the first 24 hours. However, this is not beneficial in snakebite and is obviously impractical in many undeveloped locations. Snakebite is discussed in Chapters 38 and 39.

When skin is broken, the risks of local wound infection or the transmission of systemic disease are incurred. Infection can be caused by organisms carried in the animal's saliva or nasal secretions, by human skin microbes carried into the wound, or by environmental organisms that enter the wound during or after the attack. Virtually any bacterium, virus, or fungus can become a contaminant in bite wounds. Fortunately, most wounds do not become infected.[59]

Animal bites are not clean lacerations, but are instead crush injuries that usually contain devitalized tissue. Debridement removes bacteria, clots, and soil far more effectively than does irrigation.[48] In addition, debridement creates cleaner surgical wound edges that are easier to repair, heal faster, and produce a smaller scar. Topical antiseptic ointments, such as neomycin, bacitracin, or polymyxin, are highly effective in promoting healing in minor skin wounds.[52,80] However, although topical ointments are appropriate for abrasions produced by animal bites, they may be less effective for punctures and sutured lacerations.

A sutured wound is covered by a simple, sterile, dry dressing to protect from rubbing against clothing or repetitive minor trauma. Delayed primary closure requires that the wound be kept moist; this is usually done with a wet saline dressing.

WOUND CLOSURE AND INFECTION RISK FACTORS

Three major considerations govern the decision of whether to suture a wound: cosmetics, function, and risk factors. Cosmetic appearance virtually mandates suturing all facial wounds, which usually are low risk. Similar reasons may dictate closure of wounds on other visible portions of the body. Function is of critical importance in wounds of the hand and foot, which are high-risk areas in which infection can have disastrous consequences. Thus hand wounds should generally be left open. Risk factors are many and complex and provide a useful logical framework in making the decision whether to suture, administer antibiotics, or undertake other treatments. For more information on surgical procedures, see Chapter 18.

The amount of time elapsed after wounding is a critical risk factor; the longer the interval, the more likely the chance for infection. After the first few hours, adequate wound cleansing is unlikely to be carried out. In developed countries, many victims are seen within hours of wounding, and the results are usually very good. In remote and undeveloped areas and countries, wounds commonly do not receive medical attention for half a day or more, putting them into a high-risk category that may eliminate the possibility of suturing. Certain species, including primates, wild cats, pigs, and large wild carnivores, seem to inflict infection-prone wounds, although evidence is incomplete. The presence of one or more of these risk factors may preclude suturing or may suggest the use of delayed primary closure (discussed below). However, most fresh bites can be safely sutured after proper wound preparation. Optimal conditions include prompt medical treatment, which is seldom available in remote and undeveloped areas. In those locations, leaving bite wounds open (or with a drain, although this is also controversial) is the more prudent course.

Bites of the Hand

Hand bites are common, and infection can be disastrous.[139] Therefore the hand is considered at risk for complications (Box 42-3). The hand contains many poorly vascularized structures and tendon sheaths that poorly resist infection. The fascial spaces and tendon sheaths of the hand communicate with each other, and movement seals off the wound from external drainage

---

Box 42-3   RISK FACTORS FOR INFECTION FROM ANIMAL BITE

HIGH RISK
Location

Hand, wrist, or foot
Scalp or face in patients with high risk of cranial perforation; CT or skull radiograph examination is mandatory
Over a major joint (possibility of perforation)
Through-and-through bite of cheek

Type of wound

Punctures that are difficult or impossible to irrigate adequately
Tissue crushing that cannot be debrided (typical of herbivores)
Carnivore bite over vital structure (artery, nerve, joint)

Patient

Older than 50 years
Asplenic
Chronic alcoholic
Altered immune status (chemotherapy, acquired immunodeficiency syndrome [AIDS], immune defect)
Diabetic
Peripheral vascular insufficiency
Chronic corticosteroid therapy
Prosthetic or diseased cardiac valve (consider systemic prophylaxis)
Prosthetic or seriously diseased joint (consider systemic prophylaxis)

Species

Large cat (canine teeth produce deep punctures that can penetrate joints, cranium)
Primates
Pigs (anecdotal evidence only)
Alligators, crocodiles

LOW RISK
Location

Face, scalp, ears, and mouth (all facial wounds should be sutured)
Self-bite of buccal mucosa that does not go through to skin

Type of wound

Large, clean lacerations that can be thoroughly cleansed (the larger the laceration, the lower the infection rate)
Partial-thickness lacerations and abrasions

Species

Rodents
Quokkas
Bats (although high risk for rabies)

and spreads bacteria and soil internally. Because of the unique anatomy of the hand, irrigating hand wounds adequately is often impossible.

Data on hand wound infection have been collected mostly from experience with domestic dog and cat bites. From a retrospective study in Oslo, nearly all hand bite wounds healed uneventfully when the wounds were left open, either without antibiotics or with penicillin after wound treatment.[35] In another European center, the total infection rate was 18.8% in hand bite wounds; this rose to 25% when the hand wound was closed primarily. The average time from the injury to the first medical treatment was 11 hours in infected wounds and 2 hours in noninfected ones.[2]

Because of high morbidity and permanent residual impairment from hand infections, treating them aggressively is best (see Box 42-2). Hand bite wounds should be irrigated, debrided if possible, and initially left open.[48,139] The hand should be immobilized with a bulky mitten dressing in an elevated position, and the victim usually should be started promptly on intravenous antibiotics. Specialty consultation and follow-up are mandatory for persons with an established infection, and hospitalization should be considered. Persons not hospitalized should be rechecked daily until signs of infection clear. In the patient without initial evidence of infection, 5 to 7 days of splinting and oral antibiotics should suffice if no complications develop. Radiographic examination should be performed on all significantly injured extremities.

Punctures

Punctures may occur from bites, clawings, or gorings. The infection rate is related to difficulty irrigating properly and degree of contamination, which is highest in bites. Usually, attempts to irrigate narrow punctures simply result in rapid development of tissue edema from infused saline, which does not cleanse the wound. However, if the wound is large or can be held open wide enough to permit fluid to escape, irrigation is worth the effort. Large goring-type puncture wounds up to 8 to 10 inches deep from bison have a low incidence of infection when closed primarily after irrigation and debridement.[30] For most smaller puncture wounds, irrigate or debride as well as possible, suture only if cosmetic or functional considerations require it, and treat as for high risk for infection.[48] Use delayed primary closure liberally.

Facial and Scalp Wounds

Facial and scalp wounds tend to heal rapidly with little risk of infection; in general, they may be sutured primarily and do not require prophylactic antibiotics. Typical dog bites of the face and neck (including punctures) have an infection rate of only 3%, even when sutured.[2,35,37,141] In general, cosmetic closure of facial

wounds is afforded by the lower incidence of infection, and standard of care in most cases is primary closure of an animal bite to the face.[141]

A major risk associated with facial and scalp wound victims of large carnivores is that the teeth can easily perforate the cranium, producing depressed skull fracture, brain laceration, intracranial abscess, or meningitis.[23,104] In young children with such wounds, or with adult victims of large carnivores, computed tomography (CT), or in the absence of CT, skull radiographs should be routine, looking for evidence of perforation that would mandate immediate neurosurgical consultation and admission to the hospital.

INDICATION FOR CULTURES

Cultures of animal-bite wound surfaces, whether judged quantitatively or qualitatively, are useless as predictors of infection. Some of the pathogens of greatest concern (such as *Eikenella*) can take 10 days to grow out in culture, by which time most therapeutic decisions have been made. Other organisms (such as *Pasteurella*) are fastidious, hard to identify, and frequently missed by the laboratory technician, who rarely encounters them.[53]

If the victim or wound is very high risk, or if animal bite sepsis is suspected (see the section on sepsis), obtaining cultures would be prudent to guide subsequent antibiotic therapy. In certain cases, cultures should be sent to reference laboratories, such as those in state health departments or at the Centers for Disease Control and Prevention (CDC) in Atlanta, because reference laboratories have successfully isolated more pathogens on identical samples sent to both reference and local laboratories.[127]

PROPHYLACTIC ANTIBIOTICS

Currently the weight of evidence does not support use of prophylactic antibiotics for other than high-risk wounds. The use of antibiotics is most advisable for wounds of the hand; the speed of development, frequency, severity, and complications of hand wound infections can be impressive.[48,139] Persons with other risk factors, particularly prolonged time from injury to treatment, complex wounds with massive crushing, or medical conditions, such as asplenia, diabetes mellitus, vascular insufficiency, or immune deficiency, may benefit from prophylactic antibiotics (see Box 42-3).

In bite wounds, treatment can begin only *after* wounding and bacterial inoculation; thus antibiotics are never truly prophylactic. In major surgery, prophylactic antibiotics are of proven value only in carefully selected high-risk procedures and only if begun *before* surgery.[135] Several controlled studies of dog bite wounds found no significant benefit for using prophy-

TABLE 42-3 Tetanus Prophylaxis

HISTORY OF IMMUNIZATION (DOSES)	CLEAN MINOR WOUNDS		MAJOR DIRTY WOUNDS	
	TOXOID*	TIG†	TOXOID	TIG
Unknown	Yes	No	Yes	Yes
None to one	Yes	No	Yes	Yes
Two	Yes	No	Yes	No (unless wound older than 24 hr)
Three or more				
Last booster within 5 years	No	No	No	No
Last booster within 10 years	No	No	Yes	Yes
Last booster more than 10 years ago	Yes	No	Yes	Yes

*Toxoid: Adult: 0.5 ml DT intramuscularly (IM). Child less than 5 years old: 0.5 ml DPT IM. Child older than 5 years: 0.5 ml DT IM.
†Tetanus immune globulin (TIG): 250 to 500 units IM in limb contralateral to toxoid.

lactic antibiotics in low-risk facial and scalp wounds.[38,141] Other studies recommend the use of prophylactic antibiotics only for high-risk wounds and/or patients.[35,37,59,139,141]

If used, prophylactic antibiotics must be administered early. The offending bacteria are already present in the wound when the victim is first seen. Therefore bite victims needing prophylactic antibiotic treatment should be identified early, preferably during triage on entry to the emergency department. The victim should receive immediate antibiotics by protocol; the intravenous route is by far the quickest. Although previous practice had led to prescription of prophylactic antibiotics for 7 to 10 days, current knowledge in the surgical literature is that prophylaxis is needed for only a few days after surgery. In animal bites, oral antibiotics are not expensive to continue for a few extra days; thus a maximum period of 5 days of prophylaxis should be more than sufficient with uninfected bites.

Therapy should be tailored to the largest variety of most likely pathogens for a particular type of bite. For most terrestrial mammals, the choice of antibiotic is based on experience with human, dog, and cat bites. However, with alligator or crocodile bite, or other wounds incurred in fresh water, antibiotic choice should be directed against *Aeromonas hydrophila*.[63,89]

TETANUS PROPHYLAXIS

Recently, about twice as many cases of human tetanus from animal bites have been seen each year as cases of human rabies.[13] The spores of *Clostridium tetani* are ubiquitous in soil, on teeth, and in the saliva of animals. Therefore the risk of tetanus may be present from any animal injury that penetrates the skin. Because tetanus is preventable, and many persons still do not receive tetanus immunoprophylaxis according to guidelines of the CDC, proper emergency prophylaxis against tetanus remains an important, but often underappreciated intervention.

Tetanus prophylaxis is administered in standard fashion (Table 42-3). With a clean wound that contains little devitalized tissue and that can be easily irrigated and debrided, a previous full course of immunization plus a booster within the last 10 years is sufficient. In a deep puncture or wound with much devitalized tissue that is difficult to irrigate and debride (predisposing to anaerobic growth), a full series of previous immunizations plus a booster within the last 5 years is sufficient. If there is any uncertainty regarding the status of the victim's prior immunization, a high-risk wound should prompt intramuscular injection of 250 to 500 units of tetanus human immune globulin (TIG), as well as 0.5 ml of diphtheria-tetanus (DT) toxoid booster vaccine. Because many persons do not have full prior immunization against tetanus, questioning the patient thoroughly on this point is critical. The risk of inadequate prior immunization is particularly high for elders and persons reared in underdeveloped countries. In 1995 to 1997, 35% of human tetanus cases occurred in persons 60 years and older.[11]

If the patient has not been immunized in the previous 10 years, TIG is recommended because most victims have no significant antibody response to a booster dose for at least 4 days.[13] If a definite history of prior immunization cannot be elicited, the victim must be treated with 250 to 500 units of human TIG intramuscularly in one arm and 0.5 ml of the adult DT toxoid in the other. Booster doses of tetanus toxoid are administered at 30 and 60 days after the initial injection to complete the course of immunization.

FOLLOW-UP CARE

Assuming that the possibility of major or occult trauma has been ruled out, follow-up of animal bites depends on the risk factors present (see Box 42-3) and the pa-

Box 42-4 TYPICAL AEROBIC BACTERIA FOUND IN ANIMALS' MOUTHS AND AS PATHOGENS IN INFECTED BITE WOUNDS

Acinetobacter calcoaceticus
Acinetomyces spp.
Aeromonas hydrophila
Actinobacillus lignieresii, suis
Bacillus subtilis, circulans, firmus
Bordetella spp.
Brevibacterium
Brucella canis
Capnocytophaga canimorsus, ochracea
Citrobacter amalonaticus, koseri
Clostridium perfringens
Corynebacterium, 13 spp.
Dermobacter hominis
Eikenella corrodens
Enterobacter cloacae
Enterococcus, 4 spp.
Erysipelothrix rhusiopathiae
Escherichia coli
Eubacterium
Flavimonas oryzihabitans
Flavobacterium brevis
Gemella morbillorum
Haemophilus aprophilus
Haemophilus haemolyticus
Klebsiella oxytoca, pneumonia

Lactobacillus lactis
Micrococcus spp.
Moraxella spp.
Neisseria spp.
Oerskovia
Pantoea agglomerans
Pasteurella aerogenes
Pasteurella dagmatis, canis, stomatis, multocida
Pedicoccus damnosus
Peptostreptococcus
Proteus mirabilis
Pseudomonas aeruginosa, 4 spp.
Reimerella anatispestifer
Rhodococcus
Rothia dentocariosa
Serratia marcescens
Staphylococcus, 13 spp.
Stenotrophomonas maltophilia
Stomatococcus mucilaginosus
Streptococcus, 13 spp.
Streptomyces
Weeksella virosa, zoohelcum
CDC alphanumerics:
  II-J
  EF-4a, EF-4b

tient's response to treatment. With only a superficial abrasion, infection is unlikely, and no return visit is needed. With an ordinary low-risk bite wound, one follow-up visit in 2 days, to assess any infection, is all that is needed. If the patient is very reliable and no sutures have been placed, even one visit is not necessary. Infected wounds dictate much closer follow-up, the frequency depending on the wound's response to treatment and the patient's risk factors. In a high-risk patient, the initial follow-up should be within 24 hours if the patient is not hospitalized.

COMPLICATIONS OF BITE WOUNDS

Wound Infection

Immense numbers of bacteria inhabit animals' mouths and can be inoculated into a bite wound. The exact pathogens vary depending on the biting species. The major aerobic and anaerobic bacteria are listed in Boxes 42-4 and 42-5. If inoculated in sufficiently large numbers, these microorganisms can cause localized cellulitis and abscess formation, the most common forms of infection. Wound infection is generally diagnosed on the basis of increasing redness, swelling, and tenderness of the wound margins, eventually progressing to production of pus, cell-

ulitis, lymphangitis, and local lymphadenopathy. Lymphadenitis and lymphangitis, which are much less common, occur as local defenses are overwhelmed. Systemic symptoms of infection are rare and suggest bacteremia or sepsis.

Wound infection from animal bites should be treated like infection of any other traumatic wound (i.e., elevate the wound, immobilize the affected part, remove sutures or staples if present, and provide antibiotic therapy [see Box 42-1]). Based on the 1999 Emergency Medicine Animal Bite Infection Study Group findings, recommended empiric treatment includes combining a β-lactam antibiotic and a β-lactamase inhibitor, a second-generation cephalosporin with anaerobic activity, or combination therapy with either penicillin and a first-generation cephalosporin or clindamycin and a fluoroquinolone.[127] Additional studies recommend azithromycin, trovafloxacin, or experimental ketolide antibiotics HMR 3004 or HMR 3647, which show good in vitro activity against unusual aerobic and anaerobic animal pathogens (Box 42-6).[53,56,57,127] In 1999 the Food and Drug Administration (FDA) issued a public health advisory statement recommending that the use of trovafloxacin be restricted to treatment of serious infections in hospitalized patients because of the risk of hepatic toxicity.

Box 42-5 ANAEROBIC ORGANISMS AND OTHER PATHOGENS FOUND IN ANIMALS' MOUTHS AND AS PATHOGENS IN INFECTED BITE WOUNDS

ANAEROBIC BACTERIA

Bacteroides spp.
Clostridium sordellii
Eubacterium
Filifactor villosus
Fusobacterium spp.
Lactobacillus jensenii
Leptotrichia
Peptococcus
Peptostreptococcus spp.
Porphyromonas spp.
Prevotella spp.
Propionibacterium spp.
Veillonella parvula

OTHER PATHOGENS

Cat-scratch disease organism
Cowpox and catpox virus
Hepatitis virus
Herpesvirus
Leptospira interrogans
Mycobacterium bovis
Mycobacterium marinum
Nocardia brasiliensis
Rabies virus
Rio Bravo virus
Seal finger agent
Simian herpes B virus
Spirillum minus
Sporothrix schenckii

Box 42-6 RECOMMENDED INITIAL ORAL ANTIBIOTICS FOR BITE WOUNDS

ORGANISMS KNOWN

Treat according to specific antibiotic sensitivities of cultured organisms

ORGANISMS UNKNOWN (DOG AND MOST OTHER BITES)

β-lactam antibiotic *and* β-lactamase inhibitor
or
Second-generation cephalosporin with anaerobic activity
or
Penicillin *and* first-generation cephalosporin
or
Clindamycin *and* fluoroquinolone
or
Azithromycin
or
Trovafloxacin*
or
Experimental ketolide antibiotics: HMR 3004 (RU64004) or HMR 3647 (RU 66647)

*1999 FDA recommendations restrict use to seriously ill hospitalized patients.

Extremely rare pathogens can cause infection (see Boxes 42-4 and 42-5). Culture of debrided tissue is the only reliable identification technique, and sensitivity testing may take weeks. Surgical debridement of all infected tissue is crucial. The organisms are usually sensitive to ciprofloxacin, cefoxitin, and perhaps rifampin.[107]

Septic Complications

Bacteremia and sepsis, although theoretical risks with any animal bite pathogen, have so far been reported with only a limited number of species.[4,46,76,104] Clinical manifestations include cellulitis, endocarditis, meningitis, pneumonitis, Waterhouse-Friderichsen syndrome, renal failure, shock, and death. Purpuric lesions are seen in one third of cases and may progress to symmetric peripheral gangrene and amputation. In some cases, cutaneous gangrene develops at the site of the bite, a finding unique to this species of bacteria.

Allergic Reactions

Allergic reactions to animal bites are virtually unheard of. However, up to 11% of laboratory workers have allergic reactions to laboratory animal dander, hair, and urine.[142] One case of proven hypersensitivity to rat saliva after a bite has been reported.[142] The patient was subsequently proven allergic to the saliva (presumably because of saliva proteins) and not to other portions of the rat. The bite produced lymphangitic swelling and itching that subsided within 24 hours.

Transmission of Systemic Infection

Approximately 150 systemic diseases of mammals can be transmitted in some fashion to humans. However, relatively few occur through a bite or scratch. Pathogens may be secreted in saliva, nasal secretions, or tear, or reach the animal's mouth through cleaning activities. The list includes pasteurellosis, leptospirosis, rat-bite fever, cat-scratch fever, tularemia, fish handler's disease, hepatitis A and B, monkeypox virus infection, tuberculosis, toxoplasmosis, bubonic plague, tetanus, gas gangrene, rabies, Q fever, Hantavirus infection, and sporotrichosis.[40,98] Chapter 44 reviews most of the diseases theoretically transmitted by lick, bite, or scratch. Although systemic disease is a valid consideration, 99% of mortality and morbidity arises from local wound infection, including rabies and tetanus. Chapter 44 discusses the diagnosis and treatment of zoonoses.

NEUROTROPIC DISEASE

Rabies

Rabies is discussed in detail in Chapter 44, so comments here are limited to brief remarks about epidemiology, assessment of risk in the bite victim, and local wound treatment.

Rabies is a rhabdovirus that occurs in wild and domestic animals. Migrating epidemics alternate with periods of endemicity. It is generally believed that no true reservoir host exists for rabies; that is, no species harbors a latent and nonfatal infection.

The epidemiology of rabies varies widely in different parts of the world. In the United States, western Europe, and Canada, wild animals are by far the main vectors of rabies, accounting for more than 85% of all reported cases in the past two decades.[92,99] In recent years, rabies in humans has become an extremely rare disease in the United States, with only two cases occurring in 1997.[131] Since 1980, rabies-infected bats caused 58% of the human cases of rabies diagnosed in the United States.[99] Of the more than 8000 cases of animal rabies reported in the United States in 1997, the terrestrial animals most represented were woodchucks, raccoons, skunks, foxes, and coyotes.[92] Foxes are the primary offenders in Europe, although some countries have eliminated rabies in wild populations by using innovative vaccination programs.[25]

Because of local variations in animal vectors and endemics, consultation with the state or local health department is prudent before a decision is made to initiate antirabies postexposure prophylaxis.[92] Although the number of human cases has declined, about 18,000 people per year in the United States receive postexposure prophylaxis.[47] In the rest of the world, virtually all rabies occurs in dogs. Worldwide, dogs account for 91% of all human rabies cases, cats 2%, other domestic animals 3%, bats 2%, foxes 1%, and all other wild animals only 1%.[25] Each year in India, 25,000 humans die from rabies and a half million receive antirabic vaccine.[125] In Africa, Latin America, and most of Asia, dogs are the principal vector, although jackals are also a factor. In South America and Mexico, rabid vampire bats cause occasional human infection. In recent years, disruption of the natural ecology by introduction of humans and domestic animals into the rain forest has produced epidemics of rabies caused by vampire bats. In Israel, wolves and jackals are the chief vectors, and the mon-

goose prevails in Puerto Rico. In eastern and central Europe, the raccoon dog (*Nyctereutes procynoides*) is an increasingly common vector.[25]

Judgment of risk of rabies exposure rests on several factors. The incidence of rabies in local species is important; in the United States, urban dogs and cats, domestic ferrets, rodents, and lagomorphs (rabbits and hares) are at low risk. The animal's behavior is sometimes helpful. This is easily evaluated in wild animals because most tend to shun humans. The urban appearance of a skunk, fox, or bat in broad daylight, showing no fear of human beings, is abnormal and should raise the index of suspicion.

In addition to situations involving animal bites, contact of mucous membranes with rabid saliva or an animal scratch should prompt consideration for rabies postexposure prophylaxis (PEP). If a person is found in a room with a bat and is unable to reliably report the absence of contact that could have resulted in exposure (e.g., an unattended child or sleeping or mentally incompetent adult), then rabies PEP should be administered.[99]

Thorough and rapid early treatment of wounds from animals suspected of being rabid is mandatory. Immediately cleanse all bite wounds and scratches with soap and water and a virucidal agent, such as povidone-iodine solution.[121] Evaluate all persons exposed to a possibly rabid animal for rabies immunoprophylaxis; CDC guidelines issued in 1999 recommend that for previously unvaccinated persons, *the entire dose* of rabies immune globulin, 20 IU/kg body weight should be infiltrated at the wound site if possible. Three types of rabies vaccine are currently available in the United States: human diploid cell vaccine, rabies vaccine adsorbed, and purified chick embryo cell vaccine. The chosen vaccine is given in 1-ml doses on days 0, 3, 7, 14, and 28 after exposure. Further information on rabies preexposure and postexposure prophylaxis is discussed in Chapter 44.

Other Neurotropic Infections

Although not caused by bites or wounds, oral transmission of Creutzfeldt-Jakob disease has been reported from the regionally common practice of eating the brains of wild goats, pigs, or squirrels, even when cooked. Creutzfeldt-Jakob disease is characterized by progressive dementia, ataxia, and myoclonus, and is untreatable. It is caused by a virus also identified in the brains of domestic sheep and mule deer.[71]

PSYCHIATRIC CONSEQUENCES OF ANIMAL ATTACK

Victims of traumatic or life-threatening events may develop posttraumatic stress disorder (PTSD). This syndrome has been recognized anecdotally by the author as a result of wild animal attack and is rarely reported in the scientific literature.[36] After physical recovery from an attack, the victim may be plagued by recurrent nightmares and flashbacks of the event and may have an aversion to outdoor travel. Critical incident stress debriefing and posttrauma intervention counseling may be important aspects of care for victims of animal attack.[36]

BITES OF THE WILD (BIG) CATS

Adult cats have 30 permanent teeth, arranged in rows of 16 upper and 14 lower. The upper teeth overlap the lower, resulting in an overbite.[32] This helps the animal lock its teeth into prey and exert twisting and tearing forces. The feline bite is much shorter and more rounded than that of a dog.

Big cats typically attack from behind, biting the neck and occiput of their prey and attempting to maneuver their canine teeth between the victim's cervical vertebrae and into the spinal cord.[28,114,138] Proprioceptors in the cat's tooth allow it to detect when it has encountered bone. The goal of rapidly paralyzing the prey is also accomplished by a violent shake of the cat's head, which fractures the cervical spine. In a study of fatalities from jaguar attack, 77% of victims were bitten on the nape of the neck and half of the bites were made to the base of the skull.[28] In 20% of cases, the killing bite was to the head, with at least one canine piercing the skull or ear canal. Cheetahs prefer to attack the throat of their prey, crushing the larynx and strangling the victim, a method also used by lions and leopards.[83] Big cats also claw their prey, producing deep parallel incised wounds. Several victims have died of exsanguination without evidence of strangulation or cervical spine injury.[29,114] Because of the growing propensity for people of developed countries to keep exotic animals as pets (or raise them for profit for hunting purposes), injuries by big cats can occur anywhere.

Wound care is the same as for other species, with special attention to evaluation for major internal injury. In particular, observe for penetration of deep structures of the cranium and neck, and rule out injuries of the cervical spine and deep cervical vessels (see Box 42-1).[28] One victim with an apparently trivial puncture wound after a bite to the neck from a pet cougar was discharged from the emergency department.[72] Within hours her voice was hoarse; on return, she recalled that the cougar had shaken her in its jaws when it bit her, and air was found in the prevertebral and retropharyngeal spaces on radiographic examination.

Like domestic cats, big cats usually carry *Pasteurella* as normal flora, and because of the deep penetration of their large teeth, *Pasteurella* septic arthritis, meningitis, and other serious deep infections can occur.[51,70]

Cat-scratch disease is an uncommon disease; 90% of cases are caused by scratches from domestic cats, and it has been reported in a big-cat attack victim.[33,72] The average incubation period is 3 to 10 days. The characteristic feature is regional lymphadenitis, usually involving lymph nodes of the arm or leg. In most cases, clinical diagnosis is based on finding three of the following four criteria[3]:

1. Single or regional lymphadenopathy without obvious signs of cutaneous or throat infection
2. Contact with a cat (usually an immature one)
3. Detection of an inoculation site
4. A positive skin test for cat-scratch disease.

More detailed information on the diagnosis and treatment of this disease is found in Chapter 44.

Tigers

Adult tigers are so powerful that the human victim is often killed instantly. It is not unusual for a limb to be severed with a single bite.[42,79] A swiping blow to the human head can cause a skull fracture.[108] Like many big cats, tigers typically strike without warning from behind, biting the head and neck and often shaking their heads violently to sever the victim's spinal cord.[74]

Big cats are a major threat to the lives of humans in the cats' native regions.[88] Although the number of tigers in the world is dwindling rapidly, they are still the number one animal killer of humans (see Table 42-2). Nonetheless, man killing almost invariably results from stress (wounds or old age) or lack of natural prey and habitat that forces the animal to prey on humans. A tiger subsisting solely on human meat would have to kill approximately 60 adults a year, and documented cases in selected regions have approached this rate over periods of up to 8 years. Man-eating tigers in India between 1906 and 1941 ate an estimated 125 persons each, and one had killed 436 persons. However, unlike lions, tigers are not thought to become exclusive man eaters. Some tigers have become opportunistic man eaters in lieu of plentiful natural prey, and tiger biologists hypothesize that these animals have become unafraid of man.[88]

Over the last 5 centuries, an estimated 1 million people have been eaten by tigers. In the nineteenth century, the tigers' toll in India averaged 2000 victims per year. From 1930 to 1940, the annual number never dropped below 1300. In the late 1940s, this rate dropped to abut 800 per year, where it remains. At the same time, approximately 17,000 people per year are killed in India by other wild beasts, which include nonmammalian species.

Lions

Despite their appearance and reputation, lions are not as greatly feared or respected by experienced hunters as are tigers (Figure 42-1). Lions are primarily scavengers, making fewer original kills than do hyenas. A

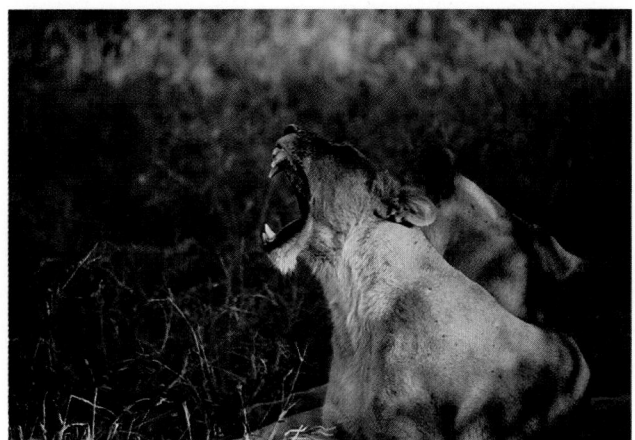

Figure 42-1   African lion. *(Photo by Cary Breidenthal, RN.)*

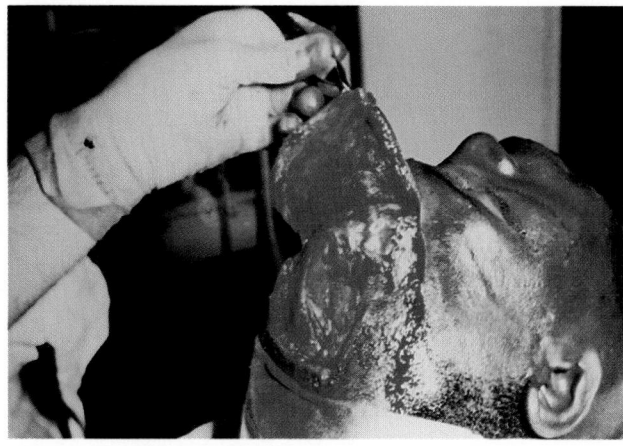

Figure 42-2   Lion attack victim. This African victim was rescued by bystanders as his head was in the lion's mouth. His only injury was a degloving scalp laceration. *(Photo by Harold P. Adolph, MD.)*

protected population of 250 Asiatic lions in India has attacked 193 humans, killing 28 between 1977 and 1991; biologists credit lion baiting for tourist shows and drought for this increasing carnage.[115]

A threatening gesture or shout may repel a lion, although a lioness guarding her cubs is more likely to attack. Experienced hunters find that when a charging lion is faced head on and confronted, it will often turn tail and run. An intended victim who flees is most likely to be attacked. Walking unarmed in lion country is usually safe; most hunters who succumb to lions are killed by wounded or sorely provoked animals, usually in dense brush (Figure 42-2). Many who survive the initial mauling die later of infection. Details of their treatment are not available. Persons who have survived attacks state that it is unwise to struggle and that the cat should be allowed to chew on an arm or other extremity. With luck, it will lose interest and leave.

Man-eating lions exist, as noted recently in South Africa, where illegal immigrants from Mozambique attempt to cross the border at night through Kruger National Park. In direct proportion to the number of immigrants on foot, the number of humans maimed or killed by lions has increased. Rangers suggest that humans on foot are an easier food source than normal prey for old or sickened lions.[95] Lions are estimated to eat 300 to 500 Africans a year and rank second to tigers among man eaters. Conversion to man eating has been blamed on drought, famine, and human epidemics in which large numbers of corpses are abandoned in the bush. Lions that become man eaters and subsist exclusively on human flesh need approximately 40 victims a year to stay alive. They usually kill instantly with one bite to the head or neck or with a swipe of the paw, which can break an ox's neck. Lions have tremendous strength and can easily carry a human victim for a mile without rest.

Although most lions in captivity become passive and dull, circus and zoo lions periodically kill attendants. Many such deaths have occurred when keepers accidentally have backed into or trod upon an animal.

Leopards

Most leopard attacks are provoked by wounds or by a dog attack. When wounded, trapped, or cornered, a leopard is unpredictable and ruthless, attacking the first person within striking distance. Unmolested and in normal health, the leopard is a shy, nervous animal with marked fear of humans. Unlike a lion or tiger, the leopard relies on fast claw work and biting. Like the jaguar, the leopard may go for the neck (in an effort to sever the spinal cord) or attempt disemboweling by raking at the victim's abdomen with the claws. The leopard seems inclined to retreat when much resistance is offered, even in encounters with baboons. There is a documented report of a man armed only with a screwdriver fighting and killing an attacking leopard.[77] Before the era of antibiotics, three fourths of people mauled by leopards died from wound infection, but modern morbidity is estimated to be less than 10%.[27]

Mauling by leopards is much more common than killing; estimated casualties are 400 per year, mostly in Africa. The leopard does not often turn into a man eater; when it does, it attacks mainly children or sick adults. In the state of Bihar in India, leopards ate 300 people in 1959 and 1960.[27] The man-eating leopard of Rudraprayag in India killed 150 people between 1918 and 1926. Becoming increasingly bold, it eventually took its prey by banging down doors, leaping through windows, or clawing its way through the walls of mud huts. Like man-eating lions, man-eating leopards completely change their normal hunting patterns when the prey becomes exclusively human.

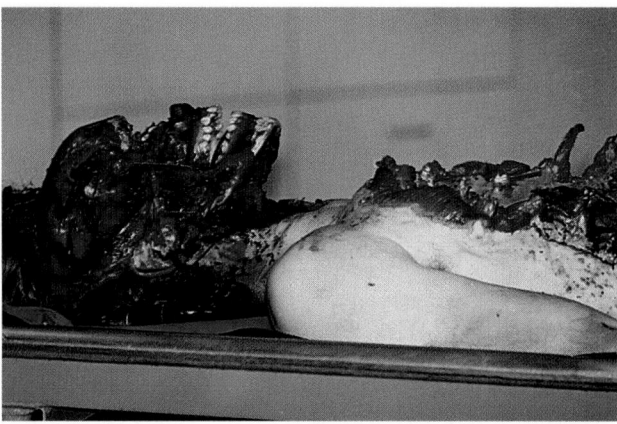

Figure 42-3 Victim of cougar predation and fatal mauling. *(Photo by Ben Galloway, MD.)*

Cougars

The North American cougar (mountain lion or puma) is a clever, basically shy cat. It is the most widely distributed large animal on the American continent. Recently, cougars are encroaching with increasing frequency into populated areas of the western United States, probably because of human expansion into the wilderness and an increased population of protected cougars.[73] The combined cougar population in California, Colorado, and Idaho is now estimated at 9000 to 12,000; humans live, exercise, or picnic in cougar country with increasing frequency.[124] Thus modern suburban dwellers (who typically are ignorant of wild animal behavior) are now in regular close contact with cougars in their homes and parks—whether they know it or not.

From 1970 to 1990, 31 cougar attacks on humans were documented, with five fatalities.[16] More people have been attacked since 1975 than over the entire previous century.[16,124,128] Most attacks occurred in the western United States and Canada. Throughout the United States, cougars took sixteenth place as an animal-related cause of death in recent years, just behind jellyfish or goats.[110] In California, no attacks occurred from 1925 until 1986, when two children were attacked in a regional park in southern California.[72] In 1991, a teenager was killed in Colorado, and a cougar killed an adult woman in California in 1994. Both victims were jogging, perhaps evoking a predatory response.[29,114] Young animals that are forced out by adults and must find their own territory are the most frequent attackers of humans.[73] Children are the preferred victims (86% of fatalities are children).[67] There has been only one alleged report of a cougar as a primary man eater, but cougars have sometimes partially eaten victims of their attacks (Figure 42-3).[29,114]

The cougar hunts like a domestic cat: crouching, slinking, sprinting, pouncing, and then breaking the prey's neck. The types of injuries to the neck are similar to those described for lions and tigers. Like many potentially dangerous wild animals, the cougar can often be scared off by the victim's aggressive behavior, even after the attack has begun.[62]

RODENTS

Rodents do not tend to bite unless severely provoked; their bites are usually small and do not cause much disability. The exact number of rodents in the world is unknown, but they probably number in the hundreds of millions, with 1500 species of laboratory and pet rodents. Despite these numbers, they account for only 1.7% to 10% of animal bites brought to medical attention.[101] Such bites are infrequent, seldom cause any problems for the victim, and often occur among lower socioeconomic groups without good access to medical attention. The other human populations at risk are owners of pet rodents and laboratory workers who handle rodents used in research. Insufficient data exist to determine any difference in outcome between wild and domestic rat bites.

Rats, Mice, and Other Small Rodents

Rat bites show an infection rate of 2% to 10%, even without treatment, and the rate is usually on the low end of this spectrum.[101] Other than bites inflicted by laboratory animals, the vast majority occur in poverty areas while the victim is sleeping and involve the face and neck, usually in infants or physically or mentally disabled adults.[100,101] There were 415 reported rat bites in New York City between 1986 and 1994.[24] Sometimes these can be severe; a week-old infant was bitten around the eyes by a rat, resulting in perforations of the globe, an estimated vascular loss of 55% of red blood cell mass (with an initial hematocrit value of 20%), and eventual blindness.[96] Despite the rat's reputation for spreading disease, however, infection did not occur. Similar bites in infants have resulted in loss of more than three fourths of the eyelids.[144]

The bacteriology of a rat bite is similar to other animal species, and the various systemic diseases transmitted by rats are discussed in Chapter 44. Sporotrichosis has been reported; this widely distributed saprophyte is found on various plants, in the soil, and on many animals.[50]

Although rodents occasionally become infected with rabies, they seldom secrete this virus in saliva; therefore they inflict extremely low-risk bites for transmission of the disease. However, local epidemics can occur, as documented in the 1980s among rodents and lagomorphs on the United States east coast.[94] In that epidemic, woodchucks constituted 80% of all rabid animals; the remainder were squirrels, beavers, rabbits (lagomorphs, not rodents), and one rat. Some of these rabid animals were very aggressive; a woodchuck attacked and knocked down an elderly woman in her garden, biting her repeatedly. Rabies was isolated from the buccal cavity of the woodchuck. A reasonable current recommendation is that a biting wild rat in the United States should be caught and examined for rabies and rabies immunoprophylaxis should be initiated only if the rabies test is positive; rabies immunoprophylaxis is probably appropriate for bites of uncaptured rodents inflicted outside the United States and Canada.[101]

A case has been reported of a cowpox virus–like infection transmitted by a probable rat bite.[141] Rodents are believed to be the natural reservoir for cowpox virus.

Rate-bite fever is an acute illness caused by *Streptobacillus moniliformis* or *Spirillum minus*, which are part of the normal oral flora of rodents, including squirrels. It may also result from bites by wild and domestic carnivores, such as weasels, dogs, cats, and pigs, which may have become infected when hunting rats and mice.[118] Carrier rates among wild rats vary from 50 to 100%.[136] Fewer than 100 cases have been reported in the North American literature; rat-bite fever is not a reportable disease in the United States.[136] Although relatively rare, cases can occur in any setting and can easily be fatal, particularly when the proper diagnosis is not suspected.[34,117,136] Further information is found in Chapter 44.

Plague is caused by the bacterium *Yersinia pestis*. Wild plague is endemic in many parts of the world, chiefly among rats, mice, moles, marmots, squirrels, hares, cats, and mongooses. One of the larger areas of endemic plague is the western United States (362 cases reported in 50 years), where voles, field mice, ground squirrels, prairie dogs, and pack rats carry the infection. The infection is usually transmitted to humans by the bite of arthropods that infest infected animals. Handling infected animals allows *Yersinia pestis* to enter cuts and abrasions, as seen in veterinarians and in hunters who skin and clean infected rabbits.[137] Transmission by bite or scratch has never been reported. The disease is mentioned here because of its historical significance and the frequency of occurrence in wild animals. Further information is found in Chapter 44.

Tularemia represents various syndromes caused by *Francisella tularensis*. This bacterium normally parasitizes about 100 different mammals and arthropods, most commonly cottontail rabbits, rodents, hares, moles, beavers, muskrats, squirrels, rats, and mice. The primary mode of transmission to humans is via a bloodsucking arthropod, such as a tick, or by skin or eye inoculation resulting from skinning, dressing, or handling diseased animals. Other routes of infection include ingestion of water contaminated by urine or feces, and inhalation of dust. Infections after bites or scratches from dogs, cats, skunks, coyotes, foxes, and hogs have been reported, although these are rare.[109] The disease is an occupational hazard of hunters, butchers, cooks, campers, and laboratory technicians. Humans are quite susceptible, and although tularemia was removed from the national notifiable disease list in 1995, 105 cases were reported in 1997 in the United States.[91] More information is found in Chapter 44.

PORCUPINES

Porcupines (a species of rodent) are virtually never reported to bite, but their quills may become embedded in the skin of humans. Because of the structure of quills, they not only embed themselves and are extremely difficult to extract, but they can migrate as much as 10 inches under the skin. The average porcupine has 30,000 quills, which range from less than an inch to 4 inches in length. The quills are barbed and their cores are spongy, so if they are not removed immediately, they absorb body fluid and expand, causing the barbs to flare even further outward. Thus each movement of the victim's body or muscles helps a quill work its way in deeper. Allegedly, such migration has led to injury to internal organs and death in humans. Infection seldom results because the quills have mild antiseptic properties, presumably to protect the porcupines themselves, which sometimes impale themselves.

No medical reports are available of appropriate treatment or complications of porcupine quill injuries, though anecdotal reports of human tetanus from porcupine quill puncture arise from Africa.[1] Most veterinarians remove quills from animals by simple extraction; the same technique is probably sufficient in humans.

BATS

Vampire bats are a vector of rabies in Central and South America; 177 cases were reported from 1980 to 1990, with 27 of those cases in Brazil.[134] Sometimes, small "epidemics" of bites occur in isolated villages in the jungle, as in one outbreak of 26 bat bites in Honoropois, Brazil; all were treated with rabies prophylaxis, and no clinical human rabies was reported.[13] Such clusters of attacks may be triggered by human destruction of wild or domestic hosts (such as pigs) of the bats.[86] Vampire bats feed at night on animal blood, including that of humans, by making an incision in the skin to lap up the blood from the victims' earlobes, forehead, fingers, or toes. One bat can eat a maximum of 1 oz of blood per night, which is clearly not enough to cause death. However, a cave of 1000 bats needs 15 gallons of blood each night, which amounts to more than 5750 gallons per year.[27,33] Protection against vampire bats is effectively provided by mosquito nets.

Insectivorous bats, such as free-tailed bats, are noteworthy for the nearly undetectable bite wounds they leave on their victims.[99] All bats should be considered high risk, and exposure—even to sick or "pet" bats that have been in captivity—should be avoided. Some situations mandating rabies prophylaxis are bizarre and reveal more about human nature than about rabies or bats. For example, rabies prophylaxis was initiated after a patient dunked a dead bat in his beer, chewed on the bat's ear, and then drank the beer.[51] In a similar case, prophylaxis was needed when a miner swallowed a live bat on a bet.[18] Most bats have small teeth that often cannot penetrate human skin, so the risk of bacterial wound infection is low.

PRIMATES

Monkeys and other primates inflict vicious bites that virtually always become infected, despite use of prophylactic antibiotics.[54] Although in developed countries this is largely an issue for laboratory workers, in tropical undeveloped countries, large apes (such as baboons) are not only common, but often aggressive. Weighing up to 90 pounds, a large baboon can be dangerous and lethal. These animals have frequent contact with humans and lose most fear of them. There have been numerous recent reports of packs of wild monkeys driven out of the jungle by hunger attacking humans who get in the way of food sources.[112,116,123]

Monkeys often bite hands and have been known to amputate parts of fingers. A literature review revealed 132 cases of simian bites in which *Bacteroides, Fusobacterium* species, and *Eikenella* corrodens were isolated from some of the wounds.[54] Three victims of simian bites with infected wounds grew diverse bacteria, including β-hemolytic streptococci, enterococci, *Staphylococcus epidermidis,* and *Enterobacteriaceae.*[54] At the present time, simian bites should be considered relatively high risk and treated as if they were human bites.

Old World macaque monkeys (rhesus macaque, cynomolgus, and other Asiatic macaque monkeys) are often infected with simian herpes virus (B virus); transmission to humans is rare but the risk is real, especially for animal control and laboratory workers.[40,98] As with rabies, local wound treatment may be important; of 61 persons bitten by probably infectious monkeys and who received wound cleansing with cetrimide and iodine solution, none became infected.[129] See Chapter 44 for additional information.

The wild gorilla, despite its reputation and appearance, is shy and avoids humans. Although it may charge in defense, it seldom attacks and can be easily confronted and forced to retreat. When a gorilla attacks, it takes one bite and runs. In Africa, gorillas are responsible for two or three attacks per year, none of which are fatal and few of which are severe. Chimpanzees occasionally attack humans, usually only if provoked or cornered. Rare instances of chimpanzees eating children and women have been reported. The baboon is responsible for one to two attacks per year, almost all in South Africa; these are usually by pets. Occasionally, man eating has been reported. The incidence of hunting and meat eating by these animals has increased over the last century, perhaps paralleling the evolution of humans into hunters and meat eaters.[27]

COYOTES, WOLVES, AND HYENAS

The coyote has not only survived the onslaught of civilization in the United States, but has thrived and multiplied. Perhaps as a result, more and more coyote attacks on people have been reported, even in urban areas such as Los Angeles and Cape Cod.[8,22,64] Occasionally, these animals are rabid, but most are not. Some attacks (especially on small children) are fatal.[69] Recently, there has been an increase in reports of attacks in national parks by animals captured and found to be disease-free.[22,65] The bite of a coyote should be treated as a dog bite regarding antibiotic and closure issues; if the animal cannot be captured and examined, rabies prophylaxis should be undertaken.

No significant problems or killings by wolves have been reported in North America, where wolves are traditionally timid. However, throughout Europe and Asia, the wolf has a well-documented history of cunning behavior, pack attacks, and human killing. European wolves tend to hunt in packs and attack women and children. Rabid wolves are seen; a substantial number of attacks by rabid wolves in Iran in the last 10 years provided the clinical population on which the human diploid cell vaccine for rabies was tested.[10] The reintroduction of wolves to wild habitat in the Yellowstone ecosystem and Idaho in 1995 has resulted in the successful proliferation of many new wolves. However, there has not yet been a negative human interaction since their release.[58]

Two other canines that traditionally hunt in packs are the cape hunting dog of Africa and the Indian "devil dog." Although both are feared in their respective environments, they are not deliberate attackers of humans.

Hyenas have tremendously strong jaws and can leave teeth marks in forged steel. The hyena frequently attacks humans in Africa. In certain areas, Africans leave the dead or dying in the bush for predators (hyenas) to eat, which accustoms the animals to the taste of human meat. Hyenas forage around campsites and villages and are wary of awake people. During the summer months when Africans sleep outside their huts, many are assaulted with one clean, massive bite that removes the face or the entire head. Young children have been dragged from their huts while sleeping when a family member leaves briefly without latching the door, and it is common for the hyena to injure or amputate the thumb of a sleeping victim as it drags the victim (by the thumb) to a more convenient place for consumption.[1] Campers are also frequently bitten on the face or limbs while they sleep at night, particularly if they have left food nearby. They usually survive but are massively disfigured. In some parts of Africa, the hyena is a more consistent man eater than the leopard or lion.

SKUNKS, FOXES, AND RACCOONS

Skunks bite readily when captured and are frequent carriers of rabies.[49] No data exist concerning the likelihood of other wound infections after skunk bite; in one series, only 21 bites were reported for the entire Untied States for a 10-year period.[111]

A skunk's most frequent means of defense is spraying the secretions of its anal sac. A skunk ready to spray directs its hindquarters to the enemy, feet firmly planted and tail straight in the air, often stamping the front feet in warning. The spray is accurate to 13 feet and, contrary to popular belief, can be discharged when the animal is lifted by the tail.

Skunk musk causes skin irritation, keratoconjunctivitis, temporary blindness, nausea, and occasionally convulsions and loss of consciousness.[49] The chief component of the musk is butyl mercaptan. This can be neutralized by strong oxidizing agents, such as sodium hypochlorite in a 5.25% solution (household bleach), further diluted 1:5 or 1:10 in water. The chlorine forms odorless sulfate or sulfone compounds by oxidizing the mercaptan and breaking the sulfur free from the carbon chain. This solution can be cleansed with tincture of green soap, followed by a dilute bleach rinse. Tomato-juice shampoo has been advocated for deodorizing hair, which can be washed and mildly bleached or cropped short.

Most human attacks by foxes are by rabid animals; fox bites have caused eyelid lacerations in children sleeping in tents and leg punctures in adults.[75,126,134] One child died of rabies from fox bites despite adequate postexposure prophylaxis.[126]

Raccoons are the definitive host of *Baylisascaris procyonis*, a zoonotic nematode parasite that may cause larva migrans syndromes in humans.[75,145] In the United States, large raccoon rabies epizootics in New England and the middle Atlantic states are spreading. Most rabies-positive animals are taken from near private homes.[120,140] Raccoons account for more than 50% of all animal rabies in the United States.

SWINE

Although domestic pigs are common, pig bites are rare in developed countries, probably because the total number of farmers in those countries is small.[12] Domestic swine can be aggressive and inflict deep goring or bite injuries, often on the posterior thigh because they tend to approach from behind.[12] Wounds are deep (particularly when the boar, with large penetrating tusks, is involved), although sometimes they can be deceptively small on the surface.[132] Carefully and thoroughly explore and debride these wounds.

Twelve percent of veterinarians have been bitten by a pig, placing it fourth in frequency behind dogs (63%), cats (81%), and horses (87%).[78] The usual wide range of bacterial pathogens is reported, including *Pasteurella aerogenes*, *Bacteroides fragilis*, *Proteus*, and α- and β-hemolytic streptococci.[60,131] Like many domestic animals, pigs often carry *Pasteurella multocida*. Unusual gram-negative bacteria have been isolated; many other poorly understood species are probably present.[55]

Wild pigs are even more likely to inflict injury. With a population of over half a million roaming the French countryside, wild pigs cause crop loss and occasionally gore and bite humans.[85] Swine wounds should be treated as high risk for infection, warranting broad-spectrum prophylactic antibiotics (perhaps parenterally) and close follow-up if the victim is not admitted to a hospital.

WILD HERBIVORES

African Buffalo

The African buffalo is a threat chiefly when provoked, but accounts for many deaths and maimings. Left alone, it does not attack; however, when shot or cornered, it charges, is difficult to avoid or stop, and can hook the victim 10 feet into the air with its horns (Figure 42-4). Buffalo that charge humans are usually old, solitary bulls that have left the safety of the large herds, most often because of wounds from poachers' snares, spears, or lion attacks. The buffalo is also wily and intelligent; wounded buffalo may lay in wait for trackers or may

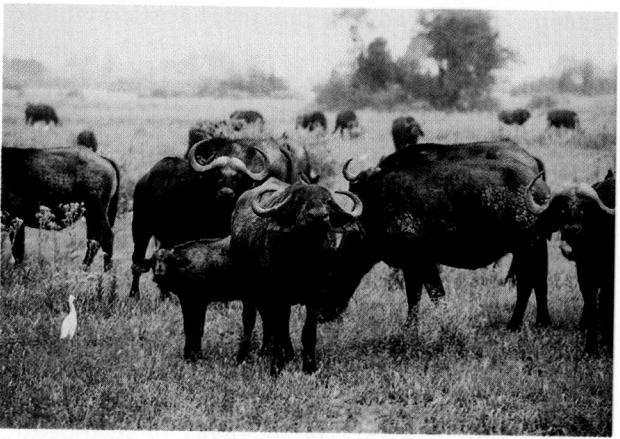

Figure 42-4 African water buffalo with calf. *(Photo by Cary Breidenthal, RN.)*

double around and come up behind them on the trail, often with fatal consequences for the humans. The buffalos' hatred of hunters is legendary in Africa; one hunter was treed but could not get his feet high enough to keep them clear of the animal. The buffalo repeatedly hooked the man's feet with his horns, eventually cutting them to ribbons so that the hunter bled to death, still hanging in the tree. In another anecdotal series, a single buffalo injured several humans in one day; all of the wounds were impaling injuries through the anus.[1]

Once the victim is prostrate, the buffalo gores into the ground with its horns and the heavy horny boss across its forehead and then whips its head from side to side, disemboweling the victim with the sharp horn tips. Such injuries are estimated to be responsible for 20 to 100 deaths per year, mostly in Africa. The horns are always covered with mud, so goring wounds may be heavily contaminated. However, victims who do not have major traumatic injuries generally do well.[119]

American Bison

Brought back from the brink of extinction, a free-ranging herd of more than 3000 North American bison (American buffalo) now lives on land in and around Yellowstone National Park and is responsible for an average of three tourist injuries per year. Fifty-six injuries and three deaths were documented from 1975 to 1993 in Yellowstone as a result of bison-human interaction.[30,31] Despite warnings to avoid approaching these animals any closer than 25 feet, most attacks involve close human approaches to obtain photographs. The mechanism of injury in bison attack is usually penetrating injury, with punctures from goring by horns and blunt injury caused by being tossed in the air and falling or being butted by the animal's massive head. Goring injuries most frequently involve the buttock or posterior thigh as the victim turns away from the bison to flee.[30,31] Gored abdomens and evisceration have been reported. Despite the inevitable contamination of these deep punctures, wound infection is rare if careful operative irrigation and debridement with closure are combined with broad-spectrum prophylactic antibiotics (cephalosporins were used in most cases in one series of reported injuries).[30]

Elephant

The elephant can be one of the most dangerous wild animals and was until recently probably the greatest killer of hunters. The annual death toll in central Africa was probably between 200 and 500.[27] In defense of the elephant, most injuries occur when humans accidentally approach elephants too closely, which the animals interpret as a threat. However, elephants turn rogue from time to time, deliberately attacking and killing humans (Figure 42-5). The incidence of such deaths might decrease as the world becomes progressively less wild, but as humans and elephants compete for the

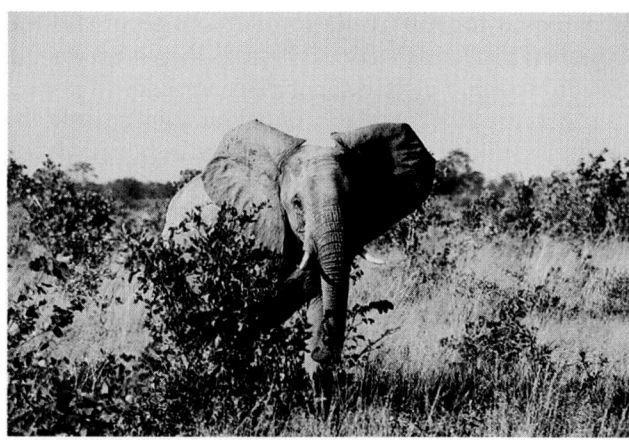

Figure 42-5 African elephant bluff-charges the photographer. *(Photo by Cary Breidenthal, RN.)*

same space and humans despoil and devastate the forests, it may also increase. In Sri Lanka, for example, such encounters force some families to sleep in trees, and at least four people a year are killed by elephants in one area with a human population of only 25,000.[5]

Elephants kill by trampling, goring with the tusks, or striking or throwing with the trunk. Once the victim has been run over or skewered with the tusks, the elephant kneels on them and crushes them. Elephants have been known to use weapons in their attacks; a villager who retreated safely up a baobab tree was hit by a tree branch the bull elephant picked up in its trunk and used as a club. Elephants frequently rip the victim's body apart and scatter the pieces, later covering them with grass and branches. Another elephant tactic is to toss the victim into the trees or straight over the pachyderm's back; a number of victims have survived this experience. Some hunters pursued by elephants have diverted them by throwing off items of clothing.

Many rogue elephants seem to be injured; others have become intoxicated by eating fermenting marula berries. Persistent hunting has made the elephant more wary and irritable than it was 100 years ago. Its traditional feeding and migration ground is increasingly invaded by farmers, leading inevitably to negative interactions. The elephant is incredibly destructive of plants and trees, and its future in this escalating conflict is in grave doubt. A few rare stories suggest that an elephant may actually be a man eater; one of these occurred in 1944 at the Zurich zoo. Elephants captive in zoos and circuses may cause deaths while temporarily deranged; since 1990, captive elephants have killed 39 and injured more than 100 humans worldwide.[105]

Hippopotamus

The hippopotamus is a frequent killer in Africa. Its placid and indolent appearance in zoos completely belies its activity and personality in the wild.

A hippopotamus can run at speeds of up to 45 mph on land and is relatively unpredictable and made irritable by people. It will attack boats and people in the water if it feels trapped (e.g., between a boat and deep water) or if its calf is threatened. With its large canine teeth, it can chop canoes (and the people in them) in half, and it does so several times a year on the Zambezi River in Zimbabwe. However, these attacks are usually in self-defense, and a hippopotamus will get out of the way if it can. Hippopotamuses graze on land and habitually run along established narrow tracks back to the river, mostly at night but also in the day. They will not change course for anything, and humans who make the mistake of staying in the tracks may be trampled.

Moose

Moose are large and potentially aggressive animals, especially during fall rutting and spring calving seasons. When moose are fed by humans, they become more aggressive when food is no longer available.[3] Moose are difficult to chase away, but it is easy to flee from a moose to a larger shelter. If the rump hairs are raised, the ears are laid back, or the moose is licking its lips, it is likely to charge. The subject of the attack should get behind a large solid object for protection. If knocked to the ground by a moose, a victim should roll into a ball, protecting the head with hands and arms and remaining still until the moose leaves.[3] A man was killed in 1995 by a moose in urban Alaska when he approached a cow with a calf who had been harassed by students throwing snowballs.[97] Moose consider dogs predatory and will attack and kill dogs without other obvious provocation.

Most human injuries caused by moose result from moose–motor vehicle collisions, which are quite hazardous in New England and in Sweden.[19,44] In a New England report, an average of two persons per year are seriously injured when their vehicle strikes a moose, usually after dark; 70% of those injured had head and facial injuries, and 26% had cervical spine injuries. The mortality in this series was 9%, and morbidity declined with use of seat belts and rear seat location.[44]

Deer and Elk

The deer population is burgeoning in parts of the United States, and as a reservoir of the tick that carries Lyme disease, it may be credited with the increasing incidence of human Lyme disease.[93] Block Island, an 11-square-mile island off Rhode Island that reintroduced one buck and 4 does to its area in 1968 now has a herd of over 1000 animals and has recorded 45 cases of Lyme disease in residents over the past 9 years. In addition, residents have been attacked by deer in their own yards.[93]

Deer rarely attack humans, but deer–motor vehicle collisions are quite common in densely populated areas. One deer jumped through a window of a law office, injuring an attorney,[7] and another buck in rut carried a man in its antlers for 45 minutes, then pinned the man on the ground until he was rescued.[17] A child was gored by a startled buck when he was feeding the animal; the antler penetrated the axilla, lacerated the pulmonary artery, and caused death by exsanguination.[43] Deer may bite, and like other ungulates may carry pasteurella as oral flora.

Similar to moose, bull elk may attack humans when in rut and cows may attack by butting and stomping when protecting their young.[103] Up to 1% of elk sampled in one study carried *Brucella abortus* and *Mycobacterium bovis*.[113]

Rhinoceros

The black rhinoceros has been represented as one of the meanest animals in Africa because it charges any moving object, including trains. The click of a camera, a gentle movement, or a scent is enough to induce a charge. Because the rhinoceros has poor eyesight but excellent hearing, it may well be running toward sounds to investigate them. Contrary to the popular belief that because of its nearsightedness it can be easily sidestepped, the rhinoceros can turn on a dime.[27] At the end of its charge, it usually hooks right and left with its horns and is generally satisfied with tossing the victim high (12 feet) in the air. However, like so many large wild animals, it probably does not desire confrontation. Rhinoceroses often flee once they have identified a sound as originating from something dangerous (such as a human), and persons who have fallen while running from a charge have been investigated with a few typical snorts and then ignored. However, severe injuries can result if the human fails to get out of the way of a rhinoceros. As with the hippopotamus, injuries and death may have more to do with being in the path of a very large, fast-moving object than with malicious intent. The white rhinoceros is docile and has killed few, if any, people.

Other Wild Herbivores

Other wild species, such as the giraffe, may turn rogue, but this is exceedingly rare. The black wildebeest has killed one or two zookeepers, as have the spiral-horned kudo and bushbuck. Other antelopes have killed or wounded hunters or zookeepers with their sharp horns.

MARSUPIALS

Opossum

The American opossum (*Didelphis virginiana*) inflicts bite injuries both when hunted for food and when accidentally provoked while handled in captivity. Aerobically cultured organisms from the mouths of seven wild opossums included streptococci, coagulase-positive and coagulase-negative staphylococci, *Aeromonas* species, *Citrobacter freundii, E. corrodens,* and *Escherichia coli.*[64] No literature is available on the bites themselves.

Quokka

One of the smallest of the wallaby family residing in western Australia, the quokka typically bites only humans who attempt to feed or pet the animal. Bites tend to occur on the finger or hand. Despite the presence of mixed coliform bacteria in quokka mouth cultures, the incidence of bite-wound infection in this series was zero.[87]

VENOMOUS MAMMALS

Only two types of venomous mammals are known. The short-tailed shrew (*Blarina brevicauda*) of the northeastern United States secretes a protein venom from its maxillary gland and injects it with the lower incisors. The venom may cause edema, a few days of burning sensation, and pain lasting up to 2 weeks.[23] No specific antivenin is available, and treatment is symptomatic. No bites have been reported since the 1930s. A similar venom is possessed by the European water shrew (*Neomys fidiens*) and the primitive Cuban insectivore (*Solenodon paradoxus*).[21] Documented bites are exceedingly rare.

A second type of venomous mammal is the male platypus *(Ornithorhynchus anatinus),* which injects venom from a hollow spur in its hind leg. This venom appears to resemble viperine snake venom and causes local pain, edema, and lymphangitis.[21] The pain can be excruciating and completely unresponsive to intravenous narcotics. Regional nerve block has been reported to be effective in combination with limb immobilization.[45] Localized edema also occurs; no specific treatment is available, and the exact pathophysiology is unknown. Functional recovery may be delayed for up to 3 months.[53] The echidna, or spiny anteater, possesses a similar spur and venom, but envenomation has not been reported.[49]

LARGE BIRDS

The ostrich is responsible for one to two deaths per year, mostly in Africa, where it is raised commercially (Figure 42-6).[6,27] Most of the fatal attacks are kicks to the head and abdomen. The ostrich can kick only forward, but when it does, a sharp toenail flicks out like a switchblade and can penetrate the abdomen. Because the ostrich can easily outrun a human being, the only protection is to lie prone to protect against disembowelment and to cover the neck to protect against pecks. Eventually, the ostrich loses interest and allows the victim to escape.

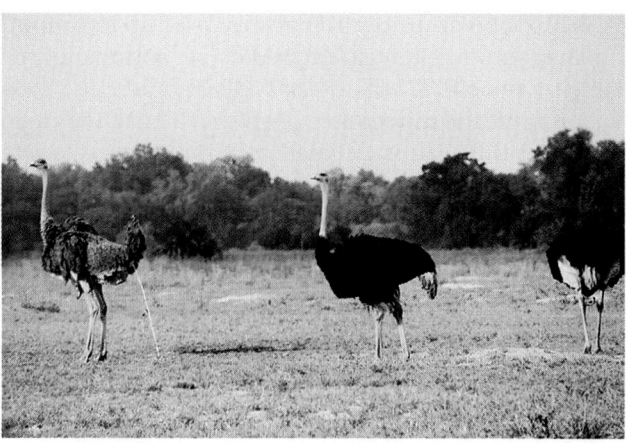

Figure 42-6 African ostrich. (*Photo by Cary Breidenthal, RN.*)

The cassowary (common in New Guinea) can easily disembowel a hunter with a single kick from its long, sharp toe claws.

Birds of paradise have been found to secrete a venom on their feathers, although cases of human toxicity from this have not been reported and the phenomenon is little studied.

The emu is a large flightless bird native to Australia that may weigh 100 to 150 lb. It is usually docile, but when cornered or frightened may lacerate a human handler by kicking.[68]

LARGE REPTILES

The Nile crocodile accounts for 1000 human deaths per year in Africa.[27] Individual crocodiles have been responsible for up to 400 deaths. Most attacks take place in the water, where crocodiles are accustomed to scavenging for the dead, sick, and deformed human babies that are tossed into the water to be disposed of by these reptiles. The crocodile has tremendous grip strength and locks this grip by slotting two lower teeth into holes in the upper jaw. When a crocodile is unable to drag the victim completely underwater, it may grasp a limb and then spin over until the limb is detached.

In a 10-year period in Australia, there were 16 attacks and four fatalities caused by crocodiles; most victims were swimming or wading at night, and alcohol ingestion was present in half.[89] Wound infections with *Aeromonas hydrophila, Pseudomonas pseudomallei, P. aeromonas,* and *Proteus, Enterococcus,* and *Clostridium* spp. were reported in 6 of 11 survivors in this series.[116] In Malawi, over a period of 4 years, 60 victims were admitted to hospitals after injury by crocodiles; (40%) had serious injuries resulting in permanent deformity, and one person died from sepsis.[133]

The American alligator is thriving in the southern United States, and its habitat is so greatly threatened by human expansion that incidents of alligators appearing in suburban backyards and swimming pools are now common. Attacks on children and pets are increasing, with 127 attacks and five deaths reported in Florida from 1973 to 1990.[63] The alligator causes crushing injuries to the torso and open extremity fractures, and may roll underwater with the victim, resulting in drowning. Blunt trauma may result from a strike by the animal's massive tail. Prevention of alligator attacks includes avoiding touching or feeding the animal or swimming at feeding time (dusk) with a dog or in waters with heavy vegetation.[31]

MEDICOLEGAL CONSIDERATIONS

In some cities and regions, animal bites must be reported to public health authorities. Reporting suspected exposure to rabies is mandatory in most regions, and failure to report could become the basis for legal action. Reporting often leads to examination of the offending animal by public health authorities and sometimes to quarantine or destruction of the animal.

Although most wild animals by definition do not have an owner, some exotic species are kept as "pets." An owner's failure to meet local regulations regarding licensure and vaccination can lead to legal action. In addition, the victim may seek compensation from the owner of the animal, with the result that the health care provided and the medical record will be reviewed in court. The injury may be related to the victim's employment, generating worker's compensation or other insurance claims. Therefore injuries and their circumstances should be documented as fully as possible, with line drawings or photographs added to the medical record whenever possible. Certain types of animal bites, particularly those of the hand, are prone to infection and can lead to permanent, litigation-associated complications. A complete medical record is the best protection against such issues and the more ordinary matter of malpractice claims made against the health care provider.

REFERENCES

1. Adolph H: Personal communication, 1999.
2. Aigner N, Konig S, Fritz A: Bite wounds and their characteristic position in trauma surgery management, *Unfallchirurg* 99:346, 1996.
3. Alaska Department of Fish and Game: What to do about aggressive moose? 1997.
4. Alberio L, Lammle B: Capnocytophaga canimorsus sepsis, *N Engl J Med* 339:1827, 1998.
5. Associated Press: Humans and elephants battle for survival: 8 people, 10 animals dead in Sri Lanka, *San Francisco Chronicle*, Sept 27, 1993.
6. Associated Press: Ostrich kicks 63 year old woman to death in South Africa, *Globe Newspaper Co*, Dec 29, 1997.
7. Associated Press: Runaway deer makes surprise visit to law firm, May 29, 1998.
8. Associated Press: Coyote attacks 3-year old boy on Cape Cod, *Boston Globe*, July 30, 1998.
9. Associated Press: White-tiger owner killed in attack, *Gainesville Sun*, Nov 22, 1998.
10. Bahmanyar M, Fayaz A, Nour-Salehi S: Successful protection of humans exposed to rabies infection, *JAMA* 236:2751, 1976.
11. Bardenheier B et al: Tetanus surveillance—United States, 1995-97, *MMWR* 47(SS-2):1, 1998.
12. Barnham M: Pig bite injuries and infection: report of seven human cases, *Epidemiol Infect* 101:641, 1988.
13. Batista-da-Costa M, Bonito RF, Nishioka SA: An outbreak of vampire bat bite in a Brazilian village, *Trop Med Parasitol* 44:219, 1993.
14. Beck AM: The epidemiology and prevention of animal bites, *Sem Veterinary Med Surg* 6:186, 1991.
15. Beck AM, Jones B: Unreported dog bite in children, *Publ Health Rep* 100:315, 1985.
16. Beier P: Cougar attacks on humans in the United States and Canada, *Wildl Soc Bull* 19:403, 1991.
17. Berner R: The St. Nick of Belle Fourche, S.D., survives raucous reindeer attack, *Wall Street Journal*, 1997.
18. Bettor eats a live bat, *San Francisco Chronicle* Aug 31, 1989, p A13.
19. Bjornstig U, Eriksson A, Ornehult L: Injuries caused by animals, *Injury* 22:295, 1991.
20. Brogan TV et al: Severe dog bites in children, *Pediatrics* 96:947, 1995.
21. Bucherl W, Buckley E, Deulofeu V: *Venomous animals and their venoms*, New York, 1968, Academic Press.
22. Carbyn LN: Coyote attacks on children in western North America, *Wildl Soc Bull* 17:444, 1989.
23. Chadwick J: New England's venomous mammals, *N Engl J Med* 281:274, 1969.
24. Childs JE et al: Epidemiology of rodent bites and prediction of rat infestation in New York City, *Am J Epidemiol* 148:78, 1998.
25. Chomel BB: The modern epidemiological aspects of rabies in the world, *Comp Immunol Microbiol Infect Dis* 16:11, 1993.
26. Clark MA et al: Fatal and near-fatal animal bite injuries, *J Forensic Sci* 36:1256, 1991.
27. Clarke J: *Man is the prey*, London, 1969, Andre Deutsch.
28. Cohle SD, Harlan CW, Harlan G: Fatal big cat attacks, *Am J Forensic Med Pathol* 11:208, 1990.
29. Conrad L: Cougar attack: case report of a fatality, *J Wild Med* 3:387, 1992.
30. Conrad L, Balison J: Bison goring injuries: penetrating and blunt trauma, *J Wild Med* 5:1, 1994.
31. Conrad L, Freer (Hallagan) L: *Wild animal attacks*, WMS Educational Slide set, 1996, The Wilderness Medical Society.
32. Constable PJ, Harrington JM: Risks of zoonoses in a veterinary service, *Br Med J* 284:246, 1982.
33. Corey L: Cat-scratch disease. In Isselbacker K, Adams R, Brauwald E, editors: *Harrison's textbook of medicine*, ed 11, New York, 1986, McGraw-Hill.
34. Cunningham BB, Paller AS, Katz BZ: Rat bite fever in a pet lover, *J Am Acad Dermatol* 38:330, 1998.
35. Dahl E: Animal bites at the casualty department of the Oslo city council, *Tidsskr Nor Laegeforen* 118:2614, 1998.
36. Denholm CJ: Survival from a wild animal attack: a case study analysis of adolescent coping, *Maternal-Child Nurs J* 23:26, 1995.
37. deMelker HE, deMelker RA: Dog bites: publications on risk factors, infections, antibiotics and primary wound closure, *Ned Tijdschr Geneeskd* 140:709, 1996.
38. Dire DJ, Hogan DE, Walker JS: Prophylactic oral antibiotics for low-risk dog bite wounds, *Pediatr Emerg Care* 8:194, 1992.
39. Dixon A: Startled tiger kills trainer, *Associated Press*, Oct 8, 1998.
40. Dreesen D: Zoonoses in animal care facilities. In *Proceedings of the 4th National Symposium on Biosafety*, April 1996.
41. Drinking man nibbles bat ear, *San Francisco Chronicle*, Sept 30, 1988.
42. Drummond A: British wildlife expert sought after Thai tiger savages boy, *Times Newspapers Ltd*, 1998.
43. Farabe B: Personal communication, 1999.
44. Farrell TM et al: Moose–motor vehicle collision: an increasing hazard in northern New England, *Arch Surg* 131:377, 1996.
45. Fenner PJ, Williamson JA, Myers D: Platypus envenomation: a painful learning experience, *Med J Aust* 157:829, 1992.
46. Findling J, Pohlmann G, Rose H: Fulminant gram-negative bacillemia (DF-2) following a dog bite in an asplenic woman, *Am J Med* 60:154, 1980.
47. Fishbein D: Rabies, *Infect Dis Clin North Am* 5:53, 1991.
48. Fleisher GR: The management of bite wounds, *New Engl J Med* 340:138, 1999.
49. Fowler M: *Restraint and handling of wild and domestic animals*, Ames, Iowa, 1978, Iowa State University Press.
50. Frean JA et al: Sporotrichosis following a rodent bite: a case report, *Mycopathologia* 116:5, 1991.

51. Garcia VF: Animal bites and *Pasteurella* infections, *Pediatr Rev* 18:127, 1997.

52. Geronemus R, Mertz P, Eaglstein W: Wound healing: the effects of topical antimicrobial agents, *Arch Dermatol* 115:1311, 1979.

53. Goldstein EJ: New horizons in the bacteriology, antimicrobial susceptibility and therapy of animal bite wounds, *J Med Microbiol* 47:95, 1998.

54. Goldstein EJ, Pryor EP, Citron DM: Simian bites and bacterial infection, *Clin Infect Dis* 20:1551, 1995.

55. Goldstein EJ et al: Recovery of an unusual Flavobacterium group IIb-like isolate from a hand infection following pig bite, *J Clin Microbiol* 28:1079, 1990.

56. Goldstein EJ et al: Activities of HMR 3004 (RU 64004) and HMR 3647 (RU 66647) compared to those of erythromycin, azithromycin, clarithromycin, roxithromycin, and eight other antimicrobial agents against unusual aerobic and anaerobic human and animal bite pathogens isolated from skin and soft tissue infections in humans, *Antimicro Agents Chemother* 42:1127, 1998.

57. Goldstein EJ et al: Trovafloxacin compared with levofloxacin, ofloxacin, ciprofloxacin, azithromycin and clarithromycin against unusual aerobic and anaerobic human and animal bite-wound pathogens, *J Antimicrob Chemother* 41:391, 1998.

58. Greater Yellowstone Coalition website: www.greateryellowstone.org, 1999.

59. Griego RD et al: Dog, cat and human bites: a review, *J Am Acad Dermatol* 33:1019, 1995.

60. Gubler JG: Septic arthritis of the knee induced by *Pasteurella multocida* and *Bacteroides fragilis* following an attack by a wild boar, *J Wild Med* 3:288, 1992.

61. Gunther K: Personal communication, Yellowstone National Park, 1999.

62. Haynes J: Wildlife encounters seldom fatal, *San Francisco Examiner,* May 24, 1992.

63. Howard RJ, Burgess GH: Surgical hazards posed by marine and freshwater animals in Florida, *Am J Surg* 166:563, 1993.

64. Howell JM, Dalsey WC: Aerobic bacteria cultured from the mouth of the American opossum *(Didelphis virginiana)* with reference to bacteria associated with bite infections, *J Clin Microbiol* 28:2360, 1990.

65. Hsu SS, Freer (Hallagan) L: Case report of a coyote attack in Yellowstone National Park, *J Wild Med* 7:170, 1996.

66. Hughes J: Tapir bites off zoo worker's arm, *Associated Press,* Nov 21, 1998.

67. Jaffe AC: Animal bites, *Pediatr Clin North Am* 30:405, 1983.

68. Jones TR: Injuries by emus, *Am J Emerg Med* 14:336, 1996.

69. Joyce M: Coyote rarely attack humans, experts say, *Mt. Democrat,* Feb 24, 1997.

70. Kadesky KM et al: Cougar attacks on children: injury patterns and treatment, *J Pediatr Surg* 33:863, 1998.

71. Kamin M, Patten B: Creutzfeldt-Jakob disease: possible transmission to humans by consumption of wild animal brains, *Am J Med* 76:142, 1984.

72. Kizer KW: *Pasteurella multocida* infection from a cougar bite: a review of cougar attacks, *West J Med* 150:87, 1989.

73. Knox ML: Close encounters of the feline kind: big cats on the prowl. *San Francisco Examiner,* Jan 6, 1991.

74. Kohout MP et al: Tiger mauling: fatal spinal injury, *Aust NZ J Surg* 59:505, 1989.

75. Koslow B: Woman recalls attack by rabid fox, *News-Journal Web Edition,* June 4, 1997.

76. Kullberg BJ et al: Purpura fulminans and symmetrical peripheral gangrene caused by *Capnocytophaga canimorsus* (formerly DF-2) septicemia: a complication of dog bite, *Medicine* 70:287, 1991.

77. LaGuardia A: Animal attack files, *Electronic Telegraph London,* Oct 2, 1998.

78. Landercasper J et al: Trauma and the veterinarian, *J Trauma* 28:1255, 1988.

79. Leonard T: Tiger bites off keeper's arm, *London Daily Telegraph,* Feb 26, 1998.

80. Leyden J, Sulzberger M: Topical antibiotics and minor skin trauma, *Am Fam Pract* 23:121, 1981.

81. Lin HH, Hulsey RE: Open femur fracture secondary to hippopotamus bite, *J Orthopaed Trauma* 7:384, 1993.

82. Lockwood R: Dog-bite–related fatalities: United States, 1995-6, *MMWR* 46:463, 1997.

83. Loefler IJ: Letter to editor, *J Trauma* 43:560, 1997.

84. Lyons R: 90's pets, the more exotic the better, *New York Times* 140:34(L) June 23, 1991.

85. MacIntyre B: Wild boars lay waste to French countryside, *Times Newspapers Ltd,* Jan 6, 1998.

86. McCarthy TJ: Human depredation by vampire bats *(Desmodus rotundus)* following a hog cholera campaign, *Am J Trop Hyg* 40:320, 1989.

87. McDonagh TJ: Quokka bites: the first report of bites from an Australian marsupial, *Med J Australia* 157:746, 1992.

88. McDougal C: The man-eating tiger in geographical and historical perspective. In Tilson RL, Seal US, editors: *Tigers of the world,* Park City, NJ, 1993, Noyes Publications.

89. Mekisic AP, Wardill JR: Crocodile attacks in the Northern Territory of Australia, *Med J Australia* 157:751, 1992.

90. *Microsoft Encarta Desktop Encyclopedia 1998,* Microsoft Corporation.

91. MMWR: Rat-bite fever: New Mexico, 1996, *MMWR* 47:89, 1998.

92. MMWR: Human rabies prevention: United States, 1999 recommendations of the ACIP, *MMWR* 48(RR-1):1, 1999.

93. Morin R: Block Island struggles with deer, *Globe Newspaper Co,* Oct 5, 1997.

94. Moro KW et al: The epidemiology of rodent and lagomorph rabies in Maryland, 1981 to 1986, *J Wildlife Dis* 27:452, 1991.

95. Munnion C: Big cats get a taste for illegal migrants, *Electronic Telegraph London,* Aug 26, 1998.

96. Myers CB, Christmann LM: Rat bite: an unusual cause of direct trauma to the globe, *J Pediatr Ophthalmol Strabismus* 28:356, 1991.

97. NBC Anchorage affiliate channel 2 evening news, Jan 9, 1995.

98. Newcomer CE: Zoonoses in animal care facilities, *Proceedings of the 4th National Symposium on Biosafety,* April, 1996.

99. Noah DL et al: Epidemiology of human rabies in the United States, 1980-1996, *Ann Intern Med* 128:922, 1998.

100. Olivarius F: Rat bites, *Cutis* 53:302, 1994.

101. Ordog G, Balasubramanium S, Wasserberger J: Rat bites: fifty cases, *Ann Emerg Med* 14:126, 1985.

102. Organization Panamericana de la Salud: Consideraciones sobre la prevencion, el control y la vigilancia epidemiologica de la rabia humana transmitida por vamiros enlas Americas, *Reunion de consulta sobre la atencion a personas expuestas a la rabia transmitida por vampiros,* Washington, DC, 1991.

103. Peaco J: Personal communication, 1999.

104. Pers C, Kristiansen J, Scheibel J: Fatal septicemia caused by DF-2 in a previously healthy man, *Scand J Infect Dis* 18:265, 1986.

105. PETA: Animal attacks: elephant attacks, *www.circuses.com,* Feb 3, 1999.

106. Phuapradit W, Saropala N: Topical application of honey in treatment of abdominal wound disruption, *Aust NZ J Obstet Gynecol* 32:381, 1992.

107. Plaus W, Hermann G: The surgical management of superficial infections caused by atypical mycobacteria, *Surgery* 110:99, 1991.

108. Prasad A, Madan VS, Buxi TB: Tiger assault: an unusual mode of head injury (letter), *Clin Neurol Neurosurg* 93:171, 1991.

109. Quenzer R, Mostow S, Emerson J: Cat-bite tularemia, *JAMA* 238:1845, 1977.

110. Rauber P: When nature turns nasty, *Sierra,* Nov/Dec 1993, p 46.

111. Reported human injuries or health threats attributed to wild or exotic animals kept as pets (1971-1981), *J Am Vet Med Assoc* 180:382, 1982.

112. Reuters: Wild monkeys wound 26 people in attacks on Japanese town, *Nando Times,* Jan 26, 1998.

113. Rhyan JC et al: Survey of free-ranging elk from Wyoming and Montana for selected pathogens, *J Wildl Dis* 33:290.

114. Rollins CE, Spencer DE: A fatality and the American mountain lion: bite mark analysis and profile of the offending lion, *J Forensic Sci* 40:486, 1995.

115. Saberwal VK et al: Lion-human conflict in the Gir Forest, India, *Conserv Biol* 8:501, 1994.

116. Sathu JN: Kashmir monkeys storm city, *Electronic Telegraph,* Feb 3, 1999.

117. Schuurman B et al: Rat bite fever after a bite from a tame pet rat, *Ned Tidjschr Geneeskd* 142:2006, 198.

118. Shackelford P: Rat bite fever. In Feigin RD, editor: *Pediatric infectious disease,* Philadelphia, 1981, WB Saunders.

119. Shattock F: Injuries caused by wild animals, *Lancet* 1:412, 1968.

120. Sinclair CL, Zhou C: Descriptive epidemiology of animal bites in Indiana, 1990-92: a rationale for intervention, *Public Hlth Rep* 110:64, 1995.

121. Smith JS et al: Unexplained rabies in three immigrants in the United States: a virologic investigation, *N Engl Med* 324:205, 1991.

122. Spence G: A review of animal bites in Delaware: 1989 to 1990, *Del Med J* 62:1425, 1990.

123. Spillius A: Hungry monkeys on rampage, *The Telegraph UK,* Nov 12, 1998.

124. Stevens WK: Survival of the big cats brings conflict with man, *New York Times,* Aug 2, 1994.

125. Sudarshan MK et al: An epidemiological study of rabies in Bangalore City, *Indian Med Assoc* 93:14, 1995.

126. Tabbara KF, Al-Omar O: Eyelid laceration sustained in an attack by a rabid desert fox, *Am J Ophthalmol* 119:651, 1995.

127. Talan DA et al: Bacteriologic analysis of infected dog and cat bites, *New Engl J Med* 340:85, 1999.

128. Tonkin MA, Negrine J: Wild platypus attack in the Antipodes, *J Hand Surg* 19B:162, 1994.

129. Tribe G, Noren E: Incidence of bites from cynomolgus monkeys in attending animal staff 1975-80, *Lab Animals* 17:110, 1983.

130. United States Department of Labor, Bureau of Labor Statistics: *Occupational injuries in the United States by industry, 1980-95,* Washington DC, 1997, the Department.

131. Van J: Ferret fad dangerous, vets warn, *Chicago Tribune,* Sept 6, 1986.

132. Van Demark RES, Van Demark REJ: Swine bites of the hand, *J Hand Surg* 16:136, 1991.

133. Vanwersch K: Crocodile bite injury in southern Malawi, *Trop Doct* 28:221, 1998.

134. Varadarajan T: Fear of US epidemic grows after young girl is bitten by rabid fox, *Times Newspapers Ltd,* Feb 25, 1998.

135. Waldvogel F et al: Perioperative antibiotic prophylaxis of wound and foreign body infections: microbial factors affecting efficacy, *Rev Infect Dis* 13(suppl):S782, 1991.

136. Washburn RG: Streptobacillus moniliformis (rat-bite fever). In Mandell GL, Bennett JE, Dolin R, editors: *Principles and practice of infectious diseases,* vol 2, New York, 1995 Churchill Livingstone.

137. Werner SB et al: Human plague: United States, 1993-1994, *MMWR* 43:242, 1994.

138. Wiens MB, Harrison PB: Big cat attack: a case study, *J Trauma* 40:829, 1996.

139. Wiggins ME, Akelman E, Weiss AC: The management of dog bites and dog bite infections to the hand, *Orthopedics* 17:617, 1994.

140. Wilson ML et al: Emergence of raccoon rabies in Connecticut, 1991-1994: spatial and temporal characteristics of animal infection and human contact, *Am J Trop Med Hyg* 57:457, 1997.

141. Wolff KD: Management of animal bite injuries of the face: experience with 94 patients, *J Oral Maxillofac Surg* 56:838, 1998.

142. Wong A: Hypersensitivity to rat saliva, *J Am Acad Dermatol* 4:606, 1984.

143. World Health Organization: *World Health Report,* Geneva, 1999, WHO.

144. Wykes WN: Rat bite injury to the eyelids in a 3-month-old child, *Br J Ophthalmol* 73:202, 1989.

145. Zagers JJ, Boersema JH: Infections with *Baylisaxcaris procyonis* in humans and raccoons, *Tijdschr Diergeneeskd* 123:471, 1998.

43 Bear Attacks

Steven P. French

Bears are one of the most widely distributed animals in the world. At least one of the eight bear species currently exists in Asia, Europe, North and South America, and the Arctic (Table 43-1). Bears in Africa became extinct several million years ago. Australia and Antarctica are the only continents where bears have never existed. The koala bear of Australia is a marsupial and not a true bear.

Bears also occupy a wide variety of habitats, including tropical forests, polar ice sheets, swamps, barren ground tundra, bamboo jungles, alpine meadows, and coniferous and deciduous forests. Their range extends from sea level up to about 6100 m (20,000 feet).

Bears are carnivores. Although some bear species practice specialized feeding in response to their habitat, all bears are also omnivores and retain the ability to feed on a variety of food types, including vegetation, insects, and meat.

Modern bears have larger brains than their extinct ancestors,[22,30] and the relative brain size for bears is larger than that of other carnivores.[14] This greater brain size probably resulted from a need to increase sensory and perceptual capacities for locating an omnivore food base with both seasonal and annual variations in distribution and abundance.[5,8,25] The larger brain size reflected the increased intelligence required by bears to develop a complex foraging strategy. Increased intelligence also allowed them to develop individual behavior, shaped by both experience and memory. Thus they possess a wide variety of behaviors and have been described as playful, lazy, doleful, entertaining, intelligent, caring, powerful, aggressive, terrifying, and vicious.[33]

The image of bears as "man-eaters" ignites our fear of them. Human injury and deaths from natural phenomena, especially wild animal attacks, are sensationalized. Bear attacks are rare, but the psychologic impact of widespread media coverage inflates their frequency and significance.[6,24] Every bear attack is traditionally referred to as a *mauling*, regardless of the extent of injuries. This term contributes to the emotional response regarding such attacks and leads to "bearanoia" in many people who visit bear country. This fear of bears may affect how people use wilderness areas with bear populations and how they view the conservation of bears and their habitat. Better understanding of bears and their behavior helps reduce bear attacks, assists physicians in treating bear attack victims, and promotes conservation of bears.

NORTH AMERICAN BEARS

Grizzly bears (*Ursus arctos horribilis*) are larger and more heavily built than most other ursids, with adults weighing 146 to 383 kg (325 to 850 pounds)[1] (Figure 43-1). Polar bears (*Ursus maritimus*) are similar in size and weight but are more elongated in shape (Figure 43-2). Black bears (*Ursus americanus*) have the same general shape of grizzly bears but are generally smaller than both polar and grizzly bears (Figure 43-3). Weights for black bears range from 63 to 135 kg (140 to 300 pounds) for adult females and 113 to 293 kg (250 to 650 pounds) for adult males.

Dentition in these three species is bunodont and reflects their omnivorous diet, although polar bears are the most carnivorous of the three (Figure 43-4). Their canine teeth are sturdy and can reach a length of 7 cm (2¾ inches). Their legs are of approximately equal length and taper to large, plantigrade feet. The fore claws of a grizzly bear are heavier, longer, and straighter than those of a black bear and can reach a length of 8.75 cm (3½ inches) measured along the external curvature[35] (Figure 43-5). A large muscular hump overlies the scapulae of grizzly bears, giving additional strength to the forelimbs for digging (Figure 43-6). The face of a brown bear tends to be more dish shaped than that of a black bear (Figure 43-7).

The physical strength of bears is tremendous, and they can run at speeds up to 65 kph (40 mph) over irregular terrain. They have a keen sense of hearing and an even keener sense of smell. Their eyesight has been described as poor,[19] although many field researchers believe that bears can see as well as humans and are especially adept at detecting movement. Evidence suggests grizzly bears have good night vision.[11]

Grizzly and black bears hibernate about 5 months during the winter, an evolutionary adaptation to reduced food availability. The hibernation of polar bears is slightly different, since their primary food (seals) is available during the winter.[28] Adult male polar bears tend to hibernate for short periods each winter in response to severe storms, whereas pregnant females have more extended hibernation. During the active (nondenning) season, all bear species wander throughout a general home range in search of seasonal foods.

The guard hairs on brown bears can be lighter in color and lend a "grizzled" appearance. Black bears can be many colors, ranging from white to black, cinnamon, brown, or "blue."[9]

TABLE 43-1. Distribution of Bear Species

COMMON NAME	SCIENTIFIC NAME	DISTRIBUTION
Panda bear	*Ailuropoda melanoleuca*	Eastern rim of China's Tibetan Plateau
Spectacled bear	*Tremarctos ornatus*	Andes Mountains in South America
Sloth bear	*Melursus ursinus*	Nepal, Bangladesh, Bhutan, northern India, Sri Lanka
Asiatic black bear	*Ursus thibetanus*	Southern Asia from Pakistan across northern India and into China and southeast Asia; separate populations in eastern Russia, Korea, Taiwan, and Japan
Sun bear	*Helarctos malayanus*	Borneo, Burma, Java, Malaysia, Sumatra, Thailand
American black bear	*Ursus americanus*	Alaska, Canada, most of lower 48 states
Brown bear	*Ursus arctos*	Eurasia, Alaska, Canada, northern Rocky Mountain states (including Wyoming, Montana, Idaho, and Washington)
Polar bear	*Ursus maritimus*	Arctic circle (circumpolar)

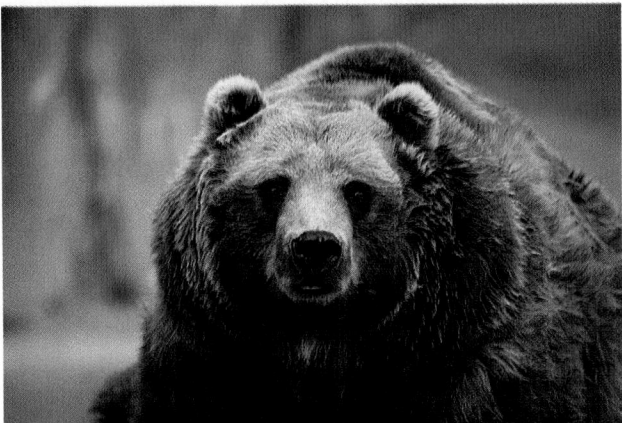

Figure 43-1   Grizzly bear. *(Courtesy Marilynn G. French.)*

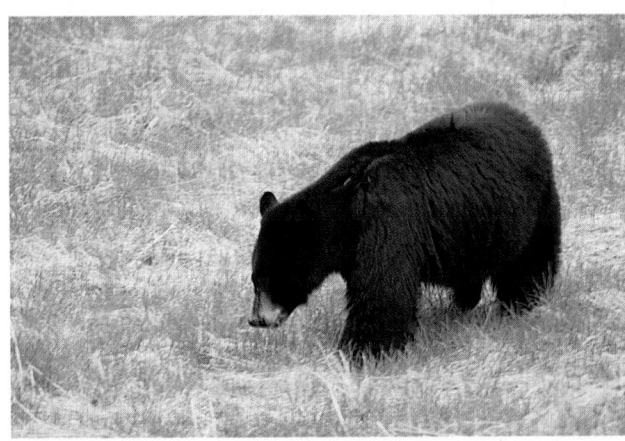

Figure 43-3   American black bear. *(Courtesy Marilynn G. French.)*

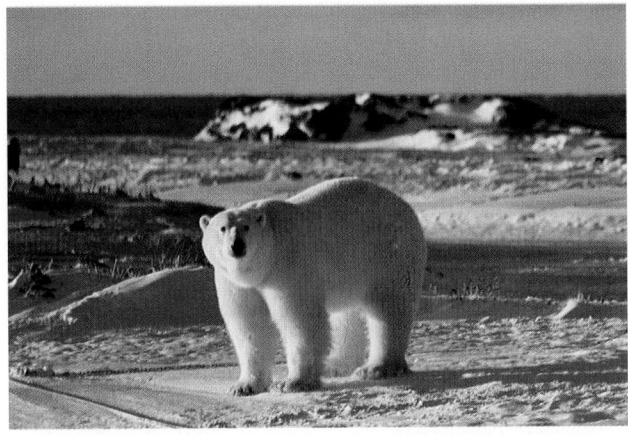

Figure 43-2   Polar bear. *(Courtesy Steven D. Evans.)*

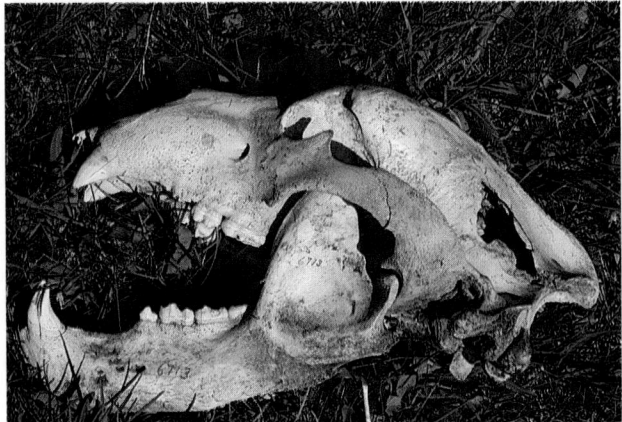

Figure 43-4   Grizzly skull, demonstrating canine teeth. *(Courtesy Marilynn G. French.)*

Grizzly Bears

The grizzly bear symbolizes wilderness in North America. In certain respects, "grizzlies" define the "wild" in wilderness. They range from Alaska down through western Canada and into the lower 48 states in remnant populations located in relatively unde-veloped federal lands, primarily in the northern Rocky Mountains.

Attacks by grizzly bears are relatively rare and spo-radic. A total of 162 bear-inflicted injuries (including deaths) were reported from 1900 through 1985 in Cana-dian and North American national parks.[19,20] From 1980

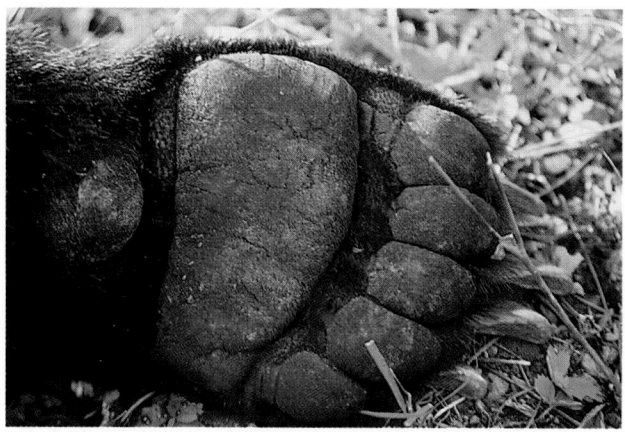

Figure 43-5 Grizzly paw with claws. *(Courtesy Marilynn G. French.)*

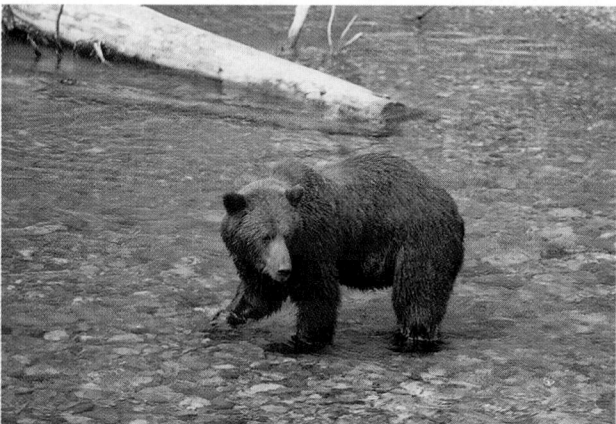

Figure 43-6 Alaskan coastal brown bear, demonstrating muscular back hump. *(Courtesy Luanne Freer.)*

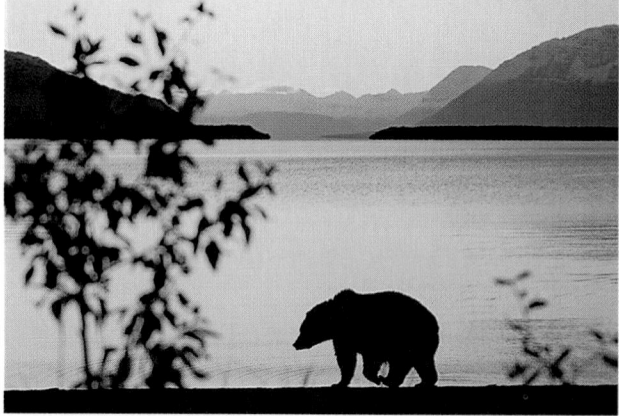

Figure 43-7 Silhouette of brown bear, demonstrating hump and "dished" face. *(Courtesy Timothy Floyd.)*

to 1994, 21 grizzly bear attacks, including two deaths, occurred in Yellowstone National Park.[18] In Alaska the number of people injured by grizzly bears in recent times,[26] possibly from increased recreational use of grizzly habitat, will probably be maintained.

Calculation of an accurate injury rate remains elusive. Earlier records were incomplete, and defining and quantifying those at risk have always been difficult. Injury rates are based on total visitation days to the national parks in Canada and North America.[20] The average number of grizzly bear–inflicted injuries is 1 in 2,260,276 visitors to these parks combined, with a high of 1 in 317,700 visitors in Kluane National Park and a low of 1 per 6,693,859 visitors in Banff. During this same period the grizzly bear–inflicted injury rate for Yellowstone National Park was 1 in 1,543,287 visitors and for Glacier National Park was 1 in 848,180 visitors.

Not every visitor to a national park is exposed to the same risk of being attacked by a grizzly bear. To calculate an injury rate more accurately for visitors with higher and more uniform exposure, similar rates are reported based on registered backcountry users. However, this method provides an inaccurate injury index because some parks do not register backcountry use and others generally underestimate it. Also, significant and perhaps most backcountry use (and therefore exposure) is by unregistered day hikers.

The number of bear attacks (both black and grizzly) increases in months when more people seek recreation in grizzly country. For national parks the incidence of bear attacks increases during the peak tourist season, July and August. For surrounding national forests another peak occurs during hunting season, September to November. With more people seeking recreation in bear country, greater opportunity exists for human-bear encounters.

Native peoples and grizzly bears occupied the same land for thousands of years in North America in what was probably a neutral coexistence, since neither had a profound influence on the other. However, the European expansion into the west after Lewis and Clark's expedition in the early 1800s tipped the scales heavily in favor of humans, both in sheer numbers and in technology, such as guns, traps, and poisons. Bears were killed in large numbers to appease fear and hatred and to protect life and property. Most of their original habitat was occupied by either people or livestock or was dramatically altered by ranching and agricultural development.

Selection pressures that began with European expansion into the grizzly bears' habitat has probably been altering their behavior. Since that early period and even today in protected areas such as national parks, aggressive bears have been removed at a higher rate than nonaggressive bears. Bears that were curious

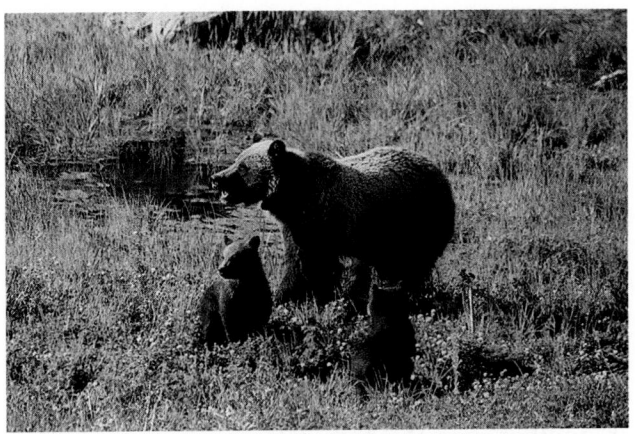

Figure 43-8 Yellowstone grizzly sow with cubs. *(Courtesy Brian Ertel.)*

about humans and human developments and those that did not readily flee the presence of humans were also removed at a higher rate. Therefore bears that avoided humans survived at a higher rate than other bears and probably passed that trait on to their offspring through genetics and learning.

A built-in safety factor exists for people entering grizzly country because the vast majority of bears now avoid a confrontation if given the opportunity, which probably explains why grizzly bear attacks on humans are so rare. Unfortunately, the available information on grizzly attacks does not always yield an accurate account of the cause-and-effect relationship. The specific sequence of events is not always known and is subjectively reconstructed, although case histories reveal certain patterns.

A sudden and close encounter with a grizzly bear is the primary event leading to human injury. From 1980 to 1994, of 21 people injured by grizzlies in Yellowstone National Park,[18] 18 resulted from people surprising a grizzly at close quarters. These attacks were often brief, and the bear generally left the area soon after the attack. Although injuries were typically described as a mauling, they were generally much less severe than the bear had the potential to inflict, and victims were rarely killed. This suggests that the bear's behavior in response to a close encounter was to remove a perceived threat.

A close encounter with a female with cubs is considered more dangerous, since she is considered to be more aggressive in defense of her young (Figure 43-8). Evidence to support this hypothesis is strong. Females with young represent about 20% of a bear population but account for more than 80% of the bears that injure humans. Another explanation, however, is that females with young are more likely to be active during daylight hours when humans are active, whereas males are active primarily in the predawn hours and after dusk.[11]

Grizzly bear attacks sometimes occur near a carcass on which the bear has been feeding. Grizzly bears may be more aggressive under these circumstances in defense of the carcass. Grizzly bears of all ages and either gender, however, may readily exit when they sense people approaching.[12] When grizzly bears injure someone near a carcass, the precipitating event may simply be a close encounter with a preoccupied bear.

Another class of attacks results from provocation, most often when a grizzly bear is shot. Once the bear is injured, its behavioral response is no longer to remove a threat but to fight for its life. These attacks tend to be more prolonged and aggressive, resulting in more severe injuries than those a resulting from a close encounter.

Provoked bear attacks can result from direct harassment by aggressive photographers. Although such incidences are rare, these attacks tend to resemble the response of an injured bear rather than one responding to a close encounter. The injuries tend to be more severe, and a disproportionate number of photographers are killed. Up to 1985, at least 10 photographers were injured, one fatally, and from 1986 to 1992, at least four were injured, two fatally.[19]

Most people attacked by grizzly bears are injured but not killed; the intent of the bear is simply to remove a perceived threat, not to prey on the individual. From 1900 to 1979, 19 human deaths resulted from grizzly attacks documented in the national parks in North America, and 22 deaths occurred in Alaska outside the parks.[19,24] Some were victims of defensive attacks and probably would have survived if current medical management techniques had been available. Some deaths, however, resulted from predatory attacks. The question is why grizzlies do not prey on humans more often. As a potential prey species, humans are predictable and abundant, easy to catch and kill, and easy for a grizzly to consume.

Little historic evidence suggests that grizzly bears routinely preyed on humans except in unusual circumstances. In 1860 a smallpox epidemic struck a small band of Stonie Indians (Assiniboin Tribe) camped in the Yarrow Creek drainage in Alberta, Canada.[32] Grizzlies began scavenging on the dead left on the ground as the tribe moved to the next drainage. Grizzlies followed them to their next encampment and began preying on survivors. For years the Indians avoided this area for fear of being eaten by grizzlies that had "learned" to prey on humans.

Since about 1900, when reasonably accurate records were first kept predatory attacks on humans by grizzly bears generally have been rare, sporadic, and isolated events.* However, a disturbing trend has begun in re-

---

*Referenes 16, 26, 27, 32, 36, 37.

cent times. Between 1967 and 1986, 12 deaths were inflicted by grizzly bears in Banff, Glacier, and Yellowstone National Parks. In each case the bear was conditioned to human foods (regularly seeking out and obtaining it) and/or habituated to human presence (not readily fleeing). Nine of the victims were partially consumed, and eight deaths were classified as predatory events.[19] During this same period, however, many bears with these same behavioral traits did not prey on humans. Conditioned and habituated behavior may predispose some grizzlies to prey on humans within their image under certain but still unknown circumstances. The relationship between conditioning and habituation appears strong but is not conclusive. The bear involved was not always known, and the terms "conditioned" and "habituation" are borrowed from learning theory and have never been precisely defined by wildlife biologists. This potential relationship, however, has significantly influenced grizzly bear management. The primary thrust currently is to prevent bears from obtaining human foods and from routinely being around people and human developments.

Grizzly bears may also mistakenly perceive a person as one of their normal prey species. Five such incidents have been documented. Two victims were killed by grizzly bears while making prey calls to lure in other predators. Two victims were attacked while field-dressing a game animal, and the fifth was attacked while carrying the hide of a deer draped over his shoulder. Clearly, persons should not look, smell, or sound like a prey species when in grizzly country.

Black Bears

Black bears are the most numerous and widely distributed of all North American bears (see Figure 43-3). They occur in more than 30 of the lower 48 states, from Maine to Florida and from California to Washington. They also occur throughout Canada and Alaska, extending up to treeline below the Arctic Circle. They are well adapted to an arboreal habitat and prefer to eat vegetation, carrion, and mast (nuts, acorns), with small mammals and insects accounting for less than 5% of the diet.[9]

Between 1960 and 1980, more than 500 people were injured by black bears, but at least 90% of these episodes resulted in minor scratches or bites inflicted by bears that were either conditioned to human foods or habituated to human presence.[19] Injuries as a result of close encounters are extremely rare, and in contrast to female grizzly (brown) bears, female black bears display little aggression in defense of their young and rarely cause injury. They have short, sharp radial claws better adapted for climbing trees than for attacking humans. They will often retreat rather than attack, even in defense; thus hunters using dogs can "tree" black bears.[9]

Whereas grizzly (brown) bears sometimes prey on humans at night, black bears occasionally prey on humans during the daytime. From 1900 through 1980, 20 people were killed by black bears, with predation considered the motivation in 18 cases. All but one case occurred in remote areas outside park boundaries, an indication that neither conditioning nor habituation was a major factor.

Since 1985, black bears attempted to prey or preyed on humans in 15 episodes, with two fatalities and 7 major injuries.[19] Details are scant, but at least four occurred at night while the victims were asleep. In one case the bear broke into a camper and pulled the victim out, and in another case the bear entered a wooden teepee ("wickiup") and dragged the victim out by her foot.[29] In most attacks, the black bears were driven away by aggressive actions by the victims and their companions, such as yelling and throwing objects.

POLAR BEARS

Polar bears are distributed in a circumpolar fashion around the Arctic Circle and subsist almost exclusively on a diet of seals (Figure 43-2). These bears feed primarily in winter on ice-covered polar seas. Some southern populations live on land during the summer in a state of waking hibernation and starvation. Polar bear–inflicted injuries are much less frequent than those by grizzly (brown) or black bears, primarily because of their remote and harsh environment with relatively little human intrusion. From 1973 to 1987, three people were injured (one fatally) in Norway,[15] and from 1965 to 1985, 20 people were injured (six fatally) by polar bears in Canada.[20] The number of injuries would probably be much higher except that most people in polar bear habitat are armed, and in the majority of aggressive encounters the bear is killed before causing injury.

Polar bear–inflicted injuries have been classified into two general categories. The major one is predation, primarily by subadult and adult males. In these instances, five of the six victims who died were probably killed instantly. The other category is injury by adult females thought to be defending their young. These episodes are typically brief and nonfatal, which supports the theory that the bear is removing a perceived threat. In more than 90% of aggressive encounters with polar bears, an attractant, such as food, garbage, or carcasses, was considered contributory.[20]

BEARS ON OTHER CONTINENTS

The available data on attacks by bears on other continents are much less complete than those for North American bears. In Europe the brown bear has coexisted with humans much longer that those in North

America. (In some parts of North America the brown bear is called a grizzly bear, but they are genetically the same species.) As a result, its behavior is less aggressive and more like that of black bears. Numbers of European brown bears are extremely low, and the animals are highly cryptic and nocturnal and thus are rarely seen or encountered. Human injury by brown bears in Europe today is almost nonexistent.

The brown bears in the former Soviet Union live in vast, relatively undeveloped areas and appear to have aggressive responses against humans similar to those of North American brown bears. Many human injuries from brown bear attacks, including deaths, may be related to bears injured by sport hunters.[4]

The panda bear (Ailuropoda melanoleuca), commonly known as the giant panda, lives in the temperate climate of the bamboo jungles distributed along the eastern rim of China's Tibetan Plateau. It is one of the most recognized bears in the world, with a distinctive white and black coloration. It is a relatively poor climber but will climb trees on occasion to avoid danger. During winter months the panda bear migrates to lower elevations where food remains plentiful, thus avoiding the need to hibernate.

The panda bear is primarily a vegetarian. About 99% of its diet consists of stalks, leaves, and shoots of only two bamboo species.[33] The panda has an enlarged wrist bone that serves as an opposable digit, much like a thumb. This evolutionary adaptation enables the panda to efficiently hold and strip bamboo stalks. Since bamboo is a poor-quality food, the panda must compensate by eating large amounts. Each day it feeds up to 12 hours. The panda bear is shy and reclusive, representing minimal threat to human safety in the wild.

The spectacled bear (Tremarctos ornatus) lives in the tropical climates of the Andes Mountains along the northwest border of South America. It is one of two bear species that live below the equator. The spectacled bear has a distinctive white coloration around its eyes. It is an excellent climber and spends most of its time in trees eating fruit. It often builds nests and rests in trees as well. Because its source of nutrition is abundant year-round, it does not hibernate. Spectacled bears are relatively small and shy. Encounters are extremely rare, and they pose very little threat to human safety.

The sloth bear (Melursus ursinus) lives in the subtropical forests of Nepal, Bangladesh, Bhutan, India, and Sri Lanka. It has a disheveled appearance because of its long, shaggy fur coat. In some of its range the sloth bear coexists with elephants, wild boars, leopards, tigers, greater one-horned rhinos, and Asiatic black bears.

The sloth bear is a special type of insectivore called myrmecophagous because it feeds primarily on ants and termites. It is uniquely adapted for this feeding behavior. Without the two upper incisors and with an elongated and raised hard palate, mobile lips, and nearly naked snout, the sloth bear can blow away dust to expose termites and create a strong sucking force to feed. It can dig out insect burrows with its long claws, and its coat protects it from insect stings.

Although the data are limited primarily to anecdotal reports, the sloth bear appears to be the most dangerous bear species in Europe or Asia, next to the Russian brown bear. Approximately one native is seriously injured or killed by a sloth bear in Chitwan National Park in Nepal each year.[13] In the remote regions of western Nepal, at least one villager is seriously injured by a sloth bear every other year. Most of these injuries are the result of a close encounter, and the victims receive wounds to the head and neck. No predatory behavior has been reported.

The aggression of the sloth bear is between that of the American black bear and grizzly bear. Sloth bear researchers in Nepal work exclusively while riding elephants because of their concern about attacks from rhinos, sloth bears, and tigers, in that order.[23]

Asiatic black bears (Ursus thibetanus) occupy the broad-leafed forests throughout a large portion of south Asia, from Pakistan across northern India and into China and Southeast Asia (Figure 43-9). Separate populations also occur in eastern Russia, Korea, Taiwan, and Japan. Some of their range overlaps with brown bears, sloth bears, and sun bears. In some localities the Asiatic black bear is called the "moon bear" or the "white-breasted bear" because of the crescent-shaped white coloration on its chest.

The Asiatic black bear is a dietary generalist and feeds on a wide variety of plants, insects, and animal matter. It is a good climber and often forages and rests in trees. Unlike pandas and spectacled bears, these bears hibernate during the winter months. They are hunted extensively for illegal trade of bear parts and rarely present a threat to human safety. There are in fact one to two attacks per year that result in significant in-

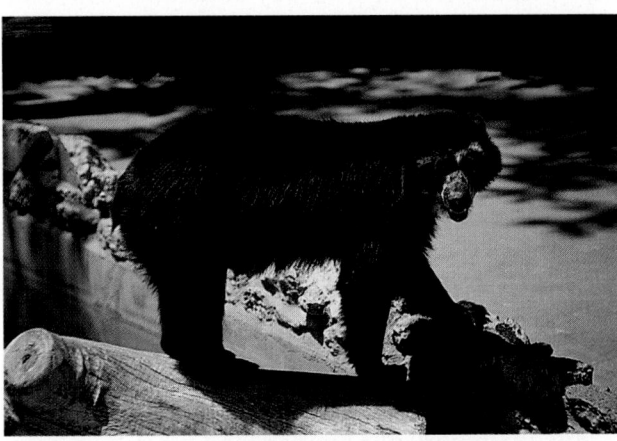

Figure 43-9 Asiatic black bear. *(Courtesy Marilynn G. French.)*

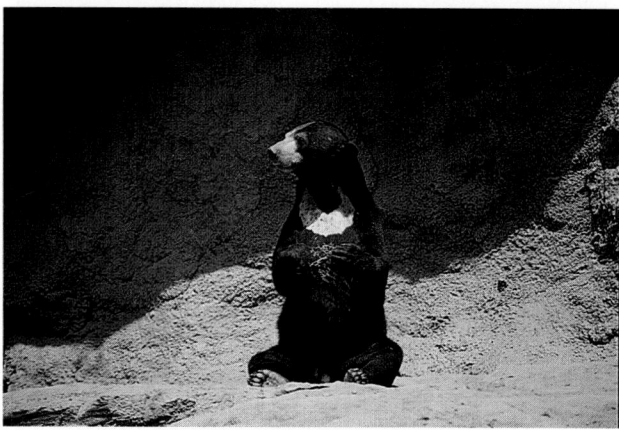

Figure 43-10 Sun bear. *(Courtesy Marilynn G. French.)*

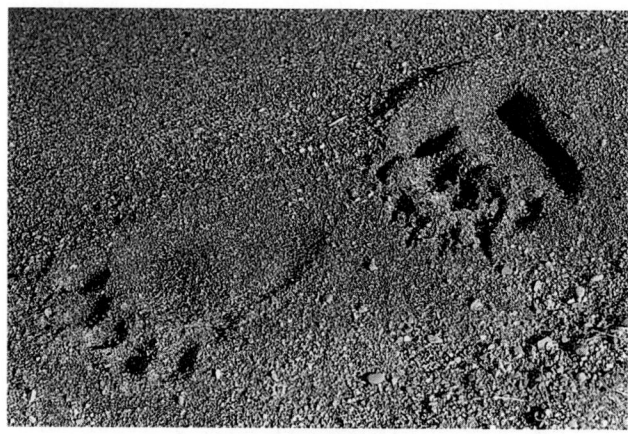

Figure 43-11 Bear prints. *(Courtesy Timothy Floyd.)*

jury requiring hospitalization. Although rare, they do occur mostly as a result of a close encounter.

The sun bear *(Helarctos malayanus)* is the smallest of all bear species, rarely weighing more than 45 kg (100 pounds) (Figure 43-10). It occupies tropical regions in Borneo, Burma, Java, Malaysia, Sumatra, and Thailand. As with the spectacled bear, the sun bear is equatorial because part of its range extends below the equator. It has a white to cream-colored, horseshoe-shaped marking on its chest, providing its common name. In some localities it is called the honey bear. It has a long slender tongue, an adaptation for extracting honey from beehives. Its claws are long and more sharply curved than those of other bears, enabling it to be a proficient tree climber, where it can easily hang upside down from a branch. The sun bear is rarely seen and represents almost no threat to humans.

PREVENTION AND RISK REDUCTION

Much literature about safety in bear country involves attack victims.[6,19,20,24,26] Such information is gathered from victims who are generally unfamiliar with bear behavior and whose interpretations of the events reflect their cultural biases. Also, victims often become instant media celebrities. In several cases the circumstances surrounding the attack changed significantly with each telling, usually reducing the victim's culpability. Because of potential litigation, some victims have told their stories only through an attorney. Caution must be used when compiling and analyzing such "data."

Recommendations for avoiding bear attacks have been drawn primarily from what attack victims did "wrong." Because most people who live, work, and regularly vacation in bear country are never injured, it is equally important to understand what they have done "right." Unlike bear attack victims, these people have successfully navigated grizzly country without

being injured. Although this information is not as readily available as attack records, it is critical to our knowledge of grizzly-human interactions.

From 1900 to 1985, 115 human injuries were reported from black, polar, and grizzly bear attacks in Alaska, but only two victims were natives.[26] This strongly suggests that the behavior of people is important in determining how to coexist with bears safely. Safety in bear country involves four levels of interaction: (1) avoiding an encounter, (2) reducing the chances of being attacked after an encounter, (3) reducing the severity of injuries received if attacked, and (4) reducing the chances of becoming prey to a bear.

Avoid an Encounter

The following actions can significantly reduce the chances of having a close encounter with a bear:

1. Make noise so that the bear knows a person is present. This only requires casual conversation to prevent startling a bear at close range. The voice may have to be amplified somewhat while traveling along a noisy stream or a windy ridge. Foghorns have been used successfully in Alaska; "bear bells" may not be sufficiently loud.

2. Remain alert in bear country and be aware that the terrain and environment may hamper a bear's ability to detect a human by sight, smell, or sound. Likewise, the terrain and environment may also hamper your ability to see or hear a bear before it discovers you. An "upwind bear" is more likely to be surprised by you, as is one in heavy forestation or near loud rushing water, in the rain, or in fog.[9] Avoid ripened berry patches, streams with spawning fish, and elk calving grounds.[9] A collection of ravens may indicate carrion and the presence of feeding bears.

3. Always use good judgment to avoid a potentially dangerous situation. If fresh bear signs are seen, such as tracks (Figure 43-11), droppings, tree scratchings (Figure 43-12), or a carcass (or even

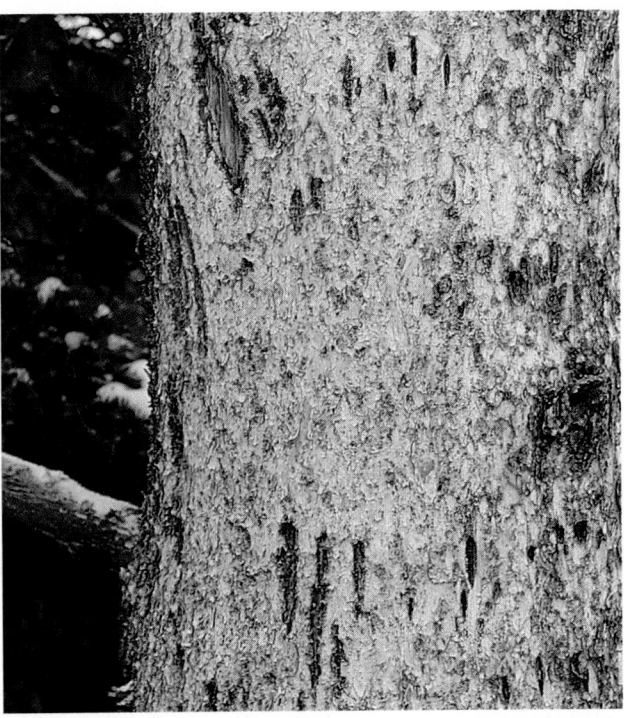

Figure 43-12   Tree scratchings from bear claws. *(Courtesy Timothy Floyd.)*

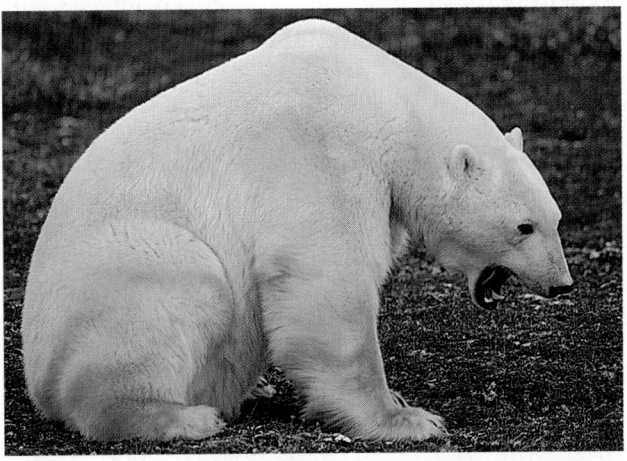

Figure 43-13   Yawning behavior may indicate agitation in a bear. *(Courtesy Timothy Floyd.)*

scavenger activity indicating that a carcass may be nearby), consider that a bear is in the vicinity and take an alternate route. If the bear is seen first, slowly and quietly retreat to safety; consider aborting the trip or taking an alternate route. Do not approach bears, or any wild animals, too closely for a better view or photograph.

Bear-bear confrontations demonstrate signs of aggression and annoyance. These include standing or turning in profile to appear larger and intimidating, vocal hissing and jaw popping, "yawning" (Figure 43-13), and head swinging (Figure 43-14).[9]

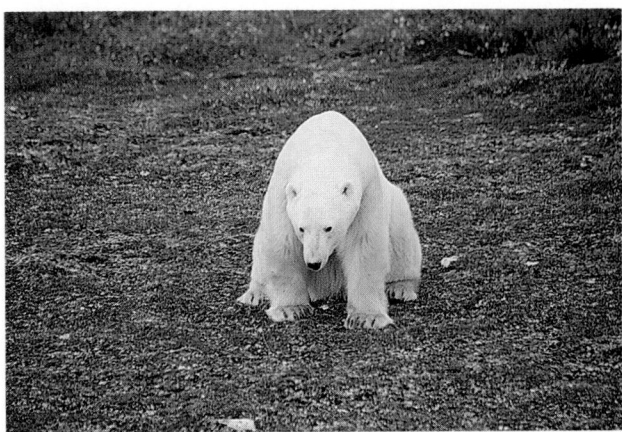

Figure 43-14   Head-swinging behavior in a polar bear. *(Courtesy Timothy Floyd.)*

Avoid Provoking an Attack

Again, the best way to avoid bear-inflicted injuries is simply to avoid surprising a bear in a close encounter situation. However, no set of known responses is guaranteed to prevent injury in a close encounter, although the following generalizations may be useful:

1. Allow the bear to know you are human and not a prey species. Step away from any visual obstruction to allow the bear to see you fully. Any attempt to hide at this point will only confuse the bear, which may approach closer to identify you, thus creating an encounter at an even closer distance. It is probably best to talk in a calm voice to allow the bear to identify you as a human.
2. Although remaining calm is difficult, do not make sudden movements or yell out, particularly with a grizzly bear. The bear may view this as an aggressive action and deal with it by an aggressive response.
3. Do not stare directly at the bear. Look to the side or stand sideways to the bear. Standing your ground is important in determining the bear's response.[35] This posture tells the bear you are willing to defend yourself if necessary, and it may prevent further aggressive behavior.
4. Do not consider climbing a tree or running away. Not only is it impossible to outrun a bear, but running may prevent the bear from correctly identifying a human and may initiate a charge. Once a bear charges, you cannot locate a climbable tree and achieve a safe height. Attempting to climb a tree may also prevent the bear from correctly identifying you as a human. Therefore the best defense during a charge is to stand quietly and nonaggressively, and allow the bear to identify you as human and not a prey species.

In most cases the bear aborts the charge after a close encounter without making contact or causing injury. At this point you should also leave the area, retreating opposite to the direction taken by the bear. If a bear continues to charge, however, resulting in physical contact, your actions should depend on the species, and information from bear attack victims is useful.

Reduce Severity and Extent of Injuries

If attacked by a bear, a victim can take several important steps to minimize injury. The actions taken immediately before, during, and after an attack will influence the type and severity of the injuries.

Humans are rarely killed during an attack precipitated by a surprise close encounter, even though bears can do so easily and quickly. During these attacks, grizzlies are only trying to remove what they perceive as a threat, and their intent is to use only as much force as necessary. When interacting with others of their species, grizzly bears are head oriented, and they usually direct their aggression toward humans in the same manner—toward the head and neck. Therefore the general rules to follow during a grizzly attack are to "help" the bear remove the perceived threat and to protect vital body parts, as follows:

1. Do not run, try to climb a tree, fight, or scream.
2. Drop to the ground and protect the head and neck by interlocking the hands behind the head (ear level) and flexing the head forward, either in the fetal position or flat on the ground face down (Figures 43-15 and 43-16). Use elbows to cover the face if the bear turns you over.
3. Do not hold out a forearm or hand to ward off the attack. Bears can readily cause significant neurovascular injuries to these structures.
4. Never try to look at the bear during an attack because it could expose you to serious facial injuries.
5. After the attack, stay down until you are sure the bear has completely left the area. This is extremely important. Victims who have gotten up

before the bear has left after the first attack generally received more severe injuries during the second one.
6. When you believe the bear has left the area, peek around while moving as little as possible, try to determine which way the bear went, evaluate options, and then leave the area.

Victims attacked from a close encounter situation who immediately protected themselves and did not try to resist typically received minor injuries treated on an outpatient basis. Victims who tried to run or fight the bear and those who left after the initial attack but before the bear had left the area typically received more severe injuries that required multiple surgical procedures, resulting in permanent cosmetic or functional disabilities.

If the attack is by a black bear, a different set of guidelines should be followed. Black bear aggression should be countered with aggression, such as shouting, yelling, throwing rocks or sticks, or whatever means are available. The victim should never lie down in a protective, submissive position because black bears are more likely to prey on humans they encounter at close range than are grizzly bears.

The data on polar bears are less complete but suggest that attacks by females with offspring are behavioral responses similar to those of grizzly females with offspring. The attacks are defensive, brief, and result in nonlethal injuries. In addition, the bear typically leaves shortly after the incident. If a polar bear is alone, however, a person should assume it is a male, whose behavioral response is predation, and should use any aggressive response available.

Prevent Predatory Behavior

The most important means of reducing the chance of being preyed on by a bear is to avoid anything that

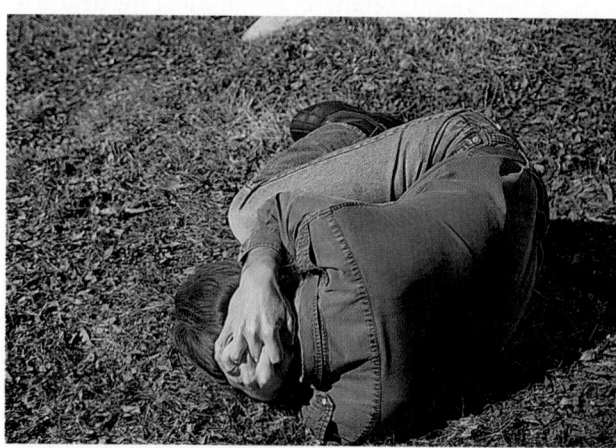

Figure 43-15 Curling into the fetal position to defend against a bear attack. *(Courtesy Marilynn G. French.)*

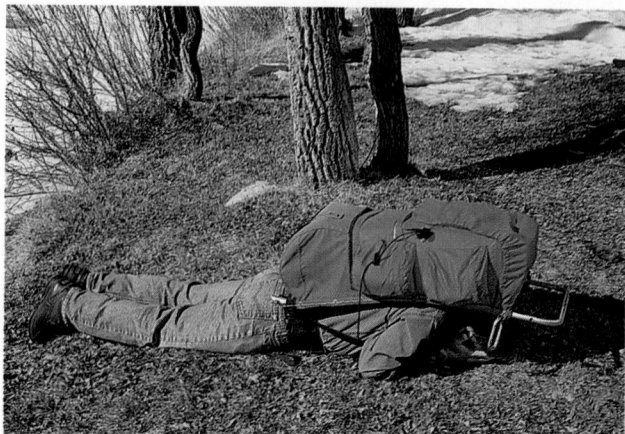

Figure 43-16 Prone position to defend against a bear attack. *(Courtesy Marilynn G. French.)*

may attract a bear to the campsite while the occupants are sleeping, as follows:

1. Avoid camping along bear travel corridors or at seasonal feeding sites.
2. Avoid campsites littered with human refuse.
3. Use proper food storage to render human food unavailable to bears. Bear-resistant food storage containers are often provided at designated campsites in bear country (Figure 43-17).
4. Reduce food odors by cooking and eating at a site away from the sleeping area. Do not sleep in clothes worn when cooking and eating.
5. Do not leave garbage or food buried or poured into the ground at the campsite. This can cause problems for future campers at this site.

The chance of a bear entering a campsite to prey on humans is small, but everyone in the camp should be familiar with a contingency plan. Everyone should know the area, even in the dark, and be aware of potential escape options, such as climbable trees or rocky ledges. Everyone should sleep in a tent because it offers a boundary of protection and may deter an inquisitive bear from walking directly to the campers. Although no study has proved its effectiveness, some people build a brush barrier around the tent to prevent a bear from readily approaching it.

Sleeping bags should be kept at least partially unzipped to facilitate a quick exit. In several instances a victim trapped inside a sleeping bag has been dragged away from a campsite by a bear.

Each tent should be equipped with a flashlight. Pepper spray is useful, as well as a firearm, unless prohibited in that area. Again, a bear that enters a tent or picks up a sleeping camper is trying to prey on that person, so all available defenses should be used.

The behavior of a predatory bear is different than that of a bear responding to a close encounter. During a close encounter a bear's response is driven by a defensive reaction, which can be aggressive and injurious. In contrast, the behavior of a predatory bear is driven by the desire for food. The bear is not looking for a confrontation or fight but rather a victim to drag from camp, usually only a few hundred feet, and consume. Predatory grizzly and black bears rarely kill their victims before consuming them. They concentrate on soft tissue or visceral consumption, and the victims frequently remain alive for an hour or more. Therefore a quick, aggressive, and unified response by companions may save the victim's life. Surprisingly, yelling, throwing rocks, or striking the bear with a stick has been effective in driving the bear away from its victim. Approaching a predatory bear in the dark while it is feeding on a human is risky, but probably the victim's only chance for survival.

In contrast, the victim of a predatory attack by a polar bear is typically killed instantaneously, so prevention of such attacks is the only chance for survival. In all predatory attacks by polar bears, all defensive measures must be considered, including guns where permitted.

Special Considerations

Menstruation. In August 1967, two women were killed in separate events on the same night by different grizzly bears in Glacier National Park. The postmortem examination showed that one had been menstruating. The assumption that menstruation may be a precipitating factor in bear attacks has unfortunately become solidly ingrained into popular opinion. Hysterical coverage by the mass media enhanced this misconception, and the scientific question was left unanswered by both scientists and government officials.[2]

A study of polar bear response to menstrual odors was published in 1983.[7] Although it was not designed to adequately test the hypothesis that menstruating women were more likely to be either attacked or preyed on by bears, the press came to this conclusion. The Interagency Grizzly Bear Committee then printed an ambivalent caution in the government's official grizzly bear pamphlet (*Bear Us In Mind*) that said, "Women may choose to stay out of bear country during their menstrual period." Fortunately, this has since been removed from the pamphlet, because no scientific evidence suggests that menstrual odors precipitate grizzly bear attacks. The attack mentioned previously is the only serious attack on a menstruating woman that has been documented in North America, and even the official investigating team at that time concluded that menstruation did not appear to have played a major role.[19]

Black bear researchers in North America report evidence of black bears attacking or being attracted to menstruating women.[31] Furthermore, no evidence links menstruation to any of the 21 grizzly bear attacks in Yellowstone National Park from 1980 to 1994.[18]

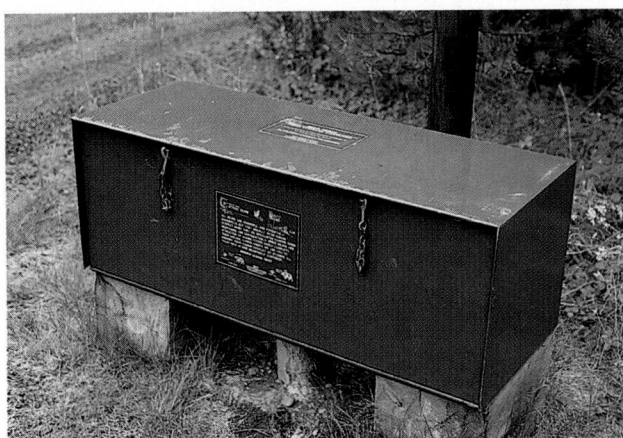

Figure 43-17 Standard government-issued bear-resistant food container. *(Courtesy Marilynn G. French.)*

Sexual Activity. A common concern among backcountry users is that sexual activity may attract bears and make them more aggressive toward campers. As with menstruation, these fears are based on hysteria and folklore. No anecdotal or scientific evidence supports this hypothesis.

Pepper Spray. Based on a concern for protection against aggressive bears, several methods were investigated for backcountry users. In the late 1970s and early 1980s, several compounds were tested for effectiveness in deterring grizzly bear attacks. The most effective method was an aerosol spray containing capsicum oleoresin, a derivative of red pepper. Captive grizzly bears were sprayed in the face at close range when they charged the researchers outside the cage. Under these controlled conditions, red pepper spray was found to be highly effective in deterring a charging grizzly bear.

Pepper spray (5% to 10% capsicum oleoresin) is commercially available as personal protection against aggressive animals. The effectiveness of pepper spray used in the field against aggressive bears has been difficult to assess. It has been used in too few cases to draw firm conclusions. Also, it is impossible to conduct scientific studies testing the effectiveness of pepper spray used in field conditions.

By 1985, pepper spray was used in the field against aggressive black and grizzly bears in 66 documented cases.[21] In general, it appeared more effective in deterring bears that charged after a close encounter than against food-conditioned bears in search of food. During the 1990s, however, most professional outfitters and guides in the northern Rocky Mountains began carrying pepper spray to deter aggressive grizzly bears, preferring spray over firearms. Although data are limited to anecdotal reports, pepper spray can be an effective and nonlethal alternative to repel aggressive grizzly bears, perhaps even more effective than firearms.

Carrying pepper spray, however, is not a substitute for knowledge of bear safety and good judgment to avoid aggressive encounters. If carried, spray must always be readily available, either in a belt-mounted holster or on a chest strap. It should be test-fired, and the user should practice drawing and firing it regularly (Figure 43-18).

Despite a manufacturer's claim that pepper spray has an effective range of 9 m (30 feet), the effective range under field conditions is significantly less due to either head winds or crosswinds. Preliminary field experience indicates that the oil-based pepper spray is more effective than water-based spray. I recommend a pepper spray that contains 10% capsicum oleoresin, has 2 million Scoville heat units, and comes in a 15-ounce pressurized aerosol container.

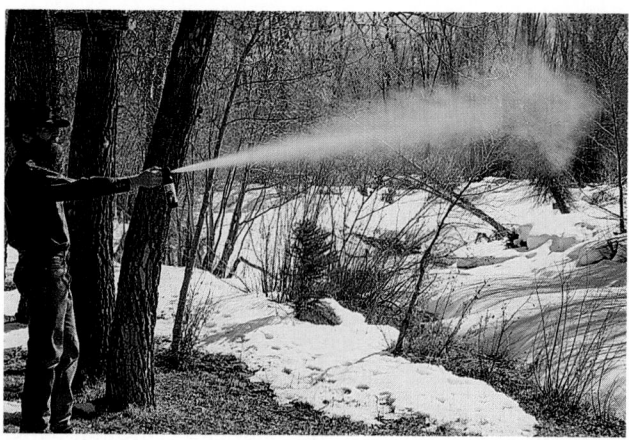

Figure 43-18 Discharging a canister of pepper spray. *(Courtesy Marilynn G. French.)*

Unfortunately, people have used pepper spray similar to mosquito spray. Despite its obnoxious and caustic smell, some sprayed it on themselves, as well as their tent, their sleeping bags, and the ground around their campsite. Once the aerosol has been released, the capsicum begins to lose its potency, and soon the active ingredient dissipates. At this point, bears may investigate the smell of pepper. Pepper spray so used thus becomes a bear attractant rather than a deterrent. One manufacturer of pepper spray (UDAP Industries, www.udap.com) provides a detailed instructional pamphlet on its proper use.

Pepper spray should be aimed toward a charging bear and discharged when the bear is within 6 to 9 m (20 to 30 feet). The person should continue spraying until the bear has stopped its charge, keeping the sprayer aimed at the bear in case it charges again. This continues until the bear has left the area. If the pepper spray is depleted, the best defense if the bear attacks is to lay down, cover the face, and offer little or no resistance. Again, there is no guarantee that pepper spray (or anything) will prevent injury by an aggressive bear.

If pepper spray is accidentally discharged into a person's face, it stimulates facial nocioreceptors and causes eyelid, ocular, and facial muscle spasms, which may result in temporary blindness. The victim should not rub the eyes (to avoid corneal abrasions) and should irrigate the eyes and skin vigorously with water for at least 15 minutes. Intraoral burning may be relieved by swishing and spitting milk or another casein-containing food product.[9]

Firearms. Many people consider carrying firearms for protection when they enter bear country. Guns can be useful in some situations. However, the target area to kill a grizzly with a shot to the head is only about 30 cm² (12 square inches). The cranial vault is narrow and sloped caudally (Figure 43-19). A bear initiating a

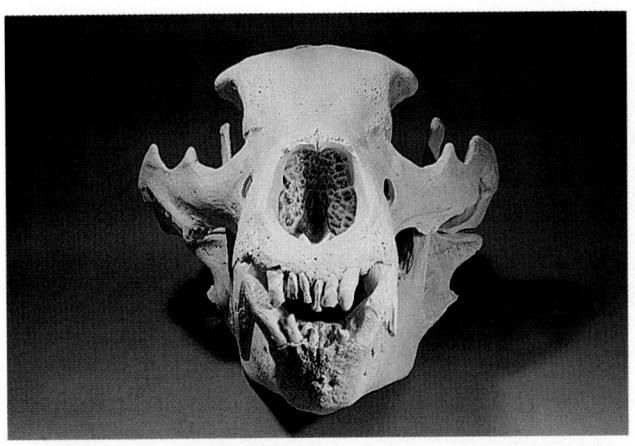

Figure 43-19 Cranial vault of a bear. *(Courtesy Timothy Floyd.)*

charge from a distance of about 45 to 55 m (50 to 60 yards) will take only 4 to 5 seconds to reach its victim.

Unless a proficient marksman, a person is unlikely to access a weapon, release the safety, aim accurately, fire, and hit a small target in a brief time under incredible emotional stress. Also, even if a shot could be fired, it probably would only wound the bear. Wounding a charging bear changes its behavior and may make its attack even more aggressive. Because of these factors, pepper spray should be considered as a nonlethal alternative to guns, especially when traveling in places where guns are not permitted, such as national parks.

According to most U.S. and Canadian wildlife agencies, the most effective firearms against grizzly bear attacks are a 12-gauge 3-inch magnum shotgun with 1-ounce slugs and a 30-06 rifle with a 200-grain bullet. A pistol is not considered to be an effective weapon against a charging grizzly. A large-caliber pistol, such as a 44-caliber magnum, can be used as a point-blank weapon to kill a bear attempting to prey. The effective range of a pistol and pepper spray is about the same, but it is easier to hit a moving target with pepper spray because of its shotgunlike aerosol pattern.

Dogs. In most national parks, dogs are not permitted in backcountry settings. Unfortunately, rare and questionable accounts report a dog stirring up a grizzly, then running back to its owner with the bear in pursuit. Most outfitters, guides, and hunters, however, report positive experiences with dogs in grizzly country. Their dogs are generally well trained and have been raised in wilderness environments. Most of these dogs can effectively deter grizzly and black bears from coming into a camp. Although no study has been conducted on the use of dogs to deter aggressive bears, most people who spend considerable time in grizzly country use their dogs for this purpose.

Horses. For individuals concerned about an aggressive bear encounter, another option is the use of horses. No one has been injured by a grizzly or black bear while riding a horse. Horses that frequently travel in bear country are the best to use, since they generally do not react unpredictably and endanger the rider when they encounter bears. Although horses may protect against aggressive grizzly encounters, riders still may be injured by the horse. People are seriously injured or killed in horse accidents each year in the northern Rocky Mountains.

Hunter Safety. Many people participate in sport hunting in bear country each year. Some are hunting for bears, but most hunt for other game species.

For hunters of bears, the risks are obvious. Bear hunters intentionally break bear safety rules to close in on their prey. The most dangerous situation, however, is after they shoot and injure a bear. They have an ethical obligation to track the wounded animal and kill it, but this is when most bear hunters are injured. This confirms that guns are not completely effective in preventing bear injury. An injured bear may take refuge in heavy cover, then charge when the hunter is at close range. With little time, a surprised hunter often cannot fire a lethal round, and even when shot, the bear can continue its attack and cause significant injury before it dies.

Hunters of other game species in bear country are at significant risk of close encounter and injury. Besides violating bear safety rules, they frequently become preoccupied with the stalk and forget they may encounter a bear. During the 1990s, more than half the people injured by grizzly bears in the Yellowstone Ecosystem have been elk hunters. Some injuries occurred during the stalk, but other factors contributed. Grizzly bears in this ecosystem have learned the association between gunfire and available food. After an elk or other game (moose, deer, bighorn sheep) has been killed, hunters field-dress their kills and leave edible remains (gut piles) on the ground. In several cases, bears approached the kill site before the hunters completed this process. In other cases, an elk or animal was field-dressed late in the evening, then hung in a nearby tree. When the hunters returned the next morning, they encountered a grizzly bear that had claimed the gut pile or the carcass. Hunters must assume that under these circumstances, at least one grizzly bear will be at the site, and they must approach cautiously, preferably on horseback.

Bow hunting represents another high-risk activity. In most states, bow hunters are not allowed to carry a firearm as a backup weapon. They also tend to violate bear safety rules to set up a shot. Elk hunters blow an artificial elk call (a bugle) to lure in bull elk. This also alerts grizzly bears that prey on adult male elk (bulls)

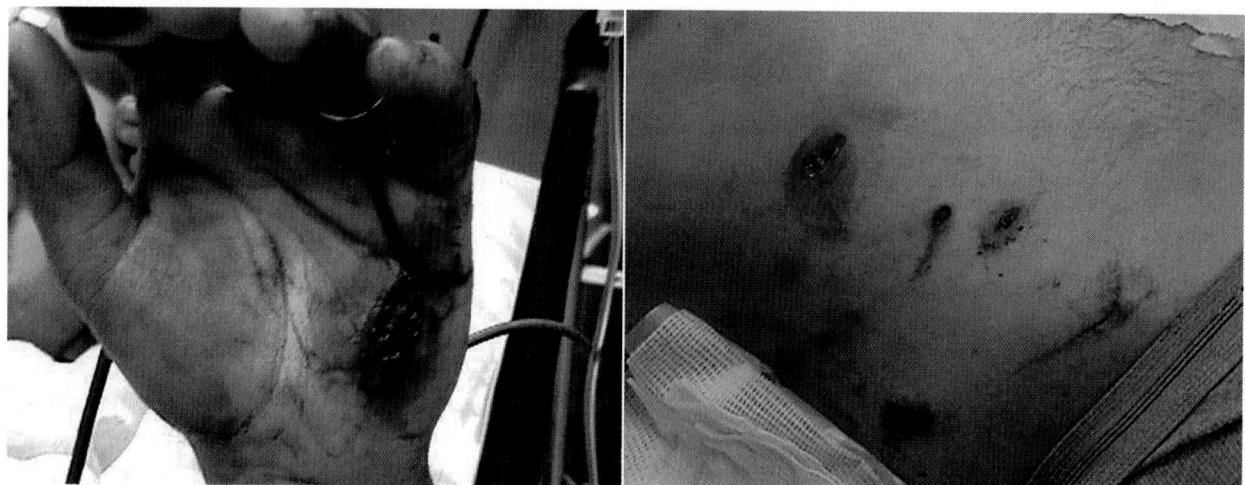

Figure 43-20 Bite wound injuries typical of a bear attack. *(Courtesy Luanne Freer.)*

during the breeding season. For protection, bow hunters should (1) hunt from a tree-stand, which provides some protection from grizzly bears, who are poor tree climbers, and (2) carry pepper spray and be prepared to use it.

BEAR-INDUCED INJURIES

Bear-inflicted injuries range from minor, treated on an outpatient basis, to complex, requiring hospitalization and surgery, typically resulting in significant cosmetic and functional disability. In this regard, bear attacks are similar to most other animal attacks, particularly those inflicted by large animals.

The character of such injuries is determined in part by the three main sources: teeth, claws, and paws. The teeth of bears, especially the canines, are large and sturdy. Although the teeth are not particularly sharp, the power of the jaw muscles allows the teeth to penetrate deep into soft tissues and fracture facial bones and bones of the hand and forearm with ease. The trauma characteristically results from punctures, with shearing, tearing, and crushing forces (Figure 43-20).

The claws are another important source of trauma. Although the claws on the front pads can be as long as human fingers, they are not particularly sharp on grizzly and polar bears. The bear's shoulders, however, provide the force and speed that allow claws to cause significant soft tissue damage in a scraping maneuver that results in deep, parallel gashes. Because black bear claws are sharper and more curved, the cuts tend to have sharper, less ragged edges.

The bear paw is capable of delivering a powerful force, resulting in significant blunt trauma, particularly to the head and neck, rib cage, and abdominal cavity, especially solid organ rupture. Therefore victims of bear attacks should be evaluated for occult blunt trauma.

Several victims of a bear attack were further injured when a companion accidentally shot them while trying to kill the attacking bear. Others were injured when they fell out of a tree while escaping a bear; some sustained long-bone fractures. At least two persons in North America have been killed by such falls, and in both incidents the bear did not attack the victims once they fell to the ground.

WOUND MANAGEMENT

The specifics of initial wound treatment are determined in part by the available medical equipment and location in which the victim is first received. Stabilization of the victim remains the primary objective. All victims of bear attacks should be considered to have major trauma and should be transported to the most appropriate facility after stabilization.

By the time most bear attack victims reach medical care, their injuries are relatively "old." Bear-inflicted injuries are often occult, producing greater tissue necrosis than initially expected. Deep structure involvement is typically more prevalent than is initially apparent. Internal injuries from either direct penetration (claws, teeth) or blunt trauma are common. Neurovascular injuries must be considered with trauma to the extremities, and neurosensory and cosmetic injuries are common with trauma to the face.

ANTIBIOTIC THERAPY

Little information is available about the organisms in bear-inflicted wounds, but anecdotal evidence suggests that bear attack victims do not develop unusual or rare septic complications from unknown pathogens. In one study, cultures of the mouths of black bears revealed a bacterial spectrum similar to that in dogs, with the ma-

TABLE 43-2. Animal Bite Risk Factors

LOCATION	TYPE OF WOUND	VICTIM CHARACTERISTICS
HIGH RISK		
Hand, wrist, or foot	Punctures	Older than 50 years
Scalp or face in infants	Tissue crushing that cannot	Asplenic
Over a major joint	be debrided	Chronic alcoholic
Through-and-through bite	Bites over vital structures	Altered immune status
of cheek	(e.g., artery, nerve)	Diabetic
		Peripheral vascular insufficiency
		Chronic corticosteroid therapy
		Prosthetic or diseased cardiac valve
		Prosthetic or seriously diseased joint
LOW RISK		
Face, scalp, ears, or mouth	Large, clean lacerations that	Younger than 50 years
Self-bite of buccal mucosa	can be cleansed	Good medical health
	Partial-thickness lacerations	
	and abrasions	

jority of species being *Micrococcus* and *Streptococcus*.[10] *Staphylococcus aureus* was found in only 8%, and *Pasteurella* and *Eikenella* were not found. In a similar study of the bacterial flora in the oral cavities of grizzly bears, *Escherichia coli* was found in 98% of the samples taken.[12]

The use of antibiotics shortly after the injury but before clinical evidence of infection remains controversial. The usual risk factors should be assessed (Table 43-2).[3] However, the blunt trauma, deep punctures, and shearing-tearing forces that are typical of bear attacks create significant tissue ischemia and necrosis that are not apparent on the initial examination. Therefore antimicrobial prophylaxis should be considered for all bear-inflicted wounds pending culture results and before clinical evidence of infection.

Before culture results are available, penicillin is suggested for relatively clean superficial injuries. A third-generation cephalosporin should be added to cover gram-negative organisms for deeper and more contaminated wounds.[10] However, adequate wound debridement and cleansing are the primary means of reducing the infection rate among these victims. Antibiotics should be administered parenterally for at least 3 days after wounding and at least 2 days after each debridement.[9]

RABIES

No case of rabies has been reported or documented in either wild or captive bears. The Centers for Disease Control and Prevention (CDC), however, recommends rabies immunization for victims attacked by wild carnivores. Therefore all victims of bear attacks should receive the standard informed-consent discussion of the risks and benefits of rabies immunization.

REFERENCES

1. Burt W, Grossenheider R: *A field guide to the mammals*, ed 2, Boston, 1964, Houghton Mifflin.
2. Byrd CP: Of bears and women: investigating the hypothesis [that] menstruation attracts bears, master's thesis, University of Montana, 1988.
3. Callaham M: Bites and injuries inflicted by mammals. In Auerbach PS, editor: *Wilderness medicine: management of wilderness and environmental emergencies*, ed 3, St Louis, 1995, Mosby.
4. Chestin I: Personal communication, 1992, University of St Petersburg, Russia.
5. Clutton-Brock TH, Harvey PH: Primates, brains, and ecology, *J Zool* 190:309, 1980.
6. Crammond M: *Killer bears*, New York, 1981, Scribner's.
7. Cushing BS: Responses of polar bears to human menstrual odors. In *Proceedings of International Conference on Bear Research and Management* 5:270, 1983.
8. Eisenberg JF, Wilson DE: Relative brain size and feeding strategies in the Chirotera, *Evolution* 32:740, 1978.
9. Floyd T: Bear inflicted human injury and fatality, *Wilderness Environ Med* 10:75, 1999.
10. Floyd T, Manville AM, French SP: Normal oral flora in black bears: guidelines for antimicrobial prophylaxis following bear attacks, *J Wilderness Med* 1:47, 1990.
11. French S, French M: Predatory behavior of grizzly bears feeding on elk calves in Yellowstone National Park, 1986-88. In *Proceedings of International Conference on Bear Research and Management* 9:335, 1990.
12. French S, French M: Unpublished data, Yellowstone Grizzly Foundation, Jackson, Wyo.
13. Garshelis DL: Personal communication, 1996, Minnesota Department of Natural Resourses.
14. Gittleman JL: Carnivore brain size, behavioral ecology, and phylogeny, *J Mamm* 67:23, 1986.
15. Gjertz I, Persen E: Confrontations between humans and bears in Svalbard, *Polar Res* 5:253, 1987.
16. Gowans F: *Mountain man and grizzly*, Orem, Utah, 1986, Mountain Grizzly Publications.
17. Gunther K: Bears and menstruating women, Yellowstone National Park, Information Paper BMO-7, 1995.
18. Gunther K, Hoekstra H: Bear-inflicted human injuries in Yellowstone, 1980-1994, *Yellowstone Sci* 4:2, 1996.
19. Herrero S: *Bear attacks: their causes and avoidance*, New York, 1985, Winchester Press.
20. Herrero S, Fleck S: Injury to people inflicted by black, grizzly, and polar bears: recent trends and new insights. In *Proceedings of International Conference on Bear Research and Management* 8:25, 1990.

21. Herrero S, Higgins A: Field use of capsaicin sprays as a bear deterrent. In *Proceedings of International Conference on Bear Research and Management 10*, 1996.

22. Hunt RM: The auditory bulla in Carnivora: anatomical basis for reappraisal of carnivore evolution, *J Morphol* 143:21, 1974.

23. Joshi AR, Garshelis DL, Smith JLD: Home ranges of sloth bears in Nepal: implications for conservation, *J Wildl Manag* 59:204, 1995.

24. Kaniut L: *Alaska bear tales*, Anchorage, Alaska, 1989, Alaska Northwest.

25. Mace GM, Harvey PH, Clutten-Brock TH: Brain size and ecology in small mammals, *J Zool* 193:333, 1981.

26. Middaugh J: Human injury from bear attacks in Alaska, 1900-1985, *Alaska Med* 29:121, 1987.

27. Mills E: *The grizzly: our greatest wild animal*, New York, 1919, Houghton Mifflin.

28. Nelson R et al: Behavior, biochemistry, and hibernation in black, grizzly, and polar bears. In *Proceedings of International Conference on Bear Research and Management* 5:284, 1983.

29. Pederson SC: Personal communication, 1997, Utah Division of Wildlife Resources.

30. Radinsky L: Evolution of brain size in carnivores and ungulates, *Am Nat* 112:815, 1978.

31. Rogers L, Scott S: Reactions of black bears to human menstrual odors, *J Wildl Manag* 55:632, 1991.

32. Russel A: *Grizzly country*, New York, 1985, Knopf.

33. Schaller G et al: *The giant pandas of Wolong*, Chicago, 1985, University of Chicago Press.

34. Shepard P, Sanders B: *The sacred paw*, New York, 1985, Viking Penguin.

35. Smith D: *Backcountry bear basics: the definitive guide to avoiding unpleasant encounters*, Seattle, 1997, The Mountaineers.

36. Storer T, Trevis L: *California grizzly*, Berkeley, Calif, 1955, University of California Press.

37. Wright W: *The grizzly bear*, Lincoln, Neb, 1977, University of Nebraska Press.

44 Wilderness-Acquired Zoonoses

Eric L. Weiss

A zoonosis is a disease of animals that may be transmitted to humans under natural conditions. There are more than 200 zoonotic pathogens. The risk of acquiring zoonoses increases proportionately with the frequency and intensity of contact. For example, hunters and trappers who handle and are exposed to the blood, viscera, secretions, and excretions of wild animals are at much greater risk than are recreational campers. Similarly, international travelers who frequent locations with a much higher density of infected animals are at greater risk for infection. The trekker in Nepal is more likely to confront rabies than the hiker in California. Disease severity is important in human infections.

This chapter emphasizes diseases in which wildlife plays a significant role in transmission to humans. Although glanders and melioidosis do not fit this pattern, they are also discussed. Zoonoses acquired primarily from domestic animals that also have a minor reservoir in wildlife are mentioned briefly; standard texts of veterinary public health[111,194,207] and infectious disease[99,139] provide further discussion.

RABIES

Rabies is one of the most ancient and feared diseases, with the first apparent reference found in the Eshnunna Code of Mesopotamia, circa 2000 BC. Aristotle (322 BC) recognized that dogs transmitted the infection to other dogs through bites, and Galen (200 AD) recommended surgical excision of bite wounds to prevent rabies. Celsus (100 AD) subsequently recommended cauterization to prevent the infection; this remained the prophylactic treatment of choice until 1885, when active rabies immunization was introduced by Louis Pasteur. In 1882 Pasteur successfully transmitted rabies experimentally, spinal cord inoculums, from one dog to another. By using the attenuation method of air drying rabbit spinal cords, he discovered that he could provide protective immunity in dogs. While hesitant to apply his findings to humans, on July 6, 1885, a 9-year-old bitten by a rabid dog was brought to his office. The boy was immunized with rabbit spinal cord vaccine and did not develop rabies. By 1886, 726 persons had similarly received "postexposure" immunization; only 10 developed rabies.

Virology

Rabies is caused by a ribonucleic acid (RNA) virus in the family Rhabdoviridae. Rhabdoviruses are bullet-shaped with RNA coiled inside an outer envelope covered with glycoprotein-containing surface spikes (Figure 44-1).[155] The rabies virus contains five proteins, including this glycoprotein and a nucleocapsid protein[192]; each has a molecular weight of 60,000. The glycoprotein induces neutralizing antibody, which can confer immunity and protection against the disease. The nucleocapsid protein induces antibodies that do not appear to be protective, but are useful diagnostically. The fluorescent antibody technique, widely used to demonstrate rabies antigen in tissues, is directed largely against the nucleocapsid protein.

Transmission

Rabies is almost always transmitted by the bite of infected animals, most often wild and domestic carnivores. Eight cases of rabies have been transmitted to the recipients of transplanted corneas from donors who subsequently died from an illness that was compatible with or shown to be rabies.[43,46,109,116,223] In two cases of rabies, transmission was by accidental aerosol in a laboratory,[231,232,283] and in two others by inhalation in a bat-infested cave.[68,69] In such caves, aerosols of rabies virus are created from the saliva, secretions, and excretions of large numbers of infected bats concentrated in a dark, humid environment that favors survival of the virus outside the host. Transmission occurs through the nasal neuroepithelium. Because the virus is sensitive to desiccation and ultraviolet light, once any contaminated materials are dry or exposed to sunlight, they can be considered noninfectious.

Carnivorous animals can acquire rabies by eating infected prey. Skunks can transmit rabies to their young transplacentally,[110] and one probable case of congenital rabies[21,72] has been reported in a calf.[146] A congenital human case has also been reported, with mother and child dying of rabies within 48 hours of delivery.[201] The mother had been bitten by a dog 33 days before she became ill. The diagnoses were made by finding Negri bodies in the brain of mother and child.

Epidemiology

Although all mammals are experimentally susceptible to rabies, the major reservoir and vectors of transmission are wild and domestic carnivores, particularly the dog (Canidae), cat (Felidae), weasel (Mustelidae), mongoose (Viveridae), raccoon (Procyonidae), and bat (Chiroptera) families. In the United States, Canada,

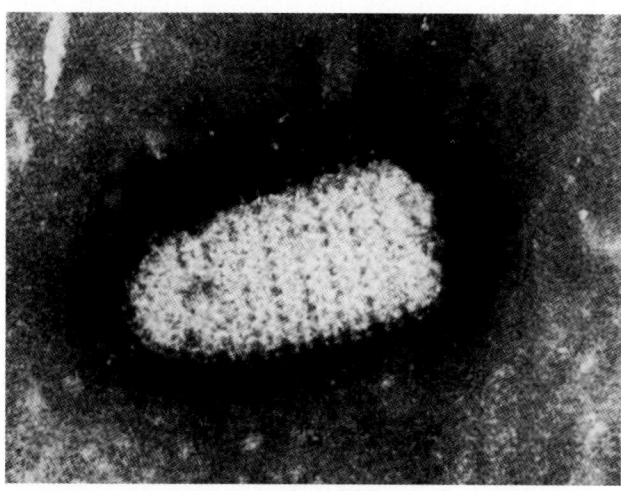

Figure 44-1 Electron micrograph of rabies virus, demonstrating the bullet shape and capsular spikes. *(Courtesy Merieux Institute.)*

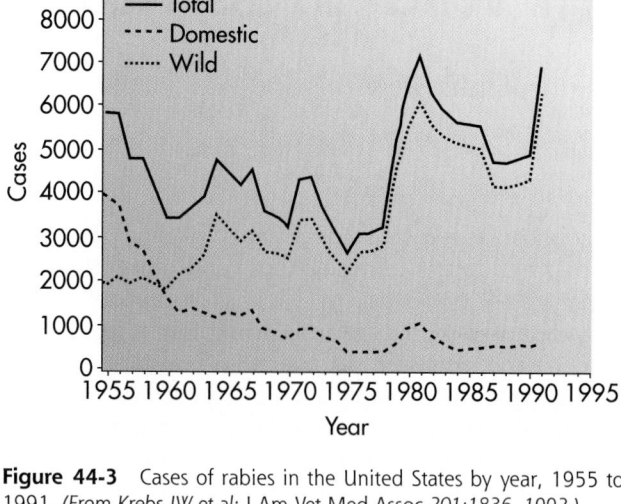

Figure 44-3 Cases of rabies in the United States by year, 1955 to 1991. *(From Krebs JW et al:* J Am Vet Med Assoc *201:1836, 1992.)*

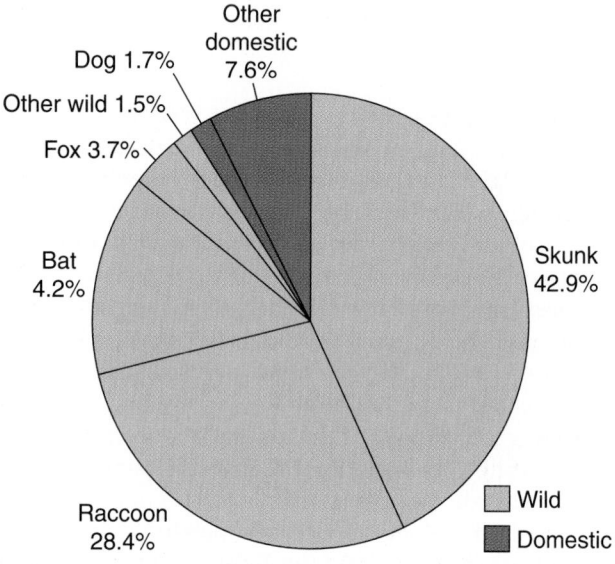

Figure 44-2 Animal rabies, United States including Puerto Rico, 1986, with 5551 cases reported. *(From Centers for Disease Control:* MMWR *36, 1987.)*

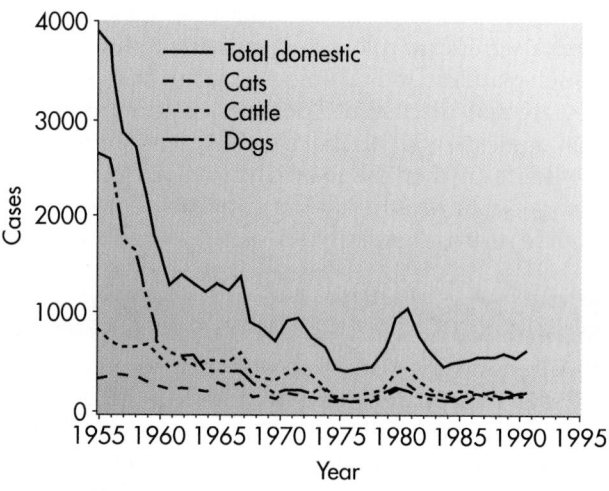

Figure 44-4 Cases of rabies in domestic animals in the United States, by year, 1955 to 1991. *(From Krebs JW et al:* J Am Vet Med Assoc *201:1836, 1992.)*

and most of Europe the principal reservoir is wildlife (Figures 44-2 and 44-3). Between 1980 and 1996, approximately 85% of rabies cases reported in the United States and Puerto Rico occurred in wild animals. In 1996, 49 states, the District of Columbia, and Puerto Rico reported 8509 cases of rabies in animals and four cases in humans to the Centers for Disease Control and Prevention (CDC). Nearly 93% (7899) were wild animals, with 7% (610) domestic species. The breakdown by species was raccoons 50.5%, skunks 24%, bats 11.3%, foxes 5.3%, cats 3.5%, dogs 1.5%, and cattle 1.4%. The epizootic of rabies in raccoons expanded into Ohio in 1997 and now includes 19 states and the District of Columbia. Only Hawaii reported no cases of rabies. The four cases in humans

resulted from infection with rabies virus variants associated with bats.[128]

Vaccination and leash law enforcement have greatly reduced the incidence of rabies in dogs in the United States and Canada. Since 1981, rabid cats have outnumbered rabid dogs in the United States (Figure 44-4).[127] In most developing countries, however, dogs remain the principal reservoir of rabies and the most common source of rabies among humans. In 1991, 81.6% of 8528 reported rabies cases in Mexico occurred in dogs.[127] Of the cases of human rabies reported to the CDC between 1980 and 1997, 12 (33%) of the 36 cases appear to have been related to rabid animals outside the United States.[60,159]

The significant wildlife reservoirs of rabies vary geographically. The mongoose is important in Puerto

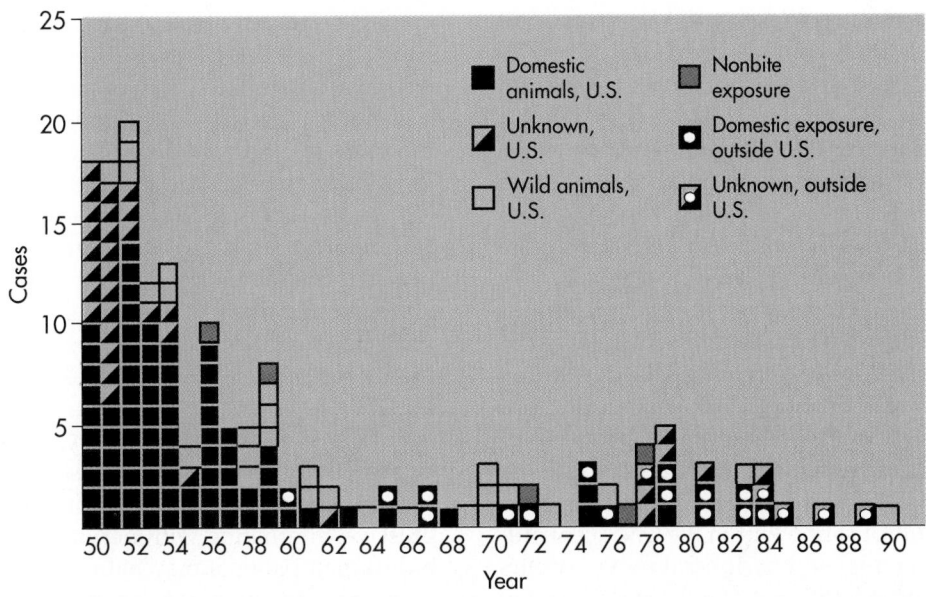

Figure 44-5 Human rabies in the United States from 1950 to 1989. Figure includes two Americans who contracted and died of rabies outside the United States (1981 and 1983). *(From Fishbein DB: Infect Dis Clin North Am 5:53, 1991.)*

Rico, jackal in much of Africa, red fox in Europe, wolf in Iran and neighboring countries, raccoon dog in Eastern and Central Europe, and vampire bat in certain Latin American countries. More than 50 countries reportedly have no rabies cases, including most islands in Pacific Oceania, most Caribbean islands, the United Kingdom, Cyprus, Finland, Iceland, Norway, Portugal, Spain, Sweden, Japan, Korea, Malaysia, Singapore, New Zealand, and Taiwan. The largest land mass reported free of rabies is Australia.[59]

Because human contact with dogs is much more intimate than with wildlife, dogs offer a greater threat of rabies transmission. Countries with significant domestic canine rabies also have the highest incidence of human rabies; 48 human cases were reported in Mexico in 1991.[127] In India, estimates of annual human rabies cases range from 15,000 to more than 25,000.[230] No more than five cases of human rabies have been reported in any year since 1960 in the United States. Twenty (36%) of the 55 human cases of rabies reported in the United States (including two Americans who acquired and died of rabies abroad) from 1960 to 1991 were acquired in foreign countries; most resulted from dog bites, with definite recollection of a bite (Figure 44-5).[92] More recently, however, most victims had no definite history of an animal bite or other event associated with rabies virus transmission. Only seven of 32 patients had a definite exposure history; six were bitten by dogs in foreign countries, and one by a bat in the United States. Rabies in the United States is rare but probably underdiagnosed, and should be considered in the differential diagnosis of any acute, rapidly pro-

gressing encephalitis, even if the patient does not recall being bitten by an animal.[159]

Mammalian species vary in their susceptibility to rabies. In general, the animals most susceptible also have the shortest course of infection. Wolves, foxes, and jackals, which are highly susceptible, generally have acute disease. Skunks and raccoons are less susceptible, and the duration of illness tends to be more prolonged. Opossums are very resistant to infection, and the only consistent way to induce rabies in them is by intracerebral inoculation.

Although rabies is considered an almost uniformly fatal infection once symptoms have developed, some cases of spontaneous recovery or of chronic, asymptomatic infection have been recorded in various wildlife species and dogs.[19,21,63,77,89] Bats that harbor and shed the virus may not be overtly ill, especially to the casual observer. This affects the practice of quarantine and observation of animals that have bitten humans as means to determine if or not they are rabid.

The pattern of human rabies reflects the epidemiology of animal bites.[17] As for animal bites in general, a disproportionately large number of rabies cases occur in males less than 18 years of age. All cases of animal bites and of rabies in people or animals should be reported to local public health authorities.

Pathogenesis

After the rabies virus is inoculated by a bite, it is first sequestered in skeletal muscle. The virus travels through neuromuscular spindles and motor end plates to the peripheral nervous system, then travels in the axons of peripheral nerves at an estimated rate of 3 mm/hr to the central nervous system (CNS). Thus, rabies resulting from a bite on the foot has an average incubation period of 60 days, but only 30 days after an infective bite to the face. The incubation period varies greatly and affects decisions about postexposure treatment of patients with a relatively distant history of an animal bite. Rabies has been described in humans more than 1 year after the infecting bite.[78]

The virus moves across synapses and multiplies within neurons. The brain may be diffusely involved or may have concentrations in different parts, depending on species, resulting in differing clinical manifestations of the disease. For example, the hippocampus is frequently involved in humans; Purkinje's cells of the cerebellum are typically involved in herbivores, such as cattle. After multiplication within the CNS, centrifugal spread along cranial and peripheral nerves occurs out to the skin, cornea, salivary glands, and other tissues. Terminally, rabies virus can be found in many organs of the body, including the nervous system, skin, eyes, salivary glands, pancreas, kidney, and myocardium. Saliva can contain up to 1 million virus particles per milliliter. Rabies is not disseminated in the body by viremia, and contact with blood of a rabid animal is not considered an exposure risk.

Clinical rabies develops in approximately half of untreated persons bitten by rabid dogs. Although controlled clinical trials are impossible, retrospective examination of situations in which rabid animals have bitten multiple persons in an environment with no available postexposure treatment provides some insight. The probability of the disease developing seems to vary with the size and depth of the inoculum, from 0.1% with salivary contamination (e.g., licking) of a minor wound to 80% after a severe rabid wolf bite.

Symptoms

The incubation period of rabies varies from as little as 9 days to more than 1 year. For the great majority of human cases, the incubation period is between 2 and 16 weeks.[21] Claims of incubation periods as long as 19 years are difficult to substantiate, but reports suggest incubation periods longer than 5 years.[24] Long incubation periods are confirmed by identifying the strain of virus as coming from an area where the patient last visited or resided years ago. For example, in three immigrants to the United States who died of rabies, the viral nucleic acid pattern matched strains from their native countries, the Philippines, Laos, and Mexico, which they had left 6 years, 4 years, and 11 months before, respectively.[204]

The initial symptoms of rabies are usually nonspecific and include malaise, fatigue, anxiety, agitation, irritability, insomnia, depression, fever, headache, nausea, vomiting, sore throat, abdominal pain, and anorexia. The only true "early" symptom is pain, pruritus, or paresthesias at the site of the bite, which occurs in approximately half of patients.

After the prodromal period, which lasts approximately 2 to 10 days, more specific neurologic symptoms develop related to localization of the infection to the limbic system, with relative sparing of the neocortex. In lower animals and in humans this can take one of two forms, either furious or paralytic (dumb) rabies. Humans are more likely to suffer from "furious" rabies with its violent outbursts, whereas dogs more commonly suffer from "dumb" rabies and become increasingly lethargic and eventually actually paralyzed. Furious rabies is characterized by increasing agitation, hyperactivity, seizures, and episodes in which the animal or person may thrash about, bite, and become aggressive, alternating with periods of relative calm. Rabid human patients may hallucinate. Between fits the victim is often aware of impending death. Severe pharyngeal spasm of respiratory muscles may occur when the individual attempts to drink. Later this reaction may be triggered merely by the sight of water, giving rise to the synonym "hydrophobia." A truly rabid patient often attempts to drink because of thirst. A hysterical patient mimicking rabies does not make the attempt. Pharyngeal spasm and choking may also occur when air is blown on the patient's face or when a breeze blows in through an open window (aerophobia).

In the initial phases of furious rabies, animals may appear unusually alert and responsive. Later they show some discomfort and restlessness and may vocalize with unusual frequency. Animals become hypersensitive and hyperresponsive to external stimuli, such as sound or touch. Certain behavioral changes develop, and wild animals that normally shun association with humans may appear unusually friendly and approach people without apparent fear. Friendly dogs or cats may begin to bite. Animals may act ferocious and may salivate excessively, "foaming at the mouth" (Figure 44-6). The key to maintenance of this infection in nature is the behavioral change in animals that causes them to bite. Skunks are particularly dangerous because they tend to bite and hold on viciously. Eventually, animals and people go into a coma and die, either from cardiac arrhythmia or secondary complications such as pneumonia, sepsis, or congestive heart failure. Untreated, the average human victim survives 8 days. With intensive supportive care, life may be extended for up to 28 days. The mortality from rabies is virtually 100%.

Dumb rabies is associated with progressive lethargy, incoordination, and ascending paralysis, starting as posterior paraplegia. In animals, cranial nerve palsies can result in protrusion of the tongue and nictitating membrane and abnormal vocalization. The tone and pitch of the animal's voice may change, probably because of involvement of laryngeal muscle innervation.

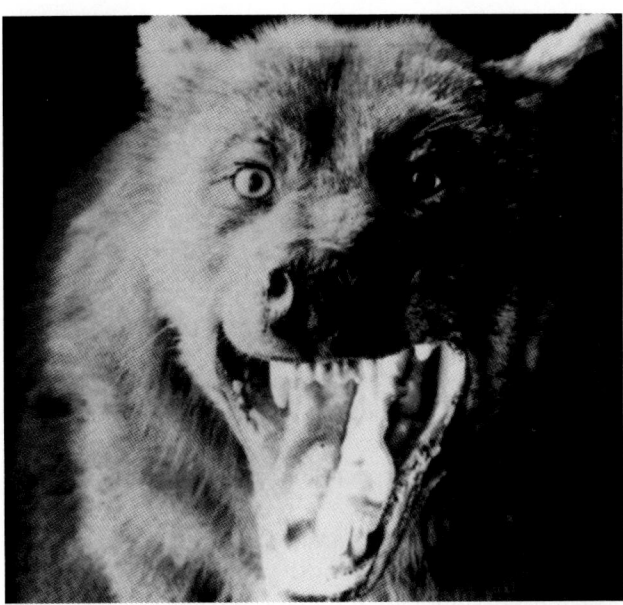

Figure 44-6 Dog-wolf cross-species from Canada with furious rabies. It has a ferocious appearance, excess salivation, and anisocoria. *(Courtesy Merieux Institute.)*

Dumb or paralytic rabies in animals and humans follows a progressive course, with eventual coma and death.

Because of progressive paralysis without biting behavior, dumb rabies is usually not transmitted further in nature. However, people may be exposed while taking care of such patients, whether animal or human, through exposure to saliva (e.g., attempting to clear oral secretions).

Preexposure Immunization of Humans

People at high risk for rabies, such as veterinarians, wildlife biologists, trappers, taxidermists, and laboratory personnel working with the virus, should be immunized before any potential exposure. Other possible candidates for preexposure immunization include spelunkers, professional hunters, and long-term travelers (especially hikers and bikers) to intensely enzootic areas. Children, especially "toddlers," are at risk because they are more likely to pet stray dogs and less likely to heed warnings. The CDC recommends preexposure rabies immunization "for persons living in or visiting (for more than 30 days) areas of the world where rabies is a constant threat."[59] This recommendation should be followed more aggressively if the individuals' activities are likely to put them at significant risk of exposure or if they are likely to have difficulty receiving appropriate medical care, including safe, effective biologics administered with a sterile needle and syringe, within a few days of exposure. If appropriate care is available, it may be more cost-effective to forgo preexposure immuniza-

tion and administer postexposure treatment to persons in need.[191] Preexposure immunization also protects against inapparent or unknown exposure.

Three vaccines have thus far been approved for human use in the United States: human diploid cell vaccine (HDCV) (Imovax), rabies vaccine adsorbed (RVA), and purified chick embryo cell vaccine (PCEC) (RabAvert). Due to concerns regarding the manufacturing process, the Food and Drug Administration (FDA) has recently suspended the production of RVA, and its future availability on the U.S. market is uncertain. All these vaccines contain virus inactivated with β-propiolactone.[55] Preexposure immunization consists of three injections given on days 0, 7, and 21 or 28. All can be given intramuscularly, 1 ml in the deltoid muscle (or anterior thigh muscle in children). An alternative route for preexposure HDCV (only) is intradermal (ID), 0.1 ml in the lateral aspect of the upper arm.[27,35,52,79] The ID dose for HDCV is significantly less expensive than the intramuscular (IM) route but may be less immunogenic. When patients are concurrently taking chloroquine phosphate for malaria prophylaxis the antibody response to ID HDCV decreases.[162] Although interference with the immune response of other antimalaria drugs, such as mefloquine, has not been studied, precautions for persons taking these medications should also be followed. IM administration of the routine series of three doses provides a sufficient immune response.[26] Also, if the ID route is used in a traveler taking chloroquine or mefloquine for malaria, a full month must pass after completing the three-dose series before beginning the antimalarial medication. Despite the cost savings, this is usually impractical, and most travelers receive the IM series. The frequency of booster doses for preexposure immunization depends on the antirabies titer of the individual and the likelihood of exposure to infection.[55,91]

Pain, erythema, or pruritus occurs at the injection site in many of those receiving primary rabies immunization.[27,55] Malaise, headache, dizziness, fever, and nausea occur in 5% to 40% of vaccinees. Marked local induration and regional lymphadenopathy are occasionally seen. Booster doses with HDCV at 1 year can cause malaise, headache, fever, myalgia, and arthralgias in 26% of recipients.[27] Boosters with HDCV can also cause an immune complex–like disease characterized by urticaria, macular rash, angioedema, or arthralgia in 10% of recipients.[80] The incidence of such delayed hypersensitivity seems to be less with the newer PCEC vaccine.[55] Immediate hypersensitivity reactions, with bronchospasm, laryngeal edema, and rashes after primary immunization with HDCV, are rare. Three cases of Guillain-Barré paralytic syndrome with complete recovery within 3 months have been reported associated with HDCV.[25,30]

Concurrent use of immunosuppressive drugs, such as corticosteroids, interferes with immunization. If possible, such drugs should not be given at the time of immunization. If preexposure immunization must be given while the person is taking an immunosuppressive drug, the vaccine should be given by the IM rather than the ID route and titers checked to determine if immunization is effective.

Postexposure Procedures

Because no specific or effective rabies treatment is available for symptomatic disease, all effort should be directed at prevention, which consists of adequate wound cleansing and prompt immunization. Evaluating exposure and the need for prophylactic immunization may be difficult, which results in considerable overtreatment.[107] Considering the prognosis and the relative safety of prophylaxis, however, overtreatment is understandable and inevitable.

Significant exposure risk is associated with bites that penetrate the epidermis or contact with saliva, other secretions, cerebrospinal fluid (CSF), or animal tissue with open wounds or mucous membranes. In general, the deeper the inoculation (e.g., by bite, scratch) and the larger the inoculum, the greater is the risk of contracting rabies.

If a dog, cat, or ferret bites an individual, the animal should be quarantined for 10 days.[157] Rabies prophylaxis can be started and discontinued if the animal remains well for 10 days. If the animal dies or neurologic symptoms develop within that time, the brain should be examined. The brain should be double bagged in plastic and sent refrigerated (e.g., on ice, not chemically fixed, frozen, or on dry ice) in a leakproof container to an appropriate diagnostic laboratory, such as that maintained by the state department of health. If quarantine is not possible or practical, the dog or cat can be killed immediately and the brain sent for examination. Any wild animal that bites a person should be killed immediately and the brain sent for diagnostic laboratory studies.[157] Wild animals are not kept under observation because their period of infectivity is usually unknown, and some species, such as skunks and bats, may shed virus in saliva for 2 weeks or more before they appear ill. If the biting animal is rabid, postexposure prophylaxis should be continued or instituted immediately.

If the biting animal is not available for examination, which is usually the case, act on the statistical probability that it was or was not rabid. If rabies is known to occur locally in that species, the person should be treated. If rabies has not occurred in the region for many years and the animal likely was not exposed to rabies, the local public health department can be consulted for regional and individual case guidelines.

Unvaccinated dogs and cats bitten by a rabid animal should be destroyed immediately. If the owner is not willing to have this done, the unvaccinated animal should be kept in strict isolation for 6 months and vaccinated 1 month before being released.[157] Dogs and cats that were currently and appropriately vaccinated before exposure should be given a booster dose immediately and kept in confinement for 45 days.[56] Local authorities will define the exact conditions of quarantine.

Domestic livestock (e.g., sheep, cattle, goats) exposed to rabid animals should be slaughtered immediately. If they are slaughtered within 7 days of being bitten, their tissues can be eaten without risk of infection, providing that the area around the bite is discarded. Animals that were exposed to rabies more than 7 days and less than 8 months previously should not be used for food. Meat, milk, or any other organ product of a clinically rabid animal should not be consumed; however, pasteurization or adequate cooking kills the virus, and inadvertent consumption of properly heated food should not be considered a rabies exposure.[157]

Although rodents are experimentally susceptible to infection, naturally acquired rabies is extremely rare in small rodents (e.g., mice, rats, gerbils, hamsters, guinea pigs, squirrels) and in lagomorphs (e.g., rabbits, hares). Exceptional cases in rabbits and a case in a squirrel have been reported.[34] With rare exceptions, a bite from a lagomorph or a small rodent should not be considered a rabies exposure, and postexposure prophylaxis should usually be withheld. Local public health officials or infectious disease specialists should be consulted about individual problem cases.

Some cases of rabies in woodchucks and beavers, which are large rodents, have been reported in the United States.[50,53] Most of these cases have occurred in the Middle Atlantic states, probably from exposure to raccoons. Bites from bats and wild carnivores, such as skunks, foxes, and raccoons in the United States and jackals, wolves, and mongooses in other enzootic countries, should be considered possible exposures. Prophylaxis should be given if the biting animal escapes.

Information about the biting animal and incident helps determine the likelihood of rabies exposure. The risk is greater if the biting incident was unprovoked. The question of provocation should be asked from the perspective of the animal rather than of the victim. For example, feeding a wild animal or attempting to separate fighting animals is likely to result in a bite. In an unprovoked attack the person did not intrude on the animal's territory or behave aggressively. The question of provocation indicates relative risk, because a provoked animal can also be rabid; a normal animal is not likely to bite unless provoked.

The animal's behavior and appearance should be described. Most rabid animals have obvious behavioral and neurologic abnormalities, such as staggering gait, excess salivation, uncontrolled rage, abnormal eye movements or pupillary reflexes (see Figure 44-6), altered vocalization, bizarre behavior (e.g., wild animals approaching humans), convulsions, or paralysis.

The physician should inquire about the animal's vaccination history. No vaccine is perfect, but the likelihood of rabies is greatly reduced if the animal was given an appropriate vaccine within the proper time frame. Rabies has occurred in immunized dogs[54] and in two people bitten by dogs that supposedly had been immunized in Nigeria[50] and Mexico.[134]

A history taken on the animal should include recent bites or involvement in a fight with another animal and travel outside the region within the past year. For example, the likelihood of a dog that stays in a nonenzootic area being rabid is small, but the risk increases if it is taken to enzootic areas to hunt.

Specific Postexposure Care. Postexposure prophylaxis consists of three steps. The first is adequate wound washing with soap (which is somewhat virucidal) and water. Studies in animals have shown that wound cleansing alone, without any other postexposure prophylaxis, can greatly reduce the likelihood of rabies.[74] This should be done as soon as possible, preferably within minutes after the bite or scratch, and definitely before seeking medical attention. Immunization can be delayed for hours or 1 to 2 days; washing a wound cannot be delayed.

The second component of postexposure prophylaxis is administration of rabies antiserum. In some parts of the world, this product may be of equine origin. Modern purified equine antirabies serum is effective, well tolerated, and approximately one-tenth the cost of human rabies immune globulin (HRIG). The incidence of adverse reactions is low (1% to 6%), and most are minor.[229] Earlier products, which were less well purified, carried a higher risk of serum sickness.[228] Equine antirabies serum in various countries may be the newer, nonreactive type or the older, more dangerous variety. Review of the package insert is recommended. It may also be advisable to test for hypersensitivity by intradermally injecting 0.1 ml of the product diluted 1:10 with saline before giving the full dose.[215]

In many Western countries, including the United States, rabies antiserum is made from the blood of immunized human donors (HRIG). HRIG contains 150 IU of neutralizing antibody per milliliter. It is given as a single dose of 20 IU/kg body weight. Recently the recommendations regarding the administration of HRIG have changed. Rather than administering half in the wound and half at a different site, the new recommendations call for the full dose of HRIG to be thoroughly infiltrated in the area around and in the wound.[62] If anatomy precludes full dosing, remaining product is injected intramuscularly at a site distant from the vaccine administration. A different syringe and different anatomic site are always used for vaccine and HRIG administration. HRIG is a safe product, not associated with anaphylaxis, serum sickness, or transmission of hepatitis or human immunodeficiency virus (HIV).

Theoretically, antiserum may be effective at any time before development of symptoms and should be given regardless of the time since the biting incident. The antiserum is given at the same time that active immunization is started, as described later. With recommended doses, no interference between passive and active immunization should take place. If HRIG was not given when active immunization was started, it can be given up to 7 days after the first vaccine dose.[55]

The third component of postexposure prophylaxis is active immunization with rabies vaccine. HDCV and PCEC are inactivated by β-propiolactone. Although ID vaccination with HDCV is acceptable for preexposure prophylaxis, this vaccine should always be administered intramuscularly, in the deltoid, for postexposure prophylaxis. PCEC should always be given in the deltoid muscle, whether used before or after exposure. HDCV or PCEC can be given in the midanterior thigh muscles of infants and small children. Either vaccine is given on days 0, 3, 7, 14, and 28 as a 1-ml dose, regardless of the age or size of the patient. The vaccines should not be given with the same syringe or in the same site as HRIG. They should *not* be given in the gluteal region, since the vaccine might be deposited in fat and be poorly immunogenic. Rabies has occurred in a person given postexposure prophylaxis using gluteal injections.[200]

After exposure, individuals previously immunized should receive booster doses of HDCV or PCEC on days 0 and 3. An effective booster response has been documented in people given primary immunization many years earlier,[87] including those given duck embryo vaccine, providing they had an appropriate immune response after the primary series. Such individuals should not receive antiserum. This is the principal advantage of receiving "preexposure" prophylaxis.

After vaccination, antirabies titers need to be checked only in individuals who may be immunosuppressed. A person who does not show a satisfactory antibody response (titer of at least 1:25 or 0.5 IU 2 to 4 weeks after immunization series) should receive additional booster doses of rabies vaccine weekly until antibody response is satisfactory. This is more important for postexposure than for preexposure immunization. Nursing and pregnancy do not contraindicate postexposure rabies prophylaxis.

In developing countries, HDCV and RVA as used in the United States may be prohibitively expensive for general use. Modified protocols for these products or other vaccines are often used to reduce the amount of vaccine and number of follow-up visits. None of these protocols is approved for use in the United States.

A purified Vero cell rabies vaccine has been used with success in Thailand.[55,92,230] This purified duck embryo cell rabies vaccine is more immunogenic and safer than the duck embryo vaccine widely used in the United States in the 1960s.[230] A purified chick embryo fibroblast rabies vaccine is used in Japan and a hamster kidney cell vaccine in China,[230] with good results.

Inactivated rabies vaccines prepared in animal brains, collectively known as Semple vaccines, are used for 93% of all postexposure rabies treatment worldwide because they are relatively cheap. They have relatively low immunogenicity and a high incidence of significant side effects, the most serious being neuroparalytic reactions because they induce antineural antibody and cellular response.[230] Earlier reports suggested a risk of such neurologic reaction in 1:3000 to 1:7000 vaccinees; however, another study from Thailand reported the rate of neurologic complications after receiving Semple vaccine to be a minimum of 8.31 cases per 1000 persons vaccinated (1:120). This complication rate was about 25 times higher than the overall complication rate of 0.33 per 1000 (1:3018) determined from 14 previous reports,[211] giving added motivation to seek preexposure immunization before travel.

Treatment of Infected Persons. Treatment of infected persons who have clinical rabies is directed toward the symptoms and consists of intensive care support of vital functions. α-Interferon, vidarabine, ribavirin, corticosteroids, inosine pranobex, multiple doses of vaccine, antithymocyte globulin, and large doses of rabies immune globulin have been used unsuccessfully in treating rabid persons.[230] The only three persons known to have survived clinically evident rabies (two with major neurologic sequelae) had received at least partial preexposure or postexposure immunization before they became symptomatic.[105,169,232]

Diagnosis

The differential diagnosis of rabies is extensive, including viral encephalitis, poliomyelitis, postinfectious encephalitis, vaccine reaction, Guillain-Barré syndrome, brain abscess, cerebrovascular accident, brain tumor, tetanus, phenothiazine toxicity, psychosis, rabies phobia, respiratory tract infection, pneumonia, sinusitis, otitis media, viral infection, gastroenteritis, myocardial infarction, hypertension, dissecting aortic aneurysm, arteritis, dehydration, lumbago, and headache.[6] Presumptive diagnosis of rabies depends on the exposure history and compatible neurologic signs, as noted earlier.

Definitive diagnosis is made by demonstration of the virus before or after death from saliva, neurologic tissue, CSF, urine sediment, or other body tissues.

One of the most reliable means of demonstrating the infection before death in the symptomatic individual is by direct immunofluorescent staining of a skin biopsy from the back of the neck. The biopsy sample should contain as many hair follicles as possible because the virus reaches the site by peripheral nerves to these follicles. Direct immunofluorescent staining of corneal impression smears may also be positive.[90] Rabies viruses can be isolated from saliva or CSF by culture on murine neuroblastoma cells or inoculation of mice.[230] These tests have great specificity but limited sensitivity. They become positive a week or more after the onset of illness.

Rabies can be indirectly diagnosed by antibody studies on serum or CSF.[90] The rapid fluorescent focus inhibition test (RFFIT), an in vitro neutralization procedure, is the standard diagnostic test used in the United States. Approximately half of persons with untreated rabies show antibody by day 8 and close to 100% by day 15. Titers resulting from actual rabies infection are generally much higher than those attained after immunization. No currently available diagnostic technique used before death can absolutely rule out rabies.

Definitive diagnosis of rabies is usually made by direct immunofluorescent antibody test on brain tissue. This test demonstrates fluorescent viral antigen particles within neurons (Figure 44-7). Confirmatory testing can be done by intracerebral inoculation of mice with saliva, brain, or other tissue from suspect human or animal patients.[90] Infected mice die in approximately 2 to 3 weeks. The diagnosis is confirmed by using direct immunofluorescent test on the brains of any mice that die or show neurologic signs. Mouse inoculation is reliable but takes time. Virus isolation on murine neuroblastoma cells takes only 24 hours but is not widely available.

Rabies can also be diagnosed by immunofluorescence and by peroxidase-antiperoxidase techniques on formalin-fixed brain tissue.[161] These methods should be used when only formalin-fixed tissues are available

Figure 44-7 Brain impression smear (direct fluorescent antibody preparation) positive for rabies from a Canadian fox. (Original magnification 400×.) *(Courtesy Centers for Disease Control and Prevention.)*

and should not be considered substitutes for the immunofluorescence technique and mouse inoculation with fresh brain tissue.

Pathology of Rabies

On gross examination, the brain may appear normal or slightly swollen and hyperemic. Histologic features include multifocal polioencephalomyelitis. Perivascular cuffing by lymphocytes is common, and there may be diffuse glial proliferation. Neurons may appear swollen, and some may be undergoing neuronophagia. Glial cells may accumulate in clusters called Babe's nodules.

Negri bodies are intracytoplasmic inclusion bodies, 0.25 to 27 μm in diameter, containing nucleocapsid material. They are diagnostic of rabies when correctly identified (Figure 44-8). They are absent in approximately 20% of cases, and some animals, such as cats, have neuronal changes associated with aging that can be mistaken for Negri bodies. Seller's stain is used to demonstrate Negri bodies in impression smears of the brain.[90] Several special stains have been used for tissue sections, but the inclusion bodies are usually demonstrable with standard hematoxylin and eosin staining.

Pathologic changes are best seen in the brainstem, including the substantia nigra, periaqueductal gray matter, and hypothalamus. The hippocampus (Ammon's horn) is commonly affected in humans and carnivores. Purkinje's cells of the cerebellum are commonly affected in ruminants. Pathologic changes are also commonly found in the gasserian ganglion. This may be a useful site for examination if the rest of an animal's brain has been destroyed.

Infection Control

Human-to-human transmission of rabies by bite, scratch, saliva, or aerosol has never been documented. Nevertheless, medical personnel should avoid contact with secretions from persons suspected of being rabid. Gloves, masks, and eye protection should be

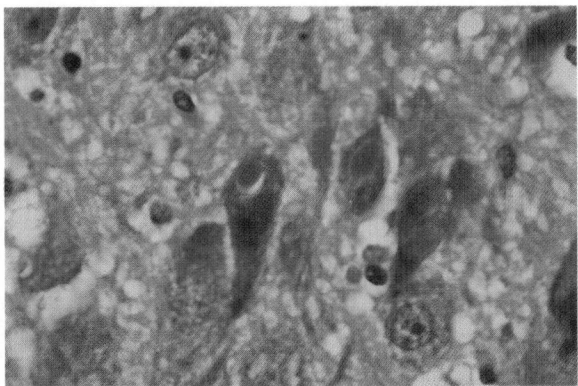

Figure 44-8 Negri bodies in the cytoplasm of neurons in the hippocampus of a dog. These inclusion bodies show some internal structure. (Hematoxylin and eosin, original magnification 1000×.) *(Courtesy Merieux Institute, Inc.)*

worn for such procedures as tracheal intubation. Rabid patients may have to be sedated and restrained if they attempt to engage in dangerous behavior, such as biting. Postexposure prophylaxis should be given only to personnel who are involved in the care of a rabies patient and had percutaneous or mucous membrane contact with saliva, respiratory secretions, tears, CSF, or tissue.[175]

LEPTOSPIROSIS

Leptospirosis is an infectious disease caused by *Leptospira interrogans* that can be acquired by animals and humans, usually by exposure to contaminated urine of wild or domestic animals. More than 170 serovars, or serologically distinct strains, are known. These serovars were given separate species status, as designated here. *Leptospira* organisms are spirochetes with hooked or curved ends, 6 to 20 μm long by 0.1 μm wide. They can grow on artificial media containing rabbit serum, such as Fletcher's semisolid and Stuart's liquid media, or on media containing albumin and fatty acids, such as Ellinghausen, McCullough, Johnson, Harris (EMJH) medium.[210]

In describing outbreaks with shared epidemiologic or clinical features, several syndromes were ascribed to different serotypes, such as Fort Bragg fever caused by *L. autumnalis,* swine herd disease caused by *L. pomona,* and Weil's disease caused by *L. icterohaemorrhagiae.* Such terms are no longer commonly used because of overlap in the symptoms and epidemiology associated with various *Leptospira* serotypes.

Adolf Weil first described the clinical picture of human leptospirosis in 1886. He described four febrile men with "particularities of an acute infectious illness with spleen tumor, jaundice, and nephritis." In addition, each had "severe nervous symptoms" and an enlarged liver. All recovered, and three had a "biphasic" clinical course with fever recurring after an afebrile period of 1 to 7 days. The term *Weil's disease* was coined by Goldschmidt in 1887. The carrier status was described in asymptomatic field mice by Ido and coworkers in 1915. Since then the infection has been recognized both as a disease and as an asymptomatic carrier state in hundreds of animal species.

Epidemiology

Leptospirosis is found throughout tropical and temperate areas of the world. It is particularly common in Southeast Asia and parts of Latin America, including some Caribbean islands.[85] Approximately 40 to 100 cases are reported annually in the United States (Figure 44-9). Undoubtedly, many cases are unreported. Active surveillance on Kauai and the east coast of the big island of Hawaii revealed a high incidence, accounting for a large proportion of flulike illness.[183] In 1996 five of 26 travelers returning from a white water rafting trip in Costa Rica developed a febrile illness and were found to have leptospirosis.[58] In 1998 leptospirosis was implicated in an outbreak of acute febrile illness among athletes from 44 states and seven countries who participated in triathlons (which involve open water swims in fresh water) in Springfield, Illinois, and Madison, Wisconsin. Eighty-four (11%) of Illinois participants and 20 (5%) of Wisconsin participants were infected and had their diagnosis confirmed by the CDC.[61] Both these reports highlight the potential risk to those with occupational, avocational, or recreational (including travel) exposure to contaminated fresh water.

Leptospirosis is a zoonosis in which certain serovars tend to have host specificity (Table 44-1). Dogs are usually associated with *L. icterohaemorrhagiae* and *L. canicola*, and swine and cattle more frequently involved with *L. pomona* and *L. grippotyphosa*, although all four of these serovars or serotypes have been isolated from each host species. The major reservoir for *Leptospira* infections for humans and domestic animals is wildlife, principally wild mammals, although the organism has also been iso-lated from frogs and snakes, and serologically positive fish and turtles have been found.[140]

Animals contaminate the environment by shedding organisms in their urine. Most human cases are environmentally acquired by contact with contaminated water or soil, and discovering the original animal source is difficult. A wet, alkaline environment favors survival, with tropical, unpolluted, nonsaline water with a slightly alkaline pH providing an optimum environment for infection. Heavy tropical rains increase infection risk by saturating soil, flushing leptospires into surface water, and drawing rodents and other small mammals into swampy areas. Infection can also be acquired by contact with infected animal blood and tissues. Factors strongly associated with acquiring leptospirosis in Hawaii include household use of rainwater catchment systems and the presence of skin cuts at the presumed time of exposure.[183]

Leptospirosis is an occupational problem for veterinary, agricultural, sewer, slaughterhouse, laboratory, and military personnel.[86,106,183] Dairy farmers are at risk in milking parlors, probably through exposure to cow's urine.[7,115] Leptospirosis poses an avocational risk for hunters, trappers, hikers, and persons who swim in fresh water, such as ponds and streams that may be contaminated with infected urine. It is acquired by ingestion or by entry through abraded skin or through the mucous membranes of the eye and mouth.

Symptoms

The incubation period is usually 7 to 12 days (range, 1 to 26 days).[182] The disease characteristically is biphasic.[117,177] The primary stage lasts 4 to 7 days and is characterized by organisms in blood, CSF, and various body tissues. During the initial phase, more than half of victims have fever, chills, severe malaise, myalgias, headache, lymph node enlargement, and conjunctival injection, usually without exudate. Nausea, vomiting, and abdominal pain may occur. A nonproductive

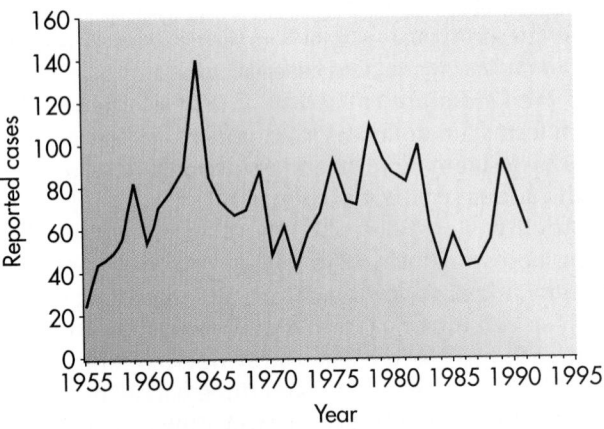

Figure 44-9 Reported annual cases of leptospirosis in the United States, 1955 through 1991. (*From MMWR 40, 1991.*)

TABLE 44-1. Leptospires Isolated from Humans in the United States, and Their Animal Reservoirs

SEROGROUP	SEROVAR	DOMESTIC ANIMALS	WILDLIFE
Icterohaemorrhagiae	*Icterohaemorrhagiae*	Dogs, cattle, swine	Brown rat, house rat, cotton rat, Pacific rat, house mouse, muskrat, gray fox, red fox, opossum, striped skunk, woodchuck, nutria
Canicola	*Canicola*	Dogs, cattle, swine	Striped skunk, raccoon, armadillo, mongoose
Pomona	*Pomona*	Dogs, cattle, swine, goats, sheep, horses	Striped skunk, raccoon, wildcat, opossum, woodchuck, red fox, deer, armadillo
Grippotyphosa	*Grippotyphosa*	Dogs, cattle, swine	Muskrat, fox squirrel, gray squirrel, bobcat, cottontail rabbit, swamp rabbit, raccoon, striped skunk, red fox, gray fox, vole, opossum
Hebdomidis	*Hardjo*	Cattle	None

Modified from Hanson LE: *J Am Vet Med Assoc* 181:1505, 1982.

cough is common. The initial clinical differential diagnosis includes meningitis, hepatitis, influenza, nephritis, encephalitis, and viral illness. The rickettsioses, typhoid fever, brucellosis, relapsing fever, toxoplasmosis, dengue fever, malaria, yellow fever, septicemia, Kawasaki syndrome, and toxic shock syndrome are also differential diagnoses.[106]

The primary stage, is usually followed by an afebrile period of 1 to 2 days. The onset of the second stage coincides with development of immunoglobulin M (IgM) antibodies. The organisms usually cannot be cultured from blood or CSF during this phase but can be isolated from urine for weeks or months. During the second stage the victim may have fever, but it is lower than in the primary stage. Headache is persistent, severe, and unresponsive to analgesics. It often heralds the onset of meningitis, one of the common complications of the secondary stage.

Myalgias, abdominal pain, nausea, and vomiting can occur in the second as well as in the primary stage. In addition to the conjunctival injection seen in the primary stage, uveitis (iridocyclitis) can be seen in the secondary stage. This can cause long-term ocular damage.[193] Occasionally, pharyngitis and a macular, purpuric, or ecchymotic rash occur (Figure 44-10). Rarely, endocarditis or myocarditis occurs. In a clinical study of leptospirosis on Barbados, cardiac arrhythmias and myocarditis occurred in 18% and pericarditis in 6% of patients.[81]

Splenic enlargement develops in approximately 20% of patients in the second stage. Hepatomegaly is sometimes found, especially if the patient is icteric.

Jaundice is a serious prognostic sign. Mortality in cases with jaundice exceeds 15% but is rare in anicteric cases. The overall case-fatality rate is approximately 5%. Mortality depends on the patient's prior condition and is higher in older individuals than in young adults. Death can occur from hemorrhagic manifestations as a result of vasculitis, renal or hepatic failure, cardiogenic shock, or myocarditis.

Diagnosis

Laboratory findings in leptospirosis include moderate leukocytosis, usually caused by an increase in neutrophils, elevated erythrocyte sedimentation rate, and thrombocytopenia. Elevated bilirubin level (up to 65 mg/dl, mainly direct bilirubin), greatly increased serum creatine kinase level (often 5 times normal), and less than fivefold increase in aspartate transaminase suggest the diagnosis. Elevated blood urea nitrogen level is a common finding. Serum amylase concentration may also be elevated.

Definitive diagnosis of leptospirosis can be made by culture of the organism on Fletcher's, Stuart's, EMJH,[210] or Tween 80–albumin medium. Blood and CSF should be cultured during the first week of illness; urine should be cultured thereafter. The likelihood of obtaining a positive culture is greatly diminished once antibiotics have been given. Oxalated blood samples can be sent to the laboratory for culture because the organisms can remain viable in oxalated blood for up to 11 days.

Some physicians have relied on darkfield examination for identification of the organisms, but this method is not considered reliable. Artifacts such as fibrin are readily mistaken for leptospires. The spirochetes can be demonstrated in tissue sections with silver stains (Figure 44-11).

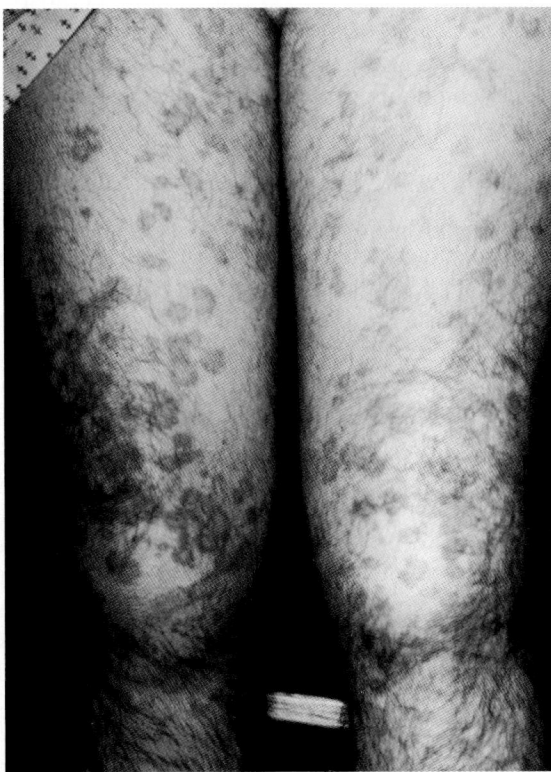

Figure 44-10 Hemorrhagic macular rash in a case of leptospirosis. *(Courtesy University of Massachusetts Medical School.)*

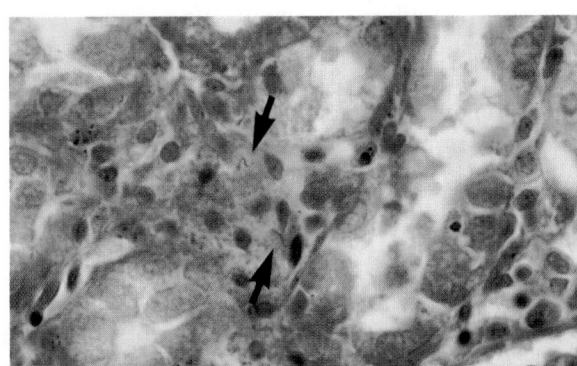

Figure 44-11 *Leptospira ictohemorrhagiae* in the kidney of an experimentally infected dog. The organisms are indicated by the arrows. (Warthin-Stany silver stain, original magnification 1000×.)

Leptospirosis can be diagnosed serologically based on demonstrating a fourfold rise in antibody titer.[221] The commercially available macroscopic slide agglutination test, using killed organisms of multiple serovars, or the complement fixation test is useful for screening purposes. The macroscopic agglutination test may become positive within the first week of illness and can persist for several months. Complement-fixing antibodies are detectable between days 10 and 21. Acute and convalescent sera should be tested 2 weeks apart because false-positive reactions can occur in single samples.

Specific serologic diagnosis of the serovar of infection can be made with the microscopic agglutination test (MAT), which uses live organisms but is available in relatively few reference laboratories. A genus-specific MAT employs a single broadly reactive antigen.[223] An IgM-specific, dot-enzyme-linked immunosorbent assay is comparable to the MAT in its ability to detect recent exposure to leptospires and is rapid and simpler.[163] Latex agglutination and indirect hemagglutination have high specificity and sensitivity and are especially useful early in the infection.[166] Although still investigational, a urine dipstick test shows promise as a rapid screening test for the diagnosis of leptospirosis.[197]

Treatment

Treatment of leptospirosis with antibiotics is most effective when begun during the first week of illness, preferably within 4 days of symptom onset. Although antibiotics were thought to have little value after this time, more recent studies indicate that they may still have some usefulness.[224] The treatment of choice is doxycycline, 100 mg orally twice a day for 7 days.[151] Alternative antibiotics include tetracycline, 2 g/day orally in three or four divided doses, or penicillin G, 3 million units/day parenterally. Amoxicillin, ampicillin, a cephalosporin, or erythromycin could also be used. Doxycycline and tetracycline should not be given to pregnant women or to children less than 9 years old.

A Jarisch-Herxheimer reaction may occur after treatment. This is a response to release of endotoxins, usually occurring within 2 to 6 hours after initiating therapy, with sudden onset of fever, chills, malaise, headache, and tachycardia. The reaction typically resolves spontaneously within 24 hours.

Other than antibiotic treatment, therapy for leptospirosis is supportive, including fluid therapy, dialysis for renal failure,[119] and transfusion for hemorrhagic complications.

Prevention

Prevention of human leptospirosis depends on avoiding infected animal tissues and areas contaminated by animal urine, blood, or tissue. Individuals who are at particularly high risk should be educated about prevention and encouraged to wear protective clothing, such as rubber gloves, when handling infective mate-

rial. Swimming in freshwater ponds and streams likely to be heavily contaminated by urine from livestock or wildlife should be discouraged.

Doxycycline, 200 mg once a week, effectively prevented infection in U.S. soldiers training in Panama.[214] Such prophylactic treatment could be given to individuals at unusually high risk.

Although *Leptospira* vaccines have been experimentally produced for human use, no product is approved and commercially available in the United States. Vaccines are available for animals. Immunization of domestic animals primarily has a veterinary benefit, in that the animals are protected from clinical disease. Immunity lasts about 6 months, but immunization does not guarantee that the animal cannot become infected. Several human cases have been traced to immunized dogs that apparently were still able to shed organisms.[88] Since then, some veterinary vaccines have been shown experimentally to reduce the renal carrier state.[120]

Veterinary Symptoms

Leptospirosis may be asymptomatic in animals, as is usually the case in wild animals, including rodents. Animals that acquire clinical disease have fever, appear depressed, lose appetite, may become jaundiced, develop hemorrhages on mucous membranes, and in late stages of the disease may have renal failure.[103] In cattle, leptospirosis can cause stillbirths, hemoglobinuria, and thickened yellowish or blood-tinged milk. Leptospires have been isolated from the milk of cattle and goats. A theoretic risk exists that leptospirosis could be transmitted by consuming such milk. Pasteurization should destroy organisms. Stillbirths or delivery of weak piglets is a common sign of leptospirosis in swine.

Cats are rarely affected by leptospirosis. They may be resistant to the disease because they are frequently exposed to infection through catching mice and other rodents.

Leptospirosis has been suspected as a cause of recurrent uveitis in horses. This is of more interest in comparative pathology than in public health, since horses infrequently transmit the infection to humans.

Prognosis

Recovery from leptospirosis apparently leaves serovar-specific immunity. Individuals can become infected with other serovars. Assuming that the infection and hemorrhagic complications can be controlled, the long-term prognosis after successful treatment is good. Renal and hepatic function usually returns, but headache and ocular damage may persist.[193]

HANTAVIRUS PULMONARY SYNDROME

Hantavirus pulmonary syndrome (HPS) is a rodent borne viral disease characterized by severe respiratory illness and a case-fatality ratio of 43%. The causative agent has been identified by serologic tests, polymerase chain reaction (PCR) to RNA, and immunohistochemistry.[61,132] The Sin Nombre virus is the primary hantavirus causing HPS in the United States, with the deer mouse (*Peromyscus maniculatus*) as its predominant carrier.[63] Other small mammals may be infected, such as piñon mice, brush mice, and western chipmunks.

Hantaviruses of the Bunyaviridae family cause the hemorrhagic fever with renal disease syndrome (HFRS). This is predominantly a disease of East Asia, where it has been called Korean hemorrhagic fever or epidemic hemorrhagic fever.[129] Wild rodents are the vectors of Hantaan, Puumala, Prospect Hill, and Seoul viruses. Hantaviruses have been isolated from the lung tissues of bats.[122]

Epidemiology

Although most cases of HPS have been clustered in the western United States, particularly the Four Corners area (Arizona, New Mexico, Colorado, and Utah), the virus may be present across the entire country.[158,170] The CDC had confirmed 217 cases of HPS in 30 states by mid-1999. From January through May 1999, seven cases of HPS were confirmed in Colorado, New Mexico, New York, and Washington. An additional 11 suspected cases with preliminary clinical and serologic evidence of HPS were reported in Arizona, California, Idaho, Iowa, Montana, New Mexico, and Washington. Eight of the confirmed and suspected cases are from Arizona, Colorado, and New Mexico. In the same 5-month period during each year from 1995 through 1998, this area averaged approximately two cases each year.[63]

Since 1994 the CDC has sponsored continuous monitoring studies of rodent populations at nine sites in Arizona, Colorado, and New Mexico. Hantavirus antibody prevalences in deer mouse populations surveyed during spring 1999 were 35% to 45% in some populations in New Mexico and up to 40% in Colorado. In comparison, prevalences during the population peaks of spring 1998 were less than 10% in New Mexico and approximately 20% in Colorado. These figures were comparable to a prevalence of 10% to 15% in deer mouse populations throughout the United States since 1993; during the 1993 outbreak, prevalences of 30% were detectecd.[64]

The hantaviruses do not cause apparent illnesses in the reservoir hosts, but the animals shed virus in saliva, urine, and feces for weeks. Human infection probably occurs when infective saliva or excreta are inhaled as aerosols, or when excreta are directly inoculated through the skin or perhaps ingested. Persons have been infected with hantavirus via rodent bite. There is no known transmission from arthropods or human to human.

Symptoms

A prodrome of fever, myalgia, and variable respiratory symptoms may include cough and shortness of breath with minimal bronchospasm. Acute respiratory distress rapidly follows. Other early phase symptoms include headache, chills, abdominal pain, nausea, and vomiting. Patients have often shown hemoconcentration and thrombocytopenia, leukocytosis, hypoalbuminemia, and lactic acidosis.

Rapid deterioration occurs, coincident with marked bilateral pulmonary infiltrates identified on chest x-ray examination. Fever, hypoxia, and hypotension may culminate in death; survivors have few or no sequelae. Autopsies have demonstrated intense pulmonary infiltration, with marked accumulations of hantavirus antigens in the endothelial cells.

Diagnosis

Laboratory evidence of acute hantavirus infection can be obtained by any of the following tests: IgM antibodies to hantavirus antigens, fourfold or greater increase in antibody titers to hantavirus antigens in paired serum specimens, positive immunohistochemical stain for hantavirus antigen in formalin-fixed tissues, or positive PCR from frozen tissue specimens (usually lungs).

Any person with a severe and sudden respiratory illness should be suspected to have been infected with hantavirus. CDC screening criteria are febrile illness in a previously healthy person characterized by unexplained adult respiratory distress syndrome *or* bilateral interstitial pulmonary infiltrates developing within 1 week of hospitalization, with respiratory compromise requiring supplemental oxygen.

Treatment

Treatment is supportive. Previously isolated hantaviruses have demonstrated in vitro sensitivity to ribavirin. The CDC has made the drug available as an investigational agent through an open-label protocol for treatment of patients with HPS. The protocol calls for administration of a 2-g loading dose of intravenous ribavirin, followed by 15 mg/kg body weight every 6 hours for 4 days and then 7.5 mg/kg every 8 hours for another 4 days. Ribavirin contributed to a patient's survival in at least one case.[172]

Prevention

According to the CDC, hantavirus transmission to humans may be epidemiologically associated with planting or harvesting field crops, occupying previously vacant dwellings, disturbing rodent-infested areas while hiking or camping, inhabiting dwellings with indoor rodent populations, or residing in an area with an increasing rodent density. Most persons with HPS who had high-risk exposures are thought to have been infected in and around their homes; limiting opportunities for domestic exposure is important. Measures to prevent HPS can be divided into four areas (Box 44-1).

TULAREMIA

Tularemia was first described in 1837 by Homma Soken, a Japanese physician who wrote of a febrile illness with generalized lymphadenopathy in persons who had eaten infected rabbit meat. In 1911 McCoy described a disease resembling plague in California ground squirrels. In the following year, McCoy and Chapin isolated the organism from rodents in Tulare County, California; this geographic site gave rise to the name of the disease. Edward Francis did much of the landmark bacteriologic and clinical investigation, and the genus of the causative organism, *Francisella*, is named after him. The role of ticks as vectors of the disease was discovered by Parker and Spencer in 1924. In 1929 they described transovarial transmission of the bacterium in ticks.

Microbiology

Francisella tularensis is a nonmotile, gram-negative coccobacillus measuring 0.2 by 0.3 to 0.7 μm. It must be grown aerobically on media containing cysteine or other sulfhydryl compounds. The organism is best grown on glucose cysteine agar with thiamine or on cysteine glucose blood agar. The organism has also been isolated in thioglycollate broth, charcoal yeast extract, and Thayer-Martin agar.

Two varieties of the organism are recognized in North America. Type A can ferment glycerol and has citrulline ureidase activity. It generally causes more severe disease than does type B, which is found in Europe and Asia as well as North America. Type B does not ferment glycerol and does not have citrulline ureidase activity. Type A is more frequently recovered from rabbits and various bloodsucking arthropods. Type B is often recovered from water, voles, muskrats, and beavers. However, the two varieties sometimes share an ecologic niche.[145]

Transmission

Before 1950, most reported cases of tularemia were associated with direct contact with rabbits. Tularemia is now most frequent transmitted by ticks.[31] Many different species of ticks are potential or proven vectors. A common vector in the United States is the dog tick, *Dermacentor variabilis*. The lone star tick, *Amblyoma americanum*, is the main vector in the southern United States. Because the infection can be transmitted transovarially, ticks are an important natural reservoir. Ticks may transmit the bacteria through their feces, since the organism has not been isolated from their salivary glands. Deerflies and other biting flies may also be suitable vectors.[124] In the United States the second most common source for human infection is rabbits. The infection can be acquired by skinning, eviscerating, or handling the tissues of infected rabbits or by eating improperly cooked infected meat. Transmission can also occur by direct contact with or ingestion of infected soil, water, or fomites. Infection can occur by inhalation of dust or water aerosol[73] or in the laboratory. Organisms remain viable in mud samples stored as long as 14 weeks, in tap water for 3 months, in dry straw for 6 months, and in salted meat for 31 days.[18]

Occasional cases of tularemia have been transmitted by cat bite[48,173] or by handling infected tissue from animals other than rabbits, such as bear,[44] deer,[41] beaver, and muskrat.[235] Person-to-person transmission is rare.

Epidemiology

Transmission by ticks and other arthropods usually occurs in the spring and summer. Transmission from rabbits most often occurs during the fall and winter hunting seasons.

The reported incidence of tularemia has been steadily decreasing in the United States since its peak at 2291 cases in 1939 (Figure 44-12). Other tick-borne infections, such as Rocky Mountain spotted fever and Lyme disease, have increased. Empiric use of antibiotics may have aborted undiagnosed cases.

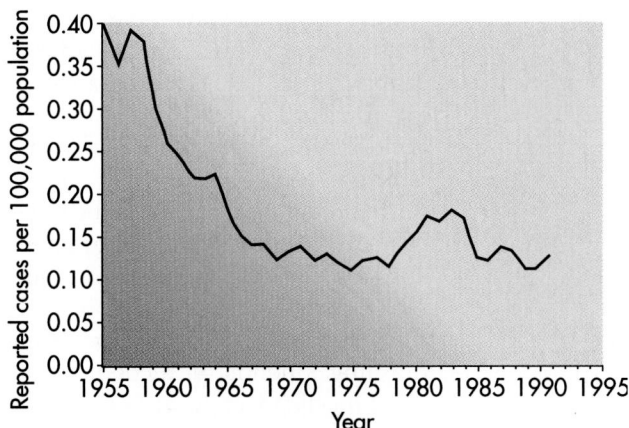

Figure 44-12 Reported cases of tularemia in the United States, 1955 through 1991. (*From* MMWR *40, 1991.*)

Most cases in the United States have been reported from the South and Midwest, particularly Arkansas, Illinois, Missouri, Oklahoma, Texas, and Tennessee. The disease is also widespread in Europe, Canada, the Middle East, Russia, and Japan.

Symptoms

Classically, tularemia occurs in one of six clinical presentations: glandular, ulceroglandular, oculoglandular, oropharyngeal, pneumonic, or typhoidal.[18,145] Evans et al[84] simplified this classification into two major categories: ulceroglandular and typhoidal. Patients are considered to have *ulceroglandular tularemia* if they have lesions of the skin or mucous membranes, with or without associated lymphadenopathy, with affected lymph nodes at least 1 cm in diameter. Patients without lesions of the skin or mucous membranes and with lesser enlargement of lymph nodes are considered to have *typhoidal tularemia.* In this classification, pharyngitis or pneumonia can occur in either the ulceroglandular or the typhoidal form of the disease.

The ulceroglandular form accounts for approximately 80% of tularemia cases. The typical skin lesion begins as an erythematous papule or nodule that indurates and ulcerates. It is frequently painful and tender. Ulcers associated with handling infected animals are usually located on the hand, with associated lymphadenopathy found in the epitrochlear or axillary regions. Infections transmitted by tick bites are usually located on the lower extremities, associated with inguinal or femoral lymphadenopathy.

So-called glandular tularemia is characterized by the presence of enlarged, tender lymph nodes without an associated skin lesion. However, the skin lesion may have healed or gone unnoticed before the development of lymphadenopathy.

In the oculoglandular form, unilateral conjunctivitis occurs with concentration of inflammatory response in and around a nodular lesion on the conjunctiva and with enlargement of the ipsilateral preauricular lymph node.[102] The oculoglandular form constitutes 1% to 2% of tularemia cases.

The typhoidal form occurs in approximately 10% of tularemia cases. It is characterized by fever, chills, and debility. As the disease progresses, weight loss may be significant. Hepatosplenomegaly can occur, especially in children.[114] Pericarditis occurs rarely.[84] Exudative pharyngitis can occur with either the typhoidal or the ulceroglandular form. There is usually associated cervical lymphadenitis.

Pneumonia is a fairly common complication of tularemia. The pulmonary infection can be acquired by inhalation of aerosol or from bacteremia. Symptoms include cough, chest pain, shortness of breath, production of sputum, and hemoptysis. Radiographic abnormalities of the chest may be found in patients without pulmonary symptoms. Chest films may reveal infiltrates, most often of the lower lobe; hilar lymphadenopathy, and pleural effusion. Tularemia patients with pneumonia are more likely to be older, less likely to have a known source of infection, and more likely to die than those without pulmonary infection.[196]

Severe complications of tularemia, such as bacteremia, pneumonia, and rhabdomyolysis, are most likely to be seen in patients with significant underlying disease, such as lymphoma, other forms of cancer, or diabetes.[165] From 1981 through 1987 the case-fatality rate of tularemia in the southwestern and central United States was 2%.[216]

Diagnosis

Ulceroglandular tularemia can be confused with cat-scratch disease, streptococcal and staphylococcal skin diseases, sporotrichosis, and plague. Typhoidal tularemia can mimic septicemic plague, brucellosis, salmonellosis, typhoid fever, other forms of Gram-negative sepsis, and leptospirosis. Tularemic pneumonia can appear similar to other forms of bacterial and nonbacterial pneumonias, including Q fever, psittacosis, and legionnaires' disease.[179,196]

Oculoglandular tularemia resembles Parinaud's syndrome (granulomatous conjunctivitis with preauricular lymphadenitis) caused by other bacteria, such as *Leptothrix* species, *Mycobacterium tuberculosis*, syphilis, and cat-scratch disease.[102]

The differential diagnosis of oropharyngeal tularemia includes infectious mononucleosis, streptococcal pharyngitis, and plague pharyngitis. The disease most likely to be confused with tularemia is plague, because both diseases occur under similar epidemiologic circumstances and are characterized by certain similar clinical syndromes.[39,202] The bacteria causing plague and tularemia share morphologic and cultural features but can be differentiated serologically and with appropriate microbiologic techniques.

Definitive diagnosis of tularemia is usually based on antibody studies.[126,213] The most common test is agglutination, either tube agglutination or microagglutination.[188] Enzyme-linked immunosorbent assay (ELISA) is also used for diagnosis. An advantage of ELISA is identifying IgM, IgA, and IgG antibodies.

Diagnosis is established serologically by demonstrating a fourfold or greater rise in titer between acute and convalescent sera taken 1 or more weeks apart. Titers of 80 or greater are generally considered significant in the agglutination test. Values rarely reach that level during the first week of infection but usually reach or exceed that by day 16 of infection. Agglutinating antibodies remain detectable for 10 to 30 years after infection. IgM, IgA, and IgG antibodies also remain detectable by the ELISA technique for at least 11 years after infection. Because of this long persistence of antibody, single titers cannot be used for definitive diagnosis.

Tularemia can also be definitively diagnosed by isolation and identification of the organism from blood or lesions. Samples for culture, however, are not routinely taken in suspect cases, and they are not encouraged because of the high frequency of contamination and infection of laboratory workers using this organism in vitro.

Treatment

Streptomycin, the drug of choice, should be given in a dose of 30 to 40 mg/kg/day, in two divided portions intramuscularly every 12 hours for 3 days, followed by half that dose for another 4 to 7 days. Rate of cure for streptomycin is 97%, with no relapses. For gentamicin and tetracycline, respectively, the rates of cure were 86% and 88%, rates of relapse 6% and 12%, and rates of failure 8% and 0. The duration of therapy with gentamicin and a delay in its initiation may have affected outcome in severe cases.[165] For chloramphenicol and tobramycin, cure rates were 77% and 50%, relapse rates 21% and 0; and failure rates 2% and 33%, respectively. Treatment with imipenem/cilastatin was successful in one case and with ciprofloxacin or norfloxacin successful in six cases; in contrast, therapy with ceftriaxone was ineffective in eight cases.[83]

Prevention

Prevention of tularemia includes avoidance of ectoparasites such as ticks and appropriate hygiene in the handling of infected animal tissues. Insect repellents should be applied when going into areas where ticks, deerflies, and other possible vectors are found. Persons walking in tick-infested brush should wear long pants, with the bottoms of trouser legs tucked into socks or boot tops. Individuals should check frequently for the presence of ticks while in the field. Ticks should be removed as quickly as possible, preferably with pointed forceps grasping the mouthparts, taking care not to break them or to squeeze the body of the tick in the removal process.

Persons handling suspect animals should wear rubber or plastic gloves. Reservoir animals such as rabbits or muskrats that appear ill should not be handled. When handling sick animals is necessary, infection control procedures should include the use of gloves, face masks, and disposable gowns.

Attempts at culturing the organism should be done only in laboratories that have appropriate containment facilities for handling such dangerous organisms. Laboratory work with *F. tularensis* should always be conducted under an appropriate microbiologic hood. Standard halogen-containing phenol or alcohol-based antiseptics can be used for disinfecting surfaces.

Although person-to-person transmission is rare, reasonable infection control measures should be taken to reduce exposure to aerosols from patients with oropharyngeal or pneumonic tularemia, and exposure to exudates should be avoided.

A live attenuated vaccine is available as an investigational new drug from the U.S. Army Medical Research Institute for Infectious Diseases at Fort Detrick, Maryland. Physicians using this vaccine must register as collaborative investigators and follow a prescribed protocol in advising the patient, administering the vaccine, and reporting on its use. The vaccine is made available only for those who are at high risk, such as laboratory personnel who frequently work with the organism. The vaccine is effective in preventing the typhoidal form of tularemia[184-187] but will not prevent cutaneous lesions forming at the site of an inoculation. The vaccine, when administered by scarification, induces humoral and cell-mediated immune responses.[220]

PLAGUE

Plague, a bacterial disease caused by *Yersinia pestis* and transmitted by the bite of infected fleas, has occurred in explosive epidemics. Probable epidemics of plague occurred during the Peloponnesian War, as described by Thucydides, in approximately 400 BC. It ravaged the Roman Empire and western Europe during the age of Justinian and continued through the seventh century. The best-known and most devastating epidemic started in 1348. Known as the Black Death, the infection spread from Asia throughout Western Europe, killing one third of the population.[95] Plague is a reportable disease under the International Sanitary Regulations.

Plague is carried by various rodent reservoir hosts and transmitted by rodent fleas. Most of the outbreaks in Europe have been ascribed to importation of plague from enzootic foci in Asia, by ships bringing infected rats and people to port cities. A matter of considerable historical and epidemiologic interest is how and why the various epidemics eventually subsided. Theories include development of mutant bacteria; changes in patterns of shipping, building, and hygiene; replacement of *Rattus rattus* by *R. norvegicus;* and development of immunity in animals and humans.[82]

Bacteriology

Y. pestis is a gram-negative, nonmotile, nonsporulating rod with a bipolar, or "safety-pin," appearance in smears stained with Giemsa's or Wayson's stain.[38] The appearance is somewhat variable by Gram's technique.

Most standard bacteriologic media support the growth of the organism aerobically or under facultative anaerobic conditions. Optimal in vitro growth occurs at 28° C (82.4° F), at which temperature colonies become visible on plain agar in approximately 48 hours.

Virulence factors encoded by the bacterial chromosome include surface capsular material that is antiphagocytic, ability to synthesize purines even if phagocytosed, and a surface component needed for iron uptake. Virulence factors mediated by a plasmid include dependence on environmental calcium for growth at 37° C (98.6° F) and production of v[83] and w[137] antigens. The relationship between calcium dependence and virulence is under investigation.[95]

Transmission

Plague is normally a flea-borne disease of rodents, although other animals, including humans, can become infected. Humans are generally infected by the bite of an infected flea; but direct contact with and percutaneous inoculation from *Yersinia pestis* organisms can lead to disease. Rarely, inhaled infective droplets cause pulmonary plague; human-to-human transmission can occur and is a threat in developing countries and in the United States.

The black rat is highly susceptible to plague and dies with severe septicemia. The concentration of organisms in the rat's blood ensures infection of the biting flea. When the rat dies, the flea leaves to seek other hosts. This cycle is unusual in that the infection kills the reservoir host and vector, but the nature of the infection in the flea and rat guarantees further transmission and survival of the microorganism. The bacteria multiply so extensively in *Xenopsylla cheopis* that they block its proventriculus, or foregut. The flea cannot feed effectively, becomes ravenously hungry, and regurgitates large numbers of bacilli when it bites.

Epidemiology

The epidemiology of plague is complex. Various fleas can transmit the infection between reservoir rodent hosts and humans. In major epidemics the prominent carriers were the tropical rat flea (*X. cheopis*) and the black rat (*R. rattus*).

Smoldering foci of infection are maintained in nature in wild rodents and their fleas. In the United States, enzootic (maintenance) hosts include deer mice (*Peromyscus maniculatus*) and various voles (*Microtus* species). Epizootic (amplifying) hosts include the prairie dog (*Cynomys* species) (Figure 44-13) and

ground squirrel (*Spermophilus* species). Other rodents and lagomorphs that maintain infection include chipmunks (*Eutamias* species), marmots (*Marmota* species), wood rats (*Neotoma* species), rabbits (*Sylvilagus* species), and hares (*Lepus* species).[168]

Enzootic foci of plague remain in parts of Asia, Africa, and South America,[36,168] as well as the western United States. The major enzootic states in the United States are New Mexico, Arizona, California, Colorado, Oregon, Nevada, and Utah. From 1944 through 1993, 362 cases of human plague were reported in the United States; approximately 90% of these occurred in Arizona, California, Colorado, and New Mexico. Seven confirmed cases of human plague were reported in 1995 (three in New Mexico, two in California, one in Arizona, and one in Oregon). Five of the seven cases were "bubonic," one was "septicemic," and one a fatal "pneumonic" case.[137] In many foreign areas the exact species of rodents and fleas involved in transmission and maintenance are not known. Vietnam is the only country considered a threat for the international introduction of plague.

Carnivorous mammals can acquire plague by ingesting infected rodents or by being bitten by their fleas. Dogs usually do not become very ill with plague, but cats can acquire severe, often fatal, forms of infection, resembling syndromes seen in humans. Bubonic plague in cats is usually manifested as severe submandibular lymphadenopathy. Cats can also acquire pneumonic plague, characterized by a subacute febrile course with cough and respiratory distress. Cats can transmit plague to humans by bite, respiratory droplets, or carrying fleas to people. Plague is an occupational risk for veterinarians who handle sick cats or their tissues.[118,178]

Although dogs are usually not as severely affected as cats, at least one human case was associated with a

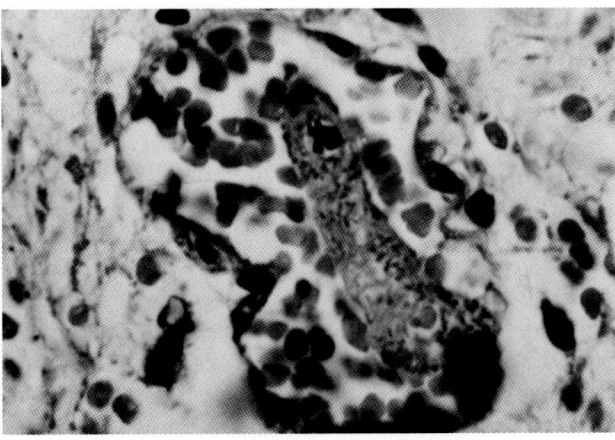

Figure 44-13 Thrombus in a vein in the subcutis of a prairie dog naturally infected with plague. Many organisms (fine stippling) are present in the thrombus. (Hematoxylin and eosin stain, original magnification 1000×.)

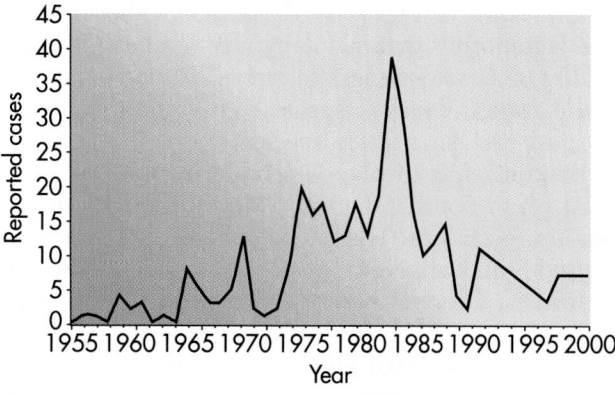

Figure 44-14 Reported cases of plague in humans in the United States, 1955 to 1999. (*Modified from MMWR 40, 1991.*)

dog that apparently died of plague.[180] Dogs may be significantly involved in the epidemiology of plague in Tanzania, as reservoirs of vector fleas or bacterial infection.[121] In the United States, one person acquired plague while skinning an infected coyote[40] and two from skinning bobcats.[45] Other carnivores, such as skunks, badgers, and raccoons, have been found with antibody to the plague bacillus and presumably were exposed while hunting infected rodents. Exposure to infected rabbits, their fleas, or both has been associated with human plague.[38] Plague is not generally recognized as a disease of farm animals in modern times, but a recent report ascribed one outbreak of plague in a Libyan village to contact with a sick camel and another to contact with two goats.[65]

In the United States the major epidemiologic factor associated with acquiring plague is living in a rural or suburban area where the enzootic disease occurs (Figure 44-14). People who hike, camp, or perform field studies in such areas are subject to this disease. Its diagnosis should be considered in anyone with a compatible history who has recently been in an enzootic area.

Symptoms

The three most common forms of plague are bubonic, pneumonic, and septicemic. Less common forms are meningeal, pharyngeal, and ophthalmic.

In the most common form, *bubonic plague,* buboes develop, which are greatly enlarged and very tender lymph nodes proximal to the point of percutaneous entry, such as a flea bite or a cut infected by handling infected tissues. Inguinal nodes are most often involved because fleas usually bite on the legs. Skinning an infected animal or handling its tissues often results in axillary buboes. Frequently, cervical, hilar, or mesenteric lymph nodes are enlarged.

The incubation period for bubonic plague is usually 2 to 6 days. In mild or early stages of infection, seeding of the blood occurs intermittently, causing a low sensi-

tivity to blood culture testing. Later, if disease becomes severe, all blood cultures are positive. Victims usually have high fever, chills, severe malaise, headache, and myalgias. Toxicity, cardiovascular collapse with shock, and hemorrhagic phenomena may occur. Blackened hemorrhagic skin lesions gave rise to the name "Black Death" during the pandemic of the fourteenth century.

Victims with bacteremia and significant symptoms but no buboes are considered to have *septicemic plague.* Such cases may be difficult to diagnose unless the physician suspects plague based on epidemiology. As with other forms of gram-negative sepsis, victims have fever, chills, malaise, headache, and gastrointestinal (GI) symptoms such as nausea, vomiting, and diarrhea, and the disease can result in cardiovascular collapse. Thrombosis (see Figure 44-13) and disseminated intravascular coagulopathy may be present. Untreated septicemic plague progresses to pulmonary involvement and death. However, transmissible pneumonic infection is estimated to occur in only 5%, since victims die before alveolar pneumonitis and the potential for droplet spread.

Pneumonic plague can result from inhalation of droplets from another pneumonic patient or by pulmonary seeding from the blood. Pneumonic plague runs an acute and fulminant course and is almost uniformly fatal if not treated. The incubation period is 2 to 3 days and disease is characterized by the sudden onset of fever, cough, bloody sputum, headache, and shaking chills. Radiographs reveal progressive consolidation of pneumonic patches in the lung, often with pleural effusion.

Of 71 cases of plague reported in New Mexico between 1980 and 1984, 18 were septicemic.[113] The victims were significantly older and more likely to die than those with bubonic plague. The white blood cell counts in the New Mexican septicemic cases were low, normal, or elevated (range, 3000 to 68,700/mm^3), but all patients had relative or absolute neutrophilia with a left shift. Bacteria were demonstrable on direct blood smears in 3 of 17 septicemic patients. Plague is most common in persons less than 40 years old, perhaps because of their greater outdoor activity, but the risk of the septicemic form increases in individuals over age 40 years. In patients with septicemic plague, mortality was greater in younger patients, perhaps because of greater delay in diagnosis and decreased likelihood that they would receive antibiotic therapy on an empiric basis.[113]

Abdominal pain was present in nearly 40% of the patients in New Mexico. Hepatosplenomegaly occurs in plague and may be a source of abdominal pain, but it was not found in the patients reported in this series. The presence of abdominal symptoms in plague should be emphasized because the disease could be mistaken for other forms of GI illness. A review of the 71 plague cases in New Mexico from 1980 to 1984 revealed that GI symptoms occurred in 57% of patients, with vomiting (39%) the most frequent symptom. Nausea (34%), diarrhea (28%), and abdominal pain (17%) were also observed.[112]

Plague should be suspected in patients who have various combinations of lymphadenopathy, high fever, malaise, tachycardia, tachypnea, hypotension, and abdominal symptoms and who have come from an endemic area. If the suspicion is reasonable, antibiotic therapy should be instituted immediately. Treatment should not be delayed to await laboratory confirmation of the diagnosis.

Rare forms of plague include pharyngeal, meningeal, and ophthalmic. Pharyngeal and ophthalmic plague can be acquired by exposure to droplets expelled by a pneumonic patient. Endophthalmitis can also be secondary to septicemia. Meningitis is acquired by direct seeding while the patient is bacteremic.

Diagnosis

Definitive diagnosis is based on culture of the organism from sputum, transtracheal aspirate, blood, or aspirates of buboes. The best staining technique to demonstrate bipolar morphology of the organism is Giemsa's or Wayson's technique.

Direct fluorescent antibody (FA) stain of aspirates and smears provides a reasonably rapid diagnostic technique. Although cross-reactions with *Yersinia pseudotuberculosis* have been recorded, and occasional strains of the plague bacillus do not stain well with FA, a positive FA test in a patient with a compatible epidemiologic and clinical picture is a reasonable basis for making a diagnosis of plague and instituting therapy.

Material from buboes should be obtained by fine-needle aspiration rather than excision or incision and drainage. This reduces risks of transmission to medical personnel and of iatrogenic septicemia.

Treatment

Patients with suspected plague should be treated immediately without awaiting definitive laboratory studies. The best available drug is streptomycin. If given too rapidly, streptomycin can cause a severe reaction as a result of rapid killing of organisms and release of endotoxin. The recommended dosage is 30 mg/kg/day intramuscularly in four divided doses every 6 hours for 5 days. A less preferred alternative to streptomycin is gentamicin, 5 mg/kg/day intravenously in four divided doses every 6 hours, reduced to 3 mg/kg/day after clinical improvement. Patients with impaired renal function should have their dosage of streptomycin or gentamicin modified appropriately.[168]

Tetracycline is often used concurrently with streptomycin. The recommended loading dose is 15 mg/kg orally, up to 1 g total dose. This is followed by 40 to 50 mg/kg in six divided doses every 4 hours on the first day. Thereafter 30 mg/kg is administered orally in four divided doses every 6 hours for 10 to 14 days. If the patient cannot tolerate treatment by mouth, tetracycline can be given intravenously, using one third of the calculated oral dose until oral therapy is tolerated.

An alternative to tetracycline is chloramphenicol, administered in a loading dose of 25 mg/kg orally, up to 3 g total, followed by 50 to 75 mg/kg orally in four divided doses for 10 to 14 days. If the patient does not tolerate oral therapy, chloramphenicol can be given intravenously, 50 mg/kg in four divided doses every 6 hours until oral therapy is tolerated. It is preferable to use chloramphenicol in the event of meningitis or endophthalmitis because of good penetration into affected tissues. Whichever drug combination is selected, antibiotic therapy should be given for at least 10 days, or for 3 or 4 days after clinical recovery.

Sulfadiazine is a less satisfactory alternative. A loading dose of 25 mg/kg is given orally, followed by 75 mg/kg orally in four divided doses every 6 hours for 10 to 14 days. Co-trimoxazole (320 mg of trimethoprim and 1600 mg of sulfamethoxazole) twice or three times a day for 10 to 17 days was found effective in treating plague[2] but much less experience has been accumulated with this medication than with other antibiotics.

Infants born to plague-infected mothers may have congenital infection. They should be treated with kanamycin, 15 mg/kg/day intravenously or intramuscularly in four divided doses every 6 hours, or streptomycin, 10 to 20 mg/kg/day in four divided doses every 6 hours.

Quarantine and Infection Control

The greatest risk of contagion is by aerosol transmission from patients with the pneumonic form of plague. All persons with suspected plague should be placed in strict quarantine and isolation for a minimum of 48 hours of specific antibiotic treatment. If no respiratory signs develop within 48 hours, wound and skin precautions will suffice for the rest of his or her hospitalization. Patients with plague pneumonia or pharyngitis should be kept under strict respiratory quarantine for at least 4 days of antibiotic treatment, until the pharyngeal culture is negative for the organism or respiratory signs abate. Contact personnel should wear gloves, gowns, masks, and eye protection. Strong[209] dramatically illustrated effective protective clothing during a pneumonic plague epidemic in Manchuria in 1911.

The greatest risk of acquiring plague from a patient with the septicemic or bubonic form is by inoculation of blood or exudate; therefore strict needle precautions should be taken. Buboes should not be incised and drained. In theory, fleas harbored by a septicemic patient should be capable of transmitting the disease, but CDC recommendations for control of plague do not cover eradication of fleas from human patients.[225] No pesticides have been FDA approved for this use. Products effective against lice may have limited effectiveness because most fleas do not remain long on a human host.

Household contacts and individuals exposed to patients with pneumonic plague should be prophylactically treated with antibiotics. Tetracycline, 500 mg orally every 6 hours for 6 days, can be given to adults. Trimethoprim-sulfamethoxazole can be given to children under 8 years of age and to pregnant women. Streptomycin, chloramphenicol, and sulfadiazine are alternative prophylactic medications, given in therapeutic doses for 1 week to 10 days.

Household contacts of individuals with bubonic plague do not have to be treated prophylactically. They should have their temperature recorded twice daily, and if it exceeds 37.7° C (100° F) orally, they should report immediately to a physician for evaluation. Careful surveillance is indicated for persons who have had face-to-face contact with patients with pneumonic plague. Their well-being should be confirmed daily.

The incubation period for primary pneumonic plague is 1 to 3 days and for pharyngeal plague 3 to 6 days. Precautionary follow-up observation of contacts should be maintained throughout this time. All cases of suspected or confirmed plague should be reported to the state health department.

Prevention

Residents and visitors to plague endemic areas should be advised of the risks of infection. They should avoid contact with rodents and other possible animal reservoirs of infection that are found sick or dead in the wild. Disposable plastic or rubber gloves should be worn when skinning or dressing a possibly infected animal. Cats and dogs should be kept indoors, leashed, or otherwise restrained. Owners of pets that have access to wild rodent populations must maintain flea control. Veterinary personnel working on animals that could have plague should follow strict infection control procedures.

Health departments in enzootic areas should maintain surveillance for plague in local reservoir species. At times of increased plague activity, insecticide sprays and powders can be applied to rodent burrows. Ectoparasite control is essential before any attempt is made to kill the rodents, because killing the rodents without control of their ectoparasites causes fleas to seek other hosts, including dogs, cats, and people.

Immunization

A killed bacterial vaccine is available in the United States but is rarely used. Its application is limited to persons who have intensive, usually occupational, exposure to the infection. Many of these persons prefer to rely on sanitation, protective clothing, and prophylactic or therapeutic treatment rather than use the vaccine, since it has short-term (6- to 12-month) efficacy and has a significant incidence of side effects, such as fever, malaise, and pain at the site of injection.[47]

Clinical and epidemiologic assistance for problems relating to plague can be obtained from the Plague Branch, Centers for Disease Control and Prevention (PO Box 2087, Fort Collins, CO 80522; 303-221-6400).

After-hours consultation can be obtained from the CDC in Atlanta (404-639-8107).

GLANDERS

Glanders, although little known in the Western world today, is one of the classic infectious diseases. Its greatest historic impact has been through its effect on cavalry horses during military campaigns, influencing battles from before the time of Christ through the Crusades and World War I.

Theories and disputes about the origin, nature, transmission, and treatment of glanders figured prominently in the development of veterinary science in Europe in the latter half of the eighteenth century. In 1795 Erik Viborg published an account that is remarkably close to our understanding of the disease today. He demonstrated that equine "farcy," characterized by cutaneous lymphangitis, and the respiratory form of the disease in horses, classically referred to as "glanders," were different manifestations of the same infection. He demonstrated that the disease was transmissible from one horse to the next by infectious exudates, and that the causative organism could be carried by fomites and killed by heat.

Transmission of glanders from horses to humans was documented in France and Germany during the first three decades of the nineteenth century. The causative organism was isolated by Loeffler and Schütz, as well as by Bouchard, Capiton, and Charrin in 1882. In 1891 Kalning and Helmann independently discovered mallein, derived from the glanders bacillus. Like tuberculin, mallein was thought to have therapeutic or prophylactic value. This turned out to be erroneous, but mallein provided a means of diagnosing the infection in clinically ill and carrier animals and provided a basis for test and slaughter techniques, which have largely eliminated glanders from most parts of the world.

Bacteriology

The causative organism is *Burkholderia mallei*, a member of the newly renamed *Burkholderia* genus, which includes *B. pseudomallei*, the cause of melioidosis, and *B. cepacia*. It is a gram-negative, nonsporulating, obligate aerobic, and nonmotile bacillus that requires glycerol for optimum growth in vitro.[174,206] In 1992 Yabuuchi et al[234] proposed that seven species formerly of *Pseudomonas* RNA group II should be transferred to a new genus, *Burkholderia*, with *B. cepacia* as the type species. The genus included *B. caryophylli, B. gladioli, B. mallei, B. pseudomallei, R. pickettii,* and *R. solanacearum;* the latter two species were transferred to the genus *Ralstonia*.[234]

Epidemiology

Glanders occurs in a few Asian and African countries, such as India, China, Mongolia, Egypt, and Mauritania.

It is primarily a disease of horses and is spread most rapidly when large numbers of horses, mules, or donkeys are kept in proximity. Many carnivorous mammals are also susceptible to infection, and outbreaks have occurred when infected horse meat was fed to lions, tigers, and other wild animals in zoos. Occasionally, infections occur in dogs, cats, sheep, and goats.

Humans are usually infected by exposure to sick horses. Infection can occur by inhalation of respiratory droplets or by contact with infected discharges. Human infections have also occurred from direct contact in the laboratory and from patients.

Symptoms

Equids. Horses may have unilateral or bilateral mucopurulent nasal discharge. There may be enlargement and induration of lymphatics, with ulceration and discharge, especially involving the legs. Nodules, pustules, and ulcers may be seen on the horse's skin. The cutaneous form of the disease is often referred to as "farcy," the thickened, inflamed lymphatics as "farcy pipes," and the enlarged lymph nodes as "farcy buds." Horses also have pneumonia, with mild respiratory embarrassment in early stages, and more severe respiratory difficulties and cachexia in later stages. Septicemia with lesions in multiple internal organs can occur.

Glanders can run an acute and fulminant course in equids, most often in donkeys and mules, or a more chronic course, more often in horses. The case-fatality rate is high, especially with more virulent strains of the organism.

Humans. The incubation period of glanders in humans can be as short as 1 to 5 days. Cases with apparent incubation periods of several months may have represented smoldering, unrecognized infection. The severity of disease can vary from mild to fatal, and the course can be acute and fulminant or chronic. Relapses can occur after quiescent periods of up to 10 years. As in horses, manifestations in humans usually involve the skin and respiratory tract. There may be pustular cutaneous eruptions, thick indurated lymphatics that may ulcerate, mucopurulent discharge from the eyes or nose, pneumonia, and metastatic abscesses in internal organs. Depending on the severity, the patient may have anorexia, fever, weight loss, headache, nausea, diarrhea, or septicemic shock. Lobar pneumonia, bronchopneumonia, or nodular densities may be seen on chest radiographs. Cases recently reported from Southeast Asia have been relatively mild, indicating that the local strain of the organism appears to have moderate pathogenicity for humans.

Diagnosis

Clinical diagnosis in horses based on symptoms can be confirmed by reaction to mallein with a cutaneous hypersensitivity test. Mallein, a filtrate derived from culture of the organism, is injected into the eyelid of a horse. A positive reaction, read 48 hours later, consists of marked local swelling and purulent conjunctivitis. Several serologic tests are also available. Complement fixation (CF) is often used. A dot-enzyme-linked immunosorbent assay is a more sensitive test.[218]

Clinical diagnosis in humans is based on compatible symptoms in an individual exposed to horses in an endemic area. The diagnosis can be confirmed by culture of the organism from lesions or by serologic testing, using CF or agglutination tests. Agglutination titers are often detectable by the second week of infection. The CF test is less sensitive but more specific than agglutination. CF tests become positive during the third week of infection.[174]

Laboratory diagnosis can be made by injection of infected material intraperitoneally into male guinea pigs or hamsters. The animals develop peritonitis that extends into the scrotal sac with severe inflammation, the Strauss reaction.

Pathology

In acute phases of the disease, abscessation occurs. Later the inflammatory focus is surrounded by a granulomatous reaction, but central karyorrhexis remains a prominent feature of the lesion. The lungs are the internal organs most typically involved (Figures 44-15 and 44-16), but septicemic glanders can involve liver, spleen, bone, or brain. With chronic infection, multiple subcutaneous and intramuscular abscesses may develop.

Treatment

Early studies indicated that sulfadiazine, 100 mg/kg/day in three divided doses given for 3 weeks, is effective. Treatment with tetracyclines and streptomycin is also recommended.[174] The organism is sensitive in vitro to sulfamethizole, sulfathiazole, trimethoprim-sulfamethoxazole, gentamicin, kanamycin, streptomycin, and tetracycline.[4] Ciprofloxacin and ofloxacin, but not norfloxacin, were found to be effective in treating experimentally infected guinea pigs and hamsters.[15] Therapy should be based on culture and sensitivity testing of isolates and on clinical response to treatment.

Prognosis

Acute untreated septicemic cases are almost uniformly fatal within 7 to 10 days.[174] The prognosis is better in chronic forms of the disease, which can last for years, but deaths are still likely without adequate treatment.

Prevention and Control

The only significant reservoir of infection in nature is equids. If the disease were eradicated in them, it would disappear. National programs should be instituted in

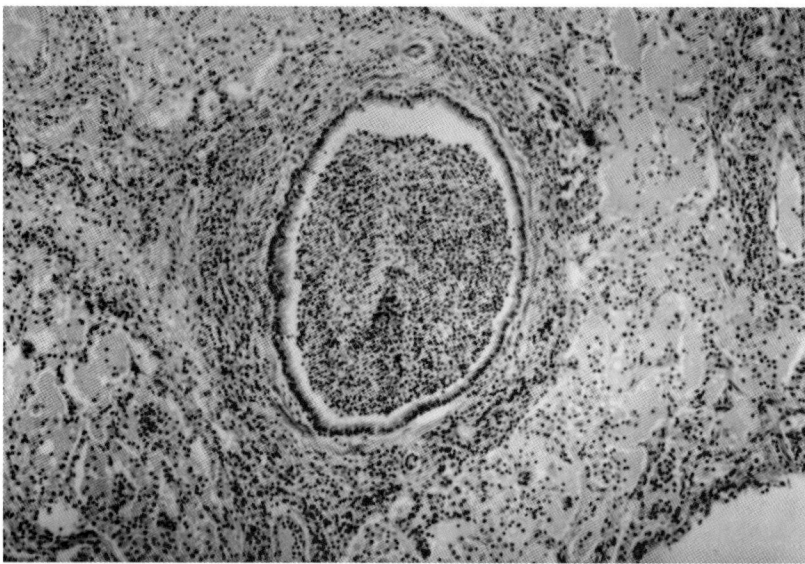

Figure 44-15 A bronchus filled and surrounded by pus in the lung of a horse with glanders. (Hematoxylin and eosin stain, original magnification 100×.)

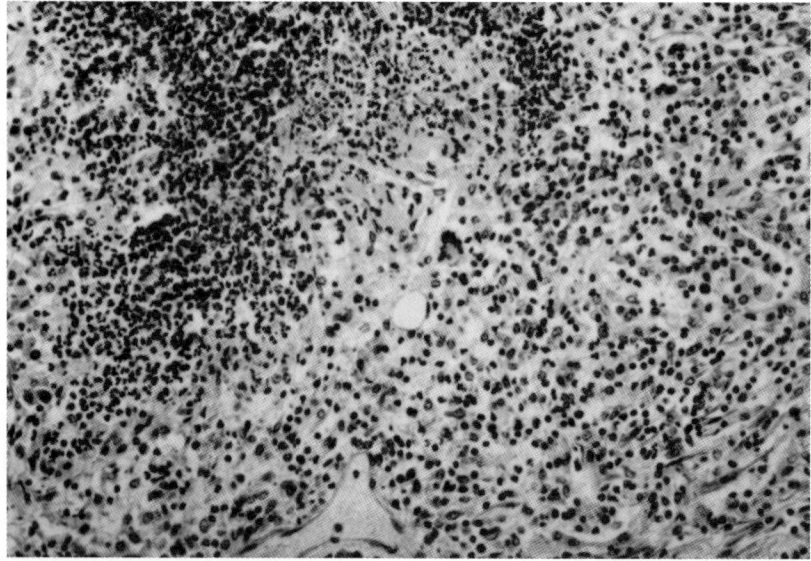

Figure 44-16 Gangrenous pneumonia with characteristic karyorrhexis in the lung of a horse with glanders. A multinucleated giant cell is in the center of the figure. (Hematoxylin and eosin stain, original magnification 250×.)

enzootic countries to eradicate the infection, by mallein or serologic tests of all horses, donkeys, and mules and slaughter of reactive animals. Persons who handle horses in enzootic countries, including trekkers who pack gear into the wilderness on these animals, should be advised of the signs of glanders in equids and warned to avoid contact with sick animals.

Glanders can be transmitted from one person to another, so strict infection control should be exercised with suspected infected patients. Personnel should avoid contact with all secretions and respiratory droplets. Transmission is also a risk in the laboratory, so if this organism is being cultured, all work should be done under appropriate microbiologic hoods.

MELIOIDOSIS

Melioidosis is an infection caused by the bacterium *Burkholderia* (formerly *Pseudomonas*) *pseudomallei*, which lives freely in soil and water.[234] Disease is spread from the environment to both humans and other animals. The causative agent and disease process in humans were first described by Whitmore and Krishnaswami[227] in Rangoon, Burma, in 1912.[131]

Bacteriology

B. pseudomallei is a bipolar, gram-negative, aerobic rod approximately 0.5 to 1 μm in width and 3 to 5 μm in length. It is readily grown on standard laboratory media at 37° C (98.6° F). After 48 to 72 hours of growth, distinctive wrinkled colonies with a "daisy head" appearance are formed. These give off a pungent, putrefactive odor.[130] The organism is oxidase positive and nonpyocyanogenic. It is resistant to colistin and gentamicin in vitro.[101] In 1992, Yabuuchi et al proposed that seven species formerly of *Pseudomonas* RNA group II should be transferred to a new genus, *Burkholderia*, with *B. cepacia* as the type species.[234]

Transmission and Epidemiology

Melioidosis is a saprozoonosis transmitted to animals and humans from the environment; transmission does not generally occur between living organisms. There is a singular case of presumed transmission by the venereal route.[152] Disease is reported much more often in adults than in children.

Most cases of melioidosis have been reported in areas between 20 degrees north and 20 degrees south of the equator.[100] A majority of cases have been reported from Southeast Asia and tropical Australia. The most heavily endemic areas include Myanmar (Burma), Malaya, Vietnam, Singapore, Cambodia, Thailand, Java, Borneo, New Guinea, and northern Australia. Occasional human and animal cases have been reported from Central India, Sri Lanka, Niger, Madagascar, Ecuador, Panama, Aruba, and Mexico. Cases from the Western Hemisphere have been reviewed.[12] *B. pseudomallei* survives during Australia's dry season in the clay layer of the soil, 25 to 30 cm below the surface, and can be brought to the surface and distributed by water seeping through this layer during the wet season.[101]

Clinical and subclinical infections occur in a variety of animals, most often sheep, goats, and swine. Infections in animals offer no direct threat to human health but are epidemiologic indicators that the organism is in a given geographic area.[100]

Transmission is thought to occur by direct percutaneous inoculation through wounds contaminated with soil or water, by ingestion, or by inhalation of infective droplets. A high incidence of pulmonary melioidosis in helicopter crew members in Vietnam was ascribed to inhalation of dust and aerosols raised by the helicopters operating in highly endemic areas.[100]

Symptoms

Most human infections are asymptomatic, as indicated by the high prevalence of seropositivity without clinical disease within endemic areas. Active disease is most likely to be seen in individuals with predisposing conditions, particularly diabetes mellitus, alcoholism, neoplasms, malnutrition, and various forms of immunodeficiency.

Clinical disease can occur in acute, subacute, or chronic forms. The lungs are the organs most frequently involved. Pulmonary melioidosis can mimic tuberculosis in that the upper lobes are most frequently involved, cough is productive, sputum often contains blood, and patients complain of chest pain and fever. However, calcifications in the lung and hilar lymph nodes typically seen in tuberculosis are rarely seen with melioidosis. An entire lobe or major segment of a lobe may be consolidated, and multiple pulmonary abscesses may be scattered in the lung parenchyma.

Septicemia can develop in the acute form of the disease and may mimic other forms of gram-negative sepsis in its manifestations. Multiple abscesses can form in skin, lungs, liver, spleen, kidney, and bone, but the CNS is rarely involved. Without treatment the case-fatality rate exceeds 90%.

In the subacute and chronic forms of disease, abscesses can form in internal organs and may drain through sinus tracts.

Melioidosis has been referred to as a "medical time bomb" because infection can lie dormant for months or years, only to become manifest when resistance is lowered. An incubation period as long as 26 years has been reported.[148] The infection should be suspected in anyone with a compatible clinical picture, including fever of unknown origin, who has resided in an endemic area.

Diagnosis

The only definitive diagnostic procedure is culture of the organism from blood, bone marrow, sputum, pus, or infected tissue. Several serologic tests are available but are not reliable, because many individuals from endemic areas have antibodies to the organism without any evidence of clinical disease. An indirect hemagglutination antibody titer of 1:40 or greater is considered compatible with infection, as is a CF titer of 1:10 or greater. Rising titers by IgM indirect FA are probably the best immunologic indication of infection.

No pathognomonic lesions are seen histologically. The abscesses consist of central areas of necrosis without unique or distinctive features permitting definitive histopathologic diagnosis.

Treatment

Combinations of antibiotics have been used, almost always including chloramphenicol, 40 mg/kg/day in adults and 50 to 75 mg/kg/day in children.[164] Even with combination therapy, however, mortality can reach 80% in disseminated septicemic melioidosis. Tetracycline is also used in adults and in children over 8 years of age, 50 mg/kg/day in four divided doses six times a day orally. Kanamycin, 15 to 20 mg/kg/day in two divided doses intramuscularly, and amikacin, 15 to 20 mg/kg/day in two divided doses every 12 hours intramuscularly, have also been recommended for treatment. Co-trimoxazole may prove useful, but experience is too limited. The antibiotic treatment should be given for several weeks in acute cases and for approximately 6 months in chronic cases. Dosage of kanamycin and amikacin should be modified appropriately if there is renal impairment.

Ceftazidine has largely replaced combination antibiotic therapy and is now generally recognized as the drug of choice.[227] It has reduced mortality in disseminated septicemic melioidosis to 35% to 40%.[130]

In vitro sensitivity tests do not always correlate with clinical response to antibiotics. Therapy must be given at sufficient dosage and long enough to avoid recurrence of infection and emergence of resistant organisms.

Prevention and Control

In the field, prevention consists of avoiding ingestion or inhalation of potentially infective soil or water. Wounds, burns, and other injuries should be thoroughly cleaned to avoid infection through contamination. No evidence exists that transmission is likely to occur from person to person, so isolation of hospitalized patients is not necessary. Reasonable care and precautions should be taken in handling purulent drainage of blood, sputum, and other materials from patients with melioidosis.

TRICHINOSIS

Trichinosis is an infection caused by nematodes in the genus *Trichinella*. In the past, only one species, *T. spiralis*, was recognized. Isoenzyme and DNA analysis indicate that the genus is polyspecific.[171] Eight gene pools, T_1 through T_8, have been identified. T_1 is classic *T. spiralis*; the principal reservoir is in domestic swine, but some wild animals can also be infected. T_2, *T. nativa*, is found primarily in terrestrial mammals such as the bear, walrus, or fox in Arctic and sub-Arctic regions. Most human infections are caused by T_1, fewer by T_2. Relatively few data are available on how frequently the other species infect people. T_3 occurs in bears (Ursidae), T_7 and T_8 in African Hyenidae and Felidae. Only T_4, *T. pseudospiralis*, can infect mammals and birds.

Unless stated otherwise, the rest of this discussion relates to trichinosis generically or to *T. spiralis* specifically.

Trichinella cysts were first noticed by Paget during an anatomic dissection in 1836 when distinct white lesions were found throughout a muscle specimen. The association of the encysted organism and the ingestion of contaminated meat was not made until 1850. In 1862 Friedreich diagnosed and described the first clinical case of acute trichinosis. Outbreaks in Germany in 1849 and 1865 were associated with mortality rates of 19% and 30%, respectively. Examination

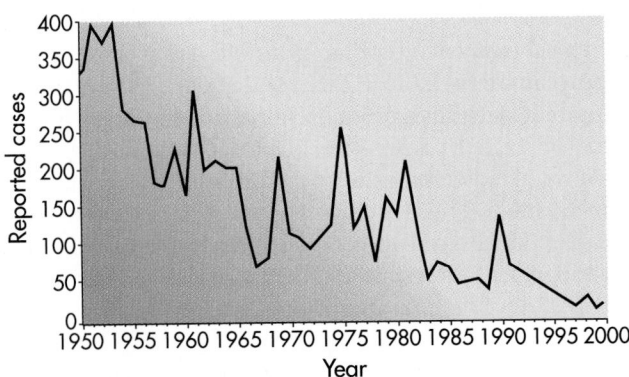

Figure 44-17 Reported cases of trichinosis in the United States, 1950 to 1999. (*Modified from MMWR 40, No. 53, 1991.*)

of diaphragmatic muscle samples in the United States between 1936 and 1941 revealed *Trichinella* organisms in 1 out of every 6 samples tested (16.7%). National reporting of trichinellosis began in 1947. The incidence of this disease has decreased significantly over time due to the passage of legislation prohibiting the feeding of raw sewage to swine (Federal Swine Health Protection Act of 1980), widespread freezing of pork, and increasing public awareness of the dangers of eating inadequately cooked pork products (Figure 44-17).

Life Cycle

The life cycle is unusual in that every host is necessarily both a definitive host, harboring the adult stage of the parasite, and an intermediate host, harboring the larval stage.

The infection is acquired by ingestion of larvae encysted in skeletal muscle. The worms mature within a few days in the small intestine. The female burrows into the mucosa and deposits larvae in the tissue, starting around the fifth day after infection. Most larvae are deposited within 4 weeks, but they can be produced for as long as 4 months. The larvae enter the circulation and invade skeletal muscle within 7 to 14 days (Figure 44-18). They become encapsulated around day 21 after infection and are then infective for the next host that ingests them.

Epidemiology

All carnivorous and omnivorous mammals are susceptible to trichinosis, but most human infections are acquired by eating raw or undercooked pork. Game animals can harbor the parasite. Trichinosis was found in 1.3% of black bears in New England.[104] It can infect other species of bears, raccoons, opossums, seals, walruses, peccaries, and wild swine.

Rodents, such as mice and rats, are commonly infected in nature. Except in certain cultures, these small

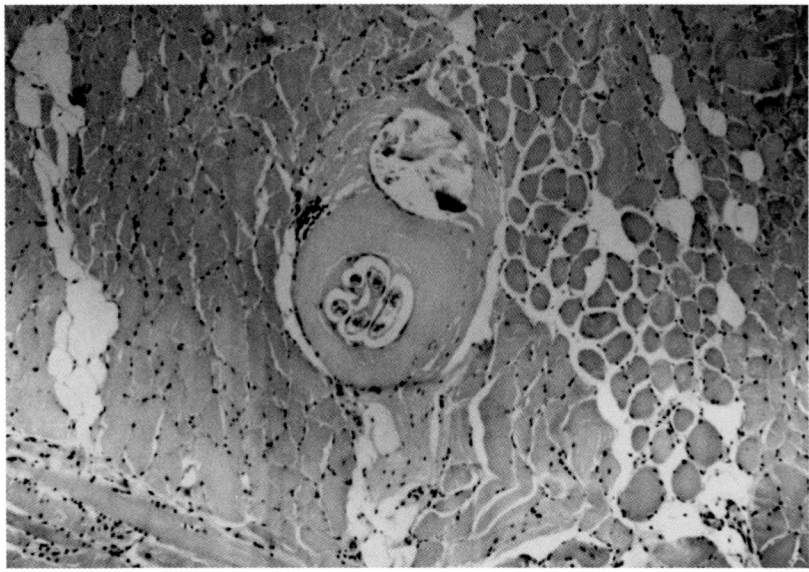

Figure 44-18 Trichinosis in a polar bear. A larva is seen within a muscle fiber in the center of the picture. The parasite found in Arctic mammals is highly resistant to freezing and has been given a separate species status, *Trichinella nativa*. (Hematoxylin and eosin stain, original magnification 100×.)

rodents are rarely eaten by people, unlike their larger cousins, squirrels, woodchucks, muskrats, agoutis, and capybaras. These larger rodents are primarily herbivorous but can still be an occasional source of human infection.

Although experimentally susceptible to trichinosis, herbivores, such as members of the deer and antelope families, are almost never infected naturally, and consumption of their flesh is not associated with this infection. Interestingly, some outbreaks of trichinosis have occurred in people who consumed horseflesh.[51] The horses could have become infected by consuming mice, dead or alive, in their feed. Alternatively, larvae passed in the stool of infected rodents could have been ingested in the horses' grain or hay.

Swine that are privately raised and slaughtered are a continuing source of human infections in many areas, including the northeastern United States.[10] Bears, walruses, and feral swine have been the principal nondomestic sources of trichinosis in the United States.[149] From 1991 to 1996, three deaths in 230 cases were reported to the CDC (average of 38 cases per year), including 14 multiple case outbreaks from 31 states and Washington, D.C. Information on the suspected food item was available for 134 (58%) of the 230 reported cases. Pork was implicated in 80 (60%) cases, bear meat in 31 (23%), walrus meat in 13 (10%), and cougar meat in 10 (7%). Sausage was the most frequently implicated pork product (i.e., 57 of the 64 cases for which the form of the pork product was identified).[154] Wild boars are a source of infections in Germany.[108]

Twenty-six cases of trichinosis reported in the United States from 1975 to 1989 were acquired during foreign travel. Seventeen of these persons had traveled to Mexico or Asia.[150]

Symptoms

The signs and symptoms of trichinosis are closely related to the activities of the parasite in its life cycle. The severity of disease is proportional to the number of adult and larval worms present. GI symptoms predominate during the first week after ingestion of infected meat. The worms mate and invade the intestinal mucosa during the first 48 hours. The female worm is capable of producing up to 1500 larvae during her lifetime. Larvae are deposited starting on approximately the fifth day after ingestion. This activity results in irritation of the bowel, with nausea, vomiting, variable diarrhea, and abdominal pain. Fever may occur. These symptoms are often mistaken for various forms of food poisoning. GI symptoms may continue until the females are cleared from the intestinal tract at approximately 4 to 6 weeks after infection.

Larval production reaches a peak during the second week after infection. The larvae start to invade skeletal muscle as early as the seventh day. During larval migration, direct capillary damage occurs, resulting in facial edema, especially involving the periorbital area, which may be accompanied by photophobia, blurred vision, diplopia, and complaints of pain on moving the eyes. Splinter hemorrhages may appear in the nailbeds, and there may be cutaneous petechiae. Hemorrhagic lesions can also occur in the conjunctivae and retinae. The temperature may reach 40.5° C (105° F).

Eosinophils start to increase in peripheral blood during the second week, often exceeding 20% of the total white blood cell count after the third week of infection.

The eosinophil count returns to normal from 6 to 12 months after infection. GI symptoms may continue during this period, until the females are cleared from the intestinal tract approximately 4 to 6 weeks after infection. During the second phase of infection, migrating larvae can cause pulmonary damage, resulting in cough, dyspnea, and pleuritic pain. There may be hemoptysis. Myocarditis can occur and may be life threatening. Damage to the brain or meninges by migrating larvae can cause encephalitic or meningitic symptoms. A spinal tap may reveal eosinophils in CSF. The third phase of infection is encystment of the larvae within skeletal muscle, starting about the second or third week after infection. This can cause significant myalgias and stiffness in affected muscle groups. The final phase of infection occurs as the larvae die and become calcified. This is a period of convalescence, which is usually asymptomatic, and typically occurs between 6 and 18 months after infection.

Trichinosis in the Inuit population of northeastern Canada, associated with eating raw walrus, is characterized by prolonged diarrhea and brief muscle symptoms. High peripheral eosinophilia and high *Trichinella* antibody titers occur. The disease is probably caused by *T. nativa,* and at least some cases may be associated with reinfection.[136]

Diagnosis

Larvae are sometimes passed in the stool in the early stages of infection, but this occurs infrequently and inconsistently and cannot be used for diagnosis.

Trichinosis is definitively diagnosed by biopsy of the gastrocnemius muscle or of clinically affected (painful, tender) muscles. The larvae are demonstrable in muscle beginning about the seventh day after infection. Diagnosis can also be made serologically, using the bentonite flocculation test (BFT), latex particle agglutination, or countercurrent immunoelectrophoresis. The BFT involves a suspension of aluminum silicate particles (bentonite) to which *Trichinella* antigen is bound and incubated with dilutions of serum from the patient. All these tests usually do not become positive until 3 to 4 weeks after infection. Newer ELISA tests are available that measure reaction by different immunoglobulin classes. Most ELISA tests offer greater specificity and sensitivity and become positive earlier than many of the other tests.[9,189,217] An ELISA IgG test, using the excretory-secretory antigen of *T. spiralis* larvae, had specificity and sensitivity of 100% at days 57 and 120 after infection but was negative at day 23.[138] An experimental "dissociated enhanced lanthanide fluoroimmunoassay" (DELFIA) can detect as little as 1 ng of antigen/ml of serum. Circulating antigen was detected in mice as early as 7 days after infection.[125]

Treatment

No satisfactory, safe, and effective drug is available for elimination of larvae, which are responsible for most of the pathologic changes and symptoms of trichinosis. Thiabendazole (25 mg/kg twice a day for 5 days, maximum 3 g/day) is effective against adult worms in the intestine. Its efficacy against larvae is questionable, however, and it can cause serious side effects, such as fever, increased edema, and myocarditis.[123] Mebendazole (200 to 400 mg three times a day for 3 days, then 400 to 500 mg three times a day for 10 days) is better tolerated,[160] but poor intestinal absorption reduces its use in extraintestinal trichinellosis. Albendazole or flubendazole are well absorbed and may be more effective, but the supporting data are scarce.

Steroids (e.g., prednisone, 30 to 60 mg/day orally for 10 to 30 days) can be given for relief of severe illness, such as myocarditis caused by migrating larvae.[123] The dose and duration of treatment are individually determined by clinical response. Steroids reduce the inflammatory response to larvae but can also interfere with rejection of adult females in the intestine, thus prolonging the period of larva deposition.

Prevention

Trichinosis is prevented by cooking meat to an internal temperature of 65.6° to 77° C (150° to 170° F). Most *Trichinella* larvae are killed by freezing. The time required depends on the thickness of the meat and the freezing temperature. Holding meat at −15° C (5° F) for 20 days, −23.3° C (−10° F) for 10 days, or −28.9° C (−20° F) for only 6 days is recommended. Salting, drying, and smoking are not always effective. Note that *T. nativa* found in Arctic mammals (Figure 44-18) is resistant to freezing.

CAT-SCRATCH DISEASE

Cat-scratch disease (CSD) is transmitted through a break in the skin (bite, scratch, or other injury) caused by a cat. First recognized by Robert Debre at the University of Paris in 1931, the disease was not officially reported until 1951. CSD is relatively rare but is probably the most common cause of unilateral lymph-adenopathy in children.[205] The current etiology of CSD is thought to be the gram-negative rod, *Bartonella henselae.*[33]

Epidemiology

About 90% of cases are caused by scratches from cats, but dog and monkey bites, as well as thorns and splinters, have also been implicated.[71] The organism may be on the claws or in the oral cavity of the offending cat. Most cases occur in children, particularly boys who tend to play more aggressively with domestic animals. CSD has been reported from all countries and in all races. An estimated 24,000 cases are recognized each year in the United States.[144] Patients are more likely than healthy cat-owning control subjects to have at least one kitten 12 months of age or younger, to have been scratched or bitten by a kitten, and to have at least one kitten with fleas.[236]

Symptoms

The average incubation period is 3 to 10 days. The characteristic feature of CSD is regional lymphadenitis, usually involving lymph nodes of the arm or leg. In one series, 54% of lymphadenopathy occurred in the axilla, with the remainder in the neck.[205] Often only one node is involved. The nodes are often painful and tender, and about 25% suppurate.[222] Adenopathy may spread proximally; occasionally, cervical adenopathy is mistaken for Hodgkin's disease. In most cases a characteristic raised, erythematous, slightly tender, and nonpruritic papule with a small central vesicle or eschar that resembles an insect bite is seen at the site of primary inoculation. Constitutional symptoms are mild, with approximately two thirds of patients manifesting fever, which is rarely greater than 38.8° C (102° F). Chills, malaise, anorexia, and nausea are common. Infrequent evanescent morbilliform and pleomorphic skin rashes lasting for 48 hours or less have been reported. This typical clinical course occurs in 88% of victims; the remainder seek medical treatment for complications such as encephalopathy, atypical pneumonia, and severe systemic disease. Parinaud's oculoglandular syndrome of granulomatous conjunctivitis and an ipsilateral, enlarged, tender preauricular lymph node occurs in about 6% of cases.[142]

Serious complications are rare and include encephalitis, seizures, transverse myelitis, osteolytic bone lesions, arthritis, splenic abscess, mediastinal adenopathy, optic neuritis, and thrombocytopenic purpura.[32,142,156,167] Although encephalopathy is rare, CSD is becoming a more common cause of encephalopathy as other viral infectious diseases disappear; the incidence of CSD-associated neurologic complications now ranks with those of varicella and herpes simplex infections, Lyme disease, Rocky Mountain spotted fever, and Kawasaki disease.[37] CSD encephalopathy should enter the differential diagnosis of patients (especially young ones) with unexplained coma or seizures (half of whom may be afebrile). The prognosis of encephalopathy generally is good.

Diagnosis

Results of routine laboratory studies, including urinalysis and complete blood cell count, are usually normal, although mild leukocytosis may be seen. An indirect FA test to *B. henselae* is now commercially available.

Immunity is thought to be largely cell mediated.[97] An intradermal skin test of 0.1 ml of CSD antigen is positive in approximately 95% of victims, although 10% of the population has a false-positive reaction. In confusing cases, biopsy of lymph nodes can yield characteristic findings of areas of granulomatous change and necrosis with central neutrophilic infiltration, a peripheral zone of histiocytic cells, and an outermost zone infiltrated by small lymphocytes and plasma cells.[141] This picture is not diagnostic, however, and is also seen in lymphogranuloma venereum (LGV), histoplasmosis, tularemia, brucellosis, sarcoidosis, and tuberculosis.

Thus lymph node biopsy is most useful to rule out malignancy. Warthin-Starry or Brown-Hopps staining of the nodes or the primary skin lesion usually demonstrates the small, pleomorphic bacilli.[142]

In most cases, clinical diagnosis is based on finding three of four criteria: (1) single or regional lymphadenopathy without obvious signs of cutaneous or throat infection, (2) contact with a cat (usually an immature one), (3) detection of an inoculation site, and (4) a positive skin test.[39]

The workup should exclude other causes of regional lymphadenopathy, such as tuberculosis, tularemia, LGV, lymphoma, brucellosis, and sporotrichosis.[190] In general, only sporotrichosis and LGV demonstrate localized unilateral lymphadenopathy; LGV usually occurs in the groin. Cat scratches are normally found on the upper extremities. Skin tests, cultures, serologic tests, and biopsies are available for the differentiation of these other diseases.

Treatment

CSD usually resolves spontaneously in weeks to months, although in 2% of persons (usually adults) the course is prolonged and involves systemic complications.[142] Systemic CSD in an adult has been successfully treated with gentamicin[133] and in a child with cefuroxime.[96] Trimethoprim/sulfamethoxazole was used in a retrospective series of 71 patients with good results; this was not the case with other antibiotics.[66] The best study, of 202 patients, is also retrospective, but found a response rate of 87% with rifampin, 84% with ciprofloxacin, 73% with IM gentamicin, and 58% with trimethoprim/sulfamethoxazole.[143] Antibiotics that were of no benefit included amoxicillin-clavulanate, erythromycin, dicloxacillin, cephalexin, tetracycline, cefaclor, ceftriaxone, and cefotaxime.

Antibiotics should be reserved for persons with severe or very prolonged disease.[143] Symptomatic treatment and reassurance that the prognosis is excellent are the best therapies. No sequelae of CSD other than the rare complications mentioned are known.

BACILLARY ANGIOMATOSIS

Bacillary angiomatosis was first described in 1983 during the early years of the acquired immunodeficiency syndrome (AIDS) epidemic and forced a reconsideration of CSD, bartonellosis, and trench fever.[208] In the early 1990s it was determined that organisms of the genus *Rochalimaea* caused a diverse array of clinical syndromes, including cutaneous bacillary angiomatosis, bacillary peliosis hepatitis, fever with bacteremia (*Rochalimaea* bacteremic syndrome) and CSD. Whether the different clinical syndromes result from subtle differences in the infecting organisms or in the response of the immune system remains unclear. Each of these conditions can be caused by the bacteria now known to be *Bartonella* (formerly *Rochalimaea*) *henselae* and *B. quintana,* also the agent of trench fever.

Epidemiology

Although clinically different from CSD, bacillary angiomatosis is also closely associated with recent cat scratch or bite. The vast majority of victims are HIV positive, but a few are not and appear otherwise well. In 34% of cases, this infection was the first one to establish the diagnosis of AIDS in a given patient. AIDS patients with bacillary angiomatosis can die if untreated, but erythromycin is usually effective.[23]

Symptoms

Most cases of bacillary angiomatosis involve cutaneous or subcutaneous lesions. The lesions are typically elevated, friable, red granulation tissue papules resembling pyogenic granulomas, numbering a few to thousands. Deeper subcutaneous nodules are seen in about half of victims. Similar lesions can occur in other body tissues.[23] Visceral lesions may be the first sign of infection; patients often have fever, weight loss, and malaise.[75] Hepatic involvement can lead to hepatic failure or even rupture (bacillary peliosis hepatitis). This usually presents with GI symptoms (nausea, vomiting, diarrhea, or abdominal distention), fever, chills, and hepatosplenomegaly. Histopathologic examination of liver biopsy specimens reveals dilated capillaries or multiple blood-filled cavernous spaces. The organism can also cause bacteremia, even in immunocompetent patients. *Rochalimaea* bacteremic syndrome is characterized by a prolonged symptom complex of malaise, fatigue, anorexia, weight loss, and recurring, ever-increasing fevers.[14,20,22] No site of focal infection is apparent. The symptoms are usually present for weeks to months before the diagnosis is finally made by isolation of the organism in blood cultures.[203]

Diagnosis

B. henselae and *B. quintana* can be isolated from blood using lysis-centrifugation blood cultures,[13,14,29] but both species have also been isolated with traditional blood culture systems.

Serologic diagnosis can also be made using techniques of indirect FA testing. Serum samples can be sent (for both *B. henselae* and *B. quintana*) to the CDC. An enzyme immunoassay for the detection of IgG antibodies to *B. henselae* is now commercially available and is reportedly 5 to 10 times more sensitive than the indirect FA test.[76] Positive results should be interpreted cautiously, taking into account the clinical context, since the meaning of positive serologic results awaits further evaluation with stricter epidemiologic methods.

Diagnosis of bacillary angiomatosis is usually made from clinical features and biopsies of lesions, with characteristic histopathologic findings in tissue sections.

Blood cultures should be obtained and incubated for a prolonged period. As more is learned about the growth requirements of the causative organisms, they may become easier to culture directly from skin lesions and lymph nodes. Serologic analysis will become an important means of diagnosis.[1]

Treatment

Treatment is with erythromycin. If patients cannot tolerate this therapy, rifampin and doxycycline or trimethoprim-sulfamethoxazole should be given. Norfloxacin, gentamicin, and ciprofloxacin are also clinically effective.[195] Penicillin and first-generation cephalosporins are not beneficial. Therapy is for a minimum of 6 weeks and may have to continue indefinitely in an immunosuppressed patient.

COWPOX AND CATPOX INFECTION

Poxviruses are large DNA viruses that are implicated in a variety of human diseases, including smallpox, monkeypox, cowpox, catpox, and molluscum contagiosum. Infection is rare because of the history of smallpox immunization. Vaccinia virus results in a local skin lesion after "vaccination" against smallpox. Because this immunization provides cross-protection against other poxviruses, cases of monkeypox, cowpox, catpox, and other infections will now increase, since smallpox has been eradicated and immunization is no longer recommended.[219]

Cowpox has been reevaluated because new epidemiologic evidence suggests that cowpox is not enzootic in cattle, that the cow has a minor role, that feline cowpox is important as a source of human infection, and that wildlife, principally rodents, are virus reservoirs.[16] Although poxvirus infection in the domestic cat has only recently been described, the incidence has increased steadily, and cats are now the most frequently reported hosts of poxvirus in Britain.[219] The infection occurs mostly among hunting cats in the late summer and early autumn; infection in humans usually is reported after close contact with or a scratch from a sick cat. The infection is manifested as an inflamed vesicular nodule with lymphadenitis, systemic symptoms (e.g., fever) and a rapid but self-limited course, similar to the orf poxvirus carried by sheep, cattle, and goats. This disease has not yet been reported in immunosuppressed persons. No effective treatment is available, but normally the disease is self-limited.

RAT-BITE FEVER

Rat-bite fever is an acute illness caused by either *Streptobacillus moniliformis* or *Spirillum minus,* which are part of the normal oral flora of rodents, including squirrels. It may also result from bites by wild and domestic carnivores, such as weasels, dogs, cats, and pigs, which may have been infected when hunting rats and mice.[199] Carrier rates among wild rats vary from none to 50%.[28,212] Fewer than 70 cases have been reported in North America, with at least half caused by *S. monili-formis* in laboratory workers. At least 10%, and up to 100%, of rats are nasopharyngeal carriers of *Strepto-bacillus*.[5,49,98] Victims of disease caused by *S. minus* are primarily children of lower socioeconomic groups with poor sanitation and heavy rodent populations.[153] Rare cases can occur in any setting and can easily be fatal, particularly when the proper diagnosis is not suspected.[153]

Streptobacillary Type

Streptobacillary rat-bite fever (Haverhill fever) is caused by *S. moniliformis,* an aerobic, nonmotile, gram-negative bacillus. The onset usually occurs within a week of the bite, but the incubation period may extend to several weeks, during which time the original wound usually heals completely. A bite need not be present, since the disease can also be transmitted by contaminated food, milk, or water.[93] It has also been transmitted by simply playing with pet rats, with no history of bite or injury.[181] Initial symptoms include fever, chills, cough, malaise, headache, and less frequently, local lymphadenitis. These are followed by a nonpruritic morbilliform or petechial rash, which frequently involves the palms and soles. Migratory polyarthritis develops in approximately 50% of victims. Generalized lymphadenitis may be present; splenomegaly and hepatomegaly are rare.[212] 25% of victims have a false-positive Venereal Disease Research Laboratories (VDRL) test. Leukocytosis with left shift is common, and agglutinating antibodies for the bacillus appear during the course of the disease. On autopsy, interstitial pneumonia, fibrinous endocarditis, mononuclear meningitis, hepatosplenomegaly, and mononuclear cell infiltrates in regional lymph nodes have been found.[198]

When a history of animal bite is lacking, the differential diagnosis must include rickettsial and viral infections. The fever and rash may suggest meningococcemia, but meningeal signs are lacking in rat-bite fever. Definitive diagnosis requires demonstration of rising antibody titers or culture of the bacillus from the blood, joint fluid, pustules, or original bite location. This can present a difficult differential diagnosis. Typically, identification by culture requires experienced laboratory workers who are seeking the organism.

Untreated, the disease runs a course of several weeks; prolongation of symptoms should raise the suspicion for endocarditis. The mortality in untreated persons is 10%, with most deaths caused by endocarditis and pneumonia. Although mortality is low, the disease can be fulminant; an infant bitten by a wild rat died 4

days after the bite and 2 days after the onset of symptoms.[198] The drug of choice is procaine penicillin, 600,000 units intramuscularly twice a day for 7 to 10 days.[212] Effective alternatives for penicillin-allergic patients are tetracycline, 30 mg/kg/day orally in four divided doses, or streptomycin, 15 mg/kg/day intramuscularly in two divided doses. Erythromycin is not effective. Complications such as endocarditis should be treated with high-dose intravenous potassium penicillin G, 10 to 20 million units a day. The organism has both a bacillary and a cell wall–deficient L phase, which is thought to account for some of the antibiotic failures. The bacterial phase responds to penicillin, streptomycin, and tetracycline, whereas the L phase is resistant to penicillin.[198]

Spirillar Type

Spirillar rat-bite fever is caused by *Spirillum minus,* a gram-negative, tightly coiled, spirillar microorganism. It is usually transmitted by infected wild rats, although cats have also been implicated. The general setting of socioeconomic deprivation in which this disease occurs is the same as in the streptobacillary form; cases in laboratory animals are unusual. The incubation period is 7 to 21 days, during which the bite lesion heals. The onset of illness is heralded by chills, fever, lymphadenitis, and a dark-red macular rash. Myalgias are common, but arthritis is absent, which helps in the differentiation from streptobacillary fever. Leukocytosis and a false-positive VDRL test are often present. The disease is episodic and relapsing, with a 24- to 72-hour cycle. The differential diagnosis includes rickettsial and viral diseases when the history of animal bite is not present. In addition to the absence of arthritis, the manifestations at the bite site are more pronounced than in the streptobacillary variety (usually involving lymphadenitis, and still present when systemic illness occurs), and the fever and illness are relapsing in nature.[212] Definitive diagnosis rests on demonstrating the presence of *S. minus* in a darkfield preparation of exudate from an infected site. The patient's blood can be inoculated into mice, which may be tested for subsequent infection. The mortality from untreated disease is considerably lower than for streptobacillary fever. The untreated course spans several months. Antibiotic therapy is the same as for streptobacillary fever.[98]

BRUCELLOSIS

Brucellosis is an anthropozoonotic disease with a broad clinical spectrum caused by a number of species of *Brucella,* a small, gram-negative bacterium. The bacterium can survive in soil for up to 10 weeks, in goat cheese for up to 180 days (at 4° to 8° C [39.2° to 46.4° F]), and in tap water up to 60 days. It is however very sensitive to heat, most disinfectants, and entirely killed by pasteurization. Brucellosis usually results from the ingestion of contaminated milk or milk products or by direct skin contact. *Brucella* organisms are carried chiefly by swine, cattle, goats, and sheep and may be recovered from almost all tissues in a sick patient. Most animals used as livestock are susceptible to brucellosis, while the occurrence in wild animals is rather small.[147]

Epidemiology

Brucella in domesticated animals tends to be species specific, with *B. abortus* infecting cattle, *B. melitensis* goats, *B. suis* swine, *B. canis* dogs, and *B. ovis* sheep. The disease is found worldwide and has an annual attack rate of approximately 500,000; U.S. cases number less than 200. Internationally, most cases are transmitted by ingestion of fresh, nonpasteurized goat cheese and raw goat's milk. The disease caused by *B. melitensis* has a higher attack rate and is more severe, whereas brucellosis in the United States is usually caused by *B. abortus* from cattle, which produces mild clinical disease and is usually occupationally acquired. A proven case of transmission by dog bite has been reported, and dogs carry their own pathogenic species.[176]

Symptoms

Many organ systems may be involved, with a wide range of disease severity and acuity.[70] The disease can be classified into three forms: acute, subacute, and chronic. In "acute" brucellosis, the victims complain of headache, weakness, diaphoresis, myalgias, and arthralgias. This is the most common presentation. Anorexia, constipation, and weight loss are often seen in the first 3 to 4 weeks. Physical examination reveals hepatomegaly and splenomegaly. Bacteremia in the early stages typically induces lesions of the viscera, bones, and joints; osteomyelitis, particularly spondylitis, is a common complication.

In *subacute,* or *undulant,* brucellosis, symptoms are milder, but with more frequent arthritis and orchitis. The clinical picture is more varied, and the diagnosis considered in any "fever of undetermined origin." In the preantibiotic era, most patients spontaneously cleared their disease in 6 to 12 months.

In chronic brucellosis, symptoms have persisted for more than 1 year. It is rare in children, but increasingly common as the patient ages. Many describe arthralgias and extraarticular rheumatism. Chronic brucellosis can mimic chronic fatigue syndrome.

Diagnosis

Brucellosis is most often diagnosed by serologic testing, including rose bengal, immunofluorescence, CFT, and ELISA.[135] After acute infection, high titers may persist for 18 months. False-positive results may be caused by *Francisella tularensis* or *Yersinia enterocolitica* infection. The isolation of *Brucella* organisms by blood culture is also used for definitive diagnosis. Blood cultures in 10% carbon dioxide is a common method, with sensitivities of 50% to 80%.[11] Bone marrow biopsy and culture can be used in patients with clinically suspected brucellosis, but negative serologic tests and blood cultures.

Treatment

Oral tetracycline, 50 mg/kg/day in four divided doses for 21 days, is used to treat brucellosis. Doxycycline may also be used. In severe cases, streptomycin, 20 to 40 mg/kg intramuscularly once a day for 1 week, is added to this regimen. The next week, streptomycin is continued at a level of 15 mg/kg. Alternatively, rifampin can be added to doxycycline.[67] The role of quinolones has been investigated.[3] The prognosis is generally excellent, with only two deaths reported in several thousand cases.[94]

ACKNOWLEDGMENT

I thank Leonard Marcus for his fine work on a previous version of this chapter.

REFERENCES

1. Adal KA, Cockerell CJ, Petri WA Jr: Cat scratch disease, bacillary angiomatosis, and other infections due to Rochalimaea, *N Engl J Med* 330:1509, 1994.
2. Ai NV et al: Co-trimoxazole in bubonic plague, *BMJ* 4:108, 1973.
3. Akova M et al: Quinolones in treatment of human brucellosis: comparative trial of ofloxacin-rifampin versus doxycycline-rifampin, *Antimicrob Agents Chemother* 37:1831, 1993.
4. Al-Izz SA, Al Bassam LS: In vitro susceptibility of *Pseudomonas mallei* to antimicrobial agents, *Compar Immunol Microbiol Infect Dis* 12:5, 1989.
5. Anderson L, Leart S, Manning P: Rat-bite fever in animal research laboratory personnel, *J Clin Microbiol* 7:223, 1978.
6. Anderson LJ et al: Human rabies in the United States, 1960 to 1979: epidemiology, diagnosis and prevention, *Ann Intern Med* 100:728, 1984.
7. Andrew ED, Marrocco GR: Leptospirosis in New England, *JAMA* 238:2027, 1977.
8. Arko RJ, Schneider LG, Baer GM: Non-fatal canine rabies, *Am J Vet Res* 34:937, 1973.
9. Au ACS et al: Study of acute trichinosis in Ghurkas: specificity and sensitivity of enzyme-linked immunosorbent assays for IgM and IgE antibodies to *Trichinella* larval antigens in diagnosis, *Trans R Soc Trop Med Hyg* 77:412, 1983.
10. Bailey TM, Schantz PM: Trends in the incidence and transmission patterns of trichinosis in humans in the United States: comparisons of the periods 1975-1981 and 1982-1986, *Rev Infect Dis* 12:5, 1990.
11. Bannatyne RM, Jackson MC, Memish Z: Rapid diagnosis of Brucella bacteremia by using the BACTEC 9240 system, *J Clin Microbiol* 35:2673, 1997.
12. Barnes PF, Appleman MD, Cosgrove MM: A case of melioidosis originating in North America, *Am Rev Respir Dis* 134:170, 1986.
13. Barry A: Clinical specimens for microbiologic exams. In Hubbert W, McCulloch W, Schnurrenberger P, editors: *Diseases transmitted from animals to man*, ed 6, Springfield, Ill, 1975, Charles C Thomas.
14. Barss P, Ennis S: Injuries caused by pigs in Papua New Guinea, *Med J Aust* 149:649, 1988.
15. Batmanov VP: Sensitivity of *Pseudomonas mallei* to fluoroquinolones and their efficacy in experimental glanders (Russian), *Antibiot Khimioter* 36:31, 1991.
16. Baxby D, Bennett M: Cowpox: a re-evaluation of the risks of human cowpox basel on new epidemiological information, *Arch Virol Suppl* 13:1, 1997.
17. Beck AM: The epidemiology of animal bite: compendium on continuing education, *Practice Vet* 3:254, 1981.
18. Bell JF: Tularemia. In Steele JH, editor: *Handbook series in zoonoses, section A: bacterial, rickettsial and mycotic diseases*, vol 2, Boca Raton, Fla, 1980, CRC Press.

19. Bell JF et al: Non-fatal rabies in an enzootic area: results of a survey and evaluation of techniques, *Am J Epidemiol* 95:190, 1972.
20. Bentley DW: Vaccinations, *Clin Geriatr Med* 8:745, 1992.
21. Beran GW: Rabies and infections by rabies-related viruses. In Steele JH, editor: *Handbook series in zoonoses, section B: viral zoonoses,* vol 2, Boca Raton, Fla, 1981, CRC Press.
22. Bergamini T et al: Combined topical and systemic antibiotic prophylaxis in experimental wound infection, *Am J Surg* 147:753, 1984.
23. Berger TG, Perkocha LA: Bacillary angiomatosis, *AIDS Clin Rev* 8:81, 1991.
24. Bernard KW, Fishbein DB: Rabies virus. In Mandell GL, Douglas RG, Bennett JE, editors: *Principles and practice of infectious diseases,* ed 3, New York, 1990, Churchill Livingstone.
25. Bernard KW et al: Neuroparalytic illness and human diploid cell rabies vaccine, *JAMA* 248:3136, 1982.
26. Bernard KW et al: Pre-exposure rabies immunization with human diploid cell vaccine: decreased antibody responses in persons immunized in developing countries, *Am J Trop Med* 34:633, 1985.
27. Bernard KW et al: Pre-exposure immunization with intradermal human diploid cell rabies vaccine: risks and benefits of primary and booster vaccination, *JAMA* 257:1059, 1987.
28. Biberstein E: Rat bite fever. In Hubbert W, McCulloch W, Schnurrenberger P, editors: *Diseases transmitted from animals to man,* ed 6, Springfield, Ill, 1975, Charles C Thomas.
29. Bloch B: Fatal fat embolism following severe donkey bites, *J Forensic Sci* 16:231, 1977.
30. Boe E, Nyland H: Guillain-Barré syndrome after vaccination with human diploid cell rabies vaccine, *Scand J Infect Dis* 12:231, 1980.
31. Boyce JM: Recent trends in the epidemiology of tularemia in the United States, *J Infect Dis* 131:197, 1975.
32. Brazis P, Stokes H, Ervin F: Optic neuritis in cat scratch disease, *J Clin Neuroophthalmol* 6:172, 1986.
33. Brenner DJ et al: Proposals to unify the genera *Bartonella* and *Rochalimaea,* with descriptions of *Bartonella quintana* comb. nov., *Bartonella vinsonii* comb. nov., *Bartonella henselae* comb. nov., and *Bartonella elizabethae* comb. nov., and to remove the family Bartonellaceae from the order Rickettsiales, *Int J Syst Bacteriol* 43:777, 1993.
34. Burridge MJ: Wildlife rabies in the United States, *Avian/Exotic Pract* 1:17, 1984.
35. Burridge MJ et al: Intradermal immunization with human diploid cell rabies vaccine: serological and clinical responses of persons with and without prior vaccination with duck embryo vaccine, *JAMA* 248:1611, 1982.
36. Butler T, Mahmoud AAF, Warren KS: Algorithms in the diagnosis and management of exotic diseases. XXV. Plague, *J Infect Dis* 136:317, 1977.
37. Carithers HA, Margileth AM: Cat-scratch disease: acute encephalopathy and other neurologic manifestations, *Am J Dis Child* 145:98, 1991.
38. Centers for Disease Control: Human plague—New Mexico, *MMWR* 23:425, 1974.
39. Centers for Disease Control: Tularemia mimicking plague—New Mexico, *MMWR* 23:299, 1974.
40. Centers for Disease Control: Human plague case—Bernalillo County, New Mexico, *MMWR* 24:90, 1975.
41. Centers for Disease Control: Tularemia—California, *MMWR* 24:126, 1975.
42. Centers for Disease Control: Trichinosis—United States, 1978, *MMWR* 28:541, 1979.
43. Centers for Disease Control: Human to human transmission of rabies via a corneal transplant—France, *MMWR* 29:25, 1980.
44. Centers for Disease Control: Tularemia acquired from a bear—Washington, *MMWR* 29:57, 1980.
45. Centers for Disease Control: Human plague—Texas, New Mexico, *MMWR* 30:137, 1981.
46. Centers for Disease Control: Human to human transmission of rabies via corneal transplant—Thailand *MMWR* 30:473, 1981.
47. Centers for Disease Control: Plague vaccine, *MMWR* 31:301, 1982.
48. Centers for Disease Control: Tularemia associated with domestic cats—Georgia, New Mexico, *MMWR* 31:39, 1982.
49. Centers for Disease Control: Rat-bite fever in a college student—California, *MMWR* 33:318, 1984.
50. Centers for Disease Control: *Rabies surveillance summary,* 1983, Atlanta, 1985, CDC.
51. Centers for Disease Control: Horsemeat associated trichinosis—France, *MMWR* 35:291, 1986.
52. Centers for Disease Control: Rabies prevention: supplementary statement on the pre-exposure use of human diploid cell rabies vaccine by the intradermal route, *MMWR* 35:767, 1986.
53. Centers for Disease Control: *Rabies surveillance, annual summary,* 1985, Atlanta, 1986, CDC.
54. Centers for Disease Control: An imported case of rabies in an immunized dog, *MMWR* 36:94, 1987.
55. Centers for Disease Control: Rabies prevention—United States, 1991: recommendations of the Advisory Committee on Immunization Practices (ACIP), *MMWR* 40:1, 1991.
56. Centers for Disease Control: Compendium of animal rabies control, *MMWR* 43:8, 1994.
57. Centers for Disease Control: Hantavirus pulmonary syndrome—United States, *MMWR* 43:45, 1994.
58. Centers for Disease Control and Prevention: Outbreak of leptospirosis among white-water rafters—Costa Rica, 1996, *MMWR* 46:577, 1997.
59. Centers for Disease Control: *Health information for international travel,* Atlanta, 1998, CDC.
60. Centers for Disease Control and Prevention: Human rabies—Texas and New Jersey, 1997, *MMWR* 47:1, 1998.
61. Centers for Disease Control and Prevention: Outbreak of acute febrile illness among athletes participating in triathlons—Wisconsin and Illinois, 1998, *MMWR* 47:585, 1998.
62. Centers for Disease Control and Prevention: Human rabies prevention—United States, 1999: recommendations of the Advisory Committee on Immunization Practices (ACIP), *MMWR* 48:1, 1999.
63. Centers for Disease Control and Prevention: Update: hantavirus pulmonary syndrome—United States, 1999, *MMWR* 48:521, 1999.
64. Childs JE et al: Serologic and genetic identification of *Peromyscus maniculatus* as the primary rodent reservoir for a new hantavirus in the southwestern United States, *J Infect Dis* 169:1271, 1994.
65. Christie AB, Chen TH, Elberg SS: Plague in camels and goats: their role in human epidemics, *J Infect Dis* 141:724, 1980.
66. Collipp P: Cat-scratch disease: therapy with trimethoprim-sulfamethoxazole, *Am J Dis Child* 146:397, 1992.
67. Colmenero JD et al: Comparative trial of doxycycline plus streptomycin versus doxycycline plus rifampin for the therapy of human brucellosis, *Chemotherapy* 35:146, 1989.
68. Conomy JP et al: Airborne rabies encephalitis: demonstration of rabies virus in the human central nervous system, *Neurology* 27:67, 1977.
69. Constantine DG: Rabies transmitted by the non-bite route, *Public Health Rep* 77:287, 1962.
70. Corbel MJ: Brucellosis: an overview, *Emerging Infect Dis* 3:213, 1997.
71. Corey L: Cat-scratch disease. In Isselbacker K, Adams R, Brauwald E, editors: *Harrison's textbook of medicine,* ed 11, New York, 1986, McGraw-Hill.
72. Correa-Giron EP, Alien R, Sulkin SE: The infectivity and pathogenesis of rabies administered orally, *Am J Epidemiol* 91:203, 1970.
73. Dahlstrand S, Ringertz O, Zetterberg B: Airborne tularemia in Sweden, *Scand J Infect Dis* 3:7, 1971.
74. Dean DJ, Baer GM, Thompson WR: Studies on the local treatment of rabies infected wounds, *Bull World Health Organ* 28:477, 1963.
75. Delahoussaye PM, Osborne EMS: Cat-scratch disease presenting as abdominal visceral granulomas, *J Infect Dis* 161:71, 1990.
76. Dellinger EP et al: Hand infections: bacteriology and treatment; a prospective study, *Arch Surg* 123:745, 1988.
77. Doege TC, Northrop RL: Evidence for inapparent rabies infection, *Lancet* 2:826, 1974.
78. Dreesen DW: A global review of rabies vaccines for human use, *Vaccine* 15:S2, 1997.
79. Dreesen DW et al: Intradermal use of human diploid cell vaccine for pre-exposure rabies immunizations, *J Am Vet Med Assoc* 181:1519, 1982.
80. Dreesen DW et al: Immune complex–like disease in two groups of persons following a booster dose of rabies human diploid cell vaccine. In *Proceedings of the 89th Annual Meeting, US Animal Health Association,* 1985.
81. Edwards CN et al: Leptospirosis in Barbados: a clinical study, *W Ind Med J* 39:27,1990.
82. Ell SR: Immunity as a factor in the epidemiology of medieval plague, *Rev Infect Dis* 6:866, 1984.
83. Enderlin G et al: Streptomycin and alternative agents for the treatment of tularemia: review of the literature, *Clin Infect Dis* 19:42, 1994.
84. Evans ME et al: Tularemia: a 30-year experience with 88 cases, *Medicine* 64:251, 1985.
85. Everard CO, Maude GH, Hayes RJ: Leptospiral infection: a household serosurvey in urban and rural communities in Barbados and Trinidad, *Ann Trop Med Parasitol* 84:255, 1990.
86. Everard CO et al: An investigation of some risk factors for severe leptospirosis on Barbados, *J Trop Med Hyg* 95:13, 1992.

87. Fayaz A et al: Booster effect of human diploid cell antirabies vaccine in previously treated persons, *JAMA* 246:2334, 1981.

88. Feigin RD et al: Human leptospirosis from immunized dogs, *Ann Intern Med* 79:777, 1973.

89. Fekadu M, Baer GM: Recovery from clinical rabies of two dogs inoculated with a rabies virus strain from Ethiopia, *Am J Vet Res* 41:1632, 1980.

90. Fekadu M, Smith JS: Laboratory diagnosis of rabies. In Fishbein DB, Sawyer LA, Winkler WB, editors: *Rabies concepts for medical professionals*, ed 2, Miami, 1986, Merieux Institute.

91. Fishbein DB: Pre-exposure and post-exposure immunization against rabies. In Fishbein DB, Sawyer LA, Winkler WG, editors: *Rabies concepts for medical professionals*, ed 2, Miami, Fla, 1986, Merieux Institute.

92. Fishbein DB: Rabies, *Infect Dis Clin North Am* 5:53, 1991.

93. Fordham JN et al: Rat bite fever without the bite, *Ann Rheum Dis* 51:411, 1992.

94. Fox M, Kaufmann A: Brucellosis in the United States, 1965-1974, *J Infect Dis* 136:312, 1977.

95. Ganem DE: Plasmids and pestilence—biological and clinical aspects of bubonic plague—Medical Staff Conference, University of California, San Francisco, *West J Med* 144:447, 1986.

96. Gerber M, Sedgwick A, MacAlister T: The aetiological agent of cat scratch disease, *Lancet* 1:1236, 1985.

97. Gerber M et al: Cell-mediated immunity in cat-scratch disease, *J Allergy Clin Immunol* 78:887, 1986.

98. Goldstein E: Rat-bite fever. In Hoeprich P, editor: *Infectious disease: a modern treatise of infectious processes*, Hagerstown, Md, 1977, Harper & Row.

99. Gorbach SL, Bartlett JG, Blacklow NR: *Infectious diseases*, Philadelphia, 1992, Saunders.

100. Groves MG: Melioidosis. In Steele JH, editor: *Handbook series in zoonoses, section A. bacterial, rickettsial and mycotic diseases*, vol 1, Boca Raton, Fla, 1979, CRC Press.

101. Guard RW et al: Melioidosis in far north Queensland, a clinical and epidemiological review of twenty cases, *Am J Trop Med* 33:467, 1984.

102. Halperin SA, Gast T, Ferrieri P: Oculoglandular syndrome caused by *Francisella tularensis*, *Clin Pediatr* 24:520, 1985.

103. Hanson LE: Leptospirosis in domestic animals: the public health perspective, *J Am Vet Med Assoc* 181:1505, 1982.

104. Harbottle JE, English DK, Schultz MG: Trichinosis in bears in northeastern United States, *HSMHA Health Rep* 86:473, 1971.

105. Hattwick MAW et al: Recovery from rabies: a case report, *Ann Intern Med* 76:931, 1972.

106. Heath CW, Alexander AD, Galton MM: Leptospirosis in the United States: analysis of 483 cases in man, 1949-1961, *N Engl J Med* 273:857, 1965.

107. Helmick CG: The epidemiology of human rabies post-exposure prophylaxis, 1980-1981, *JAMA* 250: 1990, 1983.

108. Hint E: Trichinellosis and trichinellosis control in Germany, *Southeast Asian J Trop Med Public Health* 22(suppl):329, 1991.

109. Houff SA et al: Human to human transmission of rabies virus by corneal transplant, *N Engl J Med* 300:603, 1979.

110. Howard DR: Transplacental transmission of rabies virus from a naturally infected skunk, *Am J Vet Res* 42:691, 1981.

111. Hubbert WT, McCulloch WF, Schnurrenberger PR: *Diseases transmitted from animals to man*, ed 6, Springfield, Ill, 1975, Thomas.

112. Hull HF, Montes JM, Mann JM: Plague masquerading as gastrointestinal illness, *West J Med* 145:485, 1986.

113. Hull HF, Montes JM, Mann JM: Septicemic plague in New Mexico, *J Infect Dis* 155:113, 1987.

114. Jacobs RF, Condrey YM, Yamauchi T: Tularemia in adults and children: a changing presentation, *Pediatrics* 76:818, 1985.

115. Jamieson S et al: Leptospirosis du New Zealand, *Bull Off Int Epizoot* 73:81, 1970.

116. Javadi MA et al: Transmission of rabies by corneal graft, *Cornea* 15:431, 1996.

117. Jevon TR et al: A point source epidemic of leptospirosis: description of cases, cause, and prevention, *Postgrad Med* 80: 121, 1986.

118. Kaufmann AF et al: Public health implications of plague in domestic cats, *J Am Vet Med Assoc* 179:875, 1981.

119. Kennedy ND et al: Leptospirosis and acute renal failure—clinical experience and a review of the literature, *Postgrad Med J* 55:176, 1979.

120. Kerr DD, Marshall V: Protection against the renal carrier state by a canine leptospirosis vaccine, *Vet Med Small Anim Clin* 69:1157, 1974.

121. Kilonzo BS, Makundi RH, Mbise TJ: A decade of plague epidemiology and control in the western Usambara mountains, north-east Tanzania, *Acta Trop* 50:323, 1992.

122. Kim GR, Lee YT, Park CH: A new natural reservoir of hantavirus: isolation of hantaviruses from lung tissues of bats, *Arch Virol* 134:85, 1994.

123. Klein JS: Treatment of severe trichinellosis. In Kim CW, Pawlowski ZS, editors: *Trichinellosis*, Hanover, NH, 1978, University Press of New England.

124. Klock LE, Olsen PF, Fukishima T: Tularemia epidemic associated with the deerfly, *JAMA* 226:149, 1973.

125. Ko RC: A brief update on the diagnosis of trichinellosis, *Southeast Asian J Trop Med Public Health* 28:91, 1997.

126. Koskela P, Salminen A: Humoral immunity against *Francisella tularensis* after natural infection, *J Clin Microbiol* 22:973, 1985.

127. Krebs JW et al: Rabies surveillance in the United States during 1991, *J Am Vet Med Assoc* 201:1836, 1992.

128. Krebs JW et al: Rabies surveillance in the United States during 1996, *J Am Vet Med Assoc* 211:1525, 1997.

129. LeDuc JW, Childs JE, Glass GE: The hantaviruses, etiologic agents of hemorrhagic fever with renal syndrome: a possible cause of hypertension and chronic renal disease in the United States, *Annu Rev Public Health* 13:79, 1992.

130. Leelarasame A: *Burkholderia pseudomallei*: the unbeatable foe? *Southeast Asian J Trop Med Public Health* 29:410, 1998.

131. Leelarasame A, Bovornkitt S: Melioidosis: review and update, *Rev Infect Dis* 11:413, 1989.

132. Le Guenno B: Identifying a hantavirus associated with acute respiratory illness: a PCR victory? *Lancet* 342:1438, 1993 (letter).

133. Lewis DE, Wallace MR: Treatment of adult systemic cat scratch disease with gentamicin sulfate, *West J Med* 154:330, 1991.

134. Libby J, Meislin HW: Human rabies, *Ann Emerg Med* 12:217, 1983.

135. Lucero NE et al: Competitive enzyme immunoassay for diagnosis of human brucellosis, *J Clin Microbiol* 37:3245, 1999.

136. MacLean JD et al: Trichinosis in the Canadian Arctic: report of five outbreaks and a new clinical syndrome, *J Infect Dis* 160:513, 1989.

137. Madon MB et al: O'Rullian W. An overview of plague in the United States and a report of investigations of two human cases in Kern County, California, 1995, *J Vector Ecol* 22:77, 1997.

138. Mahannop P et al: Immunodiagnosis of human trichinellosis using excretory-secretory (ES) antigen, *J Helminth* 66:297, 1992.

139. Mandell GL, Douglas RG, Bennett JE: *Principles and practice of infectious diseases*, ed 4, New York, 1995, Churchill Livingstone.

140. Marcus LC: *The veterinary biology and medicine of captive amphibians and reptiles*, Philadelphia, 1981, Lea & Febiger.

141. Margileth A: Cat scratch disease in 65 patients, *Clin Proc Child Hosp DC* 27:213,1971.

142. Margileth A, Wear D, English C: Systemic cat scratch disease: report of 23 patients with prolonged or recurrent severe bacterial infection, *J Infect Dis* 155:390, 1987.

143. Margileth AM: Antibiotic therapy for cat-scratch disease: clinical study of therapeutic outcome in 268 patients and a review of the literature, *Pediatr Infect Dis J* 11:474, 1992.

144. Margileth AM: Cat scratch disease update: etiology, diagnosis and management of 1990 patients. In *Program and abstracts of the 32nd Interscience Conference on Antimicrobial Agents and Chemotherapy*, Anaheim, Calif, 1992, American Society for Microbiology.

145. Markowitz LE et al: Tick-borne tularemia: an outbreak of lymphadenopathy in children, *JAMA* 254:2922, 1985.

146. Martell MA, Montes FC, Alcocer R: Transplacental transmission of bovine rabies after natural infection, *J Infect Dis* 127:291, 1973.

147. Matyas Z, Fujikura T: Brucellosis as a world problem, *Dev Biol Stand* 56:3, 1984.

148. Mays EE, Ricketts EA: Melioidosis: recrudescence associated with bronchogenic carcinoma 26 years following initial geographic exposure, *Chest* 68:261, 1975.

149. McAuley JB, Michelson MK, Schantz PM: Trichinosis surveillance, United States. 1987-1990, *MMWR* 40:3, 1991.

150. McAuley JB, Michelson MK, Schantz PM: *Trichinella* infection in travelers, *J Infect Dis* 164:1013, 1991.

151. McClain JBL et al: Doxycycline therapy for leptospirosis, *Ann Intern Med* 100:696, 1984.

152. McCormick JB et al: Human to human transmission of *Pseudomonas pseudomallei*, *Ann Intern Med* 83:512, 1975.

153. McHugh T, Bartlett R, Raymond J: Rat bite fever: report of a fatal case, *Ann Emerg Med* 14:1116, 1985.

154. Moorhead A et al: Trichinellosis in the United States, 1991-1996: declining but not gone, *Am J Trop Med* 60:66, 1999.

155. Murphy FA: Rabies virus morphology and morphogenesis. In Baer GM, editor: *The natural history of rabies,* vol 1, New York, 1975, Academic Press.

156. Muszynski M, Eppes S, Riley H: Granulomatous osteolytic lesion of the skull associated with cat scratch disease, *Pediatr Infect Dis J* 6:199, 1987.

157. National Association of State Public Veterinarians, Inc: Compendium of animal rabies control, 1993, *MMWR* 42, 1993.

158. Nerurkar VR et al: Genetically distinct hantavirus in deer mice, *Lancet* 342:1058, 1993 (letter).

159. Noah DL et al: Epidemiology of human rabies in the United States, 1980 to 1996, *Ann Intern Med* 128:922, 1998.

160. Ozeretskovskaya NN et al: Benzimidazoles in the treatment and prophylaxis of synanthropic and sylvatic trichinellosis. In Kim CW, Pawlowski ZS, editors: *Trichinellosis,* Hanover, NH, 1978, University Press of New England.

161. Palmer DG et al: Demonstration of rabies viral antigen in paraffin tissue sections: comparison of the immunofluorescence technique with the unlabeled antibody enzyme method, *Am J Vet Res* 46:283, 1985.

162. Pappaioanou M et al: Antibody response to preexposure human diploid-cell rabies vaccine given concurrently with chloroquine, *N Engl J Med* 314:280, 1986.

163. Pappas MG et al: Rapid serodiagnosis of leptospirosis using the IgM-specific dot-ELISA: comparison with the microscopic agglutination test, *Am J Trop Med* 34:346, 1985.

164. Patamasucon P, Urs BS, Nelson JD: Melioidosis, *J Pediatr* 100:175, 1982.

165. Penn RL, Kinasewitz GT: Factors associated with a poor outcome in tularemia, *Arch Intern Med* 147:265, 1987.

166. Petchclai B et al: Evaluation of two screening tests for human leptospirosis, *J Med Assoc Thailand* 73:64, 1990.

167. Picker R, Milder J: Transverse myelitis associated with cat-scratch disease in an adult, *JAMA* 246:2840, 1981.

168. Poland J, Barnes AL: Plague. In Steele JH, editor: *Handbook series in zoonoses,* Boca Raton, Fla, 1979, CRC Press.

169. Porras C et al: Recovery from rabies in man, *Ann Intern Med* 85:44, 1976.

170. Posson SC, Told TN, Hollar GF: Recognition of hantavirus infection in the rural setting: report of first Colorado resident to survive, *J Am Osteopath Assoc* 93:1061, 1993.

171. Pozio E, La Rosa G: General introduction and epidemiology of trichinellosis, *Southeast Asian J Trop Med Public Health* 22(suppl):291, 1991.

172. Prochoda K, Mostow SR, Greenberg K: Hantavirus-associated acute respiratory failure, *N Engl J Med* 329:1744, 1993 (letter).

173. Quenzer RW, Mostow SR, Emerson JK: Cat bite tularemia, *JAMA* 238:1845, 1977.

174. Redfearn MS, Palleroni NJ: Glanders and melioidosis. In Hubbert WT, McCulloch WF, Schnurrenberger PR, editors: *Diseases transmitted from animals to man,* Springfield, Ill, 1975, Thomas.

175. Remington PL, Shope T, Andrews J: A recommended approach to the evaluation of human rabies exposure in an acute-care hospital, *JAMA* 254:67, 1985.

176. Robertson M: Brucella infection transmitted by dog bite, *JAMA* 225:750, 1973.

177. Robertson MH: Leptospirosis, *Practitioner* 226:1552, 1982.

178. Rollag OJ et al: Feline plague in New Mexico: report of five cases, *J Am Vet Med Assoc* 179:1381, 1981.

179. Roy TM, Fleming D, Anderson WH: Tularemic pneumonia mimicking Legionnaire's disease with false positive direct fluorescent antibody stains for *Legionella, South Med J* 82:1429, 1989.

180. Ryan CP: Selected arthropod-borne diseases: plague, Lyme disease, and babesiosis. In *Zoonotic diseases,* Philadelphia, 1987, Saunders.

181. Rygg M, Bruun CF: Rat bite fever (*Streptobacillus moniliformis*) with septicemia in a child, *Scand J Infect Dis* 24:535, 1992.

182. Sanford JP: Leptospirosis—time for a booster, *N Engl J Med* 310:524, 1984.

183. Sasaki DM et al: Active surveillance and risk factors for leptospirosis in Hawaii, *Am J Trop Med* 48:35, 1993.

184. Saslaw S, Carhart S: Studies with tularemia vaccines in volunteers. III. Serological aspects following intracutaneous or respiratory challenge in both vaccinated and nonvaccinated volunteers, *Am J Med Sci* 241:689, 1961.

185. Saslaw S, Carlisle HN: Studies with tularemia vaccines in volunteers challenged with *Pasteurella tularensis, Am J Med Sci* 242:166, 1961.

186. Saslaw S et al: Tularemia vaccine study. I. Intracutaneous challenge, *Arch Intern Med* 107:121, 1961.

187. Saslaw S et al: Tularemia vaccine study. II. Respiratory challenge, *Arch Intern Med* 107:134, 1961.

188. Sato T et al: Microagglutination test for early specific serodiagnosis of tularemia, *J Clin Microbiol* 28:2372, 1990.

189. Schantz PM: Improvements in the diagnosis of helminthic zoonoses, *Vet Parasitol* 25:95, 1987.

190. Schiappacasse R, Colville J, Wong P: Sporotrichosis associated with an infected cat, *Cutis* 268, 1985.

191. Schlim DR, Schwartz E, Houston R: Rabies immunoprophylaxis strategy in travelers, *J Wilderness Med* 2:15, 1991.

192. Schneider LG, Diringer H: Structure and molecular biology of rabies virus, *Curr Top Microbiol Immunol* 75:153, 1976.

193. Schpilberg O et al: Long term follow-up after leptospirosis, *South Med J* 83:405,1990.

194. Schwabe CW: *Veterinary medicine and human health,* ed 3, Baltimore, 1984, Williams & Wilkins.

195. Schwartzman W: Infections due to *Rochalimaea:* the expanding clinical spectrum, *Clin Infect Dis* 15:893, 1992.

196. Scofield RH, Lopez EJ, McNabb SJ: Tularemia pneumonia in Oklahoma, 1982-1987, *J Okla State Med Assoc* 85:165, 1992.

197. Sehgal SC et al: LEPTO Dipstick: a rapid and simple method for serodiagnosis of acute leptospirosis, *Trans R Soc Trop Med Hyg* 93:161, 1999.

198. Sens MA et al: Fatal *Streptobacillus moniliformis* infection in a two-month-old infant, *Am J Clin Pathol* 91:612, 1989.

199. Shackelford P: Rat bite fever. In Feigin RD, editor: *Pediatric infectious disease,* Philadelphia, 1981, WB Saunders.

200. Shill M, Baynes RD, Miller SD: Fatal rabies encephalitis despite appropriate post-exposure prophylaxis: a case report, *N Engl J Med* 316:1257, 1987.

201. Sipahioghi U, Alpaut S: [Transplacental rabies in human], *Mikrbiyol Bult* 19:95, 1985 (Turkish, English abstract).

202. Sites VR, Poland JD, Hudson BW: Bubonic plague misdiagnosed as tularemia: retrospective serologic diagnosis, *JAMA* 222:1642, 1972.

203. Slater LN et al: A newly recognized fastidious gram-negative pathogen as a cause of fever and bacteremia, *N Engl J Med* 323:1587, 1990.

204. Smith JS et al: Unexplained rabies in three immigrants in the United States: a virological investigation, *N Engl J Med* 324:205, 1991.

205. Spires J, Smith R: Cat-scratch disease, *Otolaryngol Head Neck Surg* 94:622, 1986.

206. Steele JH: Glanders. In Steele JH, editor: *Handbook series in zoonoses, section A. bacterial, rickettsial and mycotic diseases,* vol 1, Boca Raton, Fla, 1979, CRC Press.

207. Steele JH: *Handbook series in zoonoses,* Boca Raton, Fla, 1979, 1980, 1981, 1982, CRC Press.

208. Stoler MH et al: An atypical subcutaneous infection associated with acquired immune deficiency syndrome, *Am J Clin Pathol* 80:714, 1983.

209. Strong RP: Studies on pneumonic plague and plague immunization. I. Introduction: the expedition to Manchuria and the conditions under which the work was performed, *Philippine J Sci* 7B:131, 1912.

210. Sulzer CR, Jones WL: *Leptospirosis: methods in laboratory diagnosis,* rev ed, Publ No (CDC) 74-8275, Washington, DC.

211. Swaddiwuthipong W et al: A high rate of neurological complications following Semple anti-rabies vaccine, *Trans R Soc Trop Med Hyg* 82:472, 1988.

212. Swartz M, Calin A: Leptospirosis, relapsing fever, rat-bite fever, and Lyme disease. In Rubenstein E, Federman D, editors: *Scientific American medicine,* New York, 1993, Scientific American.

213. Syrjala H et al: Agglutination and ELISA methods in the diagnosis of tularemia in different clinical forms and severities of the disease, *J Infect Dis* 153:142, 1986.

214. Takafuji ET et al: An efficacy trial of doxycycline chemoprophylaxis against leptospirosis, *N Engl J Med* 310:497, 1984.

215. Tantawichien T et al: Value of skin testing for predicting reactions to equine rabies immune globulin, *Clin Infect Dis* 21:660, 1995.

216. Taylor JP et al: Epidemiologic characteristics of human tularemia in the southwest-central states, 1981-1987, *Am J Epidemiol* 133:1032, 1991.

217. Van Knapen F et al: Detection of specific immunoglobulins (IgG, IgM, IgA, IgE) and total IgE levels in human trichinosis by means of the enzyme-linked immunosorbent assay (ELISA), *Am J Trop Med Hyg* 31:973, 1982.

218. Verma RD et al: Development of an avidin-biotin dot enzyme-linked immunosorbent assay and its comparison with other serological tests for diagnosis of glanders in equines, *Vet Microbiol* 25:77, 1990.

219. Vestey JP, Yirrell DL, Aldridge RD: Cowpox/catpox infection, *Br J Dermatol* 124:74, 1991.

220. Waag DM: Vaccination of human volunteers with a new lot of the live vaccine strain of *Francisella tularensis, J Clin Microbiol* 30:2256, 1992.

221. Waitkins S: Laboratory diagnosis of leptospirosis, *Lab Technol* 17:178, 1983.

222. Warwick W: Cat scratch disease. In Hubbert W, McCulloch W, Schnurrenberger P, editors: *Diseases transmitted from animals to man,* ed 6, Springfield, Ill, 1975, Charles C Thomas.

223. Watt G et al: The rapid diagnosis of leptospirosis: a prospective comparison of the dot-ELISA and genus-specific microscopic agglutination test at different stages of illness, *J Infect Dis* 157:840, 1988.

224. Watt G et al: Placebo-controlled trial of intravenous penicillin for severe and late leptospirosis: demonstration of efficacy by a double-blind, placebo-controlled study, *Lancet* 1:433, 1988.

225. White ME et al: Recommendations for the control of *Yersinia pestis* infections, recommendations from the CDC, *Infect Control* 1:324, 1980.

226. White NJ et al: Halving of mortality of severe melioidosis by ceftazidime, *Lancet* 2:697, 1989.

227. Whitmore A, Krishnaswami CS: An account of the discovery of a hitherto undescribed infective disease occurring among the population of Rangoon, *Ind Med Gaz* 47:262, 1912.

228. Wilde H, Chutivongse S: Equine rabies immune globulin: a product with an undeserved poor reputation, *Am J Trop Med* 42:175, 1990.

229. Wilde H et al: Purified equine rabies immune globulin: a safe and affordable alternative to human rabies immune globulin. *Bull World Health Organ* 67:731, 1989.

230. Wilkerson JA: Rabies: epidemiology, diagnosis, prevention and prospects for worldwide control, *J Wilderness Med* 11:31, 2000.

231. Winkler WG, Baker EF, Hopkins CC: An outbreak of non-bite transmitted rabies in a laboratory animal colony, *Am J Epidemiol* 95:267, 1972.

232. Winkler WG et al: Airborne rabies transmission in a laboratory worker, *JAMA* 226:1219, 1973.

233. World Health Organization: Two rabies cases following corneal transplantation, *Weekly Epidemiol Rec* 69:330, 1994.

234. Yabuuchi E et al: Proposal of *Burkholderia* gen. nov. and transfer of seven species of the genus *Pseudomonas* homology group II to the new genus with the type species *Burkholderia cepacia* (Palleroni and Holmes 1981) comb. nov., *Microbiol Immunol* 36:897, 1992.

235. Young LS et al: Tularemia epidemic: Vermont, 1968: forty-seven cases linked to contact with muskrats, *N Engl J Med* 280:1253, 1969.

236. Zangwill KM et al: Cat scratch disease in Connecticut: epidemiology, risk factors, and evaluation of a new diagnostic test, *N Engl J Med* 329:8, 1993.

45 Emergency Veterinary Medicine

Murray E. Fowler

The wilderness experience often involves animals other than humans. Such domestic animals as horses, llamas, elephants, camels, and yaks may be used for packing or pulling supplies, relieving hikers of this burden. Dogs may accompany owners into the wilderness as companions, as trackers of game, or in the Arctic and Antarctic as primary draft animals. Any of these animals may become injured or fatigued or fall ill with a variety of ailments that may require emergency treatment and management by trek personnel.

Observation of wild animals in their natural habitat enhances the wilderness experience, but encounters between wild animals and animals accompanying the trekkers cause problems. Healthy wild animals usually try to avoid humans, but they may show interest in domestic animals.

WILD ANIMAL ENCOUNTERS

Medical and paramedical personnel who may be called to render emergency medical care or assist in the rescue of injured or diseased humans or support animals should recognize that wild animals may be involved. Experienced trekkers can usually recognize when they are intruding into an animal's domain. Unfortunately, some people lack a sense of courtesy for animals. When trekkers in the wilderness behave as if they are entering the home of a human friend, they show appreciation for the rights of wild animals and have less risk of injury or illness to themselves or their support animals. Understanding the biology and normal behavior of wild animals known to live in the wilderness areas to be visited enhances enjoyment and diminishes exposure to potentially dangerous situations.

Others who may be at risk are wildlife biologists, hunters, and people who choose to live in remote areas. Hunters come into intimate contact with wild animals as they pursue, dress, and eat game. Plant scientists, paleontologists, geologists, and other nonanimal scientists may inadvertently encounter wild animals. Wild animal biologists conducting field investigations may capture or immobilize wild animals to collect data. Such individuals are at potential risk of injury or disease, not only as a result of wild animal contact, but also from drugs and firearms used to administer the drugs.

Chapters 42 and 43 provide more details on why and when wild animals are dangerous. Although few wild animals stalk humans, they may prey on support animals. Most wild animals fear humans and, given a choice, avoid human contact. Injuries to humans by wild animals usually result from human judgment errors, such as approaching too closely, ill-advised handling of diseased wild animals, or unlucky exposure to highly aggressive or protective animals. Such animals may be natural predators seeking food, prey species fearful for their lives or the lives of their young, or diseased and irrational animals (e.g., with rabies). Attacks on support animals usually occur at night or when humans are absent.

Animals are most likely to respond adversely if startled from sleep or if their flight distance is violated. Flight distance is that distance at which, if approached by an enemy, an animal will either fight (attack) or flee. The distance is species specific for a given region and may become greater if animals in the area have been recently hunted. Flight distance may be greater for a person walking or carrying a gun than for a person riding on horseback or in a vehicle. Cornered animals occasionally attack or risk injury trying to escape. Any animal may attack if its offspring are in danger. With any large animal, accidental or intentional positioning between a mother and her infant invites attack.

Equal danger exists for a person who comes between a territorial male and one or more females. Many wild animals are territorial. Males and females may establish feeding, breeding, and home territories. An animal may share feeding territories with other members of the same species or different species, but home territories may be defended against any intruder, including humans.

Injuries have been inflicted on hunters who approached a recently shot animal, believing it to be dead, only to have the animal revive explosively in a final effort to fight or flee.

Humans should not fraternize with wild animals. Food scraps should not be left to tempt wild animals closer for photographs. Any wild animal that will allow touching is a spoiled park animal or is diseased; neither type should be hand fed. Travelers in the wild should be observant for animal signs (e.g., feces, tracks, trails, resting areas) and should respect the behavioral characteristics of animals. Knowledge of the biology and habits of local animals obviates most avoidable close encounters and dangerous situations.

Wild animal attacks on support animals usually occur when the animal is tied on a picket line or staked out for grazing. The animal may injure itself trying to escape the attack or be bitten and mauled by its attacker. One frightened llama broke loose from a stake, but the lead rope snagged between rocks, fracturing the animal's cervical spine.

Treatment of animal-inflicted injuries that require specific therapy include lacerations, contusions, punctures, or abrasions (see Chapters 42 and 43).

SUPPORT ANIMALS

Expedition leaders and participants should consider the well-being of support animals and understand their physical capabilities, including maximal load, speed, and endurance. They should also be able to recognize signs of exertional stress.

Exertional stress is more likely to occur in horses that are ridden than in packhorses that are led. A horse can generally match or exceed the physical endurance of a hiker. Adverse metabolic conditions may develop in horses pushed beyond their limits of endurance. The type of syndrome arising from excessive exercise depends on intensity and duration, degree of prior conditioning, and nutritional status. Mules, donkeys, and llamas are less prone than horses to develop problems, because they usually refuse to be pushed to extremes of exertion.

The animal best suited to the terrain, climate, and task should be selected. Horses, mules, and donkeys are traditional beasts of burden in North America, wherever sufficient forage and water are available. Each animal has both admirable and undesirable qualities. Horses are usually the largest and can carry the heaviest loads. Mules and burros tend to be more difficult for novices to handle. No animal should be used on a trek unless at least one member of the party has considerable experience in handling and caring for the chosen animal.

In South America the llama is the beast of burden. Adventurers traveling into rugged and remote areas above 3000 m (9843 feet) will probably use llamas for support. Llamas have also become popular support animals with backpackers in North America. The llama requires less feed, can subsist better on sparse native forages, and is less damaging to the environment than is the horse.

Dogs are necessary support animals for winter travel in the Arctic. In other regions they function more as companions.

Many expeditions are mounted in countries unfamiliar to both leaders and participants. In various parts of Asia the horse is replaced by the elephant, water buffalo, Bactrian camel, or yak. In North Africa and the Middle East the dromedary camel carries the load. Each species has specialized requirements for handling, packing, and health care.

Expedition physicians may be asked to treat the ailments of support animals. Basic medical training provides the foundation necessary to diagnose and treat many conditions that may be encountered on the trail. If in doubt, expedition members should handle an ailing support animal as if it were human. With support animals carrying all or part of the load, a more sophisticated emergency medical kit may be carried.

Pretrip Animal Health Considerations

Health certificates are needed for travel and entry into the state or province of destination and possibly intervening states. Regulations are extremely variable, and inquiries should be made at least 4 weeks before departure. Each animal should receive a physical examination by a qualified veterinarian before an extended trip. Conditioning is as important for trek animals as for human participants. Training should be in terrain similar to that expected on the trek, with special attention to toughening the footpads of llamas and dogs by appropriate exercise.

Immature animals should not be taken on expeditions. Dogs should be at least 1 year old. Llamas and equids should be 3 years old. Well-conditioned and trained horses, mules, donkeys, or dogs can carry approximately 30% of their body weight. Llamas usually carry only 25% of their body weight (Table 45-1).

Frequently, arrangements are made to contract for support animal service from suppliers in the trek locale. Persons providing these services do not always understand the trek requirements and may supply animals that are poorly shod, unconditioned, poorly trained, or otherwise unsuitable for the needs of trek participants. Trek leaders must clearly describe specifications and be adamant about compliance, well in advance of the trek.

Horses, Mules, and Donkeys. A tetanus booster should have been given to equids within the past year. Vaccination against rabies is appropriate if the trek itinerary includes traveling in an endemic area. Encephalomyelitis vaccines should be used in endemic areas, especially during the insect seasons of summer and fall. Internal parasite levels should be evaluated by fecal flotation and appropriate medication given to reduce the parasite burden.

The feet should be trimmed and shod properly at least 2 weeks and not more than 4 weeks before a trek begins. Extra shoes for forefeet and hind feet of different-sized horses should be carried, along with the appropriate nails and hammer to reattach a shoe.

Llamas. Llamas should have been given a tetanus toxoid booster within the past 6 months. Other basic immunizations should include *Clostridium perfringens* toxoid, type C and D, within the past 6 months, as well as vaccinations against leptospirosis and rabies if entering an endemic area.

TABLE 45-1. Vital Statistics of Trek Animals

ANIMAL	BODY WEIGHT		HEART RATE/MIN	RESPIRATORY RATE/MIN	BODY TEMPERATURE		WEIGHT CARRIED BY WELL-CONDITIONED ANIMALS*	
	POUNDS	kg			°C	°F	kg	POUNDS
Horse	800-1200	360-540	28-40	10-14	37.2-38.0	99.0-100.5	110-136	240-300
Mule	600-1200	275-540	28-40	10-14	37.2-38.0	99.0-100.5	82-136	180-300
Donkey	300-600	136-275	28-40	10-14	37.2-38.0	99.0-100.5	40-82	90-180
Llama	300-450	136-200	60-90	10-30	37.2-38.7	99.0-101.8	34-50	75-110
Dog	20-100	9-45	65-90	15-30	37.5-38.6	99.5-101.5	3-14	6-30
Camel	880-1200	400-550	40-50	5-12	36.4-42.0	97.5-107.6	225	500
Elephant	5000-8000	2300-3700	25-35	4-6	36.0-37.0	97.5-99.0	900	2000
Yak	2200	1000	55-80	10-30	37.8-39.2	100.0-102.5	235	550

*For sustained trekking: 24 to 40 km (15 to 25 miles) per day on moderately difficult trails. This includes tack. Animals in training should be expected to carry only one half to two thirds of this weight.

Toenails should have been trimmed within the previous 2 months. Internal parasitism is debilitating in llamas. Ova levels should be checked, but treatment with an anthelminthic (ivermectin, 0.2 mg/kg subcutaneously, or fenbendazole, 5 mg/kg orally) usually is desirable within the previous 2 months.

Dogs. Dogs are routinely immunized against canine distemper, canine adenovirus, leptospirosis, and rabies. Vaccinations should be current. A check should be made for internal parasites and fleas and appropriate action taken. Although dog fleas do not permanently infest humans, they bite and may cause mild to severe local dermal reactions in sensitive individuals. Dogs should be bathed with a shampoo containing a pyrethrin insecticide before a trek. Any pyrethrin-containing dusting powder may be carried on an extended trek to relieve dogs of flea burdens. It is unlikely that the fleas involved in the sylvatic plague cycle will infest a dog, so the dog is not a source of plague infections for humans in a trek situation.

Rest

Support animals require less sleep than human trekkers. Horses can sleep while standing because they have a special locking mechanism of the tendons and ligaments of the limbs. Horses may also lie in sternal or lateral recumbency. Llamas usually rest in a sternal position but may also assume lateral recumbency. Llamas enjoy taking a "dust bath" by rolling in dirt soon after packs are removed. A few may try to roll with the pack still in place.

Watering and Feeding

All animals require daily access to potable water. It is not possible to filter or disinfect water for large animals except in extremely filthy conditions. Dogs may be susceptible to giardiasis and theoretically should drink filtered water, but no one can prevent a free-running dog from drinking from a stream or lake. Heavily mineralized or silted water may be as unpalatable for animals as for humans and may cause similar gastrointestinal problems.

The basic fluid requirement for a horse or other large trek animal is approximately 40 ml/kg/day, or 18 L (5 gallons) for a 450-kg (1000-pound) horse. Work and heavy sweating may triple the requirement. Llamas and donkeys may require one-third less water than a horse.

Llamas and donkeys tolerate dehydration better than other species, but they function better if well hydrated. The camel is noted for its ability to tolerate a number of days (2 to 7) without drinking water. Equids sweat profusely and should be given the opportunity to drink along the trail. Some llamas refuse to drink until evening.

Horses, Mules, and Donkeys. Equids consume approximately 2% to 2.5% of their body weight daily (for a 1000-pound horse, 20 to 25 pounds of total feed). When the animals are working hard, half this amount should be concentrates (grains such as rolled oats, barley, or cracked corn, or mixed grains and molasses in loose or pellet form). If forage is unavailable, alfalfa pellets should be carried. Animals should become accustomed to eating pellets before the journey begins. Concentrates should be reduced on days when the animals are not working.

Llamas. Llamas require only 1% to 1.5% of their body weight in food daily. Given the opportunity, llamas will graze and browse to satisfy their requirements. Many packers carry a supplement mixture consisting of half alfalfa pellets and half grain mix (same as for horses),

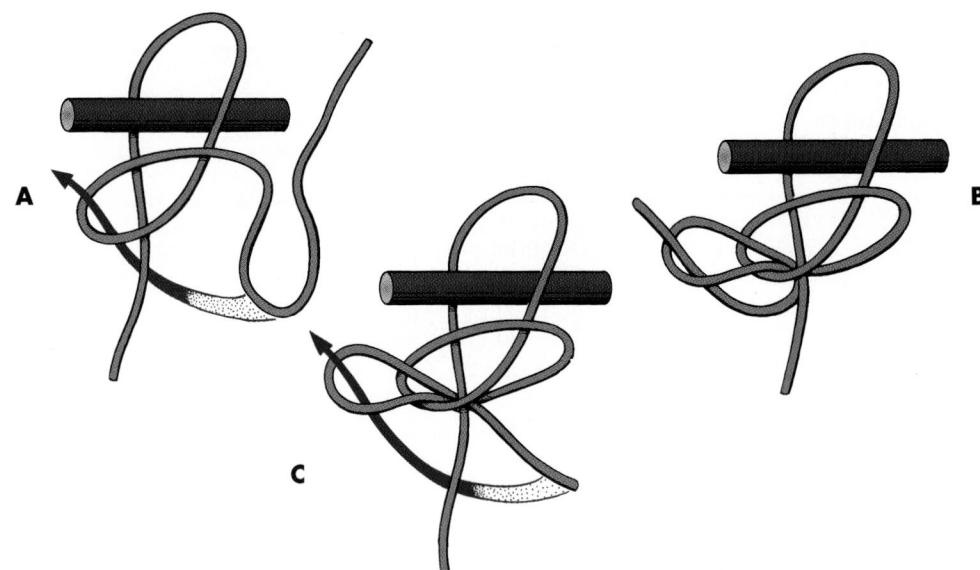

Figure 45-1 Sequence halter tie.

used as required. Some llamas are reluctant and must be trained to eat pellets or grain. Training should take place at home, not during the trek.

Dogs. A dog should be accustomed to high-quality dry dog food. The quantity fed should increase by half when the dog is exercising.

Emergency Restraint

One or (preferably) more persons on the trek should be acquainted with the general care and handling of any domestic species involved in the expedition. Methods of haltering and leading are specific for each animal. Securing animals at night may require hobbling or tethering. Skill and experience are necessary to accomplish this without risk of injury to the animal or handler. Animal handlers should be able to examine and clean the feet and hoofs of their charges. All people who deal with animals should know how to create a halter tie at rest stops and when an animal is tethered (Figure 45-1). A knowledge of temporary rope halter construction is desirable in the event of loss or breakage of halters (Figure 45-2).[7]

Horses, Mules, and Donkeys. Large animals can inflict serious or lethal injuries on people. When in pain or panicked, they may not respond even to their accustomed handlers. If a horse is down and entangled in rope, wire, or bushes, it should be approached from its back and its head held down until it can be extricated. The handler should stay out of the reach of both fore and hind limbs.[7]

A horse's defensive and offensive actions are to strike with the fore limbs, kick forward and backward with the rear limbs, and bite. The safest place to stand is close to the left shoulder. Persons examining the feet and legs of a standing horse should keep their head above the lower body line to avoid having the horse reach forward with a rear limb and strike it.

Additional restraint for painful procedures may be accomplished by grasping one or both ears of the horse. The method of "earing" a horse is as follows:

1. Stand at the left shoulder and grasp the halter or lead rope with the left hand.
2. Place the right hand palm down with the fingers together and the thumb extended, on the top of the neck.
3. Slide the hand up the neck until the thumb and fingers surround the base of the ear (Figure 45-3).
4. Squeeze tightly, but do not twist the ear.
5. The horse usually tries to pull away as the ear is grasped. Be prepared to move with the horse while maintaining a firm grip.

Llamas. Pack llamas are usually docile. Although most allow the feet to be lifted for inspection or treatment, some try to lie down. One or two people should stand on the side opposite the limb being lifted, or the llama should be placed next to a tree or large rock to prevent the animal from moving away. The limb should be firmly grasped. It may be necessary to semisupport the body if the animal tries to lie down.[7,8]

If a llama refuses to get up, the rear limbs should be pulled out behind it. If it still refuses to rise, an injury or illness that inhibits rising should be suspected.

Rarely a llama "spits" against an annoyance. The "spit" is actually stomach contents, the foul odor of which remains until thoroughly washed off. Spitting is

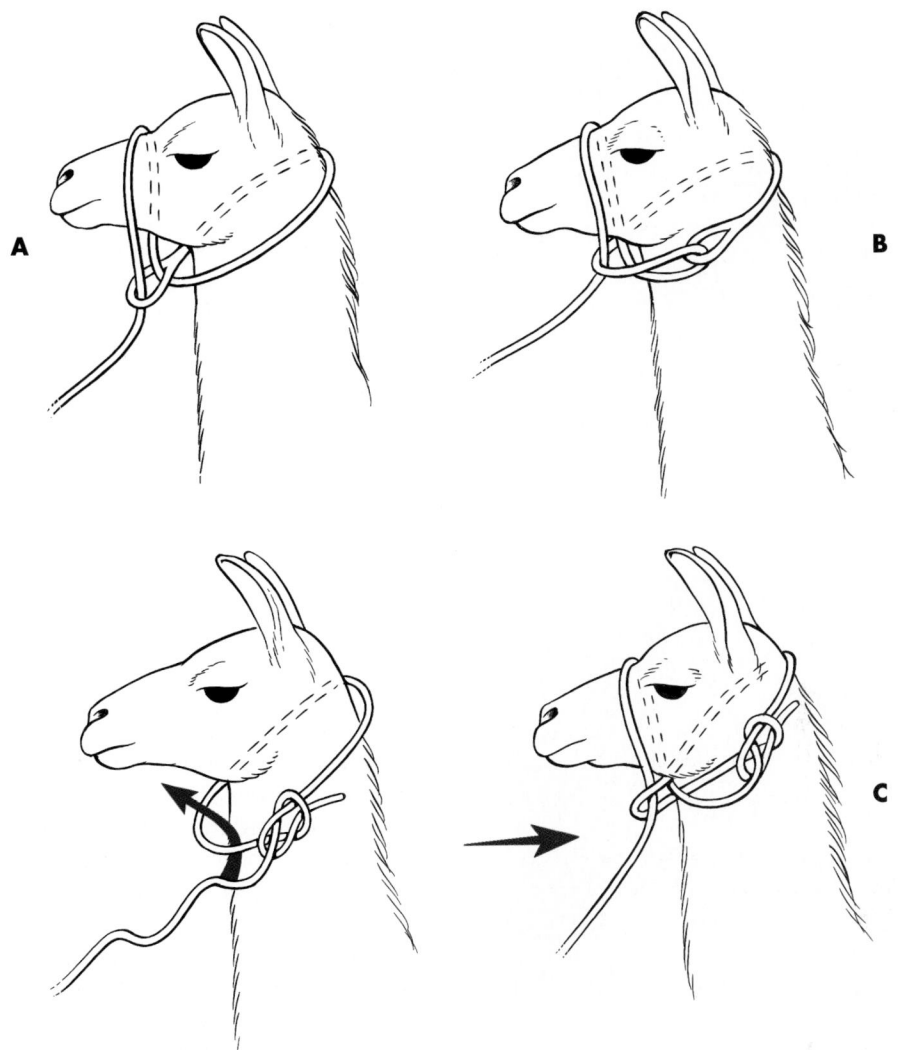

Figure 45-2 Temporary rope halters.

usually directed toward other llamas to express displeasure, but handlers may be caught in the cross fire. If a llama becomes irritated during an examination or treatment procedure, spitting can be controlled by draping a cloth over the nose and tucking the top around the nose piece of the halter. Llamas also dislike the odor of stomach contents on their noses. Llamas can be "eared" in a manner similar to horses.[8]

Dogs. Dogs usually accompany their owners, who are able to handle them under difficult circumstances. If mildly painful medical procedures must be performed, the head and mouth should be secured. The dog's body can be securely held against the handler's body by reaching across the back of the dog and grasping the base of the neck while pulling the opposite shoulder with the elbow toward the handler. The other hand should tuck the dog's head under the handler's arm.

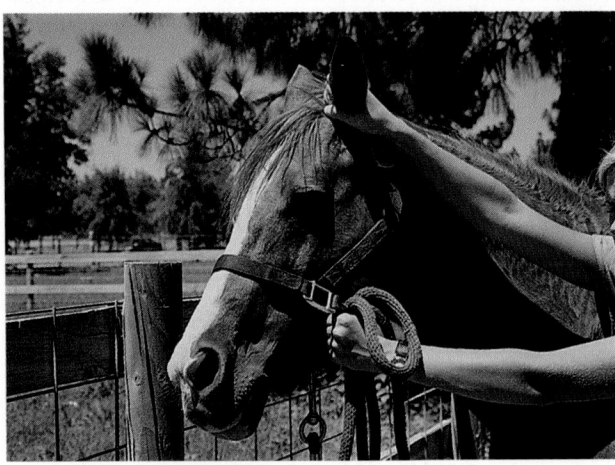

Figure 45-3 "Earing" a horse.

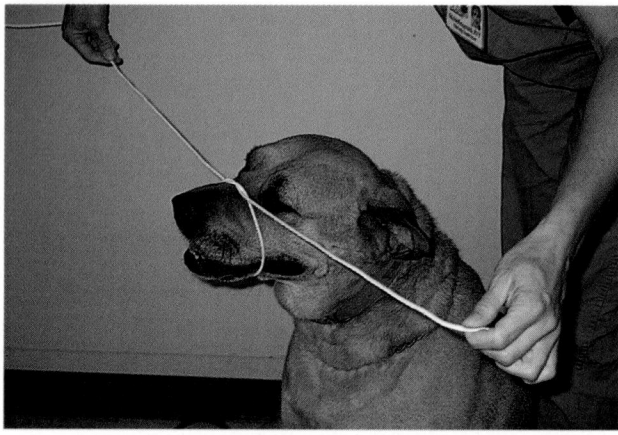

Figure 45-4 Placing a muzzle on a dog.

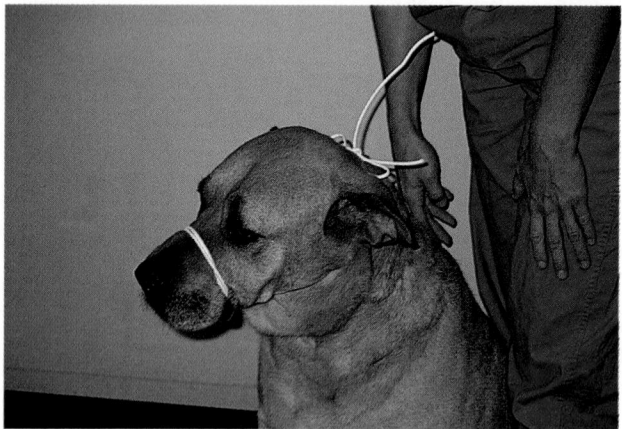

Figure 45-5 Completed muzzle on a dog.

Alternatively, a muzzle can be constructed from a nylon cord or even a shoelace. A loop should be formed with an overhand knot on one side. The loop is placed over the muzzle of the dog, with the knot on top, and tightened (Figure 45-4). The ends of the loop should be wrapped around the muzzle, crossed beneath the jaw, and tied behind the ears (Figure 45-5).

COMMON PROBLEMS

Support animals may injure each other or their human handlers, or may spread disease, such as ringworm or lice (see Chapter 41).

Trauma

Contusions, abrasions, and lacerations are the most common conditions encountered in support animals. Falls, stumbling on sharp rocks, brushing against branches, and encounters with other animals are frequent causes of injury. Such wounds should be handled similar to human injuries. Hair or wool should be trimmed from the margins of wounds before treatment or suturing to prevent matting with exudate. The skin may be sutured with any suture material suitable for humans. Antibiotics are not necessary unless vital structures, such as synovial or serosal membranes, are exposed.

Rope burns may occur in all species but are more likely to occur in horses because they tend to struggle against entanglements and their skin is quickly burned by abrasive action. Therapy is similar to that for human burns. Thermal burns are unlikely unless animals are caught in brush or forest fires.

Foot, Hoof, and Nail Problems[2]

Foot injuries may incapacitate an animal, and possibly the expedition. The hoof of the horse covers the distal extremity and third phalanx (P3). The specialized horn of the hoof and nail is analogous to the human nail. Horses are digitigrade, walking on the tip of P3. In llamas, P2 and P3 lie in a horizontal plane within the foot, with only P1 in the vertical position. The nails of the llama and dog are inconsequential in weight bearing but are extremely painful if torn or contused. The weight-bearing surface of the horse's hoof contains the firm sole and more flexible frog, overlying soft fibroelastic tissue called the digital cushion. Dogs have footpads similar to those of llamas.

The structures of the foot are subject to contusions, abrasions, lacerations, and penetration by foreign bodies (e.g., nails, stones, sticks). Segments of the hoof wall and nail may be avulsed, exposing the sensitive laminae. Infection may invade the foot and undermine the outer layers, with abscess formation. Not all lesions are visible. Stone bruises of the sole or frog of a horse may be evident only when pressure is exerted on the site of the contusion. Foreign body penetrations and abscesses may cause reluctance to place any weight on the limb. The penetrating object may have been withdrawn or may still be in place; in either case a discolored tract leads to the depth of the wound. Erosions and ulcerations of the footpads are common in unconditioned dogs and llamas. Dogs working in ice, snow, mud, and water may develop maceration, cracks, erosions, lacerations, and frostbite.

Foot and limb trauma is accompanied by varying degrees of lameness (limping). It may be difficult to establish which leg is painful, but the principles are similar to evaluation of such pain in humans, with two extra limbs to evaluate.

Cellulitis may develop on the limbs or body. The signs include heat, swelling, and redness and are the same in all species, as is therapy.

Therapy for foot injuries includes providing drainage of infected lesions, disinfection, and protection of exposed sensitive structures. Antibiotics are not indicated for most wounds unless a joint surface is exposed. It may be necessary to bandage the foot to provide protection while in camp and to fashion special shoes or boots to keep an animal functioning on the trail. Special booties are available commercially for dogs, but a temporary moccasin may be constructed from soft leather, such as that used for human moccasins.

Hyperthermia (Heat Stress, Heat Exhaustion)[8,9]

Hyperthermia is elevation of the core body temperature above normal limits. As with humans, animals on a trek may become overextended and develop hyperthermia (see Chapters 10 and 11).

Etiology. The primary cause of hyperthermia in pack animals on treks is excessive muscular exertion, especially during periods of high environmental temperatures and high humidity. Animals that struggle for prolonged periods in swampy terrain or in snow or mud may also produce excessive heat. Although high ambient temperature is a contributing factor, excessive muscle exertion in any climate may increase body temperature. Pack animals may also develop fever as a result of infectious diseases. Dehydration from inadequate supplies of potable water exacerbates the problem.

Inadequate physical conditioning is a common problem and contributes to a cumulative heat load. Other contributing factors may include lack of salt in the diet, preexisting cardiovascular insufficiency, obesity, and trauma.

Clinical Signs. Signs may vary according to species and the stage of hyperthermia, but all affected animals have an increased heart and respiratory rate, usually accompanied by open-mouth breathing. Rectal temperatures may vary from 41.1° to 43.3° C (106° to 110° F). Horses, mules, donkeys, and llamas sweat in the early stages of hyperthermia, but sweating may cease if the animal becomes severely dehydrated. Sweating is evident in horses but imperceptible in llamas because most sweating occurs on the ventral abdomen in what is known as the thermal window, where the fibers are less dense and the staple is short.

Dogs cool themselves by evaporation of respiratory fluids while panting. The mouth is held open and the tongue lolls from the mouth. The respiratory rate increases from a normal of 30 breaths/min up to 200 to 400 breaths/min. Moisture may be observed dripping from the tongue. As dehydration intensifies, salivation and dripping may slow or cease.

Hyperthermia causes a shift of blood volume from the viscera and muscles to the skin, resulting in hypovolemia and varying degrees of hypotension. Hypotension causes hypoxemia of the brain, resulting in dullness, restlessness, and incoordination. Hypoxemia may lead to convulsions and collapse. The shift of blood from the gastrointestinal tract may cause decreased motility and the potential for ileus and tympany. Colicky signs (kicking at the belly, looking back at the side, treading, attempting to lie down and roll) in horses and llamas may be noted.

A 1° C (1.8° F) rise in body temperature requires 10% more oxygen for the body's energy systems. When body temperature reaches 41° C (105.8° F), the respiratory system is no longer able to supply sufficient oxygen by normal respiration. Respiratory acidosis and electrolyte imbalances associated with sweating may produce a syndrome similar to septicemia.

Hyperthermia can affect most organ systems. The severity of the syndrome cannot be assessed in the field. It is important to recognize the conditions that lead to hyperthermia, watch for early signs of heat stress, and stop any activity that contributes to the problem. Mules and donkeys are not likely to become severely affected because they refuse to go on if stressed. Horses may be driven past their endurance and die of thermal stress.

Treatment. Cessation of excessive muscular activity may be all that is necessary if hyperthermia is mild. If streams or lakes are nearby, the animal can be walked into the water and water splashed on its underbelly. Contingencies for hyperthermia are part of all plans for capture operations for wildlife translocation and reintroduction projects. Water is carried for cooling and intravenous fluids for heat stress. Cold-water enemas are the most effective and rapid way to cool the body of a large animal.

Plant Poisoning[4,10,12,15]

Certain highly toxic plants that grow in wilderness areas of the United States should be recognized (Table 45-2) (see Chapters 48 and 49). Cooperative extension offices at federal land grant institutions frequently publish booklets on local poisonous plants.

Horses may be less at risk than llamas because horses are primarily grazers and not likely to eat trees and shrubs. Llamas eat small quantities of almost anything within reach.

Animals are not affected by poison oak (*Rhus diversiloba*) or poison ivy (*Rhus toxicodendron*). However, horses, dogs, and llamas may transmit the toxic oils of these shrubs to susceptible people through contact with contaminated hair.

Few specific antidotes are available for plant poisons. Symptomatic and supportive treatment includes removal of the poisonous material from the gastrointestinal tract by administration of a cathartic or adsorbing the toxin with a nonspecific substance such as activated charcoal (See Table 45-3).

TABLE 45-2. Poisonous Plants That May Affect Horses or Llamas on Trek

COMMON NAME	SCIENTIFIC NAME	POISONOUS PRINCIPLE	SIGNS OF POISONING	HABITAT	SPECIES	THERAPY*
False hellebore, corn lily	*Veratrum californicum*	Alkaloids	Vomiting, salivation, convulsions, fast irregular pulse	High mountains, meadows	Llama	Symptomatic
Death camas, sandcorn	*Zigadenus* spp.	Alkaloids	Foaming at mouth, convulsions, ataxia, vomiting, fast weak pulse	Hillsides, fields, meadows, in spring of year	Horse, llama	Symptomatic
Water hemlock	*Cicuta douglasii*	Resin	Frothing at mouth, muscle twitching, convulsions, death in 15-30 minutes	Standing or running water, obligate aquatic	Horse, llama	Symptomatic
Nightshade	*Solanum* spp.	Alkaloidal glycoside, solanine	Vomiting, weakness, groaning	Ubiquitous	Horse, llama	Symptomatic
Jimson weed	*Datura stramonium*	Alkaloid, atropine	Dry mucous membranes, dilated pupils, mania	Waste places	Horse, llama	Parasympathomimetics
Tobacco, tree tobacco	*Nicotiana* spp.	Alkaloid, nicotine	Stimulation of CNS, then depression; sweating, muscle twitching, convulsions	Waste places	Horse, llama	Symptomatic
Lupine, blue bonnet	*Lupinus* spp.	Alkaloid	CNS depression, dyspnea, muscle twitching, ataxia, frothing, convulsions	Ubiquitous	Horse, llama	Symptomatic
Dogbane, Indian hemp	*Apocynum cannabinum*	Cardioactive glycoside (similar to digitoxin)	Dyspnea, cardiac arrhythmias, agonal convulsions, vomiting, diarrhea	Ubiquitous	Horse, llama	Symptomatic
Oleander	*Nerium oleander*	Same as dogbane	Same as dogbane	Ornamental	Horse, llama	Symptomatic, gastrotomy
Castor bean	*Ricinus communis*	Ricin, water solution	Anaphylactic shock, diarrhea	Ornamental	Horse, llama	Treat for shock; fluids
Rhododendron	*Rhododendron* spp.	Andromedotoxin glycoside	Vomiting, colic, severe depression	Shrubs in meadows and moist places	Llama	Activated charcoal, time

CNS, Central nervous system.

*In most cases of poisoning from ingestion of poisonous plants, no specific antidote exists. Victims are treated symptomatically. The critical factor is to empty the digestive tract of the plant material with cathartics, parasympathomimetic stimulation, and enemas. Activated charcoal may be of value given orally.

Eye Injuries

An abrasion, laceration, or penetrating wound of the cornea is serious, especially in a field situation. Dust and other foreign bodies within the conjunctival sac require prompt removal to avoid more serious injury to the cornea. The management of eye problems in animals is the same as for humans, with the added difficulty of restraint for examination and therapy.

Lightning Injuries[6,9]

Lightning strike is a potential hazard in the wilderness (see Chapter 3). Animals with high head carriage, such as the horse and llama, are especially at risk, whether standing or recumbent. Animals may survive a lightning strike, but frequently a strike is lethal. Unless the strike is witnessed, it may be difficult to make a diagnosis, but signs include depression, blindness, nystagmus, paralysis of the hind limbs, and temporary unconsciousness. Linear singe marks are definitive, but lightning may kill an animal without producing burns. One llama was struck while recumbent in an open pasture, and the green grass beneath it had been singed. A single lightning strike may kill more than one animal, especially if a group has congregated under a tree for shelter. Lightning may kill so quickly that feed is still in the mouth of grazing animals.

During an electrical storm, animals should be taken to the safest environment, away from tall trees and exposed hills. Llamas may be encouraged to lie down in a small ravine, depression, or rock face, with the head tied close to the ground. A picket-line stake may be used for the tie-down. An animal should not be tied to a tree, but a small bush may be safe. Horses are more difficult because they will not lie down unless specially trained to do so.

If an animal is struck and still alive, the degree of damage to the nervous system and other vital organs will manifest over time. If the strike is witnessed and the heart has stopped, cardiac massage may be performed if conditions are safe. With the animal in lateral recumbency, the forelimb is pulled as far cranially as possible, and the chest wall is compressed just caudal to the triceps muscle. Cardiac massage may be required for several minutes.

Snakebite[5]

Venomous snakes are found in most wilderness areas of the world, except the Arctic and Antarctic. Leaders should know the species of snakes that may be encountered on the trek and should instruct all personnel on treating a bite in a human or animal. In the United States the venomous snakes most likely to be encountered are pit vipers, especially rattlesnakes of *Crotalus* species. Other members of the North American pit viper group include the copperhead, *Agkistrodon contortrix,* and the water moccasin, *Agkistrodon piscivorus* (see Chapter 38).

Llamas and young horses are curious and may extend their nose to investigate a strange animal. Thus an animal may be bitten on the nose. Leg bites may occur in any animal.

Clinical Signs. Venom injection results in pronounced swelling in the area of the bite in 1 to 3 hours. The most serious consequence of a nose bite is swelling that occludes the nostrils, making it difficult for horses and llamas to breathe. Dogs are not obligate nasal breathers, but the effects of a bite may be more severe in them than in larger animals. A rattlesnake bite on the nose is an emergency.

Treatment. A 10-cm (4-inch) segment of 1-cm-diameter, flexible plastic tubing should be in the first-aid kit. The tube should be inserted into a nostril before any swelling occurs, preventing occlusion of the nostril and providing a passageway for air. A tube cannot be inserted after swelling has developed, when the only life-saving procedure is a tracheostomy. The rescuer should *not* cut the skin and suck out the venom, since this is ineffective.

The only specific treatment for pit viper envenomation is administration of antivenin. Freeze-dried vials of antivenin may be carried and the same product is used for humans and animals. One to three vials should be administered intravenously when signs of envenomation have appeared.

Choke[8,9]

"Choke" in humans refers to lodging of food or other objects in the larynx or trachea, a life-threatening emergency. Choke in animals usually refers to lodging of food or other objects in the esophagus. The signs of choke may be alarming, but an animal will rarely die unless feed is regurgitated and inhaled into the lungs.

Etiology. Choke is most often caused by overly rapid ingestion of pellets and grain. Animals should be accustomed to any supplemental feed used on the trek. Ingestion may be slowed by placing rock pebbles in the container used to feed the animal, causing it to separate the rocks from the feed. An animal rarely swallows a metallic or wooden object. Llamas and horses are too fastidious in their eating habits to consume such objects.

Clinical Signs. Retching occurs as the animal attempts to dislodge the mass. Choked animals are able to breathe but are in obvious distress. Saliva may flow from the mouth, and the animal may cough up particles of the material (e.g., grain, pellets). A mass may be palpated on the left side of the neck if the obstruction is in the cervical area. Peristaltic waves may be observed moving up and down the left side of the neck. The mass may lodge anywhere along the esophagus but generally lies within the chest and is not visible externally.

Treatment. Water may be offered, but feed should be withheld until the problem has corrected itself. If palpations along the lower neck reveals a bulge, gentle massage will determine if it can be moved. Moderate exercise may cause the object to move toward the stomach. In some cases, passage of a stomach tube and application of gentle pressure may push the mass into the stomach. Medication may be necessary to relax esophageal muscle spasm.

Drowning[9]

Llamas, horses and dogs can swim, but circumstances may cause submersion in water and inhalation of water into the lungs. A heavy fleece is a serious detriment to a llama in water over its head. Floods may trap and drown animals.

The primary problem is to extricate the animal from its predicament, which may be extremely difficult with a large llama or a horse. It is necessary to act quickly (less than 5 minutes) to prevent death. If the animal is to revive, water must be drained from the lungs. The llama is placed on its right side with the body slanted downward to the neck and head so that water can flow out. Regurgitation is a risk in this position, but the need to remove the water from the lungs must take precedence, even though this is a desperation maneuver at best. If immersion lasted for more than 2 to 3 minutes, the heart may have stopped, making cardiac massage necessary. The action must be continued until the animal responds or is declared dead. It is highly unlikely that resuscitation will be successful in an animal that has been under water for more than 5 minutes, regardless of the water temperature.

MANAGEMENT ISSUES

Wound Dressing and Bandaging

The principles of wound dressing for animals are basically the same as those for humans. Avoid placing cotton or a bandage directly on the wound. A gauze 4 × 4-inch compress or an absorbent hydrogel pad is the best material to place against the wound. A padded or absorbent layer is then placed to collect fluids. A surface or protective bandage is applied to hold the padding in place.

A variety of bandage materials is suitable. Coban or Vetrap (bandage tape) is the most effective bandage material because it is porous, sticks to itself, and is flexible, adjusting to uneven surfaces. Other products, such as Elastikon (elastic tape) or rolled gauze bandages, also are excellent. Duct tape is satisfactory, but care should taken to avoid wrapping it too tightly, because the tape has no extensibility and may become a tourniquet.

Placement of a smooth bandage requires skill. Once the anchor roll is in place, firm but uniform pressure should be applied as the bandage unrolls. Joints require special attention. Bandaging should be done in a figure-8 pattern to provide uniform pressure over a variably shaped surface. Pressure is avoided over the point of the hock and the accessory carpal bone (back of the carpus).

The foot requires special consideration. Dress a foot wound appropriately, making certain that the space between the digits of dogs or llamas is padded with cotton. The easiest bandage to apply is a Vetrap (Coban) elastic bandage that conforms to the odd shape. If a severe foot wound occurs while trekking in the backcountry, additional protection may be necessary to allow the animal to continue on the journey. A sheet of pliable leather is used, and the dressed foot is placed in the sheet's center. The leather is gathered up around the pastern and held in place by duct tape or another bandage, forming a boot shape.

Another method of bandaging a foot uses a rolled gauze bandage. After dressing the foot, a wrap is made around the pastern, leaving a tail of gauze approximately 15 cm (6 inches) long. The tail is used as a fulcrum to change direction on the bandage as the digits are covered.

Cardiopulmonary Resuscitation[8,9]

It is unlikely that rescue breathing would be required for an animal while on trek, except in a lightning strike or drowning. The procedure is different than employed in humans because mouth-to-mouth breathing cannot be performed on an adult llama or horse, although it could be performed in a dog by clamping the mouth and lips shut and breathing through the nostrils. A llama or horse should be placed in lateral recumbency, preferably on the right side. The rescuer stands at the animal's withers (top of the shoulder) and reaches across the body to grasp and lift the arch of the rib cage. This maneuver flattens the diaphragm and expands the chest, producing inspiration. This same area is not compressed to force expiration, since this will put pressure on the stomach and possibly cause regurgitation. Instead, the area over the heart is compressed just above the elbow and caudal to the muscles of the upper limb. The rate for the horse or llama is 10 to 15 breaths/min. Rescue breathing in the dog is performed by compressing the chest at the widest segment of the thorax at a rate of 20 to 30 breaths/min.

Cardiac massage may be performed by placing the llama or horse on its right side, if not already there. An assistant pulls the upper foreleg forward and presses the chest in the area vacated by pulling the leg forward. The rescuer kneels next to the bottom of the chest, positioning the heels of both hands against the chest approximately 15 cm above the sternum, with the fingers directed toward the spine. The person presses firmly with the arms held straight and releases quickly, repeating the movement every second. After 15 compressions, check for a pulse in the saphenous artery on the medial aspect of the stifle in a llama, or listen for the heart beat with a stethoscope. After 15 heart compressions, the rescuers administer five cycles of rescue breathing, as described previously. It is futile to continue cardiac massage if no oxygen is available to the heart or the general circulation. Massage must be continued until the heartbeat returns and the animal begins to breathe, or when signs indicate that the victim is dead (pupils dilated, no response to touching the cornea).

Small or round-chested dogs are placed on their back, with compressions over the sternum. For the type of dogs likely to be on a trek, cardiac massage is performed in lateral recumbency.[1]

Disaster and Emergency Management[6]

A wilderness trek may be engulfed by a natural disaster (see Chapter 67). Attitude may be the key to human survival in a disaster situation and is also important when dealing with animals. The best assurance of a positive attitude is advance planning and preparation. Although safety and protection of people take precedence, animals should be not neglected.

Ice Storm. When rain freezes immediately on striking the ground or foliage, people and animals may have extreme difficulty walking. Animals may fall and injure themselves. In one situation a late-spring snowstorm with freezing rain halted a group of horses on a small mountain peak. Frightened by the thunder and lightning, the horses, milled around as rain and snow accumulated within their shoes, producing horses on ice skates. Fortunately, no injuries occurred before the storm abated and the feet could be cleaned out.

Fire. Fire is an ever-present risk in forests and shrubbed areas (see Chapter 12). Trek leaders should have a plan for evacuation to safety, as well as for dealing with the animals.

In brush and forest fires, wind is an important factor. Crown fires (flames racing through the tops of trees in a forest) are particularly troublesome. One should not try to outrun a fire burning up a slope. The heat generated by the fire rises and preheats the area above the fire, setting up ideal conditions for rapid spread. A hillside may seem to explode into flames because of the extensive preheating.

When llamas were caught in an advancing brush fire, they were herded into a bare ground area. In another situation, llamas were simply turned loose to fend for themselves. Owners reported that the animals adjusted quite well, without panic. When they could return, they found the animals were hungry and thirsty but with no evidence of smoke inhalation or eye damage. Llama fiber does not burn readily, but it does smolder, and some burn spots were noted in the fleece. At one ranch the only serious problem was burns on the footpads, presumably caused by animals stepping on hot coals. No one was able to observe how adult and young animals avoided the flames.

Flooding. Animals may become involved in flood conditions when they are tethered near streams or rivers that are known to generate flash floods. Animals are at the same risk as the humans in the party. Dry stream beds in many desert areas are ideally suited for flash floods that may be generated miles away, so avoid dry stream beds for camping sites. Animals should not be tethered in such locations.

Trek leaders should be aware of dams along streams, especially earth-filled dams. Heavy storms may erode a dam or fill a reservoir beyond its capacity. A llama owner in Idaho watched as a wall of water filled a gorge more than 30 m (100 feet) deep and nearly engulfed his home, barns, llamas, and farm from a burst dam a few miles upstream. Horses, llamas, and dogs can swim but may not be able to cope with the currents generated during a flood.

DISORDERS OF HORSES, MULES, AND DONKEYS

Common trail disorders encountered in horses may be classified as traumatic, metabolic, or digestive tract upsets.

Laminitis (Founder)[2,11,13,14]

Etiology. Trauma is the most likely cause of inflammation of the foot in the trek horse. Horses should have been trained in a terrain similar to that to be found on the trek. Even a trained horse, however, occasionally encounters an excessively rocky path that traumatizes its feet, especially if the rider fails to slow the pace when negotiating the trail. Leather or synthetic pads worn under the shoe may offer some protection, but new pads may be chewed off the foot by rocky trails after less than 80 km (50 miles).

Laminitis may be a sequel to severe digestive upset in a horse. Inflammation within the confines of an inflexible hoof causes malperfusion at the capillary level of the foot, which is accompanied by arteriovenous shunting.

Clinical Signs. Laminitis usually develops on both forefeet, but rear feet may also be affected in severe cases. The horse shifts its center of gravity to the hind limbs to minimize pressure on the forefeet, standing with the hind limbs forward under the body and the forelimbs extended in front of the body. The feet are hot to palpation, and the digital artery pulse is pounding. The horse is reluctant to move.

Treatment. Therapy is directed at reestablishing circulation in the foot. Proper circulation of blood within the hoof depends partially on the pumping action of the foot while walking. Mild exercise is an important aid in preventing damage to the laminae. The horse should be exercised slowly on soft ground for 10 to 15 minutes every hour for 12 to 24 hours, then exercise should be stopped. Even slow walking may be quite painful, and an analgesic (phenylbutazone, 2 to 4 g orally once daily) may be necessary. Corticosteroids are contraindicated.

Although soaking in cold water may give temporary relief to feet sore from laminitis, this practice is actually contraindicated in acute laminitis. Warm water soaks are appropriate, since they dilate the vascular tree and enhance circulation. A low volar block inhibits vascular constriction within the foot. This is accomplished by palpating the pulsating artery on the posterolateral aspect of the fetlock (Figure 45-6). The nerve lies posterior to the artery. With a 20- to 22-gauge needle, 3 ml of 2% lidocaine is injected over each nerve. It may be necessary to repeat nerve blocks two or three times daily for several days.

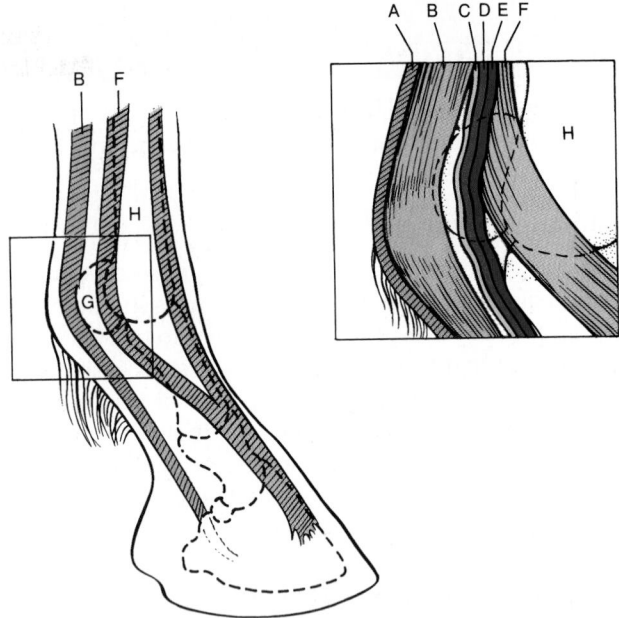

Figure 45-6 Diagram of the anatomy of the equine fetlock. *A,* Skin. *B,* Flexor tendons. *C,* Volar nerve. *D,* Palmar digital artery. *E,* Digital vein. *F,* Suspensory ligament. *G,* Sesamoid bone. *H,* Metacarpal bone (cannon).

Saddle, Cinch, and Rigging Sores[3,14]

Saddle sores are contusions, abrasions, or ulcerations of the skin and subcutis caused by friction or point pressure from the saddle, cinch, or rigging.

Etiology. Improperly fitted or maintained tack is the primary cause of saddle sores. A saddle tree may fit a horse properly at the beginning of a training period but become unsatisfactory after the horse has trimmed down.

Poorly distributed pressure is the primary cause of saddle sores. Spot pressure causes local ischemia. If pressure is prolonged, the capillary bed may be damaged. When the pressure is released rapidly, blood rushes into the blanched site and extravasation may occur, causing swelling and pain.

If the lesion is rested and treated as inflamed tissue, complete healing may occur. If the saddle is reapplied, however, it overlies a lump that is subject to abrasion. The injury can extend through the dermis, resulting in severe ulceration. Cinch and rigging sores are usually caused by friction, leading to blister formation.

Clinical Signs. Hot and tender swellings are the primary signs of acute saddle sores. The hair or epidermis may be rubbed off. General sensitivity over the back is usually caused by muscle soreness. Evidence of previous sores includes white hairs in spots over the withers or saddle bed, scars with or without hairs, thickening of the dermis, and alopecia with or without swelling.

Treatment. Prevention is better than treatment. Toughening the backs of trail horses is a major job of the trainer. Proper pads or blankets must be selected for each horse. On arrival at a rest area, the girth should be slowly loosened at intervals of 10 to 15 minutes to prevent rapid flow of blood into ischemic areas.

Once a sore has developed, the horse must be rested or the tack changed to eliminate pressure or friction on the lesion. Holes are often cut in pads to accommodate a saddle sore, but spot pressure at the ring edge may be as detrimental as the original cause of the saddle sore. Riders must keep tack cleaned and in good repair. When the saddle is removed, cold water poured over the back may minimize swelling.

Myopathy[3,11,13,14]

Exertional myopathies of horses range from simple muscle soreness, through the "tying-up" syndrome, to paralytic myoglobinuria (rhabdomyolysis, azoturia).

Etiology. Muscle integrity and function depend on proper mobilization and use of energy. Conditioned muscles may function vigorously for extended periods, but if either energy parameter is accelerated to the extreme, mild to severe muscle necrosis may occur.

Clinical Signs. Mild muscle soreness is characterized by alterations in gait that indicate muscle weakness. As severity increases, the gait becomes progressively altered until the horse is in obvious pain and reluctant to move. The horse has an anxious expression and may sweat excessively. Affected muscles are painful to palpation and may be swollen. Skin temperature over the muscle may be elevated. Muscle spasms may occur, but not consistently. Myoglobinuria is observed grossly in moderate to severe cases and should suggest stopping and resting or treating the horse.

Treatment. Rest is paramount in all cases. A rider may have difficulty differentiating the pain associated with myopathy from that seen with colic. It is disastrous to force the severely myopathic horse to walk, as is done with a suspected case of colic. If there is doubt, the horse should not be exercised.

Horses in inaccessible locations should not be walked out until all possible recovery has taken place. Horses with mild muscle soreness may improve if walked slowly, but rest from ride exertion is the primary recommended therapy.

Dehydration

Etiology. Fluid and electrolyte imbalances play a major role in all metabolic problems that develop in the horse as a result of exertional stress. The degree of dehydration is directly related to the amount of fluid loss through evaporative cooling (sweat), which in turn is related to the amount and rate of work performed and to ambient temperatures and humidity.

The horse must have an adequate amount (10 to 15 gallons) of water each day during a trek. The more strenuous the activity , the more fluids are required. Mules and especially donkeys are adapted to cope with mild dehydration.

Clinical Signs. Signs of mild dehydration (3% body weight loss) are low urine output, dry mouth, and mild loss of skin elasticity. Moderate dehydration (5% body weight loss) is characterized by marked loss of skin elasticity. The eyes become sunken. Blood pressure may fall as a result of decreased plasma volume, with weakness, fever, and a weak pulse. Sweating is not possible, even with elevated body temperature.

Marked dehydration (10% body weight loss) may involve circulatory failure from decreased plasma volume.

Treatment. During 3 hours of hard work a 450-kg (990-pound) horse may lose as much as 45 L of fluid. If this degree of dehydration is not corrected quickly, death may result. The horse should be allowed to drink along the trail if water is available. Small amounts of cool (not cold) water should be offered. If the horse refuses to drink, gastric intubation may be indicated. Fluid is also absorbed from the colon; thus enemas (2000 to 5000 ml water) are effective in rehydration.

Heat stress usually accompanies dehydration, so cooling (e.g., shade, water bath) is important. Administration of intravenous (IV) fluids, if available, is routine therapy.

Exhausted Horse Syndrome[2,11,13]

Exhausted horse syndrome (EHS) describes a complex metabolic disease occurring when horses are pushed beyond endurance limits. The syndrome has no precise characterization because the initiating mechanism may vary with the prevailing conditions. The development of EHS depends on the condition and training of the horse, the pace set by the rider, the terrain traversed, and climatic factors such as temperature, wind, and humidity.

Clinical Signs. The severely affected horse is depressed and exhibits lethargic movements, holding its head low. The ears are expressionless. Facial grimacing creates an anxious expression, which may progress to a painful expression if colic or muscle spasms accompany the syndrome. The horse takes no interest in its surroundings. Anorexia is typical, and frequently the horse has no inclination to drink, even though dehydrated. The corneas appear glazed.

Body temperature is usually elevated and may reach 41° C (106° F). The horse does not cool properly. Usually, body temperature continues to rise. Temperature measured rectally may be inaccurate in the exhausted horse, since the anal sphincter loses tone and allows air to enter the rectum.

Cardiovascular and respiratory systems are greatly affected by endurance riding. Heart and respiratory rates are elevated. The degree depends on the prior condition of the horse, pace, length of action, and amount of work performed in climbing or walking on soft footing. Heart rates may reach 150 beats/min after a grueling climb. With 10 to 15 minutes of rest the heart rate of a conditioned horse should drop to below 60 beats/min, whereas tachycardia and tachypnea may persist in the exhausted horse, which may have a respiratory rate faster than the heart rate. Respiration is shallow and inefficient. Cardiopulmonary signs also include synchronous diaphragmatic flutter, arrhythmias, murmurs, and visible jugular pulses. Auscultation of the thorax may reveal moist rales and in extreme cases frank pulmonary edema.

Severe dehydration is the most consistent sign of EHS. Loss of skin elasticity, sunken eyeballs, dry mouth, and dry mucous membranes reflect a 7% to 10% loss of body weight, after loss of 30 to 40 L of fluid. Serious electrolyte and acid-base imbalances are associated with dehydration. Alkalosis is common.

Muscular manifestations of EHS include fatigue, trembling, spasm, stiffness, muscles painful to palpation, and rarely, tying-up. Tying-up is usually a distinct entity.

Horses suffering from EHS are prone to colic, which also may occur independently. When colic accompanies EHS, it is of the spasmodic type, with diminished or absent borborygmus.

Treatment. Rest, rehydration, and electrolyte supplementation are the keys to recovery. If the horse is drinking and will take electrolytes in the water, the effect is almost as beneficial as the administration of IV fluids. Packaged electrolyte powders can be carried.

If the horse is hyperthermic, shows evidence of shock, and refuses to drink, more drastic steps must be taken. The horse may require 40 to 50 L of fluid. Besides IV fluid administration, gastric intubation may provide fluids orally. Enemas are also effective, since fluid is absorbed from the colon.

Synchronous Diaphragmatic Flutter[3,11,13]

Synchronous diaphragmatic flutter (SDF) is a clinical sign observed in endurance horses while on long-distance rides and may be seen on an expedition. It is defined as a spasmodic contraction of the diaphragm synchronous with the heartbeat. Overexertion with excessive sweating produces mild to serious metabolic alterations that may be life threatening. The development of SDF on a trek indicates that the horse should not continue.

Unlike acute exertional stress, which is characterized by acidemia, SDF is associated with alkalemia. Electrolyte imbalances may also be involved. Hypocalcemia, hypokalemia, and alkalosis probably cause equine SDF.

Clinical Signs. SDF may develop after 32 to 48 km (20 to 30 miles) of riding. There is no gender, age, or breed predilection. The primary sign is spasmodic contraction in the flank area. The "thump" is easily felt by light palpation in the flank area. Auscultating the heart while holding a hand over the dorsocaudal rib area reveals that diaphragmatic contraction is synchronous with the heartbeat. SDF may be the only clinical sign, or may be part of EHS.

The degree of thumping may vary from a barely perceptible quiver to a contraction that seems to rock the horse's body and is observable from a distance. The flutter may be continuous or intermittent, especially in degree.

Treatment. Rest and rehydration are required.

Colic

Colic is the clinical manifestation of abdominal pain, usually the result of a gastrointestinal disorder. It may also arise from the urinary system or peritoneum. Types of colic are numerous because of the unique and complex anatomy of the equine digestive system.

Etiology. Colic may be produced by gastric tympany, intestinal obstruction, or hyperspasticity. The most likely inciting causes on a trek are overeating of non-regular forages, ingestion of poisonous plants, or exhaustion. In one case a commercial packer took horses to graze in a meadow for a noon rest stop. Two hours later, at the start of the afternoon trek, two of the horses were colicky. In checking the meadow the packer saw many plants of death camas (*Zygadenus* species), some of which had been eaten. The colic was sufficiently severe to require a layover at the meadow for the rest of the day.

Clinical Signs. Horses express colic by looking back at one side, stamping the feet, getting up and down, rolling, and pressing the head against trees or rocks. The pulse rate may exceed 100 beats/min with severe pain. The conjunctival membranes are congested and cyanotic.

Treatment. Reports discuss only superficial emergency measures. Treatment depends on the anatomic location of the obstruction or spasm. Mild obstructions may be relieved by hydration and administration of a cathartic. Cold-water enemas may stimulate sluggish intestinal peristalsis and relieve impaction of the small (terminal) colon. Pain and spasms may be relieved by administration of flunixen meglumine (Banamine), 1 mg/kg intramuscularly twice a day. Walking the horse may prevent it from lying down and injuring itself by rolling.

DISORDERS OF PACK LLAMAS

Most of the medical problems of llamas have been considered under headings of disorders common to all animals. Llamas are hardy animals and unlikely to allow themselves to be pushed to exhaustion. If fatigued, they simply lie down and refuse to rise. They will not tolerate excessive loads. About 45 kg (100 pounds) is an appropriate load for a large, well-trained and conditioned llama.

Plant poisoning is more likely in llamas than in horses, but such incidents are rare. Rope burns from entanglement in tethers are less likely than in horses. The llama is less excitable, and if it becomes entangled, it usually lies quietly until help arrives.

North American venomous snakes pose minimal threat to large animals. Llamas are curious, however, and may be bitten on the nose while investigating the strange animal. Nose bites from rattlesnakes are especially hazardous to llamas because local swelling may occlude the nostrils. Llamas are primarily obligate nose breathers, so dyspnea and suffocation may ensue. Rattlesnake bites of the limbs cause edema and in severe cases, local tissue necrosis and ulceration. Many cases are diagnosed as nonspecific trauma unless the bite is observed. The signs of snakebite in llamas are essentially the same as for horses.[5,8]

Therapy for a nose bite may require tracheostomy and insertion of an improvised tube to allow breathing. Edema may persist for 2 to 3 days. If the bite is observed and progressive swelling noted, a small tube (1 cm diameter) can be inserted 15 cm (6 inches) into the ventral meatus of the nasal passage and sutured to the nares. Swelling occurs around the tube, but patency of the nasal passage is maintained.

DISORDERS OF DOGS

Exercise Stress

Sled dogs are usually conditioned for heavy work, but the inexperienced handler may push animals beyond their endurance. Dogs without adequate conditioning are frequently taken on other treks. Muscle soreness, fatigue, dehydration, and hyperthermia are common and are dealt with as for humans. Erosions of the footpads require special care. A sheet of soft leather out of which to fashion boots should be carried.

Porcupine Quills

When dogs are brought into porcupine country, the risk of an encounter is great. Some dogs fail to learn from experience and are repeatedly quilled. The dog must have physical contact with the porcupine for the introduction of quills. The muzzle and face are the usual sites of penetration, and a dog can be blinded by perforation of the eyeball.

The quills must be removed physically. A pair of pliers should be included in supplies and equipment. The process is painful and requires sedation (e.g., diazepam). The quill should not be broken because the retrograde barbs on the quill foster migration and abscess formation.

Grass Awns

Numerous species of grass awns ("foxtails") may become attached to the dog's coat or lodged in the external ear canal, nasal passage, conjunctival sac, or interdigital space. Dogs that travel when plants are mature and awns are easily dislodged from the seed head should be inspected frequently for awns in these sites.

Signs depend on the location of the foreign body. When it is within the ear canal, the dog paws at its ear and shakes its head. The head may be held tilted. Exudate may flow from the ear. Awns in the nostril cause sneezing and nasal exudate. Awns in the conjunctival sac cause lacrimation, photophobia, and corneal edema and ulceration. The dog paws at the eye. Awn penetration between the digits and at other locations through the skin is more difficult to diagnose because the awn may be some distance from the fistula.

Awns must be removed physically. Sedation, topical anesthesia, or both may be necessary. Although topical ophthalmic anesthetics are desirable in the eye, lidocaine may be used in an emergency. A pair of small alligator forceps is most suitable for reaching into otherwise inaccessible places. An otoscope may be necessary to visualize awns in the nostril or ear canal. An antibiotic ointment should be instilled after removal of the awn.

Stinging Nettle Poisoning

Stinging nettle (*Urtica* species) is common along streams and lakes in wilderness areas. Humans vary in sensitivity when the plants accidentally contact exposed skin. Leaves and stems are covered by harsh hairs, some of which have a tiny ball tip that breaks off just before penetration. The specialized hairs are hollow. A base gland produces histamines and acetylcholine, which are injected into the victim.

Short-haired dogs that move through patches of stinging nettle are at risk of poisoning from the cumulative effect of thousands of minute injections of acetylcholine. Weakness, dyspnea, and muscle tremors are characteristic of the action of acetylcholine on peripheral nerves. Parasympathomimetic effects include salivation, diarrhea, tachycardia, and pupillary dilation. Atropine sulfate (0.04 mg/kg) subcutaneously is a specific treatment.

Harness Sores

Improperly fitted harnesses of sled dogs may produce the same frictional lesions that occur in horses or llamas.

ESCAPE OF SUPPORT ANIMAL

Support animals may escape from any type of restraint imposed and run away or simply wander off. More often, animals are tied with improper knots, or poor-quality snaps and halters break when pressure is applied. A trekker may tie an animal to a shrub, bush, or branch that can be easily pulled up or broken off. Animals that are frightened by predators or other animals may bolt and exert tremendous pressure on tethers, picket lines, stakes, or branches.

Hobbling is a common technique used to allow horses and mules to graze. Trek leaders must know the habits of individual animals when hobbled. One horse may accept having the front feet hobbled together and graze peacefully, taking only the short steps possible. Another horse may learn how to gallop with the front feet hobbled. Some horses must be hobbled with three restrained legs.

Even experienced trekkers (e.g., commercial packers) may become overconfident and accept an animal's willingness to stand quietly without wandering away. They may leave just a lead rope dragging on the ground (ground tie). The animal may become frightened or bored and wander off. One llama carrying a full pack wandered off and was missing for a month. Contrary to popular belief, not all llamas are social, so they may not return to a herd that is securely tethered. As with horses and dogs, llamas have homing instincts and may set off in the presumed direction.

If a breakaway is observed, members of the party should not further frighten the animal by rushing at it. It should be given a chance to settle down and return to the group. The handlers can move around the animal to block obvious escape routes but should not try to chase it. All these animals can run faster than a human.

If the escapee has an animal "buddy" in the group or a favorite person, he or she can make an approach. A favorite treat in camp can be used to entice the animal back to the fold.

If an animal is discovered missing, the situation is assessed to determine the cause and direction taken. Generally, animals return toward the direction from which they have come. Frightened animals or those escaping at night may not adhere to any rule. A search for tracks can be made, but llamas may not leave much evidence, particularly in rocky terrain.

Scanning the surroundings may reveal the animal. It may be in the vicinity of camp resting under a tree or in a clump of bushes. Unless tracks direct otherwise, the path back toward a trailhead should be searched first. Another animal, preferably a buddy of the escapee, should be taken on the search. Even though the animal is sighted, it may not be caught unless a second animal is there to bait it in. Using vantage points, searchers should consider where they might have gone under the circumstances. Lush meadows or other areas with desirable feed should be checked.

Fellow hikers and ultimately the Forest Service or other regulatory agencies should be alerted about the missing animal.

MEDICATION PROCEDURES

Table 45-3 lists medications for animals and indications for their use; the appendix lists sources for these veterinary drugs. In the horse, intramuscular (IM) injections are given in the neck or rump. Subcutaneous (SC) injections are given by lifting a fold of skin just cranial to the scapula. IV injections are given in the jugular vein, which is easily distended along the jugular groove on the ventral aspect of the neck (Figure 45-7).

In the llama, IM injections are given in the relatively hairless area at the back of the upper rear leg, by standing against the body in front of the rear limb while facing the rear and reaching around the back of the animal to give the injection. SC injections are given in the relatively hairless area of the caudal abdomen, just in front of the rear limb. Since an inexperienced individual may have difficulty locating the jugular vein for IV administration in the llama, IM or SC routes are recommended.

In the dog, IM injections may be administered in the triceps muscles caudal to the shoulder or in the muscle masses on the upper rear limb. SC injections are made by lifting a fold of loose skin on the neck near the withers. IV administration is via the jugular or cephalic vein (Figure 45-8). For the latter, an assistant grasps the limb at the elbow to occlude the vein, which courses on the dorsal aspect of the forearm.

The vein is more visible if the hair is wetted down with water.

Euthanasia

Euthanasia may become necessary in the event of injury or illness that cannot be corrected or when the animal cannot be removed to a location where remedial action can be taken. Horses, mules, donkeys, and llamas cannot be carried out of a wilderness area manually. Large animals can be airlifted out of the wilderness by helicopter, but obtaining such help may require great time and effort. Dogs may be placed in an improvised stretcher and carried out.

Indications for euthanasia include (1) compound and comminuted fractures of long bones, (2) falling or sliding into inaccessible places from which the animal is unable to extricate itself or trek participants are unable to aid the animal, (3) lacerations exposing abdominal or thoracic organs (e.g., wild animal attacks, tree branches rammed into the body), (4) head injuries resulting in persistent convulsions or coma, and (5) protracted colicky pain unrelieved by analgesics or mild catharsis, usually associated with a pulse rate greater than 100 beats/min, rolling, and congested conjunctival membranes.

The expedition may carry a bottle of euthanasia solution, which must be given intravenously or intraperitoneally (see Table 45-3). If firearms are carried, a properly placed bullet to the head produces a fast and humane death. The shooter stands in front of the animal's head and draws an imaginary line from the medial canthus of each eye to the base of the opposite ear. The shot should be aimed where those lines cross and approximately perpendicular to the contour of the forehead (Figure 45-9). The tip of the barrel should be no more than 15 cm (6 inches) from the head. A heavy blow to the head at the same location is equally effective. The blow may be administered with the blunt edge of a single-bladed ax or hatchet. A large rock held in the hand may also be used. A less desirable but sometimes expedient method is to sever the jugular vein to allow exsanguination. This would probably be used on an animal that is already unconscious.

Some vital statistics for support animals are provided in Table 45-1. Equipment for support animals and the sources are listed in Box 45-1, Table 45-4, and the appendix.

Body Temperature

The rectal body temperature of an animal is assessed by inserting a thermometer lubricated with water or spittle through the anus with a slight twisting motion. Heavy-duty glass veterinary clinical thermometers are available, but regular human clinical thermometers are equally useful. In hot climates, clinical thermometers

Box 45-1   EQUIPMENT AND SUPPLIES FOR ANIMALS*

1. Sterile pack
   Needle forceps
   Thumb forceps
   Scissors
   Scalpel handle and blades
   Hemostats (2)
2. Alligator forceps
3. Suture material (Vicryl), swaged needles, 4 packets, various sizes (0 to 4-0)
4. Gauze sponges, 4 × 4 inch (100)
5. Roll cotton, 1 pound
6. Vetrap bandages, 3 inch, 6 rolls
7. Syringes, plastic, 12 ml (6)
8. Needles, 22-18 gauge (20)
9. Tubing
   Silastic, 1 cm outside diameter, 10 cm (4 inches) long, for endotracheal tube
   Plastic flexible stomach tube, 1 cm inside diameter, 100 cm (40 inches) long
10. Funnel, plastic, to fit into stomach tube
11. Hose, garden, 20 cm (8 inches), to serve as speculum for passage of stomach tube
12. Hoof knife
13. Hammer
14. Pliers
15. Horseshoes and nails
16. Pliable sheet of leather
17. Heavy needle and thread
18. Otoscope
19. Stomach pump

*See Table 45-4 for priorities with horses, llamas, and dogs.

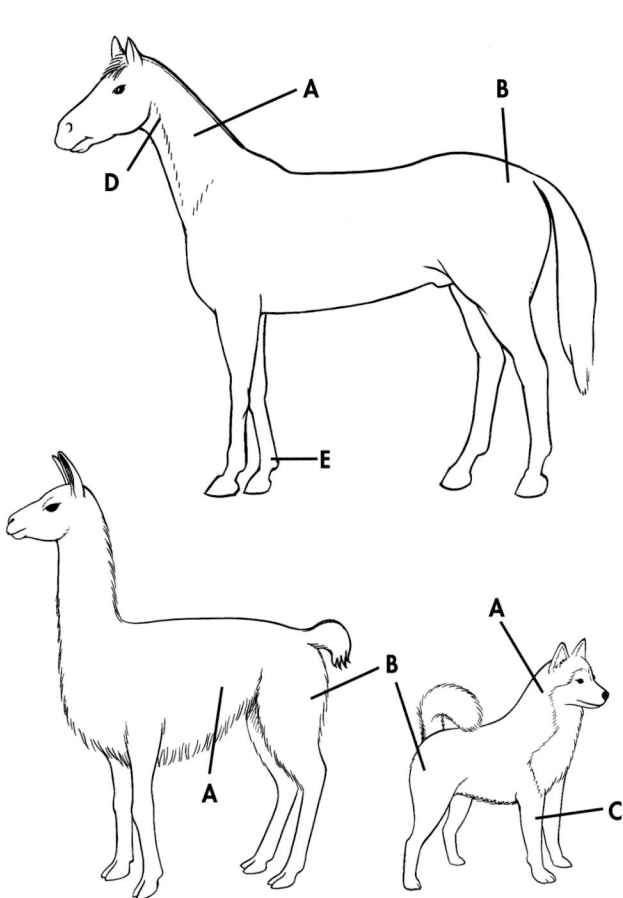

Figure 45-7   Diagrams of medication sites in the horse, llama, and dog. *A,* Subcutaneous. *B,* Intramuscular. *C,* Cephalic vein for intravenous. *D,* Jugular vein. *E,* Site for low volar nerve block.

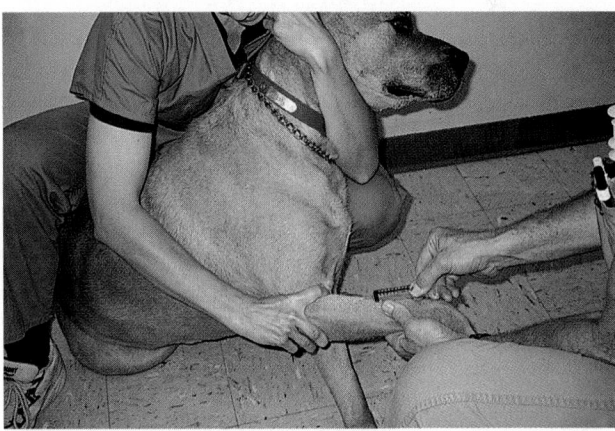

Figure 45-8   Holding a dog for administration of intravenous medication.

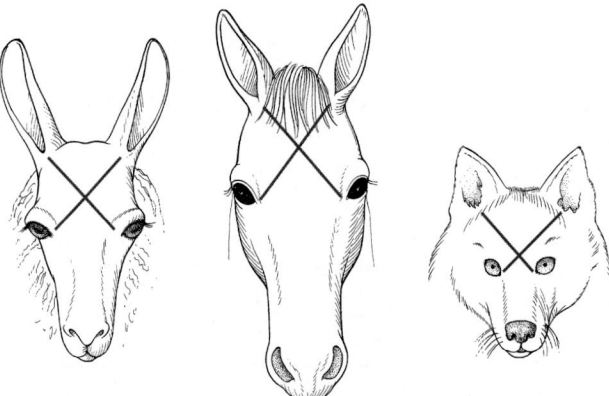

Figure 45-9   Location for euthanasia blow or shot in llama, horse, and dog.

TABLE 45-3. Medications for Trek Animals

GENERIC NAME	TRADE NAME (COMPANY)	CONCEN-TRATION IN VIAL	ROUTE OF ADMINIS-TRATION	DOSAGE AND INTERVAL			
				HORSE	LLAMA	DOG	INDICATION
Acepromazine maleate	Prom Ace (Fort Dodge)	10 mg/ml	IM or IV	0.04-0.1 ml/kg	Not indicated	0.05-0.22 mg/kg	Tranquilizer
Ampicillin sodium	Generic		IM	10-50 mg/kg qid	10-25 mg/kg tid	25 mg/kg q 6 hr	Infection
Atropine sulfate	Generic	2 mg/ml	IM, SC	0.04 mg/kg	0.04 mg/kg	0.04 mg/kg	Stinging nettle
Benzathine penicillin G	Benza Pen (Pfizer)	150,000 U/ml	IM	Not recommended	5,000-15,000 U/kg q 2 days	40,000 U/kg q 5 days	Infection
Charcoal (activated)	Generic		PO	60-250 g	100 g	3-5 g	Toxins
Dexamethasone	Azium (Schering-Plough)	2 mg/ml	IM	2-4 mg/kg	1-2 mg/kg	4 mg/kg q 8 hr	Shock
Diazepam	Generic	5 mg/ml	IV, IM	0.05-0.1 mg/kg	0.2-0.4 mg/kg	2-5 mg/kg	Sedation
Epinephrine	Generic (Bayer)	1:1000 1 mg/ml	IV, IM	0.1-0.4 mg/kg	0.1-0.5 mg/kg	0.1-0.5 mg/kg	Anaphylaxis
Fenbendazole	Panacur (Hoechst Roussel)		PO	5-20 mg/kg	10-15 mg/kg single dose	50 mg/kg	Parasites
Flunixen meglumine	Banamine (Schering-Plough)		IM	1.0 mg/kg daily	1.0 mg/kg daily	0.3 mg/kg daily	Colic pain, inflammation
Ivermectin	Ivomec (Merck AGVET)		PO, SC	0.2 mg/kg single dose	0.2 mg/kg single dose	Not indicated	Parasites
Ketamine	Vetelar (Pfizer)	100 mg/ml	IV, IM	2.0 mg/kg	2-5 mg/kg	Not indicated	Anesthesia
Lidocaine	Generic	2%	SC	As needed	As needed	As needed	Local anesthesia
Magnesium oxide	Carmilax (Pfizer)	361 g/lb	PO		10-20 g total dose		Cathartic
Magnesium sulfate	Generic		PO	20-100 g	Not indicated	8-25 g	Cathartic
Phenylbutazone	Butazolidin (Schering-Plough)	200 mg/ml 1 g tab	IV PO	1-2 g/450 kg, 2-4 g/450 kg daily	2-4 mg/kg daily	15 mg/kg q 8 hr	Pain, inflammation
Trimethoprim/ sulfamethox-azole	Tribrissen (Schering-Plough)	24%	IV, SC	2 mg/kg bid	2 mg/kg bid	2.2 mg/kg q 12 hr	Infection
Xylazine	Rompun (Bayer)	100 mg/ml	IV, IM	0.5-1.0 mg/kg	0.25-0.5 mg/kg	1.1 mg/kg	Sedation
Euthanasia Solution	T-61 (Taylor)		IV	40 ml total dose	25 ml total dose	0.3 ml/kg	Euthanasia

IM, Intramuscular; *IV*, intravenous; *PO*, oral; *SC*, subcutaneous; *q*, every; *bid*, twice daily; *tid*, 3 times daily; *qid*, 4 times daily.

TABLE 45-4. Priority of Emergency Supplies for Animals*

	DRUGS		SUPPLIES	
	PRIMARY	SECONDARY	PRIMARY	SECONDARY
Horses	1,2,3,7,9,10,12	5,11,14-17	1,3-10,12-15	19
Llamas	2,4,7-12,17	6,13,15,16	1,3,4,6-12,14	19
Dogs	3,4,7-9,12,16	11,15,17	1,2,4,6-8,14,16,17	18

*See Box 45-1 for numbered supplies.

must be kept in insulated containers; or high temperatures might render them useless.

TRANSPORTING ANIMALS[8,9]

Dogs

Dogs are easily transported in fiberglass carrying cages in common use by dog owners and for airline shipment. Appropriate opportunities for exercise and urination should be provided. Provision of food and water depends on the duration of the journey.

Horses

Horses may be transported in horse trailers or trucks. Each animal should have been trained to enter and leave the conveyance with ease. The conveyance should be covered to prevent insects and flying debris from striking animals in the face or eyes. Avoid exposure to exhaust fumes. Legs should be wrapped to support the lower limb tendons, joints, and ligaments.

Llamas

Llamas are often moved from one location to another and generally travel well. The majority lie down soon after the beginning of a journey and remain recumbent while moving; however, traveling is stressful for most lamoids whether or not they exhibit overt signs of stress. Llamas do not need to be tied within a truck or trailer, which may be hazardous. At least two fatalities have been associated with tied llamas.

Llamas are small and adaptable enough to be moved in many vehicles, including private vans, pickup trucks, livestock trucks, trailers, and commercial vans; insurance coverage should be checked. Llamas should be accustomed to the vehicle in which they are to travel.

Vehicles and trailers should be properly maintained, and exhaust fumes must not flow past the heads of the llamas.

Climatic conditions must be considered. More than one llama has died as a result of heat stress while being transported. Most trek animals will not be shipped by air, and most airlines refuse to carry live animals if daytime temperatures exceed 29.4° C (85° F) anywhere the plane lands. Caution is used when transporting in hot weather. Road conditions should be investigated, including any construction detours that may cause delays. Storms should be anticipated.

Some trailers have a small ramp leading up to the floor of the trailer for loading and unloading. Others require that the animal step up to load. Llamas prefer to step rather then walk up a ramp. It is unwise to pull or push a llama into a step-up trailer. A leg may slip beneath the floor of the trailer and be fractured if the animal lunges forward. Appropriate training eliminates such problems.

Trailer flooring must be considered. Although llamas generally can walk on smooth surfaces, it is not appropriate to leave the metal or wood floor of a trailer bare. Rubber mats or indoor/outdoor carpeting are ideal because they provide footing and insulation from both heat and cold and are softer. Straw may provide insulation in cold weather but does not provide footing. It does absorb urine. It is unwise to use straw for bedding on long journeys, especially if no feed is supplied. Hungry or bored animals may eat the straw, and if unaccustomed to it, may develop digestive upsets. Sand may be used, but wood shavings or sawdust become embedded in the fiber coat and are difficult to remove.

Llamas may be trained to use different water containers, including a flowing stream or pool. If the animal is not used to a variety of water sources, a plastic or metal bucket can be used for a few days before beginning a trip. Animals may be reluctant to drink sufficient new-source water, which may be disastrous in hot weather. The odor and taste of new water may be disguised by pretraining the animal to drink water containing two drops of vanilla extract or oil of eucalyptus. New water can then be similarly treated.

Llamas may be unwilling to defecate or urinate in a strange environment and should be provided the opportunity to stand or exit the vehicle while stopping for a rest.

Recumbent Llama. Moving a recumbent llama may be accomplished using the following technique:

1. Roll up a plastic or canvas tarp (longer than the length of the animal) on one side and place it next to the animal, which has been moved into the sternal position.
2. Do not roll the animal on its back onto the tarp; rolling may cause regurgitation and possibly inhalation pneumonia. Rather, partially roll the animal from lateral to sternal recumbency and push the roll under it.
3. Allow the animal to resume lateral recumbency so that the tarp may be unrolled beneath it.
4. Roll up both sides of the tarp to form a handhold for those who will lift and carry the animal.
5. Keep the head and forequarters higher than the rearquarters to avoid passive regurgitation.

For llamas it may be appropriate to rig a temporary sling inside a trailer or truck using a large bath towel or piece of canvas, as follows:

1. Cut four holes near the center, corresponding to the legs of the llama.
2. Gently lift a forelimb and insert the foot through one hole.
3. Repeat with the other forelimb, then repeat with the hind limbs.
4. Fasten a small rope to each corner by first folding the corner of the towel over a small rock.

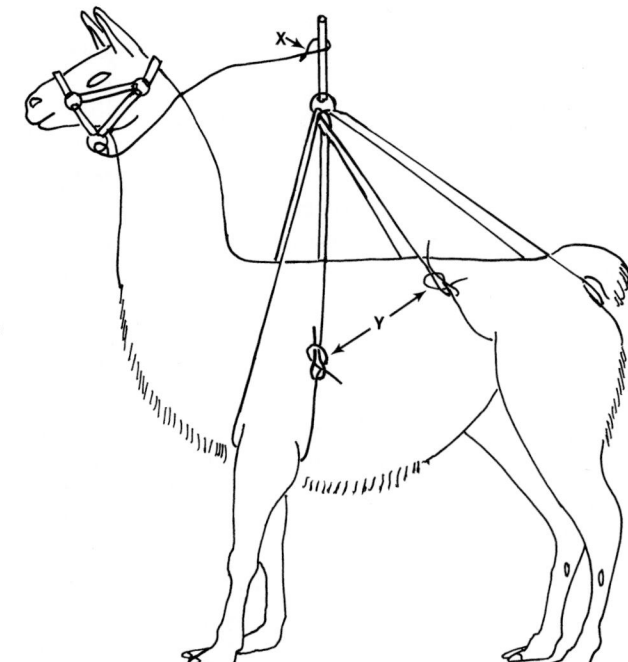

Figure 45-10 Rope sling for a llama. *X,* Halter tie; *Y,* Bowline.

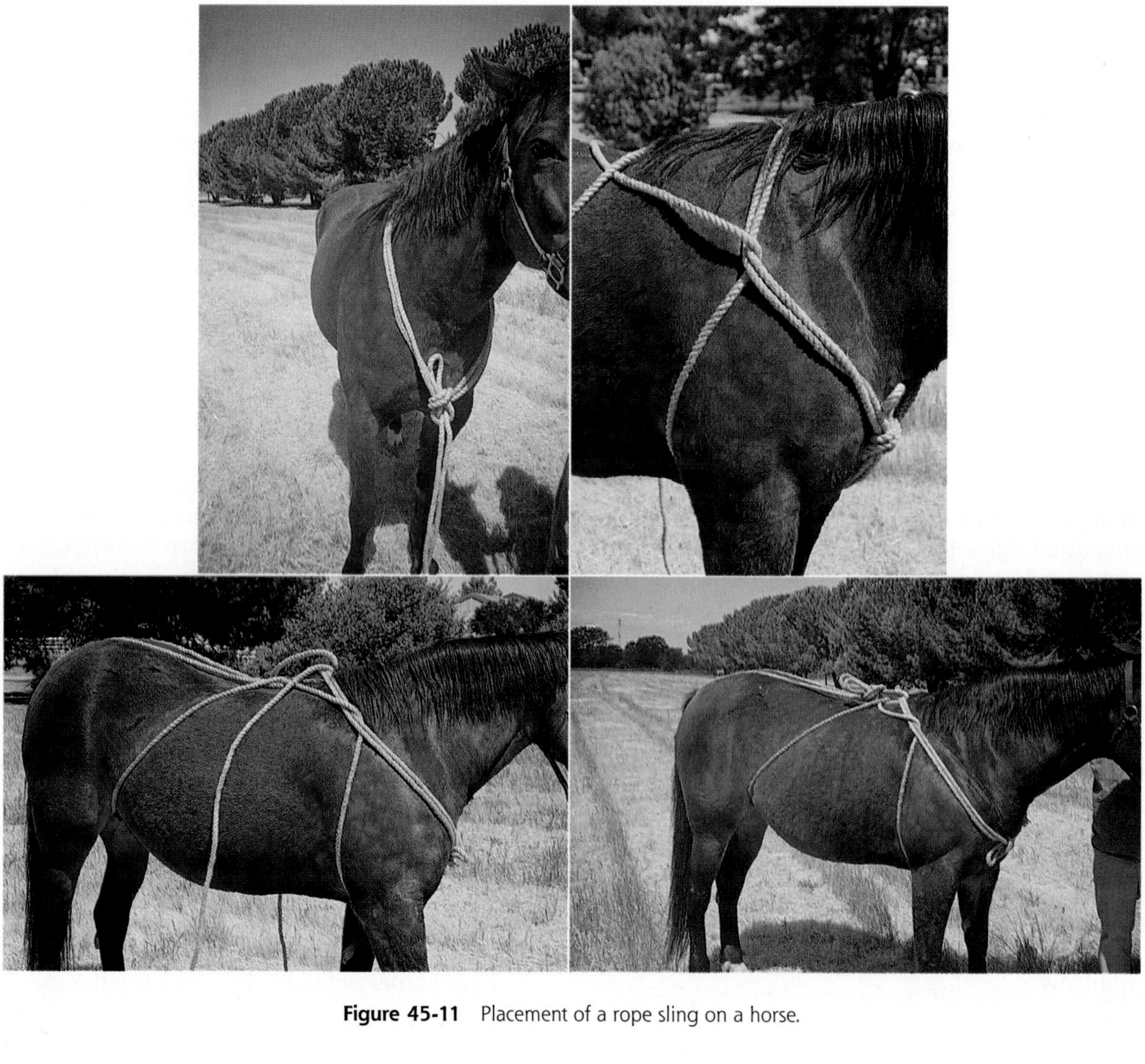

Figure 45-11 Placement of a rope sling on a horse.

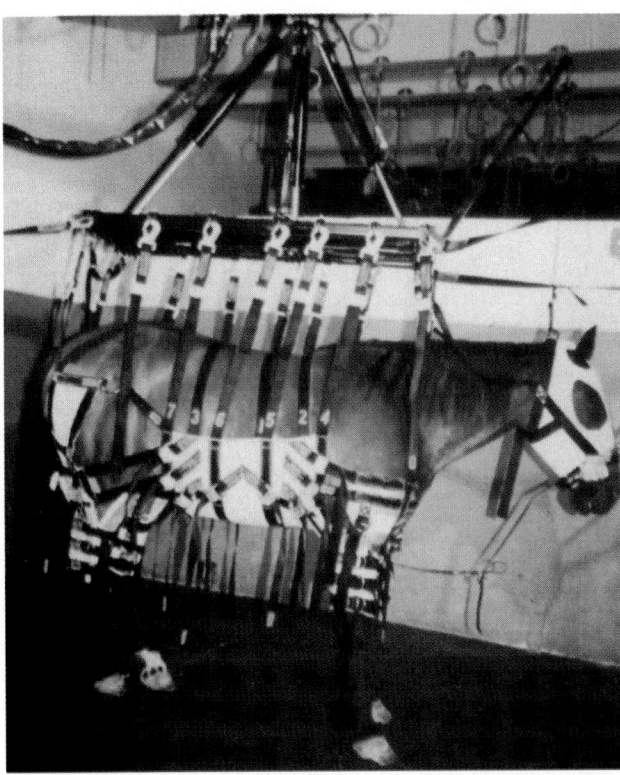

Figure 45-12 Commercial equine sling. *(Courtesy University of California, Davis, Center for Equine Health.)*

5. Tie a slipknot around the cloth and the rock and pull it tight.
6. Tie the ropes to the side of the trailer or partition.

The llama's feet should remain on the floor of the trailer, and a person should ride beside the animal.

Field Evacuation of Injured Animals

Field evacuation of injured or seriously sick trek members by helicopter has become a viable option for all but the most remote wilderness expeditions. Cost is not an important factor in evacuating humans but may have to be considered in animal evacuations.

Dogs may be taken into the cabin of a helicopter. Llamas and horses must be slung beneath the helicopter. A sling for a short journey of a llama may be fashioned with four rope loops, all brought together over the back of the llama (Figure 45-10).

A sling for a horse may be constructed from a rope. The diameter and length of the rope depend on the size of the animal; a 50-foot-long, ½-inch-wide nylon climbing rope is suitable to lift a 1000-pound horse. The technique follows:

1. Double the rope, then form a loose neck loop using a bowline knot.
2. Slip the loop over the head, and position the loop with the knot at the base of the chest.
3. Bring the running segments between the front legs and back through the corresponding side of the neck loop.

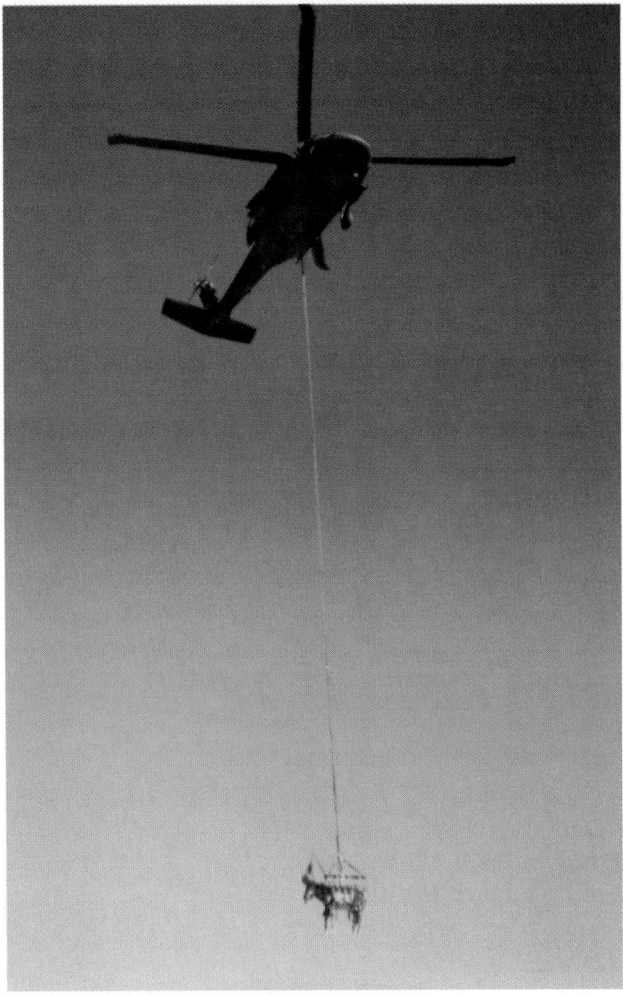

Figure 45-13 Mule transport by helicopter. *(Courtesy University of California, Davis, Center for Equine Health.)*

4. Cross the ropes over the back, then bring the ropes between the hind legs.
5. Be certain not to cross ropes underneath the animal. The ropes should pass on either side of the tail, up over the back and underneath all the ropes on the back.
6. Take all slack out of the ropes, and complete the sling by doubling the running ends back and tying with a halter tie.

An attempt should be made to place the lifting site over the approximate center of gravity of the animal (just behind the withers). Even if this is not done, however, the animal can still be lifted because each leg is in its own loop sling. The animal cannot slip out of the sling (Figure 45-11).

A more elaborate sling is available commercially* and has been used in numerous large animal rescue operations (Figures 45-12 and 45-13).

---

*CDA Products (Care for Disabled Animals), Charles Anderson, Potter Valley, Calif, 707-743-1300.

APPENDIX

Sources of Veterinary Drugs for Expeditions

Bayer Corp.
PO Box 390
Shawnee, KS 66201

Fort Dodge Laboratories
Post Office Box 518
Fort Dodge, IA 50501

Hoechst Roussel Vet
Somerville, NJ 08876

Merck AGVET
Division of Merck & Co.
PO Box 2000
Rahway, NJ 07065

Pfizer, Inc.
812 Springdale Dr.
Exton, PA 19341

Schering-Plough Corp.
Union, NJ 07033

Taylor Pharmaceutical Co.
Decatur, IL 62525

Wyeth Ayerst Laboratories
Post Office Box 8299
Philadelphia, PA 19101

REFERENCES

1. Edwards NJ, Moise NS: Cardiac emergencies. In Kirk RW, Bistner SI, Ford RB, editors: *Handbook of veterinary procedures & emergency treatment*, ed 5, Philadelphia, 1990, WB Saunders .
2. Fowler ME: Hoof, claw and nail problems in nondomestic animals, *J Am Vet Med Assoc* 177:885, 1980.
3. Fowler ME: Veterinary problems during endurance trail rides, *S Afr Vet Assoc* 51:87, 1980.
4. Fowler ME: Plant poisoning in free-living wild animals: a review, *J Wildl Dis* 19:34, 1983.
5. Fowler ME: *Veterinary zootoxicology*, Boca Raton, Fla, 1993, CRC Press.
6. Fowler ME: Management of llamas and alpacas during and following disasters and emergencies, *Llamas* 9:72, 1995.
7. Fowler ME: *Restraint and handling of wild and domestic animals*, ed 2, Ames, Iowa, 1995, Iowa State University Press
8. Fowler ME: *Medicine and surgery of South American camelids*, ed 2, Ames, Iowa, 1998, Iowa State University Press.
9. Fowler ME, Fowler AC: *First aid for llamas and alpacas*, Jackson, Calif, 1995, Clay Press.
10. Fuller T, McClintock E: *Poisonous plants of California*, Berkeley, Calif, 1987, University of California Press.
11. Hudgson DR, Rose RJ: *The athletic horse*, Philadelphia, 1994, WB Saunders.
12. James LF et al: *Plants poisonous to livestock in the western United States*, Agriculture Information Bull No 415, Washington, DC, 1980, US Department of Agriculture.
13. Jones WE, editor: *Equine sports medicine*, Philadelphia, 1989, Lea & Febiger.
14. Mansman RA, McAllister ES, editors: *Equine medicine and surgery*, ed 3, Santa Barbara, Calif, 1982, American Veterinary Publications.
15. Schmutz EM, Freeman BN, Reed RE: *Livestock-poisoning plants of Arizona*, Tucson, Ariz, 1968, University of Arizona Press.

Plants

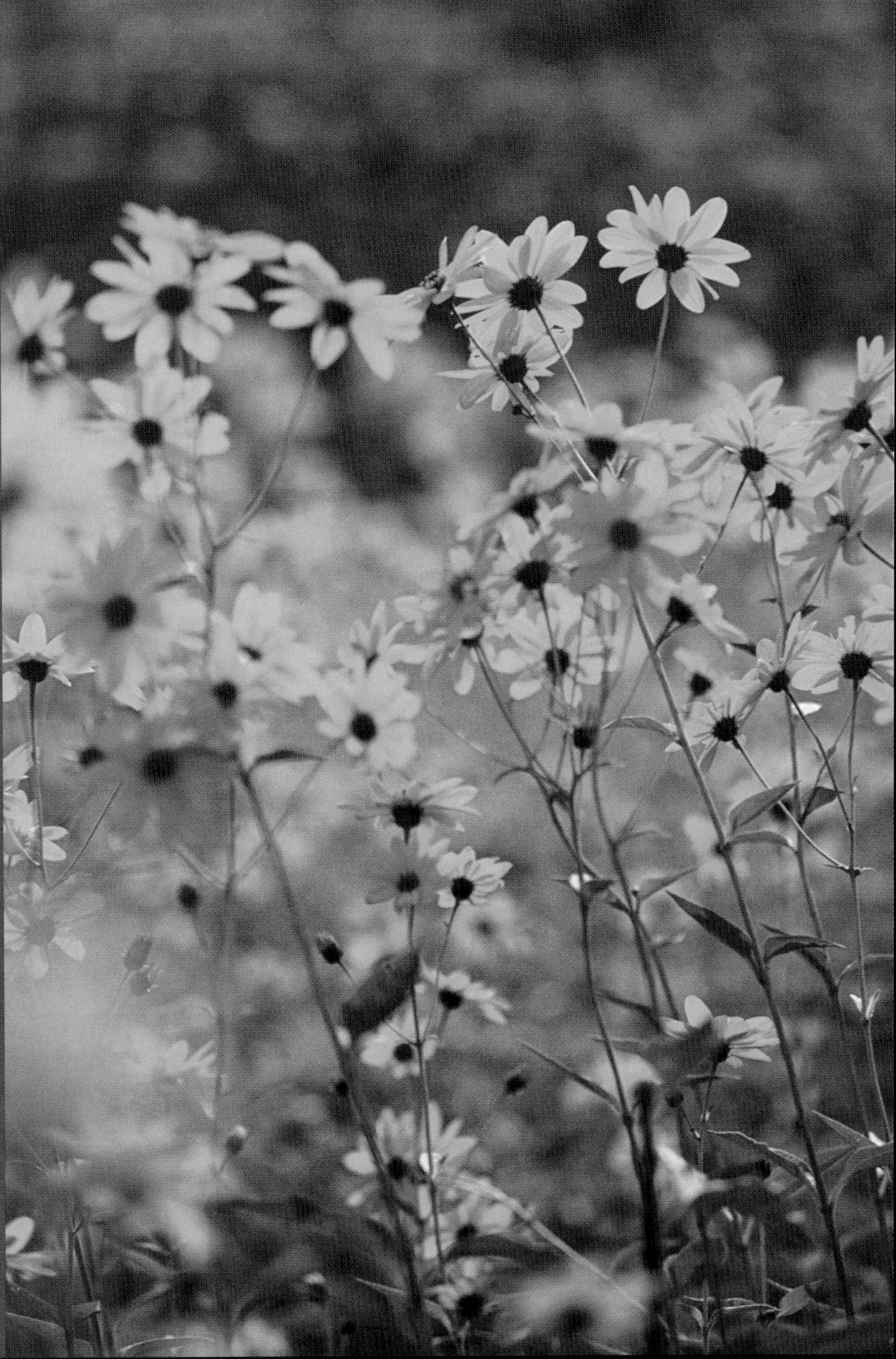

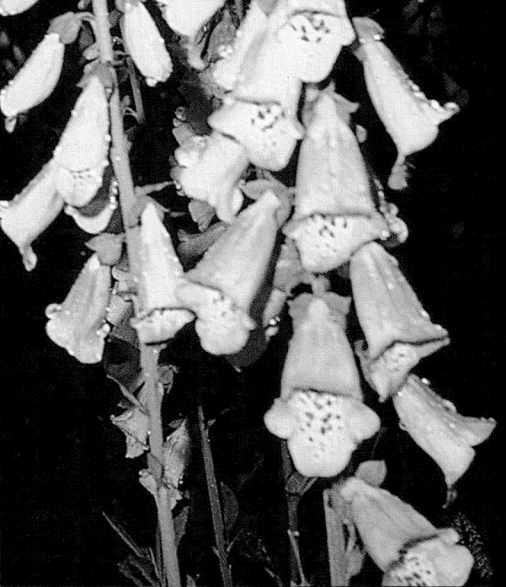

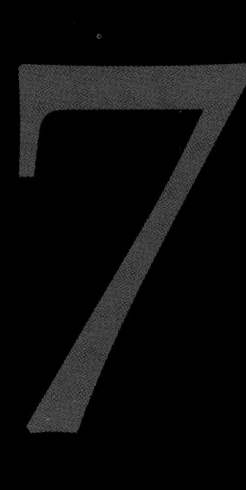

7

46 Seasonal Allergies

Naresh J. Patel and Robert K. Bush

Allergic rhinitis is the most common allergic disorder, occurring in 15% to 20% of the general population.[47] Pollens, fungi, dust mites, and animals are the most commonly implicated allergens in allergic rhinitis. Pollens and fungi are primarily responsible for inducing symptoms in the outdoors. In temperate climates, individuals with allergic rhinitis often have worsening symptoms in the warmer months, correlating with pollination of various pollen-producing plants and increase fungi growth.

Although anaphylaxis is not as common as allergic rhinitis, it represents the most severe form of allergic reaction and can lead to serious outcomes or can be fatal if not treated promptly. For example, each year about 40 deaths in the United States are attributed to anaphylaxis resulting from a bee sting.[3] Foods and drugs are the most common causes of anaphylaxis.

ALLERGIC RHINITIS

Allergic rhinitis is a chronic immunoglobulin E–mediated (IgE-mediated) inflammatory disease of the nasal mucosa. It is the most common atopic disorder, and for reasons not yet clear, its prevalence is increasing worldwide. The economic impact of allergic rhinitis is impressive; the estimated total annual cost in medications and physician visits is $3.5 billion.[52] The disease usually manifests in early childhood or adolescence and peaks in the second or third decade of life. The disease does not appear to favor any gender, ethnic group, or race. The most important risk factor for developing allergic rhinitis is a family history of atopy, especially with early onset of disease. The risk increases to 30% if one parent or sibling is atopic and 50% if both parents are affected.[35] Conversely, lack of complete concordance for atopy in identical twins emphasizes the importance of environmental factors in disease development.[5] Allergic rhinitis tends to cluster in families, as do other atopic conditions, such as asthma and atopic dermatitis.

Pathophysiology

Acute allergic reaction and late inflammatory events are important components in the pathogenesis of allergic rhinitis. Type I immediate hypersensitivity is responsible for most of the acute clinical manifestations of allergic rhinitis, and cells such as eosinophils, basophils, and T lymphocytes play important roles in late inflammatory events. Production of allergen-specific IgE (sensitization) antibodies forms the underlying basis of immediate hypersensitivity; atopy is defined as the genetic predisposition to develop allergen-specific IgE antibodies. The sensitization process requires a cooperative effort between CD4$^+$ T lymphocytes and B lymphocytes (Figure 46-1). It begins with presentation of an allergen to CD4$^+$ T lymphocytes by antigen-presenting cells (e.g., macrophages) in the context of a major histocompatibility complex. Cytokines released from CD4$^+$ T lymphocytes as a result of this interaction cause differentiation of B lymphocytes into immunoglobulin-secreting plasma cells. This differentiation leads to isotype switching (production of specific antibody types) within the plasma cells. For example, IgE switching is promoted by release of cytokine interleukin-4 (IL-4) or interleukin-13 (IL-13) from T lymphocytes.[12] Once allergen-specific IgE antibodies are produced, subsequent exposure and binding of the allergens to IgE molecules on the surface of mast cells results in cross-linking of the IgE molecules. Consequently, mast cells or basophils degranulate and release preformed and newly synthesized mediators. The prototype preformed mediator is histamine, and the newly synthesized mediators include those of the arachidonic acid pathway (leukotrienes, prostaglandins, and platelet-activating factor), neuropeptides (e.g., substance P), and cytokines (e.g., IL-4, IL-5).

The release of chemical mediators leads to various pathologic and clinical consequences. Sneezing and itching are secondary to histamine stimulation of its receptors on sensory nerve endings, rhinorrhea results from increased vascular permeability produced by all the mediators, and leukotrienes and prostaglandins are believed to play major roles in nasal congestion.[55] Our knowledge of the pathophysiology of allergic rhinitis has been greatly enhanced by nasal challenge studies.[23] It is now known that the allergic reaction consists of an early phase characterized by mast cell or basophil degranulation, and a late phase, which occurs 4 to 6 hours after the early phase (Figure 46-1). The hallmark of late-phase reaction is an influx of inflammatory cells, such as eosinophils, basophils, and T lymphocytes.[4] For example, basophils cause further histamine release and T lymphocytes release additional cytokines that enhance IgE production (via IL-4) and eosinophil activation (via IL-5). As a result of further inflammatory activity by these cells, there is recrudescence of symptoms many hours after the initial allergen exposure. Leukotrienes, prostaglandins, and cytokines released in the early-

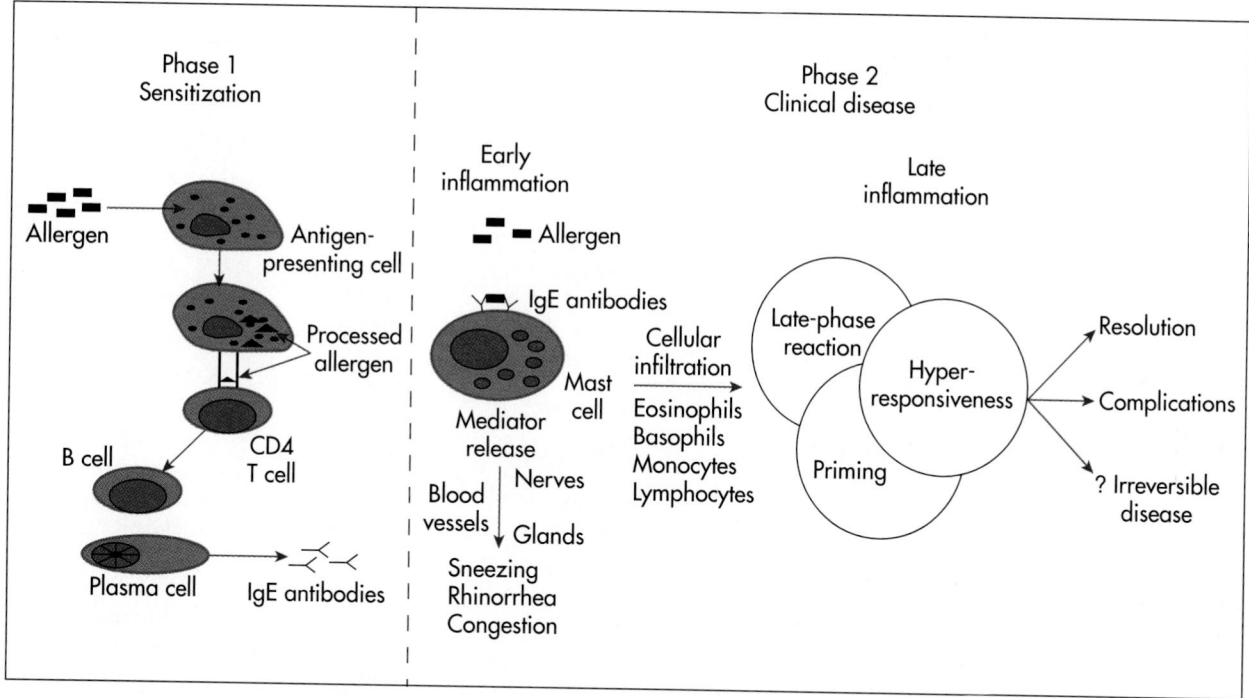

Figure 46-1 Simplified schematic representation of the natural history of allergic rhinitis. During phase 1, the individual becomes sensitized to an allergen. During phase 2, clinical disease develops. The overwhelming majority of individuals have an early response upon reexposure to the allergen. The activation of mast cells and the release of mediators dominate the early response. After the early response, most individuals have cellular infiltration of the nasal mucosa causing late inflammatory events, including the spontaneous recurrence of release of mediators (late-phase reaction), hyperresponsiveness to irritants, and increased responsiveness to the allergen (priming). The circles indicate the heterogeneity of these late inflammatory events. Inflammation can resolve spontaneously, cause a complication, or lead to an irreversible form of chronic rhinitis. (*From Naclerio R:* N Engl J Med *325:860, 1991.*)

phase reaction play an important role in recruiting the late-phase cellular milieu to the inflammatory site. Although inhaled corticosteroids block both the early- and the late-phase reactions, systemic glucocorticoids block only the late-phase reaction.

Allergens

Allergens are the etiologic agents of allergic rhinitis. Although many potential allergenic proteins exist, relatively few are clinically important and even fewer have been isolated and characterized. Allergens are low-molecular-weight proteins or glycoproteins capable of eliciting a Type I immediate hypersensitivity reaction (production of IgE antibodies). It is convenient to divide allergens into those that exist in the outdoor environment and those that exist in the indoor environment. In the outdoors, pollens of trees, grasses, and weeds and certain fungi (e.g., *Alternaria* and *Cladosporium* species) most commonly provoke allergic rhinitis symptoms. Pollen-sensitive individuals typically experience seasonal rhinitis in predictable time intervals from one season to the next. Although fungi are more ubiquitous in nature and do

not have distinct seasons like pollens, both outdoor and indoor fungi thrive in moist environments. Therefore, in temperate climates, fungi counts start to rise in spring with a peak in mid- to late summer. Indoor allergens include fungi, animals, cockroaches, and dust mites. Unlike outdoor allergens, which typically produce seasonal symptoms, indoor allergens often produce symptoms perennially; however, the symptoms are less drastic in nature, often making diagnosis more difficult.

Pollens. Pollination in higher-order plants consists of the transfer of the male gametophyte to the female gametophyte. In this process, pollen grains serve as vectors for male gametophytes. Of the different types of pollen-producing plants, flowering plants (including trees, grasses, and weeds) are the most important from an allergic standpoint. Flowering plants may be divided into those that rely on animal vectors (e.g., insects) for pollination (termed *entemophilous*) and those that depend on the wind (termed *anemophilous*). In general, only anemophilous plants (including trees, grasses, and weeds) cause allergic symptoms.[49] Pollens

TABLE 46-1. Selected Trees, Grasses, and Weeds of Allergenic Significance

REGION (STATES)	TREES	GRASSES	WEEDS
Northeast (ME, NH, VT, NY, PA, NJ, MA, RI, CT)	Birch Elm Maple Poplar Oak	Orchard Timothy June Sweet vernal Bluegrass	Sheep sorrel Plantain Russian thistle Giant ragweed Short ragweed
Mid-Atlantic (DE, MC, DC, VA, NC, SC)	Birch Elm Maple Hickory Oak	Orchard Timothy Bluegrass June Bermuda	Plantain Dock Sage Short ragweed Giant ragweed
North Central (OH, KY, WI, MI, IA, WI, northern MO, IL, IN, TN)	Ash Elm Maple Willow Box Elder	Orchard Timothy Bluegrass June	Plantain Dock Russian thistle Short ragweed Giant ragweed
Pacific Northwest (WA, NV, OR, northern CA)	Alder Birch Maple Oak Walnut	Timothy Bluegrass Fescue Rye Redtop	Dock Plantain Russian thistle Nettle Sagebrush
Plains (NE, MN, eastern MT, Dakotas)	Elm Oak Box Elder Willow Maple	Timothy Orchard Bluegrass Bermuda Redtop	Marsh-elder Russian thistle Western hemp Short ragweed Giant ragweed
Rocky Mountains (ID, WY, CO, UT, western MT)	Cedar Elm Ash Birch Oak	Timothy Orchard Fescue Redtop June	Sagebrush Russian thistle Short ragweed Giant ragweed
South (FL, GA, AL, TX, AR, southern MO)	Cedar Elm Mulberry Poplar Oak	Bermuda Orchard Timothy Saltgrass	Dock Pigweed Russian thistle Giant ragweed Short ragweed
Southwest (western TX, NM, AZ)	Cedar Ash Mulberry Oak Olive	Bermuda Johnson	Sagebrush Russian thistle Saltbush Kochia Short ragweed
Southern California	Ash Walnut Elm Oak Olive	Bermuda Saltgrass Brome	Nettle Bur ragweed Russian thistle Sage Western ragweed

From Sicherer SH, Eggleston PA: Environmental allergens. In Lieberman P, Anderson JA, editors: *Allergic diseases: diagnosis and treatment*, Totowa, NJ, 1997, Humana.
Plants are listed in the order of bloom for each region. Grasses are listed by prevalence in each region.

of entemophilous plants do not achieve high airborne concentrations. In temperate climates, pollination of trees, grasses, and weeds occurs in predictable time intervals in a given region. It is important to know the relevant local botany and the respective pollination seasons (Table 46-1 and Figure 46-2).

As shown in Figure 46-2, tree pollination marks the onset of allergy season in most parts of North America. It begins as early as mid-January in the Southwest to early April in the Northeast and terminates between early and late May. Trees of allergenic significance in various regions are listed in Table 46-1. Grass pollen,

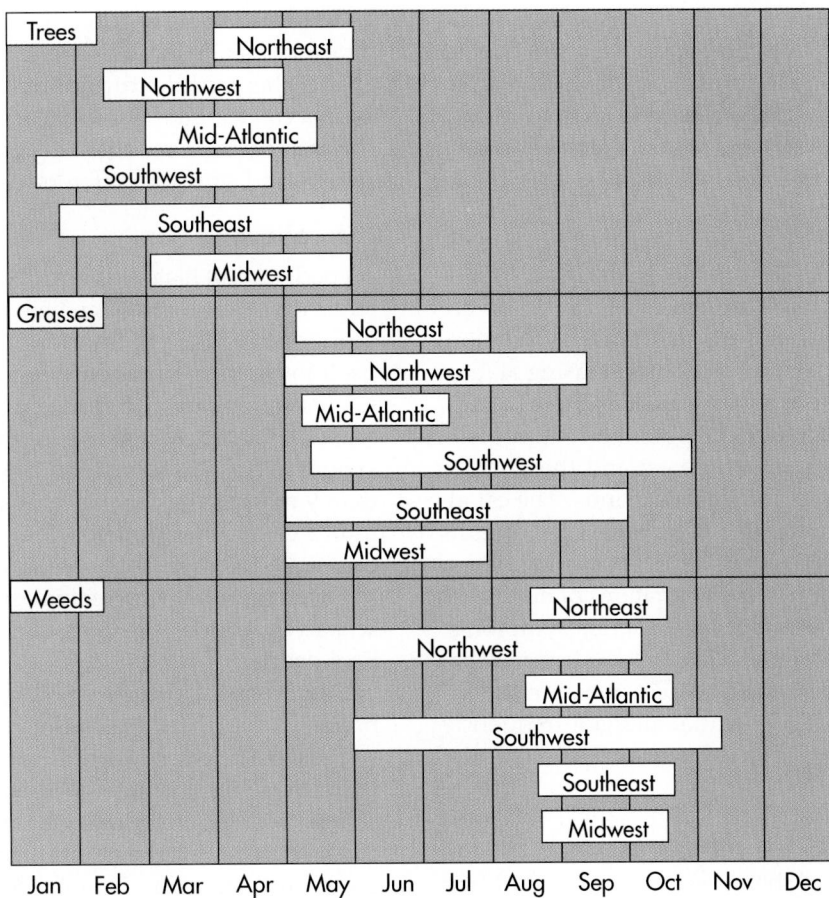

Figure 46-2 Pollen seasons by region in the continental United States. (*From Sicherer SH, Eggleston PA: Environmental allergies. In Lieberman P, Anderson JA, editors:* Allergic diseases: diagnosis and treatment, *Totowa, NJ, 1997, Humana.*)

with its worldwide distribution, is a significant source of allergen exposure and a major cause of allergic rhinitis in sensitive individuals. In frost-free areas of North America, grass pollen may be present year-round, whereas in temperate climates, grass pollination peaks between mid-May and mid-July. Important grass types are rye, timothy, Kentucky bluegrass, orchard, Johnson, and Bermuda. Unlike ragweed and tree pollen allergens, grass pollen allergens show extensive cross reactivity among different species, and allergic individuals are generally sensitive to many of these species. Weeds represent the final pollen of the season, with typical duration from mid-August through mid-October. Although a variety of weeds cause regionally significant allergies, ragweed is found in most parts of North America.

Fungi. Numerous allergenic fungi are responsible for both seasonal and perennial symptoms. The three most important classes of allergic fungi are Zygomycetes (e.g., *Rhizopus, Mucor*), Basidiomycetes (e.g., rust, smut, *Ganoderma*), and Ascomycetes (e.g., *Cladosporium, Peni-*

cillium, Aspergillus, Alternaria, Epicoccum). Among the outdoor fungi, *Caldosporium* and *Alternaria* are the most abundant, causing significant symptoms in sensitive individuals. Although fungi can survive in various climates, they grow best in warm, humid environments. The peak fungal season in many areas is in middle to late summer and fall, with a marked reduction after the first frost in temperate climates. Fungi levels may rise in spring, when decaying vegetation is uncovered after the snow has melted. Common outdoor sources of fungal growth are leaves, moist debris, and soil; therefore outdoor activities, such as raking, farming, and mowing, significantly increase exposure.

Dust Mites. Dust mites are microscopic arachnids that are close relatives of ticks and spiders. They feed on human epidermal scales and, like fungi, prefer a warm, humid environment. Dust mites are the most common indoor allergens and can cause significant perennial symptoms in sensitive individuals. Although there is no good correlation between exposure level and degree of rhinitis symptoms, a level of 10 μg/g of dust is considered a risk factor for the development of acute asthma symptoms.[38] Common indoor sources of dust mite exposure include mattresses, pillows, blankets, upholstery, and furred toys. Dust mites may proliferate in sleeping bags stored in humid environments (e.g., damp basements).

Animals. Animals, especially cats, can be highly allergenic and in sensitized individuals can cause significant rhinoconjunctivitis symptoms. Cats and dogs are the most common pets in the United States, with more than one third to one half of all homes housing at least one cat or dog.[48] Birds, rabbits, hamsters, guinea pigs, rats, and mice are some other potentially allergenic pets. The major allergens of the cat and the dog are found in their saliva and sebaceous glands. The cat allergen can remain a potential source of allergy months after its removal because of its light, sticky qualities.

Outdoors, inhalation of the emanations of moths, locusts, beetles, and flies may cause allergic symptoms. Residents of the area around western Lake Erie may experience allergic symptoms caused by the mayfly.[48] Finally the cockroach is a potential allergen frequently encountered in heavily infested, crowded, multifamily dwellings.

Functions of the Nose

The main functions of the nose—to warm, humidify, and filter air—are possible because of turbulent airflow resulting from increased surface area provided by the three turbinates (superior, middle, and inferior) on each side. The nose's functions are mainly controlled by the underlying neurovascular system. The blood supply to the nose is via the ophthalmic (branch of the internal carotid) and internal maxillary (branch of the external carotid) arteries. Neural innervations include the sensory (via the trigeminal nerve, which is responsible for the sneezing reflex) and autonomic (parasympathetic and sympathetic) nervous systems. Nasal congestion is proportionally related to the amount of blood pooling in the cavernous sinusoids (located within the turbinates) and to the degree of mucosal edema. Sinusoid filling and emptying are controlled by the autonomic nervous system. Vasodilatory parasympathetic stimulation allows the sinusoid reservoir to fill via the opening and closing of the capillary and postcapillary venule sphincters, respectively. Conversely, sympathetic stimulation contracts the capillary sphincter and relaxes the postcapillary venule sphincter, allowing the reservoir to empty.

In most people, cyclical swelling and shrinking of the turbinates between the two sides is inherent. This nasal cycle, which is approximately 1 to 4 hours in length, results from alternating sympathetic discharge and is responsible for the sensation of alternating unilateral nasal blockage experienced by allergic rhinitis sufferers.[20]

Another major function of the nose is olfaction. The olfactory area is located at the roof of the nasal cavity above the middle turbinate. Significant turbinate edema can lead to poor ventilation of this area and associated hyposmia, which is common among chronic rhinitis and sinusitis sufferers.

Clinical Evaluation

A good, careful history is crucial in the evaluation of allergic rhinitis and can often help determine whether the individual is allergic. In most cases allergy testing is used to confirm the underlying clinical suspicion. Allergic rhinitis can be divided into two main categories: seasonal (hay fever) and perennial (defined by nasal symptoms lasting more than 2 hours per day for more than 9 months of the year).[35] Seasonal rhinitis usually indicates outdoor pollen sensitivity, most commonly caused by trees, grasses, weeds, and fungi. In addition to pollens and fungi, perennial rhinitis sufferers may be sensitive to indoor allergens, such as dust mites and animal dander.

Symptoms of allergic rhinitis can range from intermittently mild to incapacitating during peak pollen season. The hallmark of allergic rhinitis is temporal correlation of symptoms with allergen exposure.[34] The most common symptoms of allergic rhinitis—sneezing, nasal congestion, rhinorrhea, and pruritus of the nose and eyes—are nonspecific. Itching and sneezing are the most distinctive complaints associated with allergic rhinitis,[35] whereas congestion seems to be more prominent in perennial rhinitis than seasonal rhinitis. In some individuals, ocular symptoms predominate over nasal symptoms. Allergic rhinitis sufferers often experience the priming effect (an increase in sensitivity to allergens after repeated exposure) and hyperresponsiveness to nonallergenic environmental stimuli, such as tobacco smoke, strong odors, pollutants, and weather changes.[10]

The timing of symptoms often helps in predicting the responsible pollens because pollination occurs at predictable intervals. For example, in the Midwest, ragweed sufferers characteristically start experiencing symptoms in mid-August. However, the specific allergen can be difficult to surmise in individuals with perennial rhinitis because other more ubiquitous allergens, such as fungi, may play a role. Other conditions of the upper respiratory tract may mimic allergic rhinitis and must be considered. Complications of allergic rhinitis include sinusitis, asthma, sleep loss, work impairment in adults, and learning difficulties in children.

In addition to nonspecific symptoms, the signs noted on physical examination are not exclusive to allergic rhinitis. Classically the nasal mucosa is pale blue and edematous, but this color change is noted in only 60% of sufferers and many individuals have erythematous mucosa.[14] In children the "allergic salute" (upward nasal rubbing) and "allergic shiners" (dark, puffy circles under the eye) may be present. Other notable signs include septal deviation, polyps, and an obvious foreign body. If congestion is profound, use of a topical decongestant, such as oxymetazoline (Afrin), may improve visualization.

Allergy Testing

Although the clinical presentation of seasonal allergic rhinitis is usually sufficient to make the diagnosis, allergy testing is recommended for individuals with perennial symptoms. Testing pinpoints various allergens and can provide useful information regarding specific avoidance measures. Allergy testing must be performed if immunotherapy is being considered.

Differential Diagnosis

There is significant overlap of rhinitis symptoms and symptoms of other upper respiratory tract disorders (Box 46-1). Rhinitis can be acute or chronic, with the most common cause of acute rhinitis being a viral infection. Allergic rhinitis may be confused with viral rhinitis; however, unlike allergic rhinitis, symptoms of viral rhinitis do not persist longer than 2 weeks unless a superseding sinusitis develops. A foreign body or

---

Box 46-1 DIFFERENTIAL DIAGNOSIS OF RHINITIS

ACUTE RHINITIS

Upper respiratory tract infection
Foreign body
Trauma

CHRONIC RHINITIS

Allergic
Nonallergic
   NARES (*non*allergic *r*hinitis with *e*osinophilia syndrome)
   Chronic sinusitis
   Systemic diseases
      Wegener's granulomatosis
      Sarcoidosis
      Hypothyroidism
      Acromegaly
   Rhinitis medicamentosa
   Mechanical-anatomic obstruction
      Nasal polyps
      Foreign body
      Tumor
      Septal deviation
   Gustatory rhinitis
   Atrophic rhinitis
   Rhinitis of pregnancy
   Cerebrospinal fluid leak
   Vasomotor (idiopathic) rhinitis

---

trauma also can cause acute rhinitis. Unilateral symptoms are the hallmark of foreign body obstruction.

NARES (*non*allergic *r*hinitis with *e*osinophilia syndrome) is characterized by (1) symptoms similar to allergic rhinitis, (2) eosinophilia noted on nasal smear, and (3) normal results of skin tests.[24] Chronic sinusitis, which can occur as a complication of allergic rhinitis, commonly produces nasal symptoms, including postnasal drip, cough, and diminished senses of smell and taste. Unlike acute sinusitis, chronic sinusitis causes symptoms that are subtle and often require radiologic evaluation, preferably computed tomography. Systemic diseases, such as Wegener's granulomatosis, have been associated with chronic sinusitis. Rhinitis medicamentosa, which usually results from overuse of topical α-adrenergic vasoconstrictors (e.g., oxymetazoline), is associated with profound nasal congestion caused by rebound effects upon withdrawal of the decongestant, usually after 5 to 7 days. Other medications implicated in rhinitis medicamentosa are birth control pills and α-blocking antihypertensives.

Mechanical and anatomic abnormalities should always be sought on physical examination. Nasal polyps are bilateral, inflammatory, and often associated with chronic sinusitis and asthma. They appear pearly, smooth, and gray (like grapes). A foreign body, tumor, or septal deviation usually causes unilateral symptoms. Moreover, unilateral growth should always heighten suspicion for a foreign body or tumor. Most people have a certain degree of septal deviation; unless symptoms are severe or sinus drainage is compromised, no treatment is warranted.

Symptoms of gustatory rhinitis are caused by cholinergic discharge that occurs after such stimuli as eating, running, and exposure to cold air. Atrophic rhinitis is a rare condition that manifests in the elderly as thick, bilateral odorous discharge with little nasal congestion.[19] Rhinitis of pregnancy should be considered in the pregnant woman with congestion, especially if there is no previous history of rhinitis. Although rare, a potentially dangerous cerebrospinal fluid leak must be considered in anyone with clear rhinorrhea and a history of central nervous system trauma. The diagnostic test is a nasal smear to detect glucose.

After all of the aforementioned conditions have been considered, many individuals are left with the diagnosis of vasomotor (idiopathic) rhinitis. These individuals typically have perennial symptoms that are often triggered by changes in weather, irritants (such as smoke or perfume), and spicy foods. Common symptoms are chronic congestion, postnasal drip, and cough. Skin tests reveal no allergies.

Treatment

Avoidance of the offending agent (or agents) is the backbone of the treatment plan for allergic rhinitis.

However, even with rigorous avoidance measures, many individuals require pharmacologic intervention. The optimal treatment plan is individualized based on the context of the disease, symptom pattern, and other comorbid conditions. The ideal medication is efficacious, cost effective, and compliance friendly, causing minimal or no side effects. Furthermore, based on the pathophysiology of allergic rhinitis, the best therapeutic agent is one that effectively addresses both early- and late-phase reactions.[50] Currently the main classes of medications available for treatment of allergic rhinitis are antihistamines, decongestants, topical or oral glucocorticoids, anticholinergics, and cromolyn. In addition, immunotherapy should be considered for a few selected individuals.

Avoidance. Although it may be difficult to avoid pollen because of its widespread distribution, certain commonsensical measures can be taken to decrease exposure. Outdoor activities should be limited or completely avoided when pollen counts are at their peaks. Pollen counts typically peak in the late morning to mid-afternoon.[60] Limiting such activities as leaf raking, lawn mowing, and farming can reduce exposure to outdoor fungi (e.g., *Alternaria* species). Because fungi thrive in moist, humid environments, important indoor control measures include dehumidification, proper ventilation, fungicide use in contaminated areas, and removal of sources of fungal growth.

Antihistamines and Decongestants. Antihistamines have been used for 50 years and are considered by many to be the first line of therapy in the treatment of allergic rhinitis.[40] They are most effective against seasonal rhinitis in which sneezing, itching, rhinorrhea, and watery eyes are the most prominent symptoms. However, only 33% to 50% of seasonal allergic rhinitis sufferers obtain complete relief with antihistamine therapy alone.[7] Antihistamines have little or no effect on nasal congestion because of the minor role of histamine in the pathophysiology of congestion. For this reason, antihistamines are usually inadequate for treatment of perennial rhinitis, in which nasal congestion is often a predominant symptom.

Antihistamines act by occupying H1 receptors on cells and thereby blocking histamine binding. In comparing first- and second-generation antihistamines, both are equally effective; however, second-generation antihistamines have gained tremendous popularity because their use is associated with a much lower incidence of sedation and fewer anticholinergic side effects. Commonly used first-generation antihistamines, most of which are available over the counter, are chlorpheniramine, diphenhydramine, brompheniramine, and clemastine. The duration of action of brompheniramine and diphenhydramine is 6 to 10 hours, whereas that of chlorpheniramine and hydroxyzine is 24 and 36 hours, respectively. All first- and second-generation antihistamines, with the exception of cetirizine and fexofenadine, are metabolized extensively in the liver via the cytochrome P_{450} system. Simultaneous administration of other medications that compete for the cytochrome P_{450} system and hepatic dysfunction may affect the metabolism of antihistamines and increase the risk of adverse effects.

Four nonsedating antihistamines are currently available (three are oral and one is intranasal) (Table 46-2). The recommended doses are given once or twice daily, depending on the medication. Cetirizine and loratadine are approved for use in children; cetirizine is recommended for children aged 2 years and older, and loratadine is for 6 those aged years and older. Azelastine (Astelin) is the only H_1 receptor antagonist available in a nasal spray; studies have shown that it is safe and

TABLE 46-2. Nonsedating Antihistamines

MEDICATION	BRAND NAME	RECOMMENDED DOSE	HOW SUPPLIED	MINIMUM AGE (YEARS)
Loratadine	Claritin	10 mg PO qd	10-mg tablets; 5 mg/tsp syrup	6
	Claritin-D 12 Hour	5 mg PO bid	5 mg loratadine and 120 mg pseudoephedrine	12
	Claritin-D 24 Hour	10 mg PO qd	10 mg loratadine and 240 mg pseudoephedrine	12
Fexofenadine	Allegra	60 mg PO bid	60-mg capsules	12
	Allegra	180 mg PO qd	180-mg capsules	12
	Allegra-D	60 mg PO bid	60 mg fexofenadine and 120 mg pseudoephedrine	12
Cetirizine	Zyrtec	5 to 10 mg PO qd	5-mg, 10-mg tablets; 5 mg/tsp syrup	2
Azelastine	Astelin	2 sprays in each nostril bid	137 µg/spray	12

PO, By mouth; *qd,* every day; *bid,* twice a day.

effective for relieving most allergic rhinitis symptoms, including nasal congestion.[27] Although all antihistamines have relatively rapid onset of action and may be used as needed, they are most effective if taken before exposure (e.g., pollen season) and if used regularly.

In some individuals the addition of a decongestant to the antihistamine may be helpful. Decongestants act by stimulating α-adrenergic receptors and thereby reducing blood supply to the sinusoids. Most are short acting (4 to 6 hours) and available over the counter with or without antihistamines. Pseudoephedrine and phenylpropanolamine are the two most commonly used decongestants. Fexofenadine and loratadine (available in 12- and 24-hour preparations) also are available with a decongestant. Insomnia and irritability are the most common side effects of decongestants, although individual tolerance varies widely. Individuals with hypertension, bladder outlet problems, glaucoma, or cardiac arrhythmias should use decongestants cautiously or preferably avoid their use altogether. Topical decongestants (e.g., oxymetazoline) have a fast onset of action (within minutes) and are therefore provide rapid relief of symptoms. Because of the risk of rhinitis medicamentosa (as described previously), topical decongestant use is limited to 5 to 7 days. Thus these medications are inappropriate for long-term therapy.

Glucocorticoids. Glucocorticoids represent the gold standard of treatment for allergic rhinitis. Numerous well-designed studies have shown that intranasal corticosteroids are superior to antihistamines and cromolyn sodium.[6,8] With the exception of ocular symptoms, nasal corticosteroids are effective in controlling all symptoms of allergic rhinitis. A glucocorticoid is often the first line of therapy for the patient with perennial rhinitis. Glucocorticoids control the rate of protein synthesis by either inducing or suppressing gene transcription within the cell.[28] The inhibitory effect of all glucocorticoids on the late-phase reaction is well established, but studies have shown that intranasal corticosteroids, unlike their oral counterparts, also inhibit the early-phase reaction.[2]

Several preparations of intranasal corticosteroids are currently available (Table 46-3). All are approximately equally effective; hence the criteria for selection depends on convenience, cost, and delivery system. Intranasal corticosteroids are given either once or twice a day in aqueous or dry powder form. Dry powder preparations are associated with a slightly greater risk of nasal irritation, burning, ulceration, and epistaxis. Because of slow onset of action, it may be 1 to 3 weeks after the initiation of therapy before the maximum benefits of inhaled corticosteroid use are achieved. For individuals with seasonal rhinitis, it is prudent to begin inhaled glucocorticoid therapy before pollen season begins. There is no role for regular use of oral glucocorticoids in the treatment of allergic rhinitis. However, a short course (7 to 10 days) of oral glucocorticoids may be appropriate when symptoms are severe (e.g., during the pollen season). In addition to providing quicker relief, oral glucocorticoids may facilitate improved delivery of intranasal corticosteroids to the nasal mucosa.

The most common side effects of intranasal corticosteroids are local irritation (reported in approximately 10% of patients) and bleeding (reported in approximately 2% of patients).[33] The incidence of side effects is higher during dry winter months. Although rare, septal perforation has been reported in patients using intranasal corticosteroids.[45] The physician must reevaluate each patient, performing a thorough nasal examination 2 to 4 weeks after initiating therapy. If significant septal ulceration and crust formation are

TABLE 46-3. Topical Nasal Corticosteroids

MEDICATION	BRAND NAME	RECOMMENDED DOSE (EACH NOSTRIL)	MICROGRAMS PER SPRAY	PREPARATION
Beclomethasone	Beconase	1-2 sprays bid	42	Dry
	Beconase AQ	1-2 sprays bid	42	Aqueous
	Vancenase	1-2 sprays bid	42	Dry
	Vancenase AQ	1-2 sprays bid	42	Aqueous
	Vancenase AQ DS	1-2 sprays qd	84	Aqueous
Budesonide	Rhinocort	2-4 sprays qd or 1-2 sprays bid	32	Dry
	Rhinocort Aqua	2-4 sprays qd or 1-2 sprays bid	32	Aqueous
Flunisolide	Nasalide	1-2 sprays bid or tid	25	Aqueous
	Nasarel	2-4 sprays bid	25	Aqueous
Fluticasone	Flonase	1-2 sprays qd	50	Aqueous
Mometasone	Nasonex	1-2 sprays qd	50	Aqueous
Triamcinolone	Nasacort	1-2 sprays qd	55	Dry
	Nasacort AQ	1-2 sprays qd	55	Aqueous

bid, Twice a day; *qd*, every day.

noted, therapy should be discontinued for a few days and nasal hygiene with saline spray should be instituted. Long-term studies have shown no evidence of mucosal atrophy associated with the use of intranasal corticosteroids.[32]

There have been recent concerns about the effects of inhaled corticosteroids on growth in children. Studies have demonstrated that the use of intranasal corticosteroids in therapeutic doses suppresses serum and urinary cortisol levels.[59] A study of 100 children (aged 6 to 9 years) receiving 168 μg of beclomethasone twice daily over 12 months showed statistically significant bone growth suppression at 1, 6, 8, and 12 months.[39] The clinical significance of these findings remains to be determined because it may be that many children's height "catches up" in adolescent years. Based on such studies, the Food and Drug Administration has considered the use of class labeling with regard to growth suppression in children for inhaled and intranasal corticosteroids.

Other Medications. Other classes of medication available for treatment of allergic rhinitis are antiasthmatics (i.e., cromolyn sodium) and topical anticholinergics. Although studies have shown the effectiveness of leukotriene antagonists, these medications currently are not approved for use in patients with allergic rhinitis.[26] Although less potent than intranasal corticosteroids, cromolyn is very safe and effective therapy for allergic rhinitis. Its mechanism of action is not completely understood, but it is believed to inhibit mast cell degranulation. For optimal relief, it requires regular use and frequent dosing (three to four times daily). It is useful as a prophylactic treatment before known exposure (e.g., visiting a family with a cat) and in such situations may be used as needed. The only indication for the use of a topical anticholinergic in the patient with allergic rhinitis is rhinorrhea. A topical anticholinergic drug, such as ipratropium (Atrovent), can be used alone if rhinorrhea is the main symptom or in addition to intranasal corticosteroids and antihistamines if symptoms persist despite these therapies. An additional benefit of anticholinergic drugs is control of postnasal drip. The recommended dose of intranasal ipratropium is one to two sprays in each nostril two to four times a day. The main side effect of intranasal ipratropium is nasal dryness.

Immunotherapy. Allergen immunotherapy is a form of immunomodulation in which a state of tolerance is achieved by injecting gradually increasing amounts of allergen extracts into a sensitized person. Although the precise mechanisms of immunotherapy are unknown, several immunologic changes have been observed, including induction of allergen-specific IgG "blocking antibodies," decreases in allergen-specific IgE, modula-

tion of mast cell or basophil function, and increases in suppressor T cells (CD8$^+$).[17]

The efficacy of immunotherapy in patients with allergic rhinitis has been well documented in numerous studies.[13,53] Most individuals who receive immunotherapy for allergic rhinitis obtain a variable degree of relief, enabling better symptom control with less medication. Immunotherapy should be considered for individuals who do not respond to avoidance measures and medical therapy and for individuals who experience significant adverse effects as a result of conventional medical therapy. In immunotherapy an initial series of weekly injections is administered, with escalating doses of allergen extracts, and is followed by monthly injections once specified maintenance doses are achieved (within 4 to 6 months). Although there are no data regarding the optimal duration of immunotherapy, the general recommendations are from 3 to 5 years.[56]

The most common adverse reactions of immunotherapy are local and include erythema, edema, and pruritus at the site of injection. However, systemic reactions may include any or all of the following: urticaria, rhinitis, bronchospasm, abdominal cramping, and hypotension. Systemic reactions to immunotherapy occur in much higher proportion in individuals with poorly controlled asthma. Therefore immunotherapy generally is not recommended for asthmatics with a forced expiratory volume in 1 second (FEV$_1$) less than 70%. Because most systemic reactions occur within 20 to 30 minutes after injection, recipients should be observed in the physician's office during this time. Patients on immunotherapy should carry epinephrine (e.g., EpiPen, Ana-Kit) for self-injection at all times to treat a possible late-onset systemic reaction. With the exception of immunotherapy against anaphylaxis resulting from an insect sting, immunotherapy should not be initiated during pregnancy. Pregnant women on maintenance doses of immunotherapy can continue treatment.

ANAPHYLAXIS

Anaphylaxis is a systemic life-threatening allergic reaction resulting from IgE-mediated mast cell and basophil degranulation (Type I hypersensitivity). It is the most severe form of Type I hypersensitivity reaction, and clinical manifestations may occur in various end organs, including the skin, upper respiratory tract, lower respiratory tract, gastrointestinal tract, and cardiovascular system. An anaphylactoid reaction is non–IgE mediated but may be clinically indistinguishable from anaphylaxis (Box 46-2). Mechanisms of anaphylactoid reactions include direct release of mediators from mast cells and basophils (e.g., opiates, radiocontrast material), disturbances in arachidonic acid metab-

---

Box 46-2   CLASSIFICATION OF ANAPHYLACTIC AND ANAPHYLACTOID REACTIONS

ANAPHYLAXIS (IgE MEDIATED)

Food

Drugs (penicillin, cephalosporins, insulin, sometimes aspirin and other NSAIDs)

Insect stings and bites

Other (exposure to antivenin or aquatic proteins)

ANAPHYLACTOID (NON–IgE MEDIATED)

Direct stimulation of mast cells

   Drugs (opiates, vancomycin)

   Radiocontrast material

   Physical stimuli (exercise, cold)

   Idiopathic

Disturbances in arachidonic acid metabolism

   Aspirin and other NSAIDs

Complement activation

   Transfusion reactions

   Immunoglobulin

IgE, Immunoglobulin E; *NSAIDs,* nonsteroidal inflammatory drugs.

olism (e.g., nonsteroidal antiinflammatory drugs [NSAIDs]),[15] and complement activation (e.g., transfusion reactions). The overall incidence of anaphylaxis is unknown. In a 1990 review of 20,064 persons admitted to a university hospital, there were nine cases of anaphylaxis (0.04%).[1] Approximately 700 to 1800 persons in the United States die each year of anaphylaxis or anaphylactoid reactions.

Etiology

The various causes of anaphylaxis can be categorized into those that are IgE antibody mediated and those that are non–IgE antibody mediated (Box 46-2). In a study by the Mayo Clinic emergency department, food was the most commonly reported cause of IgE-mediated anaphylaxis.[61] Consumption of eggs, cow's milk, peanuts (and other legumes, such as soybeans), tree nuts (e.g., hazelnuts, walnuts, cashews, almonds),[44,61] fish (e.g., cod or whitefish), and shellfish (e.g., shrimp, lobster, crab)[46] is responsible for most food-related anaphylactic reactions. In children, peanuts are probably the most frequent cause of food-induced anaphylaxis.[43] Individuals may accidentally ingest the allergenic food when it is disguised in cooking preparations or hidden by misleading labeling or contamination during the preparation process.

Drugs, especially antibiotics, may cause an anaphylactic or an anaphylactoid reaction. Penicillin and its derivatives are most often implicated, with reactions occurring in between 1 and 5 of every 10,000 courses of treatment.[22] Opiates and vancomycin cause drug reactions by directly degranulating mast cells and basophils, so prior sensitization is not required.

Aspirin and other NSAIDs can provoke allergic reactions that are either IgE or non–IgE mediated, depending on the presence or absence of underlying asthma or cutaneous diseases (e.g., chronic urticaria). In the presence of asthma and chronic urticaria, disturbance in arachidonic acid metabolism is the predominant mechanism. Aspirin and NSAIDs inhibit the cyclooxygenase pathway, leading to rapid synthesis of the lipoxygenase pathway products,[29] especially leukotrienes, which are important mediators of inflammation.

Important outdoor-related causes of anaphylaxis are envenomation (e.g., a bee sting), contact with aquatic proteins, and antivenin therapy (e.g., for snakebite). In the Mayo study mentioned earlier, bee stings were the second most common (14%) cause of anaphylaxis after consumption of allergenic foods.[61] The estimated incidence of insect sting anaphylaxis in the general population is 0.3% to 3%.[41] Bee sting anaphylactic reactions are especially common in individuals younger than 20 years but are more likely to be fatal in the elderly. In general, children's reactions are milder (e.g., urticaria only) than are adults' reactions. Individuals who experience a sting-related anaphylactic reaction have a 50% to 60% risk for suffering anaphylaxis after subsequent insect stings.[41] The offending insects vary depending on geographic location. In the United States, yellow jackets cause the most allergic reactions, whereas in Europe, honeybees and wasps caused nearly all insect sting–related reactions. Although rare, anaphylaxis can result from bites inflicted by some insects (e.g., the kissing bug *[Triatoma protracta],* the deer fly *[Chrysops discalis])*[21,58] and ticks.[9]

Physical stimuli may provoke anaphylactoid reactions. In exercise-induced reactions, symptoms typically arise after 5 minutes of moderate to heavy exercise, resolving within 30 minutes to 4 hours after exercise cessation. About 50% of affected individuals are atopic and most engage in regular vigorous exercise. A coinciting factor, such as the ingestion of an allergenic food (e.g., shellfish)[31] or NSAID, may be necessary.[37] Exercise or ingestion of a certain food or drug alone does not cause an allergic reaction. In a cholinergic anaphylactoid reaction, symptoms occur after exercise and after passive exposure to heat (e.g., hot showers, sweating, anxiety). In cold-induced anaphylactoid reactions, symptoms occur after exposure to low temperatures.

Recurrent anaphylaxis without identifiable cause is called *idiopathic anaphylaxis.* Although all the target organs of anaphylaxis may be affected, idiopathic anaphylaxis most commonly causes urticaria, angioedema, or both. Diagnosis is made by exclusion after all other possible identifiable causes have been eliminated. Individuals who suffer frequent episodes are less likely to undergo remission. Short-term treatment is the same as that for anaphylaxis resulting from other causes. Depending on the frequency of attacks, long-term treatment may require regular use of corticosteroids.

Complement activation plays a key role in anaphylactoid reactions resulting from the transfusion of blood products and immunoglobulins. Transfusion of an incompatible blood type can lead to cytotoxic anaphylactoid reactions if complement-fixing antibodies to formed elements of blood, such as red cells, white cells, and platelets, are present. In γ-globulin–related anaphylactoid reactions, immune complex aggregation occurs when antigen-antibody complexes activate complement.

Pathophysiology

Unlike the local pathologic and clinical manifestations of allergic rhinitis, the clinical consequences of Type I immediate hypersensitivity in anaphylaxis are systemic. Histamine is the most important mediator and is responsible for most clinical manifestations. Important effects of histamine include vasodilation, increased vascular permeability, smooth muscle contraction, stimulation of nerve endings, and glandular secretion. These effects lead to various clinical manifestations, including flushing, urticaria or angioedema, hypotension or shock, wheezing, abdominal cramps, and diarrhea. Arachidonic acid metabolites, such as leukotrienes, prostaglandins, thromboxane A_2, and platelet-activating factor, also are released from mast cells and basophils, causing airway smooth muscle contraction, increased vascular permeability, goblet and mucosal gland secretion, and peripheral vasodilation. Platelet-activating factor also contracts smooth muscle and enhances vascular permeability. A late-phase reaction may occur many hours after the initial event.

Clinical Features and Diagnosis

Clinical manifestations of anaphylaxis may occur in various end organs, including the skin (urticaria, angioedema, and flushing), upper respiratory tract (rhinitis, stridor, and hoarseness), lower respiratory tract (wheezing, bronchospasm, and cough), gastrointestinal tract (abdominal pain, diarrhea, and vomiting), and cardiovascular system (tachycardia, hypotension, and shock). Urticaria and angioedema are by far the most common manifestations, occurring in 83% to 90% of individuals with anaphylaxis.[25,54,57] The second most common manifestations are respiratory tract symptoms, followed by dizziness or syncope and gastrointestinal symptoms. Cardiovascular collapse with shock can occur rapidly, without any other antecedent symptoms.

Most anaphylactic reactions occur soon (within 5 minutes to 2 hours) after exposure to an inciting agent, but other patterns are possible. In bimodal anaphylaxis, symptoms begin within minutes of exposure; after transient clinical improvement the allergic reaction returns 1 to 8 hours later.[51] Protracted anaphylaxis can begin suddenly or gradually, but the clinical manifestations are prolonged, sometimes requiring hours or even days of intense resuscitation. Generally the more rapid the onset, the more severe the episode.[30] Fatalities usually result from airway obstruction, cardiovascular collapse, or both.

Treatment

Anaphylaxis is a medical emergency requiring prompt recognition and treatment. Treatment depends on the severity of the reaction and the organ system (or systems) involved. For mild anaphylactic or anaphylactoid reactions limited to the skin, antihistamines alone are effective. Individuals with cutaneous reactions should be monitored closely for signs of respiratory or cardiovascular compromise, and manifestations beyond the skin require more aggressive measures, such as administration of fluids, bronchodilators, and epinephrine.

Short-term management of anaphylaxis is detailed in Box 46-3.[50] Because most fatalities occur as a result of delayed treatment,[16] the importance of prompt administration of epinephrine cannot be overemphasized. Intravenous epinephrine may be administered if the reaction is life threatening and if the patient does not respond to subcutaneous epinephrine. However, intravenous epinephrine should be used with caution in persons older than 35 years. Aerosolized aqueous epinephrine can prevent upper airway edema, but it is inadequate to abort systemic anaphylaxis.[11] Use of over-the-counter epinephrine inhalation aerosol bronchodilators (e.g., Primatene Mist) generally is not recommended because of the lack of adrenergic specificity (i.e., it is non–β_2 selective) and the extremely short half-life. Even these agents should be used with caution, especially in individuals with a history of coronary artery disease and arrhythmias.

Repletion of intravascular volume is a mainstay of treatment for hypotension. A large volume of fluid may be necessary and should be given rapidly in either colloid or crystalloid form. Vasopressor drugs may be needed to treat hypotension if the response to subcutaneous epinephrine and fluids is inadequate. Dopamine is often the initial drug of choice. Norepinephrine, a potent vasopressor, can be used to treat severe hypotension that is unresponsive to epinephrine, dopamine, and fluids. Glucagon may be necessary to treat refractory hypotension (e.g., patients on β-blocker medica-

Box 46-3 TREATMENT OF ANAPHYLAXIS

GENERAL MEASURES

Place the individual in Trendelenburg's position.

Establish and maintain the airway. (If necessary, perform cricothyroidotomy.)

Administer oxygen as needed.

Place a venous tourniquet above the reaction site (e.g., insect sting) to decrease systemic absorption of the antigen.

Obtain intravenous access and infuse a volume expander (colloid-containing solution or normal saline) to achieve a systolic blood pressure of 90 mm Hg in an adult. Blood pressure may be briefly augmented by the application of military antishock trousers, which increases systemic vascular resistance.

EPINEPHRINE USE AND TREATMENT OF HYPOTENSION

Administer aqueous epinephrine, 1:1000, 0.3 to 0.5 ml (0.3 to 0.5 mg) subcutaneously or intramuscularly in the deltoid region. The epinephrine dose for children is 0.01 ml/kg. Repeat once or twice as necessary at 15 to 20 minute intervals to control the signs and symptoms.

If the reaction is life threatening and if the patient does not respond to subcutaneous epinephrine, administer epinephrine intravenously. Mix 0.1 ml (0.1 mg) of 1:1000 aqueous epinephrine in 10 ml of normal saline (final dilution, 1:100,000) and infuse over 10 minutes. If hypotension persists, a continuous epinephrine infusion may be started by adding 1 ml (1 mg) of 1:1000 epinephrine to 250 ml of normal saline, creating a concentration of 4 μg/ml. Infuse this solution at a rate of 1 μg/minute (15 minidrops/minute). The rate of infusion can be increased to 4 to 5 μg/minute if the clinical response is inadequate. In children and infants the starting dose is 0.1 μg/kg/minute, up to maximum of 1.5 μg/kg/minute. Intravenous epinephrine should be used with caution in persons older than 35.

If epinephrine and fluids are ineffective, intravenous dopamine infusion should be initiated. Mix 400 mg of dopamine in 500 ml of D_5W (800 μg/ml) and infuse at a rate of 2 to 20 μg/kg/minute. The rate should be titrated using the blood pressure. Norepinephrine, a potent vasopressor, can be used to treat severe hypotension that is unresponsive to the administration of epinephrine, fluids, and dopamine. Mix 4 mg of norepinephrine in 1000 ml of D_5W (4 μg/ml) and infuse at a rate of 0.5 to 1 μg/kg/minute.

In a refractory case in which the individual is not responsive to epinephrine (especially the individual on a β-blocker medication), administer a glucagon bolus at a dose of 1 to 5 mg intravenously over 2 minutes. If necessary, a continuous infusion, 1 mg in 1000 ml of D_5W (1 μg/ml), should be started at a rate of 5 to 15 μg/minute.

TREATMENT OF BRONCHOSPASM

Administer a β_2-agonist (albuterol, metaproterenol, pirbuterol, or terbutaline) via nebulization as required for bronchospasm that is not relieved by epinephrine.

Continuous nebulization may be required if bronchospasm persists.

ANTIHISTAMINES AND CORTICOSTEROIDS

Administer diphenhydramine 25 to 50 mg (1 mg/kg in children) intravenously over 3 minutes intramuscularly, or orally when the reaction is not severe. The addition of cimetidine 300 mg intravenously over 5 minutes may reverse refractory anaphylactic shock caused by the blockade of both H_1 and H_2 receptors. Transient hypotension, bradycardia, and arrhythmias have been reported after rapid intravenous administration of cimetidine.

Most authorities advocate the use of glucocorticoids to decrease the likelihood of a late-phase reaction. The standard therapy is either hydrocortisone 200 to 300 mg intravenously or prednisone 30 to 60 mg orally in milder cases.

---

tions) that is resistant to standard therapeutic regimens.[62] Glucagon is the drug of choice for patients on β-blocker medications.[18] Medical antishock trousers have been used successfully to treat refractory hypotension associated with anaphylaxis.[36]

For prominent wheezing, intermittent or continuous use (depending on severity) of an aerosolized β_2-agonist is recommended. Although antihistamines are only adjunctive therapy to epinephrine, they can relieve symptoms dramatically. Combining an H_1 antihistamine and an H_2 antihistamine may be more effective than administering either alone.[42] Most authorities recommend the use of glucocorticoids to decrease the likelihood of a late-phase reaction.

Because of possible recurrent symptoms, all individuals who suffer an anaphylactic or anaphylactoid reaction should be observed after the initial symptoms have subsided. For a mild to severe episode a period of observation between 2 and 24 hours is reasonable. Any individual with severe respiratory or cardiac compromise should be hospitalized. Persons at risk for anaphylaxis should carry a device allowing self-injection of epinephrine (Table 46-4) at all times and should wear a medical information bracelet or carry a medical information card. Finally, it is important to identify the precipitating agent for anaphylaxis so that preventive measures can be taken to reduce the risk of future reactions.

TABLE 46-4. Selected Self-Injecting Epinephrine-Containing Kits

BRAND NAME	COMPANY	DOSE (mg)	DOSES PER UNIT
Ana-Kit	Bayer-Miles	0.5	2
Ana-Guard	Bayer-Miles	0.5	2
Anahelp	Stallergenes	0.25	4
EpiPen	Dey Laboratories	0.3	1
EpiPen Jr.	Dey Laboratories	0.15	1
Fastjekt	Allergopharma	0.3	1
Min-I-Jet	IMS	1.0	1

REFERENCES

1. Amornmarn L et al: Anaphylaxis admissions to a university hospital, *J Allergy Clin Immunol* 89(suppl):349, 1992 (abstract).
2. Andersson M, Andersson P, Pipkorn U: Topical glucocorticoids and allergen-induced increase in nasal reactivity: relationship between treatment time and inhibitory effect, *J Allergy Clin Immunol* 82:1019, 1988.
3. Barnard JH: Studies of 400 Hymenoptera sting deaths in the United States, *J Allergy Clin Immunol* 52:259, 1973.
4. Bascom R et al: The influx of inflammatory cells into nasal washings during the late response to antigen challenge: effect of systemic steroid pretreatment, *Am Rev Respir Dis* 138:406, 1988.
5. Bazaral M, Orgel HA, Hamburger RN: Genetics of IgE and allergy, *J Allergy Clin Immunol* 54:288, 1974.
6. Bernstein DI et al: Comparison of triamcinolone acetonide nasal inhaler with astemizole in the treatment of ragweed-induced allergic rhinitis, *J Allergy Clin Immunol* 97:749, 1996.
7. Bousquet J, Chanez P, Michel FB: Pathophysiology and treatment of seasonal allergic rhinitis, *Respir Med* 84(suppl A):11, 1990.
8. Bronsky EA et al: Fluticasone propionate aqueous nasal spray compared with terfenadine tablets in the treatment of seasonal allergic rhinitis, *J Allergy Clin Immunol* 97:915, 1996.
9. Brown AF, Hamilton DL: Tick bite anaphylaxis in Australia, *J Accid Emerg Med* 15:111, 1998.
10. Connell JT: Quantitative intranasal pollen challenges. III. The priming effect in allergic rhinitis, *Allergy* 43:33, 1969.
11. deLage C, Irey N: Anaphylactic deaths: a clinicopathologic study of 43 cases, *J Forensic Sci* 17:525, 1972.
12. de Vries JE: The role of IL-13 and its receptor in allergy and inflammatory responses, *J Allergy Clin Immunol* 102:165, 1998.
13. Dolz I et al: A double-blind, placebo-controlled study of immunotherapy with grass-pollen extract Alutard SQ during a 3-year period with initial rush immunotherapy, *Allergy* 51:489, 1996.
14. Druce HM: Allergic and nonallergic rhinitis. In Middleton E Jr et al, editors: *Allergy: principles and practice,* ed 5, St Louis, 1998, Mosby.
15. Fischer AR et al: Direct evidence for a role of the mast cell in the nasal response to aspirin in aspirin-sensitive asthma, *J Allergy Clin Immunol* 94:1046, 1994.
16. Frazier CA et al: Anaphylaxis at school: etiologic factors, prevalence, and treatment (letter), *Pediatrics* 91:516, 1993.
17. Gleich GJ et al: Effect of immunotherapy on immunoglobulin E and immunoglobulin G antibodies to ragweed antigens: a six-year prospective study, *J Allergy Clin Immunol* 70:261, 1982.
18. Glick G, Parmley WW, Wechsler AS: Glucagon: its enhancement of cardiac performance in the cat and dog and persistence of its inotropic action despite (-receptor blockade with propranolol, *Circ Res* 22:789, 1968.
19. Goodman WS, deSouza FM: Atrophic rhinitis. In English GM, editor: *Otolaryngology,* vol 2, Philadelphia, 1987, Lippincott.
20. Hasegawa M, Kern EB: The human nasal cycle, *Mayo Clin Proc* 52:28, 1977.
21. Hoffman DF: Allergy to biting insects, *Clin Rev Allergy Immunol* 5:177, 1987.
22. Idsoe O et al: Nature and extent of penicillin side-reactions with particular reference to fatalities from anaphylactic shock, *Bull World Health Organ* 38:159, 1968.
23. Iliopoulos O: Histamine-containing cells obtained from the nose hours after antigen challenge have functional and phenotypic characteristics of basophils, *J Immunol* 148:2223, 1992.
24. Jacobs RL, Freedman PM, Boswell RN: Non-allergic rhinitis with eosinophilia (NARES syndrome): clinical and immunological presentation, *J Allergy Clin Immunol* 67:253, 1981.
25. Kemp SF et al: Anaphylaxis: a review of 266 cases, *Arch Intern Med* 155:1749, 1995.
26. Knapp HR: Reduced allergen-induced nasal congestion and leukotriene synthesis with an orally active 5-lipoxygenase inhibitor, *N Engl J Med* 323:1745, 1990.
27. LaForce C et al: Safety and efficacy of azelastine nasal spray (Astelin NS) for seasonal allergic rhinitis: a 4-week comparative multicenter trial, *Ann Allergy Asthma Immunol* 76:181, 1996.
28. LaForce C: Use of nasal steroids in managing allergic rhinitis. II. *J Allergy Clin Immunol* 103:S388, 1999.
29. Lee TH: Mechanism of bronchospasm in aspirin-sensitive asthma, *Am Rev Respir Dis* 148:1442, 1993 (editorial).
30. Lieberman P: Anaphylaxis and anaphylactoid reactions. In Middleton E Jr et al, editors: *Allergy: principles and practice,* ed 5, St Louis, 1998, Mosby.
31. Maulitz RM et al: Exercise-induced anaphylactic reactions to shellfish, *J Allergy Clin Immunol* 63:433, 1979.
32. Morrow Brown H, Storey G, Jackson FA: Beclomethasone dipropionate aerosol in treatment of perennial and seasonal rhinitis: a review of five years' experience, *Br J Clin Pharmacol* 4:2835, 1977.
33. Naclerio R: Allergic rhinitis, *N Engl J Med* 325:860, 1991.
34. Naclerio R: Clinical manifestations of the release of histamine and other inflammatory mediators. II. *J Allergy Clin Immunol* 103:S382, 1999.
35. Naclerio R, Solomon W: Rhinitis and inhalant allergens, *JAMA* 278:1842, 1997.
36. Oertel T, Loehr MM: Bee-sting anaphylaxis: the use of medical antishock trousers, *Ann Emerg Med* 13:459, 1984.
37. Okazaki M et al: Food-dependent exercise-induced anaphylaxis, *Intern Med* 31:1052, 1992.
38. Platts-Mills TAE et al: Epidemiology of acute asthma: IgE antibodies to common inhalant allergens as a risk factor for emergency room visits, *J Allergy Clin Immunol* 83:875, 1989.
39. Rachelefsky GS et al: An evaluation of the effects of beclomethasone dipropionate aqueous nasal spray (Vancenase AQ [VNS]) on long-term growth in children, *J Allergy Clin Immunol* 101:S236, 1998 (abstract).
40. Rachelefsky GS: Pharmacologic management of allergic rhinitis. II. *J Allergy Clin Immunol* 101:S367, 1998.
41. Reisman R: Insect stings, *N Engl J Med* 331:523, 1994.
42. Runge JW et al: Histamine antagonists in the treatment of acute allergic reactions, *Ann Emerg Med* 21:237, 1992.
43. Sachs M, Yunginger JW: Food-induced anaphylaxis, *Immunol Allergy Clin North Am* 11:743, 1991.
44. Sampson HA, Mendelson LM, Rosen JP: Fatal and near-fatal anaphylactic reactions to food in children and adolescents, *N Engl J Med* 327:380, 1992.
45. Schoelzel EP: Nasal sprays and perforation of the nasal septum, *JAMA* 253:2046, 1985.
46. Settipane G: Anaphylactic deaths in asthmatic patients, *Allergy Asthma Proc* 10:271, 1989.
47. Sibbald B, Strachan DP: Epidemiology of rhinitis. In Busse WW, Holgate ST, editors: *Asthma and rhinitis,* Cambridge, Mass, 1995, Blackwell Scientific.
48. Sicherer SH, Eggleston PA: Environmental allergens. In Lieberman P, Anderson JA, editors: *Allergic diseases: diagnosis and treatment,* Totowa, NJ, 1997, Humana.
49. Solomon WR, Weber RW, Dolen WK: Common allergenic pollen and fungi. In Bierman et al, editors: *Allergy, asthma, and immunology from infancy to adulthood,* ed 3, Philadelphia, 1996, WB Saunders.
50. Spector S et al: Algorithm for the treatment of acute anaphylaxis. II. *J Allergy Clin Immunol* 101:S469, 1998.
51. Spector S: Ideal pharmacotherapy for allergic rhinitis. II. *J Allergy Clin Immunol* 103:S386, 1999.

52. Stark BJ, Sullivan TJ: Biphasic and protracted anaphylaxis, *J Allergy Clin Immunol* 78:76, 1986.
53. Storms W et al: The economic impact of allergic rhinitis, *J Allergy Clin Immunol* 99:S820, 1997.
54. Varney VA et al: Usefulness of immunotherapy in patients with severe summer hay fever uncontrolled by antiallergic drugs, *Br Med J* 302:265, 1991.
55. Wade JP, Liang MH, Sheffer AL: Exercise-induced anaphylaxis: epidemiological observations, *Prog Clin Biol Res* 297:175, 1989.
56. White MV, Kaliner MA: Mediators of allergic rhinitis, *J Allergy Clin Immunol* 90:699, 1992.
57. WHO/IUIS Working Group report: Current status of allergen immunotherapy, *Lancet* i:259, 1989.
58. Wiggins CA: Characteristics and etiology of 30 patients with anaphylaxis, *Immun Allergy Prac* 13:313, 1991.
59. Wilbur RD, Evans R: An immunologic evaluation of deer fly hypersensitivity, *J Allergy Clin Immunol* 55:72, 1975.
60. Wilson AM, McFarlane LC, Lipworth BJ: Effects of repeated once daily dosing of three intranasal corticosteroids on basal and dynamic measures of hypothalamic-pituitary-adrenal axis activity, *J Allergy Clin Immunol* 101:470, 1998.
61. Wood R: Allergens. In Mygind N, Naclerio R, editors: *Allergic and non-allergic rhinitis*, Copenhagen, 1993, Munksgaard.
62. Zaloga GP et al: Glucagon reversal of hypotension in a case of anaphylactoid shock, *Ann Intern Med* 105:65, 1986.

47 Plant-Induced Dermatitis

William L. Epstein and John H. Epstein

Advertent or inadvertent exposure to plants is a common cause of skin eruptions. Because the reactions are often acute, the victims frequently seek emergency care. This subject has been reviewed in detail.[5,28] This chapter considers plant dermatitis from the acute care perspective. Although most acute, itchy eruptions share clinical features, not every rash is poison ivy dermatitis. Plant dermatitis is discussed as irritation, allergy, phytophotodermatitis, and granulomas. Similarities, distinctions, and different plans for management are emphasized. Proper recognition and adequate early treatment often lead to a cure with no further recurrence, whereas failure to diagnose and less optimal management can result in chronic, disabling dermatosis.

IRRITATION

Primary irritation is the most frequent cutaneous response to vegetation. Most of these injuries are sufficiently mild to be ignored or self-treated. Many wild plants, such as brambles and berries, have sharp thorns that can inflict significant skin trauma. The typical appearance is of linear scratches or excoriations. The area can be swollen and red with a weeping or bloody crust. Fever and adenopathy are uncommon. Pruritus, when present, is mild.

Treatment consists mostly of cool soaks or compresses with soft gauze or soft linen with aluminum acetate solution diluted 1:20 for use. The lesions usually heal in a few days. Secondary infection relates to the environment and personal hygiene. Uncommonly, these wounds allow entry of microorganisms that cause systemic diseases, such as sporotrichosis. In addition to inflicting gross mechanical damage, many plants, weeds, and fruits have fine hairs (trichomes) and barbed hairs (glochids), which cause more subtle and annoying forms of irritation. The trichome-glochid response is acute development of wheals with itching and occasionally intense pain. Large blisters may form. Although this irritation appears to have mechanical origin, the reaction is produced by natural substances in the trichomes or glochids. Low-molecular-weight acids, glycosides, proteolytic enzymes, and crystals are among the major plant chemicals that cause primary skin irritation. These lesions can occur on skin or mucous membranes and are classified as nonimmunogenic urticaria. An example is itch powder, from dried cowhage *(Mucuna pruriens),* which contains a prote-

olytic enzyme and causes intense pruritus.[117,118] Other irritant enzymes include bromelin from pineapples, papain from papaya, and ficin from figs.

Many species of flowering plants, shrubs, and trees induce primary skin irritation, but most irritant species belong to the spurge family (Euphorbiaceae). Spurge is a huge and diverse family of over 7000 species, for practical purposes classified into five subfamilies and about 50 tribes,[132] only three of which produce significant irritation in humans (Acalyphoteae, Crotonoideae, and Euphorbioideae) (Figure 47-1). Euphorbiaceae flourish primarily in tropical and subtropical climates. In rainforests, they may grow as tall trees, but usually they are found in arid areas as small trees and shrubs.[134] In North America the varieties are limited and populate mainly southern Florida and the southwestern United States; varieties grow in Europe, where they are commonly called wolfsmilk. Honey made from these plants causes burning mouth irritation accentuated by drinking water. Table 47-1 lists the more commonly recognized irritant plants of the spurge family. One of the most poisonous is the manchineel tree *(Hippomane mancinella),* or beach apple, which inhabits the Caribbean and at one time was the scourge of south Florida.[81] Every part of the plant, including the fruit, contains a milky latex that is extremely irritating and causes burning, swelling, blisters, and even blindness when rubbed into the eyes. The most irritating ingredients are diterpene esters similar to phorbol esters.[1]

Other well-known members of the spurge family are of the genus *Croton,* which contains up to 750 species distributed throughout the tropics. Croton oil is an extract of the seed of the croton plant *(Croton tiglium).* Croton oil was exported from the Caribbean and South America to the United States in the last century in large quantities to be used as a purgative and to treat warts, skin growths, and superficial fungal infections. When croton oil was purified, it was found to be a mixture of diterpenes called phorbol esters, which are well-known cocarcinogens[13] and have been used extensively in recent years in cell biology and cell differentiation experiments. Phorbol esters appear to be the irritant chemicals in most members of the genus *Croton.* Most irritating euphorbs secrete a white, milky, or viscous latex composed of a mixture of polycyclic diterpenes or triterpenes and terpenoids, which can polymerize into rubber. These complex irritant terpenes may be cocarcinogens.[58] Many are related to the phorbol esters. Poinsettia, a member of the genus *Euphorbia,* is considered by some to have relatively low irritant potential, whereas others have reported up to 10% irritant responses.[111,132]

Stinging hairs are found in many species of plants and produce injury by different mechanisms. The clinical presentation is usually an explosive onset of painful urticaria, limited or extensive, that in some geographic regions can result in tissue necrosis. In the United States the genus *Tragia* of the spurge family is a prominent offender; more than 100 species are found, mainly in southern states. The stinging mechanism is

TABLE 47-1. Some Common Irritant Plants in the Spurge Family (Euphorbiaceae)

SUBFAMILY	TRIBE/GENUS	COMMON NAMES	MECHANISMS OR IRRITANT CHEMICAL
Crotonoideae	*Croton*	Croton bush	Phorbol esters (croton oil)
	Jatropha	Coral plant	Thioglycoside (mustard oil)
	Cnidoscolus	Spurge nettle, tread softly	Stinging hairs
Euphorbioideae	*Hippomane*	Manchineel, beach apple	Diterpenes and alkaloid
	Sapium	Aurou-wood	Terpenes
	Hura	Sandbox tree	Ricinlike toxalbumin and triterpenes
	Euphorbia	Beach spurge, red spurge, milkweed, wolfsmilk, asthma plant, candelabra cactus, caper spurge, snow-on- the-mountain, crown-of-thorns	Diterpenes and triterpenes; terpenoids
	Poinsettia	Poinsettia	Phorbol esters
	Pedilanthus	Slipper bush	Terpenes?
Acalyphoideae	*Tragia*	Nose-burn	Stinging hairs

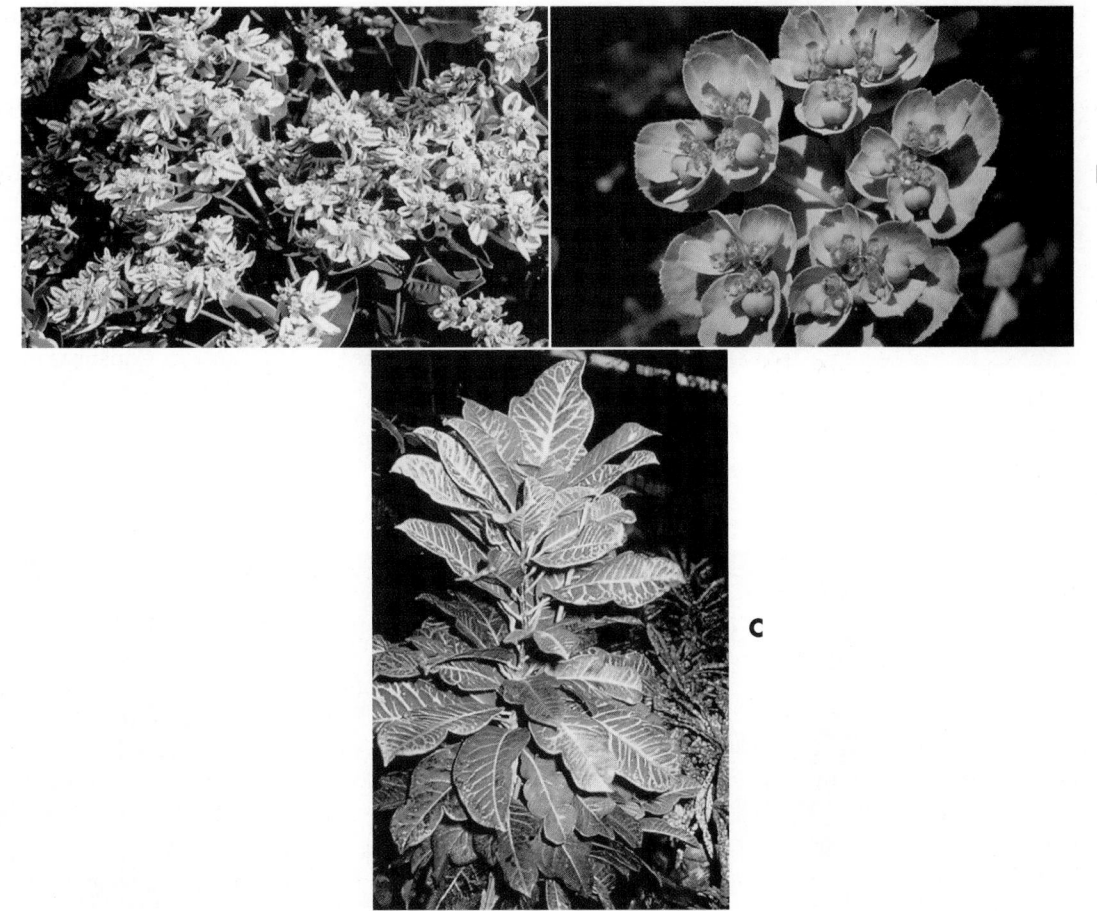

Figure 47-1 Plants that cause primary skin irritation. **A,** Snow-on-the-mountain. **B,** Wolfsmilk. **C,** Croton bush. (**C** *Courtesy Yves Sell, Institute of Botany, Louis Pasteur University, Strasbourg, France.*)

complex and involves insertion into the skin of a long crystal that releases caustic chemicals. The exact nature of the injected material remains unclear,[128] but it is considered to be a mixture of amines, possibly including histamine. Other plants with stinging hairs in the spurge family are found throughout the tropics in the genera *Cnidoscolus* and *Jatropha.* Their mechanism of stinging is similar to that of the stinging nettles, which are seen commonly in Europe and throughout North America. Plants of the genus *Urtica* produce injury when the tip of the nettle breaks off in the skin and syringelike action forces chemicals into the dermis. There is evidence that histamine and similar amines are responsible for this contact urticaria.[89,127]

Another family of irritant plants, Brassicaceae, contains the mustard seed plant radishes (Figure 47-2).

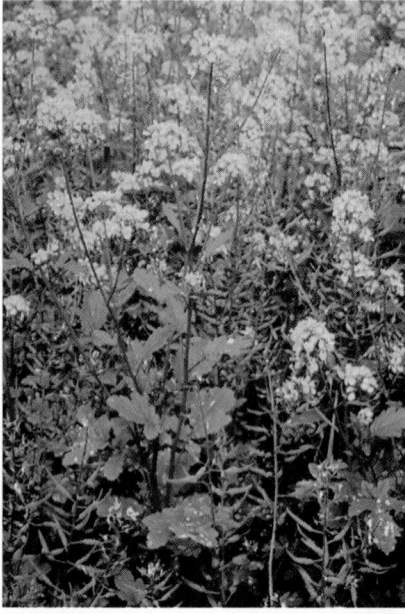

Figure 47-2 White mustard plant, an irritant of the Brassicaceae family. *(Courtesy Yves Sell, Institute of Botany, Louis Pasteur University, Strasbourg, France.)*

Contact with these odoriferous plants tends to cause blisters rather than hives. A third family of irritant plants is the buttercups (Ranunculaceae) (Figure 47-3). Table 47-2 lists common plants in this family. The irritant chemical appears to be a glycoside, ranunculin, protoanemonin, or a dimer, anemonin.[5] Many other families contain a few species of irritant plants (such as cereal grasses and dogwood leaves), which produce mechanical irritation.

The pathogenesis of primary irritation from plants has not been fully elucidated. In the case of nonimmunologic urticaria, release of histamine from mast cells with vasodilation and leakage of fluid appears to be an early direct chemical change leading to hives.[21,115] The molecular events in mast cell degranulation are thought to be similar to those described for immunogenic urticaria, with certain discrete differences. Thus there is no evidence for a selective membrane receptor, such as the high-affinity immunoglobulin E (IgE) receptor that is now well characterized and required for immunologic degranulation of mast cells.[115,122] Instead, current information suggests that a receptor-independent mode of action occurs for all nonimmunologic histamine liberators, acting directly on a pertussis toxin–sensitive G protein to initiate a signal through phospholipase C activation, which degranulates mast

TABLE 47-2. Some Irritant Plants in the Family Ranunculaceae (1900 species)

BOTANICAL NAME	COMMON NAME
Aconitum napellus	Wolfsbane
Anemone nemorosa	Windflower
Clementis vitalba	Traveler's joy
Delphinium (250 species)	Staves-acre
Helleborus niger	Christmas rose
Pulsatilla vulgaris	Pasque flower
Ranunculus (400 species)	Buttercup
Thalictrum foliosum	Meadow rue

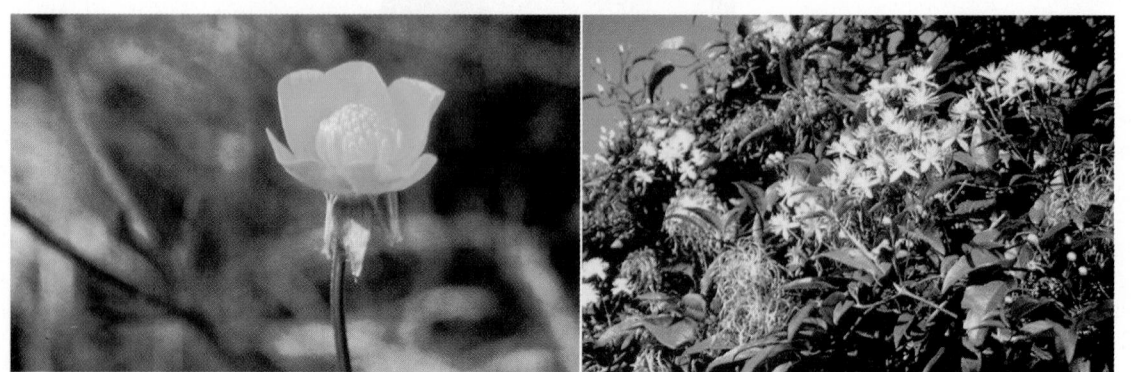

Figure 47-3 Plants of the family Ranunculaceae. **A,** Buttercup. **B,** Old Man's Beard. (**B** *Courtesy Yves Sell, Institute of Botany, Louis Pasteur University, Strasbourg, France.*)

cells of their histamine content.[82] Furthermore, there does not seem to be a requirement for methylation of the membrane phospholipids. Rather, a high intracellular calcium accumulation must occur, and the reaction is rapidly terminated without delayed mediator release.[107] Arachidonic acid metabolites are not formed in any amount.[6]

It is currently believed that both irritation and contact sensitization are mediated by epidermal derived cytokines. Thus tumor necrosis factor-α (TNF-α), interferon-γ (IFN-γ), macrophage inflammatory protein-2 (MIP-2), and granulocyte-macrophage colony-stimulating factor (GM-CSF) are produced and secreted into the tissue in response to both allergens and irritants. However, a number of other proteins are released only by allergenic stimulation. This is a continuing area of investigation.[105,136]

Treatment

Treatment of primary irritant dermatoses is often unsatisfactory. The victim must be removed from exposure to irritant chemicals and treated conservatively with rest, medicated soaks, and compresses, such as aluminum acetate solution (1:20), dilute potassium permanganate solution (1:16,000 in water), acetic acid solution (1:100), or Dalibour solution (copper and zinc sulfate and camphor, supplied commercially as Dalidane). Antihistamines usually have minimal effect. The dermatitis heals in less than 5 days if no complications develop and if tissue damage is minimal. Corticosteroids are of no use in controlling primary irritation.

ALLERGY

As with conventional contact dermatitis, irritant reactions far outnumber allergic responses elicited by vegetation. However, distinguishing irritation from allergy is important clinically because treatment varies considerably according to diagnosis. Allergic responses are more likely to evoke a reaction severe enough that the victim seeks help. Plants cause all varieties of allergic reactions. Immediate hypersensitivity reactions with angioedema, urticaria, and anaphylaxis from ingestion of foods, especially nuts, are well recognized.[10,77,109] (See Chapter 36 for management of anaphylaxis.)

Contact urticaria, or hives from exposure to plants, is fairly common and increasingly recognized as a major cause of immunogenic contact urticaria.[63] The victim has redness, itching, and swelling, which can develop as discrete wheals or widespread edema 1 to 2 hours after exposure. Usually, the eruption is linear or grouped at sites of contact, but extreme swelling and edema of an extremity can develop, depending on level of antigen exposure and the victim's degree of sensitivity, not unlike the range of responses in bee venom

hypersensitivity. Thus an oral reaction may be minimal with simple burning and tingling, especially in the mouth, or massive, with edema of the lips, oral mucous membranes, and pharynx noted after eating fruit and vegetables. Because of chronic low-grade exposure, the eruption is a prominent occupational problem of field workers, packers, grocery workers, cooks, and bakers who handle raw fruits and vegetables.[69] Long lists of offending agents have been published.[43,63] Box 47-1 is a partial list of plants and plant products that cause immunogenic contact dermatitis.

The pathogenesis of immunogenic contact urticaria is a variation of immediate type I hypersensitivity. The central cytologic reactor in skin is the mast cell, which has high-affinity IgE receptors in its membrane. An IgE molecule binds to the receptor by its Fc portion, exposing the Fab segments as recognition sites. When a divalent protein antigen appropriately bridges two IgE molecules, a series of biochemical events transpires that leads to mast cell degranulation. The plasma membrane is perturbed. Several lipids are phosphorylated and G proteins are activated, which in turn activate phospholipase C to hydrolyze phosphatidylinositol 4,5-bisphosphate (PIP_2) and yield two messengers: diacylglycerol (DG) and inositol triphosphate ($InsP_3$).[12] $InsP_3$ binds to its receptor on the endoplasmic reticulum, forming a calcium channel to release free calcium ions (Ca^{2+}) into the cytosol.[3,8,51,88] Simultaneously, DG activates protein kinase C in the plasma membrane, opening calcium channels and allowing entrance of extracellular Ca^{2+}, which further loads the cytosol with free Ca^{2+}, an important "messenger" in the stimulus secretion process.[67] G proteins interact with and release the nucleotide complexed to protein α-chains,[124] some of which probably inhibit or stimu-

Box 47-1 SOME PLANTS AND PLANT PRODUCTS CAUSING IMMUNOGENIC URTICARIA	
FRUITS	**SPICES**
Apple	Cinnamon
Carrot	Garlic
Celery	Mustard
Parsley	Rapeseed
Parsnip	
Potato	**PLANTS**
Tomato	Tulips
VEGETABLES	**TREES**
Chives	Birch pollen
Grains	Teak
Lettuce	Western red cedar
Onion	Various nuts

late cyclic adenosine phosphate and its actions as a second messenger.[12]

The result of the extensive alteration in intracellular milieu is activation of a serine proteinase and exocytosis of mast cell granule contents.[21,115] These come in three forms: preformed and rapidly released; preformed, bound to the granule matrix of heparin, and slowly released; and newly formed mediators. In addition, mast cells produce a variety of cytokines, including interleukins (ILs) IL-1, IL-3, IL-4, IL-5, and IL-6; granulocyte-macrophage colony-forming units; and TNF-α.[123] These cytokines interact with cells and structures, such as endothelium in the skin, to amplify the various inflammatory responses.[21,115,123] In acute urticaria, the rapidly released preformed mediators account for most of the signs and symptoms. These mediators include histamine, some chemotactic factors, and arylsulfatase. If the lesions persist or extend, other mediators, such as newly formed leukotrienes, heparin (or heparin fragments), cytokines, and a number of proteases, may be involved in the continuing tissue damage.

The sequence of inflammatory events leading to acute urticaria is most likely to occur in persons with an atopic background, especially those with pollen allergies.[63] This is the same group of people, mainly women and especially health care workers, who have been found in recent years to be exquisitely sensitive to latex rubber gloves[14,65,119,129] and sensitive to proteins in the natural latex from rubber trees in Asia.[83]

In the last decade, this has become an escalating problem. It now appears that there are more than 200 polypeptides produced in natural latex rubber. Many of these are contact sensitizers, so that a single antigen is not likely to be identified for a given patient. The major problem is IgE-mediated immediate type hypersensitivity and the potential for anaphylaxis. In addition to these polypeptides appearing in natural rubber latex, many are also found in a large number of plants, particularly those consumed as food. These allergens are constantly being purified and characterized. One suggestion is that these cross-reacting allergens are "defense proteins" with a role to protect the plant from attack by pathogens.[64] Whether this is true requires further investigation, but it is also possible that by plant engineering, these allergens may be genetically restricted from the foods we consume.

In addition to fruit and nuts, mustard in pizza has been implicated in anaphylaxis.[93] In less severe cases, vesicular, eczematous rashes have been noted within hours of eating mustard or rapeseed, which is used widely in production of vegetable oils and margarine.[75] Erythema multiforme–like eruptions are well recognized after contact with bracelets and ornamental necklaces made of exotic woods, such as *Dalbergia nigra*.[37] Erythema multiforme has also been seen after exposure to more common plants, such as poison ivy, primula,

and mugwort.[37] It is theorized that multiforme lesions result from vasculitis caused by deposition of immune complexes in or around the blood vessels.

Diagnosis of immunogenic contact urticaria can be confirmed by simple tests. As a use test, application of the suspected plant product to the antecubital fossa twice a day for several days may reproduce the wheal response. Open and closed patch tests, with examination of test sites in 2 to 6 hours, can be useful, as can more conventional prick, scratch, or scratch-chamber tests, in which the results are read in 15 to 20 minutes.[63] It is most important to determine whether urtication is immunologic or nonimmunologic in nature.[43,63] For complete evaluation an allergist obtains radioallergosorbent tests to quantify specific IgE in the patient's serum. More refined serologic tests include crossed radioimmunoelectrophoresis (CRIE) and CRIE inhibition.[15]

Patients with contact urticaria visit the emergency department when an eruption is extensive or extreme, or if it is associated with stridor, wheezing, and collapse. Since mast cell degranulation is the central problem, and because epinephrine stimulates cyclic adenosine monophosphate formation that opposes degranulation, it is logical to use this drug. Other supportive treatments for anaphylactic shock may be required, such as albuterol, aminophylline, oxygen, or intravenous (IV) hydrocortisone. In less severe cases, antihistamines are valuable. Intramuscular (IM) or IV diphenhydramine (Benadryl) in an adult dose of 50 to 100 mg usually stops progression of wheal formation and can be followed by oral hydroxyzine (25 to 50 mg 3 times a day) or cyproheptadine (4 to 8 mg 4 times a day) for 2 to 5 days. Pure H$_1$-blockers, such as fexofenadine (60 mg 2 to 3 times a day), are also effective and do not depress the central nervous system, although the prescriber has to be aware of any unique adverse reactions. It is important to make certain the patient has not inadvertently hidden parts of the plant on the body, in clothing, or in a towel, blanket, or knapsack. Recrudescence of the urticarial response usually can be traced to continuing unknown contact with the offending agent.

Delayed-Contact Dermatitis

Delayed hypersensitivity or type IV allergy of the contact hypersensitivity variety occurs more frequently as a result of contact with plants than does type I contact urticaria. Sensitivity to poison ivy or poison oak is undoubtedly the single most common cause of allergic skin reactions in the United States and, along with contact allergy to sesquiterpene lactones ("compositae"), probably worldwide (Figure 47-4). When a distraught young person arrives in the emergency department with an acute, edematous, and erythematous skin eruption and a history of outdoor activity, this is probably a serious bout of poison ivy or poison

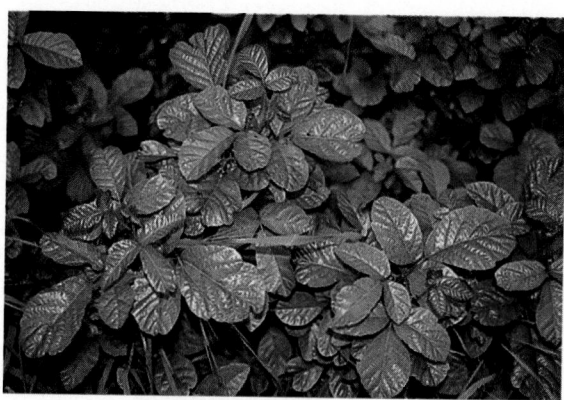

Figure 47-4 Poison oak. *(Courtesy Paul Auerbach.)*

oak dermatitis. Approximately 50% of the U.S. adult population is clinically sensitive to poison ivy, poison oak, and poison sumac. If a sensitive individual brushes against the plant or comes in contact with the heavy, nonvolatile oil in the resin canals that contains the active allergenic principle urushiol, he or she will acquire poison ivy or poison oak dermatitis. In its natural state the oil is colorless or slightly yellow. Because the oil is virtually invisible, many people fail to understand how they acquired the rash. It is not a vapor because at 315.6° C (600° F) in a fire or oven, urushiol splatters like butter. In a camp or forest fire, it attaches to smoke particles and can be carried downwind. The oil also readily coats the fur of animals, which explains why persons often get the dermatitis from their outdoor pets. On exposure to air, however, the oil oxidizes, polymerizes, and turns black. This is a way to recognize the weeds, especially in autumn when the leaves fall off.

The amount of urushiol present in poison ivy and poison oak is roughly equal year-round, even when the plants are only sticks without leaves in the winter. As the leaves turn red and start to dry up in the fall, important nutrients, including urushiol, return to the stem and roots through the subepidermal resin canals.[42] Thus the dead leaves that fall to the ground are virtually devoid of urushiol. The amount of purified urushiol required to elicit a reaction is 2 to 2.5 mg.[35] Some people (about 35%) are considered subclinically sensitive because they have negative skin test reactions to 2.5 mg urushiol but react to higher concentrations, such as 5, 10, and 50 mg.[25,35] Clinically this group is interesting because they invariably did not have poison ivy dermatitis as teenagers and often plucked the weeds with apparent impunity. However, usually in midlife after a bout of weed pulling, a rash spreads explosively. For unknown reasons, they have crossed the line into clinical sensitivity. If patch tested with dilutions of urushiol, they are often exquisitely sensitive and do not appear to lose their reactivity. The flare-up may last for

several weeks, probably because of prior contamination of the home and workplace with urushiol oil. Treatment must be aggressive and more prolonged than usual.

A smaller group (10% to 15%) does not react to the higher concentrations and cannot be sensitized by 1000 mg. This group was first detected and studied in passive transfer experiments in the 1950s.[33] These individuals are considered to be naturally tolerant, but it remains unclear whether they achieved that state by early antigenic exposure or by genetic luck. They have no inherent resistance to contact sensitization with other chemicals[34] and otherwise appear healthy. They may hold a clue to the molecular basis for immunologic tolerance.

The weeds are surprisingly fastidious. They do not grow in Alaska or Hawaii and do not survive well above 1220 m (4000 feet), in deserts, or in rainforests. They grow best along cool streams and lakes and luxuriate if it is also sunny and hot. In the California hills they grow like a forest, but in cooler, dry climates they remain isolated in small patches. Nevertheless, they are found in every state of the continental United States. The plants have different configurations in different regions, but generally, poison ivy grows east of the Rockies, poison oak grows west of the Rockies, and poison sumac grows best in the southeastern United States. Since avoidance is the best prevention, it is important to learn what the plant looks like in a given area (Figure 47-5). Once contaminated with the oil, an average person has 1 to 4 hours to wash it off to prevent dermatitis.

From a practical standpoint, only 10% to 15% of Americans (up to 40 million persons) can be categorized as exquisitely sensitive. Generally, these persons seek and need emergency medical care. They typically have had prior unpleasant experiences. Within 2 to 6 hours after exposure, swelling is accompanied by an erythematous, intensely pruritic, edematous, vesicular, and ultimately bullous eruption that can be associated with fever, malaise, and prostration. This true dermatologic emergency should be treated immediately and vigorously.

Extreme susceptibility tends to be familial; if one parent is supersensitive, children are likely to be as well. If both parents are sensitive, the chance of sensitive offspring is about 80%.[131] The level of individual sensitivity is not determined by the severity of the initial bout of dermatitis. Although almost half of patients admit to a memorable bout of dermatitis as a teenager, no more than 25% to 35% of victims at age 30 to 40 were stricken within the previous year.[25] If these subjects are patch tested with weak dilutions of urushiol, less than half react as might be expected from their histories. An individual's level of reactivity does not change appreciably if he or she is tested monthly over a year[35]; testing at less frequent intervals in very sensitive subjects

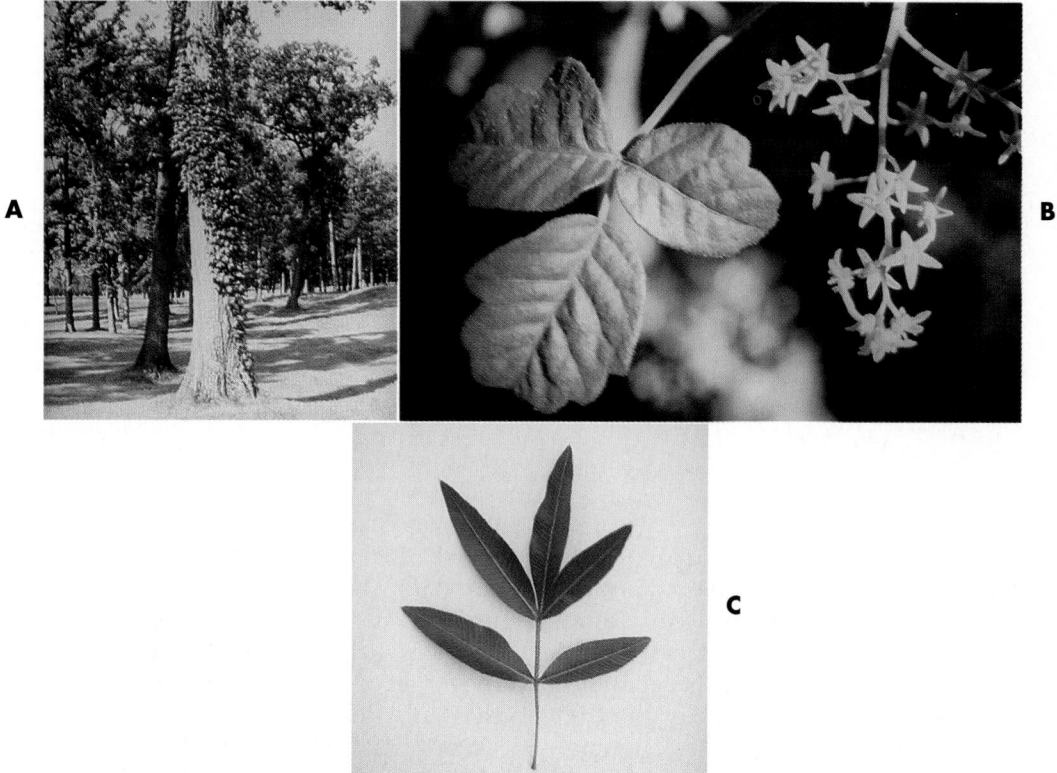

Figure 47-5 **A,** Poison ivy *(Toxicodendron radicans).* **B,** Poison oak *(Toxicodendron diversiloba).*
C, Poison sumac *(Toxicodendron vernix).*

over 3 to 4 years has shown little or no change in the level of reactivity. Repeated mild to moderate bouts of dermatitis maintain the sensitive state, whereas a single severe bout may produce a prolonged period of anergy or refractoriness,[24,25] not unlike the clinical condition of "hardening" or unresponsiveness, well described in the industrial setting.[114]

The urushiols in poison ivy, poison oak, and poison sumac differ only slightly in structure and biologically cross-react, so that a person sensitive to poison ivy may also react to poison oak and poison sumac (Figure 47-6). Plants, shrubs, and trees with cross-reacting catechols are found throughout the world, arising either indigenously or by transplantation.[27,102] The most common cross-reacting plants are mango, cashew nut shell, India marking nut, and Japanese lacquer. Increasing numbers of cross-reacting plants are reported from South America.[53] A chemical curiosity is the cross-reaction with resorcinols from cashew nut shell oil.[57] Similar cross-reacting resorcinol-containing plants have been observed in Australia[76] and Hawaii.[61] Recently, it has been confirmed that philodendron plants contain a contact sensitizing resorcinol, but it only reacts in poison oak– or poison ivy–sensitized patients who have traveled to the mainland.[62] Other studies have extended our information about the urushiol-like molecules that exists in many shrubs and small trees in South America, specifically Litre and Lithrea in Peru and Uruguay, respectively.[2,70]

IMMUNOLOGY OF POISON IVY/POISON OAK DERMATITIS

The immunologic mechanism for allergic contact dermatitis is generally conceded to be type IV cell-mediated delayed hypersensitivity.[27a] However, in skin, keratinocytes are also part of the immune surveillance system. They respond quickly to every chemical insult, either irritant or allergenic, in antigen-dependent fashion, to produce a variety of cytokines. These function mainly to amplify future inflammatory responses.[2b,87a] Early on, they secrete TNF-α and intercellular adhesion molecule.[1] Somewhat later, they release IL-1, IL-6, IL-8, and IL-10, and still later, macrophage chemotactic factor and other cytokines.[2a,43a,43b,87a,99a] These may in turn release acute-phase reactants from mast cells and endothelial cells, as seen in irritant responses.[2b,87a] Current research is attempting to identify which keratinocyte cytokines specify the allergic reaction, as distinct from simply injury. Nevertheless, it is known that the catechol molecules of poison oak and poison ivy enter the skin and bind through nucleophilic attack at benzene ring positions 4, 5, or 6 to surface proteins on antigen-presenting cells (APCs), which are primarily Langer-

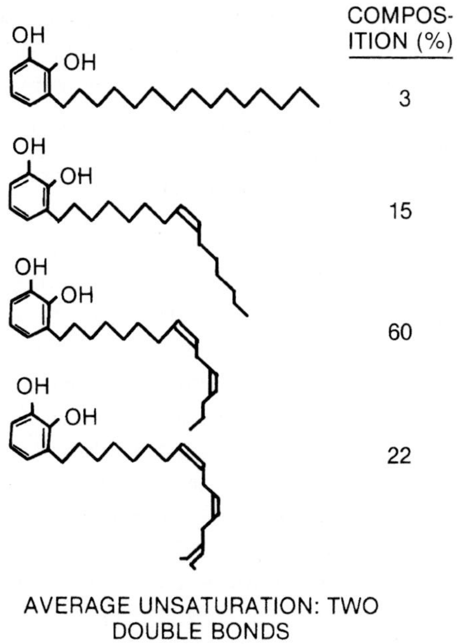

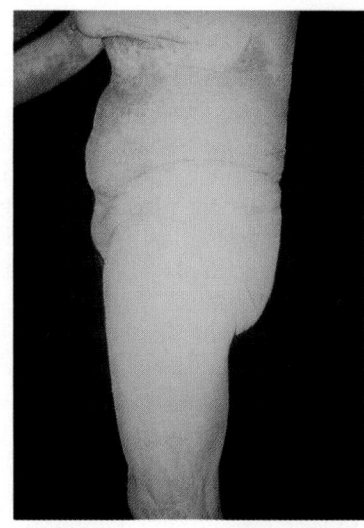

OH OH
3

OH OH
15

OH OH
60

OH OH
22

AVERAGE UNSATURATION: TWO
DOUBLE BONDS

Figure 47-6 General structure and composition of poison ivy urushiol.

Figure 47-7 Generalized poison ivy dermatitis.

hans' cells in the epidermis. The molecules are then internalized and processed in the APCs, which leave the epidermis and travel to regional lymph nodes, where they present their processed antigen on the cell surface in context with a major histocompatibility complex (MHC) class I molecule to the T cell receptor complex on a CD8 T cell. To complete the sensitization signal, another surface protein (the B7 antigen) forms a costimulary signal by binding to the CD28 ligand on the T cell. This then activates the T cell, which divides repeatedly to form a clone of urushiol-specific CD8 cells. These subsequently expand into clones of circulating activated T-effector and T-memory lymphocytes.[54a,70]

Upon a new challenge by urushiol, the CD8 lymphocytes elicit a cell-mediated cytotoxic immune response characterized by erythema, edema, and vesiculation resulting from destruction of epidermal cells and activation of the dermal vasculature. Under this scenario, the clinical reaction is driven by the CD8 cytotoxic, effector T cells, and this can be modified by CD4 T cells that may be either Th-1 or, more likely, Th-2 in nature.[54a,70] In an individual patient, this determines the severity of dermatitis after exposure to the poisonous weeds. This logical formulation, however, does not completely explain acute poison oak or poison ivy dermatitis. An acute eruption tends to begin within hours of exposure and is primarily edematous. Some have emphasized the presence of basophils in acute poison oak and poison ivy lesions and have proposed a role for basophil mediators in the pathogenesis of an early-onset acute reaction.[22] Certainly, the clinical presentation in these cases favors a late-phase reaction[65] and a mechanism possibly involving mast cell degranulation,[58a] as well as other cytokine mediators. Also possible is a CD4 T cell mediated induction of IgE reactivity.[55]

Treatment

Systemic corticosteroids are widely accepted as the first line of treatment, especially given early and in large, therapeutic doses. If the reaction is of less than 2 hours' duration, IV hydrocortisone or methylprednisolone can be curative. After a patient has suffered 4 to 6 hours with massive edema, erythema, and pruritus, IV therapy is highly effective, but it must be followed by more prolonged oral or IM administration of corticosteroids (Figure 47-7). Most patients in this category seek help after 8 to 16 hours of discomfort, at which point IV therapy is less effective. IM methylprednisolone sodium succinate (Solu-Medrol), 40 mg, combined with betamethasone sodium phosphate (Celestone), 8 to 12 mg, should give relief for 7 to 14 days. Adrenocorticotropic hormone (ACTH) gel, 80 units IM with a repeat in 8 to 12 hours, often is curative. Prednisone, 100 to 120 mg divided in four equal doses daily for 2 days, may achieve the same salubrious effect. At the same time, patients are instructed to rest at home for 3 to 4 days. If a flare-up starts, another dose of ACTH gel or a repeat regimen of prednisone is prescribed. Subsequent exacerbations are usually caused by reexposure to urushiol that has contaminated the patient's local environment, so that the patient must be warned to thoroughly wash all clothing and other articles that might have been exposed during the initial contact.

If the dermatitis has been present for more than 24 hours, the aggressive regimen is less successful (Figure 47-8). Under these circumstances, many physicians prefer a more conservative approach. Oral prednisone, 80 to 100 mg/day for 3 to 4 days with a 10- to 14-day every-other-day taper, helps many patients, but the danger lies in a sudden flare-up at the end of therapy, which becomes poorly responsive to steroids. Whenever considering systemic corticosteroids for acute allergic contact dermatitis, the physician must be certain that the patient is otherwise healthy and without active infections, vascular accidents, endocrinopathies, or a familial history of glaucoma.

When the onset of dermatitis is delayed for several days and the eruption is mild or moderate, systemic therapy offers little benefit. In this situation of a mildly to moderately sensitive patient with delayed onset, there is very little the physician can do to alleviate the signs or symptoms. Most of these patients go to the drug store and look for over-the-counter (OTC) preparations. Usually they are disappointed. It takes 7 to 10 days to heal spontaneously; their most helpful option is an inexpensive agent, such as calamine lotion, that is comforting and helps form a crust. Plain water is helpful, as are soaks with bicarbonate of soda or vinegar in water. Regardless of the option chosen, time is required for healing. Antihistamines, aspirin, or nonsteroidal an-

tiinflammatory drugs are without effect. Results of systemic corticosteroids, even in large doses, are disappointing. Topical application of soothing aluminum acetate (1:20) soaks, calamine lotion, or tepid baths, with 1 cup Aveeno oatmeal or 2 cups linnet starch per tub, relieves pruritus and allows healing to occur uneventfully. Although field workers have mentioned that aloe vera latex empirically improves wound healing, a major study in contact dermatitis showed that it was ineffective.[137] Topical lotions with anesthetics or antihistamines offer no additional benefit and may induce contact sensitization to the chemical additives. Allergic contact dermatitis is a self-healing disease that resolves over 10 to 14 days if iatrogenic influences are avoided. Secondary superficial infections may occur in children or during hospitalization. Cleanliness usually prevents this complication.

In the mildly to moderately sensitive person when the eruption is beginning (red and itchy but not yet blistered), potent, fluorinated steroids in a gel or optimized vehicle can prevent spread of the rash and speed healing. Many such preparations are available, such as fluocinonide 0.05% gel (Lidex) or clobetasol propionate gel 0.05% (Temovate). Since topical steroids are readily absorbed and can cause adrenal suppression, they should be restricted to limited amounts (less than 15 g) for a brief period (2 to 3 days). Generally, the opportu-

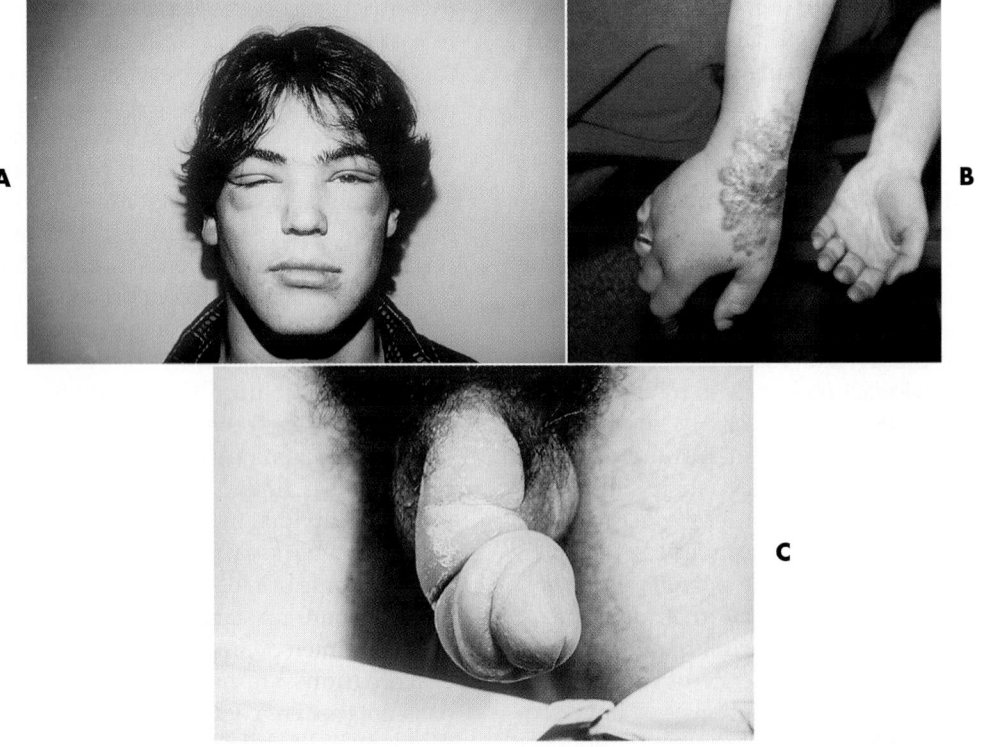

Figure 47-8 Acute poison oak dermatitis. **A,** Facial edema. **B,** Blisters. **C,** Penile edema. *(Courtesy Axel Hoke.)*

nity to use this approach does not occur in an emergency department, but it can be very effective in helping persons repeatedly exposed to poison ivy or poison oak in the course of their work.

As the dermatitis heals and scales after 10 to 14 days, the patient may note a resurgence of pruritus, which, untreated, can lead to a patch of subchronic lichenoid neurodermatitis (Figure 47-9). Judicious use of almost any steroid cream or ointment, such as triamcinolone acetonide 0.025%, desonide 0.025%, or hydrocortisone 1%, alleviates the symptoms.

The best approaches to prophylaxis come from an intimate understanding of the chemistry of urushiol and the biology of the weeds[27] and resides mainly in recognition and avoidance. Where this is not possible, protective clothing that is either disposable or washable should be worn. Water rapidly inactivates urushiol, and organic solvents such as alcohol, gasoline, and acetone can extract it from contaminated surfaces. A commercially available solvent is Tecnu, sold OTC, but it is an inexpensive solvent sold at a high price. It should not be used for therapy. The best choice is rubbing (isopropyl) alcohol, which should be applied liberally for decontamination and followed by liberal use of water wash-off to avoid spreading the oil on the skin. Use of soap is a poor excuse for better solvents. The idea of using barrier preparations has become popular again, even though in the past such creams and ointments proved disappointing.[91] The current favorite, an organoclay called Ivy-Block, was developed to protect forestry workers against these weeds during national firefighting escapades.[30] This approach was confirmed in a multicenter study.[71] The lotion can be obtained readily from a pharmacist or by major marketers. Stokogard outdoor cream, composed of a linoleic ester dimer,[92] was removed from the market for lack of U.S. Food and Drug Administration (FDA) approval but is still available in industrial supply houses that are not regulated. It also works, but when the cream is first applied, it has a foul smell, like dead fish, resulting from the release of the ester. This disappears in about 20 minutes and acts like butter to delay penetration of urushiol oil. Thus it must be washed off in 4 to 6 hours for protection.

Compositae Dermatitis

Although poison oak and poison ivy are the most common causes of allergic contact dermatitis in the United States, supremacy for this distinction worldwide is challenged by the enormous plant family Compositae. This family contains more than 20,000 species in 1000 genera and consists of many commonly recognized plants, vegetables, wildflowers, weeds, and commercially useful plants (Figure 47-10).[113] A number of these plants and species are listed in Box 47-2. Fortunately, casual exposure is usually insufficient to induce contact sensitization, or the quality of outdoor life would be greatly compromised. Most Compositae dermatitis is reported as an occupational hazard by florists, horticulturists, forestry workers, food handlers, and similar workers. However, it occasionally affects home gardeners and recreational nature enthusiasts. In India the weed *Parthenium hysterophorus* (Congress grass, feverfew), which was incidentally imported from the U.S. with loads of grain, subsequently created an epidemic of Compositae dermatitis.[69]

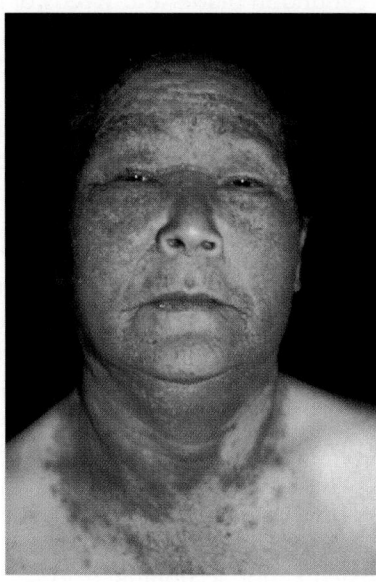

Figure 47-9 Resurgence of pruritus leading to patch of subchronic lichenoid neurodermatitis.

Box 47-2 SOME COMPOSITAE THAT CAUSE ALLERGIC CONTACT DERMATITIS

VEGETABLES
Artichoke
Chicory
Endive
Lettuce
Yarrow

WEEDS
Burweed
Cocklebur
Dog fennel
Goldenrod
Mugwort
Sneezeweed
Stinking mayweed

PERFUMERY
Costus

FLOWERS
Black-eyed Susan
Cardoon
Chamomile
Chrysanthemum
Dahlia
Daisy
Dandelion
Elecampane
Gaillardia
Mountain tobacco
Sunflower
Tansy

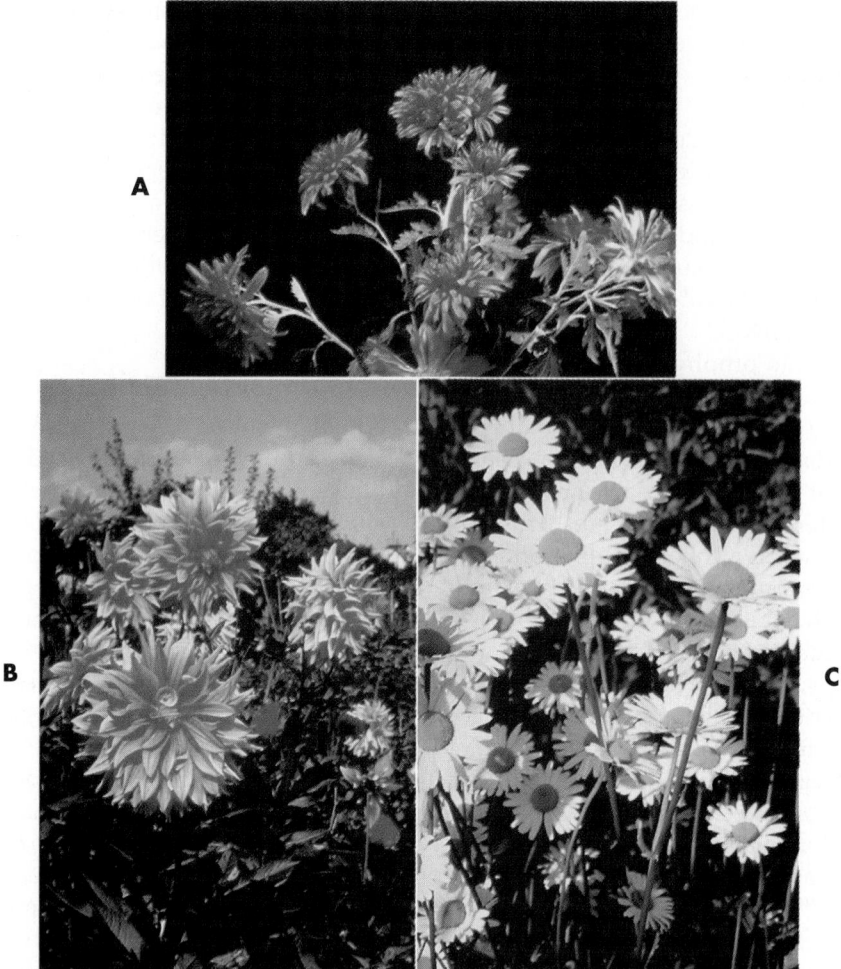

Figure 47-10 Compositae contact sensitizer. **A,** Chrysanthemum. **B,** Dahlia. **C,** Daisy. (**C** *Courtesy Yves Sell, Institute of Botany, Louis Pasteur University, Strasbourg, France.*)

The eruption generally spares children and affects predominantly young and middle-aged men. The dermatitis involves the face, neck, arms, and exposed areas in airborne or photocontact patterns, so that both allergic dermatitis and photoallergic contact dermatitis have been suggested.[50,99] When the eruption presents as acute airborne dermatitis, the victim is often severely affected and likely to seek emergency care. The dermatitis can become subacute or chronic, as has been attributed to ragweed in the Midwest and to a variety of plants in Europe.[19]

The underlying theme that links the Compositae species is the contact-sensitizing sesquiterpene lactones. More than 3000 of these 15-carbon ringed structures of complex organization with extensive ligand substitutions have been extracted from plant products. They have many important biologic properties, such as their use in antitumor, cytotoxic, anti-inflammatory, antimicrobial, and antiparasitic drugs. Only some of the structures are contact sensitizers. One problem with use of the term "Compositae dermatitis" is that cross-reacting allergens are found in plants and weeds of other plant families. Species of the Magnoliaceae, Lauraceae, and Liliaceae families have been implicated. Liliaceae is a very large family containing diverse, useful, and ornamental plants, such as aloe, asparagus, colchicum, hyacinth, and tulip. Certain species can be both irritating and sensitizing. "Hyacinth itch" is a primary irritant dermatitis probably caused by calcium oxalate crystals in the bulb scales, which may also contain an unknown sensitizer. "Tulip fingers" can be caused by irritation but usually result from contact sensitization to the sesquiterpene lactones tulipan A or tulipan B. In addition, at least three families of liverworts contain cross-reacting sesquiterpene lactones.[113] Forestry workers sensitized to frullanolide in the liverwort genus *Frullania* show cross-contact reactivity to sesquiterpene lactones in plants of the families Compositae and Asteraceae.[78]

Patterns of cross-reactivity vary extremely, so a simplistic approach is not acceptable.[106] A sesquiterpene lactone mix has proved useful in diagnosing apparent airborne or generalized eczema.[20] In a molecular analy-

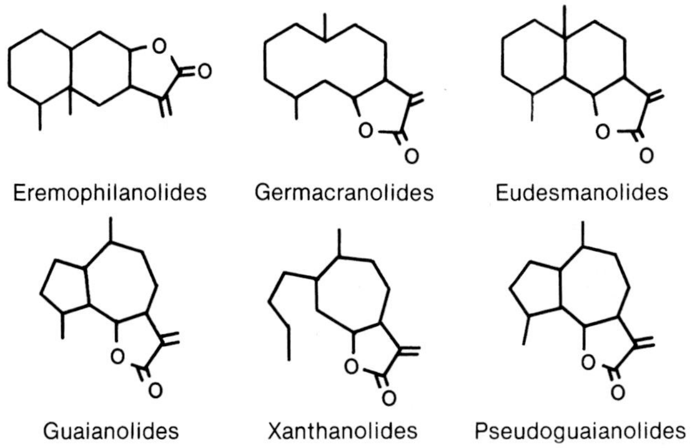

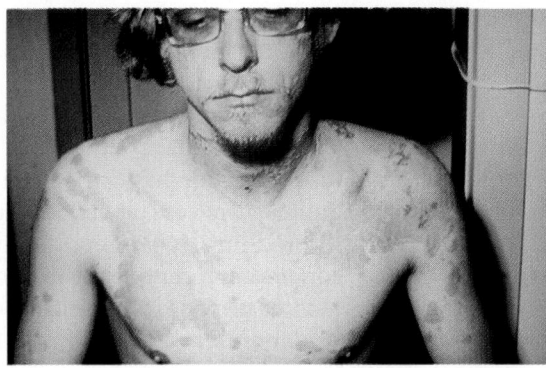

Figure 47-11 The six skeletal backbones of sesquiterpene lactones. Note the methylene configuration on the lactone ring, which is responsible for contact sensitization and contributes to other biologic activities.

Eremophilanolides   Germacranolides   Eudesmanolides

Guaianolides   Xanthanolides   Pseudoguaianolides

TABLE 47-3. Some Trees that Cause Allergic Contact Dermatitis

COMMON NAME	BOTANICAL NAME
African blackwood	*Dalbergia latifolia*
Australian blackwood	*Acacia melanoxylon*
California redwood	*Sequoia sempervirens*
Cocobolo	*Dalbergia retusa*
Mansonia	*Mansonia altissima*
Pao ferro	*Machaerium scleroxylum*
Pine	*Pinus* (about 80 species in North America)
Rosewoods	*Dalbergia* species
Silky oak	*Grevillea robusta*
Spruce	*Picea* species
Teak	*Tectona grandis*
Western red cedar	*Thuja plicata*

Figure 47-12 Wood dermatitis.

sis of the pattern of cross-reactivity in *Costus*-sensitized patients, sesquiterpene lactones with the lesser degree of oxygenated substituents close to the α-methylene–γ-butyrolactone ring gave the highest frequency of cross-reactivity.[4] Furthermore, sesquiterpene lactones belonging to any one of the six skeletal classes (Figure 47-11) contain sensitizers that would not be expected to cross-react with those from a different class; this might explain some of the discrepancies in cross-reactivity patterns described in the literature.[4] The emergency physician familiar with the Compositae family and sesquiterpene lactones may help sort out the correct offending agent in the unusual case of "poison ivy" dermatitis when that diagnosis does not clearly fit. This knowledge is critical in distinguishing between airborne and phototoxic allergic contact dermatitis.[50,99]

Toxic Woods

Toxic woods contain plant chemicals that produce allergic contact dermatitis (Figure 47-12). Most are exotic tropical woods with great commercial value.[47] They are crafted into a wide variety of common objects, such as furniture, musical instruments, boats, cabinets, walking sticks, jewelry, and art forms (Table 47-3).

The main problem with wood dermatitis occurs in an occupational setting with forestry workers, lumbar workers, carpenters, and craftspeople, but it can affect souvenir hunters or art aficionados. Chemical sensitizers in woods[46] are numerous and diverse. Many are quinones and can cause cross-sensitivity with primin found in some species of *Primula* (e.g., *P. obconica*).[5] One of the best known is Brazilian rosewood (*Dalbergia nigra*), which has been nearly depleted by its wide decorative use. The sensitizing chemical is R-4-methoxydalbergione, a complex quinone. Because of the scarcity of rosewood in recent years, it has been replaced by pao ferro wood from South America. Unfortunately, pao ferro contains an even more potent sensitizer and may be the most hazardous timber in commercial use.[47] Australian silky oak (*Grevillea robusta*) is grown as a shade tree but is also used for plywood furniture. Grevillol (5-*N*-tridecylresorcinol) is the sensitizer and may cross-react with urushiol.[76] Pines contain several terpenes that are used commercially as crude balsams or purified colophony (rosin) and turpentine. All can cause allergic contact dermatitis. California redwood (*Sequoia sempervirens*) can induce allergic alveolitis and contact dermatitis.[74] Along the Pacific coast, western red cedar (*Thuja plicata*) is a well-known cause of "cedar poisoning." It can elicit immediate hypersensitivity with allergic rhinitis, allergic alveolitis,[121] and allergic contact dermatitis.[47] The tree contains at least two quinones that act as contact sensitizers. One of these, β-thujaplicin, is reputed to be responsible for the trees' natural resistance to decay and is used in Japan to manufacture cosmetics.[40]

There are many sensitizing plants whose allergenic chemicals have not yet been identified. Prenyl chain–substituted hydroquinones called phacelioids have been identified in the family Hydrophyllaceae, a woody shrub that grows wild in the Southwest.[103] These plants produce allergic dermatitis in botanists and field workers. The phacelioids structurally resemble urushiol but do not show cross-reactivity. In humans the most potent sensitizer of the phacelioid group is geranyl hydroquinone.[103] The creosote bush, *Larrea,* is responsible for an airborne weed dermatitis rash pattern, but whether the bush is a contact sensitizer or photosensitizer is uncertain.[66] Although more than 100 chemicals have been isolated, the actual sensitizer remains unknown.[66] English ivy, a common ground cover over much of the United States, can induce allergic contact dermatitis, usually in epidemics. Recently, the principal contact-sensitizing chemical has been identified as falcarinol.[41,48]

Treatment

Treatment for plant-induced allergic contact dermatitis is the same as described for poison ivy or poison oak dermatitis. The majority of eruptions from other plant sources would be considered mild to moderate and deserve conservative, not aggressive, therapy.

PHYTOPHOTODERMATITIS

Phytodermatitis is the term used for adverse reactions to plants. *Phytophotodermatitis* denotes adverse reactions to nonionizing rays from the sun induced by plants.[59]

In general, two types of phytophotodermatitis occur. The reaction may be phototoxic or photoallergic.[23] Phototoxic reactions are much more common than photoallergic responses. They occur in anyone if sufficient amounts of offending wavelengths arrive at the skin in the presence of enough of the photosensitizing molecules. The reaction is characterized by erythema with or without edema, followed by hyperpigmentation and desquamation.

Photoallergic reactions are generally uncommon. Like all allergies, they represent an acquired altered reactivity that depends on an antigen-antibody relationship or a cell-mediated delayed hypersensitivity response. Morphologically, they are characterized by an immediate wheal and flare or a delayed papular to eczematous eruption. In general, it requires less energy to induce a photoallergic reaction than a phototoxic response.

Sun-induced plant dermatitis reactions are not rare. They may be induced by internal ingestion or topical applications of plants or plant products. The former is quite rare because of the large amount of plant material that must be eaten to sensitize an individual. However, such events have been reported with the ingestion of relatively large amounts of psoralen contained in vegetables and prolonged exposure to intense UVA radiation (long-wave ultraviolet rays between 320 and 400 nm), as would occur in a suntan salon.[68] Photoreactions to topical applications are common.

The major photoactive chemicals in plants are furocoumarins (psoralens), which are found in plant families such as Umbelliferae (e.g., celery, giant ragweed, parsnip, fennel, dill, wild carrot); Rutaceae (e.g., lime, citron, lemon, bergamot, gas plant, Persian lime); and Leguminosae (e.g., scurf-pea, bavchi) (Table 47-4) (Figure 47-13). Contact with the plant followed by exposure to UVA often leads to a phototoxic response.

The reaction is characterized by erythema with or without edema, followed by dense hyperpigmentation with unusual patterns and distribution. The lesions may be linear, irregular blotches, or confluent. All are confined to areas contacted by the plant and exposed to the sun or artificial irradiators, such as those used in UVA suntan salons (Figure 47-14).

Bullae may occur if the reaction is severe. A linear bullous eruption apparently induced by photosensitizers in "meadow grass" was described six decades ago as "dermatitis bullosa striata pratensis."[90]

Plant-induced photosensitization has caused industrial problems. For example, severe vesiculobullous eruptions involving sun-exposed areas were reported in a large number of field workers harvesting celery in Michigan in 1961.[9] The cause of this response was contact with a psoralen compound elaborated by celery infected by pink rot (*Sclerotinia sclerotinorum*) and exposure to sunlight. Normally, noninfected celery contains some 5-methoxypsoralen (5-MOP). When it is infected with the fungus, the combination produces 8-methoxypsoralen (8-MOP) and trimethylpsoralen.[100,101,104,112] The infected celery also contains higher than normal concentrations of 5-MOP.

More recently, phytophotodermatitis developed in several grocery workers handling produce in a chain of supermarkets in 13 different states.[7] This reaction apparently was induced by contact with a newly developed disease-resistant brand of celery. In at least one location, the eruption was related to handling the produce and subsequent tanning in a UVA suntan salon.[17]

Another example of industrially induced phytophotodermatitis, noted in Florida, resulted from bartenders' squeezing Persian limes (*Citrus aurantifolia*) into cocktails.[110] The rind contains a photosensitizing psoralen compound released by the squeezing.

Other persons at occupational risk are dairy workers (from plants eaten by cows), farmers, gardeners, and cannery workers who pack carrots, parsnips, figs, celery, or limes. Recently, a rare industrially related photoeruption caused by topical contact with celery was reported in a chef.[73] It should be noted that recreational exposures to limes and other plants can also induce phytophotodermatitis.[44,133]

Perfume-induced berloque dermatitis is a special form of phytophotodermatitis. It is characterized most notably by bizarre pigmentation with or without preceding erythema involving areas contacted by the perfume and exposed to the sun.[39] The name "berloque" derives from the frequent pendant configuration of the hyperpigmentation.[108]

Oil of bergamot extracted from the rind of fresh bergamot oranges (Citrus bergamia) is a common ingredient in several commercial perfumes and colognes.

This oil contains a number of furocoumarins.[72] The most potent photosensitizer appears to be bergapten, which is 5-MOP.[86,96,98] Phytophotodermatitis follows contact with offending plants and subsequent exposure to UVA. Oral plant intake rarely induces photosensitization because a very large amount of plant must be ingested to attain high blood and skin levels of the photosensitizing furocoumarins, which are also readily metabolized to nonphotosensitizing molecules.

When photosensitizing furocoumarins are raised to an excited state (usually a triplet state) by exposure to UVA, they form photoaddition products with pyrimidine bases in the cellular deoxyribonucleic acid (DNA).[86,87,96-98] The first reaction appears to be

TABLE 47-4. Common Plants Implicated in Causing Phytophotodermatitis

FAMILY	BOTANICAL NAME	COMMON NAME
Umbelliferae	Anthriscus sylvestris	Cow parsley, wild chervil
	Apium graveolens	Celery
	Heracleum mantegazzianum	
	Heracleum maximum (H. dulce)	Giant hogweed
	Pastinaca sativa (P. urens)	Parsnip (garden variety)
	Heracleum laciniatum	Tromsopalm
	Angelica sylvestris	
	Heracleum spondylium	Cow parsley
	Heracleum giganteum	Parsnip (wild parsnip)
	Foeniculum vulgare	Fennel
	Anethum graveolens	Dill
	Peucedanum oreoselium	
	Daucus carota	Wild carrot, garden carrot
	Peucedanum ostruthium	Masterwort
	Ammi majus	
	Angelica archangelica	Angelica
Rutaceae	Citrus aurantifolia	Lime
	Citrus medica (C. acida)	Citron
	Citrus sinensis	
	Citrus aurantium	Bitter orange
	Citrus limon	Lemon
	Citrus bergamia	Bergamot
	Dictamnus albus (D. fraxinella)	Gas plant, burning bush
	Ruta graveolens	Common rue
	Phebalium argenteum	Persian lime (Tahitian)
Moraceae	Ficus carica	Fig
Compositae	Achillea millefolium	Milfoil, yarrow
	Anthemis cotula	Stinking mayweed
Ranunculaceae	Ranunculus spp.	Buttercup
Cruciferae	Brassica spp.	Mustard
Convolulaceae	Convolvulus arvensis	Rindweed
Rosaceae	Argrimonia eupatoria	Agrimony
Chenopodiaceae	Chenopodium spp.	Goosefoot
Leguminosae	Psoralea corylifolia	Scurf-pea, bavchi
Hypericaceae	Hypericum perforatum	St. John's wort
Anacardiaceae	Hypericum crispum	Red quebracho
	Schinopsis quebracho-colorado (S. lorentzii)	

From Pathak MS, Worden LR, Kaufman KD: J Invest Dermatol 48:103, 1967.

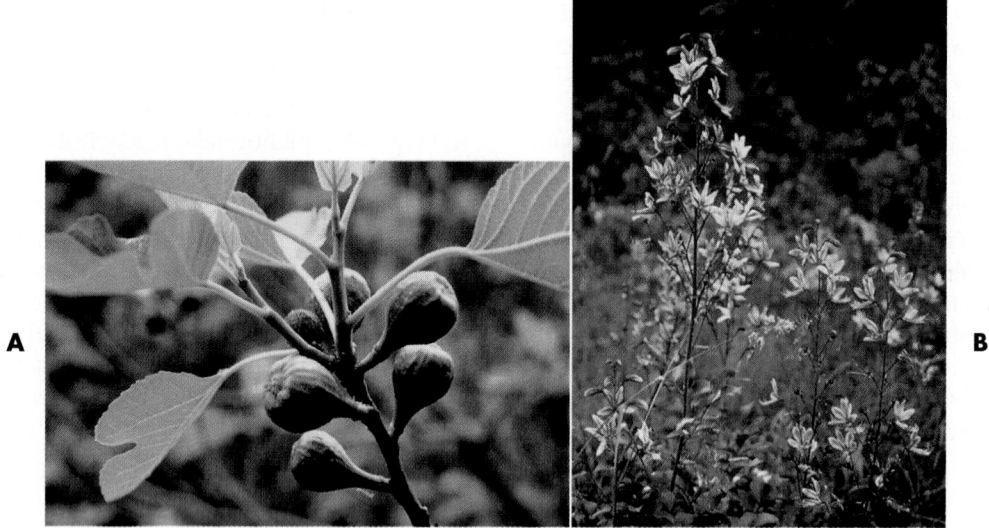

Figure 47-13 Plants that contribute to phototoxicity. **A,** Fig tree. **B,** Gas plant. (**B** *Courtesy Yves Sell, Institute of Botany, Louis Pasteur University, Strasbourg, France.*)

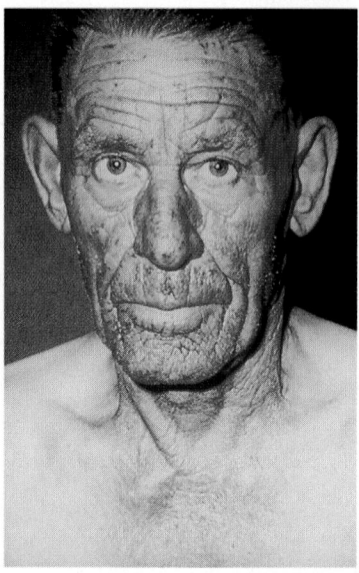

Figure 47-14 Phototoxic eczematous dermatitis caused by furocoumarins.

monoadduct formation to one strand of the DNA material, with some conversion to DNA interstrand crosslinks by a second photon reaction. This is a type I reaction that does not require oxygen.

There is evidence that a type II reaction also occurs.[94] This is a so-called photodynamic reaction, which depends on the presence of oxygen. After UVA irradiation, the psoralen compound in the triplet state induces singlet oxygen, superoxide anions, and hydroxy radicals, which are responsible for cell membrane damage, erythema, and edema. The type I reaction results in nu-

clear and ribonucleic acid (RNA) damage. Keratinocytes, Langerhans' cells, melanocytes, mononuclear cells, fibrocytes, and endothelial cells can be involved in these phototoxic events.

Photoallergic reactions are rarely induced by psoralen compounds.[58] Plant-induced photoallergic responses appear to relate to chemicals other than psoralens.[56,79]

Dense hyperpigmentation is characteristic of the psoralen-induced photoreaction. This appears to be related to increased numbers of melanocytes, melanocytic hypertrophy, increased arborization of melanocytic dendrites, increased number of melanosomes, changed pattern of melanosomes, hyperplasia of the keratinocytes, and resultant increased transfer of melanosomes into keratinocytes.[94]

A distressing eruption occurs in victims who present a clinical picture of airborne contact sensitivity but who actually have a phototoxic or even photoallergic component to the response.[38,95] These victims demonstrate a mixture of acute and subacute dermatitis with pruritic, erythematous, edematous, scaly, and lichenified eruptions distributed over the face, back of the neck, and exposed regions of the extremities. Areas shielded by glasses, the nose, and the chin often are spared, so the dermatitis in its initial presentation is fairly distinctive. However, with severe reactions, the lesions often become disseminated to the trunk and elsewhere. Thus it is important to obtain a history of the original pattern of distribution. The dermatitis can be explosive and incapacitating. The key to good care is rapid recognition and prompt institution of therapy. Unfortunately, the correct diagnosis is often not made early and the skin disease progresses to a chronic, more slowly evolving gener-

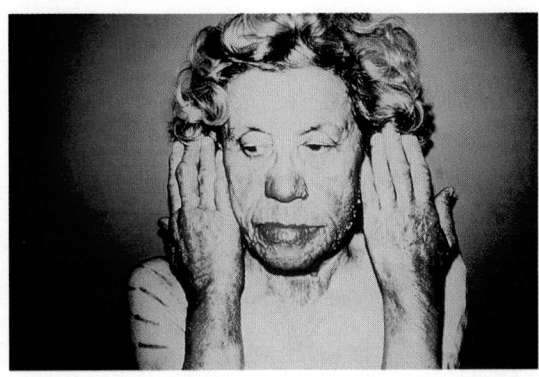

Figure 47-15 Persistent light eruptions that can eventuate from acute photoallergic contact dermatitis.

alized dermatitis with limited remissions and frequent exacerbations.

Although furocoumarins may cause the preceding type of reaction, they more often are responsible for acute reactions. More likely culprits include aromatic lichen compounds, such as usnic acid[126] and atranorin,[125] the Compositae oleoresins, and other sesquiterpene lactones, such as parthenin and ambrosin.[38] Parthenin has been demonstrated during an epidemic of airborne contact, and presumably photocontact dermatitis, after inadvertent importation of feverfew (*Parthenium hysterophorus*) into India.[69] These cases unfortunately can eventuate as persistent light reactors[16,38,52,125,126] and can even develop with granulomatous skin inflammation.[124]

The pathophysiologic mechanisms behind some phytophotodermatitis remain unresolved. The phototoxic mechanisms of furocoumarin effects have been delineated,[95] but how the aromatic lichen compounds and Compositae oleoresins effect these changes is unclear. Towers and associates[130] reported phototoxic effects of polyacetylenes and thiophene, which are present in Compositae plants. α-Terthienyl from marigold (*Tagetes erecta*, a member of the Compositae family) has been shown to act as a nonphotodynamic photosensitizer in vitro and in vivo.[54]

Rarely, cases are considered to be caused by photoallergy (Figure 47-15). It has been argued that because a relatively large number of photosensitive persons are also contact sensitive to sesquiterpene lactones, repeated exposure to these common allergens might predispose persons to become perennial and persistent light reactors.[38] This state of perennial or persistent light reactivity has become well recognized and is called chronic actinic dermatitis.[18] It is characterized by a severe eczematous eruption involving primarily sun-exposed areas but spreading to covered sites at times. This eruption predominantly affects older men, a significant number of whom are contact allergic to Com-

positae oleoresins.[38] A relationship between the contact allergy and the development of chronic actinic dermatitis has not been definitively demonstrated. However, Murphy et al[84] recently reported a gardener who progressed from a state of proven contact allergy to Compositae resins to a state of proven photosensitivity. The patient had a chronic eczematous eruption of his hands and face for 12 months with positive patch tests to sesquiterpene lactone mix and negative phototests. Six months after the initial phototesting, he was retested and found to have a significant eczematous reaction to UVA radiation, as well as being contact sensitive to Compositae resins. The authors suggest that the initial contact allergy could enable formation of an endogenous photoallergen that would be responsible for a chronic photo-induced delayed-type hypersensitivity reaction.

Treatment

The management of phytophotodermatitis depends on a number of factors, including the extent and severity of the process; the identity, amount, and potency of the photosensitizer; and the nature of the photosensitive eruption.

The initial approach is to discontinue contact with the photosensitizing plant, avoid sun exposure, or both. The vast majority of these reactions are phototoxic. Thus the offending plant is usually identified from the history of contact with a known photosensitizing plant and the distribution and character of the eruption. If the contactants are not known photosensitizers, epidemiologic and photopatch testing procedures are needed to identify the offending plant. If the problem is photoallergic in nature, photopatch testing may also be needed.

The acute inflammatory aspects of the responses are treated with appropriate dermatologic measures. The intensity of treatment depends on the severity and the extent of the dermatitis. Cool tap water wet dressings applied every 2 hours when awake for 2 to 3 days reduce inflammation and discomfort. Ice and ice water should be avoided. Topical fluorinated corticosteroids, such as fluocinonide 0.05% cream, ointment, or gel, may be useful. If the process is severe or extensive, systemic corticosteroids may be needed. Thus betamethasone suspension, 6 mg; methylprednisolone, 40 to 80 mg; or triamcinolone acetonide, 40 mg IM, are equally effective.

In general, a phototoxic event is self-limited and subsides within a week if further insult does not occur. Hyperpigmentation may persist for several months and frequently is unsightly. Topical application of 5% hydroquinone cream once or twice a day for several weeks may lighten the hyperpigmentation. Treatment of the chronic actinic dermatitis state has been most difficult. Complete elimination of light exposure temporarily ameliorates the photodermatosis. However, exacerbations generally occur with return to even minimal exposures. Photochemotherapy with 8-methoxypsoralen and UVA radiation has been helpful in a few cases.[80] However, recent studies indicate that azathioprine, generally in daily doses of 100 mg for several months, is quite effective in inducing remissions.[85] The appropriate laboratory evaluation must be performed periodically to detect azathioprine toxicity.

GRANULOMAS

Penetration and breakage of thorns, spines, and spicules in the skin can lead to foreign body granuloma.[5] When a young person has an indurated and erythematous plaque or patch on the buttocks or an exposed part of the body and gives a history of having fallen in the desert from a horse, motorcycle, or all-terrain vehicle 7 to 10 days previously, the clinical diagnosis of cactus granuloma is not difficult. However, when an urban inhabitant arrives in the emergency room during or after recovery from a prolonged domestic bout of substance abuse with grouped erythematous papulopustules on the same exposed areas, the diagnosis may not be so apparent. Cacti abound throughout urbia and conurbia.

Cactus lesions generally evolve over a matter of days to weeks but can take years to appear.[45] All lesions seem to be roughly the same age at the time of presentation. They do not develop explosively. Nevertheless, various infections must be considered, so a Gram-stained smear and microbiologic cultures are often indicated, although most lesions are aseptic. Plant-associated pathogens, such as *Mycobacterium* spp., should be considered. If the lesions are fairly firm and more papular than pustular, a biopsy should be performed. Sometimes a member of the party can provide the necessary botanical clue, but it is the essential observation that lesions are in groups or patches on extremities that leads to the suspicion that a victim might have fallen or been thrust inadvertently into a cactus. In Israel and other parts of the world, where edible cacti (prickly pears of the *Opuntia* spp.) are cultivated, a somewhat more acute papulopustular eruption is seen (Figure 47-16).[116,135] So-called sabra dermatitis is caused by implantation of detachable glochids of the cactus,[127] which can be blown by wind onto the skin, or into the eyes to cause an annoying keratoconjunctivitis.[134]

Although the basic histologic features are those of a foreign body granuloma, with periodic acid–Schiff–positive spicules detected in giant cells,[26] lesions are clearly more inflammatory than simple foreign body reactions. The predominant cells are type 1 epithelioid cells with secretory rough endoplasmic reticulum and dense lysosomal bodies in the cytoplasm.[31,32] This implies that an element of hypersensitivity also exists. Although T lymphocytes and dendritic mono-

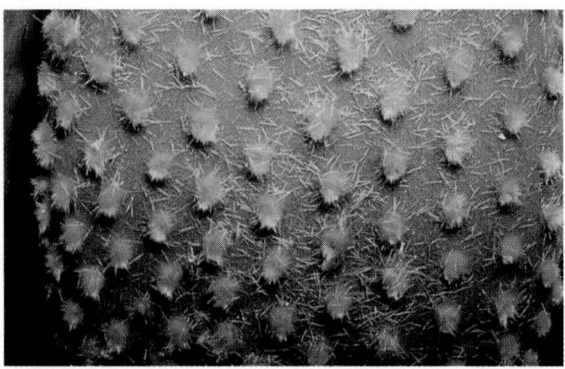

Figure 47-16 Beaver tail cactus (*Opuntia* species). *(Courtesy Eric Lewis.)*

nuclear cells are present in the area of chemically induced hypersensitivity granulomas,[29] it is not yet clear whether this type of granuloma requires an intact cell-mediated immune system to initiate granuloma formation.[29,36] However, granulomas are fully formed in the presence of a cell-mediated immune response.[11,26,29,32,135]

Treatment

Acute care treatment of cactus-induced skin lesions must remain conservative because final diagnosis cannot be achieved without histologic interpretation. Systemic corticosteroids are effective in reducing inflammation and relieving discomfort. However, failure to recognize an active infection or an infectious granuloma could lead to aggravation by overzealous corticosteroid treatment. Topical corticosteroids offer little help. The victim should be treated with cool compresses of aluminum acetate and systemic medication for pain or discomfort until a diagnosis can be made and definitive treatment (surgical, supportive, or specific) is initiated. Surgical removal of solitary or small grouped granulomas is recommended where feasible. Incision and drainage may help expose the inciting agent. If the glochids are visible in the skin, removal with sterile splinter forceps in the reverse direction of penetration usually leads to rapid healing, but this procedure can be difficult and tedious. Removal of large spines may require localization using soft tissue radiographic techniques. Small spines in groups within the skin may be peeled off using water-soluble facial gel or rubber cement, taking care to avoid contact with sensitive mucous membranes. These procedures are gratifying when they work, but they often fail. The primary reason for failure is that the tiny barbs on the glochids point backward like barbed fishhooks and hold the dart into the skin.[120] At times, watchful waiting and supportive care are all that work, and the offending agent is extruded spontaneously.[120]

REFERENCES

1. Adolf W, Hecker E: On the active principles of the spurge family. X. Skin irritants, cocarcinogens and cryptic cocarcinogens from the latex of the manchineel tree, *J Nat Prod* 47:482, 1984.
2. Alé SI et al: Allergic contact dermatitis caused by *Lithraea molleoides* and *Lithraea brasiliensis:* identification and characterization of the responsible allergens, *Am J Contact Dermat* 8:144, 1997.
2a. Bailey JM: New mechanisms for effects of anti-inflammatory glucocorticoids, *Bio Factors* 3:97, 1991.
2b. Barker JW et al: Keratinocytes as initiators of inflammation, *Lancet* 337:211, 1989.
3. Bell RM: Protein kinase C activation by diacylglycerol second messengers, *Cell* 45:631, 1986.
4. Benezra C, Epstein WL: Molecular recognition patterns of sesquiterpene lactones in *Costus*-sensitive patients, *Contact Dermatitis* 15:223, 1986.
5. Benezra C et al: *Plant contact dermatitis,* Toronto, 1985, BC Decker.
6. Benyon RC, Robinson C, Church MK: Differential release of histamine and eicosanoids from human skin mast cells activated by IgE dependent and nonimmunological stimuli, *Br J Pharmacol* 97:898, 1989.
7. Berkley SF et al: Dermatitis in grocery workers associated with high natural concentrations of furocoumarins in celery, *Ann Intern Med* 105:351, 1986.
8. Berridge MJ: Inositol triphosphate and calcium signalling, *Nature* 361:315, 1993.
9. Birmingham DJ et al: Phototoxic bullae among celery harvesters, *Arch Dermatol* 83:73, 1961.
10. Bock SA, May CD: Adverse reactions to food caused by sensitivity. In Middleton E Jr et al, editors: *Allergy: principles and practice,* ed 2, St Louis, 1993, Mosby.
11. Boros DL: Immunopathology of *Schistosoma mansoni* infection, *Clin Microbiol Rev* 2:250, 1989.
12. Bourne HR, Masters SB, Sullivan KA: Mammalian G proteins: structure and function, *Biochem Soc Trans* 15:35, 1987.
13. Boutwell RK: The function and mechanisms of promotors in carcinogenesis, *CRC Crit Rev Toxicol* 2:419, 1974.
14. Bubak ME et al: Allergic reactions to latex among health care workers, *Mayo Clinic Proc* 47:1075, 1992.
15. Carrillo T, Cuenoas M, Munoz T: Contact urticaria and rhinitis from latex surgical gloves, *Contact Dermatitis* 15:69, 1986.
16. Castro JLC et al: Musk ambrette and chronic actinic dermatitis, *Contact Dermatitis* 13:302, 1985.
17. Centers for Disease Control: Phototoxic dermatitis in grocery workers, *MMWR* 34:11, 1984.
18. Cutaneous photosensitivity, *Lancet* 1:1317, 1988.
19. Dooms-Goosens A, Deleu H: Airborne contact dermatitis: an update, *Contact Dermatitis* 25:211, 1991.
20. Ducombs G et al: Patch testing with the "sesquiterpene lactone mix": a marker for contact allergy to Compositae and other sesquiterpene-lactone-containing plants; a multicentre study of the EECDRG, *Contact Dermatitis* 22:249, 1990.
21. Dvorak AM: Human mast cells, *Adv Anat Embryol Cell Biol* 114:1, 1989.
22. Dvorak HF, Mihm MC: Basophilic leukocytes in allergic contact dermatitis, *J Exp Med* 135:235, 1972.
23. Epstein JH: Photoallergy and photoimmunology. In Stone J, editor: *Dermatologic immunology and allergy,* St Louis, 1985, Mosby.
24. Epstein WL: Rhus dermatitis, *Pediatr Clin North Am* 6:843, 1959.
25. Epstein WL: Poison oak and poison ivy dermatitis as an occupational problem, *Cutis* 13:544, 1974.
26. Epstein WL: Granulomatous inflammation in skin. In Ioachim HL, editor: *Pathology of granulomas,* New York, 1983, Raven Press.
27. Epstein WL: The poison ivy picker of Pennypack Park, *J Invest Dermatol* 88:7s, 1987.
27a. Epstein WL: Allergic contact dermatitis. In Fitzpatrick TB et al, editors: *Dermatology in general medicine,* ed 3, New York, 1987, McGraw-Hill.
28. Epstein WL: Plant-induced dermatitis, *Ann Emerg Med* 16:950, 1987.
29. Epstein WL: Mechanisms of granuloma formation. In Norris DA, editor: *Mechanisms in cutaneous disease,* New York, 1989, Marcel Dekker.
30. Epstein WL: Topical prevention of poison ivy/oak dermatitis, *Arch Dermatol* 125:499, 1989.
31. Epstein WL: Ultrastructural heterogeneity of epithelioid cells in cutaneous organized granulomas of diverse etiology, *Arch Dermatol* 127:821, 1991.
32. Epstein WL: Pathogenesis of granulomatous inflammation in skin. In Moschella SL, Hurley HJ, editors: *Dermatology,* ed 3, Philadelphia, 1993, WB Saunders.

33. Epstein WL, Kligman AM: Transfer of allergic contact-type delayed hypersensitivity in man, *J Invest Dermatol* 28:291, 1957.
34. Epstein WL, Kligman AM: The interference phenomenon in allergic contact dermatitis, *J Invest Dermatol* 31:103, 1958.
35. Epstein WL et al: Poison oak hyposensitization, *Arch Dermatol* 109:356, 1974.
36. Epstein WL et al: T-cell independent transfer of organized granuloma formation, *Immunol Lett* 14:59, 1986.
37. Fisher AA: Erythema multiforme–like eruptions due to exotic woods and ordinary plants, *Cutis* 37:101, 1986.
38. Frain-Bell W: Photosensitivity and Compositae dermatitis, *Clin Dermatol* 4:122, 1986.
39. Freund E: Uber bisher noch nicht beschribene Kunstliche Hautverfarbungen, *Dermatol Wochenschr* 63:931, 1916.
40. Fujita M, Auki T: Allergic contact dermatitis to pyridoxine ester and hinokitiol, *Contact Dermatitis* 9:61, 1983.
41. Gafner F et al: Human maximization test of falcarinol, the principal contact allergen of English ivy and Alergian ivy, *Contact Dermatitis* 19:125, 1988.
42. Gartner BL et al: Seasonal variation of urushiol content in poison oak leaves, *Am J Contact Dermat* 4:33, 1993.
43. Gollhausen R, Kligman AM: Human assay for identifying substances which induce non-allergic contact urticaria, *Contact Dermatitis* 13:98, 1985.
43a. Griffiths CEM, Nickoloff BJ: Keratinocyte intercellular adhesion molecule-1 expression precedes dermal T lymphocyte infiltration in allergic contact dermatitis (rhus dermatitis), *Am J Pathol* 135:1045, 1989.
43b. Griffiths CEM et al: Modulation of leukocyte adhesion molecules, a T-cell chemotaxin and a regulatory cytokine in allergic contact dermatitis (*Rhus* dermatitis), *Br J Dermatol* 124:519, 1991.
44. Gross TP et al: An outbreak of phototoxic dermatitis due to limes, *Am J Epidemiol* 125:509, 1987.
45. Gutierrez-Ortega MC et al: Facial granuloma caused by cactus bristles, *Med Cutan Ibero—Latin Am* 18:197, 1990.
46. Hausen BM: *Woods injurious to human health,* New York, 1981, deGruyter.
47. Hausen BM: Contact allergy to woods, *Clin Dermatol* 4:65, 1986.
48. Hausen BM et al: Allergic and irritant dermatitis from falcarinol and didehydrofalcarinol in common ivy, *Contact Dermatitis* 17:1, 1987.
49. Hjorth N, Roed-Petersen J: Occupational protein contact dermatitis in food handlers, *Contact Dermatitis* 2:28, 1976.
50. Hjorth N, Roed-Peterson J, Thomsen K: Airborne contact dermatitis from Compositae oleoresins simulating photo-dermatitis, *Br J Dermatol* 95:613, 1976.
51. Holub BJ: The cellular forms and functions of the inositol phospholipids and their metabolic derivatives, *Nutr Rev* 45:65, 1987.
52. Horio T: Actinic reticuloid via persistent light reaction from photoallergic contact dermatitis, *Arch Dermatol* 118:339, 1982.
53. Hurtado I: Poisonous Anacardiaceae of South America, *Clin Dermatol* 4:183, 1986.
54. Kagan J, Gabriel R, Reed SA: Alpha-terthienyl, a nonphotodynamic phototoxic compound, *Photochem Photobiol* 31:465, 1980.
54a. Kalish RS, Askenase PW: Molecular mechanisms of CD8+ T cell-mediated delayed hypersensitivity, *J Allergy Clin Immunol* 103:192, 1999.
55. Kalish RS, personal communication, 1999.
56. Kavli G et al: In vivo and in vitro phototoxicity of different parts of *Heracleum laciniatum,* *Contact Dermatitis* 9:269, 1983.
57. Keil H, Wasserman D, Dawson CR: Relationship of hypersensitiveness to poison ivy and to the pure ingredients in cashew nut shell liquid and related substances, *Indust Med* 14:825, 1945.
58. Kinghorn AD: Cocarcinogenic irritant Euphorbiaceae. In Kinghorn AD, editor: *Toxic plants,* New York, 1979, Columbia University Press.
58a. Kishimoto T et al: The role of basophils and mast cells in cutaneous basophil hypersensitivity reaction, *Clin Exp Immunol* 67:611, 1986.
59. Klaber R: Phyto-photo-dermatitis, *Br J Dermatol* 54:193, 1942.
60. Kligman AM: Poison ivy dermatitis, *Arch Dermatol* 77:149, 1958.
61. Knight TE: Philodendron-induced dermatitis, *Cutis* 48:375, 1991.
62. Knight TE: Resorcinols and catechols: a clinical study of cross-reactivity, *Am J Contact Dermat* 7:138, 1996.
63. Lahti A: Contact urticaria to plants, *Clin Dermatol* 4:127, 1986.
64. Lavaud F et al: Cross reactions involving natural rubber latex, *Clin Rev Allergy Immunol* 15:429, 1997.
65. Layier F et al: Prevalence of latex allergy in operating room nurses, *J Allergy Clin Immunol* 90:316, 1992.
66. Leonforte JF: Contact dermatitis from *Larrea* (creosote bush), *J Am Acad Dermatol* 14:202, 1986.

67. Linau M, Fernandex JM: IgE-mediated degranulation of mast cells does not require opening of ion channels, *Nature* 319:150, 1986.

68. Ljunggren B: Severe phototoxic burn following celery ingestion, *Arch Dermatol* 126:1334, 1990.

69. Lonker A, Mitchell JC, Calnan CD: Contact dermatitis from *Parthenium hysterophorus, Trans St Johns Hosp Dermatol Soc* 60:43, 1974.

70. Lopez CB et al: CD8+ T cells are the effectors of the contact dermatitis induced by urushiol in mice and are regulated by CD4+ T cells, *Int Arch Allergy Immunol* 117:194, 1998.

71. Marks JG, et al: Prevention of poison ivy and poison oak allergic contact dermatitis by quaternium-18 bentonite, *J Am Acad Dermatol* 33:212, 1995.

72. Marzulli FN, Maibach HI: Perfume phototoxicity, *J Soc Cosmet Chem* 21:685, 1970.

73. Maso MJ et al: Celery phytophotodermatitis in a chef, *Arch Dermatol* 127:912, 1991.

74. McCord CP: The toxic properties of some timber woods, *Indust Med Surg* 27:202, 1958.

75. Meding B: Immediate hypersensitivity to mustard and rape, *Contact Dermatitis* 13:121, 1985.

76. Menz J et al: Contact dermatitis from Grevillea "Robyn Gordon," *Contact Dermatitis* 15:126, 1986.

77. Metcalfe DD: Food hypersensitivity, *J Allergy Clin Immunol* 73:749, 1984.

78. Mitchell JC et al: Allergic contact dermatitis from Frullania and Compositae: the role of sesquiterpene lactones, *J Invest Dermatol* 54:233, 1970.

79. Moller H: Contact and photocontact allergy to psoralens, *Photoderm Photoimmunol Photomed* 7:43, 1990.

80. Morrison WL et al: Oral methosalen photochemotherapy of uncommon photodermatoses, *Acta Derm Venerol (Stockh)* 59:366, 1979.

81. Morton JF: *Plants poisonous to people in Florida and other warm areas,* ed 2, Miami, 1982, JF Morton.

82. Mousli M et al: G-proteins as targets for non-immunological histamine releasers, *Agents Actions* 33:81, 1991.

83. Mukinen-Kiljunen S et al: Characterization of latex antigens and allergies in surgical gloves and natural rubber by immunoelectrophoretic methods, *J Allergy Clin Immunol* 90:230, 1992.

84. Murphy GM, White IR, Hawk JLM: Allergic airborne contact dermatitis to Compositae with photosensitivity—chronic actinic dermatitis in evolution, *Photodermatol Photoimmunol Photomed* 7:38, 1990.

85. Murphy GM et al: Azathioprine treatment in chronic actinic dermatitis: a double-bind controlled trial with monitoring of exposure to ultraviolet radiation, *Br J Dermatol* 121:639, 1989.

86. Musajo L, Rodighiero G, Caporale G: Relation between constitution and photodynamic properties of furocoumarins (Italian), *Farmaco (Ed Sci)* 13:355, 1958.

87. Musajo L et al: Photoreactions between skin photosensitizing furocoumarins and nuclei acid. In Pathak MA et al, editors: *Sunlight and man,* Tokyo, 1974, University of Tokyo Press.

87a. Nickoloff BJ: Role of epidermal keratinocytes as key initiators of contact dermatitis due to allergic sensitization and irritation, *Contact Dermatitis* 3:65, 1992.

88. Nishizuka Y: Studies and perspectives of protein kinase C, *Science* 233:305, 1986.

89. Oliver F et al: Contact urticaria due to the common stinging nettle (Urtica dioica)—histological, ultrastructural, and pharmacological studies, *Clin Exp Dermatol* 16:1, 1991.

90. Oppenheim M: Dermatite bulleuse striee consecutive aux bains de soleil dans les pres (dermatitis bullosa striata pratensis), *Ann Dermatol Syphiligr* 3(series)7:1, 1932.

91. Orchard S: Barrier creams, *Dermatol Clin* 2:619, 1984.

92. Orchard SM, Fellman JH, Storrs FJ: Poison ivy/oak dermatitis use of polyamine salts of linoleic acid dimer for prophylaxis, *Arch Dermatol* 122:783, 1986.

93. Panconesi E et al: Anaphylactic shock from mustard after ingestion of pizza, *Contact Dermatitis* 6:294, 1980.

94. Pathak MA: *Photobiologic toxicology and pharmacologic aspects of psoralens,* Monograph 66, Washington DC, 1984, US Dept of Health and Human Services, National Institutes of Health.

95. Pathak MA: Phytophotodermatitis, *Clin Dermatol* 4:102, 1986.

96. Pathak MA, Fellman JH, Kaufman KD: The effect of structural alterations on the erythemal activity of furocoumarins, *J Invest Dermatol* 35:165, 1960.

97. Pathak MA, Kramer DM: Photosensitization of the skin in vivo by furocoumarins (psoralens), *Biochem Biophys Acta* 195:197, 1969.

98. Pathak MS, Worden LR, Kaufman KD: Effect of structural alterations on the photosensitizing potency of furocoumarins (psoralens) and related compounds, *J Invest Dermatol* 48:103, 1967.

99. Pecequerio M, Menezes-Brandae F: Airborne contact dermatitis to plants, *Contact Dermatitis* 13:277, 1985.

99a. Pequet et al: Tumor necrosis factor is a critical mediator in hapten-induced irritant and contact hypersensitivity reactions, *J Exp Med* 173:673, 1991.

100. Persone VB: The natural occurrence and uses of the toxic coumarins. In Kadis S et al, editors: *Microbial toxins,* vol 8, New York, 1972, Academic Press.

101. Persone VB, Scheel LD, Meitus RJ: A bioassay for the quantitation of cutaneous reaction associated with pink-rot celery, *J Invest Dermatol* 42:267, 1964.

102. Powell SM, Barrett DK: An outbreak of contact dermatitis from *Rhus verniciflua, Contact Dermatitis* 14:288, 1986.

103. Reynolds GW, Epstein WL, Rodriguez E: Unusual contact allergens from plants in the family Hydrophyllaceae, *Contact Dermatitis* 14:39, 1986.

104. Richards DE: The isolation and identification of the toxic coumarins. In Kadis S et al, editors: *Microbial toxins,* vol 8, New York, 1972, Academic Press.

105. Rizova H et al: Contact allergens, but not irritants alter receptor-mediated endocytosis by human epidermal langerhans cells, *Br J Dermatol* 140:200, 1999.

106. Roed-Peterson J, Hjorth N: Compositae sensitivity among patients with contact dermatitis, *Contact Dermatitis* 2:171, 1976.

107. Rosengard BR, Mahalik C, Cochrane DE: Mast cell secretion: differences between immunologic and non-immunologic stimulation, *Agents Actions* 19:133, 1986.

108. Rosenthal O: Berloque dermatitis: Berliner Dermatologische Gesellschaft, *Dermatol Z* 42:295, 1925.

109. Sach MI, Gleich GJ, Yuninger JW: Adverse reactions to food. In Franklin EG, editor: *Clinical immunology update,* New York, 1983, Elsevier.

110. Sams WM: Photodynamic action of lime oil (Citrus aurantifolia), *Arch Dermatol Syphilol* 44:571, 1941.

111. Santacci B, Picardo M, Cristaudo A: Contact dermatitis from *Euphorbia pulcherrima, Contact Dermatitis* 12:285, 1985.

112. Scheel LD et al: The isolation and characterization of two phototoxic furocoumarins (psoralens) from diseased celery, *Biochemistry* 2:1127, 1963.

113. Schmidt RJ: Compositae, *Clin Dermatol* 4:46, 1986.

114. Schwartz L: Allergic occupational dermatitis in our war industries, *Ann Allergy* 2:387, 1944.

115. Schwartz LB: Mast cells and their role in urticaria, *J Am Acad Dermatol* 25(suppl):190, 1991.

116. Shanon J, Sagher F: Sabra dermatitis, *Arch Dermatol* 74:269, 1956.

117. Shelley WB, Arthur RP: Mucunain, the active pruritogenic proteinase in cowhage, *Science* 122:469, 1955.

118. Shelley WB, Arthur RP: Studies on cowhage and its pruritogenic proteinase, mucunain, *Arch Dermatol* 72:399, 1955.

119. Smart ER, Macleod RI, Lawrence CM: Allergic reactions to rubber gloves in dental patients, *Br Dental J* 172:445, 1992.

120. Snyder RA, Schwartz RA: Cactus bristle implantation, *Arch Dermatol* 119:152, 1983.

121. Sosman AJ et al: Hypersensitivity to wood dust, *N Engl J Med* 281:977, 1969.

122. Spoerke DG, Spoerke SE: Granuloma formation induced by spines of the cactus, *Opuntia acanthocarpa, Vet Hum Toxicol* 33:342, 1991.

123. Stevens RL, Austen KF: Recent advances in the cellular and molecular biology of mast cells, *Immunol Today* 10:381, 1989.

124. Sullivan KA et al: Identification of receptor contact site involved in receptor-G protein coupling, *Nature* 330:758, 1987.

125. Thune P, Eeg-Larsen T: Contact and photocontact allergy in persistent light reactivity, *Contact Dermatitis* 11:98, 1984.

126. Thune PO, Solberg YJ: Photosensitivity and allergy to aromatic lichen acids, Compositae oleoresins and other plant substances, *Contact Dermatitis* 6:81, 1980.

127. Thurston EL: Morphology, fine structure and ontogeny of the stinging emergency of *Urtica dioica, Am J Bot* 61:809, 1974.

128. Thurston EL, Lersten NR: The morphology and toxicology of plant stinging hairs, *Bot Rev* 35:393, 1969.

129. Tomazic VJ et al: Latex-associated allergies and anaphylactic reactions, *Clin Immunol Immunopathol* 64:89, 1992.

130. Towers GNH et al: Phototoxic polyacetylenes and their thiophene derivatives (effects on human skin), *Contact Dermatitis* 5:140, 1979.

131. Walker FB, Smith PD, Maibach HI: Genetic factors in human allergic contact dermatitis, *Int Arch Allergy* 32:453, 1967.

132. Webster GL: Irritant plants in the spurge family, *Clin Dermatol* 4:36, 1986.

133. White W: Club Med dermatitis, *N Engl J Med* 314:319, 1986.

134. Whiting DA, Bristow JH: Dermatitis and keratoconjunctivitis caused by prickly pear, *South Afr Med J* 49:1445, 1975.

135. Williams GT, Jones Williams W: Granulomatous inflammation, *J Clin Pathol* 36:723, 1983.

136. Willie JJ, Kydonieus AF, Kalish RS: Inhibition of irritation and contact hypersensitivity by ethacrynic acid, *Skin Pharmacol Appl Skin Physiol* 11:279-288, 1998.

137. Zink BJ et al: The effect of jewel weed in preventing poison ivy dermatitis, *J Wilderness Med* 2:178, 1991.

48 Toxic Plant Ingestions

Kimberlie A. Graeme, George Braitberg, Donald B. Kunkel,† and Michele Adler

Plants have served as both poisons and medicines. Dioscorides listed several hundred plant species in his first *Materia Medica* in 78 BC. Galen, in second-century Rome, catalogued plants, including those containing opiates, ergotamines, and other alkaloids. Pharmacognosy was established as an independent discipline in nineteenth century Europe.[114]

Toxic plants are ingested by curious children, by foragers mistaking poisonous plants for edible fare, by herbalists mistaking poisonous plants for nontoxic remedies, by pleasure seekers attempting to attain natural highs, and by suicidal patients attempting to harm themselves. Over 122,000 plant ingestions or exposures were reported to 65 poison control centers serving more than 257 million people in 1998.[91] Plant exposures represented 5.5% of total toxic exposures reported in 1998 (fourth after cleaning substances, analgesics and cosmetics/personal care products). Approximately 7% of plant ingestions required treatment at a health care facility, with four deaths reported. More than 68% of all plant ingestions reported were in children under age 6 years.[91]

GENERAL CONSIDERATIONS

Supportive care takes priority over identification of plants ingested, but the history should include time of ingestion, amount and part of plants ingested, initial symptoms, and time between ingestion and onset of symptoms. Method of preparation (e.g., drying, cooking, boiling), number of persons who ate the same plant, and symptoms are important considerations.

Airway, breathing, and circulation are assessed, then adequacy of hydration, end-organ perfusion, and urine output. Oral administration of activated charcoal (1 g/kg) aids gastrointestinal decontamination. Laboratory studies depend on clinical presentation and suspected plant exposure. Complications of poisoning include aspiration pneumonia, rhabdomyolysis, and deep venous thrombosis.

The differential diagnosis is initially kept broad so that other illnesses, such as infection and trauma, are not missed. Table 48-1 provides signs and symptoms of toxic plant ingestions.

PLANT TOXIN PRINCIPLES

The toxic principles underlying major poisonous plant ingestions can be organized by chemical structure of plant toxins and by primary organ systems involved in toxicity. This chapter discusses plant toxins by organ system and divides toxins into chemical groups: alkaloid, glycoside, resin, oxalate, and phytotoxin.

Alkaloids

Alkaloids are nitrogen-containing organic compounds that act as bases and form salts with acids. Plant alkaloids are soluble organic acid-alkaloid salts that contain nitrogen in a ring structure that is heterocyclic, aromatic, or both. Alkaloids are generally distributed throughout the plant, so all ingested parts are toxic. Further subdivision into chemical groups is based on ring structure (Table 48-2).

Glycosides

Sugars in the form of acetals are called glycosides. In glycosides, a glycosyl group replaces an alcohol or hydroxyl group. On hydrolysis, glycosides yield sugars, or glycones, and aglycone compounds. The aglycone moiety accounts for most of the toxicity, although the sugar may enhance solubility and absorption (Figure 48-1). The glycoside-producing plants include cardioactive, cyanogenic, saponin, anthraquinone, and coumarin glycoside compounds.

Resins

Resins are highly toxic compounds of diverse chemical and plant origin united by the physical characteristics of insolubility in water, absence of nitrogen, and solid or semisolid state on extraction at room temperature. Resins are usually mixed with other compounds, such as volatile or essential oils (oleoresins), gum (gum resins), and sugars (glycoresins).

Oxalates

Oxalates occur naturally in plants as soluble (sodium and potassium) or insoluble calcium oxalates or acid oxalates. Oxalates have corrosive effects and bind serum calcium, causing hypocalcemia.

Phytotoxins

Phytotoxins, or toxalbumins, are among the most toxic substances of plant origin. They are composed of large

---

†Deceased.

TABLE 48-1 Signs and Symptoms of Plant Intoxications

		DIEFFENBACHIA, PHILODENDRON	COLCHICUM, GLORIOSA	EUPHORBIA, HIPPOMANE	ACTAEA, ANEMONE, RANUNCULUS	CONVALLARIA, DIGITALIS, NERIUM	ACONITUM	SOLANUM	PIERIS, RHODODENDRON, VERATRUM	CONIUM, LABURNUM, NICOTIANA, SOPHORA	CICUTA	TAXUS	GELSEMIUM	BRUGMANSIA, DATURA	AMARYLLIS, NARCISSUS, WISTERIA	ILEX	ABRUS, RICINUS	PRUNUS	PHYTOLACCA	PODOPHYLLUM	KARWINSKIA
MOUTH & THROAT	Burning, irritation	++	++	D	++	+	+	D	+	+											
	Increased salivation	+		D	++		+		D	+	+	D									
	Dry mouth											+	+	++							
	Dysphonia, dysphagia	+		D		±						+	+								
GASTROENTERIC TRACT	Nausea		+		+	±			D	+	+				+	+	DD				
	Vomiting		+	+	+	+	±		D	+	±	D			++	++	DD	D	++	+	
	Diarrhea		++	+	+	+		D	D	+					±		DD	D	+		
	Abdominal pain		++	++	+	+		D	D			D			+			D	+		
	Decreased bowel sounds													++						±	
CARDIOVASCULAR	Tachycardia									+				+							
	Bradycardia					+			+			D									
	Arrythmias					±	++					D									
	Conduction defects					++															
	Hypertension													+							
	Hypotension								++			D									
NERVOUS & NEUROMUSCULAR	Dizziness				±		+		+	+		+	+								
	Weakness, lethargy						+			+		D						D			
	Syncope				±																
	Delirium, psychosis				±									+							
	Tremors, convulsions				±				D±		++		±					D±			
	Depression, coma						+		D	+		D						D±		±	
	Headache								+	±			+								
	Paresthesias					++			D												
	Muscle weakness, paralysis		±						D	+			+					D±		±	DD
VISUAL	Mydriasis						+			±		+		+							
	Visual disturbances						+		D				+	+							
CUTANEOUS	Increased sweating								+	+								D	++		
	Dry skin													++							
	Flushing, rash											D		+							
	Cyanosis											D						D±			
MISC.	Hyperthermia							+						+							
	Painful, bloody micturition		+		+																

Modified from Lampe KF, McCann MA: *AMA handbook of poisonous and injurious plants,* Chicago, 1985, American Medical Association.
+, Commonly occurs; ++, pronounced or persistent; ±, occasionally reported; *D*, delayed onset; *DD*, occurrence significantly delayed.

TABLE 48-2. Plant Alkaloids and Their Structures

ALKALOID TYPE	ALKALOID STRUCTURE	EXAMPLES
Indole	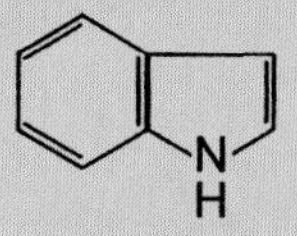	Erogonovine (ergots) Strychnine Physostigmine (calabar beans) Rauwolfia alkaloids (reserpine)
Isoquinoline	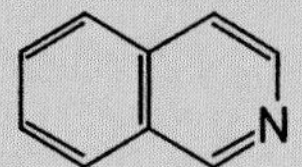	Opium alkaloids Emetine (ipecac)
Pyridine/piperidine	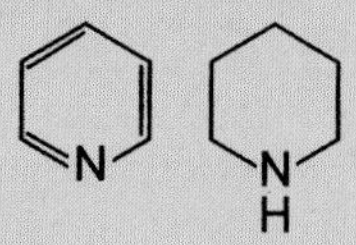	Nicotine (tobacco) Arecoline (betel nut) Lobeline (Indian tobacco)
Purine	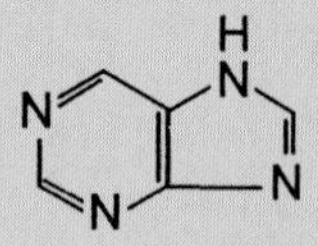	Caffeine Theobromine (cocao)
Quinoline	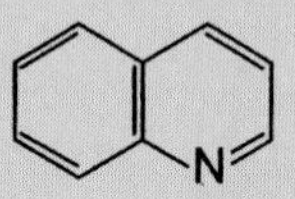	Cinchona alkaloids (quinidine)
Steroid	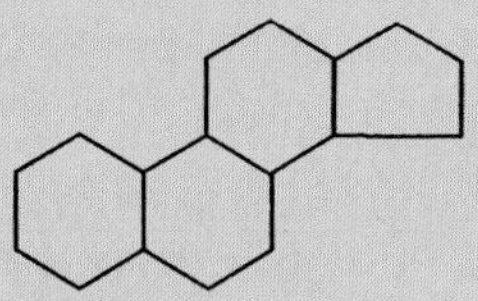	Veratrum alkaloids (false hellebore) Aconite (monkshood)
Tropane	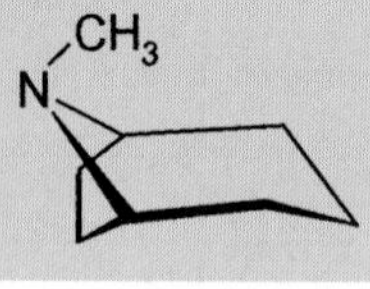	Atropine (belladonna) Hyoscyamine Hyoscine (scopolamine)

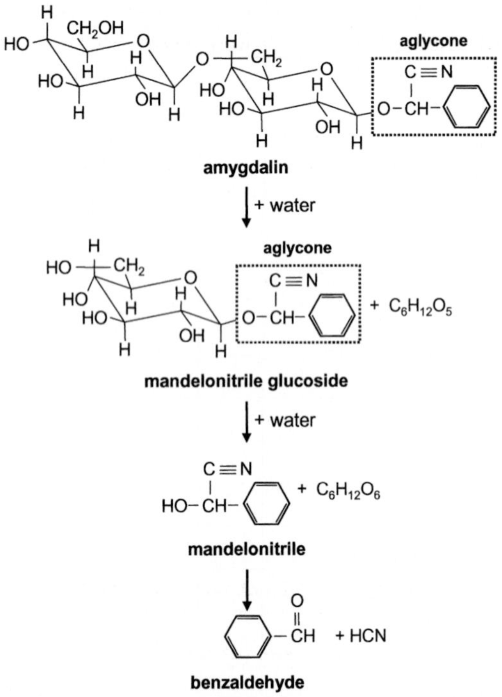

Figure 48-1 Hydrolysis of amygdalin, with its toxic aglycone group, yields hydrogen cyanide. The enzyme β-glucosidase, called emulsin, contained in plants can catalyze amygdalin hydrolysis.

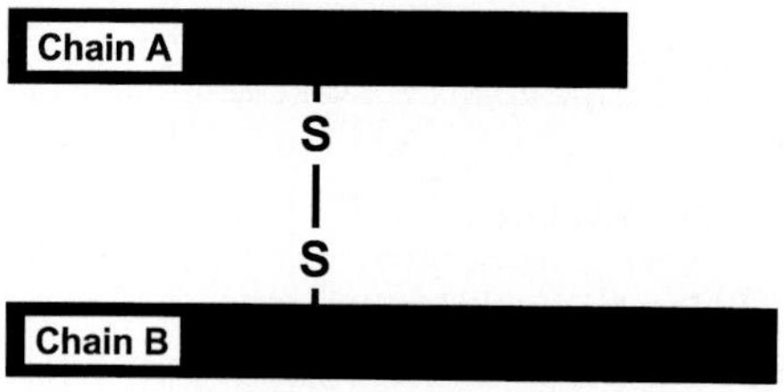

Figure 48-2 Structure of ricin, a phytotoxin isolated from the castor bean plant, is similar in structure to biologic toxins, such as botulinum. This glycoprotein is composed of two peptide chains, designated *A* and *B*, connected by a disulfide bond.

protein molecules that resemble bacterial toxins in structure and in their ability to act as antigens (Figure 48-2).

ORGAN SYSTEM PRINCIPLES

Toxic effects of certain plants can be grouped into categories designated by major effects on the central nervous, cardiovascular, gastrointestinal, renal, endocrine-metabolic, and hematopoietic systems.

Central Nervous System

Anticholinergic Plants (Tropane Alkaloids). Plants containing tropane alkaloids are often called bel-

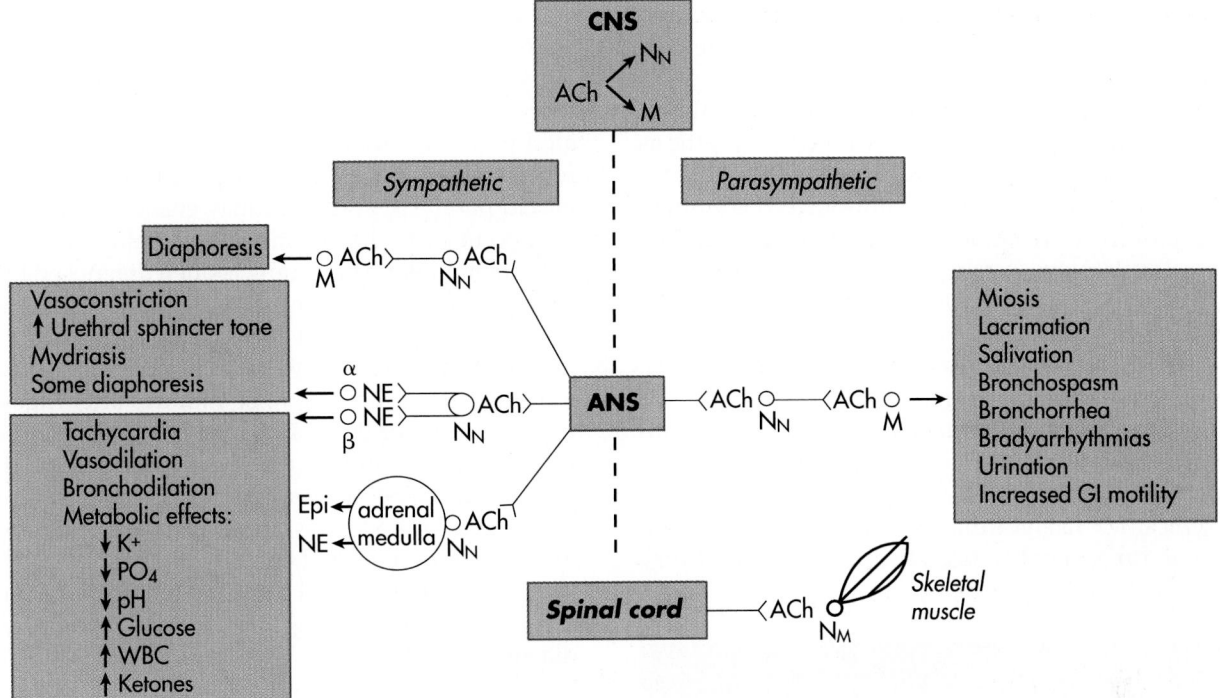

Figure 48-3 Nicotinic and muscarinic receptors of the central nervous system, autonomic nervous system, and peripheral skeletal muscles. Anticholinergic toxins (e.g., tropane alkaloids) antagonize muscarinic receptors, causing confusion, agitation, abnormal movements, hallucinations, and coma centrally and mydriasis, anhidrosis, tachycardia, urinary retention, and ileus peripherally. Direct nicotinic agonists (e.g., arecoline, coniine, cytisine, lobeline, nicotine) stimulate nicotinic receptors; however, prolonged depolarization at the receptor causes eventual blockade of nicotinic receptors. *CNS,* Central nervous system; *ANS,* autonomic nervous system; *M,* muscarinic receptor; N_N, nicotinic receptor in nervous system; N_M, nicotinic receptor at skeletal muscle; *ACh,* acetylcholine; *NE,* norepinephrine; *Epi,* epinephrine.

ladonna alkaloids and include atropine, hyoscyamine (the levorotatory isomer of atropine), and hyoscine (scopolamine).[121] Structures of the tropane alkaloids follow:

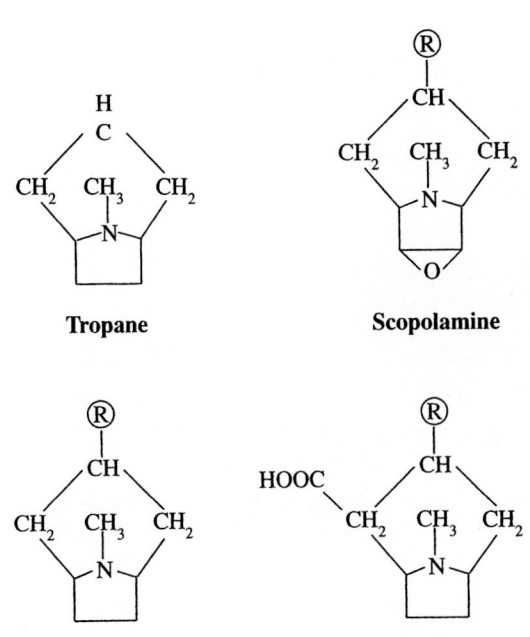

Tropane alkaloids are found in about 25 genera and 2000 species of plants. Plants causing human toxicity include *Atropa belladonna* (deadly nightshade), *Mandragora officinarum* (mandrake), *Hyoscyamus niger* (henbane), *Datura,* and *Brugmansia.*[61,121] The Solanaceae family includes *Solanum* and *Scopolia carniolica,* the source of scopolamine. *Solanum nigrum, H. niger, Cicuta minor, Datura stramonium,* and *Lactuca virosa* were used in the past to provide anesthetic solutions. Even today, poppy heads and mandrake roots are on the coat of arms of the Association of Anaesthetists.[25]

ANTICHOLINERGIC SYNDROME. Toxicity may ensue after ingesting or smoking plant parts.[28,124] The tropane alkaloids inhibit postsynaptic muscarinic receptors competitively, producing the classic anticholinergic syndrome (Figure 48-3 and Box 48-1).[55,61,121] A useful clinical sign of anticholinergic toxicity is dry axillae, without perspiration.[122] Anticholinergic findings suggesting poisoning may be remembered using the following mnemonic[123,129]:

Hot as a hare (or hot as Hades),
Blind as a bat,
Dry as a bone,
Red as a beet,
Mad as a hatter.

JIMSONWEED. *Datura* species are generally known as jimsonweed (Figure 48-4), and *Brugmansia* species are generally known as angel's trumpet.[59,61] Jimsonweed seeds contain the highest concentration of tropane alkaloids, the equivalent of 0.1 mg atropine per seed.[129] As little as one-half teaspoonful of the seeds may cause death from cardiac and pulmonary arrest.[139] Jimsonweed is thought to have derived its name from Jamestown, Virginia, where British troops were reportedly behaving bizarrely after consuming *Datura* in 1676. *Datura stramonium* has been reportedly used in Haitian zombification rituals.[28,41,59,61,139] Jimsonweed has been used to treat asthma, heralding the current use of ipratropium bromide.

Reports of abuse of *Datura* and *Brugmansia* as hallucinogens have increased in the United States and Europe.[28,61,111] Clusters of poisonings among adolescents are typical.[27,61] Tachycardia, dry mouth, agitation, nausea, vomiting, incoherence, disorientation, auditory and visual hallucinations, mydriasis, decreased bowel sounds, slurred speech, urinary retention, and hypertension have been reported.[28] Blurred vision and photophobia may be secondary to mydriasis. The associated pupillary dilation, or atropine mydriasis, is not reversed by application of 1% pilocarpine.[135] Seizures, flaccid paralysis, and coma may ensue. Hyperthermia may occur, with the victim appearing flushed.

Anticholinergic poisoning is often diagnosed by observing the victim attempting to communicate with imaginary friends, having mumbling speech, and demonstrating repetitive picking behavior.[59] Symptoms generally begin 30 to 60 minutes after ingestion and continue for 24 to 48 hours, but they may begin within several minutes and persist for several days. Patients are generally amnestic of the events. Studies may show leukocytosis, mild transient elevation of liver enzymes, elevated creatine phosphokinase (CK) levels and other evidence of rhabdomyolysis, electrocardiogram (ECG) changes consistent with tachycardia and arrhythmias.[28,61,139]

DEADLY NIGHTSHADE. Ingestion of *A. belladonna* is less common than *Datura* and *Brugmansia* ingestion. All parts of deadly nightshade contain tropane alkaloids; each berry may contain up to 2 mg of atropine. A family of eight had varying acute exposures to *A. belladonna* after eating both raw and cooked berries in a pie. The most severely poisoned patient had anticholinergic symptoms, with hypertonia, hyperthermia, respiratory failure, and coma requiring mechanical ventilation. Urine drug screens detected only atropine, but not scopolamine, which is present in much smaller quantities.[121]

In addition to poisonous or medicinal plants, a number of food staples, such as potato, tomato, eggplant,

---

Box 48-1   ANTICHOLINERGIC SYNDROME

CENTRAL	PERIPHERAL
Central nervous system excitation	Tachycardia
Agitation	Mydriasis
Hallucinations	Blurred vision
Lethargy	Inability to accommodate
Coma	Flushed skin
Respiratory depression	Hyperthermia
Mumbling speech	Absent bowel sounds
Muteness	Urinary retention
Undressing behavior	Dry mucous membranes
Repetitive picking behavior	Dry skin (particularly dry axillae)

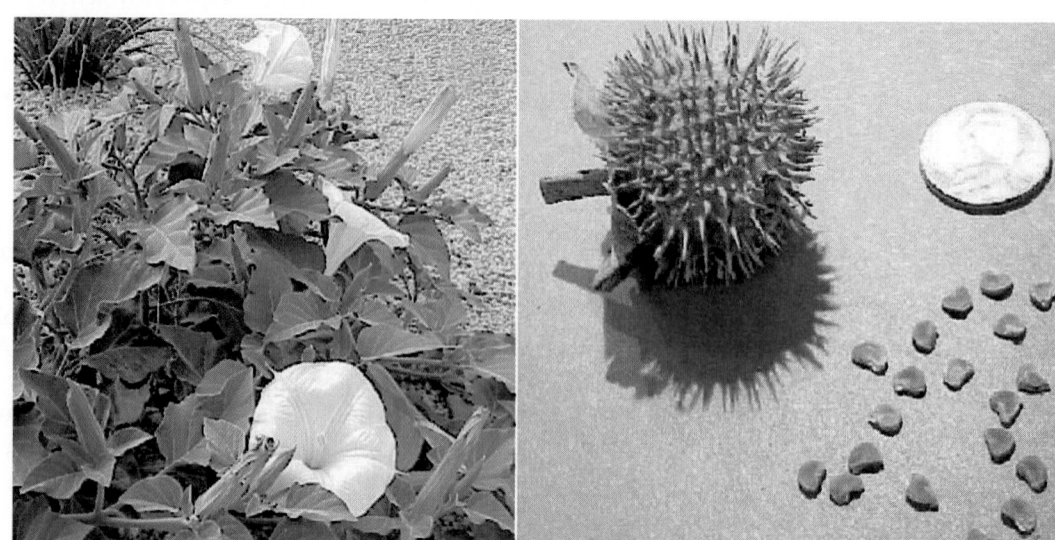

Figure 48-4 Jimsonweed (*Datura* spp.) is characterized by trumpetlike flowers **(A)** and thorny seedpods that contain numerous small kidney-shaped seeds **(B).** Nickel is shown for size comparison. *(Courtesy Kimberlie Graeme, MD, and Steven Curry, MD.)*

and chili pepper, belong to the Solanaceae family. Although atropine can be isolated from the green, unripened skins of these plants, toxicity seldom ensues.

TREATMENT. Treatment of anticholinergic plant exposure consists primarily of decontamination and supportive care, including oral administration of activated charcoal, airway protection, intravenous (IV) fluids, and vasopressors for hypotension resistant to IV fluid. Hyperthermia should be assessed and treated if significant. Agitation can be treated with careful administration of benzodiazepines. Haloperidol and phenothiazines should not be used because these agents may enhance toxicity.[55,121,124] Foley catheterization and nasogastric tube placement may be necessary if bladder distention and decreased gut motility develop, respectively.

Some recommend treating severe central anticholinergic syndrome with carefully titrated physostigmine, which is derived from the Calabar bean of *Physostigma venenosum*. This cholinesterase inhibitor blocks acetylcholine degradation; the resultant accumulation of acetylcholine overcomes the competitive inhibition of atropinic agents, such as those found in jimsonweed. Rapid reversal of peripheral and central nervous system (CNS) effects ensues. However, bradycardia, asystole, ventricular arrhythmias, hypotension, bronchospasm, bronchorrhea, and seizures have been reported after rapid IV administration of physostigmine, limiting its routine use. Persons with cardiac conduction abnormalities are particularly susceptible to these cardiac complications.[27,55,123,132,139]

Most cases of anticholinergic poisoning can be managed safely and effectively with supportive care alone.[129] We recommend consultation with a toxicologist before using physostigmine. If physostigmine is used, the recipient should be on a cardiac monitor, with pulse oximetry and a physician at the bedside slowly administrating graduated doses of the drug.[21] Risk/benefit analysis must be assessed before administration.[55] If the patient may have been exposed to tricyclic antidepressants, physostigmine should not be administered.[123,132]

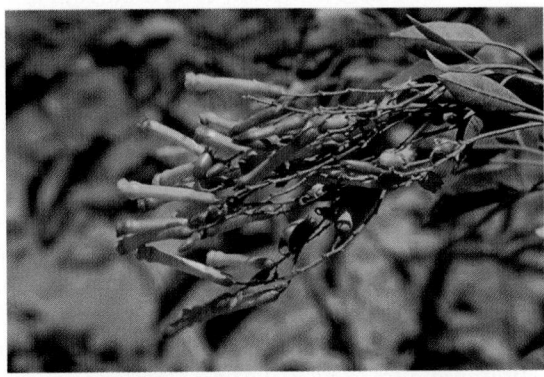

Figure 48-5 Tree tobacco *(Nicotiana glauca)*.

Nicotinic Plants (Pyridine-Piperidine Alkaloids). The pyridine-piperidine group contains the major alkaloids nicotine, coniine, lobeline, arecoline, piperine, and isopelletierine. Structures of the pyridine/piperidine alkaloids follow:

Pyridine **Nicotine**

Lobeline **Coniine**

Nicotine alkaloids are found mainly in the Solanaceae family of plants. Other families containing nicotine alkaloids include Hippocastanaceae (horse chestnut) and Asclepiadaceae (milkweed).

TOBACCO PLANTS. Tobacco contains both nicotine and related alkaloids with similar pharmacologic properties, such as the alkaloid anabasine, which is found in *Nicotiana glauca* (wild tree tobacco; Figure 48-5). Anabasine, an isomer of nicotine, may account for much of the toxicity of *Nicotiana glauca* (wild tree tobacco).[95] Other tobacco family members include *N. rustica*, *N. tabacum*, *N. trigonophylla* (desert tobacco; Figure 48-6), and *N. attenuata* (coyote tobacco). *N. tabacum* is the major source of commercial tobacco and contains between 0.5% and 9% nicotine. The kidneys excrete nicotine fairly rapidly after biotransformation in the liver and lungs. The half-life is 1 to 2 hours. The lethal dose of ingested nicotine is not well established. Two to 5 mg may cause nausea, and 40 to 60 mg may be lethal in humans. One to two cigarettes, ingested and absorbed, could be lethal to a child.

NICOTINIC SYNDROME. Peripherally, acetylcholine is a neurotransmitter for autonomic and somatic motor fibers. Acetylcholine is stored in vesicles within the presynaptic neuron and is released by calcium-dependent exocytosis into the synapse. Acetylcholine binds to receptors at the synapse and is eventually degraded by acetylcholinesterase. Acetylcholine can bind to two receptor types, nicotinic and muscarinic. Nicotinic receptors are located on postganglionic autonomic neurons (N_N receptors) and at skeletal neuromuscular junctions (N_M receptors). Direct nicotinic agonists (e.g., arecoline, coniine, cytisine, lobeline, nicotine) prolong depolarization at these receptors and eventually cause blockade of nicotinic receptors. Clinical evidence of stimulation followed by blockade is apparent. Hyper-

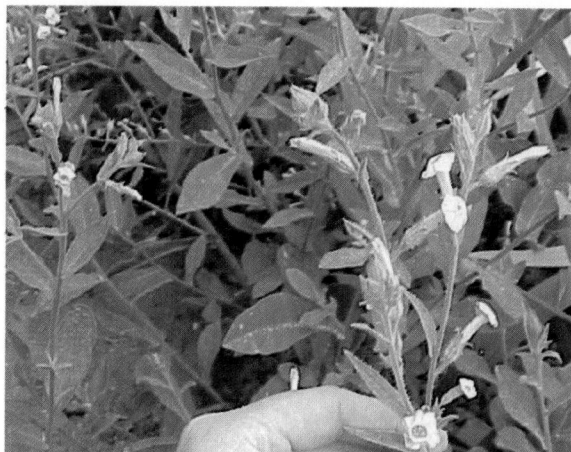

Figure 48-6 *Nicotiana trigonophylla* (desert tobacco) and other *Nicotiana* spp. are characterized by narrow tubelike flowers. *(Courtesy Kimberlie Graeme, MD, and Donald Kunkel, MD.)*

tension, tachycardia, vomiting and diarrhea, abdominal pain, salivation, bronchorrhea, muscle fasciculations and spasms, confusion, agitation, tremor and convulsions (stimulation) are followed by hypotension, bradyarrhythmias, paralysis, coma and respiratory failure (blockade)[26,38,88,95] (Box 48-2 and Figure 48-3).

Green tobacco sickness is a mild form of nicotine poisoning seen in young field workers with dermal exposure to leaves of green tobacco in wet environments. Nicotine, a water-soluble alkaloid, is absorbed dermally. The syndrome is characterized by weakness, nausea, vomiting, abdominal cramps, headache, dizziness, difficulty breathing, and occasional fluctuations in blood pressure and heart rate. The urinary nicotine metabolite, cotinine, may be helpful diagnostically.[10,88,95]

Lobeline, derived from the Indian tobacco plant, *Lobelia inflata*, is a high-affinity nicotinic ligand. It can cause nicotine-like effects (e.g., hypertension, hypotension, bradycardia) but is generally less toxic than nicotine.[40]

POISON HEMLOCK. Coniine and γ-coniceine, the principal alkaloids in *Conium maculatum* (poison hemlock), are pyridine derivatives similar to nicotine. The alkaloid is volatile and lost by drying or heating. *C. maculatum* (Figure 48-7) is also known as spotted hemlock, California or Nebraska fern, and carrot weed. It is often mistaken for an edible plant but has a mousy odor, an unpleasant bitter taste and burns the mouth and throat. The stem has purplish to reddish brown spots and is hollow. Its long taproot is solid and parsniplike. Although all plant parts are poisonous, the roots are especially toxic. Poisoning may also occur after eating birds that have consumed poison hemlock.

C. maculatum was used in ancient times for capital punishment and murder. Socrates was likely the victim of poison hemlock, suffering hypothermia, nausea, paralysis, and finally death by respiratory arrest. The primary action of the toxic alkaloids is activation then

Box 48-2 NICOTONIC SYNDROME

EARLY STAGE	LATE STAGE
Hypertension	Hypotension
Tachycardia	Bradyarrhythmias
Vomiting	Paralysis
Diarrhea	Coma
Muscle fasciculations	
Convulsions	

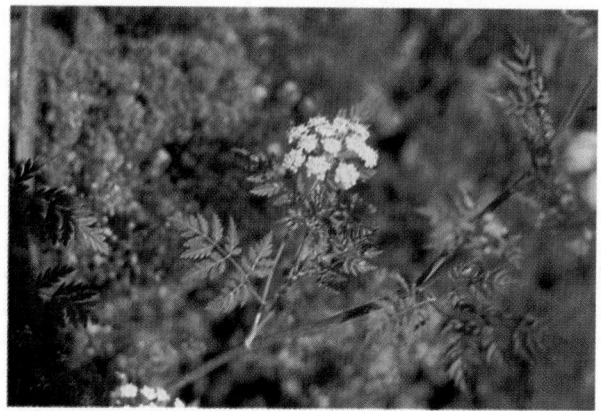

Figure 48-7 Poison hemlock (*Conium maculatum*).

blockade of nicotinic acetylcholine receptors. Initially, stimulation causes sialorrhea, nausea, vomiting, diarrhea, abdominal cramping, and tachycardia, followed by dry mucosae, gastrointestinal (GI) hypotonia, diminished cardiac contraction, and bradycardia, as with nicotinic syndrome. Muscles rapidly swell and stiffen, with multifocal necrosis of myocytes and associated muscle pain. Muscle fasciculations and flaccid paralysis may be followed by rhabdomyolysis and acute tubular necrosis with renal failure. Elevated CK and liver function tests (LFTs) may be noted. Death is usually from respiratory failure.[45,53,55,65,116]

BETEL NUT. *Areca catechu* (areca palm) produces betel nut, a common masticatory drug in the Far East, Asia, India, and the South Pacific. An estimated 10% to 25% of the world's population chews "betel quid." It is generally chewed with lime (calcium hydroxide) wrapped in leaves of betel pepper (*Piper betel*), known as "quid," "punsupari," or "pan masala." Occasionally, tobacco is added. Quid is sucked in the lateral gingival pocket. *A. catechu* contains arecoline, a volatile cholinergic alkaloid, which is hydrolyzed to the alkaloid arecaidine. Both alkaloids are nicotinic and muscarinic. Betel pepper leaves contain betel oil, which contains psychoactive phenols and cadinene that possess cocainelike properties. Clinical effects resemble nicotinic syndrome and cholinergic toxicity, including CNS effects (dizziness, euphoria, subjective arousal, altered mental sta-

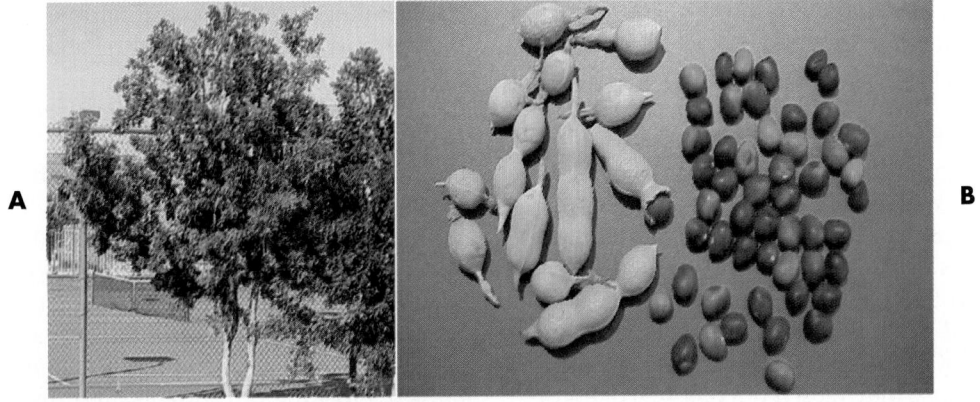

Figure 48-8 Mescal bean bush *(Sophora secundiflora)* **(A)** is characterized by bean pods that contain burnt-red seeds **(B)**. *(Courtesy Kimberlie Graeme, MD.)*

tus, hallucinations, psychosis, convulsions), cardiac effects (tachycardia, hypertension, palpitations, arrhythmias, bradycardia, hypotension), pulmonary effects (bronchospasm, dyspnea), GI effects (salivation, vomiting, diarrhea), urogenic effects (urinary incontinence), and musculoskeletal effects (weakness and paralysis). Betel nut use is also associated with flushing, diaphoresis, warm sensations, red-stained oral mucosa and saliva, and dark brown-stained teeth.[33,101,107]

QUINOLIZIDINE ALKALOIDS. Cytisine is a quinolizidine alkaloid but is often classified with the pyridine and piperidine alkaloids. Cytisine stimulates nicotinic ganglions. Common toxic plants in this group include golden chain tree *(Laburnum anagyroides)*, Kentucky coffee tree *(Gymnocladus dioica)*, necklace pod sophora *(Sophora tomentosa)*, and mescal bean bush *(Sophora secundiflora)* (Figure 48-8) (see Hallucinogenic Plants). Structures follow:

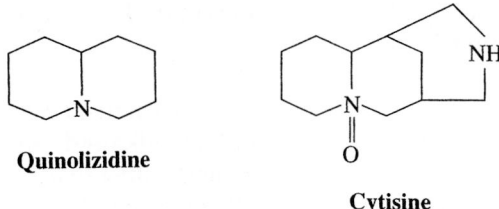

Quinolizidine

Cytisine

TREATMENT. Treatment of nicotinic syndromes consists of supportive care with particular attention to airway protection and ventilation. Administration of activated charcoal is generally recommended. Benzodiazepines and barbiturates are given for seizures. Adequate urine output is maintained, with consideration of urine alkalinization. Treating initial excessive adrenergic stimulation with phentolamine is ill advised because this complicates the nicotinic blockade that follows. Symptomatic bradycardia can be treated with atropine and hypotension with IV fluids and inotropic agents (e.g., dopamine) if needed.[88] With liver or renal failure, supportive treatment may be required for days.

Hallucinogenic Plants (Indoles, Phenylalkylamines). About 90 of the 800,000 plant species are hallucinogenic. Numerous rituals and religious ceremonies have used these plants. Many psychoactive plants are indole derivatives, which are among the most potent psychoactive compounds in nature and have the following structure:

Indole nucleus

Chemical relationships exist among serotonin, psilocybin *(Psilocybe* spp.), and *D*-lysergic acid diethylamide (LSD). LSD is synthesized from ergonovine (or ergometrine), derived from *Claviceps purpurea*. Striking structural similarities exist between the most potent psychoactive plant compounds and biochemically important neurotransmitters, as follows:

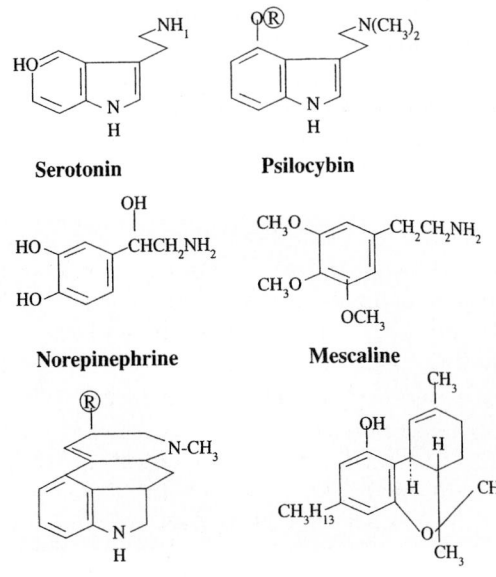

Serotonin   **Psilocybin**

Norepinephrine   **Mescaline**

Lysergic acid diethylamide   **Tetrahydrocannabinol**

ERGOT. The ergot alkaloids, ergonovine and ergotamine, are indole derivatives found in the fungus *C. purpurea* that infects rye and other grains. In the Middle Ages, epidemics of ergotism resulted from ergot-contaminated breads. Ergotism is a vasospastic condition with two forms, convulsive and gangrenous. Hallucinations can occur with both forms. In the ninth century a disease known as "St. Anthony's fire" was epidemic, consisting of burning limb pain and eventual loss of limb sensation, followed by gangrene and autoamputation of charcoal-black limbs. People migrated to St. Anthony's Order, a society of monks, and began to heal, largely because they received a diet free of ergot-contaminated grains. Neurologic ergotism manifests as diaphoresis, nausea, vomiting, formication, and convulsions. An outbreak of ergotism occurred in Ethiopia in 1977.[23,24,65,140]

Commercial grains are now inspected for the presence of ergot, and inadvertent poisoning is rare. Ergot derivatives are potent vasoconstrictors and oxytocic agents and are used medicinally for vascular headaches and for obstetric and gynecologic disorders.

MORNING GLORY. The active component of the naturally occurring hallucinogen found in the seeds of morning glory (*Ipomoea violacea*) (Figure 48-9) is ergine, or (+)-lysergic acid amide, an indole derivative.[59] About 300 seeds, or enough to fill a cupped hand, are equivalent to 200 to 300 mg of LSD, with similar systemic and hallucinatory effects. Ingestion of Hawaiian baby woodrose seeds (*Argyrlia nervosa*) presents similarly.[56]

NUTMEG. *Myristica fragrans* is used to make the spices nutmeg and mace. Mature rinds of the fruit split, revealing a bright-red fringed fleshy coating on the outside of its seed. The coating contains mace, and the seed contains nutmeg. Nutmeg contains myristicin, which has an indolelike structure and is metabolized to amphetamine-like compounds. Other alkylbenzene derivatives, such as safrole and elemicin, are also found in nutmeg. Nutmeg has been abused for its alleged hallucinogenic effects. A person who ingested one grated nutmeg (7 g)

had weakness, loss of coordination, vertigo, fainting, nausea, and paresthesias but no hallucinations.[127,141]

CANNABIS. Cannabis preparations are largely derived from the female *Cannabis sativa* plant. The primary psychoactive component is δ-9-tetrahydrocannabinol (THC), which is most concentrated in the flowering tops. Marijuana generally contains 0.5% to 5% THC; however, Sinsemilla and Netherwood varieties may contain up to 20% THC, and hashish and hashish oils have higher concentrations. Cannabinoids can be smoked or ingested. A typical marijuana cigarette contains 0.5 to 1.0 g of cannabis, and the THC delivered varies from 20% to 70%, with a bioavailability of 5% to 24%. As little as 2 mg of available THC produces effects in occasional users.[66]

Cannabinoids bind to specific cannabinoid receptors in areas of the brain involved with cognition, memory reward, pain perception, and motor coordination. Cannabinoids act as neuromodulators in the release and action of neurotransmitters (e.g., acetylcholine, glutamate).[43,66] Endogenous ligands for these receptors are endocannabinoids. The first endocannabinoid identified is anandamide, after the Sanskrit word *ananda*, which means "bliss."

Desirable effects include mild mood-altering qualities, euphoria, alteration in perceptions, time distortion, and intensification of ordinary sensory experiences (e.g., gustatory, visual, and auditory sensations). Adverse effects include impairment of short-term memory and attention, impairment of motor skills and reaction times, and anxiety. Psychotic symptoms have been reported in persons vulnerable to psychosis. Clinically, tachycardia may occur within minutes of THC exposure and may last a few hours. Minor changes in blood pressure may also occur. No confirmed deaths have been reported from cannabis poisoning.[66]

PEYOTE. The hallucinogenic peyote cactus, *Lophophora williamsii* (Figure 48-10), contains alkaloids that are phenylethylamines or isoquinolines rather than indoles. Mescaline (3,4,5-trimethoxy-β-phenylethylamine), the

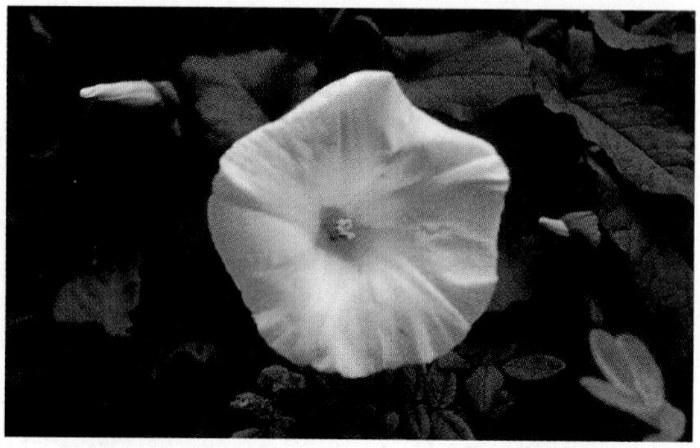

Figure 48-9 Morning glory (*Ipomoea violacea*).

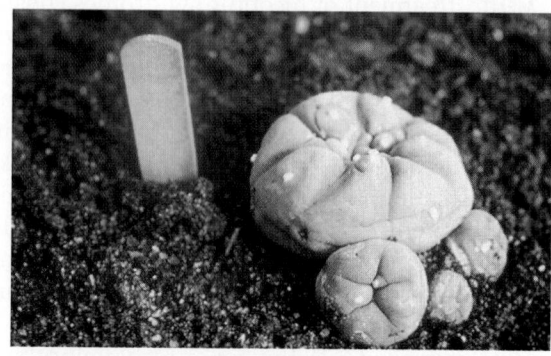

Figure 48-10 Peyote (*Lophophora williamsii*).

primary psychoactive component of peyote, is structurally similar to the neurotransmitters norepinephrine and epinephrine and to hallucinogenic amphetamines. Pharmacologically, however, mescaline is similar to hallucinogenic indoles. Mescaline may affect the action of norepinephrine and serotonin, evidenced clinically by sympathomimetic effects, followed by marked visual hallucinations. Mescaline produces a slight rise in blood pressure and heart rate, tachypnea, hyperreflexia, mydriasis, ataxia, perspiration, flushing, salivation, and urination. No deaths have been reported from peyote poisoning. Type B botulism was associated with consumption of a ceremonial tea made from peyote that was stored in a jar by members of the Native American Church. Affected members had bilaterally symmetric, flaccid weakness in all extremities, dysphagia, nasal speech, and diplopia.[4,69]

MESCAL BEAN BUSH. The mescal bean bush or Texas mountain laurel (*Sophora secundiflora*) of the pea family (Fabaceae) contains hallucinogenic dark-red beans (mescal beans; see Figure 48-8). The beans contain the toxic alkaloid cytisine, which causes nausea, convulsions, numbing sensations, hallucinations, unconsciousness, and death through respiratory failure. The beans may be boiled in water and the mixture consumed, producing a delirium or "visionary trance." The origin of mescalism in modern peyote religion is debated. Mescal beans are worn during some peyote ceremonies.[4]

KHAT. The evergreen khat tree, *Catha edulis*, grows in East Africa and Arabia. As early as 1237, khat was advocated in Arabic medical literature as a mood-elevating and hunger-suppressing agent. Khat leaves continue to be chewed for their stimulatory effects. Khat contains cathinone, cathine, and norephedrine. Cathinone (α-aminopropiophenone), a phenylalkylamine, is the major psychoactive constituent. Structurally, cathinone is similar to amphetamines, such as methcathinone synthesized from ephedrine. As with amphetamines, cathinone is an indirect sympathomimetic and induces the release of dopamine, serotonin, and norepinephrine.[76,146]

The structures of methcathinone and related drugs follow:

Methcathinone   **Cathinone**

Ephedrine

Cathinone is "diluted" in fresh plant material and must be extracted by masticating laboriously; this results in gradual absorption. As the leaf wilts, cathinone is converted to cathine, which has little activity. Because only fresh leaves produce the desired stimulatory effects, much khat use in the past was limited to countries where khat was produced (e.g., North Yemen, Ethiopia, Kenya); however, khat is now air-freighted to Europe and the United States. Freshly picked leaves are kept damp and often wrapped in banana leaves during transport.[44]

Desirable effects of khat include increased energy and alertness, feelings of increased endurance and self-esteem, and euphoria. Cathinone has both positive chronotropic and inotropic effects. Tachycardia, increased blood pressure, and mydriasis are seen. Adverse effects include hypomania, delusions, and paranoid psychosis. Khat is known to be habit-forming and has been classified as a "substance of abuse" by the World Health Organization. A person who developed abdominal pain was found to have immature *Fasciola hepatica* (fluke infestation of the biliary tree), thought to be secondary to use of contaminated khat.[2,44,76,78,146]

ANTICHOLINERGIC PLANTS. Henbane (*Hyosyamus niger*), jimsonweed (*Datura stramonium*), and mandrake (*Mandragora officinarum*) contain tropane alkaloids and can produce hallucinations, as discussed earlier.

TREATMENT. Treatment of patients exposed to hallucinogenic plants is generally supportive. First-line treatment for agitation is generally benzodiazepines.

Sedating Plants (Isoquinoline Alkaloids)

POPPY. *Papaver somniferum* flowers are large and white with purple stain at the base of each petal. They yield opium, a complex of more than 20 alkaloids, including morphine, codeine, and papaverine. Morphine was the first plant alkaloid isolated, by pharmacist Friederich Wilhelm Adam Serturner in 1806.[64] Seeds of *P. somniferum* are used in various foods and beverages, including bagels, muffins, pastries, curry sauce, rice, and teas. Ingestion of poppy seeds can result in detectable levels of morphine and codeine by urine drug screen testing; however, significant opiate-induced impairment is not apparent. Poppy dependence has been described.[15,80,96,106,138]

Convulsant Plants (Indoles, Resins)

STRYCHNINE. Strychnine, an indole found in seeds of the tree *Strychnos nux-vomica*, is a powerful CNS stimulant that competes with the inhibitory neurotransmitter glycine, producing an excitatory state with hyperreflexia, severe muscle spasm, and apparent convulsions. Children may be poisoned after accidental ingestion of rat poisons containing strychnine. Strychnine continues to be used as a suicidal and homicidal agent.[16,112] Treatment comprises decontamination and support, including activated charcoal, benzodiazepines, barbiturates, and chemical paralysis, with endotracheal intubation and mechanical ventilation for severe toxicity. Rhabdomyolysis and acidosis may occur and require treatment.[104] Occasionally, death ensues despite aggressive management.[72]

WATER HEMLOCK. Water hemlock *(Cicuta maculata)* and chinaberry *(Melia azedarach)* are two of the most toxic resin-containing plants. Chinaberry produces primarily GI symptoms (see below). The resin of *C. maculata*, an unsaturated aliphatic alcohol called cicutoxin, possesses convulsive properties and has the following structure:

$$CH_2 - CH_2 - CH_2 - (C \equiv C)_2 - (CH = CH)_3$$
$$| \qquad\qquad\qquad\qquad\qquad\qquad |$$
$$OH \qquad\qquad\qquad\qquad\qquad CH(OH)$$
$$| $$
$$C_3H_7$$

Cicutoxin

Nine subspecies of *Cicuta* of the Umbelliferae family are poisonous (Figure 48-11). *C. virosa* is common European water hemlock, whereas *C. maculata* and *C. douglasii* are found in North America. *Oenanthe crocata*, or hemlock water dropwort, also contains cicutoxin and is found in Europe and North America. Common names for *Cicuta* species include cowbane, five-finger root, snake weed, wild carrot, dead man's fingers, death-of-man, poison parsnip, wild parsnip, beaver poison, children's bane, muskrat weed, spotted hemlock, spotted cowbane, musquash root, false parsley, fever root, mockeel root, wild dill, spotted parsley, and *carottee a moreau*. Roots have a parsnip- or carrot-like odor, and *Cicuta* is often mistaken for an edible plant. Mature roots have air-filled chambers and are found on the ends of hollow stems. All parts of the plant are toxic, but the roots contain the highest concentration of cicutoxin. Ingestion of as little as 2 to 3 cm of the root may be fatal to an adult. The plant is most toxic in the spring.[29,55,131]

Early symptoms include muscarinic effects and are primarily GI, including abdominal pain, vomiting, and diarrhea; however, profuse perspiration, salivation, and respiratory distress may be seen. Nicotinic effects are less prominent (see Figure 48-3). Tachycardia and hypertension or bradycardia and hypotension may be seen. Epileptiform seizure activity or spastic and tonic movements, including opisthotonus without electroencephalographic (EEG) seizure activity, may occur with severe poisoning. Pupils may be any size. Rhabdomyolysis and renal failure have been reported. Laboratory abnormalities include metabolic acidosis, elevated CK, and elevated liver transaminases (LFTs).[7,29,55,99,116,131]

A typical clinical presentation is illustrated by a 23-year-old man who was foraging for wild ginseng in the woods of midcoast Maine. He found plants growing in a swampy area and took three bites from the root of one plant. Within 30 minutes, he vomited and began to convulse. Just over an hour after the ingestion, he was unresponsive, cyanotic, and tachycardic, with mydriasis and profuse salivation. Apnea, requiring endotracheal intubation, followed severe tonic-clonic seizures. Ventricular fibrillation occurred, and he died within 3 hours of ingesting the root later identified as *C. maculata*.[29]

TREATMENT. Treatment is symptomatic and supportive with particular attention to the airway. Activated charcoal is recommended, with benzodiazepines and barbiturates for seizure control. Adequate urine output maintenance and alkalinization of urine are initiated to treat rhabdomyolysis.[55,131]

Other Alkaloids. *Gelsemium sempervirens* (Carolina or yellow jessamine) is a woody perennial evergreen vine with fragrant yellow flowers. It contains multiple in-

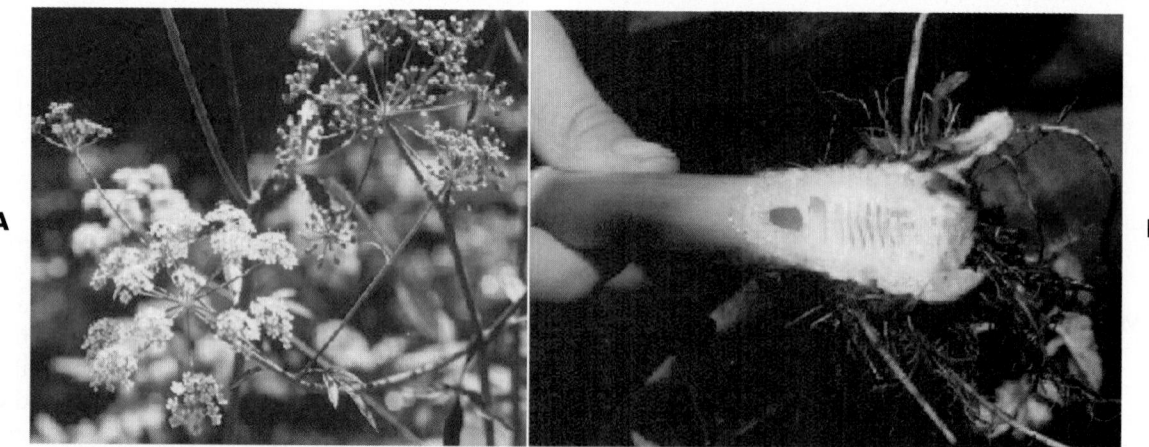

Figure 48-11 *Cicuta* species have characteristic flowering tops, typical of the Umbelliferae family **(A)**, and roots with air-filled chambers at the end of hollow stems **(B)**. *(Courtesy Steven Curry, MD.)*

dole alkaloids, including gelsemine, gelseminine, and gelsemoidin. Gelsemine binds to acetylcholine receptors at the neuromuscular junction (peripheral nicotinic acetylcholine receptors) and, to a lesser extent, at muscarinic receptors. A toddler who ate the blossoms of *G. sempervirens* experienced neuromuscular blockade with ataxia, dysarthria, facial and extremity weakness, bilateral ptosis, and transient coma. The child recovered without sequelae.[20]

Cardiovascular System (Box 48-3)

Cardiotoxins that Inhibit Na$^+$-K$^+$ ATPase (Cardiac Glycosides). More than 200 naturally occurring cardiac glycosides have been identified. Plant cardiac glycosides are composed of a steroid backbone, an attached five-membered unsaturated lactone ring (six-membered for *Helleborus*), and either a carbohydrate or sugar moiety in glycosidic linkage. The toxic aglycones are released by acid and enzymatic hydrolysis. The attached sugar moiety has no inherent cardiac action but may enhance solubility, absorption, and toxicity of the aglycone moiety. Cardiac glycosides bind to the membrane-bound enzyme, Na$^+$-K$^+$ ATPase, increasing intracellular Na$^+$ and Ca^{2+} levels and automaticity (Figure 48-12). Cardiac glycosides are found in *Digitalis purpurea* (foxglove; Figure 48-13), *D. lanata*, *Nerium oleander* (common oleander; Figure 48-14), *Thevetia peruviana* (yellow oleander; Figure 48-15), *Convallaria majalis* (lily of the valley; Figure 48-16), *Urginea maritima* (squill or sea onion; Figure 48-17), *U. indica*, *Strophanthus gratus* (ouabain), *Asclepias* species (balloon cotton, red-headed cotton-bush milkweeds), *Calotropis procera* (king's crown), *Carissa spectabilis* (wintersweet), *C. acokanthera* (bushman's poison), *Cerebera manghas* (sea mango), *Plumeria rubra* (frangipani), *Cryptostegia grandifolia* (rubber vine), *Euonymus eruopaeus* (spindle tree), *Cheiranthus, Erysimum* (wallflower), and *Hellaborus niger* (henbane).[47,49,55,63,65,87,110,137]

FOXGLOVE. Withering reported the medical use of extracts of *Digitalis purpurea* based on a recipe for treating "dropsy."[110] *Digitalis purpurea* grows wild in parts of the United States and is cultivated as a garden ornamental plant. Recently, *D. lanata* was mistakenly substituted for plantain in herbal products, with resultant human cardiotoxicity.[128] *D. lanata* contains lanatosides A, B, and C, which yield digoxin and digitoxin. *D. purpurea* contains only digitoxin, not digoxin. Digitoxin from *D. purpurea* is still used, although digoxin extracted from *D. lanata* is used more often.[19]

OLEANDER. All parts of *Nerium oleander* and *Thevetia peruviana* are toxic, but the seeds contain more glycoside than other parts of the plant.[55,87] Yellow oleander (*T. peruviana*), a native plant of tropical America, grows abundantly in the United States. Seeds of yellow oleander are known as "lucky nuts." Popular in suicidal ingestions in Sri Lanka, yellow oleander contains the

cardiac glycosides thevetin A and B, thevetoxin, neriifolin, peruviside, ruvoside, and others. Of patients admitted with *T. peruviana* poisoning in Sri Lanka, 43% had arrhythmias, many requiring temporary pacing; 6% died shortly after admission.[47] Common oleander (*N. oleander*), a native plant of the Mediterranean, grows abundantly in the United States. Common oleander contains the principal cardiac glycosides oleandrin and neriine, as well as folinerin and digitoxigenin.[19,87,110] Severe toxicity has been reported after the consumption of unprocessed common oleander leaves and prepared teas.[60,102]

SQUILL. *Urignea maritima* was used by ancient Egyptians and Romans as a diuretic, heart tonic, expectorant, emetic, and rat poison. Squill contains several cardiac

---

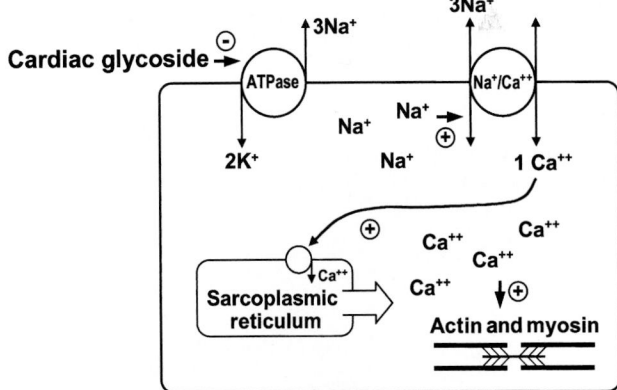

Figure 48-12 Cardiac glycosides bind to and inhibit the membrane-bound enzyme Na$^+$-K$^+$ ATPase in cardiac myocytes (shown), baroreceptor cells, and skeletal muscle cells. Inhibition of Na$^+$-K$^+$ ATPase in cardiac myocytes results in accumulation of intracellular Na$^+$, which results in accumulation of Ca^{2+} within myocytes via Na$^+$-Ca^{2+} exchangers. The resultant increase in intracellular Ca^{2+} stimulates further release of Ca^{2+} from the sarcoplasmic reticulum. The increased intracellular Ca^{2+} interacts with troponin C of the actin-myosin complex to cause increased contractions, seen as increased automaticity (e.g., premature ventricular contractions on electrocardiograms). Inhibition of membrane-bound enzyme Na$^+$-K$^+$ ATPase in baroreceptor cells and skeletal muscle cells contributes to increased vagal tone and hyperkalemia, respectively.

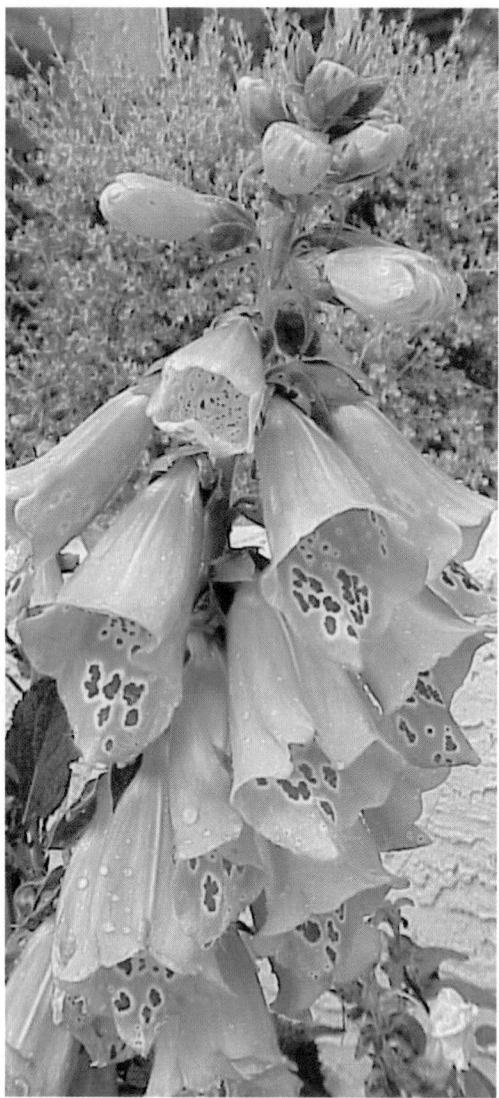

Figure 48-13 *Digitalis purpurea* (foxglove). *(Courtesy Kimberlie Graeme, MD, and Steven Curry, MD.)*

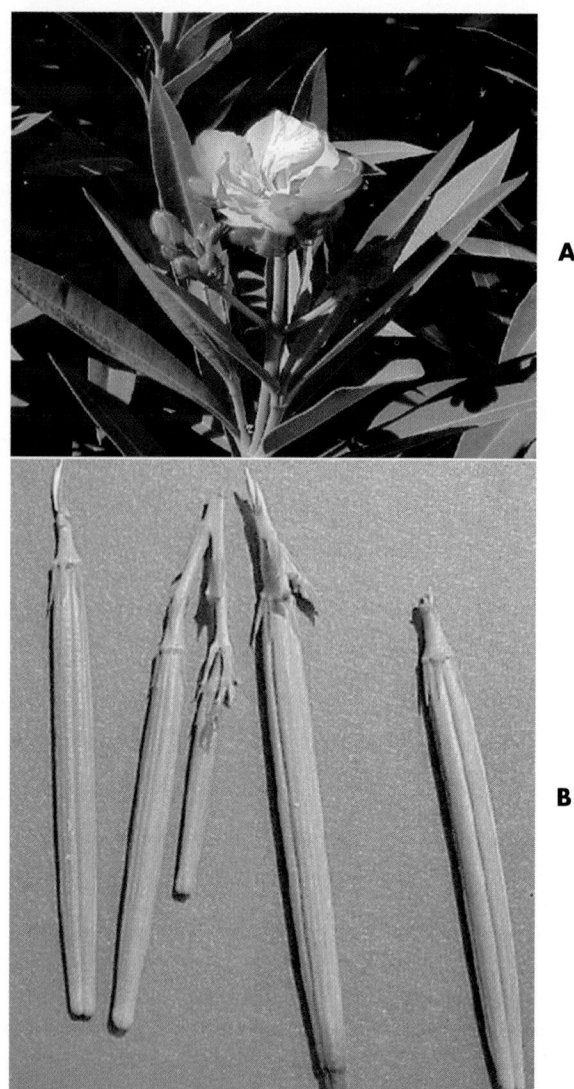

Figure 48-14 *Nerium oleander* (common oleander) plants may have white or pink flowers **(A)** and have long, narrow seedpods **(B).** *(Courtesy Kimberlie Graeme, MD.)*

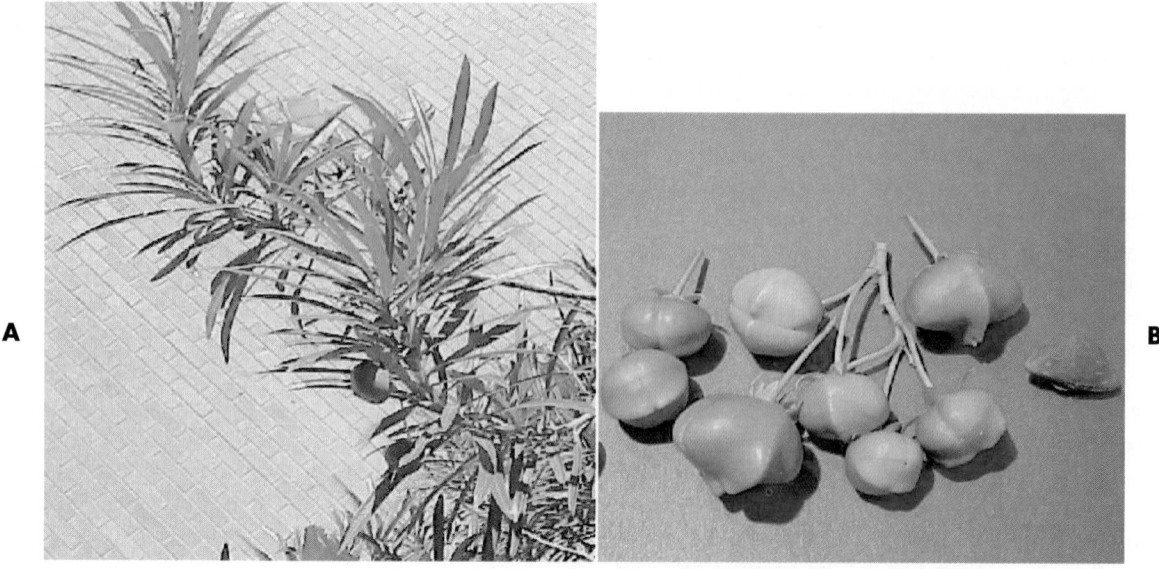

Figure 48-15 *Thevetia peruviana* (yellow oleander) has yellow flowers **(A)** with smooth seedpods, known as "lucky nuts," comprising green flesh surrounding a hard brown seed **(B).** *(Courtesy Kimberlie Graeme, MD.)*

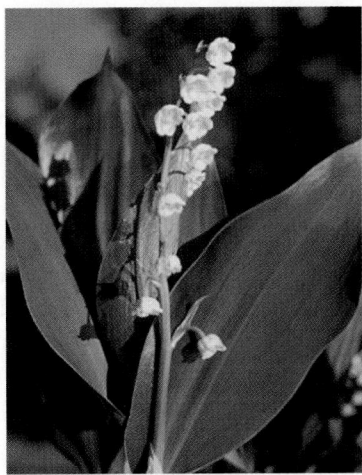

Figure 48-16 Lilly of the Valley *(Convallaria majalis). (Courtesy Donald Kunkel, MD.)*

glycosides, including scillaren A, glucoscillaren A, scillaridin A, and scilliroside.[137,143]

CLINICAL PRESENTATION. The onset and duration of action is well known for certain glycoside preparations, such as digoxin, digitoxin, and ouabain, but may vary considerably after plant ingestions. For example, oleandrin exhibits protracted binding times to cardiac myocardial tissues.[87] Generally, cardiac glycoside toxicity produces nausea, vomiting, visual changes (yellow and green colors, geometric shapes, scintillations), mental status changes (disorientation, lethargy, stupor, dysarthria, weakness, dizziness, seizures), cardiac disturbances (palpitations, bradycardia, atrioventricular block, extrasystoles, ventricular arrhythmias), hyperkalemia, and death. When death occurs, it is generally caused by cardiotoxicity. ECGs may reveal nonspecific ST-segment and T-wave changes, similar to digoxin-induced changes.[60,128] Serum digoxin levels (polyclonal digoxin immunoassays) may be elevated after exposure to plants containing cardiac glycosides, because antibody-based digoxin assays cross-react with various cardiac glycosides, nonquantitatively. Digoxin immunoassays predict only the presence of the glycoside, not the degree of toxicity.[63,87,137]

TREATMENT. Cardiac glycoside toxicity from plant ingestions have been successfully treated with activated charcoal to limit enterohepatic circulation, cardiac pacing, antiarrhythmic agents, and digoxin-specific Fab fragments (e.g., Digibind). Maintenance of fluid and electrolyte balance is important. Theoretically, administration of exogenous calcium could be harmful because of high intracellular calcium concentrations that might cause the heart to perform one final contraction without relaxation, a state termed "stone heart."[83] Phenytoin and lidocaine have been used to treat arrhythmias. In theory, digoxin-specific Fab antibody

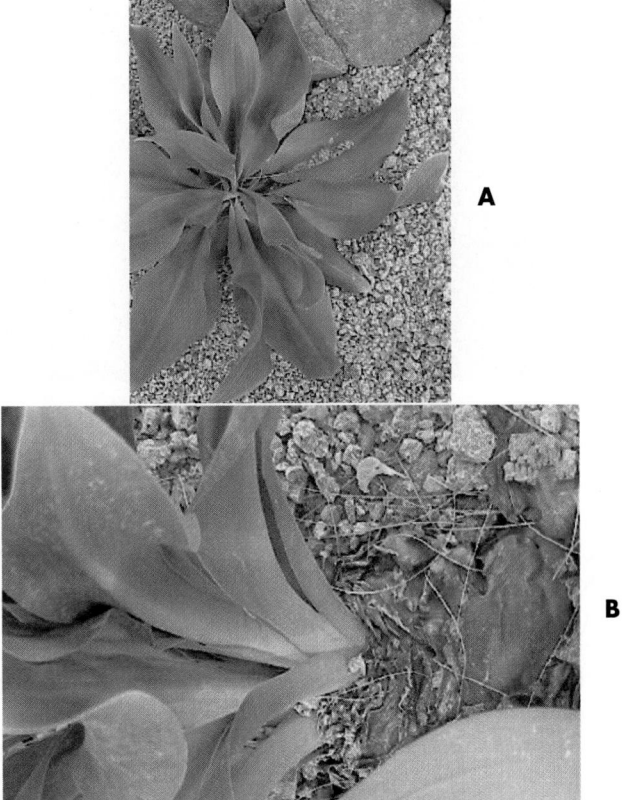

Figure 48-17 *Urginea* spp. (squill or sea onion) have broad leaves **(A)** and a red, underground bulb **(B).** *(Courtesy Kimberlie Graeme, MD, and Donald Kunkel, MD.)*

fragments could couple to circulating cardiac glycosides and limit binding of cardiac glycosides to Na^+-K^+ ATPase. The administration of digoxin-specific Fab to reverse cardiotoxicity from plant glycosides remains controversial.[34,60,87,103,113,128]

Cardiotoxins that Open Sodium Channels (Steroid Alkaloids, Resins). Steroid alkaloids form principal toxic components of several common cardiotoxic plants: monkshood (*Aconitum* spp.), American hellebore *(Veratrum viride),* and death camas (*Zigadenus* spp.). Aconite is found in *Aconitum* species, and veratrum alkaloids are found in *Veratrum viride* (false or American hellebore), *V. californicum* (skunk cabbage), *V. album* (white hellebore), *V. japonicum, Zigadenus paniculatus* (death camas), *Z. venenosus, Z. nuttallii,* and *Z. gramineus.*

ACONITE. Recently, aconite poisonings have become more common secondary to the use of *Aconitum* species in herbal products, including *A. napellus* (monkshood; Figure 48-18), *A. carmichaeli* (chuanwa), *A. brachypodum, A. vulparia,* and *A. kusnexoffii* (caowu). *Delphinium* species (larkspur) demonstrate similar toxicity. All parts of these plants are toxic. *Aconitum* species contain diterpenoid-ester alkaloids, particularly aconitine, but

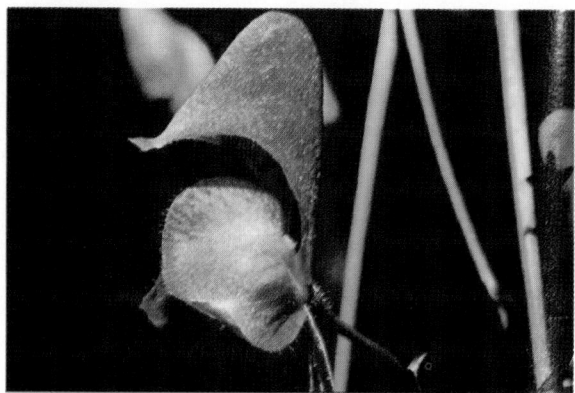

Figure 48-18 Monkshood (*Aconitum* species).

also mesaconitine and hypaconitine. Boiling these plants in water hydrolyzes aconite alkaloids into less toxic benzoylaconine and aconine derivatives.[22,31,32,55,134]

Aconite alkaloids activate sodium channels and affect excitable membranes of cardiac, neural, and muscle tissues. Enhancement of the transmembrane inward sodium current during the plateau phase of the action potential prolongs repolarization in cardiac myocytes and induces delayed and early afterdepolarizations. Delayed afterdepolarizations result in increased automaticity, such as premature ventricular beats. Early afterdepolarizations produce lengthening of the QT interval.

Symptoms begin within 3 minutes to 6 hours of ingestion and may persist for several days. Nonspecific GI symptoms (nausea, vomiting), salivation, diaphoresis, dyspnea, and restlessness are accompanied by cardiotoxicity and CNS toxicity. Cardiac effects are clinically similar to cardiac glycoside toxicity, with enhanced vagal tone, bradycardia, heart block, ectopic beats, supraventricular tachycardia, bundle branch block, junctional escape rhythms, ventricular tachycardia, bifascicular ventricular tachycardia, polymorphic ventricular tachycardia, torsades de pointes, ventricular fibrillation, asystole, and hypotension. Occasionally, death ensues, generally from ventricular arrhythmias, such as refractory ventricular fibrillation.[22,31,55,134]

Hypaconitine affects sodium channels of the nerve membrane more selectively than aconitine and is more potent than aconitine and mesaconitine in producing neuromuscular block.[32] These neurotoxins produce conduction block and paralysis through voltage-sensitive sodium channels in axons. Prolonged depolarization prevents repolarization of excitable membranes.[31] Visual impairment, dizziness, vertigo, ataxia, paresthesias (e.g., numbness of mouth and extremities), hyporeflexia, weakness, profound tetraplegia, coma, and convulsions may occur.

Elevated CK levels, without evidence of myocardial infarction, may occur. Hypokalemia, metabolic or respiratory acidosis, respiratory alkalosis, and renal and hepatic impairment may be noted.[22,134]

VERATRUM ALKALOIDS. *Veratrum* and *Zigadenus* species belong to the lily family. *Veratrum* species may be found in some sneezing powders and have been accidentally ingested when mistaken for *Gentiana lutea* and for *Phytolacca americana* (pokeweed). *Zigadenus* species have been accidentally ingested when mistaken for nontoxic wild onions. Veratrum alkaloids include protoveratrine, veratridine, and jervine, which are found within the entire plant, although the bulb and flower usually cause toxicity. These alkaloids are extremely toxic and rapidly increase the permeability of voltage-sensitive sodium channels in excitable cell membranes. This results in an initial depolarization and subsequent loss of membrane potential. Stimulation of vagal fibers may result in bradycardia and hypotension.[55,71,75,109]

Symptoms generally occur within 30 minutes to 3 hours and resolve within 24 to 48 hours. Toxicity is characterized by diaphoresis, nausea, vomiting, diarrhea, abdominal pain, hypotension, bradycardia, and shock. Scotomata, paresthesias, fasciculations, muscle spasticity, hyperreflexia, vertigo, ataxia, syncope, respiratory depression, coma, seizures, and death may also occur. ECG findings may mimic cardiac glycoside toxicity, including repolarization abnormalities (e.g., abnormal T waves and ST segments), sinoatrial and atrioventricular blocks, and prolonged QT intervals.

TREATMENT. Treatment of cardiotoxic steroid alkaloid poisoning is supportive and includes atropine, crystalloid fluids, and vasopressors. Victims may require mechanical ventilation and cardiopulmonary resuscitation.[134] Magnesium may suppress early afterdepolarizations and polymorphic ventricular tachycardia.[55]

GRAYANOTOXINS. Resins called grayanotoxins are found in rhododendrons, mountain laurels, and azaleas. Grayanotoxins produce toxicity similar to the steroid alkaloids, veratrum and aconite, by binding to myocardial sodium channels and increasing their permeability. Poisoning may result from the ingestion of leaves, flowers, or nectar; however, grayanotoxin-contaminated honey is the most common source.[86,147] The nectar of *Rhododendron* species contains the grayanotoxin *O*-acetyl-andromedol, or andromedotoxin, which is transferred to humans through consumption of honey produced by bees utilizing the nectar.[65] Poisonings still occur in the Turkish population of Central Europe. Symptoms include salivation, emesis, hypotension, bradycardia, arrhythmias, circumoral and extremity paresthesias, incoordination, and muscular weakness.

Other Cardiotoxins

TAXANE ALKALOIDS. *Taxus* species include *T. baccata* (English yew) and *T. brevifolia* (Western yew). The toxic alkaloids include taxine A, B, and C. All parts of *Taxus* plants are toxic except the pulp, or aril, which contains very little taxine. The seeds, which are surrounded by the aril, may be toxic if chewed sufficiently to allow absorption of taxine. Taxine B, believed to be the primary cardiotoxic alkaloid, inhibits both calcium and sodium transport across cell membranes.[85,89,142]

Most *Taxus* exposures occur in children, are accidental, and are not associated with significant toxicity. However, serious toxicity and death have occurred after intentional ingestions of *Taxus* species.[36] Although GI toxicity is most common, severe toxicity is characterized by arrhythmias.[85,142] Previously reported yew-induced arrhythmias are consistent with arrhythmias induced by blockade of voltage-gated sodium channels, being described as bradycardic rhythms with wide QRS complexes, despite normal electrolytes. Sodium channel blockade may be the primary cause of yew-induced arrhythmias. A patient who ingested yew plant, with severe cardiotoxicity and a wide QRS complex, responded favorably to administration of hypertonic sodium bicarbonate.[97] Lidocaine administration and cardiac pacing have also been reported to be beneficial in the treatment of yew-induced cardiotoxicity. The antineoplastic drug paclitaxel (Taxol) is made from an alkaloid extracted from the bark of the Western yew.[142] Taxol is also cardiotoxic.

PURINE ALKALOIDS. The purine alkaloids caffeine and theobromine are found in various plants, but the derivative beverages and stimulants represent a toxic risk. Theobromine is especially toxic to dogs. Even cacao bean shells contain potentially toxic quantities of theobromine, and dogs that ingest large quantities of bean shells may suffer convulsions and death.

Oral and Gastrointestinal System

Gastrointestinal Irritants (Resins, Alkaloids) (Box 48-4)
CHINABERRY TREES. *Melia azedarach* plants (Figure 48-19) are found throughout the southern United States and Hawaii. Chinaberry trees, also known as China, Texas umbrella or white cedar trees, contain tetranortriterpens (resins), identified as meliatoxins A_1, A_2, B_1, and B_2, that are enterotoxic and neurotoxic. The exact mechanisms of these toxins have yet to be determined. Gastroenteritis can occur after ingestion of any part of the plant but typically occurs after the berries are ingested by children. Immature berries are green but turn yellow and wrinkle with age. After ingestion of as little as one berry, severe gastroenteritis and often bloody diarrhea ensue. Symptoms may be rapid or delayed for several hours after ingestion. Death has been reported in children after the ingestion of the African variety of chinaberry tree.[68] Treatment is supportive, with replacement of fluids and electrolytes and administration of activated charcoal. If hypotension ensues, it generally responds to IV fluids.

SOLANUM. The *Solanum* species are the largest group of steroid alkaloid–containing plants and include

---

Box 48-4 PLANTS PRODUCING GASTROINTESTINAL SYSTEM TOXICITY

ALKALOIDS
Amine (e.g., colchicine)
Isoquinoline and quinoline (e.g., emetine in ipecac)
Pyrrolizidine
Steroid (e.g., solanine)

GLYCOSIDES
Anthraquinone
Coumarin
Saponin (e.g., phytolaccatoxin)

RESINS
Cicutoxin
Meliatoxins

PHYTOTOXINS
Abrin
Curcin
Ricin

S. tuberosum (potato), *S. gracile* (wild tomato), *S. carolinense* (horse nettle), *S. pseudocapsicum* (Jerusalem cherry), *S. dulcamara* (woody nightshade), *S. americum* (black nightshade), and other nightshade plants. *Solanum* species are used medicinally in some countries.[39,58] Solanine, a glycoalkaloid with a steroidlike moiety, is found throughout the plants but is most concentrated in unripe fruits. Solanine, which has been isolated from more than 1700 different *Solanum* species, generally produces gastroenteritis, but bradycardia, weakness, and CNS and respiratory depression may be seen.[27] Treatment is supportive, with replacement of fluids and electrolytes and administration of activated charcoal. If hypotension ensues, it generally responds to IV fluids. Atropine may be beneficial if bradycardia develops. Spontaneous recovery usually occurs in 1 to 3 days.

SAPONIN GLYCOSIDES (POKEWEED). Saponin glycosides are found throughout the plant kingdom, contained within English ivy (*Hedera helix*), pokeweed (*Phytolacca americana*), tung tree (*Aleurites* spp.), ginseng (*Panax ginseng* or *quinquefolium*), and licorice (*Glycyrrhiza glabra*).[55] Saponins may induce lysis of erythrocytes, causing hemolytic anemia. In addition, saponins are GI irritants that facilitate their own intestinal absorption. Most saponins are found in combination with other toxins, resulting in diverse clinical syndromes.

Phytolacca americana, or *P. decandra*, may be mistaken for horseradish, parsnips, or Jerusalem artichoke. Pokeweed is commonly known as Virginia poke, inkberry, pocan, pigeonberry, American cancer-root, garget, red ink, American nightshade, scoke, jalap, and redwood. *P. americana* has green leaves with red stalks. Berries are green when immature and turn deep purple with maturity. Pokeberries typically leave a purple stain. The root is the most toxic part of the plant. *P. americana* is ingested intentionally in pokeweed salad and pokeberry teas. When prepared for ingestion, leaves should be "parboiled," which entails boiling the leaves in wa-

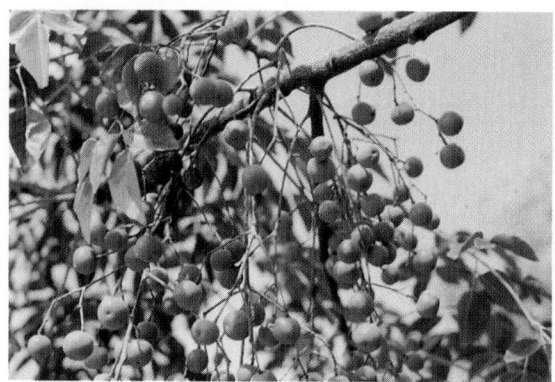

Figure 48-19 Chinaberry *(Melia azedarach). (Courtesy Donald Kunkel, MD.)*

ter that is discarded before boiling the leaves again and rinsing them with fresh water. Parboiling does not necessarily offer protection against toxicity.[55]

The saponin glycosides, phytolaccatoxin and phytolaccagenin, account for the GI injury, which manifests as fulminant gastroenteritis with vomiting and diarrhea 2 to 4 hours after ingestion. Diarrhea may appear foamy from the sudsing effect of saponin glycosides. Hypotension may follow significant GI fluid losses. Severe ingestions may result in weakness, loss of consciousness, seizures, and respiratory depression.[55]

P. americana also contains mitogenic, hemagluttinating, and antiviral proteins. Pokeweed mitogen may induce morphologic changes in lymphocytes and plasma cells. An increased number of circulating plasmablasts and proplasmacytes, eosinophilia, and thrombocytopenia can be seen after ingestion or handling of *P. americana* with broken skin. Pokeweed antiviral protein is a ribosome-inactivating protein being investigated for cancer treatment.[74]

Treatment for acute ingestion includes administration of activated charcoal and fluid replacement for dehydration secondary to GI losses. Airway support may be needed. Seizures should be treated with benzodiazepines. Hematologic changes generally resolve within weeks.[55]

ANTHRAQUINONE GLYCOSIDES. The aglycone moiety of this group is anthraquinone, which is known to have cathartic activity. Herbal teas that contain leaves, flowers, or bark of senna *(Cassia senna)*, leaves of aloe *(Aloe barbadensis)*, and bark of buckthorn *(Rhamnus frangula)* can cause severe diarrhea.[1] Treatment is supportive, emphasizing adequate volume and electrolyte replacement.

Toxins that Inhibit Protein Synthesis (Phytotoxins)

PHYTOTOXINS (RICIN, ABRIN). Phytotoxins are found in the families Fabaceae, including jequirity bean *(Abrus precatorius)*, which contains abrin, and Euphorbiaceae,

including the castor bean *(Ricinus communis)* (Figure 48-20, *A*), which contains ricin, and purging nut *(Jatropha curcas)*, which contains curcin. Poisoning results from eating or chewing on the nut or seed. Fresh, immature castor beans are encased within a soft, thorny, red seedpod. With age the seeds and surrounding seedpod become brown; seeds develop hard shells that are difficult to penetrate (Figure 48-20, *B*).[42]

Ricin, the phytotoxin found in castor beans, is a glycoprotein composed of two peptide chains, designated A and B, connected by a disulfide bond (see Figure 48-2). Chain B binds to the cell membrane, whereas chain A penetrates the cell by endocytosis and interferes with ribosomes and disrupts protein synthesis, leading to cell death.[3,30,42,79] The oral lethal dose is estimated to be 1 mg/kg, theoretically as little as one bean in a child and eight to ten in an adult.[145] Recently, a discrepancy between the serious toxicity of isolated ricin and the milder toxicity of ingested seeds of *Ricinus communis* has been recognized. A young adult consumed 10 to 15 seeds of *R. communis* and experienced severe crampy abdominal pain and vomiting 4 hours after ingestion, without GI bleeding or abdominal guarding. He received IV fluids, antiemetics, and charcoal. By the third day he had recovered completely. In contrast, a Bulgarian broadcaster who was injected with isolated ricin died from severe gastroenteritis and multiple organ failure.[3] Ingested *R. communis* is much less toxic than parenteral ricin. The degree of mastication of castor beans may determine the degree of toxicity seen with oral ingestions. Fresh seeds are likely more toxic than aged seeds that are enveloped by a hard coat. Although deaths have been reported with ingestions of a couple of seeds, toxicity is unlikely if mature seeds are swallowed whole.

Similarly, deaths have been reported after ingestion of fresh jequirity beans *(Abrus precatorius)*. Deaths occur 3 to 5 days after ingestion and are associated with cerebral edema and mucosal changes of the GI tract, including edema and hemorrhage of the Peyer's patches.[42]

Clinically, mild symptoms involve diarrhea alone. More severe symptoms include persistent vomiting, diarrhea, and abdominal pain, with associated hypovolemia and hypokalemia.[3] Hemorrhagic gastritis and bloody diarrhea may ensue. Dehydration may be associated with shock and hepatorenal dysfunction. Severely ill patients may present with hyperthermia, mental status changes, and seizures.[42] Systemic effects may be delayed as inhibition of protein synthesis occurs. Terminally, elevated serum LFTs and CK levels may be seen, indicating hepatorenal failure.[30,90,145]

TREATMENT. Treatment is supportive, including fluid and electrolyte replacement and activated charcoal administration. Patients who remain asymptomatic for 4

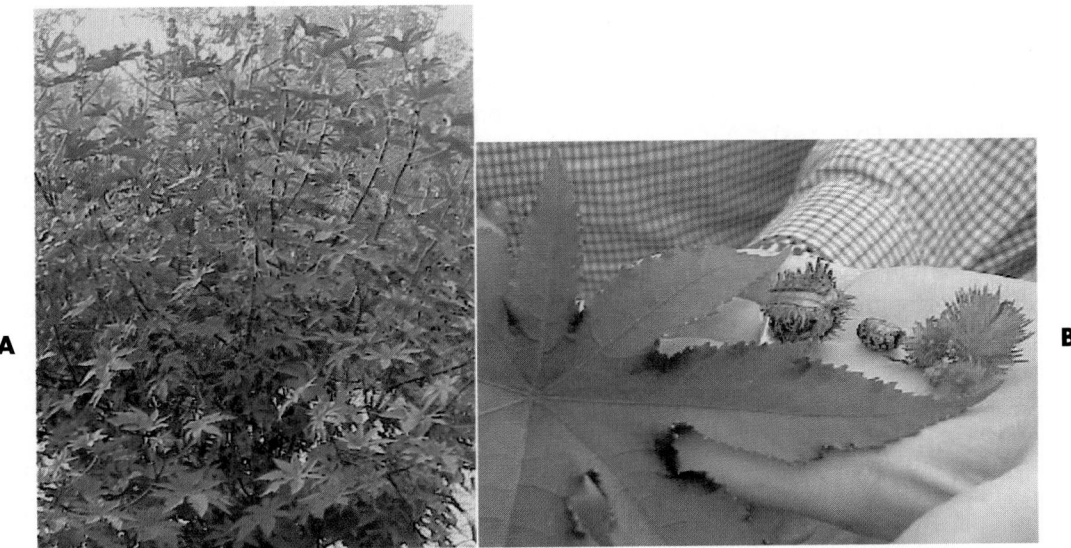

Figure 48-20 Castor bean plant *(Ricinus communis)* **(A),** which contains ricin, is characterized by broad, serrated leaves, with fresh beans encased within a soft, thorny, red seedpod. With age the seeds and surrounding seedpod become brown, and seeds develop hard shells that are difficult to penetrate **(B).** *(Courtesy Kimberlie Graeme, MD, and Donald Kunkel, MD.)*

to 6 hours after ingestion of seeds may be discharged, with instructions to return if symptoms develop. Before IV fluid resuscitation, mortality was as high as 8.1%; the rate has dropped to 0.4% since 1950.[3,30]

Toxins that Inhibit Cell Division (Amine Alkaloids)

Colchicine. *Colchicum autumnale*, from the family Liliaceae, is commonly known as autumn crocus, wild saffron, meadow saffron, naked lady, naked boy, and son-before-the-father.[73] It is found in Europe, America, and Asia. All parts of the plant contain colchicine, an amine alkaloid, but the highest concentrations are found in the underground bulb. Colchicine binds selectively and reversibly to microtubules, disrupting cell division, cell shape, mobility, and phagocytosis. Cells with the highest turnover, such as those of the GI mucosa and bone marrow, are affected most severely. Cell arrest in metaphase and abnormal nuclear morphology are seen at autopsy.[73]

Acute poisoning may occur after a latent period of several hours. Initial GI effects are severe abdominal pain, nausea, vomiting, and diarrhea, which may result in volume depletion and shock. Muscular weakness and ascending paralysis cause respiratory arrest, which may occur with a clear sensorium.[54]

Treatment. Treatment is symptomatic and supportive. Pulmonary function tests can be used to monitor respiratory function, assessing for fatigue and progressive ascending paralysis. Assisted ventilation is used as needed. Parenteral analgesics are given cautiously to relieve severe abdominal pain, since colchicine sensitizes patients to CNS depressants. Fluid and electrolyte replacement and occasionally blood component replacement may be necessary.[73] Maintain adequate urine output and assess for infection.

Hepatotoxic Agents: Pyrrolizidine Alkaloids. Plants containing pyrrolizidine alkaloids include *Senecio vulgaris* (groundsel), *S. longilobus* (gordolobo), *S. jacobaea* (tansy ragwort), *Symphytum officinale* (comfrey), *Gynura segetum*, *Ilex paraguanyensis* (mate), *Heliotropium*, *Crotalaria* (rattlebox), *Amsinckia intermedia* (fiddle neck or tar weed), *Baccharius pteronoides*, *Astragulus lentiginosus*, *Gnaphalium*, and *Adenotyles alliariae* (alpendost). These plants, especially when consumed as teas, are associated with hepatic veno-occlusive disease, hepatomegaly, cirrhosis, and Budd-Chiari syndrome. For example, *Senecio* and *Crotalaria*, which are used to make "bush tea" in Jamaica, have been associated with hepatotoxicity.[92,114,115,117,130]

Pyrrolizidine alkaloids act as alkylating agents and may be activated in the liver by cytochrome P450 and mixed-function oxidase systems to reactive pyrrolic metabolites that alkylate proteins and deoxyribonucleic acid (DNA).[98] Young victims seem more susceptible than adults. Ten milligrams of pyrrolizidine alkaloid are probably enough to produce acute or chronic veno-occlusive disease.[8] Veno-occlusive liver disease is characterized by nonthrombotic occlusion of the central veins of hepatic lobules. Histologic liver findings include central vein dilation, sinusoidal congestion, centrilobular necrosis, and fibrosis. Clinical evidence of intrahepatic portal hypertension may include ascites, painful hepatomegaly, weight gain, and jaundice.[13,114,130] Death may ensue. Treatment is supportive.

Occasionally, laparoscopic liver biopsy and hepatic and portal decompression are helpful in diagnosis and treatment, respectively.[92]

Oral Irritants (Glycosides, Oxalates)

DAPHNE. Coumarin glycosides produce effects similar to those of irritant glycoalkaloids of the steroid-alkaloid group. The only plant of significance is daphne (*Daphne mezereum*), with its fragrant succulent berries. The widely cultivated daphne represents a significant risk to curious children, in whom only a few ingested berries may be lethal.[90] The fruits contain a coumarin glycoside and a diterpene that irritate mucous membranes, with swelling of the tongue and lips. Blisters will form if berries are rubbed on the skin. Severe gastroenteritis with GI bleeding may occur.[49] In addition, progressive weakness, paralysis, seizures, and coma may develop. Treatment is supportive.

INSOLUBLE OXALATES. *Philodendron* and *Dieffenbachia* species (Araceae family) plant exposures are frequently reported.[84] These plants contain insoluble oxalates arranged in numerous needles of calcium oxalate (raphides) contained in specialized cells (idioblasts). When stimulated, as by mastication, idioblasts fire raphides that become embedded in exposed tissues, resulting in painful edema. These plants also contain trypsinlike proteases, histamine, and kininlike substances that may contribute to toxicity.[57,105]

Accidental ingestion of *Dieffenbachia* may result in painful edematous swelling, including angioedema. The victim may have dysphagia. *Dieffenbachia* is commonly known as dumbcane because of the victim's inability to speak after chewing the plant. Vesicle, bullae, or ulcer formation of the oral mucous membranes or oropharyngeal and esophageal erosions may be noted. Sudden death has been reported. Treatment is supportive, with special attention to maintaining a patent airway.[57,93,100,105]

Renal System

Soluble oxalates are found in rhubarb (*Rheum rhaponticum*) and sorrel (*Rumex*) plants. Soluble oxalates are rapidly absorbed through the GI tract. Generalized disturbance of monovalent and divalent cation metabolism occurs. Serum ionized calcium levels may drop rapidly. Weakness, tetany, hypotension, and seizures may develop. Acute renal failure may occur if calcium oxalate precipitates in urine and obstructs the renal tubules.[51,81,82,119] The structures of oxalates follow:

$$\begin{array}{ccc}
\text{COOH} & \text{COOK} & \text{COONa} \\
| & | & | \\
\text{COOH} & \text{COOH} & \text{COONa} \\
\textbf{Oxalic acid} & \textbf{Potassium oxalate} & \textbf{Sodium oxalate}
\end{array}$$

Sodium bicarbonate lavage should be avoided because of the risk of sodium oxalate formation. IV calcium gluconate is recommended for tetany, prolonged QT interval on ECG, or depressed serum ionized calcium. Urine output should be maintained to prevent deposition of calcium oxalate crystals in renal tubules.

Endocrine and Metabolic System

Plants that Induce Hypoglycemia: Ackee Fruit.

Blighia sapida, or ackee (akee) fruit, trees are indigenous to West Africa but are prevalent in the West Indies, Central America, and southern Florida. Unripe ackee fruit has a closed aril that is toxic. Ripe ackee fruit, with a spontaneously opened aril, is nontoxic. Unripe ackee fruit contains hypoglycin A, or L(R,S)-2-amino-3-methylenecyclopropylproprionic acid, a water-soluble amino acid that is converted to methylenecyclopropylacetyl–coenzyme A in vivo. Both compounds are hypoglycemic agents[94,126]; the second is a suicide inhibitor of β-oxidation of fatty acids. Inhibition of fatty acid metabolism results in microvesicular steatosis of the liver, hyperammonemia, metabolic acidosis, and hypoglycemia. Laboratory and histopathologic findings are indistinguishable from Reye's syndrome.

Ackee fruit constitutes a traditional Jamaican breakfast and has been associated with Jamaican vomiting sickness. Ingestion of unripe ackee fruit produced an outbreak epidemic of fatal encephalopathy in West Africa, primarily affecting children ages 2 to 6 years, who experienced vomiting, hypotonia, convulsions, and coma. All children died within 48 hours of onset of vomiting. Necropsy revealed massive liver steatosis and severe hypoglycemia. Urine concentrations of dicarboxylic acids were elevated. Fatal ackee fruit poisoning is more common in children than in adults; adults are more likely to present with self-resolving cholestatic jaundice.[94]

TREATMENT. Treatment is largely supportive and consists of securing an airway and administering activated charcoal and IV fluids. Before hypoglycemia was recognized, mortality rates of symptomatic unripe ackee fruit exposure approached 80%. Frequent glucose and electrolyte measurements with appropriate replacement are essential. Seizures are treated with benzodiazepines and barbiturates. Theoretically, riboflavin, glycine, and carnitine may be beneficial, although their efficacy is not established. Laboratory studies of hypoglycin poisoning in animals suggests that administration of riboflavin and glycine may be useful. Carnitine has been used for other toxins (e.g., valproate) that inhibit β-oxidation of fatty acids and may facilitate transport of fatty acids into mitochondria.[125,126]

Corticoid Plants: Licorice. Adverse effects with chronic ingestion of *Glycyrrhiza glabra* (natural licorice) result from altered steroid metabolism. *G. glabra* contains glycyrrhizic acid, which is converted to 18-β-glycyrrhetinic acid within the GI tract. Both acids inhibit 11-β-hydroxysteroid dehydrogenase, an enzyme essential to the in vivo conversion of cortisol to cortisone.[18,62] Excessive local cortisol binds to and activates mineralocorticoid receptors in the kidneys, producing a hypermineralocorticoid syndrome, characterized by water and sodium retention with potassium excretion. Signs and symptoms of chronic ingestion include hypertension, headache, edema, hypokalemia, metabolic alkalosis, paresthesias, weakness, paralysis, tetany, and muscle cramps.[48,50] Myopathy with reversible myoglobinuria has been reported.[14,46] Heart failure, arrhythmias (e.g., torsades de pointes), and cardiac arrest have been attributed to licorice root ingestion.[1]

TREATMENT. Treatment consists of discontinuing exposure to licorice, maintaining good urine output, and alkalinizing urine of patients with rhabdomyolysis. Occasionally, potassium-sparing diuretics (e.g., triamterene, spironolactone) are useful.[18] Torsades de pointes may respond to magnesium or potassium infusion.[48]

Cyanogenic Plants: Glycosides. Glycosides that yield hydrocyanic acid on hydrolysis are known as cyanogenic glycosides (see Figure 48-1). Amygdalin (D-mandelonitrile-β-D-glucoside-6-β-glucoside), which is abundant in the Rosaceae family, is the cyanogenic compound found in these plants.[133] Seeds of *Malus* species (apples) and pits of *Prunus* species, including cherries, peaches, plums, and apricots (commercial source of laetrile), are rich in amygdalin. Black or wild cherries *(P. serotina)* are considered the most dangerous. Poisonings have resulted from milkshakes that include apricot kernels and from apricot kernels sold in health food stores as snacks.[1,133] Deaths have been reported after ingestion of apricot, apple, cherry, and other fruit seeds.[90,120] Linseeds *(Linum usitatissimum)* are also cyanogenic.[118] Chronic cyanide toxicity has been reported from ingestion of cassava *(Manihot esculenta).*

Cyanide combines with and inhibits many enzymes. It possesses great affinity for the ferric iron in cytochrome oxidase of the electron transport chain, accounting for most of its toxicity (Figure 48-21). By combining with cytochrome oxidase, cyanide prevents electron transport, thereby preventing adenosine triphosphate (ATP) production by oxidative phosphorylation. Metabolic acidosis ensues. Humans detoxify cyanide by transferring sulfane sulfur to cyanide to form thiocyanate. Numerous sulfur sources are likely acted on by various sulfurtransferases to form the sulfane sulfur needed to convert cyanide to thiocyanate. Administration of exogenous sulfane sul-

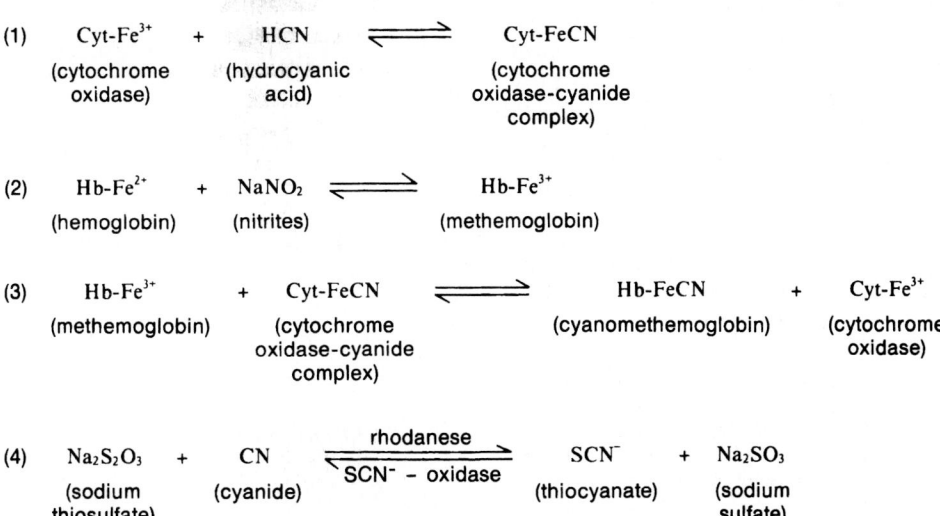

Figure 48-21 Principal steps in hydrocyanic acid poisoning and detoxification. *1,* Breakdown of cellular respiration resulting from the binding of cyanide to cytochrome oxidase. *2,* Conversion of the ferrous (Fe^{2+}) form of hemoglobin to the ferric (Fe^{3+}) form (methemoglobin) by the use of nitrites. *3,* Preferential binding of cyanide to methemoglobin, liberating cytochrome oxidase and restoring cellular respiration. *4,* Providing exogenous thiosulfate to aid in formation of the less toxic thiocyanate via various sulfurtransferases, such as rhodanese. Thiocyanate is then excreted from the body. The reaction is slowly reversible via the enzyme thiocyanate oxidase, and rebound may occur.

fur, such as sodium thiosulfate, can greatly facilitate this detoxification.[37]

Clinically, CNS changes (agitation, anxiety, excitement, weakness, numbness, hypotonia, coma, seizures), respiratory changes (hyperpnea, dyspnea, apnea), cardiovascular changes (tachycardia and hypertension followed by bradycardia and hypotension, heart block, ventricular arrhythmias, asystole), and metabolic changes (anion gap metabolic acidosis) are seen. Skin color may be pink or cyanotic, and the partial pressure of oxygen may be normal in cyanide poisoning. Arterial blood gases reveal metabolic acidosis. ECG may reveal T-on-R phenomenon due to progressive shortening of the ST segment. Multisystem organ failure and death may occur.[37]

TREATMENT. Patients with cyanide glycoside poisoning may respond to treatment with 100% oxygen and the cyanide antidote kit, which includes amyl nitrite, sodium nitrite (3% solution given intravenously based on hemoglobin and weight; generally 300 mg in a nonanemic adult), and sodium thiosulfate (12.5 g). Red blood cell or plasma cyanide levels can be determined; however, treatment should be initiated promptly, without confirmation of exposure, in patients with evidence of toxicity. Cyanide antidote kits are designed to induce methemoglobinemia through nitrite exposure. Cyanide binds preferentially to the ferric ion of methemoglobin rather than that of cytochrome oxidase in the electron transport chain. Forming methemoglobin limits inhibition of electron transport by cyanide and restores cellular respiration. Sodium thiosulfate in the cyanide kit provides exogenous sulfane sulfur groups that bind to cyanide and form thiocyanate. Although not available in the United States, hydroxocobalamin is used as antidotal therapy in some countries. Cyanide combines with hydroxocobalamin to form cyanocobalamin, which is excreted in the urine and bile.[37,133]

Chronic exposure to cyanogenic glycosides occurs with cassava consumption during droughts in areas where the bitter roots of cassava are a staple food, such as in Africa. Roots contain high concentrations of cyanogenic glucosides, specifically the cyanogenic glycoside linamarin, which produce an upper motor neuron disease known as Konzo or tropical spastic paraparesis. To remove cyanogens, roots should be soaked; however, when water is scare, this soaking process is limited. Konzo outbreaks have been reported in populations exposed chronically to cassava that is not properly soaked.[11,12]

Hematopoietic System

Plants with Anticoagulant Properties: Lactone Glycosides. *Dipteryx odoratum* and *Coumarouna* (or *Dipteryx*) *oppositofolia* (tonka bean) were among the first historically mentioned medical sources of coumarin. *Melilotus officinalis* (melilot), *Asperula odorata*, and *Galium odoratum* (woodruff) also contain significant quantities of coumarin. Occasionally, these coumarin-containing products are consumed in teas.[114] *Melilotus* (sweet clover) poisoning is caused by dicumarol, a fungal metabolite produced from substrates in sweet clover. Fungi dimerize coumarin to produce dicumarol. Dicumarol interferes with the synthesis of vitamin K–dependent coagulation factors, inducing coagulopathy. Generally, this has been problematic for livestock and not humans.[108]

Plants that Induce Hemolysis: Fava. Fava beans (*Vicia faba*) contain vicine and convicine, two metabolically inactive glycones that may be cleaved by β-glycosidase to produce divicine and isouramil. Divicine and isouramil may account for the hemolytic crisis seen in response to oxidative stress when individuals deficient in glucose-6-phosphate dehydrogenase ingest fava beans. Favism has been reported in infants who ingest breast milk from mothers who have recently ingested fava beans and in fetuses of mothers who ingest fava beans. Clinically, favism is characterized by hemoglobinuria, anemia, and jaundice.[35,70] Patients may present with complaints of malaise, weakness, lethargy, nausea, vomiting, headache, and lumbar or abdominal pain. Renal failure may ensue.[67] Supportive care is the mainstay of treatment. Occasionally, transfusions and hemodialysis are needed.

OTHER TOXINS

Oils

Irritant oils, including various mustards (*Brassica* spp.), horseradish (*Amoracia lapathifolia*), and protoanemonin from the buttercup family (Ranunculaceae), induce gastroenteritis. Essential oils, often found in combination with resins (oleoresins), are extracted commercially for use as rubefacients, salves, and liniments. Essential oils include wintergreen, eucalyptus, wormwood, and pennyroyal oils.

Wintergreen. Methyl salicylate is the methyl ester of salicylic acid, derived from *Gaultheria procumbens* (wintergreen). Widely used as an antirheumatic agent in the nineteenth century, it fell into disfavor because of its extreme side effects and the availability of more effective acetylsalicylic acid.[46] Poisoning now occurs most often in children, who are attracted to the color, smell, and flavor of wintergreen oil. Poisoning is identical to salicylism, including CNS excitation, hyperventilation, hyperthermia, and metabolic acidosis. Structures of salicylic acid and methyl salicylate follow:

Salicylic acid   **Methyl salicylate**

Eucalyptus. 1,8-Cineole is the toxic component of eucalyptus oil, derived from leaves of *Eucalyptus globulus.* Ingestion of eucalyptus oil is associated with CNS depression (hyporeflexia, coma, respiratory depression), GI upset (vomiting, diarrhea, abdominal pain), and respiratory effects (bronchospasm, pneumonitis). Hypotension and death may occur.[6,136,144]

Wormwood. Wormwood oil, from the plants *Artemisia absinthium* and *A. pontica,* was used in the liqueur absinthe, which was eventually banned because of its neurotoxicity. Wormwood oil contains α- and β-thujone and causes vomiting, vertigo, delirium, convulsions, coma, respiratory arrest, and death.[17]

Pennyroyal. Pulegone, a monoterpene, is the primary toxin of pennyroyal oil, which is derived from *Hedeoma pulegioides* or *Mentha pulegium.* Pennyroyal oil also contains several other monoterpenes. Pulegone is oxidized by hepatic cytochrome P450 enzymes to form the toxic metabolite menthofuran and other toxins. Menthofuran induces much of the hepatic and pulmonary damage. Reactive oxidative metabolites of pulegone and menthofuran bind to target cell proteins and induce cellular damage. *M. pulegium* use has caused death in women using it as an over-the-counter abortifacient and death in infants given mint teas made with *Mentha pulegium.* Hepatic and neurologic injury are generally seen. Hepatic failure followed by shock, multiple organ failure, and death may occur after ingestion. Neurologic manifestations include dizziness, obtundation, hallucinations, seizures, and cerebral edema. Laboratory studies may reveal elevated liver transaminases, coagulopathies, and metabolic acidosis. Liver histology at autopsy reveals centrilobular hepatic necrosis or confluent hepatocellular necrosis.[5,9] Treatment includes oral administration of activated charcoal and fluid and electrolyte replacement as needed. *N*-Acetylcysteine has been used for treatment because the hepatotoxicity is similar to acetaminophen-induced hepatotoxicity and is associated with glutathione depletion.[5,9]

Elements and Nitrates

Many plants absorb or accumulate metallic compounds (selenium, molybdenum, arsenic, lead, cadmium), nitrites, and nitrates. They are generally of little importance in humans but constitute a danger to grazing livestock. However, numerous cases of methemoglobinemia in infants ingesting vegetables high in nitrate content have been reported. Vegetables cited include spinach, beets, cabbage, and carrots grown in high-nitrate soils. Nitrates are converted to nitrites in the infant gut.[77]

ACKNOWLEDGEMENT

We thank Edward C. Geehr for his contributions to previous editions of this chapter.

IN MEMORIAM

This chapter is dedicated to our dear friend and mentor, Donald B. Kunkel, MD (1939-2000). Don fostered our interest in plant toxicology, and his knowledge and teachings were invaluable to the writing of this chapter.

Kimberlie A. Graeme, MD

We are saddened by the death of Don Kunkel, who was incredibly energetic and a constant mentor. His accomplishments in toxicology and the science of medicine were appreciated greatly by all who had the good fortune to know him. He made us want to be better people.

Paul Auerbach, MD

APPENDIX A

Plants: Toxic Principles and Therapeutics

COMMON NAME	GENUS	SPECIES	POISONOUS PRINCIPLE	TOXIC PARTS	DISTRIBUTION*	SECTION† THERAPEUTIC REFERENCE
Ackee (Akee)	*Blighia*	*sapida*	Hypoglycin	Fruit wall, seeds, white aril	II, S. Fla., Carib.	Hypoglycemic agents
Anemone	*Anemone*	spp.	Protoanemonin	All parts	II	Irritant and essential oils
Angel's trumpet	*Datura*	*sauveolens*	Atropine, hyoscyamine, hyoscine	Leaves, flowers	II, VI, S.E. U.S., Hi.	Tropane alkaloids
Apple of Peru	*Nicandra*	*physalodes*	Unknown	Leaves, berries	I	General considerations
Apple seeds	*Malus*	spp.	Cyanogenic glycosides	Seeds	III	Cyanogenic glycosides
Apricot pits	*Prunus*	spp.	Cyanogenic glycosides	Pits	II	Cyanogenic glycosides
Arnica	*Arnica*	*montana fulgens*	Unknown	Flowers, roots	II, N. U.S., Can.	General considerations
Autumn crocus	*Colchicum*	*autumnale*	Colchicine	Seeds, corms	II	Amine alkaloids
Azalea	(See *Rhododendron*)					
Balsam pear	*Mamordica*	*balsimia*	Saponic glycoside	Seeds, wall of fruit	I, coastal Fla. to Tex.	Saponin glycosides
Baneberry	*Actaea*	spp.	Protoanemonin, unknown glycosides	Berries, rootstock	I, widely except S.W.	Irritant and essential oils
Beech	*Fagus*	spp.	Saponic glycoside	Nuts	III	Saponin glycoside
Belladonna	(See deadly nightshade)					
Bellyache bush	*Jatropha*	*gossypiifolia*	Curcin	Fruit, seeds, sap	I, V	Phytotoxins
Betel nut	*Areca*	*catechu*	Arecoline, arecaine	Seeds	II, Fla., Hi.	Pyridine-piperidine group
Bird of paradise	*Poinciana*	*gillesii*	Unknown	Green seedpods	II	General considerations

*Distribution key:

I	Native or naturalized; found in fields, woods, and roadsides.
II	Cultivated; found in gardens and yards.
III	Found in both I and II.
IV	Common houseplants.
V	Found in decorations or as seasonal ornamentals.
VI	Found in herbal or folk remedies or used for mood alteration.
Can.	Canada
Carib.	Caribbean
Coastal Fla. to Tex.	Coastal Florida to Texas
E. N.A.	Eastern North America
Fla.	Florida
Hi.	Hawaii
Ill.	Illinois
Ind.	Indiana
Mid. W.	Midwestern United States
Minn.	Minnesota
N.A.	North America
N. Car.	North Carolina
N.E. U.S.	Northeastern United States
N. U.S.	Northern United States
Oh.	Ohio
Pac. Coast	Pacific Coast states
Roadsides	Roadsides, waste areas, and swamps
S. Cal.	Southern California
S. Can.	Southern Canada
S.E. Coastal	Southeastern coastal plain
S.E. U.S.	Southeastern United States
S. Fla.	Southern Florida
S. Tex.	Southern Texas
S.W.	Southwestern United States
Widely	Distributed throughout the United States

†See appropriate section in text.

Plants: Toxic Principles and Therapeutics—cont'd

COMMON NAME	GENUS	SPECIES	POISONOUS PRINCIPLE	TOXIC PARTS	DISTRIBUTION*	SECTION† THERAPEUTIC REFERENCE
Black cherry	*Prunus*	*serotina*	*Cyanogenic* glycoside	Bark, leaves, seeds, "tea" of leaves	I, E. N.A.	Cyanogenic glycosides
Black locust	Robinia	*pseudoacacia*	Robin, robitin (glycoside)	Inner bark, young, leaves, seeds	I, S. Can., E. N.A., Mid. W., roadsides	Phytotoxins
Black nightshade	*Solanum*	*nigrum*	Solanine	Unripened fruit	I, widely, roadsides	Steroid alkaloids
Black snake root	(See death camas)					
Bleeding heart	(See dicentra)					
Bloodroot	*Sanguinaria*	*canadensis*	Sanguinarine	All parts	I	Isoquinoline and quinoline group
Blister bush	*Phebolium*	*anceps*	Unknown	Leaves, fruit	I	General considerations
Blue cohosh	*Caulophyllum*	*thalactroides*	Unknown	Seeds, rootstock	I	General considerations
Boxwood	*Buxus*	*sempervirens*	Buxine, volatile oil	Leaves, twigs	II, V	Alkaloids, irritant and essential oils
Brazilian pepper, also: pink or red peppercorn, Florida holly	*Schinus* flowers	*terebinthifolius*	Unknown	Berries, leaves,	I, Fla.	General considerations
Broom, also: Scotch broom	*Cytisus*	*scoparius*	Cytisine	Branches	VI	Quinolizidine alkaloids
Buckeye	*Aesculus*	spp.	Aesculin	Leaves, flowers, young sprouts, seeds	III, widely	Coumarin glycosides
Buckthorn	*Rhamnus*	*cathartica, frangula*	Anthraquinones	Berries, leaves, bark	I, VI	Anthraquinone glycosides
Burning bush	*Euonymus*	spp.	Unknown	Leaves, bark, seeds	III	General considerations
Bushman's poison	*Acokanthera*	spp.	Oubain, G-strophanthin, acokantherin	All	I	Cardiac glycosides
Buttercup	*Ranunculus*	spp.	Protoanemonin	All parts	III	Irritant and essential oils
Caladium	*Caladium*	spp.	Oxalates	Leaves	II, IV	Oxalates
Candle nut (see lumbang nut)						
Caper spurge	*Euphorbia*	*lathyris*	Unknown alkaloid	Milky sap throughout plant	II	General considerations
Carolina jessamine, also: yellow jessamine	*Gelsemium*	*sempervirens*	Gelsemine, sempervirine	All parts	II	Psychoactive plants
Cassava, also: manioc, tapioca	*Manihot*	*esculenta*	Cyanogenic glycoside	Raw root	II, VI	Cyanogenic glycosides
Castor bean	*Ricinis*	*communis*	Ricin	Seeds	III	Phytotoxins
Catnip	*Nepeta*	*cataria*	Acetic, butyric and valeric acids, nepetalic acid, limonene	Leaves	VI	Psychoactive plants
Chalice vine	*Solandra*	*nitida*	(see trumpet flower)		II	
Cherry	*Prunus*	spp.	Cyanogenic glycoside	Pits	II	Cyanogenic glycosides
Chinaberry tree	*Melia*	*azederach*	Unknown resin	Fruit, tea from leaves	III	Resins

Plants: Toxic Principles and Therapeutics—cont'd

COMMON NAME	GENUS	SPECIES	POISONOUS PRINCIPLE	TOXIC PARTS	DISTRIBUTION*	SECTION† THERAPEUTIC REFERENCE
Christmas rose	*Helleborus*	*niger*	Hellebrin, helleborin, helleborein	Rootstocks and leaves	II	Cardiac glycosides
Clematis	*Clematis*	spp.	Steroid alkaloids	Seeds, young plants	II, widely	Steroid alkaloids
Coca	*Erythoxylon*	*coca*	Ecogonine	Extract of leaves	VI	Psychoactive plants
Coontie	*Zamia*	*floridana*	Unknown alkaloid	Fleshy seeds	II, S. US., Hi.	General considerations
Coral plant	*Jatropha*	*multifida*	Curcin	Fruit, seeds, sap of all parts	III, S. Fla. to Tex., Hi.	Phytotoxins
Corn cockle	*Agrostemma*	*githago*	Githagenin, sapogenin	All parts, especially seeds	I	Saponin glycosides
Cotoneaster	*Cotoneaster*	spp.	Unknown	Berries	II	General considerations
Coyotillo	*Karwinskia*	*humboldtiana*	Unknown	Fruit, seeds	I, S.W. U.S.	General considerations
Crepe jasmine	*Ervatamia*	*coronaria*	Unknown	Leaves, flowers	II	General considerations
Crownflower	*Calotropis*	*gigantea*	Unknown	All parts	II, V	General considerations
Crown of thorns	*Euphorbia*	spp.	Unknown alkaloid	Milky sap throughout plant	II, widely	General considerations
Cup of gold	*Solandra*	*cuttata*	Solanine-like alkaloids	Leaves, flowers	II	Steroid alkaloids
Cycads	(See coontie)					
Cypress spurge	*Euphorbia*	*cyparissias*	Unknown alkaloids	Milky sap throughout plant	II	General considerations
Daffodil	*Narcissus*	spp.	Lycorine	Bulb	II	General considerations
Daphne	*Daphne*	*mezereum*	Dihydroxy-coumarin, diterpene mezerein	Bark, leaves, fruit	II	Coumarin glycosides
Day jessamine	*Cestrum*	*diurnum*	Tropane alkaloids	All parts	III, Fla., Hi.	Tropane alkaloids
Deadly nightshade	*Atropa*	*belladonna*	Atropine	All parts, black berries	I	Tropane alkaloids
Death camas, also: black snakeroot	*Zigadenus*	spp.	Zygacine, zygadenine	Bulb	I, widely	Steroid alkaloids
Delphinium	*Delphinium*	spp.	Delphinine, ajacine	Seeds, young plants	III	Steroid alkaloids
Desert potato	*Jatropha*	*macrorhiza*	Phytotoxin	Plant root	I	Phytotoxins
Devil's trumpet, also: hairy thorn apple	*Datura*	*metel*	Atropine, hyoscyamine, hyoscine	Leaves, flowers	II, VI, Coastal Fla. to Tex.	Tropane alkaloids
Dicentra, also: bleeding heart, Dutchman's breeches	*Dicentra*	spp.	Protopine, apomorphine, protoberberine	All parts	I, widely	Isoquinoline and quinoline group
Dieffenbachia, also: dumbcane	*Dieffenbachia*	spp.	Oxalate, asparagine	Leaves	II, IV	Oxalates
Dogbane, also: Indian hemp	*Apocynum*	*cannabium*	Cymarin	Flowers, seeds, leaves	I, widely, roadsides	Cardiac glycosides
Duranta	(See sky flower)					
Elderberry	*Sambucus*	spp.	Unknown alkaloids	Unripe berries, leaves, wood	III, all N.A. except Pac. Coast	General considerations
Elephant ear	*Colocasia*	*antiquorum*	Oxalates	Leaves	IV	Oxalates
English bean	(See fava bean)					
English ivy	*Hedera*	*helix*	Hederogenin	Berries and leaves	II, IV, V	Saponin glycosides
False hellebore, also: Indian poke	*Veratrum*	spp.	Veratrin	Leaves	I, E.N.A., Minn.	Steroid alkaloids

Plants: Toxic Principles and Therapeutics—cont'd

COMMON NAME	GENUS	SPECIES	POISONOUS PRINCIPLE	TOXIC PARTS	DISTRIBUTION*	SECTION† THERAPEUTIC REFERENCE
False sago palm	*Cycas*	*circinalis*	Alkaloids	Seeds	II, V, S. U.S., Hi.	General considerations
Fava bean	*Vicia*	*faba*	Hemolytic anemia in glucose-6-phosphate deficiency	Bean	II	General considerations
Finger cherry	*Rhodomyrtus*	*macrocarpa*	Saponin	Fruit	S. Pacific	Saponin glycosides
Fool's parsley	*Aethusa*	*cynapium*	Unknown	Leaves	I	General considerations
Four o'clock	*Mirabilis*	*jalapa*	Unknown	Roots or seeds	II	General considerations
Foxglove	*Digitalis*	*purpurea*	Digitoxin, gitaloxin, gitoxin	Leaves	III, W. U.S.	Cardiac glycosides
Ginseng	*Panax*	*quinque-folium*	Saponin glycosides	Root	VI	Saponin glycosides
Glory lily	*Gloriosa*	*superba*	Colchicine-like alkaloids	Rhizomes	II	Amine alkaloids
Golden chain, also: golden rain	*Labrunum*	*anagyroides*	Cytisine	Flowers, seeds	II, N. U.S., S. Can.	Quinolizidine alkaloids
Golden seal	*Hydrastis*	*canadensis*	Steroid alkaloids	Seeds, young plants	I, N.E. U.S., VI	Steroid alkaloids
Ground cherry	*Physalis*	spp.	Unknown	Leaves, unripe fruit	I, widely	General considerations
Hill gooseberry	*Rhodomyrtus*	*tomentosa*	None—N.A. nontoxic (*Rhodomyrtus* spp.)		II, N. Am.	—
Holly	*Ilex*	spp.	Ilicin	Berries	III, V	General considerations
Horse bean (see fava bean)						
Horse chestnut	*Aesculus*	spp.	Aesculin	Sprouts, mature nuts	II	Coumarin glycosides
Horse nettle, also: wild tomato	*Solanum*	*carolinense*	Solanine	Fruit	I, widely	Steroid alkaloids
Horseradish	*Amoracia*	*rusticana*	Mustard oil	Roots	II	Irritant and essential oils
Hyacinth	*Hyacinthus*	*orientalis*	Narcissine-like alkaloids	Bulb	II, IV	General considerations
Hyacinth bean	*Dolichos*	*lablab*	Cyanogenic glycosides	Pods, seeds	II	Cyanogenic glycosides
Hydrangea	*Hydrangea*	spp.	Cyanogenic glycosides	Leaves, buds	III	Cyanogenic glycosides
Inkberry (See pokeweed)						
Iris (blue flag)	*Iris*	*versicolor*	Irisin, irigenin, iridin	Flowers, leaves	III	Resins
Jack-in-the-pulpit	*Arisaema*	spp.	Oxalate	Rhizome	I, N.E. U.S.	Oxalates
Jequirity pea, also: rosary pea, precatory bean	*Abrus*	*precatorius*	Abrin	Beans	I, V	Phytotoxins
Jerusalem cherry	*Solanum*	*pseudocapsicum*	Solanine	Fruit	II, V, widely	Steroid alkaloids
Jessamine	(See Carolina jessamine)					
Jessamines	*Cestrum*	spp.	Tropane alkaloids	All parts	III	Tropane alkaloids
Jetbead	*Rhodotypus*	*tetrapetala*	Cyanogenic glycosides	Berries	II, N. U.S.	Cyanogenic glycosides
Jimsonweed	*Datura*	*stramonium*	Atropine, hyoscyamine, hyoscine	Leaves, flowers	I, VI	Tropane alkaloids
Jonquil	(See daffodil)					
Kentucky coffee tree	*Gymnocladus*	*dioica*	Cytisine	Seeds, pulp	III, E. N.A., Okla.	Quinolizidine alkaloids

Plants: Toxic Principles and Therapeutics—cont'd

COMMON NAME	GENUS	SPECIES	POISONOUS PRINCIPLE	TOXIC PARTS	DISTRIBUTION*	SECTION† THERAPEUTIC REFERENCE
Lantana	*Lantana*	*camara*	Lantanin, lantadene A	Unripe fruit	II, N. U.S., S.E. U.S.	General considerations
Larkspur	(See delphinium)					
Laurel	(See mountain laurel)					
Lignum vitae	*Guaiacum*	*officinale*	Unknown	Resin in wood and fruit	II, S. Fla., S. Cal., Hi.	General considerations
Lily of the valley	*Convallaria*	*majalis*	Convallotoxin, convallarin, convallamarin	Rhizome, leaves, flowers	II, widely	Cardiac glycosides
Lobelia, also: Indian tobacco	*Lobelia*	spp.	Lobelamine, lobeline	All parts	III, IV, VI	Pyridine-piperidine group
Lumbang nut	*Aleurites*	*trisperma*	(See tung oil tree)			
Manchineel tree	*Hippomane*	*mancinella*	Unknown	Milky sap	I	General considerations
Mandrake, also: Satan's apple	*Mandragora*	*officinarum*	Hyoscyamine, scopolamine	Rhizome	VI	Tropane alkaloids
Marijuana, also: grass, dope, pot, ganja, pokololo	*Cannabis*	*sativa*	Tetrahydro-cannabinol	Leaves	III, VI	Psychoactive plants
Mayapple	*Podophyllum*	*peltatum*	Podophyllotoxin	All parts except ripe fruit	I, widely	General considerations
Mescal bean	*Sophora*	*secundiflora*	Unknown alkaloids	Seeds	III, VI	General considerations
Mexican prickly poppy	(See prickly poppy)					
Milk bush, also: pencil tree	*Euphorbia*	*tirucallii*	Unknown alkaloids	Milky sap throughout plant	I	General considerations
Mistletoe (American)	*Phoradendron*	*serotinum*	Toxalbumin	Berries	I, V	General considerations
Mistletoe (European)	*Viscum*	*album*	Viscumin	Berries	I, V	General considerations
Monkshood, also: aconite, wolfsbane	*Aconitum*	spp.	Aconitine	All parts, especially roots	III	Steroid alkaloids
Moonseed	*Menispermum*	*canadense*	Dauricine	Berries	I	Isoquinoline and quinoline group
Morning glory	*Ipomoea*	*violacea*	(+)-Lysergic acid amide	Seeds	II, VI	Psychoactive plants
Mountain ash	*Sorbus*	spp.	Unknown	Berries	I	General considerations
Mountain laurel	*Kalmia*	*latifolia*	Andromedo-toxin, arbutin, grayanotoxins	All parts	III	Steroid alkaloids
Narcissus	(See jonquil)					
Night-blooming jasmine	*Cestrum*	spp.	Tropane alkaloids	All parts	I, S. U.S.	Tropane alkaloids
Nightshade, also: woody nightshade, climbing nightshade, bittersweet	*Solanum*	*dulcamara*	Solanine	Fruit	I, V, widely	Steroid alkaloids
Nutmeg	*Myristica*	*fragrans*	Myristicine	Nut	VI	Psychoactive plants
Oak	*Quercus*	spp.	Tannin, unknown	Acorns	III, S.W.	General considerations

Plants: Toxic Principles and Therapeutics—cont'd

COMMON NAME	GENUS	SPECIES	POISONOUS PRINCIPLE	TOXIC PARTS	DISTRIBUTION*	SECTION† THERAPEUTIC REFERENCE
Ochrosia plum	*Ochrosia*	*elliptica*	Unknown	Fruit	II, Fla., Hi.	General considerations
Oleander	*Nerium*	*oleander*	Oleandrin oleandroside, nevioside	All parts	II, S. U.S., Cal., Hi., roadsides	Cardiac glycosides
Peach pits	*Prunus*	spp.	Cyanogenic glycosides	Pits	II, widely	Cyanogenic glycosides
Peyote	*Lophophora*	*williamsii*	Mescaline, lophophorine	Seeds, buttons	I, S. Tex.	General considerations, psychoactive plants
Philodendron	*Philodendron*	spp.	Oxalate	Leaves	IV	Oxalates
Physic nut, also: purging nut	*Jatropha*	*curcas*	Curcin	Fruit, seeds	II	Phytotoxins
Pigeonberry	(See pokeweed)					
Plum pit	*Prunus*	spp.	Cyanogenic glycosides	Pit	II, widely	Cyanogenic glycosides
Poinsettia	*Euphorbia*	*pulcherrima*	Unknown alkaloid	Milky sap throughout plant	II, V	General considerations
Poison hemlock	*Conium*	*maculatum*	Coniine	Seeds, roots, young leaves	I	Pyridine-piperidine group
Pokeweed, also: pokeberry, Virginia poke, scoke, garget, inkberry, caokum, American cancer, cancer jalap	*Phytolacca*	*americana*	Triterpene saponins	All parts	I	Saponin glycosides
Pongam	*Pongammia*	*pinnata*	Unknown	Seeds, roots	II, S. Fla., S. Cal., Hi.	General considerations
Potato	*Solanum*	*tuberosum*	Solanine	Unripe tubers	II, widely	Steroid alkaloids
Prickly poppy	*Argemone*	spp.	Sanguinarine, berberine, protopine	All parts, especially seeds	III, VI	Isoquinoline and quinoline group
Privet	*Ligustrum*	*vulgare, japonicum*	Unknown glycoside	Berries, leaves	II, widely	General considerations
Purging nut	(See physic nut)					
Rattlepod, also: scarlet, wisteria tree	*Sesbania*	spp.	Pyrrolizidine alkaloids	All parts	III, V, S.E. coastal, S. Cal., Hi.	Pyrrolizidine alkaloids
Rayless goldenrod	*Haplopappus*	*heterophyllus*	Tremetol	Milk of cows grazing on plant	I	Irritant and essential oils
Rhododendron, also: laurel, azalea	*Rhododendron*	spp.	Grayanotoxins	All parts	III, E. N.A., Pac. Coast	Steroid alkaloids
Rhubarb	*Rheum*	*rhabarbarum*	Oxalates	Leaves	II	Oxalates
Rock poppy	*Chelidonium*	*majus*	Sanguinarine, berberine, protopine	Leaves, seeds	I, E. N.A.	Isoquinoline and quinoline group
Rubber vine	*Cryptostegia*	*grandiflora*	Unknown	All parts	II, V, S. U.S., Hi.	General considerations
Sandbox tree	*Hura*	*crepitans*	Unknown	Milky sap	II, S. U.S.	General considerations
Senecio, also: threadleaf, groundsel	*Senecio*	*longilobus*	Pyrrolizidine alkaloids	Entire plants	I, VI	Pyrrolizidine alkaloids
Sky flower	*Duranta*	*repens*	Saponin	Berries	I	Saponin glycosides
Snow-on-the-mountain	*Euphorbia*	spp.	Unknown alkaloids	Milky sap throughout plant	II	General considerations

Plants: Toxic Principles and Therapeutics—cont'd

COMMON NAME	GENUS	SPECIES	POISONOUS PRINCIPLE	TOXIC PARTS	DISTRIBUTION*	SECTION† THERAPEUTIC REFERENCE
Spring adonis	*Adonis*	*vernalis*	Steroid alkaloids	Seeds, young plants	II	Steroid alkaloids
Spurge	*Euphorbia*	spp.	Unknown alkaloids	Milky sap	III	General considerations
Squill	*Urginea*	*maritima*	Cardiac glycosides	Bulbs	II, S. Cal., S.W.	Cardiac glycosides
Star of Bethlehem	*Ornithogalum*	*umbellatum*	Cardiac glycosides, amine alkaloids	All parts	III, V, E. N.A., Mid. W., Hi.	Cardiac glycosides, amine alkaloids
Strawberry bush	(See burning bush)					
Sweet pea	*Lathyrus*	spp.	β(λ-L-glutamyl)-aminopropioni-trile, α, λ-diamino-butryic acid	Peas	III	General considerations
Tobacco	*Nicotiana*	*tabacum*	Nicotine	Leaves	II, VI	Pyridine-piperidine group
Tomato	*Lycopersicon*	*esculenta*	Solanine	Leaves	II	Steroid alkaloids
Tree tobacco	*Nicotiana*	*glauca*	Anabasine	All parts	I, S.W., Hi., Carib.	Pyridine-piperidine group
Trumpet flower	*Solandra*	spp.	Solanine-like	Leaves, flowers	II	Steroid alkaloids
Trumpet lily	*Datura*	*arborea*	Atropine, hyoscyamine, hyoscine	Flowers, leaves	II, VI	Tropane alkaloids
Tulip bulb	*Tulipa*	*gesnariana*	Unknown	Bulb	II	General considerations
Tung oil tree	*Aleurites*	*fordii*	Saponins	Seed	II	Saponin glycosides
Virginia creeper, also: woodbine, American ivy	*Parthenocissus*	*quinquefolia*	Unknown	Berries	I, E. N.A., S.W.	General considerations
Water hemlock	*Cicuta*	*maculata*	Cicutoxin	Roots	I, widely in swamps	Resins
White snakeroot	*Eupatorium*	*rugosum*	Tremetol	Milk of cows grazing on plant	I, N. Car., Ill., Ind., Oh.	Irritant and essential oils
Wild balsam apple	*Mamordia*	*charantia*	Saponin glycoside	Seeds and wall of fruit	I	Saponin glycosides
Wild cherry	(See black cherry)					
Wisteria	*Wisteria*	spp.	Resin	Seeds	II	Resin, general considerations
Woody nightshade	(See nightshade)					
Yellow allamanda	*Allamanda*	*cathartica*	Unknown	Fruit	II, S. U.S., Hi.	General considerations
Yellow jessamine	(See Carolina jessamine)					
Yellow nightshade, also: wild allamanda	*Urechite*	spp.	Unknown	Seedpods	I, S. Fla.	General considerations
Yellow oleander, also: lucky nut	*Thevetia*	*peruviana*	Thevetin, thevetoxin	Flowers, seeds, leaves	II, Hi.	Cardiac glycosides
Yew	*Taxus*	spp.	Taxine	Berries	III, V., E. N.A., Pac. Coast	Steroid alkaloids

APPENDIX B

Nontoxic Plants*

African violet (*Saint pauliaionantha*)
Air plant (*Kalanchoe pinnata*)
Aluminum plant (*Pilea cadierei*)
Aralia, false (*Dizygotheca elegantissima*)
Aralia, Japanese (*Fatsia japonica*)
Asparagus fern (*Asparagus plumosus*), berry
Baby's breath (*Gypsophilia paniculata*)
Baby's tears (*Helxine* or *Soleirolia soleirolii*)
Begonia (*Begonia rex*)
Bird of paradise* (*Strelitzia reginae*)
Birdsnest fern (*Asplenium nidus*)
Boston fern (*Nephrolepis exaltata bostoniensis*)
Bromeliad family
California poppy (*Eschscholzia californica*)
Camellia (*Camellia japonica*)
Chinese evergreen (*Aglaonema modestrum*)
Christmas cactus (*Schlumbergera bridgesii*)
Coffee tree (*Coffee arabica*)
Coleus
Coral berry* (*Aechamea fulgens, Ardisia crispa*)
Cornstalk plant (*Dracaena fragrans*)
Crape myrtle (*Lagerstromea indica*)
Creeping Charlie* (*Pilea nummularifolia*)
Crocus*—spring-blooming only
Croton* (*Codiaeum variegatum*)
Dahlia
Dandelion (*Taraxacum officinale*)
Dogwood (*Cornus*)
Donkey's tail (*Sedum morganianum*)
Dragon tree (*Dracaena draco, marginata*)
Easter cactus (*Schlumbergera bridgesii*)
Easter lily (*Lilium longiflorum*)
Echeveria: Mexican snowball, painted lady, plush plant
Emerald ripple (*Peperomia caperata*)
Fiddleleaf fig (*Ficus lyrata*)
Fig tree, weeping (*Ficus benjamina*)
Forget-me-not (*Myosotis alpestris, sylvatica*)
Forsythia
Fuchsia
Gardenia
Geranium* (*Pelargonium*)
Gloxinia (*Sinningia speciosa*)
Grape ivy (*Cissus rhombifolia*)
Hawaiian ti plant (*Cordyline terminalis*)
Hawthorne (*Crataegus*), berry
Heavenly bamboo (*Nandina domestica*), berry
Hibiscus

Honeysuckle berry (*Lonicera*)
Ice plant
Impatiens walleriana
Jade plant (*Crassula argentea*)
Jasmine (*Jasminum rex*), Madagascar jasmine
Kalanchoe: maternity plant, monkey plant, panda bear plant
Lace plant, Madagascar (*Aponogeton senetralis*)
Lady, lady's slipper (*Cypripedium, Paphiopedilum*)
Lily of the Nile (*Agapanthus*)
Lipstick plant (*Aeschynanthus radicans*)
Maidenhair fern (*Adiantum*)
Marigold, African/American/tall (*Tagetes*)
Moon cactus (*Gymnocalycium*)
Mother-in-law's tongue or snake plant (*Sansevieria trifasciata*)
Mother of pearls (*Grapetopetalum paraguayense*)
Nandina berry
Natal plum (*Carissa grandiflora*)
Norfolk Island pine (*Araucaria heterophylla*)
Old man cactus (*Cephalocereus senilis*)
Olive tree (*Olea europaea*)
Orchid (*Cattleya, Cymbidium, Oncidium*)
Oregon grape (*Mahonia aquifolium*)
Palm: Bamboo (*Chamaedorea erumpeus*)
    Paradise (*Howea* or *Kentia forsterana*)
    Parlor (*Chamaedorea elegans* or *Kentia*)
    Sentry (*Howea belmoreana*)
Pansy flower (*Viola*)
Peanut cactus (*Chamaecereus sylvestri*)
Pellionia
Peony flower (*Paeonia*)
Peperomia
Petunia
Phlox
Piggyback plant (*Tolmiea menziesii*)
Pigmy date palm (*Phoenix roebelenii*)
Pocketbook (*Calceolaria herbeohybrida*)
Polka dot or freckle face plant (*Hypoestes sanguinolenta*)
Prayer plant (*Maranta leuconeura*)
Pussy willow (*Salix discolor*)
Pyracantha berry
Queen's tears (*Billbergia nutans*)
Rabbit's foot fern (*Davallia fejeensis*)
Rainbow plant (*Billbergia saundersii*)
Raphiolepsis
Rattlesnake plant (*Calathea insignis*)
Ribbon plant (*Dracaena sandriana*)
Rock rose (*Cistus*)
Rosary pearls (*Senecio rowleyanus*)
Rosary vine (*Ceropegia woodii*)
Roses (*Rosa*)
Rubber plant (*Ficus elastica*)
Scheffler plant (*Brassaia* or *Schefflera actinophylia*)
Sedum

From *Your guide to plant safety*, courtesy San Francisco Bay Area Regional Poison Center.
*Have not been reported to cause illness. An asterisk (*) indicates that other species may be toxic.

Sensitive plant *(Mimosa pudica)*

Silver heart *(Peperomia marmorata)*

Snake plant or mother-in-law's tongue *(Sansevieria trifasciata)*

Snapdragon *(Antirrhinum majus)*

Spider plant *(Anthericum, Chlorophytum comosum)*

Staghorn fern *(Platycerium bifurcatum)*

Starfish flower *(Stapelia)*

String of beads* *(Senecio rowleyanus* and *herreianus)*

String of hearts *(Ceropegia woodii)*

Swedish ivy *(Plectranthus australis)*

Sword fern *(Nephrolepis cordifolia, exaltata)*

Tahitian bridal veil *(Gibasis geniculata, Tripogandra multiflora)*

Umbrella tree *(Schefflera actinophylla)*

Vagabond plant *(Vriesea)*

Velvet plant, purple *(Gynura aurantiaca)*

Venus fly trap *(Dionaea muscipula)*

Violet *(Viola)*

Wandering Jew *(Tradescantia albiflora)*

Wandering Jew—Red and White *(Zebrina pendulla)*

Wax plant *(Hoya exotica)*

Yucca

Zebra plant *(Aphelandre squarrosa)*

Zinnia

REFERENCES

1. Abramowicz M, editor: Toxic reactions to plant products sold in health food stores, *Med Lett* 21:29, 1979.
2. Alem A, Shibre T: Khat induced psychosis and its medico-legal implication: a case report, *Ethiop Med J* 35:137, 1997.
3. Alpin PJ, Eliseo T: Ingestion of castor oil plant seeds, *Med J Aust* 167:260, 1997.
4. Anderson EF: *Peyote: the divine cactus,* ed 2, Tucson, 1996, University of Arizona Press.
5. Anderson IB, Mullen WH, Meeker JE: Pennyroyal toxicity: measurement of toxic metabolite levels in two cases and review of the literature, *Ann Intern Med* 124:726, 1996.
6. Anpalahan M: Deliberate self-poisoning with eucalyptus oil in an elderly woman, *Aust NZ J Med* 28:58, 1998.
7. Applefeld JJ: A case of water hemlock poisoning, *JACEP* 8:401, 1979.
8. Bah M, Bye R, Pereda-Miranda R: Hepatotoxic pyrrolizidine alkaloids in the Mexican medicinal plant *Packera candidissima* (Asteraceas: Senecioneae), *J Ethnopharmacol* 43:19, 1994.
9. Bakerink JA et al: Multiple organ failure after ingestion of pennyroyal oil from herbal tea in two infants, *Pediatrics* 98:944, 1996.
10. Ballard T et al: Green tobacco sickness: occupational nicotine poisoning in tobacco workers, *Arch Environ Health* 50:384, 1995.
11. Banea-Mayambu JP, Tylleskar T, Rosling H: Konzo and ebola in Bandundu region of Zaire, *Lancet* 349:621, 1997.
12. Banea-Mayambu JP et al: Geographical and seasonal association between linamarin and cyanide exposure from cassava and the upper motor neurone disease konzo in former Zaire, *Trop Med Int Health* 2:1143, 1997.
13. Baron F, Deprez M, Beguin Y: The veno-occlusive disease of the liver, *Haematologica* 82:718, 1997.
14. Barrella M et al: Hypokalemic rhabdomyolysis associated with liquorice ingestion: report of an atypical case, *Ital J Neurol Sci* 18:217, 1997.
15. Beer JH, Vogt A, Bernhard W: Gourmet restaurant syndrome, *Lancet* 343:1302, 1994.
16. Benomran FA, Henry JD: Homicide and strychnine poisoning, *Med Sci Law* 36:271, 1996.
17. Berlin R, Smilkstein M: Wormwood.oil@toxic.ing, *J Toxicol Clin Toxicol* 34:583, 1996.
18. Biglieri EG: Spectrum of mineralocorticoid hypertension, *Hypertension* 17:251, 1991.
19. Bisset NG, Houghton PJ: Some current trends in medicinal plant research. In Wijesekera R: *The medical plant industry,* Boca Raton, Fla, 1991, CRC Press.
20. Blaw ME et al: Poisoning with Carolina jessamine (*Gelsemium sempervirens* [L.] Ait.), *J Pediatr* 94:998, 1979.
21. Burkhart KK, Magalski AE, Donovan JW: A retrospective review of the use of activated charcoal and physostigmine in the treatment of jimson weed poisoning, *J Toxicol Clin Toxicol* 37:389, 1999.
22. But PPH, Tai YT, Young K: Three fatal cases of herbal aconite poisoning, *Vet Hum Toxicol* 36:212, 1994.
23. Carlton MW, Kunkel DB: St. Anthony's Fire: eponym misused, *Acad Emerg Med* 2:1114, 1995.
24. Carlton MW, Kunkel DB: St. Anthony's Fire: an eponym for ergotism, not erysipelas, *Am Fam Physician* 52:95, 1995.
25. Carter AJ: Narcosis and nightshade, *BMJ* 313:1630, 1996.
26. Castorena JL et al: A fatal poisoning from *Nicotiana glauca, Clin Toxicol* 25:429, 1987.
27. Ceha LJ et al: Anticholinergic toxicity from nightshade berry poisoning responsive to physostigmine, *J Emerg Med* 15:65, 1997.
28. Centers for Disease Control: Jimson weed poisoning—Texas, New York, and California, 1994, *MMWR* 44:41, 1995.
29. Centers for Disease Control: Water hemlock poisoning—Maine, 1992, *MMWR* 43:229, 1994.
30. Challoner KR, McCarron MM: Castor bean intoxication, *Ann Emerg Med* 19:1177, 1990.
31. Chan TYK, Tomlinson B, Critchley JAJH: Aconitine poisoning following the ingestions of Chinese herbal medicines: a report of eight cases, *Aust NZ J Med* 23:268, 1993.
32. Chan TYK, Tomlinson B, Critchley JAJH: Herb-induced aconite poisoning presenting as tetraplegia, *Vet Hum Toxicol* 36:133, 1994.
33. Chiang WT, Yang CC, Deng JF: Cardiac arrhythmia and betel nut chewing—is there a causal effect? *Vet Hum Toxicol* 40:287, 1998.
34. Clark RF, Selden BS, Curry SC: Digoxin-specific Fab fragments in the treatment of oleander toxicity in a canine model, *Ann Emerg Med* 20:1073, 1991.
35. Corchia C et al: Favism in a female newborn infant whose mother ingested fava beans before delivery, *J Pediatr* 127:807, 1995.
36. Cummins RO, Haulman J, Quan L: Near-fatal yew berry intoxication treated with external cardiac pacing and digoxin-specific FAB antibody fragments, *Ann Emerg Med* 19:38, 1990.
37. Curry SC, LoVecchio F: Hydrogen cyanide and inorganic cyanide salts. In Sullivan JB, Kreiger JR, editors: *Hazardous materials toxicology,* Lippincott Williams & Wilkins (in press).
38. Curry SC, Mills KC, Graeme KA: Neurotransmitters. In *Goldfrank's toxicologic emergencies,* ed 6, Stamford, Conn, 1998, Appleton & Lange.
39. Dafni A, Yaniv Z: Solanaceae as medicinal plants in Israel, *J Ethnopharmacol* 44:11,1994.
40. Damaj MI et al: Pharmacology of lobeline, a nicotinic receptor ligand, *J Pharmacol Exp Ther* 282:410, 1997.
41. Davis EW: The ethnobiology of the Haitian zombi, *J Ethnopharmacol* 9:85, 1983.
42. Davis JH: *Abrus precatorius* (rosary pea): the most common lethal plant poison, *J Fla Med Assoc* 65:189, 1978.
43. DiMarzo V et al: Endocannabinoids: endogenous cannabinoid receptor ligands with neuromodulary action, *Trends Neurosci* 21:521, 1998.
44. Doherty JF et al: Fascioliasis due to imported khat, *Lancet* 345:462, 1995.
45. Drummer OH et al: Three deaths from hemlock poisoning, *Med J Aust* 162:592, 1995.
46. Duke JA: *Handbook of medicinal herbs,* Boca Raton, Fla, 1987, CRC Press.
47. Eddleston M, Ariaratnam CA, Meyer WP: Epidemic of self-poisoning with seeds of yellow oleander tree (*Thevetia peruviana*) in northern Sri Lanka, *Trop Med Int Health* 4:266, 1999.
48. Eriksson JW, Carlberg B, Hillorn V: Life-threatening ventricular tachycardia due to liquorice-induced hypokalaemia, *J Intern Med* 245:307, 1999.
49. Everist SL: *Poisonous plants of Australia,* Sydney, 1981, Angus & Robertson.
50. Famularo G, Corsi FM, Giacanelli M: Iatrogenic worsening of hypokalemia and neuromuscular paralysis associated with the use of glucose solutions for potassium replacement in a young woman with licorice intoxication and furosemide abuse, *Acad Emerg Med* 6:960, 1999.
51. Farre M et al: Fatal oxalic acid poisoning from sorrel soup, *Lancet* 335:233, 1990 (letter).
52. Festa M et al: A case of Veratrum poisoning [Italian], *Minerva Anestesiologica* 62:195, 1996.
53. Frank BS et al: Ingestion of poison hemlock (*Conium maculatum*), *West J Med* 163:573, 1995.
54. Frohne D, Pfander HJ: *A colour atlas of poisonous plants,* London, 1984, Wolfe.
55. Furbee B, Wermuth M: Life-threatening plant poisoning, *Crit Care Clin* 13:849, 1997.

56. Furbee RB, Curry SC, Kunkel DB: Ingestion of *Argyreia nervosa* (Hawaiian baby woodrose) seeds, *Vet Hum Toxicol* 33:370, 1991.

57. Gardner DG: Injury to the oral mucous membranes caused by the common houseplant, *Dieffenbachia, Oral Surg Oral Med Oral Pathol* 78:631, 1994.

58. Giron LM et al: Ethnobotanical survey of the medicinal flora used by the Caribs of Guatemala, *J Ethnopharmacol* 34:173, 1991.

59. Graeme KA, Kunkel DB: Psychoactive plants and mushrooms, *Top Emerg Med* 19:64, 1997.

60. Graeme KA et al: Cardiotoxicity from ingestion of unprocessed *Nerium oleander* leaves treated with Fab fragments, *J Toxicol Clin Toxicol* 36:457, 1998.

61. Greene GS, Patterson SG, Warner E: Ingestion of angel's trumpet: an increasingly common source of toxicity, *South Med J* 89:365, 1996.

62. Gunnarsdottir S, Johannesson T: Glycyrrhetic acid in human blood after ingestion of glycyrrhizic acid in licorice, *Pharmacol Toxicol* 81:300, 1997.

63. Gupta A, Joshi P, Jortani SA: A case of nondigitalis cardiac glycoside toxicity, *Ther Drug Monit* 19:711, 1997.

64. Haas LF: *Papaver sominferum* (opium poppy), *J Neurol Neurosurg Psychiatry* 58:402, 1995.

65. Habermehl GG: Secondary and tertiary metabolites as plant toxins, *Toxicon* 36:1707, 1998.

66. Hall W, Solowij N: Adverse effects of cannabis, *Lancet* 352:1611, 1998.

67. Hampl JS et al: Acute hemolysis related to consumption of fava beans: a case study and medical nutrition therapy approach, *J Am Diet Assoc* 97:182, 1997.

68. Hare WR et al: Chinaberry poisoning in two dogs, *J Am Vet Med Assoc* 210:1638, 1997 (letter).

69. Hashimoto H, Clyde VJ, Parko KL: Botulism from peyote, *N Engl J Med* 339:203, 1998 (letter).

70. Hasler J, Lee S: Acute hemolytic anemia after ingestion of fava beans, *Am J Emerg Med* 11:560, 1993.

71. Heilpern KL: *Zigadenus* poisoning, *Ann Emerg Med* 25:259, 1995.

72. Heiser JM et al: Massive strychnine intoxication: serial blood levels in a fatal case, *J Toxicol Clin Toxicol* 30:269, 1992.

73. Hood RL: Colchicine poisoning, *J Emerg Med* 12:171, 1994.

74. Hur Y et al: Isolation and characterization of pokeweed antiviral protein mutations in *Saccharomyces cerevisiae*: identification of residues important for toxicity, *Proc Natl Acad Sci USA* 92:8448, 1995.

75. Jaffe AM, Gephardt D, Courtemanche L: Poisoning due to ingestion of *Veratrum viride* (false hellebore), *J Emerg Med* 8:161, 1990.

76. Kalix P: Cathinone, a natural amphetamine, *Pharmacol Toxicol* 70:77, 1992.

77. Keating JP et al: Infantile methemoglobinemia caused by carrot juice, *N Engl J Med* 288:824, 1973.

78. Khattab NY, Amer G: Undetected neuropsychophysiological sequelae of khat chewing in standard aviation medical examination, *Aviat Space Environ Med* 66:739, 1995.

79. Kinamore PA, Jaeger RW, Casro FJ: *Abrus* and *Ricinus* ingestion: management of three cases, *J Toxicol Clin Toxicol* 17:401, 1980.

80. King MA et al: Poppy tea and the baker's first seizure, *Lancet* 350:716, 1997.

81. Kingsbury JM: *Poisonous plants of the United States and Canada,* Englewood Cliffs, NJ, 1964, Prentice-Hall.

82. Kingsbury JM: Phytotoxicology. I. Major problems associated with poisonous plants, *Clin Pharmacol Ther* 10:163, 1969.

83. Kne T, Brokaw M, Wax P: Fatality from calcium chloride in a chronic digoxin toxic patient, *J Toxicol Clin Toxicol* 35:505, 1997.

84. Krenzelok EP, Jacobsen TD: Plant exposures . . . a national profile of the most common plant genera, *Vet Hum Toxicol* 39:248, 1997.

85. Krenzelok EP, Jacobsen TD, Aronis J: Is the yew really poisonous to you? *J Toxicol Clin Toxicol* 36:219, 1998.

86. Lampe KF: Rhododendrons, mountain laurel, and madhoney, *JAMA* 259:2009, 1988.

87. Langford SD, Boor PJ: Oleander toxicity: an examination of human and animal toxic exposures, *Toxicol* 109:1, 1996.

88. Lavoie FW, Harris TM: Fatal nicotine ingestion, *J Emerg Med* 9:133, 1991.

89. Lawerence RA: Poison centers and plants: more pollyanna data? *J Toxicol Clin Toxicol* 36:225, 1998.

90. Lewis W, Elvin-Lewis MPF: *Medical botany: plants affecting man's health,* New York, 1977, Wiley.

91. Litovitz TL et al: 1998 annual report of the American Association of Poison Control Centers toxic exposure surveillance system, *Am J Emerg Med* 17:435, 1999.

92. McDermott WV, Ridker PM: The Budd-Chiari syndrome and hepatic veno-occlusive disease: recognition and treatment, *Arch Surg* 125:525, 1990.

93. McIntire MS, Guest JR, Porterfield JE: Philodendron—an infant death, *J Toxicol Clin Toxicol* 28:177, 1990.

94. Meda HA et al: Epidemic of fatal encephalopathy in preschool children in Burkina Faso and consumption of unripe ackee *(Blighia sapida)* fruit, *Lancet* 353:536, 1999.

95. Mellick LB et al: Neuromuscular blockade after ingestion of tree tobacco *(Nicotiana glauca)*, *Ann Emerg Med* 34:101, 1999.

96. Meneely KD: Poppy seed ingestion: the Oregon perspective, *J Forensic Sci* 37:1158, 1992.

97. Miller MB, Eng J, Curry SC: Sodium bicarbonate for *Taxus*-induced dysrhythmia, *J Toxicol Clin Toxicol* 38:572, 2000.

98. Miranda CL et al: The microsomal function of a pyrrolic alcohol glutathione conjugate of the pyrrolizidine alkaloid senecionine, *Xenobiotica* 22:1321, 1992.

99. Mitchell MI, Routledge PA: Poisoning by hemlock water dropwort, *Lancet* 1:423, 1977 (letter).

100. Mrvos R et al: *Philodendron/Dieffenbachia* ingestions: are they a problem? *Clin Toxicol* 29:485, 1991.

101. Nelson BS, Heischober B: Betel nut: a common drug used by naturalized citizens from India, Far East Asia, and the South Pacific Islands, *Ann Emerg Med* 34:238, 1999.

102. Nishioka SA, Resende ES: Transitory complete atrioventricular block associated to ingestion of *Nerium oleander, Rev Assoc Med Brasil* 41:60, 1995.

103. Osterloh J, Herold S, Pond S: Oleander interference in the digoxin radioimmunoassay in a fatal ingestion, *JAMA* 247:1596, 1982.

104. Palatnick W et al: Toxicokinetics of acute strychnine poisoning, *J Toxicol Clin Toxicol* 35:617, 1997.

105. Pamies RJ, Powell R, Herold AH: The *Dieffenbachia* plant, *J Fla Med Assoc* 79:760, 1992.

106. Pelders MG, Ros JJW: Poppy seeds: differences in morphine and codeine content and variation in inter- and intra-individual excretion, *J Forensic Sci* 41:209, 1996.

107. Pickwell SM, Schimelpfening S, Palinkas LA: "Betelmania": betel quid chewing by Cambodian women in the United States and its potential health effects, *West J Med* 160:326, 1994.

108. Puschner B et al: Sweet clover poisoning in dairy cattle in California, *J Am Vet Med Assoc* 212:857, 1998.

109. Quatrehomme G et al: Intoxication from *Veratrum album, Hum Exp Toxicol* 12:111, 1993.

110. Radford DJ et al: Naturally occurring glycosides, *Med J Aust* 144:540, 1986.

111. Rauber-Luthy CH et al: Lethal poisoning after ingestion of a tea prepared from the Angel's Trumpet *(Datura Suaveolens)*, *J Toxicol Clin Toxicol* 37:414, 1999.

112. Reardon M, Duane A, Cotter P: Attempted homicide in hospital, *Irish J Med Sci* 162:315, 1993.

113. Rich SA, Libera JM, Locke RJ: Treatment of foxglove extract poisoning with digoxin-specific Fab fragments, *Ann Emerg Med* 22:1904, 1993.

114. Ridker PM: Health hazards of unusual herbal teas, *Am Fam Physician* 39:153, 1989.

115. Ridker PM, McDermott WV: Comfrey herb tea and hepatic veno-occlusive disease, *Lancet* 1:657, 1989.

116. Rizzi D et al: Rhabdomyolysis and acute tubular necrosis in coniine (hemlock) poisoning, *Lancet* 2:1461, 1989.

117. Roeder E, Bourauel T: Pyrrolizidine alkaloids from *Senecio leucanthemifolius* and *Senecio rodriguezii*, *Nat Toxins* 1:241, 1993.

118. Rosling H: Cyanide exposure from linseed, *Lancet* 34:177, 1993.

119. Sanz P, Reig R: Clinical and pathological findings in fatal plant oxalosis: a review, *Am J Forensic Med Pathol* 13:342, 1992.

120. Sayre JW, Kaymakcalan S: Cyanide poisoning from apricot seeds among children in central Turkey, *N Engl J Med* 270:1113, 1964.

121. Schneider F et al: Plasma and urine concentrations of atropine after ingestion of cooked deadly nightshade berries, *J Toxicol Clin Toxicol* 34:113, 1996.

122. Seldon BS, Curry SC: Anticholinergics. In Reisdorff EJ, Roberts MR, Wiegenstein JG, editors: *Pediatric emergency medicine*, Philadelphia, 1993, WB Saunders.

123. Shannon M: Toxicology reviews: physostigmine, *Pediatr Emerg Care* 14:224, 1998.

124. Shenoy R: Pitfalls in the treatment of jimsonweed intoxication, *Am J Psychiatry* 151:1396, 1994 (letter).

125. Sherratt HS, Al-Bassam SS: Glycine in akee poisoning, *Lancet* 2:1243, 1976 (letter).

126. Sherratt HSA, Turnbull DM: Methylene blue and fatal encephalopathy from ackee fruit poisoning, *Lancet* 353:1623, 1999 (letter).

127. Sjoholm A, Lindberg A, Personne M: Acute nutmeg intoxication, *J Int Med* 243:327, 1998 (letter).

128. Slifman NR et al: Contamination of botanical dietary supplements by Digitalis lanata, *N Engl J Med* 339:806, 1998.

129. Sopchak CA et al: Central anticholinergic syndrome due to jimson weed physostigmine: therapy revisited? *J Toxicol Clin Toxicol* 36:43, 1998 (letter).

130. Sperl W et al: Reversible hepatic veno-occlusive disease in an infant after consumption of pyrrolizidine-containing herbal tea, *Eur J Pediatr* 154:112, 1995.

131. Starreveld E, Hope E: Cicutoxin poisoning (water hemlock), *Neurology* 25:730, 1975.

132. Stein RD et al: Bradycardia produced by pyridostigmine and physostigmine, *Can J Anaesth* 44:1286, 1997.

133. Suchard JR, Wallace KL, Gerkin RD: Acute cyanide toxicity caused by apricot kernel ingestion, *Ann Emerg Med* 32:742, 1998.

134. Tai YT et al: Cardiotoxicity after accidental herb-induced aconite poisoning, *Lancet* 340:1254, 1992.

135. Thompson HS: Cornpicker's pupil: jimson weed mydriasis, *J Iowa Med Soc* 61:475, 1971.

136. Tibballs J: Clinical effects and management of eucalyptus oil ingestion in infants and young children, *Med J Aust* 163:177, 1995.

137. Tuncok Y et al: *Urginea maritima* (squill) toxicity, *J Toxicol Clin Toxicol* 33:83, 1995.

138. Unnithan S, Strang J: Poppy tea dependence, *Br J Psychiatry* 163:813, 1993.

139. Vanderhoff BT, Mosser MD: Jimsonweed toxicity: management of anticholinergic plant ingestion, *Am Fam Physician* 46:526, 1992.

140. Van Dongen PW, de Groot AN: History of ergot alkaloids from ergotism to ergometrine, *Eur J Obstet Gynecol Reprod Biol* 60:109, 1995.

141. Van Gils C, Cox PA: Ethnobotany of nutmeg in the Spice Islands, *J Ethnopharmacol* 42:117, 1994.

142. Van Ingen G et al: Sudden unexpected death due to *Taxus* poisoning: a report of five cases, with review of the literature, *Forensic Sci Int* 56:81, 1992.

143. Wax PM: Squill through the ages, *J Toxicol Clin Toxicol* 33:86, 1995.

144. Webb NJA, Pitt WR: Eucalyptus oil poisoning in childhood: 41 cases in southeast Queensland, *J Paediatr Child Health* 29:366, 1993.

145. Wedin GP et al: Castor bean poisoning, *Am J Emerg Med* 4:259, 1986.

146. Wilder P, Mathys K, Brenneisen R: Pharmacodynamics and pharmacokinetics of khat: a controlled study, *Clin Pharmacol Ther* 55:556, 1994.

147. Yavuz H et al: Honey poisoning in Turkey, *Lancet* 337:789, 1991 (letter).

49 Mushroom Toxicity

Sandra Schneider and Mark Donnelly

> *"Had nature any outcast face?*
> *Could she a son condemn?*
> *Had nature an Iscariot*
> *That mushroom—it is him."*
>
> Emily Dickinson

Mushrooms are often considered the vermin of the vegetable world, likened to snakes, slugs, and worms. Some are regarded as mystical and others as delicacies. The location of tasty morels is passed from generation to generation, closely guarded from strangers. Each autumn and spring, foragers scour the woods for known delicacies, and new ones untried. Some mushroom foragers search for "little brown mushrooms," not for their taste, but to evoke hallucinations.

Eating unidentified or misidentified species can be dangerous. Each year there are 10,000 to 15,000 cases of mushroom toxicity in the United States.[48] In up to 95% of these cases, the mushroom was incorrectly identified.[78] More than 40,000 species of fungi are currently described, with new ones added each year. Only a few species are toxic.

The fungi kingdom contains molds, smuts, rusts, mildews, yeast, and mushrooms, which are different from plants because they lack chlorophyll. "Toadstool" is often used to describe toxic mushrooms; this chapter differentiates toxic mushrooms by their toxins and scientific names.

The body of a fungus is a dense network of branching filaments or hyphae. The mushroom is the fruiting body of the fungus containing the spores. The hyphae and mycelia generally occur in an underground network supporting the visible mushroom. Mushrooms often grow in large rings radiating from a central network of mycelia. In the past these "fairy rings" were thought to have mystical influence. Fungi are largely saprophytic, involved with decomposition of rotting materials, usually wood. They can also be parasitic or symbiotic, living on viable materials with or without beneficial effect to the host.

As a mushroom emerges from the ground, it is covered with a membrane or veil (Figure 49-1). As the mushroom grows, the membrane breaks, leaving residual marks on the cap of the mushroom known as "warts." These warts may remain firmly attached to the mushroom, or only residual spots may remain, depending on the species of mushroom and environmental conditions. The emerging cap takes on a shape consistent with the specific species, ranging from cylindric to convex to funnel shaped.

Gills, located under the caps, contain the spore-producing bodies. Some gills are covered with a second membrane or partial veil, later pulling away to form an annulus or ring midway down the stalk of the mushroom. Gills may be attached firmly to the stalk, even running down the stalk, or only to the cap itself (free gills) (Figure 49-2). The attachment of the gills is an important aid to identification of some poisonous mushrooms, such as *Amanita phalloides* (Figure 49-3).

The stalk (stipe) begins at the cap and ends either underground or in a cup (vulva). A cup or vulva at or just below ground level often is seen with a poisonous species. The stalk is generally located in the middle of the cap and may or may not be tapered. The stalks of many poisonous species enlarge below the cap, ending in a bulb. The stalk may have a ringed membrane as evidence that the partial veil formerly protected the gills. Spores are produced by spore-forming bodies on the gills and are expelled into the air after they mature.

Spores vary in size, color, and shape but are usually unicellular. They average 5 to 10 μm in diameter. Spores are useful in identifying mushroom species. They can be obtained by cutting the stalk of a fresh specimen close to the gills, then laying the cap gill-side down on white paper for a few hours at room temperature. The initial color seen after removal of the gills is used for identification. With drying the color may fade or change. Additional information about spores can be acquired by staining with Melzer's reagent (a solution of iodine and chloral hydrate). Spores that stain blue are called *amyloid*, indicating the presence of starch. This technique may be particularly useful in spore identification from gastric aspirates. The spores of *Amanita* species are amyloid. Thin-layer chromatography of spores is a more accurate aid to identification.

Mushrooms contain approximately 90% water and 3% proteins and other nitrogen-containing compounds. The remainder is largely carbohydrate, fat, and a few vitamins. Nutritionally unimpressive, mushrooms are consumed in great quantities, primarily for their taste and texture. Wild mushrooms have the additional allure of being free. Of the many varieties of wild mushrooms, few are deadly or cause serious pathophysiologic derangement.

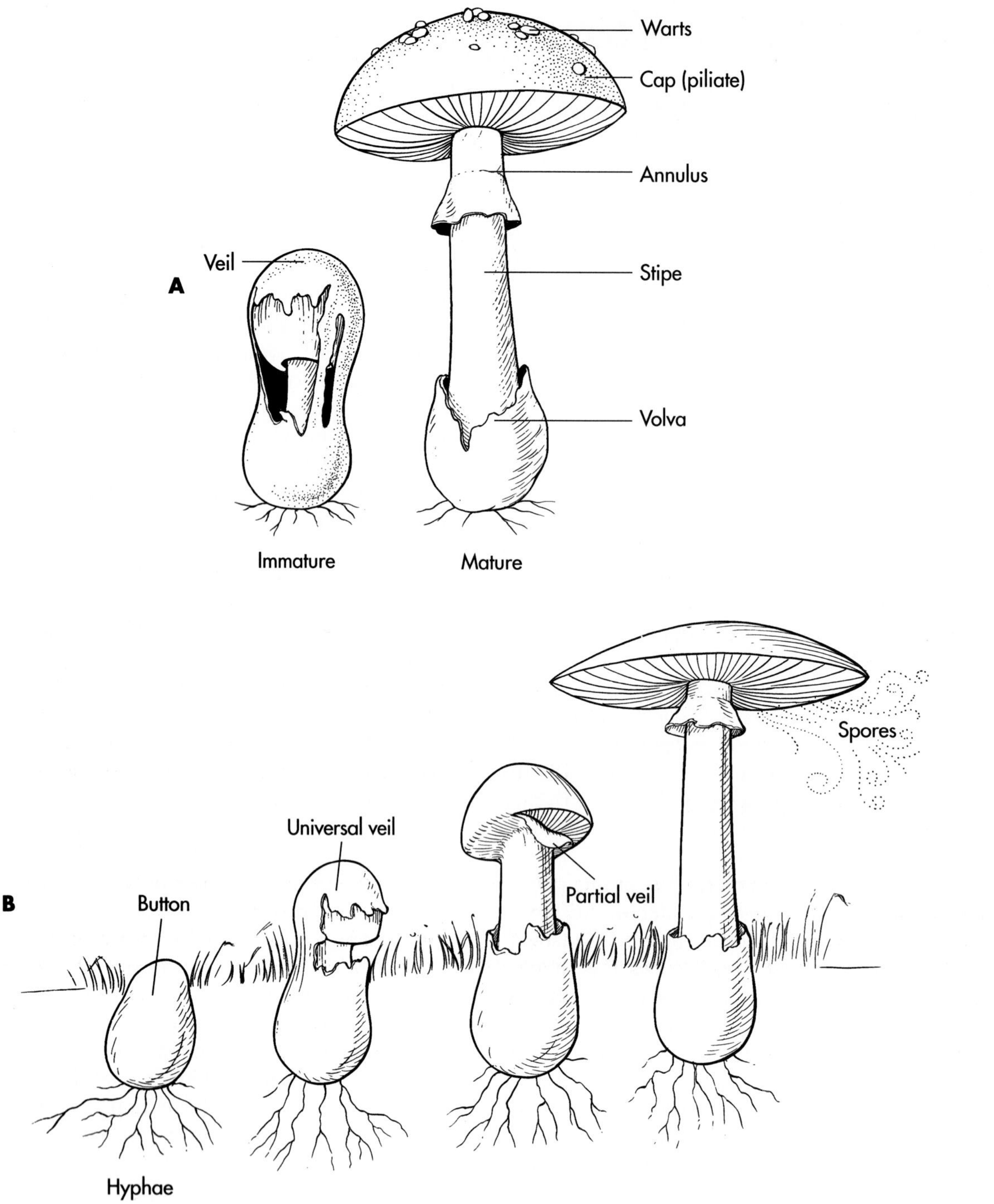

Warts

Cap (piliate)

Annulus

Veil

A

Stipe

Volva

Immature

Mature

Spores

B

Button

Universal veil

Partial veil

Hyphae

Figure 49-1 **A,** Structural characteristics, and **B,** life cycle of mushrooms.

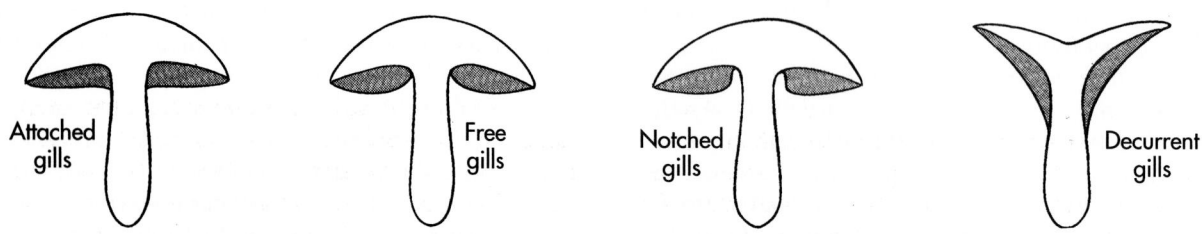

Attached gills

Free gills

Notched gills

Decurrent gills

Figure 49-2 Mushroom gill types.

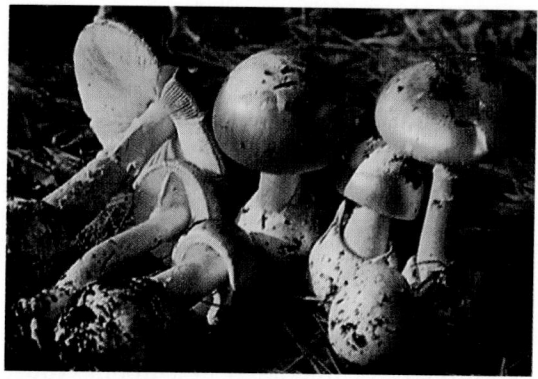

Figure 49-3 Death cap *(Amanita phalloides).*

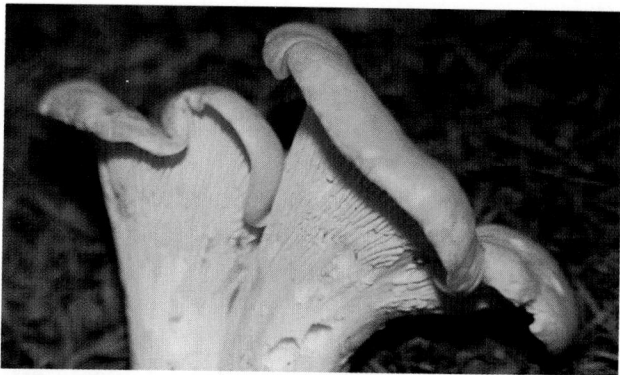

Figure 49-5 *Cantharellus cibarius.*

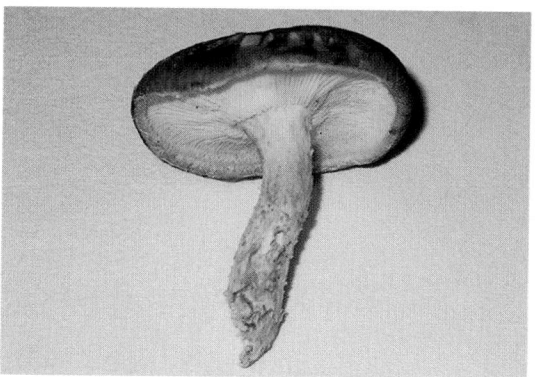

Figure 49-4 Shiitake mushroom.

Many immigrants fail to realize that the nontoxic mushrooms from their native lands have toxic look-alikes in America. This has been particularly true of Southeast Asian immigrants, who are attracted to the large *Amanita* species. Entire families have been poisoned, with many fatalities. The Russian roulette played by mushroom foragers is statistically safe. Some self-proclaimed experts are simply lucky; occasionally, they are not.

NONTOXIC MUSHROOMS

The most common commercially available mushroom in the United States is *Agaricus bisporus.* It is cultivated in abandoned mine shafts and caves. This small white mushroom with dark gills is often picked before the gills are fully exposed. Although the mushroom is considered nontoxic, hypersensitivity reactions and gastrointestinal (GI) symptoms have been reported. Researchers have tried to link carcinogenesis to *A. bisporus.*[78,97] Although tumors of the bone (osteomas, osteosarcomas) and stomach (papillomas, carcinomas) develop in mice fed large amounts of uncooked mushrooms, no direct link exists between human ingestions and cancer.[96]

A. bisporus can also be found in the wild. *Agaricus* species may be confused with the deadly *Amanita* species, as well as some *Agaricus* species that cause GI irritation.

Nontoxic mushrooms may carry environmental toxins, such as heavy metals and pesticides. Mushrooms with high lead concentrations have been gathered near highways.[35] High mercury concentrations are found in mushrooms from industrial sites.[18,35] Human toxicity has not been reported.

Mushrooms may cause allergic reactions. Acute anaphylaxis from mushroom ingestion is rare, despite the presence of haptens capable of inciting an allergic response.[56] More often, symptoms develop from inhalation of spores.[72] Victims may present with anaphylaxis or more often with chronic hypersensitivity pneumonitis. Hypersensitivity reactions are described in workers exposed to cultivation of *A. bisporus* (the most popular commercially grown mushroom in America)[63] and shiitake *(Lentinus edodes),* the popular Japanese mushroom (Figure 49-4).[85] Asthma symptoms developed in nearly 10% of shiitake-exposed workers. In one study, all workers had positive skin and inhalation challenge tests.[91] Spore counts correlate with asthma symptoms.

GI symptoms after ingestion of mushrooms may not be caused by toxins. Bacterial food poisoning may occur in foods that coincidentally contain mushrooms. Small bowel obstruction occurred in a person who consumed 500 g of the edible mushroom *Cantharellus cibarius* (chanterelle) (Figure 49-5).[36] This was largely a result of poor mastication, since entire mushrooms were recovered from the victim's intestines.

Most wild mushrooms are nontoxic, and many are delicious. Morels *(Morchella esculenta, M. deliciosa)* are highly prized delicacies. Chanterelles *(C. cibarius)* and several species of *Boletus* are particularly tasty. The chicken mushroom *(Laetiporus sulphurus)* often replaces chicken in Chinese dishes (Figure 49-6).

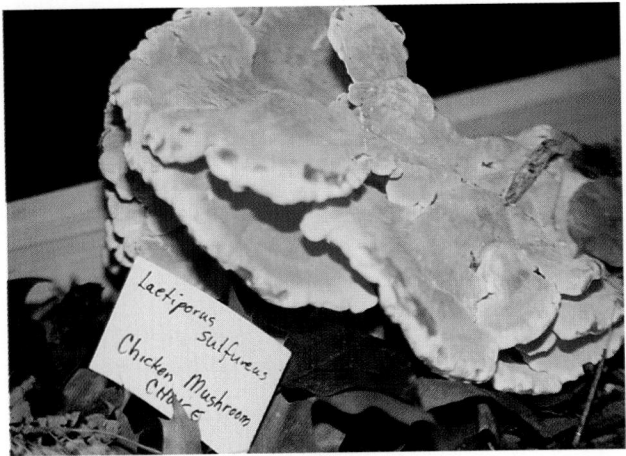

Figure 49-6 *Laetiporus sulphureus.*

GASTROINTESTINAL TOXINS

Most toxic mushrooms fall into the group of GI irritants. This large, heterogenous group of mushrooms causes GI distress—nausea, vomiting, and diarrhea—beginning 1 to 2 hours after ingestion and resolving in 6 to 12 hours. Even *A. bisporus*, the common cultivated mushroom, may cause brief gastroenteritis in some individuals.[92]

Causative Mushrooms

A large number of unrelated mushrooms cause GI symptoms with varying host response (Box 49-1). *Chlorophyllum molybdites*, also known as *Lepiota morganii*, is the most frequently reported toxic mushroom

---

Box 49-1   MUSHROOMS REPORTED TO CAUSE GASTROINTESTINAL IRRITATION

Agaricus albolutescens
Agaricus hondensis
Agaricus placomyces
Agaricus silvicola
Agaricus xanthodermus
Amanita brunnescens
Amanita chlorinosma
Amanita flavoconia
Amanita flavorubescens
Amanita frostiana
Amanita parcivolvata
Amanita spissa
Amanita spreta
Amanita volvata
Boletus luridus
Boletus pulcherrimus
Boletus satanus
Boletus sensibilis
Cantharellus bonari
Cantharellus floccosus
Cantharellus kauffmanii
Chlorophyllum molybdites (Lepiota morganii)
Entoloma (Rhodophyllus) lividum
Entoloma (Rhodophyllus) nidorosum
Entoloma (Rhodophyllus) rhodopolium
Entoloma (Rhodophyllus) salmoneum
Entoloma (Rhodophyllus) strictius
Entoloma (Rhodophyllus) vernum
Hebeloma crustuliniforme
Hebeloma fastibile
Hebeloma mesophaeum
Hebeloma sinapizans
Lactarius chrysorheus
Lactarius glaucescens
Lactarius helvus
Lactarius representaneus

Lactarius rufus
Lactarius scrobiculatus
Lactarius torminosus
Lactarius uvidus
Lepiota clypeolaria
Lepiota cristata
Lepiota lutea
Lepiota morganii
Lepiota naucina
Lycoperdon marginatum
Lycoperdon subincarnatum
Morchella angusticeps
Morchella crassipes
Morchella deliciosa
Morchella esculenta
Morchella semilibera
Naematoloma (Hypholoma) fasciculare
Omphalotus olearius
Omphalotus illudens
Omphalotus olivascens
Paxillus involutus
Ramaria (Clavaria) formosa
Ramaria (Clavaria) gelantinosa
Russula emetica (Figure 49-7)
Scleroderma aurantium (Figure 49-8)
Scleroderma cepa
Tricholoma album
Tricholoma muscarium
Tricholoma pardinum
Tricholoma pessundatum
Tricholoma saponaceum
Tricholoma sejunctum
Tricholoma sulphureum
Tricholoma venenata
Verpa bohemica

ingested in America (Figure 49-9).[14,99] Most persons who ingest *C. molybdites* confuse it with *A. bisporus*, which it closely resembles. The common name for *C. molybdites*, green-spored parasol, describes the characteristics of this summer mushroom. The whitish cap is large, 10 to 40 cm (4 to 16 inches), initially smooth and round, and becomes convex with maturity. Tan or brown warts may be present. The gills are free from the stalk, initially white to yellow, and become green with maturity. The stalk is 5 to 25 cm long, smooth, and white. The ring is generally brown on the underside. Spores are green. The mushroom is common in most of eastern and southern North America and in California. In southern California it is a common lawn mushroom.

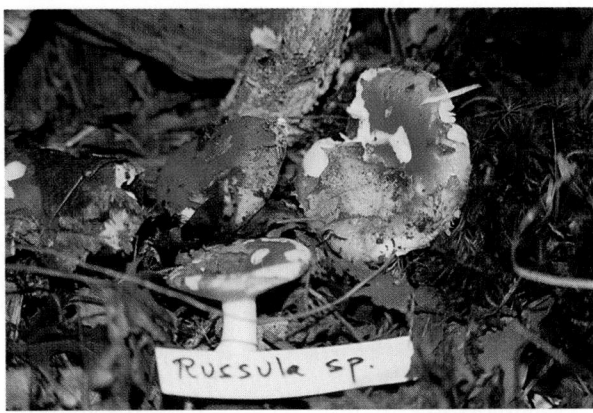

Figure 49-7   *Russula.*

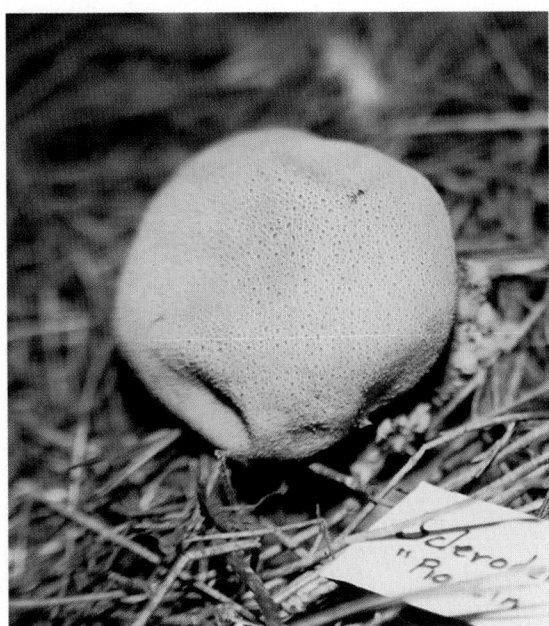

Figure 49-8   *Scleroderma.*

Another common mushroom causing GI symptoms is the jack-o'-lantern (Figure 49-10). The botanical classification is not completely settled. Most often it is referred to as *Omphalotus illudens*, *O. olearius*, or *O. olivascens*. It is a bright orange-yellow mushroom with sharp-edged gills and often grows in clusters at the base of stumps or on buried roots of deciduous trees. The cap is 4 to 16 cm in diameter on a stalk that is 4 to 20 cm long. Gills are olive to orange, with white to yellow spores. The mushroom shows characteristic luminescence lasting 40 to 50 hours after collection. Members of this family are found in both eastern and western North America, generally in autumn and early spring. They may be mistaken for the edible species *Cantharellus cibarius*. Some European reports have documented hepatic impairment and muscarinic effect after ingestion.[64,65] It is not clear whether the mushroom and its toxins are the same on both sides of the Atlantic.[3]

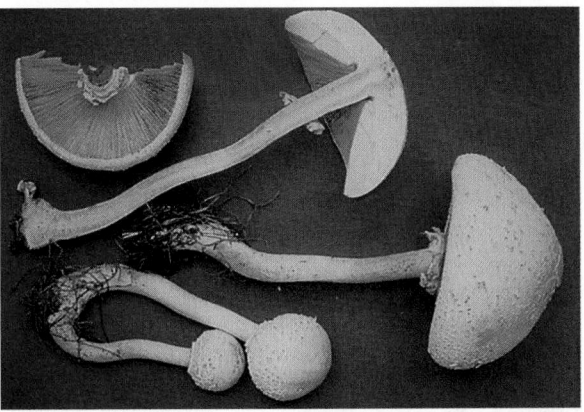

Figure 49-9   *Chlorophyllum molybdites*, gastrointestinal irritant. *(From Phillips R:* Mushrooms of North America, *Boston, 1991, Little, Brown.)*

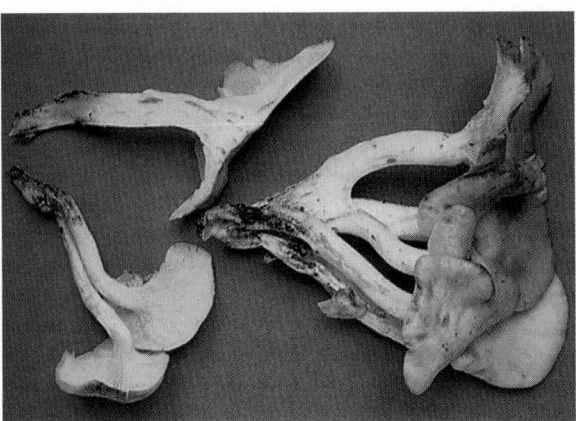

Figure 49-10   *Omphalotus olearius* (jack-o'-lantern mushroom), gastrointestinal irritant. *(From Phillips R:* Mushrooms of North America, *Boston, 1991, Little, Brown.)*

Although the genus *Amanita* is most famous for its deadly member *A. phalloides,* the genus also contains tasty nontoxic mushrooms *(A. caesarea, A. calyptrata, A. velosa).* Several *Amanita* species cause GI symptoms indistinguishable from those caused by jack-o'-lantern mushrooms or *Chlorophyllum molybdites. A. brunnescens* and *A. flavorubescens* are frequently listed as containing GI toxins, although they are occasionally listed as edible. These mushrooms resemble *A. rubescens* ("the blusher") (Figure 49-11). Both have broad yellowish to brown caps (3 to 15 cm) with loosely attached warts. The stalks are 3 to 18 cm long, enlarging toward the base with a superior ring. *A. brunnescens* stains reddish brown when bruised. As with their edible cousins, these mushrooms are found in summer or fall associated with hardwoods or conifers.

Several members of the genus *Agaricus,* particularly *A. albolutescens, A. silvaticus,* and *A. xanthodermus,* can cause GI symptoms. They resemble the cultivated mushrooms in grocery stores and are found in meadows and lawns in the summer and autumn. Table 49-1 lists the look-alike toxic and nontoxic mushrooms in this group.

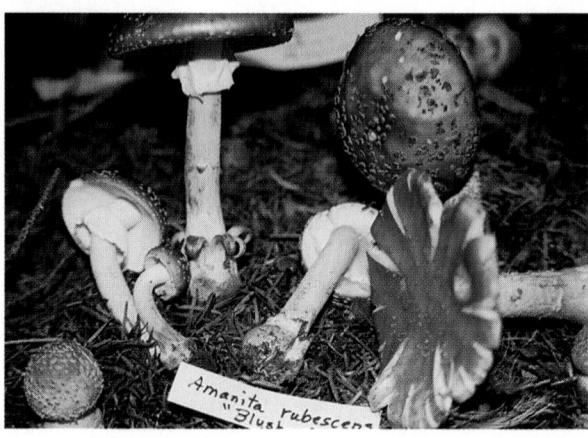

Figure 49-11 *Amanita rubescens.*

Toxins

A variety of toxins have been extracted from these mushrooms, although the structures are poorly described. Most are protein based and heat labile, although toxicity may not be completely eliminated with cooking. In some cases the toxin may be destroyed by heating, parboiling, or even preserving in salt. Host response to a toxin varies; some persons can eat such mushrooms without harm, whereas others become quite ill. Some mushrooms also contain hemolysins and toxins that cause hemorrhage and hepatitis in animals.[57,95] Human hemolysis has not been reported.[57]

Clinical Presentation

Within 1 to 2 hours of ingestion of these mushrooms, nausea, vomiting, intestinal cramping, and diarrhea develop. Stools are usually watery and occasionally bloody with fecal leukocytes. Chills, headaches, and myalgias may occur. Symptoms remit spontaneously in 6 to 12 hours. Most victims require only electrolytes and fluid replacement. The few serious cases reported in the literature have been associated with severe dehydration. In a review of 106 cases, all victims responded well to electrolyte replacement and occasional antiemetic or antidiarrheal medications.[19] Admitted patients were discharged in an average of 2 days.

Persons whose symptoms are delayed (beginning 4 hours or more after ingestion) probably have ingested a more toxic mushroom possibly *Amanita, Galerina, Lepiota,* or *Gyromitra.* These persons have severe GI distress and may develop hepatic failure. Most mushroom fatalities occur from ingestion of these mushrooms.

Recent reports of ingestion of jack-o'-lantern mushrooms describe mildly elevated liver transaminases.[101] Cases of metabolic acidosis and dehydration, and even death are attributed to *Chlorophyllum molybdites.*[14,94]

TABLE 49-1. Gastrointestinal Irritant Mushrooms Mistaken for Edible Species

GASTROINTESTINAL IRRITANT	EDIBLE SPECIES
Amanita brunnescens	*Amanita rubescens, A. inaurata*
Chlorophyllum molybdites	*Lepiota* spp., *Agaricus bisporus*
Entoloma spp.	*Pluteus cervinus, Entoloma abortivum*
Hebeloma crustuliniforme	*Rozites caperata*
Naematoloma fasciculare	*Armillariella mellea, Naematoloma sublateritium, N. capnoides*
Omphalotus olearius	*Cantharellus cibarius, Laetiporus sulphureus, Armillaria mellea*
Paxillus involutus	*Lactarius* spp.
Ramaria formosa, R. gelatinosa	*Ramaria* spp.
Scleroderma aurantium	*Lycoperdon perlatum*
Tricholoma pessundatum	*Tricholoma pessundatum*

Treatment

Treatment is largely supportive and does not depend on the type of mushroom ingested. Intravenous (IV) fluid and electrolyte replacement may be required. In a severe case an antiemetic such as prochlorperazine, 5 mg IV or 10 mg intramuscularly (IM), may prevent further emesis. Antidiarrheals are generally withheld unless diarrhea is prolonged or severe. Activated charcoal (1 g/kg) can be given orally or through a nasogastric tube, although no evidence shows that it decreases toxicity.

Care should be taken not to dismiss early GI symptoms when several types of unknown mushrooms have been ingested. Individuals may ingest both GI-irritant mushrooms *and* mushrooms containing serious toxins. Persons with prolonged gastroenteritis from unidentified mushrooms should be observed for delayed hepatic damage. Special efforts should be made to identify the ingested mushrooms.

DISULFIRAM-LIKE TOXINS

A fascinating toxicity is caused by some members of the *Coprinus* genus, known as "inky caps" (Figure 49-12). Individuals who ingest these mushrooms and subsequently ingest alcohol have symptoms similar to those of an alcohol-disulfiram (Antabuse) reaction.

Causative Mushrooms

Several members of the *Coprinus* genus may contain disulfiram-like toxins (Box 49-2), but symptoms are most common with *C. atramentarius*. The mushroom has a 2- to 8-cm cylindric cap on a thin 4- to 5-cm stalk. The cap is white, occasionally orange or yellow at the top. The mature cap often develops cracks, which turn up at its margins. The cap blackens as it matures and then liquefies ("inky cap"). A ring may be present low on the stalk. Spores are black. *C. atramentarius* grows throughout North America in clusters of three or more in grass or wood debris. It often appears overnight after a rain. Several members of the *Coprinus* genus are edible, including *C. comatus* ("shaggy mane"). All members of this genus are edible if no alcohol is ingested for the next 72 hours.

Toxin

Mushrooms causing a disulfiram reaction contain the toxin coprine, isolated from the mushroom *C. atramentarius* in 1975.[45] Coprine is distinct from disulfiram and is most likely a derivative of glutamine. It probably is not present in the raw mushroom but rather is a hydrolyte created during cooking.[59]

Coprine (or its derivative L-aminocyclopropranol) inhibits acetaldehyde dehydrogenase, similar to the action of disulfiram. Acetaldehyde accumulates, leading to β-adrenergic stimulation and the typical vasomotor response of flushing, diaphoresis, headache, tachycardia, nausea, and vomiting. Some authors believe that coprine is a relatively poor inhibitor of acetaldehyde dehydrogenase and suggest that symptoms result from altered neurotransmitter levels.[74]

Clinical Presentation

A history of wild mushroom ingestion within days before symptoms is rarely offered. Ingestion of the mushroom imparts sensitivity to alcohol, which begins 2 to 6 hours after ingestion and may last up to 72 hours. Within 15 to 30 minutes of subsequent alcohol ingestion the victim experiences severe headache, flushing, and tachycardia. Hyperventilation, shortness of breath, and palpitations may occur. Chest pain and orthostatic hypotension occur in more severe cases. Symptoms can be confused with an allergic reaction or acute myocardial infarction. Symptoms resolve spontaneously within 3 to 6 hours.

Box 49-2   MUSHROOMS SUSPECTED OR REPORTED TO CAUSE ALCOHOL-DISULFIRAM REACTION

Clitocybe clavipes
Coprinus atramentarius
Coprinus comatus
Coprinus insignis
Coprinus micaceus

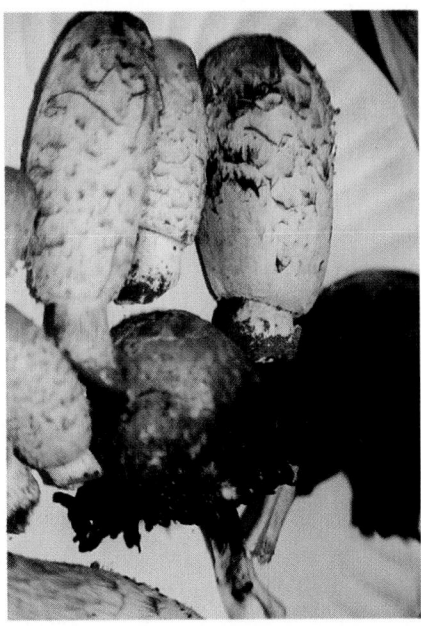

Figure 49-12 *Coprinus mushroom.*

Treatment

Supportive and symptomatic treatments are suggested. Baseline laboratory tests (blood urea nitrogen [BUN], creatinine, electrolytes, glucose) should be drawn. Urine output should be monitored. IV fluids should be given to keep urine output at 50 ml/hr (in children 1 ml/kg/hr). Activated charcoal is not beneficial. Charcoal does not adsorb alcohol; coprine has already been absorbed by the time the reaction occurs. Hypotension generally responds to IV fluid administration. Severe hypotension refractory to fluid replacement should be treated with norepinephrine (initially 4 to 8 μg/min; 1 to 2 μg/min in children and increased as necessary) rather than an indirect vasopressor, since norepinephrine stores are depleted in a true disulfiram reaction. Propranolol (0.5 to 3 mg IV; 0.01 to 0.02 mg/kg IV up to 1 mg in children) has been suggested for the treatment of supraventricular tachycardia. Propranolol may be repeated as needed after 5 to 10 minutes.

NEUROLOGIC TOXINS

Muscarine

Muscarine was first isolated from the mushroom *Amanita muscaria* more than 150 years ago. A classic muscarinic reaction includes salivation, lacrimation, urination, diaphoresis, GI upset, and emesis (SLUDGE syndrome). Buddhist adepts may have used *A. muscaria* to achieve enlightenment.[42]

Causative Mushrooms. *Amanita muscaria* has a cap 5 to 30 cm in diameter that is scarlet red with white warts (Figure 49-13). The stalk tapers upward and is white, often hollow, and grows 15 to 20 cm in length. It has a prominent cup and vulva and numerous rings. Gills are free and white, as are spores. The mushrooms grow in eastern North America and throughout much of the western United States, often near *Boletus edulis*. They grow under hardwoods and conifers from spring to autumn.

Potentially toxic amounts of muscarine are found in some members of the *Inocybe* and *Clitocybe* families (Table 49-2 and Box 49-3). The *Inocybe* family contains small brown mushrooms with conical caps up to 6 cm in diameter (Figure 49-14). Stalks are 2 to 10 cm long, covered with fine, brown to white hairs. Gills are brown and notched; spores are brown. They are found typically under hardwoods and conifers in the summer and fall. All members of this family are considered poisonous.

Box 49-3 MUSHROOMS REPORTED OR SUSPECTED TO CONTAIN MUSCARINE

Amanita gemmata	*Clitocybe dealbata*
Amanita muscaria	*Clitocybe nebularis*
Amanita pantherina	*Hebeloma crustuliniforme*
Amanita parcivolvata	*Inocybe fastigiata*
Boletus calopus	*Inocybe geophylla*
Boletus luridus	*Inocybe napipes*
Boletus pulcherrimus	*Inocybe patouillardii*
Boletus satanus	*Inocybe pudica*
Clitocybe aurantiaca	*Mycena pura*

TABLE 49-2. Look-Alikes of Mushrooms Causing Muscarine Poisoning

TOXIC SPECIES	EDIBLE SPECIES
Clitocybe dealbata	*Marasmius oreades*
Inocybe spp.	*Marasmius oreades*

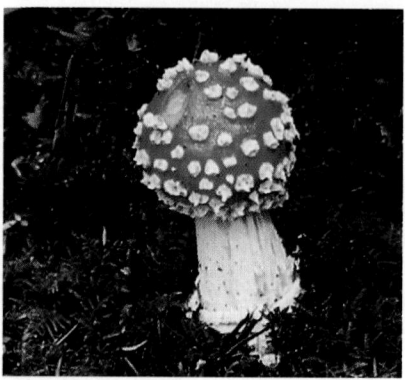

Figure 49-13 *Amanita muscaria.*

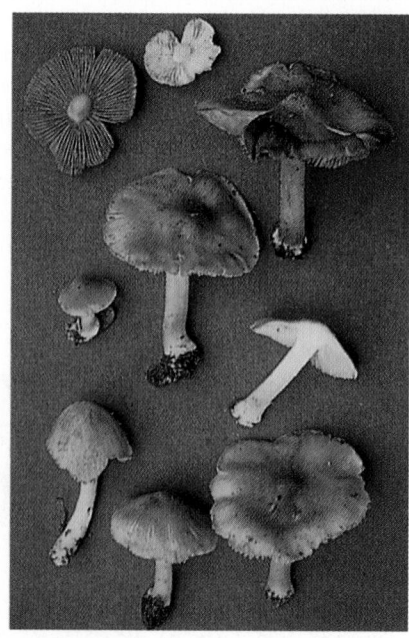

Figure 49-14 *Inocybe cookei*, which contains muscarinic toxins. (*From Phillips R:* Mushrooms of North America, *Boston, 1991, Little, Brown.*)

In contrast, many members of the *Clitocybe* family are edible. *Clitocybe* mushrooms are whitish tan to gray mushrooms with caps 15 to 33 mm long on hairless stalks 1 to 5 cm long. Gills are decurrent (run down the stalk), and spores are white. They are usually single specimens (not clustered) found on lawns in summer and fall.

Many *Inocybe* and *Clitocybe* mushrooms contain larger concentrations of muscarine than does *A. muscaria*.[13] Other toxins (e.g., ibotenic acid) are present in *A. muscaria*, and contribute to its toxicity.

Toxin. Muscarine is a quaternary trimethyl ammonium salt of 2-methyl-3-oxy-5-(amino)tetrahydrofuram. Muscarine stimulates postganglionic cholinergic receptors (muscarinic receptors), mimicking the action of acetylcholine. Muscarine stimulation of the GI tract leads to increased secretory activity, contraction amplitude, and peristalsis. Stimulation of the urinary tract leads to bladder contraction and increased peristalsis of the ureters. Stimulation of secretory tissue leads to salivation and lacrimation. Bronchoconstriction, flushing, and diaphoresis result from additional stimulation of bronchial and vascular tissues. Cardiac effects include reflex tachycardia, or more often bradycardia, and decreased atrioventricular conduction. Central nervous system (CNS) effects include headache, ataxia, and visual disturbances. The sensorium is generally not affected (except in ingestion of *A. muscaria*, which contains other CNS toxins).

Clinical Presentation. Symptoms develop within 15 to 30 minutes after ingestion of muscarine-containing mushrooms. Typical symptoms include salivation, urination, lacrimation, diarrhea, diaphoresis, abdominal pain, nausea, and emesis. Bradycardia, bronchospasm, and constricted pupils are also noted. Copious bronchial secretions may cause respiratory failure requiring mechanical ventilation.

Symptoms remit spontaneously in 6 to 24 hours. In Europe, some deaths are reported from *Inocybe patouillardii*.[59] Although this mushroom is rarely eaten, ingestion carries a mortality rate of 6% to 12%, particularly among persons with preexisting pulmonary or cardiac disease. Most deaths occur within the first 12 hours as a result of respiratory failure or cardiovascular collapse.

Treatment. Many victims require supportive care with oxygen, suctioning, and IV fluid replacement. Activated charcoal and cathartics are rarely given because of the prominent emesis and diarrhea. Atropine is a muscarine antagonist but should be used only to control secretions or profound bradycardia. It should not be given prophylactically because it may worsen the CNS effects induced by *A. muscaria*. Atropine (0.01 mg/kg IV for children, 1 mg IV for adults) can be repeated as needed until secretions are manageable. Symptoms resolve spontaneously within 24 hours.

Isoxazole Reactions

The isoxazole derivatives ibotenic acid and muscimol produce CNS symptoms, including excitement and alteration in visual perception.

Causative Mushrooms. Several mushrooms contain ibotenic acid (Table 49-3 and Box 49-4). *Amanita muscaria* is described previously. *Amanita pantherina* is 5 to 15 cm long with a cap 5 to 15 cm in diameter (Figure 49-15). The cap is generally white to pink in the young specimen but becomes reddish brown or brown, often darker at the rim, with maturity. Fragments of the universal veil form warts on the cap but may be washed

---

Box 49-4 MUSHROOMS REPORTED OR SUSPECTED TO CONTAIN IBOTENIC ACID, MUSCIMOL, AND RELATED COMPOUNDS

Amanita cokeri
Amanita gemmata
Amanita muscaria
Amanita pantherina
Panaeolus campanulatus
Tricholoma muscarium

TABLE 49-3. Look-Alikes of Mushrooms Containing Isoxazole Toxins

TOXIC SPECIES	EDIBLE SPECIES
Amanita gemmata	*Russula* spp.
Amanita muscaria	*Amanita caesarea, Amanita rubescens, Armillariella mellea*
Amanita pantherina	*Amanita rubescens*

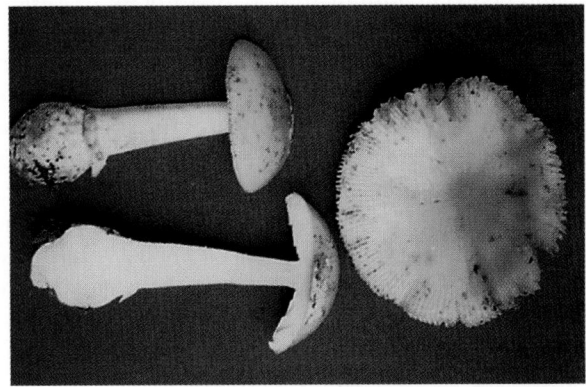

Figure 49-15 *Amanita pantherina,* which contains the neurotoxins ibotenic acid and isoxazole derivatives. (*From Phillips R:* Mushrooms of North America, *Boston, 1991, Little, Brown.*)

off by rain. The stalk has a distinct ring, with a vulva and cup at the bottom. When the flesh is cut or injured (e.g., by insect larvae), it develops a pinkish tinge. Gills are free and produce white spores. The raw mushroom has little smell and tastes very much like a raw potato. It grows from June to November in woodlands throughout North America.

Toxin. Ibotenic acid is found in the bright-red cap of *A. muscaria* and undergoes decarboxylation during drying to form muscimol, the more toxic of the compounds. The potency of the cap remains high for up to 7 years despite drying.[58] *A. muscaria* contains 0.17% to 1% isoxazole derivatives, whereas *A. pantherina* contains only 0.02% to 0.53%[44] and tends to lose potency with storage. Muscimol is a γ-aminobutyric acid (GABA) receptor agonist.[48] Muscimol increases CNS serotonin levels and decreases catecholamine levels. Ibotenic acid is a neurotransmitter agonist.

Clinical Presentation. Ingestion of 10 mg of *A. muscaria* produces mild intoxication, dizziness, and ataxia. Ingestion of 15 mg leads to pronounced ataxia and visual disturbances.[44,69] Delirium or manic behavior may develop after large ingestions. Physical activity is accelerated with inability to judge size. Visual hallucinations, seizures, and muscle twitching are common.[8] Some victims complain of residual headache.

Symptoms begin within 30 minutes of ingestion and generally last 2 hours. Rare fatalities have been reported. Some victims had ataxia and paralysis of ocular convergence.[37] In rare cases, symptoms last as long as 48 hours, depending on the dosage and individual host effect. In animals, short-acting hypnotics are potentiated by muscimol.[44] Phenobarbital or diazepam administered to treat *A. muscaria* ingestion may lead to unexpected apnea, flaccid paralysis, or both.

Treatment. Treatment consists of supportive care. Emesis caused by the toxin is unusual. Gastric emptying and charcoal administration are difficult to initiate because of the CNS disturbances and have no proven effectiveness. Appropriate sedation with IV phenobarbital (30 mg hourly, 0.5 mg/kg in children) or IV diazepam (5 mg every 10 to 15 minutes in adults as needed, 0.1 to 0.3 mg/kg in children) is often necessary but requires caution. Airway support and ventilatory assistance should be immediately available. Atropine may worsen the CNS symptoms associated with isoxazole derivatives and therefore should be withheld unless the muscarinic effects are serious.

Hallucinogenic Mushrooms

Perhaps the most sought after mushrooms are "magic mushrooms," which are available in the wild and as spores available through mail-order catalogs. These mushrooms have been used for centuries because of their hallucinogenic effects. Small stone mushroom icons believed to be 3500 years old were found in Meso-American ruins.[59] Recently, honey laced with *Psilocybe cubensis* was confiscated at the Dutch-German border. Honey with *Psilocybe* can be purchased at Dutch coffee shops.[9]

Causative Mushrooms. The most common hallucinogenic mushrooms are members of the *Psilocybe* family (Table 49-4 and Box 49-5). This family includes more than 100 species, not all of which cause hallucinations (Figure 49-16). These are "little brown mushrooms" (LBMs). The cap is 0.5 to 4 cm in diameter (depending on the species), is usually smooth, and becomes sticky or slippery when wet. The stalk is slender and 4 to 15 cm long. Gills are gray to purple gray; spores are dark, nearly black. The flesh of these mushrooms turns blue or greenish when bruised or cut. The mushrooms are often mistaken for more poisonous species (e.g., *Galerina*, *Inocybe*). These mushrooms also resemble *Agaricus bisporus*. Regular grocery store mushrooms laced with lysergic acid diethylamide (LSD) or other hallucinogens are sold on the street as *Psilocybe*. Hallucinogenic mushrooms grow in a variety of habitats and are found throughout the world.

Other mushrooms, including members of the *Panaeolus* and *Gymnopilus* genera, may contain psilocybin. *Panaeolus* mushrooms are also LBMs about the same size as *Psilocybe*. Gills are dark gray or black with black spores. They also grow on dung throughout the tropics and subtropics of North America. Unlike *Psilocybe*, their caps do not become sticky or slippery when wet. The hallucinogenic effect and quantity of toxin vary among *Panaeolus* species.

Some *Gymnopilus* species (e.g., *G. aeruginosus*) contain hallucinogens. These medium-sized mushrooms (cap, 5 to 15 cm; stalk, 5 to 12 cm) are variable in color (green, yellow, salmon, red) with yellowish gills and rusty spores. They grow on stumps or sawdust in the Pacific Northwest.

Visual hallucinations and ataxia were reported in a person ingesting *Laetiporus sulphureus*, previously thought to be harmless.[4] It is not clear whether this mushroom contained hallucinogenic material or the individual ingested an additional mushroom as well.

Toxin. Psilocybin and its somewhat unstable metabolite psilocin are indole compounds derived from tryptamine. These two toxins were first isolated by Albert Hofmann,[46] known as the father of LSD. Chemically the toxins resemble 5-hydroxytryptamine and LSD and have similar effects. They maintain their potency in dried specimens.

Box 49-5   MUSHROOMS REPORTED OR SUSPECTED TO CONTAIN EITHER PSILOCYBIN OR PSILOCIN OR BOTH

Amanita citrina
Amanita porphyria
Conocybe cyanopus
Conocybe siligineoides
Conocybe smithii
Gymnopilus aeruginosus
Gymnopilus purpuratus
Gymnopilus spectabilis
Gymnopilus validipes
Naematoloma popperianum
Panaeolus campanulatus
Panaeolus castaneifolius
Panaeolus cyanescens
Panaeolus fimicola
Panaeolus foenisecii
Panaeolus phalaenarum
Panaeolus semiovatus

Panaeolus sphinctrinus
Panaeolus subbalteatus
Psathyrella sepulchralis
Psilocybe baeocystis
Psilocybe caerulescens
Psilocybe caerulipes
Psilocybe cubensis
Psilocybe cyanaescens
Psilocybe pelliculosa
Psilocybe semilanceata
Psilocybe strictipes
Psilocybe stuntzii
Stropharia aeurginosa
Stropharia coronilla
Stropharia hornemannii
Stropharia squamosa

TABLE 49-4. Look-Alikes of Mushrooms Containing Psilocybin-Psilocin

TOXIC SPECIES	EDIBLE SPECIES
Panaeolus foenisecii	*Psathyrella candolleana, Agrocybe pediades, Marasmius oreades*
Other *Panaeolus* spp.	*Coprinus* spp.

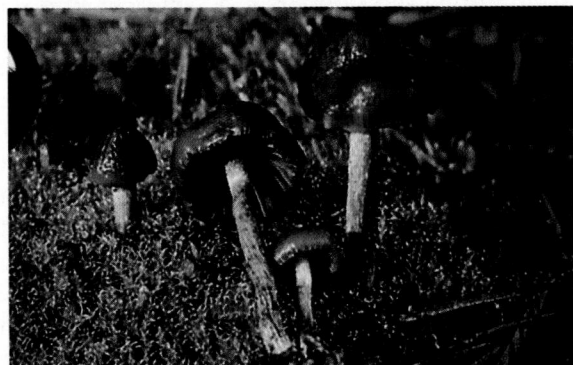

Figure 49-16   *Psilocybe caerulipes.*

Psilocybin, as well as LSD, inhibits the firing rate of serotonin-dependent neurons, particularly at the presynaptic receptors. It induces a strange euphoria, hallucinations, and a loss of time sensation. Many of these symptoms are similar to those seen with LSD. Some species contain phenylethylamine, which may be responsible for tachycardia and other adverse reactions.[6] In human volunteer studies, peak plasma levels were reached at 105 minutes.[43]

Clinical Presentation. Ingestion of 5 mg of psilocybin (10 mg of fresh *P. cubensis*) causes moderate euphoria. Ingestion of 10 mg leads to hallucinations and a loss of time sensation. Heightened imagination occurs within 15 to 30 minutes of ingestion. Hallucinations may last for 4 to 6 hours. Serious side effects are rarely seen, but fever and seizures have been reported in children.[68] Up to 50% of victims have tachycardia and hypertension.[77] A case resulting in myocardial infarction has been reported.[10] Flashbacks have been reported in some victims for up 4 months after ingestion.[7]

Treatment. Initially the victim should be placed in a quiet, supportive environment. Gastric emptying and activated charcoal administration are often impossible and may only enhance the hallucinations, but should be considered in victims with very large ingestions who are brought for treatment early. Sedation can be accomplished when necessary with a benzodiazepine (diazepam, 0.1 mg/kg IV in children, 5 mg IV in adults, repeated every 5 minutes as needed), phenobarbital (0.5 mg/kg IV in children, 30 to 60 mg IV in adults, repeated every 10 minutes as needed), chlorpromazine (50 to 100 mg IM), or haloperidol (5 mg IM). Seizures can be controlled with diazepam in the doses just listed. Hyperpyrexia, seen primarily in children, is best treated with external cooling, avoiding antipyretics.

PROTOPLASMIC POISONS

Gyromitra Toxin

False morels (*Gyromitra esculenta*) were once thought to be edible. Even today they are collected, sold fresh, canned, and exported ("morschels") in eastern and central Europe.[71] Since 1793 they have been suspected of causing toxicity and since World War II have been known to cause hepatic failure, neurologic symptoms, and death.[41] Symptoms appear 4 to 50 hours (usually 5 to 12 hours) after ingestion, with timing similar to that of *Amanita phalloides* poisoning. Since *Gyromitra* grows primarily in the spring and *A. phalloides* in the fall, however, the identity of the two mushrooms is rarely confused.

Causative Mushrooms. *Gyromitra esculenta* is approximately 5 to 16 cm in height with a reddish brown to dark-brown, irregularly shaped cap (Figure 49-17). The cap's surface is curved and folded, resembling a brain. The stalk is often as thick as the cap. The insides of the cap and stalk are hollow. This mushroom grows in the spring near pines and in sandy soil throughout North America. It is particularly common in Germany, Poland, and other eastern European countries. Mature species, particularly those with cap decay, may have increased toxicity. These mushrooms may be mistaken for morels, which are considered among the most delicious wild mushrooms (Table 49-5).

Other members of the *Gyromitra* family contain gyromitrins. None of these mushrooms has been reported to cause toxicity in humans.

Toxin. Gyromitrin (*N*-methyl-*N*-formylhydrazone) was first isolated in 1967.[61] This substance is moderately volatile and heat sensitive. Cooking thoroughly and discarding the cooking liquid may decrease or eliminate the toxin. Symptoms have occurred despite proper cooking.[38]

Once gyromitrin enters the stomach, hydrolysis yields *N*-methyl-*N*-formylhydrazine (MFH), which forms *N*-methylhydrazine or monomethylhydrazine (MH),[72] a component of rocket fuel. Workers in rocket fuel plants exposed to volatile MH develop CNS toxicity and nephrotoxicity.[54,93] MH is a competitive inhibitor of pyridoxal phosphate, which interferes with enzyme systems requiring pyridoxine as a cofactor, including decarboxylases, deaminases, and transaminases.[5] As a result, levels of GABA fall, interfering with neurotransmission.[55] This may lead to altered mental status, seizures, or both. This widely accepted theory has been questioned, since MH may cause seizures without a change in brain GABA levels.[67]

MFH and MH undergo oxidation in the liver to two highly reactive intermediates: a free methyl radical and an unstable diazonium compound.[71] These substances appear to produce local hepatic necrosis by blocking the activity of cytochrome P_{450} systems, glutathione, and other hepatic biomolecules.

Gyromitrin causes tumors in a variety of animals.[98] There are significant concerns about long-term toxicity associated with repeated consumption of *G. esculenta*. Gyromitrin has been included in the list of naturally occurring carcinogens.[51]

Each kilogram of fresh *G. esculenta* contains 3 to 100 mg of gyromitrin. Fresh mushrooms contain 50 to 300 mg of MH/kg and dried mushrooms up to 400 mg/kg.[62] The human median lethal dose (LD_{50}) is suspected to be 20 to 50 mg/kg for adults and 10 to 30 mg/kg for children, or 0.4 to 1 kg of fresh mushrooms for an adult (average 30 mushrooms) and 0.2 to 0.6 kg for a child.[71]

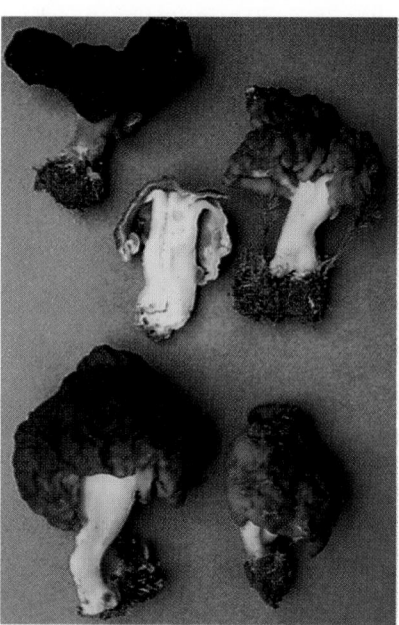

Figure 49-17 *Gyromitra esculenta*, which contains the hepatoxin gyromitrin. (*From Phillips R:* Mushrooms of North America, *Boston, 1991, Little, Brown.*)

TABLE 49-5. Look-Alike of Mushroom Containing Gyromitrin

TOXIC SPECIES	EDIBLE SPECIES
Gyromitra esculenta	*Morchella esculenta*

Clinical Presentation. Symptoms are generally delayed for 4 to 50 (average 5 to 12) hours after ingestion. Initial symptoms include nausea, vomiting, and severe diarrhea. Some victims may have dizziness, weakness, muscle cramps, and loss of muscle coordination. In a severe ingestion, delirium, seizures, and coma are present. Hepatic failure develops over several days after ingestion, although hepatic damage is generally mild. Hypoglycemia, hypovolemia, severe hepatic failure, and death may occur.

Symptoms from gyromitrin toxin, as with other mushroom toxins, depend on amount consumed, toxin concentration, nature of the mushrooms, and other factors. The variability of symptoms after ingestion of *Gyromitra* mushrooms is much greater than with other mushroom species. Some individuals can consume large quantities of *Gyromitra* with few or no symptoms. A second meal by the same person may lead to severe toxicity. Repeated consumption may increase the risk of a severe reaction.[15]

Several drugs, including isoniazid, hydralazine, and probably MH,[16] are metabolized through acetylation of a hydrazine or amino group by the liver. Individuals vary greatly in the rapidity of acetylation. Two major human groups are termed fast and slow acetylators, with slow acetylation being an autosomal recessive trait. Slow acetylators in general have greater and more prolonged toxicity after ingestion of these drugs. Similar variation in fast and slow acetylators is seen when *Gyromitra* mushrooms are ingested.

Treatment. Symptoms develop several hours after *Gyromitra* ingestion. Activated charcoal (1 g/kg orally or via gastric tube) is often given but, as with gastric emptying, is of little value. Pyridoxine has been useful in victims with neurologic disorders from MH toxicity and is of theoretic benefit in victims of gyromitrin toxicity. High-dose pyridoxine therapy may cause peripheral neuropathies.[1] Persons who ingest *Gyromitra* mushrooms and develop significant neurologic symptoms should receive pyridoxine (25 mg/kg, up to 20 kg/day, orally).[54,108] No evidence indicates that pyridoxine alters the course of hepatic disease.

Baseline measurements of alanine and aspartate transaminases (ALT, AST), prothrombin time (PT), partial thromboplastin time (PTT), BUN, creatinine, complete blood cell count (CBC), platelet count, glucose, and electrolytes should be performed. ALT/AST, PT, PTT, BUN, and creatinine should be monitored at least daily for 3 to 4 days for the development of hepatic failure. Rapid deterioration of liver function (ALT/AST levels of greater than 2000 IU, PTT > 50 secs) indicates immediate transfer to a tertiary center with transplant capability. Persons with significant hepatic failure may require monitoring of blood glucose every 2 to 4 hours and supplemental glucose administration for symptomatic hypoglycemia.

No specific antidote or treatment is available for fulminant hepatic failure. The appropriate timing or necessity of liver transplantation is uncertain. In persons with fulminant hepatic failure from infectious causes, prolonged PT (unresponsive to fresh-frozen plasma) and development of hepatorenal syndrome, grade II hepatic encephalopathy, hypoglycemia, and uncorrectable metabolic acidosis are used as signs that transplantation is needed on an emergent basis. Persons with fulminant hepatic failure from toxic ingestion, elevated bilirubin level, and young age are important indicators of a poor prognosis.[32,75] Mortality from gyromitrin poisoning is reported to be 15% to 35%.[33,76]

Renal Toxicity

Although originally thought to be an edible mushroom, *Cortinarius orellanus* was associated with 81 cases of renal toxicity in the 1950s.[40] This led to isolation of the toxin orellanine, which is found in the mushrooms *C. orellanus*, *C. speciosissimus*, and *C. gentilis*. Most cases occur in Europe and Japan.

Causative Mushroom. *C. orellanus* has a small, brown to brownish red, smooth cap 30 to 80 cm in diameter. The stalk is somewhat yellow, often darker toward the soil. Gills are orange to rust with rust-colored spores. It grows in deciduous woods, most often in sandy soil underneath oaks and birches. It is ubiquitous throughout Europe. Other *Cortinarius* species are found in the United States and may be toxic (Box 49-6).

Toxin. The two toxins isolated from *C. orellanus*, orellanine and orelline, are structurally related to paraquat and diquat. Their mechanism of action remains a mystery. These are heat-stable compounds, unaffected by cooking. The toxin appears to cause intense interstitial nephritis with early fibrosis.[47]

Amanita smithiana, which contains the nephrotoxins norleucine (aminohexadrenoic acid) and chlorocrotyl-

---

Box 49-6 MUSHROOMS REPORTED OR SUSPECTED OF CONTAINING ORELLINE OR ORELLANINE

Cortinarius gentilis
Cortinarius orellanus
Cortinarius speciosissimus
Cortinarius splendena
Cortinarius venenosus

glycine, grows in the Pacific Northwest and may be mistaken for pine mushrooms.[104] *Amanita proxima* is found in France and also causes renal failure.[17]

Clinical Presentation. Persons who ingest *C. orellanus* are generally asymptomatic for 2 to 20 days. After this latent period, acute renal failure develops. Some persons develop neurologic changes, including paresthesias, taste impairment, and cognitive disorders.

Symptoms vary greatly. One case report described 26 soldiers who ate soup made of *C. orellanus* in nearly identical quantities.[11] Acute renal failure developed in 12 on or about day 11. Eight soldiers later recovered normal renal function, whereas four required long-term dialysis or kidney transplantation. The other 14 soldiers showed no rise in BUN or creatinine levels but developed leukocyturia and hematuria that persisted for more than 1 month. Renal failure reportedly occurs in 30% to 46% of persons who ingest these mushrooms and become ill. Renal function returns in 46% to 66% of victims.

Renal biopsy in patients with orellanine-induced renal failure shows tubule lesions with epithelial necrosis and disruption of the tubular basement membrane. These biopsy changes may persist for up to 3 months.[11]

Treatment. In most persons who ingest renally toxic mushrooms, unexplained acute renal failure develops many days later. If a person presents early after eating orellanine-containing mushrooms, gastric emptying and activated charcoal administration (1 g/kg orally or via gastric tube) might prevent some absorption, decreasing the resultant toxicity. Early presentation, however, is rare.

Once acute renal failure develops, baseline and repeated monitoring of BUN, creatinine, electrolytes, CBC, differential, and urinalysis should be performed to monitor renal function. Urine output should be monitored, and if it decreases, fluid administration should be used to achieve optimal hydration. Serum potassium, calcium, and magnesium should be monitored closely. If renal failure progresses, the victim should be transferred to a facility for hemodialysis and possible renal transplantation. Renal function may return to normal after months of dialysis dependency. Steroids seem to have no effect on the course of the disease, but they may have been given too late.

Amatoxin

The mushrooms that contain amatoxins are responsible for 90% to 95% of fatalities caused by mushrooms (Table 49-6 and Box 49-7). *A. phalloides* is most common in central and eastern Europe; immigrants to the U.S. may have carried mushroom spores in wood products

---

Box 49-7 MUSHROOMS REPORTED OR SUSPECTED OF CONTAINING AMATOXINS

Amanita ocreata	*Galerina marginata*
Amanita phalloides	*Galerina venenata*
Amanita verna	*Lepiota castanea*
Amanita virosa	*Lepiota jasserandii*
Galerina autumnalis	*Lepiota helveola*

TABLE 49-6. Look-Alikes of Mushrooms Containing Amatoxin

TOXIC SPECIES	EDIBLE SPECIES
Amanita phalloides	*Amanita fulva*
Amanita virosa	*Amanita bisporus*
Amanita verna	*Lepiota flavovirens*

---

from eastern Europe. *A. verna* and *A. virosa* are more common in the United States.

Causative Mushrooms. The common names of *A. phalloides* (see Figure 49-3) and its relatives *A. verna* and *A. virosa* are death cap, death angel, and destroying angel, reflecting their association with fatal outcome. *A. phalloides* has a white to greenish cap 4 to 16 cm in diameter, often with remnants of the veil (warts). The stalk is generally thick, 5 to 18 cm long, with a large bulb at the base, often with a vulva or cup. A thin ring is usually present on the stalk. Gills are generally free and white to green in color; spores are white. The mushrooms grow under deciduous trees in the autumn.

A. virosa is more common in the United States (Figure 49-18). It resembles *A. phalloides*, but the cap is more yellow or white. *A. verna* is characteristically white. All grow in deciduous woods. Even mushroom experts have been tempted by the large white mushroom, which is tasty. The fatality rate, however, is 35% in adults and 50% in children.

Some *Lepiota* mushrooms, including *L. castanea* and *L. jasserandii*, contain high concentrations of amatoxin. Human toxicity has been reported.

Mushrooms that contain amatoxin may have a positive Meixner test. This test was first described by Wieland in 1949[107] and popularized by Meixner.[70] A drop of liquid is expressed from a fresh mushroom onto print-free (ligand-free) newspaper and allowed to dry. A drop of concentrated (10 to 12 N) hydrochloric acid is added. A blue color develops within 1 to 2 minutes in the presence of amatoxins. Control tests on newspaper without mushroom juice and paper con-

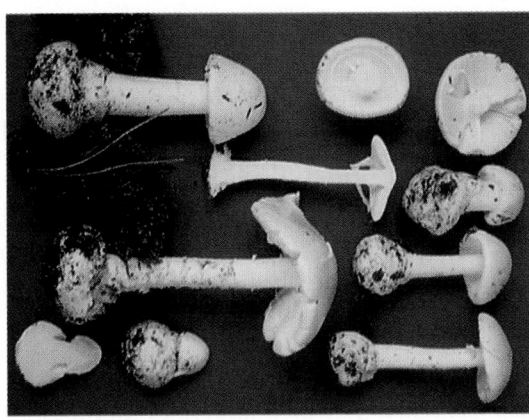

Figure 49-18 *Amanita virosa*, which causes delayed hepatotoxicity. *(From Phillips R:* Mushrooms of North America, *Boston, 1991, Little, Brown.)*

taining ligand should be conducted. False-positive results are common and can be elicited from excessive drying temperatures (greater than 63° C [145° F]) or exposure to sunlight. False-positive tests also occur from mushrooms containing psilocybin, terpenes, and bufotenin. Nearly 20% of gilled mushrooms that did not contain amatoxins tested positive in one study,[90] placing the usefulness of this technique in doubt. Thin-layer chromatography (TLC) more accurately identifies the presence of amatoxin and can be done on mushroom liquid, human serum, or urine.[81] Radioimmunoassay (RIA) of serum or urine can detect amatoxins in the body.

Toxin. The mushroom *A. phalloides* contains two groups of toxins: amatoxins and phallotoxins. Each group contains several toxins. There are now eight identified amatoxins: α-amanitin, β-amanitin, γ-amanitin, ε-amanitin, amanin, amaninamide, amanullinic acid, and amanullin.[103,105] Of these, α-amanitin is thought to be primarily responsible for human disease. α-Amanitin injected into animals produces hepatic toxicity characteristic of human ingestion of *A. phalloides*. Phallotoxins include phalloidin, phalloin, phallisin, phallacidin, phallacin, phallisacin, and prophalloin.[103] Phalloidin is the primary phallotoxin. Phallotoxins bind to F-actin, disrupting plasma membranes and causing massive efflux of calcium and potassium. Phallotoxins cause death in animals within 2 hours but are not believed to play a role in human toxicity.[34] Humans may not even absorb these toxins, which may be responsible for local gastric irritation. *A. virosa* contains amatoxins and virotoxins. Virotoxins resemble phallotoxins biochemically, and also bind F-actin and cause death within a few hours. Six different virotoxins have been isolated, but none is thought to play a role in human *Amanita* hepatotoxicity.[105]

After ingestion, amatoxins are absorbed from the gut and actively transported into the liver through transport systems shared by bile acids and xenobiotics.[106] α-Amanitin is rapidly cleared from plasma.[52] Amatoxins are not protein bound. They bind to ribonucleic acid (RNA) polymerase II and inhibit the formation of messenger RNA (mRNA).[60] This in turn inhibits transcription as the reservoir of RNA is depleted.[25] Amatoxins are excreted into the bile, where they are reabsorbed and once again transported into the liver.[12] Interruption of this enterohepatic circulation may be an important therapeutic tool.

Within the liver, α-amanitin may undergo some metabolism through the cytochrome P_{450} system. Animal studies suggest that a more toxic metabolite is produced through this metabolism.[87,89] Nuclear fragmentation and condensation of chromosomal material have been observed within 15 hours of injection.[24] Glycogen is rapidly depleted, and fatty degeneration occurs within the liver parenchymal cells.[20] Mitochondria become swollen, and microvesicules appear throughout the cytoplasm.[76] Direct renal toxicity may occur, but renal failure (10% of cases) is more likely to be caused by hepatorenal syndrome.

Clinical Presentation. Persons who ingest *A. phalloides* feel well for 4 to 16 hours. Severe nausea, vomiting, abdominal cramps, and diarrhea follow this characteristic latent period. Early complications include fluid and electrolyte imbalance (hypoglycemia, hypokalemia, elevated BUN). Persons in whom symptoms develop earlier (4 to 10 hours) are more likely to experience severe hepatotoxicity. Over the next 12 to 24 hours the victim's GI symptoms abate. The second latent period is followed by hepatic failure, which develops 48 to 72 hours after ingestion in most victims. Hepatic failure may be of varying severity; it is frequently worse in children and depends minimally on the amount of mushroom ingested.

Children have greater toxicity and higher mortality, perhaps because of the relative quantity of mushrooms ingested or the varying metabolism in young children (differing levels of P_{450}-metabolizing enzymes). Previous experiments showed that concurrent ethanol with *A. phalloides* ingestion (whole mushroom lyophilized) decreased hepatotoxicity.[30] Therefore decreased toxicity in adults could result from ingestion of ethanol with an *Amanita* mushroom dinner. More recently, however, ethanol failed to alter hepatoxicity in an animal model poisoned with α-amanitin, which raises doubts about this explanation for increased toxicity in children.[86]

In addition to hepatic failure, endocrinopathies may develop, with hypocalcemia, decreased thyroid function, and elevated insulin levels in the presence of hypoglycemia.[53] Hypocalcemia may be caused in part by loss of calcium through diarrhea or may be a direct effect on osteoclasts. Renal failure may contribute to hypocalcemia. The thyroid abnormalities probably result from decreased hormone synthesis caused by overwhelming illness and blocked peripheral conversion of thyroxine (T_4) to triiodothyronine (T_3). Thyroid-stimulating hormone (TSH) depression may result from decreased synthesis caused by the inhibition of RNA polymerase II by amatoxin. Hypothyroidism has not been clinically significant. Hypoglycemia is probably the result of several processes, including impaired hepatic gluconeogenesis, increased insulin release from the initial hyperglycemia, or tissue destruction of the pancreas.[53] Bone marrow toxicity with decreased neutrophils, lymphocytes, and platelets has been noted.[84] Disseminated intravascular coagulation and coagulopathies secondary to hepatic dysfunction are common.[84] Pancreatitis occurs in up to 50% of patients.[28] Hypophosphatemia is particularly common in children, for unknown reasons. Myopathy has been associated with *Amanita* toxicity.[39]

Hepatic biopsy shows diffuse and severe steatosis with periportal inflammation and necrosis. Extremely high levels of hepatic enzymes are seen. ALT/AST level is not helpful in predicting the victim's prognosis. A precipitous drop may occur just before death.

Treatment. Attempts to treat *A. phalloides* poisoning have ranged from scientific to purely empiric. Noting that rabbits were able to eat the *A. phalloides* mushroom with impunity, clinicians fed ground raw rabbit to victims of *Amanita* poisoning, without success.[100] Hemodialysis was long recommended but has been shown to be ineffective, since the toxin is rapidly cleared. Amatoxin is taken up in liver cells within 5 hours after IV administration.[22] In a retrospective study of 205 cases of amatoxin ingestion,[32] hemodialysis worsened the prognosis, and charcoal hemoperfusion did not improve outcome. Plasmapheresis appears to be ineffective for similar reasons.[80]

Amatoxins are enterohepatically circulated. Attempts have been made to divert the enterohepatic circulation. Although animal studies showed some benefit with this treatment,[23] it is not recommended. Multidose activated charcoal (1 g/kg orally or via gastric tube, 15 to 20 g every 4 to 8 hours with a cathartic given every second or third dose if no diarrhea) may adsorb the amatoxins and interrupt the enterohepatically circulated drug.

Antigen-binding fragment (Fab) monoclonal antibodies against amatoxin were developed by immunizing rats and fusing their spleen cells to mouse myeloma cells. The amatoxin-specific clones were selected and their immunoglobulin separated into Fab fragments. When this Fab antibody was used in α-amanitin-poisoned mice, renal toxicity was 50 times greater. All animals died of renal failure but had no hepatic damage.[21] The Fab-amatoxin compound may have dissociated in the kidney, leading to severe local damage.

Thioctic acid is used throughout Europe as a treatment for *A. phalloides* poisoning. Although its exact mechanism is unknown, it may act as a free-radical scavenger or interfere with the hepatic transport of toxin. In animal studies, thioctic acid has been ineffective against α-amanitin or extracts of the mushroom.[2] In a large retrospective study, thioctic was more frequently associated with a fatal outcome in humans.[32] Its use is not recommended.

Silymarin is the active component of the milk thistle *Silybum marianum*. A water-soluble preparation (silibinin) is effective against amatoxin in both animals and humans. Silibinin also may interrupt the enterohepatic circulation or act as a free-radical scavenger. Patients treated with silibinin were more likely to survive in one study.[50] In a retrospective study, silibinin was associated with increased survival.[32] IV silibinin is not available in the United States, but an oral form may be found in health food stores.

High-dose penicillin decreased toxicity in an animal study evaluating hemodialysis with penicillin used prophylactically.[31] The control group (penicillin alone) showed a decrease in toxicity. Other animal studies have indicated penicillin's effectiveness in reducing hepatotoxicity.[27,88] In humans, penicillin has been very effective.[32] Other antibiotics, including rifampin and cephalosporins, have been shown to protect against amatoxin poisoning.[26,73] Penicillin's exact mechanism of action is unclear. Sterilization of the intestines may lead to decreased GABA production, which may diminish ensuing cerebral encephalopathy. Penicillin may share a common transport system with amatoxin, which interferes with uptake.[29] Regardless of the mechanism, large doses of IV benzylpenicillin (300,000 to 1 million units/kg/day) are recommended. This dose may be associated with seizures.

French physicians have used hyperbaric oxygen as a treatment for *Amanita* toxicity.[57] Hyperbaric oxygen may facilitate hepatic regeneration and lessen toxicity. It is most often used with high-dose penicillin.

Animal data suggest other therapies. High-dose cimetidine (4 to 10 g/day IV in adults) appears to inhibit formation of more toxic metabolites by blocking the cytochrome P_{450} system.[87] Cimetidine has not been given in children for *Amanita* ingestion. Other drugs under investigation in animals include vitamin C,[102] zinc, and thiol compounds.[29]

Gastric aspirate or emesis can be sent for spore analysis if mushroom specimens are not available for identification. Persons with documented or suspected amatoxin ingestion should receive activated charcoal (1 g/kg orally or via gastric tube followed by 15 to 20 g every 4 to 8 hours). Repeated administration may bind drug that is enterohepatically circulated. Cathartics are generally not necessary, since diarrhea is prominent. IV normal saline or Ringer's lactate is needed to replace GI fluid losses. Electrolyte losses (particularly potassium) may be great. BUN, creatinine, CBC with differential, platelet count, electrolytes, glucose, calcium, phosphorus, magnesium, urinalysis, PT, PTT, fibrinogen, amylase, protein, and albumin should be initially measured and repeated at least daily to monitor liver and renal function. Hyperglycemia is common on the first day, but insulin is generally not required. Hypoglycemia occurs after 24 hours and may be significant, requiring concentrated IV glucose. Bedside determinations of glucose should be performed at least every 6 hours. Tests of liver function, including ALT, AST, alkaline phosphatase, PT, and PTT, should be repeated at least daily and more often if findings become abnormal. Levels rapidly rising or greater than 2000 IU for ALT/AST and 50 seconds for PTT should signal severe toxicity and the need for referral to a transplant center.

To confirm the diagnosis of amatoxin ingestion, a serum RIA is ordered for amatoxins. Urine can also be studied. The nearest laboratory performing this RIA is usually known to the regional poison information center.

Specific treatment should begin as soon as diagnosis is suspected, either by symptoms or confirmed by the fresh specimen or spores. Benzylpenicillin (penicillin G), 300,000 to 1 million U/kg/day, should be given IV in divided doses. Silibinin, if available, can be given intravenously, 20 to 40 mg/kg/day in divided doses. Hyperbaric oxygen treatments (dives to 2 atm for 30 minutes once or twice a day) can be tried. Cimetidine (4 to 10 g IV for adults for 2 days) is experimental but has few side effects.

Once liver failure begins, hypoglycemia becomes more likely. Supplemental glucose should be readily available. Dietary protein should be limited and thiamine and multivitamin supplementation given. Oral lactulose, 30 to 45 ml every 6 to 8 hours, may reduce hepatic encephalopathy. Clotting studies should be performed several times a day and vitamin K or fresh-frozen plasma (or both) used to correct abnormalities.

If hepatic failure progresses, liver transplantation may be required. The timing is highly controversial, and criteria for transplant in other forms of fulminant hepatic failure are often applied to this setting. Factors associated with poor prognosis in acetaminophen-induced hepatic damage include metabolic acidosis, elevated PT and elevated serum creatinine.[75] In viral hepatitis and other drug reactions, however, factors such as bilirubin, victim's age, and duration of jaundice before clinical encephalopathy are important.[65] In the few pertinent studies of *A. phalloides* ingestion, poor outcome was related to age less than 10 years, a short la-

tent period, and the severity of coagulopathy.[32] The largest study suggests that a person with ALT or AST level greater than 2000 IU, grade II hepatic encephalopathy, or PT greater than 50 seconds is at serious risk for death and should be considered for emergency liver transplantation.[19] Persons who met these criteria have survived.[64,82] A recent report suggests that increased reparative enzymes correlate with hepatic recovery.[49] Because hepatic failure develops rapidly, victims with significant hepatic dysfunction must be transferred early to a transplantation site. Patients undergoing liver transplantation for fulminant hepatic failure (not caused by *A. phalloides*) have a 62% survival rate. Recently a temporary liver transplant sustained a child while her liver recovered.[83]

Persons who survive acute hepatic failure without needing hepatic transplant may have persistent elevation in liver transaminases. In one study of 14 persons with severe hepatotoxicity, eight had elevated AST/ALT without normalization over a 1-year follow-up.[19] All had biopsy evidence of chronic active hepatitis, with positive anti–smooth muscle antibody and cryoglobulins. It is not known whether these persons will have an increased risk of hepatoma or develop more serious complications of chronic active hepatitis.[79] Amatoxin ingestion during pregnancy does not appear to have serious consequences to the fetus provided the mother remains healthy.

APPROACH TO THE VICTIM OF MUSHROOM POISONING

Four types of individuals develop mushroom toxicity: foragers, children, those seeking hallucinogenic "highs," and rarely, victims of attempted homicide. Most victims seek medical care after symptoms develop. Caregivers who observe small children chewing on lawn mushrooms should call the nearest poison center. Children who have ingested an entire lawn mushroom or more should receive ipecac and be observed for symptoms at home. Follow-up calls should be made to ensure that emesis has occurred and at 1, 4, and 24 hours to assess symptoms.

Persons with agitation, altered perceptions, or frank hallucinations temporally related to mushroom ingestion are probably intoxicated with isoxazole or hallucinogenic mushrooms. Whether the mushrooms are picked accidentally or ingested intentionally, the treatment and clinical course are identical.

Persons who develop muscarinic symptoms (salivation, urination, diaphoresis, GI upset, emesis) present a classic picture that is rarely confused with any other presentation. Some drugs (e.g., bethanechol) may cause similar symptoms when taken in overdose. Victims of mushroom poisoning generally remain mentally clear and should be able to relate an appropriate history.

Victims with GI symptoms can be divided into those with early and those with delayed presentations. Those with early (within 2 hours) GI symptoms generally have a benign course, *except* for persons with a mixed ingestion. Most guidebooks for mushroom hunters recommend eating only one variety of mushroom at a time, but more daring or foolish individuals mix multiple mushrooms and eat them frequently over a day. This makes diagnosis based on time of symptom onset difficult. Early onset of GI symptoms may mask more significant delayed symptoms. In these cases, identification of ingested mushrooms becomes essential to planning therapy.

Accurate botanical identification of the mushroom can be difficult. Only 800 of the 3000 species found in Europe can be identified without a microscope.[100] When multiple mushrooms are eaten together, the residual specimens may not be those causing toxicity. Cooking and refrigeration alter identifying features. Fresh mushroom specimens should be transported in a paper bag rather than a plastic container to limit the effects of humidity. Finally, precise identification of even a good specimen can be difficult and should be done by an expert. Mycologists can be contacted through a poison center, university, museum, or commercial mushroom grower.

In difficult cases, spores can be obtained from emesis or gastric emptying procedures. Specimens should be refrigerated while awaiting analysis. More specific diagnosis can be made through TLC or RIA techniques. Botanical identification may not match the victim's symptoms. The victim should be treated according to time of symptom onset and current condition when examined.

Victims with early-onset GI symptoms require supportive care with fluid and electrolyte replacement. For those with delayed GI symptoms or mixed ingestions of amatoxin or gyromitrin mushrooms, treatment should begin as soon as possible. These mushrooms generally can be differentiated by the description or by the season (spring for *Gyromitra*, autumn for *Amanita*).

Persons who have disulfiram-like reactions to alcohol should be questioned about prior mushroom ingestion. This situation is rarely diagnosed correctly, because symptoms are thought to result from panic attacks, alcohol intoxication, or even an allergic reaction. Persons rarely relate their symptoms to the dinner of mushrooms eaten days earlier.

Any person with unexplained acute renal failure should be questioned about prior wild mushroom ingestion. Although *Cortinarius orellanus* is more common in Europe and Japan, it is found with increasing frequency in the United States. Because of the long delay before the onset of renal failure (1 to 2 weeks), the history of mushroom ingestion may be missed.

REFERENCES

1. Albin RL et al: Acute sensory neuropathy-neuronopathy from pyridoxine overdose, *Neurology* 37:1729, 1987.
2. Alleva FR et al: Failure of thioctic acid to cure mushroom-poisoned mice and dogs. Presented at the 14th Annual Meeting of the Society of Toxicology, Williamsburg, Va, 1975.
3. Ammirati JF, Traquair JA, Horgen PA: *Poisonous mushrooms of Northern United States and Canada,* Minneapolis, 1985, University of Minnesota Press.
4. Appleton RE, Jan JE, Kroeger PD: *Laetiporus sulfureus* causing visual hallucinations and ataxia in a child, *Can Med Assoc J* 139:48, 1988.
5. Azar A et al: Pyridoxine and phenobarbital as treatment of aerozine-50 toxicity, *Aerospce Med* 4:1, 1970.
6. Beck O et al: Presence of phenylethylamine in hallucinogenic *Psilocybe* mushroom: possible role in adverse reactions, *J Anal Toxicol* 22:45, 1998.
7. Benjamin C: Persistent psychiatric symptoms after eating psilocybin mushrooms, *BMJ* 1:1319, 1979.
8. Benjamin DR: Mushroom poisoning in infants and children: the *Amanita pantherina/muscaria* group, *J Toxicol Clin Toxicol* 30:13, 1992.
9. Bogusz MJ et al: Honey with *Psilocybe* mushrooms: a revival of a very old preparation on the drug market? *Int J Legal Med* 111:147, 1998.
10. Borowiak KS, Ciechanowski K, Waloszczyk P: *Psilocybin* mushroom *(Psilocybe semilanceata)* intoxication with myocardial infarction, *J Toxicol Clin Toxicol* 36:47, 1998.
11. Bouget J et al: Acute renal failure following collective intoxication by *Cortinarius orellanus, Intensive Care Med* 16:506, 1990.
12. Busi C et al: *Amanita* toxins in gastroduodenal fluid of patients poisoned by the mushroom *Amanita phalloides, N Engl J Med* 300:800, 1979 (letter).
13. Catalfomo P, Eugster C: Muscarine and muscarine isomers in selected *Inocybe* species, *Helv Chim Acta* 53:848, 1970.
14. Chestnut VK: Poisonous properties of the green spored *Lepiota, ASA Gray Bull* 8:87, 1900.
15. Coulet M, Guillot J: Poisoning by *Gyromitra*: a possible mechanism, *Med Hypotheses* 8:325, 1982.
16. Coulet M et al: A propos des intoxications par *Gyromitra esculenta* Pers ex Fr, *Acta Mycol* 4:379, 1968.
17. de Haro L: [Acute renal insufficiency caused by *Amanita proxima* poisoning: experience of the Poison Center of Marseille], *Nephrologie* 19:21, 1998.
18. Falandysz J, Chwir A. The concentrations and bioconcentration factors of mercury in mushrooms from the Mierzeja Wislana sand-bar, northern Poland, *Sci Total Environ* 203:221, 1997.
19. Fantozzi R et al: Clinical findings and follow-up evaluation of an outbreak of mushroom poisoning—survey of *Amanita phalloides* poisoning, *Klin Wochenschr* 64:38, 1986.
20. Faulstich H: New aspects of *Amanita* poisoning, *Klin Wochenschr* 57:1143, 1979.
21. Faulstich H, Kirchner K, Derenzini M: Strongly enhanced toxicity of the mushroom toxin α-amanitin by an amatoxin-specific FAB or monoclonal antibody, *Toxicon* 26:491, 1988.
22. Faulstich H, Talas A, Wellhoner HH: Toxicokinetics of labeled amatoxins in the dog, *Arch Toxicol* 56:190, 1985.
23. Fauser U, Faulstich H: Beobachtungen zur therapie der Knollenblatterpilzvergiftung, *Dtsch Med Wochenschr* 98:2259, 1973.
24. Fiume L, Lachi R: Lesioni ultrastrutturali prodotte nelle cellule parenchimal epa tiche dalle phalloidina e dalla α-amanitin a, *Sperimentale* 115:288, 1965.
25. Fiume L, Stripe F: Decreased RNA content in mouse liver nuclei after intoxication with α-amanitin, *Biochim Biophys Acta* 123:171, 1976.
26. Floersheim GL: Antagonistic effects against single lethal doses of *Amanita phalloides, Naunyn-Schmiedeberg's Arch Pharmacol* 273:171, 1976.
27. Floersheim GL: Experimentille Grundlagen zur Therapie von Vergiftungen durch den grunen Knollenblatterpilz *(Amanita phalloides), Schweiz Med Wochenschr* 108:185, 1978.
28. Floersheim GL: Treatment of mushroom poisoning, *JAMA* 1985: 253:3252.
29. Floersheim G: Treatment of human amatoxin mushroom poisoning: myths and advances in therapy, *Med Toxicol* 2:1, 1987.
30. Floersheim G, Bianchi L: Ethanol diminishes the toxicity of the mushroom *Amanita phalloides, Experimenta* 40:1268, 1984.
31. Floersheim GL, Schneiberger J, Bucher K: Curative potencies of penicillin in experimental *Amanita phalloides* poisoning, *Agents Actions* 213:138, 1971.
32. Floersheim GL et al: Die Klinische Knollenblatterpilzvertigifung *(Amanita phalloides):* Prognostische faktoren und Therapeutische massahmen, *Schweiz Med Wschr* 112:1164, 1982.
33. Franke S et al: Uber die Giftigkeit der Fruhjahrslorchel *Gyromitra esculenta* Fr, *Arch Toxicol* 22:293, 1967.

34. Frimmer M: What we have learned from phalloidin, *Toxicol Lett* 35:169, 1987.

35. Garcia MA et al: Lead content in edible wild mushrooms in northwest Spain as indicator of environmental contamination, *Arch Environ Contam Toxicol* 34:330, 1998.

36. Gerber P: Pilzileus ohne vorbestehendes Passagehindernis, *Schweiz Med Wochenschr* 119:1479, 1989.

37. Gilad E, Biger Y: Paralysis of convergence caused by mushroom poisoning, *Am J Ophthalmol* 102:124, 1986.

38. Giosti GV, Carnevale A: A case of fatal poisoning by *Gyromitra esculenta, Arch Toxicol* 33:49, 1974.

39. Gonzalas J, Lacomis D, Kramer DJ: Mushroom myopathy, *Muscle Nerve* 19:790, 1996.

40. Grzymala S: Erfahrung en mit Dermacybe orellana (Fr) in Polen. B. Massenvergiftung durch den orange fuchsigen Hautkopf, *Z Pilzk* 23:137, 1957.

41. Grzymala S: Les recherches sur la frequence des intoxications par les champignons, *Bull Med Leg Toxicol Med* 2:200, 1965.

42. Hajicek-Dobberstein S: Soma siddhas and alchemical enlightenment: psychedelic mushrooms in Buddhist tradition, *J Ethnopharmacol* 48:99, 1995.

43. Hasler F et al: Determination of psilocin and 4-hydroxyindole-3-acetic acid in plasma by HPLC-ECD and pharmacokinetic profiles of oral and intravenous psilocybin in man, *Pharm Acta Helv* 72:175, 1997.

44. Hatfield GM: Toxins of higher fungi, *Lloydia* 38:36, 1975.

45. Hatfield GM, Schaumberg JP: Isolation and structural studies of Coprine, the disulfiram-like constituent of *Coprinus atramentarius, Lloydia* 38:489, 1975.

46. Hofmann A et al: Psilocybin ein psychotropen Winkstoff aus dem Mexikanischen Rauschpitz *Psilocybe Mexicana* Heim, *Experientia* 14:107, 1958.

47. Holmdahl J et al: Isolation and nephrotoxic studies of orellanine from the mushroom *Cortinarius speciosissimus, Toxicon* 25:195, 1987.

48. Honegger P, Pardo B, Monnet-Tschudi F: Muscimol-induced death of GABAergic neurons in rat brain aggregating cell cultures, *Dev Brain Res* 105:219, 1998.

49. Horn K et al: Biomarkers of liver regeneration allow early prediction of hepatic recovery following hepatic necrosis, *Am J Clin Pathol* 112:351, 1999.

50. Hruby K et al: Chemotherapy of *Amanita phalloides* poisoning with intravenous silibinin, *Hum Toxicol* 2:183, 1983.

51. International Agency for Research on Cancer: Gyromitrin (acetaldehyde formylmethylhydrazone)—on the evaluation of carcinogenic risk of chemicals to man, *IARC Monogr* 31:163, 1983.

52. Jaeger A, Jehl F, Sauder P, Kopferschmitt J: Kinetics of amatoxins in human poisoning: therapeutic implications. *J Toxicol Clin Toxicol* 31:63, 1993.

53. Kelner MJ, Alexander NM: Endocrine hormone abnormalities in *Amanita* poisoning. *Clin Toxicol* 25:21, 1987.

54. Kirklin JK et al: Treatment of hydrazine induced coma with pyridoxine. *N Engl J Med* 294:939, 1976.

55. Klosterman HJ: Vitamin B_6 antagonists of natural origin. *J Agric Food Chem* 22:13, 1974.

56. Koivikko A, Savolainen J: Mushroom allergy. *Allergy* 43:1, 1988.

57. Kretz O, Creppy EE, Dirheimer G: Characterization of bolesatine, a toxic protein from the mushroom *Boletus satanas* Lenz and its effects on kidney cells. *Toxicology* 66:213, 1991.

58. Larcan A et al: Les indications de l'oxygenotherapie hyperbare en reanimation medico-chirurgicale. *Ann Med Nancy* 13:476, 1981.

59. Lincoff G, Mitchel DH: *Toxic and hallucinogenic mushroom poisoning,* New York, 1977, Van Nostrand Reinhold.

60. Lindell TJ et al: Specific inhibition of nuclear RNA polymerase II by α-amanitin, *Science* 170:447, 1970.

61. List PH, Luft P: Gyromitrin, das Gift der Fruhjahrslorchel *Gyromitra (Helvella) esculenta* Fr, *Tetrahedron Lett* 20:1893, 1967.

62. Litovitz TL et al: 1997 annual report of the American Association of Poison Control Centers Toxic Exposure Surveillance System, *Am J Emerg Med* 16:443, 1998.

63. Lockey R: Mushroom workers' pneumonitis, *Ann Allergy* 34:282, 1974.

64. Lopez A et al: Fulminant hepatitis and liver transplantation, *Ann Intern Med* 108:769, 1988.

65. Maretic Z: Poisoning by the mushroom *Clitocybe olearia* Maire, *Toxicon* 4:263, 1967.

66. Maretic Z, Russell FE, Golobie V: Twenty-five cases of poisoning by the mushroom *Pleurotus olearius, Toxicon* 13:379, 1975.

67. Maynert EJ, Kaji K: On the relationship of brain gamma-aminobuteryric acid to convulsions, *J Pharmacol Exp Ther* 137:114, 1963.

68. McCawley EL, Brummett RE, Dana GW: Convulsions from *Psilocybe* mushroom poisoning, *Proc West Pharmacol Soc* 5:27, 1962.

69. Mendelson G: Treatment of hallucinogenic plant toxicity, *Ann Intern Med* 85:126, 1976.

70. Meixner A: Amatoxin nochwers, *Pilzen Z Mykol* 45:137, 1979.

71. Michelot D, Toth B: Poisoning by *Gyromitra esculenta*—a review, *J Appl Toxicol* 11:235, 1991.

72. Nakazawa T, Tochigi T: Hypersensitivity pneumonitis due to mushroom (*Pholiota nameko*) spores, *Chest* 95:1149, 1989.

73. Neftel K et al: Sind Cephalosporine bei der Intoxikation mit Knollenblatterpilz besser wirksam als Penicillin-G? *Schweiz Med Wochenschr* 118:49, 1988.

74. Nilsson GE, Tottmar O: Effects of disulfiram and coprine on rat brain tryptophan hydroxylation in vivo, *Neurochem Res* 14:537, 1989.

75. O'Grady JG et al: Early indications of prognosis in fulminant hepatic failure, *Gastroenterology* 97:439, 1989.

76. Orlav NI: *Sjedobuye i jadovitye griby gribenye ostravlenjia i ich profilaktica,* Megdiz, Moscow, 1953.

77. Peden NR, Pringle SD, Crooks J: The problem of psilocybin mushroom abuse, *Hum Toxicol* 1:417, 1982.

78. Pilegaard K et al: Failure of the cultivated mushroom (*Agaricus bisporus*) to induce tumors in the A/J mouse lung tumor model, *Cancer Letters* 120:79, 1997.

79. Pinson CW et al: Liver transplantation for severe *Amanita phalloides* mushroom poisoning, *Am J Surg* 158:493, 1990.

80. Piqueras J et al: Mushroom poisoning: therapeutic apheresis or forced diuresis. *Transfusion* 27:116, 1987 (letter).

81. Reick W, Platt D: High-performance liquid chromatographic method for the determination of α-amanitin and phalloidin in human plasma using the column-switching technique and its application in suspected cases of poisoning by the green species of *Amanita* mushroom (*Amanita phalloides*), *J Chromatogr* 425:121, 1988

82. Ronzoni G et al: Recovery after serious mushroom poisoning (grade IV encephalopathy) with intensive care support without liver transplantation, *Minerva Anestesiol* 57:383, 1991.

83. Rosenthal P et al: Auxiliary liver transplant in fulminant failure. *Pediatrics* 100:E10, 1997.

84. Sanz P et al: Disseminated intravascular coagulation and mesenteric venous thrombosis in fatal *Amanita* poisoning, *Human Toxicol* 7:199, 1988.

85. Sastie J et al: Respiratory and immunological reactions among Shiitake (*Lentinus edodes*) mushroom workers, *Clin Exp Allergy* 20:13, 1990.

86. Schneider SM: The effect of ethanol on alpha amanitin hepatotoxicity, *Vet Hum Toxicol* 34:352, 1992.

87. Schneider SM, Borochovitz D, Krenzelok EP: Cimetidine protection against alpha-amanitin hepatotoxicity in mice: A potential model for the treatment of *Amanita phalloides* poisoning, *Ann Emerg Med* 16:1136, 1987.

88. Schneider SM, Vanscoy GJ, Michelson EA: Penicillin and cimetidine in *Amanita* toxicity in mice, *Vet Hum Toxicol* 30:364, 1988.

89. Schneider SM et al: P_{450} inducer increases toxicity of alpha amanitin, *Vet Hum Toxicol* 32:369, 1990.

90. Seeger R: Zweitungspapiertest for Amanitin-falsch-positive Erge bnisse, *Z Mykol* 50:353, 1984.

91. Shichijo K et al: A case of bronchial asthma caused by spores of *Lentinus edodes* (Berk) Sing, *Jpn J Allergy* 18:35, 1969.

92. Simons DM: The mushroom toxins, *Del Med J* 43:177, 1971.

93. Sotaniemi E et al: Hydrazine toxicity in the human: report of a fatal case, *Ann Clin Res* 3:30, 1971.

94. Stenklyft PH, Augenstein WL: *Chlorophyllum molybdites*—severe mushroom poisoning in a child, *J Toxicol Clin Toxicol* 28:159, 1990.

95. Suzuki K et al: Purification and some properties of a hemolysin from the poisonous mushroom *Rhodophyllus rhodopolius, Toxicon* 9:1019, 1990.

96. Toth B, Erikson J: Cancer induction in mice by feeding of the uncooked cultivated mushroom of commerce *Agaricus bisporus, Cancer Res* 46:4007, 1986.

97. Toth B, Gannett P, Visek WJ, Patil K: Carcinogenesis studies with the lyophilized mushroom *Agaricus bisporus* in mice, *In Vivo* 12:239, 1998.

98. Toth B, Patel K: The tumorigenic effect of low dose levels of *N*-methyl-*N*-formyl hydrazine in mice, *Neoplasma* 27:25, 1980.

99. Trestrail JH: Mushroom poisoning in the United States—an analysis of 1989 United States Poison Center Data, *Clin Toxicol* 29:459, 1991.

100. Tyler VE: Poisonous mushrooms, *Prog Chem Toxicol* 6:339, 1963.

101. Vanden Hoek TL et al: Jack O'lantern mushroom poisoning, *Ann Emerg Med* 1991;20:550.

102. Vanscoy GJ, Schneider SM: Cimetidine and ascorbic acid in the treatment of alpha-amanitin toxicity in mice, *Vet Hum Toxicol* 30:368, 1988.

103. Vetter J: Toxins of *Amanita phalloides*, *Toxicon* 36:13, 1998.

104. Warden CR, Benjamin DR: Acute renal failure associated with suspected *Amanita smithiana* mushroom ingestions: a case series, *Acad Emerg Med* 5:808, 1998.

105. Wieland T: The toxic peptides from *Amanita* mushrooms, *Int J Peptide Protein Res* 22:257, 1983.

106. Weiland T, Faulstich H: Fifty years of amanitin, *Experientia* 47:1186, 1991.

107. Wieland TH: Uber die Gifstoffe des Knollenblatterpilzes. VII. β-Amanitin, eine dritte Komponente des Knollenblatterpilz giftes, *Justus Liebigs Ann Chem* 564:152, 1949.

108. Wright AV et al: Amelioration of toxic effects of ethylidene gyromitrin (false morel poison) with pyridoxine chloride, *J Food Safety* 3:199, 1981.

50 Ethnobotany: Plant-Derived Medical Therapy

Kevin Jon Davison

The history of ethnobotany begins before the advent of written records. In all ancient civilizations, plants served as important elements of food, shelter, dyes, ornamentation, religious rituals, and medicines. The term *ethnobotany* refers to an individual culture's use of specific plants. The medicinal use of the plant kingdom has been termed *herbalism, plant medicine, natural-based medicine,* and *phytomedicine* in its current application. The word "herb" is broadly defined as a nonwoody plant that dies down to the ground after flowering. The most commonly used interpretation, however, is any plant used for medicinal therapy, nutritional value, food seasoning, or dyeing another substance.

The precise medicinal discovery of the uses of plants by humans remains conjectural. Many scenarios probably occurred. Perhaps, in a prehistoric jungle of South America, a pool of water containing fallen plant material leached out some of the precious medicinal constituents of leaves, flowers, stems, and bark. Tannins, glycosides, sugars, and alkaloids from the bark were infused into the waters. Because of burning fever and severe dehydration, an extremely ill native drank from the pool, and his fever miraculously disappeared. The pond became known for its magical healing powers. If the water held bark from the cinchona tree, the native may have serendipitously discovered quinine.

Archeologic evidence shows that prehistoric humans used plants extensively to treat physical ailments. Instinct and trial and error led to the realization that, for example, cinchona bark controlled intermittent fevers, animals fed on ergotized grain aborted their fetuses, and latex from the opium poppy could be eaten to alleviate pain. Innumerable medicinal plant traditions that remain intact to the present originated as far back as 2700 BC. Ethnobotanically, the use of plant-based medicines represented much more than a culture's individual efforts to survive. Analyzing the methods and degrees of use of indigenous medicines reveals much about cultural philosophy, ingenuity, and sophistication. The Chinese developed an extensive and elaborate system for prescribing, classifying, and processing herbs, which dates back to the third millennium BC. The formulas identified the specific effect of each herb and interactions with other herbs. Less tolerable herbs were blended with those that would counteract undesirable effects. Formulas were custom blended, taking into account a victim's constitution and the stage of the disease. Some of the ancient knowledge from these writings is being used in many contemporary herbal preparations commercially sold as "patent" (readily available in pill form) medicines.

Many native tribes of New Guinea, Indonesia, and the Amazon use single-herb formulations as they did thousands of years ago to treat nearly all their medical conditions. In the West, written records dating to the Sumerians accurately describe the medicinal uses of specific plants.[101] In the same period of about 3000 years ago, the first Asian written record, the *Ben Tsao Gan Mu,* was compiled by the Chinese. It listed more than 360 medicinal plants and their classification, uses, contraindications, and methods of action as perceived at that time. Roman and Greek herbal remedies were described in the writings of Hippocrates and later in those of Galen, providing a pattern for the development of the Western medical tradition. Hippocrates was an advocate for using a few simple plant preparations along with fresh air, rest, and proper diet to help the body's own "life force" eliminate problems. Conversely, Galen promoted the use of direct intervention to correct the imbalances that cause disease, employing large doses of complicated "drug" mixtures that included animal, plant, and mineral ingredients.[114]

The earliest European compendium that listed the uses and properties of medicinal plants, *De Materia Medica,* was written by the Greek physician Dioscorides in the first century AD. He described about 600 plants, and his work remained the authoritative herbal medicinal resource into the seventeenth century.[41]

Herbalism was practiced in many different ways during and after the Middle Ages. There were learned traditional herbalists and lay practitioners, as well as wandering herbalists who professed pagan animism or Christian superstitions that often were more influential in healing than the herbs' properties. Little was added to the knowledge of herbalism during this period. After the Middle Ages and invention of the printing press in the 1400s, hundreds of herbal publications were compiled. Most early works were available only in Latin or Greek; it was not until the fifteenth through seventeenth centuries that the great age of herbalism was appreciated in English.[101]

Tides changed in European herbalism when a Swiss pharmacist-physician named Theophrastus Bombastis von Hohenheim, better known as Paracelsus (1490-1541), introduced a new dimension. He advocated chemistry and chemical processing and used mineral salts, acids, and other preparations in medicinal therapies. This was a departure from the plant-based medicinal methods of the past. During the latter seventeenth century, the predominance of plant medicines slowly eroded. In 1806, Freidrich Serturner, a small-town German pharmacist, became known for his efforts to isolate organic acids from plants in an attempt to find the active ingredient in opium. He discovered organic alkaloids, which became known as the first set of active plant constituents.[149] Because of their physiologic activity, the search for plant alkaloids continued into the twentieth century.

Discoveries quickly followed. The bronchodilator and antitussive ephedrine, from the herb *Ephedra sinica*, was often used in Chinese medicinal formulas for bronchial asthma. The discovery of morphine led to creation of all the narcotic analgesics. The bark of cinchona was found to contain quinine in 1819, which led to development of antimalarial drugs.

The traditional herbal extract from rhubarb (*Rheum* species) has several active compounds. These compounds mediate many of the pharmacologic effects, such as its purgative action (from sennosides); antibacterial, antifungal, and antitumor activities (from anthraquinones); antiinflammatory and analgesic activities; and improvements of lipid metabolism (from stilbenes). Treatment of leukemias from an extract of Madagascar periwinkle (*Catharanthus roseus*), known as vincristine, has been highly effective.[42]

Discoveries in the nineteenth and twentieth centuries included atropine (from belladona leaves, *Atropa belladona*) in 1831, cocaine (from coca leaves, *Erythoxylum coca*) in 1860, ergotamine (from *Claviceps purpurea*) in 1918, and tubocurarine in 1935.[114]

European settlers brought herbal knowledge and their medicinal methods to the Americas. Because of the abundance and wide use of plants on the new continents, they also learned much from the indigenous peoples. The colonists found that conditions afflicting them, such as malaria and scurvy, were treated effectively with herbs by the Native Americans.[115] In the 1700s, herbal medicine continued to have popular applications in lay circles but also was investigated by the new medical establishment. Although the creation of a small elite group of learned professionals was thought to violate the political and constitutional concepts of the early American democratic movement, the practice of medicine was carried over from England and Scotland during prerevolutionary days. Before a professional medical class was established, most illness in America was treated within the family or extended family network.

Many concepts were modified in the colonies between 1765, when the first medical school opened, and 1850, when more than 42 schools of medicine had been recognized. The inquiry into *Digitalis purpurea* (foxglove) by William Withering exemplified the change in perspective from anecdotal folk medicine to a critical examination for specific uses of botanicals from a biochemical point of view. During the early 1800s the trend was to look at the efficacy of botanicals and their intrinsic value from a more scientific perspective.

Several developments delayed the appreciation of herbalism by physicians in the colonies. For instance, Samuel Thomson promoted a system of herbal medicine by proselytizing about his patented method of herbal prescribing, which used many Native American herbs. A central theme in his approach was the advocacy of self-prescribing based on the philosophies and herbal prescriptions found in his book *New Guide to Health*. The right to sell "family franchises" for use of the Thomsonian method of healing was the basis of a widespread lay movement between 1822 and Thomson's death in 1843. Thomson adamantly believed that no professional medical class should exist and that democratic medicine was best practiced by lay persons within a Thomsonian "family unit."[39] Although his methods were considered crude and unscientific, he had over 3 million faithful followers in 1839. Founded on ignorance, prejudice, and dogma, the Thomsonian school did little to help physicians accept European and American herbal medicines. European physicians in the Thomsonian movement wished to separate themselves from the lay practitioners by creating requirements and standards for the practice of Thomsonian medicine. Thomson was adamantly against this, but a decade after his death the Thomsonian physicians formed the Eclectic School of Medicine, which attempted to unite "professional physicians," Thomsonianism, and traditional herbal medicine. The establishment of several Eclectic medical schools was a step toward validating herbal medicine, but it failed to bring herbalism into the mainstream medical establishment. The founding of the American Medical Association and the Flexner Report on medical education in 1910 thoroughly established the modern pharmaceutical industry in the medical education system.[39]

Because of the availability of pure, active constituents from plant drugs and the synthetic drugs that began to appear on the market toward the end of the nineteenth century, the prescribing habits of physicians began to change. The sensibility and predictability of administering exact doses were appealing. For example, the pure alkaloid of quinine could be prescribed for malaria rather than a foul-tasting extract of cinchona bark containing variable percentages of quinine and other alkaloids with different physiologic properties.

Many "crude drugs" were standardized for therapeutic activity. Digitalis, which still retains its status in the *United States Pharmacopeia (USP)*, is one example. Of the 200 plant drugs officially listed in the USP in 1936, about 19% are still official today.[149] An estimated 25% of all prescriptions dispensed in community pharmacies between 1959 and 1980 contained ingredients extracted from higher plants. For a significant number of synthetic drugs, natural drug products continue to serve as either models or starting points for synthesis.

EVOLUTION OF PHYTOPHARMACEUTICALS

The drive toward patenting and ownership in the pharmaceutical industry has been a strong incentive to research and develop plant-based products. Because a plant cannot be patented, however, little U.S. effort has gone into developing herbal medicines during the last century. Active principles of botanicals are investigated for their biologic activity, although in many cases the active constituent is less effective than the whole crude extract of a herb.[114]

One problem in the development of the botanical pharmaceutical industry in the United States has been quality control. In addition, lack of standardization plagues plant-based products. Quality control and standardization of crude plant extracts for herbal medicines were virtually nonexistent until recently,[114] or we might be using more botanical medicines for common ailments. In Europe and Asia, where pharmaceutical firms have been producing standardized *phytopharmaceuticals* (plant-based standardized extracts) for decades, research and development have demonstrated economic and medical sense. Europeans use phytopharmaceuticals as part of their "mainstream" medical practice. In hospitals they are used primarily as adjuvant therapies. More that 70% of general practitioners in Germany prescribe phytopharmaceuticals, and the public health insurance system pays for most of these prescriptions. The total annual market for phytopharmaceuticals in Germany alone is $1.7 billion. Beginning in 1993 the licensing procedure for German physicians required a knowledge of phytotherapy.[130]

Production and evaluation of botanical medicines have improved significantly in the past six decades. In crude plant evaluation, modern laboratory analysis can determine the percentage of active principles, as well as solubility, specific gravity, melting point, optical rotation, and water content. Scientists detect resins, alkaloids, flavonoids, enzymes, essential oils, fats, carbohydrates, and protein content. They can precisely assay using liquid, high-pressure liquid, paper, and thin-layer chromatographies; spectrophotometry; atomic absorption; and magnetic resonance imaging. These methods improve the predictability and therapeutic effectiveness of standardized crude botanical medicines, which are then evaluated for their efficacy in animal studies to determine pharmacologic potency, activity, and toxicity. U.S. and European companies have set strict quality control guidelines to ensure optimum yields of pharmacoactive principles and acceptable levels of impurities, bacterial counts, pesticides, residual solvents, and heavy metals.

Specific cultivation and harvesting techniques affect the therapeutic value of a given herb, which is related to the amount of active constituents in a specific medicinal plant. Methods of packaging, storage, and transport can dramatically affect the stability of active compounds. Both extracts and concentrates are obtained by adding appropriate solvents to raw herbs, which removes the active constituents. The most common method is infusion. As a tea bag is steeped in hot water to make a cup of tea, the water acts as a solvent. If the water were slowly evaporated, the concentrate would contain the active constituents.

Pure ethanol is an effective solvent often used to concentrate active herbal constituents. Immersing a high-quality bulk or raw herb in pure ethanol for hours or days, depending on the herb and the part used, then pressing it out, yields an herbal tincture. The alcoholic tincture is remixed with water to yield a 20% alcohol tincture. In another method, a 20% alcohol mixture is the solvent. Fluid extracts are made by distilling off some of the alcohol with vacuum distillation to avoid elevating the temperature, which may affect some of the active constituents. Another concentration process, solid extraction, yields a solid or semisolid product that can then be powdered or granulated for administration.

Once an extract is produced, qualitative and quantitative analyses can be performed to assist in standardization. The percentage of known active constituents is assayed, to obtain predictable clinical results.

An herbal infusion is generally a better source of active compounds than an air-dried or sun-dried powdered herb (Figure 50-1), but it may not be as strong in

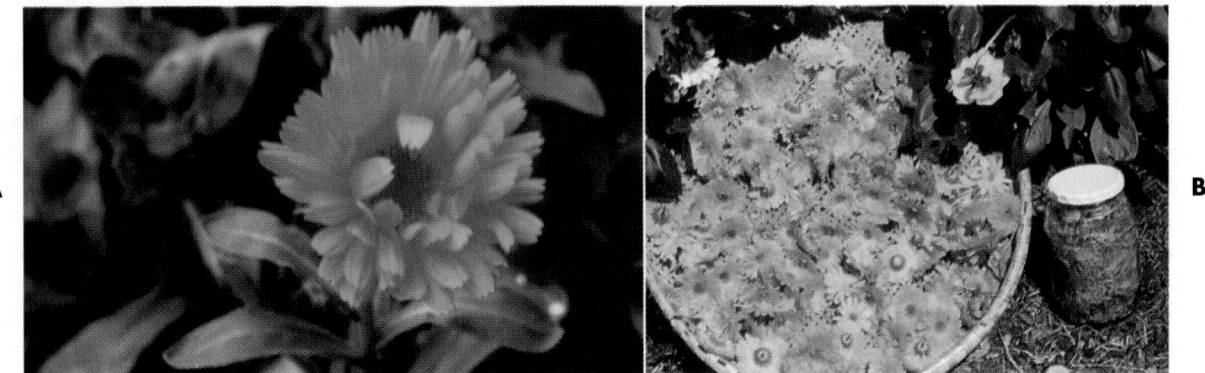

Figure 50-1 **A,** *Calendula officinalis.* **B,** *Calendula* drying and dried in a jar. *(Courtesy Cascade Anderson Geller.)*

action as concentrates such as tinctures, solid extracts, and fluid extracts. Potency of an extract can be defined by (1) percentage of active constituents or (2) concentration. Herbalists express concentration as an equivalency; a four-to-one extract is equivalent to or derived from four parts of the crude herb to yield one part extract. This is usually written as "4:1 solid extract." Longer shelf life, greater effectiveness, and higher concentration of active constituents make a more standardized (better) product than does the raw powdered herb; however, efficacy is difficult to compare.

An example of a product that is standardized to the percentage concentration of pharmacoactive glycosides is the extract of *Gingko biloba,* marketed in Europe under the trade names Tanakan, Rokan, and Tebonin. It is typically standardized as 24% flavonoid glycoside. *G. biloba* extract has been shown to prevent metabolic and neuronal disturbances of cerebral ischemia and hypoxia in experimental models.[86,96]

Quality control is addressed for many herbal products when the known clinical effectiveness can be attributed to a specific active constituent. Improved analytic methods and use of high-quality herbs (high in active principles) helps ensure standardization. In Europe the dosage is expressed in milligrams of active constituents, which favors consistency. The main difference between this method and chemical isolation or synthesis is that the extracts still contain all the synergistic cofactors that enhance the function of the active ingredient. This important aspect of herbal medicine is lost once the active constituent is removed from the whole plant.

HERBAL PREPARATIONS FOR CLINICAL AND WILDERNESS USE

Botanical preparations are readily applicable in acute prescribing for travelers and wilderness enthusiasts. Throughout the ages, botanicals have been useful adjunctive therapeutic agents. Knowing how and what preparations from the natural pharmacopeia can be used provides a sense of integration with the natural environment. Indigenous peoples who have depended on the botanical world throughout their existence hold a vast amount of untapped knowledge. Wilderness enthusiasts should help engender and preserve this understanding of the natural world and help save natural habitats. Further investigation into the plant kingdom for useful medicinal agents will aid in these efforts.

Herbal medicines can be prepared by decoction or infusion of bulk or raw herbs or by the use of extracts, concentrates, and tinctures.

Infusions are prepared like a standard tea. The soft parts of plants, flowers, stems, and leaves—are placed in a warmed pot. Boiling water is poured over the herb, and the pot is covered to prevent beneficial essential oils from evaporating. The mixture infuses for about 10 minutes, then is strained. The supernatant can be used immediately or refrigerated in an airtight container for as long as 2 days. A standard adult dose of an herbal preparation would be 1 ounce (28 g) of dried herb to 1 pint (or 500 ml) of water, or a teaspoon per cup. The amount is doubled if the herb is fresh.

Generally, it is best to take infusions hot by the cupful three times daily for a chronic problem and up to every hour or two during an acute illness. To make infusions palatable, many herbalists have added licorice, aniseed, or honey. The hard or woody parts of plants, such as bark, seeds, roots, rhizomes, and nuts, have tough cell walls that must be broken down by great heat before they can impart their constituents to water. The herbs can be broken into small pieces by chopping, crushing, or hammering.

Traditionally, a decoction was prepared in an earthen crock reserved especially for making herbal preparations. In the past, herbalists believed that some of the quality of the medicine was affected by the type of vessel or container in which the brew was prepared. Contemporary practitioners generally recommend the use of stainless steel, ceramic, or enamel and specifically discourage the use of aluminum or other alloyed metal pots. The herb is placed in an appropriate container and covered with cold water. The mixture is brought to a boil, covered, and simmered for 10 to 45 minutes, depending on the type and part of the herb being used. A decoction can be strained, flavored, or sweetened like an infusion, and it is consumed while hot.

Modern practitioners use the most efficient and predictable forms of specific herbal medicines. Concentrates in capsule form are most effective and easiest to administer. The standard herbal concentrate found in the marketplace is in the ratio of 4:1. Ease of administration and dosage and the predictable clinical effects have made this the industry standard. Herbal tinctures are extracted into a specific percentage of alcohol and can be mixed easily to make formulas tailored to personal conditions. A combination may be many times more effective than a single herb. Formula prescribing is an art. Classic formulas for common ailments have been cataloged since the first herbal compendiums were recorded centuries ago. For the purposes of this chapter, however, single herbs and their specific uses, identification, and preparation are detailed.

HOMEOPATHIC USE OF BOTANICALS

Medical pioneer Samuel Hahnemann developed a radically different system of medicine nearly 200 years ago. Homeopathy is derived from the Greek words *homoios,* which means "similar," and *pathos,* which means "disease" or "suffering." The "law of similars" states that a substance that causes a set of symptoms in pharmacologic dosages can create a cure for similar symptoms (even if the etiologic agent is different) if that substance is given in a homeopathic dilution. Most homeopathic remedies are prepared from plant, mineral, and animal products. In homeopathic medicine, there is a perfectly matched *similimum* (the most effective medicine) if the predominant symptoms of a disease or illness match the symptoms produced when the substance is taken in large doses in a healthy individual. For example, the herb *Atropa belladona,* which contains atropine, is poisonous. In excessive doses the herb causes death; in moderate doses it creates hot, feverish states; and in tiny (homeopathic) doses it can effectively treat certain types of fevers, viral syndromes, and inflammatory states.

A homeopathic dilution is created by taking a prepared tincture (mother tincture) of a botanical or an extract from nonplant sources and diluting it in a sequential or serial method. The difference in a homeopathic dilution is in its methodology. A homeopathic medicine must be succussed (shaken or agitated) mechanically or manually a prescribed number of times between each serial dilution to be effective. The succussion method originally discovered by Hahnemann is said to "dynamize" the medicine. The succussion method may affect the water molecules, creating a "memory" that the water molecules store in a lattice formation. This is similar to the storage of information on a magnetic disk or tape, except the signature resonance pattern is created from the interaction of the original tincture within the water's lattice structure. The dilution can range from a 1x potency, which is a decimal dilution of a given ingredient (one part mother tincture per nine parts solute), to a 1c (one part mother tincture to 99 parts solute), to an extremely dilute 200c (one part mother tincture per 99 solute, serially diluted 200 times). A high-potency dilution (serially diluted more than 30 times in the x potencies and more than 12 times in c potencies) would be taken much less frequently than a low-potency dilution.

To make a 30x homeopathic preparation of *Arnica montana,* one drop of the plant tincture is added to nine drops of pure water, and the mixture is succussed 50 to 100 times. Next, one drop from that solution would be added to nine drops of pure water and again succussed 50 to 100 times. This is repeated 30 times to yield the desired 30x homeopathic remedy. The number refers to the number of succussions and the letter to the ratio of the mother tincture to pure water.

The mechanisms by which homeopathy works have yet to be elucidated, even though it has been practiced effectively for several hundred years. In 1900 an estimated 15% of U.S. physicians were prescribing homeopathic remedies.[105] Recent studies have shown effective results in clinical trials using homeopathic medicines.[28,80,91] Mechanisms of action for many common pharmaceuticals also remain unknown. Many theories in medicine are still based largely on empiric observations rather than theoretic understanding.

One herbal folk remedy for bruises, sprains, strains, and rheumatism in European and native American medicine was topical application of the plant *Arnica montana* (leopard's bane). Consistent with the homeopathic principle, the toxic effects of the whole-plant extract of *Arnica* produce the same set of symptoms it is intended to cure when administered internally in a homeopathic dosage or if the tincture or oil is applied topically to the affected area.

Arnica is contained in herbal and homeopathic dosages in numerous ointments, salves, and poultices for the treatment of trauma resulting from localized sprains, strains, or contusions. Controlled studies in Germany have shown that effective products for sprains from athletic activity use an ointment that contains homeopathic *Arnica.*[158]

TOPICAL APPLICATION

The earliest method of plant administration was topical application. Although many plants contain generalized moisture-enhancing properties, some were found to be particularly effective in ameliorating specific acute conditions when applied topically. Two methods are used to apply remedies to the skin. The *endermatic method* applies medicine on the skin without friction, as when applying a compress to the dermis and epidermis after an abrasion or laceration. The *epidermatic method* uses friction and is most effective with botanical oils, liniments, ointments, and medicated warm and cold friction rubs, primarily for subdermal contusions and trauma to effect circulatory changes.[51]

Topical application of medicinal plants is useful for many conditions, including abrasions, lacerations, burns, insect bites, infections, rashes, and dermatoses. Other applications include contusions, varicosities, joint pain, inflammation, and musculotendinous aches, strains, and sprains.

Topical herbal remedies are applied with a poultice, compress, fomentation, or ointment. Probably the most common, the poultice is used to apply a remedy to a skin area with moist heat. A poultice is prepared by bruising or crushing the medicinal parts of the plant to a pulpy mass, then applying this to the affected area and covering it all with a moist heat source. If dried plants are used (or fresh plants if necessary), the materials are moistened by mixing with a hot, soft, adhesive substance such as moist flour or corn meal. A good way to apply a poultice is to spread the paste or pulp on a wet and hot cloth, which is wrapped around the affected area to help retain moisture and heat. The cloth is moistened with hot water as necessary. With irritant plants, as in a mustard "plaster," the paste is kept between two pieces of cloth to prevent direct contact with the skin. After the poultice is removed, the area is washed well with water to remove any residue. A poultice can be used to soothe, to irritate, or to draw impurities from the affected area, depending on which plants are applied.

A *fomentation* is a hot cloth soaked with an herbal infusion or decoction. Fomentations are generally less active than poultices. A cold compress is used for conditions that require an antiinflammatory cure. A cold, infusion- or decoction-soaked cloth is applied to an area and then removed when the body's circulation has warmed the cloth to body temperature. The botanicals' active principles determine what actions the external applications will impart. For example, a poultice with an astringent herb such as *Hammamelis* (witch hazel) has an entirely different effect than one made with a strong vasodilator and rubefacient, such as *Capsicum* (cayenne pepper).

Ointments are another method of topical administration. Most ointments are made in a base of petroleum jelly, stable vegetable oils, beeswax, or a combination of these. The extract from the desired botanical is suspended within the base to create a stable solid product. Topical botanical products have the same function as topical pharmaceutical ointments and are used to treat lacerations, abrasions, infections, and insect bites. Other uses for botanical topicals include hemostatic, antiinflammatory, antihistamine, rubefacient, analgesic, emollient, and circulatory stimulant actions. As with pharmaceutical topical agents, herbal poultices, compresses, and ointments deliver their active compounds transdermally.

The first uses of most medicinal plants were probably topical. In contemporary herbology, many of these plants are also used internally. Whole plants containing more than one ingredient with biologic activity generally invoke synergistic action of several components to produce the therapeutic action. Thus most botanicals have multiple applications for therapeutic purposes. Herbalists and homeopaths treat trauma of the skin, muscles, tendons, ligaments, and joint tissue with a topical agent in ointment or poultice form and give the same medicine internally in minute (homeopathic) doses to enhance the activity, as with concurrent use of *Arnica* ointment and homeopathic *Arnica*.

The major precaution in medical botany is to identify toxicity. Some of the most effective topical agents can be toxic if ingested. Most of these plants found in the wild could not be taken in sufficient doses to be fatal before causing gastrointestinal (GI) upset. A tincture, herbal concentrate, or powdered version of the plant, however, could have deadly potential.

USE OF HERBAL MEDICINE IN THE WILDERNESS

Travelers in the wilderness can choose preprocessed herbal preparations or naturally available plants in the immediate vicinity. A surprisingly large number of minor medical conditions encountered in an outdoor setting can be treated with plants in that location. North American recreational areas are home to medicinal plants that have been used by Native Americans for centuries. Recreationists in desert, alpine, and river environments can find medicinal plants in abundance. Nearly all the vegetation encountered during an alpine trek in North America has some medicinal property. Many plants in tropical and subtropical regions have medicinal properties.

Considerations for using herbal products in the wilderness are availability, ease of application, incidence of side effects, toxicity, spectrum of applicability, affordability, and effectiveness.

Availability and Application

If a condition can be improved by application of a local botanical growing in the immediate vicinity, the pharmacy is immediately available. Plants may be in season, plentiful, and easily harvested. Finding the appropriate plants can be challenging, however, depending on the location, season, the traveler's familiarity with botanicals, and the type of medical condition. During the popular mild seasons and at elevations conducive to plant growth in the continental United States, the chances of finding common plants are good. If not, standardized commercial preparations of these herbs can be carried. These are packaged for long storage life, sanitary and convenient application, and standardization of active ingredients.

Hundreds of plants can be applied topically for a variety of conditions. Most of the readily available plants, even if properly identified, require some form of processing for the active constituents to be used fully. Furthermore, expertise in the field requires years of training by a knowledgeable botanist and herbalist. It also requires knowledge of plant seasonal variation, ecologic niches, and precise plant identification. However, a non-botanist-herbalist can gain a basic understanding of a few plant medicines that have a wide spectrum of applicability and a broad range of geographic distribution.

Side Effects and Toxicity

The American Association of Poison Control Centers annually reports plant ingestion as a significant category of accidental poisoning. In 1997, 5.6% of U.S. poisonings came from plants and mushrooms. Of the substances that were involved in pediatric poisonings, plants were responsible for 7.4% of exposures.

Side effects or toxic reactions from botanicals are rarely experienced. In those covered in this chapter, toxicity is not a major consideration. Anything can be toxic when used excessively or indiscriminately. Many toxic plants produce GI distress, vomiting, or diarrhea before any severe neurologic or cardiorespiratory derangement. Often, toxic side effects are caused by one substance in a plant. When isolated, minute amounts of an alkaloid may be potentially dangerous, but when ingested in a form modified by other constituents the altered drug effect allows tolerance of larger amounts of the toxic substance or substances.

As with any medication, medicinal plants should be applied appropriately, and dosages for internal use should not exceed recommendations. Pregnancy and nursing may pose contraindications. Dosages for almost any herb can be found in numerous references.[114] Felter[51] stated that "as a rule, doses usually administered are far in excess of necessity and it is better to err on the side of insufficient dosage and trust to nature, than to overdose to the present or future harm or danger of the patient." In general, for the self-harvested herbs presented in this chapter, the dry, crushed, herbal adult dosage should be 1 teaspoon per pint of water; when the fresh herb is used, the amount should be twice that. Although no absolute law exists in administering medicines to children, Cowling's rule takes the child's age at the next birthday and divides by 24 to determine what fraction of the adult dose should be given.[51]

Spectrum of Applicability

Most herbal medicines that have been catalogued and used historically are specifically indicated for one condition, although additional therapeutic effects have been noted over time. All the botanicals covered here have multiple uses. Comfrey (*Symphytum officinale*) may be used as a topical antiinflammatory agent; it also has principles that are effective for GI conditions when taken internally.[101] *Aloe vera* gel is an excellent topical agent for abrasions and burns; taken internally, the latex portion serves as an effective laxative.[101] *Calendula officianalis* has antimicrobial properties that make it an effective topical dressing for mild infectious conditions, whereas internally it has antipyretic effects.[101]

Affordability

If the herbalist collects plants and processes them personally, the cost is minimal. The purchase price of botanicals depends on the rarity and origin. Some exotic and rare botanicals from Asia and the Amazon rainforest demand a high price on the world market. *Panax ginseng* has long been regarded by Asian peoples as a prized herbal tonic and can cost hundreds of dollars per root, depending on the size, origin, and age. *Panax quinquefolius*, or American ginseng, can cost as much as $52 per pound, and was valued at $62 million as a cash crop in 1992.[15] Many exotic herbal and animal-derived medicines from China have prices as high as those of precious metals.

Most of the herbs produced in the continental United States used for common ailments average 20 to 30 cents per dose (equivalent to 1 teaspoon of herbal tincture). Prices are not yet standardized. Quality control for production and supply and demand seem to dictate the cost of the mass-marketed herbal products.

The best way to obtain a standardized product with a good quality/price ratio is to acquire the product from a botanical company that has been in business for at least 10 years and sells only to licensed health care practitioners.

NORTH AMERICAN PLANT MEDICINES

Ephedra (Ephedra viridis)

Description and Habitat. Common names for *Ephedra* include Brigham Young weed, desert herb, Mormon tea, squaw tea, and teamsters' tea.

Ephedra species are shrubs with erect strawlike branches found in desert or arid regions throughout the world and in the southwestern deserts of the United States (Figure 50-2). The Chinese *Ephedra* called Ma Huang, *Ephedra sinica*, is found throughout Asia; *E. distacha* is found throughout Europe; *E. trifurca* or *E. viridis* (desert tea), *E. nevadensis* (Mormon tea), and *E. americana* (American *Ephedra*) are found in North America; and *E. gerardiana* (Pakistani *Ephedra*) is found in Pakistan and India. The 2- to 7-foot shrubs grow on dry, rocky, or sandy soils. The broomlike shrub has many jointed green stems with two or three small scalelike leaves that grow at the joint of stems and branches.

Pharmacology. *Ephedra* is generally utilized for its alkaloid content, which tends to be ephedrine, pseudoephedrine, and norpseudoephedrine. The various species vary significantly in both alkaloid type and content. In *E. sinica* the total alkaloid content can be from 3.3% to 20%, with 40% to 90% being ephedrine and the remainder pseudoephedrine.[46] The North American varieties, such as Mormon tea (*E. nevadensis*), are reported to contain no ephedrine.

Ephedra's pharmacology centers on the actions of ephedrine. Ephedrine and pseudoephedrine are used widely in prescription and over-the-counter drugs to treat asthma, hay fever, and rhinitis.[58]

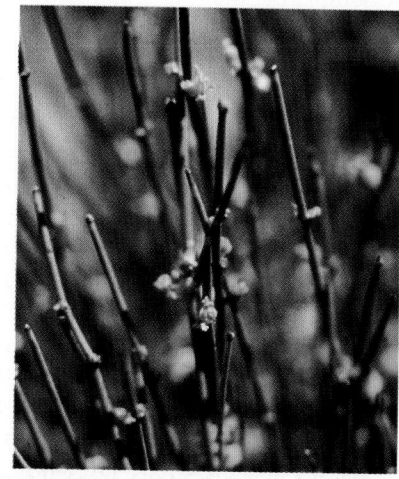

Figure 50-2 *Ephedra viridis. (Courtesy Cascade Anderson Geller.)*

The central nervous system (CNS) effects of ephedrine are similar to those of epinephrine but are much milder and longer in duration of action. The cardiovascular effects are increased blood pressure, cardiac output, and heart rate. In addition, ephedrine increases brain, heart, and muscle blood flow while decreasing renal and intestinal circulation.[58] Relaxation of bronchial, airway, and uterine smooth muscles also occurs.[58]

Pseudoephedrine has weaker CNS and cardiovascular system actions but has bronchial smooth muscle relaxation effects. Because of fewer side effects, it is used more often than ephedrine for asthma.[58] Pseudoephedrine also demonstrates significant antiinflammatory activity.[70,87] Per 100 g, the dry leaf of *Ephedra* is reported to contain 5 g protein, 5810 mg calcium, and 500 mg potassium.[46]

Native and European Medicinal Uses. *Ephedra* has been used extensively in the West and in Asia for upper respiratory conditions such as asthma, bronchitis, and hay fever. It has also been used to treat edema, arthritis, fever, hypotension, and urticaria.[34] It is said to be valuable as a diuretic, febrifuge, and tonic.[101]

The Navajo Indians used the dried, crushed, long leaf of *Ephedra* to apply to syphilitic sores, and the Hopi Indians drank a tea from the branches and twigs of a related species for the same condition.[152] Other tribes used the ground and roasted root for making bread.[46]

Mormon tea is a folk remedy for colds, gonorrhea, headache, nephritis, and syphilis.[46] Mexicans mix the leaves with tobacco and smoke them for headaches.[46]

Modern Clinical and Wilderness Applications. *Ephedra* has proved to be an effective bronchodilator for treating mild to moderate asthma and hay fever. The common preparations include other herbs that have antitussive and expectorant effects, such as licorice (*Glycyrrhiza glabra*) and grindelia (*Grindelia camporium*).

Ephedrine promotes weight loss.[114] Appetite suppression plays a role, but an increase in metabolic rate of adipose tissue is the main mechanism.[7] The weight reduction effects can be enhanced by up to 60% with the addition of methylxanthine.[47]

Clinically, standardized *Ephedra* preparations are used because of the predictable alkaloid content. *E. sinica* extracts are available with a standardized 10% ephedrine alkaloid content. The dosage of a 10% alkaloid content extract is 125 to 250 mg three times a day.

In the wilderness, specifically the desert, the raw herb Mormon tea from *E. nevadensis* or *E. viridis* can be useful for hay fever, mild asthma, bronchitis, or an upper respiratory infection (URI). These species contain minimal amounts of ephedrine and principally contain pseudoephedrine; thus they can be used without some of the unpleasant side effects of the Asian species. They can also be used for mild fevers associated with influenza or URI.

The shrubs are typically found growing on dry, rocky, or sandy slopes. The leaves can be picked fresh or sun-dried for 6 to 8 hours and can be prepared as a steeped tea or an infusion. Generally, the dose should be the equivalent volume of 1 tablespoon of dried, crushed stems per 4 ounces of water, steeped for 10 minutes. The patient should not exceed a dosage given six times per day. Once harvested, the leaves can be kept for an indefinite period for later use if stored in an airtight container.

Toxicity. According to Duke,[46] an infusion of *Ephedra* produced a "prompt and extensive contraction of uterine muscle when applied to smooth muscle strips of virgin guinea pig uteri." *Ephedra* may also elevate blood pressure. Frequent use may result in nervousness and restlessness. It should be used with caution if the patient has hypertension, heart disease, thyrotoxism, diabetes, or benign prostatic hypertrophy. Ephedrine should not be used with antihypertensive or antidepressant medications.

Goldenseal (Hydrastis canadensis)

Description and Habitat. *Hydrastis* has a perennial root or rhizome, which is tortuous, knotty, and creeping. The internal color is bright yellow, with numerous long fibers. The stem is erect, simple, herbaceous, and rounded, from 15 to 30 cm (6 to 12 inches) in height, becoming purplish and bearing two unequal terminal leaves. The leaves are alternately palmate with three to five lobes, hairy, dark green, and cordate at the base. The flowers, which are evident in early spring, are solitary, terminal, small, and white or rose colored.

The plant is a native of eastern North America and cultivated in Oregon and Washington. The parts used are the dried rhizome and roots.

Pharmacology. The alkaloids derived from *Hydrastis* are hydrastine (1.5% to 4%), berberine (0.5% to 6%), berberastine (2% to 3%), canadine, hydrastinine, and related compounds. Other constituents include meconin, chlorogenic acid, phytosterins, and resins.[114]

Native and European Medicinal Uses and Folklore. Native Americans used *Hydrastis* extensively as an herbal medicine and clothing dye. The Cherokee Indians used the roots as a wash for local inflammations and as a decoction for general debility, for dyspepsia, and to improve appetite. The Iroquois Indians used a decoction of the root for whooping cough, diarrhea, liver trouble, fever, sour stomach, flatulence, pneumonia, and heart trouble.[109]

Early European uses date back to 1793; in the *Collections for an Essay Towards a Materia Medica of the United States*, Benjamin Smith Barton noted that *Hydrastis* was useful as an eyewash for conjunctival inflammation and as a bitter tonic. In the pharmacy of the nineteenth century (1830), goldenseal was listed among the official remedies in the first revision of the New York edition of the *USP*. It was listed in the *USP* until 1926 and recognized in the *National Formulary* until 1955.[71]

Modern Clinical and Wilderness Applications. Goldenseal is among the top sellers in the American herbal medicine market. It is used as an antiseptic, hemostatic, diuretic, laxative, tonic, and antiinflammatory for inflammation of the mucous membranes. It has also been recommended for hemorrhoids, nasal congestion, sore mouth and gums, conjunctivitis, external wounds, sores, acne, and ringworm.[98]

Modern research into the active ingredients berberine and hydrastine has shown why some of the folk applications are effective. The most widely studied component is berberine. This isoquinoline alkaloid has demonstrated antibiotic, immunostimulatory, anticonvulsant, sedative, febrifugal, hypotensive, uterotonic, choleretic, and carminative activities (promoting the elimination of intestinal gas).[114] Berberine has broad-spectrum antibiotic activity. The antimicrobial activity has been demonstrated on protozoa, fungi, and bacteria, both in vitro and in vivo. Antimicrobial action has been noted against *Staphylococcus, Streptococcus, Chlamydia, Corynebacterium diphtheriae, Escherichia coli, Salmonella typhi, Vibrio cholerae, Pseudomonas, Shigella dysenteriae, Entamoeba histolytica, Trichomonas vaginalis, Neisseria gonorrhoeae* and *N. meningitidis, Treponema pallidum, Giardia lamblia, Leishmania donovani,* and *Candida albicans.*[114] Berberine inhibits the adherence of bacteria to host cells.[140]

Active ingredients in the crude botanical may be responsible for the wide-spectrum effectiveness of *Hydrastis.* The antifungal properties, for example, prevent the overgrowth of *Candida* that frequently occurs with the use of other antibiotic therapies.

Other studies have shown the immunostimulatory activity of berberine-containing plants. Berberine increases blood flow through the spleen; improved circulation may augment the immune function of this lymphoid organ.[125] Berberine also activates macrophages.[91] Historically, berberine-containing plants have been used as febrifuges, and in rat studies they have an antipyretic effect three times as potent as that of aspirin.[114]

Plants such as goldenseal are very effective in treating acute GI infections. In several clinical studies, berberine has successfully treated acute diarrhea caused by *E. coli, Shigella dysenteriae, Salmonella, Klebsiella, Giardia,* and *Vibrio cholerae.** Berberine-containing plants, in addition to their antimicrobial properties, influence the enterotoxins produced by offending pathogens.[24,141,142]

GI illness is a major concern of the traveler to areas where sanitation is questionable. Both waterborne and food-borne bacterial and protozoal infections are con-

cerns for persons in wilderness and Third World environments. Some experts recommend using a berberine-containing botanical source prophylactically at least 1 week before a visit to questionable areas and for 1 week after return.[114]

Various eye complaints involving the conjunctivae and surrounding mucous membranes have been effectively treated with forms of berberine extract. Recent studies point to the effectiveness of berberine in treating the infection caused by *Chlamydia trachomatis.* Clinical trials found that a 2% berberine solution compared favorably to sulfacetamide. Although the symptoms resolved more slowly with the berberine extract, the rate of relapse was much lower in the berberine-treated group.[9,110]

A standardized form of *Hydrastis canadensis* is beneficial for generalized digestive disorders (acute dysentery, gastritis) and infective, congestive, and inflammatory states of the mucous membranes (sinusitis, pharyngitis, stomatitis). A typical dose depends on the source and method of the extract. For the previous conditions, the following three-times-a-day dosage is recommended: dried root or as infusion, 2 to 4 g; tincture (1:5), 6 to 12 ml (1.5 to 3 teaspoons); or solid extract (4:1 or 10% alkaloid content), 250 to 500 mg. *Hydrastis* can also be used as a wash or rinse for conjunctivitis, sinusitis, and pharyngitis. Eye drops, nasal lavage, and gargle are applied in a 5% preparation of a 1:5 tincture, or 1 to 2 teaspoons of powdered herb to 8 ounces water to create an infusion for application to inflamed mucous membranes. This can be repeated three times a day.

Toxicity. Berberine and berberine-containing plants are generally nontoxic. In recommended doses, berberine-containing plants have not been shown to be toxic in clinical trials. The median lethal dose (LD_{50}) of berberine sulfate in mice is approximately 25 mg/kg, and in dogs, intravenous (IV) doses up to 45 mg/kg do not produce lethal or gross toxic effects.[125] *Hydrastis* should not be used during pregnancy, and long-term ingestion may interfere with the metabolism of B vitamins.

Arnica (Arnica montana)

Description and Habitat. *Arnica* is a perennial plant generally found in mountainous areas of Canada, the northern United States, and Europe. The plant reaches a height of 30 to 60 cm (1 to 2 feet) and generally contains from one to nine large daisylike flowerheads, which bloom during summer months (Figure 50-3).

Pharmacology. The flower is used both internally and externally for medicinal effects. The rootstock is used to make commercial preparations for tinctures and oils that are applied topically. The active principles of the plant drug are flavonoids, volatile oils, and plant pigments (carotinoids).[153] Specific constituents include ar-

---

*References 11, 37, 45, 66, 85, 126, 131

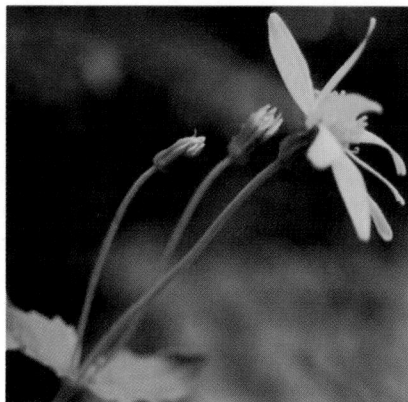

Figure 50-3 *Arnica latifolia.*

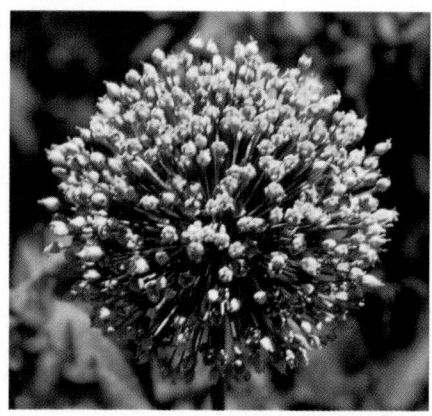

Figure 50-4 Garlic blossom (*Allium* species). *(Courtesy Cascade Anderson Geller.)*

nicine, formic acid, thymohydroquinone, lobelamine, and lobeline (piperidine alkaloid).[28]

Native and European Medicinal Use and Folklore.
The Catawa Indians administered the tea of *Arnica* roots to treat back pain. In Europe the flowerheads have been used since the sixteenth century as an application for bruises and strains.[151] European *Arnica* was included in the *USP* from the early 1800s until 1960 and was recognized for its effects on the healing of bruises and sprains.

Specific instructions given in the *American Dispensory* in 1922 listed *Arnica* as effective for "muscular soreness and pain from strain or overexertion; advanced stage of disease, with marked enfeeblement, weak circulation, and impaired spinal innervation; . . . tensive backache, as if bruised or strained; [and] . . . headache with tensive, bruised feeling and pain on movement."[51] *Arnica* in tincture (concentrated) form has been a popular but not necessarily safe medicine to treat inflammatory swellings and to relieve the soreness of myalgia and the effects of bruises and contusions. Doses above the therapeutic range cause vagal inhibition when ingested and may cause toxicity if the concentrated tincture is applied topically. Therefore the most common use has been fomentation of the flowers for topical applications in treatment of strains and sprains.

Modern Clinical and Wilderness Applications.
Contemporary use of *Arnica montana* is generally limited to topical commercially prepared ointments and salves, in conjunction with internal homeopathic (low-dose) use for the same indications. Although its alkaloid (arnicine) and volatile oil (thymohydroquinone) are both relatively toxic, the actions of these constituents are extremely useful in resolving contusions and soft tissue injury. Most ointments are found to contain a 1*x* homeopathic dilution of *Arnica* tincture, which is about 4% by volume. Oral dosage is given in homeopathic potencies of 6*x* to 200*c,* depending on the severity of the condition.

For application in the wilderness, most naturopathic first-aid kits include both the ointment and the oral homeopathic forms of *Arnica.* For direct use of the plant in treating minor sprains and strains, 2 teaspoons of the dried flower tops can be steeped in 1 cup of water for 10 minutes, and the infusion can be applied in a cold compress to the affected area. This should be repeated each 2 hours in addition to standard first-aid procedures. The infusion lasts a day if refrigerated and a few hours if not; therefore it is best to use a fresh infusion whenever possible. In addition, if available, the oral homeopathic preparation (30*x* to 200*c*) should be taken three times daily until the swelling is reduced significantly. A topical ointment can be applied every 2 to 3 hours for this condition in place of the compress.

According to Weiss,[152] *Arnica* is safe and effective for topical contusions and for stimulating granulation and epithelialization. A tablespoon of tincture is added to 500 ml of water, and the gauze compress is then placed on the wound. This stimulates local circulation and acts on the peripheral vasculature. After granulation has occurred, ointments may be applied.

Toxicity.
Arnica tincture or infusion can be toxic if the concentration is too high. Undiluted tincture should not be used internally or in compress form over an open wound. Vagus nerve inhibition is the primary toxic effect; GI irritation is also noted. Toxic reactions include gastric burning; nausea; vomiting; headache; decreased temperature; dyspnea; cardiovascular collapse; convulsions; motor, sensory, and vagal paralysis; and death.[28]

Garlic (Allium sativum)

Description and Habitat.
Garlic is a member of the lily family. It is a perennial plant cultivated worldwide (Figure 50-4). The garlic bulb is composed of individual cloves enclosed in a white skin. The medicinal herb is found in the bulb and is used either fresh or dehydrated. Garlic oil, which also has medicinal value, is ob-

tained by steamed distillation of the crushed fresh bulbs.[98]

Pharmacology. The medicinal compounds in garlic generally contain sulfur and have been the subject of most research on garlic. Two primary compounds are an odorless chemical called alliin and the enzyme allinase, which begins a cascade of chemical reactions when the garlic clove is cut, crushed, or bruised. Alliin is converted to allicin, which is responsible for the characteristic odor of garlic. Allicin is strongly antibacterial and considered to be the major source of the antimicrobial effects of garlic. Diallyl sulfide, disulfide, and trisulfide are yielded from the breakdown of allicin. Heat speeds up the reaction, so cooked garlic and steamed distilled garlic oil contain little or no allicin. Within garlic, about 0.1% to 0.36% of the volatile oil is composed of sulfur-containing compounds (e.g., allicin, diallyl sulfide, diallyl trisulfide). These volatile oils are considered to be responsible for most of the pharmacologic properties of garlic. Other constituents of garlic include s-methyl-L-cysteine sulfoxide, protein (16.8% dry weight basis), a high concentration of trace minerals (particularly selenium and germanium), vitamins, glucosinolates, and enzymes, which are composed of allinase, peroxidase, and myrosinase.[114,122]

Native and European Medicinal Use and Folklore.
Throughout history, garlic has played an important part in medicinal herbology. Clay garlic bulbs dating back to 3750 BC were found in Egypt. Preserved garlic bulbs were discovered in the tomb of Tutankhamen. An entire basket of these bulbs from the tomb of Kha at Thebes is in the Turin Museum. The Greek historian Herodotus recorded that an enormous amount of money was spent on garlic for the builders of the great pyramids. One of the earliest Sanskrit manuscripts, *The Bower Manuscript,* devotes its entire first section to garlic, describing its legendary origins. It says that garlic keeps in order the three fluids and can cure thinness, weakness of digestion, lassitude, coughs, inflammation of the skin, piles, glandular swellings in the abdomen and enlargement of the spleen, indigestion, constipation, excessive urination, worms, wind in the body (rheumatism), leprosy, epilepsy, and paralysis.

Within the traditional medical circles of Greece and Rome, medieval Europe, and the Far East, similar claims may be found. Galen, Dioscorides, and Aristotle extolled garlic as an excellent medicine. Hippocrates recommended garlic as a diuretic; to regulate digestion; to treat bowel pains, inflammations, and infections; and to regulate menstruation. Early Chinese and European herbalists used garlic for heating and drying and therefore to prevent and cure diseases arising from cold, poisons, excesses of diet and drink, and sluggish metabolism.

Pasteur noted garlic's antibiotic properties in 1858. Albert Schweitzer used garlic in Africa to treat amebic dysentery. Garlic was also used as an antiseptic to prevent gangrene during both world wars.

Modern Clinical and Wilderness Applications. The pharmacologic effects of garlic are based on its activity as a hypoglycemic and hypolipemic regulating agent,* anticoagulant,† antihypertensive,[103,124] antimicrobial,‡ detoxifier of heavy metals,[2] and immune system modulator.[82]

Animal and human studies have substantiated that garlic lowers serum cholesterol and triglyceride levels and increases the amount of high-density lipoproteins. Dietary atherosclerosis was significantly reduced in rabbits fed garlic consistently for weeks; also, extract of garlic and onions was more effective than clofibrate against hyperlipidemia and subsequent lipid deposition within the aorta.[23] After 4 months of feeding the rabbits a high-cholesterol diet, the average lipid content in the aorta of the control animals rose from 5.95 to 13.75 mg/100 g dry weight. Animals taking clofibrate for 4 months had 7.95 mg and garlic-fed animals 6.23 mg/100 g dry weight of lipid content in the aorta.[23] Other studies of experimental atherosclerosis in rabbits support these findings.[76,88] Decreased atheromatous lesions seem to be a consistent finding in rabbits fed high-cholesterol diets supplemented with garlic.

Of various sulfur-containing amino acids isolated from garlic, s-methylcysteine and s-allylcysteine exert the greatest antilipidemic effects.[74] Components of garlic can combine with the sulfhydryl group, the functional part of coenzyme A that is necessary for the biosynthesis of fatty acids, cholesterol, triglycerides, and phospholipids. The lipid-lowering effect may best be attributed to inactivation of the sulfhydryl group.[8] Both in vitro and in vivo tests show reduced conversion of acetate into cholesterol by liver tissues.[35] Since the sulfhydryl groups are involved at all levels of metabolic activity, the impact of garlic could be more extensive. Studies suggest that garlic may lower blood pressure by acting similar to prostaglandin E_1, which decreases peripheral vascular resistance.[118]

As a nutritional supplement, garlic is composed of magnesium, iron, copper, zinc, selenium, calcium, potassium chloride, germanium, sulfur compounds, amino acids, and vitamins A, B_1, and C. Garlic increases the body's capacity to assimilate thiamine by enhancing its absorption. Thiamine is a key part of the co-carboxylase enzyme system, which has beneficial effects on liver cells; this may explain why garlic offers prophylaxis against liver and gallbladder damage. In one study, garlic was shown to protect hepatocytes in tis-

---

*References 6, 8, 12, 17, 18, 20, 21, 26, 35, 36, 65, 74, 75, 78-80, 83, 84, 88, 89, 116.
†References 5, 16, 19, 24, 25, 57, 77, 102, 119, 127, 137.
‡References 3, 4, 32, 53, 93, 102, 115, 144, 146

sue culture from the damage of carbon tetrachloride.[118]

Antioxidant activity has been attributed to garlic and garlic derivatives. The free radical scavenger action of garlic may be explained by its germanium, glutathione, selenium, and zinc content. The last three are key components of the antioxidant enzyme superoxide dismutase and glutathione peroxidase. Animal studies show that feeding garlic oil enhanced physical endurance in normal rats and also reduced the decrease in physical endurance induced by isoproterenol, a synthetic catecholamine that induces necrosis of the myocardium.[129]

Garlic inhibits platelet aggregation in animals; similar effects can be demonstrated in vitro and in vivo in humans.[43,137] An antiplatelet extract of garlic, ajoene, was found to potentiate the antithrombotic effect of antiinflammatory drugs. Under fasting conditions inhibition of platelet aggregation by garlic or its extracts is dose related.[138]

The garlic effect may be linked to inhibition of thromboxane synthesis or to altered properties of the plasma membrane. Methyl (2-propenyl) trisulfide, another component of garlic, is 10 times more potent as an inhibitor of platelet aggregation than is diallyl disulfide or trisulfide.[5] Thrombocyte aggregation inhibition is enhanced by two other compounds, 2-vinyl-1,3-dithiene and allyl-1,5-hexidienyl-trisulfide.[14]

Garlic and its juice or oil also enhance fibrinolysis.[22] In a double-blind placebo-controlled trial, cycloalliin, a component of garlic, was given to volunteers and patients after myocardial infarction and significantly increased fibrinolysis 1½ hours later.[49] Chutani and Bordia[38] observed that the increase took place 6½ to 12 hours after garlic intake. Daily garlic ingestion for 1 month generated a 72% to 85% increase in fibrinolysis in patients with ischemic heart disease.[124]

The pharmacologic versatility of garlic is best reflected by its antiviral, antifungal, antiprotozoan, antiparasitic, and antibacterial activities.* Laymen are credited with being the first to describe the scientific basis for the medicinal use of garlic extract.[155] Huddleson et al[72] and Cavallito et al[33] demonstrated in 1944 that garlic juice and allicin inhibited the growth of *Staphylococcus, Streptococcus, Bacillus, Brucella,* and *Vibrio* species at low concentrations. Recent studies using serial dilutions and filter paper disk techniques have shown that fresh garlic, powdered garlic, and vacuum-dried preparations were effective antibiotic agents against many bacteria, including *Staphyloccus aureus,* α- and β-hemolytic *Streptococcus, E. coli, Proteus vulgaris, Salmonella enteritidis, Citrobacter,* and *Klebsiella pneumoniae.*[114] These studies compared the antimicrobial effects of antibiotics, including penicillin, streptomycin, chloramphenicol, erythromycin, and tetracycline, with those of garlic. Besides confirming garlic's

well-known antibacterial effects, studies demonstrated its effectiveness in inhibiting the growth of some antibiotic-resistant bacteria.[1,48,132]

Garlic has also demonstrated significant antifungal activity against a wide range of fungi.* From a wilderness perspective, inhibition of fungi that can affect the skin (*Microsporum, Trichophyton, Epidermophyton,* and *Candida albicans*) can be significant. Garlic juice applied topically is an effective alternative in treating fungal skin diseases.[3] Garlic compares well with nystatin, gentian violet, and six other reputed antifungal agents to treat *C. albicans.*[1,111,121,128]

Garlic has long been associated with prophylaxis against influenza virus. In vivo studies with mice revealed that garlic administration protected mice against intranasal inoculation with influenza viruses and enhanced reproduction of neutralizing antibodies after vaccine administration.[115] In vitro studies have shown that garlic has antiviral activity against influenza B virus and herpes hominis virus type I.[145] Preliminary studies have revealed significant enhancement of natural killer (NK) cell activity in humans administered raw or cold, aged whole-clove garlic preparations daily for 3 weeks.[82] The antiviral activity of garlic in humans may be secondary to the direct toxic effect on viruses and enhanced NK cell activity that destroys virus-infected cells.

Wilderness Medical Applications. The use of garlic in the outdoor setting can be extensive. Its use as a food should be encouraged despite its odor, particularly in people with elevated cholesterol levels, heart disease, hypertension, diabetes, asthma, fungal infections, respiratory infections, and GI disorders (intestinal parasites, dysentery). A macerated garlic poultice and garlic slices serve as topical agents for fungal infections, ulcerated wounds, pyoderma, and other skin infections. The poultice can be used directly on the dermatologic problem and as a suppository can be used to treat vaginitis, particularly infections caused by *C. albicans.* For this application, one to two fresh chopped cloves can be made into a poultice. This should be kept on the affected site for several hours and changed at least once every 6 hours with a fresh preparation. If the garlic causes epidermal irritation, its use is discontinued.

Prophylactic use during the flu season can reduce the incidence of infection. Within the first 48 hours of onset of a flu or URI, one or two cloves can be consumed with a carbohydrate source to prevent stomach irritation. Alternatively, two or three oil of garlic capsules can be taken. For persons concerned about the social segregating aspect, extracts that preserve the allicin content but remain odorless can be used.

---

*References 3, 4, 32, 53, 115, 143, 157.

*References 1, 3, 55, 73, 108, 111, 121, 128, 149.

Toxicity. For the vast majority of individuals, garlic is nontoxic at usual dosages. However, some people develop allergic contact dermatitis or irritation of the digestive tract. Apparently, they are unable to detoxify allicin and other sulfur-containing components. Prolonged consumption of large amounts of raw garlic by rats results in anemia, weight loss, and failure to grow.[117]

Ginger (Zingiber officinale)

Description and Habitat. Ginger is an upright perennial herb with tuberous rhizomes, from which grows an aerial stem to 1.5 m (5 feet) in height. It is native to southern Asia, although it is cultivated in the tropics. Extracts and dried ginger are produced from dried unpeeled ginger; peeled ginger loses much of its essential oil content.[148]

Pharmacology. Ginger is composed of a rich variety of nutrients and enzymes. The general composition is starch (50%); protein (9%); lipid (6% to 8%) composed of phosphatidic acid; lecithin; free fatty acids; triglycerides; protease (up to 2.26%); volatile oils (1% to 4%), the principal components of which are three sesquiterpenes (bisabolene, zingiberene, zingiberol); vitamins, especially niacin and vitamin A; and resins.[148]

Native and European Medicinal Use. *Zingiber officinale* is native to southern Asia and tropical Africa. Therefore it did not have a role in the early herbal preparations of European and Native American herbal medicine.

Modern Clinical and Wilderness Applications. Clinical use of ginger for antiinflammatory action, cholesterol-lowering effects, and relief of dizziness and motion sickness is noted in herbal texts.* A choleretic effect (the promotion of bile flow to the gallbladder and small intestine) and the conversion of cholesterol into bile acids are enhanced by ginger ingestion and may be responsible for its overall cholesterol-lowering effect.

An early eclectic medical text listed ginger as local stimulant, sialogogue, diaphoretic, and carminative.[51] Powdered ginger in a large quantity of cold water taken before sleep frequently "breaks up" a severe cold, and a hot infusion of ginger tea is a popular remedy for similar use to mitigate the pains of dysmenorrhea.[51] Ginger may relieve painful spasmodic contractions of the stomach and intestine. The antiinflammatory action of ginger is thought to be caused by potent inhibition of inflammatory compounds, such as prostaglandins and thromboxanes.[90] Ginger is also known to contain strong plant proteases such as bromelain, ficaine, and papain, which may explain some of its antiinflammatory action.[148]

Ginger has been used historically for major GI complaints. It is generally regarded as an excellent carminative (promotes the elimination of intestinal gas) and intestinal spasmolytic.[114] One of the most noted uses of ginger in contemporary herbal medicine that applies to wilderness medicine is its action on the symptoms of motion sickness and seasickness.[62,63,113] Ginger is also a significant antiemetic. It has long been used in the treatment of nausea and vomiting associated with pregnancy. The efficacy of ginger has been confirmed in hyperemesis gravidarum, a severe form of nausea and vomiting during pregnancy. Ginger root powder at a dose of 250 mg four times a day brought a significant reduction in both the severity of nausea and the number of attacks of vomiting during pregnancy.[52] To treat motion sickness and vertigo, two 500-mg capsules of powdered ginger root are eaten 20 to 30 minutes before the precipitating event. The same dose is used for the nausea of pregnancy during the acute attack. The raw ginger root can be grated using 1 teaspoon in 4 ounces of water, steeped for 10 minutes, and taken every 30 minutes until the symptoms of motion sickness abate.

Toxicity. There appears to be no toxicity associated with ginger root ingestion.

Comfrey (Symphytum officinale)

Description and Habitat. Comfrey is a perennial herb with a stout spreading root that is essentially divisible for propagation. Comfrey grows about 1 m (3 feet) high and has coarse, bristly, oblong, lanceolate leaves. The tubular flower can be purplish, blue, white, red, or yellow (Figure 50-5). About 25 *Symphytum* species are described; they are indigenous to countries around the Mediterranean Sea and in northern Asia. Comfrey is typically found in moist meadows and other wet places in the United States and Europe.

Pharmacology. The chemical constituents of *Symphytum officinale* roots include carbohydrate, predominantly sucrose; the amino acids serine and asparagine; the phenolic acids chlorogenic acid, caffeic acid, and

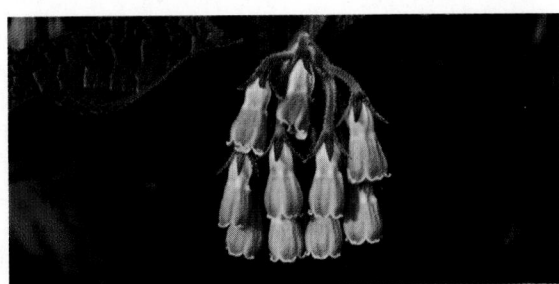

Figure 50-5 Comfrey *(Symphytum officinale). (Courtesy Cascade Anderson Geller.)*

---

*References 51, 52, 62-64, 90, 113, 134, 138, 139, 148.

p-coumaric acid; the alkaloids choline and allantoin; and the pyrrolizidine alkaloids viridiflorine, echinatine, heliosupine, symphytine, echimidine, and lasiocarpine.[150] The most concentrated (0.88% to 1.71%) alkaloid, allantoin, is generally credited with comfrey's beneficial effects.

Native and European Medicinal Uses and Folklore.
In Europe, comfrey is a common perennial grown in the garden for animal fodder. Russian comfrey is often promoted as a medicinal herb for use as a tonic. Comfrey is also cultivated in Japan as a green vegetable and tonic and has been used in American herbal medicine for hundreds of years.[95]

Comfrey has long been known as an external agent for the rehabilitation of musculoskeletal and orthopedic injuries. Its former name, "bone knit," derives from the external use of poultices of leaves and roots, which were believed to help heal burns, sprains, swellings, and bruises. Comfrey has been claimed to heal gastric ulcers and hemorrhoids, suppress bleeding, and relieve bronchial congestion and inflammation.[13] The healing action of a poultice derived from the roots and leaves is probably related to the presence of allantoin, an agent that promotes cell proliferation. The underground parts contain 0.6% to 1.3% allantoin and 4% to 6.5% tannin.[30,107] Comfrey extracts applied topically have been reported to heal wounds and bones in about half of the normal time. In herbology a general rule is that if anything is broken, use comfrey.[156] Herbalists have also found that the allantoin concentration from a fluid extract of comfrey can increase the rate of wound healing of lacerations sufficiently to avoid the use of sutures.[154]

In European folklore, comfrey was regarded as an herb having unsurpassed ability to heal any injured or broken tissue. The mucilage (gelatinous mucopolysaccharide) of the comfrey root was named "the great cell proliferator," helping new flesh and bones to grow. Comfrey was one of the main herbs found in any poultice or fomentation. European herbalists considered comfrey exceptional for coughs and soothing inflamed tissues. Comfrey is effective for treating upper respiratory inflammation and has been used successfully to treat hemorrhagic conditions of the lungs.

Modern Clinical and Wilderness Applications.
Comfrey lotions and salves containing 0.5% to 2.5% allantoin have been used for sprains, strains, and contusions. In the 1980s, comfrey became controversial because of potential hepatotoxicity. Members of the family Boraginaceae (*Heliotropium, Symphytum*) contain a variety of related pyrrolizidine alkaloids reported to cause hepatotoxicity in animals. Although no hepatotoxic episodes from the ingestion of comfrey have been reported in humans, the potential exists, so caution is advised when using comfrey for internal consump-

tion.[95] Topical use of comfrey products as yet poses no concern for toxicity.

As a topical agent after acute trauma for musculoskeletal injuries, strains and sprains, or contusions, comfrey is an exceptional medicine.[31] A prepared gel of comfrey with a standardized allantoin concentration should be carried during travel or camping expeditions in the wilderness.

The raw herb can be used if the person is in the plant's environment. The herb is readily identifiable, although it should not be confused with foxglove (*Digitalis purpurea*) and should be used with caution when taken internally in its raw state. For use in a poultice or compress, the leaves may be picked damp, macerated, and applied topically for up to 24 hours.

Toxicity.
Comfrey is not recommended for routine internal ingestion. Animal studies indicate that hepatic damage is an eventual outcome if the herb is consumed over a long period.

Aloe (Aloe vera)

Description and Habitat.
The aloe is a perennial plant native to South and East Africa and is also cultivated in the West Indies and other tropical and temperate areas. The leaves, which emerge from a central rosette produced by a central fibrous root, are 30 to 60 cm (1 to 2 feet) long, narrow, fleshy, and light green with spiny teeth on the margins (Figure 50-6). Aloe is easily cultivated as a houseplant and can be grown in a sunny warm spot with good drainage.

The genus *Aloe* comprises more than 300 species, which are members of the Liliaceae (lily) family. *Aloe* species are perennial succulents native to Africa. They are not cacti and should not be confused with American aloe, the century plant.

Pharmacology.
Two important products are derived from aloe: a gel and a latex. Aloe gel is a clear gelatinous material extracted from the mucilaginous cells found in the inner tissue of the leaf. The gel is obtained by crushing the leaves and repeated straining to re-

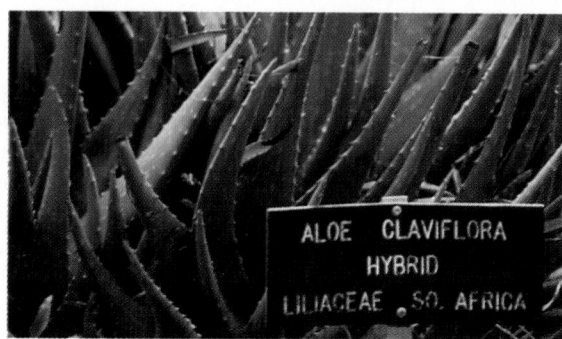

Figure 50-6 *Aloe claviflora. (Courtesy Cascade Anderson Geller.)*

move cellular debris. The result is a clear gel, which is the product most frequently used in the health food and cosmetic industries. It is generally devoid of anthraquinone glycosides. A variety of compounds have been identified in the aloe species, including polysaccharides, tannins, organic acids, enzymes, vitamins, minerals, saponins, and steroids.[95]

The bitter yellow latex of aloe contains cathartic anthraquinone glycosides, mostly barbaloin, as the active principles. The concentrations of the glycosides vary with the type of aloe, ranging from 4% to 25% of aloe in concentration. The water-soluble fraction of aloe is called aloin and is a mixture of active glycosides. Cathartics have been derived from extracts of the latex and can create strong purgative effects by stimulating the large intestine.

Native and European Medicinal Uses and Folklore.
Fresh *Aloe vera* gel is well known for its domestic medicinal values.[59,97,112,120] Aloe has been dubbed the burn plant, first-aid plant, and medicine plant. When fresh, the gel relieves thermal burns and sunburns and promotes wound healing. It also has moisturizing and emollient properties. Because of these effects, aloe is widely used as a home remedy.

Aloin and other anthraquinone derivatives of aloe are extensively used as active ingredients in laxative preparations. Aloin is also used as an antiobesity preparation.[98] Aloe or aloin extracts are also used in sunscreens and other cosmetic preparations and in drugs for moisturizing, emollient, or wound-healing purposes.

In folk medicine, aloe is used for condylomas, warts, abnormal skin growths, and cancers of the lip, anus, breast, larynx, liver, nose, stomach, and uterus.[46] Other folklore suggests that parts of the plants be chewed to purify the blood. The pulp is said to possess wound-healing hormonal activities and "biogenic stimulators" and is used for intestinal ailments, sore throat, and ulcers. In India it is used to treat piles and rectal fissures. Slukari hunters in Africa's Congo basin rubbed their bodies with the gel to eliminate the human scent, making them less likely to disturb prey. During epidemics of influenza, Lesotho natives take a public bath in an infusion of *Aloe latifolia*.[46]

Modern Clinical and Wilderness Application.
Although numerous claims have been made for aloe gel, its most common lay use is in the treatment of minor burns and skin irritations. In 1935 a report described the use of aloe in the treatment of radiation-induced dermatitis.[40] This study followed a 5-week course of topical applications of either the whole leaf or leaf macerated into gel, resulting in complete wound healing after 4 months. In 1937, studies used a calamine and lanolin-based aloe preparation to treat skin irritations resulting from burns, pruritus vulvae, and poison ivy. The results suggested that aloe stimulated tissue granulation and accelerated wound healing.[95]

Barnes[10] evaluated the effect of 5% aloe ointment on sandpaper-abraded fingertips and found that the wound-healing rate was two to three times that of control subjects, as measured by decreased electrical potential of the wound. Other studies measured tensile strength of the healed surgical wounds of mice. Healing occurred within 9 days, an improvement over the control mice.[60]

Studies of antibacterial activity of aloe extracts have been attempted several times, yielding mixed results. In 1963, studies of the antibacterial effect of macerated *Aloe vera* gel found no activity against *S. aureus* and *E. coli*.[54] Other studies have determined that *Aloe chinensis* is effective against *S. aureus*, *E. coli*, and *Mycobacterium tuberculosis*, although *Aloe vera* showed no inhibitory effect.[61] The latex possesses in vitro activity against several pathogenic strains of bacteria, although the whole leaf minus the latex from the leaf epidermis and mesophyll of aloe showed no activity.[99] Two commercial preparations of aloe gel were found to exert antimicrobial activity against gram-negative and gram-positive bacteria and *C. albicans* when used in concentrations greater than 90%.[67]

The moisturizing effect of aloe may be beneficial in the treatment of burns. The healing process may be related to mucopolysaccharides along with sulfur derivatives and nitrogen compounds in the gel, but this has not been well substantiated.[94] In attempts to document the antiinflammatory effects of aloe, a 1976 study found that *Aloe vera* had bradykinase activity in vitro, but this was not confirmed in vivo.[56]

Evidence for the internal use of aloe has been limited to studies involving mucous membrane tissue repair. Corneal ulcers treated with aloe extracts had more healing, less cellular reaction, and fewer signs of irritation than did control groups.[95] Topical application of *Aloe vera* gel after periodontal flap surgery reduced postoperative pain more than the saline control, and swelling of the treated tissue was less marked than with the control.[69]

Because of easy recognition and administration, use of the aloe plant in the wilderness environment is practical. The wild plant can yield an excellent preparation for dermal abrasions, cuts, and superficial wounds. A leaf cut from the base of a healthy plant can be conveniently carried. This allows the gel to remain intact, protected by the outer skin of the leaf. It can be squeezed from the inside through the cut portion directly onto superficial wounds with or without a gauze dressing. A standardized preparation of *Aloe vera* may be used as an antibacterial agent and an emollient for superficial wounds or dermatitis.

In the event of constipation, the mixture of aloe gel and latex can be scraped or squeezed from the leaf cortex and ingested, 1 tablespoon three times daily, or until a mild laxative effect is noted. A gel and latex mixture produces less cathartic effect than only latex. Because of the bitterness of the gel and the latex, it should be taken with food or a flavored beverage.

Toxicity. Because of its cathartic effects, oral aloe is not advised if gripping pain is associated with constipation. Aloe taken orally is contraindicated in pregnancy. Otherwise it has no reported toxicity.

Plantain (Plantago major)

Description and Habitat. The common broadleaf plantain is a familiar perennial "weed" that may be found along roadsides and in meadowlands. Plantain belongs to the order Plantaginaceae, which contains more than 200 species, 25 or 30 of which have a domestic use. The plant is a small weed with a rosette of ribbed leaves and small projecting seed stalks. Its seeds, known as psyllium seeds in North America, resemble those of another species, *Plantago psyllium.* The leaves contain 84% water, 2.5% protein, 0.2% fat, and 14% carbohydrate, trace amounts of calcium, phosphorus, iron, sodium, and potassium, as well as β-carotene, riboflavin, niacin, and ascorbic acid. Biochemically identified compounds include allantoin, adenine, baicalein, baicalin, benzoic acid, chlorogenic acid, choline, cinnamic acid, ferulic acid, L-fructose, fumaric acid, gentisic acid, D-glucose, *P*-hydroxybenzoic acid, indican, lignoceric acid, neochlorogenic acid, oleanolic acid, plantagonine, planteose, saccharose, salicylic acid, scutellarein, sitosterol, sorbitol, stachyose, syringic acid, tyrosol, ursolic acid, vanillic acid, and D-xylose.[46]

Native and European Medicinal Uses and Folklore.
Historically, plantain has been used for stings, bites, and irritations from venomous insects and reptiles. The folk medicine of the eastern United States suggests using crushed plantain leaves to stop the itching of poison ivy. It has also been reported to help relieve toothache. Ancient herbalists maintained that plantain had refrigerant (imparts a cooling sensation to the mucosa and allays thirst), diuretic, and astringent properties. When the leaves are applied to a bleeding surface wound, hemorrhage lessens. In the highlands of Scotland, plantain is still called *slan-lus,* or plant of healing.

In the United States, plantain has been known as snake weed, from the belief that it is effective for bites from venomous creatures. Felter[51] noted that "the crushed leaves were very effective for the distressing symptoms caused by puncture by the horny appendages of larvae of Lepidoptera and the irritation produced by certain caterpillars, as well as the stings of insects and bites of spiders." In native American folklore, the plant was known as "white man's foot," in reference to its trait of growing in the settlements of white men. The Shoshoni Indians heated the leaves and applied them in a wet dressing for wounds.[153]

Modern Clinical and Wilderness Applications. Plantain is readily available in the recreational areas of North America. This plant is extremely useful for various superficial wounds, abrasions, stings, and bites of mildly venomous insects. The constituents in the crushed leaves have an antihistaminic effect, and anesthetic quality. In the event of a tooth fracture, a compress or poultice of ½ teaspoon of fresh leaves may be used on the exposed nerve root of a tooth. The seeds of the plantago plant are useful for spastic colon, an effect that appears to be related to their mucilaginous properties. Psyllium seeds, known on the Asian continent as flea seed husk, are often used as a bulk laxative. The seeds are collected from the stalk, and 1 teaspoon of fresh seeds in 4 ounces of water is taken twice a day for mild constipation. Water should be ingested throughout the day to alleviate the condition and assist the laxative effect.

Because of its astringent effects, an infusion of the leaves is recommended to treat diarrhea. The preparer pours 1 pint of boiling water on 1 ounce of the herb and leaves it in a warm place for 20 minutes. After, straining and cooling, ½ cup is ingested three or four times a day.

Toxicity. No known toxicities are attributed to *Plantago.*

Chamomile (Matricaria chamomilla)

Description and Habitat. Chamomile is a low-growing perennial with a hairy prostrate branching stem. It blooms late in July through September and is found growing throughout North America and Europe. Chamomile is derived from the Greek *chamos* (ground) and *melos* (apple), which refer to the plant's low growth and the applelike scent of its fresh blooms.[135] The flower head is about 2.5 cm (1 inch) in diameter, has a conical receptacle, and is covered by yellow disk flowers surrounded by 10 or 20 white down-curving ray flowers.

Pharmacology. The most important chemicals associated with chamomile are the volatile oils containing tiglic acid esters, chamazulene, farnesene, and α-bisabolol oxide. These volatile oils are destroyed if the herb is boiled.[136]

Native and European Medicinal Uses and Folklore.
A distinction should be made between German and Roman chamomile, which have been used interchangeably for centuries. The German chamomile is preferred on the European continent, whereas the Roman chamomile has been used widely in Great Britain. In

the United States, German chamomile is by far the more widely consumed of the two species.[104]

German chamomile has a long tradition as a folk or domestic remedy. Its uses include external compresses or fomentations for gout, sciatica, inflammations, lumbago, rheumatism, and skin ailments. Infusions, decoctions, and tinctures have long been used internally to treat colic, convulsions, croup, diarrhea, fever, indigestion, insomnia, teething, toothaches, and bleeding or swollen gums. Historically, Roman chamomile was used similarly.[46,98] Chamomile is also a folk cancer remedy.

Modern Clinical and Wilderness Applications.
The biochemical constituent of chamomile is chamazulene. It is found in both species of chamomile and is reported to have antihistaminic properties.[50] Both histamine release and inhibition of histamine discharge have been considered mechanisms for the potential antiallergic action of chamazulene.

In Germany, chamomile products include tinctures, extracts, teas, and salves, widely used as antiinflammatory, antibacterial, antispasmodic, and sedative agents.[104] Studies have shown that both chamazulene and α-bisabolol have antiinflammatory activity. Chamazulene may constitute as much as 5% of the essential oil. Other studies have shown that α-bisabolol has a protective effect against peptic ulcer, as well as antibacterial and antifungal effects. α-Bisabolol has also reduced fever and shortened the healing time of skin burns in laboratory animals.[44] Most commercial European chamomile preparations have been standardized with regard to the chamazulene and a-bisabolol content.[149]

According to Rudolph Weiss,[152] one action of chamomile is to reduce gastric motility and secretions, which would alleviate colic and painful spasm. About 20 flavones and flavonols, such as apingenin, are found in the aqueous portion of the distillation process. These are three times as effective at spasmolytic activity as the opium alkaloid papaverine. Chamomile also has a significant calming effect and has been traditionally applied as a mild sedative.

Chamomile is a good botanical to have on hand when traveling or camping. For infants experiencing restlessness and discomfort from teething, one third of the adult dosage may provide relief. For the treatment of conditions that may arise from excessive nervous tension (intestinal gas, colic, peptic ulcers), 2 teaspoons (or one standard teabag) of the flower tops can be added to a cup of boiling water and infused for 5 to 10 minutes; 2 to 3 cups may be taken in 30 minutes for acute intestinal colic.

Echinacea (Echinacea angustifolia)
Description and habitat. Echinacea is a perennial herb native to the midwestern region of North America, from Saskatchewan to Texas. The plant produces a characteristic large pale-purple flower and thick hairy leaves and grows 60 to 90 cm (24 to 36 inches) high. The dried root is typically used for medicinal purposes.

Pharmacology. The compounds currently identified from *Echinacea* species are inulin, glucose, fructose, betaine, echinacin, echinacoside, trihydroxyphenyl proprionic acid, and nonspecific resins.

Native and European Medicinal Uses. This medicinal herb came to the attention of American herbalists in the late 1800s. *Echinacea* was originally used by the Indian tribes of Nebraska and the Sioux for the treatment of snakebite and as an antiseptic and analgesic. Eclectic practitioners used it externally for the same purposes but used it internally to treat "bad blood," or any condition that manifested signs of local or systemic infection, whether bacterial or viral.

Modern Clinical and Wilderness Applications. Echinacea is probably the most common botanical used and known by the public, especially in relation to its immunomodulating effects. Many have found that echinacea can reduce symptoms and derail the onset of URIs and minor influenza episodes.

Echinacea is also a good systemic adjunct to the treatment of any contusion or laceration. The polysaccharide component echinacin can maintain the structure and integrity of the collagen matrix in connective tissue and ground substance and can accelerate wound healing experimentally.[114] Echinacin also has a cortisone-like effect, with intermediate stabilization of inflammation reactions. Inulin, a major component of *Echinacea*, is a powerful activator of the immune system's alternative complement pathway. It may increase host defense mechanisms for the neutralization of viruses, destruction of bacteria, and increased action of white blood cells (lymphocytes, neutrophils, monocytes, eosinophils) within areas of infection. Extracts of the root have been shown to possess interferon-like properties. As an immune stimulant early in infection, and for posttrauma rehabilitation, dosages are taken orally three times a day: tincture (1:5), 30 to 60 drops, or solid extract (dry powdered extract 6:1), 250 to 500 mg.

Calendula (Calendula officinalis)
Description and Habitat. Calendula is found throughout Asia, North America, and Europe and is in the daisy and dandelion family. It is most often known as the marigold. The flower is generally used for the production of the tincture.

Pharmacology. Calendula's chemical constituents include flavonoids, carotenes, saponin, resin, and volatile oil. The volatile oil content is responsible for a localized increase in blood circulation and diaphoresis. The resin content is responsible for the antimicrobial and antiinflammatory action of the topical application.

Native and European Medicinal Uses. Native Americans apparently did not use calendula extensively, and the early European literature only mentions its medicinal role. Calendula, however, is one of the best topical applications for the treatment and prevention of infection and skin irritation. Early American surgeons highly regarded its ability to treat and prevent postsurgical infections.

Modern Clinical and Wilderness Applications. A fluid/water extraction or oil infusion (prepared as a tincture but using vegetable oil instead of alcohol) of *Calendula* should be used in the initial treatment of lacerations, abrasions, and scalds; immediately after any required debridement and cleaning of a wound; and for generalized inflammation of the mucous membranes. It has shown its usefulness in dermatitis and vaginal, sinus, ophthalmic, and middle and external ear infections over the decades. The application of calendula ointments, tinctures, or fluid extracts depends on the wound. The succus (fluid extract) of the flower should be applied for irrigation of wounds and in ophthalmic uses.

NATURAL PRODUCTS FIRST-AID KIT

A natural products first-aid kit should contain a variety of products that are easy to obtain and replace and that have a wide spectrum of use, including herbs (Box 50-1), homeopathic preparations, and vitamin and enzyme supplements (Table 50-1).

Homeopathic Medicines

Homeopathy can be an excellent source of relief and treatment for emergencies and general first-aid situations. Homeopathic preparations include powders,

---

Box 50-1 HERBAL MEDICINES RECOMMENDED FOR FIRST-AID KIT

Aloe gel and powder capsules
Arnica ointment
Calendula gel, ointment and tincture
Chamomile tincture
Comfrey gel or ointment
Echinacea tincture or freeze-dried powder capsules
Ephedra freeze-dried powder capsules
Goldenseal tincture or ointment
Hypericum ointment or tincture
Plantain tincture
Witch hazel fluid extract or tincture

---

tablets, tinctures, lotions, ointments, creams, and sprays. The advantages of homeopathy are the ease of administration, lack of toxicity, rapid action, and small volume of material. The disadvantages are the degree of understanding and competence required to become an effective prescriber and the lack of readily available sources of each medicine at most North American pharmacies.

A kit made exclusively of homeopathic medicines can cover most first-aid emergency situations. For the acute, straightforward injury or malady without a complex presentation, the correct similimum and rapid amelioration of symptoms are not difficult to achieve. This section discusses a few indications for the use of homeopathic medicines and the preparation most often used. Unless otherwise noted, a 6x to 12x potency in lactose pellet form should be given every 15 to 30 minutes immediately after the injury until noticeable improvement occurs. If no effect is noted after the first two doses, one must reconsider the medicine selection.

A personal experience exemplifies the relief that can be obtained from an acute injury with the appropriate homeopathic medicine. I was bitten on the lip by a small centipede while sleeping. I instantly experienced swelling and intense burning pain. Local application of ice provided no relief. I chose the homeopathic medicine *Apis mellifica* in a 6c potency because the wound was shiny and felt hot and swelling was increasing. After sublingual ingestion of two pellets I waited 1 to 2 minutes, still in excruciating pain with no change in symptoms. My next selection was *Cantharis* in a 6c potency, since a key symptom for this remedy is extreme red and hot burning pain of the face. Less than 30 seconds after administration the pain was almost undetectable. Total relief was obtained within a few minutes after being bitten. For comparison, I have had no homeopathic kit available after other centipede bites, and the pain generally lasted for hours and the residual swelling for days. Reactions from different centipedes can cause different sensations and symptoms, however, so *Cantharis* may not work for all bites.

Proper selection of the similimum or indicated homeopathic medicine requires the ability to note the subtle differences in the way the victim responds to an apparently similar traumatic or toxologic influence.

An appropriate homeopathic field guide that lists the specific indications and differentiation for each of the homeopathic remedies should accompany any first-aid kit. Unlike with Western pharmaceutical medications, it is essential to understand the specific homeopathic indications (similimum) for each of the remedies on hand. Without this, the chance of obtaining a successful outcome using homeopathics is small.

Practitioners and the homeopathic industry have realized the difficulty of single remedy prescribing, which involves understanding and memorizing the in-

TABLE 50-1. Physiologic Responses from Phytopharmaceuticals

PLANT MEDICINES	ANALGESICS	ANTIBIOTICS	ANTIFUNGALS	ANTI-INFLAMMATORIES	ASTRINGENTS	ANTISEPTICS	DECONGESTANTS	SEDATIVES
Aconitum nopellus								Homeopathic internal
Apis mellifica				Homeopathic topical, internal				
Arnica montana	Homeopathic internal Botanical topical			Homeopathic topical, internal				
Arsenicum alfum								Homeopathic internal
Bromalain				Internal				
Calendula			Botanical internal, topical	Botanical topical	Botanical topical	Botanical topical		
Chamomile	Botanical internal, topical	Botanical internal, topical		Botanical internal, topical		Botanical topical	Botanical internal	Botanical homeopathic internal
Comfrey				Botanical topical				
Echinacea	Botanical internal, topical	Botanical internal, topical	Botanical internal, topical	Botanical internal		Botanical homeopathic topical		
Ephedra							Botanical internal	
Goldenseal		Botanical internal, topical	Botanical internal, topical	Botanical topical	Botanical internal, topical	Botanical topical		
Hypericum						Homeopathic internal, topical		Homeopathic internal
Peppermint						Botanical topical	Botanical internal, topical	
Plantain					Botanical topical	Botanical topical		
Rhus toxicodendron				Homeopathic topical, internal	Botanical topical			
Witch hazel					Botanical topical			

dications for every homeopathic medicine. Therefore medicines have been developed that combine individual preparations to cover a large number of symptoms and symptom characteristics that typically accompany most ailments. These medicines, known as complex or combination homeopathic preparations, can be very helpful for the new user.

Single Preparations and Indications

ACONITE. Tincture of the whole plant with root is derived when monkshood or wolfsbane (*Aconitum napellus*) begins to flower. Aconite is indicated for acute states of emotional disturbance, including anxiety and intense fear or pain. This is one of the key remedies that should be administered after an acute injury that has dazed, shocked, or frightened the victim. Persons who are fearful or restless, cannot tolerate being touched, and have pain followed by numbness and tingling sensations are most responsive to aconite. Those with sudden onset of fever, nausea, and vomiting and who exhibit symptoms of fear, restlessness, and anxiety may also benefit.

APIS. The original tincture is manufactured from the whole honeybee and from dilutions of the venom (*Apis mellifica*). Apis is used for insect stings, particularly from bees and related insects, when the wound is swollen, shiny, and hot to the touch. Treatable symptoms from other conditions are histamine reactions (resulting in facial flushing, puffiness or swelling around the mouth, face, and eyes) sunburn, hives, burns, and early stages of abscesses and frostbite. If symptoms include a stinging, burning, or swelling quality and subside by applying cold rather than heat, *Apis* is the indicated remedy.

ARNICA. The tincture comes from the whole fresh plant, flowers, and dried roots of leopard's bane or Fallkraut (*Arnica montana*). *Arnica* is indicated for blunt traumatic wounds (resulting in both deep and superficial hematomas), contusions, swelling, and localized tenderness. This is also effective for sore muscles, as well as sprains, fractures, dislocations, and internal bleeding. I recommend taking a 6x to 30x potency every 15 minutes to 3 hours for the first few days for a severe injury. The more severe the injury, the more frequently the dosage is taken for the first day. As the symptom severity decreases, the medicine is taken less often. *Arnica* can be helpful in decreasing severity and recovery time.

ARSENICUM. Derived from arsenic trioxide, arsenicum is used for skin rashes (which feel warm but are relieved by hot applications), hay fever, asthma (especially when accompanied by notable anxiety), diarrhea, vomiting, and gastroenteritis (especially from foodborne microbes).

HYPERICUM. The tincture comes from the whole fresh plant and flowers of St John's wort (*Hypericum perforatum*). Indications include any pain that affects the peripheral or central nervous system and exhibits shooting pains that travel in a dermatomal pattern (e.g., sciatica). Wounds that affect the nerve endings, such as injuries to the fingers, toes, or teeth, are improved by *Hypericum*. Pain from dental surgery, toothaches, injuries to the coccyx, and first- and second-degree dermal burns are other indications.

LEDUM. Ledum is made from the leaves and stems of the whole fresh plant of wild rosemary (*Ledum palustre*). Homeopathic indications include puncture wounds from small, sharp objects (e.g., nails, needles) and some mosquito bites when the injured area feels cold, swollen, and numb and pain is relieved by cold application.

RHUS. This homeopathic preparation comes from the leaves and stems of the whole fresh plant of poison ivy (*Rhus toxicodendron*). This is the remedy of choice for the urticaria caused by poison ivy exposure and is also helpful for some cases of poison oak. Other skin rashes that are red, weeping, blistered, and swollen with itching can be treated with *Rhus*. It is also effective for the treatment of connective tissue irritations with swelling, stiffness, and tightness. *Rhus* is often used for overuse injuries (e.g., fasciitis, tendinitis) and some forms of arthritis, especially when the injured area feels better with warm applications and movement.

Combination Preparations for Acute Sprains and Strains. Homeopathic companies have created combination remedies for the general public that can be used without the need for in-depth understanding of homeopathic prescribing. These remedies are designed to cover a broad range of symptoms associated with acute ailments and trauma-induced medical conditions.

Traumeel (Heel Biotherapeutics, Albuquerque, NM) is a combination homeopathic formula that is effective in the treatment of trauma and inflammatory changes affecting skin, connective tissue, and muscle. The preparation comes in liquid, tablet, and ointment form. Traumeel includes remedies indicated for traumatic injuries (sprains, strains, contusions) and the resulting pain, swelling, and ecchymoses. Many German studies have demonstrated its effectiveness.[27] Traumeel may be the primary homeopathic medicine chosen for the first-aid kit because of its wide range of application and multiple delivery system.

Herbal Combination Formulas

Acute Gastroenteritis. In the tradition of Chinese herbal medicine, many formulas have been developed over the centuries to treat acute ailments. Many of these formulas were kept secret from the general populace and reserved for the nobility and ruling class. As the field of Chinese herbology developed and became more accessible to the general populace, some of the secret formulas have been mass produced into convenient pill form known as patent medicines. Many of these are extremely useful for acute conditions.

Pill Curing (Kang Ning Wan, "Healthy Quiet Pill"), botanically called Coix Formula, consists of 16 herbal medicines that are collectively effective for relieving the disturbances caused by motion sickness, food poisoning, overeating, excessive alcohol consumption (nausea, headache, vomiting) difficulty passing stool or loose stools, and GI cramping and pain. Coix Formula is currently produced in a convenient globule form (Metagenics, San Clemente, Calif). One or two capfuls of globules are swallowed with warm water every hour until symptoms improve. Relief should occur within 4 hours of administration.

Acute Hemorrhagic Conditions.

The product Yunnan Bai Yao ("Yunnan White Medicine"), produced in the western Chinese province of Yunnan, has been used for centuries as a first-line approach to trauma that results in internal or external bleeding. It is prescribed in China for excessive menstrual cramps and bleeding, bleeding ulcers, trauma-induced swelling, bleeding wounds, and allergic reactions to insect bites. It comes in powder (4-g bottles) and capsule (packets of 20) form and contains one red pellet that is to be ingested only for serious bleeding conditions. Dosage is 1 to 2 capsules four times per day. The powder can be applied externally after the wound has been properly cleaned. This product is exclusively produced in China from a proprietary formula and can be obtained from most Chinese herbal pharmacies.

Nutritional Supplements

For immune system support, antiinflammatory action, and pain relief, many natural products in the nutritional supplement category have proved to be effective agents.

Bromelain.

Bromelain is a naturally occurring proteolytic enzyme found in pineapple that is used to reduce pain and swelling after sprains and strains of soft tissues. Ingested on an empty stomach, the complex proteases in bromelain are absorbed intact and have significant antiedema, antiinflammatory, and coagulation-inhibiting effects. Bromelain shows fibrinolytic activity and acts to inhibit fibrinogen synthesis, decreasing kininogen and bradykinins.[100] For treatment of injuries and postsurgical recovery, 125 to 400 mg is ingested three times daily at 30 minutes before or 90 minutes after a meal. Bromelain is nontoxic even at high doses and is generally prepared as 100-mg tablets.

Papain.

As with bromelain, papain is a naturally occurring plant enzyme (papaya fruit) that exhibits proteolytic activity. Papain is generally used externally to neutralize bee, ant, or wasp venom. Papain is available as commercial meat tenderizer (e.g., Adolph's) or in tablet form. After removal of the stinger, a thick paste is prepared from water and tenderizer or from five or six crushed tablets and applied to the area as soon as possible.

Vitamin C.

Ascorbic acid has both wound-healing and antiinflammatory effects. Vitamin C is required for hydroxylation of proline and subsequently for the synthesis of strong collagen. Studies have shown that the stress associated with injury and wound healing results in an increased need for vitamin C.[106] For acute trauma and acute upper respiratory allergy, vitamin C in larger dosages (2 to 5 g/day in divided doses) can greatly reduce anaphylactic reactions and recovery time.[68] Therefore, for any traumatic event, high-dose vitamin C should be administered as part of the treatment.

APPENDIX

Companies

Nature's Apothecary
997 Dixon Rd
Boulder, CO 80302
800-999-7422

Small herbal kits include Dental Poultice Pac for toothaches and abscesses, Clear Eyes Eyewash Kit (including Eyebright *Euphrasia* extract), and reformulated Home Herbal Medicine Kit.

Boiron
1208 Amosland Rd
PO Box 54
Norwood, PA 19074
800-258-8823

Natural Home Health Care LeKit contains 36 single-remedy medicines in distinctive blue tubes, including the commercial flu remedy Oscillococcinum. The home kit also contains four external remedies: tinctures of *Calendula* and *Hypericum* and ointments of *Arnica* and *Calendula*. Travel LeKit is a more compact collection of single remedies (22 multidose and 16 unit-dose tubes) plus the flu remedy.

Dolisos America
3014 Rigel Ave
Las Vegas, NV 89102
702-871-7153, 800-365-4767

Single Remedy Family Kit contains 48 single remedies, a Flu-Solution remedy, *Calendula* ointment and tincture, and *Arnica* cream. The 48 combination Energy Medicine Kit includes remedies for bruises, insect bites, and poison ivy.

Biological Homeopathic Industries (BHI)
11600 Cochiti S.E.
Albuquerque, NM 87123
800-621-7644

BHI is the U.S. distributor of the German line of complex homeopathic remedies manufactured by Heel.

Books
Natural Health and Medicine

Encyclopedia of Natural Medicine by Michael Murray, and Joseph Pizzorno, Rocklin, Calif, 1991, Prima Publishing.

Health and Healing: Understanding Conventional and Alternative Medicine by Andrew Weil, Boston, 1983, Houghton Mifflin.

The Natural Remedy Bible by John Lust, and Michael Tierra, New York 1990, Pocket Books.

Herbs and Herbalism

The Healing Power of Herbs by Michael Murray, Rocklin, Calif, 1991, Prima Publishing.

Herbal Medicine by Rudolph Fritz Weiss, Beaconsfield, England, 1988, Beaconsfield Publisher.

Homeopathy Books

Boericke's Materia Medica with Repertory by William Boericke, and Oscar Boericke, New Dehli, India, 1991, B. Jain Publishing.

The Homeopathic Emergency Guide by Thomas Kruzel, Berkeley, Calif, 1992, North Atlantic Books/Homeopathic Education Services.

Homotoxicology by Hans Rekeweg, Albuquerque, NM, BHI.

Sports & Exercise Injuries: Conventional, Homeopathic & Alternative Treatments by Steven Subotnick, Berkeley, Calif, 1991, North Atlantic Books.

Further Information
Practitioners

American Association of Naturopathic Physicians
601 Valley St, Suite 105
Seattle, WA 98109
206-323-7610
www.naturopathic.org

Herbal Medicines

Herb Research Foundation
1007 Pearl St, #200F
Boulder, CO 80302
303-449-2265

Homeopathy

International Foundation for Homeopathy
2366 Eastlake Ave E, #329
Seattle, WA 98102
206-324-8230

Nutritional Products

Thorne Research
25820 Highway 2 West
PO Box 25
Dover, ID 83825
800-228-1966

Metagenics
100 Avenida La Pata
San Clemente, CA 92673
800-692-9400

PhytoPharmica
825 Challenger Dr
PO Box 1745
Green Bay, WI 54305
800-553-2370

REFERENCES

1. Adetumbi MA, Lau BH: *Allium sativum*—a natural antibiotic, *Med Hypotheses* 12:227, 1983.
2. Airolo P: *The miracle of garlic,* Phoenix, 1983, Health Plus Publisher.
3. Amer M, Taha M, Tosson Z: The effect of aqueous garlic extract on the growth of dermatophytes, *Int J Dermatol* 19:285, 1980.
4. Appleton JA, Tansey MR: Inhibition of growth of zoopathogentic fungi by garlic extract, *Mycopathologia* 67:882, 1975.
5. Ariga T, Oshiba S, Tamada T: Platelet aggregation inhibitor in garlic, *Lancet* 1:150, 1981.
6. Arora RC, Arora S: Comparative effect of clofibrate, garlic and onion on alimentary hyperlipemia, *Atherosclerosis* 39:447, 1981.
7. Astrup A et al: The effect of chronic ephedrine treatment on substrate utilization, the sympathoadrenal activity and expenditure during glucose-induced thermogenesis in man, *Metabolism* 35:260, 1986.
8. Augusti KT, Matthew PT: Lipid-lowering effect of allicin (diallyl disulphide-oxide) on long-term feeding to normal rats, *Experientia* 30:468, 1974.
9. Babbar OP et al: Effect of berberine chloride eye drops on clinically positive trachoma patients, *Indian J Med Res* 70:233, 1979.
10. Barnes: *Am J Bot* 34, 1937.
11. Bhakat MP et al: Therapeutic trial of berberine sulphate in non-specific gastroenteritis, *Ind Med J* 68:19, 1974.
12. Bhushan S et al: Effect of garlic on normal blood cholesterol level, *Indian J Physiol Pharmacol* 23:211, 1979.
13. Bianchini F, Corbetta R: *Health plants of the world,* New York, 1975, Newsweek Books.
14. Block E et al: Ajoene: a potent antithrombotic agent from garlic, *J Am Chem Soc* 106:8295, 1984.
15. Blumenthal M: Ginseng takes root in *Wall Street Journal, J Am Botan Council* 28:10, 1993.
16. Bordia A: Effect of garlic on human platelet aggregation in vitro, *Atherosclerosis* 30:355, 1978.
17. Bordia A: Effect of garlic on blood lipids in patients with coronary heart disease, *Am J Clin Nutr* 34:2100, 1981.
18. Bordia A, Bansal HC: Essential oil of garlic in prevention of atherosclerosis, *Lancet* 2:1491, 1973.
19. Bordia A, Joshi JK: Garlic on fibrinolytic activity in cases of acute myocardial infarction, Part II, *J Assoc Physicians India* 26:323, 1978.
20. Bordia AK, Verma SK: Garlic on the reversibility of experimental atherosclerosis, *Indian Heart J* 30:47, 1978.
21. Bordia A, Verma SK: Effect of garlic feeding on regression of experimental atherosclerosis in rabbits, *Artery* 7:428, 1980.
22. Bordia A et al: Effect of the essential oils of garlic and onion on alimentary hyperlipemia, *Atherosclerosis* 21:15, 1975.
23. Bordia A et al: The protective action of essential oils of onion and garlic in cholesterol-fed rabbits, *Atherosclerosis* 22:103, 1975.
24. Bordia AK et al: Effect of essential oil of garlic on serum fibrinolytic activity in patients with coronary artery disease, *Atherosclerosis* 28:155, 1977.
25. Bordia AK et al: The effectiveness and active principle of garlic and onion on blood lipids and experimental atherosclerosis in rabbits and their comparison with clofibrate, *J Assoc Physicians India* 25:509, 1977.

26. Bordia A et al: Protective effect of garlic oil on the changes produced by 3 weeks of fatty diet on serum cholesterol serum triglycerides, fibrinolytic activity, and platelet adhesiveness in man, *Ind Heart J* 34:86, 1982.

27. Bortho B, Thiel W: The treatment of recent traumatic blood effusions of the knee joint, *Biol Ther* 12:242, 1994.

28. Brinker F: *An introduction to the toxicology of common medicinal substances,* 1983, National College of Naturopathic Medicine.

29. *Br J Clin Pharmacol* 9:453, 1980.

30. *British pharmaceutical codex,* London, 1934, The Pharmaceutical Press.

31. Britz JJ et al: *J Am Osteopath Assoc* 62:731, 1963.

32. Caporaso N, Smith SM, Eng RH: Antifungal activity in human urine and serum after ingestion of garlic, *Antimicrob Agents Chemother* 23:700, 1983.

33. Cavallito CJ, Bailey JH: Allicin, the antibacterial principle of *Allium sativum.* I. Isolation, physical properties and antibacterial action, *J Am Chem Soc* 66:1950, 1944.

34. Chang HM, But PP: *Pharmacology and applications of Chinese materia medica,* vol 2, Teaneck, NJ, 1987, World Scientific.

35. Chang MLW, Johnson MA: Effect of garlic on carbohydrate metabolism and lipid synthesis in rats, *J Nutr* 110:931, 1980.

36. Chaudhuri BN et al: Hypolipidemic effect of garlic and thyroid function, *Biomed Biochim Acta* 43:1045, 1984.

37. Choudry VP, Sabir M, Bhide BN: Berberine in giardiasis, *Indian Pediatr* 9:143, 1972.

38. Chutani SK, Bordia A: The effect of fried vs. raw garlic on fibrinolytic activity in man, *Atherosclerosis* 38:417, 1981.

39. Cody G: *History of natural medicine, a textbook of natural medicine,* Seattle, 1985, John Bastyr College Publications.

40. Collins CE, Collins C: *Am J Roentgenol Rad Ther* 33:396, 1935.

41. Crellin JK, Philpott J: *Herbel medicine: past and present,* vol 2, London, Duke University Press.

42. Cunnick J, Takamoto D: Research review of bitter melon (*Momordica charantia*), *J Naturopath Med* 1:16, 1993.

43. Deboer LWV, Folts JD: Garlic extract limits acute platelet thrombus formation in canine coronary arteries, *Clin Res* 34:292A, 1986.

44. Der Marderosian AD, Liberti LE: *Natural product medicine: a scientific guide to foods, drugs, cosmetics,* Philadelphia, 1988, Stickley.

45. Desai AB, Shah KM, Shah DM: Berberine in the treatment of diarrhea, *Indian Pediatr* 8:462, 1971.

46. Duke J: *CRC handbook of medicinal herbs,* Boca Raton, Fla, 1985, CRC Press.

47. Dulloo AG, Miller DS: The thermogenic properties of ephedrine/methylxanthine mixtures: animal studies, *Am J Clin Nutr* 43:388, 1986.

48. Elnima EL et al: The antimicrobial activity of garlic and onion extracts, *Pharmazie* 38:747, 1983.

49. Ernst E: Cardiovascular effects of garlic: a review, *Pharmatherapeutica* 5:83, 1987.

50. Farnsworth NR, Morgan BM: Herb drinks: chamomile tea, *JAMA* 221:410, 1972.

51. Felter HK: *The eclectic materia medica pharmacology and therapeutics,* 1983, Eclectic Medical Publications.

52. Fischer-Tasmu S et al: Ginger treatment of hyperemesis gravidarum, *Eur J Obstet Gynecol Reprod Biol* 38:19, 1990.

53. Fliermans C: Inhibition of *Histoplasma capsulatum* by garlic, *Mycopathol Mycol Appl* 50:227, 1973.

54. Fly S, Kiem J: *Econ Bot* 14:46, 1963.

55. Fromtling R, Bulmer GS: In vitro effect of aqueous extract of garlic (*Allium sativum*) on the growth and viability of *Cryptococcus neoformans, Mycolagia* 70:397, 1978.

56. Fugita B et al: *Biochem Pharmacol* 25:205, 1976.

57. Gaffen JD, Tavares IA, Bennett A: The effect of garlic extracts on contractions of rat gastric fundus and human platelet aggregation, *J Pharm Pharmacol* 36:273, 1984.

58. Gilman AG, Goodman AS, Gilman A: *The pharmacologic basis of therapeutics,* New York, 1980, Macmillan.

59. Gjerstad, Riner TD: *Am J Pharm* 140:58, 1968.

60. Goff S, Levenstein I: *J Soc Cosm Chem* 15:509, 1964.

61. Gottshall et al: *J Clin Invest* 28:920, 1949.

62. Grontved A et al: Ginger root against seasickness: a controlled trial on the open sea, *Acta Otolaryngol* 105:45, 1988.

63. Grontved A, Hentzer E: Vertigo reducing effect of ginger root, *ORL* 48:282, 1986.

64. Gujaral S, Bhurmara H, Swaroop M: Effects of ginger oleoresin on serum and hepatic cholesterol levels in cholesterol-fed rats, *Nutr Rep Int* 17:183, 1978.

65. Gupta NN, Mehrota RML, Sircar AR: Effect of onion on serum cholesterol blood coagulation factors and fibrinolytic activity in alimentary lipemia, *Ind J Med Res* 54:48, 1966.

66. Gupta S: Use of berberine in the treatment of giardiasis, *Am J Dis Child* 129:866, 1975.

67. Haggers JP et al: *J Am Med Technol* 41:293, 1979.

68. Hatch G et al: Asthma, inhaled oxidants and dietary antioxidants, *Am J Clin Nutr* 61:6255, 1995.

69. Henry R: *Cosmetics Toiletries* 94:42, 1979.

70. Hikino H et al: Anti-inflammatory effects of ephedra herbs, *Chem Pharm Bull* 28:2900, 1980.

71. Hobbs C: Goldenseal in early American medical botany, *Pharmacy History* 32:79, 1990.

72. Huddleson IF et al: Antibacterial substances in plants, *J Am Vet Med Assoc* 105:394, 1944.

73. Hunan Medical College, China: Garlic in cryptococcal meningitis: a preliminary report of 21 cases, *Chinese Med J* 93:123, 1980.

74. Itokawa Y et al: Effect of S-methylcysteine sulfoxide, S-allylcysteine sulfoxide and related sulfur-containing amino acids on lipid metabolism of experimental hypercholesterolemic rats, *J Nutr* 103:88, 1973.

75. Jain RC: Onion and garlic in experimental cholesterol atherosclerosis in rabbits. I. Effect of serum lipids and development of atherosclerosis, *Artery* 1:115, 1975.

76. Jain RC: Onion and garlic in experimental cholesterol induced atherosclerosis, *Indian J Med Res* 64:1509, 1976.

77. Jain RC: Effect of garlic on serum lipids, coagulability and fibrinolytic activity, *Am J Clin Nutr* 30:1380, 1977.

78. Jain RC: Effect of alcoholic extraction on garlic in atherosclerosis, *Am J Clin Nutr* 31:1982, 1978.

79. Jain RC, Konar DB: Effect of garlic oil in experimental cholesterol atherosclerosis, *Atherosclerosis* 29:125, 1978.

80. Jain RC, Vyas CR: Garlic in alloxan-induced diabetic rabbits, *Am J Clin Nutr* 28:684, 1975.

81. *J Am Inst Homeopathy* 62, 1969.

82. Kadil O, Abdullah TH, Elkadi A: Garlic and the immune system in humans: its effect on natural killer cells, *Fed Proc* 46:1222, 1987.

83. Kamanna VS, Chandrasekhara N: Effect of garlic on serum lipoproteins and lipoprotein cholesterol levels in albino rats rendered hypercholesteremic by feeding cholesterol, *Lipids* 17:483, 1982.

84. Kamanna VS, Chandrasekhara N: Hypocholesteremic activity of different fractions of garlic, *Indian J Med Res* 79:580, 1984.

85. Kamat SA: Clinical trial with berberine hydrochloride for the control of diarrhoea in acute gastroenteritis, *J Assoc Physicians India* 15:525, 1967.

86. Karcher L, Zagerman P, Krieglstein K: Effect of an extract of *Ginkgo biloba* on rat brain energy metabolism in hypoxia, *Naunyn-Schmiedeberg's Arch Pharmacol* 327:31, 1984.

87. Kasahara Y et al: Anti-inflammatory action of ephedrines in acute inflammations, *Planta Med* 54:325, 1985.

88. Kritchevsky D: Effect of garlic oil on experimental atherosclerosis, *Artery* 1:319, 1975.

89. Kritchevsky D et al: Influence of garlic oil on cholesterol metabolism in rats, *Nutr Rep Int* 22:641, 1980.

90. Kuichi F, Shibuyu M, Sankawa U: Inhibitors of prostaglandin biosynthesis from ginger, *Chem Pharm Bull* 30:754, 1982.

91. Kumazawa Y et al: Activation of peritoneal macrophages by berberine alkaloids in terms of induction of cytostatic activity, *Int J Immunopharmacol* 6:587, 1984.

92. *Lancet,* Oct 18, 1986, p 885.

93. Lau BHS, Keeler WH, Adetumbi MA: Antifungal effect of garlic, *Ann Am Soc Microbiol* 387, 1983.

94. *Lawrence review of natural products,* vol 3, no 21, Collegeville, Penn, 1982, Pharmaceutical Information Associates.

95. *Lawrence review of natural products,* vol 3, nos 23/24, Collegeville, Penn, 1982, Pharmaceutical Information Associates.

96. Le Poncin S, Lafitte M, Rapin JR: Effect of *Ginko biloba* on changes induced by quantitative cerebral microembolization in rats, *Arch Int Pharmacodyn Ther* 243:236, 1980.

97. Leung AY: *Drug Cosm Ind* 120:34, 1977.

98. Leung AY: *Encyclopedia of common natural ingredients used in foods, drugs, and cosmetics,* New York, 1980, Wiley.

99. Lorenset LJ et al: *J Pharm Sci* 53:1287, 1964.

100. Lotz-Winter H: On the pharmacology of bromelain: an update with special regard to animal studies on dose dependent effects, *Planta Med* 56:249, 1990.

101. Lust J: *The herb book,* New York, 1980, Bantam.

102. Makheja AN, Vanderhoek JY, Bailey JM: Inhibition of platelet aggregation and thromboxane synthesis by onion and garlic, *Lancet* 1:781, 1979.

103. Malik SA, Siddiqui S: Hypotensive effect of freeze-dried garlic sap in dogs, *J Pakistan Med Assoc* 31:12, 1981.

104. Mann C, Staba E: The chemistry, pharmacology, and commercial formulations of chamomile. In Cracker LE, Simon JE, editors: *Herbs, spices, and medicinal plants,* vol 1, Phoenix, 1986, Oryx Press.

105. Manning C: *Bioenergetic medicines east and west,* Berkeley, Calif, 1988, North Atlantic Books.

106. Mazzotta M: Nutrition and wound healing, *J Am Podiatric Med Assoc* 84: 456, 1994.

107. *Merck Index,* ed 5, 1940, Merck.

108. Mishra SB, Dixit SN: Fungicidal spectrum of the leaf extract of *Allium sativum, Ind Phytopathol* 29:448, 1976.

109. Moerman DE: *Medicinal plants of native America,* Ann Arbor, 1986, University of Michigan.

110. Mohan M et al: Berberine in trachoma, *Indian J Ophthalmol* 30:69, 1982.

111. Moore GS, Atkins RD: The fungicidal and fungistatic effects of an aqueous garlic extract on medically important yeast-like fungi, *Mycopathologia* 69:341, 1977.

112. Morton JF: *Econ Bot* 15:311, 1961.

113. Mowrey D, Clayson D: Motion sickness, ginger, and psychophysics, *Lancet* i:655, 1982.

114. Murray M: *The healing power of herbs,* Rocklin, Calif, 1992, Prima Publishing.

115. Nagai K: Experimental studies on the preventive effect of garlic extract against infection with influenza virus, *Jpn J Infect Dis* 47:321, 1973.

116. Nagai K, Osawa S: Cholesterol-lowering effect of aged garlic extract in rats, *Basic Pharmacol Ther* 2:41, 1974.

117. Nakagawa S et al: Effect of raw and extracted-aged garlic juice on growth of young rats and their organs after peroral administration, *J Toxicol Sci* 5:9, 1980.

118. Nakayama S et al: Cytoprotective activity of components of garlic, ginseng, and ciuwjia on hepatocyte injury induced by carbon tetrachloride in vitro, *Hiroshima J Med Sci* 8:803, 1985.

119. Nasada KK et al: Effect of onion and garlic on blood coagulation and fibrinolysis in vitro, *Indian J Physiol Pharmacol* 27:141, 1983.

120. Nieberding JF: *Am Bee J* 114:15, 1974.

121. Prasad G, Sharma VD: Efficacy of garlic (*Allium sativum*) treatment against experimental candidiasis in chicks, *Br Vet J* 136:448, 1980.

122. Raj KP, Parmer RM: Garlic—condiment and medicine, *Indian Drugs* 15:205, 1977.

123. Rashid A, Khan HH: The mechanism of hypotensive effect of garlic extract, *JPMA* 35:357, 1985.

124. Ruffin J, Hunter S: An evaluation of the side effects of garlic as an antihypertensive agent, *Cytobios* 37:85, 1983.

125. Sabir M, Bhide N: Study of some pharmacologic actions of berberine, *Indian J Physiol Pharm* 15:111, 1971.

126. Sack RB, Froehlich JL: Berberine inhibits intestinal secretory response of *Vibrio cholera* toxins and *Escherichia coli* enterotoxins, *Infect Immun* 35:471, 1982.

127. Sainani GS et al: Effect of garlic and onion on important lipid and coagulation parameters in alimentary hyperlipemia, *J Assoc Physicians India* 27:57, 1979.

128. Sandrhu DK, Warraich MK, Singh S: Sensitivity of yeasts isolated from cases of vaginitis to aqueous extracts of garlic, *Kykosen* 23:691, 1980.

129. Saxena KK et al: Effect of garlic pretreatment on isoprenaline-induced myocardial necrosis in albino rats, *Indian J Physiol Pharmacol* 24:223, 1980.

130. Schilcher H: The significance of phytotherapy in Europe, an interdisciplinary and comparative study, *Z Phytother* 14:132, 1993.

131. Sharma R, Joshi CK, Gjoyal RK: Berberine tannate in acute diarrhea, *Indian Pediatr* 7:496, 1970.

132. Sharma VC et al: Antibacterial property of *Allium sativum:* in vivo and in vitro studies, *Indian J Exp Biol* 15:446, 1977.

133. Ship S: *JAMA* 238:1770, 1970.

134. Shoji N et al: Cardiotonic principles of ginger (*Zingiber officinale*), *J Pharm Sci* 10:1174, 1982.

135. Smith AW: *A gardener's book of plant names,* New York, 1963, Harper & Row.

136. Spoerke DG: *Herbal medications,* Santa Barbara, Calif, 1980, Woodbridge Press.

137. Srivastava KC: Aqueous extracts on onion, garlic and ginger inhibit platelet aggregation and alter arachidonic acid metabolism, *Biomed Biochem Acta* 43:335, 1984.

138. Srivastava KC: Effects of aqueous extracts of onion, garlic, and ginger on platelet aggregation and metabolism of arachidonic acid in the blood vascular system: in vitro study, *Prostaglandins Leukot Med* 13:227, 1984.

139. Srivastava KC, Mu S, Tafa T: Ginger and rheumatic disorders, *Med Hypotheses* 29:25, 1989.

140. Sun D, Courtney HS, Beachey EH: Berberine sulfate blocks adherence of *Streptococcus pyogenes* to epithelial cells, fibronectin, and hexadecane, *Antimicrob Agents Chemother* 32:1370, 1988.

141. Swabb EA, Tai YH, Jordan L: Reversal of cholera toxin-induced secretion in rat ileum by luminal berberine, *Am J Physiol* 248, 1981.

142. Tai YH et al: Antisecretory effects of berberine in rat ileum, *Am J Physiol* 241:253, 1981.

143. Tansye MR, Appleton JA: Inhibition of fungal growth by garlic extract, *Mycopathologia* 67:409, 1975.

144. Tariq H et al: *J Nat Med Assoc* 80:441, 1988.

145. Tsai Y et al: Antiviral properties of garlic: in vitro effects on influenza B, herpes simplex I, and Coxsackie viruses, *Planta Med* 5:460, 1985.

146. Tutakne MA et al: Sporotrichosis treated with garlic juice: a case report, *Indian J Dermatol* 28:41, 1983.

147. Tyler V: An overview: natural products and medicine, *Herbal Gram* 28:40, 1993.

148. Tyler V, Brady L, Roberts J: *Pharmacology,* ed 8, Philadelphia, 1981, Lea & Febiger.

149. Tyler VE: *The new honest herbal,* Philadelphia, 1987, Stickley.

150. University of Illinois at the Medical Center, Dept. of Pharmacognosy and Pharmacology, abstract prepared for the Herb Trade Association.

151. Weiner M: *Earth medicine, earth food,* New York, 1980, Ballantine.

152. Weiss R: *Herbal medicine,* 1991, Beaconsfield.

153. Weiss S, Weiss G: *Growing and using the healing herbs,* Emmaus, Pa, 1985, Rodale Press.

154. Willard T: *The Wild Rose scientific herbal,* Calgary, Alberta, Canada, 1991, Wild Rose College of Natural Healing.

155. Willis ED: Enzyme inhibition by allicin, the active principle of garlic, *Biochem J* 63:514, 1956.

156. Wren RC: *Potter's new encyclopaedia of botanical drugs and preparations,* Rustington, Sussex, UK, 1975, Health Science Press.

157. Yamada Y, Azuma K: Evaluation of the in vitro antifungal activity of allicin, *Antimicrob Agents Chemother* 11:713, 1977.

158. Zell J et al: Treatment of acute sprain of the ankle: a controlled double blind trial to test the effectiveness of homeopathic ointment, *Biol Ther* 7:1, 1989.

Food and
Water

8

51 Field Water Disinfection

Howard D. Backer

Waterborne disease is a risk for international travelers who visit countries that have poor hygiene and inadequate sanitation and for wilderness users relying on surface water in any country, including the United States. Natural water may be contaminated with organic or inorganic material from land erosion, dissolution of minerals, decay of organic vegetation, biologic organisms that reside in soil and water, industrial chemical pollutants, and microorganisms from animal or human biologic wastes.[38,67] Fecal pollution with enteric pathogens is the primary reason for disinfecting drinking water. However, chemical contamination of groundwater is increasing at an alarming rate in the United States and worldwide from industrial, agricultural, and individual sources. Of the 1700 million square miles of water on earth, less than 0.5% is potable.[221] According to the National Water Quality Inventory Report by the U.S. Environmental Protection Agency (EPA), as of 1994, about 40% of the nation's surveyed rivers, lakes, and estuaries are too polluted for basic uses such as fishing and swimming. Natural organic and inorganic material may not cause illness but can impart unpleasant turbidity, color, and taste to the water. Appearance, odor, and taste are not reliable to estimate water safety.

ETIOLOGY

Infectious agents in contaminated drinking water with the potential for waterborne transmission include bacteria, viruses, protozoa, and parasites (Box 51-1). The number of pathogenic microorganisms capable of waterborne transmission is more than 100 and similar to that of potential etiologic agents of travelers' diarrhea. Separating the contribution of waterborne transmission of these pathogens from food-borne and person-to-person transmission is impossible. The latter two are probably more common.

The source of fecal contamination in water may be either human or animal. Some bacterial pathogens (*Shigella, Salmonella typhosa*) occur exclusively in human feces, whereas others (*Yersinia, Campylobacter,* nontyphoidal *Salmonella*) may be present in wild or domestic animals. The enteric viruses seem to occur exclusively in human feces. No enteric viruses excreted by animals have been shown to be pathogenic to humans.[162] The major source of these enteric pathogens is fecal contamination from infected human residents. *Legionella pneu-*

mophila and *Vibrio cholerae* exist as natural organisms in water. However, the mode of transmission of *Legionella* is inhalation of aerosolized water.[194] No evidence exists of human immunodeficiency virus (HIV) transmitted via a waterborne route, and no epidemiologic evidence exists of casual transmission by fomites or by any environmentally mediated mode.[168]

Viruses

Hepatitis A virus (HAV), Norwalk virus, and rotavirus are the main viruses of concern for potable water supplies; the last two are responsible for about 77% of acute waterborne gastroenteritis.[221] In addition to HAV, waterborne transmission of hepatitis E is suspected in outbreaks among travelers from Asia.[26,100] During 1993 and 1994 an explosive waterborne epidemic of hepatitis E virus occurred in Islamabad, Pakistan, with about 4000 cases of acute icteric hepatitis.[185] Many other viruses are capable and suspected of waterborne transmission, and more than 100 different virus types are known to be excreted in human feces.[72,175] The most frequent waterborne illness (acute infectious nonbacterial gastroenteritis of unknown etiology) in the United States may be caused by undetected viruses.[43,119,189]

Protozoa

Six protozoa cause enteric disease and may be passed via waterborne transmission: *Giardia lamblia, Cryptosporidium parvum, Entamoeba histolytica, Cyclospora cayetanesis, Isospora belli,* and the microsporidia.[118] The first two are the most important for wilderness travelers. *Cryptosporidium* is a recently recognized enteric pathogen.[27] Many aspects of the epidemiology and transmission appear similar to *Giardia;* large waterborne outbreaks of *Cryptosporidium* have been documented.[25,49,78] Waterborne transmission of *E. histolytica* is common in developing countries. Cyclospora has been epidemiologically linked to waterborne transmission in the United States and in Nepal, but the reservoir and host range are not known. Unlike *Giardia* and *Cryptosporidium, Cyclospora* is not infectious when passed in feces and requires up to two weeks in the laboratory to sporulate.[187] Surface water is a common environmental source for microsporidia, however, the route of infection is unknown. *Naegleria fowleri* is a waterborne protozoan that enters the body through the nasal epithelium during swimming in contaminated surface water and causes meningoencephalitis.

Box 51-1 WATERBORNE ENTERIC PATHOGENS

BACTERIAL

Escherichia coli
Shigella
Campylobacter
Vibrio cholerae
Salmonella
Yersinia enterocolitica
Aeromonas

VIRAL

Hepatitis A
Hepatitis E
Norwalk virus
Poliovirus
Miscellaneous enteric viruses (more than 100 types: adenovirus, enterovirus, calcivirus, ECHO, astrovirus, coronavirus, etc.)

PROTOZOAL

Giardia lamblia
Entamoeba histolytica

PROTOZOAL—cont'd

Cryptosporidium
Blastocystis hominis
Isospora belli
Balantidium coli
Acanthamoeba
Cyclospora

PARASITIC

Ascaris lumbricoides (roundworm)
Ancylostoma duodenale (hookworm)
Taenia spp. (tapeworm)
Fasciola hepatica (sheep liver fluke)
Dracunculus medinensis (Guinea tapeworm)
Strongyloides stercoralis
Trichuris trichiura (whipworm)
Clonorchis sinensis (Oriental liver fluke)
Paragonimus westermani (lung fluke)
Diphyllobothrium latum (fish tapeworm)
Echinococcus granulosus (hydatid disease)

Data from Drinking Water Health Effects Task Force, US Environmental Protection Agency: *Health effects of drinking water treatment technologies,* Chelsea, Mich, 1989, Lewis; and Gelreich EE: Microbiological quality of source waters for water supply. In McFeters GA, editor: *Drinking water microbiology,* New York, 1990, Springer-Verlag.

Parasitic Organisms

Parasitic organisms other than *Giardia* and *E. histolytica* are seldom considered in discussions of disinfection. Infectious eggs or larvae of many helminths are found in sewage, even in the United States.[164,184] The frequency of infection by waterborne transmission is unknown, since food and environmental contamination or skin penetration is more prevalent.[228]

The most obvious risk is from nematodes with no intermediate hosts that are infectious immediately or soon after eggs are passed in stool. *Ascaris lumbricoides* (roundworm) is transmitted by ingestion of the eggs in contaminated food or drink. In endemic areas, 85% of the population is infected; this leads to daily global environmental contamination by 9×10^{14} eggs.[228] *Ancylostoma duodenale* (hookworm) usually infects as larvae penetrate the skin of the foot, but it also may be acquired by mouth. Oral entry of the larvae causes pulmonary (Wakana) disease. *Necator americanus* does not appear to be infectious via the oral route.

Taenia solium (pork tapeworm) is infectious to humans in cyst or egg form. Eggs passed in stool are ingested in food or water and develop into tissue cysts, often in the brain, resulting in cysticercosis.

Echinococcus granulosus (dog tapeworm) can use humans as intermediate hosts. Eggs from the feces of an infected dog or other carnivore are ingested in food and water. Hydatid disease generates cysts in the liver, peritoneum, and other sites.

Fasciola hepatica (liver fluke of herbivores and humans) is normally acquired by ingestion of encysted metacercariae on water plants or free organisms in water.

Cercariae of schistosomiasis, which live in fresh water and normally enter through skin, can enter through the oral mucosa. The cercariae are killed by stomach acid.

Dracunculus medinensis (Guinea tapeworm) is a tissue nematode of humans and causes the only such disease transmitted exclusively through drinking water.[218] *Dracunculus* larvae are released in water from subcutaneous worms on the legs of infected bathers or water-gatherers. Larvae are ingested by a tiny crustacean (*Cyclops* species), which acts as the intermediate host and releases infectious larvae when ingested by humans.

Bacterial Spores

Bacterial spores can cause serious wound and gut infections but are not likely to be waterborne enteric pathogens. *Clostridium* is ubiquitous in soil, lake sediment, tropical water sources, and the stool of animals and humans.[79,183] *C. botulinum* and *C. perfringens* type A food poisoning are not waterborne because they require germination of spores in food by inadequate cooking, then production of an enterotoxin, which is ingested. *C. perfringens* type C causes enteritis necroticans, probably through in vivo production of an enterotoxin, and thus has the potential for waterborne transmission in the tropics. However, the epidemiology of these infections, as in infant botulism, is related to food-borne sources in the United States.

Chemical Hazards

Chemical hazards are also becoming an alarming source of pollution in surface water. In the United States, chemical contamination is routinely responsible for about 30% of waterborne gastroenteritis where an etiology can be identified.[30,31] Most common sources include lead that leaches into water lines, as well as copper, nitrate, fluoride, and a variety of other chemicals. Industrialization proceeds worldwide without adequate environmental protection. A vast array of toxins are sold with little concept of safe use and no means of safe disposal. Inorganic chemicals in drinking water include common salts, heavy metals, asbestos, fluorides, nitrates, radionuclides, and some heavy metals (arsenic, copper, iron, lead, selenium). Natural organic chemicals predominate from soil runoff, forest canopy aquatic biota, and human and animal wastes. Synthetic organic matter includes pesticides, herbicides, and chemicals from industrial or human activities.[53] Major underground aquifers are becoming contaminated. Streams and rivers in rural areas are contaminated by individual carelessness, leaching landfills, and agricultural runoff. Atmospheric spread has resulted in pesticides being found in remote wilderness lakes and in the well-publicized acid rain. Numerous pesticides have been found in runoff and rivers in agricultural areas of the Midwest.[125] Wilderness users may soon need to ensure removal of chemical, as well as microbiologic, contaminants.

RISK EVALUATION

Risk of waterborne illness depends on the number of organisms consumed, which is determined by the volume of water, concentration of organisms, and treatment system efficiency.[42,89] Additional factors include virulence of the organism and defenses of the host. Infection and illness are not synonymous; the overall likelihood of illness from multiple studies for all three categories of microorganisms (bacterial, viral, protozoan) is 50% to 60%. Death is unlikely except with specific organisms (e.g., *Escherichia coli* O157:H7, *Vibrio cholerae*), hepatitis E in pregnant women, and *Cryptosporidium* with underlying malnutrition. Total immunity does not develop for most enteric pathogens and reinfection may occur.[89]

Waterborne outbreaks do not give a complete picture of the potential for waterborne illness. Most outbreaks of waterborne disease are not identified because not enough people become ill, providing an insensitive mechanism for detecting water contamination. When an outbreak is identified, it is very difficult to prove

TABLE 51-1. Estimated Infectious Dose of Enteric Organisms

ORGANISM	INFECTIOUS DOSE
Salmonella	10^5
Shigella	10^2
Vibrio	10^3
Enteric viruses	1-10
Giardia	10-100
Cryptosporidium	10-100 (?)

conclusively that the source was waterborne. The supply may have been only transiently contaminated; water samples from the time of exposure are seldom available; some organisms are difficult to detect; and almost everyone has some exposure to water.[204]

The data on concentration of microorganisms in surface water show widely varying values, but the testing is insufficient for risk assessment and dose-response models. Instead, infectious dose data and statistical techniques have been used to devise models for determining risk (Table 51-1).[89] These cannot be applied unless the microbial content of water is known. Few water sites are monitored. The excretion and loading of microbial contaminants are dynamic and change over time. Pathogenic microorganisms clearly exist in most raw source waters, especially in surface waters.[53]

Most microbiologic testing is done on community water intake sources and sewage treatment effluent. Less information is available for more remote water sources.[42,175,227] Protozoan cysts can be found even in pristine water, but their levels are a small fraction of the number in polluted water.[177]

Recreational Contact

Inadvertent ingestion during recreational water contact is a risk for swimmers and white-water boaters. The microorganisms that cause infection require only a small dose. Recreational water activities have resulted in giardiasis, cryptosporidiosis, typhoid fever, salmonellosis, shigellosis, viral gastroenteritis, and hepatitis A, as well as in wound infections, septicemia, and aspiration pneumonia due to *Legionella*.[43] From 1993 to 1994, 36 outbreaks of gastroenteritis (excluding hot tub dermatitis) from recreational water were reported. Sixteen outbreaks were caused by *Cryptosporidium*, four by *Giardia*, six by *E. coli* O157:H7, three by *Shigella sonnei*, and one by Norwalk virus.[31] Six isolated cases of primary amebic meningoencephalitis (*Naegleria fowleri*) were reported, with 100% fatality.

Underdeveloped Countries

In tropical areas and developing countries, water has a complex relationship with spread of disease. Table 51-2

TABLE 51-2. Water and Spread of Disease

TYPE	MECHANISM	EXAMPLES	PREVENTION
Waterborne	Fecal contamination of drinking water by infectious organisms	Typhoid fever, cholera, campylobacteriosis, giardiasis, hepatitis A	Sanitation and disinfection of water
Water washed	Person-to-person fecal-oral spread via direct contact, food, or water (all these are also waterborne)	Shigellosis, amebiasis, ascariasis, eye and skin infections	Handwashing and personal hygiene
Water based	Organism or agent that lives in water	Schistosomiasis, dracunculosis, parasitic worms	Prevention of exposure from bathing
Water related	Spread by insects that breed in water or collecting water	Malaria, sleeping sickness, yellow fever, dengue	Insect protection and piped water

Modified from Bradley DJ: Health aspects of water supplies in tropical countries. In Feachem R et al, editors: *Water, wastes and health in hot climates,* New York, 1977, Wiley.

presents a useful classification, and Steiner et al[195] proposed adding the category "water carried" for infections resulting from accidental ingestion in recreational water. Worldwide, 1.5 billion rural people and 200 million urban people in the world lack safe drinking water and adequate sanitation. An estimated 80% of the world's diseases are linked to inadequate water supply and sanitation. Between 10 and 25 million people die each year (28,000 to 68,000 persons each day) from diseases caused by contaminated water and unsanitary conditions. In undeveloped countries, these illnesses account for 1 billion cases of diarrhea every year and 95% of deaths in children under 5 years of age.[79,218] Of the four diseases that may cause the most morbidity and death in underdeveloped parts of the world—cholera, hepatitis, malaria, and typhoid—malaria is the only one that is not waterborne.[89]

The sanitary situation in many undeveloped countries is illustrated by current statistics from Peru evaluated during a recent cholera epidemic. Only 73% of the urban population have access to a water distribution system and only 50% to sanitation services. In rural areas, only 23% have access to a water supply and 6% to a sanitation system. In urban areas over the past 5 years the quality of water has deteriorated because of the lack of water treatment chemicals, laboratories for monitoring, and operators to control the processes. Institutional barriers impede improvements for adequate water and sanitation systems.[44] The statistics for Egypt are only slightly better.

In certain tropical countries the influence of high-density population, rampant pollution, and absence of sanitation systems means that available raw water is virtually wastewater.[35] Contamination of tap water must be assumed because of antiquated and inadequately monitored disposal, disinfection, and distribution systems. Water from springs and wells and even commercial bottled water may be contaminated with pathogenic microorganisms.

Box 51-2   ENTERIC PATHOGENS IN U.S. WILDERNESS OR RECREATIONAL WATER

OFTEN REPORTED

Giardia
Cryptosporidium

OCCASIONALLY REPORTED, WITH FIRM EVIDENCE FOR WATERBORNE

Campylobacter
Hepatitis A
Hepatitis E
Enterotoxigenic *Escherichia coli*
E. coli O157:H7
Shigella
Enteric viruses

UNUSUAL OCCURRENCES, WATERBORNE SUSPECTED

Yersinia enterocolitica
Aeromonas hydrophila
Cyclospora

United States

Waterborne pathogens account for most outbreaks of infectious diarrhea acquired in U.S. wilderness and recreation areas (Box 51-2). From 1920 to 1980, 178 waterborne outbreaks caused by use of contaminated, untreated surface water or groundwater were reported in systems serving parks, campgrounds, and recreation areas.[43] Between 1970 and 1990, gastroenteritis of undefined etiology accounted for most cases overall, while *Giardia* caused the most cases of defined etiology.[43,81] A distinct seasonal variation is seen, with the majority of cases from recreational areas occurring during summer months.[43] This is probably a result of both increased contamination and number of persons at risk. Between 1993 to 1996, *Giardia* continued to be one of the most common waterborne infections, but *Cryptosporidium* epidemics were being identified with increasing frequency in both public and surface water supplies.[78,174] An outbreak of *Cryptosporidium* in a public water supply in Milwaukee affected more than 400,000 people.[115] A surface water outbreak occurred at Lake Mead. During this period, bacteria linked to water ingestion included *Salmonella, Campylobacter, Shigella sonnei, Plesiomonas shigelloides*, and another emerging pathogen, *E. coli* O157:H7.[30,31] Enteric bacteria are still associated with 12% of waterborne outbreaks in the United States.[177]

Viruses

Testing in the United States, Europe, and developing countries shows consistent, sometimes astounding, degrees of viral contamination of drinking and surface water.* Even remote surface lakes and streams tested in California showed disturbing levels of viral contamination.[72] Widespread enteric viral contamination was found at multiple sites in a popular recreation canyon in Arizona. Viruses included poliovirus, echovirus, coxsackievirus, rotavirus, and other unidentifiable viruses, and exceeded the recommended state level for recreational water use in several areas. Virus levels correlated with human activity but not with excess levels of standard coliform indicators.[175] All surface water supplies in the United States and Canada contain naturally occurring human enteroviruses.[221] The infectious dose of enteric viruses is only a few infectious units in the most susceptible people.[119,217,227]

Protozoa

New methods to detect *Giardia* cysts in surface water have found widespread contamination[91,169,193] (Table 51-3). Cysts have been found as frequently in pristine water and protected sources as in unprotected waters.[82,176] Repeated sampling of "negative" sources invariably produced positive results.

A zoonosis with *Giardia* is known, but with at least three different species, the extent of cross-species infection is not clear.[12,225] Many of the species apparently capable of passing *Giardia* cysts to humans, including dogs, cattle, ungulates (deer), and beaver, are present in wilderness areas. Forty percent of beaver in Colorado were infected and shedding 1×10^8 cysts per animal per day. All 386 muskrats found were infected. Up to 20% of cattle examined were infected.[82] Beaver have been implicated in multiple municipal outbreaks of giardiasis. Samples from Rocky Mountain National

Park[106,128] and the California Sierra Nevada[193,197] show a direct correlation between numbers of cysts and levels of human use or beaver habitation. In Yukon, Canada, 13 of 61 scat samples from various wild animals yielded *Giardia* cysts.[170]

Ten *G. lamblia* cysts may result in infection, although the infections in this widely quoted study were asymptomatic.[165] Even with a low infectious dose, the environmental cyst recovery data indicate that the risk of ingesting an infectious dose of *Giardia* cysts is small.[230,231] However, the likely model that poses a risk to campers is pulse contamination-a brief period of high cyst concentration from fecal contamination. Beaver stool and human stool may contain 1×10^6 cysts/g. Stream contamination from a beaver has been calculated to reach 245 cysts/gallon.[91] In this instance, small amounts of water may cause infection, similar to an outbreak among lap swimmers from inadvertent water ingestion in a fecally contaminated pool.[152]

Cryptosporidium oocysts are found widespread in surface water, and the cyst is durable in the environment. A large zoonosis is evident. Environmental occurrence appears ubiquitous.[173,174] *Cryptosporidium* is now found more frequently than *Giardia* in surface water, but in smaller numbers.

Persistence of Enteric Pathogens

Once environmental contamination has occurred, a natural inactivation or die-off begins. However, enteric pathogens can retain viability for long periods (Table 51-4).[53,177] Factors promoting survival of microorganisms are pH near neutral (between 6 and 8) and cold temperatures, which explain the risk of transmission in mountain regions. In temperate and warm water, survival is measured in days, with densities of infectious agents decreasing by 90% every 60 minutes. However, tropical water differs from temperate in nutrients, creating a microbiologically rich environment. Coliform bacteria can survive several months in natural tropical river water and may even proliferate. Survival of other bacteria is also much longer (about 200 hours in tropical compared with 30 hours in temperate water). *E. coli* and *Vibrio cholerae* may occur naturally in tropical waters and are capable of surviving indefinitely.[44,79,148]

Most enteric organisms, including *Shigella*, resist freezing.[52] *Salmonella typhosa* (*typhi*) can survive for up to 5 months in frozen debris and ice.[221] HAV survives 6 months at below-freezing temperatures.[203] *Cryptosporidium* may be able to survive a week or more in home freezers.[195]

Natural Purification Mechanisms

It is widely believed that streams purify themselves and that certain water sources are reliably safe for drinking. These concepts have some truth but do not preclude the need for disinfection to ensure water quality.

---

*References 40, 67, 72, 119, 189, 227.

TABLE 51-3. Giardia Cysts and Cryptosporidium Oocysts in North American Surface Water

SOURCE	POSITIVE SAMPLES	NUMBER OF CYSTS	REFERENCE
GIARDIA			
Surface water from 301 municipalities in the U.S.	798 of 4423		176
Pristine surface waters		0.4-5 cysts/100 L	
Unprotected watersheds		0.33-104 cysts/100 L	
Rocky Mountain National Park, California Sierra Nevada	44% in high-use areas	Average 3-10 cysts/1000 L, up to 100-600 cysts/1000 L (not adjusted for 10%-30% recovery rate)	106, 128, 193, 197
3 pristine rivers and 12 tributaries in Pacific Northwest	94/224 (42%) samples over 9 months	0.1-5.2 cysts/L (adjusted for 22% recovery rate)	143
3 high-quality surface creeks in California and Washington	1.3-6 cysts/gallon		143a
Yukon Canada pristine surface water	7/22		170
CRYPTOSPORIDIUM			
Raw surface water entering U.S. treatment plants	87%		195
Surface water samples from 17 states	55% of 257 samples positive (39% from pristine sources positive)	0.43 oocysts/L	176
Western U.S.	77% rivers, 75% lakes, 28% treated drinking water samples	Average 0.02-1.3 oocysts/L; pristine areas: 0.02-0.08/L; streams and rivers: 0.58-0.91/L	143a
Yukon water	None found in pristine water but some found in water that received sewage effluent		170

TABLE 51-4. Viability of Enteric Pathogens in Water

ORGANISM	CONDITIONS	SURVIVAL	REFERENCES
Vibrio cholerae	Cold	4-5 weeks	60
	Tropical	> 1 year	148
Campylobacter	Cold	3-5 weeks	18
	Temperate stream	3-10 days	186
Escherichia coli	Temperate stream	13 hours	186
	Tropical	> 1 year	148
Salmonella	Temperate stream	Half-life 16 hours	148
Yersinia	Temperate stream	540 days	186
Shigella	Temperate stream	Half-life 22 hours	186
	Freeze/thaw	Yes	54
Enteric pathogens	Freeze/thaw	Yes	52
Salmonella typhosa	Ice/frozen debris	5 months	221
Viruses	Cold	17-130 days	182, 227
Enteric viruses	15°-25° C water	6-10 days	177
	4° C water	30 days	177
Hepatitis A virus	Cold	1 year	16, 203
	Fresh, sea, wastewater	12 weeks	16
	< 0° C	6 months	203
Giardia	Cold	2-3 months	15, 51
	15° C lake, river	10-28 days	51
Entamoeba histolytica	Cold	3 months	34
Microsporidia	4° C	> 1 year	118
Cryptosporidium	Cold	12 months	48
Ascaris eggs	Wet or dry	6-9 years	228
Hookworm larvae	Wet sand	122 days	228

Surface water is subject to frequent, dramatic changes in microbial quality as a result of activities on a watershed. Storm water causes deterioration of source water quality by increasing suspended solids, organic materials, and microorganisms. Some of these contaminants are carried by rain from the atmosphere, but most come from ground runoff. In water sources downstream from towns or villages, storms may overload sewage facilities and cause them to discharge directly into the receiving water. However, rainwater can also flush streams clean by dilution and by washing microbe-laden bottom sediments downstream.[67,79]

Every stream, lake, or groundwater aquifer has limited capacity to assimilate waste effluents and storm water runoff entering the drainage basin. Self-purification is a complex process that involves settling of microorganisms after clumping or adherence to particles, sunlight providing ultraviolet destruction, natural die-off, predators eating bacteria, and dilution. Environmental factors include water volume and temperature, hydrologic effects, acid soil contact, and solar radiation. The process is time dependent and less active during wet periods and winter conditions. Hours needed in flow time downstream to achieve a 90% bacterial kill by natural self-purification vary with pollution inflow and rate of water flow. They have been measured at approximately 50 hours in the Tennessee River in summer, 47 hours in the Ohio River in summer, and 32 hours in the Sacramento River.[67]

Storage in reservoirs or lakes also improves microbiologic quality, with sedimentation as the primary process. A 100- to 1000-fold increase in fecal coliform bacteria can be found in bottom sediments compared with overlying water. This removal must be considered temporary, influenced by recirculation of organisms trapped in bottom sediments.[51,66] In optimal conditions, 10 days of reservoir storage can result in 75% to 99% removal of coliform bacteria and 30 days can produce safe drinking water. Generally, 80% to 90% of bacteria and viruses are removed by storage, depending on inflow and outflow, temperature, and no further contamination. Cysts, with a larger size and greater weight, should settle even faster than bacteria and viruses.[3]

Groundwater is generally cleaner than surface water because of the filtration action of overlying sediments, but wells and aquifers can be polluted from surface runoff. Spring water is generally of higher quality than surface water, provided that the true source is not surface water channeling underground from a short distance above the spring.

Drawing conclusions from the preceding factors is difficult. The major factor governing the amount of microbe pollution in surface water is human and animal activity in the watershed. The settling effect of lakes may make them safer than streams, but care should be taken not to disturb bottom sediments when obtaining water.

Benefits of Water Treatment

Methods for treating water are found in Sanskrit medical lore, and pictures of apparatus to purify water appear on Egyptian walls from the fifteenth century BC. Boiling and filtration through porous vessels, sand, and gravel have been known for thousands of years. The Greeks and Romans also understood the importance of pure water.[127] Safe and efficient treatment of drinking water was one of the major public health advances of the twentieth century.[195] As the percentage of the U.S. urban population served by water treatment utilities increased after 1900, the annual death rate from typhoid decreased. Drinking water treatment processes provide enormous benefits with minimal risk. Without disinfection and filtration, waterborne disease would spread rapidly in most public water systems served by surface water.[43,53] Disinfection alters the incidence of certain enteric diseases but does not eliminate diseases. In underdeveloped countries, improving water quality decreases incidence of diarrhea and improves health status.[7,90]

Standards

Because coliforms originate primarily in the intestinal tracts of warm-blooded animals, including humans, they are used as indicators of possible fecal contamination.[79] Although compelling reasons exist for testing other organisms before determining the safety of drinking water, cost and relative difficulty in testing for viruses and protozoa are major obstacles to expanding routine water testing. Coliforms remain the worldwide standard indicator organism. Only recently have U.S. regulations stated that testing must be done for specific organisms, mainly *Cryptosporidium*. In the future, molecular probes should make this process much easier.[127]

The basic federal law pertaining to drinking water is the 1974 Safe Drinking Water Act, which was expanded and strengthened by amendments in 1977, 1986, and 1996.[127] The U.S. Public Health Service recommendations for potable water specify a mean of one coliform organism/100 ml of water, or 10 organisms/L. Absolute limits are three coliform bacteria/50 ml, four/100 ml, and 13/500 ml.[214] In 1989 the standards for detection of fecal coliform bacteria in drinking water were relaxed slightly in recognition that coliform bacteria occur in large numbers in many water distribution systems that have no problem with waterborne disease.[212] Generally the goal is to achieve a 3- to 5-log reduction in the level of microorganisms. Treatment must reduce *Giardia* by 99.9% (3 log) and enteric viruses by at least 99.99% (4 log).[161] All standards acknowledge the impracticality of trying to eliminate all microorganisms from drinking water; they allow a small risk of enteric infection.[189] Risk models are used to predict levels of illness and desired levels of reduction. For example, EPA guidelines suggest *Giardia* cyst removal with the goal of ensuring high probability that consumer risk is no more than one infection per 10,000 people per year.[162] The concept of risk is important for wilderness travelers as well, since it is impossible to know the risk of drinking the water in advance and not practical to eliminate all risk with treatment.

Definitions

Disinfection, the desired result of field water treatment, means the removal or destruction of harmful microorganisms. Technically, it refers only to chemical means such as halogens, but the term can be applied to heat and filtration. *Pasteurization* is similar to disinfection but specifically refers to the use of heat, usually at temperatures below 100° C (212° F) to kill most pathogenic organisms. Disinfection and pasteurization should not be confused with *sterilization,* which is the destruction or removal of all life forms.[107] The goal of disinfection is to achieve *potable* water, indicating only that a water source, on average over a period of time, contains a "minimal microbial hazard," so that the statistical likelihood of illness is acceptable. Water sterilization is not necessary, since not all organisms are enteric human pathogens.[84] *Purification* is the removal of organic or inorganic chemicals and particulate matter to remove offensive color, taste, and odor. It is frequently used interchangeably with disinfection, but purification may not remove or kill enough microorganisms to ensure microbiologic safety.[218]

HEAT

Heat is the oldest means of water disinfection. It is used worldwide by residents, travelers, and campers to provide safe drinking water. In countries with normally safe drinking water, it is often recommended as backup in emergencies or when water systems have become contaminated by floods or a lapse in water treatment plant efficacy. Fuel availability is the most important limitation to using heat. One kilogram of wood is required to boil 1 L of water.[35] For wilderness travelers without access to wood, liquid fuel is heavy.

Heat inactivation of microorganisms is exponential and follows first-order kinetics. Time plotted against temperature yields a straight line when plotted on a logarithmic scale.[96] Thus the thermal death point is reached in shorter time at higher temperatures, whereas lower temperatures are effective with a longer contact time. Pasteurization uses this principle to kill enteric food pathogens and spoiling organisms at temperatures between 60° and 70° C (140° and 158° F), well below boiling.[64] Therefore the minimum critical temperature is well below the boiling point at any terrestrial elevation.

Microorganisms have varying sensitivity to heat; however, all common enteric pathogens are readily inactivated by heat (Table 51-5). Bacterial spores (e.g., *Clostridium* species) are the most resistant; some can survive 100° C (212° F) for long periods but, as discussed, are not likely to be waterborne enteric pathogens.

Protozoal cysts, including *Giardia* and *Entamoeba histolytica,* are the most susceptible to heat. *Cryptosporidium* is also inactivated at these lower pasteurization levels.

Parasitic eggs, larvae, and cercariae are all susceptible to heat. For most helminth eggs and larvae, which are more resistant than cercariae and *Cyclops,* the critical lethal temperature is 50° to 55° C (122° to 131° F).[184]

Common bacterial enteric pathogens (*E. coli, Salmonella, Shigella*) are killed by standard pasteurization temperatures of 55° C (131° F) for 30 minutes or 65° C (149° F) for less than 1 minute.[64,137] Recent studies confirmed safety of water contaminated with *V. cholerae* and *E. coli* after 10 minutes at 60° to 62° C (140° to 143.6° F) or after boiling water for 30 seconds.[76,166]

Viruses are more closely related to vegetative bacteria than to spore-bearing organisms[96] and are generally inactivated at 56° to 60° C (132.8° to 140° F) in less than 20 to 40 minutes.[2,149,199] Inactivation at higher temperatures is similar to that of vegetative bacteria. Death occurs in less than 1 minute above 70° C (158° F). This has been confirmed in milk products, despite some degree of thermal protection from particles.[198]

Given its environmental stability and clinical virulence, hepatitis A virus is a special concern. It should respond to heat as do other enteric viruses, but data indicate that it has greater thermal resistance. Widely varying data probably result from different models for virus infectivity and destruction and from the use of various test media.

Boiling Time

The old recommendation for treating water is to boil for 10 minutes and add 1 minute for every 1000 feet (305 m) in elevation. However, available data indicate this is not necessary for disinfection. Evidence indicates that enteric pathogens are killed within seconds by boiling water and rapidly at temperatures above 60° C (140° F). In the wilderness the time required to heat water from 55° C (131° F) to boiling temperature works toward disinfection. Therefore any water brought to a boil should be adequately disinfected. An extra margin of safety can be added by boiling for 1 minute or by keeping the water covered and allowing it to cool slowly after boiling. Although the boiling point decreases with increasing altitude, this is not significant compared with the time required for thermal death at these temperatures (Table 51-6). The boiling time required is important when fuel is limited. In recognition of the difference between pasteurizing water for drinking purposes and sterilizing for surgical purposes, many other sources now agree with this recommendation to bring water to a boil. Because of scant data for hepatitis A the Centers for Disease Control and Prevention (CDC) and EPA still recommend boiling for 1 minute to add a margin of safety.[28] Some sources still

TABLE 51-5. Heat Inactivation of Microorganisms

ORGANISM	LETHAL TEMPERATURE (° C)/TIME	REFERENCES
Giardia	55 for 5 min	94
	100 immediately	15
	50 for 10 min (95% inactivation)	143
	60 for 10 min (98% inactivation)	
	70 for 10 min (100% inactivation)	
	55	6
Entamoeba histolytica	Similar to Giardia	
Nematode cysts, helminth eggs, larvae, cercariae	50-55	184
Cryptosporidium	45-55 for 20 min	5
	55 warmed over 20 min	
	64.2 within 2 min	59
	72 heated up over 1 min	
Escherichia coli	55 for 30 min	64
	60-62 for 10 min	76
	50 for 10 min ineffective	137
	60 for 5 min	
	70 for 1 min	
Salmonella, Shigella	65 for < 1 min	
Vibrio cholerae	60-62 for 10 min	166
	100 for 30 sec	
E. coli, Salmonella, Shigella, Campylobacter	60 for 3 min (3-log reduction)	8
	65 for 3 min (all but a few Campylobacter)	
	75 for 3 min (100% kill)	
Viruses	55-60 within 20-40 min	2
	70 for < 1 min	
Hepatitis A	98 for 1 min	105
	85 for 1 min	203
	61 for 10 min (50% disintegrated)	
	60 for 19 min (in shellfish)	150
Hepatitis E	60 for 30 min	203
Bacterial spores	>100	2

TABLE 51-6. Boiling Temperatures at Various Altitudes

ALTITUDE [ft (m)]	BOILING POINT (° C)
5000 (1524)	95
10,000 (3048)	90
14,000 (4267)	86
19,000 (5791)	81

suggest 3 minutes of boiling time at high altitude to give a wide margin of safety.[32,66,87,174]

Hot Tap Water

Although attaining boiling temperature is not necessary, it is the only easily recognizable end point without using a thermometer. Other markers, such as early bubble formation, do not occur at a consistent temperature. When no other means are available, the use of hot tap water may prevent travelers' diarrhea in developing countries. Newman[137,138] cultured samples from the hot water tap of 17 hotels in west Africa and in 15 found no coliforms, one yielded a single colony and another two colonies. Water temperature ranged from 57° to 69° C (131° to 140° F). As a rule of thumb, water too hot to touch fell within the pasteurization range. Bandres et al[8] also measured hot tap water temperature in 14 hotels in four different countries outside the United States. Most temperatures were 55° to 60° C (131° to 140° F), but one was 44° C (111.2° F), only one was 65° C (149° F), and several were 52° C (125.6° F). The authors concluded that hot water from taps would not be safe to drink. Groh et al[76] showed that tolerance to touch is too variable to be reliable, since some people found 55° C too hot to touch. If water has been sitting in a tank near 60° C for a prolonged period, enteric pathogens will be significantly reduced, likely to potable levels. Neumann's suggestion is reasonable if no other method of water treatment is available.

Solar Heat

Pasteurization has been successfully achieved using solar heating. A solar cooker constructed from a foil-lined

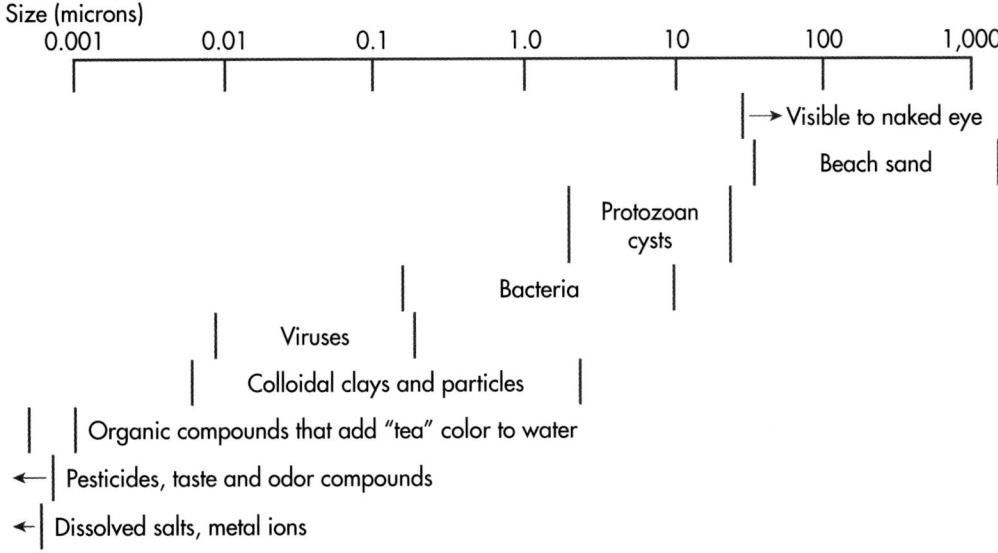

Figure 51-1 Filtration. *(Courtesy Dan Vorhis, Marathon Ceramics.)*

TABLE 51-7. Microorganism Susceptibility to Filtration

ORGANISM	AVERAGE SIZE (μm)	MAXIMUM FILTER SIZE (μm)
Viruses	0.03	N/S
Escherichia coli	0.5 × 3-8	0.2-0.4
Campylobacter	0.2-0.4 × 1.5-3.5	0.2-0.4
Microsporidia	1-2	N/S
Cryptosporidium oocyst	2-6	1
Giardia cyst	6-10 × 8-15	3-5
Entamoeba histolytica cyst	5-30 (average 10)	3-5
Cyclospora	8-10	3-5
Nematode eggs	30-40 × 50-80	20
Schistosome cercariae	50 × 100	Coffee filter or fine cloth adequate
Dracunculus larvae	20 × 500	Coffee filter or fine cloth adequate

N/S, Not specified.

cardboard box with a glass window in the lid can be used for disinfecting large amounts of water by pasteurization. Bottom temperatures of 65° C have been obtained for at least 1 hour in up to three 3.7-L jugs. Exposure to full sunshine in Kenya destroyed *E. coli* in 2-L clear plastic bottles within 7 hours if the maximum temperature reached 55° C. Inactivation in this situation was a combination of thermal and ultraviolet irradiation.[97,120] This could be a low-cost method for improving water quality, especially in refugee camps and disaster areas.

PHYSICAL REMOVAL

Filtration

Filters have the advantages of being simple and requiring no holding time. They do not add any unpleasant taste and may improve taste and appearance of water. However, they add space and weight to baggage. All filters eventually clog from suspended particulate matter (present even in clear streams), requiring

cleaning or replacement of the filter. A crack or eroded channel allows passage of unfiltered water.

Filtration is both a physical and a chemical process, so many variables influence filter efficiency. The characteristics of the filter media and the water, as well as flow rate, determine the interactions. Filtration can reduce turbidity, bacteria, algae, viruses, color, oxidized iron, manganese, and radioactive particles.[47]

The size of a microorganism is the primary determinant of its susceptibility to filtration (Table 51-7 and Figure 51-1). Filters are rated by their ability to retain particles of a certain size, which is described by two terms. *Absolute* rating means that 100% of a certain size of particle is retained. *Nominal* rating indicates that more than 90% of a given particle size will be retained. Filter efficiency is generally determined with hard particles (beads of known diameter), but microorganisms are soft and compressible under pressure.

A membrane with pore size of 0.2 μm can remove enteric bacteria. *Giardia* and *E. histolytica* cysts are easily filtered, requiring a maximum filter size of 5 μm. *Cryptosporidium* cysts are somewhat smaller than *Giardia* and more flexible; 57% are able to pass through a 3 μm membrane filter, so a filter with 1- to 2-μm pores is recommended.[174] Helminth eggs and larvae, which are much larger, can be removed by a 20-μm filter. *Cyclops* that transmits dracunculosis can be removed by passage through a fine cloth.[184]

Filters are constructed with various designs and materials, and many filters are designed for field use. Surface, membrane, and mesh filters are very thin with a single layer of fairly precise pores, whose size should be equal to or less than the smallest dimension of the organism. These filters provide little volume for holding contaminants and thus clog rapidly, but can be cleaned easily by washing and brushing without destroying the filter. Maze or depth filters depend on a long, irregular labyrinth to trap the organism, so they may have a larger pore or passage size. Contaminants adhere to the walls of the passageway or are trapped in the numerous dead-end tunnels. Granular media, such as sand or charcoal, diatomaceous earth, or ceramic filters function as maze filters. A depth filter has a large holding capacity for particles and lasts longer before clogging but may be difficult to clean effectively, since many particles are trapped deep in the filter. Flow can be partially restored to a clogged filter by back flushing or surface cleaning, which removes the larger particles trapped near the surface. For ceramic filters, surface cleaning is highly effective but destroys some of the filter medium. As a filter clogs, it requires increasing pressure to drive the water through, which can force microorganisms through the filter.

Portable filters can readily remove protozoan cysts and bacteria but may not remove viruses, which are another order of magnitude smaller than bacteria. Only the semipermeable membranes in reverse-osmosis filters are inherently capable of removing viruses. However, adsorption and aggregation reduce viruses using other mechanical filters. Virus particles may adhere to the walls of diatomite (ceramic) or charcoal filters by electrostatic chemical attraction.[58,71,163] Viruses in heavily polluted water often aggregate in large clumps and become adsorbed to particles or enmeshed in colloidal materials, making them amenable to filtration.[53,159] Thus turbidity (cloudiness from contaminants) may help remove pathogens with filtration while it inhibits halogens. In one study, however, only 10% of total virus particles detected were recovered on 3- to 5-μm pore prefilters, suggesting that most were *not* associated with the suspended sediment.[141] Furthermore, adsorbed viral particles can be subsequently dislodged and eluted from a filter.[158,206] Some filters now can remove 99% to 99.9% of viruses, but the fourth log required by water treatment units remains a challenge. Recently, the First Need filter (General Ecology, Exton,

Pa.) was able to meet the EPA standards for water purifiers, including 4-log removal of viruses. It is not clear how this filter succeeded when others have failed[71] (see Appendix). In general, however, mechanical filters should not be considered adequate for complete removal of viruses, except with special equipment.[219] Additional treatment with heat or halogens before or after filtration guarantees effective virus removal.[163] New designs and materials may overcome this limitation of microfiltration.

For domestic use and in pristine protected watersheds where pollution and viral contamination are minimal and the main concerns are bacteria and cysts, filtration can be used as the only means of disinfection. For foreign travel and for surface water with heavy levels of fecal or sewage contamination, however, most filters should not be used as the sole means of disinfection.[58] One rational use of filtration is to clear the water of sediment and organic debris, allowing lower doses of halogens with more predictable residual levels.[134] Filters are also useful as a first step to remove parasitic and *Cryptosporidium* organisms that have high resistance to halogens.

Filtration using simple, available products is of interest for use in developing countries and in emergency situations. Sand filtration is still used widely in municipal plants. A column of fine sand 60 to 75 cm deep that permits no more than 200 L/m²/hr is capable of removing turbidity and greater than 99% of organisms.[161] Rice hull ash filters are moderately effective. The United Nations International Children's Emergency Fund has devised a filter containing crushed charcoal sandwiched between two layers of fine sand that can filter 40 L/day and requires cleaning only once a year, but it has not been well tested.[35]

Reverse Osmosis. A reverse-osmosis filter uses high pressure (100 to 800 psi) to force water through a semipermeable membrane that filters out dissolved ions, molecules, and solids.[53] This process can desalinate water, as well as remove microbiologic contamination. If pressure or degradation causes breakdown of the membrane, treatment effectiveness is lost. Even *Giardia* cyst passage has been shown to occur in a compromised reverse-osmosis unit.[45]

Small hand-pump reverse-osmosis units have been developed. Their high price and slow output currently prohibit large-scale use by wilderness travelers, but they are important survival items for ocean travelers. Battery-operated units are often used on boats. The U.S. Department of Defense uses large-scale mobile reverse-osmosis units for water purification units because these are capable of producing potable water from fresh, brackish, or salt water, as well as from water contaminated by nuclear, biologic, or chemical agents. Moreover, these are considered the most fuel-efficient mobile units, producing the highest quality water from the greatest variety of raw water qualities. The units use pretreatment, filtration, and desalination, then disinfection for storage.[219]

Granular Activated Carbon (GAC). Granular charcoal has been used as an adsorbent for water purification since biblical times.[108] It is still in use for water treatment and for medical detoxification. When activated, charcoal's regular array of carbon bonds is disrupted, yielding free valences that are highly reactive and adsorb dissolved chemicals.[68,178] GAC is the best means to remove organic and inorganic chemicals from water (including disinfection byproducts) and to improve odor and taste.[53,134] Thus it is widely used in municipal disinfection plants and in home undersink devices. GAC is also a common component of field units as a filter and water purifier. GAC can be compressed into block form that acts both as a depth filter and adsorbent charcoal. The block carbon is more effective than granular because the passages are smaller, forcing closer contact with the carbon.

Many, but not all, viral particles and bacteria adhere to GAC,[134] and some cysts are trapped in the matrix.[113] However, using a bed of GAC to filter particles and microorganisms results in more rapid saturation of binding sites and clogs the bed. An alternative means of disinfection should always be used. GAC does not kill microorganisms, so it does not disinfect. In fact, bacteria colonize beds of GAC and slough off into the effluent water. Bacteria attached to charcoal are resistant to chlorination because the chlorine is adsorbed by the GAC.[53,108,134] This bacterial contamination has not been found to be harmful because the usual heterophilic bacteria are not enteric pathogens. Enteric pathogens have been shown to survive on GAC, but if an active biofilm exists, the pathogens are rapidly displaced by heterophilic bacteria and fail to become established. Therefore nonpathogenic bacterial colonization is encouraged in municipal plants.[163]

Eventually the binding sites on the carbon particles become saturated and no longer adsorb; some molecules are released as others preferentially bind.[134] Unfortunately, no reliable means are available to determine precisely when saturation is reached. Filters using charcoal in compressed block form as the filter element may clog before the charcoal is fully adsorbed. Presence of unpleasant taste or color in the water can be the first sign that the charcoal is spent. To test the charcoal, filter iodinated water or water tinted with food coloring. With regular use the lifetime of GAC is probably measured in months; it is substantially longer with infrequent use. GAC can be "recharged," but this is not practical for small-quantity use. Ingested particles of charcoal are harmless.

GAC can be used before or after disinfection. Before disinfection, GAC removes many organic impurities that result in bad odor and taste and that are precursors to trihalomethane formation. GAC is best used after chemical disinfection to make water more palatable by completely removing the halogen[134,221] and other chemical impurities. With increasing industrial and agricultural contamination of distant groundwater, final treatment of drinking water with GAC may become a necessity for wilderness users. GAC also removes radioactive contamination.

Silver Impregnation. Silver impregnation of filters neither prevents microbial contamination of the filter nor sustains its action as a bactericide in the effluent water.[11] Although silver has slow antibacterial effect on coliform organisms, filter cartridges impregnated with silver typically become colonized with heterotrophic bacteria, which increase the total bacterial count in the effluent water but have not been linked to increased illness.[11,58,68,163] In GAC filters designed to operate in line with chlorinated tap water, silver merely exerts selective pressure on the kinds of bacteria that will colonize the filter. Colonization of filters with pathogenic coliforms has not been demonstrated, but protective effect cannot be attributed to silver impregnation.[58,163]

Commercial Devices Using Mechanical Filtration. Portable water treatment products are the third highest intended purchase of outdoor equipment after backpacks and tents.[95] Some are designed as purely mechanical filters, whereas others combine filtration with GAC. Filters that contain iodine resins are considered in the discussion on halogens (see Appendix).

Environmental Protection Agency Registration. Until recently, no testing criteria were mandated for EPA registration. The EPA does not endorse, test, or approve mechanical filters; it merely assigns registration numbers.[39] However, registration requirements distinguish between two types of filters: those that use mechanical means only and those that use a chemical, designated as a pesticide. Standards were developed to act as a framework for testing and evaluation of water purifiers for EPA registration, as a testing guide to manufacturers, to assist in research and development of new units, and as a guide to consumers.[212] To be called a "microbiologic water purifier," the unit must remove, kill, or inactivate all types of disease-causing microorganisms from the water, including bacteria, viruses, and protozoan cysts, so as to render the processed water safe for drinking. An exception for limited claims may be allowed for units removing specific organisms to serve a definable environmental need, for example, removal of *Giardia* only.

The EPA standards include performance-based microbiologic reduction requirements, chemical health limits for substances that may be discharged, and stability requirements for chemical(s) sufficient for the shelf life of the device. The unit should signal the end of effective lifetime (e.g., by terminating discharge of treated water) or give simple instructions for servicing or replacing within measurable volume, throughput, or time frame. There are currently no national guidelines for the removal of chemicals by portable filters.

Challenge water seeded with specific amounts of microorganisms is pumped through the filters at given intervals during the claimed volume capacity of the filter. Between the bacteriologic challenges, different test waters without organisms are passed through the unit. Water conditions are specified to include average and worst-case conditions, which are 5° C with high levels of pollution, turbidity, and alkaline pH. Testing must be done with bacteria *(Klebsiella)*, viruses (poliovirus and rotavirus), and protozoa *(Cryptosporidium* has replaced *Giardia)*. A 3-log reduction is required for cysts, 4-log reduction for viruses, and 5- to 6-log reduction for bacteria. Testing is done or contracted by the manufacturer; the EPA neither tests nor specifies laboratories.

Filter Testing. Current registration of mechanical filters requires only that the product make reasonable claims and that the location of the manufacturer be listed; no disinfection studies are required.[24] However, many companies now use the standards as their testing guidelines. For mechanical filters the standards should be applied only for those microorganisms against which claims are made, such as protozoa and bacteria, excluding viruses. Despite criticisms of the methodology and inconsistencies and loopholes in the reporting process, the EPA standards are currently the best means to compare filters.

The ceramic filters (especially Katadyn) have been tested most extensively and generally perform well.[58,143,206] Results may not apply to all ceramic filters because efficacy depends on the characteristics of the ceramic, water quality, product engineering, and prior extent of filter use. Comparative testing of different filters is in progress. Available data are from testing organized by one filter manufacturer, so the results are not generally accepted, despite nearly all filters performing well (Table 51-8) .

Turbidity and Clarification

River, lake, or pond water is often cloudy and unappealing. Turbidity (cloudiness) is an optical measurement of light scattering as it passes through water. Visibility in water with turbidity of 10 nephelometric turbidity units (NTU) is about 30 inches and with 25 NTU is 10 inches. Turbidity is caused by suspended organic and inorganic matter, such as clay, silt, plankton, and other microscopic organisms. High turbidity is often associated with unpleasant odors and tastes, most often caused by organic compounds and metallic hy-

droxides with a much smaller particle size.[38,109] Clay-organic complexes may also carry pesticides or heavy metals. Bacteria, as well as viruses, may be adsorbed to particulate matter or be embedded in it, and in highly contaminated water, microorganisms tend to aggregate and clump. In one study, 17% of turbidity particles contained attached microbes, averaging 10 to 100 bacteria per particle.[109] Organisms in the center of these conglomerates are afforded some protection from disinfectants. Even the flocculate produced by a chlorination-flocculation tablet may harbor viable organisms.[155] Thus, removing particulate matter also decreases the number of microorganisms and halogen demand.[98,134]

Removal of turbidity and particulates may be important in preventing chemical or infectious illness. Even if turbidity is caused by benign inorganic particles, such as clay, removal is desirable for improving esthetic quality of the water. Filtration can remove larger particles, but cloudy water can rapidly clog a filter. Sedimentation and coagulation-flocculation are other clarification techniques routinely used in municipal disinfection plants that can be easily applied in the wilderness for pretreatment of cloudy water, which is then disinfected by filtration or halogenation. Coagulation-flocculation and filtration are also used to remove *Giardia* and *Cryptosporidium* cysts that are more resistant to chlorine. Early experiments with water heavily contaminated with feces containing hepatitis A virus demonstrated that filtration and sedimentation alone did not prevent infection but reduced the severity of the illness. Water pretreated with coagulation, settling, and filtration was subsequently disinfected with 0.4 ppm of residual chlorine, whereas water chlorinated to 1 mg/L without pretreatment remained infectious.[135,136]

Sedimentation. Sedimentation is the separation of suspended particles large enough to settle rapidly by gravity, such as sand and silt. The time required depends on the size of the particle. Generally, 1 hour is adequate if the water is allowed to sit without agitation. After sediment has formed on the bottom of the container, the clear water is decanted or filtered from the top. Microorganisms, especially protozoal cysts, eventually settle, but this takes longer and the organisms are easily disturbed during pouring or filtering. In one test in Tanzania, 4 days were required for sedimentation to improve microbiologic quality of the water.[35] Sedimentation should not be considered a means of disinfection.

Coagulation-Flocculation. Smaller suspended particles and chemical complexes too small to settle by gravity are called *colloids*. Most of these can be removed by coagulation-flocculation, a technique that has been used to remove unpleasant color, smell, and taste in water since 2000 BC.

Coagulation is achieved with addition of an appropriate chemical that alters the physical state of dissolved

TABLE 51-8. Performance Evaluations of Portable Filters

REFERENCE	CHALLENGE	FILTERS TESTED	RESULTS			CONCLUSIONS/COMMENTS
			BACTERIA	PROTOZOA	VIRUS	

157	Challenged Katadyn filter with 10^8 *B. subtilis* spores, 10^6 *Naegleria* cysts, 10^5 *Giardia* cysts using EPA test waters 1 and 3 (clear and cloudy) at 20° and 4° C. Survivor (reverse osmosis) tested with above plus 10^7 poliovirus and rotavirus, using EPA test water 1 and 3% seawater.	Katadyn
		  Clear
		  Cloudy
		
		Survivor 35
		  Clear
		  Sea-water
			
			Pass
			Pass 2/3
			
			Pass
			Fail
				
				Pass
				Fail 3/3
				
				Pass
				Pass
					N/A
					
					Pass
					Pass
						Katadyn filter failed unless cleaned regularly; failure was related to mechanical pump forcing organisms through a clogged filter. Recommend prefilter.
						Survivor failure was due to growth of the test organism on and throughout the filter membrane. Recommend biocide treatment of membrane.

			BACTERIA	PROTOZOA	VIRUS	

133	Condensed EPA standard testing protocol using bacteria, viruses, and *Cryptosporidium* oocysts with three test waters from average to "worst" case conditions at beginning, middle and end of claimed filter lifetime; "Pass" indicates removal of 99.9999% bacteria, 99.9% protozoa, 99.99% viruses; "N/A" indicates not applicable because no claims for virus removal.	PUR hiker
		  New
		  200 gal
		Katadyn
		  Minifilter
		
		Timberline
		  New
		  200 gal
		General Ecology
		  First Need
		Microlite
		  New
		MSR waterworks
		SweetWater
		  Guardian
		
		PUR Scout
		  New
		  200 gal
		Explorer (*See note*)
		
		SweetWater with
		  iodine (*See note*)
			
			99.96%
			99.6%
			Pass
			
			99%
			91.5%
			
			Pass
			
			99.96%
			Pass
			Pass
			
			Pass
			99.9%
			88.7%
			Pass
			
			Pass
				
				99.8% pass
				
				Pass
				
				Pass
				Pass
				
				Pass
				
				Pass
				Pass
				Pass
				
				99.8%
				99.8% pass
				
				Pass
				
				Pass
					N/A
					
					N/A
					
					N/A
					
					N/A
					
					N/A
					
					N/A
					
					N/A
					Pass
					95.2%
					85.8%
					99.7%
					
					99.7%
						This testing was sponsored by several outdoor retailers and by Sweet Water but is the best comparative testing available to date.
						Timberline made no claims for bacteria.
						
						97%-99% virus removal by this mechanical filter.
						Explorer failed to perform after only 100 gal, although claimed capacity greater. Passed tests with average case water, but failed worst case water.
						SweetWater failed viral removal at end of filter life.

			TEST 1		TEST 2	

90a	4×10^8/L *B. diminuta* bacteria; filters tested at limit of design life after passing 92-345 L high-quality river water, then tested after 4, 5, 6, and 7 L seeded water; test 2 done after passing high-turbidity water until clogged, then cleaning filters.	MSR
		  Miniworks
		  Miniworks II
		Katadyn
		  Pocket
		  Combi
		Sweet Water
		  Guardian +
		  iodine
		PUR Scout
		  Explorer
		  Hiker
			
			99.998%
			
			99.8%
			
			96.3%
			
			99.999%
			
			57.7%
					
					99.9%
					99.99999%
					
					99.6%
					99.99999%
					
					96.7%
					
					99.9999%
					99.9%
					99.999%
					97.7%
						Although independent laboratory, the testing was sponsored by MSR. Note very high levels of bacteria. PUR Scout and Explorer and SweetWater plus contain iodine resin.

and suspended solids, causing particles to stick together on contact because of electrostatic and ionic forces.[38,53] Lime (alkaline chemicals principally containing calcium or magnesium and oxygen) and alum (an aluminum salt) are commonly used, readily available coagulants. Rapid mixing is important to obtain dispersion of the coagulant. The second stage, flocculation, is a purely physical process obtained by prolonged gentle mixing to increase interparticle collisions and promote formation of larger particles. The flocculate particles can be removed by sedimentation and filtration. Coagulation-flocculation removes most coliform bacteria (60% to 98%), viruses (65% to 99%),[47,159,189] *Giardia* (60% to 99%), helminth ova (95%),[184] heavy metals, dissolved phosphates, and minerals.[38,53,113,227] Organic and inorganic compounds may be removed by forming a precipitate or by adsorbing onto aluminum hydroxide or ferric hydroxide floc particles.[53] Despite removal of most microorganisms, a subsequent disinfection step is advised.

The sequential use of coagulation and activated carbon is often beneficial. Coagulation is generally found to remove large molecules that absorb poorly on GAC. On the other hand, carbon has limited effectiveness for removing organic matter from water.[4]

To clarify water by this means in the field, add 10 to 30 mg of alum per liter of water. The exact amount is not important, so it can be done with a pinch of alum, lime, or both for each gallon of water, using more if the water is very cloudy. Next, stir or shake briskly for 1 minute to mix the coagulant, then agitate gently and frequently for at least 5 minutes to assist flocculation. Settling requires at least 30 minutes, after which the water is carefully decanted or poured through a cloth or paper filter. Finally, filtration or halogenation should be used to ensure disinfection.

TOXICITY. Questions have been raised concerning the association of aluminum with central nervous system (CNS) toxicity in mammals, but these effects have been observed only after exposures other than ingestion. Most of the aluminum in alum is removed with the floc. A report from the National Academy of Sciences concluded that aluminum in drinking water does not present a significant risk.[53] Alum is a common chemical used by the food industry in baking powder and for pickling. It can be found in some food stores or at chemical supply stores.

ALTERNATIVE AGENTS. Many substances can be used as a coagulant, including lime or potash. In an emergency, baking powder or even the fine white ash from a campfire can be used.[209] Other coagulation-flocculation agents used traditionally by native peoples include seeds from the nirmali plant in southern India and rauwaq (a form of bentonite clay) or seeds from moringa plants in Sudan.[35]

HALOGENS

Worldwide, chemical disinfection is the most widely used method for improving and maintaining microbiologic quality of drinking water. Halogens, chiefly chlorine and iodine, are the most effective chemical disinfectants. Understanding the principal factors of halogen disinfection allows intelligent and flexible use. Germicidal activity results from oxidation of essential cellular structures and enzymes.[33,107,134,139] Halogenated amines may be synthesized by white blood cells as part of the body's natural defenses to destroy microorganisms.[220] The disinfection process is determined by characteristics of the disinfectant, the microorganism, and environmental factors.[34,86,131] Dilute solutions do not sterilize water.

Variables with Halogenation

Concentration and Contact Time. The major variables in the disinfection reaction with chlorine or iodine are the amount of halogen (concentration) and the exposure time of the microorganism to the halogen disinfectant (contact time). Concentration of halogen in water is measured in parts per million (ppm) or milligrams per liter (mg/L), which are equivalent. Contact time is usually measured in minutes but ranges from seconds to hours. In field disinfection, concentrations of 1 to 10 mg/L for 10 to 60 minutes are generally effective.

Theoretically the disinfection reaction follows first-order kinetics. The rate of the reaction is determined by the initial concentration of reactants, and a given proportion of the reaction occurs in any specified interval.[86,221] This means concentration and time are inversely related, and their product results in a constant for specified disinfectant, organism, percent reduction of viable microorganisms, and given conditions of water temperature and pH: concentration $\times$ time = constant (Ct = K) (Figure 51-2).[221] When concentration and contact time are graphed on logarithmic coordinates, a straight line results. This means that concentration and time can be varied oppositely and still achieve the same result.[9] In field disinfection this can be used to minimize halogen dose and improve taste or to minimize the required contact time.

In reality the disinfection reaction deviates from first-order kinetics, and Ct values do not follow the exponential rates described by the empiric equation because microorganisms do not act as chemical reagents ($C_n t$ = K). An initial lag period may be seen before inactivation begins (e.g., because of penetration of the cyst wall), and inactivation declines for more resistant organisms or those protected by aggregation or association with other particulate matter (Figure 51-3).[77,82,86]

Contaminants. Organic and inorganic nitrogen compounds from decomposition of organisms and their

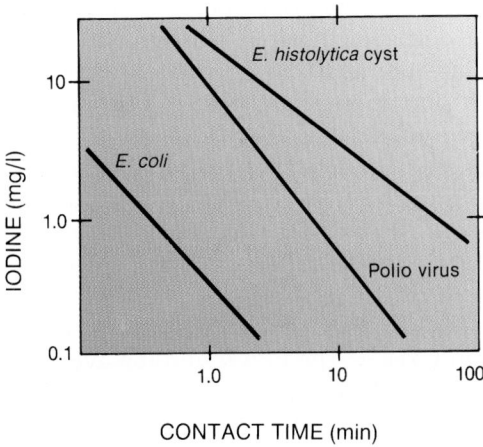

CONTACT TIME (min)

Figure 51-2 Relationship of halogen concentration and contact time for a given temperature and pH. The first-order chemical reaction results in a straight line over most values for each microorganism and halogen compound. (*Data from Change SL: J Am Pharm Assoc 47:417, 1958; and Water and Sanitation for Health [WASH] Project: Report on mobile emergency water treatment and disinfection units, WASH Field Report No 217, Arlington, Va, 1980.*)

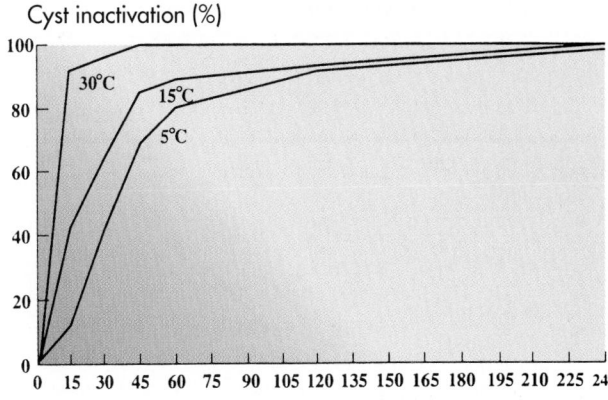

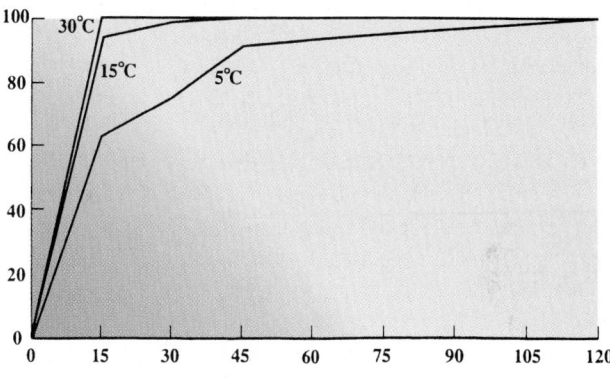

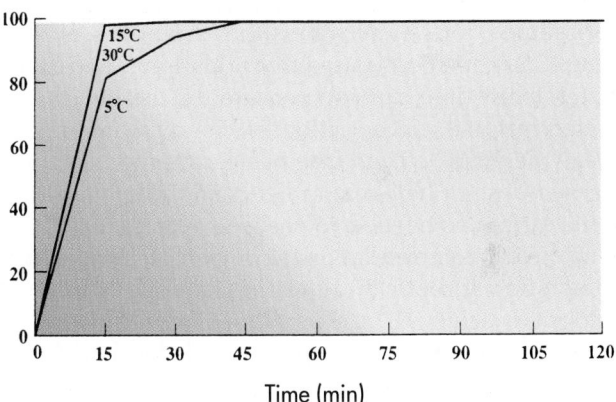

Time (min)

Figure 51-3 Effect of concentration and temperature on *Giardia* cyst inactivation by iodine. Low concentrations are effective at cold temperatures with prolonged contact time. (*From Fraker LD et al: J Wilderness Med 3:351, 1992.*)

wastes, fecal matter, and urea complicate disinfection with halogens and must be considered in field water treatment. Vegetable matter, ferrous ions, nitrites, sulfides, and humic substances also affect oxidizing disinfectants.[55,134,221] These contaminants react with halogens, especially chlorine, to form compounds with little or no disinfecting ability, effectively decreasing the concentration of available halogen.

Halogen Demand and Residual Concentration. Halogen demand is the amount of halogen reacting with impurities. Residual halogen concentration is the amount of active halogen remaining after halogen demand of the water is met. To achieve microbial inactivation in aqueous solution with a chemical agent, a residual concentration must be present for a specified contact time. Failure of chlorination in municipal systems to kill cysts or other microorganisms is usually caused by difficulty maintaining adequate residual halogen concentration and contact times, rather than by extreme resistance of the organism.[196]

Halogen demand and residual concentration of surface water are the greatest uncertainties in field disinfection. Nitrogen appears in most natural waters in varying amounts, which relate directly to the sanitary quality of water. Cysticidal dose of halogens is strongly affected by the level of contamination (cyst or viral density) in otherwise clean water.[34,75,196] Scant data are available on halogen demand for surface water (Table 51-9). Clear water is assumed to have minimal demand and cloudy water high demand. Surface water in the wilderness contains 10 times the organic carbon content

of aquifer groundwater. The green or brown color in stagnant ponds or lakes or in tropical and lowland rivers is usually caused by organic matter with considerable halogen demand. In some cases, such as runoff after storms and snowmelt, cloudy water may be caused by inorganic sand and clay that exert little halogen demand. In general, chlorine demand rises with increased turbidity.[109] In addition, particulate turbidity can shield microorganisms and interfere with disinfection.[47,98,109]

The initial dose of halogen must consider halogen demand. For clear alpine waters, 1 mg/L demand can

TABLE 51-9. Halogen Demand of Surface Water

SOURCE	HALOGEN DEMAND (mg/L)	REFERENCE
Cloudy river water, Portland, Oregon	3-4	93
Cloudy water from clay particles	None	34
Clear water with 10% sewage added	2	34
Lily pond and turbid river water	5-6	34
Colorado River, cloudy from inorganic sand, clay	0.3	207
Unspecified surface waters	2-3	46
Municipal wastewater	20-30	46
High-elevation spring	0.3	142
Western river	0.7	142
Six watersheds in western Oregon	0.4-1.6	109
Small stream, Australia	1.3	202

be assumed; for cloudy waters the assumption is 3 to 5 mg/L. If a method is used that adds 4 mg/L to clear water, extra time can compensate for the lower expected residual concentration. In cloudy water, however, where the demand may be nearly 4 mg/L, an increased dose of halogen, rather than prolonging the contact time, is needed to ensure free residual. The usual field recommendation to compensate for the unknown demand of cloudy water is a double dose of halogen (to achieve 8 to 16 mg/L). This crude means of compensation often results in a strong halogen taste on top of the taste of the contaminants. If the cause of turbidity is uncertain, the water should be allowed to sit; inorganic clay and sand will sediment, clarifying the water considerably. Other means of clarification, such as coagulation-flocculation or filtration, significantly reduce halogen demand.

Several simple color tests (most often used to test swimming pools and spas) measure the amount of free (residual) halogen in water. Testing in the wilderness for halogen residual may be reasonable for large groups but is not practical for most. Smell of chlorine usually indicates some free residual. Color and taste of iodine can be used as indicators. Above 0.6 ppm, a yellow to brown tint is noted.[221]

pH. Two other variables in the disinfection reaction are pH and temperature.[55,107,134] Halogen oxidizes water to form several compounds, each with different disinfec-

tion capabilities. The percentage of each halogen compound is determined by pH. The optimal pH for halogen disinfection is 6.5 to 7.5.[34,130] As water becomes more alkaline, approaching pH 8.0, much higher doses of halogens are required.

Although pH can be measured in the field, the relationship is too complex to allow meaningful use of the information. Most surface water pH is neutral to mildly acidic, which is within the effective range of the halogens used. Granite keeps many alpine waters mildly acidic. Unfortunately, acid rain is affecting some high mountain lakes.[122] The EPA found the average pH in western alpine lakes to be no less than 5.5; other US lakes are beginning to show lower pH levels. On the alkaline side, some surface water with pH 7.0 to 8.0 begins to affect the chemical species of chlorine, favoring less active forms.[86] Certain desert water is so alkaline that halogens would have little activity; however, these waters are usually not palatable. At this time, compensating for pH is not necessary. Tablet formulations of halogen have the advantage of some buffering capacity.

Temperature. Temperature influences the rate of the disinfection reaction. Cold water affects germicidal power and must be offset by longer contact time or higher concentration to achieve comparable disinfection.[74] The common rule is a twofold to threefold increase in inactivation rate per 10° C increase in temperature. Unusual retardation of rates as temperatures approach 0° C has not been seen.[86]

Temperature can be estimated in the field. Some treatment protocols recommend doubling the dose of halogen in cold water, but if time allows, time can be increased instead of dose. Data for killing *Giardia* in very cold water (5° C) with both chlorine and iodine indicate that contact time must be prolonged three to four times, not merely doubled, to achieve high levels of inactivation.[63,83] If feasible, raising the temperature by 10° to 20° C allows a lower dose of halogen and more reliable disinfection at a given dose.

Susceptibility of Microorganisms. The final variable is the target microorganism. Sensitivity to halogen is determined by the diffusion barrier of the cell wall or capsule and the relative susceptibility of proteins and cellular respiration to denaturation and oxidation.[33,134] Organisms, in order of increasing resistance to halogen disinfection, are enteric (vegetative) bacteria, viruses, protozoan cysts, bacterial spores, and parasitic ova (Tables 51-10 and 51-11); for example, *E. histolytica* cysts are 160 times as resistant as *E. coli* and 9 times as resistant as hardier enteroviruses to chlorine (HOCl). Virucidal residuals of I_2 and HOCl are 5 to 70 times higher than bactericidal residuals.[33,134] Relative resistance between organisms is similar for iodine and chlorine.

TABLE 51-10. Disinfection Data for Chlorine

HALOGEN*	ORGANISM	CONCENTRATION (mg/L)	TIME (min)	pH	TEMPERATURE (°C)	DISINFECTION CONSTANT (Ct)	REFERENCE
HOCl	*Escherichia coli*	0.1	0.16	6.0	5	0.016	221
FAC	*Campylobacter*	0.3	0.5	6.0-8.0	25	0.15	19
FRC	20 enteric viruses	0.5	60	7.8	2	30	22
Free Cl	6 enteric viruses	0.5	4.5	6.0-8.0	5	2.5	56
FRC	Hepatitis A virus	0.5	1	6.0	25	0.5	75
Free Cl	Hepatitis A virus	0.5	5	6.0	5	2.5†	189
HOCl	Amebic cysts	3.5	10		25	35	33
FRC	Amebic cysts	3.0	10	7.0	30	30	196
Free Cl	*Giardia* cysts	2.5	60	6.0-8.0	5	150	167
Free Cl	*G. lamblia* cysts	0.85	90	8.0	2-3	77	216
Free Cl	*G. muris* cysts	3.05	50	7.0	5	153	180
		5.87	25	7.0	5	139	180
Free Cl	*Giardia*			6.0	0.5	170	83
				6.0	5	120	83
Free Cl	*Cryptosporidium*	80	90			7200	221
FRC	Schistosome cercariae	1.0	30	7.0	28	30	228
Free Cl	Nematodes	2-3	120	(Not lethal)			134
		95-100	30	(95% lethal)			134
FRC	*Ascaris* eggs	200	20	5.0	37	2000	104

HOCl, Hypochlorous acid; *FAC*, free active chlorine; *Free Cl*, free chlorine; *FRC*, free residual chlorine.
*These represent nearly equivalent measurements of the residual concentration of active chlorine disinfectant compounds.
†Four-log reduction. Most experiments use 2- to 3-log (99% to 99.9%) reduction as the end point.

TABLE 51-11. Disinfection Data for Iodine

HALOGEN*	ORGANISM	CONCENTRATION (mg/L)	TIME (min)	pH	TEMPERATURE (°C)	DISINFECTION CONSTANT (Ct)	REFERENCE
FRI	*Escherichia coli*	1.3	1	6.0-7.0	2-5	1.3	134
I2	Amebic cysts	3.5	10		25	35	33
		6.0	5		25	30	33
		12.5	2		25	25	33
FRI	Poliovirus 1	1.25	39	6.0	25	49	13
		12.7	5	6.0	25	63	13
I2	Poliovirus 1	1	6	7.0	18	6	13
I2	Coxsackievirus	0.5	30	7.0	5	15	13
Added I2	Amebic cysts	8	10	4.0-8.0	23	80	34
	Bacteria, viruses	8	20		0-5	160	34
FRI	*Giardia* cysts	4	15	5.0	30	60†	63
		4	45	5.0	15	170†	63
		4	120	5.0	5	480†	63

*FRI (free residual iodine) and I2 (elemental iodine) are nearly equivalent measurements of the residual concentration of active iodine disinfectant compounds. Added I2 indicates initial dose.
†100% kill; viability tested only at 15, 30, 45, 60, and 120 minutes.

BACTERIA. All vegetative bacteria are extremely sensitive to halogens. Inactivation involves oxidation of enzymes on the cell membrane and does not require penetration.[221] Little modern work has focused on bacterial agents because they are more sensitive than viruses and cysts, and little difference is evident between the bacterial pathogens.[86] Although halogens were first used to disinfect water during cholera epidemics in 1850, recent cholera epidemics prompted review of data to ensure the susceptibility of *V. cholerae* to low levels of chlorine and iodine.[44] *Campylobacter* has susceptibility similar to that of other enteric pathogens.[19]

Bacterial spores, such as *Bacillus anthracis,* are relatively resistant to halogens, but with chlorine, spores are not much more resistant than *Giardia* cysts.[9,221] Quantitative data are not available for iodine solutions, but iodine does kill spores. Fortunately, sporulating bacteria do not normally cause waterborne enteric disease.[84]

VIRUSES. Enteroviruses are more resistant than enteric bacteria,[134] but they constitute such a large and diverse group of organisms that generalization is especially difficult.[33,53,107] Most studies have used poliovirus, a phage virus, or coxsackievirus. The mechanism of action for halogen inactivation of viruses has not been resolved. It is not clear whether the oxidant injures protein on the shell, a process similar to bacterial inactivation,[23] or penetrates the protein capsid by chemical transformation and then attacks the nucleic acid core, as in cyst inactivation.[221]

Most viruses tested against chlorine have shown resistance 10 times greater than that of enteric bacteria, but inactivation is still achieved rapidly (0.3 to 4.5 minutes) with low levels (0.5 mg/L) of chlorine.[56,210] Current data suggest that HAV is not significantly more resistant than other enteric viruses.[75,151,190,203] In one test using iodine tablets, HAV was inactivated under difficult conditions more readily than poliovirus or echovirus.[191] Norwalk virus may be more resistant to chlorine than several other viruses, which may account for its importance in waterborne outbreaks.[101] Powers et al[155,156] found that poliovirus was more slowly inactivated than rotavirus and *Giardia muris* by both chlorine and iodine, but this is inconsistent with other data. Clumping and association of viruses with cells and particulate matter are thought to be significant factors affecting viral disinfection, causing departure from first-order kinetics.[56,191,210] Cell-associated hepatitis A virus was 10 times more resistant than dispersed hepatitis A virus.

CYSTS AND PARASITES. Protozoal cysts are considerably more resistant than enteric bacteria and significantly more resistant than enteric viruses, probably because of cysts' physiologically inactive outer shell, which the disinfectant must penetrate to be effective.[33,221] Early

data exist for *E. histolytica,* but recent work on *G. lamblia* indicates similar sensitivity to both iodine and chlorine.[94] Higher pH and lower temperature decrease the effectiveness of halogens on *Giardia.*[82,91,191] Review literature frequently attributes exaggerated resistance of *Giardia* to halogens; Hoff[85] traced this to misquoted data. Jarrol et al[92,93] tested two chlorine methods and four iodine methods for effectiveness against *Giardia* cysts. They found all methods effective in warm water, but only two methods destroyed all cysts in cold water in recommended doses. Higher doses or longer contact times would make all these methods effective. Halogens can be used in the field to inactivate *Giardia* cysts* (see Figure 51-3). However, longer contact time is required in cold and dirty water.[73]

Cryptosporidium oocysts differ greatly from other protozoan cysts and are highly resistant to halogens. The Ct constant for *Cryptosporidium* in warm water with chlorine was estimated at 9600.[29] From 65% to 80% of *Cryptosporidium* oocysts were inactivated after 4 hours by two iodine tablets in "general case" water.[73] This implies that 3-log inactivation could have been achieved after 3 to 4 more hours. Although halogens can achieve disinfection of *Cryptosporidium* in the field, this is not practical.[48,174,221] The resistance of *Cyclospora* and microsporidia is not well studied, but the oocysts are similar to *Cryptosporidium* and thus may resemble this protozoa more than *Giardia.*

Schistosome cercariae are susceptible to low concentrations of chlorine.[223] Limited data on parasitic helminth larvae and ova indicate such high levels of resistance that chemical disinfection is not useful.[104,134,184] However, these are not common waterborne pathogens and can be readily removed or destroyed by heat, filtration, or coagulation-flocculation.

DISINFECTION CONSTANT. The best comparison of disinfection power is the disinfection constant (Ct). Disparate results may be caused by lack of standardized experimental conditions of pH, temperature, chemical species of halogen, and species of microorganism or by different techniques for concentrating, counting, and determining viability of organisms.[86,134] The latter is especially a problem for cysts and viruses, which cannot be cultured easily.[182] The end point for disinfection effectiveness is now becoming standardized by the EPA guidelines, but most older studies used 99.9% for all organisms, with some using 99% or 99.99%. Differences between laboratory and field conditions also make extrapolation from data to practice inaccurate and suggest the need for a safety factor in the field. Despite variation, Ct remains a useful and widely used concept; values provide a basis for comparing the effectiveness

---

*References 63, 83, 86, 91, 154-156, 180.

of different disinfectants for inactivation of specific microorganisms.[86] To use halogens for disinfection, a *consensus organism* (the most resistant target) determines the Ct.[86,107,221] For wilderness water this has been protozoan cysts. The resistance of *Cryptosporidium* will not raise the threshold for halogen use; rather, it will force an alternative or a combination of methods to ensure removal and inactivation of all pathogens.

Chlorine

Chlorine has been used as a disinfectant for 200 years. Hypochlorite was first used for water disinfection in 1854 during cholera epidemics in London and was first used continuously for water treatment in Belgium in 1902. It is currently the preferred means of municipal water disinfection worldwide, so extensive data support its use[221] (see Table 51-10).

Chemistry. Chlorine reacts in water to form the following compounds[55,221]:

$$Cl_2 + H_2O \leftrightarrow HOCl + H^+ + Cl^-$$

$$HOCl \leftrightarrow OCl^- + H^+$$

At neutral pH, negligible amounts of diatomic chlorine are present. The major disinfectant is hypochlorous acid (HOCl), which penetrates cell and cyst walls easily. Dissociation of HOCl to the much weaker disinfectant hypochlorite (OCl$^-$) depends on temperature and pH. In pure water at pH 6.0, 97% of chlorine is HOCl; at pH 7.5, HOCl/OCl$^-$ ratio is 1:1; and above pH 7.5, OCl$^-$ predominates.[221] The combination of these two compounds is defined as *free available chlorine.* Both calcium hypochlorite (Ca[OCl]$_2$) and sodium hypochlorite (NaOCl) readily dissociate in water, allowing the same equilibrium to form as when elemental chlorine is used.[107,221] Chloride ion (Cl$^-$, NaCl, or CaCl$_2$) is germicidally inactive. In addition, chlorine readily reacts with ammonia to form monochloramines (NH$_2$Cl), dichloramines, or trichloramines, referred to as *combined chlorine.* In field disinfection these compounds are not considered, and only free residual chlorine should be measured. However, chloramines have weak disinfecting power and are calculated as a disinfectant in municipal sewage plants.[86,130,134,221]

Toxicity. Acute toxicity to chlorine is limited; the main danger is irritation and corrosion of mucous membranes if concentrated solutions (for example, household bleach) are ingested. Numerous cases have been reported of short-term ingestion of very high residuals (50 to 90 ppm) in drinking water; one military study used 32 ppm for several months without adverse effects.[221] Animal studies using long-term chlorination of drinking water at 100 to 200 ppm have not shown toxic effects.[134]

Sodium hypochlorite is not carcinogenic; however, reactions of chlorine with certain organic contaminants yield chlorinated hydrocarbons, chloroform, and other trihalomethanes, which are considered carcinogenic.[53,134] Public health departments limit residual chlorine in public systems to decrease ingestion of trihalomethane. The concern is now fueled more by public fears than by scientific conclusion.[221] The risk of death from infectious diseases if disinfection is not used is far greater than any risk from chlorine disinfection by-products.[53] These compounds are not likely to form in clean wilderness surface water, since the organic precursors are not present.

Formulations. Chlorine is available in liquid and tablet forms for field use (Table 51-12 and 51-13).

BLEACH. Liquid household bleach is a hypochlorite solution that comes in various concentrations, usually 5.25%. This has the convenience of easy availability, low cost, high stability, and administration with a dropper. If bleach containers break or leak in a pack, the liquid is corrosive and stains clothing.

Sodium hypochlorite solutions are vulnerable to significant loss of available chlorine over time. Stability is greatly affected by heat and light. Five percent solution loses about 10% available chlorine over 6 months at 21° C (70° F) and freezes at −4.4° C (24° F).

TABLETS

Halazone. Tablets contain a mixture of monochloraminobenzoic and dichloraminobenzoic acids.[55] Each tablet releases 2.3 to 2.5 ppm of titratable chlorine.[140] These tablets have been criticized because the alkaline buffer necessary to improve halazone dissolution decreases disinfectant efficiency, requiring unacceptably high concentrations and contact times (6 tablets = 15 mg/L for 60 minutes) for reliable disinfection under all conditions.[172] Tablets have the advantage of easy administration and can be salvaged if the container breaks. However, they lose effectiveness with exposure to heat, air, or moisture. Although no significant loss of potency results from opening a glass bottle intermittently over weeks, 75% of activity is lost after 2 days of continuous exposure to air with high heat and humidity. The shelf life is 6 months; potency decreases 50% when stored at 40° to 50° C (104° to 122° F). A new bottle should be taken on each major trip or changed every 3 to 6 months. Halazone is being replaced by newer formulations of chlorine tablets.

Aquaclear and Puritabs. Each tablet contains 17 mg of sodium dichloroisocyanurate (NaDCC) in a paper/foil laminate. The effervescent tablet releases 10 mg of free chlorine (HOCl) when dissolved in 1 L of water. Fifty percent of the available chlorine remains in compound

TABLE 51-12. Water Disinfection Techniques and Halogen Doses

	ADDED TO 1 L OR QT OF WATER	
IODINATION TECHNIQUES	AMOUNT FOR 4 ppm	AMOUNT FOR 8 ppm
Iodine tabs: tetraglycine hydroperiodide EDWGT (emergency drinking water germicidal tablet) Potable Aqua Globaline	½ tab	1 tab
2% iodine solution (tincture)	0.2 ml 5 gtts	0.4 ml 10 gtts
10% povidone-iodine solution*	0.35 ml 8 gtts	0.70 ml 16 gtts
Saturated solution: iodine crystals in water	13 ml	26 ml
Saturated solution: iodine crystals in alcohol	0.1 ml	0.2 ml
CHLORINATION TECHNIQUES	AMOUNT FOR 5 ppm	AMOUNT FOR 10 ppm
Household bleach: 5% sodium hypochlorite	0.1 ml 2 gtts	0.2 ml 4 gtts
AquaClear: sodium dichloroisocyanurate		1 tab
AquaCure, AquaPure, Chlor-floc: chlorine plus flocculating agent		8 ppm/tab

Measure with dropper (1 drop = 0.05 ml) or tuberculin syringe.
*Povidone-iodine solutions release free iodine in levels adequate for disinfection, but scant data are available.

TABLE 51-13. Recommendations for Contact Time with Halogens in the Field

CONCENTRATION OF HALOGEN	CONTACT TIME IN MINUTES AT VARIOUS WATER TEMPERATURES		
	5° C	15° C	30° C
2 ppm	240	180	60
4 ppm	180	60	45
8 ppm	60	30	15

Recent data indicate that very cold water requires prolonged contact time with iodine or chlorine to kill *Giardia* cysts. These contact times have been extended from the usual recommendations in cold water to account for this and for the uncertainty of residual concentration.

and is released as free chlorine is consumed by halogen demand. NaDCC is a stable, nontoxic chlorine compound that forms a mildly acidic solution, which is optimal for hypochlorous acid, the most active disinfectant of the free chlorine compounds. To disinfect large quantities of water, tablets are also available in 340 and 500 mg of NaDCC and in screw-cap tubs.

Chlorination-flocculation. Chlor-floc, AquaPure, and AquaCure tablets were devised for the military in South Africa and are now becoming widely available in the United States. They contain alum and 1.4% available chlorine in the form of dichloroisocyanurate (sodium dichloro-s-triazinetrione) with proprietary flocculating agents. Bicarbonate in the tablets promotes rapid dissolution and acts as a buffer. One 600-mg tablet yields 8 mg/L of free chlorine. In clear water without enough impurities to flocculate, the alum causes some cloudiness and leaves a strong chlorine residual. However, this is an excellent one-step technique for cloudy and highly polluted water. After treatment, water should be poured through a special cloth to remove floc and decrease turbidity. Testing by the U.S. military demonstrated biocidal effectiveness similar to iodine tablets under most conditions.[153,155,156] Extended contact time was necessary for complete viral removal in some of the tests. Because of the ability to flocculate turbid water, the action was superior to iodine in some poor-quality water. The tablets are stable for 3 years if stored in their packaging out of the heat. (See Table 51-15.)

SUPERCHLORINATION-DECHLORINATION. The Sanitizer is a method of field chlorination that uses first superchlorination and then dechlorination. High doses of chlorine are added to the water in the form of calcium hypochlorite crystals. Concentrations of 30 to 200 ppm of free chlorine are reached at the recommended doses. These extremely high levels are above the margin of safety for field conditions and rapidly kill all bacteria, viruses, and protozoa but probably not *Cryptosporidium.* After at least 10 to 15 minutes, several drops of 30% hydrogen peroxide solution are added. This reduces hypochlorite to chloride, forming calcium chloride (a common food additive), which remains in solution, as follows:

$$Ca(OCl)_2 + 2\,H_2O \rightarrow 2\,HOCl + Ca^{++}\,(OH^-)_2$$

$$Ca(OCl)_2 + 2\,H_2O_2 \leftrightarrow CaCl_2 + 2\,H_2O + 2\,O_2$$

Excess hydrogen peroxide reacts with water to form oxygen and water. Chloride has no taste or smell. Hydrogen peroxide is also a weak disinfectant,[229] although not in common use.

The process of superchlorination-dechlorination with different reagents is used in some large-scale disinfection plants to avoid long contact times and to remove tastes and smells. High doses of chlorine remove or oxidize hydrogen sulfide and some other chemical contaminants that contribute to poor taste and odor. Chlorine bleaches organic matter, making water sparkling blue, as in swimming pools.[221]

The minor disadvantage of a two-step process is offset by excellent taste. Measurements to titrate peroxide to the estimated amount of chlorine do not need to be exact, but some experience is needed to balance the two and achieve optimal results. This is a good technique for highly polluted or cloudy water and for disinfecting large quantities. It is the best technique for storing water on boats or for emergency use. A high level of chlorine prevents growth of algae or bacteria during storage; water is then dechlorinated in needed quantities when ready to use.

The two reagents must be kept tightly sealed to maintain potency of the reagents. Properly stored, calcium hypochlorite loses only 3% to 5% of available chlorine per year. Thirty-percent peroxide is corrosive and burns skin, so it should be used cautiously.

Iodine

Iodine has been used as a topical and water disinfectant since the beginning of the twentieth century.[107] Iodine is effective in low concentrations for killing bacteria, viruses, and cysts, and in higher concentration against fungi and even bacterial spores, but it is a poor algicide[34,74,134] (see Table 51-11 and Figure 51-3). Iodine has been used successfully in low concentrations for continuous water disinfection of small communities.[103] Despite several advantages over chlorine disinfection, it has not gained general acceptance because of concern for its physiologic activity.

Chemistry. Iodine is the only halogen that is a solid at room temperature. Of the halogens, it has the highest atomic weight, lowest oxidation potential, and lowest water solubility. Its disinfectant activity in water is quite complex because of formation of various chemical intermediates with variable germicidal efficiencies. Seven different ions or molecules are present in pure aqueous iodine solutions, but only elemental (diatomic) iodine (I_2) and hypoiodous acid (HOI) play major roles as germicides. Diatomic iodine reacts in water to form the following compounds[34,74]:

$$I_2 + H_2O \leftrightarrow HOI + I^- + H^+$$

I_2 is two to three times as cysticidal and six times as sporicidal as HOI, because it more easily diffuses through the cyst wall. Conversely, HOI is 40 times as virucidal and three to four times as bactericidal as I_2, since inactivation of organisms depends directly on oxidation potential, without involving cell wall diffusion.[33] Their relative concentrations are determined by pH and concentration of iodine in solution.[34] At pH 7.0 and 0.5 ppm of iodine, the concentrations of I_2 and HOI are approximately equal, resulting in a broad spectrum of germicidal action. At pH 5.0 to 6.0, most of the iodine is present as I_2, whereas at pH 8.0, 12% is present as I_2 and 88% as HOI. At higher concentrations of iodine, more HOI is present. Under field conditions, I_2 is the major disinfectant for which doses are calculated.[34]

Other chemical species, including triiodide (I_3^-), iodate (HIO_3), and iodide (I^-), form under certain conditions but play no role in water disinfection.[34,47] Iodide is important because it readily forms when reducing substances are added to iodine solution. Iodide ion is without any effect for water disinfection and also has no taste or color, but is still physiologically active.

Toxicity. The main issue with iodine is its physiologic activity, potential toxicity, and allergenicity.[147] Acute toxic responses generally result from intentional overdoses of iodine, with corrosive effects in the gastrointestinal tract leading to hemorrhagic gastritis. Mean lethal dose is probably about 2 to 4 g of free iodine or 1 to 2 ounces of strong tincture.[62] Toxicity is limited by rapid conversion of iodine to iodide by food (especially starch) in the stomach and early reflex vomiting. Iodide is absorbed into the bloodstream but has minimal toxicity (it is used widely for radiographic imaging).

Sensitivity reactions, including rashes and acne, may occur with usual supplementation levels of iodine. Given the necessity of iodine, it is not clear why some people react to certain forms of the substance, such as iodized salt. As with other sensitivity reactions, these may occur with very low doses. Acute allergy to iodide is rare and manifests as individual hypersensitivity, such as angioneurotic and laryngeal edema.[147]

Chronic iodide poisoning, or iodism, occurs after prolonged ingestion of sufficiently high doses, but marked individual variation is seen. Symptoms simulate upper respiratory illness, with irritation of mucous membranes, mucus production, and cough.

A major disadvantage of iodine is its physiologic activity with effects on thyroid function. Iodine is an essential element for normal thyroid function and health in small amounts of 100 to 300 μg/day, but excess amounts can result in thyroid dysfunction. Maximum safe level and duration of iodine ingestion are not clearly defined, making it difficult to provide recommendations for prolonged use in water treatment.

THYROID EFFECTS OF EXCESS IODINE INGESTION. Most persons can tolerate high doses of iodine without development of thyroid abnormalities, because the thyroid gland has an autoregulatory mechanism that effectively manages excessive iodine intake. Initially, excess iodine suppresses production of thyroid hormone, but production usually returns to normal in a few days.

Iodine-induced hyperthyroidism can result from iodine ingestion by persons with underlying thyroid disease or when iodine is given to persons with prior iodine deficiency.[21,179] During the worldwide campaign to eliminate endemic goiter and cretinism, 1% to 2% of residents developed hyperthyroidism from small amounts of dietary iodine supplementation. Groups at higher risk were elderly persons, Graves' disease patients (especially after antithyroid therapy), and patients taking pharmacologic sources of iodine. Hyperthyroidism has been reported from iodine use as a water disinfectant in two travelers. Both were from iodine-sufficient areas and had antithyroid antibodies, suggesting underlying thyroiditis; one had a mother and sister with Hashimoto's thyroiditis.[111]

Iodine-induced hypothyroidism or goiter is much more common from excessive iodine intake. Hypothyroidism is attributed to prolonged suppression of thyroid hormone production induced by excess iodine levels, but the mechanism through which iodide goiter is produced is not well understood. The incidence of goiter varies and does not correlate well with quantity of iodine or with the level of hypothyroidism. Recently, goiters were discovered among a group of Peace Corps volunteers in Africa and were linked epidemiologically to the use of iodine resin water filters.[102] Forty-four (46%) of the volunteers had enlarged thyroids, but 30 of these had normal thyroid function tests.

Iodine-induced hypothyroidism or goiter may occur with or without underlying thyroid disease but is more common in several groups[21,179,224]: (1) those with underlying thyroid problems, including prior treatment for Graves' disease or subtotal thyroidectomy; (2) fetuses and infants, from placental transfer of iodide from mothers treated with iodides; (3) persons with subclinical hypothyroidism, especially elderly persons, in whom the incidence is 5% to 10%; and (4) patients with excessive iodide from medications (formerly potassium iodide; currently amiodarone).

Neonatal goiter is especially worrisome because it can lead to asphyxia during birth or hypothyroidism with mental impairment. Daily intakes as small as 12 mg have been reported to produce congenital iodide goiters, but generally much higher doses are required.

DOSE-RESPONSE OR THRESHOLD LEVEL. It is unclear what percent of the population will respond adversely to excess iodine or what should be defined as excess intake. The majority of people can tolerate high doses of iodine with no ill effects.[21] The reported incidences of goiter, hypothyroid effects, and hyperthyroid response vary so widely that they provide no clear dose limits.[147] The use of iodine for decades in the military and civilian population without reports of associated clinical thyroid problems suggests that the risks are minimal and would be outweighed by the risk of enteric disease. However, biochemical assays show that changes in thyroid function tests are common with excess iodine intake.

In controlled trials, iodine was administered to healthy volunteers, 30 to 70 mg/day for 14 to 90 days.[132,171] Two studies simulated field use of four iodine tablets (32 mg) per day.[69,110] All found the same changes in thyroid function: an increase in thyroid-stimulating hormone (TSH) and decrease in triiodothyronine (T_3) and thyroxine (T_4) within 1 to 2 weeks and persisting throughout iodine ingestion. Paul et al,[145] studied the minimum dose that would cause alterations in thyroid function and found that 1.5 mg/day decreased TSH, but not 500 and 750 μg/day. These changes were statistically significant from baseline but usually remained within the range of normal values. Even when outside the normal range, the changes in thyroid function remained subclinical. Thyroid enlargement was sometimes noted when evaluated by ultrasound. All changes reverted to normal within weeks to months without persistent thyroid disease.

Studying longer duration of ingestion, Freund[65] found minimal changes and no clinical problems when water with 1 mg/L of iodine was given to prisoners for up to 3 years. Referring to the same project, Thomas et al[201] reported that after 15 years of ongoing iodine use at 1 mg/L, iodinated water caused no decrease in serum concentrations of T_4 below normal values and no allergic reactions. Patients with prior thyroid disease had no recurrence with iodinated water; four patients with active hyperthyroidism were treated in standard fashion, and their condition remained well controlled despite the extra iodine intake. Also, 177 inmates gave birth to 181 full-term infants, and no neonatal goiters were detected.[200]

The military studied long-term toxic effects of iodine, adding sodium iodide to drinking water at a naval base for 6 months.[129] The estimated daily dose of iodine per person was 12 mg for the first 16 weeks and 19.2 mg for the next 10 weeks. No evidence of functional changes or damage in the thyroid gland, cardiovascular system, bone marrow, eyes, or kidneys was noted. No increase in skin diseases, no sensitization to iodine, and no impaired wound healing or resolution of infections was evident.

Treatment of subclinical thyroid disease is controversial, even the chronic cases found on a serologic diagnostic battery.[41,80] With a history of excess iodine ingestion, most experts would first stop the iodine intake and follow thyroid function before treating hypothyroidism.

Recommendations. The tenth edition of the recommended dietary allowances (RDAs, 1989) set the allowable dose to 1.0 mg/day for children and up to 2.0 mg/day for adults (increased from 0.5 to 1.0 mg in the ninth edition, 1980), primarily based on the data from Freund and Thomas.[147]

Possible toxicity with intermediate- to long-term use of iodine and the question of iodide toxicity remain controversial. The EPA and the World Health Organization (WHO), supported by the American Water Works Association (AWWA), have recommended iodine use for water disinfection only as an emergency measure for short periods of about 3 weeks.[218,233] However, this period of short use appears arbitrary.

The following groups should not use iodine for water treatment because of their increased susceptibility to thyroid problems:

Pregnant women

Persons with known hypersensitivity to iodine

Persons with a history of thyroid disease, even if controlled by medication

Persons with a strong family history of thyroid disease (thyroiditis)

Persons from areas with chronic dietary iodine deficiency

Available data suggests the following:

1. High levels of iodine, such as those produced by recommended doses of iodine tablets, should be limited to periods of 1 month or less.
2. Iodine treatment that produces a low residual (1 mg/L or less) appears safe, even for long periods in people with normal thyroid function. Iodine resin devices with a charcoal stage to remove residual iodine, or iodination followed by microfiltration that includes a charcoal stage, should allow prolonged use. Concern for International Space Station crew members who would be using iodin-

ated water for 6 months prompted the National Aeronautics and Space Administration (NASA) to use an exchange resin to reduce residual iodine concentration from 3 or 4 to 0.25 mg/L.[121]
3. Persons planning to use iodine for a prolonged period should have the thyroid gland examined and thyroid function measured to ensure that a state of euthyroidism exists.

Formulations. Several forms of iodine are available for field use (Tables 51-12 to 51-14).

IODINE SOLUTIONS. Iodine solutions commercially sold as topical disinfectants are inexpensive and can be measured accurately with a dropper but are staining and corrosive if spilled. These contain iodine, potassium, or sodium iodide in water, and ethyl alcohol or glycerol (Table 51-14). Iodide improves stability and solubility but has no germicidal activity and adds to the total amount of iodine ingested and absorbed into the body.

Iodophors are solutions in which diatomic iodine is bound to a neutral polymer of high molecular weight, giving the iodine greater solubility and stability with less toxicity and corrosive effect.[34,74] Povidone-iodine is a 1-vinyl-2-pyrrolidinone polymer with 9% to 12% available iodine. The iodophors are routinely used for topical disinfection, since they have less tissue toxicity than iodine solutions. Although they are not approved for water disinfection in the United States, they are used in other countries for this purpose.[10] According to the manufacturer, approval for this use in the United States was not pursued because the anticipated use did not justify the expense. Povidone is nontoxic and was used as a blood expander during World War II.

In aqueous solution, povidone-iodine provides a sustained-release reservoir of halogen; free iodine is released in water solution depending on the concentration (normally, 2 to 10 ppm is present in solution). In dilutions below 0.01%, povidone-iodine solution can be regarded as a simple aqueous solution of iodine.[74] One report found these compounds similar in germicidal efficiency to other iodine-iodide solutions.[34] Data indicate persistence of about 2 ppm of free iodine at a 1:10,000 dilution,[74] which corresponds to a 0.001% solution made by adding 0.1 ml (2 drops) to 1 L of water. However, another study found conflicting values for

TABLE 51-14. Iodine Solutions

PREPARATION	IODINE (%)	IODIDE (%)	TYPE OF SOLUTION
Iodine topical solution	2.0	2.4 (sodium)	Aqueous
Lugol's solution	5.0	10.0 (potassium)	Aqueous
Iodine tincture	2.0	2.4 (sodium)	Aqueous-ethanol
Strong iodine solution	7.0	9.0 (potassium)	Ethanol (85%)

available iodine and free iodine (measured by different techniques). Bactericidal effect on *Pseudomonas* and *Staphylococcus* bacteria increased at dilutions of 1:100, compared with 10% stock solutions, but dilutions of 1:10,000 were not bactericidal.[14] The complex chemistry of povidone-iodine solutions accounts for these conflicting data. Since free residual iodine can be measured at the concentration used for water disinfection, it should be effective. Personal and anecdotal experience of others attest to its effectiveness in field use.[10]

TABLETS. The two types of iodine tablets are those that depend on a chemical reaction to convert iodide into iodine and those in which the iodine exists as hydroperiodide.[172] The tablets used by the U.S. military and sold in the United States for water disinfection contain tetraglycine hydroperiodide, which is 40% I_2 and 20% iodide.[34,131] Tetraglycine hydroperiodide tablets are sold as Globaline, Potable Aqua, and EDWGT (emergency drinking water germicidal tablet). Each tablet releases 8 mg/L of elemental iodine into water.[34,131,140,172] An acidic buffer provides a pH of 6.5, which supports better cysticidal than virucidal capacity but should be adequate for both. Tablets have the advantages of easy handling and no danger of staining or corroding if spilled. They are stable for 4 to 5 years under sealed storage conditions and for 2 weeks with frequent opening under field conditions, but they lose 30% of the active iodine if bottles are left open for 4 days in high heat or humidity.

Tetraglycine hydroperiodide was originally developed and chosen as a preferred technique by the military for individual field use because of its broad-spectrum disinfection effect, ease of handling, rapid dissolution, stability, and acceptable taste.[34,99,131,140,154] The military requirements dictated a short contact time (10 minutes in clear, warm water)-thus the relatively high concentration of iodine (8 ppm) compared with other iodination techniques. The recommended dose has been increased to two tablets in cold water to ensure disinfection with short contact times. With adequate contact time, one tablet can be added to 2 quarts of water to yield 4 ppm of free iodine (Table 51-15).

Potable Aqua is now sold with "neutralizing" tablets made of ascorbic acid. Ascorbic acid converts iodine to iodide, removing the taste and color and stopping the disinfection action of iodine, but does not change the physiologic load of ingested iodine.

The Australian military developed the other type of iodine tablet (e.g., Afses). The tablet contains a combination of potassium iodide and potassium iodate together with an acidic material (potassium permanganate) that catalyzes a reaction to form iodine.[172] The advantage is this tablet's resistance to thermal deterioration, but it is highly sensitive to traces of moisture. It is formulated to release 8 mg/L of free iodine, but the

TABLE 51-15. Data on Microcidal Efficacy of Iodine and Chlorine Tablets

HALOGEN	DOSE	FRH (mg/L)	TIME (min)	TEMPERATURE (°C)	ORGANISM	LOG REDUCTION	REFERENCE
ChlorFloc	1 or 2 tabs	4-7	5	10-20	Bacteria	6	156
		4-14	20	10-20	*Giardia muris*	3	
			5	10-20	Rotavirus	4	
			20	10-20	Poliovirus	Inadequate	
	1 tab		12	25	Poliovirus	Inadequate	
Globaline	2 tabs		20	Various	Bacteria	6	
			45	5	*G. muris*	3	
			20	5	Rotavirus	4	
			60	5	Poliovirus	60	
AquaPure	2 tabs	7-11	40	5			155
	1 tab		30-40	15-25	Bacteria	6	
				15-25	Rotavirus	4	
				15-25	Polio virus	2	
			20	15-25	*G. muris*	2	
Globaline	2 tabs	10	60	15	*Giardia*	3	157
	1 tab		180	5	*Giardia*	3	
	2 tabs		120	5	*Giardia*	3	
Iodine	1 or 2 tabs	8-16	60	5-25	Hepatitis A	4	192
		8	60	5	Poliovirus, echovirus	Inadequate	
		16	60	5	Poliovirus, echovirus	4	

FRH, Free residual halogen.

actual amount measured in water is more variable than that released by Potable Aqua, so its biocidal performance is not as good. The tablet also contains more iodide than Potable Aqua, which contributes to potential adverse effects.[202]

CRYSTALS (SATURATED SOLUTION). Because of limited solubility in water, iodine crystals may be used for disinfection. In one technique for field use, 4 to 8 g of crystalline iodine is put in a 1- to 2-ounce bottle, which is then filled with water.[99] A small amount of elemental iodine goes into solution (no significant iodide is present); the saturated solution is used to disinfect drinking water. Water can be added to the crystals hundreds of times before they are completely dissolved.

Since the amount of iodine dissolved depends on the temperature of the solution (200 ppm at 10° C, 300 ppm at 20° C, 400 ppm at 30° C),[34,74,221] the bottle should be kept warm or the amount added to drinking water adjusted for temperature of the iodine crystal solution. In the field, it may be easier to warm the bottle in an inner pocket than to estimate temperature and adjust the dose. The supernatant should be carefully decanted or filtered to avoid ingestion of the crystals[232]; this is aided by the weight of the crystals, which causes them to sink. Many people prefer crystalline iodine because of its large disinfectant capacity, small size, and light weight. A commercial product (Polar Pure) has made iodine crystals readily available in camping supply stores.

An alternative technique is to add 8 g of iodine crystals to 100 ml of 95% ethanol.[222] Increased solubility of iodine in alcohol makes the solution less temperature dependent and allows much smaller volumes to be used (8 mg/0.1 ml), which can be measured with a 1-ml syringe or dropper (2 drops).

The stability and simplicity of iodine crystals have led to their testing for in-line systems that provide continuous water disinfection for remote households and small communities. In these designs, residual iodine is removed with GAC.[57,205]

RESINS. Iodine resins have great potential for water disinfection in individual or small systems and have been incorporated into many different filter designs available for field use. They provide many advantages over chlorination systems by eliminating the need for chemical feed systems, residual monitoring, and contact time.[218] Iodine resins are considered demand disinfectants because they are minimally insoluble in water and little iodine is released into aqueous solution. However, when a microorganism comes into contact with the resin, iodine apparently transfers to the microorganism aided by electrostatic forces, binds to the wall or capsule, penetrates and kills the organism.[116]

Iodine resins are engineered to produce low residuals in effluent water. The initial iodine residual with pentaiodide resin produces a constant 1 to 2 ppm after initial use, whereas triiodide resin produces a residual iodine concentration of less than 0.20 ppm at equilibrium.[116] The concentration in the eluent of triiodide resin is temperature dependent. Concentrations less than 1.0 ppm were obtained with water at 42.2° C (108° F), but this increased to a total iodine content of 6 to 10 ppm at 71° C (160° F). After returning to room temperature, the iodine residual returned to nominal values.[116]

Measurable iodine is attached to bacteria and cysts after resin treatment, effectively exposing the organisms to high iodine concentrations. This allows reduced contact time compared with dilute iodine solutions.[61,116] Some contact time still appears necessary.[117] Fifty percent of *Giardia* cysts were viable 10 minutes after passage through a triiodine resin. Viable *Giardia* cysts could be recovered in 4°-C (39.2°-F) water 40 minutes after passage through an iodine resin.[117] PUR Traveler cup filters failed to pass the EPA protocol for "worst-case" water unless water was passed through the filter twice. The data implied that a holding (contact) time could have achieved the same results.[70] The Canadian Health Department, challenging an in-line triiodine resin with highly polluted water, also found that a 15-minute contact time was necessary for warm water and 30-minute contact time for cold water.[57] The EPA conducted tests of triiodide resin against *E. coli* but not against other organisms, for which it relied on independent testing. It concluded that the product depends on a 0.2-ppm residual and that additional testing would be necessary below this level.

Resins are chemically and physically stable during conditions of dry storage at room temperature. Aqueous suspensions or resins retain biocidal potential for 15 years. No alteration in activity was observed after dry storage for 1 month at 50° C (122° F).[116]

Resins have proved effective against bacteria, viruses, and cysts but not against *Cryptosporidium parvum* oocysts or bacterial spores.[116] When *Cryptosporidium* oocysts were passed through a triiodide resin column, most were retained in the resin column, probably by electrostatic attraction to the resin. Of those that passed through, only a small percentage were inactivated within 30 minutes by the iodine.[208]

Despite the controversy regarding contact time, most of the testing done with iodine resins has shown high levels of effectiveness, and products have demonstrated their ability to meet the EPA guidelines for reduction of microorganisms (see Table 51-8). Recently, however, iodine resin products from two different companies (SweetWater with Viralguard and PUR filters) were withdrawn from the market when company testing showed that they failed to meet viral inactivation standards of 4-log reduction. The units had previously obtained EPA registration on the basis of successful testing contracted through a laboratory that does the majority of testing for the filter industry. This variation of test results is disconcerting for several reasons, including the source of test variability, credibility of the original laboratory, and the effectiveness of the iodine resin, which is used in the products of other manufacturers.

Iodine resin filters. Iodine resins have been incorporated into a broad line of filters for field use (see Appendix). Optimal designs incorporate two stages in addition to the iodine resin. A microfilter, generally 1 micron (micrometer), effectively removes *Cryptosporidium, Giardia,* and other halogen-resistant parasitic eggs or larva. Since iodine resins kill bacteria and viruses rapidly, no significant contact time is required for most water.[70] The addition of a third stage of activated charcoal removes dissolved residual; however, the importance of iodine residual for disinfection has not been determined.[117,205] Testing by one filter company demonstrated that a carbon block could reduce 16 mg/L of iodine to less than 0.01 mg/L for 150 gallons, which was close to the expected lifetime of its ceramic filter.[181] The effective removal of residual iodine makes the iodine resin filters safe for long-term use. For effective performance of activated charcoal, it must be replaced periodically.

In conclusion, iodine resins are effective disinfectants that can be engineered into attractive field products, including use in the space shuttle and large-scale units for international disasters. They may prove useful for small communities in undeveloped and rural areas where chlorine disinfection is technically and economically unfeasible. However, more testing is needed on specific products to ensure adequate resin contact, to define the need for contact time, and to confirm whether a residual iodine concentration is needed.

Chlorine vs. Iodine

A few investigators have reported data suggesting ineffectiveness of common halogen preparations. Jarroll et al[93,94] tested six methods of field disinfection and found that none achieved high levels of *Giardia* inactivation at the recommended dose and times. However, this failure simply reflected the need for longer contact times in cold water.[112] Ongerth et al[143] tested seven chemical treatments for *Giardia* inactivation in clear and turbid water at 10° C (50° F). None achieved 99.9% reduction in 30 minutes. All iodine-based chemical methods were effective at 8 hours, but none of the chlorine preparations was effective, even after this extended time. Although these results after 30 minutes in cold water are to be expected, the 8-hour results do not conform with other experimental data on chlorine. Unfortunately, the authors did not test for residual halogen, although initial levels achieved should have been effective, and they did not test at regular time intervals

to determine when the iodine methods had achieved the target reduction of organisms.

A large body of data proves that both iodine and chlorine are effective disinfectants with adequate concentrations and contact times (cold temperatures equate with slow disinfection time for both). Comparing effectiveness between chlorine and iodine is difficult because of the different ionic species and compounds that may exist under varying conditions.[84] Chlorine and iodine tablets have been directly compared under identical water test conditions and found to be similar in their biocidal activity in most conditions using recommended dose and contact time[153] (see Tables 51-12, 51-13, and 51-15.) Contact times in Table 51-13 are extended from the previous recommendations for treatment in cold water to provide a margin of safety and to ensure high levels of cyst destruction.

Iodine has several advantages over chlorine. Of the halogens, iodine has the lowest oxidation potential, reacts least readily with organic compounds, is least soluble, is least hydrolyzed by water, and is less affected by pH, all of which indicate that low iodine residuals should be more stable and persistent than corresponding concentrations of chlorine.[47,74,103,134]

Taste

Objectionable taste and smell are the major problems with acceptance of halogens. These depend on specific chemical compounds. Most people are familiar with the taste of chlorine (hypochlorite); tap water usually contains 0.2 to 0.5 ppm of chlorine, swimming pools 1.5 to 3.0 ppm, and hot tubs 3.0 to 5.0 ppm. Most persons note a distinct taste at 5 ppm and a strong, unpleasant taste at 10 to 15 ppm.[172] Hypochlorous acid and chloride have no taste or odor.[221] Most objectionable tastes in treated water are derived from dissolved minerals, such as sulfur, and from chlorine compounds, chloramines, and organic nitrogen compounds, even at extremely low levels.

Elemental iodine at 1 mg/L is undetectable. Most persons can detect iodine solutions at 1.5 to 2 mg/L but do not find it objectionable.[17,47,66] Eight ppm of iodine produces a distinct taste and odor; however, tablets yielding these concentrations were preferred by military personnel over tincture of iodine in equivalent doses.[34,131] Iodide ion has no color or taste.

Taste tolerance or preference for iodine over chlorine is individual. Opposite preferences have been documented when direct comparisons are done.[140,155] I believe that most persons prefer the taste of iodine to chlorine at concentrations typically used in the field. In addition, iodine forms fewer organic compounds that produce highly objectionable taste and smell.

Minimal Dosage. Taste can be improved by several means (Box 51-3). One method is to use the relationship

Box 51-3   IMPROVING THE TASTE OF HALOGENS

Decrease dose and increase contact time.
Clarify cloudy water, allowing decreased halogen.
Use iodine resin.
Remove halogen:
    Granular activated carbon
    Chemical reduction
        Ascorbic acid
        Sodium thiosulfate
        Chlorination-dechlorination (Sanitizer)
        KDF (zinc-copper) brush or media
Use alternative techniques:
    Heat
    Filtration

between halogen concentration and time and to give the minimum necessary dose, allowing a longer contact time (see Table 51-13). *Giardia* cysts and viruses can be killed with doses of chlorine or iodine of 2 ppm or less (see Figure 51-3).[63,83,107] Wilderness travelers usually can allow a longer contact time for water disinfection.

Theoretically, doubling the contact time allows a 50% reduction of halogen dose at any level. Although this relationship holds true at the higher field doses of halogens, as the levels drop, the reaction departs from mathematical models, and the straight-line graph has a "tail" (see Figure 51-2). This departure from strict first-order kinetics and the uncertainty of halogen demand in field disinfection mean that a margin of safety must be incorporated into contact times at lower doses.

Of all standard iodine doses, iodine tablets yield the highest dose (8 mg/L with an intended contact time of 10 minutes in warm water). The tablets cannot be broken in half but can be added to 2 quarts instead of 1 quart to yield concentrations consistent with the other preparations. In recommended doses the liquid preparations of iodine yield 4 mg/L. Since even clear surface water has some halogen demand, this dose of 4 mg/L should generally not be reduced. The exception would be for backing up tap water in developing countries, when the dose may routinely be cut in half for an added dose of 2 ppm with a few hours of contact time. For chlorination methods that add 5 mg/L, adding half the amount to clean surface water should be adequate if the contact time is tripled. Even less could be used for tap water. None of these concentrations will destroy *Cryptosporidium* oocysts.

Effective disinfection with low iodine residual can also be achieved by use of iodine resin filters.

Temperature and organic matter in the water may be manipulated. Increasing the temperature of the water,

especially when initially near 5° C, decreases the Ct constant (see Table 51-13 and Figure 51-2). Filtering water before adding halogen improves the reliability of a given halogen dose by decreasing halogen demand, allowing a lower dose of halogen.[134] Sedimentation or coagulation-flocculation cleans cloudy water and lowers the required halogen dosage considerably, in addition to removing many of the contaminants that contribute to objectionable taste.

Dehalogenation. Halogen can be removed from water after the required contact time. Activated charcoal removes iodine or chlorine, allowing standard or even high doses to be used without residual taste. The relative instability of chlorine in dilute solutions can be used to decrease taste over time. Chlorine residual in an open container decreases 1 mg/L in the first hour, then 0.2 mg/L in the next 5 to 8 hours, for a total of 2.0 to 2.5 mg/L in 24 hours. Ultraviolet light also depletes free chlorine.[221]

Alteration of Chemical Species (Reduction). Several chemical means are available to reduce free iodine or chlorine to iodide or chloride that have no color, smell, or taste. These "ides" have no disinfection action, so the techniques should be used only after the required contact time. The Sanitizer uses hydrogen peroxide to "dechlorinate" the water by forming calcium chloride. This reaction with hydrogen peroxide works best if calcium hypochlorite is used as a disinfectant. If bleach (sodium hypochlorite) is used, hydrogen peroxide reacts with chlorine in water to form hydrochloric acid in harmless amounts.

Two other chemicals that may be safely used with any form of chlorine or iodine are ascorbic acid (vitamin C) and sodium thiosulfate. Ascorbic acid is widely available in the crystalline or powder form. Grinding up tablets that have binders may cloud the water. Ascorbic acid is a common ingredient of flavored drink mixes, which accounts for their effectiveness in covering up the taste of halogens.[140,172]

Sodium thiosulfate similarly "neutralizes" iodine and chlorine. A few granules in 1 quart of iodinated water decolorizes and removes the taste of iodine by converting it to iodide. In reaction with chlorine, it forms hydrochloric acid, which is not harmful or detectable in such dilute concentration. Thiosulfate salts are inert in vivo and poorly absorbed from the gastrointestinal tract. Sodium thiosulfate is available at chemical supply stores.

Zinc-copper alloys act as catalysts to reduce free iodine and chlorine through an electrochemical reaction. They also remove or reduce dissolved metals, including heavy metals such as lead, selenium, and mercury. One product incorporated such an alloy into the bristles of a small brush to be stirred in the water after halogen disinfection. It is effective but slow, which limits its use to small volumes of water. Stirring for 1 minute removes 10 mg/L of chlorine from 250 ml of water.

Environmental Protection Agency Registration

Products that are used for treating municipal or private water supplies for drinking are considered pesticides and must be registered by the EPA Pesticide Branch. Registration signifies the following:

1. The composition is such as to warrant the proposed claims.
2. The labeling and other material required to be submitted comply with the requirements of the act.
3. The method will perform its intended function without unreasonable adverse effects on the environment.
4. When used in accordance with widespread and commonly recognized practice, the method will not generally cause unreasonable adverse effects on the environment.

Thus EPA registration implies only that the "pesticide" agent is not released into the water at unsafe levels.[24,39] This is less stringent than for filters that contain halogens.

MISCELLANEOUS DISINFECTANTS

Silver

Silver ion has bactericidal effects in low doses. The literature on antimicrobial effects of silver is confusing and contradictory.[88,134,221,226] Concentrations in water less than 100 parts per billion (ppb) are effective against enteric bacteria. The reaction follows first-order kinetics and is temperature dependent. Calcium, phosphates, and sulfides interfere significantly with silver disinfection. Organic chemicals, amines, and particulate or colloidal matter may also interfere, but no more than with chlorine.

Silver is physiologically active. Acute toxicity does not occur from small doses used in disinfection, but argyria, which is permanent discoloration of the skin and mucous membranes, may result from prolonged use. For this reason a maximum limit of 50 ppb of silver ion in potable water is recommended. At this concentration, disinfection requires several hours.

Experimental results indicate 18% survival of *E. coli* at 3 hours at 40 μg/L. *Salmonella typhi* was reduced more than 5 log at 50 μg/L with a 1-hour exposure; poliovirus was not reduced at 50 μg/L with a 1-hour exposure.[11]

Water disinfection systems using silver have been devised for spacecraft, swimming pools, and other settings.[221] The advantage is absence of taste, odor, and color. Persistence of residual silver concentration allows reliable storage of disinfected water. Silver can be supplied through a silver nitrate solution, desorption from silver-coated materials, or electrolysis. When coated on surfaces, silver acts as a constant-release disinfectant that produces aqueous silver ion concentrations of 0.006 to 0.5 ppm, which are sufficient to disinfect drinking water.[116] Because of this attractive feature, silver-based devices are being designed and tested in developing countries. In Pakistan a nylon bag with silver-coated sand was designed to be placed in earthenware pitchers that store water. Silver incorporated into alum is also being tested in India.[35]

Filters and granular charcoal media are sometimes coated with silver to prevent bacterial growth on the surface, but this does not maintain sterility. A slow, selective action against total coliform count is noted, but none against total bacterial count. Long-term use might overcome any bacteriostatic action initially shown.[68] In an EPA study, effluent populations from the silver-containing units were about as large as those from the units without silver.[11] Bacteria can develop resistance to silver ions through generation of silver reductase.

Large-scale use of silver for water disinfection has been limited by cost, difficulty controlling and measuring silver content, and physiologic effects. Short-term field use is limited by its marked tendency to adsorb onto the surface of any container (resulting in unreliable concentrations) and interference by several common substances. Data on silver for disinfection of viruses and cysts indicate limited effect, even at high doses.[33,134]

The use of silver as a drinking water disinfectant has been much more popular in Europe where silver tablets (MicroPur) are sold widely for field water disinfection. They have not been approved by the EPA for this purpose in the United States, but they were approved as a water preservative to prevent bacterial growth in previously treated and stored water.

Potassium Permanganate

Potassium permanganate is a strong oxidizing agent with some disinfectant properties. It was used extensively before hypochlorites as a drinking water disinfectant.[131] It is still used for this purpose and also for washing fruits and vegetables in parts of the world. It is used in municipal disinfection to control taste and odor and is usually employed in a 1% to 5% solution for disinfection.

Bacterial inactivation can be achieved with moderate concentrations and contact times (45 minutes at 2 mg/L, 15 minutes at 8 mg/L). A 1:5000 (0.5%) solution controlled *V. cholerae* and *S. typhi* contamination of fruits and vegetables. The virucidal action has been tested, but without titrations of virus that remained after various periods of contact time, so the rate of action is not known. In most instances, however, a 1:10,000 solution destroyed the infectivity of virus suspensions in ½ hour at room temperature; 30 mg/L was effective in inactivating HAV within 15 minutes.[203] Although potassium permanganate clearly has disinfectant action, it cannot be recommended for field use, since quantitative data are not available for viruses and no data are available for protozoan cysts, despite the chemical's frequent use in some parts of the world. Packets of 1 g to be added to 1 L of water are sold in some countries. A French military guide from 1940 instructed users: "To sterilize water, use a solution of 1 gram of $KMnO_4$ for 100 grams of water. Add this solution drop by drop to the water to sterilize until the water becomes pink. The operation is considered sufficient if the water remains pink for half an hour."[36] The solutions are deep pink to purple and stain surfaces. The chemical leaves a pink to brown color in water at concentrations above 0.05 mg/L. Small deposits of brown oxides settle to the bottom of the water container. A few drops of alcohol will cause this residual color to disappear.

Hydrogen Peroxide

Hydrogen peroxide is a strong oxidizing agent but a weak disinfectant.[20,134,229] Small doses (1 ml of 3% H_2O_2 in 1 L water) are effective for inactivating bacteria within minutes to hours, depending on the level of contamination. One million colony-forming units/ml of seven bacterial strains were killed overnight, with 80% kill in 1 hour. Viruses require extremely high doses and longer contact times. Although information is lacking on the effect of hydrogen peroxide on protozoa, it is a promising sporicidal agent in high (10% to 25%) concentrations.

Hydrogen peroxide was popular as an antiseptic and disinfectant in the late nineteenth century and remains popular today as a wound cleanser; for odor control in sewage, sludges, and landfill leachates; and for many other applications. It is considered safe enough for use in foods. It is naturally present in milk and honey, helping to prevent spoilage. It yields the innocuous end products oxygen and water. Solutions lose potency in time, but stabilizers can be added to prevent decomposition.[20]

Although hydrogen peroxide can sterilize water, lack of data for protozoal cysts and quantitative data for dilute solutions prevents it from being useful as a field water disinfectant. Its application in superchlorination-dechlorination is effective.

Ultraviolet Light

The germicidal effect of ultraviolet (UV) light is the result of action on the nucleic acids of bacteria and depends on light intensity and exposure time. It is well established that UV light can inactivate bacteria, viruses, and protozoans when administered in sufficient dose. However, cysts should probably be removed by filtration. UV treatment does not require chemicals and does not affect the taste of the water. It works rapidly, and an overdose to the water presents no danger; in fact, it is a safety factor. UV light has no

residual disinfection power; water may become recontaminated, or regrowth of bacteria may occur.[58] Particulate matter can shield microorganisms from UV rays.

UV disinfection units are cumbersome and require power, so they are not well adapted to use by small groups in the wilderness. However, an intriguing question is whether direct sunlight can disinfect small quantities of water. One investigation tested the ability of sunlight to disinfect oral rehydration salt solution in clear polyethylene bags or plastic containers contaminated by sewage.[1] After 1 hour in sun the coliform bacteria count was zero. UV and thermal inactivation were strongly synergistic for the solar disinfection of drinking water in transparent plastic bottles that was heavily contaminated with *E. coli* for temperatures above 45° C (113° F). Above 55° C (131° F) thermal inactivation is of primary importance.[120] Whereas thermal inactivation is effective in turbid water, UV effects are inhibited.[97] Where strong sunshine is available, solar disinfection of drinking water is an effective, low-cost method for improving water quality and may be of particular use in refugee camps and disaster areas. However, thermal effects of sunshine are probably more important than UV rays, with insufficient data to quantify UV results.

Copper and Zinc

A copper and zinc alloy (KDF) has electrochemical properties that can aid in water treatment. Its main actions are through its strong oxidation-reduction (redox) potential of 500 millivolts due to its propensity to exchange electrons with other substances. It is bacteriostatic with some bactericidal activity. Microorganisms are killed by the electrolytic field, and by formation of hydroxyl radicals and peroxide water molecules. Although KDF has been ruled a "pesticidal device" by the EPA and is used in industry to decrease bacteria levels and control bacterial growth, it should not be used as the sole means of water treatment. KDF is most often used to reduce or remove chlorine, hydrogen sulfide, and heavy metals from water. The redox reactions change contaminants into harmless components: chlorine into chloride, soluble ferrous cations into insoluble ferric hydroxide, and hydrogen sulfide into insoluble copper sulfide. Up to 98% of lead, mercury, nickel, chromium, and other dissolved metals are removed by KDF simply by bonding to the media. KDF controls the buildup of bacteria, algae, and fungi in GAC beds and carbon block filters, extending the life of carbon and improving its effectiveness. KDF media can be manufactured as brushes with wire bristles, fine steel wool-like media, or granules.

A KDF brush removes the taste of chlorine or iodine from treated water. KDF has been incorporated into a few portable field filters but has not yet gained widespread use. In series with charcoal, KDF extends the life of charcoal and increase its effectiveness. Products that claim to be purifiers, with KDF destroying all microorganisms, should be rigorously tested to prove the claims.

Ozone and Chlorine Dioxide

Ozone and chlorine dioxide are highly effective disinfectants widely used in municipal water treatment plants, but until recently, not available in stable form for field use.[221] These are the only disinfectants that have been demonstrated effective against *Cryptosporidium* in typical concentrations.[146]

Two products currently being tested may revolutionize the use of chemicals for field water disinfection. A stabilized solution of chlorine dioxide (Aquamira, McNett Corp., Bellingham, Wash.) is mixed with phosphoric acid, which activates the chemical and is then mixed with water for disinfection. EPA registration for use as a water purifier is pending. Testing data will be available from the company when EPA approval is obtained.

Developed for military use, an electrochemical process converts simple salt into a mixed-oxidant disinfectant containing free chlorine, chlorine dioxide and ozone (MIOX Corp., Albuquerque, NM).[215] The device is currently used in large- and medium-volume water treatment operations but has been reduced to a cigar-sized unit that operates on camera batteries. This will be developed for the civilian market after testing is completed.

Other Disinfection Products

Other products marketed for water disinfection for travelers cannot be recommended until more data become available. These were initially introduced into the health food market but are now being offered to the general travel market.

Citrus juice has biocidal properties. Lemon juice has been shown to destroy *V. cholerae* at a concentration of 2% (equivalent of 2 tablespoons per liter of water) with a contact time of 30 minutes. A pH less than 3.9 is essential, which depends on the concentration of lemon juice and the initial pH of the water. Its activity is greatly reduced in alkaline water.[50]

Traveler's Friend is a product marketed for water disinfection that contains citrus extract. Company-sponsored data are convincing for antibacterial and antiviral activity. However, the product was not tested against *Giardia* cysts. The active chemical disinfectant has not been identified, and a time/dose response has not been generated. Without better data, this product cannot be recommended.

Aerobic Oxygen is advertised not only as a water disinfectant, but also as a cure for headaches and tropical fish diseases. Company literature implies that the active disinfectant could be chlorine dioxide or ozone, but this is not chemically feasible. Company-sponsored

testing demonstrates activity against bacteria and viruses, but not against cysts. No dose/time response has been developed to compare the product against other disinfectants.

PREFERRED TECHNIQUE

Field disinfection techniques and their effects on microorganisms are summarized in Table 51-16. The optimal technique for an individual or group depends on the number of persons to be served, space and weight available, quality of source water, personal taste preferences, and availability of fuel (Table 51-17). The most effective technique may not always be available, but all methods will greatly reduce the load of microorganisms and reduce the risk of illness. For alpine camping with a high-quality source water, any of the primary techniques is adequate. The only limitation for halogens is *Cryptosporidium* cysts, but in high-quality pristine surface water the cysts are generally found in insufficient numbers to pose significant risk. Surface water, even if clear, in undeveloped countries where there is human and animal activity should be considered highly contaminated with enteric pathogens. Optimal protection requires either heat or a two-stage process of filtration and halogens. Iodine resin filters that combine microfiltration, halogen, and activated charcoal are a simple alternative to a two-stage process, but questions have recently surfaced concerning effectiveness against viruses under all water conditions. New techniques utilizing chlorine dioxide may prove to be highly effective.

Water from cloudy low-elevation rivers, ponds, and lakes in developed or undeveloped countries that does not clear with sedimentation should be pretreated with coagulation-flocculation, then disinfected with heat or halogens. Filters can be used but will clog rapidly with silted or cloudy water. Even in the United States, water with agricultural runoff or sewage plant discharge from upstream towns or cities must be treated to remove *Cryptosporidium* and viruses. In addition, water receiving agricultural, industrial, or mining runoff may contain chemical contamination from pesticides, other chemicals, and heavy metals. A filter containing a charcoal element is the best method to remove most chemicals. Coagulation-flocculation or KDF resin will also remove some chemical contamination.

Halogens need to be used when water will be stored, such as on a boat, in a large camp, or for disaster relief. When only heat or filtration is used before storage, recontamination and bacterial growth can occur. Hypochlorite still has many advantages, including cost, ease of handling, and minimal volatilization in tightly covered containers.[126] A minimum residual of 3 to 5 mg/L should be maintained in the water. Superchlo-

TABLE 51-16. Summary of Field Water Disinfection Techniques

	BACTERIA	VIRUSES	*GIARDIA,* AMEBAE	*CRYPTOSPORIDIUM*	NEMATODES, CERCARIAE
Heat	+	+	+	+	+
Filtration	+	±*	+	+	+
Halogens	+	+	+	−†	±‡

*Reverse osmosis is effective. Most filters make no claims for viruses; however, General Ecology claims 4-log virus removal.
†Chlorine dioxide may be effective.
‡Eggs are not susceptible to halogens but have a low risk of waterborne transmission.

TABLE 51-17. Advantages and Disadvantages of Disinfection Techniques

	HEAT	FILTRATION	HALOGENS	FILTRATION PLUS HALOGEN	CLARIFICATION (C-F) PLUS SECOND STEP
Availability	Wood can be scarce	Many commercial choices	Many common and specific products	Includes iodine resin filters	Readily available
Cost	Fuel and stove costs	Moderate expense	Inexpensive	Mainly filter costs	Depends on second stage
Effectiveness	Can sterilize or pasteurize	Most filters not reliable against viruses	*Cryptosporidium* and some parasitic eggs are resistant	Covers all organisms	Highly effective because most microbes removed by C-F
Optimal application	Clear water, but effective for cloudy water	Clear or slightly cloudy; turbid water clogs filters rapidly	Clear; need increased dose if cloudy	Clear; need increased dose if cloudy	Cloudy/turbid water
Taste	Does not change taste	Can improve taste, especially if charcoal stage	Tastes worse unless remove or "neutralize" halogen	Depends on sequence; can improve if allows reduced halogen dose or if filter has charcoal	Improves
Time	Boiling time (minutes)	Filtration time (minutes)	Contact time (minutes to hours)	Combination of two processes	Combination of two processes
Other considerations	Fuel is heavy and bulky	Adds weight and space; requires maintenance to keep adequate flow	Works well for large quantities and for water storage; some understanding of principles is optimal; damaging if spills or if container breaks	Use halogens first if filter has charcoal stage	Best means of cleaning turbid water, followed by halogen, filtration, or heat

C-F, Coagulation-flocculation.

rination-dechlorination is especially useful in this situation because high levels of chlorination can be maintained for long periods, and when ready for use, the water can be poured into a smaller container and dechlorinated. Iodine works for short-term but not prolonged storage, since it is a poor algicide. Silver has been approved by the EPA for preservation of stored water. Storage techniques can decrease risk of contamination. For prolonged storage, a tightly sealed container is best. For water access, narrow-mouth jars or containers with water spigots prevent contamination from repeated contact with hands or utensils.[188]

On oceangoing vessels where water must be desalinated during the voyage, only reverse-osmosis membrane filters are adequate. Halogens should then be added to the water in the storage tanks.

PREVENTION AND SANITATION

In remote settings in developing countries, potable water alone does not necessarily make a substantial difference in the incidence of many gastrointestinal diseases. A study in a Brazilian village showed no reduction in incidence of diarrhea with use of disinfected water. This emphasizes the importance of general hygiene, which requires education and sanitation.[35] A combination of drinking water treatment and sanitation can decrease episodes of diarrhea.[90,124]

Hygiene is also essential for wilderness travelers. A *Shigella* outbreak among river rafters on the Colorado River was investigated and assumed to be waterborne from adjacent Native American communities, but no source was found in the tributaries. It was finally traced to infected guides who were shedding organisms in the stool and contaminating food through poor hygiene.[123] Personal hygiene, mainly handwashing, prevents spread of infection from food contamination during preparation of meals.[123] Simple handwashing with soap and water purified with hypochlorite (bleach) significantly reduced fecal contamination of market-vended beverages in Guatemala.[188] No one with a diarrheal illness should prepare food.

Dishes and utensils should be disinfected by rinsing in chlorinated water, prepared by adding enough household bleach to achieve a distinct chlorine odor.

Prevention of food-borne contamination is also important in preventing enteric illness (see Chapter 52). Washing fruits and vegetables in purified water is a common practice, but little data support its effectiveness. Washing has a mechanical action of removing dirt and microorganisms while the disinfectant kills microorganisms on the surface. However, neither reaches the organisms that are embedded in surface crevices or protected by other particulate matter. When lettuce was seeded with oocysts, then washed and the supernatant examined for cysts, only 25% to 36% of *Cryptosporidium parvum* and 13% to 15% of *C. cayetanensis* oocysts were recovered in the washes. Scanning electron microscopy detected oocysts on the surface of the vegetables after washing.[144] Chlorine, iodine, or potassium permanganate are often used for this purpose. Higher concentrations can be used than would normally be palatable for drinking water. With superchlorination-dechlorination, high-chlorine concentrations are used to rinse vegetables because the chlorine can be removed with the second step. Aquaclear (NaDCC) chlorine tablet instructions suggest 20 mg/L for washing vegetables. Although effective against most microorganisms, these levels would not be effective against *Cryptosporidium* or *Cyclospora.*

The ultimate responsibility is proper sanitation to prevent contamination of water supplies from human waste. UV rays in sunlight eventually inactivate most microorganisms, but rain may first wash pathogens into a water source. In the soil, microorganisms can survive for months.[211] A Sierra Club study found more prolonged survival in alpine environments.[160] The investigator marked group latrines in alpine terrain and returned 1 to 2 years later to dig test trenches. He found a thin crust of decomposition covering unaltered raw waste with high coliform bacteria counts. Microorganisms may percolate through the soil. Most bacteria are retained within 20 inches of the surface, but in sandy soil this increases to 75 to 100 feet[209]; viruses can move laterally 75 to 302 feet.[182] When organisms reach groundwater, their survival is prolonged, and they often appear in surface water or wells.[211]

Some suggest that campers smear feces on rocks. Although desiccation occurs, UV disinfection is not reliable, and feces may wash into the watershed with rain runoff.[37] Moreover, it will be repulsive to other campers. In the Sierras, feces left on the ground generally disappeared within 1 month, but it was not known whether disinfection occurred before decomposition or whether the feces washed away, dried, or were blown in the wind.[160] Despite more rapid decomposition in sunlight rather than underground, burying feces is still preferable in areas that receive regular use. The U.S. military and U.S. Forest Service recommend burial of human waste 8 to 12 inches deep and a minimum of 100 feet from any water.[209,213] Decomposition is hastened by mixing in some dirt before burial. Shallow burying is also not recommended because animals are more likely to find and overturn the feces. Judgment should be used to determine a location that is not likely to allow water runoff to wash organisms into nearby water sources. Groups larger than three persons should dig a common latrine to avoid numerous individual potholes and inadequate disposal. To minimize latrine odor and improve its function, it should not be used for disposal of wastewater.

In some areas the number of individual and group latrines is so great that the entire area becomes contaminated. Therefore sanitary facilities (outhouses) are becoming common in high-use wilderness areas. Popular river canyons require camp toilets, and all waste must be carried out in sealed containers.

APPENDIX

Water Disinfection Devices and Products*

PRODUCT	PRICE	STRUCTURE/FUNCTION
KATADYN		
(Suunto USA, 2151 Las Palmas Dr #F, Carlsbad, CA 92009; 800-543-9124)		All filters contain a 0.2 micron ceramic candle filter, silver impregnated to decrease bacterial growth. Large units also contain silver quartz in center of filter.
Pocket Filter (Figure 51-4)	$250	Hand pump; 40-inch intake hose and strainer, zipper case; size: 10 × 2 inches; weight: 23 oz; flow: 0.75-1.0 L/min; capacity: 13,000-50,000 L.
Replacement filter element	$165	
Minifilter (Figure 51-5)	$90	Smaller, lighter hand pump; 31-inch intake hose and strainer; hard plastic enclosure and pump; size: 7 × 2.75 × 1.75 inches; weight: 9 oz; flow: 0.5 L/min; capacity: about 7000 L.
Combi (Figure 51-6)	$160	Small hand pump with ceramic filter and activated charcoal stage; can brush ceramic to clean or separately replace elements; size: 2.4 × 10.4 inches; weight: 19 oz; flow: 0.5 L/min; capacity: up to 50,000 L, 200 L for charcoal.
KFT Expedition (Figure 51-7)	$1150	Large hand pump with steel stand; size (packed in case): 23 × 6 × 8 inches; weight: 12 lb; flow: 4 L/min; capacity (per filter element): 100,000 L.
Replacement filter element	$90	

*Prices vary considerably and product lines change regularly.

Continued

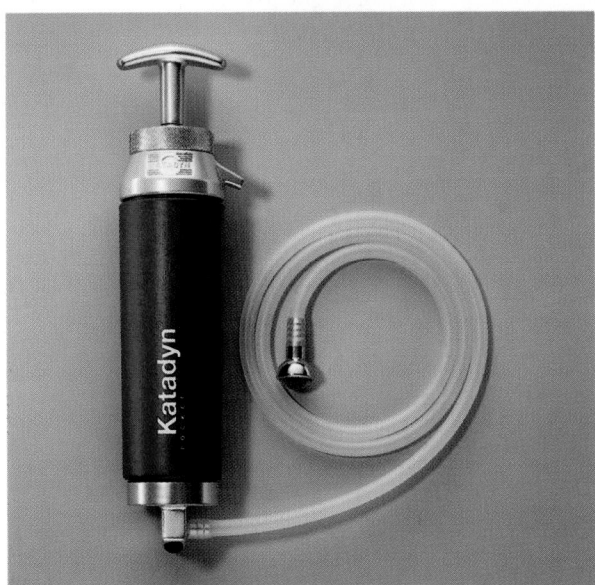

Figure 51-4 Katadyn Pocket Filter.

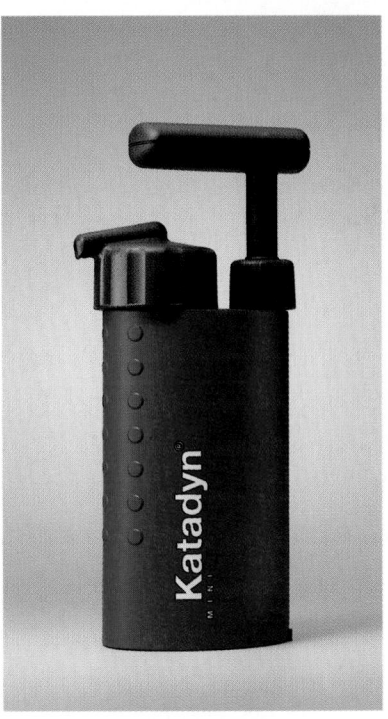

Figure 51-5 Katadyn Minifilter.

PRODUCT	PRICE	STRUCTURE/FUNCTION
KATADYN—cont'd		
Drip filter TRK (Figure 51-8)	$275	Gravity drip from one plastic bucket to another with
Replacement filter (same filter element as hand pump)	$80	3 ceramic candle filter elements; size: 18 × 11-inch diameter (26 inches high when assembled); weight: 9 lb 4 oz; flow: 1 pt/hr (10 gal/day); capacity: 100,000 L.
Syphon (Figure 51-9)	$100	Gravity siphon filter element: 12 × 2 inches; weight: 2 lb; flow: 2 gal/hr; capacity: 5000-20,000 L.

Claims

Filter removes bacterial pathogens, protozoan cysts, parasites, and nuclear debris and clarifies cloudy water. If filter clogs, brushing the filter element (which can be done hundreds of times before replacing filter element) can restore flow. Claims for removal of viruses not made in United States, although testimonials imply effectiveness in all polluted waters. Pocket Filter has a lifetime warranty.

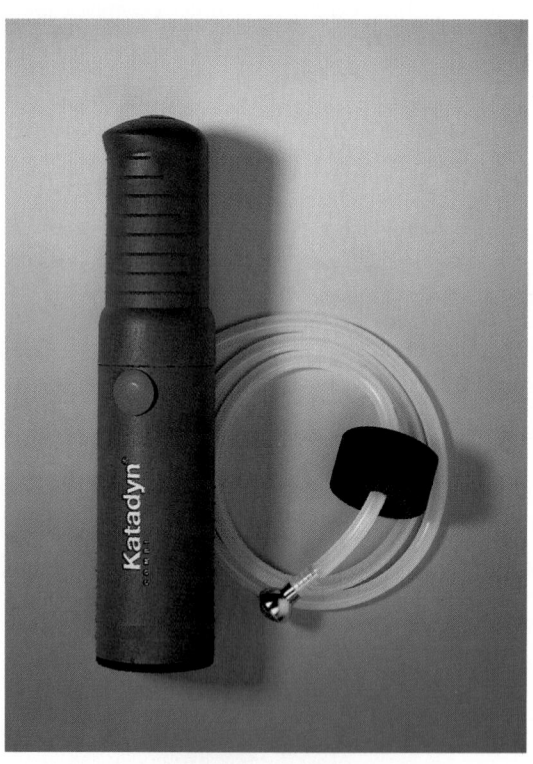

Figure 51-6 Katadyn Combi.

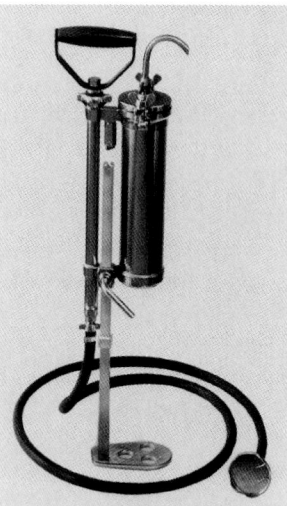

Figure 51-7 Katadyn KFT Expedition filter.

KATADYN—cont'd

Comments

Well-designed, durable products are effective for claims. However, high filter volume capacity is optimistic and not likely to be achieved filtering average surface water. Field tests found the flow comparatively slow, requiring more energy to pump and frequent cleaning. Abrading the outer surface can effectively clean ceramic filters, but the gauge must be used to indicate when filter thickness is excessively diminished.

Pocket Filter is the original, individual or small-group filter design. Metal parts make it durable but the heaviest for its size. Minifilter was designed to be lighter and more cost competitive. Expedition filter is popular for larger groups, especially river trips, where weight is not a factor. Complete virus removal cannot be expected, although most viruses clump or adhere to larger particles and bacteria that can be filtered. Silver impregnation does not prevent bacterial growth in filters.

Continued

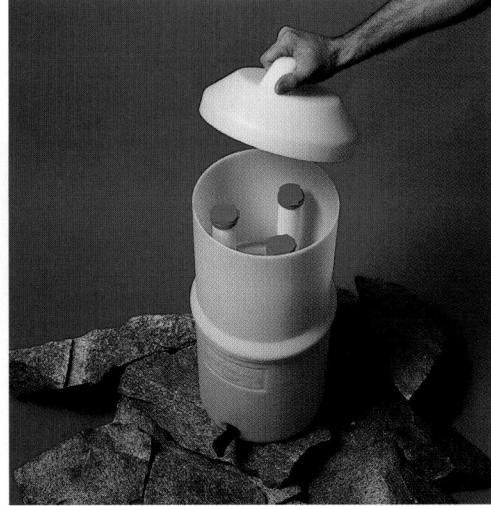

Figure 51-8   Katadyn drip filter TRK.

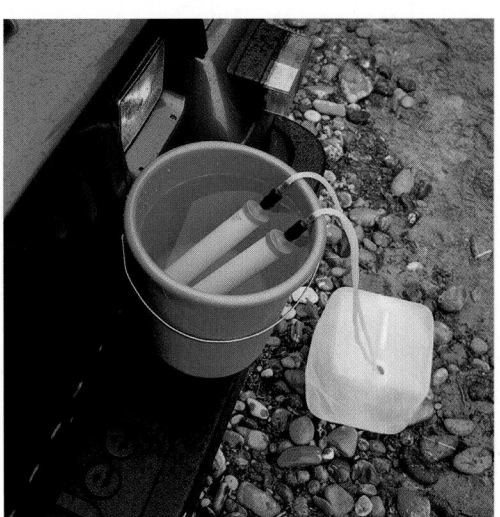

Figure 51-9   Katadyn Syphon.

PRODUCT	PRICE	STRUCTURE/FUNCTION
GENERAL ECOLOGY, INC.		
(151 Sheree Blvd, Exton, PA 19341; 610-363-7900; www.general-ecology.com)		All filters (except Microlite) contain 0.1-micron (0.4-micron absolute) Structured Matrix filter in removable canister.
First-Need Deluxe direct-connect water filter (Figure 51-10)	$70	Hand pump with intake strainer; outflow end connects directly to common water bottle; self-cleaning prefilter float; size: 6 × 6 inches, weight: 15 oz; flow: 1.6 L/min; capacity: 100-400 L.
Extra canister	$32	
Prefilter replacement	$7	
New pump assembly	$23	
Filtermate	$8	Connects older-design filter to wide-mouth Nalgene bottle.
Matrix pumping system	$9	2-L carry bag, polyethylene liners; 18-inch hose and hose adapter for creating gravity filter unit from filter elements.
Microlite (Figure 51-11)	$30	Structured Matrix filter 0.5 µm (nominal) with activated carbon; hand pump, 24-inch intake hose and strainer; attaches directly to wide-mouth or bike bottle, soda bottle, or outlet spout; size: 5.5 × 2.5 inches; weight: 8 oz; flow: 0.5 L/min; capacity: 50 L/cartridge.
Replacement cartridges (set of two)	$10	
Trav-L-Pure (Figure 51-12) (carrying case included)	$120	Filter and hand pump in rectangular housing (1.5-pt capacity); pour water into housing, then pump through prefilter and microfilter; size: 4.5 × 3.5 × 6.75 inches; weight: 22 oz; flow: 1-2 pt/min; capacity: 100-400 L.
Replacement canister	$30	
Base Camp (Figure 51-13) (carrying case included)	$500	Stainless steel casing and hand pump connected with tubing; capacity 1000 gal; canister size: 4.8 × 5.4 inches; pump: 1.5 × 10.5 inches; weight: 3 lbs; flow: 2 L/min
Replacement cartridge	$60	

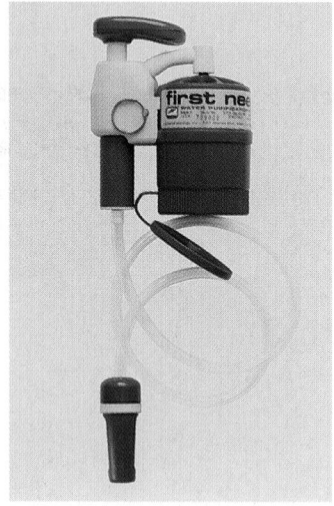

Figure 51-10 General Ecology First-Need Deluxe unit.

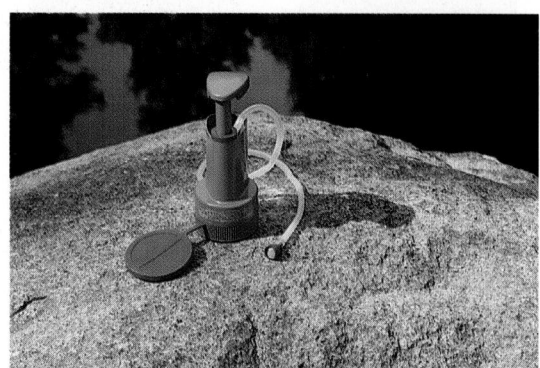

Figure 51-11 General Ecology Microlite unit.

GENERAL ECOLOGY, INC.—cont'd

Claims

First-Need filter is a proprietary blend of materials including activated charcoal. "Microfiltration removes bacteria and larger pathogens" (cysts, parasites). "Adsorption and molecular sieving": carbon absorbers remove chemicals and organic pollutants that cause color and taste; cavities in surface of adsorption material draw particles in deeper. Filter does not remove all dissolved minerals or desalinate. Proprietary process also creates ionic surface charge that removes colloids and ultrasmall particles, *including viruses,* through "electrokinetic attraction."

Microlite removes sediment, protozoan cysts, algae, and chemicals (including iodine) and improves color and taste of water. Iodine tablets are included to kill bacteria and viruses when these organisms are a concern.

Comments

Reasonable design, cost, and effectiveness. All units (except Microlite) use the same basic filter design. Most testing with *E. coli* and *Giardia* cysts show excellent removal. Charcoal matrix will remove chemical pollutants. This is the only company that claims to meet EPA standards for 4-log reduction of viruses through mechanical filtration, not inactivation. However, they do not claim to remove all viruses, since they have not been able to test with the hepatitis virus. Despite viral claims, recommend caution in highly polluted water; prior disinfection with halogen would guarantee disinfection, and carbon would remove halogen. The filter cannot be cleaned, although it can potentially be back-flushed, so it must be replaced when clogged.

Microlite is designed primarily for day use or light backpacking. Used alone, it makes microbiologic claims for protozoan cysts (*Giardia* and *Cryptosporidium*) only. Iodine tablets or solution should be used as pretreatment with this filter for all water except pristine alpine water in North America. This filter is compact, lightweight, and designed for low-volume use with inexpensive, easily changed filter cartridges. Base Camp is for large groups. It also comes with an electric pump and can be hooked up in parallel to provide large quantities of water for disaster relief.

Continued

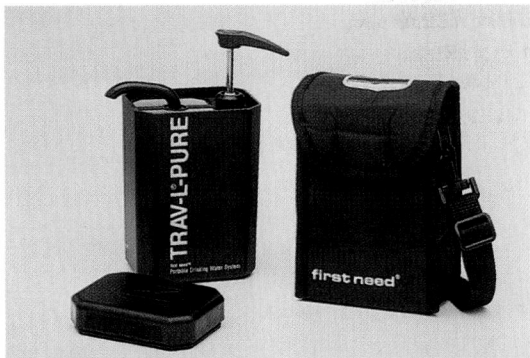

Figure 51-12   General Ecology Trav-L-Pure.

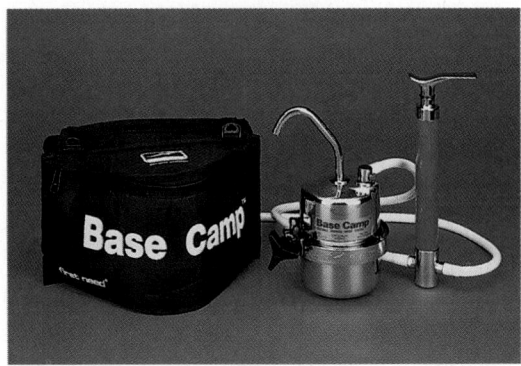

Figure 51-13   General Ecology Base Camp.

PRODUCT	PRICE	STRUCTURE/FUNCTION
STERN'S OUTDOORS (FORMERLY BASIC DESIGNS)		
(Box 1498, St Cloud, MN 56302; 800-697-5801; www.stearnsinc.com)		
High-flow ceramic water filter (B240) (Figure 51-14)	$45	Ceramic filter with 0.5-micron absolute retention size and carbon center; gravity filtration with element placed near the end of a 6-foot outflow tube connected to a 7.5-L heavy plastic collection bag, providing 2-3 lb of hydrostatic pressure through the in-line filter; packing size: 4 × 4 × 8 inches; weight: 13 oz; flow rate: 15 L/hr; capacity: 1000 L.
Replacement filter	$29	
Water carrier bag, 2.5 gal with fitting for filter output	$9	
Ceramic Filter Pump (Figure 51-15)	$22	Hand pump with ceramic cartridge at end of intake tubing and polyurethane prefilter; size: pump 8 × 1 inches, filter 4 × 3 inches, 18-inch tubing; weight: 7 oz; flow: 0.4 L/min; capacity: 500 gal.
Replacement filter	$12	

Claims

Ceramic filter removes *Giardia,* bacteria, *Cryptosporidium,* cysts, tapeworm, flukes, and other harmful pathogens larger than 1 micron. Carbon removes color, tastes, and odors. Filter can be cleaned with an abrasive pad. Pump is easily serviced in the field; ceramic cartridge is replaceable.

Comments

Ceramic candle filters are effective filtering elements, and charcoal is an effective adsorbent. No claims for virus removal. Although the pore size is larger than most filters, the low pressure depth filter increases retention of bacteria. The simple gravity design decreases cost and moving parts. Filtration rate will be slow, and this filter could clog rapidly, since there is no prefilter for larger particles. Gravity drip can be convenient after making camp, if no time restraints. The filter pump is the most practical and is reasonably priced, but the ceramic filter can break. The intake is close to the pump, which can be awkward, and the foam sleeve makes it float, requiring an extra hand to hold underwater. This filter rated poorly on field user tests. Fifteen liters per hour is not realistic for a gravity filter.

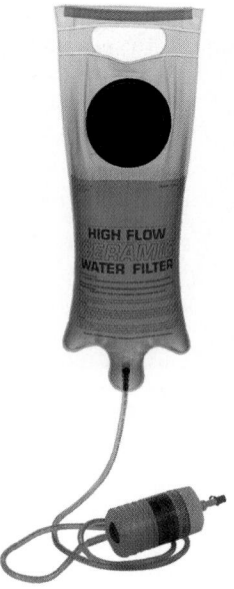

Figure 51-14 Stern's Outdoors high-flow ceramic water filter (B240).

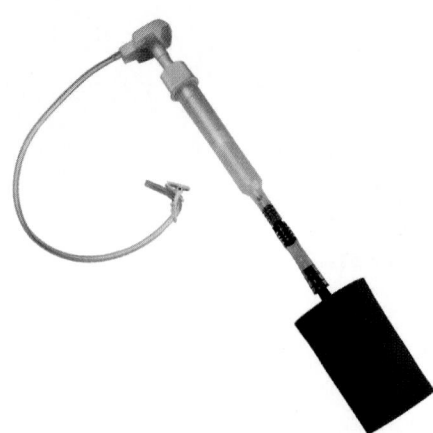

Figure 51-15 Stern's Outdoors Ceramic Filter Pump (B250).

PRODUCT	PRICE	STRUCTURE/FUNCTION
MSR AND MARATHON (3800 First Ave S, Seattle, WA 98124; 800-877-9677; www.msrcorp.com; www.marathonceramics.com)		
MSR Waterworks II (Figure 51-16) total filtration system Dromedary beverage bag (All filter elements and parts replaceable.)	$140 $20	Four filter elements of decreasing pore size: porous foam intake filter, 10-micron stainless steel wire mesh screen, cylindric ceramic filter with block carbon core, then 0.2-micron pharmacologic-grade membrane filter; pressure relief valve releases at 90-95 psi; hand pump with intake tubing; storage bag (2 or 4 L) attaches directly to outlet of pump; size: 9 × 4 inches diameter; weight: 17 oz; flow: 1 L/90 sec; capacity: 100-400 L.
Miniworks (Figure 51-17) Replacement filter	$65 $30	Similar external design to Waterworks II but slightly different ceramic filter and lacks final membrane filter; weight: 16 oz; flow rate 1 L/70 sec; capacity: 100-400 L.
Newton-Water	$249	High-retention ceramic filters with compressed block carbon core; gravity microfilter system with four ceramic filter elements; two stacked stainless steel 3-gal buckets; size: 12 × 22 inches; weight: 11 lbs; capacity: 25 gal/day.
e-water siphon filter	$35	Same filter element as above with siphon tubing; use any two containers to siphon water through filter; size: 2 × 7 ½ inches; weight 1 lb; capacity: 6-10 gal/day.
E-water Group Siphon Filter	Not yet available	Multiple ceramic filters with integral carbon block, in parallel to provide 1-2 L/min with no power or line pressure (other than gravity) required; size: 7 × 21 × 30 inches with case; weight 45 lbs.

Claims

Filter removes protozoa (including *Giardia* and *Cryptosporidium*), bacteria, pesticides, herbicides, chlorine, and discoloration. Both filters meet EPA standards for removal of cysts and bacteria. Ceramic filters reduced turbidity from 68.8 to 0.01 NTU. Carbon has been shown to reduce levels of iodine from 16 to less than 0.01 mg/L for at least 150 L. Ideal for emergency needs or for remote locations.

Comments

Excellent filter design and function. Prefilters protect more expensive inner, fine-pore filters. Effective for claims, high quality control, and extensive testing. No claims are made for viruses, although clumping and adherence remove the majority (currently 2 to 3-log removal, but not 4-log required for purifiers). The company is working on a microfilter that will effectively remove viruses. Until they succeed, the filter should not be considered reliable for complete viral removal from highly polluted waters in developing countries. Reservoir bag that attaches to outflow for filtered water storage is convenient. Design and ease of use are distinct advantages. Filter can be easily maintained in the field; maintenance kit and all replacement parts available. Ceramic filters can be effectively cleaned by abrading outer surface many times before compromising the filter. A simple caliper gauge indicates when filter has become too thin for reliable function. Miniworks was rated very highly in field tests.

Marathon ceramic products will soon be available. The gravity drip buckets are excellent products for field camps and expatriates. Iodine or chlorine can be used to ensure viral destruction, and the carbon will remove excess halogen, allowing long-term safe use of iodine. Siphon filter is inexpensive and compact.

Continued

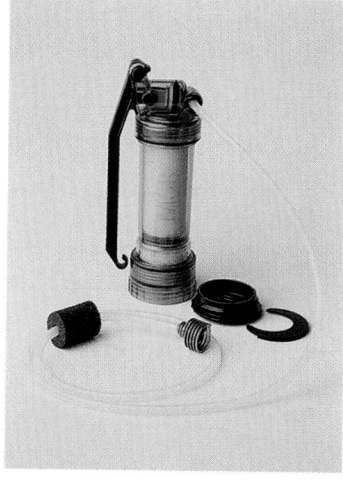

Figure 51-16 MSR Waterworks II.

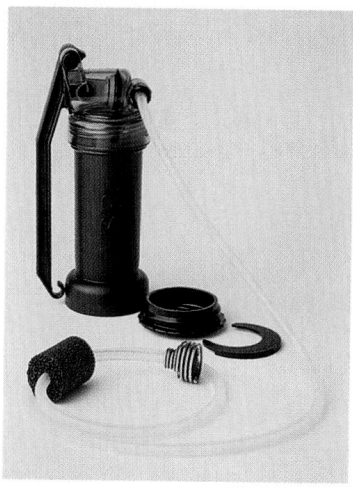

Figure 51-17 MSR Miniworks.

PRODUCT	PRICE	STRUCTURE/FUNCTION
PENTAPURE (FORMERLY WTC—WATER TECHNOLOGY CORP)		
(150 Marie Ave East, West St Paul, MN 551187; 651-450-4913; www.pentapure.com)		All products use PentaPure iodine resin.
PentaPure Sport (Figure 51-18)	$35	Drink-through sport bottle with internal (Pentacell) three-stage cartridge: 1-micron filter, iodine resin, and charcoal filter; filter and charcoal stages can be replaced independently; size: 11.5 × 3 inches; weight: 8 oz; capacity: 375 L.
Replacement cartridges		
PentaCell complete	$26	
Cysts Filter	$14	
EcoCell Filter	$9	
Spring	$25	Drink-through sport bottle with filter and charcoal, but no iodine resin; otherwise similar to Sport.

The following are considered "international" products. They are not marketed in the United States, but are available for export, which includes purchase for use outside the United States. They can be ordered from several companies, including TealBrook (800-222-6614). Availability is variable.

Penta-Pour bucket (Figure 51-19)	$170	Gravity drip bucket with 22-L storage capacity; sediment filter (30 micron), 1-micron filter; pentacide and carbon cartridge; size: 12 × 30 inches; weight: 3 kg; flow: 30 L/hr; capacity: 6500 L.
Ecomaster Outdoor Ecopour		
Travel Tap (Figure 51-20), Traveler		Pentacide and carbon cartridge; rubber cup and hose fitting on cartridge unit fits any faucet; flow: ½ gal/min; capacity: 1000 gal.
Outdoor 500 (Figure 51-21)	$1475	Expedition-size hand-lever filter with steel frame; sediment filter, iodine resin, carbon block; each can be independently replaced; size: 14 × 9.5 × 18.5 inches; weight: 7 kg; flow: 300 L/hr; capacity: 30,000 L.
Outdoor M1, Survivor		Drink-through straws; cartridge with prefilter, granular activated carbon filter sandwiched between two stages of PentPure resin; size: 5.5 inches long; weight: 1 oz; capacity: 100 gal (M1), 25 gal (Survivor).

Claims

Resin releases iodine "on demand" on contact with microorganisms; minimal iodine dissolves in water: effluent 1.0 to 2.0 ppm iodine. Charcoal removes residual dissolved iodine. Tested effective for bacteria, *Giardia*, schistosomiasis, and viruses, including hepatitis. PentaCell tested against the new EPA protocol that requires removal of 10^5 bacteria, 10^4 viruses, and 10^3 *Giardia* cysts. Charcoal stage absorbs bad tastes and odors.

Comments

Resin is essentially inexhaustible because the filter will become irreversibly clogged long before the resin is exhausted. However, the carbon filter may become fully absorbed with iodine and other impurities allowing iodine in the effluent. Although the amount of iodine in the outflow water is supposed to be low (1 to 2 ppm), higher concentrations have been measured. For long-term use, carbon filters should be changed regularly.

The company has narrowed their product line for field use and has dropped the small group hand-pump filters because of similar products on the market. They have also dropped the Travel Cup, a small pour-through plastic cup. The Sport Bottle is handy for individual use among hikers, bikers, and travelers. Pressure is generated by a combination of sucking and squeezing. Users must adapt to the effort and the slower flow compared with a regular sport bottle. Drink-through straws have limited applications, mainly survival and emergency situations. The "international" products are some of the most useful ones. Penta-Pour bucket is an excellent product for expatriates and field camps. The Outdoor series would work well for stationary or vehicle-based groups. Large units are available for large groups and disaster relief. The Traveler (formerly Travel Tap) is a small, portable unit that hooks to the end of a faucet and could be very useful for expatriates and frequent travelers.

Continued

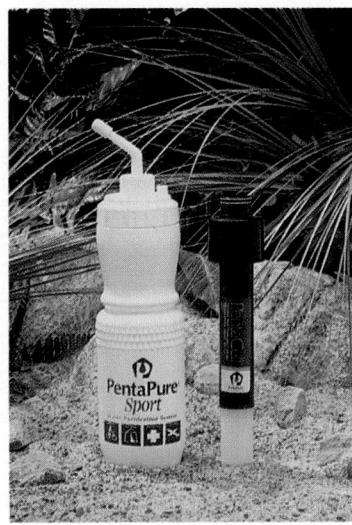

Figure 51-18   PentaPure Sport.

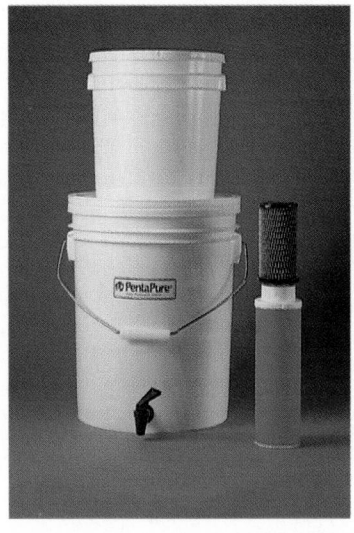

Figure 51-19   PentaPure Penta-Pour bucket.

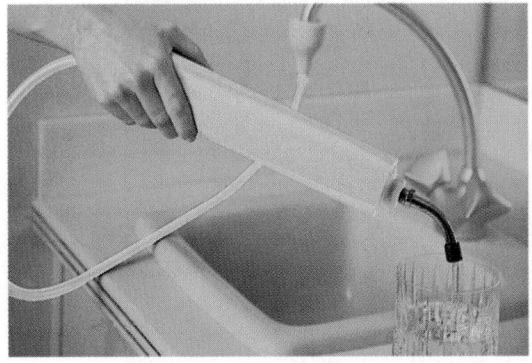

Figure 51-20   PentaPure Travel Tap.

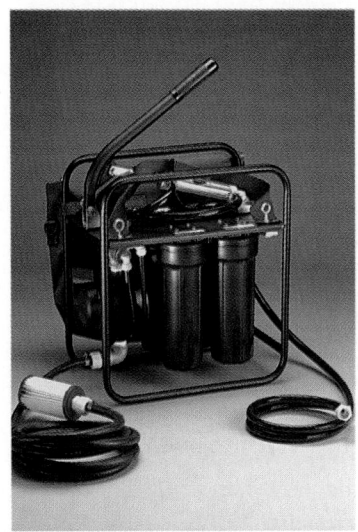

Figure 51-21   PentaPure Outdoor 500.

PRODUCT	PRICE	STRUCTURE/FUNCTION
TIMBERLINE FILTER		
(PO Box 20356, Boulder, CO, 80308; 800-482-9297)		
Timberline Eagle (Figure 51-22)	$24	1-micron fiberglass and polyethylene matrix; hand pump;
Replacement element	$12	size: 9 × 1-3 inches; weight: 6 oz; flow: 1 qt in 1.5 min.

Claims

Removes *Giardia* cysts. No claims for bacteria or viruses.

Comments

Effective for claims; intended only for high-quality North American backcountry use where *Giardia* is a possible contaminant, but should also remove *Cryptosporidium*. Lightest pump filter available. Cartridges cannot be cleaned but are replaceable. The intake is close to the pump, which can be awkward.

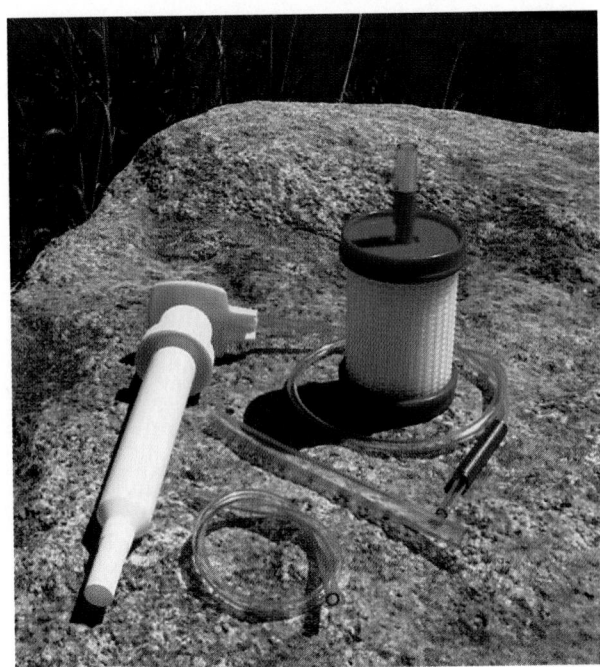

Figure 51-22 Timberline Eagle filter.

PRODUCT	PRICE	STRUCTURE/FUNCTION
PUR/RECOVERY ENGINEERING, INC.		
(9300 N 75th Ave, Minneapolis, MN 55428; 800-845-7873)		
Explorer (Figure 51-23)	$140	Hand pump with 130-micron prefilter; replaceable cartridge
Replacement parts		with 0.3-micron pleated glass-fiber filter and triiodine
Tritek cartridge	$45	resin (Tritek); internal brush cleans filter with twist of
Pump	$45	handle; combination carbon cartridge and bottle adapter
Intake filter/hose	$16	attaches to end of outflow tubing and removes residual
Carbon cartridge and bottle adapter	$15	dissolved iodine and other chemicals; size: 10.75 ×
Carbon refill pack	$6	2.25 inches; intake and output hoses: 3 ft; weight: 21 oz;
		max flow: 1.5 L/min; capacity: 100 gal/cartridge.
Scout (Figure 51-24)	$90	Hand pump with 150-micron intake filter; 0.3-micron
Replacement cartridge	$35	pleated filter and triiodine resin and carbon cartridge;
Optional carbon cartridge	$20	size: 9.5 × 2.25 inches; weight: 14 oz; max flow: 1.0 L/min
		(36 stokes/L); capacity: 100 gal/cartridge.
Pioneer (Figure 51-25)	$30	Hand pump filter (0.3-micron fiberglass disk) attaches to
Extra filters (2 pack)	$8	top of water bottle; size: 2.5 × 4.5 inches; weight: 8 oz;
		flow: 1 L/min; capacity: 20 gal.
Hiker (Figure 51-26)	$50	Hand pump with 0.3-micron pleated glass fiber with
Replacement filter	$25	160-inch^2 surface; microfilter and activated carbon core;
		size 7.5 × 2.5 × 3.5 inches; weight: 11 oz; flow: 1 L/min
		(40 stokes/L); capacity: 200 gal.
Voyageur	$70	Voyager uses same body and filter as Hiker but includes
		iodine resin; intake filter for particles; capacity: 100 gal
		until cartridge replacement.

Continued

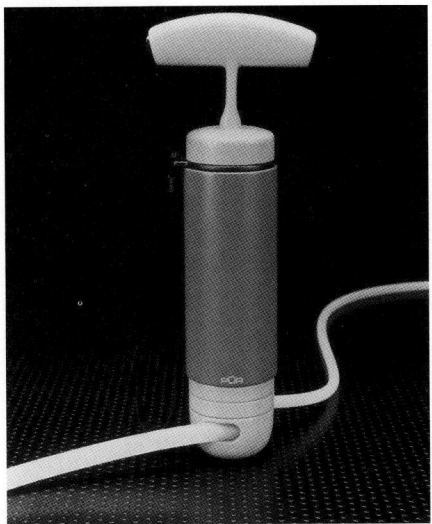

Figure 51-23 PUR Explorer.

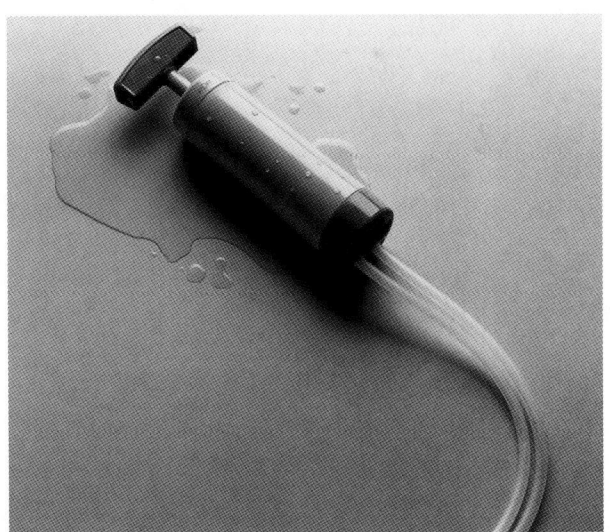

Figure 51-24 PUR Scout.

PUR/RECOVERY ENGINEERING, INC.—cont'd

Claims

Explorer, Scout, and Voyageur are purifiers that meet EPA test standards to remove or destroy all types of microorganisms. Microfilter removes cysts, and iodine resin kills bacteria and viruses on contact. Explorer has self-contained brush to clean filter without disassembling. Filter will clog before resin is exhausted. The iodine resin filters will purify (render microbiologically safe) water of any quality. However, two passages through the filter are recommended for "worst case" water (below 5° C, cloudy and highly polluted). Easily replaced carbon cartridge attaches to the outflow tubing and scavenges residual iodine. This reduces the iodine concentration from an average of 2 ppm to less than 1 ppm, leaving no iodine taste.

The Hiker and Pioneer are microfilters, without iodine resin, designed for higher quality surface water, not international travel. It will "eliminate *Giardia* and most bacteria;" activated carbon core "reduces chemicals and pesticides, plus improves taste of water." Filter surface area of 160 square inches is "guaranteed not to clog for 1 year." The Pioneer is effective against *Giardia*, *Cryptosporidium*, and most bacteria.

Comments

The Explorer is a well-designed, lightweight unit for individual or small-group use in any wilderness environment. The pumping action is very easy, and the internal brush seems to effectively restore flow. The Scout and Voyageur are smaller, less expensive, and contain the same elements except for the internal brush. The Hiker and Pioneer were designed for the domestic backpacking market with access to higher water quality, where cysts and bacteria are a threat, but viruses are less of a problem. The Hiker received top ratings for field tests evaluating user-friendliness.

Instructions for the water purifier advise passing cold, highly polluted water through this filter twice, but an alternative would be to allow 30 to 40 minutes of contact time. The company is hesitant to recommend a contact time, believing that the public expects a filter to render water safe immediately after passage, so they offer the more cumbersome recommendation of filtering twice. In fact, the conditions of worst-case water will rarely, if ever, be encountered; most would not attempt to drink such water unless desperate. NOTE: *Repeat testing of the iodine resin filters demonstrated failure to inactivate 4-log of viruses under certain conditions, leading to a product recall in 2000. The company is investigating the role of activated carbon and the need for contact time. They hope to have products back on the market early in 2001.*

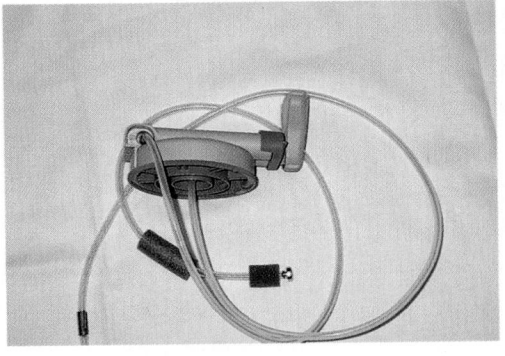

Figure 51-25 PUR Pioneer.

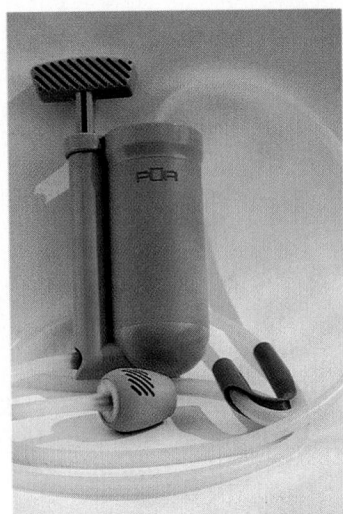

Figure 51-26 PUR Hiker.

PRODUCT	PRICE	STRUCTURE/FUNCTION
RECOVERY ENGINEERING		
Reverse-osmosis filters		
Survivor 06 (Figure 51-27)	$550	Hand pump, reverse-osmosis membrane filter with prefilter on intake line; size: 2.5 × 5 × 8 inches; weight: 2.5 lb; flow: 40 strokes/min yields 1 L/hr.
Survivor 35 (Figure 51-28)	$1425	Hand pump, reverse-osmosis membrane filter with prefilter on intake line; size: 3.5 × 5.5 × 22 inches; weight: 7 lbs; flow: 1.2 gal/hr.

Claims

Reverse-osmosis units desalinate, removing 98% salt from seawater by forcing water through a semi permeable membrane at 800 psi. In the process, bacteria are filtered out. The manual operation of these units makes them useful for survival at sea or for use in small craft without power source. Larger, power-operated units are also available.

Comments

Reverse-osmosis units are included here because sea kayaking and small boat journeys in open water are becoming more popular. Most large oceangoing boats use reverse-osmosis filters. These units can obviate the need for relying solely on stored water or can be carried for emergency survival. The military uses truck-mounted reverse-osmosis filters on land for their ability to handle brackish water and remove all levels of microorganisms. Reverse-osmosis filters could be used for land-based travel but are prohibitively expensive for most people, and the flow rates are inadequate (1 L/hr, not per minute). Desalination units will remove microorganisms, including viruses, that are larger than sodium molecules. The company does not make claims for viral removal because they assume that the membrane is imperfect and some pores will be imprecise, perhaps allowing viral passage.

Continued

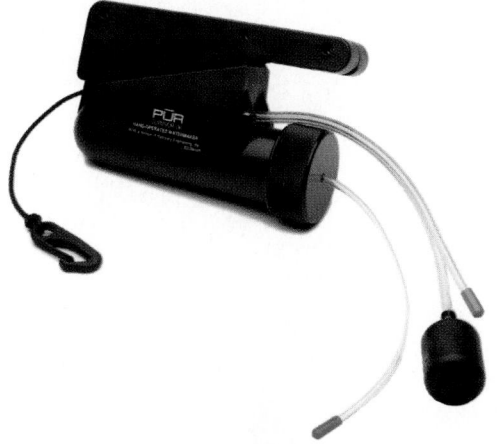

Figure 51-27 PUR/Recovery Engineering Survivor 06 filter.

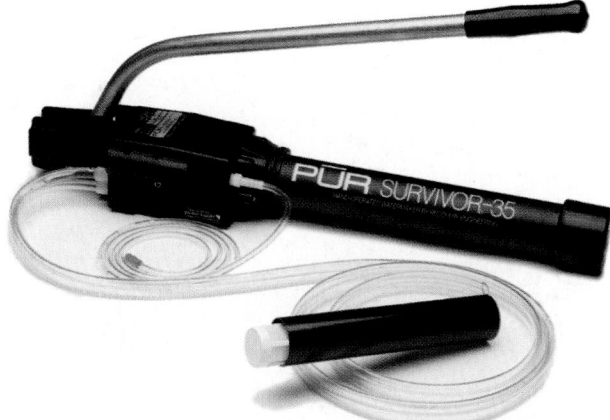

Figure 51-28 PUR/Recovery Engineering Survivor 35 filter.

PRODUCT	PRICE	STRUCTURE/FUNCTION
CASCADE DESIGNS		
(4000 1st Ave S, Seattle, WA 98134; 206-505-9500)		
SweetWater Guardian (Figure 51-29) Micro-filtration system	$50	Lexan body and pump handle; 100-micron metal prefilter; in-line 4-micron secondary filter; labyrinth filter cylinder
Replacement filter	$30	of borosilicate fibers removes pathogens to 0.2 micron;
Viral Guard iodine resin cartridge	$25	granular activated carbon (GAC); safety pressure-relief
Tap-Adapt	$10	valve; end-of-life indicator; outflow tubing has universal
Silt-stopper	$10	adapter that fits all water bottles; optional biocide
Prefilter	$9	cartridge containing iodinated resin attaches to filter—
Filter brush	$3	water passes through resin first, then filter cartridge, then
Carrying bag	$6	GAC; optional input adapter that attaches to sink faucet while traveling; size: 7.75 × 3.5 inches; weight: 11 oz; flow: 1.25 L/min (new filter); capacity: 200 gal (90 gal with Viral Guard).
Global Water Express	$90	Zipper carrying case with Guardian filter, Viral Guard cartridge, and 1-L storage bag.
Walkabout (Figure 51-30)	$35	Lightweight version with similar filter element; size: 6.5 inches high; weight: 9 oz; flow: 0.75 L/min; capacity: 125 gal.

Claims

SweetWater filter eliminates *Giardia, Cryptosporidium,* and other critical bacterial and protozoan pathogens, as well as pollutants, heavy metals, pesticides, and flavors. Kills viruses when used with the Viral Guard cartridge accessory. Lighter, more compact, and durable than comparable models, and easiest to clean or replace. Filter cartridges are recycled by the company.

Comments

Well-designed filter at a reasonable price. The three major water treatment components—filtration, GAC, and iodine resin attachment—offer broad protection and maximum flexibility. Practical design features include universal bottle adapter. Pressure-release valve indicates when filter needs cleaning, but this can be a problem as the filter clogs. A brush is provided for cleaning, and cartridges are replaceable. *NOTE: Viral Guard iodine resin was recently taken off the market due to company testing that demonstrated failure to inactivate viruses, despite prior testing in outside laboratories that passed EPA standards.*

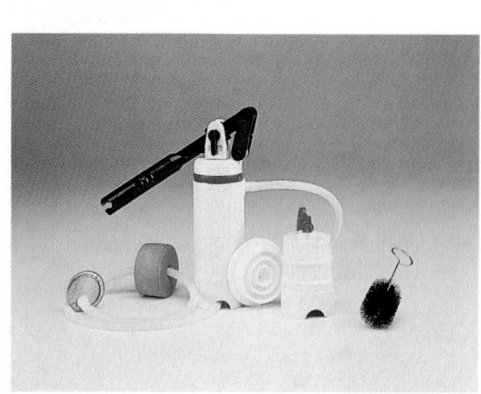

Figure 51-29 Cascade Designs SweetWater Guardian filter.

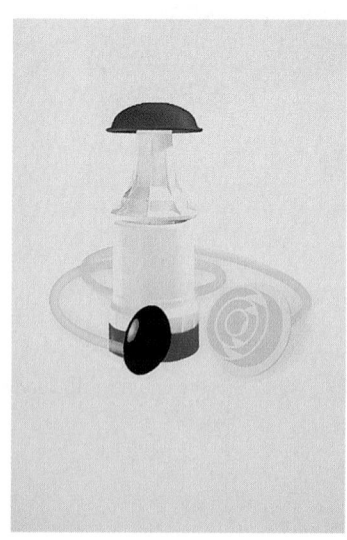

Figure 51-30 Cascade Designs Walkabout.

REFERENCES

1. Acra A et al: Disinfection of oral rehydration solutions by sunlight, *Lancet* 2:1257, 1980 (letter).
2. Alder V, Simpson R: Sterilization and disinfection by heat methods. In Russel A et al, editors: *Principles and practice of disinfection, preservation, and sterilization,* Oxford, UK, 1992, Blackwell Scientific.
3. American Water Works Association: Variance analyses and criteria for treatment regulations, *J Am Water Works Assoc* 74:34, 1986.
4. American Water Works Association: Committee report: coagulation as an integrated water treatment process, *J Am Water Works Assoc* 81, 1989.
5. Anderson B: Moist heat inactivation of *Cryptosporidium, Am J Public Health* 75:1433, 1985.
6. Aukerman R, Monzingo JD: Water treatment to inactive *Giardia, J Forestry* 18, 1989.
7. Aziz KM et al: Reduction in diarrhoeal diseases in children in rural Bangladesh by environmental and behavioural modifications, *Trans R Soc Trop Med Hyg* 84:433, 1990.
8. Bandres J et al: Heat susceptibility of bacterial enteropathogens, *Arch Intern Med* 148:2261, 1988.
9. Baumann E, Ludwig D: Free available chlorine residuals for small non-public water supplies, *J Am Water Works Assoc* 54:1379, 1964.
10. Beal C: Another method of water purification for travelers, *West J Med* 135:341, 1981 (letter).
11. Bell F: Review of effects of silver-impregnated carbon filters on microbial water quality, *J Am Water Works Assoc* 83:74, 1991.
12. Bemrick W: Some perspectives on the transmission of giardiasis. In Erlandsen S, Meyer E, editors: *Giardia and giardiasis: biology, pathogenesis and epidemiology,* New York, 1984, Plenum Press.
13. Berg G et al: Devitalization of microorganisms by iodine, *Virology* 22:469, 1964.
14. Berkelman R et al: Increased bactericidal activity of dilute preparations of povidone-iodine solutions, *J Clin Microbiol* 15:635, 1982.
15. Bingham A et al: *Giardia* sp.: physical factors of excystation in vitro and excystation vs. eosin exclusion as determinants of viability, *Exp Parasitol* 47:284, 1979.
16. Biziagos E et al: Long-term survival of hepatitis A virus and polio virus type 1 in mineral water, *Appl Environ Microbiol* 54:2705, 1988.
17. Black A et al: Use of iodine for disinfection, *J Am Water Works Assoc* 55:1401, 1965.
18. Blaser M et al: Survival of *Campylobacter fetus subsp. jejuni* in biological milieus, *J Clin Microbiol* 11:309, 1980.
19. Blaser M et al: Inactivation of *Campylobacter jejuni* by chlorine and monochlorine, *Appl Environ Microbiol* 51:307, 1986.
20. Block S: Peroxygen compounds. In Block S, editor: *Disinfection, sterilization, and preservation,* Philadelphia, 1991, Lea & Febiger.
21. Braverman L: Iodine and the thyroid: 33 years of study, *Thyroid* 4:351, 1994.
22. Briton G: *Introduction to environmental virology,* New York, 1980, Wiley.
23. Butler M: Virus removal by disinfection of effluents. In Goddard M, Butler M, editors: *Proceedings of International Symposium on Viruses and Wastewater Treatment,* Oxford, UK, 1980, Pergamon.
24. Castillo A: Federal regulation of antimicrobial pesticides and in the United States. In Block S, editor: *Disinfection, sterilization, and preservation,* Philadelphia, 1991, Lea & Febiger.
25. Centers for Disease Control: Cryptosporidiosis-New Mexico, 1986, *MMWR* 36:561, 1987.
26. Centers for Disease Control: Hepatitis E among US travelers, 1989-1992, *MMWR* 42:1, 1993.
27. Centers for Disease Control: Addressing emerging infectious disease threats: a prevention strategy for the United States, *MMWR* 43(RR-5), 1994.
28. Centers for Disease Control: Assessment of inadequately filtered public drinking water—Washington, DC, December 1993, *MMWR* 43:661, 1994.
29. Centers for Disease Control: Cryptosporidiosis infection associated with swimming pools—Dane County, Wisconsin, *MMWR* 43:561, 1994.
30. Centers for Disease Control: Surveillance for waterborne-disease outbreaks—United States, 1993-1994, *MMWR* 45(SS-1), 1996.
31. Centers for Disease Control: Surveillance for waterborne-disease outbreaks—United States, 1995-1996, *MMWR* 47:1, 1998.
32. Centers for Disease Control and Prevention: *Health information for international travel, 1999-2000,* Atlanta, 1999, US Department of Health and Human Services.
33. Chang S: Modern concepts of disinfection. In *Proceedings of National Specialty Conference on Disinfection,* 1970, American Society of Civil Engineers.
34. Chang S, Morris J: Elemental iodine as a disinfectant for drinking water, *Ind Eng Chem* 45:1009, 1953.
35. Chaudhuri M, Sattar S: Domestic water treatment for developing countries. In McFeters G, editor: *Drinking water microbiology,* New York, 1990, Springer-Verlag.
36. Chauty Y: Personal communication, Center for the Study and Practice of Survival, Pournichet, France, 1996.
37. Cilimburg A: The Scoop on poop, *NOLS* (staff newsletter), 1995.
38. Cohen J, Hannah S: Coagulation and flocculation. In American Water Works Association: *Water quality and treatment: a handbook of public water supplies,* New York, 1971, McGraw-Hill.
39. *Consumer Reports* 28, 1990.
40. Cookson J: Virus and water supply, *J Am Water Works Assoc* 66:707, 1974.
41. Cooper D: Subclinical thyroid disease: a clinician's perspective, *Ann Intern Med* 129:135, 1998 (editorial).
42. Cooper RC et al: *Infectious agent risk assessment water quality project,* UCB/SEEHRL Report No 84-4 and 84-5, Berkeley, Calif, 1984.
43. Craun G: *Waterborne disease in the United States,* Boca Raton, Fla, 1986, CRC Press.
44. Craun G et al: Prevention of waterborne cholera in the United States, *J Am Water Works Assoc* 83:40, 1991.
45. Cullimore D, Jacobsen H: The efficiency of point of use devices for the exclusion of *Giardia muris* cysts from a model water supply system. In Wallis P, Hammond B, editors: *Advances in Giardia research,* Calgary, 1988, University of Calgary Press.
46. Culp R: Breakpoint chlorination for virus inactivation, *J Am Water Works Assoc* 66:699, 1974.
47. Culp R et al: *Handbook of advanced wastewater treatment,* New York, 1978, Van Nostrand Reinhold.
48. Current W: *Cryptosporidium:* its biology and potential for environmental transmission, *CRC Crit Rev Environ Control* 17:21, 1985.
49. D'Antonio RG et al: A waterborne outbreak of cryptosporidiosis in normal hosts, *Ann Intern Med* 103:886, 1985.
50. D'Aquino M, Teves S: Lemon juice as a natural biocide for disinfecting drinking water, *Bull Pan Am Health Org* 28:324, 1994.
51. DeReigner D: Viability of *Giardia* cysts suspended in lake, river, and tap water, *Appl Environ Microbiol* 55:1223, 1989.
52. Dickens D et al: Survival of bacterial enteropathogens in the ice of popular drinks, *JAMA* 253:3141, 1985.
53. Drinking Water Health Effects Task Force, US Environmental Protection Agency: *Health effects of drinking water treatment technologies,* Chelsea, Mich, 1989, Lewis Publisher.
54. DuPont HEA: The response of man to virulent *Shigella flexneri* 2a, *J Infect Dis* 119:296, 1969.
55. Dychdala G: Chlorine and chlorine compounds. In Block S, editor: *Disinfection, sterilization, and preservation,* Philadelphia, 1991, Lea & Febiger.
56. Engelbrecht R et al: Comparative inactivation of viruses by chlorine, *Appl Environ Microbiol* 40:249, 1980.
57. Environmental Health Directorate Health Protection Branch: *Laboratory testing and evaluation of iodine releasing point-of-use water treatment devices,* Ottawa, 1979, Department of National Health and Welfare.
58. Environmental Health Directorate Health Protection Branch: *Assessing the effectiveness of small filtration systems for point-of-use disinfection of drinking water supplies (80-EHD-54),* Ottawa, 1980, Department of National Health and Welfare.
59. Fayer R: Effect of high temperature on infectivity of *Cryptosporidium parvum* oocysts in water, *Appl Environ Microbiol* 60:273, 1994.
60. Felsenfeld O: Notes on food, beverages and fomites contaminated with *Vibrio cholerae, Bull World Health Organization* 33:725, 1965.
61. Fina R et al: Virucidal capability of resin I3 disinfectant, *Appl Environ Microbiol* 44:1370, 1982.
62. Finkelstein R, Jacobi M: Fatal iodine poisoning: clinicopathologic and experimental study, *Ann Intern Med* 10:1283, 1937.
63. Fraker L et al: *Giardia* cyst inactivation by iodine, *J Wilderness Med* 3:351, 1992.
64. Frazier W, Westhoff D: Preservation by use of high temperatures. In *Food Microbiology,* New York, 1978, McGraw-Hill.
65. Freund G: Effect of iodinated water supplies on thyroid function, *J Clin Endocrinol Metab* 26:619, 1966.
66. Geldreich E: Drinking water microbiology-new directions toward water quality enhancement, *Int J Food Microbiol* 9:295, 1989.
67. Geldreich E: Microbiological quality of source waters for water supply. In McFeters G, editor: *Drinking water microbiology,* New York, 1990, Springer-Verlag.

68. Geldreich E, Reasoner D: Home treatment devices and water quality. In McFeters G, editor: *Drinking water microbiology,* New York, 1990, Springer-Verlag.

69. Georgitis W, McDermott M: An iodine load from water purification tablets alters thyroid function in humans, *Mil Med* 158:794, 1993.

70. Gerba C, Nakhforoosh M: Evaluation of iodine (I2) as tri-iodine (I3) resin for inactivation of enteric bacteria and viruses, and of microfiltration for removal of *Giardia* cysts as incorporated in the Recovery Engineering antimicrobial water purifier for world travelers: efficacy of antimicrobial agents, Tucson, 1990, University of Arizona.

71. Gerba CP, Naranjo JE: Microbiological water purification without the use of chemical disinfection, *Wilderness Environ Med* 10:12, 1999.

72. Gerba C, Rose J: Viruses in source and drinking water. In McFeters G, editor: *Drinking water microbiology,* New York, 1990, Springer-Verlag.

73. Gerba C et al: Efficacy of iodine water purification tablets against *Cryptosporidium* oocysts and *Giardia* cysts, *Wilderness Environ Med* 8:96, 1997.

74. Gottardi W: Iodine and iodine compounds, In Block S, editor: *Disinfection, sterilization, and preservation,* Philadelphia, 1991, Lea & Febiger.

75. Grabow W et al: Inactivation of hepatitis A virus and indicator organisms in water by free chlorine residuals, *Appl Environ Microbiol* 46:619, 1983.

76. Groh C et al: Effect of heat on the sterilization of artificially contaminated water, *J Travel Med* 3:11, 1996.

77. Haas C, Heller B: Kinetics of inactivation of *Giardia lamblia* by free chlorine, *Water Res* 24:233, 1990.

78. Hayes E: Large community outbreak of cryptosporidiosis due to contamination of a filtered public water supply, *N Engl J Med* 320:1372, 1989.

79. Hazen T, Toranzos G: Tropical source water. In McFeters G, editor: *Drinking water microbiology,* New York, 1990, Springer-Verlag.

80. Helfand M, Redfern C: Screening for thyroid disease: an update, *Ann Intern Med* 129:144, 1998.

81. Herwaldt B et al: Waterborne disease outbreaks, 1989-1990, *MMWR* 40(SS-3):1, 1991.

82. Hibler C, Hancock C: Waterborne giardiasis. In McFeters G, editor: *Drinking water microbiology,* New York, 1990, Springer-Verlag.

83. Hibler C et al: *Inactivation of Giardia cysts with chlorine at 0.5° C to 5.0° C,* Denver, 1987, American Water Works Association Research Foundation.

84. Hoehn R: Comparative disinfection methods, *J Am Water Works Assoc* 68:302, 1976.

85. Hoff J: Disinfection resistance of *Giardia* cysts: origins of current concepts and research in progress. In Jakubowski W, Hoff J, editors: *Waterborne transmission of giardiasis,* Cincinnati, 1979, US Environmental Protection Agency.

86. Hoff J: Inactivation of microbial agents by chemical disinfectants, Cincinnati, 1986, US Environmental Protection Agency.

87. How long to boil water, *Foreign Service Med Bull,* 1992.

88. Hurst C: Disinfection of drinking water, swimming pool water and treated sewage effluents. In Block S, editor: *Disinfection, sterilization, and preservation,* Philadelphia, 1991, Lea & Febiger.

89. Hurst C et al: Estimating the risk of acquiring infectious disease from ingestion of water. In Hurst C, editor: *Modeling disease transmission and its prevention by disinfection,* Melbourne, 1996, Cambridge University Press.

90. Huttly SR et al: The Imo State (Nigeria) Drinking Water Supply and Sanitation Project. 2. Impact on dracunculiasis, diarrhoea and nutritional status, *Trans R Soc Trop Med Hyg* 84:316, 1990.

90a. Hutton P, Ongerth J: *Performance evaluation for portable water filters.* Project report, Sept 28, 1995. Seattle, Department of Environmental Health, University of Washington.

91. Jakubowski W: Detection of *Giardia* cysts in drinking water. In Erlandsen S, Meyer E, editors: *Giardia and giardiasis: biology, pathogenesis and epidemiology,* New York, 1984, Plenum Press.

92. Jarroll E et al: *Giardia* cyst destruction: effectiveness of six small water disinfection methods, *Am J Trop Med Hyg* 29:8, 1980.

93. Jarroll E et al: Inability of an iodination method to destroy completely *Giardia* cysts in cold water, *West J Med* 132:567, 1980.

94. Jarroll E et al: Resistance of cysts to disinfection agents. In Erlandsen S, Meyer E, editors: *Giardia and giardiasis: biology, pathogenesis and epidemiology,* New York, 1984, Plenum Press.

95. Jenkins M: What's in the water? *Backpacker,* December 1996, p56.

96. Joslyn L: Sterilization by heat. In Block S, editor: *Disinfection, sterilization, and preservation,* Philadelphia, 1991, Lea & Febiger.

97. Joyce T et al: Inactivation of fecal bacteria in drinking water by solar heating, *Appl Environ Microbiol* 62:399, 1996.

98. Juranek D, MacKenzie W: Drinking water turbidity and gastrointestinal illness, *Epidemiology* 9:228, 1998.

99. Kahn F, Visscher B: Water disinfection in the wilderness-a simple, effective method of iodination, *West J Med* 122:450, 1975.

100. Kane M et al: Epidemic Non-A, Non-B hepatitis in Nepal, *JAMA* 252:3140, 1984.

101. Keswick B et al: Inactivation of Norwalk virus in drinking water by chlorine, *Appl Environ Microbiol* 50:261, 1985.

102. Kettel-Khan L et al: Thyroid abnormalities related to iodine excess from water purification units, *Lancet* 352:1519, 1998.

103. Kinman R et al: Disinfection with iodine. In *Proceedings of National Specialty Conference on Disinfection,* 1970, American Society of Civil Engineers.

104. Krishnaswami S: Effect of chlorine on *Ascaris* eggs, *Health Lab Sci* 5:225, 1968.

105. Krugman S et al: Hepatitis virus: effect of heat on the infectivity and antigenicity of the MS-1 and MS-2 strains, *J Infect Dis* 122:432, 1970.

106. Kunkle S et al: *Field survey of Giardia in streams and wildlife of the Glacier Gorge and Loch Vale basins, Rocky Mountain National Park.* Natural Resources Report Series 85-3, Fort Collins, Colo, 1985, National Park Service.

107. Laubusch E: Chlorination and other disinfection processes. In American Water Works Association: *Water quality and treatment: a handbook of public water supplies,* New York, 1971, McGraw-Hill.

108. Le Chevallier M, McFeters G: Microbiology of activated carbon. In McFeters G, editor: *Drinking water microbiology,* New York, 1990, Springer-Verlag.

109. LeChevallier M et al: Effect of turbidity on chlorination efficiency and bacterial persistence in drinking water, *Appl Environ Microbiol* 42:159, 1981.

110. LeMar H et al: Thyroid adaptation to chronic tetraglycine hydroperiodide water purification tablet use, *J Clin Endocrinol Metab* 80, 1995.

111. Liel Y, Alkan M: Travelers' thyrotoxicosis: transitory thyrotoxicosis induced by iodinated preparations for water purification, *Arch Intern Med* 156:807, 1996.

112. Lin S: *Giardia lamblia* and water supply, *J Am Water Works Assoc* 77:40, 1985.

113. Logsdon G et al: Alternative filtration methods for removal of *Giardia* cysts and cyst models, *J Am Water Works Assoc* 73:111, 1981.

114. Logsdon G: Microbiology and drinking water filtration. In McFeters G, editor: *Drinking water microbiology,* New York, 1990, Springer-Verlag.

115. MacKenzie W et al: A massive outbreak in Milwaukee of Cryptosporidium infection transmitted through the public water supply, *N Engl J Med* 331:161, 1994.

116. Marchin G, Fina L: Contact and demand-release disinfectants, *Crit Rev Environ Control* 19:227, 1989.

117. Marchin G et al: Effect of resin disinfectants I3 and I5 on *Giardia muris* and *Giardia lamblia, Appl Environ Microbiol* 46:965, 1983.

118. Marshall M et al: Waterborne protozoan pathogens, *Clin Microbiol Rev* 10:67, 1997.

119. McDermott J: Virus problems and their relation to water supplies, *J Am Water Works Assoc* 66:693, 1974.

120. McGuigan K et al: Solar disinfection of drinking water contained in transparent plastic bottles: characterizing the bacterial inactivation process, *J Appl Microbiol* 84:1138, 1998.

121. McMonigal K: Personal communication, 1999, National Aeronautics and Space Administration.

122. Melack J et al: Acid precipitation and buffer capacity of lakes in the Sierra Nevada, California. Paper presented at International Symposium on Hydrometeorology, 1982, American Water Resources Association.

123. Merson R et al: An outbreak of *Shigella sonnei* gastroenteritis on Colorado river raft trips, *Am J Epidemiol* 100:186, 1974.

124. Mertens T et al: Childhood diarrhoea in Sri Lanka: a case-control study of the impact of improved water sources, *Trop Med Parasitol* 41:98, 1990.

125. Miltner R et al: Treatment of seasonal pesticides in surface waters, *J Am Water Works Assoc* 83:43, 1989.

126. Mintz E et al: Safe water treatment and storage in the home: a practical new strategy to prevent waterborne disease, *JAMA* 273, 1995.

127. Moeller D: Drinking water and liquid waste. In *Environmental health,* Boston, 1997, Harvard University Press.

128. Monzingo D, Stevens D: *Giardia* contamination of surface waters: a survey of three selected backcountry streams in Rocky Mountain National Park, Water Resources Report No. 86-2, Fort Collins, Colo, 1986, National Park Service.

129. Morgan D, Karpen R: Test of chronic toxicity of iodine as related to the purification of water, *US Armed Forces Med J* 4:725, 1953.

130. Morris J: Chlorination and disinfection-state of the art, *J Am Water Works Assoc* 63:769, 1971.

131. Morris J et al: Disinfection of drinking water under field conditions, *Ind Eng Chem* 45:1013, 1953.

132. Namba H et al: Evidence of thyroid volume increase in normal subjects receiving excess iodide, *Endocrinol Metab* 76:605, 1993.

133. Naranjo J, Gerba C: *Evaluation of portable water treatment devices by a condensed version of the Guide of standard protocol for microbiological purifiers,* Tucson, 1995, University of Arizona.

134. National Academy of Sciences: The disinfection of drinking water, *Drinking water and health,* Washington, DC, 1980, National Academy Press.

135. Neefe J et al: Disinfection of water containing causative agent of infectious hepatitis, *JAMA* 128:1076, 1945.

136. Neefe J et al: Inactivation of the virus of infectious hepatitis in drinking water, *Am J Public Health* 37:365, 1947.

137. Neumann H: Bacteriological safety of hot tapwater in developing countries, *Public Health Rep* 84:812, 1969.

138. Neumann H: Alternatives to water chlorination, *Rev Infect Dis* 3:1255, 1981.

139. Neuwirth M et al: Effects of chlorine on the ultrastructure of *Giardia* cysts. In Wallis P, Hammond B, editors: *Advances in Giardia research,* Calgary, 1988, University of Calgary Press.

140. O'Connor J, Kapoor S: Small quantity field disinfection, *J Am Water Works Assoc* 62:80, 1970.

141. O'Connor J et al: *Removal of virus from public water supplies,* Cincinnati, 1982, US Environmental Protection Agency.

142. Ongerth J: *Giardia* cyst concentrations in river water, *J Am Water Works Assoc* 83:81, 1989.

143. Ongerth J et al: Backcountry water treatment to prevent giardiasis. *Am J Public Health* 79:1633, 1989.

143a. Ongerth JE, Stibbs HH: Identification of *Cryptosporidium* oocysts in river water, *Appl Environ Microbiol* 53:672, 1987.

144. Ortega YR et al: Isolation of *Cryptosporidium parvum* and *Cyclospora cayetanensis* from vegetables collected in markets of an endemic region in Peru, *Am J Trop Med Hyg* 57:683, 1997.

145. Paul T et al: The effect of small increases in dietary iodine on thyroid function in euthyroid subjects, *Metabolism* 37:121, 1988.

146. Peeters J et al: Effect of disinfection of drinking water with ozone or chlorine dioxide on survival of *Cryptosporidium, Appl Environ Microbiol* 55:1519, 1989.

147. Pennington J: A review of iodine toxicity reports, *J Am Diet Assoc* 90:1571, 1990.

148. Perez-Rosas N, Hazen T: In situ survival of *Vibrio cholerae* and *Escherichia coli* in a tropical rain forest watershed, *Appl Environ Microbiol* 55:495, 1989.

149. Perkins J: Thermal Destruction of microorganisms: Heat inactivation of viruses. In *Principles and methods of sterilization in health sciences,* Springfield, Ill, 1969, Charles C Thomas.

150. Peterson D et al: Thermal treatment and infectivity of Hepatitis A virus in human feces, *J Med Virol* 2:201, 1978.

151. Peterson D et al: Effect of chlorine treatment on infectivity of Hepatitis A virus, *Appl Environ Microbiol* 45:223, 1983.

152. Porter J et al: *Giardia* transmission in a swimming pool, *Am J Public Health* 78:659, 1988.

153. Powers E: *Efficacy of flocculating and other emergency water purification tablets,* TR-93/033 Natick, Mass, 1993, Natick Research, Development and Engineering Center, US Army.

154. Powers E: *Inactivation of Giardia cysts by iodine with special reference to Globaline: a review,* TR-93/022 Natick, Mass, 1993, Natick Research, Development and Engineering Center, US Army.

155. Powers E, Hernandez C: *Efficacy of Aquapure emergency water purification tablets,* TR-92/027 Natick, Mass, 1992, Natick Research, Development and Engineering Center, US Army.

156. Powers E et al: Biocidal efficacy of a flocculating emergency water purification tablet, *Appl Environ Microbiol* 60:2316, 1994.

157. Powers E et al: *Removal of biological and chemical challenge from water by commercial fresh and salt water purification devices,* TR-91-042 Natick, Mass, 1991, Natick Research, Development and Engineering Center, US Army.

158. Preston D et al: Novel approach for modifying microporous filters for virus concentration from water, *Appl Environ Microbiol* 54:1325, 1988.

159. Rao V et al: Removal of hepatitis A virus and rotavirus by drinking water treatment, *J Am Water Works Assoc* 82:59, 1988.

160. Reeves H: Human waste disposal in the Sierran wilderness. In Stanley J et al, editors *A report on the Wilderness Impact Study: the effects of human recreational activities on wilderness ecosystems with special emphasis on Sierra Club wilderness outings in the Sierra Nevada,* San Francisco, 1979, Sierra Club.

161. Regli S: Regulations on filtration and disinfection. In *Proceedings of Conference on Current Research in Drinking Water Treatment,* Cincinnati, 1988, US Environmental Protection Agency.

162. Regli S: Modeling the risk from *Giardia* and viruses in drinking water, *J Am Water Works Assoc* 83:76, 1991.

163. Regunathan P, Beauman W: Microbiological characteristics of point-of-use precoat carbon filters, *J Am Water Works Assoc* 79:67, 1987.

164. Reimers R et al: Investigation of parasites in sludges and disinfection techniques, Cincinnati, 1986, US Environmental Protection Agency.

165. Rendtorff R: The experimental transmission of human intestinal protozoan parasites. II. *Giardia lamblia* cysts given in capsules, *Am J Hyg* 59:209, 1954.

166. Rice E, Johnson C: Cholera in Peru, *Lancet* 338:455, 1991 (letter).

167. Rice E et al: Inactivation of *Giardia* cysts by chlorine, *Appl Environ Microbiol* 43:250, 1982.

168. Riggs J: AIDS transmission in drinking water: no threat, *J Am Water Works Assoc* 81:69, 1989.

169. Riggs J et al: Detection of *Giardia lamblia* by immunofluorescence, *Appl Environ Microbiol* 45:698, 1983.

170. Roach P et al: Waterborne *Giardia* cysts and *Cryptosporidium* oocysts in the Yukon, Canada, *Appl Environ Microbiol* 59:67, 1993.

171. Robison L: Comparison of the effects of iodine and iodide on thyroid function in humans, *J Toxicol Environ Health* 55:93, 1998.

172. Rogers M, Vitaliano J: Military and small group water disinfecting systems: an assessment, *Mil Med* 7:267, 1979.

173. Rose J: Occurrence and significance of *Cryptosporidium* in water, *J Am Water Works Assoc* 82:53, 1988.

174. Rose J: Occurrence and control of *Cryptosporidium* in drinking water. In McFeters G, editor: *Drinking water microbiology,* New York, 1990, Springer-Verlag.

175. Rose J et al: Occurrence of rotaviruses and enteroviruses in recreational waters of Oak Creek, Arizona, *Water Res* 21:1375, 1987.

176. Rose J et al: Survey of potable water supplies for *Cryptosporidium* and *Giardia, Environ Sci Technol* 25:1393, 1991.

177. Rose J et al: The role of pathogen monitoring in microbial risk assessment. In Hurst C, editor: *Modeling disease transmission and its prevention by disinfection,* Melbourne, 1996, Cambridge University Press.

178. Rosen A, Booth R: Taste and odor control. In American Water Works Association: *Water quality and treatment: a handbook of public water supplies,* New York, 1971, McGraw-Hill.

179. Roti E, Vagenakis A: Effect of excess iodide: clinical aspects. In Braverman L, Utiger R, editors: *Werner and Ingbar's the thyroid,* Philadelphia, 1996, Lippincott-Raven.

180. Rubin A et al: Inactivation of gerbil-cultured *Giardia lamblia* cysts by free chlorine, *Appl Environ Microbiol* 55:2592, 1989.

181. Saaski B, Bicking M: Evaluation of the Mountain Safety Research carbon and ceramic filter cartridges: iodine reduction, New Brighton, Minn, 1992, Spectrum Labs.

182. Sattar S: *Viruses, water and health,* Ottowa, 1978, Ottawa University Press.

183. Schaffner W: Gas gangrene (other *Clostridium*-associated disease). In Mandell G et al, editors: *Principles and practice of infectious disease,* New York, 1990, Churchill Livingstone.

184. Shephart M: Helminthological aspects of sewage treatment. In Feachem R et al, editors: *Water, wastes and health in hot climates,* New York, 1977, Wiley.

185. Siddiqi S et al: Water-borne hepatitis E virus epidemic in Islamabad, Pakistan: a common source outbreak traced to the malfunction of a modern water treatment plant, *Am J Trop Med Hyg* 57:151, 1997.

186. Singh A, McFeters G: Injury of enteropathogenic bacteria in drinking water. In McFeters G, editor: *Drinking water microbiology,* New York, 1990, Springer-Verlag.

187. Soave R et al: Cyclospora, *Infect Dis Clin North Am* 12:1, 1998.

188. Sobel J et al: Reduction of fecal contamination of street-vended beverages in Guatemala by a simple system for water purification and storage, handwashing, and beverage storage, *Am J Trop Med Hyg* 59:380, 1998.

189. Sobsey M: Enteric viruses and drinking water supplies, *J Am Water Works Assoc* 67:414, 1975.

190. Sobsey M et al: Inactivation of hepatitis A virus and model viruses in water by free chlorine. In *Proceedings of Conference on Current Research in Drinking Water Treatment,* Cincinnati, 1988, US Environmental Protection Agency.

191. Sobsey M et al: Inactivation of cell-associated and dispersed hepatitis A virus in water, *J Am Water Works Assoc* 83:64, 1991.

192. Sobsey M et al: Comparative inactivation of hepatitis A virus and other enteroviruses in water by iodine, *Water Sci Technol* 24:331, 1991.

193. Sorenson S et al: Isolation and detection of *Giardia* cysts from water using direct immunoflourescence, *Water Resources Bulletin* 22:843, 1986.

194. States S et al: *Legionella* in drinking water. In McFeters G, editor: *Drinking water microbiology,* New York, 1990, Springer-Verlag.

195. Steiner T et al: Protozoal agents: what are the dangers for the public water supply? *Annu Rev Med* 48:329, 1997.

196. Stringer R, Kruse C: Amoebic cysticidal properties of halogens in water. In *Proceedings of National Specialty Conference on Disinfection*, 1970, American Society of Civil Engineers.

197. Suk T et al: The relation between human presence and occurrence of *Giardia* cysts in streams in the Sierra Nevada, California, *J Freshwater Ecol* 4, 1988.

198. Sullivan R et al: Thermal resistance of certain oncogenic viruses in milk, *Appl Microbiol* 22:315, 1971.

199. Sykes G: *Disinfection and sterilization*, London, 1965, Lipincott.

200. Thomas W et al: Iodine disinfection of water, *Arch Environ Health* 19:124, 1969.

201. Thomas W et al: Effects of an iodinated water supply, *Trans Am Clim Assoc* 90:153, 1978.

202. Thomson G et al: *Evaluation of water sterilizing tablets*, AR No 004-318, Scottsdale, Tasmania, 1985, Department of Defense, Armed Forces Food Science Establishment.

203. Thraenhart O: Measures for disinfection and control of viral hepatitis, In Block S, editor: *Disinfection, sterilization, and preservation*, Philadelphia, 1991, Lea & Febiger.

204. Tillet H et al: Surveillance of outbreaks of waterborne infectious disease: categorizing levels of evidence, *Epidemiol Infect* 120:37, 1998.

205. Tobin R: Performance of Point-of-use water treatment devices. In *Proceedings of the First Conference on Cold Regions Environmental Engineering*, 1983, Fairbanks, Alaska.

206. Tobin R: Testing and evaluating point-of-use treatment devices in Canada, *J Am Water Works Assoc* 79:42, 1987.

207. Tunnicliff B et al: *Drinking water treatment and procedures for Colorado River corridor raft trips*, 1984, Grand Canyon National Park.

208. Upton S et al: Efficacy of a pentaiodide resin disinfectant on *Cryptosporidium parvum* oocysts in vitro, *J Parasit* 74:719, 1988.

209. US Army: Sanitary control and surveillance of field water supplies, Dept of Army Technical Bulletin (TB Med 577), 1986.

210. US Environmental Protection Agency: *Human viruses in the aquatic environment*, EPA-570/9-78-006, Cincinnati, 1978.

211. US Environmental Protection Agency: *Health effects of land treatment*, USEPA-600/1-82-007, Cincinnati, 1982.

212. US Environmental Protection Agency: *Guide standard and protocol for testing microbiological water purifiers*, Cincinnati, 1987.

213. US Forest Service: *Back country safety tips*.

214. US Public Health Service: *Drinking water standards*, USPHS Pub No 956, 1962.

215. Venczel L et al: Inactivation of *Cryptosporidium parvum* oocysts and *Clostridium perfringens* spores by a mixed-oxidant disinfectant and by free chlorine, *Appl Environ Microbiol* 63:1598, 1997.

216. Wallis P et al: Removal and inactivation of *Giardia* cysts in a mobile water treatment plant under field condition: preliminary results. In Wallis P, Hammond B, editors: *Advances in Giardia research*, Calgary, 1988, University of Calgary Press.

217. Ward R, Akin E: Minimum infective dose of animal viruses, *CRC Crit Rev Environ Control* 14:297, 1984.

218. Water and Sanitation for Health Project: *Water supply and sanitation in rural development*, Technical Report No 14, Washington, DC, 1981.

219. Water and Sanitation for Health Project: *Report on mobile emergency water treatment and disinfection units*, Field Report No 271, Washington, DC, 1989.

220. Weiss S et al: Long-lived oxidants generated by human neutrophils: characterization and bioactivity, *Science* 222:625, 1983.

221. White G: *Handbook of chlorination*, New York, 1992, Van Nostrand Reinhold.

222. Wilkerson J: *Medicine for mountaineering*, Seattle, 1985, The Mountaineers.

223. Witenberg G, Yoge J: Investigation on purification of water with respect to *Schistosoma cercariae*, *Trans R Soc Trop Med Hyg* 31:549, 1938.

224. Wolff J: Iodide goiter and the pharmacologic effects of excess iodide, *Am J Med* 47:101, 1969.

225. Woo P: Evidence for animal reservoirs and transmission of *Giardia* infection between animal species. In Erlandsen S, Meyer E, editors: *Giardia and giardiasis: biology, pathogenesis and epidemiology*, New York, 1984, Plenum Press.

226. Woodward R: Review of the bactericidal effectiveness of silver, *J Am Water Works Assoc* 55:881, 1963.

227. World Health Organization: *Human viruses in water, wastewater, and soil*, Geneva, 1979, WHO.

228. World Health Organization: *Intestinal protozoan and helminthic infections*, Geneva, 1981, WHO.

229. Yoshpe-Purer Y, Eylan E: Disinfection of water by hydrogen peroxide, *Health Lab Sci* 5:233, 1968.

230. Zell S: Epidemiology of wilderness-acquired diarrhea: implications for prevention and treatment, *J Wilderness Med* 3:241, 1992.

231. Zell S, Sorenson M: Cyst acquisition rate for *Giardia lamblia* in backcountry travelers to Desolation Wilderness, Lake Tahoe, *J Wilderness Med* 4:147, 1993.

232. Zemlyn S et al: A caution on iodine water purification, *West J Med* 135:166, 1981.

233. Zoeteman B: *The suitability of iodine and iodine compounds as disinfectants for small water supplies*, The Hague, 1972, WHO International Reference Centre for Community Water Supplies.

52 Infectious Diarrhea from Wilderness and Foreign Travel

Javier A. Adachi, Howard D. Backer, and Herbert L. DuPont

Acute diarrhea is one of the most common medical problems in all populations, second only to acute upper respiratory diseases. Worldwide, diarrheal diseases were reported to cause nearly 1 billion episodes of illness in 1996.[45,60,61,181] The rates of illness among children in developing areas of the world range from 5 to 15 bouts per child per year, with diarrhea being the most important cause of morbidity and mortality in many regions. Readily available oral rehydration solutions prevent great numbers of dehydration-associated deaths related to acute diarrhea, especially in developing areas, but invasive bacterial enterocolitis (caused by *Shigella* species and *Campylobacter jejuni*) and persistent diarrhea (defined as illness lasting 14 days or longer) still cause significant morbidity and mortality.[45,89,181]

Specific groups of U.S. populations with diarrhea rates similar to those in the developing world include travelers, gay males, non-toilet-trained toddlers in day-care centers, and mentally impaired residents of custodial institutions.[60,89]

This chapter provides information to help to decrease exposure to enteropathogens and risk factors, reducing the chance of acquiring illness. The clinical features of acute diarrheal illnesses often do not permit differentiation of the specific etiologic agent, but fortunately, the majority of these infections do not require etiology-specific treatment.[45,60,61] We formulate a clinical approach to self-therapy that is likely to minimize the complications and suffering caused by these illnesses. For the purpose of this discussion, "traveler" includes business or pleasure travelers as well as wilderness venturers.

GENERAL PRINCIPLES OF ENTERIC INFECTIONS

Epidemiology

Transmission. Fecal-oral contamination, through ingestion of contaminated water and food, is the usual route of transmission for enteric pathogens causing infectious diarrhea. Other, less common routes of fecal-oral transmission are through aerosols (viruses), contaminated hands or surfaces, and sexual activity. The relative importance of food and water depends mainly on location and precautions taken. Waterborne pathogens from drinking untreated surface water or from an inadvertent ingestion during water recreational activity account for most infectious diarrhea acquired in the U.S. wilderness.[89,125,131] Waterborne diarrheal diseases include typhoid fever, cholera, *Campylobacter* enteritis, cryptosporidiasis, giardiasis, and hepatitis A infection. They are usually preventable by proper sanitation and water disinfection. Enterotoxigenic *Escherichia coli*, enteroinvasive *E. coli*, *Aeromonas* species, *Plesiomonas shigelloides*, *Shigella* species, *Vibrio cholerae*, *Campylobacter jejuni*, and *Yersinia enterocolitica* can be foodborne as well as waterborne. Person-to-person transmission is seen in selected populations whose habits expose them to high levels of pathogens (e.g., infants in day-care centers, homosexuals, persons with minimal access to water); prevention of these illnesses includes adequate handwashing and personal hygiene.[45,60,61]

Location. In several areas of Africa, Asia, and Latin America, where satisfactory sanitation is lacking, diarrhea is still the leading cause of infant morbidity and mortality. Good sanitation is related to a much lower incidence of infectious diarrhea in industrialized areas of the world. Travelers to foreign countries and wilderness areas often leave behind sanitation in the form of flush toilets and safe tap water, as well as proximity to advanced medical care. Similar hygienic conditions are created in other settings.

Outbreaks of infectious diarrhea in day-care centers among non-toilet-trained toddlers are associated with *Giardia lamblia*, *Shigella*, *Campylobacter jejuni*, and *Cryptosporidium*, which have a small infectious dose. Hospitals, especially intensive care units and pediatric wards, institutions for mentally handicapped patients, and nursing homes are also locations with high incidence of diarrheal diseases. *Clostridium difficile*–associated diarrhea, *Salmonella* species, rotavirus, and enteropathogenic *E. coli* are the most common etiologic agents reported[60,89,158] (Table 52-1).

Antimicrobial Therapy. *C. difficile*–associated diarrhea is frequently related to recent use of an antimicrobial agent (or cytotoxic agent), usually during the last 2 to 4 weeks before the beginning of diarrheal illness.[30,70,104]

Age. In developing areas of the world, children below 5 years of age have higher morbidity and mortality

TABLE 52-1. Epidemiologic Associations with Enteropathogens

AGENTS	WATER-BORNE	CHILDREN*	HOSPITAL/ INSTITUTIONALIZED	HOMO-SEXUALITY	IMMUNO-COMPROMISED	ZOONOTIC
BACTERIA						
Enteropathogenic *Escherichia coli*	−	+	+	−	−	−
Enterotoxigenic *E. coli*	−	−	−	−	−	−
Enteroinvasive *E. coli*	−	−	−	−	−	−
Enterohemorrhagic *E. coli*	−	−	−	−	−	−
Enteroaggregative *E. coli*	−	+	−	−	+	−
Non-*typhi* Salmonella	−	−	+	−	−	+
Salmonella typhi	+	−	−	−	−	−
Shigella spp.	−	+	−	+	−	−
Campylobacter spp.	+	+	−	+	−	+
Vibrio cholerae	+	−	−	−	−	−
Yersinia enterocolitica	−	−	−	−	−	+
Aeromonas spp.	+	−	−	−	−	−
Plesiomonas shigelloides	−	−	−	−	−	−
Clostridium difficile	−	−	+	−	−	−
VIRUSES						
Norwalk, small round	+	−	−	−	−	−
Rotavirus	+	+	+	−	−	−
Hepatitis A	+	−	−	−	−	−
PROTOZOA						
Giardia lamblia	+	+	−	−	+	+
Entamoeba histolytica	+	−	−	−	−	+
Cryptosporidium parvum	+	−	−	+	+	+
Isospora belli	−	−	−	−	+	−
Cyclospora cayetanensis	+	−	−	−	+	−
Microsporidia	−	−	−	−	+	−
Balantidium coli	−	−	−	−	−	+
Sarcocystis	−	−	−	−	−	+
Blastocystis hominis	−	−	−	−	−	−

*In industrialized areas or day care centers.
+, Association; −, no association or unknown association.

rates related to dehydration, from an estimated five to 15 episodes of diarrhea per year, superimposed on malnutrition. The enteropathogens more common in infectious diarrhea during childhood are rotavirus, enterotoxigenic *E. coli*, enteropathogenic *E. coli*, *C. jejuni*, and *G. lamblia* (see Table 52-1). Residents in industrialized countries, such as the United States, have only one to two bouts of diarrhea per person per year, with no difference between age groups. Complications, including death, are more common in elderly persons.[45,60,76]

Reservoirs of Infection. Organisms are shed in the stools during asymptomatic and symptomatic infection and for a period after illness. Long-term shedding or chronic carrier states are reported only with typhoid fever, amebiasis, giardiasis, cryptosporidiasis, and en-

teroaggregative *E. coli* infection. These cases may act as reservoirs for spreading infection, even in areas with low risk for infection by contaminated water. A few enteric pathogens that are zoonotic (animal reservoirs) can increase the risk for certain persons (e.g., veterinarians, field biologists) and account for wilderness-acquired infections. These zoonotic organisms include *Salmonella, Yersinia, Campylobacter, Giardia, Balantidium coli, Entamoeba, Sarcocystis,* and *Cryptosporidium*[45,60] (see Table 52-1).

Incubation Period. Food intoxication caused by ingestion of preformed toxins from *Staphylococcus aureus* or *Bacillus cereus* usually has a short incubation period (7 hours or less) and may have a common source reported by multiple victims. An outbreak by any en-

TABLE 52-2. Enteropathogens Found in Tropical and Wilderness Travel

AGENTS	TRAVEL TO DEVELOPING TROPICAL REGIONS	WILDERNESS TRAVEL IN INDUSTRIALIZED REGIONS
BACTERIA		
Enteropathogenic *Escherichia coli*	Rarely	Rarely
Enterotoxigenic *E. coli*	Yes	Rarely
Enteroinvasive *E. coli*	Rarely	Rarely
Enterohemorrhagic *E. coli*	Rarely	Rarely
Enteroaggregative *E. coli*	Yes	Unknown
Salmonella spp.	Yes	Yes
Shigella spp.	Yes	Yes
Campylobacter spp.	Yes	Yes
Vibrio cholerae	Limited	No
Yersinia enterocolitica	Rarely	Limited
Aeromonas spp.	Yes	Yes
Plesiomonas shigelloides	Yes	Rarely
VIRUSES		
Norwalk, other small round	Yes	Yes
Rotavirus	Yes	Rarely
Hepatitis A	Yes	Yes
PROTOZOA		
Giardia lamblia	Yes	Yes
Entamoeba histolytica	Yes	Rarely
Cryptosporidium parvum	Yes	Yes
Isospora belli	Limited	Rarely
Cyclospora cayetanensis	Limited	Rarely
Microsporidia	Limited	Rarely
Balantidium coli	Limited	Rarely
Sarcocystis	Limited	Rarely
Blastocystis hominis	Limited	Rarely

teropathogen that must first infect the intestine usually has an incubation period of 8 or more hours.

Immunocompromised Status. Immunocompromised patients, including those infected with human immunodeficiency virus (HIV), are prone to acquire infection by a wide variety of enteropathogens, to develop infectious diarrhea, and to experience relapses or reinfections. HIV patients with advanced acquired immunodeficiency syndrome (AIDS) often experience malabsorption and chronic diarrhea because of changes in the intestinal function secondary to HIV or because of reduced immunity that allows coinfection with other enteropathogens. The agents responsible for diarrheal diseases in HIV patients are common enteric agents, *Mycobacterium avium-intracellulare* complex, *Cryptosporidium, Giardia, Isospora, Cyclospora, Microsporidium,* cytomegalovirus, herpes simplex virus and HIV. Treatment of HIV with highly active antiretroviral therapy and treatment of the enteric infec-

tion are associated with improved symptomatology and decreased rates of infection.

Etiology

Enteropathogens are the most common etiologic agents of infectious diarrhea and include bacteria, viruses, and protozoa. Fungal agents have been reported rarely. Table 52-2 lists the etiologic agents often associated with travel to developing tropical areas or with wilderness travel in an industrialized region. Foodborne illness may consist of food "poisoning" or food "infection." In food poisoning an intoxication results when toxins produced by bacteria are found in food in sufficient concentrations to produce symptoms. The major forms of intoxication result from *S. aureus* or *B. cereus*. A rare cause of food poisoning is botulism, caused when the neurotoxin of *Clostridium botulinum* is ingested. Other food borne pathogens are viruses, including rotavirus and small round viruses (Norwalk virus, astrovirus), and intestinal protozoal

TABLE 52-3. Bacterial Enteropathogens: Virulence Properties and Distribution

PATHOGEN	VIRULENCE PROPERTIES	DISTRIBUTION
Vibrio cholerae	Heat-labile enterotoxin	Endemic areas in Asia, Africa, and Latin America
Vibrio parahaemolyticus	Invasiveness (?), enterotoxin or hemolytic toxin	Endemic areas in Asia and Latin America
Enteropathogenic *E. coli*	Enteroadherence	Infants, worldwide
Enterotoxigenic *E. coli*	Heat-stable and heat-labile enterotoxins, colonization factor antigens	Developing countries, tropical areas, infants, travelers
Enteroinvasive *E. coli*	*Shigella*-like invasiveness	Worldwide, endemic in South America and Eastern Europe
Enterohemorrhagic *E. coli*	Shigalike toxin (?)	Beef, other vehicles in industrialized areas
Enteroaggregative *E. coli*	Enteroadherence	Infants, travelers, worldwide
Salmonella spp.	Cholera-like toxin, invasiveness	Worldwide
Shigella spp.	Shigalike toxin, invasiveness	Worldwide
Campylobacter jejuni	Cholera-like toxin, invasiveness	Worldwide
Aeromonas spp.	Hemolysin, cytotoxin, enterotoxin	Worldwide, especially Thailand, Australia, and Canada
Yersinia enterocolitica	Heat-stable enterotoxin, invasiveness	Worldwide, especially Canada, Scandinavia, and South Africa
Clostridium difficile	Cytotoxin A and B	Worldwide
Clostridium perfringens	Preformed toxin	Worldwide
Bacillus cereus	Preformed toxin	Worldwide
Staphylococcus aureus	Preformed toxins	Worldwide

agents, including *G. lamblia, Entamoeba histolytica,* and *Cryptosporidium.*

Pathophysiology

Three intestinal mechanisms lead to diarrhea. The most common pathophysiologic mechanism in acute infectious diarrhea is alteration of fluid and electrolyte movement from the serosal to the mucosal surface of the gut (secretory diarrhea). This alteration may occur as a result of cyclic nucleotide stimulation (as a second messenger) or by an inflammatory process that releases cytokines. The second mechanism, malabsorption or presence of nonabsorbed substances in the lumen of the bowel, and third, acceleration of intestinal motility, are more important in chronic forms of infectious and noninfectious diarrhea, such as tropical and nontropical sprue, Whipple's disease, scleroderma, malabsorption, irritable bowel syndrome, and inflammatory bowel disease. Table 52-3 shows the virulence factors of the most important enteric pathogens related to infectious diarrhea.[42,60]

In general, enteropathogens cause diarrhea by the first mechanism and can be subdivided into noninvasive and invasive groups. Noninvasive microorganisms primarily colonize the proximal small bowel and cause secretory diarrhea without disruption of the mucosal surface. The unformed stools are usually voluminous and rarely bloody, and high fever is unusual. The common pathogens in this group include *V. cholerae,* enterotoxigenic *E. coli,* preformed enterotoxins, Norwalk virus, rotavirus, *Giardia,* and *Cryptosporidium.* Dehy-

dration is the major complication, especially in the extremes of age, and without adequate therapy it can be followed by renal insufficiency. Invasive pathogens involve the distal ileum and colon, damaging the mucosa and eliciting an inflammatory response. Stools are typically liquid, small volume, and may contain blood and many leukocytes. The common microorganisms in this group are *Shigella* species, *Salmonella* species, enteroinvasive *E. coli,* enterohemorrhagic *E. coli, Y. enterocolitica, C. jejuni, Aeromonas* species, *V. parahaemolyticus,* and *E. histolytica.* Complications include dehydration and systemic involvement, especially in children with malnutrition.[42,43]

TRAVELER'S DIARRHEA

Traveler's diarrhea (TD) is the most important travel-related illness in terms of frequency and economic impact. Point of origin, destination, and host factors are the main risk determinants.[60,158] International travel is more often associated with enteric infection and diarrhea, particularly when the destination is a developing tropical region, although the same infections can be contracted domestically. The 2% to 4% rate of diarrhea for people who take short-term trips to low-endemic areas (e.g., United States, Canada, Northwestern Europe, Australia, Japan) may be related to more frequent consumption of food in public restaurants, increased intake of alcohol, or stress. This rate of diarrhea increases to about 10% for travelers from these low-endemic areas to northern Mediterranean areas, China,

Russia, or some Caribbean islands. This incidence increases as high as 40% to 50% for short-term travelers from low-risk countries to high-risk countries (developing tropical and sub-tropical regions of Latin America, southern Asia, or Africa). More than 25 million persons travel each year from these industrialized countries to high-risk areas, resulting in over 7 million travelers with diarrhea.[45,60,61] Multiple episodes of diarrhea may occur on the same trip.[158] Attack rates remain high for up to 1 year,[45,60] then decrease, but not to the levels of local inhabitants. Immunity to enterotoxigenic *E. coli* (ETEC) infection, either asymptomatic or symptomatic, occurs after repeated or chronic exposure,[141] which supports the feasibility of developing a vaccine.

TD is a syndrome, not a specific disease.[45,60,158] Although any waterborne or foodborne enteropathogen may cause TD, bacteria are the most common etiologic agents among persons traveling to high-risk areas. The bacterial flora of the bowel changes rapidly after arrival in a country with high rates of TD. At least 15% of travelers remain asymptomatic despite the occurrence of infection by pathogenic organisms, including ETEC and *Shigella*. However, most infected patients become ill.

Definition

TD refers to an illness contracted while traveling, although in 15% of sufferers symptoms begin after the return home.[44] Most studies define TD as the passage of three or more unformed stools in a 24-hour period in association with one or more enteric symptoms, such as abdominal cramps, fever, fecal urgency, tenesmus, passage of bloody, mucoid stools, nausea, and vomiting.[45,60,158]

Etiology

Since the incidence of TD reflects in part the extent of environmental contamination with feces, the etiologic agents are pathogens causing illness in local children. The list of etiologic agents changes as laboratory techniques identify new enteropathogens (Table 52-4). Twenty years ago, specific pathogens were found in only 20% of cases.[112,113] Currently, etiologic agents can be identified in up to 80% of TD episodes.[60,158] In most studies, however, causative pathogens are not identified in 20% to 40% of cases. In most of these cases, antimicrobial therapy shortens illness, suggesting that this subset of diarrhea is caused by undetected bacterial pathogens.[23,57,63,80] Overall, the major etiologic agents and their frequency of isolation are remarkably similar when one region of the world is compared with another.

Enterotoxigenic *E. coli* has proved to be the most common cause of TD worldwide,[60,141,158,178] accounting for about one third to one half of cases. *Shigella* and *Aeromonas/Plesiomonas* species are second to ETEC and

TABLE 52-4. Major Pathogens in Traveler's Diarrhea (Travel to Developing Tropical Regions)

AGENT	FREQUENCY (%)
BACTERIA	**40-80**
Enterotoxigenic *Escherichia coli*	5-40
Enteroaggregative *E. coli*	0-40
Salmonella	0-15
Shigella	0-15
Campylobacter jejuni	0-30
Aeromonas	0-10
Plesiomonas	0-5
Other	0-5
VIRUSES	**0-20**
Rotavirus	0-20
Small round viruses	0-10
PROTOZOA	**0-5**
Giardia lamblia	0-5
Entamoeba histolytica	0-5
Cryptosporidium parvum	0-5
UNKNOWN	**10-40**

cause 20% of illness. Other causes of TD include *Salmonella* (4% to 5% of cases), *Campylobacter* (3%), *Vibrio*, viruses (10%), and parasites (2% to 4%). Specific pathogens may predominate at a particular time or location. ETEC is more common in semitropical countries, including Mexico and Morocco, during rainy summer seasons and occurs less often in drier winters.[133] A recent study showed that enteroaggregative *E. coli* is the second most common etiologic organism in TD in Guadalajara (Mexico), Ocho Rios (Jamaica), and Goa (India).[3a]

Clinical Syndromes

Table 52-5 outlines the major syndromes in patients with enteric infection. The typical clinical syndrome experienced by travelers with diarrhea secondary to the major infectious causes (e.g., ETEC) begins abruptly with watery diarrhea and abdominal cramping. Most cases are mild, consisting of passage of one to two unformed stools per day associated with symptoms that are tolerable and do not interfere with normal activities. Approximately 30% of victims experience moderately severe illness, with three to five unformed stools per day and distressing symptoms that force a change in activities or itinerary. Only 10% to 20% of persons with TD experience severe illness with more than five unformed stools passed per day, incapacitating symptoms that force confinement to bed, or any number of unformed stools with concomitant fever and dysentery.[60,158] Only 4% of persons with TD consult a local

TABLE 52-5. Pathophysiologic Syndromes in Diarrheal Disease

SYNDROME	AGENT
Acute watery diarrhea	Any agent, especially toxin-mediated diseases (e.g., enterotoxigenic *Escherichia coli*, *Vibrio cholerae*)
Febrile dysentery	*Shigella*, *Campylobacter jejuni*, *Salmonella*, enteroinvasive *E. coli*, *Aeromonas* spp., noncholera *Vibrio* spp., *Yersinia enterocolitica*, *Entamoeba histolytica*, inflammatory bowel disease
Vomiting (as predominant symptom)	Viral agents, preformed toxins of *Staphylococcus aureus* or *Bacillus cereus*
Persistent diarrhea (> 14 days)	Protozoa, small bowel bacterial overgrowth, invasive or inflammatory enteropathogens (e.g., *Shigella*, enteroaggregative *E. coli*)
Chronic diarrhea (> 30 days)	Small bowel injury, inflammatory bowel disease, irritable bowel syndrome, Brainerd diarrhea

physician, and less than 1% are admitted to a local hospital while traveling. Approximately one third of travelers are confined to bed or need to alter their travel plans when a diarrheal illness develops. Although the average duration of diarrhea is 3 to 4 days, 50% of cases resolve within 48 hours, 8% to 15% last longer than 1 week, and 1% to 3% last 1 month or longer. TD is rarely life threatening.

Clinical Examination

The etiologic organism of TD cannot be diagnosed reliably based only on clinical manifestations, because illnesses caused by different microorganisms share similar clinical features.[37,60,143,158,184] Although noninvasive organisms rarely cause dysentery, invasive organisms often cause watery diarrhea without dysentery or a sequential illness beginning with watery diarrhea and progressing to bloody dysentery. If multiple people acquire the illness shortly after eating a shared meal, food poisoning caused by ingestion of preformed toxins in food should be suspected, especially if the illness has a short incubation period (8 hours or less), predominant vomiting, and resolution within 24 hours.

Investigators have studied the reliability of clinical factors to predict which persons will have a positive stool culture.[37,143,184] Bacterial pathogens are suspected when the sufferer has a large number (more than six) of stools per day, has a fever, and has had the ailment for more than 24 hours but less than 1 week. Regardless of the clinical similarities of enteropathogens causing TD, certain differences exist, with distinct clinical findings.

Dehydration. An important part of the initial assessment is to measure the level of hydration, which includes a determination of vital signs, orthostatic pulse and blood pressure, mental status, skin turgor, hydration of mucous membranes, and urine output. Dehydration is most common in pediatric and elder populations.

Fever. Fever is a reaction to an intestinal inflammatory process. High fever suggests a pathogen invasive to the intestinal mucosa, which classically includes bacterial enteropathogens such as *Shigella*, *Salmonella*, and *Campylobacter jejuni*. Fever can also be produced by enteroinvasive *E. coli*, *Vibrio parahaemolyticus*, *Aeromonas*, *Clostridium difficile*, and viral pathogens.

Vomiting. Vomiting as the predominant symptom suggests food intoxication secondary to enterotoxin produced by *Staphylococcus aureus* or *Bacillus cereus* or gastroenteritis secondary to viruses, such as rotavirus in infants or Norwalk virus in any age group.

Dysentery. Dysentery is defined as the passage of small-volume stools with gross blood and mucus. Common causes include *Shigella*, *C. jejuni*, *Salmonella*, *Aeromonas*, *V. parahaemolyticus*, *Yersinia enterocolitica*, enteroinvasive *E. coli*, enterohemorrhagic *E. coli*, *Entamoeba histolytica*, and inflammatory bowel disease. Invasive organisms most often cause dysentery. Up to 30% to 50% of cases of shigellosis or campylobacteriosis are reported to cause dysenteric diarrhea in the United States. Other enteric symptoms are tenesmus (straining without passing stools) and fecal urgency (voluntary inability to delay stool evacuation by 15 minutes), which are more common with dysentery.

Abdominal Findings. The abdominal examination in persons with TD often shows mild tenderness but should not demonstrate signs of peritoneal irritation. A rectal examination may reveal tenderness in enterocolitis, and the victim may have painful external hemorrhoids, a result of the excess stooling.

Systemic Involvement. Some of the enteric pathogens produce both diarrheal and systemic disease, such as hemolytic-uremic syndrome related to infection with shigellosis or enterohemorrhagic *E. coli*, Reiter's syndrome or glomerulonephritis related to *Y. enterocolitica*, and typhoid fever secondary to *Salmonella typhi* and *S. paratyphi*.

TABLE 52-6. Indications for Laboratory Test in Diarrheal Diseases and Possible Diagnosis

LABORATORY TEST	INDICATION	DIAGNOSIS/AGENT
Fecal leukocytes or lactoferrin	Moderate to severe cases	Diffuse colonic inflammation, invasive enteropathogen
Stool culture	Moderate to severe diarrhea, fever, persistent diarrhea, fecal leukocytes, male homosexuals, food or water outbreaks	Any bacterial enteropathogen
Blood culture	Enteric fever, sepsis	*Salmonella*, less likely *Campylobacter*, *Shigella*, *Yersinia*
Parasite examination	Persistent diarrhea, travel to specific areas, day-care centers, male homosexuals, immunocompromised persons	Any protozoan parasite
Amebic serology	Persistent diarrhea, liver abscess	*Entamoeba histolytica*
Rotavirus antigen	Hospitalized infants	
Clostridium difficile toxin	Antibiotic-associated diarrhea	*C. difficile*

Laboratory Findings

Several laboratory tests are useful in evaluating patients with diarrheal disease (Table 52-6). For most cases of TD, laboratory testing is reserved for illness continuing after the patient returns home. Persons with mild acute diarrhea usually need only clinical evaluation. An etiologic assessment is unnecessary, and treatment can be given empirically. Laboratory tests are reserved for persons with moderate to severe diarrhea and those with persistent diarrhea.

Fecal Leukocyte Test. The presence of fecal leukocytes is a reliable indicator of invasive and inflammatory distal gastrointestinal (GI) infection. For all moderate to severe illness, this is the most rapid, useful test and the ideal screening procedure. The fecal leukocyte test should be performed on a fresh sample. A mucus strand, if available, or liquid stool is stained with a drop of dilute methylene blue and observed under a microscope. The stool can be heat-fixed and examined under oil immersion or viewed as a wet-mount preparation under a coverslip with the "high dry" objective of the microscope. Leukocytes are easily seen, although they can be confused with protozoal cysts. A large number of polymorphonuclear leukocytes (PMNs) per high-power field (hpf) indicates diffuse colonic inflammation (Figure 52-1) rather than a specific etiology but correlates most significantly with invasive bacterial infection caused by *Shigella*, *Salmonella*, or *C. jejuni*. Other organisms and conditions that may lead to presence of fecal leukocytes in the stools are *C. difficile*–associated diarrhea, *Aeromonas*, *Y. enterocolitica*, *V. parahaemolyticus*, EIEC, idiopathic ulcerative colitis, and allergic colitis. Fecal leukocytes are less likely to be seen in noninvasive infections, such as diarrhea caused by

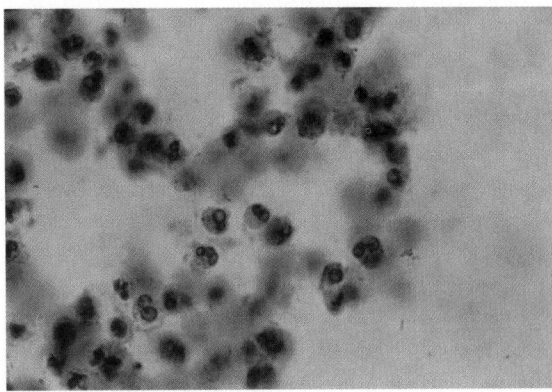

Figure 52-1   Methylene blue stain of a fecal smear from a patient with bacillary dysentery (400x). Numerous polymorphonuclear leukocytes are present, which indicates the presence of diffuse colonic inflammation.

enterotoxigenic *E. coli*, *G. lamblia*, and viral pathogens, but they are often observed in culture-negative stools.[92] Not all patients with invasive infectious diarrhea will have leukocyte-positive stools.

Stool Culture. Bacterial infection is specifically diagnosed by stool culture, although routine stool testing identifies few pathogens. A routine laboratory should be able to recover *Shigella*, *Salmonella*, and *Campylobacter* from a stool culture and, if specifically requested, *Vibrio cholerae* and *V. parahaemolyticus*, *Aeromonas*, *Y. enterocolitica*, and *C. difficile*. In the United States, only about 10% of stool cultures are positive. The percentage is higher (12% for adults, about 50% for children or travelers) among patients in developing countries when research laboratories look for all the important agents, including ETEC.[158,184] The major indications for performing a stool culture are moderate to severe diarrhea, febrile and dysenteric disease, persistent diarrhea, and presence of fecal leukocytes in fecal smears.

Blood Culture. Blood culture(s) should be performed in all patients who are hospitalized with GI symptoms or those who have enteric symptoms and high fever. Systemic infections by *S. typhi* and non-*typhi Salmonella*, *Shigella*, *Campylobacter fetus*, and *Y. enterocolitica* may be diagnosed by blood culture.

Parasite Examination. In cases of TD, direct examination of stool samples looking for a parasite infection is less useful as a routine test than is stool culture. When using microscopy to search for parasites, multiple samples may have to be examined to identify the causative agent. Immunologic techniques to detect antigens of protozoan parasites are more efficient and in common use for parasites that inhabit the duodenum (e.g., *Giardia, Cryptosporidium, E. histolytica*, microsporidia).[89,131] At times, intestinal parasites are better detected using a sample from duodenal aspiration or intestinal biopsy.[89,131] Indications to perform parasitic examination are persistent diarrhea, diarrhea during or shortly after travel within mountainous areas of the United States or Russia, diarrhea in someone who has regular contact with an infant day care center, or diarrhea in a male homosexual or immunocompromised person.

Special Tests. The Enterotest is a gelatin capsule affixed to a nylon string that is swallowed after the end of the string is taped to the cheek. After the patient consumes a meal or after the string has been attached to the cheek overnight, it is removed so that mucus and other intestinal secretions can be scraped off and studied for enteropathogens. It may be useful to sample small bowel mucus to diagnose cases of typhoid fever, giardiasis, and strongyloidiasis.

A serologic diagnostic test for typhoid fever (Widal's reaction) is only useful in endemic areas, because exposure to cross-reacting gram-negative rods other than *S. typhi* can lead to false-positive serologic results in areas where typhoid fever is not common.[136] In a patient with a typhoidlike systemic illness who has taken one or more doses of an antimicrobial, culture of bone marrow aspiration may help to identify the bacteria. Antibody-specific serologic tests are now widely used for the diagnosis of invasive amebiasis.[75]

Rotavirus antigen testing of stool is sensitive and easy to perform. It is indicated to screen infants less than 3 years of age to help guide therapy (fluids without antimicrobials are given when the test is positive).[153]

C. difficile toxin assay by tissue culture or serology is indicated for diagnosing antibiotic-associated colitis.

TABLE 52-7. Empiric Treatment of Diarrhea in Adults

CLINICAL MANIFESTATIONS	RECOMMENDATIONS
Watery diarrhea with mild symptoms (no change in itinerary)	Provide oral fluids and saltine crackers plus symptomatic treatment as needed with loperamide or bismuth subsalicylate.
Watery diarrhea with moderate symptoms (change in itinerary but able to function)	Administer symptomatic treatment with loperamide or bismuth subsalicylate.
Watery diarrhea with severe symptoms (incapacitating)	Perform stool culture and fecal leukocytes; consider antimicrobial drugs* plus loperamide.
Dysentery or fever	Perform stool culture and fecal leukocytes; consider antimicrobial drugs,* no loperamide.
Persistent diarrhea (> 14 days)	Perform stool culture and parasite examination; consider empiric trial with metronidazole.
Vomiting, minimal diarrhea	Administer bismuth subsalicylate.
Diarrhea in pregnant women	As above; administer fluids and electrolytes; consider attapulgite, no fluoroquinolones.

*Fluoroquinolones (norfloxacin, ciprofloxacin, or levofloxacin) are recommended.

Many of the commercial serologic kit tests are easier to perform, but they detect only toxin A and are less sensitive than the tissue culture procedure. Infants and children may normally carry *C. difficile* toxin in the stools, negating the value of this test.[104]

Sigmoidoscopy and Colonoscopy. In selected cases, particularly clinical colitis and diarrhea persisting for 14 days or longer, sigmoidoscopy or colonoscopy is used to study colonic lesions and collect samples for culture and microscopy. Mucosal changes may not be specific, except when pseudomembranes are sought. In homosexual male patients with acute diarrhea, examination of the distal colon may show evidence of proctitis (mucosal inflammation in the distal 15 cm of the colon), proctocolitis (inflammation beyond 15 cm), or enteritis.

Acute Diarrhea

Where routine laboratory evaluation is available, logical approaches to patients with acute diarrhea depend on the clinical syndrome. The illness, not the infection,

TABLE 52-8. Nonspecific Drugs for Prophylaxis and Therapy in Adults

AGENT	THERAPEUTIC DOSE
Attapulgite	3 g initially, then 3 g after each loose stool or every 2 hours (not to exceed 9 g/day); should be safe during pregnancy and childhood.
Loperamide	4 mg initially, then 2 mg after each loose stool (not to exceed 8 to 16 mg/day); do not use in dysenteric diarrhea.
Bismuth subsalicylate	30 ml or two 262-mg tablets every 30 minutes for 8 doses; may repeat on day 2.

should be treated, so most persons can be managed on the basis of symptoms and stool appearance. In certain situations, empiric therapy may be given without establishing an etiologic agent; in other cases, specific therapy follows laboratory confirmation of an etiologic agent (Tables 52-7 and 52-8). In patients with watery diarrhea and mild symptoms, only clinical evaluation is needed. An etiologic assessment is unnecessary, and symptomatic treatment can be given empirically. Persons with moderate to severe diarrhea, dysentery, fever, or presence of fecal leukocytes should have their stool cultured, if laboratory assessment is feasible, and should start empiric antimicrobial therapy.

Persistent and Chronic Diarrhea

Diarrhea may persist after the traveler returns home. Up to 3% of persons with TD in high-risk areas will develop persistent diarrhea. Persistent diarrhea is defined as illness lasting 14 days or longer, whereas diarrhea is considered chronic when the illness has lasted 30 days or longer.[44,60,158] The etiology of persistent or chronic diarrhea often differs from that of acute diarrhea. Important causes of persistent diarrhea include (1) protozoal parasitic agents (*G. lamblia, Cryptosporidium, Cyclospora, E. histolytica*), (2) bacterial infection (*Salmonella, Shigella, Campylobacter, Y. enterocolitica*), (3) lactase deficiency induced by a small bowel pathogen (*G. lamblia*, viral enteropathogen such as rotavirus or Norwalk virus), and (4) a small bowel bacterial overgrowth syndrome secondary to small bowel motility inhibition (as a result of enteric infection) or secondary to antimicrobial use. Occasionally, other parasitic enteric infections can cause more persistent illness. These include *Strongyloides stercoralis, Trichuris trichiura,* and severe infection by *Necator americanus* or *Ancylostoma duodenale.* In rare cases, more protracted diarrhea may be a prominent symptom in persons with schistosomiasis, *Plasmodium falciparum* malaria, leishmaniasis, or African trypanosomiasis.[44,60,158]

When chronic diarrhea occurs, the following possibilities should also be considered:

1. After eradication of microbial pathogens, bowel habits may not return to normal for several weeks. Postdysenteric colitis resembling ulcerative colitis occasionally follows infection with invasive pathogens, especially infection caused by *E. histolytica.* This could represent slow repair of the damage to the intestinal mucosa.
2. Postinfective malabsorption can persist for weeks to months after acute diarrhea; it is especially common after giardiasis.[44,61,158]
3. A poorly defined condition, tropical sprue, may explain prolonged diarrhea in a traveler. Onset usually follows an episode of acute enteritis and is associated with substandard hygiene and longer stays. The cause may involve small bowel bacterial overgrowth, since small bowel incubation may yield a heavy growth of bacteria, and patients often respond to antimicrobial therapy.
4. An underlying condition such as inflammatory bowel disease, irritable bowel syndrome, or celiac sprue may worsen after an episode of acute enteritis.
5. Brainerd diarrhea, named after a community outbreak in Brainerd, Minnesota, may be the explanation for chronic diarrhea. This condition follows the consumption of raw (unpasteurized) milk[150] or untreated water.[155] There is no diagnostic test or therapy and the diagnosis is suspected based on the epidemiologic history (exposure to unpasteurized milk or untreated water just before onset of illness).[23]

The approach to evaluate persistent or chronic diarrhea in travelers should begin with diagnostic tests for conventional bacterial pathogens in stools and at least three parasitologic evaluations in stools. Dietary modification in all cases should include avoidance of lactose. Treatment should be specific, following the results of the microbiologic tests. Because most of these chronic forms of diarrhea are self-limiting, it is unwise to keep treating these patients with multiple antibiotics, which only alters the gut ecology and encourages diarrhea. An empiric trial with metronidazole is an option if all tests are negative (see Table 52-7). If stools contain leukocytes, sigmoidoscopy or colonoscopy should be performed, along with empiric treatment for *Shigella* or *Campylobacter* infection. If there are no leukocytes, duodenal mucus should be examined for *G. lamblia,* followed by empirical treatment for *Giardia,* if metronidazole has not already been given. The next steps are tests for malabsorption and biopsy of the small bowel mucosa.

Treatment

In all cases of diarrhea, fluid and electrolyte replacement should be the primary therapy. Outpatient treatment with instructions for oral rehydration can be used in the vast majority of adults and children. Significant dehydration from diarrhea in travelers is unusual. Treatment with intravenous (IV) fluids is indicated for patients with hypotension, inability to retain oral fluids, or systemic compromise (high fever and toxicity), moderate toxicity or dehydration and a severe underlying disease, or at extremes of age. Selected patients may benefit from symptomatic therapy, and others may receive empiric antimicrobial therapy (see Table 52-7). The main goal for using therapy, such as an antimotility drug or an antimicrobial agent, is to attenuate the severity and duration of diarrhea and concomitant symptoms.

Diet and Lifestyle. Supplemental nutrition is beneficial (essential in undernourished populations) and can be given as soon as fluid deficit losses are replaced, usually after the first 4 hours. During acute diarrheal disease the intestinal tract cannot process complex dietary products, so patients are often told to avoid solid foods. As stooling decreases and appetite improves, staple foods, such as cereals, bananas, crackers, toasts, lentils, potatoes, and other cooked vegetables, are well tolerated and can be gradually added to the diet to facilitate enterocyte renewal, with progression to white meats, fruits, and vegetables. Dairy products and red meats are recommended only after diarrhea has resolved, usually after 2 to 3 days. Only foods and drinks that prolong diarrhea or increase intestinal motility should be avoided, such as those that contain lactose, caffeine, alcohol, high fiber, and fats. Breast-feeding of infants should not be suspended or should be resumed as soon as possible.[41,45,60,61,185] Patients with TD should avoid excessive physical therapy to reduce the risk of dehydration.

Fluid Treatment. The major cause of morbidity and mortality from acute diarrheal disease is depletion of body water and electrolytes. Rehydration is an essential part of therapy, especially in the extremes of age and during pregnancy. Most patients with TD do not become dehydrated, and hydration can be maintained by ingesting fluids such as sodas, juices, soup, and potable water in conjunction with a source of electrolytes (e.g., salted crackers).[23,45,60,61]

The most significant advance in the therapy of diarrhea in the past 25 years has been development of the oral rehydration concept. Oral rehydration solution (ORS) was first developed for treatment of cholera and has saved countless lives, primarily children. ORS precludes extensive use of scarce and expensive IV fluids in developing countries, and its use is the cornerstone of the World Health Organization (WHO) program to combat diarrheal diseases.[23,45,60,61] The discovery that glucose-enhanced intestinal absorption of sodium remains intact despite active diarrhea or vomiting was the key to development of

ORS.[133,170] Other electrolytes are also absorbed nonselectively when ORS is administered.

Watery diarrhea, often caused by release of an enterotoxin, has an electrolyte composition similar to plasma, varying somewhat with type of infection and age of the patient. The formula packaged and promoted by the WHO and United Nations Internations Children's Emergency Fund (UNICEF) contains powder to be mixed with 1 L of disinfected water, with the following concentrations: sodium 90 mEq, potassium 20 mEq, chloride 80 mEq, bicarbonate 30 mEq, and glucose 111 mmol. Newer formulations use trisodium citrate instead of sodium bicarbonate and complex carbohydrates instead of glucose. Cereal-based products are also available. Although this concentration of electrolytes is ideal for treating purging diarrhea associated with cholera and other dehydrating forms of diarrhea, most TD can be adequately managed with readily available soft and sport drinks, fruit juice or salt solutions, taken with salted crackers and the foods listed earlier.[23,45,60,61]

Fluid status in the field must be guided by physical signs related to hydration, including pulse, mucous membranes, skin turgor, and urine output. Urine color and volume are excellent measures. For travelers in the wilderness or tropics, fluid replacement must equal basic needs plus volume of diarrhea plus estimated sweat loss.

Nonspecific Therapy. Symptomatic medications are useful for treatment of mild to moderate diarrhea, since they decrease symptoms and allow patients to return more quickly to normal activities (see Tables 52-7 and 52-8). Nonantibiotic therapies that may be used in addition to fluids are best classified by their effects on pathophysiologic mechanisms.

ALTERATION OF INTESTINAL FLORA. Lactobacillus preparations and yogurt are safe, but evidence is insufficient to establish their value in the therapy of acute diarrhea.[23,45,60,61,94]

ADSORBENTS. Adsorbent agents bind nonspecifically to water and other intraluminal material, including bacteria and toxins, and potentially to other medications such as antibiotics. The most common medication in this group is attapulgite (see Table 52-8 for dosing), a nonabsorbable magnesium aluminum silicate that is more active than the combination of kaolin and pectin.[23] By adsorbing water, these agents give stools more form or consistency but do not decrease stool frequency, cramps, or duration of illness. They are reliable and should be safe in all persons, although adsorbents are not approved for use in young infants and pregnant women.[169]

ANTIMOTILITY DRUGS. Narcotic analogs related to opiates are the major antimotility drugs. In addition to slowing intestinal motility, these drugs alter water and electrolyte transport, probably affecting both secretion and absorption.[23,45,60,61] Compared with placebo, antimotility drugs reduce the number of stools passed and the duration of illness by about 80% during their administration.[55,56] The most frequently used product is loperamide (Imodium), 4 mg initially, followed by 2 mg after each unformed stool, not to exceed 8 to 16 mg/day. Loperamide also has a weak antisecretory effect through inhibition of intestinal calmodulin. Diphenoxylate with atropine (Lomotil) is less expensive than loperamide but has greater central opiate effects, in case of accidental overdose by a child, and more side effects without antidiarrheal benefits because of the atropine, which is added only to prevent overdoses. Tincture of opium or paregoric opium preparations are rapidly and equally effective and offer a modest relief of symptoms.

Antimotility drugs should never be used alone in patients who have dysenteric or febrile diarrhea, since inhibition of gut motility may facilitate intestinal infection by invasive bacterial enteropathogens.[23,46] However, this theoretic deleterious effect does not appear to be an issue when loperamide is used concurrently with an effective antimicrobial agent.[63,64,187] Antimotility drugs should not be given to children under age 3 years because of the danger of central nervous system (CNS) depression.[23] They are not recommended for more than 48 hours in acute diarrhea.

ANTISECRETORY DRUGS. Since increased secretion of water and electrolytes is the major physiologic derangement in acute watery diarrhea, therapy aimed at this effect is appealing. Although aspirin and other nonsteroidal antiinflammatory drugs (NSAIDs) inhibit secretion, their usefulness is limited, primarily because of mucosal toxicity.[23,61] The salicylate moiety of bismuth subsalicylate reduces the number of stools passed and duration of diarrhea by about 50%, primarily by blocking the effect of the enterotoxin on the intestinal mucosa.[23,56] Bismuth subsalicylate also has antimicrobial and antiinflammatory properties. New compounds are being developed that have antisecretory properties without motility effects.[58]

Antimicrobial Therapy. Although most enteric infections do not require antibiotics, empiric antimicrobial therapy is indicated in acute TD and febrile, dysenteric illness because of the high frequency of bacteria as etiologic agents (Table 52-9).[23,61] Therapy for specific infections is discussed in the corresponding sections. At times, treatment is indicated regardless of symptoms to prevent person-to-person spread (e.g., for food handlers, river guides, day-care workers) or to eradicate pathogenic strains and prevent conversion from asymptomatic to symptomatic illness (e.g., E. histolytica).[22,163]

Only fluoroquinolones and to a lesser extent trimethoprim/sulfamethoxazole (TMP/SMX) retain

TABLE 52-9. Antibacterial Therapy for Diarrhea in Adults

DIAGNOSIS	RECOMMENDATION
EMPIRIC THERAPY IN BACTERIOLOGICALLY UNCONFIRMED DISEASE	
Traveler's diarrhea or febrile dysenteric disease	Norfloxacin 400 mg bid, ciprofloxacin 500 mg bid, or levofloxacin 500 mg qd for 1 to 3 days
Persistent diarrhea	Trial with metronidazole 250 mg qid for 7 days
ORGANISM-SPECIFIC THERAPY IN LABORATORY CONFIRMED DIARRHEA	
Enterotoxigenic and enteroaggregative Escherichia coli diarrhea	Ciprofloxacin 1000 mg single dose or 500 mg bid for 3 days; norfloxacin 400 mg bid or levofloxacin 500 mg qd for 1 to 3 days.
Cholera	Ciprofloxacin 1000 mg single dose or 500 mg bid for 3 days; norfloxacin 400 mg bid or levofloxacin 500 mg qd for 3 days; doxycycline 300 mg single dose
Salmonellosis (typhoid fever or systemic infection)	Norfloxacin 400 mg bid, ciprofloxacin 500 mg bid, or levofloxacin 500 mg qd for 7-10 days; in patients with underlying disease or immunocompromised persons.
Salmonellosis (intestinal nontyphoid salmonellosis without systemic infection)	Antimicrobial therapy controversial (see text)
Shigellosis	Norfloxacin 400 mg bid, ciprofloxacin 500 mg bid, or levofloxacin 500 mg qd for 3 days
Campylobacteriosis	Erythromycin 500 mg qid for 5 days; azithromycin 500 mg qd, norfloxacin 400 mg bid, ciprofloxacin 500 mg bid, or levofloxacin 500 mg qd for 3 days
Enteropathogenic E. coli diarrhea	Unclear if antimicrobial therapy is necessary
Clostridium difficile colitis	Metronidazole 250 mg tid for 7 to 14 days

Bid, Twice daily; qd, daily.

enough activity against enteric pathogens to be considered useful for empiric therapy. The drug of choice for empiric therapy of TD in adults is an oral fluoroquinolone for 1 to 3 days.[23,60,61]

Fluoroquinolones, including those evaluated in TD (norfloxacin, ciprofloxacin, ofloxacin, levofloxacin), represent the treatments of choice for TD when individuals are traveling to areas where TMP/SMX resistance among bacterial enteropathogens is common or has not been determined. Potential advantages of the quinolones include a high degree of in vitro activity against virtually all bacterial etiologic agents (including *Campylobacter*) and the potential for less bacterial resistance.[23,57,63] Ciprofloxacin (500 mg twice a day) was equally effective in treating TD compared with TMP/SMX in an area where trimethoprim resistance was unusual.[63] TMP/SMX (160/800 mg) and trimethoprim (200 mg) twice a day for 5 days were equally effective in reducing the number of unformed stools, duration of illness, and abdominal symptoms compared with placebo.[51] Reduced duration of illness was reported in infections caused by ETEC or *Shigella* and also in the group without identifiable pathogens. The main problem with TMP/SMX is the increasing in vitro resistance to this antibiotic in several areas of the world.[23,60,61]

Because fluoroquinolones are not yet approved for use in children, TMP/SMX plus a macrolide, nalidixic acid, or azithromycin may be given, although a two-drug regimen is a major disadvantage. Azithromycin alone or a short course of a fluoroquinolone may soon be proven safe and efficacious.[118,168]

Travelers to high-risk regions should carry an antibacterial drug and a symptomatic drug, such as loperamide. Persons should be instructed to take an antimicrobial after passing the third unformed stool in all cases and to take loperamide only if they have no fever.[60,64,65,187] In persons who pass a third stool in less than 24 hours, illness is likely to progress without therapy. Loperamide induces more rapid relief of symptoms, and the antimicrobial exerts curative effects. The duration of antimicrobials needed in TD appears to be short. Many cases respond to single-dose treatment, and no person needs more than 3 days of treatment.[23,57,60,64]

In cases of dysenteric diarrhea the same antimicrobial regimen is given promptly. Empiric therapy should be with fluoroquinolones in adults and with TMP/SMX plus a macrolide or nalidixic acid in children. Azithromycin is an alternative antimicrobial agent under current study.

The antibiotic regimens are not effective against diarrhea caused by *Campylobacter* (in the case of TMP/SMX or trimethoprim therapy), viruses, parasites, or other noninfectious causes. Therefore antibiotics should not be continued in the face of persistent or worsening diarrhea.

Prevention and Prophylaxis

Dietary Precautions. Food and water transmit the pathogens that cause infectious diarrhea and TD.[23,45,60-62] When diarrhea occurs, however, the exact source cannot be determined. It is clear that education can play an important role in prevention of TD, but dietary habits usually cannot be rigidly controlled. Food in developing countries is often contaminated with fecal coliforms and enteropathogens.[3] *Vibrio cholerae* remains viable for 1 to 3 weeks in food,[71] and *Salmonella* can survive 2 to 14 days in water or in the environment in a desiccated state.[62]

Risk of illness appears to be lowest when most of the meals are self-prepared and eaten in a private home, intermediate when food is consumed at public restaurants, and highest when food is obtained from street vendors.[15,62] The following standard dietary recommendations for prevention are based more on known potential vehicles for transmission of illness than on strong evidence, because most of the studies evaluating risk have found little correlation between routine precaution and presence of diarrhea[45,61,62]:

1. *Avoid tap water, ice made from untreated water, and suspect bottled water.* Bottled and carbonated drinks, beer, and wine are probably safe. Boiled or otherwise disinfected water is safe. Waterborne epidemics of almost all the enteric pathogens have occurred worldwide.[62] Tap water in high-risk countries is difficult to implicate in TD, but has been shown to contain enteric bacteria and pathogenic viruses and parasites.[62,131] Tap water and occasionally even bottled water may be unsafe, but bottled carbonated beverages are considered safe because of the antibacterial effects of the low acidity. Alcohol in mixed drinks does not disinfect, so these may not be safe, but bottled beer and wine have not been found to be contaminated. Most enteric organisms can survive freezing and melting in common drinks, so ice is not considered safe unless made from treated or previously boiled water. Ice in block form is often handled with unsanitary methods.[43,62]

2. *Avoid unpasteurized dairy products.* These may be the source of infection with *Salmonella*, *Campylobacter*, *Brucella*, *Listeria monocytogenes*, *Mycobacterium tuberculosis*, and others.[161]

3. *Avoid raw food.* Raw vegetables in salads may be contaminated by fertilization with human waste or by washing in contaminated water.[62] Anything that can be peeled or have the surface removed is safe. Fruits and leafy vegetables can also be disinfected by immersion and washing in iodinated water or by exposure to boiling water for 30 seconds. Raw seafood, including that in such traditional dishes as ceviche and sashimi, has been associated with increased risk of TD. Shellfish concentrate enteric organisms from contaminated

water and can carry hepatitis A, Norwalk virus, *Aeromonas hydrophila, Y. enterocolitica, V. cholerae,* and *V. parahaemolyticus.* Raw fish can carry parasites such as *Anisakis simplex, Clonorchis sinensis,* and *Metagonimus yokogawai.* Raw meat is a source of *Salmonella* and *Campylobacter* and the vehicle for *Trichinella, Taenia saginata* and *T. solium* (beef or pork tapeworm), and *Sarcocystis.* Although adequate cooking kills all microorganisms and parasites, if food is left at room temperature and recontaminated before serving, it can incubate *Salmonella, E. coli,* or *Shigella.* Food served on an airplane, train, boat, or bus probably has been catered in the country of origin. The problems of food hygiene pertain to these forms of public transportation, even if the employees handling the food are from the United States.

Safe foods are those served steaming hot, dry foods such as bread, freshly cooked food, foods that have high sugar content (e.g., syrups, jellies), and fruits that have been peeled.[23,62]

Prophylactic Medication. Chemoprophylaxis may be useful for certain people making critical trips or for travelers with underlying medical conditions. It should only be used for 3 weeks or less and should be always approved by a physician and after a complete understanding of all risks and benefits. Despite the restrictive recommendations, 10% to 25% of European travelers to high-risk areas and up to one third of U.S. travelers to Mexico take prophylactic medication to prevent TD.[62,113] Compared with empiric therapy with a single dose of an antimicrobial agent and loperamide, chemoprophylaxis is cost-effective only when its use does not exceed a few days[62] (Table 52-10).

Several nonantimicrobial agents have been studied for prevention of TD, with some found to be minimally effective. Lactobacilli have been tested on the assumption that they are safe and favorably modify intestinal flora, but they did not invariably reduce the incidence of TD and provided protective efficacy only up to 47%.[94] Antimotility drugs, such as loperamide, have adverse effects when used for prophylaxis.[23,56,62]

Of the nonantibiotic drugs, only bismuth subsalicylate (BSS), the active ingredient of Pepto-Bismol, has been shown by controlled studies to offer reasonable protection and safety. Several studies with volunteers and in the field have demonstrated that the use of BSS gives a protection rate from 40% to 77%,[53,62] with fewer abdominal symptoms. Since the volume required is quite large with the liquid preparation, BSS in tablet form was also evaluated. The currently recommended dose of BSS is two tablets four times a day (2.1 g/day).[23,45,53,60,61] Mild side effects include constipation, nausea, tinnitus, and temporarily blackened tongue or stools. In areas where doxycycline is used for malaria prevention, concurrent BSS should be avoided because it may bind to the antimicrobial and prevent absorption.[53,62] Ninety percent of salicylate from liquid BSS is absorbed and excreted in the urine of children.[53] Whether this salicylate cross-reacts with aspirin is unknown. However, BSS should not be used by someone with a history of aspirin allergy. Caution is recommended in small children, children with chickenpox or influenza (because of the potential risk of Reye's syndrome), patients with gout or renal insufficiency, and persons taking anticoagulants, probenecid, methotrexate, or other aspirin-containing products. BSS is not approved for children under 2 years old and is not recommended as prophylaxis for more than 3 weeks. The precise mechanism by which BSS prevents diarrhea is still unknown. Salicylate released during dissociation in the stomach exhibits antisecretory activity after exposure to bacterial enterotoxin on intestinal mucosa, and bismuth salts have antimicrobial activity.[53] Adherence of bacteria to intestinal mucosa may be affected.

Since the first studies in the 1950s, a protective effect of antimicrobials in TD has been demonstrated. Several antimicrobial agents are highly effective in preventing TD when given over short periods when at risk. Protection levels of 80% to 90% have been found with antimicrobial prophylaxis, provided that enteropathogens in the area were susceptible to the agent under investigation.[45,61,62] The most experience has been obtained with doxycycline, TMP/SMX, and the fluoroquinolones. Other antimicrobials (streptomycin and sulfonamides, erythromycin, mecillinam) have shown significant protection but have not been well studied.[61,141] Studies of U.S. students in Mexico taking trimethoprim (160 mg) and sulfamethoxazole (800 mg) twice daily for 3 weeks or once daily for 2 weeks demonstrated 71% and 95% protection, respectively.[50,52]

TABLE 52-10. Prophylactic Medications for Prevention of Traveler's Diarrhea*

AGENT	PROTECTIVE EFFICACY	PROPHYLACTIC DOSE	COMMENT
Bismuth subsalicylate	65%	Two 262-mg tablets before meals and at bedtime	Safe, temporary darkening of stools and tongue
Fluoroquinolones	90%	Norfloxacin 400 mg, ciprofloxacin 500 mg, or levofloxacin 500 mg once a day	Side effects, increased bacterial resistance

*Not generally recommended for travelers, only in special situations (see text) and for no longer than 3 weeks.

The fluoroquinolones (e.g., ciprofloxacin, ofloxacin, norfloxacin, pefloxacin, fleroxacin, levofloxacin) have been shown to be highly protective when employed as prophylactic agents. Because of the emergence of resistance among enteropathogens to tetracyclines, doxycycline can no longer be recommended for prophylaxis unless the susceptibility of prevalent organisms is known. Similarly, TMP/SMX resistance has been reported in many regions of the developing world,[60,62] including areas where resistance to this agent has not been previously reported.[24] With the antibiotics evaluated, the effect lasted only as long as the drug was continued. Subjects who remained in a high-risk area experienced an increased incidence of diarrhea during the week after cessation of prophylaxis.[44,62]

Despite dramatic protection against diarrhea, investigators do not recommend widespread use of these medications for prophylaxis by travelers because of the following reasons[23,60,62]:

1. *Side effects.* These include GI symptoms, photosensitivity, and other cutaneous eruptions and reactions. Pregnant women and children should not use fluoroquinolones for this reason. With larger numbers of people using these drugs, more serious side effects (e.g., Stevens-Johnson syndrome, hemolytic or aplastic anemia, antibiotic-associated colitis, anaphylaxis) will undoubtedly result.

2. *Alteration of normal bacterial flora.* Broad-spectrum antimicrobials may increase risk of infection with other antibiotic-resistant bacteria. Severe pseudomembranous colitis caused by colonic overgrowth with *Clostridium difficile* has occurred after therapy with most antibiotics. Vaginal candidiasis and GI side effects, including diarrhea, are common with antibiotic therapy. Changes in anaerobic flora can cause long-term alterations in the metabolism of bile acids and pancreatic enzymes, although clinical effects are unknown.

3. *Development of antimicrobial resistance.* Overuse of antimicrobial agents increases the prevalence of resistant strains.[49,60,84,176]

4. *False sense of security.* Travelers taking antibiotics may relax their vigilance of dietary precautions and increase their risk of acquiring enteric infections.

5. *High cost of fluoroquinolones and rapid effectiveness of presumptive therapy,* often limiting the illness to 12 to 24 hours.

Although the consensus is that not all travelers should use antibiotic prophylaxis, this approach may be appropriate for some.[23,45,60-62] Potential candidates would be residents of a low-risk country going to a high-risk area for short stays who have one or more of the following conditions or requirements:

1. An underlying illness that increases the risk of enteric infection or morbidity, such as gastric achlorhydria (from surgery or taking proton pump inhibitors), AIDS, inflammatory bowel disease, diabetes on insulin treatment, or a cardiac, renal, or CNS disorder.

2. An itinerary that is so rigid and critical to the overall mission that travelers would not tolerate even minor schedule changes caused by illness

3. Travelers who prefer prophylaxis after hearing the pros and cons of the approach

No studies have evaluated prophylaxis of TD in young children, although they may be at higher risk for infectious diarrhea. Because of potential side effects, prophylaxis with BSS or antibiotics cannot be recommended in children under 5 years of age.

Immunoprophylaxis. Spurred by the emergence of in vitro resistance to antimicrobial agents among enteropathogens, including the fluoroquinolones, prophylaxis with vaccines is being developed to control bacterial diarrhea. Recent studies support the concept of immunoprophylaxis against rotavirus, *Shigella*, *V. cholerae*, and ETEC.[45,60,61]

BACTERIAL ENTEROPATHOGENS

Escherichia Coli

E. coli is the most prevalent facultative gram-negative rod in feces. Diarrheagenic *E. coli* is a heterogenous group of organisms that belong to one taxonomic species, but with different virulence properties, epidemiologic characteristics, and clinical features. At least six groups have been characterized, based on either genotypic or phenotypic markers.[141]

Enteropathogenic E. coli. EPEC strains were the first of the diarrheagenic *E. coli* described between the 1920s and 1940s, as causes of hospital nursery outbreaks.[141] Usually identified by serotypes, they are also characterized by a localized adherence pattern to a specialized cell line (HEp-2 cells).[194] EPEC strains have worldwide distribution, and their most accepted virulence property is enterocyte attachment with selective damage of the surface without cell invasion. They induce production of a receptor interacting with host cells' intima, and this interaction leads to intracellular changes in the enterocyte.[83,115,141]

Enterotoxigenic E. coli. ETEC strains, first identified in the 1970s, produce one or two enterotoxins that act on the small intestine through different mechanisms and time responses.[141] One of these toxins is a heat-labile cholera-like toxin (LT), a high-molecular-weight protein immunologically and physiologically similar to cholera toxin. Human ETEC strains also have a low-molecular-weight, poorly antigenic toxin that is heat stable (ST).[165] Both enterotoxins inhibit sodium reabsorption and increase secretion of anions and fluid into the intestinal lumen, resulting in secretory diarrhea without inflammatory exudate.[43,60,141] One common method for the diagnosis of ETEC is identification of specific deoxyribonucleic acid (DNA) plasmid sequences, using a hybridization technique.[141] Recently, polymerase chain reaction (PCR) has been used to improve the level of detection.[189,203] ETEC has worldwide distribution and is the major cause of TD, accounting for 20% to 50% of cases in series from all parts of the world.[60,141,158] It also accounts for a large percentage and frequently the majority of enteritis in local pediatric populations of developing countries, where contaminated food and water are the primary sources of infection.[141] Most outbreaks of ETEC in the United States have been waterborne.[141,165] Person-to-person spread is infrequent because of the large infectious dose (10^6 to 10^{10} organisms).[43,141] Contamination of different types of food with these strains has been reported.[141]

Enteroinvasive E. coli.

As with *Shigella,* EIEC strains possess the property of bowel mucosa invasion, resulting in microabscesses and ulcer formation. Because of the presence of the same invasive plasmid and other antigens of *Shigella,*[166] EIEC must be considered in the differential diagnosis of febrile dysenteric diarrhea, with *Shigella, Salmonella, Y. enterocolitica, E. histolytica, V. parahaemolyticus,* and inflammatory bowel disease. EIEC strains are found worldwide and have been associated with food-borne outbreaks, especially in areas of South America and Eastern Europe.[43,141,196]

Enterohemorrhagic E. coli.

EHEC strains are also known as verotoxin-producing *E. coli* or Shiga toxin–producing *E. coli.* They have caused outbreaks of diarrhea associated with consumption of contaminated beef, often obtained at a fast-food hamburger chain, or unpasteurized apple juice. Contact with contaminated swimming pools and exposure to farm animals have also been associated with this infection.[31,135,141,154,179] EHEC produces copious bloody diarrhea with fecal mucus (hemorrhagic colitis), but fever is either low grade or absent. The most important EHEC strain thus far identified is O157:H7. The production of Shiga or a similar toxin by these strains may be related to the hemolytic-uremic syndrome (HUS), a common complication in children infected with EHEC O157:H7 and Shiga toxin-producing *Shigella.* HUS may be life-threatening, and no evidence indicates that HUS is prevented by antimicrobial therapy of EHEC disease.[72,135,156]

Enteroaggregative E. coli.

EAEC strains are the most recent addition to the group of diarrheagenic *E. coli.* They are non-EPEC and do not produce ETEC LT or ST. EAEC adhere to HEp-2 cells in a typical aggregative pattern. The pathophysiology of these strains is uncertain; some studies suggest that they should be considered a phenotypically and genotypically heterogeneous group.[36,120,141,142] These strains have been associated with persistent illness and malnutrition in children with diarrhea, especially in the developing world, but recent studies have demonstrated their association with diarrhea in adults. EAEC is also identified as an important cause of TD,[77,80] second only to ETEC in some areas of the world.

Diffusely Adherent E. coli.

Known also as enteroadherent *E. coli,* these non-EPEC strains show a diffuse adherence pattern to HEp-2 cells. Although associated with cases of diarrhea, the pathogenicity of these isolates has not been established in outbreaks or volunteer studies. The pathophysiology and importance of these strains are still not completely understood, and some propose that they be categorized as a subtype of EAEC.[36,141,142]

Diagnosis.

Laboratory culture cannot differentiate the various diarrheagenic strains of *E. coli* from normal bowel flora or from one another. Specialized assays such as DNA probing and HEp-2 adherence technique are specifically used for research purposes.[141] New serologic techniques or PCR systems may become available in the future to help differentiate these organisms.

Treatment.

Most cases of *E. coli* diarrhea are brief and self-limited, and their therapy should be primarily supportive with oral fluid replacement and maintenance, empirically based on the clinical manifestations. Dysenteric illness is the exception and should always be treated with antibacterial drugs, whether in a developing country or an industrialized region. In developing tropical countries, TD associated with the passage of numerous watery stools is often caused by both ETEC or EAEC, and antibiotics may shorten the duration of illness, especially when started within 48 to 72 hours of symptom onset.* Because of the increasing resistance of ETEC strains to antimicrobial agents, including fluoroquinolones, new therapeutic agents are actively being sought, such as rifaximin and azithromycin.[59,84,136,141,176] Since resistance patterns vary with geographic area and season, it is necessary to monitor susceptibility of bacterial isolates in various regions of the world. Susceptibility testing is required when treating diarrhea caused by EPEC, since strains are invariably resistant to a broad range of drugs.

Immunoprophylaxis.

Oral immunization with inactivated ETEC with or without cholera toxin B subunit was shown to be safe and immunogenic in phase III trials in Egypt.[172,173] A new vaccine, using a *Salmonella typhimurium* vaccine vector expressing recombinant ETEC fimbria, elicited immunogenic response in mice.[6]

---

*References 23, 54, 65, 80, 141, 187, 197.

A live vaccine could offer advantages over a killed preparation in terms of duration and protection.

Salmonella

Salmonella infections may result in four different clinical syndromes: gastroenterocolitis, enteric (typhoid) fever, bacteremia with focal extraintestinal infection, and asymptomatic carriage,[17,171] depending on the type of organism and the host characteristics. Gastroenterocolitis is usually a mild to moderately severe, self-limited illness, with preferential involvement of the lower intestine. Enteric fever is characterized by septicemia with a prolonged toxic course if not treated. In patients infected with *Salmonella choleraesuis* strains, or with sickle cell disease or immunosuppression (e.g., splenectomy, HIV infection, malignancy, immunosuppressive therapy, newborns, elderly persons), nontyphoid salmonellae may disseminate and produce localized infection, including osteomyelitis or meningitis. A person with an abdominal aortic aneurysm is prone to develop *Salmonella* infection, leading to aneurysm perforation. As many as 1% to 3% of patients who have recovered from typhoid fever may become chronic carriers who continue to shed the organism in the intestinal tract for 1 year or longer. Characteristically, the chronic typhoid carrier is an adult woman with cholelithiasis.[17]

Microbiology. The following discussion pertains to nontyphoid *Salmonella,* unless otherwise stated. Salmonellae are nonsporulating, facultative, gram-negative rods. The genus *Salmonella* is composed of more than 2000 serotypes that infect humans and animals. Enteric fever results from infection by *Salmonella typhi* or by *S. paratyphi* A, B, and C, which usually cause milder disease. *S. typhi* and *S. paratyphi* are further distinguished by their adaptation to humans as the only host. Although numerous other serotypes are capable of causing enteric fever, illness is usually limited to gastroenteritis.[60,136,158,171] New serotypes occasionally become prominent, but most human infections are caused by only 10 serotypes, with *S. typhimurium* the most common.

Epidemiology. Nontyphoid *Salmonella* organisms infect nearly all animal species and cause zoonotic infections. They can persist in fresh water for 2 to 14 days, but they also may remain dormant in a desiccated nonsporulating state.[17] Human salmonellosis is a worldwide problem, remaining endemic in large areas of the developing world, where it is passed primarily through contaminated food and water. The Centers for Disease Control and Prevention (CDC) estimates that the 25,000 human cases of nontyphoid salmonellosis reported annually in the United States represent less than 1% of the actual number of clinical cases.[134,136] A recent report of

typhoid fever in the United States from 1985 to 1994 showed that travel to underdeveloped countries is still a risk factor for this disease.[136]

Salmonella is the most common identifiable cause of foodborne illness. Contamination may occur from the animal feed, at slaughter, or most often, during food preparation. Because the infectious dose is relatively high, averaging 10^3 to 10^6 organisms (lower in water),[17,136] the bacteria must multiply on or in food. This accounts for the high summer case incidence, when refrigeration may not be adequate.[136] The foods most commonly implicated are meat, dairy products (especially unpasteurized), poultry, and eggs. Recent outbreaks of salmonellosis have been related to different foods from toasted oat cereal to alfalfa sprouts and infant formula.[28,136,191] Person-to-person spread accounts for 10% of cases, but 20% to 35% of household contacts may become infected.[136] *Salmonella* is an occasional cause of TD, accounting for up to 15% of cases.[60,158]

Normal gastric acid, gut motility, bacterial flora, and poorly understood immune factors are elements in host resistance. Bacterial virulence factors, the vehicle of transmission, and infectious dose are the major determinants of infection.[17,136,171] Salmonellosis primarily affects children and elderly persons. Fifty-five percent of reported isolates in the United States are from persons under 5 years of age. The organism has an unexplained propensity to infect infants under 1 year of age, who may experience serious systemic infection, including sepsis and meningitis. Greater susceptibility has also been observed in patients with gastrectomy-induced hypochlorhydria, hemolytic disorders (e.g., sickle cell anemia), parasitic infections (e.g., malaria, schistosomiasis), and chronic illness (e.g., malignancies, liver disease).[134,136]

Pathophysiology. Salmonellosis involves mucosal invasion and possibly enterotoxin production.[105,171] After surviving the gastric acid barrier, the organisms reproduce in the gut, where they attach to the wall of the ileum and colon, inducing local degeneration of the microvilli. Invasion occurs through vacuolization, discharging the bacteria into the lamina propria, from where they gain entry into the bloodstream. At this point, only the strains that cause enteric fever enter and multiply within lymphatic tissue and phagocytic cells. The mechanism of diarrhea in enterocolitis is not clear. A heat-stable enterotoxin has been identified. In most cases, local inflammation of the bowel wall is not severe enough to cause mucosal sloughing and dysentery.

Recent studies of pathogenesis demonstrated that interleukin-18 and γ-interferon contribute to host resistance and that deficiency of interleukin-12 or nitric oxide is related to severity of infection.[126,132] Protection against typhoid fever is associated with the cystic fibrosis gene, called *cystic fibrosis transmembrane conductance regulator* (CFTR), similar to the protection of sickle cell against plasmodium infestation. Apparently, *S. typhi* uses this gene to invade the intestinal epithelial cells.[106,160]

Clinical Syndromes. Although the incubation period for typhoid fever is usually 1 to 2 weeks, it is only 8 to 48 hours for intestinal infections with non-typhoid *Salmonella*.[171] Nausea, vomiting, malaise, headache, and low-grade fever may precede abdominal cramps and diarrhea. Stools are usually foul, and green-brown to watery, with variable amounts of mucus, blood, and leukocytes. Cholera-like fluid loss or dysentery with grossly bloody and mucoid stools occurs less often. The acute phase lasts only a few days. Asymptomatic excretion of organisms in the stool continues for 4 to 8 weeks, and chronic carriers are rare. Infants less than 3 months of age experience longer illnesses (average 8 days) with more complications. Among all ages, transient bacteremia is common, accounting for significant isolation of *Salmonella* types from blood. Fever and malaise occurring more than 1 week after resolution of diarrhea suggest a complication or another diagnosis.[136,171] In healthy adults, *Salmonella* bacteremia occurs in 5% to 10% of infections and is not distinguishable from other causes of sepsis. Focal infections may be seen in any organ, but sites adjacent to the bowel are most common. Mortality is highest at the extremes of age, but deaths occur in all age groups.[136]

Diagnosis. Diagnosis of enterocolitis can be made by clinical manifestations and isolation of *Salmonella* organisms from stool or rectal swabs cultured onto selective media (MacConkey or *Salmonella-Shigella* agar). Blood cultures are useful to identify a systemic non-typhoidal salmonellosis. Blood cultures (or culture of bone marrow aspirates) for *S. typhi* or *S. paratyphi* are also used to diagnose enteric fever. Stool cultures are often negative early in the disease. Widal's serum test is useful for diagnosing typhoid fever in areas with high prevalence, but not in industrialized areas, because of the more frequent occurrence of cross-reaction with other gram-negative organisms.

Treatment. Supportive treatment with fluids is sufficient therapy for most cases of uncomplicated *Salmonella* enterocolitis. Antibiotics are not indicated because they do not shorten the illness, and they slightly prolong the carrier state and increase the risk of developing resistant strains.[7,136] Antimicrobial therapy is indicated for persons who have symptomatic *Salmonella* infection with fever, systemic toxicity, or bloody stools. Patients with underlying debility that may predispose to septicemia or localized infection (e.g., immunosuppression), young infants (less than 3 months), elderly

persons (more than 65 years), and sickle cell patients should be treated with antimicrobial agents. Fluoroquinolones are the treatment of choice because they shorten the duration of fever and diarrhea in salmonellosis.[7,136] Doses are the same as those recommended to treat shigellosis, although treatment is continued for 7 days (14 days if the patient is immunosuppressed).

In cases of enteric (typhoid) fever, septicemic salmonellosis, or local tissue suppuration, antibiotic therapy is indicated. The drugs of choice for enteric fever in the United States are the fluoroquinolones. These drugs can be given for a shorter duration (10 vs. 14 days), resistance to them is still low, and posttreatment carriage of *S. typhi* is reduced.[7,66] In many developing countries the drug of choice is still chloramphenicol (25 to 50 mg/kg/day in divided doses every 6 hours) because of its low price and predictable activity. Alternative empiric therapy in the United States is a third-generation cephalosporin. Other traditional options, such as ampicillin or TMP/SMX,[24] have low in vitro activity in many areas. Local suppuration may require 2 to 6 weeks of antibiotics, depending on the adequacy of surgical drainage.

As with *Shigella*, *Salmonella* species are showing increasing resistance to multiple antimicrobial agents worldwide.[81,87,136,177]

Immunoprophylaxis. Immunity to *Salmonella* is serotype specific. Vaccines have not been successful for nontyphoid *Salmonella* because of the number of serotypes. For typhoid fever, immunoprophylaxis is possible, and currently, three protective vaccines are commercially available. The traditional killed vaccine is associated with high reaction rate and has limited use in young children traveling in highly endemic areas. The two live attenuated typhoid vaccines are preferred for antityphoid immunizations. The first is a live attenuated strain Ty21a that is given as one oral dose every other day for four doses.[78] The second is a Vi polysaccharide preparation given as a single parenteral immunization.[1] Both preparations are of approximately equal cost and effectiveness. New vaccines are under evaluation. One new live attenuated *S. typhimurium* mutant is highly immunogenic and protective in animal models and induces cross-reactive antibodies to other enteric pathogens.[190]

Shigella

Microbiology. Dysentery has been described since the beginning of recorded history. At the end of the nineteenth century, Shiga first identified *Shigella dysenteriae* as the cause of an outbreak of dysenteric diarrhea in Japan, and since then, shigellosis has become synonymous with bacterial dysentery. Other bacteria and protozoa are also capable of producing the bloody and mucoid stools that define this syndrome.

Shigellae are thin, nonmotile, nonsporulating, gramnegative rods in the Enterobacteriaceae family. There are four species or groups: A (*S. dysenteriae*), B (*S. flexneri*), C (*S. boydii*), and D (*S. sonnei);* the first three contain numerous serotypes.

Epidemiology. Shigellosis occurs worldwide. *S. dysenteriae* 1 (Shiga bacillus), which causes severe disease, is most common in developing countries. In the US and in many other areas, particularly in more industrialized regions, *Shigella* remains endemic, with *S. sonnei* replacing *S. flexneri* as the most common isolate.

Humans and certain primates are the only hosts for *Shigella.* Fecal-oral contamination is the mode of spread. Common source infections occur through water or food prepared by contaminated hands. *Shigella* can survive freezing and thawing in ice cubes. With an infectious dose as low as 10 to 200 organisms, person-to-person spread is common.[54] Even in countries with good sanitation, *Shigella* accounts for persistent endemic foci and high rates of transmission, especially among groups in close physical contact (e.g., male homosexuals, children in day-care centers), groups with poor hygiene (e.g., mentally impaired patients), and those who lack sanitary facilities and water (e.g., populations in developing countries, Native Americans on reservations). Long-term carriage of *Shigella* is less common than for *Salmonella. Shigella* is a potential pathogen in the American wilderness. Environmental persistence averages 3 to 4 weeks, with best survival in cool fresh water.

Pathophysiology. The essential virulence factor of *Shigella* is invasiveness associated with a large (120- to 140-megadalton) plasmid. *Shigella* organisms invade and proliferate within the epithelium of the large bowel, producing well-demarcated ulcers with cellular infiltrates (chiefly PMNs) and overlying suppurative exudates. These organisms interact with the epithelial cells through an initial type III secretory system, with invasion of these cells and reorganization of their cytoskeleton.[40,83,144] Organisms have also been demonstrated in the small bowel, but these have reduced potential for invasion or changes in the mucosa, causing a profuse watery diarrhea, possibly mediated by an enterotoxin.[40,43]

Despite similarities in pathogenesis between EIEC and *Shigella* strains, random amplified polymorphic DNA and typing techniques were not able to characterize and differentiate them.[11,166]

Clinical Syndromes. As with most enteric pathogens, infection with *Shigella* may be asymptomatic, mild, or severe. Rarely a chronic carrier state may develop, depending on a combination of host and organism factors. Two distinct diarrheal syndromes may occur sep-

arately or sequentially in shigellosis. After a short incubation period of 1 to 3 days, illness begins with malaise, headache, nausea, fever, abdominal cramps, and watery diarrhea, representing small bowel infection. Children may present with fever, with diarrhea developing later. In the second and classic form of shigellosis, after 1 to 3 days of small bowel disease, colonic involvement causes progression to clinical dysentery. In this dysenteric form the volume of stools decreases and the frequency increases, with passage of up to 20 to 30 movements a day, containing gross blood and associated with fecal urgency and often tenesmus. Fever is common in dysenteric cases, found in up to one half of cases of shigellosis overall. Mild abdominal tenderness is also common, but without peritoneal signs.

The natural history of shigellosis is varied, with most cases resolving spontaneously within 7 days, but with others persisting for weeks.[43,47] The mortality rate is as high as 25% in developing countries when *S. dysenteriae* 1 (Shiga bacillus) diarrhea is untreated, but it decreases to less than 1% with adequate antimicrobial therapy.

Complications. Several potential complications of shigellosis may occur. Severe anemia and hypoalbuminemia may result from blood and protein losses. Febrile convulsions are seen in young children with shigellosis. Pneumonitis may complicate *Shigella* infection. A severe leukemoid reaction with white cell count up to 50,000 may result after apparent clinical improvement in patients. In some patients infected by strains that produce Shiga toxin, HUS syndrome develops, probably induced by formation of immune complexes. Reiter's syndrome has also been reported in patients with *S. flexneri* infection who are HLA B27 positive. Septicemia was found in less than 5% of *Shigella* infections, with fewer cases of metastatic abscesses.[47,54]

Diagnosis. Laboratory tests often show a mild leukocytosis with a shift to the left (increase in number of immature granulocytes). If colitis is present, microscopic examination of the stool shows countless white (PMNs) and red blood cells, but this is not specific to shigellosis. Diagnosis is made by stool culture on selective media (MacConkey or *Salmonella-Shigella* agar), which is positive in most infected patients.[47] Fresh stool or sigmoidoscopic biopsy is the best source of culture material, while rectal cotton swabs, although not as reliable, can be used if plated rapidly or placed in a holding medium. In hospitalized patients, blood cultures should be obtained.

Treatment. Therapy first involves fluid replacement. Although large-volume diarrhea is unusual, significant dehydration may occur, especially in children. Antimotility drugs are controversial in patients with signs of toxicity[46]; however, these medications are unlikely to be detrimental if antibiotics are used concurrently.[23,64,65] Patients with fever and dysentery should be treated with antimicrobial agents, since these drugs decrease duration of fever, diarrhea, and excretion of *Shigella* in stool. Antibiotic-resistant strains are emerging worldwide, with recent reports in Asia, Oceania, and Latin America,[24,81a,99,183] showing that most of the strains are resistant to ampicillin and TMP/SMX, whereas the fluoroquinolones remain active. The current recommendation for treatment is with a fluoroquinolone: norfloxacin 400 mg, ciprofloxacin 500 mg, or levofloxacin 500 mg daily, for a total of 3 to 5 days. Single-dose therapy is probably effective in milder forms of illness.[23,57,63,65,187] Fluoroquinolones currently are contraindicated in infants and children because of the possible effects on articular cartilage. However, short-course fluoroquinolone therapy appears to be safe. Alternative treatments for children in areas where TMP resistance occurs are nalidixic acid and furazolidone.[168] Other options that need further testing are azithromycin and rifaximin.[59]

Immunoprophylaxis. Temporary immunity to homologous *Shigella* strains follows natural infection.[48,145] A vaccine composed of specific polysaccharide conjugates of *S. flexneri* and *S. sonnei* has been shown to be safe and immunogenic in children.[8] Other attenuated or killed strains or specific synthetic polysaccharides have shown promise in animal studies.[32,162]

Campylobacter

Microbiology. The organism is a small, curved, gram-negative rod, initially classified as *Vibrio*. *Campylobacter jejuni* strains are widespread in the environment. The major reservoir is animals, including dogs, cattle, birds, horses, goats, pigs, cats, and sheep.[16,60,158] A reemergent species, *C. upsaliensis*, has been recently associated with diarrheal disease, persistent diarrhea in HIV patients, and a few cases of HUS.[21]

Epidemiology. Most epidemics of gastroenteritis have been caused by contaminated food. The most important source for human illness is poultry, but epidemics have also been associated with ingestion of raw milk.[16,18] *C. jejuni* has been isolated from surface water and can survive up to 5 weeks in cold water, ensuring its potential for wilderness waterborne spread. Person-to-person spread occurs but is uncommon. The prevalence of *C. jejuni* as a cause of TD varies with time of year. TD is caused by *C. jejuni* in about 3% of cases in rainy summertime and in up to 15% of cases during drier wintertime.[16,133] Studies in the United States and abroad have demonstrated that *C. jejuni* accounts for

up to 25% of patients with infectious diarrhea and is often more common than *Salmonella* or *Shigella* species.[16,19] *C. jejuni* is now the most common cause of bacterial gastroenteritis in developed countries. Rates are highest among children and young adults.[16,18]

Pathophysiology. The complete pathogenic mechanisms are unclear. All segments of the small and large intestine may be affected, accounting for the variety of diarrheal symptoms. Evidence of invasiveness includes recovery of bacteria from blood and presence of colitis, with cellular infiltration on intestinal biopsy. A heat-labile enterotoxin may play a role in disease pathogenesis.

Clinical Syndromes. The incubation period of *C. jejuni* enteritis is 2 to 7 days. Clinical symptoms are extremely variable and nonspecific. Victims often have a 1-day prodrome of general malaise and fever, followed by abdominal cramps and pain that herald the onset of diarrhea, with up to eight bowel movements a day. The diarrhea is initially watery, followed by passage of stools that are bile stained or bloody. The frequencies of reported symptoms are diarrhea (75% to 95%), cramps and abdominal pain (80% to 90%), nausea (20% to 50%), headache (50%), fever (50% to 80%), vomiting (20%), and bloody diarrhea (10% to 50%).[16] Tenesmus is unusual. Physical examination is nonspecific, with variable degrees of fever (averaging 40° C [104° F]), abdominal tenderness, and dehydration. Microscopic evaluation of stool shows blood and PMNs in 60% to 75% of samples. The enteric symptoms subside in 2 to 4 days, and the entire illness resolves spontaneously within 1 week. Organisms are shed in the stool for 3 to 5 weeks after resolution of symptoms, but chronic carrier states have not been described. Up to 20% of victims may show clinical relapse, which is usually less severe than the original symptoms.[16] Chronic diarrhea caused by *C. jejuni* has been reported in children and adults but is usually associated with significant underlying disease.

Complications. *C. jejuni* infection has been associated with Guillain-Barré syndrome.[16,139,164] *C. jejuni* infection often precedes development of the syndrome and in more severe cases is associated with axonal degeneration, slow recovery, and severe residual damage.[164]

Diagnosis. Definitive diagnosis is made by stool culture on a selective medium (e.g., Skirrow, Butzler, Campy-BAP), with isolation rates directly related to the severity of the disease. Extraintestinal sources account for 0.4% of positive *Campylobacter* cultures in the United States and usually are preceded by GI infection. Blood is the most common site, followed by the gallbladder and cerebrospinal fluid (in children), but since blood cultures are rarely drawn in the evaluation of gastroenteritis, the real frequency of bacteremia is unknown. The serologic tests available are still not well standardized and need further evaluation.

Treatment. Treatment is primarily supportive with oral fluids; dehydration is usually mild. Most patients have improved by the time the culture results return and do well without antibiotics. Antibiotic treatment does not conclusively improve *C. jejuni* gastroenteritis, but earlier therapy appears to be effective[19] and eradicates the organism from the stool within 48 hours. The antimicrobial antibiotic of choice is erythromycin or a fluoroquinolone. Fluoroquinolones are given in the same doses as for shigellosis because they are active against all the major causes of dysentery (*C. jejuni, Shigella, Salmonella*). In children, because fluoroquinolones are contraindicated, erythromycin (20 to 50 mg/kg every 6 hours for 5 days) is an option. Another alternative, in view of increased resistance to fluoroquinolones by *Campylobacter* strains,[79,176] is azithromycin, a newer macrolide that can be used in children and is active against all major bacterial enteric pathogens.[84,118]

Vibrio

Microbiology. Cholera is a severe form of watery diarrhea often associated with dehydration. The disease is caused by *Vibrio cholerae* 0 group 1 (01), a motile, curved, gram-negative rod. These microorganisms have two major biotypes, classic and El Tor, which produce similar clinical illness, and each one contains two main serotypes, Ogawa and Inaba. Non-01 *V. cholerae* strains also produce diarrheal illness, but they show less potential for epidemic disease.[107] Nine other species have been associated with human disease. *V. parahaemolyticus, V. fluvialis, V. mimicus, V. hollisae,* and *V. furnissii* are associated with GI disease. Others, mainly *V. vulnificus,* are associated with wound infections and septicemia. All are halophilic, gram-negative rods that reside in seawater and on marine organisms, and infection is acquired by ingesting infected and undercooked seafood or by contamination of a wound with infected water.[107]

Epidemiology. *V. cholerae* is endemic in areas of Asia, Africa, and the Middle East. It has accounted for seven deadly worldwide pandemics since the early 1800s. The last began in 1961 in Indonesia and spread throughout Southeast Asia, the Middle East, Africa, parts of the Pacific and Europe, and in the 1990s to Latin America. In 1973, cholera resurfaced in the United States after an absence since 1911. Since then, a small number of cases have occurred along the Gulf Coast of Louisiana and Texas. Only 10 cases of cholera were reported in travelers returning from endemic areas between 1961 and 1981. In January 1991 a new outbreak of cholera started in Latin America along the coast of Peru. Since then, this disease has become endemic in most regions of Latin America, moving as close to the United States as northern Mexico.[107] The infection is associated with consumption of uncooked or poorly handled seafood and spreads rapidly because of a highly susceptible population that has not been exposed to cholera for almost a century and because of inadequate water supply and sewage service. Cholera continues to be a disease of poor and lower socioeconomic groups, and the Indian subcontinent and southwestern Asia are still the areas with the highest prevalence.[68,107] The risk to travelers has been estimated at 1:500,000 during a journey to an endemic area,[60,158] which should be further reduced with dietary discretion.

Nonhuman reservoirs for *V. cholerae* 01 include marine or brackish waters.[68,107,158] As with other strains (*V. parahaemolyticus,* non-01 *V. cholerae*), shellfish ingest and carry these organisms. Fecal-oral spread is the major mechanism of transmission, and water is the most common vehicle, followed by food.[68] The organism remains viable for days to weeks in various foods. Because of the large infective dose of 10^6 to 10^{10} organisms,[98,158] person-to-person spread is uncommon.

Most cases of gastroenteritis caused by noncholera vibrios have been associated with ingestion of raw seafood. Cases have been reported from travelers, particularly after visits to coastal areas of Southeast Asia and Latin America. *V. parahaemolyticus* causes 70% of cases of foodborne gastroenteritis in Japan (where large amounts of raw seafood are eaten), leads to sporadic outbreaks in the United States, and is a common cause of TD in Thailand.[20]

Pathophysiology. After passing through the stomach, the organism multiplies and colonizes the small bowel. The local effects of enterotoxin account for the pathophysiology of cholera. No pathologic changes are noted in the bowel wall. The binding subunits of toxin attach to the membrane of the mucosa, after which the adenylate cyclase–activating B subunit enters the cell. The enzyme acts inside the serosal cell, enhancing production of cyclic adenosine monophosphate. This molecule produces a 70% reduction in influx of water, saline, and a wide range of other substances into the gut mucosal cells, resulting in watery diarrhea. Glucose, potassium, bicarbonate, and most significantly, absorption of sodium and water linked to glucose remain intact. Thus, although plain water worsens cholera diarrhea, the addition of glucose renders the water and essential electrolytes absorbable, forming the basis for oral rehydration therapy.[107,137,159,170] *V. cholerae* has the bacteriophage VPIphi, which encodes a receptor used by enterocytes for the phage CTXphi, which encodes the cholera toxin.[110]

Details of the pathogenesis of infection by the non-cholera vibrios remain unclear. Some strains produce an enterotoxin, but generally it is not cholera-like toxin. In the case of *V. parahaemolyticus,* a hemolytic toxin was thought to explain its effects, but the dysenteric illness that typically develops implies invasion. Another enterotoxin has been found in some strains.[20]

Clinical Syndromes. Some cholera infections are asymptomatic, and 60% to 80% of clinical cases are presented as mild diarrhea that never raise suspicion for cholera.[98,158] After an incubation period of 2 days (range 1 to 5 days), fluid accumulates in the gut, causing intestinal distention and diarrhea. Diarrhea may begin as passage of brown stools but soon assumes the translucent gray watery appearance known as "rice water" stools. In serious cases, stool volume may reach 1 L/hr, leading to severe dehydration, acidosis, shock, and death. Vomiting may occur as a result of gut distention or acidosis.[107]

The clinical syndrome caused by noncholera vibrios is not characteristic. Intestinal illness is associated with diarrhea, abdominal cramps, and fever, with nausea and vomiting in about 20% of cases. Diarrhea may be severe, with up to 20 to 30 watery stools per day. In outbreaks of *V. parahaemolyticus* infection, explosive diarrhea associated with abdominal cramps and nausea is often described, with vomiting in about 50% and fever in about 30% of cases. In Asia, a dysentery-like syndrome with mucoid bloody diarrhea is often seen.[20] Infections are usually brief, lasting an average of 3 days, with spontaneous resolution.

Diagnosis. Diagnosis for any of the vibrio diarrheas can be made by stool culture on suitable media (e.g., thiosulfate-citrate-bile salts-sucrose or TCBS agar). Vibrios can survive for 1 week on a stool-saturated piece of filter paper sealed in a plastic bag, before placing it in the culture media.[107] In the case of *V. cholerae,* another way to diagnose infection is using a darkfield microscopic examination of fresh stools, which may reveal the characteristic helical vibrio motion.

Treatment. Aggressive replacement of fluid and electrolytes is the cornerstone of therapy for cholera, especially in severe cases. Severe untreated cholera has a 50% mortality, which may be reduced to 1% with appropriate treatment. Children are at higher risk for complications and death.

With fluid replacement, most cases of cholera last 3 to 5 days, with the peak fluid losses 24 hours after the onset of illness. When hypotension or persistent vomiting is present, IV fluids are necessary, but as soon as initial rehydration is complete, ORS is used for maintenance. Less than 5% of patients require IV maintenance after initial rehydration, and ORS alone is successful in 90% of cholera cases without shock. With voluminous losses,

ORS can be given by nasogastric tube to continue fluids during the night. A normal or light diet should be resumed early in the course of treatment, after initial rehydration. Success of fluid replacement therapy was clearly demonstrated by the low mortality rate seen during the cholera outbreak in Peru, where principles of rehydration were applied.[68,107]

Antibiotics shorten the duration of diarrhea and excretion of organisms in severe cholera and reduce fluid losses but they are not as important as fluid therapy. Oral antibiotics can be started within a few hours of initial rehydration. The drug of choice is doxycycline, 300 mg single dose in adults or 50 mg/kg/day in four divided doses for children. This is perhaps the only indication for the use of tetracycline in children because a short course (2 to 4 days) is unlikely to stain teeth. Furazolidone (100 mg every 6 hours for adults and 5 mg/kg/day in four divided doses for children) for 2 days is an alternative. *Vibrio* strains are also susceptible to fluoroquinolones, but these medications are more expensive.[23,45,60,107]

Treatment of patients infected with noncholera vibrios should also focus on fluid replacement. Little information exists on the benefit of antibiotic therapy for GI disease, but antimicrobials may be reasonable in dysentery-like cases or prolonged illness. The same antimicrobial agents used in cholera could be used against this infection.

Immunoprophylaxis. Temporary immunity to homologous, but not to heterologous, strains of cholera develop after infection.[107] The current parenteral vaccine has no antitoxin activity and is only about 50% effective in reducing attack rates over a 3- to 6-month period for those living in endemic areas. It is recommended for persons who live and work under poor sanitary conditions in highly endemic areas and for those with known achlorhydria. It is not recommended for travelers to endemic areas.[107]

A recent advance was the development of transgenic potatoes that synthesized cholera toxin subunit B without requiring a cold chain. This is a promising option for an inexpensive, effective vaccine for the developing world. New vaccines are in different stages of evaluation. Two studies in adult volunteers, one using a polysaccharide-cholera toxin conjugate and the other using a new El Tor strain that was CTXphi negative and hemagglutinin/protease defective, have shown promising results. A study of CVD103-HgR strain in Austrian travelers confirmed the tolerance of this oral vaccine. Finally, a bivalent (CVD103-HgR plus CVD 111) oral vaccine has been shown to be more effective than the monovalent one.[13,90,188]

Yersinia Enterocolitica

Microbiology. *Y. enterocolitica* is a facultative anaerobic, gram-negative rod in the Enterobacteriaceae family, with different serogroups found to cause human infection.

Epidemiology. The major natural reservoir of the organism is wild, farm, and domestic animals. In the United States and Europe the organism resides in surface and unchlorinated well waters. Evidence indicates that persistence in warm water ranges from days to weeks, with longer survival at colder temperatures. Human isolates of *Y. enterocolitica* are found worldwide, but with preference for colder regions such as Canada and Northern European countries, with an incidence equal to or greater than those of *Salmonella* and *Shigella*.[130,158] Transmission occurs from fecal-oral contamination, through food and water, and probably through person-to-person or animal-to-person contact.[130,158,192] Raw milk and oysters have also been implicated as vehicles of transmission. The infectious dose and attack rate are not well studied, but yersiniosis is suspected to be caused by ingestion of a large infectious dose based on a common source of transmission. The incubation period averages from 3 to 7 days. Patients with β-thalassemia show a greater risk for acquisition of yersiniosis.[4]

Pathophysiology. Illness caused by *Y. enterocolitica* may involve three pathogenic mechanisms: bowel mucosal invasion, release of a heat-stable enterotoxin similar to that produced by ETEC, and elaboration of a cytotoxin.[43,130] The organism multiplies in the small bowel and characteristically invades the mucosa in the region of the terminal ileum and colon. The mucosa may be diffusely inflamed with small and shallow ulcerations. Also, some bacteria migrate through lymphatics to mesenteric lymph nodes, producing adenitis with focal areas of necrosis.

Clinical Syndromes. The most common clinical presentation in yersiniosis is gastroenteritis, characterized by diarrhea, fever, and abdominal pain, with nausea and vomiting in 20% to 40% of cases and dysentery (passage of bloody stools) in 10% to 25%.[130,192] Fever or abdominal pain without important diarrhea may be the most prominent sign, mimicking appendicitis in 20% of patients with positive stool cultures.[10] Although acute appendicitis has been associated with serologic evidence of *Y. enterocolitica* infection, the usual surgical findings are mesenteric adenitis or terminal ileitis. Severe colitis rarely results in septicemia, extensive necrosis, or perforation. Numerous extraintestinal manifestations of *Y. enterocolitica* infection include skin rash (erythema nodosum or maculopapular) and arthritis, probably related to an immune reaction. Extraintestinal infection involving lung, joints, lymph nodes, wounds, or septicemia may occur with or without enteritis. In the majority of intestinal infections, illness is mild and self-limited, with duration averaging 1 week, but some patients experience prolonged symptoms.[130,192] Excretion of the organism in stool continues for a few weeks to months. Complications may be related to particularly severe disease and a misdiagnosis of Crohn's disease or appendicitis and development of Reiter's disease or collagenous colitis.[128]

Diagnosis. The diagnosis of yersiniosis is usually made by stool culture, but it can grow also from blood or surgical samples. The organism grows better at lower (22° to 25° C [71.6° to 77° F]) temperatures, which inhibit most other enteric bacteria. Abnormalities related to ileitis or colitis seen on contrast radiography and colonoscopy may be mistaken for other causes of colitis.[10,130] Serologic tests are also diagnostic and especially helpful to diagnose *Yersinia* arthritis.

Treatment. Tetracyclines have been suggested as the drug of first choice for chronic or fulminant infections,[10,23] but *Yersinia* is also susceptible *in vitro* to streptomycin, chloramphenicol, aminoglycosides, fluoroquinolones, and trimethoprim/sulfamethoxazole. Most are resistant to penicillins and cephalosporins and variably resistant to erythromycin and sulfonamides.[23,130]

Aeromonas Species and Plesiomonas Shigelloides

Aeromonas species and *P. shigelloides* are gram-negative, facultatively anaerobic, nonsporulating rods. Their normal habitats are water and soil, and these bacteria have been implicated in a variety of human illnesses, most often gastroenteritis.[60,96,97,101,158,195]

Aeromonas was previously part of the Vibrionaceae family, until the family Aeromonadaceae was established to include the 14 species so far identified. Only five species (*A. hydrophila, A. caviae, A. veronii, A. jandaei,* and *A. schubertti*) have been associated with a variety of human diseases, including gastroenteritis, soft tissue infections, HUS, burn-associated sepsis, and respiratory infections.[101,195] *A. hydrophila* is the most commonly isolated species, but its real prevalence is still uncertain. *A. hydrophila* has been associated with diarrheal illness in the United States, Australia, India, and southwestern Asia.[96,101,195] Association of illness with drinking untreated spring or well water was demonstrated in the United States. Pathogenicity includes production of cytotoxin, enterotoxin, and proteases, as well as the capacity of adhesion and invasion, but the exact mechanisms of disease pathogenicity remain controversial.[101,174]

Clinical illness associated with enteric infection by *A. hydrophila* varies from acute to chronic diarrhea and from passage of watery stools to dysentery with colitis.[101,195] Median duration of diarrhea is 2 weeks, with occasional cases that persist a month or longer. Asymptomatic carriers have been identified. Non-GI infections, such as those of soft tissue and septicemia, have been associated with exposure of wounds to water. *Aeromonas* strains are susceptible to chloramphenicol, tetracycline, TMP/SMX, fluoroquinolones, and aminoglycosides but are resistant to ampicillin and erythromycin.[101]

P. shigelloides has been isolated from patients with gastroenteritis, both in sporadic cases and outbreaks.[60,97,158] Infection has been associated with recent travel and ingestion of raw or inadequately cooked shellfish. *Plesiomonas* may cause dysenteric illness suggestive of an invasive organism, but its pathogenic mechanisms remain poorly defined.[97]

Miscellaneous Bacterial Agents

Klebsiella pneumoniae and *K. oxytoca* have been reported to occasionally cause diarrhea, but they are usually commensals of the GI flora.[88] Another cause of severe diarrhea in hospitalized (usually postoperative) patients receiving antibiotics is *Staphylococcus aureus*. The causative organism may be methicillin-resistant *S. aureus*.[175]

VIRAL ENTERIC PATHOGENS

Recent studies have identified viruses as major causes of acute nonbacterial GI infections.[15,29,93] The most important defined agents are Norwalk virus and other caliciviruses, enteric adenoviruses, astrovirus, and rotavirus. Usually they cause vomiting with or without mild and self-limiting watery diarrhea. Transmission occurs through fecal-oral contamination or person-to-person transmission. Respiratory symptoms are common in patients with viral gastroenteritis.

Caliciviruses and astroviruses are similar to Norwalk virus in structure and clinical presentation. They generally infect in early childhood and provide apparently lifetime immunity.[151,152]

Norwalk and Norwalk-like Viruses

Norwalk virus was the first well-described etiologic agent in nonbacterial gastroenteritis outbreaks; an elementary school outbreak occurred in Norwalk, Ohio.[108] Soon after, several other small round viruses were identified as causes of nonbacterial gastroenteritis.[151,152]

Norwalk virus and the related viruses are nonsymmetric, single-stranded ribonucleic acid (RNA) viruses, recently classified within the family Caliciviridiae.[103,119] They are the main cause of outbreaks of epidemic nonbacterial GI illness worldwide. They also cause "winter vomiting disease" because of their wintertime predisposition and common association with vomiting.

These viruses are highly infective (10 to 100 organisms per inoculum), and the infection is spread by common-source vehicles with a propensity for secondary person-to-person spread (high secondary attack rate).[93,119] Humans are the only known carriers of these viruses. Outbreaks have been recognized in family settings, health care facilities, nursing homes, schools, and travel settings, characteristically affecting both children and adults in the United States. They are found less often in neonates and toddlers. Contaminated water supplies, drinking water in cruise ships, recreational swimming pools, and commercial ice cubes have been implicated in outbreaks.[93,119] Also, vehicles identified for food-borne outbreaks may be contaminated shellfish, salads, bakery products, cold foods, cooked meat, and fresh fruits.[152] Between 20% to 67% of outbreaks of Norwalk virus have been associated with food.[26,147]

After invasion of the enterocytes, the viral particles replicate inside, resulting in damage of the villi and crypt cell hyperplasia.[151] Malabsorption of fat, lactose, and xylose occurs with these histologic changes. The exact mechanisms of diarrhea production in viral gastroenteritis are not completely understood. Small numbers of viral particles are shed in stool during the acute illness, but prolonged carrier states are not seen.

In the United States, antibodies in stools typically appear during late adolescence, but in tropical, developing countries, children acquire antibodies at a young age. Although antibodies persist in most people, they do not provide protection from clinical illness.[151]

Transmission is followed by an incubation period of 24 to 48 hours, and illness begins abruptly with vomiting, abdominal cramps, and diarrhea. Stools are watery and usually do not contain blood or leukocytes. Other common symptoms include low-grade fever, malaise, myalgias, respiratory symptoms, and headache. Illness is almost always mild and self-limited, lasting 1 to 2 days. Complications and mortality are extremely rare and usually involve elderly and debilitated patients. Some malabsorption of fats and disaccharides persists after the acute illness. Supportive treatment with oral fluids and electrolytes is sufficient in the vast majority of cases.[151]

Historically, and because of the difficulty or impossibility of growing these viruses in cell culture, electron microscopy was the initial means of detecting these viruses. Currently, there are immunoassays and molecular techniques (reverse-transcription PCR) available for detection of these small round RNA viruses in stool.[85,102,140,151]

Vaccine development is not currently feasible because of difficulties culturing the virus and lack of animal models.

Rotavirus

Rotaviruses are 70-nm double-stranded RNA viruses that are classified by the capsid antigens, with group A and serotype G1 being the most common in human infections worldwide. Most severe infections in children are caused by serotypes G1 to G4.[14,153] Rotavirus is the most common enteric pathogen in children causing diarrhea worldwide, resulting in up to 800,000 deaths per year.[29,93,153] Infection tends to be endemic, with peak incidence during winter months in temperate climates. Transmission is by person-to-person contact or as a result of common-source outbreaks. Viral shedding occurs in stools, and particles can retain infectivity for months. Rotaviruses have been found in almost every animal species, and in general, animal strains have reduced virulence for humans.[14,29]

Rotavirus infects humans repeatedly, at any age. It is the most frequently isolated pathogen in infantile diarrhea and is responsible for a disproportionate amount of hospitalization for dehydration.[14,153] The majority of symptomatic infections occurs in children under 3 years old, with peak incidence in children 6 months to 2 years of age. Rotavirus can also cause illness in adults, usually associated with secondary spread within a family.[14]

Nonspecific pathologic changes are seen in small bowel epithelial cells, with particles identified intracellularly. The exact mechanism of diarrhea is unknown, but a net secretion of water, sodium, and chloride occurs during the illness. Diarrheal losses contain 30 to 40 mEq/L each of sodium and potassium. Lactose malabsorption may persist for 1 to 2 weeks, associated with continued viral excretion in stool. Large numbers of viral particles are shed in the stool of ill patients, but prolonged excretion is unusual.[153]

After an incubation period of 24 to 72 hours, illness begins with vomiting, followed by diarrhea associated with abdominal cramps, low-grade fever, and malaise. Vomiting usually resolves within 2 days (range 1 to 5), but the diarrhea may last 3 to 8 days or longer. Natural infection reduces the incidence and severity of subsequent episodes. Serum antibody levels are demonstrated within the first few years of life and in almost all adults but appear to be nonprotective. Severity of illness usually decreases with age. Adults are more likely to have asymptomatic or mild illness with less vomiting. Dehydration frequently occurs in children, accounting for appreciable mortality in developing countries. Fortunately, oral fluid and electrolytes can be successfully used in most cases.[153]

The first rotavirus vaccine approved by the U.S. Food and Drug Administration (FDA) in 1998 is a tetravalent rhesus-human strain that provides coverage against the four common G serotypes of human rotavirus.[146,153,193] In clinical trials in industrialized countries, this vaccine provided 50% to 70% protection (up to 60% to 100% in severe cases). The recommendation was to give this vaccine to all children by mouth at 2, 4, and 6 months of age,[146] but concerns of vaccine-associated intussusception will delay routine use. The vaccine's efficacy and cost-effectiveness in developing countries and travelers should be further evaluated.

INTESTINAL PROTOZOA

Protozoal infections may be pathogenic or commensal (little or no effect) to the human host. Most protozoal infections are suspected on the basis of subacute or chronic GI symptoms, which may fluctuate over time. Although acute self-limited diarrheal illness may occur, the symptoms are nonspecific, and the diagnosis is often made on stool examination.

Several factors have increased the prevalence of intestinal parasites in the Unites States and worldwide: increase in immunocompetent persons who frequently become infected by these organisms, improvement in diagnostic techniques, changes in social behaviors (increased use of day care and nursing homes, more frequent international travel), and in the United States, increased immigration of people from Asia, Africa, and Latin America.[60,89,109,158]

As with enteric bacteria, symptoms from infection by intestinal protozoa depend on the level of bowel colonized. Those colonizing the small intestine, such as *Giardia* and coccidia, cause a wide spectrum of GI complaints, including malabsorption (foul stools and flatulence) and weight loss in persistent infections. Although many protozoa are capable of superficial mucosal invasion, only *Entamoeba histolytica* and *Balantidium coli*, which colonize the colon, can ulcerate the bowel wall, cause dysentery, and spread to other tissues.[89]

All intestinal protozoa are transmitted by the fecal-oral route, so infection rates are highest in areas and groups with poor sanitation, close contact, or particular customs favoring transmission. These reemerging infections have been related to large outbreaks of communicable diseases in the United States, often secondary to water contamination. Protozoal parasites were the most frequent etiologic agent detected in waterborne outbreaks from 1991 to 1994.[116,131,138] In addition to spread by food, water, and person-to-person contact, mechanical vectors such as flies may spread these organisms. Transmission of intestinal protozoa is favored by a hardy cyst, which is passed in the feces of an infected host. In addition to an infective cyst, the life cycle for most intestinal protozoa includes a trophozoite, which is responsible for reproduction and pathogenicity. Only a single host is required, except for *Sarcocystis*, which requires ingestion of raw meat from an intermediate host. Zoonotic spread to humans has been documented for *Giardia, Cryptosporidium, Entamoeba polecki,* and *B. coli*. Treatment of intestinal protozoan infections is summarized in Table 52-11.

Giardia Lamblia

G. lamblia is a flagellate protozoan that was first observed in 1681 by Leeuwenhoeck. In the last 30 years it

TABLE 52-11. Antiparasitic Therapy for Infectious Diarrhea in Adults

DIAGNOSIS	RECOMMENDATION
Giardiasis	Metronidazole 250 mg tid (15 mg/kg/day for children), Albendazole 400 mg qd, or quinacrine* 100 mg tid for 7 days, or tinidazole* 2000 mg single dose
Entamoeba histolytica excretion (asymptomatic)	Iodoquinol 650 mg tid for 20 days or paromomycin 500 mg tid for 7 days
E. histolytica diarrhea	Metronidazole 750 mg tid for 5 to 10 days or tinidazole* 1000 mg bid for 3 days, followed by iodoquinol 650 mg tid for 20 days or paromomycin 500 mg tid for 7 days
Cryptosporidiosis	None; in severe cases or AIDS patients, consider paromomycin 500-750 mg tid or qid for about 2 weeks or azithromycin 1200 mg qd for 4 weeks
Cyclosporidiosis	TMP/SMX 160 mg/800 mg bid for 7 days, followed by 160 mg/800 mg 3 times/week in AIDS patients
Isosporiasis	TMP/SMX 160 mg/800 mg qid for 10 days, followed by 160 mg/800 mg bid for 3 weeks, or pyrimethamine 75 mg qd with folinic acid 10 mg qd for 2 weeks
Microsporidiosis	Albendazole 400 mg bid for 2 to 4 weeks, followed by chronic suppression for AIDS patients

TMP/SMX, Trimethoprim and sulfamethoxazole; *tid,* 3 times a day; *qd,* daily; *qid,* 4 times a day; *bid,* twice daily.
*Not available in the United States.

has gained recognition as an important human pathogen.[67,123] The classification of *Giardia* species remains controversial.

The life cycle of *Giardia* involves two stages. Active trophozoites are responsible for symptomatic illness. The organisms attach to the mucosa of the duodenum and proximal jejunum, where they multiply rapidly through binary division. Trophozoites are rarely infective because they rapidly die outside the body and are less resistant to gastric acidity. Responding to unknown stimuli, some trophozoites encyst during passage through the colon and are eliminated in the stools of infected hosts. Cysts are infectious as passed in the host stool; no period of maturation or intermediate development stage is required. Furthermore, they are very hardy in the external environment. When ingested by a potential host, excystation is stimulated by passage through the stomach, and the motile trophozoite migrates to the small bowel to complete the cycle.[67,123,148]

Giardia is the most common protozoal intestinal parasite isolated worldwide. All age groups are affected.[67,109,148] Giardiasis usually represents a zoonosis, with cross-infectivity from animals to humans, and vice versa. *Giardia* has been found in stools of beavers, cattle, dogs, cats, rodents, and sheep.[148]

The infective dose of *Giardia* for humans is low: 10 to 25 cysts caused infection in eight of 25 subjects; more than 25 cysts caused infection in 100%.[148] Person-to-person spread may be the most common means of transmission for humans. Twenty-five percent of family members with infected children become infected.[67] Areas and populations with poor hygiene and close physical contact have higher rates of infection. Venereal transmission occurs among homosexuals through di-

rect fecal-oral contamination.[67] Epidemics and carrier rates of 30% to 60% have been found among children in day-care centers and in Native American reservations. Water is a major vehicle of infection in community outbreaks.[131] Cysts retain viability in cold water for as long as 2 to 3 months. In the United States from 1964 to 1984, 90 outbreaks (24,000 cases) of giardiasis were linked epidemiologically to water, and it is still the most frequently identified cause of waterborne diarrhea outbreaks. Most of these occurred in small water systems that used untreated or inadequately treated surface water.[121,122,131] Clear and cool mountain water has been so often associated with giardiasis that the illness has been called "backpacker's diarrhea" or "beaver fever" (although fever is not usually seen). An outbreak in Aspen, Colorado, in 1964 was the first well-documented waterborne outbreak in the United States, and recent outbreaks around the same area indicate that this area remains endemically infected with *Giardia*. In the northeastern states, large outbreaks have occurred in the mountain communities of Rome, New York, and Berlin, New Hampshire. Every U.S. region has experienced waterborne outbreaks, but the western mountain regions (Rocky Mountains, Cascades, Sierra Nevada) have reported the majority, where giardiasis must be considered endemic.[67,131,148]

Giardia accounts for a small percentage of TD.[60,158] It has been identified in a large percentage of cases among travelers to St. Petersburg, Russia, where tap water is the usual source. Because of the relatively long incubation period and persistent symptoms, *Giardia* is more likely to be found as the cause of diarrhea that occurs or persists after returning home from travels to any developing region.[42,60,158]

The pathophysiologic mechanisms of diarrhea and malabsorption in giardiasis are poorly understood.[148] Reversible malabsorption of fats, vitamins A and B, folate, and disaccharides has been demonstrated in some patients with diarrhea. Malabsorption may result from (1) physical blockade by large numbers of trophozoites blanketing the intestinal mucosa; (2) deconjugation of bile acids; (3) bacterial or fungal overgrowth in the small intestine; (4) increased turnover of cells on the mucosa of the villi, which do not absorb normally; and (5) epithelial damage. Altered gut motility and hypersecretion of fluids, perhaps through increased adenylate cyclase activity, may play a role. Histologic changes of villous atrophy and inflammatory infiltrates with epithelial cell destruction have been observed. In some series, these changes correlated with degree of malabsorption and reverted to normal after treatment. However, most small bowel biopsies in human patients demonstrate minimal or no changes, with only occasional mucosal invasion (with trophozoites found intracellularly and extracellularly) and no local inflammatory response.[67] Enterotoxins have not been found. More than one mechanism is probably involved. Infectivity apparently depends on both host and parasite factors.[148]

Most infections are asymptomatic, and in endemic areas, *Giardia* is found in healthy people. The attack rate for symptomatic infection in the natural setting varies from 5% to 70%.[148] Asymptomatic carrier states with high numbers of cysts excreted in stools are common. Correlation between inoculum size and infection rates has been noted, but not with numbers of cysts passed or severity of symptoms. Hypochlorhydria, certain immunodeficiencies, blood group A, and malnutrition apparently predispose to symptomatic infection.[67,148]

The incubation period averages 1 to 2 weeks, with a mean of 9 days and a wide clinical presentation. A few people experience abrupt onset of explosive watery diarrhea accompanied by abdominal cramps, foul flatus, vomiting, low-grade fever, and malaise. This typically lasts 3 to 4 days before transition into the more common subacute syndrome. In most patients the onset is more insidious and symptoms are persistent or recurrent. Stools become mushy, greasy, and malodorous. Watery diarrhea may alternate with soft stools and even constipation. Upper GI symptoms, typically exacerbated postprandially, accompany stool changes but may be present in the absence of soft stool. These include mid-abdominal and upper abdominal cramping, substernal burning, acid indigestion, sulfurous belching, nausea, distention, early satiety, and foul flatus. Constitutional symptoms of anorexia, fatigue, and weight loss are common.[67,148] Unusual presentations include allergic manifestations, such as urticaria, erythema multiforme, and bronchospasm. Some *Giardia* infections are associated with a chronic illness. Adults may have a longstanding malabsorption syndrome and marked weight loss, and children may have a failure-to-thrive syndrome.[44,148]

Laboratory confirmation of giardiasis can be difficult. Stool examination remains the primary means of diagnosis (Figure 52-2) but is being replaced by newer immunodiagnostic tests. Trophozoites may be found in fresh, watery stools but disintegrate rapidly. Although trophozoites remain in fresh stools for at least 24 hours, stools should be preserved in a fixative such as polyvinyl alcohol or a formalin preparation if not immediately examined. Cyst passage is extremely variable and not related to clinical symptoms.[148] In the office, fresh stool can be mixed with an iodine solution (e.g., Gram's iodine) or methylene blue and examined for cysts on a wet mount. Many antibiotics, enemas, laxatives, and barium studies mask or eliminate parasites from the stools, so examinations should be delayed for 5 to 10 days after these interventions. Trichrome stain is better than the formalin-ether concentration technique for identification of protozoal cysts and trophozoites.[75] The current recommendation is to examine three samples taken at intervals of 2 days. Another noninvasive office test is duodenal mucus sampling, using a string test (Enterotest), which has a reported sensitivity of 10% to 80%.[75,148] Duodenal biopsy is rarely necessary but may be the most sensitive test.[75]

A commercial enzyme immunoassay (EIA) has shown the same sensitivity as microscopic examination, but has 100% specificity, making it a convenient screening method. EIA is much easier and requires less experience than microscopy, but can not differentiate between cysts and trophozoites.[5] Immunofluorescent techniques using monoclonal antibodies can detect low numbers of organisms in short time but require centrifugation of the sample.[74] Molecular techniques need further development.[148,199]

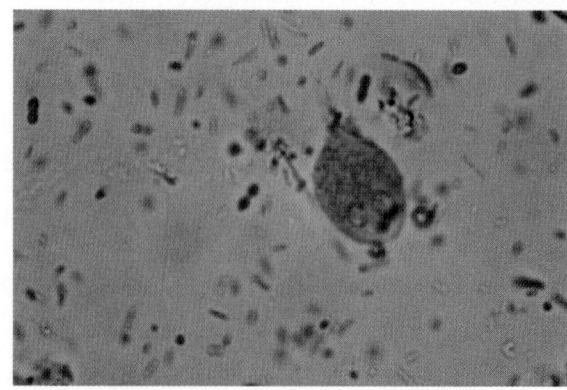

Figure 52-2 *Giardia lamblia* trophozoite seen by methylene blue wet mount staining under oil (1000x). The finding of cysts or trophozoites in a patient with diarrhea is sufficient to make a tentative diagnosis of giardiasis.

Immunologic responses to *Giardia* infection are complex. Epidemiologic studies show acquired resistance, with lower rates of infection and illness (1) among residents of endemically infected areas compared with visitors and (2) among adults compared with children. However, reinfection does occur. Levels of IgG antitrophozoite antibodies rise with both symptomatic and asymptomatic infections, helping to clear the infection. Hypogammaglobulinemic patients have a higher incidence of symptomatic giardiasis, implying an important protective function of immunoglobulins.[67,148] Effects of mucosal secretory antibodies in humans have not been clearly demonstrated, although mouse studies show a protective effect of IgA secretory antibodies. Both cellular and humoral responses to *Giardia* have been demonstrated. Immunologic responses are effective in the majority of infections because spontaneous clinical recovery is common with or without the disappearance of organisms. Average duration of symptoms in all ages ranges from 3 to 10 weeks.[44,148]

Given the difficulty and expense of confirming the diagnosis in some patients, a therapeutic trial of drugs may be attempted when suspicion is high. Imidazole derivatives, (e.g., metronidazole) affect bacterial flora as well, so they are less specific but still better for empiric (unproven diagnosis) therapy because of their wide activity.

Symptomatic patients should be treated for comfort and to prevent the development of chronic illness. Asymptomatic carriers in nonendemic areas should be treated when identified because they may transmit the infection or develop symptomatic illness. No drug is effective in all cases. In resistant cases, longer courses of two drugs taken concurrently have been suggested. Relapses occur up to several weeks after treatment, necessitating a second course of the same medication or an alternative drug. Malabsorption usually resolves with treatment, but persistent diarrhea may result from lactose intolerance or a syndrome resembling celiac disease rather than treatment failure.[148]

Three groups of drugs are currently being used: nitroimidazoles (metronidazole, tinidazole, albendazole, ornidazole, nimorazole), nitrofuran derivatives (furazolidone), and acridine compounds (mepacrine, quinacrine). Metronidazole (Flagyl, 250 mg three times a day for 5 days for adults) is often used in the United States. Cure rates of 85% to 90% are comparable to those with quinacrine, but with better tolerance. Tinidazole (Fasigyn, 2000 mg single dose) has the same success rate with better compliance but is not available in the United States. Quinacrine (Atabrine, 100 mg three times a day for 5 days for adults and 7 mg/kg/day in three divided doses for children for 5 days), with cure rates of about 95%, has been considered the drug of choice in adults. Unfortunately, quinacrine is no longer available in the United States because it produces more frequent side effects, especially in children. No pediatric liquid form is always available. In severely symptomatic individuals, paromomycin (Humatin, 25 to 30 mg/kg in three divided doses for 5 to 10 days) has been effective.[67,123,148]

Entamoeba

Lösch described the trophozoite form of *Entamoeba* in 1875 and Quincke and Ross the cyst form in 1893. Recently molecular biologic studies confirmed the existence of an invasive parasite *(Entamoeba histolytica)* and a noninvasive, commensal organism *(E. dispar)*.[100,124] Isoenzyme analysis has recognized 22 different zymodemes of *E. histolytica*, which may explain the pathogenic and commensal strains and the geographic differences in rates of invasive disease.[22,124,163]

The life cycle of *E. histolytica* involves two forms and one host. The reproductive form is the trophozoite, which resides in the large intestine of the host and can cause illness. Encystment occurs in the gut, and cysts pass in the stool. The early cyst matures within the host or externally by undergoing two nuclear divisions. Usually the cysts are infectious when passed. Although sensitive to boiling, adequate chlorination, and complete desiccation, cysts may survive drying or freezing and persist for months in a moist environment. After cysts are ingested, they undergo nuclear division in the small intestine, resulting in eight trophozoites per cyst.[22,124] Humans are the primary reservoir of *E. histolytica*. Infected individuals may pass up to 45 million cysts per day.

E. histolytica is found worldwide. Approximately 12% of the world's population is infected.[163] The higher prevalence in tropical countries (30% to 50%) is related to increased risk of fecal-oral contamination, which depends on sanitation, cultural habits, crowding, and socioeconomic status.[22,124] It is the third most important cause of death by parasitic infection worldwide. Similar conditions create pockets of endemic infection in the United States among institutional inmates, Native Americans on reservations, and homosexuals. Importation of infections by travelers and immigrants accounts for most cases in the United States and other temperate countries.[117] Attack rate and prevalence are difficult to determine because the majority of infections are asymptomatic, and screening with single stool samples is likely to identify only 20% to 50%.[22,124] The 10% to 15% of the U.S. population once infected with *E. histolytica* has decreased to 1% to 5% overall, primarily because of adequate water and sewage treatment.[109,117] Between 1946 and 1980, six waterborne outbreaks of amebiasis were reported in the United States.[131,125] Amebiasis accounts for less than 1% of TD.[60,124,158]

Pathogenicity of *E. histolytica* is not well understood.[124] Invasion may be a function of motility or lytic enzymes. The cecum and ascending colon are most frequently involved, followed by the rectum and sigmoid colon. Five different lesions of increasing severity can be distinguished in the colon: (1) diffuse inflammation with cellular infiltrate and an intact epithelium, (2) superficial erosions, (3) early invasion followed by shallow ulceration, (4) late invasive lesions forming the classic flask ulcers with skip lesions, and (5) loss of mucosa and muscularis, resulting in exposure of underlying granulation tissue. Extraintestinal spread is hematogenous. Abscesses containing acellular debris develop primarily in the liver but may involve the brain and lung.[124]

Although 80% to 99% of infections result in asymptomatic carriers, a spectrum of GI diseases may result. The incubation period ranges from 1 to 4 months, depending on the area of endemicity. Most often, colonic inflammation without dysentery causes lower abdominal cramping and altered stools, sometimes containing mucus and blood.[124,163] Weight loss, anorexia, and nausea may be present. Symptoms commonly fluctuate and continue for months. The subacute infection may evolve into a chronic, nondysenteric bowel syndrome, with intermittent diarrhea, abdominal pain, weight loss, and flatulence. Dysentery may develop suddenly after an incubation period of 8 to 10 days or a period of mild symptoms. Affected persons may have frequent passage of bloody stools, tenesmus, moderate to severe abdominal pain and tenderness, and fever. There is considerable variation in severity.[124]

Humoral antibodies increase with invasive disease and persist for long periods. Although they do not protect against reinfection or bowel invasion, they show antiamebic action in vitro and may prevent recurrent liver infection, which is uncommon. Once the infection is cleared, recurrence is unusual, but asymptomatic cyst shedding and active GI illness may persist for years, indicating lack of consistent immune response in the intestinal lumen.[124,163]

The fatality rate for amebic dysentery and its complications is about 2%. Complications of intestinal involvement develop in 2% to 20% of cases and include perforation, toxic megacolon, and ameboma. An ameboma is an annular inflammatory lesion of the ascending colon containing live trophozoites. It may be improperly diagnosed as a pyogenic abscess or a carcinoma. A postdysenteric syndrome can occur in patients with acute amebic dysentery and can be confused with ulcerative colitis.

The diagnosis of intestinal amebiasis is made by identification of cysts or trophozoites in stool. Mucus from fresh stools or sigmoidoscopic scrapings and aspirates mixed with a drop of saline may show trophozoites if examined within an hour. For delayed examination, stool must be preserved in polyvinyl alcohol or other fixative and may later be examined with trichrome stain.[75,124] The same limitations and problems discussed with *Giardia* apply to *E. histolytica*. Fecal shedding of cysts is irregular. Three stools on alternate days identify most infections. Overdiagnosis may result from misidentification of leukocytes. Sigmoidoscopy or colonoscopy is useful for viewing the pathologic lesions and obtaining selective samples of mucus and biopsies of mucosal ulcers, which usually contain organisms.[75] Finding cysts does not confirm the diagnosis of symptomatic intestinal amebiasis. The key to establish the diagnosis is finding motile trophozoites with ingested red blood cells. Culture techniques have been developed that identify infection in some cases when small numbers of cysts are missed in stool examinations, but culture techniques are expensive and time-consuming.[75] Serologic tests are not useful for identifying asymptomatic carriers but are positive in 85% to 95% of patients with dysentery and 90% to 100% of patients with liver abscess.[75,91,157] Also, new antigen detection techniques can differentiate between *E. histolytica* and *E. dispar*.[100,111] Recently, PCR techniques have been developed, showing greater than 95% sensitivity and specificity.[2,199]

Treatment of amebiasis is based on the location of infection and degree of symptoms. Medications are divided into tissue amebicides, which are well-absorbed drugs that combat invasive amebiasis in the bowel and liver (e.g., metronidazole, tinidazole, emetine, dehydroemetine, chloroquine), and poorly absorbed drugs for luminal infections (e.g., iodoquinol, paromomycin, diloxanide furoate). In general, treatment is effective for invasive infections but disappointing for intestinal colonization. U.S. guidelines suggest that asymptomatic carriers should be treated, since a cyst passer represents a potential health hazard to others and reinfection in the United States is uncommon. Routine screening of asymptomatic persons of high-risk groups is not cost-effective, except perhaps for food handlers.[124]

The current drug of choice for asymptomatic carriers is iodoquinol (650 mg 3 times a day for adults and 40 mg/kg/day in three divided doses for children for 20 days). Side effects are mild and consist of abdominal pain, diarrhea, and rash. Diloxanide furoate (Furamide) is another drug of choice (500 mg 3 times a day for adults and 20 mg/kg/day in three divided doses for children for 10 days), but in the United States it is classified as an investigational drug, available only through the CDC. Side effects are limited to flatulence and other mild GI symptoms.[124] Paromomycin is also effective (500 mg 3 times a day for adults and 30 mg/kg/day in three divided doses for children for 7 days). Although metronidazole has been used in asymptomatic carriers with 90% success, most reserve this drug for invasive and symptomatic infections.

Invasive disease is treated with a tissue-active drug, followed by a luminal agent (in the same doses as just listed). For oral therapy, metronidazole is the drug of choice (750 mg 3 times a day for adults and 50 mg/kg/day in three divided doses for children for 5 to 10 days), followed by iodoquinol. Tinidazole (1000 mg twice daily for 3 days), is not available in the United States but appears to be effective and is well tolerated for intestinal and hepatic amebiasis. Emetine and dehydroemetine (1 mg/kg/day, maximum 90 mg/day) are used parenterally in severe cases of amebiasis, primarily extraintestinal, followed by iodoquinol for 20 days. These two drugs have frequent systemic side effects, including the development of cardiac arrhythmias requiring hospitalization for cardiac monitoring. Since this class of drugs is related to ipecac, they also cause vomiting.[23,124]

Another species, *Entamoeba polecki,* although usually nonpathogenic, has been suspected of causing lower intestinal symptoms in sporadic cases involving heavy infection.[167] Cysts are passed in stool and may be confused with *E. histolytica,* which they closely resemble. Successful resolution of symptoms has been reported with metronidazole followed by diloxanide furoate in the same doses as for amebiasis and balantidiasis.

Cryptosporidium

Cryptosporidium is a coccidian parasite that belongs to the phyla Sporozoa. It is a reemergent enteric pathogen in humans. *Cryptosporidium parvum,* the only human pathogen of this genus, was originally described in 1912 but first identified in humans in 1976.[34,35,86]

Ingested thick-walled oocysts release sporozoites, which invade small bowel enterocytes, then develop into trophozoites that reside intracellularly but are extracytoplasmic (beneath the host cell membrane, similar to a vacuole). Trophozoites divide by asexual multiplication into merozoites (type I meront), with each one containing six to eight nuclei. From this stage they continue with asexual multiplication as type I meronts, which can infect other enterocytes (merogonic or schizogonic stage), or they develop into a type II meront and initiate sexual multiplication and oocyst development (sporogonic or gametogonic stage). About 80% of zygotes develop into thick-walled oocysts (each with four sporozoites) that are released in the stool, while the rest develop into thin-walled oocysts that participate in autoinfection of the host.[82]

C. parvum is a ubiquitous zoonosis with a worldwide distribution. *Cryptosporidium* infects a wide variety of young animals, including domestic calves, birds, piglets, horses, pigs, kittens, puppies, and wild mammals, such as raccoons, beavers, squirrels, and coyotes.[86] Prevalence of infection in human populations varies from 0.1% to 3% in cooler, developed countries (Europe, North America) to 0.5% to 10% in warmer areas (Africa, Asia). The infection has been described in those who have contact with animals, such as veterinarians and farmers; infants in day-care centers; travelers to endemic areas; and AIDS or other immunocompromised patients. It may infect large numbers of individuals in community-wide waterborne outbreaks.[35,86,131] The infective dose of *Cryptosporidium* for humans is low, similar to *Giardia* species. Sporulated oocysts are infective as passed in the stool, so fecal-oral contamination is the mode of transmission.[86] The different routes of transmission are waterborne, especially in large community outbreaks; person to person, especially in day-care centers, custodial institutions, and hospitals; food-borne disease, through apple cider, uncooked sausage, and raw milk; sexual, with no association with specific behavior; and zoonotic.[73,86,121,122] In 1993 in Milwaukee, *Cryptosporidium* caused the largest waterborne outbreak of protozoal parasites in the United States.[127] The pathophysiologic mechanisms of diarrhea and malabsorption are not completely understood. The initial invasion of parasites may activate cellular and humoral immune and inflammatory responses, leading to cell damage with villi atrophy and crypt hyperplasia, ultimately producing malabsorption and osmotic diarrhea.[82,86]

The clinical manifestations depend on immune status, but asymptomatic infection occurs in both normal and immunocompromised hosts.[86] In immunocompetent persons the usual incubation period of *Cryptosporidium* is from 5 to 28 days. Symptoms consist of watery diarrhea associated with cramps, nausea, flatulence, and at times, vomiting and low-grade fever. The syndrome is generally mild and self-limited, with a duration of 5 to 6 days in some groups (range 2 to 26 days). In contrast, immunocompromised hosts experience more frequent and prolonged infections, with profuse chronic watery diarrhea, malabsorption, and weight loss lasting months to years. Fluid losses can be overwhelming in a fulminant cholera-like illness, with high mortality. Cyst passage in stool usually ends within 1 week of symptom resolution but may persist for up to 2 months after recovery. Reinfection of an immunocompetent person has been documented.

Rarely, *Cryptosporidium* can infect the respiratory system, which may be fatal in the immunocompromised host. The other extraintestinal manifestations relate to involvement of the liver and biliary system, particularly in immunocompromised persons. Cholangitis may not respond to common luminal agents used to treat intestinal cryptosporidiasis, requiring sphincterotomy for therapy.[86]

Diagnosis in initial case descriptions was made by small bowel biopsy, but oocysts can be found in the stools routinely in intestinal infections, even though shedding may be intermittent. Concentration techniques, such as formalin-ether or sucrose flotation, and subsequent staining with modified acid-fast, Giemsa, or Ziehl-Neelsen techniques facilitate identification of

Cryptosporidium oocysts. The Enterotest is also useful in the diagnosis of cryptosporidiosis. Newer immunologic techniques are faster and have adequate sensitivity and excellent specificity. Several other methods (flow cytometry using monoclonal antibodies, PCR, RFLP analysis) have been developed, but their efficacy in the clinical setting is not yet known.[25,74,86,114]

No clearly effective treatment has been found for cryptosporidiosis. Because this disease is usually mild and self-limited in immunocompetent hosts, only supportive care is needed. Anticryptosporidial agents, such as paromomycin (500 to 750 mg 3 or 4 times a day for 2 weeks) and azithromycin (1200 mg daily for 4 weeks) may be used in immunocompetent persons with persistent infection and in immunocompromised patients. Paromomycin, azithromycin, roxithromycin, ionophores, sulfonamides, mefloquine, and nitazoxanide have been tested against cryptosporidiosis, especially in AIDS patients with chronic diarrheal disease, with variable but generally positive effects.[86,180,201] Further studies with these and other new agents, including clinical trials using immunotherapy options, are in progress.[33,86]

Isospora belli

I. belli is also a coccidian protozoal parasite. The first description of *Isospora* was in 1915. More recently, *I. belli* was identified as the pathogenic species for humans. It is an uncommon cause of diarrhea in humans, but as with *Cryptosporidium,* its prevalence has been increasing in immunocompromised patients.[33,82,129,131,200]

Humans are the only host, and infections are transmitted by fecal-oral contamination through direct contact of food and water. *I. belli* is endemic in areas of South America, Africa, and Asia. The prevalence is not precisely known but it ranges from 0.2% to 3% in United States AIDS patients and 8% to 20% in Haitian and African AIDS patients. This parasite has also been associated with outbreaks in custodial institutions, in day-care centers, and among immigrants. Infection rates in otherwise healthy persons with diarrhea are usually low. Most cases have been identified in tropical regions among natives, travelers, and the military.[82,131]

Life cycle and pathogenesis of *I. belli* are similar to *Cryptosporidium.* The organism invades mucosal cells of the small intestine, causing an inflammatory response in the submucosa and variable destruction of the brush border.[82]

In immunocompetent persons, the *I. belli* infection may be asymptomatic or cause mild transient diarrhea and abdominal cramps. Other symptoms include profuse watery diarrhea, flatulence, anorexia, weight loss, low-grade fever, and malabsorption.[82] Generally infection is self-limited, ending in 2 to 3 weeks, but some persons have symptoms lasting months to years, clinically similar to giardiasis. Recurrences are common. Infections in immunocompromised patients tend to be

more severe and follow a more protracted course.[129] Rarely, acalculous cholecystitis or reactive arthritis has been reported in isosporiasis.[12]

Diagnosis can be made by identification of immature oocysts in fresh stool. However, excretion may occur sporadically and in small numbers, so concentration techniques are usually required. Staining with modified Ziehl-Neelsen and auramine-rhodamine are also useful. When stools are negative, the organism can be recovered from the jejunum through a biopsy or string test. Unlike the other intestinal protozoa, *I. belli* may cause eosinophilia.[75]

Successful treatment has been reported with TMP/SMX (160/800 mg 4 times a day for 10 days, then 2 times a day for 3 weeks in normal hosts). Other options are pyrimethamine (75 mg daily for 14 days) with folinic acid, and metronidazole (for patients allergic to sulfonamides). In HIV patients, chronic lifetime suppression therapy is indicated with either TMP/SMX (160/800 mg 3 times a week) or pyrimethamine (25 mg) plus folinic acid (5 mg) daily.[82,129]

Cyclospora Cayetanensis

Cyclospora species were first discovered in moles in 1870 and were identified as human pathogens in 1979. They were initially thought to be blue-green algae (cyanobacteria-like organism).[149,182,202] The life cycle and pathogenesis of *C. cayetanensis* are not completely understood.

The organism has shown to be an important cause of acute and protracted diarrhea. *C. cayetanensis* is endemic in many developing countries in all continents, with the highest rates occurring in Nepal, Haiti, and Peru. In the United States, most of the native outbreaks have been from areas east of Rocky Mountains, usually associated with ingestion of contaminated imported raspberries.[27,82] Fecal-oral transmission also occurs through water and soil.[182] *Cyclospora* infection is closely associated with diarrhea in travelers to endemic areas.[82,95,131,202]

The onset of diarrhea is usually abrupt with symptoms lasting up to 7 weeks or even longer.[82] In AIDS patients the duration may be longer and the severity greater.[129] Small spheric organisms can be detected in fresh or concentrated stool, and they show variable staining with acid-fast methods. *C cayetanensis* stains best with carbolfuchsin.[202] Phase-contrast microscopy and autofluorescence are also useful in the diagnosis.[75] A PCR method is still used only for research.[131]

The treatment of choice is TMP/SMX (160/800 mg 4 times a day for 10 days). This treatment provides more rapid clinical and parasitologic cure, with fewer recurrences.[82,182] In AIDS patients, chronic suppression with TMP/SMX may be required.[129]

Miscellaneous Parasitic Agents

Microsporidia. More than 100 genera and 1000 species of microsporidia exist in the phylum Microspora. Most species infect insects, birds, and fish. Since the first description in humans in 1985, only 12 species have been reported to infect humans: *Enterocytozoon bieneusi,* three *Encephalitozoon* species, three *Nosema* species, two *Trachipleistophora* species, *Pleistophora, Vittaforma corneae,* and *Microsporida* species. Microsporidians cause a wide spectrum of disease, but only two, *E. bieneusi* and *E. intestinalis,* have been found to cause diarrhea.[38,82,198,200]

Transmission is thought to be fecal-oral or urinary-oral[38] and the infection zoonotic. Waterborne transmission also occurs.[131] Prevalence of microsporidiosis in AIDS patients with chronic diarrhea is 7% to 50%.[9,198]

The clinical manifestations of intestinal microsporidiosis are chronic diarrhea, loss of appetite, weight loss, malabsorption and fever.[9,198] Acute self-limited diarrhea has been reported in immunocompetent hosts. Other infections include keratoconjunctivitis, hepatitis, peritonitis, myositis, CNS infection, urinary tract infections, sinusitis and disseminated disease. Diagnosis involves trichrome staining of concentrated stools or intestinal biopsy sampling, but electron microscopy is considered the gold standard. Immunologic and molecular biologic techniques are still under evaluation.[69,198]

The most effective drug is albendazole (400 mg twice a day for 2 to 4 weeks). It is effective against most species, but results are variable with diarrhea from *E. bieneusi.*[39] Other drugs show different efficacy and include thalidomide, fumagillin, atovaquone, metronidazole, furazolidone, azithromycin, itraconazole, and sulfonamides.[38]

Sarcocystis. Few human infections with *Sarcocystis* have been reported. Infection may be asymptomatic or associated with diarrhea, abdominal pain, nausea, and bloating. Symptoms typically improve within 48 hours of onset of illness. Diagnosis is based on identification of cysts in concentrated feces. No specific treatment has been established, but TMP/SMX and furazolidone have had variable efficacy.[200]

Balantidium. *Balantidium coli* is a rare pathogen in humans.[186,200] Although many aspects of the epidemiology are unclear, pigs appear to be the primary reservoir and source of human infection. Clinical features also resemble amebiasis, with a spectrum including asymptomatic infection, chronic intermittent diarrhea of variable intensity, acute dysentery with mucosal invasion, and rarely, metastatic abscesses. Diagnosis is made by observing the organism in stool. Trophozoites are seen much more often than are cysts. Recommended treatment is tetracycline (500 mg 4 times a day for 10 days) or metronidazole (750 mg 3 times a day for 10 days).[200]

Blastocystis. The role of *Blastocystis hominis* in diarrheal disease is still controversial, although it is often identified in stool samples. *B. hominis* has not been di-

rectly correlated with symptoms,[200] which could be caused by other undetected pathogens. When found in large numbers as the sole pathogen, *B. hominis* is suspected as the potential etiologic agent of diarrheal illness.

Dientamoeba. *Dientamoeba fragilis* occasionally causes diarrhea, occurring characteristically in residents of or visitors to developing tropical regions. It may be found in stools of persons without enteric symptoms. Because cyst forms have not been identified, the mode of transmission remains unknown. Illness caused by the parasite typically resembles giardiasis, but treatment of these two parasitic infections is different. Iodoquinol and tetracyclines are effective against *D. fragilis.*[200]

REFERENCES

1. Acharya IL et al: Prevention of typhoid fever in Nepal with the Vi capsular polysaccharide of *Salmonella typhi, N Engl J Med* 317:1101, 1987.
2. Acuna-Soto RJ et al: Application of the polymerase chain reaction to the epidemiology of pathogenic and nonpathogenic *Entamoeba histolytica, Am J Trop Med Hyg* 48:58, 1993.
3. Adachi JA et al: Fecal contamination of sauces served in public restaurants in Guadalajara, Mexico. Abstract presented at the 36th Annual Meeting of the Infectious Diseases Society of America, Denver, 1998.
3a. Adachi A et al: Enteroaggregative *Escherichia coli* as a major etiologic agent in travelers' diarrhea in three regions of the world (in press).
4. Adamkiewicz TV et al: Infections due to *Yersinia enterocolitica* in a series of patients with beta-thalassemia: Incidence and predisposing factors, *Clin Infect Dis* 27:1362, 1998.
5. Addiss DG et al: Evaluation of commercially available enzyme-linked immunosorbent assay for *Giardia lamblia* antigen in stool, *J Clin Microbiol* 29:1137, 1991.
6. Ascon MA et al: Oral immunization with a *Salmonella typhimurium* vaccine vector expressing recombinant enterotoxigenic *Escherichia coli* K99 fimbriae elicits elevated antibody titers for protective immunity, *Infect Immun* 66:5470, 1998.
7. Aserkoff B, Bennett JV: Effect of antibiotic therapy in acute salmonellosis on the fecal excretion of salmonellae, *N Engl J Med* 281:636, 1969.
8. Ashkenazi S et al: Safety and immunogenicity of *Shigella sonnei* and *Shigella flexneri* 2a O-specific polysaccharide conjugates in children, *J Infect Dis* 179:1565, 1999.
9. Asmuth DM et al: Clinical features of microsporidiosis in patients with AIDS, *Clin Infect Dis* 18:819, 1994.
10. Attwood SEA et al: *Yersinia* infection and acute abdominal pain, *Lancet* 1:529, 1987.
11. Bando SY et al: Characterization of enteroinvasive *Escherichia coli* and *Shigella* strains by RAPD analysis, *FEMS Microbiol Lett* 165:159, 1998.
12. Benator DA et al: *Isospora belli* infection associated with acalculous cholecystitis in a patient with AIDS, *Ann Intern Med* 121:663, 1994.
13. Benitez JA et al: Preliminary assessment of the safety and immunogenicity of a new CTXPhi-negative hemagglutinin/protease-defective El Tor strain as a cholera vaccine candidate, *Infect Immun* 67:539, 1999.
14. Bishop RF: Natural history of human rotavirus infection, *Arch Virol Suppl* 12:119, 1996.
15. Blacklow NR, Greenberg HB: Viral gastroenteritis, *N Engl J Med* 325:252, 1991.
16. Blaser MJ: Epidemiologic and clinical features of *Campylobacter jejuni* infections, *J Infect Dis* 176 (suppl 2):S103, 1997.
17. Blaser MJ, Newman LS: A review of salmonellosis. I. Infective dose, *Rev Infect Dis* 4:1096, 1982.
18. Blaser MJ et al: *Campylobacter* enteritis: clinical and epidemiological features, *Ann Intern Med* 91:179, 1979.
19. Blaser MJ et al: *Campylobacter* enteritis in the United States: a multicenter trial, *Ann Intern Med* 98:360, 1983.
20. Bolen JL, Zamiska SA, Greenough WB: Clinical features in enteritis due to *Vibrio parahaemolyticus, Am J Med* 57:638, 1974.
21. Bourke B, Chan VL, Sherman P: *Campylobacter upsaliensis:* waiting in the wings, *Clin Microbiol Rev* 11:440, 1998.
22. Bruckner DA: Amebiasis, *Clin Microbiol Rev* 5:356, 1992.

23. Caeiro JP, DuPont HL: Management of travelers' diarrhea, *Drugs* 56:73, 1998.

24. Carrillo C et al: In vitro antimicrobial susceptibility of *Vibrio cholerae*, *Salmonella typhi* and *paratyphi*, *Shigella* spp. and *Brucella* to several antibiotics, Lima, Peru. Abstract presented at the 34th Interscience Conference on Antimicrobial Agents and Chemotherapy, American Society of Microbiology, Orlando, Fla, 1994.

25. Casemore DP: Laboratory methods for diagnosis cryptosporidiosis, *J Clin Pathol* 44:445, 1991.

26. Caul EO: Viruses in food. In Spencer RC, Wright EP, Newsom SWB, editors: *Rapid methods and automation in microbiology and immunology*, Andover, NH, 1994, Intercept Ltd.

27. Centers for Disease Control and Prevention: 1996 update: outbreaks of *Cyclospora cayetanensis* infections—United States and Canada, *MMWR* 45:611, 1996.

28. Centers for Disease Control and Prevention: Multi-state outbreak of *Salmonella* serotype Agona infections linked to toasted oats cereal—United States, April-May, 1998, *JAMA* 280:411, 1998.

29. Christensen ML: Human viral gastroenteritis, *Clin Microbiol Rev* 2:51, 1989.

30. Cleary RK: *Clostridium difficile*–associated diarrhea and colitis: clinical manifestations, diagnosis and treatment, *Dis Colon Rectum* 41:1435, 1998.

31. Cody SH et al: An outbreak of *Escherichia coli* O157:H7 infection from unpasteurized commercial apple juice, *Ann Intern Med* 130:202, 1999.

32. Coster TS et al: Vaccination against shigellosis with attenuated *Shigella flexneri* 2a strain SC602, *Infect Immun* 67:3437, 1999.

33. Crabb JH: Antibody-based chemotherapy of cryptosporidiosis, *Adv Parasitol* 40:121, 1998.

34. Current WL: *Cryptosporidium parvum:* household transmission, *Ann Intern Med* 120:518, 1994.

35. Current WL, Garcia LS: Cryptosporidiosis, *Clin Microbiol Rev* 4:325, 1991.

36. Czeczulin JR et al: Phylogenetic analysis of enteroaggregative and diffusely adherent *Escherichia coli*, *Infect Immun* 67:2692, 1999.

37. DeWitt TG: Clinical predictors of acute bacterial diarrhea in young children, *Pediatrics* 76:551, 1985.

38. Didier AE: Microsporidiosis, *Clin Infect Dis* 27:1, 1998.

39. Dieterich DT et al: Treatment with albendazole for intestinal disease due to *Enterocytozoon bieneusi* in patients with AIDS, *J Infect Dis* 169:178, 1994.

40. Dorman CJ, Porter ME: The *Shigella* virulence gene regulatory cascade: a paradigm of bacterial gene control mechanism, *Mol Microbiol* 29:677, 1998.

41. Duggan C, Nurko S. "Feeding the gut": the scientific basis for continued enteral nutrition during acute diarrhea, *J Pediatr* 131:801, 1997.

42. DuPont HL: Infectious diarrhea, *Aliment Pharmacol Ther* 8:3, 1994.

43. DuPont HL: Pathogenesis of traveler's diarrhea, *Chemotherapy* 41(suppl 1):33, 1995.

44. DuPont HL, Capsuto EG: Persistent diarrhea in travelers, *Clin Infect Dis* 22:124, 1996.

45. DuPont HL, Ericsson CD: Prevention and treatment of travelers' diarrhea, *N Engl J Med* 328:1821, 1993.

46. DuPont HL, Hornick RB: Adverse effect of Lomotil therapy in shigellosis, *JAMA* 226:1525, 1973.

47. DuPont HL et al: The response of man to virulent *Shigella flexneri* 2a, *J Infect Dis* 119:296, 1969.

48. DuPont HL et al: Immunity in shigellosis. II. Protection induced by oral live vaccine or primary infection, *J Infect Dis* 125:12, 1972.

49. DuPont HL et al: Comparative susceptibility of Latin American and United States students to enteric pathogens, *N Engl J Med* 295:1520, 1976.

50. DuPont HL et al: Prevention of travelers' diarrhea with trimethoprim-sulfamethoxazole, *Rev Infect Dis* 4:533, 1982.

51. DuPont HL et al: Treatment of travelers' diarrhea with trimethoprim/sulfamethoxazole and with trimethoprim alone, *N Engl J Med* 307:841, 1982.

52. DuPont HL et al: Prevention of travelers' diarrhea with trimethoprim-sulfamethoxazole and trimethoprim alone, *Gastroenterology* 84:75, 1983.

53. DuPont HL et al: Prevention of travelers' diarrhea by the tablet formulation of bismuth subsalicylate, *JAMA* 257:1347, 1987.

54. DuPont HL et al: Inoculum size in shigellosis and implications for expected mode of transmission, *J Infect Dis* 159:1126, 1989.

55. DuPont HL et al: A randomized, open-label comparison of nonprescription loperamide and attapulgite in the symptomatic treatment of acute diarrhea, *Am J Med* 88(suppl 6A):20S, 1990.

56. DuPont HL et al: Comparative efficacy of loperamide hydrochloride and bismuth subsalicylate in the management of acute diarrhea, *Am J Med* 88(suppl 6A):15S, 1990.

57. DuPont HL et al: Five versus three days of ofloxacin therapy for traveler's diarrhea: a placebo-controlled study, *Antimicrob Agents Chemother* 36:87, 1992.

58. DuPont HL et al: Zaldaride maleate (Zm), an intestinal calmodulin inhibitor, in the therapy of travelers' diarrhea, *Gastroenterology* 104:709, 1993.

59. DuPont HL et al: Rifaximin: a nonabsorbed antimicrobial in the therapy of travelers' diarrhea, *Digestion* 59:708, 1998.

60. Ericsson CD: Travelers' diarrhea: epidemiology, prevention and self-treatment, *Infect Dis Clin North Am* 12:285, 1998.

61. Ericsson CD, DuPont HL: Travelers' diarrhea: approaches to prevention and treatment, *Clin Infect Dis* 16:298, 1993.

62. Ericsson CD, Rey M: Prevention of travelers' diarrhea: risk avoidance and chemoprophylaxis. In DuPont HL, Steffen R, editors: *Textbook of travel medicine and health*, Hamilton, Ontario, Canada, 1997, Decker.

63. Ericsson CD et al: Ciprofloxacin or trimethoprim-sulfamethoxazole as initial therapy for travelers' diarrhea, *Ann Intern Med* 106:216, 1987.

64. Ericsson CD et al: Treatment of travelers' diarrhea with sulfamethoxazole and trimethoprim and loperamide, *JAMA* 263:257, 1990.

65. Ericsson CD et al: Single dose ofloxacin plus loperamide compared with single dose or three days of ofloxacin in the treatment of travelers' diarrhea, *J Travel Med* 4:3, 1997.

66. Eykyn SJ, Williams H: Treatment of multiresistant *Salmonella typhi* with oral ciprofloxacin, *Lancet* 2:1407, 1987.

67. Farthing MJ: Giardiasis, *Gastroenterol Clin North Am* 25:493, 1996.

68. Faruque SM, Albert MJ, Mikalanos JJ: Epidemiology, genetics and ecology of toxigenic *Vibrio cholerae*, *Microbiol Mol Biol Rev* 62:1301, 1998.

69. Fedorko DP, Hijazi YM: Application of molecular techniques to the diagnosis of microsporidial infection, *Emerg Infect Dis* 2:183, 1996.

70. Fekety R: Guidelines for the diagnosis and management of Clostridium difficile–associated diarrhea and colitis. American College of Gastroenterology, Practice Parameters Committee, *Am J Gastroenterol* 92:739, 1997.

71. Felsenfeld O: Notes on food, beverages and fomites contaminated with *Vibrio cholerae*, *Bull World Health Organ* 33:725, 1965.

72. Feng P et al: Genotypic and phenotypic changes in the emergence of *Escherichia coli* O157:H7, *J Infect Dis* 177:1750, 1998.

73. Fricker CR, Crabb JH: Water-borne cryptosporidiosis: detection methods and treatment options, *Adv Parasitol* 40:241, 1998.

74. Garcia LS et al: Evaluation of a new monoclonal antibody combination reagent for direct fluorescence detection of *Giardia* cysts and *Cryptosporidium* oocysts in human fecal specimens, *J Clin Microbiol* 30:3255, 1992.

75. Garcia LS et al: *Diagnostic medical parasitology*, Washington, DC, 1993, American Society for Microbiology.

76. Garthwright W, Archer D, Kvenberg J: Estimates of incidence and cost of intestinal infectious diseases in the United States, *Public Health Rep* 107, 1988.

77. Gascon J et al: Enteroaggregative *Escherichia coli* strains as a cause of traveler's diarrhea: a case-control study, *J Infect Dis* 177:1409, 1998.

78. Germanier R, Fürer E: Isolation and characterization of *galE* mutant Ty21a of *Salmonella typhi:* a candidate strain for a live oral typhoid vaccine, *J Infect Dis* 131:553, 1975.

79. Gibreel A et al: Rapid emergence of high-level resistance to quinolones in *Campylobacter jejuni* associated with mutational changes in gyr4 and parC, *Antimicrob Agents Chemother* 177:951, 1998.

80. Glandt M et al: Enteroaggregative *Escherichia coli* as a cause of travelers' diarrhea: clinical response to ciprofloxacin, *Clin Infect Dis* 29:335, 1999.

81. Glynn MK et al: Emergence of multidrug-resistant *Salmonella enterica* serotype *typhimurium* DT 104 infections in the United States, *N Engl J Med* 338:1333, 1998.

81a. Gomi H et al: In-vitro antimicrobial susceptibility testing among bacterial enteropathogens causing travelers' diarrhea in four areas of the world (in press).

82. Goodgame RW: Understanding intestinal spore-forming protozoa: Cryptosporidia, Microsporidia, Isospora, and Cyclospora, *Ann Intern Med* 124:429, 1996.

83. Goosney DL et al: Enteropathogenic *E. coli*, *Salmonella* and *Shigella*: Masters of host cell cytoskeletal exploitation, *Emerg Infect Dis* 5:216, 1999.

84. Gordillo ME et al: In vitro activity of azithromycin against bacterial enteric pathogens, *Antimicrob Agent Chemother* 37:1203, 1993.

85. Green J et al: Recent developments in the detection and characterization of small round structured viruses, *PHLS Microbiol Dig* 12:219, 1995.

86. Griffiths JK: Human cryptosporidiosis: epidemiology, transmission, clinical disease, treatment and diagnosis, *Adv Parasitol* 40:37, 1998.

87. Gross U et al: Antibiotic resistance in *Salmonella enterica* serotype *typhimurium*, *Eur J Clin Microbiol Infect Dis* 17:385, 1998.

88. Guerin F et al: Bloody diarrhea caused by *Klebsiella pneumoniae*: a new mechanism of bacterial virulence? *Clin Infect Dis* 27:648, 1998.

89. Guerrant Rl, Bobak DA: Bacterial and protozoal gastroenteritis, *N Engl J Med* 325:327, 1991.

90. Gupta RK et al: Phase I evaluation of *Vibrio cholerae* O1, serotype Inaba, polysaccharide-cholera toxin conjugates in adult volunteers, *Infect Immun* 66:3095, 1998.

91. Haque RL et al: Rapid diagnosis of *Entamoeba* infection by using *Entamoeba* and *Entamoeba histolytica* stool antigen detection kits, *J Clin Microbiol* 33:2558, 1995.

92. Harris JC, DuPont HL, Hornick RB: Fecal leukocytes in diarrheal illness, *Ann Intern Med* 76:697, 1972.

93. Hedberg CW, Osterholm MT: Outbreaks of food-borne and waterborne viral gastroenteritis, *Clin Microbiol Rev* 6:199, 1993.

94. Hilton E et al: Efficacy of *Lactobacillus* GG as a diarrheal preventive in travelers, *J Travel Med* 1:41, 1997.

95. Hoge CW et al: Epidemiology of diarrhoeal illness associated with coccidian-like organism among travelers and foreign residents in Nepal, *Lancet* 341:1175, 1993.

96. Holmberg SD et al: *Aeromonas* infections in the United States, *Ann Intern Med* 105:683, 1986.

97. Holmberg SD et al: *Plesiomonas* infections in the United States, *Ann Intern Med* 105:690, 1986.

98. Hornick RB et al: The Broad Street pump revisited: response of volunteers to ingested cholera vibrios, *Bull NY Acad Med* 47:1181, 1971.

99. Hossain MA et al: Increasing frequency of mecillinam-resistant *Shigella* isolates in urban Dhaka and rural Matlab, Bangladesh: a 6-year observation, *J Antimicrob Chemother* 42:99, 1998.

100. Jackson TF: *Entamoeba histolytica* and *Entamoeba dispar* are distinct species: clinical, epidemiological and serological evidence, *Int J Parasitol* 18:181, 1998.

101. Janda JM, Abbott SL: Evolving concepts regarding the genus *Aeromonas*: an expanding panorama of species, disease presentation, and unanswered questions, *Clin Infect Dis* 27:332, 1998.

102. Jiang X et al: Expression, self-assembly, and anteginicity of the Norwalk virus capsid protein, *J Virol* 66:6527, 1992.

103. Jiang X et al: Sequence and genomic organization of Norwalk virus, *Virology* 195:51, 1993.

104. Johnson S, Gerding DN: *Clostridium difficile*–associated diarrhea, *Clin Infect Dis* 26:1027, 1998.

105. Jones MA et al: Secreted effector proteins of *Salmonella dublin* act in concert to induce enteritis, *Infect Immun* 66:5799, 1998.

106. Josefson D: CF gene may protect against typhoid fever, *BMJ* 316:1481, 1998.

107. Kaper JA et al: Cholera, *Clin Microbiol Rev* 8:48, 1995.

108. Kapikian AZ et al: Visualization by immune electron microscopy of a 27-nm particle associated with infectious nonbacterial gastroenteritis, *J Virol* 10:1075, 1972.

109. Kappus KD et al: Intestinal parasitism in the United States: update on a continuing problem, *Am J Trop Med Hyg* 50:705, 1994.

110. Karaolis DK et al: A bacteriophage encoding a pathogenicity island, a type-IV pilus and a phage receptor in cholera bacteria, *Nature* 399:375, 1999.

111. Katzwinkel-Waldarsh ST et al: Direct amplification and differentiation of pathogenic and nonpathogenic *Entamoeba histolytica* DNA from stool specimens, *Am J Trop Med Hyg* 51:115, 1994.

112. Kean BH: The diarrhea of travelers to Mexico, *Ann Intern Med* 59:605, 1963.

113. Kean BH: Travelers' diarrhea: an overview, *Rev Infect Dis* 8(suppl 2):111, 1986.

114. Kehl KS at al: Comparison of four different methods for detection of *Cryptosporidium* species, *J Clin Microbiol* 33:416, 1995.

115. Kenny B et al: Enteropathogenic *E. coli* (EPEC) transfers its receptor for intimate adherence into mammalian cells, *Cell* 91:511, 1997.

116. Kramer MH et al: Surveillance for waterborne disease outbreaks—United States, 1993-1994, *MMWR* 45:1, 1996.

117. Krogstad DJ et al: Amebiasis: epidemiologic studies in the United States, 1971-1974, *Ann Intern Med* 88:89, 1978.

118. Kuschner R et al: Use of azithromycin for the treatment of *Campylobacter* enteritis in travelers to Thailand, *Clin Infect Dis* 21:536, 1995.

119. Lambden PR et al: Sequence and genome organization of a human small round-structured (Norwalk-like) virus, *Science* 259:516, 1993.

120. Law D, Chart H: Enteroaggregative *Escherichia coli*, *J Appl Microbiol* 84:685, 1998.

121. LeChevallier MW et al: Occurrence of *Giardia* and *Cryptosporidium* spp. in surface water supplies, *Appl Environ Microbiol* 57:2610, 1991.

122. LeChevallier MW et al: *Giardia* and *Cryptosporidium* spp. in filtered drinking water supplies, *Appl Environ Microbiol* 57:2617, 1991.

123. Lewis DJ, Freedman AR: *Giardia lamblia* as an intestinal pathogen, *Dig Dis* 10:102, 1992.

124. Li E, Stanley SL Jr: Protozoa, amebiasis, *Gastroenterol Clin North Am* 25:471, 1996.

125. Lippy EC, Waltrip SC: Waterborne disease outbreaks—1946-1980: a thirty-five year perspective, *J Am Water Works Assoc* 76:60, 1984.

126. MacFarlane AS et al: In vivo blockage of nitric oxide with aminoguanidine inhibits immunosuppression induced by an attenuated strain of *Salmonella typhimurium*, potentiates *Salmonella* infection, and inhibits macrophage and polymorphonuclear leukocyte influx into spleen, *Infect Immun* 67:891, 1999.

127. Mackenzie WR et al: A massive outbreak in Milwaukee *Cryptosporidium* infection transmitted through the public water supply, *N Engl J Med* 331:161, 1994.

128. Makinen M et al: Collagenous colitis and *Yersinia enterocolitica* infection, *Dig Dis Sci* 43:1341, 1998.

129. Mannheimer SB, Soave R: Protozoal infections in patients with AIDS: cryptosporidiosis, isosporiasis, cyclosporiasis and microsporidiosis, *Infect Dis Clin North Am* 8:483, 1994.

130. Marks MI et al: *Yersinia enterocolitica* gastroenteritis: a prospective study of clinical, bacteriologic and epidemiologic features, *Pediatrics* 96:26, 1980.

131. Marshall MM et al: Waterborne protozoal pathogens, *Clin Microbiol Rev* 10:67, 1997.

132. Mastroeni P et al: Interleukin 18 contributes to host resistance and gamma interferon production in mice infected with virulent *Salmonella typhimurium*, *Infect Immun* 67:478, 1999.

133. Mattila L et al: Seasonal variation in etiology of travelers' diarrhea, *J Infect Dis* 165:385, 1992.

134. McCarron B: A 3-year retrospective review of 132 patients with Salmonella enterocolitis admitted to a regional infectious diseases unit, *J Infect* 37:136, 1998.

135. Mead PS, Griffin PM: *Escherichia coli* O157:H7, *Lancet* 352:1207, 1998.

136. Mermin JH et al: Typhoid fever in the United States, 1985-1994: changing risks of international travel and increasing antimicrobial resistance, *Arch Intern Med* 158:633, 1998.

137. Michell AR: Oral rehydration for diarrhoea: symptomatic treatment or fundamental therapy, *J Comp Pathol* 118:175, 1998.

138. Moore AC et al: Surveillance for waterborne disease outbreaks—United States, 1991-1992, *MMWR* 42:1, 1993.

139. Nachamkin I, Allos BM, Ho T: *Campylobacter* species and Guillain-Barré syndrome, *Clin Microbiol Rev* 11:555, 1998.

140. Nakata S et al: Detection of human calicivirus antigen and antibody by enzyme-linked immunosorbent assays, *J Clin Microbiol* 26:2001, 1988.

141. Nataro JP, Kaper JB: Diarrheagenic *Escherichia coli*, *Clin Microbiol Rev* 11:401, 1998.

142. Nataro JP, Steiner T, Guerrant RL: Enteroaggregative *Escherichia coli*, *Emerg Infect Dis* 4:231, 1998.

143. Nelson JD, Haltalin KC: Accuracy of diagnosis of bacterial diarrheal disease by clinical features, *J Pediatr* 78:519, 1971.

144. Nhieu GT, Sansonetti PJ: Mechanism of *Shigella* entry into epithelial cells, *Curr Opin Microbiol* 2:51, 1999.

145. Noreiga FR et al: Strategy for cross-protection among *Shigella flexneri*, *Infect Immun* 67:782, 1999.

146. Offit PA: The rotavirus vaccine, *J Clin Virol* 11:155, 1998.

147. Okada SS et al: Antigenic characterization of small, round-structured viruses by immune electron microscopy, *J Clin Microbiol* 28:1244, 1990.

148. Ortega YR, Adam RD: *Giardia*: overview and update, *Clin Infect Dis* 25:545, 1997.

149. Ortega YR et al: A new coccidian parasite (Apicomplexa: Eimeridae) from humans, *J Parasitol* 80:625, 1994.

150. Osterholm MT et al: An outbreak of a newly recognized chronic diarrhea syndrome associated with raw milk consumption, *JAMA* 256:484, 1986.

151. Owen CE: Viral gastroenteritis: small round structured viruses, caliciviruses and astroviruses. Part I. The clinical and diagnostic perspective, *J Clin Pathol* 49:874, 1996.

152. Owen CE: Viral gastroenteritis: small round structured viruses, caliciviruses and astroviruses. Part II. The epidemiological perspective, *J Clin Pathol* 49:959, 1996.

153. Parashar UD et al: Rotavirus, *Emerg Infect Dis* 4:561, 1998.

154. Parry SM et al: Risk factors and prevention of sporadic infections with vero cytotoxin (shiga toxin) producing *Escherichia coli* O157, *Lancet* 351:1019, 1998.

155. Parsonnet J et al: Chronic diarrhea associated with drinking untreated water, *Ann Intern Med* 110:985, 1989.

156. Paton JC, Paton AW: Pathogenesis and diagnosis of shiga toxin–producing *Escherichia coli* infections, *Clin Microbiol Rev* 11:450, 1998.

157. Patterson M, Healy GR, Shabot JM: Serologic testing for amoebiasis, *Gastroenterology* 78:136, 1980.

158. Peltola H, Gorbach SL: Travelers' diarrhea: epidemiology and clinical aspects. In DuPont HL, Steffen R, editors: *Textbook of travel medicine and health,* Hamilton, Ontario, Canada, 1997, Decker.

159. Phillips RA: Water and electrolyte losses in cholera, *Fed Proc* 23:705, 1964.

160. Pier GB et al: *Salmonella typhi* uses CFTR to enter intestinal epithelial cells, *Nature* 393:79, 1998.

161. Potter ME et al: Unpasteurized milk: the hazards of a health fetish, *JAMA* 252:2050, 1984.

162. Pozsgay V et al: Protein conjugates of synthetic saccharides elicit higher levels of serum IgG lipopolysaccharide antibodies in mice than do those of the O-specific polysaccharide from *Shigella dysenteriae* type 1, *Proc Natl Acad Sci USA* 96:5194, 1999.

163. Reed SL: Amebiasis: an update, *Clin Infect Dis* 14:385, 1992.

164. Rees JH et al: *Campylobacter jejuni* infection and Guillain-Barré syndrome, *N Engl J Med* 333:1374, 1995.

165. Roels TH et al: Clinical features of infections due to *Escherichia coli* producing heat-stable toxin during an outbreak in Wisconsin: a rarely suspected cause of diarrhea in the United States, *Clin Infect Dis* 26:898, 1998.

166. Rolland K et al: *Shigella* and enteroinvasive *Escherichia coli* strains are derived from distinct ancestral strains of *E. coli, Microbiology* 144:2667, 1998.

167. Salaki JS, Shirey JL, Strickland GT: Successful treatment of symptomatic *Entamoeba polecki* infection, *Am J Trop Med Hyg* 28:190, 1979.

168. Salam MA et al: Randomized comparison of ciprofloxacin suspension and pivmecillinam for childhood shigellosis, *Lancet* 352:522, 1998.

169. Samuel BU, Barry M: The pregnant traveler, *Infect Dis Clin North Am* 12:325, 1998.

170. Santosham M et al: Oral rehydration therapy for diarrhea: an example of reverse transfer of technology, *Pediatrics* 100: E10, 1997.

171. Saphra I, Winter JW: Clinical manifestation of salmonellosis in man, *N Engl J Med* 256:1128, 1957.

172. Savarino SJ et al: Safety and immunogenicity of an oral, killed enterotoxigenic *Escherichia coli*–cholera toxin B subunit vaccine in Egyptian adults, *J Infect Dis* 177:796, 1998.

173. Savarino SJ et al: Oral, inactivated, whole cell enterotoxigenic Escherichia coli plus cholera toxin B subunit vaccine: results of the initial evaluation in children, *J Infect Dis* 179:107, 1999.

174. Schiavano GF et al: Virulence factors in *Aeromonas* spp. and their association with gastrointestinal disease, *New Microbiol* 21:23, 1998.

175. Schiller B et al: Methicillin-resistant staphylococcal enterocolitis, *Am J Med* 105:164, 1998.

176. Segreti J et al: High level quinolone resistance in clinical isolates of *Campylobacter jejuni, J Clin Infect Dis* 165:667, 1992.

177. Shannon K, French G: Multiple-antibiotic-resistant *Salmonella, Lancet* 352:490, 1998.

178. Shore EG et al: Enterotoxin-producing *Escherichia coli* and diarrheal disease in adult travelers: a prospective study, *J Infect Dis* 129:577, 1974.

179. Slutsler L et al: A nationwide case-control study of *Escherichia coli* O157:H7 infection in the United States, *J Infect Dis* 177:962, 1998.

180. Smith NH et al: Combination drug therapy for cryptosporidiosis in AIDS, *J Infect Dis* 178:900, 1998.

181. Snyder JD, Merson MH: The magnitude of the global problem of acute diarrhoeal disease: a review of active surveillance data, *Bull World Health Organ* 60:605, 1982.

182. Soave R: *Cyclospora:* an overview, *Clin Infect Dis* 13:429, 1997.

183. Sohail M, Sultana K: Antibiotic susceptibilities and plasmid profiles of *Shigella flexneri* isolates from children with diarrhoea in Islamabad, Pakistan, *Infect Immun* 66:838, 1998.

184. Stoll BJ et al: Value of stool examination in patients with diarrhea, *BMJ* 286:2037, 1983.

185. Sullivan PB: Nutritional management of acute diarrhea. *Nutrition* 14:758, 1998.

186. Swartzwelder JC: Balantidiasis, *Am J Dig Dis* 17:173, 1950.

187. Taylor DN et al: Treatment of travelers' diarrhea: ciprofloxacin plus loperamide compared with ciprofloxacin alone: a placebo-controlled, randomized trial, *Ann Intern Med* 114:731, 1991.

188. Taylor DN et al: Expanded safety and immunogenicity of a bivalent, oral, attenuated cholera vaccine, CVD 103-HgR plus CVD 111, in United States military personnel stationed in Panama, *Infect Immun* 67:2030, 1999.

189. Tsen HY, Jian LZ: Development and use of a multiplex PCR system for the rapid screening of heat-labile toxin I, heat-stable toxin II and shiga-like toxin I and II genes of *Escherichia coli* in water, *J Appl Microbiol* 84:585, 1998.

190. Valentine PJ et al: Identification of three highly attenuated *Salmonella typhimurium* mutants that are more immunogenic and protective in mice than a prototypical aroA mutant, *Infect Immun* 66:3378, 1998.

191. Van Beneden CA et al: Multinational outbreak of *Salmonella enterica* serotype Newport infections due to contaminated alfalfa sprouts, *JAMA* 281:158, 1999.

192. Verhaegen J et al: Surveillance of human *Yersinia enterocolitica* infections in Belgium: 1967-1996, *Clin Infect Dis* 27:59, 1998.

193. Vesikari T: Rotavirus vaccines against diarrhoeal disease, *Lancet* 350:1538, 1997.

194. Vial PA et al: Comparison of two assay methods for patterns of adherence to HEp-2 cells of *Escherichia coli* from patients with diarrhea, *J Clin Microbiol* 28:882, 1990.

195. Von Graevenitz A, Mensch AH: The genus *Aeromonas* in human bacteriology, *N Engl J Med* 278:245, 1968.

196. Wanger AR et al: Enteroinvasive *Escherichia coli* in travelers' diarrhea, *J Infect Dis* 158:640, 1988.

197. Wanke CA et al: Successful treatment of diarrheal disease associated with enteroaggregative *Escherichia coli* in adults infected with human immunodeficiency virus, *J Infect Dis* 178:1369, 1998.

198. Weber R et al: Human microsporidial infections, *Clin Microbiol Rev* 7:426, 1994.

199. Weiss JB: DNA probes and PCR for diagnosis of parasite infections, *Clin Microbiol Rev* 8:113, 1995.

200. Weiss LM, Keohane EM: The uncommon gastrointestinal protozoa: Microsporidia, *Blastocystis, Isospora, Diantamoeba* and *Balantidium, Curr Clin Top Infect Dis* 17: 147, 1997.

201. White AC et al: Paromomycin for cryptosporidiosis in AIDS: a prospective, double-blind trial, *J Infect Dis 170:419, 1994.*

202. Wurtz R: *Cyclospora:* a newly identified intestinal pathogen of humans, *Clin Infect Dis* 18:620, 1994.

203. Yavzori M et al: Detection of enterotoxigenic *Escherichia coli* in stool specimens by polymerase chain reaction, *Diagn Microbiol Infect Dis* 31:503, 1998.

53 Nutrition, Malnutrition, and Starvation

E. Wayne Askew

How does it feel to starve? A test subject in the Minnesota Starvation Study made the following observation after 24 weeks of semistarvation (1570 kcal/day, 24% weight loss)[35]:

I am hungry. I am always hungry . . . at times I can almost forget about it but there is nothing that can hold my interest for long . . . I am cold . . . my body flame is burning as low as possible to conserve precious fuel and still maintain my life processes . . . I am weak. I can walk miles at my own pace in order to satisfy laboratory requirements, but often I trip on cracks in the sidewalk. To open a heavy door it is necessary to brace myself and push or pull with all my might. I wouldn't think of throwing a baseball and I couldn't jump over a twelve inch railing if I tried. This lack of strength is a great frustration. It is often a greater frustration than the hunger . . . And now I have edema. When I wake up in the morning my face is puffy . . . Sometimes my ankles swell and my knees are puffy . . . Social graces, interests, spontaneous activity and responsibility take second place to concerns about food . . . I lick my plate unashamedly at each meal even when guests are present . . . I can talk intellectually, my mental ability has not decreased, but my will to use my ability has.

Nutrition is essential to proper human physiology and daily functioning but is often unappreciated in wilderness expedition planning. Many enthusiasts do not consider food as critical as gear and equipment, medical supplies, physical fitness, and other logistical considerations. In temperate environments, where food and water are plentiful and resupply is feasible, the importance of nutrition diminishes. When a stressful physical environment is superimposed on physically demanding wilderness tasks, however, the role of nutrition becomes crucial to maintain performance and prevent disease and injury, as evidenced from the description of Napoleon's disastrous 1812 winter retreat from Moscow by Baron D.J. Larrey[50]:

The ice and deep snow with which the plains of Russia were covered, impeded . . . calorification in the capillaries and pulmonary organs. The snow and cold water, which the soldiers swallowed for the purpose of allaying their hunger or satisfying their thirst . . . contributed greatly to the destruction of these individuals by absorbing the small portion of heat remaining in the viscera. The agents produced the death of those *particularly who had been deprived of nutriment.*

Although they usually have food, misfortune can strike the best-prepared adventurers. A wrong turn on the trail, injury, unanticipated terrain, an unexpected storm, or a downed airplane can isolate a victim from anticipated food sources. Food is often the most important item in a survival situation, particularly as the supply is exhausted. Although a concern, a shortage of food does not necessarily mean disaster. Humans are remarkably adaptable and can subsist on non-ideal dietary patterns for prolonged periods without disastrous effects on health and performance. A baseline level of energy intake ensures a minimal intake of vitamins and minerals, forestalling malnutrition and nutrient deficiency states. Hunger is uncomfortable and may hinder performance, but a food-deprived individual can still function for an extended time.

This chapter discusses three nutritional states or situations in terms of wilderness environments: (1) nutrition for optimal or effective functioning in environmental extremes; (2) malnutrition or suboptimal nutrition; and (3) starvation, or lack of nutrition. Preventive dietary planning for wilderness expeditions and emergency nutrition measures after rescue from starvation will be discussed.

ENVIRONMENTAL STRESS AND NUTRIENT REQUIREMENTS

The physical environment plays a significant role in determining survival time in the absence of food or water. The most important nutrient is water.[9] If an adequate supply of water is not available, death occurs from dehydration before depletion of energy stores. Humans can survive complete food deprivation for weeks or even months depending on body fat. A nonobese adult fasting in a clinical setting can live as long as 60 to 70 days, with loss of all their body fat and one-third their lean body mass.[32] One climber survived 43 days and was near death when rescued from a cave in the Himalayas with water but no food.[55] Time to death after complete water deprivation is 6 to 14 days, depending on the rate of water loss. Death from starvation in nonobese individuals is imminent if approximately 50% of body weight has been lost. This discussion on energy restriction assumes an adequate supply of water (see Chapters 10 and 11).

Modern camping foods and military field rations can support health and performance in a variety of temperate environments.[41] The situation may change rapidly, however, in wilderness environments characterized by more extreme temperatures and terrain.[40,42]

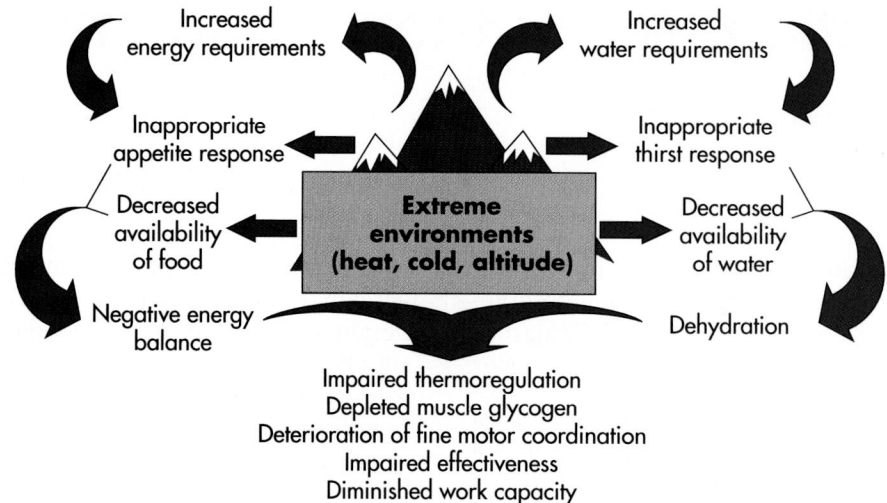

Increased energy requirements

Increased water requirements

Inappropriate appetite response

Inappropriate thirst response

Decreased availability of food

Extreme environments (heat, cold, altitude)

Decreased availability of water

Negative energy balance

Dehydration

Impaired thermoregulation
Depleted muscle glycogen
Deterioration of fine motor coordination
Impaired effectiveness
Diminished work capacity

Figure 53-1 Influence of extreme wilderness environments on food and fluid intake and physical and mental performance. (*From Askew EW: Nutrition and performance under adverse environmental conditions. In Hickson JF Jr, Wolinski I, editors: Nutrition in exercise and sport, Boca Raton, Fla, 1989, CRC Press.*)

Stress, whether heat, cold, altitude, level of exertion, or food restriction, influences nutrient requirements.[7,53] Superimposed stressors, such as extreme altitude or sleep deprivation, jeopardize both physical and mental performance[10,26,40,42,43] (Figure 53-1).

Energy and fluid deficits arising from the interaction of environment and nutrition can potentially negatively impact both physical[27] and mental[43] performance.

Energy Needs

Cold and altitude stress and its influence on macronutrient and vitamin requirements have been a major focus of military and civilian research.[8] Vitamin and mineral requirements are not significantly increased by cold exposure, although caloric requirements for thermogenesis may be elevated.[42] Work in cold environments can be adequately supported by combinations of fat, carbohydrate, and protein, although certain macronutrients may be more beneficial.[4] The macronutrient source is not as important as consuming enough total calories to support activity and thermogenesis. When wilderness activities shift from sea-level cold weather to moderate or high altitude, however, the importance of the macronutrient mixture should be reconsidered. Fat is an efficient energy source during cold weather activities at sea level but is not as well tolerated at altitude.[5]

The substitution of carbohydrate for fat and partly for protein can help an individual's oxygen economy while working at altitude.[3] Carbohydrate is more efficient fuel at altitude than fat because it is already partially oxidized and requires less oxygen to combust its carbon skeleton to CO_2. The metabolism of carbohydrate for energy requires approximately 8% to 10% less

inspired oxygen than that required to process a similar amount of calories from fat. A high-carbohydrate diet can reduce the symptoms of acute mountain sickness, enhance short-term high-intensity work as well as long-term submaximal efforts,[3,11,24] and "lower the effective elevation" as much as 300 to 600 m (about 1000 to 2000 feet) by requiring less oxygen for metabolism. Initial altitude exposure results in anorexia and subsequently reduces energy and carbohydrate intake.[20] Food intakes usually improve with time and acclimatization but, depending on the altitude, may never match those at sea level. Weight loss and performance decrements are common under these conditions.

Carbohydrate supplementation of the diet at elevations exceeding 2200 m (7218 feet) is usually an effective method to increase carbohydrate and total energy intakes.[3,20,25] Carbohydrate supplementation at altitude may reduce symptoms caused by acute altitude exposure,[24] but not all studies have demonstrated this benefit.[62] The most effective form of carbohydrate supplementation is usually liquid beverages; people will drink even when they are reluctant to eat.[20,25] Also, increasing fluid intake is beneficial at high altitudes, where increased fluid losses occur with diuresis and respiration in the dry atmosphere.[9]

Nutritional requirements for males in environmental extremes are well studied, but little research has been done on female requirements.[36] Studies in the late 1960s reported that female soldiers deployed to moderate to high altitude would require supplemental dietary iron for optimal support of the hematopoietic response to hypoxia.[30] Subsequent research on iron requirements and the thermogenic response to cold identified iron as a key micronutrient for females in a cold environment.[17,39] Females usually consume less total food calories than males because of their reduced body size and therefore are at increased risk for reduced vitamin and mineral intakes. Fortunately, the need for these vitamins and minerals (except iron) is related to lean body mass, and females usually have less lean body mass than males.

Performance across a broad spectrum of backcountry tasks is not always severely degraded by suboptimal energy and carbohydrate intakes. Soldiers can maintain relatively normal work capacities for short periods (less than 10 days) of food restriction.[26] The Minnesota starvation studies conducted during World War II demonstrated that energy deficits resulting in less than 10% body weight loss did not impair physical performance; however, underconsumption of calories for longer periods with continued body weight loss produced significant deficits in physical performance.[63]

Restricted energy and dietary carbohydrate content over 30 days supported light to moderate activity level without evidence of greatly impaired physical performance capabilities.[12] On the other hand, longer periods of caloric restriction (8 weeks) and higher levels of energy expenditure have been associated with significantly reduced physical performance capacity.[48]

It is difficult to derive a closely predictable relationship between energy deficit and performance. Some indicators of performance, such as grip strength, appear to be well preserved until nutritional status is severely compromised, whereas other measures, such as the maximal lift test, maximal jump height, isometric leg extension, and maximal oxygen uptake, appear to be more sensitive predictors of impaired performance.[34] Nonobese individuals seem to maintain strength with up to 5% body weight loss. Aerobic capacity and strength are reduced when body weight loss exceeds 10%. Friedl[26] concluded that changes in oxygen capacity in response to modest caloric restriction influence performance less than reductions in muscle strength in response to weight loss. The primary concern with weight loss from inadequate energy during extended wilderness activities may be loss of muscle strength, which is significant with 5% to 10% body weight loss. Significant declines in aerobic capacity can also occur after weight losses of this magnitude, but the decline in aerobic capacity appears to have relatively little effect on individual performance at moderate (less than 50% oxygen capacity) sustainable workload levels.[26] Thus a prior food restriction with significant loss of body weight may not preclude a gradual trek to the summit, but a short-term rigorous push for the summit to avoid impending bad weather might be compromised.

The effects of energy restriction on performance involve other factors besides strength and aerobic capacity. Weight losses up to 6% over 10 to 45 days generally do not significantly impair cognitive performance, but

habitual or forced consumption resulting in a 50% loss of energy requirements may degrade cognition.[43] Reduced food intake coupled with other stressors, such as high rates of energy expenditure and sleep deprivation, can also impair immune function.[37,45]

Carbohydrate

Both the time provided for dietary adaptation to carbohydrate restriction and the level of carbohydrate in the diet can influence the level of aerobic endurance.[2] Performance can be reduced by 40% after only 4 days on a calorie-adequate but low-carbohydrate (10% of kcal) diet.[29] Another calorie-adequate low-carbohydrate (5% of kcal) diet for 2 weeks also reduced performance, but only by 15%, presumably because of metabolic adaptations to the shift in energy sources.[52]

More than any macronutrient other than water, reduced carbohydrate intake can negatively influence muscle glycogen levels and endurance.[2] Certain types of performance, such as backpacking, cross-country skiing, and climbing, may be influenced by an acute shortage of carbohydrate in the diet, depending on the intensity of the workload. Inadequate carbohydrate and successive days of intense prolonged exercise may result in gradual reduction of glycogen stores, deterioration of performance, and perception of fatigue. Furthermore, perceived exertion for certain wilderness activities, such as load bearing, may be assumed to be a function of the dietary carbohydrate and its effect on muscle glycogen levels. Carbohydrates may extend or enhance performance when ingested before, during, and after moderate to intense aerobic exercise.[33] This requires daily consumption of approximately 500 to 550 g of carbohydrate. Typical dietary carbohydrate intakes of male soldiers fed a variety of rations during 18 field studies in temperate, hot, and cold environments ranged from 244 to 467 g/day.[15] It is also probable that daily carbohydrate intakes for wilderness activities would be less than the 500 to 550 g/day recommended for optimal physical performance, since total caloric intake during outdoor work is often less than that required to maintain energy balance.[41] Most people do not selectively consume low-carbohydrate diets during wilderness activities; however, total carbohydrate intake is often low because of its relationship to total energy intake and to limited food choices. In the short term, lack of energy (calories) is not as significant to performance as lack of carbohydrate.[26]

Definitive field studies demonstrating a positive effect of dietary carbohydrate supplements on performance are lacking.[6] When field conditions can be modeled under well-controlled laboratory settings, results suggest that carbohydrate supplementation benefits performance. One study tested the concept that soldiers would benefit from carbohydrate supplementation under conditions simulating field operations.[47]

Supplemental carbohydrate permitted a higher level of physical performance or aerobic power. Run times to exhaustion were increased approximately 6% with single carbohydrate feeding and 17% with divided doses. The ingestion pattern influenced performance, indicating that a supply of easily consumed carbohydrate supplement or food item ingested before, during, and after field activities is an effective method to sustain or boost physical performance.

Protein

Considerable discussion of the proper amount of protein to maintain muscle mass, prevent "wasting," and maintain performance under conditions of physical stress exists in the literature. However, despite all the controversies, recommendations concerning the amount of protein in the diet have changed little since World War I, as evidenced by reviewing a 1919 report by Murlin and Miller[46]: "The amount of protein . . . sufficient to repair all of the wastes of the body and to supply an adequate reserve is 13% of the total energy intake. It seems a matter of indifference to the muscles whether they receive their energy from carbohydrate or from fat . . . Hard muscular work, therefore can be done on a diet high in carbohydrate or upon a high fat diet. It is of general experience, however, that muscular work is done with less effort if there is a plentiful supply of carbohydrate."

"Thirteen percent" of the energy intake translates to an intake of 65 g of protein on an energy-restricted intake of 2000 kcal/day, or 130 g of protein for a 4000-kcal diet. This quantity of dietary protein is easy to obtain (e.g., one stick of beef jerky or one serving of peanut butter contains 6 to 8 g of protein). Although dietary protein is important, the quantity of carbohydrate in a food-restricted diet is more closely related to nitrogen balance or the preservation of lean body mass than to the absolute amount of protein. Carbohydrates apparently "spare" amino acids derived from dietary protein from subsequent deamination and oxidation for energy. Approximately 40 g of dietary protein seems to be a *minimum* daily amount required to prevent excessive nitrogen loss under food restriction.

Vitamins

Vitamins are coenzymes of important biochemical reactions in energy metabolism. Vitamins E and C and the precursor of vitamin A (β-carotene) also exert important protective actions as antioxidants. Oxidative stress may be significant during work in environmental extremes.[7]

Prevention of vitamin deficiencies is poorly understood in short-term and long-range nutrition planning. Body stores of some vitamins (primarily the water-soluble vitamins) are limited, and, vitamin deficiencies

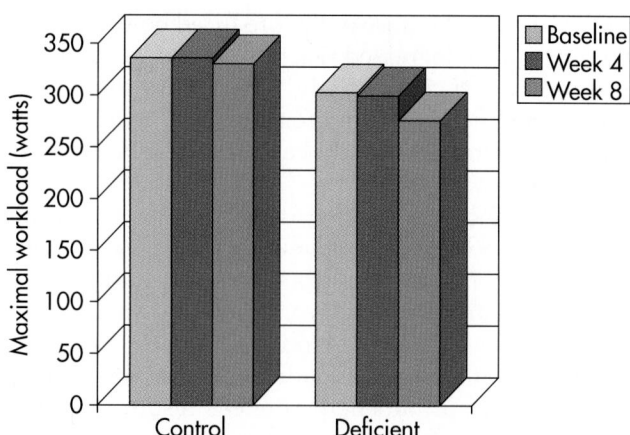

Figure 53-2 Impact of restricted vitamin intake on functional performance. Experimental conditions: diet, 3070 kcal; % U.S. RDA: thiamin 28%, riboflavin 31%, vitamin B₆ 16%, vitamin C 10%; performance test—incremental cycle ergometer. (*Data from van der Beek EJ:* Marginal deficiencies of thiamin, riboflavin, vitamin B₆, and vitamin C: prevalence and functional consequences in man, *Amsterdam, 1992, TNO.*)

can occur with prolonged periods of dietary restriction. Tissue depletion of thiamin, riboflavin, and pyridoxine can occur in 11 weeks with a calorie-adequate but vitamin deficient, experimental diet composed of common food products.[66] Van der Beek et al[65-67] studied the maintenance of human physical performance with varying degrees of vitamin restriction. With vitamin intakes significantly less than the recommended dietary allowances (RDAs), vitamin deficiencies manifested slowly in terms of physical performance impairments. Restricted intakes (percent U.S. RDA) of thiamin (28%), riboflavin (31%), pyridoxal phosphate (16%), and ascorbate (vitamin C, 10%) resulted in less than a 20% decrease in cycle ergometer performance (maximum workload) after 8 weeks at this level of restriction (Figure 53-2).

The effect of vitamin restriction on performance contrasts with the more immediate effects of acute or long-term dietary carbohydrate restriction. Physical performance impairment is much more sensitive to the amount of dietary carbohydrate in the short term (1 to 3 days) than to dietary vitamin, protein, or fat in the long term (6 to 8 weeks).[2]

A vitamin deficiency is a progressive process with four stages and a spectrum of physiologic manifestations (Box 53-1).

The possibility that certain nutrients might help people "adapt" or in some manner function more efficiently in stressful environments has intrigued explorers and scientists for years. Perhaps the most thorough exploration of this possibility was conducted in 1953 in the "Medical Nutrition Laboratory Army Winter Project: Vitamin Supplementation of Army Rations Under Stress Conditions in a Cold Environment—The Pole

---

Box 53-1   FOUR STAGES IN DEVELOPMENT OF A VITAMIN DEFICIENCY

1. PRELIMINARY STAGE

Inadequate amount from poor dietary patterns or altered availability in the diet

Often occurs after short-duration wilderness activities (<30 days) with poor nutritional planning

Consequence: none, except progressing to stage 2

2. BIOCHEMICAL DEFICIENCY

The body's pool of the vitamin is decreased

May occur after long-term wilderness activities (> 30 days) accompanied by suboptimal daily nutrient intakes

Consequence: rates of enzyme-catalyzed reactions may be slightly altered

3. PHYSIOLOGIC OR "SUBCLINICAL" DEFICIENCY

Can be detected by some functional tests

May occur after extended periods of consuming foods low in vitamins or periods of food restriction

Consequence: performance may be impaired slightly

4. CLINICAL DEFICIENCY

Specific symptoms manifested; detectable in a clinical setting

May occur after starvation or extended periods of food deprivation

Both health and performance may be impaired

Box 53-2   CONDITIONS THAT MAY REQUIRE VITAMIN SUPPLEMENTATION

Energy intake less than 1200 to 1600 kcal/day

Meals routinely missed

Poor or bizarre eating habits

Increased oxidative stressors (ultraviolet light exposure, high rates of energy expenditure, lack of fruits and vegetables)

Mountain Study." The objective of this study was to determine if supplementation with large quantities of ascorbic acid and B-complex vitamins would influence the physical performance of soldiers engaged in high levels of physical activity in a cold environment, both with and without caloric restriction.[8] The investigators concluded that supplementing the diet of men engaged in high levels of physical activity in the cold, with or without caloric restriction, did not result in significantly better physical performance.[8]

The vitamin concerns for wilderness exertions are not as critical as total energy and carbohydrate provision. Vitamin supplementation is recommended in certain situations under conditions of environmental extremes and food restriction (Box 53-2).

Certain vitamins, such as E and C, may have important functions beyond their conventional essential roles, such as preventing degradation of the immune response and maintaining red blood cell flexibility and oxygen delivery under conditions of increased oxidative stress. In light of uncertainties regarding the quantity and quality of food and oxidative stressors encountered during wilderness activities, it seems prudent to include a multivitamin supplement with the food supplies.

Minerals

The mineral content of the diet is usually of secondary concern, provided that a mixed diet is consumed daily in amounts close to energy requirements. Adequate dietary sodium is usually the mineral of primary concern because of its loss in sweat, especially in hot environments (see Chapters 10 and 11). Appropriate acclimatization to the heat and sodium conservation by the kidney reduce the amount of sodium required for work. Laboratory studies have shown that heat acclimatization can occur with as little as 4 to 8 g of sodium chloride (NaCl) ingested per day.[1] Whether this is adequate NaCl for safe work in the heat depends on degree of acclimatization and amount of sweating. Altered dietary patterns or excessive sweating can influence sodium balance. Starvation can lead to plasma volume depletion because of insufficient sodium in the circulation to enable osmotic forces to retain water.[32] Acute exposure of nonacclimatized humans to simultaneous food restriction and high sweat rates can result in excessive loss of sodium, leading to dizziness, syncope, and even collapse. These problems can be avoided by ensuring that extra salt is included in the food provisions and is used during and after high sweat losses.

Another form of sodium deficit is dilutional hyponatremia caused by overhydration and low sodium intake. Hyponatremia from overconsumption of fluids rarely occurs when regular meals are consumed. As a complication of overhydration when food is often neglected, hyponatremia has been described for hot and cold wilderness environments.[13,68] Calorie deprivation can alter sodium requirements. In addition to reduced intake of sodium in food, severe caloric restriction leads to marked natriuresis. The increased loss of sodium in turn leads to fluid volume depletion, impaired cardiovascular function, and reduced work capacity, separate from the effects of energy restriction. The accompanying increased aldosterone levels in response to reduced plasma volume can also lead to accelerated potassium wasting.[51]

MALNUTRITION AND STARVATION

There is little uniformity in the terminology used to describe the physiology of human starvation. Hoffer[32] has suggested the following definitions:

Fasting: total absence of food intake.

Starvation: physiologic condition that develops when macronutrient content is inadequate for a prolonged time.

Semistarvation or food restriction: more commonly encountered condition of insufficient energy and protein provision.

Malnutrition: general term for the condition resulting from longstanding inadequate consumption of nutrients, abnormal absorption of nutrients, or unusual demands on certain nutrients, usually accompanied by suboptimal food intake and/or consuming food of poor nutrient density, resulting in micronutrient and macronutrient deficiencies.

Protein-energy malnutrition (PEM): inadequate intake of energy, protein, or both for prolonged periods. Two specific types of interrelated PEM are *marasmus,* primarily an energy deficiency, and *kwashiorkor,* primarily a protein deficiency; they occur across a spectrum of conditions and share many of the same symptoms. PEM frequently results from starvation, but all starvation does not necessarily lead to PEM. The development of PEM depends on body energy reserves, length of the fast, age, and presence or absence of disease.

Cachexia: more specific term referring to the wasting that results from metabolic stress; sometimes called *cytokine-induced malnutrition* to distinguish from simple food deprivation in the absence of stress. The inanition of advanced-stage cancer patients is an example of cachexia.

Various metabolic and physiologic consequences of starvation or energy restriction might be encountered in wilderness settings. Unplanned emergencies may result in shortage of food, and wilderness rescue operations may involve victims of unintentional starvation. In these settings the duration of food restriction is usually shorter than that associated with famine, war, crop failures, and disease.

Solomons[59] has stated that malnutrition simply means "bad" nutrition and has listed six possible causes of nutrient deficiencies leading to malnutrition: (1) reduced intake, (2) decreased absorption, (3) decreased utilization, (4) increased destruction, (5) increased wastage, and (6) increased requirement. Primary malnutrition is caused by reduced intake of food, the most common cause of malnutrition in wilderness

settings. Reduced intake and increased requirement contribute to the development of nutrient deficiencies during expeditions in environmental extremes. Secondary causes of nutrient deficiencies can contribute significantly if disease or illness strikes the wilderness traveler. Impaired immune function, decreased resistance to infection, and prolonged recovery from injury are consequences of long-term food restriction.[22,27,37,57,58]

Starvation can be acute or chronic and total or partial. Different forms of starvation are similar but not identical. Two major sequences of metabolic adaptations occur in the progression of starvation: metabolic responses during acute energy restriction and metabolic changes in chronically undernourished individuals as a result of long-term low energy intakes.[56]

Acute Energy Restriction

A rapid progression of events occurs in response to acute energy inadequacy, such as a 50% shortfall of food during the second week of a 2-week backpacking trip. The body reacts quickly to an energy shortage by utilizing readily available muscle and liver glycogen stores. When the body's carbohydrate stores have been depleted, the glucagon level rises, the insulin level falls, and the process of gluconeogenesis accelerates, converting noncarbohydrate precursors such as lactate, glycerol and amino acids into glucose to maintain blood glucose and prevent hypoglycemia (Figure 53-3).

The reduction in carbohydrate intake during food restriction is compensated largely by accelerated gluconeogenesis. About 100 g of protein from endogenous tissue sources can provide approximately 55 g of carbohydrate. The glycerol from 100 g of mobilized fat can yield 10 to 15 g of carbohydrate through gluconeogenesis.[19] Simultaneous with glycogen depletion, cate-

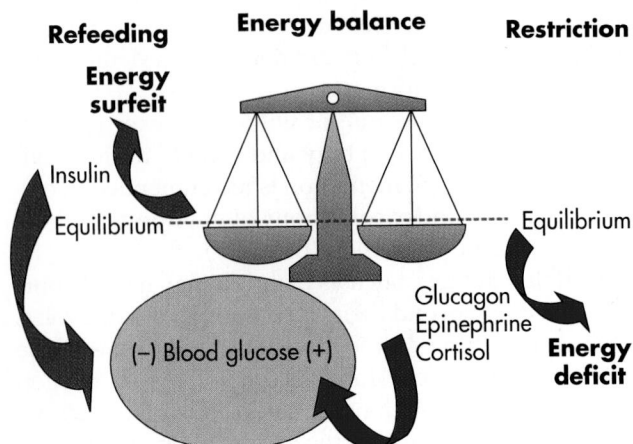

Figure 53-3 Influence of energy balance on hormonal control of blood glucose. When food is consumed, insulin is released, lowering blood glucose. When no food is consumed, gluconeogenic hormones are released, raising blood glucose.

cholamine production rises, facilitating fatty acid mobilization from adipose depots. Once mobilized, fatty acids are taken up by muscle in proportion to their concentration in the blood and are oxidized for energy. Figure 53-4 shows the metabolic events of a short-term fast.

Long-Term Energy Restriction

A fast longer than 2 to 3 days exhausts liver glycogen and uses up about half the muscle glycogen stores.[32] Thereafter, glucose utilized by the body (in the absence of food consumption) must be synthesized from endogenous precursors through gluconeogenesis.

Ketone bodies in the blood, breath, and urine result from the low insulin/glucagon ratio accompanying a prolonged fast. Ketone bodies are a metabolic consequence of vigorous fatty acid oxidation from adipose tissue engendered by starvation in the absence of significant carbohydrate intake. During fasting, production of acetoacetate and β-hydroxybutyrate increases greatly during the first 7 to 10 days and stabilizes after 2 to 3 weeks.[18] Ketone bodies can be increasingly used for energy by muscle and brain as energy restriction becomes prolonged. Even a short-term fast elicits a significant production of ketone bodies (see Figure 53-4). Ketone body production may stop, however, if 150 g of carbohydrate is ingested daily to supply the brain with glucose for energy.[19,32] Normally, in the fed state,

ketone body oxidation accounts for less than 3% of total energy requirement. Longer periods (7 to 10 days) of fasting are accompanied by greatly increased ketone bodies, which can provide as much as 40% of the total energy expenditure and greater than 50% of the brain's glucose requirement. The switch to using ketone bodies for energy by the brain is controlled by the concentration of ketone bodies in the blood rather than by a direct hormonal effect on the brain.[18] Figure 53-5 shows metabolic changes during a long-term fast (about 30 days).

With increasing duration of the fast and depletion of muscle and liver glycogen, ketones and glucose derived from gluconeogenesis of amino acids contribute to the energy requirements of the brain. As starvation is prolonged, less and less glucose is used, thereby reducing the amount of protein that must be catabolized to support gluconeogenesis. Blood levels of branched chain amino acids (leucine, isoleucine, valine) are preferred amino acid substrates for muscle energy metabolism and double by 3 to 5 days of fasting, but levels fall during prolonged fasting. These branched chain amino acids are believed to augment gluconeogenesis until fat metabolism has adapted to fasting.[18]

The amino acid glutamine has special importance during fasting as a precursor of glucose, an energy source, and a transporter of amino acid nitrogen in the

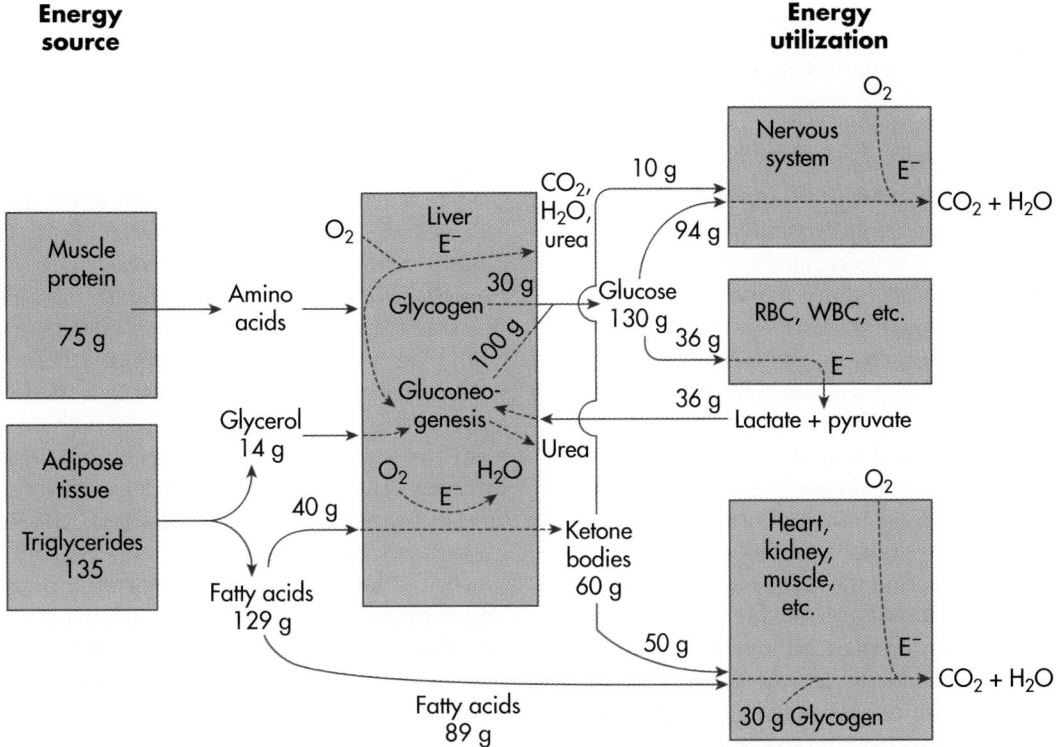

Figure 53-4   Fuel utilization in short-term starvation. Metabolic rates in grams per day after a 24-hour fast, with energy expenditure of 1800 kcal/day. *RBC, WBC,* red and white blood cells. (*Adapted from data published in Bursztein S et al:* Energy metabolism, indirect calorimetry, and nutrition, *Baltimore, 1989, Williams & Wilkins.*)

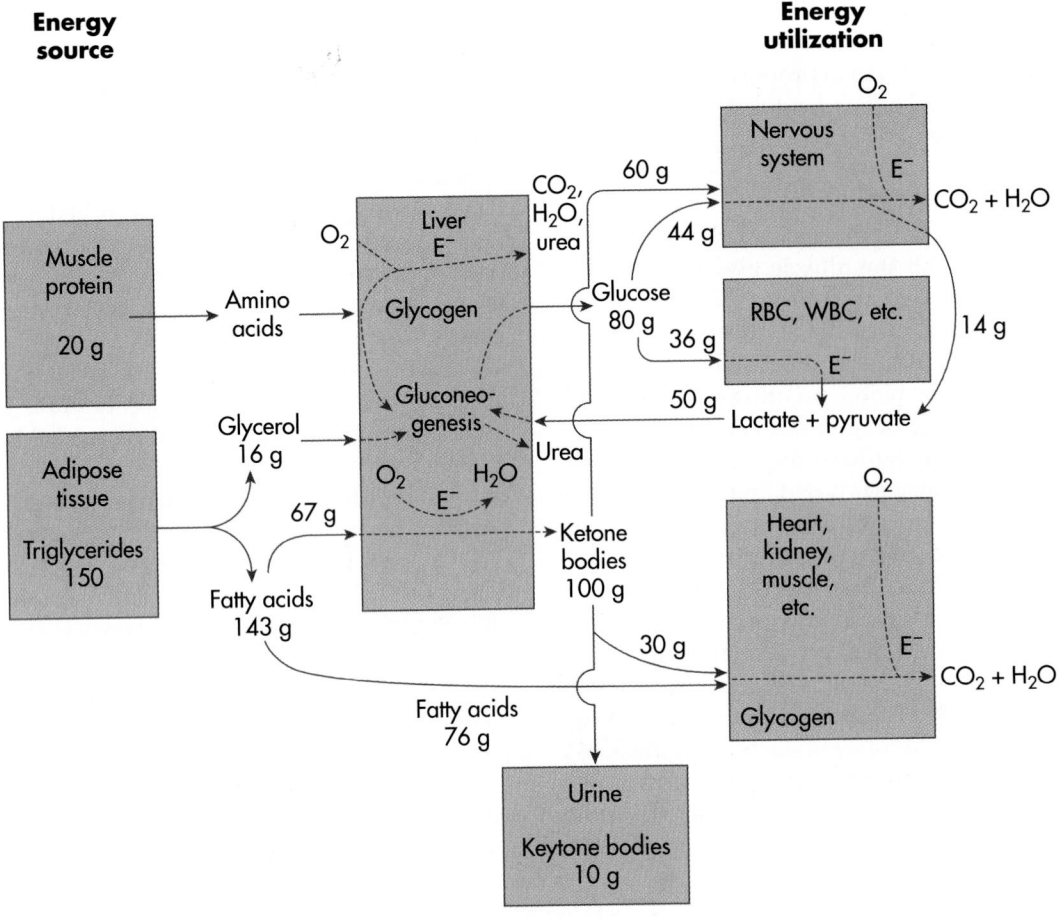

Figure 53-5 Fuel utilization in long-term starvation. Metabolic rates in grams per day after a prolonged fast of 5 to 6 weeks, with energy expenditure of 1450 kcal/day. (*Adapted from data published in Bursztein S et al: Energy metabolism, indirect calorimetry, and nutrition,* Baltimore, 1989, Williams & Wilkins.)

form of ammonia to the kidney for excretion. Urea is the major nitrogen excretory product in the urine during the fed state but is greatly reduced as the fast progresses. Ammonia nitrogen increases in the urine during a fast as urea nitrogen decreases. The increase in ammonia nitrogen is believed to buffer ketoacids during their excretion in the urine. Glutamine is released from muscle during fasting (NH_3 formed from amino acid deamination by muscle is transaminated to glutamate to form glutamine) and serves as a special energy source for the gut and as a gluconeogenic substrate for the kidney. With increasing ketone body production the liver reduces its rate of gluconeogenesis, and the kidney becomes the major organ of gluconeogenesis, producing more than half the body's glucose requirement. Glutamine is the predominant substrate for kidney gluconeogenesis and provides the ammonia required to buffer ketoacid excretion produced by ketogenesis from fat oxidation.[18]

Fortunately, muscle proteolysis does not continue at the high initial rate indicated by negative nitrogen balances of 10 to 12 g/day during the first 7 to 10 days of fasting. After this time, adaptation in the nitrogen economy of the body reduces nitrogen loss in the urine to less than half the initial rate.[32] The "signal" that causes muscle to reduce its catabolic rate is probably related to the shift to ketone body utilization by the brain and to the shift to fatty acid oxidation by muscle. When adaptation to food restriction is not successful or food restriction is too severe, nitrogen can be lost from both the central (visceral) and the peripheral (skeletal muscle) sites. Development of central protein deficiency can lead to anergy and hypoalbuminemia. Reduced plasma albumin lowers plasma oncotic pressure, which allows fluid to migrate out of the vasculature into the extracellular space, resulting in edema of the extremities. Edema is not present in all victims of starvation, but its presence indicates severe metabolic stress and central protein deficiency, and edema is a potentially dangerous condition.[32]

The net result of short-term and long-term metabolic adaptations in energy restriction is an increased efficiency of the body's metabolism. Over 14 days, during which body weight decreases 8% to 10%, the basal metabolic rate (BMR) can decrease about 21%. This short-term decrease in BMR is greater than would be predicted from the decrease in metabolically active lean tissue mass. Bines[18] suggests that the reduction in BMR during energy restriction occurs in two different phases. The initial decrease in BMR is not attributable to changes in body weight or body composition. Then, with continued energy restriction, BMR is further reduced by loss of metabolically active tissue. Several physiologic mechanisms operate to down-regulate metabolic activity in the active tissue mass and increase its metabolic efficiency. The decreased energy flux reduces activity of the sympathetic nervous system and lowers secretion and activity of three thermogenic hormones: catecholamines, triiodothyronine (T_3), and insulin. Other activities that require energy activities, such as the sodium-potassium pump and "futile" metabolic cycling (e.g., phosphorylating and dephosphorylating metabolic intermediates), may also be reduced during starvation.

Tissue Utilization during Starvation

A hierarchy of fuel sources is used during starvation. During extended fasting, muscle mass is more likely to be reduced than the viscera.[56] Important internal organs, such as the liver, show no evidence of dysfunction after 7 days of fasting,[54] whereas muscle cell mass decreases in a linear fashion with the severity and duration of a fast.[56] Adipose mass decreases along with muscle but not as rapidly, perhaps due to the energy density of the fat depot and the low amount of associated water. The body may "defend" a certain amount of body fat as essential for nerve sheath insulation, brain neurolipids, cell membrane integrity, and hormone synthesis. Figure 53-6 shows the general progression of energy source utilization.

The largest energy reserves are found in the largest organs of the body, specifically muscle (about 28 kg) and adipose tissue (15 kg) (Table 53-1). Critical internal organs, such as the liver, brain, heart, and kidneys, have a collective mass of less than 9 kg and are not good fuel source candidates, since they begin to lose function (decompensation) as they become energy sources during starvation. Sex hormone synthesis is depressed during extended periods of food restriction,[27,28] since reproduction is not a high priority during starvation. As the fast progresses, eventually visceral organs are utilized as the body decompensates, or "feeds on itself." Organ failure and death ultimately result unless nutritional intervention occurs before decompensation (internal organ catabolism, loss of integration of bodily systems, deterioration of homeostasis).

Limits of Human Starvation

The following are James Scott's observations near the end of a 43-day period of starvation while lost in the Himalayas[55]:

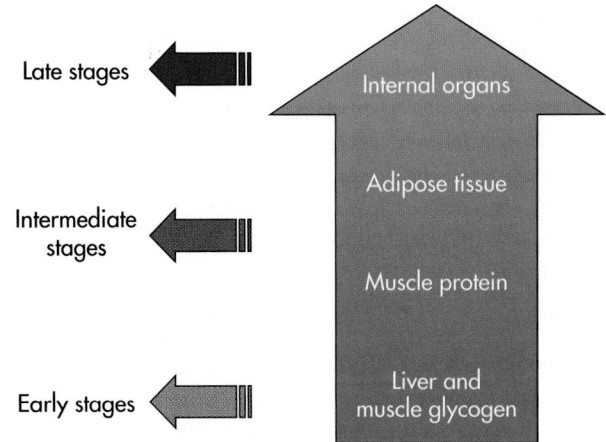

Figure 53-6 Hierarchy of energy sources utilized during progressive stages of starvation.

TABLE 53-1. Utilizable Energy Stores in Sedentary 70-Kg Man

ENERGY SOURCE	MASS (kg)	ENERGY (kj)
Fat (adipose tissue)	15	590
Protein (muscle)	6	100
Glycogen (muscle)	0.15	2.51
Glycogen (liver)	0.075	1.25
Plasma glucose	0.020	0.33
Plasma free fatty acids	0.0003	0.012
Plasma triglycerides	0.003	0.125

From Cahill GF: *N Engl J Med* 282:668, 1970.

There were horrific changes in my body. My buttocks were bones jutting against skin. I could no longer warm my hands by nestling them between my thighs. Now I could push a clenched fist between my legs without touching either thigh. I continually felt nauseated. The nausea became so severe I retched uncontrollably. This went on night after night. Death was closing in. My body was conceding defeat.

Body fat of nonobese humans can be considered "beneficial" fat when viewed in the context of surviving starvation.[49] Body fat level approaching 6% indicates impending lean body mass deterioration in the fasting individual.[28] Essential fat stores (fat in bone marrow, heart, lungs, liver, kidneys, intestine, muscle cell membranes, and the central nervous system) are necessary to maintain of life and prevent decompensation. Essential fat stores constitute 3% to 4 % of body weight. Total body fat depletion in previously nonobese individuals occurs at approximately 50% body weight loss. In fasting uncomplicated by disease the time until death is largely determined by the size of fat stores and the time to reach the 3% level of essential fat. Low fat stores are not the cause of death, but their diminution contributes to breakdown of homeostasis and impairment of physiologic function. Fat stores protect function. Typical fat stores in humans are 10 to 15 kg (including 2.1 kg of "essential" fat), or approximately 27% of body weight. A well-nourished adult has sufficient fat stores to sustain life for 60 to 70 days. Death has been reported sooner in voluntary hunger strikers and may be related to simultaneous fluid restriction and the lack of "will to live."

A loss of greater than 50% of the lean body mass is also predictive of death. Remaining body fat and protein reserves are difficult to measure accurately. The body mass index (BMI, weight in kg divided by height in m^2) is a convenient method to assess risk of mortality in severely starved individuals. Before the unfortunate war and famine in Somalia, the lowest BMI compatible with life was thought to be 13 in males and 11 in females.[31] Collins[23] found that a BMI of 10 could be compatible with life under conditions of specialized hospital care. A BMI of 10 may be compatible with life among certain somatotypes in a warm climate, but other races in colder climates may face death before reaching the low BMI level noted in Somalia.

Age and Gender Differences

Persons possessing the most limited amount of body reserves, such as the elderly and the very young, are at increased risk for early mortality during extended periods of starvation. Children have increased nutrient requirements for growth and develop deficiency symptoms rapidly when faced with severe food restriction.

Evidence of unintentional situational starvation in both men and women indicates that women may possess certain metabolic advantages over men that may lead to reduced mortality from severe starvation. Wartime and famine observations demonstrate the disproportionate survival of women over men.[26,49] Earlier observations of the survivors of the Mormon handcart trek[16] and the Donner party[60] support the conclusion that women are at lower risk for mortality under nutritionally stressful situations. McCurdy[44] examined the mortality pattern in the Donner party, who became trapped without adequate food supplies in the Sierra Nevada mountains during the winter of 1846-1847 (Table 53-2). Very young children and males were at the highest risk of mortality during starvation. Women generally have lower body mass and less lean body mass to maintain than do men, as well as more subcutaneous fat, which may have insulative value during cold exposure. Gender-related behavior, such as the performance of strenuous and high-risk tasks by men, may also explain the reduced mortality rate among women during prolonged starvation.

The "gender effect" during starvation may be caused by certain metabolic advantages, such as females' higher initial level of body fat and subsequent reduced loss of protein and lean body mass during fasting. Lowell and Goodman[38] proposed that protein

TABLE 53-2. Demographic Characteristics and Mortality Rate of the Donner Party, 1846-1847

CHARACTERISTIC	FREQUENCY (%)	MORTALITY RATE (%)
Total party	90 (100)	42/90 (47)
AGE (YEARS)		
Less than 5	19 (21)	11/19 (58)
6-14	21 (23)	2/21 (10)
5-34	24 (38)	16/34 (47)
Greater than 35	14 (16)	11/14 (79)
GENDER		
Male	55 (61)	32/55 (58)
Female	35 (39)	10/35 (29)

Data from McCurdy SA: *West J Med* 160:338, 1994.

sparing in skeletal muscle during prolonged starvation depends on the availability of lipid fuels, which may provide energy and attenuate the rise in catabolic hormones during starvation. Also, fatty acids may specifically modulate the breakdown of myofibrillar protein, independent of their oxidation as a fuel, thus causing direct muscle-sparing effect during prolonged starvation.

REALIMENTATION OF STARVATION VICTIMS

With sophisticated communication and highly trained search and rescue teams, a person lost or injured in a wilderness environment is usually rescued quickly.[61] One only has to compare the length of time involved in the rescue of the starving Donner party from the Sierra Mountains in 1847[44] (4 months) with the evacuation of nutritionally depleted Mike Stroud and Ranulph Fiennes[61] from Antarctica in 1993 (1 day). Although Stroud and Fiennes voluntarily prolonged their period of starvation before requesting evacuation, most individuals usually do not have to spend longer than a weekend or, at the most, a few days longer than anticipated in uncomfortable circumstances. It is likely that a certain amount of food will be available to the stranded person, since most people do not enter the wilderness totally unprepared. The individual may have consumed the initial food supply and then fasted for several days before rescue or, if disciplined, may have restricted or rationed food intake for a period of several days. Helicopter evacuation can place the rescued individual in a hospital setting within hours. The worst-case scenario would be the rescue of a severely injured or ill person who had not eaten for an extended period and could not be evacuated by helicopter. Refeeding victims of short-term starvation does not involve the complications of prolonged starvation.[55]

The specific physiologic and metabolic effects induced by refeeding depend on the individual's existing metabolic state and body composition, as well as the composition of the refeeding diet.[32] The rescuer can offer normal food to most victims of short-term starvation (3 to 5 days). The most common problem may be that the individual wants to eat too much too soon, which is usually self-correcting. The victim should first be reassured and then checked for injuries, illness, and dehydration. Juices, soups, instant oatmeal, granola bars, and small piece of jerky slowly chewed along with the fruit juice are all good choices to prime the digestive system for again processing food. Frequent small feedings are best. Sports drinks are often a good choice for simultaneous rehydration, providing carbohydrates for energy and electrolytes that may be needed for plasma volume expansion.

The priority for realimentation of individuals lost in the wilderness for an extended time is to correct fluid and electrolyte imbalance and halt ongoing protein catabolism. Oral rehydration solutions similar to those used to treat diarrheal disease can be used in wilderness rescue for extremely dehydrated individuals.[14] Intravenous saline and dextrose may be needed for individuals unable to eat because of shock, injury, or vomiting. Water-borne or food-borne illness may be encountered in backcountry scenarios. Rescued victims may have diarrheal disease as well as starvation. The World Health Organization (WHO) oral rehydration solution is composed of the following (g/L): glucose (20), NaCl (3.5), potassium chloride (1.5), and trisodium citrate (2.9) (osmolality, 310).* If trisodium citrate is not available, 2.5 g of common baking soda can be substituted.

Fluids should be continued until the victim is able to urinate every 2 to 3 hours. If the individual does not seem to be especially dehydrated, dilute fruit juices or sports drinks containing 5% to 10% carbohydrate and about 20 mEq (1.2 g) Na^+/L are reasonable rehydration fluids. Water is always appropriate, and additional sodium can be provided by liberally salting the solid food offered. A simple rehydration solution can be made by adding ½ tsp of table salt and 3 to 4 tsp of sugar to a quart or liter of water. Sports drinks usually contain 10 to 25 mEq of Na^+ and 2 to 5 mEq of K^+ per liter. Bouillon cubes are a good source of sodium and convenient. One bouillon cube contains about 1000 mg of Na^+ (44 mEq). Providing sodium to a moderately depleted individual is beneficial for restoring plasma volume but should be approached more cautiously in victims with severe malnutrition to avoid overly rapid expansion of plasma volume, which can lead to congestive heart failure.[32] Bananas are excellent sources of

K^+ (450 mg/banana) but are perishable and seldom available. Dried banana chips are a good alternative (152 mg K^+/ounce).

After correcting for hydration status and electrolyte balance, the victim should be placed on a high-protein, high-energy diet as soon as solid food is comfortably ingested. Some diets are more appropriate for realimenting starvation victims. For example, a diet high in sodium and carbohydrate fed to a severely malnourished individual may rapidly increase extracellular volume, resulting in peripheral edema and fluid accumulation in the heart and lungs. A low-protein, high-energy diet may be beneficial at first but, if continued, may increase fat mass without the desired increase in lean tissue mass. A high-protein diet may halt nitrogen loss but will not lead to simultaneous replenishment of fat stores. An easy-to-prepare high-protein, high-energy liquid food for initial refeeding of severely malnourished and starving individuals consists of powdered cow's milk (140 g), sucrose (100 g), oil (40 g), and water (900 ml), which provides 3 to 4 g protein/dl.[64]

Victims of prolonged starvation may have hyponatremia, hypocalcemia, hypomagnesemia coupled with severe anemia, and impaired membrane and cardiovascular function. These victims should be realimented cautiously to avoid sudden expansion of intravascular fluid volume. Cardiac failure may develop if high-protein/energy feedings are instituted too soon. Increased sodium and albumin levels from refeeding greatly expand the circulatory volume, leading to pulmonary edema, congestive heart failure, and possibly secondary pulmonary infection (Boxes 53-3 and 53-4).

NUTRITIONAL PLANNING

Nutritional planning for wilderness activities is often limited by space and weight constraints of gear. In general a daily food ration of 4000 kcal for men and 3500

> **Box 53-3 STEPS IN REFEEDING SEVERELY MALNOURISHED INDIVIDUALS**
>
> 1. Normalize and maintain fluid and electrolyte parameters.
> 2. Provide a mixed diet at the maintenance level to establish tolerance and avoid the refeeding syndrome.
> 3. Slowly increase energy intake to achieve positive energy balance and promote fat and protein gain.
> 4. Provide protein intakes of 1.5 to 2.0 g/kg to promote rapid repletion of body protein at any refeeding energy level.

Modified from Hoffer J: Metabolic consequences of starvation. In Shils ME et al, editors: *Modern nutrition in health and disease,* Baltimore, 1999, Williams & Wilkins.

---

*Preparation information available at www.rehydrate.org/html/ors.htm; commercially available from Jianas Bros Packaging Co, 2533 SW Blvd, Kansas City, MO 64108.

Box 53-4 HOMEOSTATIC RESTORATION OF NUTRITIONAL STATUS IN SEVERELY MALNOURISHED INDIVIDUALS

1. Resolve life-threatening conditions first.
2. Initiate restoration of nutrition as soon as possible.
3. Replace nutrient tissue deficits as rapidly and as safely as possible.
4. Begin slowly to avoid metabolic disruptions.
5. Schedule frequent feedings of small amounts every 4 hours.
6. Provide diets that derive 60% to 75% of their energy from fat, which are usually well tolerated.
7. Ensure that protein source is of high biologic value (milk, eggs, meat, fish, soy isolates).
8. Supplement diets to provide K^+, Mg^{++}, Zn^+, and Cu^{++}. Begin Fe^{++} supplementation 1 week after the start of diet therapy. Maintain sodium at low levels initially, until peripheral edema has disappeared.
9. Introduce normal foods gradually when edema has disappeared, skin lesions have improved, and appetite has been restored.

Modified from Torun B, Chew F: Protein-energy malnutrition. In Shils ME et al, editors: *Modern nutrition in health and disease*, Baltimore, 1999, Williams & Wilkins.

TABLE 53-3. Approximate Daily Calorie Guidelines*

| BODY WEIGHT (pounds) | LIGHT HIKING | BACKPACKING | |
		LIGHT	HEAVY
100-120	2000	2500	3500
130-150	2500	3000	4000
160-180	3000	3500	4500
180-200	3500	4000	5000

*Target calorie levels for food item selection; modify according to weight and work level and prior experience.

kcal for women adequately covers most situations (Table 53-3). If the task is hard physical work in the cold, 4000 to 6000 kcal/day may be needed. An allowance of 45 to 55 kcal/kg body weight/day generally covers energy needs for most moderate to moderately heavy levels of exertion (e.g., for a 70-kg individual anticipating moderate work levels: 50 kcal/kg/day × 70 kg body weight = 3500 kcal/day). These are only approximate guidelines because of differences in gender, body size, workload, and environment.

The actual macronutrient composition of the food is usually less important than the total energy content, except for efforts over short periods (2 to 3 days), when carbohydrate content may be the most important con-

sideration. If a high level of performance is anticipated (e.g., sustained or repeated high levels of power generation, working at greater than 60% oxygen capacity for prolonged periods), carbohydrate should be emphasized over fat. Approximately 50% to 60% of the daily calories should come from carbohydrate. If weight of the provisions is an overriding consideration, maximum caloric density may be important. Lower levels of power generation (e.g., working at a slow, steady, sustained rate less than 50% oxygen capacity) can usually be supported by higher levels of dietary fat (about 50% of daily calories). Individuals with diets containing greater than 50% of the energy from fat usually require about 2 weeks to adjust to the high level of dietary fat. Most trail rations (food for 1 day) consisting of typical macronutrient content (50% carbohydrate, 35% fat, 15% protein) weigh approximately 3 to 6 pounds, depending on the degree of dehydration. The protein content of the diet should be 12% to 15% of the calories, or about 60 to 100 g/day. Higher levels of protein are feasible, but may be an inefficient source of energy and may require more water if the amino acids of the protein are deaminated, the nitrogen is excreted as urea, and the carbon skeletons are used for energy.

Palatable and nutritious arrays of backpacking foods are available at most outdoor stores specializing in camping gear. A simpler approach is to purchase packaged military food such as the Meal, Ready-to-Eat (MRE). These packaged military meals contain a balanced macronutrient, vitamin, and mineral profile. A typical MRE contains 1275 kcal (12% protein, 36% fat, 52% carbohydrate) and weighs about 1.25 pounds.* For outdoor "minimalists," commercial food bars are much better than candy bars and other "junk food" items.

Food Bars

The modern equivalents of the early explorer's pemmican are food bars. Although food bars are not as energy dense as pemmican (dried meat pulverized with fat and sometimes berries), they are more palatable and nutritious. Most bars contain 200 to 300 kcal, with significant amounts of carbohydrate and protein (Table 53-4). Most are low in fat, since they are aimed at replenishing glucose and glycogen supplies during and after physical performance. Because the market is competitive, some manufacturers include "unique" nutrients or herbal compounds, the nutritional merit of which is often more fanciful than efficacious. These additions include vitamins and minerals, medium-chain triglycerides (alternate energy source), branched-chain amino acids (special fuel for muscle), soy protein (anti-

---

*Specific nutrient information about the MRE can be found at www.usariem.army.mil/mre/mre17.htm.

TABLE 53-4. Key Nutritional Components of Food Bars

COMPONENT	AMOUNT	FUNCTION
Carbohydrate	30 to 40 g/bar	Replenish glycogen stores.
Fiber	3 to 5 g/bar	Fiber-rich foods are scarce on the trail; prevents constipation.
Protein	5 to 10 g/bar	High-quality protein such as casein or soy may be useful in emergencies when other protein sources not available.
Fat	Variable	Usually not critical; bars with more fat are more calorie dense.
Vitamins	Greater than 30% RDA	Not normally needed but can provide "insurance"; antioxidant vitamins E and C are most important.
Minerals	Greater than 30% RDA	Ca^{++}, Mg^{++}, and Zn^{++} are most important; males may want to choose bars without Fe^{++} (possible promotion of oxidative stress), whereas females may benefit more from Fe^{++}, especially at altitude.
Temperature stability	Low melting point in heat, but chewable in cold	These factors must be determined by trial and error; frozen bars not easily consumed.
Palatability	Should "taste good"	Taste fatigue can set in rapidly with food bars; variety helps increase food intake.

RDA, Recommended dietary allowance.

cancer effect), ginseng (for "stress"), and gingko biloba and choline (to improve concentration).

Emergency Food Supplies

Emergency food supplies of 250 to 350 kcal/day should be included in addition to food for calculated caloric needs. These supplies should be packed separately in case the main food supply is lost or destroyed. Individually packaged food bars, jerky, dehydrated soup mixes, and hard candy should be included, as well as a bottle of multivitamins, extra salt packets, and water disinfection supplies. These small emergency food considerations may not seem important during preparation, but perceptions rapidly change during an emergency. Finally, the most carefully planned food supply is useless unless it is eaten; foods should be palatable and comforting to the traveler, and a hot meal prepared on the trail can boost morale.

REFERENCES

1. Armstrong LE et al: Responses of soldiers to 4-gram and 8-gram NaCl diets. In Marriott BM, editor: *Nutritional needs in hot environments*, Washington, DC, 1993, National Academy Press.
2. Askew EW: Effect of protein, fat, and carbohydrate deficiencies on performance. In *Predicting decrements in military performance due to inadequate nutrition*, Washington, DC, 1986, National Academy Press.
3. Askew EW: Nutrition and performance under adverse environmental conditions. In Hickson JF, Jr, Wolinski I, editors: *Nutrition in exercise and sport*, Boca Raton, Fla, 1989, CRC Press.
4. Askew EW: Nutrition for a cold environment, *Physician Sportsmed* 17:77, 1989.
5. Askew EW: Nutrition and performance at environmental extremes. In Wolinski I, Hickson JF Jr, editors: *Nutrition in exercise and sport*, Boca Raton, Fla, 1994, CRC Press.
6. Askew EW: Nutritional enhancement of soldier performance at the U.S. Army Research Institute of Environmental Medicine, 1985-1992. In Marriott BM, editor: *Food components to enhance performance*, Washington, DC, 1994, National Academy Press.
7. Askew EW: Environmental and physical stress and nutrient requirements, *Am J Clin Nutr* 61:631S, 1995.
8. Askew EW: Cold-weather and high-altitude nutrition: overview of the issues. In Marriott BM, Carlson SJ, editors: *Nutritional needs in cold and high-altitude environments*, Washington, DC, 1996, National Academy Press.
9. Askew EW: Water. In Ziegler EE, Filer LJ, Jr, editors: *Present knowledge in nutrition*, Washington, DC, 1996, ILSI Press.
10. Askew EW: Nutrition and performance in hot, cold, and high altitude environments. In Wolinski I, editor: *Nutrition in exercise and sport*, Boca Raton, Fla, 1997, CRC press.
11. Askew EW et al: Metabolic effects of dietary carbohydrate supplementation during exercise at 4100 m altitude, Technical Report No T12-87, Natick, Mass, 1987, US Army Research Institute of Environmental Medicine.
12. Askew EW et al: Nutritional status and physical and mental performance of Special Operation soldiers consuming the Ration, Lightweight or the Meal, Ready-to-Eat ration, Technical Report No T7-87, Natick, Mass, 1987, US Army Research Institute of Environmental Medicine.
13. Backer HD, Shopes E, Collins SL: Hyponatremia in recreational hikers in Grand Canyon National Park, *J Wilderness Med* 4:391, 1993.
14. Backer HD et al: *Wilderness first aid*, Sudbury, Mass, 1998, Jones & Bartlett.
15. Baker-Fulco CJ: Overview of dietary intakes during military exercises. In Marriott BM, editor: *Not eating enough*, Washington, DC, 1995, National Academy Press.
16. Bartholemew R, Arrington LJ: *Rescue of the 1856 Handcart Companies*, Salt Lake City, 1995, Charles Redd.
17. Beard JL, Borel MJ, Derr J: Impaired thermoregulation and thyroid function in iron deficiency anemia, *Am J Clin Nutr* 52:813, 1990.
18. Bines J: Starvation and fasting. In Sadler MJ, Caballero B, editors: *Encyclopedia of human nutrition*, New York, 1999, Academic Press.
19. Bursztein S, Elwyn DH, Askanazi J, Kinney JM: *Energy metabolism, indirect calorimetry, and nutrition*, Baltimore, 1989, Williams & Wilkins.
20. Butterfeld G: Maintenance of body weights at high altitudes: in search of 500 kcal/day. In Marriott BM, Carlson SJ, editors: *Nutritional needs in cold and high-altitude environments*, Washington DC, 1996, National Academy Press.
21. Cahill GF: Starvation in man, *N Engl J Med* 282:668, 1970.
22. Chandra RK: Nutrition and immune response: what do we know? In *Military strategies for sustainment of nutrition and immune function in the field*, Washington, DC, 1999, National Academy Press.
23. Collins S: The limit of human adaptation to starvation, *Nat Med* 1:810, 1995.
24. Consolazio CF et al: Effects of high carbohydrate diet on performance and symptomatology after rapid ascent to high altitude, *Fed Proc* 28:937, 1969.
25. Edwards JSA et al: Nutritional intake and carbohydrate supplementation at high altitude, *J Wilderness Med* 5:20, 1994.
26. Friedl KL: When does energy deficit affect soldier physical performance? In Marriott BM, editor: *Not eating enough*, Washington, DC, 1995, National Academy Press.

27. Friedl KL: Variability of fat and lean tissue loss during physical exertion with energy deficit. In Kinney JM, Tucker HN, editors: *Physiology, stress and malnutrition: functional correlates, nutritional intervention,* Philadelphia, 1997, Lippincott-Raven.

28. Friedl KL et al: Lower limits of body fat in healthy active men, *J Appl Physiol* 77:933, 1994.

29. Galbo H, Holst JJ, Christensen NT: The effect of different diets and insulin on hormonal response to prolonged exercise, *Acta Physiol Scand* 107:19, 1979.

30. Hannon JP, Shields JL, Harris CW: Effects of altitude acclimatization on blood composition of women, *J Appl Physiol* 26:540, 1969.

31. Henry CKJ: Body mass index and the limits of human starvation, *Eur J Clin Nutr* 44:329, 1990.

32. Hoffer J: Metabolic consequences of starvation. In Shils ME et al, editors: *Modern nutrition in health and disease,* Baltimore, 1999, Williams & Wilkins.

33. Ivy JL: Food components that may optimize physical performance: an overview. In Marriott BM, editor: *Food components to enhance performance,* Washington, DC, 1994, National Academy Press.

34. Johnson MJ et al: Loss of muscle mass is poorly reflected in grip strength performance in healthy young men, *Med Science Sports Exerc* 26:235, 1999.

35. Keys A et al: *The biology of human starvation,* vol 2, Minneapolis, 1950, University of Minnesota Press.

36. King N, Askew EW: Nutrition issues of women in the U.S. Army. In Wolinski I, Klimis-Tarvantzis DJ, editors: *Nutritional concerns of women,* Boca Raton, Fla, 1996, CRC Press.

37. Kramer TR et al: Effects of food restriction in military training on T-lymphocyte responses, *Int J Sports Nutr* 18:S84, 1997.

38. Lowell BB, Goodman MN: Protein sparing in skeletal muscle during prolonged starvation, *Diabetes* 36:14, 1987.

39. Lukaski HC, Hall CB, Nielsen FH: Thermogenesis and thermoregulatory function of iron-deficient women without anemia, *Aviat Space Environ Med* 61:913, 1998.

40. Marriott BM, editor: *Nutritional needs in hot environments,* Washington, DC, 1993, National Academy Press.

41. Marriott B, editor: *Not eating enough,* Washington, DC, 1995, National Academy Press.

42. Marriott BM, Carlson SJ, editors: *Nutritional needs in cold and high-altitude environments,* Washington, DC, 1993, National Academy Press.

43. Mays M: Impact of underconsumption on cognitive performance. In Marriott BM, editor: *Not eating enough,* Washington, DC, 1995, National Academy Press.

44. McCurdy SA: Epidemiology of disaster—the Donner party, *West J Med* 160:338, 1994.

45. *Military strategies for sustainment of nutrition and immune function in the field,* Washington, DC, 1999, National Academy Press.

46. Murlin JR, Miller CW: Preliminary results of nutritional surveys of United States Army camps, *Am J Public Health* 9:401, 1919.

47. Murphy TC et al: Performance enhancing ration components program: Supplemental carbohydrate test, Technical Report No T95-2, Natick, Mass, 1994, US Army Research Institute of Environmental Medicine.

48. Nindl B et al: Physical performance and metabolic recovery among lean, healthy men following a prolonged energy deficit, *Int J Sports Med* 18:1, 1997.

49. Norgan NG: The beneficial effects of body fat and adipose tissue in humans, *Int J Obesity* 21:738, 1997.

50. Paton B: Hypothermia and warfare, Napoleon's retreat from Moscow, 1812, *Newslett Wilderness Medical Society* 12, 1995.

51. Phinney S: The functional effects of carbohydrate and energy underconsumption. In Marriott BM, editor: *Not eating enough,* Washington, DC, 1995, National Academy Press.

52. Pruett EDR: Glucose and insulin during prolonged work stress in men living on different diets, *J Appl Physiol* 28:199, 1970.

53. Rodahl K, Issekutz B Jr: Nutritional effects on human performance in the cold. In Vaughn L, editor: *Nutritional requirements for survival in the cold and at altitude,* Ft Wainwright, Ark, 1965, Arctic Aeromedical Laboratory.

54. Savendahl L et al: Prolonged fasting in humans results in diminished plasma choline concentrations but does not cause liver dysfunction, *Am J Clin Nutr* 66:622, 1997.

55. Scott J, Robertson J: *Lost in the Himalayas,* Port Melbourne, 1993, Lothian.

56. Shetty PS: Overview of adaptive responses to malnutrition. In Sadler MJ, Cabellero B, editors: *Encyclopedia of human nutrition,* New York, 1999, Academic Press.

57. Shippee RL: Physiological and immunological impact of U.S. Army special operations training. In *Military strategies for sustainment of nutrition and immune function in the field,* Washington, DC, 1999, National Academy Press.

58. Shippee R et al: Nutritional and immunological assessment of ranger students with increased caloric intake, Technical Report No T95-5, Natick, Mass, 1994, US Army Research Institute of Environmental Medicine.

59. Solomons NW: Secondary malnutrition. In Sadler MJ, Caballero B, editors: *Encyclopedia of human nutrition,* New York, 1999, Academic Press.

60. Stewart GR: *Ordeal by hunger—the story of the Donner party,* Boston, 1988, Houghton-Mifflin.

61. Stroud M: *Shadows on the wasteland,* Woodstock, NY, 1993, Overlook Press.

62. Swenson ER et al: Acute mountain sickness is not altered by a high carbohydrate diet nor associated with elevated circulating cytokines, *Aviat Space Environ Med* 68:503, 1997.

63. Taylor HL et al: Performance capacity and effects of caloric restriction with hard physical work on young men, *J Appl Physiol* 10:421, 1957.

64. Torun B, Chew F: Protein-energy malnutrition. In Shils ME et al, editors: *Modern nutrition in health and disease,* Baltimore, 1999, Williams & Wilkins.

65. Van der Beek EJ: *Marginal deficiencies of thiamin, riboflavin, vitamin B-6, and vitamin C: prevalence and functional consequences in man,* Amsterdam, 1992, TNO.

66. Van der Beek EJ et al: Thiamin, riboflavin, and vitamins B-6 and C: impact of combined restricted intake on functional performance in man, *Am J Clin Nutr* 48:1451, 1988.

67. Van der Beek EJ et al: Thiamin, riboflavin and vitamin B-6: impact of restricted intake on physical performance in man, *J Am Coll Nutr* 13:629, 1994.

68. Zafren K: Hyponatremia in a cold environment, *Wilderness Environ Med* 9:54, 1998.

54 Seafood Toxidromes

Karen B. Van Hoesen and Richard F. Clark

At least three quarters of the world's population lives within 10 miles of the coast. One of the many reasons why populations congregate near the sea is the abundance of food beneath the ocean's waters. Seafood provides a significant percentage of the protein in diets of many cultures; at present, 200 to 240 million tons of fish are harvested each year, with 50% of the total coming from coastal regions. Only the depth at which we can harvest seafood restricts the variety of organisms that are edible. Americans consume 15 pounds of fish per person per year. It is becoming increasingly clear that the ocean is one of our last great food resources.

Toxic seafood was described in the Bible. Humans have recognized that toxic seafood has been associated throughout time with seasons of the year, phases of the moon, water temperature, weather conditions, waterfowl mortality, and the color of the waves that wash into shore, along with many other things. Unfortunately, none of these methods has proven entirely successful at predicting when seafood poisoning will occur.

Marine creatures that are poisonous to eat include dinoflagellates, coelenterates, mollusks, echinoderms, crustaceans, fishes, turtles, and mammals. Most marine biotoxins are naturally occurring poisons derived directly from marine organisms, including phytotoxins (plant poisons) or zootoxins (animal poisons). Ingestible toxins may be classified by specific toxin or by the donor organ of origin ingested by the victim. *Ichthyosarcotoxin* is a general term for poison derived from the fresh flesh (muscle, viscera, skin, or slime) of any fish. This is further defined by specific organ system. Geographic location, dietary and clinical histories, and appropriate index of suspicion figure prominently in the diagnosis and treatment.

Data on food-borne disease outbreaks in the United States demonstrate that seafood is the third most reported category according to vehicle of transmission (unknown vehicles ranked first and multiple vehicles ranked second).[71] Some 90% of the outbreaks of seafood-related illnesses and 75% of individual cases come from contaminated raw molluscan seafood (e.g., oysters and clams), histamine poisoning (scombroid) and ciguatoxin found in reef fish species.[299]

MONITORING PROGRAMS FOR PHYCOTOXIN-PRODUCING MARINE ALGAE AND SEAFOOD POISONINGS

Despite the increasing risk of human intoxication from contaminated seafood, standards and methods of screening and law enforcement vary throughout the world.[430] According to the U.S. Department of Agriculture, imports account for more than 55% of total U.S. seafood consumption. The largest source of seafood imports comes from Canada, Asia, and Latin America. The U.S. Food and Drug Administration (FDA) has been criticized for inadequate inspection of all food imports.[299] In 1995 the FDA switched to a new program for seafood safety known as the Hazard Analysis and Critical Control Point (HACCP) system. This program became mandatory for the seafood industry on December 18, 1997.[137] HACCP focuses on the identification of sources and points of contamination, levels, transmission, rate and transport of microorganisms, and the possibility of exposure of the consumer to the contaminant. HACCP focuses on preventing hazards rather than relying on spot-checks and random sampling of products. The most effective control strategies can then be implemented. For shellfish- and viral-associated diseases, the data suggest that harvesting from unapproved sources is associated with more than 30% of the outbreaks.[256] For imports the biggest risks relate to histamines and scombroid poisoning, mainly from tuna and mahimahi that is imported from Argentina, Taiwan, and Ecuador. For these foods traveling great distances, refrigeration is the most critical control point.

The United States is the second largest importer of shrimp in the world. Shrimp aquaculture currently accounts for approximately 30% of the world's supply. Antibacterials are routinely used outside the United States for shrimp aquaculture.[311] Irradiation of seafood products is still being considered for approval by the FDA, although it is currently used in Asian and European markets, especially for shrimp.[10]

Molluscan poisoning is mainly a problem with domestic seafood. In 1991, California was the first state to require restaurants that serve or sell Gulf Coast oysters to warn prospective customers about possible deleterious effects from *Vibrio* contamination, particularly *Vibrio vulnificus*.[329] Florida and Louisiana have adopted these warning regulations. Additionally, fishermen are now required to refrigerate oysters within 6 hours after harvesting from the Gulf of Mexico. Regulations require oyster lot tagging, labeling, and record retention to facilitate trace back investigations of outbreaks. The United States and Canada allow the sale of oysters if there are less than 10,000 colony-forming units (CFU) per gram of *Vibrio parahaemolyticus*. However, in recent outbreaks in the Pacific Northwest in 1997 and New York in 1998, oysters had less than 200 *V. parahaemolyticus* CFU/g of oyster meat, suggesting that human illness can occur at lower levels.[73,75]

Approximately a third of U.S. shellfish beds carry bans or limitations on harvesting because of high levels of fecal coliform bacteria. The fecal indicator system for shellfish-harvesting waters has been effective in protecting consumers against general types of bacteria fecal contamination. However, several pathogenic bacteria are not predicted by the system. The efficacy of methods for virus recovery may range from 2% to 47%.[447] The most promising of the new detection methods are based on molecular techniques. Deoxyribonucleic acid (DNA) hybridization and the polymerase chain reaction (PCR) have an advantage of specificity for particular pathogens, sensitivity, and speed (most assays are completed within a few hours). PCR has been used in shellfish to detect *Salmonella*, *Vibrio* species, and viruses, including hepatitis A virus and Norwalk virus.* Phycotoxin-producing marine algae are responsible for the syndromes of paralytic, neurotoxic, and diarrhetic shellfish poisoning. The closure of fisheries (product harvest areas) depends on the density of algae. In some cases the decision to close a fishery is based on the toxicity level in shellfish; in others, algae in the water and toxin in shellfish must both be found. In Florida, more than 5000 cells per liter of *Ptychodiscus breve* must be detected before fisheries are closed. The quarantine level of saxitoxin ranges across countries from 40 to 80 mg of toxin per 100 g of seafood.[21] The upper number, as determined by mouse bioassay, is used in the United States, as monitored by the Interstate Shellfish Sanitation Conference and the FDA.

The maximum acceptable concentration of diarrhetic shellfish toxin, okadaic acid, also varies between countries because of the lack of precise analytic methods for quantification. Countries with established regulations apply 4 to 5 mouse units or 20 to 25 microgram equivalents of okadaic acid as an acceptance limit. In the United Kingdom the Ministry of Agriculture, Fisheries and Food (MAFF) shellfish surveillance program tests shellfish harvested weekly from April to October and sporadically during the winter for the presence of toxins.[357] The United States, Canada, and Portugal monitor for domoic acid (cause of amnesic shellfish poisoning)

and use 2 mg/100 g of seafood as the threshold. Ciguatoxins are monitored infrequently because of difficulties associated with the assay. In French Polynesia, 0.06 ng/g of seafood of ciguatoxin as determined by mosquito bioassay is considered toxic; in the United States, detection of the toxin at any level by immunoassay (Florida, Hawaii) renders the fish unsaleable.

Two features render toxin surveillance difficult: the performance problems of the assays and the impracticality of surveying every fish. As mentioned above, PCR holds the most promise for rapid, specific, and sensitive detection of pathogens.

ICHTHYOSARCOTOXISM

The term *ichthyosarcotoxism* describes a variety of conditions arising as the result of poisoning by fish flesh. The toxins are generally not destroyed by heat or gastric acid. Various toxins may be contained in the musculature, viscera, blood, skin, and mucus secretions. Further classification can be divided into poisoning based on the specific organ system and includes ichthyocrinotoxins (glandular secretions), ichthyohemotoxins (blood poisoning), ichthyohepatotoxins (liver), ichthyootoxins (toxic gonads), ichthyoallyeinotoxins (hallucinatory fish poisoning), and gempylotoxins.

Ichthyocrinotoxication

Ichthyocrinotoxic fish poisoning is induced by the ingestion of glandular secretions not associated with a specific venom apparatus; this usually involves skin secretions, poisonous foams, or slimes. Examples of toxic fish are certain file fish, puffer fish, porcupine fish, trunk fish, box fish, cow fish, lampreys, moray eels, and toadfish (Box 54-1). Cyclostome poisoning results from ingestion of the slime and flesh of certain lampreys and hagfishes. Pahutoxin and homopahutoxin have been isolated from the secretion of the Japanese boxfish *Ostracion immaculatus*.[143]

Ichthyotoxic skin secretions may cause a bitter taste.[159] Ingestion of ichthyocrinotoxins causes gastrointestinal symptoms within a few hours of ingestion and is characterized by nausea, vomiting, dysenteric diarrhea, tenesmus, abdominal pain, and weakness. Most victims recover within 24 hours; however, some individuals may have symptoms for up to 3 days. Therapy is supportive and based on symptoms. Additionally, some slime, such as "grammistin" from the soap fish (*Rypticus saponaceous* of the family Grammistidae), can cause a contact irritant dermatitis.[184] The dermatitis is managed with cool compresses of aluminum sulfate and calcium acetate (Domeboro).

All suspect fish should be washed carefully with water or brine solution and skinned before eaten. Puffer skin is extremely toxic. Care must be taken to avoid toxin contact with the eyes.

---

*References 15, 16, 18, 23, 95, 243, 318, 353.

Box 54-1   REPRESENTATIVE ICHTHYOCRINOTOXIC FISH HAZARDOUS TO HUMANS

Phylum Chordata
  Class Agnatha
    Order Myxiniformes: hagfishes, lampreys
      Family Myxinidae
        Myxine glutinosa: Atlantic hagfish
        Petromyzon marinus: sea lamprey, large nine-eyes
  Class Osteichthyes
    Order Anguilliformes: eels
      Family Muraenidae
        Muraena helena: moray eel
    Order Perciformes: perchlike fishes
      Family Serranidae
        Grammistes sexlineatus: golden striped bass
        Rypticus saponaceus: soapfish
    Order Tetrodontiformes: triggerfishes, puffers, trunkfishes
      Family Canthigasteridae
        Canthigaster jactator: sharp-nosed puffer
      Family Diodontidae
        Diodon hystrix: porcupinefish
      Family Ostraciontidae
        Lactoria diaphana: trunkfish
        Lactoria fornasini: trunkfish, boxfish
      Family Tetraodontidae
        Arothron hispidus: puffer, toadfish, blowfish, rabbitfish
        Fugu xanthopterus: puffer
    Order Batrachoidiformes: toadfishes
      Family Batrachoididae
        Opsanus tau: oyster toadfish
        Thalassophryne maculosa: toadfish

Box 54-2   REPRESENTATIVE POISONOUS SHARKS (ELASMOBRANCHS) HAZARDOUS TO HUMANS

Phylum Chordata
  Class Chondrichthyes
    Order Squaliformes: sharks
      Family Carcharhinidae
        Carcharhinus melanopterus: blacktip reef shark
        Carcharhinus menisorrah: gray reef shark
        Galeocerdo cuvieri: tiger shark
        Prionace glauca: blue shark
      Family Dalatiidae
        Somniosus microcephalus: Greenland shark, sleeper shark, nurse shark
      Family Hexanchidae
        Hexanchus griseus: cow shark, gray shark, mud shark
      Family Isuridae
        Carcharodon carcharias: white shark
      Family Scyliorhinidae
        Scyliorhinus caniculus: dogfish, lesser-spotted cat shark
      Family Sphyrnidae
        Sphyrna diplana: hammerhead
      Family Squatinidae
        Squatina dumeril: monkfish, angel shark
      Family Triakidae
        Triaenodon obesus: white-tip houndshark

Ichthyohemotoxication

Ichthyohemotoxic fish are perfused with "poisonous blood," the toxicity of which is usually inactivated by heat and gastric juice. Examples are various eels, such as morays, anguilliformes, and congers. The syndrome is predominantly gastrointestinal and should be treated according to symptoms. Hematologic complications are rare. The risk of intoxication is increased by ingestion of raw or undercooked fish.

Ichthyohepatotoxication

Ichthyohepatotoxic fish carry the toxin predominantly in the liver. The remainder of the fish may be nontoxic. Fish that are always toxic fall into two basic groups: (1) Japanese perchlike fish (e.g., mackerel, sea bass, porgy, sandfish); and (2) tropical sharks (e.g., requiem fish, sleeperfish, cowfish, great white shark, catfish, hammerhead, angelfish, Greenland fish, dogfish).[315] In addition, some skates and rays, which share a similar phylogeny with sharks, harbor ichthyohepatotoxins.

Ingestion of the Japanese perchlike fish group causes onset of symptoms within the first hour, with maximum intensity over the ensuing 6 hours.[382] Symptoms include nausea, vomiting, headache, flushing, rash, fever, and tachycardia. No fatalities have been reported. Delayed (24 to 48 hours) necrodermolysis is rare.

Ingestion of tropical shark liver (and occasionally of the musculature), such as that of the Greenland shark *(Somniosus microcephalus),* results in "elasmobranch poisoning" (Box 53-2).[28] Symptoms are noted within 30 minutes of ingestion and include nausea, vomiting, diarrhea, abdominal pain, malaise, diaphoresis, headache, stomatitis, esophagitis, muscular cramps, arthralgias, paresthesias, hiccups, trismus, hyporeflexia, ataxia, incontinence, blurred vision, blepharospasm, delirium, respiratory distress, coma, and death. Recovery varies from several days to weeks. If only the flesh is eaten, the symptoms are mild and gastroenteric, with spontaneous resolution.

In 1993, 200 people in Madagascar were poisoned after ingesting a single shark identified as *Carcharhinus leucas.* The attack rate was 100% with a case fatality ratio of 30%. Two liposoluble toxins were isolated from the shark liver and named carchatoxin-A and -B.[46] Trimethylamine oxide, which is found in shark liver and flesh, has also been implicated in shark poisoning.[13] A similar syndrome occurs in sled dogs that ingest large quantities of shark flesh.

Therapy is supportive and based on symptoms. If the victim is treated within 60 minutes of ingestion of shark liver or other viscera, gastric emptying or lavage followed by administration of activated charcoal (50 to 100 g) may be of value. Fish liver should not be eaten; indeed, neither should any shark viscera. Drying the flesh properly may minimize the toxicity.

Ichthyootoxication

Ichthyootoxic fish possess toxic gonads, which may vary in toxicity with the reproductive cycle. The musculature is generally nontoxic. Examples are the sturgeon, alligator gar, salmon, pike, minnow, carp, catfish, killifish, perch, and sculpin. Sea urchins may be toxic during the reproductive period.[28] This toxicity is exemplified by *Paracentrotus lividus* (Europe), *Tripneustes ventricosus* (West Africa), and *Diadema antillarum* (West Indies).

Symptoms begin within an hour of ingestion and include nausea, vomiting, diarrhea, headache, dizziness, fever, thirst, xerostomia, bitter taste, tachycardia, seizures, migraine, paralysis, hypotension, and death. Treatment is supportive and based on symptoms. The roe of any fish should not be eaten during the reproductive season. Heat will not inactivate the toxin.

Ichthyoallyeinotoxication

Ichthyoallyeinotoxic fish induce hallucinatory fish poisoning. These fish are predominantly reef fish of the tropical Pacific and Indian reefs, which carry the heat-stable toxins mainly in the head parts, brain, and spinal cord, and in lesser amounts in the musculature. Typical species include surgeonfish, chub, mullet, unicornfish, goatfish, sergeant major, grouper, rabbitfish, rock cod, drumfish, rudderfish, and damselfish. Hallucinatory mullet poisoning has been described as a seasonal condition that occurs only during the summer months in restricted areas on the Hawaiian islands of Kauai and Molokai.[186] Dangerous species include the mullet, surmullet or goatfish, rudderfish, and surgeonfish.

Symptoms can develop within 5 to 90 minutes of ingestion and include dizziness, circumoral paresthesias, diaphoresis, weakness, incoordination, auditory and visual hallucinations, nightmares, depression, dyspnea, bronchospasm, brief paralysis, and pharyngitis.[28]

No fatalities have been reported. Various toxins including indoles akin to lysergic acid diethylamide (LSD) have been implicated with sources in algae and plankton eaten by the fish.[374]

Therapy is supportive and based on symptoms. Haloperidol may be used as an antipsychotic agent if the victim is psychotic and violent. Mild agitation may be eased with small graded doses of diazepam, particularly if the victim also suffers anticholinergic symptoms. The victim should be observed until a normal mental status is regained. The head, brain, or spinal cord of any tropical fish should not be eaten. Heat does not inactivate the toxin.

Gempylotoxication

Gempylotoxic fishes are the pelagic mackerels, which produce an oil with a pronounced purgative effect. The "toxin" is contained in both musculature and bones. No particular characteristic distinguishes a gempylotoxic fish from a nontoxic fish of the same species. The castor oil fish (*Ruvettus pretiosus*) is named for its purgative properties.

The victim suffers from abdominal cramping, bloating, mild nausea, and diarrhea, usually within 30 to 60 minutes of ingestion. The disorder is self-limited and resolves over 12 to 18 hours. The diarrhea often occurs without concomitant systemic effects. Fever, bloody or foul-smelling stools, or protracted vomiting suggest infectious gastroenteritis. No specific antidote is recommended. If the victim cannot tolerate oral fluids because of nausea or severe abdominal cramping, intravenous fluid supplementation may be initiated. Antimotility agents, such as diphenoxylate with atropine, are not recommended unless the diarrhea is debilitating because inhibition of peristalsis prolongs the transit time of the toxin through the gut and may increase the duration of the disorder.

SPECIFIC FISH-RELATED TOXIC SYNDROMES

Two specific toxic syndromes related to fish consumption are scombroid poisoning and tetrodotoxin (pufferfish poisoning) (Table 54-1). Carp gallbladder poisoning is also discussed below.

Scombroid Poisoning

Scombroid fish poisoning, the most commonly reported seafood poisoning in the United States, occurs when certain species of fish are improperly handled and stored after catch. These most often consist of fish from the family Scombridae that includes albacore, bluefin and yellowfin tuna, mackerel, saury, needlefish, wahoo, skipjack, and bonito (Figure 54-1). Nonscombroid fish that produce scombroid poisoning include mahimahi (dolphin), kahawai, sardine, black marlin, pilchard, anchovy, herring, amberjack (yellowtail or kahala), and the Australian ocean salmon *Arripis truttaceus*.[273,364,379,407] In Hawaii the most commonly implicated fish is the dolphin *Coryphaena hippurus*. In the northeastern United States, bluefish (*Pomatomus saltratix*) has recently been linked to scombrotoxism.[321] Scombroid poisoning accounts for 5% of food-related outbreaks reported to the Centers for Disease Control and Prevention (CDC) in Atlanta.[409] Because greater numbers of nonscombroid fish are now recognized as "scombrotoxic," Prescott[321] has suggested that the syndrome be more appropriately called *pseudoallergic fish poisoning*.

Pathophysiology. During conditions of inadequate preservation or refrigeration (optimal temperatures for bacterial growth of 37° to 43° C [98.6° to 109.4° F]), the musculature of dark-fleshed or red-muscled fish undergoes bacterial decomposition.[33,315] The normal piscine surface bacteria *Proteus morganii, Klebsiella pneumoniae, Aerobacter aerogenes, Escherichia coli, Alcaligenes metalcaligenes,* and others have been implicated in the putrefactive process, which includes the decarboxylation of the amino acid L-histidine to histamine and saurine (histamine PO_4 and histamine HCl).[407] The term *saurine* originated because of the association of scombrotoxism with saury, a Japanese dried fish delicacy.[193] Because of this process, "scombrotoxin" was initially thought to be histamine, which is commonly found in large amounts in the flesh of usually implicated fish. Evidence initially suggesting that histamine may be the causative toxin of scombroid fish poisoning was presented in an investigation of a small outbreak.[286] The urinary excretion of histamine and its metabolite, *N*-methylhistamine, was measured in three persons who had scombrotoxism after ingestion of marlin. The marlin contained levels of histamine from 842 to 2503 mmol per 100 g of tissue. Urine samples collected 1 to 4 hours after fish ingestion demonstrated histamine and *N*-methylhistamine levels 9 to 20 times and 15 to 20 times the normal mean, respectively. The authors failed to measure any increase in the principal metabolite of prostaglandin D_2, a mast cell secretory product considered to indicate release of histamine from mast cells. This supported the hypothesis that the excess histamine was from the fish rather than endogenously produced in the victims. Histamine levels greater than 20 to 50 mg/100 g are frequently noted in scombrotoxic fish, and it is not unusual to record levels in excess of 400 mg/100 g. Normal fresh fish contains less than 1 mg/100 g of histamine.[364] Affected fish typically have a sharply metallic or peppery taste but may be normal in appearance, color, and flavor. However, not all persons who eat a scombrotoxin- or histamine-contaminated fish become ill, possibly because of uneven distribution of decay within the fish. It is possible that some other compound may be responsible for scombroid symptoms, since the syndrome cannot be reproduced solely by the administration of equal or even massive doses of histamine by the oral route. Histamine is rapidly inactivated by enzymes in the gastrointestinal tract and on first pass through the liver, with very little reaching systemic circulation. It has been speculated that some other compound, such as cadaverine or putrescine, may be present in the decomposed fish flesh that either facilitates the absorption or inhibits the gastrointestinal or hepatic degradation of histamine.[345,407] The toxin is heat stable and not destroyed by cooking.

Clinical Presentation. The effects of scombroid fish poisoning occur within minutes of consumption of the fish. Although not an allergic reaction, the symptoms are similar and typically include headache, diffuse erythema, a sense of warmth without elevations in core temperature, nausea, vomiting, diarrhea, abdominal cramps, conjunctival injection, pruritus, dizziness, and a burning sensation in the mouth and oropharynx.[220,273] Flushing of the head, neck and upper torso is characteristic and may be exacerbated by ultraviolet light. Severe effects, such as bronchospasm, generalized urticaria, hypotension, palpitations, and arrhythmias, have been reported but are not frequent.[155,193] In most healthy victims the syndrome is self limited, resolving within 8 to 12 hours. In patients with preexisting respiratory or cardiac disease, the effects of the poisoning can precipitate a more severe illness.[48,273] Scombroid reactions may be markedly more severe in patients concurrently ingesting isoniazid (INH) because of this compound's blockade of gastrointestinal tract histaminase.[428] Death has never been reported after scombroid poisoning.

Treatment. The use of emesis or other methods of gastric decontamination for scombroid poisoning is not indicated because symptoms occur rapidly, vomiting can be a primary effect of the toxin, and induced emesis has not been demonstrated to be helpful. The oral administration of activated charcoal may be beneficial, although this has not been studied. Symptoms can be lessened or controlled with the administration of histamine-1 (H_1) receptor antagonists, such as diphenhydramine or hydroxyzine, administered initially in doses of 25 to 50 mg orally or intravenously. The use of histamine-2 (H_2) receptor antagonists (e.g., cimetidine, famotidine) has also been shown to relieve most of the symptoms, and perhaps a combination of H_1 and H_2 receptor antagonists may be most effective.[44,168] Gastroenteritis is usually controlled by an antihistamine but occasionally requires the addition of a specific antiemetic, such as prochlorperazine. The persistent headache of scombroid poisoning may respond to cimetidine or a similar drug if standard analgesics are not effective.[19] Intravenous fluids and inhaled bronchodilators should be used as needed. Vasopressors are rarely necessary because hypotension is usually mild.

TABLE 54-1. Summary of Fish- and Algae-Related Toxic Syndromes

TOXIDROME	SEAFOOD INVOLVED	AREAS COMMONLY SEEN	CAUSATIVE ORGANISMS	TOXIN PRODUCED
FISH-RELATED TOXIC SYNDROMES				
Scombroid	Albacore, tuna, wahoo, mackerel, skipjack, bonito, mahimahi	Worldwide	Bacteria within the fish transform histidine to histamine	Histamine, saurine
Tetrodotoxin	Puffer fish, "fugu," porcupine fish, sunfish	Tropical and subtropical	? *Pseudomonas* species	Tetrodotoxin
ALGAE BLOOM–RELATED TOXIC SYNDROMES				
Ciguatera	Tropical and semi-tropical reef fish such as barracuda, grouper, snapper, jack	Worldwide, most common in Indian Ocean, South Pacific, Caribbean	*Gambierdiscus toxicus* and other species	Ciguatoxin, maito-toxin, GT1-4, palytoxin
Clupeotoxin	Herring, sardines, anchovies, tar-pons, bonefish	Caribbean, Indo-Pacific, Africa	*Ostreopis siamensis*	Palytoxin
PSP	Shellfish	NE and NW coast of US, Philippines, Alaska, North Sea	*Protogonyaulax, Alexandrium catarella, Pyrodinium, Saxidomus, Gonyaulax*	Saxitoxin, neosaxitoxins, gonyautoxins
NSP	Shellfish	Gulf of Mexico, Florida, Texas, North Carolina, New Zealand	*Ptychodiscus breve*	Brevetoxins
DSP	Shellfish	Japan, Spain, Netherlands, Chile	*Dinophysis, Prorocentrum*	Okadaic acid and others
Domoic acid	Shellfish	Canada, Japan, NE and NW USA	*Nitzschia pungens, Pseudonitzschia australis*	Domoic acid
***Pfiesteria* syndrome**	Estuarine fish	Coastal waterways in eastern USA and Gulf coast	*Pfiesteria piscicida*	Unidentified
Haff disease	Buffalo fish	USA, Russia, Sweden	? Blue-green algae	Unknown

IVF, intravenous fluid; *ATPase*, adenosine triphosphatase; *PSP*, paralytic shellfish poisoning; *AV*, atrioventricular; *NSP*, neurotoxic shellfish poisoning; *DSP*, diarrhetic shellfish poisoning.

MECHANISMS OF ACTION	CLINICAL MANIFESTATIONS	SYMPTOM ONSET AFTER INGESTION	DURATION OF ILLNESS	TREATMENT
Histamine response	Diffuse erythema, flushing, nausea, vomiting, pruritus, headache, urticaria, bronchospasm	Rapid, minutes	Resolves 8-12 hr	Histamine-1 and -2 blockers, antiemetics
Na$^+$ channel blocker, blocks axonal transmission	Paresthesias of lip and tongue, hypersalivation, weakness, ataxia, tremor, dysphagia, seizure, bronchospasm, hypotension, nausea, vomiting, diarrhea, death	10 min to 4 hr	Hours to days	Supportive Aggressive airway management, IVF, inotropic agents, ?anticholinesterase
Na$^+$ channel blocker	Gastroenteritis followed by neurologic symptoms: dysesthesias, hot/cold reversal, weakness, respiratory paralysis	2-6 hr	Days to months	Supportive, ? IV mannitol
Inhibits Na$^+$-K$^+$ ATPase	Metallic taste, nausea, vomiting, diarrhea, paresthesias, hypotension, death	Rapid onset, 30-60 min	Days	Supportive, ? early gastric emptying
Na$^+$ channel blocker, may suppress AV nodal conduction	Paresthesias of face and extremities, numbness, dysphonia, dysphagia, ataxia, weakness, paralysis, death from respiratory failure	30-60 min	Weeks	Supportive, charcoal, ventilatory support
Modulate Na$^+$ channel	Circumoral paresthesias, ataxia, GI symptoms if aerosolized, may cause conjunctivitis, bronchospasm	Minutes to hours	Several hours to a few days	Supportive
Phosphatase A$_1$ and A$_2$ inhibitor	Acute gastroenteritis	Rapid, 30 min to 2 hr	2-3 days	Supportive
Glutamate antagonist	Gastroenteritis, seizures, coma, anterograde memory disorder	1-24 hr	24 hr to 12 wk	Supportive, benzodiazepines for seizures
Unknown	Headache, skin lesions, eye irritation, respiratory irritation, learning and memory deficits, cognitive impairment	Within 2 wk of exposure	Improve within 3-6 mo	No treatment, cholestyramine for persistent symptoms
Unknown	Severe muscle pain, rhabdomyolysis, weakness, tachycardia, hypotension	6-12 hr	Days	Supportive, IVF, ? diuretics

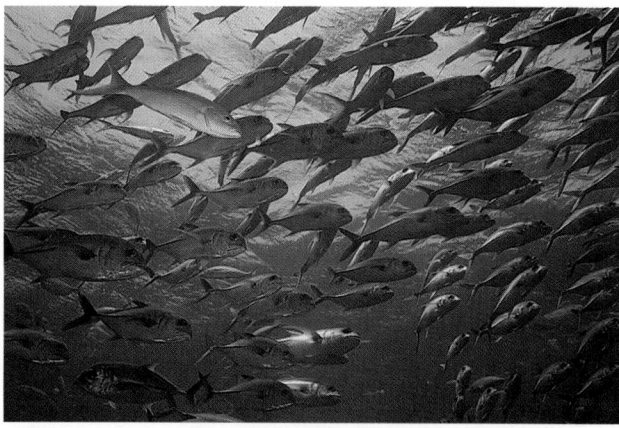

Figure 54-1 Schooling jacks. This type of fish can cause scombroid poisoning. *(Karen Van Hoesen, MD.)*

Prevention. Scombroid fish poisoning is a preventable illness and can be avoided if the offending fish species are promptly refrigerated below 15° C (59° F) or iced after catch and maintained until the fish is cooked or processed for storage. Recreational fishermen must pay particular attention to their coolers. No fish should be consumed if it has been handled improperly or has the smell of ammonia. Fresh fish generally has a sheen or oily rainbow appearance; "dull" packaged fish should be avoided. If an episode of scombroid poisoning is recognized, it is important to report it promptly to local public health authorities to prevent exposure of additional people, particularly if the food was served in a public eating establishment.[194]

Tetrodotoxin Fish Poisoning

Tetrodotoxin (TTX) is a potent neurotoxin found in a variety of creatures and has been isolated from animals of four different phyla, including puffer fish, the California newt, the blue-ringed octopus, poison dart frogs, the ivory shell, and the trumpet shell. The puffer fish, also known as the blowfish or globefish, is one of the better-recognized species that contains TTX. These species of fish can be found in both freshwater and salt water.[173] In humans the most common exposure to TTX is through the ingestion of fugu, a specially prepared species of puffer fish. Human TTX poisonings have also occurred after consumption of gastropod mollusks.[461] Envenomation from the blue-ringed octopus is rare.[135]

Puffer fish poisoning has been recognized for millennia. Ancient Oriental literature documents the dangers of eating puffer fish.[173] There are references to puffer fish in hieroglyphics of the ancient Egyptian dynasty of 2700 BC. Scholars suggest this fish was known to be poisonous during Egyptian times. Mosaic sanitary laws against eating fish without fins and scales may have been derived to avoid fish containing TTX;

the TTX containing fish in the region inhabited by the Israelites were scaleless.[173]

Captain Cook recorded in 1774 his experience after eating a piece of liver from a puffer fish purchased from a native fisherman.[438] Before preparing the fish for eating, it was described and drawn. Cook tasted the liver and described a vivid feeling of extraordinary weakness and numbness.[173] There has been some contention that TTX ("puffer powder") was used as a component of Haitian voodoo potion in the zombie ritual.[421] This has been challenged on grounds, among others, that under the usual conditions of extreme alkaline storage, any TTX in a "zombie potion" would be decomposed irreversibly into pharmacologically inactive products.[217,464]

Tetrodotoxin was named around 1911 after searching for the active ingredient in fugu ovaries.[140] Isolation of the chemical was achieved in the 1950s. In 1964, tarichatoxin, a nonprotein neurotoxin, was confirmed to be the same molecule as TTX.[287] This compound is found in the California and Japanese newts (e.g., *Taricha granulosa, Notophthalmus viridescens, Cynops ensicauda*); international salamanders of the family Salamandridae (e.g, *Triturus, Pleurodeles, Cynops, Paramesotriton, Tylototriton*); the skin of central American frogs of the genus *Atelopus*; the goby *Gobius criniger*; shellfish (ivory shell, *Babylonia japonica*; lined moon shell, *Natica lineata*; calf moon shell, *Natica vitellus*; bladder moon shell, *Polinices didyma*; and trumpet shell, *Charonia sauliae*); the starfish *Astropecten polyacanthus*; the ribbon worm *Cephalothrix linearis*; the flatworm *Planocera multitentaculata*; the crab *Atergatus floridus*; the horseshoe crab *Carcinoscorpius rotundicanda*; and the Australian blue-ringed octopus (*Hapalochlaena maculosa*).[135,140,173,395,461] In the 1970s the major toxin in certain poison dart frogs was identified as TTX. In 1978, isolation of crystalline TTX was performed.

Fugu. TTX is characteristic of the order Tetraodontiformes.[395] The suborder Tetrodontoidei contains three families of fish (Tetraodontidae, Diodontidae, and Canthigasteridae), including pufferfish (Figure 54-2) (toadfish, blowfish, globefish, swellfish, balloonfish, toado) and porcupine fish. Sunfish (*Mola* species) are members of the suborder Moloidei. Pufferfish are tropical and subtropical, some of which are prepared as delicacies called fugu.[70] Pufferfish can inflate their bodies to a nearly spherical shape using air or seawater (Figure 54-3). At least 50 of the more than 100 species of these fish have been involved in poisonings of humans or may be intermittently toxic.[344]

Chefs must undergo a rigorous certification process before they are allowed to prepare fugu. The filet of the puffer fish contains very minute concentrations of TTX. Fugu is served raw with paper-thin slices placed into an ornate configuration. The presence of small

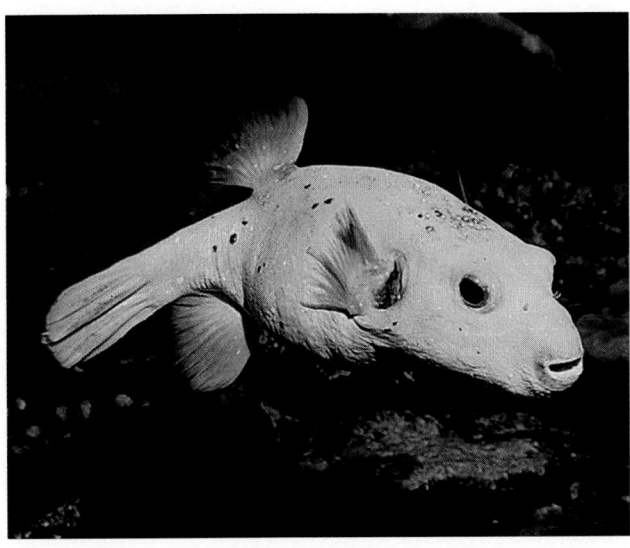

Figure 54-2 Pufferfish (French Polynesia). *(Courtesy Carl Roessler.)*

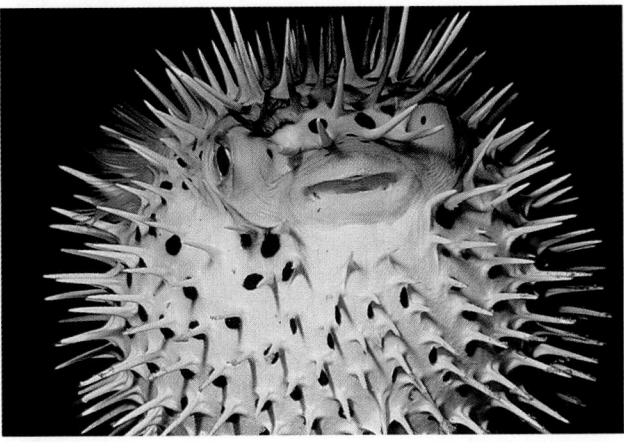

Figure 54-3 Porcupine fish inflated with seawater. *(Karen Van Hoesen, MD.)*

quantities of TTX gives the desired effect of slight oral tingling. Importation of fugu into the United States is illegal; however, smuggling has resulted in cases of poisoning.

The precise origin of the toxin may be production by *Pseudomonas* species that live on the skin of the puffer fish.[470] This would explain transmittal of toxicity between toxic and nontoxic fish through skin contact. Other investigators have found the production of tetrodotoxin by *Vibrio* and other species isolated from the intestines of puffer fish.[443] Radiolabeled tetrodotoxin injected into a puffer accumulated most in skin, liver, intestines, and muscle; however, the toxin is concentrated in the liver, viscera, gonads, and skin of the fish. Female fish are considered more toxic than males especially because there are high concentrations

of TTX in ovaries. Musculature is less toxic but still may contain a significant amount of TTX. The toxin is heat stable and is not inactivated by freezing. Seasonal variation of TTX concentration occurs with peak levels during spawning season.

Pathophysiology. Tetrodotoxin has a unique nonprotein structure and is widely used as a research tool to study sodium channels. Mouse bioassays demonstrate that the minimal lethal dose of TTX by intraperitoneal injection is 8 to 20 µg/kg.[287] Tetrodotoxin blocks sodium channels during the rising phase of the action potential.[216] The interaction of TTX with the sodium channel is thought to be stoichiometric with each TTX molecule interfering with one channel. Tetrodotoxin affects the spike generating process of sodium channels, not the resting or steady state voltage.[216]

TTX interferes with both central and peripheral neuromuscular transmission. Although it is not a depolarizing agent, in animals it causes depression of the medullary respiratory mechanism, intracardiac conduction, and myocardial and skeletal muscle contractility. At the microcellular level the mechanism of action of TTX is linked to the axon, rather than to the nerve endplate. TTX blocks axonal transmission by interfering with sodium conductance within the depolarized regions of the cell membrane, perhaps by acting at a metal cation binding site in the sodium channel, without affecting the presynaptic release of acetylcholine or its effects on the neuromuscular junction.[5,188] Saxitoxin, implicated in paralytic shellfish poisoning, has essentially the same action as tetrodotoxin on the nerve membrane, although it is believed to have a discrete receptor.[219] There is no apparent effect on potassium permeability.[342] The LD50 for mice is 10 mg/kg when TTX is administered by intraperitoneal, intravenous, or subcutaneous routes.[419]

Animal studies suggest that TTX has a peripheral effect that results in vasodilation independent of α or β receptors.[216,219] Further studies suggest a dose-dependent action. At low doses, systemic blood pressure is lowered, although perfusion pressure is initially maintained. Higher doses of TTX result in a profound fall in blood pressure.[216] Experiments with animal models using TTX from blue-ringed octopi demonstrate a similar profound hypotension. α-Agonists have been the most effective agents in raising blood pressure in models of TTX poisoning.[135]

Clinical Presentation. The onset of symptoms after TTX administration can be as rapid as 10 minutes or delayed up to 4 hours, but usually occurs within 30 minutes of ingestion. Death has been recorded within 17 minutes of exposure. The extent and type of symptoms vary according to the individual and the amount of TTX ingested. Paresthesias of the lips and tongue initially occur and may be rapidly followed by hypersalivation, diaphoresis, lethargy, headache, weakness, ataxia, incoordination, tremor, paralysis, cyanosis, aphonia, dysphagia, seizures, dyspnea, bronchorrhea, bronchospasm, respiratory failure, coma, and hypotension. Gastrointestinal symptoms can be severe and include nausea, vomiting, diarrhea, and abdominal pain.[375] Paresthesias advance to the extremities often with severe numbness that has been described as a feeling of the body "floating." Hypersalivation with diaphoresis is common. Motor paralysis may occur with the onset of weakness, incoordination, hyporeflexia, and cranial nerve dysfunction. Weakness and paralysis may appear in the upper extremities and descend to the lower extremities.[344] Early miosis may progress to mydriasis with poor pupillary light reflex.[419] A disseminated intravascular coagulation–like syndrome may occur and is heralded by petechial skin hemorrhages that can progress to bullous desquamation and diffuse stigmata of prolonged coagulation. Hypotension can be profound and may be refractory to treatment. Respiratory distress and insufficiency can occur. Bradycardia and atrioventricular node conduction abnormalities may be present. Complete cardiovascular collapse with respiratory paralysis precedes death. Normal consciousness may be maintained until shortly before death.[140] Sixty percent of victims may die, most of these within the first 6 hours. Survival past 24 hours is a good prognostic sign.

Treatment. Treatment of TTX is primarily supportive with aggressive airway management and assisted ventilation. Decontamination should be considered with a dose of activated charcoal given on early presentation. Since the toxin may be partially inactivated in alkaline solutions, gastric lavage with at least 2 L of 2% sodium bicarbonate in 200-ml aliquots has been recommended. However, the efficacy of this therapy has never been studied, and since many patients will have gastroenteritis before presentation to a health care facility, this practice is unlikely to be of much benefit. Atropine may be used to treat bradycardia in conjunction with adequate oxygenation. Intravenous fluid resuscitation should be initiated for hypotension; however, use of inotropic agents may be required to maintain perfusion. α-Agonists such as phenylephrine or norepinephrine are more likely to be effective.

Anticholinesterase agents such as edrophonium have been used to treat victims of TTX poisoning with mixed success. There have been case reports that suggest subjective improvement in the neurologic symptoms after administration of anticholinesterase agents.[83,419] Other case reports noted no improvement after infusion of these compounds.[263,416] A review of earlier studies shows that TTX is not antagonized by anticholinesterase agents since the toxin interrupts neuromuscular transmission on motor neurons and muscle membranes and not the motor endplate.[215] The administration of veratrine-like agents, which prolong skeletal muscle contraction without dependence on intact neuromuscular transmission, provides prophylactic protection against the action of TTX on sciatic nerve anterior tibial muscle preparations from rats.[342] Applicability of this to human clinical situations is unclear. Antihistamines and steroids have also been utilized with no clear benefit.[263]

No antidote is currently available to treat TTX poisoning; however, studies are ongoing. TTX has been conjugated to keyhole limpet hemocyanin and the conjugate used as an immunogen in rabbits and mice. Mice immunized with the conjugate were protected from a lethal dose of toxin, and passive protection experiments using rabbit antiserum exhibited a dose-related therapeutic activity after toxin challenge.[141] The shore crab *Hemigrapsuss sanguineus* is highly resistant to TTX by virtue of a toxin-binding substance.[368] Whether this natural phenomenon can be applied to the human situation remains to be seen.

A minor intoxication with TTX may be limited to paresthesias and mild dysphagia. In such a case the victim should be observed in the emergency department or intensive care unit for at least 8 hours to detect deterioration, particularly in respiratory function. The victim should not be discharged until the symptoms are clearly improving. Although water soluble, TTX is very difficult to remove from fish, even by cooking. It is wisest to avoid all puffers, even when prepared by an expert.

Grass Carp Gallbladder Poisoning

Ingestion of the Asian freshwater grass carp (*Ctenopharyngodon idellus*) or other similar fishes (*Cyprinus carpio*) can lead to serious illness, attributed to the nephrotoxic and hepatotoxic properties of a toxin found in the bile.[78] The structure of the toxin in *C. carpio* has recently been characterized as 5μ-cholestane-3μ, 7μ, 12μ, 26,27-pentol 26-sulfate.[17] Most cases have occurred in Hong Kong, Taiwan, and South Korea. Two recent cases were reported in the United States in immigrants who ate raw gallbladders from carp caught in Maryland.[68] One of the patients required hemodialysis for acute renal failure. His renal and hepatic function gradually improved.

People eat the raw gallbladder for its putative antirheumatologic properties. Several hours after ingestion, abdominal pain, nausea, vomiting, and watery diarrhea develop, which can be accompanied by marked elevations in concentrations of liver enzymes (aspartate and alanine aminotransferases). The hepatitis is transient and to date has not led to hepatic failure. Nephrotoxicity may be profound, leading to oliguric or nonoliguric renal failure within 48 to 72 hours after ingestion. Renal biopsy demonstrates acute tubular necrosis without evidence of rhabdomyolysis. Therapy is supportive and based on symptoms. Hemodialysis may be necessary until renal function improves.

POISONINGS ASSOCIATED WITH ALGEAL BLOOMS

Although there are thousands of species of microalgae that form the base of the food chain, less than 60 species are toxic or harmful. These toxic species can cause significant kills of fish and shellfish, mortality among seabirds and marine mammals, and human illnesses and death. In the United States, harmful algae blooms now threaten virtually every costal state with increasing numbers of toxic species. Several distinct clinical syndromes exist: ciguatera fish poisoning, clupeotoxic fish poisoning, paralytic shellfish poisoning, neurotoxic shellfish poisoning, diarrhetic shellfish poisoning, domoic acid intoxication, *Pfiesteria* syndrome, and Haff disease (see Table 54-1).

Ciguatera Fish Poisoning

Worldwide, ciguatera accounts for more cases of fishborne illness than any other type of ichthyosarcotoxicosis.[59] Ciguatera is most commonly seen in the Indian Ocean, South Pacific, and Caribbean. In the United States, ciguatera poisoning is the most common nonbacterial food poisoning associated with fish, with cases having been reported in many states.[148,190,284,440] Outbreaks of ciguatera poisoning are greatest between the months of April and August. In endemic areas the incidence is estimated to be between 500 and 600 cases per 10,000 people.[237] Worldwide, it has been estimated that ciguatera poisoning may affect over 50,000 persons each year. Most cases in the United States occur in Hawaii and Florida, with the incidence in Florida estimated to be five cases per 10,000 people.[125] Outbreaks of ciguatera poisoning have been associated with the ingestion of warm water reef–dwelling fish caught between +35 and −35 degrees latitude; however, there have been recent reports of ciguatoxic fish being caught in waters at +33 degrees latitude.[30,174] In addition, the advent of flash freezing and shipping of fish around the world has accounted for several cases of ciguatera in nonendemic areas.[190]

More than 400 species of benthic fish have been implicated in ciguatera poisoning, with the greatest concentration in the Caribbean Sea, in the Pacific Ocean around the Indo-Pacific islands, and along the continental tropical reefs. The most frequently implicated reef fishes include the families Muraenidae (moray eels), Mugilidae (mullets), Serranidae (groupers) (Figure 54-4), Lutjanidae (snappers), Sparidae and Lethrinidae (porgies), Carangidae (jacks), Labridae (wrasses), Scaridae (parrotfishes), Acanthuridae (surgeonfishes), Balistidae (triggerfishes), and Sphyraenidae (barracuda).[157] Of reported cases, 75% (except in Hawaii) involve the barracuda, snapper, jack, or grouper. Hawaiian carriers of the toxin include the

parrot-beaked bottom feeders and surgeonfishes, particularly those inhabiting waters with high dinoflagellate populations, such as those with disturbed coral reefs.[202] Other fish that have been reported as ciguatoxic are listed in Box 54-3. Recently, ciguatera poisoning has been

---

Box 54-3 SOME FISH KNOWN TO BE CIGUATOXIC

Albulidae (ladyfishes)
Chanidae (milkfishes)
Clupeidae (herrings)
Elopidae (tarpon)
Engraulidae (anchovies)
Synodontidae (lizardfishes)
Congridae (true eels)
Ophichthyidae (snake eels)
Belonidae (needlefishes)
Exocoetidae (flying fishes)
Hemiramphidae (halfbeaks)
Aulostomidae (trumpetfishes)
Syngnathidae (seahorses)
Holocentridae (squirrelfishes)
Apogonidae (cardinalfishes)
Arripidae (sea perches)
Chaetodontidae (butterfly fishes)
Cirrhitidae (hawkfishes)
Coryphaenidae (dolphins)
Gempylidae (oilfishes)
Gerridae (silverfishes)
Gobidae (gobies)
Istiophoridae (sailfishes)

Kuhliidae (bass)
Kyphosidae (rudderfishes)
Mullidae (goatfishes)
Pempheridae (sweeperfishes)
Pomacentridae (damselfishes)
Pomadasyiidae (grunts)
Priacanthidae (snapper)
Scatophagidae (spade fishes)
Sciaenidae (croakers)
Scombridae (tunas)
Scorpaenidae (scorpionfish)
Siganidae (rabbitfishes)
Xiphiidae (swordfishes)
Zanclidae (moorish idol)
Bothidae (flounders)
Aluteridae and Monacanthidae (filefishes)
Ostraciontidae (trunkfishes)
Batrachoididae (toadfishes)
Antennariidae (sargassumfish)
Lophiidae (goosefish)
Ogcocephalidae (longnose batfish)

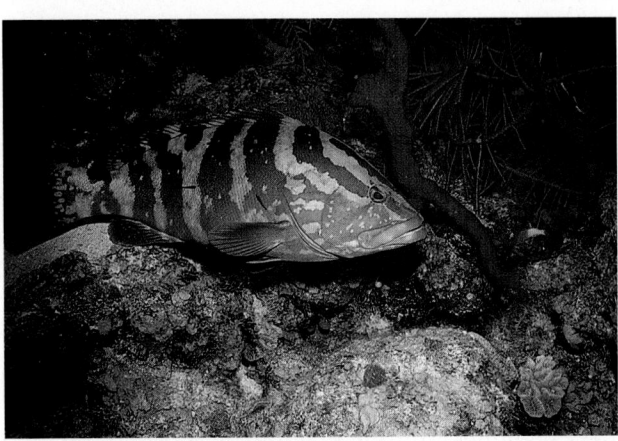

Figure 54-4 Groupers are often implicated in ciguatera fish poisoning. *(Karen Van Hoesen, MD.)*

reported after the ingestion of farm-raised salmon.[113] There is one report of ciguatera from the consumption of jellyfish.[473]

The name *ciguatera* is derived from the Spanish name "cigua" for the sea snail *Turbo pica* found in the Caribbean Spanish Antilles.[27,414] This neurotoxic syndrome has been recognized throughout history with one of the earliest cases likely reported in the fourth century, when Alexander the Great refused to allow his soldiers to eat fish, and also during the Tang Dynasty in China.[388] One of the earliest written records of suspected ciguatera poisoning is from the journal of Captain William Bligh, who described symptoms consistent with ciguatera on June 10, 1789, after eating dolphin fish (mahimahi).[388] In addition, it was also quite possibly ciguatera fish poisoning that was illustrated by Captain James Cook while sailing on the *Resolution* in the South Pacific in 1774.[312] In this episode, several of his officers were poisoned after eating fish from the island Malicolo in the Pacific nation of Vanuatu.

Pathophysiology. The blue-green algae and free algae dinoflagellate, *Gambierdiscus toxicus,* is thought to be responsible for producing ciguatoxins.[388] *Gambierdiscus toxicus* adheres to dead coral surfaces and marine algae, which are consumed by smaller herbivorous fish.[157,237] Although *Gambierdiscus toxicus* is likely responsible for the majority of ciguatoxins encountered in fish, the cyanobacterium *Trichodesmium erythraeum* can elaborate water- and lipid-soluble precursors to the toxins that may generate ciguatera syndrome.[124] Other dinoflagellates, such as *Prorocentrum concavum, P. mexicanum, P. rhathymum, Gymnodinium sanguineum,* and *Gonyaulax polyedra,* may generate toxins that play a role in ciguatera syndrome.[324,417]

Larger reef fish eat the contaminated smaller fish, thereby becoming vectors as ciguatoxin is bioconcentrated up the food chain. As the fish within the food chain become larger and older, the toxin is accumulated.[93,184,193,315] Experimental induction of ciguatera toxicity in surgeonfish (*Acanthurus xanthopterus*) has been achieved by a diet of ciguatoxic red snapper (*Lutjanus bohar*).[187] Although the entire fish is toxic, the viscera (particularly the liver) and roe are considered to carry the highest concentrations of toxin.[29] No plankton feeders have so far been reported to be ciguatoxic.

It has been suggested that the proliferation of toxic algae may be triggered by contamination of the water from a number of sources, including industrial wastes, golf course runoff, metallic compounds, ship wreckage, or other pollutants.[174] In the Marshall Islands (Micronesia), consequent to nuclear testing, the incidence of toxin-producing plankton has tripled.[333] Similar observations have been made with respect to various military activities (dumping and explosives) in the Line and Gilbert Islands (Kiribati, Central Pacific), Hao Atoll

(Tuamotu Archipelago, French Polynesia), Gambier Islands (French Polynesia), and others.[341] Yet another cause for toxic dinoflagellate proliferation may be the transfer and dumping of ballast water in large ocean-going vessels.

Ciguatera fish poisoning is associated with more than five toxins, including fat-soluble quaternary ammonium compounds (ciguatoxins), a water-soluble component (maitotoxin, from the Tahitian vernacular name *maito* for the surgeonfish *Ctenochaetus striatus*), a maitotoxin-associated hemolysin (lysophosphatidylcholine, or lysolecithin), and a ciguatoxin-associated adenine triphosphatase (ATPase) inhibitor.[177,245,251,350] Scaritoxin (isolated from *Scarus gibbus*) is similar to the fat-soluble component and is specific to parrotfishes.[87] Lipid-extracted toxins from *Gambierdiscus toxicus* have been designated GT-1, GT-2, and GT-3; a water-soluble toxin is designated GT-4.[109,278] Chemical analysis of ciguatoxins demonstrates that they closely resemble brevetoxin C (from *Ptychodiscus brevis*) and okadaic acid, isolated from marine sponges and the dinoflagellate *Prorocentrum lima*.[133,290] The identification of okadaic acid from the Caribbean dinoflagellate *Prorocentrum concavum* lends support to the notion that this toxin may be more significant in ciguatera poisoning than previously thought. Another compound named prorocentrolide has also been found in reef-dwelling fish with okadaic acid and has been implicated in diarrhetic shellfish poisoning, another common fish-borne illness.[133,192]

Three major ciguatoxins are usually found in the flesh and viscera of ciguateric fishes. They are labeled CTX-1, CTX-2, and CTX-3. Each is found in variable concentrations, which may account for the inconsistency of reported clinical signs and symptoms.[251] CTX-2 is a diastereomer of CTX-3.[254] Ciguatoxins may result from the oxidation of gambiertoxins, possibly through the cytochrome system in the liver of fish.[253] The lipid components have been characterized as crystalline, colorless, heat-stable compounds of approximate molecular weight 1100 daltons, with functional hydroxyl and quaternary nitrogen groups. CTX is excreted in bodily fluids and toxicity can be transmitted by both semen and breast milk.[58,283]

Ciguatoxins activate voltage-dependent Na+ channels.[250] One mechanism of their action may be by falsely occupying calcium receptor sites that modulate sodium pore permeability in neural, muscle, and myocardial membranes.[35] This effect could allow increased membrane permeability to sodium and cause sustained depolarization. Electrophysiologic studies of the sural and common peroneal nerves in humans with ciguatera poisoning demonstrating reduced light touch, pain, and vibratory sensation in the extremities showed prolongation of the absolute refractory, relative refractory, and supernormal periods. These findings indirectly suggest that CTX may abnormally prolong sodium channel opening in nerve membranes.[60] This influx of sodium is antagonized by the presence of tetrodotoxin.[40]

In vitro studies have also shown that scaritoxin causes the release of norepinephrine and acetylcholine and increases sodium channel permeability.[405] Maitotoxin as well may trigger the release of norepinephrine and stimulate cellular uptake of calcium and has been hypothesized to stimulate cholinergic receptors by inhibiting acetylcholinesterase.[40,374] However, evidence suggests that highly purified ciguatoxin preparations may not have anticholinesterase effects in vivo.[244]

Palytoxin is an extremely poisonous nonprotein agent of low molecular weight that has been isolated from various zoanthid "soft" corals of the genus *Palythoa*, although its true origin is unknown.[169] In animal models it causes a fast potassium outflow from erythrocytes, increases the permeability of cell membranes to sodium and potassium but not calcium, and inhibits sodium-potassium ATPase. Although palytoxin is presumed to originate in coelenterates or even bacteria, there has been some suggestion that it can be a causative agent for ciguatera poisoning.[230,275,304] Ingestion in humans reportedly causes abdominal cramps, nausea, diarrhea, paresthesias of the extremities, muscle spasm, and respiratory distress. Of this cluster of symptoms, the predominant physical findings appeared to be respiratory distress and extreme tonic muscle contractions with massive accumulation of serum creatine kinase and myoglobinuria. Palytoxin has been found in mackerel (*Decapterus macrosoma*), triggerfish (*Melichtys vidua*), and crab (*Demania reynaudii*).[7,142,230] Since a rapid and sensitive hemolysis neutralization assay for palytoxin is now available, its presence in toxic seafood, and perhaps its role in ciguatera poisoning, should become easier to determine.[41]

Hypertension occurring with ciguatera poisoning can be suppressed in animal models with phentolamine, suggesting α-receptor sympathomimetic activity. Although purified ciguatoxin appears to have cardiac stimulatory effects (increasing heart rate and output), maitotoxin is a myocardial depressant in vitro, which may explain the variation in clinical presentation. Isolated human atrial trabeculae show concentration-dependent positive inotropy with CTX-1, which is not reversed with mannitol.[250] Cardiac calcium conduction effects have been implicated in the activity of maitotoxin because its action is inhibited in the presence of verapamil, magnesium ions, or low-calcium solutions. In mice, injection of maitotoxin can induce a marked increase in total calcium content of the adrenal glands and a rise in plasma cortisol concentration.[412] When injected into mice, ciguatoxin targets the heart, adrenal glands, and autonomic nervous system.[414] Ciguatoxin and CTX-4c (a derivative) administered in

repeated doses cause the mouse heart to suffer septal and ventricular interstitial fibrosis, accompanied by bilateral ventricular hypertrophy.[410] Ciguatoxin is a potent substance, with an LD_{50} in mice of 0.45 mg/kg in purified form. In most toxic fish flesh the concentration is 0.5 to 10 parts per billion. Maitotoxin is even more potent, with an LD_{50} of 0.13 mg/kg in mice. It is interesting to note that ciguatoxins can become toxic to fish in higher concentrations, thus potentially limiting the levels of these compounds carried by a fish.[249] However, the toxin or toxins may reside in the skeletal muscle or other tissues of the fish in association with proteins that may be protective of the carrier.[170]

All toxins associated with ciguatera identified to date are unaffected by freeze-drying, heat, cold, and gastric acid and do not affect the odor, color, or taste of the fish. There is some evidence that cooking methods can alter the relative concentrations of the various toxins. For example, boiling fish flesh will remove water-soluble toxins, but frying or grilling the flesh may increase toxicity of lipid-soluble toxins as a result of releasing lipid-soluble components from cellular compounds to which they are normally bound.[123]

Clinical Presentation. The meal containing ciguatera is generally unremarkable in taste and smell. Symptoms may develop within minutes of ingestion, although they generally occur within 2 to 6 hours after the meal. Almost all victims develop symptoms by 24 hours, and the toxicity can generally be ruled out if the onset is delayed longer than this time.[27,125] The severity of symptoms seems to follow a dose-dependent fashion, with victims eating larger portions of ciguatoxic fish experiencing more severe symptoms (Box 54-4).

The most common initial symptoms reported in cases of ciguatera poisoning include acute gastroenteritis, with abdominal cramps, nausea, vomiting, and diarrhea.[27] These symptoms rarely persist for longer than 24 hours but may require fluid resuscitation.[125] A myriad of other symptoms have been reported in ciguatoxic patients and are listed in Box 54-4. Headache is a common symptom, and victims often complain of experiencing a metallic taste. An overall death rate of 0.1% to 12% has been reported with ciguatera poisoning, but the lower percentage seems more likely with modern supportive care. Death is usually attributed to respiratory paralysis.[211] In a well-described clinical outbreak affecting a group of scuba divers who consumed coral trout (*Cephalopholis miniatus*), the most common symptoms were weakness, cold sensitivity, paresthesias, a taste sensation of "carbonation," and myalgias.[3] Two men suffering from ciguatera poisoning had painful ejaculation with urethritis, which in turn induced dyspareunia (pelvic and vaginal burning) in their female partners after intercourse.[238] The variations in symptoms of ciguatera poisoning may result from different concentrations

Box 54-4 SIGNS AND SYMPTOMS ASSOCIATED WITH CIGUATERA POISONING

Abdominal pain
Nausea
Vomiting
Diarrhea
Chills
Paresthesias (particularly of the extremities and circum-
  oral region)
Pruritus (particularly of the palms and soles)
Tongue and throat numbness or burning
A sensation of "carbonation" during swallowing
Odontalgia or dental dysesthesias
Dysphagia
Dysuria
Dyspnea
Weakness
Fatigue
Tremor
Fasciculations
Athetosis
Meningismus
Aphonia
Ataxia

Vertigo
Pain and weakness in the lower extremities
Visual blurring
Transient blindness
Hyporeflexia
Seizures
Nasal congestion and dryness
Conjunctivitis
Maculopapular rash (erythematous, with occasional
  desquamation)
Skin vesiculations
Dermatographia
Sialorrhea
Diaphoresis
Headache
Arthralgias
Myalgias (particularly in the lower back and thighs)
Insomnia
Bradycardia
Hypotension
Central respiratory failure
Coma

of specific toxins in different fish.[229] Characteristics associated with a severe attack include ingestion of a carnivorous fish and a history of previous ciguatoxism.[158] Neurologic symptoms seem to develop after initial gastrointestinal symptoms. Paresthesias and myalgias are typically seen within the first 24 hours and usually resolve by 48 to 72 hours after ingestion of ciguatoxins, although there have been reports of neurologic symptoms persisting for weeks to months.[26,242]

Many case reports of ciguatera poisoning describe symptoms of a sensory perception of "hot and cold reversal," and loose, painful teeth. Although the presence of these symptoms is suggestive of ciguatera poisoning, their absence does not exclude the possibility of the disease.[26] There have also been reports of a paradoxical reversal to temperature perception only resulting in cold feeling hot rather than hot feeling cold.[26] However, other reports demonstrated that gross temperature discernment remains intact and the description of paradoxical heat perception may be misleading.[59] These authors describe the symptoms as intense, painful tingling or "electric shock" rather than true reversal of hot and cold perception.[59] This peculiar symptom may have a delay in onset of 2 to 5 days, may last for months after ingestion, and is only otherwise seen with neurotoxic shellfish poisoning (brevetoxins), caulerpicin (from the green alga *Caulerpa*) toxicity, or turban shell poisoning.[115,463] Pruritus is another vague but often described sensation in victims of ciguatera poisoning. The onset of pruritus may be delayed for more than

24 hours but is rarely, if ever, seen in the absence of other symptoms.[133,242] Pruritus may persist for weeks and be exacerbated by any activity that increases skin temperature (blood flow), such as exercise or alcohol consumption.[242] Ciguatera-induced pruritus may occasionally become severe and may improve after treatment with histamine receptor antagonists. Delayed symptoms may also include hiccups.

Tachycardia and hypertension are often described in ciguatera poisoning, in some cases after what can be severe transient bradycardia and hypotension.[80] Hallucinations, flushing, flaccid paralysis, and fever are uncommon. More severe reactions tend to occur in persons previously stricken with the disease. Severely affected persons may report intermittent symptoms for up to 6 months, with a gradual diminution in frequency and intensity. There may be some regional variability to the symptoms of presentation.[26,283] Persons who have ingested parrotfish (scaritoxin) have been reported to suffer from classic ciguatera poisoning, as well as a "second phase" of toxicity 5 to 10 days after the initial onset, consisting of ataxia, dysmetria, and a resting or kinetic tremor.[86] Whether ciguatoxin crosses the placenta is not known, but exposures during pregnancy have resulted in normal fetal outcomes.[360]

In small children, the symptoms of ciguatera poisoning may be no more specific than irritability, sleep disturbance, nausea, and vomiting.[448] Other reported symptoms have included carpopedal spasm, ptosis, and inconsolability.

Diagnosis. The diagnosis of ciguatera poisoning is based on clinical symptoms. The differential diagnosis includes paralytic shellfish poisoning, eosinophilic meningitis, type E botulism, organophosphate insecticide poisoning, tetrodotoxin poisoning, and psychogenic hyperventilation.[26,340] Unreliable folklore used in the past to aid in predicting ciguateric seafood includes the advice that a lone fish (separated from the school) should not be eaten; that ants and turtles refuse to eat ciguatoxic fish; that a thin slice of ciguatoxic fish does not show a rainbow effect when held up to the sun; and that a silver spoon tarnishes in a cooking pot with ciguatoxic fish.[92] Ciguatoxin may be detected in the flesh of fish by two immunoassay techniques, a mouse bioassay where a sample of the fish is injected intraperitoneally into a mouse and a "rapid" IgG assay.[190] Rapid immunoassays have largely replaced determination of ciguatera toxicity by injection of fish tissue extracts into mice or by traditional tests of feeding fish to a mongoose or cat to observe for neurologic symptoms or death. High-performance liquid chromatography (HPLC) is also available for ciguatoxins and okadaic acid. Unfortunately, tests for ciguatoxin are still of limited clinical benefit because most institutions do not have the equipment needed for their performance.

Treatment. If possible, a piece of the implicated fish should be obtained in the event that analysis for ciguatoxins can be performed. The treatment of ciguatera poisoning is primarily supportive. Intravenous hydration with crystalloid and electrolyte replacement may be necessary for dehydration. Severe or refractory hypotension may require a vasopressor such as dopamine. Antiemetics such as droperidol, prochlorperazine, and metoclopramide may be beneficial. Atropine has been shown to be effective in patients with symptomatic bradycardia or excess cholinergic stimulation.[133] Ipecac-induced emesis or gastric lavage is rarely indicated since presentation is usually delayed and gastroenteritis is usually already present. Activated charcoal may bind some of the toxin in the gastrointestinal tract but is rarely useful given the expected time of presentation.

Many traditional remedies have been used for centuries in the treatment of ciguatera poisoning. Edrophonium, neostigmine, corticosteroids, pralidoxime, ascorbic acid, pyridoxine (vitamin B_6), and salicylic acid–colchicine–vitamin B complex have all been tried with variable success; however, there is no current clinical support for these modalities.[283] Local anesthetics (e.g., lidocaine, tocainide) have also been administered for treatment of ciguatera.[61,239] These agents are effective blockers of sodium influx and may antagonize the sodium channel effects of ciguatoxin. In addition, amitriptyline has been used for its sodium channel

blocking effects, as well as its potent antimuscarinic effects.[53,58,103] Nifedipine has been used to counteract the cellular uptake of calcium caused by maitotoxin and to relieve headache.[58] Although there is limited experience with most of these therapies, they may be beneficial in cases refractory to supportive care alone.

Recently, mannitol has become the most widely applied therapy in severe cases of ciguatera poisoning.[51,389] Most of the reports of success with the use of mannitol are based on limited data with small numbers of patients.[118,309,313,449] One series described successful treatment in 24 victims of ciguatera poisoning who received mannitol. Each was infused up to 1g/kg of a 20% mannitol solution intravenously over 30 minutes. None of the victims received more than 250 ml.[309] The mechanism by which mannitol might be effective in abating the neurologic symptoms from ciguatera poisoning is unknown, but suggested theories have included acting as a free radical scavenger, acting as a competitive inhibitor of ciguatoxin at the cell membrane, and promoting a decrease in Schwann cell edema.[313,449] It is also possible that the osmotic action of mannitol may render ciguatoxin inert.[309,313] Curiously, mannitol therapy seems to have no beneficial effect on mice administered a sublethal intraperitoneal dose of ciguatoxin (CTX-1).[252] In humans the empiric observation is that mannitol has greater benefit if administered early in the course of the illness. One concern with the administration of mannitol in the setting of ciguatoxin is that patients may present dehydrated. In these cases, patients should be adequately rehydrated before the administration of mannitol. During recovery from ciguatera poisoning, it is recommended that victims exclude fish, shellfish, alcoholic beverages, and nuts and nut oils, which may result in an exacerbation of the syndrome.[373]

Prevention. For travelers, common sense dictates avoiding any fish the local fisherman and residents do not eat, or fish caught in known ciguatera-endemic areas. Because of the accumulation of toxin, all oversized fish of any predacious reef species (such as jack, snapper, barracuda, grouper, or parrot-beaked bottom feeder) should be suspected toxic. Moray eels should never be consumed. Internal organs of implicated fish seem to concentrate the toxin and should therefore be avoided. Natural events such as hurricanes and earthquakes have been associated with an increased incidence of ciguatera, presumably because of reef disturbance. The recent El Niño storms may also affect the incidence of ciguatera in the Pacific.[30]

Clupeotoxin Fish Poisoning

Clupeotoxic fish poisoning involves plankton-feeding fish, which ingest planktonic blue-green algae and dinoflagellates. The poisoning is distinguished from ciguatera based on its severity and high fatality rate and the implicated clupeoid fish. These fish of the order Clupeiformes are found in tropical Caribbean, Indo-Pacific, and African coastal waters. Examples include the families Clupeidae (herrings and sardines), Engraulidae (anchovies), Elopidae (tarpons), Albulidae (bonefishes), and Pterothrissidae (deep-sea slickheads).[28,277] Toxicity is reported to increase during the warm summer months. Viscera are considered to be highly toxic.

Previously, the toxin has been poorly characterized as a result of the infrequency of the syndrome and rare access to toxic animals. Recently the first case to shed light on clupeotoxism was reported in a Madagascar woman who died after eating a sardine, *Herklotsichthys quadrimaculatus*. The causative toxin was identified as palytoxin or its analog, which distinctly differed from ciguatoxin. The benthic dinoflagellate *Ostreopsis siamensis* was presumed to be the probable toxin source.[307,462] This same sardine has been implicated in clupeotoxism in Fiji and the Philippines.[465,467]

Clinical Presentation. The onset of symptoms is rapid and characterized as "violent," often within 30 to 60 minutes of ingestion and rarely prolonged beyond 2 hours. Initial signs and symptoms include a marked metallic taste, xerostomia, nausea, vomiting, diarrhea, and abdominal pain. These symptoms are followed by chills, headache, diaphoresis, severe paresthesias, muscle cramps, vertigo, malaise, tachycardia, peripheral cyanosis, hypotension, delirium and death, with a mortality of up to 45%. Severe debility leading to death may occur within 15 minutes of the onset of symptoms.[174] A postmortem examination in one case after ingestion of *Sardinella marquesensis* (Marquesan sardine) flesh and viscera demonstrated enterocolitis and the sequelae of hypotension and acute heart failure.[277] As with ciguatera toxin, the poison does not impart any unusual appearance, odor, or flavor to the fish.

Treatment. Therapy is supportive and based on symptoms. Because of the severe nature of the intoxication, early gastric emptying is desirable; however, the disease is so unusual and so rarely suspected (because of a lack of history) that gastric emptying is not often carried out. Aggressive management and early intensive care are essential.

Prevention. Clupeotoxic fish should be avoided, especially during summer months, in fish indigenous to the Caribbean, African coastal, or Indo-Pacific waters. The viscera of suspicious fish can be fed to experimental animals to see if an illness is generated.

Paralytic Shellfish Poisoning

Shellfish have been implicated in poisonings for centuries, if not millennia. Epidemics of shellfish toxicity have been linked to the proliferation of dinoflagellates and other small marine organisms that are responsible for "red tides" or "blooms" in oceans around the world. The Bible refers to red tides in Exodus 7:20-21, where "the waters that were in the rivers were turned into blood, and the fish that was in the rivers died; and the river stank . . ." The Red Sea was so named by ancient Greeks for its red appearance in certain seasons when red tides occurred. Red tides are described in the *Iliad* and were first recognized by North American Indians as luminescence or "flickering" of ocean waves.[65]

The first published description in the western world of a patient with clinical findings suggestive of paralytic shellfish toxicity probably dates back to 1689. An article from a French journal named *Ephemeredes des curieux de la nature* described a young woman who had ingested mussels.[82,172] The description notes that her symptoms included fever, chest pain, respiratory insufficiency, nausea, seizures, and tachycardia. She had emesis induced, bringing up the mussels, and eventually recovered. For years after this report, the incidence and cause of paralytic shellfish toxicity were undocumented throughout the world, but epidemics were known to occur in certain seasons and under certain conditions. Improvements in monitoring and public health reporting have demonstrated patterns of occurrence. Gessner[149] described 54 outbreaks of paralytic shellfish poisoning (PSP) in Alaska occurring in 117 individuals between 1973 and 1992. The California Paralytic Shellfish Poisoning Prevention Program has been so successful that it has been used as a model of surveillance for many other countries.[322] PSP has been a reportable condition in California since 1927, with more than 500 cases and 30 deaths reported since that time. In California there is an annual 6-month quarantine (May through October) on mussels, clams, and oysters of local harvest.

Several types of neurologic diseases occur after ingestion of shellfish. PSP is one of the most common. This syndrome is most frequently reported during the summer months when water temperature is highest but has been recorded from May to November.[160,172] Some authors suggest that the toxin responsible for paralytic shellfish poisoning may be of significant concentration in some shellfish, such as the Alaska butter clam, in some areas year round, and that shellfish harvested from untested areas of these regions never be consumed.[149] The most commonly implicated varieties of shellfish include mussels, clams, oysters, and scallops.[149,172]

Pathophysiology. The unicellular (*Protogonyaulax* is 0.03 mm in diameter) phytoplankton (phylum Protozoa, class Mastigophora, order Dinoflagellata) is the foundation of the ocean food chain, and in warm summer months these organisms are noted to "bloom" rapidly in nutrient-rich coastal temperate and semitropical waters. They rank second in abundance to diatoms and are extremely important producers of marine carbohydrates, fats, and proteins. Typical species include *Alexandrium* species and *Gymnodinium catenatum*.

Dinoflagellates produce a number of toxins, the most commonly identified of which is saxitoxin. If a single organism predominates, it can discolor the water, creating a black, blue, pink, red, yellow, brown, or luminescent "tide."[88] Organisms can multiply rapidly from a concentration of 20,000 per liter to over 20,000,000 per liter. These plankton can release massive amounts of toxic metabolites into the water, at times leading rapidly to enormous mortality in various bird and marine populations, including large mammals such as dolphins and even whales. Large numbers of dead animals on the beach suggest a colored tide. The trend to increased numbers and magnitude of blooms is attributed empirically to many factors, including coastal development, dumping of sewage, fertilizer runoff, and ocean warming. Kills by the dinoflagellate *Ptychodiscus* (formerly *Gymnodinium*) *breve* are estimated at 100 tons of fish per day. The problem is increasing remarkably in Europe.[431]

A limited number out of approximately 1200 species of dinoflagellates have been implicated in human toxic syndromes.[349] PSP has been linked to the dinoflagellate *Protogonyaulax*, species *catanella* (U.S. Pacific coast) and species *tamarensis* var. *excavata* (U.S. Atlantic coast and Europe).[272,406] In northwestern Spain, the organism that generates the toxins causing this syndrome is *Gymnodinium catenatum*. These creatures are relatively fastidious and prefer warm, sunlit water of low salinity in which to bloom. Some algal organisms may release their toxin in the form of microscopic cysts, which can overwinter at the sediment-water interface. In mollusks, the greatest concentration of toxin is found in the digestive organs (dark "hepatopancreas"), gills, and siphon.[362] Toxic benthic dinoflagellate cysts may be transported by dredging operations and potentially introduce a dinoflagellate population into a new region.[468]

Although the origin of PSP toxins is assumed to be dinoflagellates, the toxins have been isolated in both marine and freshwater bivalves that are not associated with dinoflagellates. It has not been determined how this has occurred.[302] The bacterium *Moraxella* isolated from *Protogonyaulax tamarensis* has been shown to produce PSP toxins in culture. Toxin production can increase in nutritionally deficient environments.[231] The paralytic shellfish toxins identified to date are 18 related tetrahydropurine compounds produced mainly by the dinoflagellates of the genus *Alexandrium*. The best characterized is saxitoxin. Saxitoxin ($C_{10}H_{17}N_7O_4$) takes its name from *Saxidomus giganteus*, the Alaskan butter clam. *Ptychodiscus breve* is a toxic dinoflagellate

that produces a milder toxin. Other dinoflagellates considered poisonous to animals or humans include *Gonyaulax acatenella*, *Pyrodinium phoneus*, *Pyrodinium bahamense* var. *compressa*, *Gonyaulax monilata*, *Gonyaulax polyhedra*, *Gymnodinium veneficum*, and *Exuviaella ariaelebouriae*.[308] The taxonomic differentiation of *Protogonyaulax* from *Gonyaulax* species has only recently been appreciated, as has the relationship to the genus *Gessnerium*.[406] *S. giganteus* and the Washington clam (*S. nutalli*) may carry the toxin in their neck parts for up to 2 years; however, no physical characteristic distinguishes a carrier animal.

Unfortunately, a direct human serum assay to identify the toxin responsible for PSP is not as yet readily available to the clinician. Paralytic shellfish poison is assessed in foodstuff using the mouse bioassay, in which a 20-g mouse is injected with 1 ml of an acid extract of the shellfish, and the time taken for the animal to die is recorded. One mouse unit (mu) or 0.18 mg is the amount of injected saxitoxin that kills a test mouse in 15 minutes.[431] In most countries the action level for closure of a fishery is 400 mu/100 g shellfish. Polyclonal enzyme-linked immunosorbent assays (ELISAs) that measure saxitoxin, neosaxitoxin, and gonyautoxins 1 and 3 may be refined soon as reasonable screening techniques. Other testing methods under investigation include a sodium channel blocking assay, spectrometry, thin-layer chromatography, and HPLC. An automated tissue culture (neuroblastoma cell) bioassay may become a valid alternative to live animal testing.[207]

Saxitoxin and related compounds are water-soluble and heat- and acid-stable. Twelve derivatives of saxitoxin (such as neosaxitoxin) that originate from dinoflagellates of the genus *Protogonyaulax* are formed by the addition to saxitoxin of N-1-hydroxyl, 11-hydroxysulfate, and 21-sulfo groups.[171] Like tetrodotoxin, they can be destroyed to a certain extent in an alkaline medium but not by ordinary cooking. Saxitoxin acts by blocking sodium channels in nerve and muscle cells.[127,216] Inhibition of sodium flow in these cells arrests impulse conduction along neurons. In addition, saxitoxin may suppress atrioventricular nodal conduction, directly depress the medullary respiration center, and progressively reduce peripheral nerve excitability. Because of the similarity of the clinical syndrome to tetrodotoxin poisoning, it has been inferred that the same receptors may be blocked. Although the illness-causing levels for humans are not definitively known, it has been suggested that ingestion of 200 to 500 μg would cause at least mild symptoms, 500 to 2000 μg moderate illness, and more than 2000 μg serious or fatal illness. However, serious symptoms have been reported after ingestion of less than 100 μg of saxitoxin in adults. During peak red tide seasons, mussels may accumulate up to 50,000 mu each of saxitoxin. Muscle concentrations of saxitoxin have been recorded to be too high for consumption when seawater dinoflagellate counts are as few as 200/ml.[362] A saxitoxin concentration of greater than 75 to 80 μg/100 g foodstuff is considered hazardous to humans. In the 1972 New England red tide, the concentration of saxitoxin in blue mussels exceeded 9000 μg/100 g foodstuff. More recently, after cases of paralytic shellfish poisoning in Massachusetts, saxitoxin concentrations of 24,400 μg/100 g were recorded in raw mussels. With oral ingestion of saxitoxin, the LD_{50} for mice is 263 μg/kg. It has been estimated that as little as 0.5 to 1 mg of saxitoxin can be fatal in humans.[362]

Neither steaming nor cooking affects the potency of the toxin. Commercial processing of shellfish does not eliminate the toxin or the potential for toxicity; therefore public health agencies in the United States and Canada strictly monitor these canning industries.

Clinical Presentation. The onset of symptoms of paralytic shellfish poisoning is rapid. Within 30 to 60 minutes of ingesting toxic shellfish, victims complain of paresthesias, numbness, vertigo, and tingling of the face, tongue, and lips. Cranial nerve dysfunction, including dysarthria, dysphonia, dysphagia, and even blindness, can occur.[149,172,193,272] Other early symptoms include lightheadedness, "floating," ataxia, weakness, hyperreflexia, incoherence, sialorrhea, thirst, abdominal pain, nystagmus, dysmetria, headache, diaphoresis, a sensation of loose teeth, chest pain, and tachycardia. Neurologic symptoms progress to involve the extremities and trunk over the first 1 to 2 hours. Weakness of the limbs may begin anytime after the sensory changes, and gradually progresses to ataxia, inability to use the extremities, and finally paralysis. Reflexes are frequently normal throughout progression of the disease, and patients remain awake and alert. Death results from respiratory failure with diaphragmatic and chest wall muscle paralysis.

Although some victims have nausea, vomiting, or diarrhea, the lack of gastroenteritis and thus early self-decontamination may in part explain why mortality from paralytic shellfish poisoning approaches 25% in some older series.[27] More recent reports cite a lower incidence of fatalities, likely resulting from improvements in respiratory care. Hypotension can result from direct action of the compound on vascular smooth muscle.[216] Toxicity is never delayed more that 10 to 12 hours, with a median onset of 3 hours. Prognosis is good for individuals surviving past 12 hours, but weakness can persist for weeks after recovery. Children seem to be more sensitive to saxitoxins than adults, based on mortality figures from recent outbreaks. In milder cases, alcohol ingestion appears to increase toxicity.

Treatment. There are currently no antidotes for saxitoxin or paralytic shellfish poisoning. The victim should be closely observed in the hospital for at least 24 hours for respiratory insufficiency. Airway patency and respiratory support are of utmost importance, and even patients with severe symptoms of PSP often do well if expeditiously supported with mechanical ventilation. Although gastric emptying has been advocated by some authors when shellfish suspected of containing saxitoxin are ingested, airway loss can be rapid and emesis should *not* be attempted in most cases.[193] These toxins bind well to charcoal, and an oral dose of charcoal should be administered if this can be done safely.[328] Some authors suggest that atropine administration may worsen symptoms of paralytic shellfish poisoning and should be avoided since saxitoxin and its derivatives may have some antimuscarinic effects.[361] Several studies have also suggested that acidity may enhance the potency of saxitoxin, leading some authors to speculate that serum alkalinization might be of benefit to victims, although the efficacy of this practice has yet to be established.[8,183,268,310] Current research is directed at the development of polyclonal and monoclonal antibodies directed against saxitoxin and neosaxitoxin, for the purposes of diagnosis and therapy. Antivenin raised in rabbits against a saxitoxin-bovine serum albumin conjugate is curative in mice, but the product has not yet been used in humans.

At least one human case report and animal data have implied that dialysis or hemoperfusion may benefit some victims of severe PSP.[27,328] More recent reports are less optimistic and other in vitro trials have demonstrated that dialysis is not effective in removing saxitoxin.[119] Some authors have suggested enhancing renal clearance with diuresis, but again no study supports this practice. Maintaining urine output in normal quantities should suffice in most cases.

Prevention. The most important aspect of managing paralytic shellfish poisoning is prevention. Although leeching of shellfish in freshwater for several weeks followed by vigorous cooking may remove up to 70% of the toxin, such procedures are recommended only for persons stranded on desert islands. It has been said that one should not eat shellfish in the Northern Hemisphere in months that contain the letter "r." It has become more apparent with changing ocean conditions that shellfish in many parts of the world may be contaminated throughout the year resulting from high water concentrations of *Gonyaulax*. Because fin fish do not accumulate the toxins in their muscle tissue, there is no risk of PSP from their consumption.[446] Most coastal agencies monitor dinoflagellate concentrations off the shores of developed countries and restrict shellfish harvesting during high-risk periods. Many recent outbreaks of this illness have occurred on isolated islands where public health monitoring is infrequent and intensive care medicine resources scarce.

Neurotoxic Shellfish Poisoning

Ptychodiscus breve is a toxic dinoflagellate that can "bloom" and create a colorful tide. Ingestion of shellfish contaminated with *P. breve* can induce a milder version of paralytic shellfish poisoning, known as neurotoxic shellfish poisoning (NSP). The condition resembles ciguatera toxin poisoning in symptoms and does not have a major paralytic component. Death has not been reported in humans. Symptoms include circumoral paresthesias and paresthesias of the extremities, dizziness and ataxia, muscle aches, and gastrointestinal symptoms. The median incubation time is 3 hours; the illness lasts several hours to a few days.[285] Most NSP outbreaks have occurred on the Gulf of Mexico, the west coast of Florida, coastal Texas, North Carolina, and New Zealand.[285,380]

Unlike other shellfish poisons, NSP can cause a respiratory irritation syndrome. When large blooms of *P. breve* occur near the shoreline, wind and wave action can aerosolize the toxin; if sea breezes blow the aerosolized toxin onshore, rapidly reversible conjunctivitis, rhinorrhea, and bronchospasm with nonproductive cough can occur in sensitive individuals.[193] Severe respiratory distress is uncommon. The effects are similar to those of muscarinic stimulation.

P. breve produces at least 10 toxins, known as brevetoxins.[24,25] Brevetoxins (designated PbTx-1 to PbTx-10) are potent lipid-soluble cyclic polyether compounds that bind to and modulate voltage-gated sodium channel activity. Brevetoxins produce acute neuronal injury and death in rat cerebellar neurons.[38] In a canine model, brevetoxins produce depolarization of tracheal and bronchial smooth muscle.[334] Intratracheal brevetoxin instillation in rats resulted in systemic distribution of brevetoxin, which suggests that the initial respiratory irritation and bronchoconstriction may be only part of the toxicologic syndrome with brevetoxin inhalation.[36] The brevetoxins are potent ichthyotoxins and are associated with large numbers of dead birds, fish, and mammals. In 1996, 149 manatees died along the southwest Florida coast; brevetoxin was implicated as the primary etiology for the epizootic.[49] Signs and symptoms of intoxication in fish include violent twisting and corkscrew swimming, defecation and regurgitation, pectoral fin paralysis, caudal fin curvature, loss of equilibrium, quiescence, vasodilation, convulsions, and fatal respiratory failure.[25] An enzyme immunoassay has been developed to detect these brevetoxins, based on antibodies to PbTx-3.[422] A newer micellar electrokinetic capillary chromatography (MEKC) detection method allows measurement of brevetoxin at trace levels and is 100-fold better than previous chromatographic or electrophoretic methods.[365] Brevetoxin A has recently been synthesized and is now synthetically available, allowing for further biochemical studies.[300]

Diarrhetic Shellfish Illness

Ingestion of shellfish contaminated with the dinoflagellates belonging to the genus *Dinophysis* (*D. fortii*, *D. acuminata*, *D. norvegica*, and *D. acuta*) or *Prorocentrum* (*P. lima* and *P. minimum*) causes diarrhetic shellfish poisoning (DSP). The lipid-soluble toxins accumulate in shellfish fatty tissues and the hepatopancreas of mussels. They exert their effects mainly on the small intestine, leading to diarrhea and degenerative changes of the absorptive epithelium.[270,431] Symptoms include rapid onset (30 minutes to 2 hours) of diarrhea, nausea, vomiting, abdominal pain, and chills. Rarely, symptoms are delayed up to 12 hours. The syndrome is self-limited and resolves after 2 to 3 days. During the period 1976 to 1982, DSP was diagnosed in at least 1300 persons in Japan, particularly in the northeastern regions. The period of greatest toxicity appears to be May to August. In 1981, more than 5000 cases were reported in Spain.[466] Other outbreaks have occurred in the Netherlands and Chile.[176] In 1993, a particularly bad episode occurred in Spain with unusual symptoms; analyses revealed a complex toxin profile with both PSP and DSP toxins present.[144]

DSP toxins include okadaic acid (OA), OA diolester, dinophysistoxins (DTX-1 to DTX-4), pectenotoxins and yessotoxin.[21,267,429,451,466] OA was first isolated from a sponge in the Pacific (*Halichondria okadai*).[397] OA is a specific and potent inhibitor of protein synthesis and inhibits phosphatases A_1 and A_2 in vitro. OA induces diarrhea because of phosphorylation of proteins either controlling the sodium secretion of intestinal cells or influencing the permeability of cell membranes.[91,108] It is a potent tumor promoter in mouse cells and can act as a genotoxic.[131] Other DSP toxins exert various effects in experimental animals: pectenotoxins induce liver necrosis, and yessotoxins (from the Japanese scallop *Patinopecten yessoensis*) induce intracytoplasmic edema in cardiac muscle.[411,413] Minimum doses of OA and DTX-1 necessary to cause DSP symptoms are 40 µg and 36 µg, respectively.[178] Metals (e.g., aluminum, copper, lead, mercury, cadmium) in concentration ranges at or below acceptable levels in mussels synergistically increase the cytotoxicity of low concentrations of OA in cultured cells.[423]

Increasing incidences of phytoplankton blooms with the danger of toxin release have necessitated the search for new diagnostic methods that can detect toxin quickly and reliably. A variety of techniques, including a radioimmunoassay using antibodies raised in rabbits, a competitive ELISA, idiotypic anti-idiotypic competitive immunoassay, rapid tissue culture assays, and cytotoxicity assays, can identify the presence of OA.[84,94,248,366,427] A unified bioscreen for the detection of diarrhetic shellfish toxins and microcystins (as from cyanobacteria *Microcystis aeruginosa* blooms) uses capillary electrophoresis coupled with a liquid chromatography–linked protein phosphatase bioassay.[47] A protein phosphatase 2A inhibition assay has been shown to be rapid, accurate, and reproducible; it can detect concentrations as low as 0.063 ng/ml in aqueous solutions and 2 ng/g in mussel digestive glands.[426] The Japanese quarantine standard is 200 ng of OA per gram of shellfish tissue. Four times this amount of toxin has been identified recently in northeastern Pacific Ocean mussels.

Domoic Acid Intoxication

Domoic acid is an excitatory neurotransmitter first described in Japan in 1958 isolated from the red algae *Chondria armata*.[403] The first documented human outbreak of poisoning with this compound was in 1987 from Prince Edward Island, Canada, when more than 100 people became ill after ingesting cultured blue mussels, *Mytilus edulis*, later found to be contaminated with domoic acid.[316,408,460] Three of these individuals died, and the clinical description of persistent memory impairment in many survivors prompted the nickname of "amnestic shellfish poisoning."[134] The source of the toxin in these cases was found to be *Nitzschia pungens*, a pennate diatom that had been ingested by the mussels before human consumption.[31,392] The mussels concentrate the toxin in the hepatopancreas.

Epidemics of domoic acid poisoning have been more prominent in other marine life, especially sea birds.[445,457,458] A large number of dead and distressed pelicans and cormorants were noted in Monterey Bay, California, in September 1991.[457,458] Autopsies performed on the dead birds demonstrated they had consumed large quantities of anchovies from the bay. Subsequent testing showed the anchovies contained high levels of domoic acid. This was the first report documenting the presence of domoic acid in the United States. Further studies of mussels taken during the same period from Monterey Bay also revealed the presence of domoic acid.[445] Water samples taken in the area identified significant quantities of the diatom *Pseudonitzschia australis*, which when grown in a laboratory environment were able to produce domoic acid.[147,457] Three species of *Pseudonitzschia* are now known to produce domoic acid.

Domoic acid has also been detected in Gulf shellfish (Gulf coast oyster, *Crassostrea virginica*) and phytoplankton in the Gulf of Mexico, although no outbreaks of amnestic shellfish poisoning have been recorded in this region. The toxic *N. pungens* forma *multiseries* has also been confirmed in Korea; Japan; Oslofjord, Scandinavia; the northeastern and northwestern United States; eastern and western Canada; and eastern South America.[110]

In the fall of 1991, the latest reported epidemic of domoic acid poisoning occurred in Washington State.[224] Over 20 people who consumed razor clams were involved. Subsequent testing confirmed the presence of domoic acid in razor clams along the coasts of both Washington and Oregon, although mussels tested in these areas were virtually free of toxin. Dungeness crabs collected from these waters were also found contaminated with domoic acid.

Pathophysiology. After the 1987 epidemic of domoic acid poisoning, significant evaluation was undertaken of the surviving victims. Chemical analysis at various laboratories ruled out all other known toxic causes of the symptoms displayed by the patients.[460] Intraperitoneal injection of extracts of the implicated mussels into mice produced a syndrome characterized by reproducible scratching followed eventually by death.[316,408] The toxin was finally identified as domoic acid.

Domoic acid is a glutamate agonist. After its discovery in 1958, it was investigated for potential use as an antihelminthic in children in Japan at doses of about 0.6 mg/kg, significantly lower than that ingested by affected individuals in Canada.[460] Domoic acid has also been tested for its insecticidal properties with disappointing results.

Domoic acid is structurally related to kainic acid, a potent neurotoxic amino acid.[306,354,408,460] This group of compounds is excitatory and acts on three types of receptors in the central nervous system, with the hippocampus being the most sensitive. Domoic acid seems to work by activating kainate receptors in the brain more potently than kainic acid itself. The result of this stimulation is extensive damage to the hippocampus in victims of the poisoning, as well as less severe injury to portions of the thalamic and forebrain regions.[356,378,408]

It was estimated that mussels implicated in the Canadian outbreak of amnestic shellfish poisoning contained a total amount of domoic acid in excess of 6 kg, with most being concentrated in the digestive glands.[160,460] When the same toxic blue mussels were placed into tanks of clean water, they rapidly purged themselves of the toxin over several weeks. Other organisms known to produce domoic acid include the phytoplankton *Alsidium corallinum* and *Chondria armata*. Subsequent research suggests that other phytoplankton, such as *Amphora coffaeformis* can also produce domoic acid. Scientists continue to monitor shellfish and marine microorganisms to determine the presence of other sources.

Clinical Presentation. Rats injected with high concentrations of domoic acid develop hippocampal seizures and die within several days.[316] Surviving rats exhibit difficulty in remembering maze pathways they had previously encountered, signifying retrograde amnesia. In these same rats injected with domoic acid, prior maze learning skills are also not retained, suggesting an additional effect on anterograde memory.[316,408] These effects are similar to that of intraperitoneally injected kainic acid. Interestingly, pelicans reportedly poisoned by domoic acid containing anchovies in 1991 exhibited a similar "scratching behavior" demonstrated in laboratory rats after domoic acid injection.[294]

Humans involved in the Canadian epidemic of amnestic shellfish poisoning had initial symptoms of nausea, vomiting, abdominal cramps, and diarrhea 1 to 24 hours after ingestion.[316,408] Neurologic symptoms initiated by memory loss began within 48 hours after ingestion and progressed in some victims to seizures, hemiparesis, ophthalmoplegia, and coma. Some victims displayed purposeless grimacing and chewing. Follow-up neuropsychologic testing on affected patients displayed predominantly an anterograde memory disorder, with most other cognitive functions preserved.[316] The most severely affected individuals also had some retrograde amnesia. A labile blood pressure and cardiac arrhythmias were recorded in a few individuals. Elevations in blood urea nitrogen (BUN) and creatine phosphokinase were also noted in many victims and have been recorded in animals suffering domoic acid poisoning, possibly resulting from exertional myopathies or tremors.[316,458]

The onset of symptoms in victims of the Prince Edward Island epidemic ranged from 15 minutes to 38 hours, with the average approaching 5 hours.[316,408] Most fatalities occurred in the oldest victims, with postmortem findings suggesting neuronal loss or necrosis, accompanied by astrocytosis.[316] The most severe damage was to the hippocampus and amygdala areas. Lesions were also noted in the claustrum, septal, and olfactory regions. No lesions were found in the motor nuclei of the brainstem. Hippocampal lesions in victims at autopsy resembled those seen in the brains of animals injected with kainic acid.[316,356,378] A follow-up study done on patients from the Montreal area suggested that bronchial secretions became so profuse in the hours after mussel ingestion that half of the severely affected individuals required endotracheal intubation.[316] Pupillary dilation or constriction and piloerection were also common findings. Approximately 10% of the involved patients demonstrated either persistent memory loss or other neuropathies. Of those patients exhibiting neurologic toxicity, maximal effects were noted within the first 3 days of mussel ingestion, and maximal improvement in the neurotoxicity occurred in 24 hours to 12 weeks after ingestion.

Treatment. As with most other shellfish toxins, no antidote exists for amnestic shellfish poisoning. Based on the alleged mechanism of action of both domoic and kainic acid, it is possible that benzodiazepines may be beneficial in controlling some of the excessive hippocampal activity and seizures.[306,458] Animal studies have suggested a lowered mortality in groups in which benzodiazepines are used after domoic acid exposure. Government agencies continue to observe coastal areas for outbreaks of domoic acid toxicity and for the presence of phytoplankton known to produce the compound. "Blooms" of organisms such as *Nitzschia pungens* and *Pseudonitzschia australis* are closely monitored and reported.

Pfiesteria Syndrome

Pfiesteria piscicida is a toxic dinoflagellate that inhabits estuarine and coastal waters of the eastern United States and has been associated with fish kills and human illness. Since 1991, *P. piscicida* and other *Pfiesteria*-like species have been implicated in massive fish kills in estuaries of North Carolina, Maryland, and Chesapeake Bay.[156,162,370] *P. piscicida* is responsible for a fish disease formally known as *ulcerative mycosis*. *Pfiesteria* is primarily a benthic organism but can exist in at least 24 different life stages. When fish swim into an area with *Pfiesteria*, toxin is produced by the dinoflagellate. These fish develop characteristic ulcerative lesions and erratic swimming behavior. *Pfiesteria* have now been found in coastal waterways extending from Delaware to the Gulf Coast of Alabama.

The first report of adverse health effects in humans was described after accidental laboratory exposure in which investigators working with *Pfiesteria* developed respiratory and eye irritation, skin rashes, and cognitive and personality changes.[156] During the 1990s, commercial fishermen who were exposed to waterways with *Pfiesteria* species reported similar symptoms.[162,164,165,370] The route of exposure is unknown, although it is thought to be either by prolonged direct skin contact with toxin-laden water or via aerosols after breathing the air over areas where fish are dying from toxic *Pfiesteria*.

Individuals with high exposure complain of headache, skin lesions, skin burning on contact with water, eye irritation, upper respiratory irritation, muscle cramps, and neuropsychologic symptoms, including increased forgetfulness and difficulties with learning and higher cognitive function.[164] No consistent physical findings or laboratory abnormalities have been found. When skin lesions appear, they are erythematous, edematous papules on the trunk or extremities and resolve within a few days to a week after exposure. Thorough neuropsychologic testing has documented deficits in higher cognitive function and learning and functional memory.[164] The severity of the cognitive dysfunction was directly related to the degree of exposure. The exact nature of the neurocognitive deficit is unknown; however, rats exposed to water containing *Pfiesteria* toxins have shown significant learning impairments.[246,247] Deficits may be expected to improve significantly within 3 to 6 months after cessation of exposure to affected waters. The natural history of *Pfiesteria* syndrome is improvement in most symptoms without treatment; however, cholestyramine has been successfully used in five patients with persistent symptoms.[371]

Diagnosis of *Pfiesteria* syndrome is difficult because the specific toxins at fault have not yet been identified and a biomarker of exposure has not been developed. Current recommendations for diagnosis include (1) developing symptoms within 2 weeks after exposure to estuarine water, (2) memory loss or confusion of any duration and/or three or more symptoms from the complex as described above, and (3) no other cause for symptoms identified.[76] Currently, a multiplex PCR is being developed for rapid identification of *P. piscicida* and other toxic *Pfiesteria* species.[282] *Pfiesteria* syndrome is not infectious and has not been associated with eating fish or shellfish caught in waters where *P. piscicida* has been found. No deaths have been associated with exposure to *Pfiesteria* species. People should avoid areas with large numbers of diseased, dying, or dead fish.

Haff Disease

Haff disease is a syndrome characterized by severe muscle pain and rhabdomyolysis after consuming fish; it was first described in 1924 around the shores of the Bay of Konigsburg Haff on the Baltic Sea.[474] Further outbreaks have occurred in Sweden and Russia.[37,372,381] Twelve cases have been reported in the United States; all have been associated with eating buffalo fish (*Ictiobus cyprinellus*), a bottom-feeding species found in the Mississippi River and its tributaries. Haff disease is most likely the result of a heat-stable toxin in blue-green algae that is eaten by fish; however, the toxin is unidentified.[74]

Haff disease presents as generalized muscle pain and tenderness, rigidity, weakness, and rhabdomyolysis. Tachycardia, hypertension, tachypnea, and a drop in temperature can also occur. Elevated serum creatine kinase occurs with leukocytosis, myoglobinuria, and elevation of lactate dehydrogenase and other muscle enzymes. Symptoms generally appear approximately 18 hours after eating fish (range: 6-21 hours).[74] Pathologically, there is neuromyodystrophy with necrosis in motor neurons of the brain and spine, coagulation necrosis of muscle, and myoglobinuric nephrosis. Treatment includes large volumes of intravenous fluids and diuretics to prevent renal failure from myoglobin toxicity. Diagnosis is based on clinical presentation, laboratory data, and food history.

Blue-Green Algae

Blue-green algae are worldwide freshwater cyanobacteria that may proliferate rapidly in a bloom, discoloring the surface of the water and spoiling its odor and taste. Terrestrial, fresh, brackish, and sea-water cyanobacteria produce toxins that cause acute and chronic hazards to human and animal health and are responsible for isolated, sporadic animal fatalities each year. Typical algal species include *Microcystis aeruginosa*, *Anabaena flos-aquae*, *Nodularia spumigena*, *Nostoc*, *Oscillatoria agardhii*, and *Aphanizomenon flos-aquae*.[90,126,295,343]

During conditions of a bloom (warm stagnant water, frequently enhanced by phosphorus and nitrogen fertilizers), the toxins are concentrated to a degree to become a significant hazard to wild and domestic animals and have been responsible for the death of livestock and dogs.[90,122,181,297,432] In most species of toxic cyanobacteria, the toxins are cyclic heptapeptides called microcystins, or cyanoginosins. More than 60 cyanobacterial toxins have been isolated from blue-green algae.[90,376] The toxins are of multiple configurations and include alkaloids, polypeptides, and lipopolysaccharides (endotoxins).[386]

Anatoxin-a and homoanatoxin-a are potent nicotinic agonists that act as postsynaptic, depolarizing neuromuscular blocking agents. These toxins along with saxitoxin cause animals to collapse quickly from neuromuscular paralysis, with features of staggering, muscle fasciculations, gasping, and convulsions.[180] Anatoxin-a(s) is an anticholinesterase that causes demonstrable cholinergic toxicity in animals.[64,180] Anatoxin-a and anatoxin-a(s) are both derived from *Anabaena flos-aquae*. Nodularins and microcystins cause hepatotoxicosis. Cylindrospermopsin is a protein synthesis inhibitor and induces necrotic tissue injury of multiple organs. Cyanobacterial lipopolysaccharide endotoxins are responsible for gastroenteritis and skin irritations.[90] In mice, administration of microcystin-LR causes rapid hepatocellular necrosis with hemorrhagic shock.[98,415]

Human exposure to blue-green algae blooms has resulted in allergic reactions, skin irritations, gastroenteritis, pulmonary consolidation, and liver damage.[90,317] A person who swims through a bloom may suffer local effects, such as conjunctivitis, facial swelling, or papulovesicular dermatitis. Ingestion of contaminated water causes a dysenteric diarrhea, with green slimy stools. This may or may not be associated with elevation of γ-glutamyl-transpeptidase and alanine aminotransferase. Inhalation of toxins is a likely exposure route; microcystin-LR and anatoxin-a cause significant toxicity in mice via intranasal aerosol exposure.[134]

In 1996, more than 50 people died at a hemodialysis clinic in Brazil with associated liver damage. Microcystins are thought to have been present in the water used for hemodialysis.[90,117]

Treatment is supportive in humans and animals. Recently, cyclosporine A has been shown to inhibit the fatal effects of microcystins administered to mice. In humans, no special treatment is recommended other than fluid and electrolyte supplementation as needed, since all related afflictions appear to be self-limited.

OTHER SHELLFISH AND INVERTEBRATE POISONINGS

Callistin Shellfish Poisoning

The Japanese *Callista* clam (*C. brevisiphonata*) is toxic during the spawning months of May to September, at which time cholinergic compounds in the ovaries are increased. The intoxication resembles cholinergic crisis, with both muscarinic and nicotinic components. Within an hour of ingestion of the heat-stable toxin, generalized pruritus, urticaria, erythema, facial numbness and paralysis, hypersalivation, diaphoresis, fever, chills, nausea, vomiting, diarrhea, bronchorrhea, bronchospasm, and constrictive dyspnea develop.[28] Therapy is supportive, and recovery is usually complete within 2 days. In severe cases of cholinergic crisis, particularly with marked bradycardia, atropine (0.5 mg intravenously every 5 minutes to a total dose of 2 mg) may be administered.

Venerupin Shellfish Poisoning

The Japanese lake-harvested oyster (*Crassostrea gigas*) and clam (*Tapes semidecussata*) occasionally feed on toxic dinoflagellate species of the genus *Prorocentrum*, posing the greatest risk during the months of December through April.[28,175] The heat-stable toxin induces the rapid onset of gastrointestinal distress, headache, and nervousness, which are followed over 48 hours by hepatic dysfunction, manifested by elevation of liver enzymes, leukocytosis, jaundice, and profound coagulation defects. Delirium and coma may ensue, with death occurring in 33% of victims. Therapy is supportive and based on symptoms. Any victim who shows the early symptoms of gastroenteritis should be placed on a low-protein diet and observed for 48 to 72 hours for signs of liver failure. There is not yet clinical experience with exchange transfusion, chemotherapy, hemoperfusion, or liver transplantation in the management of profound liver failure associated with this disorder.

Tridacna Clam Poisoning

Giant clams of the species *Tridacna maxima* are eaten in French Polynesia.[28] This species can cause a poisoning characterized by nausea, vomiting, diarrhea, paresthesias, tremor, and ataxia. Severe cases can be fatal. The toxin appears to be concentrated in the mantle and viscera of the clam. Therapy is supportive.

Whelk Poisoning

In Japan, poisoning has followed ingestion of mollusks of the genera *Neptunea, Buccinum,* and *Fusitriton* (whelks, or ivory shells). The toxin is located in the salivary glands and has been characterized as tetramine.[12] Tetramine (trimethylammonium) is a naturally occurring quaternary ammonium compound that has been identified in anemones, gorgonians, jellyfishes, and mollusks.[11] Symptoms include headache, dizziness, nausea, vomiting, blurred vision, and dry mouth. No fatalities have been reported. Therapy is supportive.[28]

Ivory Shell Poisoning

Human intoxications have followed consumption of the ivory shell, *Babylonia japonica,* which is widely distributed along the coastline of Japan. The toxin, surugatoxin, located in the midgut of the animal, is reputed to be produced by a gram-negative bacterium on which the snail feeds. Surugatoxin and IS-toxin appear to have autonomic ganglionic blocking action. Symptoms include abdominal pain, diarrhea, nausea, vomiting, oral paresthesias, syncope, and seizures.[176] Tetrodotoxin has been identified in *B. japonica.*

Abalone Poisoning

Abalone poisoning follows ingestion of the viscera of certain Japanese abalone (tsunowata, or tochiri), particularly from the Island of Hokkaido, where *Haliotis discus* and *Haliotis sieboldi* are found. Symptoms include severe urticaria, erythema, pruritus, edema, and skin ulceration. The reaction appears to be of a photosensitive nature, since the lesions are confined to areas of ultraviolet exposure. The toxin may be derived from chlorophyll contained in the seaweeds on which the abalone feed.[28] Therapy is supportive.

Cephalopod Poisoning

In certain areas of Japan, intoxications have resulted from ingestion of squid and octopus. Symptoms develop within 10 to 20 hours and consist of nausea, vomiting, diarrhea, abdominal pain, headache, weakness, paralysis, and seizures. Although most victims recover within 48 hours, deaths have occurred.[28] Therapy is supportive.

Sea Cucumber Poisoning

Sea cucumbers are eaten throughout Asia and in some Pacific islands, where they are known as trepang, sea slugs, cucumbers, erico, or hai shen. Gastroenteritis is induced by saponins of the triterpinoid variety, such as holothurin. The disorder consists chiefly of abdominal pain, nausea, and diarrhea and is self-limited.

Sea Hare Poisoning

Sea hares are marine gastropod mollusks prevalent in certain South Pacific waters, including Fiji. *Aplysia* species have been considered to be toxic since Roman times. *A. juliana* secretes an antibacterial and antineoplastic protein found in the water-soluble fraction of a fetid secretion lethal to crabs. Human poisoning has been reported after ingestion of *Dolabella auricularia* ("veata").[347,384] The symptoms began approximately 30 minutes after eating and included prickling skin sensation, vomiting, diarrhea, shaking, tremors, fasciculations, arthralgias, dyspnea, visual disorientation, altered sensorium, and fever. The course of illness exceeded a week. It has been suggested that sea hare poisoning in humans might be a form of subacute organobromine intoxication.

Ingestion of the sea hare *A. kurodai* was associated with acute liver damage with sustained elevations of aminotransferases. Microscopic findings in a liver biopsy specimen revealed characteristic apoptotic hepatocytes accompanied by mitotic hepatocytes. Bioactive substances in the sea hare might induce such apoptosis of hepatocytes in the liver.[348]

Anemone Poisoning

In the South Pacific, ingestion of the green or brown anemones *Radianthus paumotensis* or *Rhodactis howesii* (*mata-malu samasama*) has been associated with severe illness and death. Accidental deaths generally involve small children, whereas adults may be the unfortunate recipients of improperly cooked anemone or even be intentionally stricken in acts of suicide. The toxic substances are found in the nematocysts and the tentacular tissues. Anemones have been used for criminal purposes in the South Pacific.[28] *Physiobranchia douglasi* is poisonous eaten raw but is reputedly safe if cooked.[176]

Ingestion of the raw anemone induces altered mental status within 30 minutes, often immediately after the ingestion. The victim becomes agitated or confused, delirious, and then comatose. Other symptoms reported include fever, seizures, myalgias, abdominal pain, respiratory failure, hypotension, and death. Contact with the skin, particularly mucous membranes, is extremely painful with rapid inflammation and vesiculation.

Treatment is symptomatic and supportive. Because of the rapid onset in symptoms the rescuer must be prepared to provide advanced life support within the first hour after ingestion.

A toxic protein has been isolated from the sea anemone *Urticina piscivora*. It is a potent cardiac stimulatory protein and a potent hemolysin on erythrocytes of rat, guinea pig, dog, pig, and human, causing toxicity as low as 10^{-10} M.[89]

Crab Poisoning

Human intoxications have followed ingestion of crabs in many Indo-Pacific islands. Most of the toxic crab species are members of the family Xanthidae and include the genera *Demania, Carpilius, Atergatis, Platypodia, Zosimus, Lophozozymus,* and *Eriphia*. Clinical symptoms develop 15 minutes to several hours after ingestion and include nausea, vomiting, diarrhea, perioral and extremity paresthesias, ataxia, aphasia, respiratory distress, altered mental status, coma, and rapid death.

A number of toxins have been isolated from crab species, and there is a marked similarity to PSP and TTX poisoning. Saxitoxin, neosaxitoxin, and gonyautoxins have been isolated from crab species in Okinawa and from *Eriphia sebana* and *Atergatis floridus* off Australian coral reefs.[257-260] Tetrodotoxin and palytoxin have also been characterized from poisonous crabs.[7] Tetrodotoxin was responsible for an epidemic of 71 persons with 2 deaths in Thailand who ate the toxic eggs of the horseshoe crab *Carcinoscorpius rotundicauda*.[214] The poisonous mosaic crab *Lophozozymus pictor* from the Indo-West Pacific region has caused several fatalities in the Philippines and Singapore. The toxins were concentrated in the gut and hepatopancreas, whereas the muscle was less toxic. Captive crabs lose toxicity such that it almost completely gone by 24 days.

Coconut crab (*Birgus latro*) poisoning is manifested as nausea, vomiting, headache, chills, myalgias, and exhaustion, with occasional deaths. Asiatic horseshoe crabs (*Carcinoscorpius rotundicauda*) are eaten in Thailand, where they cause mimi poisoning. Symptoms include nausea, vomiting, diarrhea, abdominal cramps, dizziness, palpitations, weakness, lower extremity paresthesias, aphonia, perioral burning, pharyngitis, sialorrhea, syncope, paralysis, and death. Again, the toxin appears highly similar to saxitoxin.[81]

Crab lung has followed the aspiration of tiny fragments of North American blue crab shells into the lung, necessitating removal with fiberoptic bronchoscopy. The diagnosis of occult aspiration should be considered in anyone with an unexplained cough who has recently consumed cracked crab, particularly while intoxicated.

Freshwater crabs are a potential source of human paragonimiasis, a parasitic disease that was prevalent in Asia until the 1960s.[85] Paragonimiasis usually causes pulmonary disease with a productive cough and bloody sputum. Central nervous system involvement has also been reported.[323] The disease is contracted by eating raw crab infected with the metacercariae of *Paragonimus* species. Areas known to be endemic are Vietnam, China, Japan, Korea, Equador, and Liberia.*

BACTERIAL AND VIRAL PATHOGENS IN SEAFOOD

Bacterial and viral contamination of shellfish, particularly bivalve mollusks, is implicated more than any other marine animal in seafood-related human illness.[256] As filter feeders, bivalve mollusks filter large quantities of water unselectively to gather plankton and extract oxygen, which allows concentration of bacteria and viruses (along with biologic toxins, pesticides, industrial chemicals, radioactive wastes, toxic metals, and hydrocarbons). They are sessile invertebrates that generally inhabit shallow waters close to shore and pol-

---

*References 6, 85, 96, 296, 323, 346, 437.

lution sources. Standard depuration in purified (with ultraviolet light or ozone) water for 48 to 72 hours may not significantly reduce these contaminants, nor does it appear to remove viruses.[209,353] Disease and deaths resulting from viruses and naturally occurring bacteria are now of greatest concern because they are the most common causative agent. The greatest risk of death caused by consumption of raw shellfish is among people with underlying health conditions.

Bacteria Associated with Fecal Contamination

Bacterial pathogens associated with fecal contamination have accounted for only 4% of the shellfish associated gastroenteritis outbreaks in the United States.[336] Important bacteria include *Salmonella, Shigella, Campylobacter, Yersina, Listeria, Clostridium, Staphylococcus,* and *Escherichia coli.*[200] The incidence of enteric bacteria in seafood has greatly reduced with the development of surveillance programs and standards to minimize fecal contamination.[336] However, infections continue to occur in other parts of the world.

Salmonella typhi was the most common cause of bacteria-associated shellfish disease until the 1950s. The incidence of *S. typhi* in shellfish has dramatically declined and the risk of infection in the United States is very low.[336,450] However, *S. typhi* is still responsible for outbreaks of illness in other countries.[390,391] Nontyphoidal *Salmonella* species, including *S. paratyphi* and *S. enteritidis,* have been detected in shrimp and bivalves. Eight *Salmonella* shellfish infections were reported in the United States between 1984 and 1993, and *S. enteritidis* phage type 19 was responsible for a recent outbreak of infections from cockles in the United Kingdom.[166,452] *Shigella* was responsible for 111 shellfish cases and 4 outbreaks in the United States.[336] *Shigella* has a low infectious dose and long survival time in clams and oysters.

Campylobacter species have been isolated from shellfish; however, their role in seafood infections is not known.[450] *Listeria monocytogenes* has been identified in high rates in isolates from fresh and processed fish and shellfish.[199] Listeria seafood-borne infections are probably underreported in the United States. *Yersinia enterocolitica* has also been identified in fish and shellfish; however, most *Yersinia* infections are not associated with seafood.[200,336] *Escherichia coli* has not been an important source of seafood-related illness, although *E. coli* is found in shellfish.[57]

Viruses Associated with Fecal Contamination

Most infections associated with consumption of shellfish are viral in origin. Over 120 enteric viruses can be found in human sewage. These viruses can produce a variety of symptoms, including gastroenteritis, meningitis, paralysis, myocarditis, and hepatitis. Compared with other food-borne illnesses, those caused by viruses are less severe and seldom fatal. Viruses that have been isolated from seafood include hepatitis (A, non-A, and non-B), enteroviruses (echovirus, poliovirus, coxsackie A and B), adenoviruses, rotaviruses, and small round viruses (Norwalk, calicivirus, Snow Mountain agent, and small rounded structured viruses [SRSV]).

Harvest areas are surveyed and closed for fecal contamination. However, the relative absence of fecal coliform bacteria in areas of shellfish harvesting does not indicate freedom from viral contamination. Recent outbreaks of Norwalk virus and calicivirus were due to oyster harvesters discharging their sewage overboard.[72] In addition, shellfish depuration processes that eliminate bacteria do not necessarily remove viral contaminants.[353] Steamed clams probably pose a significant risk because household cooking techniques are often insufficient to kill viruses. Although it takes 4 to 6 minutes of pressure-cooker steaming for the internal temperature of soft-shell clams ("steamers") to reach 100° to 106° C (212° to 222.8° F), it requires only 60 seconds for the shells to open, at which point they may appear cooked.[223] Poliovirus can survive (7% to 13%) in oysters that are steamed, fried, baked, or stewed.[112]

New methods using PCR amplification of target viral genomes provide a rapid, specific, and sensitive test for detection of viruses. The amplification of viral ribonucleic acid (RNA), DNA, and complementary DNA (cDNA) has shown a high prevalence of human viruses that would not be detected by the use of classical techniques.[318] PCR has been used to detect the presence of hepatitis A virus in oysters and scallops during an outbreak and SRSV, adenovirus, enterovirus, and Norwalk virus in shellfish.*

Hepatitis Viruses. Oysters, mussels, and clams harvested from raw sewage contaminated waters are the most frequent cause of food-borne viral hepatitis A. Often there is a long incubation period of 2 to 8 weeks, so it is common for hepatitis A to occur 3 to 4 weeks after gastroenteritis following consumption of shellfish.[336] Symptoms include fever, jaundice, nausea, and abdominal pain, whereas diarrhea is rare. Treatment is supportive.[42]

Enteroviruses. Enteroviruses are commonly isolated from marine water and shellfish. In the United States, up to 63% of shellfish in areas closed for harvesting, and up to 40% of shellfish in areas open for harvesting were positive for enteroviruses.[339] In contaminated waters in Venezuela, 40% of harvested shrimp contained enteroviruses.[50] Enterovirus outbreaks have not been characterized, and the impact of enteroviruses on public health is not fully appreciated.[256]

---

*References 15, 16, 18, 95, 243, 318, 353.

Small Round Viruses. Small round viruses include Norwalk virus, calicivirus, Snow Mountain agent, and SRSV. These viruses are a major cause of shellfish-associated gastroenteritis.* Caliciviruses are small, single-stranded RNA and have been responsible for a number of oyster-related gastroenteritis outbreaks in Louisiana.[72,77] Norwalk virus has been located both in and outside the shellfish alimentary tract and is poorly depurated using conditions favorable for *E. coli* depuration. Reverse transcription PCR (RT-PCR) assay can easily detect Norwalk virus in contaminated water, shellfish, and stool from infected people.[233,353] The virus may be excreted in the feces of food handlers and harvesters for 48 hours after recovery from the infection.[43] Symptoms including nausea, vomiting, fever, abdominal cramps, and nonbloody diarrhea appear 24 to 48 hours after ingesting contaminated shellfish and resolve over 1 to 2 days. Antibodies to Norwalk virus have been measured in serum of patients with gastroenteritis, and electron microscopy or RT-PCR can detect virus in stool.[233] Treatment is supportive, and complications are rare.

Vibrio Poisoning and Septicemia

Over the last few decades, naturally occurring bacteria are becoming a more important cause of shellfish illness, particularly the bacteria belonging to the family Vibrionaceae. *Vibrio* organisms can cause gastroenteric disease and soft tissue infections, which can lead to bacteremia and death, particularly in immunocompromised hosts, after the consumption of raw shellfish. Between 1988 and 1996, 422 infections from *Vibrio vulnificus* were reported to the CDC; 61% of patients with primary septicemia died.[363]

Vibrio species are the most potentially virulent halophilic organisms that flourish in the marine environment. In general, they are not associated with fecal contamination, hence surveillance methods as mentioned above for bacteria and viruses do not correlate with the presence of *Vibrio*. *Vibrio* species proliferate in warmer water; infections seem to cluster during the summer months, which may be related to increased numbers of people at the seashore.[280] *Vibrio* species are mesophilic organisms and grow best at temperatures of 24° to 40° C (75.2° to 104° F), with essentially no growth below 8° to 10° C (46.4° to 50° F).[57] *Vibrio* species can grow in brackish waters and require less sodium for maximal growth than do other more fastidious marine organisms, a factor that allows explosive reproduction in the 0.9% saline environment of the human body. *V. parahaemolyticus* has also been identified in freshwater habitats.[20]

Gastrointestinal illness has been associated with *V. cholerae* 0 group 1, non-01, *V. parahaemolyticus, V. flu-*vialis, *V. mimicus, V. hollisae, V. furnissii, V. alginolyticus,* and *V. vulnificus.** Septicemia, with or without an obvious source, has been attributed to infections with *V. cholerae* non-01, *V. parahaemolyticus, V. alginolyticus, V. vulnificus, V. hollisa,* and *V. metschnikovii.*†

Whenever a *Vibrio* species is suspected, the microbiology laboratory must be alerted to use an appropriate selective culture medium for stool cultures, such as thiosulfate–citrate–bile salts–sucrose (TCBS) agar or Monsur taurocholate-tellurite-gelatin agar.[262,281] Pathogenic *Vibrio* species generally grow on MacConkey agar. The stool specimen should be collected if possible within the first 24 hours of illness and before the administration of antibiotics; specimens should not be allowed to dry. The specimen may be transported in the semisolid transport medium of Cary and Blair; buffered glycerol-saline is not satisfactory because glycerol is toxic to vibrios. Tellurite-taurocholate-peptone broth is adequate. All *Vibrio* species grow in routine blood culture mediums and on nonselective mediums, such as blood agar.

Key characteristics that aid in the separation of *Vibrio* species from other medically significant bacteria (*Enterobacteriaceae, Pseudomonas, Aeromonas, Plesiomonas*) are the production of oxidase, fermentative metabolism, requirement of sodium chloride for growth, and susceptibility to the 0/129 vibriostatic compound.[204] Species that cannot be identified in the hospital microbiology laboratory may be referred to a state laboratory or the CDC. Multiple PCR methods are now used to detect various strains of *Vibrio* species in oyster tissue and water samples that are sensitive and reliable.[34,256,436]

Vibrio Vulnificus. *Vibrio vulnificus* is a free-living, motile halophilic gram-negative bacillus that causes septicemia, gastroenteritis, and wound infections that occur 12 hours to 7 days after the ingestion of contaminated raw or undercooked seafood, particularly raw oysters. Persons with compromised immune systems and liver disease are at a significantly high risk for fatal septicemia. *V. vulnificus* has a rapid onset and the highest mortality rate of any of the *Vibrio* species. *V. vulnificus* is naturally present in marine environments; it has a worldwide distribution and is found throughout the United States.[336,363]

The growth of *V. vulnificus* is favored in waters with an intermediate salinity of 5 to 25 ppt. The optimal temperature for growth (doubling time 15 minutes) for *V. vulnificus* is 35° C (95° F). Below 10° C (50° F), *V. vulnificus* enters a nonculturable state and is viable but ceases to replicate.[305] The number of *V. vulnificus* found in the marine environment and in shellfish increases

---

*References 72, 77, 116, 233, 387, 393.

*References 62, 73, 163, 326, 330, 363, 400, 452.
†References 1, 45, 79, 163, 206, 227, 228, 236, 261, 363.

and peaks during the summer months, as does the incidence of *V. vulnificus* infections.[288]

V. vulnificus may appear as one of two morphotypes; opaque and virulent, or translucent and less virulent. The opacity of the virulent morphotype is due to an acidic mucopolysaccharide capsule (opaque colony) that increases the resistance of the organism against bactericidal activity of human serum and phagocytosis and thus renders the organism more virulent. At extremely low frequency, some strains can shift between unencapsulated and capsulated serotypes.[469] The encapsulated isolates are sensitive to iron. The organism is unable to use transferrin-bound iron for growth. In patients with iron overload and transferrin saturation greater than 75%, free iron is available for use. Additionally, virulent isolates can use iron in hemoglobin and hemoglobin-haptoglobin complexes.[54,56,472] *V. vulnificus* can bind specifically to human intestinal cells and quickly induce cytotoxic effects.[235] In vivo studies show that 4 hours after inoculation in the duodenum, the organism is found in the systemic circulation via bacterial translocation.[191] The severity of *V. vulnificus* infections is related to both bacterial characteristics as described above and host factors. In patients with liver disease, chronic cirrhosis, and alcoholism, portal hypertension allows shunting of the organism around the liver. These patients also have reduced phagocytic acidity, chemotaxis, opsonization, and complement levels, thus promoting the virulence of *V. vulnificus*.[325] Persons with high serum iron levels (from chronic cirrhosis, hepatitis, thalassemia major, or hemochromatosis) are at increased risk for infection as described above.[56,236,441] Any individual with impaired immunity (e.g., malignancy, human immunodeficiency virus [HIV] infection, diabetes, long-term corticosteroids) is at greater risk for fulminant bacteremia.[398] Based on the prevalence of predisposing diseases in the general population, 3.8% of the general population is at risk of having *V. vulnificus* septicemia if they contact this organism.[104]

CLINICAL PRESENTATION. *V. vulnificus* infection occurs as two clinical syndromes: primary septicemia and wound infection. The syndrome consists of flulike malaise, fever, vomiting, diarrhea, chills, hypotension, and early skin vesiculation that evolves into necrotizing dermatitis, with vasculitis and myositis (see Chapter 60 for discussion of *Vibrio* wound infections). Primary septicemia occurs when *V. vulnificus* is acquired through the gastrointestinal tract. Blood cultures are positive for the organism in 97% of patients. Septic shock, disseminated intravascular coagulation, and death may occur.[441] The mortality of patients with primary septicemia is 56% and increases to 92% when septic shock occurs.[189]

Gastroenteritis was previously thought to exist as an isolated entity in 10% of cases. However, it is more likely that other enteric pathogens are the causal agent and *V. vulnificus* illness has been erroneously attributed to the asymptomatically carried organism.[203]

V. vulnificus is also implicated in other infectious presentations, including meningitis, spontaneous bacterial peritonitis, corneal ulcers, epiglottitis, osteomyelitis, rhabdomyolysis, endocarditis, and infections of the testes and spleen.* *V. vulnificus* endometritis has been reported after an episode of intercourse in the water of Galveston Bay, Texas.[418]

TREATMENT. Early recognition of *V. vulnificus* infection is essential for effective treatment. Blood and wound cultures should precede immediate and aggressive antibiotic and supportive treatment. Current recommendations include doxycycline (100 mg IV q12h) and ceftazidime (2 g IV q8h) or ciprofloxacin 400 mg IV q12h).[152] Other antibiotics that have been suggested include imipenem/cilastatin, trimethoprim/sulfamethoxazole, carbenicillin, tobramycin, gentamicin, and many third-generation cephalosporins. Supportive care includes crystalloid and pressor agents for hypotension.

Vibrio Parahaemolyticus. *Vibrio parahaemolyticus* is a halophilic gram-negative rod that can cause gastroenteritis when consumed in raw or partially cooked seafood and has been reported in temperate, subtropical and tropical coastal regions.[32,73,75,182,271] The organisms are found in marine and estuarine waters along the entire coastline of the United States. The concentration of *V. parahaemolyticus* in seawater increases with rising water temperature and corresponds with an increased incidence of clinical disease in warm summer months when the organism is commonly found in zooplankton.[189] The optimal growth temperature of *V. parahaemolyticus* is 35° to 37° C (95° to 98.6° F). *V. parahaemolyticus* has also been isolated from colder waters. The largest reported outbreak in North America of culture confirmed *V. parahaemolyticus* infections occurred during July-August 1997 in the Pacific Northwest; 209 persons became ill and one person died after eating raw or undercooked oysters.[73] *V. parahaemolyticus* has been recovered at frequencies up to 25% in frozen peeled shrimp.[455]

Ingestion of raw or partially cooked *V. parahaemolyticus*-contaminated shrimp, oysters, crab, or fish is followed in 6 to 76 hours by explosive diarrhea, nausea, vomiting, headache, abdominal pain, fever, chills, and prostration. In immunocompetent persons, *V. parahaemolyticus* causes mild to moderate gastroenteritis with

---

*References 111, 130, 221, 276, 424, 434, 441, 456.

a mean duration of illness of 3 days. Serious illness and death can occur in persons with underlying disease (pre-existing liver disease, diabetes, iron overload states, or compromised immune system).[227] The stools may contain blood and classically demonstrate leukocytes on methylene blue staining. The syndrome generally resolves spontaneously in 24 to 72 hours but may be of a severity sufficient to cause significant fluid and electrolyte depletion. Stool cultures should be obtained before the initiation of antibiotic therapy. Panophthalmitis requiring enucleation occurred in a man who suffered a corneal laceration.[399] A course of oral ciprofloxacin, trimethoprim/sulfamethoxazole, or tetracycline may shorten the course of severe gastroenteritis.

Vibrio Mimicus. *Vibrio mimicus* is a motile, non-halophilic, gram-negative, oxidase-positive rod with a single flagellum. It can be distinguished from *V. cholerae* by its inability to ferment sucrose, inability to metabolize acetylmethyl carbonyl, sensitivity to polymyxin, and negative lipase test.[102] Multiple toxins are produced by *V. mimicus,* including cholera-like toxin, enterotoxin, and hemolysin.[326,367,436] *V. mimicus* causes a syndrome of gastroenteritis (diarrhea, nausea, vomiting, abdominal cramps, fever, and headache) following the ingestion of raw oysters, crawfish, crab, or shrimp. *V. mimicus* was identified by PCR in 11 individuals with gastroenteritis from eating raw turtle eggs.[62] Nonfatal bacteremia resulting from *V. mimicus* has been reported.[228] The median incubation period is 24 hours, with delayed diarrhea noted up to 3 days after ingestion of contaminated seafood. Isolates are sensitive to tetracycline, ciprofloxacin, and norfloxacin.[280]

Vibrio Alginolyticus. *Vibrio alginolyticus* can cause gastroenteritis in immunocompetent individuals and bacteremia in immunosuppressed patients.[261,330] More commonly, it is implicated in soft tissue infections (such as those caused by coral cuts or surfing scrapes), sinusitis, and otitis media and externa.[146,261,331,425]

Vibrio Cholerae. In developing countries, cholera caused by toxigenic *V. cholerae* is a major public health problem. The last several cholera pandemics were caused by the consumption of fecal contaminated water.[459] *V. cholerae* is commonly linked to ingestion of raw or inadequately cooked mollusks and crustaceans and is responsible for the third highest number of shellfish-related illnesses behind other noncholera *Vibrio* species and Norwalk virus.[213,452] Toxigenic 01 *V. cholerae* infections are associated with a secretory, profuse watery diarrhea, nausea, and vomiting. Since the stool is virtually isotonic, large amounts of fluid and electrolytes are lost, which leads to rapid dehydration, shock, acidosis, and renal failure. The treatment consists of aggressive fluid replacement, intravenous if available, combined

with oral rehydration. In a recent outbreak in Italy, all strains were resistant to tetracycline but the patients responded to ciprofloxacin.[264] Untreated, the disease remits in 3 to 8 days.

Nontoxigenic, non-01 *V. cholerae* strains cause gastroenteritis and septicemia.[200] Self-limited (24 to 48 hours) nausea, vomiting, abdominal cramping, and invasive diarrhea with blood and fecal leukocytes are typical. Spontaneous non-01 *V. cholerae* bacteremia and peritonitis have been reported in patients with cirrhosis after eating raw oysters.[255,319,338] Meningitis and death have also been associated with non-01 *V. cholerae.*[79,227]

Other Vibrios. *Vibrio metschnikovii* has caused bacteremia in a patient with cholecystitis; the authors postulated that it may have been associated with long-term carriage after seafood ingestion.[206] *Vibrio cincinnatiensis* has caused meningitis; a relationship to foreign travel, seawater exposure, or seafood ingestion has not been established.[45] *Vibrio fluvialis,* previously designated as enteric group EF-6 or group F, is common in the marine environment. It causes diarrheal disease associated with vomiting, abdominal pain, dehydration, and fever.[400] Fatal gastroenteritis has been reported.[228] It can be mistaken easily in the microbiology laboratory for *Aeromonas hydrophila,* from which it can be distinguished by growth in 6% to 7% sodium chloride. *Vibrio hollisae* and *V. furnissii* have both been linked to gastroenteritis after seafood ingestion and *V. hollisae* has been associated with septicemia.[1,163]

PREVENTION. Persons who are immunosuppressed or chronically ill, particularly with hepatic insufficiency, should not eat raw or partially cooked shellfish. All seafood should be cooked thoroughly, protected from cross-contamination after cooking, and eaten promptly or stored at temperatures above 60° C (140° F) or below 4° C (39.2° F) to prevent multiplication of *Vibrio* species.

The FDA has prepared a series of four booklets for subpopulations of persons with altered immunity who may be susceptible to *Vibrio* infections. One set of booklets on seafood safety for high-risk individuals is available to health professionals free of charge from: FDA, Seafood Brochures, HFI-40, 5600 Fishers Lane, Rockville, MD 20857.[136]

Botulism

Botulism is a paralytic disease caused by the potent natural toxin of *Clostridium botulinum.* Seven toxins (A to G) have been identified, but only A, B, E, F, and G cause human illness.[383] Seafood-related botulism can be caused by raw, parboiled, salt-cured, or fermented meats from marine mammals (seal, walrus, whale) or fish products (particularly salmon and salmon roe).[185] Toxin type E spores are found in mud and sediment in northern coastal areas and inland lakes, accounting for the prevalence of type E toxin in fish-borne botulism (although types A and B may also be involved). Improperly preserved (smoked, dried, or canned) foods are at high risk for *C. botulinum* toxin proliferation. The technique of "hanging" meat for decomposition (flavor and texture improvement) supports growth of the nonproteolytic, psychotolerant forms of *C. botulinum*, which may grow at temperatures as low as 4° C (39.2° F).[185]

In the last four decades in the United States, over 10% of outbreaks of food-borne botulism have been related to the consumption of fish. Using quantitative PCR analysis, the prevalence of *C. botulinum* type E gene was 10% to 40% in raw fish samples and 4% to 14% in fish roe samples in Finland.[196] In 1991, 91 patients were hospitalized in Cairo with botulism intoxication associated with eating faseikh (uneviscerated salted mullet fish); *C. botulinum* type E was isolated.[444]

C. botulinum spores germinate in an environment of appropriate pH (greater than 4.6), warm temperature (higher than 10° C [50° F]), sufficient moisture, and an anaerobic environment. The toxins are proteins of approximate molecular weight 150,000 daltons and are absorbed in the proximal gastrointestinal tract.

Clinical Presentation. The toxin affects the presynaptic cholinergic neuromuscular junction, where it blocks the release of acetylcholine and causes flaccid paralysis.[29] Signs and symptoms develop within 12 to 36 hours of ingestion and include nausea, vomiting, abdominal pain, and diarrhea, followed by dry mouth, dysphonia (hoarseness), difficulty swallowing, facial weakness, ptosis, nonreactive or sluggishly reactive pupils (third cranial nerve), mydriasis, blurred or double vision (sixth cranial nerve), descending symmetric muscular weakness leading to paralysis, and bulbar and respiratory paralysis. With adequate ventilatory support, mentation frequently remains normal. Death occurs in 10% to 50% of cases, depending on the availability of antitoxin.

If botulism is suspected, a careful food history should be obtained and the suspected food items collected. Laboratory confirmation of botulism is achieved when botulinal toxin or viable *C. botulinum* is detected in the food, toxin is demonstrated in the victim's serum or stool, or the organism is cultured from the stool. Toxin types are distinguished using type-specific antitoxin.[29] To determine the clinical need for botulism antitoxin, a number of tests may be helpful. Electromyography should be performed using repetitive stimulation at 40 Hz or greater; a positive test shows diminished amplitude of the muscle action potential with a single supramaximal stimulus, and facilitation of action potentials using paired or repetitive stimuli.[29] Cerebrospinal fluid may be examined for white blood cells and protein (to rule out infectious etiologies), and edrophonium (Tensilon) challenge test may be per-formed to rule out myasthenia gravis. Vital capacity should be monitored as a sensitive indicator of clinical deterioration.

Treatment. Ventilatory support should be provided at the first sign of respiratory inadequacy. Cathartics are recommended to eliminate residual toxin in the gastrointestinal tract. Equine trivalent antitoxin A, B, E should be administered as soon as possible to any person with symptoms, before irreversible neural dysfunction.[401] Each 8-ml vial of trivalent antitoxin contains 7500 IU type A, 5500 IU type B, and 8500 IU type E antitoxin.[29] A physician who seeks antitoxin should first contact the state health department. If this is unsatisfactory, the CDC may be telephoned at 404-329-2888 (24 hours). The trivalent antitoxin is administered as an initial dose of 16 ml (two vials) every 2 to 4 hours for 3 to 5 doses or longer if symptoms persist.[29] Before administration the victim should be skin tested for hypersensitivity to horse serum. If horse serum test material is not available, 0.1 ml of a 1:10 dilution of antitoxin in saline may be used. The antitoxin should not be stored at a temperature greater than 37° C (98.6° F).

An adjunct to therapy may be administration of guanidine, which increases the release of acetylcholine from nerve endings. The dosage is 15 to 50 mg/kg/day orally in four divided doses.

Prevention. Prophylaxis with antitoxin is not currently recommended, nor is general pentavalent (A to E) toxoid immunization.[9] The best prevention is public health education with respect to food preparation and avoidance of improperly stored food products. Since the spores are frequently detected in fish intestines, it is important to clean fish properly and to avoid consumption of the viscera, even in salt-cured products. To eliminate spores in food, heat or irradiation may be used. Types A and B may survive boiling for several hours (particularly at the lower temperatures associated with higher altitude) and generally require pressure heating at 120° C (248° F) for 30 minutes; type E spores are killed at 80° C (176° F) after 30 minutes. Preformed toxin is inactivated after heating for 20 minutes at 80° C or 10 minutes at 90° C (194° F). Germination is inhibited by acidification, refrigeration, freezing, drying, or the addition of salt, sugar, or sodium nitrate; however, heating remains the most reliable technique.[29]

PARASITES IN SEAFOOD

Most parasites of marine animals are of little public health concern to humans. However, there are 50 species of helminths worldwide from fishes, crabs, crayfishes, and bivalves that can cause human infections. With the increasing consumption of raw seafood such as sushi and sashimi, the number of documented human infections is increasing. The overall risk of human infection is small.

Fish Tapeworm

In the United States the consumption of raw fish (sushi) is increasingly popular, which has led to more frequent recognition of infestation with the fish tapeworm, *Diphyllobothrium latum*. Salmon appears to be a popular culprit.[97,121,195,420] Diphyllobothriasis is also reported from eating raw flesh of redlip mullet.[86] The fish tapeworm has a complex life cycle, in which a gravid egg released into freshwater releases a ciliated coracidium, which is eaten by a crustacean intermediate host. The coracidium penetrates the intestinal wall of the crustacean and then develops into a procercoid larva. A fish eats the small crustacean, and the procercoid larva migrates through the intestinal wall of the fish into fish muscle, where it changes into a plerocercoid larva. It is this final larval stage that is ingested by a human and that subsequently attaches to the intestine, where it grows into a mature tapeworm.

Classic symptoms include subacute abdominal pain, nausea, vomiting, diarrhea, and weight loss. Proglottids may be passed in the stool. Chronic *D. latum* infestation may induce megaloblastic anemia, as the tapeworm splits the vitamin B_{12}–intrinsic factor complex and prevents absorption of the vitamin.[161] The diagnosis can be made by examination of the stool for typical proglottids or operculate egg forms, which measure 60 to 75 μm in length. Proper identification of the eggs is important in the differentiation from the ova of trematodes endemic in Southeast Asia, such as *Paragonimus westermani*, which may be carried by refugees to the United States.[114] For documented *D. latum* infestation, praziquantel 10 mg/kg in one dose for adults or children is the recommended treatment.[154,303] Magnesium sulfate as a purgative has been used to help expel the worm.[420] Niclosamide can also be used for treatment.[314] Because a worm may not be identifiable if expulsion is delayed or follows a purge, stool analysis should be repeated at 3 months to confirm successful therapy.

Fish tapeworm infection can be avoided by cooking fish until the parts for consumption reach a temperature of at least 56° C (133° F) for 5 minutes or freezing the fish to −18° C (0° F) for 24 hours or −10° C (14° F) for 72 hours.[454]

Trematodes

Humans can acquire an intestinal infection from the trematode *Nanophyetus salmincola*, which infests salmonid fishes, such as steelhead trout or salmon.[120] Canine infection with this fluke is a well-known phenomenon in the Pacific Northwest of the United States.

Humans ingest the flesh of fish infested with the metacercariae, which excyst in the host and attach to the upper small bowel. The worms release eggs that are detected in the stool approximately 1 week after ingestion of infected fish.

Symptoms of nanophyetiasis include diarrhea, peripheral blood eosinophilia, abdominal discomfort, bloating, nausea and vomiting, weight loss, and fatigue. Although symptoms may resolve spontaneously over a period of months, antihelminthic treatment is recommended. Praziquantel 25 mg/kg orally 3 times a day for 1 day is the first-line treatment.[2] Other regimens have included bithionol 50 mg/kg orally for two doses, niclosamide 2 g orally for three doses, or mebendazole 100 mg orally bid for 3 days. A similar syndrome has been caused by intestinal infection with *Heterophyes heterophyes*, which was successfully treated with praziquantel.[2]

Numerous other trematode infections are the cause of enormous morbidity worldwide as the liver and intestinal flukes cause distinct medical syndromes. For instance, in Southeast Asia, opisthorchosis caused by the liver fluke *Opisthorchis viverrini* is quite serious. The cercariae are ubiquitous in cyprinid fish.[150] Clonorchiasis occurs when humans eat raw or undercooked freshwater fish harboring the metacercariae of *Clonorchis sinensis*.[358]

Anisakiasis

Approximately 5000 restaurants serve sushi in the United States. Many of these do so without specific knowledge of the various parasites that can infest their fare. For instance, many serve raw salmon, squid, shrimp, and mackerel.

The first report of acute gastric anisakiasis caused by penetration of the *Anisakis* larvae through the gastric mucosa was by Van Thiel in 1960.[433] It is a rare problem in the United States but increasingly noted in Japan, where raw fish is more commonly eaten.[225,394] In a Japanese series the fish consumed included predominantly mackerel; less common perpetrators included horse mackerel, bream, squid, sardines, and bonito.[394] In the United States, anisakine nematodes are present in many commercial fish intended for raw or semiraw consumption, such as Pacific herring (thus "herring worm disease"), sablefish, Pacific cod (thus "codworm disease"), arrowtooth flounder, petrale sole, coho salmon, Pacific ocean perch, silvergray rockfish, yellowtail rockfish, and bocaccio.[295] In rare cases the anisakine worm can be present in tuna or yellowtail. The preservation of marine mammals along the West Coast of the United States has been linked to greater worm burdens in fishes associated with these mammals, such as Pacific rockfish, red snapper, and salmon.[274]

Life and Habits. Anisakine nematodes, members of the order Ascarida (suborder Ascaridae), are found in great numbers in the viscera and muscles of fish.[291]

There are 30 genera in the family Anisakidae, including *Anisakis* and *Pseudoterranova* (or *Phocanema*). Adult worms infest the stomachs of marine mammals, burrowing in clusters into the mucosal surface. Eggs passed in the stool embryonate and hatch in seawater to produce second-stage larvae, which are ingested by crustaceans, which are in turn eaten by squid or fish. In these hosts the larvae migrate through the gut wall and encyst in the viscera or musculature.[348] The fish may then pass the parasite to other fish, to humans, or back to another marine mammal. The coiled *Anisakis* larva grows to approximately 2.5 to 3 cm in length and 0.5 to 1 mm in diameter. Thus fish are usually the intermediate (transport) host for larval anisakines.

The definitive host for *Phocanema decipiens* is the seal; the *Anisakis* larvae grow to maturity in the whale. Shellfish are not infested. Only four genera of anisakine nematodes have been implicated in human anisakiasis: *Anisakis*, *Phocanema*, *Porrocaecum*, and *Contracaecum*. In the United States, all cases are related to the larval stages of *Anisakis simplex* and *Phocanema decipiens*.[274]

Clinical Aspects. Symptoms from ingestion of *Anisakis* may begin within 1 hour of ingestion of raw fish and include severe epigastric pain, nausea, and vomiting. The presentation may mimic an acute abdomen. Asymptomatic gastroduodenal anisakiasis has also been a cause of acute urticaria and severe anaphylaxis in sensitized patients.[100,139,145] If the anisakine worms (such as *Phocanema*) do not implant and the infection is luminal without tissue penetration, the worms may be coughed up, vomited, or defecated, generally within 48 hours of the meal.[99] If the worm is felt in the oropharynx or proximal esophagus, the "tingling throat syndrome" is described.[274] An anisakine worm has been documented in the tonsil of a 6-year-old girl with recurrent tonsillitis.[39]

Intestinal anisakiasis is more often delayed in onset (up to 7 days after ingestion) and marked by abdominal pain, nausea, vomiting, diarrhea, fever, eosinophilia (particularly with gastric anisakiasis), and occult blood in the stool.[99] This may be easily confused with appendicitis, regional enteritis, gastric ulcer, colonic or other gastrointestinal carcinoma, or most commonly, other causes of small bowel inflammation with partial obstruction.[52,210,369,402] In one study, 29% of patients with Crohn's disease had detectable specific total immunoglobulin (IgG), IgM, and IgA antibodies against *A. simplex*.[167]

Diagnosis and Treatment. The definitive diagnosis of anisakiasis is usually made on the basis of morphologic characteristics of the whole worm when the creature is expelled by the patient or removed from the stomach after endoscopic examination.[348] In gastrointestinal tract X-rays, threadlike gastric filling defects approximately 30 mm in length are typical, with a circular or ringlike shape.[52,394] Edema of the mucosa and pseudotumor formation are also seen. Ultrasound can be useful in identifying intestinal anisakiasis.[197] If the worms have migrated to extragastric sites, the diagnosis can be difficult.

Early fiberoptic gastroscopy is recommended for patients in whom acute gastric anisakiasis is suspected and for those who have eaten raw fish within 6 to 12 hours before the onset of gastric symptoms. *Anisakis* is usually found in the greater curvature of the stomach, often associated with severe mucosal edema.[212] Worms may penetrate the wall of the intestine.

The larvae of *Anisakis* can be visualized on endoscopy and removed with biopsy forceps. Fourth-stage larvae of *Anisakis simplex* and *Pseudoterranova (Phocanema) decipiens* are found in the intestine and stomach of humans.[226] The larva is visible in the mucosa or buried within the submucosa, surrounded by an intense inflammatory granulomatous response.

When laparotomy is performed for presumed appendicitis, the diagnosis is based on identification of the worm in an inflamed segment of appendix, cecum, small intestine, mesentery, or omentum.[63,105] The only effective therapy for inflamed bowel is resection.

Antibodies to the ileal worm have been detected by radioallergosorbent test (RAST), ELISA, and immunofluorescent antibody assay, but these laboratory methods are not widely available.[167] Physical removal by endoscopy or surgery is the treatment of choice. Mebendazole 200 mg po bid for 3 days is also recommended.[154]

Prevention. The larvae are extremely difficult to spot in fish flesh, since they are colorless and normally tightly coiled in a spiral of approximately 3 mm. Only cooked (above 60° C [140° F]) or previously frozen (to −20° C [−48° F] for 24 hours) fish should be eaten. Smoking (kippering), marinating, pickling, brining, and salting may not kill the worms.[99] Candling is an inadequate method of surveillance, particularly in dark-fleshed fish infested with *Anisakis* larvae. Fish should be gutted as soon as possible after they are caught to limit the migration of worms from the viscera into the muscle.

The irradiation of fish to limit their infectivity is controversial because of potential generation of long-lived free radicals within the fish, as well as germination of spores of *Clostridium botulinum*.[453] To date, this practice is not legal for seafood in the United States, although it is used in other countries.

Eustrongylides

Eustrongylides is a genus of roundworms that can invade fish in its larval form and thus be consumed by humans in their quest for sushi and sashimi. *Eustrongylides* may also parasitize bait minnows, which are swallowed whole by fishermen. The worms are released into the human gastrointestinal tract, where they attain lengths of 15 to 30 cm and penetrate the intestinal wall to enter the peritoneal cavity. Symptoms include unexplained abdominal pain, peritonitis, and fever in a live-bait fisherman. Surgical intervention may be required in pursuit of the acute abdomen, at which time the characteristically bright red worm is identified.[454]

OTHER SEAFOOD-RELATED POISONINGS

Poisoning by Environmental Contamination

In the process of concentrating fish proteins as a food source, a variety of protein-bound, non–water-soluble, or non–alcohol-soluble toxic compounds may be preserved. These include organic mercurials, hydrocarbons, dioxins, polychlorinated dibenzofurans, chlorinated pesticides, and heavy metals (e.g., antimony, arsenic, cadmium, chromium, cobalt, lead, phosphorus, mercury, nickel, zinc).[23,92,396] The overall public health risk for environmental contamination is concerning; however, the true risk of exposure is unknown.

Higher concentrations of polychlorinated biphenyls (PCBs) and dioxin-like compounds are found in Inuit people in the Arctic because of their traditional diet, which includes large quantities of sea mammal fat.[23] Data suggest that there is an elevated risk of multiple myeloma in groups with high consumption of dioxin-contaminated fish from the Baltic Sea, Alaska, and accidental exposure in Italy.[355] Dioxin has been found in Dungeness crabs in Humboldt Bay, California.

In Taiwan, high levels of copper, zinc, and arsenic concentrations were found in oysters. The long-term exposure of metals from seafood consumption is potentially dangerous, although the real risk is unknown.[179] Urine arsenic levels have been shown to increase 2 to 7 times after consumption of certain types of seafood (mackerel, herring, crab, and tuna).[14] Consumption of fish rich in amines has been shown to increase the excretion of N-nitrosodimethylamine in the urine, demonstrating increased formation of carcinogenic N-nitrosamines.[435]

Mercury is found in marine organisms in the form of methylmercury (MeHg) and is concentrated in the food chain. Increased fish consumption is associated with higher blood levels of mercury.[265] MeHg is neurotoxic and crosses the placenta and blood-brain barrier; prenatal poisoning causes mental retardation and cerebral palsy. The risk from seafood is unclear. High blood and hair concentration of mercury have been found in fishermen of coastal villages, and adverse effects have been reported.[292,332] Controversy exists over the fetal risk from exposure to low-dose MeHg from maternal consumption of fish.[22] A recent study on children exposed to MeHg from seafood in a Madeira fishing community did not show any mercury-associated deficits.[289] A longitudinal cohort study of children showed no adverse outcome with either prenatal or postnatal MeHg exposure.[101]

Spills of toxic chemicals and petroleum by-products will certainly continue to expand the list of carcinogens to which humans are becoming exposed through the marine environment. Although radiation exposure is not known to induce production of new marine poisons, the ingestion of radioactive fish poses a potential radiation hazard. Divers are exposed to a variety of environmental contaminants while exploring polluted waters. These hazards include solvents, nuclear wastes, herbicides, chemical effluents, and sewage.

Red Seaweed

Seaweed is a common component in the diet of individuals living in the Pacific Islands and the Pacific Rim. It can be eaten raw or cooked. Most *Gracilaria* species are nontoxic and edible. A number of poisonings and deaths have been reported in Japan, Guam, and Hawaii. Ingestion of the red seaweeds *G. verrucosa* (ogonuri) and *G. chordai* (tsurushiramo) are associated with a toxic syndrome, including gastroenteritis and death.[301] It is commonly referred to as Japanese "ogonuri poisoning."

In 1991 in Guam, 13 individuals became ill and 3 died after ingesting the red algae *Polycavernosa tsudae* (formerly *Gracilaria tsudae* or *edulisi*).[177] Symptoms consisted of diarrhea, abdominal cramping, vomiting, generalized numbness, perioral and extremity paresthesias, numbness of the fingertips, diaphoresis, jaw aching, muscle spasm, tremors, and hypotension. *G. lemanaeformis* may have been responsible for three illnesses in California in 1992.[69] In Japan, two people became ill with nausea, vomiting, and hypotension and one died after ingestion of *G. verrucosa*. Prostaglandin E_2 is suggested as the toxic component of *G. verrucosa*, and polycavernosides, which are glycosidic macrolides, are the probable toxins in *G. tsudae*.[301,471]

An outbreak of acute gastroenteritis from the ingestion of the red alga *G. coronopifolia* occurred in Hawaii in 1994, in which seven individuals reported symptoms of diarrhea, nausea, vomiting, and a burning sensation in the mouth and throat.[69] Aplysiatoxin and debromoaplysiatoxin have been isolated as the causative agents.[293] These toxins probably are produced by blue-green algae that are found on the surface of *G. coronopifolia* and are known to cause contact dermatitis in swimmers in Hawaii. Aplysiatoxin and debromoaplysiatoxin experimentally cause edema and bleeding of the small intestine, leading to hemorrhagic shock and diarrhea in the large intestine.[201]

Sea Turtle Poisoning (Chelonintoxication)

A variety of tropical Pacific, particularly Japanese, marine turtles are toxic when ingested (Box 54-5).[385] The term chelonintoxication comes from the Order Chelonia. All portions of the turtle are toxic; the freshness of the meat is irrelevant. In Madagascar, 60 people became ill after eating sea turtle in 1994. The mortality rate was 7.7%.[327] Lyngbyatoxin A has been isolated from the meat of a green turtle, *Chelonia mydas,* that was involved in a fatal intoxication.[462] The source of the toxin was suspected to be a blue-green algae belonging to the genus *Lyngbya.* The sea turtle may feed on sea grass contaminated with this algae.

Symptoms develop from 1 to 48 hours after ingestion and include ulcerative glossitis and stomatitis, pharyngitis, diaphoresis, hypersalivation, nausea, vomiting, diarrhea, abdominal pain, vertigo, icterus, desquamative dermatitis, hepatosplenomegaly, centrilobular hepatic necrosis with fatty degeneration, renal failure, somnolence, and hypotension. The mortality rate can be as high as 28% to 44%. Therapy is supportive and based on symptoms.

A variety of *Salmonella* serotypes have been isolated from pet turtles (*Pseudemys* [or *Chrysemys*] *scripta elegans*) imported into and from the United States.[107,232,266] Pet-associated salmonellosis was a significant problem in the 1970s. In 1975, Canada banned the importation of turtles, and in the same year, the FDA prohibited the sale of small turtles in the United States. However, the popularity of iguanas and other reptiles is increasing; these reptiles can also transmit salmonella to humans. Reptile-associated salmonellosis causes febrile gastroenteritis, septicemia, and meningitis; one death has been reported due to myocarditis from *S. virchow* in a small child.[67,107,298]

Liver Poisoning—Hypervitaminosis A

Hypervitaminosis A can occur with the ingestion of the livers of certain polar bears, seals, sea lions, whales, dolphins, walruses, husky dogs, and Pacific sharks. The vitamin A content of shark liver can attain 100,000 IU/g. A typical ingestion involves the administration of more than 1 million (and occasionally up to 3 to 8 million) IU of vitamin A (the recommended daily allowance is 4000 to 5000 IU). Symptoms of hypervitaminosis A include formication, headache, apathy, drowsiness, giddiness, irritability, photophobia, nausea, vomiting, diarrhea, polyarthralgia, seizures, desquamative dermatitis, ophthalmoplegia, and raised cerebrospinal fluid pressure with a pseudotumor cerebri–type presentation (acute or chronic, the latter with headache, lip fissuring, papilledema, decreased visual acuity, and tinnitus).[128,279] Elevated levels of serum glutamic oxaloacetic transaminase and serum vitamin A (markedly in excess of 70 mg%) may be measured. A normal serum β-carotene level excludes the possibility of a plant source (for example carrots or mangoes) for the vitamin.[279] The syndrome is rarely fatal and resolves in 2 to 8 weeks.

AMEBIC INFECTIONS

Free-living, amphizoic amebas belonging to the genera *Naegleria, Acanthamoeba,* and *Balamuthia* can cause significant central nervous system (CNS) pathology in human beings. Approximately 350 cases of human infection have been reported to date.[269,337] These amebas are ubiquitous in nature; they are found in soil, lakes, ponds, swimming pools, hot springs, and warm water around the world. Human infection caused by amebas has significantly increased over the last 10 years.[269]

Free-living amebas are responsible for three disease entities: (1) primary amebic meningoencephalitis (PAM) produced by *Naegleria fowleri,* (2) granulomatous amebic encephalitis (GAE) caused by *Acanthamoeba* species and *Balamuthia mandrillaris,* and (3) *Acanthamoeba* keratitis (AK), caused by *Acanthamoeba* species.

Primary Amebic Meningoencephalitis

PAM is a fulminant, rapidly progressive CNS infection produced by *N. fowleri.* It was first described in 1965 by Malcolm Fowler and Rodney Carter in four human cases of meningoencephalitis from *N. fowleri.*[138] Worldwide, approximately 180 cases of PAM have been reported, with over 80 cases reported in the United States alone.* *N. fowleri* multiplies and grows between 40° and 45° C (104° and 113° F). In response to adverse environmental conditions, such as cold temperature, the ameba encysts and remains in the sediment in the bottom of lakes, rivers, and pools.

---

*References 66, 106, 240, 269, 337, 439.

Infections occur in healthy children and adults who contact the ameba while swimming in polluted water in human-made lakes, ponds, and swimming pools, or the ameba may be inhaled from the dust and air.[269] Infection is more common during summer months. The amebas enter the CNS through the nasal mucosa and olfactory neuroepithelium. The amebic trophozoites travel up the unmyelinated fila olfactoria of the olfactory nerves and through the cribriform plate to the subarachnoid space.[208] They proliferate and penetrate into the CNS, causing edema and necrosis. The incubation period is from 1 to 15 days. Symptoms include severe headache, fever, nausea, vomiting, and stiff neck. Rapid neurologic deterioration accompanied by signs of fulminant meningitis with seizures, coma, and death follows within 2 to 3 days.

Diagnosis is made by the direct visualization of trophozoites in the cerebrospinal fluid along with polymorphonuclear pleocytosis, elevated protein, and low glucose. *Naegleria* trophozoites typically measure 8 to 12 microns in diameter with indistinct cytoplasm, a round nucleus, and a perinucleolar halo.[269] *N. fowleri* causes acute leptomeningitis and hemorrhagic necrosis of the orbitofrontal cortex, olfactory bulbs, and base of the brain with edema of the cerebral hemispheres and cerebellum. Computed tomography (CT) scan of the brain shows nonspecific cerebral edema.[222,351] Early detection and treatment is essential, since this disease carries a very poor prognosis with a mortality rate of 98%. To date, there are six cases of successful treatment of PAM in individuals who were treated very early in the clinical course.[55,320,359,442] Treatment includes high-dose intravenous and intrathecal amphotericin B alone or in combination with miconazole.[153] Oral ketoconazole and rifampicin have been used in addition to amphotericin B.[320]

PAM should be suspected in any previously healthy individual who has been exposed to fresh warm water within 7 days of onset of illness and who has clinical findings of bacterial meningitis with a basilar distribution of exudate by brain CT.[66]

Granulomatous Amebic Encephalitis

Several species of *Acanthamoeba* and *B. mandrillaris* are pathogenic opportunistic amebas that cause GAE, mainly in victims who are immunocompromised, debilitated, diabetic, or alcoholic. GAE has been reported in patients with systemic lupus, acquired immunodeficiency syndrome (AIDS), and bone marrow transplantation.[4,129,234,404] However, two recent cases of GAE caused by *B. mandrillaris* occurred in apparently immunocompetent individuals.[337] Approximately 170 cases of GAE have been reported worldwide.[269]

Acanthamoeba species are ubiquitous in nature; they have been found in ocean water, ponds, sewage, rivers, air-conditioner filters, cooling towers, eye wash stations, and dust. Some of the *Acanthamoeba* opportunis-

tic species include *A. castellanii, A. hatchetti, A. culbertsoni, A. astronyxis, A. polyphaga, A. rhysodes,* and *A. mauritaniensis.*[269] *B. mandrillaris* has not been isolated from the environment, although it probably exists in cyst form similar to *Acanthamoeba.* The trophozoites and cysts can enter through the lungs and ulcerations in the skin. The olfactory neuroepithelium may also act as a portal of entry.[205,269] The incubation period is unknown but is probably weeks.

Both *Acanthamoeba* species and *B. mandrillaris* produce a chronic granulomatous encephalitis. The clinical presentation may mimic tuberculous meningitis or viral encephalitis. Symptoms include headache, fever, seizures, personality changes, cranial nerve palsies, hemiparesis, and coma. There may be ulcerations of the skin. The amebas cause hemorrhagic necrosis and foci of encephalomalacia in occipital, parietal, temporal, and frontal lobes. The lesions are multifocal and most numerous in the basal ganglia, midbrain, brainstem, and cerebral hemispheres.[269] Angiitis can occur, and trophozoites are often found invading the vascular walls.[335] The amebas multiply and can disseminate throughout the body; other organs involved (at the time of autopsy) include liver, lungs, kidneys, adrenals, pancreas, lymph nodes, and heart.[4,404]

CT scans and magnetic resonance imaging (MRI) have shown multiple enhancing lesions in the cerebral hemispheres and cerebellum; however, the scans are nondiagnostic.[222,335,351] Diagnosis is difficult, since amebas are rarely observed in the CSF. Examination of the CSF shows a moderate mononuclear pleocytosis, elevated protein, and low glucose. Definitive diagnosis is made by direct visualization of amebic trophozoites and cysts within brain tissue. Unfortunately, there is no effective treatment for GEA, and mortality is 100% in immunocompromised patients.[269] Although pentamidine isethionate, propamidine, sulfadiazine, and ketoconazole are effective in vitro, these drugs do not appear to be useful because of the underlying immunosuppression of most of these patients.[269] Based on tissue-culture studies, pentamidine isethionate appears to be the best choice for treatment of *B. mandrillaris* encephalitis.[352] Only one case of widespread granulomatous skin lesions in an immunocompromised patient resulting from *A. rhysodes* was successfully treated with intravenous pentamidine isethionate for 4 weeks, topical chlorhexidine gluconate, and ketoconazole cream followed by oral itraconazole.[377]

Acanthamoeba Keratitis

Acanthamoeba keratitis is caused by *Acanthamoeba* species; over 700 cases have been reported worldwide.[269] *Acanthamoeba* enters the corneal stroma through minor trauma or abrasion, causing chronic inflammation of the cornea, which can impair vision and lead to vascularized corneal scarring, perforation, and loss of the eye. The use of soft contact lenses and homemade saline solutions are the greatest risks for AK. Symptoms include severe eye pain, photophobia, conjunctival inflammation, and blurred vision. Diagnosis is by identification of the trophozoites or cysts by corneal scrapings or biopsies. The treatment of choice for AK is 0.02% polyhexamethylene biguanide (PHMB) or propamidine 0.1% with topical polymyxin B, gramicidin, or neomycin.[151,241] Penetrating keratoplasty and corneal grafting have been used.[132] Contact lens wearers should use sterile solutions for lenses and should consider not wearing contacts while engaged in water sports.[198]

REFERENCES

1. Abbott SL, Janda JM: Severe gastroenteritis associated with *Vibrio hollisae* infection: report of two cases and review, *Clin Infect Dis* 18:310, 1994.
2. Adams KO et al: Intestinal fluke infection as a result of eating sushi, *Am J Clin Pathol* 86:688, 1986.
3. Adams MJ: An outbreak of ciguatera poisoning in a group of scuba divers, *J Wilderness Med* 4:304, 1993.
4. Anderlini P: *Acanthamoeba* meningoencephalitis after bone marrow transplantation, *Bone Marrow Transplant* 14:459, 1994.
5. Agnew WS et al: Purification of the tetrodotoxin-binding component associated with the voltage-sensitive sodium channel from *Electrophorus electricus* electroplax membranes, *Proc Natl Acad Sci USA* 75:2606, 1978.
6. Aka NA et al: [Epidemiological observations on the first case of human paragonimiasis and potential intermediate hosts of *Paragonimus sp.* in Benin], *Bulletin de la Societe de Pathologie Exotique* 92:191, 1999.
7. Alcala AC et al: Human fatality due to ingestion of the crab *Demania reynaudii* that contained a palytoxin-like toxin, *Toxicon* 26:105, 1988.
8. Anderson DM, Sullivan JJ, Reguera B: Paralytic shellfish poisoning in Northwest Spain: the toxicity of the dinoflagellate *Gymnodinium catenatum*, *Toxicon* 31:371, 1991.
9. Anderson JH, Lewis GE: Clinical evaluation of botulinum toxoids. In Lewis GE, editor: *Biomedical aspects of botulism*, New York, 1981, Academic Press.
10. Andrews LS et al: Food preservation using ionizing radiation, *Rev Environ Contam Toxicol* 154:1, 1998.
11. Anthoni U et al: Tetramine: occurrence in marine organisms and pharmacology, *Toxicon* 27:707, 1989.
12. Anthoni U et al: The toxin tetramine from the "edible" whelk *Neptunea antiqua*, *Toxicon* 27:717, 1989.
13. Anthoni U et al: Poisonings from flesh of the greenland shark *Somniosus microcephalus* may be due to trimethylamine, *Toxicon* 29:1205, 1991.
14. Arbouine MW, Wilson HK: The effect of seafood consumption on the assessment of occupational exposure to arsenic by urinary arsenic speciation measurements, *Journal of Trace Elements and Electrolytes in Health and Disease* 6:153, 1992.
15. Arnal C et al: Comparison of seven RNA extraction methods on stool and shellfish samples prior to hepatitis A virus amplification, *J Virol Methods* 77:17, 1999.
16. Arnal C et al: Quantification of hepatitis A virus in shellfish by competitive reverse transcription-PCR with coextraction of standard RNA, *Appl Environ Microbiol* 65:322, 1999.
17. Asakawa M et al: Structure of the toxin isolated from carp (*Cyprinus carpio*) bile, *Toxicon* 28:1063, 1990.
18. Atmar RL et al: Detection of Norwalk virus and hepatitis A virus in shellfish tissues with the PCR, *Appl Environ Microbiol* 61:3014, 1995.
19. Auerbach PS: Persistent headache associated with scombroid poisoning: resolution with cimetidine, *J Wilderness Med* 1:279, 1990.
20. Auerbach PS et al: Bacteriology of the freshwater environment: implications for clinical therapy, *Ann Emerg Med* 16:1016, 1987.
21. Aune T: Health effects associated with algal toxins from seafood, *Arch Toxicol Suppl* 19:389, 1997.
22. Axtell CD et al: Semiparametric modeling of age at achieving developmental milestones after prenatal exposure to methylmercury in the Seychelles child development study, *Environmental Health Perspectives* 106:559, 1998.
23. Ayotte P et al: PCBs and dioxin-like compounds in plasma of adult Inuit living in Nunavik (Arctic Quebec), *Chemosphere* 34:1459, 1997.

24. Baden DG: Brevetoxins: unique polyether dinoflagellate toxins, *FASEB J* 3:1807, 1989.
25. Baden DG et al: Brevetoxin binding: molecular pharmacology versus immunoassay, *Toxicon* 26:97, 1988.
26. Bagnis R, Kuberski T, Langier S: Clinical observations on 3009 cases of ciguatera fish poisoning in the South Pacific, *Am J Trop Med Hyg* 28:1067, 1979.
27. Bagnis R et al: Origins of ciguatera fish poisoning: a new dinoflagellate, *Gambierdiscus toxicus* Adachi and Fukuyo, definitely involved as a causal agent, *Toxicon* 18:199, 1965.
28. Bagnis R et al: Problems of toxicants in marine food products, *Bull WHO* 42:69, 1970.
29. Bartlett JC: Botulism. In Wyngaarden JB, Smith LH, editors: *Textbook of medicine*, ed 16, Philadelphia, 1982, WB Saunders.
30. Barton ED et al: Ciguatera fish poisoning. A southern California epidemic. *West J Med* 163:31, 1995.
31. Bates SS et al: Pennate diatom *Nitzschia pungens* as the primary source of domoic acid, a toxin in shellfish from eastern Prince Edward Island, Canada, *Can J Fish Aquat Sci* 46:1203, 1989.
32. Bean NH et al: Crayfish: a newly recognized vehicle for *vibrio* infections. *Epidemiology and Infection* 121:2691998.
33. Behling AR, Taylor SH: Bacterial histamine production as a function of temperature and time of incubation, *J Food Sci* 47:1311, 1982.
34. Bej AK et al: Detection of total and hemolysin-producing *Vibrio parahaemolyticus* in shellfish using multiplex PCR amplification of tl, tdh and trh, *J Microbiol Methods* 36:215, 1999.
35. Benoit E, Legrand AM, Dubois JM: Effects of ciguatoxin on current and voltage clamped frog myelinated nerve fiber, *Toxicon* 24:357, 1986.
36. Benson JM, Tischler DL, Baden DG: Uptake, tissue distribution, and excretion of brevetoxin 3 administered to rats by intratracheal instillation, *J Toxicol Environ Health* 57:345, 1999.
37. Berlin R: Haff disease in Sweden, *Acta Med Scand* 129:560, 1948.
38. Berman FW, Murray TF: Brevetoxins cause acute excitotoxicity in primary cultures of rat cerebellar granule neurons, *J Pharmacol Exp Ther* 290:439, 1999.
39. Bhargava D et al: Anisakiasis of the tonsils, *J Laryngol Otol* 110:387, 1996.
40. Bidard JN et al: Ciguatoxin is a novel type of Na+ channel toxin, *J Biol Chem* 259:8353, 1984.
41. Bignami GS: A rapid and sensitive hemolysis neutralization assay for palytoxin, *Toxicon* 31:817, 1993.
42. Bishai WR, Sears CL: Food poisoning syndromes, *Gastroenterol Clin North Am* 22:579, 1993.
43. Blacklow NR, Greenberg HB: Viral gastroenteritis, *N Engl J Med* 325:252, 1991
44. Blakesley ML: Scombroid poisoning: prompt resolution of symptoms with cimetidine, *Ann Emerg Med* 12:104, 1983.
45. Bode RB et al: A new *Vibrio* species, *Vibrio cincinnatiensis*, causing meningitis: successful treatment in an adult, *Ann Intern Med* 104:55, 1986.
46. Boisier P et al: [Fatal ichthyosarcotoxism after eating shark meat. Implications of two new marine toxins], *Archives de L Institut Pasteur de Madagascar* 61:81, 1994.
47. Boland MP et al: A unified bioscreen for the detection of diarrhetic shellfish toxins and microcystins in marine and freshwater environments, *Toxicon* 31:1393, 1993.
48. Borysiewicz L, Krikler D: Scombrotoxic atrial flutter, *Brit Med J* 282:1434, 1981.
49. Bossart GD et al: Brevetoxicosis in manatees (*Trichechus manatus latirostris*) from the 1996 epizootic: gross, histologic, and immunohistochemical features, *Toxicol Pathol* 26:276, 1998.
50. Botero L, Montiel M, Porto L: Enteroviruses in shrimp harvested from contaminated marine water, *Int J Environ Health Res* 6:103, 1996.
51. Bourdy G et al: Traditional remedies in the western Pacific for the treatment of ciguatera poisoning, *J Ethnopharmacol* 36:163, 1992.
52. Bouree P, Paugam A, Petithory JC: Anisakidosis: report of 25 cases and review of the literature, Comparative Immunology, *Microbiol Infect Dis* 18:75, 1995.
53. Bowman PB: Amitriptyline and ciguatera, *Med J Aust* 140:802, 1984.
54. Brennt CE et al: Growth of *Vibrio vulnificus* in serum from alcoholics: association with high transferrin iron saturation, *J Infect Dis* 164:1030, 1991.
55. Brown RL: Successful treatment of primary amebic meningoencephalitis [see comments], *Arch Intern Med* 151:1201, 1991.
56. Bullen JJ et al: Hemochromatosis, iron and septicemia caused by *Vibrio vulnificus*, *Arch Intern Med* 151:1606, 1991.

57. Burkhardt WD, Watkins WD, Rippey SR: Seasonal effects on accumulation of microbial indicator organisms by *Mercenaria mercenaria*, *Appl Environ Microbiol* 58:826, 1992.

58. Calvert GM, Hryhorczuk DO, Leiken JB: Treatment of ciguatera fish poisoning with amitriptyline and nifedipine, *J Toxicol Clin Toxicol* 25:423, 1987.

59. Cameron J, Capra MF: The basis of the paradoxical disturbance of temperature perception, *J Toxicol Clin Toxicol* 31:571, 1993.

60. Cameron J, Flowers AE, Capra MF: Electrophysiological studies on ciguatera poisoning in man (Part II), *J Neurol Sci* 101:93, 1991.

61. Cameron J, Flowers AE, Capra MF: Modification of the peripheral nerve disturbances in ciguatera poisoning in rats with lidocaine, *Muscle Nerve* 1993 16:782, 1993.

62. Campos E et al: *Vibrio mimicus* diarrhea following ingestion of raw turtle eggs, *Appl Environ Microbiol* 62:1141, 1996.

63. Cancrini G, Magro G, Giannone G: [1st case of extra-gastrointestinal anisakiasis in a human diagnosed in Italy], *Parassitologia* 39:13, 1997.

64. Carmichael WW: Cyanobacteria secondary metabolite—the cyanotoxins, *J Appl Bac* 72:445, 1992.

65. Carson RL: The changing year. In Carson RL, editor: *The sea around us,* New York, 1961, Oxford University Press.

66. Centers for Disease Control: Primary amebic meningoencephalitis—North Carolina, 1991, *MMWR* 41:437, 1992.

67. Centers for Disease Control: Reptile-associated salmonellosis—selected states, 1994-1995, *MMWR* 44:347, 1995.

68. Centers for Disease Control: Acute hepatitis and renal failure following ingestion of raw carp gall bladders, *MMWR* 44:565, 1995.

69. Centers for Disease Control: Outbreak of gastrointestinal illness associated with consumption of seaweed—Hawaii, 1994, *MMWR* 44:724, 1995.

70. Centers for Disease Control: Tetrodotoxin poisoning associated with eating puffer fish transported from Japan, *MMWR* 45:389, 1996.

71. Centers for Disease Control: Surveillance for foodborne disease outbreaks—United States, 1988-1992, *MMWR* 45(Surveillance Summary 5), 1996.

72. Centers for Disease Control: Viral gastroenteritis associated with eating oysters—Louisiana, December 1996-January 1997, *MMWR* 46:1109, 1997.

73. Centers for Disease Control: Outbreak of *Vibrio parahaemolyticus* infections associated with eating raw oysters—Pacific Northwest, 1997, *MMWR* 47:457, 1998.

74. Centers for Disease Control: Haff disease associated with eating buffalo fish—United States, *MMWR* 47:1091, 1998.

75. Centers for Disease Control: Outbreak of *Vibrio parahaemolyticus* infection associated with eating raw oysters and clams harvested from Long Island Sound—Connecticut, New Jersey, and New York, 1998, *MMWR* 48:48, 1999.

76. Centers for Disease Control: Notice to readers possible estuary-associated syndrome, *MMWR* 48:381, 1999.

77. Chalmers JW, McMillan JH: An outbreak of viral gastroenteritis associated with adequately prepared oysters, *Epidemiol Infect* 115:163, 1995.

78. Chan DWS, Yeung CK, Chan MK: Acute renal failure after eating raw fish gall bladder, *BMJ* 290:897, 1985.

79. Chan HL, Ho HC, Kuo TT: Cutaneous manifestations of non-01 *Vibrio cholerae* septicemia with gastroenteritis and meningitis, *J Am Acad Dermatol* 30:626,1994.

80. Chan TYK, Wang AYM: Life-threatening bradycardia and hypotension in a patient with ciguatera fish poisoning, *Trans R Scoc Trop Med Hyg* 87:71, 1993.

81. Chen DZK et al: Identification of protein phosphatase inhibitors of the microcystin class in the marine environment, *Toxicon* 31:1407, 1993.

82. Chevallier A, Duchesne EA: Memoire sur les empoisonements par les huitres, les moules, les crabes, et par certains poissons de mer et de riviere, *Ann Hyg Publi (Paris)* 46:108, 1851.

83. Chew SK et al: Anticholinesterase drugs in the treatment of tetrodotoxin poisoning, *Lancet* 2:108, 1984.

84. Chin JD et al: Screening for okadaic acid by immunoassay, *J AOAC Int* 78:508,1995.

85. Cho SY, Kong Y, Kang SY: Epidemiology of paragonimiasis in Korea, *Southeast Asian J Trop Med Public Health* 28(suppl 1)1:32, 1997.

86. Chung PR et al: [Five human cases of *Diphyllobothrium latum* infection through eating raw fish flesh of redlip mullet, *Liza haematocheila*], *Korean J Parasitol* 35:283, 1997.

87. Chungue E et al: Isolation of two toxins from a parrotfish *Scarus gibbus*, *Toxicon* 15:89, 1977.

88. Clark RB: Biological causes and effects of paralytic shellfish poisoning, *Lancet* 2:770, 1968.

89. Cline EI et al: Toxic effects of the novel protein UpI from the sea anemone *Urticina piscivora*, *Pharm Res* 32:309, 1995.

90. Codd GA, Ward CJ, Bell SG: Cyanobacterial toxins: occurrence, modes of action, health effects and exposure routes, *Arch Toxicol Suppl* 19:399, 1997.

91. Cohen P, Holms CFB, Tsukitani Y: Okadaic acid: a new probe for the study of cellular regulation, *Trends Biochem Sci* 98, 1990.

92. Connell DW et al: Fate and risk evaluation of persistent organic contaminants and related compounds in Victoria Harbor, Hong Kong, *Chemosphere* 36:2019, 1998.

93. Craig CP: It's always the big ones that should get away, *JAMA* 244:272, 1980.

94. Croci L et al: A rapid tissue culture assay for the detection of okadaic acid and related compounds in mussels, *Toxicon* 35:223, 1997

95. Cromeans TL, Nainan OV, Margolis HS: Detection of hepatitis A virus RNA in oyster meat, *Appl Environ Microbiol* 63:2460, 1997.

96. Cui J et al: An outbreak of paragonimiosis in Zhengzhou city, China, *Acta Tropica* 70:211, 1998.

97. Curtis MA, Bylund G: Diphyllobothriasis: fish tapeworm disease in the circumpolar north, *Arctic Medical Research* 50:18, 1991.

98. Dabholkar AS, Carmichael WW: Ultrastructural changes in the mouse liver induced by hepatotoxin from the freshwater cyanobacterium *Microcystis aeruginosa* strain 7820, *Toxicon* 25:285, 1987.

99. Dailey MD, Jensen LA, Hill BW: Larval anisakine roundworms of marine fishes from southern and central California, with comments on public health significance, *California Fish and Game* 67:240, 1981.

100. Daschner A et al: Gastric anisakiasis: an underestimated cause of acute urticaria and angio-oedema? *Br J Dermatol* 139:822,1998.

101. Davidson PW et al: Effects of prenatal and postnatal methylmercury exposure from fish consumption on neurodevelopment: outcomes at 66 months of age in the Seychelles Child Development Study [see comments], *JAMA* 280:701, 1998.

102. Davis BR et al: Characterization of biochemically atypical *Vibrio cholerae* strains, and designation of a new pathogenic species, *Vibrio mimicus, J Clin Microbiol* 14:631, 1981.

103. Davis RT, Villar LA: Symptomatic improvement with amitriptyline in ciguatera fish poisoning, *N Engl J Med* 315:65, 1986.

104. Dayal HH, Trieff NM, Dayal V: Preventing *Vibrio vulnificus* infections: who should bear the responsibility? *Am J Prev Med* 9:191, 1993.

105. Del Olmo Escribano M et al: [Anisakiasis at the ileal level], *Revista Espanola De Enfermedades Digestivas* 90:120, 1998.

106. DeNapoli TS: Primary amoebic meningoencephalitis after swimming in the Rio Grande, *Tex Med* 92:59, 1996.

107. Dessai S, Sanna C, Paghi L: Human salmonellosis transmitted by a domestic turtle, *Eur J Epidemiol* 8:120, 1992.

108. Dho S et al: Phosphatase inhibition increases tight junctional permeability in cultured human intestinal epithelial cells, *J Cell Biol* 11:410A, 1990.

109. Dickey RW, Miller DM, Tindall DR: Extraction of a water-soluble toxin from a dinoflagellate, *Gambierdiscus toxicus*. In Ragelis EP, editor: *Seafood toxins*, Washington, DC, 1984, American Chemical Society.

110. Dickey RW et al: Detection of the marine toxins okadaic acid and domoic acid in shellfish and phytoplankton in the Gulf of Mexico, *Toxicon* 30:355, 1992.

111. DiGaetano M, Ball SF, Strauss JG: *Vibrio vulnificus* corneal ulcer, *Arch Ophthalmol* 107:323, 1989.

112. DiGirolamo R, Liston J, Matches JR: Survival of virus in chilled, frozen and processed oysters, *Appl Microbiol* 20:58, 1970.

113. DiNubile MJ, Hokama Y: The ciguatera poisoning syndrome from farm-raised salmon, *Ann Intern Med* 122:113, 1995.

114. Dooley JR: Diphyllobothriasis in Americans and Asians, *JAMA* 247:2230, 1982.

115. Doty MS, Aguilar-Santos G: Caulerpicin, a toxic constituent of *Caulerpa*, *Nature* 211:990, 1966.

116. Dowell SF et al: A multistate outbreak of oyster-associated gastroenteritis: implications for interstate tracing of contaminated shellfish, *J Infect Dis* 171:1497, 1995.

117. Dunn J: Algae kills dialysis patients in Brazil, *BMJ* 312:1183, 1996.

118. Eastaugh JA: Delayed use of intravenous mannitol in ciguatera (fish poisoning), *Ann Emerg Med* 28:105, 1996.

119. Eastaugh J, Shepherd S: Infectious and toxic syndromes from fish and shellfish consumption: a review, *Arch Intern Med* 149:1735, 1989.

120. Eastburn RL, Fritsche TR, Terhune CA: Human intestinal infection with *Nanophetus salminicola* from salmonid fishes, *Am J Trop Med Hyg* 36:586, 1987.

121. Ebe T et al: [Eight cases of diphyllobothriasis]. *Kansenshogaku Zasshi* 64:328, 1990.

122. Edwards C et al: Identification of anatoxin-A in benthic cyanobacteria (blue-green algae) and in associated dog poisonings at Loch Insh, Scotland, *Toxicon* 30:1165, 1992.

123. Endean R et al: Variation in the toxins present in ciguateric narrow-barred Spanish mackerel, *Scomberomorus commersoni*, *Toxicon* 31:723, 1993.

124. Endean R et al: Apparent relationships between toxins elaborated by the cyanobacterium *Trichodesmium erythraeum* and those present in the flesh of the narrow-barred Spanish mackerel *Scomberomorus commersoni*, *Toxicon* 31:1155, 1993.

125. Engleberg NC et al: Ciguatera fish poisoning: a major common source outbreak in the US Virgin Islands, *Ann Intern Med* 98:336, 1983.

126. Eriksson JE et al: Preliminary characterization of a toxin isolated from the cyanobacterium *Nodularia spumigena*, *Toxicon* 26:161, 1988.

127. Evans MH: Cause of death in experimental paralytic shellfish poisoning (PSP), *Br J Exp Pathol* 46:245, 1965.

128. Farris WA, Erdman JW: Protracted hypervitaminosis A following long-term, low-level intake, *JAMA* 247:1317, 1982.

129. Feingold JM: *Acanthamoeba* meningoencephalitis following autologous peripheral stem cell transplantation, *Bone Marrow Transplant* 22:297, 1998.

130. Fernandez A, Justiniani FR: Massive rhabdomyolysis: a rare presentation of primary *Vibrio vulnificus* septicemia, *Am J Med* 89:535, 1990.

132. Fessard V et al: Okadaic acid treatment induces DNA adduct formation in BHK21 C13 fibroblasts and HESV keratinocytes, *Mutat Res* 361:133, 1996.

132. Ficker LA, Kirkness C, Wright P: Prognosis for keratoplasty in *Acanthamoeba* keratitis, *Ophthalmology* 100:105, 1993.

133. Fiorentini C et al: Okadaic acid induces changes in the organization of F-actin in intestinal cells, *Toxicon* 34:937, 1996.

134. Fitzgeorge IR, Choice A, Hosja W: Routes of intoxication. In *Detection methods for cyanobacterial toxins*, Cambridge, UK, 1994, The Royal Society of Chemistry.

135. Flachsenberger WA: Respiratory failure and lethal hypotension due to blue-ringed octopus and tetrodotoxin envenomation observed and counteracted in animal models, *Clin Toxicol* 24:485, 1986.

136. Food and Drug Administration: *Med Bull* 23:6, 1992.

137. Food and Drug Administration: Procedures for the safe and sanitary processing and importing of fish and fishery products. Final Rule, 21 CFR 123, *Federal Register* 60(242):65095, 1995.

138. Fowler M, Carter RF: Acute pyogenic meningitis probably due to *Acanthamoeba* sp: a preliminary report, *BMJ* 2:740, 1965.

139. Fraj Laazaro J et al: Anisakis, anisakiasis and IgE-mediated immunity to Anisakis simplex, *J Invest Allergol Clin Immunol* 8:61, 1998.

140. Fuhrman FA: Tetrodotoxin, tarichatoxin, and chiriquitoxin: historical perspectives, *Ann NY Acad Sci* 479:1, 1986.

141. Fukiya S, Matsumura K: Active and passive immunization for tetrodotoxin in mice, *Toxicon* 30:1631, 1992.

142. Fukui M et al: Occurrence of palytoxin in the triggerfish *Melichtys vidua*, *Toxicon* 25:1121, 1987.

143. Fusetani N, Hashimoto K: Occurrence of pahutoxin and homopahutoxin in the mucus secretion of the Japanese boxfish, *Toxicon* 25:459, 1987.

144. Gago-Martinez A et al: Simultaneous occurrence of diarrhetic and paralytic shellfish poisoning toxins in Spanish mussels in 1993, *Nat Toxins* 4:72, 1996.

145. Garcaia-Labairu C et al: Asymptomatic gastroduodenal anisakiasis as the cause of anaphylaxis, *Eur J Gastroenterol Hepatol* 11:785, 1999.

146. Garcaia-Martos P, Benjumeda M, Delgado D: [Otitis externa caused by *Vibrio alginolyticus*: description of 4 cases], *Acta Otorrinolaringologica Espanola* 44:55. 1993.

147. Garrison DL et al: Confirmation of domoic acid production by *Psudonitzschia australis (Bacillario-phyceae)* cultures, *J Phycol* 28:604, 1992.

148. Geller RJ, Olson KR, Senécal PE: Ciguatera fish poisoning in San Francisco, California, caused by imported barracuda, *West J Med* 155:639, 1991.

149. Gessner BD, Middaugh JP: Paralytic shellfish poisoning in Alaska: a 20-year retrospective analysis, *Am J Epidemiol* 141:766, 1995.

150. Giboda M et al: Human Opisthorchis and Haplorchis infections in Laos, *Trans R Scoc Trop Med Hyg* 85:538, 1991.

151. Gilbert DN, Moellering RC, Sande MA: *The Sanford guide to antimicrobial therapy*, ed 29, p 9, 1999.

152. Gilbert DN, Moellering RC, Sande MA: *The Sanford guide to antimicrobial therapy*, ed 29, p 38, 1999.

153. Gilbert DN, Moellering RC, Sande MA: *The Sanford guide to antimicrobial therapy*, ed 29, p 89, 1999.

154. Gilbert DN, Moellering RC, Sande MA: *The Sanford guide to antimicrobial therapy*, ed 29, p 95, 1999.

155. Gilbert RJ et al: Scombrotoxic fish poisoning: features of the first 50 incidents to be reported in Britain (1976-9), *BMJ* 281:71, 1980.

156. Glasgow HB Jr et al: Insidious effects of a toxic estuarine dinoflagellate on fish survival and human health, *J Toxicol Environ Health* 46:501, 1995.

157. Glazious P, Legrand AM: The epidemiology of ciguatera fish poisoning, *Toxicon* 32:863, 1994.

158. Glazious P, Martin PMV: Study of factors that influence the clinical response to ciguatera fish poisoning, *Toxicon* 31:1151, 1993.

159. Goldberg AS, Duffield AM, Barrow DK: Distribution and chemical composition of the toxic skin secretions from trunkfish (family Ostraciidae), *Toxicon* 26:651, 1988.

160. Goldfrank LR et al: *Toxicologic emergencies*, ed 5, Norwalk, Conn, 1994, Appleton & Lange.

161. Goldmann DR: Hold the sushi, *JAMA* 253:2495, 1985.

162. Golub JE et al: Pfiesteria in Maryland: preliminary epidemiologic findings, *Md Med J* 47:137, 1998.

163. Gras-Rouzet S et al: First European case of gastroenteritis and bacteremia due to *Vibrio hollisae*, *Eur J Clin Microbiol Infect Dis* 15:864, 1996.

164. Grattan LM et al: Learning and memory difficulties after environmental exposure to waterways containing toxin-producing *Pfiesteria* or *Pfiesteria*-like dinoflagellates, *Lancet* 352:532, 1998.

165. Grattan LM et al: Neurobehavioral complaints of symptomatic persons exposed to *Pfiesteria piscicida* or morphologically related organisms, *Md Med J* 47:127, 1998.

166. Greenwood M, Winnard G, Bagot B: An outbreak of *Salmonella* enteritis phage type 19 infection associated with cockles, *Communicable Disease and Public Health* 1:35, 1998.

167. Guillaen-Bueno R et al: Anti-anisakis antibodies in the clinical course of Crohn's disease, *Digestion* 60:268, 1999.

168. Guss DA: Scombroid fish poisoning: successful treatment with cimetidine, *Undersea and Hyperbaric Medicine* 25:123, 1998.

169. Habermann E: Palytoxin acts through Na+, K+-ATPase, *Toxicon* 27:1171, 1989.

170. Hahn ST, Capra MF, Walsh TP: Ciguatoxin-protein association in skeletal muscle of Spanish mackerel *(Scomberomorus commersoni)*, *Toxicon* 30:843, 1992.

171. Hall S, Reichardt PB: Cryptic paralytic shellfish toxins. In Ragelis EP, editor: *Seafood toxins*, Washington, DC, 1984, American Chemical Society.

172. Halstead BW: *Poisonous and venomous marine animals of the world*, vol 1, Washington, DC, 1965, United States Government Printing Office.

173. Halstead BW: *Poisonous and venomous marine animals of the world*, vol 2, Washington, DC, 1967, United States Government Printing Office.

174. Halstead BW: Marine pollution and the pharmaceutical scientist, *Am J Pharmacol Ed* 37:267, 1978.

175. Halstead BW: *Current status of marine biotoxicology—an overview*, Colton, Calif, 1980, International Biotoxicological Center, World Life Research Institute.

176. Halstead BW: Miscellaneous seafood toxicants. In Ragelis EP, editor: *Seafood toxins*, Washington, DC, 1984, American Chemical Society.

177. Halstead BW, Haddock RL: A fatal outbreak of poisoning from the ingestion of red seaweed *Gracilaria tsudae* in Guam—a review of the oral marine biotoxicity problem, *J Nat Toxins* 1:87, 1992.

178. Hamano Y, Kinoshita Y, Yasumoto T: Suckling mice assay for diarrhetic shellfish toxins. In Anderson DM, White AW, Baden DG, editors: *Toxic dinoflagellates*, New York, 1985, Elsevier.

179. Han B et al: Estimation of target hazard quotients and potential health risks for metals by consumption of seafood in Taiwan, *Arch Environ Contam Toxicol* 35:711, 1998.

180. Harada K-I et al: A new procedure for the analysis and purification of naturally occurring anatoxin-a from the blue-green alga *Anabaena flos-aquae*, *Toxicon* 27:1289, 1989.

181. Harding WR et al: Death of a dog attributed to the cyanobacterial (blue-green algal) hepatotoxin nodularin in South Africa, *J S Afr Vet Assoc* 66:256, 1995.

182. Hariharan J et al: Bacteriological studies on mussels and oysters from six river systems in Prince Edward Island, Canada, *J Shellfish Res* 14:527, 1995.

183. Hartigan-Go K, Bateman DN: Redtides in the Phillipines, *Hum Exp Toxicol* 13:824, 1994.

184. Hashimoto Y, Kamiya H: Occurrence of a toxic substance in the skin of a sea bass *Pogonoperca punctata*, *Toxicon* 7:65, 1969.

185. Hauschild AHW, Gauvreau L: Food-borne botulism in Canada, 1971-84, *Can Med Assoc J* 133:1141, 1985.

186. Helfrich P: Fish poisoning in Hawaii, *Hawaii Med J* 22:361, 1963.

187. Helfrich P, Banner AH: Experimental induction of ciguatera toxicity in fish through diet, *Nature* 197:1025, 1963.

188. Henderson R, Ritchie JM, Strichartz GR: Evidence that tetrodotoxin and saxitoxin act at a metal cation binding site in the sodium channels of nerve membrane, *Proc Natl Acad Sci USA* 71:3936, 1974.

189. Hlady WG, Klontz KC: The epidemiology of *Vibrio* infections in Florida, *J Infect Dis* 173:1176, 1996

190. Ho AM, Fraser IM, Todd ECD: Ciguatera poisoning: a report of three cases, *Ann Emerg Med* 15:1225, 1986.

191. Howard RJ, Bennett NT: Infections caused by halophilic marine *Vibrio* bacteria, *Ann Surg* 217:525, 1993.

192. Hu T et al: Isolation and structure of prorocentrolide B, a fast-acting toxin from *Prorocentrum maculosum*, *J Nat Prod* 59:1010,1996.

193. Hughes JM, Merson MH: Fish and shellfish poisoning, *N Engl J Med* 295:1117, 1976.

194. Hughes JM, Potter ME: Scombroid-fish poisoning: from pathogenesis to prevention, *N Engl J Med* 324:766, 1991.

195. Hutchinson JW et al: Diphyllobothriasis after eating raw salmon, *Hawaii Med J* 56:176, 1997.

196. Hyytiea E, Hielm S, Korkeala H: Prevalence of *Clostridium botulinum* type E in Finnish fish and fishery products, *Epidemiol Infect* 120:245, 1998.

197. Ido K et al: Sonographic diagnosis of small intestinal anisakiasis, *J Clin Ultrasound* 26:125, 1998.

198. Illingworth CD et al: *Acanthamoeba* keratitis: risk factor and outcome, *Br J Ophthalmol* 79:1078, 1995.

199. Iida T et al: Detection of *Listeria monocytogenes* in humans, animals and foods, *J Vet Med Sci* 60:1341, 1998.

200. Institute of Medicine: *Seafood safety*, Washington, DC, 1991, National Academy Press.

201. Ito E, Nagai H: Morphological observations of diarrhea in mice caused by aplysiatoxin, the causative agent of the red alga *Gracilaria coronopifolia* poisoning in Hawaii, *Toxicon* 36:1913, 1998.

202. Iwaoka W et al: Analysis of *Acanthurus triostegus* for marine toxins by the stick enzyme immunoassay and mouse bioassay, *Toxicon* 30:1575, 1992.

203. Janda JM: A lethal leviathan—*Vibrio vulnificus*, *West J Med* 155:421, 1991.

204. Janda JM et al: Current perspectives on the epidemiology and pathogenesis of clinically significant *Vibrio* spp, *Clin Microbiol Rev* 1:245, 1988.

205. Janitschke, K: Animal model *Balamuthia mandrillaris* CNS infection: contrast and comparison in immunodeficient and immunocompetent mice: a murine model of "granulomatous" amebic encephalitis, *J Neuropathol Exp Neurol* 55:815, 1996.

206. Jean-Jacques W et al: *Vibrio metschnikovii* bacteremia in a patient with cholecystitis, *J Clin Microbiol* 14:711, 1981.

207. Jellett JF et al: Paralytic shellfish poison (saxitoxin family) bioassays: automated endpoint determination and standardization of the in vitro tissue culture bioassay, and comparison with the standard mouse bioassay, *Toxicon* 30:1143, 1992.

208. John DT: Primary amebic meningoencephalitis and the biology of *Naegleria fowleri*, *Ann Rev Microbiol* 36:101,1982.

209. Jones SH, Howell TL, O'Neill KR: Differential elimination of indicator bacteria and pathogenic *Vibrio* spp from Easter oysters (Crassostrea virginica Gmelin, 1791) in a commercial controlled purification facility in Maine, *J Shellfish Res* 10:105, 1991.

210. Juglard R et al: [Anisakiasis, rare pseudotumor colonic involvement. Apropos of a case], *J Radiol* 79:883, 1998.

211. Juranovic LR, Park DL: Foodborne toxins of marine origin: ciguatera, *Rev Environ Contam Toxicol* 117:51, 1991.

212. Kakizoe S et al: Endoscopic findings and clinical manifestation of gastric anisakiasis, *Am J Gastroenterol* 90:761, 1995.

213. Kam KM et al: Outbreak of *Vibrio cholerae* 01 in Hong Kong related to contaminated fish tank water, *Public Health* 109:389, 1995.

214. Kanchanapongkul J, Krittayapoositpot P: An epidemic of tetrodotoxin poisoning following ingestion of the horseshoe crab *Carcinoscorpius rotundicauda*, *Southeast Asian J Trop Med Public Health* 26:364, 1995.

215. Kao CY: Tetrodotoxin, saxitoxin, and their significance in the study of excitation phenomena, *Pharmacol Rev* 18:997, 1966.

216. Kao CY: Pharmacology of tetrodotoxin and saxitoxin, *Fed Proc* 31:1117, 1972.

217. Kao CY, Yasumoto T: Tetrodotoxin in "zombie powder," *Toxicon* 28:129, 1990.

218. Kao CY, Yeoh PH: Different receptors for saxitoxin and tetrodotoxin, *Proc Physiol Soc* 284:88P, 1982.

219. Kao CY et al: Vasodilatory effects of tetrodotoxin in the cat, *J Pharmacol Exp Ther* 178:110, 1971.

220. Kasha EE, Norins AL: Scombroid fish poisoning with facial flushing (letter), *J Am Acad Dermatol* 18:1363, 1988.

221. Katz BZ: *Vibrio vulnificus* meningitis in a boy with thalassemia after eating raw oysters, *Pediatrics* 82:784, 1998.

222. Kidney DD, Kim SH: CNS infections with free-living amebas: neuroimaging findings, *Am J Roentgenol* 171:809, 1998.

223. Kirkland KB et al: Steaming oysters does not prevent Norwalk-like gastroenteritis, *Pub Health Rep* 111:527, 1996.

224. Kizer KW: Domoic acid poisoning, *West J Med* 161:59, 1994.

225. Kliks MM: Anisakiasis in the western United States: four new case reports from California, *Am J Trop Med Hyg* 32:526, 1983.

226. Kliks MM: Human anisakiasis: an update, *JAMA* 255:2605, 1986.

227. Klontz KC: Fatalities associated with *Vibrio parahaemolyticus* and *Vibrio cholerae* non-01 infections in Florida (1981 to 1988), *South Med J* 83:500, 1990.

228. Klontz KC et al: Fatal gastroenteritis due to *Vibrio fluvialis* and nonfatal bacteremia due to *Vibrio mimicus*: unusual vibrio infections in two patients (letter), *Clin Infect Dis* 19:541, 1994.

229. Kodama AM, Hokama Y: Variations in symptomatology of ciguatera poisoning, *Toxicon* 27:593, 1989.

230. Kodama AM et al: Clinical and laboratory findings implicating palytoxin as cause of ciguatera poisoning due to Decapterus macrosoma (mackerel), *Toxicon* 27:1051, 1989.

231. Kodama M et al: Production of paralytic shellfish toxins by a bacterium *Moraxella* sp. isolated from *Protogonyaulax tamarensis*, *Toxicon* 28:707, 1990.

232. Kodjo A et al: Isolation and identification of *Salmonella* species from chelonians using combined selective media, serotyping and ribotyping, *Zentralbl Veterinarmed (B)* 44:625, 1997.

233. Kohn MA et al: An outbreak of Norwalk virus gastroenteritis associated with eating raw oysters. Implications for maintaining safe oyster beds (published erratum appears in JAMA 273:1492, 1995), *JAMA* 273:466, 1995.

234. Koide J et al: Granulomatous amoebic encephalitis caused by *Acanthamoeba* in a patient with systemic lupus erythematosus, *Clin Rheumatol* 17:329, 1998.

235. Krovacek K et al: Detection of potential virulence markers of *Vibrio vulnificus* strains isolated from fish in Sweden, *Comp Immunol Microbiol Infect Dis* 17:63, 1994.

236. Kumamoto KS, Vukich DJ: Clinical infections of *Vibrio vulnificus*: a case report and review of the literature, *J Emerg Med* 16:61, 1998.

237. Lange WR: Ciguatera fish poisoning, *Am Fam Phys* 50:579, 1994.

238. Lange WR, Lipkin KM, Yang GC: Can ciguatera be a sexually transmitted disease? *Clin Toxicol* 27:193, 1989.

239. Lange WR et al: Potential benefit of tocainide in the treatment of ciguatera: report of three cases, *Am J Med* 84:1087, 1988.

240. Lares-Villa F: Five cases of primary amebic meningoencephalitis in Mexicali, Mexico: study of the isolates, *J Clin Microbiol* 31:685, 1993.

241. Larkin DFP, Kilvington S, Dart JKG: Treatment of *Acanthamoeba* keratitis with polyhexamethylene biguanide, *Ophthalmol* 99:185, 1992.

242. Lawrence DN et al: Ciguatera fish poisoning in Miami, *JAMA* 244:254, 1980.

243. Le Guyader F et al: Detection and analysis of a small round-structured virus strain in oysters implicated in an outbreak of acute gastroenteritis, *Appl Environ Microbiol* 62:4268, 1996.

244. Legrand AM, Bagnis R: Mode of action of ciguatera toxins. In Ragelis EP, editor: *Seafood toxins*, Washington, DC, 1984, American Chemical Society.

245. Legrand AM, Galannier M, Bagnis R: Studies on the mode of action of ciguateric toxins, *Toxicon* 20:311, 1982.

246. Levin ED et al: Persisting learning deficits in rats after exposure to *Pfiesteria piscicida*, *Environ Health Perspect* 105:1320, 1997.

247. Levin ED et al: *Pfiesteria* toxin and learning performance, *Neurotoxicol Teratol* 21:215, 1999.

248. Levine L et al: Production of antibodies and development of a radioimmunoassay for okadaic acid, *Toxicon* 26:1123, 1988.

249. Lewis RJ: Ciguatoxins are potent ichthyotoxins, *Toxicon* 30:207, 1992.

250. Lewis RJ, Hoy AWW, McGiffin DC: Action of ciguatoxin on human atrial trabeculae, *Toxicon* 30:907, 1992.

251. Lewis RJ, Sellin M: Multiple ciguatoxins in the flesh of fish, *Toxicon* 30:915, 1992.

252. Lewis RJ, Wong Hoy AW, Sellin M: Ciguatera and mannitol: in vivo and in vitro assessment in mice, *Toxicon* 31:1039, 1993.

253. Lewis RJ et al: Purification and characterization of ciguatoxins from moray eel (*Lycodontis javanicus*, Muraenidae), *Toxicon* 29:1115, 1991.

254. Lewis RJ et al: Ciguatoxin-2 is a diastereomer of ciguatoxin-3, *Toxicon* 31:637, 1993.

255. Lin CJ et al: Non-O1 *Vibrio cholerae* bacteremia in patients with cirrhosis: 5-yr experience from a single medical center, *Am J Gastroenterol* 91:336, 1996.

256. Lipp EK, Rose JB: The role of seafood in foodborne diseases in the United States of America, *Revue Scientifique et Technique* 16:620, 1997.

257. Llewellyn LE, Endean R: Toxic coral reef crabs from Australian waters, *Toxicon* 26:1085, 1988.

258. Llewellyn LE, Endean R: Toxins extracted from Australian specimens of the crab, *Eriphia sebana* (Xanthidae), *Toxicon* 27:579, 1989.

259. Llewellyn LE, Endean R: Toxicity and paralytic shellfish toxin profiles of the xanthid crabs, *Lophozozymus pictor* and *Zosimus aeneus,* collected from some Australian coral reefs, *Toxicon* 27:596, 1989.

260. Llewellyn LE, Endean R: Paralytic shellfish toxins in the xanthid crab *Atergatis floridus* collected from Australian coral reefs, *J Wilderness Med* 2:118, 1991.

261. Lopes CM et al: A case of *Vibrio alginolyticus* bacteremia and probable sphenoiditis following a dive in the sea (letter), *Clin Infect Dis* 17:299, 1993.

262. Lotz MJ, Tamplin ML, Rodrick GE: Thiosulfate–citrate–bile salts–sucrose agar and its selectivity for clinical and marine vibrio organisms, *Ann Clin Lab Sci* 13:45, 1983.

263. Lyn PCW: Puffer fish poisoning: Four case reports, *Med J Malaysia* 40:31, 1985.

264. Maggi P et al: Epidemiological, clinical and therapeutic evaluation of the Italian cholera epidemic in 1994, *Eur J Epidemiol* 13:95, 1997.

265. Mahaffey KR, Mergler D: Blood levels of total and organic mercury in residents of the upper St. Lawrence River basin, Quaebec: association with age, gender, and fish consumption, *Environ Res* 77:104, 1998.

266. Mallaret MR et al: [Human salmonellosis and turtles in France], *Revue D Epidemiologie et de Sante Publique* 38:71, 1990.

267. Manowitz NR, Rosenthal RR: Cutaneous-systemic reactions to toxins and venoms of common marine organisms, *Cutis* 23:450, 1979.

268. Maramba NPC, Panganiban LCR, Hartigan-Go KY: *Algorithm of common poisoning,* Manila, Philippines, National Science and Technology Authority, pp 99-102, 1991.

269. Martinez, AJ, Visvesvara, GS: Free-living, amphizoic and opportunistic amebas, *Brain Pathol* 7:583, 1997.

270. Matias WG, Traore A, Creppy EE: Variations in the distribution of okadaic acid in organs and biological fluids of mice related to diarrhoeic syndrome, *Hum Exp Toxicol* 18:345, 1999.

271. Matte GR et al: Distribution of potentially pathogenic Vibrios in oysters from a tropical region, *J Food Prot* 57:540, 1994.

272. McCollum JPK et al: An epidemic of mussel poisoning in northeast England, *Lancet* 2:767, 1968.

273. McInerney J et al: Scombroid poisoning, *Ann Emerg Med* 28:235, 1996.

274. McKerrow JH, Sakanari J, Deardorff TL: Anisakiasis: revenge of the sushi parasite (letter), *N Engl J Med* 319:1228, 1988.

275. Mebs D: Occurrence and sequestration of toxins in food chains, *Toxicon* 36:1519, 1998.

276. Mehtar S et al: Adult epiglottitis due to *Vibrio vulnificus, BMJ* 296:827, 1988.

277. Melton RJ et al: Fatal sardine poisoning: a fatal case of fish poisoning in Hawaii associated with the Marquesan sardine, *Hawaii Med J* 43:114, 1984.

278. Miller DM, Dickey RW, Tindall DR: Lipid-extracted toxins from a dinoflagellate, Gambierdiscus toxicus. In Ragelis EP, editor: *Seafood toxins,* Washington, DC, 1984, American Chemical Society.

279. Misbah SA, Peiris JB, Atukorala TMS: Ingestion of shark liver associated with pseudotumor cerebri due to acute hypervitaminosis A, *J Neurol Neurosurg Psychiatry* 47:216, 1984.

280. Mitra U et al: Acute diarrhoea caused by *Vibrio mimicus* in Calcutta (see comments), *J Assoc Phys India* 41:487, 1993.

281. Morris GK et al: Comparison of four plating media for isolating *Vibrio cholerae, J Clin Microbiol* 9:79, 1979.

282. Morris JG, Jr: Pfiesteria, "the cell from hell," and other toxic algal nightmares, *Clin Infect Dis* 28:1191, 1999.

283. Morris JG et al: Clinical features of ciguatera fish poisoning: a study of the disease in the US Virgin Islands, *Arch Intern Med* 142:1090, 1982.

284. Morris PD, Campbell DS, Freeman JI: Ciguatera fish poisoning: an outbreak associated with fish caught from North Carolina coastal waters, *South Med J* 83:379, 1990.

285. Morris PD et al: Clinical and epidemiological features of neurotoxic shellfish poisoning in North Carolina, *Am J Public Health* 81:471, 1991.

286. Morrow JD et al: Evidence that histamine is the causative toxin of scombroid-fish poisoning, *N Engl J Med* 324:716, 1991.

287. Mosher HS et al: Tarichatoxin-tetrodotoxin: A potent neurotoxin, *Science* 144:1100, 1964.

288. Motes ML et al: Influence of water temperature and salinity on *Vibrio vulnificus* in Northern Gulf and Atlantic Coast oysters (Crassostrea virginica), *Appl Environ Microbiol* 64:1459, 1998.

289. Murata K et al: Delayed evoked potentials in children exposed to methylmercury from seafood, *Neurotoxicol Teratol* 21:343, 1999.

290. Murata M et al: Structures and configurations of ciguatoxin from the moray eel *Gymnothorax javanicus* and its likely precursor from the dinoflagellate *Gambierdiscus toxicus, J Am Chem Soc* 112:4380, 1990.

391. Myers BJ: Anisakine nematodes in fresh commercial fish from waters along the Washington, Oregon and California coasts, *J Food Prot* 42:380, 1979.

292. Myers GJ, Davidson PW: Prenatal methylmercury exposure and children: neurologic, developmental, and behavioral research, *Environ Health Perspect* 106(suppl 3):841, 1998.

293. Nagai H, Yasumoto T, Hokama Y: Aplysiatoxin and debromoaplysiatoxin as the causative agent of a red alga *Gracilaria coronopifolia* poisoning in Hawaii, *Toxicon* 37:753, 1996.

294. Nakajima S, Potvin JL: Neural and behavioral effects of domoic acid, and amnestic shellfish toxin, in the rat, *Can J Psychology* 46:569, 1992.

295. Namikoshi M et al: Isolation and structures of microcystins from a cyanobacterial water bloom (Finland), *Toxicon* 30:1473, 1992.

296. Nawa Y: Recent trends of *Paragonimiasis westermani* in Miyazaki Prefecture, Japan, *Southeast Asian J Trop Med Public Health* 22(suppl):342, 1991.

297. Negri AP, Jones GJ, Hindmarsh M: Sheep mortality associated with paralytic shellfish poisons from the cyanobacterium *Anabaena circinalis, Toxicon* 33:1321,1995.

298. Neuwirth C et al: Myocarditis due to *Salmonella virchow* and sudden infant death (letter), *Lancet* 354:1004, 1999.

299. New system for seafood safety, *Environ Health Perspect* 106: A475, 1998

300. Nicolaou KC et al: Total synthesis of brevetoxin A, *Nature* 392:264, 1998.

301. Noguchi T et al: Poisoning by the red alga 'ogonori' (*Gracilaria verrucosa*) on the Nojima Coast, Yokohama, Kanagawa Prefecture, Japan, *Toxicon* 32:1533, 1994.

302. Ogata T, Sato S, Kodama M: Paralytic shellfish toxins in bivalves which are not associated with dinoflagellates, *Toxicon* 27:1241, 1989.

303. Ohnishi K, Murata M: Single dose treatment with praziquantel for human *Diphyllobothrium nihonkaiense* infections, *Trans R Scoc Trop Med Hyg* 87:482, 1993.

304. Okano H et al: Rhabdomyolysis and myocardial damage induced by palytoxin, a toxin of blue humphead parrotfish, *Intern Med* 37:330, 1998.

305. Oliver JD et al: Entry into, and resuscitation from, the viable but nonculturable state by *Vibrio vulnificus* in an estuarine environment, *Appl Environ Microbiol* 61:2624, 1995.

306. Olney JW: Excitotoxicity: an overview, *Can Dis Weekly Rep* 16(suppl):47, 1990.

307. Onuma Y et al: Identification of putative palytoxin as the cause of clupeotoxism, *Toxicon* 37: 55, 1999.

308. Oshima Y et al: Paralytic shellfish toxins in tropical waters. In Ragelis EP, editor: *Seafood toxins,* Washington, DC, 1984, American Chemical Society.

309. Palafox NA et al: Successful treatment of ciguatera fish poisoning with intravenous mannitol, *JAMA* 259:2740, 1988.

310. Park DL et al: Variability of mouse bioassay for determination of paralytic shellfish poisoning toxins, *J Assoc Anal Chem* 69:547, 1986.

311. Park ED, Lightner DV, Park DL: Antimicrobials in shrimp aquaculture in the United States: regulatory status and safety concerns, *Rev Environ Contam Toxicol* 138:1, 1994.

312. Pearn J: Ciguatera—an early report (letter), *Med J Aust* 151:724, 1989.

313. Pearn JH et al: Ciguatera and mannitol: experience with a new treatment regimen, *Med J Aust* 151:77, 1989.

314. Pearson RD, Hewlett EL: Niclosamide therapy for tapeworm infections, *Ann Intern Med* 102:550, 1985.

315. Pepper SJ, Smith HM: Toxic fish and mollusks, Information Bulletin No 12, Maxwell AFB, Alabama, Air Training Command/Experimental Information Division.

316. Perl T et al: An outbreak of toxic encephalopathy caused by eating mussels contaminated with domoic acid, *N Engl J Med* 322:1775, 1990.

317. Pilotto LS et al: Health effects of exposure to cyanobacteria (blue-green algae) during recreational water-related activities, *Aust NZ J Public Health* 21:562, 1997.

318. Pina S et al: Viral pollution in the environment and in shellfish: human adenovirus detection by PCR as an index of human viruses, *Appl Environ Microbiol* 64:3376, 1998.

319. Poulos JE et al: Non 0-1 *Vibrio cholerae* septicemia and culture negative neutrocytic ascites in a patient with chronic liver disease, *J Fla Med Assoc* 81:676, 1994.

320. Poungvarin N, Jariya P: The fifth nonlethal case of primary amoebic meningoencephalitis, *J Med Assoc Thai* 74:112, 1991.

321. Prescott BD: "Scombroid poisoning" and bluefish: the Connecticut connection, *Conn Med* 48:105, 1984.

322. Price DW, Kizer KW, Hansgen KH: California's Paralytic Shellfish Prevention Program, 1927-89, *J Shellfish Res* 10:119, 1991.

323. Queuche F, Cao Van V, Lae Dang H: [Endemic area of paragonimiasis in Vietnam], *Sante* 7:155, 1997.

324. Ragelis EP: Ciguatera seafood poisoning: overview. In Ragelis EP, editor: *Seafood toxins*, Washington, DC, 1984, American Chemical Society.

325. Rajkovic IA, Williams R: Abnormalities of neutrophil phagocytosis, intracellular killing and metabolic activity in alcoholic cirrhosis and hepatitis, *Hepatology* 6:252, 1986.

326. Ramamurthy T et al: *Vibrio mimicus* with multiple toxin types isolated from human and environmental sources, *J Med Microbiol* 40:194, 1994.

327. Ranaivoson G et al: [Mass food poisoning after eating sea turtle in the Antalaha district], *Archives de L Institut Pasteur de Madagascar* 61:84, 1994.

328. Rand PW et al: The application of charcoal hemoperfusion to paralytic shellfish poisoning, *J Maine Med Assoc* 68:147, 1977.

329. *Raw oyster warning and tag and label requirements*. 17 Calif Code Reg #13675..

330. Reina J, Fernandez-Baca V, Lopez A: Acute gastroenteritis caused by *Vibrio alginolyticus* in an immunocompetent patient, *Clin Infect Dis* 21:1044,1995.

331. Reina Prieto J, Hervas Palazaon J: [Otitis media due to *Vibrio alginolyticus*: the risks of the Mediterranean Sea (letter)], *Anales Espanoles de Pediatria* 39:361, 1993.

332. Renzoni A, Zino F, Franchi E: Mercury levels along the food chain and risk for exposed populations, *Environ Res* 77:68, 1998.

333. Reppun JIF: Ciguatera poisoning in the Pacific, *Hawaii Med J* 47:462, 1988.

334. Richards IS et al: Florida red-tide toxins (brevetoxins) produce depolarization of airway smooth muscle, *Toxicon* 28:1105, 1990.

335. Riestra-Castaneda JM: Granulomatous amebic encephalitis due to *Balamuthia mandrillaris* (Leptomyxiidae): report of four cases from Mexico, *Am J Trop Med Hyg* 56:603, 1997.

336. Rippey SR: Infectious diseases associated with molluscan shellfish consumption, *Clin Microbiol Rev* 7:419, 1994.

337. Rodrâiguez R et al: [Central nervous system infection by free-living amebas: report of 3 Venezuelan cases, *Revista de Neurologia* 26:1005, 1998.

338. Rodraiguez Ramos C et al: Spontaneous non-O1 *Vibrio cholerae* peritonitis after raw oyster ingestion in a patient with cirrhosis, *Eur J Clin Microbiol Infect Dis* 17:362, 1998.

339. Rose JB, Sobsey MD: Quantitative risk assessment for viral contamination of shellfish and coastal waters, *J Food Protec* 56:1042, 1993.

340. Rosen L et al: Studies on eosinophilic meningitis. 3. Epidemiologic and clinical observations on Pacific Islands and the possible etiologic role of *Angiostrongylus cantonensis*, *Am J Epidemiol* 85:17, 1967.

341. Ruff TA: Ciguatera in the Pacific: a link with military activities, *Lancet* 1:201, 1989.

342. Rump S, Rabsztyn T: Effects of some veratrine-like agents on the muscular blocking action of tetrodotoxin, *Toxicon* 15:521, 1977.

343. Runnegar MTC, Jackson ARB, Falconer IR: Toxicity of the cyano-bacterium *Nodularia spumigena mertens*, *Toxicon* 26:143, 1988.

344. Russell FE: Comparative pharmacology of some animal toxins, *Fed Proc* 26:1206, 1967.

345. Russell FE, Maretic Z: Scombroid poisoning: mini-review with case histories, *Toxicon* 24:967, 1986.

346. Sachs R, Cumberlidge N: Distribution of metacercariae in freshwater crabs in relation to Paragonimus infection of children in Liberia, West Africa, *Ann Trop Med Parasitol* 84:277,1990.

347. Sakamoto Y et al: Acute liver damage with characteristic apoptotic hepatocytes by ingestion of *Aplysia kurodai*, a sea hare, *Intern Med* 37:927, 1998.

348. Sakanari JA et al: Intestinal anisakiasis: a case diagnosed by morphologic and immunologic methods, *Am J Clin Pathol* 90:107, 1988.

349. Schantz EJ: Historical perspective on paralytic shellfish poison. In Ragelis EP, editor: *Seafood toxins*, Washington, DC, 1984, American Chemical Society.

350. Scheuer PJ et al: Ciguatoxin: isolation and chemical nature, *Science* 155:1267, 1967.

351. Schumacher et al: Neuroimaging findings in rare amebic infections of the central nervous system, *Am J Neuroradiol* 4(suppl):930, 1995.

352. Schuster FL, Visvesvara GS: Axenic growth and drug sensitivity studies of *Balamuthia mandrillaris*, an agent of amebic meningoencephalitis in humans and other animals, *J Clin Microbiol* 34:385, 1996.

353. Schwab KJ et al: Distribution of Norwalk virus within shellfish following bioaccumulation and subsequent depuration by detection using RT-PCR, *J Food Protec* 61:1674, 1998.

354. Schwarcz R, Scholz D, Coyle JT: Structure-activity relations for the neurotoxicity of kainic acid derivatives and glutamate analogues, *Neuropharmacology* 17:145, 1978.

355. Schwartz GG: Multiple myeloma: clusters, clues, and dioxins (see comments), *Cancer Epidemiol Biomarkers Prev* 6:49, 1997.

356. Schwob JE et al: Widespread patterns of neuronal damage following systemic or intracerebral injections of kainic acid: a historical study, *Neurosciences* 5:991, 1980.

357. Scoging A, Bahl M: Diarrhetic shellfish poisoning in the UK (letter), *Lancet* 352:117, 1998.

358. Scully RE: Case records of the Massachusetts General Hospital, *N Engl J Med* 323:467, 1990.

359. Seidel JS et al: Successful treatment of primary amebic meningoencephalitis, *N Engl J Med* 306:346, 1982.

360. Senecal P-E, Osterloh JD: Normal fetal outcome after maternal ciguateric toxin exposure in the second trimester, *Clin Toxicol* 29:473, 1991.

361. Seven MJ: Mussel poisoning, *Ann Intern Med* 48:891,1958.

362. Shantz EJ: Poisonous red tide organisms, *Environ Lett* 9:225, 1975.

363. Shapiro RL et al: The role of Gulf Coast oysters harvested in warmer months in *Vibrio vulnificus* infections in the United States, 1988-1996. Vibrio Working Group, *J Infect Dis* 178:752, 1998.

364. Shaw JFE et al: Restaurant-associated scombroid fish poisoning—Alabama, Tennessee, *MMWR* 35:264, 1986.

365. Shea D: Analysis of brevetoxins by micellar electrokinetic capillary chromatography and laser-induced fluorescence detection, *Electrophoresis* 18:277, 1997.

366. Shestowsky WS, Quilliam MA, Sikorska HM: An idiotypic-anti-idiotypic competitive immunoassay for quantitation of okadaic acid, *Toxicon* 30:1441, 1992.

367. Shi L et al: Detection of genes encoding *Cholera* toxin (ct), *Zonula occludens* toxin (zot), accessory *Cholera* enterotoxin (ace) and heat-stable enterotoxin (st) in *Vibrio mimicus* clinical strains. *Microbiol Immunol* 42:823, 1998.

368. Shiomi K et al: Occurrence of tetrodotoxin-binding high molecular weight substances in the body fluid of shore crab (*Hemigrapsus sanguineus*), *Toxicon* 30:1529, 1992.

369. Shirahama M et al: Colonic anisakiasis simulating carcinoma of the colon (letter), *AJR* 155:895, 1990.

370. Shoemaker RC: Diagnosis of *Pfiesteria*-human illness syndrome, *Md Med J* 46:521, 1997.

371. Shoemaker RC: Treatment of persistent *Pfiesteria*-human illness syndrome, *Md Med J* 47:64, 1998.

372. Sidorova LD et al: Kidney lesions in dietary and toxic paroxysmal myoglobinuria (Iuksovsk-Sartlansk disease), *Ter Arkh* 57:120, 1985.

373. Sims JK: The diet in ciguatera fish poisoning, *Communicable Diseases Report*, Hawaii State Department of Health, p 4, April 1985.

374. Sims JK: A theoretical discourse on the pharmacology of toxic marine ingestions, *Ann Emerg Med* 16:1006, 1987.

375. Sims JK, Ostman DC: Pufferfish poisoning: emergency diagnosis and management of mild human tetrodotoxication, *Ann Emerg Med* 15:1094, 1986.

376. Sivonen K et al: Isolation and structures of five microcystins from a Russian *Microcystis aeruginosa* strain CALU 972, *Toxicon* 30:1481, 1992.

377. Slater CA et al: Brief report: Successful treatment of disseminated *Acanthamoeba* infection in an immunocompromised patient, *N Engl J Med* 331:85, 1994.

378. Sloviter RS, Damiano B: On the relationship between kainic acid-induced epileptiform activity and hippocampal neuronal damage, *Neuropharmacology* 20:1003, 1981.

379. Smart DR: Scombroid poisoning: a report of seven cases involving the western Australian salmon, *Arripis truttaceus*, *Med J Aust* 157:748, 1992.

380. Smart DR: Clinical toxicology of shellfish poisoning. In Meier J, White J, editors: *Handbook of clinical toxicology of animal venoms and poisons*, Boca Raton, Fla, 1995, CRC Press.

381. Smirnov VV et al: Myoglobinuria caused by food poisoning, *Klin Med (Mosk)* 65:97, 1987.

382. Smith HM: Toxic fish and mollusks. *Information Bulletin No 12*. Maxwell Air Force Base, Alabama, 1975, Air Training Command, Environmental Information Division.

383. Sonnabend O et al: Isolation of *Clostridium botulinum* type G and identification of type G botulinal toxin in humans: report of five sudden unexpected deaths, *J Infect Dis* 143:22, 1981.

384. Sorokin M: Human poisoning by ingestion of a sea hare (*Dolabella auricularia*), *Toxicon* 26:1095, 1988.

385. Southcott RV: Australian venomous and poisonous fishes, *Clin Toxicol* 10:291, 1977.

386. Spoerke DG, Rumack BH: Blue-green algae poisoning, *J Emerg Med* 2:353, 1985.

387. Stafford R et al: An outbreak of Norwalk virus gastroenteritis following consumption of oysters, *Comm Dis Intell* 21:317, 1997.

388. Steinfeld AD, Steinfeld HJ: Ciguatera and the voyage of Captain Bligh, *JAMA* 228:1270, 1974.

389. Stewart MPM: Ciguatera fish poisoning: treatment with intravenous mannitol, *Trop Doct* 21:54, 1991.

390. Stroffolini T et al: Typhoid fever in the Neapolitan area: a case-control study, *Eur J Epidemiol* 8:539, 1992.

391. Styliads S, Borczyk A: Typhoid outbreak associated with consumption of raw shellfish—Ontario, *Can Comm Dis Rep* 20:63, 1994.

392. Subba Rao DV, Quillan MA, Pocklington R: Domoic acid—a neurotoxic amino acid produced by the marine diatom *Nitzschia pungens* in culture, *Can J Fish Aquat Sci* 45:2076, 1988.

393. Sugieda M, Nakajima K, Nakajima S: Outbreaks of Norwalk-like virus-associated gastroenteritis traced to shellfish: coexistence of two genotypes in one specimen, *Epidemiol Infect* 116:339, 1996.

394. Sugimachi K et al: Acute gastric anisakiasis: analysis of 178 cases, *JAMA* 253:1012, 1985.

395. Sutherland SK: *Australian animal toxins*, Melbourne, Australia, 1983, Oxford University Press.

396. Svensson B-G et al: Exposure to dioxins and dibenzofurans through the consumption of fish, *N Engl J Med* 324:8, 1991.

397. Tachibana K et al: Okadaic acid, a cytotoxic polyether from two marine sponges of the genus *Halichondria*, *J Am Chem Soc* 103:2469, 1981.

398. Tacket CO, Brenner F, Blake PA: Clinical features and an epidemiological study of *Vibrio vulnificus* infections, *J Infect Dis* 149:558, 1984.

399. Tacket CO et al: Panophthalmitis caused by *Vibrio parahaemolyticus*, *Clin Microbiol* 16:195, 1982.

400. Tacket CO et al: Diarrhea associated with *Vibrio fluvialis* in the United States, *J Clin Microbiol* 16:991, 1982.

401. Tacket CO et al: Equine antitoxin use and other factors that predict outcome in type A foodborne botulism, *Am J Med* 76:794, 1984.

402. Takabe K et al: Anisakidosis: a cause of intestinal obstruction from eating sushi, *Am J Gastroenterol* 93:1172, 1998.

403. Takemoto T, Daigo K: Constituents of *Chondria arata*, *Chem Pharm Bull* 6:578, 1958.

404. Tan B et al: *Acanthamoeba* infection presenting as skin lesion in patients with acquired immunodeficiency syndrome, *Arch Pathol Lab Med* 117:1043, 1993.

405. Tatsumi M et al: Potent excitatory effect of scaritoxin on the guinea-pig vas deferens, taenia caeci and ileum, *J Pharmacol Exp Ther* 235:783, 1985.

406. Taylor FJR: Toxic dinoflagellates: taxonomic and biogeographic aspects with emphasis on *Protogonyaulax*. In Ragelis EP, editor: *Seafood toxins*, Washington, DC, 1984, American Chemical Society.

407. Taylor SL. Histamine food poisoning: toxicology and clinical aspects, *CRC Crit Rev Toxicol* 17:91, 1986.

408. Teitelbaum HS et al: Neurologic sequelae of domoic acid intoxication due to the ingestion of contaminated mussels, *N Engl J Med* 322:1781, 1990.

409. Tennessee Department of Health and Environment: *Tennessee Communicable Diseases Bulletin* 18:7, 1986.

410. Terao K, Ito E, Yasumoto T: Light and electron microscopic studies of the murine heart after repeated administrations of ciguatoxin or ciguatoxin-4c, *Nat Toxins* 1:19, 1992.

411. Terao K et al: Histopathological studies on experimental marine toxin poisoning. I. Ultrastructural changes in the small intestine and liver of suckling mice induced by dinophysistoxin-1 and pectenotoxin-1, *Toxicon* 24:1141, 1986.

412. Terao K et al: Histopathological studies on experimental marine toxin poisoning. 4. Pathogenesis of experimental maitotoxin poisoning, *Toxicon* 27:979, 1989.

413. Terao K et al: Histopathological studies on experimental marine toxin poisoning. 5. The effects in mice of yessotoxin isolated from Patinopecten yessoensis and of a desulfated derivative, *Toxicon* 28:1095, 1990.

414. Terao K et al: Light and electron microscopic studies of pathologic changes induced in mice by ciguatoxin poisoning, *Toxicon* 29:633, 1991.

415. Theiss WC et al: Blood pressure and hepatocellular effects of the cyclic heptapeptide toxin produced by the freshwater cyanobacterium (blue-green alga) *Microcystis aeruginosa* strain PCC-7820, *Toxicon* 26:603, 1988.

416. Tibballs J: Severe tetrodotoxic fish poisoning, *Anaesth Intens Care* 16:215, 1988.

417. Tindall DR et al: Ciguatoxigenic dinoflagellates from the Caribbean Sea. In Ragelis EP, editor: *Seafood toxins*, Washington, DC, 1984, American Chemical Society.

418. Tison DL, Kelly MT: *Vibrio vulnificus* endometritis, *J Clin Microbiol* 20:185, 1984.

419. Torda TA, Sinclair E, Ulyatt DB: Puffer fish (tetrodotoxin) poisoning: clinical record and suggested management, *Med J Aust* 1:599, 1973.

420. Torres P et al: [New records of human diphyllobothriasis in Chile (1981-1992), with a case of multiple *Diphyllobothrium latum* infection], *Boletin Chileno de Parasitologia* 48:39, 1993.

421. Tosteson TR, Ballantine DL, Durst D: Seasonal frequency of ciguatoxic barracuda in southwest Puerto Rico, *Toxicon* 26:795, 1988.

422. Trainer VL, Baden DG: An enzyme immunoassay for the detection of Florida red tide brevetoxins, *Toxicon* 29:1387, 1991.

423. Traorae A et al: Synergistic effects of some metals contaminating mussels on the cytotoxicity of the marine toxin okadaic acid, *Arch Toxicol* 73:289, 1999.

424. Truwit JD et al: *Vibrio vulnificus* bacteremia with endocarditis, *South Med J* 80:1457, 1987.

425. Tsakris A, Psifidis A, Douboyas J: Complicated suppurative otitis media in a Greek diver due to a marine halophilic *Vibrio* sp, *J Laryngol Otol* 109:1082, 1995.

426. Tubaro A et al: A protein phosphatase 2A inhibition assay for a fast and sensitive assessment of okadaic acid contamination in mussels, *Toxicon* 34:743, 1996.

427. Tubaro A et al: Suitability of the MTT-based cytotoxicity assay to detect okadaic acid contamination of mussels, *Toxicon* 34:965, 1996.

428. Uragoda CG: Histamine poisoning in tuberculous patients after ingestion of tuna fish, *Am Rev Respir Dis* 121:157, 1980.

429. Vale P, Sampayo MA: Estersof okadaic acid and dinophysistoxin-2 in Portuguese bivalves related to human poisonings, *Toxicon* 37:1109, 1999.

430. van Egmond HP, Speyers GJA, van den Top HJ: Current situation on worldwide regulations for marine phycotoxins, *J Nat Toxins* 1:67, 1992

431. van Egmond HP et al: Paralytic and diarrhetic shellfish poisons: occurrence in Europe, toxicity, analysis and regulations, *J Nat Toxins* 2:41, 1992.

432. Van Halderen A et al: Cyanobacterial (blue-green algae) poisoning of livestock in the western Cape Province of South Africa, *J S Afr Vet Assoc* 66:260, 1995.

433. Van Thiel PH: A nematode parasitic to herring causing acute abdominal syndromes in man, *Trop Geogr Med* 2:97, 1960.

434. Vartian CV, Septimus EJ: Osteomyelitis caused by *Vibrio vulnificus*, *J Infect Dis* 161:363, 1990.

435. Vermeer IT et al: Volatile N-nitrosamine formation after intake of nitrate at the ADI level in combination with an amine-rich diet, *Environ Health Perspect* 106:459, 1998.

436. Vicente AC, Coelho AM, Salles CA: Detection of *Vibrio cholerae* and *V. mimicus* heat-stable toxin gene sequence by PCR, *J Med Microbiol* 46:398, 1997.

437. Vieira JC et al. Paragonimiasis in Ecuador: prevalence and geographical distribution of parasitisation of second intermediate hosts with *Paragonimus mexicanus* in 438. Esmeraldas province, *Trop Med Parasitol* 43:249, 1992.

438. Vietmeyer ND: The preposterous puffer, *National Geographic* 166:260, 1984.

439. Viriyavejakul P, Rochanawutanon M, Sirinavin S: *Naegleria* meningomyeloencephalitis, *Southeast Asian J Trop Med Public Health* 28:237, 1997.

440. Vogt RL, Liang AP: Ciguatera fish poisoning—Vermont, *MMWR* 35:263, 1986.

441. Vollberg CM, Herrera JL: *Vibrio vulnificus* infection: an important cause of septicemia in patients with cirrhosis, *South Med J* 90:1040, 1997.

442. Wang A et al: Successful treatment of amoebic meningoencephalitis in a Chinese living in Hong Kong, *Clin Neurol Neurosurg* 95:249, 1993.

443. Watabe S et al: Distribution of tritiated tetrodotoxin administered intraperitoneally to pufferfish, *Toxicon* 25:1283, 1987.

444. Weber JT et al: A massive outbreak of type E botulism associated with traditional salted fish in Cairo, *J Infect Dis* 167:451, 1993.

445. Wekell JC et al: Occurrence of domoic acid in Washington state razor clams (*Siliqua patula*) during 1991-1993, *Nat Toxin* 2:197, 1994.

446. White AW: Paralytic shellfish toxins and finfish. In Ragelis EP, editor: *Seafood toxins*, Washington, DC, 1984, American Chemical Society.

447. Williams FP, Fout GS: Contamination of shellfish by stool-shed viruses: methods of detection, *Environ Sci Technol* 26:689, 1992.

448. Williams RK, Palafox NA: Treatment of pediatric ciguatera fish poisoning (letter), *Am J Dis Child* 144:747, 1990.

449. Williamson J: Ciguatera and mannitol: a successful treatment, *Med J Aust* 153:306, 1990.

450. Wilson IG, Moore JE: Presence of *Salmonella* spp. and *Campylobacter* spp. in shellfish, *Epidemiol Infect* 116:147, 1996.

451. Windust AJ: Comparative toxicity of the diarrhetic shellfish poisons, okadaic acid, okadaic acid diol-ester and dinophysistoxin-4, to the diatom *Thalassiosira weissflogii, Toxicon* 35:1591, 1997.

452. Wittman RJ, Flick GJ: Microbial contamination of shellfish: prevalence, risk to human health, and control strategies, *Annu Rev Public Health* 16:123, 1995.

453. Wittner M, Tanowitz HB, Ash LR: Safe sushi (reply) (letter), *N Engl J Med* 321:901, 1989.

454. Wittner M et al: Eustrongylidiasis—a parasitic infection acquired by eating sushi, *N Engl J Med* 320:1124, 1989.

455. Wong H-C, Chen L-L, Yu C-M: Occurrence of *Vibrios* in frozen seafoods and survival of psychrotrophic *Vibrio cholerae* in broth and shrimp homagenate at low temperatures, *J Food Protec* 58:263, 1995.

456. Wongpaitoon V et al: Spontaneous *Vibrio vulnificus* peritonitis and primary sepsis in two patients with alcoholic cirrhosis, *Am J Gastroenterol* 80:706, 1985.

457. Work TM et al: Domoic acid intoxication of brown Pelicans *(Pelecanus occidentalis)* in California. Newport, RI: *Abstract 5th Int Conf Toxic Marine Phytoplanton*, Oct 28-Nov 1, p 33, 1991.

458. Work TM et al: Epidemiology of domoic acid poisoning in Brown's pelican *(Pelecanus occidentalis)* and Brant's cormorants *(Phalacrocorax penicillatus)* in California, *J Zoo Wildlife Med* 24:54, 1993.

459. World Health Organization: *Emerging and other communicable disease (EMC) cholera fact sheet*, Fact sheet N107, Geneva, March 2, 1996.

460. Wright JLC et al: Identification of domoic acid, a neuroexcitatory amino acid, in mussels from eastern Prince Edward Island, *Can J Chem* 67:481, 1989.

461. Yang CC et al: An outbreak of tetrodotoxin poisoning following gastropod mollusk consumption, *Hum Exp Toxicol* 14:446, 1995.

462. Yasumoto T: Fish poisoning due to toxins of microalgal origins in the Pacific, *Toxicon* 36:1515, 1998.

463. Yasumoto T, Kanno K: Occurrence of toxins resembling ciguatoxin, scaritoxin, and maitotoxin in a turban shell, *Bull Jpn Soc Sci Fish* 42:1399, 1976.

464. Yasumoto T, Kao CY: Tetrodotoxin and the Haitian zombie, *Toxicon* 24:747, 1986.

465. Yasumoto T, Ray U, Bagnis R: *Seafood poisoning in Tropical regions*, publication from the Laboratory of Food Hygiene, Faculty of Agriculture, Tohoky University, 74, 1984.

466. Yasumoto T et al: Diarrhetic shellfish poisoning. In Ragelis EP, editor: *Seafood toxins*, Washington, DC, 1984, American Chemical Society.

467. Yasumoto T et al: *Studies on tropical fish and shellfish infected by toxic dinoflagellate*, publication from the Laboratory of Food Hygiene, Faculty of Agriculture, Tohoky University, 53, 1985

468. Yentson CM: Paralytic shellfish poisoning: an emerging perspective. In Ragelis EP, editor: *Seafood toxins*, Washington, DC, 1984, American Chemical Society.

469. Yoshida S, Ogawa M, Mizuguchi Y: Relation of capsular materials and colony opacity to virulence of *Vibrio vulnificus, Infect Immun* 47:446, 1985.

470. Yotsu M et al: Production of tetrodotoxin and its derivatives by *Pseudomonas* sp. isolated from the skin of a pufferfish, *Toxicon* 25:225, 1987.

471. Yotsu-Yamashita M et al: Four new analogs of polycavernoside A, *Tetrahedron Lett* 36:5563, 1995.

472. Zakaria-Meehan Z et al: Ability of *Vibrio vulnificus* to obtain iron from hemoglobin-haptoglobin complexes, *Infect Immun* 56:275, 1988.

473. Zlotnick BA et al: Ciguatera poisoning after ingestion of imported jellyfish: diagnostic application of serum immunoassay, *Wilderness Environ Med* 6:288, 1995.

474. Zu Jeddeloh B: Haffkrankheit (Haff disease), *Erg Inn Med* 57:138, 1939.

55 Seafood Allergies

Susan L. Hefle and Robert K. Bush

True seafood allergies are immunoglobulin E (IgE)–mediated reactions. Although allergic reactions can occur to all classes of seafoods, accurate epidemiologic data are difficult to obtain. Crustacean allergies are one of the most common types of food allergy in the U.S. adult population[62]; codfish allergy is probably the most common form of food allergy in Scandinavian countries.[2]

BIOLOGIC CLASSIFICATION

An understanding of the taxonomic relationships among different species of marine animals is important. Although many seafood species may be allergenic, most allergic patients are not sensitive to all species. The degree of allergic cross-reactivity among the different fish species varies widely among patients. Thus selective avoidance diets are possible. The biologic classification of the edible species of fishes is given in Table 55-1. Most edible fishes belong to class Osteichthyes, although sharks are in a different class. The most common fishes consumed belong to only a few orders: Salmoniformes (salmons, trout, whitefishes, smelts, and pikes), Perciformes (basses, perches, dolphins, snappers, groupers, redfishes, mackerels, and tunas), Gadiformes (codfishes, pollocks, haddocks, and hakes), Pleuronectiformes (flounders, halibuts, and soles), Clupeiformes (herrings, sardines, anchovies, shad, menhadens, and alewives), Cypriniformes (carps and catfishes), and Scorpaeniformes (rockfishes). Many of the edible fish species belong to the orders Salmoniformes, Perciformes, and Gadiformes (Tables 55-2 to 55-4).

The physician should be alert to the confusing common names of fishes. For instance, king mackerel may be sold as cero, silver cero, black salmon, cavalla, or kingfish. Kingfish can also mean king whiting, which itself is sold as ground mullet, whiting, gulf whiting, surf whiting, southern whiting, sand whiting, or silver whiting. Whiting may be a name used to describe hake. The identification of fish is often erroneous, particularly when performed by sport fishermen.

Crustacea are classified as arthropods with spiders, centipedes, and insects. At least 30 edible species of crustacea are consumed in the United States. The Mollusca include clams, mussels, oysters, cockles, snails, cuttlefish, limpets, abalone, and squid and octopus (Tables 55-5 to 55-7).

CLINICAL MANIFESTATIONS

The symptoms of seafood allergy are the same as those caused by other allergenic foods. The symptoms are often related to the method of exposure, whether ingestion, inhalation, or physical contact. With ingestion, symptoms may occur first in the mouth and on the face, including localized or general pruritus, urticaria, laryngeal edema, and angioedema.[84] Atopic dermatitis may be exacerbated by seafood allergies.[92] Gastrointestinal (GI) symptoms such as nausea, vomiting, diarrhea, and cramps may occur as a result of ingestion. Some reports indicate severe asthma and bronchospasm as primary symptoms after consumption of certain mollusks[16,26] and fish.[85] In some individuals, seafood can cause anaphylaxis. Symptoms of anaphylaxis may include these symptoms in addition to hypotension, electrocardiogram (ECG) changes, and cardiovascular collapse. Symptoms of food allergy usually occur within an hour after ingestion.[1,14,15,23] However, delayed reactions (3 to 24 hours after ingestion) have been noted with fish,[85] cuttlefish,[94] abalone,[72] and limpets.[80] With food-dependent exercise-induced anaphylaxis, persons in the resting state can eat food without difficulty. However, exercise within 2 to 4 hours after ingestion can bring on the symptoms of anaphylaxis. Shrimp, mollusks, and squid are among the implicated foods.[52,76,77]

Occupational reactions can include dermatitis, urticaria, angioedema, rhinitis, conjunctivitis, asthma, and hypersensitivity pneumonitis. Employees in the fishing and seafood processing industries are at risk of developing occupational allergy. Although asthma is the most prominent symptom, anaphylaxis has been reported with occupational exposure.[74] Physical contact with seafood can elicit allergic symptoms in sensitive individuals, and urticaria, contact dermatitis, angioedema, and asthma have been reported after contact with shellfish[22,37,96,106,108] and fish.[8,22,30] Most of these contact reactions occur as part of occupational exposure, but consumers can also be affected.[84] Inhalation reactions are most often associated with occupational exposure, such as in cleaning and cooking seafood, but can also occur when seafood is cooked at home or in restaurants. Seafoods implicated in occupational asthma include oysters,[83] clams,[29] shrimp,[29,63] prawns,[38] fish,[20,32] snow and king crabs,[17,86] lobsters,[63,91] sea squirts,[53] abalone,[19] powdered marine

TABLE 55-1. Taxonomic Relationships Among the Edible Fishes

	TAXONOMIC CLASSIFICATION	
CLASS	SUBCLASS OR ORDER	COMMON NAME
Chondrichthyes	Elasmobranchii	Sharks
Osteichthyes	Acipenseriformes	Sturgeons, paddlefishes
	Elopiformes	Tarpons, ten-pounders, bonefishes
	Anguilliformes	Common eels, morays
	Clupeiformes	Herrings, sardines, alewives, shad, menhaden, anchovies
	Salmoniformes	Trouts, salmons, whitefishes, graylings, discoes, pikes, lake herrings, pickerels, muskelunges, euchalons, capelins, smelts, saugers
	Gonorynchiformes	Milkfishes, awa
	Cypriniformes	Minnows, carps, suckers, catfishes
	Beloniformes	Sauries, needlefishes, flying fishes
	Mugiliformes	Mullets, barracudas, silversides, threadfishes
	Lambridiformes	Opah, mariposas
	Tetradontiformes	Pufferfishes, boxfishes, trunkfishes
	Pleuronectiformes	Flounders, halibuts, soles, dabs, turbots
	Perciformes, suborder Percodei	Basses, crappies, bluegills, sea basses, sunfishes, perches, bluefishes, jacks, pompanos, dolphins, snappers, groupers, scups, grunts, porgies, pomfrets, sheepsheads, snooks, robalos, bigeyes, catalugas, croakers, spots, redfishes, tautogs, butterfly fishes, wrasses, spadefishes, goatfishes, mojarras, rudderfishes, surffishes, weakfishes, roaches, drums, cichlids
	Perciformes, suborder Scombroidei	Mackerels, tunas, cutlassfishes, albacores, bonitos, kingfishes
	Perciformes, suborder Xiphoidei	Swordfishes, marlins, sailfishes, spearfishes
	Perciformes, suborder Ammodytoidei	Sand lances (sand eels)
	Perciformes, suborder Stromateoidei	Butterfishes
	Scorpaeniformes	Rockfishes, scorpionfishes, greenlings
	Gadiformes	Codfishes, ling cods, pollocks, haddocks, tomcods, hakes, codlings
	Percopsoidei	Trout-perches, sand rollers

TABLE 55-2. Taxonomic Relationships Among Salmoniformes

		TAXONOMIC CLASSIFICATION	
SUBORDER	FAMILY	GENUS	COMMON NAME
Salmonoidei	Salmonidae	*Coregonus*	Whitefishes, ciscoes, bloaters, lake herrings
		Onchorhynchus	Pacific salmons
		Salmo	Trouts, Atlantic salmon
		Salvelinus	Chars, brook trout, Dolly Varden trout, lake trout
		Thymallus	Grayling
	Osmeridae	*Osmerus*	Smelts
		Mallotus	Capelins
		Thaleichthys	Euchalon
Esocoidei	Escidae	*Esox*	Pikes, saugers, pickerels, muskelunges

TABLE 55-3. Taxonomic Relationships Among Perciformes

	TAXONOMIC CLASSIFICATION	
SUBORDER	FAMILY	COMMON NAME
Percoidei	Centraranidae	Largemouth bass, black basses, breams, bluegill, sunfishes, crappie, Sacramento perch
	Percichthyidae	Striped bass, white bass, white perch, yellow bass
	Serranidae	Groupers, sea basses, jawfishes
	Percidae	Pikes, saugers, yellow perch, river perch
	Centropomidae	Snooks, robalos
	Priacanthidae	Cataluras, bigeyes
	Pomatomidae	Bluefish
	Coryphaenidae	Dolphin fish (mahi mahi)
	Carangidae	Jacks, pompanos, cavallas, moonfishes, scads, jack mackerel
	Bramidae	Pomfret
	Pomadasyidae	Grunts
	Lutjanidae	Snappers, mutton fish, rabirubias
	Chaetodontidae	Butterflyfishes
	Ephippidae	Spadefishes
	Labridae	Wrasses, tautog
	Cichlidae	Cichlids
	Sciaenidae	Drums, redfish, croakers, weakfishes, kingfishes
	Mullidae	Goatfishes
	Sparidae	Porgies, scups, spots, sheepsheads
	Gerridae	Mojarras
	Kyphosidae	Rudderfishes, sea chubs
	Embiotocidae	Surffishes
Scombroidei	Scombridae	Mackerels, tunas, bonitos, Spanish mackerels, sierra, kingfish, cero, cavalla, petos
	Trichiuridae	Cutlassfishes
Xiphiodei	Xiphiidae	Swordfishes
	Istiophoridae	Marlins, sailfishes, spearfishes
Ammodytoidei	Ammodytidae	Sand lances (sand eels)
Stromateoidei	Stromateidae	Butterfishes

TABLE 55-4. Taxonomic Relationships Among Gadiformes

		TAXONOMIC CLASSIFICATION	
SUBORDER	FAMILY	GENUS	COMMON NAME
Gadoidei	Merlucciidae	*Merluccius*	Pacific hake
	Gadidae	*Pollachius*	Pollock
		Theragra	Walleye pollock
		Gadus	Codfishes
		Microgadus	Tomcods
		Lota	Turbot
		Melanogrammus	Haddock
		Urophycis	Atlantic hake, red hake, Gulf hake

TABLE 55-5. Taxonomic Relationships Among Edible Mollusks and Crustacea

		TAXONOMIC CLASSIFICATION	
PHYLUM	CLASS	SUBCLASS	COMMON NAME
Mollusca	Gastropoda	Prosobranchi	Marine snails, abalone, periwinkles, whelks
		Pulmonata	Freshwater snails
	Bivalvia	Lamellibranchii	Mussels, cockles, oysters, scallops, clams
	Cephalopoda	Coleoidea	Squid, octopus
Arthropoda	Crustacea	Malacostraca	Shrimp, crabs, lobsters, crayfish

TABLE 55-6. Edible Bivalves and Cephalopods

GROUP	COMMON NAME	SCIENTIFIC NAME
Clams	Surf or bar clam	*Mactra solidissima*
	Soft clam	*Mya arenaria*
	Hard clam or quahog	*Venus mercenaria*
	Atlantic razor clam	*Ensis directus*
	Pacific razor clam	*Siliqua patula*
	Stout razor clam	*Tagelus gibbus*
	Butter clam	*Saxidomus nuttali*
	Little neck clam	*Tapes staminea*
	Geoduck clam	*Panope generosa*
	Freshwater clam	*Coribula leana*
	Pismo clam	*Tivela stultorum*
	Short-necked clam	*Venerupis japonica*
	Jackknife clam	*Tagelus californianus*
Mussels	European or Atlantic mussel	*Mytilus edulis*
	Pacific mussel	*Mytilus californianus*
	South Asian green mussel	*Mytilus smaragdinus*
Cockles	Common cockle	*Cardium corbis*
	Red cockle	*Cardium echinatum*
	Spiny cockle	*Caridum aculateum*
Scallops	Common scallop	*Pecten gibbus borealis*
	Deep water scallop	*Placopecten megallanicus*
	Japanese scallop	*Pecten yessoensis*
Oysters	Pacific oyster	*Cassostrea gigas*
	Atlantic oyster	*Crassostrea virginica*
	Japanese oyster	*Crassostrea laperousei*
	Coon oyster	*Ostrea frons*
Squid	North American squid	*Loligo paeleii*
	North American squid	*Loligo opalescens*
	Japanese squid	*Ommastrephes sloani pacificus*
Octopus	Common octopus	*Octopus vulgaris*

TABLE 55-7. Edible Crustacea

GROUP	COMMON NAME	SCIENTIFIC NAME
Lobsters	Atlantic lobster	*Homarus vulgaris*
	European lobster	*Homarus gammarus*
	Northern lobster	*Homarus americanus*
	Spiny lobster	*Pancilirus argus*
Crabs	Blue crab	*Callinectis sapidus*
	Deep sea blue crab	*Portunus pelagicus*
	Dungeness crab	*Cancer magister*
	Jonah crab	*Cancer borealis*
	King crab	*Paralithodes camtschatica*
	Snow crab	*Chinoectes bairdi*
	Tanner crab	*Chinoectes tanneri*
	Spider crab	*Talvia maticum*
	Stone crab	*Menippe mercenaria*
Prawns and shrimp	Common prawn	*Palaemon serratus*
	Deep water prawn	*Pandalus bortalis*
	Pink Maine shrimp	*Pandalus borealis*
	Coon stripe shrimp	*Pandalus hypsinotus*
	Brown shrimp	*Panaeus aztecus*
	Pink shrimp	*Panaeus duorarum*
	White shrimp	*Panaeus indicus*
	Gamba shrimp	*Panaeus longirostris*
	Karuma prawn	*Panaeus japonicus*
	Giant tiger prawn	*Panaeus monodon*
	Common tiger prawn	*Panaeus esculentus*
	Indian prawn	*Panaeus indicus*
	Eastern king prawn	*Panaeus plebejus*
	Banana prawn	*Panaeus merguiensis*
	Brine shrimp	*Artemia salina*
	Rock shrimp	*Silyomia brevirostris*
	Sea bob shrimp	*Xiphophenaeus kroyeri*
	Royal red shrimp	*Hymenopenaeus robustus*
	Freshwater prawn	*Macrobrachium carcinus*

sponges,[7] cuttlefish,[95] and clam liver extract.[54] Mollusk shell dust has been found to cause hypersensitivity pneumonitis.[87,88]

DIAGNOSIS

Medical History

The diagnosis of food allergy may be simple or extremely complex. With seafood it is particularly important to identify the offending food correctly to determine if cross-reaction patterns can be established. An estimate of the quantity of the food needed to elicit the reaction may help to distinguish intolerance from a true seafood allergy.

Skin Testing and Radioallergosorbent Test

The skin prick test is extremely useful, but commercial extracts are not available for all individual seafood species. Often, mixed extracts are used. Some risk exists for patients who have experienced severe anaphylactic reactions. As with other food allergen extracts, fish skin prick tests have superior sensitivity and negative predictive accuracy, but poor positive predictive value and specificity.[9] Some commercial fish skin test extracts may contain relatively high levels of histamine,[102] which could be a contributing factor; however, the person often fails to distinguish the species causing the allergy. Allergists generally recommend removing all edible fish from a person's diet, including both Osteichthyes (bony fish) and Chondrichthyes (shark), when the person has a history of allergic reaction to any fish or a positive skin test or radioallergosorbent test (RAST) to a fish extract. However, research using double-blind placebo-controlled fish (food) challenges[9] (DBPCFCs) and other tests[2,28] in fish-allergic children has shown that they are not uniformly sensitive to all species. Hypersensitivity to one species does not automatically warrant dietary elimination of all fish. Fish challenges in children with negative skin tests were negative; therefore skin testing may be advisable first.[9] Seafood extracts are available for skin prick testing and as reagents for CAP-RAST (Box 55-1). CAP-RAST is reserved for persons who have had severe reactions to skin testing.

Double-Blind Placebo-Controlled Food Challenges

The ultimate test to verify that a particular food causes a reaction is the DBPCFC.[11,12] This should not be performed in persons who have experienced life-threatening reactions and should be undertaken only under close physician supervision. Dried or freeze-dried foods are encapsulated in opaque, dye-free capsules, and appropriate identical placebo capsules are pre-

---

Box 55-1 COMMERCIALLY AVAILABLE SEAFOOD EXTRACTS FOR SKIN AND RADIOALLERGOSORBENT TESTING

SKIN TEST

Fish: anchovy, bass, catfish, codfish, flounder, haddock, halibut, herring, mackerel, perch, pickerel, salmon, sardine, smelt, snapper, sole, swordfish, trout, tuna, whitefish

Fish mixtures
 1. Codfish, flounder, mackerel, tuna
 2. Codfish, halibut, mackerel, perch, salmon, trout, tuna

Crustacea: crab, lobster, shrimp

Mollusks: clam, oyster, scallop

Shellfish mixtures
 1. Clam, crab, oyster, scallop, shrimp
 2. Clam, crab, lobster, oyster, shrimp, scallop

RADIOALLERGOSORBENT TEST (CAP-RAST)

Fish: anchovy, cod, eel, hake, halibut, herring, jack mackerel, mackerel, chub mackerel, megrim (whiff), plaice, trout (rainbow), salmon, sardine, swordfish, tuna

Crustacea and mollusks: crab, lobster, shrimp (pink), lobster (spiny), mussel (blue), octopus, oyster, snail, squid

---

pared. Although such testing is time-consuming and expensive, DBPCFC permits a precise diagnosis.

Elimination Diets

When a certain type of seafood is suspected of producing symptoms, it may be eliminated from the diet. After the initial complaints have resolved, the person then reintroduces the food to see if the reaction recurs. Elimination diets should only be used in persons who have not experienced life-threatening symptoms as a manifestation of seafood allergy.

Controversial Techniques

A number of clinical and laboratory tests are unreliable predictors of the presence of seafood allergy. These include pulse index, in vitro cytotoxic food tests, intracutaneous provocation, sublingual provocation, basophil degranulation, and sublingual neutralization.[5]

Occupational Asthma

Although the measures described previously are useful in diagnosing cutaneous, GI, or systemic manifestations of food allergy, the diagnosis of occupational asthma requires a different approach. If the person notes the onset of asthma symptoms related to work exposure, then improves on weekends or while on vacation, occupational asthma should be suspected. Asthma is verified by appropriate pulmonary function tests, such as spirometry with and without bronchodilators. If the history is suggestive but not corroborated by physical examination or simple spirometry, performing provocation with inhaled methacholine or histamine may be necessary to document airway hyperreactivity. The diagnosis depends ultimately on the provocation of asthma by a bronchial inhalation challenge with the suspected allergen. Such evaluation should occur under close observation in a hospital setting.

TREATMENT

The treatment for seafood allergies is the same as for other allergic reactions. Avoidance should encompass both consumption and inhalation of cooking vapors from the appropriate species. To avoid unnecessary dietary restrictions, proper diagnosis is extremely important.

IDENTIFICATION AND CHARACTERIZATION OF SEAFOOD ALLERGENS

Fish

Of the seafood allergens that have been isolated and purified, the best characterized is the major allergen of codfish, *Gad c* 1, which belongs to a group of muscle tissue proteins known as parvalbumins.[34] *Parvalbumins* are responsible for mediating the concentration of calcium in muscle. *Gad c* 1 is an acidic protein with a molecular weight of 12,328 daltons, is composed of 113 amino acids and 1 glucose molecule, and has an isoelectric point of 4.75. It comprises three domains: AB, CD, and EF, consisting of three helices interspaced by one loop.[35] Each of the loops of the CD and EF domains coordinates one Ca^{+2} binding site; these sites correspond to IgE binding sites. It is stable to heat, extremes of pH, and mild proteolysis. The allergenicity of *Gad c* 1 is decreased by acetylation or polymerization of the tyr-30 residue,[6] modification of the arg-75 residue, or dechelation of the two calcium ions,[33] but these methods cannot be used commercially.

Another codfish allergen was identified in an in vitro study with cod-allergic patient sera to have a molecular size of 41 kilodaltons (kD), in addition to six other bands at 13, 21, 27, 47, and 58 kD.[39] The 41-kD allergen had an isoelectric point estimated at 5.8. The 13-kD band was a major allergen for all subjects in the study. The 13- and 41-kD bands were recognized by antiparvalbumin monoclonal antibodies specific for the first calcium binding site, as were the bands at 28 and 49 kD. No correlation exists between the amino acid composition of the 41-kD allergen and other cod allergens previously described in the literature.[39] In another study investigating IgE binding in sera of fish-allergic patients, prerigor cod muscle was found to contain IgE binding bands of 12, 22, 30, 45, 60, 67, 104, and 130 kD.[31]

A major IgE binding band for all sera was at 12 kD; the 30- and 67-kD bands also possessed good IgE binding activity. The bands at 104 and 130 kD were thought to be aggregates of smaller bands. When the cod had been dead for several days, new IgE binding bands of 18, 41, and 80 kD appeared, and the relative content of IgE binding proteins was increased. The action of naturally occurring proteases could have opened up sections of the peptides and made them more accessible to IgE binding during this period. The codfish antiparvalbumin monoclonal antibody was also found to bind to all IgE binding bands identified in this study, indicating that all peptides shared similar structures.

Protamine sulfate, a sperm protein of salmon, herring, trout, and other species belonging to the families Salmonidae and Clupeidae, has been identified as an allergen in some persons with sensitivities to salmon, herring, and related fish.[56] It is a low-molecular-weight protein widely used as a heparin antagonist. Surimi, a collection of one or many different varieties of small fish that are minced and washed extensively, gave a single band at 63.5 kD that bound IgE from all sera of fish-allergic patients in one study.[75] Although many fish-allergic patients are allergic to multiple fish species, monospecificity has been reported to tuna, cod, and swordfish. In these studies, subjects with multiple allergies to fish species showed IgE binding to 12- to 13-kD bands, whereas the monospecifically sensitive subjects showed IgE binding to unique bands at 40 kD in tuna and 25 kD in swordfish.[51,55]

Structurally related parvalbumins in divergent fish species may explain cross-reactivity to fish species in certain allergic individuals. Hansen et al[43] noted that in adults with clinical sensitivity to cod, reactions were reported to mackerel, herring, and plaice, and in vitro results showed IgE binding to a single band in the 11- to 14-kD region of mackerel, herring, and plaice extracts. An IgE binding protein from salmon, *Sal s* 1, was identified by in vitro analyses and shown to be salmon parvalbumin.[71] In one study, almost 50% of cod-allergic patients had clinical sensitivity to salmon.[3] *Sal s* 1 has two bands at 12 and 14 kD and therefore has at least two isotypic variants.[71] While tuna-allergic individuals have been noted to have IgE binding to the 12-kD *Gad c* 1 codfish allergen,[13] one study noted that raw tuna extracts seemed to lack the IgE binding bands in the parvalbumin size range that were present in extracts of catfish, cod, and snapper.[53] However, Park et al[89] described IgE binding in sera from fish-allergic persons to tuna proteins at 12-13 kD. Sera from fish-allergic patients possessed IgE to bands at 12 to 13 kD in mackerel, pollock, and cod and showed unique binding to a band at 19 kD from saury and 37 kD from tuna. In one study, canned tuna did not present problems for five fish-allergic children[10]; canning may decrease the allergenicity of cod. Amino acid sequencing has shown, however, that the 12 to 13-kD band from tuna does not have the same sequence as cod, which may explain why tuna does not cross-react extensively with other species.[9,46,90]

Although many studies have shown skin prick test reactivity and in vitro reactivity between multiple species of fish, Glazzaz et al[40] found that amounts of parvalbumin in different fish extracts did not affect skin prick tests in fish-allergic subjects. An important verification tool is the oral challenge (DBPCFC). Bernhisel-Broadbent et al[9] found that in 11 subjects demonstrating in vitro allergy to fish, positive DBPCFC occurred only to one species in seven subjects, to two species in one subject, and to three in two others. Other studies using DBPCFC confirm this observation.[51] Different species of fish have shared allergenic determinants, and some fish-allergic patients are sensitive to multiple species of fish. Aas[1] found that of 61 fish-allergic children challenged with fish, 34 reacted to all species tested, and 27 could tolerate one or more types of fish. Other studies have found that subjects clinically react to multiple fish.[44,51,70] Negative skin prick tests are an excellent predictor of lack of allergy. Skin prick testing is an important tool, but DBPCFC should follow to determine the species that fish-allergic patients can tolerate.

Crustacea

The crustacean family includes shrimp, prawns, crabs, lobsters, and crayfish[107] and is a common reported cause of food hypersensitivity. Research indicates that crustacea share allergenic and antigenic determinants,[42,61] although some reactions are species specific.[59,79] Also, qualitative differences in the allergenic determinants of different shrimp extracts have been reported[79]; therefore use of extracts from more than one species for skin testing and CAP-RAST is recommended. Presence of IgE to either unique or shared allergens may explain an individual's clinical sensitivity to one or more members of this taxonomic class.

Shrimp is the most thoroughly studied of the crustacea in regard to allergens. Hoffman et al[47] were the first to characterize allergens from shrimp. Antigen I, isolated from raw shrimp, was an acidic, heat-labile protein composed of two noncovalently bound 21-kD polypeptide chains. Antigen II, isolated from cooked shrimp, was an acidic heat-stable 38-kD glycoprotein with an isoelectric point of 4.5 composed of 341 amino acid residues and 4% carbohydrate. Antigen II appeared to be a major allergen for the subjects in this study.

An allergenic transfer ribonucleic acid (tRNA) moiety from cooked prawns has been described.[81] The researchers could not isolate a preparation completely devoid of protein, however, so the allergenicity may have been caused by RNA-associated proteins. Further

work by this group[82] yielded the description of two allergenic polypeptides from cooked shrimp; SA-I, at 8.2 kD, was not analyzed further. The second allergen, SA-II, at 34 kD, was composed of 301 amino acid residues and appeared similar to antigen I isolated by Hoffman and colleagues.

The major shrimp allergen of 36 kD, readily isolated from the boiling water and meat of cooked shrimp, is *tropomyosin*, a muscle protein.[24] The allergen is composed of 312 amino acid residues and 2.4% carbohydrate. Monoclonal antibodies directed against the 36-kD shrimp allergen, *Pen a* 1 reacted to a 36-kD protein in crayfish, crab, and lobster extracts.[24] Antigen I, SA-II, and *Pen a* 1 appear to be the same protein. A tropomyosin is the major allergen, identified as SA-II, of two additional shrimp species, *Par f* 1 (*Parapenaeus fissurus*)[69] and *Met e* 1 (*Metapenaeus ensis*).[64,93] Lin et al[69] identified a 74-kD component in shrimp with IgE binding in 40% of subjects with allergy to shrimp and positive skin prick tests. Minor components of 41, 47, 50, and 86 kD bound to IgE in 10% to 20% of the sera. A monoclonal antibody made against *Par f* 1 also reacted to a 39 kD component in crab, and the two bands had similar amino acid compositions. *Par f* 1, at 39 kD, has an isoelectric point of 5.1 to 5.6.

Crab

Leung et al[66] describe the identification of a crab allergen, *Cha f* 1, from the crab species *Charybdis feriatus* from a constructed complementary deoxyribonucleic acid (cDNA) library screened with crab-allergic sera. Recombinant *Cha f* 1, at 34 kD, was identified as a tropomyosin. Snow crab also causes allergic sensitization in occupational settings.[17,45] Heat-labile and stable allergens have been found in snow crab extract; snow crab–specific IgE bound more to boiled crab than to raw crab.[45] The most prominent bands were at 37 to 42 kD in crab cooking water and extracts of cooked crab meat. In contrast to findings by Leung et al,[66] however, a 14-kD protein seemed to be the most prominent IgE binding protein, indicating that in cases of sensitization through the inhalation route, the responsible allergens might be different than those for the ingestion route.

Lobster

Leung et al[67] screened a library made from *Panulirus stimpsoni*, the spiny lobster, with sera from crustacea-allergic subjects. A recombinant IgE binding protein was designated *Pan s* 1, at 34 kD. The researchers also found a similar protein in *Homarus americanus*, the American lobster, which was designated *Hom a* 1. *Hom a* 1 possesses cross-reactive IgE epitopes in lobster and shrimp and has significant homology to *Pen a* 1 and *Met e* 1, with the major shrimp allergen. Similar IgE binding sites are found in *Met e* 1, *Pan s* 1, and *Hom a* 1. Although the size of *Hom a* 1 was not directly reported, the work described a 60-kD fusion protein, which would make *Hom a* 1 approximately 34 kD in size. Wiley and Griffin[101] demonstrated two IgE binding proteins of 35 to 37 and 97 kD in extracts of lobster in pooled sera from subjects with respiratory symptoms to Norwegian lobster *(Nephrops norvegicus)*. In native form the allergens were greater than 800 kD in size and were recognized by more than 80% of the serum samples involved, making them major respiratory allergens.

Mollusks

The mollusks are a diverse group. Squid and octopus are cephalopods, whereas clam, cockles, scallops, mussels, and oysters are bivalves. Abalones, conches, limpets, snails, and whelks are gastropods.

Squid

Allergic reactions have been documented in sensitive subjects after ingestion of squid or inhalation of vapors from cooking squid.[15] Almost all these victims also experienced symptoms after ingesting shrimp and demonstrated strong positive skin test reactions to boiled squid extracts and various commercial crustacea extracts. Immunoassay studies showed cross-reactivity between shrimp and squid allergens, although cross-reactivity was not demonstrated between squid and octopus or squid and other mollusks. Miyazawa et al[78] have described the major squid allergen as a 38-kD heat-stable protein, designated *Tod p* 1. Cross-reactivity between *Tod p* 1 and shrimp allergens was demonstrated by in vitro IgE binding studies and with monoclonal antibodies. The amino acid sequence of *Tod p* 1 showed marked homology with tropomyosin from the blood fluke (a snail) and was identified as squid tropomyosin.

Oyster

Two allergens, *Cra g* 1 and 2, were isolated from the oyster *Crassostrea gigas*.[48] They are both 86-kD glycoproteins with a carbohydrate content of about 5% and have 35-kD subunits. The allergic reactivity of the two allergens was equivalent in oyster-allergic patients. Studies on molecular characteristics and amino acid composition suggested that they are oyster tropomyosin. The allergenicity is apparently heat-stable, as is that of *Pen a* 1, shrimp tropomyosin. Partial digestion with a peptidase gave a protein sequence different from that for IgE binding characteristics of *Pen a* 1. *Cra g* 1 has 76% protein sequence homology with mussel tropomyosin, 74% with the gastropod tropomyosin *Haliotis rufescens*, and 58% with *Metapenaeus ensis* (shrimp) tropomyosin.[50]

Limpet and Abalone

Limpet and abalone can cause moderate to severe anaphylactic reactions and occasionally fatalities.[14,18,73,80]

Sensitive subjects usually have positive skin tests and RASTs to extracts of the offending shellfish. In one study, five patients were monospecifically allergic to limpet and presented with symptoms of severe asthma after ingestion; 43 other patients in the study were cross-reactive to several species of shellfish and showed a range of allergic symptoms after ingestion.[18] Another study noted that all six limpet-allergic subjects developed severe bronchospasm as their primary symptom after ingestion.[16] The major IgE binding proteins of grand keyhole limpet appear to have molecular weights of 38 and 80 kD.[73] Another research group[72] found a unique 49-kD major IgE binding protein (*Hal m* 1) and another component of 38 kD that bound IgE in abalone. Although most subjects in the study (38) had immediate reactions to abalone, 13 had delayed (up to 7 hours) reactions after ingestion. Only 17 of these sera were positive by RAST to abalone. The abalone-allergic subjects primarily had bronchial symptoms, and those reporting delayed reactions predominantly showed respiratory and cutaneous symptoms.

Snail

In a study of 10 subjects allergic to snails, eight experienced bronchial symptoms, and six reported no skin or GI symptoms. All subjects could ingest cephalopods and bivalves without adverse reaction.[27] In another study, asthma symptoms were reported after ingestion of snails by 15% of the subjects, and six different IgE binding protein bands, with molecular weight of 12 to more than 66 kD, were found in boiled snail extract. Keyhole limpet hemocyanin did not provoke cross-reactive responses in these subjects. Specific IgE binding was exhibited to bands at 12, 15, 24, and 66 kD, but these peptides were not characterized further.[4] Many reports of severe anaphylactic reactions to snails involve bronchial symptoms and previous sensitization to dust mites (see Seafood-Insect Cross-Reactions).

Horned Turban Mollusk

One study has reported the major allergen of the gastropod *Turbo cornutus*, a horned turban mollusk and popular food item in Japan. The major allergen, *Tur c* 1, was identified as a tropomyosin of 35 kD. However, *Tur c* 1 has an IgE binding epitope in the c-terminal region that is dissimilar to those in *Cra g* 1 (oyster) and *Pen a* 1 (shrimp).[50] *T. cornutus* also causes exercise-induced anaphylaxis.[52]

Shellfish Cross-Reactions

Shrimp-sensitive patients often report clinical histories of allergic reactions to several species of crustacea.[100] Clinical and in vitro evidence for cross-reactions has been shown between mollusks and crustacea.[58,59,60,100] Leung et al[65] found that IgE from subjects who were anaphylactic to shrimp recognized proteins from other crustaceans and also mollusks; tropomyosin was determined to be the cross-reactive allergen. In a study of crustacea-sensitive subjects, specific IgE binding was observed to six crayfish components and four spiny lobster components.[42] One study found clinical association between clam and mussel, but not among clam and mussel and crustacea.[18] No association was found between in vitro IgE binding and clinical history for shellfish. Squid-allergic IgE is cross-reactive with other mollusks.[15] Clinical association can occur within the same and different phyla, reflecting common allergenic epitopes.[18] The presence of IgE to unique and shared class allergens may explain an individual's clinical sensitivity to one or more members of a class.

Seafood-Insect Cross-Reactions

Insects belong to the Arthropoda, as do the crustacea. Patients allergic to chironomids (nonbiting midges) also often demonstrate positive skin tests to crustacea. Chironomid extracts have been found to inhibit RAST with shrimp, and vice versa,[36] although other researchers report low cross-reactivity.[105] Allergic reactions were reported among aquarists and fish-food factory workers when exposed to chironomids.[68] Symptoms reported most often were conjunctivitis, rhinitis, asthma, and urticaria, and other reports indicate atopic dermatitis on exposure to chironomids in pet foods.[104] The invertebrate hemoglobin (erythrocruorin) molecule might be involved in the reported cross-reactivity of caddis fly and mollusk allergy. It is a potent allergen for chironomid-allergic individuals, and serum from caddis-sensitive persons in one study reacted with a component of similar molecular weight in mollusk and bee venom extracts.[57] Thus individuals exposed to caddis fly antigens could develop allergic reactions during their first exposure to shellfish or their first bee sting.

Tropomyosins may be the major cross-reactive allergens between insects and shellfish. Shared antigenic and allergenic determinants between shrimp *Pen a 1* and fruitfly extract have been found, with *Pen a 1* sharing 87% homology with fruit fly tropomyosin.[25] In vitro IgE cross-reactivity has been found between boiled Atlantic shrimp and the German cockroach,[21] showing binding in both types of extracts between 30 and 43 kD. Leung et al[65] found that IgE from shrimp-allergic subjects bound to a 38-kD band in grasshopper, cockroach, and fruit fly preparations.

Castillo et al[18] found an unexpectedly high prevalence of cockroach sensitivity among limpet-allergic subjects sensitive to crustacea and cephalopods. Crustacea and cockroaches are arthropods, but limpets are cephalopods and are less closely related, so this observation is most likely not caused by cross-reactive IgE, but by concomitant allergies. In six individuals with anaphylactic reactions to limpet, five experienced severe systemic reactions during dust mite immunotherapy. Since the limpet filter-feeds on sea mites and other small animals, the limpets could be contaminated with mites and thus cause a reaction.[16] However, no mite allergen was found in the limpet extracts used. No significant cross-reaction occurs between abalone and dust mites.[72]

Cross-reactions may be serious between mites and snails because severe reactions to snail ingestion are common in persons allergic to dust mites.[26,41,98,99] The sensitizing agent may be the dust mite for most snail-allergic patients.[97] Allergy to snails may have been induced in individuals receiving immunotherapy for treatment of dust mite allergy; IgE from the subjects was cross-reactive for snails. Large increases of in vitro IgE reactivity to shrimp and snail were observed in some patients, and two patients developed oral symptoms after eating shrimp. The IgE response to mite allergens did not increase. The average IgE response to snail increased, and two of 17 patients converted from negative to positive for snails.[97] Mite-allergic patients had no IgE reactivity to tropomyosin, but shrimp-allergic patients possessed IgE against mite extract,[103] and tropomyosin appeared to be a major allergen for this latter group.[97] However, tropomyosin was not found to be the major cross-reactive allergen in snail-allergic subjects.

REFERENCES

1. Aas K: Studies of hypersensitivity to fish: a clinical study, *Int Arch Appl Immunol* 29:23, 1966.
2. Aas K: Studies of hypersensitivity to fish: allergological and serological differentiation between various species of fish, *Arch Allergy* 30:257, 1966.
3. Aas K: Fish allergy and the cod fish allergen model. In Brostoff J, Challacombe SJ, editors: *Food allergy and intolerance*, London, 1987, Bailliere Tindall.
4. Amoroso S et al: Antigens of *Euparipha pisana* (snail). I. Identification of allergens by means of in vivo and in vitro analysis, *Int Arch Allergy Appl Immunol* 85:69-75, 1988.
5. Anderson JA, Sogn DA, editors: *Adverse reactions to foods*, Bethesda, Md, 1984, Public Health Service, National Institutes of Health, US Department of Health and Human Services.
6. Apold J, Elsayad S: The effect of amino acid modification and polymerization on the immunochemical reactivity of cod allergen M, *Mol Immunol* 16:559, 1979.
7. Baldo BA, Krills S, Taylor KM: IgE-mediated acute asthma following inhalation of a powdered marine sponge, *Clin Allergy* 12:179, 1982.
8. Beck HI, Nissen BK: Contact urticaria to commercial fish in atopic persons, *Acta Derm Venereol Stockh* 63:257, 1983.
9. Bernhisel-Broadbent J, Scanlon SM, Sampson HA: Fish hypersensitivity. I. In vitro and oral challenge results in fish-allergic patients, *J Allergy Clin Immunol* 89:730, 1992.
10. Bernhisel-Broadbent J, Straus D, Sampson HA: Fish hypersensitivity. II. Clinical relevance of altered fish allergenicity caused by various preparation methods, *J Allergy Clin Immunol* 90:622, 1992.
11. Bernstein M, Day JH, Welsh A: Double-blind food sensitivity in the adult, *J Allergy Clin Immunol* 70:205, 1982.
12. Bock SA et al: Double-blind, placebo-controlled food challenge (DBPCFC) as an office procedure: a manual, *J Allergy Clin Immunol* 82:986, 1988.
13. Bugajska-Schretter A et al: Parvalbumin, a cross-reactive fish allergen, contains IgE-binding epitopes sensitive to periodate treatment and Ca2+ depletion, *J Allergy Clin Immunol* 101:67, 1998.
14. Carrillo T et al: Allergy to limpet, *Allergy* 46:515, 1991.
15. Carrillo T et al: Squid hypersensitivity: a clinical and immunologic study, *Ann Allergy* 68:483, 1992.

16. Carillo T et al: Anaphylaxis due to limpet ingestion, *Ann Allergy* 73:504, 1994.

17. Cartier A et al: Occupational asthma in snow crab–processing workers, *J Allergy Clin Immunol* 74:261, 1984.

18. Castillo R et al: Shellfish hypersensitivity: clinical and immunological characteristics, *Allergol Immunopathol* 22:83, 1994.

19. Clarke PA: Immediate respiratory hypersensitivity to abalone, *Med J Aust* 1:623, 1979 (letter).

20. Crespo JF et al: Allergic reactions associated with airborne fish particles in IgE-mediated fish hypersensitive patients, *Allergy* 50:257, 1995.

21. Crespo JF et al: Cross-reactivity of IgE-binding components between boiled Atlantic shrimp and German cockroach, *Allergy* 1995:918, 1995.

22. Cronin E: Dermatitis of the hands in caterers, *Contact Dermatitis* 17:265, 1987.

23. Daul CB et al: Immunologic evaluation of shrimp-allergic individuals, *J Allergy Clin Immunol* 80:716, 1987.

24. Daul CB et al: Common crustacea allergens: identification of B cell epitopes with shrimp-specific monoclonal antibodies. In Kraft D, Sehon A, editors: *Molecular biology and immunology of allergens*, Boca Raton, Fla, 1993, CRC Press.

25. Daul CB et al: Identification of the major brown shrimp (*Penae aztecus*) allergen (*Pen a* 1) as the muscle protein tropomyosin, *Int Arch Allergy Immunol* 105:49, 1994.

26. De Bernardi G et al: Near fatal asthma after snail ingestion, *Allergy* 53(suppl 43):149, 1998.

27. De la Cuesta CG et al: Food allergy to *Helix terrestre* (snail), *Allergol Immunopathol* 17:337, 1989.

28. De Martino M et al: Allergy to different fish species in cod-allergic children: in vivo and in vitro studies, *J Allergy Clin Immunol* 86:909, 1990.

29. Desjardins A et al: Occupational IgE-mediated sensitization and asthma caused by clam and shrimp, *J Allergy Clin Immunol* 96:608, 1995.

30. Diaz Sanchez C et al: Protein contact dermatitis associated with food allergy to fish, *Contact Dermatitis* 31:55, 1994.

31. Dory D et al: Recognition of an extensive range of IgE-reactive proteins in cod extract, *Allergy* 53:42, 1998.

32. Douglas JD et al: Occupational asthma caused by automated salmon processing, *Lancet* 346:737, 1995.

33. Elsayad S, Apold J: Immunochemical analysis of cod fish allergen M: locations of the immunoglobulin binding sites as demonstrated by the native and synthetic peptides, *Allergy* 38:449, 1983.

34. Elsayad S, Bennich H: The primary structure of allergen M from cod, *Scand J Immunol* 4:203, 1975.

35. Elsayad S et al: The structural requirements of epitopes with IgE binding capacity demonstrated by three major allergens from fish, egg, and tree pollen, *Scand J Clin Lab Invest* 204(suppl):17, 1991.

36. Erikkson NE, Ryden F, Jonsson P: Hypersensitivity to larvae of chironomids (non-biting midges), *Allergy* 44:305, 1989.

37. Freeman S, Rosen RH: Urticarial contact dermatitis in food handlers, *Med J Austr* 155:91, 1991.

38. Gaddie J, Legge JS, Friend JAR: Pulmonary hypersensitivity in prawn workers, *Lancet* 2:1350, 1980.

39. Galland AV et al: Purification of a 41 kDa cod-allergenic protein, *J Chromatogr B Biomed Sci Appl* 27:63, 1998.

40. Glazzaz SS et al: Reactivity to finfish: correlation of skin tests with parvalbumin content, *J Allergy Clin Immunol* 93:303, 1994.

41. Grembiale RD et al: Snail ingestion and asthma, *Allergy* 51:361, 1996.

42. Halmepuro L, Salvaggio JE, Lehrer SB: Crawfish and lobster allergens: identification and structural similarities with other crustacea, *Int Arch Allergy Immunol* 84:165, 1987.

43. Hansen TK et al: Codfish allergy in adults: IgE cross-reactivity among fish species, *Ann Allergy Asthma Immunol* 78:187, 1997.

44. Haydel R et al: Food allergy: challenge studies of fish allergic subjects, *J Allergy Clin Immunol* 91:344, 1993.

45. Hefle SL et al: Snow crab allergy: identification of IgE-binding proteins, *J Allergy Clin Immunol* 95:332, 1995.

46. Helbling A et al: Immunopathogenesis of fish allergy: identification of fish-allergic adults by skin test and radioallergosorbent test, *Ann Allergy Asthma Immunol* 77:48, 1996.

47. Hoffman DR, Day ED, Miller JS: The major heat stable allergen of shrimp, *Ann Allergy* 47:17, 1981.

48. Ishikawa M et al: Isolation and properties of allergenic proteins in the oyster *Crassostrea gigas*, *Fish Sci* 63:610, 1997.

49. Ishikawa M et al: Purification and IgE-binding epitopes of a major allergen in the gastropod *Turbo cornutus*, *Biosci Biotechnol Biochem* 62:1337, 1998.

50. Ishikawa M et al: Tropomyosin, the major oyster *Crassostrea gigas* allergen and its IgE-binding epitopes, *J Food Sci* 63:44, 1998.

51. James JM et al: Comparison of pediatric and adult IgE antibody binding to fish proteins, *Ann Allergy Asthma Immunol* 79:131, 1997.

52. Juji F et al: A case of food-dependent exercise-induced anaphylaxis possibly induced by shellfish (*Sulculus supertexta* and *Turbo cornutus*), *Arerugi* 39:1515, 1990.

53. Jyo T et al: Sea squirt asthma—occupational asthma induced by inhalation of antigenic substances contained in the sea squirt body fluid, *Allergy Immunol* 21:425, 1974.

54. Karlin JM: Occupational asthma to clam's liver extract, *J Allergy Clin Immunol* 63:197, 1979.

55. Kelso JM et al: Monospecific allergy to swordfish, *Ann Allergy* 77:227, 1996.

56. Knape JTA et al: An anaphylactic reaction to protamine in a patient allergic to fish, *Anaethesiology* 55:324, 1981.

57. Koshte VL, Kagen SL, Aalberse RC: Cross-reactivity of IgE antibodies to caddis fly with arthropoda and mollusca, *J Allergy Clin Immunol* 84:174, 1989.

58. Laffond E et al: Seafood hypersensitivity: clinical and immunological characteristics, *Allergy* 53(suppl 43):85, 1998.

59. Lehrer SB: The complex nature of food antigens: studies of cross-reacting crustacea allergens, *Ann Allergy* 57:267, 1986.

60. Lehrer SB, McCants ML: Reactivity of IgE antibodies with crustacea and oyster allergens: evidence for common antigenic structures, *J Allergy Clin Immunol* 80:133, 1987.

61. Lehrer SB, McCants M, Salvaggio J: Identification of crustacea allergens by crossed radioimmunoelectrophoresis, *Int Arch Allergy Appl Immunol* 77:192, 1985.

62. Lemanske RJ Jr, Taylor SL: Standardized extracts, foods, *Clin Rev Allergy* 5:23, 1987.

63. Lemiere C et al: Occupational asthma to lobster and shrimp, *Allergy* 51:272, 1996.

64. Leung PSC et al: Cloning, expression, and primary structure of Metapenaeus ensis tropomyosin, the major heat-stable shrimp allergen, *J Allergy Clin Immunol* 94:882, 1994.

65. Leung PSC et al: IgE reactivity against a cross-reactive allergen in crustacea and mollusca: evidence for tropomyosin as the common allergen, *J Allergy Clin Immunol* 98:954, 1996.

66. Leung PS et al: Identification and molecular characterization of *Charybdis feriatus* tropomyosin, the major crab allergen, *J Allergy Clin Immunol* 102:847, 1998.

67. Leung PSC et al: Molecular identification of the lobster muscle protein tropomyosin as a seafood allergen, *Mol Marine Biol Biotechnol* 7:12, 1998.

68. Liebers V, Hoernstein M, Baur X: Humoral immune response to the insect Chi t 1 in aquarists and fish-food factory workers, *Allergy* 48:236, 1993.

69. Lin RY et al: Identification and characterization of a 30 kD major allergen from *Parapenaeus fissurus*, *J Allergy Clin Immunol* 92:837, 1993.

70. Lin HY et al: Fish induced anaphylactic reaction: report of one case, *Chung Hua Min Kuo Hsaio Erh Ko I Hsueh Hui Tsa Chih* 39:200, 1998.

71. Lindstrom CDV et al: Cloning of two distinct cDNAs encoding parvalbumin, the major allergen of Atlantic salmon (*Salmo salar*), *Scand J Immunol* 44:334, 1996.

72. Lopata AL et al: Characteristics of hypersensitivity reactions and identification of a unique 49 kd IgE-binding protein (Hal-m-1) in abalone (*Haliotis midae*), *J Allergy Clin Immunol* 100:642, 1997.

73. Maeda S et al: Eleven cases of anaphylaxis caused by grand keyhole limpet (abalone-like shellfish), *Arerugi* 40:1415, 1991.

74. Malo JL, Cartier A: Occupational reactions in the seafood industry, *Clin Rev Allergy* 11:223, 1993.

75. Mata E et al: Surimi and native codfish contain a common allergen identified as a 63-kDA protein, *Allergy* 49:42, 1994.

76. Maulitz RM, Pratt DS, Schocket AL: Exercise-induced anaphylactic reaction to shellfish, *J Allergy Clin Immunol* 63:433, 1979.

77. Miyake T et al: A pediatric case of food-dependent exercise-induced anaphylaxis, *Arerugi* 37:53, 1988.

78. Miyazawa H et al: Identification of the first major allergen of squid (*Todarodes pacificus*), *J Allergy Clin Immunol* 95:948, 1996.

79. Morgan JE et al: Species-specific shrimp allergens: RAST and RAST-inhibition studies, *J Allergy Clin Immunol* 83:1112, 1989.

80. Morikawa A et al: Anaphylaxis to grand keyhole limpet (abalone-like shellfish) and abalone, *Ann Allergy* 65:415, 1990.

81. Nagpal S, Metcalfe DD, Rao PV: Identification of a shrimp-derived allergen as tRNA, *J Immunol* 138:4169, 1987.

82. Nagpal S et al: Isolation and characterization of heat-stable allergens from shrimp (*Penaeus indicus*), *J Allergy Clin Immunol* 83:26, 1989.

83. Nakashima T: Studies on bronchial asthma observed in culture oyster workers, *Hiroshima J Med Sci* 18:41, 1969.

84. O'Neill C, Lehrer SB: Seafood allergy and allergens: a review, *Food Technol* 49:103, 1995.

85. O'Neill C et al: Allergic reactions to fish, *Clin Rev Allergy* 11:183, 1993.

86. Orford RR, Wilson JT: Epidemiologic and immunologic studies in processor of king crab, *Am J Ind Med* 7:155, 1985.

87. Orriols R et al: Mollusk shell hypersensitivity pneumonitis, *Ann Int Med* 113:80, 1990.

88. Orriols R et al: High prevalence of mollusk shell hypersensitivity pneumonitis in nacre factory workers, *Eur Respir J* 10:780, 1997.

89. Park KH et al: Pediatric IgE antibody binding to the most common seafood proteins in Korea, *J Allergy Clin Immunol* 101:S90, 1998.

90. Pascual C et al: Fish allergy: evaluation of the importance of cross-reactivity, *J Pediatr* 121:S29, 1992.

91. Patel PC, Cockcraft DW: Occupational asthma caused by exposure to cooking lobster in the work environment: a case report, *Ann Allergy* 68:360, 1992.

92. Sampson HA: Role of immediate food hypersensitivity in the pathogenesis of atopic dermatitis, *J Allergy Clin Immunol* 71:473, 1983.

93. Shanti KN et al: Identification of tropomyosin as the major shrimp allergen and characterization of its IgE-binding epitopes, *J Immunol* 151:5354, 1993.

94. Shibasaki M et al: Late anaphylactic reaction to cuttlefish, *Ann Allergy* 63:421, 1989.

95. Tomaszunas S et al: Allergic reactions to cuttlefish in deep-sea fisherman, *Lancet* 1:116, 1988.

96. Valseechi R et al: Contact urticaria from *Loligo japonica, Contact Dermatitis* 35:367, 1996.

97. Van Ree R et al: Asthma after consumption of snails in house-dust-mite-allergic patients: a case of IgE cross-reactivity, *Allergy* 51:387, 1996.

98. Van Ree R et al: Possible induction of food allergy during mite immunotherapy, *Allergy* 51:108, 1996.

99. Vuitton DA: Cross-reactivity between terrestrial snail (*Helix* species) and house-dust mite *(Dermatophagoides pteronyssinus).* I. In vivo study, *Allergy* 53:144, 1998.

100. Waring N et al: Hypersensitivity reactions to ingested crustacea: clinical evaluation and diagnostic studies in shrimp-sensitive individuals, *J Allergy Clin Immunol* 76:440, 1985.

101. Wiley K, Griffin P: Characterisation and purification of allergens from Norwegian lobster, *Clin Exp Allergy* 24:175, 1994.

102. Williams PB et al: The histamine content of allergen extract, *J Allergy Clin Immunol* 89:738, 1992.

103. Witteman AM et al: Identification of a cross-reactive allergen (presumable tropomyosin) in shrimp, mites, and insects, *Int Arch Allergy Immunol* 105:56, 1994.

104. Wuthrich B: Atopic dermatitis flare provoked by inhalant allergens, *Dermatologica* 178:51, 1989.

105. Yamashita N et al: Allergenicity of Chironomidae in asthmatic patients, *Ann Allergy* 63:423, 1989.

106. Yamura T, Kurose H: Oyster-shucker's dermatitis, *Arerugi* 15:813, 1966.

107. Yuninger JW: Food antigens in food allergy. In Metcalfe DD, Sampson HA, Simon RA, editors: *Food allergy: adverse reactions to foods and food additives,* Boston, 1991, Blackwell.

108. Zhoutyi VR, Borozov MV: Dermatitis in workers processing mussels, *Vestn Dermatil Venerol* 47:71, 1973.

Marine
Medicine

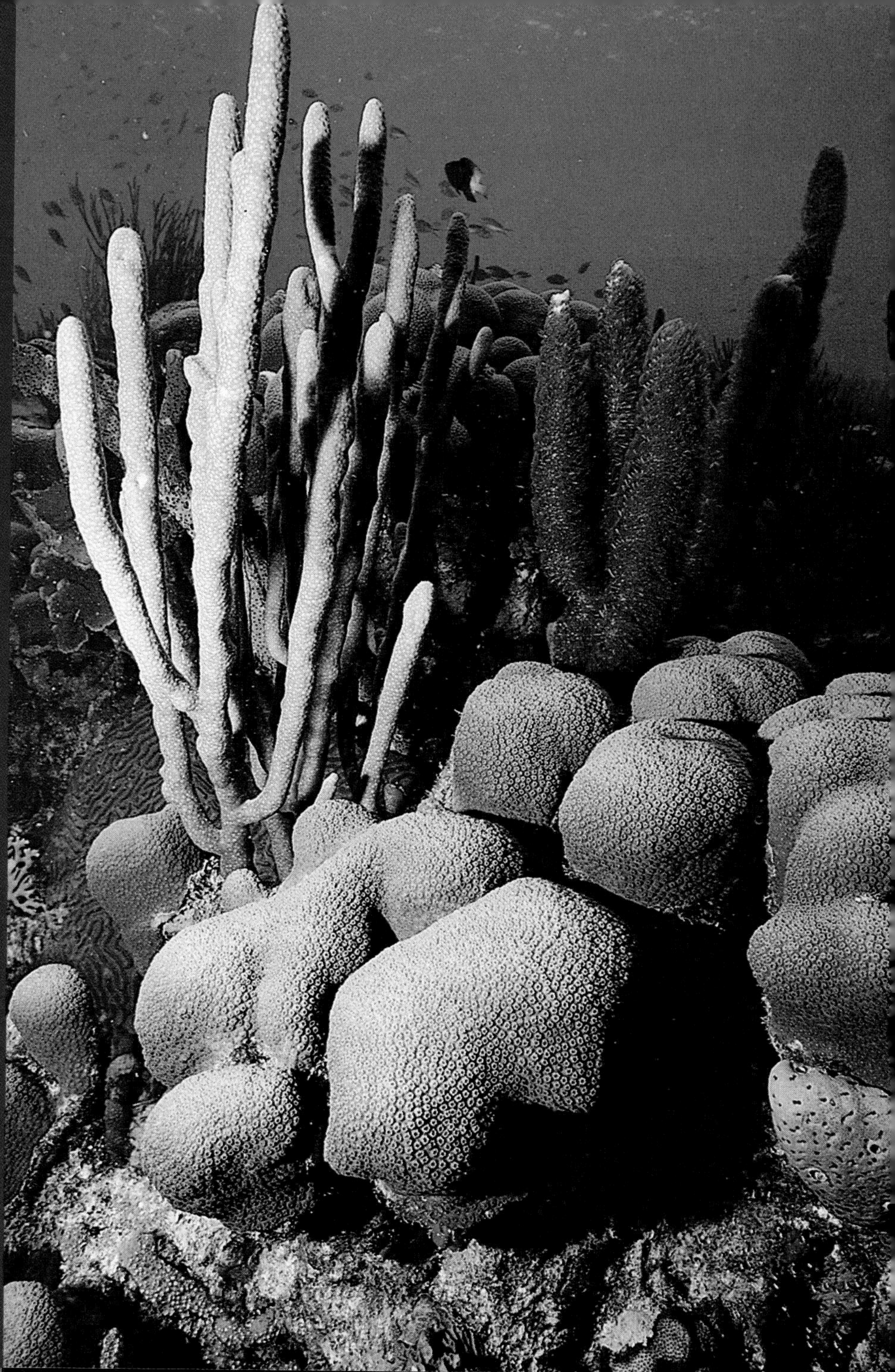

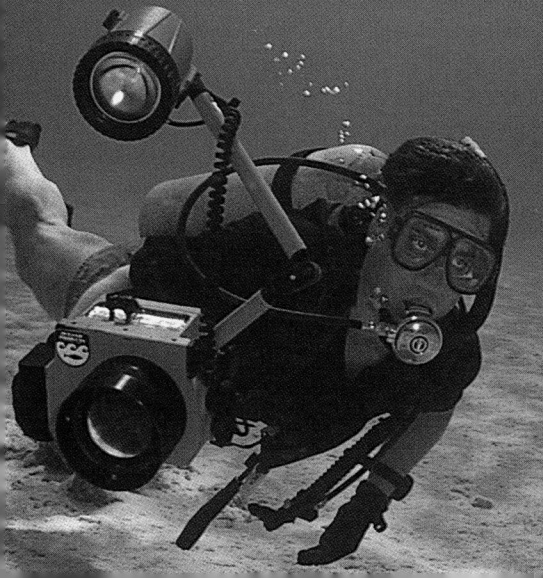

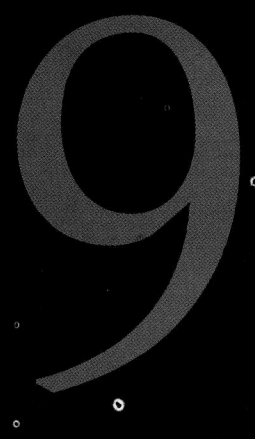

56 Submersion Incidents

Andrew B. Newman

A man who is not afraid of the sea will soon be drowned, he said, for he will be going out on a day he shouldn't. But we do be afraid of the sea, and we do only be drowned now and again.

John Millington Synge, *The Aran Islands*

Humans' ancestral home was the water, and we are often drawn back to the aquatic environment. Three fourths of our planet's surface is water, and the earliest records of human perception of life in and under the oceans indicate both fascination and fear. In eighteenth-century Europe, sudden death by drowning sparked the interest of humanitarians, who thought actions could be taken to restore life. The incidence of drowning on commercial waterways was probably high, since roads were nearly nonexistent and swimming as recreation was unknown among the general populace. Drowning became a significant public health issue.[11] In response to this fashionable humanitarian cause, the Society for the Recovery of Persons Apparently Drowned was formed in 1774. Their activities included research, public education, and treatment of victims. The organization survives today as the Royal Humane Society.[109] Techniques for resuscitating drowning victims developed after groups with a special interest in the problem of drowning were established. A 1796 work describes mouth-to-mouth ventilation and tactile endotracheal intubation.[97]

During the 1990s, greater understanding of the pathophysiology and natural history of submersion incidents has allowed revised approaches to therapy, confirmed the importance of immediate care to eventual outcome, and permitted adoption of more optimistic medical attitudes.[53,167]

PREVENTION

Prevention is as important as any action that can be taken after drowning or near drowning. Anyone who will be on or near the water should have swimming, rescue, and lifesaving skills, including a working knowledge of cardiopulmonary resuscitation (CPR). Prevention of near drowning must focus on several areas (Box 56-1). Water sport participants need to maintain adequate health and training for their possible levels of performance. Water knowledge includes readiness for an accident and self-assessment of skills.

Open water activities should always be done with partners and with plans for self-rescue. Careful attention to the location, weather, and environment before the initiation of aquatic activities can prevent harmful events.[53]

Swimming pools should be completely enclosed by a 5-foot fence with self-closing and self-latching locks above the reach of small children. Lifesaving equipment should be close at hand. Every pool should be equipped with a life preserver and a long pole for rescue attempts.[129]

Parents should always be present to supervise children when they are in the water. After swimming, children should be dressed in clothing to discourage unsupervised returns to the swimming area. Children in families that have a pool or anticipate water-oriented vacations should have early swimming lessons.[92] People prone to syncope or seizures should always be with someone when in or near the water. In addition, even a little alcohol may prove fatal in the marine environment.

Everyone on a boat or raft should have a U.S. Coast Guard–approved life vest or life jacket that will support the person with the head above water, even if the person becomes unconscious. Travelers on water should be aware of lifeboat and raft availability. Courses on safe boating, rescue, and navigation are offered by the local Coast Guard.

Emergency medical services (EMS) systems in areas with lake, river, or ocean access should consider adopting a plan for a water rescue unit prepared to respond and deal immediately with accidents. These units include improved boat access and paramedics who are master divers.[233]

Physicians may help in their local areas by increasing drowning awareness among their patients or by teaching community-based CPR or emergency care classes.[132] Medical schools may be able to improve preventive care by increasing education on drowning during training. Physicians should provide drowning prevention instruction and materials to all their patients with children or who engage in water-related activities.[168]

TERMINOLOGY

Thirty-five years ago in a classic monograph on drowning, David Green succinctly summarized the problem:

Box 56-1   PREVENTION OF NEAR DROWNING

PERSONALITY

Water skills
Health
    Acute conditions
    Chronic conditions
Water knowledge

PERSONNEL

Water partners
Supervisors
Rescuers
Cardiopulmonary resuscitators

ENVIRONMENT

Water condition
    Sea state
    Temperature
    Visibility
Objects in water
Proximity to shore
Proximity to care

Modified from *Near drowning: forty-seventh workshop of the Undersea and Hyperbaric Medical Society,* Kensington, Md, 1997, the Undersea and Hyperbaric Medical Society.

drowning is the process by which air-breathing animals succumb on submersion in a liquid. In the evolutionary process, water-living species adapted to terrestrial life, lost their ability to breathe under water, and became susceptible to drowning.[85] *Near drowning* is a term introduced by Modell[146] to indicate submersion with at least temporary survival.

Drowning syndromes comprise the continuum from minimal aspiration of water to overwhelming lung injury and death. Several terms are used to describe different points in the continuum.[55,127] *Delayed drowning* or *secondary drowning* occurs when a victim appears to have survived an episode but then subsequently dies from respiratory failure (adult respiratory distress syndrome, or ARDS) or infectious complications that often originate with pneumonia. Submersion incidents or near drowning may also be classified with modifiers about aspiration of water or other liquid. Postimmersion syndromes include illnesses that occur after an immersion episode.

The use of a more neutral term without the implication of time, prognosis, or retrospective analysis is necessary to avoid confusion and to simplify classification. A person who is adversely affected by being submersed in water has experienced a *submersion incident.* The term is descriptive, implies no particular prognosis, and can therefore be used in immediate care without the considerations of time or outcome.

A new classification is based on severity of disease, and with the following six categories of illness focusing on the pulmonary findings on clinical examination:

Grade 1: normal examination with cough
Grade 2: rales in some fields
Grade 3: acute pulmonary edema
Grade 4: pulmonary edema with arterial hypotension
Grade 5: isolated respiratory arrest
Grade 6: cardiopulmonary arrest

In conjunction with this classification system, 1831 drowning cases were analyzed to show an increase in mortality from 0% with grade 1 to 93% with grade 6.

INCIDENCE

It is difficult to estimate accurately the total number of submersion incidents, since such accidents are not reportable. Two of the largest and most densely populated countries do not report statistics to the World Health Organization (WHO), and little has been written about the morbidity of persons after submersion.[56] Retrospective studies are beginning to quantify the problem and suggest directions for prevention and management. Drowning is second only to motor vehicle accidents as the most common cause of accidental death. In states with seat belt laws, drowning has become the leading cause of accidental death in children.[28,29,143] An estimated 140,000 deaths occur worldwide annually from drowning.[138,187] Of an estimated 80,000 submersion incidents, 9000 deaths occur each year in the United States.[10] These statistics probably underestimate the problem, since many incidents are unreported or classified in other categories, such as motor vehicle accidents, acute illnesses, and suicide.[15] Drowning kills mainly the young; 64% of all victims are less than 30 years of age, and 26% are under age 5.[73,171] The incidence of near drowning may be 500 to 600 times the rate of drowning.[113] Submersion incidents increase in areas with abundant recreational waterways, although the home swimming pool or even the bathtub can be the site of a lethal event. Recent catastrophic natural disasters, such as floods and tsunamis, have drawn media attention to drowning as a cause of death.

RISK FACTORS

The problem of submersion incidents can often be related to risk factors (Box 56-2) or to certain behaviors or groups. This is particularly true of children.[180] Understanding these factors can help in planning and instituting preventive measures and practices.

Age

Age appears to be an indicator of risk. Drowning is a young person's accident. The most important age group is toddlers, with children under 1 year of age having the highest drowning rate, followed by teenage males.[107] In 1989, 1200 deaths occurred in the 10- to 19-year-old group.[204] In a survey of 9420 primary school children in South Carolina, up to 10% of children under age 5 experienced a "serious threat" of near drowning.[213] The highest risk of near drowning is in the age group of 15 to 24 years, and the lowest risk is in persons over age 65.[27,28,193,199,220]

Toddlers are at risk because of their inquisitive nature and because they are often unsupervised, especially at home. Children frequently drown while bathing with a younger sibling without an adult present.[107] The high risk of a submersion incident among teenage boys reflects their mobility and adventuresome nature and the absence of adult supervision. The low risk of a serious submersion incident in the older age group reflects decreased exposure to water environments, increased experience, and mature judgment.

Gender

Males predominate among drowning victims. In all age groups, males account for more than half of cases, with a male-to-female ratio of 12:1 for boat-related drownings and 5:1 for non-boat-related drownings.[10] For males the peak drowning incidence occurs at age 2 years, decreases until the age of 10, and then rises rapidly to a peak at age 18. The incidence in females peaks at age 1 year, then falls off and does not rise again.[10,60]

A study of aquatic activity participation in 3042 households suggests that males may be more at risk for drowning because of higher exposure rates to aquatic activities, higher alcohol consumption while at the waterfront, and more risk-taking behavior.[103]

Location

Drowning, that is, death by asphyxia resulting from submersion, is not necessarily a recreational accident. Incidents and deaths occur not only in the backyard swimming pool and in the ocean, but also in the unsupervised bath and the cleaning bucket.* In rural areas,

having a home well increases by sevenfold the risk of a young child drowning. Water barrels, courtyard pools, and underground cisterns are also hazardous sites.[26] A survey of deaths in California from drowning in 1993 showed that they resulted in $5.2 million in hospital charges.[61] The location of the submersion incident is often determined by the geography and social aspects of the community. In water-oriented areas such as Florida, California, and Australia, submersion incidents are common year-round and often occur in home swimming pools. The great majority of drowning deaths in children under age 4 years occur at home.[199]

Domestic swimming pools are especially dangerous, particularly for young children. Approximately 300 children drowned in home swimming pools in the United States in 1981, and in 1983 about 2000 children were seen in emergency departments after submersion incidents.[228] Two of three victims of swimming pool drownings were under 3 years of age. Whereas black children tend to drown in lakes, canals, and quarry sites, white children die more frequently in backyard swimming pools. Public or motel pools are implicated infrequently. Despite ordinances defining safe operation of home swimming pools, safety features may be faulty or ignored. Although all but 3% of home swimming pools in a Florida community were properly fenced and protected, 70% of the locks were found to be unfastened or nonfunctioning.[199] In a study of 700 pool owners in Florida, more than 40% did not know how to perform CPR.[129] In an Australian study of drowning incidents, only 1 of 66 swimming pool barriers was considered adequate, and in 76% of the incidents there was no fence.[187] The risk of drowning is almost 4 times greater in unfenced pools.[185] The level of water in the pool may be important in the etiology of some deaths. The average distance from the water to the poolside lip is 12 to 14 inches (30 to 35 cm). This distance provides a significant barrier to young children who have fallen into a pool; they may reach the side but be unable to pull themselves out of the water. Some recommend raising the level of water in swimming pools.[199]

Illegal immigrants who attempt to enter countries by crossing canals or bodies of water at night to escape detection are also at extreme risk for drowning episodes.[1]

Although the incidence of drownings tends to be greater in coastal communities oriented to large bodies of water and the aquatic environment in general, most surveys indicate that drownings in salt water are relatively rare. Notable exceptions to this are in cold water fishing communities, such as in Alaska, Nova Scotia, Maine, western New Zealand, and the North Sea, where the annual fatality rate may be as high as 415 drownings per 100,000 fisherman.[165,211] Submersion incidents that do not result in death or even in hospitalization may be common in these communities.[187] In my

---

*References 108, 110, 114, 137, 182, 214.

experience, this is particularly true in Australia and California. This may be a result, at least in part, of effective surveillance and rescue efforts at public beaches by lifeguards and surf lifesaving societies.[138]

Race

Evidence shows that race is a factor in the increased risk of exposure to submersion incidents, particularly in children. The incidence of both drownings and near drownings appears to be greater in black children. The drowning rate of black male children has been estimated to be as much as 3 times that of white males.[212] In the United States, unsupervised swimming or accidental falls into unattended canals or quarries accounted for a large percentage of deaths in black males.[199] Such statistics probably reflect socioeconomic conditions in the affected communities.

Ability to Swim

The ability to swim does not appear to be consistently related to drowning rates unless gender differences are considered. White males have a higher incidence of drowning than white females but reportedly have better swimming ability. On the other hand, black females are reported to have the lowest swimming ability but a very low rate of drowning.[212] In Florida, nonswimmers or beginners accounted for 73% of drownings in home swimming pools and 82% of incidents in canals, lakes, and ponds.[199]

Parental example is an important determinant of whether children can swim. Children whose parents can swim are most likely to be strong swimmers; those with parents who cannot swim are likely to be nonswimmers. Parents of white children are much more likely to be swimmers than are the parents of black children.[212]

Drugs

Alcohol is the chief drug implicated in submersion incidents; the danger of its use in the aquatic environment cannot be overemphasized.[20,135] An Australian study reported that 64% of males who drowned had measurable levels of alcohol in blood samples taken after death, and 53% of those over age 26 had blood alcohol levels greater than 100 mg/dl.[187] Although it cannot be stated definitively that alcohol was the cause of these tragedies, the common association of intoxication with drowning argues strongly against the use of alcohol near the water.[51] Despite the sobering statistics, a Massachusetts survey revealed that 36% of men and 11% of women had consumed alcoholic beverages during their most recent aquatic activities.[2,102] Loss of judgment from use of intoxicants most likely explains the frequent association with drowning incidents. In addition, alcohol increases heat loss, decreases laryngeal reflexes, and increases the incidence of vomiting—all factors that worsen the prognosis in submersion incidents.[56] Drugs such as phencyclidine (PCP), lysergic acid diethylamide (LSD), and marijuana alter the sensorium, increasing the risk of accidents in the water. Up to 30% of adult drownings occur because of boating accidents in which occupants demonstrated poor judgment: overcrowding, speeding, use of boats for purposes not intended, failure to wear life jackets, and reckless handling of the craft. The incidence of drug use in these episodes is not known, but it can be assumed that intoxicants play a role in many such accidents.[51,187]

Underlying Disease or Injury

Underlying injury or illness can account for loss of life in the water. Hypoglycemia, myocardial infarction, cardiac arrhythmias, depression and suicide, and syncope predispose to drowning incidents.[30,77,196,209] Persons with a history of seizures must be supervised at all times while on boats or swimming and should be encouraged to shower (not take a bath) in a nonglass cubicle in an unlocked bathroom.[47,117,174] A search for an underlying cause of the tragedy should be made, particularly in persons who are evaluated in the hospital after rescue.

Cervical spine injuries and head trauma should be suspected in all unwitnessed incidents, particularly in those involving surfers and in victims found near diving boards or rafts in shallow water. Possible damage to the cervical spine should be a consideration in both immediate on-scene and ED management.

Child Abuse

Attention has been drawn to the problem of submersion incidents as a manifestation of child abuse. All suspicious incidents must have a thorough social service and legal investigation consistent with the laws of each community.[86,121,126] Frequently, however, this does not occur. In a study of 95 drownings and near drownings in Seattle, only 28% of the cases had a social service evaluation, and only eight drownings were reported to children's protective services.[65] A study of children sustaining bathtub near drownings between 1982 and 1992 found that 67% had historical or physical findings compatible with a diagnosis of abuse or neglect.[125] Child abuse should be considered in any bathtub child drowning unless epilepsy or a developmental problem is present.[118] Children who have been previously abused are also much more likely to be purposeful drowning victims.[75,210]

Hypothermia (see Chapters 6 and 8)

Recent reports of victims surviving after submersion periods of as long as 30 minutes in very cold water have elicited medical and lay hypotheses regarding survival after prolonged submersion.[30,57,104]

Drowning may result directly from hypothermia.[36,100] Experiences with persons shipwrecked even in relatively warm water have shown that the body temperature of victims can be lowered to the point at which hypothermia threatens survival. Thermal conductivity of cold water is approximately 25 to 30 times that of air.[100,126,128] Water at 33° C (91.4° F) is thermally neutral, the point at which heat loss equals heat production for a swimmer without clothes. Any water colder than this will lead to ongoing heat loss. Thus, in very cold water, hypothermia may ensue rapidly and lead to drowning. This is particularly true in children, who have less subcutaneous fat and relatively greater body surface area than adults.[126] Cooling may occur by a combination of conductive heat loss directly into the water and circulatory cooling from chilled venous blood returning to the circulation. Survivors of a Canadian boating tragedy painted a vivid picture of the effects of hypothermia that resulted in the deaths of an instructor and 12 of his students: "Gradually we could feel the sensation going out of our limbs, and we heard some of the boys starting to get paranoid about being in the water . . . Some started to talk nonsense and then, one by one, their voices faded away as they lost consciousness."[227]

Death in submersion-associated hypothermia can be attributed to the basic mechanisms discussed next.

Immersion Syndrome. Immersion syndrome is defined as cardiac arrest secondary to massive vagal stimulation.[78,115,126]

Excessive Fatigue and Confusion. The combination of hypothermia, exertion, panic, and confusion leads to poor judgment, which causes victims to endanger themselves further by swimming away from help, leaving an overturned canoe, or misjudging the distance to shore.

Direct Hypothermia. At or below a core temperature of 28° C (82° F), ventricular fibrillation is a real risk[93,160,219] (see Chapter 6). It has been estimated that at a water temperature of 0° C (32° F), the victim of submersion cannot survive for more than 1 hour; at a water temperature of 15° C (59° F), survival is not common after 6 hours.[35,76] However, several Canadian cases temper blind acceptance of any particular dogma. In one incident, a pilot and passenger ditched their plane into a lake on final approach to an island airport.[142] Air temperature was 2.2° C (36° F) and water temperature 4° C (39.2° F). Both men were similarly clothed and in the water for 60 minutes before being rescued. The passenger, a 48-year-old man, weighed 101 kg, was 190 cm in height, and had a core temperature of 32° C (89.6° F) on admission to the hospital. He was alert, complained only of being cold, was actively rewarmed, and left the

hospital the next day. The pilot, a previously healthy 38-year-old man, was of medium body habitus and had little subcutaneous fat. He was admitted to the same regional trauma unit in ventricular fibrillation with a core temperature of 29.1° C (84.2° F). Despite core rewarming and vigorous resuscitative measures over 4 hours, he could not be revived. In view of the identical environmental conditions, clothing worn, and time in the water, the authors concluded that skinfold thickness was the most important discriminating factor in the outcome.[149]

A second case illustrates that preparation and protective clothing may lengthen survival time in cold water.[141] A married couple, both experienced sailors, began to take on water in their boat about 11 km from shore in a Canadian lake.[226] The boat sank after 40 minutes, during which time they were able to prepare for abandoning ship by lashing together life preservers and donning heavy parkas and special survival gear carried in the boat. The month was August, but a storm had developed with gale-force winds of 60 km/hr and high waves. Water temperature was estimated to be 18° C (64° F). Both persons spent over 18 hours in the water before rescue and helicopter transport to the regional trauma unit. Both were mildly hypothermic on admission; the husband's rectal temperature was 32° C (89.6° F), and the wife's was 36.4° C (97.5° F). Both were discharged the next day without complications, with survival attributed to survival preparedness and protective clothing.

In victims kept afloat by life preservers or other means, death may result directly from hypothermia. Although some people may appear to be dead after rescue, efforts to resuscitate and rewarm them may be rewarded with recovery. Still, the absolute effect of hypothermia on eventual survival after a submersion incident remains in doubt. In certain cases, hypothermia appears to be protective, as in the case of the Norwegian child who survived neurologically intact after being rescued from an ice-laden stream in which he had been submerged for 40 minutes.[217] His temperature on admission to the hospital was 24° C (75° F), and after 1 hour of resuscitation, spontaneous circulation returned. He was discharged from the hospital 8 days later. Similar cases have involved submersion under ice with eventual survival.

Orlowski[171] reviewed the world literature on prolonged submersion with good outcomes. He reported 17 victims, most of whom were younger than 19 years of age and male. He concluded that no one factor correlated well with outcome. These factors included water temperature, core temperature, rewarming techniques, and duration of resuscitation. He further cautioned against assuming a good prognosis in victims submerged in very cold water, citing several cases of children who, despite hypothermia and appropriate treatment, had poor outcomes.[238] Some children may survive after long periods of submersion in very cold water because the "diving reflex" present in lower mammals may be operative.[37,79,141] The mammalian diving reflex, especially impressive in seals, slows heart rate, shunts blood to the brain, and closes the airway. However, recent evidence suggests that the diving reflex present in seals is active in only 15% to 30% of human subjects. This response, with its potential for improved brain circulation, may be a significant factor in why some persons survive and others drown.[80,91] After a study of breath-holding and bradycardia in children and adults, one group concluded that the diving reflex in children is weak and may not contribute significantly to survival after cold water submersion.[192]

Immersion in cold water may lead quickly to hypothermia because of surface heat loss and core cooling. In addition, swallowing or aspiration of cold water may contribute to rapid cooling.[91,171] Rapid onset of hypothermia during freshwater drowning may result from core cooling from pulmonary aspiration and rapid absorption of cold water. Significant cerebral cooling is therefore likely before cessation of circulation.[38]

If the diving reflex is discounted, the most likely explanation for survival after prolonged submersion in cold water is that rapidly induced hypothermia reduces tissue oxygen demand and protects the brain. Catecholamine release may be blunted in victims who quickly become hypothermic in very cold water, lessening the propensity to ventricular fibrillation that accompanies warm water submersion incidents.[171] Muscle movement is probably less in persons exposed suddenly to very cold water, further reducing oxygen demand.

In contradistinction to the possible protective effect of hypothermia in submerged victims, hypothermia can create serious problems for the victim struggling to survive in cold water. Specific patterns of heat loss can be demonstrated in subjects placed in water at temperatures as low as 4.5° C (40.1° F).[35] In these studies, thermograms have graphically recorded heat loss from various parts of the body, demonstrating preferential loss from the head and neck (up to 50%), thoracic cage, and inguinal area. Movement of any kind increases heat loss.

Collis[35] compared several options available to victims faced with the dilemma of cold water survival. He concluded that methods of survival that require much movement would be "suicidal" and, based on the observations of heat loss, devised preferred means of conserving body heat while immersed in cold water. These methods have been approved and adopted by the U.S. Coast Guard (Department of Transportation).

As summarized in Figure 56-1, treading water, swimming, and drown-proofing all resulted in reduced survival time (less than 2 hours) at a water temperature

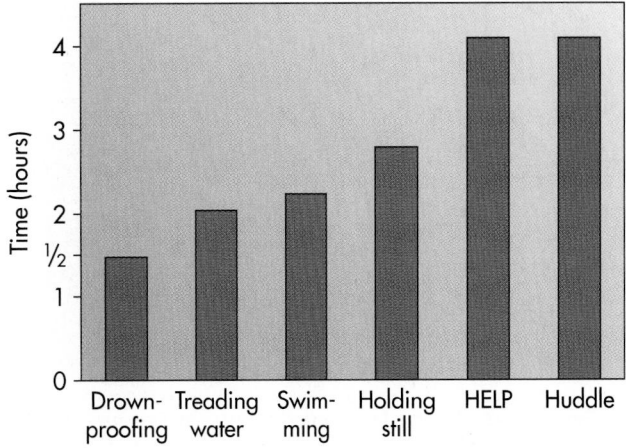

Figure 56-1 Survival times in cool (10° C [50° F]) water using various techniques in several situations. (*Data from Collis ML:* Survival behaviour in cold water immersion. *In* Proceedings of the Cold Water Symposium, *Toronto, 1976, Royal Life-Saving Society of Canada.*)

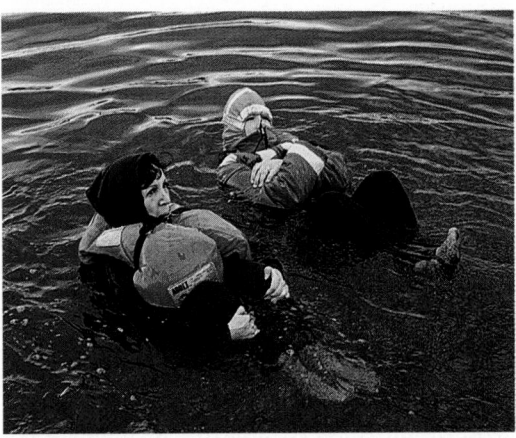

Figure 56-2 Heat escape lessening posture (HELP). *(Courtesy Alan Steinman, MD.)*

of 10° C (50° F). Survival time was estimated to double if victims assumed a position designed to protect areas of body heat loss. In this position, termed the *heat escape lessening posture* (HELP), the arms are folded across the chest and pressed to the sides, the knees are drawn up to the chest, and the legs are crossed at the ankles. In this position the victim attempts to keep still, maintaining the head out of water. To assume this position, the victim must be wearing a life jacket (Figure 56-2). When this position was tested on members of the swim team at the University of Pittsburgh, they reported it as fatiguing at best.

If two or more persons are in the water, the *huddle position* is recommended to lessen total body heat loss. Since children become hypothermic much more quickly than adults, they should be placed in the mid-

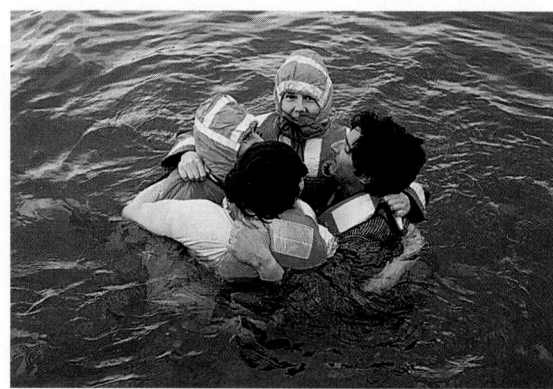

Figure 56-3 Huddle technique. *(Courtesy Alan Steinman, MD.)*

dle of the huddle. In this position, life jackets are tied behind the back to press together the groin and lower body regions (Figure 56-3).[35]

Because hypothermia alters the therapeutic approach to victims of submersion incidents, core temperatures should be determined in all potentially hypothermic victims brought to the ED. Resuscitation efforts must persist until normal core temperature is approached.[176,219] No decision on survival should be made until the patient is nearly euthermic (see Chapters 6 and 8).

Type of Water

Drowning may occur in almost any type of fluid, and victims of submersion may aspirate salt or fresh water, sewage, wash water, or tap water.[41,155,156,225] Most victims aspirate impurities or foreign materials, including algae, bacteria, sewage, chemicals, and sand.[82] In animal experiments the osmolarity of water has been shown to cause biochemical changes in nonsurvivors. Although the difference between saltwater and freshwater submersion is not of immediate clinical importance, knowledge of the effect of aspiration of several kinds of fluids helps in the interpretation of laboratory and clinical findings.[201]

Theoretically, the changes that occur after aspiration of salt water and fresh water should be different, and the biochemical abnormalities secondary to such aspiration should play a role in management. This has not proved to be the case. The amount of water aspirated, not the type, is of prime importance.[32,153,155,156]

Orlowski et al[173] studied pulmonary injury and the ability to resuscitate dogs after "drowning" produced by instilling fluids of varied tonicity into the lungs. The six fluids used were sterile water and 0.225%, 0.45%, 0.9%, 2%, and 3% sodium chloride solutions. Each of these solutions was tested with and without additional chlorine. The dogs were anesthetized, intubated, and ventilated with room air; 20 ml/kg of each fluid was in-

stilled into the endotracheal tube, which was then clamped for 5 minutes before resumption of ventilation with 100% oxygen and 10 cm of positive end-expiratory pressure (PEEP). Three control dogs were made anoxic for 5 minutes by occlusion of the endotracheal tubes, without fluid instillation.

When judged by the effect on pulmonary variables (A-a oxygen pressure difference, intrapulmonary shunt fraction, and PaO_2/FIO_2 ratio), the 0.225% saline solution was less disruptive to lung function, particularly when compared with sterile water, with or without chlorine. Sterile water was found to be the most damaging to the lungs, whether chlorinated or not. No differences between solutions were seen in the ability to resuscitate dogs with cardiac arrest. The authors suggested that swimming pool water be salinated to 0.225% normal sodium chloride solution to reduce pulmonary injuries of persons who suffer submersion injuries. These studies clearly indicate that the cardiovascular changes that occur with drowning are really from anoxia and do not depend on tonicity of the aspirated fluid.[175]

Freshwater Aspiration

Freshwater is hypotonic to plasma and passes readily out of the alveolus into the circulation. Theoretically, if a sufficient volume is aspirated (more than 22 mg/kg), blood volume can increase and hemolysis can result. Hemolysis, along with hypoxia, can lead to hyperkalemia, high levels of circulating free hemoglobin, and lowered hematocrit value. Expansion of blood volume caused by fluid shifts from the alveoli to the intravascular compartment lowers the concentrations of serum sodium chloride, calcium, and magnesium.[155,156]

Hypokalemia has also been reported,[69] but this may be caused by other factors, such as administration of epinephrine, glucose, and bicarbonate during resuscitation.[34] Despite theoretic changes, few near drowning victims (survivors) have electrolyte abnormalities serious enough to warrant therapy. In survivors of a submersion injury, biochemical and blood volume changes are corrected quickly and should be considered transient.[149,153,201] Management efforts in both freshwater and saltwater submersion should be directed primarily toward the effects of aspiration on the lungs.

Aspiration of fresh water induces pulmonary changes, the most important of which is the washout of surfactant.[159] This leads to atelectasis, with consequent ventilation-perfusion imbalance and hypoxia.[151,157] In addition, direct destruction of alveolar cells may lead to accumulation of fluid within the lungs and decreased compliance. Thus the overwhelming insult in the initial management of submersion injury is hypoxia.

Seawater Aspiration

Seawater has an osmolarity three to four times that of blood. Aspiration of this hypertonic fluid results in a rapid shift of plasma fluid into the alveoli and interstitial spaces of the lung parenchyma, resulting in severe pulmonary edema.[32,126,151,156] Theoretically, loss of fluid from the circulation should produce a blood volume decrease and rise in serum electrolytes because of high concentrations of sodium, potassium, and magnesium in seawater. However, as with freshwater aspiration, electrolyte changes do not appear to be important in the early management of submersion casualties.[149,171]

Unusual exceptions to this rule occur. Near drownings from bodies of water with high electrolyte content, such as the Dead Sea, are characterized by significant changes in concentrations of serum electrolytes, particularly calcium and magnesium. Yagil et al[236] confirmed these findings and a high mortality rate (50%) in eight treated patients. Experts still stress the importance of hypoxia and pulmonary injury caused by aspiration in the deaths of all victims of submersion.[148,179]

In a case of seawater aspiration, pulmonary edema results quickly, with outpouring of protein-rich fluid into the alveoli and interstitium, reduction of compliance, and direct parenchymal damage.[159] Hypoxia and metabolic acidosis remain the immediate concerns.

Contaminants

Most water in which submersion incidents occur contains chemicals, contaminants, or particulates that may produce further pulmonary injury.[100,151] Calcium salts, frequently used near oil drilling equipment, may render near-drowned divers hypercalcemic.[70] Although some maintain that pool water containing chlorine may be irritating to the tracheobronchial tree, animal studies indicate that the hypotonicity of the fluid, rather than the chlorine, causes the damage.[173] Water contaminated with chemical wastes, cleaning solvents, detergents, or disinfectants may induce further fluid accumulation in the already edematous lung.[155,214] Inhalation of mud, sand, and other particulates may require bronchoscopy to cleanse the airway. Although uncommon in survivors, "sand bronchograms" have been described on chest films and computed tomography (CT) scans of surfers and others who aspirated radiopaque calcium carbonate sand.[19,54]

Persons submerged in fresh water may be exposed to microbes, such as *Aeromonas hydrophila*, that are resistant to common antibiotics.[132,136,139] In patients who develop lung infection, culture and sensitivity testing is essential to identify the causative agents and to choose the appropriate antibiotic(s).[63,64,195] Cerebral infection with *Pseudallescheria* mycosis, as well as disseminated aspergillosis, has also been reported as a complication of near drowning.[202] Table 56-1 provides an extensive list of possible pathogens.[24,53]

TABLE 56-1. Organisms Associated with Infection in Near Drowning Victims*

	TYPE OF WATER
BACTERIA	
Klebsiella oxytoca	FW
Herellea spp.	FW
Neiserria meningitidis	FW
Pseudomonas aeruginosa	FW
Listeria monocytogenes	FW
Plesiomonas shigelloides	FW
Edwardsiella tarda	FW
Chromobacterium violaceum	FW
Aeromonas hydrophila	SW, FW
Escherichia coli	SW, FW
Proteus mirabilis	SW, FW
Staphylococcus aureus	SW, FW
Neiserria mucosa	Brackish
Pseudomonas putrefaciens	SW
Francisella philomiragia	SW
Vibrio parahaemolyticus	SW
FUNGI	
Pseudallescheria boydii	FW
Aspergillus fumigatus	FW

Modified from Brown SD, Piantadosi CA: Near drowning: hospital management. In *Near drowning: Forty-seventh workshop of the Undersea and Hyperbaric Medical Society*, Kensington, Md, 1997, the Undersea and Hyperbaric Medical Society.
FW, Fresh water; *SW*, salt water.
*Organisms isolated from sputum or blood of clinically infected near drowning victims soon after admission. This list does not include organisms recovered from infected wounds.

CLASSIFICATION AND TYPES OF DROWNING

Death by submersion, or drowning, has historically been classified according to pathophysiology. Such classifications are usually made after the fact and are of little use in immediate management.

Wet vs. Dry Drowning

The term *wet drowning* refers to the great majority of patients who aspirate water; the lungs are wet, with pulmonary derangements resulting from the effect of the fluid. An estimated 85% to 90% of victims fall into this category.[100,151,179] The remaining 10% to 15% do not aspirate to a significant degree and have "dry" lungs. Such *dry drowning* victims may develop laryngospasm in response to the cold water stimulus, mechanical irritation of swallowed water, or initial inhalation of fluid.[73,146] Although one might assume that victims who do not aspirate will respond better to resuscitation measures, no evidence supports this notion. The response to resuscitation depends more on rapid reversal of hypoxia than on the type of submersion injury.

Acute and chronic responses of the lungs to various amounts and types of fluids may range from mild to severe, as discussed later. Persons with preexisting pulmonary disease are at greater risk for decompensation if they have a submersion incident.

Shallow Water Blackout

The phenomenon known as shallow water blackout predisposes to drowning in persons who hyperventilate before entering the water for an endurance underwater swim, a training method sometimes attempted by competitive swimmers. Hyperventilation substantially reduces arterial carbon dioxide pressure ($PaCO_2$) without increasing oxygen storage. Vigorous underwater muscular activity may use the available stored oxygen, causing hypoxia before sufficient CO_2 accumulates in the blood to provide a stimulus to return to the surface to breathe. Without sufficient hypercapnia to stimulate breathing, consciousness can be lost because of hypoxia, and the victim may drown. Apparent shallow water blackout affected one author, who spent several days in his own intensive care unit.[235] Another clinician warns against hyperventilation during training.[99]

Immersion Syndrome and Diving Reflex

Immersion syndrome is sudden death after contact with very cold water, presumably a result of vagal stimulation[78] and resultant cardiac arrest.[115] The exact mechanism of this phenomenon is not understood, but in the past it has been attributed to the mammalian diving reflex, also present in seals and lower mammals. Investigation into the nature of this reflex was reported in the early 1960s. Cold water stimulation of cutaneous receptors appears to trigger shunting of blood to the brain and heart from the skin, gastrointestinal tract, and extremities. Bradycardia results from the reflex vagal response to increased central volume. This allows increased cerebral circulation with longer breath-holding times because of lower peripheral oxygen use. The diving reflex does not occur to the same extent in all people. Work in humans suggests that the diving reflex is part of the mechanism of survival in cold water for all near drownings and may be a significant factor for the 10% to 20% of victims who have a profound diving reflex response, helping them survive.* Studies indicate that less arterial desaturation occurs during nonexertional breath-holding in water than while not immersed and that the extent of the diving response may respond to training. Korean and Japanese pearl divers, as well as other trained breath-holding divers, exhibit more diving-related bradycardia than their nondiving counterparts.[6,208,222] This probably prolongs breath-holding dive times.

---

*References 80, 91, 101, 151, 171, 177, 191, 192, 223.

Postimmersion Syndrome

"Postimmersion syndrome" is an unsatisfactory term referring to delayed development of ARDS, which is preceded by a relatively asymptomatic interval of several hours to several days.[72] The term "secondary drowning" has been used to refer to delayed-onset pulmonary failure, but continued use of this term adds little to understanding submersion injury.

PATHOPHYSIOLOGY OF SUBMERSION

The effects of submersion on mammals were first reported in the scientific literature in the late 1800s. In his classic monograph, Greene noted that, "inundation of the upper airway, the bronchial tree and segments of the alveolar spaces blocks gas exchange in the lung and produces asphyxia. Thus drowning involves the rapid development of hypoxia, hypercapnia and acidosis with the associated sequence of hypertension, bradycardia, arrhythmias, hypotension, hyperpnea, apnea, and terminal gasping." Findings in animals were consistent with drowning episodes later observed in humans.[100,133,163] The initial response in humans to submersion, particularly in cold water, includes a period of panic, accompanied by hyperventilation caused by stimulation of thermal receptors in the skin. Breath-holding may be attempted, but at some point in breath-holding, the breaking point is reached. This is the point at which no voluntary efforts will prevent respiration and is determined by both CO_2 and oxygen levels. Hyperventilation before diving or swimming may prolong this point, which is also responsible for blackout in swimmers attempting long underwater swims.[127] Hyperventilation is usually uncontrollable by the victim and can result in aspiration of significant quantities of water. If the water is very cold, such aspiration probably hastens the onset of hypothermia and may explain the "protection" apparent in some cases of cold water immersion. Swallowing large amounts of water may lead to vomiting and subsequent aspiration of gastric contents.[126,141] This may present difficulties to initial rescuers; gastric distention may make ventilation more difficult, and regurgitation is a constant danger.

In most victims of submersion, violent struggling occurs before loss of consciousness; exercise-induced acidosis leads to greater hyperventilation and risk of aspiration of water (Figure 56-4).

The common denominator of submersion is hypoxia, caused by either laryngospasm or water aspiration. Once the victim is unconscious, all airway reflexes are abolished, and fluid is passively introduced into the airway. Cardiac arrest follows this sequence of events. Hypoxia and acidosis lead to derangements in many organ systems in victims of serious incidents.[100]

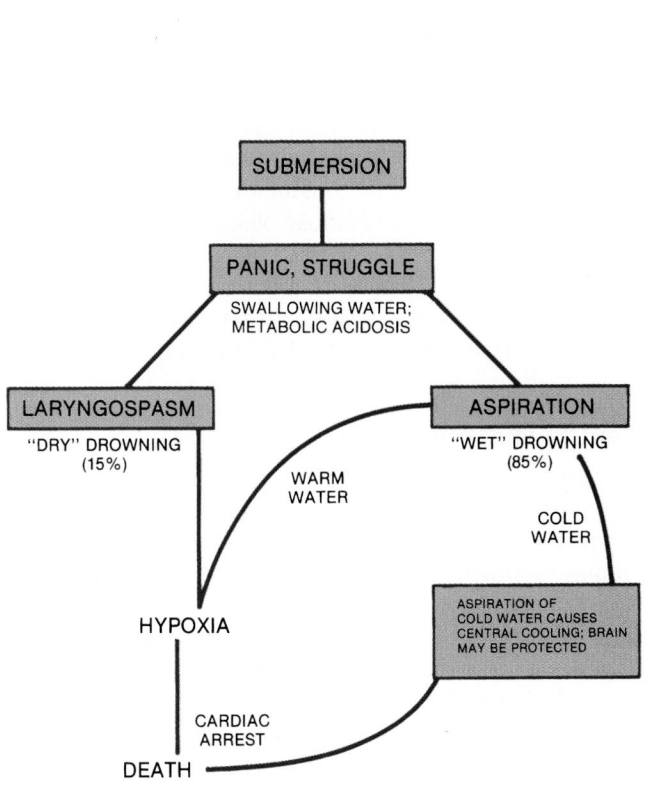

Figure 56-4 Progression of the drowning incident.

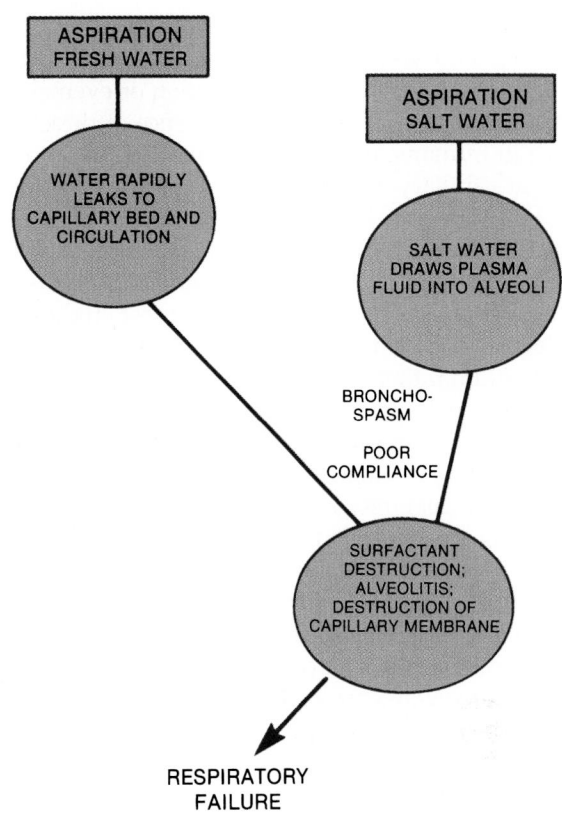

Figure 56-5 Pulmonary effects of water aspiration.

Pulmonary System

The target organ in submersion episodes is the lung (Figure 56-5). Once aspirated, water evokes vagally mediated pulmonary vasoconstriction and pulmonary hypertension.[33,34] Neurogenic pulmonary edema may also occur at this time.[203] In cases of freshwater aspiration, fluid moves quickly across the alveolar-capillary membrane into the microcirculation, surfactant destruction or washout occurs, and high surface tensions in the lung lead to reduced compliance and atelectasis. Marked ventilation-perfusion mismatching occurs, with as much as 75% of blood flowing through hypoventilated lung tissue.[14,100,113,159] Seawater aspiration also leads to surfactant destruction and produces rapid exudation of protein-rich fluid into the alveoli and pulmonary interstitium, reduced compliance, and direct capillary damage.[105] These changes usually lead quickly to serious hypoxia. In some cases of near drowning, this may not occur until hours later, when alveolitis, atelectasis, and shunting show clinical effects.

Even in survivors of near drowning, it may be days before normal ventilation-perfusion matching returns.[127] Normal lung function depends on alveoli that expand easily with inspiration (low surface tension) and recoil efficiently. These properties are facilitated by the presence of surfactant, a layer of fluid lining the alveolar walls. Fifty percent or more of this substance is dipalmitoyl phosphatidylcholine, a phospholipid; the rest is composed of other phospholipids and proteins. Surfactant is manufactured by alveolar epithelial type II cells, and its metabolism is under hormonal control as well as control through the interaction of β-adrenergic agonists, cyclic adenosine monophosphate, and prostaglandins.[119] Alveolar aspiration of water appears to destroy or "dilute" pulmonary surfactant.[73,74] When the substance is absent or does not function properly, atelectasis occurs and stiff, noncompliant lungs result. The consequence in the nearly drowned patient is severe shunting and hypoxia.[100]

An important development in the treatment of premature infants who are surfactant deficient has been instillation of exogenous surfactant through an endotracheal tube.[71] The surfactant, which was first derived from bovine or human amniotic fluid, is now produced from artificial sources. Dramatic results have been reported, with pulmonary function and oxygenation improving within hours of treatment.[145] Theoretically this therapy should benefit the injured lung in near drowning.[9]

Inhalation of particulate matter, contaminants, bacteria, or chemicals can produce irritation that results in more tracheobronchial fluid deposition or even alveolar destruction.[153,215] Despite the absence of direct evidence in humans, it is suspected that damage to the alveolar-capillary membrane may be produced by coagulation defects, platelet breakdown, microembolization, and other adverse effects initiated by fluid aspiration or hypoxia. Although alveolar and surfactant destruction has been emphasized in most studies, the initial pulmonary insult may be damage to the vascular endothelium rather than the alveolar cells.[112]

Hypoxia in humans after submersion incidents is the result of fluid in the alveolar and interstitial spaces, loss of surfactant, proteinaceous material in the alveoli and tracheobronchial tree, damage to the alveolar-capillary membrane and vascular endothelium, and hypoxia-initiated central nervous system (CNS) reflex mechanisms.[100,126,146] Acute respiratory failure follows, with reduced compliance and increased ventilation-perfusion mismatching, resulting in enhanced shunt.[56,100] The difference in oxygen tension between alveoli and arterial blood is increased with pulmonary failure after submersion. In normal subjects breathing 100% oxygen the difference is about 35 mm Hg; in human victims of submersion, differences as high as 600 mm Hg with 100% oxygen have been reported.[100]

In cases of prolonged submersion or significant aspiration, pulmonary derangements occur rapidly. In lesser insults the onset of symptoms may be delayed for as long as 24 hours. This phenomenon probably represents delayed onset of the initial insult rather than severity of the injury or a different disease entity or syndrome.[147,189]

The type of water aspirated during a submersion incident may determine the extent of lung damage and degree of resultant hypoxia. In animal models, sterile water has produced the most profound changes in pulmonary function.[84,158] Isotonic sodium chloride solution (0.9%) has been shown to produce injury, but not as great as that produced by sterile water.[173] The presence of chlorine in a concentration of 1 to 2 ppm apparently does not influence the degree of pulmonary injury or dysfunction.

Cardiovascular System

Cardiovascular derangements in cases of serious submersion injury are usually secondary to hypoxia, acidosis, or other indirect causes, rather than being caused by actual fluid aspiration. In the past, death was thought to be caused by induction of ventricular fibrillation by electrolyte changes, but this is not the case. Cardiac dysrhythmias and depression of myocardial function are caused by acidosis and hypoxia resulting from pulmonary injury.[89,100]

Supraventricular tachycardias are common.[56] Karch[111] reported that the myocardia of rabbits subjected to aspiration of fresh and salt water demonstrated focal areas of eosinophilia and disruption of some myocardial elements. The lesions resembled those produced in hearts exposed to very high levels of catecholamines. Cardiac derangements seen in near drowning may result from increased catecholamines secondary to the stress of the incident.[58,111]

Management requires close observation of the cardiovascular system. A delicate balance often exists between pulmonary function and oxygenation vs. cardiac output and right-sided heart return. This has particular relevance when PEEP is used to improve oxygenation.

Central Nervous System

The end point of successful resuscitation of victims of submersion incidents once was restoration of adequate perfusion and pulmonary function. With development of more sophisticated monitoring capabilities, however, attention is now directed toward preserving CNS function and preventing further damage once vascular perfusion has been restored. "Cerebral resuscitation" is well studied, but most pharmacologic interventions are still experimental. The most important step in cerebral preservation is rapid institution of rescue measures and basic life support, without which later measures may be futile.

Insults to the CNS include hypoxia and trauma to the spine and spinal cord. A search for other causes of CNS dysfunction is mandatory in persons who remain comatose after submersion incidents. All patients should be investigated for expanding intracranial lesions secondary to trauma or for damage to the spinal cord, which may occur in surfing mishaps, in platform diving accidents, or during horseplay.

The initial insult to brain tissue is hypoxia and ischemia, but evidence suggests that tissue damage can continue after restoration of cerebral blood flow.[40,206] Dysfunction of the CNS occurs rapidly after the onset of hypoxia; flattening of the electroencephalogram takes place within 20 seconds of total cerebral ischemia. Continued CNS injury after resuscitation results from edema, elevated intracranial pressure (ICP), and increased cerebral vascular resistance, which compromise oxygenation.[100,206] Hyperpyrexia that accompanies drowning increases cerebral oxygen consumption and tissue insult.[39,40]

Methods to monitor ICP are often promoted as essential guides to the success of measures directed toward cerebral resuscitation, but this has not been demonstrated definitively. Attempts to prevent postresuscitation cerebral injury may play a prominent role in management of patients who remain comatose after serious submersion accidents.[152,154,171] Magnetic resonance spectrography may help to provide treatment indices and to help determine progress and outcome. A spectrographic prognosis index has been proposed based on ratios of metabolites.[123] Loss of *N*-acetylaspartate and increases in glutamine/glutamate and lactate were worrisome. Generalized brain edema, indistinct lentiform nuclei margins, and basal ganglia hyperintensity were all predictors of poor outcome.

Renal System

Acute renal failure is not common in victims of submersion incidents. When it occurs, the most frequent cause is destruction of tubules secondary to hypoxia. Reduced blood flow secondary to shock and acidosis increases the incidence of renal failure.[100,126]

Metabolic Changes

Electrolyte changes in a survivor of a submersion incident do not appear to be either consistent or important in initial management. An unusual exception is near drowning in water with extremely high electrolyte concentrations, such as in the Dead Sea.[236] Sodium concentrations are three times as high (1493 vs. 531 mmol/L) in the Dead Sea as in the Mediterranean Sea; chloride 6092 vs. 630 mmol/L; potassium 970 vs. 11 mmol/L; calcium 1709 vs. 48 mmol/L; and magnesium 6987 vs. 273 mmol/L.

Drowning in hot springs baths may also result in elevated levels of calcium from absorption of calcium in the spring water.[134]

Elevations of potassium levels in victims who have aspirated fresh water have been ascribed to hemolysis. Few patients who survive aspirate sufficient water to pose any problem; aspiration of quantities that would cause serious electrolyte imbalance usually results in death.[36,72] This applies equally to the aspiration of fresh and salt water. Postmortem measurements of electrolytes in experimental animals have uncovered increases in serum sodium, chloride, calcium, and potassium, presumably a result of the high concentrations in seawater. Again, these problems are not seen consistently in survivors of submersion incidents.

Respiratory acidosis is the main immediate problem in patients.[100,149,171,176] In most patients, severe metabolic acidosis develops, in part because of pulmonary failure with resultant cellular anaerobic metabolism. Persistent acidosis depresses myocardial function and leads to lethal arrhythmias.

Hematologic Changes

Hemolysis has been described in both freshwater and saltwater aspiration, more often in the former, with levels of circulating free hemoglobin ranging from 8 to 500 mg/dl.[155] There is no consistent change in the level of hemoglobin or hematocrit after submersion in humans. Low values should initiate a search for underlying trauma with hemorrhage or a bleeding disorder. Disseminated intravascular coagulation has been de-

scribed with submersion and aspiration.[43,100] Contributing to the genesis of this disorder are hypoxia, acidosis, sepsis, hemolysis, and low-perfusion states.

PREDICTING OUTCOME

It would be helpful to be able to predict the future course of victims, particularly those with severe injuries. Previous attempts to predict outcome were thwarted by lack of uniformity of terminology and of a standard classification of patients' conditions. Recent attempts have been more successful. The importance to eventual survival of rapid rescue and immediate CPR has been recognized by almost all authorities on the subject of near drowning.* The extent of cerebral recovery can be related to age and gender, hypothermia, submersion time, initial resuscitation, and critical care with special measures of cerebral salvage.[3,44,106,170]

Predicting the outcome of patients is based largely on initial and serial examinations of cerebral function. Orlowski[170,171] developed a "score" that, in conjunction with the Glasgow Coma Scale (GCS), permits a fairly accurate estimate of the likely outcome (Box 56-3). Unfavorable prognostic factors include young age and severe acidosis. With one or two adverse factors present, a 90% change of recovery is indicated; three or more reduce the chances to less than 5%.

Prolonged attempts to resuscitate victims who have not been hypothermic and who did not initially have vital signs may result in more deaths or more survivors with persistent vegetative states.[16] The importance of initial assessment to predicting outcome cannot be overemphasized. Victims who are alert on admission, are in sinus rhythm, and have reactive pupils should do well, whereas those who are in coma with absent brainstem reflexes, unreactive pupils in the ED, or a GCS score of less than 5, as well as those who have been submerged more than 10 minutes and had resuscitation durations of more than 25 minutes, have a less than 5% chance of recovery.[68,80,116,124]

---

*References 62, 149, 171, 176, 180, 195.

Box 56-3 UNFAVORABLE PROGNOSTIC FACTORS FOR VICTIMS OF NEAR DROWNING

Age 3 years or less
Estimated submersion time longer than 5 minutes
No resuscitation attempts for at least 10 minutes after rescue
Patient in coma on admission to emergency department
Arterial blood gas pH 7.1 or less

Modified from Orlowski JP: *J Am Coll Emerg Phys* 8:176, 1979.

Unconscious victims who have not regained normal spontaneous purposeful movements and brainstem functions, including pupillary light reflexes, oculovestibular reflexes, corneal reflex, and respiratory pattern, carry a grave prognosis.[22,23,31,87]

MANAGEMENT

Immediate Care

The scene of the submersion incident is often characterized by general chaos. Modell[151] notes that persons on the scene of the event rarely report seeing someone who was "flailing and screaming for help" while they "struggled to remain on the surface of the water." Instead, they found victims floating on the surface of the water or saw swimmers suddenly become motionless or dive under water and never surface. Attempts at rescue must consider the safety of rescuers so that multiple drownings do not occur. The Red Cross recommends that whenever possible, safety devices should be used to tow in the victim, or life preservers should be tossed to people in trouble before a human lifesaver actually enters the water in a boat or on a board to attempt a rescue. Well-intentioned but ill-advised heroic efforts can create additional victims and compound the tragedy.

Recovery of victims still submerged should be the responsibility of professional or volunteer workers trained specifically in water retrieval and rescue. Water rescue demands special equipment and expert personnel and may be carried out in extremely adverse circumstances, especially in winter weather[169] (Figure 56-6). Australian studies indicate much higher levels of success in resuscitations closer to lifeguard stands.[66] An EMS physician should be involved in consultation early during the incident, particularly when cold weather rescue and hypothermia are involved.

Until evidence shows that aggressive on-scene resuscitation does not help prevent loss of life, no effort

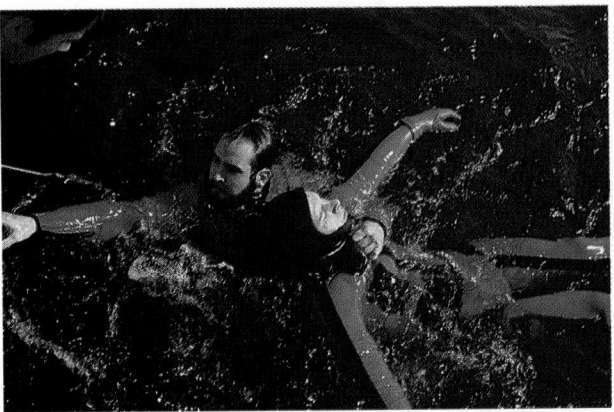

Figure 56-6 Cold water rescue; both victim and rescuer are dressed in wet suits. *(Courtesy Alan Steinman, MD.)*

should be withheld. Prehospital care workers should be given definitive guidelines that insist on prompt application of life support to all victims of submersion unless hypothermia is not present and the duration of submersion has been long. Thus rescuers must begin resuscitative measures and present the patient to the in-hospital team, which can decide on therapy. This is especially true in the case of winter or cold water conditions. The decision to withhold or cease resuscitation attempts is rarely made in the field, except in a remote wilderness area. Transport of the near-drowned victim from remote terrain has been made more expeditious with wider availability of helicopter evacuation.

Estimates of time under water are notoriously inaccurate when made by bystanders, parents, and even trained rescuers.[154] The history can be crucial in this regard. In one case, rescuers delayed instituting life support to a victim of submersion in a river with a water temperature of 11.7° C (53° F).[186] Later it was found that the initial radio message relayed from the first unit receiving the call did not include information that the woman was struggling as she floated down the river. The rescuers removing her from the water assumed she had been submerged for some time and did not begin CPR until a rhythm was detected on the electrocardiogram. The victim was hypothermic, responded almost immediately to resuscitative measures, and survived to leave the hospital.

Specific Therapy

Initial evaluation and resuscitation of any victim must include complete examination for obvious trauma, with appropriate stabilization and repeated examination. Thorough examination should minimize death from unrecognized trauma, such as ruptured spleen or fractured cervical spine. Appropriate intensive care monitoring should be part of the management routine.

The victims of submersion incidents may be classified into four groups: (1) the asymptomatic patient, (2) the symptomatic patient, (3) the patient in cardiopulmonary arrest, and (4) the obviously dead or still-submerged patient.

Asymptomatic Patient. The patient who has experienced a period of submersion or a near drowning episode and who remains asymptomatic presents a particular dilemma. The history is of prime importance. A description of the incident, an estimate of submersion time, and the past medical history of the patient should be obtained. All patients with possible history of submersion who manifest shortness of breath (however slight) should be considered hypoxic; oxygen by simple face mask at 8 to 10 L/min should be given. It may be better to err on the safe side and administer oxygen to any patient seen in the field with a history of submersion, regardless of the time submerged or the absence of symptoms.

It has been frequently recommended that all patients with a history of submersion be treated as if a lung insult had occurred and that admission to a hospital for a period of observation be mandatory.[141,171,195] This recommendation is often made in the belief that in patients sustaining a near drowning episode with apparently successful resuscitation, an asymptomatic period sometimes precedes the onset of respiratory failure, a condition termed secondary drowning. Close examination of the patients on whom this belief is based indicates that persons with significant pulmonary insults rarely fail to show signs or symptoms immediately after rescue and initial resuscitation.

In a survey of 52 swimmers who had submersion incidents on California beaches, 31 declined medical attention and left the beach.[189] Telephone follow-up of 26 persons indicated that none had sought medical care subsequent to the incident and that all returned to a normal state of health. Of 21 persons evaluated in a hospital, respiratory distress was manifested within 4 hours. Despite its obvious limitations and uncontrolled nature, this report suggests guidelines for the emergency management of the asymptomatic or minimally symptomatic patient with a history of near drowning (Table 56-2).

Secondary drowning probably represents evolution of preexisting lung injury rather than sudden and unexpected occurrence in a patient exposed to near drowning. Most injured patients can be identified through careful evaluation and a 4- to 6-hour observation period in the ED combined with a plan for careful follow-up. Asymptomatic survivors of a submersion incident should not be sent home from the site of the incident. All potential victims should be taken to a hospital for competent medical evaluation, or at least strongly encouraged to seek medical advice.[189]

Symptomatic Patient. Any victim who shows signs of distress (anxiety, tachypnea, dyspnea, syncope, persistent cough, or vital sign change) at the scene has had a significant submersion injury until serial observations in the hospital prove otherwise (Table 56-3). Two immediate problems will be hypoxia and acidosis. Correction involves respiratory manipulation. The airway must be kept patent, which can be a problem in persons who are vigorously vomiting. Emesis is frequent in submersion victims, especially in persons who have swallowed large amounts of seawater. If transport time is long, diarrhea caused by the laxative effect of swallowed seawater may add insult to injury.

SUPPLEMENTAL OXYGEN. If the victim is breathing spontaneously, high flow rates should be provided by face mask (12 to 15 L/min via a nonrebreathing mask) or by demand valve, which gives 100% oxygen at the valve outlet. If available, pulse oximetry may be used to mon-

TABLE 56-2. On-Scene Management of the Asymptomatic Patient*

HISTORY	EXAMINATION	INTERVENTION
Time submerged	Appearance	Oxygen by face mask, 8-10 L/min
Description of incident	Vital signs	Intravenous line at "keep-open" rate
Complaints	Chest examination	Reexamine patient as needed
Past health	Electrocardiographic monitor	Transport patient

*Patients refusing treatment should have telephone number and address taken and arrangement for follow-up made.

TABLE 56-3. Field Approach to the Symptomatic Patient*

HISTORY	EXAMINATION	INTERVENTION
Description of incident	General appearance	Oxygen via mask (8-10 L/min) by demand valve
Time submerged, water temperature, water contamination, vomiting, type of rescue	Level of consciousness	Intravenous line at "keep-open" rate; consider intubation if patient is tachypneic or dyspneic with cyanosis or depressed mental status
Symptoms	Vital signs, electrocardiographic monitor	Transport patient

*Be prepared for vomiting. Take measures to prevent hypothermia and shivering. Treat cardiac arrhythmias as they arise, keeping in mind that hypoxia may be the underlying cause.

itor oxygen saturation. Persons in respiratory distress who breathe spontaneously might benefit from continuous positive airway pressure (CPAP) using a tight-fitting mask. No prehospital experience has yet been reported with the use of this modality.

Body temperature should not decrease. All wet clothing must be removed and the patient wiped dry. If the patient continues to shiver, carefully wrapped hot packs may be placed in the axillae and inguinal areas and near the scalp and neck (see Chapters 6 and 8).

Attention to potential metabolic acidosis is given after establishment of a patent airway, oxygenation, and access to the intravascular space. Metabolic acidosis can exist even in relatively asymptomatic victims of submersion.[100,171] The first line of treatment is adequate ventilation and correction of hypoxia.[169] Administration of sodium bicarbonate has been advocated in patients with adequate circulation who are tachypneic or dyspneic with cyanosis.[144] Recommendations do not support this practice, particularly in the field environment.[149] Administration of bicarbonate should follow vigorous attention to ventilation and oxygenation and generally awaits arterial blood gas (ABG) analysis.

For the most part, other drugs are administered in the hospital. Cardiac irritability usually responds to correction of hypoxia and acidosis. If significant ventricular irritability persists, judicious field use of lidocaine by multibolus technique is justified, using an initial dose of 1 mg/kg over 2 minutes and 0.5 mg/kg every 5 to 10 minutes, not to exceed a total dose of 225 mg.

PATIENT IN CARDIOPULMONARY ARREST. Vigorous CPR can be initiated immediately, even with the victim in the water (Box 56-4). This is the most important survival factor in drownings.[143] Mouth-to-mouth ventilation should be attempted during extrication, but this may be difficult, depending on the strength of the rescuer and demands of the environment (Figure 56-7). As soon as the shore, jetty, shallow water, surfboard, or boat is reached, mouth-to-mouth ventilation should begin in earnest.

Some suggest initiating closed-chest compressions in the water as soon as the victim is reached.[140] Trials in which a recording manikin was ventilated and compressed, using a modified ventilator and posterior grasp position, demonstrated adequate chest compression and ventilation. However, these trials did not measure blood flow achieved when the patient was held in a nearly upright position. The likelihood of providing any circulation or keeping such a victim afloat is remote. Other factors that argue against this technique include frigid water and rescuer fatigue; dangers from wave, surge, and current; wet suit and scuba apparatus obstruction; and the delay to definitive out-of-water CPR.[120,122] No reports have been published regarding the successful use of this technique in an actual submersion incident.

Box 56-4 FIELD INTERVENTION IN VICTIMS IN CARDIOPULMONARY ARREST*

BEGIN VENTILATION AND COMPRESSION
Use mouth-to-mouth, mouth-to-mask (preferably with oxygen supplementation), or bag-valve-mask (preferably with balloon mask or two-rescuer) ventilation
Use supplemental oxygen

ENDOTRACHEAL INTUBATION
Positive end-expiratory pressure at 5 to 10 cm may be useful
Intravenous line at "keep-open" rate

IF COPIOUS DRAINAGE FROM LUNGS OR STOMACH
Suction through endotracheal (ET) tube
Pass nasogastric tube
Apply abdominal thrusts between ventilations if ET tube in place and copious drainage persists

*Sodium bicarbonate ordered on advice of physician or according to protocol of the system. Treat dysrhythmias in standard fashion. If cervical injury is suspected, use collar and sandbags, etc.

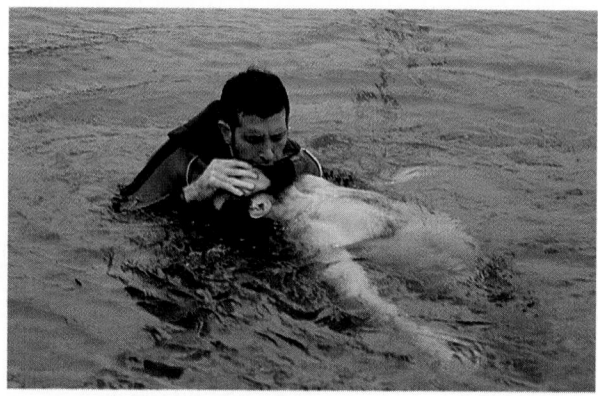

Figure 56-7 Mouth-to-mouth ventilation in the water is difficult in the best of circumstances. *(Courtesy Alan Steinman, MD.)*

As soon as the victim is extracted from the water, he or she should be placed on a firm surface (float board, backboard, jetty, or boat deck) and appropriate resuscitation measures continued. Basic care given at the scene is thus far the most important treatment factor in determining survival.* A trial of CPR with a pneumatic device appeared to produce better blood flow than did traditional CPR. Additional trials with this technique will suggest if it should become a new standard.[91] If rescue is performed on a sloping beach, the victim should be placed parallel to the water's edge (neither

*References 67, 149, 171, 176, 180, 195.

head up nor head down), theoretically to prevent a decrease in forward blood flow during chest compressions in the head-up position or an increase in intracranial pressure in the head-down position.

An adequate airway provides access not only for positive-pressure ventilation but also for clearing of copious secretions. This can be achieved only by prompt insertion of an endotracheal tube, which should be placed after good initial ventilation. When only tank oxygen with a delivery hose, nasal cannula, or face mask is available, mouth-to-mouth or mouth-to-mask ventilation may be supplemented with oxygen by applying the nasal prongs to the rescuer (at 6 to 8 L/min). This increases the delivered oxygen concentration from 21% to 40%.[101] CPR using a bag valve mask, laryngeal mask or combitube provides a safe format for mouth-to-mouth resuscitation and also prevent the possibility of AIDS transmission.[48,169] If a bag-valve-mask ventilator is used, it must have an oxygen reservoir to increase the percentage of oxygen delivered to the patient. This reservoir should be of the soft inflatable type with a capacity of at least 2.5 L.[4,25] It should be fitted with a balloon mask that provides a tight seal on the patient's face and reduces leak.[224] Without this mask, bag-valve-mask devices are not the preferred method of applying positive-pressure ventilation in a field setting because of the difficulty in achieving a mask seal and because of operator fatigue, both of which inevitably reduce delivered volumes.[4,59,90]

LUNG DRAINAGE. Frequent airway clearing is necessary with most victims of submersion. Vomiting and copious drainage from the lungs and stomach can occur. The issue of lung drainage is historically and currently controversial. Draining the lungs is reasonable, since submerged victims have been estimated to aspirate up to 2 L,[176] as well as to accumulate pulmonary edema fluid. The concept of draining water from the lungs dates back to the seventeenth and eighteenth centuries. The Dutch method consisted of rolling the victim over a barrel; another method advised flinging the victim over the back of a horse, which was then made to trot.[131] In 1975, Dr. Henry Heimlich introduced an abdominal compression maneuver (Heimlich maneuver), advocated for victims of food choking.[94] In the initial and subsequent reports, he suggested its use in the victims of drowning.[95,96]

Evidence for the effectiveness of the maneuver in drowning is anecdotal at best. Abdominal compression in victims of submersion may predispose to induced emesis of large amounts of swallowed water, thus exposing the patient to further aspiration, this time of gastric contents.[172]

Although one study demonstrated greater survival rates in animals subjected to drainage techniques,[159] the dogs used apparently did not require closed-chest CPR. It was concluded that drainage techniques were useful only in victims of seawater aspiration. Studies at the University of Pittsburgh demonstrated no difference in canine survival in groups treated without drainage, with the Heimlich maneuver, or with Trendelenburg positioning.[234] As far back as 1962, efforts to drain water from the lungs were condemned as "of no practical use" and "a waste of valuable time" in applying mouth-to-mouth ventilation.[200] The same investigators showed in cadavers that only small amounts of the 1 L of 1% saline solution instilled into the lungs could still be recovered by prone positioning, "jackknifing," or thoracic compression. A delivered volume of up to 2 L of air could still be accomplished with higher ventilating pressures.

No human studies of lung drainage in submersion have been reported, and descriptions of drainage procedures refer to *gastric* drainage.[206] The technique in these cases was to place the patient on the side and compress the abdomen, or to place the patient in a prone position, grasp him or her about the abdomen, and lift ("breaking" the victim, in older lay language). Whether these maneuvers led to drainage of water from the stomach or lungs is not clear.

Gastric drainage may be required in persons who have swallowed large amounts of water, since gastric distention may interfere with ventilation. If gastric distention is a problem, abdominal compression with adequate suction available (or gravity drainage) may suffice. Abdominal compression accomplishes drainage without the need to interrupt cardiac compressions or ventilation for as long a time as other methods. Whatever the method, it must be performed quickly so that basic life support can continue. A nasogastric tube is preferred to all other methods. Most clinicians, the American Heart Association, and the Institute of Medicine advise against the Heimlich maneuver except when the airway is obviously blocked with foreign material.[4,190,197] None of the methods suggested for gastric drainage should precede initial attempts at ventilation.

ENDOTRACHEAL INTUBATION AND POSITIVE END-EXPIRATORY PRESSURE. Endotracheal intubation controls the airway by reducing dead space, providing protection against aspiration, and facilitating pulmonary toilet. In apneic submersion patients requiring positive-pressure ventilation, PEEP has been demonstrated to be useful.[113,180,199,205,229] Although there is no decrease or is even an increase in total lung water, PEEP acts in several ways to improve ventilation patterns in the noncompliant lung: (1) by shifting interstitial pulmonary water into capillaries; (2) by increasing lung volume through prevention of expiratory air space collapse; (3) by increasing the diameter of large and small airways to improve ventilation distribution; and (4) by decreasing alveolar-capillary blood flow and providing better alveolar ventilation, with improved ventilation-perfusion ratio and PaO_2.

The use of PEEP in the field situation is possible with a small apparatus adaptable to manual self-inflating bag ventilation devices.[130] Experience with field PEEP is limited, and clinicians must be thoroughly familiar with its drawbacks. These include reduced venous return to the right side of the heart, increased fluid retention in an already stressed lung, increased pulmonary artery pressure, decreased cardiac output, and, at high levels, increased ICP.[7,46,161,216] High-frequency jet ventilation in the intensive care unit may prevent further pulmonary barotrauma to an injured lung.[218]

DRUGS. In the past, standard drug therapy in CPR emphasized prompt attention to sodium bicarbonate administration. Severe metabolic acidosis may exist in a submersion victim because of circulatory arrest and preceding muscular activity in the struggle for survival.[157] Administration of bicarbonate has potential disadvantages, including increased sodium concentration with resultant fluid load, which may not be beneficial to patients whose cardiovascular reserve is already limited.[221,232] Other problems include impairment of oxygen delivery to the tissues, paradoxical increase in lactate production, and increase in CO_2 production, which can worsen already profound metabolic and respiratory acidosis.[113,221,232] The possible inappropriateness of bicarbonate administration in cardiac arrest has led to reconsideration of this practice.[4,17] The decision to administer bicarbonate should be made by the in-hospital team after more data are available on which to base a decision. The most likely problems leading to acid-base imbalance are hypoxia and respiratory acidosis, which require effective ventilation before consideration of sodium bicarbonate.

OBVIOUSLY DEAD OR STILL-SUBMERGED PATIENT. "Obviously dead" refers to any patient who has a normal temperature and demonstrates asystole, absent respirations, postmortem lividity, or rigor mortis. If rescue operations have been in progress for more than 30 minutes, victims who are retrieved from warm water during summer months or in warm southern waters may be considered dead on the scene. Because cold water submersion for more than 40 minutes has been associated with neurologic survival,[217] rescue crews must institute life support measures in all persons who are not obviously dead, who may be hypothermic, and whose histories suggest recent signs of life.

When persons are obviously dead or still submerged, the rescue team must comfort the family and friends and participate in body recovery. Once retrieved, the victim should be covered immediately and treated with proper dignity. Family members and friends should be escorted from the scene, if possible, before recovery. Most drownings are medical exam-

TABLE 56-4. Classification of Near Drowning Victims*

CATEGORY	DESCRIPTION
A	Awake—fully oriented
B	Blunted—arousable; purposeful response to pain
C	Comatose—not arousable; abnormal response to pain
C_1	Flexor response to pain
C_2	Extensor response to pain
C_3	Flaccid
C_4	Arrested

Modified from Conn AW, Barker GA: *Can Anaesth Soc J* 31:S38, 1984.
*Assessment is made in emergency department within 1 hour of rescue.

iner cases, since the possibility of foul play must be investigated.

In-Hospital Management. Once the victim reaches the hospital, a brief but pertinent description of the event, an estimate of time submerged, and the extent of field intervention will provide team members with important information bearing on further treatment, as well as offer some basis for expectation of outcome.

CLASSIFICATION OF PATIENTS. Patients may be classified on admission in a manner similar to that used in the field setting: asymptomatic, symptomatic, in cardiac arrest, or obviously dead (Table 56-4). In 1980, Modell and Conn[152] suggested an ABC classification of patients based on presenting neurologic examination. This system has undergone revision, with the time of initial examination being changed to the ED after initial resuscitation, and usually within 1 hour of rescue. More aggressive resuscitation led to the introduction of a fourth subgroup under "C." Under this system, patients were "A"—alert, "B"—blunted in consciousness, or "C"—comatose. The comatose patients were further categorized according to their abnormal neurologic responses: C_1—flexor response; C_2—extensor response; or C_3—flaccid. A C_4 category was added to include patients in whom vigorous CPR was being applied that might result in a change in condition and therefore prognosis.[38]

In their series on children, Conn et al[39,40] reported that all patients in category A survived and were normal and that all but one patient survived in category B. The patients in coma were most likely to benefit from therapy while being most at risk. The C group showed various responses, with increasingly poor outcomes. Similar studies in adults have not yet been reported.

Graf et al[81] studied 194 submersion victims and found that four variables could predict unfavorable outcome: comatose state, lack of pupillary light reflex, male gender, and initial blood glucose level greater

TABLE 56-5. Pediatric Risk of Mortality (PRISM) Score

VARIABLE	AGE RESTRICTIONS AND RANGES		SCORE
Systolic BP (mm Hg)	*Infants*	*Children*	
	130-160	150-200	2
	55-65	65-75	
	>160	>200	6
	40-54	50-64	
	<40	<50	7
Diastolic BP (mm Hg)	>110		6
HR (beats/min)	*Infants*	*Children*	
	>160	>150	4
	<90	<80	
Respiratory rate (breaths/min)	*Infants*	*Children*	
	61-90	51-70	1
	>90	>70	5
Pao_2/Fio_2*		200-300	2
		<200	3
$Paco_2$† (mm Hg)		51-65	1
		>65	5
Glasgow Coma Score‡		<8	6
Pupillary reactions	Unequal or dilated		4
	Fixed and dilated		10
PT/PTT	1.5 × control		2
Total bilirubin (mg/dl)	>3.5 (>1 mo)		6
Potassium (mEq/L)	3-3.5		1
	6.5-7.5		
	<3		5
	>7.5		
Calcium (mg/dl)	7-8		2
	12-15		
	<7		6
	>15		
Glucose (mg/dl)	40-60		4
	250-400		
	<40		8
	>400		
Bicarbonate§ (mEq/L)	<16		3
	>32		

Modified from Pollack MM et al: *Crit Care Med* 16:1113, 1998.
BP, Blood pressure; *HR*, heart rate; *Pao₂/Paco₂*, arterial oxygen/carbon dioxide pressure; *Fio₂*, fraction of inspired air; *PT/PTT*, prothrombin/partial thromboplastin time.
*Cannot be assessed in patients with intracardiac shunts or chronic respiratory insufficiency; requires arterial blood sampling.
†May be assessed with capillary blood gases.
‡Assessed only if there is known or suspected CNS dysfunction; cannot be assessed in patients during iatrogenic sedation, paralysis, anesthesia, etc. Scores <8 correspond to coma or deep stupor.
§Use measured values.

than 200 mg/dl on presentation. Some studies suggest the use of the pediatric risk of mortality (PRISM) score to predict outcome. Victims with PRISM scores greater than 20 died or survived with severe neurologic deficits.[66,87] (Table 56-5.)

ASYMPTOMATIC PATIENTS. Victims may arrive in the ED with little or no evidence of submersion injury (Box 56-5). It is widely believed that respiratory complications develop in some victims of submersion incidents 12 to 72 hours after the event.[176,178] This has led many to recommend that even asymptomatic patients be admitted for observation for this period. Almost all these patients had a history of severe insult (cardiopulmonary arrest requiring resuscitation) or had shown some abnormalities on arrival at the ED. Victims with minor symptoms who decline on-scene medical help probably do not deteriorate.[189] Most acute care clinicians, faced with a reliable history of submersion, elect to perform a physical examination, obtain ABG measurements, and acquire a chest x-ray study on even asymptomatic or minimally symptomatic victims of a

---

Box 56-5 IN-HOSPITAL MANAGEMENT OF ASYMPTOMATIC VICTIMS OF SUBMERSION INCIDENTS

CHECK AIRWAY

Supplemental oxygen: nonrebreathing mask at 12 to 15 L/min or via demand valve pending oximetry or arterial blood gas determinations

Obtain history and estimate severity of incident, look for possible underlying causes, e.g., cerebrovascular accident, epilepsy, drugs, myocardial infarction, arrhythmia

TAKE VITAL SIGNS AND EXAMINE PATIENT

Draw and hold blood samples for complete blood count, electrolytes, blood urea nitrogen, platelets, prothrombin time, partial thromboplastin time; send if indicated

Arterial blood gases; consider pulse oximetry; consider blood alcohol level and toxicology screen

Urinalysis

Chest radiograph

DISPOSITION

Observe all patients for 4 to 6 hours; discharge home if completely asymptomatic and adequate telephone or medical follow-up can be guaranteed

---

Box 56-6 IN-HOSPITAL APPROACH TO SYMPTOMATIC VICTIMS OF SUBMERSION INCIDENTS

CHECK AIRWAY

Supplemental oxygen: nonrebreathing mask at 12 to 15 L/min or via demand valve

CONSIDER ENDOTRACHEAL INTUBATION

For comatose patients

For patients unable to maintain a PaO_2 above 90 mm Hg on high-flow oxygen (nonrebreathing mask at 12 to 15 L/min), or unable to maintain a $PaCO_2$ below 45 mm Hg

CHECK VITAL SIGNS

Start intravenous line: draw blood for complete blood count, electrolytes, blood urea nitrogen, platelets, prothrombin time, partial thromboplastin time

Arterial blood gas studies

Urinalysis

Administer bicarbonate according to blood gas results if acidosis is severe and cannot otherwise be corrected

Chest radiograph

Cervical spine radiograph if any doubt about circumstances of incident

Nasogastric tube

Indwelling urinary catheter if necessary

DISPOSITION

Admit all patients with abnormal vital signs, abnormal radiologic signs, or abnormal findings on blood gas measurements

Completely asymptomatic patients with no findings may be discharged after 4 to 6 hours observation if adequate telephone or other medical follow-up can be guaranteed

---

near drowning.[122,149,171,180] Persons who show abnormalities or who deteriorate within 4 hours of admission to the ED should be admitted for observation and further management.[171]

Supportive therapy. The patient who remains asymptomatic may need attention because of the psychologic trauma of the near tragedy. This is frequently important when others have been involved in the incident, particularly when fatalities resulted. Survivors frequently suffer from posttraumatic stress syndrome with depression and disturbances of sleep and concentration.[49]

Radiographic studies. Radiographic examination of the chest is performed on all persons with a history of submersion. The findings vary widely with the severity of the incident and other factors. The usual pattern seen in persons with a significant insult is similar to that of noncardiogenic pulmonary edema. In mild cases, fine alveolar infiltrates are found, predominantly in the periphery. Persons who become symptomatic often demonstrate changes consistent with diffuse or localized intraalveolar or interstitial infiltrates, segmental atelectasis, or "shock lung." Air bronchograms are frequently seen in severely affected patients, and the lungs may appear opaque. An initial normal chest radiograph does not rule out a significant pulmonary insult. Depending on the duration of submersion, findings are usually seen within several hours of the incident, but changes have been delayed for as long as 24 hours after the patient became symptomatic.[105,198]

Spinal injury should be suspected in victims who have been platform diving or surfing or who may have fallen from a height into the water. A full radiographic series of all seven cervical vertebrae is standard before neck manipulation.

SYMPTOMATIC PATIENTS. Patients complain of combinations of coughing, sore throat, burning in the chest, and dyspnea (Box 56-6). Patients who are dyspneic are almost always hypoxic and if severely affected (with cyanosis) are likely to be acidotic. Intervention must be aggressive and planned. Initial ABG and serum chemistry measurements should be performed. A chest radiograph may be taken by portable machine unless the patient receives priority in the main radiology department.

ABG determinations or pulse oximetry can be carried out rapidly in most EDs and usually guide therapy. Oxygen is administered by demand valve (100%) or through a nonrebreathing mask at a rate of 12 to 15 L/min. This will suffice if the PaO_2 can be maintained at or above 90 mm Hg at an FIO_2 of 0.50 or less.[73] Maintaining positive pressure in the airway during expiration can be valuable. This is particularly indicated if the PaO_2/FIO_2 ratio is 300 or less.[171] In some patients who are able to hold a mask, CPAP can be provided via the tight-fitting mask, and intubation may be avoided.[83,216] Although experience with this method is growing, patients must be carefully chosen. In selected cases in the intensive care unit, use of mask CPAP has delayed or eliminated the need for intubation.[83] When provided by experienced personnel, it is an acceptable adjunct to ED therapy. Inability to maintain a PaO_2 of 55 mm Hg on an FIO_2 of 0.50 is one criterion for use of this method.[151] In addition, the patient must be able to respond to verbal commands and control his or her airway and must be nonhypercarbic ($PaCO_2$ less than 45 mm Hg).[216] Pressures used within the system, as well as the FIO_2, vary according to the clinical and ABG response. Pressures may range from 0 to 4 cm H_2O on inspiration and 4 to 14 cm H_2O on expiration. Experience with this method is insufficient for it to be recommended definitively in the prehospital environment.

Irritation of the tracheobronchial tree by inhaled water and particles may evoke cough and bronchospasm. Bronchospasm may worsen hypoxia; aggressive management is essential in symptomatic patients. Aerosolized albuterol is the drug of choice for initial treatment of bronchospasm in the ED. It is a relatively selective β_2-adrenergic agonist, rapid acting, and with minimal side effects.[13,194] It is administered to spontaneously breathing patients via a nebulizer fitted with mouthpiece or face mask. The average dose for a single treatment is 1.25 to 2.5 mg (0.25 to 0.50 ml) diluted in 2 to 5 ml or more of sterile normal saline or sterile water. With severe bronchospasm the first dose may be increased to 5 mg, or the initial lower dose may be repeated if necessary. Albuterol may be administered to intubated patients using a nebulizer attached to a T-piece hooked to the endotracheal (ET) tube. Ipratropium (Atrovent) nebulizer solution may be combined with β-agonists to try to decrease mucus and spasm. Aminophylline, in an intravenous (IV) loading dose of 5.6 mg/kg over 20 to 30 minutes, may be added if bronchospasm is not relieved.[166,194] This is useful predominantly for persons who are already taking the medicine and in whom subtherapeutic blood levels are determined.

The decision to perform ET intubation is made on the basis of ABG determinations and the following: (1) comatose patient unable to handle secretions; (2) comatose patient who requires a nasogastric tube; or (3) patient with a PaO_2 of 90 mm Hg or less on high-flow oxygen by

---

Box 56-7   PROGNOSTIC SIGNS IN SUBMERGED VICTIMS

GOOD

Alert on admission
Hypothermic
Older child or adult
Brief submersion time
On-scene basic or advanced life support (probably most
    important)
Good response to initial resuscitation measures

POOR

Age less than 3 years
Fixed, dilated pupils in emergency department
Submerged longer than 5 minutes
No resuscitation attempts for more than 10 minutes
Preexisting chronic disease
Arterial pH 7.10 or less
Coma on admission to emergency department

---

nonrebreathing mask at 12 to 15 L/min or with a $PaCO_2$ greater than 45 mm Hg.[96] A trial of nasal CPAP (continuous positive airway pressure) may help avert intubation.[50] CPAP delivers positive pressure to the airways by a pressurized face mask from a ventilator circuit.

An IV line should be placed, as well as an external cardiac monitor, indwelling urinary catheter (as needed), and nasogastric tube.

Comatose Patients or Patients in Cardiac Arrest

PROGNOSTIC SIGNS. Guidelines on predicting outcomes offer a uniform approach to management, allow for realistic expectations based on measurable data, and propose common terminology and nomenclature.[38,171] Despite advances, resuscitating patients who face serious CNS deficits may carry a poor prognosis. In some pediatric studies, 21% of children who survived had severe encephalopathy.[183] Others report that the outlook, particularly in children, is good, with morbidity ranging from 3.5% to 5%.[39,154,181,231]

In the absence of profound hypothermia, the neurologic status of a victim on admission to the ED is crucial in determining the patient's course. Persons who are alert when admitted should seldom die.[3,44,106,154,170] Prognostic indicators, particularly in pediatric patients, have included the Glasgow Coma Scale[44] and the presence of spontaneous respirations.[52,81,106,123] The duration of submersion, because of its unreliability, is not a helpful gauge of the outcome of resuscitation attempts. Full recovery of some patients with initial fixed and dilated pupils tempers the tacit acceptance of all factors historically outlined as prognostic signs. However, good and poor signs can significantly affect the chances of recovery (Box 56-7).

For ED personnel, initiation and continuation of resuscitation begun in the field should be automatic, except in the most unusual circumstances. Termination of efforts is entertained only after standard methods have been used.

HOSPITAL MANAGEMENT. The airway is reevaluated (Box 56-8). If the patient does not already have an ET tube in place and is comatose without gag or cough reflexes, a nasotracheal or ET tube should be inserted after initial hyperventilation with 100% oxygen via bag-valve device. ABGs should be measured immediately. Cervical spine precautions should be observed.

If the patient is not breathing spontaneously, 100% oxygen should be administered by volume ventilator. The object in these patients is to increase the functional residual capacity and to reduce ventilation-perfusion mismatching. PEEP may be necessary, beginning at

---

Box 56-8 IN-HOSPITAL MANAGEMENT OF PATIENTS IN COMA OR CARDIAC ARREST*

AIRWAY CONTROL

Endotracheal tube; nasotracheal preferred
Supplemental oxygen or mechanical ventilation with intermittent mandatory ventilation (IMV), continuous positive airway pressure, or IMV with positive end-expiratory pressure
Bicarbonate therapy guided by arterial blood gas values
Treatment of cardiac arrhythmias according to protocol

DIAGNOSTIC

Arterial blood gases
Blood for complete blood count, electrolytes, coagulation baseline
Urinalysis
Chest x-ray examination
Cervical spine films (if indicated)
Electrocardiographic monitoring
Computed tomography or magnetic resonance imaging suggested in patients who remain comatose
No antibiotics
No steroids

FURTHER INTENSIVE CARE MEASURES

Arterial line
Swan-Ganz catheterization when fluid status in doubt
Diuretics
H_2 antagonists
Paralysis (pancuronium, 0.1 mg/kg IV prn)
Maintain blood pressure: fluids if needed and vasopressors: dopamine, 1-20 µg/kg/min; dobutamine, 2-15 µg/kg/min

*Routine hypothermia is not recommended. Barbiturates after cardiac arrest are not proven effective. Intracranial pressure monitoring may be considered.

---

5 cm H_2O to increase the ratio of PaO_2/FIO_2 to 300 or greater.[171] Respiratory acidosis is managed with appropriate airway measures, including intubation, pulmonary toilet, and PEEP. Metabolic acidosis is often severe. Despite recent reluctance to administer bicarbonate during states of cardiac arrest,[4,221] most clinicians advise administration of sodium bicarbonate if the pH is less than 7.25 and not improving with vigorous respiratory management.[151] One formula for calculating the dose of bicarbonate is: sodium bicarbonate (mEq) = patient weight (kg) × base deficit × 0.2.[149] One-half the calculated dose is given initially and the effect on ABGs observed.

Hypoglycemia may be present as a result of marked fatigue and alcohol ingestion.[56] After initial resuscitation, treatment is directed toward correcting derangements in specific organ systems, including pulmonary, cardiovascular, and central nervous systems.

PULMONARY SYSTEM. The major insult to the lung follows reduction of surfactant and accumulation of intrapulmonary and interstitial fluid.[73,74,100,126] The treatment of pulmonary failure caused either by salt or fresh water is mechanical ventilation with or without some form of CPAP. The aim is to maintain a balance between adequate oxygenation, cardiac output, and reduction in intrapulmonary shunting. Continuous mechanical ventilation is appropriate for apneic patients or those who are spontaneously breathing but are unable to maintain a PaO_2 of at least 90 mm Hg while wearing a face mask delivering an FIO_2 of 0.50. Patients with a PaO_2/FIO_2 ratio less than 300 need positive airway pressure in addition to oxygen.[171] In comatose patients this requires endotracheal intubation.

The most desirable form of ventilation in severely affected patients is intermittent mandatory ventilation, in which spontaneous breaths between mechanical inflations improve venous return and ensure adequate cardiac output. Most consultants recommend maintaining the $PaCO_2$ at 40 mm Hg and the pH above 7.35[100] unless hyperventilation is undertaken for control of intracranial hypertension. The airway pressures required to provide a PaO_2 of at least 60 mm Hg with an FIO_2 of 0.45 vary according to the severity of the pulmonary insult and individual factors in different patients.[45,126]

In intubated patients whose ventilation is being controlled, PEEP may be used and should be maintained at a level that will ensure a balance between cardiac output and a reduction of shunt. After an adequate level of oxygenation is achieved, PEEP or CPAP should be maintained for at least 24 hours to foster the regeneration of surfactant.[126,176] Airway pressures with PEEP must be carefully monitored in postsubmersion patients, since increasing intrathoracic pressure leads to elevations in ICP.

Care must be exercised in removing patients from ventilatory support. Some respond dramatically to controlled ventilation, but 2 to 4 days may be required to replenish surfactant and resolve the problem of atelectasis. Premature removal from the ventilator may be followed by deterioration in pulmonary status, which could require reintubation and reintroduction of mechanical ventilation.[126] Generally, when a Pao_2 of 60 mm Hg or above can be supported with an Fio_2 of 0.40 or less in the absence of PEEP, the patient can be removed from the ventilator.

The use of steroids to prevent deterioration of lung function after submersion injury has few advocates.[100,149,171] No evidence shows a benefit in pulmonary failure, and good data suggest the progression of chemical aspiration to bacterial pneumonitis.[151,153] Intratracheal instillation of surfactant may help patients not responding to maximal medical therapy. Experimental studies are now investigating the use of butyl alcohol vapor or surfactant as an adjuvant to traditional respiratory support.[23,230]

Prophylactic antibiotics are not recommended. Daily Gram's stain of sputum and frequent blood, urine, and sputum cultures may be required in the long-term management of these patients.

CARDIOVASCULAR SYSTEM. Cardiac dysrhythmias and arrest during the course of resuscitation often are corrected by improvements in oxygenation and acid-base status. An arterial pressure cannula is helpful to monitor cardiovascular status and ABGs.

The use of Swan-Ganz catheters is advisable in patients who develop hemodynamic instability or who require high levels of CPAP or PEEP to maintain oxygenation.[149] When shock is evident, pulmonary artery wedge pressures and cardiac output determinations allow a more rational approach to fluid administration. The Swan-Ganz catheter allows measurement of mixed venous oxygen saturation and can provide some information on oxygen transport and cardiac output. Pressor agents, such as dopamine and dobutamine, may be required if arterial hypotension and reduced cardiac output persist after adequate hydration is ensured. In most animal studies, cardiac output is best supported by fluids rather than inotropic agents.[56] The cause of most cases of postsubmersion pulmonary edema is altered permeability rather than pump failure. However, dopamine (2 to 20 μg/kg/min) and dobutamine (2 to 15 μg/kg/min) have been effective in some patients.[98] Sepsis and shock are constant threats.

RENAL AND METABOLIC FUNCTION. In victims of significant submersion injury, renal blood flow may decrease as a result of hypovolemia or hypotension. This can be detected by close attention to urine output. Renal failure is usually caused by hypoxia and acidosis with tubular damage.[82,111] Deposition of hemoglobin in the tubules from hemolysis of red blood cells is rarely a cause of renal failure. Maintenance of adequate circulating blood volume and restoration of renal perfusion are the best insurance against renal damage. An indwelling urinary catheter should be placed and urine production monitored and maintained at a minimum of 50 ml/hr. Mannitol in a dose of 0.25 g/kg intravenously has been used to maintain adequate urine flow and prevent obstruction of the tubules. This is given only after adequate intravascular volume is obtained.

CEREBRAL RESUSCITATION. Until recently, therapeutic measures were exclusively directed toward stabilizing the cardiovascular and pulmonary systems. Patients who were restored to adequate levels of cardiopulmonary function often died later from brain failure. Although some measures to protect the brain from postischemic insults are still experimental, the outlook for patients with severe initial defects is improving.[38-40,45,152] Measures directed toward cerebral salvage began with observations of the effect of hypothermia on brain metabolism. The initial enthusiasm and expectations for barbiturate cerebral resuscitation after cardiac arrest have not been justified in international multicenter studies.[21,162,237]

The most important approach to CNS resuscitation in postsubmersion patients is provision of an adequate airway and attention to ventilation and oxygenation. Patients who respond promptly to such measures are unlikely to require methods of cerebral preservation, probably because the cerebral insult has not been severe. Patients who remain comatose and who may have head trauma should be examined with computed tomography (CT) or magnetic resonance imaging (MRI) as soon as practical. Scanning may reveal intracranial or intracerebral hemorrhage and provides an early picture of the extent of cerebral edema.

When the victim does not respond immediately to vigorous resuscitation measures, one practical protocol for management requires control of several elements, including ventilation, hydration, temperature, brain metabolism and edema, and muscular activity.[38,40,152]

VENTILATION. Hyperventilation is maintained to achieve a $Paco_2$ of about 30 mm Hg to balance cerebral vasoconstriction with cerebral blood flow. PEEP is used to maintain a high Pao_2 (150 mm Hg), since it is thought that this facilitates cerebral oxygen transport.

HYDRATION. Diuresis is promoted with a loop diuretic (furosemide, 0.5 to 1 mg/kg). Fluid restriction is guided by laboratory and clinical measurements such as blood pressure, pulmonary wedge pressure, and occasionally blood volume measurements.

TEMPERATURE. Normothermia should be maintained and hyperpyrexia prevented with the use of cooling mattresses if necessary. The routine use of induced hypothermia is not recommended, particularly because hypothermia can induce neutropenia and lead to sepsis.[18,179,180] In the case of ICP uncontrolled by other measures, some clinicians advise reduction of core temperature to 30° C (86° F) while paralyzing the patient to combat shivering.[40] Revisions of this opinion urge caution, since the effect on outcome is uncertain.[149,150]

CEREBRAL METABOLISM AND EDEMA. Control of cerebral metabolism and reduction of edema are difficult and controversial areas of management. Patients who remain comatose and do not respond to adequate fluid balance and hyperventilation should have the management of presumed ICP elevation guided by clinical examination and direct monitoring using an epidural transducer, ventricular catheter, or subarachnoid bolt.

The use of barbiturates for cerebral protection after cardiac arrest has not been encouraging, but the ability of these drugs in certain circumstances to reduce ICP by cerebral vasoconstriction can be helpful to patients with an ICP above 20 cm H_2O.[150] A direct "protective" effect of barbiturates on nerve tissue has not been demonstrated. Difficulties with instituting barbiturate therapy and maintaining patients on the regimen include hypotension and inability to evaluate the patient clinically. Conn et al[39,40] used phenobarbital for a minimum of 4 days in children (50 mg/kg on day 1 in three divided doses, then half that dose subsequently), with daily determinations of barbiturate levels. Reports of equivocal results in children treated with barbiturates and hypothermia indicate that these measures should not be used routinely.[18,171]

If barbiturates are used, the patient should be placed in an intensive care unit with staff fully skilled in the use of these agents. When pentobarbital is used, a constant infusion technique is guided by monitoring arterial pressure, ICP, and cardiac output. If blood pressure falls, the infusion rate should be decreased or an inotropic agent (dopamine, dobutamine) used to support myocardial function.[98,100] Whenever barbiturate therapy is considered, mass intracranial lesions should first be ruled out by CT or MRI because any clinical signs caused by these lesions might be masked by the barbiturate. Sudden increases in ICP can be managed by hyperventilation and the use of mannitol (0.5 to 1 g/kg IV bolus). No comparative studies have demonstrated the success of therapy directed at reducing ICP and maintaining cerebral perfusion pressure.

Because postischemic brain insult was associated with high intraneuronal calcium ion concentration, calcium channel blocking agents were used to ameliorate the effects of ischemia on the CNS.[162,207] The use of these agents remains under investigation.

Some clinicians have used corticosteroids because steroid use improved the CNS function of patients with primary or secondary brain tumors,[12] apparently by reducing cerebral reaction and swelling around the mass lesions.[11] In an attempt to duplicate this beneficial effect in patients with acute intracranial hemorrhage, large doses of corticosteroids were administered to patients with head injury. No benefit was seen,[42] and most clinicians no longer recommend corticosteroids for the reduction of ICP and for cerebral protection after ischemic brain insults.[38,149] Steroids in high doses appear to be beneficial in selected cases of spinal cord injury.

MUSCULAR ACTIVITY. Complete muscular paralysis is advocated by Conn et al[40] to facilitate control of ventilation and to prevent ICP increase induced by muscle rigidity and restlessness. Muscle paralysis is achieved with pancuronium (0.1 mg/kg intravenously) hourly or as needed.

GENERAL MEASURES. Other measures for patient support during intensive postsubmersion therapy include placement of a nasogastric tube and selective administration of antacids or a histamine-2 antagonist, such as cimetidine, to prevent gastric hemorrhage.[171,184]

REFERENCES

1. Agocs MM et al: Activities associated with drownings in Imperial County, CA, 1980-90: implications for prevention, *Public Health Rep* 109:290, 1994.
2. Alcohol and aquatic activities—Massachusetts, 1988, *MMWR* 39(20), 1990.
3. Allman FD et al: Outcome following cardiopulmonary resuscitation in severe pediatric near-drowning, *Am J Dis Child* 140:571, 1986.
4. American Heart Association: Standards and guidelines for cardiopulmonary resuscitation and emergency cardiac care, *JAMA* 255:2841, 1986.
5. Andersson J, Schagatay E: Arterial oxygen desaturation during apnea in humans, *Undersea Hyper Med* 25:21, 1998.
6. Anker AL et al: Artificial surfactant administration in an animal model of near drowning, *Acad Emerg Med* 2:204, 1995.
7. Ashbaugh DG, Petty TL: Positive end-expiratory pressure—physiology, indications and contraindications, *J Thorac Cardiovasc Surg* 65:165, 1973.
8. Auerbach PS et al: Bacteriology of the freshwater environment: implications for clinical therapy, *Ann Emerg Med* 16:1016, 1987.
9. Avery ME, Taeusch HW, Floros J: Surfactant replacement, *N Engl J Med* 315:825, 1986.
10. Baker SP, O'Neill B, Karpf RD: *The injury fact book*, Lexington, Mass, 1984, Heath.
11. Bartecchi CE: Cardiopulmonary resuscitation—an element of sophistication in the 18th century, *Am Heart J* 100:580, 1980.
12. Beks JWF, Doorenbos H, Walstra GJM: Clinical experiences with steroids in neurosurgical patients. In Reuben HJ, Schurmann K, editors: *Steroids and brain edema*, Berlin, 1972, Springer-Verlag.
13. Bennett P, Elliott D: *The physiology and medicine of diving*, ed 4, Philadelphia, 1993, Saunders.
14. Bergquist RE et al: Comparison of ventilatory patterns in the treatment of freshwater near-drowning in dogs, *Anesthesiology* 52:142, 1980.
15. Bierens JJLM et al: Submersion cases in the Netherlands, *Ann Emerg Med* 18:4, 1989.
16. Biggart MJ, Bohn DJ, Desmond J: Effect of hypothermia and cardiac arrest on outcome of near-drowning accidents in children, *J Pediatr* 117:179, 1990.
17. Bishop RL, Weisfeldt MZ: Sodium bicarbonate administration during cardiac arrest: effect on arterial pH, PCO_2 and osmolality, *JAMA* 235:506, 1976.

18. Bohn DJ et al: Influence of hypothermia, barbiturate therapy, and intracranial pressure monitoring on morbidity and mortality after near-drowning, *Crit Care Med* 14:529, 1986.

19. Bonilla-Santiago J, Fill WL: Sand aspiration in drowning and near-drowning, *Radiology* 128:301, 1978.

20. Borges G et al: Male drinking and violence-related injury in the emergency room, *Addiction* 93:103, 1998.

21. Brain Resuscitation Clinical Trial I Study Group: Randomized clinical study of thiopental loading in comatose survivors of cardiac arrest, *N Engl J Med* 314:440, 1986.

22. Bratton SL et al: Serial neurologic examinations after near drowning and outcome, *Arch Pediatr Adolesc Med* 148:167, 1994.

23. Braun R, Krishel S: Environmental emergencies, *Emerg Med Clin North Am* 15:451, 1997.

24. Brown SD, Piantadosi CA: Near drowning: hospital management. In *Near drowning forty-seventh workshop of the Undersea and Hyperbaric Medical Society*, Kensington, Md, 1997, The Society.

25. Campbell TP et al: Oxygen enrichment of bag-valve-mask units during positive pressure ventilation: a comparison of various techniques, *Ann Emerg Med* (in press).

26. Celis A: Home drowning among preschool age Mexican children, *Inj Prev* 3:252, 1997.

27. Centers for Disease Control: Drowning—Georgia, 1981-1983, *MMWR* 34:281, 1985.

28. Centers for Disease Control: Drownings in a private lake—North Carolina, 1981-1990, *MMWR* 41:329, 1992.

29. Child drownings and near drownings associated with swimming pools, Maricopa County, Arizona, 1988 and 1989, *JAMA* 264(6), 1990.

30. Chochinov AH et al: Recovery of a 62-year-old man from prolonged cold water submersion, *Ann Emerg Med* 31:127, 1998.

31. Christensen DW et al: Outcome and acute care hospital costs after warm water near drowning in children, *Pediatrics* 99:715, 1997.

32. Cohen DS et al: Pulmonary edema associated with salt water near-drowning: new insights, *Am Rev Respir Dis* 146:794, 1992.

33. Colebatch HJH, Halmagyi DFJ: Reflex pulmonary hypertension of freshwater aspiration, *J Appl Physiol* 18:179, 1963.

34. Colebatch HJH, Halmagyi DJP: Effect of vagotomy and vagal stimulation on lung mechanics and circulation, *J Appl Physiol* 18:881, 1963.

35. Collis ML: Survival behaviour in cold water immersion. In *Proceedings of the Cold Water Symposium*, Toronto, 1976, Royal Life-Saving Society of Canada.

36. Conn AW: The role of hypothermia in near-drowning. In *Proceedings of the Cold Water Symposium*, Toronto, 1976, Royal Life-Saving Society of Canada.

37. Conn AW: Near-drowning and hypothermia, *CMA J* 120:397, 1979 (editorial).

38. Conn AW, Barker GA: Freshwater drowning and near-drowning—an update, *Can Anaesth Soc J* 31:S38, 1984.

39. Conn AW, Edmonds JF, Barker GA: Cerebral resuscitation in near-drowning, *Pediatr Clin North Am* 26:691, 1979.

40. Conn AW et al: Cerebral salvage in near-drowning following neurological classification by triage, *Can Anaesth Soc J* 27:201, 1980.

41. Conn AW et al: A canine study of cold water drowning in fresh versus salt water, *Crit Care Med* 23:2029, 1995.

42. Cooper PR et al: Dexamethasone and severe head injury: a prospective double-blind study, *J Neurosurg* 51:307, 1979.

43. Culpepper RM: Bleeding diathesis in freshwater drowning, *Ann Intern Med* 83:675, 1975 (letter).

44. Dean MJ, Kaufman ND: Prognostic indicators in pediatric near-drowning: the Glasgow Coma Scale, *Crit Care Med* 9:536, 1981.

45. DeNicola LK et al: Submersion injuries in children and adults, *Crit Care Clin* 13:477, 1997.

46. Dick W et al: The influence of different ventilatory patterns on oxygenation and gas exchange after near-drowning, *Resuscitation* 7:255, 1979.

47. Diekema DS, Quan L, Holt VL: Epilepsy as a risk factor for submersion injury in children, *Pediatrics* 91:612, 1993.

48. Doerges V et al: Airway management during cardiopulmonary resuscitation—a comparative study of bag-valve-mast, laryngeal mask airway and a combitube in a bench model, *Resuscitation* 41:63, 1999.

49. Dooley E, Gunn J: The psychological effects of disaster at sea, *Br J Psychiatry* 167:233, 1995.

50. Dottorini M et al: Nasal-continuous positive airway pressure in the treatment of near-drowning in freshwater, *Chest* 110:1122, 1996.

51. Drinking and drowning, *Br Med J* 2:1284, 1978 (editorial).

52. Dubowitz DJ et al: MR of hypoxic encephalopathy in children after near drowning: correlation with quantitative proton MR spectroscopy and clinical outcome, *AJNR Am J Neuroradiol* 19:1617, 1998.

53. Dueker CW: Introduction. In *Near drowning: forty-seventh workshop of the Undersea and Hyperbaric Medical Society*, Kensington, Md, 1997, The Society.

54. Dunagan DP et al: Sand aspiration with near-drowning: radiographic and bronchoscopic findings, *Am J Respir Crit Care Med* 156:292, 1997.

55. Edmonds, C: Drowning syndromes: the mechanism, *SPUMS J* 28:2, 1998.

56. Edmonds C, Lowry C, Pennefather J: Drowning. In *Diving and subaquatic medicine*, ed 3, Newton, Mass, Butterworth-Heinemann.

57. Edwards ND et al: Survival in adults after cardiac arrest due to drowning, *Intensive Care Med* 16:336, 1990.

58. Eliot RS, Todd GL, Pieper GM: Pathophysiology of catecholamine-mediated myocardial damage, *J SC Med Assoc* 75:513, 1979.

59. Elling R, Politis J: An evaluation of emergency medical technicians—ability to use manual ventilation devices, *Ann Emerg Med* 12:765, 1983.

60. Ellis AA, Trent RB: Hospitalizations for near drowning in California: incidence and costs, *Am J Public Health* 85:1115, 1995.

61. Ellis AA, Trent RB: Swimming pool drownings and near-drownings among California preschoolers, *Public Health Rep* 112:73, 1997.

62. Emergency Cardiac Care Committee and Subcommittees, American Heart Association: Guidelines for cardiopulmonary resuscitation and emergency cardiac care. IV. Special resuscitation situations, *JAMA* 268:2242, 1992.

63. Ender PT et al: Near-drowning-associated Aeromonas pneumonia, *J Emerg Med* 14:737, 1996.

64. Ender PT, Dolan MJ: Pneumonia associated with near-drowning, *Clin Infect Dis* 25:896, 1997.

65. Feldman KW, Monastersky C, Feldman GK: When is childhood drowning neglect? *Child Abuse Negl* 17:329, 1993.

66. Fenner PJ et al: Success of surf lifesaving resuscitations in Queensland, 1973-1992, *Med J Aust* 163:580, 1995.

67. Fields AI: Near-drowning in the pediatric population, *Crit Care Clin* 8:113, 1992.

68. Fisher B, Peterson B, Hicks G: Use of brainstem auditory-evoked response testing to assess neurologic outcome following near drowning in children, *Crit Care Med* 20:578, 1992.

69. Frank BS: Hypokalemia following fresh-water submersion injuries, *Pediatr Emerg Care* 3:158, 1987.

70. Fromm RE: Hypercalcemia complicating an industrial near drowning, *Ann Emerg Med* 20:669, 1991.

71. Fujiwara T et al: Artificial therapy in hyaline membrane disease, *Lancet* 1:55, 1980.

72. Fuller RH: Drowning and the post-immersion syndrome: a clinicopathologic study, *Milit Med* 128:22, 1963.

73. Giammona ST: Drowning: pathophysiology and management, *Curr Probl Pediatr* 3:3, 1971.

74. Giammonna ST, Modell JH: Drowning by total immersion: effects on pulmonary surfactant of distilled water, isotonic saline, and seawater, *Am J Dis Child* 114:612, 1967.

75. Gillenwater JM et al: Inflicted submersion in childhood, *Arch Pediatr Adolesc Med* 150:298, 1996.

76. Golden FS: Accident hypothermia, *R Naval Med Serv* 58:196, 1972.

77. Golden FS et al: Immersion, near-drowning and drowning, *Br J Anaesth* 79:214, 1997.

78. Goode RC, Duffin J, Miller R: Sudden cold water immersion, *Respir Physiol* 23:301, 1975.

79. Gooden BA: Drowning and the diving reflex in man, *Med J Aust* 2:583, 1972.

80. Gooden BA: Why some people do not drown: hypothermia versus the diving response, *Med J Aust* 157:629, 1992.

81. Graf WD et al: Predicting outcome in pediatric submersion victims, *Ann Emerg Med* 26:312, 1995.

82. Grausz H, Amend WJC Jr, Earley LE: Acute renal failure complicating submersion in seawater, *JAMA* 217:207, 1971.

83. Greenbaum DM et al: Continuous positive airway pressure without tracheal intubation in spontaneously-breathing patients, *Chest* 69:615, 1976.

84. Greenberg MI et al: Effects of endotracheally administered distilled water and normal saline on the arterial blood gases of dogs, *Ann Emerg Med* 11:600, 1982.

85. Greene DG: Drowning. In *Hanbook of physiology*, vol II, Washington, DC, 1965, American Physiological Society.

86. Griest KJ, Zumwalt RE: Child abuse by drowning, *Pediatrics* 83(1), 1989.

87. Habib DM et al: Prediction of childhood drowning and near-drowning morbidity and mortality, *Pediatr Emerg Care* 12:255, 1996.

88. Halperin HR et al: A preliminary study of cardiopulmonary resuscitation by circumferential compression of the chest with use of a pneumatic vest, *N Engl J Med* 329:762, 1993.

89. Harries MG: Drowning in man, *Crit Care Med* 9:407, 1981.

90. Harrison RR, Maull KI, Keenan RL: Mouth-to-mouth ventilation: a superior method of rescue breathing, *Ann Emerg Med* 11:74, 1982.

91. Hayward JS et al: Temperature effect on the human dive response in relation to cold water near-drowning, *J Appl Physiol* 56:202, 1984.

92. Hazinski MF et al: Pediatric injury prevention, *Ann Emerg Med* 22:456, 1993.

93. Hegnauer HA, Angelakos ET: Excitable properties of the hypothermic heart, *Ann NY Acad Sci* 80:336, 1959.

94. Heimlich HJ: A life-saving maneuver to prevent food-choking, *JAMA* 234:398, 1975.

95. Heimlich HJ: Subdiaphragmatic pressure to expel water from the lungs of drowning persons, *Ann Emerg Med* 10:476, 1981.

96. Heimlich HJ, Hoffman KA, Canestri FR: Food-choking and drowning deaths prevented by external subdiaphragmatic compression, *Ann Thorac Surg* 20:188, 1975.

97. Herholdt JD, Rafn CG: *Life-saving measures for drowning persons*, Copenhagen, 1796, Tikiob.

98. Hess D, Kapp A, Kurtek W: The effect on delivered oxygen concentration of the rescuer's breathing supplemental oxygen during exhaled gas ventilation, *Respir Care* 30:691, 1985.

99. Higgins P, Siminski J, Pearson RD: "Hypoxic" lap swimming—a cause of near-drowning, *N Engl J Med* 315:1552, 1986 (letter).

100. Hoff BH: Multisystem failure: a review with special reference to drowning, *Crit Care Med* 7:310, 1979.

101. Hong SK: Physical and physiologic adaptations to breath-hold diving in humans: a review. In *Proceedings of the 9th International Symposium on Underwater and Hyperbaric Physiology*, Bethesda, Md, 1987, Undersea and Hyperbaric Medical Society.

102. Howland J et al: A pilot survey of aquatic activities and related consumption of alcohol, with implications for drowning, *Public Health Rep* 105:415, 1990.

103. Howland J et al: Why are most drowning victims men? Sex differences in aquatic skills and behaviors, *Am J Public Health* 86:93, 1996.

104. Huckabee HC et al: Near drowning in frigid water: a case study of a 31-year-old woman, *J Int Neuropsychol Soc* 2:256, 1996.

105. Hunter TB, Whitehouse WM: Freshwater near-drowning: radiological aspects, *Radiology* 112:51, 1974.

106. Jacobsen WK et al: Correlation of spontaneous respiration and neurologic damage in near-drowning, *Crit Care Med* 11:487, 1983.

107. Jensen LR et al: Submersion injuries in children younger than 5 years in urban Utah, *West J Med* 157:641, 1992.

108. Joseph MM, King WD: Epidemiology of hospitalization for near-drowning, *South Med J* 91: 253, 1998.

109. Julian DG: Cardiac resuscitation in the eighteenth century, *Heart Lung* 4:6, 1975.

110. Jumbelic MI, Chambliss M: Accidental toddler drowning in 5 gallon buckets, *JAMA* 263(14), 1990.

111. Karch SB: Pathology of the heart in near-drowning, *Arch Pathol Lab Med* 109:176, 1985.

112. Karch SB: Pathology of the lung in near-drowning, *Am J Emerg Med* 4:4, 1986.

113. Karkal MB, Rasch DK, Gilbert J: Optimizing salvage in drowning and near drowning victims, *Emerg Med Rep* 10(16), 1989.

114. Kasian GF, O'Farrell NM, Linwood ME: Bathtub near-drowning of an infant in a flotation device, *CMAJ* 136, 1987.

115. Keating WR, Hayward MG: Sudden death in cold water and ventricular arrhythmia, *J Forensic Sci* 26:459, 1981.

116. Kemp AM, Sibert JR: Outcome in children who nearly drown: a British Isles study, *Br Med J* 302:931, 1991.

117. Kemp AM, Sibert JR: Epilepsy in children and the risk of drowning, *Arch Dis Child* 68:684, 1993.

118. Kemp AM et al: Accidents and child abuse in bathtub submersions, *Arch Dis Child* 70:435, 1994.

119. King RJ: Pulmonary surfactant, *J Appl Physiol* 53:1, 1982.

120. Kizer KW: Resuscitation of submersion casualties, *Emerg Med Clin North Am* 1:643, 1983.

121. Knopp R: Near drowning, *J Am College Emerg Phys* 7:249, 1978.

122. Kram JA, Kizer KW: Submersion injury, *Emerg Med Clin North Am* 2:545, 1984.

123. Kreis R et al: Hypoxic encephalopathy after near-drowning studied by quantitative 1H- magnetic resonance spectroscopy, *J Clin Invest* 97:1142, 1996.

124. Lavelle JM, Shaw KN: Near drowning: is emergency department cardiopulmonary resuscitation or intensive care unit cerebral resuscitation indicated? *Crit Care Med* 21:368, 1993.

125. Lavelle JM et al: Ten-year review of pediatric bathtub near-drownings: evaluation for child abuse and neglect, *Ann Emerg Med* 25:344, 1995.

126. Levin DL: Near drowning, *Crit Care Med* 8:590, 1980.

127. Levin DL et al: Drowning and near-drowning, *Pediatr Clin North Am* 40:321, 1993.

128. Levinson R et al: Comparison of the effects of water immersion and saline infusion on central hemodynamics in man, *Clin Sci Mol Med* 52:343, 1977.

129. Liller KD et al: Risk factors for drowning and near-drowning among children in Hillsborough County, Florida, *Pub Health Rep* 108:346, 1993.

130. Lilly JK: An inexpensive portable positive end-expiratory pressure system, *Anesth Analg* 58:53, 1979.

131. Liss HP: A history of resuscitation, *Ann Emerg Med* 15:65, 1986.

132. Losonsky G: Infections associated with swimming and diving, *Undersea Biomed Res* 18:181, 1991.

133. Lougheed DW, James JM, Hall GE: Physiological studies in experimental asphyxia and drowning, *CMAJ* 40:423, 1939.

134. Machi T et al: Severe hypercalcemia and polyuria in a near-drowning victim, *Intern Med* 34:868, 1995.

135. Mackie I: Alcohol and aquatic disasters, *Med J Aust* 1:652, 1978.

136. Mangge H et al: Late-onset miliary pneumonitis after near drowning, *Pediatr Pulmonol* 15:122, 1993.

137. Mann NC, Weller SC, Rauchschwalbe R: Bucket-related drownings in the United States, 1984 through 1990, *Pediatrics* 89:1068, 1992.

138. Manolios N, Mackie I: Drowning and near-drowning on Australian beaches patrolled by life-savers: a 10-year study, 1973-1983, *Med J Aust* 148:165, 1988.

139. Manser TJ, Warner JF: *Neisseria mucosus* septicemia after near drowning, *South Med J* 80:1323, 1987.

140. March NF, Matthews RC: New techniques in external cardiac compressions: aquatic cardiopulmonary resuscitation, *JAMA* 244:1229, 1984.

141. Martin TG: Near-drowning and cold water immersion, *Ann Emerg Med* 13:263, 1984.

142. McCallum AL et al: Two cases of accidental hypothermia with differing outcomes under identical conditions, *Aviat Space Environ Med*, 1988.

143. Mebane GY: Drowning in a sea of tears, *Alert Diver* 4:8, 1993.

144. Medical news, *JAMA* 210:1683, 1969.

145. Merritt TA et al: Reduction of lung injury by human surfactant treatment in respiratory distress syndrome, *Chest* 83:27S, 1983.

146. Modell JH: *Pathophysiology and treatment of drowning and near-drowning*, Springfield, Ill, 1971, Charles C Thomas.

147. Modell JH: Drown versus near-drown: a discussion of definitions, *Crit Care Med* 9:351, 1981 (editorial).

148. Modell JH: Serum electrolyte changes in near-drowning victims, *JAMA* 253:557, 1985 (editorial).

149. Modell JH: Near-drowning. In Callaham ML, editor: *Current therapy in emergency medicine*, St Louis, 1986, Mosby.

150. Modell JH: Treatment of near-drowning: is there a role for H.Y.P.E.R. therapy? *Crit Care Med* 14:593, 1986.

151. Modell JH: Drowning, *N Engl J Med* 328:253, 1993.

152. Modell JH, Conn AW: Current neurological considerations in near-drowning, *Can Anaesth Soc J* 27:197, 1980 (editorial).

153. Modell JH, Graves SA, Ketover A: Clinical course of 91 consecutive near-drowning victims, *Chest* 10:231, 1976.

154. Modell JH, Graves SA, Kuck EJ: Near-drowning: correlation of level of consciousness and survival, *Can Anaesth Soc J* 27:211, 1980.

155. Modell JH, Moya F: Effects of volume of aspirated fluid during chlorinated fresh-water drowning, *Anesthesiology* 27:663, 1966.

156. Modell JH et al: The effects of fluid volume in seawater drowning, *Ann Intern Med* 67:68, 1967.

157. Modell JH et al: Blood gas and electrolyte changes in human near-drowning victims, *JAMA* 203:99, 1968.

158. Modell JH et al: Changes in blood gases and A-aDO$_2$ during near-drowning, *Anesthesiology* 29:456, 1968.

159. Modell JH et al: Effects of ventilatory patterns on arterial oxygenation after near-drowning in seawater, *Anesthesiology* 40:376, 1974.

160. Mortensen E et al: Changes in ventricular fibrillation threshold during acute hypothermia: a model for future studies, *J Basic Clin Physiol Pharmacol* 4:313, 1993.

161. Neuman TS: Near drowning. In Bove AA, editor: *Bove & Davis' diving medicine*, ed 3, Philadelphia, 1997, Saunders

162. Newberg LA: Cerebral resuscitation: advances and controversies, *Ann Emerg Med* 13:853, 1984.

163. Noble CS, Sharp N: Drowning: its mechanism and treatment, *CMAJ* 89:402, 1963.

164. Noonan L et al: Freshwater submersion injuries in children: a retrospective review of seventy-five hospitalized patients, *Pediatrics* 98:368, 1996.

165. Norrish AE, Cryer PC: Work related injury in New Zealand commercial fishermen, *Br J Ind Med* 47:726, 1990.

166. Nowak RM: Acute adult asthma. In Rosen P et al, editors: *Emergency medicine: concepts and clinical practice*, St Louis, 1988, Mosby.

167. Oakes DD et al: Prognosis and management of victims of near-drowning, *J Trauma* 2:544, 1982.

168. O'Flaherty JE, Pirie PL Prevention of pediatric drowning and near-drowning: a survey of members of the American Academy of Pediatrics, *Pediatrics* 99:169, 1997.

169. Olshaker JS: Near drowning, *Emerg Med Clin North Am* 10:339, 1992.

170. Orlowski JP: Prognostic factors in drowning and near-drowning, *J Am Coll Emerg Phys* 8:176, 1979.

171. Orlowski JP: Drowning, near-drowning and ice-water submersions, *Pediatr Clin North Am* 34:75, 1987.

172. Orlowski JP: Vomiting as a complication of the Heimlich maneuver, *JAMA* 258:512, 1987.

173. Orlowski JP, Abulleil MM, Phillips JM: Effects of tonicities of saline solutions on pulmonary injury in drowning, *Crit Care Med* 15:126, 1987.

174. Orlowski JP, Rothner AD, Lueders H: Submersion accidents in children with epilepsy, *Am J Dis Child* 136:777, 1982.

175. Orlowski JP et al: The hemodynamic and cardiovascular effects of near drowning in hypotonic, isotonic, or hypertonic solutions, *Ann Emerg Med* 18:1044, 1989.

176. Ornato JP: The resuscitation of near-drowning victims, *JAMA* 256:75, 1986.

177. Pan AW et al: Blood flow in the carotid artery during breath-holding in relation to diving bradycardia, *Eur J Appl Physiol* 75:338, 1997.

178. Pearn JH: Secondary drowning in children, *Br Med J* 281:1103, 1980.

179. Pearn J: The management of near-drowning, *Br Med J* 291:1447, 1985.

180. Pearn J: Why children drown, *Aust J Paediatr* 22:161, 1986.

181. Pearn JH, Bart RD, Yamaoka R: Neurologic sequelae after childhood near-drowning: a total population study from Hawaii, *Pediatrics* 65:187, 1979.

182. Pearn J, Nixon J: Bathtub immersion accidents involving children, *Med J Aust* 1:211, 1977.

183. Peterson B: Morbidity of childhood near-drowning, *Pediatrics* 59:364, 1977.

184. Peura DA, Johnson LF: Cimetidine for prevention and treatment of gastroduodenal mucosal lesions in patients in an intensive care unit, *Ann Intern Med* 103:173, 1985.

185. Pitt WR, Balanda KP: Childhood drowning and near-drowning in Brisbane: the contribution of domestic pools, *Med J Aust* 154:661, 1991.

186. *Pittsburgh Press*, May 8, 1987, p 1.

187. Plueckhahn VD: Drowning: community aspects, *Med J Aust* 2:226, 1979.

188. Pollack MM et al: Pediatric risk of mortality (PRISM) score, *Crit Care Med* 16:1110, 1998.

189. Pratt FD, Haynes BE: Incidence of "secondary drowning" after saltwater submersion, *Ann Emerg Med* 15:1084, 1986.

190. Quan L: Drowning issues in resuscitation, *Ann Emerg Med* 22:366, 1993.

191. Quan L, Kinder D: Pediatric submersions: prehospital predictors of outcome, *Pediatrics* 90:909, 1992.

192. Ramey CA, Ramey DN, Hayward JS: The dive response of children in relation to cold water near-drowning, *J Appl Physiol* 63:665, 1987.

193. Riley MD et al: Drowning fatalities of children in Tasmania: differences from national data, *Aust NZ J Public Health* 20:547, 1996.

194. Robertson C, Levison H: Bronchodilators in asthma, *Chest* 87:64S, 1985.

195. Robinson MD, Seward PN: Submersion injury in children, *Pediatr Emerg Care* 3:44, 1987.

196. Rockett IR, Smith GS: Covert suicide among elderly Japanese females: questioning unintentional drownings, *Soc Sci Med* 36:1467, 1993.

197. Rosen P et al: The use of the Heimlich maneuver in near drowning: Institute of Medicine report, *J Emerg Med* 13:397, 1995.

198. Rosenbaum HT, Thompson WL, Ruller RH: Radiographic pulmonary changes in near-drowning, *Radiology* 83:306.

199. Rowe MI, Arango A, Allington G: Profile of pediatric drowning victims in a water-oriented society, *J Trauma* 17:587, 1977.

200. Ruben A, Ruben H: Artificial respiration: flow of water from lung and stomach, *Lancet* 1:780, 1962.

201. Rubenstein E: Water-related accidents, *Sci Am Med* 8:1, 1986.

202. Ruchel R, Wilichowski E: Cerebral Pseudallescheria mycosis after near-drowning, *Mycoses* 38:473, 1995.

203. Rumbak MJ: The etiology of pulmonary edema in fresh water near-drowning, *Am J Emerg Med* 14:176, 1996.

204. Runyan CW, Gerken EA: Epidemiology and prevention of adolescent injury, *JAMA* 262(16), 1989.

205. Rutledge RR, Flor RJ: The use of mechanical ventilation with positive end-expiratory pressure in the treatment of near-drowning, *Anesthesiology* 38:194, 1973.

206. Safar P: *Cardiopulmonary cerebral resuscitation*, Stavanger, Norway, 1981, Laerdal.

207. Safar P: Recent advances in cardiopulmonary cerebral resuscitation: a review, *Ann Emerg Med* 13:856, 1984.

208. Schagatay E, Andersson J: Diving response and apneic time in humans, *Undersea Hyper Med* 25:13, 1998.

209. Schmidt P, Madea B Death in the bathtub involving children, *Forensic Sci Int* 72:147, 1995.

210. Schmidt P, Madea B Homicide in the bathtub, *Forensic Sci Int* 72: 135, 1995.

211. Schnitzer PG, Landen DD, Russell JC: Occupational injury deaths in Alaska-s fishing industry, 1980 through 1988, *Am J Public Health* 83:685, 1993.

212. Schuman SH et al: The iceberg phenomenon of near-drowning, *Crit Care Med* 4:127, 1976.

213. Schuman SH et al: Risk of drowning: an iceberg phenomenon, *J Am Coll Emerg Phys* 6:139, 1977.

214. Scott PH, Eigen H: Immersion accidents involving pails of water in the home, *J Pediatr* 92:282, 1980.

215. Segarra F, Redding RA: Modern concepts about drowning, *CMAJ* 110:1057, 1974.

216. Shelhamer JH, Nathanson C, Parilloje: Positive end-expiratory pressure in adults, *JAMA* 251:2692, 1984.

217. Siebke H et al: Survival after 40 minutes submersion without cerebral sequelae, *Lancet* 1:1275, 1975.

218. Smith DW et al: High-frequency jet ventilation in children with the adult respiratory distress syndrome complicated by pulmonary barotrauma, *Pediatr Pulmonol* 15:279, 1993.

219. Southwick FS, Dalglish PH: Recovery after prolonged asystolic arrest in profound hypothermia, *JAMA* 243:1250, 1980.

220. Spack L et al: Failure of aggressive therapy to alter outcome in pediatric near- drowning, *Pediatr Emerg Care* 13:98, 1997.

221. Stacpoole PW: Lactic acidosis: the case against bicarbonate therapy, *Ann Intern Med* 105:276, 1986 (editorial).

222. Stanket KS et al: Continuous pulse oximetry in the breath-hold diving women of Korea and Japan, *Undersea Hyperb Med* 20:297, 1993.

223. Sterba JA, Lundgren CEG: Breath-hold duration in man and the diving response induced by face immersion, *Undersea Biomed Res* 15:361, 1988.

224. Stewart RD et al: Influence of mask design on bag-mask ventilation, *Ann Emerg Med* 14:403, 1985.

225. Swann HG, Spafford NR: Body salt and water changes during fresh and sea water drowning, *Texas Rep Biol Med* 9:356, 1951.

226. *Toronto Star*, Aug 10, 1987, p 1.

227. *Toronto Sun*, June 16, 1978, p 2.

228. US Consumer Product Safety Commission and National Spa and Pool Institute: *National Pool and Spa Safety Conference: final report*, May 14, 1985.

229. Van Herringen JR et al: Treatment of the respiratory distress syndrome following nondirect pulmonary trauma with positive end-expiratory pressure, with special emphasis on near-drowning, *Chest* 66:305, 1974.

230. Waugh WH: Potential use of warm butyl alcohol vapor as adjunct agent in the emergency treatment of sea water wet near-drowning, *Am J Emerg Med* 11:20, 1993.

231. Wegener FH, Edwards RM: Cerebral support for near-drowned children in a temperate environment, *Med J Aust* 2:135, 1980.

232. Weil MH et al: Difference in acid-base state between venous and arterial blood during cardiopulmonary resuscitation, *N Engl J Med* 315:153, 1986.

233. Weiss LD et al: The development of a water rescue unit in an urban EMS system, *Ann Emerg Med* 18:884, 1989.

234. Werner JZ et al: No improvement in pulmonary status by gravity drainage or abdominal thrusts after sea water near-drowning in dogs, *Anesthesiology* 57:A81, 1982.

235. Westacott P: A most unlikely patient, *Med J Aust* 2:157, 1980.

236. Yagil Y et al: Near drowning in the Dead Sea: electrolyte imbalance and therapeutic implications, *Arch Intern Med* 145:50, 1985.

237. Yatsu F: Cardiopulmonary-cerebral resuscitation, *N Engl J Med* 314:440, 1986 (editorial).

238. Young RSK, Zalneraitis EL, Dooling EC: Neurological outcome in cold water drowning, *JAMA* 244:1233, 1980.

57 Diving Medicine

Kenneth W. Kizer

More than 70% of Earth's surface is covered by water, but less than 5% of this underwater wilderness has ever been seen by man. Only recently has this last frontier of the planet begun to be explored in a systematic way. Much of this exploration has been possible because of the development of scuba diving.

Scuba diving is an exhilarating and generally safe activity for persons who are healthy, well trained, well conditioned, well equipped and "water wise." It can, however, be a demanding and even dangerous sport because of intrinsic hazards of the underwater environment.

The hazards of scuba diving include the generic problems found in other aquatic activities, such as near drowning, hypothermia, immersion-related skin disorders, water-borne infectious diseases, and hazardous marine life, as well as several relatively unique problems related to the increased atmospheric pressure found under water and the effects of various breathing gases at elevated pressure.

Currently there are many millions of recreational scuba divers around the world, and hundreds of thousands of new divers are certified each year. Scuba diving is conducted in lakes, rivers, quarries, oceans, and almost every other imaginable aquatic setting. Despite the extent of diving activity, scuba-diving fatalities and serious injuries are relatively infrequent. In 1997 the 270 recompression chambers worldwide reporting to the Divers Alert Network reported a total of 972 diving injury cases and 82 fatalities from recreational scuba diving that year.[36] The total number of injuries was roughly similar to other recent years, whereas the number of fatalities was down from 104 in 1995 (but up from 67 in 1991) and less than the 10-year average of 89 deaths per year. Notwithstanding this apparent downward trend in fatalities, concern about the safety of diving continues because of the changing character of the sport-diving population and what is considered to be recreational diving.

In the past 40 years the nature of the scuba-diving population has substantially changed. Scuba divers of the 1950s and 1960s were generally "water people"—well-trained, vigorous athletes experienced in breath-hold diving and competitive swimming. To don a scuba tank and regulator was a natural extension of familiar activity. These early scuba divers seldom encountered problems that required the attention of the general medical community. However, as scuba diving

equipment became more available, adventure-minded persons from all walks of life became attracted to the sport. The popularization of scuba diving in recent years has attracted participants who may be poorly conditioned, have little or no experience in aquatic or other sports, are of advanced age, or have significant underlying medical conditions. Because of the arduous and unforgiving nature of the aquatic environment, such persons may be at increased risk of a diving-related injury or illness. Certain medical conditions are an absolute contraindication to diving.

In the last decade recreational divers have increasingly sought more technically complicated diving in efforts to increase the amount of time they can spend underwater or the depth to which they can dive. Although these diving techniques have been long used in commercial and military diving under controlled conditions, there are significant concerns about the safety of "technical" diving in the much less controlled recreational diving setting.

All primary care physicians should be prepared to answer basic questions about fitness for diving and to initially manage diving-related medical emergencies. Likewise, every emergency medical treatment facility should be prepared to evaluate, provide urgent care and, if needed, arrange transport to a hyperbaric treatment facility (recompression chamber) if a diver is suspected to have decompression sickness or arterial gas embolism.

This chapter focuses primarily on the pressure-related diving syndromes collectively known as *dysbarism;* other conditions relevant to diving are discussed in other chapters (e.g., immersion hypothermia in Chapter 8, hazardous marine life in Chapters 60 to 62, and near-drowning in Chapter 56).

HISTORICAL PERSPECTIVE

Human beings did not evolve for an aquatic existence and are not well adapted for function in the aquatic environment. Nonetheless, they have been breath-hold diving to gather food and other natural resources from the oceans for thousands of years. There is archaeologic evidence that Neanderthal man breath-hold dived 40,000 years ago. The Ama of Japan and Hae-Nyu of Korea have been breath-hold diving to collect edible mollusks and seaweed for about 6000 years. The Indians of southern Patagonia engaged in similar diving practices, and fires along the shores of the Straits of Magellan built to warm these native American divers are believed to be the source of the name "Tierra del Fuego" (Land of Fire) given to the area by Ferdinand Magellan.

Written records of diving for salvage and military purposes date back to around 500 BC, when the Greek historian Herodotus recorded the feats of Scyllis as he dived in the Mediterranean Sea for the Persian king Xerxes during the 50-year war between Greece and Persia. Other colorful accounts of military and salvage divers dot the history of Roman and other early cultures. However, human underwater exploits remained limited to breath-hold diving until about 300 years ago, when a series of technologic developments began to expand human underwater activity. These developments principally involved the use of different types of external air supply to prolong submergence.

In the seventeenth century, primitive bells containing air were carried from the surface, allowing Swedish divers to stay underwater longer than a single breath and to salvage cannons from Stockholm's harbor.[97] In 1690 Sir Edmund Halley devised a leather tube to carry surface air to barrels, which resupplied air to manned bells at a depth of 60 feet. These barrels were submerged, and the air they contained was compressed.[34]

The first practical diving suit was fabricated by Augustus Siebe in 1837.[2,34,97] Atmospheric air was supplied to the diver as compressed air from a manually powered pump on the surface. By 1841 French engineers had developed the technique of using compressed air to keep water and mud out of caissons sunk to the bottom of riverbeds for bridge footings and tunnels. Soon thereafter it was noted that people working in a compressed-air environment sometimes suffered joint pains, paralysis, and other medical problems soon after leaving the caisson. This poorly understood condition was called "caisson's disease" and was the first recognition of what is now known as *decompression sickness*.[98]

Underwater diving remained an esoteric activity having limited commercial and military utility until the 1930s. By that time, and increasingly during World War II, the military importance of submarines and other undersea activities became evident to navies throughout the world. With the development of submarine forces came the need to train men to escape from submarines that became disabled at depth (an all too frequent occurrence in the early days of submarines). Given the shallow operational depths of these early boats, it was usually possible to escape by simply exiting the vessel and ascending to the surface. It was noted early that failure to exhale while ascending through the water led to pulmonary over-pressurization accidents and a new and dramatic syndrome that we now know to be *arterial gas embolism*.

In 1865 the French engineers Rouquayrol and Denayrouse developed a device that could supply air on demand at ambient pressures different from the 1 atm of pressure found at sea level. These inventors were able to supply air on demand at appropriate breathing pressure to persons underwater with a "demand regulator," as it subsequently became known. This device originally required a surface air supply connection.[2] The demand valve regulator was later modified to supply auxiliary oxygen for pilots operating at high altitude. In 1943, while working with the French resistance against Nazi Germany, Jacques-Yves Cousteau and Emile Gagnon combined a demand valve regulator with a compressed air tank, giving rise to what they called "*self-contained underwater breathing apparatus*," or *scuba*.

The potential military usefulness of scuba was immediately recognized and led to a considerable amount of investigation during World War II. As initially configured, scuba was used in an open-circuit mode in which exhaled air was just vented into the water. This was wasteful of the compressed air supply and had other disadvantages for military uses. Further work led to refinement of rebreather scuba devices (both closed and semiclosed circuit systems), such as Lambertsen's amphibious respiratory unit.[8] These rebreather systems conserved the breathing gas by using a carbon dioxide scrubber and recirculating all or part of each exhalation (see rebreather section below). These specialized scuba systems were useful for military purposes because they allowed longer submergence times and could be used in clandestine operations or when disarming pressure-sensitive explosive devices. However, they had a greater risk of mishap, so rebreather systems were not widely used.

After World War II the development and marketing of open-circuit scuba equipment to the general public made the underwater world accessible to growing numbers of people. In the last four decades, scuba diving has opened the underwater world to millions of divers and hundreds of millions of cinema observers. Scuba is now used as a basic tool with myriad commercial, military, scientific, and recreational applications (Box 57-1).[5] The growth of sport diving has been especially noteworthy. For example, since scuba was first introduced into the United States in 1951, it is estimated that over 7 million Americans have been certified as recreational or sport divers.

TYPES OF DIVING AND DIVING EQUIPMENT

There are five general types of diving, each using different equipment and having different logistical support needs. From the least to the most sophisticated equipment used, the types of diving are breath-hold or free diving, scuba diving, surface-supplied or tethered diving, saturation diving, and one atmosphere diving.

Box 57-1 TYPES OF COMMERCIAL DIVING

Harvest of natural resources
    Oil and natural gas
    Minerals
    Fish and shellfish
    Pearls, corals, and shells
    Algae
    Wood (underwater logging)
    Aquaculture
Salvage and recovery operations
Maintenance and construction
    Ship hulls
    Nuclear power plants
    Bridges and tunnels
    Piers and jetties
    Aquariums
    Water treatment plants
    Dams
Underwater photography and motion picture productions
Marine studies
    Biology
    Geology
    Archeology
    Other sciences
Rescue operations
Sport-diving instructors and tour guides

Modified from Kizer KW: Medical aspects of scuba diving. In Noble J, editor: *Textbook of general medicine and primary care*, Boston, 1987, Little, Brown.

Breath-Hold or Free Diving

Breath-hold diving—also known as *free diving, skin diving,* or *snorkeling*—is the simplest and oldest form of underwater diving. It uses no external supply of air, so submergence time is limited to the length of time the diver can hold his or her breath. Generally, the breath-hold diver uses a face mask to facilitate underwater vision, fins for propulsion, a snorkel to breathe air while swimming face down on the water's surface, some sort of attire for thermal protection (e.g., a neoprene wet suit), and sometimes lead weights to counterbalance the positive buoyancy of a wet suit or one's innate positive buoyancy.

Scuba Diving

Scuba diving uses a tank fitted with a pressure regulator that supplies compressed air to the diver at a pressure equal to ambient water pressure. In sport diving, the diver's scuba tank usually contains either 72 or 90 cubic feet of filtered, oil-free compressed air pressurized to about 2200 or 3300 pounds per square inch gauge (PSIG). The regulator employs two stages. The first stage is attached to the tank and makes an initial reduction in pressure to the lower-pressure second stage, which is attached to the diver's mouthpiece and from which the diver actually breathes.

Like the snorkeler, the scuba diver wears a face mask covering the eyes and nose to allow underwater vision, fins for propulsion, snorkel for surface swimming, weight belt, buoyancy-compensating vest to adjust buoyancy under water and for flotation in case of an emergency, diving watch and depth gauge (or a diving computer) to track time and depth underwater, compass, and tank pressure gauge to monitor air consumption. Because of the higher thermal conductivity of water, divers typically wear neoprene wet suits in all but warm tropical waters. These suits maintain a layer of water warmed by body heat between the skin and suit. A nonpermeable "dry suit" and warm undergarments are usually worn when diving in colder water (e.g., colder than 10° C [50° F]).

In addition to the preceding basic equipment, additional equipment may be needed for safety, navigation, communication, or other special purposes (e.g., camera, spear gun, or game bags). All of these objects increase the diver's resistance to movement underwater and decrease efficiency of movement.

Although recreational scuba diving is mostly done using compressed air in an open-circuit mode, special types of scuba gear may be used for mixed-gas diving (see below) or to achieve semiclosed or closed-circuit diving.

Surface-Supplied or Tethered Diving

Surface-supplied or tethered diving includes several different diving technologies, all of which share the common characteristic of the diver's breathing gas (compressed air or mixed gas) being supplied to the diver by hoses from a surface supply or from a diving bell at a pressure equal to water pressure.

The best known form of surface-supplied diving is classic *hardhat diving*, which is sometimes called *mud diving* because it is often done in harbors (which typically have very muddy bottoms). In this type of diving, the diver wears a large bronze helmet with face plates, a canvas suit, weight belt and weighted shoes, and other gear. The gear alone weighs 192 pounds for the typical helmet diver. Surface-supplied diving is most often used for commercial or military purposes. It is frequently performed in very arduous environments having zero visibility (i.e., the diver operates in total darkness, often against a current or surge, performing tasks primarily by feel).

The diving techniques of surface-supplied diving are quite different than those of scuba and they are not further discussed here; however, the unique physiologic and medical problems of surface-supplied divers are identical to those encountered in scuba diving.

Saturation Diving

Once under water, the diver begins to absorb increased amounts of nitrogen or other inert gas, depending on the breathing medium, until a new equilibrium is established according to the pressure of the depth of submergence. In certain deep-diving scenarios, the time needed to off-gas, or "decompress," this inert gas on returning to normal atmospheric pressure may be much greater than the time spent at depth.

In the late 1950s, experiments by U.S. Navy diving medical officers George Bond and Robert Workman coincided with those of Jacques-Yves Cousteau and Edward Link in the commercial sector, all of whom were working on ways to stay under water at great depths long enough to perform useful work.[2] The need for prolonged decompression after deep diving led to the development of saturation diving.

The basic concept of saturation diving is that after approximately 24 hours at any given depth, the diver's tissues have established equilibrium with the gases in the breathing mixture. From that point, the decompression obligation remains the same no matter how long the diver remains at that depth. If the diver can be kept "at pressure" for a prolonged period, the decompression is the same as if he or she were there for only a short time.

Modern saturation complexes allow divers to live for days in large chambers at the pressure of a given work site and to be transported to the underwater site by locking into a personal transfer capsule (PTC) or sealed diving bell. When depth is reached, the water pressure equals the gas pressure within the capsule and divers may exit the PTC into the water while breathing gas supplied by umbilical hoses. To maintain the diver's thermal balance in the very cold water found at great depths, heated water is circulated in special hot-water suits.

Another application of saturation diving, used primarily for scientific purposes, is characterized by the use of underwater habitats (i.e., steel chambers situated at a given depth of water and pressurized with a compressed gas atmosphere at the same pressure as the surrounding water). Divers may live for days or weeks in the habitat, leaving the chamber with scuba equipment to perform studies or observe marine life in its natural state. In this specialized type of diving, rigorous precautions are taken to avoid inadvertent surfacing, thermal stress, and skin and ear infections during prolonged stays in the continuously moist environment of the habitat. Prolonged saturation decompression schedules, often taking several days, are required to return

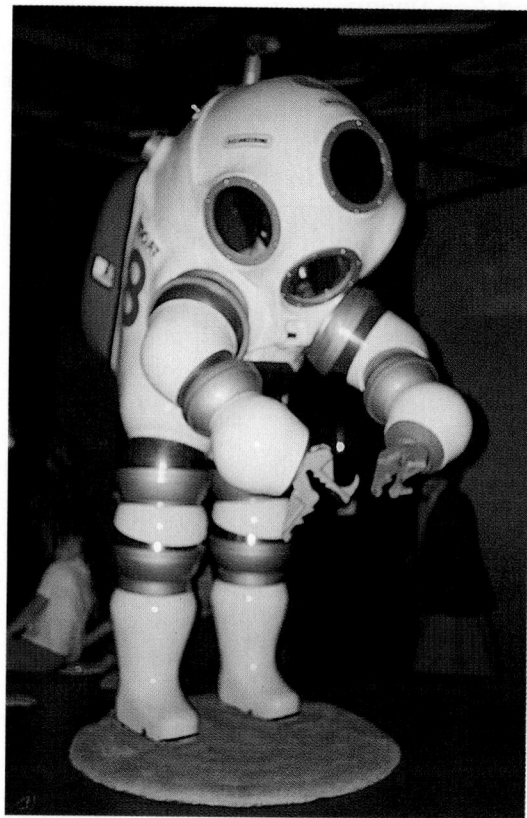

Figure 57-1 JIM diving suit. The diver remains at sea level pressure inside the suit and can work for prolonged periods of time at extreme depths underwater.

divers safely to sea level pressure on completion of the underwater mission.

One-Atmosphere Diving

In recent years it has become clear that humans cannot reliably or safely function at the greatly elevated pressure of deep water, and this has become the limiting factor in human exploration of the ocean depths. This has led to numerous developments in one-atmosphere diving systems. Leonardo de Vinci drafted schematic drawings that look similar to modern one-atmosphere diving systems, but these systems had to await late twentieth century advances in metallurgy, engineering, and communications.

One-atmosphere absolute (ATA) diving systems are, in essence, small submarines with various types of propulsion systems and manipulators that allow the operator to work at great depth. The interior of the unit is maintained with environmental control systems to retain safe physiologic parameters. These systems range from one-person ATA suits in which a diver can "walk" (Figure 57-1) to submersibles that accommodate two or more occupants.

Mixed-Gas Diving

Diving can be done using either compressed air or "mixed gas." Compressed air is most commonly used, especially with scuba, but there are a number of settings where mixed gas is needed or preferred.

Mixed-gas diving refers to diving using a breathing medium other than compressed air (i.e., a gas mixture in which the concentrations of nitrogen and oxygen have been changed or in which a different inert gas [e.g., helium] is substituted for nitrogen). Mixed-gas diving can be used in surface-supplied, saturation, or scuba diving modes, although historically it has been used most often in surface-supplied or saturation diving operations.

Mixed-gas diving has been used for many decades, but because of the greater logistical support it requires and its greater expense and hazards it has been used primarily in commercial and military diving operations. That has changed in the past decade as "technical" sport divers have sought to go deeper and stay down longer.

Enriched Air Nitrox. Nitrox is a breathing-gas mixture containing oxygen and nitrogen in concentrations different from those found in air. More than a dozen different such mixtures have been used by recreational divers, all of which are lumped under the heading "nitrox," but the two most commonly used mixtures are the ones labeled by the National Oceanographic and Atmospheric Administration (NOAA) as Nitrox I (a gas mixture containing 32% oxygen and 68% nitrogen) and Nitrox II (a gas mixture containing 36% oxygen and 64% nitrogen). Each nitrox mixture, or blend, requires its own set of decompression tables and has its own bottom time limits. Only Nitrox I is approved for recreational diving use, and subsequent reference to enriched air nitrox in this chapter is to this mixture.

Of note, the term "nitrox" historically was used to refer to gas mixtures having less than 21% oxygen. These mixtures were used in diving habitats or other saturation diving situations in which one wanted to avoid, or at least lesson, the risk of oxygen toxicity. Technically, if the oxygen percentage is adjusted to greater than 21%, the mixture is called "enriched air nitrox" (EAN), or "oxygen enriched air" (OEA), although "EAN" and "nitrox" are used interchangeably in common diver's parlance.

Beginning in the 1980s an increasing number of recreational divers began using EAN to reduce decompression risk or to extend bottom time (compared with what was possible using compressed air) without incurring additional decompression risk. Although many thousands of recreational EAN divers have been certified over the past decade, its use continues to be closely observed because of safety concerns.

EAN diving enthusiasts typically claim that nitrox is safer than compressed air because it has less risk of decompression sickness (compared with compressed air) for equivalent bottom times. In particular, at depths between 50 and 130 feet of sea water (fsw), EAN allows up to twice the bottom time without required decompression when compared with compressed air. However, this rationale does not constitute a complete analysis of the situation.

Although diving with nitrox may lessen the risk of decompression sickness compared with diving with compressed air, it does not eliminate the risk, and EAN presents additional risks of its own. The main concern is with central nervous system (CNS) oxygen toxicity, which usually manifests suddenly (with few, if any, prodromal symptoms) by loss of consciousness and onset of convulsions. Because of the risk of CNS oxygen toxicity, EAN should not be used below 130 fsw.

A diver can still suffer decompression sickness diving with EAN if he or she stays down too long, surfaces too fast, bypasses a required decompression stop, or uses the wrong nitrox decompression table for the particular breathing medium. Further, although nitrox may increase a diver's allowable no-decompression bottom time, this is usually irrelevant because a diver's bottom time is as much a function of gas supply as the decompression limit. The average scuba diver would exhaust his gas supply long before reaching the no-decompression limit.

Overall, nitrox diving for recreational purposes is still in its infancy, Clearly, it has advantages and disadvantages (Box 57-2), with the advantages being most likely realized in a setting that ensures strict discipline and adherence to safety.

Heliox. Other than nitrox, the most commonly used mixed gas is heliox, or oxy-helium, a mixture of helium and oxygen. Helium is used as the inert gas, replacing nitrogen and part of the oxygen. Use of heliox eliminates nitrogen narcosis and allows the oxygen level to be controlled to reduce the risk of oxygen toxicity. As with nitrox, *heliox* is a generic term that applies to a number of different gaseous blends or mixtures of helium and oxygen.

Because it causes negligible, if any, narcosis and is easier to breathe at greater depths (because of its lesser density), heliox is the preferred gas used in commercial diving at depths over 130 fsw. The major problems with helium are its expense, which precludes its widespread use in recreational diving, and hindrance of speech. In commercial and military settings, helium speech unscramblers are typically used.

Tri-Mix. *Tri-mix* is another generic term, in this instance referring to any mixture of helium, nitrogen, and

Box 57-2   ADVANTAGES AND DISADVANTAGES OF ENRICHED OXYGEN NITROX DIVING COMPARED WITH COMPRESSED AIR AT DEPTHS BETWEEN 50 AND 130 FSW

ADVANTAGES

- Decreased risk of decompression sickness
- Decreased occurrence of nitrogen narcosis
- Reduced residual nitrogen time
- Shorter surface interval times
- Reduced decompression times if maximum bottom time limits are exceeded
- Reduced surface intervals between diving and flying

DISADVANTAGES

- Requires special training
- Requires equipment dedicated for use with nitrox only
- Increased oxidation of scuba cylinders
- Possible increased rate of deterioration of equipment
- Increased fire hazards
- Inability to use air-based dive computers
- Potential for nitrox mixing and filling problems
- Risk of CNS oxygen toxicity

oxygen. This breathing medium was developed by the military for diving operations at depths greater than those possible with air. Helium replaces some of both the nitrogen and oxygen in an effort to eliminate or minimize nitrogen narcosis and to prevent CNS oxygen toxicity. The precise concentrations of helium, nitrogen, and oxygen used in tri-mix vary according to the specific depth profile of the dive. Obviously, in deep diving operations, the percentage of both nitrogen and oxygen will be much less than in air, which means that a "travel" gas mixture is needed for breathing in the shallower depths that must be traversed to get to the depth at which the tri-mix will be used. Currently, the U.S. Navy specifies the use of tri-mix for diving at depths greater than 190 fsw, and tri-mix is typically used in extreme-depth (e.g., greater than 600 fsw) commercial diving.

A spin-off of tri-mix that has begun to be used in recreational diving is oxygen-enriched tri-mix, or *helitrox*. A tri-mix blend commonly used in this setting is 26% oxygen, 17% helium, and 57% nitrogen (TX 26/17). Helitrox advocates promote its use for diving to depths of up to 150 fsw, using either helitrox to decompress or switching to pure oxygen at the 20-fsw decompression stop.

A number of untimely deaths of sport divers have been associated with the use of tri-mix, and its use in recreational diving remains controversial. However, its use is expected to grow in the years ahead, as has occurred with nitrox.

Rebreather Diving

Although most people connect the first self-contained underwater diving with scuba, it was actually first done with the assistance of a rebreather in the 1880s. Rebreathing devices for diving were perfected over the years, but with the advent of scuba in the 1940s, rebreathers were relegated to use in only a few special commercial and military situations. Beginning in the 1990s, however, rebreathers have started to be used increasingly in recreational diving (especially for underwater photography and cave diving).

Conceptually, rebreathers are devices that capture and recirculate a diver's exhaled breath, removing the carbon dioxide added by the body's metabolism and replacing the oxygen extracted by the body before giving the air back to the diver to once again breathe. As a diving technology, rebreathers are much more efficient than open-circuit scuba, and they allow one to dive to greater depths and stay underwater longer than is possible with conventional open-circuit scuba. They are also very useful when exhaled bubbles may be problematic (e.g., when studying or photographing marine life or when disarming a mine). However, they can be quite hazardous if not maintained and operated properly.

All rebreathers have certain elements in common, and all fall into one of four general categories of devices[6]:

1. Closed-circuit oxygen rebreather
2. Closed-circuit mixed-gas rebreather
3. Semiclosed-circuit rebreather using premixed gas
4. Semiclosed-circuit rebreather that mixes the breathing gas on board.

There are many different rebreather designs available, and new systems continue to be developed. Therefore a diver must be individually trained on the use of each rebreather.

SPECIAL DIVING SITUATIONS

Diving in general, and scuba diving in particular, has become a tool that allows humans to engage in a wide array of underwater activities (see Box 57-1). There are a number of special diving situations.

Under-Ice and Cold-Water Diving

Diving under the ice in extremely cold environments is done for exploration, search and rescue, salvage, inspections, research, and other work. This takes place in lakes, rivers, and polar regions. Besides meticulous preparation and provision of thermal protection for the diver under ice, extremely low temperature, wind, and snow above water at the dive site necessitate careful planning for topside shelter. For diving in such cold water, dry suits or hot-water suits are used. Dry suits are made of closed-cell foam neoprene, rubber, or rubberized canvas and fit loosely on the body, with seals at the wrists, ankles, and neck to keep the diver and insulating underwear dry and to allow admission of air to maintain equal suit volume during the dive. Free-flooding hot-water suits are loosely fitted, closed-cell foam neoprene suits with hoses inside to allow warm water to flow continuously over the diver's body and exit at the wrist and neck.[109] In this specialized type of diving, other considerations are provision of breathing regulators that are not likely to freeze, planning for immediate rescue and rapid rewarming of an individual who might fall into the frigid water without adequate protection, maintenance of adequate nutrition and hydration, and total prohibition of alcoholic beverages or mind-altering drugs at the dive operation because these activities permit little margin for error.

Cave and Cavern Diving

The advent of scuba has allowed exploration of many underwater caverns and cave systems, leading to important archaeologic and geologic discoveries. However, cave diving is the most dangerous form of diving.[54]

To trained, experienced, and properly equipped cave divers, the number of cave-diving fatalities (over 300 in Florida alone since 1960) is distressing, although generally explainable. Most fatalities have involved inexperienced recreational scuba divers who were never formally trained in cave diving. Most often, the divers became lost and ran out of air while in a cave. The National Association of Cave Divers (NACD) and the National Speleological Society-Cave Diving Section (NSS-CDS) are the recognized training organizations for cave diving.

Because cave divers are separated from the outside world and cannot simply surface in case of an emergency, specific equipment and procedures are required. These include double tanks, meticulous planning of air consumption, backup lights, and guide cables to avoid becoming lost. No one should attempt cave diving without completing formal training approved by either the NACD or the NSS-CDS.

River Diving

Diving in rivers is often done by public safety personnel in search of evidence or to retrieve bodies (usually drowning victims). Because of the typically poor visibility, strong currents, and potential for entanglement in debris, this type of diving should be done only by persons who have been trained in the special techniques of river diving and who have proper surface support.

Miscellaneous Other Settings

Diving is undertaken for a variety of special purposes in settings that pose unique hazards. Examples of these settings include nuclear power plants, harbors with toxic chemical or infectious disease contamination, water treatment facilities, and dams generating electric power. Each of these settings requires special diving techniques, health monitoring, and safety precautions.

DYSBARISM

Divers encounter many adverse environmental conditions underwater. These include cold, changes in light transmission and sound conduction, lack of air to breathe, increased density of the surrounding environment, and increased atmospheric pressure. Not surprisingly, diverse medical problems are related to diving (Box 57-3).

Of the various environmental factors affecting divers, pressure is by far the most important because it contributes either directly or indirectly to the majority of serious diving-related medical problems.

Box 57-3 MEDICAL PROBLEMS OF SCUBA DIVERS

Environmental exposure problems
  Motion sickness
  Near drowning
  Hypothermia
  Heat illness
  Sunburn
  Phototoxic and photoallergic reactions
  Irritant and other dermatitides
  Infectious diseases
  Mechanical trauma
Dysbarism
  Barotrauma
  Dysbaric air embolism
  Decompression sickness
  Dysbaric osteonecrosis
  Dysbaric retinopathy
  Hyperbaric cephalgia
Breathing gas-related problems
  Inert gas narcosis
  Hypoxia
  Oxygen toxicity
  Hypercapnia
  Carbon monoxide poisoning
  Lipoid pneumonitis
Hazardous marine life
Miscellaneous
  Hyperventilation
  Hearing loss
  Carotid-related blackout
  Panic and other psychologic problems

Therefore understanding the basic physics and physiologic effects of pressure is essential to treating the pressure-related maladies that fall under the general term *dysbarism*.

Definitions and Terminology

Dysbarism is a term that encompasses all the pathologic conditions caused by altered environmental pressure. These disorders primarily affect divers and persons who work in compressed-air environments, who are also exposed to increased atmospheric pressure; however, some of the conditions may also occur in aviators, astronauts, and certain types of industrial workers as a result of abrupt exposure to the reduced pressure found at actual or simulated high altitude.

Dysbarism most often develops acutely because of problems caused by the mechanical effects of pressure on closed air spaces *(barotrauma)* or problems caused by breathing gases at elevated partial pressure (such as *nitrogen narcosis* or *decompression sickness).* Less often, clinical effects are delayed for months or years, as in the case of dysbaric osteonecrosis; the pathophysiology of these conditions is less well understood.

Pressure is defined as force per unit area. *Atmospheric pressure* is the pressure exerted by the air above the earth's surface. Atmospheric pressure varies with altitude. At sea level, atmospheric pressure is 760 millimeters of mercury (mm Hg) or 14.7 pounds per square inch (PSI). The barometric pressure at sea level is generally referred to as 1 atmosphere (atm). *Absolute pressure* is the total barometric pressure at any point. With pressure gauges calibrated to read zero at sea level, gauge pressure is the amount of pressure greater than atmospheric pressure. In general, gauge pressure is 1 atm less than absolute atmospheric pressure. It is always important to specify whether pressure is expressed in terms of gauge or absolute pressure. Except in situations requiring laboratory precision, the following units are commonly used to express water pressure:

- Feet of seawater (fsw)
- Feet of fresh water (ffw)
- Atmospheres absolute (ATA)
- Pounds per square inch gauge (psig)
- Pounds per square inch absolute (psia)

As a diver descends under water, absolute pressure increases much faster than in air. Each foot of seawater exerts a force of 0.445 psig. Therefore if the 14.7 psi pressure of 1 atm is divided by 0.445 psi per foot of seawater, at 33 fsw the absolute pressure will have doubled. In the ocean, each 33 feet of depth adds one additional atmosphere of pressure. The gauge pressure at 33 fsw is 14.7 psig (in excess of atmospheric pressure), and the absolute pressure is 29.4 psia.

Because of the weight of solutes in seawater, it is slightly heavier than fresh water. In fresh water, 34 feet equals one additional atmosphere of pressure.

Pressure change with increasing depth is linear, although the greatest relative change in pressure per unit of depth change occurs nearest the surface. Table 57-1 lists commonly used units of pressure measurement in seawater.

When a diver submerges, the force of the tremendous weight of the water above is exerted over the entire body. Except for air-containing spaces such as the lungs, paranasal sinuses, intestines, and middle ears, the body behaves as a liquid. The law that describes the behavior of pressure in liquids is named for the seventeenth century scientist Blaise Pascal. Pascal's law states that a pressure applied to any part of a fluid is transmitted equally throughout the fluid. Thus when a diver reaches 33 fsw, the pressure on the surface of the skin and throughout the body tissues is 29.4 psia or 1520 mm Hg (Figure 57-2). The diver's body is generally unaware of this pressure, except in the air-containing spaces of the body. The gases in these spaces obey Boyle's law (Figure 57-3), which states that the pressure of a given quantity of gas for which temperature remains unchanged varies inversely with its volume. Thus air in the middle ear, paranasal sinuses, lungs, and gastrointestinal tract is reduced in volume during compression or descent under water. Inability to maintain gas pressure in these body spaces equal to the surrounding water pressure leads to various untoward mechanical effects, which are discussed later.

Because of the weight of the water exerting pressure over the chest wall, humans can breathe surface air through a snorkel or tube connected to the surface for only a short distance underwater, typically only to a depth of 1 to 2 feet. Attempts to breathe at greater depths through the tube are not only impossible but

TABLE 57-1. Commonly Used Units of Pressure in the Underwater Environment

DEPTH (fsw)	PSIG	PSIA	ATA	mm Hg (ABSOLUTE)
Sea level	0.0	14.7	1	760
33	14.7	29.4	2	1520
66	29.4	44.1	3	2280
99	44.1	58.8	4	3040
132	58.8	73.5	5	3800
165	73.5	88.2	6	4560
198	88.2	102.9	7	5320
231	102.9	117.6	8	6080
264	117.6	132.3	9	6840
297	132.2	147.0	10	7600

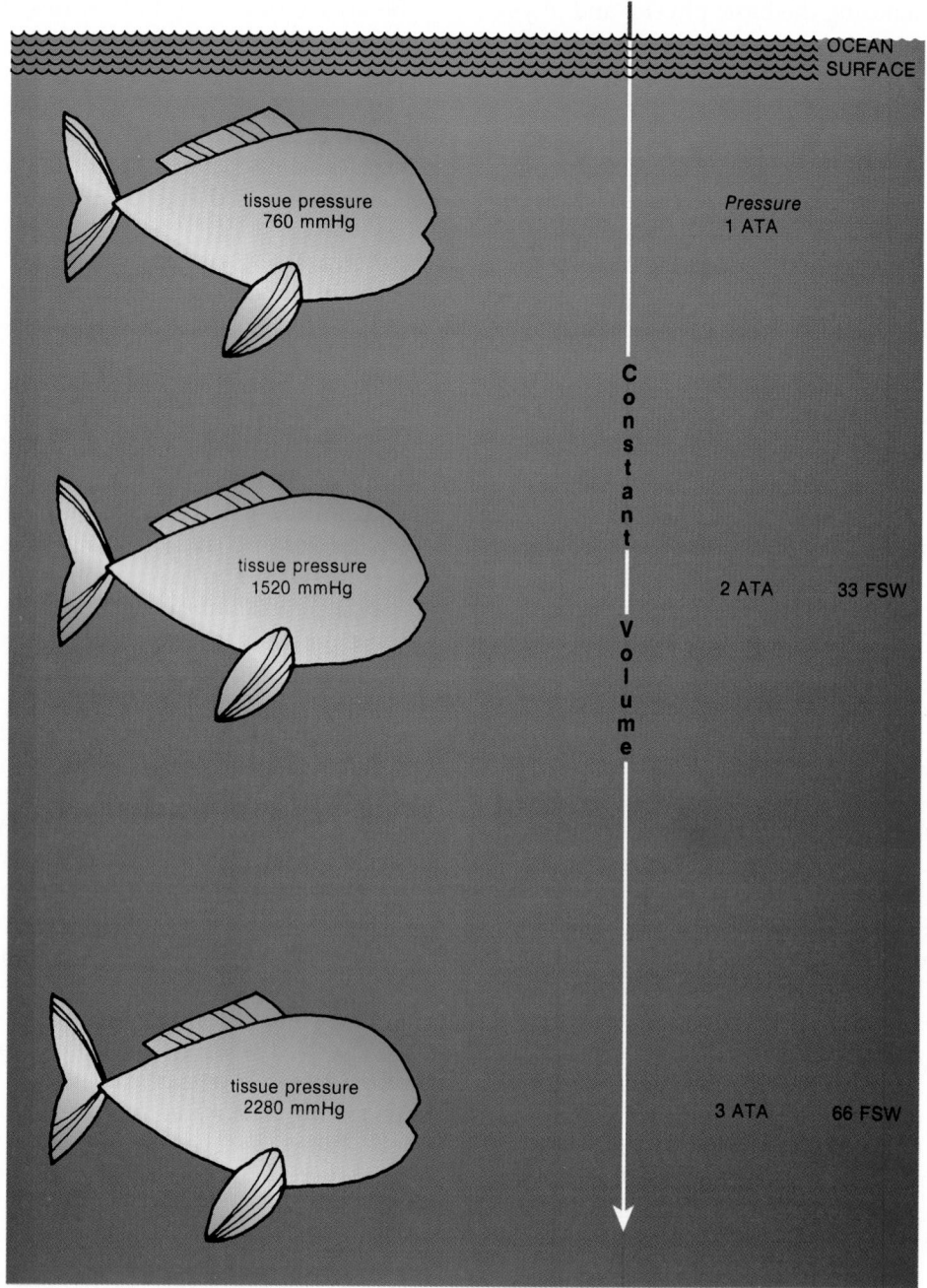

Figure 57-2 Pascal's law. Pressure applied to any part of a fluid is transmitted equally throughout the fluid.

dangerous, because the respiratory effort greatly augments the already physiologic negative-pressure breathing. In other words, when the respiratory muscles are relaxed at sea level, alveolar pressure is equal to surrounding air pressure. At a depth of 1 foot, the total water pressure on the chest wall is nearly 200 pounds. Because of the loss of normal chest expansion and the pressurization of intraalveolar air, the diver has to use forceful negative-pressure breathing to draw surface air into the lungs through the tube. Even at a depth of 1 foot, the great respiratory effort required is rapidly fatiguing, and respiration becomes impossible at further depths of only a few inches. Forced negative-pressure breathing can ultimately result in pulmonary capillary damage, with intraalveolar edema or hemorrhage. Symptoms include dyspnea and hemoptysis. Should this occur, there is no specific treatment; therapy is purely supportive.

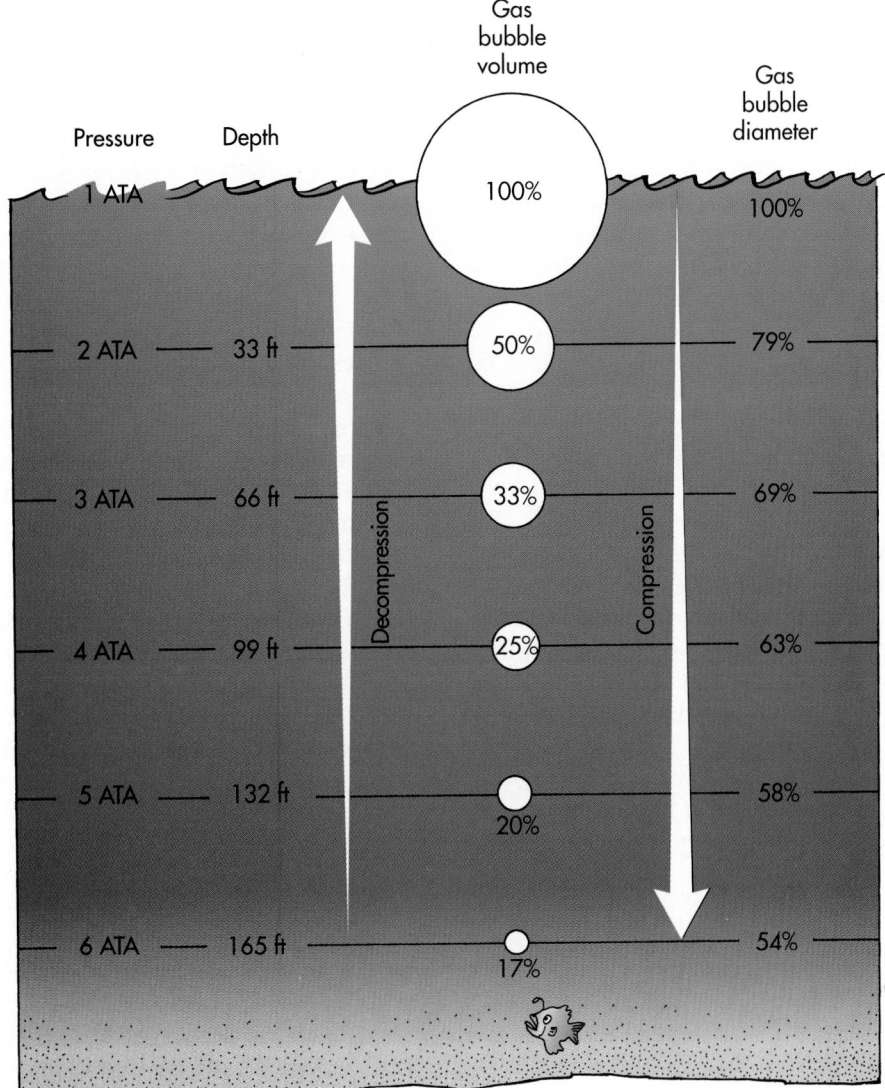

Figure 57-3 Boyle's law. The volume of a given quantity of gas at constant temperature varies inversely with pressure: $P_1V_1 = P_2V_2$.

BAROTRAUMA

Gas pressure in the various air-filled spaces of the body is normally in equilibrium with the environment. However, if anything obstructs the passageways of gas exchange for these spaces and a change in ambient pressure occurs, a pressure disequilibrium develops. The tissue damage resulting from such pressure imbalance is known as *barotrauma*.

Overall, barotrauma is the most common medical problem in scuba diving, potentially involving any structure or combination of structures that leads to entrapment of gas in a closed space. This may include skin trapped under a fold in a dry suit, the portion of the face under a face mask, ears, paranasal sinuses, lungs, and gastrointestinal tract.

Specific Types of Barotrauma

Mask Squeeze. For humans to see underwater, an airspace must be present between the eye and water. In scuba diving, this is created by use of a face mask consisting of tempered safety glass in a soft malleable mask that seals across the forehead, on the sides of the face, and under the nose to allow nasal exhalations to maintain air pressure inside the mask equal to water pressure during descent. If inexperience or inattention causes the diver to forget to maintain this balance, negative pressure in the mask can rupture capillaries, causing skin ecchymoses and conjunctival hemorrhage. This condition is known as *mask squeeze* (see Figure 22-19). Such a pressure imbalance could be especially dangerous after keratotomy because of the slow healing rate of corneal incisions.[30]

Ear Canal Squeeze. A tight-fitting wet-suit hood can trap air in the external auditory canal and potentially lead to a painful *external ear squeeze* during descent as the volume of air is reduced according to Boyle's law. This problem can be prevented by remembering to break the seal to allow water to fill the external ear canal before descent. External ear squeeze also can occur if the canal is blocked by cerumen, exostoses, or ear plugs (which should never be worn when diving).

Symptoms and signs of ear canal squeeze include pain, swelling, erythema, petechiae, or hemorrhagic blebs of the ear canal wall. In very severe (and very rare) cases, the tympanic membrane can rupture from the negative pressure in the ear canal. If this occurs, further diving is contraindicated until the membrane has healed (as discussed below).

Barotitis Media or Middle Ear Squeeze. Referred to in diver parlance as ear *squeeze*, barotitis media is the most common medical problem in scuba diving, probably affecting more than 40% of divers.[53] The problem is a direct application of Boyle's law (Figure 57-4), potentially compounded by the structure of the eustachian tube.

As previously noted, Boyle's law describes the inverse relationship of pressure and volume in an enclosed airspace. It also explains why the greatest relative volume change for a given depth change occurs near the surface, which is why the greatest risk of middle ear squeeze occurs near the surface.

Because each foot of seawater exerts a pressure of about 23 mm Hg, a diver who descends 2.5 feet and does not equalize the pressure in his or her middle ear will develop a relative vacuum in the middle ear because of the contraction of air volume in the ear. Typically the diver notices slight pain at a 60-mm Hg pressure differential between air in the middle ear and ambient water pressure. This pressure differential causes the tympanic membrane to stretch and bulge inward, causing increasing discomfort and eventually severe pain. At a depth of 4 feet, a 90-mm Hg pressure differential is generated, and the unsupported, flutter-valve medial third of the eustachian tube collapses and becomes obstructed. At this point, attempts to autoinflate the middle ear by Valsalva or Frenzel maneuvers may be unsuccessful. The diver must ascend to equalize middle ear pressure with ambient environmental pressure.

The Valsalva maneuver involves blowing with an open glottis against closed lips and nostrils to increase pressure in the nasopharynx to inflate the middle ear through the eustachian tube. This may force open a collapsed eustachian tube. The Frenzel maneuver is performed by swallowing with a closed glottis while the lips are closed and the nostrils are pinched.

If a diver does not heed the symptoms of barotitis media and allows the pressure differential to reach 100 to 400 mm Hg (i.e., at depths of 4.3 to 17.4 feet), the pressure imbalance may be unsatisfactorily resolved by rupture of the tympanic membrane.[50] In such a case, the problem for the diver may be compounded by entry of cold water into the middle ear. This may cause severe vertigo. Before this event, serum may have been drawn into the middle ear by the relative vacuum, causing serous otitis media.

Prevention is the key in dealing with barotitis media. Divers who understand the sequence just described generally take steps to inflate the middle ear immediately on submerging and thereby avoid the entire sequence as they descend in the water. If middle ear pressure is kept equal to or greater than water pressure, no problem should occur. However, if the diver forgets to inflate the middle ear or suffers from eustachian-tube dysfunction (caused by mucosal congestion secondary to upper respiratory infection, allergies, smoking, mucosal polyps, excessively vigorous autoinflation maneuvers, or previous maxillofacial trauma), middle ear barotrauma may occur. This most often happens just after the diver leaves the surface, with the diver complaining of ear fullness or pain. Generally, the pain rapidly becomes so severe that the diver either corrects the problem or aborts the dive.

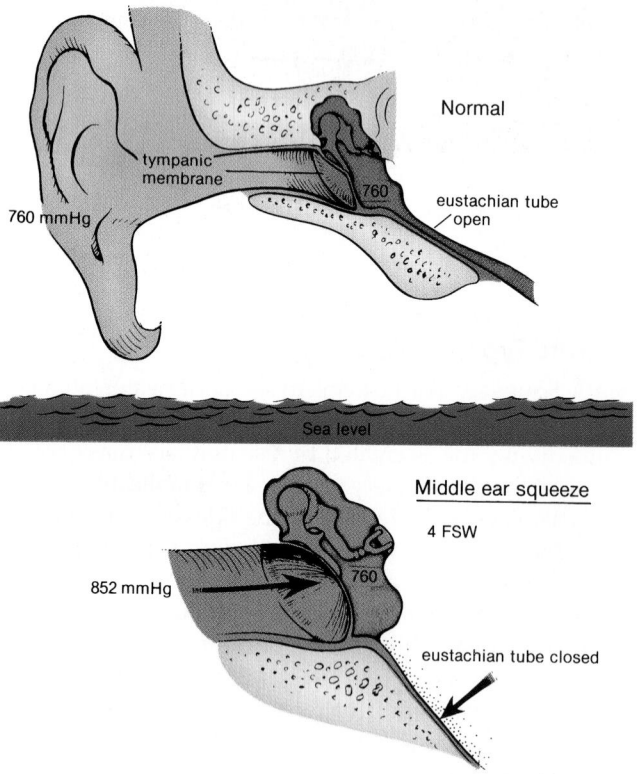

Figure 57-4 Middle ear barotrauma. Symptoms include fullness and pain caused by stretching of the tympanic membrane.

The otoscopic appearance of the tympanic membrane in cases of barotitis media varies with the severity of the injury. A commonly used grading scheme is the Teed classification, which grades the severity according to the amount of hemorrhage in the tympanic membrane.[45] Grade 0 is for symptoms only (i.e., pain without any physical stigmata); grade 1 is for erythema over the malleus; grade 2 is for erythema of the malleus plus mild or spotty hemorrhage within the tympanic membrane; grade 3 is for gross hemorrhage throughout the tympanic membrane; grade 4 is for free blood in the middle ear; and grade 5 is for free blood in the middle ear plus perforation of the tympanic membrane. Each higher grade tends to be more painful than the preceding one, except for grade 5, which may be relatively painless. With grade 5, the cessation of pain corresponds with the membrane tearing, which immediately equalizes the pressure in the middle ear with the external environment. Use of this grading scheme facilitates communication when describing these injuries.

In addition to having an abnormal-appearing tympanic membrane, persons with barotitis media occasionally have a small amount of bloody drainage around the nose or mouth and mild conductive hearing loss.

Middle ear squeeze should be treated with decongestants and analgesics. Antihistamines may be used if the eustachian-tube dysfunction has an allergic component. Divers should abstain from diving until the condition has resolved. Combining an oral decongestant with a long-acting topical nasal spray (such as 0.5% oxymetazoline or phenylephrine) for the first few days is usually most effective. Repeated gentle autoinflation of the middle ear by use of the Frenzel maneuver also can help to displace any collection of middle ear fluid through the eustachian tube. Antibiotics (such as amoxicillin-clavulanic acid) should be used when there is a tympanic membrane rupture or preexisting infection. If the tympanic membrane has ruptured, no diving should be done until it is fully healed or a surgical repair is successful, and until eustachian-tube function allows easy autoinflation.

Most cases of barotitis media resolve without complication in 3 to 7 days, although occasionally it takes longer. The condition can be prevented if a diver refrains from diving when unable to easily equalize pressure in the ears and heeds the warning symptoms of ear pain.

Barosinusitis. Barosinusitis, or *sinus squeeze*, results from essentially the same mechanism as barotitis media but is less common (Figure 57-5). If there is inability to maintain the air pressure in any paranasal sinus during descent, a relative vacuum develops in the sinus cavity. This initially produces intense pain, then damage to the sinus wall mucosa, with bleeding into the sinus. Less commonly, a reverse sinus squeeze can occur on ascent in the water. In this condition, pain is produced by relatively high air pressure in the sinus. This usually occurs in the setting of a diver who has an upper respiratory infection or severe allergies and who has taken a decongestant some time before diving but in whom the vasoconstricting effect wears off while at depth.

Prevention of barosinusitis requires avoidance of diving with an upper respiratory infection or while allergic rhinitis is causing edema of the mucosa about the sinus orifices, and when sinusitis, nasal polyps, or any other condition is present that impairs free flow of air from sinus cavity to nose. Treatment involves use of systemic (e.g., pseudoephedrine) and topical (e.g., phenylephrine or oxymetazoline) vasoconstrictors, analgesics, abstinence from diving until resolved, and antihistamines if needed. Antibiotics may be needed in the event of a severe squeeze with bleeding into the sinus cavity or in cases of frontal sinusitis.

Barodontalgia. One of the most infrequent yet dramatic types of barotrauma is *barodontalgia*, or *tooth squeeze*; this is sometimes called *aerodontalgia*. This painful condition is caused by entrapped gas in the interior of a tooth or in the structures surrounding a

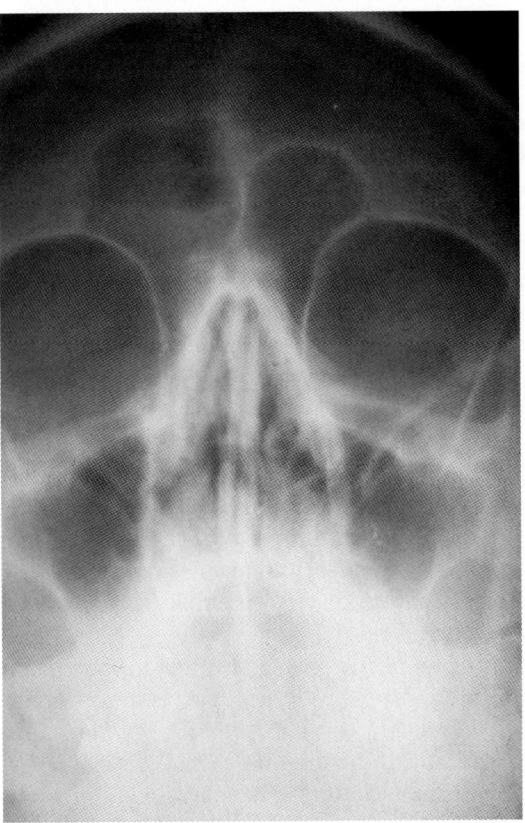

Figure 57-5 Frontal sinus barotrauma 3 days earlier. Note the persistent air-fluid level. *(Kenneth W. Kizer, MD.)*

tooth. The confined gas develops either positive or negative pressure relative to ambient pressure, which exerts force on the surrounding sensitive dental structures and causes pain.

Barodontalgia may be caused by an array of dental conditions, including caries, defective restorations, oral tissue lacerations, recent extractions, periodontal abscesses, pulpal or apical lesions or cysts, and endodontal (root canal) therapy. If a pocket of trapped air remains at sea level pressure while ambient pressure increases during descent, the tooth can implode or the cavity can fill with blood. Conversely, air that is forced into a tooth during descent can expand during ascent, causing the tooth to explode. To prevent barodontalgia, a diver should wait at least 24 hours after dental treatment (including fillings) before diving.

Other causes of tooth pain associated with pressure changes are less well understood. Pulpitis or other dental infections can produce pain during a dive. Of course, upper tooth pain associated with pressure changes should raise a question about a pathologic condition in the maxillary sinus.

Labyrinthine Window Rupture. A serious but relatively unusual form of aural barotrauma is *inner ear barotrauma* causing *labyrinthine window rupture*. This is the most serious form of aural barotrauma because of possible injury to the cochleovestibular system that may lead to permanent deafness or vestibular dysfunction.[43,49]

Inner ear barotrauma results from rapid development of markedly different pressures between the middle and inner ear, such as may occur from an overly forceful Valsalva maneuver or an exceptionally rapid descent, during which middle ear pressure is not adequately equalized. The pressure disequilibrium may cause several types of injury to the cochleovestibular apparatus, including hemorrhage within the inner ear; rupture of Reissner's membrane, leading to mixing of endolymph and perilymph; fistulation of the oval or round window, with development of a perilymph leak; or a mixed injury involving any or all of these things.[95]

The classic triad of symptoms indicating inner ear barotrauma is roaring tinnitus, vertigo, and hearing loss. In addition, a feeling of fullness or "blockage" of the affected ear, nausea, vomiting, nystagmus, pallor, diaphoresis, disorientation, or ataxia may be present in varying degree.

Symptoms of inner ear barotrauma may develop immediately after the injury or may be delayed for hours, depending on the specific damage and the diver's activities during and after the dive. Vigorous isometric exercise after a dive may complete an incipient or partial membrane rupture. Findings on physical examination may be normal or may reveal signs of middle ear barotrauma or vestibular dysfunction. Audiometry may demonstrate mild to severe sensorineural hearing loss.

Hemorrhage within the inner ear is usually associated with findings of middle ear barotrauma, absent or transient vestibular symptoms, and diffuse mild to severe sensorineural hearing loss. Patients should be treated with bed rest (with the head elevated to 30 degrees), avoidance of any strenuous activity, and symptomatic measures as needed. There is a good prognosis for full recovery of hearing in 3 to 12 weeks. Patients with a tear in Reissner's membrane have manifestations similar to those with inner-ear hemorrhage, although there will be persistent localized sensorineural hearing loss commensurate with the area of membrane tear. The management is the same.

A patient with a perilymph fistula usually has high-frequency sensorineural hearing loss or marked cochleovestibular dysfunction and little evidence of middle ear barotrauma. Initially, he or she should be treated with bed rest, avoidance of strain, and symptomatic measures, although some authorities advocate immediate tympanotomy if severe symptoms are present. In all cases, however, deterioration of hearing, worsening of vestibular symptoms, or persistence of significant vestibular symptoms after a few days heralds the need for detailed otolaryngologic evaluation and probable surgical exploration and repair.

A diagnostic dilemma exists whenever a diver complains of vertigo, tinnitus, and hearing loss associated with a dive. These symptoms are classic for labyrinthine rupture, in which case recompression is contraindicated because of the potential for further barotrauma to worsen the injury. Conversely, these symptoms may indicate a diagnosis of inner ear decompression sickness, which requires expeditious treatment in a hyperbaric chamber. In such cases the most important differential feature for diagnostic use on a dive boat or other diving site is a careful history as to time of onset and dive activities preceding the onset of symptoms. If symptom onset was during descent and ear clearing was difficult or impossible, requiring forcible Valsalva maneuvers, perilymph fistula is more likely. If the onset was during or after a decompression dive, decompression sickness must be assumed and chamber treatment sought. In some cases, however, it simply is not possible to rule out decompression sickness, or rarely, air embolism, and a "trial of pressure" in the recompression chamber may be necessary.

Alternobaric Vertigo. An unusual type of aural barotrauma is *alternobaric vertigo* (ABV). This usually occurs with ascent and is caused by sudden development of unequal middle ear pressure, which causes asymmetric vestibular stimulation and resultant pronounced vertigo.[83] Although usually only transient and requiring no treatment, ABV may precipitate a panic response leading to near drowning, pulmonary barotrauma and resultant air embolism, or other serious injury. Rarely, alternobaric vertigo lasts for several hours or days, in which case it should be treated symptomatically after excluding inner ear barotrauma.

Suit Squeeze. If an area of the diver's skin becomes trapped under a fold or wrinkle of a dry suit, causing a closed airspace, the pressure-induced contraction of air under the fold, and resulting partial vacuum, can cause transudation of blood through the skin. This is unusual and generally benign, although the resultant skin ecchymosis may have a dramatic appearance. *Suit squeeze* requires no treatment and resolves in a few days to a couple of weeks.

Lung Squeeze. *Lung squeeze* is a very unusual form of barotrauma that has been observed with breath-hold diving. Persons having this syndrome complain of shortness of breath and dyspnea after surfacing from a deep (greater than 100 FSW) breath-hold dive. The diver may cough up frothy blood, and a chest radiograph may show pulmonary edema. The condition is treated with supplemental oxygen and respiratory support as needed. Symptoms typically resolve within a few days.

The classic understanding of lung squeeze is that it occurs when a diver descends to a depth at which total lung volume (TLV) is reduced to less than residual volume (RV), at which point transpulmonic pressure exceeds intraalveolar pressure, causing transudation of fluid or frank blood (from rupture of pulmonary capillaries) and the overt manifestations of pulmonary edema and hypoxemia.

According to this scenario, a breath-hold diver with a TLV of 6000 ml and an RV of 1200 ml could dive to only 6000/1200 or 5 ATA (equal to 132 FSW) before lung squeeze would occur. However, breath-hold divers have dived much deeper without apparent problem.

In 1968 Schaefer and associates[104] reported that breath-hold divers pool their blood centrally, accumulating a central volume increase of as much as 1047 ml at 90 FSW. If it is assumed that this adjustment in pulmonary blood volume reduces the RV, then theoretically it should be possible for the diver with a TLV of 6000 ml to breath-hold to 6000/(1200 to 1047) or almost 40 ATA. Although Gianluca Grenoni's 1997 world record breath-hold dive to 395 FSW seems to support the beneficial effect of central pooling of blood, cases of lung squeeze continue to occur at much shallower depths. The exact pathophysiology of this condition remains unclear. Fortunately, it occurs very infrequently.

Underwater Blast Injury. Barotrauma can be caused by underwater explosions. Shock waves from a blast are propagated farther in the dense medium of water than in air.[24] Underwater explosions may result from ordnance or ignition of explosive gases during cutting or welding operations.

Underwater blasts can cause serious injuries to divers. Air-containing body cavities such as the lungs, intestines, ears, and sinuses are most vulnerable. Pneumothorax, pneumomediastinum, and air embolism may result from laceration of the lung and pleura.[62] There may be intestinal perforation, subserosal hemorrhage, and subsequent peritonitis. The occurrence of air embolism at depth, which worsens with decompression, requires treatment by recompression, if possible. Otherwise, management of underwater blast injuries is no different than for terrestrial blast injury.

Gastrointestinal Barotrauma. Because the intestines are pliable, contraction of intraluminal bowel gas during descent does not cause barotrauma. In unusual situations, however, expanding gas can become trapped in the gastrointestinal tract during ascent and cause gastrointestinal barotrauma, which is also known as *aerogastralgia*, or gas in the gut.[26,82] This infrequent condition has been noted most often in novice divers, who are more prone to aerophagia; in divers who repeatedly perform the Valsalva maneuver in the head-down position, which may force air into the stomach, or who chew gum while diving; and in divers who consume large quantities of carbonated beverages or legumes shortly before diving.

Divers with gastrointestinal barotrauma typically complain of abdominal fullness, colicky abdominal pain, belching, and flatulence. Rarely, syncope has been reported and is presumed to result from a combination of decreased venous return and vagal reflexes. Most often the physical examination of divers having symptoms of gastrointestinal barotrauma is normal because the condition typically resolves by the time medical care is obtained. However, abdominal distention, tympany, and abdominal tenderness may be seen. In extreme cases there may even be signs of cardiovascular compromise as a result of obstruction of venous return.[44]

Gastrointestinal barotrauma is most often self-remedied by elimination of the excess gas. Recompression may be necessary in severe cases, but this is exceedingly rare.

Pulmonary Barotrauma of Ascent (Pulmonary Over-Pressurization Syndrome). The most serious type of barotrauma is pulmonary barotrauma of ascent, which results from expansion of gas trapped in the lungs. If a diver does not allow the expanding gas to escape, it ruptures alveoli, producing a spectrum of injuries collectively referred to as *pulmonary overpressurization syndrome* (POPS), or burst lung. Basically, POPS is a dramatic clinical demonstration of Boyle's law.

Divers suffering pulmonary overpressurization typically give a history of rapid and uncontrolled ascent to the surface before the onset of symptoms (e.g., as a result of running out of air, panic, or sudden development of uncontrolled positive buoyancy, such as a dropped weight belt or inadvertent inflation of the buoyancy compensator). However, localized overinflation of the lung from focally increased elastic recoil may also occur in divers who ascend at a proper rate.[25]

It is important to remember that the purpose of all diving regulators is to keep intrapulmonic pressure equal to surrounding water pressure, thus avoiding negative-pressure breathing. As long as these pressures are equal, the diver is relatively unaware of the surrounding crushing water pressure and no problems occur. In this regard, three additional factors have clinical importance:

1. There is significant change in barometric pressure in shallow water. Boyle's law dictates greater volume changes for a given change in depth near the surface than at greater depths. Thus shallow depths are the most dangerous for breath-holding ascents.
2. A pressure differential of only 80 mm Hg (alveolar air) above ambient water pressure on the chest wall, or about 3 to 4 feet of depth, is adequate to force air bubbles across the alveolar-capillary membrane.
3. Fatal pulmonary overpressure accidents have occurred from breath-holding during ascent from a depth as shallow as 4 feet of water.

If a given intrapulmonary gas volume is trapped by forcible breath-holding or a closed glottis, or even in a small portion of the lung by bronchospasm during ascent, intrapulmonary volume increases (according to Boyle's law) until the elastic limit of the chest wall is reached. After that, intrapulmonary pressure rises until, at a positive differential pressure of about 80 mm Hg, air is forced across the pulmonary capillary membrane. This air usually enters either the pulmonary interstitial spaces or the pulmonary capillaries.

The diagnosis of POPS is based on the development of characteristic symptoms after diving. The actual clinical manifestations may take several forms, including pneumomediastinum, subcutaneous emphysema, pneumopericardium, pneumothorax, pneumoperitoneum, and pulmonary interstitial emphysema. Diffuse alveolar hemorrhage has been described as a rare manifestation of pulmonary barotrauma.[3] Systemic arterial gas embolism resulting from gas leaking into ruptured pulmonary veins is the most feared complication of POPS.

The specific clinical manifestations of POPS depend on the location and amount of air that escapes into an extraalveolar location.

Mediastinal Emphysema. Mediastinal emphysema is the most common form of POPS, resulting from pulmonary interstitial air dissecting along bronchi to the mediastinum. In these cases the diver usually has gradually increasing hoarseness, neck fullness, and substernal chest pain several hours after diving. Subcutaneous emphysema may be present. In severe cases, the diver may complain of marked chest pain, dyspnea, and dysphagia. Syncope may occur. Radiographs may show extraalveolar air in the neck, mediastinum, or both, although radiographs are rarely necessary to make the diagnosis.

Treatment of mediastinal emphysema and most other forms of POPS is conservative, consisting of rest, avoidance of further pressure exposure (including flying in commercial aircraft), and observation. Supplemental oxygen administration may be useful in severe cases. Recompression is indicated only in extraordinarily severe cases because it carries a risk of causing further barotrauma and worsening the situation.

Pneumothorax. Pneumothorax is an infrequent manifestation of diving-related pulmonary overpressurization because it requires that air be vented through the visceral pleura, a path generally having greater resistance than air tracking through the interstitium. Despite being infrequent, pneumothorax must be considered and excluded whenever POPS is suspected.

In cases of diving-related pneumothorax, the diver usually complains of pleuritic chest pain, breathlessness, and dyspnea, just as in cases of pneumothorax from any other cause. Radiographs may confirm the diagnosis. It is treated in the standard fashion with tube thoracostomy in all but trivial cases.

A diver with an untreated pneumothorax should not be recompressed except in dire circumstances, and then only if tube thoracostomy will be completed before decompression begins. Because the intrapleural gas of a pneumothorax cannot be vented to the environment, it may convert to a lethal tension pneumothorax during depressurization from hyperbaric treatment.

ARTERIAL GAS EMBOLISM

Arterial gas embolism (AGE), also known as *dysbaric air embolism* and *cerebral air embolism*, is the most feared complication of POPS. AGE is one of the most dramatic and serious injuries associated with compressed-air diving and is a major cause of death and disability among sport divers.[72]

AGE results from air bubbles entering the pulmonary venous circulation from ruptured alveolae. When air is introduced into the pulmonary capillary blood, gas bubbles are showered into the left atrium, to the left ventricle, and subsequently into the aorta, where bubbles may enter the coronary arteries and produce myocardial infarction or cardiac arrest secondary to vessel occlusion.[19] Gas embolization to the coronary arteries also may induce arrhythmias, which may be exacerbated by or independently generated by cerebral air embolism.[48,68]

Most of the bubbles entering the aorta pass into the systemic circulation, lodging in small arteries and occluding the more distal circulation. Bubbles most often travel up the carotid arteries to embolize the brain. They may also embolize the vertebral arteries, causing sudden cardiopulmonary arrest from brainstem ischemia.

Depending on the site or sites of circulatory occlusion, AGE produces myriad and often disastrous consequences. The neurologic pattern may be confusing as showers of bubbles randomly embolize the brain's circulation, producing ischemia and infarction of diverse brain regions. Combined carotid and vertebral artery embolization may produce severe, diffuse brain injury (Figure 57-6).[72]

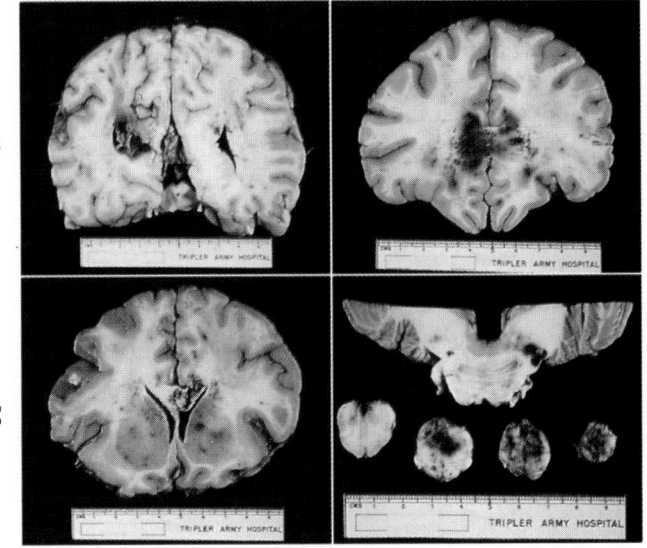

Figure 57-6 **A** to **D,** Cross sections of the brain of a 31-year-old male sport diver who suffered an arterial gas embolism, dying 4 days after the accident and extended hyperbaric oxygen treatment. Bubble-induced infarcts are found throughout the brain in the distribution of both the carotid and vertebral arteries. *(Kenneth W. Kizer, MD.)*

Arterial gas embolism typically develops immediately after the diver surfaces, at which time the high intrapulmonary pressure resulting from lung overpressurization is relieved, allowing bubble-laden pulmonary venous blood to return to the heart and pass into the systemic circulation. It is axiomatic that symptoms of AGE develop within 10 minutes of surfacing from a dive, although most often they are clearly evident within the first 2 minutes. Sudden loss of consciousness on surfacing from a dive should be considered to represent air embolism until proven otherwise.

In a pulmonary overpressure accident, as soon as normal breathing resumes at the surface of the water, the pressure differential that drives air bubbles into the pulmonary capillaries is equalized. From this point on, usually no further intraarterial air is introduced.

Clinical Manifestations of Arterial Gas Embolism

Clinical manifestations of cerebral air embolism are sudden, dramatic, and often life threatening. Many diver deaths officially listed as drowning probably have been cases of cerebral air embolism. Unfortunately, the accident investigation and postmortem evaluation of many diving-accident victims are insufficient to establish the precise cause of death. Autopsies of diving-accident victims should be performed according to special procedures.[33]

Neurologic manifestations of AGE are typical of an acute stroke, although hemiplegia and other purely unilateral brain syndromes are infrequent. Loss of consciousness, monoplegia or asymmetric multiplegia, focal paralysis, paresthesias or other sensory disturbances, convulsions, aphasia, confusion, blindness or visual field defects, vertigo, dizziness, or headache are most often observed (Table 57-2).[38,48,72,88,93]

The physical findings of AGE are extremely variable and depend on the specific site or sites of vascular occlusion. Neurologic findings generally dominate the clinical picture because of the frequency of cerebral involvement. All patients with suspected AGE should be carefully examined for neurologic deficits. Specific manifestations of POPS (such as subcutaneous or me-

TABLE 57-2. Pulmonary Overpressure Accident: Typical Symptoms and Signs

CONDITION	SYMPTOMS	SIGNS
Arterial gas embolism	Seizure (focal or general), unconsciousness, confusion, headache, visual disturbances, bloody sputum	Hemiplegia, monoplegia, altered level of consciousness, blindness, visual motor deficit, focal motor or sensory loss
Mediastinal-subcutaneous emphysema	Substernal pain, "brassy voice," neck swelling, dyspnea, bloody sputum	Subcutaneous crepitus, gas patterns on radiograph of mediastinum and neck
Pneumothorax	Chest pain, dyspnea, bloody sputum	Loss of breath sounds, hyperresonant chest percussion, tracheal shift

diastinal emphysema) may or may not be present but should always be carefully sought.

Rarely, air bubbles may be visualized in the retinal arteries, or sharply circumscribed areas of glossal pallor (Liebermeister's sign) may be noted, but these findings cannot be relied on to make the diagnosis. The diagnosis of dysbaric air embolism is clinical and based on the diving history and symptoms.

Treatment of Arterial Gas Embolism

All cases of suspected AGE must be referred for recompression treatment (hyperbaric oxygen therapy) as rapidly as possible. This is the primary and essential treatment for the condition.[42]

Before recompression, whether in the field, emergency department, or clinic, or during transport to a recompression chamber, the affected diver should be given supplemental oxygen at a high flow rate (e.g., 6 to 8 L/min by mask) with other necessary supportive measures as indicated by the specific clinical condition.

Historically, much attention was directed toward keeping the AGE patient in the Trendelenburg position in the field. This was based on anecdotal reports and limited experimental data.[75] The rationale for keeping the patient with AGE head down was the belief that the weight of the column of blood would force bubbles through the cerebral capillary bed, that the buoyancy of the bubbles would keep them in the aorta or heart, and that the weight of the spinal fluid might compress bubbles in the cord. These benefits were never well demonstrated or experimentally confirmed, and a relatively recent study showed that the Trendelenburg position did not keep bubbles from being distributed to the systemic circulation.[16] Likewise, it is more difficult to oxygenate persons in a head-down position, and if one is maintained in this position for longer than 30 to 60 minutes, it may cause or worsen cerebral edema. Therefore, in contrast to former recommendations, it is now recommended that AGE patients be maintained in the supine position, both in the field and during transport to an emergency medical treatment facility or recompression chamber.

Because the AGE event so often occurs while the victim is in the water, he or she frequently suffers concomitant near drowning. Thus the rescuer must be prepared to provide cardiopulmonary resuscitation (CPR) and to protect the airway from aspiration of gastric contents secondary to vomiting.

While life support measures are being instituted, a member of the diving or rescue team should telephone the nearest civilian or military recompression chamber and contact an air ambulance if air evacuation is required. Aircraft selection is crucial because the stricken diver should not be exposed to a significantly lower atmospheric pressure in the aircraft. Ideally, the diver should be transported by aircraft pressurized to sea level so that existing intraarterial bubbles do not expand further. In the case of helicopter evacuation or in the event that an unpressurized aircraft is required, the flight altitude must be maintained as low as possible, not to exceed 1000 feet above sea level, if possible.

An intravenous infusion of isotonic solution should be started, and urine output maintained at 1 to 2 ml/kg/hr.[29] It is important to maintain adequate intravascular volume because inert gas cannot be effectively eliminated from tissues or from intravascular bubbles at the arteriolar-capillary level unless adequate capillary perfusion is maintained.

The AGE-affected diver should be transported to the recompression chamber as quickly as possible. Delay prolongs cerebral ischemia and cellular hypoxia, resulting in significant cerebral edema, which typically leads to a more difficult course of therapy. Conversely, transport should still be undertaken even if delay is unavoidable. Remarkable improvement has been seen in cases in which treatment was delayed for more than 24 hours after the onset of neurologic manifestations.[69]

If the AGE-stricken diver is first seen at a hospital emergency department or clinic, and if transport to a hyperbaric treatment facility will not be delayed, baseline laboratory, radiographic, and other diagnostic tests (such as electrocardiography) should be obtained before the patient is sent to the chamber. Computed tomography (CT) or magnetic resonance imaging (MRI) of the brain should be deferred until after initial hyperbaric treatment unless intracranial hemorrhage, carotid artery dissection,[91] or other nondiving injury is strongly suspected.

Hyperbaric treatment consists of rapidly increasing ambient pressure (recompression) to reduce intravascular bubble volume and to restore tissue perfusion, using oxygen-enriched breathing mixtures to enhance bubble resolution and to supply oxygen to hypoxic nervous tissue, and then providing slow decompression to avoid the reformation of bubbles.[15,29,32] Additional details about the hyperbaric regimens used for treating AGE are provided in Chapter 59. Ideally, these patients should be treated in multiplace hyperbaric chambers (Figure 57-7) capable of being pressurized to 6 ATA and in which both air and oxygen can be administered to the patient. There is growing evidence that recompression to 2.8 ATA on 100% oxygen may be more effective treatment than initial pressurization to 6 ATA for sports divers because of the typical several-hour delay in getting to a chamber and, thus, less need for the higher pressure to resolubilize bubbles (and perhaps a greater immediate need for tissue oxygenation).[24,39,71,72,78,79]

Although the majority of victims with AGE have neurologic deficits when examined, the initial manifestations may spontaneously resolve by the time the victim is seen by medical personnel. Occasionally a person has symptoms but no reproducible neurologic

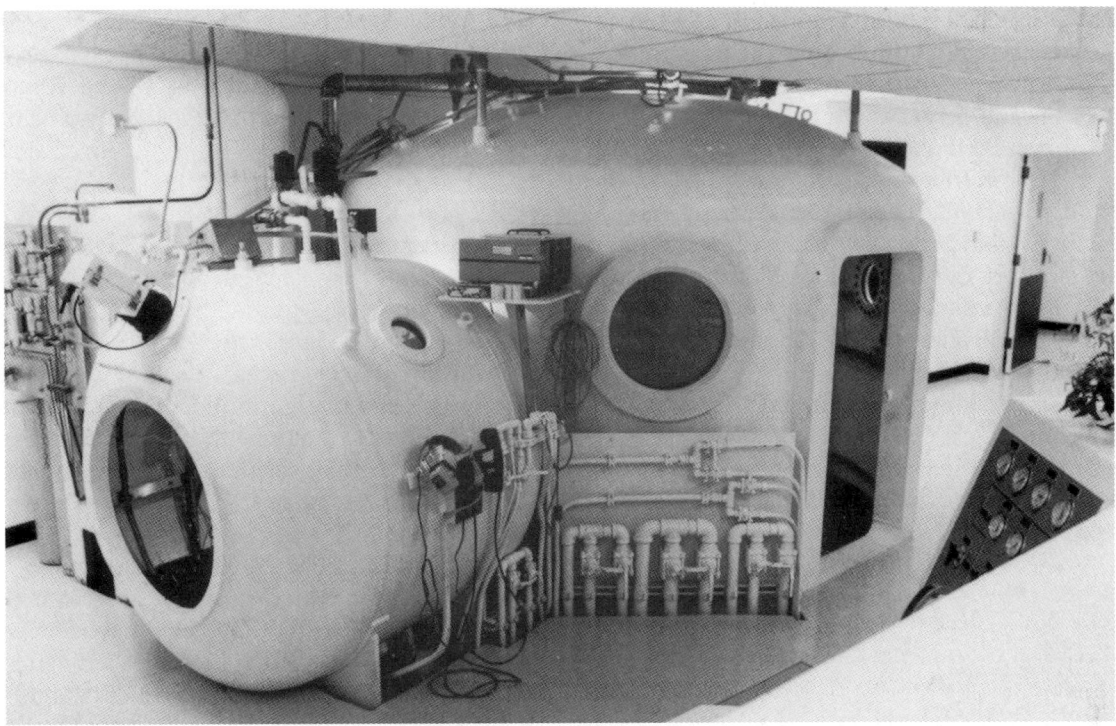

Figure 57-7 An example of a large modern hyperbaric chamber. Preferably, a hyperbaric chamber for treating decompression sickness or arterial gas embolism should have a pressure capability of at least 6 ATA (165 fsw) and should have space for an attendant to provide ongoing "hands-on" care and repeated neurologic examinations. It must have provisions for supplying 100% oxygen and other gases for treatment of the stricken diver.

deficits on physical examination.[72,77] Nonetheless, all patients must be referred for diving medicine consultation and hyperbaric treatment if the history is suggestive of AGE because neurologic impairment is impossible to exclude in the acute care setting, and waiting to complete definitive diagnostic studies may allow subtle neurologic injuries to become irreversible.[93]

Prevention of Pulmonary Overpressure Accidents

In view of the potentially catastrophic consequences of POPS, one of the key goals of scuba-diving training is to prevent pulmonary overpressure accidents. Divers must be warned of the potentially great intrathoracic volume changes that can occur at shallow depths and trained to keep an open airway during ascent, particularly through the last 10 feet to the surface. If equipment malfunction or depletion of air supply at depth makes this impossible, the diver must make every attempt to exhale continuously during an "emergency swimming ascent." This is an attempt to vent the increasing volume of air in the lungs. With a satisfactory air supply the diver should simply breathe normally on ascent to the surface, taking care to ascend slowly near the surface.

INDIRECT EFFECTS OF PRESSURE

Several diving-related problems may develop as a result of breathing gases at higher than normal atmospheric pressure. Chief among these are nitrogen narcosis, oxygen toxicity, and decompression sickness.

Dalton's Law of Partial Pressures

Dalton's law of partial pressures states that the total pressure exerted by a mixture of gases is the sum of the pressures that would be exerted by each of the gases if it alone occupied the total volume. The partial pressure of a gas in a mixture is the pressure exerted by that gas alone. The symbols for partial pressure of oxygen, nitrogen, carbon dioxide, and water vapor are P_{O_2}, P_{N_2}, P_{CO_2}, and P_{H_2O}, respectively. Dalton's law states that in an air mixture the total pressure $(P_T) = P_{N_2} + P_{O_2} + P_{H_2O} + P_{other}$. The partial pressure of each gas in the mixture is found by multiplying the percentage of that gas present by the total pressure. In Figure 57-8, a mixture of air, nitrogen is assumed to be present in a proportion of 78%, oxygen at 21%, carbon dioxide at 0.03%, and the balance composed of water vapor and other trace gases.

The partial pressures of inspired gases in a gas mixture, not their percentages, are of prime importance in diving. For example, it has been shown that in hyperbaric chamber treatment of decompression sickness, 100% oxygen can be safely used at depths to 60 fsw (2.8 ATA) for 20-minute periods with the subject at rest in the dry chamber. On the other hand, with 21% oxygen in a helium-oxygen mixture at 600 fsw (20 ATA), the diver would breathe $(0.21) \times (20 \text{ ATA})$, or 4.2 ATA of oxygen, which would rapidly produce CNS oxygen poisoning. This type of problem is avoided in deep diving by reducing the oxygen percentage in the gas mixture to between 0.35 and 0.50 ATA, so that the P_{O_2} will be between 266 and 380 mm Hg.

The scuba diver who uses open-circuit compressed air is subject to the effects of the component gases in the air according to their partial pressures. Thus, even though the gas mixture is simply air with normal percentages of oxygen and nitrogen, the increases in par-

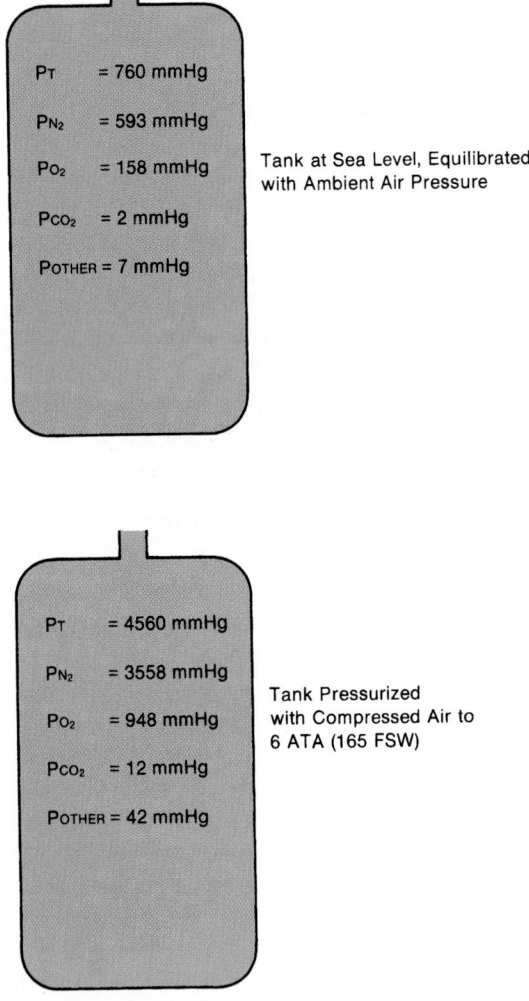

PT   = 760 mmHg

PN₂   = 593 mmHg

PO₂   = 158 mmHg

PCO₂   = 2 mmHg

POTHER = 7 mmHg

Tank at Sea Level, Equilibrated with Ambient Air Pressure

PT   = 4560 mmHg

PN₂   = 3558 mmHg

PO₂   = 948 mmHg

PCO₂   = 12 mmHg

POTHER = 42 mmHg

Tank Pressurized with Compressed Air to 6 ATA (165 FSW)

Figure 57-8 Dalton's law of partial pressures. The total pressure exerted by a mixture of gases is the sum of the pressures that would be expected by each of the gases if it alone were present and occupied the total volume.

tial pressures of these gases and those of the trace contaminants at sea level create numerous potential breathing medium–related problems. Most notable among these for scuba divers is the problem of nitrogen narcosis.

Nitrogen Narcosis

Nitrogen narcosis, also known as *rapture of the deep, inert gas narcosis*, or the *narcs*, is development of increasing intoxication as the partial pressure of nitrogen in inspired compressed air increases at depth. Nitrogen narcosis is important to divers because it causes anesthetic-like euphoria, overconfidence, and deterioration in judgment and cognition, all of which can lead to serious errors in diving techniques, accidents, and drowning. Many divers have died as a consequence of nitrogen narcosis.

During the 1930s Behnke and associates[8,9] first suggested that the mood changes described by divers breathing compressed air at 200 fsw were caused by high inspired P_{N_2}. Much has been learned since that time, and a complete compilation of data on inert gas narcosis has been provided by Bennett.[11-13] The subject was more recently reviewed by Hamilton and Kizer.[56]

Theories to explain the mechanism by which nitrogen causes its intoxicating effects center on the effects of gaseous anesthetics in general. According to currently accepted theory, an alteration in electrical properties of cellular membranes is effected by absorption of gas molecules into their lipid component. Supporting this theory is the observation that the greater the lipid solubility of a given gas, the greater its narcotic potency. Thus higher partial pressures of pure nitrogen are required to produce an anesthetic effect than can be achieved by a much lower partial pressure of nitrous oxide, which is much more soluble in lipid than is nitrogen. Helium's lack of narcotic effect is in accord with its low lipid solubility. Indeed, substitution of helium for nitrogen as the inert gas in the diver's breathing gas prevents nitrogen narcosis and is the main reason helium-oxygen mixtures are used for deep diving.

Typically, a scuba diver breathing compressed air develops symptoms of nitrogen narcosis at depths between 70 and 100 fsw. These symptoms include lightheadedness, loss of fine sensory discrimination, giddiness, and euphoria. Symptoms progressively worsen at deeper depths. At depths over 150 fsw, a diver becomes severely intoxicated, manifesting increasingly poor judgment and impaired reasoning, overconfidence, and slowed reflexes. At depths of 250 to 300 fsw, auditory and visual hallucinations may occur, along with feelings of impending blackout. Most divers will lose consciousness when they reach a depth of 400 fsw.

Of note, individual and diurnal variability occur in the depth of onset and severity of symptoms in nitrogen narcosis. Also, some degree of acclimatization allows experienced divers to work more safely at greater depths than can inexperienced divers. Nonetheless, nitrogen narcosis is a major problem for all compressed-air divers at depths greater than 100 fsw. This is one of the factors that led to the general recommendation that sport divers not dive deeper than 100 fsw.

Treatment of nitrogen narcosis requires ascent to a shallower depth (usually less than 70 to 100 fsw), where symptoms promptly clear. Of course, the condition is prevented by avoiding deep dives. In commercial diving, where there may be good reasons to dive deeper than 100 fsw, the problem is prevented by using heliox.

Oxygen Toxicity

Although oxygen is essential for most life-forms on Earth, it becomes a poison at elevated partial pressures, so *oxygen toxicity* is another indirect effect of pressure that divers need to understand. Oxygen toxicity in divers can affect either the central nervous or the pulmonary system.

High inspired P_{O_2} can occur in diving in two ways. Breathing 100% oxygen in underwater or hyperbaric chambers is one. The second results from Dalton's law of partial pressures. If a normal 21% oxygen-gas mixture is breathed at 300 fsw (10 ATA), an inspired P_{O_2} of 2.1 ATA is generated, equivalent to breathing 100% oxygen at 36 fsw. Again, it is the partial pressure of a gas that determines its biologic effects.

Pulmonary Oxygen Toxicity. Retrolental fibroplasia in premature infants and pulmonary oxygen toxicity in adults are well-known problems associated with the use of therapeutic oxygen. Pulmonary oxygen toxicity is induced by breathing an above normal, but relatively low P_{O_2} for prolonged periods. The limit for indefinite exposure without demonstrable lung damage is generally considered to be a P_{O_2} of about 0.5 ATA. On a time-dose curve, it is generally considered safe to breathe 100% oxygen at 1 ATA for up to about 20 hours, or at 2 ATA for up to 6 hours. This time can be lengthened significantly by using intermittent exposures, such as interspersing a 5-minute air break between every 20 minutes of oxygen breathing.[58] At 2.8 to 3 ATA (60 to 66 fsw), at which 100% oxygen is used to treat decompression sickness and gas gangrene, pulmonary oxygen toxicity is rarely a problem because CNS manifestations usually intervene before sufficient time elapses to induce pulmonary damage. This subject has been thoroughly reviewed by Clark and Lambertsen.[22] Use of hyperbaric oxygen according to U.S. Navy Treatment Table 6 (as is used in treating decompression sickness; see Chapter 59) does not produce clinical manifestations of pulmonary oxygen toxicity. However, animal studies with more extreme oxygen exposures have shown a pathologic sequence of alveolar capillary endothelial damage, with increased permeability leading to pulmonary edema and hemorrhage. While species variation in susceptibility occurs, interruption of exposure usually results in reversal of these pathologic changes.[19]

The most common clinical manifestation of pulmonary oxygen toxicity is substernal discomfort on inhalation. If exposure continues, this can progress to severe burning substernal pain and persistent coughing. Reduction of inspired oxygen partial pressure to 0.21 to 0.5 ATA usually results in prompt relief. Severe cases of pulmonary oxygen toxicity may require endotracheal intubation and positive end-expiratory pressure (PEEP) ventilation to achieve adequate arterial oxygenation at the required lower partial pressures of inspired oxygen.

Central Nervous System Oxygen Toxicity. During the 1880s the French physiologist Paul Bert described convulsions in animals breathing 100% oxygen at elevated chamber pressures. The same phenomena were observed in humans in the 1930s by Behnke and others. Donald's classic observations on divers were published in 1947 and provide much of the current knowledge on predisposing factors and clinical manifestations of CNS oxygen toxicity.[40,41]

In brief, Donald found that, at a given duration and pressure of oxygen, a diver in the water was more susceptible to oxygen-induced seizures than was the same diver in a warm, dry hyperbaric chamber. Based on this observation, a limit of 25 fsw was imposed for military special operations dives using 100% oxygen.

Most people can tolerate breathing 100% oxygen for 30 minutes at rest at 2.8 ATA in a dry chamber, although some manifest toxicity even at this exposure. Common symptoms and signs of CNS poisoning are shown in Box 57-4. Unfortunately, some persons may have no warning symptoms, and the first manifestation of CNS oxygen toxicity may be a generalized convulsion.

Box 57-4 TYPICAL MANIFESTATIONS OF CENTRAL NERVOUS SYSTEM OXYGEN POISONING

Apprehension
Feeling of air hunger
Sweating
Nausea
Focal muscle twitching
Isolated jerking of a limb
Auditory changes (such as "bells ringing")
Tunnel vision
Diaphragmatic flutter
Convulsion

Treatment for CNS oxygen toxicity in a hyperbaric chamber involves removal of the oxygen mask, maintenance of the airway, and keeping the patient from injuring himself or herself. Of note, chamber pressure should be kept constant until the seizure activity ceases to prevent a possible pulmonary overpressure accident.

After a postictal period, the patient who has had an oxygen-induced seizure recovers without sequelae. Although anticonvulsant drugs theoretically should suppress oxygen-induced seizures, none has been tested to determine efficacy or therapeutic dosage.

Anticonvulsant therapy is not usually considered necessary for persons who have had oxygen-induced seizures because termination of oxygen breathing routinely stops the seizure and recurrent seizures are exceedingly rare. Removing oxygen at the first sign of CNS toxicity (e.g., when feelings of apprehension are noted or when sweating, nausea, or twitching are observed) has to date prevented any documented permanent CNS damage after an oxygen-induced seizure. Importantly, there is no reason for a person who has had an oxygen-induced seizure not to receive normobaric 100% oxygen if it is medically indicated.

Contaminated Breathing Gas

As breathing-gas cylinders are pressurized or filled, the sea level partial pressure of each gaseous component is multiplied. Thus any contaminant in the air source can potentially become dangerous to the diver at the elevated pressure found underwater. Compressor motors must be free of oil that could be pumped into tanks; otherwise, the oil mist in the air may cause the diver to suffer lipoid pneumonitis.[73]

Compressed air inlets should always be situated so that they avoid engine exhaust from the compressor, parking lots, or other combustion sources that produce carbon monoxide. Because carbon monoxide is colorless, odorless, and tasteless, the diver cannot detect it unless it is accompanied by other contaminants. The first warning of carbon monoxide poisoning may be headache, nausea, or dizziness during the dive. Examination at the surface may show lethargy, mental dullness, and nonspecific neurologic deficits, which may be confused with those accompanying decompression sickness or air embolism. The cherry-red skin color often mentioned in standard medical texts is actually rarely observed in carbon monoxide poisoning. Fortunately, the treatment of choice for serious acute carbon monoxide poisoning, decompression sickness, and air embolism is hyperbaric oxygen.

Another potential breathing-gas problem involves carbon dioxide. Alveolar partial pressure of carbon dioxide (Pa_{CO_2}) reflects arterial P_{CO_2}; thus even as ambient pressure increases at depth, Pa_{CO_2} remains constant at about 40 mm Hg unless environmental or physiologic changes occur. Hypercapnia can occur because of increased P_{CO_2} in the breathing gas or decreased pulmonary ventilation. Unless there is regulator malfunction or contaminated breathing gas, hypercapnia is exceptionally rare in open-circuit scuba diving. Hypercapnia can occur in helmet or chamber diving if these closed spaces are inadequately ventilated or the breathing gas becomes contaminated by carbon dioxide, and in closed-circuit scuba diving if there is failure of the CO_2-absorbent (scrubbing) material.

At sea level, a concentration of 5% to 6% inspired CO_2 leads to dyspnea, increased respiratory rate, and mental confusion. At 10% inspired CO_2, pulse rate and blood pressure may fall to the point that unconsciousness occurs. With prolonged exposure to 12% to 14% inspired CO_2, such that Pa_{CO_2} exceeds 150 mm Hg, central respiratory and cardiac depression can be fatal. Because elevated Pa_{CO_2} causes vasodilation, hypercapnia potentially increases susceptibility to nitrogen narcosis, oxygen toxicity, and possibly decompression sickness.

Hyperventilation

Hypocapnia can result from *hyperventilation* during or before diving. The well-known symptoms of hyperventilation—dizziness and paresthesia—have been postulated to cause unconsciousness among divers, but whether this actually occurs is unclear. In contrast, unconsciousness associated with hyperventilation before a breath-hold dive is caused by hypoxia, rather than hypocapnia.

In what is commonly described as *shallow water blackout,* a diver hyperventilates before a dive, lowering alveolar P_{CO_2} to 20 to 30 mm Hg. However, because hemoglobin is nearly saturated with oxygen during normal respiration, there is little gain in arterial P_{O_2}. In an underwater swim, even in a shallow swimming pool, exercise-induced hypoxia sufficient to cause unconsciousness may occur before arterial P_{CO_2} reaccumulates to provide sufficient stimulus to breathe.[7]

In a deep breath-hold dive the problem is compounded. In addition to the initial depression of arterial P_{CO_2} secondary to hyperventilation, elevations in alveolar and arterial P_{O_2} occur. During the dive these serve to suppress the respiratory response to hypercarbia. During descent in the water, Pa_{CO_2} increases from the increased pressure, but after oxygen consumption at depth, depressurization on return to the surface causes a dramatic drop in alveolar and arterial P_{CO_2}. Even if Pa_{CO_2} rises to the stimulatory breakpoint during ascent, hypoxemia may cause unconsciousness and near drowning. An expansion of Edmonds' *Commonest Causes of Unconsciousness in Divers* is presented in Box 57-5.[44]

Box 57-5 CAUSES OF UNCONSCIOUSNESS IN DIVERS

BREATH-HOLD DIVING

Underwater hypoxemia after hyperventilation before the dive ("shallow-water blackout")
Near drowning

COMPRESSED GAS EQUIPMENT

Hypoxic breathing gas
Contaminated breathing gas (such as carbon monoxide)
Equipment failure or exhaustion of breathing gas
Near drowning
Inert gas narcosis
Oxygen toxicity
Pulmonary overpressure accident with arterial gas embolism

REBREATHING EQUIPMENT

Carbon dioxide toxicity
Oxygen poisoning

DECOMPRESSION SICKNESS

In the mid-nineteenth century, tunnel and bridge workers who labored in caissons pressurized with compressed air were sometimes observed to suffer joint pains, paralysis, and various other medical problems after decompression. The condition was not understood and became dubbed as *caisson disease* or *compressed air illness*.[98] Of course, these early high-pressure workers were experiencing the same symptoms that were later observed in divers and aviators and that we now know to be decompression sickness (DCS).

For many decades caisson disease remained a medical curiosity, but because of its occurrence in increasingly important areas of activity in the twentieth century, considerable research has been directed toward its causes and treatment in the past several decades.

Today, we know that DCS is caused by the formation of bubbles of inert gas (such as nitrogen) within the intravascular and extravascular spaces after a reduction in ambient pressure. This may occur during or after decompression from being underwater or in a caisson or hyperbaric chamber in which pressures are greater than at sea level, or in aviators, astronauts, or hypobaric (high-altitude) chamber workers who travel rapidly from sea level to pressures less than 0.5 ATA. Although DCS is a major concern in commercial divers who breathe heliox, this discussion concentrates on compressed-air diving situations likely to be encountered by recreational scuba divers.

Etiology of Decompression Sickness

To understand the etiology of DCS, one must understand the temporal uptake and elimination of inert gases supplied in the diver's breathing medium. Clearly, if it were possible for a diver to breathe 100% oxygen while underwater, there would be no problems with decompression sickness because oxygen is rapidly metabolized by the body and for all practical purposes does not contribute to bubble formation on ascent from depth. Unfortunately, pure oxygen breathing at increased atmospheric pressure causes CNS toxicity and thus cannot be used in sport diving. The requirement to have an inert gas diluent (nitrogen) in the diver's breathing medium is the crux of the problem in DCS.

As alveolar air pressure increases at depth, partial pressures of inspired gases increase. At 99 FSW (4 ATA), the absolute pressure is 3040 mm Hg (see Table 57-1). Seventy-nine percent of this pressure is nitrogen (2400 mm Hg, as compared with 600 mm Hg P_{N_2} at sea level). Accounting for water vapor and carbon dioxide, this results in an alveolar partial pressure of nitrogen (Pa_{N_2}) of about 2360 mm Hg. This Pa_{N_2} is rapidly reflected across the alveolar-capillary membrane to the arterial blood, where (according to Henry's law) nitrogen becomes physically dissolved in the blood. Henry's law states that the amount of gas dissolved in a liquid at any given temperature is a function of the partial pressure of the gas in contact with the liquid and the solubility coefficient of the gas in that particular liquid. As nitrogen-laden blood is presented to tissues at the capillary level, a complex set of variables dictated by perfusion, diffusion, and inert gas solubility results in a family of nitrogen uptake curves similar to the pharmacokinetic drug uptake curves commonly displayed for medications. Thus tissue nitrogen saturations on any given dive are a function of depth (i.e., pressure) and time.

Clinical Manifestations of Decompression Sickness

DCS is a multisystem disorder caused by a rapid decrease in ambient atmospheric pressure such that inert gas (e.g., nitrogen) comes out of solution, causing the formation of bubbles in tissue and venous blood. Conceptually, DCS is the same illness whether it occurs in high-altitude aviators or deep-sea divers, although there are some differences in the symptoms of the disease depending on whether it is caused by hyperbaric or hypobaric exposure.

The physiologic sequelae of bubble formation in tissue and venous blood are myriad. These effects include cellular distention and rupture; mechanical stretching of tendons or ligaments, producing pain; and intravascular or intralymphatic occlusion, resulting in congestive ischemia and infarction or lymphedema.

Intravascular bubbles also cause multiple biophysical effects at the blood-bubble surface interface because bubbles are viewed by the immune system as foreign matter and incite an inflammatory reaction. The key step in the process is activation of Hageman factor, which in turn activates the intrinsic clotting, kinin, and complement systems, producing platelet activation, cellular clumping, lipid embolization, increased vascular permeability, interstitial edema, and microvascular sludging. The overall effect is decreased tissue perfusion and ischemia.

As with arterial gas embolism, the diagnosis of DCS is a clinical diagnosis based on the history of diving with compressed air and subsequent development of characteristic symptoms and signs. The majority of patients with DCS become symptomatic in the first hour after surfacing from a dive, with most of the rest noticing symptoms within 6 hours after diving. A very few DCS patients (1% to 2%) may not note their symptoms until 24 to 48 hours after diving.

The clinical manifestations of DCS are protean (Table 57-3), with the neurologic and musculoskeletal systems being most often affected. Symptoms of DCS are often categorized into *types I and II,* with type I referring to the mild forms of DCS (cutaneous, lymphatic, and musculoskeletal) and type II including the neurologic and other serious forms. In addition, some investigators in recent years have advocated for use of the term *type III decompression sickness*

to refer to combined AGE and DCS with neurologic symptoms.[92] Other numerical classification schemes have also been espoused.

Although the categorization of DCS as types I and II is firmly entrenched in the literature, its use is not advocated. It is clinically more meaningful to refer to the body systems affected when discussing patients with DCS, especially in light of the growing awareness that all DCS must be considered serious and treated vigorously.

Musculoskeletal Decompression Sickness. Musculoskeletal DCS, or *the bends,* is periarticular joint pain associated with DCS. It is the most common symptom of DCS, occurring in about 70% of patients. This form of DCS is often referred to as *limb bends, joint bends,* or *pain-only bends.*

The term *bends* originated at the beginning of the twentieth century when caisson workers on the Brooklyn Bridge who were suffering from DCS of the hips were noted to walk stiffly, bending forward at the hips.[98] Co-workers would describe the stricken men as walking as if they were trying to do the "Grecian bend," a forward bending, stiff-at-the-hips way that stylish women of the day would walk because of their tight corsets. Over time the term became shortened to just "bends."

The shoulders and elbows are the joints most often affected by DCS in scuba divers, but any joint may be

TABLE 57-3. Common Symptoms and Signs of Decompression Sickness

CONDITION	SYMPTOMS	SIGNS
Musculoskeletal decompression sickness, limb bends	Severe joint pain, single or multiple joints involved, paresthesia or dysesthesia about joint, lymphedema (uncommon)	Tenderness, which may be temporarily relieved by local pressure with blood pressure cuff; pain worsened by movement of joint
Neurologic decompression sickness		
Spinal cord	Back pain, girdling abdominal pain, extremity heaviness or weakness, paralysis, paresthesia of extremities, fecal incontinence, urine retention	Hyperesthesia or hypoesthesia, paresis, anal sphincter weakness, loss of bulbocavernosus reflex, urinary bladder distention
Brain	Visual loss, scotomata, headache, dysphasia, confusion	Visual field deficit, spotty motor or sensory deficits, disorientation or mental dullness
Fatigue	Profound generalized heaviness or fatigue	May precede signs of other forms
Cutaneous manifestations	Intense pruritus	No visible signs, mottling, local or generalized hyperemia or marbled skin (cutis marmorata)
Chokes	Dyspnea, substernal pain that is worsened on deep inhalation, nonproductive cough	Cyanosis, tachypnea, tachycardia
Vasomotor decompression sickness (decompression shock)	Weakness, sweating, unconsciousness	Hypotension, tachycardia, pallor, mottling, hemoconcentration, decreased urine output

involved. Conversely, the hips and knees are most commonly affected in saturation divers, caisson workers, and aviators. The reason for the different anatomic predilection is not known.

The pain of joint bends is usually described as "boring" or a dull ache deep within the joint, although it may also be characterized as sharp or throbbing. It is sometimes described as "tearing" or feeling like tendinitis or bursitis. It may radiate to surrounding areas. Movement of the joint worsens the pain, so the joint is usually held immobile. An area of vague numbness or dysesthesia may surround the affected joint, but this typically does not conform to any anatomic distribution and should not be confused with neurologic involvement. There also may be erythema around the joint, and it may be mildly swollen. The joint may also be tender to touch.

Sometimes divers will complain of having a "niggle" after a dive. This is mild pain in a single joint that improves 10 to 15 minutes after the onset of pain and then disappears without treatment. Whether niggles should be treated with recompression is controversial, but the safest approach is to treat them with at least a U.S. Navy Treatment Table 5.

The differential diagnosis between limb bends and trauma may be aided by inflation of a sphygmomanometer cuff placed around the joint to 150 to 250 mm Hg.[102] By reducing the gas volume in tendons and ligaments, this may immediately relieve the pain directly under the cuff if the pain is caused by DCS. This relief suggests that the mechanism of pain is gas expansion (i.e., bubbles) in tendons and ligaments that stretches nerve endings. The pain of limb bends recurs when the cuff is deflated. The test is helpful when it is positive. Failure to respond to the application of local pressure, however, should not be used to rule out the presence of DCS; this must be done with a "test of pressure" in a hyperbaric chamber. Importantly, most often there may be neither abnormal physical signs (other than splinting or stiffness from pain) nor abnormal radiographic findings.

Limb bends pain itself is not immediately threatening to life or function but indicates that bubbling may be occurring in venous blood. Often, patients who begin with musculoskeletal DCS and are not treated progress to more serious forms of DCS. Likewise, as discussed later, untreated DCS may lead to osteonecrosis of the major joints.

Fatigue. Profound fatigue that is out of proportion to the activity performed underwater, or otherwise while under pressure, may be an early manifestation of DCS. Although its etiology is unknown, a feeling of severe fatigue after diving demands careful evaluation for other manifestations of DCS and may in and of itself justify a "test of pressure."

Skin Bends or Cutaneous Decompression Sickness. DCS may present a variety of cutaneous manifestations, including scarlatiniform, erysipeloid, or mottled rashes, pruritus, and formication. Occasionally, localized swelling or peau d'orange may result from lymphatic obstruction, and rarely, an entire limb may become edematous.

Skin manifestations are relatively uncommon, and in and of themselves are usually not serious. However, mottling or marbling of the skin (cutis marmorata) is often a harbinger of more severe DCS. The exact physiologic basis of the mottled skin lesion is unknown. Skin bends should be easily distinguished from cutaneous barotrauma, "wet suit dermatitis,"[76,103] marine envenomation, or other skin rashes often seen in divers.

Itches, or *the creeps,* is a type of skin bends seen during decompression in hyperbaric chamber workers when the skin is exposed to the high partial pressure of nitrogen in compressed air. This is a highly pruritic skin reaction most intensely felt on body parts exposed to the compressed air. The sensation is often described as feeling like ants crawling over one's body.

In hyperbaric chambers, inert gas from the external environment is absorbed directly into skin, and itches represents bubble formation in the skin during decompression. The concentrations of dissolved gases in ocean water are essentially constant at all depths, so the skin is not exposed to elevated partial pressures of inert gases under water.

Chokes or Pulmonary Decompression Sickness. The *chokes* is an unusual but very serious form of DCS characterized by burning substernal pain (especially on inhalation), cyanosis, dyspnea, and nonproductive cough. Animal studies have demonstrated gas bubbles or foam in the pulmonary arteries, right atrium, and right ventricle after unsafe decompression. Chokes probably represents massive pulmonary gas embolism with mechanical obstruction of the pulmonary vascular bed by bubbles. Typically, symptoms of pulmonary venous air embolization begin when 10% or more of the pulmonary vascular bed is obstructed. Patients with chokes can progress rapidly to profound shock and/or neurologic DCS. The specific clinical and radiologic manifestations of the chokes are similar to those seen with venous gas embolism (VGE) from other causes.[74]

Symptoms of VGE include air hunger, dyspnea, cough, and chest pain. Findings may include pallor, diaphoresis, tachypnea, tachycardia, hypotension, cyanosis, expiratory wheezing, neurologic signs, and a "mill wheel" heart murmur. Victims may also exhibit increased central venous or pulmonary artery pressure, electrocardiographic changes of ischemia or cor pulmonale, decreased end-tidal carbon dioxide fraction, and precordial Doppler sounds of circulating gas bubbles. Rarely, air may be visualized in the main pulmonary artery on chest radiographs; this is pathognomonic for pulmonary air embolism.[62,74]

Neurologic Decompression Sickness. Neurologic impairment may occur as the sole manifestation of DCS or as part of a larger dysbaric syndrome. Neurologic DCS is manifested by a myriad of symptoms and signs because of the random nature by which DCS affects the nervous system. Although any level of the CNS may be affected, the most commonly involved site in divers is the spinal cord, specifically in the lower thoracic and lumbar regions. The peripheral nervous system also may be involved.[64]

Based on military experience, neurologic DCS was believed to occur in only 10% to 20% of DCS cases,[100] but neurologic manifestations of DCS have been found in 50% to 60% of scuba-diving casualties treated in Hawaii[47,65] and have been reported in similarly high frequencies in other populations of sport divers.[29,38]

Classically, dysbaric spinal cord injury occurs in the lower thoracic, lumbar, and sacral portions of the cord, producing low back pain, subjective "heaviness" in the legs, paraplegia or paraparesis, lower extremity paresthesia or dysesthesia, and possible bladder or anal sphincter dysfunction. General malaise or fatigue is often noted as well. Involvement of the cervical and thoracic cord may cause chest or abdominal pain and weakness or sensory disturbances in the upper extremities. Absence of the bulbocavernosus reflex, elicited by gently squeezing and pulling the glans penis to seek reflex contraction of the anal sphincter, often foretells a poor prognosis, as does absence of the superficial anal reflex, which can be elicited in the male or female by stroking the perianal region.

The mechanism of spinal cord DCS is multifactorial, involving autochthonous inert gas bubble formation in the cord[52,96] and in the epivertebral venous system (Batson's plexus), with resulting congestive infarction of the spinal cord,[55] and other mechanisms that are not well understood.[59,96]

DCS of the brain produces a variety of symptoms, most of which are indistinguishable from AGE. These include dizziness, vertigo, altered mentation or level of consciousness, generalized weakness, and visual deficits (e.g., diplopia, scotoma, visual field defects and blindness). Involvement of the cerebellum or inner ear may produce ataxia and loss of balance.

Inner Ear or Vestibular Decompression Sickness. The *staggers* is another classic DCS syndrome. In this case, the inner ear is primarily affected, and the name derives from the unsteady gait that results from the vestibular damage. Other manifestations include dizziness, vertigo, nystagmus, tinnitus, nausea, and vomiting. It is most often seen in saturation divers when

there is a rapid ascent on heliox, or when switching gases on ascent during very deep dives.

Vasomotor Decompression Sickness. Vasomotor DCS, or *decompression shock,* is a rare, life-threatening form of DCS. The pathogenesis of this shock syndrome is not completely understood, but it is believed to be caused by a rapid shift of fluid from intravascular to extravascular spaces secondary to diffuse bubble embolization, ischemia, and hypoxia.[21] Hypotension may also result from massive venous air embolization of the lungs.

Despite vigorous intravenous fluid replacement, the hypotension of decompression shock may not respond until recompression is undertaken. Unfortunately, the condition is highly lethal, and many patients do not survive to undergo recompression unless a hyperbaric chamber is immediately available.

Long-Term Sequelae of Decompression Sickness

Although DCS is the most overt manifestation of inadequate decompression after diving, it has now been clearly established that there may be long-term sequelae of diving related to inadequate decompression, even if the diver never manifests overt DCS. The best characterized of these problems is dysbaric osteonecrosis.

Dysbaric Osteonecrosis. *Dysbaric osteonecrosis* (DON) is a form of avascular or aseptic necrosis of bone associated with pressure changes. The major joints (i.e., shoulders, elbows, hips, and knees) are most often affected, although any bone can be involved.[20,46,87]

DON was first recognized in compressed-air workers in the early 1900s.[94] Since then its incidence in professional divers has been found to range from less than 1% to over 80%, depending on the age of the diver and the type of diving done. Its occurrence correlates well with deep diving, decompression diving, the occurrence of DCS, and missed decompression.[35,46,63,87,107] Most diving medicine experts consider DON a long-term sequel to inadequate decompression. Interestingly, fossil evidence of avascular necrosis has been found in some species of marine mosasaurs of the Cretaceous period, suggesting that at least some of these extinct giant marine lizards dived deeply.[101]

Dysbaric Retinopathy. Infrequently, DCS affects the eyes, producing a wide array of acute ophthalmic effects, including homonymous hemianopsia, cortical blindness, central retinal artery occlusion, retinal hemorrhage, nystagmus, convergence insufficiency, and optic neuropathy.[17,18] Some long-term ophthalmic findings in divers also have been observed.

A retinal fluorescein angiography survey of asymptomatic divers found a higher incidence of retinal pigment epithelium than in nondivers and various capillary changes at the fovea.[99] The significance of these abnormalities is unclear because none of the divers had visual loss. Similarly, the cause of such changes is unclear, although they are postulated to be the result of small bubble microembolization.

Diagnosis of Decompression Sickness

A variety of laboratory abnormalities may be demonstrated in DCS, but most have little or no usefulness in the immediate management of patients. Two tests that may be useful, however, are measurement of the urine specific gravity and hematocrit because intravascular volume depletion and hemoconcentration are common in serious DCS because of increased vascular permeability caused by endothelial damage and release of kinins. The results of these tests can help guide replacement fluid therapy. Hematocrit percentages are commonly in the high 50s or 60s in serious DCS.

As with laboratory tests, radiographic evaluation of patients with suspected DCS may yield various findings, but the radiographs are rarely useful in acute management of the patient. Bone radiographs of patients with acute joint bends do not show abnormalities. Months to years later, they may demonstrate findings of DON. Noncardiogenic pulmonary edema may be seen on chest radiographs of persons with pulmonary or vasomotor DCS.

Both CT and MRI have been used to evaluate neurologic DCS injury, although conventional CT suffers from poor sensitivity of early lesions and its inability to image spinal cord lesions.[60,67] Limited clinical data support the feasibility and efficacy of MRI of these conditions,[80,108] especially when intracranial injury is suspected, although the exigency of obtaining recompression treatment makes these modalities useful primarily in the postrecompression evaluation of residual deficits.

Treatment of Decompression Sickness

All persons with suspected DCS must be referred to a hyperbaric treatment facility as quickly as possible because recompression is the primary and essential treatment for this condition. The physician must have a high index of suspicion when diagnosing DCS, because the often diverse manifestations of DCS may present a very confusing clinical picture. The history of the dive profile is helpful if the diver knowingly violated decompression procedures, but DCS may occur on dives that should be safe according to current decompression schedules.[1] Likewise, the reported depth and time of the dive are often not accurate.

Management of DCS must be commenced as soon as the condition is suspected.[29] Sport divers are usually far from a recompression chamber when their symptoms develop, so treatment is often initiated in the field or at an outpatient acute care facility. One hundred percent oxygen should be administered by a tight oronasal mask to provide a favorable gradient for nitrogen washout. Of equal importance is maintenance of intravascular volume to ensure capillary perfusion for elimination of microvascular inert gas bubbles and for tissue oxygenation. An intravenous infusion of isotonic solution should be started and run at a flow rate sufficient to maintain urine output at 1 to 2 ml/kg/hr. With spinal cord involvement, an indwelling urinary catheter may be needed because of sacral nerve root dysfunction. Intractable vomiting or vertigo should be treated with appropriate parenteral agents. Diazepam has been quite effective in providing relief from the vertigo associated with labyrinthine DCS when other agents have failed. Oral aspirin (5 to 10 grains) also may be useful for its antiplatelet activity. Of course, advanced life support measures should be undertaken appropriate to the patient's clinical condition.

While these measures are undertaken, someone should arrange for emergency transportation to the nearest recompression chamber. Because of the large number and frequently changing status of recompression chambers, no list is provided here. Instead, refer to the national Divers Alert Network (DAN) at Duke University (Figure 57-9). Help with the treatment of dive-related incidents may be obtained 24 hours a day by calling 919-684-8111 and requesting DAN. This telephone number should be readily available to all divers and medical facilities. DAN's diving medicine experts provide help with diagnosis and immediate care of the patient and provide information about the location of the nearest hyperbaric chamber.

Before a patient is transferred to the hyperbaric treatment facility, it is imperative to contact the chamber to determine its availability. The chamber may be out of service or tied up with the treatment of another patient. The physician should never send a patient without first discussing the transfer with the hyperbaric treatment personnel.

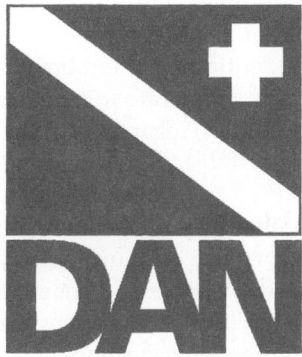

Figure 57-9 Logo for Divers Alert Network. *(Courtesy Divers Alert Network.)*

If airborne evacuation is required, it is critical to obtain an aircraft that can maintain sea level cabin pressurization during flight. Examples of such aircraft are the military C9 and C-130 Hercules, Learjet, and Cessna Citation. In the case of helicopters (which cannot be pressurized), the crew must maintain the lowest possible flight altitude, and preferably never greater than 1000 feet above the starting elevation. This is always problematic in evacuations from mountain lakes. All resuscitative measures must be maintained in flight.

At the recompression chamber, one of several standard hyperbaric treatment protocols is followed. In a multi-lock compressed air chamber, the patient and an attendant can be pressurized with compressed air and the patient given 100% oxygen by mask.

As with AGE, hyperbaric treatment of decompression sickness has undergone significant evolution during the past two decades and is discussed in more detail in Chapter 59. It is most often successful, but the likelihood of success is difficult to predict for any given diver. In general, the sooner after the onset of symptoms that treatment begins, the better the outcome.[4] In one series of 92 sport scuba divers treated after a significant delay between the offending dive and the start of recompression treatment, 85% had good results when standard U.S. Navy treatment tables were followed.[29] Similar results were achieved in another series of 50 patients.[70] Such treatment is usually given according to U.S. Navy Tables 5 and 6 (Figure 57-10). Any patient with neurologic or pulmonary DCS requires treatment with at least the protocol in Table 6 (Figure 57-10, *B*), with extension of the hyperbaric oxygen periods depending on how the patient responds.

Monoplace hyperbaric chambers are used to treat decompression sickness and air embolism,[57,71] but the "conventional wisdom" is to use a multiplace chamber whenever possible because of the free access to the patient possible in these larger chambers and the flexibility in treatment schedules, if needed.

U.S. Navy Treatment Table 7 is an option for serious DCS cases; however, this treatment table should be reserved for patients with major deficits because of its length and commitment of resources. The diver and attendant are held at 2.8 ATA for at least 12 hours, and longer if needed, with the patient breathing oxygen in 30-minute periods as tolerated. A final, slow, 32-hour decompression follows, regardless of the time spent at 2.8 ATA. Details of Table 7 are found in the U.S. Navy Diving Manual.[37]

Another potentially useful recommendation for dealing with the recurrence of neurologic symptoms and signs after apparently successful chamber treatment of neurologic DCS has been advanced by Edmonds.[44] Frequent postrecompression recurrence of neurologic manifestations led him to institute multiple 30-minute sea level oxygen-breathing periods with 30-minute air breaks for 6 to 8 hours during posttreatment hospital observation, rechecking vital capacity frequently to detect and prevent pulmonary oxygen toxicity.

Although experimental proof of their efficacy is lacking, high-dose parenteral corticosteroids have been widely recommended and used in the past as an adjunct to recompression treatment of both neurologic DCS and AGE. Rapid-acting hydrocortisone hemisuccinate (1000 mg) or methylprednisolone sodium succinate (125 mg) followed by dexamethasone, 4 to 6 mg every 6 hours, with continuation of the dexamethasone for 72 hours, has been the standard regimen.

The use of steroids became prevalent based on the belief that they were beneficial in the treatment of cerebral edema, shock, and other conditions pertinent to DCS, although their benefit in many of these conditions is uncertain. Anecdotal data suggesting that steroids were beneficial in combination with hyperbaric oxygen treatment have been reported,[29,66,77] but there have been no published clinical series or controlled trials demonstrating their efficacy. In contrast, controlled studies of high-dose parenteral dexamethasone and methylprednisolone in DCS-affected dogs showed that the use of glucocorticoids as an adjunct to conventional hyperbaric oxygen therapy produced no benefit, and even suggested that the steroid-treated animals did less well.[51] Thus the benefit and role of steroids in the treatment of DCS continue to be a matter of controversy. Similarly, the value of intravenous lidocaine is speculative.[23]

Because the outcome of recompression treatment is influenced by the time interval from onset of symptoms to the initiation of treatment, every emergency department and every diver should know the location of the nearest recompression chamber. Spinal cord decompression sickness treated after a few hours delay may result in residual deficits ranging from mild weakness or sensory changes to permanent paraplegia or worse. On the other hand, dramatic improvements have been witnessed even in persons arriving at a chamber many days after the insult.

Prevention of Decompression Sickness

Ever since DCS was first recognized, efforts have been directed at preventing its occurrence. Such efforts have utilized all manner of intervention, but to date the only effective way to prevent DCS is to limit the time a diver spends at increased pressure (i.e., depth) and/or to ensure that decompression from increased pressure is slow enough, or staged, so that the body's burden of excess inert gas is eliminated without forming bubbles. Such depth/time ascent schedules have given rise to a variety of decompression tables.

Decompression Tables. Navies and commercial diving companies around the world have developed vari-

DEPTH/TIME PROFILE

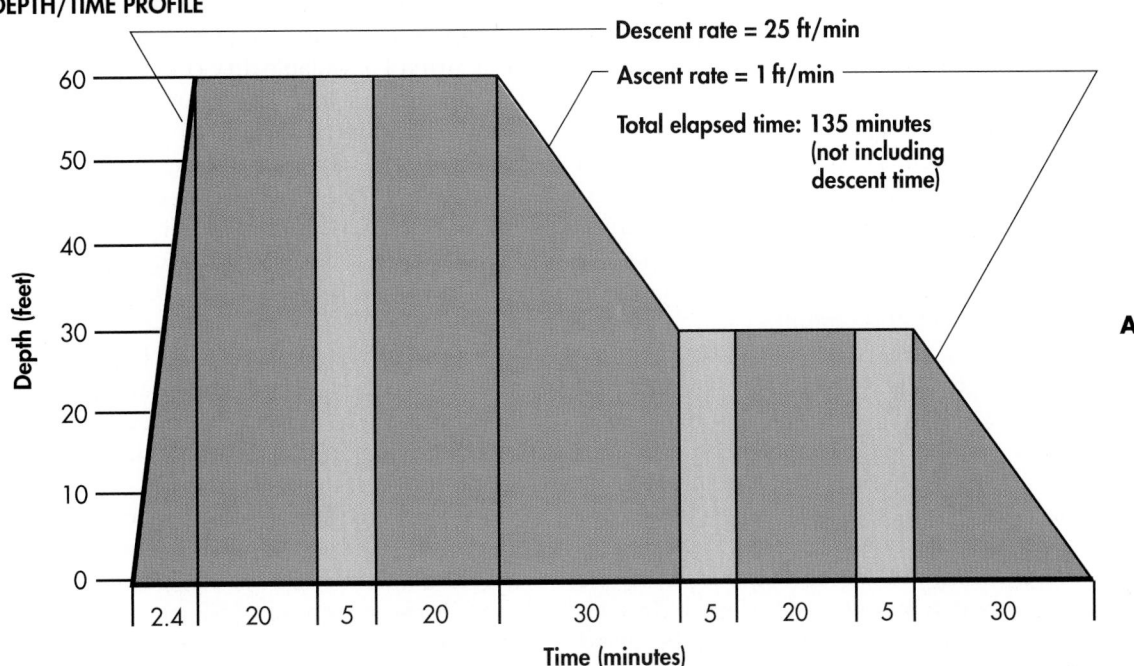

DEPTH/TIME PROFILE

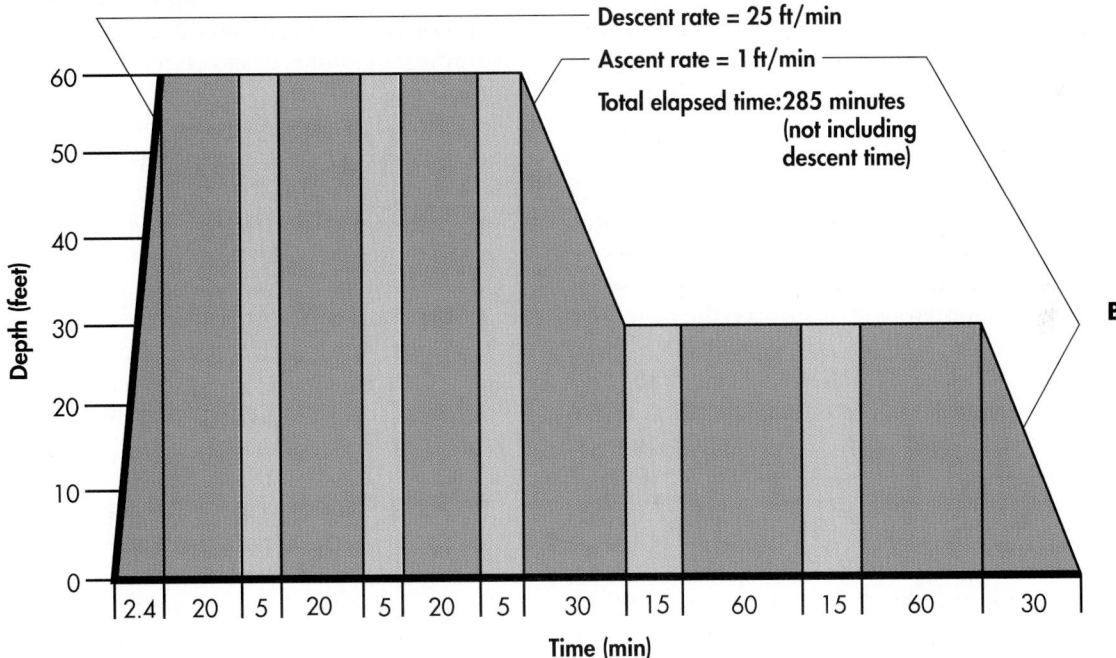

Figure 57-10 Examples of U.S. Navy decompression tables. Dark shading represents oxygen breathing; light shading represents air breathing. **A,** USN Treatment Table 5, oxygen treatment of type-1 decompression sickness. **B,** USN Treatment Table 6, oxygen treatment of type-2 decompression sickness. (*Modified from Department of the Navy: U.S. Navy diving manual, vol 2, rev 2, Flagstaff, Ariz, 1988, Best Publishing Company.*)

ous decompression schedules based on calculations and actual testing (animal and human) that allow divers to avoid exceeding safe rates of decompression after specified depth-time dive profiles. These listings of "safe" depth-time diving profiles are generally referred to as *decompression tables.* Many different sets of decompression tables exist, with the U.S. Navy Standard Air Decompression Tables being the most widely used.[37] Decompression tables continue to be the subject of considerable scientific controversy, however, resulting in periodic revision and continual search for improved safety.

Over the years, the U.S. Navy Standard Decompression Tables have been the ones most often used in recreational diving. Various rearrangements or modifications of these tables have been promulgated by sport diving groups in recent years in efforts to improve the safety of recreational diving, which is qualitatively different from military diving (for which the Navy decompression tables were developed). In general, these sport-diving modifications have involved applying various safety factors to the standard Navy protocols.

Recent "multilevel" dive tables also have been developed to address the depth fluctuations that typically occur in sport diving because the diver ranges from shallow to deep repetitively during the course of a dive. These multilevel tables give the diver decompression "credit" for the time spent at shallower depths, as opposed to the Standard U.S. Navy tables, which require the diver to use the maximum depth of the dive to select no-decompression limits or decompression schedules and repetitive-dive group designations. The reason for doing this has been the belief that the U.S. Navy tables are too restrictive and excessively limit the diver's time underwater. Multilevel tables allow a diver to spend more time underwater, although there continues to be concern that they provide less safety margin.

Dive Computers. Automatic decompression meters that measure and record time and pressure underwater give the diver an indication of decompression status.[105] These "dive computers" track the exact dive profile and then calculate a decompression requirement according to the actual dive profile. The devices have used different physiologic and decompression models and technologies. Early automated decompression meters presented problems because their use was associated with an unacceptable rate of DCS. More recent technologic innovations, however, have overcome many of the earlier difficulties. The most recent generation of dive computers is considerably more advanced than the initial devices.[61,81] The sport scuba diver now has access to a variety of devices that offer the convenience of automatic and accurate depth-time recording,

together with accurately computed multilevel decompression schedules.

Currently available dive computers typically use microprocessors with decompression tables stored in memory. The microprocessor in the dive computer quickly reads a pressure transducer (which converts pressure into electrical impulses) and applies nitrogen uptake and elimination algorithms to this information every few seconds. The computer tracks a diver's exact profile and calculates decompression requirements accordingly.

Use of dive computers has become the norm, although concerns about their safety remain. Clearly, these computers are accurate depth-time recorders and are convenient because they obviate the clerical aspect of diving (i.e., the need to write down the depth and time of all dives, consult the decompression tables, calculate and record residual nitrogen time and surface intervals, and so on). Dive computers also offer advantages for some types of diving over use of the standard U.S. Navy decompression tables. They are especially useful in multilevel diving because they give bottom-time credit for time spent underwater at depths shallower than the deepest depth attained. However, it must be remembered that dive computers calculate decompression status based on models designed to simulate nitrogen uptake and release in a diver's body. These models may not accurately predict gas flow into and out of a given diver's tissues. Human physiology is not always as predictable as the computer model, and many factors can influence the actual rate of inert gas uptake and elimination. Also, most computers have no built-in safety margin to compensate for the difference between predicted and actual gas uptake and elimination, in contrast to decompression tables, which usually contain an inherent safety margin and require "rounding up" intermediate depths and times, providing a further safety factor.

Because of the multiple-tissue compartment modeling that dive computers use, another concern with their use is that they integrate the entire depth-time profile, so that in cases of repetitive diving (multiple dives per day, or multiple successive days of diving), dive computers would be more liberal than the Navy tables, allowing more time under water and potentially allowing a gradual unsafe accumulation of nitrogen in slow tissues. In such settings the risk of developing DCS may be greater.

Other notable concerns associated with the use of dive computers are their allowance of multiple reverse-profile dives (shallow, then deep dives—an inherently risky way to dive), risk of equipment failure (such as battery failure or flooding of the battery compartment), loss of information by inadvertently turning off the computer, or failure to turn on the computer at the beginning of a dive. In the last three scenarios, the safety of the dives done after the one in which the problem occurred would be jeopardized.

Despite the widespread use of dive computers in recent years, it is not possible, at this time, to say whether they are more or less safe than the U.S. Navy Standard Decompression Tables when the tables are actually followed. The fact that substantial numbers of divers treated for DCS in recent years (more than half of diving casualties treated at some recompression chambers) were using dive computers underscores that they do not inherently protect a diver from getting the bends.[39,85,86] Based on experience, dive computers appear to be relatively safe when used as directed.

SAFE SCUBA DIVING

Sport scuba divers are fortunate that the most colorful marine life and abundant natural light exist at shallow depths. This obviates the need to dive deep. Indeed, 100 fsw should be considered a deep dive for sport diving and, for all intents and purposes, the maximum depth for recreational diving.

Recreational diving is usually done hours to days away from the nearest recompression chamber, so the occurrence of DCS or AGE usually necessitates a major effort to evacuate an afflicted diver to the chamber. This often requires the use of special aircraft. Unfortunately, the delay between symptom onset and treatment may cause the damage to be poorly responsive to hyperbaric treatment. Therefore divers should do their best to avoid developing AGE or DCS.

The need to take a conservative approach to depth and time is even clearer when one considers that individual variability in DCS susceptibility, workload during the dive, water temperature, and ill-advised post-dive exercise or altitude exposure may confound any set of decompression tables or dive computers. Indeed, the potentially devastating consequences of DCS, even with the most vigorous hyperbaric treatment, mandate that divers always dive with the prevention of this disease foremost in their minds.

The following safe diving recommendations should be adhered to by recreational or sport divers:

- Dive within the limits of "no-decompression" ("no-D") tables. When a decompression computer is used, do not approach the limits of no-decompression diving.
- When using the decompression tables, always use the next greater depth to determine the "no-D" limits, then "jump" tables. For example, a 37-minute dive with maximum depth of 68 feet is considered a 70-foot dive and the "no-decompression limit" should be determined for the next jump, or in this case, that of an 80-foot dive for 40 minutes. Ascent toward the surface at a rate no faster than 1 foot per second should begin at the end of the prescribed limit (40 minutes in this example), regardless of how much time was actually spent at shallower depths. This "penalty" for dive time spent at shallower depth is an important safety factor.
- After any dive deeper than 60 fsw, and at the conclusion of all repetitive dives, make at least a 3- to 5-minute safety stop at 10 to 15 fsw.
- When using the decompression tables, use the surface-to-surface time or "total time of dive" in selecting the repetitive group designation.
- Carefully plan any repetitive dive so that it will be shallower than the previous dive and so that you stay well within "no-decompression" limits.
- Remember that any device or table that allows prolonged time at shallow depths after a deeper excursion also allows continued uptake of inert gas.
- Maintain hydration during diving days to ensure normal capillary perfusion for inert gas exchange. Remember that immersion diuresis and topside sweat loss in tropical regions can result in significant dehydration, which is often not overtly apparent. Keep the urine "clear and copious" on diving days.
- Do not engage in heavy exercise, such as jogging or wind surfing, for at least 6 hours after a dive.
- Do not fly, even in the pressurized cabin of commercial airlines, for at least 12 hours after "no-decompression" diving. If decompression stops were required, wait at least 24 hours before flying. If aircraft cabin altitude (e.g., an unpressurized airplane) will exceed 8000 feet, wait 24 hours before flying after any compressed gas dive.

Diving in mountain lakes requires significant adjustments in decompression tables to account for the decreased atmospheric pressure at the surface of the lake. Dive computers must be calibrated for altitude. Boni and associates[14] pointed out that for the same depth and the same bottom time of a dive, surfacing at a lower ambient air pressure than sea level necessitates longer decompression times. Several decompression tables for altitude diving have been calculated and tested in the field.[10,27,90] The U.S. Navy Standard Decompression Tables can be used up to an altitude of 2300 feet.

Even when these safe diving practices are followed, unexplained DCS cases sometimes occur.[1] Two mechanisms are postulated to account for these cases. After an otherwise safe dive, one well within the specified decompression procedure, elevated inert gas tensions exist in tissues and venous blood, which carry gas to the lungs for elimination. If all else is normal and conservative depths and times have been followed, the inert gas remains in solution or, at worst, "silent" or asymptomatic volumes of venous gas emboli are returned to the lungs. If a physiologically patent foramen ovale (PFO) allows intermittent retrograde flow from the right to the left atrium, bubbles can become arterial gas emboli. The potential for this type of paradoxical gas embolism to occur has been demonstrated in recent years for both PFO and other types of intracardiac shunts.[28,89,106] Whether the presence of a PFO should disqualify someone from diving is currently unclear because conflicting data have been found as to the association of a PFO and the occurrence of neurologic DCS.[28,89,106,111-113]

Another plausible explanation for DCS occurring after safe diving postulates that focal pulmonary barotrauma, or inadvertent breath-holding during decompression, produces local air trapping during ascent and releases "microbubbles" into the systemic circulation. These microscopic "seed" bubbles in arterialized blood then pass through the capillary bed to become bubble nuclei in venous blood, precipitating overt bubble formation and the classic manifestations of DCS.

DIVE ACCIDENT INVESTIGATION

When investigating a dive accident, whether for treatment purposes or as part of a forensic evaluation in the case of a fatal accident, the investigator begins by taking a detailed dive-accident history. A number of specific details must be determined about the patient's diving activities, the time of symptom onset, and the nature and progression of the symptoms, in addition to past medical history and other information that should be obtained on any patient. The diving-related history should specifically solicit information in the following areas[70]:

1. *The type of dive and equipment used.* Inquire specifically as to whether a decompression computer, diving watch, and depth gauge were used. Was compressed air or mixed gas used, and what was the source of the gas? Was a rebreather used?

2. *The number, depth, bottom or total dive time, and surface interval or intervals between dives for all dives in the 72 hours preceding symptom onset.* This information will be needed by the diving medicine consultant because it allows calculation of any omitted decompression and thus helps decide the likelihood of the patient having DCS or other problems. Unfortunately, the diver's interpretation of whether required decompression was omitted cannot be the sole source of data; this is notoriously unreliable. If a decompression computer was used, it should be checked for information about the need for recompression and whether it was worn on all dives.

3. *Whether in-water decompression was taken and if so, how much.* This is relevant to the likelihood of the diver having DCS. If a decompression computer was used, the diver should be asked whether the specified decompression profile was followed.

4. *Whether in-water recompression with compressed air was attempted after the onset of symptoms.* For all practical purposes, this should never be done because it almost always leaves the diver in a worse condition and is fraught with other hazards. (Of note, special protocols for in-water recompression treatment using 100% oxygen have been developed for emergency situations in exceptionally remote places.)

5. *The site of diving (e.g., ocean, lake, or quarry) and the environmental conditions (such as water temperature or presence of current or surge) associated with the dive.* These factors enter into the differential diagnosis and may raise the possibility of the symptoms being caused by something other than a bubble-related problem. For example, DCS is more common after diving in cold water, other things being equal, or motion sickness may develop in a diver swimming back to shore on a choppy sea even if there was no problem with seasickness before or during the dive.

6. *Primary diving activity (such as spearfishing, underwater photography, or shell collecting).* Like knowledge of environmental conditions, this helps in the differential diagnosis. For example, DCS is more likely after an arduous dive such as may occur with spearfishing than a dive to take photographs.

7. *Presence of predisposing factors for DCS.* A number of factors have been associated with an increased risk of DCS, including dehydration, vigorous exercise under water, advanced age, obesity, poor physical conditioning, local physical injury, and multiple repetitive dives in unacclimatized individuals.

8. *Whether the dive was complicated by running out of air, an untoward marine animal encounter, trauma, or other unexpected event.* For example, low back pain suggestive of DCS may be caused by a muscle strain from lifting the scuba tank or climbing into the dive boat, and tingling or numbness in an extremity may be caused by jellyfish envenomation.

9. *Whether the patient flew in an airplane, went jogging, or engaged in any other particular activity after diving but before the onset of symptoms.* If so, the effect of the activity on the symptoms should be ascertained. Some activities (such as flying in an unpressurized aircraft or vigorously exercising immediately after diving) may precipitate DCS in someone who might otherwise not be affected, or trivial dysbaric symptoms may become severe after similar activities.

10. *Time of symptom onset.* Symptoms that began soon after getting in the water (e.g., nausea from motion sickness), even if they worsen afterward, are not likely to be from DCS.

In fatal diving accidents, information gathered from the diving accident history should be supplemented with an appropriate diving accident autopsy, thorough evaluation of the diving equipment used, and detailed environmental history.[33] Environmental factors, such as weather, currents, wave action, visibility, water temperature, potential for entanglement, and dangerous marine life, must be also be considered. The diving equipment should be carefully studied for proper function and amount of compressed air in the tanks, and the air should be analyzed for contaminants. The diver's medical and psychologic histories should be sought because they may contain clues to a coincidental medical event that led to the diver's death but was unrelated to the dive. Aside from the obvious psychosocial risk factors such as alcoholism, drug abuse, or propensity to panic, the use of a scuba dive for suicide or homicide must be considered.

Unique aspects of the diving-victim autopsy should include a careful search for subcutaneous emphysema or other physical signs of POPS and a search for signs of marine envenomation. For example, before the surface of the body is washed, it should be examined for evidence of nematocysts from coelenterate stings. In addition, in contrast to the thoracic incision being made first, the calvarium should be opened before other incisions to prevent accidental introduction of air into the intracranial circulation. A finding of gas bubbles in intracranial vessels may result from AGE or DCS. Postmortem introduction of gas into the cerebral veins can be avoided if the calvarium is opened under water.[33] Likewise, the initial thoracic incision must be made with care to determine whether pneumothorax is present. A careful search should be made for gas bubbles in the major blood vessels and the heart. The middle ear should be examined for the presence of blood, and the tympanic membrane and paranasal sinuses should be examined for evidence of barotrauma.

Meticulous investigation of dive accidents is important to find equipment, procedural, or medical causes that could be useful in improving the safety of diving and to gather information for legal procedures that often follow diving accidents.

MEDICAL FITNESS FOR DIVING

General Considerations

Persons who want to take up scuba diving should first be cleared medically. The diving examination should focus on the pulmonary, otolaryngologic, cardiac, neurologic, and integumentary systems, as well as the person's psychological stability.

Many medical conditions are contraindications for diving because of the changes in pressure that occur with excursions underwater; the physical and sometimes psychological stress of diving; the potential for nitrogen narcosis, altered sensory stimulation, and other factors to interact with pharmaceuticals; and the inherent nature of being underwater. In general, these can be divided into five categories. Persons falling into any of these categories are at increased risk for a diving-related problem:

1. Persons who are unable to equalize pressure in one or more of the body's air spaces are at increased risk for barotrauma.
2. Persons who have a medical or psychiatric condition that may become manifest underwater or at a remote diving site and endanger the diver's life because of the condition itself, because it occurs in the water, or because inadequate medical help is available.
3. Persons who have impaired tissue perfusion or diffusion of inert gases and thus have an increased risk of DCS.
4. Persons who are in poor physical condition and thus at increased risk of DCS or exertion-related medical problems. The factors compromising physical condition may be physiologic or pharmacologic.
5. Women who are pregnant, because the fetus may be at increased risk of dysbaric injury.

Disqualifying Conditions

In accordance with the likelihood of causing a diving problem and the potential seriousness of the problem, conditions falling into one of the preceding five categories may be absolutely, relatively, or temporarily disqualifying for scuba diving.

Absolutely Disqualifying Conditions. Based on the opinion of a multispecialty panel of diving medicine experts,[30,31] the following conditions are considered to be absolute, or near absolute, disqualifications for diving:

1. *History of epilepsy or other seizure disorder.* Seizures occurring underwater essentially always result in a catastrophic outcome. After head injury, diving should not be allowed during that period of time when the patient is at increased risk of seizures.
2. *Insulin-dependent diabetes mellitus.* The risk of a hypoglycemic reaction underwater is increased by the possible need for sudden bursts of energy expenditure in emergencies. Underwater incapacitation due to hypoglycemia not only endangers the life of the individual but may also risk the lives of other persons during rescue attempts. Sport diving sometimes may be possible

for persons with diabetes that can be controlled by diet and exercise or, in special situations, diabetics who are well controlled on insulin, used to vigorous physical exercise, kowledgable about their condition, and dive with prepared buddies.

3. *Symptomatic coronary artery disease.* In addition to the need for cardiac reserve in an in-water emergency, carrying tanks, donning equipment, and swimming against current entail significant physical stresses. A history of myocardial infarction is considered a disqualification for sport diving, except in cases of exceptional rehabilitation after revascularization or comparable procedures.

4. *Sickle-cell disease or trait.* The chances that a sport diver will breathe a hypoxic gas mixture are remote, but it is possible. Other concerns are heavy exertion in cold water or local compromise of microvascular blood flow by bubble evolution during decompression, which could lead to sickling and a vicious cycle of hypoxia with further sickling.

5. *Unexplained syncope.*

6. *Inability to equalize pressure in the middle ear by autoinflation.* Of note, this may be caused by a correctable problem, such as polyps, allergic rhinitis, nasal septal deviation, or coryza, in which case the diver can be reevaluated after successful treatment.

7. *Bullous lung disease.* Air-containing pulmonary blebs or cysts can trap air and lead to local pulmonary overpressure accidents during decompression. If a ball-valve or flutter-valve effect allows such a bleb or cyst to equalize with the elevated breathing pressure during compression or descent, but blocks the escape of air during decompression, rupture could cause POPS and air embolism.

8. *Significant pulmonary obstructive disease.*

9. *Substance abuse.*

10. *Reactive airway disease (asthma).* Because of the risk of local air trapping and pulmonary overpressure accidents, persons having asthma should not dive. Although scuba air is generally free of pollens, other stresses in diving (such as cold, heavy exertion, or psychologic stress) could precipitate bronchospasm at depth, with resultant local air trapping during ascent. If there is any suggestion of bronchospastic tendencies, pulmonary function studies should be performed. Even minimal air trapping at sea level takes on great significance at depth.

11. *Spontaneous pneumothorax.* Even without the pressure variations of diving, a history of previous spontaneous pneumothorax carries a significant incidence of recurrence, and the candidate must be advised against compressed-gas diving. A pneumothorax that occurs while the diver is still at pressure underwater or in a recompression chamber can become a life-threatening tension pneumothorax as the pleural cavity air expands (Boyle's law) during ascent. Persons who have had traumatic or surgical pneumothorax may be cleared for diving, depending on the specific circumstances.

12. *Perforation of the tympanic membrane.* Until the eardrum is fully healed or successfully repaired and eustachian tube function is good, diving is contraindicated.

Possibly Disqualifying Conditions. The following disorders require special consideration; whether they are disqualifying for diving is controversial among diving physicians.

1. *Migraine and other vascular headaches.* Scintillating scotomas and other neurologic symptoms associated with migraines may be confused with DCS. A migraine after diving could be misinterpreted, causing unnecessary recompression treatment. Because commercial diving generally requires constant readiness to dive, migraine is often viewed as disqualifying for commercial diving.

2. *Middle ear surgery with placement of a prosthesis in the conduction chain.* The risk of displacement during pressure change and ear clearing is the determining factor in these cases.

3. *History of overpressure accident in previous diving.* The circumstances of the offending dive weigh heavily in these cases. For instance, if a diver suffers a "physiologically undeserved" or unexplained episode of POPS (i.e., the diver breathes normally to the surface, yet suffers an air embolism), risk of recurrence would be of greater concern. On the other hand, a diver who suffers a pulmonary overpressure accident that is considered "physiologically deserved" (e.g., rapid ascent after inadvertent inflation of a buoyancy compensator) could be considered for a return to diving after full neurologic recovery and with the determination of normal pulmonary function. However, some argue that even this diver is at greater risk because of potential pulmonary scarring and the inability to detect small airway air trapping.

4. *Hypertension.* The suitability of a hypertensive person for diving is based largely on the therapy required for blood pressure control. Diving has little effect on blood pressure, and when a regimen of weight control, diet, and mild diuretics is successful, diving usually can be allowed. If more potent antihypertensive agents are needed, diving may be contraindicated.

5. *Decreased visual acuity.* In sport diving, corrective lenses can be mounted in scuba face masks or contact lenses can be worn, so this is no longer as much a concern as in the early days of scuba diving. Soft contact lenses are preferable for diving.

Temporarily Disqualifying Conditions.

The following disorders are temporary disqualifications for diving:

1. *Coryza or bronchitis.* These conditions may cause inability to equalize pressure in the ears, sinuses, or lungs because of mucosal edema, mucus plugs, or bronchospasm.
2. *Pregnancy.* At present, there is near consensus that a woman who is or may be pregnant should suspend compressed-air diving until after delivery. Animal studies have produced conflicting results in different species and laboratories, but the possibility of bubble formation in fetal or placental tissues is a concern, even on a dive that is safe for the mother.
3. *Abdominal hernias.* These present a potential risk of trapping expanding gas in a herniated loop of bowel during ascent. In general, diving should be suspended until surgical repair is completed.
4. *Poor physical fitness.* Sport scuba diving is deceptively easy until an emergency occurs that requires swimming against a current, rescue of a buddy diver, or other vigorous activity. The diver should be capable of performing strenuous activity before entering the water. Regular swimming or other exercise programs to ensure cardiovascular fitness are encouraged.

Selection and Training of Disabled Divers

In recent years, many persons with limb amputations or other serious orthopedic impairment, spinal cord injury, cerebral palsy, or similar physical condition have sought to participate in scuba diving. Some of these persons were accomplished athletes or divers before an accident changed their physical status. For others, scuba diving is a completely new experience, being offered as part of a rehabilitation program. Whatever the case, it is clear that persons having "disabilities" can enjoy diving as much as anyone else if they are properly trained, understand their condition and the limitations it causes them, and make appropriate adjustments, when necessary, for their condition.[36] Indeed, when done in this context, scuba diving can open exciting new vistas for some disabled persons. Williamson and co-workers[110] demonstrated significant improvement in self-concept and body image among a group of young people with disabilities ranging from post-head injury brain damage, congenital deafness, blindness, and spinal cord dysfunction to major limb amputations. They were examined according to standard diving medicine practice regarding pulmonary

and ear, nose, and throat status and detailed psychological testing. Motivation proved to be an important predictor of success. The subjects were given extensive scuba-diving training with at least one-on-one instructor attention.

In any of these situations, the diver and his or her buddy need to fully understand the concerns attendant to his or her condition (e.g., autonomic dysreflexia, skin breakdown, personal hygiene, and a possible increased risk of DCS) and the wisdom of taking a conservative no-decompression approach to diving.

FLYING AFTER DIVING

Because diving is often done at remote destinations, the question of when it is safe to fly after diving often comes up. Flying too soon after diving can seriously jeopardize decompression safety, leading to development of DCS during or after the flight because of the reduced atmospheric pressure present in most commercial aircraft.

The normal commercial aircraft cabin pressure is equivalent to an altitude exposure of 5000 to 8000 feet, which is sufficient pressure reduction to cause dissolved nitrogen to come out of solution and form intravascular bubbles. (Depending on the age and maintenance of the aircraft, the internal cabin pressure may be equivalent to an even higher altitude.) The Divers Alert Network reports that 5% to 7% of divers with DCS contacting them in recent years reported flying before the onset of their symptoms. (The actual significance of these statistics is uncertain because the total number of divers who flew after diving is unknown, but the total is estimated to be very large compared with the number who developed DCS.)

With the continued growth of the dive-travel vacation industry, the issue of when it is safe to fly after diving has become even more important. Unfortunately, not enough experimental or detailed experiential data on the subject are available to precisely quantitate the risks, or to establish precise surface intervals for various types of diving profiles. However, this matter has been the subject of a number of workshops sponsored by the Undersea and Hyperbaric Medical Society and other concerned groups.

At present the generally accepted guidelines for flying after recreational diving are as follows:

1. Observe a minimum surface interval of 12 hours between the last dive and flying in a commercial jet.
2. Divers who make daily, multiple dives for several days, or who make dives that require decompression stops should exercise special caution and wait for an extended surface interval beyond 12 hours before flying in a commercial airliner. (Exactly what this extended surface interval should be is less well quantified, but many authorities

suggest at least 24 hours.) The longer the interval between diving and flying, the less the likelihood of DCS.

Having noted the above, it is important to emphasize that no rule about flying after diving can be guaranteed to prevent DCS. These are guidelines that represent the best estimate of a safe surface interval for the majority of sport scuba divers.

REFERENCES

1. Aharon-Peretz J et al: Spinal cord decompression sickness in sport diving, *Arch Neurol* 50:753, 1993.
2. Bachrach AJ: A short history of man in the sea. In Bennett PB, Elliott DH, editors: *The physiology and medicine of diving*, ed 3, London, 1982, Bailliere-Tindall.
3. Balk M, Goldman JM: Alveolar hemorrhage as a manifestation of pulmonary barotrauma after scuba diving, *Ann Emerg Med* 19:930, 1990.
4. Ball R: Effect of severity, time to recompression with oxygen, and re-treatment on outcome in 49 cases of spinal cord decompression sickness, *Undersea Hyperbaric Med* 20:133, 1993.
5. Barsky SM, Barsky KC, Damico RL: *Careers in diving*, Flagstaff, Ariz, 1994, Best Publishing Company.
6. Barsky S, Thurlow M, Ward M: *The simple guide to rebreather diving*, Flagstaff, Ariz, 1998, Best Publishing Company.
7. Bayne GC: Breath-hold diving. In Davis JC, editor: *Hyperbaric and undersea medicine*, vol 1, San Antonio, Tex, 1981, Medical Seminars Publishing.
8. Behnke AR: The history of diving and work in compressed air. In Davis JC, editor: *Hyperbaric and undersea medicine*, vol 1, San Antonio, Tex, 1981, Medical Seminars Publishing.
9. Behnke AR, Thomson RMA, Motley EP: Psychological effects from breathing air at four atmospheres pressure, *Am J Physiol* 112:554, 1935.
10. Bell R, Borgwordt R: The theory of high-altitude corrections to the U.S. Navy Standard Decompression Tables: the Cross corrections, *Undersea Biomed Res* 3:1, 1976.
11. Bennett PB: *Psychometric impairment in men breathing oxygen-helium at increased pressures*, Rep No 251, 1965, Medical Research Council, RN Personnel Research Committee, Underwater Physiology Subcommittee.
12. Bennett PB: The physiology of nitrogen narcosis and the high pressure nervous syndrome. In Strauss RH, editor: *Diving medicine*, New York, 1976, Grune & Stratton.
13. Bennett PB: Inert gas narcosis. In Bennett PB, Elliott DH, editors: *The physiology and medicine of diving*, ed 4, London, 1993, W.B. Saunders.
14. Boni M et al: Diving at diminished atmospheric pressure: air decompression tables for different altitudes, *Undersea Biomed Res* 3:189, 1976.
15. Bove AA et al: Successful therapy of cerebral air embolism with hyperbaric oxygen at 2.8 ATA, *Undersea Biomed Res* 9:75, 1982.
16. Butler BD et al: Effect of the Trendelenburg position on the distribution of arterial air emboli in dogs, *Ann Thorac Surg* 45:198, 1988.
17. Butler FK: Ocular manifestations of decompression sickness. In Gold D, Weinstein T, editors: *The eye in systemic disease*, Philadelphia, 1990, JB Lippincott.
18. Butler FK: Decompression sickness presenting as optic neuropathy, *Aviat Space Environ Med* 62:346, 1991.
19. Cales RH et al: Cardiac arrest from gas embolism in scuba diving, *Ann Emerg Med* 10:539: 1981.
20. Chryssanthou CP: Dysbaric osteonecrosis, *Clin Orthop* 130:94, 1978.
21. Chryssanthou CP et al: Studies on dysbarism. II. Influences of bradykinin and "bradykinin-antagonists" on decompression sickness in mice, *Aerospace Med* 35:741, 1964.
22. Clark JM, Lambertson CJ: Pulmonary oxygen toxicity: a review, *Pharmacol Rev* 23:37, 1971.
23. Cogas WB: Intravenous lidocaine as adjunctive therapy in the treatment of decompression illness, *Ann Emerg Med* 29:284, 1997.
24. Cole RH: *Underwater explosions*, New York, 1965, Dover Publications.
25. Colebatch HJH, Smith MM, Ng CKY: Increased elastic recoil as a determinant of pulmonary barotrauma in divers, *Respir Physiol* 55:64, 1976.
26. Cramer FS, Heimback RD: Stomach rupture as a result of gastrointestinal barotrauma in a scuba diver, *J Trauma* 22:238, 1982.
27. Cross ER: Technifacts: high altitude decompression, *Skin Diver Magazine*, Nov 1970, p 17.
28. Cross SJ et al: Safety of subaqua diving with a patent foramen ovale, *Br Med J* 304:481, 1992.
29. Davis JC, editor: *Treatment of serious decompression sickness and arterial gas embolism*, Pub No 34, Bethesda, Md, 1979 Undersea Medical Society.
30. Davis JC: Hyperbaric medicine: critical care aspects. In Shoemaker WC, editor: *Critical care: state of the art*, Aliso Viejo, Calif, 1984, The Society of Critical Care Medicine.
31. Davis JC: *Medical examination of sport scuba divers*, San Antonio, Tex, 1986, Medical Seminars Publishing.
32. Davis JC, Youngblood DH: Definitive treatment of decompression sickness and arterial gas embolism. In Davis JC, editor: *Hyperbaric and undersea medicine*, vol 1, San Antonio, Tex, 1981, Medical Seminars Publishing.
33. Davis JH: The autopsy in diving fatalities. In Davis JC, editor: *Hyperbaric and undersea medicine*, vol 1, San Antonio, Tex, 1981, Medical Seminars Publishing.
34. Davis RH: *Deep diving and submarine operations*, ed 6, London, 1955, Siebe Gorman.
35. Decompression Sickness Central Registry and Radiological Panel: Aseptic bone necrosis in commercial divers, *Lancet* 2:384, 1969.
36. Degnan F: *A guide for teaching scuba to divers with special needs*. Flagstaff, Ariz, 1998, Best Publishing Company.
37. Department of the Navy: *U.S. Navy diving manual*, vol 1, rev 2, Flagstaff, Ariz, 1988, Best Publishing Company.
38. Dick APK, Massey EW: Neurological presentation of decompression sickness and air embolism in sport divers, *Neurology* 35:667, 1985.
39. Divers Alert Network: *1999 report on decompression illness and diving and fatalities*, Durham, NC, 1999, DAN.
40. Donald K: *Oxygen and the diver*, Worcester, UK, 1992, published by Kenneth Donald in conjunction with the Self Publishing Association, Ltd.
41. Donald KW: Oxygen poisoning in man, *Br Med J* 1:667, 1947.
42. Dutka AJ: A review of the pathophysiology and potential application of experimental therapies for cerebral ischemia to the treatment of cerebral gas embolism, *Undersea Biomed Res* 12:403, 1985.
43. Edmonds C, Freeman P, Tonkin F: Fistula of the round window in diving, *Trans Am Acad Ophthalmol Otolaryngol* 78:444, 1974.
44. Edmonds C, Lowry C, Pennefather J: In *Diving and subaquatic medicine*, ed 3, Oxford, UK, 1992, Butterworth-Heinemann.
45. Edmonds C et al: *Otological aspects of diving*, Glebe, New South Wales, Australia, 1973, Australian Medical Publishing.
46. Elliott DH, Harrison JAB: Bone necrosis: an occupational hazard of diving, *J R Navy Med Serv* 56:140, 1970.
47. Erde A, Edmonds C: Decompression sickness: a clinical series, *J Occup Med* 17:324, 1975.
48. Evans DE et al: Cardiovascular effects of cerebral air embolism, *Stroke* 12:338, 1981.
49. Farmer JC: Diving injuries to the inner ear, *Ann Otol Rhinol Laryngol* 86(suppl 36, no 1, pt 3):1, 1977.
50. Farmer JC, Thomas WG: Ear and sinus problems in diving. In Strauss RH, editor: *Diving medicine*, New York, 1976, Grune & Stratton.
51. Francis TJR, Dutka AJ: Methylprednisolone in the treatment of acute spinal cord decompression sickness, *Undersea Biomed Res* 16:165, 1989.
52. Francis TJR et al: Is there a role for the autochthonous bubble in the pathogenesis of spinal cord decompression sickness? *J Neuropath and Exper Neur* 47:475, 1988.
53. Green SM et al: Incidence and severity of middle ear barotrauma in recreational scuba diving, *J Wilderness Med* 4:270, 1993.
54. Grey HV: Cave diving hazards and challenges, *Pressure* 16:5, 1987.
55. Hallenbeck JM: Cinematography of dog spinal vessels during cord-damaging decompression sickness, *Neurology* 26:190, 1976.
56. Hamilton RH, Kizer KW, editors: *Nitrogen narcosis*, Bethesda, Md, 1985, Undersea Medical Society.
57. Hart GB, Strauss MB, Lennon PA: The treatment of decompression sickness and air embolism in a monoplace chamber, *J Hyperbaric Med* 1:1, 1986.
58. Hendricks PL et al: Extension of pulmonary oxygen tolerance in man at 2 ATA by intermittent oxygen exposure, *J Appl Physiol* 42:593, 1977.
59. Hills BA: Spinal decompression sickness: hydrophobic protein and lamellar bodies in spinal tissue, *Undersea & Hyperbaric Med* 20:3, 1993.
60. Hodgson M, Beran RG, Shirtley G: The role of computed tomography in the assessment of neurologic sequelae of decompression sickness, *Arch Neurol* 45:1033, 1988.
61. Huggins KE: Underwater decompression computers: actual vs. ideal. In Lang MA, editor: *Proceedings of the Eighth Annual Scientific Diving Symposium*, Costa Mesa, Calif, 1988, American Academy of Underwater Sciences.

62. Huller T, Buzini Y: Blast injuries of the chest and abdomen, *Arch Surg* 100:24, 1970.

63. Hunter WL et al: Aseptic bone necrosis among U.S. Navy divers: survey of 934 randomly selected personnel, *Undersea Biomed Res* 5:25, 1978.

64. Isakov AP et al: Acute carpal tunnel syndrome in a diver: evidence of peripheral nervous system involvement in decompression sickness, *Ann Emerg Med* 28:90, 1996.

65. Kizer KW: Dysbarism in paradise, *Hawaii Med J* 39:109, 1980.

66. Kizer KW: Corticosteroids in the treatment of serious decompression sickness, *Ann Emerg Med* 10:485, 1981.

67. Kizer KW: The role of computed tomography in the management of dysbaric diving accidents, *Radiology* 140:705, 1981.

68. Kizer KW: Ventricular dysrhythmia associated with serious decompression sickness, *Ann Emerg Med* 9:580, 1981.

69. Kizer KW: Delayed treatment of dysbarism: a retrospective review of 50 cases, *JAMA* 247:2555, 1983.

70. Kizer KW: Management of dysbaric diving casualties, *Emerg Med Clin North Am* 1:659, 1983.

71. Kizer KW: Monoplace chamber treatment of dysbaric diving diseases, *J Hyperbaric Med* 1:137, 1986.

72. Kizer KW: Dysbaric cerebral air embolism in Hawaii, *Ann Emerg Med* 16:535, 1987.

73. Kizer KW, Golden JA: Lipoid pneumonitis in a commercial abalone diver, *Undersea Biomed Res* 14:545, 1987.

74. Kizer KW, Goodman PG: Radiographic manifestations of venous air embolism, *Radiology* 144:35, 1982.

75. Kruse CA: Air embolism and other skin diving problems, *Northwest Med* 62:525, 1963.

76. LaCour JP et al: Diving suit dermatitis caused by *Pseudomonas aeruginosa*: two cases, *J Am Acad Dermatol* 31:1055, 1994.

77. Leitch DR, Green RD: Pulmonary barotrauma in divers and the treatment of cerebral arterial gas embolism, *Aviat Space Environ Med* 57:931, 1986.

78. Leitch DR, Greenbaum LJ, Hallenbeck JV: Cerebral arterial air embolism. I. Is there benefit in beginning HBO treatment at 6 bar? *Undersea Biomed Res* 11:221, 1984.

79. Leitch DR, Greenbaum LJ, Hallenbeck JM: Cerebral arterial air embolism. III. Cerebral blood flow after decompression from various pressure treatments, *Undersea Biomed Res* 11:249, 1984.

80. Levin HS et al: Neurobehavioral and magnetic resonance imaging findings in two cases of decompression sickness, *Aviat Space Environ Med* 60:1204, 1989.

81. Lippman J: Dive computers, *SPUMS J* 18:126, 1988.

82. Lundgren CEG, Ornhagen H: Nausea and abdominal discomfort: possible relation to aerophagia during diving: an epidemiologic study, *Undersea Biomed Res* 2:155, 1975.

83. Lundgren CEG, Tjernstrom O, Ornhagen H: Alternobaric vertigo and hearing disturbances in connection with diving: an epidemiologic study, *Undersea Biomed Res* 1:251, 1974.

84. McAniff JJ: *U.S. underwater diving fatality statistics, 1983-1984,* Washington, DC, 1986, US Dept of Commerce, NOAA Undersea Research Program.

85. McGough EK, De Santeles DA, Gallagher TJ: Dive computers and decompression sickness: a review of 83 cases, *J Hyperbaric Med* 5:159, 1990.

86. McGough EK, De Santeles DA, Gallagher TJ: Performance of dive computers during single and repetitive dives: a comparison to the U.S. Navy diving tables, *J Hyperbaric Med* 5:163, 1990.

87. Medical Research Council: Decompression sickness and aseptic necrosis of bone, *Br J Industr Med* 28:1, 1971.

88. Miller J: Management of diving accident: author's reply, *Emerg Med* 13:23, 1981.

89. Moon RE, Camporesis EM, Kisslo JA: Patent foramen ovale and decompression sickness in divers, *Lancet* 1:513, 1989.

90. Morris B, McClellan M: *Practical altitude diving procedures,* Incline Village, Nev, 1986, Altitude Concepts.

91. Nelson EE: Internal carotid artery dissection associated with scuba diving, *Ann Emerg Med* 25:103, 1995.

92. Neuman TS, Bove AA: Severe refractory decompression sickness resulting from combined no-decompression dives and pulmonary barotrauma: type III decompression sickness. In Undersea and Hyperbaric Medical Society: *Ninth international symposium on underwater and hyperbaric physiology,* Bethesda, Md, 1987, The Undersea and Hyperbaric Medical Society.

93. Neuman TS, Hallenbeck JM: Barotraumatic cerebral air embolism and the mental status examination: a report of four cases, *Ann Emerg Med* 16:220, 1987.

94. Ohta Y, Matsunaga H: Bone lesions in divers, *J Bone Joint Surg* 56B:3, 1974.

95. Parell GJ, Becker GD: Conservative management of inner ear barotrauma resulting from scuba diving, *Otolaryngol Head Neck Surg* 93:393, 1985.

96. Palmer AC: Nature and incidence of bubbles in the spinal cord of decompressed goats, *Undersea Hyperbar Med* 24:193, 1997.

97. Paterson M: Underwater archeology. In Idyll CP, editor: *Exploring the ocean world,* New York, 1977, Thomas Y. Crowell.

98. Phillips JL: *The bends: compressed air in the history of science, diving and engineering,* New Haven, Conn, 1998, Yale University Press.

99. Polkinghorne PJ et al: Ocular fundus lesions in divers, *Lancet* 2:1381, 1988.

100. Rivera JC: Decompression sickness among divers: an analysis of 935 cases, *Milit Med* 129:314,1964.

101. Rothschild B, Martin LD: Avascular necrosis: occurrence in diving Cretaceous mosasaurs, *Science* 236:75, 1991.

102. Rudge FW, Stone JA: The use of the pressure cuff test in the diagnosis of decompression sickness, *Aviat Space Environ Med* 62:266, 1991.

103. Saltzer KR et al: Diving suit dermatitis: a manifestation of Pseudomonas folliculitis. *Cutis* 59:245, 1997.

104. Schaefer KE et al: Pulmonary and circulatory adjustments determining the limits of depths in breath-hold diving, *Science* 162:1020, 1968.

105. Stubbs RA, Kidd DJ: Computer analogies for decompression. In Lambertson CJ, editor: *Proceedings of the Third Underwater Physiology Symposium,* Baltimore, 1967, Williams & Wilkins.

106. Vik A, Jenssen BM, Brubakk AO: Arterial gas bubbles after compression in pigs with patent foramen ovale, *Undersea Hyperbaric Med* 20:121, 1993.

107. Wade CE et al: Incidence of dysbaric osteonecrosis in Hawaii's diving fishermen, *Undersea Biomed Res* 5:137, 1978.

108. Warren LP et al: Neuroimaging of scuba diving injuries to the CNS, *AJR* 142:1003, 1988.

109. Webb P: Thermal problems. In Bennett PB, Elliott DH, editors: *The physiology and medicine of diving,* ed 3, London, 1982, Bailliere-Tindall.

110. Williamson JA et al: Selection and training of disabled persons for scubadiving, *Med J Aust* 141:414, 1984.

111. Wilmhurst PT, Byrne JC, Webb-Peploc MM: Neurological decompression sickness, *Lancet* 1:731, 1989.

112. Wilmhurst PT, Byrne JC, Webb-Peploc MM: Relation between interatrial shunts and decompression sickness in divers, *Lancet* 2:1302, 1989.

113. Wilmhurst PT, Ellis BG, Jenkins BS: Paradoxical gas embolism in a scuba diver with an atrial septal defect, *Br Med J* 293:1277, 1986.

58 Emergency Oxygen Administration

Kimberley P. Walker

Emergency medical oxygen (O_2) administration is a critical part of emergency medical care of the ill and injured. Every provider of emergency medical care must be familiar with O_2, its therapeutic value, indications, and hazards. Equipment and techniques associated with its administration must also be well understood. O_2 is a colorless, odorless, and tasteless gas that is necessary for cellular metabolism. It makes up 21% of Earth's atmosphere, and although it is not flammable by itself, it is necessary to support combustion. O_2 utilized for respiration is diatomic and is obtained commercially by fractional distillation of air.[4,5] In the case of an ill or injured person suffering from hypoxia or anoxia, supplemental O_2 is used regularly as first aid (before emergency medical service personnel arrive), prehospital, or in-hospital emergency medical treatment.

THERAPEUTIC VALUE OF SUPPLEMENTAL OXYGEN

The therapeutic value of supplemental O_2 is to treat hypoxia and anoxia by increasing the amount of dissolved O_2 in the plasma and bound to hemoglobin, thereby increasing cellular perfusion by oxygenated blood. In addition, O_2 is a mild vasoconstrictor and may in certain circumstances help to limit edema generation.

INDICATIONS

Indications for the use of supplemental O_2 include (but are not limited to) the following[2,6]:
- Shock, hypoxia
- Hypoxemia
- Trauma
- Medical emergencies (asthma, anaphylaxis, acute myocardial infarction, cerebrovascular accident)
- Decompression illness (DCI), including both decompression sickness (DCS) and arterial gas embolism (AGE)
- Acute mountain sickness (AMS)
- High altitude pulmonary edema (HAPE)
- High altitude cerebral edema (HACE)
- Carbon monoxide (CO) poisoning
- Respiratory or cardiopulmonary arrest

CONTRAINDICATIONS

In an acutely hypoxic patient there is no contraindication to the administration of high concentrations of supplemental O_2 for a limited time. O_2 should not be withheld out of fear of suppressing respiration when hypoxia is suspected.[10] However, a person with a history of chronic obstructive pulmonary disease (COPD) who is not acutely hypoxic or in need of emergency prehospital care and transport to an emergency department should not be administered more than his or her prescribed flow rate of supplemental O_2.

Pulmonary Oxygen Toxicity

In situations in which high concentrations of supplemental O_2 administration may be carried out for many hours, there exists a concern for possible pulmonary O_2 toxicity. Prolonged exposure to high concentrations of O_2 is associated with intratracheal and bronchial irritation, with substernal or retrosternal burning, chest tightness, cough, and dyspnea. Continued exposure may result in adult respiratory distress syndrome (ARDS). Early pulmonary changes associated with pulmonary O_2 toxicity are reversible with cessation of O_2 therapy.[12]

At a fraction of inspired oxygen (FIO_2) of 0.5 to 1.0 (constant with no air breaks) and at normobaric or hypobaric ambient pressure, signs and symptoms of pulmonary O_2 toxicity may begin to appear in approximately 10 to 18 hours. Avoidance of the onset of symptoms may be accomplished by the use of periodic "air breaks," during which the patient breathes air for 5 to 10 minutes.[7,12]

Central Nervous System Oxygen Toxicity

Central nervous system (CNS) O_2 toxicity is of concern when a person is exposed to O_2 at ambient pressures greater than one atmosphere (sea level) and where FIO_2 exceeds 1.0, such as while scuba diving or in a hyperbaric O_2 chamber. It is not of concern to persons at normobaric or hypobaric ambient pressure. Signs and symptoms may appear at FIO_2 of greater than 1.6 and include (but are not limited to) sweating, bradycardia, mood changes, visual field constriction, twitching, syncope, and seizures. During hyperbaric O_2 therapy the likelihood of CNS O_2 toxicity is reduced by the use of periodic air breaks.[12]

EQUIPMENT

Cylinders

Medical O_2 cylinders or tanks are made of aluminum or steel and come in a variety of sizes (Table 58-1). In the United States, any pressure vessel that is transported on public roads is subject to U.S. Department of Transportation (US DOT) regulations. The US DOT requires that cylinders be visually and hydrostatically tested every 5 years and either be destroyed if they fail or be stamped and labeled appropriately if they pass.[15] Gas suppliers will not fill cylinders that have not been appropriately tested and stamped. The working pressure of steel medical O_2 cylinders is 2015 psi. The working pressure of aluminum O_2 cylinders is either 2015 psi or 2216 psi, depending on the type.

Valves

Valves for medical O_2 cylinders sold in the United States are designed to accept only medical O_2 regulators to avoid the possibility of using a medical O_2 regulator with an incompatible gas such as acetylene. The two types of valves available in the United States are the CGA-870 and the CGA-540. The CGA-870 is also known as the *pin-index valve* and is used on smaller portable cylinders (e.g., D, E). The CGA-540 is used primarily on larger, nonportable cylinders, such as those mounted in ambulances (e.g., H, M).

There a number of other valve types manufactured and used with medical O_2 throughout the world. For example, there are adapters available to make a U.S. pin-index regulator fit on an Australian bull-nose valve, but it must be noted that the use of adapters is discouraged by the U.S. Compressed Gas Association (CGA).

Regulators

The device that mounts directly to the cylinder is the regulator. Its function is to regulate the flow rate of the O_2 by reducing the pressure of the O_2 from either 2015 psi or 2216 psi to a usable flow rate. Regulators primarily have three types: constant flow only, demand/flow restricted oxygen-powered ventilator (FROPV) only, or multifunction, which has both constant flow and demand/FROPV capability.

The regulator mounts to the cylinder with a matching-type valve. A pressure gauge allows the user to monitor the amount of O_2 in the cylinder. Other features may include a diameter index safety system (DISS) fitting for an FROPV, a constant flow controller device (either knob or gauge), or both, as in the case of the multifunction regulator.

Devices for Ventilation of Nonbreathing Patients

All of the following devices keep direct patient contact at a minimum to reduce the risk of disease transmission. Other body substance isolation equipment (e.g., gloves, goggles) and practices should be observed as well.

In addition, when used on a nonintubated patient, all of the devices discussed below depend on adequate mask seal to be able to deliver adequate ventilations and ensure adequate respiration. The single most common cause of inadequate ventilation and respiration is poor mask seal.

FROPV/Positive Pressure Demand Valve.
Older style positive pressure demand valves (PPDVs) such as the LSP 063-05 or Elder CPR Demand valve (both manufactured by Life Support Products/Allied Health Care) function both in positive pressure mode (pushing the button to ventilate a nonbreathing patient) and in demand mode.

When used in demand mode, the recipient simply holds the mask to his or her face. When he or she inhales, negative pressure in the mask and demand valve opens the valve, and gas flows. The flow of gas stops when the person stops inhaling or exhales, similar to other demand regulators such as scuba and aviation regulators.

TABLE 58-1. Common Portable Medical Oxygen Cylinder Specifications

CYLINDER SIZE	ALLOY	WORKING PRESSURE (lbs/sq inch or psi)	VOLUME (L, cu ft)	LENGTH (in, cm)	DIAMETER (in, cm)	WEIGHT (lb, kg)
M9	Aluminum	2015	246.3, 8.7	10.9, 27.7	4.4, 11.1	3.9, 1.8
D	Aluminum	2015	424.7l, 15	16.5, 41.9	4.4 , 11.1	5.5, 2.5
D*	Steel	2015	410.4, 14.5	16.75, 42.5	4.4, 11.1	7.5, 3.4
Jumbo D	Aluminum	2216	648.3, 22.9	17, 43.2	5.3, 13.3	9.0, 4.1
E	Aluminum	2015	679.4, 24	25.6, 65.0	4.4, 11.1	8.0, 3.6
E*	Steel	2015	682.0, 24.1	25.75, 65.4	4.4, 11.1	10.5, 4.8

NOTE: Aluminum cylinder specifications provided by Luxfer Inc.
*Steel cylinder specifications provided by Pressed Steel Tank Co.

There has been a misconception that a PPDV will easily cause pulmonary overpressurization injury, and thus they have fallen out of favor with some health care providers. In fact, in positive pressure mode, all PPDVs manufactured in the United States are required to have an overpressure relief valve that stops the flow of gas at a pressure of 55 to 65 cm H_2O (a little more than half the pressure required to overpressurize a human lung). This was done to avoid pulmonary overpressurization injury. The most recent model introduced in 1993, the MTV-100 FROPV (LSP/Allied) has two overpressure relief valves, the first set at 60 cm H_2O and the second at 65 to 80 cm H_2O.*

With respect to the positive pressure mode, earlier PPDVs were originally designed to meet the Emergency Cardiac Care Committee (ECC) cardiopulmonary resuscitation (CPR) guidelines before 1986, which called for "four quick initial breaths and then two quick breaths after every 15 compressions."[10] This faster rate of ventilation was equivalent to 160 L/min (liters per minute).

In 1986 CPR standards were changed to "two slow breaths, each one and one-half seconds in duration."[10] The standard changed again in 1992 to the current one of "two slow, full breaths, with a duration of 1½ to 2 seconds each" (equivalent to 40 L/min).[10] This was changed to reduce the possibility of gastric insufflation, regurgitation, and aspiration of gastric contents. To meet this guideline of a 1½- to 2-second breath, the manufacturers of PPDVs added a restricting orifice that limited the flow rate to 40 L/min. Unfortunately, this created increased breathing resistance to the demand feature.

In 1993 a new style PPDV, called a *flow restricted oxygen-powered ventilator* (FROPV) (MTV-100, manufactured by LSP/Allied) was introduced. Its specifications include a flow rate of 40 L/min while being used in positive pressure mode and 115 L/min in demand mode, eliminating the difficulties of the earlier models.

The mask adapter is a standard 15-mm fitting that fits a variety of masks and can also be used directly with an endotracheal tube. The disadvantages of the FROPV are that a supply of O_2 is required for its use and that in intubated patients the health care provider will not be able to "feel" decreased lung compliance.

Bag-Valve-Mask. The bag-valve mask (BVM) consists of a mask, bag, and valves that control or direct the flow of air and O_2. Like the FROPV, the mask can be changed to different styles to accommodate different faces or can be used directly with an endotracheal tube. The volume of the bag is 1000 to 1200 ml, depending on the manufacturer. Some have an outlet and reservoir for use with supplemental O_2.

An advantage to the BVM is that although it works best with supplemental O_2, it will function on room air if the O_2 supply is depleted. In addition, in intubated patients, some health care providers are able to "feel" decreased lung compliance.

The primary disadvantage is that it requires training and practice to effectively use a BVM, and even with much practice, many find it is difficult to maintain adequate mask seal and ventilate sufficient volumes when only one rescuer is available to use it. Even with proper training, few individuals can maintain adequate mask seal and a patent airway with one hand while squeezing the bag fully to achieve the 800 to 1200 ml standard volume. The US DOT National Standard Curricula for First Responder to Paramedic recommend the BVM be used first with two rescuers (one maintaining mask seal and patency of the airway, the other squeezing the bag). The NSC recommends that a BVM with one rescuer be the last choice (after all other devices and techniques) in ventilating a patient.[15] In addition, there is no overpressurization relief valve. This is rarely a concern in unintubated patients because of the aforementioned difficulties in achieving even minimally acceptable ventilatory volumes, but it is of concern in intubated patients.

Resuscitation Mask

The pocket-type resuscitation mask consists of a clear, flexible plastic mask designed to fit over the mouth and nose of the victim while the health care provider ventilates by exhaling through the "chimney." There is usually a one-way valve that directs the rescuer's breath into the victim while at the same time directing the exhaled breath of the victim away from the rescuer. It is a relatively simple device that requires minimal training, is lightweight, and is more likely to be available when equipment is at a minimum. It is available both with and without an outlet for supplemental O_2.

The pocket-type mask is most effective when used with supplemental O_2. It will also function on room air and does not have an overpressurization relief valve.

Constant Flow Devices for Adequately Breathing Patients. The nonrebreather mask is the first choice when considering constant flow supplemental O_2 in an acute medical emergency. It consists of a mask, reservoir bag, and two or three one-way valves, one separating the reservoir from the mask and the other one or two on the sides of the mask. Oxygen flows into the reservoir bag so that when the patient inhales, he or she inhales O_2 from the reservoir. The one-way valves on the sides of the mask keep air from coming into the mask and diluting the O_2. When the patient exhales, expired air goes out of the mask through the one or two valves on the face and is prevented from entering the reservoir.

---

*Specifications from Allied Healthcare, Inc./Life Support Products.

The efficiency of this mask depends on the mask fit and seal and proper functioning of the valves. Under ideal conditions this mask (when fitted with all three valves) may deliver an FIO_2 of up to 0.95. Field studies show it may deliver FIO_2 as low as 0.60, but it is still the most effective constant flow device available (except for O_2 rebreathers).[14]

To use the mask, it is attached to the O_2 supply at a flow rate of 10 to 15 L/min. The reservoir bag must be inflated or "primed" before placing it on the patient. This can be accomplished by placing a thumb or fingers on the valve between the reservoir and mask while the reservoir inflates. Care must be taken to not allow the O_2 supply to be depleted while the mask is on the patient. Because of the one-way valves, if there is no O_2 supply, suffocation may result. The mask is available with either two one-way valves on the sides or with only one (labeled as "with safety outlet"). If the mask has only one valve on the side of the mask, it will deliver reduced FIO_2.

The advantage of the nonrebreather mask is that it provides the highest FIO_2 of the constant flow devices. However, it also wastes O_2 and may not deliver a high FIO_2 under less than ideal conditions. Care must be taken to monitor the patient and O_2 supply closely to avoid allowing the tank to empty while the mask is still on the patient's face.

The only other recommended constant flow device for prehospital emergency O_2 administration is the nasal cannula.[15] This is recommended when the patient will absolutely not tolerate any kind of mask, such as a person with a long history of COPD. In this case it is believed that some supplemental O_2 is better than none. It must be understood that a nasal cannula is capable of only delivering FIO_2 of 0.24 to 0.29.[14] In wilderness medicine, the nasal cannula should rarely warrant consideration.

Flow rates for a nasal cannula are limited to 1 to 6 L/min. To use the nasal cannula, place the prongs in the patient's nares and loop the tubing over the top of the ears to hold it in place. Adjust the tightness at the neck to a comfortable level. Flow rates exceeding 6 L/min are extremely uncomfortable for the patient and may result in drying of the nasal mucosa.

Other constant flow masks, such as the partial rebreather mask, the simple face mask, and the venturi mask, are not recommended for use in prehospital emergency medicine because of low levels of delivered FIO_2.[14,15]

Oxygen Rebreathers

One of the problems with long transports commonly seen in the case of wilderness or remote emergency medical care is that all of the previously discussed O_2 delivery devices waste O_2 and require multiple portable or large nonportable cylinders if the transport time exceeds 1 hour. Breathing room air, a person inhales 21% O_2 and exhales 16% O_2. If a person inhales (under ideal conditions) 100% O_2, the exhaled gas will contain 95% O_2 and 5% CO_2. The theory of the design of a rebreather is to remove CO_2 from the exhaled gas, supplement for the 5% O_2 that was metabolized, and reuse the exhaled O_2.

There are several manufacturers of rebreathers for emergency medical O_2 administration and they all have the same basic components. There is a mask, a breathing circuit (similar to anesthesia equipment), and a canister with an absorbent chemical, usually soda lime or Sodasorb.*

The soda lime chemically removes CO_2 from the exhaled gas, allowing for the O_2 to be rebreathed.† Supplemental O_2 is added at flow rates of less than 2 Lpm to replace the metabolized O_2, and thus the cylinder that can last 45 minutes with a nonrebreather mask or a little more than 1 hour on demand now lasts more than 6 hours, and the patient (with proper technique) will still receive FIO_2 of 0.85 to 0.99. In a situation in which equipment is limited because of size and weight, this device may prove invaluable.

Different manufacturers recommend beginning the patient on O_2 during assembly, setting up the unit, flushing the system of air, applying it to the patient, and considering air breaks to minimize the risk of pulmonary oxygen toxicity.

Thermal considerations are important because of the chemical reaction that takes place with the soda lime. The reaction produces heat and water, so it provides warmed and humidified O_2. In cold climates, this is an advantage, but in hot climates it may be a disadvantage. If one is in a hot climate, it is recommended to pass the breathing circuit hoses through cold or ice water to cool the gas. Rebreather set-ups are typically lightweight and allow high FIO_2 (>0.80) at constant flow rates of less than 2 L/min, thereby extending the life of the cylinder.

Disadvantages are the training requirement and that the breathing circuit and absorbent canister containing the soda lime are typically "single-patient use." Like other O_2 delivery devices, the rebreather also depends on an adequate mask seal to function effectively. Poor mask seal results in dilution of inhaled gas with air and lower FIO_2. There may also be an increase in breathing resistance when compared with a constant-flow mask.

The most common types of resuscitators available on the market today are the American DAN $REMO_2$ system, two German systems (the Wenoll and the Circulox), and an Australian system (OXI-Saver Resuscitator).[11,13]

---

*Sodasorb is manufactured by W.R. Grace, Inc. and is most commonly NaOH.
†$2NaOH + CO_2 = Na_2CO_3 + H_2O + heat$, from W.R. Grace, Inc.

Airways

See Chapter 17.

CONCERNS INVOLVING VENTILATING OR ASSISTING VENTILATIONS IN NONBREATHING OR INADEQUATELY BREATHING PATIENTS

Concerns for ventilating nonbreathing patients include rate (breaths per minute), volume, flow rate or speed, pressure, and oxygenation. The rate of ventilations per minute is 12 per minute for an adult (over 8 years old) and 20 per minute for children and infants.[10]

The recommended volume for ventilations for an adult is 800 to 1200 ml. If a ventilation device or technique does not have an over-pressure relief valve and greater volumes are administered, pulmonary barotrauma (pulmonary overpressurization injury) may result. Ventilatory volumes less than 800 ml may not be sufficient to inflate the alveoli, and thus gas exchange will be inadequate. Each ventilation should be at least 1½ to 2 seconds in duration (equivalent to 40 L/min). Faster ventilation rates or speeds force open the esophagus and then force air into the stomach rather than the lungs. Increased gastric insufflation greatly increases the risk of regurgitation and aspiration of gastric contents.[10]

It has been demonstrated that a differential pressure of as little as 90 to 110 cm H_2O has been sufficient to rupture alveolar septa and to allow gas to escape into interstitial spaces.[1,2,8] Care must be taken to not exceed these pressures when ventilating a patient. Humans can easily generate pressures exceeding 120 cmH_2O by exhaling forcefully, and thus according to ECC CPR guidelines, one should "blow until the chest rises" to accommodate various sizes of patients. The only device for ventilating adult patients that has an overpressure relief valve is the PPDV/FROPV.

The primary goal of ventilation is oxygenation of the patient. With mouth-to-mouth or mouth-to-mask breathing without supplemental O_2, FIO_2 will be the same as exhaled gas, which is 0.16, or 16% O_2. Adding O_2 at a flow rate of 15 L/min may increase the FIO_2 with a pocket mask to up to 50%. A BVM on room air is 0.21, and with O_2 at 15 L/min up to 0.9, depending on the equipment and the skill of the ventilator. A FROPV delivers close to 1.0, or 100% O_2.[2,10]

Both the volume and oxygenation achieved by ventilations depend on the quality of the mask seal and patency of the airway. The single most common cause of inadequate ventilation in a nonintubated patient is poor mask seal. Great care must be taken to ensure that the airway is fully patent and that there is a good mask seal with each ventilation. If the patient is not intubated, an oropharyngeal, nasopharyngeal, or a combination airway should be used if available.

Because a FROPV delivers the highest FIO_2, is the only device that is limited to 40 L/min flow rate (1½ to 2 seconds in duration) and has an overpressure relief valve, it may be the best choice for ventilating a person in respiratory arrest, whether or not they are intubated. A BVM unit used by rescuers (one to maintain the mask seal, and the other to squeeze the bag) is the best alternative. This method of ventilation is the first choice for ventilating a person in respiratory arrest, according to the US DOT National Standard Curricula for EMTs (1994), First Responders (1995), and Paramedics (1998).[9,15] According to these same curricula, the following is the order of preference in ventilating a person in respiratory arrest:

1. BVM unit with two rescuers and supplemental O_2
2. Pocket mask with supplemental O_2
3. FROPV
4. BVM unit with one rescuer and supplemental O_2
5. Last choice, and not an option for the professional rescuer, is mouth-to-mouth breathing, because of the risk of disease transmission

HAZARDS

Oxygen alone or in a vacuum is not flammable. However, in the presence of flammable substances, combustion can be very vigorous. It is imperative to use O_2 only in open, well-ventilated areas and not in the presence of burning materials. Care must be taken when handling O_2 equipment to avoid allowing contaminants such as petroleum products to come into contact with the regulator, particularly in or around the orifices on the cylinder or regulator through which O_2 flows. Cylinders should not be exposed to temperatures above 52° C (125° F).

LEGAL ISSUES

The United States Food and Drug Administration (FDA) regulations regarding O_2 administration equipment state that to qualify as "emergency medical oxygen administration equipment" the device must "be capable of administering a flow rate of at least 6 L/min for a period of at least 15 minutes."* Equipment not meeting this minimum standard may not be sold in the United States as emergency medical O_2 administration equipment.

To fill a medical O_2 cylinder, the FDA states, "For emergency use only when administered by properly trained personnel for O_2 deficiency and resuscitation. For all other medical applications, Caution: Federal law prohibits dispensing without prescription."†

---

*FDA website: *http://www.fda.gov/cdrh/indexlo.html#0*
†Human Drug CGMP Notes (December 1996), Section 503(b)(4) of the Food Drug and Cosmetic Act; 21 CFR Sections 201(b)(1) and Reference: 211.130; website: *http://www.fda.gove/cder/compliance/gaswhat.htm*

REFERENCES

1. Bennett PB, Elliott D: *The physiology and medicine of diving,* ed 4, Philadelphia, 1993, WB Saunders.
2. Bledsoe BE, Porter RS, Shade BR: *Paramedic emergency care,* Upper Saddle River, NJ, 1994, Prentice Hall.
3. Bove A, Davis J: *Diving medicine,* ed 3, Philadelphia, 1998, WB Saunders.
4. Corry JA: Setting the record straight: oxygen delivery and the injured diver. In Bennett PB, Moon RE, editors: *Diving accident management,* Bethesda, Md, 1990, UHMS.
5. Corry JA: *Student workbook for emergency oxygen administration and field management of scuba diving accidents workshop, rev,* Montclair, Calif, 1990, NAUI.
6. Cummins RO, editor: *Advanced cardiac life support,* Dallas, 1997, American Heart Association.
7. Donald K: *Oxygen and the diver,* Hanley Swan, Great Britain, 1992, self-published.
8. Edmonds C, Lowry C, Pennefeather J: *Diving and subaquatic medicine,* ed 3, Woburn, Mass, 1992, Butterworth-Heinemann.
9. Elling R: An evaluation of emergency medical technician's ability to use manual ventilation devices, *Ann Emerg Med* 12:765, 1983.
10. Emergency Cardiac Care Committee: Guidelines for emergency cardiac care, *JAMA* 268, 1992.
11. Hobbs GW et al: Evaluation of commercially available closed circuit rebreather systems, Duke University Medical Center.
12. Kindwall EP, editor: *Hyperbaric medicine practice,* Flagstaff, Ariz, 1995, Best Publishing Co.
13. Lippmann J: *DAN Australia Closed Circuit Resuscitator Training Manual,* DAN SEAP, 1996.
14. Tsing GCC et al: *Oxygen provision by first-aid equipment: what FIO_2s?,* Townsville, Australia, 1998, Hyperbaric Technicians and Nurses Association.
15. United States Department of Transportation: National Standard Curricula (US DOT NSC) for First Responder (1995), EMT-Basic (1994), EMT-I (1999), EMT-Paramedic (1998), website: *http://www.nhtsa.dot.gov/people/injury/ems/nsc.htm*

59 Principles of Hyperbaric Oxygen Therapy

Claude A. Piantadosi

Hyperbaric oxygen therapy (HBOT) is defined as the inhalation of oxygen at a partial pressure greater than the normal barometric pressure at sea level of 760 mm Hg (one atmosphere absolute [atm]). HBOT is used as a treatment in which a patient breathes pure oxygen inside a pressurized chamber to help resolve certain difficult or refractory medical problems. Most treatments are performed at 2 to 3 atm; these pressures are equivalent to 33 to 66 feet of seawater (FSW).

HBOT may be used as either a primary therapeutic modality (e.g., for decompression sickness [DCS]) or as an adjunctive modality (e.g., for clostridial myonecrosis). The therapeutic effects of hyperbaric oxygen (HBO) are related to specific physical, physiologic, and biochemical effects of high partial pressures of oxygen (PO_2) in the blood and tissues of the body. The conditions for which HBOT has a sound scientific rationale and demonstrated clinical efficacy are relatively few but encompass a heterogeneous body of disorders, indicating that its pharmacologic effects are not mediated by a single mechanism of action. Currently, HBOT is widely recommended for only 13 medical conditions (Table 59-1); these constitute the indications approved by the Undersea and Hyperbaric Medical Society.[3]

BIOLOGIC EFFECTS OF HYPERBARIC OXYGEN

The biologic effects of HBO are related to changes in physicochemical processes in the body by molecular oxygen. These processes include gas diffusion, convective transport of oxygen and inert gases, and chemical reactions involving oxygen, including generation of reactive oxygen species. The physiologic effects of HBO are related primarily to the first two of these processes, diffusion and convection, which allows substantial increases in the PO_2 of arterial blood and in certain body tissues under hyperbaric conditions. Diffusion is also necessary to facilitate movement of bubbles of inert gas (such as nitrogen) in the blood and tissues in the resolution after decompression from a higher-pressured to a lower-pressured environment. The third process, the chemical activity of oxygen, determines the effects of HBO on normal metabolic events, as well as the manifestations of oxygen toxicity.

Transport of oxygen from the ambient environment to the tissues depends on a gradient of partial pressures between the air spaces of the lung and the cells of the body. This gradient, known as the oxygen cascade, nor-

mally begins during air breathing at sea level with inspired PO_2 of about 150 mm Hg. From the lungs, oxygen diffuses into the pulmonary capillaries, where it is carried in arterial blood out to the tissues. Hyperbaric oxygen produces profound effects on gas exchange by the lungs, oxygen transport to tissues, and PO_2 in the tissues.

Gas Exchange by the Lungs

Normal oxygen exchange begins in the alveoli of the lungs after inspired gas is warmed to body temperature, humidified and diluted with carbon dioxide (CO_2) leaving the body through ventilation. These factors are taken into account by subtracting the partial pressures of water vapor (47 mm Hg) and CO_2 ($PACO_2$, normally 40 mm Hg) from total gas pressure in the alveoli. These relationships are described by the alveolar air equation:

$$PAO_2 = FIO_2 (PB - PH_2O) - PACO_2 \times [FIO_2 + (1 - FIO_2)/R]$$

where PAO_2 is the partial pressure of oxygen in the alveoli; PB and PH_2O are the barometric and water vapor pressure, respectively; FIO_2 is the fractional concentration of oxygen in inspired air; and R is the respiratory quotient (usually 0.8). During air breathing at FIO_2 of 0.21 and assuming R value of 0.8, the equation can be simplified to:

$$PAO_2 = 0.21 (Pb - 47) - 1.25(PaCO_2)$$

where $PACO_2$ has been replaced by the arterial PCO_2 ($PaCO_2$). Therefore PO_2 in the ideal alveolus at sea level is $0.21(760 - 47) - 1.25(40)$ or $(150 - 50)$ or 100 mm Hg. Alveolar PO_2 is slightly higher than the value in arterial blood because of the presence of small shunts and regions of ventilation-perfusion mismatch. Areas of shunt, where ventilation is zero but blood flows from right to left or left to left circulations, occur normally in the thebesian veins of the heart and the bronchial circulation. This shunt amounts to 2% to 5% of cardiac output and produces arterial PO_2 in normal adults of approximately 90 mm Hg. The difference between the ideal alveolar and the actual arterial PO_2 is called the alveolar to arterial oxygen difference ($AaDO_2$). This difference widens to about 100 mm Hg during 100% oxygen breathing; however, the ratio of PaO_2 to PAO_2 (a/A ratio) remains constant over this range of partial pressures because it is the slope of the

TABLE 59-1. Approved Indications for Hyperbaric Oxygen Therapy

INDICATION	RECOMMENDED PROTOCOL	NUMBER OF TREATMENTS*
Arterial gas embolism	U.S. Navy Table 6 or 6A	1-10
Carbon monoxide poisoning	2.4-3 atm for 90-120 min	1-5
Clostridial myonecrosis	2.4-3 atm for 90 min	3-10
Compromised skin grafts	2-2.5 atm for 90-120 min	10-40
Crush injuries	2-2.5 atm for 90-120 min	3-12
Decompression sickness	U.S. Navy Table 5 or 6	1-10
Delayed radiation injury	2-2.5 atm for 120-140 min	30-60
Exceptional blood loss	2.5-3 atm for 120-240 min	—
Intracranial abscess	2-2.5 atm for 60-90 min	10-20
Necrotizing infections	2-2.5 atm for 90-120 min	3-30
Problem wounds	2-2.5 atm for 90-120 min	10-30
Refractory osteomyelitis	2-2.5 atm for 90-120 min	20-40
Thermal burns	2-2.5 atm for 90-120 min	20-50

*The higher numbers are limits for utilization recommended by the Undersea and Hyperbaric Medical Society.

line describing the relationship between arterial and alveolar P_{O_2}.

The arterial P_{O_2} that can be achieved during exposure to HBO has been studied in healthy individuals and patients and found to be predictable from the a/A ratio measured at 1 atm. With the help of the following equation, Pa_{O_2} can be predicted for a patient breathing hyperbaric oxygen:

$$Pa_{O_2} \text{ (predicted)} = (Pa_{O_2}/PA_{O_2})[(760 \text{ atm} - 47) - Pa_{CO_2}]$$

where the atm is the ambient pressure in atmospheres. In general, Pa_{O_2} values of greater than 1000 mm Hg are needed to produce therapeutic effects during HBOT.

Hyperbaric oxygen has significant effects on ventilation and CO_2 excretion. HBO affects ventilation by reducing carotid chemoreceptor activity. It also increases the density of the breathing gas in direct proportion to the ambient pressure and increases the CO_2 content of the tissues. The latter effect is due to "arterialization" of venous blood under hyperbaric conditions (see below), which prevents CO_2 from binding to hemoglobin as the carbamino compound. This additional load of oxygen causes the P_{CO_2} of venous blood to increase by about 5 mm Hg and produces mild respiratory acidosis. The net effect of these responses is a small increase in resting ventilation during HBO. This increase in ventilation allows a normal Pa_{CO_2} to be maintained. However, Pa_{CO_2} may rise rapidly with exertion under hyperbaric conditions.

Oxygen Transport to Tissues and the Effects of HBO

Oxygen is transported in the blood by two physical processes. Most oxygen is chemically bound to the hemoglobin molecule and thereby transported by red blood cells. Hemoglobin accounts for more than 98% of the oxygen content of normal blood. The remaining oxygen is carried in plasma in physically dissolved form. The oxygen transport system is described by the Fick equation:

$$V_{O_2} = Q(Ca_{O_2} - Cv_{O_2})$$

where V_{O_2} is the oxygen consumption rate of the body (ml/min), Q is cardiac output (L/min) and Ca_{O_2} and Cv_{O_2} are the arterial and mixed venous oxygen content values (ml/dl), respectively. Oxygen delivery is the product of Q and Ca_{O_2}. The basal oxygen consumption rate is approximately 250 ml/min. Oxygen extraction, the difference between arterial and venous oxygen content (AV_{DO_2}), is approximately 5 ml/dl.

The oxygen content of blood is the sum of oxygen carried by hemoglobin and oxygen dissolved in the blood plasma. The oxygen content of hemoglobin is determined by multiplying hemoglobin concentration by the oxygen saturation and the oxygen carrying capacity of the molecule. Each gram of hemoglobin can carry 1.34 ml of oxygen when fully saturated. At a normal concentration of 15 g/dl, hemoglobin carries 20 ml/dl of oxygen. The oxygen content of blood plasma is determined by the solubility of O_2 in plasma at 37° C, which is (0.0031 ml/mm Hg) times the P_{O_2}, which at 100 mm Hg results in oxygen in solution of only 0.31 ml/dl. Once hemoglobin has combined fully with oxygen, increases in P_{O_2} can only increase the oxygen content of blood by increasing the amount of oxygen in solution. At P_{O_2} values above 100 mm Hg, the oxygen content increases in direct proportion to P_{O_2} in the blood (Figure 59-1).

During hyperbaric oxygen therapy, P_{O_2} will increase approximately 700 mm Hg and Ca_{O_2} will increase approximately 2.1 ml/dl for every atmosphere of pressure for patients with normal pulmonary gas exchange. At

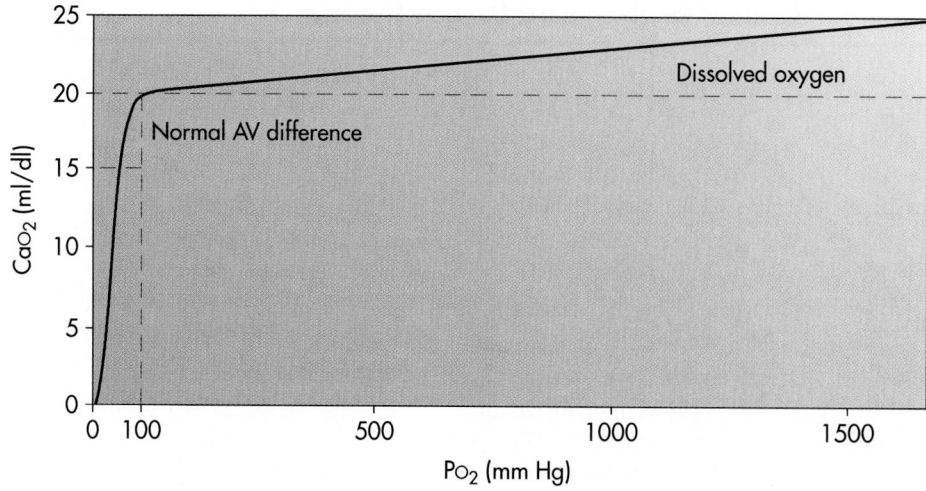

Figure 59-1 Effects of hyperbaric oxygen on the oxygen content of arterial blood. The blood oxygen content (CaO_2) under normal conditions is approximately 20 ml/dl and is carried almost exclusively by hemoglobin. The normal oxygen extraction (AV difference) is approximately 5 ml/dl or about one quarter of the total CaO_2. During HBOT, dissolved O_2 in plasma can be increased to provide the entire AV difference without unloading O_2 from hemoglobin.

the partial pressures of oxygen used for clinical HBO treatments (2 to 3 atm), the amount of oxygen in physical solution in the blood approaches or exceeds the 5 ml/dl needed to meet the oxygen requirement of the body at a normal cardiac output. Hence, the heart can deliver enough oxygen in plasma under hyperbaric conditions to avoid any unloading of oxygen from hemoglobin.

Tissue Effects of HBO and Assessment of Tissue Oxygenation

In the systemic capillaries, oxygen is released by hemoglobin into the plasma, where it diffuses down a concentration gradient into cells to be consumed in mitochondria by an irreversible, enzymatic reaction. The enzyme cytochrome c oxidase is the final member of the respiratory chain that reduces oxygen to water. This reaction accounts for more than 90% of oxygen consumed by the body. Although mitochondria can respire at very low values of PO_2, if oxygen concentration falls too low, the rate of respiration becomes limited by oxygen availability, the cell becomes hypoxic, and production of high-energy metabolites (e.g., adenosine triphosphate [ATP]) is compromised. Normally, tissue oxygenation can be regulated only by changes in blood flow or changes in oxygen extraction. Changes in local oxygen demand (metabolic rate) are met by these two processes singly or in combination.

Hyperbaric oxygen has at least two obvious advantages for maintaining oxygen availability in tissues. First, as noted above, convective delivery of oxygen to systemic capillaries is greater than normal at any cardiac output owing to the increase in arterial oxygen content. Second, large increases in CaO_2 result in a higher PO_2 at both the arterial and venous ends of the capillaries for any oxygen consumption rate. The resulting increase in tissue oxygen concentration has important physiologic and biochemical effects in both normal and diseased tissue.

Oxygen directly alters organ blood flow by adjusting vessel caliber. Remarkable decreases in tissue blood flow have been observed when arterial PO_2 rises to above 500 mm Hg. Oxygen-induced vasoconstriction occurs in both the arterial and venous sides of the circulation; its mechanisms are complex and not yet understood completely. In humans, decreases in cerebral, retinal, and renal blood flow have been demonstrated during HBOT. Even in the presence of vasoconstriction, however, HBO readily oxygenates both normal and diseased tissues, provided that blood flow through major arteries has been preserved. HBO can produce tissue PO_2 values in the range of several hundred mm Hg as measured by indwelling PO_2 electrodes or transcutaneous oxygen measurements.

HYPERBARIC CHAMBERS AND PROCEDURES

Hyperbaric oxygen treatments can be conducted in either a multiplace or a monoplace chamber facility. Each type of chamber has specific advantages and disadvantages. In general, either device is suitable for the routine treatment of stable patients. Critically ill patients, however, are more easily and safely managed in multiplace chambers, where nurses and other medical personnel can attend the patients immediately. In recent years, portable monoplace recompression cham-

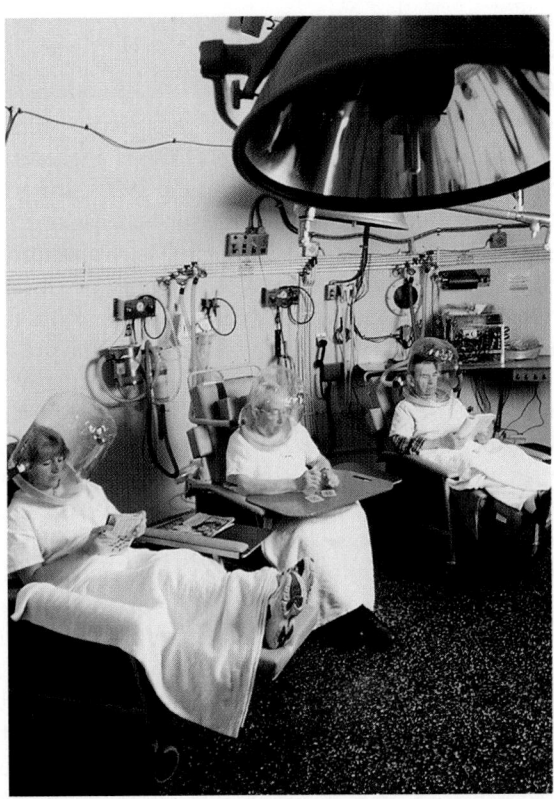

Figure 59-2   Multiplace hyperbaric chamber. Multiplace chambers allow more than one patient at a time to receive hyperbaric oxygen. Attendants may accompany the patients during treatments. *(Courtesy Duke University Photography. Photo by Les Todd.)*

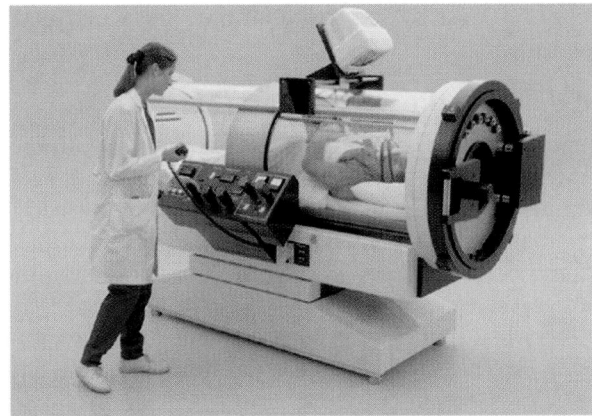

Figure 59-3   Monoplace hyperbaric chamber. Monoplace chambers hold a single patient, usually in an environment of pure oxygen. Attendants remain outside the chamber during treatment.

bers with limited capabilities have been developed for remote diving sites and high-altitude expeditions to relatively inaccessible regions of the world.

Multiplace Chambers[7]

Multiplace hyperbaric chambers hold two or more people, including patients, nurses, respiratory therapists, and other attendants (often known as tenders). The chamber is pressurized to the treatment depth with air, and the patient breathes 100% oxygen by mask or head tent or through an endotracheal tube. Large chambers are capable of treating a dozen or more patients at the same time (Figure 59-2).

Monoplace Chambers[10]

Monoplace chambers accommodate a single patient and are generally pressurized with pure oxygen that the patient breathes directly (Figure 59-3). Air breaks are given by mask or with a scuba regulator. Alternatively, the monoplace chamber may be pressurized with air and the patient supplied with oxygen from a mask, regulator, or other built-in breathing system (BIBS). The monoplace chamber must be decompressed for attendants to have direct access to the patient.

Portable Recompression Chambers

Portable recompression chambers can be either rigid or collapsible. Rigid chambers tend to have greater versatility but are more cumbersome to transport than collapsible chambers. Portable chambers usually rely on compression with ambient air, and for collapsible chambers, internal pressure and inspired PO_2 can only be increased by a few tenths of an atmosphere. Collapsible systems, for example, the Gamow bag or the Certec chamber, are most often used on high-altitude expeditions for temporary treatment of serious high altitude–related illness when descent is not feasible or is delayed unavoidably. The extent to which simulated descent can be achieved in a collapsible chamber depends on the altitude at which it is used. For instance, the Gamow bag has a nonadjustable pressure "pop-off" valve at 2 psi (0.13 atm). The Certec chamber can operate at a slightly higher pressure (0.22 atm). The beneficial effects of these small increases in pressure on altitude sickness are transient. Furthermore, some patients, such as those with high-altitude pulmonary edema, may not tolerate lying down inside a small tube. If available, administration of supplemental oxygen while awaiting descent is logistically easier and preferred to recompression in a collapsible chamber for treatment of serious altitude illness (see Chapter 1).

Portable, or "fly-away," systems also have been used to treat decompression illness in divers. Use of these systems is expensive and requires a considerable degree of technical expertise and logistic support. These systems are available primarily in the U.S. Navy and to commercial diving contractors. Therefore routine emergency treatment for all forms of decompression illness at sites of remote diving operations is administration of high-flow supplemental oxygen by mask (or endotracheal tube) until the victim can undergo recompression in a fully-equipped facility. Treatment of decompression illness by recompressing in the water is not recommended.

Patient Care Procedures and Monitoring[7,10]

Proper control of chamber atmosphere is essential for comfort, safety, and therapeutic efficacy during HBO administration. The most important variables affecting hyperbaric environments are the temperature, humidity, and concentrations of oxygen, CO_2, and contaminant gases.

The ideal inspired oxygen concentration is 100%; however, 98% O_2 or above is an attainable practical goal. The recommended maximum ambient CO_2 concentration is 3.18 mm Hg, which is 0.5% surface equivalent concentration. This recommendation is designed to avoid stimulation of ventilation and to minimize the risk of central nervous system (CNS) O_2 toxicity. The concentrations of contaminant gases, such as carbon monoxide, methane, and other hydrocarbons, in the gas supply should be monitored periodically and kept below accepted air purity standards. The relative humidity recommended for oxygen-enriched breathing gases is 50% to 70% for patient comfort and fire safety considerations.

A variety of standard patient monitoring and support devices can be used in hyperbaric environments with appropriate safety precautions. Available monitoring devices include electrocardiogram (including defibrillator), electroencephalogram, vascular pressure monitors, and evoked potential recorders. Support devices, including intravenous (IV) infusion pumps (using flexible IV bags) and mechanical ventilators, can be adapted successfully for chamber use. It has long been standard practice to minimize the number of electrical and electronic devices inside the chamber by plumbing electrical connections, including patient monitoring cables, through the chamber wall. This practice has proven to be an effective fire prevention method in hyperbaric chambers.

Hyperbaric Chamber Safety

Hyperbaric chambers are quite safe, and catastrophic failures are extremely rare. The most serious safety concern in hyperbaric environments is the risk of fire. Fires in oxygen-rich environments are far more dangerous than those occurring in normal atmospheres because of the ability of O_2 to support combustion. At ambient O_2 concentrations above 25% by volume, electrical sparks or chemical ignition can lead to explosive combustion and ultrarapid incineration of any flammable materials in the chamber. Of the more than two dozen chamber fires reported over the past 40 years, approximately half were caused by ignition sources, such as cigarette lighters and hand warmers, brought into the chamber by patients. Stringent precautions to avoid sources of combustion and flammable materials in the chamber should be taken at all times.

INDICATIONS FOR HYPERBARIC OXYGEN THERAPY

Reference to the therapeutic use of hyperbaric pressure can be found in the medical literature as early as the mid-seventeenth century, but until the 1920s, the treatment was largely restricted to caisson disease (decompression sickness, or DCS). In the 1920s, Cunningham advocated hyperbaric air to treat a variety of ailments for which HBOT had no scientific rationale. When the American Medical Association condemned this practice in 1928, the treatment fell out of favor until after World War II. The use of HBOT reemerged in the 1950s and 1960s after scientific reports supported its potential efficacy as a treatment for decompression illness, carbon monoxide poisoning, and gas gangrene. In 1976 the Undersea and Hyperbaric Medical Society established a multidisciplinary committee to review research and clinical data and provide recommendations about the safety and efficacy of HBOT. From the work of this committee has come a list of 13 indications currently accepted in the United States for the clinical application of HBO (Table 59-1).[3] The rationale and approach to treatment of the most common conditions are briefly summarized below.

Decompression Sickness

The earliest therapeutic use of hyperbaric chambers was to recompress divers with DCS, also known as the bends. When divers suffering from mild to moderate cases of bends were recompressed promptly on air, complete relief of symptoms usually could be obtained. More severe types of DCS, such as those involving significant neurologic injury, responded less well to air recompression. The development of oxygen recompression tables, however, has substantially improved the clinical outcome for all types of DCS.[6]

DCS arises from ascending too rapidly from underwater diving, flying after diving, or ascent in an unpressurized aircraft. It is also encountered after an exposure to increased pressure in a hyperbaric chamber or on exposure to decreased pressure in a hypobaric chamber. During decompression, bubbles of inert gas (nitrogen) form when the rate of ascent exceeds the rate at which diffusion and perfusion reduce the inert gas partial pressure in tissues. Inert gas bubbles may be formed in sufficient quantities to interfere with organ function by occluding blood flow or disrupting tissue, or they may produce biochemical events that damage tissue.[2] The latter events include platelet aggregation, activation of coagulation, complement activation, leukocyte adhesion, endothelial damage, and capillary leakage.

The clinical manifestations produced by DCS vary by type and severity (see Chapter 57). Historically, they have been categorized into two types. Type I DCS involves pain only, usually in one or more joints ("limb bends"), whereas type II DCS involves more severe symptoms, usually involving the nervous system or the cardiorespiratory system. The latter condition is known as "chokes." In severe cases, shock and death may occur. Other systems, however, may be involved, including the audiovestibular, skin, and lymphatic systems. Extreme fatigue after diving can also be a manifestation of serious DCS.

Two main points in differential diagnosis must be considered in evaluating a person for treatment of possible DCS. For limb pain the possibility of unrecognized trauma or strain injury is an important diagnostic consideration; however, in practice this distinction can be difficult. Under such circumstances, a trial of pressure in the chamber can be helpful. For patients with more serious DCS, distinguishing between DCS and arterial gas embolism (AGE) can be difficult, and the two conditions may coexist. This distinction, however, may not be as clinically useful as once believed because the same recompression tables may be appropriate for both conditions.

Treatment of DCS is based on the twin principles of reducing bubble size with recompression and hastening inert gas elimination with oxygen (Figure 59-4). The most widely used oxygen recompression tables for treatment of DCS are U.S. Navy Tables 5 and 6.[9] These tables require compression to 60 FSW (2.8 atm) and intermittent O_2 breathing for varying periods of time (Figure 59-5). Table 5 is used for mild DCS that re-

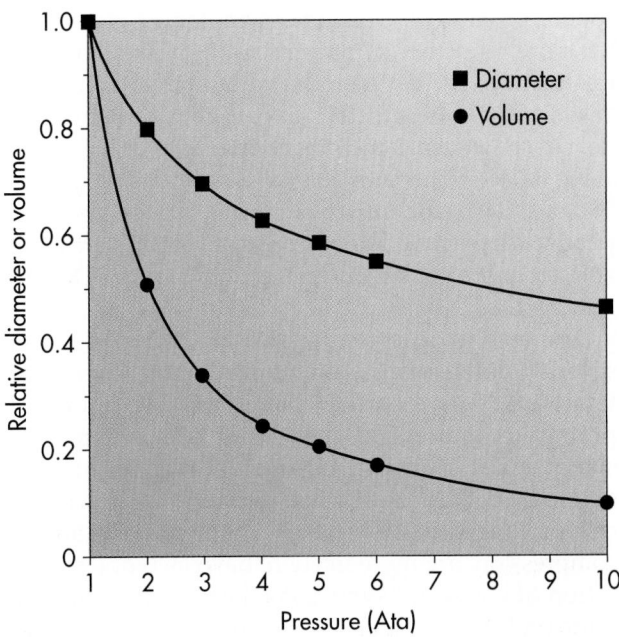

Figure 59-4 Effects of recompression therapy on gas bubble size. The relative bubble volume and diameter are plotted as a function of recompression depth (pressure in atm). The greatest effect occurs on bubble volume during the initial 2- to 3-atm pressure change. As the volume of the bubble decreases, the partial pressure of nitrogen (P_{N_2}) rises inside it. This allows N_2 to diffuse more rapidly down its concentration gradient into the tissue, where the P_{N_2} is lower. The addition of O_2 breathing lowers P_{N_2} in the tissue, thereby increasing the gradient for N_2 elimination.

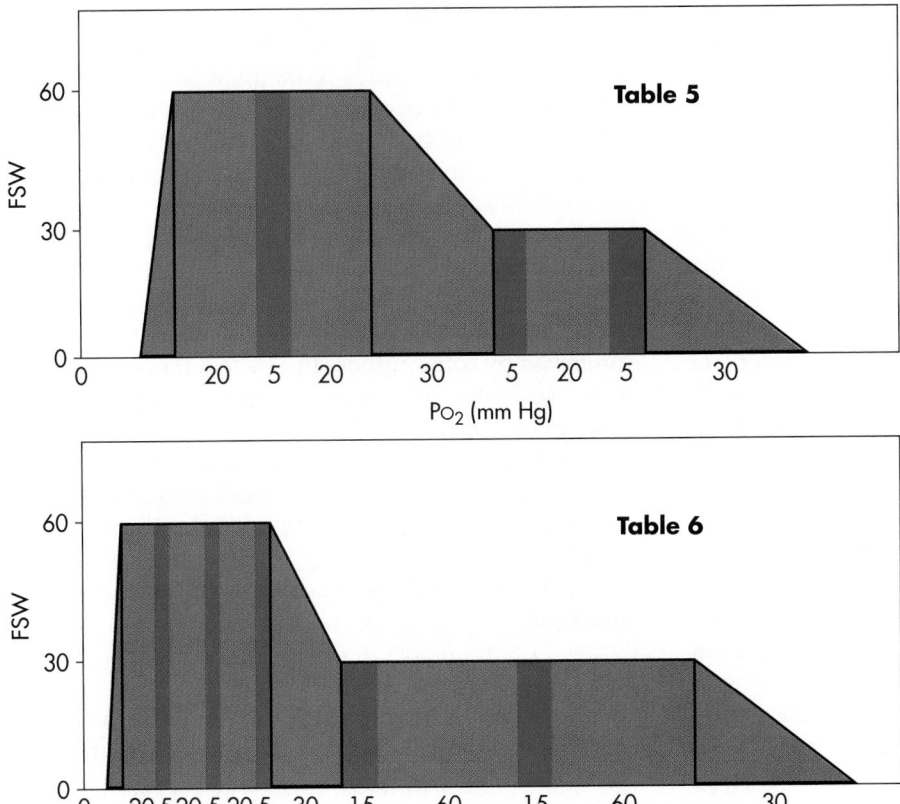

Figure 59-5 U.S. Navy oxygen recompression tables for treatment of DCS. Oxygen breathing periods are indicated in green; air breaks are shown in blue. The rate of compression to 60 FSW is 25 feet/min (2.4 min). US Navy Table 5 requires 135 minutes and Table 6 requires 285 minutes, excluding time of compression. U.S. Navy Table 6 may be extended up to two O_2 cycles at 60 FSW and two O_2 cycles at 30 FSW.

sponds promptly to recompression. Table 6 is designed for more refractory symptoms and is also suitable for treatment of AGE. When the volume of intravascular gas after AGE is sufficient to cause major neurologic deficits, however, some practitioners prefer U.S. Navy Table 6A with compression to 165 FSW using air or a 50% N_2/O_2 (nitrox) mixture. Longer oxygen treatment tables with extended decompression profiles are available for more severe and refractory cases of DCS involving the CNS.

The results of recompression therapy depend on severity of illness and delay to treatment. Three quarters of patients with DCS have pain only, and with prompt recompression, they obtain complete relief of symptoms after a single treatment. Patients with more severe DCS, particularly that involving the spinal cord or a prolonged delay between symptom onset and recompression, are more likely to have incomplete resolution of signs and symptoms. Such victims may require prolonged or repetitive treatments. Some patients with spinal cord DCS continue to show benefit from repetitive daily recompression tables for several days. In general, treatments are continued until the patient shows no further improvement during the treatment period. Alternatively, some multiplace facilities have the capacity to perform prolonged "saturation" treatments during which the patient remains at pressure for several days. During such treatments the patient continues to receive intermittent periods of O_2 breathing. Saturation treatments are expensive and logistically difficult for both the patient and medical personnel. However, they occasionally result in rapid, dramatic clinical responses in victims with serious neurologic injuries.

Adjunctive treatment for serious DCS is relatively limited. Immediate management includes high-flow supplemental oxygen (e.g., by face mask). Relief of symptoms of milder forms of DCS with oxygen alone is not uncommon; however, surface O_2 is not a substitute for recompression therapy. Aggressive oral or IV hydration is important in the first 24 to 48 hours. IV lidocaine, 2 mg/kg bolus followed by 1 to 2 mg/hr for 12 to 24 hours, has been recommended for treatment of spinal cord DCS. Lidocaine is relatively safe and easy to administer, but its benefit has not been proven in a controlled trial. The use of large doses of corticosteroids is also unproven and has produced variable results in experimental animal models of DCS. Therefore routine use of corticosteroids is not recommended for treatment of serious DCS.

The probability of complete relief of symptoms and return of function after treatment in patients with neurologic DCS is difficult to predict. In general, immediate improvement is expected during the first recompression table unless the delay to treatment has been many hours. Some patients will suffer relapse of symptoms during decompression from the treatment table or between repetitive treatments; however, such recurrences generally respond to additional recompression treatments. A small number of patients are left with long-term neurologic deficits, including leg weakness, sensory changes, and bowel or bladder dysfunction. These deficits may either be permanent or improve gradually over 6 to 12 months.

Arterial Gas Embolism

Another mechanism by which gas may be introduced into the vasculature is rupture of a gas-containing space (e.g., the air spaces of the lungs) into a blood vessel (see Chapter 57). In compressed gas divers this can be caused by rapid ascent from depth, and in aviators, by explosive aircraft decompression. In compressed gas diving, gas embolism may occur with ascent from less than 1 m of water in the presence of breath-holding or an obstructive airway lesion. The rapid expansion of gas may cause pulmonary overdistension and disruption of the alveolar capillary membrane, allowing gas to enter the pulmonary veins and traverse the left heart to the systemic circulation.

AGE may occur under circumstances in which the rate and magnitude of ascent are insufficient to release enough gas to bubble out of physical solution to cause DCS. AGE, however, may coexist with DCS in divers undergoing rapid uncontrolled ascents, such as in the condition sometimes known as "blow-up." Under this circumstance the amount of gas released into the circulation can be massive, resulting in loss of consciousness, seizures, focal neurologic deficits, cardiac ischemia, and arrhythmias. AGE is a true medical emergency and requires immediate recompression to obtain clinical recovery. Delays to recompression of more than 1 to 2 hours are associated with a poor clinical outcome, including permanent neurologic impairment and death.

The treatment of AGE is similar to that of DCS. Recompression on U.S. Navy Table 6, Table 6A, or equivalent tables is usually recommended. Deeper recompression tables with nitrox treatment gases are preferred by some authors but have not been shown to provide better treatment outcomes than shallower treatment tables.

The Divers Alert Network (DAN) offers a free consultative service in triage and treatment of diving accidents worldwide. In the United States this service is available 24 hours a day, 7 days a week by calling (919) 684-8111 and asking for the on-call DAN team member.

Carbon Monoxide Poisoning[8]

Exposure to carbon monoxide (CO) gas is the most frequent cause of accidental poisoning in the United States and accounts for approximately 1000 deaths per year. CO is a toxic by-product of incomplete combustion of hydrocarbons, and CO exposure occurs primarily from inhalation of fumes from faulty gas furnaces, smoke from fires, and exhaust from internal combustion engines. CO poisoning has been reported in recreational boaters and campers who use internal combustion engines and fossil fuel heaters in enclosed spaces.

Tissue damage caused by CO has been viewed primarily as a hypoxic stress (CO hypoxia) caused by the formation of carboxyhemoglobin (COHb). CO binds to hemoglobin with an affinity of more than 200 times that of oxygen. This tight binding of CO to hemoglobin prevents hemoglobin from binding oxygen and increases the affinity of oxygen for remaining unoccupied heme sites. The result of this interaction is to shift the oxygen dissociation curve (ODC) to the left, leading to greater difficulty unloading oxygen to the tissues at any Po_2. The decrease in O_2 content and leftward shift of the ODC produced by COHb leads to tissue hypoxia and its untoward consequences. These consequences are most pronounced in organs that require a continuous supply of oxygen, such as the brain and heart. In addition, tissue hypoxia facilitates movement of CO into cells, where it has deleterious effects. These include binding to critical heme proteins (e.g., myoglobin, cytochrome oxidase), generation of oxidative stress, and interference with normal cell signaling processes.

Standard treatment for CO poisoning is administration of high concentrations of inspired oxygen. Oxygen hastens dissociation of CO from hemoglobin and its removal from tissue stores. This process is greatly accelerated by HBO (Figure 59-6). In addition, HBO but not normobaric oxygen can ameliorate certain pathologic processes in the CNS associated with CO poisoning, such as delayed neurologic syndrome. The delayed syndrome occurs in 10% to 30% of persons with severe CO poisoning and is characterized by deterioration in cognitive and/or motor function, beginning a few days to several weeks after the initial event.

HBOT is usually recommended for victims of poisoning with COHb levels of 25% and greater, loss of consciousness, or any evidence of cardiac or neuropsychiatric disturbances regardless of COHb level. The COHb level serves primarily as an indicator of significant poisoning, but it correlates poorly with the extent of neurologic impairment.

Patients who receive HBOT within 2 to 6 hours of CO poisoning usually show return of normal cognitive function after a single 90-minute treatment at 2.4 to 3 atm. These victims also have a reduced risk of developing the delayed neurologic syndrome after a single HBOT treatment. The response to HBOT is less certain and recovery is less predictable when treatment is delayed more than 6 hours or when CO exposure has been particularly long or intense. Dramatic clinical responses should not be expected when treating comatose or severely poisoned patients after delays of more than 6 to 12 hours, although anecdotal reports have indicated significant cognitive improvement of severely poisoned patients who receive HBOT after delays of 24 hours or more.

Clostridial and Other Necrotizing Soft Tissue Infections[3]

Necrotizing soft tissue infections are acute, invasive, and potentially fatal bacterial infections of the subcutaneous tissues, fascia, and muscle. They are usually distinguished on the basis of microbiologic etiology and anatomic location and often involve anaerobic bacteria (e.g., clostridial myonecrosis, myositis). Common organisms include *Clostridium perfringens* (gas gangrene), group B streptococci, and *Escherichia coli*. Very often, infections of soft tissue occur that involve one or more aerobic and anaerobic bacteria. Such mixed infections appear in a variety of clinical settings, particularly after trauma, in surgical wounds, or in the vicinity of a foreign body. The patient is often compromised in some way, for example, with diabetes, malignancy, or vasculopathy.

HBOT for gas gangrene or other necrotizing soft tissue infections is adjunctive to surgical debridement and antibiotics. However, it is effective in blocking α-toxin production by clostridial species and inhibiting the growth of anaerobic bacteria. HBO may be limb saving and tissue sparing when used early in the course of these infections. In general, three treatments at 2.5 to 3 atm are recommended in the first 24 hours, and 5 to 10 total treatments over 3 to 5 days for maximum benefit.

Selected Problem Wounds

The adjunctive use of HBO in the treatment of wounds that fail to respond to routine medical and surgical

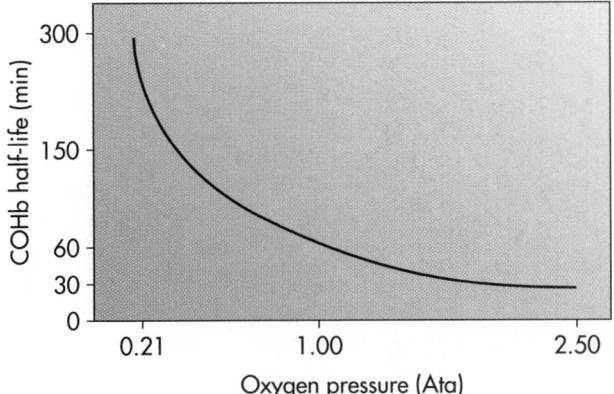

Figure 59-6 The effects of oxygen on the dissociation of CO from carboxyhemoglobin (COHb). Oxygen breathing at 1.0 atm decreases the half-life of COHb to 60 minutes from approximately 300 minutes in air. HBO at 2.5 atm reduces the half-life to 30 minutes, allowing most of the COHb to be removed from the body within 90 minutes.

treatment has had substantial success, particularly in tissues with compromised blood flow and oxygen supply.[3] Such wounds are usually hypoxic and have tissue oxygen tensions of only a few mm Hg. This hypoxia interferes with collagen deposition, angiogenesis, and immune function necessary for proper wound healing. Restoration of tissue P_{O_2} into the normal range with HBO accelerates healing in these problem wounds. HBOT has been particularly useful in treating diabetic ulcers, where controlled trials have shown more rapid and complete healing when adjunctive HBOT is used. In general, however, these wounds are slow to heal and may require 40 to 60 treatments.

One type of wound of special interest is that caused by the bite of the brown recluse spider (*Loxosceles reclusa*). This spider releases a venom that can cause severe dermatonecrosis and a painful ulcer that enlarges progressively over 7 to 14 days. These ulcers have been reported to respond to HBOT at 2 to 3 atm when administered early in the course of the injury. A strong scientific rationale for HBOT is lacking for treatment of brown recluse spider bites in normal individuals.[5] In addition, clinical reporting on HBOT for spider bites is anecdotal and uncontrolled.

Delayed or Late Radiation Injury of Soft Tissue and Bone[4]

Delayed radiation injury is a long-term complication of radiation therapy, usually involving soft tissues and bone. It generally develops after a latent period of 6 or more months and is characterized by obliterative endarteritis, fibrosis, and tissue hypoxia. HBOT has been utilized prophylactically before oral surgery in a radiated tissue field and to treat delayed radiation tissue injury. In patients who have received radiation doses of 4500 Gy or greater, HBOT has been shown to be cost effective when used before oral surgery to prevent soft tissue breakdown and osteoradionecrosis of the mandible. It is also effective in combination with surgery for treatment of established osteoradionecrosis. HBOT also has been used successfully to treat soft tissue radionecrosis of the head and neck, larynx, chest wall, pelvis, bladder, and bowel. HBO enhances neovascularization in irradiated tissues, thereby improving tissue oxygen tension and tissue viability.

OXYGEN TOXICITY

Clinical applications of HBOT are limited primarily by the toxic effects of oxygen.[1] Oxygen toxicity is related to the inspired oxygen concentration and duration of exposure. If exposure is sufficiently intense, molecular O_2 is eventually toxic to all living cells. Some tissues (e.g., lungs, premature retina) are susceptible to oxygen toxicity at partial pressures of O_2 in the normobaric range, whereas others (e.g., brain) require exposure to oxygen

under hyperbaric conditions. Despite its potential for toxicity, oxygen is the most widely used therapeutic gas, and its safe use at high partial pressures, including those in the hyperbaric range, requires familiarity with its toxicity.

Mechanisms of Oxygen Toxicity

The susceptibility of any tissue to oxygen toxicity depends on its oxygen supply, metabolic activities, biochemical makeup, and antioxidant defenses. Each tissue therefore has a unique dose-response curve that describes the relationship between O_2 concentration and the duration of exposure necessary to produce toxicity. In general, these relationships can be described by a family of rectangular hyperbolas. Examples of such curves for pulmonary and CNS oxygen toxicity are illustrated in Figure 59-7. The limit, or asymptote of the curve, for the lung occurs at approximately 0.5 atm, whereas that for the brain is reached at approximately 1.4 atm.

Tissue injury from oxygen is mediated by reactive oxygen species (ROS) generated by elevated P_{O_2}. These ROS include superoxide anion (O_2^-), hydrogen peroxide (H_2O_2), and hydroxyl radical ($OH \cdot$). ROS are produced by both intracellular and extracellular chemical reactions involving single electron transfers to molecular oxygen or its metabolites. The sites and reactions that produce ROS in the cell involve many intracellular structures, including mitochondria, peroxisomes, endoplasmic reticulum, and nuclear and plasma membranes. These reactions usually depend on oxygen concentration; they proceed more rapidly as P_{O_2} is raised. As P_{O_2} increases, ROS production may overwhelm endogenous antioxidant defenses, resulting in lipid peroxidation, protein oxidation, sulfhydryl depletion, and

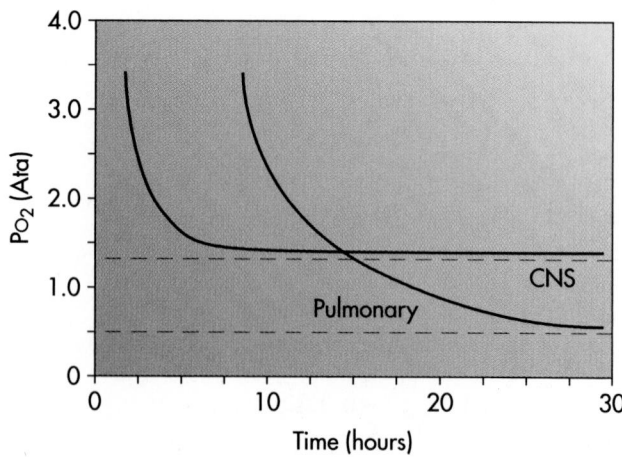

Figure 59-7 Hyperbolic relationship between oxygen concentration and time in tissue oxygen toxicity. Typical pressure-time curves for the CNS and lung are shown for comparison. The threshold for CNS toxicity is approximately 1.4 atm and for pulmonary toxicity is approximately 0.5 atm.

oxidation of nucleic acids. In addition, many extracellular sources of ROS and cellular inflammatory responses amplify oxygen toxicity. Most notably, the oxidative damage produced by inflammatory cells, such as neutrophils and macrophages, contributes to later phases of pulmonary oxygen toxicity.

Certain physiologic factors can amplify O_2 toxicity, particularly for manifestations involving the CNS. In diving, these factors include immersion, exercise, and elevated PCO_2. In clinical settings, fever, thyrotoxicosis, adrenal stress, hypercapnia, and acute cerebral injury can exacerbate CNS O_2 toxicity. In addition, certain drugs are associated with an increased risk of CNS O_2 toxicity. These include catecholamines, such as dopamine and norepinephrine.

Clinical Manifestations of Oxygen Toxicity

The clinical manifestations of oxygen toxicity are diverse and difficult to predict. Signs and symptoms of O_2 toxicity related to the lungs, CNS, and eye are well described (see below). Hemolysis has been reported rarely, primarily in vitamin E–deficient patients. In addition, experimental studies of hyperoxia have reported evidence of cellular toxicity to cardiac, renal, and hepatic tissues. In clinical practice, however, HBO causes toxicity primarily to the lungs and CNS.

Pulmonary Oxygen Toxicity. Clinical symptoms of pulmonary oxygen toxicity usually begin after 12 to 18 hours of continuous exposure to O_2 at 1 atm and within 3 to 6 hours of exposure to 2 atm. The initial symptoms are mild substernal irritation and dry cough that become more intense with continued exposure. The substernal irritation becomes painful and exacerbated by inspiration. Changes in mechanical airway function occur relatively early; these are characterized primarily by airflow obstruction. These airway changes are followed by parenchymal injury, leading to progressive impairment of pulmonary gas exchange. This is characterized by increased shunt fraction, ventilation-perfusion mismatch, and lung edema, which cause progressive hypoxemia.

CNS Oxygen Toxicity. The symptoms of CNS O_2 toxicity are nonspecific and unpredictable. They only occur during O_2 exposures of 1.4 atm or greater and may include irritability, tinnitus, dizziness, tunnel vision, nausea, vomiting, and seizures. Oxygen seizures may occur without warning and are not distinguishable from other types of grand mal seizures. Oxygen seizures are self-limited and usually respond immediately to dis-

continuing oxygen. They have not been associated with long-term neurologic sequelae. Because O_2 seizures are rare and self-limited, anticonvulsants are not generally recommended for prevention of seizures during HBOT.

OXYGEN TOLERANCE

Although high concentrations of oxygen produce conditions that can damage cells, most cells and tissues contain adequate antioxidant defenses to deal with the short-term effects of HBOT.[1] These defenses, including antioxidant enzymes such as catalase and superoxide dismutase and low-molecular-weight scavengers such as glutathione and vitamin E, limit the damaging effects of ROS production at elevated PO_2. Although most HBOT treatment tables and schedules are designed to avoid O_2 toxicity, it is also possible to improve O_2 tolerance, thereby decreasing the risk of toxicity. For instance, vitamin E supplements have been used for many years in Europe as an adjunctive therapy to lessen free radical damage during HBOT. In the typical clinical setting, however, there is significant variability in O_2 tolerance among individuals, and for any individual, variability in tolerance to repetitive exposures to the same HBO profile. The most useful proven way to extend O_2 tolerance is to introduce brief periods of air breathing (air breaks) during hyperbaric oxygen treatments. This is usually accomplished by interspersing 5-minute air breaks between each 20- to 30-minute O_2 breathing period for treatment pressures in excess of 2 atm and durations in excess of 2 hours.

REFERENCES

1. Clark JM: Oxygen toxicity. In Bennett PB, Elliott DH, editors: *The physiology and medicine of diving*, ed 4, Philadelphia, 1993, WB Saunders.
2. Francis TJR, DF Gorman: Pathogenesis of the decompression disorders. In Bennett PB, Elliott DH, editors: *The physiology and medicine of diving*, Philadelphia, 1993, WB Saunders.
3. Hampson NB: *Hyperbaric oxygen therapy: 1999 committee report*, Kensington, Md, 1999, Undersea and Hyperbaric Medical Society.
4. Marx RE: Radiation injury to tissue. In: Kindwall EP, editor: *Hyperbaric medicine practice*, Flagstaff, Ariz, 1995, Best Publishing.
5. Maynor ML et al: Brown recluse spider envenomation: a prospective trial of hyperbaric oxygen therapy, *Acad Emerg Med* 4:184, 1997.
6. Moon RE, Sheffield PJ: Guidelines for the treatment of decompression illness, *Aviat Space Environ Med* 68:234, 1997.
7. Moon RE, Hart BB: Operational use and patient monitoring in a multiplace hyperbaric chamber, *Resp Care Clin N Am* 5:21, 1999.
8. Piantadosi CA: Diagnosis and treatment of carbon monoxide poisoning, *Respir Care Clin N Am* 5:183, 1999.
9. Thalmann ED: Principles of US Navy recompression treatments for decompression sickness. In Moon RE, Sheffield PJ, editors: *Treatment of decompression illness*, Kensington, Md, 1996, Undersea and Hyperbaric Medical Society.
10. Weaver LK: Operational use and patient care in the monoplace hyperbaric chamber, *Respir Care Clin N Am* 5:51, 1999.

60 Injuries from Nonvenomous Aquatic Animals

Paul S. Auerbach and Bruce W. Halstead

The expanses of ocean and freshwater that cover the earth are the greatest wilderness. Seventy-one percent of the earth's surface is composed of ocean, the volume of which exceeds 325 million cubic miles. Within the undersea realm exists four fifths of all living organisms.

The opportunity for direct encounters with aquatic organisms is constantly increasing because of recreational, industrial, scientific, and military oceanic and riverine activities. The underwater recovery of historical artifacts and treasures will accelerate in the new millennium. As fishermen harvest their catches, they handle animals that bite and sting in self-defense.

Nearly 80% of the world's population resides in coastal regions. It is estimated that 127 million U.S. citizens will live along the coasts by the year 2010. A significant proportion of this population will be directly involved as entrants into the aquatic world. Millions of sport scuba enthusiasts will venture into the undersea realm in the next decade. Therefore it is imperative that clinicians be familiar with hazards unique to the aquatic environment.

Although noxious marine organisms are concentrated predominantly in warm temperate and tropical seas, particularly in the Indo-Pacific region, hazardous animals may be found as far north as 50° latitude. Increasing numbers of saltwater aquaria in private homes and public settings, intercontinental seafood shipping, and accessibility of air travel for sport divers create additional risks.

Like the rainforest, the ocean depths have the potential to reveal virtually limitless active pharmaceutical agents. For example, genetically engineered reproduction of the adhesive protein of the marine mussel *Mytilus edulis* has created a tissue adhesive agent that may one day prove superior to cyanoacrylic compounds. Toxins isolated from ascidians (tunicates or sea squirts) include cyclic peptides, some of which (esteinascidin 743, aplidine) have undergone evaluation for cancer chemotherapy; others (e.g., thiocoralina and kahalide F) may follow. Investigative techniques continue to improve. In pursuit of anatomic information that can elucidate the biology and ecology of fish, evolution, cellular physiology, and aquatic models of human disease, nuclear radiologists have performed in vivo nuclear magnetic resonance imaging (MRI) and spectroscopy of anesthetized (tricaine methsulfonate [MS222]) aquatic organisms.[14]

Despite the wondrous nature of the deep, jeopardy exists. The ubiquity of hazardous creatures and their propensity to appear at inopportune times make it imperative to be aware of them, to respect their territorial rights, and to avoid needless unpleasant contact with them.

DIVISIONS AND DEFINITIONS

Dangerous aquatic animals are divided into four groups: (1) those that bite, rip, puncture, or shock without envenomation; (2) those that sting (envenom), discussed in Chapters 61 and 62; (3) those that are poisonous on ingestion (see Chapter 54); and (4) those that induce allergies (see Chapter 55). Aquatic skin disorders are discussed in Chapter 63.

IN DEFENSE OF THE FISH

A word must be written in defense of the fish. As in all nature (except for humans), indiscriminate aggression is rarely involved when injuries are inflicted by aquatic animals. Most injuries result from gestures of warning or self-defense; with the exception of some sharks, few aquatic creatures attack humans without provocation. Attacks are made in defense of young, in territorial dispute, or to procure food. It is hoped that better understanding will foster caution when dealing with potentially injurious aquatic creatures.

GENERAL PRINCIPLES OF FIRST AID

The physician must adhere to fundamental principles of medical rescue. Although many injuries and envenomations have unique clinical presentations, the cornerstone of therapy is immediate attention to the airway, respiration, and circulation. Along with specific interventions directed against a particular venom or poison, the rescuer must simultaneously be certain that the victim maintains a patent airway, breathes spontaneously or with assistance, and is supported by an adequate blood pressure. Because marine attacks and envenomations may affect a scuba diver, the rescuer should anticipate near drowning (see Chapter 56), immersion hypothermia (see Chapter 8), and decompression sickness or arterial air embolism (see Chapter 57). Any victim rescued from the ocean should be thoroughly examined for external signs of a bite, puncture, or sting.

WOUND MANAGEMENT

Whether the injury is a bite, abrasion, or puncture, meticulous attention to basic wound management is necessary to minimize posttraumatic infection.

Wound Irrigation

All wounds acquired in the natural aquatic environment should be vigorously irrigated with sterile diluent, preferably a normal saline (0.9% sodium chloride) solution. Seawater is not a favorable irrigant because it carries a hypothetical infection risk. Sterile water or hypotonic saline is acceptable. Tap water (preferably disinfected) appears to be a suitable irrigant and should be used when the alternative is delay to irrigation.[3] Irrigation should be performed before and after debridement to maximize the benefits. A 19-gauge needle or 18-gauge plastic intravenous (IV) catheter attached to a syringe that delivers a pressure of 10 to 20 psi will dislodge most bacteria without forcing irrigation fluid into tissue along the wound edges or deeper along dissecting tissue planes. Convenient ring-handle syringes with blunt irrigation tips and IV tubing that connects to standard IV bags are available. At least 100 to 250 ml of irrigant should be flushed through each wound. If a laceration is from a stingray, proteinaceous (and possibly) heat-labile venom may be present in the wound. In such a case the irrigant should be warmed to 45° C (113° F).[6]

An antiseptic may be added to the irrigant if the wound appears to be highly contaminated. Povidone-iodine solution in a concentration of 1% to 5% may be used with a contact time of 1 to 5 minutes.[63,90] When antiseptic irrigation is completed, the wound should be thoroughly irrigated with normal saline or tap water to minimize tissue toxicity. Antiseptics that are particularly harmful to tissues include full-strength hydrogen peroxide, povidone-iodine scrub solution, hexachlorophene detergent, and silver nitrate.

Scrubbing should be used to remove debris that cannot be irrigated from the wound. Sharp surgical debridement is preferable to sponge scrubbing, which may increase infection rates, particularly when applied with harsh antiseptic solutions. Poloxamer 188 (Pluronic F-68) is a nontoxic nonionic surfactant skin wound cleanser that may be used to irrigate or scrub wounds. It does not offer any significant advantage over traditional sterile saline irrigation.

Wound Debridement

Debridement is more effective than irrigation at removing bacteria and debris. Crushed or devitalized tissue should be removed with sharp dissection to provide clean wound edges and encourage brisk healing with minimal infection risk. The limitations are those imposed by anatomy, specifically skin tautness or the presence of vital structures. Anesthesia of wound edges may be attained by regional nerve block or local infiltration with lidocaine, which do not damage local tissue defenses. A topical anesthetic mixture of tetracaine, epinephrine, and cocaine may be less desirable because of the vasoconstrictive effect of epinephrine and theoretical infection-potentiating effects. Definitive wound exploration, debridement, and repair should be undertaken in the most appropriate sterile environment. It is inappropriate to explore complex wounds in the emergency department. Whenever necessary, operating loupes should be used to inspect the wound for residual foreign material, such as sand, seaweed, teeth, spine fragments, or integumentary sheath shards. Standard radiographs, static soft tissue techniques, MRI, or fluoroscopy may be used preoperatively or perioperatively to localize spines or teeth.

Wound Closure

The decision to close a wound weighs the cosmetic result against the risk of infection. The incidence of infection is high in wounds acquired in natural bodies of water because such wounds may be contaminated with venom, potentially virulent microorganisms, or both; because early adequate irrigation and debridement are often unavailable; and because definitive care is often delayed. Tight wound closure restricts drainage and promotes bacterial proliferation. Wounds at high risk in this regard include those on the hands, wrists, or feet; punctures and crush injuries; wounds into areas of fat with poor vascularity; and wounds to victims who are immunosuppressed. Whenever possible, the use of sutures to close dead space in contaminated wounds should be avoided because the absorbable sutures act as foreign bodies.

Prophylaxis against Tetanus

Any wound that disrupts the skin can become contaminated with *Clostridium tetani*. Anaerobic bacteria, predominantly of the genus *Clostridium*, have been isolated in shark tissue and as part of the oral flora of alligators and crocodiles. Proper immunization with tetanus toxoid virtually eliminates the risk of disease. However, although it was previously accepted that the protective level of toxin-neutralizing antibody is 0.01 antitoxin unit/ml, it appears that clinical tetanus can develop despite an antibody level many times that amount. Therefore it is imperative to provide an early and adequate booster injection. If the victim is over 50 years of age, is from an underdeveloped country, or cannot provide a definite history of tetanus immunization, it is more likely that circulating toxin-neutralizing antibody will be suboptimal. Prophylaxis should be provided according to the scheme in Table 18-3.

BACTERIOLOGY OF THE AQUATIC ENVIRONMENT

Wounds acquired in the aquatic environment are soaked in natural source water and sometimes contaminated with sediment. Penetration of the skin by the spines or teeth of animals, the razor edges of coral or shellfish, or the blades of a boat propeller may inoculate pathogenic organisms into a wound. Sports activities, such as surfing, snorkeling, and diving, lead to ubiquitous abrasions and minor lacerations that heal slowly and with marked soft tissue inflammation. Wounds acquired in the aquatic environment tend to become infected and may be refractory to standard antimicrobial therapy. Not infrequently, indolent or extensive soft tissue infections develop in the normal or immunocompromised host.[10,68] A clinician faced with a serious infection after an aquatic injury frequently needs to administer antibiotics to a patient before definitive laboratory identification of pathogenic organisms.

Marine Bacteriology

Marine Environment. Ocean water provides a saline milieu for microbes. The salt dissolved in ocean water (3.2% to 3.5%) is 78% sodium chloride (sodium 10.752 g/kg; chlorine 19.345 g/kg). Other constituents include sulfate (2.791 g/kg), magnesium (1.295 g/kg), potassium (0.39 g/kg), bicarbonate (0.145 g/kg), bromine (0.066 g/kg), boric acid (0.027 g/kg), strontium (0.013 g/kg), and fluorine (0.0013 g/kg). The temperature of the surface waters varies with latitude, currents, and season. Tropical waters are warmer and maintain a more constant temperature than temperate and subtropical waters, which are subject to substantial meteorologic variation. Shallow and turbulent coastal waters are generally richer in nutrients than the open ocean, which is reflected in the diversity of life that can be identified in the intertidal zone. Although the greatest number and diversity of bacteria are found near the ocean surface, diverse bacteria and fungi are found in marine silts, sediments, and sand. In ocean waters having marked differences in density, the greatest concentration of bacteria is noted at the thermocline, where changes in both temperature and salinity are usually found.[73] This effect is lost in active coastal waters, where the constant admixture creates an even distribution of sediments, microbes, salinity, and temperature. Microbes are most abundant in areas that have the greatest numbers of higher life-forms. Marine bacteria are generally halophilic, heterotrophic, motile, and gram-negative rod forms. Growth requirements vary from species to species with respect to use of organic carbon and nitrogen sources, requirements for various amino acids, vitamins and cofactors, sodium, potassium, magnesium, phosphate, sulphate, chloride, and calcium. Most marine bacteria are facultative anaerobes, which can thrive in oxygen-rich environments. Few are obligatory aerobes or anaerobes. Some marine bacteria are highly proteolytic, and the proportion of proteolytic bacteria seems to be greater in the oceans than on land or in freshwater habitats.[73]

Diversity of Organisms. Unique conditions of nutrient and inorganic mineral supply, temperature, and pressure have allowed the evolution of unique, highly adapted marine microbes.[99,100] In addition, numerous other bacteria, microalgae, protozoa, fungi, yeasts, and viruses have been identified in or cultured from seawater, marine sediments, marine life, and marine-acquired or marine-contaminated infected wounds or body fluids of septic victims. In their natural environment the bacteria presumably serve to scavenge and transform organic matter in the intricate cycles of the food and growth chains. Some of these bacteria are listed in Box 60-1. Enteric pathogenic bacteria have been isolated from sharks.[32] A shark attack victim in South Africa who sustained serious injuries to his lower

---

Box 60-1 BACTERIA AND FUNGUS ISOLATED FROM MARINE WATER, SEDIMENTS, MARINE ANIMALS, AND MARINE-ACQUIRED WOUNDS

Achromobacter	*Mycobacterium marinum*
Acinetobacter lwoffi	*Neisseria catarrhalis*
Actinomyces	*Pasteurella multocida*
Aerobacter aerogenes	*Propionibacterium acnes*
Aeromonas hydrophila	*Proteus mirabilis*
Aeromonas sobia	*Proteus vulgaris*
Alcaligenes faecalis	*Providencia stuartii*
Alteromonas espejiana	*Pseudomonas aeruginosa*
Alteromonas haloplanktis	*Pseudomonas cepacia*
Alteromonas macleodii	*Pseudomonas maltophila*
Alteromonas undina	*Pseudomonas putrefaciens*
Bacillus cereus	*Pseudomonas stutzeri*
Bacillus subtilis	*Salmonella enteritidis*
Bacteroides fragilis	*Serratia*
Branhamella catarrhalis	*Staphylococcus aureus*
Chromobacterium violaceum	*Staphylococcus epidermidis*
Citrobacter	*Streptococcus*
Clostridium botulinum	*Vibrio alginolyticus*
Clostridium perfringens	*Vibrio carchariae*
Clostridium tetani	*Vibrio cholerae*
Corynebacterium	*Vibrio damsela*
Edwardsiella tarda	*Vibrio fluvialis*
Enterobacter aerogenes	*Vibrio furnissii*
Erysipelothrix rhusiopathiae	*Vibrio harveyi*
Escherichia coli	*Vibrio hollisae*
Flavobacterium	*Vibrio parahaemolyticus*
Fusarium solani	*Vibrio mimicus*
Klebsiella pneumoniae	*Vibrio splendidus I*
Legionella pneumophila	*Vibrio vulnificus*
Micrococcus sedentarius	

extremities was reported to have developed a fulminant infection attributed to *Bacillus cereus* shown to be sensitive to fluoroquinolones, amikacin, clindamycin, vancomycin, and tetracyclines and resistant to penicillin and cephalosporins (including third generation). In another report, one shark (presumed bronze whaler) attack victim in Australia grew both *Vibrio parahaemolyticus* and *Aeromonas caviae* from his wounds, whereas another grew *Vibrio alginolyticus* and *Aeromonas hydrophila* from his wound.[74]

For practical purposes, most marine isolates are heterotrophic (require exogenous carbon and nitrogen-containing organic supplements) and motile gram-negative rods. Previous opinions that enteric pathogens (associated with the intestines of warm-blooded animals) deposited into marine environments ultimately succumbed to sedimentation, predation, parasitism, sunlight, temperature, osmotic stress, toxic chemicals, or high salt concentration may be untrue.[31] Pathogens may accumulate in surface water in association with lipoidal particulates, from which they are rapidly dispersed toward shore by wave and wind activity. In addition, dredging, storms, upwellings, and other benthic disturbances may churn enteric organisms into the path of wastewater nutrients.

Wound Infections Caused by Vibrio Species. *Vibrio* organisms can cause gastroenteric disease (gastroenteric *Vibrio* infections are discussed in Chapter 54) and soft tissue infections, particularly in immunocompromised hosts. Extraintestinal infections may be associated with bacteremia and death. *Vibrio* species are the most potentially virulent halophilic organisms that flourish in the marine environment. The teeth of a great white shark have been swabbed and yielded *V. alginolyticus*, *V. fluvialis*, and *V. parahaemolyticus*.[16] Mako shark tooth culture has yielded *V. damsela*, *V. furnisii*, and *V. splendidus I.*[4] *V. parahaemolyticus* has also been identified in freshwater habitats.[7] Water that is brackish (salinity of 15 to 25 parts per thousand) allows the growth of *Vibrio* species if appropriate nutrients are present; *V. vulnificus* infection has been documented after exposure to waters with salinities of 2 and 4 ppt. The optimal season for disease appears to be summer, when water temperatures encourage bacterial proliferation. In most studies reported, infections seem to cluster during the summer months; this may be related to increased numbers of people at the seashore. This has been corroborated to some degree by the observation that *V. parahaemolyticus* cultured from marine mammals was recovered only in the warmer months of the year in the Northeast or in animals from subtropical regions. Sharks appear to develop some immunity to autochthonous *Vibrio* species, as suggested by the detection of a binding protein similar to the immunoglobulin M (IgM) sub-class of immunoglobulin. Allochthonous (for the shark) *Vibrio* species, such as *V. carchariae*, may be the agents of elasmobranch disease when the animal is under stress.

Vibrio species are halophilic, gram-negative rods that are facultative anaerobes capable of using D-glucose as their sole or principal source of carbon and energy.[22] They are part of the normal flora of coastal waters not only in the United States but also in many exotic locations frequented by recreational and industrial divers and seafarers. Vibrios are mesophilic organisms and grow best at temperatures of 24° to 40° C (75.2° to 104° F), with essentially no growth below 8° to 10° C (46.4° to 50° F). Other marine bacteria are facultative psychrophiles, barophiles, or both. *Vibrio* species seem to require less sodium for maximal growth than do other more fastidious marine organisms, a factor that allows explosive reproduction in the 0.9% saline environment of the human body. At least 11 of the 34 recognized *Vibrio* species have been associated with human disease.[22] Wound infections have been documented to yield *V. cholerae* 0 group 1 and non-01, *V. parahaemolyticus*, *V. vulnificus*, *V. alginolyticus*, and *V. damsela*. Septicemia, with or without an obvious source, has been attributed to infections with *V. cholerae* non-01, *V. parahaemolyticus*, *V. alginolyticus*, *V. vulnificus*, and *V. metschnikovii*.

VIBRIO PARAHAEMOLYTICUS. *Vibrio parahaemolyticus* is a halophilic gram-negative rod. The organisms are found in waters along the entire coastline of the United States. Generally the incidence of clinical disease is greatest in the warm summer months when the organism is commonly found in zooplankton. *V. parahaemolyticus* absorbs onto chitin and to minute crustacean copepods that feed on sediment. It has been postulated that unusual warm coastal currents (such as El Niño) may contribute to increased proliferation of *Vibrio* species. The optimal growth temperature of *V. parahaemolyticus* is 35° to 37° C (95° to 98.6° F); under ideal conditions the generation time has been estimated at less than 10 minutes, with explosive population growth from 10 to 10^6 organisms in 3 to 4 hours.

Extraintestinal wound infections are most common in persons who suffer chronic liver disease or immunosuppression. Although over 95% of *V. parahaemolyticus* strains associated with human illness are positive, the relationship to pathogenicity of the Kanagawa reaction (production of a cell-free hemolysin on high salt-mannitol [Wagatsuma] agar), caused by a heat-stable direct hemolysin, is not yet clear. Furthermore, most marine strains are not Kanagawa positive. Some primary soft tissue infections previously attributed to *V. parahaemolyticus* may theoretically be attributed to misidentified *V. vulnificus*. Panophthalmitis requiring enucleation occurred in a man who suffered a corneal laceration.

VIBRIO VULNIFICUS. *Vibrio vulnificus* (formerly known as a "lactose [fermenting]-positive" vibrio) is a halophilic gram-negative bacillus. *V. vulnificus* ("wounding") is found in virtually all U.S. coastal waters and has been reported to cause infection worldwide.[8] It prefers salinity of 0.7% to 1.6%; although it prefers a habitat of warm (at least 20° C [68° F]) seawater, it can be found in much colder water. It does not appear to be associated with fecal contamination of seawater. It has been shown to exist in Chesapeake Bay with bacterial counts comparable with those reported from the Gulf of Mexico.[97]

The organism may or may not have an acidic polysaccharide capsule (opaque colony), which confers protection against bactericidal activity of human serum and phagocytosis and thus renders the organism more virulent in animals. At extremely low frequency, some strains can shift between unencapsulated (avirulent; translucent colony) and capsulated (virulent) serotypes. The encapsulated isolates show exquisite (positive) sensitivity to iron. Virulent isolates can use 100% but not 30% saturated (normal for humans) transferrin as an iron source, as well as iron in hemoglobin and hemoglobin-haptoglobin complexes. *V. vulnificus* exhibits enhanced growth and virulence in the presence of increased serum iron concentration and/or saturated transferrin-binding sites.[1] *V. vulnificus* is classified in two biotypes: biotype 1 (pathogenic for humans) and biotype 2 (pathogenic for fish).[22]

Infection evolves rapidly after the initiation of symptoms and has been noted most frequently in men over 40 years of age with preexisting hepatic dysfunction, leukopenia, or impaired immunity (malignancy, human immunodeficiency virus [HIV] infection, diabetes, long-term corticosteroids), although it has been reported in young, previously healthy individuals. Preexisting liver disease is a predictor of death, with 50% of such individuals succumbing to the illness in one series.[36] Persons with high serum iron levels (from chronic cirrhosis, hepatitis, thalassemia major, hemochromatosis, multiple transfusions [such as are given for aplastic anemia]) or achlorhydria (low gastric acid; may be iatrogenically induced with H_2 blockers) may be at greater risk for fulminant bacteremia.[1,81,88] This has been attributed in part to the protective effect of gastric acid, the iron requirement of the organism, and the effects of liver disease (decreased polymorphonuclear leukocyte and macrophage activity, flawed opsonization, shunting of portal blood around the liver). *V. vulnificus* produces a siderophore ("vulnibactin") and a protease that may enhance pathogenicity.[1]

The syndrome consists of flulike malaise, fever, vomiting, diarrhea, chills, hypotension, and early skin vesiculation that evolves into necrotizing dermatitis and fasciitis, with vasculitis and myositis (Figures 60-1 and 60-2).[98] Hematogenous seeding of vibrios to secondary cutaneous lesions is probable. Primary wound

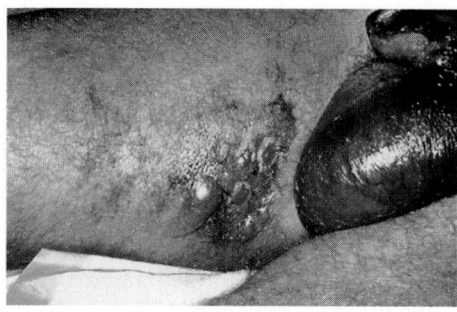

Figure 60-1 Echthyma gangrenosum associated with *Vibrio vulnificus* sepsis. *(Courtesy Edward J. Bottone, MD., Dept. of Microbiology, Mt. Sinai Hospital, N.Y.)*

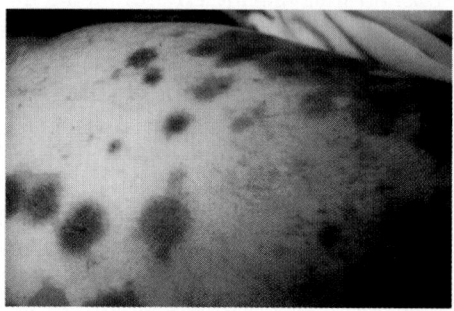

Figure 60-2 Torso of a victim with *Vibrio vulnificus* sepsis.

infections (approximately 30% of cases) rapidly show marked edema, with erythema, vesicles, and hemorrhagic or contused-appearing bullae, progressing to necrosis. This may require radical surgical debridement or amputation. Up to 25% of these victims may have sepsis. When this *Vibrio* species is recovered from the blood of a victim with sepsis attributable to a wound infection, the case fatality rate may exceed 30%.[36] Extracellular elastin-lysing proteases elaborated by the organism, as well as a potent collagenase, probably contribute to the rapid invasion of healthy tissue. *V. vulnificus* also produces a cytotoxin-hemolysin and phospholipases. Cytolysin produced by most pathogenic strains of *V. vulnificus* is extremely toxic to mice when injected IV and results in severe perivascular edema and neutrophil infiltration in lung tissues.[64] The precise roles of these and other factors (pili, mucinase, chondroitinase, hyaluronidase) in the in vivo pathogenicity of the organism have yet to be determined. Bleeding complications (which may include gastrointestinal hemorrhage and disseminated intravascular coagulation) are common and may be attributed in part to thrombocytopenia. Gastroenteritis is more common (15% to 20%) with the septicemic presentation than with primary wound infection and may exist as an isolated entity (approximately 10% of cases), although it is debated that illness has been erroneously attributed to the asymptomatically carried organism. *Vibrio vulnificus* endometritis has been reported after an episode of intercourse in the water of Galveston Bay, Texas. Other presentations of *Vibrio vulnificus* infections have included meningitis, spontaneous bacterial peritonitis, corneal ulcers, epiglottitis, and infections of the testes, spleen, and heart valves.

The explosive nature of the syndrome can lead to gram-negative sepsis and death, reportedly in up to 50% of cases. The mortality rate may be as high as 90% in victims who become hypotensive within 12 hours of initial examination by a physician. Appropriate antibiotics should be administered as soon as the infection is suspected (see below). In one report, *V. vulnificus* sepsis was treated with antibiotic therapy, debridement of necrotic tissues, and direct hemoperfusion using polymyxin B immobilized fiber, which serves as an artificial reticuloendothelial system and removes endotoxin from the circulating blood.[75] For wound infections from all *Vibrio* species, the organism may only be recovered from blood specimens in less than 20% of victims.[36] In an immunocompetent victim who acquired a *V. vulnificus* hand infection from peeling shrimps, treatment with oral ciprofloxacin was successful. In a series of seven patients treated for primary skin and soft tissue infections secondary to *V. vulnificus*, prompt operative exploration and debridement were correlated with a decrease in the intensive care unit and hospital length of stay, particularly if the surgery occurred within 72 hours from the time of infection.[35] The authors noted that all patients had necrosis of underlying subcutaneous tissue, while some did not demonstrate skin necrosis.

VIBRIO MIMICUS. *Vibrio mimicus* is a motile, non-halophilic, gram-negative, oxidase-positive rod with a single flagellum. It can be distinguished from *V. cholerae* by its inability to ferment sucrose, inability to metabolize acetylmethyl carbonyl, sensitivity to polymyxin, and negative lipase test. An ear infection may follow exposure to ocean water. Isolates are sensitive to tetracycline. Physicians who collect stool samples for culture to identify suspected *V. mimicus* must alert the laboratory to use appropriate culture media (thiosulfate-citrate-bile salts-sucrose [TCBS] agar).

VIBRIO ALGINOLYTICUS. *Vibrio alginolyticus*, found in seawater, has been implicated in soft tissue infections (such as those caused by coral cuts or surfing scrapes), sinusitis, and otitis, particularly after previous ear infections or a tympanic membrane perforation. Although bacteremia has been reported in immunosuppressed patients and patients with burns, *V. alginolyticus* does not generally carry the virulent potential of *V. vulnificus*. Typical symptoms include cellulitis, with seropurulent exudate.

VIBRIO DAMSELA. *Vibrio damsela*, formerly enteric group EF-5 and so named because it is pathogenic for the damselfish, causes wound infections similar to those attributed to other vibrios. Rapidly progressive infection leading to muscle necrosis or to sepsis and death may transpire in an immunosuppressed victim. This may be related to an extracellular cytolysin or other unidentified enzymes. It has been proposed that *V. damsela* be placed into the new genus *Listonella*.

VIBRIO CHOLERAE. A case of necrotizing fasciitis and septic shock caused by *V. cholerae* non-O1 (not agglutinated in cholera polyvalent O1 antiserum) acquired in San Diego, California, has been described.[92] The victim suffered from preexisting diabetes mellitus complicated by chronic plantar ulceration of the affected limb.

Growth in Culture. Although plating on standard clinical laboratory media may detect only 0.1% to 1% of the total number of microorganisms found in seawater or marine sediment, most marine bacteria that are pathogenic to humans can be readily recovered on standard media. Although pathogenic *Vibrio* species can grow on conventional blood agar media, other marine bacteria may require saline-supplemented media and incubation at 25° C (77° F) instead of the standard 35° to 37° C (95° to 98.6° F). In culture, marine bacteria may grow at a slower rate than terrestrial bacteria, which delays identification. Pleomorphism in culture may be attributed to adaptation to small concentrations of nutrients in seawater. Most organisms require sodium, potassium, magnesium, phosphate, and sulfate for growth; a few require calcium or chloride.

TCBS agar is selective and recommended for the detection of marine *Vibrio* organisms, although cellobiose-polymyxin B-colistin (CPC) agar may be as good or better.[12,50] An alternative is Monsur taurocholate-tellurite-gelatin agar. A large clinical laboratory near the ocean might consider the use of TCBS or CPC agar routinely. Pathogenic vibrios generally grow on Mac-Conkey agar. All species except *V. cholerae* and *V. mimicus* require sodium chloride for growth. Enrichment broth (alkaline peptone water with 1% NaCl) is recommended for isolation of vibrios from convalescent and treated patients. Another enrichment broth that may be more effective is 5% peptone, 1% NaCl, and 0.08% cellobiose (PNC) at pH 8.0.[38] All *Vibrio* species grow in routine blood culture mediums and on nonselective mediums, such as blood agar. A recent comparison of strategies for the detection and recovery of *V. vulnificus* from marine samples of the western Mediterranean coast determined that the best strategy consisted of the combination of culture-based methods (3-hour enrichment in alkaline-saline peptone water at 40° C [104° F], followed by culture on CPC agar) and deoxyribonucleic acid (DNA)-based procedures (specific polymerase chain reaction [PCR] amplification of the presumptive colonies with primers Dvu 9V and Dvu 45R).[4]

Key characteristics that aid in the separation of *Vibrio* species from other medically significant bacteria (Enterobacteriaceae, *Pseudomonas, Aeromonas, Plesiomonas*) are the production of oxidase, fermentative metabolism, requirement of sodium chloride for growth, and susceptibility to the 0/129 vibriostatic compound. *Vibrio vulnificus* can be cultured from the blood, wounds (bullae), and stool. The laboratory must be cautioned to use selective culture media with a high salt content (3% NaCl) for prompt identification. Suggestive features include positive fermentation of glucose, positive oxidase test, positive indole test, positive reaction for both lysine and ornithine decarboxylase, positive *o*-nitrophenyl–β-d-galactopyranoside, and inability to ferment sucrose. A useful identification scheme for pathogenic *Vibrio* species is found in the chapter on *Vibrio* in the most recent edition of the American Society for Microbiology's *Manual of Clinical Microbiology.*

Because growth of *V. vulnificus* in culture generally requires 48 hours, current research is directed at a more rapid diagnostic test. Direct identification of *V. vulnificus* in clinical specimens by nested PCR has been accomplished utilizing serum specimens and bulla aspirates from septicemic patients.[49] A nested PCR method for rapid and sensitive detection of *V. vulnificus* in fish, sediments, and water has been developed.[5]

Mycobacteria must be cultured in media such as Middlebrook 7H10 or 7H11 agar or Lowenstein-Jensen medium; fungi require a medium such as Sabouraud dextrose or brain-heart infusion/Sabhi agar. Antibiotic susceptibility testing can be performed using established procedures, except for the addition of NaCl 2.3% to the Mueller-Hinton broth or agar used for disk diffusion. Certain commercial test kits may not accurately identify marine organisms. In the setting of wound infection or sepsis, the clinician should alert the laboratory that a marine-acquired organism may be present. If a laboratory does not have the time or resources to perform a complete identification, the bacteria may be sent to a reference laboratory. Marine bacteria are kept in the American Type Culture Collection. Because of the diversity of species, complete agreement has not yet been reached on comprehensive taxonomic criteria for identification.

Antibiotic Therapy. The objectives for the management of infections from marine microorganisms are to recognize the clinical condition, culture the organism, and provide antimicrobial therapy. Management of marine-acquired infections should include therapy against *Vibrio* species. Third-generation cephalosporins (cefoperazone, cefotaxime, or ceftazidime) provide variable coverage in vitro; first- and second-generation products (cefazolin, cephalothin, cephapirin, cefamandole, ce-

fonicid, ceforanide, or cefoxitin) appear to be less effective in vitro. The organism has been reported in some cases to be resistant in vitro to third-generation cephalosporins, mezlocillin, aztreonam, and piperacillin.[66] A combination of cefotaxime and minocycline seems to be synergistic and extremely effective against *V. vulnificus* in vitro.[23] Oral cultures taken from two captive moray eels at the John G. Shedd Aquarium in Chicago, Illinois, demonstrated *V. fluvialis, V. damsela, V. vulnificus,* and *Pseudomonas putrefaciens* sensitive to cefuroxime, ciprofloxacin, tetracycline, and trimethoprim/sulfamethoxazole.[30] Imipenem/cilastatin is efficacious against gram-negative marine bacteria, as are trimethoprim/sulfamethoxazole and tetracycline. Gentamicin, tobramycin, and chloramphenicol have tested favorably against *P. putrefaciens* and *Vibrio* strains. Nonfermentative bacteria (such as *Alteromonas, Pseudomonas,* and *Deleya* species) appear to be sensitive to most antibiotics. In a mouse model, combination therapy with minocycline and cefotaxime was more effective than either drug alone.[24]

Quantitative wound culture has no advantage before the appearance of a wound infection. Pending a prospective evaluation of prophylactic antibiotics in the management of marine wounds, the following recommendations are based on the indolent nature and malignant potential of soft tissue infections caused by *Vibrio* species:

1. Minor abrasions or lacerations (such as coral cuts or superficial sea urchin puncture wounds) do not require prophylactic antibiotics in the normal host. Persons who are chronically ill (as with diabetes, hemophilia, or thalassemia) or immunologically impaired (as with leukemia or acquired immunodeficiency syndrome [AIDS], or undergoing chemotherapy or prolonged corticosteroid therapy), or who suffer from serious liver disease (such as hepatitis, cirrhosis, or hemochromatosis), particularly those with elevated serum iron levels, should be placed immediately after the injury on a regimen of oral ciprofloxacin, trimethoprim/sulfamethoxazole, or tetracycline because these persons appear to have an increased risk of serious wound infection and bacteremia. Preliminary experience suggests that cefuroxime may be a useful alternative. Penicillin, ampicillin, and erythromycin are not acceptable alternatives.[58,60] Norfloxacin may be less efficacious against certain vibrios.[59,70] Other quinolones (ofloxacin, enoxacin, pefloxacin, fleroxacin, lomefloxacin) have not been extensively tested against *Vibrio;* they may be useful alternatives, but this awaits definitive evaluation. The appearance of an infection indicates the need for prompt debridement and antibiotic therapy. If an infection develops, antibiotic coverage should be chosen that will

also be efficacious against *Staphylococcus* and *Streptococcus* because these are still the most common perpetrators of infection. In general, the fluoroquinolones, which are particularly effective for treating gram-negative bacillary infections, may become less and less useful against resistant staphylococci.[87] If *Staphylococcus* is a β-lactamase–producing strain, a semisynthetic penicillin (nafcillin or oxacillin) should be chosen, with a cephalosporin such as cefazolin or cephalothin used if there is a history of delayed-type penicillin allergy. Vancomycin is recommended in the event of methicillin resistance.[51]

2. Serious injuries from an infection perspective include large lacerations, serious burns, deep puncture wounds, or a retained foreign body. Examples are shark or barracuda bites, stingray spine wounds, deep sea urchin punctures, scorpaenid spine envenomations that enter a joint space, and full-thickness coral cuts. If the victim requires hospitalization and surgery for standard wound management, recommended antibiotics include gentamicin, tobramycin, amikacin, ciprofloxacin, and trimethoprim/sulfamethoxazole. Cefoperazone and cefotaxime may or may not be effective. There is a recommendation in the literature advocating the use of ceftazidime (in combination with tetracycline).[44] Chloramphenicol is an alternative agent less commonly used because of hematologic side effects. Imipenem/cilastatin is an extremely powerful antibiotic that should be used in a circumstance of sepsis or treatment failure. Patients who simultaneously receive imipenem or ciprofloxacin and theophylline may have an increased tendency to seizures.[77]

   If the victim is managed as an outpatient, the drugs of choice to cover *Vibrio* are ciprofloxacin, trimethoprim/sulfamethoxazole, or tetracycline. Cefuroxime is an alternative. It is a clinical decision whether oral therapy should be preceded by a single intravenous or intramuscular loading dose of a similar or different antibiotic, commonly an aminoglycoside.

3. Infected wounds should be cultured for aerobes and anaerobes. Pending culture and sensitivity results, the patient should be managed with antibiotics as described previously. In a person who has been wounded in a marine environment and has rapidly progressive cellulitis or myositis, *Vibrio parahaemolyticus* or *V. vulnificus* infection should be suspected, particularly in the presence of chronic liver disease. If a wound infection is minor and has the appearance of a classic erysipeloid reaction (*Erysipelothrix rhusiopathiae*), penicillin, cephalexin, or ciprofloxacin should be administered (see Chapter 63).

Freshwater Bacteriology

Diversity of Organisms. Although it has not been as extensively studied as the marine environment, the natural freshwater environment of ponds, lakes, streams, rivers, lagoons, harbors, estuaries, and artificial bodies of water is probably as hazardous as the ocean from a microbiologic standpoint. Waterskiing accidents, propeller wounds, fishhook punctures, lacerations from broken glass and sharp rocks, fish fin or catfish stings, and crush injuries during white-water expeditions are commonplace. A large number of bacteria have been identified in water, sediments, animals, and wounds. In fringe areas of the ocean that carry brackish water (NaCl content below 3%), marine bacteria, salt-tolerant freshwater bacteria, and brackish-specific bacteria, such as *Agrobacterium sanguineum*, are noted. The combined effects of human and animal traffic and waste disposal increase the risk for coliform contamination. In Great Britain, antibiotic-resistant *Escherichia coli* have been documented in rivers and coastal waters.[80] Coxsackievirus A16 has been isolated from children stricken ill after bathing in contaminated lake water.[26] Of particular note is the presence of virulent species, such as *Chromobacterium violaceum*, *Vibrio parahaemolyticus*, and *Aeromonas hydrophila*, associated with serious and indolent wound infections.[56,91] The last can be cultured from natural bodies of water, as well as from the mouths of domesticated aquarium fish, such as the piranha.[72] Biologic control agents, such as guppy fish bred in wells to control mosquito proliferation, can carry bacterial pathogens, such as *Pseudomonas*.[21]

One investigation sampled water, inanimate objects, and animals from freshwater environments in California, Tennessee, and Florida.[7] Bacteria isolated were predominantly gram-negative and included *Aeromonas hydrophila*, *Flavobacterium breve*, *Pseudomonas* species, *Vibrio parahaemolyticus*, *Serratia* species, *Enterobacter* species, *Plesiomonas shigelloides*, *Bacillus* species, *Acinetobacter calcoaceticus*, and *Alcaligenes denitrificans*.

Wound Infections Caused by Aeromonas Species.

Aeromonas hydrophila ("gas producing and water loving") is a gram-negative, facultatively anaerobic, polarly flagellated, non-spore-forming, and motile rod member of the family Vibrionaceae that commonly inhabits soil, freshwater streams, and lakes.[2,9] *Aeromonas* species are widely distributed and found at wide ranges of temperature and pH. Three species (*A. hydrophila*, *A. sobria*, and *A. caviae*) have been associated with human disease; there are seven or more distinct genotypes. *A. hydrophila* is pathogenic to amphibians, reptiles, and fish. Soft tissue and gastroenteric human infections occur predominantly during the period from May to November. Virulence factors elaborated by *Aeromonas* species include hemolysin, cytotoxin, enterotoxin, cholera toxin–like factor, and hemagglutinins.[15,89]

A wound, particularly of the puncture variety, immersed in contaminated water may become cellulitic within 24 hours, with erythema, edema, and a purulent discharge.[96] The lower extremity is most frequently involved. This usually occurs from stepping on a foreign object or being punctured underwater. The appearance may be indistinguishable from a typical streptococcal cellulitis, with localized pain, lymphangitis, fever, and chills. Untreated or managed with antibiotics to which the organism is not susceptible, this may rarely progress to a severe gas-forming soft tissue reaction, bulla formation, necrotizing myositis, or osteomyelitis. Appearance similar to ecthyma gangrenosum caused by *Pseudomonas aeruginosa* has been reported in *Aeromonas* septicemia.

Fever, hypotension, jaundice, and chills are common manifestations of septicemia.[43] Additional clinical manifestations include abdominal pain or tenderness, altered consciousness, acute renal failure, and coagulopathy. In a manner analogous to the pathogenicity of virulent *Vibrio* species, the chronically ill or immunocompromised host (chronic liver disease, neoplasm, diabetes, uremia, corticosteroid therapy, extensive burns, etc.) is probably at greater risk of a severe infection and/or complication, such as meningitis, endocarditis, or septicemia. Freshwater aspiration may result in *Aeromonas hydrophila* pneumonitis and bacteremia. Infection has followed the bite of an alligator. A 15-year-old boy suffered *A. hydrophila* wound infection after a bite from his pet piranha. For unknown reasons there is a marked preponderance of male victims. This may represent the phenotypic variation of critical bacterial adhesins. Corneal ulcer caused by *A. sobria* was reported after abrasion by a freshwater reed.[19]

In the microbiology laboratory, *Aeromonas* species may be identified on the basis of positive oxidase reaction, no growth on TCBS agar, growth on MacConkey agar, and resistance to the vibriostatic compound 0/129.[43]

Gram's stain of the purulent discharge may demonstrate gram-negative bacilli, singly, paired, or in short chains. Given the appropriate clinical setting (after a wound acquired in the freshwater environment), this should not be casually attributed to contamination.[41] *Aeromonas hydrophila* is generally sensitive to chloramphenicol, aztreonam, gentamicin, amikacin, tobramycin, trimethoprim/sulfamethoxazole, cefotaxime, cefuroxime, moxalactam, imipenem, ceftazidime, ciprofloxacin, and norfloxacin. In one case, culture of a severe wound infection demonstrated the presence of two species, *Aeromonas hydrophila* and *A. sobria*. Notably, the latter was resistant to tetracycline in vitro. Initial therapy for a severe infection that includes an aminoglycoside provides coverage against concomitant *Pseudomonas* or *Serratia* infection. As has been demonstrated with *Vibrio* species, the first-generation cephalosporins, penicillin, ampicillin, and ampicillin/sulbactam are not efficacious,

perhaps because of the production of a β-lactamase by the organism. *Aeromonas* species are capable of producing chromosomally encoded β-lactamases induced by β-lactam antibiotics. This leads to resistance to penicillins, cephalosporins, and monobactams. The β-lactamase inhibitors, such as clavulanate, are not effective against these β-lactamases, so that amoxicillin-clavulanate may not kill *Aeromonas*.[65] Because of the microbiologic similarity of *Aeromonas* on biochemical testing to members of the Enterobacteriaceae family, such as *Escherichia coli* or *Serratia* species, it is important to alert the laboratory to the clinical setting.

Initial therapy of a severe soft tissue infection related to *Aeromonas* should include aggressive wound debridement to mitigate the potentially invasive nature of the organism. In one case of severe cellulitis unresponsive to debridement, fasciotomy, and antibiotic therapy, treatment with hyperbaric oxygen was felt to contribute to successful infection control.[53]

Curiously, medicinal leeches can harbor *Aeromonas* in their gut flora; soft tissue infections related to this phenomenon have been reported. The genus *Plesiomonas* also belongs to the family Vibrionaceae; it has been definitively linked with aquarium-associated infection complicated by watery diarrhea and fever.

Infections Caused by a Fish Pathogen, Streptococcus iniae. *Streptococcus iniae* is a pathogen of fish, noted to cause subcutaneous abscesses in Amazon freshwater dolphins (*Inia geoffrensis*) kept in captivity.[94] Epizootic fatal meningoencephalitis in fish species caused by streptococci has been observed in outbreaks affecting tilapia, yellowtail, rainbow trout, and coho salmon. Persons who handle these fish are at risk for bacteremic illness, which can be manifest as cellulitis or sepsis. Endocarditis, meningitis, and arthritis have been noted to accompany *S. iniae* infection.

The tilapia (*Oreochromis* species) is also known as St. Peter's fish or Hawaiian sunfish. The surface of this commonly aquacultured fish may be colonized with *S. iniae*. Persons of Asian descent have been identified as prone to infection, probably because they often prepare this fish with the intent to dine. Typically, the victim recalls puncturing the skin of the hand with a fin, bone, or implement of preparation. Cellulitis with lymphangitis and fever is common, without skin necrosis or bulla formation.[94]

In culture, *S. iniae* shows β-hemolysis. However, it may appear to be α-hemolytic because the narrow zone of β-hemolysis is ringed by more prominent zone of α-hemolysis. Therefore it may be misidentified as a viridans streptococcus and therefore considered a contaminant. A reasonable approach to antibiotic therapy includes penicillin, cefazolin, ceftriaxone, erythromycin, clindamycin, or trimethoprim/sulfamethoxazole. In one series, ciprofloxacin showed slightly less efficacy in vitro.

A General Approach to Antibiotic Therapy. Management of freshwater-acquired infections should include therapy against *Aeromonas* species. First-generation cephalosporins provide inadequate coverage against growth of freshwater bacteria. Third-generation cephalosporins provide excellent coverage, whereas second-generation products are less effective. Ceftriaxone may not be efficacious against *Aeromonas* species. Ciprofloxacin, imipenem, ceftazidime, gentamicin, and trimethoprim/sulfamethoxazole are superb antibiotics against gram-negative microorganisms. Trimethoprim alone may be inefficacious, as is ampicillin.

Whether to begin antimicrobial therapy before establishment of a wound infection is controversial. Pending a prospective evaluation of prophylactic antibiotics in freshwater-acquired wounds, the following recommendations are based on the potentially serious nature of soft tissue infections caused by *Aeromonas* species:

1. Minor abrasions or lacerations do not require the administration of prophylactic antibiotics in the normal host. Persons who have chronic illness, immunologic impairment, or serious liver disease, particularly those with elevated serum iron levels, should be placed immediately on a regimen of oral ciprofloxacin or norfloxacin (first choice), trimethoprim/sulfamethoxazole (second choice), or doxycycline/tetracycline (third choice—use only in the setting of allergy to the first two choices, since resistance to *Aeromonas* species has been observed) because these persons appear to have an increased risk of serious wound infection and bacteremia. Penicillin, ampicillin, erythromycin, and trimethoprim do not appear to be acceptable alternatives. The appearance of an infection indicates the need for prompt debridement and antibiotic therapy. If an infection develops, antibiotic coverage that will also be efficacious against *Staphylococcus* and *Streptococcus* should be chosen, since these are still probably the most common perpetrators of infection.

2. If the victim requires surgery and hospitalization for wound management, recommended antibiotics include ciprofloxacin, gentamicin, or trimethoprim/sulfamethoxazole. Imipenem/cilastatin is an extremely powerful antibiotic that should be used in a circumstance of sepsis or treatment failure. If the victim is to be managed as an outpatient, the oral drug of choice is trimethoprim/sulfamethoxazole, or tetracycline or doxycycline. It is a clinical decision whether oral therapy should be preceded by a single intravenous or intramuscular loading dose of a similar or different antibiotic, commonly an aminoglycoside.

3. Infected wounds should be cultured. Pending culture and sensitivity results, the patient should be managed with antibiotics as outlined previously. If fever or rapidly progressive cellulitis characterized by bullae and large areas of necrosis develops, *Aeromonas hydrophila* infection should be suspected. Less rapidly progressive *Aeromonas* infections may have the appearance of streptococcal cellulitis.[42]

SHARKS

Myth and folklore surround sharks, the most highly feared of all sea creatures. These occasionally savage animals are the subjects of many behavioral investigations, but until more reproducible data are available, a degree of mystery will remain. Shark attacks on humans have always held enormous fascination for scientists, adventurers, and clinicians. H. David Baldridge prepared a special technical report, *Shark Attack Against Man,* for the U.S. Navy Bureau of Medicine and Surgery in 1973. The International Shark Attack File, initiated by Perry W. Gilbert and Leonard P. Schultz in 1958 for the American Institute of Biological Sciences and the Office of Naval Research and formerly maintained at the Mote Marine Laboratory in Sarasota, Florida, is now housed at the University of Florida at Gainesville, where it is maintained by the International Elasmobranch Society and the Florida Museum of Natural History.[17] It remains an authoritative collection of analyzed data, containing a series of approximately 3000 individual investigations from the mid-1500s to the present. Mote Marine Laboratory (www.mote.org) is an independent, nonprofit marine research institution that operates The Center for Shark Research, focused on behavioral and medicine-related research. The Shark Research Institute (www.njscuba.com) publishes that it maintains a database that "contains more than 2,000 incidents involving divers, surfers, swimmers and fisherman," with a "network of investigators throughout the world that actively investigates attacks." Other records of shark attacks are maintained by the California Department of Fish and Game and the Waikiki Aquarium in Honolulu, Hawaii.

Although dreaded, sharks are among the most graceful and magnificent denizens of the deep. Sharks may be found in oceans, tropical rivers, and lakes. The bull shark *Carcharhinus leucas* is a frequent river inhabitant. Sharks range in size from 10 to 15 cm (*Squaliolus laticaudus*) to over 15 m and more than 18,144 kg (the whale shark *Rhincodon typus,* fortunately a plankton feeder).

The world's shark population is in danger from overfishing. Each year, more than 100 million animals, or 10 million sharks for each human shark-related fatality, are mutilated or slaughtered. This occurs in large part for the heinous practice of finning, in which a shark is captured, its fins are sliced off, and then it is returned to the water.[52] The fins are sold for the extraction of putative aphrodisiacs or to make shark-fin soup, which is extremely popular in Asia. Shark flesh is a major food source (commonly the "fish" in "fish and chips"), particularly since, to date, sharks do not appear to carry ciguatera toxin except in the liver. Innumerable animals are ground into fertilizer. Although at least 7150 tons of sharks were harvested commercially in U.S. coastal waters in 1989, more than 90% of captured sharks were discarded. In addition, vast numbers of sharks are caught in fishing nets as "by-catch" and meet an untimely end. This activity may double the estimated shark kill figures. (The National Marine Fisheries Service estimates that 20 million metric tons of marine wildlife are killed and thrown back into the sea as by-catch.) In Tahiti and other Polynesian locations, sharks are mercilessly killed to acquire their teeth for jewelry manufacture. In 1991 the South African government declared the great white shark a protected species within 200 miles of its coast. The U.S. government has lowered allowable fishing quotas in Atlantic waters. Great white sharks are protected off Australia, the southern coastline of Africa, the Maldives, and parts of the United States. Still, the populations of these and other shark species are declining, and unless there are further interventions, extinctions are likely.

Life and Habits

Sharks have inhabited the oceans for at least 400 million years. They appeared on the planet during the Devonian period, approximately 200 million years before the dinosaurs. Ancestral sharks may have been enormous; *Carcharodon megalodon* probably grew to a length of more than 15 m, with teeth longer than 3.2 cm. This was a predator of astronomic proportions.

Some 32 of the currently known 375 (approximate) species of sharks have been implicated in the 100 to 150 shark attacks upon humans that are estimated to occur annually worldwide, and another 35 to 40 species are considered potentially dangerous. U.S. coastal waters may be the setting for nearly one quarter of the attacks. Between 6 and 10 deaths from shark attacks are reported worldwide each year. The most frequently implicated offenders are the larger animals, such as the great white (Figure 60-3), bull, tiger (*Galeocerdo cuvieri*), and oceanic whitetip sharks. Sporadic attackers include the gray reef, blue (Figure 60-4), shortfin mako, dusky, hammerhead (Figure 60-5), lemon, Ganges River, Galápagos, spinner, sand, nurse, blacktip, blacknose, blue, bronze whaler, and ragged tooth sharks.[61] Tiger sharks were identified in a cluster of attacks around the Hawaiian Islands in the winter of 1993.

Sharks are carnivorous; many are apex predators. Their danger to humans results from the combination of size, aggression, and dentition. Some sharks, such as the giant whale shark (the largest fish at 50 feet in

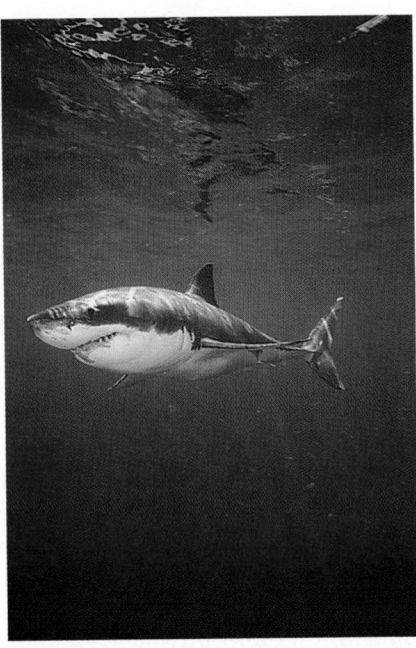

Figure 60-3 Great white shark *(Carcharodon carcharias)*. The most dangerous of sharks, this animal has been implicated in many attacks on humans. *(Photo by Howard Hall.)*

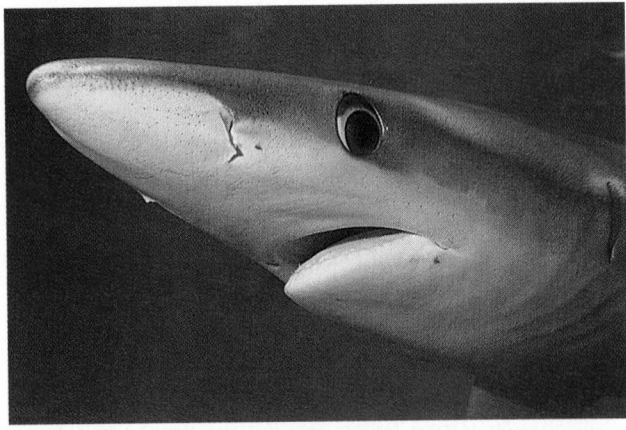

Figure 60-4 Blue shark, considered a dangerous species. *(Photo by Marty Snyderman.)*

length and more than 40,000 pounds), eat plankton and use their teeth as filters (Figure 60-6). Even small sharks can be powerful and destructive. The white shark is responsible for more attacks than any other species, particularly in the waters of southern Australia, the east coast of South Africa, the middle Atlantic coast of North America, and the American Pacific coast north of Point Conception, California. Attacks by great white sharks off the coast of northern California have led to the designation of a "red (or bloody) triangle" bordered on the north by Point Reyes and Tomales Bay through the Farallon Islands to the west and down south to Año Nuevo and Point Sur facing the Monterey Bay. This is a

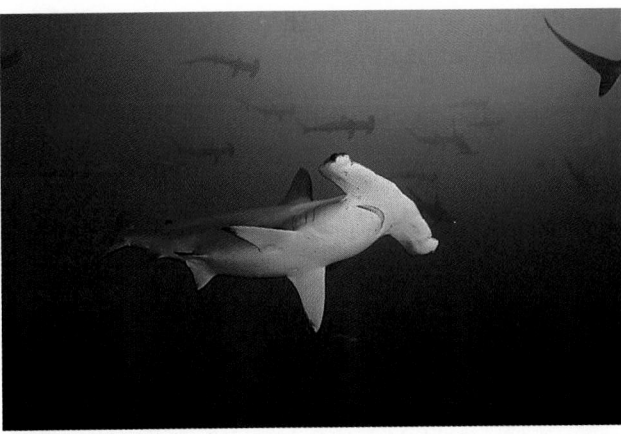

Figure 60-5 Hammerhead sharks, schooling off Cocos Island. The positioning of the eyes is reputed to increase the peripheral vision of these apex predators. *(Photo by Howard Hall.)*

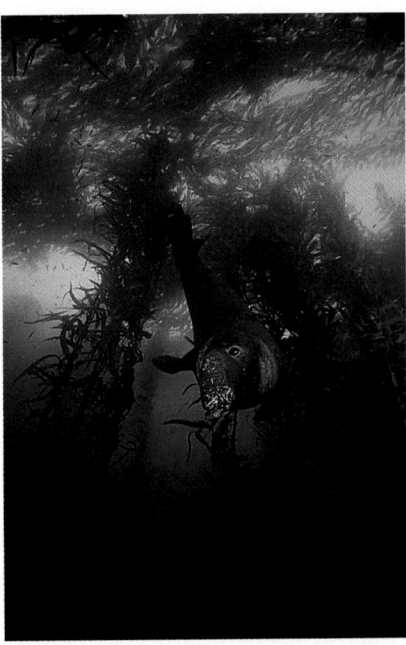

Figure 60-7 The elephant seal, shown here swimming through a kelp bed, is a favorite food for the great white shark. *(Photo by Howard Hall.)*

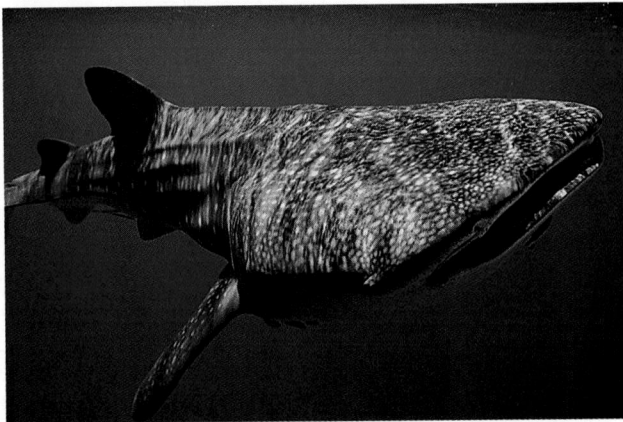

Figure 60-6 Whale shark *(Rhincodon typus)*, the largest fish in the sea, is fortunately a plankton eater. *(Photo by Norbert Wu.)*

breeding area for elephant seals *(Mirounga angustirostris)* (Figure 60-7), which yield 200-pound pups, perfect food for the immense predators.

The tiger *(Galeocerdo cuvieri)* (up to 18 feet and 2000 pounds) and bull *(Carcharinus leucas)* sharks are the next most dangerous with regard to attacks on humans. The great hammerhead *(Sphyrna mokarran)* (see Figure 60-5) has a reputation as a man-eater in equatorial waters. Scattered over its entire undersurface, the hammerhead has ampullae sensitive to electromagnetic fields, which in combination with its highly developed sense of smell may make it a superior predator.

In an analysis of California attacks, Miller and Collier[57] attributed unprovoked attacks north of San Miguel Island to white sharks, while those south of this area involved members of the families Carcharhinidae (requiem sharks), Sphyrnidae (hammerheads), and possibly Squatinidae (angel sharks).

Sharks are members of the class Chondrichthyes, or cartilaginous fish, which also includes skates, rays, and chimaeras, comprising approximately 780 species.[20] Unlike many bony fish, sharks are not buoyant because they do not possess swim bladders for flotation. In certain species, a large liver contributes to buoyancy. Thus sharks must stay in constant motion to keep from sinking and to drive water past the gills. Only a few bottom-dwelling species rest. Although sharks are not highly intelligent, they are endowed with remarkable sensory systems. Their color vision is poor but well compensated for by the acute perception of motion; the eye musculature is adapted for fixation with any body motion. The *tapetum lucidum* (responsible for the eye shine seen at night) is a series of reflecting plates containing silver guanine crystals in the choroidal layer behind the retina, which reflects light from a photoreceptor back along the same optical path to increase the sensitivity of the eye. This is present in sharks that are active in low-light environments.[84] The eyes are protected by upper and lower eyelids and the nictitating membrane (except for the great white shark, which does not have the membrane; it rotates its eyes in the sockets to avoid injury). Keen olfactory and gustatory chemoreceptors permit taste and the recognition of blood, urine, or peritoneal fluid in the water (in some cases, 1 part blood in 100 million parts of water). Sharks are most sensitive to chemicals that are similar to those produced by normal prey, such as amino acids, amines, and small fatty acids.[61] Up to two thirds of the shark brain can be devoted to smell. The nostrils are the openings of the olfactory organs and do not take part in breathing, which is accomplished by oxygen extraction from the water through a series of five to seven gill slits. Additionally, sharks possess skin chemoreceptors that detect chemical irritants. The lateral line system extending from the back along the side to the tail responds to sonic vibrations or pulsed low-frequency (20 to 60 cycles/sec) sound waves.[20] The lateral line organs are small holes along the sides of the shark's body that register motion in the water. These systems allow the shark to locate struggling fish, swimmers, or divers. Perhaps the most important series of telereceptors is located about the head, within the jelly-filled ampullae of Lorenzini, which are extremely sensitive to electrical voltage gradients (generated by the muscle contractions of fish; down to a $1/10^9$ volt per cm). Continuing research is directed at delineating the piscine ability to recognize electric fields. For instance, the common smooth dogfish (*Mustelus canis*) can detect an electrical voltage gradient of 5/1000 of a microvolt. Sharks also have extremely sensitive hearing, which may detect prey underwater from a distance of 914 m (3000 feet).

Research has in the past focused on isolation of antineoplastic agents from shark cartilage, organs, and body fluids.[48,67] For instance, sphyrnastatins have been isolated from the hammerhead shark *Sphyrna lewini*.[67] "Squalamine," produced by the spiny dogfish, is a broad-based antibiotic with antibacterial and antifungal properties. Shark cartilage (which does not appear to have significant antineoplastic activity) is used in the creation of artificial skin for humans, and shark blood and liver oil are being investigated for hematologic and immunologic properties. The latter is used in preparations to shrink hemorrhoids.

Shark Feeding and Attack

As previously noted, sharks are well equipped in the sensory aspects of feeding. They seem particularly able to avoid detection by potential prey, by virtue of coloration and a stealthy approach. Sharks feed in two basic patterns: (1) normal or subdued, with slow, purposeful group movements; and (2) frenzied or mob, as the result of an inciting event. The latter is precipitated by the sudden presentation of commotion or food/blood in the water. Frenzied behavior is enhanced by the proximity of other sharks in large numbers. In a frenzy, sharks become fearless and savage, snapping at anything and everything, including each other. After a shark decides to attack, it "postures," swimming erratically with elevated snout, arched back, pectoral fin depression, stiff lateral bending of the body, and rapid tail motion, in contrast to its normal sinuous and graceful swimming style.[40] In bursts of speed a shark can use its powerful caudal fin muscles and attain speeds in the water of 20 to 40 miles (32 to 64 km) per hour. As the Carchariniform shark prepares to strike, it rapidly

opens and closes its jaws (up to three times each second), depresses the pectoral fins in a braking action, and elevates the head. During a bite, the shark shakes its head and forebody in an effort to tear flesh from the victim. The shark may bite and spit to mortally wound the victim before eating it. Sharks swallow food whole without chewing it. Analysis of human remains recovered from a tiger shark indicate that the human victim was dismembered and then swallowed and digested.[39] It is difficult to postulate hunger as the sole attack motive, since more than 70% of victims are bitten only once or twice. Hit-and-run attacks are most common. Usually the lower teeth are used first in feeding; solitary upper tooth slashes might indicate attacks unrelated to feeding. Up to 60% of wounds involve only the upper teeth. At the moment of the strike the shark rolls its eyes back in the socket and uses the ampullae of Lorenzini to home in on the victim.

Sharks are selective feeders with clear dietary preferences. They commonly attack young, old, injured, or sick prey. Sea turtles, squid, penguins, seals, and stingrays are consumed in preference to humans. Sharks often eat other sharks. The great white shark cruises along the bottom of the ocean preparing to launch an attack on an unsuspecting surface animal. It can strike with enough force to lift the animal out of the water and breach itself, tearing a 50-pound chunk of flesh from its victim or even decapitating the animal (Figure 60-8). The cookiecutter (or cigar) shark *Mirounga angustirostris* or *Isistius brasiliensis* (Figure 60-9) creates a circular craterlike wound approximately 5 to 6 cm in diameter when it attacks its pinniped prey. Sharks have short intestines, seem to be able to selectively digest ingested foodstuffs, and may be able to keep portions of what they ingest intact for prolonged periods of time, perhaps as a method to regulate nourishment.

It is difficult to generalize about shark attacks on humans. Current explanations suggest that frightened

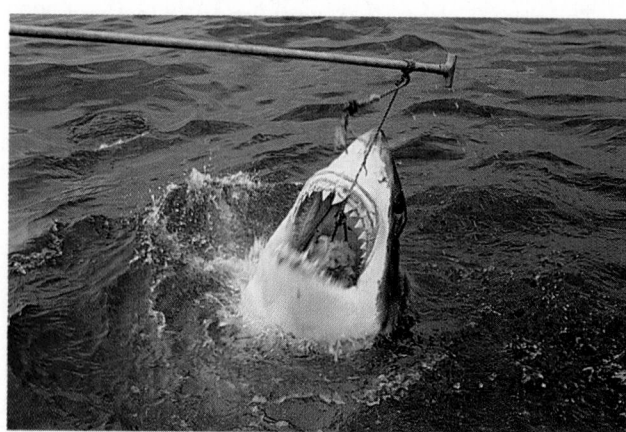

Figure 60-8 The great white shark advances its upper jaw in the act of biting to feed. *(Photo by Pete Romano, Images Unlimited, Inc.)*

persons are more likely to be targets of aggression. This has been demonstrated in the case of the gray reef shark, *Carcharhinus amblyrhynchos*. Aggression may be aggravated by purely anomalous behavior, the violation of courtship patterns, or territorial invasion. More docile behavior tends to be the rule with other reef sharks, such as the silvertip *(Carcharinus albimarginatus)*, blackfin *(C. melanopterus)*, or whitetip *(Triaenodon obesus)* (Figure 60-10). The legs and buttocks are most commonly bitten (Figure 60-11), perhaps an indication of dangling legs or buttocks displayed by an abalone diver facing a rock or ledge. Since sharks do not chew

their food, their method of biting and rolling or thrashing allows flesh to be stripped from the victim. Teeth may be embedded in prey (Figure 60-12), but fractured bones are surprisingly rare.[39] A large shark can attack and sink a boat but may wait to return and consume the human boaters.

The great white shark *(Carcharodon carcharias)* is a man-attacker but probably not a man-eater. This statement reflects the observation that this highly feared animal (which has been observed at a length of 19.5 feet and an estimated weight of 4500 pounds; it is claimed, but not proven, that it can attain a length of 25 feet and a weight of 5500 pounds) usually releases its victim following a single "inquisitory" bite, after it recognizes that a mouthful of neoprene, fiberglass, or lead weights is not normal dietary fare. This is small consolation to the unfortunate victim, who may have an entire

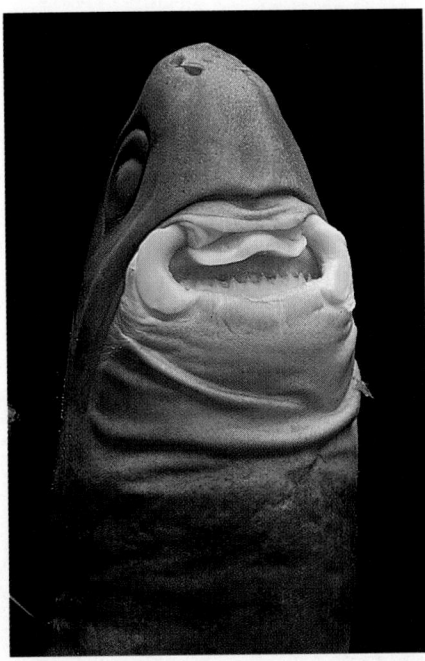

Figure 60-9 The cookie cutter shark *(Isistius brasiliensis)* cuts pieces of flesh off its prey with its unusual tooth configuration. *(Photo by Norbert Wu.)*

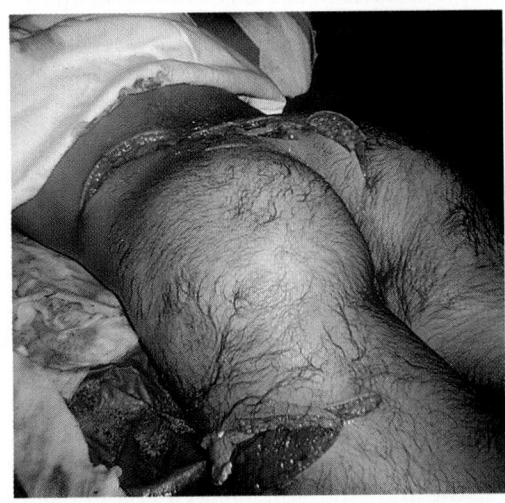

Figure 60-11 Shark bite of the buttocks. *(Courtesy T. Hattori, MD.)*

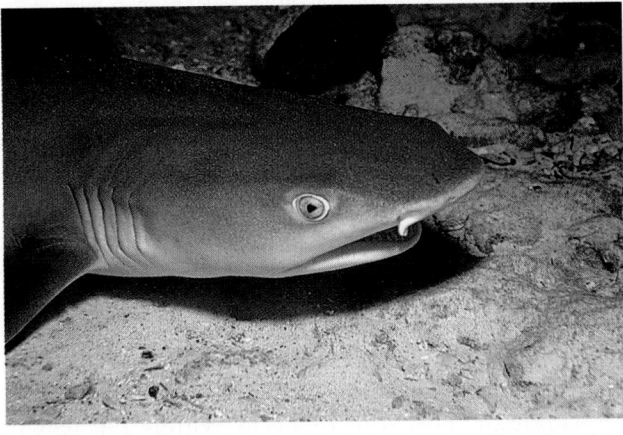

Figure 60-10 Whitetip reef shark. This species tends to be fairly docile.

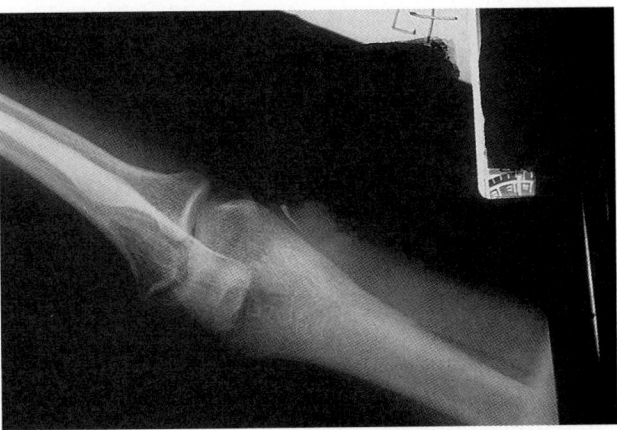

Figure 60-12 The presence of a shark tooth in the arm is revealed by x-ray examination.

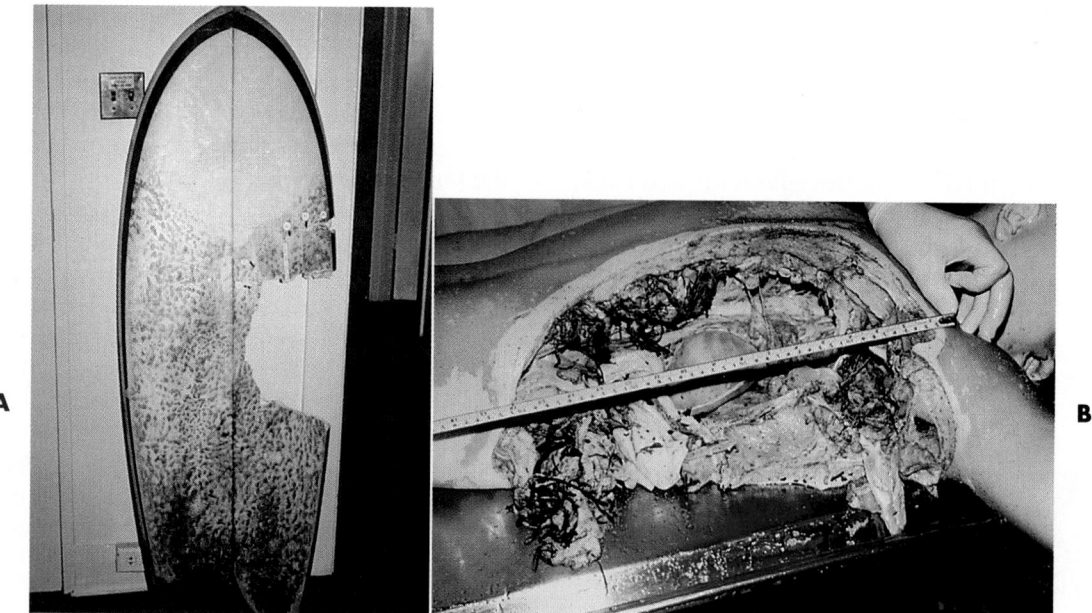

Figure 60-13 Victim of great white shark attack. **A,** Damaged surfboard ridden by the victim. **B,** Massive thoracic injury after a single bite. It was estimated that the shark was 20 feet long. *(Courtesy P. Crossman, Coroner's Division, Salinas, Calif.)*

hemithorax or limb removed (Figure 60-13). The great white shark has only recently been closely observed in the wild and is thus the subject of much speculation about predation strategies.[55] The feared trait of the great white sharks is they initiate contact with humans.[28] Their unpredictable nature ranges from a seemingly docile approach to a research boat to a powerful attack on a surface sea lion. Adults feed largely on pinnipeds; the bite-and-spit behavior is considered a means of avoiding injury from struggling prey (Figure 60-14). One theory is that a shark that largely consumes a human victim does so because the victim was solitary in the water.[29] Breath-hold diver behavior and the similarity of the silhouette of a contemporary surfboard to that of a surface seal may be responsible for attacks on humans. Most attacks on humans occur at the water's surface. One fatal attack in 1989 with two victims was on sea kayakers off the coast of southern California. At the time of this writing, there have been (since 1876) approximately 250 documented attacks by great white sharks upon humans, with approximately 65 fatalities.

Shark attacks have occurred from the upper Adriatic Sea to southern New Zealand, with most between latitudes 46° N and 47° S. The odds of being attacked by a shark along the North American coastline are approximately 1 in 5 million. The danger is greater during the summer months (more persons in the water), in recreational areas, during late afternoon and nighttime feeding, and in murky, warm (20° C [68° F]) water. White sharks frequently venture into colder water, and attacks

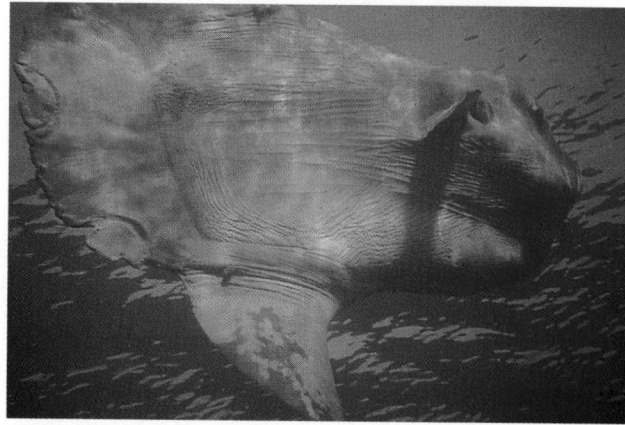

Figure 60-14 Giant sunfish *(Mola mola)*. Note the shark bites on the posterior end of the fish. *(Photo by Paul S. Auerbach, MD.)*

have occurred in waters as cold as 10° C [50° F]. The frequency of shark attacks off the northern California coastline appears to be increasing, particularly with respect to the great white shark. Contrary to the findings of worldwide shark attack analysis, attacks in northern California occur more frequently in clearer water at temperatures of less than 16° C [60° F].[57] Shark attacks in Hawaiian waters are relatively rare, with the exception of recent events.[93]

Although most attacks occur within 100 feet of shore, it is believed that the danger is greater further out, in deep channels or drop-offs. Because of their abil-

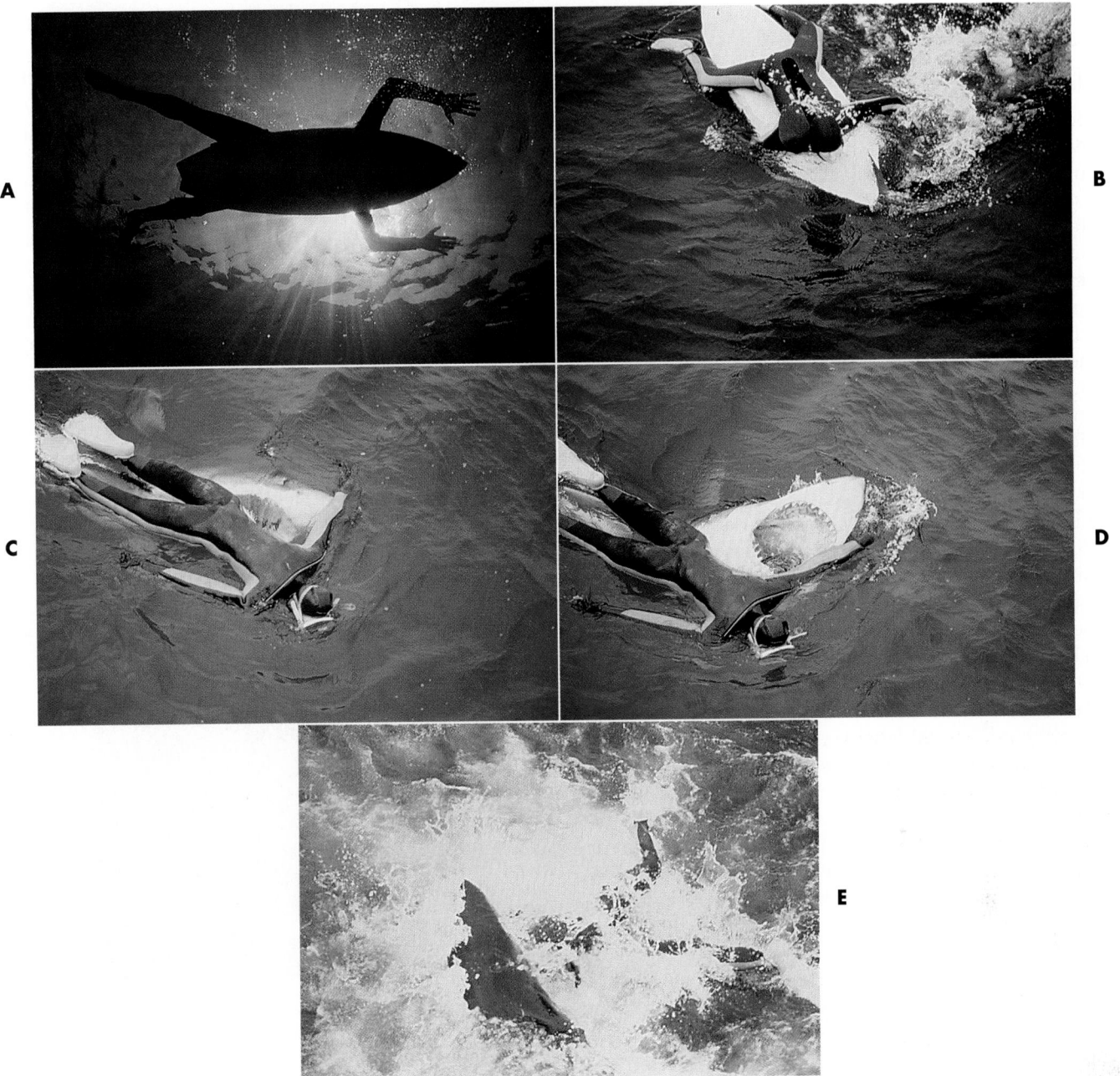

Figure 60-15   A, Silhouette of diver on surfboard to demonstrate similarity in shadow and contour to a sea lion at the surface. **B,** A great white shark passes underneath a dummy on a surfboard before making an attack. **C,** The shark begins to elevate its head from the water. **D,** With jaws wide, the shark attacks the dummy. **E,** With great commotion, the dummy and surfboard are dragged beneath the surface. *(All photos courtesy of Images Unlimited, Inc.* **A,** *Al Giddings.* **B,** *Rosemary Chastney.* **C** *to* **E,** *Walt Clayton.)*

ity to detect contrasts, sharks have a predilection to attack bright, contrasting, or reflective objects. Movement is an added attraction to sharks, which have been known to bite surfboards, boats, and buoys. Recent shark attacks in northern California coastal waters involved swimmers on surfboards (black on white) who entered migratory elephant seal (shark food) habitats (Figure 60-15).

Most victims are attacked by single sharks, violently and without warning. In the majority of attacks the victim does not see the shark before the attack. The first contact may be a bumping, which is an attempt by the shark to wound the victim before the definitive strike. Severe skin abrasions from the shark skin (shagreen) placoid scales (denticles) are produced in this manner. These microscopic appendages have the same origin as teeth, with a pulp cavity, dentine, and vitreodentine ("enamel") covering.

Clinical Aspects

The jaws of the major carnivorous sharks are crescent-shaped and contain up to five or six rows or series of razor-sharp ripsaw triangular teeth, which are replaced every few weeks by advancing inner rows (Figure 60-16). Each species has distinctively shaped teeth.[84] However, a study of the teeth of the great white shark revealed no consistent pattern of size or arrangement of the marginal serrations that was sufficiently characteristic within an individual shark to serve as a reliable index of identification of a tooth as originating from that particular shark. However, the serrations are sufficiently distinctive to enable the potential identification of an individual tooth as having been the cause of a particular bitemark.[62] Although normal tooth replacement takes 7 to 10 days, in some species a lost tooth can be replaced within 24 hours. Amazingly, some sharks produce up to 25,000 teeth in a lifetime. The upper jaws generally have larger cutting teeth, whereas the sharp lower teeth are designed to fasten onto and hold prey during capture.[33] The teeth are cartilaginous, strengthened by the deposition of calcium phosphate crystals (apatite) in a protein matrix, all covered by an enameloid substance. They are considered to be as hard as granite and as strong as steel. In a great white shark, the largest serrated triangular teeth can grow to 2.5 inches. There are 26 upper and 24 lower teeth exposed in the front row. The height of the enamel of the largest tooth in the upper jaw is proportional to the animal's length, so a body length of up to 25 feet may be possible. The upper jaw is advanced forward and protruded to allow its participation in the biting action (Figure 60-17). The biting force of some sharks is estimated at 18 tons per square inch. Severe shark bites result acutely in massive tissue loss, hemorrhage, shock, and death. Even a smaller animal, such as a lemon shark, can bite with bone-crushing force.[34] The potential for destruction is unparalleled in the animal kingdom.

The human leg (or legs) is most frequently bitten, followed by the hands and arms, as the victim attempts to fend off the shark. Proximal femoral artery disruption carries a poor prognosis because of the torrential hemorrhage (Figure 60-18). Although fractures are not common, broken ribs often accompany intrathoracic, intraperitoneal, and retroperitoneal injuries. Because the victim is generally far from medical assistance, blood loss may be profound. The wounds have historically been fatal in 15% to 25% of attacks, with major causes of death listed as hemorrhage and drowning. Rapid response and prehospital care seem to be somewhat improving this statistic.

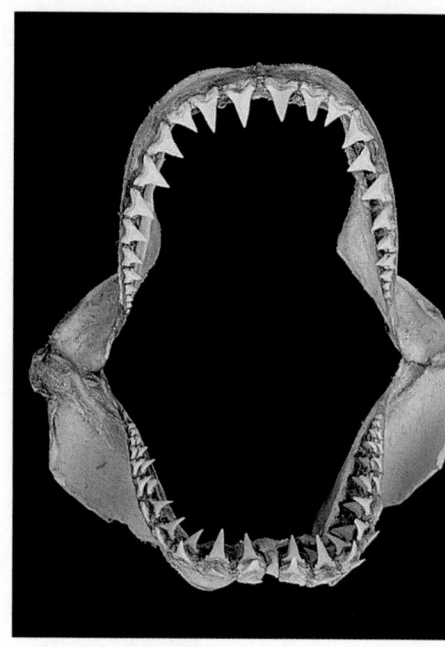

Figure 60-17 Jaw of a great white shark. *(Photo by Norbert Wu.)*

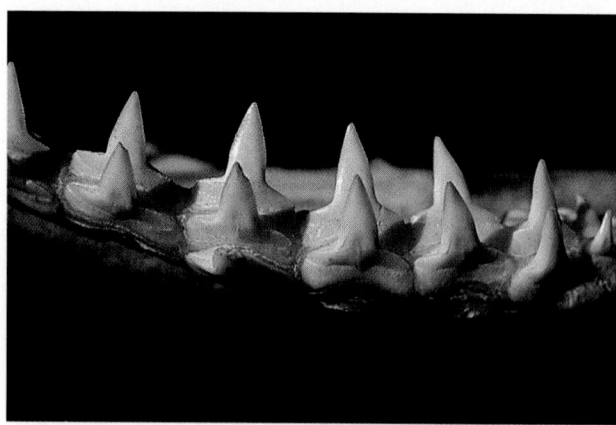

Figure 60-16 Teeth of bull shark *(Carcharhinus leucas). (Photo by Norbert Wu.)*

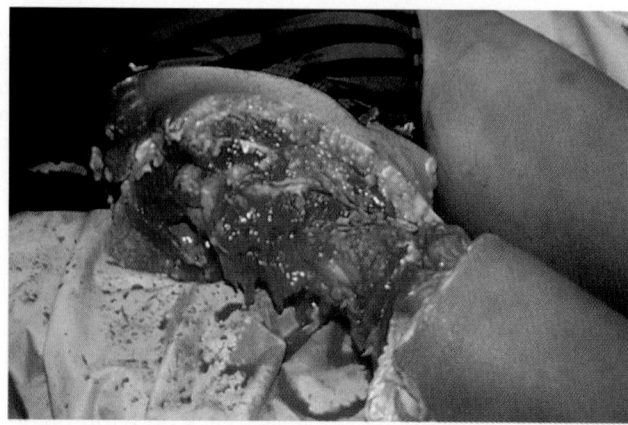

Figure 60-18 Shark bite of the proximal thigh. This unfortunate victim exsanguinated from a disrupted femoral artery. *(Courtesy Kenneth W. Kizer, MD.)*

Treatment

In most cases the immediate threat to life is hypovolemic shock. Thus it is occasionally necessary to compress wounds or manually to constrict arterial bleeding while the victim is in the water. As soon as the victim is out of the water, all means available must be used to ligate large, disrupted arteries or to apply compression dressings. If possible, the injudicious use of pressure points or tourniquets should be avoided. If intravascular volume must be replaced in large quantities, at least two large-bore IV lines should be inserted into the uninvolved extremities to deliver crystalloid (lactated Ringer's solution, normal saline, or hypertonic saline), colloid, or blood products.[63,85] Central venous cannulation should be reserved for the emergency department.

The victim should be kept well oxygenated and warm while being transported to a facility equipped to handle major trauma. Blood losses should be replaced with whole blood or packed red blood cells and fresh-frozen plasma.[86] The precise ratio of crystalloid to blood products and proper mean arterial blood pressure endpoint of primary resuscitation in the presence of a major vascular injury are the subjects of ongoing investigations.[82] The victim should be thoroughly examined for evidence of cervical, intrathoracic, and intraabdominal injuries. Because *Clostridium* can be cultured from ocean water, tetanus toxoid 0.5 ml intramuscularly (IM) and tetanus immune globulin (Hyper-Tet, Cutter) 250 to 500 units IM must be given. The administration of prophylactic antibiotics is more controversial. The victim of a shark bite should be treated with an IV third-generation cephalosporin, trimethoprim/sulfamethoxazole, an aminoglycoside, ciprofloxacin, or some reasonable com-

bination of these agents. Imipenem/cilastatin should be reserved for established wound infections or early indications of septicemia, particularly in the setting of immunosuppression. The rationale for prophylactic antibiotics is that shark wounds are prone to heavy contamination with seawater, sand, plant debris, shark teeth, and shark mouth flora. After a clinical infection is recognized, wounds should be cultured for aerobes and anaerobes by insertion of sterile swabs deeply into available lesions.

Proper operative intervention is mandatory. It is inappropriate to attempt emergency department exploration of what often prove to be extensive and complicated wounds. In the operating room, devitalized tissue should be widely debrided and the wound irrigated copiously to remove all foreign material (Figure 60-19). An x-ray may reveal one or more shark teeth in the wound (see Figure 60-12). Unless it is absolutely necessary to achieve tight closure, the wound should be closed loosely around multiple drains (preferably closed systems) or packed open to await delayed primary closure. Although there is debate about whether to use internal or external fixation of grossly open and contaminated fractures, it seems logical to recommend surgical stabilization to facilitate vascular and soft tissue repair. In the pediatric population, damage to the physis and future limb length discrepancy should be anticipated.[34]

The abrasion associated with a shark "bumping" should be managed like a second-degree burn, with daily debridement and application of antiseptic ointment.

A reasonable "shark pack" should be available in emergency facilities and rescue vehicles near shark-infested waters. This must be portable and should in-

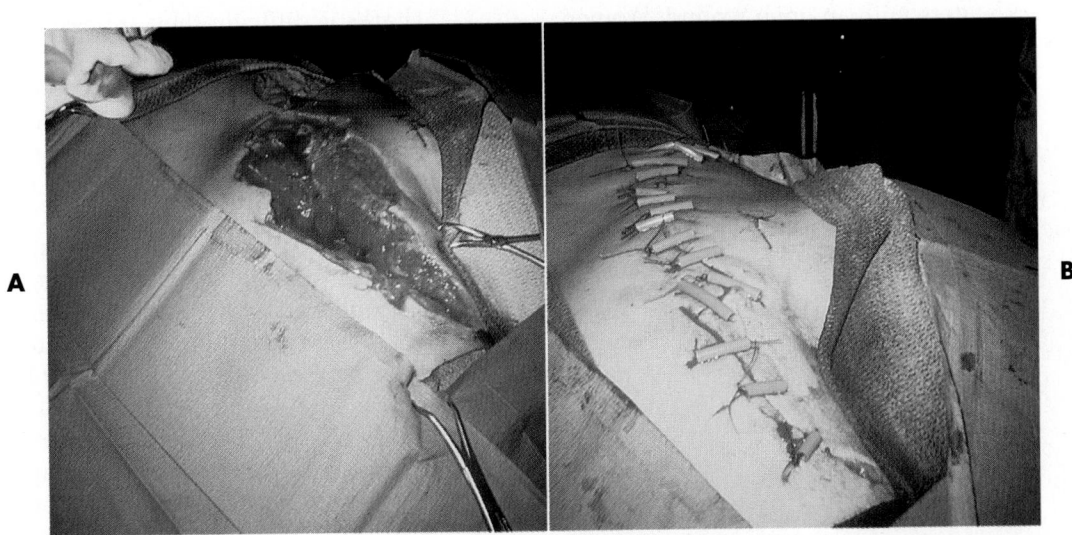

Figure 60-19 Operative repair of shark bite wound shown in Figure 60-11. **A,** Debridement and exploration of the wound in the operating room. **B,** Proper closure technique with tension-releasing sutures. *(Courtesy T. Hattori, MD.)*

clude items necessary to control hemorrhage and initiate IV therapy.

Prevention

Every precaution should be taken to avoid shark attack, beginning with an intimate knowledge of the local waters. The following is precautionary advice and a list of alternatives for action in the event of a confrontation:

1. Avoid shark-infested water, particularly at dusk and at night. Do not swim through schools of bait fish. Do not enter posted waters. Do not wander too far from shore. Surfers are generally at greater risk than divers. Do not disguise yourself as a pinniped (seal). Do not swim with animals (such as dogs or horses) in shark waters. Shark behavior can be unpredictable, so it is best not to remain in the water with sharks, particularly if you are fearful. Although some persons believe that sharks can be domesticated, there is no such thing as a friendly shark. Photograph hazardous sharks from within the confines of a protective cage (Figure 60-20), rather than from an unprotected position.

2. Swimmers should remain in groups. Isolation creates a primary target and eliminates companion surveillance. When diving, maintain constant vigilance.

3. Turbid water, drop-offs, deep channels, breeding inlets, and sanitation waste outlets are areas frequented by larger sharks and should be avoided. However, it appears that sharks attack at least half the time in clear water. Humans are most often attacked in shallow water or beyond the breakers.

4. Blood and other body fluids (including peritoneal fluid) attract sharks. No person should be in shark waters with an open wound. Women have historically been advised to avoid diving during menstruation, although there are no data to support attraction of sharks to the discharge of menstruation.

5. Brightly colored swimwear or diving equipment and shiny snorkeling gear attract certain sharks. Bright (international) orange appears to be particularly attractive to sharks. Flat black is probably the least attractive color. There is scant evidence that sharks are more attracted to light-skinned bathers.

6. Captured fish must be tethered at a distance from any divers. There is no greater chemical attractant for a shark than fish blood. Divers who harvest abalone should be aware that the banging and prying noise of an "abalone iron" may attract sharks.

7. The presence of porpoises in the water does not preclude the presence of sharks. Be alert for the presence of a shark whenever schools of fish behave in an erratic manner.

8. Do not tease or corner a shark. This is particularly true with captive animals. Do not pull on a shark's tail. Do not chase after a shark. If a shark begins to act in an erratic manner, do not photograph it at close range using a strobe flash apparatus.

9. If a shark appears in shallow water, swimmers should leave the water with slow, purposeful movements, facing the shark if possible and avoiding erratic behavior that could be interpreted as distress. If a shark approaches in deep water, the diver should remain submerged, rather than wildly surface to escape. The diver should move to defensive terrain with posterior protection to fend off, as best as possible, a frontal attack. It is inadvisable to trap a shark so that it must attack to obtain freedom. Fighting sharks is difficult; they are best repulsed with blunt blows to the snout, eyes, or gills. If possible, the bare hand should not be used, to avoid severe abrasions or lacerations. A stream of air bubbles from a scuba regulator directed into the face of a shark may be sufficient deterrent. Although spears, knives, shotgun shell– or 30-.06–loaded powerheads ("bang sticks" [Figure 60-21]), strychnine-filled spears, and carbon dioxide darts can kill small sharks, they can worsen the situation if they are misapplied or their application promotes frenzy in a school of sharks.

Do not splash on the surface or create a commotion in a manner that might cause a shark to interpret your behavior as that of a struggling fish. Surface chop and perhaps the sounds created by helicopter rotor wash attract sharks. During a helicopter rescue, exit the water as soon as possible.

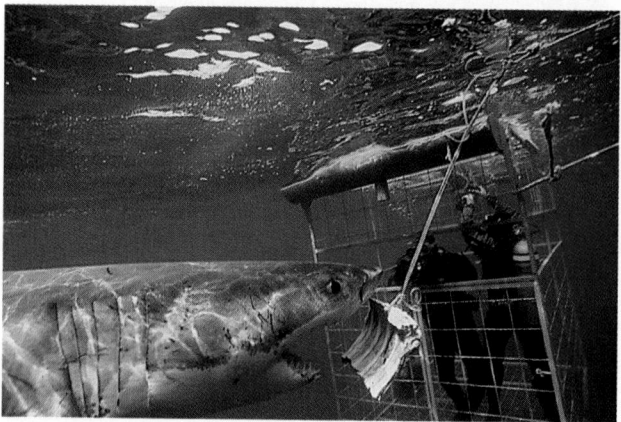

Figure 60-20 Caged divers view an inquisitive great white shark. *(Photo by Carl Roessler.)*

10. Shark defense techniques and repellents are constantly evolving. In response to shark attacks on downed airmen and sailors during World War II, copper acetate blended with a water-soluble wax and nigrosine dye was packaged as a slowly dissolving waxy cake for deployment as "Shark Chaser" by the Office of Naval Research of the U.S. Navy.[11] It was theorized that the acetate resembled the decaying carcasses of sharks and sharks would thus be repelled. Unfortunately, while a morale booster, this was and is not a reliable deterrent. Its use was discontinued by the Navy in 1976. Limited progress has been made since that time. Recreational beaches in Australia and South Africa are protected with extensive gill net systems ("meshing") to trap overly curious animals. These work to a certain degree but are not foolproof. Electric shark barriers ("cable device") using 0.8-msec pulses 15 times per second to create a field of 4 volts per meter seem to generate a fright response in sharks longer than 1.2 m and are being investigated.[18,79] Their benefits include repulsion rather than shark capture or destruction. However, some sharks respond weakly to these stimuli. Abalone divers in South Australia work from one-person, self-propelled shark cages.

Experimental devices for individuals include chain-mesh diving suits, inflatable dull-colored plastic protective bags (yellow is easy for aircraft to spot, but most attractive to sharks), acoustic and hand-held electrical field transmitters, surfactants and other chemical repellents (such as firefly and the Red Sea and western Indian Ocean Moses sole [flatfish; *Pardachirus marmoratus*] glandular extract [pardaxin]).[25] Pardaxin is an excitatory polypeptide neurotoxin that forms voltage-gated pores and triggers neurotransmitter release.[47] The ichthyotoxic secretion from the fish, which appears as a milky substance from a series of glands located along the dorsal and anal fins, also contains shark repellent lipophilic constituents that appear to be steroid monoglycosides.[69,83] It appears that in sharks, the gills and/or pharyngeal cavity are the target organ(s) for the repellent action. However, it has been estimated that about 24 kg of any effective drug would have to be contained in the volume of water through which a slowly approaching shark might swim as it attacked a human in the ocean.[11] For the exudate from the Moses sole, concentrations of 10 to 25 g/m^3 are needed to elicit an immediate indication of repellency. For more common synthetic detergents (sodium dodecyl sulfate), the concentration needed is 800 g/m^3. These findings show that a chemical carried in a life jacket cannot be reliably useful against sharks, since it would have to be instantaneously effective at a concentration of no greater than 100 parts per billion. There is no question that shark avoidance is the most reliable maneuver.

The SharkPOD (Figure 60-22) is a personal device marketed to recreational, commercial, and scientific divers with an output of 90 volts of 75 minutes duration on a rechargeable battery that has been evaluated in both startle (turn the device on when the shark is within 1-m distance) and exclusion (turn on when the shark is out of range of the electrical field) tests on a variety of shark species, including the great white shark. The effective electrical field created by the device is approximately 7 feet in diameter. Observations have included that sharks already in the process of feeding may not be repelled by the device, so the current

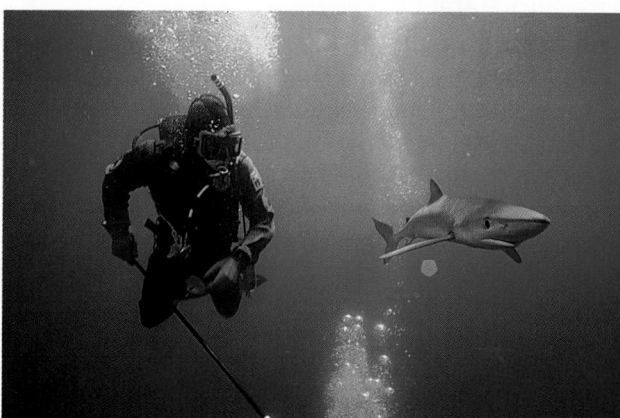

Figure 60-21 Diver carrying a "bang stick" in the presence of a blue shark. *(Photo by Howard Hall.)*

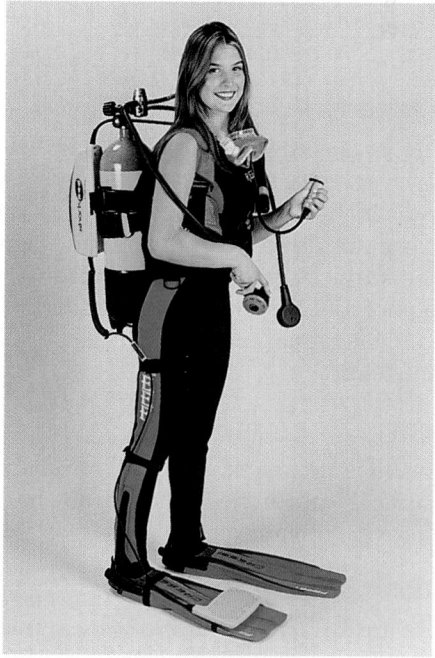

Figure 60-22 SharkPOD shark repellent device.

thought is that the device should be turned on at the beginning of a dive to create a situation of "exclusion." A wand-type unit is currently being evaluated.

BARRACUDA

To many divers, the barracuda appears more sinister than the shark, and it is more highly feared. Barracuda are distributed from Brazil north to Florida, and in the Indo-Pacific from the Red Sea to the Hawaiian Islands. Of the 22 species of barracuda, only the great barracuda (*Sphyraena barracuda*) has been implicated in human attacks.

Life and Habits

The great barracuda is encountered in all tropical seas and can grow to 2.5 m and 50 kg but is rarely sighted at a length greater than 1.5 m (Figure 60-23). A solitary swimmer, the fish is extremely swift and swims in a disconcerting darting fashion. The barracuda possesses an elongated narrow mouth filled with large knifelike teeth, similar in appearance to those of canines (Figure 60-24). Smaller fish may be found in large schools.

Although great barracuda seldom attack divers, they do so rapidly and fiercely, often out of confusion in murky waters. More commonly the fish charges through or leaps from shallow water to bite the dangling legs of a boater, particularly if a shiny anklet (which resembles a fishing lure) is worn. Persons have been bitten on the scalp while wearing a barrette or on the face when trying to feed a barracuda by holding a dead fish bait in their mouths. Considering the great frequency with which barracuda are encountered and the low number of reported attacks, they do not pose nearly the hazard of sharks.

Clinical Aspects

Barracuda jaws contain two nearly parallel rows of teeth, which produce straight or V-shaped lacerations, in contradistinction to the crescent-shaped bite of the shark. Except for this difference and the magnitude of injury, the surgical problems generated by the barracuda do not differ from those of the shark. The clinician encounters tissue loss, moderate hemorrhage, and wound infections.

Treatment

Barracuda bites are treated identically to shark bites. If a barracuda is captured, it should not be eaten in ciguatera toxin–endemic regions.

Prevention

Barracuda are attracted to turbid waters, underwater commotion, irregular motion, surface splashing, shiny objects, and tethered fish. These should all be avoided.

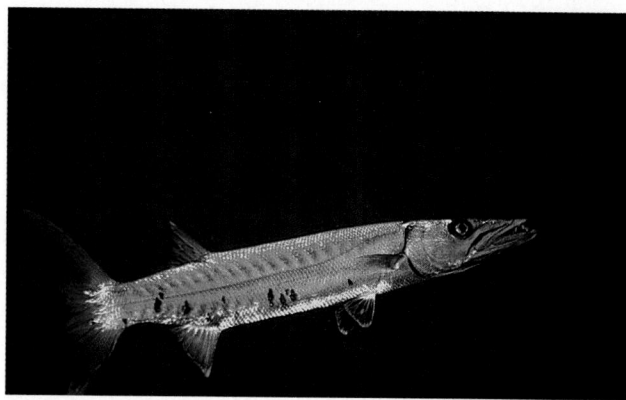

Figure 60-23 Great barracuda *(Sphyraena barracuda)*. *(Photo by Paul S. Auerbach, MD.)*

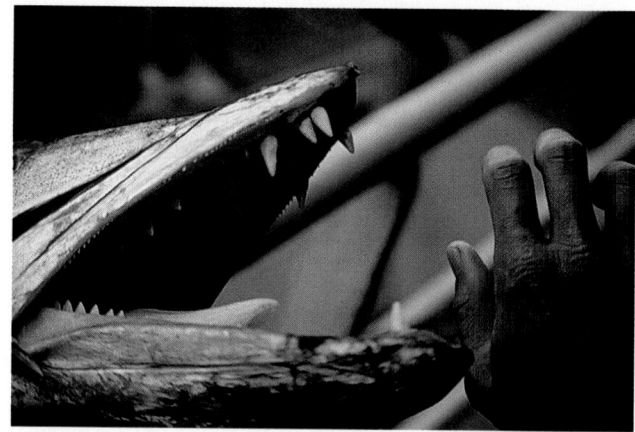

Figure 60-24 Jaws of the great barracuda, with canine-configured teeth next to the author's hand.

It is unwise to dangle a body part adorned with reflective jewelry before the jaws of a barracuda.

MORAY EELS

Life and Habits

Moray eels are found in tropical, subtropical, and some temperate waters. In the family Muraenidae, some individuals of the larger species may attain lengths of 3.5 m and diameters of more than 35 cm. Morays are muscular, powerful, and savage bottom dwellers, residing in holes or crevices or under rock and coral. They have a snakelike appearance and rarely have scales or pectoral fins. The distinguishing feature of the morays is the small, round gill opening. The skin of the moray eel is leathery and mucus coated, not easily lacerated with a knife. Fortunately, the eel usually evades confrontation unless cornered or provoked. Bites occur when a diver intentionally probes into a coral bed or cave, or a fisherman reaches into a net and offers a

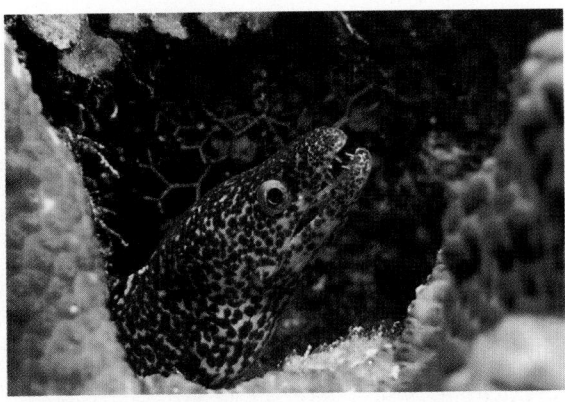

Figure 60-25 Moray eel, demonstrating the sharp teeth and biting potential. *(Photo by Paul S. Auerbach, MD.)*

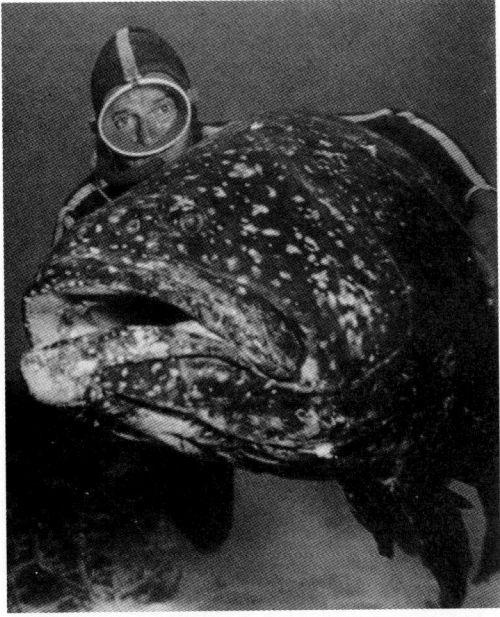

Figure 60-26 Diver alongside a giant grouper. *(Courtesy Bruce Halstead, MD.)*

hand to a feeding eel. Aquarium-housed morays may strike when handled improperly. Most moray eels are easily intimidated and avoid confrontation unless cornered. An aggressive eel may strike out in competition for prey, particularly lobster. Elderly, vision-impaired eels may attack without specific provocation, especially at night. In U.S. coastal waters, the most prevalent species are the California, green, and spotted morays.

Clinical Aspects

Morays are forceful and vicious biters that can inflict severe puncture wounds with their narrow and vise-like jaws, which are equipped with long, sharp, retrorse, and fanglike teeth (Figure 60-25). Molar-type teeth are present in some species. A moray eel has the tenacity of a bulldog and will hold on to a victim, rather than strike and release. Multiple small puncture wounds are common after the bite of smaller eels, with the hand most commonly involved. If the eel is ripped forcefully from the victim, the resulting lacerations may be extensive.

Treatment

Moray bites are treated in a manner analogous to that of shark bites. If the eel remains attached to the victim, the jaws may need to be broken or the animal decapitated to effect release. The primary wound should be irrigated copiously and explored to locate any retained teeth. The risk of infection is high, particularly in bites to the hand. The puncture wounds should be left unsutured to allow drainage and the victim given appropriate prophylactic antibiotics. If the wound is extensive and more linear in configuration (resembling a dog bite), the wound edges may be debrided and loosely approximated with nonabsorbable sutures or staples, and antibiotics may be administered. In all cases, it is prudent to inspect the wound at 24 and 48 hours to detect the onset of infection.

Prevention

It is unwise for a snorkeler or diver to place a hand underneath unexplored coral or rock unless it has been probed or otherwise disturbed specifically in search of an eel. All fishing nets should be handled carefully. A dive guide who feeds moray eels by holding a loaf of bread or bait fish in his mouth is offering his nose and mouth as a meal for an unpredictable eel.

GIANT GROUPERS

Some of the larger species of sea bass or grouper (family Serranidae) may grow to exceed 3.6 m and 227 kg (Figure 60-26). Distributed in both tropical and temperate seas, they are curious, pugnacious, and voracious feeders. Although not aggressive like a shark, a giant grouper should be respected for its fearlessness, bulk, and cavernous mouth. Groupers can be found frequenting shipwrecks; swimming in caves, caverns, and holes; and lurking behind large rocks and coral outcroppings. They are territorial and may become aggressive while protecting their domain. Bite wounds may be ragged with extensive maceration and are treated the same as shark bites. Large groupers should not be eaten in ciguatera toxin–endemic regions. It is always wise to visually survey an underwater cave before entering or exiting. The diver should not block the exit if a grouper is attempting to escape and should not carry speared fish. Many scare tactics used against sharks are of no avail with groupers.

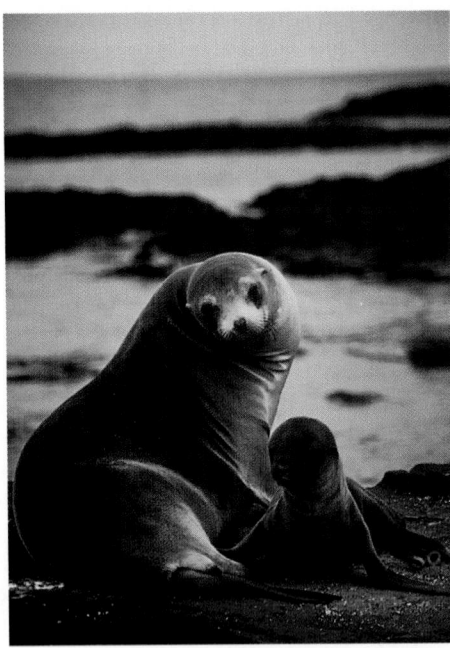

Figure 60-27 Sea lion and pup. Parents of both genders aggressively protect their young. *(Photo by Paul S. Auerbach, MD.)*

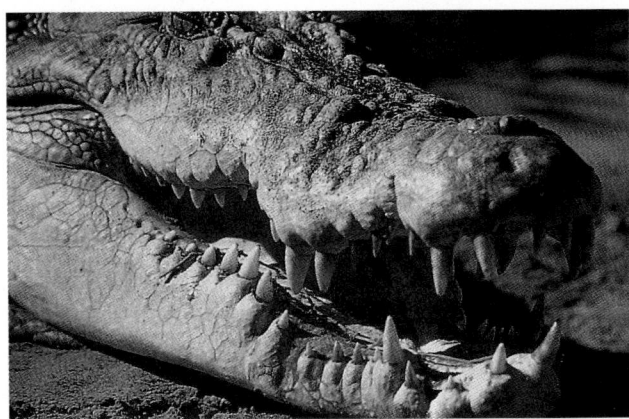

Figure 60-28 The jaws of a saltwater crocodile. *(Courtesy Allan P. Mekisic.)*

SEA LIONS

Sea lions (family Otaridae) and seals (family Phocidae) are mild-mannered mammals except during the mating season, when the males may become aggressive, and the breeding season, when both genders attack in defense of their newborn pups (Figure 60-27). Divers have been seriously bitten and therefore should avoid ill-tempered and abnormally aggressive animals. There is nothing unique about the clinical aspects of these injuries, except for the posttraumatic infections. The bites are treated the same as shark bites.

"Seal finger" (speck finger, blubber finger) follows a bite wound from a seal or from contact of even a minor skin wound with a seal's mouth or pelt. The affliction is characterized by swelling of the digit, with or without articular involvement. There may be lymphadenopathy and involvement of adjacent joints. No particular organism has been consistently cultured from these injuries, but there has been suggestion that in addition to *Staphylococcus* and *Streptococcus*, *Erysipelothrix rhusiopathiae* may an inciting pathogen (see Chapter 63).

CROCODILES AND ALLIGATORS

Crocodiles (genus *Crocodylus*) and alligators (genus *Alligator*) are long-bodied loricates with reputations as ferocious aquatic reptiles. Considered to be less sluggish than alligators, crocodiles (*C. niloticus* in the Nile and the larger estuarine *C. porosus* of eastern Asia and the Pacific islands) may attack and severely injure a human. *C. porosus*, which ranges over an extensive geographic area, including India, Sri Lanka, southern China, the Malay Archipelago, Palau, the Solomon Islands, and northern Australia, has been claimed to be a prolific man-eater. Estimates of human fatalities may be exaggerated based on isolated reports of atrocities committed by this beast. An adult crocodile devours prey much larger in size than a human. According to one report, the stomach of an Australian estuarine crocodile contained the remains of an aborigine and a 4-gallon drum containing two blankets. At a length greater than 20 feet and a weight exceeding 2500 pounds, the crocodile can travel in water at a speed of 20 mph and can charge a short distance over land at 15 to 30 mph. The enormous jaws and canine teeth (Figure 60-28) can bite with sufficient force to sever an outboard boat propeller. However, the teeth are not well suited for tearing apart or chewing, so most prey is allowed to rot, which makes them easier to swallow. Most crocodiles are content to eat fish, turtles, kangaroos, and wild pigs. However, excursions into freshwater rivers and onto land have introduced them to cows, horses, and humans. A crocodile attacks by grasping the victim in its powerful jaws and dragging it underwater, where it drowns and dismembers the victim with a constant twirling motion ("death rolls"). In a series of 16 crocodile attacks reported from the Northern Territory of Australia, four fatalities involved transection of the torso or decapitation.[56] Most attacks (fatal and nonfatal) were on persons swimming or wading in shallow water. In riverine areas of Tanzania, crocodiles are a considerable health hazard. In the Korogwe District from 1990 to 1994, 51 human and 49 crocodile deaths were reported. The attacks are attributed to increased waste products in the water, which reduces the crocodiles' primary food sup-

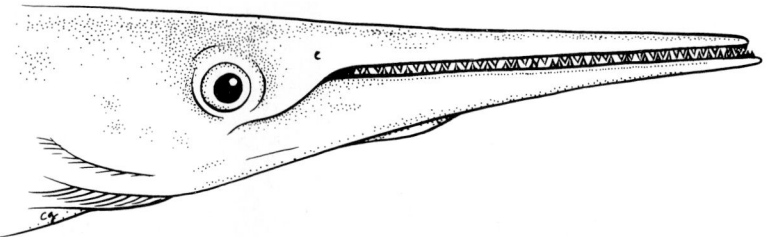

Figure 60-29 Needlefish beak, capable of causing a penetrating injury.

ply. In addition, "tamed" crocodiles are not hunted for fear of reprisal by witchcraft and because of local superstitions.[76] The American alligator *Alligator mississippiensis* most commonly attacks in the water but will also attack on land. These attacks seem to be motivated by feeding.

Crocodile bites produce large crush injuries and lacerations. Surgical wound management is similar to that for dog bites. The bacteriologic considerations have not been extensively studied but should be assumed to be the same as for other animals that reside in the aquatic environment. Wound infections should be anticipated in the largely contaminated extensive crush injuries. Prophylactic antibiotics to cover *Aeromonas hydrophila, Pseudomonas,* and *Vibrio* should be administered. Coverage against anaerobes, such as *Bacteroides,* is prudent. Antitetanus primary or booster immunization is mandatory.

NEEDLEFISH

Marine needlefish (family Belonidae) are slender, tubular, silver, and lightning-quick surface swimmers found in tropical seas. They resemble, but are not related to, the freshwater gar and may attain streamlined lengths of up to 2 m. Possessed of an elongated pointed snout, which comprises one quarter the length of the fish and contains small pointed teeth, the fish moves rapidly, often leaping out of the water in fear or when attracted to lights or windsurfers (Figure 60-29). The needlefish, or garfish, is an occupational hazard for persons who fish from small canoes at night in tropical Indo-Pacific ocean waters.[13] On occasion they have flown into people, spearing them in the chest, abdomen, extremities, head, and neck. In one reported case a fish caused brain injury with an internal carotid–cavernous sinus fistula after orbitocranial perforation.[54] In another case, the calcified elongated jaws of a needlefish embedded in a woman's neck were retained for over a month before removal.[95] In another, penetration of the knee by *Tylosurus crocodilus* occurred in an ocean surface swimmer in New Caledonia.[45] Exsanguination from a neck wound has been anecdotally reported from Papua New Guinea. A chest wound can be accompanied by a pneu-

mothorax. Death may occur from chest or abdominal penetration. Treatment is according to the nature of the injury. All wounds should be debrided and irrigated, followed by a search for foreign material. Radiographs appropriate to identify foreign bodies should be obtained. A small superficial wound may cause the physician to underestimate an internal injury. The major risk is wound infection. Injury prevention is difficult, although it has been suggested that canoes be positioned in a circle to allow spearing of fish in a central pool of light. Other species of flying fish pose less risk, since they have blunt heads.

Many other fish leap from the water, but injuries are extremely uncommon. A single case of a wahoo (150 cm; 22.5 kg), family Scombridae, leaping from the water and biting a victim on the upper extremity has been reported.[37] The razor-sharp teeth generated extensor tendon lacerations on the dorsal hand and forearm that required surgical repair. A careless fisherman can easily be cut by a wahoo when extracting a fishing lure. As previously described, barracuda exit the water in pursuit of shiny metallic objects that resemble fishing lures. Bluefish *(Pomatomus saltatrix)* school and feed in a frenzy, but most bites occur as the fish are handled out of the water; in-water attacks on humans are theoretic.[46] The fish has sharp, conical canine teeth in both the upper and lower jaws and can grow to 1.2 m and over 12 kg.

The sailfish sports an elongated bill. Although not considered a predator, a sailfish has on at least a few occasions driven its bill into a human victim (Figure 60-30), in one case causing a colon perforation in a snorkeler.

KILLER WHALES

The killer whale, *Orcinus orca,* is probably not the ferocious killer it is reputed to be. The largest of the living mammalian dolphins, these magnificent animals (Figure 60-31) grow to 33 feet and 10 tons and are found in all oceans. They usually travel in pods of up to 40 individuals. Swift and enormously powerful creatures, they feed on squid, fish, birds, seals, walruses, and other whales. Their powerful jaws are equipped with cone-shaped teeth directed back into the throat, designed to

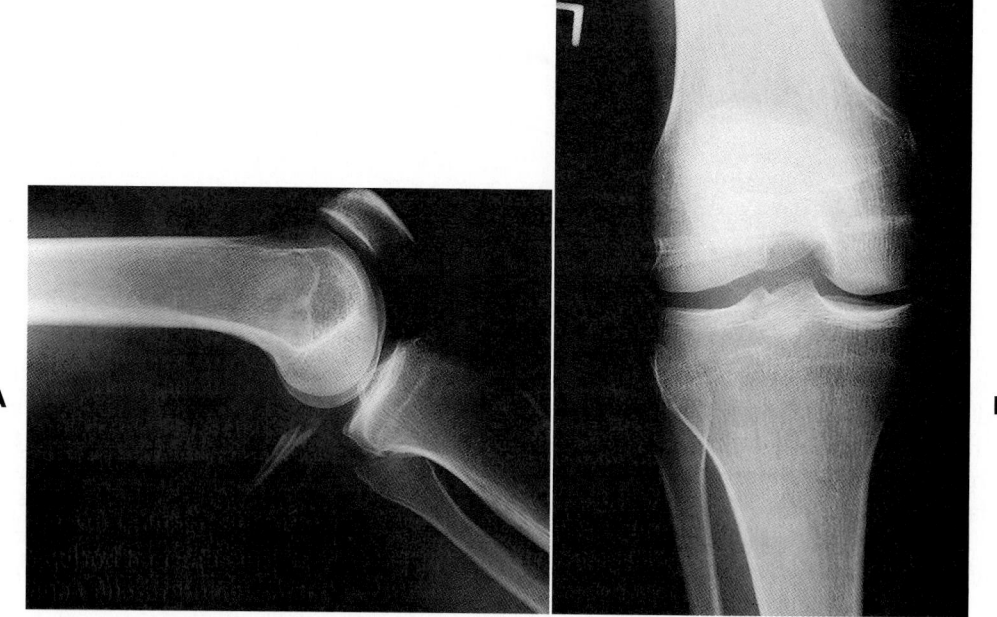

Figure 60-30 Sailfish bill lodged in the posterior knee. **A,** Lateral view. **B,** Anterior view.

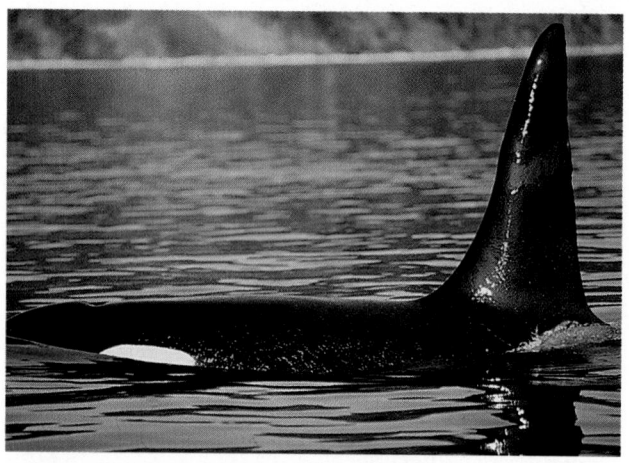

Figure 60-31 Distinctive markings of a killer whale near the San Juan Islands, Washington State. *(Photo by Norbert Wu.)*

grasp and hold food. The killer whale can generate enough crushing power to bite a seal or porpoise in two with a single snap.

In captivity, killer whales are playful creatures and seem intelligent, without the primal behavior of sharks. Nonetheless, although killer whales are believed not to prey on humans, they should be regarded with respect and at a distance in their natural habitat. Mistaken for a sea lion, a human would be a nice snack for a killer whale.

Other whale species, such as the finback, have rammed boats, theoretically in defense of their young. Territorial behavior should be anticipated and respected.

GIANT CLAMS

Although many adventure stories describe divers being caught in the clamp of a giant clam (family Tridacnidae), there are no verifiable reports of such a calamity resulting in a major injury. *Tridacna gigas* can attain a length of 1 m (Figure 60-32) and weigh as much as 300 kg. The hazard to divers is hypothetic.

GIANT SQUID

The giant decapod (10 arms) squid (Figure 60-33), possibly *Architeuthis*, grows to a length in excess of 20 m and weight of 38,000 kg, with long (10 m) menacing tentacles, eyes of nearly 35 cm (Figure 60-34), and a razor-sharp beak that it uses to eat prey. The tentacles are armed with chitinous serrated rings equipped with teeth on each of the suckers (Figure 60-35). Sperm whales have been examined with sucker wounds of diameter 46 cm, which would extrapolate to a monstrous squid measuring at least 60 m in length. The battles between sperm whales and giant squid are legendary, but humans are unlikely to encounter this awesome animal, which is found at depths far beyond the range of a sport scuba diver.[27] With increased deep sea exploration by small submersibles, we may learn more about this fascinating creature. It is possible that a hungry giant squid

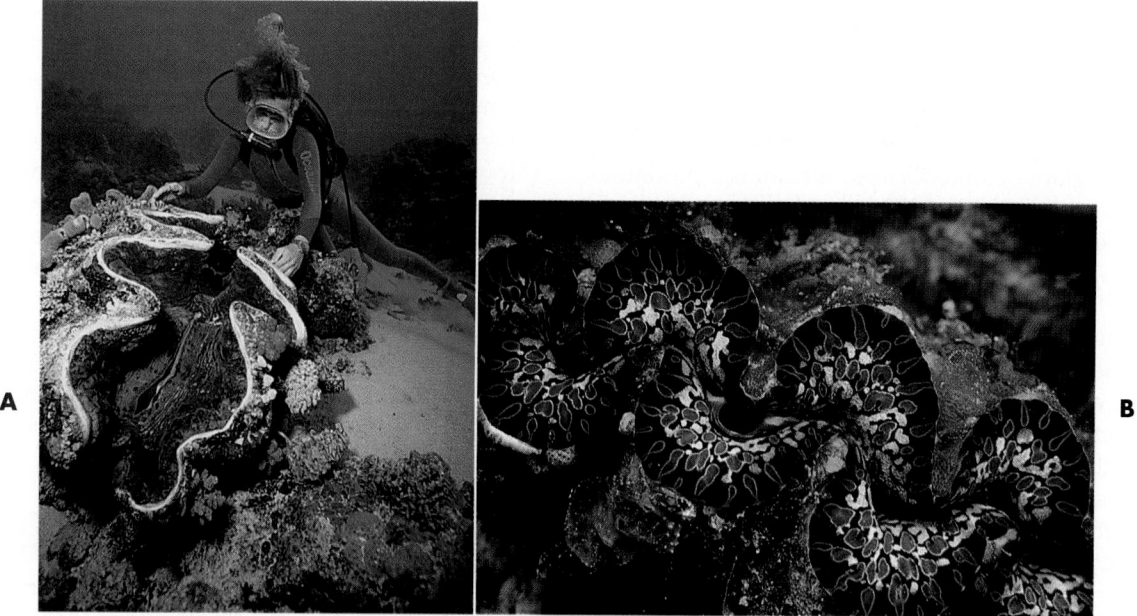

Figure 60-32   Giant clams. **A,** Giant clam with diver. **B,** Giant clam mantle (*Tridacna* sp.) obtains its coloration from algae utilized for photosynthesis. *(**A,** Photo by Howard Hall. **B,** Photo by Norbert Wu.)*

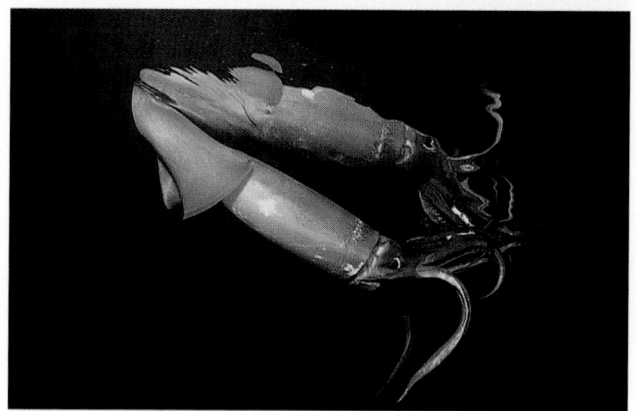

Figure 60-33   Giant Humboldt squid *(Dosidicus gigas)* attains a length of 15 feet and weight of 50 pounds. It is a voracious carnivore. *(Photo by Norbert Wu.)*

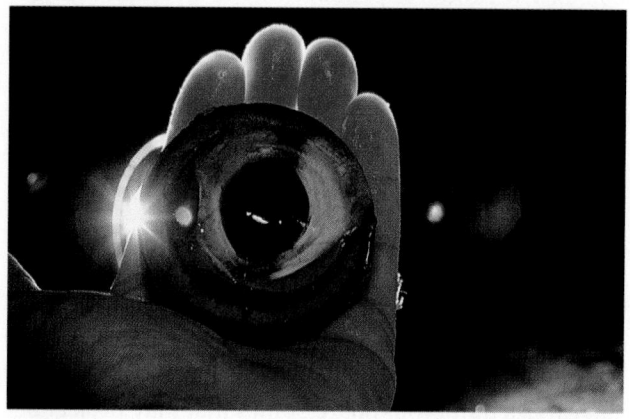

Figure 60-34   Eyeball of a giant Humboldt squid cut up by local fishermen. *(Photo by Norbert Wu.)*

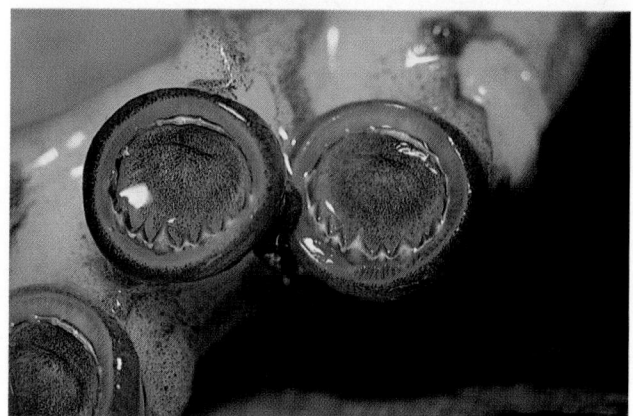

Figure 60-35   Suckers of the giant Humboldt squid are lined with razor-sharp teeth. *(Photo by Norbert Wu.)*

might ingest a human, but this has not yet been observed.

GIANT OCTOPUS

The Pacific giant octopus *Octopus dofleini* is a predator that has been captured at 272 kg with an arm span of over 30 feet. It ranges off the western North American coast from northern California to Alaska and off eastern Asia southward to Japan. The cephalopod is armed with suckers on eight arms and a parrotlike chitinous mouth located centrally underneath the head. Although it exhibits curiosity, it does not exhibit aggression directed against humans. However, it possesses the strength and agility to easily overwhelm a human. Anecdotes from the South Pacific tell of native breath-hold divers being subdued and drowned by angered captive octopuses.

GIANT MANTA RAY

The giant manta ray *Manta birostris* can have a wing span of more than 6 m and a weight of 1600 kg (Figure 60-36). The caudal appendage carries a vestigial stinger that poses no threat to humans. However, the coarse dermal denticles can create severe abrasions, which generally occur when divers attempt to ride these gentle and accommodating creatures.

MANTIS SHRIMP

The mantis shrimp (e.g., *Gonodactylus bredini, Hemisquilla ensigera californiensis*) is not a true shrimp but resembles a large flattened shrimp or miniature lobster (up to 36 cm) and is equipped with a pair of legs that serve as specialized jackknife claws (Figure 60-37). The tail carries numerous sharp spines that may project beyond the edge of the sturdy tail fin. Lacerations may be induced by either the front raptorial (prey-acquiring) claws or the tail, particularly when the shrimp attacks an unwary victim. It has been claimed that an attacking mantis shrimp struck with enough force to crack a diver's face mask. In the Caribbean, the stomatopod ("foot-mouth") mantis shrimp is known as "thumb splitter." *Odontodactylus scyllarus* from the Indo-Pacific can be afflicted with a disease that digests areas of its dorsal cuticle and eventually is lethal. This may explain one anecdotal report of a human finger wound (which led to amputation) characterized by cartilage destruction and from which no pathogenic organism could be cultured. The mantis shrimp is a superb predator, in part because it has the most highly developed eyes of any crustacean.

PIRANHA

South American characins include the piranha *Serrasalmus natterei*, equipped with a formidable set of razor-sharp teeth. These small fish (Figure 60-38) attack

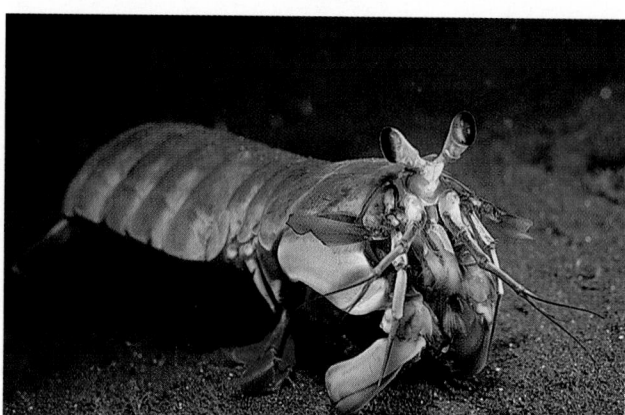

Figure 60-37 Mantis shrimp, ready to strike with its claws. *(Photo by Norbert Wu.)*

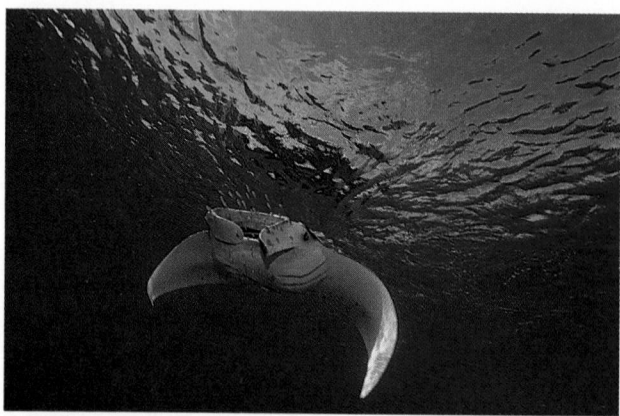

Figure 60-36 Giant manta ray. The sting on the caudal appendage is vestigial, but the "wings" can slap and abrade the unwary individual. *(Photo by Paul S. Auerbach, MD.)*

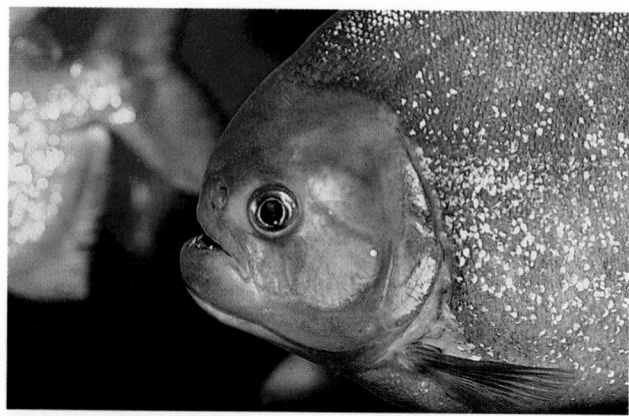

Figure 60-38 Piranha. *(Photo by Norbert Wu.)*

in schools of several hundred and can theoretically reduce a human to a shiny skeleton in short order. They are attracted by blood or commotion.

TRIGGERFISH

The triggerfish are usually shy and unimposing, but during mating season the females of at least two species (*Pseudobalistes fuscus* and the "giant" *Balistoides viridescens*) can become extremely territorial in guarding a nest and thus aggressive, inflicting painful bites. The former can grow to 55 cm and the latter to 75 cm. The strong jaws each carry eight long, protruding, and chisel-like teeth (Figure 60-39) in an outer row, backed by an inner row of six teeth.[71] Usually the fish "bites and runs," but the orange-striped triggerfish *Balistoides undulatus* has been reported to bite and not release. It is common to have to strike the fish in some manner to get it to release. In the Gilbert Islands a release technique is to bite the fish on the top of the head.

STONY CORALS

Life and Habits

The anthozoan Madreporariae, or true (stony) corals, exist in colonies that possess calcareous outer skeletons (the origin of calcium carbonate, or limestone) with pointed horns, razor-sharp edges, or both (Figure 60-40). There are nearly 1000 species of corals. Corals live in waters at temperatures of 20° C (68° F) or higher, generally at depths of up to 20 fathoms. A "coral head" is actually a colony of individual polyps. Rare species have been noted at depths of more than 6000 fathoms. Certain coral species, such as *Plexaura hommomalla*, are under investigation as sources of prostaglandins and other pharmaceutical precursors to treat conditions as diverse as asthma, leukemia, and infections. Pieces of coral have been evaluated for use as bone grafts.

Coral reefs are under pressure worldwide from climatic changes (e.g., El Niño), chemical poisons (e.g., cyanide used for fishing), natural predators (e.g., crown-of-thorns sea star), and mechanical destruction (e.g., ship anchors and explosives).

Clinical Aspects

Snorkelers and divers, particularly photographers and spear fishermen, frequently handle or brush against these living reefs, resulting in superficial cuts and abrasions on the extremities (Figure 60-41). Coral cuts are probably the most common injuries sustained underwater. The initial reaction to a coral cut is stinging pain, erythema, and pruritus, most commonly on the forearms, elbows, and knees. Divers without gloves frequently receive cuts to the hands. A break in the skin may be surrounded within minutes by an erythematous wheal, which fades over 1 to 2 hours. The red, raised welts and local pruritus are called coral poisoning. Low-grade fever may be present and does not necessarily indicate an infection. With or without prompt

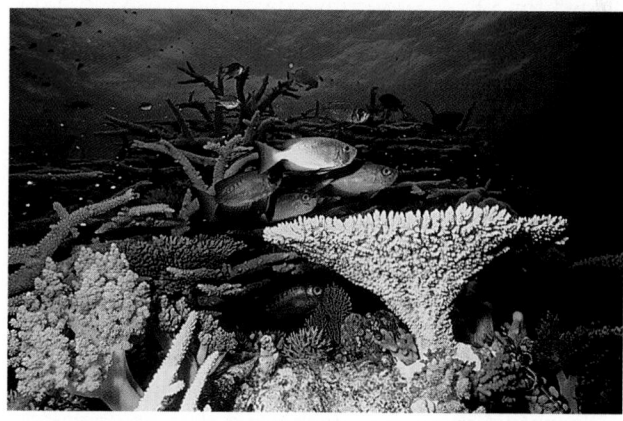

Figure 60-40   Coral garden. *(Photo by Paul S. Auerbach, MD.)*

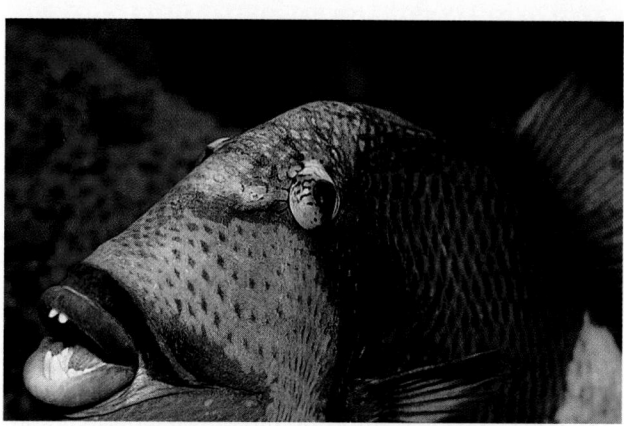

Figure 60-39   Triggerfish. *(Photo by John Randall.)*

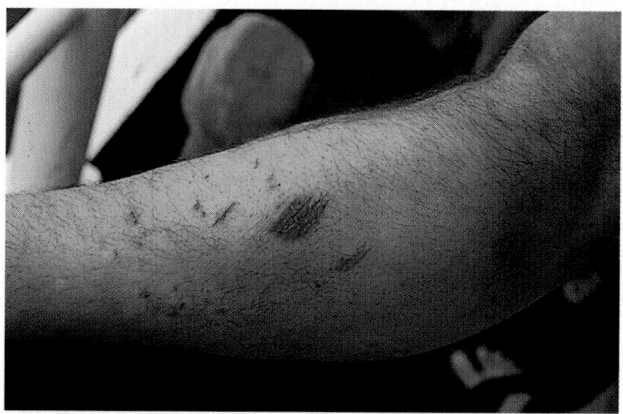

Figure 60-41   Abrasions of the leg from bumping against sharp coral. *(Photo by Paul S. Auerbach, MD.)*

treatment, the wound may progress to cellulitis with ulceration and tissue sloughing. These wounds heal slowly (3 to 6 weeks) and result in prolonged morbidity. In an extreme case the victim develops cellulitis with lymphangitis, reactive bursitis, local ulceration, and wound necrosis.

Treatment

Coral cuts should be promptly and vigorously scrubbed with soap and water, then irrigated copiously with a forceful stream of freshwater or normal saline to remove all foreign particles. Using hydrogen peroxide to bubble out "coral dust" is occasionally helpful. Any fragments that remain can become embedded and increase the risk for an indolent infection or foreign body granuloma. If stinging is a major symptom, there may be an element of envenomation by nematocysts (see Chapter 61). A brief rinse with diluted acetic acid (vinegar), papain solution, or isopropyl alcohol 20% may diminish the discomfort (after the initial pain from contact with the open wound). If a coral-induced laceration is severe, it should be closed with adhesive strips rather than sutures if possible; preferably it should be debrided for 3 to 4 consecutive days and closed in a delayed fashion.

A number of approaches can be taken with regard to subsequent wound care. One method is to apply twice-daily sterile wet-to-dry dressings, using saline or a dilute antiseptic (povidone iodine 1% to 5%) solution. Alternatively, a nontoxic topical antiseptic or antibiotic ointment (mupirocin, bacitracin, or polymyxin B-bacitracin-neomycin) may be used sparingly and covered with a nonadherent dressing (e.g., Telfa). Secondary infections are dealt with as they arise. A final approach is to apply a full-strength antiseptic solution, followed by a powdered topical antibiotic, such as tetracycline. An "alternative medicine" technique that has been reported to me to be effective is to apply Tibet Red Flower Seed Oil (brand "Dragon" is authentic) 4 times a day, noting that the application will cause burning pain for a short period of time. No method has been supported by any prospective trial.

Despite the best efforts at primary irrigation and decontamination, the wound may heal slowly, with moderate to severe soft tissue inflammation and ulcer formation (Figure 60-42). All devitalized tissue should be debrided regularly using sharp dissection. This should be continued until a bed of healthy granulation tissue is formed. Wounds that appear infected should be cultured and treated with antibiotics as previously discussed.

The victim who demonstrates malaise, nausea, and low-grade fever may have a systemic form of coral poisoning or be manifesting early signs of a wound infection. It is prudent at this point to search for a localized infection, procure wound cultures or biopsy specimens as indicated, and initiate antibiotics pending confirma-

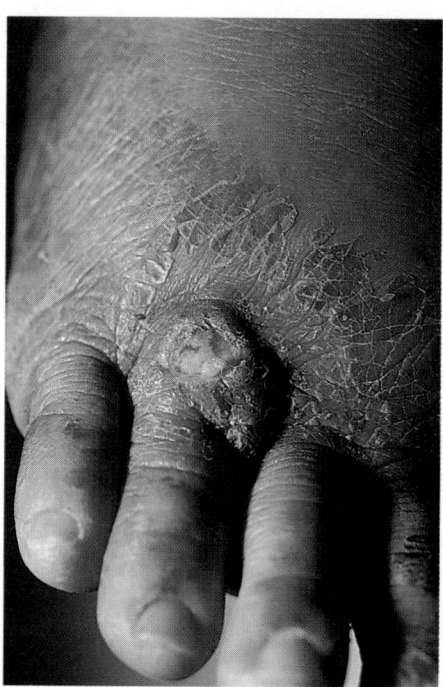

Figure 60-42 Poorly healing wound following coral cut. *(Photo by Paul S. Auerbach, MD.)*

tion of organisms. If the victim is started on an antibiotic and does not improve, a supplemental trial of a systemic glucocorticoid (prednisone 80 mg tapered over 2 weeks) is not unreasonable. In the absence of an overt infection, the natural course of the wound is to improve spontaneously over a 4- to 12-week period.

Prevention

Divers exploring near coral reefs must take every care to avoid coral cuts. Protective clothing and gloves should be impenetrable. Snorkelers and underwater photographers in shallow water should wear adequate hand, elbow, and knee protection.

SHOCKING MARINE AND FRESHWATER ANIMALS

Only two groups of electric fish are marine; the remainder are freshwater animals. They rarely pose a health hazard but rather are curious creatures surrounded by superstition and folklore. The marine electric fish include the stargazers (*Astroscopus*) (Figure 60-43) and the electric rays (*Torpedo*). The electric eel is a freshwater Amazonian animal.

Electric rays are found in temperate and tropical oceans. Of the class Chondrichthyes, they are round bodied, with short tails and thick bodies (compared with stingrays). In California, *Torpedo californica* (Figure 60-44) attains a length of 4 feet and weight of 80 to 90 pounds. It swims slowly and sluggishly and is usually

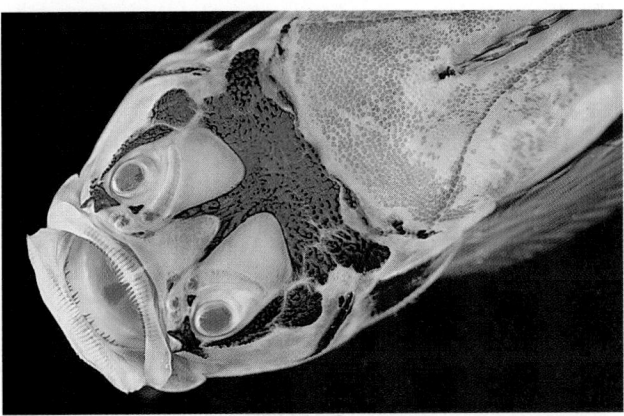

Figure 60-43 Stargazer *(Astroscopus zephyreus)* with electric plates above each eye. *(Photo by Norbert Wu.)*

A

B

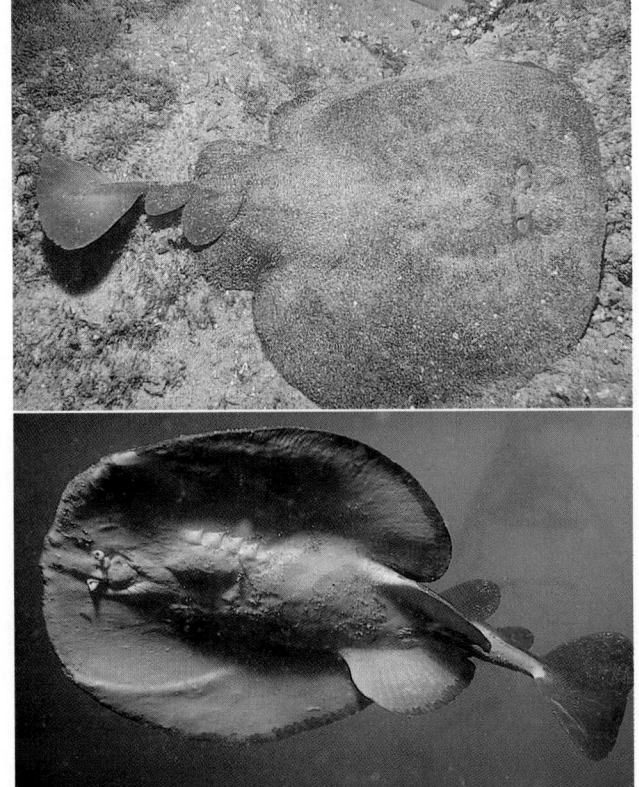

Figure 60-44 Electric ray *(Torpedo californica)*. **A,** Dorsal view. **B,** Ventral view. *(Photos by Norbert Wu.)*

found partially buried in bottom mud and sand. Well camouflaged, its dorsal surface is multicolored and the ventral surface creamy white. The externally visible electric organs are located on each side of the anterior part of the disk between the anterior extension of the pectoral fin and the head, extending from above the level of the eye backward past the gill region onto the

ventral surface. The electric organs are composed of a honeycomb network of modified muscles organized into columnar prismlike structures and connective tissue, which generate an electrical charge by neuromuscular activity. The muscle cells ("electroplaques") are stacked 500 to 1000 deep, creating up to 500 cm^2 of surface area. The electroplaques depolarize in series and in parallel simultaneously, producing amperage sufficient to stun prey. Species in the tropical eastern Pacific include the lesser ray, *Narcine entemedor*, and the bullseye ray *Diplobatis ommata*.

Generally the ventral surface of the ray is negative and the dorsal side is positive. An electrical discharge is reflexively produced on contact, often in a series exhaustive for the fish. This necessitates a period of recharging. Electricity is delivered in doses of 8 to 220 volts. The Atlantic *Torpedo nobiliana* produces 180 to 220 volts. Although the shock is of low amperage, it is sufficient to stun a grown man and might induce drowning. Recovery from the shock has been reported anecdotally to usually be uneventful. An electric ray should not be handled. The energy generated by skates is considerably less, measured in millivolts to 1 to 2 volts.

REFERENCES

1. Albanyan EA, Morad AB, Vallejo JG: *Vibrio vulnificus* sepsis in a child with Diamond-Blackfan syndrome, *Pediatr Infect Dis J* 16:818, 1997.
2. Albreski DA, Huey C, Spadone SJ: *Aeromonas hydrophila.* A fresh water pathogen and its pedal manifestations, *J Am Podiatr Med Assoc* 86:135, 1996.
3. Angerås MH et al: Comparison between sterile saline and tap water for the cleaning of acute traumatic soft tissue wounds, *Eur J Surg* 158:347, 1992.
4. Arias CR et al: A comparison of strategies for the detection and recovery of *Vibrio vulnificus* from marine samples of the western Mediterranean coast, *Syst Appl Microbiol* 21:128, 1998.
5. Arias CR, Garay E, Aznar R: Nested PCR method for rapid and sensitive detection of *Vibrio vulnificus* in fish, sediments, and water, *Appl Environ Microbiol* 61:3476, 1995.
6. Auerbach PS: Clinical therapy of marine envenomation and poisoning. In Tu AI, editor: *Handbook of natural toxins*, vol 4, *Marine toxins and venoms*, New York, 1988, Marcel Dekker.
7. Auerbach PS et al: Bacteriology of the freshwater environment: implications for clinical therapy, *Ann Emerg Med* 16:1016, 1987.
8. Auerbach PS et al: Bacteriology of the marine environment: implications for clinical therapy, *Ann Emerg Med* 16:643, 1987.
9. Badhour LM: Extraintestinal *Aeromonas* infections—looking for Mr. Sandbar, *Mayo Clin Proc* 67:496, 1992.
10. Bailey JP et al: *Mycobacterium marinum* infection: a fishy story, *JAMA* 247:1314, 1982.
11. Baldridge HD: Shark repellent: not yet, maybe never, *Mil Med* 155:358, 1990.
12. Barry AL, Thornberry C: Susceptibility tests: diffusion test procedures. In Lennette EH et al, editors: *Manual of clinical microbiology*, Washington, DC, 1985, American Society for Microbiology.
13. Barss PG: Injuries caused by garfish in Papua New Guinea, *BMJ* 284:77, 1982.
14. Blackband SJ, Stoskopf MK: In vivo nuclear magnetic resonance imaging and spectroscopy of aquatic organisms, *Magn Reson Imaging* 8:191, 1990.
15. Bloch S, Monteil H: Purification and characterization of *Aeromonas hydrophila* beta-hemolysin, *Toxicon* 27:1279, 1989.
16. Buck JD, Spotte S, Gadbaw JJ: Bacteriology of the teeth from a great white shark: potential medical implications for shark bite victims, *J Clin Microbiol* 20:849, 1984.
17. Burgess GH, Callahan MT, Howard RJ: Sharks, alligators, barracudas, and other biting animals in Florida waters. *J Fla Med Assoc* 84:428, 1997.

18. Campbell GD, Smith ED: The problem of shark attack upon humans, *J Wilderness Med* 4:5, 1993.

19. Carta F et al: Corneal ulcer caused by *Aeromonas* species, *Am J Ophthalmol* 118:530, 1994.

20. Castro JI: *The sharks of North American waters,* College Station, Tex, 1983, Texas A & M University Press.

21. Chadee DD: Bacterial pathogens isolated from guppies *(Poecilia reticulata)* used to control *Aedes aegypti* in Trinidad, *Trans R Soc Trop Med Hyg* 86:693, 1992.

22. Chakraborty S, Nair GB, Shinoda S: Pathogenic vibrios in the natural aquatic environment, *Rev Environ Health* 12:63, 1997.

23. Chuang Y-C et al: In vitro synergism between cefotaxime and minocycline against *Vibrio vulnificus, Antimicrob Agents Chemother* 41:2214, 1997.

24. Chuang Y-C et al: Minocycline and cefotaxime in the treatment of experimental murine *Vibrio vulnificus* infection, *Antimicrob Agents Chemother* 42:1319, 1998.

25. Clark E, Chao S: A toxic secretion from the Red Sea flatfish *Pardachirus marmoratus* (Lacepede), *Bull Sea Fish Res Sta (Haifa)* 60:53, 1973.

26. Denis RA et al: Coxsackie A16 infection from lake water, *JAMA* 228:1370, 1974.

27. Ellis R: *The search for the giant squid,* New York, 1998, The Lyons Press.

28. Ellis R, McCosker JE: *Great white shark,* New York, 1991, HarperCollins.

29. Engaña AC, McCosker JE: Attacks on divers by white sharks in Chile, *Calif Fish Game* 70:173, 1984.

30. Erickson T et al: The emergency management of moray eel bites, *Ann Emerg Med* 21:212, 1992.

31. Grimes DJ et al: The fate of enteric pathogenic bacteria in estuarine and marine environments, *Microbiol Sci* 3:324, 1985.

32. Grimes DJ et al: Vibrios as autochthonous flora of neritic sharks, *Syst Appl Microbiol* 6:221, 1985.

33. Gruber SH: Why do sharks attack humans? *Naval Res News* 90:2, 1988.

34. Guidera KJ et al: Shark attack: a case study of the injury and treatment, *J Orthop Trauma* 5:204, 1991.

35. Halow KD, Harner RC, Fontenelle LJ: Primary skin infections secondary to *Vibrio vulnificus:* the role of operative intervention, *J Am Coll Surg* 183:329, 1996.

36. Hlady WG, Klontz KC: The epidemiology of *Vibrio* infections in Florida, 1981-1991, *J Infect Dis* 173:1176, 1996.

37. Hoffman J, Hack GR, Clark B: The man did fine, but what about the wahoo? *JAMA* 267:2039, 1992 (letter).

38. Hsu W-Y, Wei C-I, Tamplin ML: Enhanced broth media for selective growth of *Vibrio vulnificus, Appl Environ Microbiol* 64:2701, 1998.

39. Iscan MY, McCabe BQ: Analysis of human remains recovered from a shark, *Forensic Sci Int* 72:15, 1995.

40. Johnson RH, Nelson DR: Agonistic display in the gray reef shark, *Carcharhinus menisorrah,* and its relationship to attacks on man, *Copeia* 1:76, 1973.

41. Joseph SW et al: *Aeromonas* primary wound infection of a diver in polluted waters, *J Clin Microbiol* 10:46, 1979.

42. Katz D, Smith H: *Aeromonas hydrophila* infection of a puncture wound, *Ann Emerg Med* 9:529, 1980.

43. Ko W-C, Chuang Y-C: *Aeromonas* bacteremia: review of 59 episodes, *Clin Infect Dis* 20:1298, 1995.

44. Kumamoto KS, Vukich DJ: Clinical infections of *Vibrio vulnificus:* a case report and review of the literature, *J Emerg Med* 16:61, 1998.

45. Labbe J-L, Bordes J-P, Fine X: An unusual surgical emergency: a knee joint wound caused by a needlefish, *Arthroscopy* 11:503, 1995.

46. Lange WR: The perils of bluefish: handle with care! *Md Med J* 37:475, 1988.

47. Lazarovici P et al: Secondary structure, permeability and molecular modeling of pardaxin pores, *J Nat Toxins* 1:1, 1992.

48. Lee A, Langer R: Shark cartilage contains an inhibitor of tumor neovascularization. In Colwell RR, Sinskey AJ, Pariser ER, editors: *Biotechnology in the marine sciences,* Proceedings of the First Annual MIT Sea Grant Lecture and Seminar, New York, 1984, John Wiley & Sons.

49. Lee SE et al: Direct identification of Vibrio vulnificus in clinical specimens by nested PCR, *J Clin Microbiol* 36:2887, 1998.

50. Lotz MJ, Tamplin ML, Rodrick GE: Thiosulfate-citrate-bile salts-sucrose agar and its selectivity for clinical and marine vibrio organisms, *Ann Clin Lab Sci* 13:45, 1983.

51. Lowy FD: *Staphylococcus aureus* infections, *N Engl J Med* 339:520, 1998.

52. Manire CA, Gruber SH: Anatomy of a shark attack, *J Wilderness Med* 3:4, 1992.

53. Mathur MN et al: Cellulitis owing to *Aeromonas hydrophila:* treatment with hyperbaric oxygen, *Aust NZ J Surg* 65:367, 1995.

54. McCabe MJ et al: A fatal brain injury caused by a needlefish, *Neuroradiology* 15:137, 1978.

55. McCosker J: White shark attack behavior: observations of and speculations about predator and prey strategies, memoir No 9, *Calif Acad Sci* 9:123, 1985.

56. Mekisic AP, Wardill JR: Crocodile attacks in the Northern Territory of Australia, *Med J Aust* 157:751, 1992.

57. Miller DJ, Collier RS: Shark attacks in California and Oregon, *Calif Fish Game* 67:76, 1980.

58. Morris JG, Tenney J: Antibiotic therapy for *Vibrio vulnificus* infection, *JAMA* 253:1121, 1985.

59. Morris JG, Tenney JH, Drusano GL: In vitro susceptibility of pathogenic *Vibrio* species to norfloxacin and six other antimicrobial agents, *Antimicrob Agents Chemother* 28:442, 1985.

60. Morse DL et al: Widespread outbreaks of clam- and oyster-associated gastroenteritis: association of Norwalk virus, *N Engl J Med* 314:678, 1986.

61. Moss SA: *Sharks: an introduction for the amateur naturalist,* Englewood Cliffs, NJ, 1984, Prentice-Hall.

62. Nambiar A, Brown KA, Bridges TE: Forensic implications of the variation in morphology of marginal serrations on the teeth of the great white shark, *J Forensic Odonto Stomatology* 14:2, 1996.

63. Nakayama S et al: Small volume resuscitation with hypertonic saline (2400 mOsm/liter) during hemorrhagic shock, *Circ Shock* 13:149, 1984.

64. Park J-W et al: Pulmonary damage by *Vibrio vulnificus* cytolysin, *Infect Immun* 64:2873, 1996.

65. Paterson DL: Antibiotic-induced antimicrobial resistance in *Aeromonas* spp., *Med J Aust* 166:165, 1997.

66. Penman AD et al: *Vibrio vulnificus* wound infections from the Mississippi gulf coastal waters: June to August 1993, *South Med J* 88:531, 1995.

67. Pettit GR, Ode RH: Antineoplastic agents L: isolation and characterization of sphyrnastatins 1 and 2 from the hammerhead shark *Sphyrna lewini, J Pharm Sci* 66:757, 1977.

68. Pien FD et al: Bacterial flora of marine penetrating injuries, *Diagn Microbiol Infect Dis* 1:229, 1983.

69. Primor N: Pharyngeal cavity and the gills are the target organ for the repellent action of pardaxin in shark, *Experientia* 41:693, 1985.

70. Qadri SM, Lee G, Brodie L: Antibacterial activity of norfloxacin against 1700 relatively resistant clinical isolates, *Drugs Exp Clin Res* 15:349, 1989.

71. Randall JE, Millington JT: Triggerfish bite a little-known marine hazard, *J Wilderness Med* 1:79, 1990.

72. Revord ME, Goldfarb J, Shurin SB: *Aeromonas hydrophila* wound infection in a patient with cyclic neutropenia following a piranha bite, *Pediatr Infect Dis J* 7:70, 1988.

73. Rheinheimer G: *Aquatic microbiology,* New York, 1974, John Wiley & Sons.

74. Royle JA et al: Infections after shark attacks in Australia, *Ped Infect Dis J* 16:531, 1997.

75. Sato T et al: Endotoxin removal column containing polymyxin B immobilized fiber is useful for the treatment of the patient with *Vibrio vulnificus* septicemia, *Artif Organs* 22:705, 1998.

76. Scott R, Scott H: Crocodile bites and traditional beliefs in Korogwe district, Tanzania, *BMJ* 309:1691, 1994.

77. Semel JD, Allen N: Seizures in patients simultaneously receiving theophylline and imipenem or ciprofloxacin or metronidazole, *South Med J* 84:465, 1991.

78. Semel JD, Trenholme G: *Aeromonas hydrophila* water-associated wound infections: a review, *J Trauma* 30:324, 1990.

79. Smith ED: Electric shark barrier: initial trials and prospects, *Power Engineer J,* July 1991, p 167.

80. Smith HW: Incidence of R+ *Escherichia coli* in coastal bathing waters of Britain, *Nature* 234:155, 1971.

81. Stabellini N et al: Fatal sepsis from *Vibrio vulnificus* in a hemodialyzed patient, *Nephron* 78:221, 1998.

82. Stern SA et al: Effect of blood pressure on hemorrhage volume and survival in a near-fatal hemorrhage model incorporating a vascular injury, *Ann Emerg Med* 22:155, 1993.

83. Tachibana K, Gruber SH: Shark repellent lipophilic constituents in the defense secretion of the Moses sole *(Pardachirus marmoratus), Toxicon* 26:839, 1988.

84. Taylor L: *Sharks of Hawaii: their biology and cultural significance,* Honolulu, 1993, University of Hawai'i Press.

85. Traverso LW, Lee WP, Langford MJ: Fluid resuscitation after an otherwise fatal hemorrhage. I. Crystalloid solutions, *J Trauma* 26:168, 1986.

86. Traverso LW et al: Fluid resuscitation after an otherwise fatal hemorrhage. II. Colloid solutions, *J Trauma* 26:176, 1986.

87. Trucksis M, Hooper DC, Wolfson JS: Emerging resistance to fluoro-quinolones in staphylococci: an alert, *Ann Intern Med* 144:424, 1991 (editorial).

88. Tsuzuki M et al: *Vibrio vulnificus* septicemia in a patient with severe aplastic anemia, *Int J Hematol* 67:175, 1998.

89. Vadivelu J et al: Possible virulence factors involved in bacteraemia caused by *Aeromonas hydrophila, J Med Microbiol* 42:171, 1995.

90. Viljanto J: Disinfection of surgical wounds without inhibition of normal wound healing, *Arch Surg* 155:253, 1980.

91. Voss LM, Rhodes KH, Johnson KA: Musculoskeletal and soft tissue *Aeromonas* infection: an environmental disease, *Mayo Clin Proc* 67:422, 1992.

92. Wagner PD et al: Necrotizing fasciitis and septic shock caused by *Vibrio cholerae* acquired in San Diego, California, *West J Med* 163:375, 1995.

93. Welch K, Martini FH: Non-fatal shark attack on Maui, *Hawaii Med J* 40:95, 1981.

94. Weinstein MR: Invasive infections due to a fish pathogen, *Streptococcus iniae, N Engl J Med* 337:589, 1997.

95. Wolf M et al: Penetrating cervical injury caused by a needlefish, *Ann Otol Rhinol Laryngol* 104:248, 1995.

96. Wolff RL, Wiseman SL, Kitchens SC: Aeromonas hydrophila bacteremia in ambulatory immunocompromised hosts, *Am J Med* 68:238, 1980.

97. Wright AC et al: Distribution of *Vibrio vulnificus* in the Chesapeake Bay, *Appl Environ Microbiol* 62:717, 1996.

98. Yip KMH, Fung KSC, Adeyemi-Doro FAB: Necrotizing fasciitis of the foot caused by an unusual organism, *Vibrio vulnificus, J Foot Ankle Surg* 35:222, 1996.

99. ZoBell CE, Johnson FH: The influence of hydrostatic pressure on the growth and viability of terrestrial and marine bacteria, *J Bacteriol* 57:179, 1949.

100. ZoBell CE, Morita RY: Barophilic bacteria in some deep sea sediments, *J Bacteriol* 73:563, 1957.

61 Envenomation by Aquatic Invertebrates

Paul S. Auerbach

This chapter discusses envenomation by aquatic invertebrate life-forms. Chapter 62 discusses envenomation by aquatic vertebrate life-forms.

See Chapter 60 for a discussion of infections associated with aquatic wounds and the relevant antimicrobial therapy. Standard wound care measures, such as antitetanus immunization, should be undertaken whenever there is penetration of the skin.

The science of poisons, biotoxicology, is divided into plant poisons, or phytotoxicology, and animal poisons, or zootoxicology. "Toxinology" connotes the science of toxic substances produced by or accumulated in living organisms, their properties, and their biologic significance for the organisms involved.[77] Animals in which a definite venom apparatus is present are sometimes called phanerotoxic, whereas animals whose body tissues are toxic are termed cryptotoxic.[97] Naturally occurring aquatic zootoxins may be designated as oral toxins (which are poisonous to eat and include bacterial poisons and products of decomposition), parenteral toxins (venom produced in specialized glands and injected mechanically [by spine, needle, fang, fin, or dart]), and crinotoxins (venom produced in specialized glands and administered as slime, mucous, and gastric secretion). Within these three subdivisions, further classifications are by phylogeny, chemical structure, and clinical syndrome.

Although all venoms are poisons, not all poisons are venoms. According to the theory that offensive venoms are generally oral (mouth and fang) and defensive venoms are aboral (tail and sting) or dermal (barb and secretion), the majority of marine venoms are defensive. In the evolutionary scheme, it appears that venomous fish seek specific self-defense, whereas poisonous fish are noxious in a nonspecific manner.[4] A brief comparison of the features of venoms and poisons shows that poisons produced in skin, muscle, blood, or organs are generally heat stable (46° to 49° C [115° to 120° F]), gastric acid stable, and carry seasonal toxicity. They are not "released" and may lack a well-defined biologic function. Venoms are more commonly heat labile, gastric acid labile, and nonseasonal in toxicity. They can be released in varying amounts and have evolved for conquest and defense.

In snakes, the latency, toxicity, and duration of a venom effect are related to the route of envenomation. Intravascular injection is significantly more lethal than intraperitoneal or transcutaneous injection, as determined by the measured lethal dose of 50% survival of the group (LD$_{50}$). This principle is not commonly applied to marine venoms because few encounters involve direct intravascular invasion.

Most venoms are high-molecular-weight amalgams of vasoactive amines, proteolytic enzymes, and other biogenic compounds. These substances denature membranes, catabolize cyclic 3',5'-adenosine monophosphate, degranulate mast cells, provoke histamine release, initiate arachidonate metabolism, accelerate coagulopathy, interfere with cellular transport mechanisms, disrupt metabolic pathways, impede neuronal transmission, and evoke anaphylaxis and shock. Frustratingly, although many marine venoms are composed of protein and polypeptide subunits, they lack sufficient immunogenicity to allow development of antitoxins or antivenoms. Poisons represent metabolic by-products and are usually of smaller molecular weight.

Taxonomy of marine animals can sometimes be confusing. The hierarchical distinctions are made in descending order: kingdom, phylum, class, order, family, genus, and species.

ANAPHYLAXIS

An envenomation or administration of antivenom can elicit an allergic reaction. In the previously sensitized individual, the antigen (venom, aquatic protein, or animal serum) complexes with immunoglobulin E (IgE) and perhaps with IgG homocytotopic antibodies or activated complement cleavage products attached to the membranes of mast cells and basophils. This induces membrane permeability, which allows degranulation or membrane production of histamine, serotonin, kinins, prostaglandins, platelet-activating factor, eosinophil and neutrophil chemotactic factors, leukotrienes, and other bioactive chemical mediators.[6]

The signs and symptoms of anaphylaxis may occur within minutes of exposure and include hypotension, bronchospasm, tongue and lip swelling, laryngeal edema, pulmonary edema, seizures, cardiac arrhythmia, pruritus, urticaria, angioedema, rhinitis, conjunctivitis, nausea, vomiting, diarrhea, abdominal pain, gastrointestinal bleeding, and syncope. Most severe allergic reactions occur within 15 to 30 minutes of envenomation, and nearly all occur within 6 hours. Fatalities are related to airway obstruction or hypotension. Acute elevated pulmonary vascular resistance may contribute to hypotension that results from generalized arterial vasodilation.[7,9]

Treatment

Decisive treatment should be instituted at the first indication of hypersensitivity. Specific treatment recommendations for anaphylaxis are found in Box 46-3.

ANTIVENOM ADMINISTRATION

A number of marine envenomations, such as those by the box-jellyfish and certain sea snakes, may require the administration of specific antivenom. Marine antivenoms are raised in sheep and horses and therefore are antigenic in humans, inducing both immediate and delayed hypersensitivity. Most authorities recommend that a skin test be performed for sensitivity to horse serum, if the clinical situation permits, after a sea snake envenomation. (There is rarely time for a skin test with a *Chironex* envenomation, which requires immediate intervention.) This should be done only after deciding to administer antivenom and not to determine whether antivenom is necessary. The purpose of sensitivity testing is to allow adequate prophylaxis against anaphylaxis. The skin test is performed with an intradermal injection into the upper extremity of 0.02 ml of a 1:10 dilution of horse serum test material in saline, with 0.02 ml saline in the opposite extremity as a control. Erythema and pseudopodia are present in 15 to 30 minutes in a positive response. Because antivenom contains many times the protein content of horse serum used for skin testing, the use of antivenom for skin testing may increase the risk of anaphylactic reaction. If the skin test is positive, the antivenom intended for intravenous (IV) infusion should be diluted in sterile water to a 1:100 concentration for administration. Successive vials should be less dilute if the allergic reaction is minimal (controlled by antihistamines and epinephrine). A negative skin test does not preclude the possibility of an anaphylactic response to antivenom administration.

The rationale for administering antivenom is to provide early and adequate neutralization of the toxin at the tissue site of entry before it gains systemic dominance. Except for stonefish antivenom, the product should preferentially be administered intravenously, taking care to provide adequate doses for children and the elderly, who have a decreased volume of distribution and increased sensitivity to venom effects. The antivenom intended for IV administration should always be diluted with normal saline, Ringer's lactate, or dextrose 5% in water.

Marine antivenoms are produced and distributed in the Indo-Pacific regions. They include the following:

1. *Chironex fleckeri* (box-jellyfish) antivenom, from Commonwealth Serum Laboratories (CSL), Melbourne, Australia. A hyperimmune sheep globulin preparation, this may be used to neutralize the stings of *Chironex fleckeri* and *Chiropsalmus quadrigatus*.
2. *Enhydrina schistosa* (beaked sea snake) sea snake antivenom, from CSL. A hyperimmune horse globulin preparation, this may be used to neutralize the bites of most sea snakes. It is prepared by immunizing horses with venom from *E. schistosa* and the Australian tiger snake *Notechis scutatus*.
3. *Notechis scutatus* (tiger snake) antivenom, from CSL. This is the antivenom of second choice against the bites of most sea snakes.
4. *Enhydrina schistosa* (beaked sea snake) monovalent antivenom, from the Haffkine Institute in Bombay, India. This may be used to neutralize the bites of most sea snakes; it is most effective against the bite of *E. schistosa*.
5. *Synanceja trachynis* (stonefish) antivenom, from CSL. A hyperimmune horse globulin preparation, this may be used to neutralize the stings of stonefish and more virulent scorpionfish species.

A person who is known to be sensitive to horse or sheep serum, has a positive skin test, or develops signs of an allergic reaction or anaphylaxis during antivenom therapy requires aggressive medical management. A recipient of antivenom should be pretreated with 50 to 100 mg of IV diphenhydramine (1 mg/kg in children). After this, the initial dose of antivenom is administered at a rate no faster than one vial each 5 minutes. If no allergic manifestation ensues, the antivenom can be administered at a more rapid rate. If signs of anaphylaxis develop, usually heralded by an urticarial eruption or pruritus, 0.1 to 0.2 ml aliquots of antivenom should be alternated with 3 to 10 ml (0.03 to 0.1 mg) IV doses of aqueous epinephrine 1:100,000 (infused over 5 to 10 minutes). Alternatively, an epinephrine drip may be prepared as previously described in the discussion on anaphylaxis. The victim should be managed in an intensive care unit, with electrocardiographic and blood pressure monitoring. The dose of epinephrine should not exceed that which elevates the pulse rate above 150 beats/min. The administration of IV epinephrine may cause transient hypokalemia as potassium is driven intracellularly; cessation of the epinephrine infusion may create a transient hyperkalemia as the potassium regains entry into the extracellular space. If a victim is highly allergic to antivenom, serious consideration should be given to supportive therapy (including hemodialysis) without antivenom administration.

In one series, stonefish antivenom was administered to 24 victims in a dose of one or two ampules by the intramuscular (IM) route, without any "immediate reactions" reported.[112] In this same report, six victims received box-jellyfish antivenom by the IV route without immediate or delayed reactions.

Serum Sickness

The formation of IgG antibodies in response to antigens present in antivenom (heterologous serum) results in the deposition of immune complexes in many tissue sites, notably in the walls of blood vessels. These complexes induce vascular permeability, activate the complement cascade and chemotactic factors, degranulate mast cells, and trigger the release of proteolytic enzymes. Decreased levels of C_3 and C_4 are accompanied by increased C_{3a}/C_{3a} des-arginine, a split product C_3.[45,64] Although immune complexes can be measured by various tests (Raji-cell IgG assay and C_{1q}-binding assay), levels of immune complexes may not correlate with the clinical presentation.[45,82] Dermal biopsy of lesional skin may reveal leukocytoclastic vasculitis.

Symptoms are generally present within 8 to 24 days and include fever, arthralgias, malaise, urticaria, lymphadenopathy, urticarial and morbilliform skin rashes, peripheral neuritis, and swollen joints. It is not uncommon for the primary urticarial lesion to be noted at the injection site. Serum sickness is managed with the administration of corticosteroids. An initial loading dose of prednisone (40 to 60 mg for adults; 2 to 5 mg/kg, not to exceed 50 mg, for children) should be administered and maintained daily until symptoms markedly resolve. The corticosteroid should be tapered over a 2- to 3-week course to avoid induction of adrenal insufficiency. Aspirin or other nonsteroidal antiinflammatory agents are rarely helpful and may be contraindicated because of circulating immune complex-induced platelet dysfunction.

STINGING ANIMALS

The stinging animals constitute a large collection of marine organisms containing invertebrates and vertebrates (see Chapter 62), ranging from primitive to extremely sophisticated organisms. Aggregated, stinging animals pose the most frequent hazards for swimmers and divers.

INVERTEBRATES

Sponges

Life and Habits. There are approximately 5000 species of sponges (phylum Porifera; predominately class Desmospongiae), which are supported by horny, but elastic, internal collagenous skeletons of "spongin," some forms of which we use as bath sponges. Sponges are without digestive, excretory, respiratory, endocrine, circulatory, and nervous systems. Embedded in the connective tissue matrices and skeletons are spicules of silicon dioxide (silica) or calcium carbonate ("calcite"), by which some sponges can be definitively identified. In general, sponges are stationary acellular animals that attach to the sea floor or coral beds and may be colonized by other sponges, hydrozoans, mollusks, coelenterates, annelids, crustaceans, echinoderms, fish, and algae. These secondary coelenterate inhabitants are responsible for the dermatitis and local necrotic skin reaction

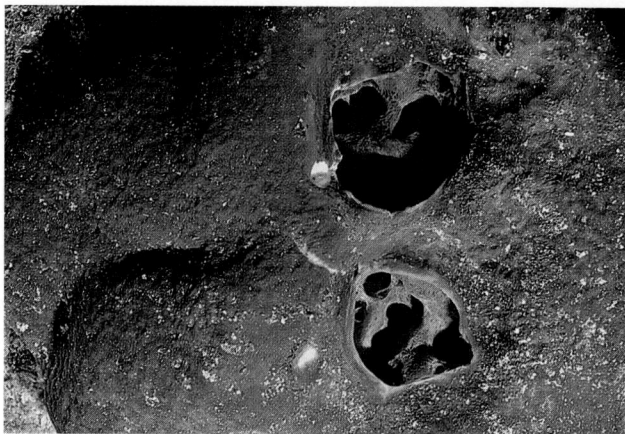

Figure 61-1 Pacific fire sponge. *(Photo by Norbert Wu.)*

termed sponge diver's disease (maladie des plongeurs).[107] In recognition of a medicinal property, the ancient Greeks burnt sea sponges and inhaled the vapors in prophylaxis against goiter.[31] Sponges harbor various biodynamic substances, with possible antineoplastic, antibacterial, growth-stimulating, antihypertensive, neuropharmacologic, psychopharmacologic, and antifungal properties. A number of sponges produce crinotoxins that may be direct dermal irritants, such as subcritine, halitoxin (*Haliclonia* species), p-hydroxybenzaldehyde, and okadaic acid. These may be present in surface or internal secretions. Murine monoclonal antibodies against okadaic acid intended for use in an assay system for the detection of diarrhetic shellfish poisoning have been prepared from the sponge *Halichondria okadai*.[119]

Clinical Aspects. Two general syndromes, with variations, are induced by contact with sponges. The first is a pruritic dermatitis similar to plant-induced allergic dermatitis, although the dermatopathic agent has not been identified. Rarely, erythema multiforme or an anaphylactoid reaction may be present. A typical offender is the friable Hawaiian (Figure 61-1) or West Indian fire sponge (*Tedania ignis*), a brilliant yellow-vermilion-orange (Figure 61-2) or reddish-brown organism with a crumb-of-bread appearance found off the Hawaiian Islands and the Florida Keys.[100,105] This sponge grows in thick branches, which are easily broken off, extending from a larger base. Other culprits include *Fibula* (or *Neofibularia*) *nolitangere*, the "poison bun sponge" (Figure 61-3) (and the related sponge *N. mordens*), and *Microciona prolifera*, the red moss sponge (found in the northeastern United States).[61] *F. nolitangere* is found in deeper water and grows in clusters, with holes (oscula) large enough to admit a diver's finger. It is brown (Figure 61-4) and bready in texture, so it may crumble in the hands.

Within a few hours, but sometimes within 10 to 20 minutes after skin contact, the reactions are charac-ter-

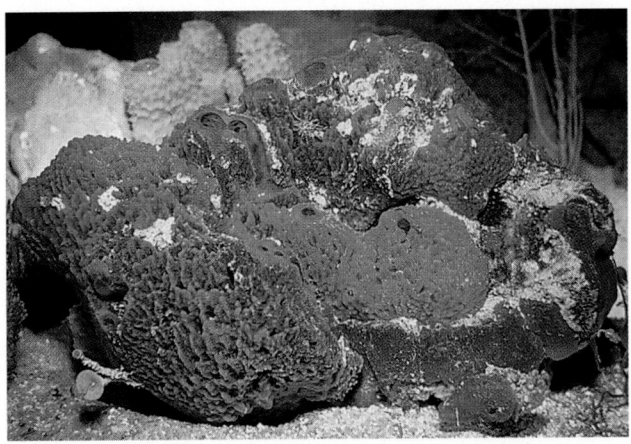

Figure 61-2 Atlantic fire sponge. *(Photo by Dee Scarr.)*

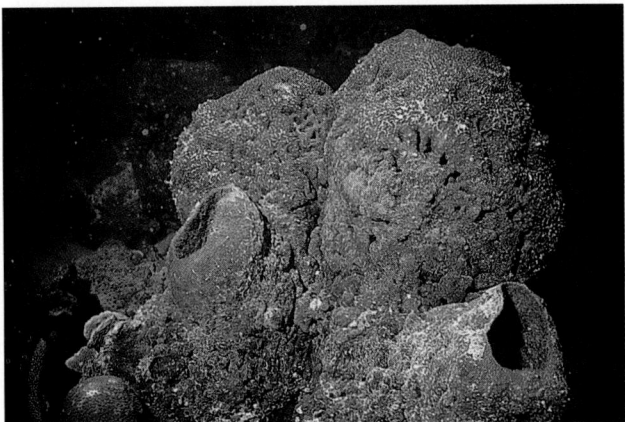

Figure 61-3 Poison bun sponge *Neofibularia nolitangere*. *(Photo by Dee Scarr.)*

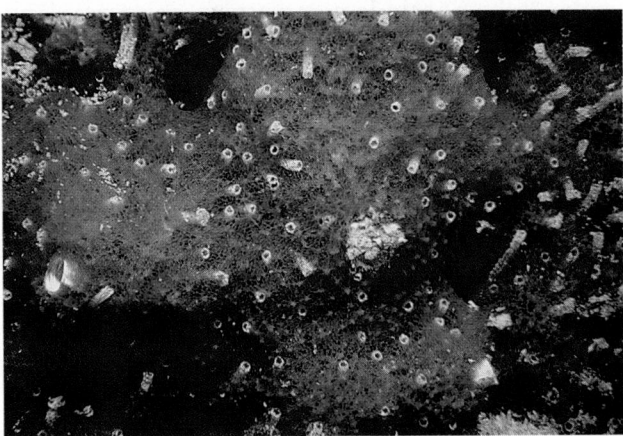

Figure 61-4 "Crumb-of-bread" appearance of poison bun sponge. *(Photo by Dee Scarr.)*

ized by itching and burning, which may progress to local joint swelling, soft tissue edema, vesiculation, and stiffness, particularly if small pieces of broken sponge are retained in the skin near the interphalangeal or metacarpophalangeal joint. Most victims of sponge-induced dermatitis have hand involvement, since they handle sponges without proper gloves. In addition, abraded skin, such as that which has been scraped on stony coral, may allow more rapid or greater absorption of toxin(s).[97] When the sponge is penetrated, torn, or crumbled, the skin is exposed to the toxic substances. Untreated, mild reactions subside within 3 to 7 days.[50] When large skin areas are involved, the victim may complain of fever, chills, malaise, dizziness, nausea, muscle cramps, and formication. Bullae induced by contact with *Microciona prolifera* may become purulent. Systemic erythema multiforme or an anaphylactoid reaction may develop a week to 14 days after a severe exposure.[133] The skin may become mottled or purpuric, occasionally after a delay of up to 10 days.[105]

The second syndrome is an irritant dermatitis and follows the penetration of small spicules of silica or calcium carbonate into the skin. Most sponges have spicules; toxic sponges may possess crinotoxins that enter microtraumatic lesions caused by the spicules.

In severe cases, surface desquamation of the skin may follow in 10 days to 2 months. No medical intervention can retard this process. Recurrent eczema and persistent arthralgias are rare complications.

Treatment. Because distinguishing clinically between the allergic and spicule-induced reactions is usually impossible, it is reasonable to treat for both. The skin should be gently dried. Spicules should be removed, if possible, using adhesive tape, a thin layer of rubber cement, or a facial peel. As soon as possible, dilute (5%) acetic acid (vinegar) soaks for 10 to 30 minutes 3 or 4 times a day should be applied to all affected areas.[105,108,132] Isopropyl alcohol 40% to 70% is a reasonable second choice. Although topical steroid preparations may help relieve the secondary inflammation, they are of no value as an initial decontaminant. If they precede the vinegar soak, they may worsen the primary reaction. Delayed primary therapy or inadequate decontamination can result in the persistence of bullae, which may become purulent and require months to heal.

Erythema multiforme may require the administration of a systemic glucocorticoid, beginning with a moderately high dose (prednisone 60 to 100 mg) tapered over 2 to 3 weeks. Anecdotal remedies for the management of sponge envenomation that have been suggested without demonstration of efficacy include antiseptic dressings, broad-spectrum antibiotics, methdilazine, pyribenzamine, phenobarbital, diphenhydramine, promethazine, and topical carbolic oil or zinc oxide cream.[105]

After the initial decontamination, a mild emollient cream or steroid preparation may be applied to the skin. If the allergic component is severe, particularly if there is weeping, crusting, and vesiculation, a systemic glucocorticoid (prednisone 60 to 100 mg, tapered over 2 weeks) may be beneficial. Severe itching may be controlled with an antihistamine.

Because *Clostridium tetani* has been cultured from sea sponges, they should not be used to pack wounds. Proper antitetanus immunization should be part of sponge dermatitis therapy. Frequent follow-up wound checks are important because significant infections sometimes develop.[62] Infected wounds should be cultured and managed with antibiotics (see Chapter 60). If sponge poisoning induces an anaphylactoid reaction, standard resuscitation using epinephrine, bronchodilators, corticosteroids, and antihistamines should be undertaken.[133]

As mentioned previously, sponge diver's disease is not caused by any toxin produced by the sponge, but rather is a stinging syndrome related to contact with the tentacles of the small coelenterate anemone *Sagartia rosea* (family Sagartiidae) or anemones from the genus *Actinia* (family Actiniidae) that attach to the base of the sponge. Treatment should include that for coelenterate envenomation.

Prevention. All divers and net handlers should wear proper gloves. Sponges should not be broken, crumbled, or crushed with bare hands. If the victim brings a specimen, the physician should take care to document its appearance. Dried sponges may remain toxic.

Coelenterates (Cnidaria)

Coelenterates are an enormous group, comprising approximately 10,000 species, at least 100 of which are dangerous to humans. Coelenterates that possess the venom-charged stinging organoids commonly called nematocysts are known as cnidaria (nettle); those without nematocysts are acnidaria. For practical purposes the cnidaria can be divided into three main groups: (1) hydrozoans, such as the Portuguese man-of-war; (2) scyphozoans, such as true jellyfish; and (3) anthozoans, such as soft corals (alcyonarians), stony corals, and anemones. Gorgonians (order Gorgonacea, class Anthozoa, subclass Alcyonaria) secrete mucinous exudates having toxic effects in experimental animals that can be characterized as hemolytic, proteolytic, cholinergic, histaminergic, serotonergic, and adrenergic.[43] Fenner divides jellyfish into three main classes: schyphozoans (true jellyfish), with tentacles arising at regular intervals around the bell; cubozoans (e.g., "box" jellyfish), with tentacles arising only from the corners—these may be further divided into carybdeids (e.g., Irukandji), with only one tentacle (except in rare cases) arising from each lower corner of the bell, and chirodropids, which have more than one tentacle in each corner of the bell; and other jellyfish, such as the hydrozoans (e.g., *Physalia* species).

Morphology, Venom, and Venom Apparatus. Coelenterates ("hollow gut") are predators that feed on

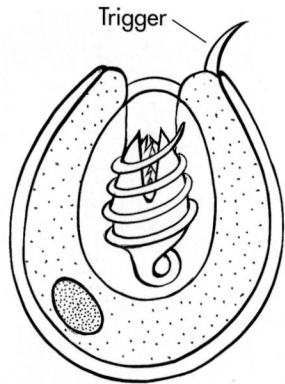

Figure 61-5 Nematocyst before discharge.

other fish, crustaceans, and mollusks. They are radially symmetric animals of simple structure (95% water) and exist in two predominant life-forms, either as sedentary, asexual polyps (hydroids) or as free-swimming and sexual medusae.[57] They are the lowest form of life organized into different layers.[97] Generally, the polyps are saclike creatures attached to the substrate at the caudal (aboral) end, with a single orifice or mouth at the upper end surrounded by stinging tentacles (dactylozooids). This form predominates in the hydrozoans and anthozoans. The medusa is a bell-shaped creature, with a floating gelatinous umbrella from which hang an elongated tubular mouth and marginal nematocyst-bearing tentacles. This form predominates in the scyphozoans and is also found in the hydrozoans.

Cnidocytes are living cells that encapsulate the nonliving intracytoplasmic stinging organoids called cnidae (which include nematocysts, spirocysts, and ptychocysts). The cnidocytes are located on the outer epithelial surfaces of the tentacles or near the mouth and are triggered by contact with the victim's body surface. The nematocyst is contained within an outer capsule called the cnidoblast, to which is attached a single pointed "trigger," or cnidocil. The nematocyst (3 to 10 μm in diameter) is filled with fluid and contains a hollow, sharply pointed, coiled or folded "thread" tubule (nema) (Figure 61-5). This tubule may attain lengths of 200 to 850 μm and is sufficiently hardy to penetrate a surgical glove. In the undischarged state, the toxin is located in the folds and invaginations of the tubule's membrane. The tubule is lined with hollow barbs, which help it penetrate and anchor into the victim. In the undischarged state, the barbs occupy the lumen of the twisted and folded tubule. When the cnidocil is stimulated, either by physical contact or by a chemoreceptor mechanism, it causes the opening of a trapdoor (operculum) in the cnidoblast, and the venom-bearing tubule is everted (Figure 61-6) within 3 microseconds. This exocytosis has been hypothesized to occur because

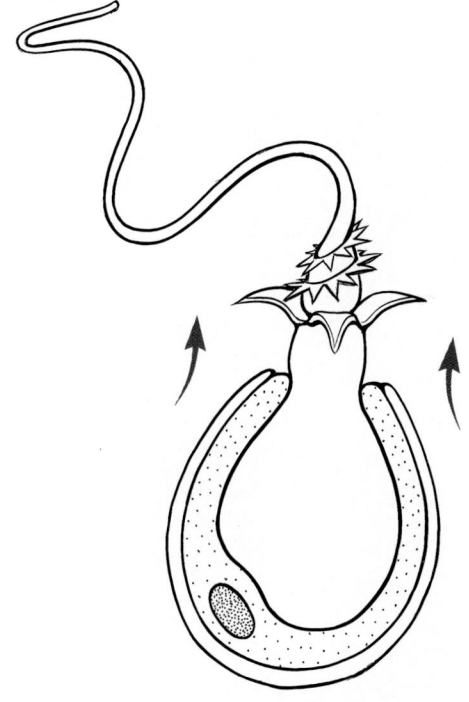

Figure 61-6 Nematocyst after discharge.

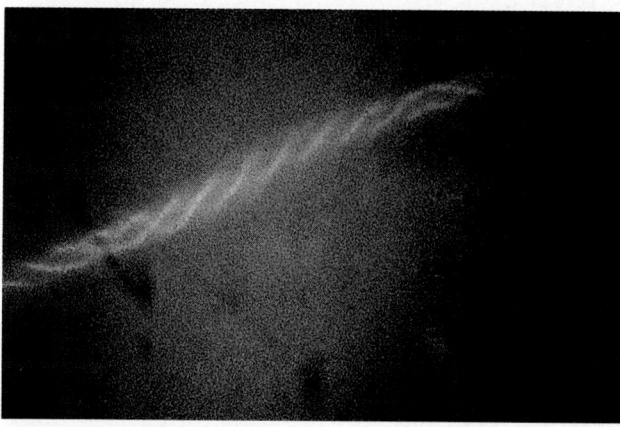

Figure 61-7 Helical arrangement of barbs on the tubule of a nematocyst. *(Photo by Amit Lotan.)*

of osmotic swelling of the capsular matrix caused by influx of water (leading to a hydrostatic pressure of up to 150 atm), release of intrinsic tensile forces (up to 375 MPa on the inner capsule wall), or deformation of the wall-induced internal pressure. The sharp tip of the thread tube enters the victim's skin and envenomation occurs as toxin is translocated by hydrostatic forces from the surface of the everted and extended tubule through the now helically arranged (Figure 61-7) and extended hollow barbs.[66,67] It has been estimated that the velocity of ejection attains 2 m/sec, which corresponds to an acceleration of 40,000 g, with an estimated skin striking force of 2 to 5 psi.[32,95] A human encounter

with a large Portuguese man-of-war could conceivably trigger the release of several million stinging cells. The thread penetrates the epidermis and upper dermis, where the venom diffuses into the general circulation. The agitated victim moves about and assists the venom's distribution by the muscle-pump mechanism. Based on mouse studies, it appears that the rapid death of a victim is related to discharge of venom directly into capillaries, as opposed to that which must diffuse into the bloodstream from the dermis.

In the case of the Indo-Pacific box-jellyfish *Chironex fleckeri*, which may carry up to 59 tentacles bearing millions of nematocysts, it is the cigar-shaped microbasic p-mastigophores that are most important in human envenomation (Figure 61-8). The capsule of the structure holds a hollow coiled tube and granular matrix. The thread tube has a thick butt end that is attached to the operculum. The tube contains three rows of helically arranged spines. When the nematocyst fires into the human victim, the tube everts through the opercular end of the nematocyst, with the butt anchoring first to keep the nematocyst adherent to the victim. The thread then everts through the hollow butt and uncoils, presenting the spines and accompanying toxins to the living tissue. Although the major toxic fractions appear to be present in the nematocysts, there appears to be toxic material present in tentacles denuded of such organelles.[14] The largest nematocysts of *C. fleckeri* can penetrate human skin to a depth of 0.9 mm.[77]

Coelenterate venoms are viscous mixtures of proteins, carbohydrates, and other nonproteinaceous components. To date, they have been difficult to fractionate. Although they are heat labile in vitro, this does not seem to apply in the clinical setting. The primary difficulties encountered in jellyfish venom purification are the lack of stability and the tendency of active toxins to adhere to each other and to support matrices.[86] Cytolytic toxins have been characterized from *Physalia physalis*, *Rhizostoma pulmo*, *Chironex fleckeri*, and *Carybdea marsupialis*.[96] Many jellyfish and marine animal venoms generate autonomic neurotoxicity.[25] This may be a result of their ability to affect ion transport (sodium and calcium in particular), induce channels or pores in nerve and muscle cell membranes, alter membrane configurations, and release mediators of inflammation. Coelenterate venoms can target the myocardium, Purkinje fibers, atrioventricular (AV) node, and aortic ring, as well as injure the hepatic P-450 enzyme family.

Clinical Aspects. For clinical purposes, a considerable phylogenetic relationship exists among all stinging species, so that the clinical features of the coelenterate syndrome are fairly constant, with a spectrum of severity. This is related to the season and species (venom potency and configuration of the nematocyst), the number of nematocysts triggered and the size of the animal

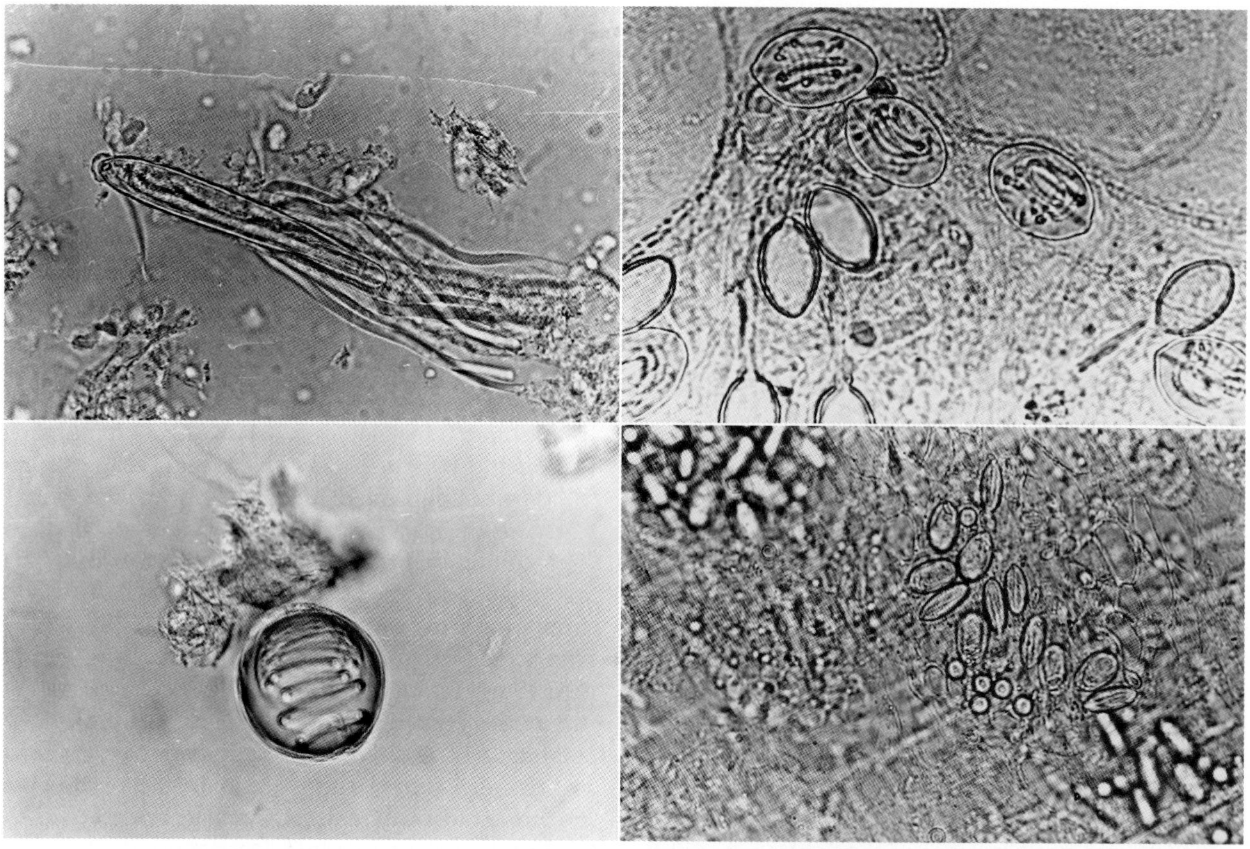

Figure 61-8 Nematocyst identification guide. **A,** Microbasic p-mastigophore (undischarged) of *Chironex fleckeri*. Capsule length 75 µm. **B,** Same (discharged and undischarged) of Irukandji. **C,** Isorhiza (undischarged) of "bluebottle"—*Physalia physalis*. **D,** Clustered isorhizas and uryteles on tentacle of "hair jelly"—*Cyanea*. (**A** to **D** *courtesy Bob Hartwick.*)

(venom inoculum), the size and age of the victim (the very young and old and the smaller person tend to be more severely affected), the location and surface area of the sting, and the health of the victim. The wise clinician suspects a coelenterate envenomation in all unexplained cases of collapse in the surf, diving accidents, and near drownings. Any victim in distress pulled from marine waters should be carefully examined for one or more cutaneous lesions that may provide the clue to a coelenterate envenomation.

Mild envenomation may result only in an annoying dermatitis, whereas severe envenomation can progress rapidly to involve virtually every organ system, resulting in significant morbidity and mortality. Clinical envenomation is described here by severity, with the understanding that there is a fair amount of overlap.

MILD ENVENOMATION. The stings caused by the hydroids and hydroid corals, along with lesser envenomations by *Physalia, Velella vellela, Drymonema dalmatinium* (stinging cauliflower), *Olindias sambaquiensis* (endemic to Blanca Bay area south of Buenos Aires province), scyphozoans, and anemones, result predominantly in skin irritation.[63] There is usually an immediate pricking or stinging sensation, accompanied by pruritus, paresthesias, burning, throbbing, and radiation of the pain centrally from the extremities to the groin, abdomen, and axillae. The area involved by the nematocysts becomes red-brown-purple, often in a linear whiplike fashion, corresponding to tentacle prints. Other features are blistering, local edema, angioedema, and wheal formation, as well as violaceous petechial hemorrhages. The papular inflammatory skin rash is strictly confined to the areas of contact and may persist for up to 10 days. Areas of body hair appear to be somewhat more protected from contact than hairless areas. If the envenomation is slightly more severe, the aforementioned symptoms, which are evident in the first few hours, can progress over a course of days to local necrosis, skin ulceration, and secondary infection. This is particularly true of certain anemone (*Sagartia, Actinia, Anemonia, Actinodendron,* and *Triactis*) stings. A painless "jellyfish sting," in which there is a pattern of hyperpigmented linear streaks, might represent the occurrence of phytophotodermatitis (e.g., from citrus juice spilled on skin and later exposed to light).[13]

Untreated, the minor to moderate skin disorder resolves over 1 to 2 weeks, with occasional residual hyperpigmentation for 1 to 2 months. Rubbing can cause lichenification. Local hyperhidrosis, fat atrophy, and contracture may occur.[18] Facial swelling with sterile abscess formation has been reported.[114] Permanent scarring or keloids may result. Persistent papules or plaques at the sites of contact may demonstrate a predominantly mononuclear cell inflammatory infiltrate, which may represent a delayed hypersensitivity response to an antigenic component of the coelenterate nematocyst or venom. This may be accompanied by localized arthritis and joint effusion. It has been suggested that sensitization may occur without a definite history of a previous sting, since coelenterates may release antigenic and allergenic venom components into the water. Granuloma annulare, which is usually both a sporadic and a familial inflammatory dermatosis, has been associated with a *Physalia utriculus* envenomation.[70] Gangrene has been observed.

MODERATE AND SEVERE ENVENOMATION. The prime offenders in this group are the anemones, *Physalia* species, and scyphozoans. The skin manifestations are similar or intensified (as with *Chironex*) and are compounded by the onset of systemic symptoms, which may appear immediately or be delayed by several hours:

1. Neurologic: malaise, headache, aphonia, diminished touch and temperature sensation, vertigo, ataxia, spastic or flaccid paralysis, mononeuritis multiplex, Guillain-Barré syndrome, parasympathetic dysautonomia, plexopathy, radial-ulnar-median nerve palsies, brainstem infarction (not a confirmed relationship), delirium, loss of consciousness, convulsions, coma, and death[27,37,78,89]
2. Cardiovascular: anaphylaxis, hemolysis, hypotension, small artery spasm, bradyarrhythmias (including electromechanical dissociation and asystole), tachyarrhythmias, vascular spasm, deep venous thrombosis, congestive heart failure, and ventricular fibrillation
3. Respiratory: rhinitis, bronchospasm, laryngeal edema, dyspnea, cyanosis, pulmonary edema, and respiratory failure
4. Musculoskeletal or rheumatologic: abdominal rigidity, diffuse myalgia and muscle cramps, muscle spasm, fat atrophy, arthralgias, reactive arthritis (sero-negative symmetric synovitis with pitting edema),[122] and thoracolumbar pain
5. Gastrointestinal: nausea, vomiting, diarrhea, dysphagia, hypersalivation, and thirst
6. Ocular: conjunctivitis, chemosis, corneal ulcers, corneal epithelial edema, keratitis, iridocyclitis, elevated intraocular pressure, synechiae, iris depigmentation, chronic unilateral glaucoma, and lacrimation[46,47]
7. Other: acute renal failure, lymphadenopathy, chills, fever, and nightmares

The extreme example of envenomation occurs with *Chironex fleckeri*, the dreaded box-jellyfish. *Physalia* and anemone stings, although extremely painful, are rarely fatal. Death after *Physalia* stings has been attributed to primary respiratory failure or cardiac arrhythmia, which may have reflected an element of anaphylaxis.[21,109] Confirmed deaths after coelenterate envenomation have been attributed to *Chironex fleckeri, Chiropsalmus quadrigatus,* and *Chiropsalmus quadrumanus.*[77] *Stomolophus nomurai* (the sand jellyfish) has caused at least eight deaths in the South China Sea.[33] Although there have been other deaths, the animals have not been definitively identified.

Clinical reports and studies on the serologic response to jellyfish envenomation suggest that allergic reactions may play a significant pathophysiologic role in humans. When crude or partially purified nematocyst venom and an antigen are used in an enzyme-linked immunosorbent assay (ELISA), both IgG and IgE can be detected.[44,98] Elevated specific anti-jellyfish IgG and IgE may persist for several years, recurrence of the clinical cutaneous reaction to jellyfish stings may occur within a few weeks without additional contact with the tentacles, and serologic cross-reactivity between the sea nettle (*Chrysaora quinquecirrha*) and *Physalia physalis* occurs. In a case of significant envenomation by the moon jellyfish *Aurelia aurita*, the victim developed significant cross-reacting antibodies to *Chrysaora quinquecirrha* antigens.[20]

Persons with extracutaneous or anaphylactoid responses to a coelenterate sting have been noted to have higher specific IgG and IgE antibody levels.[98] However, elevated persistent specific anti-jellyfish serum IgG concentrations are not protective against the cutaneous pain resulting from a natural sting.[23] A false-positive ELISA serologic test to venom may occur, as demonstrated by negative skin testing.

A person recently stung by *Physalia physalis* may have recurrent cutaneous eruptions for 2 to 3 weeks after the initial episode, without repeated exposure to the animal. This may take the form of lichenification, hyperhidrosis, angioedema, vesicles, large bullae, nodules that resemble erythema nodosum, granuloma annulare, or a more classic linear urticarial eruption.[5,22,71] Recurrent eruptions have also followed a solitary envenomation by the cnidarian *Stomolophus meleagris*.[17] In a histologic study of delayed reaction to a Mediterranean Sea coelenterate, skin biopsy demonstrated grouping of human leukocyte antigen-DR-positive cells with Langerhans' cells and helper/inducer T lymphocytes, which indicates the possibility of a type IV immunoreaction.[90]

Venom-specific IgG antibodies appear to persist for longer periods than IgM antibodies. The binding of brown recluse spider venom and purified cholera toxin to anti-*Chrysaora* and anti-*Physalia* monoclonal antibodies indicates that there may be a common or cross-reacting antigenic site or sites between these toxic substances and certain coelenterate venoms.[85]

Acute regional vascular insufficiency of the upper extremity has been reported after jellyfish envenomation. It can be manifested by acral ischemia, signs and symptoms of compartment syndrome, and massive edema.[129]

Treatment. Therapy is directed at stabilizing major systemic decompensation, opposing the venom's multiple effects, and alleviating pain.

SYSTEMIC ENVENOMATION. Generally, only severe *Physalia* or Cubomedusae stings result in rapid decompensation. In both cases, supportive care is based on the signs and symptoms. Hypotension should be managed with the prompt IV administration of crystalloid, such as lactated Ringer's solution. This must be done in concert with detoxification of any nematocysts (particularly those of *Chironex* or *Chiropsalmus*) that are still attached to the victim, to limit the perpetuation of envenomation. Hypotension is usually limited to very young or elderly victims who suffer severe and multiple stings, the effects of which are worsened by fluid depletion that accompanies protracted vomiting. Hypertension is an occasional side effect of a cubomedusan envenomation, such as that of *Carukia barnesii*. Excessive catecholamine stimulation is one putative cause, which has prompted clinical intervention with phentolamine, an α-adrenergic blocking agent (5 mg intravenously as an initial dose, followed by an infusion of up to 10 mg/hr). Bronchospasm may be managed as an allergic component. If the victim is in respiratory distress with wheezing, shortness of breath, or heart failure, arterial blood gas measurement may be used to guide supplemental oxygen administration by face mask. Seizures are generally self-limited but should be treated with IV diazepam for 24 to 48 hours, after which time they rarely recur.

Any victim with a systemic component should be observed for a period of at least 6 to 8 hours because rebound phenomena after successful treatment are not uncommon. All elderly victims should undergo electrocardiography and be observed on a cardiac monitor, with frequent checks for arrhythmias. Urinalysis demonstrates the presence or absence of hemoglobinuria, indicating hemolysis after the putative attachment of *Physalia* venom to red blood cell membrane glycoprotein sites.[49] If this is the case, the urine should be alkalinized with bicarbonate to prevent the precipitation of pigment in the renal tubules, while a moderate diuresis (30 to 50 ml/hr) is maintained with a loop diuretic (such as furosemide or bumetanide) or mannitol (0.25 g/kg intravenously every 8 to 12 hours). In rare instances of acute progressive renal failure, peritoneal dialysis or hemodialysis may be necessary.

If there are signs of distal ischemia or an impending compartment syndrome, standard diagnostic and therapeutic measures apply. These include Doppler ultrasound, angiography, or both for diagnosis, regional thrombolysis for acutely occluded blood vessels, measurement of intracompartmental tissue pressures to guide fasciotomy, and so forth. Reversible regional sympathetic blockade may be efficacious if vasospasm is a dominant clinical feature. However, the vasospasm associated with a jellyfish envenomation may be severe, prolonged, and refractory to regional sympathectomy and intraarterial reserpine or pentoxifylline.[1]

A small child may pick up tentacle fragments on the beach and place them into his or her mouth, resulting in rapid intraoral swelling and potential airway obstruction, particularly in the presence of exceptional hypersensitivity. In such cases an endotracheal tube should be placed before edema precludes visualization of the vocal cords. In no case should any liquid be placed in the mouth if the airway is not protected. In 1999, a lifeguard in Cairns, Australia, drank from a container containing 4-day-old *Chironex fleckeri* tentacles. He fortunately suffered only a sore throat and transient shortness of breath.

Chironex fleckeri, the box-jellyfish, produces the only coelenterate venom for which a specific antidote exists. To date, the venoms of *Physalia* and *Chrysaora* species have not been sufficiently purified as antigens to permit the production of an antitoxin. Antivenom administration may be lifesaving and should accompany the first-aid protocol previously described.

PAIN CONTROL. Often the pain can be controlled by treating the dermatitis. However, if pain is excruciating and there is no contraindication (such as head injury, altered mental status, respiratory depression, allergy, or profound hypotension), the administration of a narcotic (morphine sulfate, 2 to 10 mg intravenously; nalbuphine, 2 to 10 mg intravenously; or intramuscularly; meperidine, 50 to 100 mg, with hydroxyzine, 25 to 50 mg intramuscularly; or meperidine, 15 to 30 mg, with promethazine, 12.5 to 25 mg, or prochlorperazine, 2.5 mg intravenously) is often indicated. Severe muscle spasm may respond to 10% calcium gluconate (5 to 10 ml IV slow push), diazepam (5 to 10 mg intravenously), or methocarbamol (1 g, no faster than 100 mg/min through a widely patent IV line).

TREATMENT OF DERMATITIS. If a person is stung by a coelenterate, the following steps should be taken:

1. Immediately rinse the wound with seawater, not with freshwater. Do not rub the wound with a towel or clothing to remove adherent tentacles. Nonforceful freshwater rinsing or a rubbing vari-

ety of abrasion (the latter in the absence of simultaneous application of a decontaminant such as papain or vinegar) is felt to stimulate any nematocysts that have not already fired. Surf life savers (lifeguards) in the United States and Hawaii have reported that a freshwater hot shower applied with a forceful stream may decrease the pain of an envenomation. If this is successful, one theoretic explanation is that the mechanical effect of the water stream (that dislodges tentacle fragments and/or stinging cells) supercedes the deleterious (sting-stimulating) effect of the hypotonic water. Remove any gross tentacles with forceps or a well-gloved hand. In an emergency, the keratinized palm of the hand is relatively protected, but take care not to become envenomed.

Commercial (chemical) cold or ice packs applied over a thin dry cloth or plastic membrane have been shown to be effective when applied to mild or moderate *Physalia utriculus* ("bluebottle"—see below) stings.[32] Whether the melt-water from ice applied directly to the skin can stimulate the discharge of nematocysts has not been determined. Applications of hot packs or gentle rinses with hot water are not recommended because they may worsen the pain of the envenomation.

2. Acetic acid 5% (vinegar) is the treatment of choice to inactivate *Chironex fleckeri* toxin. Vinegar will not alleviate the pain from a *Chironex* sting but interrupts the envenomation. It may not be extremely effective against *Chrysaora* or *Cyanea*. The detoxicant should be applied continuously for at least 30 minutes or until the pain is relieved. A sting from the Australian *Physalia physalis*, a relatively recently differentiated species, should not be doused with vinegar, since this may cause discharge of up to 30% of nematocysts.[36]

For a sting from *Chironex fleckeri*, if the pressure-immobilization technique for venom sequestration is going to be used, the bandage should be applied as soon as possible (see below). If vinegar is immediately available, a liberal dousing should occur and at least 30 seconds should pass before removing the tentacles. After the tentacles are removed, proceed at once with pressure-immobilization. If vinegar is not available, remove the tentacles before applying pressure-immobilization.[34] A venolymphatic occlusive tourniquet should be considered only if a topical detoxicant and pressure-immobilization is unavailable, the victim suffers from a severe systemic reaction, and transport to definitive care is delayed.

For stings from other species, there are substances that may be more specific and therefore more effective. Depending on the species, these include isopropyl alcohol (40% to 70%), dilute ammonium hydroxide, sodium bicarbonate (particularly for stings of the sea nettle *Chrysaora quinquecirrha*), olive oil, sugar, urine, and papain (papaya latex [juice] or unseasoned meat tenderizer powdered or in solution). The last is supposed to work by cleaving active polypeptides into non-toxic amino acids. Ammonia has been noted to be relatively ineffective for stings of *Carybdea marsupialis* in the Adriatic Sea.[88]

Perfume, aftershave lotion, and high-proof liquor are not particularly efficacious and may be detrimental. Other substances mentioned to be effective at one time or another, but which are to be condemned on the basis of inefficacy and toxicity, are organic solvents such as formalin, ether, and gasoline.

There is recent evidence that alcohol may stimulate the discharge of nematocysts in vitro; the clinical significance is as yet undetermined. The rescuer must remember that pain relief may not equate with nematocyst inhibition.[77]

A commercial aqueous solution of aluminum sulfate 20% and 11% anionic surfactant in aqueous solution (Stingose) has sometimes been mentioned as effective on the basis that the aluminum ion interacts with proteins and long-chain polysaccharide components to denature and inactivate venom. Prior treatment with topical alcohol or methylated spirits reduces the effectiveness of aluminum sulfate solution. This product seems to have fallen out of favor with clinician jellyfish experts in Australia.

3. No systemic drugs (other than antivenom for a *Chironex* envenomation) are of verifiable use. Ephedrine, atropine, calcium, methysergide, and hydrocortisone have all been touted at one time or another, but no proof exists that they help. Antihistamines may be useful if there is a significant allergic component. The administration of epinephrine is appropriate only in the setting of anaphylaxis.

4. Immersing the area in hot water is generally not recommended; the hypotonic solution causes nematocysts to discharge.

5. Once the wound has been soaked with a decontaminant (e.g., vinegar), remaining (and often "invisible") nematocysts must be removed. The easiest way to do this is to apply shaving cream or a paste of baking soda, flour, or talc and to shave the area with a razor or similar tool. If sophisticated facilities are not available, the nematocysts should be removed by making a sand or mud paste with seawater and using this to help scrape the victim's skin with a sharp-edged shell or piece of wood. The rescuer must take care not to become envenomed; bare hands must be rinsed fre-

quently. If a scrub brush or pad has been used to treat the envenomation, this step may not result in as much, if any, clinical improvement.

6. A topical anesthetic ointment (lidocaine, 2.5%) or spray (benzocaine, 14%), antihistaminic cream (diphenhydramine or tripelennamine), or mild steroid lotion (hydrocortisone, 1%) may be soothing. These are used after the toxin is inactivated. Paradoxical reactions to benzocaine are rarely noted.

7. Victims should receive standard antitetanus prophylaxis.

8. Prophylactic antibiotics are not automatically indicated. Each wound should be checked at 3 and 7 days after injury for infection. Any ulcerating lesion should be cleaned 3 times a day and covered with a thin layer of nonsensitizing antiseptic ointment, such as mupirocin. A jellyfish sting to the cornea may cause a foreign body sensation, photophobia, and decreased or hazy vision. Ophthalmologic examination reveals hyperemic sclera, chemosis, and irregularity of the corneal epithelium with stromal edema. Depending on the extent of the wound, the anterior chamber may demonstrate the inflammatory response of iridocyclitis (flare with or without cells).[131] The victim should be referred to an ophthalmologist, who may prescribe steroid-containing eye medications, such as prednisolone acetate 1% with hyoscine 0.25%. Applying a traditional skin detoxicant directly to the cornea is not recommended, since it is likely to worsen the tissue injury.

DELAYED REACTION. A delayed reaction, similar in appearance to erythema nodosum, may be noted in areas of skin contact, and be accompanied by fever, weakness, arthralgias, painful joint swelling, and effusions. This may recur multiple times over the course of 1 to 2 months. The treatment is a 10- to 14-day taper of prednisone, starting with 50 to 100 mg. Prednisone administration may need to be prolonged or repeated with each flare of the reaction.

PERSISTENT HYPERPIGMENTATION. Postinflammatory hyperpigmentation is common after the stings of many jellyfish and other lesser coelenterates. A solution of 1.8% hydroquinone in a glycol and alcohol base (70% ethyl alcohol and propylene glycol mixed at a 3:2 ratio) twice a day as a topical agent for 3 to 5 weeks has been used successfully to treat hyperpigmentation after a *Pelagia noctiluca* sting.

PERSISTENT CUTANEOUS HYPERSENSITIVITY. Persistent local dermal hypersensitivity may occur after a jellyfish sting, such as that from the Hawaiian box-jellyfish *Carybdea alata*.[116] This is characterized by erythematous papulonodular lesions in the pattern of the original sting, which may persist for months. Treatment, which may be unsatisfactory, consists of topical and intralesional steroids.

Prevention. A protocol has been developed to establish the effectiveness of topical agents to block firing of nematocysts.[26] Current research is directed at a combination jellyfish sting inhibitor–sunscreen lotion that may prevent discharge of more than 90% of nematocysts that contact protected skin. Failed topical barriers include petrolatum, mineral oil, silicone ointment, cocoa butter, and mechanic's grease.

If jellyfish are sighted, they should be given a wide berth because the tentacles may trail great distances from the body. All swimmers and divers in hazardous areas should be on constant alert. Persons should not dive headfirst into jellyfish-infested waters; it is far safer to walk in. Bathers should wear protective clothing in infested areas. This includes "stinger suits" or a double thickness of panty hose. If "stinger enclosures" are present, bathers should stay within the netted barriers .

Divers concerned about jellyfish tentacles dangling from the surface or congregations of creatures at the surface should remain deeper than 20 feet and should always check snorkel and regulator mouthpieces for tentacle fragments before entering the water in endemic areas. In areas inhabited by anemones and hydroid corals, protective gloves should be worn when handling specimens. Beached dead jellyfish or tentacle fragments washed up after a storm can still inflict serious stings. Any person stung by a jellyfish should leave or be assisted from the water because of the risk of drowning.

The International Consortium for Jellyfish Stings was formed to gather reports and encourage prospective investigations. At the time of this writing, a marine sting or bite report form can be obtained from Joseph W. Burnett, M.D., Department of Dermatology, 6th Floor, University of Maryland Hospital, 405 West Redwood Street, Baltimore, MD 21201-1703.

Hydrozoa. The hydrozoans range in configuration from the feather hydroids and sedentary *Millepora* hydroid coral to the free-floating siphonophore *Physalia* (Portuguese man-of-war). These are perfect examples of the class Hydrozoa.

HYDROIDS. Hydroids are the most numerous of the hydrozoans. The feather hydroids of the order Leptomedusae, typified by *Lytocarpus philippinus* ("fire weed" or "fire fern"), are featherlike or plumelike (Figure 61-9) animals that sting the victim who brushes against or handles them.[93] After a storm the branches may be fragmented and dispersed through the water, so that merely diving or swimming in the vicinity

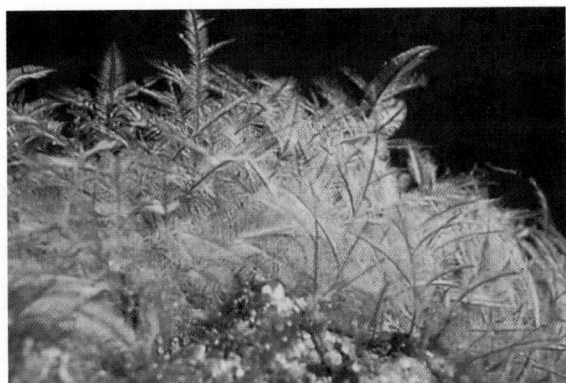

Figure 61-9 Coelenterate hydroid. *(Photo by Paul Auerbach, MD.)*

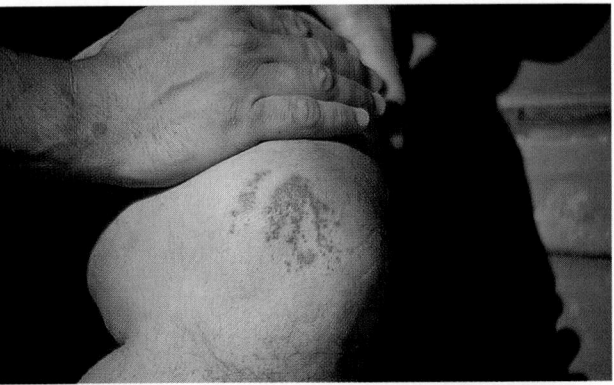

Figure 61-11 Fernlike hydroid "print" on the knee of a diver. *(Photo by Paul Auerbach, MD.)*

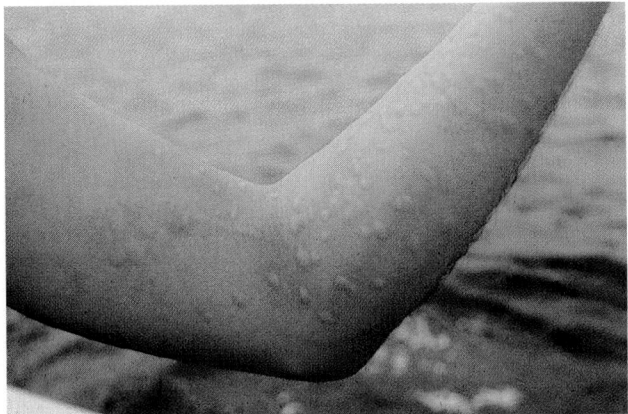

Figure 61-10 Hydroid sting on the arm of a diver. *(Photo by Neville Coleman.)*

causes itching and burning and may induce visible skin irritation.

Clinical aspects. Contact with the nematocysts of a feather hydroid induces a mild reaction, which consists of instantaneous burning, itching, and urticaria. If the exposure is brief, the skin rash may not be noticeable or it may consist of a faint erythematous and miliary irritation (Figure 61-10). A second variety of envenomation consists of a delayed papular, hemorrhagic, or zosteriform reaction (Figure 61-11) with onset 4 to 12 hours after contact. Rarely, erythema multiforme or a desquamative eruption may develop. In turbulent waters or in a strong current, fragments may be washed into a diver's mask or regulator mouthpiece; this will be evident as a burning sensation in the conjunctivae or oral mucous membranes. Systemic manifestations (such as abdominal pain, nausea, vomiting, diarrhea, muscle cramps, and fever) are rarely reported and are associated with large areas of surface involvement. Allergic sensitization and subsequent anaphylaxis have been proposed.

Treatment. The skin should be rinsed with seawater and gently dried without abrasive activity. Application of freshwater and brisk rubbing are strictly prohibited because they encourage any nematocysts remaining on the skin to discharge and thus worsen the envenomation. Acetic acid 5% (vinegar) or isopropyl alcohol 40% to 70% has been traditionally recommended for application to the skin for 15 to 30 minutes to relieve the cutaneous reaction. In an in vitro evaluation, vinegar and urine caused discharge of a few nematocysts in 10% to 15% of defensive tentacle polyps; methylated spirits were found to cause gross discharge of microbasic mastigophores in all defensive polyps.[93] Freshwater did not cause discharge. On the basis of this study the authors recommended that freshwater irrigation and the application of ice be used to treat acute stings. However, the clinical correlation remains to be described.

Alternative topical agents are discussed in the larger discussion on therapy for coelenterate stings. After pain relief is achieved, a mild steroid cream (hydrocortisone 1%) or moisturizing lotion may be applied.

FIRE CORAL. The stony, hydroid, and coral-like *Millepora* species (for example, *M. alcicornis*), or fire corals, are not true corals. They are widely distributed in shallow tropical waters. Sessile creatures, they are found attached to the bottom in depths of up to 1000 m (3281 feet). They are often mistaken for seaweed because they attach to pilings, rocks, shells, or coral. Although smaller segments resemble Christmas trees or bushes 3 to 4 inches in height, they may attain heights of 2 m. The color ranges from white to yellow-green, with pale yellow (Figure 61-12) most common. Rare purple fire corals exist. Fire coral is structured on a razor-sharp lime carbonate exoskeleton, which is an important component in the development of coral reefs. The outcroppings assume upright, clavate, bladelike, honeycomb, or branching calcareous growth structures that form encrustations over coral and objects such as sunken vessels.

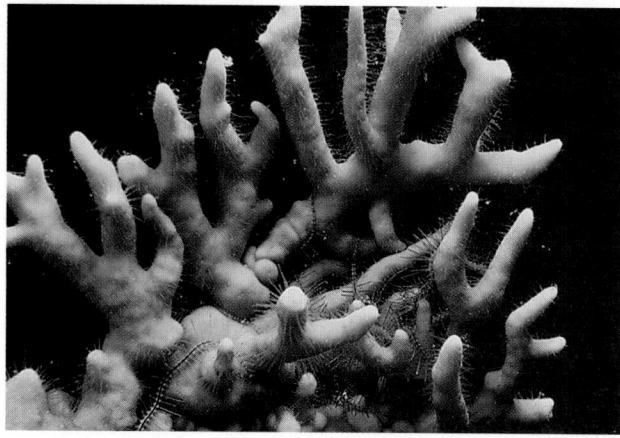

Figure 61-12 Fire coral. *(Photo by Paul Auerbach, MD.)*

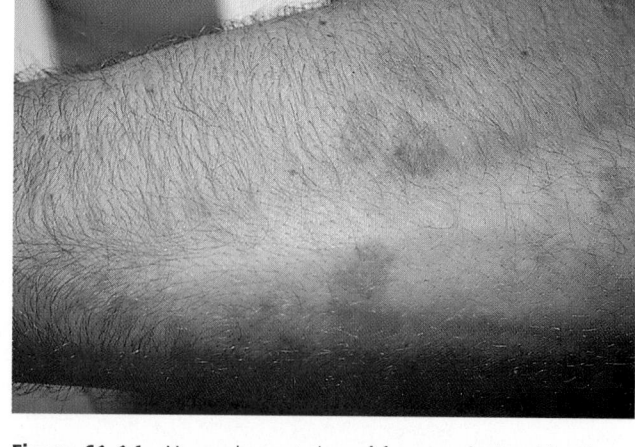

Figure 61-14 Hyperpigmentation of forearm depicted in Figure 61-13 following a fire coral sting. *(Photo by Kenneth Kizer, MD.)*

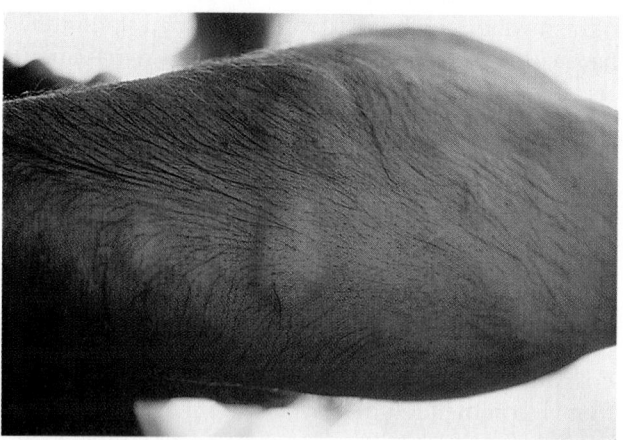

Figure 61-13 Fire coral sting of the author. *(Photo by Kenneth Kizer, MD.)*

From numerous minute surface gastropores protrude tiny nematocyst-bearing tentacles, wherein lies the stinging apparatus. *M. alcicornis* probably accounts for more coelenterate envenomations than any other species. Unprotected and unwary recreational scuba enthusiasts handle, kneel, or lean on this marine stinger.

Clinical aspects. Immediately after contact with fire coral, the victim suffers burning or stinging pain, rarely with central radiation. Intense and painful pruritus follows within seconds, which frequently induces the victim to rub the affected area vigorously, worsening the envenomation. Over the course of 5 to 30 minutes, urticarial wheals develop, marked by redness, warmth, and pruritus (Figure 61-13). The wheals become moderately edematous and reach a maximum size in 30 to 60 minutes. Untreated, they flatten over 14 to 24 hours and resolve entirely over 3 to 7 days, occasionally leaving an area of hyperpigmentation (Figure 61-14) that may require 4 to 8 weeks to disappear. The pain generally resolves without treatment in 30 to 90 minutes. In the case of multiple stings, regional lymph nodes may become inflamed and painful. This does not necessarily indicate a secondary infection. Long thoracic mononeuritis with serratus anterior muscle paralysis has been described after *Millepora* sting, confirmed by demonstrated presence of immune-specific IgG.[79]

Treatment. The skin should be rinsed liberally with seawater and then immediately soaked with acetic acid 5% (vinegar) or isopropyl alcohol 40% to 70% until pain is relieved. Alternative topical agents are discussed in the larger coelenterate treatment section. Residual dermatitis is generally not very severe and can be managed in a fashion similar to that after a feather hydroid sting. If the rash becomes eczematous and indolent, it may respond to a course of systemic corticosteroids (prednisone 60 to 100 mg, tapered over 2 weeks). Divers should avoid touching with bare skin anything resembling coral. For instance, the underwater statue of Jesus at John Pennycamp Park in Key Largo, Florida, is encrusted with fire coral, so posing divers have been envenomed.

PHYSALIA (MAN-OF-WAR). The Atlantic Portuguese man-of-war (*Physalia physalis*) of the phylum Coelenterata, order Siphonophora, is a pelagic (open sea) polymorphic colonial siphonophore that inhabits the surface of the ocean. It is constructed of a blue or pink-violet and iridescent floating sail (pneumatophore), nitrogen and carbon monoxide filled and up to 30 cm in length, from which are suspended multiple nematocyst-bearing tentacles, which may measure up to 30 m (98 feet) in length (Figure 61-15). It has recently been reported that an Australian version of *Physalia physalis* is present in north Australian waters.[36] This jel-

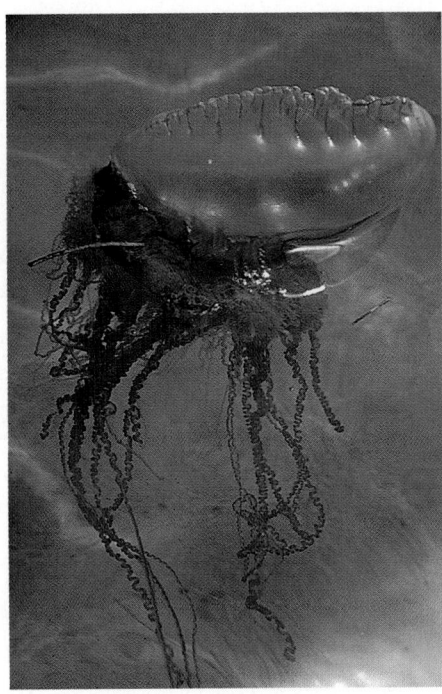

Figure 61-15 Atlantic Portuguese man-of-war. *(Photo by Norbert Wu.)*

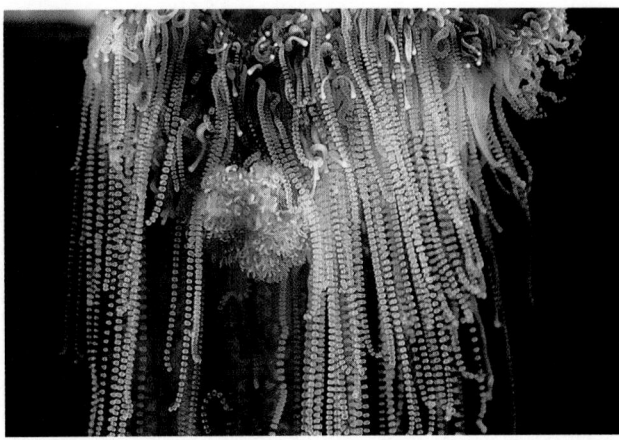

Figure 61-16 Tentacles of the Atlantic Portuguese man-of-war. Nematocysts may number in the hundreds of thousands on tentacles coiled into "stinging batteries." *(Courtesy Larry Madin, Woods Hole Oceanographic Institution.)*

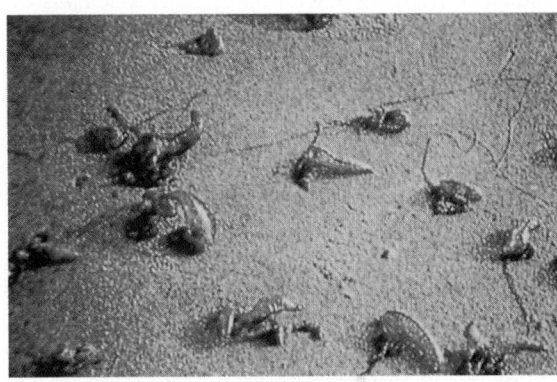

Figure 61-17 Pacific man-of-war washed ashore may retain their stinging potency for weeks. *(Courtesy John Williamson, MD.)*

lyfish is characterized by float lengths of up to 15 cm, up to five thick dark blue "main" tentacles, and up to 10 other long, thin, and pale-colored tentacles. The smaller Pacific bluebottle *(Physalia utriculus)* usually has a single fishing tentacle, which attains lengths of up to 15 m. In some species the sail can be deflated to allow the animal to submerge in rough weather.

The physaliae depend on the winds, currents, and tides for movement, traveling as individuals or in floating colonies that resemble flotillas. They are widely distributed but seem to abound in tropical waters and in the semitropical Atlantic Ocean, particularly off the coast of Florida and in the Gulf of Mexico. Envenoming has been reported as far south as the coast of Brazil.[29] Their arrival at surf's edge can transform a halcyon vacation into a stinging nightmare. Unfortunately, peak appearance time for both the man-of-war and sea nettle is July through September, which is prime beach season.

As with icebergs, the scene above water conceals much of the story. Because the tentacles are nearly transparent, they pose a hazard to the unwary. As the animal moves in the ocean, the tentacles rhythmically contract, sampling the water for potential prey. If the tentacle strikes a foreign object, the nematocysts are stimulated and discharge their contents into the victim. Each tentacle in a larger specimen may carry more than 750,000 nematocysts. To increase the intensity of the "attack," the remainder of the tentacle shortens in such a way as to create loops and folds, presenting a greater surface

area and number of nematocysts for offensive action in what are called "stinging batteries" (Figure 61-16).

Detached moistened tentacles, often found by the thousands fragmented on the beach, carry live nematocysts capable of discharging for months. Air-dried nematocysts may retain considerable potency, even after weeks (Figure 61-17). The loggerhead turtle *(Caretta caretta)* (Figure 61-18) feeds on *Physalia.* Like the clownfish with the sea anemone, the brightly colored fish *Nomeus gronovii* has a unique symbiotic relationship with the man-of-war, living freely among the tentacles. Two species of nudibranch (sea slug), *Glaucus atlanticus* and *G. glaucilla,* eat the tentacles and nematocysts of *P. physalis.* The nematocysts are not digested and ultimately reside in the dorsal papillae of the nudibranchs, where they may sting on contact. Other nudibranchs are also able to ingest hydroids and store their stinging cells in the cerata, or flesh appendages. Dermatitis can also result from contact with water containing venom that has already been released from stimulated nema-

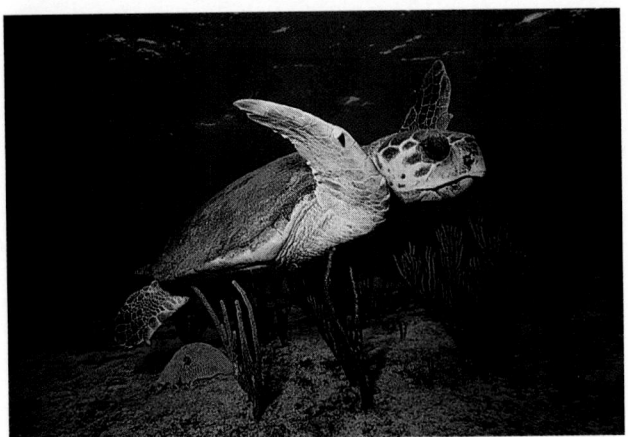

Figure 61-18 The loggerhead turtle sometimes dines on jellyfish tentacles. *(Photo by Howard Hall.)*

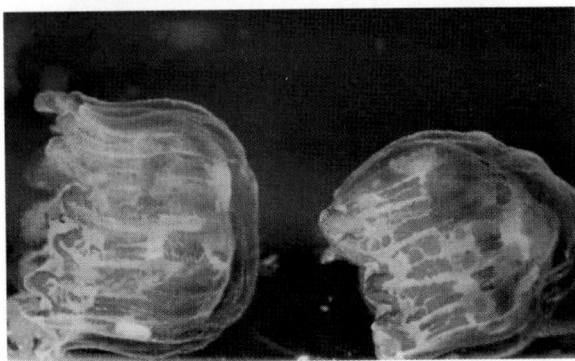

Figure 61-19 Mature *Linuche unguiculata*, the causative agents of seabather's eruption. The planula or larvae of these coelenterates were collected from plankton tows and grown to maturity at the University of Miami Marine school. Slightly smaller than their brethren found in the open ocean, these specimens are approximately 2 cm in diameter when open and 1 cm when contracted. *(Courtesy David Taplin and Terri L. Meinking.)*

tocysts. The Mediterranean octopus *Tremoctopus violaceous* stores intact dactylozooid segments in its suckers for later use.[22]

GONIONEMUS SPECIES. These small hydrozoans are distributed worldwide but have only been reported as causing severe envenomation in the Sea of Japan near Vladivostock, Russia, and the northwest shores of Honshu Island, Japan.[33] It is a small creature of 5 to 15 mm in diameter across the bell, with a symmetric, right-angled cross visible in the transparent part.

When the reaction is painful, the victim suffers muscle, joint, chest, and pelvic pain for up to 3 days. There may be muscle fasciculations. In a respiratory presentation, the victims suffer rhinitis, tearing, hoarseness, cough, and shortness of breath. In addition, there may be a combination of symptoms, with or without sore throat, tachycardia, vomiting, and mild hypertension. Psychiatric depression and hallucinations may occur.[83]

It has been noted that envenomation may occur beneath a bathing suit. In addition, a similar syndrome was reported after ingestion of raw seaweed, to which was presumably attached the jellyfish.[33]

Seabather's Eruption. Seabather's eruption, commonly termed "sea lice" ("pika-pika" around the Belize barrier reef; "sea poisoning," "sea critters," and "ocean itch" are other names), refers to a dermatitis that results from contact with ocean water.[57] It has become a seasonal problem afflicting oceangoers in south Florida and across the Caribbean. It predominantly involves covered areas of the body and is commonly caused by pinhead-sized (0.5 mm) greenish-brown to black larvae of the thimble jellyfish *Linuche unguiculata* (Figure 61-19), which breeds in Caribbean waters throughout the summer with a peak in May.[118] *L. unguiculata* exists in three other forms during its life cycle: schyphistomae (polyp), ephyra (first swimming stage), and adult medusa. It is likely that the

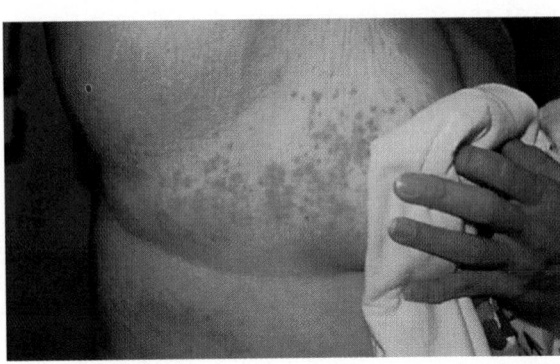

Figure 61-20 Seabather's eruption. *(From Wong DE et al: J Am Acad Dermatol 30:399, 1994.)*

adult and ephyra *L. unguiculata* can also initiate the eruption.[91] Another culprit off Long Island, New York, has been the planula larval form (visible at 2 to 3 mm) of the sea anemone *Edwardsiella lineata*, which carries hundreds of nematocysts.[38,39] Given the number of coelenterates that inhabit the oceans of the world and the cross-reactivity of antigens, it is likely that etiologic organisms are numerous.

A swimmer who encounters the stinging forms usually complains of cutaneous discomfort soon after contact, often while in the water or soon after exiting. Application of fresh water may intensify the sting. The eruption occurs a few minutes to 12 hours after bathing and consists of erythematous and intensely pruritic wheals, vesicles, or papules that persist for 2 to 14 days and then involute spontaneously. When a bathing suit has been worn by a woman, the areas commonly involved include the buttocks, genital region, and breasts (Figure 61-20). A person at the water's surface (com-

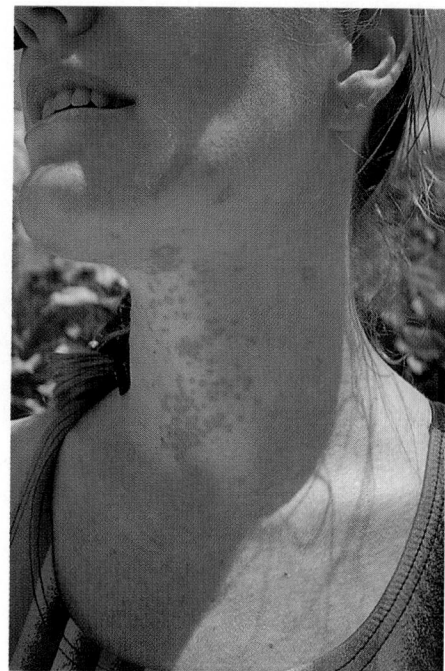

Figure 61-21 Seabather's eruption on the neck of a diver in Cozumel, Mexico. *(Photo by Paul Auerbach, MD.)*

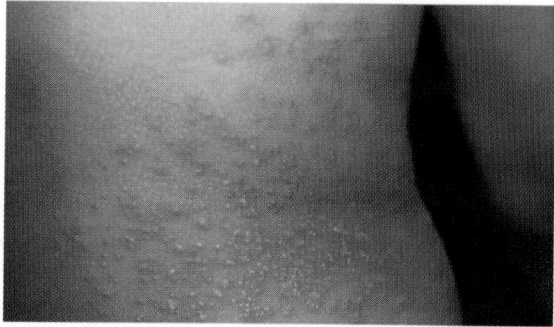

Figure 61-22 Seabather's eruption in an area under the weight belt. *(Courtesy Doug Wong, MD.)*

monly a person who surfaces after a dive) may suffer stings to the exposed neck (Figure 61-21), particularly if there has been recent motorboat activity in the vicinity, which may disturb and fragment the causative jellyfish. Nematocysts adherent to scalp hair may sting the neck as the hair hangs down. Coalescence indicates a large inoculum. Individual lesions resemble insect bites. Surfers develop lesions on areas that contact the surfboard (chest and anterior abdomen). The rash may also be seen under bathing caps and swim fins or along the edge of the cuffs of wet suits, T-shirts, or "stinger suits" (Figure 61-22).[118] In children with extensive eruptions, fever is common. Other symptoms can include headache, chills, fatigue and malaise, vomiting, conjunctivitis, and urethritis. Itching is often pronounced at night and awakens the victim from sleep. Burnett and Burnett[12] reported blurred vision and left arm weakness in a teenager stung by adult *Linuche.* Persons who note a stinging sensation during the primary contact while still in the water may have a higher incidence of previous sensitization to the antigen or antigens. Persons who wear clothing that has been contaminated with the larvae may suffer recurrent reactions. Prior sensitization may precede prolonged (up to 6 weeks) reactions (rash and pruritus).

Elevated IgG levels specific for *Linuche unguiculata* can be measured by ELISA in the sera of victims who have suffered from seabather's eruption. The extent of the cutaneous eruption or sting severity appears to correlate with the antibody titer.[24] In an evaluation of

southeast Florida victims envenomed by *L. unguiculata,* histopathologic examination of inflammatory papules demonstrated superficial and deep perivascular and intersitital infiltrate consisting of lymphocytes, neutrophils, and eosinophils.[130]

Field management is identical to that for any coelenterate sting (see above), with the empirical observation that topical papain may be more effective as an initial decontaminant than vinegar, isopropyl alcohol, or other substances. This may be more effective if applied with a mildly abrasive scrub pad. On the basis of anecdotal reports, this approach appears to be effective field therapy for seabather's eruption. Whether the pain relief is due to nematocyst inactivation or counterirritation is not yet known. Substances that are believed to be ineffective include hydrogen peroxide, garlic, antifungal spray, anti–head lice medication, petroleum distillates, fingernail polish, and citrus juice.

The skin eruption is self-limited and usually remits within 10 days. However, in a severe envenomation, the rash may persist for up to 4 weeks and leave atrophic scars.[69] Further treatment is palliative and consists of calamine lotion with 1% menthol. Because the lesions rarely extend into the dermis, a potent topical corticosteroid may be helpful in mild cases, but benefit is not invariably attained. In a more severe case, an oral or parenteral antihistamine or systemic corticosteroid may be used. A thorough soap and water scrub (not a casual rinse) on leaving the water provides partial prophylaxis. Avoidance logically includes advice to ocean bathe in abbreviated swimwear (which may expose a person to other stings), to maintain tightly occlusive cuffs on dive skins and wet suits, to change swimwear as soon as possible after leaving the water, and to use caution during high season for *L. unguiculata* (April to July off south Florida) or *E. lineata* (August to November off Long Island) and when there are strong onshore winds. Swimwear worn and suspected to be contaminated with nematocysts should be washed in detergent and freshwater and dried before wearing.[100]

As mentioned previously, current research is directed at a specific topical jellyfish sting inhibitor. The first such product to be commercialized is Safe Sea ("jellyfish safe sun block") by Nidaria Technology Ltd, Jordan Valley, Israel. DermaShield (Benchmark Enterprises, Salt Lake City, Utah) is a barrier topical formulation that contains lanolin, aloe vera, and vitamin E. According to the manufacturer, this chemically inert (1-vinyl-2-pyrrolidione) protectant is hydrophobic (dimethicone and stearic acid) and does not wash off but is shed as the epithelium sloughs naturally. It has been reported anecdotally by ocean bathers to protect against the agents of seabather's eruption. To my knowledge, no prospective evaluation of the use of DermaShield to protect against any coelenterate stings has been published. Smerbeck et al were assigned a U.S. Patent in 1999 for a method and composition containing polymeric quaternary ammonium salts for protecting the skin from jellyfish stings.

True sea lice (see Chapter 63) are parasites on marine creatures and do not cause this disorder.

Scyphozoa. This group of animals comprises the larger medusae or jellyfish, including the deadly box-jellyfish and sea wasps (e.g., *Chironex, Cyanea,* and *Chiropsalmus*). These creatures are armed with some of the most potent venoms in existence. Jellyfish are mostly free-swimming pelagic creatures; however, some can be found at depths of more than 2000 fathoms. They may be transparent or multicolored and range in size from a few millimeters to more than 2 m (6½ feet) in width across the bell, with tentacles up to 40 m (131 feet) in length. Like physaliae, the scyphozoans depend on the wind, currents, and tides for transport and are widely distributed. Some vertical motion may be produced by rhythmic contractions of the gelatinous bell, from which originate the feeding tentacles.

Some jellyfish contain less than 5% solid organic matter. Regardless, they can withstand remarkable temperature and salinity variations, although they do not fare well with violent activity and thus may descend to the depths during stormy surface weather. Some scyphozoans avoid sunlight; others follow an opposite pattern. Certain jellyfish have adapted to local nutrient (largely algal) supply and lost their ability to sting humans (Figure 61-23).

In the eastern coastal waters of the North American continent, the creatures appear to grow larger as they progress north (Figure 61-24), so that true giant jellyfish, typified by *Cyanea capillata* (lion's mane), are found in arctic waters (Figure 61-25). Tentacles (which may number up to 1200) of larger specimens may exceed 30 m (100 feet) in length.[22] *Pelagia* species (purple-striped or "mauve"-pink stingers) are commonly found in large numbers off the California coast and appear in the Mediterranean Sea in abundance every 10 to 12 years.[92] *P. noctiluca* (Figure 61-26) phosphoresces at

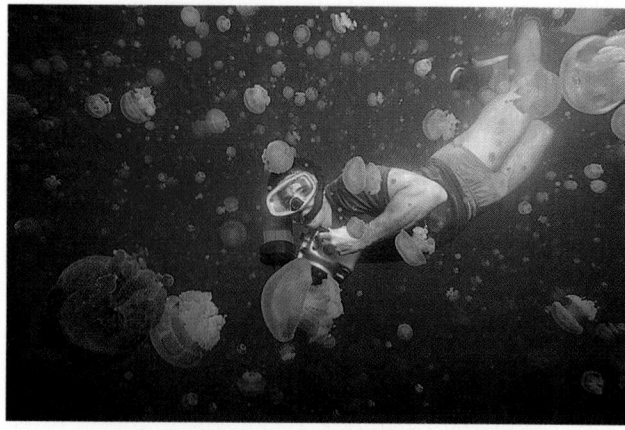

Figure 61-23 The author snorkels in "Jellyfish Lake" in Palau. The jellyfish have evolved to subsist on algae and thus no longer pose a stinging hazard to humans. *(Photo by Avi Klapfer.)*

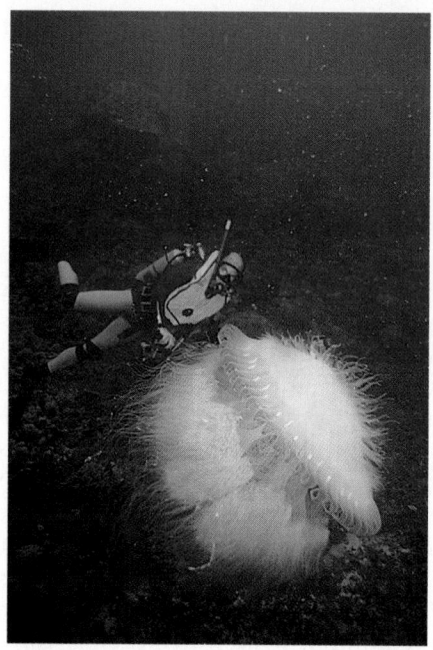

Figure 61-24 Lion's mane jellyfish *(Cyanea capillata). (Photo by Carl Roessler.)*

night, hence its name.[77] *Olindias sambaquiensis* is a jellyfish that stings bathers in South American coastal waters. *Rhopilema nomadica* is a tropical jellyfish that has invaded the eastern Mediterranean.[34,65,66] As a further example, stings from *Stomolophus nomurai* in the Bohai waters of China produce severe pulmonary edema, coma, convulsions, psychoses, and death. Australian jellyfish include the blubber jellyfish (*Catostylus* species), hair jellyfish (*Cyanea* species), little mauve stinger (*Pelagia noctiluca),* and the cuboid-shaped jellyfish (*Chironex fleckeri* and *Chiropsalmus quadrigatus*). A

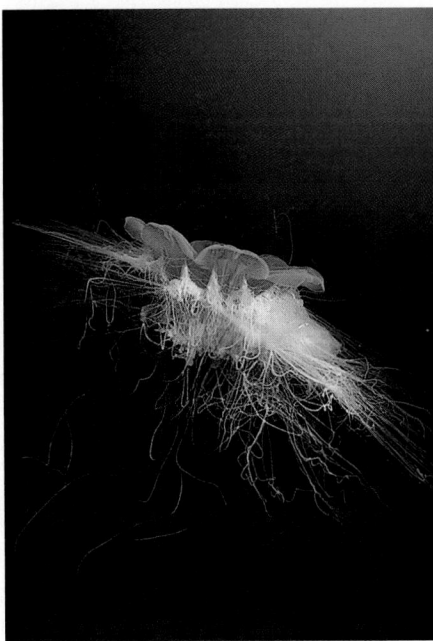

Figure 61-25 Lion's mane jellyfish *(Cyanea capillata)* can reach 3 m (10 feet) in diameter in Arctic waters. *(Photo by Norbert Wu.)*

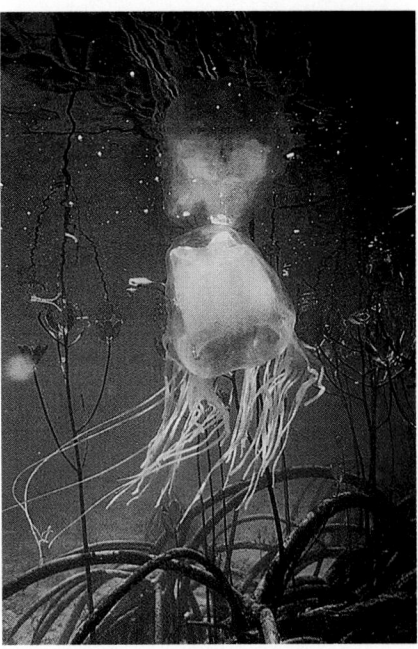

Figure 61-27 Box-jellyfish *(Chironex fleckeri)*, swimming just beneath the surface of the water. *(Courtesy John Williamson, MD.)*

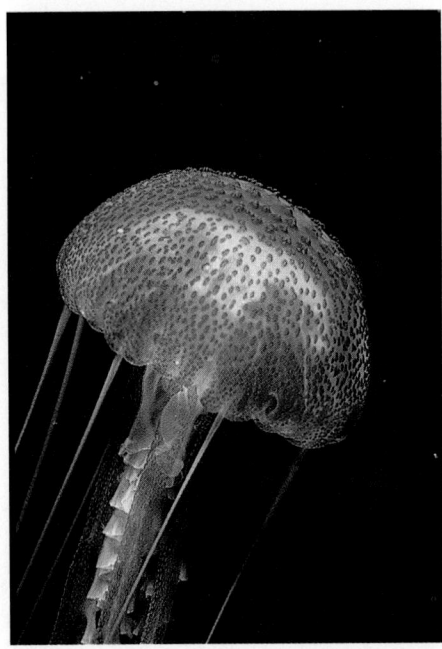

Figure 61-26 Mauve stinger *(Pelagia noctiluca)*. *(Courtesy Larry Madin, Woods Hole Oceanographic Institution.)*

number of cubomedusan ("box-shaped jellyfish") scyphozoans of highly toxic nature inhabit Indo-Pacific and, less frequently, Caribbean waters. These include *Carybdea rastoni* (jimble) and *C. marsupialis* (sea wasp), *Chiropsalmus quadrumanus* (box-jellyfish or sea wasp), *C. quadrigatus* (sea wasp), and *Chironex fleckeri* (box-

jellyfish). The "carybdeids" of order Carybdeidea have four tentacles only, whereas the "chirodropids" of order Chirodropidea may have up to 60 tentacles. All are frequently called "box-jellyfish."

CHIRONEX (BOX-JELLYFISH). The dreaded chirodropid box-jellyfish *(Chironex fleckeri* Southcott), often misnamed the "sea wasp," is the most venomous sea creature and can induce death in less than 60 seconds with its potent sting. Like all other scyphozoans, it is a carnivore, adapted to deal rapidly with prey. It is a member of the group of Cubomedusae jellyfish and ranges in size from 2 to 30 cm across the bell. Although these creatures seem to prefer quiet, protected, and shallow areas, chiefly in the waters off northern Queensland, Australia, they can be found in the open ocean. A seasonal alternation of polypoid and medusoid generations from winter to summer, respectively, appears to account for the shift in preferred habitat from tidal estuaries to the open eulittoral zone.[52] The "stinger season" in the Northern Territory of Australia is from October 1 to May 31.[28] Its presence precludes swimming and bathing in littoral and estuarine waters of Indonesia, Malaysia, and Northern Australia during this season, which coincides with the hottest tropical months in the southern hemisphere.[87] *Chironex* are fragile and photosensitive and thus are found submerged in bright sunlight (Figure 61-27), seeking the surface in the early morning, afternoon, and evening. They are swift and graceful travelers, capable of sailing along at a steady 2 knots.

An adult *Chironex* carries up to 15 broad tentacles (Figure 61-28) in each corner of its bell (up to 60 tentacles total, each with a length of up to 3 m [10 feet]) and has enough venom (in excess of 10 ml) to kill three adults.[110] Two fractions have been isolated from the venom: a "lethal" fraction of molecular weight 150,000, and a lethal-hemolytic-dermatonecrotic fraction of molecular weight 79,000. At least 72 fatalities have been verified in Australian and Southeast Asian waters, with greater numbers probably lacking official documentation. Thus the box-jellyfish is a much greater true hazard than the more fearsome shark. Other jellyfish, such as *Carybdea rastoni* and *Pelagia noctiluca,* infrequently cause severe prolonged reactions and have rarely been reported to lead to death but are capable of causing dramatic immediate reactions. Sudden death in a child has followed envenomation by *Chiropsalmus quadrumanus* in the Gulf of Mexico at Crystal Beach, Texas.[10] Death was attributed to acute arrhythmia after a catecholamine surge, followed by cardiogenic shock and pulmonary edema.

Clinical aspects. The extreme example of envenomation occurs with the chirodropid *Chironex* ("the assassin's hand") *fleckeri* (after Dr. Hugo Flecker).[87] Death is attributed to hypotension, profound muscle spasm, muscular and respiratory paralysis, and subsequent cardiac arrest. The overall mortality after box-jellyfish stings may approach 15% to 20% in selected locales.

Most commonly, bathers are stung, frequently aboriginal children in shallow and remote coastal waters who do not recognize the small, semitransparent, and submerged creature, which may approach as a member of a small armada. Most stings are minor; severe reactions or death follows skin contact with tentacles longer than 6 or 7 m (20 to 23 feet), although 10 cm of tentacle is capable of delivering a lethal dose of venom.[87,111] The sting is immediately excruciatingly painful, and the victim usually struggles purposefully for only a minute or two before collapse. The toxic skin reaction may be intense, with rapid formation of wheals, vesicles, and a darkened reddish brown or purple whiplike flare pattern with stripes 8 to 10 mm in width (Figure 61-29). With major stings, skin blistering occurs within 6 hours, with superficial necrosis in 12 to 18 hours (Figure 61-30). The skin defect(s) that result from a severe envenomation can be profound (Figure 61-31). On occasion a pathognomonic "frosted" appearance with a transverse cross-hatched pattern may be present (Figure 61-32). More severe reactions and increased mortality in women and small children have been attributed to greater hairless body surface area and smaller body mass.

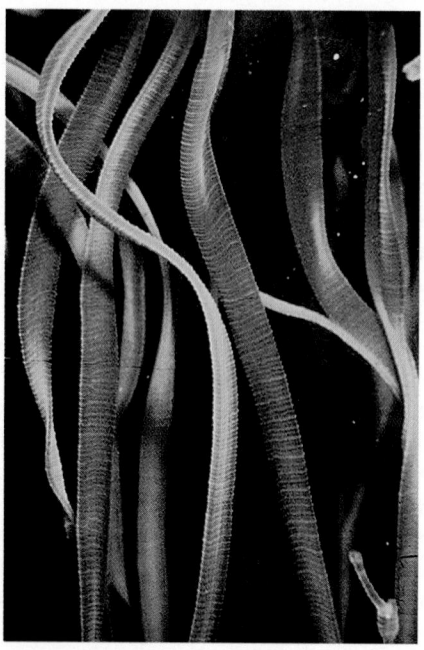

Figure 61-28 Close-up of the tentacle mass of an adult box-jellyfish *(Chironex fleckeri). (Courtesy Bob Hartwick.)*

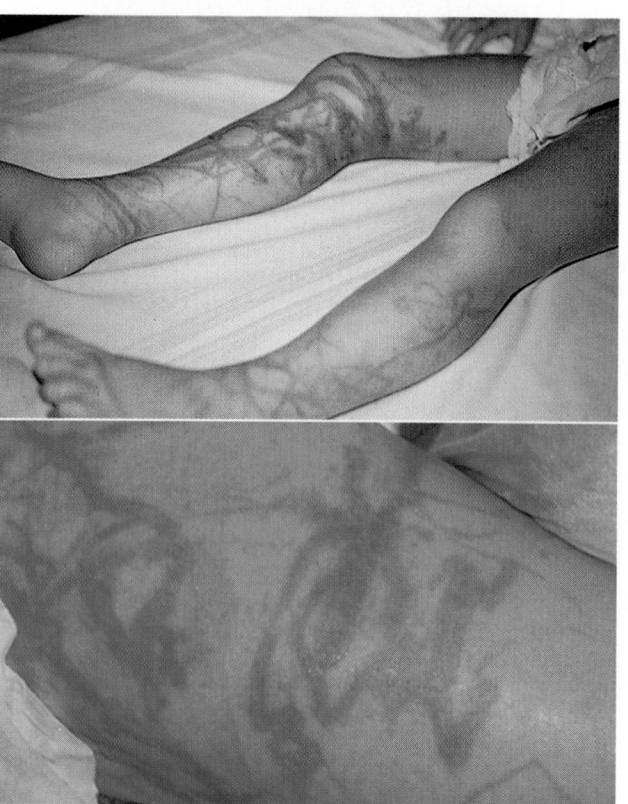

Figure 61-29 Intense necrosis (here at 48 hours) is typical of a severe box-jellyfish *(Chironex fleckeri)* sting. **A,** Involvement of nearly an entire limb. **B,** Skin darkening can be rapid with cellular death. *(A and B courtesy John Williamson, M.D.)*

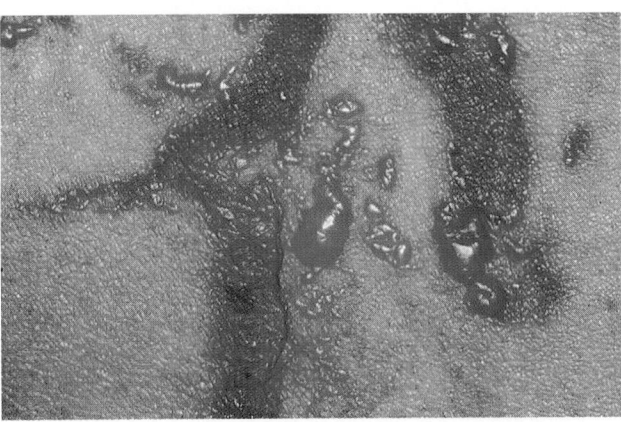

Figure 61-30 Incipient necrosis and blistering within 24 hours of box-jellyfish *(Chironex fleckeri)* envenomation. *(Courtesy John Williamson, MD.)*

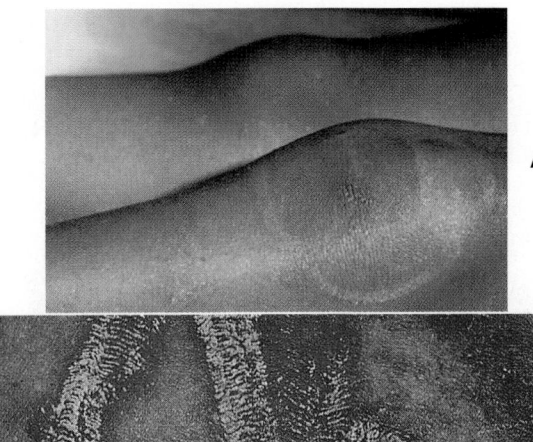

A

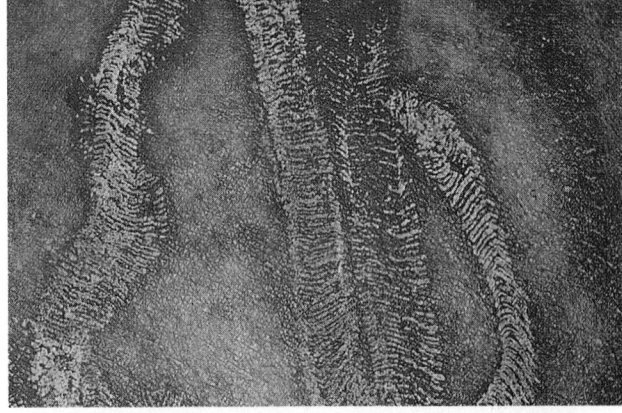

B

Figure 61-32 Frosted cross-hatched pattern pathognomonic for a box-jellyfish envenomation. **A,** The victim of this sting expired rapidly. **B,** The enhanced "frosted" appearance is a result of application of a spray of aluminum sulphate. (**A** and **B** *courtesy John Williamson, MD.)*

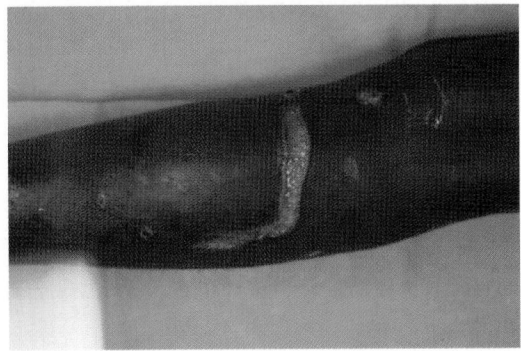

Figure 61-31 Skin destruction 3 weeks after an untreated box-jellyfish *(Chironex fleckeri)* envenomation. *(Courtesy John Williamson, MD.)*

Treatment. In the case of a known or suspected box-jellyfish envenomation, the victim must be assessed rapidly for adequacy of breathing and supported with an airway and artificial ventilation if necessary. The victim should be moved as little as possible. It is essential to immediately and liberally flood the skin surrounding any adherent tentacles with acetic acid 5% (vinegar) before any attempt is made to remove them; this paralyzes the nematocysts and avoids worsening the envenomation (Figure 61-33). Significant pain relief should not be expected from this maneuver. Although most nematocysts cannot penetrate the thickened skin of the human palm, the rescuer should pay particular attention to his or her own skin protection. If acetic acid is not available, aluminum sulfate surfactant (Stingose) may be used in substitution, although its efficacy has not been well demonstrated for a *Chironex* envenomation. A number of experts recommend that isopropyl alcohol not be used as a topical decontaminant for a box-jellyfish envenomation, based on in vitro observations of ineffi-

cacy and nematocyst discharge after application of this detoxicant.[53,111]

The pressure-immobilization bandaging technique (see Figure 39-2) can be used to prevent the absorption of *Chironex* venom and is applied after vinegar has been used to inactivate the nematocysts.[110,126] Pressure-immobilization is applied by taking a cloth or gauze pad of approximate dimensions 6 to 8 cm by 6 to 8 cm by 2 to 3 cm (thickness) and placing it directly over the bite. The pad is then held firmly in place by a circumferential bandage 15 to 18 cm wide applied at lymphatic-venous occlusive pressure (40 to 70 mm Hg for the upper extremity; 55 to 70 mm Hg for the lower extremity).[127] If the pad is not available, the wrap is applied without it. The arterial circulation should not be occluded, as determined by the detection of arterial pulsations and proper capillary refill. One hypothesis holds that the pressure-immobilization technique devascularizes the area immediately below the pad and prevents the distribution of venom into the general circulation.[5] After the wrap is applied, the limb should be splinted to prevent motion. The bandage should be released after the victim has been brought to proper medical attention and the rescuer is prepared to provide systemic support. It should be noted that pressure-immobilization is not uniformly recommended through-

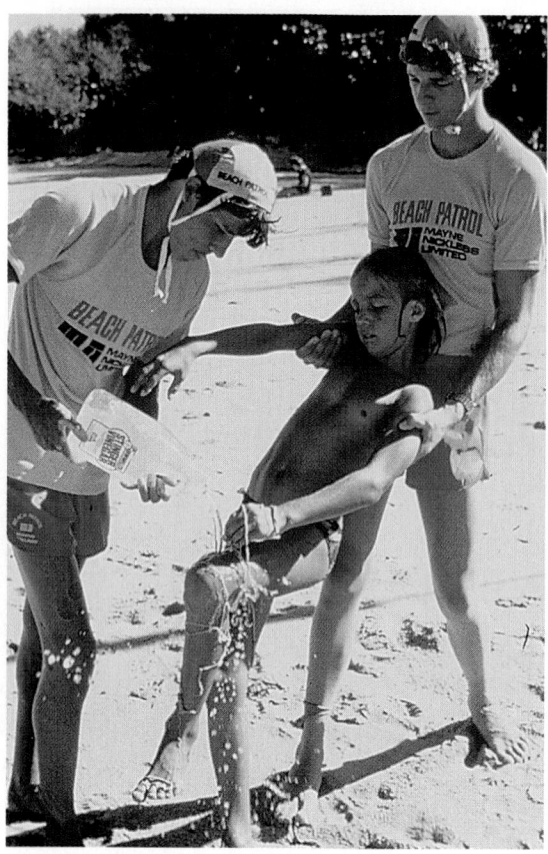

Figure 61-33 Surf lifesavers pour vinegar on the leg of a simulated box-jellyfish envenomation. Note how they restrain the victim's arms to prevent him from handling the harmful tentacles. *(Courtesy John Williamson, MD.)*

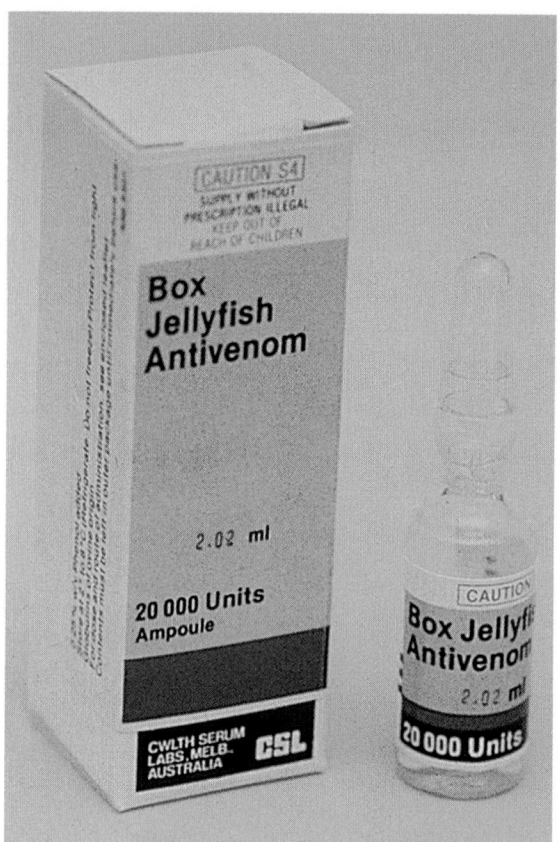

Figure 61-34 Box-jellyfish antivenom. *(Courtesy John Williamson, MD.)*

out Australia, since some have questioned its efficacy and have noted the fact that large affected skin surfaces cannot be effectively bandaged.

In the absence of the ability to apply a pressure-immobilization bandage, a rescuer might apply a constriction bandage proximal to the site of an extremity sting, to impede lymphatic and superficial venous return. Such a bandage should be loosened for 90 seconds every 10 minutes and should be completely removed after 1 hour. In no case should an arterial tourniquet be applied. Use of a proximal constriction band has not been proven to be helpful.

Chironex antivenom should be administered intravenously as soon as possible. The intramuscular route is less preferred. The antivenom is supplied in ampoules of 20,000 units by CSL (Figure 61-34). The initial dose is one ampoule (diluted 1:5 to 1:10 in isotonic crystalloid; dilution with water is not recommended) administered intravenously over 5 minutes, or three ampoules intramuscularly. This has been administered successfully over the years by members of the Queensland Surf Life-Saving Association and the Queensland Ambulance Transport Brigade. Although the an-

tivenom is prepared by hyperimmunizing sheep and adverse reactions reported to date have been rare and mild, the prudent physician is always prepared to treat anaphylaxis or serum sickness.[28] It cannot be overemphasized that the timely administration of antivenom can be lifesaving.[125] In addition to its lifesaving properties, the early administration of antivenom may markedly reduce pain and decrease subsequent skin scarring.[128] Antivenom administration may be repeated once or twice every 2 to 4 hours until there is no further worsening of the skin discoloration, pain, or systemic effects. A large sting in an adult may require the initial administration of up to three ampoules IV. The antivenom may also used to neutralize the effects of a *Chiropsalmus* envenomation.[110] The antivenom should be stored in a refrigerator at 2° to 10° C (35.6° to 50° F) and must not be frozen.[22] The concomitant administration of a glucocorticoid (such as hydrocortisone 200 mg intravenously) is often recommended for its antiinflammatory activity but is no substitute for the administration of antivenom.

Even with successful treatment, skin irritation may persist for months, marked by discolored striae, intermittent desquamation, and pruritus. Burnett and Calton[16] discovered that verapamil can prolong the life of mice challenged with box-jellyfish, sea nettle, or Portuguese man-of-war venom. It was considered to be inactive or deleterious in anaesthetized laboratory pigs envenomed with box-jellyfish venom.[117] To date, extrapolation of these data to the human condition is as yet untested. Although there is logic to using verapamil from a theoretic pharmacologic perspective (venom affects calcium influx through voltage-dependent channels), the suitability of using verapamil as an adjunct to therapy in humans has been questioned because of the perceived problem of administering a hypotensive agent during an episode of cardiac decompensation.[55] Further information and opinions about the use of verapamil will undoubtedly be forthcoming.

IRUKANDJI. *Carukia barnesii,* the carybdeid jellyfish known as "Irukandji," is a small (1 to 2.5 cm across the bell) translucent jellyfish with four thin nematocyst-covered tentacles (2.5 to 4.5 cm in length at rest, and up to 65 cm extended) found off the coast of northern Australia in both inshore and open waters.[8,106] Most stings occur near shore and during the afternoon.[3,87] Because the jellyfish tend to aggregate, victims often present in clusters. After causing a severe immediate skin reaction characterized by pain and erythema without wheal formation, the venom may induce muscle pain and spasm, back pain, abdominal pain, parasympathetic dysautonomia, respiratory difficulty, headache, nausea, and vomiting, which progress to profound weakness and collapse.[40] Localized piloerection and sweating have been reported. Generally the discomfort remits in 6 to 24 hours; however, it occasionally recurs. The "Irukandji syndrome" presupposes massive catecholamine release, with abdominal and chest pain, vomiting, diaphoresis, hypertension (diastolic blood pressure to 140 mm Hg), tachycardia, severe pulmonary edema, and hypokinetic heart failure.[35,72] This resembles what might be seen with a pheochromocytoma. Papilledema and coma in a child have been described. Although the systemic syndrome can be quite distinctive, there can be minimal cutaneous signs of envenomation.[50] To date, death has not been reported. It is interesting to note that many Irukandji-like stings occur inside "stinger enclosures" (bathing nets) designed to exclude *Chironex fleckeri.* Other carybdeid medusae that envenom with lesser severity include the jimble (*Carybdea rastoni*) and fire jelly (*Tamoya haplonema*). The morbakka is a stinging creature that resembles the Irukandji but is larger. The bell, which measures up to 16 by 12 cm, is covered with clumps of nematocysts and may be as dangerous to handle as the meter-long tentacles. This animal may have been previously misidentified as *Tamoya.*

CHRYSAORA (SEA NETTLE). Sea nettles (such as *Chrysaora quinquecirrha* and *Cyanea capillata*) are considerably less lethal animals and can be found in both temperate and tropical waters, particularly in Chesapeake Bay, where they are found in seasonal "plague" proportions.[77] Not as dangerous as the Indo-Pacific box-jellyfish, they are still capable of inducing a moderately severe sting. *Chrysaora quinquecirrha* and similar species carry a proteinaceous venom that contains at least seven enzymes, with at least one antigenic and thermolabile component that is cardiotoxic, neurotoxic, and dermatonecrotic. The venom also contains histamine, histamine releasers, prostaglandins, serotonin, and kininlike factors; the last mentioned have also been found in venoms of *Chironex fleckeri* and *Physalia physalis.*[14] Large intradermal injections of crude sea nettle venom in normal saline produced immunosuppression (T cells) for several days, which was homologous against the same coelenterate antigen and heterologous against antigens contained within vaccinia and herpes simplex viruses and tetanus bacillus.[120]

Clinical aspects. The clinical presentation of a sea nettle envenomation is similar to that of *Physalia* species, with perhaps a greater incidence of systemic complications. Death is exceedingly rare. Elevated levels of serum anti–sea nettle venom IgM, IgG, and IgE may persist for years in victims who suffer exaggerated reactions to *Chrysaora quinquecirrha* stings. These antibodies cross-react with *Physalia* venom and have been postulated to be of value in identifying victims at risk for a severe reaction.[15] Currently this technique is not widely available or frequently used, and its reliability and reproducibility require further verification.

The reaction after a sting by the blubber jellyfish (*Catostylus* species) is relatively mild, with the formation of wheals, erythema, and pruritus limited to the areas of contact. Systemic effects are exceedingly rare. *Cyanea* species carry long thin tentacles that induce a similar effect, with occasional muscle aching, nausea, and drowsiness, particularly in small children. Pelagia species also induce wheals, which are more circinate or irregularly shaped and may not follow a linear pattern. The venom is sufficiently toxic to cause severe generalized allergy, with bronchospasm and pruritus.

Treatment. Treatment for a sea nettle envenomation is similar to that for the sting of *Physalia* species. Baking soda may be the most effective commonly available initial detoxicant.[35] Monoclonal antibodies to jellyfish venoms have been developed that demonstrate cross-reactivity among venoms of a variety of coelenterates, which may allow the development of a single protective antivenom or vaccine.

Anthozoa. The class Anthozoa includes the sea anemones, stony (true) corals (Zooantharia), and the soft corals (Alcyonaria). The anemones are considered here because they envenom.

ACTINARIA (ANEMONES). Actinarians (sea anemones) are abundant (1000 species) multicolored animals with sessile habits and a flowerlike appearance. They are composed of stalked, fingerlike projections capable of stinging and paralyzing passing fish. Their sizes range from a few millimeters to more than 0.5 m; they are found at depths of up to 2900 fathoms. The insides of some anemones can be eaten after they are dried.

Anemones can be colorful creatures and found in tidal pools, where the unwary brush up against them or inquisitively touch them. Other anemones burrow into bottom mud or sand. Like other coelenterates, they possess tentacles loaded with one of two variations of the nematocyst, either the sporocyst or the basitrichous isorhiza (basitrich). These wreak havoc once stimulated by an unfortunate victim. Some sporocysts are adhesive and act to hold and to envenom the prey. When an exposed anemone wishes to present a greater number of nematocysts to the victim, it inflates the tentacles by filling them with water. Many anemones also secrete mucous, which covers the anemone's body and may contain cytolytic and hemolytic protein toxins. These may serve to repel potential predators.

Although a number of sea animals, such as clownfish (anemonefish) of the genera *Amphiprion* and *Premnas*, live in symbiosis with certain anemones (*Heteractis* spp., *Stichodactyla* spp., *Macrodactyla doreensis*, *Entacmaea quadricolor*, and *Cryptodendrum adhaesivum*), humans are not so fortunate and are frequently stung when attempting to handle these not so delicate "flowers." The clownfish have evolved resistance to the anemone's sting by repeated contact and development of a mucous coat (Figure 61-35), and perhaps by immunity.[75]

Sea anemones contain biologically active substances, including neurotoxins (sodium channel interaction), cardiotoxins, hemolysins (for erythrocytes and platelets), and proteinase inhibitors.[76,102] A cytolytic toxin has been isolated from the Indo-Pacific sea anemone *Stoichactis kenti*.[11] The anemone *Actinia equina* elaborates cytolytic polypeptide toxins known as equinatoxins, which may induce hemolysis and cardiorespiratory arrest in animals, attributed by some to coronary vasospasm.[68] Tenebrosin-C from the anemone *Actinia tenebrosa* is a positive inotrope that can be inhibited by the cyclooxygenase blockers indomethacin and aspirin, a lipooxygenase blocker and leukotriene antagonist, and mepacrine (a phospholipase A_2 inhibitor).[41] Potassium channel toxins have been isolated from the sea anemones *Bundosoma granulifera* and *Stichodactyla helianthus*.[54] Cytolytic toxins elaborated by anemones include "cytolysins," which are thought to

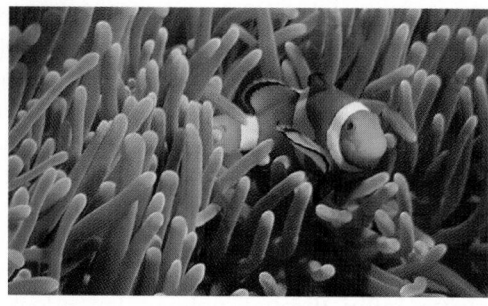

Figure 61-35 Clownfish in peaceful coexistence with a sea anemone. (Photo by Kenneth Kizer, MD.)

exert their effect by damaging membranes via pore or channel formation.

Clinical aspects. Most victims are stung when they handle or accidentally brush against an anemone in shallow water. Nudists may acquire genital injuries; small children may accidentally or intentionally ingest tentacles. The dermatitis caused by contact with an anemone is similar in all regards to that from fire coral or a small man-of-war; it is often likened to a bee sting. The variation in skin reaction is related to the specific toxicity of the venom, so that although *Actinia* species produce painful urticarial lesions, *Anemonia* species induce paresthesias, edema, and erythema.[64] Most commonly the initial skin lesion is centrally pale with a halo of erythema and petechial hemorrhage. This is soon followed by edema and diffuse ecchymosis. If the envenomation is severe, intense local hemorrhage, vesiculation, necrosis, skin ulceration, and secondary infection may occur, particularly after the stings of certain species (*Sagartia, Actinia, Anemonia, Actinodendron,* and *Triactis*). In Floridian waters, the turtle grass anemone *Viatrix globulifera*, translucent-white and less than 1 inch in diameter, is very hazardous, particularly for fishermen wading on grass flats. The Hell's fire sea anemone (*Actinodendron plumosum*) is aptly named. Systemic reactions are less likely after the sting of an anemone than after that of a man-of-war; reactions include fever, chills, somnolence, malaise, weakness, nausea, vomiting, and syncope. Fulminant fatal hepatic failure 3 days after a sea anemone sting of approximately 3 cm diameter upon the scapula and complicated by coma, severe coagulopathy, and renal failure has been attributed to *Condylactis* (Figure 61-36; commonly found in reefs and lagoons of south Florida, the Bahamas, and the Caribbean) on the basis of a positive serum test of IgG by ELISA at a dilution of 1:450.[42]

In most cases, mild envenomations resolve within 48 hours. More severe reactions, characterized by discoloration and vesicle formation, may become indolent, with eschar leading to residual hyperpigmentation, hypopigmentation, or keloid formation.

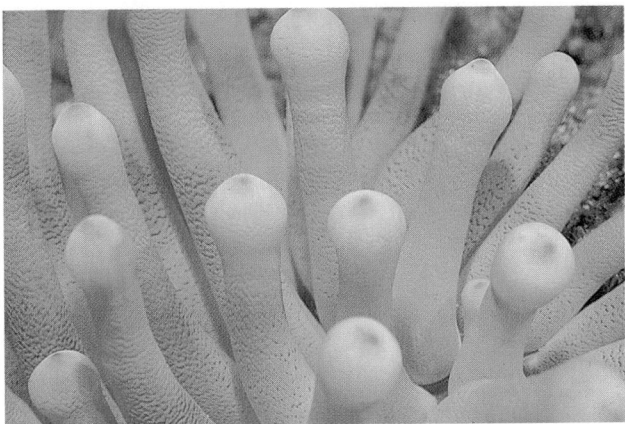

Figure 61-36 Giant anemone *(Condylactis gigantea). (Photo by Norbert Wu.)*

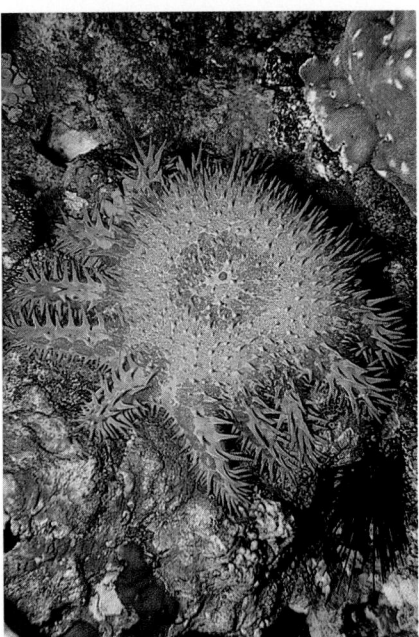

Figure 61-37 Crown-of-thorns starfish *(Acanthaster planci). (Photo by Paul Auerbach, MD.)*

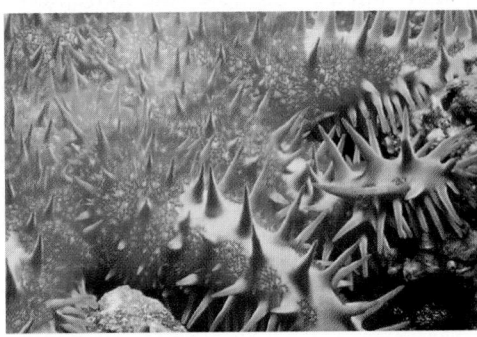

Figure 61-38 Spines of the crown-of-thorns starfish *(Acanthaster planci). (Photo by Paul Auerbach, MD.)*

Sponge fisherman's (diver's) disease is caused by contact with an anemone *(Sagartia* or *Actinia)* that attaches itself symbiotically to the base of a sponge. A few minutes after contact with the sponge, the victim's skin begins to itch and burn, with development of erythema and small vesicles. As described previously, this transforms to a darkened purple appearance, with frequent systemic components (headache, nausea, vomiting, fever, chills, and muscle spasm).

Treatment. Treatment for an anemone envenomation is similar to that for the sting of *Physalia* species. The dermatitis is frequently more severe and may require prolonged wound care consisting of debridement and antibiotic therapy for secondary infection. The healing process is generally slower after an anemone sting than after a man-of-war envenomation.

Echinodermata

The phylum Echinodermata ("spiny skin") has five classes: sea lilies, brittle stars, starfish, sea urchins, and sea cucumbers. Only the last three are of human medical interest, although some brittle stars carry toxins capable of causing paralysis and death in small animals.

Starfish

LIFE AND HABITS. Starfish are simple, free-living, and stellate echinoderms covered with thorny spines of calcium carbonate crystals held erect by muscle tissue. The creatures move upon the ocean floor by means of tube feet located under the arms (rays). They eat other echinoderms, mollusks, coral, worms, and poisonous shellfish. Starfish proliferation and destruction of coral beds within the Great Barrier Reef off the coast of Australia is a conservation issue of international concern. The starfish everts its membranous stomach through its mouth and secretes digestive enzymes that destroy coral polyps. Only the stark white coral skeleton remains. The crown-of-thorns starfish *(Acanthaster planci)* is found in the coral reef communities of the Great Barrier Reef, throughout the Pacific and Indian Oceans, in the Red Sea, and in the Gulf of California.

VENOM AND VENOM APPARATUS. Glandular tissue interspersed in or underneath the epidermis (integument) produces a slimy venomous substance. The carnivorous *Acanthaster planci* is a particularly venomous species normally 25 to 35 cm in diameter, which attains sizes of up to 70 cm in diameter, with 7 to 23 arms (Figure 61-37). The sharp, rigid, and venomous aboral spines of this animal may grow to 4 to 6 cm (Figure 61-38). Potentially toxic saponins and histamine-like compounds have been isolated from the spine surfaces; crude venom extracts demonstrate hemolytic, capillary permeability increasing, myotoxic (phospholipase A_2), myonecrotic, and anticoagulant effects. *A. planci* lethal factor is a potent hepatotoxin in laboratory animals.[103] "Plancinin" is an anticoagulant purified from the crown-of-thorns starfish. This peptide shows activity in mice that suggests a longer duration of action than heparin.[60] Severe systemic hypotension, thrombocytopenia, and leukopenia were induced by *A. planci* venom in dogs.[104] Indomethacin, a cyclooxygenase inhibitor, suppressed the hypotension. *A. planci* venom caused smooth (uterine) muscle contraction in rats, which was blocked by inhibitors of prostaglandin synthesis but not by atropine.[59]

Other starfish that might envenom humans are those of genus *Echinaster*. The slime (cushion) star *Pteraster tessalatus*, which inhabits Pacific coastal waters from Puget Sound to Alaska, generates the unique defense of copious gelatinous or rubbery, poisonous mucus to repel natural enemies. No human injuries have been reported to date.

CLINICAL ASPECTS. The ice pick–like spine of *Acanthaster planci* can penetrate the hardiest of diving gloves. Most spines are composed of porous crystalline magnesium calcite, articulated at the base and extremely sharp, with three raised cutting edges at the tips. As the spine enters the skin, it carries venom into the wound, with immediate pain, copious bleeding, and mild edema. The pain is generally moderate and self-limited, with remission over a period of $1/2$ to 3 hours. The wound may become dusky or discolored. Multiple puncture wounds may result in acute systemic reactions, including paresthesias, nausea, vomiting, lymphadenopathy, and muscular paralysis. If a spine fragment is retained, a granulomatous lesion may develop akin to that from a sea urchin puncture wound. If the victim has been previously sensitized, he or she may suffer a prolonged reaction lasting for weeks and consisting of local edema and pruritus. Contact with other less injurious starfish may induce a pruritic papulourticarial eruption (irritant contact dermatitis).

TREATMENT. Immersion therapy may provide some relief from the pain. The wound should immediately be immersed into nonscalding hot water to tolerance (45° C [113° F]) for 30 to 90 minutes or until there is significant pain relief. The pain is rarely severe enough to require local anesthetic infiltration. The puncture wound should be irrigated and explored to remove all foreign material. Because of the stout nature of the spines, it is rare to retain a fragment. However, if any question of a foreign body exists, a soft tissue radiograph often identifies the fractured spine. Not infrequently the victim suffers an indolent contact dermatitis from handling a starfish, such as *Solaster papposus*, the sun (Figure 61-39)

or rose star. The dermatitis may be managed in standard fashion with topical solutions, such as calamine with 0.5% menthol, or a corticosteroid preparation. Systemic therapy is supportive. Granulomas from retained spine fragments may require excision. Starfish that have ingested poisonous shellfish are themselves toxic on ingestion.

Sea Urchins

LIFE AND HABITS. Sea urchins are free-living echinoderms that have an egg-shaped, globular, or flattened body. A hard skeleton (test) comprised of fused calcareous plates surrounds the viscera and is covered by regularly arranged spines and triple-jawed (pincerlike) pedicellariae, the latter of which (globiferous, or glandular) are sometimes used for defense. Urchins are nocturnal and omnivorous (mostly in pursuit of algae) eaters yet are shy, nonaggressive, and slow-moving animals found on rocky bottoms or burrowed in sand and crevices (Figure 61-40). Their bathymetric range extends from the intertidal zone to great depths. The raw or cooked gonads of several species are eaten as great delicacies by humans.

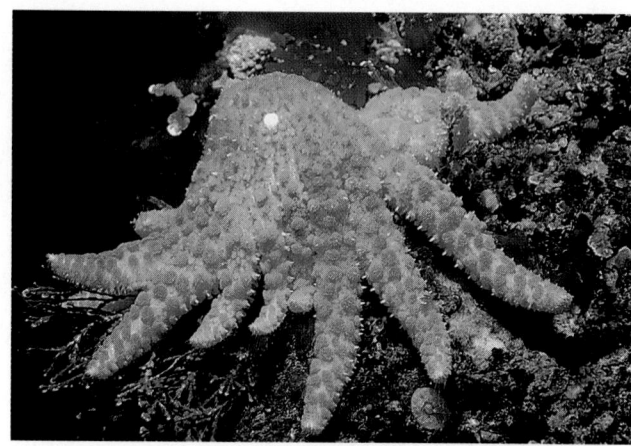

Figure 61-39 Sun starfish *(Solaster)*. *(Photo by Norbert Wu.)*

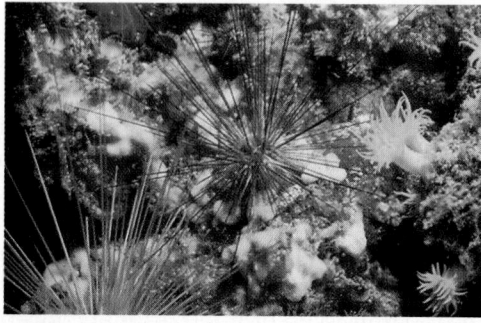

Figure 61-40 Needlelike spines of sea urchins in their natural habitat. *(Photo by Kenneth Kizer, MD.)*

VENOM AND VENOM APPARATUS. The venom apparatuses of sea urchins consist of the hollow, venom-filled spines and the triple-jawed globiferous pedicellariae. Venom may also be released from within a thin integumentary sheath on the external surface of the spines of certain urchins.

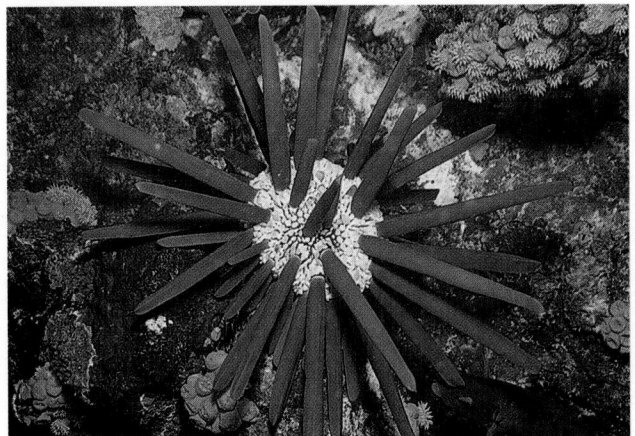

Figure 61-41 Nontoxic "pencil" urchin with blunt, rounded tips. *(Photo by Paul Auerbach, MD.)*

The spines of sea urchins, formed by the calcification of a cylindrical projection of subepidermal connective tissue, may either be non–venom-bearing, with solid blunt and rounded tips (Figure 61-41), or venom-bearing (such as families Echinothuridae and Diadematidae), with hollow, long, slender, and sharp needles (Figure 61-42). These are extremely dangerous to handle; the spines, which are attached to the shell with a modified ball-and-socket joint, are brittle and break off easily in the flesh, lodging deeply and making removal difficult. They are keen enough to penetrate rubber gloves and fins. *Diadema setosum* (black sea urchin) spines may exceed 1 foot in length. *Echinothrix* species also carry lengthy spines. The purple sea urchin *Strongylocentrotus purpuratus* (Figure 62-43) of California has much shorter spines. The genera *Asthenosoma* and *Aerosoma* have special venom organs (sacs) on the sharp tips of the aboral spines, which introduce the potent venom.

Pedicellariae are small, delicate seizing organs attached to the stalks scattered among the spines. These are considered to be modified spines with flexible heads.[97] Globiferous pedicellariae are typified by those found in *Toxopneustes pileolus* (flower urchin) (Figure

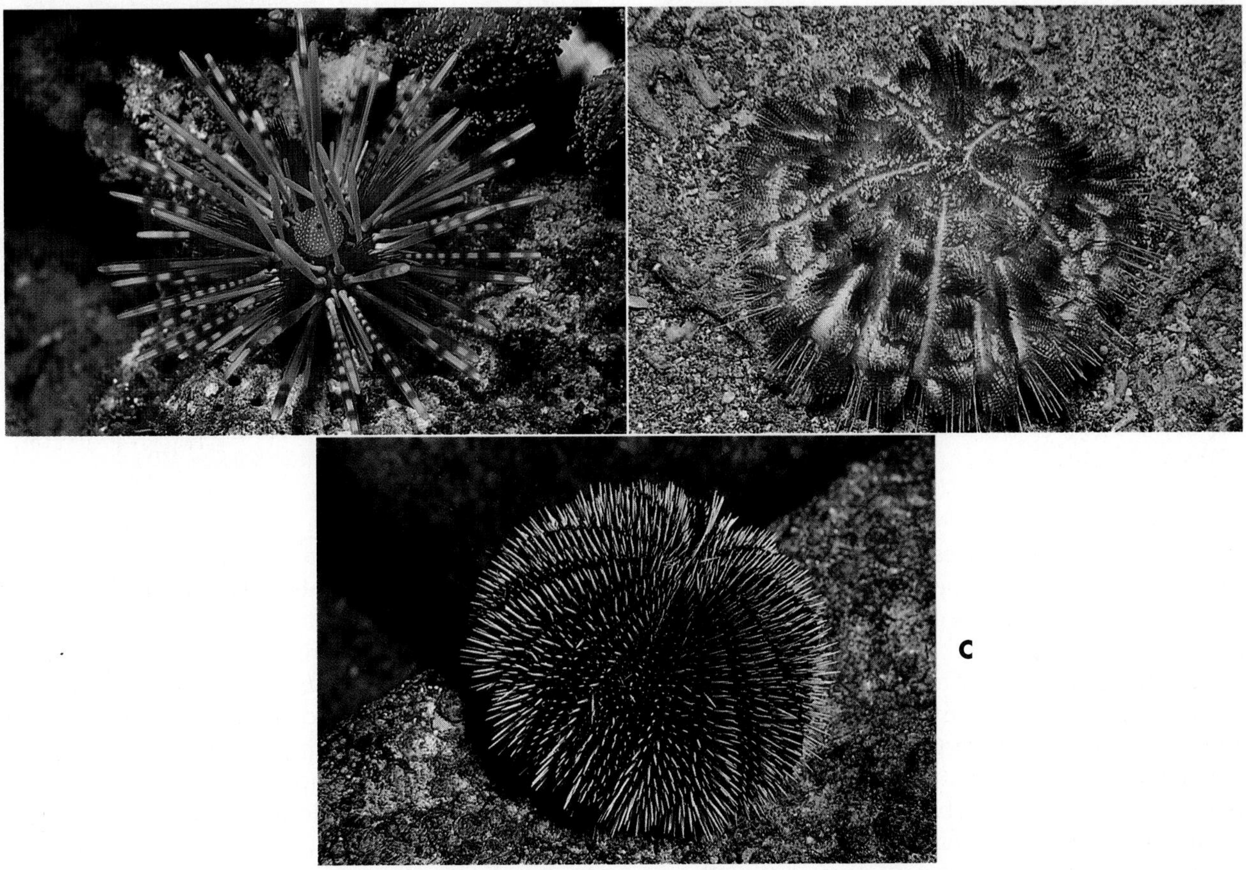

Figure 61-42 Three examples of sharp-spined (venomous) sea urchins. *(Photos by Paul Auerbach, MD.)*

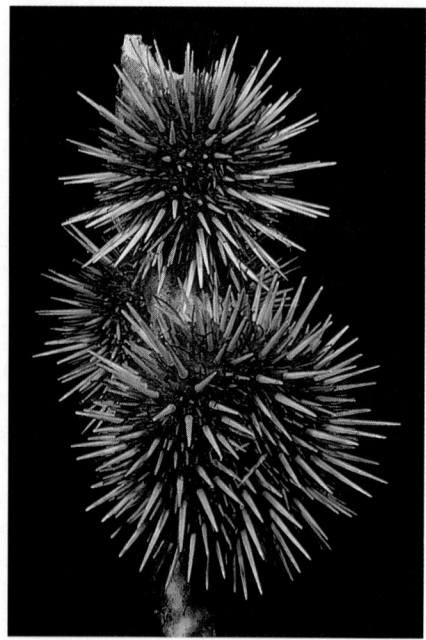

Figure 61-43 Purple sea urchins. *(Photo by Howard Hall.)*

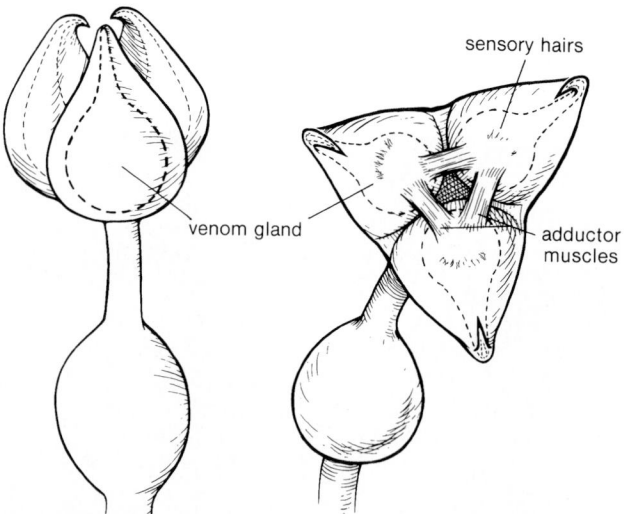

Figure 61-45 Globiferous pedicellaria of a sea urchin, used to hold and envenom prey.

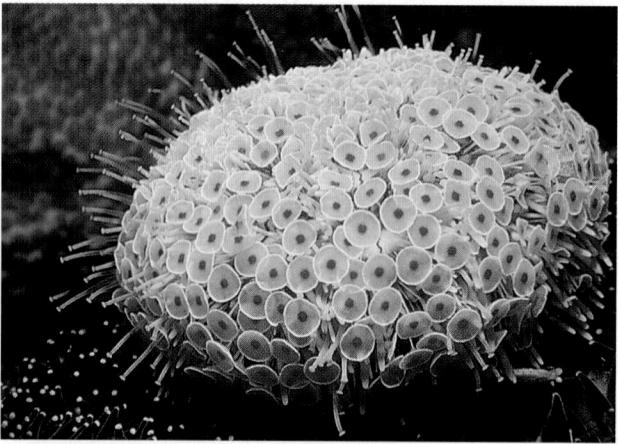

Figure 61-44 Flower urchin *(Toxopneustes pileolus)*. *(Photo by Ken Kizer, MD.)*

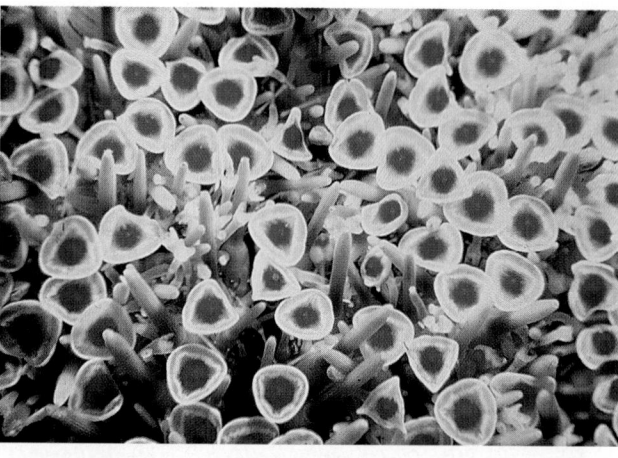

Figure 61-46 Close-up of opened flower urchin *(Toxopneustes pileolus)* pedicellariae seeking prey. *(Photo by Ken Kizer, MD.)*

61-44) and *Tripneustes* species and have globe-shaped heads which contain the venom organs (Figure 61-45). The terminal head, with its calcareous pincer jaws (2 to 4; usually 3), is attached by the stalk to the shell plates of the sea urchin. The outer surface of each opened "jaw" is covered by a large venom gland, which is triggered to contract with the jaw on contact. When the sea urchin is at rest in the water, the jaws are extended, slowly moving about (Figure 61-46). Anything that touches them is seized. As long as the object is moving, the pedicellariae continue to bite and envenom. Once a pedicellaria attaches to a victim, it will be torn from the shell rather than let go. Detached pedicellariae may remain active for several hours. The *Toxopneustes* sea urchin also has solid spines, but these are nonvenomous.

The venom of sea urchins contains various toxic fractions, including steroid glycosides, hemolysins, proteases, serotonin, and cholinergic substances. The Pacific *Tripneustes* urchin carries a neurotoxin with a predilection for facial and cranial nerves. A toxic substance from the sea urchin *Toxopneustes pileolus* induces histamine release from rat peritoneal mast cells.[115] Contractin A from the pedicellariae of the same species causes contraction of isolated guinea pig tracheal smooth muscle.[81]

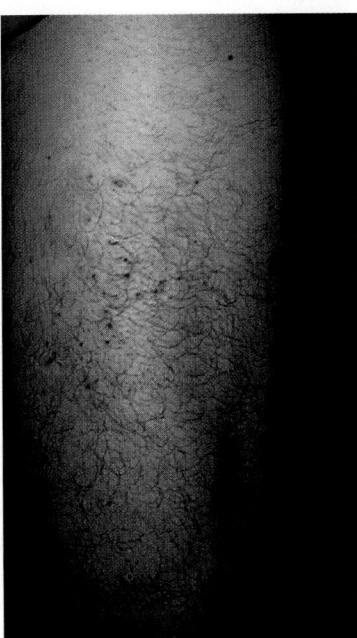

Figure 61-47 Thigh of the author demonstrating multiple sea urchin punctures from black sea urchins *(Diadema).* Within 24 hours, the black markings were absent, indicative of spine dye without residual spines. *(Photo by Ken Kizer, MD.)*

CLINICAL ASPECTS. Most victims are envenomed when they step on, handle, or brush up against a sea urchin. Because the creatures tend to be nocturnal, divers are most commonly injured in dark waters during night diving activities, particularly in small caves or in shallow turbulent waters. Young inquisitive children who explore tidepools frequently handle urchins incorrectly and may be injured. If a diver moves his or her hand slowly toward a spiny (venomous) sea urchin, the spines may align to offer the greatest defense.

Venomous spines inflict immediate and intensely painful stings. The pain is initially characterized by burning, which rapidly evolves into severe local muscle aching with visible erythema and swelling of the skin surrounding the puncture site or sites. Frequently a spine breaks off and lodges in the victim. Some sea urchin spines (such as those of *Diadema setosum* or *Strongylocentrotus purpuratus*) contain purplish dye, which may give a false impression of spines left in the skin (Figure 61-47). Soft tissue density x-ray techniques or magnetic resonance imaging may reveal a radiopaque foreign body. If a spine enters a joint, it may rapidly induce severe synovitis. If multiple spines have penetrated the skin, particularly if they are deeply embedded, systemic symptoms may rapidly develop, including nausea, vomiting, paresthesias, numbness and muscular paralysis, abdominal pain, syncope, hypotension, and respiratory distress. The presence of a frank neuropathy may indicate that the spine has lodged in contact with a peripheral nerve. The pain from multiple stings may be sufficient to cause delirium. Secondary infections and indolent ulceration are common. A delayed hypersensitivity-type reaction ("flare-up") at the site of the puncture(s) has been described, in which the victim demonstrates erythema and pruritus in a delayed fashion (7 to 10 days) after primary resolution from the initial envenomation.[3] The sensitizing antigen in such cases has yet to be identified.

Two separate unusual cases were reported in 1993 to me by neurologists. In each case the victim sustained multiple punctures from one or several black sea urchins in Hawaiian waters. The immediate clinical reaction was typical, but it was followed in 6 to 10 days by severe bulbar polyneuritis with respiratory insufficiency. In one case the victim was hyporeflexic and appeared to suffer a Guillain-Barré variation with elevated protein levels in cerebrospinal fluid; in the other, the victim manifested meningoencephalitis documented by magnetic resonance imaging. The relationship to the urchin stings suggests an autoimmune phenomenon.

A spine that enters a finger in proximity to the nail apparatus may cause a subungual or periungual granulomatous nodular lesion. Excision may cause permanent nail plate dystrophy.

The stings of pedicellariae are often of greater magnitude, causing immediate intense radiating pain, local edema and hemorrhage, malaise, weakness, paresthesias, hypesthesia, arthralgias, aphonia, dizziness, syncope, generalized muscular paralysis, respiratory distress, hypotension, and, rarely, death. In some cases the pain may disappear within the first hour, whereas the localized muscular weakness or paralysis persists for up to 6 hours.

TREATMENT. The envenomed body part should immediately be immersed in nonscalding hot water (upper limit 45° C [113° F]) to tolerance for 30 to 90 minutes in an attempt to relieve pain. Any pedicellariae still attached to the skin must be removed or envenomation will continue. This may be accomplished by applying shaving foam and gently scraping with a razor. Embedded spines should be removed with care because they easily fracture. Black or purplish discoloration surrounding the wound after spine removal is often merely spine dye and therefore may be of no consequence. Although some thin venomous spines may be absorbed within 24 hours to 3 weeks, it is best to remove those that are easily reached. All thick spines (calcium carbonate, magnesium carbonate, and silica) should be removed because of the risk of infection, foreign body encaseation granuloma, or dermoid inclusion cyst. External percussion to achieve fragmentation may prove disastrous if a chronic inflammatory process is initiated in sensitive tissue of the hand or foot. If the spines have acutely entered joints or are closely aligned to neurovascular structures, the surgeon should take advantage of an operating microscope in an appropriate setting to remove all spine fragments. The extraction should be performed as soon as possible after the injury. If the spine has entered an interphalangeal joint, the finger should be splinted until the spine is removed to limit fragmentation and further penetration. This also may control the fusiform finger swelling (Figure 61-48) commonly noted after a puncture in the vicinity of the middle or proximal interphalangeal joint. It is inappropriate to rummage about in a hand wound in the emergency department, virtually looking for a needle in a haystack. If the presence of a spine is in question, soft tissue density radiographic techniques for a radiopaque foreign body may be diagnostic. Magnetic resonance imaging (Figure 61-49) may be quite useful to locate spine fragments. Although the calcium carbonate is relatively inert, it is accompanied by slime,

bacteria, and organic epidermal debris. Therefore secondary infections are common (Figure 61-50) and deep puncture wounds are an indication for prophylactic antibiotics.

Some sea urchin spines are phagocytosed in the soft tissues and ultimately dissolve. The granulomas caused by retained sea urchin spine fragments have sarcoidal histologic features and generally appear as flesh- or dye-colored surface or subcuticular nodules 2 to 12 months after the initial injury (Figure 61-51).[95] In thin-skinned areas these nodules are erythematous and rubbery, painless, and infrequently umbilicated. In thicker-skinned areas (palms, soles, and knees) that are frequently abraded, they have a keratinized appearance. Although necrosis and microabscess formation may be evident microscopically, suppuration is unusual. Rarely, the destructive nature of the inflamma-

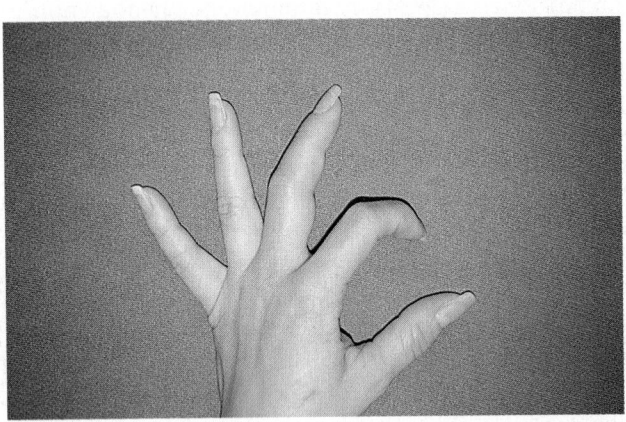

Figure 61-48 Finger swelling from sea urchin puncture. A single spine entered the palm over the mid third metacarpal bone. Swelling was severe in the second and third digits. *(Photo by Paul Auerbach, MD.)*

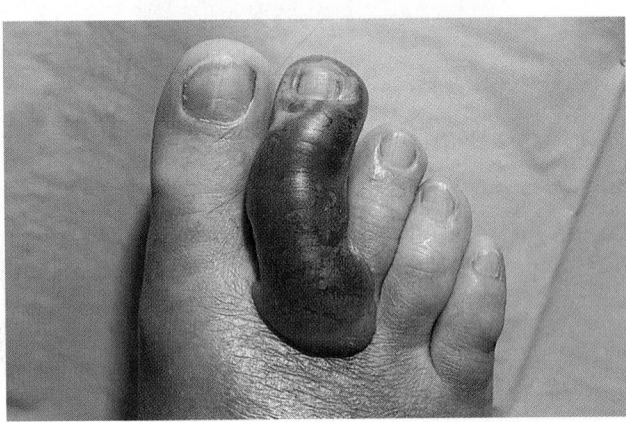

Figure 61-50 Infection after sea urchin puncture. The rapid onset, gas-containing hemorrhagic blister, and severe cellulitis with sepsis are common features of infection with *Vibrio* species. *(Photo by Paul Auerbach, MD.)*

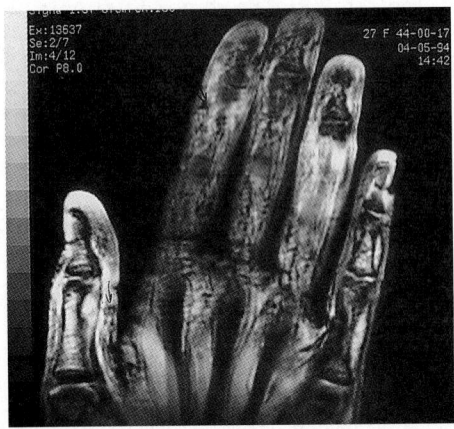

Figure 61-49 Magnetic resonance imaging of the hand of a victim of multiple sea urchin spine punctures, demonstrating the presence of spine fragments in the soft tissues. *(Photo by Paul Auerbach, MD.)*

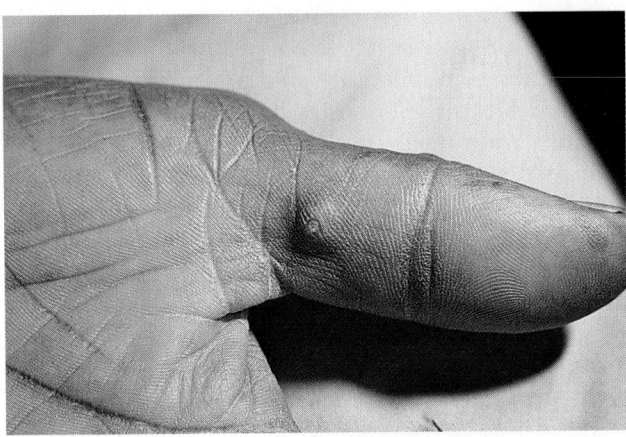

Figure 61-51 Subcuticular nodule after sea urchin puncture. *(Photo by Paul Auerbach, MD.)*

tory process may be severe enough to necessitate amputation of a digit. If a spine cannot be removed and becomes a nidus for cyst or granuloma formation, the lesion may be removed surgically. Intralesional injection with a corticosteroid (triamcinolone hexacetonide 5 mg/ml) is less efficacious but may be successful. Systemic antiinflammatory drugs may be minimally helpful but are not substitutes for removal of the spine. A diffuse delayed reaction, consisting of cyanotic induration, fusiform swelling in the digits, and focal phalangeal bony erosion, may be treated with a systemic corticosteroid and antibiotics.

Sea Cucumbers

LIFE AND HABITS. Sea cucumbers are free-living worm- or sausage-shaped bottom feeders of diverse external patterns (Figure 61-52) and coloration that are essentially scavengers. They are cosmopolitan in distribution, found in both shallow and deep waters. Cucumbers are harvested as a food (trepang, bêche-de-mer) in the South Pacific.

VENOM AND VENOM APPARATUS. Cucumbers produce in their body walls a visceral cantharidin-like liquid toxin ("holothurin"). Holothurin is concentrated in the tentacular organs of Cuvier, which can be projected and extended anally when the animal mounts a defense (Figure 61-53). Toxic genera include *Actinopyga*, *Stichopus*, and *Holothuria*. Some cucumbers dine on nematocysts and thus can secrete coelenterate venom as well.

CLINICAL ASPECTS. Holothurin may induce contact dermatitis when the tentacular organs directly contact the skin. Generally the substance is diluted in the surrounding ocean water and the reaction is minimal. However, persons who dissect sea cucumbers topside

in the preparation of food products may inadvertently handle the toxin and develop a papular skin irritation. The major risk underwater is to the corneas and conjunctivae, which may become intensely inflamed if directly contacted by tentacular fragments or high concentrations of the toxin. This may occur if the mask is cleared in the immediate vicinity of recent sea cucumber manipulation. A severe reaction may lead to blindness. Holothurin is a potent cardiac glycoside and may cause severe illness or death on ingestion.

TREATMENT. The management of holothurin-induced contact dermatitis is similar to that for starfish dermatitis. A topical or systemic corticosteroid may be necessary to manage a severe reaction. Because cucumbers that dine on nematocysts may secrete coelenterate venom, the initial skin detoxification should include topical application of 5% acetic acid (vinegar), papain, or 40% to 70% isopropyl alcohol. If an eye is involved, it should be anesthetized with 1 or 2 drops of proparacaine 0.5% and then irrigated with 100 to 250 ml of normal saline to remove any residual foreign matter. The cornea should then be stained with fluorescein to identify corneal defects. A proper slit-lamp examination is optimal to determine whether inflammation extends into the anterior chamber or involves the iris. If there is no sign of infection, a moderate approach to the inflammatory keratitis includes regular instillation of cycloplegic, mydriatic, and corticosteroid ophthalmic solutions. Prompt referral to an ophthalmologist is essential.

Annelid Worms

LIFE AND HABITS. There are 6200 species of segmented marine worms (phylum Annelida, class Polychaeta), either free moving or sedentary. Some members of the former group are considered toxic and may attain 1

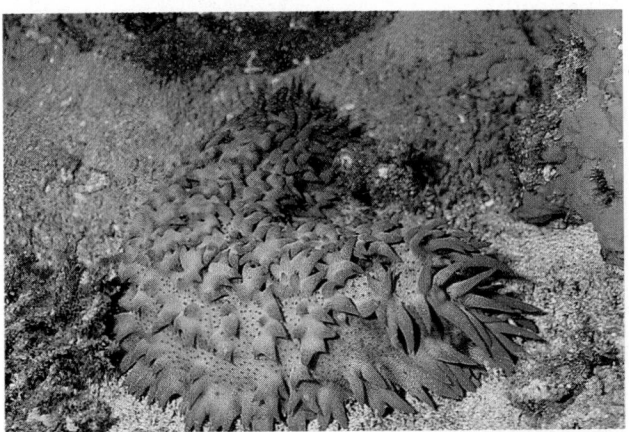

Figure 61-52 Sea cucumber. *(Photo by Paul Auerbach, MD.)*

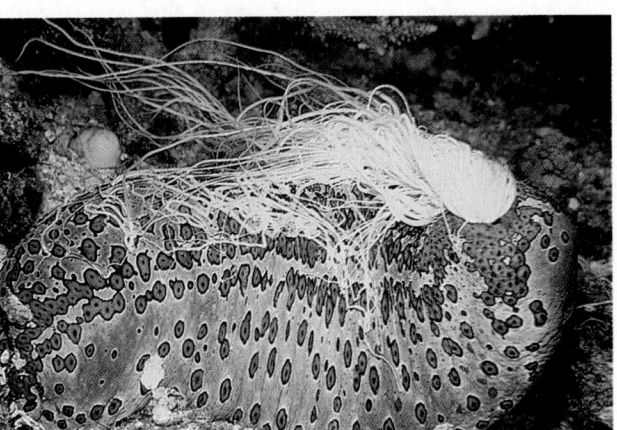

Figure 61-53 Extruded tentacular organs of Cuvier from within a sea cucumber. *(Photo by Paul Auerbach, MD.)*

foot in length. The worms are predominantly carnivorous and exist in the tidal zone to depths of 5000 m (16,405 feet), mostly as bottom feeders. Each segment of the worm possesses paddlelike appendages (parapodia) for locomotion. From these project numerous silky or bristlelike setae, which are capable of puncturing the victim (Figure 61-54).

The chitinous urticating bristles are arranged in soft rows about the body. When a worm is stimulated, its body contracts and the bristles are erected. There are no associated venom-producing cells. Easily detached, the bristles penetrate skin like cactus spines and are difficult to remove. The ubiquitous bottom-dwelling bristleworm *Hermodice carunculata* is frequently handled in Floridian and Caribbean waters by snorkelers and divers. This worm can attain a length of 1 foot and a width of 1 inch. It is found on coral, under rocks, and moving among sponges. The body is green or reddish with tufts of white bristles. *Chloeia flava* is found along the Malayan coast, *Chloeia viridus* in the West Indies, Gulf of California, and Gulf of Mexico south to Panama, and *Euythoe complanata* in Australia and other tropical seas. Other worms, such as *Chloeia euglochis ehlers,* are free swimming. Some marine worms possess strong chitinous jaws with pharyngeal teeth and can inflict painful bites.

CLINICAL ASPECTS. The bite or sting of an annelid worm may induce intense inflammation typified by a burning sensation with a raised, erythematous, and urticarial rash, most frequently on the hands and fingers (Figure 61-55). Edema and papules ensue, with rare necrosis. The setae are easily fractured into the skin and are generally not visible on external inspection, although the victim may report a sensation of pricking or abrasion. Untreated, the pain is generally self-limited over the course of a few hours, but the inflammatory component of erythema and urticaria may last for 2 to 3 days, with total resolution of the skin discoloration over 7 to 10 days. With multiple stings, marked local soft tissue edema and pruritus may develop. Secondary infections and cellulitis may occur if the eczematous component is severe.

TREATMENT. All large visible bristles should be removed with forceps. The skin should be dried (without scraping, to avoid breaking or embedding the spines further into the skin) so that a layer of adhesive tape may be applied to remove the remaining smaller spines, which are too tiny for individual extraction. Application of tape may force spines into the tissue, causing pain. Alternatively, a facial "peel" or thin layer of rubber cement may be applied and removed. After this maneuver, acetic acid 5% (vinegar), isopropyl alcohol 40% to 70%, dilute ammonia, or a paste or solution of unseasoned meat tenderizer (papain) or application of a papain scrub brush may provide some pain relief. If the inflammatory reaction becomes severe, the victim may benefit from the administration of a topical or systemic corticosteroid.

Mollusks

The phylum Mollusca (45,000 species) encompasses a group of unsegmented, soft-bodied invertebrates, many of which secrete calcareous shells. Generally a muscular foot is present with various modifications. There are five main classes, of which three predominate in their hazard to humans: the pelecypods (such as scallops, oysters, clams, and mussels), the gastropods (such as snails and slugs), and the cephalopods (such as squids, octopuses, and cuttlefish). Mollusks are often implicated as the transvectors in poisonous ingestions.

Cone Snails ("Cone Shells")

LIFE AND HABITS. There are approximately 300 species of these circumtropical, beautiful, yet potentially lethal, univalve and cone-shaped shelled mollusks of the class Gastropoda, family Conidae, genus *Conus* (Figure

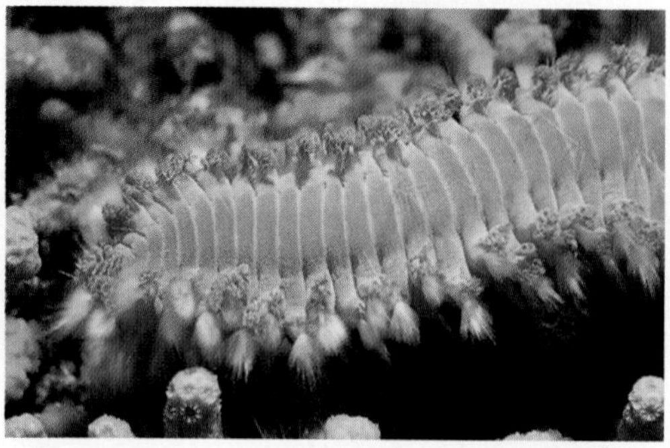

Figure 61-54 The chitinous spines of a bristleworm are easily dislodged into the skin of an unwary diver. *(Photo by Paul Auerbach, MD.)*

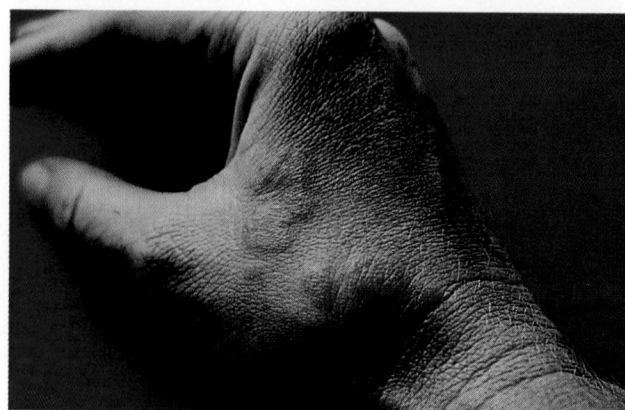

Figure 61-55 Skin rash caused by a bristleworm. *(Photo by Paul Auerbach, MD.)*

61-56). Most of these carnivores carry a highly developed venom apparatus, and at least 18 species have been implicated in human envenomations, with occasional fatalities (approximately 16 to 30 have been recorded).[48] These include *Conus aulicus* (court), *C. geographus* (geographer), *C. gloria-maris* (glory of the sea), *C. omaria* (marbled), *C. striatus* (striated), *C. textile* (textile), and *C. tulipa* (tulip).

Most harmful cone snails ("cones") are creatures of shallow Indo-Pacific waters; the variance in feeding habits and venom production accounts for the varying toxicity. Atlantic species, such as *C. ermineus* (turtle) are less toxic. *Conus regious* (crown or queen) and *C. spurius* (Chinese alphabet) are found in Florida waters. Apparently, cones that feed on fish or mollusks are the most dangerous. Less toxic stings are attributed to cones that feed on marine worms. Predominantly nocturnal creatures, cones burrow in the sand and coral during the daytime, emerging at night to feed.

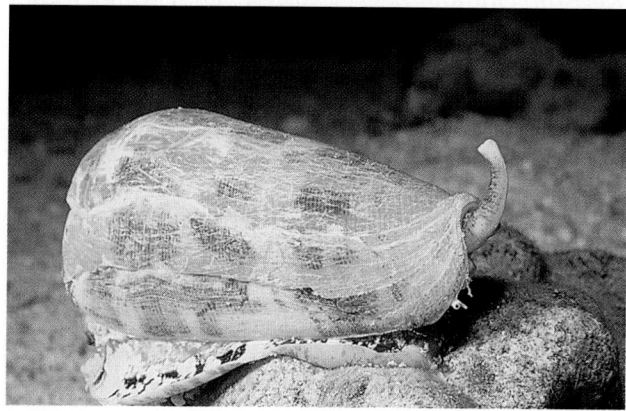

Figure 61-56   Cone snail found in the Red Sea. *(Photo by Norbert Wu.)*

VENOM AND VENOM APPARATUS. Cone snails are predators that feed by injecting rapid-acting venom by means of a detachable, dartlike radular tooth ("radula"). To do this, the head of the animal must extend out of the shell. The venom apparatus is composed of a set of minute, harpoonlike, chitinous, and hollow radular teeth associated with a venom bulb, long convoluted duct, and radular sheath (Figure 61-57).[77] The barbed teeth, which may attain a length of 1 cm, are housed within the radular sheath. The act of envenomation is performed by the release of a radular tooth from the sheath into the pharynx, where it is "charged" with venom from the venom duct and then transferred to the extensible proboscis. This appendage, which may extend in some species as far back as the spire of the shell, grasps the venom-impregnated and barbed tooth and thrusts it into the flesh of the victim. The venom is composed of biologically active peptides (to date, more than 100 "conotoxins" have been identified) of 13 to 35 amino acids in length.[84] Smaller peptides are probably strategic from an evolutionary perspective because of the speed of diffusion through a poisoned fish. The venom targets are neuromuscular transmission and ion channels.[48] At the same site as tetrodotoxin and saxitoxin, μ-conotoxins bind and modify muscle sodium channels.[51,81] Voltage-dependent calcium uptake at the presynaptic cleft and cholinergic transmission in avian and mammalian neuromuscular junctions are inhibited by ω-conotoxins like that from *Conus geographus*.[30] These ω-conotoxins bind to neuronal (N-type) rather than the cardiac (L-type) calcium channels, which prevents the calcium influx necessary for neurotransmitter release. Ziconatide is a conotoxin under investigation at the time of this writing as a potent analgesic intended for human application directly to the spinal cord and to prevent cell death in the brain after head trauma and ischemic events. The α-conotoxins

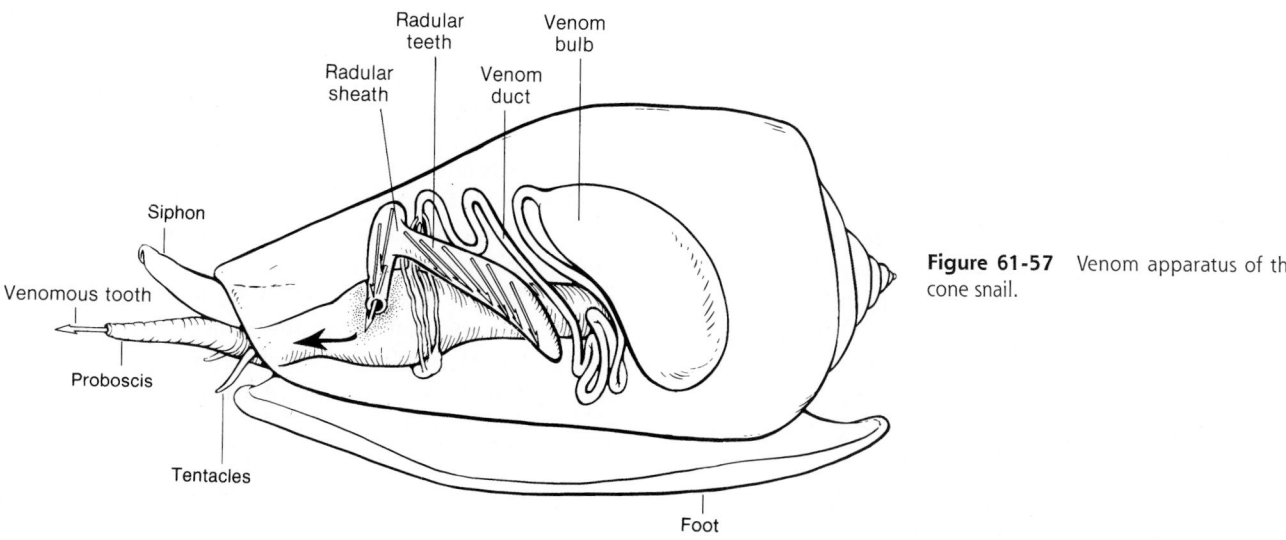

Figure 61-57   Venom apparatus of the cone snail.

block the nicotinic acetylcholine receptor.[48,81] A sleeper peptide in *C. geographus* venom causes test animals to enter a deep sleeplike state.[48] If the observation that certain contoxins target *N*-methyl-D-aspartate (NMDA) receptors can be translated into an effective drug, this may lead to another approach to the treatment of epilepsy. Serotonin is present in venom from the cone snail *C. imperialis,* which is a worm feeder.[74] In the act of envenomation, milky venom from the venom duct is transformed into a clear product, which may indicate conversion from an ineffective to effective toxin.

CLINICAL ASPECTS. Most stings occur on the fingers and hand, as the unknowledgeable fossicker incorrectly handles a hazardous specimen. Mild stings are puncture wounds that resemble bee or wasp stings, with associated burning or sharp stinging sensation. The initial pain is followed by localized ischemia, cyanosis, and numbness in the area surrounding the wound. Numbness may occur without preceding pain, or in a rare case, the envenomation may be without any specific dermal sensation. More serious envenomations induce paresthesias at the wound site, which rapidly encompass the limb and then become perioral before generalized. Partial paralysis transitions to generalized muscular paralysis causing diaphragmatic dysfunction and respiratory failure; bronchospastic respiratory distress is not commonly seen. Coma has been observed, and death is attributed to diaphragmatic paralysis or cardiac failure. Other symptoms include dysphagia, syncope, weakness, failing coordination, areflexia, aphonia, dysarthria, diplopia, ptosis, absent gag reflex, blurred vision, and pruritus. The bite of *C. geographus* may be rapidly toxic, with progression to cerebral edema, coma, respiratory arrest, and cardiac failure within a few hours, perhaps even 1 hour. Although mild stings may cause symptoms of nausea, blurred vision, malaise, and weakness for only a few hours, a severe envenomation may induce symptoms that require 2 to 3 weeks to achieve total resolution. *C. textile* and *C. marmoreus* have been reported to kill humans. A fatality has been attributed to *C. gloria-maris,* but this has not yet been confirmed.[77]

TREATMENT. No antivenom is available for a cone shell envenomation. Numerous therapies have been recommended, including the pressure-immobilization technique, application of a proximal lymphatic-venous occlusive bandage, incision and suction, soaking in nonscalding hot water to tolerance (upper limit 45° C [113° F]) until pain is relieved, injection of a local anesthetic (lidocaine 1% to 2% without epinephrine), and local excision. The pressure-immobilization technique makes sense and should be applied.

Cardiovascular and respiratory support are the usual priorities after a severe envenomation. The wound should be inspected for the presence of a foreign body (radula). Edrophonium (10 mg intravenously in an adult) has been suggested as empirical therapy for paralysis. A rational approach would be to administer an edrophonium (Tensilon) test to determine effectiveness. The clinician should choose a weak muscle group for which strength can be objectively measured, then inject edrophonium 2 mg IV. If there is improvement, this is followed by edrophonium 8 mg IV. Adverse reactions to edrophonium (anticholinesterase inhibitor) include salivation, nausea, diarrhea, and muscle fasciculations. These can be ameliorated with atropine 0.6 mg IV.

Cone shells should be handled only when wearing proper gloves; if the proboscis protrudes, the cone should be dropped. If the animal must be carried, it should always be lifted by the large posterior end of the shell, although this does not afford complete protection. A collector should never carry a live cone inside a wet suit, clothing pocket, or buoyancy compensator pocket.

Octopuses

LIFE AND HABITS. Octopuses and cuttlefish are cephalopods that are usually harmless and retiring. On occasion, they are noted to manifest "curiosity" or "play behavior," by navigating mazes or manipulating objects without intent to feed or create a habitat. True octopuses are inhabitants of warmer waters and have little tolerance for extremes in salinity. They prefer rocky bottoms and rock pools in the intertidal zones. The entertainment media have created the image of a giant creature that envelops its victim in a maze of tentacles and suction cups. The truth is that most dangerous (envenoming) creatures are smaller than 10 to 20 cm and do not squeeze their victims at all. However, there are reports in the South Pacific of breath-hold spearfishermen drowned while hunting octopuses. The method used to kill the animals was to allow an octopus to cling to a diver, who would bite the animal between the eyes as the combatants surfaced. Apparently, the octopuses were large enough (4-m [13-foot] tentacle span) to resist the technique.

Octopus bites are rare but can result in severe envenomations. Fatalities have been reported from the bites of the Australian blue-ringed (or "spotted") octopuses, *Octopus (Hapalochlaena) maculosus* and *O. (H.) lunulata.* These small creatures, which rarely exceed 20 cm in length with tentacles extended, are found throughout the Indo-Pacific (Australia, New Zealand, New Guinea, Japan) in rock pools, under discarded objects and shells, and in shallow waters, posing a threat to curious children, tidepoolers, fossickers, and unwary divers.[113] Divers rarely spot them in water deeper than

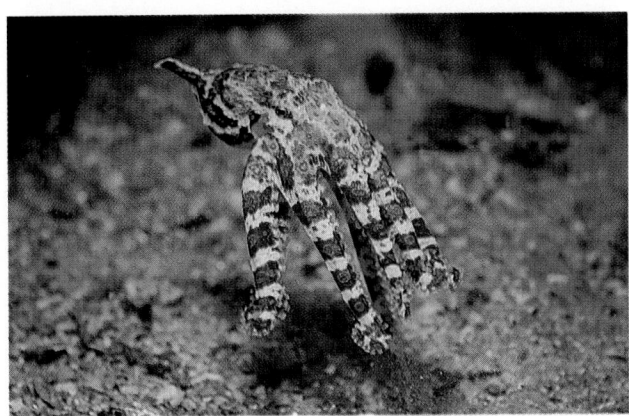

Figure 61-58   Blue-spotted octopus. *(Photo by Norbert Wu.)*

3 m. In Australian waters, *H. maculosa*, the southern species, is smaller and yellow. *H. lunulata* is found in the north; larger, darker, and predominantly brownish, it favors the warmer tropical water. When either animal is at rest, it is covered with dark brown to yellow-ochre bands over the body and arms, with superimposed blue patches or rings.[110] When the animal is excited or angered, the entire body darkens and the blue circles or stripes glow iridescent peacock blue, a trait shared by other animals, such as the peacock flounder *(Bothus lunatus).* The colorful appearance is attractive to small children, who can easily handle the 25- to 90-g animal (Figure 61-58). The smallish *Octopus joubini* of the Caribbean, which lives in small shells and empty containers, such as submerged bottles, is dangerous to a lesser degree; envenomation causes pain followed by numbness, fever, and nausea. The large common octopus *O. vulgaris* is nontoxic. Many octopuses can release inky fluid into the water, which is used to confuse attackers; this mechanism is not present in the blue-ringed octopus. The chameleon-like changing of colors to match the surroundings is accomplished with pigment cells (chromatophores).

VENOM AND VENOM APPARATUS. The venom apparatus of the octopus consists of the anterior and posterior salivary glands, salivary ducts, buccal mass, and beak. The mouth is located ventrally and centrally at the base of the tentacles and is surrounded by a circular lip fringed with fingerlike papillae, leading into a muscular pharyngeal cavity. This anatomic complex (buccal mass), concealed by the tentacles, is fronted by two parrotlike, powerful, and chitinous jaws (the "beak"), which bite and tear with great force at food held by the suckers. The salivary glands, particularly the posterior, secrete maculotoxin (or cephalotoxin) via the salivary ducts into the pharynx. This venom, normally released into the water to subdue crabs, may be injected into the victim with great force through the dermis down to the muscle fascia.[113] Only the venom of *H. maculosa* has been extensively studied. The toxin, maculotoxin (molecular weight less than 5000), contains at least one fraction identical to tetrodotoxin ($C_{11}H_{17}O_8N_3$) of molecular weight 319.3, which blocks peripheral nerve conduction by interfering with sodium conductance in excitable membranes.[101] This paralytic agent rapidly produces neuromuscular blockade, notably of the phrenic nerve supply to the diaphragm, without any apparent direct cardiotoxicity. It has been estimated that enough venom (25 g) may be present in one adult octopus to paralyze 750 kg of rabbits or 10 adult victims.[110,113] An adult blue-ringed octopus can inject a second fatal dose of toxin after a 1-hour interval. The venom is active on ingestion or by parenteral administration, the latter being much more effective. Other components of the venom, which include hyaluronidase, histamine, 5-hydroxytryptamine, tyramine, serotonin, and "hapalotoxin" (still not confirmed as being present), are not thought to be major contributors to the clinical effects of an octopus bite.[159] Because most venoms and toxins with molecular weights less than 30,000 are poor antigens, octopus venom elicits no good antivenom.[113]

CLINICAL ASPECTS. Most victims are bitten on the hand or arm, as they handle the creature or "give it a ride." No blue-ringed octopus bites have yet been reported from an animal in the water.[124] An octopus bite usually consists of two small puncture wounds produced by the chitinous jaws. The bite goes unnoticed or causes only a small amount of discomfort, described as a minor ache, slight stinging, or a pulsating sensation. Occasionally the site is initially numb, followed in 5 to 10 minutes by discomfort that may spread to involve the entire limb, persisting for up to 6 hours. Local urticarial reactions occur variably, and profuse bleeding at the site is attributed to a local anticoagulant effect or may rarely be a harbinger of coagulation abnormalities. Within 30 minutes, considerable erythema, swelling, tenderness, heat, and pruritus develop. By far the most common local tissue reaction is absence of symptoms, a small spot of blood, or a tiny blanched area.[123] More serious symptoms are related predominantly to the neurotoxic properties of the venom. Within 10 to 15 minutes of the bite, the victim notices oral and facial numbness, rapidly followed by systemic progression.[124] Voluntary and involuntary muscles are involved, and the illness may rapidly progress to total flaccid paralysis and respiratory failure. Other symptoms include perioral and intraoral anesthesia (classically, numbness of the lips and tongue), diplopia, blurred vision, aphonia, dysphagia, ataxia, myoclonus, weakness, a sense of detachment, nausea, vomiting, peripheral neuropathy, flaccid muscular paralysis, and respiratory failure, which may lead to death. Ataxia of cerebellar configuration may occur after an envenomation that does not

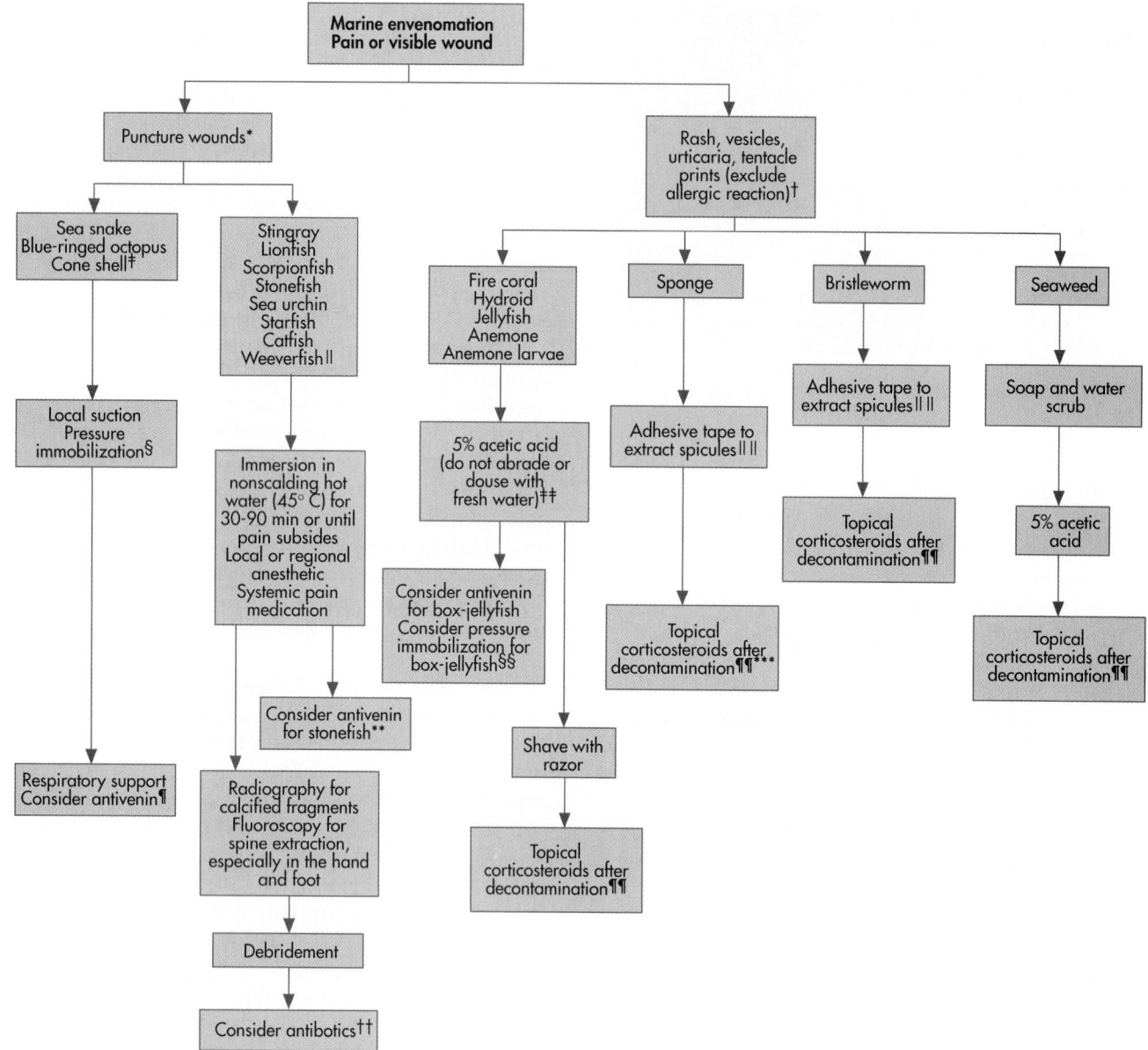

Figure 61-59 For legend see opposite page.

progress to frank paralysis. The victim may collapse from weakness and remain awake, so long as oxygenation can be maintained. When breathing is disturbed, respiratory assistance may allow the victim to remain mentally alert, although paralyzed. Cardiac arrest is probably a complication of the anoxic episode.[121] Although tetrodotoxin is a potent vascular smooth muscle depressant, it does not appear to often produce significant hypotension in humans. However, hypotensive crisis has been mentioned in the literature as a complicating factor.

TREATMENT. First aid at the scene might include the pressure-immobilization technique described in the section on treatment of box-jellyfish envenomation, although this is as yet unproven for management of octopus bites. A monoclonal rabbit serum antibody IgG has been effective against tetrodotoxin injected into mice.[73,94] This raises the possibility of the practical use of passive immunotherapy in the event of tetrodotoxin poisoning.

Treatment is based on the symptoms and is supportive. Prompt mechanical respiratory assistance has by far the greatest influence on the outcome. Respiratory demise should be anticipated early, and the rescuer should be prepared to provide artificial ventilation, including endotracheal intubation and the application of a mechanical ventilator. The duration of intense clinical venom effect is 4 to 10 hours, after which the victim who has not suffered an episode of significant hypoxia shows rapid signs of improvement.

Figure 61-59 Algorithmic approach to marine envenomation.

*A gaping laceration, particularly of the lower extremity, with cyanotic edges suggests a stingray wound. Multiple punctures in an erratic pattern with or without purple discoloration or retained fragments are typical of a sea urchin sting. One to eight (usually two) fang marks are usually present after a sea snake bite. A single ischemic puncture wound with an erythematous halo and rapid swelling suggests scorpionfish envenomation. Blisters often accompany a lionfish sting. Painless punctures with paralysis suggest the bite of a blue-ringed octopus; the site of a cone shell sting is punctate, painful, and ischemic in appearance.

†Wheal and flare reactions are nonspecific. Rapid (within 24 hours) onset of skin necrosis suggests an anemone sting. "Tentacle prints" with cross-hatching or a frosted appearance are pathognomonic for box-jellyfish (*Chironex fleckeri*) envenomation. Ocular or intraoral lesions may be caused by fragmented hydroids or coelenterate tentacles. An allergic reaction must be treated promptly.

‡Sea snake venom causes weakness, respiratory paralysis, myoglobinuria, myalgias, blurred vision, vomiting, and dysphagia. The blue-ringed octopus injects tetrodotoxin, which causes rapid neuromuscular paralysis.

§If *immediately* available (which is rarely the case), local suction can be applied without incision using a plunger device, such as The Extractor (Sawyer Products, Safety Harbor, Fla.). As soon as possible, venom should be sequestered locally with a proximal venous-lymphatic occlusive band of constriction or (preferably) the pressure immobilization technique, in which a cloth pad is compressed directly over the wound by an elastic wrap that should encompass the entire extremity at a pressure of 9.33 kPa (70 mm Hg) or less. Incision and suction are not recommended.

¶Early ventilatory support has the greatest influence on outcome. The minimal initial dose of sea snake antivenin is one to three vials; up to ten vials may be required.

‖The wounds range from large lacerations (stingrays) to minute punctures (stonefish). Persistent pain after immersion in hot water suggests a stonefish sting or a retained fragment of spine. The puncture site can be identified by forcefully injecting 1% to 2% lidocaine or another local anesthetic agent without epinephrine near the wound and observing the egress of fluid. Do not attempt to crush the spines of sea urchins if they are present in the wound. Spine dye from already-extracted sea urchin spines will disappear (be absorbed) in 24 to 36 hours.

**The initial dose of stonefish antivenin is one vial per two puncture wounds.

††The antibiotics chosen should cover *Staphylococcus, Streptococcus,* and microbes of marine origin, such as *Vibrio*.

‡‡Acetic acid 5% (vinegar) is a good all-purpose decontaminant and is mandated for the sting from a box-jellyfish. Alternatives, depending on the geographic region and indigenous jellyfish species, include isopropyl alcohol, bicarbonate (baking soda), ammonia, papain, and preparations containing these agents.

§§The initial dose of box-jellyfish antivenin is one ampule intravenously or three ampules intramuscularly.

¶¶If inflammation is severe, steroids should be given systematically (beginning with at least 60 to 100 mg of prednisone or its equivalent) and the dose tapered over a period of 10 to 14 days.

***An alternative is to apply and remove commercial facial peel materials.

‖‖An alternative is to apply and remove commercial facial peel materials followed by topical soaks of 30 ml of 5% acetic acid (vinegar) diluted in 1 L of water for 15 to 30 minutes several times a day until the lesions begin to resolve. Anticipate surface desquamation in 3 to 6 weeks.

If no period of hypoxia occurs, mentation may remain normal. Complete recovery may require 2 to 4 days. Residua are uncommon and related to anoxia rather than venom effects.

Management of the bite wound is controversial. Some clinicians recommend wide circular excision of the bite wound down to the deep fascia, with primary closure or an immediate full-thickness free skin graft, whereas others advocate observation and a nonsurgical approach. Because the local tissue reaction is not a significant cause of morbidity, excision is recommended, presumably to remove any sequestered venom. Kinetic studies of radiolabeled venom absorption are necessary to track the movement of octopus bite–introduced tetrodotoxin. As previously mentioned, there is no antivenom. Granuloma annulare of the hand developing over a 2-week period after an octopus (presumed to be *Octopus vulgaris* of the Florida Gulf Coast) bite of the hand has been reported.[40] On biopsy, histologic sections demonstrated superficial and deep dermal foci of altered dermis surrounded by histiocytes, lymphocytes, and fibroblasts. Intralesional triamcinolone acetonide injections were temporarily successful in treating the primary lesion.

PREVENTION. All octopuses, particularly those less than 20 cm in length (including *Octopus joubini* of the Caribbean), should be handled with gloves. Divers need to be familiar with the lethal creatures in their domain. Giving an octopus a ride on the back, shoulder, or arm is not recommended.

SUMMARY

A summary algorithmic approach to marine envenomation can be followed when the causative agent cannot be positively identified (Figure 61-59). Once the physician has made a commitment to a course of treatment based on a presumption of what creature has caused the injury, the subtleties of therapy can be utilized.

REFERENCES

1. Abu-Nema T et al: Jellyfish sting resulting in severe hand ischaemia successfully treated with intra-arterial urokinase, *Injury* 19:294, 1988.
2. Anker RL et al: Retarding the uptake of mock venom in humans: comparison of three first-aid treatments, *Med J Aust* 1:212, 1982.
3. Asada M et al: A case of delayed hypersensitivity reaction following a sea urchin sting, *Dermatologica* 180:99, 1990.
4. Auerbach PS: Marine envenomations, *N Engl J Med* 325:486, 1991.
5. Auerbach PS, Hays T: Erythema nodosum following a jellyfish sting, *J Emerg Med* 5:487, 1987.
6. Bach MK: Mediators of anaphylaxis and inflammation, *Annu Rev Microbiol* 36:371, 1982.
7. Barach EM et al: Epinephrine for treatment of anaphylactic shock, *JAMA* 251:2118, 1984.
8. Barnes JH: Cause and effect in Irukandji stingings, *Med J Aust* 1:897, 1964.
9. Barsan WG et al: A hemodynamic model for anaphylactic shock, *Ann Emerg Med* 14:834, 1985.
10. Bengston K et al: Sudden death in a child following jellyfish envenomation by *Chiropsalmus quadrumanus*, *JAMA* 266:1404, 1991.
11. Bernheimer AW, Lai CY: Properties of a cytolytic toxin from the sea anemone, *Stoichactis kenti*, *Toxicon* 23:791, 1985.
12. Burnett HW, Burnett JW: Prolonged blurred vision following coelenterate envenomation, *Toxicon* 28:731, 1990.
13. Burnett JW: *Jellyfish newsletter number 16*, International Consortium for Jellyfish Stings, page 4, correspondence 1, Jan 1997.
14. Burnett JW, Calton GJ: The chemistry and toxicology of some venomous pelagic coelenterates, *Toxicon* 15:177, 1977.
15. Burnett JW, Calton GJ: Use of IgE antibody determinations in cutaneous coelenterate envenomations, *Cutis* 27:50, 1981.
16. Burnett JW, Calton GJ: Response of the box-jellyfish (*Chironex fleckeri*) cardiotoxin to intravenous administration of verapamil, *Med J Aust* 2:192, 1983.
17. Burnett JW, Calton GJ: Recurrent eruption following a solitary envenomation by the cnidarian *Stomolophus meleagris*, *Toxicon* 23:1010, 1985.
18. Burnett JW, Calton GJ: Jellyfish envenomation syndromes updated, *Ann Emerg Med* 16:1000, 1987.
19. Burnett JW, Calton GJ, Burnett HW: Jellyfish envenomation syndromes, *J Am Acad Dermatol* 14:100, 1986.
20. Burnett JW, Calton GJ, Larsen JB: Significant envenomation by *Aurelia aurita*, the moon jellyfish, *Toxicon* 26:215, 1988.
21. Burnett JW, Gable WD: A fatal jellyfish envenomation by the Portuguese man-o-war, *Toxicon* 27:823, 1989.
22. Burnett JW et al: Local and systemic reactions from jellyfish stings, *Clin Dermatol* 5:14, 1987.
23. Burnett JW et al: Serological diagnosis of jellyfish envenomations, *Comp Biochem Physiol* 91C:79, 1988.
24. Burnett JW et al: The antibody response in seabather's eruption, *Toxicon* 33:99, 1995.
25. Burnett JW et al: Autonomic neurotoxicity of jellyfish and marine animal venoms, *Clin Auton Res* 8:125, 1998.
26. Burnett JW et al: A protocol to investigate the blockade of jellyfish nematocysts by topical agents, *Contact Dermatitis* 40:56, 1999.
27. Chand RP, Selliah K: Reversible parasympathetic dysautonomia following stinging attributed to the box-jellyfish (*Chironex fleckeri*), *Aust NZ J Med* 14:673, 1984.
28. Currie B: Clinical implications of research on the box-jellyfish *Chironex fleckeri*, *Toxicon* 32:1305, 1994.
29. De Freitas JC, Schiozer WA, Malpezzi ELA: A case of envenoming by Portuguese man-of-war from the Brazilian coast, *Toxicon* 33:859, 1995.
30. De Luca A et al: Differential sensitivities of avian and mammalian neuromuscular junctions to inhibition of cholinergic transmission by ω-conotoxin GVIA, *Toxicon* 29:311, 1991.
31. Dormandy TL: Trace element analysis of hair, *BMJ* 293:975, 1986.
32. Exton DR, Fenner PJ, Williamson JA: Cold packs: effective topical analgesia in the treatment of painful stings by *Physalia* and other jellyfish, *Med J Aust* 151:625, 1989.
33. Fenner PJ: Dangers in the ocean: the traveler and marine envenomation. I. Jellyfish, *J Travel Med* 5:135, 1998.
34. Fenner PJ, Williamson JA: Worldwide deaths and severe envenomation from jellyfish stings, *Med J Aust* 165:658, 1996.
35. Fenner PJ et al: The Irukandji syndrome and acute pulmonary edema, *Med J Aust* 149:150, 1988.
36. Fenner PJ et al: First aid treatment of jellyfish stings in Australia: response to a newly differentiated species, *Med J Aust* 158:498, 1993.
37. Filling-Katz MR: Mononeuritis multiplex following jellyfish stings, *Ann Neurol* 15:213, 1984.
38. Freudenthal AR: Seabather's eruption: range extended northward and a causative organism identified, *Rev Int Oceanographic Med* 137, 1991.
39. Freudenthal AR, Joseph PR: Seabather's eruption, *N Engl J Med* 329:542, 1993.
40. Fulghum DD: Octopus bite resulting in granuloma annulare, *South Med J* 79:1434, 1986.
41. Galettis P, Norton RS: Biochemical and pharmacological studies of the mechanism of action of tenebrosin-C, a cardiac stimulatory and haemolytic protein from the sea anemone, *Actinia tenebrosa*, *Toxicon* 28:695, 1990.
42. Garcia PJ, Schein RM, Burnett JW: Fulminant hepatic failure from a sea anemone sting, *Ann Intern Med* 120:665, 1994.
43. Garcia-Alonso I et al: Biological activity of secretions and extracts of gorgonians from Cuban waters, *J Nat Toxins* 2:27, 1993.
44. Gaur PK, Calton GJ, Burnett JW: Enzyme-linked immunosorbent assay to detect anti sea nettle venom antibodies, *Experientia* 37:1005, 1981.
45. Gilliland BC: Serum sickness and immune complexes, *N Engl J Med* 311:1435, 1984.
46. Glasser DV et al: Ocular jellyfish stings, *Ophthalmology* 92:1414, 1992.
47. Glasser DV et al: A guinea-pig model of corneal jellyfish envenomation, *Toxicon* 31:808, 1993.
48. Gray WR, Olivera BM, Cruz LJ: Peptide toxins from venomous *Conus* snails, *Annu Rev Biochem* 57:665, 1988.
49. Guess HA, Saviteer PL, Morris RC: Hemolysis and acute renal failure following a Portuguese man-of-war sting, *Pediatrics* 70:979, 1982.
50. Hadok JC: "Irukandji" syndrome: a risk for divers in tropical waters, *Med J Aust* 167:649, 1997.
51. Hahin R et al: Alterations in sodium channel gating produced by the venom of the marine mollusc *Conus striatus*, *Toxicon* 29:245, 1991.
52. Hartwick RF: Distributional ecology and behaviour of the early life stages of the box-jellyfish *Chironex fleckeri*, *Hydrobiologia* 216/217:181, 1991.
53. Hartwick R, Callahan V, Williamson J: Disarming the box-jellyfish, *Med J Aust* 1:15, 1980.
54. Harvey AL, Aneiros A, Casaneda O: Potassium channel toxins from marine animals, *Toxicon* 31:504, 1993 (abstract).
55. Hodgson WC: Pharmacological action of Australian animal venoms, *Clin Exp Pharmacol Physiol* 24:10, 1997.
56. Holstein T, Tardent P: An ultrahigh-speed analysis of exocytosis: nematocyst discharge, *Science* 233:830, 1984.
57. Jefferies NJ: Caribbean itch: eight cases and one who didn't (exercise blue calypso diamond), *J R Army Med Corps* 143:163, 1997.
58. Kao CY: Tetrodotoxin, saxitoxin, and their significance in the study of the excitation phenomena, *Pharmacol Rev* 18:997, 1966.
59. Karasudani I, Omija M, Aniya Y: Smooth muscle contractile action of the venom from the crown-of-thorns starfish, *Acanthaster planci*, *J Toxicol Sci* 21:11, 1996.
60. Karasudani I et al: Purification of anticoagulant factor from the spine venom of the crown-of-thorns starfish, *Acanthaster planci*, *Toxicon* 34:871, 1996.
61. Kizer KW: Marine envenomations, *J Toxicol Clin Toxicol* 21:527, 1984.
62. Kizer KW, Auerbach PS: Marine envenomations: not just a problem of the tropics, *Emerg Med Rep* 6:129, 1985.
63. Kokelj F et al: Dermatitis due to *Olindias sambaquiensis*: a case report, *Cutis* 51:339, 1993.
64. Lawley TJ et al: A prospective clinical and immunologic analysis of patients with serum sickness, *N Engl J Med* 311:1407, 1984.
65. Lotan A, Fine M, Ben-Hillel R: Synchronization of the life cycle and dispersal pattern of the tropical invader scyphomedusan *Rhopilema nomadica* is temperature dependent, *Mar Ecol Prog Ser* 109:59, 1994.
66. Lotan A, Fishman L, Zlotkin E: Toxin compartmentation and delivery in the cnidaria: the nematocyst's tubule as a multiheaded poisonous arrow, *J Exp Zool* 275:444, 1996.
67. Lotan A et al: Delivery of a nematocyst toxin, *Nature* 375:456, 1995.
68. Maček P, Lebez D: Isolation and characterization of three lethal and hemolytic toxins from the sea anemone *Actinia equina* L, *Toxicon* 26:441, 1988.
69. MacSween RM, Williams HC: Seabather's eruption—a case of Caribbean itch, *BMJ* 312:957, 1996.
70. Mandojana RM: Granuloma annulare following bluebottle jellyfish (*Physalia utriculus*) sting, *J Wilderness Med* 1:220, 1990.
71. Mansson T et al: Recurrent cutaneous jellyfish eruptions without envenomation, *Acta Derm Venereol Suppl (Stockh)* 65:72, 1985.

72. Martin JC, Audley I: Cardiac failure following Irukandji envenomation, *Med J Aust* 153:164, 1990.

73. Matsumura K: *In vivo* neutralization of tetrodotoxin by a monoclonal antibody, *Toxicon* 33:1239, 1995.

74. McIntosh JM et al: Presence of serotonin in the venom of *Conus imperialis*, *Toxicon* 31:1561, 1993.

75. Mebs D: Anemonefish symbiosis: vulnerability and resistance of fish to the toxin of the sea anemone, *Toxicon* 32:1059, 1994.

76. Mebs D et al: Hemolysins and proteinase inhibitors from sea anemones of the Gulf of Aqaba, *Toxicon* 21:257, 1983.

77. Meier J, White J: *Handbook of clinical toxicology of animal venoms and poisons*, Boca Raton, Fla, 1995, CRC Press.

78. Meyer PK: Seastroke: a new entity? *South Med J* 86:777, 1993.

79. Moats WE: Fire coral envenomation, *J Wilderness Med* 3:284, 1992.

80. Mulcahy R, Little M: Thirty cases of Irukandji envenomation from far north Queensland, *Emerg Med* 9:297, 1997.

81. Nakagawa H, Tu AT, Kimura A: Purification and characterization of contractin A from the pedicellarial venom of sea urchin, *Toxopneustes pileolus*, *Arch Biochem Biophys* 284:279, 1991.

82. Neale TJ, Theofilopoulos AN, Wilson CB: Methods for the detection of soluble circulating immune complexes and their application, *Pathobiol Annu* 9:113, 1979.

83. Ohtaki N et al: Cutaneous reactions caused by experimental exposure to jellyfish, *Carybdea rastonii*, *J Dermatol* 17:108, 1990.

84. Olivera BM et al: Conotoxins and other biologically active peptides in *Conus* venoms, *Toxicon* 28:256, 1990 (abstract).

85. Olson CE et al: Interrelationships between toxins: studies on the cross-reactivity between bacterial or animal toxins and monoclonal antibodies to two jellyfish venoms, *Toxicon* 23:307, 1985.

86. Othman I, Burnett JW: Techniques applicable for purifying *Chironex fleckeri* (box-jellyfish) venom, *Toxicon* 28:821, 1990.

87. Pearn J: The sea, stingers, and surgeons: the surgeon's role in prevention, first aid, and management of marine envenomations, *J Pediatr Surg* 30:105, 1995.

88. Peca G et al: Contact reactions to the jellyfish *Carybdea marsupialis*: observation of 40 cases, *Contact Dermatitis* 36:124, 1997.

89. Peel N, Kandler R: Localized neuropathy following jellyfish sting, *Postgrad Med* 66:953, 1990.

90. Piérard GE, Letot B, Piérard-Franchimont C: Histologic study of delayed reactions to coelenterates, *J Am Acad Dermatol* 22:599, 1990.

91. Puertas LS, Burnett JW, Heimer de la Cotera E: The medusa stage of the coronate scyphomedusa, *Linuche unguiculata* ('thimble jellyfish') can cause seabather's eruption, *Dermatology* 198:171, 1999.

92. Querel P, Bernard P, Dantzer E: Severe cutaneous envenomation by the Mediterranean jellyfish *Pelagia noctiluca*, *Vet Hum Toxicol* 38:460, 1996.

93. Rifkin JF, Fenner PJ, Williamson JAH: First aid treatment of the sting from the hydroid *Lytocarpus philippinus*: the structure of, and in vitro discharge experiments with its nematocysts, *J Wilderness Med* 4:252, 1993.

94. Rivera VR, Poli MA, Bignami GS: Prophylaxis and treatment with a monoclonal antibody of tetrodotoxin poisoning in mice, *Toxicon* 33:1231, 1995.

95. Rocha G, Fraga S: Sea urchin granuloma of the skin, *Arch Dermatol* 85:406, 1962.

96. Rottini G et al: Purification and properties of a cytoloytic toxin in venom of the jellyfish *Carybdea marsupialis*, *Toxicon* 33:315, 1995.

97. Russell FE, Nagabhushanam R: *The venomous and poisonous marine invertebrates of the Indian Ocean*, New Dehli, 1996, Oxford and IBH Publishing Co.

98. Russo AJ, Calton GJ, Burnett JW: The relationship of the possible allergic response to jellyfish envenomation and serum antibody titers, *Toxicon* 21:475, 1983.

99. Savage IVE, Howden MEH: Hapalotoxin, a second lethal toxin from the octopus, *Hapalochlaena maculosa*, *Toxicon* 15:463, 1977.

100. Schwartz S, Meinking T: Venomous marine animals of Florida: morphology, behavior, health hazards, *J Fla Med Assoc* 84:433, 1997.

101. Sheumack DD et al: Maculotoxin: a neurotoxin from the venom glands of the octopus *Hapalochlaena maculosa* identified as tetrodotoxin, *Science* 199:188, 1978.

102. Shiomi K et al: Isolation and characterization of a lethal hemolysin in the sea anemone *Parasicyonis actinostoloides*, *Toxicon* 23:865, 1985.

103. Shiomi K et al: Liver damage by the crown-of-thorns starfish (*Acanthaster planci*) lethal factor, *Toxicon* 28:469, 1990.

104. Shiroma N et al: Haemodynamic and haematologic effects of *Acanthaster planci* venom in dogs, *Toxicon* 32:1217, 1994.

105. Sims JK, Irei MY: Human Hawaiian marine sponge poisoning, *Hawaii Med J* 9:263, 1979.

106. Southcott RV: Revision of some Carybdeidae (Scyphozoa/Cubomedusae), including a description of the jellyfish syndrome responsible for the Irukandji syndrome, *Aust J Zool* 15:651, 1967.

107. Southcott RV: Human injuries from invertebrate animals in the Australian seas, *Clin Toxicol* 3:617, 1970.

108. Southcott RV, Coulter JR: The effects of the southern Australian marine stinging sponges, *Neofibularia mordens* and *Lissodendoryx* sp, *Med J Aust* 2:895, 1971.

109. Stein MR et al: Fatal Portuguese man-o'-war (*Physalia physalis*) envenomation, *Ann Emerg Med* 18:312, 1989.

110. Sutherland SK: *Venomous creatures of Australia*, Melbourne, 1981, Oxford University Press.

111. Sutherland SK: *Australian animal toxins*, Melbourne, 1983, Oxford University Press.

112. Sutherland SK: Antivenom use in Australia. Premedication, adverse reactions and the use of venom detection kits, *Med J Aust* 157:734, 1992.

113. Sutherland SK, Lane WR: Toxins and mode of envenomation of the common ringed or blue-banded octopus, *Med J Aust* 1:893, 1969.

114. Tahmassebi JF, O'Sullivan EA: A case report of an unusual mandibular swelling in a 4-year-old child possibly caused by a jellyfish sting, *Int J Paed Dentistry* 8:51, 1998.

115. Takei M et al: A toxic substance from the sea urchin *Toxopneustes pileolus* induces histamine release from rat peritoneal mast cells, *Agents Actions* 32:224, 1991.

116. Tamanaha RH, Izumi AK: Persistent cutaneous hypersensitivity reaction after a Hawaiian box jellyfish sting (*Carybdea alata*), *J Am Acad Dermatol* 35:991, 1996.

117. Tibballs J, Williams D, Sutherland SK: The effects of antivenom and verapamil on the haemodynamic actions of *Chironex fleckeri* (box jellyfish) venom, *Anaesth Intens Care* 26:40, 1998.

118. Tomchik RS et al: Clinical perspectives on seabather's eruption, also known as sea lice, *JAMA* 269:1669, 1993.

119. Usagawa T et al: Preparation of monoclonal antibodies against okadaic acid prepared from the sponge *Halichondria okadai*, *Toxicon* 27:1323, 1989.

120. Wachsman M, Aurelian L, Burnett JW: Human immunosuppression induced by sea nettle (*Chrysaora quinquecirrha*) venom, *Toxicon* 29:386, 1991.

121. Walker DG: Survival after severe envenomation by the blue-ringed octopus (*Hapalochlaena maculosa*), *Med J Aust* 2:663, 1983.

122. Weinberg SR: Reactive arthritis following a sting by a Portuguese man-of-war, *J Fla Med Assoc* 75:280, 1988 (letter).

123. Williamson JA: The blue ringed octopus, *Med J Aust* 140:308, 1984.

124. Williamson JA: The blue-ringed octopus bite and envenomation syndrome, *Clin Dermatol* 5:127, 1987.

125. Williamson JA, Callahan VI, Hartwick RF: Serious envenomation by the northern Australian box-jellyfish (*Chironex fleckeri*), *Med J Aust* 1:13, 1980.

126. Williamson JA et al: Acute management of serious envenomation by box-jellyfish (*Chironex fleckeri*), *Med J Aust* 141:851, 1984.

127. Williamson JA, Fenner PJ, Burnett JW: *Venomous and poisonous marine animals: a medical and biological handbook*, Sydney, 1996, University of New South Wales Press.

128. Williamson JA et al: Box-jellyfish venom and humans, *Med J Aust* 140:444, 1984.

129. Williamson JA et al: Acute regional vascular insufficiency after jellyfish envenomation, *Med J Aust* 149:698, 1988.

130. Wong DE et al: Seabather's eruption, *J Am Acad Dermatol* 30:399, 1994.

131. Wong SK, Matoba A: Jellyfish sting of the cornea, *Am J Ophthalmol* 100:739, 1985.

132. Yaffee HS: Irritation from red sponge, *N Engl J Med* 282:51, 1970.

133. Yaffee HS, Stargardtner F: Erythema multiforme from *Tedania ignis*, *Arch Dermatol* 87:601, 1963.

62 Envenomation by Aquatic Vertebrates

Paul S. Auerbach

See Chapter 60 for a discussion of infections associated with aquatic wounds and the relevant antimicrobial therapy.

STINGRAYS

The stingrays are the most commonly incriminated group of fish involved in human envenomations. They have been recognized as venomous since ancient times, known as "demons of the deep" and "devil fish." Aristotle (384-322 BC) made reference to their stinging ability.

Stingrays are members of the class Chondrichthyes (cartilaginous fish), subclass Elasmobranchii (plates and gills; with sharks and chimaeras), order Rajiformes (which contains stingrays [Dasyatidae], guitarfish [Rhinobatidae], skates [Rajidae], electric rays [Torpedinidae], eagle rays [Myliobatidae], mantas [Mobulidae], and freshwater rays [Potamotrygonidae]). There are 22 species of stingrays found in U.S. coastal waters, 14 in the Atlantic and 8 in the Pacific. The family Dasyatidae includes most of the species that cause human envenomation. Skates are harmless. It is likely that at least 2000 stingray injuries take place each year in the United States. On the west coast of the United States, the round stingray *(Urolophus halleri)* is a frequent stinger; along the southeastern coast, it is the southern stingray *(Dasyatis americana)*. Most attacks occur during the summer and autumn months, as vacationers venture into the surf that may be laden with congregating (for spawning purposes) rays. Freshwater species do not inhabit U.S. waters. They are found in South America, Africa, and Southeast Asia.

Life and Habits

Stingrays are usually found in tropical, subtropical, and warm temperate oceans, generally in shallow (intertidal) water areas, such as sheltered bays, shoal lagoons, river mouths, and sandy areas between patch reefs.[35] Rays can enter brackish and fresh waters, as well. Although rays are generally found above moderate depths, at least one deep-sea species has been discovered.

Rays are small (several inches) to large (up to 12 feet by 6 feet) creatures observed lying on top of the sand and mud or partially submerged, with only the eyes, spiracles, and part of the tail exposed (Figure 62-1). Their flattened bodies are round-, diamond-, or kite-shaped, with wide pectoral fins that look like wings (Figure 61-2). Rays are nonaggressive scavengers and bottom feeders that burrow into the sand or mud to feed on worms, mollusks, and crustaceans. The mouth and gill plates are located on the ventral surface of the animal (Figure 62-3).

Venom and Venom Apparatus

The venom organ of stingrays consists of one to four venomous stings on the dorsum of an elongate, whiplike caudal appendage. There are four different anatomic types of stingray venom organs, based on their adaptability as a defense organ (Figure 61-4). Thus the stinging ability of rays may be divided into four categories: the gymnurid type (butterfly rays, or Gymnuridae), with a poorly developed sting of up to 2.5 cm placed at the base of a short tail; the myliobatid type (eagle and bat rays, or Myliobatidae), with a sting of up to 12 cm placed at the base of a cylindrical caudal appendage that terminates in a long whiplike tail; the dasyatid type (stingrays and whiprays, or Dasyatidae), with a sting of up to 37 cm placed at the base or further out on the caudal appendage that terminates in a long whiplike tail; and the urolophid type (round stingrays, or Urolophidae), with a sting of up to 4 cm located at the base of a short, muscular, well-developed caudal appendage. The efficiency of the apparatus is related to the length and musculature of the tail and to the location and length of the sting. Eagle rays and some mantas (Atlantic *Mobular mobular* and Pacific *Mobula japanica*) have a stinging apparatus, but it is less of a threat because the spine is located at the base of the tail and is not well adapted as a striking organ. Although the manta may grow to a width of 6 m (20 feet) and weight of 3000 pounds, it dines on small fish, crustaceans, and microorganisms (Figure 62-5). Many divers have "hitched" a ride on the wings of a manta; there are no reports of envenomation. However, manta skin is rough and can abrade unprotected human skin. A stingray "hickey" is a mouth-bite, created by powerful grinding plates, that produces superficial erosions and ecchymosis in an oral pattern. Persons who hand feed stingrays may incur this type of injury.[15] The suction force generated by a stingray is sufficient to pull in a large amount of soft tissue, say, from a thigh. This may result in a large and painful contusion and/or hematoma.

In all cases, the venom apparatus of stingrays consists of a bilaterally retroserrate spine or spines and the enveloping integumentary sheath or sheaths. The elongate and tapered vasodentine spine is firmly attached

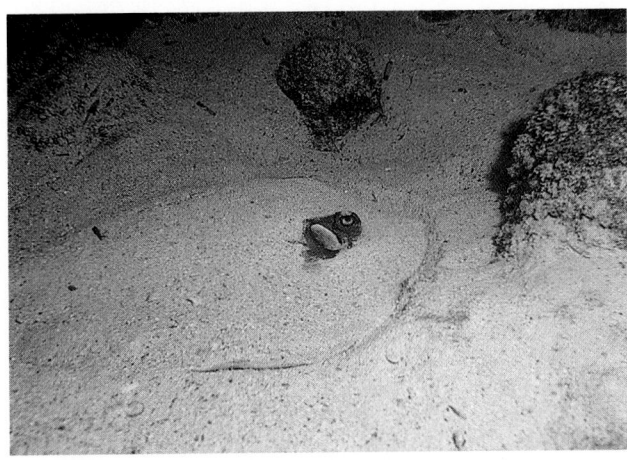

Figure 62-1 Stingray nestled in the sand. Only the eyes and spiracles are visible. *(Photo by Paul Auerbach, MD.)*

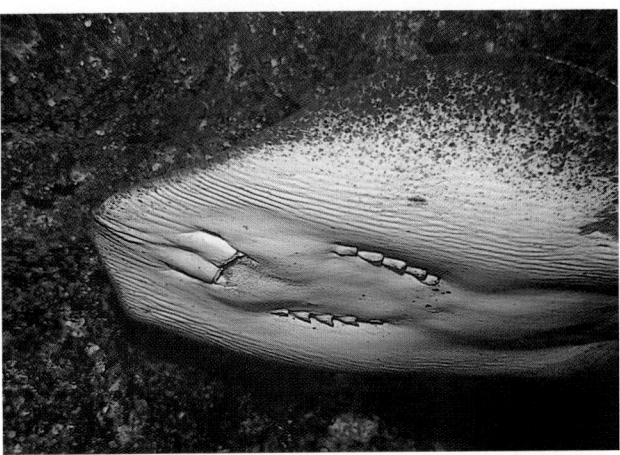

Figure 62-3 Ventral surface of a stingray, demonstrating mouth and gill plates. *(Photo by Paul Auerbach, MD.)*

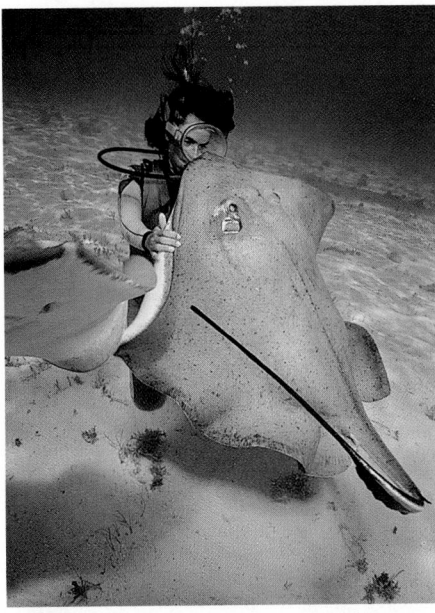

Figure 62-2 Diver cavorting with a large stingray. *(Photo by Howard Hall.)*

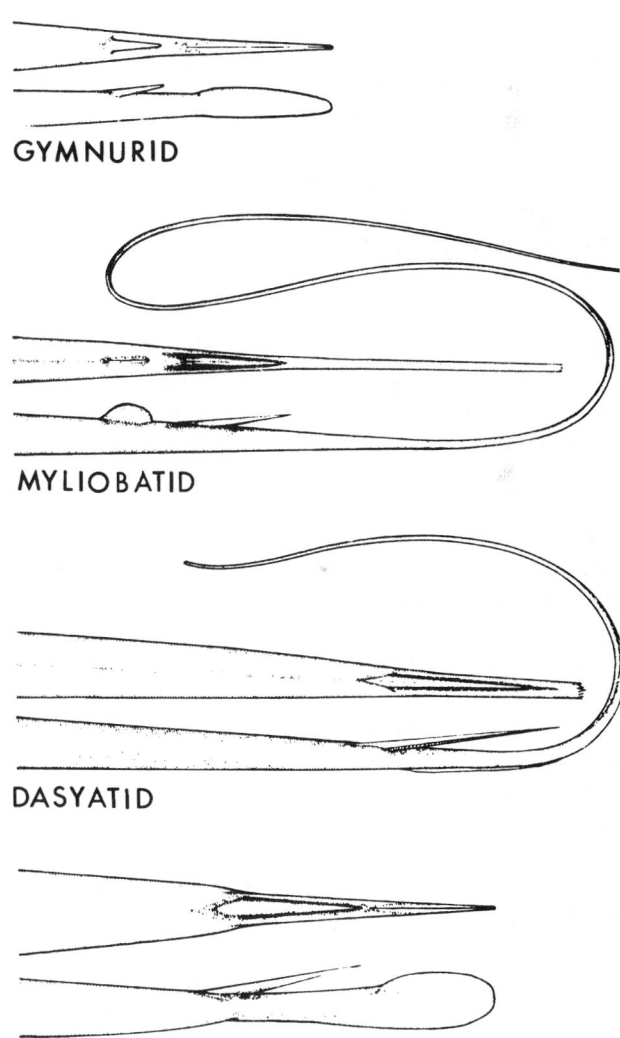

GYMNURID

MYLIOBATID

DASYATID

UROLOPHID

Figure 62-4 Four anatomic types of stingray venom organs.

to the dorsum of the tail (whip) by dense collagenous tissue and is edged on either side by a series of sharp retrorse teeth. Along either edge on the underside of the spine are the two ventrolateral glandular grooves, which house the soft venom glands. The entire spine is encased by the integumentary sheath, which also contains some glandular cells. The sting is often covered with a film of venom and mucus. The spine is replaced if detached.

The venom contains various toxic fractions, including serotonin, 5'-nucleotidase, and phosphodiesterase. Russell[43] investigated the pharmacologic properties of stingray venoms. In animal studies he demonstrated

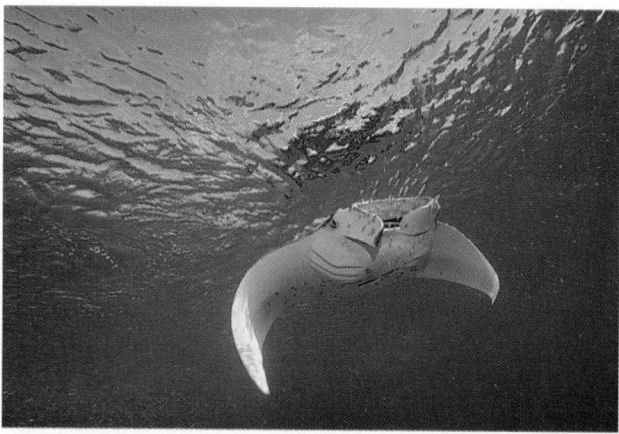

Figure 62-5 Manta ray. (Photo by Paul Auerbach, MD.)

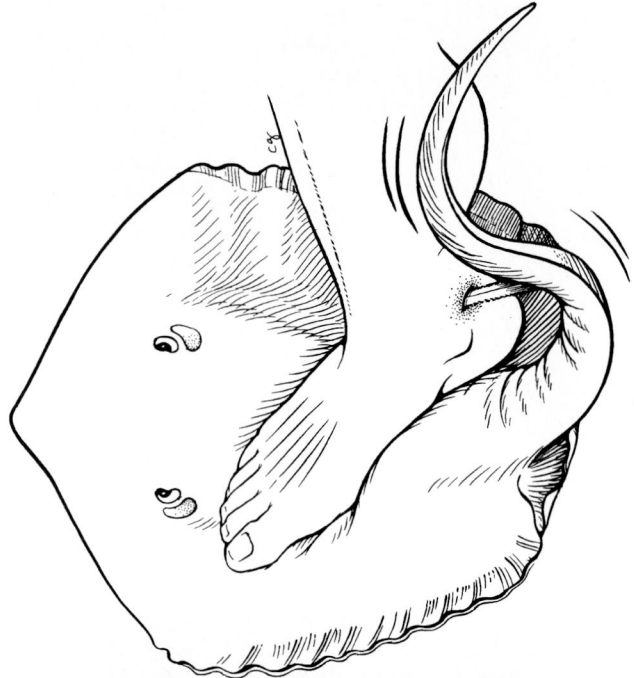

Figure 62-6 The stingray lashes its tail upward into the leg and generates a deep puncture wound.

significant venom-induced peripheral vasoconstriction, bradycardia, atrioventricular block, ischemic ST-T wave abnormalities, asystole, central respiratory depression, seizure activity, ataxia, coma, and death. The venom did not appear to be a paralytic neuromuscular agent. Research on stingray venom from the 1950s observed that heating the venom to a temperature above 50° C (122° F) diminished some biologic effects.

Clinical Aspects

Stingray "attacks" are purely defensive gestures that occur when an unwary human handles, corners, or steps on a camouflaged creature while wading in shallow waters. The tail of the ray reflexively whips upward and accurately thrusts the caudal spine or spines into the victim, producing a puncture wound or jagged laceration (Figure 62-6). The integumentary sheath covering the spine is ruptured and venom is released into the wound, along with mucus, pieces of the sheath, and fragments of the spine. On occasion the entire spine tip is broken off and remains in the wound (Figure 62-7).[44] "Domesticated stingrays," such as those that congregate at "Stingray City" in the waters of Grand Cayman Island, are habituated to the presence of humans and apparently pose less hazard.

Thus a stingray wound is both a traumatic injury and an envenomation. The former involves the physical damage caused by the sting itself. Because of the retrorse serrated teeth and powerful strikes, significant lacerations can result. Secondary bacterial infection is common. Osteomyelitis may occur if the bone is penetrated. Most injuries occur when the victim steps on a ray; another common cause is handling a ray during its extraction from a fishing net or hook. The lower extremities, particularly the ankle and foot, are involved most often, followed by the upper extremities, abdomen, and thorax. In a rare case, the heart was directly injured.[42] Fatalities have occurred after abdominal or

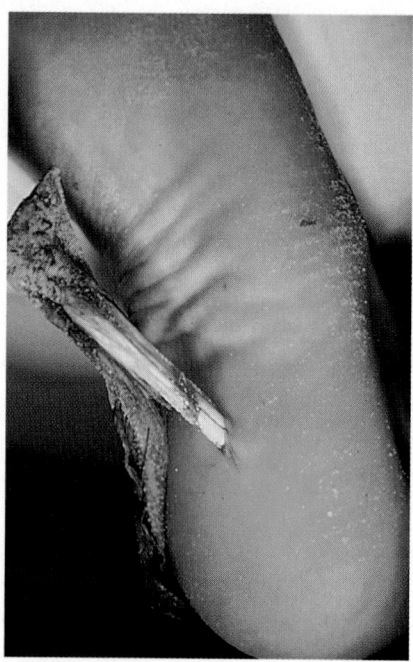

Figure 62-7 Stingray spine tip broken off into the heel of a victim. (Photo by Robert D. Hayes.)

thoracic (cardiac) penetration, and from exsanguination from the femoral artery. Another death has been attributed to tetanus complicating a leg wound. A spine partially or totally denuded of its sheath and venom glands may not cause an envenomation.[16]

The envenomation classically causes immediate local intense pain, edema, and variable bleeding. The pain may radiate centrally, peaks at 30 to 60 minutes, and may last for up to 48 hours. The wound is initially dusky or cyanotic and rapidly progresses to erythema and hemorrhagic discoloration, with rapid fat and muscle hemorrhage and necrosis.[6] If discoloration around the wound edge is not immediately apparent, within 2 hours it often extends several centimeters from the wound. Minor stings may simulate bacterial cellulitis. Systemic manifestations include weakness, nausea, vomiting, diarrhea, diaphoresis, vertigo, tachycardia, headache, syncope, seizures, inguinal or axillary pain, muscle cramps, fasciculations, generalized edema (with truncal wounds), paralysis, hypotension, arrhythmias, and death.[23,26] The paralysis may represent spastic muscle contractures induced by pain, which are a tremendous hazard for a diver or swimmer.

Treatment

The success of therapy is largely related to the rapidity with which it is undertaken. Treatment is directed at combating the effects of the venom, alleviating pain, and preventing infection. If hot water for immersion and irrigation (see below) is not immediately available, the wound should be irrigated immediately with nonheated water or saline. If sterile saline or water is not available, tap water may be used. This removes some venom and mucus and may provide minimal pain relief.

As soon as possible, the wound should be soaked in nonscalding hot water to tolerance (upper limit 45° C [113° F]) for 30 to 90 minutes. This might attenuate some of the thermolabile components of the protein venom (although this has never been proven in vivo) and/or interrupt nerve impulse transmission, and, in some envenomations, relieves pain. There is no indication for the addition of ammonia, magnesium sulfate, potassium permanganate, or formalin to the soaking solution. Under these circumstances they are toxic to tissue and may obscure visualization of the wound. During the hot water soak (or at any time, if soaking is not an option), the wound should be explored and debrided of any readily visible pieces of the sting or its integumentary sheath, which would continue to envenom the victim. Cryotherapy is disastrous, and no data yet support the use of antihistamines or steroids. One local remedy, application of half a bulb of onion directly to the wound, has been reported to decrease the pain and perhaps inhibit infection after a sting from the blue-spotted stingray *Dasyatis kuhlii* (Figure 62-8).[48] The author noted that this approach is used in the Northern Territory of Australia for other fish spine stings, and that the medicinal use of the Liliaceae plant family has been recorded in many cultures. No other folk remedy, such as the application of macerated cockroaches, cactus juice,

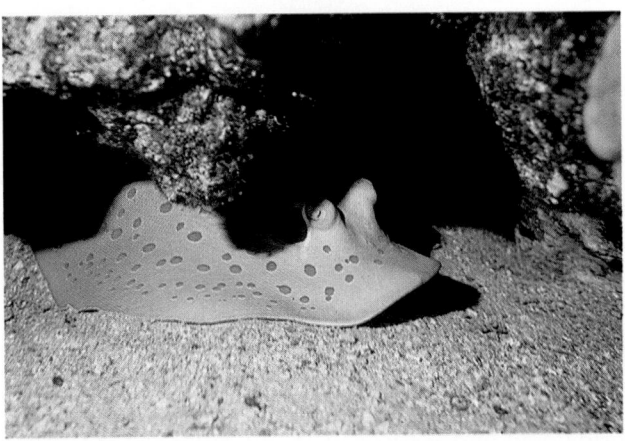

Figure 62-8 Blue-spotted stingray. *(Photo by Paul Auerbach, MD.)*

"mile-a-minute" leaves, fresh human urine, or tobacco juice, has been proven effective.[37]

Local suction, if applied in the first 15 to 30 minutes, has been suggested by some clinicians to be of potential value (this is controversial), as may a proximal constriction band (also controversial) that occludes only superficial venous and lymphatic return. This should be released for 90 seconds every 10 minutes to prevent ischemia.

Pain control should be initiated during the first debridement or soaking period. Narcotics may be necessary. Local infiltration of the wound with 1% to 2% lidocaine (Xylocaine) or bupivacaine 0.25% (not to exceed 3 to 4 mg/kg total dose in adults; not approved in children under the age of 12 years) without epinephrine may be useful. A regional nerve block may be necessary.

After the soaking procedure, the wound should be prepared in a sterile fashion, reexplored, and thoroughly debrided. Wounds should be packed open for delayed primary closure or sutured loosely around adequate drainage in preference to tight closure, which might increase likelihood of wound infection. Another approach that has been mentioned is wound excision followed by packing with an alginate-based wick dressing.[17,37] Prophylactic antibiotics are recommended because of the high incidence of ulceration, necrosis, and secondary infection. Necrotizing fasciitis caused by *Vibrio alginolyticus* has followed stingray injury in a victim with preexisting hepatic cirrhosis.[25] If the abdominal cavity is penetrated, the victim should receive cefoxitin or clindamycin-gentamicin intravenously in addition to any antibiotic(s) chosen to cover marine microbes.

If the treatment plan is to treat and release, the victim should be observed for at least 3 to 4 hours for systemic side effects.

Wounds that are not properly debrided or explored and cleansed of foreign material may fester for weeks or months. Such wounds may appear infected, when what really exists is a chronic draining ulcer initiated by persistent retained organic matter. Within the first few weeks after an envenomation, a foreign body can sometimes be observed by soft tissue radiograph, ultrasound, or magnetic resonance imaging. After a few weeks, exploration may reveal erosion of adjacent soft tissue structures and the formation of an epidermal inclusion cyst or other related foreign body reaction.[7] As with other marine-acquired wounds, indolent infection should prompt a search for unusual microorganisms. A case of invasive fusariosis (*Fusarium solani*) after stingray envenomation responsive to sequential debridement and ketoconazole (the latter of indeterminate effect) has been reported.[24] Necrotizing fasciitis due to *Photobacterium damsela* (formerly *Vibrio damsela*) followed a leg laceration caused by a stingray. Notably, the patient had the wound sutured primarily and was not prescribed an antibiotic at the time of the repair.[5a]

Prevention

A stingray spine can penetrate a wet suit, leather or rubber boot, and even the side of a wooden boat; therefore a wet suit or pair of sneakers is not adequate protection. Persons walking through shallow waters known to be frequented by stingrays should shuffle along and create enough disturbance to frighten off any nearby animals.

SCORPIONFISH

Scorpionfish are members of the family Scorpaenidae and follow stingrays as perpetrators of piscine stings. Distributed in tropical and less commonly in temperate oceans, several hundred species are divided into three groups typified by different genera on the basis of venom organ structure: (1) *Pterois* (zebrafish, lionfish, and butterfly cod), (2) *Scorpaena* (scorpionfish, bullrout, and sculpin), and (3) *Synanceja* (stonefish). All have a bony plate (stay), which extends across the cheek from the eye to the gill cover. Each group contains a number of different genera and species; at least 80 species of the family Scorpaenidae have been implicated in human injuries or studied anatomically, biochemically, or physiopharmacologically.

Other venomous fish that sting in a manner similar to scorpionfish include the Atlantic toadfish (family Batrachoididae and genus *Thalassophryne*), with two venomous dorsal fin spines, and the Pacific ratfish (*Hydrolagus colliei*) (Figure 62-9) and European ratfish (*Chimaera monstrosa*), both with a single dorsal venomous spine. Toadfish hide in crevices and burrows, under rocks and debris, or in seaweed, sand, or mud. They may change coloration rapidly and remain superbly camouflaged. Rabbitfish (family Siganidae) and leatherjacks (leatherbacks or leatherjackets, family

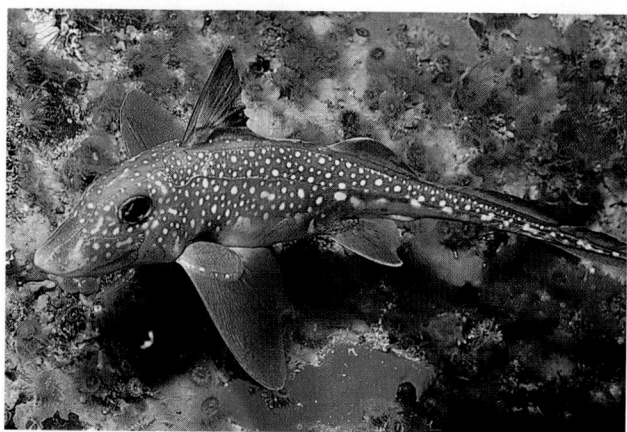

Figure 62-9 Ratfish *(Hydrolagus colliei). (Photo by Howard Hall.)*

Carangidae) carry venomous spines or fins and pose additional risks. Stargazers (family Uranoscopidae) have spines but do not appear to be venomous.

Life and Habits

Zebrafish (lionfish, firefish, or turkeyfish) are beautiful, graceful, and ornate coral reef fish generally found as single or paired free swimmers or hovering in shallow water (Figure 62-10). They are increasingly popular as aquarium pets and are imported illegally as part of the "underground zoo."

Scorpionfish proper (Scorpaena) dwell on the bottom in shallow water, bays, coral reefs, and along rocky coastlines, to a depth of 50 fathoms. Their shape and coloration provide excellent camouflage, allowing them to blend in with the ambient debris, rocks, and seaweed (Figure 62-11). They can be captured by hook and line and serve as important food fish in many areas. The protective coloration and concealment in bottom structures make scorpionfish difficult to visualize. Some species bury themselves in the sand, and most dangerous types lie motionless on the bottom. In many regions, scorpionfish are valuable as food fish. In the United States, they are found in greatest concentration around the Florida Keys and in the Gulf of Mexico, off the coast of southern California, and in Hawaii.

Stonefish live in shallow waters, often in tide pools and among reefs (Figure 62-12). They frequently pose motionless and absolutely fearless under rocks, in coral crevices or holes, or buried in the sand or mud. They are so sedentary that algae frequently take root on their skin (Figure 62-13). They are usually 15 to 20 cm in length. Stonefish are not indigenous to North American coastal waters.

Venom and Venom Apparatus

The venom organs are the 12 or 13 (of 18) dorsal (Figure 62-14), 2 pelvic, and 3 anal spines, with associated venom glands. Although they are frequently large,

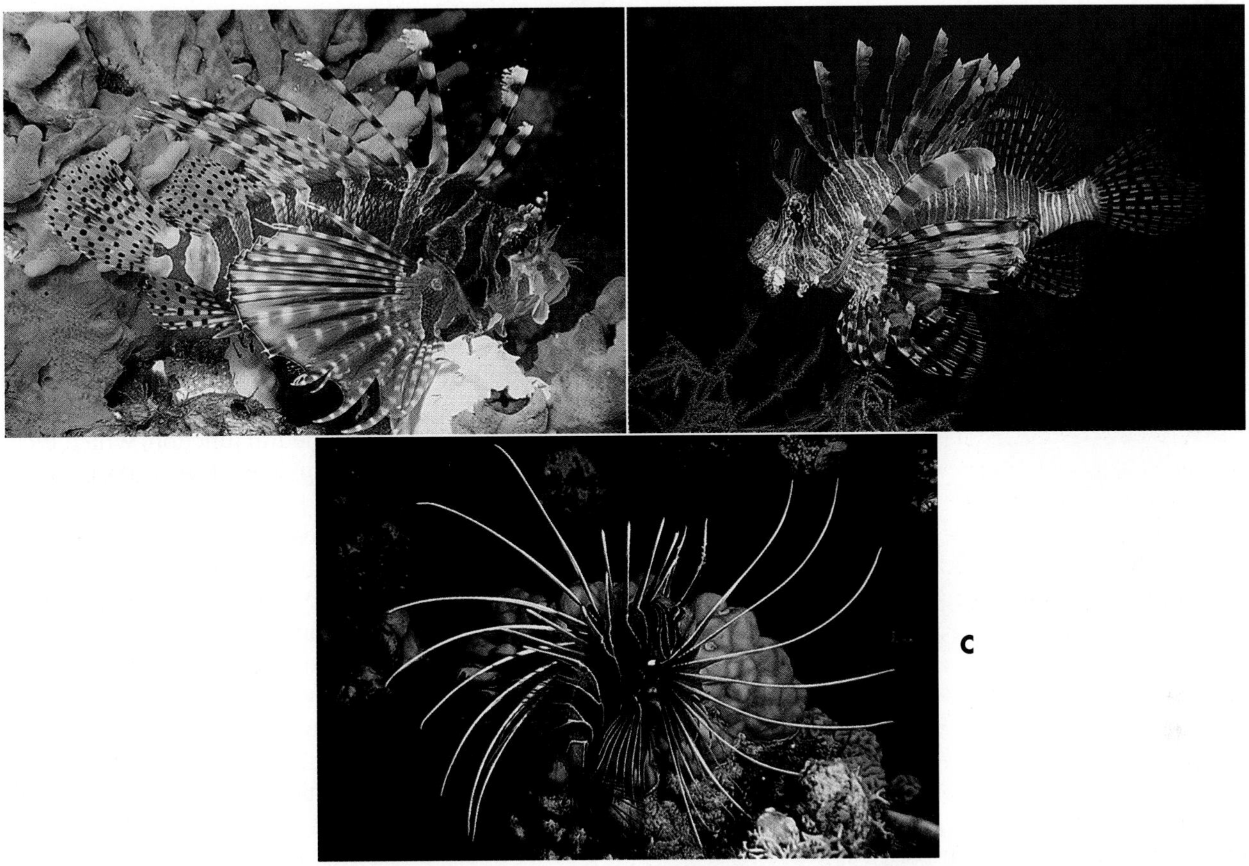

Figure 62-10 Three examples of lionfish. **A,** Juvenile lionfish from Sulawesi, Indonesia. **B,** Adult lionfish. **C,** Lionfish from the Red Sea. *(Photos by Paul Auerbach, MD.)*

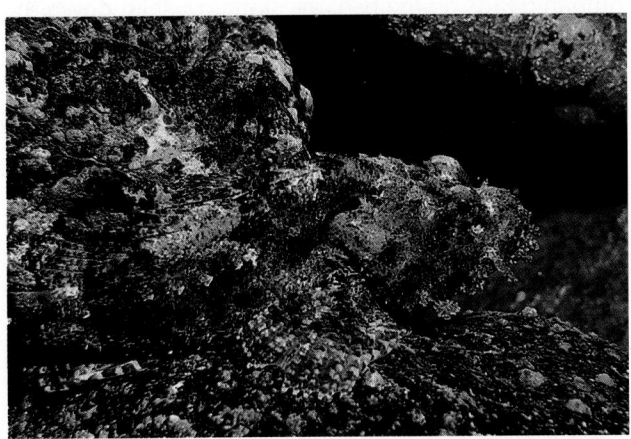

Figure 62-11 Scorpionfish assuming the coloration of its surroundings. *(Photo by Paul Auerbach, MD.)*

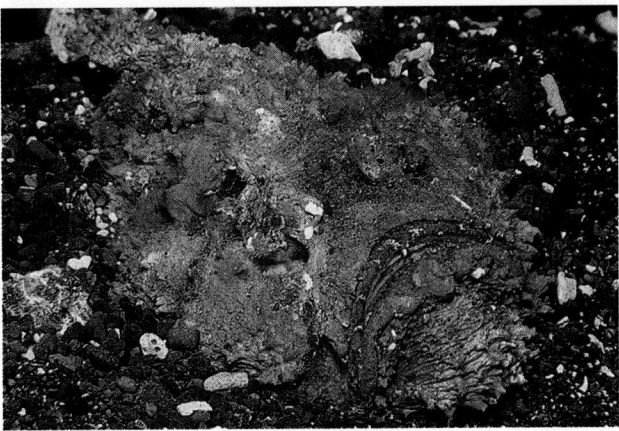

Figure 62-12 The deadly stonefish *(Synanceja horrida). (Photo by Paul Auerbach, MD.)*

plumelike, and ornate, the pectoral spines are not associated with venom glands. Each spine is covered with an integumentary sheath, under which venom filters along grooves in the anterolateral region of the spine from the paired glands situated at the base or in the midportion of the spine. It is estimated that the two

venom glands of a dorsal stonefish spine carry 5 to 10 mg of venom, closely associated with antigenic proteins of high molecular weight (between 50,000 and 800,000).[11] Scorpionfish venom contains multiple toxic fractions and, in the case of stonefish venom, has been likened in potency to cobra venom. The major toxic component

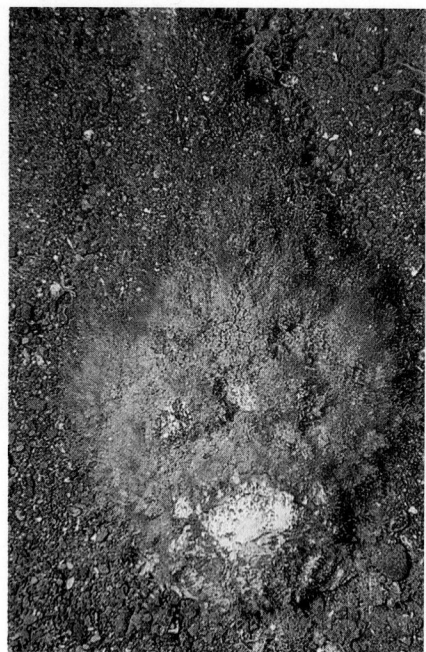

Figure 62-13 Some stonefish are so sedentary that algae grow on their skin. *(Photo by Paul Auerbach, MD.)*

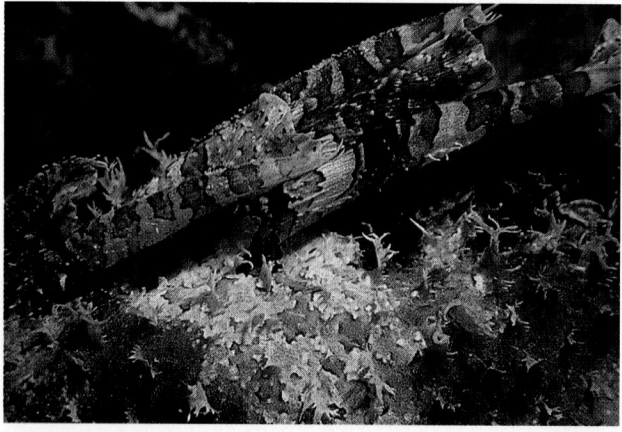

Figure 62-14 Scorpionfish spines. *(Photo by Kenneth Kizer, MD.)*

of *Synanceja* venom (stonustoxin) is a protein of molecular weight 148,000 (comprised of alpha and beta subunits of molecular weight 71,000 and 79,000, respectively) that is both antigenic and heat labile. The principal action of stonefish venom appears to be direct muscle toxicity, resulting in paralysis of cardiac, involuntary, and skeletal muscles.[21] In one analysis of biologic activity, stonefish (*Synanceja horrida*) venom exhibited edema-inducing, hemolytic, hyaluronidase, thrombinlike, alkaline phosphomonoesterase, 5'-nucleotidase, acetylcholinesterase, phosphodiesterase, arginine esterase, and arginine amidase activities.[27] In a recent evaluation, chromatographic analysis with electrochemical detection showed the presence of substances co-migrating with norepinephrine, dopamine, and tryptophan. Serotonin was not detected.[20] Crude venom of the stonefish *Synanceja verrucosa* possesses numerous enzymatic properties, including hyaluronidase, 8 esterases, and 10 aminopeptidases.[19] Stonefish venom causes pulmonary edema in laboratory animals, which may reflect a general vascular permeability.[27,30] It also causes species-restricted (nonhuman) hemolysis and platelet aggregation.[28] Profound endothelial relaxation may contribute directly to hypotension.[33] The neuromuscular toxicity appears to be a consequence of the venom's dose-dependent presynaptic and postsynaptic actions at the myoneural junction, which include release and depletion of neurotransmitter from the nerve terminal, followed by irreversible depolarization of muscle cells and microscopically observable muscle and nerve damage.[31] The nondialyzable opalescent venom retains full potency for at least 24 to 48 hours after the death of a scorpionfish.[29]

Pterois species carry long, slender spines with small venom glands covered by a thin integumentary sheath. An extract of lionfish spine tissue contains acetylcholine and a toxin that affects neuromuscular transmission.[12] *Scorpaena* species carry longer heavy spines with moderate-sized venom glands covered by a thicker integumentary sheath. *Synanceja* species carry short, thick spines with large, well-developed venom glands covered by an extremely thick integumentary sheath (Figures 62-15 and 62-16). However, the skin over the venom gland is loosely attached, so when a human treads on the fish, the skin is pushed down the spine and the venom gland is compressed by the crumpled sheath. The pressure forces the venom gland to empty up the paired narrow ducts so that venom and glandular tissue spurt into the wound.[22]

When any of these fish is removed from the water, handled, stepped on, or otherwise threatened, it reflexively erects the spinous dorsal fin and flares out the armed gill covers and pectoral and anal fins. If provoked while still in the water, it actually attacks. The venom is injected by a direct puncture wound through the skin, which tears the sheath and may fracture the spine, in a manner analogous to that of a stingray envenomation.

Clinical Aspects

Native residents of the Indo-Pacific islands have great fear of a sting from the dreaded venomous stonefish, such as the Tahitian "nohu" ("nofu" or "no'u") or the Australian "warty ghoul." The presentation of the injury is similar to that of the stingray envenomation, in that the unwary diver or fisherman steps on or handles the fish. In the United States, marine aquarists and beneficiaries of illegal importation of tropical animals are increasingly envenomed as they unknowledgeably

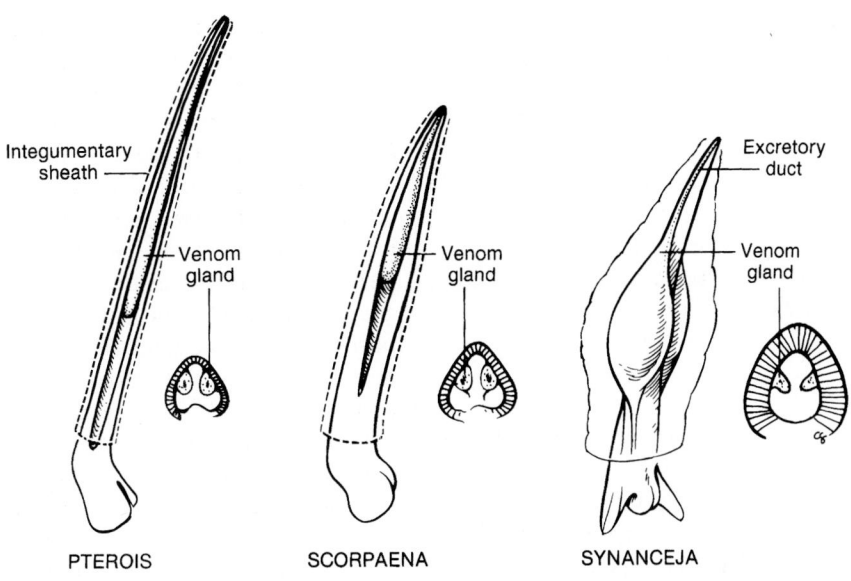

Figure 62-15   Lionfish, scorpionfish, and stonefish spines with associated venom glands.

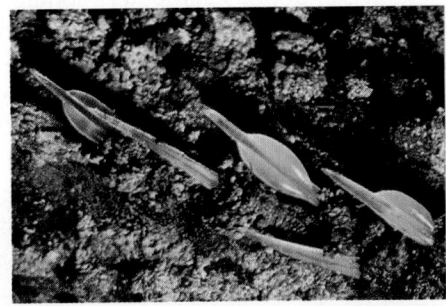

Figure 62-16   Spines of the venomous stonefish, demonstrating venom glands. *(Courtesy John Williamson, MD.)*

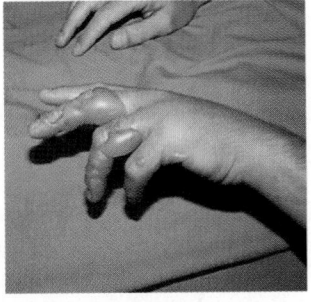

Figure 62-17   Vesiculation of the hand 48 hours after the sting of a lionfish. *(Photo by Howard McKinney.)*

handle *Pterois volitans, P. radiata,* or *Scorpaena guttata.* In Indo-Pacific waters, envenomations of the foot and lower extremity are more commonly caused by the stonefish, such as *Synanceja horrida, S. trachynis,* or *S. verrucosa.* Scorpionfish stings vary according to the species, with a progression in severity from the lionfish (mild) through the scorpionfish (moderate to severe) to the stonefish (severe to life threatening).

The severity of the envenomation depends on the number and type of stings, species, amount of venom released, and age and underlying health of the victim. Pain is immediate and intense, with radiation centrally. Untreated, the pain peaks at 60 to 90 minutes and persists for 6 to 12 hours. With a stonefish envenomation, the pain may be severe enough to cause delirium and may persist at high levels for days. The wound and surrounding area are initially ischemic and then cyanotic, with more broadly surrounding areas of erythema, edema, and warmth. Vesicles may form (Figure 62-17).

Human (hand) vesicle fluid after the sting of the lionfish *Pterois volitans* was analyzed for mediators of inflammation and demonstrated an appreciable quantity of prostaglandin $F_{2\alpha}$; thromboxane B_2, prostaglandin E_2, and 6-keto-prostaglandin $F_{1\alpha}$ were present in negligible quantities. Whether or not residual venom is present in blister fluid is a matter of conjecture. Rapid tissue sloughing and close surrounding areas of cellulitis, with anesthesia adjacent to peripheral hypesthesia, may be present within 48 hours. Necrotic ulceration is rare, but may occur, after a lionfish envenomation.[41] Severe local tissue reaction is more common after the sting of a scorpionfish or stonefish. Systemic effects include anxiety, headache, tremors, maculopapular skin rash, nausea, vomiting, diarrhea, abdominal pain, diaphoresis, pallor, restlessness, delirium, seizures, limb paralysis, peripheral neuritis or neuropathy, lymphangitis, arthritis, fever, hypertension, respiratory distress, bradycardia, tachycardia, atrioventricular block, ventricular fibrillation, congestive heart failure, pericarditis, hypotension, syncope, and death. Pulmonary edema is a bona fide sequela.[32] Death in humans, which is extremely rare, usually occurs within the first 6 to 8 hours. The wound is indolent and may require months to heal, only to leave a cutaneous granuloma or marked tissue defect, particularly after a secondary infection or deep abscess. Mild pain may persist for days to weeks. After successful therapy, paresthesias or numbness in the affected extremity may persist for a few weeks.

Treatment

As soon as possible, the wound or wounds should be immersed in nonscalding hot (upper limit 45° C [113° F]) water to tolerance. This may inactivate at least one of the thermolabile components of the protein venom that might otherwise induce a severe systemic reaction. Platelet aggregation in blister fluid is inhibited by heat treatment, which suggests that the venom or some other active component is neutralized. The soak should be maintained for a minimum of 30 minutes and may continue for up to 90 minutes. Recurrent pain that develops after an interval of 1 to 2 hours may respond to a repeat hot water treatment. As soon as is practical, all obvious pieces of spine and sheath fragments should be gently removed from the wound. Vigorous irrigation should be performed with warmed sterile saline to remove any integument or slime. If pain is severe or inadequately controlled (in terms of degree or rapidity or relief) by hot water immersion, local tissue infiltration with 1% to 2% lidocaine without epinephrine or regional nerve block with an anesthetic such as 0.25% bupivacaine may be necessary. After injection with a local or regional anesthetic, the hot water immersion should be discontinued or closely observed to avoid inadvertent creation of a burn wound in the now insensate body part. Infiltration with emetine, hydrochloride, potassium permanganate, or Congo red has been largely abandoned, despite reports of favorable experiences with acidic emetine. The biochemical bases for the success of folk remedies, such as the application of meat tenderizer, mangrove sap, or green papaya (papain), have yet to be confirmed. The effectiveness of alternative remedies may be related to the protein behavior of the venom, which is inactivated by heat, extremes of pH (it is partially inactivated at pH of greater than 8.6 and completely at a pH of less than 4), hydrogen peroxide, iodine, and potassium permanganate (which is, unfortunately, tissue toxic). Until further notice, no data are available to support the topical administration of empirical remedies, such as mineral spirits, organic dye, ground liver, or formalin. Cryotherapy is absolutely contraindicated, to avoid an iatrogenous cold-induced injury.

Although the spine rarely breaks off into the skin, the wound should be explored to remove any spine fragments, which will otherwise continue to envenom and act as foreign bodies, perpetuating an infection risk and poorly healing wound. If the spine has penetrated deeply into the sole of the foot, surgical exploration should be performed in the operating room with magnification. Vigorous warmed saline irrigation should be performed. Wide excision and debridement are unnecessary. Because of the nature of the puncture wound, tight suture or surgical tape closure should not be undertaken; rather, the wound should be allowed to heal open with provision for adequate drainage. If the puncture wound is high risk (deep, into the hand or foot or both), a prophylactic antibiotic(s) should be administered. It is probably wise to remove blister fluid using aseptic technique.

A stonefish antivenom is manufactured by the Commonwealth Serum Laboratories (CSL), Melbourne, Australia (Figure 62-18). In cases of severe systemic reactions from stings of *Synanceja* species, and rarely from other scorpionfish, it is administered intramuscularly. The antivenom is supplied in ampoules containing 2 ml (2000 units) of hyperimmune Fab$_2$ horse serum active against *Synanceja trachynis*, with 1 ml capable of neutralizing 10 mg of dried venom.[13] After skin testing to

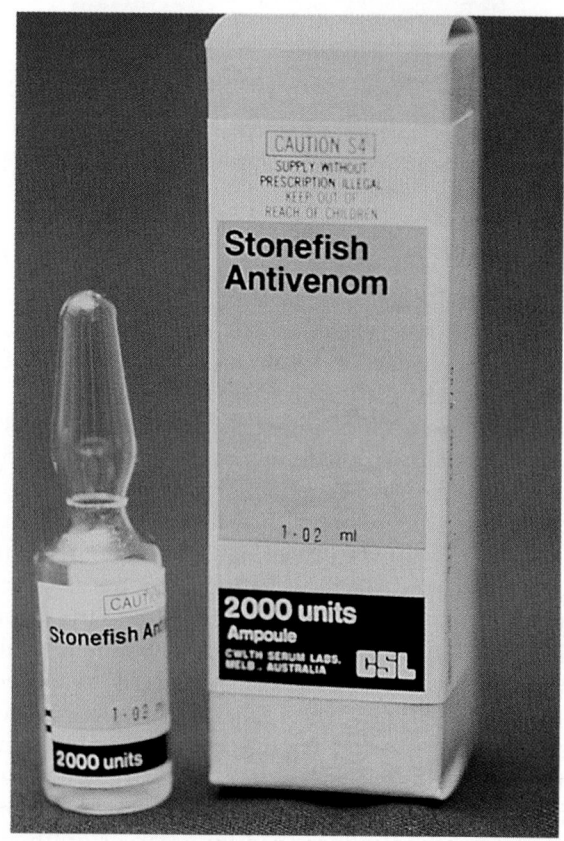

Figure 62-18 Stonefish antivenom. *(Courtesy John Williamson, MD.)*

estimate the risk for an anaphylactic reaction to equine sera, the antivenom should be given intramuscularly, since this is the only currently recommended route for this particular antivenom. However, review of the literature failed to identify any adverse effect attributable to intravenous (IV) administration other than the risk of anaphylaxis. As a rough estimate, one ampoule should neutralize one or two significant stings (punctures). For one or two puncture wounds, administer 1 ampoule; for three or four puncture wounds, 2 ampoules; for more than four puncture wounds, administer 3 ampoules. One or more additional ampoules may be necessary if there is recurrent severe pain. General guidelines for administration of antivenom have been previously discussed. When not in use, the antivenom should be protected from light and stored at 0° to 5° C (32° to 41° F), never frozen. Unused portions should be discarded.

Prevention

The most effective way to prevent envenomation is to avoid handling a scorpionfish. A diver should make a careful inspection before setting down on the bottom. Amateur aquarists should be exceedingly cautious when handling exotic tropical fish. Seemingly dead fish may yield an unpleasant surprise for the unwary.

CATFISH

Life and Habits

Approximately 1000 species of catfish inhabit both fresh and salt waters; many of these are capable of inflicting serious stings. Marine animals include *Plotosus lineatus* (oriental catfish), which lurks in tall seaweed and can inflict extremely painful stings, the larger sailcat *(Bagre marinus)*, and the common sea catfish *(Galeichthys felis)*, which hovers along the sandy bottom. The coral catfish *(Plotatus lineatus)* has also been reported to sting humans.[45] Ocean catfish, particularly juveniles, "swarm" and feed along the bottom (Figure 62-19). Freshwater catfish of North America include the brown bullhead *(Noturus nebulosus)*; Carolina madtom *(N. furiosus)*; and channel *(N. punctatus)*, blue *(N. furcatus)*, and white *(N. catus)* catfish.

The catfish derives its name from the well-developed sensory barbels ("whiskers") surrounding the mouth. Catfish possess a slimy skin without any true scales. Marine catfish, unlike freshwater catfish, frequently travel in large schools. Most freshwater catfish are bottom feeders noted for their junkyard diet. They are poor swimmers and not very evasive.

The South American astroblepins have flattened suctorial lips that allow them to scale cliffs. Tiny South American (Amazonian) catfish of the genus *Vandellia* are known as "urethra fish" in English, "candirú" by Brazilians, and "canero" by Spanish speakers.[8] Approxi-

mately an inch long, they carry short spines on their gill covers (Figure 62-20). The fish is putatively attracted to urine (water motion, warmth) and can swim up the human urethra or other urogenital apertures, where it extends the gill covers and thus becomes embedded, preventing removal by pulling on the fish's tail. Within the urethra, it causes extreme pain and inflammation. Since the animal normally seeks the outflow stream from a larger fish's gills, perhaps it is not urinophilic, but merely swimming upstream. Natives wear pudendal shields when urinating in natural bodies of water. A tight-fitting bathing suit is certainly prudent.

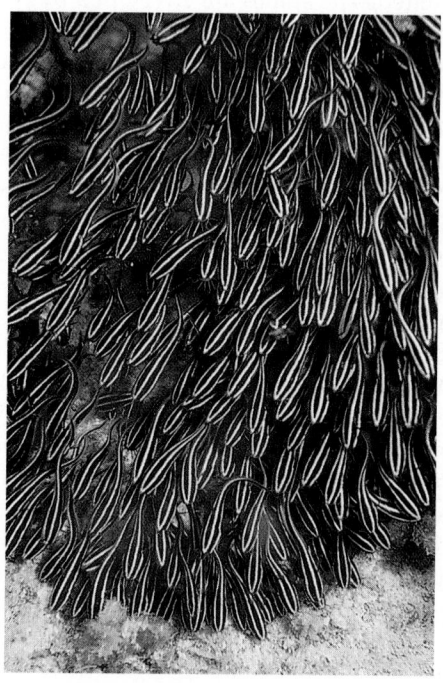

Figure 62-19 Juvenile ocean catfish. *(Photo by Norbert Wu.)*

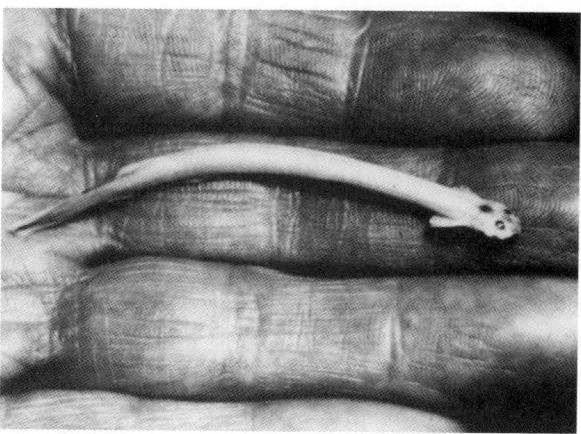

Figure 62-20 Amazonian catfish (candirú), which can enter the human urethra.

At best, extraction is painful. Amputation of the penis by natives has been described in the older literature. Ingestion of the green fruit of the jagua tree or buitach apple (*Genipa americana* L.) as a concoction (tea) apparently works to dispel the urethra-lodged candirú by the action of a large quantity of citric acid (megadose vitamin C), which softens calcium spines.

Venom and Venom Apparatus

The venom apparatus of the catfish consists of the single dorsal and two pectoral fin spines ("stings") and the axillary venom glands. Both the dorsal and pectoral spines are exquisitely sharp and can be locked into an extended position by the fish when it is handled or becomes excited. The spines are enveloped by glandular tissue within an integumentary sheath; some spines have sharp retrorse teeth. Scattered reports note envenomation in persons who handled only the tail of the fish, such as the Arabian Gulf catfish (*Arius thalassinus*), which suggests the presence of a toxic skin secretion (crinotoxin). Other observers note that toxin released from epidermal skin cells can cause throbbing pain, tissue necrosis, and perhaps muscle fasciculations.[18] Oriental catfish toxin, which is poorly antigenic, contains vasoconstrictive, hemolytic, edema-forming, dermatonecrotic, and other biogenic fractions.[46] It behaves in vivo much like a milder version of stingray venom. In contrast, the crinotoxin of the Arabian Gulf catfish contracts smooth muscle and stimulates the release of prostaglandins; pretreatment with atropine and indomethacin attenuates the response.[1,45] Furthermore, wound healing responses are accelerated by repeated local application of preparations from the epidermal secretions of another Arabian gulf catfish (*Arius bilineatus* Valenciennes).[2]

Clinical Aspects

Most stings are incurred when a fish is handled, which creates an injury out of proportion to the mechanical laceration. When the spine penetrates the skin, the integumentary sheath is damaged and the venom gland exposed. Catfish stings are described as instantaneously stinging, throbbing, or scalding, with central radiation up the affected limb. Normally the pain subsides within 30 to 60 minutes, but in severe cases it can last for up to 48 hours. The area around the wound quickly appears ischemic, with central pallor that gradually becomes cyanotic before the onset of erythema and edema. Swelling can be severe and secondary infections are frequent; gangrenous complications have been reported. Common side effects include local muscle spasm, diaphoresis, and fasciculations. Bleeding from the puncture wounds may be more severe than expected. Less common sequelae are peripheral neuropathy, lymphedema, adenopathy, lymphangitis,

weakness, syncope, hypotension, and respiratory distress. Death is extremely rare. The sting of the marine catfish is usually more severe than that of its freshwater counterparts and may have a propensity to more local hemorrhage.[36] Infection risk (see Chapter 60) is similar to that for any aquatic-acquired wound, in that *Vibrio* and *Aeromonas* species may be pathogens and the infection may be polymicrobial.[39] Other organisms that have been reported to be associated with marine or freshwater catfish-related injuries include *Edwardsiella tarda, Citrobacter freundii, Fusobacterium mortiferum, Morganella morganii, Providencia rettgeri, Enterococcus faecalis, Pseudomonas aeruginosa, Mycobacterium terrae,* and *Enterobacter cloacae*.[39] *E. tarda* is a gram-negative bacillus of the family Enterobacteriaceae that is mainly associated with aquatic environments and the animals that inhabit them, particularly catfish and other cold-blooded animals.[3,5] It may be a pathogen for eels and catfish. If *E. tarda* infection is determined, it is sensitive in vitro to ampicillin, aminoglycosides, β-lactamase stable cephalosporins, quinolones, tetracycline, and trimethoprim/sulfamethoxazole.[5]

Treatment

There are no specific antidotes. As with stingray and scorpionfish envenomations, the success of therapy is related to the rapidity with which it is undertaken. With catfish envenomations, in contrast to those of stingrays, constriction bandages have not been shown to be of value. The wound should be immediately immersed in nonscalding hot water to tolerance (upper limit 45° C [113° F]) for 30 to 90 minutes or until there is significant pain relief. This may inactivate heat-labile components of the venom and perhaps helps to reverse local toxin-induced vasospasm. There is no evidence that adding mineral salts, solvents, antiseptics, or other chemicals to the water is of additional benefit. Cryotherapy is inefficacious. A popular and unstudied local (U.S. rural) remedy is to rub the sting with skin mucus (slime) from the catfish. If the hot water soak is not sufficient to control pain, local infiltration of the wound with buffered (alkalinized) bupivacaine or lidocaine without epinephrine or a regional nerve block may be necessary. It has been theorized that the pH alteration offered by the alkalinized local anesthetic may neutralize venom.[34] The wound should be explored surgically to remove all spine and sheath fragments. Standard radiographs or soft tissue exposures may locate a radiopaque foreign body (Figure 62-21). The wound should be left unsutured to heal, to allow adequate drainage and minimize the risk of infection. All wounds must be carefully observed for infection until healed. If the puncture wound is high risk (deep, into the hand or foot or both), a prophylactic antibiotic(s) should be administered.

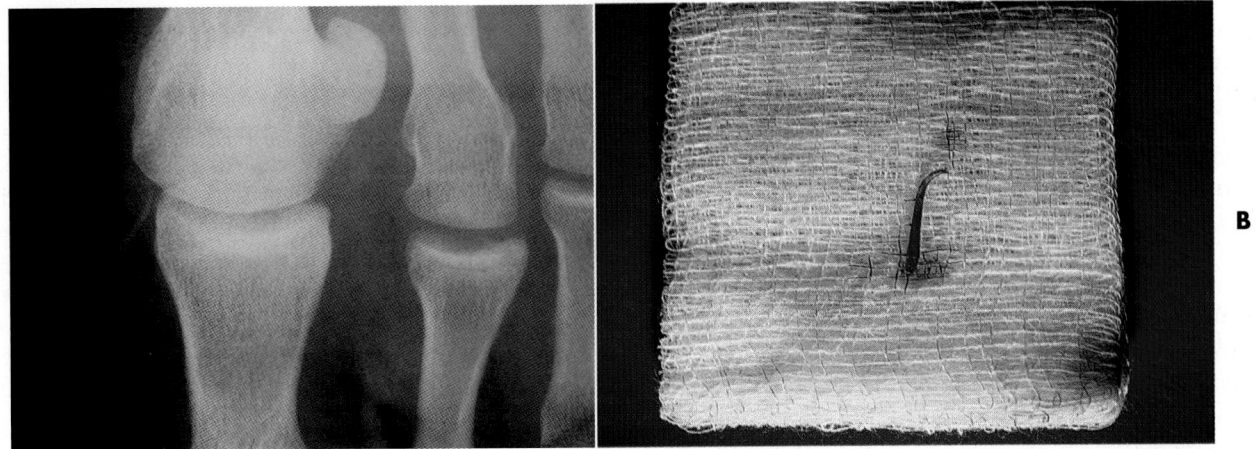

Figure 62-21 Catfish spine lodged in the foot. **A,** Radiograph demonstrating the presence of a foreign body. **B,** The spine removed. (**A** and **B** by Paul Auerbach, MD.)

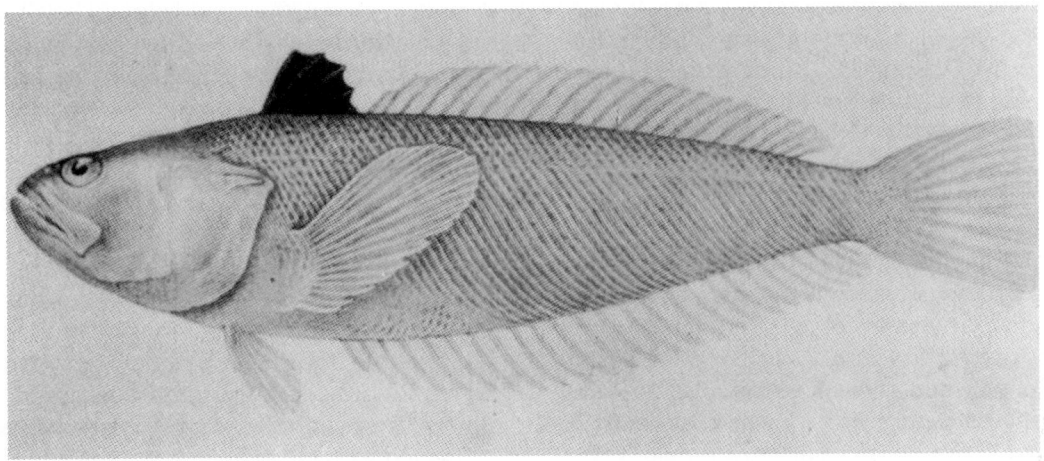

Figure 62-22 Lesser weeverfish.

Prevention

Catfish should be handled without grabbing the dorsal or pectoral fins, preferably by using a mechanical instrument or gaff. If possible, *Plotosus lineatus* should not be handled at all.

WEEVERFISH

Life and Habits

The weeverfish (*Echiichthys* species, formerly named *Trachinus*) (Figure 62-22) is the most venomous fish of the temperate zone. It is found in the Black Sea, Mediterranean Sea, eastern Atlantic Ocean, North Sea, and European coastal areas. Common names for the weeverfish include the adderpike, sea dragon, sea cat, and stang. Weeverfish are small (10 to 53 cm) marine

creatures that inhabit flat sandy or muddy bays, usually burying themselves in the soft bottom with only the head partially exposed. They lead sedentary lives but when provoked can strike out with unerring accuracy. Weevers are terrors to fishermen working in shallow sandy areas.

Venom and Venom Apparatus

The venom apparatus consists of four to eight elongate and needle-sharp dorsal (up to 4.5 cm in length) and two opercular and daggerlike dentinal spines, associated holocrine glandular tissue, and the thin enveloping stratified squamous epithelium integumentary sheath. When excited, the fish extends the dorsal fin and expands the operculum, projecting the opercular spine out at a 35- to 40-degree angle from the longitudinal axis of the body. Weeverfish survive for hours out of the water, and the toxin remains potent for hours in dead animals, particularly when they are well refrigerated. Although incompletely characterized, the unstable (heat-labile) protein venom (ichthyoacanthotoxin) contains several peptides, at least one protein of high molecular weight (324,000), and possibly 5-hydroxytryptamine, epinephrine, norepinephrine, histamine, and mucopolysaccharide components. To date, serotonin has not been identified in weeverfish venom. The greater weeverfish (*Echiichthys draco*) releases a protein venom, dracotoxin, which has membrane depolarizing and hemolytic activities. It appears to be a single polypeptide of molecular weight 105,000.[10] Other weeverfish of significance include *E. draco*, *E. vipera*, *E. radiatus*, and *E. lineatus*.

Clinical Aspects

Weeverfish stings usually afflict professional fishermen or vacationers who wade or swim along sandy coastal areas. The thrust of the spine is sufficient to penetrate a leather boot and creates a substantial puncture wound. The integumentary sheath is torn, and venom is injected into the wound. The onset of pain is instantaneous, described as intensely burning or crushing, and spreads rapidly to involve the entire limb. The pain usually peaks at 30 minutes and subsides within 24 hours but can last for days. Its intensity can induce irrational behavior and syncope; even narcotics are poorly effective. The puncture wound bleeds little and often appears pale and edematous initially. The sting of *E. vipera* may bleed freely. Over the course of 6 to 12 hours the wound becomes erythematous, ecchymotic, and warm. The edema may increase for 7 to 10 days, causing the entire limb to become markedly swollen. Secondary bacterial infections are common, and gangrene has been reported. The indolent wound may require months to heal, depending on the nature of the sting and underlying health of the victim. Raynaud's phenomenon in an envenomed digit occurring a few weeks after a weeverfish sting has been reported.[9] Persistent edema has been noted to last for more than 1 year.

Systemic symptoms associated with weeverfish envenomation include headache, delirium, aphonia, fever, chills, dyspnea, diaphoresis, cyanosis, nausea, vomiting, seizures, syncope, hypotension, and cardiac arrhythmias. Deaths have been reported but remain to be confirmed.

Treatment

The wound should immediately be immersed in nonscalding hot water to tolerance (upper limit 45° C [113° F]) for 30 to 90 minutes, or until there is significant pain relief. This may inactivate heat-labile com-

ponents of the venom and perhaps helps reverse local vasospasm that might contribute to local sequestration of venom and the inhibition of free bleeding. The addition of mineral salts, ammonia, vinegar, urine, or other substances to the water is of no proven value. Immersion in hot water is often a less successful therapy for a weeverfish sting than for that of a scorpionfish. When the heat inactivation method is inadequate to control pain, it is necessary to infiltrate the wound with a local anesthetic (1% to 2% lidocaine without epinephrine) or perform a regional nerve block. The liberal use of narcotics is often required. Cryotherapy is contraindicated.

Rarely, a spine breaks off into the skin. The wound should be gently explored, all fragments of sheath removed, and vigorous warmed saline irrigation performed. Wide excision and debridement are unnecessary. Because of the nature of the puncture wound, tight suture or surgical tape closure should not be undertaken; rather, the wound should be allowed to heal open with provision for adequate drainage. If the puncture wound is high risk (deep, into the hand or foot or both), a prophylactic antibiotic(s) should be administered. No commercial antivenom is currently available. An effective experimental antivenom was created at the Institute of Immunology in Zagreb, Yugoslavia, but is no longer available.

Prevention

Weeverfish hide in bottom sand and mud; thus persons must shuffle along with adequate footwear. These fish are easily provoked and should be avoided by scuba divers. They should never be handled alive and must be treated with extreme caution even when dead. Weeverfish survive for hours out of the water, and careless handling of a seemingly dead fish may result in an envenomation.

VENOMOUS (HORNED) SHARKS

Life and Habits

Horned sharks are species that possess dorsal fin spines. In the United States the group is essentially limited to the spiny dogfish (*Squalus acanthias*) (Figure 62-23). These and similar animals are distributed throughout sub-Arctic, temperate, tropical, and sub-Antarctic seas. The Port Jackson shark *Heterodontus portusjacksoni* is particularly dangerous.

The fish are sluggish and prefer cooler water and shallow protected bays. They are erratic in their migration and may be found singly or in schools. Voracious feeders, they eat other fish, coelenterates, mollusks, crustaceans, and worms.

The venom apparatus consists of a spine anterior to each of two dorsal fins and the associated venom glands.

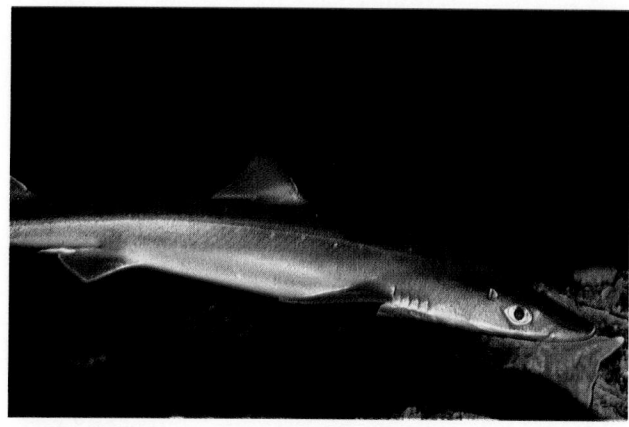

Figure 62-23 Spiny dogfish *(Squalus acanthias). (Photo by Norbert Wu.)*

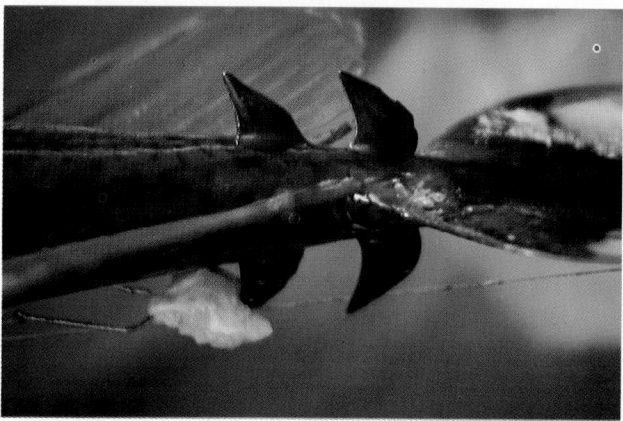

Figure 62-24 Surgeonfish "blades." *(Photo by Paul Auerbach, MD.)*

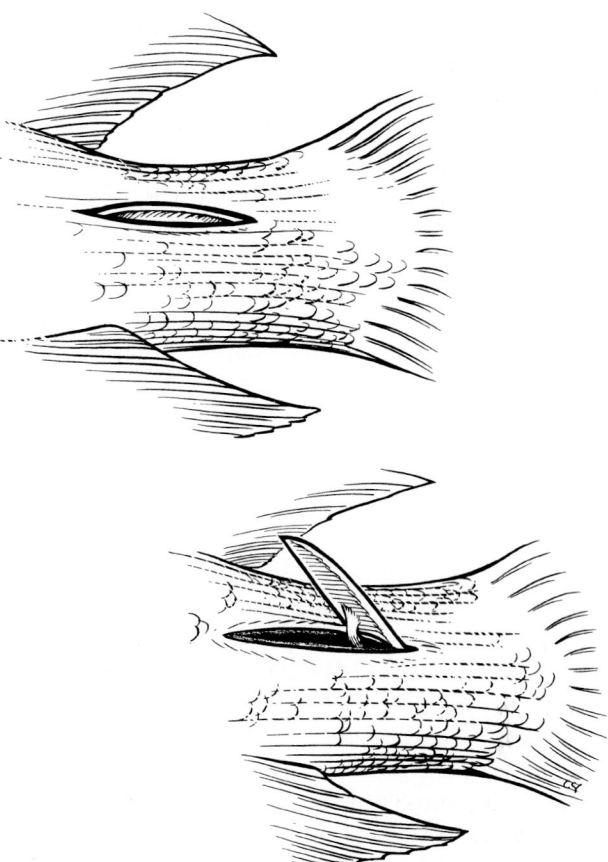

Figure 62-25 "Blade" mechanism of the surgeonfish.

Clinical Aspects

As with other vertebrate stings, there is immediate intense stabbing pain that may last for hours and is accompanied by erythema and edema. Although systemic side effects are rare, fatalities are possible.

Treatment

Treatment is the same as for stingray envenomation.

SURGEONFISH

Life and Habits

The surgeonfish (doctorfish, or "tang") is a tropical reef fish of the family Acanthuridae that carries one or more retractable jackknifelike epidermal appendages ("blades") on either side of the tail (Figure 62-24). When the fish is threatened, the blade may be extended out at a forward angle, where it serves to inflict a laceration (Figure 62-25). There does not appear to be any associated envenomation.

Clinical Aspects

A victim cut by a surgeonfish notes a laceration or deep puncture wound that is immediately painful; it usually bleeds freely. The pain is moderate to severe and of a burning nature. Systemic reactions are infrequent and consist of nausea, local muscle aching, and apprehension.

Treatment

The wound should be irrigated and then soaked in nonscalding hot water to tolerance (upper limit 45° C [113° F]) for 30 to 90 minutes or until pain is relieved, although this may be of variable efficacy. It should be scrubbed vigorously to remove all foreign material and watched closely for the development of a secondary infection. Unless absolutely necessary for hemostasis, sutures should not be used to close the wound.

PLATYPUS

Venom and Venom Apparatus

The platypus *Ornithorhynchus anatinus* is a furry venomous mammal that inhabits riverine systems of eastern Australia between northern Queensland and southern Tasmania.[14] These strange, fat animals have bills like a duck, webbed feet, a paddlelike tail, and claws on the feet. The male animal has an erectile keratinous spur on each hind limb linked via a distensible duct to a venom gland. The spur attains a length of 15 mm in mature animals. There is a duct on each side that connects the spur to a venom gland situated under the thigh muscles. The venom appears to have components that mediate a type I hypersensitivity reaction with mast cell degranulation, which is consistent with the clinical presentation of soft tissue edema. Other venom fractions include a natriuretic peptide, proteases, and hyaluronidase. Venom-induced local edema in laboratory rats is attenuated by ketanserin and, to a lesser degree, by cimetidine, which may indicate a role of 5-hydroxytryptamine and histamine.

Clinical Aspects

Normally, the platypus is a shy creature. However, when provoked, it grasps its opponent with the hind legs and thrusts a spur or spurs into the victim. From 2 to 4 ml of venom may be released. When a human is envenomed, symptoms include immediate severe pain, tissue edema, and prolonged local sensitivity to painful stimuli. Movement, even remote (such as coughing), worsens the pain. The pain and hyperesthesia may generalize for several days before the pain recedes back to the envenomed limb. The pain may last for weeks, and in a severe case, muscle mass may be lost.

Treatment

Therapy is supportive and includes pain medication, wound care, and physical therapy after the acute episode. Hot water immersion does not appear to be of benefit acutely. Short-term corticosteroid therapy has been suggested to diminish pain and mitigate swelling, but there is no proof that antiinflammatory agents are definitively useful.

SEA SNAKES

Life and Habits

Sea snakes (Figure 62-26) of the family Hydrophiidae (subfamilies Hydrophiinae [genera *Hydrelaps, Kerilia, Thalassophina, Enhydrina, Acalytophis, Thalassophis, Kolpophis, Lapemis, Astrotia, Pelamis,* and *Microcephalophis*] and Laticaudinae [genera *Laticauda, Aipysurus,* and *Emydocephalus*]) are probably the most abundant reptiles on earth. There are at least 52 species, all venomous. Species implicated in serious envenomations or human fatalities include *Astrotia stokesii, Enhydrina schistosa, Hydrophis ornatus, Hydrophis cyanocinctus, Lapemis hardwickii, Pelamis platurus,* and *Thalassophina viperina.*

The snakes are distributed in the tropical and warm temperate Pacific and Indian Oceans, with the highest number of envenomations occurring along the coast of Southeast Asia, in the Persian Gulf, and in the Malay Archipelago. No sea snakes live in the Atlantic Ocean or

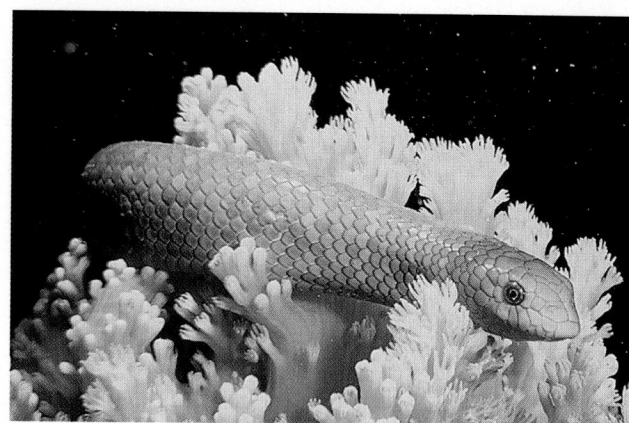

Figure 62-26 Olive sea snake. *(Photo by Michele Hall.)*

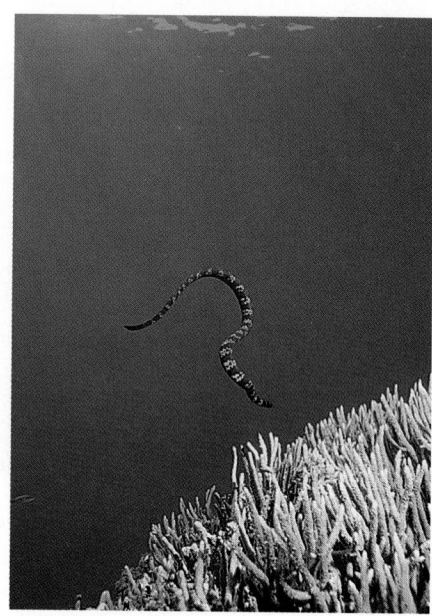

Figure 62-27 Sea snake in the Coral Sea. *(Photo by Carl Roessler.)*

in the Caribbean Sea. Hawaii is the only U.S. state that has sea snakes (predominantly *Pelamis platurus*). The Pacific snakes usually inhabit sheltered coastal or coral reef waters and congregate about river mouths, and only on rare occasion venture into the open ocean. *Pelamis platurus*, the most widely distributed sea snake, is pelagic and may be found in the Pacific coastal waters of Central and South America (see Figure 39-13). It does not migrate to the Caribbean because of the freshwater barrier of Gatun Lake in the center of the Panama Canal.

Although sea snakes have the general appearance of land snakes, true sea snakes and sea kraits have valvelike nostril flaps and rudimentary ventral plates, without gills, limbs, ear openings, sternum, or urinary bladder. Most species of sea snakes are 0.9 to 1.2 m (3 to 4 feet) long, but some attain lengths of up to 2.7 m (9 feet). They are sinuous scaled creatures whose bodies are compressed posteriorly into a flat, paddle-shaped tail designed for marine locomotion (Figure 62-27). They swim in an undulating fashion and can move backward or forward in the water with equal speed. On land, however, they are awkward and do not survive readily. They may be brightly colored, as is the yellow-bellied sea snake, *Pelamis platurus*. With a single lung the sea snake is capable of diving to 100 m (328 feet) and remaining submerged for 2 hours. The sea snake can be distinguished from a sea eel by the presence of scales and the absence of gills and fins.

Sea snakes use an air retention mechanism in the lung to control buoyancy. Their food, small fish swallowed whole, is captured underwater, usually around bottom rocks and coral. In general, sea snakes are docile creatures and flee when approached. However, when cornered or handled, they may become aggressive and strike out. During the reproductive season, some males adopt more irritable attitudes. The banded sea snake (sea krait) *Laticauda semifasciata* is served as a food (raw, smoked, or cooked) in certain Asian countries, notably Japan and the Philippines.

Venom and Venom Apparatus

The well-developed venom apparatus consists of two to four hollow maxillary fangs and a pair of associated venom glands. Fortunately, because the fangs are short and easily dislodged from their sockets, most bites (approximately 80%) do not result in significant systemic envenomation. Most fangs, except for those of *Astrotia stokesii* and *Aipysurus laevii*, are not long enough to penetrate a wet suit. The venom yield of sea snakes varies with species and is largely related to the size of the venom glands.

The protein venom is highly toxic and includes stable peripheral neurotoxins more potent than those of terrestrial snakes. Neuromuscular transmission is blocked predominantly at the postsynaptic membrane and caused by attachment of toxin to the α subunit of the acetylcholine receptor. Presynaptic toxin in sea snake venom has been less well studied but appears to be related to inhibition of transmitter release by blocking resynthesis of acetylcholine from choline. It seems probable that the action of *Laticauda semifasciata* venom on excitable membranes is to alter ionic permeability, particularly that of sodium and chloride, without effect on Na^+, K^+-dependent adenosine triphosphatase activity. Calcium transport abnormalities are currently under investigation. Among other fractions of the venom are phospholipases, nerve growth factors, capillary permeability factor, anticomplement-active factor, enzymes (including acetylcholinesterase, hyaluronidase, leucine aminopeptidase, 5'-nucleotidase, phosphomonoesterase, phosphodiesterase), and hemolytic and myotoxic compounds, which result in skeletal muscle necrosis, intravascular hemolysis, and renal tubular damage. Myonecrosis is related to phospholipase A, which may inhibit calcium uptake into the sarcoplasmic reticulum. Neurotoxins are thought to ex-

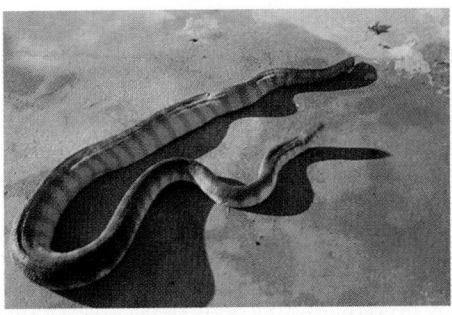

Figure 62-28 Beaked sea snake *(Enhydrina schistosa)*. A common sea snake of Southeast Asia, the average length is about 1 m (3 feet). This creature inflicts a high proportion of the sea snake bites recorded in Asian coastal waters. *(Photo by Sherman Minton, MD.)*

ert their toxicity by binding in a nondepolarizing fashion to the nicotinic acetylcholine receptor and blocking neuromuscular transmission.[40]

The venoms of sea snakes are similar, as is reflected in positive reactions during immunodiffusion, immunoelectrophoresis, cross-neutralization by antivenom against heterologous venoms, and amino acid composition and sequences of neurotoxins. This is a reflection of phylogenetic relationships and is a logistic aid in the preparation of effective antivenom.

Although large venom yields have been obtained from *Astrotia stokesii*, *Enhydrina schistosa* is considered the most dangerous sea snake (Figure 62-28). *E. schistosa* is the most widely distributed sea snake in the Arabian sea. *Aipysurus duboisii* and *Acalyptophis peronii* from the Coral Sea have recently been shown to carry venoms of high human lethality potential. In an evaluation of poisonous land and sea snakes representative of those encountered in Saudi Arabia, sea snakes were noted to have an average lethal dose in dogs of 0.05 mg/kg, in comparison with the average lethal dose of vipers (1.13 mg/kg) and elapids (0.69 mg/kg).[47] Deaths were attributed to respiratory paralysis and failure.

Clinical Aspects

Bites are usually the result of accidental handling of snakes snared in the nets of fishermen, or of accidentally stepping on a snake while wading. Most sea snake poisonings occur in remote fishing villages and in boats engaged in fishing. Nearly all bites involve the extremities.

The diagnosis of sea snake bite is based on the following:

1. Location. A person must have been in the water or handling a fishing net containing a sea snake to have been bitten. Some snakes may foray briefly onto land, particularly in areas of heavy mangrove growth, but it is quite unusual for a bite to occur out of the water. Because snakes may inhabit sheltered coastal waters and frequently congregate near river mouths, a bite can occur in an estuarine setting, up to 5 km inland.

2. Absence of pain. Initially, a sea snake bite does not cause great pain and may resemble no more than a pinprick.

3. Fang marks. These are multiple pinhead-sized, hypodermic-like puncture wounds, usually 1 to 4, but potentially up to 20. If the skin is not broken, envenomation cannot occur. In some cases, particularly with a superficial injury through the arm or leg of a neoprene wet suit, the fang marks may be difficult to visualize because of the lack of a localized reaction.

4. Identification of the snake. Snakes should be captured or killed carefully with a nonmacerating blow behind the head and retained for identification by an expert.

5. Development of characteristic symptoms. These include painful muscle movement, lower extremity paralysis, arthralgias, trismus, blurred vision, dysphagia, drowsiness, vomiting, and ptosis. Neurotoxic symptoms are rapid in onset and usually appear within 2 to 3 hours. If symptoms do not develop within 6 to 8 hours, there has been no envenomation.

Envenomation by sea snakes characteristically shows an evolution of symptoms over a period of hours, with the latent period being a function of venom volume and victim sensitivity. The onset of symptoms can be as rapid as 5 minutes or as long as 8 hours. There is no appreciable local reaction to a sea snake bite other than the initial pricking sensation. The first complaint may be euphoria, malaise, or anxiety. Over 30 to 60 minutes, classic muscle aching and stiffness (particularly of the bitten extremity and neck muscles) develop, along with a "thick tongue" and sialorrhea, indicative of speech and swallowing dysfunction. Within 3 to 6 hours, moderate to severe pain is noted with passive movements of the neck, trunk, and limbs. Ascending flaccid or spastic paralysis follows shortly, beginning in the lower extremities, and deep tendon reflexes diminish and may disappear after an initial period of spastic hyperreactivity. Nausea, vomiting, myoclonus, muscle spasm, ophthalmoplegia, ptosis, dilated and poorly reactive pupils, facial paralysis, trismus, and pulmonary aspiration of gastric contents are frequent complications. Occasionally, bilateral painless swelling of the parotid glands develops.

Severe envenomations are marked by progressively intense symptoms within the first 2 hours of symptoms. Victims become cool and cyanotic, begin to lose vision, and may lapse into coma. Failing vision is reported to be a preterminal symptom. If peripheral paralysis predominates, the victim may remain conscious if hypoxia is avoided. Leukocytosis may exceed 20,000 white blood cells per milliliter; elevated plasma creatine kinase is variable. Elevated glutamic oxaloacetic transaminase reflects hepatic injury. Pathog-nomonic myoglobinuria becomes evident about 3 to 6 hours after the bite and may be accompanied by albuminuria and hemoglobinuria. Cerebrospinal fluid is normal. Respiratory distress and bulbar paralysis, pulmonary aspiration related hypoxia, electrolyte disturbances (predominantly hyperkalemia), and acute renal failure (attributed in part to myonecrosis and pigment load) all contribute to the ultimate demise, which can occur hours to days after the untreated bite. Preterminal hypertension may occur. The mortality is 25% in victims who do not receive antivenom and 3% overall.

It is interesting to note the effects of sea snake (*Aipysurus laevis*) venom on prey fish.[49] The prey are subdued in six stages, which correlate roughly to certain aspects of a human envenomation: stage 1, increased ventilatory rate; stage 2, loss of mouth control, fin control, coordination, and buoyancy; stage 3, depressed ventilation, weakness, ineffective swimming; stage 4, apnea; stage 5, near paralysis, body color darkening; and stage 6, death.

Treatment

If possible, the offending snake should be captured for identification, taking care not to increase the number of victims. The therapy for bites by snakes of the family Hydrophiidae is similar to that for terrestrial snakes of the family Elapidae. The affected limb should be immobilized and maintained in a dependent position while the victim is kept as quiet as possible. The pressure-immobilization technique (see above) for venom sequestration should be applied. If the bite is on a digit where a compression bandage cannot be applied, a loose constriction bandage that constricts only the superficial venous and lymphatic flow may be applied proximal to the wound. This should be released for 90 seconds every 10 minutes and should be completely removed after 4 to 6 hours. If the bite is older than 30 minutes, neither technique may be very effective.

There is little clinical enthusiasm for the perpetuation of incision and suction therapy, which has just about been universally relegated to therapeutic history.

The victim must be kept warm and as still as possible. As with terrestrial snakebite, cryotherapy (immersion into ice water) is inefficacious and potentially harmful.

With any evidence of envenomation, sea snake antivenom (an equine pepsin-digested immunoglobulin from CSL) prepared against the venom of *Enhydrina schistosa* and the Australian tiger snake *Notechis scutatus* should be administered IV after appropriate skin testing for equine serum hypersensitivity. If this is not available, tiger snake (*Notechis scutatus*) antivenom should be used. As a last resort, CSL polyvalent snake antivenom can be used. Sea snake antivenom is specific and absolutely indicated in cases of envenomation. Supportive measures, although critical in management, are no substitute. The administration of antivenom should begin as soon as possible and is most effective if initiated within 8 hours of the bite. The minimum effective adult dosage is one ampoule (1000 units), which neutralizes 10 mg of *E. schistosa* venom. The victim may require 3000 to 10,000 units (3 to 10 ampoules), depending on the severity of the envenomation. The proper administration of antivenom is clearly described on the antivenom package insert.

Sea snake envenomation may induce severe physiologic derangements that require intensive medical management. Urine output and measured renal function should be closely monitored because hemolysis and rhabdomyolysis release hemoglobin and myoglobin pigments into the circulation, which precipitates acute renal failure. If hemoglobinuria or myoglobinuria is detected, the urine should be alkalinized with sodium bicarbonate and diuresis promoted with a loop diuretic (furosemide or bumetanide) or mannitol, as previously described for management of *Physalia* venom induced nephropathy. Acute renal failure may necessitate a period of peritoneal dialysis or hemodialysis. Hemodialysis offers an alternative therapy that may be successful if antivenom is not available.

Respiratory failure should be anticipated as paralysis overwhelms the victim. Endotracheal intubation and mechanical ventilation may be required until antivenom adequately neutralizes the venom effects. Serum electrolytes should be measured regularly to guide the administration of fluids and electrolyte supplements. Hyperkalemia related to rhabdomyolysis and renal dysfunction must be promptly recognized and treated.

As previously mentioned, symptoms usually occur within 2 to 3 hours after envenomation. If there is no early evidence of envenomation, the victim should be observed for 8 hours before discharge from the hospital.

SUMMARY

A summary algorithmic approach to marine envenomation can be followed when the causative agent cannot be positively identified (see Figure 61-59).[4] Once the physician has made a commitment to a course of treatment based on a presumption of what creature has caused the injury, the subtleties of therapy can be utilized.

REFERENCES

1. Al-Hassan JM et al: Vasoconstrictor components in the Arabian Gulf catfish *(Arius thalassinus)* proteinaceous skin secretion, *Toxicon* 24:1009, 1986.
2. Al-Hassan JM et al: Acceleration of wound healing responses induced by preparations from the epidermal secretions of the Arabian gulf catfish *(Arius bilineatus, Valenciennes)*, *J Wilderness Med* 2:153, 1991.
3. Ashford RU, Sargeant PD, Lum GD: Septic arthritis of the knee caused by *Edwardsiella tarda* after a catfish puncture wound, *Med J Aust* 168:443, 1998.
4. Auerbach PS: Marine envenomations, *N Engl J Med* 325:486, 1991.

5. Banks AS: A puncture wound complicated by infection with *Edwardsiella tarda*, *J Am Podiatr Assoc* 82:529, 1992.
5a. Barber GR, Swygert JS: Necrotizing fasciitis due to *Photobacterium damsela* in a man lashed by a stingray, *N Engl J Med* 342:824, 2000.
6. Barss P: Wound necrosis caused by the venom of stingrays, *Med J Aust* 141:854, 1984.
7. Bendt RR, Auerbach PS: Foreign body reaction following stingray envenomation, *J Wilderness Med* 2:298, 1991.
8. Breault JL: Candirú: Amazonian parasitic catfish, *J Wilderness Med* 2:304, 1991.
9. Carducci M et al: Raynaud's phenomenon secondary to weever fish stings, *Arch Dermatol* 132:838, 1996.
10. Chhatwal I, Dreyer F: Isolation and characterization of dracotoxin from the venom of the greater weever fish *Trachinus draco*, *Toxicon* 30:87, 1992.
11. Choromanski JM, Murray TF, Weber LJ: Responses of the isolated buffalo sculpin heart to stabilized venom of the lionfish *(Pterois volitans)*, *Proc West Pharmacol Soc* 27:229, 1984.
12. Cohen AS, Olek AJ: An extract of lionfish *(Pterois volitans)* spine tissue contains acetylcholine and a toxin that affects neuromuscular transmission, *Toxicon* 27:1367, 1989.
13. Cooper NK: Stone fish and stingrays some notes on the injuries that they cause to man, *J R Army Med Corps* 137:136, 1991.
14. De Plater G, Martin RL, Milburn PJ: A pharmacological and biochemical investigation of the venom from the platypus *(Ornithorhynchus anatinus)*, *Toxicon* 33:157, 1995.
15. Evans LA, Evans CM: Stingray hickey, *Cutis* 58:208, 1996.
16. Evans RJ, Davies RS: Stingray injury, *J Accid Emerg Med* 13:224, 1996.
17. Fenner PJ: Stingray envenomation: a suggested new treatment, *Med J Aust* 163:655, 1995.
18. Frederette SR, Derk FF, Nardozza AJ: Catfish spine injury of the foot, *J Am Podiatr Med Assoc* 87:187, 1997.
19. Garnier P et al: Enzymatic properties of the stonefish *(Synanceia verrucosa* Bloch and Schneider, 1801) venom and purification of a lethal, hypotensive and cytolytic factor, *Toxicon* 33:143, 1995.
20. Garnier P et al: Presence of norepinephrine and other biogenic amines in stonefish venom, *J Chromatogr B Biomed Sci Appl* 685:364, 1996.
21. Goetz CG: Pharmacology of animal neurotoxins, *Clin Neuropharmacol* 5:231, 1982.
22. Gopalakrishnakone P, Gwee MCE: The structure of the venom gland of stonefish *Synanceja horrida*, *Toxicon* 31:979, 1993.
23. Grainger CR: Occupational injuries due to sting rays, *Trans R Soc Trop Med Hyg* 74:408, 1980.
24. Hiemenz JW, Kennedy B, Kwon-Chung KJ: Invasive fusariosis associated with an injury by a stingray barb, *J Med Vet Mycol* 28:209, 1990.
25. Ho P-K et al: Necrotizing fasciitis due to *Vibrio alginolyticus* following an injury inflicted by a stingray, *Scand J Infect Dis* 30: 192, 1998.
26. Ikeda T: Supraventricular bigeminy following a stingray envenomation: a case report, *Hawaii Med J* 48:162, 1989.
27. Khoo HE et al: Biological activities of *Synanceja horrida* (stonefish) venom, *Nat Toxins* 1:54, 1992.
28. Khoo HE et al: Effects of stonustoxin (lethal factor from *Synanceja horrida* venom) on platelet aggregation, *Toxicon* 33:1033, 1995.
29. Kizer KW, McKinney HE, Auerbach PS: Scorpaenidae envenomation: a five-year poison center experience, *JAMA* 253:807, 1985.
30. Kreger AS: Detection of a cytolytic toxin in the venom of the stonefish *(Synanceja trachynis)*, *Toxicon* 29:733, 1991.
31. Kreger AS et al: Effects of stonefish *(Synanceia trachynis)* venom on murine and frog neuromuscular junctions, *Toxicon* 31:307, 1993.
32. Lehmann DF, Hardy JC: Stonefish envenomation, *N Engl J Med* 329:510, 1993 (letter).
33. Low KSY et al: Stonustoxin: effects on neuromuscular function *in vitro* and *in vivo*, *Toxicon* 32:573, 1994.
34. Mann JW, Werntz JR: Catfish stings to the hand, *J Hand Surg* 16A:318, 1991.
35. Manowitz NR, Rosenthal RR: Cutaneous-systemic reactions to toxins and venoms of common marine organisms, *Cutis* 23:450, 1979.
36. McKinistry DM: Catfish stings in the United States: case report and review, *J Wilderness Med* 4:293, 1993.
37. Meyer PK: Stingray injuries, *Wild Environ Med* 8:24, 1997.
38. Midani S: Vibrio species infection of a catfish spine puncture wound, *Pediatr Infect Dis J* 13:333, 1994.
39. Murphey DK, Septimus EJ, Waagner DC: Catfish-related injury and infection: report of two cases and review of the literature, *Clin Infect Dis* 14:689, 1992.

40. Pachner AR, Ricalton N: In vitro neutralization by monoclonal antibodies of +-bungarotoxin binding to acetylcholine receptor, *Toxicon* 27:1263, 1989.

41. Patel MR, Wells S: Lionfish envenomation of the hand, *J Hand Surg* 18A:523, 1993.

42. Ronka EKF, Roe WF: Cardiac wound caused by the spine of the stingray (suborder Masticura), *Mil Surg* 97:135, 1945.

43. Russell FE: Comparative pharmacology of some animal toxins, *Fed Proc* 26:1206, 1967.

44. Russell FE et al: Studies on the mechanism of death from stingray venom: a report of two fatal cases, *Am J Med Sci* 235:566, 1958.

45. Shepherd S, Thomas SH, Stone CK: Catfish envenomation, *J Wilderness Med* 5:67, 1994.

46. Shiomi K et al: Toxins in the skin secretion of the oriental catfish *(Plotosus lineatus):* immunological properties and immunocytochemical identification of producing cells, *Toxicon* 26:353, 1988.

47. Vick JA: Medical studies of poisonous land and sea snakes, *J Clin Pharmacol* 34:709, 1994.

48. Whiting SC, Guinea ML: Treating stingray wounds with onions, *Med J Aust* 168:584, 1998.

49. Zimmerman KD, Gates GR, Heatwole H: Effects of venom of the olive sea snake, *Aipysurus laevis,* on the behaviour and ventilation of three species of prey fish, *Toxicon* 28:1469, 1990.

Vicki Mazzorana

Dermatitis acquired from the aquatic environment can be related to exposure to diving equipment, chemicals, or animal or plant irritants. Hypersensitivity reactions to water have been documented. Bacteria, algae, and parasites can be the etiologic agents of a variety of aquatic infections. Wounds resulting from stings, bites, punctures, and suction may result from inadvertent contact with marine life.

CONTACT DERMATITIS

Diving Equipment

Diving Wet Suits. An allergic reaction to wet suits may reflect sensitivity to either the rubber or thiourea compounds within the suit.[1,66,69] N/N-diethylurea is a chemical compound used within the wet suit to bond the nylon lining to the rubber. It can cause contact dermatitis of the neck, trunk, and extremities in sensitive individuals.[1,22,66,123] The rash varies from generalized redness to severe, itchy papulovesicles. Wearing a tight diving suit may produce irritant skin lesions at the pressure points. Antihistamine use is recommended to provide symptomatic relief from the pruritus. Systemic corticosteroids may be necessary in the treatment of severe reactions. The rash should be observed because secondary cellulitis may occur.

Diving Masks, Goggles, and Mouthpieces. The facial condition termed *mask burn* has been described as a reddish imprint of the mask on the face and was initially thought to be a requisite annoyance of snorkeling and scuba diving.[1,4,66] More severe reactions, consisting of painful, disabling eruptions characterized by vesiculation, weeping, and crusting, have been described. Mouthpieces attached to regulators and snorkels may cause minor oral irritation described as a mild burning sensation. Persons who become sensitized to the constituents of the mouthpiece may suffer severe intraoral ulceration and inflammation accompanied by vesiculation of the oral mucosa, gingiva, and tongue.[4] Neoprene swim goggles can cause raccoonlike periorbital contact dermatitis in sensitive individuals.[6,80] Chemical constituents in the equipment may be the causative agents.

Rubber mouthpieces and masks contain antioxidants similar to those that cause contact dermatitis in surgeons who are allergic to rubber gloves. Mercaptobenzothiazol, tetraethylthiuram, and isopropyl paraphenylene diamine have been implicated in such reactions.[69] N-isopropyl-N-phenyl-paraphenylenediamine, a rubber antioxidant used in scuba masks, can cause facial dermatitis.[153,240] Use of diving equipment can result in both irritant and allergic reactions.[65,68] Acute facial dermatitis may be treated with the application of cool compresses containing Burow's solution and the administration of oral systemic corticosteroids, such as prednisone, beginning with a supraphysiologic dose and tapered over 7 to 10 days. For serious intraoral reactions, rinsing twice daily with a mouthwash consisting of equal parts antihistamine, such as diphenhydramine elixir, and milk of magnesia may be efficacious.[69] Individual sores may be coated twice daily and again at bedtime with triamcinolone acetonide (0.1%) dental paste (Kenalog in Orabase) for 5 to 7 days. The problem may be avoided at the outset by using silicone rubber hypoallergenic masks and mouthpieces.

Rubber Swim Gear. Nose clips, ear plugs, and swim fins produce allergic contact dermatitides in some individuals.[69] Nonallergenic equipment is available. Mercaptobenzothiazole, which is a constituent of some bathing caps, also can cause contact dermatitis.[69] Silicone swim caps are available for persons who are allergic to standard bathing caps.

Chemical Irritants

Sulfur Springs. Contact dermatitis has not been noted to occur in persons who bathe in hot springs. Skin lesions consisting of numerous pea-sized areas of raised erythema have been attributed to bathing in green sulfur springs.[230] The lesions develop within 24 hours after bathing and are distributed over the trunk and limbs. No microorganisms that could cause the rash have been found in the water or the lesions. The most important characteristics of green sulfur springs that may account for the irritant reaction are the water's high soluble chloride and sulfur content and its extreme acidity.

Chlorinated Water. Chlorinated pool or spa water rarely causes irritant dermatitis or an allergic reaction. It may produce contact urticaria. Nitrogen trichloride, which is produced when chlorine is added to water containing ammonia, has a pungent odor and may cause eye and nose irritation.[67,176]

Bromine. Bromine-based disinfectants are used in swimming pools and spas. They are more effective than chlorine-based disinfectants against pseudomonads at high temperatures.[72] Bromine rash is described as a pruritic, generalized, eczematous irritant contact dermatitis arising within 24 hours of exposure to a spa or pool recently disinfected with 1 bromo-3-chloro-5, 5-dimethylhydantoin (Halobrome).[199] The rash resolves spontaneously once spa use is discontinued. Treatment is symptomatic.

Algaecides. Copper solutions or quaternary ammonium compounds may be used to combat algae growth in pools and spas. Copper algaecide solutions used to treat pool and spa water can cause greenish discoloration of the scalp hair in blondes.[138] Wetting the hair with fresh water before immersion in pool or spa water decreases the incidence and severity of hair discoloration. Shampooing decreases the green tint, and immersing the hair in 3% peroxide solution removes the green in a couple of hours.

Animal or Plant Irritants

Sea Cucumbers. Sea cucumbers (see Chapter 61) are invertebrates that extrude sticky, white tentacular organs used to entangle prey. Humans who come into contact with these moplike strands suffer dermatitis. Cutaneous erythema, pain, and pruritus may occur. The skin manifestations are self-limited. Prompt washing with soap and water appears to remove any toxins.[154]

Ichthyocrinotoxic Fish. A number of fish possess glands that secrete skin toxins (crinotoxins) but do not have venomous defense organs, such as spines. These fish include soapfish, trunkfish, gobies, sole, toadfish, clingfish, and pufferfish.[90] The toxins can be extremely powerful, but resulting dermatitides are poorly documented. The soapfish (family Grammistidae), *Rypticus saponaceus* (Figure 63-1), receives its name from the soapy mucus it releases when handled or disturbed. Fisherman in the Caribbean know that holding a soapfish in a restricted volume of seawater with other fish results in death of the other fish.[95] Human contact results in dermatitis. The skin irritant is called *grammistin;* similar substances have been isolated from boxfish and sea bass species.[29,95,187]

Cool compresses of Burow's solution, aluminum sulfate and calcium acetate (Domeboro), or colloidal oatmeal alleviate the burning and itching caused by soap-

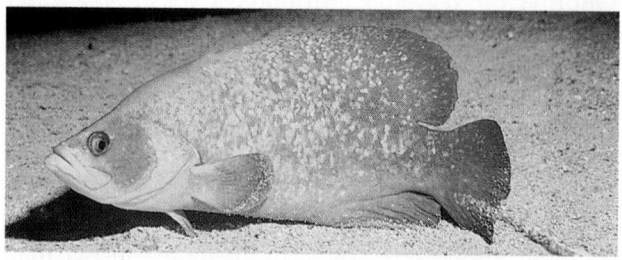

Figure 63-1 Soapfish (*Rypticus saponaceus*). Skin contact with soapy mucus causes dermatitis. *(Photo by Carl Roessler.)*

fish dermatitis. In severe cases topical corticosteroids are beneficial. Systemic corticosteroids are rarely required. Wearing protective clothing and gloves when handling fish prevents these dermatitides. Washing protective wear with soap and water after use is required to remove toxins.

Sea Moss Dermatitis and Dogger Bank Itch. Dogger Bank itch is an eczematous dermatitis caused by a plant (*Fragilaria striatula*) and bryozoarian animals referred to as *sea chervils (Alcyonidium hirsutum* and *Alcyonidium gelatinosum).*[154] This irritant contact dermatitis is most common among fishermen of the North Sea. These fishermen contact sea mosses or sea mats that are drawn up within fishnets. The irritation first appears on the palms and forearms and often disappears when the fisherman goes ashore.[171] Recurrent exposure causes subsequent attacks to be more severe. The cutaneous reaction initially consists of erythema but may progress to vesiculated, edematous eruptions of the hands, arms, legs, and face. It is controversial as to whether or not this is an allergic reaction or an irritant dermatitis. Reactions to patch tests performed with an extract from the causative source and lack of reaction in controls support an allergic etiology.

Treatment is symptomatic. Application of dilute (26%) isopropyl alcohol in calamine lotion may provide relief. Severe reactions may require the use of oral antihistamines and corticosteroids or topical fluorinated corticosteroids. Wearing proper protective clothing may prevent this self-limited disorder.

Red Tide Dermatitis. A "red tide" occurs when large numbers of unicellular microscopic free-swimming dinoflagellate organisms are present in the water. A variety of plant life proliferations, such as *Ptychodiscus breve,* have been implicated as causative agents of red tides. These unicellular algae reproduce at an alarming rate when conditions are favorable. They secrete toxins that can cause dermatitis, conjunctivitis, and respiratory symptoms in humans (see Chapter 54). Swimming during a red tide may result in an acute urticarial papular eruption. Massive blooms of toxic phytoplankton are toxic to fish. Avoidance of affected areas, especially during windy conditions, is the best prevention. Symptomatic treatment is provided after the victim has exited the water.

Ciguatera Dermatitis. Blooms of toxic dinoflagellates, such as *Gambierdiscus toxicus,* synthesize toxins that become incorporated into the food chain.[262] Ciguatera toxins are extremely harmful to humans (see Chapter 54). The dermatologic manifestations include an intense generalized pruritus associated with a diffuse maculopapular eruption leading to blisters and desquamation. Other manifestations include hair and nail loss, intense diaphoresis leading to dehydration, cyanosis, and urticarial reactions. Symptom severity depends on factors such as geographic location.[262]

Seaweed Dermatitis Caused by Algae. Seaweed dermatitis is almost always secondary to irritation resulting from contact with algae, of which more than 25,000 species are known. Algae are loosely defined as chlorophyll-bearing or colorless organisms that are thallous (without true roots, stems, or leaves). They vary in size, shape, and color. Some are equipped with flagella and propel themselves through the water.[235] Algae range from microscopic diatoms (1 μm in length) to kelp plants (100 m in length). Algae are found in all marine environments and are extremely adaptive to temperature and depth variation. For instance, one form of blue-green algae thrives at hot spring temperatures of 71° C (160° F); others dwell in frigid Arctic water. Although sunlight can penetrate only to a depth of 900 feet in the ocean, some blue-green algae exist at depths up to 12,000 feet.

MICROCOLEUS LYNGBYACEUS. *Microcoleus lyngbyaceus,* formerly known as *Lyngbya majuscula Gomont,* is a blue-green saltwater alga that has strains of varying toxicity, often within geographic proximity. The "stinging seaweed" is dark green or olive, drab, and finely filamentous, occurring in abundance at depths of up to 100 feet.[212,213,218] It grows in hairlike masses or mats throughout the Pacific and Indian Oceans and Caribbean Sea, although large epidemics have been reported in Hawaii and Okinawa, Japan.[111] Outbreaks of *Microcoleus* organism–induced dermatitis occur between March and September in Florida and between June and September in Hawaii. In Hawaii the largest reported series involved windward beaches.[84] The assumption is that strong currents and winds dislodge the alga from its normal habitat, fragment it, and blow the fragments into the surf line.[111] The alga produces a dermatonecrotic and potent inflammatory agent called *debromoaplysiatoxin,* as well as an indole alkaloid dermatitis-producing toxin called *lyngbyatoxin A.*[37,168,218] An indole stain identifies the presence of lyngbyatoxin A; a radioimmunoassay is under development.[111] *Vibrio alginolyticus* and *Vibrio parahaemolyticus* have been cultured from marine specimens of *M. lyngbyaceus* collected from the beaches of Hawaii. Typically the affected individual swam in turbid water infested with plant life and did not remove his or her bathing suit after leaving the water. Within minutes to hours a pruritic, burning, moist, and erythematous rash develops in a bathing suit distribution, followed by bullous escharotic desquamation in the genital, perineal, and perianal regions.[213] Lymphadenopathy, pustular folliculitis, and local infections occur in some individuals. It may be difficult to differentiate this reaction from sea bather's eruption (which is attributed to thimble jellyfish or larval anemone organisms). There also are occasional out-

breaks of similar skin reactions after exposure to freshwater blue-green algae.[43,99] Oral and ocular mucous membrane lesions, facial rash, conjunctivitis, and perhaps interstitial pulmonary edema have been attributed to *M. lyngbyaceus.*[111,212]

Treatment of dermatitis caused by *M. lyngbyaceus* consists of copious irrigation with soapy water, followed by isopropyl alcohol rinses and application of topical steroids. Severe cases may require oral administration of a systemic corticosteroid, such as prednisone, tapered over 2 weeks. Treatment of seaweed dermatitis is preventive. Prevention is accomplished by showering with soapy water and removing all swimwear immediately upon leaving the water. Avoid swimming in areas laden with seaweed.

SARGASSUM NATANS. *Sargassum* species algae collect as seaweed masses in great numbers off the southeastern coast of Florida. Breezes blow the algae toward the coast in the winter. The algae are generally considered to be harmless to man. After *Sargassum* species seaweed was placed in the swimwear of two children at play, they both developed an erythematous skin eruption with urticarial lesions. The rash disappeared within 4 hours.[33]

Blue-Green Algae of Freshwater. In freshwater environments, warm weather can cause rapid growth of blue-green algae (group Cyanophyta) in a "bloom."[222] During conditions of a bloom, toxins are concentrated and become a significant hazard.[54,58] Species such as *Microcystis aeruginosa, Aphanizomenon flos-aquae, Nodularia spumigena, Nostoc* species, *Oscillatoria agardhii, Anabaena spiroides,* and *Anabaena flos-aquae* have been implicated in the acute poisoning and death of wild and domestic animals.[169,198] In most species of toxic cyanobacteria, the toxins are cyclic heptapeptides called *microcystins* or *cyanoginosins.*[215,226] More than 40 microcystins have been isolated from blue-green algae.[215] The toxins are of multiple configurations and include alkaloids, polypeptides, and lipopolysaccharides (endotoxins).[222] The rapid-acting "death factors" resemble saxitoxin and tetrodotoxin. Animals may collapse quickly and appear to suffer neuromuscular paralysis, with features of staggering muscle fasciculations, gasping, and convulsions.[93] A different dominant symptom complex includes gastrointestinal hemorrhage and hepatic failure. Although ingestion of contaminated water may cause considerable animal mortality, human exposures to date have resulted primarily in local effects, including allergic reactions, conjunctivitis, ear infection, facial swelling, lip swelling, papulovesicular dermatitis, and gastroenteritis.[26,143] Therapy is supportive in both animals and humans because all afflictions appear to be self-limited. Cyclosporin A has been shown to inhibit the fatal effects of microcystins administered to mice.

HYPERSENSITIVITY REACTIONS

Aquagenic Urticaria

Aquagenic urticaria is a rare condition that occurs when skin contacts water at any temperature, resulting in an urticarial rash at the site of exposure (Figure 63-2).[178,180,206] The appearance of the urticarial rash is usually preceded by itching. The rash is characterized by pruritic, punctate, and perifollicular wheals 1 to 2 mm in diameter that develop as soon as 10 minutes after contact with water and persist for up to 60 minutes. The rash is usually confined to the neck, upper trunk, and arms. The face, hands, legs, and feet are spared.[178] An episode is usually followed by a refractory period lasting several hours. No systemic complications have been reported. This entity usually occurs in postpubescent individuals, and it is reported more frequently in women than in men.[150] There may be a family history of atopy.[24] The coexistence of other forms of physical urticaria has been demonstrated in some patients.[48,156]

The pathogenesis of this phenomenon has been studied but is not completely understood. Histamine involvement is supported by the finding of elevated local histamine levels and suppression of the rash by various antihistamines.[46,48,209,254] Dermographism typically is not present, and serum IgE levels usually are normal.[209] In some cases prophylaxis with antihistamines fails to prevent the urticarial response to contact with water, suggesting a mechanism in the development of aquagenic urticaria unrelated to the release of

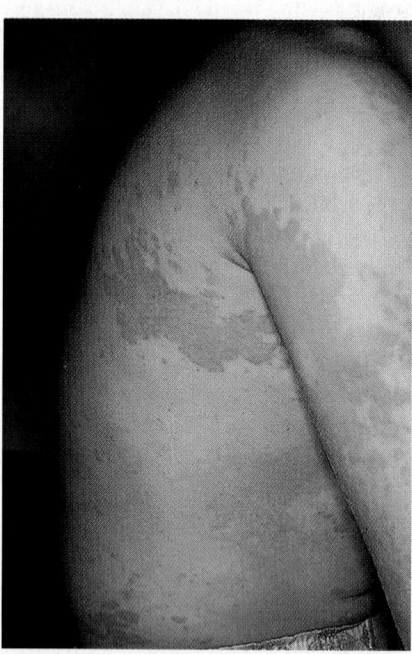

Figure 63-2 Aquagenic urticaria. Pruritic, punctate, and perifollicular wheals characteristic of the rash of aquagenic urticaria. *(Courtesy Edgar Maeyens, MD.)*

histamine. Some have suggested that water may react with a component of sebum on the stratum corneum, forming a toxic substance that diffuses through the skin and may either directly cause urticaria or stimulate mast cells to release histamine, resulting in urticaria.[46,206] Another theory is that there is a change in the osmotic pressure in the skin around hair follicles, allowing for passive permeation of water through the skin.[254] In some victims there is a significant increase in acetylcholinesterase activities, suggesting that the pathogenesis of aquagenic urticaria may be related to the release of acetylcholine in the nerve fibers of sebaceous glands.[209] The ability of anticholinergics to suppress the hypersensitivity reaction in some individuals suggests that aquagenic urticaria is acetylcholine mediated.[162] Aquagenic urticaria must be differentiated from other forms of physical urticaria, which can be induced by pressure, exercise, cold, or stress.[156] Clinically the morphology and distribution of the rash are similar to those of cholinergic urticaria. Aquagenic urticaria can be differentiated from cholinergic urticaria by pretreating the skin with topical atropine, which does not prevent wheal formation in aquagenic urticaria but prevents the rash of cholinergic urticaria.[209] Aquagenic urticaria also must be differentiated from aquagenic pruritus, in which exposure of skin to water elicits intense pruritus without cutaneous lesions.[87] Before the diagnosis of aquagenic urticaria can be made, other physical urticarias must be ruled out and the patient must respond to a water provocation test.[156]

Aquagenic urticarial reactions can be inhibited by applying petroleum ointment to the skin before water exposure.[209] There may be a role for prophylaxis with antihistamines and anticholinergics. Exposure to ultraviolet (UV) light (psoralen plus UVA [PUVA] and UVB) may be considered as an alternative treatment if others fail.[122,155,180] PUVA and UVB radiation may cause immunosuppression or inhibit mast cell response to the application of water. UV light treatment may thicken the epidermis, inhibiting the penetration of water. There is a case report in which a patient with aquagenic urticaria responded well to treatment with the anabolic steroid, stanozolol. At a dose of 10 mg/day, symptoms of aquagenic urticaria were controlled.[63]

Aquagenic Pruritus

Transient itching of the skin after exposure to water is not unusual. Common etiologies of nonspecific water-mediated itching include eczema, xerosis, cold urticaria, heat urticaria, vibratory urticaria, cholinergic urticaria, symptomatic dermographism, polycythemia rubra vera, aquagenic urticaria, aquagenic pruritus of the elderly, and aquagenic pruritis.[224] Aquagenic pruritus, in which contact with water at any temperature consistently induces intense, disabling itching without any visible cutaneous changes, is uncommon.[52,70,87] The condition is characterized by generalized skin discomfort provoked by contact with water. It is a distinct clinical entity with clearly described diagnostic criteria. Criteria for the diagnosis of aquagenic pruritus include: (1) severe pruritus, prickling, stinging, or burning that consistently develops after skin contact with water, regardless of water temperature or salinity; (2) lack of visible cutaneous lesions; (3) reaction within minutes of exposure and lasting between 10 minutes and 2 hours; (4) lack of a concurrent skin disease, internal disorder, or medication use to account for the reaction; and (5) exclusion of all other physical urticarias, symptomatic dermographism, and polycythemia ruba vera.[52,224,225] Symptoms may occur only in areas exposed to water. Typically the head, palms, soles, and mucosa are spared.[225] The disabling nature of this intense, unrelenting skin discomfort may account for the mood changes demonstrated by more than half of patients.

Aquagenic pruritus is slightly more prevalent in males, can occur at any age, and may have a familial component.[52,147,190] Aquagenic pruritus has been associated with haematoproliferative conditions, including polycythemia rubra vera, myelodysplasia, and hypereosinophilic disorders. Recently an association between histiocytic disorders, such as juvenile xanthogranuloma, and aquagenic pruritus has been established.[91]

The pathogenesis of aquagenic pruritus is poorly understood, but it has been demonstrated that water, not other liquids, elicits the symptom complex. Increased mast cell degranulation (with an increase in circulating histamine), release of acetylcholine, and increased cutaneous fibrinolytic activity have all been implicated as potential etiologies for the hypersensitivity component of aquagenic pruritus.[70,87,148] Topical application of capsaicin, the spicy component within the hot pepper plant, induces release of neuropeptides, including substance P, and reversibly suppresses the axon reflex in the skin.[96,147] This finding suggests that neuropeptides could play a significant role in the pathophysiology of pruritus.

Treatment for aquagenic pruritus has been disappointing. Preventive alkanization of water and application of petroleum ointment have had limited success. Administration of antihistamines, anticholinergics, aspirin, iron, serotonin antagonists, propanolol, recombinant interferon-alpha, and triamcinolone is under investigation and has produced inconclusive results.[86,96,164,190] The use of UV radiation and psoralen photochemotherapy has had promising results. It is postulated that UV irradiation is effective because it may reduce end-organ responsiveness by producing ultrastructural changes within nerves or by raising sensory nerve thresholds.[96,164,217] It may stabilize mast cells at nerve endings, inhibiting the release of histamine. Complete avoidance of water exposure is the only guaranteed effective therapy for aquagenic pruritus.

INFECTIOUS DERMATITIS

Freshwater Bacteria

Pseudomonas Aeruginosa. Numerous cases of "hot tub" or "whirlpool" dermatitis have been described.[39,202,253] Eruptions occur after the use of heated recreational water sources, such as whirlpools, hot tubs, swimming pools, and water slides.* Family bathtubs, contaminated bath toys, loofah sponges, moisturizing creams, and diving suits have been implicated in cases of pseudomonal folliculitis.[25,71,75,105,163]

Pseudomonas aeruginosa is the most common microbe causing skin disorders in occupational saturation divers and can occur after recreational use of diving suits.[2,136,201] *P. aeruginosa* (predominantly serotype 0-11) is a ubiquitous, motile, nonfermentative, obligate aerobic, gram-negative bacillus.[105,163] It is a fastidious organism, surviving in extremes of temperature, under hostile conditions, and with minimal nutritional support. It infects humans, other vertebrates, animals, and plants. Extracellular toxins and enzymes produced by *P. aeruginosa* contribute to its virulence and are responsible for cutaneous manifestations, including necrotizing subcutaneous nodules, cellulitis, ecthyma gangrenosum, and hemorrhage. *P. aeruginosa* infects healthy, moistened skin. No unusual host factors have been identified. The high water temperature, hydration of the skin, high concentration of organisms, and chemical irritants in the water all contribute to this dermatitis. In several outbreaks deficiencies in disinfection have been noted.

The follicular rash appears within 48 hours of exposure and resolves within 7 days without treatment. Biopsy specimens demonstrate folliculitis. There is minimal change in the epidermis, but there are perforations in the follicular epithelium, with inflammatory infiltrates. The eruption is most pronounced in areas covered by bathing garments, and the head and neck are spared unless they are submerged. Other symptoms include external otitis; conjunctivitis; tender breasts; enlarged, tender lymph nodes; fever; and malaise.[105,203] Serious infections arise in immunosuppressed and debilitated individuals. The erythematous, maculopapular, and vesiculopustular eruption usually is accompanied by pruritus.

The eruption is self-limited (7 to 14 days), and thus treatment can be conservative. Papules or abscesses can reappear for up to several months without reexposure. Skin lesions heal without scarring but can cause postinflammatory hyperpigmentation that clears with time. The pruritus may be managed with drying lotions, such as calamine, or with oral antihistamines. "Whirlpool" folliculitis is usually self-limited, and treatment is not required. Local infections may be treated with ap-

---

*References 57, 89, 106, 112, 160, 183, 202, 203, 208, 221, 234, 266.

plications of antimicrobial ointments, such as polymyxin B or gentamicin, until resolved. Rapid progression to severe systemic disease, manifested by hemorrhagic bullae, pneumonia, or septicemia, suggests immunosuppression.[57,79,195,220] *P. aeruginosa* is resistant to many antibiotics. Systemic infection may be treated with an aminoglycoside or ciprofloxacin. Prevention of *P. aeruginosa* infection requires either use of adequate disinfectant or avoidance of recreational closed-water systems, and reservoirs and vehicles of transmission should be disinfected. Showering does not appear to prevent the disorder.[203]

Other infections that have been acquired in closed-cycle recreational water systems include eczema herpeticum and molluscum contagiosum. Whether diminished host resistance resulting from skin hyperhydration or an unusual presentation of pathogens causes viral afflictions after water exposure remains to be determined.

Aeromonas Hydrophilia. *Aeromonas hydrophilia* is a gram-negative, facultatively anaerobic, polarly flagellated, non–spore-forming, motile rod member of the family Vibrionaceae that commonly inhabits soil, freshwater streams, and lakes.* *Aeromonas* species are widely distributed and found at wide ranges of temperature and pH.[98,249] Three species (*Aeromonas hydrophila*, *Aeromonas sobia*, and *Aeromonas caviae*) have been associated with human disease.

Although *A. hydrophilia* may produce soft tissue infections or cellulitis in normal hosts, serious infections are more commonly noted in immunocompromised persons.[157,216,257,263] *A. hydrophila* may cause gastroenteritis, endocarditis, peritonitis, meningitis, and septicemia. Soft tissue and gastroenteric human infections occur predominantly between May and November.[113,249,258] A wound (frequently of the lower extremity) immersed in contaminated water may become cellulitic within 24 hours, with erythema, edema, and a purulent discharge.[257,260] The wound is usually sustained when the individual steps on a foreign object or suffers a laceration or puncture wound while in water.[126,205] The symptoms may be indistinguishable from those of streptococcal cellulitis, with localized pain, lymphangitis, fever, and chills. If managed with inappropriate antibiotics or if untreated, this infection may progress to a severe gas-forming soft tissue reaction, bullae formation, necrotizing myositis, or osteomyelitis.† The appearance of aeromonad septicemia is reportedly similar to that of ecthyma gangrenosum caused by *P. aeruginosa*.[263] In a manner analogous to the pathogenicity of virulent *Vibrio* species, the chronically ill or immunocompromised host probably is at greater risk for severe complications, such as meningitis, endocarditis, or sep-

ticemia.* In the individual who has aspirated freshwater, *A. hydrophila* can cause pneumonitis and bacteremia.[189] Infections also have occurred after individuals have been bitten by an alligator or a pet piranha.[191,197] For unknown reasons there is a marked preponderance of male patients,[11] which may reflect the phenotypic variation of critical bacterial adhesions.

A Gram's stain of the purulent discharge may demonstrate gram-negative bacilli. Given the appropriate clinical setting (after a wound has been acquired in the freshwater environment), this finding should not be casually attributed to contamination.[126] *A. hydrophila* generally is sensitive to tetracycline, chloramphenicol, gentamicin, tobramycin, trimethoprim/sulfamethoxazole, cefotaxime, moxalactam, imipenem, ceftazidime, and ciprofloxacin.[10,60,125,177] However, it is typically resistant to penicillin. In one case, culture of a severe wound infection demonstrated the presence of two species—*A. hydrophila* and *A. sobia*.[121] Notably the latter species was resistant to tetracycline in vitro. Initial therapy for a severe infection should include an aminoglycoside to provide coverage against concomitant *Pseudomonas* or *Serratia* species infection.[92] As has been demonstrated with *Vibrio* species, the first-generation cephalosporins, penicillin, and ampicillin are not effective against *A. hydrophila*, perhaps because of the production of a β-lactamase by the organism.[10,32,60,62,177] Because of the microbiologic similarity of *Aeromonas* species on biochemical testing to members of the Enterobacteriaceae family, such as *Escherichia coli* and *Serratia* species, it is important to alert the laboratory to the clinical setting. A case of *A. hydrophilia* cellulitis that did not respond to antimicrobials and surgical debridement responded successfully to adjunct hyperbaric oxygen therapy.[44,157] High oxygen concentrations may suppress virulence factors and inhibit or kill anaerobic organisms.[44]

In addition to antibiotic therapy, initial treatment of a severe soft tissue infection related to *Aeromonas* organisms should include aggressive wound debridement and adequate drainage to mitigate the potentially invasive nature of the organism. Medicinal leeches can harbor *Aeromonas* species in their gut flora; soft tissue infections related to leech attachment have been reported.[251] The genus *Plesiomonas* also belongs to the family Vibrionaceae; it has been definitively linked with aquarium-associated infection complicated by watery diarrhea and fever.[237]

Chromobacterium Violaceum. *Chromobacterium violaceum* is a mesophilic (prefers a temperature of 20° C to 37° C [68° F to 98° F]), saprophytic, facultatively anaerobic, and gram-negative rod. It is motile, with both polar and lateral flagella. This bacterium produces a violet pigment (violacein) with oxidative and fermentative

---

*References 76, 92, 121, 125, 197, 250.
†References 49, 76, 125, 140, 216, 257.

*References 50, 76, 125, 140, 145, 216, 257, 263.

glucose use. It is an abundant inhabitant of tropical and subtropical freshwater rivers and soil, especially in the southeastern United States, and is generally considered nonpathogenic.[109,166] The infection usually presents after the organism enters an individual's body through a minor skin injury or after the individual ingests contaminated water.[114,166,172,186,223] Sepsis is sometimes a feature of this infection. Bacteremia leads to diffuse pustular dermatitis, with *C. violaceum* cultured from both blood and skin pustules.[223] Other skin manifestations include vesicles, ecchymotic maculae, a maculopapular rash, ulcers, subcutaneous nodules, cellulitis, lymphangitis, and digital gangrene.[151] Additional manifestations are secondary to systemic disease and include suppurative lymphadenitis; osteomyelitis; urinary tract infection; sinusitis; orbital cellulitis; lung, kidney, and liver abscesses; and meningitis.[151,166,223,239,247] Persons with chronic granulomatous disease, which is characterized by the inability of granulocytes and monocytes to convert oxygen into hydrogen peroxide and other oxygen metabolites necessary for microbicidal activity, are at particular risk for severe infection.[82,116,151] Fortunately, *C. violaceum* infection, which is potentially fatal and associated with a high mortality rate, is rare. Of 34 reported cases, 65% were fatal.[186] The interval between the onset of the illness and death ranged from 7 to 15 months. Although most patients with *C. violaceum* infection are not immunocompromised, the presence of immunodeficiency, such as that caused by chronic granulomatous disease, can be a predisposition to infection.

Treatment consists of antibiotics and prompt surgical drainage of purulent collections. The organism is generally sensitive to imipenem, carbenicillin, ciprofloxacin, chloramphenicol, tetracycline, gentamicin, kanamycin, tobramycin, and trimethoprim/sulfamethoxazole. Resistance to cephalosporins, penicillins, and aztreonam has been reported.[166,223,228] Southeastern physicians should be highly suspicious when caring for a septic patient with a history of exposure to stagnant water and typical skin lesions, organ abscesses, or both.

Marine Bacteria

Mycobacterium Marinum. Cutaneous granulomas, referred to as *swimming pool granulomas* or *fish tank granulomas*, caused by *Mycobacterium marinum* were first described in 1954 by Linell and Norden.[5,142] The lesions resembled tuberculosis verrucosa cutis (Figure 63-3). *M. marinum* is a so-called atypical (anonymous or unclassified) bacterium. Typical mycobacteria are animal pathogens that cannot multiply outside the animal host, whereas atypical mycobacteria are free-living soil and water saprophytes, rarely pathogens. *M. marinum* is an acid-fast and rod-shaped bacillus, a Runyon group 1 photochromogen that produces yellow-orange pigment after light exposure. It grows optimally at 31° C to 33° C (88° F to 91° F). Therefore human infec-

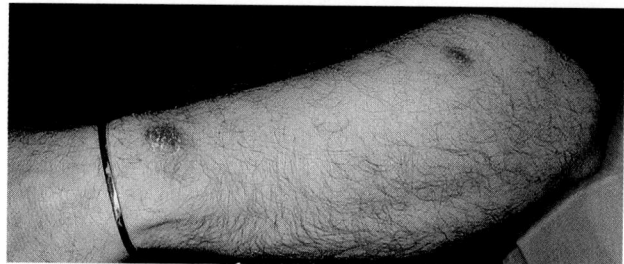

Figure 63-3 *Mycobacterium marinum.* Cutaneous granulomas on the forearm of a patient with *Mycobacterium marinum. (Courtesy Edgar Maeyens, MD.)*

tions are limited to cooler acral skin and rarely involve deeper, warmer lymphatic or lymph node structures. Swimming pool chlorination provides little protection because the organism is relatively resistant to chlorine. *M. marinum* is an opportunistic pathogen found in aquatic (freshwater and saltwater) environments.[27,81,85,193] This lesion tends to be associated with trauma or exposure to fresh water, salt water, or marine life.[5,31,135] Fish may develop disseminated granulomatous disease. Human infection is typically limited to cutaneous granulomatous lesions, although deeper infections, including bursitis, tenosynovitis, septic arthritis, and osteomyelitis, may result.* *M. marinum* may be rapidly invasive, leading to sepsis in both healthy and immunocompromised individuals.[64,108] Infections may occur after exposure to fresh, salt, or brackish water and are reported by commercial fish handlers, aquarium tenders, pool cleaners, and dolphin trainers.† *M. marinum* invades tissues through a preexisting skin lesion. Three types of lesions may occur: ascending lymphatic sporotrichin lesions, a solitary granulomatous verrucous papule or nodule that may ulcerate and express purulent drainage, and rare cutaneous disseminated lesions.[81,185] In one variety of penetration, 7 to 10 days after the individual sustains a puncture wound or laceration, particularly of a cooler distal extremity, a localized area of cellulitis develops. In the absence of appropriate treatment, this area of cellulitis may progress to localized arthritis, bony erosion, formation of subcutaneous nodules, and superficial desquamation.[12,104,133,261] Aspiration of a joint effusion may reveal the acid-fast bacilli. Alternatively, within 3 to 4 weeks of the primary inoculation, a red papule develops and slowly grows, becoming a hard purple nodule. This nodule often is scaly, ulcerated, and verrucous with a violaceous base, resembling tuberculosis verrucosa cutis.[65,132,146,204,211] The lesion may enlarge to 6 cm in diameter, although a diameter of 1 to 2 cm is more common. New lesions may develop in a pattern that resembles sporotrichosis, with dermal granulomas in a

*References 5, 15, 41, 94, 137, 207, 219.
†References 31, 45, 51, 73, 117, 135, 137, 219.

linear distribution along the superficial lymphatics. The granuloma may become secondarily infected, resulting in cellulitis or lymphangitis. The differential diagnosis should include sporotrichosis, cutaneous leishmaniasis, psoriasis, verrucous lichen planus, verruca vulgaris, iodine and bromine granulomas, sarcoidosis, paratuberculosis, syphilis, gout, other cutaneous mycobacteriosis, and chronic pyogenic infections.[115]

The diagnosis of *M. marinum* is frequently overlooked, resulting in significant delays in treatment, because there is no characteristic skin lesion. The diagnosis is confirmed by a skin biopsy or wound culture. The diagnosis of *M. marinum* granuloma is confirmed bacteriologically by isolation of the organism from a homogenized skin biopsy (minimum 4-mm punch) specimen on standard mycobacterial culture medium (Lowenstein-Jensen) at 31° C to 33° C (88° F to 91° F), rather than the standard 37° C (98° F).[5,78,115,135,259] Acid-fast bacilli are visualized directly in only 10% to 13% of biopsies, and approximately 50% of cultures are positive.[59] Cutaneous intradermal skin tests show cross reactivity between *M. marinum* and *M. tuberculosis*. Risk factors for the development of atypical cutaneous mycobacterial infection include immunosuppression secondary to lymphoma, leukemia, human immunodeficiency virus infection, and medical therapy.

The literature does not reflect consensus on treatment. Conservative therapy, aggressive surgical excision, and multiple antibiotic therapies have been described.* Because most lesions are self-limiting and heal spontaneously within a few months to 3 years, generally leaving some scarring and residual pigmentation, some advocate conservative therapy. Small lesions often are easily excised but may be complicated by local recurrences. Although there have been few reports of prompt diagnosis and successful treatment with antibiotics before surgical biopsy, the astute physician may recognize the initial presentation before surgical intervention.[12] The optimum treatment of cutaneous *M. marinum* infection, which may ultimately resolve spontaneously, is equally unclear. *M. marinum* is susceptible to many antibiotics. Those used previously with inconsistent results include amoxicillin/clavulanate, azithromycin, amikacin, kanamycin, clarithromycin, minocycline, tetracycline, levofloxacin, trimethoprim/sulfamethoxazole, and tuberculostatic drugs, such as streptomycin, isoniazid, ethambutol, and rifampin.† Because clinical evidence regarding the most efficacious treatment of *M. marinum* is lacking, the current recommendation is to treat the patient empirically with one of the aforementioned antibiotics until sensitivities are obtained.[31] Drug sensitivities of the isolated organisms

should be determined.* Susceptibility testing of *M. marinum* is usually delayed for several weeks after treatment has begun and therefore does not have a role in directing initial treatment.[137] Recent reports favor the use of trimethoprim/sulfamethoxazole or ethambutol plus rifampin as first-line therapy.[53,135,137] Trimethoprim/sulfamethoxazole is safe, efficacious, and inexpensive.[135] Subsequent treatment should be based on the sensitivity and clinical response. All studies agree that antibiotic treatment should be long term, with the duration of treatment varying from months to years.[53,81] Although the organism is sensitive to heat, heat therapy is no longer recommended. Intralesional steroids are contraindicated.[56]

Vibrio Vulnificus. The genus *Vibrio* is classified in the family Vibrionaceae, along with the genera *Photobacterium*, *Aeromonas*, and *Plesiomonas*.[9] *Vibrio vulnificus* is a part of normal marine flora but is recognized as a virulent pathogen in the United States and other parts of the world (see Chapter 54). Two distinct clinical syndromes result from infection. Ingestion of raw or undercooked shellfish contaminated with *V. vulnificus* may result in fatal septicemia. *V. vulnificus* contamination of minor wounds can result in virulent, necrotizing cellulitis with bullous skin lesions that require surgical debridement.[182] The lesions may be attributed to proteolytic, collagenolytic, and elastase activity. The organism has been isolated in warm (20° C [68° F] or warmer) coastal water and in water with salinity of 0.7% to 1.6%.[173,182] It has been found in brackish inland waters. Inoculation results from contamination of minor skin wounds, lacerations, and punctures by contaminated objects or from skin trauma suffered while exposed to contaminated water. Victims frequently report that they had been handling shellfish or fish in a marine environment when they obtained a small wound. The wound rapidly progresses to an edematous, erythematous or ecchymotic, cellulitic, and painful infection.[20] What begins as an erythematous lesion may develop into hemorrhagic bullae or vesicles with distal satellite lesions. Lesions may advance rapidly to necrotizing vasculitis or myositis, with acute sepsis.[127] Hematogenous seeding is thought to be responsible for "hallmark" lesions.[20]

Because of the severity and rapid progression of *V. vulnificus* wound infection, prompt diagnosis and antimicrobial treatment, along with early surgical debridement, are mandated.[182] Antimicrobial therapy may include doxycycline, ciprofloxacin, chloramphenicol, gentamicin, imipenem/cilastatin, third-generation cephalosporins, amikacin, tobramycin, aztreonam, and trimethoprim/sulfamethoxazole. Multiple antimicrobials may be required. Despite prompt diagnosis and

---

*References 5, 36, 53, 81, 137, 139, 241.
†References 15, 23, 31, 41, 51, 53, 65, 74, 78, 110, 128, 132, 134, 137, 139, 146, 179, 188, 204, 211, 219, 241, 255.

*References 15, 23, 41, 51, 53, 65, 74, 78, 110, 128, 132, 134, 137, 139, 146, 179, 188, 204, 211, 219, 241, 255.

treatment, the mortality rate remains high, especially in persons who are medically or immunologically compromised.

Erysipelothrix Rhusiopathiae.

Erysipeloid is an acute infection of traumatized skin caused by the slender gram-positive bacillus (rod) *Erysipelothrix rhusiopathiae* (formerly *Erysipelothrix insidosa*) (Figure 63-4). The infection occurs in fishermen, butchers, and others who handle raw fish, poultry, or meat products. Also called *speck finger, fish handler's disease, blubber finger,* and less commonly *erysipeloid of Rosenbach,* the condition is noted most often in coastal regions where workers handle crabs and live fish.[77,88,196] The bacillus is facultatively aerobic and nonmotile and has no spores or capsules. It is hardy enough to survive saltwater or freshwater exposure, drying, salting, pickling, and smoking and survives 12 days in direct sunlight, 4 months in putrefied flesh, and 9 months in a buried carcass.[88]

Erysipelothrix organisms enter the skin through a puncture wound or abrasion, usually on the finger or hand. Between 1 and 7 days later, a hallmark lesion develops. The puncture wound takes on the appearance of a minor purple-red skin irritation or infected paronychia, with edema and a small amount of purulent discharge. This lesion is surrounded by an area of relative central fading or noninvolvement ("clearing"), which in turn in surrounded by a classical, centripetally advancing, raised, well-demarcated, and marginated erythematous or violaceous ring. Usually the lesion, which is located on the finger or hand, is warm and tender, with characteristic progression up the dorsal edge of the finger into the web space and descent along the adjoining finger (Figure 63-5).[256] The lesion is painful and often pruritic, and regional lymph nodes may be inflamed. Pitting and suppuration are absent.[88] The infection seldom affects the palm. Although the infection is generally limited to the hand, it may spread to the wrist or forearm.[130] Low-grade fever and malaise are not uncommon. In the diffuse cutaneous form the local lesion enlarges, and dissemination results in multiple satellite lesions distant from the original site, occasionally with vesiculation or formation of large bullae.[55] Bacteremia, severe generalized cutaneous infections, systemic infections, and endocarditis are rare.[65,88]

E. rhusiopathiae may be cultured from the erysipeloid lesion by excising a punch biopsy or by injecting sterile (not bacteriostatic) saline into the edge of the lesion and then reaspirating without withdrawing the needle.[256] For transport, the specimen should be immediately placed into an infusion broth containing 1% glucose. The microbiology laboratory should be alerted to the possible presence of *E. rhusiopathiae* because it is closely related bacteriologically to *Listeria monocytogenes* and *Corynebacterium* species and may be easily confused with streptococci or diphtheroids.[88] Without treatment, erysipeloid usually is self-limited and runs its course within 3 weeks. For isolated skin involvement, penicillin VK or cephalexin (250 to 500 mg by mouth four times daily) or ciprofloxacin (500 to 750 mg by mouth twice daily) is rapidly effective.[14] Erythromycin is no longer recommended. *E. rhusiopathiae* is resistant to aminoglycoside antibiotics.[210] If arthritis, septicemia, or endocarditis is present, aqueous penicillin G should be administered in a dose of 2 to 4 million units intravenously every 4 hours for 4 to 6 weeks.

Shewanella Putrefaciens.

Shewanella putrefaciens, formerly known as *Pseudomonas putrefaciens,* is a ubiquitous bacterium isolated from sea water, soil, fish, and oily foodstuffs. It is a rare human pathogen that has been associated with lower limb ulceration, otitis media in divers, peritonitis, and bacteremia. Direct contact with sea water and inoculation of a preexisting wound are potential mechanisms of infection. Infection manifests as cellulitic ulcerations. Complications include phlegmon formation and sepsis. *S. putrefaciens* has been documented to produce the extracellular enzymes lecithinase, lipase, and DNase. These enzymes may cause the necrosis of the skin and subcutaneous tissue. Ciprofloxacin has been successfully used to treat this infection.[179]

Algae

Human and animal infections have been caused by achlorophyllic mutants of the green alga *Chlorella*

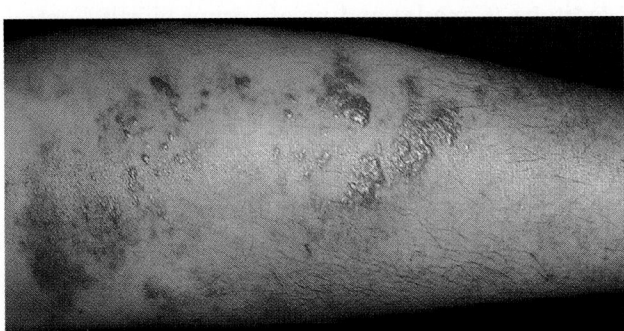

Figure 63-4 *Erysipelothrix rhusiopathiae. (Courtesty Edgar Maeyens, MD.)*

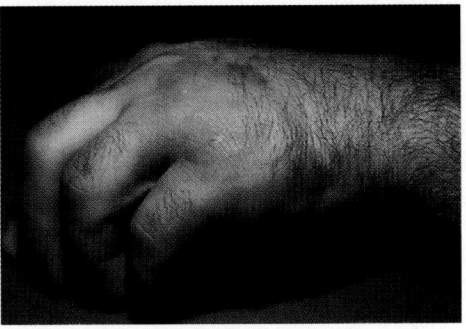

Figure 63-5 Typical appearance of *Erysipelothrix rhusopathiae* skin infection. *(Photo by Paul Auerbach, MD.)*

pyrenoidosa. The genus *Protheca* consists of nonpigmented algae from the family Chlorellaceae. Three species of *Protheca* are recognized: *Protheca stagnora, Protheca wickerhamii,* and *Protheca zopfii.* Only *P. zopfii* and *P. wickerhamii* are demonstrated pathogens in humans.[28,47,131,252] These organisms are ubiquitous and have been isolated in fresh and marine water, streams, lakes, sewage treatment systems, the slime flux of trees, and animal feces.* Prothecae are unicellular, aerobic, and achlorophyllic spherical organisms with hyaline sporangia that reproduce asexually. They are unable to produce energy from photosynthesis and therefore exist as saprophytes.[28] They are distinct from fungi and bacteria in size, morphology, and method of reproduction. They resemble *Chlorella* organisms and probably represent a mutation of this genus.[28,232] Prototothecosis can present after recreational exposure in swampy areas or after aquarium management.[28] It results from contamination of preexisting wounds with dirty water and soil or exposure of skin to contaminated water. Percutaneous inoculation with contaminated water after trauma is the most common mechanism of infection.[232,252]

Clinical manifestations include chronic subcutaneous or cutaneous lesions, olecranon bursitis, and rarely systemic infection involving several internal organs.[28,165,167,233,252] Although widespread visceral disease has been noted in animals, infections in humans have been limited to the skin, subcutaneous tissue, and regional lymphatics. Most victims cannot identify the portal of entry. Prototothecosis has been reported in humans worldwide.

Prototothecosis takes two forms: a papular or eczematoid dermatitis in immunosuppressed individuals or a localized infection of the olecranon bursa in individuals with a healthy immune system.[170,233,252] Infections are nontransmissible, exogenous, and occasionally associated with an episode of trauma or contact with contaminated water. In cases associated with a traumatic episode the initial lesion is a nodule or tender red papule, which enlarges, becomes pustular, and ulcerates. A purulent, malodorous, and blood-tinged discharge may be present. Satellite lesions usually develop and frequently become confluent. The lesions may become verrucous and resemble chromomycosis. Regional lymph nodes may develop metastatic granulomas. The lesions develop centrifugally and occasionally disseminate. In the olecranon bursitis form the infection develops several weeks after an elbow injury and is localized to the bursa and overlying sinus tracts.[170] The diagnosis is made based on histologic sections and culture. The organisms are spherical, basophilic, and gram positive; they vary in diameter from 3 to 15 μm (*P. wickerhamii*) or 7 to 30 μm (*P. zopfii*) and stain well with Grocott-Gomori methenamine silver nitrate, col-

loidal iron for acid mucopolysaccharides, and periodic acid-Schiff. Larger organisms have thick walls and characteristic internal septation. *Protheca* organisms grow on Sabouraud agar, blood agar, or brain-heart infusion agar at an optimum temperature of 30° C to 32° C (86° F to 90° F). The colonies are cream colored, yeastlike, and microaerophilic and reproduce in 1 to 2 days.[17,124] Antisera for identification of species of *Protheca* can be used on fresh or formalin-fixed tissues.[229]

Prototothecosis and chlorellosis are chronic and progressive diseases. At least one case of chlorellosis has occurred, with the report of a granulomatous reaction of the human foot.[118] Effective therapy has not been established. Localized lesions can be excised, which may be curative.[159,181] Topical medications are unsatisfactory. Algaecidal agents, including ketoconazole, itraconazole, fluconazole, miconazole, fluorocytosine, and tetracycline, may inhibit or kill the organisms in optimal conditions. There is early indication that parenteral therapy with amphotericin B combined with oral tetracycline may be effective.*

Parasites

Schistosomiasis. There are three types of cutaneous manifestations of schistosomiasis, reflecting the trematode lifecycle.[61] "Swimmer's itch" presents when humans become abnormal, accidental hosts for nonhuman schistosomes.[61,107,248] This condition frequently is caused by avian, rodent, or ungulate schistosomes (of the genera *Trichobilharzia, Ornithobilharzia, Gigantobilharzia, Orientobilharzia, Austrobilharzia,* and *Bilharziella*).[8,103,152,200] It is a reaction to penetration of the cercariae through the skin. The cercariae are immature, usually microscopic, larval forms of the parasitic flatworms. The condition's geographic distribution is worldwide, occurring in Arctic, temperate, and tropical zones and in fresh and salt water.[144] Although serious infestation is uncommon in North America, cercarial dermatitis is a vexing problem in certain U.S. locations and has been documented in Massachusetts, Rhode Island, Connecticut, New York, Florida, Louisiana, California, Texas, Oregon, Washington, North Dakota, Nebraska, Iowa, Wisconsin, Minnesota, Michigan, and Ohio.[13] Most commonly, snails and birds that inhabit the lakes of Wisconsin, Michigan, Manitoba (Canada) and neighboring North Central states are the intermediate hosts for these trematodes.[161] Any body of water that is infested with either the definitive or the intermediate host of the schistosome is a potential source of infection. Cercarial dermatitis has been noted in an aquarist who kept an aquarium containing watersnails.[16] Various synonyms, including *Pearl Harbor itch, sawah itch, el Caribe, Koganbyo, lakeside disease, clam digger's itch, swimmer's itch, collector's itch,* and *sea bather's eruption,* are used interchangeably with

---

*References 129, 167, 170, 233, 236, 238, 252.

*References 28, 129, 158, 159, 165, 167, 184, 232, 233, 238, 245, 252, 246.

the term *cercarial dermatitis*. However, there is a clear distinction between swimmer's itch and sea bather's eruption (see Chapter 61), limiting the former to eruptions caused by cercariae and the latter to dermatitis caused by larvae of cnidaria.[16] Abundant submerged vegetation, seaweed in the surf, strong shoreward winds, and high temperatures favor human exposure to schistosomes.[13]

Cercarial dermatitis results when humans become interlopers in the complex life cycle of the schistosome. Adult schistosomes are blood parasites that live in birds and mammals. Schistosome eggs are excreted in animal feces. Swimming miracidia hatch from these eggs and then infest certain species of snails, which serve as intermediate hosts. After incubation in a snail and passage through two sporocyst stages, approximately 200,000 fork-tailed cercariae (infective larvae) are released into the water.[13] The parasites then enter a specific warm-blooded host and mature in the vascular system, unless humans accidentally intrude into the life cycle at the cercariae stage. When the adult worms produce eggs, the cycle restarts. The severity of the dermatitis and the time of onset depend on the number of cercariae involved and whether the victim has been previously exposed.[61] Although the cercariae may penetrate the skin while the host is still in the water, penetration usually occurs when the film of water on the skin evaporates. The cercariae penetrate the epidermis but cannot travel beyond the papillary dermis. Histologic examination reveals intraepithelial burrows and abscesses surrounded by an infiltrate of eosinophils, polymorphonuclear leukocytes, and lymphocytes.[264] The cercariae are walled off and destroyed within 10 to 20 hours of entering the epithelial layers of the skin, where they initiate the destructive inflammatory reaction.[13] Cercariae are not evident in serial histologic sections if the biopsy is taken more than 24 hours after penetration.[30]

Swimmer's itch triggers an immune response in the human, an unnatural host. This sensitization phenomenon is suggested by the more severe reactions in individuals who have been previously exposed. The victim initially experiences a prickling sensation. Itching occurs 4 to 60 minutes after the cercariae penetrate the skin and is accompanied by erythema and mild edema. The initial urticarial reaction subsides within 60 minutes, leaving red macules that become papular and more pruritic over the next 10 to 15 hours. Discrete and highly pruritic papules 3 to 5 mm in diameter that are surrounded by a zone of erythema are typical of this disorder. Vesicles, which may become pustules, frequently form within 48 hours. These lesions may persist for 7 to 14 days.[103] The eruption occurs primarily on exposed body areas. Excoriation leads to pustulation, crusting, and secondary infection. The inflammatory response peaks within 3 days and subsides slowly over 1 to 2 weeks. In mild cases application of iso-

propyl alcohol or equal parts of isopropyl alcohol and calamine lotion controls the itching. Severe cases may require systemic corticosteroids (prednisone, 20 to 60 mg, tapered over 2 weeks). Secondary bacterial infections, which are most often caused by *Staphylococcus aureus* or *Streptococcus* species, may be managed with topical antiseptic ointments (mupirocin or bacitracin) or systemic antibiotics (such as erythromycin sustained release, 333 mg three times daily for 8 to 10 days). Cercarial dermatitis is diagnosed based on a detailed history and the clinical presentation. The cercariae are not evident on biopsy specimens because they are destroyed before medical attention can be obtained.

The avoidance of areas where there is submerged and dense vegetation allowing snails to flourish decreases the incidence of human infestation. Recently the study of lakes' limnologic characteristics has demonstrated a potential association between water temperature, lake depth, and algae levels and the risk of cercarial dermatitis.[141] The identification of potential risk factors for the disease may result in better preventive recommendations for recreational bathers.[40,141] Briskly rubbing with a rough, dry towel immediately after leaving the water removes water droplets that harbor the cercariae and may provide some protection against the condition. Washing the skin with rubbing alcohol or soapy water after bathing is not effective.[13] Previously, copper sulfate was used as a molluscicide in cercariae-infested lakes, but this substance is now recognized as an environmental hazard.[13] Niclosamide does not contain heavy metals and is applied as a molluscicide in 5% granular form to areas exposed during bathing.[175] Preliminary experiments indicate that niclosamide applied to the skin prevents penetration of cercariae.[13] Treatment is symptomatic. Antipruritic medications and antihistamines provide some relief.

Dermatitis schistosomia is a similar reaction resulting from human schistosome cercarial skin penetration. When human blood flukes penetrate the skin during the invasive stage of visceral schistosomiasis, an eruption that mimics the purely cutaneous syndrome occurs.[61] Both the nonhuman and human schistosomes produce skin manifestations consisting of pruritic, erythematous macules and papules. The human blood flukes *Schistosoma mansoni*, *Schistosoma japonicum*, and *Schistosoma haematobium* cause local skin reactions and serious systemic disorders referred to as *visceral schistosomiasis* or *bilharziasis*.

Bilharziasis or schistosomiasis is a cutaneous manifestation caused by either the presence and migration of human schistosomes or the production and release of eggs. It is a hypersensitivity, immune complex–mediated response. An urticarial eruption is present and is associated with eosinophilia and frequently headache, fever, cough, and diarrhea.[61,248]

Bilharziasis cutanea tarda is a rare disorder that occurs when ova are ectopically deposited within the dermis. It most frequently is caused by *S. haematobium* and affects the genital area.[61,248] Eggs reach this site by direct spread of adult flukes or eggs through anastomoses between the superficial veins and pelvic venous plexuses. Clinically, erythematous papules are observed. These papules may become erosive, nodular, vegetative, hypertrophic, or fistulous. Biopsy specimens demonstrate eggs surrounded by granulomatous infiltrates.

WOUNDS

Cutaneous Larva Migrans

Cutaneous larva migrans ("creeping eruption") is a cutaneous eruption caused by the larvae of various nematode parasites for which humans are an abnormal final host. *Ancylostoma braziliensis,* a hookworm of wild and domestic cats and dogs, is the most common helminthic infection affecting humans in the Western Hemisphere.[101] Other less commonly reported species that can cause this condition are *Ancylostoma caninum, Gnathostoma spinigerum, Uncinaria stenocephala,* and *Bunostomum phlebotomum.*[192] A transient creeping eruption also results from infestation with the larvae of the human hookworms *Ancylostoma duodenale* and *Necator americanus.* Humans can become accidental hosts when they contact soil that has been contaminated with the feces of parasitically infected animals. Eggs are eliminated in the feces, and the ova that are deposited in the soil hatch into larvae, which can penetrate human skin. Soil in sandy, warm, and shady areas is most favorable for larvae. Persons commonly affected include ocean bathers, children, gardeners, farmers, and those who work under buildings. Athletes also have been affected.[19]

In humans the larvae penetrate the skin but not the dermis. Erythematous papules and petechiae develop at the site of the infection. The larvae migrate between the dermis and the epidermis, producing superficial linear serpiginous tunnels called *lava currents.* The feet and buttocks are involved most commonly. Some larvae remain quiescent for a few weeks or months, and then migration is manifested by a wandering, thin, linear, raised, and tunnel-like lesion 2 to 3 mm in width. Older lesions become dry and crusted. Nonspecific symptoms include pruritus, urticaria, and a maculopapular exanthem. A case of cutaneous larva migrans complicated by a systemic inflammatory disorder (erythema multiforme) has been documented.[244] The larvae move between a few millimeters and a few centimeters each day. Larva migrans may be associated with eosinophilia (in 10% to 35% of cases) and Löffler's syndrome.

Larva currens is a special form of cutaneous larva migrans caused by *Strongyloides stercoralis.* Usually the eruption is associated with intestinal strongyloidiasis and begins in the perianal skin. It may involve the but-

tocks, thighs, back, and shoulders, but the genitalia are spared. Pruritus is intense, and the lesions spread rapidly, covering between 5 and 10 cm each hour. The larvae leave the skin, enter the bloodstream, and later settle in the intestinal mucosa, and the rash fades.

Treatment of cutaneous larva migrans includes cryotherapy and other physical modalities (application of liquid nitrogen and carbon dioxide with ethyl chloride), topical thiabendazole, and systemic administration of oral thiabendazole (25 to 50 mg/kg) for 2 to 4 days, albendazole (400 mg daily) for 7 days, or ivermectin (12 mg) as a single dose.* Oral albendazole is an effective treatment, reducing the number of side effects, recurrences, and failures.[120,174] Secondary infection sometimes occurs and may require incision and drainage of pustules or furuncles and the use of topical and systemic antibiotics.

In endemic areas, precautions include (1) not sitting or lying on damp soil or sand, especially during rainy seasons; (2) not walking barefoot or using water shoes with fenestrated fabric[231]; (3) draping the ground with impenetrable material before crawling in the dirt; and (4) covering sandboxes with a tarpaulin to prevent contamination by prowling cats.

Leeches

Leeches are members of the phylum Annelida, class Hirudinea. These segmented worms are found in freshwater and marine environments. Their biting jaws allow them to attach to the unsuspecting victim's skin. The freshwater leech may attach without causing significant pain, whereas the marine leech may produce a significant sting upon attachment, perhaps even drawing blood.[154] Upon attachment of the leech, anticoagulants (hirudin and fibrinase) are released into local tissues, which causes moderate painless bleeding at the site after leech removal. A substance that has local analgesic qualities also may be released.[83] The release of such a substance could account for the absence of significant pain during freshwater leech attachment. Leeches feed on their host until they become so engorged that they fall off.

Leeches are still used for medicinal and therapeutic purposes throughout the world.[97,214] The hyaluronidase, collagenase, and aspartase released may play a role in degrading connective tissue and increasing capillary permeability.[214] Future benefits of therapeutic leech attachment may include the prevention of hypertrophic scar formation and venous congestion in skin transplant recipients.[97] Symptoms and signs of leech attachment include local pain, redness, swelling, pruritus, and evidence of puncture wounds (caused by the leech's fangs).[154] The wounds may bleed for a pro-

---

*References 21, 38, 149, 192, 194, 243.

longed time, heal slowly in unsensitized individuals, and become secondarily infected. Previous sensitization to leeches may lead to a more severe reaction. Leech bites can cause serious systemic allergic reactions, including anaphylaxis.[100] The wound may become necrotic, urticarial, or bullous.

Leeches must be carefully removed from the skin. If a leech is ripped from the skin, its fangs may break off and remain embedded, which induces phagedena. Leech removal is facilitated by the application of a few drops of alcohol, vinegar, or brine. An alternative removal method involves the application of a lit match at the site of attachment.[65] After the leech has been removed, the site is carefully inspected to ensure that the fangs are absent. Hemostasis can be achieved by applying direct pressure and using a styptic pencil, oxidized regenerated cellulose absorbable hemostat, or topical thrombin solution. The wound should be cleansed thoroughly with an antiseptic agent several times daily to prevent infection. To prevent leech bites, avoid wading through waters infested with leeches. Individuals who must enter these waters should wear protective clothing and cover all exposed skin.

Parasitic Sea Lice (Cymothoidism)

Sea lice (cymothoids) are small marine crustaceans of the order Isopoda, suborder Cymothoidra. Water skiers, skin divers, and swimmers who frequent coastal and estuarine waters of temperate and tropical seas may encounter these free-swimming crustaceans.[18] Sea lice may live as parasites on invertebrates and fish. Sea lice bites are commonly reported along the coast of southern California. Cymothoids are usually buried in sandy bottoms below water level, but they attack any creature that encroaches upon their space.[69] They typically attack marine animals but may injure humans. They are equipped with a biting apparatus that readily allows them to attach to fish or to human skin.[18] The bite is rapid and sharp, causing punctate hemorrhagic wounds referred to as *sea lice dermatitis* (cymothoidism). The wounds should be cleansed initially with hydrogen peroxide or a brisk soap and water scrub. A topical antiseptic ointment (neomycin or bacitracin) should be applied, and the wound should be inspected daily for secondary infection. The injury resolves over 5 to 7 days with appropriate care.

Crab Larvae

An unusual sensation and irritation described as "pine needles sticking in the skin" is reported when crab larvae contact exposed skin.[34] This sensation resolves upon removal of the larvae. The larvae, found floating on the water's surface, are described as "floating sand particles or small, gray seeds." These larvae have small, translucent gray bodies with no glandular structures.

Calcified spines induce traumatic injury upon contact with skin.[69] Contact does not produce urticaria or any other form of dermatitis.

Other

For a discussion of the wounds inflicted by bristleworms, sponges, and coelenterates, see Chapter 61.

DIVING-RELATED LESIONS

Diver's Hand

Diver's hand affects most long-term occupational saturation divers at one time or another. The condition is described as extensive peeling and scaling of the upper skin layers covering the palms of the hands and occasionally the soles of the feet.[3] Victims complain that their skin peels off in large flakes, and they suffer palmar fissures. The peeling starts at the fingers and continues proximally. There are no vesicles, papulae, or hyperkeratosis. Secondary infection rarely occurs. The dermatitis continues for 1 to 2 weeks, but the skin remains sore and thin with fissures for 2 to 4 weeks. Victims complain of increased sensitivity to nonspecific toxic agents. Diver's hand may occur in divers without any previous skin problems. Skin biopsies reveal the formation of horizontal clefts in the upper two thirds of the stratum corneum. The absence of inflammatory components and infectious organisms might indicate that physical or chemical factors are of etiologic relevance. Diver's hand is theorized to develop in all phases of saturation (compression, bottom time, and decompression), as well as after the end of saturation. Divers without diver's hand may have several other skin symptoms, including *P. aeruginosa* infection and otitis externa, during a saturation period.[2,3] There is no effective protection or treatment available.

Mask Squeeze

Divers can experience bilateral subconjunctival hemorrhages and may sustain pressure marks in the shape of the diving mask if they are unable to equalize pressure within the mask as they descend (see Figure 22-19).

Nitrogen Rash

If scuba divers linger longer than the recommended time at depth, oversaturation of nitrogen under pressure in the subcutaneous tissue can rarely cause transient dermatitis. Nitrogen rash is manifested by pruritic, tender, and erythematous lesions involving primarily the flanks and elbows.[154] Diving should be discontinued until all symptoms and signs resolve.

Decompression Rash

If a diver surfaces too rapidly after being at depth, decompression sickness (see Chapter 57) may result. Cutaneous manifestations of decompression sickness include pruritus, erythema, mottling, and pallor.[154] Recompression therapy is mandated.

AQUATIC SPORTS-RELATED DERMATOSES

Otitis Externa

Infection of the external ear canal is the most common of all aquatic dermatoses (Figure 63-6). It causes extreme discomfort and interferes with participation in aquatic activities. The duration of exposure to water is directly related to the incidence of otitis externa. Otitis externa is referred to as *swimmer's ear* because swimmers and scuba and deep-sea divers frequently are afflicted with this problem. As described by Strauss, the adult ear canal is a cul-de-sac lined with stratified squamous epithelium approximately 5 mm in diameter and 25 mm in length. The outer third of the ear has a physiologic barrier to infection, consisting of an acidic waxy mantle with sloughed epithelial cells. However, this barrier is not present to the same degree on the thinner and more delicate epithelium of the inner two thirds of the ear.[227]

The pathophysiology of otitis externa involves the interaction of moisture retention, moderate to high temperatures, and infection. Other factors that predispose a diver to the development of otitis externa include canal occlusion (e.g., exostoses, cerumen plugs, entrapped particles of sand, earplugs), trauma related to mechanical attempts to clean the ear canal, intrinsic dermatoses (e.g., allergic conditions, eczema, psoriasis, contact and seborrheic dermatitis, neurodermatitis), cerumen degradation, and pH variation (normal pH is 4 to 5). The initial symptoms of otitis externa include itching of the ear canal, pain, pressure or fullness within the ear, and diminished hearing. As the inflammatory process within the ear canal progresses, the pain becomes more intense. Pain is noted upon applying pressure to the external auditory meatus or the tragus and upon pulling the ear lobe. A severe infection may develop into otitis media, canal occlusion, cervical lymphadenopathy, headache, nausea, fever, toxemia, and cellulitis with associated purulent discharge. Infection can spread to the periauricular soft tissues, parotid gland, and temporomandibular joint. A secondary periauricular irritant contact dermatitis may occur when suppuration in the ear canal discharges toward the surrounding skin. The usual bacterial pathogens responsible for otitis externa are *P. aeruginosa* and *S. aureus*.[102,265] Otitis externa is polymicrobial, so other isolates include *Acinetobacter calcoaceticus, Proteus mirabilis, Enterococcus faecalis, Bacteroides fragilis,* and *Peptostreptococcus magnus*.[42,102,265] Otitis externa does not appear to be associated with bacterial indicators of recreational water quality, such as fecal coliform bacteria, enterococci, or *Pseudomonas* organisms.[35] A recent

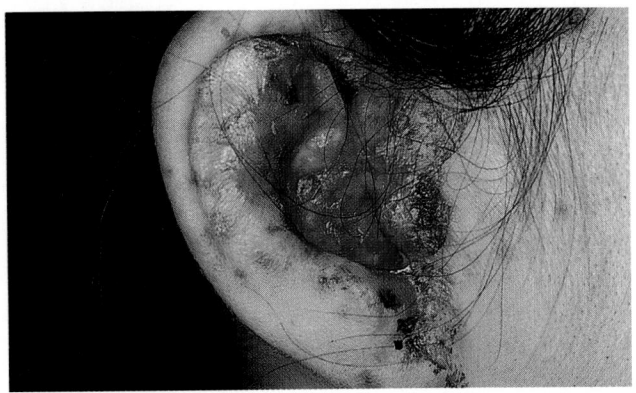

Figure 63-6 Malignant otitis externa. *(Courtesy Edgar Maeyens, MD.)*

study showed that even when current water standards for recreational aquatic activities are met, swimming can increase an individual's risk of otitis externa because of exposure to *P. aeruginosa*.[242]

Treatment is directed at changing the environment within the ear canal. The goals of topical therapy are reacidification and desiccation of the ear canal and are accomplished by the topical administration of a mixture of alcohol and acetic acid (vinegar) or Burow's solution (aluminum sulfate and calcium acetate [Domeboro]). Mild otitis externa characterized by slight pain and itching can be treated with eardrops alone. An excellent topical preparation is nonaqueous acetic acid with or without hydrocortisone 1% (VoSol otic). If suppuration occurs, antibiotic eardrops, such as hydrocortisone 1%, polymixin B, and neomycin (Cortisporin otic) or ofloxacin otic, are indicated.[119] Products not currently recommended include benzocaine, antipyrine, camphor, ichthammol, and thymol.[227] If the ear canal is so swollen that drops cannot be instilled, a gauze wick should be placed and continually soaked with the topical agent for 24 to 72 hours. Systemic antibiotics, such as oral trimethoprim/sulfamethoxazole or amoxicillin/clavulanate, are indicated if cellulitis, adenopathy, profuse purulent discharge, or fever is present. Intravenous antibiotics are indicated when the infection worsens or does nor resolve rapidly. In patients who do not respond to the standard antimicrobial management, a course of antibiotics that cover anaerobic bacteria is warranted.[42] Fortunately, otitis externa rarely progresses to the life-threatening condition of malignant otitis externa. When the condition does not respond to other treatment measures, some suggest that hyperbaric oxygen can be effective. Analgesics are required for pain control. Systemic steroids should be avoided unless an underlying dermatosis exists because they may interfere with the host's response to infection. Oily suspensions or moisturizers must be avoided.

To prevent otitis externa, the individual must take prophylactic measures intended to inhibit moisture accumulation within the external ear canal. Head shaking, tilting, and fanning; use of a blow dryer; and use of desiccating and acidifying agents all prevent moisture accumulation and decrease the incidence of otitis externa. Cotton-tipped applicators should not be used to extract moisture or remove cerumen because they may damage the ear lining or press cerumen deeper into the canal. Cerumen softening products are not useful because they only soften hardened or impacted cerumen without removing it. If warranted, a trained professional may remove cerumen with irrigation or curettage. Earplugs should not be used because they produce ischemia of the ear canal lining. Oily substances, such as petroleum jelly, should not be used to form a water-tight seal because they will act as a moisture trap for debris, increasing the incidence of otitis externa.

REFERENCES

1. Adams RM: Contact allergic dermatitis due to diethylthiourea in a wet suit, *Contact Dermatitis* 8:277, 1982.
2. Ahlen C, Mandal LH, Iversen OJ: Identification of infectious Pseudomonas aeruginosa strains in an occupational saturation diving environment, *Occup Environ Med* 55:480, 1998.
3. Ahlen C et al: Diver's hand: a skin disorder common in occupational saturation diving, *Occup Environ Med* 55:141, 1998.
4. Alexander JE: Allergic reactions to mask skirts, regulator mouthpieces, and snorkel mouthpieces, *Pressure* 5:10, 1976.
5. Alloway JA, Evangelisti SM, Sartin JS: Mycobacterium marinum arthritis, *Semin Arthritis Rheum* 24:382, 1995.
6. Alomar A, Vilaltella I: Contact dermatitis to dibutyl-thiourea in swimming goggles, *Contact Dermatitis* 13:348, 1985.
7. Ancona A, de la Torre RS, Macotela E: Allergic contact dermatitis from povidone-iodine, *Contact Dermatitis* 13:66, 1985.
8. Appleton CC: Schistosome dermatitis: an unrecognized problem in South Africa? *S Afr Med J* 65:467, 1984.
9. Auerbach PS: Natural microbiologic hazards of the aquatic environment, *Clin Dermatol* 5:55, 1987.
10. Auerbach PS et al: Bacteriology of the freshwater environment: implications for clinical therapy, *Ann Emerg Med* 16:1016, 1987.
11. Baddour LM: Extraintestinal Aeromonas infections: looking for Mr. Sandbar, *Mayo Clin Proc* 67:496, 1992.
12. Bailey JP et al: Mycobacterium marinum: a fishy story, *JAMA* 247:1314, 1982.
13. Baird JK, Wear DJ, Connor DH: Cercarial dermatitis: the swimmer's itch, *Clin Dermatol* 5:88, 1987.
14. Barber M, Nellen M, Zoob M: Erysipeloid of Rosenbach: response to penicillin, *Lancet* 1:125, 1946.
15. Barton A et al: Mycobacterium marinum infection causing septic arthritis and osteomyelitis, *Br J Rheum* 36:1207, 1997.
16. Bastert J et al: Aquarium dermatitis: cercarial dermatitis in an aquarist, *Dermatology* 197:84, 1998.
17. Berkhoff HA, Connelly MR, Lockett LJ: Differential microbiological diagnosis of prototheccosis from nonhuman sources. *Am J Med Technol* 48:609, 1982.
18. Best WC, Sablan RG: Cymothoidism (sea louse dermatitis), *Arch Dermatol* 90:177, 1964.
19. Biolcati G, Alabiso A: Creeping eruption of larva migrans: a case report in a beach volley athlete, *Int J Sports Med* 18:612, 1997.
20. Blake PA et al: Disease caused by a marine vibrio: clinical characteristics and epidemiology, *N Engl J Med* 300:1, 1979.
21. Blaum JM, Omura EF: Cutaneous larva migrans, *N Engl J Med* 338:1733, 1998.
22. Boehncke WH et al: Allergic contact dermatitis from diphenylthiourea in a wet suit, *Contact Dermatitis* 36:271, 1997.
23. Bonnet E et al: Clarithromycin: a potent agent against infections due to Mycobacterium marinum, *Clin Infect Dis* 18:664, 1994.
24. Bonnetblanc JM et al: Familial aquagenic urticaria, *Dermatologica* 158:468, 1979.
25. Bottone EJ, Perez AA II, Oeser JL: Loofah sponges as reservoirs and vehicles in the transmission of potentially pathogenic bacterial species to human skin, *J Clin Microbiol* 32:469, 1994.
26. Bourke ATC, Hawes RB: Freshwater cyanobacteria (blue-green algae) and human health, *Med J Aust* 1:491, 1983.
27. Boyce SH: Fish tank granuloma: an unusual cause of skin infection, *J Accid Emerg Med* 14:400, 1997.
28. Boyd AS, Langley M, King LE Jr: Cutaneous manifestations of Protheca infections. I, *J Am Acad Dermatol* 32:758, 1995.
29. Boylan DB, Scheuer PJ: Pahutoxin: a fish poison, *Science* 155:52, 1967.
30. Brackett S: Pathology of schistosome dermatitis, *Arch Dermatol* 42:410, 1940.
31. Brady RC et al: Facial sporotrichoid infection with Mycobacterium marinum, *J Pediatr* 130:324, 1997.
32. Bugler RJ, Sherris JC: The clinical significance of Aeromonas hydrophila: a report of two cases, *Arch Intern Med* 118:562, 1966.
33. Burnett JW, Burnett HW, Burnett MG: Sargassum dermatitis, *Cutis* 59:303, 1997.
34. Burnett JW, Cargo DG: Cutaneous irritation induced by crab larvae, *J Am Acad Dermatol* 1:42, 1979.
35. Calderon R, Mood EW: An epidemiological assessment of water quality and swimmer's ear, *Arch Environ Health* 37:300, 1982.
36. Califano L et al: Verrucous nodule of the finger, *Arch Dermatol* 134:365, 1998.
37. Cardellina JH, Marner FJ, Moore RE: Seaweed dermatitis: structure of lyngbyatoxin A, *Science* 204:193, 1979.
38. Caumes E et al: Efficacy of ivermectin in the therapy of cutaneous larva migrans, *Arch Dermatol* 128:994, 1992.
39. Centers for Disease Control and Prevention: Pool-associated rash illness: North Carolina, *MMWR* 24:349, 1975.
40. Chamot E, Toscani L, Rougemont A: Public health importance and risk factors for cercarial dermatitis associated with swimming in Lake Leman at Geneva, Switzerland, *Epidemiol Infect* 120:305, 1998.
41. Clark RB et al: Osteomyelitis and synovitis produced by Mycobacterium marinum in a fisherman, *J Clin Microbiol* 28:2570, 1990.
42. Clark WB et al: Microbiology of otitis externa, *Otolaryngol Head Neck Surg* 116:23, 1997.
43. Cohen SG, Reif CB: Cutaneous sensitization to blue-green algae, *J Allergy* 24:452, 1953.
44. Cohn GH: Hyperbaric oxygen therapy. Promoting healing in difficult cases, *Postgrad Med* 79:89, 1986.
45. Cott RE, Carter DM, Sall T: Cutaneous disease caused by atypical mycobacteria, *Arch Dermatol* 95:259, 1967.
46. Czarnetzki BM, Breetholt KH, Traupe H: Evidence that water acts as a carrier for an epidermal antigen in aquagenic urticaria, *J Am Acad Dermatol* 15:623, 1986.
47. Davies RR, Spencer H, Wakelin PO: A case of human prototheccosis, *Trans R Soc Trop Med Hyg* 58:448, 1964.
48. Davis RS et al: Evaluation of a patient with both aquagenic and cholinergic urticaria, *J Allergy Clin Immunol* 68:479, 1979.
49. Davis WA, Kane JH, Garagusi VF: Human Aeromonas infections: a review of the literature and a case report of endocarditis, *Medicine* 57:267, 1978.
50. Dean HM, Post RM: Fatal infection with Aeromonas hydrophila in a patient with acute myelogenous leukemia, *Ann Intern Med* 66:1177, 1967.
51. Dorronsoro I et al: Cutaneous infections by Mycobacterium marinum: description of three cases and review of the literature, *Enferm Infecc Microbiol Clin* 15:82, 1997.
52. Du Peloux Menage H, Greaves MW: Aquagenic pruritus, *Semin Dermatol* 14:313, 1995.
53. Edelstein H: Mycobacterium marinum skin infections: report of 31 cases and review of the literature, *Arch Intern Med* 154:1359, 1994.
54. Edwards C et al: Identification of anatoxin-A in benthic cyanobacteria (blue-green algae) and in associated dog poisonings at Loch Insh, Scotland, *Toxicon* 30:1165, 1992.
55. Ehrlich JC: Erysipelothrix rhusiopathiae infection in man, *Arch Intern Med* 78:565, 1944.
56. Ekerot I, Jacobsson L, Forsgren A: Mycobacterium marinum wrist arthritis: Local and systemic dissemination caused by concomitant immunosuppressive therapy, *Scand J Infect Dis* 30:84, 1998.
57. El Baze P et al: Pseudomonas aeruginosa 0-11 folliculitis, *Arch Dermatol* 212:873, 1985.
58. Eriksson JE et al: Preliminary characterization of a toxin isolated from the cyanobacterium Nodularia spumigena, *Toxicon* 26:161, 1988.

59. Even-Paz Z et al: Mycobacterium marinum skin infections mimicking cutaneous leishmaniasis, *Br J Dermatol* 94:435, 1976.

60. Fainstein V, Weaver S, Bodey GP: In vitro susceptibilities of Aeromonas hydrophila against new antibiotics, *Antimicrob Agents Chemother* 22:513, 1982.

61. Farrell AM et al: Ectopic cutaneous schistosomiasis: extragenital involvement with progressive upward spread, *Br J Dermatol* 135:110, 1996.

62. Fass RJ, Barnishan J: In vitro susceptibilities of Aeromonas hydrophila to 32 antimicrobial agents, *Antimicrob Agents Chemother* 19:357, 1981.

63. Fearfield LA, Gazzard B, Bunker CB: Aquagenic urticaria and human immunodeficiency virus infection: treatment with Stanozol, *Br J Dermatol* 137:620, 1997.

64. Feddersen A et al: Infection of the upper extremity by Mycobacterium marinum in a 3-year-old boy: diagnosis by 16S-rDNA analysis, *Infection* 24:47, 1996.

65. Fisher AA: *Atlas of aquatic dermatology*, New York, 1978, Grune & Stratton.

66. Fisher AA: Water related dermatoses, *Cutis* 25:132, 1980.

67. Fisher AA: Dermatitis from chlorine and certain chlorinated products, *Cutis* 33:20, 1984.

68. Fisher AA: *Contact dermatitis*, ed 3, Philadelphia, 1986, Lea & Febiger.

69. Fisher AA: Contact dermatitis to diving equipment, swimming pool chemicals, and other aquatic denizens, *Clin Dermatol* 5:36, 1987.

70. Fisher AA: Aquagenic pruritus, *Cutis* 51:146, 1993.

71. Fisher AA: Folliculitis from the use of a "loofah" cosmetic sponge, *Cutis* 54:12, 1994.

72. Fitzgerald DA et al: Spa pool dermatitis, *Contact Dermatitis* 33:53, 1995.

73. Flowers DJ: Human infection due to Mycobacterium marinum after a dolphin bite, *J Clin Pathol* 23:475, 1970.

74. Forsgren A: Antibiotic susceptibility of Mycobacterium marinum, *Scand J Infect Dis* 25:779, 1993.

75. Frenkel LM: Pseudomonas folliculitis from sponges promoted as beauty aids, *J Clin Microbiol* 31:2838, 1993.

76. Fulghum DD, Linton WR Jr, Taplin D: Fatal Aeromonas hydrophila infection of the skin, *South Med J* 71:739, 1978.

77. Gilchrist TC: Erysipeloid, with a record of 322 cases, of which 239 were caused by crab bites or lesions produced by crabs, *Journal of Cutaneous Disease* 22:507, 1904.

78. Gluckman SJ: Mycobacterium marinum, *Clin Dermatol* 13:273, 1995.

79. Goett KD, Fowler V: Hot tub acquired Pseudomonas septicemia, *Journal of the Association of Military Dermatologists* 10:40, 1984.

80. Goette DK: Racoon-like periorbital leukoderma from contact with swim goggles, *Contact Dermatitis* 10:129, 1984.

81. Goldhagen M, Nunberg S, Freeman AM: Right hand and arm rash, *Acad Emerg Med* 2:919, 1995.

82. Good RA et al: Fatal (chronic) granulomatous disease of childhood: a hereditary defect of leukocyte function, *Semin Hematol* 5:215, 1968.

83. Graham CE: Leeches, *BMJ* 310:603, 1995.

84. Grauer FH, Arnold HL: Seaweed dermatitis: first report of a dermatitis-producing marine alga, *Arch Dermatol* 84:720, 1961.

85. Gray S et al: Fish tank granuloma, *BMJ* 300:1609, 1990.

86. Greaves MW, Handfield-Jones SE: Aquagenic pruritus pharmacological findings and treatments, *Eur J Dermatol* 122:103, 1990.

87. Greaves MW et al: Aquagenic pruritus, *BMJ* 282:2008, 1981.

88. Grieco MH, Sheldon C: Erysipelothrix rhusiopathiae, *Ann NY Acad Sci* 174:523, 1970.

89. Gustafson TL et al: Pseudomonas folliculitis: an outbreak and review, *Rev Infect Dis* 5:1, 1983.

90. Halstead BW: *Poisonous and venomous marine animals of the world*, Princeton, NJ, 1978, Darwin Press.

91. Handfield-Jones SE et al: Aquagenic pruritus associated with juvenile xanthogranuloma, *Clin Exp Dermatol* 18:253, 1993.

92. Hanson PG et al: Freshwater wound infection due to Aeromonas hydrophila, *JAMA* 238:1053, 1977.

93. Harada K-I et al: A new procedure for the analysis and purification of naturally occurring anatoxin-a from the blue-green alga Anabena flos-aquae, *Toxicon* 27:1289, 1982.

94. Harth M, Ralph ED, Faraawi R: Septic arthritis due to Mycobacterium marinum, *J Rheumatol* 21:957, 1994.

95. Hashimoto Y, Kamiya H: Occurrence of a toxic substance in the skin of a sea bass Pogonoperca punctata, *Toxicon* 7:65, 1969.

96. Hautmann G, Teofoli P, Lotti T: Aquagenic pruritus, PUVA and capsaicin treatments, *Br J Dermatol* 131:920, 1994.

97. Hayden RE, Phillips JG, McLear PW: Leeches. Objective monitoring of altered perfusion in congested flaps, *Arch Otolaryngol Head Neck Surg* 114:1395, 1988.

98. Hazen TC et al: Prevalence and distribution of Aeromonas hydrophila in the United States, *Appl Microbiol* 36:731, 1978.

99. Heise HA: Symptoms of hay fever caused by algae, Microcystis: another form of algae-producing allergenic reactions, *Ann Allergy* 9:100, 1951.

100. Heldt TJ: Allergy to leeches, *Henry Ford Hospital Medical Journal* 9:498, 1961.

101. Hendrix CM et al: Cutaneous larva migrans and enteric hookworm infections, *J Am Vet Med Assoc* 209:1763, 1996.

102. Hoadley AF, Knight DE: External otitis among swimmers and non-swimmers, *Arch Environ Health* 30:445, 1975.

103. Hoeffler DF: Cercarial dermatitis: its etiology, epidemiology, and clinical aspects, *Arch Environ Health* 29:225, 1974.

104. Hoffman GS et al: Septic arthritis associated with Mycobacterium avium: a case report and literature review, *J Rheumatol* 5:199, 1978.

105. Hogan PA: Pseudomonas folliculitis, *Australas J Dermatol* 38:93, 1997.

106. Hopkins RS, Abbott DO, Wallace LE: Follicular dermatitis outbreak caused by Pseudomonas aeruginosa associated with a motel's indoor swimming pool, *Public Health Rep* 96:246, 1981.

107. Horak P et al: Cercaria-schistosomulum surface transformation of Trichobilharzia szidati and its putative immunological impact. II, *Parasitology* 116:139, 1998.

108. Horsburgh CR: Epidemiology of disease caused by nontuberculous mycobacteria, *Semin Respir Infect* 11:244, 1996.

109. Huffam SE, Nowotny MJ, Currie BJ: Chromobacterium violaceum in tropical northern Australia, *Med J Aust* 168 335, 1998.

110. Iijima S, Saito J, Otsuka F: Mycobacterium marinum skin infection successfully treated with levofloxacin, *Arch Dermatol* 133:947, 1997.

111. Izumi AK, Moore RE: Seaweed (Lyngbya majuscula) dermatitis, *Clin Dermatol* 5:92, 1987.

112. Jacobson JA: Pool-associated Pseudomonas aeruginosa dermatitis and other bathing-associated infections, *Infect Control* 6:398, 1985.

113. Janda JM, Bottone EJ, Reitano M: Aeromonas species in clinical microbiology: significance, epidemiology, and speciation, *Diagn Microbiol Infect Dis* 1:221, 1983.

114. Johnson WM, Disalvo AP, Steuer RR: Fatal Chromobacterium violaceum septicemia, *Am J Clin Pathol* 56:400, 1971.

115. Johnston JM, Izumi AK: Cutaneous Mycobacterium marinum infection ("swimming pool granuloma"), *Clin Dermatol* 5:68, 1987.

116. Johnston RB, Baehner RL: Chronic granulomatous disease: correlation between pathogenesis and clinical findings, *Pediatrics* 48:730, 1971.

117. Johnston RG, Fung J: Bacterial flora of wild and captive porpoises, *J Occup Med* 11:276, 1969.

118. Jones J et al: Green algal infection in a human, *Am J Clin Pathol* 80:102, 1983.

119. Jones RN, Milazzo J, Seidlin M: Ofloxacin otic solution for treatment of otitis externa in children and adults, *Arch Otolaryngol Head Neck Surg* 123:1193, 1997.

120. Jones S et al: Oral albendazole for the treatment of cutaneous larva migrans, *Br J Dermatol* 122:99, 1990.

121. Joseph SW et al: Aeromonas primary wound infection of a diver in polluted waters, *J Clin Microbiol* 10:46, 1979.

122. Juhlin L, Malmros-Enander I: Familial polymorphous light eruption with aquagenic urticaria: successful treatment with PUVA, *Photodermatology* 3:346, 1986.

123. Kanerva L, Estlander T, Jolanki R: Occupational allergic contact dermatitis caused by thiourea compounds, *Contact Dermatitis* 31:242, 1994.

124. Kapica L: First case of human prototothecosis in Canada: laboratory aspects, *Mycopathologia* 73:43, 1981.

125. Karam GH, Ackley AM, Dismukes WE: Posttraumatic Aeromonas hydrophila osteomyelitis, *Arch Intern Med* 143:2073, 1983.

126. Katz D, Smith H: Aeromonas hydrophila infection of a puncture wound, *Ann Emerg Med* 9:529, 1980.

127. Kelly MT, McCormick WF: Acute bacterial myositis caused by Vibrio vulnificus, *JAMA* 246:72, 1981.

128. Kim R: Tetracycline therapy for atypical mycobacterial granuloma, *Arch Dermatol* 110:299, 1974.

129. Kim ST et al: Successful treatment with fluconazole of prototothecosis developing at the site of an intralesional corticosteroid injection, *Br J Dermatol* 135:803, 1996.

130. Klauder JV: Erysipeloid as an occupational disease, *JAMA* 111:1345, 1938.

131. Klintworth GK, Fetter BF, Nielson HS Jr: Prototothecosis, an algal infection: report of a case in man, *J Med Microbiol* 1:211, 1968.

132. Knox JM et al: Atypical acid-fast organism of the skin, *Arch Dermatol* 84:386, 1961.

133. Kozin SH, Bishop AT: Atypical mycobacterium infections of the upper extremity, *J Hand Surg* 19A:480, 1994.

134. Kuhn SM et al: Treatment of Mycobacterium marinum facial abscess using clarithromycin, *Pediatr Infect Dis J* 14:631, 1995.

135. Kullavanijaya P, Sirimachan S, Bhuddhavudhikrai P: Mycobacterium marinum cutaneous infections acquired from occupations and hobbies, *Int J Dermatol* 32:504, 1993.

136. Lacour JP et al: Diving suit dermatitis caused by Pseudomonas aeruginosa: two cases, *J Am Acad Dermatol* 31:1055, 1994.

137. Laing RB et al: Antimicrobial treatment of fish tank granuloma, *J Hand Surg* 22:135, 1997.

138. Lampe RM, Henderson AC, Hansen GH: Green hair, *JAMA* 237:2092, 1977.

139. Lee MW, Brenan J: Mycobacterium marinum: chronic and extensive infections of the lower limbs in south Pacific islanders, *Australas J Dermatol* 39:173, 1998.

140. Levin ML: Gas-forming Aeromonas hydrophila in a diabetic, *Postgrad Med* 54:127, 1973.

141. Lindblade KA: The epidemiology of cercarial dermatitis and its association with limnological characteristics of a northern Michigan lake, *J Parasitol* 84:19, 1998.

142. Linell F, Norden A: Mycobacterium balnei: a new acid fast bacillus occurring in swimming pools and capable of producing skin lesions in humans, *Acta Tuberc Scand Suppl* 33:1, 1954.

143. Lippy EC, Erb J: Gastrointestinal illness at Sewickley, Pennsylvania, *Journal of American Water Works Associations* 68:606, 1976.

144. Loken BR, Spencer CN, Granath WO Jr: Prevalence and transmission of cercariae causing schistosome dermatitis in Flathead Lake, Montana, *J Parasitol* 81:646, 1995.

145. Lopez JF, Quesada J, Saied A: Bacteremia and osteomyelitis due to Aeromonas hydrophila, *Am J Clin Pathol* 50:587, 1968.

146. Loria PR: Minocycline hydrochloride treatment for atypical acid-fast infection, *Arch Dermatol* 112:517, 1976.

147. Lotti T, Teofoli P, Tsampau D: Treatment of aquagenic pruritus with topical capsaicin cream. I, *J Am Acad Dermatol* 30:232, 1994.

148. Lotti T et al: Increased cutaneous fibrinolytic activity in a case of aquagenic pruritus, *Int J Dermatol* 23:61, 1984.

149. Loughrey MB et al: Cutaneous larva migrans: the case for routine oral treatment, *Br J Dermatol* 137:155, 1997.

150. Luong KV, Nguyen LT: Aquagenic urticaria: a report of a case and review of the literature, *Ann Allergy Asthma Immunol* 80:483, 1998.

151. Macher AM, Casale TB, Fauci AS: Chronic granulomatous disease of childhood and Chromobacterium violaceum infections in the southeastern United States, *Ann Intern Med* 97:51, 1982.

152. Mahmoud AAF: Schistosomiasis. In Warren KS, Mahmoud AAF, editors: *Tropical and geographical medicine*, New York, 1984, McGraw-Hill.

153. Maibach H: Scuba diver facial dermatitis: allergic contact dermatitis to N-isopropyl-N-phenyl paraphenylenediamine, *Contact Dermatitis* 1:330, 1975.

154. Mandojana RM, Sims JK: Miscellaneous dermatoses associated with the aquatic environment, *Clin Dermatol* 5:134, 1987.

155. Martinez-Escribano JA et al: Treatment of aquagenic urticaria with PUVA and astemizole, *J Am Acad Dermatol* 36:118, 1997.

156. Mathelier-Fusade P et al: Association of cold urticaria and aquagenic urticaria, *Allergy* 52:678, 1997.

157. Mathur MN et al: Cellulitis owing to Aeromonas hydrophila: treatment with hyperbaric oxygen, *Aust N Z J Surg* 65:367, 1995.

158. Matsumoto Y et al: Two cases of protothecosis in Nagoya, Japan, *Australas J Dermatol* 37(suppl 1):S42, 1996.

159. McAnally T, Parry EL: Cutaneous protothecosis presenting as recurrent chromomycosis, *Arch Dermatol* 121:1066, 1985.

160. McCausland WJ, Cox PJ: Pseudomonas infection traced to motel whirlpool, *J Environ Sci Health* 37:455, 1975.

161. McMullen DB, Brackett S: Distribution and control of schistosome dermatitis in Wisconsin and Michigan, *Am J Trop Med* 21:725, 1941.

162. Medeiros M Jr: Aquagenic urticaria, *J Investig Allergol Clin Immunol* 6:63, 1996.

163. Meislich D, Long SS: Invasive Pseudomonas infection in two healthy children following prolonged bathing, *Am J Dis Child* 147:18, 1993.

164. Menage HD et al: The efficacy of psoralen photochemotherapy in the treatment of aquagenic pruritus, *Br J Dermatol* 129:163, 1993.

165. Mendez CM, Silva-Lizama E, Logemann H: Human cutaneous protothecosis, *Int J Dermatol* 34:554, 1995.

166. Midani S, Rathore M: Chromobacterium violaceum infection, *South Med J* 91:464, 1998.

167. Monopoli A, Accetturi MP, Lombardo GA: Cutaneous protothecosis, *Int J Dermatol* 34:766, 1995.

168. Mynderse JS et al: Antileukemia activity in the Oscillatoriaceae: isolation of debromo-Aplysiatoxin from Lyngbya, *Science* 196:538, 1977.

169. Namikoshi M et al: Isolation and structures of microcystins from a cyanobacterial water bloom (Finland), *Toxicon* 30:1473, 1992.

170. Nelson AM, Neaflie RC, Connor DH: Cutaneous protothecosis and chlorellosis, extraordinary opportunistic "aquatic-borne" algal infections, *Clin Dermatol* 5:76, 1987.

171. Newhouse ML: Dogger bank itch: survey of trawlermen, *BMJ* 1:1142, 1966.

172. Ognibene AJ, Thomas E: Fatal infection due to Chromobacterium violaceum in Vietnam, *Am J Clin Pathol* 54:607, 1970.

173. Oliver JD, Warner RA, Cleland DR: Distribution of Vibrio vulnificus and other lactose-fermenting vibrios in the marine environment, *Appl Environ Microbiol* 45:985, 1983.

174. Orihuela AR, Torres JR: Single dose of albendazole in the treatment of cutaneous larva migrans, *Arch Dermatol* 126:398, 1990.

175. Osment LS: Update: seabather's eruption and swimmer's itch, *Cutis* 18:545, 1976.

176. Osmundsen P: Contact dermatitis due to sodium hypochlorite, *Contact Dermatitis* 4:177, 1978.

177. Overman TL: Antimicrobial susceptibility of Aeromonas hydrophila, *Antimicrob Agents Chemother* 17:612, 1980.

178. Panconesi E, Lotti T: Aquagenic urticaria, *Clin Dermatol* 5:49, 1987.

179. Papanaoum K et al: Concurrent infection due to Shewanella putrefaciens and Mycobacterium marinum acquired at the beach, *Australas J Dermatol* 39:92, 1998.

180. Parker RK, Crowe MJ, Guin JD: Aquagenic urticaria, *Cutis* 50:283, 1992.

181. Pegram PS et al: Successful ketoconazole treatment of protothecosis with ketoconazole-associated hepatotoxicity, *Arch Inter Med* 143:1802, 1983.

182. Penman AD et al: Vibrio vulnificus wound infections from the Mississippi Gulf coastal waters: June to August 1993, *South Med J* 88:531, 1995.

183. Perrotta DM et al: An outbreak of Pseudomonas folliculitis associated with a waterslide: Utah, *JAMA* 250:1259, 1983.

184. Phair JP et al: Phagocytosis and algicidal activity of human polymorphonuclear neutrophils against Protheca wickerhamii, *J Infect Dis* 144:72, 1981.

185. Phillips SA et al: Mycobacterium marinum infection of the finger, *J Hand Surg* 20B:801, 1995.

186. Ponte R, Jenkins SG: Fatal Chromobacterium violaceum infections associated with exposure to stagnant waters, *Pediatr Infect Dis J* 11:583, 1992.

187. Randall JE et al: Grammistin, the skin toxin of soapfishes, and its significance in the classification of the Grammistidae, *Publications of the Seto Marine Biological Laboratory* 19:157, 1971.

188. Rastogi N et al: Spectrum of activity of levofloxacin against nontuberculous mycobacteria and its activity against the mycobacterium avium complex in combination with ethambutol, rifampin, roxithromycin, amikacin, and clofazimine, *Antimicrob Agents Chemother* 40:2483, 1996.

189. Reines HD, Cook F: Pneumonia and bacteremia due to Aeromonas hydrophila, *Chest* 30:264, 1981.

190. Reinhold U et al: Treatment of aquagenic pruritus using recombinant interferon-alpha, *Br J Dermatol* 137:324, 1997.

191. Revord ME, Goldfarb J, Shurin SB: Aeromonas hydrophila wound infection in a patient with cyclic neutropenia following a piranha bite, *Pediatr Infect Dis J* 7:70, 1988 (letter).

192. Richey TK et al: Persistent cutaneous larva migrans due to Ancylostoma species, *South Med J* 89:609, 1996.

193. Ries KM, White GL, Murdock RT: Atypical mycobacterial infection caused by Mycobacterium marinum, *N Engl J Med* 322:633, 1990.

194. Rizzitelli G, Scarabelli G, Veraldi S: Albendazole: a new therapeutic regimen in cutaneous larva migrans, *Int J Dermatol* 36:700, 1997.

195. Rose HD et al: Pseudomonas pneumonia associated with use of a home whirlpool spa, *JAMA* 250:2027, 1983.

196. Rosenbach FJ: Experimentelle morphologische und blinische studie uber die krankheitserregenden microorganismen des schweinrotlaufs, des erysepiloids und der mausesepsis, *Hyg Infectionschr* 63:343, 1909.

197. Rosenthal SG, Bernhardt HE, Phillips JA III: Aeromonas hydrophila wound infection, *Plast Reconstr Surg* 53:77, 1974.

198. Runnegar MTC, Jackson ARB, Falconer IR: Toxicity of the cyanobacterium Nodularia spumigena Mertens, *Toxicon* 26:143, 1988.

199. Rycroft RJG, Penny PT: Dermatoses associated with brominated swimming pools, *BMJ* 287:462, 1983.

200. Sabha GH, Malek EA: Dermatitis caused by cercariae of Orientobilharzia turkestanicum in the Caspian Sea of Iran, *Am J Trop Med Hyg* 28:912, 1979.

201. Saltzer KR et al: Diving suit dermatitis: a manifestation of Pseudomonas folliculitis, *Cutis* 59:245, 1997.
202. Sausker WF: Pseudomonas aeruginosa folliculitis ("splash rash"), *Clin Dermatol* 5:62, 1987.
203. Sausker WF et al: Pseudomonas folliculitis acquired from a health spa whirlpool, *JAMA* 239:2362, 1978.
204. Schaeffer WB, Davis CL: A bacteriologic and histopathologic study of skin granuloma due to Mycobacterium balnei, *American Review of Respiratory Disease* 844:837, 1961.
205. Semel JD, Trenholme G: Aeromonas hydrophila water-associated traumatic wound infections: a review, *J Trauma* 30:324, 1980.
206. Shelley WB, Rawnsley HM: Aquagenic urticaria: contact sensitivity reaction to water, *JAMA* 189:895, 1964.
207. Shih JY et al: Osteomyelitis and tenosynovitis due to Mycobacterium marinum in a fish dealer, *J Formos Med Assoc* 96:913, 1997.
208. Shirtcliffe P, Robinson GM: A case of severe Pseudomonas folliculitis from a spa pool, *Aust N Z J Med* 111(1075):389, 1998.
209. Sibbald RG et al: Aquagenic urticaria: evidence of cholinergic and histaminergic basis, *Br J Dermatol* 105:297, 1981.
210. Simerkoff MS, Rahal JJ Jr: Acute and subacute endocarditis due to Erysipelothrix rhusiopathiae, *Am J Med Sci* 266:53, 1973.
211. Sims JK: Dangerous marine life. In Shilling CW, Carlson CB, Mathias RA, editors: The physician's guide to diving medicine, New York, 1984, Plenum Press.
212. Sims JK, Zandee Van Rilland RD: Escharotic stomatitis caused by the "stinging seaweed" Microcoleus lyngbyaceus (formerly Lyngbya majuscula): a case report and review of the literature, *Hawaii Med J* 40:243, 1981.
213. Sims JK et al: Vibrio in stinging seaweed: potential infection, *Hawaii Med J* 52:274, 1993.
214. Siragusa M, Batolo D, Schepis C: Anetoderma secondary to the application of leeches, *Int J Dermatol* 35:226, 1996.
215. Sivonen K et al: Isolation and structures of five microcystins from a Russian Microcystis aeruginosa strain CALU 972, *Toxicon* 30:1481, 1992.
216. Smith CA, Hall FA: Cellulitis due to Aeromonas hydrophila, *Journal of the Medical Association of the State of Alabama* 51:45, 1982.
217. Smith RA, Ross JS, Staughton RC: Bath PUVA as a treatment for aquagenic pruritus, *Br J Dermatol* 131:584, 1994.
218. Solomon AE, Stoughton RB: Dermatitis from purified sea algae toxin (debromoaplysiatoxin), *Arch Dermatol* 114:1333, 1979.
219. Speight EL, Williams HC: Fish tank granuloma in a 14-month-old girl, *Pediatr Dermatol* 14:209, 1997.
220. Spiers ASD, Tattersall MHN, Goya H: Indications for systemic antibiotic prophylaxis in neutropenic patients, *BMJ* 4:440, 1974.
221. Spitalny KC, Vogt RL, Witherall LE: National survey on outbreaks associated with whirlpool spas, *Am J Public Health* 74:725, 1978.
222. Spoerke DG, Rumack BH: Blue-green algae poisoning, *J Emerg Med* 2:353, 1985.
223. Starr AJ et al: Chromobacterium violaceum presenting as a surgical emergency, *South Med J* 74:1137, 1981.
224. Steinman HK: Water-induced pruritus, *Clin Dermatol* 5:41, 1987.
225. Steinman HK, Greaves MW: Aquagenic pruritus, *J Am Acad Dermatol* 13:91, 1985.
226. Stoner RD et al: Cyclosporine A inhibition of microcystin toxins, *Toxicon* 28:569, 1990.
227. Strauss MB, Dierker RL: Otitis externa associated with aquatic activities (swimmer's ear), *Clin Dermatol* 5:103, 1987.
228. Suarez AE et al: Nonfatal chromobacterial sepsis, *South Med J* 79:1146, 1986.
229. Sudman MS, Kaplan W: Identification of Protheca species by immunofluorescence, *Appl Microbiol* 25:981, 1973.
230. Sunn CC, Sue MS: Sulfur spring dermatitis, *Contact Dermatitis* 32:31, 1995.
231. Swanson JR, Melton JL: Cutaneous larva migrans associated with water shoe use, *J Eur Acad Dermatol Venereol* 10:271, 1998.
232. Tang WY et al: Cutaneous protothecosis: a report of a case in Hong Kong, *Br J Dermatol* 133:479, 1995.
233. Tejada E, Parker CM: Cutaneous erythematous nodular lesion in a crab fisherman, *Arch Dermatol* 130:244, 247, 1994.
234. Thomas P et al: Pseudomonas dermatitis associated with a swimming pool, *JAMA* 253:1156, 1985.
235. Tiffany HL: Algae: the grass of many waters, Springfield, IL, 1968, Charles C Thomas.

236. Tindal JP, Fetter BF: Infection caused by achloric algae (protothecosis), *Arch Dermatol* 104:490, 1911.
237. Tippen PS, Meyer A, Blank EC: Aquarium-associated Plesiomonas shigelloides infection: Missouri, *MMWR* 38:617, 1989.
238. Tsuji K et al: Protothecosis in a patient with systemic lupus erythematosus, *Intern Med* 32:540, 1993.
239. Tucker RF, Winter WG, Wilson HD: Osteomyelitis associated with Chromobacterium violaceum infection, *Bone Joint Surg* 61A:949, 1979.
240. Tyup E, Mitchell JC: Scuba diver facial dermatitis, *Contact Dermatitis* 9:334, 1983.
241. Utrup LJ et al: Susceptibilities of nontuberculous mycobacterial species to amoxicillin-clavulanic acid alone and in combination with antimycobacterial agents, *Antimicrob Agents Chemother* 39:1454, 1995.
242. Van Asperen IA et al: Risk of otitis externa after swimming in recreational fresh water lakes containing Pseudomonas aeruginosa, *BMJ* 311(7017):1407, 1995.
243. Van den Enden E, Stevens A, Van Gompel A: Treatment of cutaneous larva migrans, *N Engl J Med* 339:1246, 1998.
244. Vaughan TK, English JC III: Cutaneous larva migrans complicated by erythema multiforme, *Cutis* 62:33, 1998.
245. Venezio FR et al: Progressive cutaneous protothecosis, *Am J Clin Pathol* 77:485, 1982.
246. Vernon SE, Goldman LS: Protothecosis in the southeastern United States, *South Med J* 76:949, 1983.
247. Victoria B, Baer H, Ayoub EM: Successful treatment of systemic Chromobacterium violaceum infection, *JAMA* 230:578, 1974.
248. Visser LG, Polderman AM, Stuiver PC: Outbreak of schistosomiasis among travelers returning from Mali, West Africa, *Clin Infect Dis* 20:280.
249. Von Graevenitz A: Aeromonas and Plesiomonas. In Lennett EH et al, editors: *Manual of clinical microbiology,* Washington, DC, 1985, American Society for Microbiology.
250. Von Graevenitz A, Mensch AH: The genus Aeromonas in human bacteriology: report of 30 cases and review of the literature, *N Engl J Med* 278:245, 1968.
251. Voss LM, Rhodes KH, Johnson KA: Musculoskeletal and soft tissue Aeromonas infection: an environmental disease, *Mayo Clin Proc* 67:422, 1992.
252. Walsh SV, Johnson RA, Tahan SR: Protothecosis: an unusual cause of chronic subcutaneous and soft tissue infections, *Am J Dermatopathol* 20:379, 1998.
253. Washburn J et al: Pseudomonas aeruginosa rash associated with a whirlpool, *JAMA* 235:2205, 1976.
254. Wasserman D, Preminger A, Zlotogorski A: Aquagenic urticaria in a child, *Pediatr Dermatol* 11:29, 1994.
255. Watt B, Rayner A, Harris G: Comparative activity of azithromycin against clinical isolates of mycobacteria, *J Antimicrobial Chemother* 38:539, 1996.
256. Weaver RE: Erysipelothrix. In Lennette EH et al, editors: *Manual of clinical microbiology,* Washington, DC, 1985, American Society for Microbiology.
257. Weinstock RE et al: Aeromonas hydrophila: a rare and potentially life-threatening pathogen to humans, *J Foot Surg* 21:45, 1982.
258. Werner SB: Aeromonas wound infections associated with outdoor activities: California, *MMWR* 39:334, 1990.
259. Williams CS, Riordan DC: Mycobacterium marinum (atypical acid-fast bacillus) infections of the hand, *J Bone Joint Surg Am* 55:1042, 1973.
260. Winslow DL, Jones R: Severe cellulitis due to Aeromonas hydrophila following immersion injury, *Del Med J* 56:361, 1984.
261. Winter FE, Ruyon EH: Prepatellar bursitis caused by Mycobacterium marinum (balnei), *J Bone Joint Surg Am* 47:375, 1965.
262. Withers N: Ciguatera research in the northwest Hawaiian islands: laboratory and field studies on ciguatoxigenic dinoflagellates in the Hawaiian archipelago. In Grigg RW, Tanoue KY, editors. Proceedings of the second symposium on resource investment in the northwest Hawaiian islands, Honolulu, *UH Sea Grant College Program* 1:144, 1984.
263. Wolff RL, Wiseman SL, Kitchens CS: Aeromonas hydrophila bacteremia in ambulatory immunocompromised hosts, *Am J Med* 68:238, 1980.
264. Wood MG, Srolovitz H, Schetman D: Schistosomiasis: paraplegia and ectopic skin lesions as admission symptoms, *Arch Dermatol* 112:690, 1976.
265. Wright DN, Alexander JM: Effect of water on the bacterial flora of swimmer's ears, *Arch Otolaryngol* 99:15, 1974.
266. Zacherle BJ, Silver DS: Hot tub folliculitis: a clinical syndrome, *West J Med* 137:191, 1982.

64 Survival at Sea

Michael E. Jacobs

It is difficult for us to grasp the idea that parts of our planet remain in an almost primordial state of wildness and isolation. There are only a few places left on earth where merely getting across them is an achievement: Antarctica . . . the Sahara . . . the Southern Ocean . . . the wilderness of ice or sand or water or terrible places where nature retains power over humans to terrify and diminish.

Derek Lundy, *Godforsaken Sea*

The greatest wilderness on earth is the sea. It covers two thirds of the planet and, with the exception of the sun, has the greatest influence on global weather patterns. Although it may take hours to days to succumb in other environments, death at sea can happen in less than a minute. Compared with desert heat, high-altitude hypoxia, and polar subzero temperatures, water is the most hostile and life-threatening natural environment for inadequately equipped survivors.

The 1979 Fastnet Race distinguished itself as the worst disaster in the 100-year history of ocean yacht racing. When a killer storm approached the Irish Sea between southwest England and southern Ireland, it exploded without warning in the midst of the Fastnet racing fleet. Suddenly, 2700 men and women in 303 ocean sailing yachts unwittingly became participants in a study of survival at sea. With winds up to 55 knots and seas to 50 feet, waves knocked down one third of the fleet and completely capsized one fourth. Despite a massive response of personnel and equipment, 15 sailors drowned, 24 crews abandoned ship (five eventually sank), and 136 people were rescued from disabled yachts. The inquiry noted, "The common link between all 15 deaths was the violence of the sea, an unremitting danger faced by all who sail."

Mastering seamanship and survival skills requires training and experience. The ultimate challenge for every mariner is to confront and handle the fears that render a person helpless in a survival situation. Survival therefore depends on both a philosophic and a psychologic orientation, as well as skills and knowledge of equipment. This chapter discusses some of the basics for survival at sea.

EMERGENCIES AT SEA

The Decision to Abandon Ship

The only time a crew should abandon ship is when the vessel is about to sink. Sinking is generally caused by flooding, fire, or collision. "Always step *up* to the life raft" means that it is usually unnecessary to abandon the vessel before the decks are awash. Leaving a ship prematurely often places the crew at greater risk than remaining with the disabled craft. Many flooded boats fill with water and then remain partially submerged on the sea surface because of the positive flotation integral to the hull's design and structure.

With rare exception, a floating disabled yacht is a much safer place than a life raft. The vessel is always the number-one life boat. The boat provides a more visible rescue platform from both the air and the sea compared with a small life raft. The vessel is more likely to withstand wind and waves because it is stronger than most life rafts. The equipment and provisions necessary for communication and survival are generally more extensive aboard the well-stocked mother ship than those found in the life raft. Conditions will be much worse in a life raft.

Flooding

Before abandoning ship, a quick assessment of the damage should be made. Time is the limiting factor. The crew's level of training, experience, and expertise will be decisive to prevent loss of the ship. Having the proper tools and repair materials to respond quickly and efficiently is equally important. Box 64-1 lists the recommended contents of a damage control kit suitable for an offshore sail or power boat.

Flooding is the most common disaster at sea. It can result from material failure, system failure, accidents, and hull and rigging damage caused by extremely violent weather (Box 64-2).

Early detection of flooding is the critical first step to mounting an effective response. Frequent and regular visual inspections should be made of the bilge, engine room, galley, and head while underway. A backup bilge alarm is useful between inspections, and automatic bilge pumps are essential for unattended boats.

If flooding occurs, the following actions are recommended:

1. Alert the crew and put on life jackets.
2. Turn on the electric bilge pumps and start the engine to run the engine-driven pumps.
3. Send out a distress message.

The captain should try to transmit a distress call before the electric system short-circuits from water rising in the cabin. The call can always be canceled should the vessel be saved.

Box 64-1 DAMAGE CONTROL KIT

Assorted hose clamps
Extra through-hull conical wooden plugs
3-M 5200 or equivalent sealant/glue (cartridge and gun)
Collision mat with 15-foot lines in corners
Water-activated fiberglass repair fabric ("Syntho-Glass")
Hacksaw with spare blades
Bolt and rigging cutters
Drifts matching size of clevis pins
Duct tape
Two 12- to 16-inch plywood squares for hole patches
Self-tapping screws (1 to 2 inches)
Hammer and large screwdriver
Shoring materials and wood wedges
Portable VHF emergency ship antenna
Emergency single-sideband (SSB) coaxial antenna
Vise-grip pliers
Hand drill and bits
Extra canvas buckets
Extra dry chemical fire extinguishers

Box 64-2 SOURCES OF FLOODING

1. Failure of through-hull fittings involving the following systems: head, galley, wash basins, shower sump, bilge pumps, centerboard pins and cables, engine exhaust, engine cooling, deck and cockpit drains, bait box, drain plugs (for small boats), knot meter sensor, depth sounder sensor, propeller shaft stuffing box, shaft struts shaft log, rudder post
2. Failure of hose connections, clamps, pipes, and fittings
3. Open hatches, portholes, and ventilators
4. Siphoning of sea water back into the boat because of poor system design or failure of a check valve
5. Collision with large floating or submerged objects
6. Structural failure in hull, deck, or rigging
7. Punctured hull from overboard broken spars (e.g., dismasting)
8. Ruptured on-board water tanks (a boat will not sink from leaking internal water tanks)

The next three tasks are to (1) locate the source of flooding, (2) stop or reduce the inflow, and (3) repair the damage. The volume of water coming in depends on the size of the opening and its depth below waterline. A typical ½-inch-diameter open seacock located 2 feet below waterline will admit 62 gallons per minute (gpm), and the same opening 4 feet down will allow 87 gpm. A 1-inch hole 2 feet below the waterline will bring water on board at the rate of almost 300 gpm and a 6-inch hole at 1000 gpm.

A boat equipped with the largest manual double-action twin-diaphragm bilge pump can only pump a maximum of 42 gpm. It is important to locate and stop the leak rather than fight a losing battle trying to bail a boat with hand-operated pumps. A bucket has a capacity of 3 gallons and weighs about 20 pounds. A bucket brigade may be effective for a limited time until the source is located.

As the water rises, it becomes more difficult to locate the leak. The rate of flooding slows as water rises above the hole and the pressure gradient is reduced. Inflow of water steadily decreases as the depth of water in the boat increases. The inherent buoyancy of the boat as it settles in the water may help attain a point of zero net flooding. Therefore the ship is not abandoned at the first sign of flooding. Many small wood and fiberglass boats float when fully flooded, or the rate slows sufficiently to allow pumps to handle the volume. Most small boats under 20 feet constructed in the United States after July 1972 are required to have sufficient built-in flotation to remain afloat when swamped. Every effort should be made to plug the hole and keep the pumps working, even if this is only partially effective, until help arrives or the leak is sealed. A diagram showing the location of all through-hull fittings with the routes of connecting hoses should be readily available. A tapered wood plug sized to fit a leaking through-hull fitting can serve indefinitely as an adequate seal. Any soft pliable material, such as blanket, towel, cushion, clothing, or foam pad, can be used as a plug to slow water rushing through a jagged break in the hull. It should be backed with a board or other firm solid material and shored in place with a stick or pole. Heeling the boat away from the area of damage to raise the hole will decrease water pressure and flow, and reducing forward speed decreases water coming in from the bow.

Flooding after a capsize is usually the result of massive structural damage breaching the watertight integrity of the hull. Broken spars (mast or boom) that are overboard must be cut away before they puncture the hull. Large holes in the hull can be overlaid with a collision mat placed outside the hull to supplement the interior patch. The mat is a piece of heavy canvas with grommets and lines that enable it to be positioned and secured on the outside surface. It is held in place by the water pressure and lines. These mats can be purchased or improvised by using a small sail or awning material. An umbrella-like device called a "Subrella" can be pushed through the damaged area from the inside and then opened on the outside of the hull by pulling it sharply back. The water pressure automatically spreads the patch over the hole to form an effective seal and holds it in place.

If on scene the Coast Guard can supply a portable gasoline-powered dewatering pump. If the pump is dropped into the sea from an aircraft, a retrieving line will be lowered to crew on deck. The pump is simple to operate and comes in a waterproof barrel with hoses, gasoline, and operating instructions. It usually takes two people to lift the barrel from the sea onto the deck. A standard dewatering pump can pump 140 gpm.

Some oceangoing recreational boats are built with watertight compartments to confine flooding to a limited area. The crew must know the locations of watertight doors and how to operate them.

Finally, if the circumstances permit, the captain might consider intentionally running the boat onto shore, where it can be repaired and salvaged later.

Fire

Approximately 7500 pleasure boat fires and explosions occur annually, with at least 10% of the boats declared total losses. More than half the fire-related injuries occur on small, open motor boats. Extrapolating from the U.S. Coast Guard's recreational casualty statistics, 2700 serious injuries occur annually, with 3 to 13 fatalities.

Common causes of onboard fires include fuel leakage in the engine compartment, faulty electric wiring, leaking hydrogen battery gas, faulty or careless use of galley stoves and their fuels, improper stowage of paints and solvents, careless smokers, and lightning. Box 64-3 lists ways to prevent fires.

The explosive potential of fuels depends in part on their vapors and where they accumulate in the enclosed, unventilated spaces in a boat. Hazardous liquids are classified according to their *flash points*, the lowest temperature at which a liquid releases enough vapor to sustain burning. Flammable liquids, such as gasoline, turpentine, lacquer thinner, and acetone, have flash points below 38° C (100.4° F), which means they release enough vapor at common ambient temperatures to form burnable and explosive mixtures. Combustible liquids, such as diesel oil, kerosene, and hydraulic fluid, have flash points above 38° C.

Most boat fires start in the engine compartment. The best protection and first priority is to install a properly sized automatic discharging extinguisher system. Some new products are designed to monitor the compartment and sound an alarm if they detect an open flame. They work by sensing ultraviolet radiation. Others incorporate a high temperature sensor that activates when the temperature exceeds 66° C (150.8° F).

Fuel leakage in the engine compartment and bilge is a common cause of boat fires. Gasoline ignites when it spills onto hot engine parts or from the heat within the enclosed space. A teaspoon of gasoline can vaporize and cause an explosion; a cup of gasoline has the explosive potential of several sticks of dynamite. Vaporized gasoline is heavier than air and accumulates in the lowest part of an enclosed compartment. Diesel fuel is much less explosive and dangerous. Other fuels, such as charcoal, can spontaneously ignite in a damp and unventilated locker.

Box 64-3 FIRE PREVENTION AT SEA

1. Sniff the engine compartment before starting a gasoline engine and before starting the electric bilge blower.
2. Ventilate the bilge and run the bilge blower for at least 4 minutes before starting a gas engine.
3. Periodically inspect wiring for cracks and check electric motors for sparks.
4. Ventilate the battery compartment, and never create sparks around a battery until the surrounding space has been ventilated. Inspect and tighten battery cable connections. Never smoke around a battery.
5. Install a lightning protection system.
6. Observe all precautions when taking on fuel. Close all hatches and ports before filling the tanks, and extinguish all flames.
7. Use portable kerosene and alcohol heaters with caution and only when someone is on board.
8. Never leave the stove unattended while in use.
9. Store extra fuel on deck in approved plastic containers.
10. Store any outboard motor and its fuel tank on deck.
11. Transfer gasoline and other flammable liquids from one container to another on deck or off the boat.
12. Inboard engines require meticulous inspection and maintenance. Become an expert in examining and repairing all components of the fuel system.
13. Install a heat-activated automatic fire-extinguishing system in the engine compartment, together with smoke and flame detectors.
14. Properly store fuels, solvents, paints, brushes, and combustibles in a deck storage locker. Keep all rags in metal containers with the lid tightly closed. Do not keep oily rags below decks or in the engine compartment.
15. Place fire extinguishers away from the intended area of use so that they are accessible, and have them inspected and maintained annually.
16. Read the extinguishers' instructions periodically, and practice on a controlled fire away from the boat.

Another highly flammable and potentially explosive gas is hydrogen. This gas is generated while batteries are charging and thus accumulates in the battery compartment or in the compartment overhead, because the gas is lighter than air. Overcharging batteries produces excess hydrogen gas, and a spark from a nearby electric system can set off an explosion.

Used in galley stoves, liquefied petroleum gas (LPG) is also heavier than air, and a leak in the system can lead to accumulation of highly explosive gas in the bilge. Leaks in gas lines can be detected with an electronic gas detector installed beneath the stove and in the bilge. The main purpose of a pressure gauge is to demonstrate leaks, not to indicate fuel levels. After rough weather the system is tested by opening the cylinder valve with the solenoid switched on and recording the gauge reading. Next, only the cylinder valve is closed to see if pressure drops, indicating a leak. To avoid accidents, after cooking, the solenoid is switched off first, and the burner continues to flame until the line is free of gas. Once the flame is extinguished, the burner is turned off and the cylinder valve closed. Both the cylinder and the solenoid valves should be closed whenever the stove is not in use or the boat is left unattended. The stove should not be used as a cabin heater. The open flame can deplete a tightly closed cabin of oxygen and cause asphyxiation of the sleeping crew.

Stove alcohol is also potentially hazardous. Alcohol stoves become especially dangerous if one burner is accidentally extinguished and liquid alcohol pours onto the stove and is subsequently ignited by another flaming burner. A nonpressurized burner can also reignite if it is refilled while still hot. An alcohol fire can be extinguished with a fire blanket or wet towel. A grease fire on the stove can also be extinguished with these items or by liberally sprinkling the fire with baking soda. A kettle of water placed on the burner when first igniting an alcohol stove helps to contain any large flames from the excess alcohol used in priming the burner.

All recreational vessels are required to have portable fire extinguishers. The standard multipurpose dry chemical extinguisher is useful on all types of fires, class A, B, or C. It smothers a fire by preventing access to oxygen. The disadvantages are the powdery mess and destruction of circuitry in electronic equipment. Crew should know in advance how to operate the extinguisher, because it will completely discharge in a few precious seconds. The nozzle is directed to the base of the fire and the powder discharged with a sweeping, side-to-side motion. If all on board extinguishers are depleted, fires involving common combustible materials can still be brought under control by cooling with large amounts of water. Fires involving flammable or combustible liquids can be smothered to remove the oxygen (using a fire blanket if available), and electrical fires can often be controlled by cutting the electric power (Box 64-4).

Collision

Collisions are responsible for approximately half of all recreational boating accidents reported to the U.S. Coast Guard. Only capsizing and crew falling overboard cause more fatalities. Collision with another boat or with a fixed or floating object is responsible for the greatest number of nonfatal injuries and accounts for more than three times as many injuries as any other type of marine accident. The most common injuries are fractures, head, brain and neck injuries, and lacerations. Two thirds of water craft involved in collisions are open motorboats under 26 feet in length and jet-ski personal

---

Box 64-4 GUIDELINES FOR FIRE AT SEA

1. Attack the fire immediately at the source. Detection and reaction time must be within a few minutes, before the fire burns out of control. Prepare a plan that has been shared with the crew so that everyone knows the location of equipment and their responsibilities.
2. Initiate a mayday call immediately. The purpose is to alert ships in the area that the crew may have to abandon ship.
3. Put on life jackets. Ensure that the life raft is away from the fire, and prepare to abandon ship.
4. Slow the boat to reduce relative wind, and steer to keep smoke and flames clear of the crew and vessel. Keep the fire on the downwind side of the ship, exposing the smallest amount of the boat's structure to the flames.
5. Position personnel between the fire and a clear escape route.
6. Cut off the source(s) of the fire (e.g., fuel supply, electric current). Turn off blowers, and stop the engine immediately.
7. Close the hatches, doors, and vents to all compartments free of people.
8. If you must open a hatch to discharge a portable extinguisher, beware of burning your hands or face. As fresh air enters the compartment, the fire will rise to the air source and flare up. The safest way to open a hatch is to wear gloves and stand on the hinged side of the hatch while pulling it open.
9. If the fire is too large or out of control, abandon ship before the fuel tanks explode.

---

watercraft (PWC). Even though PWC are involved in more accidents, more than six times as many fatalities occur with open motorboats. Since 75% of fatalities result from drowning, the wearing of life jackets by PWC riders may explain the lower number of fatalities in this group. Approximately 80% of all reported boating accidents involve operator-controllable factors, not equipment or environmental factors. The boats generally have no major mechanical problems, and fair weather with good visibility and calm seas are the rule.

The operator factors responsible for collisions include inattention and inexperience, carelessness, recklessness, excessive speed, improper lookout, and lack of boating safety education. Alcohol consumption in reported accidents accounts for at least 27% of fatalities.

The majority of recreational boating accidents occur on inland or near coastal waters, which corresponds to the commonly used areas of recreational boating.

For adventurous boaters cruising the world's oceans, collisions have become a major hazard. Encounters with whales may be the most memorable, but they are rare occurrences. The major threats to small boat cruisers are collisions with partially submerged objects or being run down by a huge commercial ship in a standard shipping route.

Regulations to prevent collisions at sea, referred to as COLREGS, define the responsibility of ships when collision is possible between two boats, as when crossing each other, overtaking, or meeting head on. Although the privileged vessel, which has the right of way over the burdened vessel, is permitted to hold course and speed, the rules require that both ships take whatever actions necessary to avoid an imminent collision. In the presence of large ships, small boats must be extra vigilant and defensive. The visibility from the pilothouse of a large vessel may be partially obstructed, so a small craft may not be seen by the lookout, show up on radar, or be granted right of way. Unfortunately, both commercial ships and solo ocean racers often run on autopilot without a lookout on deck. This is a clear violation of rule 5 of the COLREGS: "Every vessel shall at all times maintain a proper lookout by sight and hearing . . ."

Radar is invaluable in poor visibility. At night or in fog the unit can be used to identify other ships, hazards to navigation, squalls, and other local weather phenomena that may endanger a vessel.

Many affordable small radar units are available for recreational boaters. One problem common to units on small boats is that during storm conditions, large commercial ships and yachts may be lost on the radar screen because of the mass of echoes from nearby tall waves. The intense reflection of radar signals from the sea is called *sea clutter.* Fiberglass and wooden boats are nearly invisible to radar. Regardless of construction, all boats should have a radar reflector mounted when in busy shipping traffic lanes, on the open sea, or under conditions of reduced visibility. Ideally, a reflector should provide consistent reflective performance in all directions; in general, the larger the reflector, the better the reflection.

To make a vessel the brightest reflection on the other vessel's radar screen, an active transponder can be used. Mounted on the masthead, this device receives the radar signal and then transmits the signal back to the radar unit with a signal electronically enhanced and stronger than one from a passive reflector.

Another useful function of radar is the ability to maintain an electronic guard zone. The radar scans this zone, which is preset as a circle of a given radius. The radar sounds an alarm when a new target enters the guard zone. Box 64-5 reviews measures to prevent collisions at sea.

Partially submerged objects, especially floating logs and cargo containers, are difficult to detect. An estimated 1000 or more shipping containers fall from the decks of merchant ships every year during storms at sea, and about half of them continue to float. The most

---

Box 64-5   PREVENTING COLLISIONS AT SEA

1. Post a lookout with a 360-degree view of the horizon.
2. Know the rules for steering and right of way.
3. Use radar.
4. Use Collision Avoidance Detection Radar (CARD) if available.
5. Use a radar reflector, and place it as high as possible.
6. Do not assume other boats have operational or unobstructed running lights.
7. Observe rule 7 of the COLREGS: "When a vessel has any doubt as to whether a risk of collision exists, she shall assume it does and avoid it."
8. Ask yourself, "Can I be seen?" Do not assume you are seen, even in daylight. The height of the steering station of a large commercial vessel makes it difficult if not impossible to see a small boat near the bow or alongside the ship.
9. If you hear a foghorn, stop and let the other ship steer around you.
10. If a collision threatens, sound the danger signal (five or more short blasts on the horn), and take whatever actions necessary to save your boat.
11. Maintain radio contact with other ships in the area. VHF channel 13 is the bridge-to-bridge channel. Use channel 16 if there is no response.
12. Avoid shipping routes if possible, and avoid navigating in the harbor's incoming and outgoing traffic separation lanes designated for commercial traffic.
13. When your boat is in the way of another vessel, the right of way does not automatically grant you safe passage.
14. To avoid collision with another vessel, make early and recognizable changes in course and/or speed.
15. Give large ships a wide berth.
16. Observe the bearing of an approaching vessel (the direction relative to you). If the bearing does not change, and if the distance between the two boats is decreasing, you are on a collision course.

---

common shipping container is 40 feet long and 8 feet wide; constructed of aluminum, steel, or wood; and capable of carrying up to 50,000 pounds of cargo. A refrigeration container weighs about 4 tons empty and may float partially submerged, even with the doors ajar, because of its thick insulation.

The sea is rapidly becoming littered with other types of floating cargo. A 425-foot log transport carrying 12,000 tons of 40-foot white spruce logs to British Columbia recently dumped 90% of its cargo into the Gulf of Alaska during a storm. In the same weather pattern, a Pacific storm overwhelmed four container ships en route from Japan to Seattle, causing them to lose 400 containers overboard.

Massive stumps and log debris float in the coastal waters of northern California, Oregon, and Washington as a result of logging practices in northern river watersheds. The waterlogged stumps flow down the rivers, enter the ocean, and float just below the surface.

The sinking of the 19-ton, 43-foot schooner Lucette in the Pacific after attack by three killer whales reminds all sailors that yachts can be destroyed in unprovoked attacks. Cruising at 10 knots and accelerating underwater to speeds up to 30 knots, there is little time for a whale to reconnoiter and reevaluate its target while attacking torpedo style. Other attacks may be a reprisal by a whale accidentally rammed while sleeping at the surface. This is probably what occurred to the cruise ship Royal Majesty, which arrived in Bermuda with a dead 60-foot finback whale balanced atop its bow.

Sailors crossing the North Atlantic in summer along a great circle route to Europe need to beware of colliding with icebergs. Every year from February to July, more than 10,000 icebergs are separated from Greenland glaciers. At least 1000 of them drift in the Labrador current south and east of Newfoundland and become a hazard to mariners above 41° north latitude. Navigation around icebergs is complicated by dense fog often present over the Grand Banks region and the difficulty of detecting icebergs with radar. Radar is 60 times less likely to pick up an iceberg than to detect a ship of the same size. Iceberg reports are broadcast twice daily by U.S. and Canadian Coast Guards. The International Ice Patrol broadcast times and frequencies can be obtained by calling 203-441-2626.

Seasickness

During storm conditions, mariners frequently consider seasickness a medical emergency and justification for medical evacuation. Each year, dozens of yachts are abandoned while still seaworthy because their exhausted and despondent crew have lost their collective will to persevere.

At the very least, seasickness (mal de mer) may be moderately disabling; it can also lead to rapid deterioration with progressive dehydration, loss of manual dexterity, ataxia, loss of judgment, and loss of the will to survive.

The underlying mechanism of mal de mer involves a conflict of sensory inputs processed by the brain to orient the body's position. Below decks the eyes oriented to the cabin sole and ceiling detect no tilt from vertical, while fluid in the inner ear's vestibular organs constantly shifts. Position sensors in the neck, muscles, and joints send additional signals depending on how persons shift and secure themselves from falling. This mix of sensory data from the eyes, inner ear, and position sensors creates a neural mismatch that activates responses and stimulates the vomiting center in the brain.

The balance center has the ability to adapt to the new environments; this is called "getting your sea legs." Medication is more effective in preventing symp-

toms than in reversing them after seasickness is fully symptomatic, so antimotion sickness medication should be used early before leaving port. The traveler should begin the trip well hydrated, avoid alcohol, which impairs vestibular function, and eat light meals. Many anecdotal reports favor eating carbohydrates rather than protein, but no conclusive study favors any particular food or diet. Ginger is often recommended as an antiemetic. It is safely and effectively used by women to curb nausea and vomiting in the first trimester of pregnancy. Ginger is available in 500-mg capsules; the suggested dose is 1000 mg every 6 hours. The capsules can be supplemented with gingersnap cookies, ginger ale, and candied ginger.

Both field and laboratory experiments have documented the efficacy of acupressure in preventing seasickness. One small trial at sea showed that acustimulation suppresses the symptoms of motion sickness. Pressure should be applied on the Neiguan P6 point of the forearm. This is found two fingerbreadths proximal to the wrist joint between the two prominent finger flexor tendons. The easiest way to accomplish this is with commercially available elastic wrist straps with buttons, called "seasickness bands." The ReliefBand is a watchlike device worn over the P6 area on the ventral side of the wrist to deliver transcutaneous electrical stimulation to the median nerve. It can be used before or after the start of symptoms and offers an alternative to people sensitive to the side effects of medication. Preliminary reports suggest this modality may be as effective as commonly used drugs.

Recommendations for prevention of mal de mer include the following. Limit the time below decks. Equipment, provisions, and the galley arrangement should all facilitate the preparation of quick and easy meals. Have one or two simple meals prepared so you can stay out of the galley the first day. Keep personal items easily accessible.

After departure, stay on deck and amidships (center) or aft (toward the stern), where the pitching and rolling is less severe. Look out and obtain a broad view of the horizon using peripheral vision. This provides a stable and level point of reference. Avoid close focused visual tasks such as prolonged reading, writing, and navigation. Stay out of areas with fumes and odors that can stimulate nausea. Continue any medication for seasickness at regular intervals, and begin to taper the dose after the first day.

The early signs and symptoms of seasickness are yawning, sighing, dry mouth or salivating, drowsiness, headache, dizziness, and lethargy. Pallor, cold sweats, belching, flatulence, nausea, dry heaves, and vomiting occur after the illness has developed. The window of opportunity for early intervention is often missed because early signs are not recognized or the symptoms are denied.

TABLE 64-1. Medications for Seasickness

MEDICATION	DOSE	INTERVAL
Dimenhydrinate (Dramamine)	50-mg liquid/capsule/ chewable tablet	4-6 hr
Meclizine (Antivert) (Bonine)	12.5/25-mg tablet 25-mg chewable tablet	4-6 hr 4-6 hr
Cyclizine (Marezine)	50-mg tablet	4-6 hr
Cinnarizine (Sturgeron)	15-mg tablet	6-12 hr
Scopolamine (Transderm-Scop)	1.5-mg skin patch	72 hr
Promethazine (Phenergan)	12.5/25/50-mg tablet, suppository, injection	6-12 hr
Phenergan plus ephedrine	25-mg tablet of each	6-12 hr

One of the best tactics is to take the wheel and steer at the first sign of seasickness. Use the waves, clouds, horizon and distant marks as reference points. Sit or stand in the cockpit and actively posture to anticipate the boat's motion and "ride" the waves. Keep head and chest balanced over the hips.

If symptoms progress, lie down in a secure, well-ventilated bunk, face up and head still, then close your eyes and try to sleep. Parenteral antinausea medication may help. Take small amounts of water, crackers, and hard candy.

Debilitated seasick persons can easily fall or be washed overboard. They should wear a safety harness while on deck, and someone should be designated to monitor them. In storm conditions the safest place is to be secured below in a bunk. Table 64-1 lists medications available for motion sickness. Time-release forms and longer-acting drugs may be preferable when storms are expected to last a few days.

Transdermal scopolamine is available by prescription. One adhesive patch is placed behind the ear several hours before departure. Scopolamine is delivered into the bloodstream at a constant rate to provide a therapeutic blood concentration for up to 3 days, with minimal side effects. The most common adverse effects are dry mouth (66%) and drowsiness (17%). The patch is contraindicated for children, persons with glaucoma, and men with prostatic hypertrophy.

Over-the-counter antihistamines have potential side effects, including drowsiness, dry mouth, blurred vision, irritability, urinary retention, dizziness, and headache. NASA astronauts use a combination of intramuscular promethazine with oral ephedrine to counter the drowsiness. A nonprescription substitute for ephedrine that is equally effective is pseudoephedrine, which is available in 30- to 100-mg tablets.

THUNDERSTORMS AND ASSOCIATED WEATHER EVENTS

Lightning is one of nature's most destructive phenomena (see Chapter 3). Boating, fishing, and swimming rank second only to playing sports on an open field as the most dangerous activities associated with a lightning strike. Although the odds that an individual will be struck and killed by lightning are about one in three million, the odds for a boat being struck are greater. A cruising sailor in Florida, the lightning capital of America, can expect at least one strike to his boat in its lifetime. Although there is no lightning-proof boat, it is possible to reduce the likelihood of a lightning strike and provide a high degree of protection for the boat and people and equipment on board.

A single thunderstorm is a small unit, generally less than 2 miles in diameter. It is brief, lasting about 30 minutes, with marked fluctuations in wind, temperature, and barometric pressure. *Waterspouts*, which are the equivalent of tornadoes at sea, may form (see later). A *squall line* is a fast moving row of violent thunderstorms. The line may be more than 100 miles long and arrives 40 to 300 miles ahead of an intense cold front. It contains most of the gusting winds and rain normally found in the front itself. It is visible on radar and to the naked eye appears as a wall of boiling black clouds arising from the sea.

Rapid growth of cumulus clouds is the primary signal indicating formation of a thunderstorm. The faster the clouds build, the more violent the resulting storm, because the steep pressure gradients within the cloud generate high winds.

Within the thunderhead are columns of rapidly sinking air, called *downdrafts*. Downdrafts along the leading edge of the thunderstorm form the gust front. This zone of advancing cold air is characterized by a sudden increase in wind speed. Very strong and highly localized downdrafts are called *downbursts*, the smallest of which are *microbursts*. Airplane pilots refer to these as *wind shear*. Downbursts are extremely intense concentrations of sinking air. On reaching the surface, they fan out radially in all directions, often generating winds at the gust front in excess of 150 knots. They are short-lived, typically lasting less than 15 minutes, and are concentrated in an area less than 3 miles across.

A single thunderstorm can produce a series of downdrafts affecting an area several miles long and can persist an hour or more. Blowing spray under or slightly ahead of the storm may be the only indicator of its presence. The gust front often precedes the microburst. The combination of these two extremely strong and shifting wind systems can blow equipment and personnel off the deck and capsize small craft.

In the United States, squalls occur predominantly during the spring and summer in association with thunderstorms or towering cumulus clouds. Occasionally, they may form with the building of the cloud and not be associated with the typical rain, thunder, and lightning. These violent winds are called *white squalls.* The only warning may be the sudden appearance of a cold shifting wind with an increase in its velocity.

To avoid or prepare for the potential fury of a thunderstorm, the mariner must be aware of local weather conditions. The best source of up-to-date weather information for coastal waters is the continuous 24-hour National Weather Service (NWS) broadcast (Box 64-6). This US National Oceanographic and Atmospheric Administration (NOAA) VHF-FM radio transmission repeats recorded messages every 4 to 6 minutes. They are updated every 2 to 3 hours with the latest local information. The broadcasts can usually be received 20 to 60 miles from the transmitting antennas, which are located at 66 different locations in the United States.

The NWS uses specific terminology to broadcast a severe weather warning. These warnings can be heard on the NOAA radio transmissions (Box 64-7). Many of the newer VHF radios have a Weather Alert function, known as Weather Watch. When the radio receives a special warning signal from NOAA, it sounds a special alerting tone, signifying an urgent NOAA weather forecast. Some radios automatically tune to the active weather channel, whereas others require manual tuning.

For offshore sailors, single-sideband (SSB) high-frequency radios can receive a variety of high-seas marine weather broadcasts. The time schedules and frequencies for these transmissions can be found in the U.S. Defense Mapping Agency (DMA) Publication 177, *Radio Navigation Signals.* A less comprehensive list for specific locations can be found in *Reed's Nautical Almanac.*

Forecasts are compiled by the NWS and broadcast by high-frequency radio facsimile via the U.S. Coast Guard from their East, Gulf, and West Coast communication centers. These marine weather charts are updated every 6 hours and available within 3½ hours of the valid time. The NWS has an Internet page at http://www.nws.noaa.gov, where all weather charts broadcast over SSB can be found. This site contains text forecasts, ocean current and surface analysis charts, wave charts, buoy reports, and prognosis charts for weather outlooks of 12, 24, 36, 48, and 96 hours. An onboard cellular connection, modem, and laptop computer are required to obtain this information. Beyond cellular range, a dedicated weather fax unit or SSB/laptop/weather fax module is needed. Details on what charts are available can be obtained from the U.S. Government publication, *Selected Worldwide Marine WX Broadcasts,* available at NOAA chart dealers.

Visualization of characteristic cloud formations at night can be accomplished with radar or night-vision binoculars. With experience a person can learn to recognize a squall line, the cloud sequence of an approaching cold and warm front, and the growth of cumulus to cumulonimbus clouds with the characteristic anvil head. In the daytime a band of low, dark, smooth tubular clouds can often be seen at the leading edge of a squall. This is a roll cloud preceding the cold front. The faster a roll cloud approaches, the stronger the wind is likely to be, and the more agitated the sea under it. When the sea can be observed beneath the roll cloud, it is about 2 miles away, and since the clouds typically move at about 25 mph, the face will arrive in

---

Box 64-6 NATIONAL WEATHER SERVICE BROADCASTS

NOAA WEATHER RADIO CHANNELS

WX-1 162.55 MHz
WX-2 162.40 MHz
WX-3 162.475 MHz

CANADA

Canadian Channel 21 161.65 MHz

WEATHER WARNINGS BY RADIO

National Bureau of Standards: WWV in Fort Collins, Colo, and WWVH in Hawaii broadcast time signals and weather warnings on 5, 10, and 15 MHz. WWV broadcasts at 8, 10, and 12 minutes after the hour. WWVH broadcasts at 47, 49, and 50 minutes after the hour.

U.S. COAST GUARD BROADCASTS

USCG VHF Voice: Broadcasts coastal and offshore forecasts and storm warnings on VHF channel 22A after an initial call on VHF channel 16.
USCG MF Voice: Broadcasts offshore forecasts and storm warnings on 2670 kHz following an initial call on 2182 kHz.

Box 64-7 STORM WARNINGS

Small craft advisory: generally associated with sustained winds 18 to 33 knots (19 to 38 mph) and/or sea conditions dangerous to small boats.
Gale warning: sustained winds 34 to 47 knots (39 to 54 mph).
Storm warning: sustained winds over 48 knots (55 mph). If winds are associated with a tropical cyclone, the storm warning display indicates forecast winds of 48 to 63 knots (55 to 73 mph).
Hurricane warning: sustained winds of 64 knots (74 mph) and greater as the result of a tropical cyclone.
Special marine warning: winds of 35 knots or more generally lasting less than 2 hours. These are usually associated with an individual thunderstorm or an organized series of thunderstorms, as in a squall line.

about 3 minutes. Another early warning of an approaching thunderstorm is a sharp drop in barometric pressure of about 1.5 millibars for 1 to 4 hours. Large ocean swells precede a heavy weather system, whereas chop without swells often reflects a local, more isolated, and temporary disturbance.

An excellent early-warning device is the SkyScan Lightning and Severe Storm Warning unit. This unit has a sophisticated receiver for listening to the characteristics of lightning and can detect and report air-to-ground lightning strikes in four different ranges of 0 to 3, 3 to 8, 8 to 20, and 20 to 40 miles. The unit can calculate the distance of a ground strike to within 1 mile 97% of the time.

Because it is often impossible to predict the power of a thunderstorm, mariners should always prepare for the worst and initiate defensive tactics (Box 64-8).

Box 64-8   DEFENSIVE MEASURES IN THUNDERSTORMS*

1. Alert everyone on board of the imminent storm threat.
2. When boating on a small pond or lake, return to shore and exit the boat.
3. If practical and time permits, take evasive action and set a course perpendicular to the expected thunderstorm track. In rough water a small boat is most stable going downwind with the seas on the stern quarter (about 45 degrees to the back of the boat).
4. Ascertain position, and identify any shoals, rocks, and other boats in the immediate area that may pose a hazard to navigation if visibility becomes severely reduced.
5. If practical, seek shelter from wind and waves in the lee (downwind) side of a land mass.
6. Secure all loose gear on deck and below, and verify that lockers, cabinets, and drawers are properly secured.
7. Close all hatches, ventilators, ports, and lazarettes to prevent flooding in the event of a knockdown or capsize. Close all seacocks not immediately required. Secure doors or boards to companionways leading below.
8. Reef the sails (reduce sail area) or lower them completely, and start the engine.
9. Pump the bilge dry, and be sure the pumps are ready for operation. Water shifting in the bilge can adversely affect the boat's stability.
10. All crew and passengers should wear foul weather gear and life jackets.
11. All crew on watch should be secured with a safety harness.
12. All remaining personnel should go below with clear knowledge of how to egress in the event of a capsize.
13. Safety gear, communication (hand-held VHF radio), and visual distress devices should be readily available.

*Measures are listed in sequence, as storm approaches.

Tall and narrow objects, with highly charged and focused electric fields, are likely to attract lightning. Structures such as a sailboat mast, radio antenna, fishing outrigger, fishing rod, and even a person standing in a motorboat make good targets. In an anchorage or marina the boat with the tallest mast is most vulnerable to a lightning strike. Satellite data have documented that storms at sea generate more lightning than previously realized, especially lightning within the clouds themselves. The most critical factor initiating the streamer is not only the height of the boat's mast, but also its electric potential. The pale-blue or green light sometimes seen in a ship's rigging, called St. Elmo's fire, is visible static electricity induced by nearby thunderclouds.

Many boats struck by lightning are destroyed by fires and explosions. A strike exiting through the bilge can instantly vaporize trapped bilge water and raise it to explosive pressures. Many boats sink or are seriously damaged by ruptured through-hull fittings or large exit holes burned in the hull. The structural integrity of the boat must be protected by providing a path of least resistance for the major current to travel through and off the boat into the water. Protection from a side flash (see later) is accomplished by taking precautions to equalize the electric potential of all the metal objects aboard. By understanding the different components of a lightning protection system (LPS), the mariner can appreciate how best to protect the boat and crew.

Metal boats are rarely damaged by lightning, because the high conductivity of the metal hull in direct contact with the water permits rapid dissipation of the electric charge. By contrast, nonconductive fiberglass and wooden boats, especially sailboats, do not provide the automatic grounding protection offered by metal hull craft.

The traditional way to protect a boat is to mount a rod on the highest part of the vessel to attract and control a strike, then safely discharge it down a path to a ground plate, usually a metal plate attached to the hull below the waterline. The more advanced systems, such as static dissipators, are designed to decrease the probability of a strike. The dissipator prevents the charge from building so that it will not attract the "leaders" approaching from a storm cloud.

On a sailboat the masthead is the obvious location to place the dissipator. On a powerboat without a dominant high structure, a special mast (air terminal) can hold an LPS. The grounded air terminal or mast will theoretically create an electrically safe zone called the *cone of protection*. The apex of this cone is the top of the mast, and the base is a circle around the boat with a radius equal to the mast height. Without additional precautions, the cone of protection does not guarantee safety from lightning strikes.

Commercial units are designed to accept and disperse the static charge accumulating on the boat. The two most common types are a single, sharply pointed spike and a device that resembles a brush with wire bristles. However, the LPS still may be unable to keep the voltage difference between the boat and the cloud base lower than the breakdown resistance of the air gap. To protect the boat from a lightning strike, it is necessary to guide the current from the masthead containing the dissipator in as straight, direct, and short a route as possible to an underwater ground on the bottom of the hull. Without grounding, a bolt will find its way to the sea from the base of the mast, usually through the hull. The path to the ground must be of a highly conductive material of low resistance so that the current passing through will not create heat sufficient to melt the conductor itself. Copper wire with a minimum of 4 AWG (not 8 AWG, as previously suggested) is required, and a ground plate ideally made of solid copper or bronze with a dimension of at least 1 square foot is recommended. A lead keel on a sailboat makes an excellent ground plate only if it is properly connected to the base of the mast and if it is not encapsulated with fiberglass. Some motor and auxiliary sailboats use the exposed surface of the engine prop and shaft to act as a ground plate. With engine grounding, damage may occur from the heat generated by a powerful strike. Boats constructed of aluminum or metal are already grounded to the surrounding water.

Lightning can also generate a *side flash,* which is the secondary flow of current from the surrounding charged areas to some object near the path the strike follows to the water. This current is equally destructive and especially dangerous to the crew members. Grounding prevents major hull damage but does not prevent side flashes. After the current in a strike follows a designated path to the ground, another electric potential is created between the ground system and the objects surrounding it. The entire boat becomes high voltage, so the secondary electric current, the side flash, is created. The key to preventing secondary current flows is to equalize the voltages of all the metallic objects on board by establishing a common electrical ground for the entire boat, a system called *bonding.* Any area capable of collecting a large static charge, each piece of metal equipment on board, and all electronic instruments and radio equipment must be grounded to the same discharge system used to protect the boat from the effects of the initial lightning strike. This is accomplished by connecting copper wire from all metal objects to the common ground. Metal through-hull fittings are also capable of building a static charge and require connection to the ground plate. Box 64-9 outlines the general principles to protect the boat from lightning damage.

Crew members may also become part of the current path if they are in contact with or come between two different metal objects that are not interconnected. The best protection in the event of a direct lightning strike, even if the boat is grounded and bonded, is to remain low in the boat (preferably in a cabin) and far away

---

Box 64-9 PROTECTING BOATS FROM LIGHTNING DAMAGE

1. Install a lightning protection system (LPS), and have it tested for conductivity from masthead to grounding plate by a marine electronic specialist.
2. Install temporary lightning protection for motorized dinghies and open small boats. Battery jumper cables connected to a railing and dropped into the water will work.
3. Keep water out of the bilge, and consider adding a large-capacity manual bilge pump. Pump the bilge dry when a thunderstorm approaches.
4. Place cone-shaped plugs next to all through-hull fittings in case of blowout. Have a handy diagram of the hull indicating location of all through-hull fittings.
5. Conduct a regular maintenance and inspection schedule. All ground pathways and bonding connections must be clean, secure, electrically sound, and free of corrosion.
6. During a severe thunderstorm, do not do anything that will alter the boat's electric potential profile, such as dropping anchor.
7. Lower, remove, or tie down the radio antenna and other similar upright devices if they are not part of the LPS.

---

from metal objects, wiring, and the electric conductors (Box 64-10).

Waterspouts are the maritime version of tornadoes. Although less common than lightning and downbursts, they are generated by the same dynamic forces found in the squall line at the leading edge of an advancing cold front, or in a rapidly building summer afternoon thunderstorm. The danger inherent in a waterspout lies in the powerful revolving winds, which may exceed 200 mph, and the very low pressure at its center, which may cause tightly enclosed spaces to explode. Waterspouts are visible during the day, when the majority of them occur, and can also be located and tracked by radar. The earliest visible sign of a waterspout is an area of boiling water in the distance, with the spray rising upward that joins with a funnel cloud and its characteristic snakelike, gyrating appendage. Waterspouts move rapidly and usually last only 30 to 60 minutes. Preparation of the boat and crew is similar to that for a thunderstorm. Because a waterspout is relatively narrow, steering a course perpendicular to its projected path is a realistic avoidance tactic.

The best tactic for dealing with the fury of hurricanes and cyclones is to avoid them. Although recommendations include placing the boat in the so-called safe or navigable semicircle and avoiding the strongest winds surrounding the eye of the hurricane, the safest course is to stay out of their path. In the Northern Hemisphere the wind blows counterclockwise around

Box 64-10 PROTECTING CREWS FROM LIGHTNING INJURY

1. Get out of the water. If possible, get off the water and away from the water.
2. Get off the beach. If stranded, squat down and place legs and ankles together. Keep surface area of the body in contact with the ground to a minimum. Spread people out to maximize the possibility that some will survive a lightning strike.
3. If possible, get off the boat, including boats at anchor or in a marina.
4. Remove wet suits and other wet clothing. Put on dry clothing and foul weather gear, hat and boots, and a personal flotation device. Wet bodies make good electric conductors, but wet foul weather gear may provide protection by lowering surface resistance and guiding the current around you.
5. Remove all metal articles , especially jewelry, scuba tanks, and weight belts.
6. Avoid direct contact with all metal objects, including handrails, engine, stove, rigging, and spars.
7. Do not touch any of the boat's installed electrical equipment, including navigation instruments and radios. Use a hand-held VHF radio for emergency communications during the storm.
8. Avoid contact with objects connected to the lightning protection system. Do not simultaneously touch two components connected to the system, such as the engine throttle and spotlight handle.
9. Stay away from the mast, stays, shrouds, and wet sails.
10. Stay out of areas where bridging between two highly charged areas, or side flashes, may occur. These areas include the foredeck, between the mast and the headstay, or a seat between an outboard engine and the portable metal fuel tank or steering wheel.
11. Stay within the cone of protection, a distance (the radius of a circle) from the base of the highest mast equal to the height of the mast.
12. If caught in a storm while on a sailboard, lower the sail and mast and sit down on the board.
13. If fishing or trawling, stop and lay the rods and trawls horizontal in the boat.
14. Put nonessential crew and passengers below decks, in the center of the cabin. Stay out of the companionway, engine room, and head. If there is no cabin, stay low in the boat.
15. Place the boat on autopilot to minimize contact with a metal wheel.
16. Avoid activity that may suddenly alter your electric potential profile, such as stepping into a dinghy or stepping onto a beach from a small boat.

the eye. Facing into the wind and stretching the right arm back 120 degrees will point at the eye of the hurricane. In the Southern Hemisphere the wind blows clockwise around the eye. Facing into the wind and stretching the left arm back 120 degrees will point to

the eye. In the Northern Hemisphere the strongest winds are to the right side of the hurricane's path, where the forward movement over the water adds to the local wind speed; this is the more dangerous semicircle. In the Southern Hemisphere the strongest winds are on the left side of the path.

Hurricane track forecasting has acknowledged limits and errors. The expected track error for a hurricane is 100 miles either side of the predicted track for each 24-hour forecast period. For a 72-hour forecast, an error of 300 miles to the left or right of the predicted forecast track can be expected, and for 96 hours, 400 miles to either side is applied. That would make the storm's potential swath for destruction 800 miles wide, a considerable area to avoid if a vessel can only travel at 6 to 7 knots in storm conditions. In order to take meaningful evasive action, a hurricane needs to be monitored at least every 6 hours, which is the official forecast interval for the NWS Tropical Prediction Center. The National Hurricane Center in Coral Gables, Florida, provides advisory updates on developing tropical storms and hurricanes 24 hours a day. Voice recordings can be heard by calling 305-229-4483 or information obtained via the Internet at http://www.nhc.noaa.gov.

EMERGENCY COMMUNICATIONS AND DISTRESS SIGNALS

Cellular Telephones

Sailors frequently use cellular phones rather than marine radios to call for assistance. A variety of emergency services, including regional Coast Guard stations, can be called directly, and in some coastal areas, the Coast Guard can be accessed immediately by dialing *CG.

The cellular phone has several disadvantages when used in search and rescue (SAR). Currently, 10 miles is the average effective range of cellular phones, and use is restricted to high traffic areas where there are both cellular antennas and relay stations. Private cellular phone communication, in contrast to the more public broadcast over very-high-frequency (VHF) radio, excludes potential rescuers who might be in the immediate vicinity. In SAR operations, no practical way exists to maintain continuous communication with a number of rescue craft via cellular phone. The Coast Guard is unable to use a radio direction finder to locate a cellular signal, as it can with the VHF-FM signal.

Since cellular ultrahigh-frequency (UHF) signals are transmitted along line of sight, both reception and transmission can be strengthened by using an external antenna placed as high as possible on the boat. A hand-held phone's range can also be improved by standing in a high location, such as the cabin top. Signal strength can also be improved by reprogramming the phone for the best reception in a specific location using wireline (B-side) or nonwireline carriers.

In the future, cellular phones will be linked to low-earth-orbit (LEO) satellites, giving them a worldwide range from anywhere at sea.

If a cellular phone is the only communications link on board, extra charged phone batteries and a waterproof pouch are needed. A comprehensive list of emergency phone numbers should include local hospitals and physicians, regional Coast Guard stations, harbormasters, and maritime towing services.

The newest communication system is the Globalstar satellite phone system. It consists of 48 LEO satellites operating at an altitude of 876 miles. When fully operational, coverage will extend from 70 degrees north latitude to 70 degrees south latitude, covering 80% of the earth's surface. The compact and portable 13-ounce handsets easily switch from terrestrial cellular telephony to satellite telephony as required.

Marine Radios

The VHF-FM radio transceiver is the most popular, user friendly, and reliable form of marine communication. The VHF signal range is limited to line of sight and therefore depends on the height of both the transmitting and the receiving antennas. The Coast Guard places antennas along the coast, connects them with land lines to their operations centers, and is able to monitor and communicate with all vessels that have a masthead-mounted aerial and are within 25 miles of the coast. The range may even extend up to 300 miles when communicating with an aircraft. The VHF radio is ideal for near-shore emergency communication. Communication is not private, which is a distinct advantage in SAR. VHF is the open party line connecting all vessels within the signal range. Any boat in the area monitoring distress channel 16 (which they automatically do if the radio is turned on) will receive the distress call. Rescue boats and aircraft are equipped with radio direction-finding equipment that can home in on a boat's VHF-FM signal and precisely locate the caller.

The more powerful permanently installed radio is used for the initial distress call. A transmission range of approximately 15 miles can be expected between boats having masthead-mounted antennas. If a sailing vessel becomes dismasted, the VHF will be inoperable because the antenna is usually mounted at the mast top. Therefore a small folding emergency antenna should be carried that can be inserted into the VHF radio jack to allow short-range communication.

The portable hand-held radio is used for special circumstances and is taken when boarding the life raft. The range of the portable unit is up to 5 miles. To conserve batteries, the user should transmit only when a ship is in sight and whenever a message is received, even if the calling ship is not in sight. Transmission uses 15 times more battery power than does listening. Although the range is less than a high-power fixed-

Box 64-11	USEFUL MARINE CHANNELS
06	Intership safety communications
12	Port operations, traffic advisories
13	Intership navigation safety
14	Port operations and some Coast Guard (CG) shore stations
16	Distress, safety, and calling
22	Working CG ships and shore stations, CG marine information broadcasts
24-28	VHF marine operator
68-69	Noncommercial intership and ship to coast
70	Noncommercial only, ship to ship
71	Noncommercial intership and ship to coast
72	Noncommercial intership
78	Noncommercial intership and ship to coast
WX 1 to 3	Weather broadcast

installation VHF radio, reliable communication can be established with any visible aircraft or vessel. If other ships are nearby, transmit a mayday message every 30 minutes on the hour and at the half hour for 3 minutes on channel 16. The new multichannel VHF survival radios are designed to be packed into a life raft or life boat. They are completely waterproof, submersible down to 10 feet, and float. The antenna, circuitry, and power are tuned for maximum range. The operating life with the lithium battery is a minimum of 8 hours.

The most important channel on the VHF band is channel 16, the distress and safety frequency (156.8 MHz). This calling frequency is used to initiate contact between any two vessels and is the only frequency constantly monitored by the Coast Guard. When a radio is not active on another channel, it is eavesdropping for distress calls on channel 16. Box 64-11 lists other VHF-FM channels often used by pleasure craft.

VHF can also be used to place a direct phone call with a marine operator. MariTEL Marine Communications System has its own network of marine VHF radio towers covering coastal waters, inland rivers, and the Great Lakes. Outgoing calls are private and not monitored by other marine VHF radios. The effective ship-to-shore calling range is 50 miles, in contrast to the much shorter cellular range. To make a call, set your VHF radio to the selected MariTEL channel for the area, key your mike (depress the VHF microphone button for 6 seconds), follow the short recorded instructions, and stand by for a marine operator. Routine transmissions and distress messages can be transmitted with relative ease (Boxes 64-12 and 64-13).

When receiving a Mayday call, listen and do not interrupt. If the Coast Guard or another vessel does not respond, acknowledge the Mayday call as follows:

- Repeat the name of the distressed vessel three times.

4125 kHz (Ch. 450), 6215.5 kHz (Ch. 650), 8291.0 kHz (Ch. 850), 12,290.0 kHz (Ch. 1250), and 16,420 kHz (Ch. 1650) have all been designated for distress and safety calls. The high-frequency transceivers can call and receive voice and digital communications to and from anywhere in the world. The best method to select an optimum emergency frequency is to listen to the quality of a radio broadcast. A station that your radio receives loud and clear will also provide good reception for your broadcast at that time. SSB is also an excellent receiver for voice weather and weather fax broadcasts.

On Feb. 28, 1999, AT&T closed its high-seas radio telephone stations. WLO in Mobile, Alabama, is presently the sole provider of worldwide ship-to-shore SSB high-frequency radiotelephone service in the United States. Complete information regarding their radiotelephone channels can be obtained by calling 334-666-5110 or via the Internet at www.wloradio.com.

Global Maritime Distress and Safety System

As of Feb. 1, 1999, a ship or coast station has no legal requirement to monitor the traditional distress frequencies, such as VHF channel 16 or 2182 kHz. Until the new Global Maritime Distress and Safety System (GMDSS) is in use, however, the Coast Guard and many recreational and commercial ships will continue a radio watch on these frequencies. A complete transition to the new GMDSS is not expected until at least the year 2003. The GMDSS is a worldwide infrastructure, controlled from a shore-based communications center, to coordinate the assistance of vessels in distress. This fully automated system uses satellite and digital communication techniques. New radio equipment and dif-

- Transmit your name three times and then say, "Received Mayday."
- Listen to see if any other vessel is closer and preparing to offer assistance. If not, recontact the vessel and give your position and estimated time of arrival.
- If you are able to contact the Coast Guard or another ship in the vicinity, transmit "Mayday-relay, mayday-relay, mayday-relay," then give your vessel name and location and the information you have received.

For communication beyond the VHF range, a more powerful and elaborate SSB radio transmitter is required. Depending on the radio frequency band used, communication may be extended over thousands of miles. The international distress and calling frequency is 2182 kHz; located in the medium-frequency range, 2182 kHz is used for distances from 20 to 100 miles day or night. The frequency 2670 kHz is designated for distress and safety communications with the U.S. Coast Guard. On the high-frequency bands the frequencies

ferent communication protocols are required. GMDSS will simplify routine communications at sea and facilitate regular weather forecasts, navigation warnings, and distress relays in the form of maritime safety information (MSI). Digital selective calling (DSC) technology permits a VHF radio to call another radio selectively using digital messages, similar to the modem on a computer. As with a direct-dial telephone call on land, only the vessel called receives the message. The usual VHF "party line" connecting boats in the area capable of monitoring the message is eliminated.

Every vessel has its own unique maritime mobile service identity (MMSI). The vessel's MMSI is manually coded into the DSC radio. Part of that number may characterize a particular group, so calls made to a group MMSI will alert everyone in the group. The digital information is carried on a designated channel; for VHF digital radios, this is channel 70. The dialing signal is also able to carry other essential information, such as the caller's identity and location and the nature of the call.

Distress messages can be sent automatically. The vessel's identity is permanently coded into the unit, and its position can be determined from the data output of a global positioning satellite (GPS) receiver linked to the radio. On a DSC-equipped radio the receiver sounds an alarm if it receives an "all ships call" (distress or otherwise), a group call, or a call specifically to that vessel. All other DSC calls are ignored.

A distress alert (equivalent to Mayday) can be sent automatically as a digital signal to a shore-based rescue coordination center (RCC). Once the alert has been sent, the radio will automatically repeat at intervals between 3½ and 4½ minutes until the RCC acknowledges receipt of the message on channel 70. Subsequent communication should continue on channel 16 or another selected frequency for voice transmission. A verbal Mayday can also be sent immediately on channel 16 after the first alert, since DSC equipped transceivers can listen simultaneously on channel 70 for DSC and Channel 16 or other channels for voice transmission. A verbal Mayday follows the same sequence as outlined in Box 64-13 and includes the MMSI as part of the vessel's identification.

To make a ship-to-ship or ship-to-shore call on DSC, the nine-digit MMSI number of the station to be called must be keyed in on the radio together with a proposed working radio telephone channel for voice communication. This announcement is transmitted on channel 70 and should be acknowledged on channel 70. Four VHF channels are available for special use within the GMDSS: channel 06 is for SAR coordination, channel 13 for intership safety of navigation (bridge to bridge), channel 16 still for distress and safety, and channel 70 for DSC alerting.

The GMDSS utilizes satellite communication links such as the International Maritime Satellite Organization (INMARSAT M) to provide long range global communication. Geostationary (geosynchronous) INMARSAT satellites cover the whole world between 70° north and 70° south latitude. The satellites pass over the equator at an altitude of 22,500 miles with an orbital period of 24 hours, allowing them to remain stationary over fixed points on Earth. They provide high-quality worldwide speech, data, and facsimile communication as well as reliable distress alerting and follow-up communication within the GMDSS. Presently the size of the equipment and power consumption make this system unsuitable for smaller recreational craft. INMARSAT Mini-M uses small units with tracking antennas that weigh a mere 15 pounds, designed for smaller commercial boats and yachts over 45 feet.

INMARSAT C offers digital data messaging (no voice) and is the only two-way marine satellite data message system approved for GMDSS safety at sea. The hardware is small enough to fit any boat. It can send a distress signal at the touch of a button and can easily be integrated with a GPS receiver. Pressing the distress key sends a message with the ship's identity and location to the nearest RCC.

NAVTEX is a worldwide land-based radio navigation warning service transmitting text messages in English to a compact onboard receiver. The unit can be programmed to receive both specific stations and message categories; it can print out area weather forecasts, gale warnings, navigation warnings, ice warnings, and distress relay messages on the assigned frequency 518 kHz. Vital messages (e.g., gale warnings, SAR information) activate an alarm in the receiver as the message is being printed.

In the field of hand-held satellite communications, the ORBCOMM LEO system, utilizing 36 LEO satellites, can provide e-mail and data transfer coverage to most of the world. The Magellan portable data-messaging radio is designed to send brief text messages using this system in a cost-effective way. It is also a fully functioning GPS receiver. The unit with a built-in telescoping antenna weighs 37 ounces and uses two AA batteries.

Emergency Beacons

Emergency position indicating radio beacons (EPIRBs) are handheld portable radio transmitters that can transmit a signal interpreted as a Mayday call (Figure 64-1). It is the satellite-linked equivalent of a 911 call for mariners in distress. In the absence of a marine radio, EPIRB is the most important piece of signaling equipment. This radio should be used only as a last resort when all other means of communication have failed to establish contact and when there is a life-threatening emergency.

EPIRB signals are transmitted on established distress frequencies 121.5/243.0 MHz or 406/121.5 MHz. The

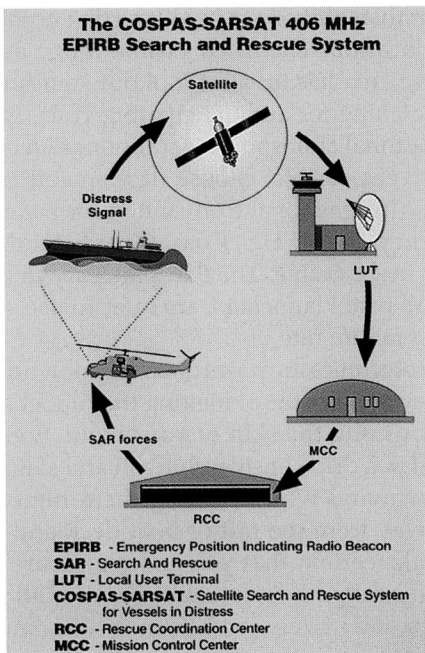

Figure 64-1 Anatomy of a rescue. The 406-MHz emergency position indicating radio beacon (EPIRB) sends a digitally coded signal to low-earth-orbit satellite, which relays the signal to a nearby ground receiving station (LUT). The location of the EPIRB is calculated and forwarded to the nearest mission control center, which matches the EPIRB user's registration with the specific signal. These data are relayed to the local rescue coordination center, which initiates the search and rescue. *(Courtesy ACR Electronics.)*

signals are monitored by the global COPAS-SARSAT (search and rescue satellite-aided tracking) satellite system coordinated by the United States, Canada, France, and Russia. This system consists of a constellation of polar orbiting and geostationary satellites fitted with transponders to receive the distress signal and locate the activated beacon. The polar satellites orbit 600 miles above the earth and have an orbital time of 105 minutes.

The first-generation 121.1/243.0 EPIRBs, which are still in use, can also be monitored by SAR ground stations, aircraft, and ships with appropriate receivers.

The second-generation 406-MHz EPIRB provides the most reliable worldwide coverage. Satellites with 406-MHz transponders can store the signal in memory until a ground station is in view and then can retransmit the signal. The LEO satellites therefore can receive EPIRB transmissions from virtually anywhere in the world. These satellites are 500 miles above the earth and circle the globe every 99 minutes. The distress signal is quickly relayed to a ground station called a local user terminal (LUT), passed on to the mission control center (MCC), and relayed to the appropriate maritime rescue coordination center (MRCC). The satellites are able to compute the position of the beacon within 2 km. The 406-MHz EPIRB transmits a digital signal with a unique identification code. It can then be instantly identified through an NOAA encoded-transmission program. If the unit is properly registered with NOAA, vital information regarding the vessel can be passed on to SAR units. All registered EPIRBs are issued a dated decal that provides proof of registration and includes a unique 15-character hexadecimal code, registration expiration date, and the vessel's eight-digit registration code.

Failure to register can lead to unnecessary and tragic delays. NOAA receives many EPIRB signals daily, some in error and some justified. The signals are processed by computer and matched by updated information provided by the owner on a biannual schedule. The signals from unregistered EPIRBs are considered questionable and are not given top priority. The 406-MHz EPIRB will be required aboard all commercial vessels operating 3 or more nautical miles from shore.

The newest generation of EPIRB is the 406-MHz unit with a GPS interface. The GPIRB transmits its exact location, obtained using GPS latitude and longitude coordinates, with the emergency EPIRB signal. It utilizes the polar orbiting satellites and the new geostationary search and rescue (GEOSAR) satellites in high earth orbit. The satellites receive the signal as soon as the beacon is activated. Position information is continually updated and stored every 20 minutes in the unit as long as it maintains a direct connection to the GPS receiver. The battery has a minimum operating life of 48 hours and operates longer in temperate climates. With this unit, accuracy is within 100 m.

All EPIRBs have a homing signal at 121.5 MHz. This is the homing frequency used by SAR vessels equipped with radio direction-finding equipment to locate precisely the craft in distress. Once activated the EPIRB is left on until the emergency is over. To update a position, it must broadcast continuously. EPIRB radio signals cannot penetrate water, wood, metal, or fiberglass, but the signals will be received from inside a life raft, on deck, or on the water's surface. A fully charged EPIRB battery will allow transmission for at least 48 hours.

A rescue team will not appear immediately after the EPIRB is activated. It may take hours or days to mobilize rescue craft. Potential delays justify carrying a second 406-MHz EPIRB when cruising in isolated areas of the ocean and far offshore. While the EPIRB is activated, it is appropriate to continue signaling by all the other methods available. EPIRBs with lithium batteries have a shelf life of 10 years, making it practical to store one in the life raft; the prudent sailor puts a second unit in the survival pack.

Visual and Sound Distress Signals

In an age dependent on electronic navigation and sophisticated electronic and satellite communication, the simplest signaling strategies and devices are often over-looked (Box 64-14).

Visual pyrotechnic distress signals have a high failure rate and age rapidly, so they require replacement according to the labeled expiration date.

Hand-held flares have varying effectiveness for attracting attention during daylight. Luminosity ratings range from 500 candlepower (CP) to 15,000 CP. The lowest rated flares are virtually invisible in daylight at ¼ mile, and the highest rated flares are only slightly more visible. For daytime use, orange smoke devices are the most effective way to attract attention. Smoke canisters are superior to hand-held smoke flares. They float and emit orange smoke for 2 to 5 minutes. Immediately after ignition the canister should be thrown in the water downwind of the craft. Smoke signals have a visible range of 1 to 3 miles in daylight, depending on the dissipating effects of the prevailing wind. Helicopter pilots find the smoke signal especially useful to indicate the strength and direction of the wind at sea level.

When using flares after sunset, consider luminosity, burn time, and altitude. Use an aerial flare (meteor or parachute) to attract attention at night, then ignite a hand-held flare to guide a rescue craft to your location. Due to the curvature of the earth, sighting distances are limited. A high-altitude flare enables a ship beyond your line of sight to be alerted. The greater the height, the longer and further the signal can be seen by a distant viewer. A parachute flare at 1000-foot (305-m) altitude is seen as a brief flash of light on the horizon from a distance 40 miles away, but from 20 miles, it appears to be at about 500 feet above the horizon and is visible for a longer time. Luminosity and burn time are more important than altitude to help assisting craft home in on your location. The rated visible range assumes a ship in the area has an alert lookout standing on the bridge watching for and anticipating your signal on a night of optimal atmospheric conditions and calm seas.

Whenever possible, choose flares meeting SOLAS standards (International Convention for Safety of Life at Sea). They exceed U.S. Coast Guard standards and are much more visible. The flares are easy to ignite, do not require pistol launchers, are safer to use, and have the lowest failure rate.

All pyrotechnics are hazardous and potentially injurious. They are capable of melting the rubber of the life raft and burning the skin of your hand. Some hand-held red flares drip considerable ash and slag, so point them downwind while holding them high at arm's length, away from the raft or boat deck and over the water. Make certain that you are in a secure position and that the raft or boat is stable. Remove all adhesive fastenings and covers, and be sure you know from which end the rocket or flare will exit. After the signal is activated, turn your face away to protect your eyes from the intense glare. If a rocket or flare fails to ignite immediately, it may not ignite at all or there may be a lag time before firing. Hold your position and count to sixty. If there is still no ignition, throw the flare into the sea. Never look into a flare tube to see why it failed, and never put it back in the raft. Treat it as an activated and live explosive.

The parachute flare is designed to attract the attention of potential rescuers out of sight over the horizon. For practical purposes, a parachute flare has a useful range of about 10 miles regardless of its rated range or altitude. These red flares drop slowly beneath a nonflammable parachute and burn for 45 seconds. The SOLAS models burn the brightest and longest. They should be fired downwind at an angle just slightly less than vertical. The main body of the rocket is contained within the launch tube. After activating the firing mechanism, hold the tube with both hands to prevent the tube from slipping due to recoil. Use gloves or a dry cloth if your hands are wet.

The red meteor (aerial) hand-launched or pistol-launched flare should be launched downwind approximately 80 degrees above the horizon. These flares are less effective than the parachute flares because of their short burn time of 5 to 9 seconds. It is best to fire them in pairs, the first one to attract attention, the second about 10 seconds later to confirm distress and general position. They are also visible for 12 to 15 miles.

Do everything possible to attract attention with signal mirrors, flashlights, kites, or any other means before using flares. Do not fire flares in the direction of high-flying commercial aircraft. They cannot see your signal when they are flying at 30,000 feet (9144 m). Do not waste all the flares when the first ship or low-

---

Box 64-14 VISUAL AND SOUND DISTRESS SIGNALS AT SEA

1. If other vessels are in sight, stand in an unobstructed area and slowly and repeatedly raise and lower outstretched arms as though you are flapping wings.
2. Sound a foghorn or blow a whistle continuously, or sound out SOS.
3. At night, point a flashlight at another boat and flash SOS (dot dot dot, dash dash dash, dot dot dot) repeatedly.
4. Fly the ship's ensign upside down, or fly the recognized distress flag: an orange flag with a black square under a black ball. Any square flag with a ball shape above or below is also a recognized distress signal.
5. Wave any brightly colored clothing or foul weather gear attached to a paddle or pole.
6. Use controlled flames or smoke on the vessel, or pour a dye marker in the sea near the vessel.

flying aircraft appears, since it might pass close by without seeing your signals.

A signal mirror is an inexhaustible device and is definitely more effective than flares in daylight. Mirrors are especially useful when trying to attract the attention of aircraft, even those flying at high altitudes. Aim the signal at the front end of the fuselage while the airplane is still far in the distance and coming toward your vessel. The flash from a signal mirror can be seen up to 40 miles from the air on a clear day. If you hear a plane, begin signaling with the mirror, because the flashing light can be seen before you can see the plane. The mirror is also useful at night; as with reflector tape, it can reflect back a ship's searchlight, thereby making the raft or ship much easier to locate in the dark. Other shiny materials that can be used as reflectors include foil space blankets, jewelry, eating utensils, fishing lures, and credit cards.

Radar is used by rescue ships and aircraft to accurately locate a life raft or vessel in distress. Visibility on the radar screen can be improved by using an electronic radar reflector known as a *search and rescue transponder* (SART). Once activated by an incoming radar signal (the interrogating radar), it is capable of sending back an electronic signal to any commercial radar located on a ship within a 10-mile radius and up to 50 miles on the radar screen of an aircraft flying at 3000 feet (914 m). It is much more effective than a simple radar reflector. When activated by interrogating radar, a line of 12 intense blips will appear on the radar screen radiating outward from the position of the SART. As the search vessel approaches, these blips widen to form a series of concentric circles around the transponder's position on the screen. In standby mode, the batteries have an operating life of 96 hours. The life is more than 8 hours in the operational mode. As with a radar reflector, a SART should be mounted at the highest possible point. On a raft the telescopic pole normally provided or the man overboard pole can be used as a mast to support the SART. Alternatively, it can be lashed to the top of the raft. If a radar reflector is supplied with the life raft, it should not be deployed at the same time, since it will block some of the SART signals.

Fluorescent dye marker is designed to be seen by airplanes and has a daytime visibility of 2 to 5 miles. In moderate weather it will last for a half hour; in rough weather it will rapidly dissipate. Use it whenever an aircraft is expected or if you believe you are beneath a flight path. The sea anchor will keep your drift rate the same as that of the dye.

Hand-held waterproof strobe flashers are 10 times brighter than the brightest parachute flare and can flash for hours on a single replaceable battery. Although they are not an internationally recognized distress signal, when supplemented with other recognized distress signals, they are very effective.

CREW OVERBOARD

Personal Flotation Devices

About 600 boaters drown every year because they were not wearing a personal flotation device (PFD). Drownings usually occur in less than a minute. Time is always the critical factor for survival.

Very cold water, 10° C (50° F) or less, is the great equalizer for all mariners, regardless of their swimming ability (see Chapter 8). Cold swimmers lose strength and coordination, making movement difficult. Sailors who survive a fall overboard into cold water are often too weak to climb back into the boat. Hypothermic sailors may have difficulty climbing up the cargo net or ladder of the rescue boat because of weak arms and legs.

Few boaters routinely wear PFDs and most people put them on only in stormy weather. The main reasons for veteran sailors not wearing PFDs are discomfort and inconvenience. All the type I offshore life jackets and type II near-shore life vests are bulky, uncomfortable, and awkward to wear. The common type III vest is comfortable and wearable but has poor reserve buoyancy and freeboard (distance from the water to the mouth); it cannot turn the unconscious victim face up (righting ability) and cannot support the head (body angle). It is suitable only for calm water and should be worn only by active boaters who are able to swim.

The new inflatable vests have a flat and lightweight design that allow them to lie flush against the body so they do not restrict movement. When inflated, they achieve excellent flotation. The offshore model can be purchased with an integral safety harness (Figure 64-2). Inflatable vests provide as much as 35 pounds of buoyancy, compared with 22½ pounds in type I and 15½ pounds in type III. In most cases this buoyancy floats

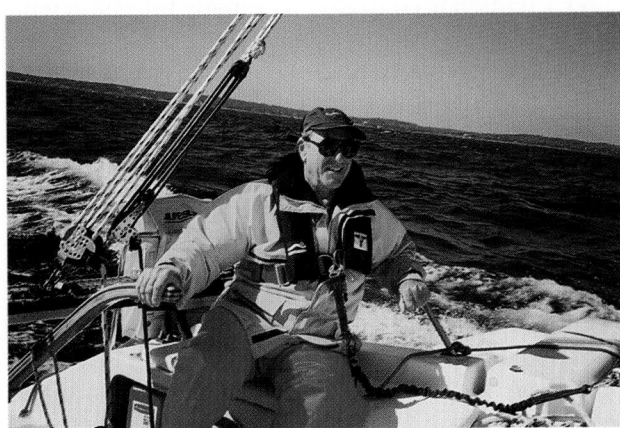

Figure 64-2 Comfortable, lightweight, and convenient integrated safety harness and automatic inflatable life vest. It is Coast Guard approved and features both a backup rip cord and an oral inflation system.

the head higher and makes it easier to breathe. By keeping the head and chest higher out of the water, it is easier to adopt the heat escape lessening position (HELP; see Chapter 56). With buoyancy high on the chest, there is also better righting ability and head support.

The U.S. Coast Guard has approved the manual inflation models of these vests. These are ripcord-activated carbon dioxide (CO_2) inflation systems. The automatic inflatable PFDs, despite lack of Coast Guard approval, have an extremely reliable water-activated mechanism and can always be inflated by pulling the ripcord or by oral inflation if necessary. Automatic inflation is an obvious advantage if the person entering the water is injured, semiconscious, or disoriented. The disadvantages would occur in much less likely scenarios, such as when a boat capsizes and the inflated vest impedes the exit by pinning the person to the cabin sole (which is now the ceiling), thus preventing a dive down to the open companionway. Autoinflation vests should be worn at all times by nonswimmers, because they may panic when falling overboard, and by children who may not understand or have difficulty with a manual device.

Boaters who resist wearing any type of vest may tolerate the offshore inflatable vest in a compact belt pack. It is the least cumbersome of any PFD because it is worn on the waist. After inflation, it is donned while in the water as a conventional life vest and offers 22 pounds of buoyancy.

When boating in cold weather, a float coat may be worn instead of a regular jacket. Besides providing floatation, the coat protects against hypothermia. An inflatable jacket is also highly effective for the same reasons.

Whatever style of PFD is chosen, it is important to test and wear it in the HELP position. You should float in a slightly reclining position with the water rising no higher than armpit level. The PFD should be close fitting with small arm holes to prevent it riding up on the chest. Children need to have a properly fitted size with crotch straps so they do not submerge if the vest slips up over their arms and head. Never buy an oversized PFD that a child will "grow into" over time.

An immersion suit is the ultimate protection from hypothermia and drowning. It is a combination life raft and dry suit. The suit has a watertight full-length zipper, watertight hood, face seal for wind and water protection, detachable mitts, neoprene wrist seals, integral boots, inflatable head pillow for optimum flotation angle, water-activated safety light, whistle, and buddy line. Their general bulkiness (one size fits a 110- to 300-pound person) and built-in gloves, however, make them impractical for continued wear while actively working aboard ship.

Safety Harness

A safety harness should always be worn in rough weather, at night, whenever alone on deck, or if work-ing on deck out of sight of the crew. In heavy weather, harnesses should also be used even when steering in the relative protection of the cockpit. The harnesses should be adjusted to fit snugly around the chest and 1 to 2 inches below the armpits. They should be constructed with webbing at least ½ inch in width with a breaking strength exceeding 3300 pounds. Tethers connect the harness to a through-bolted deck fitting or to a strong line, wire, or webbing running fore and aft. Each of these must have a breaking strength of over 4950 pounds. These specifications are based on the calculation that the force generated by a 150-pound body falling 12 feet is more than 3000 pounds. Being dragged in the water by a safety harness can be a bruising experience. Therefore tethers should be no more than 6 feet in length and fitted with highest quality snap shackles at both ends. The shackles should be easy to disconnect for quick release from a capsized boat.

Don the harness before going on deck, and secure the tether while still in the companionway. When on deck and under sail, always hook on the windward (uphill, upwind) side. If you fall, you will fall downhill the length of the tether and land on deck. If you hook onto the leeward side (downhill, downwind) you will probably be thrown overboard and dragged through the water.

Women should be careful not to wear the chest strap below their breasts. Injury may occur from the upward force that is placed on the harness when it suddenly comes under tension. Women should wear harnesses specifically designed for them. Safety harnesses are also available with an integrated inflatable vest. This convenient combination may be the most important piece of personal safety gear at sea.

Remaining Aboard

Falling overboard is the most common cause of marine fatalities in recreational boating and commercial shipping. In stormy weather the safest location is in the cabin. Virtually all "man overboard" incidents can be prevented by following these rules:

1. Remain sober, especially if you expect to go on deck for any reason.
2. Wear nonskid footwear when working on deck.
3. Walk in a crouched position with a low center of gravity and wide-based stance when the boat is rolling, heeling, or pitching.
4. If the boat's motion is too violent to stand, crawl or slide along the deck.
5. Use a safety harness as a "third hand," secured to a strong attachment point.
6. Use a safety harness whenever going aloft in the rigging or climbing any superstructure.
7. Avoid leaning overboard with all your weight on a lifeline or stanchion.
8. Know the location of secure handholds and grab rails so you can find them at night.

9. Know the safe routes to avoid tripping on deck hardware, vents, and hatches, especially at night.
10. Do not urinate from the afterdeck in rough weather unless you are kneeling and attached with a safety harness.
11. Wear a safety harness whenever seasick, and vomit into a bucket rather than leaning overboard.
12. In heavy weather, sleep in your harness and be ready to attach the tether quickly if called on deck for an emergency.
13. In heavy weather, stay below in the cabin unless absolutely needed on deck.

Recovery of Crew Overboard

If you suddenly find yourself in the water without a safety harness, maintain a positive attitude about your survival and rescue. The will to live makes all the difference. In cold water, be prepared for violent shivering and intense pain. Do not undress. Clothing traps air, which provides insulation and buoyancy, and the trapped water next to the skin retards heat loss, as in a wet suit. If possible, cover your head, neck, and hands. Move slowly to decrease heat loss. Slowly tread water just enough to keep your head out of the water. Assume the HELP position if wearing a life jacket. If a short swim is your best chance of survival, remove extra clothing and footwear, and try to keep your head out of the water using a breast stroke or dog paddle. Up to 50% of the body's heat loss is from the head. Allow the vessel to come to you. Do not swim to the boat unless it is completely disabled and cannot return to you. Conserve your strength for the rescue. When possible, get out of the cold water and stay out of it, no matter how low the air temperature. Keep on all clothing to reduce windchill. If given the opportunity, always reboard or climb on top of a swamped or capsized boat and await rescue.

Time is the critical factor in recovering a person overboard. A well-rehearsed rescue under expert leadership with clear communication is the rescue most likely to succeed. When someone is observed falling overboard, shout "man overboard" and sound the all stations alarm (a continuous blast of the ship's whistle supplemented by continuous ringing of the general alarm bell for not less than 10 seconds, or three short whistle blasts). One or more crew members should be designated to spot and point to the victim continuously. Floating objects should be thrown overboard, including buoyant cushions, horseshoe buoys, ring buoys, and extra life jackets, in order to litter the water surrounding the victim. The gear may provide extra flotation and will help mark the area for the spotter. Unfortunately, most of these objects will drift faster in winds over 10 knots than a person can swim, so the person cannot expect to receive a PFD after falling overboard.

Special equipment is designed for locating and retrieving a person overboard. A crew overboard pole is a 12-foot flagpole that is ballasted to remain upright in rough seas. Without the drogue accessory, it will quickly drift away from the designated area. A man overboard module (MOM) automatically deploys a CO_2-activated horseshoe buoy and a 6-foot inflatable locator pole equipped with a drogue and water-activated lithium-powered light.

A variety of lights have been developed to serve as rescue beacons. The overboard marker strobe marks the site and illuminates the scene for the rescuers. It automatically activates when thrown into the water. Waterproof personal rescue strobe lights attached to a PFD can flash for 8 hours at 1-second intervals and are visible 1 mile away. Other personal strobe lights can last up to 60 hours, with variable rates to conserve battery power. A U.S. Navy whistle has a special flat design to prevent the whistle body from holding water and dampening the sound. One should be attached to every life vest.

The water-activated UHF radio transmitter and strobe unit (ALERT) attaches to a life jacket and sets off an overboard alarm inside the boat. When the wearer falls overboard, the transmitter activates the onboard receiver, which triggers a loud alarm. The ALERT receiver can also shut down the engine and mark a position on a compatible GPS.

All onboard GPS units have an overboard function, which, if activated, will pinpoint the latitude and longitude of the person at the time of the fall. It will then give the reciprocal course to steer, the bearing, and distance back to the victim. The GPS is a powerful SAR tool, but is not a substitute for maintaining strict visual contact and using visual signal lights and markers. The inherent small degree of error with GPS is magnified in heavy winds, large seas, and strong currents, because the person may drift while the boat returns to the scene.

GPS receivers on board receive signals from U.S. Air Force satellites and then compute the location accurately to within 10 m. It may be close to impossible to locate the person in rough seas or during reduced visibility.

Rather than rely on the ship's emergency locator beacon, sailors can wear their own. A small unit can be worn by a crew member as a *personal locator beacon* (PLB). Weighing as little as 17 ounces, it also transmits on the 406- and 121.5-MHz frequencies; the battery life for this compact unit exceeds 24 hours.

The goal in overboard recovery is to return as quickly as possible to the victim using the simplest maneuver. Motorboats should reduce speed and return in a simple circle. Sailboats under power alone can return by simply circling back and approaching downwind of the victim. Establish contact by using a heaving line, such as a floating polypropylene line in a throw bag. If the boat is drifting downwind, slowly advance forward to complete the recovery over the windward side. Placing the boat upwind of the victim entails the risk of drifting onto the person. Sailboats under sail can choose from a variety of options. The "quick stop" is designed for rapid overboard recovery. This method enables the boat to reduce speed immediately by turning into the wind while trimming in the mainsail and keeping the headsail (jib) aback. Thereafter the helmsman keeps the boat turning downwind while maneuvering to remain close to the victim. After passing abeam (to one side of the vessel at a right angle to the boat's centerline) of the victim, the boat heads into the wind to stop two to three boat lengths away from the victim at an angle of 60 degrees to the wind, with the sails luffing. The technique is similar to picking up a mooring under sail. The boat can also be left beam to wind with the sails luffing while contact is made with the victim. The engine can be started and left in neutral, ready to be used if needed in the final approach. Rescuers must ensure all lines are aboard before engaging the engine to avoid fouling the propeller, returning to neutral when close to the victim. The main danger to the victim is being sucked under the stern while the prop is turning and the boat is moving forward under power.

The direction of approach to the victim used by the rescue boat is controversial and involves judgment based on many variables, including the sea state, wind strength, drift of the boat relative to the victim, and maneuverability of the boat. An injured or unconscious person requires assistance by a rescue swimmer who should be tethered to the boat.

The goal is to have the victim back on board as quickly as possible. Practice the different techniques and decide which method and modifications work best on your boat. The Lifesling, developed to enable one person to retrieve a person overboard, is a floating collar that doubles as a hoisting sling. The collar is deployed from a bag hung on the stern pulpit and is delivered to the victim in the water by repeatedly circling in smaller circles, similar to the way a ski boat would maneuver to deliver the tow rope to a fallen water skier. After securing the horseshoe over the head and under the arms, the victim is pulled back to the boat and hoisted in the apparatus with the assistance of a halyard and winch. If you lose sight of and are unable to find the victim, immediately call for assistance. A Mayday call on VHF-FM channel 16 will notify the Coast Guard and simultaneously alert all ships in the area monitoring this channel. The last known position should be obtained using GPS or reference to any navigational buoys and landmarks on shore. Repeat searches of the area, since it is easy to miss someone in poor visibility or choppy seas. The chances for recovery are close to 100% if the victim has a well-equipped high-visibility (orange or yellow) PFD with a personal strobe light, reflective tape, loud whistle, packet of waterproof self-launching meteor flares (Skyblazer), a pouch of fluorescent dye marker, and a personal EPIRB.

HOW TO ABANDON SHIP

Before abandoning ship, the first priority is to dress warmly and put on a life jacket. Layer on as much warm and quick-drying clothing as possible. If a survival suit is available, wear that instead of a life jacket, but bring the jacket for later use in the raft. One crew member should man the radio and broadcast a Mayday message on VHF-FM channel 16 (good up to a 20-mile range) or on SBB 2182 kHz (good beyond 50-mile range). Simultaneously, other crew should launch the life raft and locate the "abandon ship bag" (a survival kit). To guarantee that the critical survival items (VHF radio, EPIRB, SART, water maker, medical kit, signal pack) remain together with the life raft, these items should be packed into the life raft itself before departure, or they can be packed into a waterproof bag securely attached by a short line to the raft.

Each crew member should have an easily accessible prepacked waterproof bag containing extra dry clothing, personal medications, passport, prescription glasses and sunglasses, personal strobe, safety harness and tether, wallet, and any other personal valuables and necessities. If the ship's bag has been properly stocked, little else is needed from the sinking ship except synthetic blankets (not down sleeping bags, which will never dry), jerry jugs of fresh water, extra food (especially high-energy sports bars), and navigation tools. If time permits, additional communication and signaling equipment is collected from the stricken vessel, even if equipment was already placed in the bag or raft. This includes a 406-MHz EPIRB, a SART, and a waterproof hand-held VHF radio. In a life raft, a person can never have too many EPIRBs, radios, flares, and fishhooks (Box 64-15).

There are three classes of life rafts: ocean, offshore, and coastal. This classification refers to the areas in which the vessel normally operates and reflects the differences in size, design, construction, quantity of survival stores, and kinds of equipment. Another practical way to categorize life rafts is in terms of performance. A poor life raft will keep its occupants from drowning until they die of hypothermia or heatstroke. A mediocre life raft will protect the survivors from dying of exposure until they succumb to thirst and starvation. The best life raft will provide food and water, have a means of replenishing both, and be sufficiently equipped to sustain life and facilitate rescue.

Box 64-16 lists the gear found in a six-man inflatable life raft approved by SOLAS for ocean service (SOLAS A). The SOLAS B raft is designated for limited service. It carries no food, water, or fishing kit. These rafts also

Box 64-15 ABANDON SHIP BAG FOR OCEAN PASSAGE

SIGNALS AND COMMUNICATION

Registered 406-MHz class II COPAS/SARSAT emergency position indicating radio beacon (EPIRB) (carry two if one is not packed in life raft)

Waterproof and submersible portable VHF hand-held radio transmitter with spare batteries

Search and Rescue Transponder (SART)

Flares, smoke signals, horn

Kite, dye marker, signal mirror

Radar reflector

"Cyalume" chemical light sticks

Underwater flashlight with extra batteries

Strobe flasher with spare batteries

PROTECTION

Survival suits, gloves

Expanded medical pack with extra seasick medications, SAM splints, narcotics, sunscreen, lip balm

Backup sea anchor and line

SUSTENANCE

Portable reverse-osmosis desalinator

Solar still

Fishing harpoon, spear gun with spare heads, extra fishing gear, including fishing line, wire leaders, assorted barbed hooks, sinkers, lures

Knife, sharpening stone, small cutting board, scissors, storage bags, eating utensils, nylon mesh bag, waterproof bags

Collapsible bucket, urine bottle

Comprehensive survival manual, fish identification book, cards, reading material

Collapsible water container

TOOLS

Small ax, pliers, and screwdriver

Dive mask

Duct tape

Raft patching clamps

Box 64-16 LIFE RAFT EQUIPMENT (OCEAN SERVICE)

Inflation pump with hose

Two 4-foot paddles

Two sea anchors (one stowed inside ready for use, one outside automatically deployed)

Two bailers

Two sponges

Drogue and cord

Repair kit containing sealing clamps, patches, cement

100-foot buoyant heaving line with quoit

Floating sheath knife

Scissors

Can openers

Thermal protection bags

Provisions

Water ($\frac{1}{2}$ quart of water per person)

Graduated drinking vessel

First-aid kit (primarily for wound management)

Seasickness pills (6 per person)

Fishing kit

Survival instructions

Operating instructions

Two red parachute flares (hand held, rocket propelled, red)

Six hand-held flares (stowed in watertight container)

Signaling mirror and whistle

Signal flashlight with spare batteries and spare bulb

Two smoke canisters

carry half the number of flares and smoke signals found in SOLAS A life rafts. An ocean-service raft is designed for use in rough offshore conditions. It is constructed with two complete, stacked inflation chambers. One flotation chamber is sufficient to support the number of people for which the raft is rated.

Careful thought must be given to stowage of the life raft. The raft should be securely stowed either on deck, with hardware capable of withstanding the shearing forces in a capsize, or below in the cabin. The lid on a deck locker or lazarette is likely to open in a knockdown or capsize, making these poor storage areas for such vital gear.

If the boat has a dinghy, prepare to tow it behind the raft. It is useful for storing additional supplies and can be used with an improvised sailing rig. Although a solid dinghy is less seaworthy in a storm than a life raft, it is far more durable against shark attack and is immune to chafe. A dinghy has more maneuverability and strength than a raft.

To launch the raft, the canister should be thrown overboard on the downwind (leeward) side of the boat and then inflated. It is dangerous to inflate a life raft with the CO_2 cartridge aboard the ship because it may become wedged in the rigging of the sinking ship or accidentally punctured. If the raft fails to inflate in the water, however, it must be brought aboard to be inflated with the hand pump.

A sharp jerk on the outstretched line coming out of the canister (the painter) triggers the CO_2 cartridge and inflates the raft. If the first pull is unsuccessful, give a second stronger tug. The painter should be attached to the boat before the raft is inflated. In the confusion surrounding an emergency, this critical step is sometimes forgotten, and after the raft inflates, it drifts away. One person with a knife should be stationed by the painter prepared to cut the line. Another safety knife is located in a pocket by the entrance of the raft to cut the painter if the ship begins to sink after the crew has entered the raft.

Once everyone is aboard, get clear of the sinking vessel as quickly as possible by letting out all of the painter line. Risks include being struck from below by surfacing wreckage and becoming entangled with the boat's rigging as it rolls and sinks. If the boat does not sink, stay close by attaching a quick release line to it. The wreckage is always easier to spot than a small life raft, and the boat may be salvaged later.

Large-capacity rafts, usually found on commercial ships, are often mounted in a cradle with an automatic disconnect device called a hydrostatic release mechanism (Figure 64-3). This mechanism can be manually activated by pressing a button, which releases the straps holding the canister to the cradle. The canister can then be dropped overboard. In the event the boat begins to sink before the life raft is launched, a hydrostatic release mechanism will open when the vessel sinks to a depth of 10 to 15 feet, allowing the canister to float up to the surface. As the vessel sinks to the end of the painter's length, it will jerk the painter and initiate inflation. The specially designed "weak link" on the cradle where the painter is attached is designed to break and free the raft from the vessel completely before it is pulled under by the sinking boat. An unoccupied inflated raft will be blown downwind very quickly, much faster than someone in a life jacket can swim; a person in the water while a raft inflates must hold onto the raft or painter.

You can enter the raft before it is fully inflated by crawling under the collapsed canopy. When possible, try to remain dry and enter it directly from the sinking

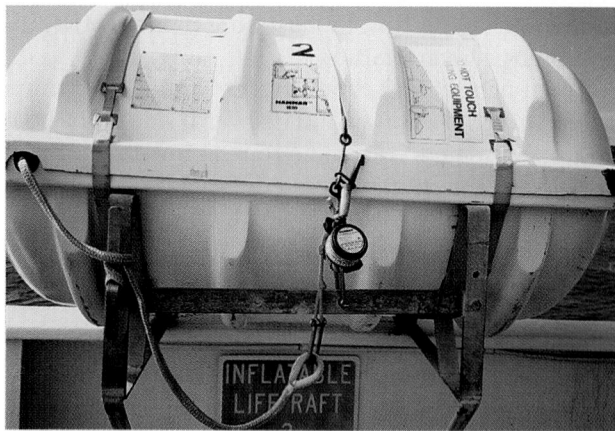

Figure 64-3 This inflatable life raft will float free if the vessel sinks. The packing bands are designed to break when the raft is inflated. The rope painter, which is attached to the "weak link," must be secured to a cleat if the raft is manually deployed overboard. The disk-shaped hydrostatic release is set to release the raft from the cradle at water depths of 5 to 15 feet, with a button for manual release.

boat rather than from the water. All rafts are strong and stable enough so that you can jump directly onto the canopy and supporting arch tube when entering the raft. Be careful not to jump on top of the occupants or tear the canopy. The canopy serves to collect rainwater, helps to keep the raft dry, and shields survivors from the elements. When entering from the water, use the automatically deployed boarding ladder and handholds at the entrance to the raft. If the crew is forced to enter from the water, the first person into the raft should throw the heaving line to the others. The line has a rubber donut (quoit) attached to the end and will allow a person to hold on firmly. It is important to get everyone out of the water quickly. If you must swim away from the raft to help a crewmate, be certain you are attached to the craft with a safety line.

The hissing sound heard after inflation does not signify a leaking or defective raft. The relief valve is simply releasing excess gas pressure. Immediately after the release of the CO_2/nitrogen mixture into the raft's interior space, ventilate the life raft thoroughly and periodically thereafter. The floor is inflated separately with the manual pump and provides insulation from the cold sea. Because the craft is so vulnerable to capsize (see later), it is extremely important to inventory and then secure all equipment as it comes aboard. Then check the life raft for any damage or leaks and the crew for any life-threatening injuries. Activate the EPIRB immediately and leave it on.

The first medical action should be distribution of seasickness medication. In a life raft, everyone is susceptible to seasickness, especially in the first 24 hours. Make the raft as dry as possible, and remove wet clothing. Close the door, and huddle together to conserve heat. Do everything possible to conserve body heat, strength, and spirit as you prepare for rescue.

Life rafts have ballast pockets under the floor to trap sea water and thereby increase stability. Unfortunately, if the wind gets under the craft as it rises on a wave, it can still capsize. A capsize is most likely immediately after launching when the raft is empty. The raft may even initially inflate upside down; most rafts can be properly righted from the deck of the boat without entering the water.

No immediate danger exists if the raft capsizes with crew inside, since sufficient air is available in the space under the canopy. It is necessary to enter the water in order to right the raft, however, since it is unlikely to right itself unless rolled again by successive waves. With the raft empty, it can be righted by pulling on the righting straps at the bottom. Kneel on the downwind side with feet braced on the CO_2 cylinder, and lean back. The raft will then right itself easily when the wind catches it.

To prevent recurrent capsizes in heavy wind and seas, additional measures need to be taken. Every raft is equipped with a cone-shaped sea anchor. This device is essential in rough weather. It provides stability in high winds, helps to prevent capsizing in rough seas, is an aid in directional control of the raft, and helps to reduce drift. The benefit of reducing drift in storm conditions is controversial, since the raft may become sluggish with the sea anchor deployed. If sea room is sufficient, the occupants may be more comfortable and the raft less likely to capsize if it is allowed to drift at the same rate as the waves. Deployment of the sea anchor is automatic on some rafts. Stream the sea anchor after the raft is clear of the sinking vessel. It should be trailed somewhere in the trough between wave crests while the raft is sitting on a crest. Check that the rope does not become entangled, and protect the raft from chafe at the point where the rope is attached. Weight distribution is also critical to avoid capsize. Position most of the crew on the windward side, the same side from which the sea anchor is deployed, to act as ballast. Weight on the windward side reduces the chance of the raft being lifted and flipped over by the wind. In seas with high wave crests, be prepared to maintain the raft's balance and quickly shift as needed to prevent capsize in the other direction.

Since a survivor can quickly become separated from a capsized raft, have everyone attach a line to the handholds if capsize is possible. Whenever a craft capsizes, gather the crew in the water and check that no one is under the overturned raft. Everyone should return as quickly as possible to avoid hypothermia and to conserve precious energy.

PREPARATION FOR RESCUE: LIFE IN THE RAFT

Having successfully abandoned ship and secured both crew and equipment in the life raft, the task of preparing for rescue begins. Panic, fear, helplessness, and hopelessness can easily defeat the best-equipped and most experienced crew. Optimistic persons are most likely to survive. The leader can set the example and improve morale by staying calm and formulating an active strategy to be rescued. Assigning meaningful duties to everyone and structuring the work and rest time will instill in the crew some sense of control over their destiny. In Pornichet, France, the Center for the Study and Practice of Survival proposes the following "seven tools of the mind to help you survive":

1. *Size* up the situation rationally. Analyze and evaluate all options and plan the best course of action. Consider the resources available, the time frame, and risks.
2. *Understand* and control. Get in touch with your feelings. Identify and acknowledge your fears; own and control them.
3. *Risk* the least, achieve the most. Evaluate and estimate the risks of any course of action. Ask what

can be done to lessen the risk, and consider if the crew can handle the increased stress.
4. *Value* your reason for living. Find your own personal reason for wanting to survive. It will motivate you and powerfully counter any urge to give up.
5. *Imagine* new ways to do things. Use unconventional, lateral thinking. Improvise and try imaginative, creative solutions to problems. Trust your intuition.
6. *Victory* comes with time. Time is your asset, and problems often resolve themselves if given the opportunity. Avoid looking for quick solutions. Rushing a task often leads to failure.
7. *Enrich* yourself with a permanent positive mental attitude. Appreciate that you are alive, and keep your sense of humor.

Review how to use each type of distress signal. Take inventory of the signaling devices available, and agree on priorities for their use. Turn on the EPIRB and leave it on. The battery is good for 48 hours, during which time the signal should have activated an SAR operation and transmitted an updated location.

The most important duty aboard the raft is to maintain a continuous and effective lookout for rescue boats and airplanes. A watch schedule should be devised to rotate the duties every 2 hours. It is the lookout's responsibility to monitor changes in the weather, wind, and sea and look for signs of nearby land. Other crew members need to look after the well-being of the sleeping survivors. Their duties may include providing first aid and comfort to injured victims, fishing, making potable water, organizing the stores, keeping the log, bailing, and maintaining the raft.

The raft is subject to tears, punctures, chafe, and structural deterioration, which can cause leaking air chambers and loss of watertight integrity. If the raft deflates, it begins to flex and chafe. The buoyancy chambers should be kept taut with no apparent folds. To prevent overinflation, the pressure relief valves must be operational during the daytime to let off heated expanding air, especially in the tropics. As the temperature drops at night, the raft should be reinflated with the manual pump.

The raft must be protected against sharp, pointed, and abrasive objects such as knives, tools, fishhooks, spears, fish bones and teeth, shells, belt buckles, jewelry, and pens. All pointed tools must be kept sheathed or wrapped except when in use.

Attached to the canopy are internal and external dome lights. These help survivors find the raft at night when abandoning ship and provide interior lighting. These battery-operated lights last 12 to 24 hours, so turn them off when not in use. They are not intended to be rescue lights.

Except for seasickness, probably no other condition is more debilitating than chronic sleep deprivation.

Sleep deprivation causes decreased alertness with apparent blackouts of attention, which become increasingly prolonged and frequent. A groggy, inattentive lookout can easily miss the opportunity to observe and signal a passing ship. Conversely, the person may begin to hallucinate and see ships and planes. Impaired responsiveness to new situations and inability to make decisions rapidly further jeopardize the rescue.

Whenever possible, lie down and rest. Stretch out to relax muscles that are constantly working to keep the body stable in the raft. It is important to insulate the recumbent body against heat loss, especially from the cold floor of the raft. Always keep the double bottom of the floor of the raft fully inflated, and make every effort to keep the raft dry. Line the floor with sails, tarps, and extra clothing. The double layer floor also protects against the bumps of sharks, dorados, and other fish. Dry clothing protects the skin from painful saltwater boils. Apply an emollient to knees, hands, elbows, and buttocks to decrease skin abrasion. Common lubricants that moisturize the skin are petrolatum, mineral oil, and baby oil. Any area of skin breakdown should be smeared with an antiseptic or antibiotic cream and covered with a dry dressing.

Hypothermia becomes a threat with an air temperature of 0° to 10° C (32° to 50° F) or with repeated immersion in cold water (see Chapters 6 and 8). This is likely if the raft repeatedly capsizes. Sustained uncontrollable shivering is the earliest clinical sign of a drop in core temperature. Other early clues of hypothermia are alterations in motor skills and changes in mental status. Manual dexterity, balance, and strength are impaired. Ability to climb back into the raft may become impossible. Changes in mental status may involve judgment and cognitive skills.

Recognition of the early signs of hypothermia is critical. Prompt treatment usually prevents progression to profound hypothermia, which is likely to be fatal since it is untreatable in the raft. Treatment consists of preventing further heat loss by sheltering the victim from the wind, sea spray, or rain. Whenever possible, remove all wet clothing and dry the skin completely, then dress the victim in multiple layers of dry clothing. If a change of clothing is impossible, provide a vapor barrier with foul weather gear, a sail bag, or sleeping bag. If only a sail or blanket is available, wrap up the victim, covering the head, neck, and face. Let the victim shiver; if the shivering is vigorous, the heat generated internally provides the most effective method of rewarming. Calories from simple sugars and carbohydrates and ample water are necessary for the muscles to continue the shivering response.

A new SOLAS requirement for survival craft is a thermal protection suit for each crew member. These suits are ideal for keeping a person warm and dry in the survival craft. Foil space blankets are useful as sun reflectors on the canopy, and they effectively prevent heat loss from radiation. However, the major heat loss in raft survivors is by conduction through the raft floor, against which a foil blanket affords little protection.

To prevent heat-related illness (see Chapters 10 and 11) and dehydration, it is imperative to drink water at regular intervals. If possible, keep drinking until the urine is clear. Mechanisms for obtaining water are discussed later.

Keep clothing on and damp to help reduce fluid losses and prolong the cooling effect. Wear long-sleeved shirts, trousers, and a hat. Clothing also protects the skin from sunburn and reduces passive heating from solar radiation. Apply a waterproof sun protection cream to exposed areas of the face, hands, arms, neck, and feet. Stay in the shade of the raft canopy, but make sure the raft is well ventilated. The best rafts have a double canopy with an air layer in between that acts as insulation from the heat of the sun. Space blankets with a reflective surface may also be tied over the canopy to reflect the sun's rays. Deflating the raft's floor chambers helps to cool the raft. It may be tempting to take a dip in cool sea water if you feel very hot. Be sure you have the strength and ability to climb back aboard and have someone watch you.

The body's requirement for water depends on body weight, individual physiology, amount of exertion, diet, ambient humidity, and temperature. The average person at rest can survive for about 12 days without consuming water; the person remains fit for only 5 to 6 days, then may become delirious. A half liter of fresh water per day doubles the survival time, and a liter a day permits almost unlimited survival. By contrast, the body can go several weeks without food (see Chapter 53), provided there is enough fresh water to drink. On a restricted diet, the human body at sea level, in the shade, and at a maximum temperature of 25° C (77° F) requires an estimated 1.3 to 1.6 quarts of water per day; at 35° C (95° F), 5 quarts are needed. Evaporative loss from the action of sunlight in an open boat in the tropics is estimated at 5 pints per day if the body is at rest. The required water supplied aboard a life raft in tins is only 1.5 quarts per person for 2 days. A minimum daily survival ration of water is considered to be 600 ml (20 ounces, or 1.25 pints).

Hand-operated, portable reverse-osmosis desalination units contain a semipermeable membrane made of three different synthetic polymers. One of the polymers, polyamide, is layered on the membrane and is responsible for the semipermeable properties. Polyamide contains negatively charged carbolic acid side chains that project out from the surface of the polymer; these serve to repel any negatively charged chlorine ions that may try to cross the membrane. As a result, no positive cations (sodium) can pass either, because both anions and cations must pass together to maintain the charge balance on both sides of the membrane. Application of pressure to the sea water forces the water through the membrane against an osmotic gradient (reverse osmosis), creating fresh water. These units can produce 98% salt-free water from sea water at a rate of 1 ounce every 2 minutes, up to 1.2 gallons an hour. An added benefit is that the units remove bacteria, viruses, protozoa and other contaminants.

With malfunction or loss of the desalinator, solar stills can evaporate fresh water from salt water. The solar still was included in survival kits used by naval aviators during World War II. It provides about a quart of fresh water daily in temperate climates with sunshine. When inflated, the 24-inch ball containing a saltwater-soaked cloth collects fresh water after it condenses on the inner surface of the ball. The still is reusable and requires no chemicals. Unfortunately, most older solar stills are fragile and will not work in rough weather.

Rainwater can be collected with the canopy of the life raft. An exterior gutter collects and routes the water to a large container for storage. Daily washing of the canopy with sea water whenever practical helps to remove the buildup of salt deposits. In a heavy sustained downpour, the rain should rinse the canopy before the water is collected.

Ingestion of protein produces urea, and the kidneys must excrete the solute with water. Therefore, when water is in short supply, a diet rich in carbohydrates is preferred. Do not eat if water is unavailable. With 2 quarts a day or more, however, eat as desired. Fish and other sea creatures contain water with extremely low salt content in their eyes, flesh, and cerebrospinal fluid. Fish blood has a high salt concentration and is not recommended. Juices can be pressed out of the flesh by twisting pieces of fish in a cloth. The blood from sea birds and turtles is a reliable source of hydration for castaways.

Sea water is not potable. After exposure, drinking sea water is believed to be the major cause of death of life raft occupants. Ingesting sea water may hasten death rather than prevent it. Sea water is hyperosmotic at about 1000 mOsmol/L. The salt content ranges from 28 to 35 parts per thousand, whereas blood is about 8 parts per thousand. Drinking sea water usually causes immediate vomiting. If one is unlucky enough to hold it down, it increases the osmolarity of the blood and causes a shift of free water from the intracellular space into the blood and other extracellular fluids.

In the high latitudes, old sea ice is a good source of water. Sea ice loses its salt content after 1 year. The ice is brittle, bluish in color, and has round edges. New sea ice is gray, salty, opaque, and hard. Melting the ice allows tasting and judging the salinity. If the temperature drops to freezing, sea water can be collected in a can and allowed to freeze. Fresh water freezes first. Therefore the salt concentrates in the center, forming slush surrounded by ice containing very little salt. Sea ice

should not be confused with ice from an iceberg. Water from melted iceberg chunks is glacial fresh water. Chewing a piece of gum or cloth also helps to moisten the mouth and reduce thirst.

Unless survivors are assured of an early rescue or have a reverse-osmosis desalinator, they should not ingest water in the first 24 hours. After the first day, they can start drinking a minimum of 6 ounces three times a day from the water rations in the raft.

Nutrition is the last priority for survival. If the rescue will be delayed for days or weeks, plan to eat very little for the first 3 days. Thereafter, begin the lifeboat rations of carbohydrates and sugar. Save some rations until rescue is imminent, when extra energy will be needed.

Fish are usually the mainstay of a diet at sea once a survival routine has been established. The raft casts a dark shadow beneath the surface, which appears as a safe haven for a variety of fish, especially dorado ("school dolphin"). With practice and patience, fish can be taken near the sea surface with a harpoon, gaff, or spear gun. Care must be taken not to puncture the raft with these devices.

Successful fishing with a spear gun requires proficiency. Refraction makes it difficult to accurately hit the fish, so it is advised to minimize these effects by aiming straight down at the target, rather than obliquely. The ideal area to strike is located just behind the gill cover. Attach all fishing gear to the raft with a lanyard to avoid losing it. Fish away from the raft can be caught by trailing a line with a baited hook. Bait can be obtained from the first fish caught by using its guts, stomach contents, or thin strips of flesh. Lures can be made from any shiny object.

At night, fish are attracted to bright lights. Instead of a flashlight, try a signal mirror or any other shiny surface to reflect moonlight onto the water.

When bringing a fish aboard the raft, use a cloth or piece of canvas to wrap the fish. Both dolphin and wahoo, which have serrated teeth, thrash wildly when they come out of the water. Wounds from fish heal poorly and can easily become infected. Have a cutting board ready to kill the fish quickly by cutting through its spine right behind the head. A large fish can be stunned with a blow to the top of the head at eye level, and simply covering its eyes will calm it down sufficiently to position it for a quick kill.

Special care is required when bringing a shark aboard. A paddle or stick should be thrust in its mouth, and the fish held on its back over the flotation chamber tail first, until it is dead. The jaws should be cut out and thrown over the side before the fish is dressed.

Certain fish are inherently poisonous (see Chapter 62); these are usually located around shoals and reefs in shallow waters. These include pufferfish, porcupine fish, and the ocean sunfish (mola). Any fish with spines or bristles instead of scales should not be eaten.

As a general rule, do not eat any fish that smells bad. If uncertain about the safety of a fish, test it first for edibility. If it burns, stings, or tastes bad on the tip of your tongue, do not eat it. If it has an acceptable taste, try a small piece every hour for 3 to 4 hours initially, and if there are no ill effects after 12 hours, you can assume the food is edible. To save fish for future meals, cut the flesh into thin strips about an inch wide and half inch thick, and spread it out to dry in the sun on a flat surface. If you cut the strips with the fibers running the long way, the strips can be hung on a piece of string and allowed to dry in the open air under the raft canopy. Fish spoils within hours in the heat, so start drying some as soon as it is caught. Fresh-caught fish (except tuna), as well as dried turtle and bird meat, are good for days when the heat and humidity are not too high. Most ocean fish can safely be eaten raw. Freshwater fish should not be eaten raw, because they harbor parasites.

Seaweed is valuable in two ways. As a floating nest, it can harbor a variety of small edible creatures, including small fish, barnacles, crabs, and other crustaceans. All kelp and almost all brown and green seaweed are edible. Red seaweed is highly toxic, and any seaweed that tastes bitter may be one of the rare poisonous varieties. Leafy green seaweed can be dried for storage. Before eating seaweed, wash it in fresh water to eliminate any toxic plankton and salt that may be adhering to the weed. Seaweed must be chewed well and swallowed only after it becomes a soft paste. It has limited nutritive value because the carbohydrates are not digestible and the cellulose has laxative properties.

Plankton also has a high cellulose and chitin content and cannot be ingested in large quantities. Some toxic plankton are difficult to detect. The red tides that cause paralytic shellfish poisoning result from the blooms of dinoflagellates (see Chapter 54).

Many creatures follow a raft. There are reports of killer whales attacking small boats, but no documented accounts of attacks on life rafts. Other dolphins and whales may accompany the boat but are not likely to harm the survivors in a raft. Sharks can be a menace as they swim about the raft for days or even weeks and drive away other potentially edible fish. The shark's habit of frequently bumping a raft with its abrasive skin causes wear on the flotation chambers. Every effort should be made to avoid attracting sharks. Take special care to dispose of blood and offal at night, preferably when the raft is moving. Try not to create a waste trail for the sharks to follow, and bring hooked or speared fish aboard as quickly as possible.

Sea turtles' sharp claws and beaks can damage a raft or cause lacerations, so always bring them aboard cautiously by holding the hind flippers, then flipping them over onto their backs. The sea turtle can easily be killed by severing the vital arteries on the underside of the neck, with the spurting blood collected in a cup. The blood must be consumed immediately, because it coagulates in about 30 seconds. Draining the blood also preserves the quality of the meat for storage and future use. The eggs, heart, and bone marrow are edible, but the liver should not be eaten. Dry whatever meat is not immediately eaten. The bones inside the flippers have tasty marrow. Turtle eggs are rich in protein and fat. If the liver is crushed, the skimmed oil can be used as a skin oil. The shell can be used to bail the raft.

All seabirds are edible, but catching them may be more luck than skill. Their beaks and wings can be dangerous, so grab them by the feet. Float a baited hook on the water (fish guts are best), and let the bird hook itself. After the bird is hooked, throw a piece of canvas or article of clothing over the bird. With the head and beak well covered, compress the chest to suffocate the animal, or twist and quickly pull its neck. Rather than plucking the bird, slit the skin over the breastbone and peel off the skin with the feathers intact. The entire bird, except for the intestines and the small green gallbladder, is edible. The flesh may contain bioluminescent substances from ingested plankton, giving the dead bird a ghostlike glow at night, but it is nontoxic. The forewings and legs make excellent bait, and the feathers can be made into fishing lures.

RESCUE AND EVACUATION OF SICK AND INJURED SURVIVORS

Transferring personnel from a boat or a life raft to a rescue ship or helicopter entails risk for everyone involved. Rescue of personnel from a vessel in distress or from a life raft may be the most dangerous aspect of the survival ordeal.

The Automated Mutual Assistance Vessel Rescue System (AMVERS) provides resources to help any vessel in distress on the high seas. AMVERS is the only worldwide safety network available to all authorized RCCs. Participation is free, voluntary, and available to ships of all nations. More than 2700 vessels participate by being available to respond to emergencies at sea. The positions of all these ships around the world's oceans are tracked by computer and continuously updated. With these data, AMVERS creates a "surface picture" with the location of the ships in any given area. This vital information is then transmitted to the RCCs that deploy ships nearest the scene of the emergency. These ships are not designed for SAR, and their crew may have no experience or training in recovering survivors from small boats or life rafts under storm conditions.

In ship-to-ship rescue, collision between the vessels is the greatest risk. The typical scenario is a large merchant ship with limited maneuverability approaching a smaller vessel in distress, which usually has no maneuverability. Unless the rescue craft is highly maneuverable, the captain and crew experienced, and the seas relatively calm, it is much safer to use a smaller, more maneuverable craft to transfer personnel between the boats. This might include a rigid-hull inflatable boat (RHIB), a lifeboat, or even a life raft. In rough seas, a boat or raft is never secured to the rescue vessel. The constant battering of the two hulls is likely to damage and possibly sink the smaller craft. Whether to approach the rescue vessel upwind or downwind depends on the wind, sea, and size and relative drift of the two vessels. The advantages and disadvantages are similar to those for retrieving a person overboard. Becoming pinned and capsizing are risks when sitting in the lee (downwind) side of a large, rolling ship.

The transfer of personnel between ships is also hazardous if it requires the sick, injured, or exhausted crew to climb a cargo net or pilot ladder. Under the best of circumstances, it can be extremely difficult, and hypothermia is often the major obstacle.

A large rescue ship most often approaches upwind of the survival craft unless the ship's rate of drift is greater than that of the craft. This provides a calmer sea in the lee side of the rescue vessel as it slowly drifts down to the survivors' craft. If the sea anchor is deployed, be sure to pull it in to prevent entanglement in the rescue vessel's propeller. Remain calm, and do not rush to board the ship. Wait to see if a life boat or rescue swimmer is lowered to facilitate the transfer. If the raft must be lifted aboard with injured survivors, the floor must be fully inflated. Attach the lifting lines to the towing bridles on both sides of the raft, and attach two steadying lines to each side as well.

Never attempt to climb a scrambling net or pilot ladder without someone holding you on a safety line. The best way to board a rescue ladder is to wait until the craft being departed is on the crest of a wave. At that moment, transfer to the ladder. This drops the survival craft down while you are climbing up and eliminates the danger of the raft being raised up by a wave and hitting you. The safest procedure is being hoisted up to the deck in a harness by a crane.

Helicopter emergency evacuation and rescue has now become commonplace within 300 miles of the coastline. A detailed briefing is radioed to the crew when the helicopter is en route to the vessel in distress. All loose gear onboard must be well secured, including cockpit cushions, coils of line, winch handles, dive gear, hats, and clothing. Any gear not secured on deck may become a flying missile in the 100-mph winds generated by the helicopter. This debris may be sucked into the intake of the helicopter's engine or become tangled in the rotor blades.

All crew on deck should wear life jackets. Add extra clothing layers because the helicopter's downdraft creates a windchill effect. Avoid shining flashlights on the helicopter because the light may blind the pilot and rescue team; for the same reason, never fire aerial flares in the vicinity of a helicopter.

The transfer device is either a rescue basket or a Stokes litter. Selection depends on the victim's medical condition and the necessity to remain horizontal during the hoist. The horizontal position is particularly important for persons with profound hypothermia. A basket is the preferred device for lifting. It is easy to enter, especially in rough weather, and has positive flotation so that it will not sink. Just climb in it and fasten the straps. The basket will settle on the sea surface, enabling someone in the water to float into it.

A "horse collar" sling is a padded loop that is placed over the body around the back and underneath the armpits. The hoist is made with the line in front of the face. Always wear a PFD when entering the basket or hoist, and follow the directions for securing the safety straps.

The helicopter builds up static electricity traveling to the scene, and this is transferred down the cable to the basket. Allow the basket to touch the deck or the water first to discharge any static electricity. The electric shock is strong but nonlethal. The orange steadying line, which is dropped first, can be handled safely and will not produce any shock.

Unhook the hoist cable only if it becomes necessary to move a litter below decks, then set the cable free to be hauled back. When it is lowered again, allow the hook to ground on the vessel, then reattach it to the rescue device. Never attach the hoist cable or the steadying line to any part of the vessel or life raft, even temporarily.

If a helicopter picks up survivors from a life raft, the downdraft from the chopper's blades may capsize it, especially if the raft has relatively small ballast pockets. Similarly, a raft loaded to capacity with crew becomes increasingly unstable as the occupants are removed and winched aboard the helicopter. The survivors should sit on the roof and on the inflated support arch to decrease the amount of surface exposed to the downdraft. The strongest persons in the raft should be evacuated last.

The raft may also be used as an intermediate rescue platform between the distressed vessel and the helicopter. This is especially useful if the boat's mast and rigging interfere with the positioning of the helicopter or threaten to entangle the basket hoist. In this situation the raft is allowed to drift downwind attached to the distressed vessel by a line. The helicopter pilot cannot see the raft directly below. The winch operator therefore guides the rescue operation. When being winched up by cable and harness, follow directions to secure yourself properly, and keep on your life jacket. With an integrated safety harness and inflatable life vest, it is much easier to put on the helicopter's rescue harness when not encumbered by a bulky life vest. It may be preferable to leave the vest uninflated when being hoisted from the ship.

The helicopter has enormous potential for safe and effective SAR. The new H-60 Jayhawk can fly 300 nautical miles offshore, remain on scene for 45 minutes, hoist up to six people on board, and return to base at 140 knots. Use this form of evacuation judiciously, especially if it is for transfer of sick or injured victims. Communicate medical data accurately so that the appropriate method of evacuation is selected. The C-130 Hercules is the largest of the U.S. Coast Guard SAR fleet, with a range in excess of 1000 miles. It can air drop an enormous amount of lifesaving equipment, including dewatering pumps, life rafts, and survival and signaling equipment. The most recognizable airplane is the Falcon jet. This medium-range, fast-response plane flies at 350 knots and has a 2000-nautical-mile range. Sophisticated onboard electronics, including infrared scanners and surface search radar, allow the jet to fly a variety of search patterns on autopilot.

SUGGESTED READINGS

Are dangerous objects lying ahead? *Ocean Voyager* 74:19, 1996.

Armstrong R: The current, *Soundings* 36:4, 1999.

Auerbach PS, Donner HJ, Weiss, EA: *Field guide to wilderness medicine,* St Louis, 1999, Mosby.

Bailey M, Bailey M: *117 days adrift,* Dobbs Ferry, NY, 1997, Sheridan House.

Bernon B: When it all goes wrong, *Cruising World* 23:5, 1997.

Biewenga B: How to access the latest weather information, *Cruising World* 21:71, 1995.

Boating statistics—1994 to 1997: US Coast Guard.

Boyd W: Doctor on call, *Ocean Voyager* 97:52, 1999.

Braden T, editor: Chartroom chatter, *Ocean Navigator* 93:5, 1996.

Braden T, editor: Chartroom chatter: floating hazards threaten yacht, *Ocean Navigator* 94:8, 1998.

Braden T, editor: Chartroom chatter: dying of thirst? Try turtle blood, *Ocean Navigator* 98:8, 1999.

Brandt RP: *Survival at sea,* Boulder, Colo, 1994, Paladin Press.

Brown J: Trial by storm, *Cruising World* 24(10), 1998.

Buchanan A: Interview: a Sydney-Hobart survival story, *Sailing* 33:14, 1999.

Callahan S: *Adrift: seventy-six days lost at sea,* Boston, 1986, Houghton.

Cargal M: *The captain's guide to life raft survival,* Dobbs Ferry, NY, Sheridan House.

Carlin D: Best medical books, *Ocean Navigator* 82:79, 1997.

Carr M: Understanding waves, *Sail* 29:38, 1998.

Cayard P: Learn to expect the worst: Sydney-Hobart, *Seahorse International Sailing,* March 1999.

Center for the Study and Practice of Survival: *A practical guide to lifeboat survival,* Annapolis, Md, 1997, Naval Institute Press.

Chapman piloting, ed 62, New York, 1996, Hearst Marine Books.

Chisnell M: *Risk to gain,* Stockholm, 1998, Bokförlaget Max Ström Skeppsholmen.

Clemmetsen A: *GMDSS for small craft,* West Sussex, UK, 1997, Fernhurst Books.

Containers float! *Ocean Navigator* 76:8, 1996.

Coote JH: *Total loss,* Dobbs Ferry, NY, 1996, Sheridan House.

Craighead FC, Craighead JJ: *How to survive on land and sea,* Annapolis, Md, 1984, Naval Institute Press.

Darcy M : Lightning protection, *Cruising World,* April 1994.

Date S: Passagemaking: weather on a budget, *Sail* 27:30, 1996.

Day G: Single sideband: don't leave home without it, *Cruising World* 21:63, 1995.

Diels J et al: Investigating electricity in the sky, *Sci Am* 277:50, 1997.

Dove T: Making the cellular connection, *Sail* 27:28, 1996.

Edles P: Stoves that go to sea, *Sail* 26:72, 1995.

Efficacy of a portable acustimulation device in controlling seasickness, *Aviat Space Environ Med* 66:1155, 1995.

Electronics and the voyager, *Ocean Voyager* 74:50, 1996.

Flame alarms: firebuoy vs flameseeker, *Practical Sailor* 21:8, 1994.

Flannery J: Mitch's toll, *Soundings,* January 1999:10.

Focus on IMO, *Proc Marine Safety Council,* 54:62, 1997.

Forgey W: *Wilderness medicine,* Merrillville, Ind, 1994, ICS Books.

Fox J: Man overboard! *Cruising World* 20:73, 1994.

Frederiksen P: Safety net, *Yachting* 185:28, 1999.

Giles D: Hell in the Bass Strait, *Sailing* 33:56, 1999.

Gill PG: *The onboard medical handbook,* Camden, Me, 1997, International Marine.

Greenwald M: *Survivor,* San Diego, 1995, Blue Horizons Press.

Herzog C: Building skills: rules of the road, *Sail* 30:20, 1999.

Houghton D, Sanders F: *Weather at sea,* Camden, Me, 1988, International Marine.

Howe RF: The deep end of the sea, *Time* 153: 60, 1999.

Hu S et al: P6 acupressure reduces symptoms of vection-induced motion sickness, *Aviat Space Environ Med* 66:631, 1995.

Huck MV: *Lightning and boats: a manual of safety and prevention,* Brookfield, Wisc, 1995, Seaworthy Publications.

Huck MV: Living with lightning, *Sail* 29:24, 1998.

Huff R, Farley M: *Sea survival: the boatman's emergency manual,* Blue Ridge Summit, Pa, 1989, Tab Books.

Husick C: Electronics: using radar, *Sail* 29:36, 1998.

Husick C: AT&T ends its SSB-phone link, *Cruising World* 25:18, 1999.

Johnson D, Smith J: Red sky at night, *Cruising World* 21:31, 1995.

Kaufman J: Watermarkers reduce water supply worries, *Ocean Voyager* 97:35, 1999.

Knox S: After a knockdown, *Ocean Navigator* 95:64, 1999.

Lee ECB, Lee K, editors: *Safety and survival at sea,* London, 1990, Greenhill Books.

Lembo E: Cell phone's for chat, not trouble, *Cruising World,* February 1999:12.

Leonard B: Commonsense cruising: cooking on the move, *Sail* 30:63, 1999.

Lightning protection, *Practical Sailing,* December, 1993.

Linskey T: What really happened to Melinda Lee, *Sail* 30:82, 1999.

Lundy D: *Godforsaken sea,* Toronto, 1998, Knopf.

Marquez GG: *The story of a shipwrecked sailor,* New York, 1989, Vintage International.

McAllister D: Cold water: friend or foe? *Cruising World* 20:77, 1994.

McDowell JS: Take a look inside a thunderstorm, *Cruising World* 23:27, 1997.

McKenna L: The schedule method of collision avoidance, *Ocean Navigator* 87:34, 1998.

Medical resources, *Ocean Voyager* 97:58, 1999.

Mellor J: You can learn to pilot through fog, *Cruising World* 21:57, 1995.

Meurn RJ: *Survival guide for the mariner,* Centreville, Md, 1997, Cornell Maritime Press.

Minick J: Talkin' about a revolution in the way we communicate, *Cruising World* 22:66, 1996.

More on lightning protection, *Practical Sailing,* June 1994.

Mundle R: A black day, *Seahorse International Sailing,* March 1999.

Mundle R: Hell and high water: Sydney-Hobart, *Sailing World* 38:26, 1999.

Murphy T: Shoreline, *Cruising World* 25:8, 1999.

Olton T: Overcoming fear at sea, *Sail* (26):75, 1996.

Payson H: Abandoned ship, *Sail* 29:16, 1998.

Queeney T: Automation is key for VHF marine operators, *Ocean Navigator* 79:17, 1997.

Robertson D: *Survive the savage sea,* London, 1973, Elek Books.

Ross B: Racing: Sydney-Hobart, *Sail* 30:74, 1999.

Rousemaniere J: *Fastnet force 10,* New York, 1980, Norton.

Safety at sea, *Cruising World* 22:58, 1996.

Sherman E et al: Electronics review, *Cruising World* 25:74, 1999.

Taking the hurricane threat more seriously, *Ocean Voyager* 74:10, 1996.

Textor K: Downloads for daysailors, *Sail* 29:30, 1998.

The end of self reliance? *Ocean Voyager* 74:50, 1996.

Tilton B: Health, *Paddler* 13:28, 1993.

Trimmer JW: *How to avoid huge ships,* Centreville, Md, 1994, Cornell Maritime Press.

$200 lightning detection device? *Practical Sailor* 22:14, 1996.

von Haeften D: *How to cope with storms,* Dobbs Ferry, NY, 1997, Sheridan House.

Waters J: *A guide to small boat emergencies,* Annapolis, Md, 1993, Naval Institute Press.

Watts A: Understanding airmasses, *Sail* 28:32, 1997.

Watts A: Weather: windshifts, *Sail* 28:60, 1997.

Watts A: *Instant weather forecasting,* Dobbs Ferry, NY, 1998, Sheridan House.

West G: Communications: single-sideband channels, *Sail* 28:36, 1997.

Williams M: *The boater's weather guide,* Centreville, Md, 1990, Cornell Maritime Press.

Willis C, editor: *Rough water: stories of survival from the sea,* New York, 1999, Balliett & Fitzgerald/Thunder's Mouth Press.

Worsley FA: *Shackleton's boat journey,* New York, 1977, Norton.

Wright CH: *Survival for yachtsmen,* Glasgow, 1985, Brown, Son & Ferguson.

Travel, Environmental Hazards, and Disasters

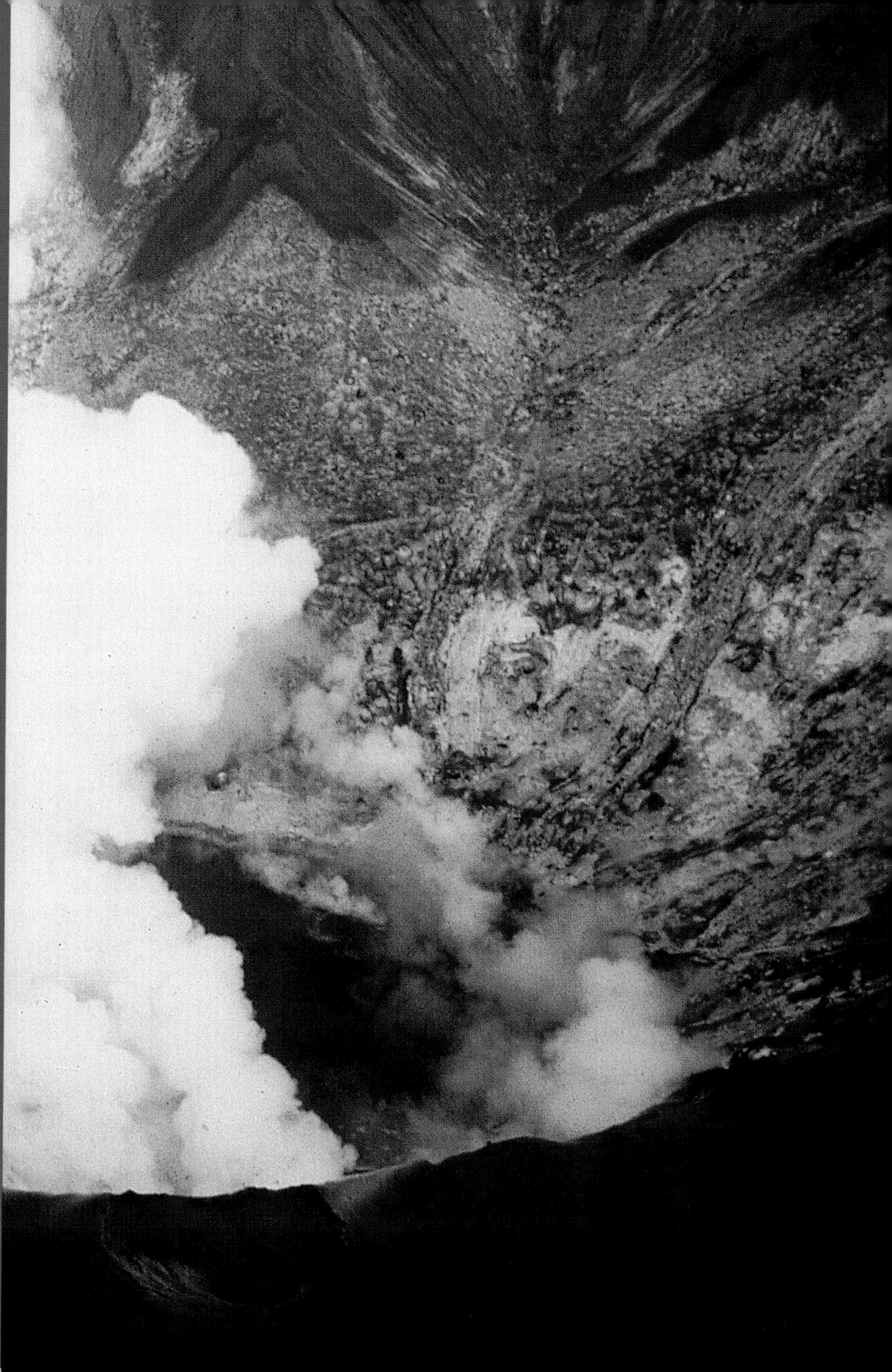

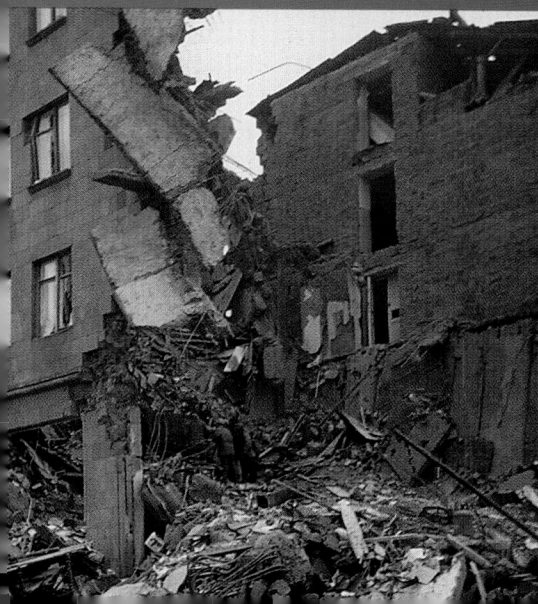

10

65 Travel Medicine

Elaine C. Jong

International travelers have unique health needs based on a person's underlying health, purpose of the trip, style of travel, and geographic destination. When individuals and groups travel to foreign locales to participate in wilderness and outdoors activities, exposure to unfamiliar people, food, sanitation, and environments may have a deleterious effect on health and interfere with the purpose and enjoyment of the trip. The multidisciplinary specialty of travel medicine uses selected principles from the fields of public health, infectious diseases, tropical medicine, and environmental and wilderness medicine, integrated with geographic and chronologic data, to formulate an approach to health risk assessment for a given journey. This chapter serves as a basic introduction to travel medicine and focuses on public health and communicable diseases. Closely related topics are covered extensively in other chapters in this book.

SOURCES OF INFORMATION

A publication of the Centers for Disease Control and Prevention (CDC), *Health Information for International Travel* (the "yellow book"), is the authoritative source of information on travel medicine and is updated annually. Two other periodicals published by the CDC and available by subscription, the *Morbidity and Mortality Weekly Report* (MMWR) and *Summary of Health Information for International Travel* (the "blue sheet," published biweekly), provide updated information on the status of worldwide disease outbreaks and changes in health conditions. However, the best way to obtain current and reliable travel health information, including vaccine requirements, malaria chemoprophylaxis, and disease outbreaks for various regions of the world is to consult the CDC Database of Health Information for International Travel website (*www.cdc.gov/travel.index.htm*). This website also contains links to the U.S. State Department Consular Information Sheets, for nonmedical information of interest to the traveler.

Professional societies, foundations, and private publishers are additional sources of telephone advice, topical brochures and information sheets, newsletters containing information on travel medicine topics, schedules of travel medicine meetings and continuing education courses, and other information, including lists of travel medicine clinics in the United States and abroad and English-speaking physicians worldwide. A list of resources for travel medicine information is given in the Appendix at the end of the chapter.

Standard textbooks on infectious diseases and tropical medicine and a number of monographs on travel medicine provide in-depth information on travel medicine–related subjects; many of these resources are listed in the suggested readings at the end of the chapter. A number of computer-based interactive programs for travel medicine clinics are commercially available. They are not listed here because the software and vendors are rapidly changing; the best sources of current information on travel medicine software are published reviews and "hands-on" demonstrations at medical and scientific meetings.

American travelers abroad who experience an emergency of any sort should contact the nearest U.S. consulate or embassy or call the U.S. Department of State Citizen's Emergency Center (see Appendix). If an extended stay in a given country is planned, the Citizen's Emergency Center suggests that the traveler register with the consulate or embassy shortly after arrival in the country.

Travelers should ascertain several months in advance of departure whether their regular health insurance policy covers the costs of treatment and hospitalization for illness or injuries occurring abroad, and the costs of emergency medical evacuation back to the United States, if necessary. Medicare usually covers only health care expenses arising in the United States and its territories. Some credit card services provide worldwide medical referrals and arrangements for emergency transportation for their cardholders but do not actually cover the costs incurred. What the traveler needs is a short-term health insurance policy that specifically covers medical expenses and medical evacuation during foreign travel. Depending on the insurer, chronic medical conditions may be excluded, or covered only if they are certified to be under control for 60 to 90 days before departure. Travelers more than 70 years old may find it more difficult to get medical insurance of this kind.

TRAVEL HEALTH RISK ASSESSMENT

Pretravel medical preparation appropriate for a given traveler and trip is determined by a review of the geographic destinations, duration of the trip, style of travel, purpose of the trip, underlying health of the traveler, and access to medical care during the trip (Box 65-1). In this context, immunizations, malaria chemoprophylaxis, traveler's diarrhea, and parasitic infections must be addressed. Prevention and treatment of common ailments such as jet lag, motion sickness, sun exposure, altitude illness, insect bites, and animal bites should be reviewed. Some attention should be given to personal safety, sexually transmitted diseases, prevention of motor vehicle injury, and emergency medical evacuation. Information about the level of sanitation and environmental hazards at the destinations can be used to identify special health concerns in tropical climates and areas of extreme weather conditions, high altitude, or aquatic activities.[38,39]

Multiple destinations in several countries and travel lasting more than 3 weeks both tend to increase the complexity of the medical preparation with regard to vaccination and malaria recommendations. In addition, the content of the travel medical kit becomes more inclusive as a greater number of health needs over time are anticipated. The style of travel is an important factor in travel risk assessments. Travelers staying in urban air-conditioned hotels or well-developed resorts have less exposure to mosquitoes carrying malaria and other diseases than those living among residents in small villages or camping. If accommodations in malarious areas are likely to be in unscreened rooms, travelers should plan to take with them portable bed nets and insect repellents against mosquitoes and other biting insects. The purpose of the trip is another factor that influences exposure of the traveler to potential health hazards. Teachers, students, missionaries, relief workers, agricultural consultants, field biologists, and adventure travelers are more likely than persons on standard tourist packages and business travelers to be exposed to endemic infectious diseases transmitted by the local residents (such as hepatitis B, tuberculosis, and meningitis), insect borne diseases (such as malaria, yellow fever, leishmaniasis, filariasis, plague, and ty-phus), and diseases associated with animal exposure (such as rabies, leptospirosis, and anthrax).

All travelers, however, should be cautioned about the infectious hazards of sexual activity with new partners during travel, especially with commercial sex workers in host countries. Gonorrhea and chlamydia are common in the industrialized world and also have a worldwide distribution. Other sexually transmitted diseases, such as human immunodeficiency virus (HIV) infection, syphilis, chancroid, and lymphogranuloma venereum, are more prevalent in the developing world.[36,45]

Although surveys and case reports of returned travelers confirm that attention to vaccine-preventable diseases (e.g., diphtheria, measles, polio, hepatitis, typhoid fever, and cholera) and exotic infectious diseases (e.g., malaria, schistosomiasis, leishmaniasis, and trichinosis) is appropriate, the importance of the traveler's underlying health and accidental injuries must also be emphasized.* Cardiovascular diseases, motor vehicle accidents, and injuries accounted for more morbidity and mortality among American travelers and expatriates than did infectious diseases.[28,29]

Most international travelers should begin pretravel medical preparation 4 to 6 weeks before the date of departure so immunization schedules can be adequately spaced and appropriate medications and special supplies can be obtained (Table 65-1). Although the medical preparation for an international trip may be straightforward for people in good health, advance planning and consultation with a travel medicine expert are recommended for people with allergies, special health needs (pregnancy, infancy, advanced age, handicaps), or chronic or underlying health conditions (such as cardiovascular disease, respiratory conditions, compromised immune status, diabetes, renal failure, organ transplants, and seizure disorders).

---

*References 4, 7, 8, 12, 13, 25, 31, 33, 48, 58, 63, 71.

Box 65-1 APPROACH TO MEDICAL PREPARATION FOR TRAVEL

TRAVEL INFORMATION

Geographic itinerary (countries in order of travel)
Month(s) and duration of travel in each country
Urban versus rural travel
Style of travel (hotel or resort versus hut or camping)
Purpose of travel
Access to medical care during travel

PERSONAL HEALTH

General health status
Allergies to drugs and vaccines

PERSONAL HEALTH—cont'd

Age and weight
Pregnant or lactating
Impaired immune response resulting from disease,
    medications, or treatment
Medications taken on a regular basis
History of previous immunizations
Medical or physical conditions requiring special care

Modified from Jong EC: *Med Clin North Am* 76:1277, 1992.

TABLE 65-1. Vaccine Interactions

VACCINE	INTERACTION	PRECAUTION
Immune globulin	Measles/mumps/rubella (MMR) vaccine	Give these vaccines at least 2 wk before immune globulin (IG) or 3-5 mo after IG, depending on dose received
Oral typhoid vaccine	Antibiotic therapy	Do not take antibiotics concurrently
Oral typhoid vaccine	Mefloquine malaria chemoprophylaxis	Schedule an interval of at least 8 hr between oral typhoid dose and mefloquine dose
Oral typhoid vaccine	Oral polio vaccine	Oral polio vaccine (OPV) should not be taken at same time as OTV; OPV can be given 7-10 days before or 10-14 days after OTV
Rabies vaccine (HDCV) intradermal series	Chloroquine malaria chemoprophylaxis	Complete rabies vaccine (intradermal series) at least 3 wk before starting chemoprophylaxis with chloroquine; use rabies vaccine intramuscular series if 3-wk interval is not possible
Virus vaccines, live (MMR, OPV, yellow fever vaccine)	Other live virus vaccines	Give live virus vaccines on same day, or separate doses by at least 1 mo
Virus vaccines, live (MMR, OPV, yellow fever vaccine)	Tuberculin skin test (PPD)	Do skin test on same day as receipt of a live virus vaccine, or 4-6 wk after, because virus vaccines can impair the response to PPD skin test
Yellow fever	Cholera vaccine	Give the two vaccines on same day or at least 3 wk apart

From Jong EC: Immunizations for international travelers. In *The travel medicine advisor,* Atlanta, 1993, American Health Consultants.

IMMUNIZATIONS FOR TRAVEL

Immunizations may be divided into three categories: routine, required, and recommended.[38] Primary vaccine schedules and booster intervals are given in Tables 65-2 and 65-3. The international traveler should have all current immunizations recorded in *The International Certificates of Vaccination* as approved by the World Health Organization (WHO), a document in booklet form printed on yellow paper.[37] The booklet has a special page for official validation of the yellow fever vaccine. Recent copies of the document (after 1988) do not contain a separate page for cholera vaccine validation because the WHO officially removed cholera vaccination from the International Health Regulations in 1973. If given, the cholera vaccination can be recorded in the space provided for "Other Vaccinations" in the newer booklets. In general, live virus vaccines and attenuated bacterial vaccines are contraindicated during pregnancy and in persons with altered immunocompetence.[15]

Required Travel Immunizations

The required immunizations refer to those regulated by the WHO. Yellow fever vaccine may be required for entry into member countries according to current WHO regulations. Smallpox vaccine and cholera vaccine are no longer required for international travel according to WHO regulations.

Yellow Fever Vaccine. Yellow fever is a viral infection transmitted by *Aedes aegypti* mosquitoes in equatorial South America and Africa. The endemic zones are shown in Figure 65-1. The yellow fever (YF) vaccine is a live attenuated viral vaccine that is highly immunoprotective (YF Immune, Connaught). The YF vaccine is given as a single dose for primary immunization; the booster interval is 10 years. The vaccine is contraindicated in infants less than 4 months of age because of the age-related risk of encephalitis after immunization. If possible, YF immunization should be delayed until the infant is 9 months of age or older. The vaccine is generally not recommended during pregnancy except when travel to a highly endemic area cannot be avoided or postponed by the pregnant traveler and the risk of the actual disease is thought to be greater than the theoretical risk of adverse effects from the vaccine.

Additional contraindications to receiving the vaccine include immunosuppression caused by underlying disease (e.g., malignancy, HIV infection, congenital immune deficiency) or by medical therapy (e.g., corticosteroids, cancer chemotherapy, radiation therapy, organ transplant therapy). The vaccine virus is cultured in eggs and is contraindicated in persons with a history of severe allergy to eggs (anaphylaxis). The package insert contains instructions for skin-testing persons with an uncertain history of allergy to eggs.

If a person for whom the vaccine is contraindicated must travel to a country where yellow fever vaccine is

TABLE 65-2. Dosage Schedules for Routine Immunizations

VACCINE	PRIMARY SERIES	BOOSTER INTERVAL
Diphtheria and tetanus toxoids and pertussis vaccine adsorbed (DTP) (use in children <7 yr old)	4 doses* IM of vaccine: first 3 doses given 4-8 wk apart; dose 4 given 6-12 mo after dose 3	Booster at 4-6 yr of age
Haemophilus B conjugate (Hib conjugate vaccines are not considered interchangeable for the primary immunization series)		
PRP-HbOC	3 doses* IM or SC at 2, 4, 6 mo	Booster at 15 mo
PRP-OMP	2 doses* IM or SC at 2, 4 mo	Booster at 15 mo
PRP-D, PRP-HbOC, or PRP-OMP	1 dose* IM or SC at 15 mo up to 5th birthday	None
Hepatitis B (Engerix B) (accelerated schedule)	3 doses at 0, 30, and 60 days (1 ml IM in deltoid area)	4th dose is recommended at 12 mo if still at risk for hepatitis B exposure
Hepatitis B (Engerix B or Recombivax) (standard schedule)	3 doses at 0, 1, and 6 mo (1 ml IM in deltoid area)	Need for booster not determined
Influenza virus	1 dose* IM or SC annually	
Measles/mumps/rubella (MMR)†	1 dose* SC at 15 mo of age or older	Boost measles vaccine at school age; boost measles vaccine *once* in adult life before international travel for people born after 1957 and before 1980
Pneumococcus (23-valent)	1 dose* SC	None (see text)
Poliomyelitis, enhanced inactivated (E-IPV) (killed vaccine, safe for all ages)	Give doses* 1 and 2 SC or IM 4-8 wk apart; give dose 3 6-12 mo after dose 2; give dose 4 to children 4-6 yr of age	Give dose *once* to persons (all ages) before travel in areas at risk
Poliomyelitis, oral (OPV) (attenuated live virus)†	Give doses* 1 and 2 po 6-8 wk apart; give dose 3 at 6 wk after dose 2 (customarily at 8-12 mo after dose 2); give dose 4 to children 4-6 yr of age	Give dose *once* to people less than 18 yr before travel in areas of risk
Tetanus and diphtheria toxoids adsorbed (Td) (for children >7 yr of age and for adults)	3 doses (0.5 ml SC or IM), doses 1 and 2 given 4-8 wk apart, dose 3 6-12 mo later	Routine booster dose every 10 yr

Modified from Jong EC: Immunizations for international travelers. In *The travel medicine advisor*, Atlanta, 1993, American Health Consultants.
IM, Intramuscularly; *SC*, subcutaneously.
*See manufacturer's package insert for recommendations on dosage.
†May be contraindicated in patients with any of the following conditions: pregnancy, leukemia, lymphoma, generalized malignancy, immunosuppression from HIV infection or treatment with corticosteroids, alkylating drugs, antimetabolites, or radiation therapy.

required for entry, a signed statement on letterhead stationery that the yellow fever vaccine could not be given to the traveler because of medical contraindications will be accepted in lieu of the vaccination statement, according to WHO regulations.

Cholera Vaccine. The injectable cholera vaccine in current use is not highly efficacious, even when the primary series of two doses given a week or more apart is received. The WHO no longer endorses a requirement for this vaccine for entry into any country. Nonetheless, some countries still require a cholera vaccine for travelers arriving from cholera-endemic areas.[26] If this situation is anticipated, a single cholera dose should meet this requirement and should be recorded in the traveler's *International Certificates of Vaccination* (see earlier discussion).

Travelers going to cholera-endemic or cholera-epidemic areas are encouraged to follow food and water precautions to prevent all forms of travel-associated diarrhea. A new oral cholera vaccine is presently available in Western Europe and Canada (Orachol, Swiss Serum Institute; Mutachol, Berna). At present, there are no standardized recommendations for use of this vaccine, although health care workers and relief workers going to outbreak areas might be suitable candidates.

TABLE 65-3. Dosage Schedules for Travel Immunizations

VACCINE	PRIMARY SERIES	BOOSTER
Cholera (parenteral)	2 doses 1 wk or more apart (0.5 ml SC or IM); pediatric dose 0.3 ml for 5-10 yr of age, 0.2 ml for 6 mo-4 yr of age	6 mo
Hepatitis A, inactivated	3 doses given at 0, 1, and 6-12 months	None recommended
Immune globulin (hepatitis A protection)	1 dose IM in gluteus muscle (2-ml dose for 3 mo protection; 5-ml divided dose for 5 mo); pediatric dose 0.02 ml/kg for 3-mo trip, 0.06 ml/kg for 5-mo trip	Boost at 3- to 5-mo intervals depending on initial dose received
Japanese encephalitis	3 doses given on days 0, 7, and 30 (1 ml SC ≥3 yr old; 0.5 ml SC <3 yr old)	Booster dose may be given after 2 yr
Meningococcus (A/C/Y/W-135)	1 dose* SC	None (variable immunogenic response in children <4 yr of age: revaccination for this group recommended after 2-4 yr for those who continue to be at high risk).
Plague	1st dose (1 ml IM); 2nd dose (0.2 ml IM) 4 wk later; dose 3 (0.2 ml IM) 3-6 mo after dose 2	Boost if risk of exposure persists: give first 2 booster doses (0.1-0.2 ml) 6 mo apart, then give 1 booster dose at 1- to 2-yr intervals as needed
Rabies, human diploid cell vaccine (HDCV)	3 doses (0.1 ml ID) on days 0, 7, and 21 or 28	Boost after 2 yr or test serum for antibody level (must not use chloroquine prophylaxis until 3 wk after completion of ID vaccine series)
Rabies (HDCV, RVA, or PCEC)	3 doses (1 ml IM in the deltoid area) on days 0, 7, and 21 or 28	Boost after 2 yrs or test serum for antibody level
Tick-borne encephalitis	3 doses given SC on days 0, 30, and 180 days	Boost at 3- to 5-year intervals
Tuberculosis (BCG vaccine)†	1 dose percutaneously with multiple-puncture disk; half strength for infants <1 mo old	Revaccination after 2-3 mo in those who remain tuberculin negative to 5 TU skin test
Typhoid, whole-cell parenteral	2 doses (0.5 ml SC or IC) 4 or more wk apart; pediatric dose (<10 yr old) 0.25 ml	Boost after 3 yr for continued risk of exposure
Typhoid Ty21A, oral	1 capsule po every 2 days for 4 doses (>6 yr old)	5 yr
Typhoid Vi Polysaccharide	1 dose SC*	2 yr
Yellow fever†	1 dose (0.5 ml SC); pediatric dose 0.5 ml SC for >6 mo old	10 yr

Modified from Jong EC: Immunizations for international travelers. In *The travel medicine advisor*, Atlanta, 1993, American Health Consultants.
ID, Intradermally; *IM*, intramuscularly; *po*, orally; *SC*, subcutaneously.
*See manufacturer's package insert for recommendations on dosage.
†Caution, may be contraindicated in patients with any of the following conditions: pregnancy, leukemia, lymphoma, generalized malignancy, immunosuppression from HIV infection or treatment with corticosteroids, alkylating drugs, antimetabolites, or radiation therapy.

Some practitioners recommend that travelers to cholera endemic areas who have underlying gastric conditions, such as achlorhydria or partial gastric resection, either of which may increase susceptibility to cholera infection, be immunized with cholera vaccine.

Smallpox Vaccine. Although the last case of smallpox acquired through natural transmission was reported in 1977 and the requirement for smallpox vaccine for international travel was removed from the WHO regulations in 1982, health care providers still receive sporadic inquiries about smallpox vaccine. The vaccine is no longer available commercially. Limited supplies are released on a case-by-case basis from the CDC based on individual review. Research scientists and health care workers who work with the smallpox and closely related viruses are candidates for immunization.[14]

Recommended Travel Vaccines

The recommended vaccines are those given to travelers depending on the travel health risk assessment. Vaccines in this category include those for hepatitis A, hepatitis B, typhoid fever, meningococcal meningitis, Japanese encephalitis B virus, and rabies. Immuniza-

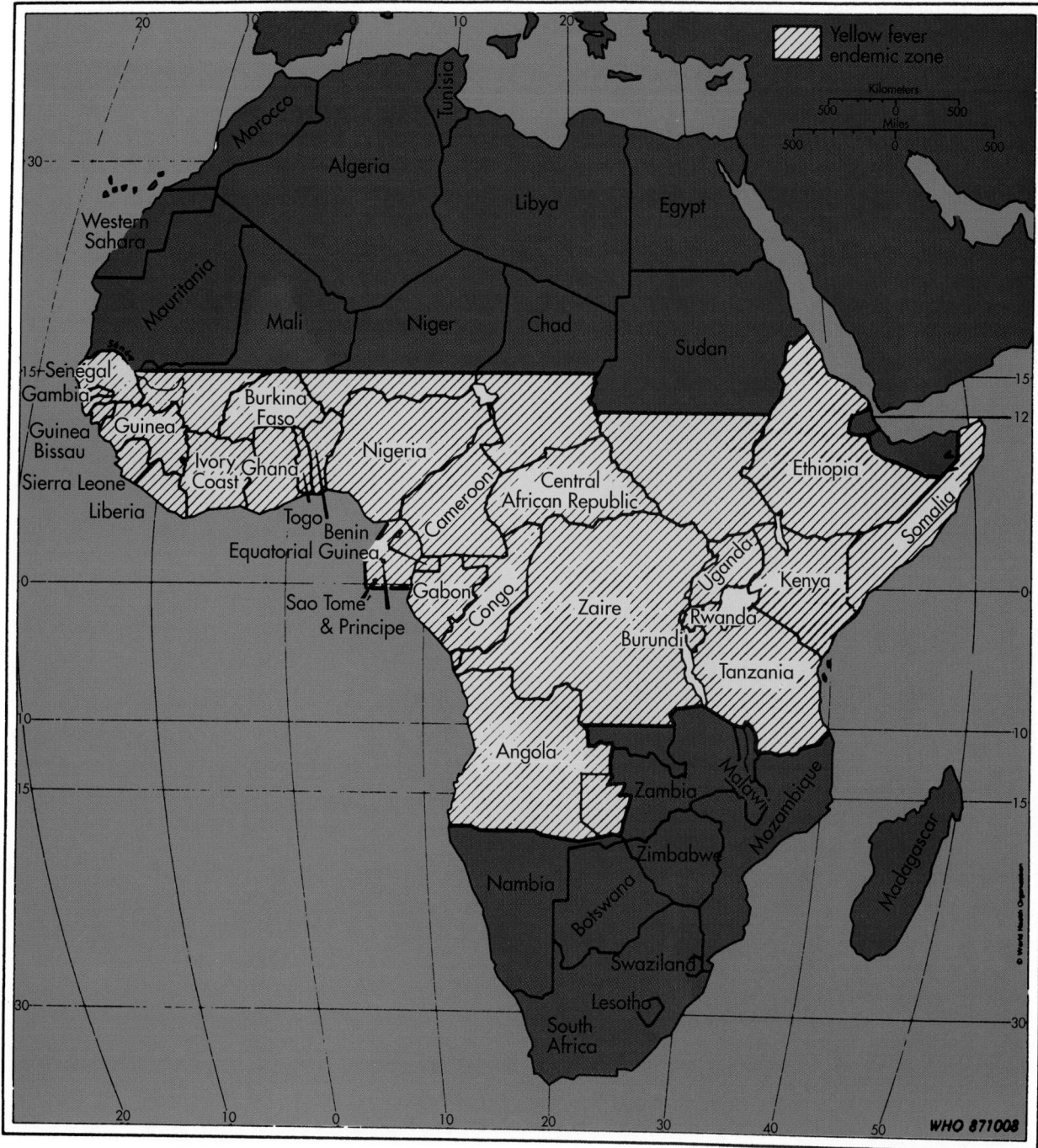

Figure 65-1 Yellow fever endemic zones. (*From Centers for Disease Control:* Health information for international travel, 1999-2000, *Washington, DC, 1999, US Government Printing Office.*)

Continued

tion against tick-borne encephalitis and tuberculosis (bacillus Calmette-Guerin [BCG] vaccine), or a tuberculosis skin test (purified protein derivative [PPD]), may also be recommended for some travelers. The vaccine against plague is associated with a prolonged immunization schedule and is not readily obtained. Persons at risk are usually prescribed a standby regimen of antibiotic treatment.

Hepatitis A Vaccine. Hepatitis A is the leading vaccine-preventable disease among international travelers to the developing world. Hepatitis A is a serious viral infection with a transmission similar to polio, cholera, typhoid, and traveler's diarrhea (i.e., fecal contamination of food and water). Although up to 60% of adults over 40 years of age from industrialized countries may have immunity to hepatitis A through clinical or sub-

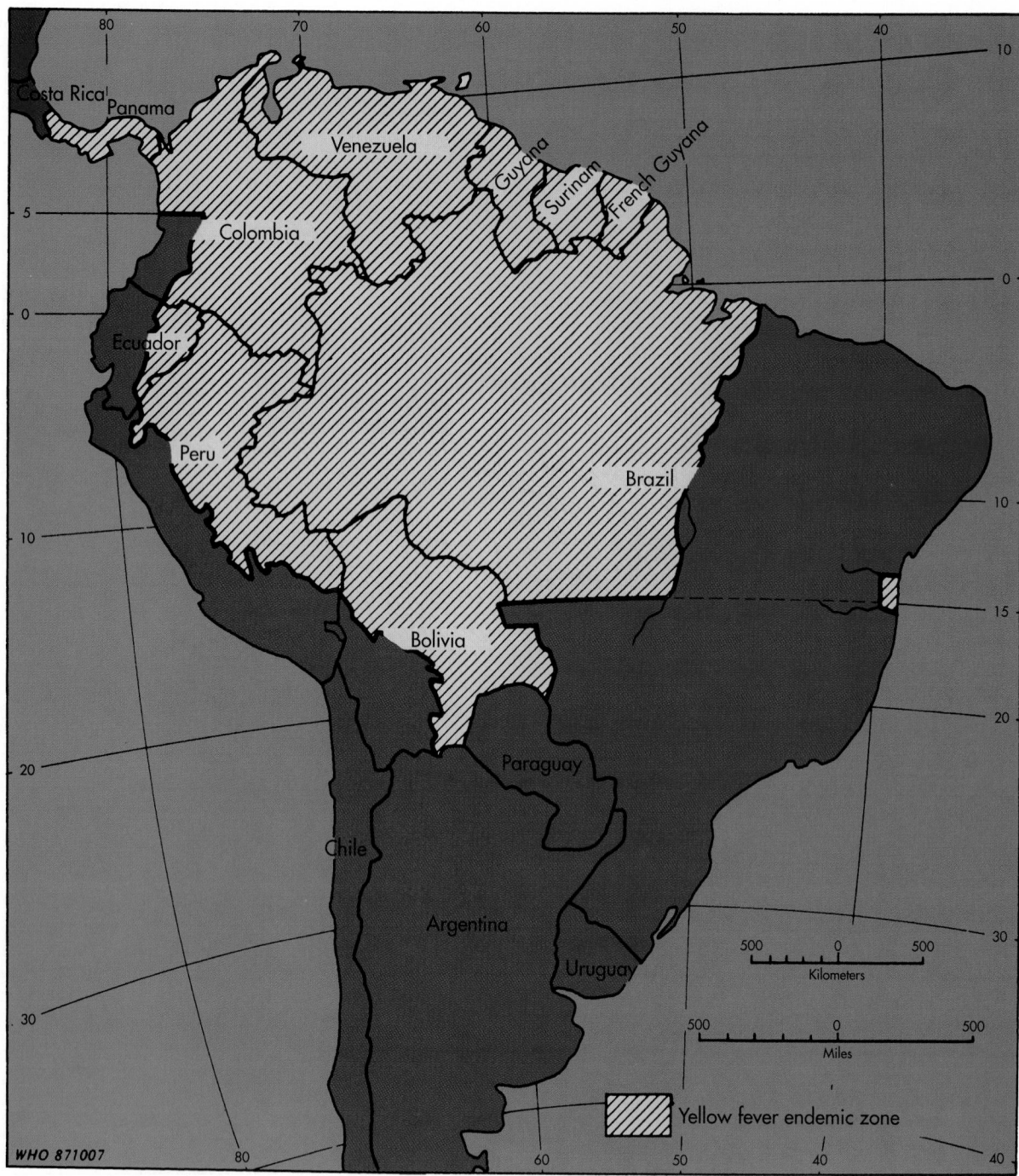

Figure 65-1, cont'd See legend on p. 1559 *(From Centers for Disease Control: Health information for international travel, 1999-2000, Washington, DC, 1999, US Government Printing Office.)*

clinical infection, most travelers less than 40 years old are susceptible.[49] (For more information, see the CDC website: *www.cdc.gov/nicidod/diseases/hepatitis*.) Adventure travelers who venture off usual tourist routes may be at increased risk compared with other groups of travelers. Two new hepatitis A inactivated viral vaccines became licensed in the United States during the 1990s: Havrix (SmithKline Beecham) in 1994 and

VAQTA (Merck) in 1996. Both vaccines are safe, efficacious, and produce long-lasting immunity. Each vaccine is given by intramuscular injection into the deltoid muscle. Within 2 to 4 weeks after the first hepatitis A vaccine dose, 98% to 99% of vaccine recipients develop protective levels of antibodies. A second dose, constituting a booster dose, is given 6 to 18 months after the first dose (according to package directions), and based on mathematical modeling, it will elicit immunity lasting approximately 15 to 20 years.

Protection against hepatitis A can be obtained from immune globulin (gamma globulin) containing preformed antibodies against hepatitis A. Depending on dosage, 0.02 mL to 0.06 mL/kg body weight given by deep intramuscular injection into the gluteus maximus creates 3 to 5 months' protection respectively from this passive form of immunization. If time allows, a serum test for hepatitis A antibody should be performed in people who travel frequently, who are of foreign birth, or who are over age 40; unnecessary immunization may be avoided if a person has protective antibodies from an inapparent hepatitis A infection in the past.

Hepatitis B Vaccine. Hepatitis B vaccine was added to the list of vaccines recommended for routine immunization of children in the United States in 1991.[10,17] However, American adults who are at high risk for exposure to hepatitis B infection because of occupation, personal activities (travel, close contact with infected people, institutionalization), or medical treatment with blood or blood-derived products are also targeted for immunization.

In many parts of Asia and Africa, up to 15% of the general population may be asymptomatic carriers of hepatitis B virus. Travelers to countries in Asia and Africa who will live and work among the residents, such as missionaries, volunteer relief workers, teachers, students, adventure travelers, and other travelers who might have intimate or sexual contact with the residents, should consider immunization against hepatitis B.

Two recombinant vaccines are available, Recombivax (Merck) and Engerix B (SmithKline Beecham). The standard dosage for both vaccines consists of injected doses at 0, 1, and 6 months. Engerix B vaccine has an approved accelerated dosage schedule of 0, 1, and 2 months. This may allow full immunization of a traveler with limited time before departure; however, a booster dose at 12 months is recommended if risk of infection continues.[10,13] A combined hepatitis A and hepatitis B vaccine (Twinrix, SmithKline Beecham) is available in Western Europe and Canada. This vaccine is pending Food and Drug Administration (FDA) approval and release in the United States.

Typhoid Fever Vaccine. The incidence of typhoid fever among American travelers is relatively low (58 to 174 cases per 1 million travelers), but among reported cases in the United States, 62% were acquired during international travel.[58] Mexico, Peru, India, Pakistan, and Chile are countries in which the risk of transmission appears particularly high. Sub-Saharan Africa and Southeast Asia are also regarded as areas of increased risk for typhoid fever.

Avoidance of potentially contaminated food and drink during travel is important, even if the typhoid vaccine is received. The parenteral heat-phenol-inactivated whole-cell typhoid vaccine requires two doses given by injection 4 weeks apart for primary immunization, and a booster dose after 3 or more years. The protection against typhoid fever afforded by immunization with the parenteral whole cell vaccine ranges from 51% to 76%. The vaccine has been associated with troublesome side effects; most recipients complain of soreness at the injection site, headache, low-grade fever, and general malaise for 1 or 2 days after immunization.

The use of the parenteral whole-cell typhoid vaccine has been mostly supplanted by use of either of two modern typhoid vaccines, the oral Ty21A typhoid vaccine (Vivotif, Berna) and the parenteral purified Vi polysaccharide typhoid vaccine (Typhim Vi, Pasteur Merieux Connaught). The oral typhoid vaccine contains a live attenuated strain of *Salmonella typhi* bacteria (Ty21A). The vaccine is in capsule form and is recommended for individuals 6 years of age and older. Both the primary and booster immunization consist of a series of four capsules, one taken every other day over the course of a week. The booster interval is 5 years. A liquid suspension form of this vaccine is expected in the near future; this will facilitate administration of the vaccine to young children and to others who have difficulty swallowing capsules. Persons who have previously received the parenteral whole-cell typhoid vaccine and who now desire immunization with the oral vaccine should receive the full four-capsule series because only limited data on alternative regimens are available. Although protection rates of 43% to 96% were reported in field trials with the oral live-attenuated typhoid vaccine among residents of endemic areas, limited data are available for protection rates in people from nonendemic areas who travel to endemic areas.[8]

The purified Vi polysaccharide typhoid vaccine consists of a single dose given by injection, and the booster interval is 2 years in the United States (3 years in Canada and abroad). The vaccine may be used in persons 2 years of age and older, and has an efficacy range in clinical field trials similar to that observed for the oral typhoid vaccine. The purified Vi polysaccharide typhoid vaccine is preferred for persons who have difficulties with swallowing capsules, who have a limited time before departure (10 days), who may be poorly compliant with the multidose outpatient regimen for oral typhoid vaccine, or who have a medical condition that is a contraindication for taking the live attenuated oral Ty21A typhoid vaccine.

Meningococcal Vaccine. Vaccine protection against meningococcal meningitis is recommended for people going to countries or regions where outbreaks have been reported. Meningococcal vaccine is required for travel to Saudi Arabia during the time of the annual religious pilgrimage (the hajj) to Mecca in late spring. The vaccine is also recommended for people going to live and work in certain areas of Africa (sub-Saharan) and South America (Brazil), where outbreaks of the disease are frequent among the residents.

Meningococcal polysaccharide vaccine (Menomune, Aventis) is a quadrivalent vaccine inducing immunity against serogroups A, C, Y, and W-135. A single dose appears to provide immunity for at least 3 years. Vaccine efficacy is variable in young children, and a second dose of vaccine after 2 or 3 years is recommended for children living in high-risk areas who received the first vaccine dose at less than 4 years of age.

Japanese Encephalitis Virus Vaccine. Japanese encephalitis (JE) is a viral infection transmitted by *Culex* mosquitoes in Asia and Southeast Asia. Transmission is year round in the tropical and subtropical areas and during the late spring, summer, and early fall in temperate climates. Pigs and some species of birds are natural reservoirs of the virus, whereas the mosquito vectors breed extensively in flooded rice fields and irrigation projects. JE virus is not considered a risk for short-term travelers visiting the usual tourist destinations in urban and developed resort areas. For visitors to rural areas during the transmission season, the estimated risk for JE during a 1-month period is 1:5000, or 1:20,000 per week.[16]

The risk of infection can be greatly decreased by personal measures that prevent mosquito bites: wearing protective clothing, using insect repellents, and sleeping under bed nets. Nonetheless, because JE has been acquired by short-term travelers to endemic rural areas, and agricultural projects bordering on urban areas can bring infected mosquitoes into the proximity of susceptible urban dwellers, the vaccine should be offered to travelers going on trips of any length to rural areas (especially areas of pig farming), and to expatriate workers, missionaries, and students who plan to live in endemic areas.[68]

An inactivated viral vaccine (JE Vax, Biken, licensed and distributed in the United States by Connaught) consisting of three doses given by injection over the course of a month is available for administration to travelers determined to be at significant risk. A schedule consisting of doses at 0, 7, and 30 days appears to result in a higher seroconversion rate and geometric mean titer of antibody among recipients than does a 2-week accelerated schedule consisting of doses at 0, 7, and 14 days.[3,16,56,68] A booster dose of vaccine may be given 2 to 3 years after the primary immunization for continued risk of exposure.

Adverse reactions to JE vaccine include local pain and swelling at the injection site in about 20% of recip-

ients, systemic symptoms (fever, headache, malaise, rash) in about 10% of recipients, and hypersensitivity reactions (mainly urticaria, angioedema, or both) in 15 to 62 per 10,000 American vaccinees. The hypersensitivity reactions reported occurred after the first, second, or third dose of vaccine, either almost immediately afterward or with delays of up to 2 weeks after receipt of the vaccine dose. Limited data suggest that persons who have had urticarial reactions to *Hymenoptera* envenomation and to other stimuli might be at greater risk of JE vaccine–induced hypersensitivity reactions. The CDC recommends that vaccinees be directly observed for 30 minutes after receipt of JE vaccine and that they not depart on their travel until 10 days after the last dose, so that delayed adverse reactions can be detected and treated.[16]

Rabies Vaccine. Animal bites, especially dog bites, present a potential rabies hazard to international travelers who travel to rural areas in Central and South America, the Middle East, Africa, and Asia.[11,70] Preexposure rabies immunization is recommended for rural travelers, especially adventure travelers who go to remote areas, and for expatriate workers, missionaries, and their families living in countries in which rabies is a recognized risk.

There are three modern tissue culture–derived inactivated virus rabies vaccines available in the United States for preexposure and postexposure immunization: human diploid cell vaccine (HDCV) (RabImmune, Aventis), rabies vaccine adsorbed (RVA) (Michigan Department of Public Health, distributed by SmithKline Beecham), and purified chick embryo cell vaccine (PCEC) (RabAvert, Chiron). Preexposure rabies immunization consists of three doses (1.0 mL each) of tissue culture–derived vaccine given over the course of 1 month by intramuscular injection into the deltoid muscle. The usual booster interval for rabies vaccine is 2 years; however, if time permits, serologic testing may show persistence of protective levels of antibody and therefore the booster dose may be delayed to 3 or even 4 years after the last dose on the basis of annual testing. This sparing of vaccine doses received could be beneficial to recipients who have a long-term need for protection (veterinarians, field biologists, laboratory workers, and expatriates living in high-risk areas). The three vaccine preparations are considered interchangeable for booster doses.

Only the HDCV vaccine has an intradermal (0.1-ml dose) injection preexposure immunization schedule approved by the FDA. The smaller doses used for the intradermal series are less expensive than the intramuscular doses, but the intradermal series requires advance planning; vaccine efficacy is compromised if chloroquine prophylaxis against malaria is started within 3 weeks after the third dose of intradermal vaccine.[55] If there is not sufficient time before departure, one of the intramuscular vaccines should be given.

Mild local reactions to rabies vaccine are common and consist of erythema, pain, and swelling at the injection site. Mild systemic symptoms—headache, dizziness, nausea, abdominal pain, and myalgia—may develop in some recipients. In approximately 5% of people receiving booster doses of HDCV for preexposure prophylaxis and in a few receiving postexposure immunization, a serum sickness-like illness characterized by urticaria, fever, malaise, arthralgias, arthritis, nausea, and vomiting may develop 2 to 21 days after a vaccine dose is received. The RVA vaccine is derived from virus grown in tissue culture cells in medium free of human albumin and is not associated with a serum sickness-like vaccine-associated reaction. The RVA vaccine is approved for intramuscular administration only. Data are accumulating on the incidence of reactions after immunization with this preparation. The PCEC vaccine is also prepared from tissue culture cells in medium free of human albumin.

For postexposure rabies immunization, see Chapter 44.

Tick-Borne Encephalitis Vaccine.

Tick-borne encephalitis (TBE) is a viral disease spread by ticks in Europe (Austria, the Czech Republic, Slovakia, Germany, Hungary, Poland, and Switzerland) and the newly independent states of the former Soviet Union during the months of April through August. TBE is transmitted to humans by bites from infected *Ixodes ricinus* ticks, usually found in forested areas of endemic regions. However, systemic infection after ingestion of unpasteurized dairy products from infected cows, goats, or sheep can also occur.[50]

Vaccination against TBE is not available in the United States. An inactivated TBE vaccine manufactured by Immuno (Vienna, Austria) is available in Europe and in Canada. The vaccine is produced in chick embryo cell cultures; primary immunization consists of three doses given by subcutaneous injection over 6 months. The limited availability of the vaccine and the relatively long immunization schedule mean that most travelers from North America who anticipate a need for protection against TBE will not be able to obtain the vaccine. An inactivated TBE vaccine, Encepur, manufactured by Chiron (Behring, Germany) has a rapid immunization schedule, with primary doses given on 0, 7, and 21 days, with booster doses at 12 to 18 months and at 3 to 5 years. This vaccine is not currently available in North America.[3,50]

Travelers planning outdoor activities (hiking, biking, camping) in areas where TBE is endemic need to rely on personal measures to prevent tick bites. They should wear protective clothing when outdoors, use insect repellents containing *N,N*-diethyl-meta-toluamide (DEET) on exposed areas of skin, and treat their outer clothing with a permethrin-containing insecticide. All travelers to such areas should be advised to avoid ingestion of unpasteurized dairy products.

Tuberculosis (BCG Vaccine).

Persons going on short trips for tourism or business to countries in which tuberculosis is much more common among the general population than in the United States are not considered to be at great risk of contracting this infection, which is commonly spread from person to person by inhalation of infected respiratory droplets in closed environments. However, travelers who will live among foreign residents or who will work in foreign orphanages, schools, hospitals, or other facilities may be at significant risk of exposure to infection with tuberculosis. Such travelers should be skin tested with tuberculin (PPD) and control antigens (such as *Candida* and *Trichophyton*) before the trip, and afterward if the original test was negative. People who convert to test positivity on the skin test can be treated with isoniazid or other drugs to prevent tuberculosis.[6]

The BCG vaccines around the world were originally derived from in vitro attenuation of a bovine tubercle bacillus (*Mycobacterium bovis*) strain in the early 1900s in France. Subsequently, the organisms have been maintained by several laboratories under varying conditions, so currently available vaccines are not considered microbiologically identical. The BCG vaccines are used widely all over the world for childhood immunization against tuberculosis, although this has never been a public health policy in the United States. There is no consensus on the protective efficacy of BCG vaccines, and estimates of protection have varied from study to study. BCG strain differences, regional differences in mycobacterial ecology, and differences in trial methods have all contributed to the observed variation in studies of vaccine efficacy.[6,24]

Epidemiologic data suggest that the vaccine may be more useful in protecting children from disseminated extrapulmonary complications of tuberculosis than in protecting adults from primary pulmonary infection. Persons immunized with BCG vaccine test positive on PPD skin tests for many years afterward, regardless of the degree of protection conferred by the vaccine. As a result, the PPD skin test cannot be used as a reliable indicator of infection in recipients, and this situation can contribute to a delay in diagnosis in people who have contracted tuberculosis infection despite BCG vaccination.

Occasionally, children in families going abroad for extended residence are requested by the receiving country to provide proof of BCG vaccination to qualify for a visa. A BCG vaccine is commercially available in the United States and is approved by the American Academy of Pediatrics Committee on the Control of Infectious Diseases for use in children going to live in areas in which tuberculosis is prevalent or there is a likelihood of exposure to adults with active or recently arrested tuberculosis. The vaccine is also recommended for children of tuberculous mothers. The vaccine might be considered appropriate in the case of uninfected (PPD skin test negative) health care workers who are going to work in areas where there is a high endemic prevalence of tuberculosis in the population and who will have limited access to medical diagnosis and treatment.[6] Like other live attenuated vaccines, BCG vaccine is contraindicated in people with immunosuppression caused by congenital conditions, chemotherapy, radiation therapy, HIV infection, or another condition resulting in impaired immune responses. Pregnancy is considered a relative contraindication.[15]

Plague Vaccine. Plague, a bacterial disease caused by *Yersinia pestis,* is enzootic among wild rodents in countries of Africa, Asia, and the Americas. Plague is transmitted to humans by fleas or direct contact with infected animals. Person-to-person spread is common through respiratory secretions. International travelers following on standard tourist itineraries to countries in which plague is reported are unlikely to be at risk. Persons who are at high risk of exposure include field biologists and persons who plan to work or camp in rural mountainous or upland areas, where avoidance of rodents and fleas is difficult.

Plague vaccine is a killed bacterial vaccine with poorly documented protective efficacy. Primary immunization consists of three doses of vaccine given by intramuscular injection over 10 months. Side effects include pain, redness, and induration at the site of injection. Systemic symptoms consisting of fever, headache, and malaise may occur after repeated doses. An alternative to plague vaccination is the use of prophylactic tetracycline (500 mg by mouth four times a day) during periods of active exposure to plague-infected animals or humans. The efficacy of using tetracycline prophylaxis is unproven by controlled clinical trial, but inferred from use of the drug in the treatment of plague.

Routine Immunizations

Routine immunizations are those customarily given in childhood and updated in adult life, usually regardless of travel.[13,17] The assessment of immunization needs for international travel provides an opportunity for individuals to receive "missed" booster doses of the routine immunizations. This is a special concern among middle-aged and older people.[34,40]

The routine vaccines currently recommended in childhood include those against tetanus, diphtheria, pertussis, measles, mumps, rubella, poliovirus, *Haemophilus influenzae* type b (Hib), and hepatitis B.[13,17] After 7 years of age, booster doses for tetanus, diphtheria,

measles, and poliovirus are given as indicated below. The recommendation for universal pediatric immunization against hepatitis B is relatively recent (see previous section on hepatitis B vaccine).[10] Recommendations for immunization against viral influenza and pneumococcal pneumonia are based on underlying health and age.

Tetanus and Diphtheria Vaccine. The tetanus/diphtheria vaccine (Td) is used for primary immunization and booster doses in older children and adults. Booster doses of Td vaccine given at 10-year intervals throughout life are recommended to maintain immunity. The diphtheria-pertussis-tetanus vaccine is used for immunization of children less than 7 years of age and contains different proportions of the tetanus and diphtheria vaccine antigens than those present in Td.[9,13]

Poliomyelitis Vaccine. Poliomyelitis vaccine is usually not boosted after childhood in the United States, except for anticipated high-risk exposure through work or travel to areas in which polio is endemic or epidemic. Although the risk of polio transmission is greatest in the developing countries, sporadic outbreaks have occurred in industrialized countries among unvaccinated subpopulations, usually religious groups.

A combination of two inactivated (killed) virus polio vaccine (IPV) doses and two attenuated live-virus oral polio vaccine (OPV) doses, or an all-IPV regimen is recommended for a primary immunization series given before 18 years of age. IPV is recommended for primary immunization and for booster doses in people 18 years of age and older because of a higher risk of complications associated with OPV in older patients.[13]

Measles, Mumps, and Rubella Vaccine. A single dose of measles, mumps, and rubella (MMR) vaccine is recommended for all infants at 15 months of age. The Immunization Practices Advisory Committee recommends a second dose of measles vaccine in childhood on entry into grade school, middle school, or high school; this is required by law in many states. Also, persons born after 1957 should receive a second dose of measles vaccine. The second dose of measles vaccine is usually administered as MMR vaccine.[13,17] MMR vaccine is a live attenuated virus preparation, and it is contraindicated in pregnancy and in persons with compromised immunity. Transmission of naturally-occurring measles is higher among populations in developing countries than in the United States, thus travelers are at higher risk of exposure.

Haemophilus Influenzae B Vaccine. The risk for invasive *H. influenzae* disease, including meningitis, is greatest in children less than 7 years old, and the infection is common among children in the developing world. Primary immunization is recommended at 2 months of age or as soon as possible thereafter. Three different conjugate vaccines are commercially available against *H. influenzae* type b (Hib). The vaccines contain the antigenic polyribosyl-ribitol (PRP) moiety conjugated to a carrier protein. Two doses of PRP-OMP vaccine, or three doses of HbOC vaccine given 2 months apart, are recommended for all children less than 12 months of age. After 12 months of age, a single dose of either vaccine is sufficient for immunization. The third Hib conjugate vaccine, PRP-D, is approved for use only in children 15 months or older and is given as a single dose.

Influenza Vaccine, Pneumococcal Vaccine. Annual immunization against viral influenza is recommended for all people over 65 years of age. Influenza vaccine is also recommended for groups of persons at increased risk from complications of viral influenza. These persons include those with chronic respiratory disease (emphysema, asthma), ischemic heart disease, transplanted organs, renal failure, and impaired immune response from congenital conditions, acquired illness, or immunosuppressive therapy. The 23-valent polysaccharide vaccine against pneumococcal pneumonia consists of a single dose and is recommended for the same groups. A booster dose at 3 to 5 years after the initial dose is recommended for certain risk groups.[13]

In addition to the elderly and ill, this vaccine is also recommended for all health care workers and for international travelers, because prolonged air travel and exposure to crowded or extreme environments predispose them to respiratory infections.

Malaria

Malaria is a mosquito-transmitted, blood-borne, parasitic infection present throughout tropical and developing areas of the world, including Mexico, Haiti, Central and South America, Africa, the Middle East, the Indian subcontinent, Asia, Southeast Asia, and Oceania (Figure 65-2). The estimated worldwide incidence of malaria is 280 million cases per year. Approximately 1000 cases per year are reported in the United States to the CDC. Although the risk to travelers is relatively low compared with other medical problems (e.g., diarrhea, respiratory problems) in travelers, malaria infection causes a severe febrile illness that is potentially fatal.

Four species of malaria commonly cause disease in humans: *Plasmodium vivax* (worldwide distribution), *P. falciparum* (worldwide distribution), *P. ovale* (western Africa), and *P. malariae* (worldwide distribution). The protozoan malaria parasites are transmitted by female *Anopheles* mosquito vectors, which tend to bite between dusk and dawn.

The incubation period for malaria is usually 1 or more weeks after the mosquito injects malaria sporozoites into the human host during a blood meal. The malaria parasites incubate, then multiply in hepatocytes. The infected hepatocytes rupture, releasing thousands of malaria merozoites into the bloodstream. The merozoites invade circulating red blood cells (RBCs) and develop into the next developmental stage, trophozoites. Ring-shaped trophozoites within RBCs can be seen on peripheral blood smears, as can later parasite stages: schizonts (asexual reproduction) or male and female gametocytes (sexual reproduction). Diagnosis of malaria is based on

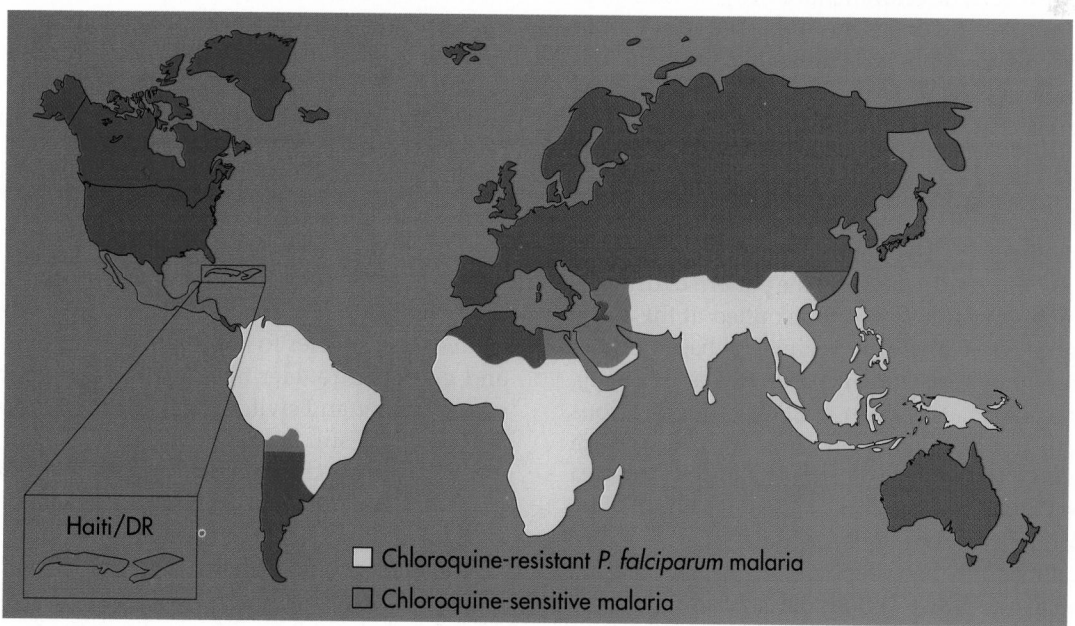

Haiti/DR

☐ Chloroquine-resistant *P. falciparum* malaria
☐ Chloroquine-sensitive malaria

Figure 65-2 Map of worldwide malaria transmission. (*From Centers for Disease Control:* Health information for international travel, 1999-2000, *Washington, DC, 1999, US Government Printing Office.*)

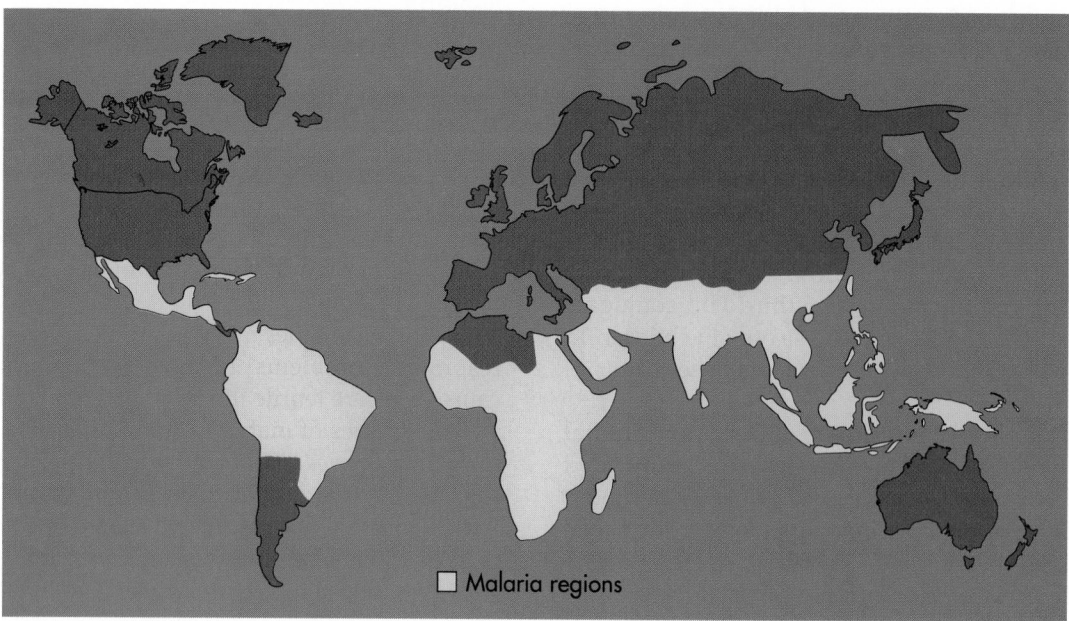

Figure 65-3 Malaria regions of the world.

recognition of characteristic trophozoites, schizonts, and gametocytes on peripheral blood smears. Schizonts rupture, releasing new crops of merozoites that can infect other RBCs. Male and female gametocytes are taken up by the female mosquito during a blood meal and propagate infection in the mosquito.[35,73]

Malaria Chemoprophylaxis. Travelers to malarious areas are usually prescribed one of several drug regimens to prevent malaria (chemoprophylaxis). However, in *P. falciparum* strains, development of drug resistance to chloroquine and other drugs has made the selection of appropriate chemoprophylaxis difficult for certain high risk destinations.[35,41,43,72] Drug allergies, contraindications, drug toxicity, drug interactions, underlying medical conditions, access to recommended drugs, and compliance with recommended regimens all contribute to the problem.[2,46,54,69]

Selection of malaria chemoprophylaxis is determined by the geographic destination and the pattern of drug resistance among malaria strains transmitted at the destination (Figure 65-3). The drug regimen is based on the risk of chloroquine-resistant falciparum malaria (CRPF). Chloroquine phosphate (Aralen, and others) is efficacious and relatively nontoxic in the few areas in which malaria is still sensitive to the drug, currently Central America west of the Panama Canal Zone, Mexico, Haiti, the Dominican Republic, and most of the Middle East. Chloroquine resistance has been reported in Yemen, Oman, Saudi Arabia, and Iran. Mefloquine (Lariam), doxycycline (Vibramycin, and others), and atovaquone/proguanil (Malarone) are considered the drugs of choice for malaria chemoprophylaxis in CRPF areas; however, in some places, such as certain border areas in Thailand where CRPF strains have developed resistance to mefloquine, doxycycline or atovaquone/proguanil are recommended for prophylaxis against CRPF.[35,47,72,73] Chloroquine-resistant *P. vivax* has been reported in Irian Jaya and Sumatra, Indonesia, and Papua, New Guinea.[1,59,61] Mefloquine, doxycycline, or atovaquone/proguanil chemoprophylaxis recommended for the CRPF present in these areas is also adequate for resistant *P. vivax*. Primaquine phosphate is considered another effective alternative for prevention of CRPF, providing that a glucose-6-phosphate-dehydrogenase (G-6-PD) screening test can be done before prescribing, since the drug causes severe hemolytic anemia in G-6-PD–deficient individuals. Doses and schedules for drugs commonly used in malaria chemoprophylaxis are given in Table 65-4.

Travelers should start taking antimalarials (chloroquine or mefloquine) with a weekly dosing regimen at least 1 or 2 weeks before departure. This allows time for familiarity with the side effects of the drug while the drug builds up to steady-state levels in the body, enables the traveler to habituate to the timing of doses, and gives the traveler time to contact his or her health care provider and switch to an alternative drug, if necessary, while still at home. Antimalarial drugs with a daily dosing schedule (doxycycline, atovaquone/proguanil, or primaquine phosphate) can be started 1 to 2 days before entering the area of malaria risk.

Travelers should be warned not to switch antimalarial regimens during the trip without the specific advice of a knowledgeable health care provider. Casual advice given by travelers from other countries or recommendations by personnel in foreign drugstores in which

TABLE 65-4. Malaria Chemoprophylaxis*

DRUG	DOSE
ADULTS	
Chloroquine phosphate (Aralen)	250 mg, 2 tablets/wk
	500 mg, 1 tablet/wk
Mefloquine (Lariam)	250 mg, 1 tablet/wk
Doxycycline (Vibramycin)	100 mg, 1 tablet daily
Atovaquone/proguanil (Malarone)†	250 mg/100 mg, 1 tablet daily
Primaquine phosphate	30 mg base daily
Proguanil (Paludrine) (in addition to weekly chloroquine)	100 mg, 2 tablets/day
CHILDREN	
Chloroquine phosphate	8.3 mg/kg/wk po
Mefloquine	15-19 kg: ¼ tablet/wk po
	20-30 kg: ½ tablet/wk po
	31-40 kg: ¾ tablet/wk po
Proguanil (Paludrine) (in addition to weekly chloroquine)	<2 yr: 50 mg/day po
	2-6 yr: 100 mg/day po
	7-10 yr: 150 mg/day po
	>10 yr: 200 mg/day po
Atovaquone/proguanil (Malarone Pediatric)†	62.5 mg/25 mg,
	11-20 kg: 1 Malarone Pediatric tablet daily
	21-30 kg: 2 Malarone Pediatric tablets daily
	31-40 kg: 3 Malarone Pediatric tablets daily
	>40 kg: 4 Malarone Pediatric tablets daily (equal to 1 Malarone tablet [250 mg/100 mg])

From Jong EC, McMullen R: *The travel and tropical medicine manual,* ed 2, Philadelphia, 1995, WB Saunders.
*See general remarks and precautions in the text.
†Malarone product information, Glaxo Wellcome Inc., Research Triangle Park, NC, July 2000.

many antimalarial drugs are available over the counter should not be the basis for medication changes.

The usual incubation periods for malaria are 8 to 11 days for *P. falciparum,* 10 to 17 days for *P. vivax* and *P. ovale,* and 18 to 40 days for *P. malariae.* Prolonged latent incubation times of up to 3 years or more have been reported rarely, especially with the *P. malariae* species. Among cases reported in Americans, over 90% of *P. falciparum* infections and 50% of *P. vivax* infections cause clinical attacks during the first 4 to 8 weeks after return from a malaria area. Current recommendations are that chloroquine, mefloquine, and doxycycline chemoprophylactic regimens should be continued for 4 weeks after the traveler leaves a malaria area to prevent attacks of malaria in the immediate posttravel period. Atovaquone/proguanil should be continued for 7 days after leaving a malaria area, and primaquine should be taken for 2 days after leaving; both drugs appear to have activity against latent incubating hepatic stages of the malaria parasites.

Rapidly developing drug resistance among malarial parasites worldwide means that no current antimalarial drug regimen can be considered to provide complete protection. Use of personal insect precautions (repellents, protective clothing, and bed nets) and behavioral modification (limiting time outdoors) are two important adjuncts to malaria chemoprophylaxis.

Some regimens against CRPF recommended by experts are not licensed or available in the United States; even if these are not standard recommendations, the alternative regimens may be considered in special cases. For instance, mefloquine is not recommended for use in the first trimester of pregnancy, and doxycycline is contraindicated for use in pregnant women. Although mefloquine may be used in weight-adjusted dosages in children weighing less than 15 kg, doxycycline is not recommended for children less than 8 years of age. Atovaquone/proguanil is not recommended during pregnancy due to lack of data (pregnancy category C) and is not recommended for use in children less than 11 kg. In travelers unable to take any of these drugs, a combination of weekly chloroquine plus daily proguanil may provide some protection (suboptimal) against CRPF, and this alternative regimen is considered safe in pregnant women and young children. Proguanil is not licensed or marketed in the United States and must be purchased abroad.

Another approach for travelers to CRPF areas who are unable to take the optimal chemoprophylactic drugs would be to take weekly chloroquine prophy-

TABLE 65-5. Malaria Drugs for Standby Treatment*

DRUG	ADULT DOSE	PEDIATRIC DOSE
Pyrimethamine 25 mg/ sulfadoxine 500 mg (Fansidar)	3 tablets po as single dose	2-11 mo: ¼ tablet 1-3 yr: ½ tablet 4-8 yr: 1 tablet 9-14 yr: 2 tablets >14 yr: 3 tablets po as single dose
Mefloquine, 250 mg tab (Lariam)	2 tablets as single dose, followed by 2 tablets after 8-12 hr; reduce second dose to 1 tablet for adults <60 kg	15 mg/kg po as single dose (do not use in infants <15 kg)
Atovaquone/proguanil, 250 mg/ 100 mg (Malarone)	4 tablets as a single dose daily for 3 consecutive days	11-20 kg: 1 tablet daily × 3 days 21-30 kg: 2 tablets as a single dose daily × 3 days 31-40 kg: 3 tablets as a single dose daily × 3 days >40 kg: 4 tablets as a single dose daily × 3 days
Quinine sulfate tablets	650 mg 3 times a day for 3 days (continue for 7 days in Southeast Asia)	10 mg/kg 3 times a day for 3 days (continue for 7 days in Southeast Asia)
Plus tetracycline	250 mg 4 times a day for 7 days	>8 yr of age: 5 mg/kg of body weight po four times a day for 7 days
Or plus doxycycline	100 mg twice a day po for 7 days	>8 yr of age: 2 mg/kg of body weight po twice a day for 7 days
Or plus clindamycin *Or* plus Fansidar	10 mg/kg three times a day for 5 days Fansidar dose above	10 mg/kg three times a day for 5 days Fansidar dose above
Halofantrine, 250 mg tab (Halfan)	2 tablets in one dose +2 tablets after 6 hr + 2 tablets after 6 more hr (total dose of 6 tablets in 12 hr); *repeat therapy in 7 days in nonimmune patients*	
Halofantrine, 2% suspension (Halfan)		8 mg/kg po for three doses, each dose 6 hr apart; *repeat therapy in 7 days in nonimmune patients*

Modified from Jong EC, McMullen R: *The travel and tropical medicine manual,* ed 2, Philadelphia, 1995, WB Saunders.
*See general remarks and precautions in the text.

laxis, use good personal insect precautions, and carry standby drug treatment for CRPF malaria (see later discussion). Chemoprophylactic regimens using proguanil plus sulfonamide, proguanil plus dapsone, and mefloquine plus sulfadoxine-pyrimethamine have been studied in areas in which there is intense transmission of multidrug-resistant falciparum malaria, but there are limited data about the efficacy and tolerance of these regimens in civilian travelers.[42,53,63]

Standby Drug Treatment For Malaria. In some cases a prescription for standby drug treatment for CRPF malaria, in addition to chemoprophylaxis, should be given to travelers, especially adventure and outdoor travelers going to remote areas known to have highly resistant strains of malaria. Standby drug treatment should also be given to other travelers who for any reason must take a regimen of malaria chemoprophylaxis that is suboptimal for the geographic region. Drugs and doses used for standby treatment of malaria are given in Table 65-5.

Travelers need to familiarize themselves with the signs and symptoms of the clinical illness so they can recognize a possible attack of malaria and treat themselves if necessary (Table 65-6). In case of an illness accompanied by high fever similar to a bad case of viral influenza, the traveler should seek immediate medical care. A traveler who becomes ill while remote from health care should be instructed to use standby malaria treatment as prescribed. Because of drug resistance among *P. falciparum* parasites from most malarious areas of the world, the standby treatment (regardless of which drug regimen is selected) may result only in temporary or partial improvement from a malaria attack, thus allowing evacuation from a distant area. However, further definitive treatment of malaria as soon as possible may be necessary to eradicate the infection.

TABLE 65-6. Clinical Illness in Malaria and Dengue Fever

SIGNS AND SYMPTOMS	MALARIA	DENGUE FEVER
Fever	+++	+++
Chills	+++	++
Headache	+++	+++
Malaise		++
Anorexia		++
Nausea, vomiting	++	++
Abdominal pain	++	
Myalgia	++	++
Arthralgia		++
Backache	+	
Dark urine	+	

+++, >90% of patients; ++, >50% of patients; +, <10% of patients.

Pyrimethamine plus sulfadoxine (Fansidar) is currently recommended by the CDC as a standby treatment for a malaria attack and can be used if the person is not allergic to sulfa drugs. Although serious and potentially fatal hypersensitivity reactions were reported in travelers taking this drug combination for CRPF prophylaxis on a weekly basis (1 case per 5000 to 8000 users), the remote risk of a significant adverse effect after taking a single treatment dose would be outweighed by the seriousness of an untreated CRPF attack. Thailand is reported to have a high prevalence of *P. falciparum* infections resistant to Fansidar, so other drugs should be considered for standby treatment of malaria acquired there.

Mefloquine may be used in treatment doses as a standby regimen if the traveler is not already taking mefloquine for malaria chemoprophylaxis. Serious adverse side effects, including seizures and cardiac arrest, have been reported rarely for mefloquine given at treatment doses, but again, the remote risk of a significant adverse effect after taking the drug in treatment doses would be outweighed by the seriousness of an untreated CRPF attack.[69] Mefloquine-resistant *P. falciparum* infections are being reported sporadically from countries in Southeast Asia and Africa but appear to be of most concern along the Thai-Burma (Myanmar) border.

Atovaquone/proguanil is highly efficacious in the treatment of acute, uncomplicated *P. falciparum* malaria and has been shown to be effective in areas where resistance to chloroquine, mefloquine, halofantrine, mefloquine, and amodiaquine is reported. It may be considered an alternative to Fansidar for emergency self-treatment of malaria especially in regions where *P. falciparum* strains are multi-drug resistant and are resistant to both Fansidar and mefloquine.

The regimen of oral quinine sulfate plus a second drug (tetracycline, doxycycline, clindamycin, or Fansidar) remains one of the most effective treatments for CRPF. However, this regimen should not be recommended to travelers as a standby treatment if other options are available. The development of cinchonism (ringing in the ears, headache, nausea, visual disturbance) from quinine is almost predictable during the first 3 days of treatment, and many travelers would be unable to complete the 7-day therapeutic quinine course (recommended for malaria acquired in Southeast Asia) in the field without medical assistance and supportive therapy.

Halofantrine, which is not presently available in the United States, is available in some countries of Western Europe, Africa, and Asia. Halofantrine is an effective oral drug for treatment of CRPF and Fansidar-resistant CRPF and may be prescribed as a standby treatment. The incidence of side effects is low. These include abdominal pain, pruritus, vomiting, diarrhea, headache, and rash. The drug is contraindicated in pregnant women because animal data show embryotoxic effects. Higher-than-conventional doses of halofantrine appear to be required for successful treatment of mefloquine-resistant *P. falciparum* strains being reported along the Thailand-Cambodia (Democratic Kampuchea) and the Thailand-Burma (Myanmar) borders. However, recent reports of cardiac conduction disturbances with prolongation of the PR and QT intervals on electrocardiograms of malaria patients treated with halofantrine, especially after mefloquine treatment failure, have raised concerns about the drug's safety.[54] Some experts recommend that physicians obtain a pretravel electrocardiogram from travelers who will be prescribed halofantrine standby treatment to document that there is no underlying conduction defect that might be exacerbated by the drug.

Qinghaosu (artemisinin) and its derivatives artemether, artesunate, and arteether are a group of antimalarial drugs derived from a Chinese medicinal herb, *qing hao*. The compounds have shown remarkable efficacy during clinical trials in the treatment of severe chloroquine-resistant falciparum malaria and can rapidly clear parasites without apparent significant toxicity. Artemisinin compounds are available for clinical use in China, Vietnam, and other malarious areas of Southeast Asia.[32]

Artesunate may be given by intravenous or intramuscular injection, artemether can be given by intramuscular injection only, and various artemisinin compounds are available for administration by mouth or by suppository. At the time of writing, dosage and toxicity parameters for the oral compounds are still under investigation, so the artemisinin compounds cannot be considered in the category of standby treatment for malaria. Travelers developing severe febrile illness in multidrug-resistant malarious areas of Asia who reach medical assistance might be treated effectively with artemisinin compounds, however.[32,35]

Personal Insect Precautions. Personal insect precautions are just as important as drugs for preventing malaria, especially if the traveler must take one of the suboptimal antimalarial drug regimens. Prevention of itching skin lesions caused by insect bites (and the possibility of secondary skin infections) and prevention of other insect-borne infections for which there are no prophylactic drugs or vaccines are other considerations. In regard to malaria prevention, exposure to mosquito vectors of malaria can be decreased by limiting time outdoors between dusk and dawn, by wearing protective clothing while outdoors, and by applying insect repellents to exposed areas of skin while outdoors.

The most effective insect repellents for skin application contain *N,N*-diethyl-meta-toluamide (DEET). Older formulations of repellents containing DEET depended on high concentrations and frequent applications to the skin for effectiveness. Concerns about DEET toxicity and the inconvenience of frequent applications led to development of repellent formulations that rely on new molecular entrapment technology to keep repellent chemicals on the surface of the skin for longer periods. It is claimed that newer insect repellents that have lower concentrations of DEET and a longer duration of adherence to the surface of the skin have decreased absorption through the skin. A wide variety of DEET-containing insect repellents are available commercially, and often may be sampled at sporting goods stores. If skin protection against the sun and insects must be used simultaneously, the sunscreen should be applied to the skin first, followed by the insect repellent.

Mosquito bed nets should be used when sleeping in unscreened rooms. The protection afforded by bed nets can be increased by application of a pyrethrum-based insecticide. Pyrethrums are insecticides related to naturally occurring alkaloids in the chrysanthemum plant family. Permethrin is a chemical derivative and is relatively nontoxic. Permethrin insecticides are suitable for treatment of external clothing and mosquito nets but are not recommended for direct skin application because they may induce skin hypersensitivity reactions.

Bed nets and external clothing can be treated by spraying or soaking with a permethrin solution and letting it air dry before use (Figure 65-4; Box 65-2). Treated bed nets and clothing retain residual insecticide activity for weeks (sprayed) to months (soaked).[62] In addition to repelling mosquitoes, permethrin insecticides are effective against gnats, ticks, chiggers, bedbugs, scorpions, centipedes, beetles, and flies (see Chapter 32). Permethrin insecticide coils and electric vaporizers can augment the use of bed nets indoors.

Dengue Fever. Dengue fever is a mosquito-transmitted viral infection that occurs worldwide in tropical and subtropical zones. The areas of dengue virus trans-

---

Box 65-2   PERMETHRIN-CONTAINING INSECTICIDES*

Permanone Tick Repellent: Contains permethrin in a pressurized spray can; repels ticks, chiggers, mosquitoes, and other bugs (Coulston International Corp., Easton, PA 18044)

Duranon Tick Repellent: Contains permethrin in a formula lasting up to 2 weeks; supplied in a pressurized spray can (Coulston International Corp., Easton, PA 18044)

PermaKill 4 Week Tick Killer: 13.3% permethrin liquid concentrate supplied in 8-oz bottle; can be diluted (⅓ oz permethrin concentrate in 16 oz water) to be used with a pump spray bottle, or be diluted 2 oz in 1½ cups of water to be used to impregnate outer clothing, bed nets, and curtains (see Figure 65-4) (Coulston International Corp., Easton, PA 18044)

Modified from Jong EC, McMullen R: *The travel and tropical medicine manual*, ed 2, Philadelphia, 1995, WB Saunders.
*Brand names are given for identification purposes only and do not constitute an endorsement.

---

mission overlap malaria endemic areas in many parts of the world, although the vector mosquitoes are different: *Aedes aegypti* and *Aedes albopictus*. An attack of dengue fever may be clinically indistinguishable from a malaria attack, especially as self-diagnosed by travelers in the field. Acute dengue fever is characterized by high fever, headache, and severe myalgias and arthralgias, similar to malaria. Thus if a traveler is stricken while in a malarious area with an illness accompanied by a high fever, he or she should be instructed to seek medical care for diagnosis and treatment of possible malaria, or to take standby drug treatment for malaria if remote from medical care. No specific treatment is recommended for dengue fever, but if the cause of the febrile illness is malaria, early medication with antimalarial drugs may be lifesaving.

The true incidence of dengue fever and other arboviral infections acquired by travelers abroad is not known because the stricken travelers may not have come to medical attention or have been accurately diagnosed. Many arboviral illnesses are mild and self-limited. However, diagnosis and treatment in returned travelers with a febrile illness who do seek medical attention can be hampered by limited diagnostic tools (serologic tests, cultures) and a lack of specific therapeutic agents.[3,5,45,68]

Of the more than 530 arboviruses registered in the International Catalogue of Arboviruses, more than 150 are known to infect humans. Effective vaccines are available for yellow fever, Japanese encephalitis, and tick-borne encephalitis. Vaccines for other arboviral infections have been produced but are limited to investi-

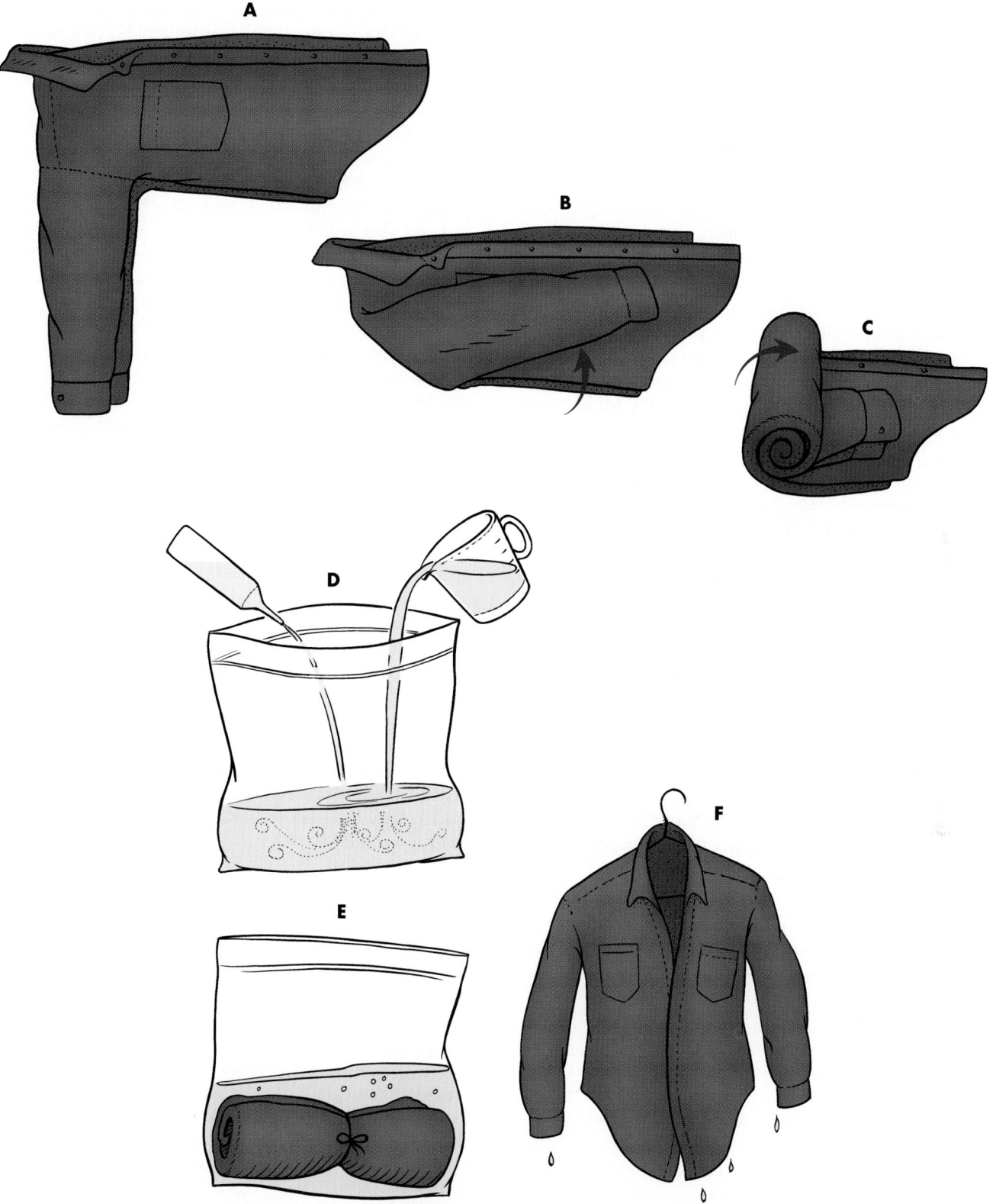

Figure 65-4   Technique for impregnating clothing or mosquito netting with permethrin solution. **A** to **C,** Lay jacket flat and fold it shoulder to shoulder. Fold sleeves to inside, roll tightly, and tie middle with string. For mosquito net, roll tightly and tie. **D,** Pour 2 oz of permethrin into plastic bag. Add 1 quart water. Mix. Solution will turn milky white. **E,** Place garment or mosquito netting in bag. Shut or tie tightly. Let rest 10 minutes. **F,** Hang garment or netting for 2 to 3 hours to dry. Fabric can also be laid on clean surface to dry. (*Redrawn from Rose S:* International travel health guide, *Northampton, Mass, 1993, Travel Medicine.*)

gational use. Personal behavior and practices that limit exposure to arthropod vectors (see earlier discussion of insect precautions) are important health measures for all travelers.

TRAVELER'S DIARRHEA

The term *traveler's diarrhea* usually refers to an acute syndrome of watery diarrhea, which may be accompanied by nausea, loss of appetite, abdominal cramps, low-grade fever, and malaise (see Chapter 52). The risk of traveler's diarrhea is high (20% to 50%) among short-term travelers going from industrialized areas and northern temperate zones to tropical and developing areas. The risk of traveler's diarrhea is high wherever food storage, fuel for cooking, and sanitation are inadequate. Latin America, the Caribbean, the Middle East countries, Africa, India, Asia, the South Pacific, and the newly independent states of the former Soviet Union are recognized high-risk areas for acquisition of traveler's diarrhea. Seasonal or climatic factors may also contribute to the risk of traveler's diarrhea.

Diarrhea associated with travel can result from any of multiple causes, including a change in the normal diet, food poisoning (toxins), and infection with viruses (rotavirus and Norwalk virus), bacteria (enterotoxigenic *Escherichia coli*, *Shigella*, *Campylobacter*, *Aeromonas*, *Salmonella*, and *Vibrio*, among others), and parasites (including *Giardia lamblia*, *Entamoeba histolytica*, and *Cryptosporidium*). The worldwide prevalence of *Cyclospora*, the recently described cyanobacterium-like microorganism, as a causative agent of traveler's diarrhea is unknown.[18,20,27]

Traveler's diarrhea usually runs a self-limited course lasting less than a week. In one study, only 8% to 15%

of persons had an episode of illness lasting longer than 1 week.[20] Recovery without antimicrobial treatment is usual in healthy adults; however, most travelers want to avoid the inconvenience and discomfort of diarrhea and ask for medications to terminate an attack as soon as possible. Dehydration from loss of fluids and decreased oral intake is the biggest risk to health, and young children and debilitated or older people are most susceptible to this complication.[20,23,30,65]

Food and water precautions recommended against traveler's diarrhea aim to decrease the risk of diarrhea from all possible causes. Antimicrobial therapy is directed against the bacterial pathogens implicated most often in cases of traveler's diarrhea. Presumably such antimicrobial therapy will not alter the course of illness if the cause is toxin, virus, or parasite. If the antimicrobial used for empirical treatment of traveler's diarrhea is active against the bacteria involved, a rapid recovery may be obtained.

Prevention Of Traveler's Diarrhea

Prevention of traveler's diarrhea can be divided into three categories: food and water precautions, bismuth subsalicylate prophylaxis, and antimicrobial prophylaxis (Table 65-7). Food and water precautions include drinking only disinfected water or bottled carbonated or canned beverages; eating well-cooked foods served piping hot, baked goods, or fruits with thick skins that can be peeled by the traveler; avoiding ice cubes in beverages; and not eating salads, raw or undercooked fish and shellfish, or cheese and dairy products made from unpasteurized milk. Despite good intentions, most travelers eventually face situations in which they have no choice but to eat and drink whatever is available.

TABLE 65-7. Prevention of Traveler's Diarrhea: Drug Regimens for Adults

DRUG	DOSAGE	COMMENTS
Bismuth subsalicylate (Pepto-Bismol)	2 tablets qid	Less effective than antibiotic prophylaxis; contraindicated in people allergic to aspirin, in people on other salicylate-containing drugs, and during pregnancy; not recommended for children
Trimethoprim 160 mg and sulfamethoxazole 800 mg (Bactrim, Septra)	1 tablet/day	Contraindicated in people allergic to sulfa; may not be as effective as the quinolones in some parts of the world
Doxycycline 100 mg (Vibramycin, Doryx, etc.)	1 tablet/day	Contraindicated in pregnancy, age <8 yr; efficacy shown in Africa only
Norfloxacin 400 mg (Noroxin)	1 tablet/day	Contraindicated in pregnancy, age <18 yr, and in people allergic to quinolones; drug interaction with theophylline and caffeine
Ciprofloxacin 500 mg (Cipro)	1 tablet/day	Contraindicated in pregnancy, age <18 yr, and in people allergic to quinolones; drug interaction with theophylline and caffeine

Modified from Jong EC, McMullen R: *The travel and tropical medicine manual*, ed 2, Philadelphia, 1995, WB Saunders.

Bismuth subsalicylate (BSS) can be used to prevent traveler's diarrhea by persons going on trips of 3 weeks or less. A regimen of two tablets of BSS four times a day appears to significantly reduce the incidence of diarrhea among travelers to Mexico. Disadvantages to this regimen include cost, the bulk of the BSS in luggage, the risk of salicylism, development of a black tongue, and possible constipation.[18,20]

Some experts concede that taking a broad-spectrum antibiotic during travel can be an effective way to avoid becoming ill; this might be a reasonable strategy for a traveler who is taking a brief trip (1 week or less) to a high-risk area and cannot afford to be ill for even a single day. Travelers falling into this category might include competitive athletes, politicians, sales representatives, and people going to special events.[18,20,52] However, prophylaxis with antimicrobials might be considered unnecessary in most cases because more recent studies have shown that relief of diarrhea within a few hours can be obtained after a high dose of an oral antibiotic taken immediately after the onset of symptoms.[19,22,67]

The antibiotics trimethoprim-sulfamethoxazole (Bactrim, Septra), norfloxacin (Noroxin), ciprofloxacin (Cipro), and ofloxacin (Floxin) have been studied as prophylactic agents. Table 65-8 summarizes antibiotic doses. The quinolone antibiotics are contraindicated in pregnancy and in persons less than 18 years of age.

Symptomatic Treatment Of Traveler's Diarrhea

Fluid replacement is the cornerstone of therapy for traveler's diarrhea. Correcting dehydration significantly lessens the general malaise of the stricken person regardless of whether antimicrobial therapy is used. Oral fluid intake should be pushed to approximate fluid losses in the stools. Maintenance of normal urine frequency, color, and volume can serve as a marker of adequate rehydration. Generally, fruit juices or flavored mineral water can be used for oral rehydration during mild to moderate diarrhea. Packets of oral rehydration salts, which can be reconstituted to make oral rehydration solution according to WHO guidelines, are increasingly available in pharmacies

TABLE 65-8. Drugs for Adult Self-Treatment of Traveler's Diarrhea

DRUG	DOSAGE*	COMMENTS†
Bismuth subsalicylate (Pepto-Bismol)	30 ml (or 2 tablets) every 30 min for eight doses	Maximum recommended dose is 240 ml (16 tablets) per day
Diphenoxylate plus atropine (Lomotil)	2 tablets for first dose, then 1 after each loose bowel movement; do not exceed 8 tablets in 24 hr	Antiperistaltic drug; do not use in dysentery; available by prescription
Loperamide (Imodium)	2 caplets (2 mg each) for first dose then 1 after each loose bowel movement; do not exceed 8 caplets (16 mg) in 24 hr	Antiperistaltic drug; do not use in dysentery; sold over the counter; liquid form available for pediatric doses—use dose adjusted for weight as described on package insert
Tetracycline	2.5 g as a single oral dose	Antibiotic; do not use during pregnancy or for children <8 yr old
Doxycycline (Vibramycin, Doryx, etc.)	100 mg po every 12 hr for six doses	Antibiotic; do not use during pregnancy or for children <8 yr old
Trimethoprim/sulfamethoxazole (Bactrim, Septra)	160 mg/800 mg tablet (one double-strength tablet) every 12 hr for six doses	Antibiotic; do not use in sulfa-allergic patients
Norfloxacin (Noroxin)‡	400 mg tablet every 12 hr for six doses	Antibiotic; do not use during pregnancy or for teenagers <18 yr old
Ciprofloxacin (Cipro)	500 mg tablet every 12 hr for six doses	Antibiotic; do not use during pregnancy or for teenagers <18 yr old
Ciprofloxacin (Cipro)‡	750 mg tablet once at start of diarrhea symptoms	Antibiotic; do not use during pregnancy or for teenagers <18 yr old
Levofloxacin (Levoquin)	500 mg tablet every 24 hr for three doses	Antibiotic; do not use during pregnancy or for teenagers <18 yr old
Furazolidone	100 mg qid for 7-10 days	Antibiotic; also has activity against *Giardia*

Modified from Jong EC, McMullen R: *The travel and tropical medicine manual*, ed 2, Philadelphia, 1995, WB Saunders.
*Adult doses given.
†See comments in Table 65-7.
‡Unlabeled use.

throughout the world. Sports electrolyte solutions also provide adequate replacement if diluted to approximately one half to two thirds strength.

BSS in large doses (30 ml of BSS liquid or two BSS tablets by mouth every 30 minutes for eight doses) has been reported to relieve diarrhea and cramps.[18,20] A recent study suggests that in infants and young children with acute watery diarrhea, BSS at weight-adjusted doses (100 or 150 mg/kg body weight/day for up to 5 days) may be a useful adjunct to oral rehydration therapy.[23]

The over-the-counter antiperistaltic drug loperamide (Imodium) or the combination drug diphenoxylate plus atropine (Lomotil) available by prescription may offer some relief to people with watery diarrhea and cramps but should be avoided in those with blood or mucus in the stool or with signs of serious illness (high fever, recurrent vomiting, and increasingly severe abdominal pain).

Antibiotic Treatment of Traveler's Diarrhea

Traveler's diarrhea can be relieved within hours after empirical antibiotic therapy is instituted, with or without the concurrent use of the antiperistaltic drug loperamide. The drug regimens studied included the antibiotics trimethoprim-sulfamethoxazole and ciprofloxacin. With reports of increasing resistance to trimethoprim-sulfamethoxazole among bacterial enteropathogens such as *Shigella* species and *Campylobacter jejuni,* many experts recommend ciprofloxacin, levofloxacin, or one of the other quinolones as the drug of choice for empirical diarrhea treatment. Recommended dosages are shown in Table 65-8.[18-22,65-67] If the traveler has started initial treatment of watery diarrhea with BSS therapy, at least 8 hours should elapse before antimicrobial therapy because BSS can impair absorption of the orally administered antimicrobial.[57]

If blood or mucus is present in the stool, travelers should be advised to take the antibiotic prescribed for diarrhea but to refrain from using an antiperistaltic medication. If the diarrhea is caused by a susceptible bacterial species, the patient may obtain relief within a few hours after empirical treatment but should continue to take the given antibiotic for a minimum of 3 days to prevent relapse.

If the patient is ill with a bacterial pathogen resistant to the antibiotic taken, with a viral or parasitic infection, or with toxin-induced gastroenteritis, the antibiotic therapy usually does not alter the outcome of the illness, although the possible risk of antibiotic-associated side effects must always be considered. Travelers who do not respond to empirical antibiotic treatment or who have persistent diarrhea of more than 1 week's duration should have a complete work-up for bacterial and parasitic pathogens so that specific treatment may be instituted.

TRAVEL MEDICAL KIT

Traveling patients are advised to prepare a travel medicine kit appropriate to their itinerary (see Chapter 69). Such a kit should contain adequate supplies of all prescription medications normally taken, the medications for malaria and diarrhea as discussed previously, and some remedies for common problems such as headache, musculoskeletal pain, allergies, nasal and sinus congestion, cough, jet lag, and constipation. Persons prescribed one of the jet-lag drugs should be warned not to ingest alcoholic beverages concomitantly.[51] Travelers should be instructed to carry their prescription medications in their hand-held luggage to avoid loss, and to carry copies of their prescriptions in case replacements are needed.[39]

Depending on the travel itinerary, insect repellent, sunscreen, topical antibiotic ointment, antifungal cream or powder, and medications for motion sickness, allergic reactions, and high-altitude illness might be included. Female travelers should be reminded to carry personal sanitary supplies; disposable tampons and pads may be difficult to obtain in developing countries. Sexually active travelers of both sexes should take along a supply of high-quality latex condoms; those available abroad may be of lesser quality and more susceptible to leaks and rupture.

FOLLOW-UP AFTER TRAVEL

Travelers should be reminded of the importance of continuing malaria chemoprophylaxis for 4 weeks after leaving a malarious area to decrease the possibility of a clinical attack. Travelers should be instructed to alert their health care providers about the possibility of malaria in case a severe illness accompanied by high fever develops weeks, months, or even years after travel in a malaria-endemic area. Many physicians in geographic areas in which malaria is not endemic are unfamiliar with the clinical signs and symptoms of a primary malaria attack and may fail to include malaria in the differential diagnosis.[25,44,71] A person who has traveled in a malaria-endemic area and who has taken malaria chemoprophylaxis may not donate blood for 3 years, according to current blood-banking practice.

Diarrhea or any change in normal bowel habits that persists after empirical treatment for traveler's diarrhea should prompt a thorough diagnostic workup. Drug-resistant bacterial infections, intestinal parasites, dietary changes, or hepatitis may account for the prolonged symptoms after return home.[4,7,27,48] However, coincidental manifestations of biliary tract disease, inflammatory bowel disease, or intestinal malignancy must be considered in cases of gastrointestinal illness that elude diagnosis after the first round or two of diagnostic tests have been done.

Unusual skin lesions in returned travelers are often misdiagnosed in medical facilities that do not routinely see immigrants, refugees, and returned travelers. Common exotic infections in returned travelers seeking medical care include cutaneous myiasis (subcutaneous fly larvae), cutaneous larva migrans (migrating dog or cat hookworm larvae), and cutaneous and mucocutaneous leishmaniasis (protozoan parasitic infection).

Secondary bacterial infection is common with all of these conditions, and the appearance of the skin lesion may initially seem to improve after institution of standard antibiotic therapy for bacterial skin infection. However, if the skin lesion fails to completely resolve, consultation with a tropical medicine specialist might be helpful. In a series of cases reported to the CDC of cutaneous leishmaniasis in American returned travelers, the average time between seeking initial medical care for a nonhealing skin lesion and the correct diagnosis was 5 months.[31]

Intestinal parasites, especially helminthic or worm infections, can manifest their presence by spontaneous passage of adult worms from the rectum after dwelling for months in an unsuspecting, asymptomatic host. However, a systemic parasitic infection may have signs and symptoms that are not referable to a particular organ system: fever, headache, myalgia, malaise, fatigue, and nausea. The initial differential diagnosis may be broad and includes viral, bacterial, and parasitic infections. The differential diagnosis can be narrowed after the clinician takes into account incubation time, geographic area, immunizations received, malaria chemoprophylaxis taken, dietary habits, insect and rodent exposure, animal bites, and intimate or sexual contact with foreign residents or fellow travelers.

SUMMARY

Although the potential for travel-acquired illness during or after travel exists, it appears that pretravel medical preparation and behavior modification can promote travel in good health by reducing risk of many health hazards and enabling the traveler to cope with common traveler's ailments, thus increasing the overall enjoyment of the trip.

APPENDIX

Resources for Travel Medicine Information

Telephone Information, Hotlines, and Audio Libraries

- Centers for Disease Control and Prevention (CDC) Traveler's Health Hotline: 404-332-4559

- United States Department of State Citizen's Emergency Center: 202-647-5225

Official References

- Centers for Disease Control: *Health information for international travel, 1999-2000*, Washington, DC, US Government Printing Office (revised annually). Telephone: 202-738-3238.
- World Health Organization: *International travel and health, vaccination requirements and health advice, 1999*, World Health Organization Publications Center USA, 49 Sheridan Avenue, Albany, NY 12210 (revised annually).

Directories and Periodicals

- *Directory of Travel Medicine Clinics:* American Society of Tropical Medicine and Hygiene, American Academy of Clinical Tropical Medicine and Traveler's Health; website: www.astmh.org.
- *IAMAT Directory of English-Speaking Physicians:* International Association for Medical Assistance to Travellers, 40 Regal Road, Guelph, Ontario, N1K 1B5. Telephone 519-836-0102; FAX 519-836-3412.
- *International Register of Travel Clinics and Advisors:* International Society of Travel Medicine; website: www.istm.org.
- *Morbidity and Mortality Weekly Report,* Centers for Disease Control and Prevention, Atlanta, GA 30333. Subscriptions are available through the Massachusetts Medical Society, P.O. Box 9120, Waltham, MA 02254-9120, or through the website: www.cdc.gov.
- *Travel Health Online,* Shoreland Inc.; website: www.travelhealthonline.com.
- *The Travel Medicine Advisor Update:* Bia F, editor, American Health Consultants, P.O. Box 740056, Atlanta, GA 30374. Telephone 404-262-7436; FAX 404-262-7837.

REFERENCES

1. Baird JK, Basri H, Purnomo: Resistance to chloroquine by *Plasmodium vivax* in Irian Jaya, Indonesia, *Am J Trop Med Hyg* 44:547, 1991.
2. Bern JL, Kerr L, Stuerchler D: Mefloquine prophylaxis: an overview of spontaneous reports of severe psychiatric reactions and convulsions, *J Trop Med Hyg* 95:167, 1992.
3. Brandt WE: From the World Health Organization: development of dengue and Japanese encephalitis vaccines, *J Infect Dis* 162:577, 1990.
4. Centers for Disease Control: Enterically transmitted non-A non-B hepatitis: Mexico, *MMWR* 36:597, 1987.
5. Centers for Disease Control: Management of patients with suspected viral hemorrhagic fever, *MMWR* 37(S-3):1, 1988.
6. Centers for Disease Control: Use of BCG vaccines in the control of tuberculosis: a joint statement by the ACIP and the Advisory Committee for Elimination of Tuberculosis, *MMWR* 37:663, 1988.
7. Centers for Disease Control: Acute schistosomiasis in U.S. travelers returning from Africa, *MMWR* 39:140, 1990.
8. Centers for Disease Control: Typhoid immunization: recommendations of the Immunization Practices Advisory Committee (ACIP), *MMWR* 39(RR-10):1, 1990.
9. Centers for Disease Control: Diphtheria, tetanus, and pertussis: recommendations for vaccine use and other preventive measures: recommendations of the Immunizations Practices Advisory Committee (ACIP), *MMWR* (RR-10):1, 1991.

10. Centers for Disease Control: Hepatitis B virus: a comprehensive strategy for eliminating transmission in the United States through universal childhood vaccination: recommendations of the Immunization Practices Advisory Committee (ACIP), *MMWR* 40:1, 1991.

11. Centers for Disease Control: Rabies prevention—United States, 1991: recommendations of the Immunization Practices Advisory Committee (ACIP), *MMWR* 40(RR-3):1, 1991.

12. Centers for Disease Control: Update: cholera—Western hemisphere, 1991, *MMWR* 40:860, 1991.

13. Centers for Disease Control: Update on adult immunization: recommendations of the Immunization Practices Advisory Committee (ACIP), *MMWR* 40(RR-12):1, 1991.

14. Centers for Disease Control: Vaccinia (smallpox) vaccine. Recommendations of the Immunization Practices Advisory Committee (ACIP), *MMWR* 40(RR-14):1, 1991.

15. Centers for Disease Control and Prevention: Committee on Immunization Practices (ACIP): use of vaccines and immune globulins in persons with altered immunocompetence, *MMWR* 42(RR-4):1, 1993.

16. Centers for Disease Control and Prevention: Inactivated Japanese encephalitis virus vaccine: recommendations of the Advisory Committee on Immunization Practices (ACIP), *MMWR* 42(RR-1):1, 1993.

17. Centers for Disease Control and Prevention: Standards for pediatric immunization practices recommended by the National Vaccine Advisory Committee, approved by the U.S. Public Health Service, *MMWR* 42(RR-5):1, 1993.

18. DuPont HL, Ericsson CD: Prevention and treatment of traveler's diarrhea, *N Engl J Med* 328:1821, 1993.

19. DuPont HL et al: Five versus three days of ofloxacin therapy for traveler's diarrhea: a placebo-controlled study, *Antimicrob Agents Chemother* 36:87, 1992.

20. Ericsson CD, DuPont HL: Travelers' diarrhea: approaches to prevention and treatment, *Clin Infect Dis* 16:616, 1993.

21. Ericsson CD et al: Ciprofloxacin or trimethoprim-sulfamethoxazole as initial therapy for traveler's diarrhea, *Ann Intern Med* 106:216, 1987.

22. Ericsson CD et al: Treatment of traveler's diarrhea with sulfamethoxazole and trimethoprim and loperamide, *JAMA* 63:257, 1990.

23. Figueroa-Quintanilla D et al: A controlled trial of bismuth subsalicylate in infants with acute watery diarrheal disease, *N Engl J Med* 328:1653, 1993.

24. Fine PEM, Rodrigues LC: Modern vaccines: mycobacterial diseases, *Lancet* 335:1016, 1990.

25. Froud JRL et al: Imported malaria in the Bronx: review of 51 cases recorded from 1986-1991, *Clin Infect Dis* 15:774, 1992.

26. Gellert G, Wagner G, Ehling LR: Risks of cholera immunisation at port of entry, *Lancet* 337:552, 1991.

27. Guerrant RL, Bobak DA: Bacterial and protozoal gastroenteritis, *N Engl J Med* 325:327, 1991.

28. Hargarten SW, Baker SP: Fatalities in the Peace Corps: a retrospective study: 1962-1983, *JAMA* 254:1326, 1985.

29. Hargarten SW, Baker T, Guptill K: Overseas fatalities of United States citizen travelers: an analysis of deaths related to international travel, *Ann Emerg Med* 20:622, 1991.

30. Hayani KC, Ericsson CD, Pickering LK: Prevention and treatment of diarrhea in the traveling child, *Semin Pediatr Infect Dis* 3:22, 1992.

31. Herwaldt BL, Stokes SL, Juranek DD: American cutaneous leishmaniasis in U.S. travelers, *Ann Intern Med* 118:779, 1993.

32. Hien TT, White NJ: Qinghaosu, *Lancet* 341:603, 1993.

33. Hill D: Illness associated with travel to the developing world. In Lobel HO, Steffen R, Kozarsky P, editors: *Travel medicine 2*, Atlanta, 1992, International Society of Travel Medicine.

34. Hilton E et al: Status of immunity to tetanus, measles, mumps, rubella, and polio among U.S. travelers, *Ann Intern Med* 115:32, 1991.

35. Hoffman SL: Diagnosis, treatment, and prevention of malaria, *Med Clin North Am* 76:1327, 1993.

36. Holmes KK: The changing epidemiology of HIV transmission, *Hosp Pract* 11:153, 1991.

37. *International certificates of vaccination*, Washington, DC, US Government Printing Office.

38. Jong EC: Immunizations for international travelers, *Med Clin North Am* 76:1277, 1992.

39. Jong EC, McMullen R: General advice for the international traveler, *Infect Dis Clin North Am* 6:275, 1992.

40. Jong EC, McMullen R: Immunization needs of Americans attending a university-based travel medicine clinic from July 1980 to June 1990. In Lobel HO, Steffen R, Kozarsky P, editors: *Travel medicine 2*, Atlanta, 1992, International Society of Travel Medicine.

41. Kamolratanakul P et al: The effectiveness of chemoprophylaxis against malaria for non-immune migrant workers in eastern Thailand, *Trans R Soc Trop Med Hyg* 83:313, 1989.

42. Karwacki JJ et al: Proguanil-sulphonamide for malaria chemoprophylaxis, *Trans R Soc Trop Med Hyg* 84:55, 1990.

43. Lackritz EM et al: Imported *Plasmodium falciparum* malaria in American travelers to Africa: implications for prevention strategies, *JAMA* 265:383, 1991.

44. Laga M: Risk of HIV infection and other STDs for travelers. In Lobel HO, Steffen R, Kozarsky P, editors: *Travel medicine 2*, Atlanta, 1992, International Society of Travel Medicine.

45. LeDuc JW: Epidemiology of hemorrhagic fever viruses, *Rev Infect Dis* 11(suppl 4):S730, 1989.

46. Lobel HO et al: Effectiveness and tolerance of long-term malaria prophylaxis with mefloquine: need for a better dosing regimen, *JAMA* 265:361, 1991.

47. Looareesuwan S et al: Malarone: a review of its clinical development for treatment of malaria, *Am J Trop Med Hyg* 60:533, 1999.

48. McAuley JB, Michelson MK, Schantz PM: Trichinella infection in travelers, *J Infect Dis* 164:1013, 1991.

49. McMullen R, Jong EC: Incidence of antibody to hepatitis A among employees of a multinational corporation: implications for immunoglobulin prophylaxis. In Steffen R et al, editors: *Travel medicine*, Berlin, 1989, Springer-Verlag.

50. McNeil JG et al: Central European tick-borne encephalitis: assessment of risk for persons in the armed services and vacationers, *J Infect Dis* 152:650, 1985.

51. Morris HH, Estes ML: Traveler's amnesia: transient global amnesia secondary to triazolam, *JAMA* 258:945, 1987.

52. National Institutes of Health Consensus Development Conference: Travelers' diarrhea, *JAMA* 253:2700, 1985.

53. Navaratnam U et al: Chemosuppression of malaria by the triple combination mefloquine/sulfadoxine/pyrimethamine: a field trial in an endemic area in Malaysia, *Trans R Soc Trop Med Hyg* 83:755, 1989.

54. Nosten F et al: Prospective electrocardiogram study of Karen patients with falciparum malaria, *Lancet* 341:1054, 1993.

55. Pappaioanou M et al: Antibody response to pre-exposure human diploid cell rabies vaccine given concurrently with chloroquine, *N Engl J Med* 314:280, 1986.

56. Poland JD et al: Evaluation of the potency and safety of inactivated Japanese encephalitis vaccine in US inhabitants, *J Infect Dis* 161:878, 1990.

57. Radandt JM, Marchbanks CR, Dudley MN: Interactions of fluoroquinolones with other drugs: mechanisms, variability, clinical significance, and management, *Clin Infect Dis* 14:272, 1992.

58. Ryan CA, Hargrett-Brown NT, Blake PA: *Salmonella typhi* infections in the United States, 1975-1984: increasing role of foreign travel, *Rev Infect Dis* 11:1, 1989.

59. Schuurkamp GJ, Spicer PE, Kereu RK: Chloroquine-resistant *Plasmodium vivax* in Papua New Guinea, *Trans R Soc Trop Med Hyg* 86:121, 1992.

60. Schwartz E, Regev-Yochay G: Primaquine as prophylaxis for malaria for nonimmune travelers: a comparison with mefloquine and doxycycline, *Clin Infect Dis* 29:1502, 1999.

61. Schwartz IK, Lackritz EM, Patchen LC: Chloroquine-resistant *Plasmodium vivax* from Indonesia (letter), *N Engl J Med* 324:927, 1991.

62. Sexton JD et al: Permethrin-impregnated curtains and bed-nets prevent malaria in western Kenya, *Am J Trop Med Hyg* 43:11, 1990.

63. Shanks GD et al: Malaria chemoprophylaxis using proguanil/dapsone combination on the Thai-Cambodian border, *Am J Trop Med Hyg* 46:643, 1992.

64. Steffen R et al: Health problems after travel to developing countries, *J Infect Dis* 156:84, 1987.

65. Swerdlow DL, Ries AA: Cholera in the Americas: guidelines for the clinician, *JAMA* 267:1495, 1992.

66. Tauxe RV et al: Antimicrobial resistance of Shigella isolates in the USA: the importance of international travelers, *J Infect Dis* 162:1107, 1990.

67. Taylor DN et al: Treatment of travelers' diarrhea: ciprofloxacin plus loperamide compared with ciprofloxacin alone, *Ann Intern Med* 114:731, 1991.

68. Tsai TF: Arboviral infections: general considerations for prevention, diagnosis, and treatment in travelers, *Semin Pediatr Infect Dis* 3:62, 1992.

69. Weinke T et al: Neuropsychiatric side effects after the use of mefloquine, *Am J Trop Med Hyg* 45:86, 1991.

70. Wilde H et al: Rabies in Thailand: 1990, *Rev Infect Dis* 13:644, 1991.

71. Winters RA, Murray HW: Malaria—the mime revisited: fifteen more years of experience at a New York City teaching hospital, *Am J Med* 93:243, 1991.

72. Wyler D: Malaria chemoprohylaxis for the traveler, *N Engl J Med* 329:31, 1993.

73. Wyler D: Malaria: Overview and update, *Clin Infect Dis* 16:449, 1993.

SUGGESTED READINGS

Freedman D, editor: Travel medicine, *Infect Dis Clin North Am* vol 12, June, 1998.

Jong EC, editor: Travel medicine, *Med Clin North Am* vol 83, June, 1999.

Jong EC, McMullen R, editors: *The travel and tropical medicine manual,* ed 2, Philadelphia, 1995, WB Saunders.

Strickland GT: *Hunter's tropical medicine,* Philadelphia, 1999, WB Saunders.

Wilson ME: *A world guide to infections,* New York, 1991, Oxford University Press.

Wolfe MS, editor: *Health hints for the tropics,* ed 12, 1998, American Society of Tropical Medicine and Hygiene.

66 Non–North American Travel and Exotic Diseases

Ian J. Woolley and James W. Kazura

Travelers to tropical and subtropical areas of the world where hygienic conditions may be poor may encounter infectious agents that are uncommon or are not transmitted in temperate areas of North America.[72,128] The most important consideration in the management of this problem, which is increasing as international travel expands, is appropriate preventive measures through counsel with a travel medicine specialist and prophylaxis using safe drugs and vaccines. This chapter is concerned primarily with infectious diseases that are not common in North America and with which most health professionals in North America have scant familiarity. Other chapters give specific details relevant to tick-borne diseases (Chapter 33), infectious diarrhea (Chapter 53), and travel medicine (Chapter 65). The infectious diseases considered in this chapter should not be considered a complete listing. This is especially important to keep in mind in an era when diseases once thought to be eliminated or nonexistent in North America are emerging or reemerging coincidental with large-scale movements of human and vector populations.

MAJOR VIRAL INFECTIONS

A vast number of viruses may cause disease. This section describes selected viral infections that may be acquired outside North America and for which there are effective preventive or therapeutic measures. These include the viral hemorrhagic fevers, viral hepatitis, and Japanese B encephalitis.

Major Viral Hemorrhagic Fevers

A diverse group of ribonucleic acid (RNA) viruses can produce the hemorrhagic fever syndrome (Box 66-1). Although clinical presentations vary with different etiologic agents, fever, headache, myalgias, and malaise usually characterize the syndrome, which develops over several hours to 3 to 4 days. In the full-blown hemorrhagic fever syndrome, these early disease manifestations are followed by hemorrhagic signs, including petechiae and bleeding from the gums and gastrointestinal tract.[61,83] Loss of plasma volume is usually manifested by increased hematocrit value, although hypotension and shock may occur in some individuals. Elevated blood urea nitrogen and creatinine levels herald renal dysfunction. Death most often follows in-

tractable hypotension, bleeding, electrolyte disturbances, and renal failure. Other viral causes of this syndrome exist (e.g., Rift Valley fever) but are not discussed here. In general, the management principles are the same and largely consist of supportive therapy.

Yellow Fever

European physicians did not recognize the clinical syndrome now known as yellow fever until the late 1490s. Initially described by Columbus in the West Indies, large-scale epidemics were later observed throughout the Americas and tropical Africa in the 1700s and 1800s.[99] After epidemic yellow fever in Texas, Louisiana, and Tennessee caused 20,000 deaths in the 1880s, the Yellow Fever Commission was organized to study the problem. Identification of the mosquito vector, *Aedes aegypti,* was followed by massive campaigns to eradicate breeding sites. This led to virtual elimination of urban yellow fever from the Americas. The last case of yellow fever acquired in the continental United States was reported in 1911. Since it is difficult if not impossible to eliminate jungle reservoirs, there continue to be 50 to 300 and 100 to 200 cases reported annually from South America and tropical Africa, respectively.[101,148] Larger outbreaks secondary to resurgent vector populations have occurred in recent years in tropical West Africa.[94,145]

Virology and Pathophysiology. Yellow fever is a single-stranded RNA flavivirus. Strain differences are of little clinical relevance, although they may be of use in epidemiologic studies. The pathophysiologic mechanisms operating in viral hemorrhagic fevers are not well defined. In general, viral replication occurs at the site of inoculation. After the virus spreads to lymph nodes and monocyte-rich organs, further reproduction results in massive viremia.

The liver is the principal target organ. Pathologic studies show coagulative necrosis of hepatocytes and the appearance of various markers of cell involvement (Councilman and Torres bodies). However, the degree of physiologic derangement is usually much more severe than expected for the extent of hepatic damage seen on pathologic examination. Perivascular edema and occasional focal bleeding occur in the kidney, heart, and brain, but these changes are less severe than expected for the degree of clinical disease.

Yellow fever
Dengue fever
Hemorrhagic fever and renal syndrome nephropathia epidemica
Lassa fever; Argentine and Bolivian hemorrhagic fevers
Ebola virus
Marburg virus
Crimean-Congo hemorrhagic fever

Ecology and Epidemiology. In the Americas, primates in the forest canopy serve as hosts for the yellow fever virus. Mosquitoes of the genus *Haemogogus* transmit infection. Since this vector does not travel far from the forest, jungle yellow fever occurs when humans enter jungle areas or the forest border zones. Urban yellow fever involves a different vector, *A. aegypti*. This mosquito is highly anthropophilic, lives in and around human habitations, and prefers domestic water storage containers for breeding. The presence of a large population of *A. aegypti* places an urban area at significant risk for epidemic spread of yellow fever once the virus is introduced from a nearby forest area. In Africa the presence of larger numbers of mosquito species that can serve as vectors has hindered complete understanding of the ecology of the disease.

At present, both the Americas and Africa have a constant low level of jungle yellow fever because of the inability to eradicate either the monkey reservoir or the mosquito vector. Overall there are about 2000 cases per year in Africa and 200 per year in the Americas.[132] Some suggest that these rates are underestimated by at least tenfold.[83,94,148] Persons at risk include workers or travelers in or near the tropical rainforest canopy. The recent death of an American traveler to Brazil emphasizes the need for vaccination among those at risk.[87] Urban yellow fever had been reduced in the Western Hemisphere through massive anti-*Aedes* campaigns. However, the benefits of these campaigns have declined and there is currently an increased threat of further outbreaks of disease. Introduction of *Aedes albopictus,* an aggressive anthropophilic dengue vector from Southeast Asia, and reemergence of *A. aegypti* into the Americas[31,93] raise the specter of increased yellow fever transmission in the Western Hemisphere. Less intense vector control measures and a more complex ecology have made eradication of urban yellow fever in Africa even more difficult.

Clinical Presentation. Although yellow fever may appear as an undifferentiated viral syndrome, classic dis-

ease is characterized by a triphasic pattern. The infection phase begins with sudden onset of headache, fever, and malaise, often accompanied by bradycardia and conjunctival suffusion. After approximately 3 to 4 days, victims often experience brief remission. Within 24 hours, however, the intoxication phase develops, characterized by jaundice, recrudescent fever, prostration, and, in severe cases, hypotension, shock, oliguria, and obtundation. Hemorrhage is usually manifest as hematemesis; however, bleeding from multiple sites may occur. Signs of a poor prognosis include early onset of the intoxication phase, hypotension, severe hemorrhage with disseminated intravascular coagulation (DIC), renal failure, shock, and coma. Death occurs in between one quarter and one half of all cases.[132] Diagnosis in the infection phase is difficult. With development of the classic syndrome, the differential diagnosis narrows somewhat but still includes malaria, leptospirosis, typhoid fever, typhus, Q fever, viral hepatitis, and other viral hemorrhagic fevers. The standard means of diagnosis is evaluation for neutralizing antibodies in acute and convalescent sera (available through state health departments in the United States). Several new systems for early detection of immunoglobulin M (IgM) or viral antigen are now being evaluated for more rapid diagnosis.[95] A specimen of whole blood (at $-70°$ C [$-57°$ F] on dry ice) should be sent to the state health laboratory for isolation. Growth of the virus is possible in a number of systems, including Vero cells and infant mice. The virus is most easily isolated during the first 4 days of fever.

Management. Appropriate management of viral hemorrhagic fevers requires awareness of the geographic distribution of the disease and travel history of the victim. In the first several days of infection, differentiation of a viral hemorrhagic fever from other infectious diseases is nearly impossible. However, the occurrence of an undifferentiated febrile syndrome in a traveler from a yellow fever-endemic area warrants a careful physical examination, thick and thin blood smears to rule out malaria, and blood cultures for bacterial pathogens *(Salmonella typhi).* In recently returned travelers, dengue serology should be considered. Progression to the intoxication phase or any sign of volume disturbance, renal failure, or hemorrhage mandates immediate admission to an intensive care unit.

There are no effective antiviral therapies for yellow fever. Supportive care should address several important problem areas. Fever should be controlled with acetaminophen, not with salicylates. Evaluation of volume status should include Swan-Ganz or central venous pressure monitoring to direct volume expansion and use of vasopressor agents. Calculation of fractional excretion of urinary sodium may help differentiate prerenal azotemia (for which volume expansion is appropriate) from acute tubular necrosis (which may require temporary dialysis). Plasma volume loss may contribute to serious electrolyte disturbances, necessitating close observation of serum electrolytes and arterial blood gases. Rapid correction of these abnormalities, which commonly include hyperkalemia and acidosis, is essential. Hypoglycemia is presumably a result of impaired hepatic gluconeogenesis.

Serial coagulation studies (including platelet count, prothrombin time, partial thromboplastin time, fibrinogen, and fibrin degradation products) should be obtained.[7,28,38] Whole blood or fresh-frozen plasma is indicated to maintain the prothrombin time and hematocrit value at near-normal levels. If DIC is documented, the use of heparin may be considered. No controlled trials have documented the effectiveness of heparin in yellow fever, but the benefit of heparin was suggested in a small number of patients with DIC.[7,120] This approach remains controversial. To reduce the risk of upper gastrointestinal hemorrhage, H_2 blockers have been suggested. Although the efficacy of intensive care treatment has not been studied for victims of yellow fever, clinical experience with dengue shock syndrome suggests that similar benefits might be obtained.

Prevention. Avoidance of this potentially fatal infection is possible through use of the yellow fever vaccine. The vaccine strain 17D is an attenuated live virus grown in chicken embryos. Greater than 95% of persons vaccinated achieve significant antibody levels. Repeat vaccinations are recommended every 10 years, although persistent antibody titers have been detected as long as 30 to 40 years after vaccination.[25] Yellow fever vaccine is well tolerated, with headache or malaise occurring in less than 10% of those vaccinated. Rare allergic side effects occur primarily in persons with hypersensitivity to eggs. The vaccine is not recommended in the first 6 months of life or in other situations where live virus vaccines are contraindicated. Although pregnant women have received the vaccine without adverse effect to themselves or their infants, it is not recommended for use in this group because of possible teratogenic effects. Other means of reducing the risk of yellow fever (and any mosquito-borne disease) include liberal use of mosquito repellent and netting in endemic areas.

Treatment of severe yellow fever is difficult and often unsuccessful. Avoidance through mosquito protection measures and administration of the highly effective vaccine before entry into endemic areas is of utmost importance.

Dengue

Dengue fever has been reported since the late 1700s. Since World War II, increased attention has focused on the dengue virus, largely as a result of recognition of dengue hemorrhagic fever (DHF) and dengue shock syndrome (DSS). First noted in Southeast Asia, DHF and DSS have attained worldwide distribution in the last 30 years.[20,31,61]

Virology and Pathophysiology. The etiologic agent is a single-stranded RNA flavivirus, which may be one of four serotypes, denoted dengue 1 through 4. As with yellow fever, local viral replication is followed by dissemination to lymphocyte- and macrophage-rich areas, where most of the reproductive activity occurs. Infection with one virus serotype provides long-lasting protection against that type only. For the dengue 2 serotype, previous infection with a heterologous serotype may result in a more severe clinical course than noted in those experiencing dengue 2 infection without such a history. Nonneutralizing antibodies produced in response to infection with other dengue serotypes aid entrance of the virus into host macrophages.[76] Although cases of DHF and DSS may result from "immune enhancement,"[60] severe DHF and DSS also occur with other serotypes in the absence of previous infection with a heterologous dengue virus serotype.[96,116,117] Pathologic studies of DHF and DSS show hemorrhage, congestion, and perivascular edema of multiple organs. The liver may show areas of focal necrosis. As with yellow fever, the extent of pathologic findings does not correspond to severity of the clinical course.

Ecology and Epidemiology. *A. aegypti* is the principal vector for dengue viruses worldwide. In the Americas and Asia, viral transmission is maintained through a mosquito-human cycle without a major animal reservoir. Monkey carriers have been identified in Africa and Asia, but their importance in transmission is unclear. *A. albopictus,* an anthropophilic dengue vector from Southeast Asia, has also been recognized recently in the Western Hemisphere. Both of these mosquitoes are capable of large-scale transmission to humans in endemic areas. At present, dengue is endemic in tropical and subtropical Asia, Africa, South America, and the Caribbean basin. In the early 1920s, large epidemics occurred in Texas, where dengue infections were reported in 500,000 inhabitants. In the last 30 years, endemic transmission on the mainland United States has been documented only in Texas; however, between 1986 and 1992, 157 cases of dengue were confirmed in American travelers by the Centers for Disease Control and Prevention (CDC).[31]

Clinical Presentation. Most dengue infections appear after an incubation period of 2 to 14 days either as an undifferentiated viral syndrome with fever and mild respiratory or gastrointestinal symptoms or as dengue ("break-bone") fever with bone pain, generalized myalgia, and severe headache. After 1 to 3 days a quiescent period may ensue. There may be a subsequent second episode of fever accompanied by a maculopapular or morbilliform rash that spreads outward from the chest and that ultimately desquamates. Lymphadenopathy and leukopenia occur during this phase of the illness. A distinct severe form of dengue disease referred to as either DHF or DSS may occur around the usual time of recovery. These syndromes are classified grades I to IV, according to World Health Organization (WHO) guidelines.[143] In cases of grade I DHF the only hemorrhagic manifestation is a positive tourniquet test, in which inflation of a tourniquet to midway between systolic and diastolic pressure leads to development of petechiae distal to the tourniquet. A complete blood cell count classically shows a decreased platelet count and an increase in hematocrit value. Grade II DHF is defined as the above plus hemorrhage from any site. DSS (grade III) includes clammy skin, hypotension, or a narrow pulse pressure (less than 20 mm Hg) in a patient with DHF. An undetectable blood pressure defines grade IV DHF and DSS. Most studies have noted DHF and DSS primarily in infants and young children, usually with a history or serologic evidence of previous heterologous dengue infection.[61] Two cases of DSS in American travelers involved young children (ages 7 years and 16 months).[96,116,117] However, DHF and DSS may occur in adults. Of the 10 cases in the 1986 Puerto Rico outbreak, four were in adults, and of the two deaths, one was an adult.[20]

Management. Awareness of the local epidemiology of DHF and DSS, especially the occurrence of other cases, is important in establishing the diagnosis. The diagnosis may be confirmed by a fourfold change in antibody titer between acute and convalescent sera or by presence of anti-dengue IgM antibodies. In the United States, isolation of the virus from serum scan be arranged through state health departments.[31] Management is symptomatic. In the dengue fever syndrome, acetaminophen may be given for fever and myalgia. Salicylates should not be used. Hydration should be vigorously maintained.

Selected victims of grade I or II DHF may be managed as outpatients. However, outpatient care requires careful monitoring of hematocrit value, platelets, and electrolytes. If significant bleeding develops, hospitalization is appropriate for rapid and continuous assessment. Progression to DSS (grade III or IV) is a medical emergency and requires immediate hospitalization. There is no specific antiviral chemotherapy. Supportive measures described in the section on treatment of severe yellow fever are appropriate.

Lassa Fever

Four viral hemorrhagic fevers—Lassa, Marburg, Ebola, and Crimean-Congo—have been associated with out-breaks of fatal person-to-person spread.[23,49] Although the overall number of clinical cases in travelers caused by these viruses is small, they represent potentially significant threats as emerging diseases. They have also achieved a certain notoriety as a group as a result of media interest. Lassa fever was first recognized in 1969, when several nurses caring for febrile patients at a mission hospital in Nigeria became ill.[46] Since that time, seroepidemiologic studies have established a large area of endemicity and a broad spectrum of clinical manifestations of infection.

Epidemiology. The principal animal host for this virus is a rat, *Mastomys natalensis,* which prefers living in and around human dwellings. The rodents become chronically infected, secreting viral particles for long periods. Natural infection in humans occurs after rodent contamination of food and drink, inhalation of aerosolized rodent secretions, or contact with rodent material through skin abrasions. Lassa fever has been reported in several areas of sub-Saharan West Africa, and large outbreaks have been noted in Nigeria, Sierra Leone, and Liberia.[83,86] Complete seroprevalence data are lacking, making definition of an endemic area impossible at this time. Secondary human infection has been reported and may occur after contact with infected secretions.

Virology and Pathophysiology. Lassa virus is a single-stranded RNA arenavirus. Proliferation and dissemination presumably occur after initial replication at the inoculation site. As with the flaviviral diseases, the extent of end organ involvement noted at autopsy does not account for the rapid death of infected patients. Recent work in an animal model provides evidence for platelet dysfunction and an endothelial cell defect in shock caused by Lassa fever virus.[42,43] DIC, believed to be a major cause of bleeding and death in patients with other viral hemorrhagic fevers, appears to play a relatively minor role in arenavirus infections.[7,35]

Clinical Presentation. Most seroconversions to Lassa virus are not accompanied by obvious symptoms.[87] Only 5% to 14% of seroconverters experienced a febrile illness, and the fatality/infection ratio was 1:100 to 2:100. Patients hospitalized with Lassa fever show a distinct clinical syndrome. Fever, malaise, and purulent pharyngitis often develop after the insidious onset of headache. Retrosternal chest pain, possibly a result of pharyngitis and esophagitis, suggests the diagnosis. A case-control study found the combined presence of retrosternal chest pain, fever, pharyngitis, and proteinuria to be the best predictor of Lassa fever.[85] Hemorrhagic complications (hematemesis, vaginal bleeding, hematuria, lower gastrointestinal bleeding, and epistaxis) were seen in less than 25% of patients with Lassa fever. Non-fatal disease usually begins to resolve in 8 to

10 days. The combined presence of fever, sore throat, and vomiting was associated with a poor prognosis (relative risk of death equals 5.5). Terminal stages of fatal disease were accompanied by hypotension, encephalopathy, and respiratory distress caused by stridor (presumably secondary to laryngeal edema). Laboratory indicators of a poor prognosis include an admission serum aspartate aminotransferase (AST) of greater than 150 IU/L (55% death rate) and viremia greater than 10^4 $TCID_{50}$ ($TCID_{50}$ is the titer at which sera containing the virus infects 50% of tissue culture test plates).

Diagnosis. Establishing an accurate diagnosis is extremely difficult during the early phase of the infection. As the classic clinical syndrome develops, differentiation from other viral hemorrhagic fevers depends on serologic confirmation. Serologic diagnosis is made by indirect fluorescent antibody analysis of acute and convalescent sera or detection of Lassa-specific IgM antibody. Clotted whole blood may be sent to the CDC for viral culture if handled appropriately. If the diagnosis is suspected, the CDC should be contacted immediately for assistance in diagnosis, isolation, and management.

Management. As mentioned above, Lassa fever has been associated with outbreaks of fatal person-to-person spread.[23,126] Secondary infection occurs through direct contact with infected persons or their secretions. The role of aerosols in person-to-person spread is unclear. Blood and body fluids should be considered infectious. In light of the potentially fatal outcome of Lassa fever and the relative ease of transmission, the CDC has published specific recommendations for management of possible or confirmed cases.[23] If a person has (1) a compatible clinical syndrome (especially pharyngitis, vomiting, conjunctivitis, diarrhea, and hemorrhage or shock); (2) a relevant travel history, including time spent in an endemic area; and (3) prior contact within 3 weeks of presentation with a person or animal from an endemic area suspected of having a viral hemorrhagic fever, he or she should be isolated and local, state, and federal (CDC) health officials contacted. Ideally, an isolation unit with negative air pressure vented outside the hospital should be used. However, lack of a negative-pressure room alone is not a reason for transfer to another medical care facility.

The probability of transmission of Lassa fever virus to medical and nursing staff can be reduced by the use of routine blood and body fluid precautions as well as strict barrier nursing.[63] Barrier nursing includes wearing gloves, gown, mask, shoe covers, and, if there is risk of splashing fluids, goggles whenever entering the patient's room. Decontamination of solid articles and rooms may be accomplished with 0.5% sodium hypochlorite solution. Full recommendations for the management of patients with viral hemorrhagic fever have been published by the CDC.[23]

Supportive care as described for the treatment of severe yellow fever is indicated for patients with signs and symptoms suggestive of a poor prognosis, including hemorrhage, volume disturbance, or hypotension. In addition to supportive measures, an effective antiviral compound, intravenous (IV) ribavirin, is available.[84] This drug should be administered as soon as the diagnosis is suspected and is significantly more effective if given during the first 6 days of fever. Ribavirin should be administered as a 30 mg/kg IV loading dose, followed by 16 mg/kg IV every 6 hours for 4 days. Then, 8 mg/kg is given IV every 8 hours for 6 days. Persons having significant contact with a patient with Lassa fever (mucous membrane contact or a penetrating wound contaminated with infected material) should receive prophylactic ribavirin, 250 mg by mouth 3 times a day for 10 days.[24]

Argentine and Bolivian hemorrhagic fevers are endemic to the pampas of Argentina and the Bolivian plateau, respectively.[83,92] Both are arenaviruses causing infection of humans through contact with infected rodents. Disease occurs primarily in rural areas. The clinical symptoms are similar to those of other viral hemorrhagic fevers. Management guidelines given for yellow fever may be followed. Person-to-person spread has not been significant. Strict isolation (such as is suggested for Lassa, Ebola, Marburg, and Crimean-Congo hemorrhagic fevers) is not required. Routine blood and enteric precautions are nevertheless advisable.

Ebola and Marburg Viruses

Ebola and Marburg viruses are closely related large RNA viruses known as filoviruses. They cause severe viral hemorrhagic fever syndromes with high mortality rates. Both are endemic in focal areas of central and southern Africa. Ebola virus seropositivity has been noted in Sudan, Democratic Republic of the Congo, the Central African Republic, Cote d'Ivoire, and Kenya. A strain of Ebola known as Ebola Reston has been found in monkeys imported into the United States from the Philippines. More recently, there have been outbreaks involving more than 100 deaths in Gabon and the Democratic Republic of Congo.[4] Marburg disease is found in South Africa, Zimbabwe, and Kenya. Although Marburg disease was associated with contact with African green monkeys during the initial outbreak in 1967,[89] no animal reservoir has been defined for either virus. Person-to-person transmission has been well documented, primarily through contaminated needles and contact with infected individuals.[3,64,89]

Pathophysiology and Clinical Presentation. Marburg and Ebola viruses are presumed to act through pathophysiologic mechanisms similar to other viral hemorrhagic fevers. Work with a primate model of Ebola virus infection found no evidence for DIC and suggested the possibility of platelet dysfunction and endothelial cell defects as important in the creation of a capillary leak syndrome leading to multisystem failure.[43]

Patients present after an incubation period of 4 to 10 days with fever, headache, and myalgias. Diarrhea and abdominal pain occur commonly. In many victims, rash, conjunctivitis, sore throat, and chest pain appear early in the disease. As in other hemorrhagic fevers, hemorrhage, hypotension, shock, and electrolyte abnormalities mark fatal courses. The high mortality reported in various outbreaks (25% for Marburg virus and 55% to 88% for Ebola virus) emphasizes the importance of intensive supportive care.

Diagnosis and Treatment. If these diseases are suspected, strict isolation procedures should be instituted and the local health authorities and CDC notified immediately. Diagnosis may be made on a serologic basis or by polymerase chain reaction (PCR). There appears to be no serologic cross reactivity between the two viruses. Although anecdotal reports suggest the efficacy of immune sera in therapy, this has not been consistently observed in experimental studies. There are currently no specific antiviral therapies for Marburg or Ebola virus infection.[23] Care is supportive, and the therapeutic considerations given for treatment of severe yellow fever should be followed. Two patients with documented DIC and Marburg virus infection were given heparin and survived.[49]

Crimean-Congo Hemorrhagic Fever

Virology and Epidemiology. The etiologic agent of Crimean-Congo hemorrhagic fever (CCHF) is a bunyavirus. Ixodid ticks serve as both reservoirs and vectors of the virus. Infection in humans results from tick bites or direct contact with infected secretions from crushed ticks, animals, or humans. Most cases occur in individuals with occupations or living conditions that bring them in contact with domestic goats, sheep, or cattle on which ticks feed.[32,55] The disease has been observed in southeastern Europe, south central Asia, the Middle East, and much of Africa.[2,55] Nosocomial transmission through contact with infected body fluids has been well documented.[2,134]

Pathophysiology and Clinical Presentation. Pathophysiologic mechanisms are presumably similar to those of other hemorrhagic fevers. One in five infections results in clinical disease.[55] Among those clinically ill, mortality ranges from 15% in sporadic cases to 70% in rare hospital outbreaks.[2,55]

Diagnosis. The diagnosis can be confirmed with acute and convalescent serologic evaluation for a fourfold rise in IgG antibody titers. The virus can be cultured from whole blood if it is drawn during the first week of symptoms and kept on dry ice (or at −70° C [−57° F]) during shipment to the CDC.

Management. Initial management is similar to that for Lassa, Marburg, and Ebola virus infections, with strict patient isolation and notification of health authorities. Supportive therapy should be instituted as discussed for yellow fever. Although not confirmed in clinical trails, ribavirin has good activity in vitro against CCHF virus. The CDC recommends that patients believed to have CCHF receive IV ribavirin in the doses suggested for treatment of Lassa fever.[23] Persons in contact with CCHF patients should receive prophylactic ribavirin as suggested for Lassa fever contacts. Treatment with oral ribavirin has been successfully used in a nosocomial setting when IV therapy was not available.[44]

Hemorrhagic Fever with Renal Syndrome/ Hantavirus Pulmonary Syndrome

Hemorrhagic fever with renal syndrome (HFRS) first came to the attention of Western medical science during the Korean War, when febrile illness accompanied by bleeding and renal failure developed in 3000 United Nations troops.[144] Mortality ranged from 5% to 10%. A similar although less severe syndrome ("nephropathia epidemica") had been recognized in Scandinavia since the 1930s. More recent investigations have resulted in the identification of a group of RNA viruses, known as hantaviruses, as a cause of this syndrome. A novel infection associated with a new hantavirus, the Muerto Canyon or Sin Nombre virus, was described after a cluster of deaths in the Southwestern United States in 1993. This is hantavirus pulmonary syndrome, in which a nonspecific febrile illness is followed by shock and alveolar pulmonary edema.[40]

Epidemiology. The agent of HFRS causes chronic nondebilitating infections of rodents. Human infection is initiated by contact with rodent secretions or inhalation of aerosolized rodent material. The disease occurs most commonly in rural areas, although occasional urban outbreaks, presumably with the common house rat as vector, have been described.[80,144] Cases have been described most frequently from the Far East, including China, Korea, Japan, and the Soviet Union, but the disease also occurs in Eastern Europe. A recent epidemiologic study from China found the highest rates of infection in men who engaged in heavy farm work and slept on the ground (rather than on raised wooden beds).[147] The Sin Nombre agent appears to cause a chronic infection of the deer mouse, *Peromyscus maniculatus*, which is the main reservoir of the virus in the United States. Since the initial outbreak, additional cases have been described across the United States and South America.[52]

The risk of infection is likely to be related to rodent exposure, but transmission is infrequent.

Virology and Pathophysiology. The etiologic agent of HFRS is the prototype hantavirus, Hantaan virus, a member of the bunyavirus family. A related hantavirus, the Puumala agent, is the apparent cause of the more benign nephropathia epidemica. Other closely related viruses can cause similar, although less frequently recognized, syndromes. Seoul virus causes a milder form of HFRS in the Far East, and a recently described severe HFRS-like syndrome in Eastern Europe has been attributed to a related virus.[89] As described above, Sin Nombre virus is the usual cause of hantavirus pulmonary syndrome (HPS) in the United States, but other hantaviruses probably cause the same syndrome.

Clinical Presentation. As with most viral hemorrhagic fevers, infection may be asymptomatic or accompanied by a mild nonspecific illness. In the classic severe form, an initial febrile phase is associated with petechiae, proteinuria, and abdominal pain. After 3 to 5 days, a hypotensive phase occurs, with decreased platelet counts and more severe hemorrhagic phenomena. An oliguric phase follows with concomitant electrolyte abnormalities. Subsequently, a diuretic phase develops. This usually commences 10 days after the onset of illness. Death occurs from hemorrhage, hypotension, and pulmonary edema, presumably secondary to fluid overload and renal failure. With modern management, the case-fatality rate of classic HFRS is about 5%.[144] The more benign nephropathia epidemica syndrome has a case-fatality rate of less than 1%. In this disease, hypotension, shock, and hemorrhagic manifestations are rare.

With HPS, there is usually a prodromal illness with fever and mild respiratory or gastrointestinal symptoms, followed by shock and pulmonary edema. The tempo of the disease at this stage may be rapid and require respiratory and circulatory support in an intensive care unit.

Diagnosis. The diagnosis of HFRS, nephropathia epidemica, and HPS is confirmed by indirect fluorescent or enzyme-linked immunosorbent assay (ELISA) for antibodies in acute and convalescent sera. IgM antibody determination may also be helpful. Virus isolation is difficult, but PCR and immunohistochemical staining may be useful in affected tissues.

Management. Care of patients with HFRS is supportive and should follow the guidelines given for yellow fever. With HFRS, renal dysfunction occurs early and may require institution of dialysis soon after diagnosis to prevent fluid overload and to correct electrolyte disturbances. Patients' secretions should be handled with care, and enteric precautions (but not strict isolation)

are prudent. It is not clear whether person-to-person transmission of the virus through direct inoculation occurs. For the hantaviruses, viremia recedes and antibody levels rise as the clinical phase appears. Accordingly, nosocomial transmission or hematogenous transmission with hantavirus infections has not been frequently documented, although presumed nosocomial transmission has been reported.[139,147]

Japanese B Encephalitis

Japanese B encephalitis has been recognized in Japan since the nineteenth century. It is the only arboviral encephalitis for which an effective inactivated vaccine has been developed. Vaccine use in Japan and elsewhere since the 1960s has resulted in a significant decrease in the disease rate. However, there is concern regarding the routine use of the vaccine for travelers because of the description of several adverse reactions described in Western countries. These tend to occur on the day after vaccination.[29] Therefore use of the vaccine depends on a risk-benefit analysis. Relevant considerations include the duration of travel (minimum of at least 30 days), travel in an endemic area during the transmission season, and the likelihood of exposure to mosquitoes. A history of adverse reactions to the vaccine is a contraindication to its use.

Epidemiology. Rice field–breeding mosquitoes serve as the vectors for Japanese B encephalitis. In addition to humans, birds and pigs can be infected. Pigs play an important role as amplifying hosts because they develop high-grade viremia from which large numbers of mosquitoes may be infected. Most infections in endemic areas occur in children, whereas all age groups of previously unexposed populations are at risk. Transmission of Japanese B encephalitis currently occurs in India, Southeast Asia, China, Korea, Indonesia, the Western Pacific region, eastern Russia, and Japan.[133]

Virology and Pathophysiology. Japanese B encephalitis is caused by a neurotropic flavivirus. After initial replication near the mosquito bite, viremia occurs, which if prolonged may seed infection to the brain.[12] The cytopathologic effect of the flavivirus is believed to cause nerve cell destruction and necrosis.

Clinical Presentation. Most infections do not cause clinical illness, and it has been suggested that only 1 in 300 infections results in encephalitis. Many patients recall a mild undifferentiated febrile illness, which probably coincides with the viremic phase of infection. Patients with encephalitis often report a similar prodrome. The encephalitis syndrome is not easily distinguishable from other arboviral encephalitides. The patient usually complains of headache, lethargy, fever, and confusion and may display tremors or seizures. Reported mortality of persons with clinical encephalitis ranges from 10% to 50%.[133] One clinical series suggested that the presence on admission of (1) unresponsiveness to pain, (2) low levels of anti–Japanese B encephalitis virus IgG or IgM antibodies (in serum or cerebrospinal fluid [CSF]), or (3) virus in CSF culture was associated with death.[12] Of the 16 patients with fatal disease, all died within 7 days of hospitalization.

Diagnosis. Acute and convalescent sera for antibody determination (virus neutralization or hemagglutination inhibition assays) provide the only reliable method of diagnosis. Paired sera should be sent for these assays through state health departments. Sensitive assays for determinations of IgG and IgM antibodies in serum and CSF have been developed[10,11] but are not yet widely available. Since most patients seek treatment long after the viremic phase, blood cultures are rarely positive for the virus and CSF cultures are often positive only in patients with a poor prognosis.

Management. There is no specific therapy. The main interventions are prophylactic: vaccination and reduced arthropod exposure. Supportive care may require an intensive care unit. Since the virus is present in body fluids, especially CSF, blood and body fluid precautions should be considered. Japanese B encephalitis is only one of several of arthropod-borne viruses that may cause encephalitis in different areas of the world, for example, Murray Valley encephalitis in Australia; tick-borne encephalitis in Europe (for which a vaccine exists); and Lacrosse, West Nile, and St. Louis encephalitis in the United States.

Named Hepatitis Viruses

Although infectious hepatitis has been a well-known clinical entity for hundreds of years, it is only in the last few decades that identification of specific viral pathogens has been possible. The causes of hepatitis may be divided into two groups. Firstly, the so-called named, or more accurately, lettered viruses now include hepatitis A to G. These are associated with defined clinical syndromes and elevated liver function tests. Second, other organisms cause hepatitis as part of a more systemic infection, including Epstein-Barr virus, cytomegalovirus, toxoplasmosis, and leptospirosis. Only the former group is discussed here.

Epidemiology. Hepatitis A virus is transmitted primarily by the fecal-oral route by either person-to-person contact or ingestion of contaminated food or water. Food items commonly associated with outbreaks are raw or undercooked clams and shellfish. Homosexual men have higher rates of seropositivity than the population at large. Occasional cases are associated with exposure to nonhuman primates. Transmission by blood transfusion has been reported,[98] but this is an uncommon source of infection. Hepatitis A is endemic worldwide, but underdeveloped nations have higher prevalences than those in North America. Most persons in these areas show serologic evidence of past infection with hepatitis A virus. Several recent studies suggest that hepatitis is the most common serious viral infection occurring in travelers and that hepatitis A virus is the most common identifiable cause.[34,54,58]

Virology and Pathophysiology. Hepatitis A virus is a picornavirus with a single-stranded RNA genome. Although the pathophysiologic mechanism has not been delineated, most infections begin with introduction of viral particles into the proximal gastrointestinal tract. Brief viremia precedes seeding of hepatocytes, where viral replication has been documented.[54] With replication, hepatocellular necrosis is accompanied by lymphocytic infiltration. In the vast majority of cases, hepatic regeneration occurs after acute disease and no significant sequelae are observed.

Clinical Manifestations. The incubation period ranges from 2 to 7 weeks. The infection may be asymptomatic or mild, especially in children, but also in a minority of adults. The classic syndrome includes initially anorexia, followed by nausea, vomiting, fever, and abdominal pain. These symptoms may be accompanied by hepatosplenomegaly. AST and alanine aminotransferase (ALT) levels rise within a few days of the onset of symptoms. In children, AST and ALT return to normal levels in 2 to 3 weeks, whereas in adults resolution of elevated serum aminotransferase levels may take several months. The bilirubin level rises shortly after AST and ALT elevations. Jaundice usually follows gastrointestinal symptoms by several days to a few weeks. Resolution of jaundice may take another 3 to 4 weeks. The syndrome is occasionally preceded by arthralgias and rash, but these prodromal symptoms are uncommon.[71] Resolution of acute disease is permanent in most instances, but rare cases of relapse have been noted.[106] It has become clear in recent years that death after acute hepatitis A is not as rare as initially believed.[54] The fatality rate in cases reported to the CDC is 0.6%.[24] Anti–hepatitis A antibody (primarily IgG) is detectable in the blood for many years after infection. The presence of the antibody confers immunity. Accordingly, reinfection with hepatitis A virus is not believed to occur.

Diagnosis. The clinical presentation of hepatitis A is usually milder than other types of viral hepatitis. Consequently, the symptoms are not distinctive enough to allow a firm diagnosis, which requires detection of hepatitis A antigen in the stool or serologic evaluation for hepatitis A–specific IgM or total anti–hepatitis A virus antibody. Stool hepatitis A antigen is maximal before the onset of symptoms but may be detected as long as 2 weeks after the onset of disease. A more practical test is measurement of hepatitis A–specific IgM antibody, which is usually present by the time symptoms are recognized and generally absent 6 months later. Measurement of anti–hepatitis A antibodies may be helpful in evaluating possible causes of past icteric episodes or for seroepidemiologic studies, but their presence does not differentiate recent from past infection.

Management. No specific therapy exists for hepatitis A. Affected persons are usually managed as outpatients and should be instructed on enteric precautions to avoid transmission to others. Although infectivity drops sharply soon after the onset of jaundice, it is prudent to maintain enteric and blood-drawing precautions for about 2 weeks after jaundice appears. Nosocomial transmission has also been documented, but most spread probably occurs before jaundice and diagnosis.[56]

Prevention. Active immunization with hepatitis A vaccine is recommended for most travelers to at-risk areas. There are two inactivated hepatitis A vaccines available in the United States. Both have excellent safety and efficacy profiles. Two doses of vaccine 6 to 12 months apart appear to provide adequate antibody responses for at least 10 years. Although no specific therapy is available for hepatitis A, additional prophylactic measures may be considered.[24] Human immunoglobulin (IG) is effective for both preexposure and postexposure prophylaxis. IG is concentrated human immunoglobulin prepared by ethanol fractionation of pooled human sera. Although human immunodeficiency virus (HIV) contamination is a theoretic risk, epidemiologic studies show no increased risk of acquired immunodeficiency syndrome (AIDS) in recipients of IG, and laboratory evaluations confirmed that the IG manufacturing process inactivates HIV.[21] Thus IG is safe for use as prophylaxis.

Hepatitis B

The spread of hepatitis by parenteral means was noted in 1885. Recognition in the 1960s of specific viral particles (the Australia antigen) in the serum of hepatitis patients led to identification of the responsible agent.

Epidemiology. With the widespread use of serologic markers for hepatitis B disease, it became apparent that spread occurs through exchange of blood, semen, or, rarely, saliva of infected people. Although spread is possible from persons with acute disease, the primary sources of viral particles are chronic carriers. Persons are defined as carriers if blood samples obtained 6 months apart contain hepatitis B surface antigen particles (HBsAg). The carrier state follows acute infection in up to 90% of infected infants and 10% of adults.[47] Risk factors

for acquisition of hepatitis B infection in the United States include IV drug use, homosexual activity, and working in health care. In the United States, most victims are adults, and the carrier rate in the general population is less than 0.5%. In many areas of the developing world, most infections occur in infancy or childhood, and chronic carriers may comprise as much as 10% to 20% of the total population. Thus travelers are more likely to be exposed to carriers than is the nontraveling population. The risk is higher in persons regularly exposed to body fluids, including medical personnel and persons with frequent sexual partners.

Virology and Pathophysiology. Hepatitis B virus is a deoxyribonucleic acid (DNA) virus unrelated to the agent responsible for hepatitis A. Infection occurs naturally in humans and can be induced easily in some nonhuman primates. The virus cannot be grown in vitro. Most hepatitis B infections are subclinical. In those resulting in clinical disease, entry of the virus into the liver is followed by viral replication and hepatocyte necrosis. HBsAg, a viral particle, appears in the bloodstream within 3 months of infection. In most cases, IgM antibody to the core antigen appears first, followed by anti-HBsAg antibody. Antibody to a third hepatitis antigen, the e antigen (HBeAg), is present for variable periods. The course of the disease varies widely, depending on a number of factors that are not well defined. In brief, most cases are self-limited and resolve in 4 to 6 months. In these patients, anti-HBsAg or anti-HBcAg IgG antibodies can be detected for years after the episode of hepatitis. Chronic carriers do not develop anti-HBsAg antibody, but rather maintain measurable levels of HBsAg. Similarly, carriers with persistent HBeAg detectable in blood samples appear to be more infectious than carriers without circulating HBeAg. The intricate network of antibody-antigen relationships in hepatitis B is believed to play a role not only in development of acute and chronic hepatitis but also in the many extrahepatic syndromes associated with hepatitis B.[106] Immune complex formation has been suggested as etiologic in hepatitis B–associated arthritis, rash, arteritis, and renal disease.[53]

Clinical Presentation. The incubation period for hepatitis B ranges from 7 to 22 weeks; however, the patient may be antigenemic for a large portion of that time. The manifestations of hepatitis B infection are similar to hepatitis A, including fever, anorexia, nausea, vomiting, and abdominal pain. In addition, a prodrome of rash, arthralgia or arthritis, and fever is seen in up to 20% of hepatitis B patients compared with their rarity in hepatitis A. Glomerulonephritis is occasionally seen. Jaundice usually appears a short time after the onset of gastrointestinal symptoms. In the self-limited disease, recovery is complete by 6 months. Some infections follow a fulminant course; case-fatality rates are 2% or less in most series. In addition to complete resolution or death, three other sequelae are possible with acute hepatitis B. A person may become an asymptomatic chronic carrier and remain HBsAg positive but have no detectable active hepatitis. Chronic persistent hepatitis is a term used to describe persistent, but not progressive, hepatic inflammation (usually monitored by serum transaminase levels), often with HBsAg in the serum. Persons with chronic active hepatitis may be HBsAg positive and have progressive hepatitis, which may result in cirrhosis and death directly related to liver disease. Any of these three conditions results in the presence of hepatitis B viral particles in the blood.

Diagnosis. A variety of antigen and antibody tests have been developed for the diagnosis and monitoring of hepatitis B disease. The most practical and widely available test for diagnosis of acute disease is the assay for HBsAg. Antigen is usually present before the onset of symptoms and persists during symptomatic disease. Occasionally, HBsAg may be undetectable in patients with clinical disease caused by hepatitis B. In these cases, antibody to HBcAg is often present. Later, antibody to HBsAg will appear, but this is often long after the episode of clinical hepatitis.

Management. Management is similar to that of hepatitis A. Prolonged viremia makes blood and body fluid precautions necessary until the absence of HBsAg antigen and the presence of antibody to HBsAg are established.[24] For patients with chronic infection, therapy with interferon-α (IFN-α) involving three injections per week for 6 months is recommended. Even in individuals with good prognostic indicators, the response rate in terms of long-term clearance of virus and seroconversion approaches only 30%.

Prevention. Travelers to highly endemic areas who stay for 6 or more months or have close contact with inhabitants should be vaccinated. Two types of vaccine have been available. The first vaccine was prepared from pooled human plasma using several biochemical and physical procedures that result in a suspension of HBsAg particles. The processes used in manufacturing this vaccine inactivate blood-borne human viruses,[21,24] including HIV. This vaccine is no longer produced in the United States, and its use is generally restricted to persons with allergies to yeast and severely immunocompromised hosts. The newer hepatitis B vaccines are produced using recombinant DNA technology by introduction of a plasmid containing the gene for HbsAg into baker's yeast. After the yeast has grown, the cells are lysed and HBsAg is separated from the lysate. The recombinant HBsAg is suspended to a concentration of 10 mg/ml. The recommended dose is 1 ml (10 mg) in-

tramuscularly, with repeat doses at 1 and 6 months. Immunogenicity is similar for both vaccine preparations if used as directed by the manufacturer.[24] Injections into subcutaneous fat are poorly immunogenic, so the vaccine should be given in the deltoid muscle.[138] Hepatitis B immune globulin (HBIG) is available for postexposure situations. HBIG is prepared from pooled sera by ethanol fractionation and contains high titers of antibody to HBsAg. In brief, if an unvaccinated person is exposed to blood or has sexual contact with a person known to be HBsAg positive, he or she should receive HBIG (0.06 ml/kg body weight, intramuscularly) and the complete vaccine series (first injection in a different site from the HBIG) within 7 days of exposure. If only HBIG is available, the initial HBIG dose should be followed in 1 month by another HBIG injection. This second dose of HBIG is not required if the patient is given the vaccine series.

The remaining recommendations assume availability of vaccine. If the exposed person has been vaccinated and serologic testing is available, nothing need be done if anti-HBsAg antibody is adequate. If levels of this antibody are inadequate, a routine dose of HBIG and a booster dose of vaccine (1 ml, intramuscularly) should be given. If there is uncertainty of the HBsAg status of the source, HBsAg testing should be done. In the unvaccinated person, the vaccine series should be given immediately, and if the source proves to be HBsAg positive, HBIG should be administered as previously described. In vaccinated persons with an adequate vaccine response, no action should be taken. If the vaccine response was inadequate and the source was HBsAg positive, HBIG and a booster vaccine should be given. If the source was unknown, the vaccine series should be given to the unvaccinated individual, and nothing need be done for the vaccinated person.[24] Risk reduction, such as advice regarding the practice of safe sex when traveling, is equally important.

Delta Hepatitis

Hepatitis with the delta agent was first suspected in 1977, when cases of severe hepatitis B disease and exacerbations of hepatitis were being evaluated.

Epidemiology. Delta virus infection is found only in patients concomitantly or previously infected with hepatitis B.[113] Transmission follows a pattern similar to hepatitis B.[114] In the United States, affected populations are IV drug abusers and multiply transfused hemophiliacs.[115] Serologic evidence of delta virus disease has been documented in the Mediterranean basin, West Africa, and parts of South America.[113]

Virology and Pathophysiology. The delta agent has been termed a "defective" virus because it requires hepatitis B virus activity for its own replication.[112,115]

The agent is a single strand of RNA and a 68-kD protein enclosed in a protein coat of HBsAg. The delta agent infects cells at approximately the same time as hepatitis B virus (coinfection), or it may be introduced later in the course of persistent hepatitis B infection (superinfection). In coinfected patients the clinical picture may not differ from hepatitis B, but a higher percentage of such patients develop severe disease than those with hepatitis B alone. Patients superinfected with the delta agent develop flare-ups of hepatitis, which may become fulminant. After the acute infection, the delta agent can cause progressive disease in previously stable hepatitis B patients. In general, infection with the delta agent worsens the prognosis of hepatitis B disease. The diagnosis can be made by detection of antibody to the delta antigen in the serum[114] or less commonly by detection of free delta antigen in serum.[112]

Management and Prevention. Management of acute hepatitis consists of supportive care. Precautions against transmission are the same as for hepatitis B. There is no specific vaccine or IG for the delta agent. The best preventive measure is to be vaccinated for hepatitis B because delta agent infection cannot occur in the absence of the former virus.

Hepatitis C

As serologic methods for the diagnosis of hepatitis A, hepatitis B, and delta agent were developed, it became apparent that there was a group of persons with hepatitis for which no etiologic agent had been identified. This syndrome was previously termed non-A, non-B (NANB) hepatitis and thought to be caused by a heterogeneous group of etiologies.[123,129,149] It is now clear that a majority of such cases were due to hepatitis C.

Epidemiology. Risk factors for hepatitis C include IV drug use and, before routine testing, transfusion of blood products.[74,75] Nonparenteral routes of infection are less important than for hepatitis B. Hepatitis C is a global problem. Approximately 80% of exposed individuals develop chronic infection, which may lead to cirrhosis in 20% of subjects and hepatocellular carcinoma in up to 5% of this subset of infected persons. Rates of infection vary from 1% to 5% in most Western countries to 20% in parts of the Middle East, such as Egypt.[142]

Virology and Clinical Manifestations. Hepatitis C is a single-stranded RNA virus of the *Flaviviridae* family. It was discovered in the late 1980s.[33] Transition to chronic hepatitis after an insidious asymptomatic infection is the usual pattern. Chronic hepatitis may be asymptomatic or associated with nonspecific symptoms, such as lethargy, nausea, and abdominal discomfort. The patterns of cirrhosis and hepatocellular carcinoma

when they occur do not differ significantly from that of other conditions. Extrahepatic syndromes associated with hepatitis C infection include porphyria cutanea tarda, membranous glomerulonephritis, and mixed cryoglobulinemia.

Diagnosis. Diagnosis of hepatitis C has been a vexing problem. First-generation ELISA tests available soon after the discovery of the virus led to a significant number of false positives. These tests have subsequently become more sensitive and specific, and radioimmunoassays (RIA or RIBA) have become available and are useful in confirmatory testing. To clarify the significance of a positive screening test, it should be repeated, and if possible, a second confirmatory test should be done (usually a RIBA). Interpretation of the significance of such tests should be tempered by the presence or absence of risk factors for infection. PCR tests for hepatitis C may also provide further evidence of infection and a direct measure of viral replication. If the PCR results are positive, it should be interpreted with several caveats. First, a minority of infected individuals clear the virus, so a negative test does not exclude past infection. Second, the serum PCR may be negative in the face of viral replication in the liver. Third, performance of PCR is operator dependent, so an experienced laboratory should be used.[1,103]

Management and Prevention. Prevention of hepatitis C is largely dependent on risk reduction, especially with respect to drug use. Pooled immunoglobulin has been used after exposure, but this should be procured from donors screened for hepatitis C. It is, however, not generally recommended. Unlike hepatitis B, protective antibody responses have not been demonstrated. Treatment of acute hepatitis C is supportive. Treatment of chronic infection is with IFN-α, though the overall results are disappointing and side effects significant. Response rates increase to approximately 40%, however, when IFN-α is used in combination with ribavirin.[88]

Hepatitides E, F, and G

Hepatitis E is an RNA virus provisionally placed in the *Caliciviridae* family. It is the second most common cause of viral hepatitis transmitted via the enteric route. The epidemiologic characteristics are similar to hepatitis A. This group of infections is especially important in the Indian subcontinent, the Middle East, and Africa. The incubation period varies between 2 and 6 weeks. The disease is usually self-limited but may be associated with severe illness in pregnant women.

Diagnosis in travelers from endemic areas can be made on the basis of IgM antibody to hepatitis E in serum or testing of stool for viral antigen. PCR for hepatitis E may be available in some centers. In the United States, testing for hepatitis E is best undertaken in returned travelers with clinical hepatitis who are negative in testing for hepatitides A, B, and C. No specific therapy is of benefit. There is no association with chronic hepatitis, although a more severe illness may occur in persons with underlying liver disease. Vaccines are under development but not yet available. Prophylaxis is appropriate advice to travelers regarding ingestion of food and water in endemic areas.

Hepatitis F is a putative hepatitis virus of uncertain significance first described in France. Hepatitis G is a member of the flavivirus family with limited homology to hepatitis C. Its significance as a cause of hepatitis is also unclear.[130]

MAJOR BACTERIAL INFECTIONS

This section reviews several bacterial diseases of relevance to the overseas traveler, including typhoid fever, meningococcal disease, pertussis, diphtheria, and tetanus. Other chapters deal with bacterial causes of gastroenteritis and diarrhea, tick-borne diseases, and zoonoses.

Typhoid Fever

Typhoid fever was recognized as a clinical entity in the 1800s and first associated with transmission by the fecal-oral route in the 1870s. Although effective treatment with chloramphenicol became possible in 1948, the disease continues to be a major cause of morbidity and mortality in the developing world.[41]

Epidemiology. Typhoid fever occurs worldwide, but its prevalence and attack rates are much higher in underdeveloped countries. Humans are the only host for *Salmonella typhi,* the most common cause of the typhoid fever syndrome. Nearly all cases are contracted through ingestion of contaminated food or water. Transmission occurs through a variety of mechanisms, the most common of which include contact with a chronic carrier of the organism, especially food handlers, or ingestion of untreated waste material or sewage. One expert has estimated an incidence rate of 12.5 million cases a year in the developing world (excluding China).[41] Improved sewage and tracking of chronic carriers have markedly reduced the incidence in developed countries, although several hundred cases a year are reported to the CDC in the United States. Evaluation of cases reported between 1975 and 1984 revealed that 62% of typhoid fever cases in the United States were acquired during foreign travel. The highest attack rates occurred in persons traveling to India, Pakistan, Peru, and Chile (58 to 174 cases per 1 million travelers).[119]

Bacteriology and Pathophysiology. *Salmonella* species are gram-negative enteric bacilli. *S. typhi* is the prime cause of typhoid fever, but other species, including many of the *S. enteritidis* serotypes and some non-*Salmonella* enteric organisms such as *Yersinia* or *Campylobacter,* may cause a typhoid fever–like syndrome. *Salmonella* species are easily grown on routine bacterial culture plates, but if multiple organisms are present, media with selective growth inhibitors may be needed for optimal sensitivity. After ingestion of food or water containing the pathogen, organisms are subjected to the acid stomach environment, which results in significant bacterial killing. If the organisms get through the small intestine, several processes may occur. The bacteria may simply pass through, causing few clinical symptoms. If the bacteria multiply and invade the mucosa, a gastroenteritis-like syndrome will result. Typhoid fever requires penetration of the intestinal mucosa and intestinal lymphatics, where replication of *S. typhi* occurs intracellularly. Soon thereafter, bacteria seed the bloodstream and are transported to reticuloendothelial cells throughout the body, where further intracellular replication can take place. After the acute episode of infection is over, *Salmonella* species may remain and asymptomatically reproduce in scarred or chronically inflamed tissues. Persons may shed organisms from such foci for years and serve as a source of outbreaks while they themselves are asymptomatic. The most common site for such colonization is the chronically diseased gallbladder.

Clinical Presentation. After exposure to the pathogen, 10 to 14 days usually passes before the onset of clinical illness. Some patients may experience gastroenteritis early in the course of disease, and abdominal pain or diarrhea may be present at the time the classic typhoid fever picture develops. Fever is usually the first sign of disease. Fever increases slowly over several days[70] and may remain constant for 2 to 3 weeks, after which time defervescence begins. With antibiotic therapy, fever resolves more rapidly, often within 3 to 4 days.[70] Relative bradycardia may accompany fever. Most victims also report headache, malaise, and anorexia. Rose spots (2- to 4-mm maculopapular blanching lesions) are classically described on the trunk, although they are not seen in the majority of patients. Hepatomegaly and splenomegaly have been reported in a large number of patients.[69,110] Laboratory investigations early in the course may show a high white blood cell (WBC) count, anemia, and mild elevations of serum hepatic enzyme levels, including AST, lactate dehydrogenase, and alkaline phosphatase.[69] Later in the course of the disease, leukopenia (WBC < 3500/mm³) develops.

Uncomplicated and untreated typhoid fever resolves in 3 to 4 weeks. Several complications may herald or contribute to death. Intestinal perforation, presumably secondary to necrosis of lymphoid areas of the bowel wall, may lead to peritonitis and death. Significant gastrointestinal hemorrhage may occur but rarely is fatal.

Secondary pneumonia is common. A subgroup of patients has more severe disease, which may include myocardial involvement, mental status changes, hyperpyrexia, and multisystem failure. The overall case fatality rate has ranged from 12% to 32% in the developing world but is less than 2% in industrialized nations.[41]

Diagnosis. Culture of a bacterial species associated with the syndrome (most likely *S. typhi*) from a normally sterile fluid makes the diagnosis. Multiple studies have evaluated the usefulness of various diagnostic tests. In general, bone marrow culture is the most sensitive method, detecting up to 90% of cases, whereas blood cultures are less sensitive.[41] Both methods are most useful in the first week of disease. Stool cultures (and string test cultures) may be positive later in the course of disease but provide only circumstantial evidence of the causative agent. Work is currently being done on serodiagnostic methods, but no clear consensus has been reached on the relative usefulness of any test.[41]

Management. Chloramphenicol had been the mainstay of treatment for typhoid fever since the late 1940s. Ampicillin and trimethoprim/sulfamethoxazole were the traditional alternatives. In the last decade, there has been increasing multiple drug resistance so that ciprofloxacin is now the first-line antibiotic. Unfortunately, increasing resistance to quinolones has been observed, especially from the Indian subcontinent. In cases of quinolone resistance, either laboratory or clinical, ceftriaxone or other third generation cephalosporins are indicated.[118,139] Other treatment modalities include fluid support and adequate nutrition. Corticosteroids have been used empirically for many years. A single randomized double-blind study showed that administration of high-dose dexamethasone (3 mg/kg for the first dose, followed by 1 mg/kg every 6 hours for eight more doses) with chloramphenicol resulted in significantly lower mortality in patients with severe typhoid fever than in those treated with chloramphenicol alone.[68] Severe typhoid fever was defined in this study was defined by the presence of obtundation, delirium, stupor, coma, or shock (systolic blood pressure less than 90 mm Hg for those 12 years or older and less than 80 mm Hg in children). High-dose steroids were not recommended for those with less severe disease and should be used cautiously in those with severe disease.[37]

Prevention. Three vaccines exist for prophylactic use. The oldest in use is a heat-killed, acetone-precipitated vaccine. Efficacy in Americans, however, is only about 50%, and significant incidences of local inflammatory reactions and febrile responses occur in persons receiving the vaccine. Two doses of 0.5 ml are given subcutaneously separated by a 4-week interval. An oral vaccine was licensed for use in the United States in 1989. The vaccine contains the Ty21a strain of *S. typhi* and is associated with minimal side effects. The Ty21a vaccine is given as a four-dose series, with 2 days between each dose.[141] Immunosuppression, antibiotic use, and gastroenteritis are contraindications to the use of this vaccine. A newer parental vaccine contains the Vi (virulence) polysaccharide of *S. typhi* purified from formalin-killed bacteria. It is administered as a single intramuscular injection and is therefore most useful when vaccination is required at short notice. A booster is required every 2 years.[36] Even when the vaccine is given before travel, it is important to observe routine precautions for ingestion of food and water to prevent typhoid fever and acquisition of other pathogens by the fecal-oral route.

Meningococcal Disease

Classically, meningococcal meningitis attacks children and young adults and is often seen in epidemic form. Although the advent of effective antibiotic therapy and a useful vaccine have greatly improved the ability to deal with this disease, it remains a major problem in many parts of the world.

Epidemiology. Cases of meningococcal disease occur sporadically worldwide, with epidemic disease generally limited to developing nations. Epidemic situations clearly pose the greater health problem to both travelers and resident populations. Since 1970, large outbreaks have occurred in Brazil, China, the Sahel region of sub-Saharan Africa (from Mali and Burkina Faso to Ethiopia and northwestern Somalia), New Delhi, India, and Nepal.[35] Particularly in sub-Saharan Africa and China, the disease demonstrates yearly incidence peaks and periodic massive outbreaks, the exact determinants of which are unknown. Transmission of the organism occurs by exchange of respiratory secretions; contact is believed to be important in the spread of the disease. Asymptomatic transient nasopharyngeal carriage of the meningococcus, occurring with a baseline prevalence of 5% to 10%,[9] may increase during epidemic periods and in close contacts of cases. The secondary attack rate among household contacts of patients with sporadic disease is 2:1000 to 4:1000, whereas that in epidemics ranges from 11:1000 to 45:1000 household contacts.[90]

Bacteriology and Pathogenesis. *Neisseria meningitidis* is a gram-negative diplococcus that grows easily on several common media, including chocolate and blood agar. The organism is characterized further on the basis of serologic analysis of capsular antigens. The most common serogroups are A, B, C, Y, and W135. Serogroups A and C are often associated with epidemic disease, whereas serogroup B is the major cause of sporadic disease in the United States.[25] Asymptomatic persons may carry various serotypes of *N. meningitidis* in the nasopharynx for short periods of time. An antibody response is often generated to these strains during asymptomatic carriage. The conditions that cause one person to become clinically ill with invasive disease while another carrier remains healthy are not well understood. The route of entrance of the organism to the bloodstream and central nervous system (CNS) is presumably through the nasopharynx or respiratory tract.

Clinical Presentation. Meningococcal disease may appear in a variety of forms, including, but not limited to, bacteremia with septic shock; meningitis, often accompanied by bacteremia; and pneumonia. Sustained meningococcemia may lead to severe toxemia with hypotension, fever, and DIC. In the fulminant presentation, adrenal hemorrhage may lead to Waterhouse-Friderichsen syndrome, and death may follow intractable shock. In the United States the case-fatality rate for sustained meningococcemia is generally higher than for meningococcal meningitis.[140] There is also a clinical syndrome of chronic meningococcemia with a much more insidious onset.

Meningitis caused by *N. meningitidis* classically begins with fever, headache, and a stiff neck. It may also be accompanied by bacteremia and any of several skin manifestations, including petechiae, pustules, or maculopapular rash. In either meningitis or bacteremia, progression of petechiae to broad ecchymoses is a poor prognostic sign. As with septic meningococcemia, severe meningitis may progress with mental status deterioration, hypotension, congestive heart failure, DIC, and death. The case-fatality rate of meningococcal meningitis with or without bacteremia is now estimated to be about 10%.[140] In classic cases of meningitis or bacteremia with sepsis, the peripheral WBC count is elevated, with polymorphonuclear cell predominance. CSF typically is purulent, usually with more than 500 polymorphonuclear cells/mm[3]. There may be a more heterogeneous cell population and fewer cells if CSF is obtained early in the course or if the patient has been treated with antibiotics. The CSF glucose level is usually low and protein high, as in other bacterial meningitides. Gram's stain of CSF may show the gram-negative diplococci. Meningococcal pneumonia is a well-known but less common clinical entity,[109] most recently described in military recruit populations involving serogroup Y organisms.[77]

Diagnosis. The presumptive diagnosis in an epidemic can be made on the basis of clinical presentation and purulent spinal fluid. The presence of characteristic bacterial forms on Gram's stain is also suggestive. A definitive diagnosis requires culture of the organism from CSF or a normally sterile fluid (usually peripheral blood). This may be impossible in the case of a patient who was previously treated. Several commercial kits for measuring meningococcal antigen are now available for use on CSF or blood samples.

Management. Treatment of meningococcal meningitis or sepsis is a medical emergency. Fortunately, the organism remains sensitive to a large number of antibiotics. The treatment of choice is penicillin G, 300,000 units/kg/day (up to 24 million units a day), given intravenously in divided doses every 2 hours. Between 7 and 10 days of therapy for serious disease is appropriate. Ceftriaxone is an alternative antimicrobial agent. If the patient is allergic to penicillin, chloramphenicol (100 mg/kg/day) may be given, although the emergence of chloramphenicol-resistant strains of *N. meningitidis* is of great concern.[48] Notably, antibiotic treatment before culture or hospital referral is recommended in clinically suspected cases.

Supportive care should include close monitoring for hypotension and cardiac failure. Fluids and vasoactive and cardioselective agents may be important. This type of support necessitates invasive monitors and intensive care unit technology. Development of DIC is an ominous sign. The role of heparin in this disease is still debated. Although focal bleeding and adrenal necrosis may lead to acute adrenal insufficiency, the role of replacement steroids in the treatment of Waterhouse-Friderichsen syndrome is unclear.[5] Since the infectious agent has been found in household contacts and in those with exposure to oral secretions, contacts should receive prophylaxis to eradicate the organism. Rifampin, 600 mg by mouth every 12 hours for four doses, is standard adult prophylaxis. Children should receive 10 mg/kg of rifampin every 12 hours for four doses if they are older than 1 month and 5 mg/kg every 12 hours for four doses if they are less than 1 month of age.[17] More recently, alternate regimens using ceftriaxone and ciprofloxacin have also been proven to be efficacious, although rifampin remains the standard.

Prevention. An effective meningococcal vaccine that has been available in the United States for several years contains purified polysaccharide from the bacterial capsule of *N. meningitidis* serogroups A, C, Y, and W135. No vaccine is effective for group B disease. The recommended dose is one injection of 0.5 ml subcutaneously.[17] Clinical efficacy of more than 65% is maintained for at least 3 years in persons immunized at 4 years of age or older, although protection wanes more rapidly in children vaccinated at less than 4 years of age.[111] The incidence of meningococcal disease in the United States is so low that mass administration of the vaccine is inappropriate; however, vaccination is recommended for persons without spleens, with specific complement deficiencies, or those planning to travel to high-risk areas.[16,17] Epidemics have occurred since 1980 in sub-Saharan Africa; New Delhi, India; Nepal; and Saudi Arabia. Since the areas in which epidemic meningococcal disease occurs change from time to time, it is prudent to check with appropriate authorities to determine current recommendations for meningococcal vaccination before travel.

Pertussis

Pertussis, or whooping cough, was first recognized as a major threat in the 1500s. After the introduction of a vaccine in the 1940s, the incidence of pertussis dropped sharply among immunized populations. However, since recognition of rare side effects to pertussis vaccine, immunization rates have fallen. The age-specific incidence of pertussis in all age groups increased between 1981 and 1985 in the United States, with rates in persons 20 years and older increasing by thirteenfold during that period.[22]

Epidemiology. Pertussis is found throughout the world. The incidence is currently highest in undeveloped countries, where immunization rates are low and socioeconomic conditions predispose to many communicable diseases. Pertussis is highly infectious, with attack rates of greater than 90% in unvaccinated household contacts. In the United States, most infections and the most severe disease occur in children under 5 years old. Transmission is by airborne particles from respiratory secretions of infected persons.

Bacteriology and Pathophysiology. *Bordetella pertussis* is a gram-negative coccobacillus. The organism produces several toxins when present in the respiratory tract. Pertussigen stimulates lymphocytosis and hemagglutination. Dermonecrotic toxin and tracheal cytotoxins damage respiratory epithelium. In addition, endotoxin is produced. During the course of the somewhat protracted disease, complications can occur that may cause death. The most serious of these are secondary pneumonia or fulminant encephalopathy. In addition, fits of coughing often result in pneumothorax, hemorrhage (facial, conjunctival, and CNS), and aspiration.

Clinical Presentation. Classic pertussis develops after an incubation period of 7 to 10 days. The disease appears in three stages: catarrhal, paroxysmal, and convalescent. The catarrhal stage lasts 1 to 2 weeks and resembles an undifferentiated upper respiratory tract infection with cough and mild fever. Progression of the cough to yield the classic whoop (which results when the patient gasps for breath after a prolonged coughing episode) marks the paroxysmal stage, which again can last as long as 2 weeks. During this stage, the peripheral white blood cell count may show marked lymphocytosis. Finally, cough resolves during the convalescent

stage. Death may occur from pertussis alone or from complications such as aspiration pneumonia. Recent case-fatality rates for Americans were 0.4% for all persons and 1% for patients less than 1 year old.[22] The disease in adults is often milder, although it may show a severe classic pattern.[81] Some investigators believe mild or atypical disease in adults may serve as a reservoir for infection of susceptible children.[97]

Diagnosis. Culture of the organism from a nasopharyngeal swab is the most efficient way to diagnose pertussis; however, the culture is positive most frequently early in the illness, and late cultures (after the second week of illness) are rarely helpful. For optimal recovery, Bordet-Gengou media should be used, with methicillin added to reduce overgrowth by other bacteria present in the nasopharyngeal flora. Direct fluorescent antibody techniques may also be used to evaluate nasopharyngeal swabs or sputum samples for the presence of organisms.

Management. Treatment with antibiotics, unless begun in the incubation or catarrhal period, has little effect on the course of the disease. Antibiotics can reduce subsequent transmission to contacts, however, and should be instituted as soon as the diagnosis is made. Erythromycin, the drug of choice, should be given for at least 2 weeks. Other useful agents include doxycycline, trimethoprim/sulfamethoxazole, and chloramphenicol. In patients with severe disease, corticosteroids may provide some improvement.[150] Perhaps more important than specific antibiotics is supportive care, including hydration, nutrition, care to maintain adequate ventilation, and supplemental oxygen. In addition, external stimuli, which seem to exacerbate symptoms, should be kept to a minimum.

Prevention. Immunization of children with diphtheria-pertussis-tetanus (DPT) vaccine is recommended by the CDC, since the benefits of immunization are greater than the risk of neurologic damage from the vaccine.[26,66,67] Introduction of new acellular pertussis vaccines may reduce this risk even further.[27] Vaccination is not recommended for persons older than 7 unless there is specific risk. The goal of treatment is to reduce secondary transmission. Close contacts under 7 years old who are unimmunized should be immunized, and persons who have not had a dose of DPT in 3 years should receive one. Furthermore, all close contacts under 1 year old should receive a 14-day course of erythromycin or trimethoprim/sulfamethoxazole, as should unimmunized contacts under 7 years old.[26]

Diphtheria

Diphtheria, once a highly feared cause of morbidity and mortality in young people, can be controlled with appropriate use of a vaccine. However, according to some surveys, waning immunity has left more than 40% of American adults (18 years or older) with inadequate circulating levels of antitoxin against diphtheria. Of 15 cases of respiratory diphtheria occurring in the United States between 1980 and 1983, 11 occurred in persons 20 years of age or older.[27] Endemic diphtheria is present in the developing world and a cause for concern among travelers. A recent outbreak in the Russian Federation and other former states of the Soviet Union, primarily involving persons older than 14, highlights the need for up-to-date immunization in travelers.[28]

Epidemiology. Humans are the natural host for *Corynebacterium diphtheriae*. Person-to-person spread occurs through contact with respiratory secretions or diphtheritic skin lesions. A carrier state exists in which people who have either been immunized or previously infected harbor the organism and asymptomatically transmit it to others. Evidence suggests that diphtheria can be transmitted through food or water, but this is not a major route of transmission.

Bacteriology and Pathogenesis. *C. diphtheriae* is a gram-positive, club-shaped bacillus. On Gram's stain, the clustered bacteria have the characteristic "Chinese letter" configuration. The organisms grow on standard media, but to avoid overgrowth of other oral flora, selective media (Löffler's culture medium or cysteine-tellurite agar) are suggested. The presence of a lysogenic bacteriophage in some *C. diphtheriae* organisms induces production of diphtheria toxin. The toxin is produced as a single molecule with two subunits, fragments A and B. Fragment B facilitates attachment to the cell membrane of host cells, and after attachment, fragment A enters the cell. Cell death results from large-scale disruption of protein synthetic capabilities.

Clinical Presentation. The most important manifestation of diphtheria is respiratory tract infection. Illness begins after an incubation period of about a week with nonspecific symptoms of malaise, fatigue, mild sore throat, and slight fever. The classic lesion is exudative pharyngitis progressing to a greenish-gray membrane that is difficult to dislodge. This membrane may spread over the posterior pharynx, tonsils, and uvula and down the respiratory tree to involve the larynx and trachea. Any one of these areas may be involved selectively, and the severity of illness is to some extent related to the area grossly involved.

In severe disease, swollen tissues may result in a bull neck appearance. Major complications include obstruction of the respiratory tract, which may result from direct parapharyngeal swelling or laryngeal involvement in young children, and sloughing of the tracheobronchial membrane in older patients. In addition to respiratory tract damage, toxin directly injures myocardial and neural tissue. Endocarditis occurs in some patients. Early signs in the first week of disease include ST-T wave depression and atrioventricular conduction abnormalities on the electrocardiogram. Congestive heart failure and cardiac enlargement may develop. Neurologic deficits usually begin with pharyngeal and cranial nerve paralysis. Cranial nerve paralysis may progress to bilateral motor paralysis, which generally resolves over a period of 3 to 6 months.[59] In the tropics, cutaneous diphtheria is seen frequently. The skin lesions are not consistent in appearance and range from very superficial impetigo-like lesions to deep ulcers. In most cases of cutaneous disease, absorption of toxin is not great enough to cause the multisystem involvement seen in respiratory tract disease. The prevalence of skin lesions increases the overall likelihood of coming in contact with toxigenic *C. diphtheriae*.

Diagnosis. Reliable isolation of the organism requires a selective medium and several days of culture. Treatment should be started as soon as the patient is evaluated and is guided by clinical manifestations.

Management. Since the toxin and not the organism mediates life-threatening clinical manifestations of diphtheria per se, neutralization of absorbed toxin is crucial.[59] A horse-derived antitoxin is available and should be administered as soon as the diagnosis is seriously considered. A 0.1 ml test dose of intradermal antitoxin diluted to a 1:1000 concentration (with a saline control) is observed for 20 minutes. If no reaction occurs, full doses can be given intravenously. Antitoxin should be diluted to 1:20 in saline and given no faster than 1 ml/min. For mild cases, 20,000 units may be adequate, 40,000 units for moderate cases, and as much as 80,000 to 120,000 units for severely ill patients. Erythromycin or penicillin may be given to eradicate the carrier state, although their use has no effect on the clinical course of disease. Close observation is crucial to evaluate the need for respiratory support, especially in young children. Serial electrocardiograms and neurologic evaluation establish the onset of complications. If significant conduction abnormalities are present, continuous heart monitoring should be undertaken. Strict bed rest is recommended for all patients for 2 to 3 weeks.

Prevention. Close contacts of patients with respiratory diphtheria should receive diphtheria vaccine if they have not received at least three doses previously or if 5 or more years have elapsed since the last dose.[26] In addition, unimmunized or partially immunized contacts should receive either intramuscular benzathine penicillin (600,000 units if younger than 6 years old, 1.2 million units if older than 6 years old) or 7 to 10 days of erythromycin (40 mg/kg/day for children or 1 g/day for adults, in four divided doses). Antitoxin is not recommended for contacts. The most important way to prevent diphtheria in adults, however, is to ensure that all adults receive a booster dose of diphtheria-tetanus toxoid every 10 years.

Tetanus

Tetanus was recognized by the early Greeks and is still a cause of infant and adult mortality. Today, the mortality approaches 90% and 40% for untreated infants and adults, respectively.[122] Tetanus toxoid immunization has drastically reduced the incidence of disease in populations with high coverage rates.

Epidemiology. The bacterium and its spores are ubiquitous. Approximately 10% of people in the general population carry *Clostridium tetani* in fecal flora.[108] Person-to-person spread is not important in this disease. Disease occurs when the organism is introduced into an environment suitable for its growth, specifically, wound sites with an anaerobic environment. In the United States, most of the 75 to 90 cases each year occur in persons over 50 years old.[124] In the developing world, the vast majority of cases are in neonates as a result of umbilical stump infections.

Bacteriology and Pathophysiology. *C. tetani* is a gram-positive, anaerobic, spore-forming rod. The spores are hardy and can occasionally survive boiling for short periods. After proliferating in an appropriate anaerobic environment, *C. tetani* releases the toxin, tetanospasmin, which, in generalized disease, reaches the spinal column and CNS by hematogenous spread. The toxin is taken up by inhibitory neurons, where it interferes with release of inhibitory neurotransmitters, resulting in disinhibition of motor groups. Disinhibition of the sympathetic nervous system neurons occurs through a similar mechanism. The result is muscular spasm of varying severity and signs of sympathetic nervous system hyperactivity, including tachycardia, sweating, arrhythmias, and high blood pressure.

Clinical Presentation. A tetanus-prone wound precedes most adult disease, which may not be evident at the time of presentation. Localized tetanus, with spasm of a focal set of muscle groups, may occur and remain localized for weeks, then slowly resolve. This form of tetanus is much less common than the generalized form, which often begins with trismus, or spasm of the masticator muscle group. Gradual onset of spasm of other muscle groups usually involves the trunk and extremities. Since the posterior muscles are stronger during spasms, the victim exhibits lumbar lordosis, with the neck and legs extended and arms flexed at the elbows (opisthotonos). Spasms seem to be exacerbated by external stimuli, such as sudden sound or light. The primary danger is loss of ability to breathe, especially during prolonged spasms. Respiratory failure is the main cause of death. The clinical picture in neonatal tetanus is similar, but begins with restlessness and failure to nurse, with progression to tetany and sympathetic overactivity. There is no definitive laboratory test to confirm the diagnosis of tetanus, but the clinical picture is adequate in the majority of cases.

Management. Emergency medical treatment of tetanus patients should include (1) excision of the wound, (2) administration of human tetanus IG (at least 500 units,[6] but a range of 500 to 3000 units is commonly used), and (3) administration of an antibiotic effective against *C. tetani*, such as penicillin or metronidazole.[121] Depending on the severity of the disease, different levels of supportive care and sedation may be appropriate. Diazepam may be given to mildly affected patients for sedation. Patients should be evaluated carefully for dysphagia. If dysphagia is present or other respiratory difficulties arise, endotracheal intubation or a tracheostomy should be performed. With prolonged spasms, hypoxia and cyanosis may occur; mechanical ventilation with pharmacologic paralysis is appropriate. At the same time, attention must be given to fluid balance and nutrition. Enteral feeding by a nasogastric tube is the least invasive way to supply both. Beta-blockers have been suggested to relieve symptoms of autonomic overactivity, such as tachycardia and hypertension, but there is no proven benefit to their prophylactic use. Sources of sensory stimulation should be reduced when the spasms are uncontrolled.

Prevention. Although rare cases of tetanus have occurred in previously immunized persons,[102] immunization is considered at least 99.9% effective.[26] Several vaccine formulations are now available in the United States. Children under 7 years old may receive either DPT or DT (diphtheria and tetanus toxoid only) vaccine. A third vaccine, Td, is manufactured for use in persons at least 7 years old and consists of tetanus toxoid and a smaller amount of diphtheria toxoid than is present in the pediatric vaccines. A reduced amount of diphtheria toxoid is used in the adult preparation, since both the amount of toxoid and increasing age were found to be associated with more severe reactions to vaccination. Adults who are unimmunized should be given a series of three doses (0.5 ml intramuscularly) of Td, with the second dose 4 to 8 weeks after the first, and the third dose 6 to 12 months after the second. A booster should be given every 10 years thereafter. All travelers should know their primary immunization and stay up to date with booster doses. From the standpoint of tetanus prevention, care of wounds is crucial. The tetanus-prone wound, contaminated with dirt or feces or caused by puncture, crush, avulsion, or frostbite, should be cleaned and debrided appropriately. Persons with tetanus-prone wounds should receive 250 to 500 units of human tetanus IG if their immunization history is unknown or their immunization series is incomplete. These persons should also receive a dose of Td and complete an immunization series. Persons fully immunized and given an appropriate booster before a tetanus-prone wound should not receive tetanus IG. If they have not received a booster within 5 years, however, they should get a dose of Td.[3]

MAJOR PROTOZOAN INFECTIONS

Malaria

Malaria, or "ague" in previous centuries, is a major cause of childhood mortality in developing countries. Travelers who are not immune (i.e., most North Americans and Europeans) are at great risk for the disease.

Epidemiology. The four major human malaria parasites, *Plasmodium falciparum, P. vivax, P. ovale,* and *P. malariae,* are found in most tropical developing countries where the appropriate anopheline mosquito vector exists. The degree of endemicity in a specific region may be judged by the proportion of residents who have enlarged spleens. The degree varies from a hypoendemic area, in which less than 10% of children have enlarged spleens, to hyperendemic, in which more than 50% of children have enlarged spleens.

Persons are inoculated by sporozoites when a mosquito releases the parasite during a blood meal. Sporozoites rapidly invade liver cells, where they proliferate into multiple merozoites. After 1 to 2 weeks, merozoites rupture from hepatocytes and invade red blood cells. A proportion of *P. vivax* and *P. ovale* organisms may enter a dormant phase in the liver and cause recrudescence of disease months to years later. *P. falciparum* does not enter this dormant phase. After merozoites enter a red blood cell, they may undergo asexual proliferation (schizogony) to eventually form more merozoites (which may invade other red blood cells) or sexual differentiation to form gametocytes. Merozoites cause red blood cell lysis, whereas gametocytes must be ingested by mosquitoes to continue the parasite life cycle. Development of fertilized eggs in the mosquito to form infective sporozoites takes 10 to 14 days. Travelers may be infected and develop disease from one sporozoite; cases of malaria have been reported in individuals who presumably had contact only with mosquitoes that entered an aircraft in transit through endemic areas.

Pathogenesis and Clinical Manifestations. Rupture of erythrocytes by asexual schizonts containing merozoites is associated with fever, nausea, and severe myalgias.[127] Cerebral malaria and other evidence of organ dysfunction, such as renal failure in falciparum malaria, are presumably related to sludging in the microvasculature by poorly deformable red blood cells or erythrocytes with parasite-induced surface molecules that adhere to the endothelium. Anoxia of surrounding tissue results.[127] Anemia induced by all *Plasmodium* species is secondary to hemolysis and ineffective erythropoiesis.

Clinical manifestations of malaria may first be evident within 1 to 2 weeks after the victim enters an endemic area, or sooner if infected blood obtained by transfusion or use of shared needles is the source. Although there are no pathognomonic signs, many subjects report paroxysms of chills, followed by high fever and sweating. These may last several hours and recur every 2 to 3 days. Classic periodic attacks are often not observed in severe falciparum malaria, and fever may be constant. In addition, abdominal cramps and diarrhea may be presenting symptoms. Cerebral malaria, associated with high levels of parasitemia (usually more than 10% of red blood cells infected) is characterized by high fevers, confusion, and eventually coma and death.

Diagnosis. Malaria can be definitively diagnosed only by the presence of malaria parasite–containing red blood cells. Prophylactic medications do not exclude the possibility of being infected. Thick and thin blood smears should be made and stained with Giemsa stain for microscopic inspection. Thin films are prepared in a standard manner. Thick films are prepared by spreading a drop of blood in a 1-cm-diameter circle. The blood is allowed to dry, red blood cells are lysed with water, and the slide is stained with Giemsa stain. Various intraerythrocytic forms (schizonts, trophozoites, merozoites) should be identified. Blood smears should be obtained on initial contact with the patient and every 12 hours until they show positive results. Speciation of malaria is important when falciparum infection is a possibility because this parasite may be resistant to chloroquine and cause lethal disease. Several assays for detection of malaria antigens in blood (e.g., "dipstick" assays) may be useful in situations where expertise in microscopic detection of the parasite is not readily available.

Management

PLASMODIUM FALCIPARUM. A major issue involved in treating falciparum malaria is sensitivity of the parasite to chloroquine.[107] Chloroquine-resistant strains of *P. falciparum* are found in all endemic areas of the world except Central America west of the Panama Canal, islands in the Caribbean Sea, and the Middle East, including Egypt. Since no laboratory test can distinguish between sensitive and resistant strains, all persons diagnosed as having *P. falciparum* acquired outside these areas should be treated as having chloroquine-resistant malaria. There are multiple useful drug regimens. A commonly used regimen for adults is quinine sulfate, 600 mg orally 3 times per day for 7 days, plus tetracycline, 250 mg every 6 hours for 7 days. The dose of quinine salt for children is 10 mg/kg body weight. Pregnant women and children under 8 years should not be given tetracycline. In some parts of the world, mefloquine (Lariam) at a single dose of 1250 mg (or 15 mg base per kg) is used (the drug should not be administered if quinine has been given in the previous 12 hours). In persons believed to have chloroquine-sensitive *P. falciparum* infection, chloroquine phosphate, 1000 mg initially, should be followed by 500 mg 6 hours later and 500 mg/day for an additional 2 days. In persons with severe and complicated *P. falciparum* infection, such as those with cerebral malaria, IV quinine should be used. For quinine a loading dose of 16.7 mg base (suspended in isotonic saline) per kilogram of body weight is given intravenously over 4 hours. This is followed by 8.3 mg base per kg every 8 hours until oral medications can be taken and a full 3- or 7-day course (if infection was acquired in Southeast Asia) is completed. The loading dose is decreased to 8.3 mg/kg if mefloquine or quinine has been taken within the previous 12 hours. If IV quinine is unavailable, quinidine gluconate may be substituted. The loading dose is 10 mg/kg given in saline over 1 hour followed by continuous infusion of 0.02 mg/kg/min for up to 3 days. The patient should be switched to oral quinine as soon as possible. These medications should be administered in an intensive care unit with continuous cardiac monitoring. Exchange transfusion to lower the level of parasitemia may also be useful in this setting. Corticosteroids are contraindicated, since controlled studies show that mortality is higher when they are given.[136]

PLASMODIUM VIVAX, P. OVALE, AND P. MALARIAE. These infections are treated as described for chloroquine-sensitive *P. falciparum*. Since *P. vivax* and *P. ovale* may have dormant hepatic forms, primaquine phosphate, 26.3 mg daily for 14 days, should follow administration of chloroquine to eliminate extraerythrocytic hypnozoites. Individuals given primaquine should first be screened for the presence of glucose-6-phosphate dehydrogenase (G-6-PD) deficiency, since this drug may cause oxidant-induced hemolysis. If G-6-PD deficiency is severe, primaquine should not be administered and the patient should be monitored periodically for symptoms of malaria. Individuals with mild G-6-PD deficiency may be given primaquine under close supervision because hemolysis is self-limited.

Proper precautions include avoidance of contact with mosquitoes through the use of nets, sprays, and long-sleeved clothing. Travelers to endemic areas should take prophylactic medications[18] (see Chapter 65).

African Trypanosomiasis

Trypanosoma brucei rhodesiense and *T. brucei gambiense* have provided remarkable insights into the importance of antigenic variation as a strategy used by parasites to avoid the immune response.[135] *T. brucei gambiense* causes African sleeping sickness, and *T. brucei rhodesiense* causes an acute disease that may end in heart failure. The parasites are transmitted to humans by tsetse flies (*Glossina* species) in sub-Saharan Africa. Metacyclic promastigotes are injected into the bloodstream through the saliva of the biting tsetse fly and divide into long slender forms in the bloodstream. These eventually differentiate into short stumpy forms, which are taken up in the blood meal of the tsetse. Once in the fly, the parasite differentiates into procyclic forms. It takes approximately 3 weeks for the protozoa to develop into infective metacyclics within the tsetse fly.

Clinical Manifestations. In nonimmune individuals the initial sign of infection is a nodule at the site of the tsetse fly bite. This lesion becomes erythematous and painful over a period of 1 week and recedes after several days. Dissemination of the trypanosome throughout the body causes clinical symptoms, notably fever, headache, and severe malaise. On physical examination, enlarged supraclavicular and posterior cervical lymph nodes are noted. This phase of illness lasts several days and is followed by an asymptomatic period of several weeks. The acute phase may then recur. In the case of *T. brucei gambiense* infection, symptoms are less severe and evolve into a syndrome characterized by behavioral changes and chronic somnolence. *T. brucei rhodesiense* infections cause severe anemia, frequent episodes of fever, and eventual heart failure and severe CNS involvement.

Diagnosis. Definitive diagnosis depends on identification of parasites in the blood, lymphatics, or CSF. Thick blood smears and buffy coat preparations should be stained with Giemsa stain and examined for the presence of trypanosomes. The CSF should be subjected to centrifugation and the sediment examined for parasites. Associated laboratory abnormalities include anemia, monocytosis, and elevated serum and CSF IgM levels.[45]

Management. Suramin* should be used for treatment of early *T. brucei rhodesiense* infection, although the drug may cause proteinuria.[39] A test dose of 100 mg intravenously is first given to detect possible idiosyncratic reactions. If tolerated, 1 g should be given on the initial day of treatment and 3, 7, 14, and 21 days later. If CNS involvement is diagnosed or strongly suspected (CSF

---

*Available in the United States from the Parasitic Diseases Division of the CDC.

lymphocytosis and elevated IgM), melarsoprol (available from the CDC) should also be administered.[39] This drug is given at an initial dose of 1.5 mg/kg of body weight, with gradually increasing doses (e.g., increase every 48 hours to 3.6 mg/kg in 2 weeks). After a week with no drug given, additional injections of 3.6 mg/kg are given every other day 3 times. This arsenical compound is toxic, causing encephalopathy and exfoliative dermatitis, and should be used only in a controlled hospital setting. For early *T. brucei gambiense* infection, pentamidine (4 mg/kg body weight intramuscularly, up to 300 mg/kg given over 7 days) is the treatment of choice. Eflornithine, 100 mg/kg every 6 hours for 14 days, should be used for more advanced cases of this infection.

South American Trypanosomiasis (Chagas' Diseases)

T. cruzi is transmitted to humans by triatomids that live in the cracks of mud-built homes in Central and Latin America. These insects are particularly common in areas of Brazil, Venezuela, and Argentina with poor socioeconomic development. The infection has been reported as far north as the southern United States. Affected individuals generally do not recall initial contact with the insects, during which time the protozoan organisms deposited on broken skin or mucous membranes in triatomid feces multiply within local macrophages. The macrophages rupture and elicit an inflammatory reaction characterized as a nodule with slightly painful satellite nodules or draining lymph nodes. A symptomatic phase, characterized by fever and diffuse lymph node enlargement, develops subsequently. Hepatosplenomegaly may also occur. In severe cases, acute myocarditis, pericarditis, or endocarditis is seen. After several months, the acute phase resolves and chronic disease appears, characterized by cardiomyopathy, megaesophagus, or megacolon.[78] It is rare for the traveler to develop these signs and symptoms. Diagnosis during the acute phase may be made by demonstration of parasites in leukocytes in Giemsa-stained blood smears. Amastigotes of *T. cruzi* may also be present in biopsy specimens of lymph nodes or muscle. Elevated IgM antibody titers to *T. cruzi* (performed by the CDC) also support the diagnosis. In the chronic phases of Chagas' disease, the clinical findings of cardiomyopathy, megaesophagus, or megacolon, in concert with isolation of *T. cruzi* from blood, support the diagnosis. To detect trypanosomes in blood, uninfected triatomids are permitted to feed on the patient's forearm for 30 minutes. The insects are then kept for 30 days and the intestinal contents of the insects examined for *T. cruzi*. If negative, the examination may be repeated after 60 days. This test is positive in about 50% of cases. Serologic tests, including complement fixation for anti–*T. cruzi* antibodies (done at the CDC), are also

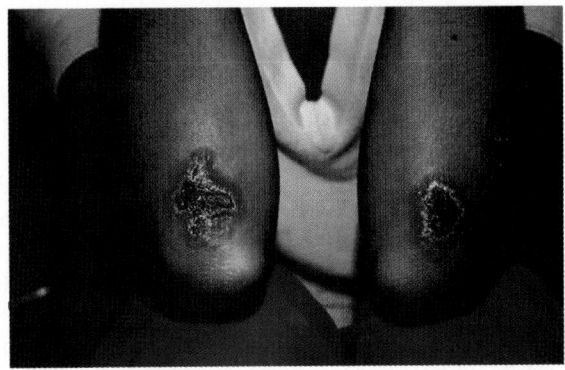

Figure 66-1 Old world leishmaniasis. *(Courtesy Richard Kaplan, MD.)*

useful but may be positive in long-term residents of endemic areas. Acute Chagas' disease is treated with nifurtimox, 8 to 10 mg/kg orally per day in four divided doses for 120 days. The drug is available from the CDC.

Leishmaniasis

Humans may be infected by *Leishmania* species that cause skin, mucocutaneous, or visceral disease.[146] These intracellular parasites are transmitted by phlebotomine sandflies. Various forms of the infection occur throughout Latin and Central America, Africa, the Middle East, and Asia (Figure 66-1). Cutaneous lesions caused by *L. tropica* and *L. tropica major* are referred to as "Oriental sores" in Asia and the Middle East. In Central and South America, *L. mexicana* and *L. braziliensis* cause skin lesions characterized in the chronic phase as nonhealing ulcers that frequently become secondarily infected by bacteria. *Espundia*, or mucocutaneous leishmaniasis caused by *L. braziliensis*, begins as a single nodule and eventually involves the oropharyngeal or nasal mucosa, where it causes severe destruction. This disease occurs primarily in residents of the Amazon basin in Brazil. *Kala-azar*, or visceral leishmaniasis, is caused by *L. donovani* in Africa and Asia. Affected individuals generally do not recall an initial skin lesion. Several months after inoculation, fever, abdominal discomfort, and weakness develop and become progressively more severe. Nausea and vomiting are protracted, the skin becomes dry and dark, and abdominal distention with hepatosplenomegaly eventually appears. This disease is rare in travelers and nonresidents of endemic areas.

MAJOR HELMINTHIC INFECTIONS

Worm infections are common among travelers to developing countries, especially among persons who spend time in rural areas. However, unlike many viral or protozoan infections, helminths rarely cause life-threatening disease and infested persons are often asymptomatic.

Schistosomiasis

Three major species of schistosomes infect humans: *Schistosoma mansoni*, *S. haematobium*, and *S. japonicum*. *S. mansoni* infection occurs in South America and Africa. *S. haematobium* infection occurs primarily in Africa, especially Egypt and East Africa. *S. japonicum* infection is present exclusively in the Far East. Schistosomiasis is transmitted by freshwater snails. These snails release cercariae that penetrate the skin of humans. The cercariae rapidly transform into schistosomulae, which migrate to the lungs and eventually the portal (in the case of *S. mansoni* and *S. japonicum*) or vesical (in the case of *S. haematobium*) venous system to differentiate into adult worms. Fecund female worms release eggs, which may be passed in feces or urine. Miracidia released from this stage may then infect snails in water used for bathing, washing clothes, or other communal activities.

Signs and symptoms of infection vary among the three schistosome species. The initial presentation of *S. mansoni* infection reported in Puerto Rico includes fever, anorexia, weight loss, and abdominal pain.[65] Hepatomegaly and splenomegaly were observed in 33% and 20% of subjects, respectively. This unusual symptom complex, which occurs in individuals with heavy infection, has been referred to as Katayama fever and appears 18 to 60 days after exposure. Travelers with light or moderate exposure, however, usually have no specific signs or only mild local dermatitis associated with contact with cercariae, the infective stage of the parasite released by snails. In persons with established infections the prevalence of clinical manifestations is low. Most individuals have no signs specifically attributable to *S. mansoni* infection. Hepatomegaly or splenomegaly, attributable to portal hypertension after granulomatous reactions to eggs deposited in the liver, occurs in 15% of subjects.[125] Eggs may also embolize to the lungs and induce granulomatous lesions and cor pulmonale. Those at greatest risk are persons who have the heaviest intensity of infection as judged by fecal egg counts. These complications may ultimately result in esophageal and gastrointestinal varices, which cause acute blood loss. The manifestations of schistosomiasis japonicum are similar to schistosomiasis mansoni, except that Katayama fever appears to be more frequent. In addition, there is a unique manifestation of *S. japonicum* infection attributable to embolization of eggs to the brain. Generalized or Jacksonian seizures are the major signs of cerebral schistosomiasis. Since *S. haematobium* adult worms inhabit the venous system of the genitourinary tract, the signs and symptoms of this helminth infection are primarily secondary to granulomatous reactions to eggs present in the ureters and bladder wall. Dysuria and hematuria have been reported in many individuals who reside in endemic areas. The frequency and severity of hematuria and dysuria and associated complications (such as calcifi-

cation of the bladder and lower ureters and hydronephrosis) correlate directly with the intensity of infection, as judged by urinary egg output. It should be stressed that these complications are unusual in the traveler who spends little time in freshwater in endemic areas.[137]

All these species of schistosome infections are diagnosed by identification of eggs in urine, feces, or tissue sections. In the cases of *S. mansoni* and *S. japonicum*, microscopic inspection of feces by the Kato or formol-ether methods is most widely available in hospital laboratories.[105] *S. haematobium* eggs may be seen in urinary sediment or by more sensitive filtration techniques.[105] Treatment of all three species of schistosome infections is with praziquantel (40 mg/kg body weight in two divided doses for *S. haematobium* and *S. mansoni*, 60 mg/kg for *S. japonicum*). To avoid infection, travelers should be advised against swimming in freshwater lakes and rivers in endemic areas.

Filariases

Three major types of human filariasis exist. Infections caused by *Onchocerca volvulus* are manifest primarily as skin and eye disease. *Brugia malayi* and *Wuchereria bancrofti* cause lymphatic filariasis. Loa loa infection may cause skin disease. Each of these is described separately, since their ecologies and manifestations are distinctive.

Onchocerciasis. *O. volvulus* is transmitted to humans by *Simulium* species of blackflies in Central America and West and Central Africa. Infective, or third-stage, larvae eventually develop into adult worms contained in deep subcutaneous nodules that are asymptomatic and may be palpable. Microfilariae are released from adult female worms and cause dermatitis as they migrate through the skin. In Central and West Africa, the organisms have a propensity to invade the eye (especially the anterior chamber and cornea), where they cause blindness. Diagnosis is based on prolonged residence in an endemic area (e.g., Peace Corps volunteers) and parasitologic identification in skin snips or slit-lamp examination of the eye.[109]

Lymphatic Filariasis. *B. malayi* and *W. bancrofti* are transmitted by mosquitoes. Infective larvae eventually develop into lymphatic-dwelling adult worms, which release microfilariae into the bloodstream. Although chronic infection and recurrent exposure are associated with a wide variety of clinical manifestations, including tropical pulmonary eosinophilia, acute lymphangitis, and elephantiasis, these manifestations are rare in nonresidents of endemic areas.[100] The only definitive diagnostic test is identification of parasites in the bloodstream. Since nonresidents and many residents who are infected may not have detectable parasitemia, other laboratory studies (eosinophilia, elevated serum IgE level) must be used as aids in diagnosis. Diethylcarbamazine (cumulative dose of 72 mg/kg body weight given over 2 weeks) is the treatment.[62]

Loiasis. *Loa loa* is transmitted to humans by the bites of tabanid flies that live along river edges in Central and West Africa. Microfilariae migrate in the bloodstream, whereas adult worms migrate in cutaneous tissues. The major disease manifestation is calabar swellings, which are characterized as egg-sized or smaller raised lesions, predominantly over the extremities, that are tender and surrounded by edematous skin. They may migrate and last several days. Their pathogenesis may be related to migration of adult worms or release of antigens that elicit immunologic hypersensitivity reactions. Treatment is with diethylcarbamazine at a dose of 9 mg/kg body weight/day for 3 weeks.[62] Retreatment is occasionally required.

Intestinal Helminth Infections

Ascariasis. Approximately 25% of the world's population is infected with *Ascaris lumbricoides*.[79] Although this nematode contributes significantly to morbidity in children with poor nutrition, it generally does not cause significant health problems for the traveler. The helminth is transmitted by eggs contained in ingested pieces of soil, such as may be found on vegetables grown in many countries with poor hygienic conditions. It is not limited to tropical climates and occurs in North America and Europe. Ingested eggs enter the small intestine. Larvae leave the eggshell to penetrate the mucosa and eventually enter the bloodstream and lymphatics. Between 1 and 5 days after infection, they enter the liver and, at about 14 days, the lungs. The larvae then rupture through the alveoli, ascend the trachea, and return to the intestine on being swallowed. In the small intestine, adult males and females develop into macroscopic worms (12 to 25 cm long). Eggs passed via feces continue the life cycle. Ascaris infection is often totally asymptomatic, but several syndromes are associated with tissue and intestinal phases of infection. Persons who are recurrently exposed may develop pulmonary ascariasis, characterized by cough, wheezing, eosinophilia, and fleeting pulmonary infiltrates on chest x-ray examination.[104] Children may suffer from intestinal or biliary tract obstruction if they repeatedly ingest eggs. Intestinal symptoms are seen mainly in persons with heavy infection, an uncommon situation in the traveler.

Diagnosis of ascariasis may be made by identification of one of several parasite stages. Adult ascarids occasionally migrate from the mouth or anus. *Ascaris* larvae may rarely be observed in sputum or gastric washings. The most common means of diagnosis is identification of eggs in feces. Eggs are ovoid, 35 to 70 mm in diameter, and consist of an outer white shell and brownish ovum internally. The eggs are not produced

until approximately 9 weeks after infection. Intestinal ascariasis is treated with mebendazole, 100 mg twice daily for 3 days. An alternative regimen that avoids the use of benzimidazoles (e.g., for treatment of pregnant women) is pyrantel pamoate (11 mg/kg body weight to a maximum of 1 g).

Hookworm. *Ancylostoma duodenale* and *Necator americanus* infections occur most commonly in the tropics but also in temperate climates where sanitation is poor.[91] Hookworm is second only to *Ascaris* in terms of the number of people infected. Humans are infected percutaneously by third-stage larvae in the soil. The larvae enter the bloodstream, pass to the lungs, and rupture the alveolar lining to eventually ascend the trachea and descend the esophagus to differentiate into adult worms. These stages contain cutting plates on the anterior end and feed on host blood obtained through their attachment sites in the upper small intestine. It has been estimated that each *N. americanus* causes 0.03 ml of blood loss per day,[76] whereas *A. duodenale* consumes 0.26 ml per day. Iron deficiency anemia, especially in persons with low iron intake, is the major clinical manifestation of hookworm infection.[50] The diagnosis may be made by identification of hookworm eggs in feces. The eggs are round, 40 to 60 mm in diameter, and have a "smoother" shell than do *Ascaris* eggs. Although multiple drugs are effective in treatment, mebendazole (300 mg for the first dose, followed by 100 mg twice daily for 2 days) is most readily available. Supplemental iron should be given to persons when necessary. Infection with hookworm is rare in the traveler from a developed country.

Strongyloidiasis. *Strongyloides stercoralis* infection occurs in tropical and temperate regions. The infection is initiated by contact with soil containing infective third-stage larvae. The helminth follows a route within the host similar to that described for hookworms. In addition, there is an autoinfection cycle in which larvae released in the intestine may penetrate the mucosa directly and then migrate through the liver and lungs. This occurs only in immunocompromised individuals.[122]

Many persons with *S. stercoralis* infection are asymptomatic. Some persons, however, have cutaneous or intestinal manifestations. The former are urticarial lesions around the buttocks and waist that last 1 to 2 days.[59] These are secondary to penetration of larvae present in the feces. Other symptoms include indigestion, abdominal cramps, and diarrhea. Diagnosis is made by identification of larvae in fresh stools or gastrointestinal washings. Rhabditiform larvae with a length of 250 mm and a width of 10 to 20 mm are most commonly observed, although filariform larvae (500 mm long) may also be present. Treatment is with thiabendazole at a dose of 25 mg/kg body weight twice daily for 2 days.

Enterobiasis. Enterobiasis, or pinworm infection, exists in all parts of the world. Eggs are passed from female worms in the colon. Infection is transmitted by ingestion of *Enterobius vermicularis* eggs, which develop into gravid adult female worms in the large bowel. The infection is especially common in crowded settings where sanitation is poor. The diagnosis may be made by identification of adult worms migrating along the perianal area or by eggs deposited in the same area. Eggs are detected by applying a piece of sticky cellophane tape to the area and inspecting it microscopically.[82] Treatment is with a single 100-mg dose of mebendazole.

REFERENCES

1. Allain J-P: The status of hepatitis C screening, *Transfusion Med Rev* 12:46, 1998.
2. Al-Tikriti SK et al: Congo/Crimean haemorrhagic fever in Iraq, *Bull WHO* 59:85, 1981.
3. Baron RC, McCormick JB, Zubeir OA: Ebola virus disease in southern Sudan: hospital dissemination and intrafamilial spread, *Bull WHO* 61:997, 1983.
4. Beer B, Kurth R, Bukreyev A: Characteristics of Filoviridae: Marburg and Ebola viruses, *Naturwissenschaften* 86:8, 1999.
5. Belsey NA, Hoffpauir CW, Smith MHD: Dexamethasone in the treatment of acute bacterial meningitis: the effect of study design on the interpretation of results, *Pediatrics* 44:503, 1969.
6. Blake PA et al: Serological therapy of tetanus in the United States, 1965-1971, *JAMA* 235:42, 1976.
7. Borges APA et al: Estudo da coagulacao sanguinea na febre amarela, *Rev Patol Trop* 2:143, 1973.
8. Broome CV: The carrier state: *Neisseria meningitidis*, *J Antimicrob Chemother* 18(suppl A):25, 1986.
9. Buck AA et al: Onchocerciasis: some new epidemiologic and clinical findings, *Am J Trop Med Hyg* 18:217, 1969.
10. Burke DS, Nisalak A: Detection of Japanese encephalitis virus immunoglobulin M antibodies in serum by antibody capture radioimmunoassay, *J Clin Microbiol* 15:353, 1982.
11. Burke DS, Nisalak A, Ussery MA: Antibody capture immunoassay for detection of Japanese encephalitis virus immunoglobulin M and G antibodies in cerebrospinal fluid, *J Clin Microbiol* 16:1034, 1982.
12. Burke DS et al: Fatal outcome in Japanese encephalitis, *Am J Trop Med Hyg* 34:1203, 1985.
13. Cahill KM et al: Preparing patients for travel, *Patient Care*, p 217, June 15, 1987.
14. Centers for Disease Control: Bacterial meningitis and meningococcemia, United States, 1978, *MMWR* 28:277, 1979.
15. Centers for Disease Control: Dengue—Texas, *MMWR* 29:451, 1980.
16. Centers for Disease Control: Epidemic meningococcal disease: recommendations for travelers to Nepal, *MMWR* 34:119, 1985.
17. Centers for Disease Control: Meningococcal vaccines, *MMWR* 34:121, 1985.
18. Centers for Disease Control: Revised recommendations for preventing malaria in travelers to areas with chloroquine-resistant *Plasmodium falciparum*, *MMWR* 34:185, 1985.
19. Centers for Disease Control: Dengue in the Americas, *MMWR* 35:732, 1986.
20. Centers for Disease Control: Dengue hemorrhagic fever—Puerto Rico, *MMWR* 35:779, 1986.
21. Centers for Disease Control: Safety of therapeutic immune globulin preparations with respect to transmission of human T-lymphotropic virus type III/lymphadenopathy-associated virus infection, *MMWR* 35:231, 1986.
22. Centers for Disease Control: Pertussis surveillance, United States, 1984 and 1985, *MMWR* 36:168, 1987.
23. Centers for Disease Control: Management of patients with suspected viral hemorrhagic fever, *MMWR* 37:1, 1988.
24. Centers for Disease Control: Recommendations for protection against viral hepatitis, *MMWR* 39(RR-2):1, 1990.
25. Centers for Disease Control: Yellow fever vaccine, *MMWR* 39(RR-2):1, 1990.
26. Centers for Disease Control: Diphtheria, tetanus and pertussis: guidelines for vaccine use and other preventive measures, *MMWR* 40(RR-10):1, 1991.
27. Centers for Disease Control: Pertussis vaccination: acellular pertussis vaccine for reinforcing and booster use—supplementary ACIP statement, *MMWR* 41(RR-1):1, 1992.
28. Centers for Disease Control: Diphtheria outbreak—Russian Federation, 1990-1993, *MMWR* 42:840, 1993.
29. Centers for Disease Control: Inactivated Japanese Encephalitis virus vaccine. Recommendations of the advisory committee on immunization practices, *MMWR* 42(No RR-1), 1993.
30. Centers for Disease Control: Inactivated Japanese encephalitis virus vaccine, *MMWR* 42(RR-1):1, 1993.
31. Centers for Disease Control: Dengue surveillance—United States, 1986-1992, *MMWR* 43(SS-2):7, 1994.
32. Chapman LE et al: Risk factors for Crimean-Congo hemorrhagic fever in northern Senegal, *J Infect Dis* 164:686, 1991.
33. Choo Q-L et al: Isolation of a cDNA clone derived from a blood-borne non-A, non-B viral hepatitis genome, *Science* 244:359, 1989.
34. Christenson B: Epidemiological aspects of acute viral hepatitis A in Swedish travelers to endemic areas, *Scand J Infect Dis* 17:5, 1985.
35. Cochi SL et al: Control of epidemic group A meningococcal meningitis in Nepal, *Int J Epidemiol* 16:91, 1987.
36. Conrad JA, Jenson HB: New and improved vaccines. Promising weapons against varicella, hepatitis A, and typhoid fever, *Postgrad Med* 113:113, 1996.
37. Cooles P: Adjuvant steroids and relapse of typhoid fever, *J Trop Med Hyg* 89:229, 1986.
38. Cosgriff TM et al: Studies of the coagulation system in arenaviral hemorrhagic fever—pichinde virus in guinea pigs, *Am J Trop Med Hyg* 36:416, 1987.
39. Drugs for parasitic infection, *Med Lett* 24:5, 1982.
40. Duchin JS et al: Hantavirus pulmonary syndrome: clinical description of a disease caused by a newly recognized hemorrhagic fever virus in the southwestern United States, *N Engl J Med* 330:949, 1994.
41. Edelman R, Levine MM: Summary of an international workshop on typhoid fever, *Rev Infect Dis* 8:329, 1986.
42. Fisher-Hoch SP et al: Pathophysiology of shock and hemorrhage in a fulminating viral infection (Ebola), *J Infect Dis* 152:887, 1985.
43. Fisher-Hoch SP et al: Physiological and immunologic disturbances associated with shock in a primate model of Lassa fever, *J Infect Dis* 155:465, 1987.
44. Fischer-Hoch SP et al: Crimean-Congo-Hemorrhagic fever treated with oral ribavirin, *Lancet* 346:472, 1995.
45. Foulkes JR: Human trypanosomiasis in Africa, *BMJ* 283:1172, 1981.
46. Frame JD et al: Lassa fever, a new virus disease of man from West Africa. I. Clinical description and pathological findings, *Am J Trop Med Hyg* 19:670, 1970.
47. Francis DP et al: Occurrence of hepatitis A, B, and non-A/non-B in the United States, *Am J Med* 76:69, 1984.
48. Galimand M et al: High level chloramphenicol resistance in *Neisseria meningitidis*, *N Engl J Med* 339:868, 1998.
49. Gear JSS et al: Outbreak of Marburg virus disease in Johannesburg, *BMJ* 4:489, 1975.
50. Gilles HM, Watson-Williams EJ, Ball P: Hookworm infection and anemia, *Q J Med* 33:1, 1964.
51. Gimson AE et al: Clinical and prognostic differences in fulminant hepatitis type A, B, and non-A non-B, *Gut* 24:1194, 1983.
52. Glass GE: Hantaviruses, *Curr Opin Infect Dis* 10:362, 1997.
53. Gocke DJ: Immune complex phenomena associated with hepatitis. In Vyas GN, Cohen SN, Schmidt R, editors: *Viral hepatitis: a contemporary assessment*, Philadelphia, 1978, Franklin Institute Press.
54. Gocke DJ: Hepatitis A revisited, *Ann Intern Med* 105:960, 1986.
55. Goldfarb LG: An epidemiological model of Crimean hemorrhagic fever, *Am J Trop Med Hyg* 29:260, 1980.
56. Goodman RA et al: Nosocomial hepatitis A transmission by an adult patient with diarrhea, *Am J Med* 73:220, 1982.
57. Grove DI: Strongyloidiasis in Allied ex-prisoners of war in Southeast Asia, *BMJ* 280:598, 1980.
58. Hall SM, Mortimer PP, Vanderveld EM: Hepatitis A in the traveler, *Lancet* 2:1198, 1983.
59. Halsey NA, Smith MHD: Diphtheria. In Warren KS, Mahmoud AAF, editors: *Tropical and geographical medicine*, New York, 1984, McGraw-Hill.
60. Halstead SB: The pathogenesis of dengue: molecular epidemiology in infectious disease, *Am J Epidemiol* 114:632, 1981.

61. Halstead SB: Selective primary health care: strategies for control of disease in the developing world. XI. Dengue, *Rev Infect Dis* 6:251, 1984.

62. Hawking F: Diethylcarbamazine and new compounds for the treatment of filariasis, *Adv Pharmacol Chemother* 16:129, 1979.

63. Helmick CG et al: No evidence for increased risk of Lassa fever infection in hospital staff, *Lancet* 2:1202, 1986.

64. Heymann NL et al: Ebola hemorrhagic fever: Tandala, Zaire, 1977-78, *J Infect Dis* 142:371, 1980.

65. Hiatt RA et al: Factors in the pathogenesis of acute schistosomiasis mansoni, *J Infect Dis* 139:659, 1979.

66. Hinman AR, Koplan JP: Pertussis and pertussis vaccine: reanalysis of benefits, risks and costs, *JAMA* 251:3109, 1984.

67. Hinman AR, Koplan JP: Pertussis and pertussis vaccine: further analysis of benefits, risks and costs, *Dev Biol Stand* 61:419, 1985.

68. Hoffman SC et al: Reduction of mortality in chloramphenicol-treated severe typhoid fever by high-dose dexamethasone, *N Engl J Med* 310:116, 1984.

69. Hoffman TA et al: Waterborne typhoid fever in Dade County, Florida: clinical and therapeutic evaluations of 105 bacteremic patients, *Am J Med* 59:481, 1975.

70. Hornick RB et al: Typhoid fever: pathogenesis and immunologic control, *N Engl J Med* 283:686, 1970.

71. Inman RD et al: Arthritis, vasculitis and cryoglobulinemia associated with relapsing hepatitis A infection, *Ann Intern Med* 105:700, 1986.

72. Jones TC: Health advice and immunizations for travelers. In Remington JS, Swartz MN, editors: *Current topics in infectious diseases,* New York, 1985, McGraw-Hill.

73. Kalkofen UP: Intestinal trauma resulting from feeding activities of *Ancylostoma caninum, Am J Trop Med Hyg* 23:1046, 1974.

74. Khuroo MS: Study of epidemic of non-A, non-B hepatitis: possibility of another human hepatitis virus distinct from post-transfusion non-A non-B type, *Am J Med* 68:818, 1980.

75. Khuroo MS et al: Failure to detect chronic liver disease after epidemic non-A, non-b hepatitis, *Lancet* 2:260, 1980.

76. The known and the unknown about dengue fever, *Lancet* 1:488, 1987 (editorial).

77. Koppes GM, Lellenbogen C, Gephart RJ: Group Y meningococcal disease in United States Air Force Recruits, *Am J Med* 62:661, 1977.

78. Laranja FS et al: Chagas' disease: a clinical epidemiologic and pathologic study, *Circulation* 14:1015, 1956.

79. Lawlowski SW: Ascariasis: host pathogen biology, *Rev Infect Dis* 4:806, 1982.

80. Lee HW et al: Isolation of Hantaan virus, the etiologic agent of Korean hemorrhagic fever, from wild urban rats, *J Infect Dis* 146:638, 1982.

81. Linneman CC Jr, Nasenbeny J: Pertussis in the adult, *Annu Rev Med* 28:177, 1977.

82. Mayers CP, Pervis RJ: Manifestations of pinworms, *Can Med Assoc J* 103:489, 1970.

83. McCormick JB: Viral hemorrhagic fevers. In Warren KS, Mahmoud AAF, editors: *Tropical and geographical medicine,* New York, 1984, McGraw-Hill.

84. McCormick JB et al: Lassa fever: effective therapy with ribavirin, *N Engl J Med* 304:20, 1986.

85. McCormick JB et al: A case-control study of the clinical diagnosis and course of Lassa fever, *J Infect Dis* 155:445, 1987.

86. McCormick JB et al: A prospective study of the epidemiology and ecology of Lassa fever, *J Infect Dis* 155:437, 1987.

87. McFarland JM et al: Imported yellow fever in a US citizen, *Clin Infect Dis* 25:1143, 1997.

88. McHutchinson JG et al: Interferon alfa-2b alone or in combination with ribavirin as initial treatment for chronic hepatitis C, *N Engl J Med* 339:1485, 1998.

89. McKee KT, Le Duc JW, Peters CJ: Hantaviruses. In Belshe RB, editor: *Textbook of virology,* ed 2, St Louis, 1991, Mosby.

90. Meningococcal Disease Surveillance Group: Meningococcal disease secondary attack rate and chemoprophylaxis in the United States, 1974, *JAMA* 235:261, 1974.

91. Miller TA: Hookworm infection in man, *Adv Parasitol* 17:315, 1979.

92. Molinas FC, de Bracco MME, Maiztegui JI: Coagulation studies in Argentine hemorrhagic fever, *J Infect Dis* 143:1, 1981.

93. Monath TP: *Aedes albopictus,* an exotic mosquito vector in the United States, *Ann Intern Med* 105:449, 1986.

94. Monath TP: Yellow fever: a medically neglected disease, report on a seminar, *Rev Infect Dis* 9:165, 1987.

95. Monath TP et al: Indirect fluorescent antibody test for the diagnosis of yellow fever, *Trans R Soc Trop Med Hyg* 75:282, 1981.

96. Morens DM et al: Dengue shock syndrome in an American traveler with primary dengue 3 infection, *Am J Trop Med Hyg* 36:424, 1987.

97. Nelson JE: The changing epidemiology of pertussis in young infants, *Am J Dis Child* 132:371, 1978.

98. Noble RC et al: Post-transfusion hepatitis A in a neonatal intensive care unit, *JAMA* 253:2711, 1984.

99. Noguiera P: Early history of yellow fever. In *Yellow fever: a symposium in commemoration of Juan Carlos Finlay,* Philadelphia, 1955, Jefferson Medical College.

100. Ottesen EA: Immunopathology of lymphatic filariasis in man, *Semin Immunopathol* 2:373, 1980.

101. Pan American Health Organization: Present status of yellow fever: memorandum from a PAHO meeting, *Bull WHO* 64:511, 1986.

102. Passen EL, Anderson BR: Clinical tetanus despite a "protective" level of toxin-neutralizing antibody, *JAMA* 255:1171, 1986.

103. Pawlotsky J-M et al: What strategy should be used for the diagnosis of hepatitis C virus infection in clinical laboratories? *Hepatology* 27:1700, 1998.

104. Pawlowski ZS: Ascariasis, *Clin Gastroenterol* 7:157, 1982.

105. Peters PA, Kazura JW: Update on diagnostic methods for schistosomiasis. In Mahmoud AAF, editor: *Balleire's clinical tropical medicine and communicable diseases,* London, 1988, WB Saunders.

106. Peters RL: Viral hepatitis: a pathologic spectrum, *Am J Med Sci* 270:17, 1975.

107. Phillips RE: Management of *Plasmodium falciparum* malaria, *Med J Aust* 141:511, 1984.

108. Press E: Desirability of routine use of tetanus toxoid, *N Engl J Med* 239:50, 1948.

109. Putsch RW, Hamilton JD, Wolinsky E: *Neisseria meningitidis,* a respiratory pathogen, *J Infect Dis* 121:48, 1970.

110. Ramachandran S, Godfrey JJ, Perera MVF: Typhoid hepatitis, *JAMA* 230:236, 1974.

111. Reingold AL et al: Age-specific differences in duration of clinical protection after vaccination with meningococcal polysaccharide A vaccine, *Lancet* 2:114, 1985.

112. Reyes GR et al: Isolation of a cDNA from the virus responsible for enterically transmitted non A, non B hepatitis, *Science* 247:1335, 1990.

113. Rizzetto M, Canese MG: Hepatitis delta virus disease, *Prog Liver Dis* 8:417, 1986.

114. Rizzetto M et al: Incidence and significance of antibodies to delta antigen in hepatitis B virus infection, *Lancet* 2:986, 1979.

115. Robinson WS: Delta agent hepatitis. In Remington JS, Schwartz R, editors: *Current clinical topics in infectious diseases,* vol 8, New York, 1987, McGraw-Hill.

116. Rosen L: The emperor's new clothes revisited, or reflections on the pathogenesis of dengue hemorrhagic fever, *Am J Trop Med Hyg* 26:337, 1977.

117. Rosen L: The pathogenesis of dengue hemorrhagic fever, *S Afr Med J* 70s:41, 1986.

118. Rowe B, Ward LR, Threfall EJ: Multidrug-resistant Salmonella typhi: a worldwide epidemic, *Clin Infect Dis* 24(suppl 1): S106, 1997.

119. Ryan CA, Hargrett-Bean NT, Blake PA: *Salmonella typhi* infections in the United States, 1975-1984, *Rev Infect Dis* 11:1, 1989.

120. Santos F et al: Intravascular disseminada aguda na febre amarela: dosagem dos factores da coagulacao, *Brasilia Med* 9:9, 1973.

121. Schofield F: Selective primary health care: strategies for control of disease in the developing world. XXII. Tetanus: a preventable problem, *Rev Infect Dis* 8:144, 1986.

122. Schumaker JD et al: Thiabendazole treatment of severe strongyloidiasis in a hemodialysed patient, *Ann Intern Med* 89:655, 1978.

123. Shih W-K, Estebon Mur JI, Alter HJ: Non-A non-B hepatitis: advances and unfulfilled expectations of the first decade, *Prog Liver Dis* 8:433, 1986.

124. Simonsen O et al: Immunity against tetanus and response to revaccination in surgical patients more than 50 years of age, *Surg Gynecol Obstet* 164:329, 1987.

125. Siongok TKA et al: Morbidity in schistosomiasis mansoni in relation to intensity of infection: study of a community in Machakos, Kenya, *Am J Trop Med Hyg* 35:273, 1976.

126. Speed BR et al: Viral haemorrhagic fevers, *Med J Aust* 164:79, 1996.

127. Spitz S: The pathology of acute falciparum malaria, *Mil Surg* 99:555, 1946.

128. Steffen R et al: Health problems after travel to developing countries, *J Infect Dis* 156:84, 1987.

129. Tabor L et al: Additional evidence for more than one agent of human non-A, non-B hepatitis: transmission and passage studies in chimpanzees, *Transfusion* 24:224, 1983.

130. Tepper ML, Gully PR: Viral hepatitis: know your D, E, F and Gs, *Can Med Assoc J* 156:1735, 1997.

131. Threfall EJ, Ward LR. Skinner JA: Ciprofloxacin-resistant Salmonella typhi and treatment failure, *Lancet* 353:1590, 1999.

132. Tsai TF: Yellow fever, *Bull WHO* 76(suppl 2):158, 1998.

133. Umenai T et al: Japanese encephalitis: current worldwide status, *Bull WHO* 63:625, 1985.

134. Van Eeden PJ et al: A nosocomial outbreak of Crimean-Congo haemorrhagic fever at Tygerberg Hospital. A. Clinical features, *S Afr Med J* 68:711, 1985.

135. Vickerman K: Antigenic variation in trypanosomes, *Nature* 273:613, 1978.

136. Warrel DA et al: Dexamethasone proves deleterious in cerebral malaria, *N Engl J Med* 306:313, 1982.

137. Warren KS: Regulation of the prevalence and intensity of schistosomiasis in man: immunology or ecology? *J Infect Dis* 127:595, 1973.

138. Weber DJ et al: Obesity as a prediction of poor antibody response to hepatitis B plasma vaccine, *JAMA* 254:3187, 1985.

139. Wells RM et al: An unusual hantavirus outbreak in southern Argentina: person to person transmission? *Emerg Infect Dis* 3:171, 1997.

140. Wenger JD et al: Bacterial meningitis in the United States, 1986: report of a multistate surveillance study, *J Infect Dis* 162:1316, 1990.

141. Woodruff BA, Pavia AT, Blake PA: A new look at typhoid vaccination: information for the practicing physician, *JAMA* 265:756, 1991.

142. Woolley I, Boom WH: Viral hepatitis. In Tan JT, editor: *Experts' guide to the management of common infectious diseases,* Philadelphia, American College of Physicians (in press).

143. World Health Organization: Hemorrhagic fever with renal syndrome: memorandum from a WHO meeting, *Bull WHO* 61:269, 1983.

144. World Health Organization: *Dengue hemorrhagic fever: diagnosis, treatment and control,* Geneva, 1986, WHO.

145. World Health Organization: Yellow fever virus surveillance in western Africa, *Weekly Epi Rec* 69:93, 1994.

146. Wyler DJ, Marsden PA: Leishmaniasis. In Warren KS, Mahmoud AAF, editors: *Tropical and geographical medicine,* New York, 1984, McGraw-Hill.

147. Xu ZY et al: Epidemiological studies of hemorrhagic fever with renal syndrome: analysis of risk factors and mode of transmission, *J Infect Dis* 152:137, 1985.

148. Yellow fever in Africa, *Lancet* 2:1315, 1986 (editorial).

149. Yoshizawa H et al: Demonstration of two different types of non-A, non-B hepatitis by reinjection and cross challenge studies in chimpanzees, *Gastroenterology* 81:107, 1981.

150. Zoombaulakis D et al: Steroids in the treatment of pertussis: a controlled clinical trial, *Arch Dis Child* 48:51, 1973.

67 Natural Disaster Management

Eric K. Noji

Throughout history, natural disasters have exacted a heavy toll of death and suffering (Tables 67-1 and 67-2). During the past 25 years they have claimed more than 3 million lives worldwide, have adversely affected the lives of at least 800 million more people, and have resulted in property damage exceeding $50 billion.[73,80,103,117] Recent natural catastrophes have included earthquakes in Los Angeles (1994)[67] and Kobe, Japan (1995),[88,116,148,149] a series of devastating hurricanes in the Caribbean in 1998 (including hurricanes Mitch and Georges), severe flooding in the central United States in 1993 and California in 1998,[33-35,39] tornadoes in Oklahoma and Texas (1999), global adverse weather conditions related to the El Niño phenomenon in 1997 and 1998, and the volcanic eruption of Mt. Soufriere on the island of Montserrat (1997).

The future appears to be even more frightening. Increasing population density in floodplains and in earthquake- and hurricane-prone areas points to the probability of future catastrophic natural disasters with millions of casualties.[75,154,163] Many natural disasters of large magnitude occur in remote areas, far from towns and hospitals. The roads frequently become impassable, bridges collapse, and inclement weather adds to the difficulties. The more remote the area, the longer it takes for external assistance to arrive, and the more the community will have to rely on its own resources, at least for the first several hours, if not days. Friends, neighbors, and relatives conduct the initial search and rescue of victims, provide basic first aid, and transport injured victims to the nearest health care facilities.

Good disaster management must link data collection and analysis to an immediate decision-making process.[15] The overall objective of disaster management from a public health perspective is to assess the needs of disaster-affected populations, match available resources to those needs, prevent further adverse health effects, implement disease control strategies for well-defined problems, evaluate the effectiveness of disaster relief programs, and improve contingency plans for various types of future disasters.[57]

The effects of disasters on the health of populations are quantifiable.[39] Common patterns of morbidity and mortality follow certain disasters.[162] Better epidemiologic knowledge of the causes of death and types of injuries and illnesses caused by natural disasters is essential to determine the relief supplies, equipment, and personnel needed to respond effectively.[2,15,72] In addition, results of disaster research provide informed advice about the probable health effects of future disasters, establish priorities for action by emergency medical services, and emphasize the need for accurate information as the basis for relief management decisions.[15,63]

Proper planning and execution of disaster medical aid programs require knowledge of the types of disasters and resulting morbidity, mortality, and medical care needs. Emergency responders should be experts on how to handle the type of disaster most prevalent in their own communities because each type of disaster is characterized by different morbidity and mortality patterns and has different health care requirements.[15,113] For example, hospitals along the Gulf Coast of the United States should plan for hurricanes, whereas those in California should plan for earthquakes.[43,72,85]

In addition, specific types of medical and health problems tend to occur at different times after a natural disaster's impact. With earthquakes, for example, the problem of severe injuries that require immediate trauma care must be handled mainly at the time and place of impact. The problem of increased risk of disease transmission can be handled later, however, because it takes longer to develop, and the greatest danger occurs with crowding and poor sanitation. Effective emergency medical response depends on anticipating the different medical and health problems and delivering the appropriate interventions when needed most.[140]

NATURE OF DISASTER

The World Health Organization (WHO) defines *disaster* as a sudden ecologic phenomenon of sufficient magnitude to require external assistance.[124,165] At the community level, this can be defined operationally as any community emergency that seriously affects people's lives and property and that exceeds the community's capacity to respond effectively.[83]

The essence of a disaster is substantial environmental damage, which may be accompanied by large numbers of casualties. This chapter refers to limited incidents creating relatively small numbers of casualties and slight environmental disturbance as *multiple casualty incidents*. The term *disaster* is reserved for incidents that cause great disruption of the physical and social environments and that require extraordinary resources and special medical care, even in the absence of mass casualties.

TABLE 67-1. Mortality Estimates by Type of Disaster

	DEATHS			
DISASTER TYPE	1960-1969	1970-1979	1980-1989	1990-1999
Floods	28,700	46,800	38,598	103,870
Cyclones/hurricanes	107,500	343,600	14,482	201,790
Earthquakes	52,500	389,700	53,740	98,678
Other disasters			1,011,777	2,686
TOTAL			1,119,860	407,204

From Office of US Foreign Disaster Assistance: *Disaster history: significant data on major disasters worldwide, 1900-present,* Washington, DC, 1990, Agency for International Development; and Walker P, Walter J: *World disasters report: focus on public health,* Geneva, 2000, International Federation of Red Cross and Red Crescent Societies.

TABLE 67-2. Selected Natural Disasters of the Twentieth Century*

YEAR	EVENT	LOCATION	APPROXIMATE DEATH TOLL	YEAR	EVENT	LOCATION	APPROXIMATE DEATH TOLL
1900	Hurricane	USA	6,000	1962	Earthquake	Iran	12,000
1902	Volcanic eruption	Martinique	29,000	1963	Tropical cyclone	Bangladesh	22,000
1902	Volcanic eruption	Guatemala	6,000	1963	Volcanic eruption	Indonesia	1,200
1906	Typhoon	Hong Kong	10,000	1963	Landslide	Italy	2,000
1906	Earthquake	Taiwan	6,000	1965	Tropical cyclone	Bangladesh	17,000
1906	Earthquake/fire	USA	1,500	1965	Tropical cyclone	Bangladesh	30,000
1908	Earthquake	Italy	75,000	1965	Tropical cyclone	Bangladesh	10,000
1911	Volcanic eruption	Philippines	1,300	1968	Earthquake	Iran	12,000
1915	Earthquake	Italy	30,000	1970	Earthquake/ landslide	Peru	70,000
1916	Landslide	Italy, Austria	10,000				
1919	Volcanic eruption	Indonesia	5,200	1970	Tropical cyclone	Bangladesh	300,000
1920	Earthquake/ landslide	China	200,000	1971	Tropical cyclone	India	25,000
				1972	Earthquake	Nicaragua	6,000
1923	Earthquake/fire	Japan	143,000	1976	Earthquake	China	250,000
1928	Hurricane/flood	USA	2,000	1976	Earthquake	Guatemala	24,000
1930	Volcanic eruption	Indonesia	1,400	1976	Earthquake	Italy	900
1932	Earthquake	China	70,000	1977	Tropical cyclone	India	20,000
1933	Tsunami	Japan	3,000	1978	Earthquake	Iran	25,000
1935	Earthquake	India	60,000	1980	Earthquake	Italy	1,300
1938	Hurricane	USA	600	1982	Volcanic eruption	Mexico	1,700
1939	Earthquake/ tsunami	Chile	30,000	1985	Tropical cyclone	Bangladesh	10,000
				1985	Earthquake	Mexico	10,000
1945	Flood/landslide	Japan	1,200	1985	Volcanic eruption	Columbia	22,000
1946	Tsunami	Japan	1,400	1988	Hurricane Gilbert	Caribbean	343
1948	Earthquake	USSR	100,000	1988	Earthquake	Armenia SSR	25,000
1949	Flood	China	57,000				
1949	Earthquake/ landslide	USSR	20,000	1989	Hurricane Hugo	Caribbean	56
				1990	Earthquake	Iran	40,000
1951	Volcanic eruption	Papua New Guinea	2,900	1990	Earthquake	Philippines	2,000
				1991	Tropical cyclone	Bangladesh	140,000
1953	Flood	North Sea coast	1,800	1991	Volcanic eruption	Philippines	800
				1991	Typhoon/flood	Philippines	6,000
1954	Landslide	Austria	200	1991	Flood	China	1,500
1954	Flood	China	40,000	1992	Hurricane Andrew	USA	52
1959	Typhoon	Japan	4,600	1993	Earthquake	India	10,000
1960	Earthquake	Morocco	12,000	1995	Earthquake	Japan	6,000
1961	Typhoon	Hong Kong	400	1998	Hurricane Mitch	Central America	10,000
1962	Landslide	Peru	5,000				

Data from Office of US Foreign Disaster Assistance: *Disaster history: significant data on major disasters worldwide, 1900-Present,* Washington, DC, 1999, Agency for International Development; and National Geographic Society: *Nature on the rampage, our violent earth,* Washington, DC, 1987, National Geographic Society.
*Disasters selected to represent global vulnerability to rapid-onset disasters.

True disasters affect a community in numerous ways. Roads, telephone lines, and other transportation and communication links are often destroyed. Public utilities and energy supplies may be disrupted. Substantial numbers of victims may be rendered homeless. Portions of the community's industrial or economic base may be destroyed or damaged. Casualties may require medical care, and damage to food sources and utilities may create public health threats.

PAST PROBLEMS IN NATURAL DISASTER MANAGEMENT

In ancient times, little mitigation was possible against the effects of disaster. Today, communications inform us rapidly of disasters and allow us to provide effective medical aid to victims. This requires adequate planning and brisk execution. Medical aid in many previous disasters has been well intentioned but poorly organized, with limited benefits.[57,124]

Health decisions made during emergencies are often based on insufficient, nonexistent, or even false information, which results in inappropriate, insufficient, or unnecessary health aid, waste of health resources, or countereffective measures.[140] For example, large amounts of useless drugs and other consumable supplies are frequently sent to a disaster site. After the 1976 earthquake in Guatemala, 100 tons of unsorted medicines were airlifted to the country from foreign donors.[48,50] Of these supplies, 90% were of no value because they consisted of medications that had expired, were already opened, or carried labels written in foreign languages. A similar situation occurred after the 1988 Armenian earthquake, when international relief operations sent at least 5000 tons of drugs and consumable medical supplies. Because of the difficulties with identification and sorting, only 30% of the drugs were immediately usable by the health workers in Armenia; 11% were useless, and 8% had expired. Ultimately, 20% of all the drugs provided by international aid had to be destroyed.[4] Other examples of inappropriate aid include sending mobile hospitals and teams of specialized trauma or emergency medicine specialists that arrive much too late and sending unprepared medical volunteers when nonmedical relief workers (e.g., sanitation engineers) would be more appropriate. The arrival of unprepared and inexperienced foreign personnel may damage the relief effort by tying up communication, transportation, and housing. These problems are all compounded in the vacuum created by the disaster, including the lack of communication, transportation, local supplies and support, and a decision-making structure. Because these relief operations are often conducted under the watchful eye of the media, medical relief efforts are often pejoratively called *the second disaster*.[89,114]

INFORMATION MANAGEMENT SYSTEMS FOR DISASTER RESPONSE

Over the past several years, efforts have been made to develop rapid and valid disaster damage assessment techniques.[152,166] These techniques must be able to define quickly the overall effects of the disaster impact, the nature and extent of the health problems, groups in the population at particular risk for adverse health events, specific health care needs of the survivors, local resources to cope with the event, and the extent and effectiveness of the response to the disaster by local authorities.[83,145] Guha-Sapir and Lechat[71-73] have developed indicators for needs assessment in earthquakes ("quick and dirty" surveys), highlighting simplicity, speed of use, and operational feasibility. The techniques employed (e.g., systematic surveys, simple reporting systems) are methodologically straightforward. With suitable personnel and transport, estimates of relief needs can be quickly obtained.[32] Problems may arise, however, with the interpretation of data, particularly incomplete data, and in developing countries in which predisaster health and nutritional levels are unknown.

The ultimate goal of surveillance is to prevent or reduce the adverse health consequences of the disaster itself, as well as to optimize the decision-making process associated with management of the relief effort. These epidemiologic objectives can be simply defined as the *surveillance cycle*: the collection, analysis, and response to data.[57] The surveillance cycle must be repeated many times: immediately, with rapid assessments of problems using the most rudimentary data collection techniques; then short-term assessments involving the establishment of simple but reliable sources of data; and subsequently, ongoing surveillance to identify continuing problems and monitor response.

Field surveillance methods vary greatly by disaster setting and by the personnel and time available. Early field surveys must be simple and provide immediate answers that will directly prevent loss of life or injury. Subsequently, surveys can address issues such as the availability of medical care, assessment of the need for specific interventions, and epidemic control (a rumor clearinghouse), each of which demands more careful investigation. Surveillance must determine whether the effort is having a tangible impact on the population, or whether new strategies are needed.[147] Surveillance becomes an iterative, cycling process in which simple health outcomes are constantly monitored and interventions assessed for efficacy.

Finally, linking postdisaster information to a decision-making process is important.[72] In the rapid evolution of a disaster relief program, major decisions regarding relief are made early, hastily, and often irreversibly, so reliable early data to assist in making these decisions are vital. Organized data collection in disaster situations can greatly improve decision making. Adaptable questionnaires can assist in an efficient data collection operation.

Operational decisions depend on the phase of the disaster. In the early phase of relief, basic needs of water, food, clothing, shelter, and medical care must be met, after which the long-term process of rebuilding proceeds. Relief aid can often be squandered by overreacting to minor problems when excitement is great, needs are extensive, and scrutiny by the media is omnipresent.[140] Because everyone in the disaster area has needs and experiences loss, the challenge of early assessment is to decide where initial interventions will prevent the greatest loss of life or severe morbidity. The postimpact phase requires information on long-term rehabilitation and restoration of health services. Epidemiologic assessment, prioritization of needs, and ordering an appropriate response can have a major impact on the community's ability to return to normalcy in both the short and longer term.

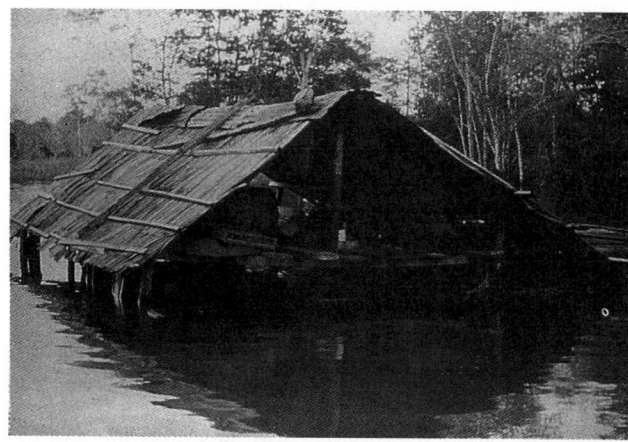

Figure 67-1 During summer 1988, monsoon rains resulted in the most severe flooding ever recorded in Bangladesh. Water covered three fourths of the land area of Bangladesh, displacing up to 40 million persons from their homes. *(Courtesy Centers for Disease Control and Prevention and US Public Health Service.)*

HEALTH CARE NEEDS IN SPECIFIC NATURAL DISASTERS

Natural hazards that can cause substantial property damage, economic dislocation, and medical problems include earthquakes and associated phenomena, volcanic eruptions, and extreme weather incidents, such as heat waves and blizzards. Accounts of morbidity and mortality recorded after previous disasters can predict the medical care needs of future disaster victims and provide a foundation for disaster response planning.

Floods

Floods are the most common natural disasters. They affect more people worldwide and cause greater mortality than any other type of natural disaster.[73,118,163] They occur in almost every country, but 70% of all flood deaths occur in India and Bangladesh[103] (Figure 67-1). In the United States, floods cause more deaths than any other natural disaster, with most fatalities resulting from flash floods.[60]

Fast-flowing water carrying debris such as boulders and fallen trees accounts for the primary flood-related injuries and deaths. The main cause of death from floods is drowning, followed by various combinations of trauma, drowning, and hypothermia with or without submersion.[11] Persons submerged in cold water for up to about 40 minutes have been successfully resuscitated with 100% recovery of neurologic function.[118] Unfortunately, such resuscitations from clinical death require technologically advanced measures, which may not be available for days after a flood, even in a highly developed country such as the United States.

Among flood survivors, the proportion requiring emergency medical care is reported to vary between 0.2% and 2%.[139,146] Most injuries requiring urgent med-

ical attention are minor and include lacerations, skin rashes, and ulcers.[124] However, flood-associated lacerations are frequently contaminated, so primary wound closure should be done with caution. Primary closure without careful evaluation of the wound almost always requires reopening the wound and additional treatment within 24 to 48 hours.[11]

Increased incidence of snakebites was reported after floods in India and the Philippines.[158] In India, most snakebites were by cobras that had been driven by rising water to seek higher ground near towns and villages.

For some floods, substantial numbers of casualties caused by fire have been documented.[118] Fast-flowing water can break oil or gasoline storage tanks. If the film of oil is ignited, the fire may spread to buildings on land.

From a public health viewpoint, floods may disrupt water purification and sewage disposal systems, cause toxic waste sites to overflow, or dislodge chemical containers stored above ground.[51] In addition, makeshift evacuation centers with insufficient sanitary facilities may become substantially overcrowded.[125] The combination of these events may contribute to increased exposure to highly toxic biologic and chemical agents. Examples include the potential for waterborne disease transmission of such agents as enterotoxigenic *Escherichia coli, Shigella, Salmonella,* and hepatitis A virus.[139] The risk of transmission of malaria and yellow fever may be increased because of enhanced vector-breeding conditions.[124] In 1973 Ussher[158] reported that the most serious problems encountered after a flood in the Philippines were viral upper respiratory tract infections, which were probably caused by crowded conditions in temporary shelters.

Despite the potential for communicable diseases to follow floods, mass vaccination programs are counterproductive for a variety of reasons. They not only di-

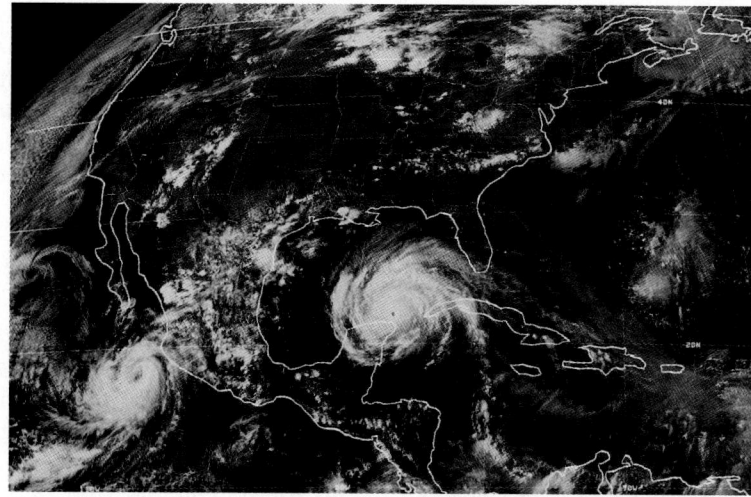

Figure 67-2   Satellite image of a hurricane and a cyclone striking Mexico simultaneously. *(Courtesy World Health Organization and Office of the UN Disaster Relief Coordinator.)*

vert limited personnel and resources from other critical relief tasks, but also may create a false sense of security and cause persons who have been vaccinated to neglect basic hygiene.[49] Unfortunately, after floods the public often demands typhoid vaccine and tetanus toxoid, although no epidemic of typhoid after a flood has ever been documented in the United States.[95] In addition, antibodies to typhoid after immunization take several weeks to develop, and even then, vaccination protects only moderately. Likewise, mass tetanus vaccination programs are not indicated. Management of flood-associated wounds should include appropriate evaluation of the injured person's tetanus immunization history, and the person should be vaccinated only if indicated.

The proper approach to the problem of communicable diseases is to set up an epidemiologic surveillance system so that an increase in cases of communicable diseases in the flood-stricken area can be identified quickly. Particular attention should be given to diseases endemic to the area. For example, when floods occur in areas with endemic arthropod-borne encephalitides, arthropods known to transmit the disease should be monitored and areas should be sprayed if the vector population increases significantly after the flood.

Tropical Cyclones (Hurricanes or Typhoons)

Cyclones, hurricanes, and typhoons have killed hundreds of thousands and injured millions of people during the last 30 years (Figure 67-2).[75,117] From 1900 to 1999 more than 14,000 people lost their lives in hurricanes in the United States (Table 67-3).[56] The greatest natural disaster in U.S. history occurred on Sept. 8, 1900, when a hurricane struck Galveston, Texas, and killed more than 6000 persons.[59,103] In 1970 deaths resulting from a single tropical cyclone striking Bangladesh were estimated to exceed 250,000. As population

TABLE 67-3. Hurricanes Causing More Than 100 Deaths in the United States, 1900-1982

STORM/AREA	YEAR	DEATHS
Texas (Galveston)	1900	6000
Florida (Lake Okeechobee)	1928	1836
South Texas, Florida (Keys)	1919	600-900*
New England	1938	600
Florida (Keys)	1935	408
Audrey/Louisiana, Texas	1957	390
Northeast United States	1944	390†
Louisiana (Grand Isle)	1909	350
Louisiana (New Orleans)	1915	275
Texas (Galveston)	1915	275
Camille/Mississippi, Louisiana	1969	256
Florida (Miami)	1926	243
Diane/Northeast US	1955	184
Florida (Southeast)	1906	164
Mississippi, Alabama, Florida (Pensacola)	1906	134
Agnes/Northeast US	1972	122

From French JG: Hurricanes. In Gregg MB, editor: *The public health consequences of disasters*, Atlanta, 1986, Centers for Disease Control.
*Includes more than 500 persons lost on ships at sea.
†Includes 344 persons lost on ships at sea.

growth continues along vulnerable coastal areas, deaths and injuries resulting from tropical cyclones will increase.[70,141]

Although hurricane winds do great damage, wind is not the primary killer in a hurricane. Hurricanes are classic examples of disasters that trigger secondary effects such as tornadoes and flooding that, together with storm surges, can cause extraordinarily high rates of morbidity and mortality. This was seen after the 1991 cyclone and sea surge in Bangladesh, in which 140,000 persons drowned, and during Hurricane Mitch in Central America in 1998, with thousands of drowning deaths.[66] Nine of 10 hurricane fatalities are drownings associated with storm surges.[58,59,123] The major rescue problem is locating persons stranded by rising waters and evacuating them to higher land. Other causes of deaths and injuries include burial beneath houses collapsed by wind or water, penetrating trauma from broken glass or wood, blunt trauma from floating objects or debris, or entrapment by mud slides that may accompany hurricane-associated floods.[31,74] Many of the most severe injuries occur to persons who are in mobile homes during the storm, or those who are injured or electrocuted during postdisaster cleanup.[28,29,127]

Most persons who seek medical care after hurricanes do not require sophisticated surgical or intensive care services and can be treated as outpatients.[107,132] The majority have lacerations caused by flying glass or other debris[74]; a few have closed fractures and other, mostly penetrating, injuries.[36,42] Longmire et al[91,92] studied injuries associated with hurricanes Frederic (1984) and Elena (1985). They found a statistically significant increase in lacerations, puncture wounds, chain saw injuries, burns, gasoline aspiration, gastrointestinal complaints, insect stings, and spouse abuse in the 2 weeks after the hurricane. The authors concluded that minor trauma treated in the outpatient setting created an urgent demand for primary care physicians and nurses skilled in managing minor surgical emergencies. In addition, although the number of chain saw injuries was small, the time-consuming nature of treating such wounds increased significantly the demands placed on remaining emergency department personnel to treat those with other injuries. As with flood-related wounds, emergency medical care providers should be aware that wounds may contain highly contaminated material such as soil or fecal matter.[122,126] Because of this danger, primary wound closure should be done with caution.

Storm shelters are often severely crowded.[30] As with flood disasters, this crowding increases the probability of disease communication through aerosol or fecal-oral routes, particularly when sanitary facilities are insufficient.[16]

Trauma after a cyclone is not usually a major public health problem when compared with the need for water, food, clothing, sanitation, and other hygienic measures.[146] Studies demonstrate that sending fully equipped mobile hospitals and specialized surgical teams that arrive much too late at the disaster site is an ineffective response to a cyclone disaster. Nonmedical relief (e.g., epidemiologists, sanitation engineers, shelter, food, agricultural supplies) is probably more effective in reducing mortality and morbidity. On the other hand, field hospitals and emergency medical teams from outside the disaster-affected area may be useful in providing ongoing primary health care services to the community when all other health care facilities

have been destroyed or severely damaged.[76] This was the case in St. Croix after hurricane Hugo[132] and in south Florida after hurricane Andrew.[157] These situations reemphasize the importance of conducting rapid assessments of public health needs before sending relief personnel and materials to a disaster.[125]

Tornadoes

Tornadoes are among the most violent of all natural atmospheric phenomena, as has been witnessed after recent devastating tornadoes in Oklahoma, Texas, and Alabama (Figure 67-3).[103] Although almost 700 tornadoes occur in the United States each year, only about 3% result in severe injuries requiring hospitalization.[90] Of 14,600 tornadoes studied between 1952 and 1973, only 497 caused fatalities, and 26 of these events accounted for almost half of the fatalities.[61] The Centers for Disease Control and Prevention (CDC) has reviewed the public health impact of tornadoes in great detail.[90]

The destruction caused by tornadoes results from the combined action of strong rotary winds and the partial vacuum in the center of the vortex.[102] For example, when a tornado passes over a building, the winds twist and rip at the outside. Simultaneously, the abrupt

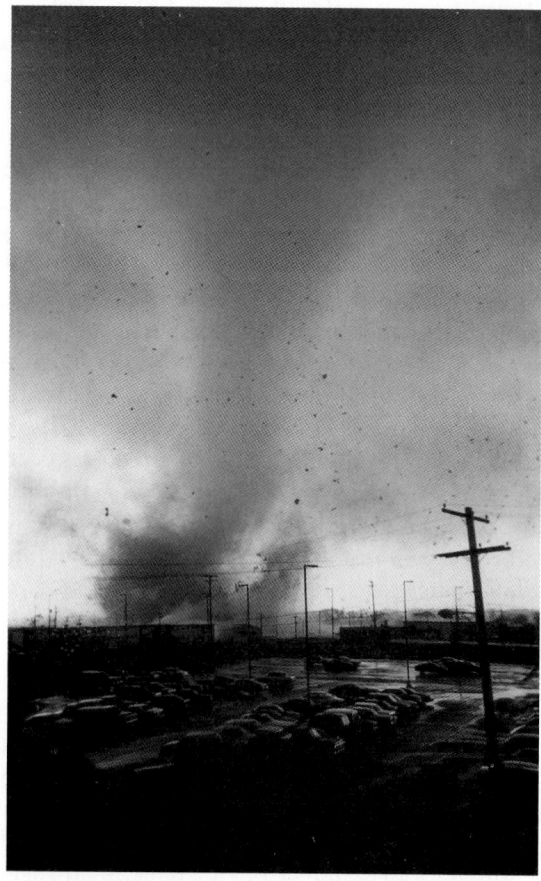

Figure 67-3 Tornado striking McConnell Air Force Base, Kansas, April 26, 1991. *(Courtesy US Air Force.)*

pressure reduction in the tornado's eye causes explosive pressures inside the building. Walls collapse or topple outward, windows explode, and the debris from this destruction can be driven as high-velocity missiles through the air. Buildings made of unreinforced masonry, wood frame buildings, and those with large window areas will likely have the most extensive damage.[87] Building practices may be largely responsible for the severity of injury resulting from tornadoes.[20]

In the last 50 years, tornadoes have been responsible for more than 9000 deaths in the United States.[65] About 4% of all injuries sustained were fatal. For every person seriously injured or killed, approximately 44 others required some emergency medical attention.[68]

Victims of tornado disasters show characteristic patterns of fatal and nonfatal injuries. The leading cause of death is craniocerebral trauma,[18,96] followed by crushing wounds of the chest and trunk.[6,139] Fractures are the most frequent nonfatal injury. Lacerations, penetrating trauma with retained foreign bodies, and other soft tissue injuries also frequently occur. A high percentage of wounds among tornado casualties are heavily contaminated.[19,77] In many instances, foreign materials such as glass, wood splinters, tar, dirt, grass, and manure are deeply embedded in areas of soft tissue injury.[96] Wound contamination appears to be a major factor contributing to the high rate of postoperative sepsis for tornado victims who require surgery, even under conditions in which patients receive highly skilled and prompt surgical debridement. Sepsis is common in both minor and major injuries; sepsis affects one half to two thirds of patients with minor wounds.[6] In 1956 Hight et al[77] examined the postoperative course of patients after the Worcester tornado and found sepsis in 12.5% to 23.0% of orthopedic and neurosurgical patients with lacerations, three cases of gas gangrene, but no cases of tetanus.

Three studies have looked specifically at the species of bacteria that contaminate wounds sustained during tornadoes.[19,62,81] These revealed frequent infection with aerobic gram-negative bacilli, presumably derived from soil.

Volcanic Eruptions

Volcanic eruptions have claimed more than 266,000 lives in the past 400 years, with fatalities occurring in about 5% of eruptions.[17,144] Some of the more catastrophic eruptions in history include the eruption of Krakatoa (Indonesia), which caused 36,000 deaths; of Mt. Pelee in 1902, which caused the destruction of St. Pierre in Martinique and the deaths of 28,000 persons; of Nevado del Ruiz in Colombia, which claimed 25,000 lives; and of Mt. Pinatubo in the Philippines, with effects still ongoing because of persistent mudflows. The U.S. Geological Survey has identified about 35 volcanoes in the western United States and Alaska that are likely to erupt in the future. Most of these are in remote rural areas and are not likely to result in disaster. A few, such as Mt. Hood, Mt. Shasta, Mt. Rainier, and the volcano underlying Mammoth Lakes in California, are near population centers.[5,12] Because of the increasing population density in areas of volcanic activity, volcanic hazards are of growing concern.[44,75,86,103]

Eruptions have immediate life-threatening health effects through suffocation from inhalation of massive quantities of airborne ash, scalding from blasts of superheated steam, and surges of lethal gas (Table 67-4).[10,13] Pyroclastic flows and surges are particularly lethal.[8] These are currents of extremely hot gases and particles that flow down the slopes of a volcano at tens to hundreds of meters per second and cover hundreds of square kilometers. Because of their suddenness and speed, pyroclastic flows and surges are difficult to escape.

TABLE 67-4. Principal Health Effects Caused by Volcanic Eruptions

ERUPTIVE EVENT	CONSEQUENCE	HEALTH EFFECT
Explosions	Lateral blast, rock fragments	Trauma, skin burns
	Air shock waves	Lacerations from broken windows
Hot ash release	Glowing avalanches	Skin and lung burns
	Ashflows and ashfalls	Asphyxiation
	Lightning	Electrocution
	Forest fires	Burns
Melting ice, snow, and rain accompanying eruption	Mudflows, floods	Engulfing, drowning
Lava	Forest fires	Burns
Gas emissions: sulfur dioxide, carbon monoxide, carbon dioxide, hydrogen sulfide, hydrogen fluoride	Pooling in low-lying areas and inhalation	Asphyxiation, airway constriction
Radon	Radiation exposure	Lung cancer
Earthquakes	Building damage	Trauma

From Baxter PJ, Bernstein RS, Buist AS: *Am J Public Health* 76(suppl):84, 1986.

Mudflows, or lahars, account for at least 10% of volcano-related deaths.[161] These are flowing masses of volcanic debris mixed with water. The mud is sometimes scalding hot, and entrapped persons may sustain severe burns. A relatively minor eruption of snow-capped Nevado del Ruiz in 1985 triggered lahars from the volcano's icecap that buried more than 22,000 persons in Colombia, South America.[144]

An indirect effect of volcanic activity is accumulation of toxic volcanic gases in deep crater lakes.[119,143] Sudden release of these gases can be catastrophic; carbon dioxide released from Lake Monoun and Lake Nyos in Cameroon in 1984 and 1986, respectively, claimed 1800 lives. Other toxic effects of these gas releases include pulmonary edema, irritant conjunctivitis, joint pain, muscle weakness, and cutaneous bullae. In the rare event of a ground-level release of toxic gases or aerosols (e.g., from a vent opening to the atmosphere from the side of the volcano), equipment for monitoring atmospheric concentrations of sulfur dioxide, hydrogen sulfide, hydrofluoric acid, carbon dioxide, and other gases should be available.[10,13]

A volcanic eruption may also generate tremendous quantities of ashfall.[101,133] Buildings have been reported to collapse from the weight of ash accumulating on roofs, resulting in severe trauma to the occupants.[97] Ash can also be irritating to eyes (causing corneal abrasions), mucous membranes, and the respiratory system.[94] Upper airway irritation, cough, and bronchospasm, as well as exacerbation of chronic lung disease, are common findings in symptomatic patients.[8] In extremely high concentrations, as in the path of a pyroclastic flow or near the volcanic vent during an ashfall, volcanic ash may cause severe tracheal injury, pulmonary edema, and bronchial obstruction, leading to death from acute pulmonary injury or suffocation.[97] After the eruption of Mt. St. Helens in 1980, 23 immediate deaths were reported (Figure 67-4). Postmortem examinations revealed that 18 of these resulted from asphyxia.[54] In most asphyxiated victims, the ash mixed with mucus and formed plugs, obstructing the trachea and main bronchi. Finally, delayed onset of ash-induced mucus hypersecretion or obstructive airway disease may occur.[9]

Victims who recover from volcano-generated mudflows may have severe dehydration, burns, and eye infections.[55] Reports of surgical care after the volcanic eruption in Colombia in 1985 showed that primary closure of wounds contaminated by mud and other volcanic material resulted in major complications.[120] These complications included gangrene necessitating amputation, osteomyelitis, compartment syndrome, and sepsis.

Most volcanic deaths are caused by immediate suffocation and, to a lesser extent, by burns or blunt trauma. Advanced cardiac and trauma life support capabilities, even if immediately available, would probably arrive too late to save asphyxiated victims. Persons who may de-

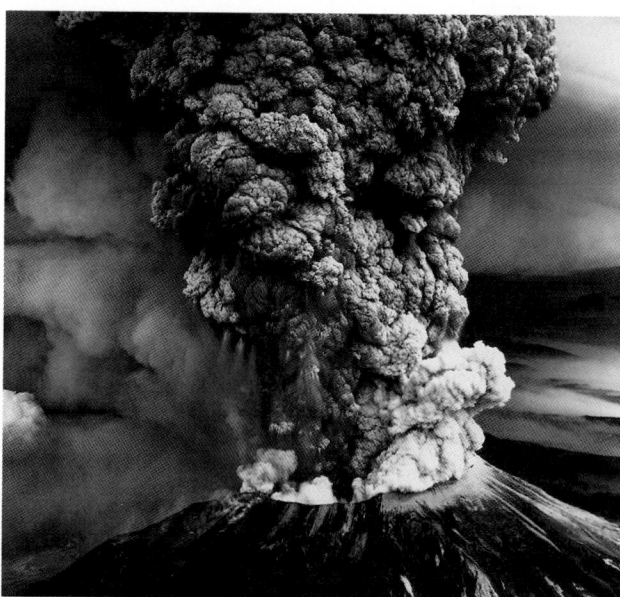

Figure 67-4 Eruption of Mt. St. Helens, Washington State, May 18, 1980. *(Courtesy of the US Geological Survey.)*

velop severe respiratory distress syndrome should be admitted to an intensive care unit (ICU) for appropriate respiratory supportive measures, ranging from continuous positive airway pressure to mechanical ventilation with positive end-expiratory pressure.[97] Hospitals in the vicinity of both active and dormant volcanoes should be prepared to deal with a sudden influx of victims with severe burns and lung damage from inhalation of hot ash, as well as multiple varieties of trauma.[8,13]

Earthquakes

An earthquake of great magnitude is one of the most destructive events in nature. During the past 20 years, earthquakes have caused more than a million deaths and injuries worldwide.[117] In the United States, approximately 1600 deaths attributed to earthquakes have been recorded since colonial times, of which more than 1000 have occurred in California (Figure 67-5).[109,142] Hospitals and other health care facilities are particularly vulnerable to the damaging effects of an earthquake. Because of loss of power and water supply, equipment (e.g., x-ray and kidney dialysis machines, ventilators, blood analyzers) and hospital facilities (e.g., ICUs and surgical theaters) cannot function normally when they are most needed.[3,112,130]

Disaster medical planners should note injury type and/or diagnostic classification among survivors to determine the medical care needed. The primary cause of death and injury from earthquakes is the collapse of buildings that are not adequately designed for earthquake resistance, are built with inadequate materials, or are poorly constructed (Figure 67-6).[64,93] Factors determining the number of people killed when a building collapses include how badly trapped they are, how

four measures: simplifying care (austerity); rationing care (adopting a triage ethic); calling for outside help; and in circumstances of catastrophe, instituting mass care measures typical of battlefield medicine. Many compromises in work methods eliminate attention to details that would be required in less urgent situations. Physicians and nurses often perform procedures beyond the scope of their usual practices. Professional functions and roles are widely shared among physicians, nurses, and paramedics. These adaptations allow available resources to serve more victims.[160]

Austerity

To be effective, disaster medical care must be confined to basic measures that preserve life and function. Examinations, techniques, appliances, and drugs that are not essential to patient survival or preservation of function are luxuries. It may be necessary to perform fracture reductions and other minor surgical procedures with oral narcotic analgesia only. Orthopedic devices are often improvised. Outdated drugs are better than no drugs. The level of austerity is determined by the health care personnel, supplies, and equipment available at the disaster treatment site.

Triage And Rationing

Initial management of mass casualties includes triage, basic field stabilization, and transportation. In general, *triage* can be defined as the prioritization of patient care based on severity of injury or illness, prognosis, and availability of resources.[134,135] The goal of triage is to select those patients in greatest need of immediate medical attention and to arrange for that treatment. It is a concept born on the world's battlefields, by which victims are classified and treated based on the seriousness of their injuries. Military surgeons recognized that the number of victims produced in battle could overwhelm medical resources. Some persons suffer injuries that would be fatal even under ideal circumstances in which resources are unlimited. Attempts at salvaging mortally wounded individuals with heroic measures under conditions of limited personnel and supplies may deprive other victims of care for life-threatening but correctable conditions. The "walking wounded" sustain injuries that are survivable even if the provision of definitive medical care is significantly delayed. Thus, in the humanitarian interest of providing the greatest good for the greatest number of persons, methods of classification have been developed that facilitate treatment prioritization. The first victims treated are those with life-threatening injuries that can be readily stabilized without the expenditure of massive amounts of limited resources. The next priority is persons who have sustained injuries likely to cause significant morbidity, which would be appreciably lessened by early intervention. Catastrophically injured patients (e.g., those with burns involving 95% body surface area) who have

a minimal chance for survival despite optimal medical care are provided comfort measures and may need to be left to die (Box 67-1). Spending time on patients who are not likely to live leaves other patients who might be saved awaiting care. If too much time intervenes, these patients also may become nonsalvageable. In addition to the nature and urgency of the patient's systemic condition, triage decisions must be sensitive to factors affecting prognosis, such as age, general health, physical condition of the patient, the qualifications of the responders, and availability of key supplies and equipment.[131]

Triage procedures are routinely used in civilian multiple or mass casualty incidents and are essential in disaster incidents. Prioritization of victims may be needed with smaller numbers of casualties when environmental conditions, remote settings, or unusual circumstances limit availability of medical care or ease of evacuation. The decision to evacuate persons with a reasonable chance of survival before mortally injured victims may be necessary in mountain and cave rescues, or with overland transport from isolated wilderness regions. Effective triage is critical to the success of any disaster care operation and should be performed by a senior and knowledgeable provider. The essential differentiation is "now" versus "not now." In disaster triage the moribund victim unlikely to survive is classified as "not now," when in ordinary circumstances he or she would be "immediate."

Triage methods can be qualitative and quantitative.[82,98,155] *Qualitative methods* classify patients into subjective categories (e.g., immediate, delayed, minor, expectant). Two-tier, three-tier, four-tier, and five-tier systems have been described (Box 67-2). Any qualitative triage method can be used successfully in a disaster. Each ranks patients relative to others and to the available care, and each requires periodic reconsideration for treatment.

Quantitative methods assign an objective score to each patient based on initial clinical status. Various systems based on anatomic indicators of injury severity, physiologic measurements, and mechanisms of injury have been developed to predict outcomes, including the Trauma Score.[37,38] Many emergency medical systems use the revised Trauma Score for field triage and as a guide for patient routing in tiered trauma treatment systems.[37] Although experienced physicians frequently rely on their best medical judgment to triage patients, medically inexperienced personnel may benefit from such an algorithmic approach to assessment and triage. Suppose that several members of an isolated mountain village were injured during an earthquake, that the village had only one health care worker, and that evacuation and treatment resources were limited. Decisions would have to be made regarding who would be evacuated first and who would be treated first. A trauma assessment based on physiologic variables could provide a relatively objective evaluation of the victim's condition and a rational basis for the allocation of scarce re-

Box 67-1   TRIAGE CATEGORIES BY INJURY TYPE

SIMPLE TRIAGE

Immediate (Priority I)

Asphyxia
Respiratory obstruction from mechanical causes
Sucking chest wounds
Tension pneumothorax
Maxillofacial wounds in which asphyxia exists or is likely
   to develop
Shock caused by major external hemorrhage
Major internal hemorrhage
Visceral injuries or evisceration
Cardiopericardial injuries
Massive muscle damage
Severe burns over more than 25% of body surface area
Dislocations
Major fractures
Major medical problems readily correctable
Closed cerebral injuries with increasing loss of
   consciousness

Delayed (Priority II)

Vascular injuries requiring repair
Wounds of the genitourinary tract
Thoracic wounds without asphyxia
Severe burns over less than 25% of body surface area
Spinal cord injuries requiring decompression
Suspected spinal cord injuries without neurologic
   signs
Lesser fractures
Eye injuries
Maxillofacial injuries without asphyxia
Minor medical problems
Victims with little chance of survival under the best
   conditions

**MASS CASUALTY TRIAGE WITH AN OVERWHELMING
NUMBER OF INJURIES**

Immediate (Priority I)

Asphyxia
Respiratory obstruction from mechanical causes
Sucking chest wounds
Tension pneumothorax
Maxillofacial wounds in which asphyxia exists or is likely
   to develop
Shock caused by major external hemorrhage
Dislocations
Severe burns over less than 25% of body surface area*
Lesser fractures*
Major medical problems that are readily treatable

Delayed (Priority II)

Major fractures (if able to stabilize)*
Visceral injuries or evisceration*
Cardiopericardial injuries*
Massive muscle damage*
Severe burns over more than 25% of body surface area*
Vascular injuries requiring repair
Wounds of the genitourinary tract
Thoracic wounds without asphyxia
Closed cerebral injuries with increasing loss of
   consciousness*
Spinal cord injuries requiring decompression*
Suspected spinal cord injuries without neurologic signs
Eye injuries
Maxillofacial injuries without asphyxia
Complicated major medical problems*
Minor medical problems
Victims with little chance of survival under the best
   conditions

Data from Office of Emergency Services, State of California.
*Conditions that have changed categories.

Box 67-2   TRIAGE RATING SYSTEM

FIVE-TIER SYSTEM (USED IN MILITARY TRIAGE)

Dead or will die
Life threatening—readily correctable
Urgent—must be treated within 1 to 2 hours
Delayed—noncritical or ambulatory
No injury—no treatment necessary

FOUR-TIER SYSTEM

Immediate—seriously injured, reasonable chance of
   survival
Delayed—can wait for care after simple first aid
Expectant—extremely critical, moribund
Minimal—no impairment of function, can either treat self
   or be treated by a nonprofessional

THREE-TIER SYSTEM

Life threatening—readily correctable
Urgent—must be treated within 1 to 2 hours
Delayed—no injury, noncritical, or ambulatory

TWO-TIER SYSTEM

Immediate—life-threatening injuries that are readily
   correctable on scene, and those that are urgent
Delayed—no injury, noncritical injuries, ambulatory
   victims, moribund, and dead

sources. The use of such standardized scoring systems for triage decisions, however, remains to be studied in the disaster setting. Triage methods founded on scoring systems require familiarity with the scoring systems. They cannot be used by disaster medical personnel unfamiliar with their application or modification.

Mechanics of the Triage Process

Triage should begin as soon as trained medical personnel arrive on the scene. A rapid survey is performed, noting the number of victims, hazards to victims and rescuers, and the need for additional help. This information should be relayed rapidly to the communication centers responsible for the dispatch of emergency services so additional help can be mobilized as early as possible. The most qualified medical person present should be designated the provisional triage officer. The triage officer should not be assigned other duties and should not become extensively involved in patient care. During the initial survey, each victim is rapidly assessed for immediately correctable life-threatening problems, such as airway obstruction, vigorous hemorrhage, or nonfatal penetrating chest injuries. Initial care should be limited to correction of these problems; resuscitation and definitive care have no role at this stage. Care should be limited to manually opening airways and controlling external hemorrhage.[136] Physical

hazards may influence the decision to provide further care on site or delay additional therapy until victims are transported a safe distance to a casualty collection point. As additional experienced emergency medical personnel arrive, the role of triage officer should be assumed by the most experienced and knowledgeable person present. Advanced medical knowledge is an asset in minimizing triage errors. However, field-experienced physicians are relatively rare. Successful disaster triage under mock conditions can be performed by appropriately trained advanced emergency medical technicians or by experienced nurses. Triage is a dynamic process. Continued clinical deterioration or improvement may change the initial decision to evacuate or treat a victim. Triage should be performed whenever the responsibility for a victim's care is transferred.[159]

Adjuncts to Triage

A triage tag is a paper tag intended to show the triage category in which a patient has been classified. Most bear color codes designating triage category. All enforce the use of the particular scheme of categorization for which they were designed, such as "immediate," "delayed," "minor," and "expectant," depending on injury severity and prognosis. Most are deliberately simple, such as the METTAG (Figure 67-7, *A*), and bear only minimal information to identify the patient and indi-

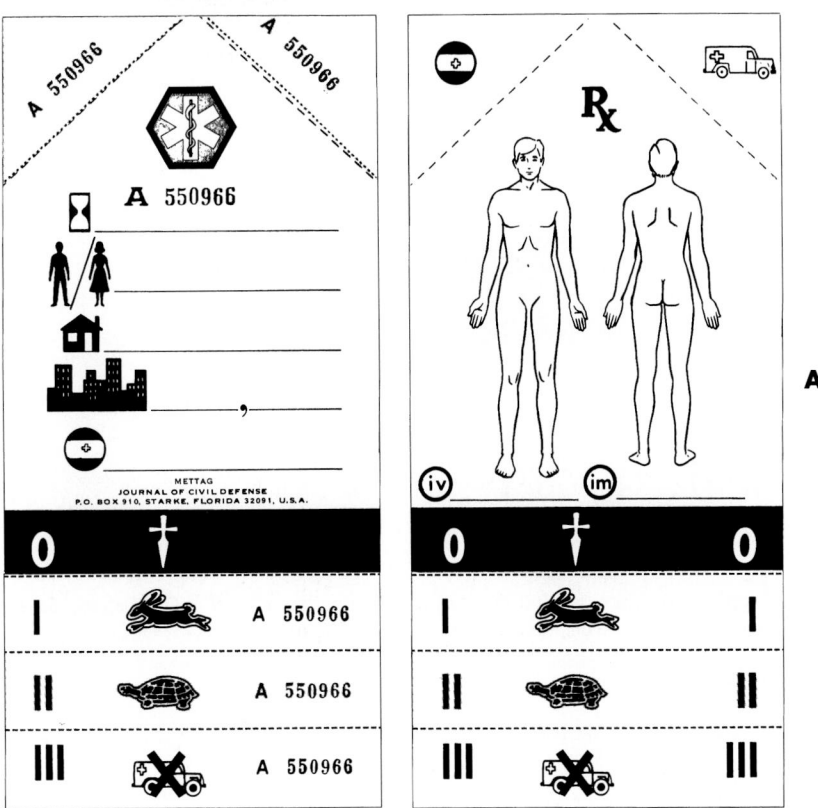

Figure 67-7 Examples of disaster tags. **A,** METTAG. *Continued*

Figure 67-7, cont'd B, More detailed disaster tag. (**A,** Courtesy *Journal of Civil Defense, Starke, Fla.* **B,** Courtesy *Precision Graphics Division, Precision Dynamics Corp., Burbank, Calif.*)

cate triage class and site of injury. Others carry more information and serve as an abbreviated medical record (Figure 67-7, *B*). Vayer et al[159] reported that the tags had been used effectively in only a few multicasualty incidents. These authors recommend that triage tags be abandoned and replaced by a system of "geographic triage" that sorts casualties into areas reserved for patients of similar priority for treatment. Simultaneously, some disaster medical systems are recasting their "triage tags" as "victim tracking tags" in an elaborate evacuation system.

On-Site Medical Care

The amount and type of care administered at disaster sites depend on several factors.[121] If the number of patients is small and sufficient prehospital personnel and transportation resources are available, on-site medical care can proceed normally, with rapid stabilization and transportation to nearby hospitals. When extrication is prolonged, potentially lifesaving interventions, such as intravenous fluids for hypovolemic shock, should be instituted.[136] On the other hand, early rapid transportation with minimal treatment should be practiced in circumstances such as danger to rescuers and casualties from fire, explosion, falling buildings, hazardous materials, and extreme weather conditions.[45]

With an overwhelming number of casualties that exceed transportation capacities, advanced field medical treatment may be beneficial because hours may pass before seriously injured patients can be evacuated.[7] This may necessitate the establishment of field hospitals with operating theater capabilities.[100] Such a field hospital may be set up in a large building such as a school or church. Casualties are brought to the field hospital from the disaster site for further assessment and initial treatment of injuries. After observation and stabilization, they are either sent home or transported to a hospital.

Evacuation of slightly injured and ambulatory persons may rapidly overwhelm local hospitals before the arrival of more severely injured victims.[129] Under these conditions, local treatment may be preferable to evacuation of the severely injured victims.

Communication From Disaster Site to Hospital

Local emergency communications or the disaster operations center should alert hospitals in the affected area of a possible mass or multiple casualty situation. This report should include number of injured and, specifically, number of seriously injured and number for whom ambulatory treatment is sufficient.[22] Hospitals should report the following information to the local emergency communications center:

1. Bed availability
2. Number of casualties received thus far
3. Number of additional casualties that the hospital is prepared to accept
4. Specific items in short supply

Specific Clinical Issues

Wound infections may occur in virtually all types of disasters. Infected wounds and gangrene were major problems after the Armenian earthquake.[111] In hurricanes or tornadoes, persons may be cut by flying glass and other potentially highly contaminated material.[124,165] Because of this, all wounds should be copiously flushed with saline. Primary closure of heavily contaminated wounds may result in major complications, as occurred after the Armero volcanic eruption in Colombia. If lacerations are old (more than 6 to 12 hours) or appear contaminated, they should be treated by debridement and left open for primary delayed closure for a 3-day period.[21] This allows an opportunity to observe the wound for the development of infection. For tetanus prophylaxis, all patients should receive a tetanus booster, and if the wound is highly contaminated, tetanus immune globulin (Hypertet) should be administered.

Victims with blunt trauma, such as those trapped by rubble for several hours or days, should be watched closely for signs and symptoms of crush syndrome, such as cardiac arrhythmias and renal failure.[116] Fulminant pulmonary edema from dust inhalation may also be a delayed cause of mortality for victims of building collapse.[111]

PUBLIC HEALTH PROBLEMS

Epidemics

Natural disasters are often followed by rampant rumors of epidemics, such as typhoid, cholera, or rabies, or unusual conditions, such as increased snakebites and dog bites. Such unsubstantiated reports gain great public credibility when printed as facts in newspapers or reported on television or radio. After disasters in developing countries, any disruption of the water supply or sewage treatment facilities is usually accompanied by rumors of outbreaks of cholera or typhoid. Such rumors may well reflect psychologic fears and anxieties about a disastrous event rather than an imminent problem. Although natural disasters do not usually result in outbreaks of infectious disease, they may increase disease transmission.[1,140] In addition, information on disease incidence in most developing countries is poor, and some outbreaks may have been missed by public health authorities.[13,49] The most frequently observed increases in communicable disease are caused by fecal contamination of water and by respiratory spread, such as measles in refugee camps.[26,27]

During the past 60 years, outbreaks of communicable disease after natural disasters have been unusual.

Disasters can contribute to transmission of disease, however, and persons responsible for managing disaster relief operations should establish a surveillance system and institute appropriate sanitary and medical measures to prevent outbreaks.[15,63,69,140,164] Mass vaccination programs are rarely necessary.[25] A clearinghouse for rumors is helpful not only in developing countries, but also in disasters occurring in urban settings of industrialized countries.

Disposition of Dead Bodies

The public and government authorities are usually greatly concerned about the danger of disease transmission from decaying corpses (Figure 67-8). Responsible health authorities should recognize, however, that the health hazards associated with unburied bodies are minimal, particularly if death resulted from trauma.[79] Such bodies are unlikely to cause outbreaks of diseases such as typhoid, cholera, or plague, although they may transmit agents of gastroenteritis or food poisoning to survivors if the bodies contaminate streams, wells, or other water sources.[124] Despite the negligible health risk, dead bodies represent a delicate social problem. Demands for mass burial or cremation are certainly not justified on public health grounds, and mass cremations require tremendous quantities of fuel.

Health Effects

Table 67-5 outlines short-term health effects from natural disasters that require effective emergency medical care with an appropriate public health response. The overall objective of disaster management is to assess the needs of disaster-affected populations, to match resources to needs efficiently, to prevent further adverse health effects, to evaluate relief program effectiveness, and to plan for future disasters.[108]

All natural disasters are unique in that each affected region of the world has different social, economic, and health backgrounds. Recognition of similarities among the health effects of different natural disasters, however, can ensure that health and emergency medical relief and limited resources are well managed.[72]

TABLE 67-5. Short-Term Effects of Major Natural Disasters

EFFECTS	EARTHQUAKES	HIGH WINDS (WITHOUT FLOODING)	TSUNAMIS	FLOODS/FLASH FLOODS
Deaths	Many	Few	Many	Few
Severe injuries requiring extensive care	Overwhelming	Moderate	Few	Few
Increased risk of communicable diseases	Potential (but small) risk after all major disasters (probability rises as overcrowding increases and sanitation deteriorates)			
Food scarcity (may occur because of factors other than food shortage)	Rare	Rare	Common	Common
Major population movements (may occur in heavily damaged urban areas)	Rare	Rare	Common	Common

Modified from *Emergency health management after natural disaster*, Office of Emergency Preparedness and Disaster Relief Coordination, Scientific Publication No 407, Washington, DC, 1981, Pan American Health Organization.

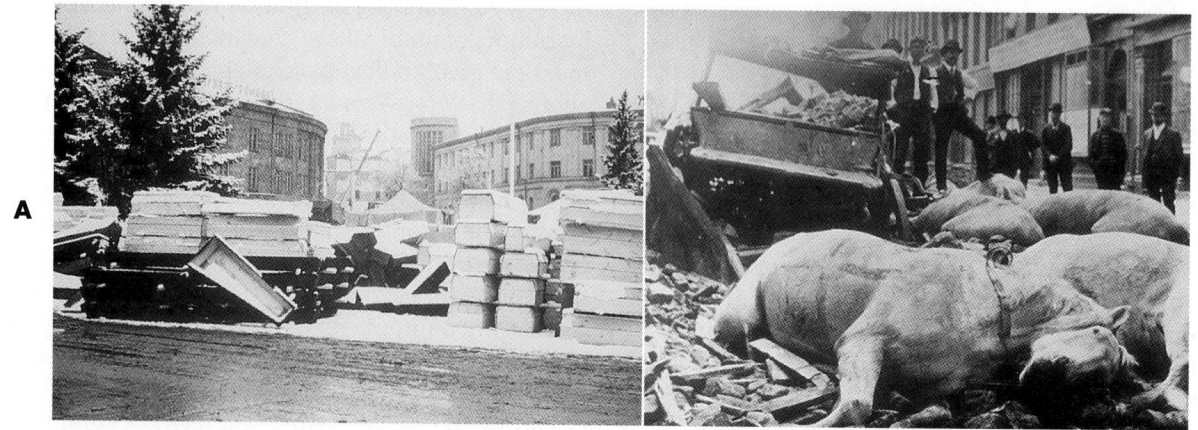

Figure 67-8　**A,** Coffins lining the street in the city of Leninakan after the 1988 earthquake in Armenia. (Eric K. Noji photo.) **B,** Three horses were killed as a result of falling debris during the 1906 San Francisco earthquake. (**A,** *Courtesy Eric K. Noji.* **B,** *Courtesy Eric Swenson, US Geological Survey.*)

REFERENCES

1. Aghababian RV, Teuscher J: Infectious diseases following major disasters, *Ann Emerg Med* 21:362, 1992.
2. Armenian HK: Methodologic issues in the epidemiologic studies of disasters. In *Proceedings of the international workshop on earthquake injury epidemiology: implications for mitigation and response*, Baltimore, 1989, Johns Hopkins University.
3. Arnold C, Durkin M: *Hospitals and the San Fernando earthquake of 1971: the operational experience*, San Mateo, Calif, 1983, Building Systems Development.
4. Autier P et al: Drug supply in the aftermath of the 1988 Armenian earthquake, *Lancet* 335:1388, 1990.
5. Bailey RA et al: *The Volcano Hazards Program: objectives and long-range plans*, US Geological Survey Open-File Report 83-400, 1983.
6. Bakst HJ et al: *The Worcester County tornado: medical study of the disaster*, Washington, DC, 1954, National Research Council, Committee on Disaster Studies.
7. Baskett P, Weller R: *Medicine for disasters*, London, 1988, Wright.
8. Baxter PJ: Volcanoes. In Noji EK, editor: *The public health consequences of disasters*, New York, 1997, Oxford University Press.
9. Baxter PJ, Bernstein RS, Buist AS: Preventive health measures in volcanic eruptions, *Am J Public Health* 76(suppl):84, 1986.
10. Baxter PJ et al: Medical aspects of volcanic disasters: an outline of the hazards and emergency response measures, *Disasters* 6:268, 1982.
11. Beinin L: *Medical consequences of natural disasters*, Berlin, 1985, Springer-Verlag.
12. Bernstein RS, Baxter PJ, Buist AS: Introduction to the epidemiological aspects of explosive volcanism, *Am J Public Health* 76(suppl):3, 1986.
13. Bernstein RS et al: Immediate public health concerns and actions in volcanic eruptions: lessons from the Mt. St. Helens eruptions, May 18-October 18, 1980, *Am J Public Health* 76(suppl):25, 1986.
14. Better OS, Stein JH: Early management of shock and prophylaxis of acute renal failure in traumatic rhabdomyolysis, *N Engl J Med* 322:825, 1990.
15. Binder S, Sanderson LM: The role of the epidemiologist in natural disasters, *Ann Emerg Med* 16:1081, 1987.
16. Bissell R: Delayed-impact infectious disease after a natural disaster, *J Emerg Med* 1:59, 1983.
17. Blong RJ: *Volcanic hazards: a sourcebook on the effects of eruptions*, North Ryde, Australia, 1984, Academic Press.
18. Brenner SA, Noji EK: Head injuries and mortality in tornado disasters, *Am J Public Health* 82:1296, 1992 (letter).
19. Brenner SA, Noji EK: Wound infections after tornadoes, *J Trauma* 33:643, 1992 (letter).
20. Brenner SA, Noji EK: Risk factors for death and injury in tornadoes: an epidemiologic approach. In Church C et al, editors: *The tornado: its structure, dynamics, prediction, and hazards*, Washington, DC, 1993, American Geophysical Union.
21. Burkle FM, Sanner PH, Wolcott BW, editors: *Disaster medicine*, New York, 1984, Medical Examination Publishing.
22. Butman AM: *Emergency training: responding to the mass casualty incident: a guide for EMS personnel*, Westport, Conn, 1982, Educational Direction.
23. Butman A: The challenge of casualties en masse, *Emerg Med* 15(7):110, 1983.
24. Byrd TR: Disaster medicine: toward a more rational approach, *Milit Med* 145:270, 1980.
25. Centers for Disease Control: Current trends in flood disasters and immunization—California, *MMWR* 32:171, 1983.
26. Centers for Disease Control: Outbreak of diarrheal illness associated with a natural disaster—Utah, *MMWR* 35:662, 1986.
27. Centers for Disease Control: Health assessment of the population affected by flood conditions—Khartoum, Sudan, *MMWR* 38:785, 1989.
28. Centers for Disease Control: Medical examiner/coroner reports of deaths associated with Hurricane Hugo—S. Carolina, *MMWR* 38:754, 1989.
29. Centers for Disease Control: Update: work-related electrocutions associated with Hurricane Hugo, *MMWR* 38:718, 1989.
30. Centers for Disease Control: Surveillance of shelters after Hurricane Hugo—Puerto Rico, *MMWR* 39:41, 1990.
31. Centers for Disease Control: Medical examiner reports of deaths associated with Hurricane Andrew—Florida: preliminary report, *MMWR* 41:641, 1992.
32. Centers for Disease Control: Rapid health needs assessment following Hurricane Andrew—Florida and Louisiana, *MMWR* 41:696, 1992.
33. Centers for Disease Control and Prevention: Flood-related mortality—Missouri, 1993, *MMWR* 42:836, 1993.
34. Centers for Disease Control and Prevention: Morbidity surveillance following the Midwest flood—Missouri, 1993, *MMWR* 42:797, 1993.
35. Centers for Disease Control and Prevention: Public health consequences of a flood disaster—Iowa, 1993, *MMWR* 42:653, 1993.
36. Centers for Disease Control and Prevention: Deaths associated with Hurricanes Marilyn and Opal—United States, September-October 1995, *MMWR* 45:32, 1996.
37. Champion HR: Trauma triage, *J World Assoc Emerg Disaster Med* 3(2):1, 1987.
38. Champion HR et al: The trauma score, *Crit Care Med* 9:672, 1981.
39. Chartoff SE, Gren JM: Survey of Iowa emergency medical services on the effects of the 1993 floods, *J Prehosp Disaster Med* 12:210, 1997.
40. Coburn AW, Hughes RE: Fatalities, injury and rescue in earthquakes. In *2nd Conference of the Development Studies Association*, Manchester, England, 1987, University of Manchester.
41. Coburn AW, Murakami HO, Ohta Y: *Factors affecting fatalities and injury in earthquakes: engineering seismology and earthquake; disaster prevention planning internal report*, Hokkaido, Japan, 1987, Hokkaido University.
42. Cohen SP, Raghavulu CV: *The Andhra Pradesh cyclone of 1977*, New Delhi, India, 1979, Vikas.
43. Contzen H: Preparations in hospital for the treatment of mass casualties, *J World Assoc Emerg Disaster Med* 1:118, 1985.
44. Cuny F: *Disasters and development*, Oxford, England, 1983, Oxford University Press.
45. Currance PL, Bronstein AC: *Emergency care for hazardous materials exposure*, St Louis, 1988, Mosby.
46. de Bruycker M, Greco D, Lechat MF: The 1980 earthquake in southern Italy: morbidity and mortality, *Int J Epidemiol* 14:113, 1985.
47. de Bruycker M et al: The 1980 earthquake in southern Italy: rescue of trapped victims and mortality, *Bull World Health Organ* 61:1021, 1983.
48. de Ville de Goyet C, Jeannee E: Epidemiological data on morbidity and mortality following the Guatemala earthquake, *IRCS Med Sci Soc Med* 4:212, 1976.
49. de Ville de Goyet C, Zeballos JL: Communicable diseases and epidemiological surveillance after sudden natural disasters. In Baskett P, Weller R, editors: *Medicine for disasters*, London, 1988, Wright.
50. de Ville de Goyet C et al: Earthquake in Guatemala: epidemiologic evaluation of the relief effort, *Pan Am Health Organ Bull* 10:95, 1976.
51. Dietz VJ et al: Health assessment of the 1985 flood disaster in Puerto Rico, *Disasters* 14:164, 1990.
52. Disaster epidemiology, *Lancet* 336:845, 1990 (editorial).
53. Dubouloz M: An introduction to disaster medicine, *Bull Int Civil Defence*, 8:25, 1983.
54. Eisele JW et al: Death during the May 18, 1980, eruption of Mount St. Helens, *N Engl J Med* 305:931, 1981.
55. Falk H et al: *Mount St. Helens volcano health report*, Atlanta, 1980, CDC.
56. Federal Emergency Management Agency: *Principal threats facing communities and local emergency management coordinators: a report to the US Senate Committee on Appropriations*, Washington, DC, 1992, FEMA Office of Emergency Management.
57. Foege WH: Public health aspects of disaster management. In Last JM, editor: *Public health and preventive medicine*, Norwalk, Conn, 1986, Appleton-Century-Crofts.
58. Frazier K: *The violent face of nature: severe phenomena and natural disasters*, New York, 1979, Morrow.
59. French JG: Hurricanes. In Gregg MB, editor: *The public health consequences of disasters*, Atlanta, 1989, CDC.
60. French JG et al: Mortality from flash flood: a review of National Weather Service Reports, *Public Health Rep* 98:584, 1983.
61. Galway G: Relationship of tornado deaths to severe weather watch areas, *Monogr Weather Rev* 103:737, 1975.
62. Gilbert DN et al: Microbiologic study of wound infections in tornado casualties, *Arch Environ Health* 26:125, 1973.
63. Glass RI, Noji EK: Epidemiologic surveillance following disasters. In Halperin WE, Baker EL, Monson RR, editors: *Public health surveillance*, New York, 1992, Van Nostrand Reinhold.
64. Glass RI et al: Earthquake injuries related to housing in a Guatemalan village, *Science* 197:638, 1977.
65. Glass RI et al: Injuries from the Wichita Falls tornado: implications for prevention, *Science* 207:734, 1980.
66. Glass RI et al: Health effects of the 1991 Bangladesh cyclone: report of a UNICEF evaluation team, New York, 1992, UNICEF.
67. Goltz JD: *The Northridge, California earthquake of January 17, 1994: general reconnaissance report*, Buffalo, NY, 1994, National Center for Earthquake Engineering Research.
68. Gordon PD: *Special statistical summary—deaths, injuries and property loss by type of disaster, 1970-1980*, Washington, DC, 1982, FEMA.

69. Gregg M: *Management of surveillance operations following a disaster,* Atlanta, 1979, CDC.

70. Gross EM: The hurricane dilemma in the United States, *Episodes* 14:36, 1991.

71. Guha-Sapir D: Rapid needs assessment in mass emergencies: review of current concepts and methods, *World Health Stat Q* 44:17, 1991.

72. Guha-Sapir D, Lechat MF: Information systems and needs assessment in natural disasters: an approach for better disaster relief management, *Disasters* 10:232, 1986.

73. Guha-Sapir D, Lechat MF: Reducing the impact of natural disasters: why aren't we better prepared? *Health Policy Planning* 1:118, 1986.

74. Gurd CH, Bromwich A, Quinn JV: The health management of Cyclone Tracy, *Med J Aust* 1:641, 1975.

75. Hagman G: *Prevention better than cure,* Stockholm, 1984, Swedish Red Cross.

76. Henderson AK et al: Disaster medical assistance teams: providing health care to a community struck by Hurricane Iniki, *Ann Emerg Med* 23:726, 1994.

77. Hight D et al: Medical aspects of the Worcester tornado disaster, *N Engl J Med* 254:267, 1956.

78. Hingston RA, Hingston L: Respiratory injuries in earthquakes in Latin America in the 1970s: a personal experience in Peru (1970); Nicaragua (1972-3); and Guatemala (1976), *Disaster Med* 1:425, 1983.

79. Hooft PJ, Noji EK, Van de Voorde HP: Fatality management in mass-casualty incidents, *Forensic Sci Int* 40:3, 1989.

80. IDNDR Secretariat: *The international decade for natural disaster reduction: action plan for 1998-1999,* Geneva, 1998, UN Office for the Coordination of Humanitarian Assistance.

81. Ivy JH: Infections encountered in tornado and automobile accident victims, *J Ind Med Assoc* 61:1657, 1968.

82. Jacobs L et al: An emergency medical system approach to disaster planning, *J Trauma* 19:157, 1979.

83. Jenkins AL, van de Leuv JH,: *Disaster planning in emergency department organization and management,* ed 2, St Louis, 1978, Mosby.

84. Katsouyanni K, Kogevinas M, Trichopoulos D: Earthquake-related stress and cardiac mortality, *Int J Epidemiol* 15:326, 1986.

85. Katz LB, Pascarelli EF: Planning and developing a community hospital disaster program, *Emerg Med Serv,* 9/10:70, 1978.

86. Kerr RA: Volcanoes to keep an eye on, *Science* 221:634, 1983.

87. Kindel S: Penny-wise, pound-foolish, *Forbes* 17:170, 1985.

88. Kunii O, Akagi M, Kita E: Health consequences and medical and public health response to the great Hanshin-Awaji earthquake in Japan: a case study in disaster planning, *Med Global Survival* 2:32, 1995.

89. Lechat MF: Updates: the epidemiology of health effects of disasters, *Epidemiol Rev* 12:192, 1990.

90. Lillibridge DR: Tornadoes. In Noji EK, editor: *The public health consequences of disasters,* New York, 1997, Oxford University Press.

91. Longmire AW, Burch J, Broom LA: Morbidity of Hurricane Elena, *South Med J* 81:1343, 1988.

92. Longmire AW, Ten Eyck RP: Morbidity of Hurricane Frederic, *Ann Emerg Med* 13:334, 1984.

93. Malilay J: Medical and healthcare aspects of the 1992 earthquake in Egypt. In *Report of the Earthquake Engineering Research Institute Reconnaissance Team,* Oakland, Calif, 1992, Earthquake Engineering Research Institute.

94. Malilay J: *Volcanic eruption of Cerro Negro, Nicaruagua, April, 1992,* Washington, DC, 1992, Emergency Preparedness and Disaster Relief Coordination Unit, Pan American Health Organization.

95. Malilay J: Floods. In Noji EK, editor: *The public health consequences of disasters,* New York, 1997, Oxford University Press.

96. Mandelbaum I, Nahrwold D, Boyer DW: Management of tornado casualties, *J Trauma* 6:353, 1966.

97. Manni C, Magalini S, Proietti R: Volcanoes. In Baskett P, Weller R, editors: *Medicine for disasters,* London, 1988, Wright.

98. Marian JF, Bougarte W: Disaster preparedness. In Schwartz GR et al, editors: *Principles and practice of emergency medicine,* Philadelphia, 1978, WB Saunders.

99. Memarzadeh P: The earthquake of August 31, 1968, in the south of Khorasan, Iran. In *Proceedings of the joint IHF/IUA/UNDRO/WHO seminar,* Manila, 1978, World Health Organization Regional Office.

100. Nancekievill D, Finch P: The role of hospital mobile medical teams at a major accident. In Cowley RA, editor: *Proceedings of mass casualties: a lessons learned approach,* Baltimore, June 1982, Maryland Institute for Emergency Medical Service System.

101. Nania J, Bruya TE: In the wake of Mount St. Helens, *Ann Emerg Med* 11:184, 1982.

102. National Oceanic and Atmospheric Administration, US Department of Commerce: *Tornado,* Washington, DC, 1973, US Government Printing Office.

103. National Research Council: *Confronting natural disasters: an international decade for natural disaster reduction,* Washington, DC, 1987, National Academy Press.

104. Noji EK: Prophylaxis of acute renal failure in traumatic rhabdomyolysis, *N Engl J Med* 323:550, 1990 (letter).

105. Noji EK: Medical consequences of earthquakes: coordinating medical and rescue response, *Disaster Management* 4:32, 1991.

106. Noji EK: Acute renal failure in natural disasters, *Renal Failure* 14:245, 1992.

107. Noji EK: Analysis of medical needs in disasters caused by tropical cyclones: the need for a uniform injury reporting scheme, *J Trop Med Hyg* 96:370, 1993.

108. Noji EK: Progress in disaster management, *Lancet* 343:1239, 1994.

109. Noji EK: Earthquakes. In Noji EK, editor: *The public health consequences of disasters,* New York, 1997, Oxford University Press.

110. Noji EK: *The public health consequences of disasters,* New York and Oxford, 1997, Oxford University Press.

111. Noji EK, Armenian HK, Oganessian A: Issues of rescue and medical care following the 1988 Armenian earthquake, *Int J Epidemiol* 22:1070, 1993.

112. Noji EK, Jones NP: Hospital preparedness for earthquakes. In Tomasik KM, editor: *Emergency preparedness: when disaster strikes,* Oakbrook Terrace, Ill, 1994, Joint Commission on the Accreditation of Healthcare Organizations.

113. Noji EK, Sivertson KT: Injury prevention in natural disasters: a theoretical framework, *Disasters* 11:290, 1987.

114. Noji EK, Toole MJ: Public health and disasters: the historical development of public health responses to disasters, *Disasters* 21:369, 1997.

115. Noji EK et al: The 1988 earthquake in Soviet Armenia: a case study, *Ann Emerg Med* 19:891, 1990.

116. Oda Y et al: Crush syndrome sustained in the 1995 Kobe, Japan earthquake: treatment and outcome, *Ann Emerg Med* 30:507, 1997.

117. Office of US Foreign Disaster Assistance: *Disaster history: significant data on major disasters worldwide, 1900-present,* Washington, DC, 1999, Agency for International Development.

118. Orlowski J: Floods, hurricanes, and tsunamis. In Baskett P, Weller R, editors: *Medicine for disasters,* London, 1988, Wright.

119. Othman-Chande M: The Cameroon volcanic gas disaster: an analysis of a makeshift response, *Disasters* 2:96, 1987.

120. Oxtoby MJ, Broome C V, Pinzon MR: Late mortality in Nevado del Ruiz victims. In *The volcanic eruption in Colombia, November 13, 1985,* Washington, DC, 1986, Pan American Health Organization.

121. Oyen O: The on-scene medical organization, *J World Assoc Emerg Disaster Med* 1(2):115, 1985.

122. Pan American Health Organization: *The effects of Hurricane David, 1979, on the population of Dominica,* Washington, DC, 1979, the Organization.

123. Pan American Health Organization: *Report on disasters and emergency preparedness for Jamaica, St. Vincent and Dominica,* Washington, DC, 1980, the Organization.

124. Pan American Health Organization: *Emergency health management after natural disaster,* Washington, DC, 1981, Emergency Preparedness and Disaster Relief Coordination Unit, the Organization.

125. Pan American Health Organization: *Assessing needs in the health sector after floods and hurricanes,* Washington, DC, 1987, the Organization.

126. Pan American Health Organization: *Hurricane Gilbert in Jamaica, September, 1988,* Washington, DC, 1989, the Organization.

127. Philen RM et al: Hurricane Hugo—1989, *Disasters* 15:177, 1992.

128. Pointer JE et al: The 1989 Loma Prieta earthquake: impact on hospital care, *Ann Emerg Med* 21:1228, 1992.

129. Quarantelli EL: *Delivery of emergency medical services in disasters: assumptions and realities,* New York, 1983, Irvington.

130. Reitherman R: How to prepare a hospital for an earthquake, *J Emerg Med* 4:119, 1986.

131. Roding H: Triage and its ethical problems, *J World Assoc Emerg Disaster Med* 3(3):10, 1987.

132. Roth PB et al: The St. Croix disaster and the National Disaster Medical System, *Ann Emerg Med* 20:391, 1991.

133. Rubin CH, Noji EK: Impact of the eruption of Mt. Hudson on livestock in Argentina, *Bull Global Volcanism Network* 16:5, 1991.

134. Rund D, Rausch T: *Triage,* St Louis, 1981, Mosby.

135. Rutherford WH: Sorting patients, sometimes called triage, *Disaster Med* 1(1):121, 1983.

136. Safar P: Resuscitation potentials in mass disasters, *J World Assoc Emerg Disaster Med* 2:34, 1986.

137. Safar P, Pretto EA, Bircher NG: Resuscitation medicine including the management of severe trauma. In Baskett P, Weller R, editors: *Medicine for disasters,* London, 1988, Wright.

138. Schultz CH, Koenig KL, Noji EK: A medical disaster response to reduce immediate mortality after an earthquake, *N Engl J Med* 334:438, 1996.

139. Seaman J: Epidemiology of natural disasters, *Contrib Epidemiol Biostat* 5:1, 1984.

140. Seaman J: Disaster epidemiology: or why most international disaster relief is ineffective, *Injury* 21:5, 1990.

141. Sheets RC: *The United States hurricane problem: an assessment for the 1990s,* Miami, 1994, National Hurricane Center.

142. Shoaf KI et al: Injuries as a result of California earthquakes in the past decade, *Disasters* 22:218, 1998.

143. Sigurdsson H: Gas bursts from Cameroon crater lakes: a new natural hazard, *Disasters* 12:131, 1988.

144. Sigurdsson H, Carey S: Volcanic disasters in Latin America and the 13th November 1985 eruption of Nevado del Ruiz volcano in Colombia, *Disasters* 10:205, 1986.

145. Smith GS: Development of rapid epidemiologic assessment methods to evaluate health status and delivery of health services, *Int J Epidemiol* 18(suppl):S2, 1989.

146. Sommer A, Mosley WH: East Bengal cyclone of November, 1970, *Lancet* 1:1029, 1972.

147. Surmieda RS et al: Surveillance in evacuation camps after the eruption of Mt. Pinatubo. In *Public health surveillance and international health,* Atlanta, 1992, CDC.

148. Tanaka K: The Kobe earthquake: the system response—a disaster report from Japan, *Eur J Emerg Med* 3:263, 1996.

149. Tatemachi K: Acute diseases during and after the Great Hanshin-Awaji earthquake. In *Proceedings of the WHO symposium on earthquakes and people's health, 27-30 January 1997,* Kobe, Japan, 1997, WHO Center for Health Development.

150. Thiel CC et al: 911 EMS process in the Loma Prieta earthquake, *Prehosp Disaster Med* 7:348, 1992.

151. Toole MJ: Communicable disease epidemiology following disasters, *Ann Emerg Med* 21:418, 1992.

152. Toole MJ, Tailhades M: Disasters: what are the needs? How can they be assessed? *Trop Doct* 219(suppl):18, 1991.

153. Trichopoulos D, Katsouyanni K, Zavitsanos X: Psychological stress and fatal heart attack: the Athens 1981 earthquake natural experiment, *Lancet* 1:441, 1983.

154. UN General Assembly: *International decade for natural disaster reduction: report of the Secretary-General,* New York, 1988, United Nations.

155. US Air Force: *Medical planning for disaster and casualty control,* Washington, DC, 1967, US Air Force Medical Service.

156. US National Committee for the Decade for Natural Disaster Reduction, National Research Council: *A safer future: reducing the impacts of natural disasters,* Washington DC, 1991, National Academy Press.

157. US Public Health Service: *Hurricane Mitch,* Rockville, Md, 1998, US Public Health Service.

158. Ussher JH: Philippine flood disaster, *J Res Naval Med Serv* 59:81, 1973.

159. Vayer JS, Ten Eyck RP, Cowan ML: New concepts in triage, *Ann Emerg Med* 15:927, 1986.

160. Waeckerle JF et al: Disaster medicine: challenges for today, *Ann Emerg Med* 23:715, 1994.

161. Walker GPL: Volcanic hazards, *Interdisc Sci Rev* 7:148, 1982.

162. Western K: *The epidemiology of natural and man-made disasters: the present state of the art,* London, 1972, University of London, dissertation.

163. Wijkman A, Timberlake L: *Natural disasters: acts of God or acts of man,* New York, 1984, Earthscan.

164. Woodruff B et al: Disease surveillance and control after a flood—Khartoum, Sudan, 1988, *Disasters* 14:151, 1990.

165. World Health Organization: Emergency care in natural disasters: views of an international seminar, *WHO Chron* 34:96, 1980.

166. World Health Organization: *Rapid health assessment protocols,* Geneva, 1999, WHO.

167. Yong S: Medical support in the Tangshan earthquake: a review of the management of mass casualties and certain major injuries, *J Trauma* 27:1130, 1987.

68 Natural and Human-Made Hazards: Mitigation and Management Issues

Sheila B. Reed

The term *hazard* is usually applied to rare or extreme events in the natural or human-made environment. Hazards can adversely affect human life or property to the extent of causing a disaster, or major disruptive situation. *Natural hazards* are caused by biologic, geologic, seismic, hydrologic, or meteorologic processes in the natural environment and include drought, flood, earthquake, volcanic eruption, and severe storms. When natural hazards affect vulnerable human settlements, structures, and economic assets, they can be disastrous, disrupting the normal functioning of a society and necessitating extraordinary emergency interventions to save lives and the environment.

Human-made hazards are derived from human interactions with the environment, human relationships and attitudes, and the use of technology. For example, transportation accidents, petrochemical explosions, mine fires, building collapses, oil spills, hazardous waste leaks, and nuclear power plant failures are disasters where the principal and direct causes are human actions. Many hazards have both natural and human components. Desertification results from arid conditions, erosion, and overgrazing; landslides may occur from poorly planned construction on unstable hillsides, and flooding may be caused by dam failures.

The distinction between many natural causes of hazards and contributions of humans to disastrous situations is becoming increasingly blurred. As populations grow and expand, pressure on land resources may force settlement in vulnerable areas, where hazards such as volcanic eruptions, earthquakes, or floods can become major disasters. Pest infestations may lead to famine in food-deficient areas, incidences of disease might become an epidemic because of overcrowding, and drought may become famine where food shortages result from combinations of lack of rainfall and displacement of people. The recent focus on global warming emanates from studies of the effects of climatic conditions and environmental pollution. Variables in these studies form such complex interactions that even computerized models have difficulty predicting the outcomes. Hazards with a combination of causes result in complex disasters and often in complex emergencies. Whatever their causes, disasters have serious political, economic, social, and environmental implications. In less developed areas, disasters can severely set back or reverse development efforts.

DISASTER MANAGEMENT

This chapter focuses on hazards with a significant geophysical component, from a disaster management perspective. Disaster management encompasses all aspects of planning for and responding to disasters, including predisaster and postdisaster activities. It refers to the management of both the risks and the consequences of disasters. Components of disaster management include vulnerability and risk assessment, disaster mitigation and preparedness, and disaster assessment. Selection of management options depends on the type of hazard and whether the onset is likely to be slow or rapid.

Box 68-1 lists the elements usually found in a disaster preparedness plan for sudden-onset hazards, such as earthquakes, volcanic eruptions, tropical cyclones, and floods. Preparedness measures for slow-onset disasters, such as drought, include early warning systems that alert authorities to precursory conditions and allow preparations to avert famine and displacement.

Slow-Onset vs. Rapid-Onset Hazards

Hazards may develop gradually and persist for a long time or may arise suddenly and be resolved rapidly. Rapid-onset hazards often occur with violent intensity and have profound effects on the surrounding environment, resulting in measurable numbers of casualties and damage. Slow-onset climatic changes brought on by deforestation, drought, desertification, or environmental pollution change the suitability of different parts of the world to agriculture and also affect the flora and fauna. The effects of slow-onset disasters are often insidious, and their impact can be measured only through environmental studies and in terms of reduction in quality of life and productivity for the affected population. The study of disaster management, which formerly focused on natural hazards, now encompasses a range of slow-onset and rapid-onset disasters and their natural and human causes.

Conservatively, an estimated 1.5 to 2 million people have been killed in rapid-onset disasters since 1946, or an average annual death toll of 35,000 to 50,000. The primary killers are earthquakes, tropical cyclones, and floods. Most deaths are concentrated in a relatively small number of communities, predominantly in poorer nations of Asia, Latin America, and Oceania. In comparison, North America, Europe, Japan, and Australia have average annual death tolls that rarely exceed a few hundred persons.

Although no comprehensive data are available for economic losses from rapid-onset hazards, a few examples illustrate the scale of the problem. Annual worldwide losses from tropical cyclones are estimated at between $6 and $7 billion. For landslides the comparable figure exceeds $1 billion. These figures only hint at the human impact of destruction. The eruption of Colombia's Nevado del Ruiz volcano in 1985 killed approximately 22,000 people and left 10,000 more homeless. Hurricane Andrew's impact on Florida in 1992 destroyed 30,000 homes, damaged 60,000, and left 350,000 people homeless, with damage estimates of $16 billion. An earthquake in south-central India in October 1993 claimed at least 30,000 lives.

The relative human, economic, and social impacts of rapid-onset disasters are usually greatest in small, poor nations. The 1985 earthquake in Mexico City caused economic losses equivalent to about 3.5% of Mexico's gross national product (GNP). Hurricane Allen in 1980 caused losses in St. Lucia equivalent to 89% of the nation's GNP and destroyed 90% of the nation's banana crop, which normally accounts for 80% of the country's agricultural output. One of the strongest storms in recent history, Hurricane Mitch in 1998 devastated the economies and infrastructure of Honduras and Nicaragua.

Economic losses from rapid-onset hazards are increasing at a fast pace. In the United States, damage to buildings from earthquakes, tropical cyclones, and floods was estimated to increase from approximately $6 billion in 1978 to more than $11 billion in 2000 without additional loss reduction measures. A major earthquake in Tokyo would probably kill more than 30,000 people, cause the collapse of 60,000 houses, and set fire to more than 400,000 homes.

Slow-onset disasters take an even greater toll, but precise figures are difficult to find. Drought currently affects more people than any other disaster; worldwide, droughts have been estimated to affect more than 18 million people each year during the 1960s, more than 24 million people during the 1970s, and 101 million from 1980 to 1989. During the early 1980s, drought affected up to 30 million people in Africa alone. Droughts have led to famines, resulting in large numbers of deaths and displacements. Increasing desertification in arid areas may be contributing to droughts. *Desertification*, or decline in biologic productivity, extends to 70% of total productive arid lands or 3.6 billion acres worldwide and may adversely affect the quality of life for 10% of the world population, including urban dwellers.

Possible global warming is predicted in the next century from increased atmospheric carbon dioxide caused by burning of fossil fuels, deforestation, and generation of methane. If this occurs, sea levels will rise and coastal cities worldwide will be inundated. A rise of 1 m (3⅓ feet) in sea level could flood 15% of arable land in Egypt's Nile Delta and completely submerge the tiny islands of the Maldives, inhabited by 200,000. Hundreds of millions of people will also be affected if increased ultraviolet radiation is delivered to the earth's surface as a result of stratospheric ozone depletion caused by continued release of chlorofluorocarbons.

Although global warming and ozone depletion are threats to the future, other forms of environmental pollution, such as water and air pollution, affect life today. Massive oil spills make headlines, and adverse health effects are seen from contamination and smog. Deforestation, particularly in the tropical rainforests, is highly significant. In addition to its contribution to possible global warming, it increases vulnerability to droughts, landslides, and floods.

Assessing Vulnerability and Risk

Not all hazards become disasters. Whether or not a disaster occurs depends on the magnitude, intensity, and duration of the event and the vulnerability of the community. For example, a severe earthquake is not a disaster unless it significantly disrupts a community by creating large numbers of casualties and substantial destruction. Effective disaster management requires information about the magnitude of the risk faced and how much importance society places on the reduction of that risk. Risks are often quantified in aggregated ways (e.g., a probability of 1 in 23,000 per year of dying in an earthquake in Iran). The importance placed on risk of a hazard is likely to be influenced by the nature of the risks faced on a daily basis. In Pakistan, where communities are regularly affected by floods, earthquakes, and landslides, people use their meager resources to protect against what they perceive to be greater risks, such as disease and irrigation failure. In California, where risk of disease is low, communities choose to initiate programs against natural disasters.

Vulnerability is often measured as the susceptibility of buildings, infrastructure, economy, and natural resources to damage from hazards. Many aspects of vulnerability, however, cannot be described in monetary terms and should not be overlooked, such as personal loss of family, home, and income and related human suffering and psychosocial problems. Although communities in developed nations may be as prone to hazards as communities in poor nations, the wealthier communities are often less vulnerable to damage. Although southern California and Managua, Nicaragua, are both prone to earthquakes, California is less vulnerable to damage because of strictly enforced building codes, zoning regulations, earthquake preparedness training, and sophisticated communications systems. In 1971 the San Fernando earthquake in California measured 6.4 on the Richter scale but caused minor damage and 58 deaths, whereas an earthquake of similar magnitude struck Managua 2 years later and reduced the center of the city to rubble, killing approximately 6000 people. Similarly, in wealthy countries, drought and resulting loss of food production and groundwater are managed by use of food surpluses and treated water, but drought in poor nations often leads to deaths from famine and to sickness and death from contaminated water supplies.

Disaster Mitigation Strategies

Mitigation involves not only saving lives and reducing injury and property losses, but also reducing the adverse consequences of hazards to economic activities and social institutions. Where resources are limited, they should be directed toward protecting the most vulnerable elements. *Vulnerability* also implies a lack of resources for rapid recovery.

For most risks associated with natural geophysical hazards, such as volcanic eruptions, tsunamis, and tropical cyclones, little or no opportunity is available to reduce the hazard itself. In these cases the emphasis must be placed on reducing the vulnerability of the elements at risk. However, for technologic and human-made hazards or slow-onset hazards such as environmental pollution and desertification, reducing the hazard is likely to be the most effective mitigation strategy.

Actions by planning authorities to reduce vulnerability can be *active*, where desired actions are promoted through incentives, or *passive*, where undesired actions are prevented by use of controls and penalties. Mitigation options are discussed next.

Engineering and Construction. Engineering measures range from large-scale engineering works to strengthening individual buildings and implementing small-scale community-based projects to incorporate better protection into traditional structures, such as buildings, roads, and embankments.

Physical Planning Measures. Careful location of new facilities, particularly community facilities such as schools, hospitals, and infrastructure, plays an important role in reducing settlement vulnerability. In urban areas, *deconcentration* of elements especially at risk is an important principle. Specific procedures include hazard mapping and development of a master plan containing land use control guidelines. Hazard occurrence probabilities can be extrapolated from historical data and used to create hazard maps to show regional variation. Hazard mapping can be detailed by an inventory of people or things that are exposed or vulnerable to the hazard. In France, the Zones Exposed to Risks of Movements of the Soil and Subsoil (ZERMOS) plan produces landslide hazard maps at scales of 1:25,000 or larger that are used as tools for mitigation planning. The maps portray degrees of risk of various types of landslides, including activity, rate, and potential consequences.

Economic Measures. The linkages among different sectors of the economy may be more disrupted than the physical infrastructure. Diversifying and strengthening the economy are important ways to reduce risk. Within a strong economy, governments can use economic incentives to encourage individuals or institutions to take disaster mitigation actions.

Management and Institutional Measures. Building disaster protection takes time and requires support from programs of education, training, and institution building to provide the professional knowledge and competence required. Development of forecasting and warning systems are important protective measures.

Societal Measures. Mitigation planning should aim to develop a "safety culture" in which all members of society are aware of the hazards they face, know how to protect themselves, and support the protection efforts of others and communities as a whole. Specifically, these include conducting community education programs and planning and practicing evacuation procedures.

Disaster Assessment and Postdisaster Needs

Assessments regularly conducted during the recovery process help to identify needs that lead to appropriate types of assistance. In the cases of slow-onset hazard types such as desertification, deforestation, and environmental pollution, a distinct postdisaster period usually does not exist; thus ongoing impact assessment is vital. The initial response to a rapid-onset hazardous event includes the following steps by local authorities:

1. Evacuation
2. Emergency shelter
3. Search and rescue
4. Medical assistance
5. Provision of short-term food and water
6. Water disinfection and purification
7. Epidemiologic surveillance
8. Provision of temporary lodging
9. Reopening of roads
10. Reestablishment of communications networks and contact with remote areas
11. Brush and debris clearance
12. Disaster assessment
13. Provision of inputs for recovery and rehabilitation

Nature of Hazards

Many types of natural hazards and many hazards partially rooted in natural systems exist. Many of these occur infrequently or affect only small populations. One example is the eruption of toxic gases from several volcanic lakes in Cameroon that killed 2000 people in 1984 and 1986. Other rare events such as meteor impacts may occur only once every few centuries. Other widespread but minor phenomena that damage property but do not generally cause loss of life include land subsidence and sinkholes. Some hazards, such as snowstorms, often occur in areas that are prepared to deal with them so that they rarely become disasters.

This chapter discusses 12 hazards that affect large populations and that can be categorized as follows:

Geologic hazards—(1) earthquakes, (2) tsunamis, (3) volcanic eruptions, (4) landslides
Climatic hazards—(5) tropical cyclones, (6) tornadoes, (7) floods, (8) drought, (9) winter storms
Environmental hazards—(10) environmental pollution, (11) deforestation, (12) desertification

To plan appropriate responses to implement emergency medical care and other measures to save or restore physical and mental health of affected populations, officials first need to understand the causal phenomena, characteristics, and predictability of the hazards and the factors that contribute to vulnerability. Examination of the hazard's effects on humans, property, and the environment can promote measures to prevent or lessen casualties and destruction.

EARTHQUAKES

Earthquakes are among the most destructive and feared of natural hazards. They may occur at any time of year, day or night, with sudden impact and little warning. They can destroy buildings in seconds, killing or injuring the inhabitants. Earthquakes not only destroy entire cities but may destabilize the government, economy, and social structure of a country.

Causal Phenomena

The earth's crust is a rock layer of varying thickness from a depth of about 10 km under the oceans to 65 km under the continents. The theory of plate tectonics holds that the crustal plates, varying in size from a few hundred to many thousands of kilometers, ride on the mobile mantle. When the plates contact each other, stresses arise in the crust. Stresses occur along the plate boundaries by pulling away from, sliding alongside, and pushing against one another. All these movements are associated with earthquakes.

The areas of stress at plate boundaries that release accumulated energy by slipping or rupturing are known as *faults. Elastic rebound* occurs when the maximum point of supportable strain is reached and a rupture occurs, allowing the rock to rebound until the strain is relieved (Figure 68-1). Usually the rock rebounds on both sides of the fault in opposite directions. The point of rupture is called the *focus* and may be located near the surface or deep below it. The point on the surface directly above the focus is termed the *epicenter* (Figure 68-2).

The energy generated by an earthquake is not always released violently and can be small or gradual. Minor earth tremors are recorded daily in the United States, but whether they are caused by the same processes that can level a city is not known. Most damaging earthquakes are associated with sudden ruptures of the crust.

Characteristics

The actual rupture process may last from a fraction of a second to a few minutes for a major earthquake. Seismic (from the Greek *seismos,* meaning "shock" or "earthquake") waves are generated that last from less than a tenth of a second to a few minutes and cause ground shaking. The seismic waves propagate in all directions, causing vibrations that damage vulnerable structures and infrastructure.

There are three types of seismic waves. The body waves (P, or primary, and S, or secondary) penetrate the body of the earth, vibrating fast (Figure 68-3). *P waves* travel at about 6 kilometers per second (kps) and provide the initial jolt that causes buildings to vibrate up and down. *S waves* travel about 4 kps in a movement similar to the snap of a whip, causing a sharper jolt that

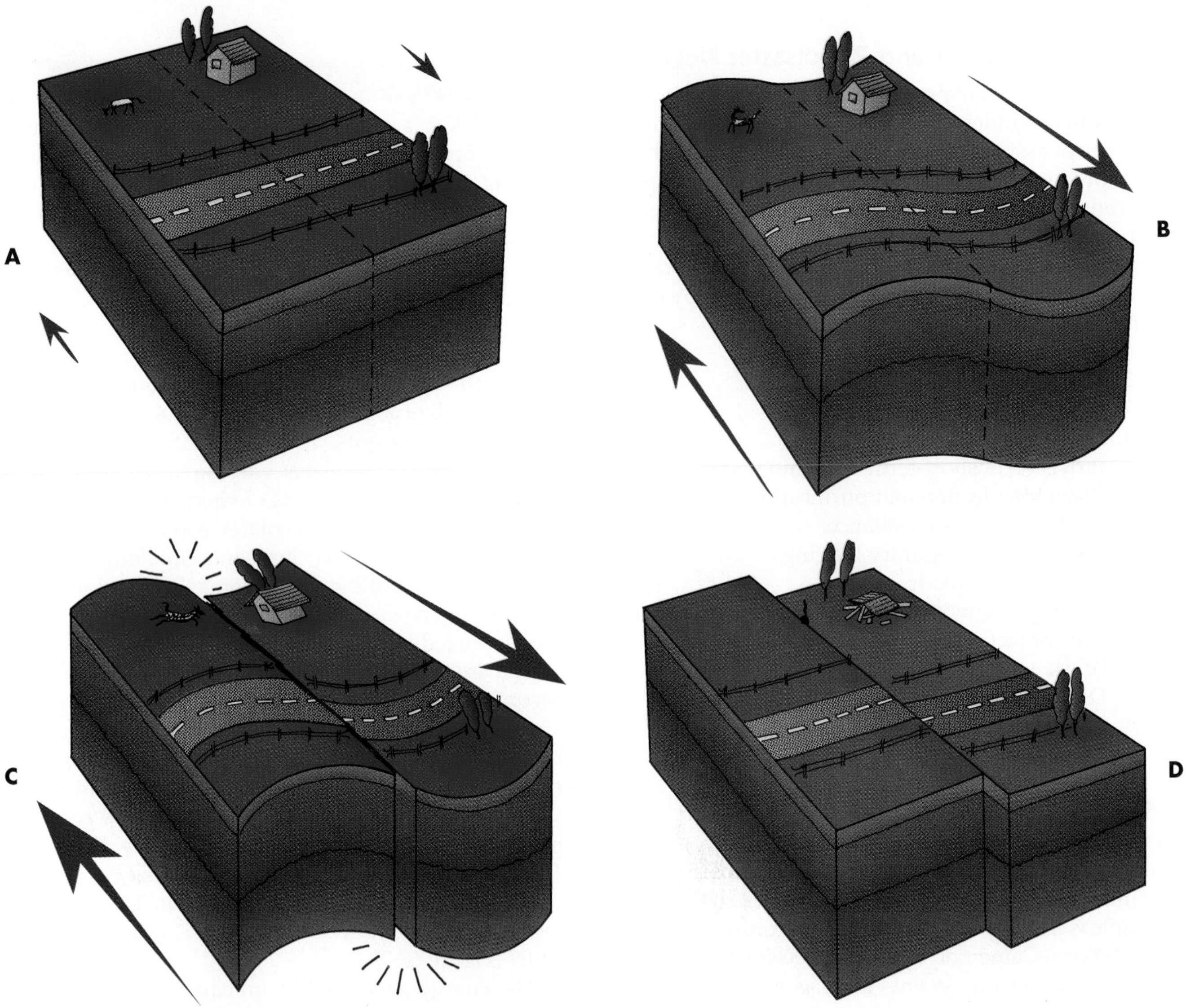

Figure 68-1. Elastic rebound in earthquake. **A,** Forces build up over time. **B,** Crust deforms. **C,** Crust snaps. **D,** Plates slide.

Figure 68-2. Motion of the earth's plates causes increased pressure at faults where the plates meet. Eventually the rock structure collapses and movement occurs along the fault. Energy is propagated to the surface above and radiates outward. Waves of motion in the earth's crust shake landforms and buildings, causing damage. *(Courtesy Disaster Management Center, University of Wisconsin.)*

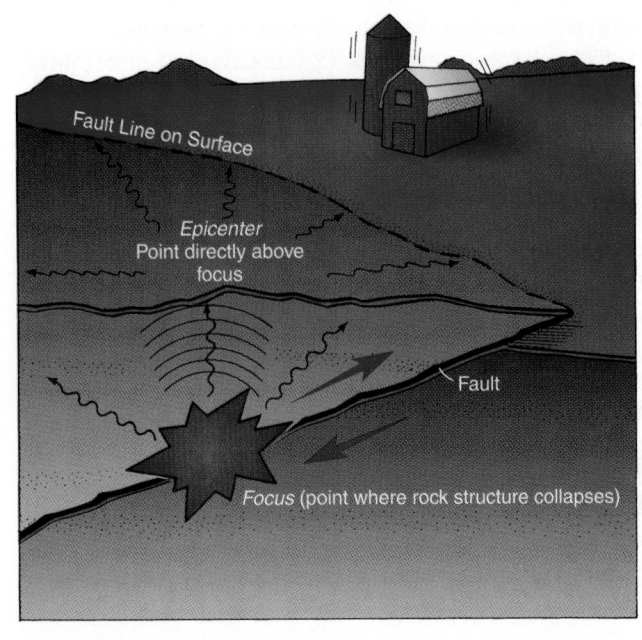

Fault Line on Surface

Epicenter
Point directly above focus

Fault

Focus (point where rock structure collapses)

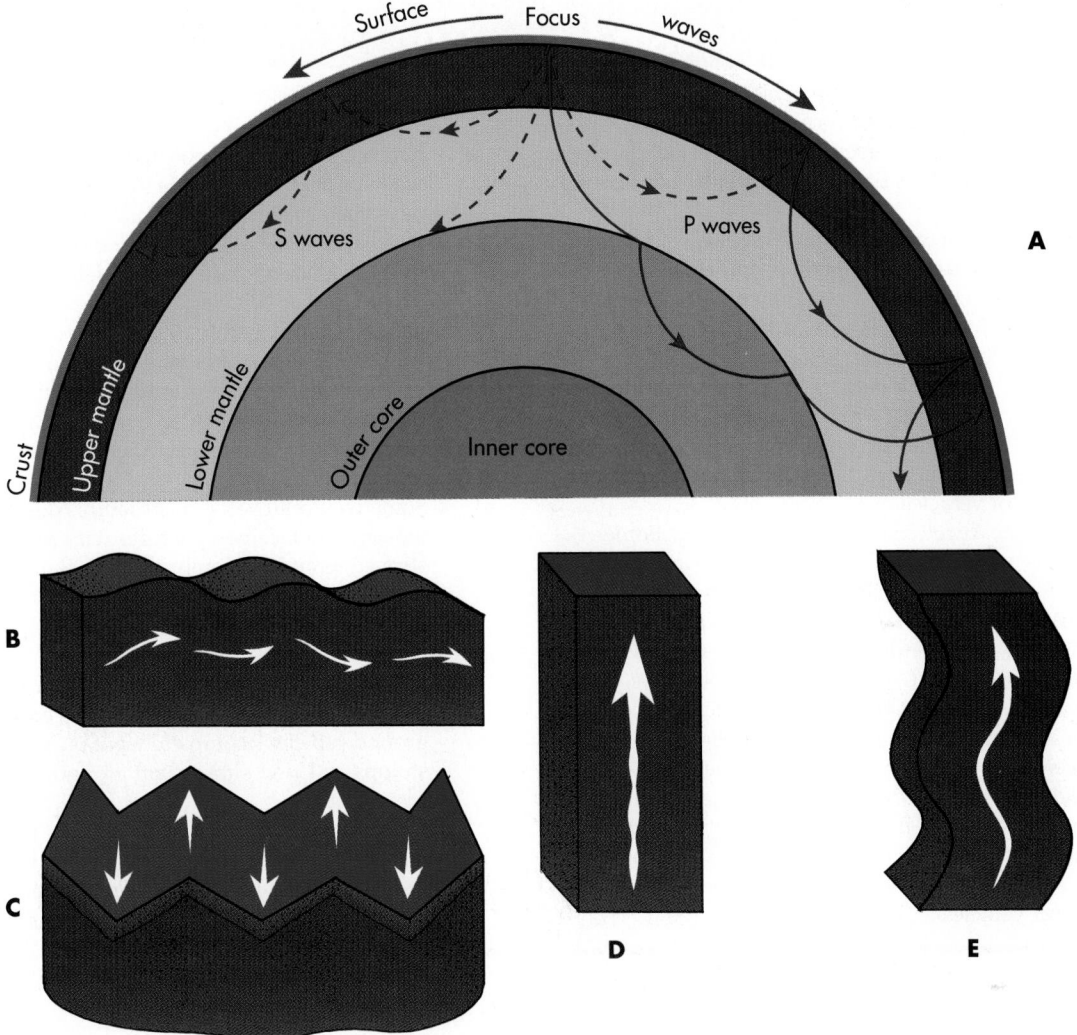

Figure 68-3. A, Propagation of seismic waves in an earthquake. Surface waves vibrate the ground horizontally (**B** and **C**) and vertically (**D** and **E**).

vibrates structures from side to side and usually resulting in the most destruction. *Surface waves,* the third type, vibrate the ground horizontally and vertically and cause swaying of tall buildings, even at great distances from the epicenter.

Earthquake *focus depth* is an important factor in determining the characteristics of the waves. The focal depth can be deep (from 300 to 700 km) or shallow (less than 60 km). Shallow-focus earthquakes are extremely damaging because of their proximity to the surface. The earthquake may be preceded by preliminary tremors and followed by aftershocks of decreasing intensity.

Earthquake Scales

Earthquakes can be described by use of two distinctly different scales of measurement demonstrating magnitude and intensity. Earthquake *magnitude,* or

amount of energy released, is determined by use of a seismograph, which records ground vibrations. The Richter scale mathematically adjusts the readings for the distance of the instrument from the epicenter. The Richter scale is logarithmic; an increase of one magnitude signifies a tenfold increase in ground motion, or about 30 times the energy. Thus an earthquake with a magnitude of 7.5 releases 30 times more energy than one with 6.5 magnitude. The smallest quake to be felt by humans is of magnitude 3. The largest earthquakes that have been recorded under this system are 9.25 (Alaska, 1969) and 9.5 (Chile, 1960).

The earthquake intensity scale measures the effects of the earthquake where it occurs. The most widely used scale of this type is the modified Mercalli scale, which expresses the intensity of earthquake effects on people, structures, and the earth's surface in values

---

Box 68-2 MODIFIED MERCALLI INTENSITY SCALE OF 1931

I Not felt except by very few persons under especially favorable circumstances.

II Felt only by a few persons at rest, especially on upper floors of buildings. Delicately suspended objects may swing.

III Felt quite noticeably indoors, especially on upper floors of buildings, but many people do not recognize it as an earthquake. Standing motor vehicles may rock slightly. Vibration similar to passing of truck. Duration estimated.

IV During the day felt indoors by many but outdoors by few. At night some awakened. Dishes, windows, doors disturbed; walls make creaking sound. Sensation resembles heavy truck striking building. Standing motor vehicles rocked noticeably.

V Felt by nearly everyone; many awakened. Some dishes, windows, etc., broken. A few instances of cracked plaster. Unstable objects overturned. Disturbances of trees, poles, and other tall objects sometimes noticed. Pendulum clocks may stop.

VI Felt by all; many frightened and run outdoors. Some heavy furniture moved; a few instances of fallen plaster or damaged chimneys. Damage slight.

VII Everybody runs outdoors. Damage negligible in buildings of good design and construction, slight to moderate in well-built ordinary structures, considerable in poorly built or badly designed structures. Some chimneys broken. Noticed by persons driving motor vehicles.

VIII Damage slight in specially designed structures, considerable in ordinary substantial buildings with partial collapse, great in poorly built structures. Panel walls thrown out of frame structures. Fall of chimneys, factory stacks, columns, monuments, and walls. Heavy furniture overturned. Sand and mud ejected in small amounts. Changes in well water. Persons driving motor vehicles disturbed.

IX Damage considerable in specially designed structures. Well-designed structures thrown out of plumb, greatly in substantial buildings with partial collapse. Buildings shifted off foundations. Ground cracked conspicuously. Underground pipes broken.

X Some well-built wooden structures destroyed. Most masonry and frame structures with foundations destroyed; ground severely cracked. Rails bent. Landslides considerable from river banks and steep slopes. Shifted sand and mud. Water splashed (slopped) over banks.

XI Few, if any, (masonry) structures remain standing. Bridges destroyed. Broad fissures in ground. Underground pipelines completely out of service. Earth slumps and land slips in soft ground. Rails bent greatly.

XII Damage total. Practically all works of construction are damaged greatly or destroyed. Waves seen on ground surface. Lines of sight and level are distorted. Objects are thrown upward into the air.

---

from I to XII (Box 68-2). Another, more explicit scale used in Europe is the Medvedev-Sponheuer-Karnik (MSK) scale.

Location and Predictability

Most earthquakes (95%) occur in well-defined zones near the boundaries of the tectonic plates. These areas bordering the Pacific Ocean are called the *circum-Pacific belt*. Areas traversing the East Indies, the Himalayas, Iran, Turkey, and the Balkans are called the *Alpide belt*. Earthquakes also occur along the ocean trenches, such as around the Aleutians, Tonga, Japan, and Chile and within the eastern Caribbean. Some earthquakes occur in the middle of the plates, possibly indicating where earlier plate boundaries might have been. These include the New Madrid earthquake in 1811 and the Charleston earthquake in 1816 in the United States, the Agadir earthquake in 1960 in Morocco, and the Koyna earthquake in 1967 in India.

Earthquake prediction was a constant preoccupation for early astrologers and prophets. Some signs noted by observers were buildings gently trembling, animals and birds becoming excited, and well water turning cloudy and smelling bad. Although some modern scientists claim ability to predict earthquakes, the methods are still controversial. For example, the 1995 earthquake in Kobe, Japan, which killed more than 5000, was not predicted. However, mechanical observation systems make it possible to issues warnings to nearby populations immediately after detection of an earthquake. Reasonable risk assessments of potential earthquake activity can be made with confidence based on the following:

1. Knowledge of seismic zones or areas most at risk, gained through study of historical incidence and plate tectonics
2. Monitoring of seismic activity by use of seismographs and other instruments (U.S. Geological Survey monitors 80 countries)
3. Use of community-based, scientifically sound observations, such as elevation and turbidity of water in wells and radon gas escape into well water

Earthquake Hazards

Earthquakes produce many direct and sometimes indirect effects. Landslides, flooding, and tsunamis are considered secondary hazards and are also discussed separately in this chapter.

Fault Displacement and Ground Shaking. Fault displacement, either rapid or gradual, may damage foundations of buildings on or near the fault area or may displace the land, creating troughs and ridges. Ground shaking causes more widespread damage, particularly to the built environment. The extent of the damage is related to the size of the earthquake, the closeness of the focus to the surface, the buffering power of the area's rocks and soil, and the type of buildings being shaken. Aftershocks may cause further damage and may recur for weeks or even years after the initial event.

Ground Failure and Liquefaction. Seismic vibrations may cause settlement beneath buildings when soils consolidate or compact. Certain types of soil, such as alluvial or sandy soils, are more vulnerable to failure. Liquefaction is a type of ground failure that occurs when saturated soils lose strength and collapse or become liquefied. During the 1964 earthquake in Nigata, Japan, the ground beneath earthquake-resistant buildings became liquefied, causing the buildings to lean up to 45 degrees from the vertical. Most of these buildings were later jacked back into an upright position and reoccupied.

Lateral Spreads and Flow Failure. Lateral spreads involve the lateral movement of large blocks of soil as a result of liquefaction in a subsurface layer. Lateral spreads generally develop on gentle slopes with horizontal movement of 10 to 15 feet. However, where conditions are favorable and duration of ground shaking is extended, movements can be 100 to 150 feet. During the 1964 Alaska earthquake, more than 200 bridges were damaged or destroyed by lateral spreading of flood plain deposits toward river channels. In the 1906 San Francisco earthquake, a number of major pipelines were broken by lateral spreading, hampering efforts to fight fires, which caused most of the damage to the city. In 1989 the Marina District in San Francisco, built on soft landfill, was damaged from lateral spreading.

Flow failure, in which either a layer of liquefied soil rides on top of another layer or blocks of intact material ride on top of liquefied soil, can be catastrophic. Flow failures usually form in loose, saturated sands or silts on slopes greater than 3 degrees. They can originate either on land or underwater. Some of the most damaging flow failures have occurred underwater in coastal areas, carrying away large sections of port facilities and generating large sea waves. Some flow failures on land have been as much as a mile in length and breadth, such as those induced by the 1920 earthquake in Kansu, China, which killed 200,000 people.

Landslides and Avalanches. Slope instability may cause landslides and snow avalanches during an earthquake. Steepness, weak soils, and presence of water may contribute to vulnerability from landslides. Liquefaction of soils on slopes may lead to disastrous slides. The most abundant types of earthquake-induced landslides are rock falls and rock slides, usually originating on steep slopes.

Flooding. Tsunamis may be generated by undersea or near-shore earthquakes and may break over the coastline with great destructive force. Other flooding may be caused by seiches (back-and-forth wave action in bays) or by failures in dams and levees.

Typical Adverse Effects

Ground shaking can damage human settlements, buildings and infrastructure (particularly bridges), elevated roads, railways, water towers, water treatment facilities, utility lines, pipelines, electrical generating facilities, and transformer stations. Aftershocks can do great damage to already weakened structures. Significant secondary effects include fires, dam failures, and landslides, which may block waterways and cause flooding. Damage may occur to facilities using or manufacturing dangerous materials, resulting in chemical spills. Communications facilities may break down. Destruction of property may have a serious impact on shelter needs, economic production, and living standards of the affected community. Depending on their level of vulnerability, many people may be homeless in the aftermath of an earthquake.

The casualty rate is often high, especially when earthquakes occur in areas of high population density, particularly when streets between buildings are narrow, buildings are not earthquake resistant, the ground is sloping and unstable, or adobe or dry stone construction is used, with heavy upper floors and roofs.

Casualty rates may be high when quakes occur at night because the preliminary tremors are not felt during sleep and people are not tuned in to receive media warnings. In daytime, people are particularly vulnerable in large unsafe structures such as schools and offices. Casualties generally decrease with distance from the epicenter. As a rule of thumb, quakes result in three times as many injured survivors as persons killed. The proportion of dead may be higher with major landslides and other secondary hazards. In areas where houses are of lightweight construction, especially with wood frames, casualties are generally much fewer, and earthquakes may occur regularly with no serious, direct effects on human populations.

The most widespread medical problems are fracture injuries. Other health threats may occur with secondary flooding, when water supplies are disrupted (earthquakes can change levels in the water table) and contaminated water is used or water shortages exist, and when people are living in high-density relief camps, where epidemics may develop or food shortages exist.

In the aftermath of the Colombia earthquake of January 1999, which most heavily affected Armenia, the death toll was 1185, and 160,000 people were homeless, most in urban areas. About 90,500 homes in the central coffee-growing region had been affected. In Armenia, 60% to 70% of homes had been destroyed, movement was restricted by fallen debris, and unemployment rose from 12% to 35%. People were living in unsatisfactory shelters made with plastic sheeting. Many migrated from the area to other places, which may not be able to absorb them. Although international response to aid Colombia was strong, the overwhelming need continued to pose problems. Five weeks after the earthquake, supplies of food, clean drinking water, and shelter materials were still urgently required. Communities were clamoring for support to inform them of official policies and to organize a response to the temporary shelter problem. Hygiene and sanitation services and essential medicines were badly needed. Social services were required to work toward normalizing the lives of victims, especially children.

TSUNAMIS

Tsunami is a Japanese word meaning "harbor wave." Although tsunamis are sometimes called "tidal waves," they are unrelated to the tides. The waves originate from undersea or coastal seismic activity, landslides, and volcanic eruptions. They ultimately break over land with great destructive power, often affecting distant shores.

Causal Phenomena and Characteristics

The geologic movements that cause a tsunami are produced in three major ways (Figure 68-4). The foremost cause is fault movement on the sea floor, accompanied by an earthquake. The second most common cause is a landslide occurring underwater or originating above the sea and then plunging into the water. The highest tsunamis ever reported were produced by a landslide at Lituya Bay, Alaska, in 1958. A massive rock slide produced a wave that reached a high water mark of 530 m (1740 feet) above the shoreline. A third cause of a tsunami is volcanic activity, which may uplift the flank of the volcano or cause an explosion.

Tsunamis differ from ordinary deep ocean waves, which are produced by wind blowing over water. Normal waves are rarely longer than 300 m (984 feet) from crest to crest. Tsunamis, however, may measure 150 km (90 miles) between successive wave crests. Tsunamis travel much faster than ordinary waves. Compared with normal wave speed of around 100 kilometers per hour (kph), tsunamis in the deep water of the ocean

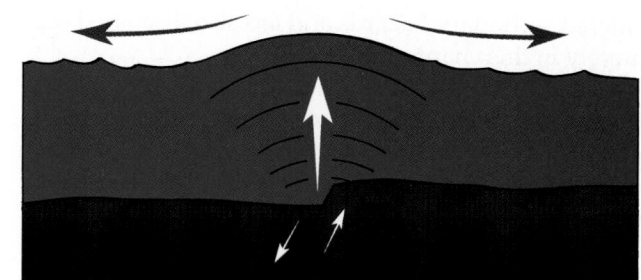
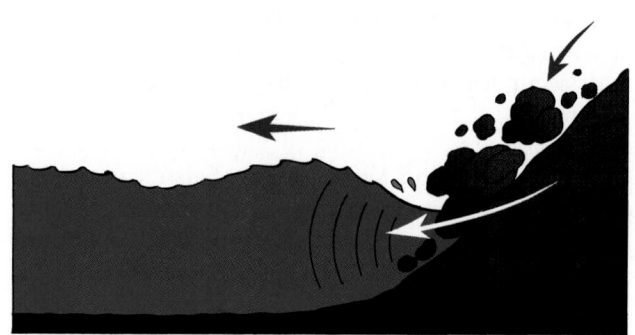
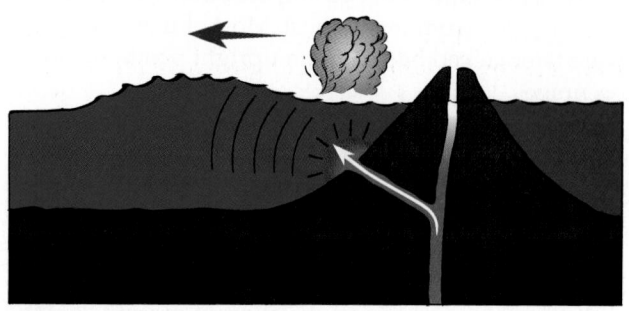

Figure 68-4. Tsunamis are produced in three ways. **A.** Fault movement on the sea floor. **B.** Landslide. **C.** Submarine explosion from volcanic eruption.

may travel at the speed of a jet airplane—800 kph. Despite their speed, tsunamis increase the water height only 30 to 45 cm and often pass unnoticed by ships at sea. In 1946 a ship's captain on a vessel lying offshore near Hilo, Hawaii, claimed he could feel no unusual waves beneath him, although he saw them crashing on the shore.

Contrary to popular belief, the tsunami is not a single giant wave. A tsunami can consist of 10 or more waves, termed a *tsunami wave train*. The waves follow each other in 5- to 90-minute intervals. As tsunamis approach the shore, they travel progressively slower. The final wave speed depends on the water depth. Waves in 18 m (59 feet) of water travel about 50 kph. The shape of the near-shore sea floor influences how tsunami waves will behave. Where the shore drops off quickly into deep water, the waves are smaller. Areas with long shallow shelves, such as the major Hawaiian islands, allow formation of very high waves. In the bays and estuaries, seiches where the water sloshes back and forth can amplify waves to some of the greatest heights ever observed.

On shore, the initial sign of a tsunami depends on what part of the wave first reaches land; a *wave crest* causes a rise in the water level, and a *wave trough* causes a recession. The rise may not be significant enough to be noticed by the general public. Observers are more likely to notice the withdrawal of water, which may leave fish floundering on the sea floor. A tsunami does not always appear as a vertical wall of water, known as a *bore*, as typically portrayed in drawings. More often, the effect is that of an incoming tide that floods the land. Normal waves and swells may ride on top of the tsunami wave, or the tsunami may roll across relatively calm inland waters.

The flooding produced by a tsunami may vary greatly from place to place over a short distance, depending on submarine topography, shape of the shoreline, reflected waves, and modification of waves by seiches and tides. The Hilo tsunami of 1946, originating in the Aleutian Trench, produced 18-m waves in one location and only half that height a few miles away. The sequence of the largest wave in the tsunami wave train also varies, and the destructiveness is not always predictable. In 1960 in Hilo, many people returned to their homes after two waves had passed, only to be swallowed up in a giant bore that in this case was the third wave.

Predictability

Tsunamis have occurred in all oceans and in the Mediterranean Sea, but the great majority of them occur in the Pacific Ocean. The zones stretching from New Zealand through East Asia, the Aleutians, and the western coasts of the Americas all the way to the South Shetland Islands are characterized by deep ocean trenches, explosive volcanic islands, and dynamic mountain ranges.

Since 1900 the effects of tsunamis recorded included casualties and significant damage only locally, and nine struck areas throughout the Pacific. The Tsunami Warning System (TWS) was developed in Hawaii shortly after the 1946 Hilo tsunami and is headquartered in the Pacific Warning Center in Honolulu. It has been improved and expanded and now consists of 62 tide stations, 77 seismic stations, and hundreds of points for dissemination of information. There are 24 member countries in the Pacific basin.

The TWS works by monitoring seismic activity from a network of seismic stations. A tsunami is almost always generated by an undersea earthquake of magnitude 7 or greater. Therefore special warning alarms

sound when a quake measuring 6.5 or over occurs anywhere near the Pacific. A tsunami watch is declared if the epicenter is close enough to the ocean to be of concern. Government and voluntary agencies are then alerted, and local media are activated to broadcast information. The five nearest tide stations monitor their gauges, and trained observers watch the waves. With positive indicators a tsunami warning is issued.

The TWS met with general success in saving lives during the tsunamis of 1952 and 1957 in Hawaii. In 1960, however, two major earthquakes occurring a day apart rocked the coast of Chile in South America. The first registered 7.5 on the Richter scale and produced a small but noticeable wave in Hilo Bay. The second registered a stunning 8.5, more than 30 times the energy of the first, and authorities predicted generation of a large, destructive tsunami. When the waves hit Hilo, 15 hours after the earthquake, not all the public had taken the warnings seriously, and 61 people were killed. About 7 hours later the tsunami struck Japan, killing 180. When information of conditions in Chile reached TWS, three giant waves had destroyed villages along a 500-mile stretch of coastal South America, arriving only 15 minutes after the earthquake.

The Chilean government in recent years has experimented with use of satellite technology to provide nearly immediate warnings of potentially tsunamigenic earthquakes. Project THRUST (Tsunami Hazards Reduction Utilizing Systems Technology) can provide lifesaving tsunami hazard information in an average elapsed time of 2 minutes within its communication radius. In conjunction with this satellite communications network, historical data, model simulations, and emergency operations plans are used.

Vulnerability

The following major factors contribute to vulnerability to tsunamis:

1. Growing world population, increasing urban concentration, and larger investments in infrastructure, particularly on the coastal regions, with some settlements and economic assets on low-lying coastal areas
2. Lack of tsunami-resistant buildings and site planning
3. Lack of a warning system or lack of sufficient education for the public to create awareness of the effects of a tsunami and unpredictable intensity

Having observed relatively moderate tsunamis in 1952 and 1957, citizens at Hilo in 1960 actually converged on the coast to watch the waves come in, with catastrophic results.

Typical Adverse Effects

The force of water in a bore can raze everything in its path with pressures of up to 10,000 kg/m². The flooding from a tsunami, however, affects human settlements most, by water damage to homes and businesses, roads, and infrastructure.

Withdrawal of tsunami waves also causes significant damage. As the waves are dragged back toward the sea, bottom sediments are scoured out, collapsing piers and port facilities and sweeping out foundations of buildings. Entire beaches have disappeared and houses have been carried out to sea. Water levels and currents may change unpredictably, and boats of all sizes may be swamped, sunk, or battered.

Casualties and Public Health. Deaths occur principally from drowning as water inundates homes or neighborhoods. Many people may be washed out to sea or crushed by the giant waves. Some injuries occur from battering by debris. Little evidence exists of tsunami flooding directly causing large-scale health problems. Malaria mosquitoes may increase because of water trapped in pools. Open wells and other groundwater may be contaminated by salt water and debris or sewage. Normal water supplies may be inaccessible for days because of broken water mains.

Crops and Food Supplies. Flooding and damage by tsunami waves may result in the following:
1. The harvest may be lost, depending on time of year.
2. Land may be rendered infertile from saltwater incursion from the sea.
3. Food stocks not moved to high ground are damaged.
4. Animals not moved to high ground may perish.
5. Farm implements may be lost, hindering tillage.
6. Boats and fishing nets may be lost.

In July 1998 an earthquake of magnitude 7 occurred close to the northwest coast of Papua New Guinea. Although the tremor was felt over a large area, no earthquake damage was reported. Only 10 minutes after the quake, however, the first of three 7 to 10 m waves came ashore in Sandaun Province. The tsunamis struck at high speed after dark and penetrated up to 1 km inland, totally destroying villages and vegetation along 50 km of the coast. Of the 9000 people affected, more than 2000 died, mainly from being battered by debris as they were swept away in the wave.

VOLCANIC ERUPTIONS

A volcano is a vent or chimney to the earth's surface from a reservoir of molten rock, called magma, deep in the earth's crust. Approximately 600 volcanoes are active (have erupted in recorded history) in the world today, and many thousands are dormant (could become active again) or extinct (are not expected to erupt again). On average, about 50 volcanoes erupt every year. Since 1000 AD, more than 300,000 people have been killed directly or indirectly by volcanic eruptions, and at present about 10% of the world's population lives on or near potentially dangerous volcanoes.

Volcanology, the study of volcanoes, has experienced a period of intensified interest after five major eruptions in the 1980s and early 1990s: Mt. St. Helens in the United States (1980), El Chichon in Mexico (1982), Galunggung in Indonesia (1982), Nevado del Ruiz in Colombia (1985), and Mt. Pinatubo in the Philippines (1991). Although the Mt. St. Helens eruptions were predicted with remarkable accuracy, predictive capability on a worldwide basis for more explosive eruptions has not been achieved. No recognized immediate precursors to the eruption of El Chichon were known. It caused the worst volcanic disaster in Mexico's history. Ineffective implementation and evacuation measures despite sufficient warnings resulted in more than 22,000 deaths from the eruption of Nevado del Ruiz. Galunggung erupted for 9 months, disrupting the lives of 600,000 people. Despite a major evacuation effort from Mt. Pinatubo, 320 people died, mainly from collapse of ash-covered roofs. A study of these eruptions underscores the importance of predisaster geoscience studies, volcanic hazard assessments, volcano monitoring, contingency planning, and enhanced communications between scientists and authorities. The world's most dangerous volcanoes are in densely populated countries where only limited resources exist to monitor them.

Causal Phenomena

The basic ingredients for a volcanic eruption are magma and an accumulation of gases beneath an active volcanic vent, which may be either on land or below the sea. Magma is composed of silicates containing dissolved gases and sometimes crystallized minerals in a liquidlike suspension. Driven by buoyancy and gas pressure, the magma, which is lighter than surrounding rock, forces its way upward. As it reaches the surface, the pressures decrease, enabling the dissolved gases to effervesce, pushing the magma through the volcanic vent as they are released.

The chemical and physical composition of magma determines the amount of force with which a volcano erupts. Magmas that are less viscous allow gas to be released more easily. More viscous magma, perhaps containing a greater concentration of solid particles, may confine these gases longer, allowing greater pressures to build up. This greater pressure may lead to more violent eruptions.

Types

Volcanic eruptions may be described as follows in descending order of intensity (Figure 68-5).

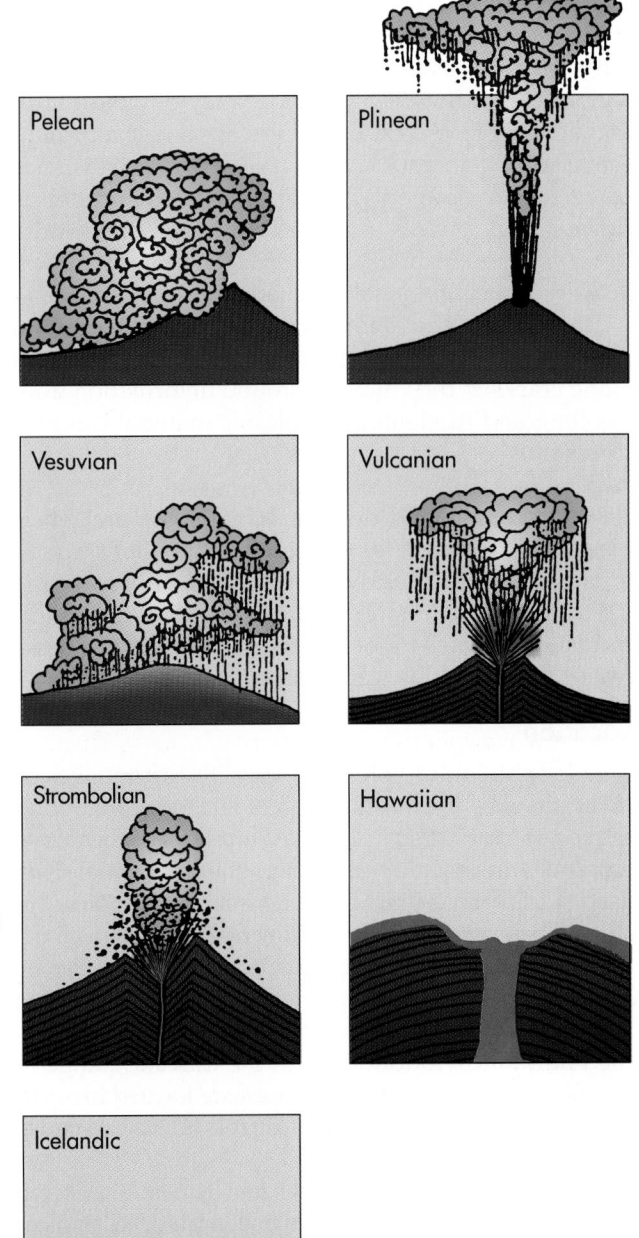

Figure 68-5. Eruption types. **A,** Pelean. **B,** Plinean. **C,** Vesuvian. **D,** Vulcanian. **E,** Strombolian. **F,** Hawaiian. **G,** Icelandic. (*Modified from Introduction to hazards, ed 3, New York, Disaster Management Training Programme, United Nations Development Program, UN Organization for Coordination of Humanitarian Assistance.*)

Pelean. This is the most disastrous type of eruption. The hardened plug at the volcano's throat forces the magma to blast out through a weak spot in the volcanic flank. The great force of the blast devastates most objects in its path, as occurred in the Mt. St. Helen's eruption of 1980.

Plinean. As the pressure on the magma is released, a violent upward expulsion of gas can extend far into the atmosphere. In 1991, Mt. Pinatubo sent a plume of tephra 30 km above the surface.

Vesuvian. As in the eruption of Mt. Vesuvius in Italy in 79 AD, this type is very explosive and occurs infrequently. The explosion of built-up magma discharges a cloud of ash over a wide area.

Vulcanian. Lava forms a crust over the volcanic vents between eruptions, building up the volcano. Subsequent eruptions are more violent and eject dense clouds of material. The Paracutin, Mexico, volcano originated in a cornfield in 1943 and eventually covered 260 square km. A major eruption occurred in 1947.

Stombolian. Gases escape through slow-moving lava in moderate explosions that may be continuous. Volcanic "bombs" of clotted lava may be ejected into the sky, as occurred in the 1965 eruption of Irazu in Costa Rica.

Hawaiian. The lava is mobile and flows freely. Gases are released quietly, as in the Kilauea, Hawaii, volcano, which has continued to erupt since 1983.

Icelandic. Similar to the Hawaiian type, lava flows from deep fissures and forms sheets spreading out in all directions, as in the Laki, Iceland, eruption of 1783.

Characteristics

No international scale exists to measure the size of volcanic eruptions. The volcanic explosivity index (VEI) estimates the energy released in a volcanic eruption, based on measurements of the ejected matter, height of the eruption cloud, and other observations. The VEI scale ranges from 0 to 8. The largest eruption recorded was in Tambora, Indonesia, in 1815, which was a VEI of 7.

The primary volcanic hazards are associated with products of the eruption: pyroclastic flows, air-fall tephra, lava flows, and volcanic gases. The most destructive secondary hazards include lahars, landslides, and tsunamis.

Pyroclastic Flows. Pyroclastic (meaning "fire-broken" in Greek) flows are the most dangerous of all volcanic phenomena because there is virtually no defense against them. They are horizontally directed explosions or blasts of gas containing ash and larger fragments in suspension. They travel at great speed and burn everything in their path. The flows move like a snow or rock avalanche because they contain a heavy load of dust and lava fragments that are denser than the surrounding air. Gas continues to be released as they travel, creating a continuously expanding cloud.

Pyroclastic flows are responsible for the majority of deaths associated with volcanic eruptions. The pyroclastic flows from the Mt. St. Helens eruption in 1980 moved at rates up to 870 kph, and pyroclastic deposits found 2 days after the blast at the foot of the mountain registered temperatures of more than 700° C. The greatest distance recorded by such flows in historical times is 35 km.

Air-Fall Tephra. Tephra smaller than 2 mm is classified as ash. Almost all volcanoes emit ash, but emissions vary widely in volume and intensity. Heavy ashfalls can cause complete darkness or drastically reduce visibility. Fine material from great eruptions may travel around the world and affect world climate. Clouds of dust and ash can remain in the air for days or weeks and spread over large distances, causing difficulty in driving and breathing as well as contributing to building collapse and air traffic disruption. The largest tephra are rocks or blocks, sometimes called "bombs," which have been known to travel more than 4 km. Tephra may be hot enough to start fires when it lands on structures or vegetation.

Lava Flows. Lava flows are formed by hot, molten lava flowing from a volcano and spreading over the surrounding countryside. Depending on the viscosity, a flow may move a few meters per hour. It is usually slow enough that living creatures can move to safety. Sometimes the edges break off, causing small hot avalanches.

Volcanic Gases. Gas is a product of every eruption and may also be emitted by the volcano during periods of inactivity, either intermittently or continually. Volcanic gas is composed mostly of steam, although often present are large amounts of toxic sulfur dioxide, hydrogen sulfide, and smaller but measurable amounts of toxic hydrochloric and hydrofluoric acid gases. Carbon dioxide is often a major component of volcanic gas and is an asphyxiant because it is much denser than air and tends to travel to and through low-lying areas and valleys. Several mountain climbers and skiers in Japan were overcome by hydrogen sulfide fumes in a valley near the Kusatsushirane volcano, and eventually an alarm system was installed. In 1986 about 1800 people were asphyxiated by gas bursts from crater lakes in Cameroon.

Lahars and Landslides. Enormous quantities of ash and larger fragments (tephra) accumulate after an eruption on the steep slopes of a volcano, sometimes to a depth of several meters. When mixed with water, the volcanic debris is transformed into a material resembling wet concrete that flows easily downhill. *Lahar* is an Indonesian word for debris flows or mudflows. A primary debris flow is caused by eruptive activity, such as melting of snow and ice by hot volcanic materials, and a secondary debris flow results when heavy rainfall saturates the deposits.

The rate of flow is affected by the volume of mud and debris, the viscosity, and the slope and character of the terrain. Velocity may reach 100 kph, and distance traveled may exceed 100 km. Mudflows and debris flows can be very destructive. They have buried entire towns, such as Armero, Colombia. They can silt up waterways, causing floods and changing river courses.

Landslides and debris avalanches are common where stress from intruding magma causes fractures along cracks in the volcano. Ground deformation from swelling and hardening of volcanic material can produce landslides.

Tsunamis. Tsunamis, described previously, are generated by movement of the ocean floor, possibly caused by a volcano. In a study of volcanic eruptions in the past 1000 years, human fatalities resulting from indirect tsunami wave hazards were as significant as those from pyroclastic flows and primary mudflows.

Location

The distribution of volcanoes, as with earthquakes, is determined by the location of geologic forces involving the tectonic or crustal plates. About 80% of the active volcanoes are located near subduction boundaries. *Subduction volcanoes* occur where denser crustal plates are shoved beneath less dense continental plates, which occurs in most of the Pacific Ocean, known as the Pacific Ring of Fire. Subduction volcanoes are found in the Aleutian Islands stretching from Alaska to Asia, Japan, the Philippines, Indonesia, and the Cascade Range in the United States. Many volcanoes are located beneath the ocean, and submarine eruptions may cause tsunamis and other effects.

Rift volcanoes occur at divergent zones where two distinct plates are slowly being separated. Rift volcanoes, such as those in Iceland and East Africa, account for about 15% of active volcanoes. *Hot spot volcanoes* are located where crustal weaknesses allow molten material to penetrate, but not necessarily on the plate boundaries. These isolated regions of volcanic activity exist in about 100 places in the world. The Hawaiian islands, in the middle of the Pacific plate, and Yellowstone Park, within the North American plate, are good examples.

Predictability

Systematic surveillance of volcanoes, begun early in the twentieth century at the Hawaiian Volcano Observatory, indicates that most eruptions are preceded by measurable geophysical and geochemical changes. Short-term forecasts of future volcanic activity in hours or months may be made through volcano monitoring techniques that include seismic monitoring, ground deformation studies, and observations and recordings of hydrothermal, geochemical, and geoelectric changes. By carefully monitoring these factors, scientists were able to issue a high confidence forecast of the 1991 Mt. Pinatubo eruption, allowing a largely successful evacuation. The best basis for long-term forecasting (within a year or longer) of a possible eruption is through geologic studies of the past history of each volcano. Each past eruption has left records in the form of lava beds. These are deposits and layers of ash and tephra that can be studied to determine the extent of the flows and length of time between eruptions.

Problems in Eruption Forecasting and Prediction.
Although significant progress has been made in long-term forecasting of volcanic eruptions, monitoring techniques have not progressed to the point of yielding precise predictions. For the purposes of warning the public and avoiding false alarms that create distrust and chaos, ideal predictions should provide precise information concerning the place, time, type, and magnitude of the eruption. The importance of enhanced communications between scientists and authorities is also emphasized. Despite sufficient warning, evacuation orders were not issued by local authorities, which resulted in more than 22,000 deaths from lahars produced by Nevado del Ruiz. The eruption of Mt. St. Helens was adequately monitored and forecasted, but the main explosion surprised authorities because the volcano did not exhibit expected signs before eruption and the blast was lateral rather than vertical; 57 people who remained in the danger area were killed.

The greatest constraint to predictability is lack of baseline monitoring studies, which depict the full range of characteristics of the volcano. Interpretation of baseline data enables differentiation of the precursory pattern of an actual eruption from other volcanic activity, such as intrusion of magma under the surface, which is sometimes termed *aborted eruption*. Before the 1982 eruption of El Chichon, virtually nothing was known of its history of frequent and violent eruptions. No monitoring was conducted before or during the brief eruption.

Developing countries suffer the greatest economic losses from volcanic eruptions. More than 99% of eruption-caused deaths since 1900 have been in developing countries. Because of shortages of funds and trained personnel, monitoring is also poorest in these countries.

Vulnerability
Rich volcanic soils and scenic terrains attract people to settle on the flanks of volcanoes. These people are more vulnerable if they live downwind from the volcano, in the path of historical channels for mudflows or lava flows, or close to waterways likely to flood because of

silting. Structures with roof designs that do not resist ash accumulation are vulnerable even miles from a volcano. All combustible materials are at risk.

Typical Adverse Effects
Casualties and Health. Deaths can be expected from pyroclastic flows and mudflows and to a much lesser extent from lava flows and toxic gases. Injuries may occur from impact of falling rock fragments and from being buried in mud. Burns to the skin, breathing passages, and lungs may result from exposure to steam and hot dust clouds. Ashfall and toxic gases may cause respiratory difficulties for people and animals. Nontoxic gases of densities greater than air, such as carbon dioxide, can be dangerous when they collect in low-lying areas. Water supplies contaminated with ash may contain toxic chemicals and cause illness. Deaths have also occurred indirectly from starvation and from tsunami waves.

Settlements, Infrastructure, and Agriculture. Complete destruction of everything in the path of pyroclastic or lava flows should be expected, including vegetation, agricultural land, human settlements, structures, bridges, roads, and other infrastructure. Structures may collapse under the weight of ash, particularly if the ash is wet. Falling ash may be hot enough to cause fires. Flooding may result from waterways filling up with volcanic deposits or from melting of large amounts of snow or glacial ice. Rivers may change course because of over-silting. Ashfall can destroy mechanical systems by clogging openings such as those in irrigation systems and airplane and other engines. Communication systems could be disrupted by electrical storms developing in the ash clouds. Transportation by air, land, and sea may be affected. Disruption in air traffic from large ash eruptions can have serious effects on emergency response.

Crops in the path of flows are destroyed, and ashfall may render agricultural land temporarily unusable. Heavy ash loads may break the branches of fruit or nut trees. Livestock may inhale toxic gases or ash. Ash containing toxic chemicals, such as fluorine, may contaminate the grazing lands.

The Caribbean island of Montserrat has undergone volcanic activity for years. In June 1997 the famous Soufriere Hills volcano erupted, causing at least nine deaths. The resulting pyroclastic flows buried and destroyed seven villages. Only one third of the island is now considered relatively safe.

LANDSLIDES

Landslides are a major threat each year to human settlements and infrastructure. *Landslide* is a general term covering a wide variety of landforms and processes involving the downslope movement of soil and rock. Although landslides may occur with earthquakes, floods, and volcanoes, they are much more widespread and over time cause more property loss than any other geologic event.

Causal Phenomena

Landslides result from sudden or gradual changes in the composition, structure, hydrology, or vegetation of a slope. These changes may be natural or caused by humans and disturb the equilibrium of the slope's materials. A landslide occurs when the strength of the material in the slope is exceeded by the downslope stress. The resistance in a slope may be reduced by the following:

- Increase in water content, caused by heavy rainfall or rising ground water.
- Increase in slope angle, for new construction or by stream erosion
- Breakdown or alteration of slope materials, from weathering and other natural processes, placement of underground piping for utilities, or use of landfill

The downslope stress may be caused by the following:

- Vibrations from earthquakes (triggering some of the most disastrous landslides), blasting, machinery, traffic, or thunder
- Removal of lateral support by previous slope failure, construction, or excavation
- Removal of vegetation from fires, logging, overgrazing, or deforestation that causes loosening of soil particles and erosion
- Loading with weight from rain, hail, snow, accumulation of loose rock or volcanic material, weight of buildings, or seepage from irrigation and sewage systems

Characteristics

Landslides usually occur as secondary effects of heavy storms, earthquakes, and volcanic eruptions. The materials that compose landslides are divided into two classes: bedrock and soil (earth and organic matter debris). A landslide may be classified by its type of movement (Figure 68-6).

Falls. A fall is a mass of rock or other material that moves downward by falling or bouncing through the air. These are most common along steep road or railroad embankments, steep escarpments, or steeply undercut cliffs, especially in coastal areas. Large individual boulders can cause significant damage.

Slides. Resulting from shear failure (slippage) along one or several surfaces, the slide material may remain intact or break up.

Topple. A topple is caused by overturning forces that rotate a rock out of its original position. The rock sec-

tion may have settled at a precarious angle, balancing itself on a pivotal point from which it tilts or rotates forward. A topple may not involve much movement, and it does not necessarily trigger a rockfall or rock slide.

Lateral Spread. Large blocks of soil spread out horizontally by fracturing off the original base. Lateral spreads occur generally on gentle slopes, usually less than 6%, and typically spread 3 to 5 m but may move from 30 to 50 m where conditions are favorable. Lateral spreads usually break up internally and form numerous fissures and scarps. The process can be caused by liquefaction, in which saturated loose sands or silts assume a liquefied state. A lateral spread is usually triggered by ground shaking (as with an earthquake). During the 1964 Alaskan earthquake, more than 200 bridges were damaged or destroyed by lateral spreading of floodplain deposits near river channels.

Flows. Flows move as a viscous fluid, sometimes very rapidly, and can cover several miles. Water is not essential for flows to occur; however, most flows form after periods of heavy rainfall. A mudflow contains at least 50% sand, silt, and clay particles. A lahar is a mudflow that originates on the slope of a volcano and may be triggered by rainfall, sudden melting of snow or glaciers, or water flowing from crater lakes. A debris flow is a slurry of soils, rocks, and organic matter combined with air and water. Debris flows usually occur on steep gullies. Very slow, almost imperceptible flows of soil and bedrock are called *creeps*. Over long periods, creeps may cause telephone poles or other objects to tilt downhill.

Predictability

The velocity of landslides varies from extremely slow (less than 0.06 m/year) to extremely fast (greater than 3 m/sec), which might imply a similar variation in predictability. In absolute terms, however, predicting the actual occurrence of a landslide is extremely difficult, although situations of high risk, such as forecasted heavy rainfall or seismic activity combined with landslide susceptibility, may lead to estimation of a time frame and possible consequences.

Estimation of landslide hazard potential includes historical information on the geology, geomorphology (study of landforms), hydrology, and vegetation of a specific area. Structural features that may affect stability include sequence and type of layering, lithologic changes, planes, joints, faults, and folds. The most important geomorphologic consideration in the prediction of landslides is the history of landslides in a given area.

The source, movement, amount of water, and water pressure must be studied. Climatic patterns combined with soil type may cause different types of landslides. For example, when monsoons occur in tropical regions, large

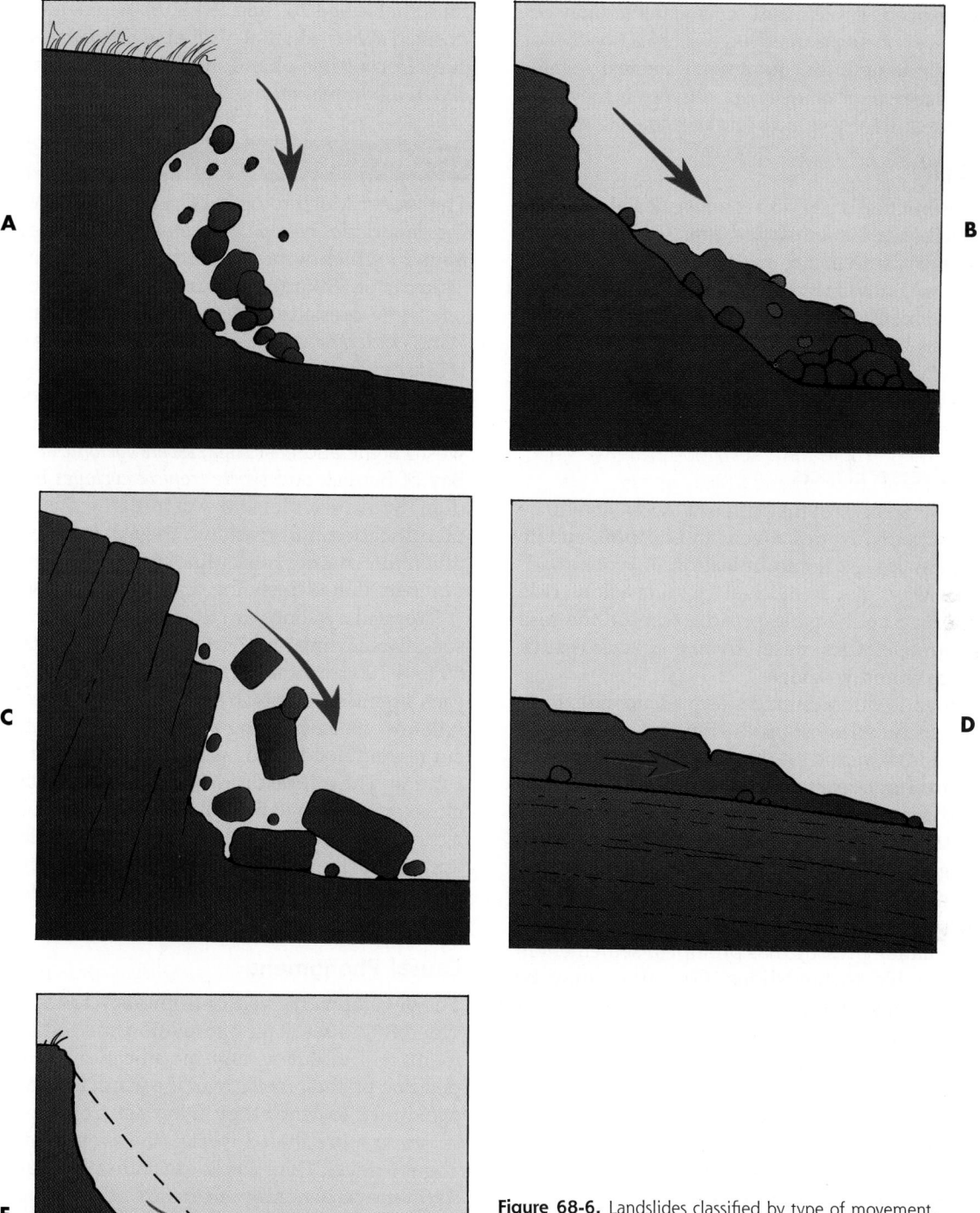

Figure 68-6. Landslides classified by type of movement. **A,** Fall. **B,** Slide. **C,** Topple. **D,** Lateral spread. **E,** Flow.

debris slides of soils, rocks, and organic matter may occur. Plant cover on slopes may have either a positive or negative stabilizing effect. Roots may decrease water runoff and increase soil cohesion, or conversely they may widen fractures in rock surfaces and promote infiltration.

Vulnerability

Settlements built on steep slopes, in weak soils, on cliff tops, at the base of steep slopes, on alluvial outwash fans, or at the mouth of streams emerging from mountain valleys are all vulnerable. Roads and communication lines through mountainous areas are in danger. In most types of landslides, damage may occur to buildings even if foundations have been strengthened. Infrastructural elements, such as buried utility lines or brittle pipes, are vulnerable.

Typical Adverse Effects

Anything on top of or in the path of a landslide will be severely damaged or destroyed. In addition, rubble may damage lines of communication or block roadways. Waterways may be blocked, creating a flood risk. Casualties may not be widespread, except in the case of massive movements caused by major hazards such as earthquakes and volcanoes.

In addition to direct damage from a landslide, indirect effects include loss of productivity of agricultural or forest lands (if buried), reduced real estate values in high-risk areas and lost tax revenues from these devaluations, adverse effects on water quality in streams and irrigation facilities, and secondary physical effects, such as flooding.

Casualties. Fatalities have resulted from slope failure where population pressure has prompted settlement in areas vulnerable to landslides. Casualties may be caused by collapse of buildings or burial by landslide debris. Worldwide, approximately 600 deaths occur per year, mainly in the circum-Pacific region. The estimate for loss of life in the United States is 25 lives per year, greater than the average loss from earthquakes. Catastrophic landslides have killed many thousands of persons, such as the debris slide on the slopes of Huascaran in Peru triggered by an earthquake in 1970, which killed more than 18,000 people. In January 1989, only 6 weeks after an earthquake killed 25,000 people in Armenia, another quake struck the republic of Tadjikistan, 50 km southwest of the capital city of Dushanbe. This quake registered 5.8 on the Richter scale. The earthquake triggered a landslide of hillside soils that had become wet with melted snow. The liquefied soil spilled downhill and eventually covered an area about 8 km long and 1 km wide. The total volume of mud was more than 10 million m^3. The epicenter of the earthquake was located in the village of Sharora. This village and several others were engulfed with mud that killed 200 and left 30,000 homeless. Mud deposits reached a height of 25 m in Sharora, causing rescue efforts to be abandoned. Later the area was declared a national monument.

TROPICAL CYCLONES

The World Meteorological Organization (WMO) uses the generic term *tropical cyclone* to cover weather systems in which winds exceed *gale force* (minimum of 34 knots or 63 kph). Tropical cyclones are rotating, intense low-pressure systems of tropical oceanic origin. Winds of *hurricane force* (63 knots or 117 kph) mark the most severe type of tropical storm. They are called *hurricanes* in the Caribbean, the United States, Central America, and parts of the Pacific; *typhoons* in the northwest Pacific and east Asia; *severe cyclonic storms* in the Bay of Bengal; and *severe tropical cyclones* in south Indian, South Pacific, and Australian waters. For easy identification and tracking, the storms are generally given alternating masculine and feminine names or numbers that identify the year and annual sequence.

Tropical cyclones are the most devastating of seasonally recurring rapid-onset natural hazards. Between 80 and 100 tropical cyclones occur around the world each year. Devastation by violent winds, torrential rainfall, and accompanying phenomena, including storm surges and floods, can lead to massive community disruption. The official death toll in individual tropical cyclones reached 140,000 (Bangladesh, 1991), and damages approached $10 billion in Hurricane Gilbert (1988) and Hurricane Hugo (1989). The damages from Hurricane Andrew in Florida and Louisiana in 1992 totaled $16 billion.

Causal Phenomena

The development cycle of tropical cyclones may be divided into three stages: formation and initial development, full maturity, and modification or decay. Depending on their tracks over the warm tropical seas and proximity to land, they may last from less than 24 hours to more than 3 weeks (the average duration is about 6 days). Their tracks are naturally erratic but initially move generally westward, then progressively poleward into higher latitudes, where they may make landfall, or into an easterly direction as they lose their cyclonic structure.

Formation and Initial Development Stage. Four atmospheric and oceanic conditions are necessary for development of a cyclonic storm (Figure 68-7), as follows:

1. A warm sea temperature (greater than 26° C [78.8° F] to a depth of 60 m [197 feet]) provides abundant water vapor in the air by evaporation.
2. High relative humidity (degree to which the air is saturated by water vapor) of the atmosphere to a

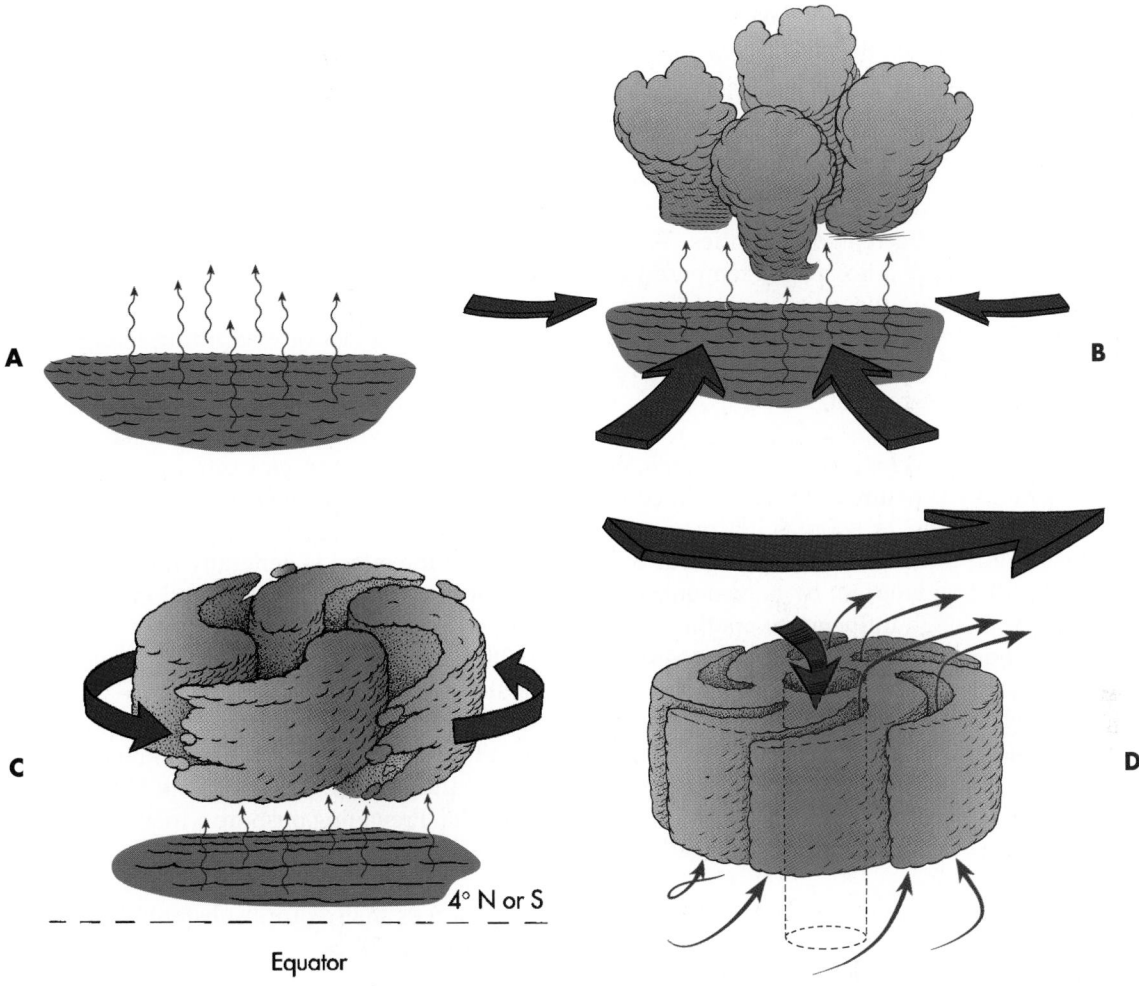

Figure 68-7. Cyclone formation. **A,** Warm seas (greater than 26° C [78.8° F]) cause rising humid air. **B,** Cooler high-altitude temperatures cause formation of cumulonimbus clouds. The surrounding air moves toward the central low-pressure area. **C,** Cumulonimbus clouds form into spiraling bands. The Coriolis effect causes winds to swirl around the central low-pressure area. **D,** High altitude dispels the top of the cyclonic air system. Dry high-altitude air flows down the "eye." Hurricane force winds circle around the eye.

height of about 7000 m (23,000 feet) facilitates condensation of water vapor into water droplets and clouds, releases heat energy, and induces a drop in barometric pressure.

3. Atmospheric instability (an above-average decrease of temperature with altitude) encourages considerable vertical cumulus cloud convection when condensation of rising air occurs.

4. A location of at least 4 to 5 latitude degrees from the equator allows the influence of the forces as the earth's rotation (Coriolis force) takes effect and induces cyclonic wind circulation around a low-pressure center.

The atmosphere can usually organize itself into a tropical cyclone in 2 to 4 days. This process is characterized by increasing thunderstorms and rain squalls at sea. Meteorologists can monitor these processes with weather satellites and radar from as far as 400 miles

away from the storm. The existence of favorable conditions for cyclone development determines the cyclone season for each monitoring center. In the Indian and south Asian region the season is divided into two periods, from April to early June and from October to early December. In the Caribbean and United States, tropical storms and hurricanes reach their peak strengths in middle to late summer. In the Southern Hemisphere, the cyclone season extends from November to April or May, but occasionally cyclones occur in other months in lower latitudes.

Maturity Stage. As viewed by weather satellites and radar imagery, the main physical feature of a mature tropical cyclone is a spiral pattern of highly turbulent, giant cumulus thundercloud bands. These bands spiral inward and form a dense, highly active central cloud core that wraps around a relatively calm and cloud-free "eye." The eye, where light winds occur, typically has a diameter of 20 to 60 km and appears as a black hole or dot surrounded by white clouds.

In contrast to the light wind conditions in the eye, the turbulent cloud formations extending outward from the eye accompany winds of up to 250 kph, sufficient to destroy or severely damage most nonengineered structures in the affected communities. These strong winds are caused by a horizontal temperature gradient that exists between the warm core of the cyclone (up to 10° C higher than the external environment) and the surrounding areas, resulting in a correspondingly high-pressure gradient.

Decay Stage. A tropical cyclone begins to weaken, in terms of its central low pressure, internal warm core, and extremely high winds, as soon as its sources of warm moist air begin to ebb or are abruptly cut off. This would occur during landfall, by movement into higher latitudes, or through influence of another low-pressure system. The weakening of a cyclone does not mean that danger to life and property is over. When the cyclone hits land, especially over mountainous or hilly terrain, widespread riverine and flash flooding may last for weeks. The energy from a weakening tropical cyclone may be reorganized into a less concentrated but more extensive storm system causing widespread violent weather.

Characteristics

Tropical cyclones are characterized by their destructive winds, storm surges, and exceptional level of rainfall, which may cause flooding.

Destructive Winds. The strong winds generated by a tropical cyclone circulate clockwise in the Southern Hemisphere and counterclockwise in the Northern Hemisphere, while spiraling inward and increasing toward the cyclone center. Wind speeds progressively increase toward the core as follows:

1. 150 to 300 km from the center of a typical mature cyclone, winds of 63 to 88 kph
2. 100 to 150 km from the center, storm force winds of 89 to 117 kph
3. 50 to 100 km from the center, winds in excess of hurricane force, 117 kph or greater
4. 20 to 50 km from the center, the edge of the inner core containing winds 250 kph or greater

As the eye arrives, winds fall off to become almost calm, but they rise again just as quickly as the eye passes and are replaced by hurricane force winds from a direction nearly the reverse of those previously blowing.

The Beaufort scale is used to classify the intensity of the storms. It estimates the wind velocity by observations of the effects of winds on the ocean surface and familiar objects. Both the United States (Saffir-Simpson Potential

Hurricane Damage Scale) (Box 68-3) and Australia (Cyclone Severity Categories) use country-specific scales that estimate potential property damage in five categories. The Philippines recently increased its typhoon warning signal numbers from three ranges of wind speeds to four in order to take into account the lower standards of building structures and regional variations.

Storm Surges. The storm surge, defined as the rise in sea level above the normally predicted astronomic tide, is frequently a key or overriding factor in a tropical storm disaster. As the cyclone approaches the coast, the friction of strong onshore winds on the sea surface, in combination with the "suction effect" of reduced atmospheric pressure, can pile up sea water along a coastline near a cyclone's landfall well above the predicted tide level for that time. In cyclones of moderate intensity the effect is generally limited to several meters, but exceptionally intense cyclones can cause storm surges up to 8 m.

Of the countries experiencing cyclonic storms, those most vulnerable to storm surges are those with low-lying land along the closed and semi-enclosed bays facing the ocean. These countries include Bangladesh, China, India, Japan, Mexico, the United States, and Australia. Prevailing onshore winds and low pressures from winter depressions in nontropical latitudes, as in countries bordering the North Sea, are also subject to storm surges that require substantial mitigation measures, such as dikes.

Rainfall Events. The world's highest rainfall totals over 1 to 2 days have occurred during tropical cyclones. The highest 12- and 24-hour totals, 135 cm and 188 cm, respectively, have both occurred during cyclones at La Reunion Island in the southwestern Indian Ocean. The very high specific humidity condenses into exceptionally large raindrops and giant cumulus clouds, resulting in high precipitation rates. When a cyclone makes landfall, the rain rapidly saturates even dry catchment areas, and rapid runoff may explosively flood the usual water courses as it creates new ones.

The relationship between rainfall and wind speed is not always proportional. For instance, if the atmosphere over land is already saturated with moisture, rainfall will be strongly enhanced, and the cyclone will weaken slowly. If the atmosphere is dry, the rainfall will be greatly reduced, and the cyclone will decay faster. Thus landfall of even a relatively weak tropical cyclone may result in extensive flooding.

Predictability

Tropical cyclones form in all oceans of the world except the South Atlantic and South Pacific east of 140° W longitude. Nearly one quarter form between 5° and 10° latitude of the equator and two thirds between 10° and

Box 68-3   SAFFIR-SIMPSON POTENTIAL HURRICANE DAMAGE SCALE

SCALE NO. 1

Winds of 74 to 95 mph. Damage primarily to shrubbery, trees, foliage, and unanchored mobile homes. No real damage to other structures. Some damage to poorly constructed signs. And/or storm surge 4 to 5 feet above normal. Low-lying coastal roads inundated, minor pier damage, some small craft in exposed anchorage torn from moorings.

SCALE NO. 2

Winds of 96 to 110 mph. Considerable damage to shrubbery and tree foliage; some trees blown down. Major damage to exposed mobile homes. Extensive damage to poorly constructed signs. Some damage to roofing materials of buildings; some window and door damage. No major damage to buildings. And/or storm surge 6 to 8 feet above normal. Coastal roads and low-lying escape routes inland cut by rising water 2 to 4 hours before arrival of hurricane center. Considerable damage to piers. Marinas flooded. Small craft in unprotected anchorages torn from moorings. Evacuation of some shoreline residences and low-lying island areas required.

SCALE NO. 3

Winds of 111 to 130 mph. Foliage torn from trees; large trees blown down. Practically all poorly constructed signs blown down. Some damage to roofing materials of buildings; some window and door damage. Some structural damage to small buildings. Mobile homes destroyed. And/or storm surge of 9 to 12 feet above normal. Serious flooding at coast and many smaller structures near coast destroyed; larger structures near coast damaged by battering waves and floating debris. Low-lying escape routes inland cut by rising water 3 to 5 hours before hurricane center arrives. Flat terrain

5 feet or less above sea level flooded inland 8 miles or more. Evacuation of low-lying residences within several blocks of shoreline possibly required.

SCALE NO. 4

Winds of 131 to 155 mph. Shrubs and trees blown down; all signs down. Extensive damage to roofing materials, windows, and doors. Complete failure of roofs on many small residences. Complete destruction of mobile homes. And/or storm surge 13 to 18 feet above normal. Flat terrain 10 feet or less above sea level flooded inland as far as 6 miles. Major damage to lower floors of structures near shore due to flooding and battering by waves and floating debris. Low-lying escape routes inland cut by rising water 3 to 5 hours before hurricane center arrives. Major erosion of beaches. Massive evacuation of all residences within 500 yards of shore possibly required, and of single-story residences on low ground within 2 miles of shore.

SCALE NO. 5

Winds greater than 155 mph. Shrubs and trees blown down; considerable damage to roofs of buildings; all signs down. Very severe and extensive damage to windows and doors. Complete failure of roofs on many residences and industrial buildings. Extensive shattering of glass in windows and doors. Some complete building failures. Small buildings overturned or blown away. Complete destruction of mobile homes. And/or storm surge greater than 18 feet above normal. Major damage to lower floors of all structures less than 15 feet above sea level within 500 yards of shore. Low-lying escape routes inland cut by rising water 3 to 5 hours before hurricane center arrives. Massive evacuation of all residential areas on low ground within 5 to 10 miles of shore possibly required.

From National Oceanic and Atmospheric Administration: *Tropical cyclones of the North Atlantic Ocean, 1871-1977*, Asheville, NC, 1978, National Climatic Center.

20° latitude. It is rare for a tropical cyclone to form south of 20° to 22° latitude in the Southern Hemisphere; however, they occasionally form as far north as 30° to 32° in the more extensive warmer water of the Northern Hemisphere. They are mainly confined to the warmer 6 months of the year but have occurred in every month in the western North Pacific.

The locations, frequencies, and intensities of tropical cyclones are well known from historical observations and, more recently, from routine satellite monitoring. Tropical cyclones do not follow the same track except coincidentally over short distances. Some follow linear paths, others recurve in a symmetric manner, and still others accelerate or slow down and seem stationary for a time. For this reason, predicting when, where, and if a storm will hit land is often difficult, especially with islands. In general, the difficulty in forecasting in-

creases from lower to higher latitudes, whereas the margin of error in determining the cyclone center decreases as landfall approaches.

Special warning and preparedness strategies for evacuation from offshore facilities or closure of industrial plants must relate the costs and benefits of those strategies against the uncertainties of precision in the forecasts. For general community purposes that require a minimum 12 hours of preparedness time, the imprecision in forecasting the location of landfall within 24 hours should be generally tolerable, bearing in mind that highly adverse cyclonic weather usually commences about 6 hours before landfall of the cyclone.

Regrettably, progress in reducing forecasting errors has remained slow in the last two decades despite huge investments in monitoring systems. However, substantial progress has been made in the organization of warning and dissemination systems, particularly through regional cooperation. The activities of national meteorologic services are coordinated at the international level by the WMO. Forecasts and warnings are prepared within the framework of the WMO's World Weather Watch (WWW) program. Under this program, meteorologic observational data are provided nationally, and data from satellites and information provided by the regional centers are exchanged around the world. The WWW system includes 8500 land stations, 5500 merchant ships, aircraft, special ocean weather ships, automatic weather stations, and meteorologic satellites. A tropical cyclone is first identified and then followed from satellite pictures. A global telecommunications system relays the observations.

Ultimately, however, national services are responsible for providing forecasts and warnings to the local population regarding tropical cyclones and the associated winds, rains, and storm surges. Unfortunately, many of the less developed countries, where most deaths from tropical cyclones occur, do not possess state-of-the-art warning systems.

Vulnerability

Human settlements located in exposed, low-lying coastal areas are vulnerable to the direct effects of a cyclone, such as wind, rain, and storm surges. Settlements in adjacent areas are vulnerable to floods, mud slides, or landslides from the resultant heavy rains. The death rate is higher where communications systems are poor and warning systems are inadequate.

The quality of structures determines resistance to the effects of the cyclone. Those most vulnerable are lightweight structures with wood frames, older buildings with weakened walls, and houses made of unreinforced concrete block (Figure 68-8). Infrastructural elements particularly at risk are telephone and telegraph poles, fishing boats, and other maritime industries. Hospitals may be damaged, reducing access to health care and essential drugs.

Typical Adverse Effects

Structures are damaged and destroyed by wind force, through collapse from pressure differentials, and by flooding, storm surge, and landslides. Severe damage can occur to overhead power lines, bridges, embankments, nonweatherproofed buildings, and roofs of most structures. Falling trees, wind-driven rain, and flying debris cause considerable damage.

Casualties and Public Health. Relatively few fatalities occur because of the high winds in cyclonic storms, but many people may be injured and require hospitalization. Storm surges may cause many deaths but usually few injuries among survivors. Because of flooding and possible contamination of water supplies, malaria or-

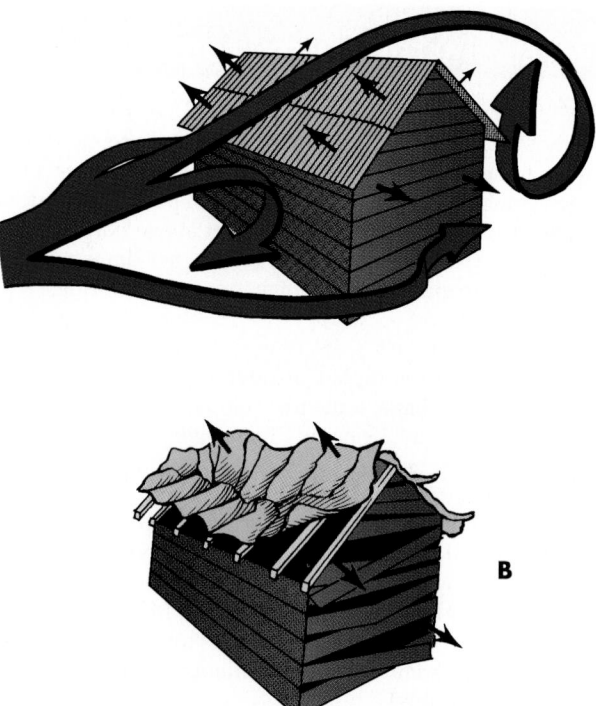

Figure 68-8. How high winds damage buildings. **A,** Wind blowing into a building is slowed at the windward face, creating high pressure. The airflow separates as it spills around the building, creating low pressure or suction at the end walls, roof, and leeward walls. **B,** The roof may lift off and the walls blow out if the structure is not specially reinforced. *(Courtesy Disaster Management Center, University of Wisconsin.)*

ganisms and viruses may be prevalent several weeks after the flooding.

Water Supplies. Open wells and other groundwater supplies may be temporarily contaminated by flood waters and storm surges. They are considered contaminated by pathogenic organisms only if dead people or animals are lying in the sources or if sewage is present. Normal water sources may be unavailable for several days.

Crops and Food Supplies. The combination of high winds and heavy rains, even without flooding, can ruin standing crops and tree plantations. Food stocks may be lost or contaminated if the structures in which they were held have been destroyed or inundated. Salt from storm surges may also be deposited on agricultural lands and increase groundwater salinity. Fruit, nut, and lumber trees may be damaged or destroyed by winds, flood, and storm surges. Plantation-type crops, such as bananas, are extremely vulnerable. Erosion can occur from flooding and storm surges. Food shortages may occur until the next harvest. Tree and food crops may be blown down or damaged and must be harvested prematurely.

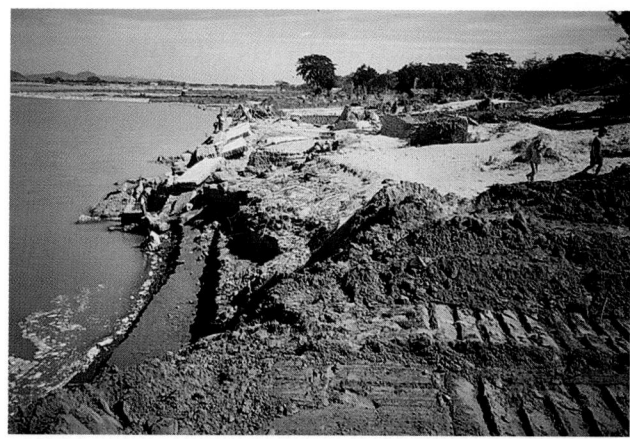

Figure 68-9. Aftermath of Hurricane Mitch in Honduras in 1998. *(Courtesy Paul Thompson, InterWorks.)*

Communications and Logistics. Communications may be severely disrupted as telephone lines, radio antennas, and satellite dishes are brought down, usually by wind. Roads and railroad lines may be blocked by fallen trees or debris, and aircraft movements may be curtailed for at least 12 to 24 hours after the storm. Modes of transportation, such as trucks, carts, and small boats, may be damaged by wind or flooding. The cumulative effect of all damage is to impede information gathering and transport networks.

Preparedness Measures in India

Tropical cyclones twice struck the same coastal areas of the Indian state of Andhra Pradesh. In 1978 10,000 people perished. In 1990, despite significant increases in population, fewer than 1000 died. A program of improved monitoring and warning dissemination had been developed by the Indian government. This included use of a domestic satellite, an upgraded cyclone contingency preparedness plan, and enhanced community awareness. Widespread evacuation procedures were initiated by the state counterdisaster committee 48 hours ahead of forecasted landfall. A total of 651,865 people were evacuated from 546 villages to 1098 emergency relief camps by 2019 evacuation teams using 745 transport vehicles. People had also been instructed by the media to go to the camps before the commencement of the cyclonic weather.

1998's Deadly Hurricane Season

The 1998 Atlantic hurricane season, from June 1 to Nov. 30, was one of the deadliest in 200 years, killing more than 10,000 people in eight countries and causing billions of dollars in damage. Fourteen named storms, four more than average, formed in the Atlantic Ocean, Caribbean Sea, and the Gulf of Mexico. Of these, 10 became hurricanes. Hurricane Bonnie hit the North Carolina coast and prompted disaster declarations in three

states. Hurricane Georges followed a path across the U.S. Virgin Islands, Puerto Rico, the Dominican Republic, Haiti, and Cuba, killing more than 500 and causing $5 billion in damages. Hurricane Mitch moved across Central America, killing an estimated 10,000 in Honduras and wiping out the country's infrastructure (Figure 68-9). Mitch regenerated as a tropical storm and then passed over southern Florida.

TORNADOES

Tornadoes are the most dramatic example of a class of storms, often called *severe local storms,* which includes thunderstorms and hailstorms. Severe local storms a few miles to a few tens of miles in diameter are often accompanied by unusually strong, gusty winds that can cause severe damage, by heavy local rain that can cause flash floods, and by lightning, hail, and sometimes tornadoes. These intense vortices may be only a few hundred feet in diameter but can contain winds in excess of 300 mph, capable of tearing roofs off houses and lifting houses, trees, and vehicles hundreds of feet through the air. Tornadoes have been known to occur in swarms, with as many as several dozen affecting an area of hundreds of thousands of square miles in a single day. A new 1-day record was set in the United States on Jan. 21, 1999, when 38 tornadoes were hatched in Arkansas, surpassing the previous record of 20 statewide.

Causal Phenomena

Tornadoes and other severe local storms result from intense, local atmospheric instability, usually caused by solar heating of the earth's surface, which causes intense convective columns. A tornado is a vortex in which air spirals inward and upward. It is frequently, but not always, visible as a funnel cloud hanging part or all of the way from the generating storm to the ground. The upper portion of the funnel consists of water droplets, and the lower portion usually consists of dust and soil being sucked up from the ground. The funnel size may range from a few meters to a few hundred meters in diameter and from 10 m to several kilometers high. The funnel may undergo changes in appearance during the tornado's lifetime. There may be a single well-defined funnel, multiple funnels, or funnels that appear to consist of several ropelike strands. Tornadoes may be as loud as the roar of a freight train.

Tornadoes are the most violent event associated with thunderstorms. They occur in many parts of the world but are most frequent and fierce in the United States. As many as 1000 may strike the United States each year, mostly in the central plains and southeastern states, although they have occurred in every state, mostly in the spring and summer. Of all the natural hazards in the United States, thunderstorms with associated winds, rain, hail, lightning, and tornadoes rank first in number of deaths, second in number of injuries, and third in property damage.

The most common type of tornado is small and lasts only a minute or two, causing minor damage over a track often less than 300 feet wide and 1 to 2 miles long. Most tornado-related deaths, injuries, and property damage are caused by relatively infrequent, large, and long-lasting tornadoes with paths more than 1 mile wide and more than 100 miles long over several hours.

Predictability

Although conditions favorable to tornado formation can often be predicted a number of hours in advance, the areas in which these conditions are found may cover hundreds of thousands of square miles. It is impossible to predict where individual tornadoes will occur. When a warning is issued, a tornado has already formed and the threatened population may have only a few minutes to take cover. In the United States, when tornadoes are considered likely within a well-defined region, a tornado watch is issued. When a tornado is actually detected, either visually or on radar, a tornado warning is issued.

Vulnerability

Most injuries from tornadoes are caused by flying or falling debris, usually from destroyed structures. The quality of structures will determine resistance to the effects of the cyclone. Those most vulnerable are light-weight structures with wood frames, older buildings with weakened walls, mobile homes, and houses made of unreinforced concrete blocks. Thorough education regarding taking shelter from flying debris is essential to reduce deaths and injuries.

Examples of Tornado Outbreaks

In March 1925 a tornado struck Missouri, Illinois, and Indiana, killing 689 people. On April 11, 1965, an outbreak of at least 37 tornadoes struck Iowa, Wisconsin, Illinois, Indiana, Michigan, and Ohio, killing 271 people, injuring more than 3000, and causing $300 million in damage. On April 3 and 4, 1974, an outbreak of 147 tornadoes struck Illinois, Indiana, Michigan, Ohio, West Virginia, Virginia, Kentucky, Tennessee, North Carolina, South Carolina, Georgia, and Alabama, killing 335 people, injuring more than 5500, affecting more than 27,000 households, and causing more than $600 million in damage. More than half the deaths were caused by less than 5% of the tornadoes. The worst of these struck Xenia, Ohio. It cut a swath of destruction half a mile wide and 16 miles long, killed 34 people, injured 1150, and damaged or destroyed 2400 homes. On May 31, 1985, 43 tornadoes struck Ohio, Pennsylvania, New York, and southern Ontario, killing 87 people. The 1999 tornado damage season began early with multiple tornadoes in Arkansas in January. In early May, tornadoes hit Oklahoma and Kansas, killing 43, the largest number in more than a decade.

FLOODS

Throughout history, people have been attracted to the fertile lands of the floodplains, where their lives have been made easier by virtue of proximity to sources of food and water. Ironically, the same river or stream that provides sustenance to the surrounding population also renders humans vulnerable to disaster by periodic flooding. Flooding occurs when surface water covers land that is normally dry or when water overflows normal confinements. The most widespread of any hazard, floods can arise from abnormally heavy precipitation, dam failures, rapid snow melts, river blockages, or even burst water mains. However, floods can provide benefits without creating disaster and are necessary to maintain most river ecosystems. They replenish soil fertility, provide water for crop irrigation and fisheries, and contribute seasonal water supplies to support life in arid lands.

Every year in Bangladesh, large tracts of land are submerged during the monsoon season, a normally beneficial process that deposits a rich layer of alluvial soil. The floods originate from three great river systems in the Himalayan mountains: the Ganges, the Brahmaputra, and the Meghna. In summer 1988 the rivers reached their highest levels in history, and 60% of the land was flooded. At least 1500 people died in the floods, and 49 million were affected by crop loss and damaged homes.

In the aftermath of the flooding, cases of diarrheal diseases reached epidemic proportions, with 50,000 cases reported daily. The risk of other diseases, such as hepatitis, typhoid fever, and measles, was elevated because of contaminated water supplies. Destruction of almost 4 million hectares of crops and partial damage to 3 million hectares left a shortfall in annual grain requirements of 1 million tons and placed the population at risk of famine. In the flood of 1974 in Bangladesh, affecting 50% of the land, 27,500 persons perished from subsequent disease and starvation. Fortunately, timely arrival of food aid in 1988 averted a famine crisis.

Causal Phenomena

The most important cause of floods is excessive rainfall. Rain may be seasonal occurring over wide areas, or may form localized storms that produce the highest intensity rainfall. Some storms are attributed to atmospheric and oceanic processes such as the El Niño Southern Oscillation (ENSO) or strong jet streams. Melting snow is another major contributor.

Types

Flash. These are usually defined as floods that occur within 6 hours of the beginning of heavy rainfall. This type of flooding requires rapid localized warnings and immediate response by affected communities if damage is to be mitigated. Flash floods are normally a result of runoff from a torrential downpour, particularly if the catchment slope is unable to absorb and hold a significant part of the water. Other causes of flash floods include dam failure or sudden breakup of ice jams or other river obstructions. Flash floods are potential threats particularly where the terrain is steep, surface runoff is high, water flows through narrow canyons, and severe rainstorms are likely.

River. River floods are usually caused by precipitation over large catchment areas, by melting of the winter accumulation of snow, or sometimes by both. The floods take place in river systems with tributaries that may drain large geographic areas and encompass many independent river basins. In contrast to flash floods, river floods normally build up slowly, are often seasonal, and may continue for days or weeks. Factors governing the amount of flooding include ground conditions (the amount of moisture in the soil, vegetation cover, depth of snow, cover by impervious urban surfaces such as concrete) and size of the catchment basin (Figure 68-10).

Coastal. Some flooding is associated with tropical cyclones (also called hurricanes and typhoons). Catastrophic flooding from rainwater is often aggravated by wind-induced storm surges along the coast. Salt water may flood the land by one or a combination of effects from high tides, storm surges, or tsunamis. As in river floods, intense rain falling over a large geographic area will produce extreme flooding in coastal river basins.

Contribution by Humans

Floods are naturally occurring hazards but can become disasters when they affect human settlements. The

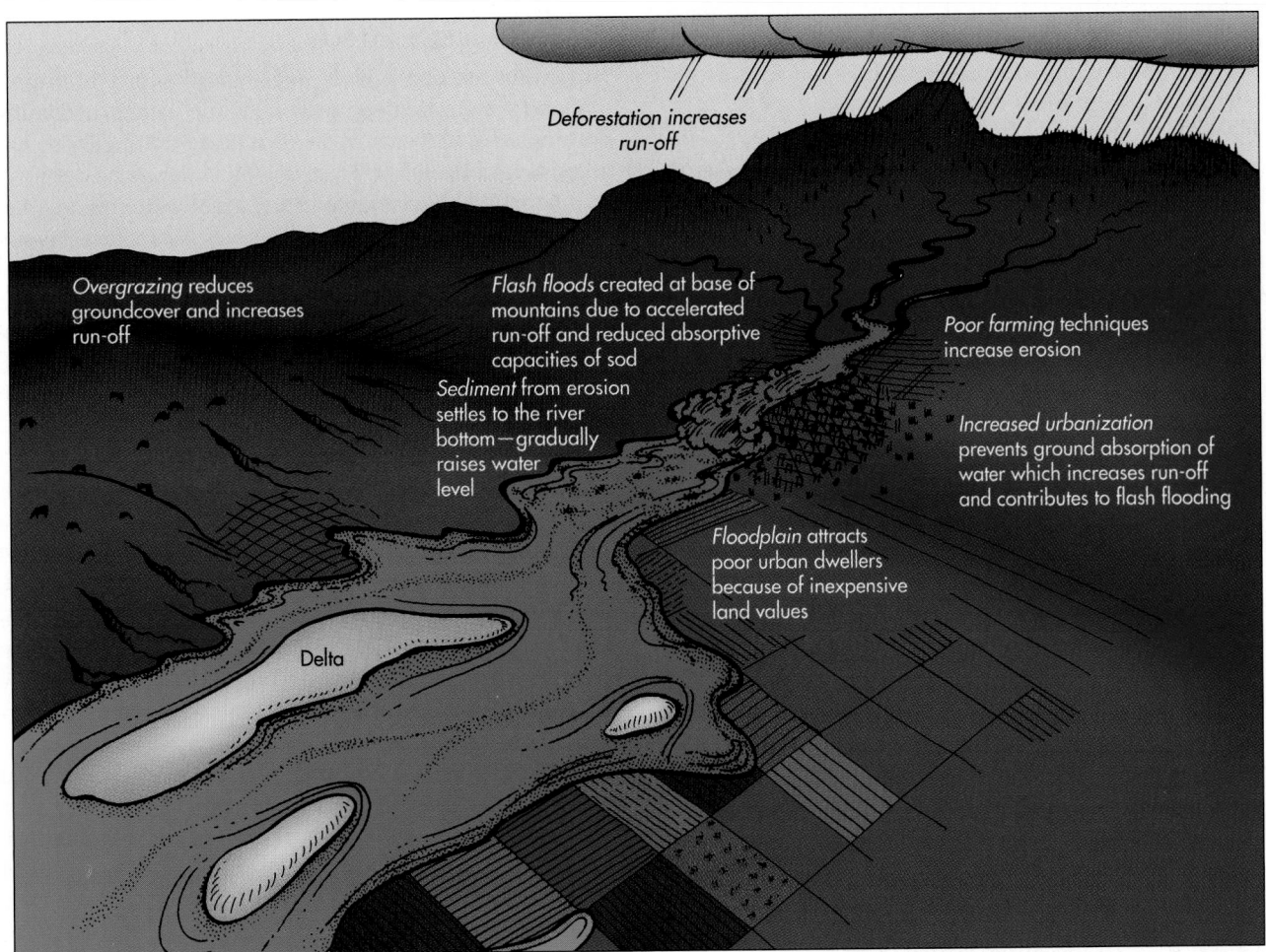

Figure 68-10. Flooding and its causes. *(Courtesy Disaster Management Center, University of Wisconsin.)*

magnitude and frequency of flooding often increase because of human actions. Settlement on floodplains contributes to flooding disasters by endangering humans and their assets. However, the economic benefits of living on the floodplain outweigh the dangers for some societies. Population pressure is now so great that people have accepted the risk associated with floods because of the greater need for a place to live. In the United States, billions of dollars have been spent on flood protection programs since 1936. Despite this, the annual flood hazard has become greater because people have built on floodplains faster than engineers can design better flood protection.

Urbanization contributes to urban flooding. Roads and buildings prevent infiltration of water, so runoff forms artificial streams. The network of drains in urban areas may deliver water and fill natural channels more rapidly than natural drainage routes, or drains may be insufficient and overflow. Natural or artificial channels may become constricted by debris or obstructed by river facilities, impeding drainage and overflowing the catchment areas. Failure to maintain or manage drainage systems, dams, and levees in vulnerable areas also contributes to flooding.

Deforestation and removal of root systems increase runoff. Subsequent erosion causes sedimentation in river channels, which decreases their capacity.

Predictability

Riverine flood forecasting estimates river level stage, discharge, time of occurrence, and duration of flooding, especially of peak discharge at specific points along river systems. Flooding resulting from precipitation, snow melt in the catchment system, or upstream flooding is predictable from 12 hours to as much as several weeks ahead. Forecasts issued to the public result from regular monitoring of the river heights and rainfall observations. Flash flood warnings, however, depend solely on meteorologic forecasts and knowledge of local geographic conditions. The very short lead time for the development of flash floods does not permit useful monitoring of actual river levels for warning purposes.

For comparison with previous flood events and conversion to warning information, assessment of the following elements should be included: flood frequency analysis, topographic mapping and height contouring around river systems with estimates of water-holding capacity of the catchment area, precipitation and snow melt records, soil filtration capacity, and (if in a coastal area) tidal records, storm frequency, topography, coastal geography, and breakwater characteristics.

An effective means of monitoring floodplains is through remote sensing techniques. The images produced by satellites can be interpreted to map flooded and flood-prone areas. Other efforts to improve forecasting are being implemented by United Nations or-

ganizations, such as the WMO, using WWW and the Global Data Processing System. These systems are strategic when flood conditions exist across international boundaries. The great majority of river and flash flood forecasts, however, depend on observations made by national weather services for activation of flood alert warnings.

Vulnerability

At notable risk in floodplain settlements are buildings made of earth or with soluble mortar, buildings with shallow foundations, or buildings that are nonresistant to water force and inundation. Infrastructural elements at particular risk include utilities such as sewer systems, power and water supplies, and machinery and electronics belonging to industry and communications. Of great concern are food stocks and standing crops, confined livestock, irreplaceable cultural artifacts, and fishing boats and other maritime industries.

Other factors affecting vulnerability are lack of adequate refuge sites above flood levels and accessible routes for reaching those sites. Also, lack of public information about escape routes and other appropriate response activities renders communities more vulnerable.

Typical Adverse Effects

Structures are damaged by receiving the force of impact of flood waters, floating away on rising waters, becoming inundated, collapsing because of undercutting by scouring or erosion, and being struck by waterborne debris.

Damage is likely to be much greater in valleys than in open, low-lying areas. Flash floods often sweep away everything in their path. In coastal areas, storm surges are destructive both on inward travel and on outward return to the sea. Mud, oil, and other pollutants carried by water are deposited and ruin crops and building contents. Saturation of soils may cause landslides or ground failure.

Casualties and Public Health. Currents of moving or turbulent water can knock down and drown people and animals in relatively shallow depths. Major floods may result in large numbers of deaths from drowning, particularly among young and weak persons, but generally inflict few serious but nonfatal injuries requiring hospital treatment. Slow flooding causes relatively few direct deaths or injuries but often increases the occurrence of snakebites.

Endemic disease will continue in flooded areas, but little evidence exists of floods directly causing any large-scale additional health problems besides diarrhea, malaria, and other viral outbreaks 8 to 10 weeks after the flood.

Water, Crops, and Food Supplies. Open wells and other groundwater supplies may be contaminated temporarily by debris carried by flood waters or by salt water brought in by storm surges. They are contaminated by pathogenic organisms, however, only if bodies of people or animals are caught in the sources or if sewage is present. Normal sources of water may not be available for several days.

An entire harvest may be lost along with animal fodder, resulting in long-term food shortages. Food stocks may be lost by submersion of crop storage facilities, resulting in immediate food shortages. Grains quickly spoil if saturated with water, even for a short time. Most agricultural losses result from the inundation of crops or stagnation by standing water, as in the 1988 Bangladesh flood.

Large numbers of animals, including draught animals, may be lost if they are not moved to safety. This may reduce the availability of milk and other animal products and services, such as preparation of the land for planting. These losses, in addition to possible loss of farm implements and seed stocks, may hinder future planting efforts.

Floods bring mixed results in terms of their effects on the soil. In some cases, land may be rendered infertile for several years after a flood because of erosion of the topsoil or salt permeation, as in the case of a coastal flood. Heavy silting may have adverse effects or may significantly increase fertility of the soil.

In coastal areas, where fish provide a source of protein, boats and fishing equipment may be lost or damaged.

On the positive side, floods may flush out pollutants in the waterways. Other positive effects include preserving wetlands, recharging groundwater, and maintaining the river ecosystems by providing breeding, nesting, and feeding areas for fish, birds, and wildlife.

DROUGHT

Of all natural disasters, droughts potentially have the greatest economic impact and affect the greatest number of people. They invariably have a direct and significant impact on food production and the overall economy. Due to the slow onset of droughts, their effects may accumulate over time and linger for many years. Their impact may be less obvious than that of other natural hazards but may be spread over a wider geographic area. Because of the pervasive effects of droughts, assessing their impact and planning assistance become more difficult than with other natural hazards.

No universal definition exists for drought. In general, drought is a temporary reduction in water or moisture availability that is significantly below the normal or expected amount for a specified period. Because droughts occur in nearly all regions of the world and have varying characteristics, however, working definitions must be regionally specific and focus on the impacts, which result from discrepancies between the supply and demand for water.

Droughts are most often associated with low rainfall and semiarid climate. However, they also occur in areas with normally abundant rainfall. Humans tend to stabilize their activities around the expected moisture environment. Thus, after many years with above-average rainfall, people may perceive the first year of average rainfall as a drought. A rainfall level that meets the needs of a pastoralist may constitute a serious drought for a farmer growing corn. To define drought in a region, it is necessary to understand both the meteorologic characteristics and the human perception of drought.

Types

Meteorologic. Meteorologic drought results from a shortfall in precipitation and is based on the degree of dryness relative to the normal or average amount and on the duration of the dry period. This comparison must be region specific and may be measured against daily, monthly, seasonal, or annual rainfall amounts.

Hydrologic. Hydrologic drought involves a reduction of water resources, such as streams, groundwater, lakes, and reservoirs. It involves data on availability and offtake rates in relation to the normal operations of the system (domestic, industrial, irrigated agricultural) being supplied. One impact is competition between users for water in these storage systems.

Agricultural. Agricultural drought is the impact of meteorologic and hydrologic droughts on crops and livestock production. It occurs when soil moisture is insufficient to maintain average plant growth and yields. The impact of agricultural drought is difficult to measure because of the complexity of plant growth and the possible presence of other factors that may reduce yields, such as pests, weeds, low soil fertility, and low crop prices. *Famine drought* can be regarded as an extreme form of agricultural drought in which food shortages are so severe that large numbers of people become unhealthy or die. However, famine disasters usually have complex causes, such as political conflict. Although scarcity of food is the main factor in a famine, death can result from other complicating influences, such as disease or lack of access to water and other services.

Socioeconomic. Socioeconomic drought correlates the supply and demand of goods and services with the three other types of drought and emphasizes the relationship between drought and human activities. When the supply of some goods or services, such as water, hay, or electric power, is weather dependent, drought may cause shortages.

Causal Phenomena

The reasons for lack of rain are not well understood. Displacement of the normal path of the jet stream may steer rain-bearing storms elsewhere. Recent research has focused on *teleconnection,* or linkages to global interactions, between the atmosphere and the oceans. Sea surface temperature anomalies (SSTAs) influence heat and moisture, such that warm surface water may create air conditions favorable for a cyclone formation. A large-scale SSTA is linked to ENSO events in the Pacific. These involve the periodic (every 2 to 7 years) invasion of warm surface waters into the normally colder waters off the coast of South America. Droughts of 1982-1983 in Africa, Australia, India, Brazil, and the United States coincided with a major El Niño.

Human causes of drought that include land use practices that give rise to desertification, such as deforestation, overcultivation, overgrazing, and mismanagement of irrigation, are thought to result in greater persistence of drought. Traditional drought coping systems in Africa, such as pastoralists' use of seasonal grazing lands and farmers' use of fallow periods, have been reduced because of population pressures and economic policies (see Desertification).

Droughts vary in terms of intensity, duration, and coverage. Droughts tend to be more severe in drier areas of the world because of low mean annual rainfall and longer duration of dry periods. In dry areas, drought builds up slowly over several years of poor rainfall. Dry conditions in the African Sahel over a 16-year period led to widespread famine in 1984-1985. The quarter century of drought conditions in the Sahel was interrupted by heavy rains in 1994. The area affected by drought in a country has important implications for food security. Larger countries, such as India and Brazil, are rarely completely affected by drought, but smaller countries may be totally affected (Figure 68-11). Worldwide food availability may be adversely affected by drought in grain-exporting nations.

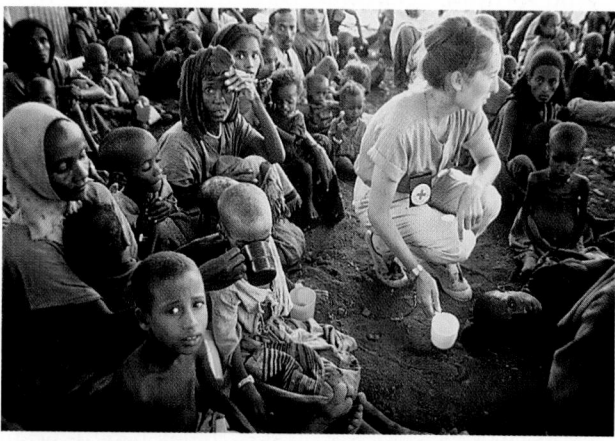

Figure 68-11. Victims of drought in Ethiopia. *(Courtesy United Nations.)*

Predictability

Modern meteorologic monitoring and telecommunications systems can prevent casualties from drought-induced food shortages. The slow onset of drought allows a warning time between the first indications, usually several months, and when the population will be affected. In 1987, satellite imagery and rainfall reports indicated areas within Ethiopia with below-normal moisture and allowed timely intervention to avert a major food shortage. Longer-term prediction requires analysis of a century of rainfall data, which do not exist for some parts of the world.

Satellite Data. Satellite remote sensing is a powerful tool for detecting the characteristics of drought from a distance. In addition to the unique vantage point and condensed view, remote sensing provides a permanent and historical record. The National Oceanic and Atmospheric Administration (NOAA) satellites use the Advanced Very High Resolution Radiometer (AVHRR) to provide twice-daily coverage of the planet's surface. These data are available at many receiving stations around the world. NOAA has developed crop-monitoring technology for large areas of the Sahel. The Normalized Difference Vegetation Index (NDVI) use the satellite data to indicate areas of stressed vegetation, which can help predict food shortages when combined with local weather data and crop information.

Vulnerability

Although drought is more likely in dry areas with limited rainfall, physical factors such as the moisture retention of soil and timing of rains influence the degree of crop loss. Dependency on rain-fed agriculture increases vulnerability. Farmers unable to adapt with repeated plantings may experience crop failure. Livestock-dependent populations without adequate grazing territory are also at risk. Those dependent on stored water resources or irrigation are more vulnerable to water shortages and may face competition for water.

Drought-related effects are more severe in countries with yearly food deficiencies and in largely subsistence-level farming and pastoralist systems. Food shortages have the greatest impact where malnutrition already exists. Most food shortage–related deaths occur in the semiarid countries of sub-Saharan Africa, whereas in more developed countries the consequences are largely economic. Adverse effects may be more serious where drought response has not been adequately planned and where assistance measures may be poorly targeted or ineffective.

Typical Adverse Effects

The effects of drought can be grouped as economic, environmental, and social. Economic effects include losses in crops, dairy and livestock, timber and fisheries, national economic growth, and income for farmers and others. Decreased tourism, loss of hydroelectric power and increased energy costs, increased food prices, unemployment, and losses of revenue to governments are other economic effects. Environmental losses include damage to animals, fish, and plant species and habitat; wind and water erosion of soils; reduced water quality or altered salination; and reduced air quality from dust and pollutants. Social effects include food shortage (malnutrition, famine), loss of human life, conflict between water users, health problems from decreased water flow, decline in living conditions, increased poverty, social unrest, and population migration for employment.

WINTER STORMS

Winter storms feature strong winds, extreme cold, ice storms, and heavy snowstorms. These are often deceptive killers because most deaths are indirectly related to the storm, such as from traffic accidents and hypothermia. In the United States, for deaths related to ice and snow, about 70% occur in automobiles, and 25% are people caught out in a storm. The majority are males over 40 years old. For deaths related to cold, 50% are people over 60 years old, more than 75% are males, and about 20% occur in the home.

When temperatures are below freezing, everyone is at potential risk from winter storms. In areas of the world where roads are rarely maintained to mountainous areas, such as in Lebanon, Iraq, and Russia, local populations cope by storing provisions for the winter months. In more heavily populated areas, individual and societal precautions must be taken to avoid the effects of winter storms. The cost of cleaning up after winter storms and loss of business during the storm can have significant economic impact.

Causal Phenomena

Cold air and below-freezing temperatures in the clouds and near the ground are necessary to make snow and ice. Moisture is needed to form clouds and precipitation. The source of moisture may be air blowing across a body of water, such as a large lake or the ocean. *Lift*, or the required force needed to raise the moist air to form the clouds and cause precipitation, can occur when warm air collides with cold air and is forced to rise over the cold dome. The boundary between the warm and cold air is called a *front*. Lift might also occur from air flowing up a mountainside.

Strong Winds.

Strong winds that sometimes accompany winter storms can create blizzard conditions with blinding wind-driven snow, severe drifting, and dangerous windchill factor. Strong winds with these intense storms and cold fronts can knock down trees, util-

ity poles, and power lines. Storms near the coast can cause coastal flooding and beach erosion, as well as sink ships at sea. Winds descending from mountains can gust to 100 mph or more, damaging roofs and other structures.

The windchill factor is based on the rate of heat loss from exposed skin caused by combined effects of wind and cold. As the wind increases, heat is carried away from the body at an accelerated rate, driving down the body temperature. Animals are also affected by windchill.

Extreme Cold. Extreme cold often accompanies a winter storm or is left in the aftermath. What constitutes extreme cold varies in different areas. For example, in areas unaccustomed to winter weather, cold may be extreme only at the freezing mark. Freezing temperatures can cause severe damage to citrus fruit crops and other vegetation.

Prolonged exposure to cold can cause frostbite (damage to body tissue caused by tissue being frozen) or hypothermia (low body temperature) (see Chapters 6 and 7). Infants and elders are most susceptible.

Ice Storms. Even a small amount of ice poses a significant hazard to motorists and pedestrians. Accumulations of ice can bring down trees, electrical wires, telephone poles and lines, and communication towers. Communication and power can be disrupted for days while utility companies work to repair extensive damage.

Snowstorms. Snow may fall as flurries, showers, squalls, blowing snow, or blizzards, where winds over 35 mph and blowing snow reduce visibility. Sleet (raindrops that freeze into ice pellets before reaching the ground) can accumulate and cause problems. Heavy snow can immobilize a region and paralyze a city. Travelers can be stranded and emergency services disrupted. In rural areas, homes and farms may be cut off for days, and livestock may die if unprotected. The probability of avalanches increases in the mountains.

Predictability

Although winter storm patterns are known in most areas of the world, predicting the intensity and characteristics of winter storms is not an exact science. The effects of El Niño on the winter storm patterns of 1998 are still being debated. Typical U.S. storm patterns include the "Nor'easter," which affects the mid-Atlantic coast to New England from low-pressure areas off the Carolina coast. Research is continuously underway to improve forecasting tools and techniques. For example, the Stormscale Research and Application Division of the National Severe Storms Laboratory at the University of Oklahoma provides feedback for the National Weather Service, NASA, and the Department of Defense.

The capacities of most national weather services allow individuals and public services to prepare for winter storms. Winter storm watches and warnings and winter weather advisories are normally issued in most vulnerable areas.

Vulnerability

Lack of a preparedness plan by individuals and communities or lack of understanding of the effects of winter storms, increases vulnerability. Failure to heed warnings lack of communication facilities to receive warnings, and insufficient preparation to cope with the cold or possible isolation from heavy snow can lead to casualties. For example, a person stranded in a vehicle or home during a winter storm without a storm survival kit or with inadequate heat or food and water may become hypothermic or dehydrated. Lack of protection for infrastructure, utilities, and houses can result in damage, loss of service, and roof collapse from heavy snow. Downed trees may cause later forest fires. Motorists unaccustomed to driving in winter storms cause more accidents. People living in uninsulated or unheated buildings are at greater risk for hypothermia.

The 1998 Ice Storm

A storm of unprecedented impact began on January 5, 1998, and ultimately damaged about 18 million acres of rural and urban forests throughout Maine, New Hampshire, Vermont, upstate New York, and southeastern Canada. The storm severely impacted the dairy industry, maple sugar industry, small businesses, public facilities, and infrastructure. Power outages lasted for up to 23 days. Thousands of people required shelter for an extended period, and nine people died in the United States.

The causal factors of the storm were a combination of natural and human made. Population and urbanization had recently increased in the area. Cold surface temperatures were overrun by a warm moist tropical air mass, resulting in record rainfall of 2 to 6 inches. Below-freezing temperatures caused the rain to freeze on contact, producing ice accumulations of more than 3 to 4 inches. These factors were intensified by the long duration and significant scope of the storm, resulting in severe flooding and ice damage. Much of the damage could not be assessed until the spring thaw. As a result of the storm, the Federal Emergency Management Agency (FEMA) reviewed the mitigation measures in place and made new recommendations.

ENVIRONMENTAL POLLUTION

The world population is expected to be 8.3 billion by 2050, increasing by 86 million people annually. Despite the pressures placed on natural resources by the expanding population, many poor countries still desperately need the benefits accompanying industrialization and economic growth. In general, people in developing countries are much more vulnerable to the effects of environmental degradation because they are poorer and depend more directly on the land.

Causal Phenomena

Various parts of the environment are subjected to the effects of toxic (poisonous) chemicals produced in manufacturing, such as paint and metal production, and the burning of fossil fuels, such as gasoline, coal, and oil. Some of these chemicals are heavy metals, such as lead, which are essentially nondegradable. Other toxic compounds, such as pesticides, are purposely introduced into the environment. Toxic chemicals may accumulate and affect the quality of air and water. Other pollutants of importance are from biologic sources, such as human wastes, soil sediments, and decaying organic matter.

Air Pollution. Much of the world's urban population breathes polluted air at least part of the time. Sulfur dioxide, a major pollutant, is a corrosive gas harmful to humans and the environment. Electricity generation using fossil fuels is the key source of this compound in industrialized countries. In developed countries the burning of fossil fuels also contributes. Other air pollutants include nitrogen oxides, carbon dioxide (CO_2), and lead, mainly from vehicle exhaust.

Marine Pollution. Sewage is the major cause of ocean pollution. Raw sewage containing human excreta and domestic wastes is disposed of in large quantities directly into the ocean. In the summer of 1993, thousands of ocean beaches were closed in the United States because of high levels of pathogens from human and animal wastes. Industrial effluents are also piped into the ocean. Other pollutants include marine litter, oil spills, and dumped chemical compounds, such as those containing mercury and radioactive substances.

Freshwater Pollution. Human waste and other domestic wastewaters are often discharged directly into nearby bodies of water, particularly in urban areas. In developing countries this waste may be completely untreated. Industrial effluents from papermaking, chemical, metalworking, textile, and food-processing industries reach bodies of water by direct discharge or by leaching from dumps.

Clearing the land for agriculture and using irrigation, fertilizers, and pesticides have seriously affected water quality in many countries. Unprecedented deforestation has led to soil erosion, causing accelerated runoff and sediment deposits in riverbeds. The sediment level in rivers may increase 100-fold in deforested areas during rainy seasons.

Runoff of nitrogen from fertilizers, particularly in industrialized nations, renders some water unfit to drink without treatment. Use of irrigation systems may lead to increased salinity of water sources and saltwater intrusion on coastal areas where water is withdrawn. Approximately 25% of the world's pesticide production is used in developing countries, mainly on cash crops. Accumulations of pesticide toxins are found in food, soil, and water. Although data on Africa are lacking, studies in Asia indicate that rivers and lakes in Indonesia and Malaysia have very high levels of polychlorinated biphenyls (PCBs) and some pesticides.

Ozone Depletion

Ozone is a form of oxygen composed of three atoms of oxygen. Most atmospheric ozone is concentrated in the upper atmosphere, or stratosphere. The ozonosphere, or the ozone layer, is 11 to 24 km above the earth. Ozone screens out harmful wavelengths of ultraviolet radiation (UV-B) that originate from the sun, protecting life on Earth (see Chapter 14). Ultraviolet light is associated with increased non-melanoma skin cancer, ocular cataracts, and deterioration of the retina and cornea. In addition, oceanic phytoplankton are reduced, with damage to fish larvae and young fish. Since fish provide 14% of the animal protein consumed worldwide (60% of that in Japan), the impact could be significant. Thinning of the ozone layer is caused by chlorofluorocarbons (CFCs), chemicals used in refrigeration, foam products, and aerosol propellants. The CFCs that damage the ozone layer may also contribute to global warming. Although they compose a fraction of greenhouse gases, they account for 20% of the warming trend caused by radioactive trapping potential (10,000 times greater than that of CO_2).

Global Warming

Global temperatures appear to be higher today than they have been since 1862, when temperatures were first recorded by instrumentation. The last 15 years include the six hottest temperatures ever recorded. One explanation for this increase is perhaps a global warming caused by the greenhouse effect.

The term *greenhouse effect* is used to describe the role of atmospheric gases, such as CO_2, methane, and water vapor, in trapping radiation that would otherwise leave the atmosphere. Without this canopy of gases and clouds, the temperature of the earth would be extremely cold. The atmospheric gases therefore behave similarly to a greenhouse.

Since the beginning of the Industrial Revolution in the late eighteenth century, CO_2 in the atmosphere has increased by almost 25%, mainly from combustion of coal, oil, natural gas, and gasoline. A strong scientific consensus states that buildup of greenhouse gases is warming the global atmosphere. Computer models used to examine the climatic effects of increasing CO_2 suggest that if it doubles, global temperatures would increase on average by 3° to 5° C.

Trees play a vital role in recycling CO_2 by taking it in, transforming it chemically, storing the carbon, and releasing oxygen into the air. When trees are cut down, left to decay, or burned, they release stored carbon to the air as CO_2. Recently in Central Africa, virgin rainforests were found to have air pollution levels comparable to those in industrial areas. A major cause of this pollution is the fires that rage for months across huge stretches of land to clear shrubs and trees for the production of crops and grasses. Deforestation has been estimated to account for 20% of total atmospheric content of CO_2. The effects of acid rain (pollutants that are held in the clouds and fall back to Earth in rainwater) and air pollution in Europe, Canada, and the United States also contribute to the increase of CO_2.

Another greenhouse gas is methane. *Methane* is generated by bacteria as they break down organic matter. It is emitted largely by landfills, cattle, and fermenting rice paddies. The concentration of methane gas in the atmosphere has doubled in the past 200 years, mainly because of expanded animal husbandry and rice cultivation, more landfills, and leaking natural gas pipelines.

The greenhouse effect is still a subject of controversy in the scientific community. Both the magnitude and the timing the warming and future climatic changes are uncertain. The status can be summarized as follows:

Fact: Greenhouse gases are responsible for keeping the planet warmer than it would be otherwise.

Fact: Concentrations of greenhouse gases are increasing at unprecedented rates.

Theory: Continued greenhouse gas emissions will lead to global warming.

Characteristics and Typical Adverse Effects

Air Pollution. Pollution of the troposphere (lower atmosphere) is damaging to agricultural crops, forests, aquatic systems, buildings, and human health. Primary pollutants often react to form secondary pollutants (acidic compounds), a frequent cause of environmental damage. The following effects are possible:

1. Crop and vegetation damage by injury to plant tissue, increasing susceptibility to disease and drought
2. Decline in forests caused by leaf damage by acidic compounds, acidic soils, and stresses of multiple pollutants

3. Damage to aquatic ecosystems so that they no longer support life
4. Degradation of building materials, such as metal, stone, and brick
5. Adverse impact on human health by damage to respiratory tracts

Marine Pollution. Marine pollution has the following major effects:
1. Spread of pathogens from human wastes, including viruses and protozoa that cause hepatitis, cholera, typhoid, and other infectious diseases
2. Release of undegradable materials, such as plastics and netting, that may injure marine mammals
3. Oil pollution from oil spills
4. Spread of hazardous chemicals and radioactive substances into the marine ecosystem where they may accumulate in seafood

Freshwater Pollution. Freshwater pollution results in the following adverse effects:
1. Untreated wastewater carries viruses and bacteria from human feces into human drinking water, which can result in illness or even in infant mortality
2. *Eutrophication,* or decay of organic matter, which decreases oxygen levels in water, upsetting the balance of the aquatic ecosystem
3. Adverse health effects in persons drinking untreated water from tainted sources
4. Water acidification, which reduces water's capacity to support aquatic life
5. Runoff sediment from eroded soil deposits in drainage basins, reducing the basins' capacity and exacerbating flooding
6. Salinization from irrigation, with harmful effects on downstream agriculture
7. Pesticides and fertilizer chemicals, which accumulate in water and affect tissues in living organisms

Global Warming. The impacts of global warming are still uncertain. Computer models are unable to make reliable predictions of regional changes. The following changes *may* occur.

RISE IN SEA LEVEL. Melting of the Arctic ice sheets and alpine glaciers could cause the seas to expand and sea levels to rise. Depending on the degree of global warming, the seas may rise 30 cm to 2 m by 2075, jeopardizing coastal settlements and marine ecosystems. A rise of 1 m in sea level could flood 15% of arable land in Egypt's Nile Delta and would flood 12% of Bangladesh, displacing 11 million people. The tiny island of the Maldives, inhabited by 200,000, would be submerged.

CLIMATE CHANGE. Natural disasters such as superhurricanes could become common. A temperature increase of a few degrees in tropical seas can intensify hurricane production. The warmer oceans may increase the El Niño phenomenon near the coast of Peru. ENSO inhibits phytoplankton growth, causes fish and shellfish to migrate or die, and forces higher forms of life (e.g., birds, humans) dependent on these sealife to migrate or die.

Other climatic changes could lead to warmer and drier conditions in middle latitudes, higher temperatures in semitropical and tropical areas, and higher rates of evaporation. Rainfall patterns may also change. The combined effects of increased CO_2 and climate changes may alter plant and animal productivity. Plants may grow faster and larger but may have reduced nutritive value.

CHANGES IN ECOSYSTEMS. In warmer climates, grasslands, savannas, and deserts may expand, rendering them vulnerable to increased degradation through erosion and fire. Animal species that do not adapt to the temperature increases may have to relocate to survive, which would be difficult, given population pressures on land. Plant species unable to adapt would perish.

PUBLIC HEALTH IMPACT. Global warming may affect mortality because of heat stress and may increase the incidence of respiratory diseases, allergies, and reproductive illnesses. Geographic ranges of vector-induced diseases (e.g., mosquito-borne malaria, yellow fever) and parasitic diseases might increase.

Measurement

Air and Water Pollution. Pollutants are measured worldwide, but to a much lesser degree in developing countries. The most comprehensive data collection system is the Global Environment Monitoring System (GEMS) of the United Nations Environmental Programme (UNEP), which provides data on sulfur dioxide and particulate matter in urban air and contaminants in water resources. Pollution production is related to per capita consumption, so that as countries develop, pollution also tends to increase.

Ozone Depletion. Ozone levels are regularly monitored each year, especially in the Southern Hemisphere, where a seasonal ozone hole opens over Antarctica every year. Twenty million tons of CFCs were manufactured and have either escaped or will escape to the atmosphere.

Greenhouse Effect. Greenhouse gas emissions are regularly measured throughout the world. Even if the exact levels of future greenhouse emissions were available, however, predicting the effects on global climate would be difficult. Climatic models are used to study climate change, but the models differ in their interpretation of the various interactions in the earth's systems, partly because information put into the system is incomplete or poorly understood.

Risk Reduction Measures

Air and Water Pollution. Most nations are acting individually to control air pollution. Basic requirements are (1) to set ambient air quality standards that measure pollutants away from the source and set controls on acceptable levels and (2) to require that every source of an air pollutant meet certain emission limits. In some cases, humans may have to develop the technologies to make the latter possible.

Pollution control of coastal areas in the past has proved that recovery is possible to some extent. The banned pesticide DDT, which was present in many forms of marine life, is now decreasing in concentration. Most strategies for protecting the oceans must address broader ranges of pollutants from sewage to industrial effluents. More national and international efforts should focus on establishing policy for protection of coastal areas.

Improvement of soils can decrease the possibility of water contamination by toxic chemicals and decrease runoff, thereby lessening silting and sedimentation of waterways. Establishing terraces and contour bounds, stabilizing sand dunes, building check dams, and planting trees and shrubs can help to stabilize soil. Watershed mapping, management, and protection are also of vital importance in ensuring a safe and plentiful drinking water supply. Proper systems to dispose of human waste should be promoted.

Regulations must be established and enforced by government agencies to protect citizens against the toxic effects of pesticides and other chemicals. Improvement of soils will also help to absorb and degrade toxins. Further studies must be made on the effects of pesticide residues. Farmers may use crop types resistant to pests or an integrated approach to pest management requiring less pesticide.

Ozone Depletion. International cooperation to limit CFC emissions should reduce production and use of CFCs in industrialized nations by 50% from 1986 levels, with developing countries allowed to increase their use slightly. Research is addressing the need for CFC substitutes, for minimizing loss to the atmosphere, and for recycling. Countries can regulate import and use of aerosols and disposal of refrigeration units.

Global Warming. Since burning of fossil fuels (at least in theory) is the primary cause of global warming, developed countries are mainly at fault, and poorer countries are more likely to be the victims. Scientists estimate that 20% of greenhouse gases (mainly CO_2) are generated by deforestation, however, a trend occurring at a devastating rate in developing countries, particularly in tropical rainforests. Since global warming could affect the entire planet, steps can be taken to prepare for its effects and to prevent its acceleration, as follows:

1. Reduce the rate of deforestation. Plant trees to solve community needs for wood, such as fuel wood, or to provide profits for individual farmers with agroforestry.
2. Increase energy production and use. Promote energy efficiency in urban areas, and support renewable energy sources, such as wind, water, geothermal, and solar power. These may be of great use in areas where no electricity sources exist.
3. Develop regulations to curb pollution from traffic emissions and industry in urban areas.

Education is a vital tool for environmental awareness. By understanding the relationships of ecosystems and the long-term effects of degradation, people are motivated to act. Women's groups in India have established a tree protection lobby. Their motto is "trees are not wood," a concept that promotes trees as a vital part of the ecosystem involving CO_2 exchange to the air and a root system to hold down the soil. Education regarding the environment should begin in the early grades. Education for adults may take place in farmers' cooperatives, women's cooperatives, and village settings or may accompany programs to distribute seeds and tools.

Trying to Save the Black Sea

The Black Sea, named for the dark clouds and fierce storms that affect its shores each autumn, faces an even darker future. The residues of modern agriculture and industry now threaten its marine life and the air quality of its bordering countries of Bulgaria, Romania, Turkey, and parts of the new Commonwealth of Independent States. The Black Sea is particularly vulnerable to pollution, since it collects 10 times more water per square meter of surface area than any other sea or ocean. It is fed by several major rivers, which deposit many of the pollutants. The most important is the Danube, which flows through eight highly industrialized countries, all using chemically intensive agricultural practices.

In addition, the Black Sea has natural pollutants—organic matter collected over thousands of years, now decaying and diminishing the supply of oxygen in the water vital to life. In the unique two-stratum structure of the sea, where salt water from the Mediterranean forms a bottom layer and fresh water a top layer, toxic hydrogen sulfide from the decomposing matter remains on the bottom layer, where oxygen is not present. Construction of irrigation works and dams has reduced the flow of fresh water into the Black Sea, so the toxic layer that was previously 200 m below the surface has now risen to a depth of only 80 to 100 m.

Further deterioration of the Black Sea and air pollution from industries around it could be economically disastrous to the surrounding countries that depend on it to draw tourists. The resource-poor country of Bulgaria has developed a 20-year plan to save the sea and to bolster tourism, as follows:

1. A total ban on discharge of any pollutants into the sea
2. Regulation of development of concentrated industrialization in the coastal zone
3. Environmental monitoring by 20 different institutions in coordination with UNEP
4. Restricting the inflow of fertilizers and the building of dams
5. Proliferation of blue mollusks to eat plankton, which use up the precious oxygen; shellfish cultivation also a possibility
6. Holding a convention to assess the sea's environmental problems and develop a plan that would be closely linked to the international effort to address the pollution problems of Europe's major rivers

DEFORESTATION

Deforestation is the removal or damage of vegetation in a region that is predominantly tree covered. Deforestation is a slow-onset hazard that may contribute to disasters caused by flooding, landslides, and drought. Deforestation reaches critical proportions when large areas of vegetation are removed or damaged, harming the land's protective and regenerative properties. The rapid rate of deforestation in some parts of the world is a driving force in the yearly increase of flood disasters in these areas.

Approximately 17 million hectares of tropical forests and woodlands are converted into agriculture, pasture lands, or other uses every year. This includes 7.3 million hectares of tropical forest (6.1 million hectares of moist forest) and 3.8 million hectares of open and savanna woodland. Less than 10% of the land being deforested is replanted every year. Although the amount of forest land coming under protection or conservation is growing, the future still poses problems because of rapidly increasing pressures of development and exploitation.

Causal Phenomena

The spread of agriculture, firewood collection, and unregulated timber harvesting are the principal and immediate reasons for deforestation. Beneath the obvious causes are fundamental problems in development, such as the use of inefficient agricultural practices, insecure land tenure, rising unemployment, rapid population growth, and failure to regulate and preserve forest lands.

Farming. The major cause of forest loss is the spread of farming. Land may be cleared for commercial ventures such as sugarcane, coffee, or rubber plantations, which is a principal cause of deforestation in Central America. In tropical rainforests, both legal and illegal colonists are trying to farm the former jungle lands, where soil conditions are fragile. Up to 90% of the nutrients are in vegetation rather than in the soil. When the forest is cut and burned, a nutrient surge occurs in the soil, lending initial fertility. After cropping and exposure to sun and rain, however, soil fertility rapidly declines, and the area becomes unproductive, perhaps prompting the farmer to slash and burn new forest areas.

Many traditional people in the Amazon Basin, Central Africa, and Southeast Asia still practice shifting cultivation techniques, allowing fallow periods between cropping for soils to regenerate. This practice becomes unsustainable if populations increase to the extent of forcing people into smaller areas. Insecure land tenure or fixed land titles may also force overuse of the land.

Because of crowded conditions in cities and farm areas, many people migrate to areas of marginal fertility, where they must keep moving their fields to produce sufficient food. Where this occurs, the migrant farmer may damage timber, wildlife, and human resources. In Venezuela, which has a high rate of unemployment and rising numbers of landless peasants, 30,000 families live and farm in national parks, forest reserves, and other legally protected areas. An influx of cultivators who settled on the watershed above the Panama Canal has caused increased silting of a major reservoir that supplies Panama City.

Grazing. In Central and South America, large areas of tropical forest have been cleared to create grazing lands. A major portion of this can be attributed to economic enterprises designed for meat production. The Brazilian government has granted large land concessions to both domestic and foreign corporations wanting to raise cattle in the Amazon area. In Central America, virgin forest is being destroyed by ranchers who intend to export beef to the United States.

Firewood Collection. Firewood collection can contribute to the depletion of tree cover, particularly in lightly wooded areas. Because of a lack of alternative fuels and fuel-efficient stoves, this is especially a problem in Africa and in Asian highland countries such as Nepal. In areas of dense woods, dead material may fill local requirements for fuel. The outright destruction of trees for fuel occurs most commonly around cities and towns, where commercial markets for firewood and charcoal exist. Well-organized groups and individuals bring fuel wood by vehicle, pack animal, and cart into many cities, hastening local deforestation.

Fuel Wood Crisis. About 100 million people in developing countries cannot meet their minimum needs for energy, and almost 1.3 billion consume fuel wood resources faster than they are being replenished. In parts of West Africa today, some urban families spend one fourth of their income on wood or charcoal for cooking. In India, firewood is subsidized for the poor to prevent starvation.

Logging. Extensive logging in humid tropical forests, particularly in Asia and in temperate and mountainous forests, is conducted by large multinational corporations for export or to fill building needs in cities. The procedure usually involves either "clear cutting" or "creaming," or selective logging, of the forest's small proportion of valued species. Creaming, even though a less radical alternative to clear cutting, still causes significant damage to vegetation and wildlife that is not apparent from the statistics. A study in Indonesia revealed that logging operations damaged or destroyed about 40% of trees left behind. The roads created by logging operations may encourage settlers to enter the forest and begin slash and burn agriculture, so that eventually even more of the forest is lost.

Characteristics

Trees play a vital role in regulating the earth's atmosphere, ecosystems, and weather systems. They recycle CO_2, a gas now increasing in the atmosphere and thought to contribute to global warming. They release moisture to the air, thus contributing to rainfall and moderating local and global climate. Their roots trap nutrients, improve soil fertility, and trap pollutants, keeping these from the water supply. They provide habitats for species, engendering diversity. They nurture traditional cultures by giving shelter, wood, food, and medicinal products. These benefits are lost as trees are destroyed.

The root systems of vegetation help retain water in the soil, anchor the soil particles, and provide aeration to keep soil from compacting. When vegetation dies, the nutrients go back to the soil. When root systems are removed, soil becomes destabilized. Water tends to flow off the top of the soil instead of percolating in, and it carries valuable topsoil along with it. This soil eventually forms sediment in the drainage basins.

Deforestation poses the most immediate danger by its contribution to the following hazards:

1. Destabilized soils are more susceptible to landslides and may increase the landslide risk in areas vulnerable to earthquakes and volcanoes.

2. Loss of moisture from deforestation may contribute to drought conditions, which in turn may trigger famines. Soil nutrients may also be lost through erosion of topsoil, resulting in decreased food production and possible chronic food shortages.

3. Erosion and dry conditions, combined with loss of vegetation and soil compaction, result in desertification and unproductive lands.

4. Dryness may accelerate the spread of fires.

5. Loss of CO_2 from dying trees and fires may add to global warming.

6. Deforestation of watersheds, especially around smaller rivers and streams, can increase the severity of flooding, reduce stream flows, evaporate springs in dry seasons, and increase the amount of sediment entering waterways.

Of all the hazards associated with deforestation, flooding may be the most serious. Usually, curative measures, such as dredging and dam building, are taken over preventive measures to solve flooding problems. As flooding worsens in developing countries, more attention is given to protection of watersheds. In India, flood damages between 1953 and 1978 averaged $250 million per year. Today, even more people live in flood-prone areas. Flood problems may not be lessened without reforestation of the increasingly denuded hills of northern India and Nepal.

Predictability

Measurement and monitoring of forested areas may be conducted through ground-level sampling and aerial or satellite surveys. Each method has drawbacks. Ground sampling is tedious and difficult to extrapolate, aerial surveys are expensive, and satellite imagery poses difficulty in distinguishing forest from other vegetation. Combinations of methods usually produce the best results. Vague definitions in the study of deforestation still make exact determinations and forecasting difficult. Three different prediction methods follow:

1. One type of study predicts future deforestation rates by extrapolating present rates of deforestation into the future. If the present rate of deforestation at 6.1 million hectares per year were to continue, the tropical moist forests would be completely cleared in 177 years. Where deforestation is more acute, the losses will be more serious. Cote d'Ivoire and Nigeria annually lose about 5.2% of their forests, and Costa Rica, Sri Lanka, and El Salvador lose between 3.2% and 3.6%. Each of these countries could lose all forests between the years 2007 and 2017.

2. Another forecast for 43 tropical countries was made using a mathematical model, which assumed that when forests in a country fell to a crit-

ical level, governments would take action to prevent further deforestation. Considerably more optimistic, the results predicted deforestation rates to decrease to between 0.9 and 3.7 million hectares per year in 2030.

3. Perhaps the bleakest theoretic forecast incorporates the effects of population growth and increasing consumption, which might be assumed to increase the rate of deforestation worldwide. However, growth of economies and technologies at the same time may assist to curtail the deforestation process if governments take appropriate action.

Typical Adverse Effects

The specific impacts of deforestation include the following:

1. Loss of soil fertility in the tropics and loss of productive capacity
2. Soil erosion and deposition of sediment
3. Increased runoff
4. Reduction in rainfall and increase in temperature
5. Destruction of biodiversity and traditional cultures
6. Loss of "free" goods, such as fuels, food, and medicines
7. Exacerbation of other disasters

Economic Impact. Most developing countries are already importers of forest products, especially paper. Because the amount of wood and wood products available per person in the world is falling and thus increasing in price, combined with shortages of foreign currencies, import of forest products may be increasingly prohibitive for these countries. Commercially marketed firewood is becoming more scarce, and prices are climbing. Wood for construction is also scarce in many countries, which adversely affects the availability of housing.

Risk Reduction Measures

Various types of forest management, reforestation, and community participation can reduce deforestation. Most governments now recognize the vital importance of national forestry programs. Foresters help people meet their basic needs for forest products, and not always from the traditional forest or concentrated woodlot. For instance, forestry practiced by many farmers on their lands has been shown to be more environmentally effective. Reforestation has become intrinsically interwoven with other government policies that affect the population. Forestry therefore should be considered an integral part of land use and natural resource planning sectors of government.

Forests should be viewed by governments as capital resources to be managed. Management of the system should discourage concessionaires or other land users from practices that are not sustainable. Good management encourages highly selective harvesting without undue waste of remaining trees, especially in tropical forests. For any country to address its loss of forests and ensure that forests will yield economic benefits well into the future, the following steps must be taken:

1. Forest law or basic forest policy must be written that clearly states the objective of long-term sustainable management of the forest.
2. Forest regulations or management guidelines must be written and followed.
3. Sufficient financial and human resources must be allocated.

Forest management must be considered in the broadest sense of land use planning to include solutions for people as well as for trees. Compromises between complete destruction of the forests and complete conservation might entail regulated clearing of forests for shifting cultivation, habitation, or hunting; voluntary and intentional protection of forests or individual species by designating areas for reserves or national parks; and enrichment of the forest with species from other places. The last option may be considered risky, since pests and other species-specific problems may accompany introduction of new species.

Many unresolved scientific issues in forest management remain. How can the ever-expanding areas of secondary vegetation and degraded soils be managed to be more productive for the local people? Since most primary forests have disappeared, what type of forest can be established that would be stable and productive and that would ensure the conservation of biologic diversity? What further types of basic ecologic research are needed to manage natural forests?

Social Forestry in Thailand

A project was begun in 1980 by Thailand's Royal Forestry Department (RFD) aimed at restoring the depleted forests. In just one generation since 1960, Thailand's forests had been reduced by half as its population doubled. The challenge facing the government was to restore the forests while permitting the expanding population to earn a living through farming.

The 8000 Thais living on 10,000 hectares near Nakhon Ratchasima on the Khorat Plateau had used slash-and-burn agriculture for years, destroying the forest. To develop the project, a survey was conducted for an entire year to determine the cropping patterns of the settlers and their expectations for the future. The RFD discovered that most wanted to remain on the land and farm. The 60% of the land suitable for farming would be used as incentive to encourage permanent settlement. The remaining 40% would be reforested by the RFD to prevent erosion of the hillsides and destruction of watersheds. The plan called for village councils to be formed and infrastructural inputs provided, such as roads, schools, and health centers.

The trees planted by RFD grew rapidly and prompted villagers to plant 3.5 million seedlings. Complementary projects were initiated, including beekeeping, cottage industries, and crop diversification. The RFD provided training to its own staff, including experience with successful social forestry programs in other countries.

Many problems remain in Thailand. During the past 30 years the total amount of forest replanted is equivalent to only 1 year of cutting. Much timber is being harvested for profit without permits. Relentless population growth and poverty place constant pressure on forest resources. However, the government is committed to future projects of this kind. The national policy in Thailand is to return 40% of the country to forest, which is crucial if Thailand is to become a major exporter of timber again.

DESERTIFICATION

Desertification is defined as land degradation in arid, semiarid, and dry subhumid areas resulting mainly from human actions. Poor land use is a significant contributing factor, but desertification can also be caused by natural cycles of climate change. It affects both developed and developing regions, including Africa, the Middle East, India, Pakistan, China, Australia, the Commonwealth of Independent States, the central and southwestern United States, and many Mediterranean countries. A slow-onset disaster, desertification worsens conditions of poverty, brings malnutrition and disease, and destabilizes the social and economic bases of affected countries.

Causal Phenomena

Role of Climate. Vulnerability to desertification and the severity of its impact are partially governed by climatic conditions of an area. The lower and more uncertain the rainfall, the greater is the potential for desertification. Other influencing factors are seasonal patterns of rainfall and high temperatures that increase evaporation, land use, and the type of vegetation cover.

The world's drylands are found in two belts centered approximately on the Tropic of Cancer and the Tropic of Capricorn (23.5 degrees north and south of the equator, respectively) and cover one third of the earth's surface. More than 80% of the total area of drylands is found on three continents: Africa (37%), Asia (33%), and Australia (14%). The drylands can be further classified into hyperarid, arid, and semiarid zones, depending on the average amount of rainfall received per year. Other factors, such as temperature and soil conditions, must be considered when determining the dryness ratio.

Both natural and human-derived climatic changes may contribute to desertification. Natural effects, such as long-term climatic cycles and the basic Earth-sun geometry, have resulted in drier conditions in the Sahara. Human influence is associated with the predicted global warming trend and local climatic changes, in which deforestation has reduced the moisture-holding capacity of soil and has decreased cloud formation. The result is less rainfall and higher temperatures.

Despite the common misperception that desertification is caused by the desert advancing itself, land degradation can occur at great distances from deserts. Desertification usually begins as a spot on the land where land abuse has been excessive; from that spot, land degradation can spread outward with continued abuse (Figure 68-12). Desertification does not cause drought but may result in greater persistence or susceptibility to drought. Drought, on the other hand, contributes to desertification and increases the rate of degradation. When the rains return, however, well-managed lands recover from droughts with minimal adverse effects. Land abuse during periods of good rains and its continuation during periods of deficient rainfall contribute to desertification.

Role of Land Use Management. Desertification can be caused by five main types of poor land use: overcultivation, cash cropping, overgrazing, deforestation, and poor irrigation practices.

OVERCULTIVATION. Overcultivation damages the structure of the soil or removes vegetation cover, leaving the soil vulnerable to erosion. Reasons for overcultivation include drought, increasing demand for food because of population growth, cropping on marginal range lands unsuitable for long-term production, land tenure restrictions confining sectors of the population to marginal lands, mechanized farming, and expansion of cash cropping.

CASH CROPPING. Although a large part of agricultural production in developing countries fills subsistence needs, some cash crops are grown for foreign exchange. A feature of most cash crops, however, is their extreme demand for nutrients and optimum conditions. Degradation of land occurs directly through improper management of such crops and indirectly by displacing subsistence crops and pastoralism to marginal lands.

OVERGRAZING. Overgrazing is a major cause of desertification (range lands account for 90% of desertified lands) and occurs when too many animals are pastured. The number of cattle in Niger, for example, increased an estimated 450% between 1938 and 1961 and an additional 29% by 1970, when the majority were killed by starvation. Livestock density increases when

Healthy region

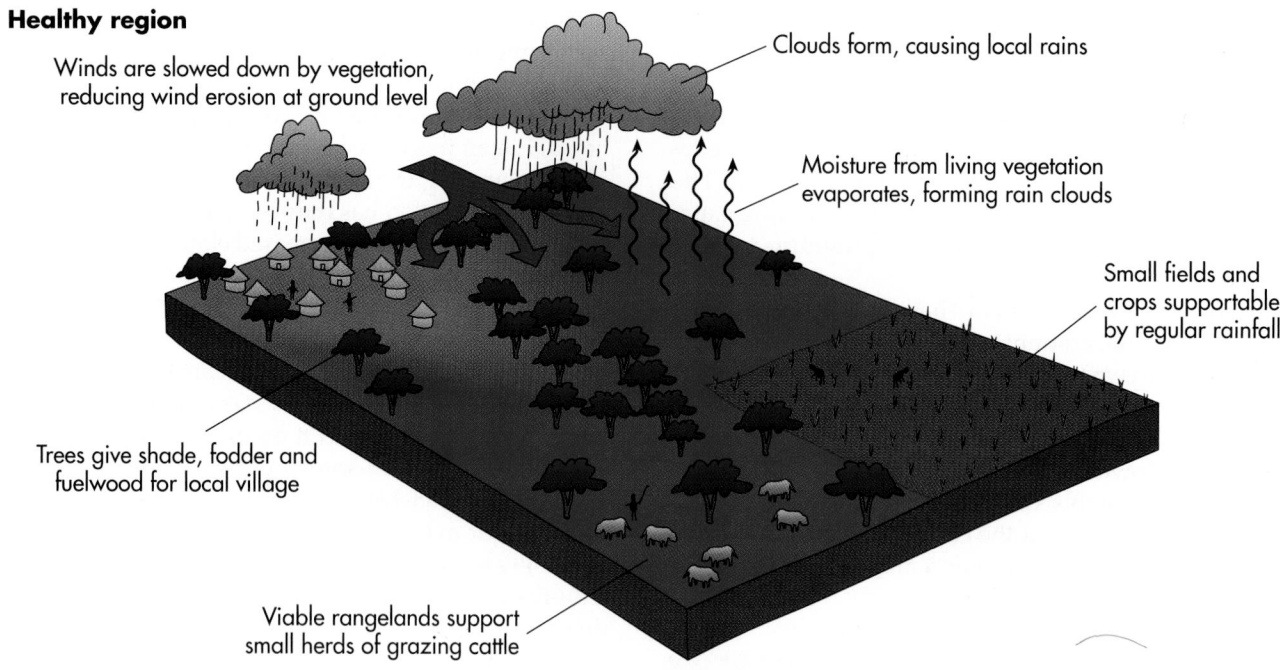

Winds are slowed down by vegetation, reducing wind erosion at ground level

Clouds form, causing local rains

Moisture from living vegetation evaporates, forming rain clouds

Small fields and crops supportable by regular rainfall

Trees give shade, fodder and fuelwood for local village

Viable rangelands support small herds of grazing cattle

Desertified region

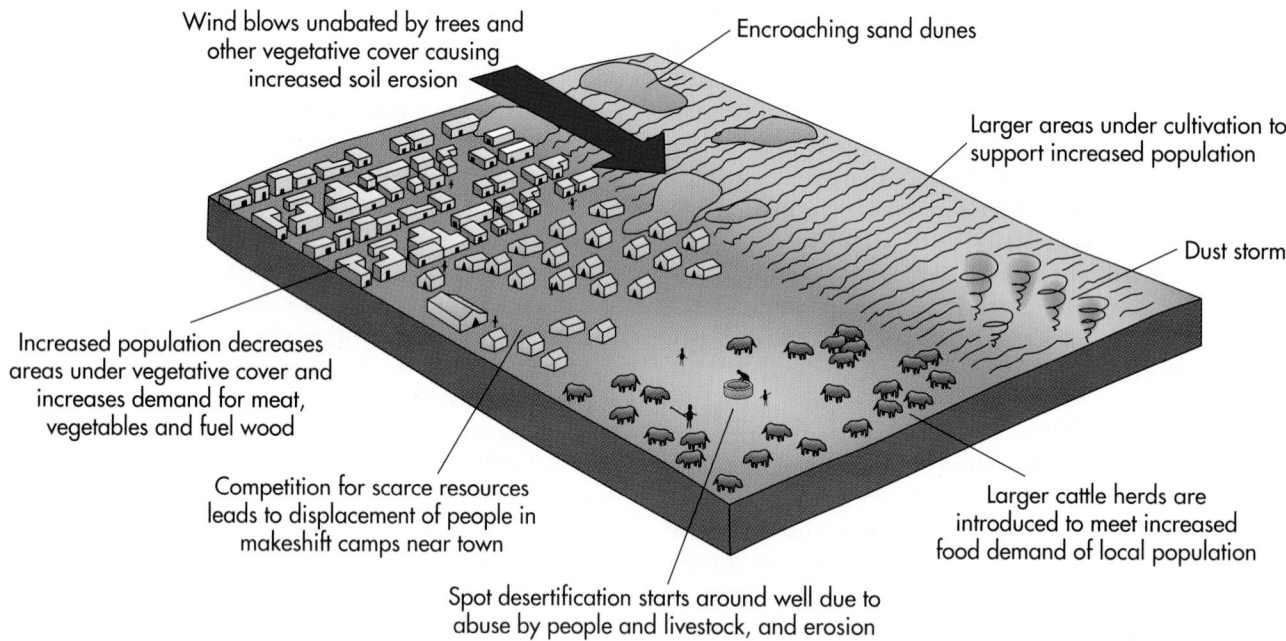

Wind blows unabated by trees and other vegetative cover causing increased soil erosion

Encroaching sand dunes

Larger areas under cultivation to support increased population

Dust storm

Increased population decreases areas under vegetative cover and increases demand for meat, vegetables and fuel wood

Competition for scarce resources leads to displacement of people in makeshift camps near town

Spot desertification starts around well due to abuse by people and livestock, and erosion

Larger cattle herds are introduced to meet increased food demand of local population

Figure 68-12. Comparison of healthy and desertified regions. (*Modified from* Introduction to hazards, *ed 3, New York, 1997, Disaster Management Training Programme, United Nations Development Program, UN Organization for Coordination of Humanitarian Assistance.*)

herd sizes grow too large in wet years and cannot be sustained in dry years. Lucrative markets for meat, such as Nigeria and the Middle East, have resulted in cattle ranches, where concentrated activity threatens land, with poor returns for the investment.

Better veterinary care has decreased mortality rates. Deep wells increase availability of water, allowing

larger, less mobile herds that congregate in the well area and degrade the vegetation and soil.

DEFORESTATION. Land is cleared for agriculture, livestock, and fuel wood production. Deforestation is the first step toward desertification, removing vegetative barriers and exposing land to sun, wind, and rain. In

Africa, demands for fuel wood and charcoal exert considerable stress on wood resources.

POOR IRRIGATION MANAGEMENT. The concept of using irrigation to ward off the threat of crop failure during drought has been promoted by many development agencies. Ironically, poor management of irrigation projects has been a cause of desertification. In some cases, productivity falls and soils become salinized, alkalized, or waterlogged. The major problem is usually inadequate drainage, and damage may be irreversible. A key example is the Greater Mussayeb irrigation project in Iraq, begun in 1953. By 1969, waterlogging was widespread, and two thirds of the soil was saline. In 1970 a project to reclaim the salinized land was begun, but by 1976, because of technical and organizational limitations, the project still had not been successful. Egypt, Iraq, and Pakistan have lost more than 25% of their irrigated areas to salinization and waterlogging.

Role of Government Policy. Population growth and economic expansion also contribute to desertification. As populations grow, government and multilateral policies must promote increased food production through appropriate technologies that prevent soil degradation and erosion. Government policy should also address the causes of poverty, or disadvantaged peoples will place more stress on land to obtain needed resources. Some governments choose to expand cash crop cultivation to improve foreign currency holdings rather than promote food security for the poor, or they fail to resolve conflicts over scarce resources. Policies may mandate land uses that are difficult to enforce and that result in breakdown of customary land tenure or natural resource management institutions.

Characteristics

The two main characteristics of desertification, the degradation of soil and degradation of vegetation, have the same result: reduction of productivity.

Degradation of Vegetation. Vegetation in arid lands adapts to the cycle of water availability by adjusting its growth. The drier the area, the farther apart plants grow. Some plants grow only during the rainy seasons. Degradation of vegetation occurs initially in the early stages of desertification with deforestation but continues after soil fertility declines.

The two main forms of vegetation degradation are (1) overall reduction of density of the vegetation cover, or biomass, and (2) a more subtle change in types of vegetation to less productive forms. For example, range land perennial grasses may be replaced by less palatable annual varieties, or more saline-tolerant crops, such as barley, may be substituted for traditional crops because of low yields from waterlogging and salinization.

Degradation of Soil. Soil degradation occurs in four major ways: water erosion, wind erosion, soil compaction, and waterlogging, which results in salinization and alkalinization.

WATER EROSION. Vegetation normally protects soil from being washed away by rain and also from splash erosion by raindrops. The raindrops move the soil particles and pack them together on the surface, sealing the pores and thereby decreasing infiltration and increasing runoff. *Sheet erosion* is a more serious form of erosion in which fine layers of topsoil carrying soil nutrients are washed away. Unless the nutrients are replenished artificially, crop yields decline. Gullies are created by the runoff and, unless reclaimed by conservation measures, render the land unusable.

WIND EROSION. Wind erosion occurs when finer components of the soil, such as silt, clay, and organic matter that contain most of the nutrients, are blown away, leaving behind the less fertile sand and coarse particles. Sand itself may start to drift, forming dunes, but this accounts for a minor proportion of the effects of wind erosion. Strong winds may form dust storms that damage crops by shredding leaves.

SOIL COMPACTION. Nearly complete compaction can occur when soil of poor structure is compressed by heavy machinery or by hooves of large herds of animals. A less serious form of compaction, called *surface crusting*, results when high-speed mechanical cultivation or dry season cultivation turns particles into thin powder, which then forms a crust when pelted with raindrops. Crusting and compaction make the soil less permeable for germination of new plants.

WATERLOGGING (SALINIZATION AND ALKALINIZATION). These effects result from poor management of irrigation and water supplies in general. When the soil is waterlogged, the upward movement of saline in groundwater leaves salt on the surface when the water evaporates.

Predictability

Desertification is a direct socioeconomic threat to more than 200 million people and a less direct threat to 700 million, but data are still insufficient to quantify the extent of the problem and its progression. Databases are incomplete or do not exist for many countries. More information is needed on the characteristics and status of dryland ecosystems. An understanding of climatic changes, including the effects of possible global warming, is crucial to predictability.

Socioeconomic indicators showing trends in human health, income, and welfare must be collected to understand related issues.

The International Soil Reference Centre and UNEP support the Global Assessment of Soil Degradation (GLASOD), which uses a geographical information system (GIS) to access data for different areas of the world and estimate land degradation.

Rate and Scope

Although the numbers remain controversial, yearly losses to desertification are estimated at 1.0 to 1.3 million hectares of irrigated land, 3.5 to 4.0 million hectares of rainfed cropland and 4.5 to 5.8 million hectares of range land. These estimates represent an increase from estimates in 1994 of 3.4% and indicate that the situation is worsening.

Desertification affects drylands in more than 100 countries but is concentrated in Asia and Africa, which account for 70% of all desertified land. Scientists have tried to quantify the areas desertified on a worldwide basis. The physical damage can be measured in reduced productivity of soils and loss of vegetation. The number of casualties cannot be scientifically extrapolated, but deaths occur, directly from famine or indirectly from reduced standards of living.

ACKNOWLEDGMENTS AND RESOURCES

This chapter draws on several publications, especially *Introduction to Hazards*, third edition, 1997, a teaching module prepared for the Disaster Management Training Programme of the United Nations Development Program (UNDP) and UN Organization for Coordination of Humanitarian Assistance (OCHA). Another background document is *Natural Hazards: Causes and Effects,* published by the Disaster Management Center of the University of Wisconsin. I would like to thank Paul Thompson and Jim Good of InterWorks for their collaboration on this project and Robert L. Southern of Weather Associates for his input on the tropical cyclone section.

Websites and e-mail addresses for more information on hazards include the following:

Federal Emergency Management Agency: www. fema.gov

Global Information and Early Warning System on Food and Agriculture: GIEWS@fao.org

Hazlit Data Base, University of Colorado: www.colorado.edu/hazard/litbase

International Tsunami Information Center: itic@itic.noaa.gov

National Earthquake Information Center: quake@gldfs.urgs.gov

National Oceanic and Atmospheric Association website: www.noaa.gov

Relief Web: www.reliefweb.int

United Nations Environmental Program: www.unep.ch

SUGGESTED READINGS

Disaster history: significant data on major disasters worldwide, 1900-95, 1996, Washington, DC, Office of Foreign Disaster Assistance.

Dregne HM, Rozanov B: A new assessment of the world status of desertification, *Desertification Control Bull* 20, 1991.

Dudley WC, Lee M: *Tsunami!* Honolulu, 1988, University of Hawaii Press.

Earthquakes and volcanoes, 1989, United States Geological Survey.

El-Baz F, Hassan MHA, editors: *Physics of desertification,* Amsterdam, 1986, Martinus Nijhoff.

Erikson J: *Volcanoes and earthquakes,* Blue Ridge Summit, Pa, 1988, Tab Books.

Forest resources assessment 1990: global synthesis, Rome, 1995, Food and Agriculture Organization.

Global perspectives on tropical cyclones, Geneva, 1995, World Meteorological Organization.

Grainger A: *The threatening desert: controlling desertification,* London, 1990, Earthscan.

Hanley ML: Can the Black Sea be saved? *World Dev* 3:6, 1990.

International Federation of Red Cross and Red Crescent Societies: *World disaster report 1995,* Amsterdam, 1996, Martinus Nijhoff.

Lorca E: Integration of the THRUST project into the Chile Tsunami Warning System, *Nat Hazards* 4:293, 1991.

Mitigating natural disasters, phenomena, effects and options, New York, 1991, United Nations Disaster Relief Organization.

Natural hazards primer, Washington, DC, 1990, Organization of American States.

Nuhfer E, Proctor R, Moser P: *The citizen's guide to geologic hazards,* 1993, American Institute of Professional Geologists.

Smith K: *Environmental hazards: assessing risk and reducing disaster,* London, 1996, Routledge.

Tilling RI: Volcanic hazards and their mitigation: progress and problems, *Rev Geophys* 27:237, 1989.

Tsunami—the great waves, 1995, International Tsunami Information Center.

Vickers DO: Tropical cyclones, *Nature Resources* 27:31, 1991.

Volcanic emergency management, New York, 1985, United Nations Disaster Relief Organization.

Wernly D: *The roles of meteorologists and hydrologists in disaster preparedness,* Geneva, 1995, World Meteorological Organization.

Wilhite DA: *Preparing for drought: a guidebook for developing countries,* New York, 1992, Earthwatch Climate Unit, United Nations Environmental Programme.

Wilhite DA, Glantz MH: Understanding the drought phenomenon: the role of definitions, *Water Int* 10:111, 1985.

World Resources Institute: *World resources 1988-89, New York,* 1988, Basic Books.

World Resources Institute: World resources 1996-97, *Oxford, UK,* 1996, Oxford University Press.

Equipment and Special Knowledge

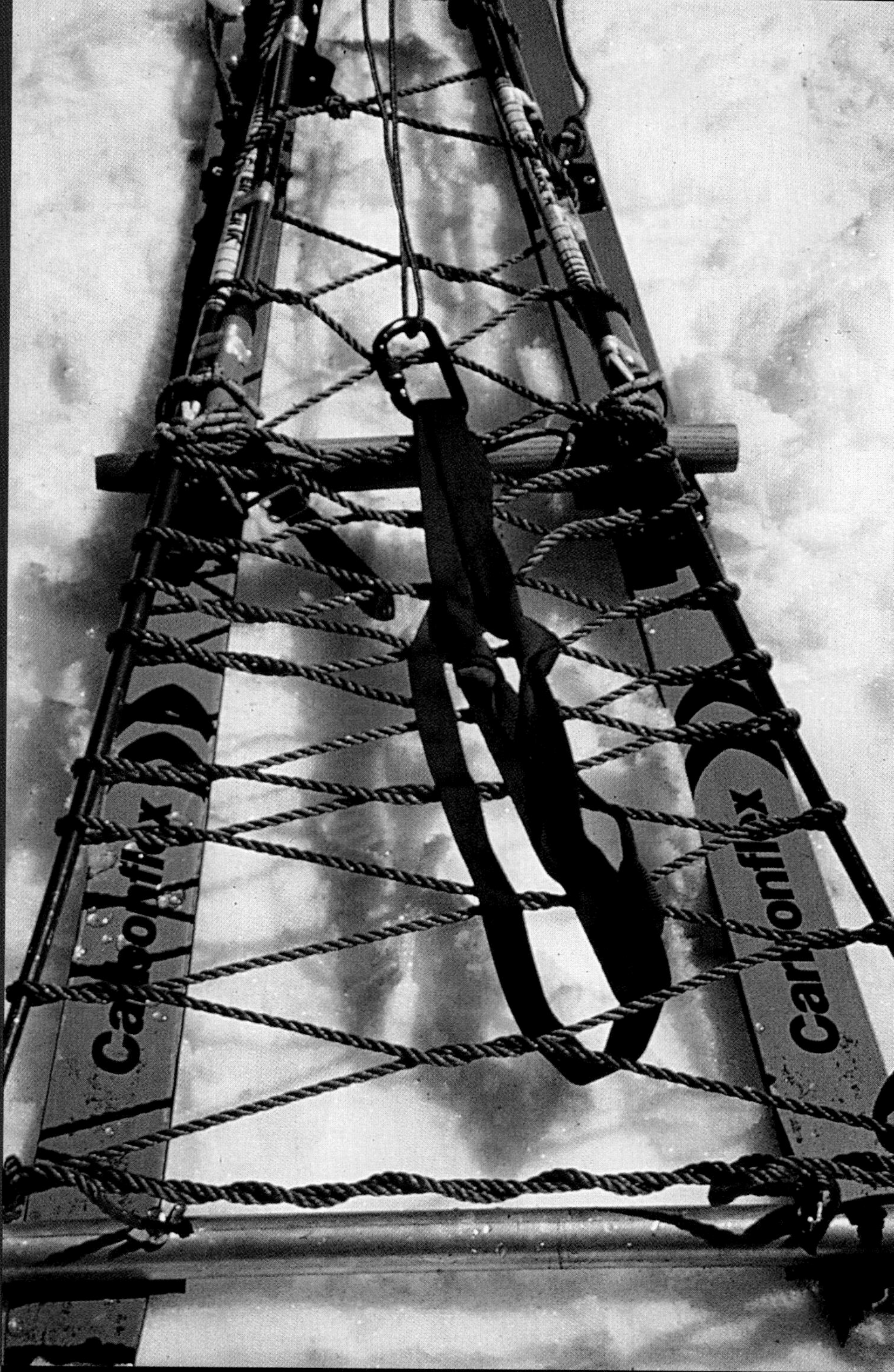

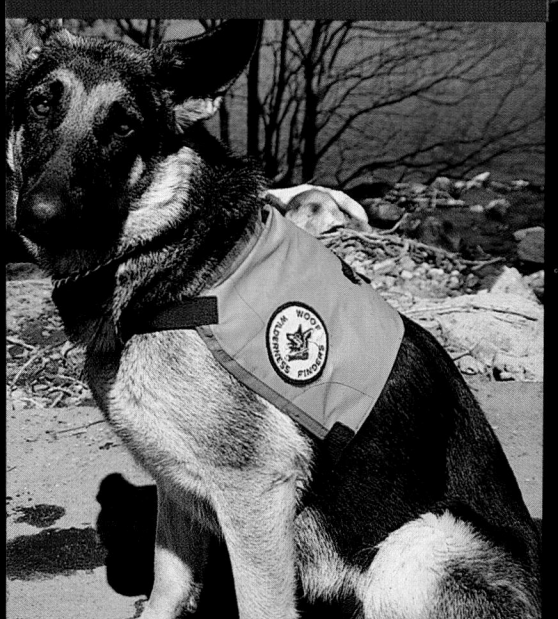

11

69 Wilderness Preparation, Equipment, and Medical Supplies

Steven C. Zell and Philip H. Goodman

The foremost challenges of wilderness recreation are the prevention and management of injury and illness. Medical care may be greatly delayed for the injured person many hours from civilization. Unnecessary suffering can be minimized by educating the traveler, planning each trip carefully, and carrying appropriate medical and nonmedical emergency supplies.

Large expeditions usually enlist experienced medical professionals in logistic planning. Unfortunately, most smaller groups trekking into the wilderness do not have access to this expertise. Even when a physician is a party member, he or she is usually not specifically trained in wilderness medicine. This text details medical management in the wilderness setting. This chapter is intended to complement that material by summarizing recommendations for selecting medical provisions for a variety of wilderness experiences. The first part of the chapter is an overview of important preventive measures and risk factors for wilderness travel. The second part highlights assembly of the medical kit, providing recommendations for its comprehensive, basic components. The latter is primarily directed toward persons engaging in low-risk wilderness travel lacking medical expertise. The index for expedition travel (see Figure 69-2) is intended specifically for groups having persons with medical experience. Based on defined categories of travel risk, which is a function of trip duration and remoteness from medical care, prescription medical supplies appropriate to the task at hand are denoted to allow a more sophisticated selection. The chapter concludes with an update describing specific high-technology items that are not standard to the basic wilderness medical kit but that may be necessary as a function of a group's outdoor interest and activities.

Before any travel in the wilderness, it is important to understand the epidemiology of wilderness injuries. However, it is difficult to make statements on the precise statistical risk of injuries and illness associated with outdoor travel. In the absence of any required reporting of medical problems, information has come from special interest groups and providers of emergency medical services (EMS) in national parks. Hopefully, future wilderness epidemiologic data will characterize injuries and illness patterns.

Despite such limitations, the proportion of accidental injuries to illness occurring during travel is remarkably constant. Data on outdoor travel suggest that traumatic injury, generally of a minor nature, exceeds medical illness of participants by roughly threefold. When reviewing injury patterns, most are attributable to soft tissue damage (e.g., abrasions, contusions, lacerations), sprains, or strains; serious dislocations or bony fractures account for less than 5% of all trauma. The lower extremities are by far the most likely to be involved in minor orthopedic injury, emphasizing the importance of appropriate footwear selection.

Most medical illnesses reported by wilderness travelers are attributable to nonspecific syndromes, such as gastroenteritis or upper respiratory illness. Both may result from crowded conditions, precluding adequate preemptive hygiene measures. Other commonly reported medical problems include headache (exacerbated by high altitude), dyspepsia resulting from local food intolerance, dermatitis, sunburn, dehydration or heat-related illness from inadequate fluid intake, and allergic reactions, mostly related to insect stings.

The outdoor travel literature shows that most deaths are attributable to sudden cardiac arrest, likely a function of the number of older travelers venturing outside. After excluding deaths from cardiac causes, drowning remains the number one cause of accidental death among outdoor participants. Ice and rock climbing has a unique array of injuries, including rare traumatic death from severe head trauma. Environmental issues predominantly relate to high altitude and extremes of temperature. A participant's awareness of environments and events is critical to make certain that appropriate first-aid equipment, not routinely found in most kits, is available to deal with relevant emergencies. Recommendations for such unique supplies are covered in the section on specific equipment purchases.

PREPARING FOR TRAVEL

General Preparedness

The trip coordinator is responsible for assessing the health limitations of the group (see Appendix A). The coordinator should confidentially but frankly discuss medical problems with each candidate and require a medical evaluation if uncertainty exists. Safety of the individual and the group are the coordinator's first priorities. Boxes 69-1 to 69-3 give checklists for general preparedness.

Box 69-1 CHECKLIST FOR GENERAL PREPAREDNESS

Physical conditioning
Immunizations (especially tetanus)
Planning of potential rescue and evacuation routes and leaving an itinerary with person to initiate rescue if group does not return on time
Proper clothing and equipment
Medical-alert medallion or card (illness, allergy, medication)

Water disinfection (chemicals or devices)
Sunglasses, sunscreen, and adhesive blister pads
Historical appraisal of weather conditions: National Climatic Data Center (http://www.ncdc.noaa.gov)
Precipitation and temperature short-term forecasts: National Weather Service (http://www.nws.noaa.gov)
Immediate weather updates/current conditions: The Weather Channel (http://www.weather.com)

Box 69-2 CHECKLIST OF PRETRAVEL MEASURES FOR DEVELOPING COUNTRIES

Predetermine local sources of medical help
Important phone numbers for obtaining up-to-date travel warnings
   Centers for Disease Control and Prevention: International Traveler's Hotline (http://www.cdc.gov)
   Department of State Citizens Emergency Center 202-647-5225
Immunization information and advice
Local health department/travel medicine clinics
   International Society of Travel Medicine (ISTM) Clinic Directory—available by request (contact: Secretariat/ISTM 770-736-7060)
   USPHS booklet: *Health information for international travel, 1999-2000 ed*, U.S. Government Printing Office, Washington, DC (item #017-023-00202-3), 202-512-1800

Required immunizations as defined by the World Health Organization
   Yellow fever: listing of countries requiring this vaccine found in USPHS publication above
Immunizations requiring an update
   Tetanus-diphtheria
   Measles (if born after 1956 and unvaccinated), mumps, and rubella
   Polio
   Influenza/pneumococcal (for elderly and immuno-compromised)
Immunizations for special circumstances
   Hepatitis A immune globulin or vaccine
   Hepatitis B
   Rabies
   Meningococcal vaccine
   Typhoid fever
   Japanese encephalitis

Box 69-3 GUIDELINES DURING TRAVEL PERIODS IN UNDERDEVELOPED COUNTRIES

General recommendations
   Contact U.S. embassy on arrival.
   Avoid ice, unboiled or unbottled water, and uncooked food.
   Avoid wading or swimming in lakes and canals of populous regions.
   Avoid blood transfusions and use of needles. Adhere to safe sex guidelines, especially in Africa and Southeast Asia.

Take necessary precautions against insects, especially mosquitoes:
   Avoid nocturnal travel.
   Use a repellent containing DEET.
   Sleep in a well-screened area.
Initiate recommended chemoprophylaxis based on travel itinerary.
   Malaria: On return, continue medications for another 4 weeks.
   Traveler's diarrhea.

Fitness

HEALTHY PARTICIPANTS. Active, healthy individuals should begin a graduated exercise program at least 2 months before departure to minimize the deleterious effects of muscular, metabolic, and mental fatigue. This is especially important for persons going to high altitude; aerobic capacity in a sedentary person drops about 4% for each 300 m (1000 feet) above the 1200-m (4000-foot) level, but the loss is only half as great in an aerobically fit individual (see Chapter 1). Careful stretching of muscle groups may increase efficiency and lessen the likelihood of soft tissue injury during exertion and minor accidents.

If excessive environmental heat (see Chapters 10 and 11) is anticipated, preparatory exercise in a hot, humid environment (simulated with sweat clothing) for 1 hour daily for at least 7 days before departure will increase plasma volume (aldosterone effect) and sweat rate while lowering myocardial oxygen demand and sweat sodium content. This acclimatization will be lost within a week if not maintained.

PERSONS WITH PREEXISTING MEDICAL PROBLEMS. Participants with preexisting cardiopulmonary disease and those with a few selected medical problems delineated below deserve special attention.

Persons with asthma and chronic obstructive pulmonary disease (COPD) may experience difficulty as a result of hypoxia from high altitude or secondary to reactive airway disease from noxious stimuli. Wheezing during travel may be triggered by exercise undertaken in cold, dry air. Poor air quality, a by-product of fossil fuel burning, along with winds that can "stir up" larger particulate matter such as dust or sand, can be irritating. Besides carrying a β-agonist metered dose inhaler, asthmatic travelers should carry a 2-week course of an oral steroid (e.g., prednisone) plus a broad-spectrum oral antibiotic.

For persons with COPD, concerns relate to outdoor travel at high altitude and alveolar hypoxia. Studies of aircraft pressurized to 8000-foot altitude reveal that persons with moderately severe COPD (forced expiratory volume in 1 second [FEV_1] of less than 50% at sea level) may have significant dyspnea; this serves as an indication regarding the altitude to which such persons can safely travel. Absolute contraindications to high-altitude travel include persons with pulmonary hypertension and cor pulmonale, recent pulmonary embolism, sickle cell disease, and sleep apnea. Persons with mild to moderate COPD who have adequate pulmonary reserve should be advised to not sleep above 3048 m (10,000 feet) because of nocturnal desaturation.

Outdoor adventure travel adversely limits exercise endurance and can provoke angina in persons with underlying heart disease. There is great debate concerning the evaluation and advice a physician should provide to persons with cardiovascular disease. Persons with predictable angina of mild to moderate level may engage in outdoor travel if able to exercise by Bruce protocol for at least 9 minutes; however, such individuals must pace themselves proportionately to the expected declines in available oxygen that limits work capacity at higher altitude (see Chapter 1). As a guideline, activity levels should be titrated to not exceed a heart rate that is roughly 75% of one's ischemic threshold. For persons with unstable angina, congestive heart failure, or valvular disease such as aortic stenosis, vigorous adventure travel is contraindicated.

Other disorders deserve comment. A person with a history of transient ischemic attacks can participate in outdoor travel with attention to proper hydration and use of aspirin to maintain desirable blood viscosity. A person taking a proton pump inhibitor for management of acid reflux has an increased risk for acquiring water-borne enteric infections. As a result, meticulous attention to water quality is essential; dubious drinking water should be both filtered and disinfected (see Chapter 51), with consideration given to carrying a fluoroquinolone to treat diarrhea empirically. Outdoor travel often disrupts normal meal schedules of diabetics. During air travel, an insulin-dependent diabetic should take his or her daily dose of insulin and eat according to the local time (departure) schedule. For a diabetic traveling eastbound across multiple time zones, the day is effectively shortened, so on arrival, the person should eat and administer insulin according to local time but reduce the dose by one third. For travel westbound, the days will be lengthened. A second dose of insulin after 18 hours of travel may be administered following glucose monitoring, if indicated (glucose > 240 mg/dl). Human immunodeficiency virus (HIV) infection should not preclude outdoor travel so long as an HIV-positive person pays meticulous attention to water disinfection and receives immunizations against pneumonia, influenza, hepatitis A, and hepatitis B.

Many prescription drugs predispose to heat, cold, and altitude-related illnesses. Diuretics contract intravascular volume and may thus impair heat transfer to the skin or may exacerbate dehydration and hypokalemia resulting from fluid loss from exertion or diarrhea. Such persons should carry a packaged electrolyte replacement (oral rehydration solution) and a source of potassium (dried orange slices or bananas). The anticholinergic action of antihistamines, phenothiazines, and tricyclic antidepressants may result in hypothalamic dysfunction and diminished sweating. Whenever possible, alternative preparations should be considered for use during wilderness travel. Alcohol should generally be avoided because it induces peripheral vasodilation and may lead to net heat gain in hot environments and excessive heat losses in cool, windy, or wet conditions. In addition, alcohol's effects on judgment and sensory perception may result in failure to acknowledge early symptoms of environmental illness.

Patients with serious medical allergies or active illnesses should have an appropriate medical identification bracelet, anklet, medallion, or wallet card and store their personal medications in a protected but accessible location in their pack. Persons with cardiac disease should carry a copy of their most recent electrocardiogram. Everyone should carry a complete medicine list in some form during foreign travel.

Oral Hygiene and Health. Mild sore throat and a foul taste are common when traveling in the mountains and in cool weather, probably because of mouth breathing and enhanced loss of moisture from the upper respiratory tract. Carry a supply of hard candies or medicated lozenges (e.g., Cepacol, Chloraseptic). Saline spray may be used to keep nasal passages hydrated.

Since treatment of early caries and loose fillings (which may trap expanding air) can prevent this, each party member should have a dental examinations before the trip. On the trail, frequent brushing may be impractical; flossing after meals, rinsing well with water, and chewing sugar-free gum will help maintain oral hygiene en route. Toothache is common at high altitude. Temporary filling materials, such as Cavit (see Chapter 23), can be obtained in small squeeze tubes and applied to a tooth with a wet cotton applicator to prevent sticking.

Urine containers may be appropriate if prolonged adverse weather is a possibility. Funnel-like devices that connect to urine containers (e.g., Lady-J, available from Campmor; see Appendix B) are helpful for women. Groups camping in a delicate ecology or when close to a lake or river should use a lightweight, portable commode with disposable plastic holding bags.

Hikers whose feet sweat excessively may benefit from talc or medicated powder (e.g., tolnaftate; see Table 69-2). Keeping feet and socks dry minimizes the tendency to blister formation and reduces heat loss in the cold.

Travelers to cold and aquatic environments are especially prone to dry skin. Regular application of a lubricating lotion such as Eucerin, Lubriderm, or Keri lotion may help forestall microtrauma and epidermal cracking.

Education in First Aid and Wilderness Safety. Participants should be encouraged to take general courses in first aid and wilderness safety. Agencies that offer general and specialized training in skiing, mountaineering, river-rafting, and other types of wilderness medicine are listed in Appendix C. Locally organized programs may be found through the American Red Cross, sporting goods stores, and continuing education departments of local colleges.

Before departure, the trip coordinator should review the emergency supplies with the rest of the group. The proper use of mechanical devices should be demonstrated, and indications for the use of medications should be discussed. Groups planning an extended or high-risk outing may wish to conduct an exercise of mock injury evaluation and management.

Factors in Trip Planning

The primary considerations in planning a trip relate to: (1) the maximum anticipated delay in obtaining medical assistance, (2) duration of an outing, (3) risks imposed by environmental extremes, and (4) hazardous recreational activities that require use of specialized equipment and supplies.

Availability of Medical Care. The longer the maximum anticipated delay in obtaining advanced medical assistance, the more likely the irreversible loss of neurologic function, limb, or life. The anticipated delay must take into account that in very rural areas, the nearest physician or hospital may not be equipped to handle a major wilderness injury or illness. An extreme case example is the planning of emergency access to a recompression chamber for members of a deep-sea diving expedition. A more typical example is a deeply penetrating arm laceration. As the hours pass, the likelihood of infection grows. If the victim can reach advanced medical help within an hour, it will suffice to control bleeding and apply a sterile dressing held in place by improvised cravats or tape. If definitive care is several hours away, irrigation with water containing a topical disinfectant is desirable. If the delay in care will be over 6 hours, a decision will have to be made whether to close the wound in the field or to evacuate the victim to medical care (see Chapter 18). The estimate of the anticipated delay depends on the type of rescue services, method of contact, terrain and weather, and number of able (carrying) persons. Party members should agree in advance on simple emergency distress signals, such as whistle or flashlight bursts in groups of three. Usually, uninjured party members have to make contact with outside agencies.

Manually evacuating the victim is an option but requires a relatively mobile victim or at least six carriers if the victim is immobilized. In this regard, it is important to know whether other groups might be trekking in the same vicinity. If access is controlled by permit, the administering agency should be asked about the itinerary of neighboring parties. The decision to carry a victim out must be based on a realistic appraisal of the hours it would take messengers to reach aid vs. a manual evacuation effort to traverse the greatest distance or worst foreseeable weather and terrain.

Trip Duration. The likelihood of mishap rises as the trip duration increases. This is partly attributable to unpredictable weather and the cumulative effects of fatigue and overuse syndromes. In addition, long trips usually involve extensive planning, significant financial investment, and time away from work. Party members are therefore reluctant to cut the trip short and are more willing to continue in the face of mild medical disability and equipment failure. Groups planning to be away from civilization for more than a week should have a maximally diversified list of medical and contingency items.

Environment and Risk of Activities. Weather, terrain, and activity interact and increase the risk of illness or injury. Particularly hazardous combinations include winter climbing, mountaineering, skiing, and white-water kayaking. The anticipated ranges of weather and terrain must be figured into estimates of the maximum delay to medical assistance (see earlier discussion). U.S. and global historical summary data indicating temperature ranges, winds, and duration, type, and amount of precipitation can be obtained from the National Climatic Data Center (see Box 69-1 and Appendix C). State and national park services and state climatology offices are also sources of such information about their territories. The National Weather Service office nearest the travel site can provide short-term forecasts and in many regions broadcasts weather information between 162.40 and 162.55 MHz VHF (see Appendix C).

Expedition Travel: Special Equipment and Supplies for High-Risk Groups. Medically trained individuals traveling with a group at high risk of trauma or illness may wish to carry supplies requiring special expertise for proper use (Boxes 69-4 and 69-5). Some of the necessary skills may be acquired in advanced first aid, paramedic, or nursing classes. Intramuscular and intravenous (IV) medications should be administered only by those with formal training in the indications, dosing, and risks of those drugs. Inclusion of a limited supply of emergency oxygen or IV saline may be reasonable to carry for a high-risk expedition. Adequate rehydration can generally be accomplished in a conscious person with a motile bowel using commercially available oral rehydration packets. Thus a comprehensive supply and variety of IV solutions (e.g., antibiotics, pain medicines, dextrose in saline) is predominantly a component of either a medical base support camp or for situations of search and rescue (see Chapter 25). Items such as surgical tools, chest tubes, and mechanical suction devices would be appropriate only for extremely high-risk expeditions and military excursions.

Box 69-4   CHECKLIST FOR HIGH-RISK OUTINGS: DEVICES REQUIRING SPECIAL MEDICAL TRAINING

Airway, nasopharyngeal (impaired mental status; resuscitation)

Cricothyrotomy cannula or catheter (e.g., Abelson cannula—see Appendix B)

Chest tube set (chest trauma; empyema—practical only on major expeditions)

Glucose testing strips and buccally absorbed glucose preparation (if diabetic on trip; strips must be protected from freezing)

Ophthalmoscope with blue filter and fluorescein strips to stain corneal lesions (retinal hemorrhages; anterior eye examination—practical only on expeditions)

Oxygen (hypoxemia, shock, cerebral/pulmonary edema, impaired mental status)

Sphygmomanometer (aneroid, plastic housing—practical only on expeditions)

Stethoscope

Suction device (mechanical) (clearing oral cavity; chest tube drainage—practical only on expeditions)

Surgical tools (practical only on remote expeditions)

Box 69-5   CHECKLIST FOR HIGH-RISK OUTINGS: MEDICATION REQUIRING SPECIAL MEDICAL TRAINING

GENERAL USE

Intravenous (IV) solutions (isotonic) and tubing (for hydration, route for IV medications)

Needles and syringes (for IV hydration and emergency injectables)

Antibiotic, potent oral with wide-spectrum coverage (e.g., ciprofloxacin)* or injectable (ceftriaxone)*

β-Agonist metered-dose inhaler (for asthma, anaphylactic reaction)*

Ophthalmic anesthetic*

HIGH RISK OF INSECT BITES/ALLERGIES

EpiPen*

Diphenhydramine oral (for allergic reaction, mild sedation/insomnia)

Oral corticosteroid*

HIGH RISK OF TRAUMA

Fentanyl patch (Duragesic) applied to skin on chest when mental status precludes oral narcotics*

Alprazolam (Xanax) for sedation*

HIGH RISK OF ALTITUDE ILLNESS

Acetazolamide for mountain sickness*

Corticosteroid oral or injection (e.g., dexamethasone) (cerebral edema)*

Furosemide tablets for pulmonary edema*

Nifedipine for pulmonary edema*

HIGH RISK OF SNOWBLINDNESS

Ophthalmic cycloplegic (e.g., cyclopentolate 1%) (for pain from snowblindness)*

Ophthalmic corticosteroid-antibiotic combination (e.g., Maxitrol) (recommended for short-term use in snowblindness *only* if blue filter ophthalmoscopic examination using fluorescein stain rules out herpetic keratitis)*

---

*See Tables 69-2 and 69-3 for comments on considerations of dispensing medication.

A host of recreational activities have inherent risks that may dictate specialized equipment beyond a basic medical kit. Mountain climbing not only poses a risk from traumatic injury but also subjects the climber to high-altitude illness, thus requiring portable oxygen or a pressure (Gamow) bag for treatment of victims suffering the ill effects of extreme altitude. Extreme cold exposure might dictate the need for technical devices to provide warmed IV fluids and humidified oxygen. Adventures in white-water sports place the participants at risk from freshwater drowning, and such expeditions might consider carrying adjuncts for airway management. Cycling poses soft tissue injuries from abrasions that require occlusive water-based gel dressings for optimal wound care. Travel to underdeveloped nations in which mosquitoes transmit deadly infectious diseases requires specialized equipment, such as protective netting for sleeping and chemical insecticides or repellents. Table 69-1 lists common recreational activities and identifies specialized equipment that may be considered for high-risk expeditions (see Box 69-8).

ASSEMBLING THE MEDICAL KIT

Organizational Levels

The emergency kit may be broken down into five components (see Boxes 69-6 to 69-10): (1) a personal medical kit, (2) a more comprehensive community medical kit, (3) medical kits for expeditions and the medically trained, (4) specialized equipment and supplies to deal with environmental and recreational hazards, and (5) items stored in the vehicle. The components of a well-equipped first-aid medical kit designed for the management of trauma and common medical problems are itemized in Box 69-6. Such a kit consists of nontechnical items that promote wound management and permit stabilization of extremity injuries, while including useful over-the-counter medicines to deal with common medical complaints. For persons without the time or desire to create such a comprehensive medical kit, consideration can be given to a host of commercially packaged wilderness first-aid kits (see Figure 69-1 and Appendix B). Experienced groups involved in high-risk expedition travel having participants with medical knowledge may wish to consider carrying the basics recommended in Box 69-7. Further tailoring of this medical kit may be achieved via the index for expedition travel (Figure 69-2) that helps guide selection of prescription medicines as a function of trip duration and remoteness from medical care.

Items Carried on the Person. The purpose of carrying a minimum amount of items on one's person relates to the ever-present danger of separation from travel partners. A sudden fall, avalanche, or swamping can quickly separate victim and gear. In anticipation of this, experienced wilderness travelers need to carry a bare minimum of items on their person at all times (see Box 69-9). Such supplies provide protection from the elements, permit self-treatment of minor traumatic injuries, and help signal for help for purposes of search and rescue. These typically include assorted adhesive compress strips, knife or razor blade, butane lighter or matches (preferably the waterproof, strike-anywhere type), plastic whistle, small reflective mirror, length of thin nylon

TABLE 69-1. Recreational Activities Requiring Specialized Equipment

RECREATIONAL ACTIVITY	SPECIALIZED EQUIPMENT					
	HIGH ALTITUDE	COLD EXPOSURE	WATER SPORTS	BICYCLING	CLIMBING AND HIKING	THIRD WORLD TRAVEL
Backpacking		X	X		X	
Mountain climbing and expeditions	X	X	X		X	X
Rock climbing					X	
Winter backcountry camping and skiing		X			X	
Cycling				X		
Water sports			X			X
Fishing			X		X	
Hunting		X	X		X	
Search and rescue		X	X		X	
International travel and trekking			X		X	X

Recommended specialized equipment for each recreational activity is denoted by an X in the appropriate column and itemized in Box 69-8. Lists are comprehensive and intended for groups at a distance from medical help or involved in a high-risk adventure; not all items may be needed for low-risk travel. Purchase of specialized equipment should be based on the foundation of a comprehensive medical kit as highlighted in Box 69-6.

Box 69-6 CONTENTS OF A COMPREHENSIVE MEDICAL KIT

WOUND MANAGEMENT

Irrigation syringe with 18-gauge needle
Povidone-iodine solution USP 10%
Wound closure strips
Butterfly closures
Tincture of benzoin
Alcohol pads
Moleskin
Antiseptic towelettes
Scalpel with no. 11 or 15 blade
Latex or non-latex surgical gloves

OVER-THE-COUNTER MEDICATIONS

Acetaminophen (Extra Strength Tylenol)
Ibuprofen 200 mg (Nuprin)
Diphenhydramine (Benadryl)
Pseudoephedrine (Sudafed)
Ranitidine (Zantac 75)
Simethicone (Mylanta II antacid)
Loperamide (Imodium AD)
Rectal glycerine suppositories
Saline eye wash
Glutose paste
Hydrocortisone cream 1%
Tinactin antifungal cream
High-SPF sunscreen and lip balm

Aloe vera gel
Neosporin ointment

BANDAGING MATERIALS

Lamino Trauma Dressing
4 × 4 sterile dressing pads
Eye pad
Cotton-tipped applicators
Nonadherent sterile dressing
Elastic bandage wrap with Velcro closure
Adhesive cloth tape
Band-Aids
3-inch sterile gauze bandage

MISCELLANEOUS EQUIPMENT

Folding scissors
Forceps for removal of splinters and ticks
Thermometer
Cavit temporary dental filling
SAM splint
Triangular bandage and safety pins
Plastic resealable (Zip-Lock) bags

PRESCRIPTION MEDICINES*

Selection function of trip duration/interval to care

*See Tables 69-2 and 69-3.

Box 69-7 CONTENTS OF A MEDICAL KIT FOR EXPEDITIONS AND THE MEDICALLY TRAINED

Comprehensive first-aid kit for the management of trauma (see Box 69-6)
Medical devices requiring specialized training (see Box 69-4)
Appropriate prescription medications for general illness (see Tables 69-2 and 69-3)

Prescription medications for specific injuries/illness (see Box 69-5)
Repair materials (see Table 69-4)
Indicated equipment based on recreational and environmental hazards (see Box 69-8)

Box 69-8 SPECIALIZED EQUIPMENT FOR RECREATIONAL AND ENVIRONMENTAL ACTIVITIES

HIGH ALTITUDE

Gamow Bag and accessories
  Gamow Tent
  Breathing Bladder
  Portable air compressor
EPAP mask with headstrap
Sportstat portable pulse oximeter

COLD EXPOSURE

External thermal stabilizer bag
Res-Q-Air
Hot-Sack IV Warmer
Grabber Warmers
Hotronic Foot Warmers
Space Thermal Reflective Survival Bag
Low-reading thermometer
Adhesive climbing skins
Life-link adjustable ski/probe pole
AvaLung avalanche vest
Tracker DTS (digital transceiving system) avalanche beacon

WATER SPORTS

CPR Microshield
Katadyn or MSR WaterWorks filter

BICYCLING

All-Terrain Cyclist Kit
Hydrogel occlusive dressing

MOUNTAIN CLIMBING AND HIKING

SAM Splint
Air-Stirrup ankle brace

TROPICAL AND THIRD WORLD TRAVEL

Sawyer Extractor
Permethrin repellent
TropicScreen mosquito net
Oral rehydration salts packets

Box 69-9 CONTENTS OF A PERSONAL MEDICAL KIT

ON-PERSON ITEMS

Identification/pencil and notepad
Hat and sunglasses
Topographical map/compass
Swiss Army knife or razor blade
Nylon cord
Whistle and small reflective mirror
Lighter or waterproof matches
Poncho and space blanket
Adhesive compress and tape

Bandanna
Nonperishable high-carbohydrate energy bar

IN-PACK ITEMS

Personal first-aid and hygiene material
Survival guide/first-aid booklet
Prescription medications, labeled (in plastic or water-proof aluminum box)
Over-the-counter medications noted in the comprehensive first-aid kit (see Box 69-6)

Box 69-10 CHECKLIST: RECOMMENDED IN-VEHICLE EMERGENCY SUPPLIES

FIRST-AID KIT

As for trail, but include large burn dressings
Boards for splint construction
Backboard, short or folding long (e.g., Junkin—see Appendix B)

RESCUE AND SURVIVAL

Avalanche probe poles, collapsing*
Bags, large plastic
Blankets, wool and "space" blankets
Climbing rope and hardware†
Candles, long-burning
Flashlight
Food and water (in canteen)
Ice ax†
Matches (waterproof) or lighter
Radio, citizens band
Rope
Saw with metal-cutting blade
Small stove, pot or coffee can, and utensils

Ski climbing skins, snowshoes*
Tarp, plastic
Toilet paper

AUTOMOTIVE

Aluminum foil to cover windows (minimizes heat loss or gain)
Cables to jump battery
Chains with tighteners (with repair links and special pliers)*
Fire extinguisher
Flares, 10-minute (at least six) (can also serve as fire starter)
Gloves
Oil, extra can
Shovel, metal or Lexan with short or collapsing handle
Tool kit (consider inclusion of a small ax)
Tow chain or cable
Wheel chock or wedgeblocks

*Winter weather supplies.
†Mountain terrain supplies (special training needed).

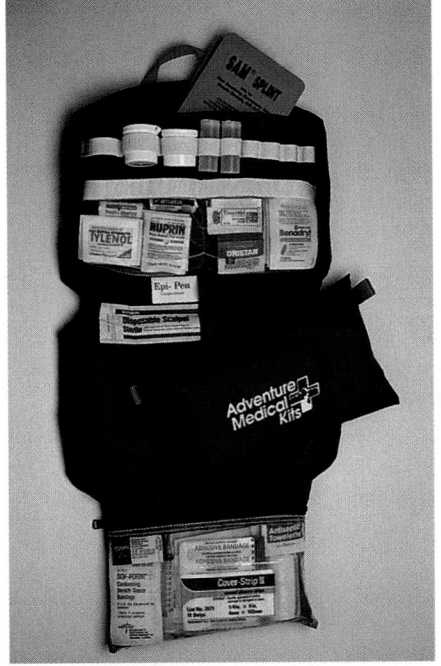

Figure 69-1 Prepackaged wilderness first-aid kits are available from many manufacturers. Kits are neatly organized and rugged, with detachable inner pouches that are useful for day trips. Bags are water resistant to allow for white-water use. A surprisingly large amount of first-aid material can be carried, as shown in the illustration.

Maximal interval to medical care or rescue	Duration of outing: Day outing	2-3 days	>3 days
<4 hours	Topical 1 Systemic 1	Topical 1,2 Systemic 1-3	
4-12 hours	Topical 1 Systemic 1	Topical 1-3 Systemic 1-5	Topical 1-5 Systemic 1-9
>12 hours		Topical 1-4 Systemic 1-6	Topical 1-7 Systemic 1-16

Figure 69-2 Recommendations for prescription medicines for expedition travel based on the duration of outing (vertical columns) and the maximum interval to medical care (horizontal rows). Itemized numbers refer to recommended topical and systemic medicines found in Tables 69-2 and 69-3, respectively.

cord, and bandanna (which can double as a cravat or sling). A nonperishable source of quick high-energy food may be of value during isolation to maintain strength. These items can be compactly stored inside a plastic bag or small stuff sack and may be carried in either a pocket or a small fannypack (zippered, passport-size waist belts are comfortable and inexpensive). As noted previously, all travelers should carry some form of identification, and those with serious medical allergies or active illnesses should have an appropriate medical alert bracelet, anklet, medallion, or wallet card. Those with a history of bee, wasp, or other anaphylactic allergy should carry at least two preloaded syringes of 1:1000 aqueous epinephrine solution (EpiPen; Ana-Kit) in a cool dark compartment and should inform others in the party of the medicine's location and proper usage.

Personal Items Carried in the Pack. Certain basic contingency "essentials" should be carried on virtually every venture. In addition to one's personal first-aid, hygiene, and clothing items, a flashlight, coins for telephone calls, and extra pair of sunglasses are recommended. Extra clothing, food, and water should be carried in proportion to the risk associated with the trip.

A host of over-the-counter medications may be useful for wilderness travel, especially for low-risk outings of short duration. Some commonly required nonprescription items that may be of value are listed in Box 69-6. Of prime importance is the control of pain associated with trauma. For mild to moderate pain, aspirin, acetaminophen, or a nonsteroidal antiinflammatory drug is effective. Decongestants are helpful in treating symptoms associated with upper respiratory infections, and their antihistaminic effects are useful for the treatment of allergies and insomnia. Gastrointestinal complaints necessitate antacids and an antidiarrheal agent.

Saline eyewash is helpful for irritated eyes and in removing foreign objects. Antiseptic cream or ointment is useful in treating superficial infections of the skin, and a steroid ointment is of value for treatment of certain rashes or contact dermatitis. Aloe vera gel is useful for treatment of frostbite and injuries from burns or excessive sun exposure.

Frequently needed first-aid material and personal medications are carried in stuff sacks or plastic box containers. Medication containers should be stored in an accessible but thermally and physically protected location in each individual's pack because capsules and suppositories may melt if exposed to extreme heat. Dressings, bandages, and adhesive materials should be kept in a plastic bag within their container to protect them from moisture.

Medications should be stored in unit dose sheets or screw-top plastic bottles labeled with the patient's and physician's names, generic and trade drug names, dispensing information, and expiration date. Medications requiring a prescription with directions for their use (Tables 69-2 and 69-3) should be secured in a watertight plastic or aluminum box. The trip coordinator should ask each member of the party to check that any expired medications are replaced and that capsules and suppositories are intact.

Community Supplies Carried in the Pack. As mentioned previously, traumatic injuries represent the greatest concern during wilderness travel. A comprehensive medical kit is the most important community item (see Box 69-6). Emphasis is placed on the management of wounds and stabilization of injuries through appropriate bandaging. Suture material is not recommended on the list of items because of the likelihood of subsequent infection. Large wounds are best treated with sterile pressure dressings.

Bulky and heavy items, including most stock first-aid and contingency supplies, should be labeled and distributed among the members of the group for storage and transport. A cross made from strips of tape or cloth should be placed on the pack overlying the compartment containing the first-aid items. This allows ready access by any member of the party in an emergency situation. Repair materials are best kept in clearly labeled stuff sacks, or aluminum or plastic boxes independent of the first-aid and medical supplies.

Items Stored in the Vehicle. A complete emergency kit in the vehicle (see Box 69-10) is highly recommended. It will facilitate further stabilization of an injured person evacuated to a trailhead. The vehicle kit should also provide material necessary to deal with accidents encountered along the highway and to cope with the environment if the occupants are stranded by automotive trouble or natural disaster. Several large burn dressings and a neckboard with strapping will fit in a standard trunk or other recess. Although only large vehicles can accommodate the usual full-length backboard, a folding backboard is now available from Junkin Safety Appliance Co. (see Appendix B). The remaining contents of an emergency kit will fit in a medium (6 inches W × 12 inches L × 9 inches H) or large (8 inches W × 18 inches L × 14 inches H) war surplus ammunition box or a toolbox of similar size.

Selecting Contingency Supplies: Advanced Expedition Planning

Individuals with medical training involved with risky wilderness travel may opt to tailor their own medical kit. Adventurous expeditions may wish to include a host of prescription medications that require advanced knowledge (see Box 69-5) and carry special devices requiring medical training (see Box 69-4). In addition, specialized equipment to handle expected environ-

mental and recreational hazards should be considered (see Box 69-8). An appropriate emergency kit is adequate in content but not too heavy or bulky. Attempting to carry all possible medical supplies and equipment to handle any conceivable emergency is not practical.

An alternative approach is as follows: Assess the group's trip risk on the basis of proximity to support (a function of interval to medical care) and comfort level of handling unanticipated traumatic injury or medical illness (cumulative probability related to trip duration). Figure 69-2 itemizes recommended prescription medicines as highlighted in boxes formed by the intersection of the latter two factors in bold. Specialized equipment purchases (Box 69-8) are then added on as dictated by unique recreational activities (Table 69-1).

Using a Wilderness Index. The wilderness index for expedition travel serves to assist group participants with advanced first aid or medical training in the selection of appropriate prescription medications. The latter serve to augment the contents of the comprehensive medical kit that includes only over-the-counter medicines. In Figure 69-2 a unique "square" of recommended prescription medicines is found at the intersection of the horizontal row "Duration of Outing" and the vertical column "Maximum Interval to Medical Care." Numbers refer to specific medical items, topical and systemic, found in Tables 69-2 and 69-3, respectively. The drug doses listed in Table 69-3 are intended for nonpregnant, young, or middle-aged adults in good health. Reduced doses are often necessary for children, the elderly, and those with end-organ disease (especially renal, hepatic, and cardiac). The personal physician should modify the doses appropriately.

The rationale for medicine selection among a host of prescribed items is based on one's expected time frame for support and rescue in the event of unexpected injury and the cumulative likelihood of experiencing a medical illness as trip duration increases. A low-risk outing (e.g., a day hike) is one in which the interval to medical care is short (<4 hours) and trip duration (<1 day) places one at low likelihood of acquiring a medical illness. Therefore expectations for a prompt rescue and medical support preclude the need to carry most prescription medicines, since traumatic injury or a life-threatening allergic reaction become of prime concern. In such circumstances, pain control and management of anaphylaxis take precedence. A moderate-risk trek (e.g., a 1-day "ski-in" with 2 nights winter camping) will have an interval to medical care that is longer (4 to 12 hours) and a trip duration that increases chances for medical illness. With a "ski-out" time of 4 to 12 hours plus added time to return with organized help, expectations are that an ill group member will not receive sophisticated rescue efforts until the following day. In such instances,

TABLE 69-2. Topical Medications for Wilderness Travel

CLASSIFICATION*	RECOMMENDED	EXAMPLES/ BRANDS	INDICATIONS	CONTRA- INDICATIONS
1. Corticosteroid cream, potent topical	High-potency fluorinated compounds (e.g., betamethasone, fluocinolone, halcinonide)	Synalar-HP 0.2% Diprosone 0.05% Lidex 0.05%	Rash, swelling due to plant (poison oak, ivy) contact and insect bites	Minimize application to skin of face and groin
2. Antibiotic, ophthalmic	Sulfonamide-containing preparation	Sulamyd 10% ointment	Conjunctivitis; snowblindness; corneal abrasion	Known allergy to sulfonamides
3. Corticosteroid-antibiotic combination, ophthalmic ointment	Dexamethasone with neomycin and polymyxin	Maxitrol	To reduce inflammatory pain due to snowblindness; to temporarily control disabling allergic conjunctivitis	
4. Cycloplegic, ophthalmic	Cyclopentolate 1%	Cyclogyl 1%	To reduce pain (relaxes iris) due to snowblindness	
5. Antibiotic/ antiinflammatory, ear canal	Antimicrobial plus hydrocortisone 1%	Acetic acid 2% plus hydrocortisone 1% (VoSol HC)	Ear pain (worsened by pulling, itching, discharge)	Allergy to ingredients (R); suspected perforation of eardrum (R in adults)
6. Anesthetic, ophthalmic	Proparacaine 0.5%	Ophthaine, Ophthetic	To facilitate eye examination for foreign body, abrasion, or burn	
7. Fluorescein strips, ophthalmic	Fluorescein	Fluoro-I-Strip	To distinguish herpetic keratitis, foreign body, corneal abrasions, and corneal burn (snowblindness)	

C, Common, >10%; O, occasional, 1%-10%; R, rare, <1%; D, dose-related.
*Numbers refer to the classification scheme in Figure 69-2.

narcotics to control pain, an antibiotic to prevent infection from soft tissue injuries, and antiemetics or antidiarrheals to control gastrointestinal upset and preserve fluid and electrolyte balances become paramount. A high-risk outing (e.g., a weeklong expedition with mountain climbing) precludes seeking formal help within a 12-hour period and has a long trip duration, with the added challenge of encountering bothersome medical illness. With such an expedition, nonthreatening problems (e.g., athlete's foot, infected blisters, dermatitis, asthma, bronchitis, sinusitis) are apt to occur, limiting performance and enjoyment. Besides carrying those medicines noted above for low- and moderate-risk treks, one should have treatments to manage more persistent medical illness, to include a full course of oral antibiotics for upper respiratory, abdominal, and soft tissue infections, oral and potent topical steroids for dermatologic problems, and assorted ophthalmic and otic medications to deal with bothersome infections or allergic reactions of vital sensory organs.

SIDE EFFECT	DOSAGE (ADULT)	QUANTITY	ALTERNATIVE DRUGS	COMMENTS
Worsening of some infections (short-term)	Rub in thoroughly 2-3 times daily while skin is still moist after washing, as needed for itching	15 g per 4-6 people (group)	Oral antihistamines; also apply cold compress or soaks	Not helpful for sunburn; if rash worsens, discontinue corticosteroid and consider fungus; consider oral steroid for contact dermatitis involving face, groin, or more than 25% of body surface
Transient stinging (C); allergic reaction (R)	Deposit inside lower lid every 4 hr and at bedtime	Smallest tube (individual)	Polymixin B-bacitracin (Polysporin)	Avoid topical preparation of systemic drugs (e.g., penicillins, tetracycline, gentamicin) and neomycin because sensitization could lead to future reaction
Short-term use only (1-2 days) to minimize risk of superinfection	Instill in eye(s) 2-3 times daily for pain control	Tube (group)	TobraDex (dexamethasone plus tobramycin)	Neosporin may sensitize to some systemic antibiotics
	One drop in eye(s) 1-3 times daily for pain control	Bottle (group)		
Local irritation, allergic reaction (R)	Four drops into ear (keep upward for 5 min) 4 times daily for 7 days	10-ml bottle (individual)	Antibacterial (usually Neosporin-HC combinations) (Corticosporin; otic Neo-Cort-Dome; Coly-Mycin)	Neosporin may sensitize to some systemic antibiotics
Allergic reaction (R); corneal toxicity with repeated use	One to two drops onto eye	Bottle (group)	Tetracaine 0.5%	
Systemic reaction (R)	Moisten fluorescein strips with sterile water and place inside lower lid; close the eyelid tightly until staining achieved, then remove strip	Several strips (group)		Need a blue-filtered penlight to best detect the bright-green fluorescence of exposed tissue

A Sample Journey. The month is April and the goal is a 21-mile round-trip cross-country ski tour to the top of Mt. Whitney (elevation 4418 m [14,495 feet]) in the Sierra Nevada mountains. The team consists of four cross-country skiers who have completed an American Red Cross advanced first-aid course and an avalanche seminar offered to the public by the National Ski Patrol System. The trip duration will be 3 days and 2 nights, depending on weather and snow conditions. The base camp will be at 3810 m (12,500 feet). Were a skier to be-come disabled en route, one of the others would remain with the victim while the remaining two would ski out to the nearest telephone or source of help (no longer than an 8-hour downhill ski from the farthest point along the route). Helicopter evacuation to the nearest hospital would usually be accomplished within the next 2 to 4 hours, making the maximum interval to medical care within 12 hours. The trip poses risks related to trauma, cold injury, avalanche danger, snow-blindness, and high-altitude illness. With the possibility

Text continued on p. 1678

TABLE 69-3. Systemic Medication for Wilderness Travel

CLASSIFICATION*	RECOMMENDED	EXAMPLES/ BRANDS	INDICATIONS	CONTRAINDICATIONS†
1. Epinephrine, intramuscular	Auto-injecting epinephrine for injection; a single dose delivered from the auto-injector	EpiPen	Emergency intramuscular use to treat anaphylactic reaction to stinging insects, medication, or foods	None for short-term use in indicated setting
2. Acetazolamide	Acetazolamide	Diamox	Prevention and treatment of acute mountain sickness (headache, sleep disturbance, lassitude, nausea, incoordination)	Concurrent diuretic medications; sulfa allergy *Caution:* Toxicity (confusion, lethargy, incontinence) may develop with the concomitant use of aspirin or Pepto-Bismol
3. Corticosteroid, oral	Prednisone	Prednisone, generic	Anaphylaxis or severe or disseminated allergic reactions (including contact dermatitis); severe asthma; moderate cerebral edema	None for short-term use in indicated setting
4. Analgesic, oral narcotic	Acetaminophen 500 mg with hydrocodone (5 or 7.5 mg)	Vicodin, Lortab	Moderate to severe pain; severe cough	Respiratory difficulty, head injury; other sedative drugs or alcohol; narcotic allergy
5. Antibiotic, oral for skin, respiratory, or urinary infection	Amoxicillin 500 mg with clavulanate 125 mg	Augmentin	Infection: skin, respiratory, urinary	If allergic to penicillin, consider cephalexin, trimethoprim/ sulfamethoxazole, or levofloxacin
6. Antibiotic, oral, for traveler's diarrhea	Ciprofloxacin 750 mg	Cipro	Prolonged loose stooling and cramps, fever and weakness	
7. Antiemetic/ antinausea, rectal suppository	Promethazine 25 mg suppository	Phenergan	Severe nausea, vomiting	Hypothermia; heavy sedation from injury, illness, or other drugs; high fever; known phenothiazine allergy
8. Sedative, oral	Alprazolam 0.125 mg	Xanax	Sleeplessness; anxiety, severe jet lag; muscle spasm	Coexisting sedation from alcohol, drugs, illness

C, Common, <10%; O, occasional, 1%-10%; R, rare, <1%; D, dose-related.
*Numbers refer to the classification scheme in Figure 69-2.
†Allergy, pregnancy, and breast-feeding are always assumed contraindications, unless otherwise indicated.
‡Doses listed in Table 69-3 are intended for nonpregnant, young, or middle-aged adults in good health. In all situations, the traveler's personal physician should recommend appropriate doses.
§Traveler's diarrhea is usually mild and subsides spontaneously within 4 days—reserve antibiotics for indications above and for treatment of dysentery (blood and mucus). During diarrhea, avoid milk products and solids, but maintain fluid intake and electrolytes—the U.S. Public Health Service recommends drinking alternately from each glass: (1) 8 oz fruit juice with ½ tsp honey, corn syrup, or sugar with a pinch of table salt, and (2) 8 oz carbonated or boiled water with ¼ tsp baking soda. Alternatively, packets of electrolyte powder (to mix with water) may be useful for isolated, high-risk travel.

SIDE EFFECTS	DOSAGE (ADULT)‡	QUANTITY (PER TRIP)	ALTERNATIVE DRUGS	COMMENTS
Tremulousness, agitation, palpitations, arrhythmia	Each autoinjection contains 0.3 mg (0.3 ml) of epinephrine 1:1000; inject into deltoid or anterior thigh, every 1-2 hr as needed.	1 (individual)	Antihistamine (e.g., diphenhydramine) for mild reaction with no history of prior anaphylaxis	
Tingling (C); fatigue, drowsiness, nausea (O)	*Prevention:* 62.5-125 mg every 12 hr, or 500 mg sustained action capsule, for 1 day before and 1-2 days into ascent *Treatment:* 250 mg every 8-12 hr as needed for up to 48 hr	10-12 tablets (individual)	Oxygen is helpful but not curative; potent diuretics not recommended for acute mountain sickness	Best treatment for severe acute mountain sickness is descent by at least 2000 feet
Agitation, mood disturbance, fluid retention (O); others (R) with short-term use	Prednisone 10-mg tablets in a tapering fashion: 4-6 tablets once to twice daily for 2-3 days, dropping by half every 2-3 days, depending on severity of illnes	40 tablets (individual)	Methylprednisolone 4 mg, dexamethasone 1 mg	Drug treatment for cerebral edema does *not* substitute for prompt descent of at least 2000 feet
Respiratory depression and hypotension (D); drowsiness, vomiting, constipation (C); rash (R)	1-2 tablets every 4-6 hr as needed	12-24 tablets (individual)	Other acetaminophen/opiate combinations	
Abdominal pain, nausea, diarrhea, delayed vaginal infection (O)	1-2 tablets every 8 hr for at least 5 days	21 tablets (individual)	Cephalexin 500 mg 4 times daily, trimethoprim/ sulfamethoxazole DS twice daily, or levofloxacin 500 mg twice daily	
	1 twice daily for 3-5 days	10 tablets (individual)	Trimethoprim/ sulfamethoxazole DS twice daily	See footnote§
Sedation (D); dry mouth, blurred vision (O)	25 mg suppository per rectum every 8 hr as needed	6 suppositories (individual)	Prochlorperazine 25 mg or trimethobenzamide 200 mg suppositories	Keep suppositories protected from heat and pressure
Drowsiness, dizziness (D); loss of coordination (O); anterograde amnesia (R)	1-4 tablets every 6 hr as needed	12 tablets (individual)	Other short-to-medium duration benzodiazepines	

TABLE 69-3. Systemic Medication for Wilderness Travel—cont'd

CLASSIFICATION*	RECOMMENDED	EXAMPLES/ BRANDS	INDICATIONS	CONTRAINDICATIONS†
9. Asthma inhaler	Albuterol MDI	Proventil; Ventolin (17-g metered-dose inhalers)	Wheezing, cough in setting of cold air or bronchitis	None for short-term use in indicated setting
10. Antibiotics, extended spectrum	Ceftriaxone for intramuscular injection; ciprofloxacin (above) plus metronidazole (below)	Rocephin injectable; Cipro (above); Flagyl	Severe infection with fever, change in mental status, overwhelming infection	None for short-term use in indicated setting
11. Corticosteroid, for intravenous injection	Dexamethasone	Decadron phosphate, 4 mg/ml in prefilled 2.5-ml syringes	High-altitude cerebral edema; anaphylaxis in poorly responsive person	None for short-term use in indicated setting
12. Diuretic, for intravenous injection	Furosemide	Lasix, 10 mg/ml in 4-ml syringes	High-altitude cerebral edema or pulmonary edema	Known sulfa allergy; severe dehydration, volume loss, or hemorrhage
13. Nifedipine	Nifedipine	Procardia or generic, 30-mg sustained-release tablets	High-altitude pulmonary edema (lowers pulmonary artery pressure by causing arterial dilatation)	Severe dehydration, volume loss, or hemorrhage
14. Amphetamine stimulant	Dextroamphetamine 5 mg	Dexedrine	Life-threatening mental fatigue	None in indicated setting
15. Opiate analgesic patch	Fentanyl patch	Duragesic Transdermal System, 20 cm² patch containing 5 mg of fentanyl (releasing 50 µg/hour)	Severe, prolonged (>24 hr) painful disorder or injury	Bowel obstruction, preexisting respiratory depression or difficulty breathing, head injury with impaired consciousness
16. Antibiotic for giardiasis and amebiasis	Metronidazole 500 mg	Flagyl	Profuse diarrhea delayed >2 weeks (*Giardia* suspected), or dysentery in areas endemic for *Entamoeba histolytica* (amebiasis suspected)	None for short-term use in indicated setting

C, Common, <10%; *O*, occasional, 1%-10%; *R*, rare, <1%; *D*, dose-related.

SIDE EFFECTS	DOSAGE (ADULT)	QUANTITY (PER TRIP)	ALTERNATIVE DRUGS	COMMENTS
Tremulousness, palpitations (D)	2 inhalations every 4 hr as needed	1 inhaler (individual)	Metaproterenol metered-dose inhaler	Long-acting metered-dose inhalers not recommended for this situation
Nausea/vomiting, abdominal pain, diarrhea (O); rash, other reactions (R) NOTE: avoid ceftriaxone in those with history of immediate allergy to pencillins	Rocephin: into 1 g powder vial inject 3.6 ml of sterile water or 1% lidocaine (without epinephrine); inject 1-2 g every 24 hr deeply into gluteus or lateral thigh muscles	Ceftriaxone: 4-8 vials (group)	Combination of oral amoxicillin-clavulanate and metronidazole; imipenem-cilastatin 750 mg powder vial diluted with 3 ml 1% lidocaine, given twice daily intramuscularly	Consider Rocephin for remote expeditions
Agitation, mood disturbance (O); others (R) with short-term use	2.5 ml (10 mg) intravenously every 6-8 hr as needed	8 syringes (group)		Requires medical, nursing, or paramedic training for direct intravenous injection
Dehydration, low sodium and potassium (potential cardiac irritability) (D)	1 to 4 ml (10 to 40 mg) intravenously every 6-8 hr as needed	4 tablets (group)	Ethacrynic acid (nonsulfa); bumetanide (neither available in pre-filled syringes)	Requires medical, nursing, or paramedic training for direct intravenous injection
Hypotension (especially if volume depleted), flushing, weakness, headache, syncope, palpitations, dizziness, lightheadedness (D)	*Prevention:* 1 tablet every 12 hr for first 72 hr of ascent *Treatment:* 1 tablet every 8 hr times three	24 tablets (group)		Treatment of high-altitude pulmonary edema with nifedipine is only recommended if descent is not immediately possible, for limited periods (24 hr) with monitoring of blood pressure required
Stimulation (D); anorexia (C); GI disturbance (C); tremors and headache (O)	5-10 mg every 4-6 hr as needed	6 tablets (individual)	Methylphenidate (Ritalin) 5 mg tablets	Only for high-risk conditions in remote regions
Respiratory depression, constipation (D); sinus bradycardia and hypotension, nausea/vomiting, itching (O)	1-2 patches applied every 3 days to a nonirritated, clean and dry area on the upper torso	4 patches (individual)		May require a full day to become effective, so rely on short-acting opiates during first day
Nausea; vomiting, metallic taste (C) abdominal discomfort (O)	*Giardiasis:* 1 tablet 3 times daily for 5 days *Amebiasis:* 750 mg 3 times daily for 10 days (followed by 3 weeks of iodoquinol 650 mg 3 times daily)	15-90 tablets (individual)	*Giardiasis:* albendazole (400 mg daily for 5 days)	In areas of ascariasis, hookworm, and trichuriasis: mebendazole (100 mg twice daily for 3 days); for strongyloidiasis: thiabendazole (25 mg/kg twice daily for 3 days); for common tape-worms: niclosamide (1 g, repeat in 1 hr)

TABLE 69-4. Repair Supplies to Consider for Wilderness Travel

ITEM	DESCRIPTION, QUANTITY, WEIGHT*	COMMENT
Needle or sewing awl	With heavy thread (1 oz)	Clothing, pack repair
Screwdrivers	Flat and Phillips No. 2 (3-6 oz)	For skis, No. 3 "posidrive" (or filed-down No. 2 Phillips)
Tape, duct or reinforced strapping	1-2 inches wide, 5 yards (2 oz) (per person per trip)	
Wire	Braided steel, 3-6 ft (2 oz)	Repair of binding, boot, snowshoe, and pack
Awl	On multifunction knife (2 oz) (per person per trip)	Repair of clothing, pack, shelter
Visegrip pliers	5-inch (5-8 oz)	
Glue	Two-component epoxy, or meltable nylon glue stick (1 oz)	
Spare bale and screws	Two	Repair of ski binding
"P-tex" ski base stick	Meltable No. 1 (1 oz)	Repair of plastic ski base
Spare ski tip	Plastic or aluminum (3-5 oz)	
Spare crampon wrench	No. 1 (one)	
Knife sharpener	Diamond-bar, ceramic, or stone (2-3 oz)	

*Quantity is per group unless specified; weight given is per individual item, in ounces (35 oz = 1 kg = 2.2 lb).

of an overnight stay until rescue arrives, medicine selection focuses on pain control for traumatic injury. Appropriate topical medicines include those for managing corneal injury from snowblindness. Systemic medicines of value include a limited supply of antibiotics to prevent infection of soft tissue injuries plus specialized medicines for prevention and treatment of acute mountain sickness. The following steps refer to the index for expedition travel (see Figure 69-2).

1. Determine the maximum interval to medical care. In the example given, "4-12 hours" would be found at the left of the figure, representing the square denoting the intersecting horizontal row.
2. Determine the trip duration. In the example, "2-3 days" would be found at the figure's top and denote the corresponding vertical column of intersection.
3. Find the "square" itemizing recommended topical and systemic medicines. On the index, the intersection of the horizontal and vertical columns defines a square suggesting prescription items. Note the reference numbers listed and find the suggested medicines in the tables recommended in the figure legend.

Finally, emphasis must be placed on the recreational and environmental hazards likely to be encountered during travel. In this example, the dangers relate mainly to high altitude and cold exposure. Specialized equipment that may be of value under the conditions described is listed in Box 69-8. Because of proximity to a medical center able to provide prompt helicopter evacuation, a Gamow Bag would not be mandated for

the treatment of high-altitude illness. In addition, the need to carry technical equipment to provide warmed IV solutions or humidified oxygen is offset by a prompt helicopter rescue. However, frostbite can occur rapidly, and an individual might wish to carry a Grabber Warmer because of its low weight and ease of packing (see section for product descriptions). Additionally, certain repair equipment should be carried, as denoted in Table 69-4.

Eyewear (see also Chapter 22)

The appropriate use of sunglasses and goggles will protect eyes from sunlight, wind, and dust. The major variables to consider when buying sunglasses are durability and safety, light transmission, photochromicity (darkening with increasing sun intensity), and polarization. Lenses for aquatic, desert, snow, and high-altitude use should absorb 85% to 95% of visible light and essentially all (greater than 99%) ultraviolet (UV) radiation. This degree of visible light absorption can be easily achieved with polycarbonate, glass, or plastic lenses. (The wilderness trekker may need to carry another, less dark pair for use while driving a vehicle.) Most outdoor equipment retailers offer a wide selection of nonprescription lenses. In addition, customized lens/frame combinations can be obtained from an eye-care specialist in nonprescription or prescription configurations. Soft contact lenses that absorb UV radiation are also available.

Although plastic lenses are lightweight, they scratch more readily than other materials (despite improved coatings) and are generally not recommended for extensive wilderness trekking. Glass lenses are available with the best photochromic properties and can be coated for greater than 99% UV absorption, but they are heavy, susceptible to breakage, and moderately susceptible to scratching. The most durable lenses are made of polycarbonate and are lightweight and shatterproof. In addition, polycarbonate lenses absorb greater than 99% of UV light and, in just the past few years, have become available with photochromicity, polarization, and antireflective coatings. For these reasons, polycarbonate is presently the preferred material for serious wilderness sports. Polycarbonate models that absorb at least 99% UV are manufactured under such brand names as All Weather, Bolle, Coyote (polarized), Gargoyles, Gentex, Learjet, Ski-Optics, Suncloud, Transitions (photochromic), and Wings.

Polarization decreases reflected solar glare from horizontal water, snow, and ice surfaces and is highly desirable for winter mountaineering, skiing, and aquatic wilderness sports. Polarized lenses are now available in many colors. An external clip-on flip-up plastic polarizer can be added to any lenses. These clip-on polarizers absorb an additional 50% of the remaining transmitted light (increasing visible light absorption from, say, 90% to 95%) and may be of additional benefit in very bright conditions.

Frame construction is an important feature for extended wilderness travel. Frames should be composed of nylon, Lexan, silicone-graphite, or metal, rather than plastic. High-impact frames (such as RecSpecs) with polycarbonate lenses are available for hazardous sports, such as climbing, white-water venturing, and hang-gliding. Frames with springs are break-resistant and self-adjusting. Frame hinges should have a bolt and nut rather than a pin. For extended wilderness use, nuts should be sealed with Locktite and pins sealed with cyanoacrylate glue.

Other considerations include optical gradient and mirroring, frame construction, color, peripheral features, and price. Gradient lenses may be darker (or mirrored) at the top or bottom to preferentially block direct or reflected sunlight, respectively. This feature is desirable for aquatic, desert, and high-altitude travel but probably unnecessary for most backpacking activity. The choice of lens color is based largely on personal preference. Although yellow or rose lenses may appear to enhance contrast or hazy (flat) light conditions, research studies have found no consistent benefit. Sunglass models with side shields and nose protectors are recommended for snow, desert, and aquatic terrain. Retention (neck) straps are recommended for any activity involving climbing or skiing. For water sports, a lanyard may be attached from the frame over the back to a belt loop. A pair of high-quality sunglasses from an outdoor retailer generally costs between $50 and $170 (the more expensive models are often priced for their fash-ionable appearance rather than optical merit). Sunglasses with a custom configuration from an eyecare specialist can cost up to $250.

Because the technology is rapidly evolving, the serious outdoor traveler may have difficulty finding an outdoor retailer with the "ideal" pair of sunglasses: polycarbonate lens with 100% UV and greater than 85% visible light absorption, polarization, photochromicity, antireflective coating, and springing nylon frame. It may be worthwhile to consult an eyecare specialist to research the latest products and customize the features to suit your needs.

Medical Supplies

Wound Care Material. Needles and other surgical tools may be crudely "sterilized" by being rubbed vigorously with a prepackaged towelette containing alcohol, chlorhexidine (Hibistat), povidone-iodine (Betadine), or benzalkonium chloride. After the instruments are rubbed with alcohol or Hibistat towelettes, the residual alcohol can be ignited for additional effect. Flame sterilization to red hot may also be acceptable. A less efficient method is to immerse the tool in boiling water for about the same duration recommended to disinfect water for drinking.

Forcefully ejecting irrigant solution from a 20- or 35-ml syringe through an 18- or 19-gauge needle generates pressures adequate to dislodge bacteria and microscopic particles from contaminated wound surfaces. Unfortunately, the literature does not specify how "clean" an irrigant solution must be. Since the primary goal of irrigation is the removal of debris, it seems reasonable that water pure enough to drink should be adequate for irrigation, especially if povidone-iodine solution to achieve a 1% to 10% concentration is added.

Significant advances in wound care include Tegaderm adhesive dressings and Spenco 2nd Skin. Tegaderm is a transparent 3×3-inch adhesive covering for clean wounds that provides a barrier to water, dust, and dirt while allowing oxygen to penetrate. It can be left in place for several days provided that no wound complications arise. Spenco 2nd Skin is a polyethylene oxide gel laminate for placement over blistering skin and burns. 2nd Skin reduces friction damage to the underlying skin and may offer additional protection by redistributing pressure and absorbing exudate. It is an excellent product to carry, especially for bicycling, in which abrasion injuries are common.

Topical Medications. Sweat, water, wind, dirt, and friction inherent in wilderness travel diminish the efficacy of topical sunscreens and corticosteroids. For this reason, sunscreen products containing methoxycinnamates in combination with oxybenzones are recommended to provide high substantivity, or "staying power" (see Chapter 14). A sunscreen sun protection factor (SPF) of at least 15 is recommended for wilderness travel by anyone even mildly susceptible to sunburn, since the goal is to prevent the burn entirely.

Topical corticosteroids are especially useful for contact dermatitis and insect bites. They may alleviate suffering and obviate the need for systemic drugs. Maximally potent fluorinated corticosteroid preparations (e.g., betamethasone, fluocinolone, fluocinonide, halcinonide) are recommended (see Table 69-2) for use under the harsh circumstances of wilderness travel; it is extremely unlikely that any complications would result from short-term use.

Intravenous and Classified Drugs. Injectable drugs are rarely needed for the management of wilderness-associated trauma and illness, as most emergencies can be managed by either oral or transdermal application of medicines. IV medications are temperature sensitive, fragile, expire quickly, and require monitoring of vital signs because of potency and immediate onset of action. Narcotic analgesics should be used to treat pain only if mild analgesics such as aspirin and acetaminophen are inadequate, mental status is not clouded (as might occur with head trauma), and respiratory distress is not present (unless it is due solely to discomfort). Oral narcotic–containing products are appropriate for moderately severe pain. If indicated by the circumstances, more potent dermal delivery systems of narcotics can be achieved (e.g., fentanyl patch) when oral administration is not possible. A short-acting central nervous system amphetamine stimulant (see Table 69-3) may be justifiably carried during extremely high-risk activity, such as winter mountaineering, in which the participant might have to overcome fatigue to assist in a rescue effort or to reach aid. The small quantity prescribed on a one-time basis is unlikely to be associated with abuse.

Specific Equipment Purchases

This section reviews specialized items that are not basic to the comprehensive medical kit but may be needed for certain high-risk recreational activities. Box 69-8 itemizes such equipment. Descriptions of products, usage, and indicated circumstances are given here. Suppliers and their unique products are listed in Appendix B.

High-Altitude Exposure (see also Chapter 1). The Gamow Bag (Figure 69-3) is a portable hyperbaric chamber resembling a large sleeping bag with a window. It has been shown to be effective for the treatment of high-altitude pulmonary and cerebral edema. Constructed of nylon, the bag is foldable and has a packing weight of 14.5 pounds. Inflated, it is 7 feet long and has

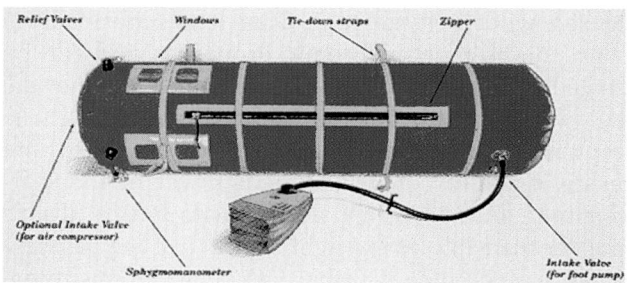

Figure 69-3 Gamow Bag. Attached is the foot pump required to pressurize the compartment to 2 pounds per square inch. Four windows are strategically located to permit observation. Entry is via a lengthwise zipper.

a diameter of 21 inches. The bag is pressurized with a foot pump at a rate of 10 to 20 strokes per minute and has relief valves pressurized to 2 pounds per square inch, allowing the venting of expired air. In a situation such as a remote clinic with electricity, a mechanical compressor can be used to avoid the fatiguing task of foot pumping.

A Breathing Bladder has been introduced. One end of this large nylon bag connects to a face mask, and the other to one of the pressure relief valves of the Gamow Bag. The patient inhales uncontaminated air from the Gamow Bag, and the exhaled air flows down a plastic tube into the bladder. This obviates the need for manual foot pumping of the bag for a 15- to 30-minute period until the bladder becomes full. It is then necessary to operate the foot pump again to repressurize the bag. The bladder is an excellent alternative for expeditions at very high altitude that are far from medical evacuation and when a prolonged period of resuscitation is anticipated.

The recently developed Gamow Tent operates on the same principles as the Gamow Bag. It is nearly 50% larger, and the added height allows a victim to sit upright.

The aforementioned devices are expensive and intended for expeditions going to extreme altitude (greater than 4267 m [14,000 feet]) or in dangerous situations that prevent an easy, rapid descent (e.g., ice climbing on a steep glacial crevasse).

Cold Exposure (see also Chapters 6 and 7). Equipment purchases for cold exposure relate to the stabilization and resuscitation of victims with accidental exposure hypothermia. For most travel, removal of an individual from exposure and prevention of further heat loss are sufficient measures when medical assistance is nearby. Persons engaging in low-risk travel can use a sleeping bag wrapped with a space emergency blanket to provide a capsule that preserves heat and allows

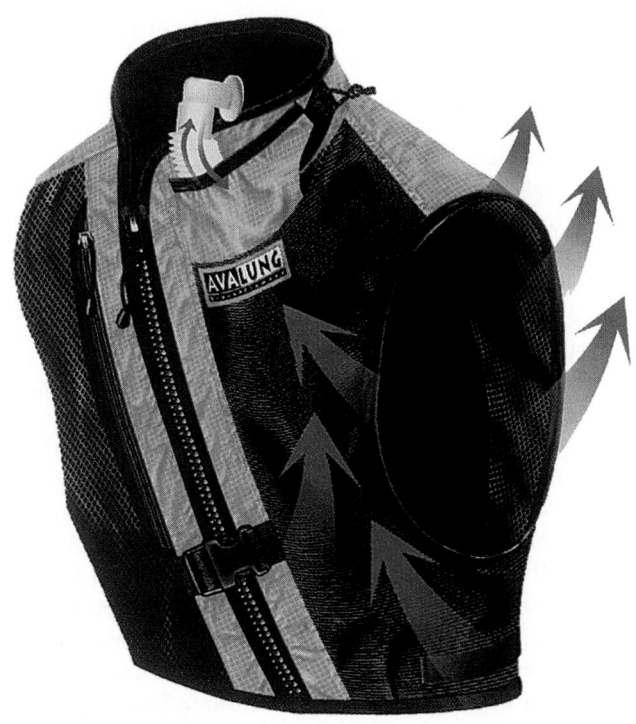

Figure 69-4 The AvaLung (Black Diamond, Ltd.). A lightweight vest designed to improve avalanche survival. Victims are able to draw air from even a dense snowpack via the front using an air exchange mouthpiece. A one-way valve permits exhalation of carbon dioxide expelled through the vest back.

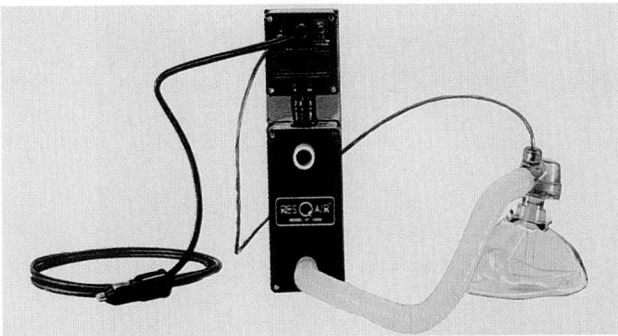

Figure 69-5 The Res-Q-Air system for delivery of warm, saturated air. The unit is portable and battery run for use in the field. Its use requires minimal training. Temperature is adjusted by a single control dial.

thermal recovery. The latter product is made of a lightweight material capable of reflecting and retaining over 80% of radiated body heat. Another helpful product is the Grabber Warmer. Useful in the prevention of frostbite, this small pad undergoes a chemical reaction on exposure to the air, producing heat. Grabber Warmers can maintain a temperature of 66° C (150° F) for 7 hours or more. They can be placed in gloves, shoes, and pockets for the prevention of frostbite.

For more serious expeditions involving high-risk travel or distant from medical rescue or assistance, several highly sophisticated products may be of value. Of value in circumstances of high avalanche danger is a lightweight vest with a breathing tube that permits extraction of oxygen and release of carbon dioxide when trapped under snow (Figure 69-4). Such a device can significantly prolong survival chances until the victim is found by another person appropriately manned with an avalanche beacon and/or extendable ski pole. For victims of severe exposure hypothermia, elevation of core temperature and prevention of further body heat loss may be critical. Inhalation of warm, humidified air provides an excellent method of heat exchange and is now possible with portable field units. The Res-Q-Air (Figure 69-5) provides warm, saturated air by using a

battery-operated device that requires a small amount of water and delivers heat for inhalation via an attached hose and face mask. The unit is simple to operate, has a temperature control valve, and runs for 1 hour on battery power. It is small (9 × 3 × 2 inches), weighs 4½ pounds, and is portable. In the event that emergency IV fluids may be required, an IV bag warmer, the Hot-Sack, can be used. This product comes in a soft, rugged portable case and has its own battery power source. Temperature within the bag remains at 37° C (98° F) so that IV fluids are kept warm. The bag has a protective sleeve to place over IV tubing to maintain warmth.

Advanced expeditioners and persons involved in cold water search and rescue should consider the purchase of a Hypothermic Stabilizer Bag. This product consists of an internal, high-pile fabric that wicks water to allow quick drying of hypothermic victims. The thermal properties far exceed those of an equivalent-thickness conventional down sleeping bag, and the product requires no additional insulation underneath for support and comfort. A key feature involves the ability to perform complete cardiopulmonary resuscitation through an access window over the chest. The stabilizer's outer cover is made of water-resistant material and has carrying handles to allow for safe transport of the victim (Figure 69-6).

Water Disinfection (see also Chapter 51)**.** The key design features of a filtration system that produce acceptable water for consumption are (1) adequate pore size of the filter to remove bacteria and protozoan cysts (0.2 mm or less), (2) filter element that either has activated charcoal or is impregnated with silver or iodine for local antibacterial action, (3) pump-feed mechanism that forces water through the filter housing, (4) device that can be easily disassembled and cleaned for proper maintenance, and (5) product having durability and simplicity of use. Noteworthy fil-

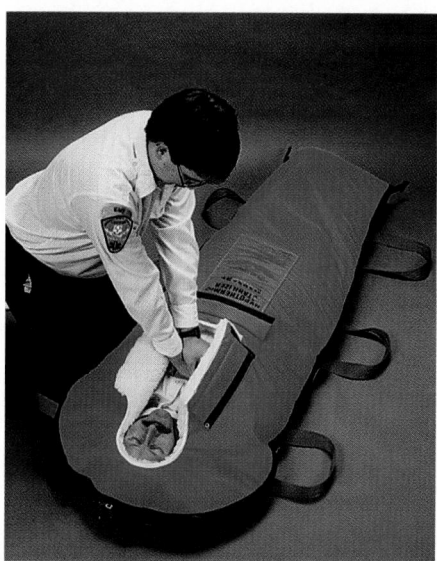

Figure 69-6 Hypothermic Stabilizer bag. This excellent prehospital transport device allows passive rewarming of victims suffering from cold exposure and is especially useful in cold water immersion because of the drying ability of its high-pile fabric. The unit weighs only 12 pounds and measures 12 × 13 inches when packaged in a portable case.

ters that have most of the desirable features include the Katadyn water filter, PUR filter, and MSR Water-Works.

Bicycling. Several prepackaged medical kits for the cyclist can be purchased. Persons who want to upgrade a basic first-aid kit to treat cycling injuries should consider the abrasions and minor burns likely to be encountered. Proper wound management requires a protective pad that is nonadherent, cools the skin, and absorbs exuded fluids. A number of breathable water-based gels, such as Spenco 2nd Skin, exist for this purpose.

Mountain Climbing and Hiking. In wilderness travel above the treeline or on shipboard, the inclusion of more advanced splinting products should be considered. The SAM splint weighs only 4 ounces. Its coated aluminum strip unfolds to provide rigid longitudinal support. It can also be configured as a cervical collar,

although the injured neck may require additional immobilization. At least two SAM splints are needed to stabilize an entire extremity. More elaborate devices include an air-stirrup ankle brace having an inner liner of adjustable air cells blown up through a valve. If activity will predispose to high risk of femoral fracture and a traction splint is desirable, the Kendrick traction device should be considered.

Third World Travel. Travelers to underdeveloped countries are at risk of infection from a host of diseases transmitted by insect bites. For travel outside of urban areas, the risks are especially great when sleeping unprotected in the outdoors. A lightweight bed net that can enclose two persons should be carried. Further protection against mosquitoes can be achieved by spraying the nets with permethrin. For bites from certain insects and snakes, the Sawyer Extractor may be of value. Several topical medications that combine an anesthetic (benzocaine) along with a cooling agent (menthol), such as Sawyer's Sting Aid or Itch Balm Plus, may be helpful in dealing with bites or minor allergic rashes. Because of the high risk of traveler's diarrhea, oral rehydration packets should be carried. Commercially prepackaged units contain essential elements that allow oral rehydration when combined with 1 L of disinfected water.

SUMMARY

The trip coordinator for travel in the outdoors should review the health status and experience of potential participants, emphasize preventive measures, and carefully review risk factors imposed by environmental extremes and recreational activities. An array of supplies to deal with potential problems can be appropriately tailored to augment the contents of the basic medical kit. Based upon trip duration and remoteness from medical care, specific prescription medications may be chosen and dispensed by knowledgeable and responsible individuals. Such efforts may forestall serious disability or discomfort while one awaits search and rescue efforts, or permit a sick group member to continue travel in the setting of non–life-threatening medical illness.

APPENDIX A

Health Questionnaire for Wilderness Travel

TRIP COORDINATOR: _____   Dates of trip: _____

Trip Location: _____   Major type of activity: _____

Please provide the following information (use another sheet of paper if necessary): (All information will be used *confidentially* by the coordinator to promote the safety of the party)

Name _____   Age _____   Height _____   Weight _____

Address _____   What is your overall HEALTH? (circle one)

_____   Poor   Fair   Good   Excellent

Phone ( )_____

Person to contact in EMERGENCY:

Contact's Name _____   What is your overall PHYSICAL condition? (circle one)

Contact's Phone ( )_____   Poor   Fair   Good   Excellent

MEDICAL DATA

 1. Allergies (drug, pollen, food, etc.—be specific) .... (YES)   (NO)
 2. Allergies (insect bites—be specific) .... (YES)   (NO)
 3. Diabetes .... (YES)   (NO)
 4. Epilepsy, Seizures, or Convulsions .... (YES)   (NO)
 5. Heart Problems .... (YES)   (NO)
 6. Kidney Problems .... (YES)   (NO)
 7. Injuries or Problems with Joints: (Specify which side, EXPLAIN problem)
    A. Ankle .... (YES)   (NO)
    B. Knee .... (YES)   (NO)
    C. Hip .... (YES)   (NO)
    D. Fingers/Toes .... (YES)   (NO)
    E. Wrist .... (YES)   (NO)
    F. Elbow .... (YES)   (NO)
    G. Shoulder .... (YES)   (NO)
    H. Back/Spine .... (YES)   (NO)
    I. Other .... (YES)   (NO)
 8. Have you ever had: (EXPLAIN problem)
    A. Mountain sickness .... (YES)   (NO)
    B. Cerebral edema .... (YES)   (NO)
    C. Pulmonary edema .... (YES)   (NO)
    D. Heatstroke .... (YES)   (NO)
    E. Sun/snow blindness .... (YES)   (NO)
    F. Frostbite .... (YES)   (NO)
    G. Hypothermia/exposure .... (YES)   (NO)
    H. Immersion foot .... (YES)   (NO)
    I. Excessive nosebleeds .... (YES)   (NO)
    J. Asthma .... (YES)   (NO)
    K. Ulcers .... (YES)   (NO)
    L. Bowel problems .... (YES)   (NO)
    M. Broken bones .... (YES)   (NO)

 9. List any medical problems, illnesses, injuries, or chronic conditions that you have presently or have had in the last 3 years (be as specific as possible):

10. List any MEDICATIONS that you are currently taking (include the dosing, if possible):

Modified from Green P: *The outdoor leadership handbook*, Tacoma, Wash, 1982, Emergency Response Institute.

Suppliers Listed in Text and Tables

Many of the products cited in this chapter can be found in outdoor equipment retail stores or pharmacies. The sources listed below provide specialized products referred to in the text.

1. **Adventure Medical Kits,** P.O. Box 43309, Oakland, CA 94624; 800-324-3517. Web site: www.adventuremedicalkits.com. Supplier of well-designed medical kits that are prepackaged for a range of specific recreational activities, such as bicycling, white-water rafting, and backcountry travel.

2. **Black Diamond Equipment, Ltd.,** 2084 East 3900 South, Salt Lake City, UT 84124; 801-278-5552. Web site: www.avalung.com. Manufacturer of the AvaLung, which is the first and only active avalanche safety device that may enable the avalanche victim to breathe while waiting to be excavated.

3. **Campmor,** P.O. Box 700, Saddle River, NJ 07458; 800-226-7667. Web site: www.campmor.com. Lady-J urinal guide.

4. **Chinook Medical Gear, Inc.,** 3455 Main Ave., Durango, CO 81301; 800-766-1365. Web site: www.chinookmed.com. The most complete catalog retailer for wilderness medical supplies; carrier of the Gamow Bag; good beginning source for the person in need of a wide variety of medical supplies.

5. **Gilbert Surgical Instruments, Inc.,** P.O. Box 458, Bellmawr, NJ 08031; 609-933-2770. Abelson Emergency Cricothyrotomy Cannula.

6. **Grabber Performance Group,** 4600 Danvers Drive SE, Grand Rapids, MI 49512; 616-940-1940. Manufacturer of a variety of packaged miniheaters with accessories useful for preventing cold-related injuries of the hands, feet, and face.

7. **Junkin Safety Appliance Co.,** 3121 Millers Ln., Louisville, KY 40216; 502-775-8303. Folding aluminum full-length backboard, 15 lb.

8. **MARSARS/Great Eastern Marine, Inc.,** 205 Myrtle St., Shelton, CT 06484-4015; 203-924-7315. Manufacturer of water and ice rescue equipment; a hypothermic stabilizer bag and additional accessory heat packs are available.

9. **Mountain Safety Research,** P.O. Box 24547, Seattle, WA 98124; 206-624-7048. Web site: www.msrcorp.com. Manufacturer of high-performance and lightweight stoves, as well as the WaterWorks filtration system.

10. **National Ski Patrol System, Inc.** (NSP), 133 S. Van Gordon, Ste. 100, Lakewood, CO 80228; 303-988-1111. Various first-aid supplies and equipment for winter skiing and mountaineering sold by catalog to NSP members.

11. **Outdoor Research,** 1000 1st Ave. S, Seattle, WA 98134; 800-421-2421. Web site: www.orgear.com. Diverse array of tote bags, medical travel kits, and stuff sacks useful for international travel.

12. **Patagonia, Inc.,** P.O. Box 150, Ventura, CA 93002; 805-643-8616. Web site: www.patagonia.com. Capilene underclothing; variety of outdoor clothing.

13. **Recreational Equipment, Inc.** (REI), 800-426-4840. Web site: www.rei.com. Thermax underclothing; variety of sunglasses, outdoor gear and clothing.

14. **Res-Q Products, Inc.,** P.O. Box 661, Quathiaski Cove, BC, Canada V0P 1N0. Contact: Robert Douwens. Web sites: www.hypothermia.org (educational site) or www.hypothermia-ca.com. Res-Q-Air and IV HOT-SACK plus accessories; sophisticated equipment for the serious expedition traveler to areas of extreme cold.

15. **Seaberg Co.,** 4909 South Coast HWY #245, Newport, OR 97365; 541-867-4726. Web site: www.samsplint.com. SAM folding splint, 4 oz.

16. **Travel Medicine Inc.,** 351 Pleasant St., Suite 312, Northampton, MA 01060; 800-872-8633. Web site: www.travmed.com. Specializing in educational books and handy supplies for international travel; source of insect repellents, clothing, and nets for mosquito protection.

Sources of Information about Wilderness Emergencies

1. **American River Touring Association,** 24000 Casa Loma Rd., Groveland, CA 95321; 800-323-2782. Web site: www.arta.org. Nonprofit organization that sponsors basic and leadership courses for river-rafting and kayaking.

2. **Emergency Response Institute,** 1819 Mark Street N.E., Olympia, WA 98506; 360-491-7785. Publishes books and sponsors symposia on search and rescue, emergency preparedness, survival, and outdoor leadership.

3. **Forest Laboratories Inc.,** NY; attention: Dr. J.M. Schor; 909 3rd Avenue, New York, NY 10022; 212-421-7850. Information on the availability of buccal morphine sulfate preparation.

4. **National Association for Search and Rescue** (NASAR), 4500 Southgate Pl. #100, Chantilly, VA 20151; 703-222-6277. Web site: www.nasar.org. Educational association that provides conferences, symposia, and training in search and rescue and emergency response, including communications; sponsors *Rescue* magazine (JEMS

Communications, 1947 Camino-Vida Roble, Suite 200, Carlsbad, CA 92008; 619-431-9797).

5. **National Climatic Data Center,** 151 Patten Avenue #120, Asheville, NC 28801-5001; 828-271-4800. Web site: www.ncdc.noaa.gov. Provides historical weather summaries for U.S. and many foreign cities; small fee for materials. Telephone first to determine availability of relevant data.

6. **National Ski Patrol System, Inc.** (NSP), 133 S. Van Gordon, Ste. 100, Lakewood, CO 80228; 303-988-1111. Web site: www.nsp.org. Sponsors training programs in winter emergency care, avalanche, and ski mountaineering, some that are open to the public; sells equipment and first-aid supplies through catalog to NSP members.

7. **National Weather Service** in city near region of travel; for further information, write: Attn. W/OM 15 × 2, Silver Spring, MD 20910. Web site: www.nwss.noaa.gov. The NWS nearest the travel site can provide forecasts and in many regions provides broadcasts over NOAA Weather Radio on frequencies between 162.40 and 162.55 mHz, including 3- to 5-day forecasts and avalanche warnings.

8. **Outward Bound Training Institute,** 800-477-2627. Web site: www.cobs.org. Nonprofit educational organization that uses the mountain, river, and ocean wilderness settings to provide stimuli for personal development; separate leadership training courses available.

9. **Sierra Club,** P.O. Box 52968, Boulder, CO 80321-2968; 415-977-5522. Web site: www.sierraclub.org.

10. **Undersea and Hyperbaric Medical Society,** 10531 Metropolitan Ave., Kensington, MD 20895: 301-942-2980. Web site: www.uhms.org. Nonprofit organization that sponsors workshops and meetings on the prevention and treatment of diving injuries and illnesses treatable with hyperbaric oxygen. Publishes bimonthly newsletter, *Pressure,* and two research publications, *Undersea Biomedical Research* and *Journal of Hyperbaric Medicine.*

11. **Wilderness Education Association,** Department of Recreation Resources, Colorado State University, Fort Collins, CO 80523; 970-491-6591. Nonprofit educational organization that sponsors, in conjunction with colleges, a 5-week National Standards Program for Outdoor Leadership Certification.

12. **Wilderness Medical Society,** 3595 E. Fountain Blvd. Ste A1, Colorado Springs, CO 80910: 719-572-9255. Web site: www.wms.org. Nonprofit organization of medical and related professionals interested in the prevention and treatment of wilderness injuries and illnesses. Publishes

quarterly newsletter, *Wilderness Medicine Letter,* covering wilderness medicine meetings, literature review, field management, and position statements. Publishes *Wilderness and Environmental Medicine* (formerly *Journal of Wilderness Medicine*), the official academic publication of the society.

SUGGESTED READINGS

Adventurous Traveler Bookstore, 245 South Champlain St., P.O. Box 64769, Burlington, VT 05406-4769; 800-282-3963. Web site: www.adventurestraveler.com. A complete source of outdoor travel books, maps, videos and CD-ROMs.

American Red Cross: *Emergency response,* ed 3, St Louis, 1999, Mosby Staywell (available from local offices of the ARC). Accepted guidelines for advanced first aid, best reviewed in a classroom format before travel.

Auerbach PS: *Medicine for the outdoors,* ed 3, New York, 1999, Lyons Press. Web site: www.lyonspress.com (800-836-0510). This is the "bible" on wilderness medicine for laypersons. It covers all situations and environments and is meant to be carried by anyone who will treat an illness or injury outdoors.

Backer H: Medical limitations to wilderness travel, *Emerg Med Clin North Am* 15:17, 1997.

Backer HD et al: *Wilderness first aid,* Sudbury, Mass, 1998, Jones and Bartlett. A layman's wilderness first-aid guide written as a collaborative effort between the Wilderness Medical Society and the National Safety Council.

Bowman W: *Outdoor emergency care: comprehensive first aid for non-urban settings,* ed 3, Lakewood, Colo, 1998, NSPS (133 S. Van Gordon, Lakewood, CO 80228; 303-988-1111). Web site: www.nsp.org. Developed for ski patrollers, provides an up-to-date, comprehensive guide to the prevention, recognition, and management of injuries and illness encountered in nonurban settings. Highly recommended reading for participants in all varieties of skiing.

Darvill F: Mountaineering medicine, ed 14, Berkeley, Calif, 1998, Wilderness Press (2440 Bancroft Way, Berkeley, CA 94704; 510-843-8080). Web site: www.wildernesspress.com. Lightweight, easily carried, reminder of the principles of first aid and basic medical care for the mountain environment.

Gentile DA et al: Wilderness injuries and illnesses, *Ann Emerg Med* 21:853, 1992.

Hackett P: *Mountain sickness: prevention, recognition and treatment,* New York, American Alpine Club (113 E. 90th Street, New York, NY 10028). Thorough review. Recommended reading for travelers to high altitude.

Lentz M et al: *Mountaineering first aid,* ed 4, Seattle, 1996, The Mountaineers (306 Second Ave West, Seattle, WA 98119; 800-553-4453). Web site: www.mountaineers.org. Good review of mountaineering first aid, most appropriate for classroom or individual reading in advance of departure.

Montalvo R et al: Morbidity and mortality in the wilderness, *West J Med* 168:248, 1998.

Olsen LD: *Outdoor survival skills,* La Vergne, Tenn, 1998, Ingram Trade. Chapters on shelter, fire, water, plants and special skills on how to build a lean-to, and how to harvest and prepare plants in the wild.

Wilderness Medicine Letter (3595 E. Fountain Blvd. Ste A1, Colorado Springs, CO 80910; 719-572-9255). Web site: www.wms.org. The newsletter of the Wilderness Medical Society. Reviews of recent publications, notification of events and meetings, official position statements, and commentary by experts in the field. Highly recommended reading for physicians serving as advisors to travelers.

Wilkerson J, editor: *Medicine for mountaineering and other wilderness activities,* ed 4, Seattle, 1992, The Mountaineers (306 Second Ave. West, Seattle, WA 98119: 800-553-4453). Web site: www.mountaineers.org. Comprehensive coverage of the prevention, recognition, and advanced field management of mountaineering injuries and illnesses. Many sections are easily understood by general readers, but chapters on medical illness require familiarity with medical terminology and concepts, and a working knowledge of basic first aid is assumed. Recommended that a single copy be carried by the person responsible for medical care of a large group on an extended or high-risk mountaineering outing.

Wilkerson J, Bangs C, Hayward J: *Hypothermia, frostbite and other cold injuries,* Seattle, 1986, The Mountaineers (306 Second Ave. West, Seattle, WA 98119; 800-553-4453). Web site: www.mountaineers.org. Excellent overview that explains, in lay terms, the metabolic disturbances underlying cold injury, as well as practical methods of preventing and treating these disorders. Especially welcome is the chapter on immersion injuries containing valuable information for persons involved in aquatic sports. Highly recommended reading for all travelers to cold weather, mountain, and aquatic wilderness environments.

Zell SC: Common questions: environmental and recreational hazards associated with adventure travel, *J Travel Med* 4:94, 1997.

70 Selection and Use of Outdoor Clothing

John Gookin

The Inuit people do not have a word for *luck* because leaving things to chance is not part of their mind-set. They travel prepared for whatever conditions they might encounter and are particularly meticulous about mending and replacing clothing. In a blizzard, they can remain warm until the storm passes.

What to wear and what to carry are strategic issues. You can decide whether to carry everything needed to remain comfortable in any extreme or to use a "travel light, freeze at night" strategy. To gain competency in this skill area, you need quality clothing and must know a multitude of ways to use layers with finesse. Experience and the ability to adjust are more dependable than specialized gear, so learn how to use your gear well instead of buying new "perfect" gear.

BASIC CONSIDERATIONS

The expected length of the expedition affects the selection of an outdoor wardrobe. If you are merely ducking outdoors in nonextreme weather to grab an armload of firewood, cotton clothing is an excellent choice because it absorbs sweat once you are back inside. When you are outside and initiate aerobic activities combined with rest, your metabolic rate alternately increases and decreases, which calls for adjustable insulation. For example, a cross-country skier usually wears little more than undergarments and wind gear while skiing but adds an inch or two of insulation while resting. Clothing must be durable enough to last the entire expedition.

Level of activity is another important factor. For instance, carrying a backpack is always aerobic exercise. The more aerobic the activities, the more versatile clothes need to be. The ideal situation is to regulate layers and activity so that you work at peak performance without wasting moisture and energy to sweating or shivering.

PRINCIPLES OF CLOTHING USE

Choose clothing appropriate to the local climate (explained in Clothing Systems for Different Climates). Choose fabrics for properties such as insulation and breathability (explained in Material Properties of Outdoor Clothing). Carry enough layers that you can adapt to different work levels and climatologic extremes. Climatologic data can be obtained from a variety of sources. You can use such information in selecting gear that will allow you to be comfortable during average highs and lows; however, you should also prepare to survive the extremes.

Dress in layers because many thin layers are easier to fine-tune than one or two thicker garments. Layers need to fit comfortably on top of one another without binding. Use an outer layer that will protect you from the environment. In hot weather, one layer may be all you need. In cooler weather, choose inner layers of appropriate thicknesses so that you can continuously adjust them. For instance, at $-29°$ C ($-20°$ F) alongside a fjord (a wet, cold environment), you should wear expedition-weight undergarments, two or three insulation layers, and a snow-proof parka and pants.

Anticipate changes in body temperature and climate and adjust layers accordingly. As you begin to walk up a steep hill, remove layers and ventilate (open) zippers *before* you overheat. Expose more skin around the head, neck and wrists. Take off your gloves. Walk in the shade instead of the sun. Turn your head slightly so that you face into the breeze. Do what you can to keep from sweating.

You do more than avoid discomfort when you prevent sweating in cold conditions. You keep your insulation drier, fluffier, and warmer for when you slow down. Garments remain cleaner for extended use. Experienced expeditioners know that this strategy is not just for peak performance during work cycles; it helps achieve a lower metabolic rate and therefore conserves energy and water.

Add clothing layers as you head over a windy pass or downhill. Always add insulation to trap heat before resting in cold weather. If you begin to feel cold and begin shivering or feel a chill, add one or more layers.

In a warm climate, as the temperature rises, adjust layers before becoming overheated or sunburned. Plan a sun-exposed hike for the hours of the day when the angle of the sun is least and ultraviolet radiation (UVR) is filtered by more atmosphere. If necessary and if it is safe, hike at night, when it is not as hot.

MATERIAL PROPERTIES OF OUTDOOR CLOTHING

Outdoor clothing is made from various fabrics woven of various fibers. A fiber is a single strand of threadlike material. Sometimes, fabrics encase loose fill of down or synthetic fibers. Certain fleece fabrics contain a woven layer with bulky fibers attached on one side, like a pile rug. The following four material properties pertain to fibers and fabrics:

1. The thicker the material, the greater the insulative value, as long as the material stays dry. Thickness of an inch or more in any layer is rarely needed with modern materials.
2. The following qualities of fiber reaction to moisture are important:
   a. Ease of "wicking" action: hydrophilic fabric transfers moisture from the body surface *to* the material; hydrophobic fabric transfers moisture from the body surface *across* the fabric to other clothing or to the air.
   b. Evaporative ability: rate of drying.
   c. "Moisture regain": amount of moisture a material can absorb before it feels cold. With a higher moisture regain, the fabric will be more functional for high levels of activity in cold or wet environments.
   d. Amount of insulative value a material retains when wet.
3. The less the thermal conductance, the better the insulation.
4. Tighter weaves and coated fabrics help block wind, which decreases convective cooling but allows more perspiration to accumulate in insulation layers.

Commonly used clothing materials for outdoor activities are nylon, polyester, polypropylene, wool, cotton, and down and synthetic fiber fill. The four important properties are different for each of these materials.

Wool is a good insulator because it is a poor conductor of heat. It has moderate affinity for absorbing moisture but can absorb a great deal—about 35% to 55% saturation—before it feels wet. Its evaporative ability (speed of drying) is poor compared with that of polypropylene, but its fiber structure allows it to suspend water vapor without decreasing insulation. In summary, wool does not absorb water easily, is warm when damp, but when dripping wet feels cold.

Cotton feels great in summer when, for example, a hiker is struggling up a steep grade with a heavy pack and there is a light breeze. However, cotton may do more harm than good in any environment where conservation of heat is needed. In fact, mountaineers say, "Cotton kills." Cotton loses up to 90% of its insulative value when wet; it is hydrophilic, and its moisture regain is poor. (Hence, it makes a great towel.) On the plus side, cotton is excellent for abrasion resistance, it blocks UVR to a certain degree (wet white cotton transmits considerable UVR), and it helps keep a person cool. It is also quiet, making it quite useful for hunters and soldiers.

Polypropylene, like cotton, wicks moisture well, but unlike cotton, it has very low thermal conductance and is hydrophobic. These properties make it popular as an underlayer material for active outdoor enthusiasts. Great versatility of form, smooth feel, and easy maintenance have elevated polypropylene to a favored underwear material. Many of the new polyester fibers, such as Capilene and Thermax, perform just as well.

Polyester is justifiably the most widely used material in outdoor clothing. The fibers can be formed into several thicknesses and configurations, thereby fashioning underwear garments, insulation layers such as the popular fleece jackets, and even outer-layer wind- and moisture-protective gear. New "windstopper" fabric adds both insulation and wind protection in one simple layer. Polyesters are poor heat conductors (good insulators), high in moisture regain (absorb water without feeling cold), and hydrophobic. Polyester has replaced wool as the principal insulative layer material, usually as zippered or pullover jackets. Styles with longer fleece offer better protection against the wind. When polyester is designed as an outer (protective) layer, fibers are woven more densely, and a water- or wind-repellent sheath, often made of nylon and Lycra, is laminated to it. The outer surface can be sprayed with a water-repellent substance such as Ultrex. Some 80% of polyester fleece used in outdoor gear is processed from recycled plastic bottles.

Cotton/polyester blends are used for a great deal of nonexpedition outdoor gear. This combination provides a good fabric for temperate climates because it blends the properties of both fabrics. It does not perform well in either very hot or very cold climates. In particular, this fabric is used by many people who routinely work outdoors and who desire the comfort of cotton blended with the higher performance of polyester; for example, it is used in the uniforms of park rangers.

Nylon absorbs little water, so it allows moisture to evaporate quickly. It also has good moisture regain. Because of durability, it is often the material preferred for outerwear. However, unless nylon is tightly knit, it does not screen wind and water well. It can be coated to provide more wind and water repellency but at the expense of breathability. In any type of material, protection against moisture and ability to breathe become a trade-off. No material can do both in ideal fashion when intensity of activity exceeds 50% of maximum oxygen consumption, the level that a fit person can sustain for hours. W.L. Gore Company's high-profile Gore-Tex Teflon base was first laminated to nylon in outerwear garments that were breathable as well as water resistant.

Down is an excellent insulator when dry. Goose down has a great loft rating (measured in cubic inches of fill power per ounce). Down with a higher loft rating is composed of more pure down and fewer feathers. However, as with cotton, moisture regain is very low. Down is hydrophilic, and its drying rate is dis-mally slow. Down is even worse than cotton in a cold, wet environment because the loft all but disappears when it is soaked. It is nearly impossible to dry a soaked down sleeping bag in the field.

Synthetic fiber fill has many of the insulating benefits of down, but it is hydrophobic and has a high moisture regain and good evaporative qualities. Synthetics lose loft over time because the fibers break down with use and washing; synthetic fiber clothing and sleeping bags should be stored in a noncompressed state. Synthetic fibers are more dense than down. Some fiber fill, such as Qualofil, is less dense than other synthetics, but in general the denser fiber fills are more durable, retaining their loft for longer periods.

TYPES OF LAYERS

There are three types of layers based on function. Outer layers protect from direct contact with the elements, such as thorns, rain, wind, and sun. A base layer is used against the skin for a small amount of insulation combined with vapor transport away from the body. Insulation layers are generally added as needed between the inner and outer layers.

Base Layer

Long Underwear. Polypropylene and polyesters are preferable because of low cost, good insulating ability, and evaporative ability. Wool is still an excellent choice for long underwear but is harder to find and more difficult to care for. Fabrics containing cotton are hydrophilic and do not transport vapor well. Cotton is inappropriate for the base layer. A fabric with some stretch is needed so that it will flex with motion. In general, the softer the fabric, the faster it wears out. Long johns come in three weights: light, medium, and expedition (heavy). These weights are discussed in Clothing Systems for Different Climates.

Socks. Wool with 10% to 15% nylon added for strength is an excellent choice for socks. A small amount of Spandex adds stretch that assists with fit. Polyester fleece socks are an alternative to wool; they perform better in damper conditions but generally wear out faster. Fit your boots with two pairs of socks for a more comfortable fit and more insulation, if that is what you need. An additional pair of very thin polypropylene socks worn next to the skin can help wick moisture and lessen friction on the skin. The entire sock combination needs to be comfortable and matched perfectly to the fit of the boots. Carry two changes of socks while backpacking and one spare pair of wool socks so that you can wear dry socks in camp and in the sleeping bag. If you must routinely wade through water, neoprene socks, Seal Skin socks, or fleece socks function better than wool.

Gloves. Light polypropylene, wool, silk, or fleece gloves work well when the conditions are moderately cold or when finger dexterity is required. Fingerless versions are also available. Gloves of polyester/Lycra combinations provide a tighter, more conforming fit to enhance fine finger movements. Synthetic gloves come in many weights. In colder temperatures, mittens provide more efficient insulation. Thin glove liners are often used in combination with an insulating mitten layer and mitten shells.

Mittens come in polypropylene, fleece (pile), wool, or nylon-lined synthetic fiber fill (which works like a sleeping bag). Mittens are more efficient insulators than gloves because they expose less surface area around the fingers. You can add a layer of mittens on top of light "glove liners" so that you can use your fingers without baring them directly to the elements. Mittens used as a layer on top of polypropylene gloves do not need to be particularly thick.

Insulation Layers

Shirts, jackets, and sweaters should be made of suitable synthetic material, which can be woven or fleece. Vests can be used, but most layers should have long sleeves. Wool shirts work well. Large pockets with buttons or Velcro are handy for carrying items such as sunglasses or a compass. Shirts should open completely in the front or at least have a half-zipper for ventilation. A turtleneck protects the neck, as do neck warmers and mufflers. Be sure that insulation layers fit comfortably on top of all other layers so that when worn together, they allow freedom of movement. Fleece jackets have become a common insulating layer because of their versatility. A fleece jacket, pulled fuzzy-side out and wrapped around some clothes, also makes a nice pillow.

Pants made of fleece work well, but wool is acceptable. The advantages of wool pants are that they tend to have pockets and they stay up better. Fleece pants should have reinforcements at the knees and buttocks. Full or partial lateral leg zippers are convenient for changing pants over boots. Consider using suspenders with fleece pants if they tend to slide down over other clothing.

Hats are used for shade or insulation. Hats used for shade should have at least a 4-inch brim and be made of material that blocks UVR. In windy conditions, hats need to be tied onto the head. Hats used for insulation should be made of pile, Orlon, polypropylene, wool, or wool-polypropylene and should be large enough to cover the ears. A small bill helps shade the eyes. "Bomber" caps with bills and pull-down earflaps are popular. A balaclava covers the entire head and neck but has a large hole for the face. You should also protect your face from cold wind; a balaclava configuration, a scarf, or a neoprene face mask does this. One useful combination is a ski hat with a neck warmer (a tubular scarf that rings the neck) that can be pulled up to cover most of the lower face. On expeditions, some people carry a thin polypropylene balaclava for sleep and a thick fleece balaclava to wear during the day. The fleece balaclava can also be rolled up and worn like a stocking cap. Be certain that any cold-weather hat system works in combination with your glasses and goggles without collecting moisture that fogs lenses. Although these small layers for your head may seem trivial, strategically it is much more important to cover bare skin than it is to add insulation elsewhere.

Outer Layer

Parka. A noninsulated nylon parka is often used on top of clothing systems. If it is uncoated, it is called a *wind jacket* or *wind shirt*. If it is coated with urethane or rubber, it is called a *rain jacket*. Parkas made with Gore-Tex or one of the other selectively permeable membranes are common because they are versatile. The parka should have a hood with a drawstring, a two-way zipper down the front with an overlying weather flap closed with snaps or Velcro, a cloth flap to protect the chin from the metal zipper pull, and enough pockets to contain frequently needed items.

Zippered ventilation openings at the armpits make a parka more versatile. It helps even more if the armpit openings are large enough so that the parka can be converted into a vestlike garment during warm conditions by inserting the arms through the openings and tucking the sleeves inside the parka.

Nylon Pants. Uncoated nylon pants are called *wind pants* and work best in dry conditions. Coated nylon pants, called *rain pants*, work best in wet conditions but trap perspiration. Gore-Tex is a good choice in many conditions because of its versatility, but do not expect it to perform as well in environmental extremes. Long, zippered side openings are useful for donning pants without removing the boots, as well as for ventilation.

Mitten Shells. Mitten shells are nylon shells that fit over mittens or gloves. They are very light and add a layer of wind or water protection. For many travelers, this is the first hand layer they add to their pack as conditions get colder because they are light and add such versatility to the clothing system. Some people ski wearing mitten shells over bare hands so that they can dissipate heat but retain a snow and wind barrier.

Boots. Boot selection depends on the planned activity, the expected foot hazards (such as sharp rocks and cactus spines), and the anticipated environmental temperatures. For light hiking, when no more than a day pack is carried, a light boot with good ankle support is sufficient. In hot weather, high-topped trail-running shoes

might be ideal. Boots made of leather or fabric such as Gore-Tex are light and adequate for trail hiking but not durable enough for rocky terrain. Backpacking boots have shanks in the midsoles. A shank is a stiffener for the foot platform. For moderate terrain or loads up to 30% to 40% of body weight, choose sturdy leather hiking boots with a steel or fiberglass half-length shank and lug soles. For loads over 50% of body weight, use a boot with a three-quarter-length or full-length shank to help support the feet. A full-length shanked boot is stiff and is considered to be a very specialized boot. Most backpackers are fine carrying a heavy load in rough terrain with a high-quality boot with a three-quarter-length shank.

A high-quality boot has fewer seams, making it easier to seal. It is made of excellent leather; some manufacturers use only specific pieces of cowhide, offering a more consistent product. It is sufficiently soft on the inside, so that it "breaks in" quickly. Beware of boots that are so stiff that they do not mold to the shape of the foot: these boots feel harder than others when flexed.

Fit is crucial to boot selection. Different brands are built on different lasts (forms) based on regional foot norms. European lasts are often narrower, German lasts are wider, and American lasts are moderate. Once you find a specific brand of boot that fits well, there is a good chance their other models will also fit the same foot shape. A boot needs to be roomy enough to accommodate the desired numbers of socks. Boots must be long enough so that the toes do not strike the front of the boot during downhill walking. Test this fit by walking down a steep ramp or kicking a wall in the boot shop. If your toes hit the front on the first kick, the boot is either too short or laced too loosely. Boots should be laced tightly enough that the heel does not move up and down much, but not so tightly that circulation is restricted and the toes cannot be wiggled easily.

In extreme cold, the Canadian type of pak-boot (such as the Sorel) with a removable inner felt liner is a good choice for light snowshoeing and other nontechnical outdoor activities. On extremely cold expeditions, consider replacing the felt liner with a nylon-clad polyester fiber fill booty with a closed cell foam sole. These dry much more easily than the felt liners and last for years.

Special double ski boots are available for ski touring or for skiing at ski areas. These consist of an outer shell and an inner liner. The shells are leather or plastic; leather shells flex more, whereas plastic shells are hydrophobic. The liners are leather or foam; leather liners last longer but are not as warm, whereas foam liners are hydrophobic and are used by many professionals. Foam liners are warm, but they weigh more. Plastic and foam boots are easier to manage while camping in the snow because you do not have to keep them from freezing when they are off the feet. Double ski boots offer tremendous insulation and ankle support but are too warm for many skiing conditions.

Plastic hiking boots with foam or leather liners were originally designed for snow and ice mountaineering. They are an excellent option in wet, cold conditions. Lighter, more flexible versions of plastic boots have been developed, so some people are now using them instead of leather boots for hiking in temperate climates. They are water resistant and warm but sometimes too warm; sweat accumulation can occur.

Care of leather boots is critical to continued fit and insulation. Such boots should stay sealed with commercial sealants to keep the leather waterproof and supple. Dry leather tends to get hard, absorb more water, and shrink more than well-oiled leather. Nikwax and Biwell are good sealants if the boot manufacturer has no specific recommendations. An inner seal that treats leather on the inside of boots helps keep them softer and increases their longevity.

Gaiters and Overboots. Gaiters are long nylon tubes that cover the lower leg and upper part of the boot. They are designed to keep snow, sand, and gravel out of boots and socks. They extend to just below the knee, open at the side or in front with a zipper or Velcro, and have a strap that fits under the boot sole to keep them snug on the boots and drawstrings at the top to hold them up. Gaiters with a front opening closed by a wide Velcro flap are easy to put on and take off. Shorter versions that extend to just above the ankle are adequate for summer hiking. A simple, durable gaiter design is the tube gaiter, which is merely a tube of nylon slipped on your ankle before you pull your boots on. However, tube gaiters are not as convenient as other gaiters because the boots need to be removed before the gaiters.

Special insulated overboots or lined gaiters are especially warm for their weight. A "supergaiter" is a gaiter that attaches along the seam between the sole and the boot, covering the entire top of the boot, and is insulated. Supergaiters need to be matched exactly to the boot to stay on in typical mountaineering conditions.

Vapor Barrier Systems

Vapor barrier systems involve the use of waterproof garments and sleeping bag liners close to the skin to prevent the saturation of outer clothing and sleeping bags with sweat (with a resulting reduction in insulating value), reduce sweating, and decrease the body's water requirement. Vapor barriers seem to work better in very cold weather than at moderate temperatures. A light garment of polypropylene or similar material should be worn next to the skin with the waterproof garment layered over this. People with hyperhidrosis and those who object to a clammy feeling next to the skin may not like a vapor barrier system.

CLOTHING SYSTEMS FOR DIFFERENT CLIMATES

Different systems are needed in different climates. The climates addressed here will merely be called *hot, temperate,* or *cold* in combination with *dry* or *wet* (Table 70-1). *Extreme* is used to address rare cases that go beyond the norms experienced by most outdoor enthusiasts. *Hot* is any temperature warmer than 38° C (100° F). *Extremely hot* is a temperature above 46° C (115° F). *Temperate* includes temperatures from 0° to 38° C (32 to 100° F), roughly from the freezing point of water to normal human body temperature. *Cold* is any temperature below 0° C (32° F). *Extremely cold* is any temperature below −29° C (−20° F).

Wet refers to the maritime climate, common to coastal areas, where humidity is generally high, averaging well above 50%. Insulation does not dry easily in this environment. *Dry* refers to a more continental climate, where the humidity is generally low, averaging at or below 50%. Insulation dries more easily in this environment.

TABLE 70-1. General Climates

	TEMPERATURE	WET*	DRY†
Extremely hot	High above 46° C (115° F)	Rare because water lessens temperature extremes	Desert in summer
Hot	High above body temperature	Rainforest	Desert in summer
Temperate	Temperature between freezing and body temperature	Deciduous forest	Inland mountain
		Coastal forest	Forest
		Maritime mountain	Desert in winter
Cold	Low below freezing temperature of water	Coast at high latitude	Inland mountain
		Coastal mountain	Tundra
Extremely cold	Low below −29° C (−20° F)	Rare because cold air cannot carry much moisture	Alpine winter
			High latitude and altitude

*Humidity usually above 50%.
†Humidity usually below 50%.

Another significant climatologic factor in clothing performance is wind. Wind chills and heats humans more quickly than calm air because of convection. A wet wind can drive the rain into and under clothing layers, whereas a dry wind is the ultimate drying tool for clothing.

Clothing systems for hot, dry weather protect against the sun and wind; thin layers are chosen for cover from UVR. These may be certain blends of cotton or treated synthetics. Long cotton pants and shirts promote cooling by trapping perspiration and protect from sun and thorns. Loose layers allow better air circulation. Hats with brims on all sides provide shade for the head and neck. A large bandanna can be draped over a hat to shade the sunny or windward side of the head and face.

During exercise in moderate heat, short sleeves and pants may be appropriate. Choose short pants before short sleeves while hiking because the legs generate considerable heat. Hot weather climbers have adopted the type of clothing worn by gymnasts, whereas many backpackers wear runners' gear. Nylon shorts and Lycra or cotton sports bras are standard for backpackers in moderately hot weather.

Hot, wet conditions are more challenging because humidity reduces evaporative cooling. Clothing needs to allow maximal cooling, and activities need to be regulated until you are adequately acclimatized to the heat. Use strategies such as seeking shade when possible; pouring water over the wrists, head, or clothing; and donning long loose-fitting clothes for shade if one must be in the sun.

In extremely hot conditions, clothing considerations become subordinate to changes in behavior. Avoid the most intense heat of the day, particularly when you are active. Indigenous people in extremely hot climates habitually rest or sleep during the middle of the day but are active during the beginning and end. They have adapted to the realities of the heat.

Hot environments are often also dusty. Eye protection should include sunglasses that are scratch resistant and block 100% of UVR. In dusty conditions, goggles are essential; ski goggles converted to desert goggles work better if the lens is replaced with clear plastic. The goggles need a carrying case and a spare lens; use the old lens as much as possible and save the new lens for special situations when the most visibility is needed.

Temperate conditions require a clothing system that allows you to be active in warm, sweat-producing conditions but that still provides warmth during cool nights. Many backpackers wear nylon shorts and cotton tee-shirts while hiking in these conditions. These clothes are rugged. The nylon shorts dry quickly. The cotton shirts may need to be taken off after a hike if the moisture feels wet and cold. In a more maritime climate, the outerwear needed is coated nylon rain gear.

In a cold rainforest, a long raincoat, such as an anorak or a cagoule with a rubber coating, may be preferable. Wind gear (uncoated nylon) may suffice for dry conditions. Many people choose Gore-Tex outerwear for temperate conditions because it keeps them reasonably dry in rainstorms but does not collect sweat unless it is soaked. Polypropylene long johns and a thin fleece jacket or a heavy polyester shirt are often sufficient insulation in temperate conditions. If more than this is needed, it is often more versatile to carry thin polypropylene gloves and a balaclava than to carry an extra jacket. In general, it is more efficient to cover bare skin before adding more insulation to areas already covered.

If you need to wear pants because of brush, consider hiking in uncoated nylon wind pants. Sweatpants or anything else with a loose weave snags and tears in heavy brush. A good option is to wear work pants of a cotton/polyester blend. These are the same pants worn by many park rangers. Compared with jeans or canvas pants, they dry quickly, yet are very durable. The cotton pockets do not dry very quickly.

Cold conditions require an inner layer of long johns, an outer layer of nylon, and several insulation layers. The thickness of the long johns depends on the ambient temperature and level of activity. Since undergarments are not a layer repeatedly put on or taken off during normal activities, a weight that is thin enough in which to comfortably work should be chosen. If you cool easily, conditions are damp, and it is windy, err on the side of heavier long johns. Some people carry two different weights on an expedition and wear the expedition-weight clothes in cooler conditions but switch to the medium-weight or lightweight clothes in warmer weather. The practice of carrying different weights adds versatility, but eventually you should be able to predict what clothing will be needed to keep a lighter pack on shorter trips. It is so easy to fine-tune a cold-weather clothing system to insulate or ventilate that the weight of long johns is not critical. Outerwear can consist of uncoated wind gear in cold, dry conditions. Use Gore-Tex or coated nylon in cold wet conditions but pay special attention to ventilating layers when necessary to evaporate perspiration.

Extreme cold tends to be dry because air below $-40°$ C $(-40°$ F) holds no moisture. Exceptions include high-latitude coastlines and some areas with "ice-fog" from hot springs or wood smoke. Dry conditions make it easier to insulate in many ways. Gear tends to stay dry and "fluffed up" at temperatures below $-23°$ C $(-10°$ F). This advice is for living and moving in the range of $-23°$ to $-40°$ C $(-10$ to $-30°$ F) in snowy conditions. When temperatures fall below this, when conditions are also wet, or when it is also windy, it takes superb gear, considerable experience, and absolute discipline to keep body parts from quickly freezing.

Clothing systems for extreme cold do not include an easy option of adding layers in the middle of the system. Use a system like that described for dry, cold weather but add a second down or fiber fill insulation layer that can be worn on the outside. This outer insulation system needs to be cut large enough to allow freedom of movement when worn over every other layer. It can usually be covered with thin nylon, but for working in brush, it needs to be tear resistant. This extra layer supplements rather than replaces the cold-weather system. This is important because if you purchase a parka meant to work by itself at −29° C (−20° F), it will be challenging to use it in combination with a cold-weather clothing system. The additional layers should be 1 to 2 inches thick, not 4 to 6 inches thick.

The parka should be insulated with a thin layer of down or synthetic fill. It should be cut so that it does not allow a cold draft on the torso. Some parkas have waist-level snow-guards with drawstrings (like a draft tube on a sleeping bag but not insulated) that control this draft, but other parkas are cut longer (thigh to knee length) and intentionally allow air to circulate, helping keep you drier. Both strategies work fine, but the shorter parkas with the snow-guards are lighter. The sleeves should be longer than normal to help cover the wrists better. Wrists should be protected with a system that is snug but not tight, since tight fits can impair both circulation and function. The parka hood should move with the head, have at least one drawstring, cover the neck, and have a "snorkel" or "tunnel" to keep the wind off the face. (It is called a *snorkel* because it creates a tube through which to look that moves with the head.) Fur or fleece edges on the tunnel provide more wind protection and conduct less heat when touched. Outside pockets should be big enough to carry overmitts. Many outer pockets have two compartments: one inside the insulation for warming hands and another outside the insulation for storing gear. Inner pockets should be large enough to store lots of clothing so that it can be dried out while walking around camp. This drying system works quickly in extreme cold and dry, cold conditions because the ambient air is so dry and the temperature differential drives the moisture out of the clothing. It is critical that the parka be donned while the wearer is still warm, not only to trap heat but also to supply enough heat to warm up the parka.

Insulated overpants should be rugged enough for the local conditions, should be long enough to overlap the booty system (explained later), and should have coated seat and knee patches to protect the pants from wear and moisture when you sit or kneel. The nylon layers of overpants tend to slide over one another so easily that it is hard to keep them up. Suspenders are better than belts or cord-locks for this purpose. Some pants come with integral cord-locks: if this cord-lock slips, replace it with the flat style of cord-lock that does not slip. Full-length zippers allow you to pull pants on and off, even while wearing skis. Half-length zippers may allow pants to go on and off over boots; this is the minimal standard for extreme cold-weather overpants. Some people use fleece pants as overpants in extreme cold. This works, but they collect snow more easily. Again, pants need to go on and off without removing any other layers.

Insulated overmitts can be fleece or synthetic fiber fill with nylon covers on all sides of the mittens. Thin nylon is usually fine on the back, but a coarser weave of nylon in the palm helps prevent wear and adds friction for grabbing objects. Some mitts use textured vinyl on the palm, although the vinyl tends to crack and wear. Fleece is usually more durable, but synthetic fill (which works like a hand-sized sleeping bag) is warmer. Gauntlet length helps seal the wrists; adjustments in the hand and wrist areas allow a custom fit and scoop up less of the fluffy snow common in these conditions. Fur or fleece on the back of one mitt is nice for wiping your nose without cooling it down as much. Some overmitts are partially leather; be sure this is treated with oil or silicone, or it will collect moisture that will allow it to freeze.

You should be able to wear insulated overboots over your work boots (such as leather ski boots) and over fiber fill booties when not wearing your work boots. Some overboots allow walking, skiing, or snowshoeing. These boots are nearly all nylon on the outside with synthetic fiber-fill insulation. The outside requires a durable coarse-weave sole so that you do not slide on snow as easily. The upper part needs to overlap any insulated pants and attach like an insulated gaiter to the top of the calf. The upper part does not need to be thick, but it does need some insulation. The key to keeping this insulated gaiter up usually is not the drawstring at the top; it is mostly the drawstrings around the foot and ankle. Inner booties can be worn in one or two layers inside the overboots. Booties with closed cell foam insoles often work as one layer. Some people prefer to use two layers of booties without integrated insoles so that they can sleep in the booties. (Booties with foam insoles accumulate sweat in a sleeping bag.) In this case, people tend to cut insoles out of old closed-cell foam sleeping pads to fit in the overboots. The best way to do this is to put a piece of notebook paper inside each overboot, then put them on over your booties. Walk around the room, then pull the papers out to use as patterns. The patterns will be much larger than your feet, providing better coverage inside the overboots. This booty system is very comfortable to wear around camp, offering the opportunity to dry out both feet and leather boots. If the parka does not have a place to store boots inside it, tie the laces together and hang the boots around your neck, keeping them near your chest. Once they are dry, they can either be put back on or stored wrapped in a sleeping bag.

71 Backcountry Equipment for Health Care Professionals

John Gookin

BASIC PRINCIPLES FOR CHOOSING OUTDOOR EQUIPMENT

Backcountry equipment can be crucial on an expedition or during an evacuation. Health professionals who operate in the backcountry need reliable gear. They need to know how to use it well, maintain it, and repair it. These tools must be used routinely for them to become valuable.

Choices can be overwhelming. When outfitting yourself, use these basic principles:

- *Reliability is always important.* Choose equipment that breaks less, uses readily available maintenance supplies, is rebuildable, comes with spare parts, and is simple to use.
- *Maximal performance level is rarely important.* A common error is to dwell on finding a tool that puts out 5% more performance but is more complicated (less reliable). Those last few percentage points rarely matter. Choose high-end gear, but do not be overly concerned about absolute peak performance.
- *Lightweight gear breaks more easily.* Backpacking and mountaineering equipment needs to be cared for better than car camping equipment. Either carry lightweight gear and be careful with it or carry heavy gear and be less careful with it.
- *Experience is more important than having the perfect tool.* If you purchase a $200 headlamp and leave it on a shelf so that it will not get dirty, you will gain no experience in how to use it. Choose tools that you will be willing to use routinely.
- *Simple tools work better and are less problematic.* A Swiss army knife or intricate pocket multitool performs many tasks but may be inadequate. The knife on a multitool probably performs only half as well as a simple lockback knife for most camp tasks. (Performance includes how easy it is to cut things, how easy it is to maintain control of the instrument, and how easy it is to keep it clean.) The pliers on a multitool typically have 5% to 50% of the torque (depending whether you are grabbing a tent pole or a nut) of the 6-inch channel locks that many mountaineers choose for pot grips.
- *People perform in crises the same as in training.* When a crisis puts you in fight-or-flight mode, it is important to have access to equipment that is part of your routine if you want to perform well.
- *Everyone does not need the same gear.* There can be strength in diversity on a team. If everyone has different tools on an expedition, then the team has a greater selection of tools to match to the more challenging tasks.

HEADLAMPS, NIGHT VISION GEAR, AND LANTERNS

When light is needed in the backcountry, electric headlamps are the only reasonable tool. Some headlamps are brighter than others but consume batteries faster; others feature better light distribution, durability, water resistance, and maintenance. A simple reliable headlamp is easy to find. However, the perfect headlamp does not exist because every choice has trade-offs.

The brightest headlamps available are too bulky for expeditions. Many lightweight headlamps are designed for expedition use. Search-and-rescue groups may have access to Wheat Lamps, TAG Lights, or other lights that use small automotive batteries; these are excellent lights with roughly ten times the light output of lightweight headlamps. There are many excellent headlamps with bright lights.

A good headlamp has a spare bulb stored in it, is weather resistant, and has smooth light distribution. If you are comparing lights in a shop, take them into a dark room and walk around. If the lamp zooms (a nice option) walk around with the lamp zoomed out to about 30 degrees (a third of a quarter of the space around you). Look for even light distribution instead of a small bright spot. It is even preferable to have a light with many bright spots and lines (projected from the filament) than it is to have just one ultrabright spot. A good field of illumination provides even lighting in front of you and well into your peripheral vision. A poor field of illumination provides one bright spot; the two problems with this are lack of illumination in your periphery and overintensity of the bright spot, making it harder for your eyes to catch details in the shadows.

Weatherproof headlamps perform well in most conditions. If submerged, they should be taken apart in the sun to dry out the interior. The Petzl zoom is an example of a weatherproof lamp used by many "wet cavers," but some hard-core cavers think waterproof is the required level of performance. Waterproof lamps have O-rings or other gaskets to make them submersible. Some inexpensive waterproof headlamps, such as the Eveready Waterproof Headlamp, are available; they are very waterproof but do not provide the zoom feature.

Dive headlamps can be very reliable light sources. Some of the headlamps breaking into the backpacking market were originally developed as dive lights. However, many have narrow beams that not only give poor peripheral vision but also feature a concentrated bright spot that significantly diminishes the ability to see detail in darker areas. (They work great if you are only looking through a facemask.) Some dive lights require special tools just to change a bulb. If you carry a light like this, carry a spare headlamp that you can use until it is convenient to service your dive light. Be sure to occasionally lubricate the O-rings on the light. If the O-rings begin to show cracks from age, replace them early before they leak.

Batteries

AA batteries are common in lightweight headlamps. If you are doing things where you constantly need light, such as caving or winter expeditioning, consider larger batteries to keep costs down. If a brighter light is needed to search for a lost child in the chaparral, then a bigger, brighter light that uses bigger batteries is necessary. C batteries are much lighter in weight than D batteries, but cost about the same. D batteries are much less expensive to run per lumen-hour, but their weight necessitates an external battery pack and a wire connection.

Lithium batteries put out a lot of light per weight of the battery, but they are expensive, and their odd voltage (a lithium D-cell is 3 volts instead of the traditional 1.5 volts) can require a different bulb. In cold conditions, lithium batteries work much better than alkaline batteries. Headlamps with remote battery compartments worn inside the parka, like the Petzl Mega, seem to work fine with ordinary alkaline cells at −40° C (−40° F). Some people use the "hands-free" model of headlamp made by Easter Seal, run a lithium 3-volt D cell in it for bright use, and then switch in a 1.5-volt alkaline D cell for finding things in their pack and other low-light tasks. Using a dim light better preserves night vision, and an alkaline D cell lasts a long time when burning at such low wattage.

Battery compartments can be mounted on the head or torso. Torso-mounted batteries keep batteries warmer for better performance in subfreezing temperatures, but the wire can be a nuisance.

On an expedition, disposable alkaline cells yield roughly double the light per weight of rechargeable batteries. Rechargeable batteries make sense only with a reliable charging system. Before you buy a solar charging system, learn from others how many charge cycles their rechargeable batteries have lasted and whether they have to run down the cells before recharging.

Buy "big name" alkaline cells. Cheap brands tend to have fewer and less consistent amp hours.

Carry an inexpensive battery voltmeter to test any loose (unpackaged) battery going into a headlamp or radio. Even when you use fresh batteries out of a sealed container, it is not a bad idea to test the batteries. One poor battery causes reduced performance in the entire set. Be sure to keep batteries in sets that do not mix new and old.

Light Bulbs

Bulbs dictate brightness and battery consumption. Halogen bulbs emit whiter light than tungsten and krypton filaments but usually consume power at much higher rates. Bright bulbs consume batteries faster, and when the bulbs fade, they do so quickly. A fading 4AA headlamp with a ½-watt bulb provides less than a minute of dimming time before going to total darkness, whereas less "hot" bulbs allow up to half an hour of dimming light that might allow you to reach a convenient location before changing batteries. Some headlamps, such as the Petzl "Duo," have a cool bulb and a hot bulb that can be switched on and off quickly. This is a very nice feature that has the benefit of adding the redundancy of two bulbs.

Light-Emitting Diodes and Fluorescent Lights

There are new lights with light-emitting diodes (LEDs) and fluorescent tubes as bulbs. These are potentially the best lights for smooth light and efficient battery use. LEDs are almost indestructible, but fluorescent tubes are impact sensitive. Custom prototypes of each cost hundreds of dollars but perform well. LED headlamps may become the new state of the art.

Lightless Travel

Any serious outdoor enthusiast should become familiar with night travel in certain conditions without artificial light. On snow-covered or moonlit nights, you can sometimes see more by not using a headlamp. One person with a headlamp can ruin night vision for everyone else, especially when it is shone at close range once in a while. It takes 30 minutes for the iris, rods, and brain to completely adapt to low light. For a brief moment of light to view a map, some options that save night vision are to: (1) use a red filter, (2) cover the light with your hand and let only a little light sneak out between your fingers, (3) close one eye but be ready for some short-term depth perception problems, (4) squint your eyes enough that little light gets inside, or (5) let someone else look at the map and you keep the bright light from ruining your night vision. Nautical charts are often labeled "red light readable" specifically so that a red light can be used to look at the chart. This is done by adding blue to the red ink; otherwise, a red light would make the red parts look like the white parts. If you have never tried using a red light for occasional use, learn its strengths and limitations. It is hard to beat a full-moon hike down a canyon, but it is not good to accidentally ski off a drop with a full pack and sled. Practice but be careful.

Night Vision Gear

Night vision gear can aid distant observation during a search, especially on a moonlit night. It can also be used to travel, with significant limitations. You can walk faster with a $10 headlamp than with a $5000 night vision device (NVD). Climbing or skiing with night vision equipment is problematic and unsafe unless stealth is preferable to wearing a headlamp for military reasons.

NVDs are small video cameras and TV screens that amplify existing light. Some have infrared (IR) LEDs for use in total darkness, but typical IR LEDs work effectively only to a range of 1 to 2 m. You can (tediously) read instructions in a booklet with these LEDs but not much else.

Night vision gear comes in monocular and binocular versions. Some of the monoculars are telescopic, like a rifle scope. Monoculars are better for sitting in one place and observing; they preserve night vision in the "off" eye and are simpler, lighter and less expensive. Binoculars, or night vision goggles (NVGs), are made for use while traveling; they fit on the head like an oversized dive mask. Despite being binocular, they do not offer depth perception. They work very well on a starry night as long as the forest cover does not shadow the starlight. You can climb rocks with NVGs but need to constantly alter the focus from near to far. The greatest limitation of traveling with NVGs is in flat light, especially on sand or snow because you cannot see the telltale shadows that define terrain. It is easy to walk off a cliff when traveling with NVGs in flat light or full darkness.

American NVDs evolved through different generations. First-generation NVDs from the Vietnam era had good optics, but the electronics could not handle changing light intensities, so the light amplification had to be constantly adjusted. Most are no longer available because the screens burned out when a bright spot overilluminated them. Second-generation devices automatically adjust to light levels but very slowly. A second-generation unit is a functional choice if you are not in a hurry to see things. Be certain to observe how the unit operates to be sure that there are no dead spots on the screen, and if possible, compare several units before selecting the one that works best. Third-generation devices are quick to respond to light levels and have noticeably better clarity. They are light-overload protected, so a bright spot will not burn out part of the TV screen. Rebuilt third-generation military models may be purchased for high-end performance. New models generally are not as rugged as the rebuilt military units refitted with new sensors.

Russian-surplus NVGs are available at bargain-basement prices, but their performance is poor and inconsistent. They are better than nothing, but lack optical clarity, and the poor response to overillumination makes them problematic for practical functions.

Accessories are important. A dust-proof case and lens cap are invaluable. Some night vision gear uses uncommon batteries. An important accessory in cold conditions is an Arctic battery adapter that allows you to keep the battery in your pocket so that it will function better. Sometimes lithium batteries can be used in the cold, but an Arctic adapter allows the use of less expensive and more readily available batteries. Lithium batteries deliver more hours of use with an Arctic adapter in the cold.

The new thermal imagers are very sensitive in the IR range but do not capture the visible light spectrum. They are better than classic NVDs at spotting lost people, since they highlight objects (such as people) that are warmer than the environment. However, they are very expensive. Thermal imagers are available in handheld modes that weigh about 5 pounds and are also fitted on some helicopters used by the military, fire fighters, and power companies. These are often referred to as FLIRs (forward-looking IR). For a major search operation, a handheld thermal imager may be borrowed from the state emergency management coordinator or local military security team. Basic training on use of the device is important before sending it into the field. Have the operators sit on one side of a valley while you direct "lost" people to walk around across the valley. Have the wanderers sit behind different types of bushes and mimic other possible situations so that the operators can learn the patterns. A handheld thermal imager on a cool night can image a human being from 5 to 10 km. In hot weather, use this device in the morning, before the sun starts heating things up. You will quickly notice that south-facing rocks look warmer than north-facing rocks and that humans glow brightly.

Lanterns are valuable for base camp–type operations and on long trips in dark winter conditions. Coleman Peak 1 lanterns burn Coleman fuel, which yields more light per pound of fuel than any battery-powered lamp. It makes sense to use the same fuel for stoves and lanterns. There are small lanterns that burn unleaded gasoline, but they are not as small as the Peak 1 lantern. If you carry a gas lantern, be sure to carry plenty of spare mantles and use the plastic case. These cases come apart easily; many people buy a piece of stout bungee cord and tie it around the case, from top to bottom, to help it stay together in a pack or sled.

Electric fluorescent lamps or lanterns burn more efficiently and provide a smoother, more useable light. Solar rechargeable lamps are a great idea as long as plenty of sunlight is available for charging. Most solar rechargeable lamps do not function well during travel because they need to be held at a proper solar angle during the same hours that one tends to be doing other things.

STOVES AND COOKING GEAR

Camp stoves are valuable for heating water, improve nutrition and hydration, and help keep spirits up in rough weather. The general standard is to burn white gas in a self-cleaning multifuel stove. White gas is also sold as Coleman fuel, stove fuel, or naphtha in different parts of the world. White gas burns hot; it can be argued that some liquid fuels burn hotter than others, but the differences are minor. Liquid-fuel backpacking stoves burn significantly hotter than small propane stoves. A hot stove is faster and is more reliable in bad weather. Multifuel stoves tend to work better in cold weather because they have fuel preheating loops in the fuel line. A self-cleaning stove has an internal cleaning needle that reams out the gas jet. A stove that requires a handheld external cleaning needle is a poor choice because it requires more maintenance to operate. Although it is easy to rationalize that occasional maintenance is not a problem, these clogged jets are more problematic in tough conditions when there is a greater need for the stove to perform at higher levels of heat and reliability.

Gas cartridge stoves are a quick and easy option for three-season use (anytime but winter.) They are turned on and lit like a gas range. However, the typical gas stove puts out roughly half the heat of a good liquid fuel stove. This is a great first stove for a backpacker because it is virtually maintenance free. Hotter fuels are available in some countries.

Kerosene stoves do not burn as clean as white gas stoves, so they need more frequent cleaning. They are harder to light in the cold but still light at subzero temperatures. This fuel is "thicker," so it is more stable (off-gasses less and ignites at a higher temperature) than white gas.

Multifuel stoves can burn many liquid fuels but generate more soot with fuels other than white gas. Although you may have heard all sorts of precautions about burning lower-grade fuels in these stoves, in the short run this is no problem. At $-29°$ C ($-20°$ F), it may take some priming to get #2 diesel fuel to burn blue, but it works once the burner head and preheating loop are warm.

Types of stoves include free-standing models and the lighter models that attach to a fuel bottle. Recent advances in the attached stoves have made them stable

and reliable enough to capture most of the backpacking market. Be sure to choose a stove that simmers well. If you do not want to research which stove is better at simmering than the rest, buy a top-of-the-line MSR multifuel stove. The model chosen is not as important as how well the stove is used and maintained.

Stove Hazards

Burns are the most common stove or cooking injury. Backpacking stoves often tip over. Burns commonly come from spilled pots of scalding water, from using bare hands near a flame or frying pan, and occasionally directly from burning stove fuel. To minimize spills, do the following:

1. Supervise the stove area so that no one tips over a pot.
2. Do not allow people to sit in the impact area around a burning stove.
3. Use a ladle instead of pouring from the pot.
4. Do not carry a pot of boiling water over humans.
5. Do not pour boiling water into a cup that is in someone's hand.

All stoves generate noxious fumes. While a stove is being primed, the cold fuel burns poorly and creates a black cloud that should be avoided. Do not prime a stove in an enclosed sleeping area. Indoor cooking is reasonable in a well-ventilated tent or snow cave as long as the stove is primed outdoors first. Even then, the stove fumes give some people headaches.

Fatalities from cooking in closed tents have been related to carbon monoxide. This is avoidable with ventilation, even though ventilation may be hard to accomplish when, for example, you are leaning against the side of the tent to keep it from collapsing from wind pressure while your tentmate is melting snow to drink.

Burns from spilled fuel are usually related to open fuel bottles near lit stoves in warm weather. Unfortunately, people tend to push or throw a burning fuel bottle instead of merely setting the cap back on to quickly extinguish the flame. Once the burning bottle is spilled, the fire grows quickly.

Stove Accessories

Fuel bottles come in many sizes and materials. A 1-L aluminum bottle is standard. On long expeditions, carry full gallon cans of stove fuel rather than a bag full of aluminum bottles. Carry at least one aluminum bottle for controlled pouring or to attach to the stove. Save space by crushing the empty gallon can. Plastic fuel bottles lack the durability of aluminum and do not attach to newer, lightweight stoves.

A windscreen is a valuable accessory in bad weather. A wildland fire fighter may be able to provide an old "shake 'n' bake" (aluminum/fiberglass blanket). In a raging blizzard, use a square meter of the blanket to completely enclose the stove and bake using a "backcountry microwave" technique in full blizzard conditions. In deep snow, you can build a small snow kitchen that keeps the wind and snow away from the stove, decreases cooking time, saves fuel, and decreases wear and tear on the stove.

A stove base can help stabilize a stove, keep it from sinking into the snow, and protect the ground from heat and fuel. An after-market stove base can be purchased or constructed from an 8-inch square of thin plywood. Set the stove on the pad and trace the footprints. Drill holes halfway into the wood for the stove feet. Some people glue a thin layer of tin or aluminum to the top to make it fireproof. In very cold conditions, glue a piece of an old closed cell foam pad to the bottom of the base, and consider making the base wider to serve as a better snowshoe for the stove.

Fuel and time are wasted when you cook a pot of food and then set it on the cold snow or ground. An extra piece of plain closed cell foam is useful as a pot trivet when cooking in the snow. Pot grips should be substantial. A 6-inch pair of channel locks are the best grips used to prevent dropping a pot.

Repair kits are critical. Stopping to sew a small pant leg tear from a crampon might keep a person from tripping later. Replacing the bulb in a headlamp might allow the group to move twice as fast. Maintenance habits affect what spare parts are carried in a repair kit. If all the gaskets and O-rings are replaced on each stove and headlamps are replaced every year, you will not need to carry those spare parts. If maintenance is performed only when equipment breaks, then it will be necessary to carry a complete expedition repair kit. To learn which parts are usually needed, ask the manufacturer or speak to someone who repairs stoves and lamps for an outfitter.

Cooking dishes vary from an unused pot at home to specialized nesting backpacker ware. On an extended trip, stainless steel pots are durable and easy to clean. Good aluminum and titanium pots are available, but stainless steel is the common standard. Nesting pots pack better for larger groups, and also offer more versatile sizes. Nonstick coatings are attractive on frying pans, but since little soap is used when backpacking for environmental reasons, expect sand and grit to wear down the nonstick coatings. Cooking utensils can include pot grips (6-inch channel locks), a serving spoon, a ladle for dishing out hot water, and a spatula. Stainless steel tools are more durable, but lighter weight plastic and aluminum utensils are available. As with any gear, lighter weight equipment needs more care and cannot be used for as many tasks as heavy duty gear. Most people that go on a lot of expeditions do not skimp on utensils.

Eating utensils need to be simple, durable, and easy to clean. They need to be able to withstand an occasional boiling to keep them clean. A spoon is the eating utensil of choice among backpackers. Lexan spoons are very light. Stainless steel spoons are more durable and can also help scrape a pot or unscrew a large-slotted screw. Bowls should be of a large enough volume so that when the meal is divided, you receive a full portion so that the pot can be used for its next function. Some travelers prefer a Tupperware-type bowl with a lid to carry leftovers as trail food. Mugs should carry at least 16 ounces. In hot weather, when hot drinks are not usually fixed, it may work to carry one dish to use as cup and bowl and drink only from a water bottle.

Fire-Starting Tools

Starting fires can be challenging. Catalogs are full of flints and steels, and all sorts of equipment. The smartest device to carry and use is a cigarette lighter. Break off the childproof plastic barrier by the striker in cold weather; this barrier can eat a hole under your thumbnail as you try to strike the lighter. Carry the primary lighter in a handy location. Carry a spare lighter deep in the pack where it cannot get wet. For all-weather reliability, carry an electronic piezo lighter. Some of these lighters have waterproof caps and should last a long time. Cheaper lighters still work but work only a few months after exposure to saltwater.

KNIVES, MULTITOOLS, SAWS, AND SHOVELS

Expedition tools should include a Swiss army knife, a pocket multitool with pliers, or both devices. The more a tool is hybridized, the less it can perform any single function. To reattach ski bindings, you want a real screwdriver to apply the torque and control. A good tool kit includes duct tape, baling wire, an awl (to drill holes), a standard screwdriver, a Phillips screwdriver, and channel locks or pliers.

Knives need to be simple, durable, strong, and easy to clean. An excellent choice is a Swiss Army brand model that is all metal and only has 4 blades: knife, awl, and two flat screwdrivers with bottle and can openers. An all-metal Swiss Army knife can be dropped in the pot during routine sterilization of camp utensils. This sterilization involves taking every utensil (already thoroughly cleaned) and dropping it in a pot of boiling water. Once the pot begins to boil again, the bacteria on the utensils are killed. Knives with plastic covers tend to lose their plastic parts when boiled.

An alternative knife choice is a simple ultralight lockback knife with a 3-inch blade. Larger blades are too big for most camp chores, and smaller blades cannot adequately perform certain tasks, such as cutting cheese. Smaller blades also tend to allow food to penetrate the hinge and thus are harder to keep clean. "Ultralight" knives are light because their cases are made of composite resins; they are strong, durable, and easy to clean. Locking knives are illegal to carry on some international flights. Pack knives in checked luggage or expect them to be temporarily confiscated by the airlines.

Knife maintenance starts with keeping a knife clean. Even the best stainless steel corrodes if food or dirt is left on it. When a knife becomes dirty, it should be cleaned quickly. Occasional sterilization keeps it even cleaner. Occasional lubrication with a Teflon-based lubricant (the kind used on camming devices and fishing reels) helps tools open easier and minimizes corrosion in the joints. If a tool is immersed in salt water, it should be rinsed in fresh water and the joints relubricated. The lubrication not only greases the joint but also displaces water. Joints are more prone to corrosion because of electrolysis between different metals in the tool. Clean knives work better than dirty ones.

Knives should be sharpened as needed. Ceramic sticks are good for a quick sharpening because they reform just the edge of the blade rather than grinding it down. Sharpening with a whetstone too often leads to thinning and reshaping of the blade.

Multitools come in many configurations and sizes. Full-sized multitools work much better than smaller ones. Microtools may look appealing, but they lack the torque and control to do many tasks well. A multitool should have all the tools already mentioned. Brand names such as Buck, Gerber, Leatherman, Schrade, SOG, and Victorinox have stronger steel, better machining, and tighter rivets. Cheap tools are available but do not perform well or last long.

Choose the multitool that fits your specific needs by performing these comparisons with different models at the same time:

1. Open all accessories. Blades that lock open are generally more controllable than nonlocking blades. Blades that are difficult to open when new may be impossible to open after a few expeditions.
2. Determine which tools will really be used. Having more little tools usually is inconsequential. The blades are much more important.
3. Tightly grip the pliers of each and crank on a 1-inch piece of wood or around a fat tent pole, torquing one set of pliers against the other. Some tools have sharper handle corners than others: the smoother edges often allow a better grip, providing more control, better fit, and less pain. In general, there is more torque with a larger tool or with the compound leverage of some pliers such as the SOG. In general, a torque wrench shows no measurable difference between the pliers of different full-sized multitools.

Once you purchase a multitool, practice performing some household tasks with it. It takes a lot of finesse and composure to use these tools; for example, practice bolting a pack frame back together tightly so that you will not strip the nuts, practice using the awl to drill a neat hole in a tent pole, and practice whittling a new spoon.

Saws are used for improvising splints and litters out of local wood, clearing trails, or cutting firewood. Some Swiss Army knives have saws, but they can cut only small wood. Another simple saw is a little cable saw, which is lightweight and works in an emergency but is not the tool of choice for extended wood cutting because it is hard to use and wears out. Some backpacker-type saws fold up. These devices use conventional saw blades, as on a bow saw (thin, flat steel with big teeth.) When assembled and tightened securely, these saws can cut big pieces of wood quickly. In general, the triangular Sven-Saw with an all-metal frame is a reliable saw for the trail. For an emergency, a cable saw or Swiss Army knife saw will work fine.

Shovels are used for digging cat holes for human waste and building fires. Small, folding shovels, such as the Udigit, work well and are very durable. A cheaper option is a simple plastic gardening trowel, but they are not very rugged, especially once they have been used a year or two. If something bigger is needed, the Boy Scout shovel with the oak handle or a military entrenching tool (E tool) works well. If you will be moving snow, consider the small but unbreakable Life Link Lexan shovels or the larger, extendable aluminum ski-touring shovels such as the Voilé shovel.

WATER CONTAINERS

Carry 1 to 2 L of water storage on any hike, and add 5 to 10 L of water storage per day for "dry camping." *Dry camping* means camping away from a water source, such as in the desert or high on a ridge. Since water weighs roughly 2 pounds/L, most people camp near water and use their larger water containers to keep a ready supply in the "kitchen."

A clean 1-L IV bottle is an excellent personal water bottle. It packs well and is lightweight, and the price is right. Many serious adventurers use these as their primary water bottles on short expeditions. On long expeditions, the use of something more durable, such as a Nalgene bottle, is standard. Narrow-mouthed bottles work, but wide-mouthed bottles fill faster and are easier to deal with if the liquid is frozen.

Larger quantities of water can be carried in large inexpensive plastic water containers available at any camping store. The accordion styles are generally more durable than the square plastic ones. These containers are used only for hauling water from the stream to the kitchen and not for long-range transport.

A more rugged option is an MSR Dromedary or another nylon water bag, which can be stuffed inside a pack. A 5-L dromedary is an excellent addition to the pack, even if you only need to carry an extra liter or two of water. The advantage of a nylon water bag over a case of water bottles is that the nylon container collapses, making it more versatile.

There are medium-sized (2- to 3-L) heavy duty plastic water vessels that are not expedition grade like the nylon vessels. However, they are especially handy in hot weather because they hold an amount of water that is between the classic 1-L bottle and the big water tanks needed for dry camping.

A drinking tube can be obtained for many of these bags so that you can sip while walking without having to open the pack. Drinking tubes freeze quickly in very cold conditions but are very helpful in hot, dry conditions. Neoprene sleeves help minimize, but not eliminate, freezing in drinking tubes.

In cold weather, some people put their water bottles in insulated sleeves. If you buy one, be sure it encloses the whole bottle. Foam sleeves can be made from old sleeping pads and contact cement or can be fashioned from a large insulated mitten or booty. It helps to pack water near the body to capitalize on body heat. This works down to $-20°$ C ($-29°$ F), but in even lower temperatures, it is best to carry a minimum of water, since frozen water makes not only the water but also the container unavailable. Thawing frozen water bottles is a painfully slow process and uses a lot of fuel. Frozen containers often break because people try to chip out the ice or they try to warm the plastic near a fire, melting the plastic too. Thaw a frozen water container by putting it in a pot of hot water. Once part of the ice in the container melts, pour cold water out of and hot water into the bottle.

Disinfect all drinking water (see Chapter 51). This holds true for the containers as well. If you use a filter instead of iodine or chlorine, you must occasionally disinfect the water containers or bacterial growth may occur. Water bottles that have carried sugar drinks support bacterial growth in warm weather. Drinking tubes and the threads on bottle lids are especially prone to bacteria. Between trips, clean glass and hard plastic water containers by running them through the dishwasher. Soft nylon water containers can be run through the washing machine. Soft plastic containers need to be scrubbed by hand. Before long-term storage, rinse with super-chlorinated water (one teaspoon of bleach in a liter of water) and dry thoroughly to minimize mold and bacterial growth. Before using a stored water container, quickly rinse it with tap water to get rid of distasteful odors.

BACKPACKS

Internal-frame packs are the current standard and an excellent choice for many situations. With careful packing, internal-frame packs are easier to carry than the older external-frame packs. Choose a volume that you will use often. Packing all of your gear takes a lot of care; if the pack is overloaded, it does not handle well.

External-frame packs are easier and faster to load. Some people can carry a heavy load (more than 50% of body weight) more easily with an external-frame pack. Many people attach a daypack as a top storage compartment so that it can be detached for lesser loads in camp. Although many soft (internal-frame) packs have top pockets that detach as fanny packs, they are smaller and perform less well compared with a good standalone daypack. External-frame packs are generally easier for finding specific items such as tools, clothing, or food during a hike because the packing system is more compartmentalized.

Size is the first consideration. A total of 3000 to 4000 in³ is a great size for a day pack. For packing overnight gear, 5000 in³ is a better size. For a week's journey, 6000 in³ is preferable. On an extended expedition, at least 7000 in³ is needed. In winter, allow more storage space for extra clothing layers. If you carry medical equipment plus gear, you will need a large pack. Extra volume makes it easier to pack and to find things. One can always add pockets to some packs, but this should be done primarily to make access more convenient, not to carry more weight. Pockets tend to flop around on packs and are a less efficient way to carry heavy items. (The flopping causes slight jolting with every step.) Slightly bigger packs have as many advantages as disadvantages; choose a general size range and then shop for a style you really like.

Suspension systems vary from a simple webbing belt and shoulder straps (inadequate) to well-padded systems that wrap around the torso. For full loads (more than 40% of body weight) choose a system that comfortably rests the weight on the hips but snugly pulls the load toward the back. Choose thick padding on the hips and shoulders, and a fit that easily adjusts while walking to take the pressure off hot spots. Carrying heavy loads is never easy, but a good suspension system makes carrying them more bearable (Figure 71-1).

Comfort features on packs include adjustable stays (straps that position the load), a lumbar pad, and a hip suspension system to fit the body. Trying on a pack is essential. Put in as much weight as intended for the expedition and hoist the pack up and over obstacles and especially down some stairs. If you cannot make the pack fit comfortably, try another, perhaps one with more adjustments. Certain adjustments, such as shoulder strap height, can be fitted once and then not changed much, but other features, such as side stays (load adjustment straps), need to be easily adjustable while walking down the trail because they can help distribute weight better, making it less fatiguing to haul the load. A sternum strap holds the shoulder straps together, helping them wrap around the torso better. On men, the sternum strap should cross the nipples.

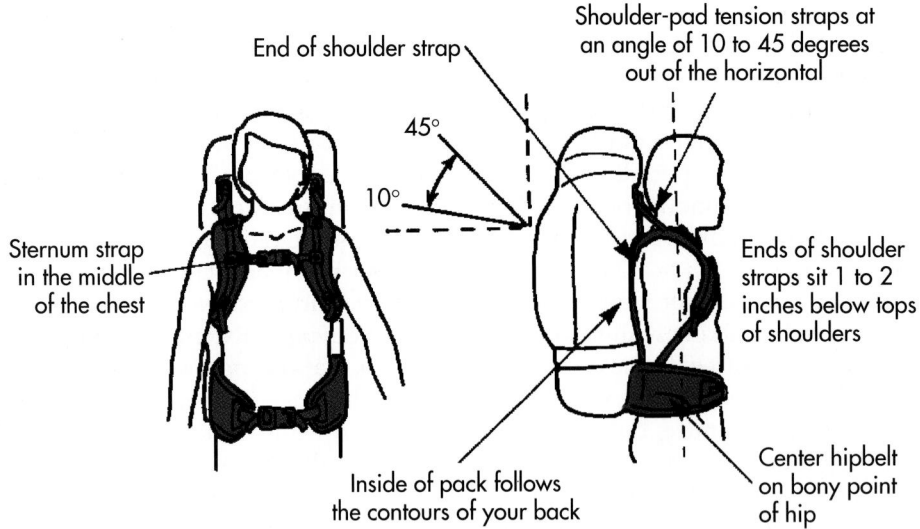

Figure 71-1 Backpack suspension system. (*Redrawn from Harvey M:* The National Outdoor Leadership School's wilderness guide: the classic handbook, *New York, 1999, Fireside.*)

Women need to position this strap above or below the breasts for comfort. This is obviously a function of personal anatomy and the angle of the shoulder straps and can only be determined by active trial. Basic comfort may seem like a luxury, but on the trail, how well one carries a load has direct bearing on how much energy can be put into hauling essential gear and how much energy remains to enjoy the wilderness.

Pack Accessories

Extra pockets can be great additions. These are left at home for lighter trips or when hauling a pack up a big wall. Some packs come with integral map pockets, water bag holders, crampon straps, ice tool straps, and other pockets. If these accessories are used, then the weight is justifiable. However, they can diminish the basic comfort that encourages use of the pack. One should carry ¾" nylon tape lash straps for attaching things like sleeping pads to the pack. Fastex buckles make these lash straps easier to use. Buy the straps 50% longer than you think you need so that they can be used for other applications. Lash points allow attachment of items such as ice axes and foam pads without squeezing them inside. Lash points do not weigh much and add a lot of versatility to any pack.

Stuff sacks should be used to compartmentalize the gear. They should be slightly oversized so that they can change shape more easily when packing. Thin, coated nylon is a good material for stuff sacks; in general, thinner is better because of weight and stuffability. The heavy stuff sacks on the market are soft luggage and entirely too heavy to use as backpack compartments. Mesh bags offer good options for a see-through bag; even a mosquito head net can be used for a stuff sack in the day pack and can double as a bug net. Use a large

(18 × 12 × 12 inch) stuff sack for clothes, a medium to large size for food (actual size depends on whether you need to carry food for 1 or 10 days), and two small sacks for toiletries and for the "possible bag." A possible bag has all of the little items needed during the day: compass, pocket knife, lip balm, sunscreen, insect repellent, and such. While most of these stuff sacks usually fit into the main compartment of a pack, the possible bag is typically carried in the small pocket of the day pack so that it is always available.

Packing a backpack is as important as choosing one. Pack heavy objects low and forward to avoid having to lean further forward to balance the hoisted load. Pack fuel below food because sooner or later, the fuel will leak. Avoid lashing loose objects on the outside of the pack; rattling hardware is a nuisance and causes routine jolting. Balance the pack so that left and right are equal. Stuff items such as sleeping bags into "compression stuff sacks," or stuff sleeping bags and parkas into the bottom of the pack. Internal-frame packs do not allow very good accessibility, so pack carefully. A nice option is to choose a pack that has a large top pocket that becomes a fanny pack. Keep items needed for short day hikes in the fanny pack so that they are readily accessible. In cold weather, shed a big clothing layer as the hike begins but put it back on before resting. Therefore you should leave room in the packing system for such practicalities. In wet climates, consider waterproofing the pack by lining it with a tough garbage bag.

Adjust the pack to fit comfortably. It is best to store the pack with the straps "adjusted out" so that they will not become misshapen. When donning the pack, adjust the hip belt to get the pack to the correct height and to rest the weight on the hips. Then adjust the shoulder strap length and tighten the adjusters that pull the pack forward to the shoulders. With slight increases and decreases in these adjusters, you can shift pressure for more comfort. If you do not follow this routine, you will put more pressure on the shoulders than necessary.

TENTS

Tents can be as simple as centered-pole tarps, such as Black Diamond's Megamid or Mountain Hardware's Kiva, which work fine in most environments. In bug seasons, use a tent with mosquito netting. In muddy conditions, a tent with a floor is important. Choose a name-brand manufacturer from a reliable outfitter. Traditionally, North Face and Sierra Designs have offered state-of-the-art tents for decades, but some of the new lines, such as Mountain Hardware, are proving to be more innovative with the same quality workmanship. Less expensive brands may be fine for family camping but are not as high-quality as the other tents typically used by mountaineers above tree-line. Plan on purchasing a tent for a decade's use.

Tent fabrics range from cotton to Gore-Tex, with nylon being the norm. Cotton tents are heavy but are not considered expedition gear, even when dry. Gore-Tex is a fine option for traveling light but never breathes as well or lasts as long as a classic fly-canopy system. Many large expeditions use Gore-Tex tents to control weight. Most people purchase a tent with an uncoated canopy (the fabric that is the ceiling) and a urethane-coated rainfly (the fabric on the top.) This provides ventilation by allowing perspiration to move through the canopy while keeping the occupant dry. Check for coating on a fabric by trying to suck air through it; uncoated nylon allows air to pass through easily. One fabric option sometimes available by special order is an "expedition" or "outfitter" floor. This heavier fabric strengthens the most vulnerable part of the tent.

For extra convenience and room, get a top-end state-of-the-art dome tent with a vestibule, such as a North Face VE-25. Use aluminum poles because they are lighter and stronger than fiberglass poles. Avoid pole sleeves; get a tent that has pole clips on the canopy. A rain fly with adjustable bottom straps is welcome in cold conditions when the nylon gets stiff and tight. You can cook in the vestibule with extreme care about fuel and fumes. The tent should be easy to set up in dark or windy conditions.

Backpacking tents are small. Expect space to be tight if teammates are large or there is a lot of gear. Try a tent for size before buying. Fill it with pads and sleeping bags and some extra gear, and use it for a while before committing to it.

Accessories can make a tent more versatile. A thin nylon ground cloth under the tent keeps the bottom cleaner and more waterproof and helps protect it from rocks and sticks. A nice accessory is a mesh shelf across the top, or mesh pockets on the sides. These help keep loose gear organized, making it easier to move in and get comfortable without the frustration of losing items such as glasses and mitten shells. A single vestibule is an obvious accessory, but some tents can handle two vestibules. This is excellent for base camping.

Choose tent stakes according to the ground into which they will be driven. In hard dirt, thin aluminum stakes work fine. In softer dirt, larger-diameter plastic stakes hold much better. In sand or snow, long stakes reach down into the more compressed damp sand, or very large stakes act as "dead men." A dead man is a stick or stake about a foot long, buried sideways with a string looped around it. The stake needs to be at a right angle to the direction of the string. Compress the sand or snow and let it set up for a few minutes so that it will hold. If you use a disposable stick and tie it off above ground, the dead man can be left in the ground. This is especially nice in snow because the snow "sinters" (crystallizes together), making it hard to dig out the stick. In windy conditions, it takes more than tent stakes to hold down a tent. You may need to tie the sides of the tent to rocks, logs, and bushes or may even need to sit in the tent to hold it down as a front passes through.

To set up a tent, tie it down so that it is taut and make the knots adjustable. A trucker's hitch (see Chapter 72) is the first knot to be mastered if you wish to excel at setting up tents. As the fabric stretches as a result of heat or moisture, retighten the knots. Tie the tent to stakes, trees, rocks, or dead men. In inclement weather, how tightly the tent is secured controls the flapping that can eventually shred any tent.

Care of a tent includes routine seam-sealing of the outside of the rainfly and tent bottom. Seam-sealer prevents the capillary action that allows water to seep into the tent through the threads and seams. Routine seam-sealing does not mean adding more sealant every time the tent is used. Rather, sealant should be reapplied as it is noticed to crack and wear. You need to apply seam sealer to a dry tent; it will not adhere to moisture. Keeping a tent out of the sun and gently cleaning it after use makes the nylon fabric last longer. Storing the tent in a cool, dry place minimizes mildew and fabric rot. Keeping zippers clean on a daily basis and lubricating them helps them last longer. Lubricate them with a commercial product or in a pinch use lip balm or candle wax. Zippers are often the first thing to fail; careful attention to not stressing zippers can postpone this inevitable failure point. Carry a spare zipper slider, a spare zipper "stop," and nylon repair tape.

SLEEPING BAGS

Materials for sleeping bags include only a few options. Insulation can be one of the spins of polyester fiber fill, or it can be goose down. Fiber fill bags are often referred to as *synthetic bags*. Covers can be uncoated nylon or Gore-Tex. The most common bag is fiber fill with an uncoated cover, but there is no need to be limited by convention.

Down bags are lighter and stuff much better than synthetic bags. In a continental climate (away from the oceans), a down bag can be both luxurious and practical, especially in dry, cold conditions. Once soaking wet, however, a down bag will not regain full insulation until tumbled in a cool dryer with a tennis shoe to fluff it up. Name-brand manufacturers usually provide high-quality goose down; other brands may provide more feathers and less fill power (rated in cubic inches per ounce of down.)

Fiber fill or synthetic bags include Polarguard 3D, Polarguard HV, Lite Loft, Thinsulate, and Qualofil fibers. Polarguard HV is one of the tougher fiber fills because it has a casing of "scrim" around the bats, like a sausage casing: it handles repeated washings better than others. Polarguard 3D is lighter and stuffs better but is not as resilient, losing more fluff than Polarguard HV after repeated washings. Qualofil performs almost as well as down when new because it has four hollow tubes running down its core, providing a structure that fluffs it up; however, it does not withstand repeated washings. A sample of 200 Polarguard HV bags, which are some of the toughest fiber fill bags, used continuously for 6 months and washed once a month, appear to have roughly half to two thirds the thickness of a new bag. This represents a decade of use for a typical weekend hiker.

Uncoated nylon breathes better than Gore-Tex but also absorbs moisture from rain or the ground more quickly. Some people prefer a Gore-Tex cover on a down bag, but more people use a Gore-Tex bivouac sack on their bags so that they have the option of adding that extra layer for warmth or leaving it at home.

Bag warmth is rated by temperature, which has no commonality from one manufacturer to another. One retailer might rate a bag at −7° C (20° F) (meaning it ought to keep you warm on such a night when new), and another retailer might sell the identical bag with it labeled as a −1° C (30° F) bag. Use any temperature rating to get in the ballpark, and choose a temperature rating that is conservatively below what is necessary. To compare one bag to another, it needs to be the same style; for instance, compare the insulation weight, with three pounds of Dacron being significantly warmer than two pounds of the same insulation.

Shape can be as important as thickness. Any decent bag has a differential cut, meaning the nylon on the outside is cut bigger than the nylon on the inside. This detail is one of the fundamental differences between a top-brand sleeping bag and a discount bag. An efficient bag is mummy shaped, just like the human body. A bag

that has too much extra space will be hard to heat and will have cold spots as you shift during the night. You will be unable to comfortably maneuver in a bag that fits too tightly. Most people cannot easily change socks while zipped up in a sleeping bag. Draft tubes make a bag much more efficient. One draft tube runs along the zipper. When testing a bag, see whether that draft tube naturally lays across the cold zipper, or if it only ends up there when you wake up and move it there. A draft tube between the chest and neck helps keep the torso's body heat in the bag as you roll around; it requires an adjustable draw cord to work well. Even in a summer-weight bag, this adjustable option is smarter to carry than the equivalent weight in insulation. The last draft tube encircles the face. This also needs an adjustable draw cord. In very cold conditions, you will draw this cord so tightly that only the mouth and nose are exposed; make sure the draw cord works easily at that range because when you wake up too cold or too hot in the middle of the night, you do not want a desperate struggle to adjust the cord. Most important, a bag needs to fit the body, with no pressure on the toes, but a minimum of extra space.

Sleeping pads add warmth and comfort to a sleeping system. A simple closed cell foam pad (closed cell foam does not allow air to pass through it), such as a Ridge Rest, insulates a person from the ground and is very reliable. An open cell foam pad is inadequate for backpacking because it absorbs water. In cold weather, it makes sense to have two pads under the torso. Tests at the Teton Science School have shown that a typical "three-season" bag is improved more by adding ground insulation than by adding more loft to the bag. Many winter campers carry a full-length pad and an extra half-pad that is their "sit-upon" during the day and serves to double-insulate the torso at night. An inflatable pad, such as a Thermarest, is a very effective insulator because it is constructed of open cell foam but is waterproof with a coated nylon cover. Cheap inflatable air mattresses with no foam grow cold quickly because of convective cooling to the ground. The risk with the best inflatables is puncture; a slow leak can be devastating. Always carry a repair kit; many expeditioners carry Shoe Goo (a "liquid rubber" compound) seam-grip instead of the contact cement that comes in a Thermarest repair kit because these substances hold better when applied in the marginal gluing conditions typical to an expedition.

Bivouac sacks are not essential but increase the number of options and provide a quick tent substitute for a short trip. The classic style has a coated nylon bottom, Gore-Tex top, and zipper with a small rain cover over it and is cut big enough to contain a sleeping pad and bag. Some have small wands (poles) to hold them up. For camping in a maritime (wet) climate, the wands are important. If you use this sack just to keep a down bag off the snow in a snow cave, it does not require wands. Mosquito netting adds an important option for sleeping out on a warm night when you do not wish to be zipped tightly in the bag.

Using a sleeping bag carefully is important. If you become too warm, loosen the draft tubes and unzip a bit of the bottom of the zipper first. Compared with being too cold, being too warm at night is not a problem for most people. Increase warmth by going to bed warm, even if you have to go for a short run or dig snow for a while. Close the draw cords tighter, until you reach the limits of good breathing. Breathing inside a bag provides short-term heat but adds water vapor that diminishes insulation and causes evaporative cooling. Many bags have just as much insulation on the top as on the bottom. You can sleep in a bag placed upside down to use the mummy hood to trap the heat around the head; this is much warmer. Add clothing layers to increase warmth: it is obvious that an extra pile jacket will keep you warmer but this works only if it fits loosely and does not impair circulation. Any clothing that covers bare skin has a pronounced warming effect, so gloves and a hat help contain body heat. Specialized gear, such as Dacron booties and pile balaclavas, are simple but very effective ways to help sleep warmer. Sleeping strategies, such as overlapping sleeping pads to prevent cold spots or even cuddling together, are often overlooked. Hydration and nutrition are essential to sleeping warmer on a cold night. You can also place hot water bottles in the groin area to help maintain warmer body temperature on a cold night, but most people first try simpler maneuvers.

72 Ropes and Knot Tying

Loui H. Clem and Steve Hudson

Although ropes are among the oldest tools known to man, the evolution of ropes for different purposes has been a long and complex process. From aboriginal peoples twisting a few plant fibers together to make a cord to the multitude of rope materials and designs available today, ropes have been a part of our lives for thousands of years. The foundation for selecting a rope is being able to assess the characteristics required for its intended use.

No rope should ever be used to support a human life unless it has been specifically built for that purpose. Stories abound of towropes being used (fatally) as climbing ropes, utility ropes coming apart when used as handlines, and natural fiber ropes rotting away to nothing. One good way to be certain that a rope is designed for life-safety purposes is to check whether it is certified to any life-safety standards, such as the Union of International Alpine Associations (UIAA), Cordage Institute (CI), American Society for Testing and Materials (ASTM), or National Fire Protection Association (NFPA).

Options for life-safety ropes include dynamic ropes for lead climbing falls, low-stretch ropes for low fall factors (see Fall Factors), and static ropes for minimal fall factors. Each rope construction type and material has pros and cons for specific applications. It is important to understand the performance characteristics of rope types to be able to select the right rope for the job.

ROPES

Rope Construction Types

Rope construction types historically found in life-safety applications include laid, eight-strand plaited, double-braid, and kernmantle. Kernmantle can be further broken down into more specific designs of static, low stretch, and dynamic.

Laid Rope. Although laid ropes have largely been replaced by newer technology, it is one of the oldest and most familiar designs and may still be found on rescue trucks, especially in rural areas. Laid ropes are manufactured by twisting bundles of fiber (usually three) around one another and resemble the design of the old manila ropes. These ropes tend to untwist slightly under loading, which causes them to spin and kink. They also tend to have high elongation properties, which can be a disadvantage when trying to position a constant load. More important, in laid rope construction, the supporting fibers are directly exposed to grit and abrasion. There is no protective covering to help reduce wear on the load-bearing strands (Figure 72-1).

Eight-Strand Plaited Rope. Eight-strand plaited ropes are not heavily used in rescue, but because plaited ropes were marketed to rescuers for a time and because some may still be in service, it is prudent to recognize their existence. Interweaving eight bundles of rope yarn creates an eight-strand plaited rope. Because these ropes are woven together loosely, they are very easy to handle. However, for the same reason, they are limp, knots tend to jam, and they do not hold up well. Their popularity was short lived because they are very susceptible to abrasion and "picking" (snagging) of bundles against rocks and building edges (Figure 72-2).

Double-Braid Rope. A double-braid rope consists of a braid of rope inside a larger, hollow braided rope. Because of the rather soft construction, this is an easy rope to splice or with which to tie knots and is therefore popular for marine use. Double-braid ropes are susceptible to abrasion and to picking of the individual bundles. It is also easy for grit and other material to penetrate to the rope's interior. The outer sheath braid of this rope sometimes slips on the inner core braid when a person is rappelling or climbing (Figure 72-3).

Kernmantle Rope. The German word *kernmantle* means "core" *(kern)* and "sheath" *(mantle).* Kernmantle rope sheaths are braided around the core and their design is crucial to the hand, knotability, and abrasion resistance of the rope. A tightly woven sheath will prove more durable than a loose one, but this feature must be finely balanced to maintain knotability. Other variables include fiber denier, number of strands in the braid, and angle of weave.

The core of a kernmantle rope primarily determines the elongation, force absorption, and strength properties of the rope. In the following descriptions of three common constructions, it should be noted that the terms "dynamic," "low stretch," and "static" are technically misnomers, in that all the ropes are "dynamic" at least to some degree. However, these are the industry-standard terminology and are quite useful in relating the degree of elongation inherent in each type of rope.

DYNAMIC KERNMANTLE ROPE. A well-designed dynamic rope is a must for "lead climbing" or in other situations

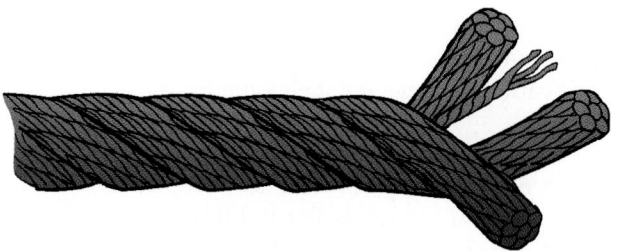

Figure 72-1   Laid rope.

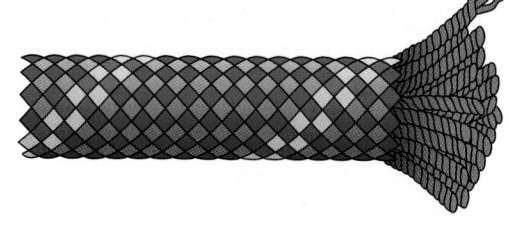

Figure 72-4   Dynamic kernmantle rope.

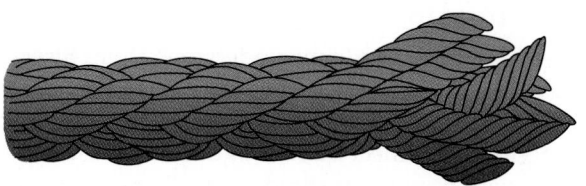

Figure 72-2   Eight-strand plaited rope.

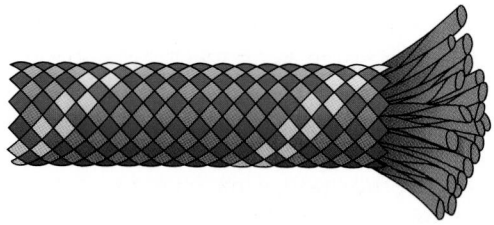

Figure 72-5   Static kernmantle rope.

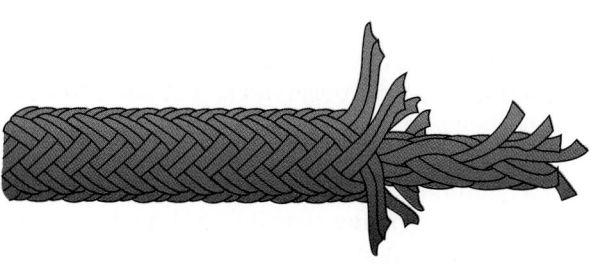

Figure 72-3   Double-braid rope.

in which there is a numerically high fall factor. This rope is designed to absorb the shock load in such a fall, thereby reducing the effects of the fall. This translates to the rope being very stretchy: as much as 30% elongation at 10% of minimum breaking strength (see Rope Strength).

Thus a dynamic kernmantle rope would be very difficult to use effectively for positioning heavy loads (such as a rescue load), contending with changing loads (i.e., loading a patient midface on a rock wall), or rigging into a haul system (in which energy would be wasted with each pull because of the inherent elongation). It would also be very difficult to use effectively under high tension (as in a highline). Dynamic kernmantle ropes also tend to have a lower tensile strength than static or low-stretch kernmantle ropes because of the same design characteristics that allow it to stretch. Furthermore, dynamic kernmantle designs are often softer and have a lower percentage of sheath than sta-

tic kernmantle ropes, making them more susceptible to abrasion and wear (Figure 72-4).

Static Kernmantle Rope. A static kernmantle rope is designed to be very strong and to have minimal stretch: as little as 3% to 6% at 10% of minimum breaking strength. For consistent strength, inner bundles run continuously and unbroken throughout the length of the rope, usually in a near-parallel manner to reduce stretch and spin. This load-carrying core is protected from dirt, abrasion, and cutting by a tightly braided outer sheath. Static kernmantle ropes are ideal for lowering and raising heavy loads (as in rescue), work positioning, and fall protection. Static ropes should not be subjected to a fall factor greater than 0.25 unless additional force absorption provisions are made in the system (Figure 72-5).

Low-Stretch Kernmantle Rope. Low-stretch kernmantle ropes elongate 6% to 10% at 10% breaking strength, fulfilling the needs not met by highly dynamic climbing ropes or very stable static kernmantle designs. This is achieved using a different core construction and a better sheath/core relationship and typically gives such ropes a softer profile than static lines. However, these same characteristics decrease abrasion resistance and make it a less desirable rope for positioning. Low-stretch ropes are often used for belaying heavy loads, especially where low fall factor potential exists.

Fall Factors

Fall factors can be calculated by dividing the fall distance by the length of the rope between the load and the anchor or belay. Thus a 3-foot fall on a 10-foot rope would be a fall factor of 0.3, a 3-foot fall on a 3-foot rope would be a fall factor of 1.0, and a 3-foot fall on a 100-foot rope would be a fall factor of 0.03. This formula assumes that the fall takes place in free air without rope drag across the rock face or through intermediate equipment (Figure 72-6).

The danger of a high fall factor on a low-stretch or static rope is not that the rope will break but that the high-impact forces may subject the person to great discomfort and possible injury or death. A static rope transfers more of a shock load to the anchors than a dynamic rope, increasing damage potential there as well.

Another concern in any impact load situation is the effect such forces have on equipment such as belay devices, rope grabs, or ascenders. Some of these devices can damage a rope when subjected to relatively low-impact forces. The study of impact forces and ways that different pieces of equipment relate to different constructions of rope when subjected to such forces is fairly complicated. Two general rules of thumb are to

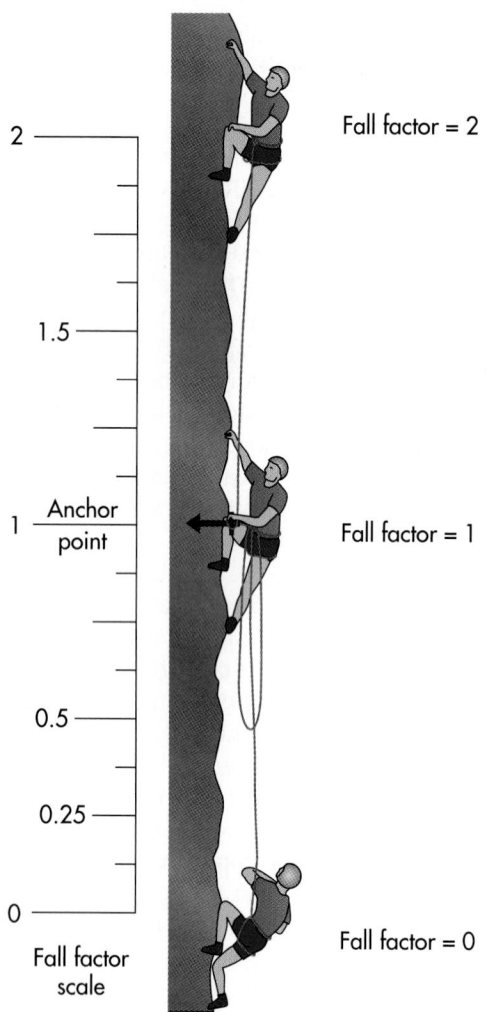

Figure 72-6 Fall factors.

(1) design and operate your rope systems to minimize the potential for high-impact forces and (2) exercise great caution in selecting belay methods.

Rope Size

Just as no single type of rope is appropriate for all activities, no single size fits all conditions. Purchasing the largest rope in the hope that it will fit all situations because it is so strong could lead to problems in working with the rope and the auxiliary equipment. Rope strength and elongation are actually the more critical determinations, and size considerations should follow.

Rope Strength

Rope strength is a fairly misunderstood topic. Strength of life safety rope is usually referred to as *minimum breaking strength*. Unfortunately, reported numbers do not necessarily reflect numbers adequate for comparison. Variations in test methods, as well as in analysis of results, provide marketing fodder that can create great confusion.

One way to report strength is as the rope's "ultimate, or maximum, breaking strength," which is the highest score of a given rope in a series of tests. An alternative is to list the "average breaking strength" of several tests. A more conservative method is to define *breaking strength* at a value two or three standard deviations below the average test result. Another method is to list a "minimum breaking strength" and then define *minimum* as not greater than 10% below the average. Often, figures for tensile or breaking strength are reported without any explanation as to whether they are average or minimum or whether some other measure was used. Simply stated, "breaking strength" might refer to any one of these reporting methods, or even to another.

To add to the confusion, a number of factors affect test results. The rate at which the pull is applied to the rope, the temperature, the humidity, the diameter of the object to which the rope is attached, and other factors all have an effect on test results. Thus unless ropes are tested in exactly the same way, results cannot be meaningfully compared.

One common test method that has been adopted by several standards organizations is "CI-1801" from the Cordage Institute (CI). CI-1801 for life-safety rope is specific and gives a common baseline from which to attain results. This standard also calls for a very conservative reporting method, wherein *minimum breaking strength* is defined as three standard deviations below the mean of several break tests. This helps normalize the results. In addition to type of construction, the strength of a rope comes from the amount of nylon used to make it; similar rope constructions of the same diameter should have similar strengths if they have the same amount and quality of nylon.

Results from laboratory tests may differ greatly from rope performance in real-world applications, which cannot be consistently and accurately quantified. A knotted rope loaded over a building edge, for example, may not come close in strength to a rope loaded in a laboratory tensile test machine.

It is clear that a rope should be stronger than the force of the intended load, but how much stronger? The ratio of a rope's strength to load is often called a *design factor*. If the strength of a rope is 2500 pounds and the load is 500 pounds, then the design factor is 5:1. The design factor takes into consideration only the new condition of an item as it is designed to perform. When translating a design factor into a system safety factor, factors such as age, wear and tear, dry/wet condition, and system rigging should be considered.

A rope system is only as strong as its weakest link. The ratio between the weak link in a system and the load to be applied is known as the *system safety factor*. System safety factors also take into account the way that loads are applied to a system. For instance, redirectional pulleys, rigging angles, and mechanical advantage systems can all increase the forces within a system.

Generally, component design factors tend to be very high, often as high as 15:1. Once the real world is factored into an actual system, the remaining system safety factor may be half that value. As a rule, the higher the probability of and consequences of failure, the higher the safety factor should be.

Rope Fiber

Before the development of synthetic fiber ropes, the standard for many years was rope made of natural fibers, such as manila. Natural-fiber rope degrades in strength even when carefully stored, lacks the ability to absorb shock loads, lacks continuous fiber along the length of the rope, and has low strength compared with certain artificial fibers. For these reasons, natural-fiber ropes are no longer considered appropriate for life-safety applications. Synthetic fibers, including polyolefin, aramids, ultra-high-modulus polyethylene (UHMPE), polyester, and nylon, are more commonly used in modern-day rope making.

Polyolefin. Polyolefin (polypropylene or polyethylene) fiber ropes are used when their flotation property is desired, such as in water rescue. They also have good resistance to most acids. However, polyolefin fibers rapidly degrade, especially under ultraviolet exposure. Because the fiber has low abrasion resistance, strength, life expectancy, and melting point, it is a poor choice for most life-safety applications.

Aramids. Aramids, commonly known by the trade name *Kevlar*, are extremely strong fibers and resist high temperatures. However, aramid is very susceptible to internal and external abrasion. Because it cannot absorb dynamic energy and breaks if bent too tightly (such as in a knot or rappel device), it is dangerous to use in life-safety applications.

UHMPE. UHMPE, more commonly known by trade names *Spectra* and *Vectran*, is a newer type of high-modulus lightweight fiber. It has better abrasion resistance than aramid but still has too little stretch to absorb dynamic energy. UHMPE fibers also have too low a melting point to safely be used with most rappelling equipment. In addition, they tend to be very slippery and do not hold knots well under high tension.

Polyester. Polyester fibers are used in many ropes. Dacron (DuPont) has a melting point of about 249° C (480° F), which is in the range of nylon 6.6 and above the melting point for nylon 6. Polyester fiber has a high tensile strength even when wet, low elongation at break, and can be as effectively UV stabilized as nylon. These factors make polyester rope well suited for marine applications, such as for boat rigging lines, and makes it an interesting choice for life safety. However, polyester fiber has low dynamic energy absorption, which means that the fiber cannot handle shock loads or repeated loading as well as nylon fiber.

Nylon. Nylon is the most common and most suitable fiber for general life-safety use. Nylon is approximately 10% stronger than polyester, but nylon fiber may lose as much as 10% to 15% of its strength when wet. However, it regains its strength when it dries. Nylon can handle about twice as much shock loading per pound as polyester when both are wet.

Nylon strongly resists most chemicals, but certain alkalis, acids, or bleaches can cause degradation, especially in high concentrations. For the high-angle technician, the source of most damaging acids are batteries, including lead acid and so-called "sealed" or dry-cell batteries. Users must scrupulously protect ropes from direct contact with batteries or exposure to acid fumes or residues that might be found in vehicle storage compartments, trunks, and garage floors. Industrial users should take special storage and handling precautions because of chemicals used in their rescue environments.

Service Life

The service life of a rope cannot be determined in advance. How long a rope lasts depends on a large number of variables, including individual care, frequency of use, type of hardware used, speed of descent on rappels, exposure to abrasion, local climate, and type of loading. DuPont claims at least a 10-year shelf life for nylon, and rope tests have confirmed that an unused rope can last up to 10 years without significant strength loss. Used ropes degrade more quickly.

Any rope can fail after poor care or under extreme conditions, such as shock loading and sharp edges. A shock load of 0.25 fall factor for a static rope or 1.5 fall factor for a dynamic rope will likely cause internal, invisible damage to the rope, although damage may also be caused under lower fall factors. Regardless of how long it has been in service, you should immediately discard a rope when it becomes cut, when abrasion has caused significant wear to the sheath, after a hard shock load, when you suspect chemical contamination, or any time you are in doubt about the rope.

KNOTS

The medical professional encounters many knots in the course of his or her career. From the square knot in a stitched laceration to neck ties at administrative functions, practical and symbolic representations of knots abound.

In modern society, knots are used as a form of expression, in art, as mathematical structures, and for security purposes. Determination of "good" vs. "bad" in the analysis of a knot lies solely in the knot's ability to achieve the purpose for which it was created. Therefore you may find that several of the good and clever knots you have learned are useless when it comes to functioning in the wilderness.

Uses

Knots are applied in several ways in the wilderness environment. They are used to stake out tents or shelters, tie flies to fishing lines, create suspended "bear-proof" gear caches, and occasionally to tie things together.

In wilderness medical evacuation, knots take on great significance. Many medical professionals find themselves working alongside rescue technicians in steep terrain where knots are used for the safety of rescue personnel and for patient evacuation. Improvisational medical techniques often involve knots. Knotted rope or fabric can be used to secure a splint, create a hasty patient-transport device, or provide secure shelter to persons in precarious environmental situations.

How Knots Work

The theory behind a "lotta knot" is that if you cannot tie it right, at least tie it big. In a lotta knot, the greater the mass of rope and the more twists and turns it takes in relation to itself, the higher the probability that the knot will hold.

Eventually the rope user learns that certain types of twists and bends hold better than others; the reason the lotta knot works is because the larger mass increases the odds of getting a bend to hold in the mix. There are many disadvantages to the lotta knot, however. It takes up a lot of rope and is very difficult to tension. The varying twists and turns are not conducive to tightening the knot or positioning it properly. Finally the lotta knot often fails to perform altogether.

The internal friction of a knot is essentially what holds the lotta knot together. This friction can be attained by the rope taking twists and turns around itself or from friction against another object, such as a capstan or another rope.

The serious professional should take knot tying seriously because in a wilderness rescue, lives may depend on this skill. One should be able to select the correct knot without hesitation, tie knots correctly the first time, and be able to tie knots with gloved hands, on muddy or icy rope, in the dark, and under stress. Finally, one should be able to ascertain by looking at a knot whether it is tied correctly.

Categories of Knots

The most practical way to select a particular knot is to first evaluate what role that knot is expected to perform. For the purposes of this book, knots are addressed based on five basic functions: stopper knots, end-of-line knots, midline knots, knots to join two ropes, and safety knots.

There are subsets of knots for the terminology purist. A knot that is tied around something (e.g., a tree, a standing rope, or the rail of a litter), that conforms to the shape of the object around which it is tied, and that does not keep its shape when the object around which it is tied is removed is called a *hitch*. In its simplest form, a *loop* is a section of rope that crosses itself. A *tied loop* is a knot that forms a fixed eye or loop in the end of a rope. Regardless of the name or the way in which the terminology applies, there are basic rules that apply to any of these ties.

When working with rope, it is critical to be aware of the type of material into which the knot is tied. Some fibers have a low coefficient of friction and require special considerations in knot tying. Knots that are effective on rope do not always perform well in webbing or sling material.

Anatomy of a Knot. Common baseline terminology follows:

The *working end* of the rope is the section used to tie or rig the knot.

The *standing part* (or *end*) of the rope is the section not actively used to form the knot or rigging.

The *running end* (or simply the *end*) is the free end of the rope.

A *line* is a rope in use. For example, a rope used to rappel is a rappel line.

A *bight* of rope is formed when the rope takes a U-turn on itself so that the running end and standing end run parallel to each another. The U portion, where the rope bends, is referred to as the *bight*.

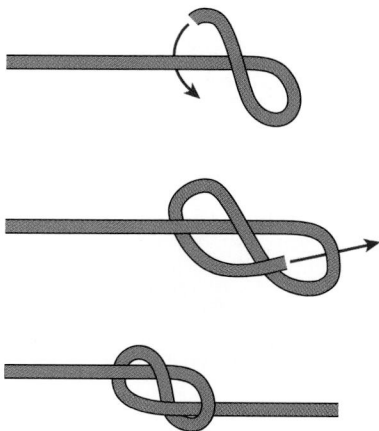

Figure 72-7 Figure-8 knot.

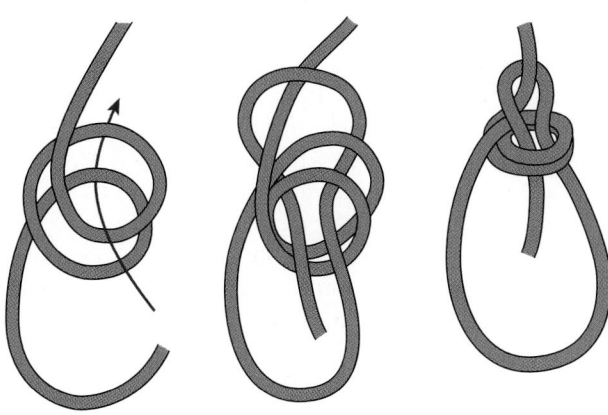

Figure 72-9 Double bowline.

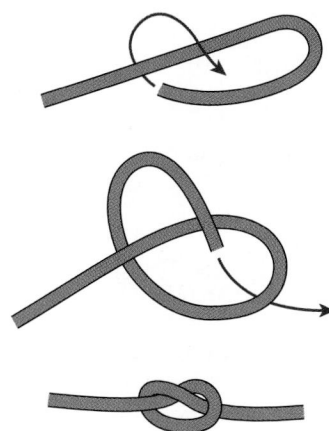

Figure 72-8 Overhand knot.

A *loop* of rope is made by crossing a portion of the standing end over (or under) the running end. Note that a loop closes, as compared to a bight. Thus many knots that form a loop from a bight in the standing part of the rope are named *something on a bight,* such as *figure 8 on a bight.*

The *tail* of a rope is the (usually short) unused length of rope that is left over once the knot is tied.

Stopper Knot. A stopper knot is often used in rappelling. Before an end of the rope is thrown down for the rappel, a stopper knot is tied into the end to prevent the rappeller from rappelling off the end should the rope not reach the ground. Stopper knots are also used in other applications to perform a similar function.

The most common stopper knot is a figure 8 (Figure 72-7). When two ropes are used in tandem, the stopper knot should be tied into both lines together. A simple overhand knot (Figure 72-8) may also be used for this

purpose, but its relatively low bulk makes it less desirable than a figure 8.

End-of-Line Knot. Perhaps the most common use of a knot is to make a loop in the end of a rope to anchor, tie in, or attach the rope to something. Borrowed from mariners, bowlines have been used by mountaineers for years. However, this knot can "capsize" into a slip-knot quite easily when the tail is pulled; therefore the "double bowline" (or high-strength bowline) is preferred (Figure 72-9).

Many people prefer to use forms of the figure 8 for multiple applications on the theory that they have to learn only one knot. This may prove limiting to a technician who would like to become a rope professional. Some people feel that the figure 8 is easier to tie and easier to check than other knots. In truth, the redundant nature of the figure 8 retrace can make it deceiving to visually inspect, a factor that has resulted in accidents.

Midline Knot. Knots are often used to form loops in the middle of the rope, for clipping into, for grasping, or for bypassing a piece of damaged rope. A figure 8 on a bight (Figure 72-10) is often used for this purpose and works well as long as the load is attached to the bight. However, if the rope below the knot is loaded, the knot deforms and weakens.

More preferable by far is the butterfly knot (Figure 72-11). The butterfly can be pulled effectively either from the loop or from below the knot without negative effect. Caution must be taken with this knot, however, because if the loop is not big enough and not loaded, it can pull out under tension.

Knots To Join Two Ropes. Tying a knot that will not untie itself is very important when joining two ropes, particularly since the knotted ends are unlikely to be in a place where they can be constantly monitored. The overhand bend is proclaimed by many in the climbing

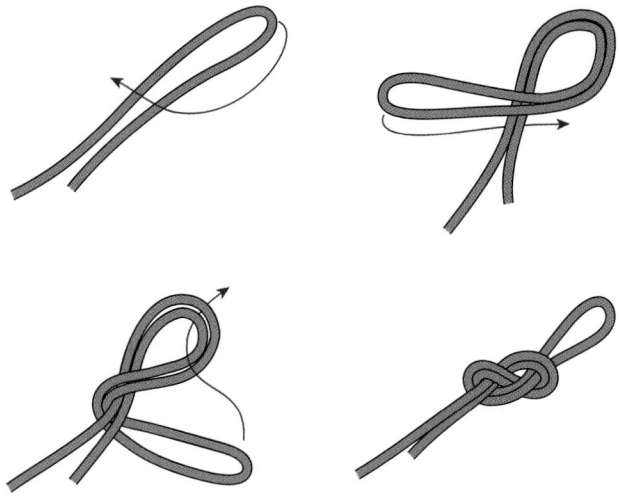

Figure 72-10 Figure 8 on a bight.

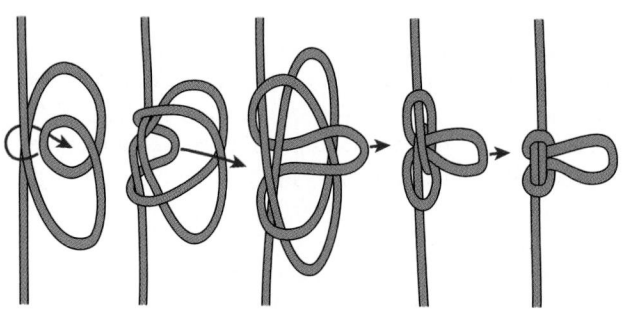

Figure 72-11 Butterfly knot.

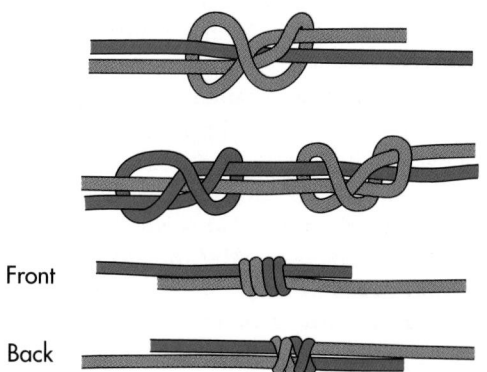

Figure 72-12 Double fisherman's bend.

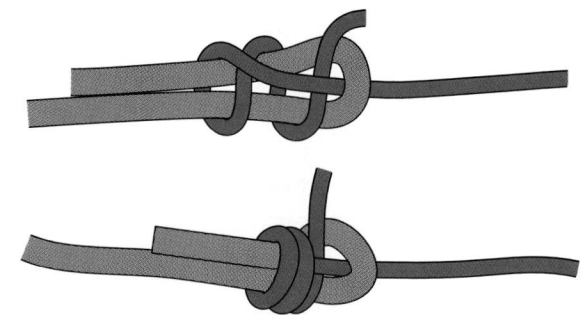

Figure 72-13 Double-sheet bend.

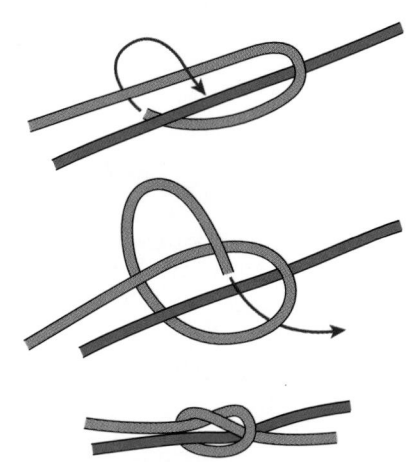

Figure 72-14 Single-sheet bend.

community to be the preferred choice for joining two ropes. However, this knot may untie while in use and is not deemed secure enough for rescue purposes. Instead, the more secure double fisherman's bend (Figure 72-12) should be used. This bend is very effective for joining ropes of relatively equal diameter. Care should be taken to ensure that the two halves of the bend nestle against each other and that there is enough tail protruding from the knot to keep the knot from unraveling. This knot is also used to join two ends of a short length of cordage for use as a Prusik (see Hitches).

When ropes of unequal diameter are joined, the double-sheet bend (Figure 72-13) is a more effective tie. This is a bulkier alternative, and although perhaps not quite as strong, it can be easier to untie and in the case of joining ropes of different diameters, is preferred.

Knot Safety

Every knot should be checked (preferably by someone other than the person who tied it) to ensure that it is tied properly and monitored at intervals thereafter. Many knots have a tendency to loosen, and some can even change forms, for instance, into a slipknot.

A safety knot can help prevent mishaps. A safety knot is an overhand knot (Figure 72-14) or barrel knot (Figure 72-15) tied into the tail of the rope after the knot is tied. This safety knot is placed to keep the knot from deforming or unraveling.

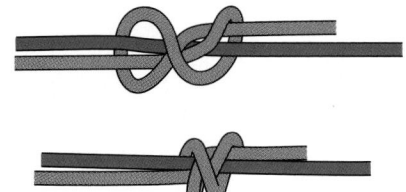

Figure 72-15   Barrel knot.

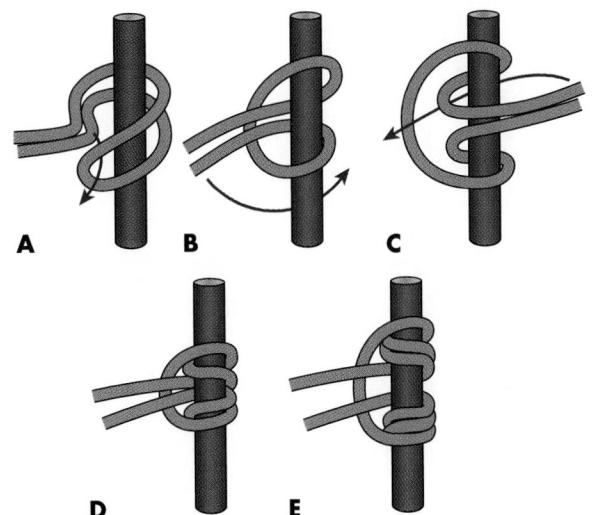

Figure 72-16   Prusik hitch. **A** to **C,** Tying sequence for the Prusik knot. **D,** Two-wrap Prusik knot. **E,** Three-wrap Prusik knot.

Hitches

Hitching refers to a method of tying a rope around itself or an object in such a way that the object is integral to the support of the hitch. Hitches are seldom used in rescue and should be considered for use only by a skilled technician because there are severe consequences when a hitch comes untied. Specifically, the disintegration of a hitch results in immediate release of whatever load it is holding.

One of the most commonly used hitches is the Prusik hitch (Figure 72-16). A Prusik is a sliding hitch by which a cord can be attached to a rope and slid up and down the rope for positioning. However, under tension, the hitch will not slide. A Prusik is created by tying a length of cordage into a loop by means of a double fisherman's bend. Wrapping the loop around the main rope and through its own loop two or three times and then pulling it tight forms the hitch.

Another fairly common hitch used in climbing and rescue applications is the clove hitch. This hitch can be useful when trying to shorten the distance between two objects, such as the climber's belay and the climber or the litter rail and the rescuer.

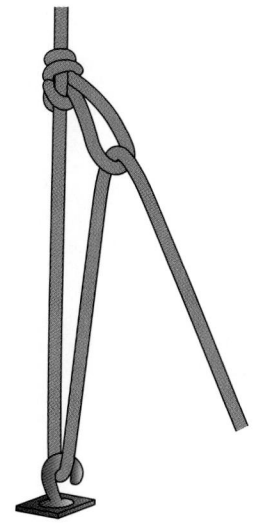

Figure 72-17   Trucker's hitch.

No discussion of knots would be complete without mention of the trucker's hitch, useful for pulling a cord tight across something, such as a load in the bed of a pickup truck (hence the name), or securing a patient snugly into a litter (Figure 72-17).

KNOT AND ROPE STRENGTH

Knots inevitably reduce the strength of a rope to some degree. Knot strength is affected by the tightness of bends as well as by the "pinching" effect that a knot has on itself.

The strength of any given knot is directly proportional to the strength of the material into which it is tied. Knot strengths are usually expressed in terms of "efficiency ratio." That is, a knot rated at 85% efficiency is said to maintain about 85% of the reported breaking strength of the rope.

Some individuals and agencies have reported that any knot reduces the strength of a rope by at least 50%. This information is erroneous because the efficiency of any knot depends on which knot is used, which rope it is tied into, whether it is tied correctly, and how it is cared for. Most knots recommended for use in wilderness rescue reduce the strength of a typical rescue rope to no less than 65% of that rope's minimum breaking strength. Most commonly used knots are even more efficient, in the range of 80%.

Unfortunately, accurate data on knot efficiencies are hard to find. Comprehensive testing that takes into account statistically significant sampling, differences between rope fibers, construction and diameter, static vs. dynamic loading, and other variables is virtually nonexistent.

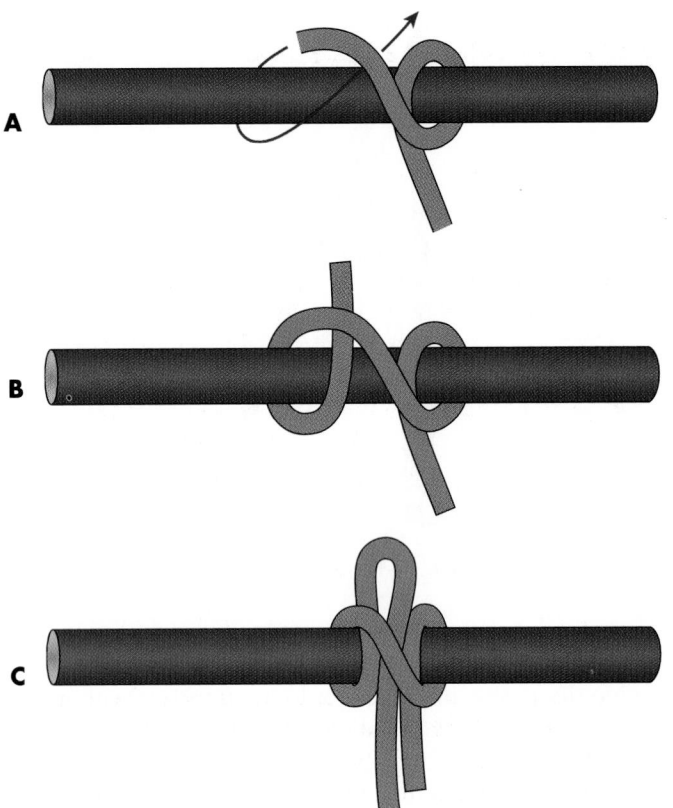

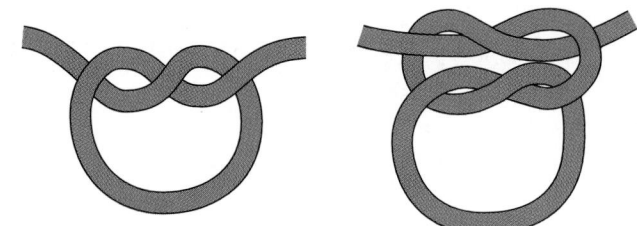

Figure 72-19 Reef knot, or square knot.

Figure 72-18 **A** and **B,** Clove hitch. **C,** Clove hitch with draw loop for temporary attachment.

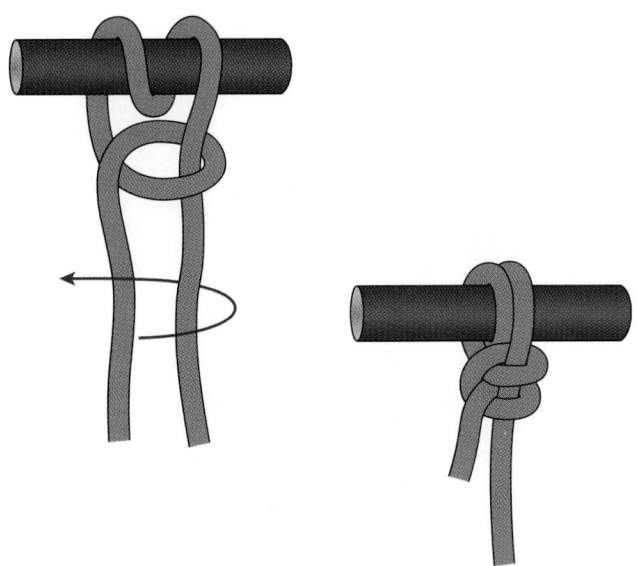

Figure 72-20 Round turn and two half-hitches.

The following data, taken from many different sources and reflecting limited testing, should be referenced for trend information only.

The relative breaking strength of kernmantle design ropes with knots follows:

Double fisherman's bend	65%-70%
Bowline	70%-75%
Figure 8 on a bight	75%-80%
Overhand knot	60%-65%

The best way to know the strength of a knot on a given rope is to actually test the type of knot you use on the types of rope you use and test enough samples using statistical analysis to provide a reasonable margin of error.

ADDITIONAL KNOTS

See Figures 72-18 to 72-20 for additional knots.

LEARNING MORE ABOUT ROPES AND KNOTS

For more information on using ropes to move patients, we suggest the second edition of *High-Angle Rescue Techniques* by Hudson and Vines, supplemented by training through a respectable course. A good basic vertical class on rappelling and ascending a rope requires a minimum of 2 to 3 days. After a basic rope skills class is completed, regular practice is required to maintain proficiency. Many excellent advanced classes in patient movement by rope or vertical rescue are offered. Figure on at least a week of training for a beginning class on rope rescue.

SUGGESTED READINGS

Vines T, Hudson S: *High-angle rescue techniques,* ed 2, St Louis, 1999, Mosby.
PMI product catalogs, LaFayette Ga, 1997, 1998, Pigeon Mountain Industries.

Wilderness Navigation Techniques

Steven C. Carleton

Many environmental illnesses occur as a consequence of becoming lost. Even well-prepared individuals may suffer hypothermia, heat stroke, frostbite, immersion foot, sunburn, dehydration, starvation, and a variety of other conditions if they become separated from the resources of their expedition or have an unanticipated extension of their time outdoors. This chapter discusses use of the magnetic compass for route finding, application of celestial navigation techniques for determination of direction and position, navigation with the global positioning system (GPS), and use of alternative methods for recovering when lost.

All of navigation boils down to two processes: determination of direction and establishment of position. In the wilderness setting the determination of direction and fixing of position are challenging. Generally, routes and landmarks are provided by a map, but local knowledge from memory may have to suffice. Usually, direction is derived from a magnetic compass, but other methods of direction finding can be exploited when the compass is forgotten, lost, damaged, or unreliable. Generally, *lines of position* (LOPs) are established by trails or by bearings to identifiable landmarks; however, shorelines, firebreaks, power lines, altimeter readings, and relative bearings to celestial bodies or radio sources can substitute. Finally, position can be fixed through the use of technologies such as GPS or with the time-tested methods of celestial navigation and triangulation of bearings. None of these navigational techniques is prohibitively expensive or so equipment-intensive as to be incompatible with a hiker's kit. Each method requires an understanding of its practice and limitations. Nothing substitutes for preparation, but effective wilderness navigation can be practiced using nothing more than the clues offered by the environment and the wits of the navigator.

COMPASS NAVIGATION AND DEAD RECKONING

The directional properties of lodestone (magnetite) were recognized by a variety of civilizations in ancient times. References to the use of a directional magnetized needle at sea appear in Chinese literature dating from the twelfth century. Descriptions of the magnetic compass in European writings followed in the thirteenth century, by which time it was noted that a needle stroked on lodestone pointed to the vicinity of the North Star.[1,29] Discovery of the magnetic compass was a seminal event in the exploration of the planet; the compass allowed reasonably accurate steering in all weather and permitted development of a fundamental process in navigation, the process of *dead (deduced) reckoning*. Dead reckoning is the estimation of current location based on knowledge of the direction, rate, and time of travel from a known starting point. Whenever traveling in the wilderness, dead reckoning should be practiced so that a general awareness of position is never lost. Estimates of time of travel, rate of travel, and direction of travel should be recorded whenever possible.

Magnetic Dip, Deviation, and Declination

The directional properties of the compass result from the interaction between magnetized iron in the compass needle and the magnetic lines of force generated by metals in the Earth's core. These lines of force have vertical and horizontal components. The vertical component is termed *magnetic inclination,* or *dip*. Dip causes a compass needle to incline downward from horizontal, potentially to a degree that interferes with the ability of the needle or card to pivot freely. Dip is 90° at the magnetic poles and 0° at the magnetic equator. Most modern compasses are manufactured to compensate for the average dip likely to be encountered in the region of intended use. Others allow a small weight to be moved along the indicator needle to compensate for dip in any region of use.[27]

The horizontal component of the magnetic lines of force causes the compass needle to point to the Earth's north magnetic pole. Unfortunately, the Earth's magnetic and geographic poles do not correspond in location, and the Earth's magnetic lines of force are not straight lines but meander in an irregular fashion dictated by irregularities in the density of the core. The irregular directionality of the Earth's magnetic field is called *magnetic declination*. The compass needle is also influenced by local magnetic forces. These forces may result from natural sources such as ore deposits, or from artificial sources such as ferromagnetic metals in vehicles, equipment, and clothing fasteners. The displacement of the compass needle resulting from local magnetic influences is termed *deviation*. As a result of magnetic declination and deviation, compasses point to geographic north only when used with care in selected locations. In general, compasses point northward but not exactly due north.

Direction in compass navigation is expressed in three ways: (1) *true direction,* or direction measured in reference to the Earth's meridians and geographic poles; (2) *magnetic direction,* or direction measured in reference to the Earth's magnetic poles; and (3) *compass direction,* or direction as measured by the magnetic compass. Magnetic direction varies from true direction by the sum of declination and deviation. Compass direction varies from magnetic direction by the quantity of deviation.[5,22] The definitions of magnetic and compass direction point out the necessity for minimizing preventable sources of compass deviation when taking bearings. For practical purposes, when preventable sources of deviation are minimized and the compass is used with caution, magnetic direction and compass direction can be considered the same.

Wandering lines of points with equal magnetic declination can be graphed on representations of the Earth's surface. These are called *isogonic lines.* Lines representing points on the surface of the Earth where the magnetic declination is zero, and magnetic north and true north are aligned, are termed *agonic lines.* In the Americas an agonic line follows a relatively straight, slanting course extending from the east coast of Victoria Island in north-central Canada through western Lake Superior, along the east coast of Florida, and traversing South America from the Gulf of Venezuela to the southeastern coast of Brazil. At locations east of the agonic line, the compass needle declines to the west (counterclockwise) of true north; at points west of the agonic line, the compass needle declines to the east (clockwise) of true north. By convention, magnetic declination is given a positive sign when east and a negative sign when west (Figure 73-1). Declination is quan-

tified as the number of degrees of arc between true and magnetic north.

For example, in southwestern Ohio, the current magnetic declination is negative 4.5°, or 4.5° west. This means that a compass needle actually points 4.5° to the west of true north, and that the true bearing given by the needle is 355.5°. When the needle is aligned to 360° on the compass rim, any magnetic bearing taken with a compass will be 4.5° greater than the true bearing. To correct from magnetic to true, 4.5° must be subtracted from any indicated magnetic bearing.

The mnemonic "declination east, compass bearing least; declination west, compass bearing greatest" may be helpful in converting magnetic direction to true direction when taking a bearing. Restated, to convert from magnetic to true while taking a bearing from the compass, add east declination to the compass bearing, or subtract west declination from the compass bearing. If converting from a true bearing taken from map to a magnetic bearing on the compass, subtract east declination from the compass bearing, or add west declination to the compass bearing. The interconversion between magnetic and true bearings is an essential skill in compass navigation. Failure to recognize the relationship will result in significant errors when following a map route by compass because directional references on the map are based on true direction. At a location where the magnetic declination is 10°, travel over a straight course derived from a map and guided by compass bearings will result in a 0.18-mile error for each mile traveled if the declination is not considered.[14]

Magnetic declination for any location can be determined by reference to the *Isogonic Chart for Magnetic Declination* produced every 5 years by the United States Geologic Survey (USGS). In the United States, magnetic declination varies from +23° in Washington state to −22° in Maine[23] (see Figure 73-1). On standard USGS 7½-minute and 15-minute squares, magnetic declination is indicated by a pointer next to the pointer indicating true north at the bottom of the map. Without recourse to an *Isogonic Chart,* declination for any location in the Northern Hemisphere can be empirically determined with reasonable accuracy by comparing the magnetic bearing of north with the true bearing as indicated by a line pointing to the star Polaris. Polaris lies up to 45 minutes of arc (0.75°) away from true north at most times of day, but this offset is negligible for wilderness navigation situations. Declination at any location also can be determined by comparing the magnetic bearing of a prominent landmark with the true bearing between the observer's known location and the location of the landmark as read from a map.[3]

Compass Types

The three compass types used in land navigation are the fixed-dial compass, magnetic card compass, and

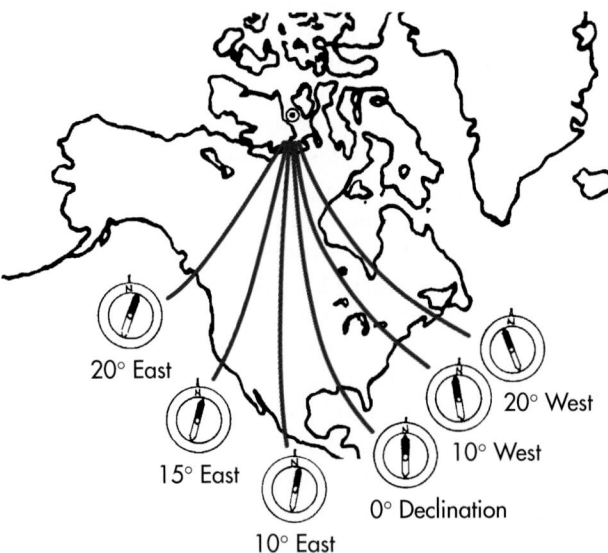

Figure 73-1 Schematic representation of North America showing declination at various locations as the difference between true north ("N" on the compass rim) and magnetic north (tip of the compass needle). (*From Seidman D: The essential wilderness navigator, Camden, Me, 1995, Ragged Mountain Press.*)

baseplate compass (Figure 73-2). The simplest compass is the fixed-dial, which utilizes a magnetized needle balanced on a pivot and enclosed in a case that is graduated around its periphery into 360°. The magnetic card compass utilizes a magnetized needle or wire fixed to a circular card that is graduated around its periphery from 0° to 360°. The housing of the compass is marked with a line, the lubber line, that allows magnetic bearings to be determined when the line is pointed at an object of interest. The lensatic compass used by the military, which has a lens for magnification of the compass card and sights for alignment to distant objects, is a magnetic card compass. The most useful compass for land navigation is the baseplate compass,[14,17,25,28] which consists of a fixed-dial compass (or capsule) mounted to a baseplate in a manner that allows the capsule to rotate in relation to the baseplate. The baseplate is marked with a line used to indicate the direction of travel. This line functions in a manner identical to the lubber line of the magnetic card compass. The capsule of the compass has an orienting arrow inscribed on its lower surface that points to the graduation denoting north on the capsule rim. On different models, this graduation may be labeled "0°," "360°," or "N." Rotation of the capsule such that the compass needle is superimposed on the orienting arrow and points to "N" on the capsule rim allows the user to easily read the magnetic bearing indicated by the direction-of-travel line. As long as the direction-of-travel line is followed and the needle remains superimposed on the orienting arrow, the user is assured of maintaining the desired magnetic bearing during travel.

Many baseplate compasses allow the orienting arrow to be adjusted relative to the rim of the capsule to compensate for magnetic declination. When this feature is present, the orienting arrow is rotated such that the "N" graduation on the capsule rim points to true north when the orienting arrow points to magnetic north. When the adjusted compass is rotated to align the needle with the orienting arrow, bearings as read on the capsule rim will represent true, rather than magnetic, bearings. Baseplate compasses have other features particularly suited for use with a map, including plotting scales, a straight edge, and often a protractor and magnifier.[28]

Correction for declination when using a fixed-dial or magnetic card compass requires addition or subtraction of the declination, as appropriate, from the magnetic bearing indicated by the compass rim or lubber line.

Compass Use

The magnetic compass is most useful for determining the cardinal directions and for establishing bearings for use in route finding and back-bearings for use in returning to a known starting location. A *back-bearing* is the reciprocal of the bearing followed on the out-bound leg of a journey (out-bound bearing minus 180°). Any route can be subdivided into legs that can be defined by magnetic bearing lines. Ideally, each leg should pass between prominent, identifiable landmarks that will remain recognizable even in the dark or in poor weather. However, even when weather or lighting conditions prevent visual acquisition of the landmark from a distance, careful compass work should permit the user to reach the objective. Early in the course of travel over each leg, the observer should visually check the back-bearing of the direction of travel to become familiar with the view of the starting point as it will appear on the return journey. If possible, the bearing and back-bearing of each leg of a route, and the landmarks defining each leg, should be recorded on paper rather than trusted to memory.

Use of the compass in this manner permits the user to easily return to the desired direction of travel if an obstacle to the intended route is encountered. The course around the obstacle is recorded as a series of legs of known direction and estimated (by stride) length. When permitted by the terrain, right-angle detours are the simplest to follow. The user returns to the intended route by traveling the reciprocal of the course of the detour for the same lateral distance as that required to bypass the obstacle[5] (Figure 73-3). Return to the intended course is greatly augmented by using *natural ranges*. A natural range is formed by two landmarks lying along the same bearing line, one of intermediate distance from the viewer and one of greater distance—for example, a large tree or rock formation several kilometers distant, and the silhouette of a hill or mountain on the horizon. As the traveler deviates from the intended course, the near and far landmarks will fall out of line. When the traveler returns to the

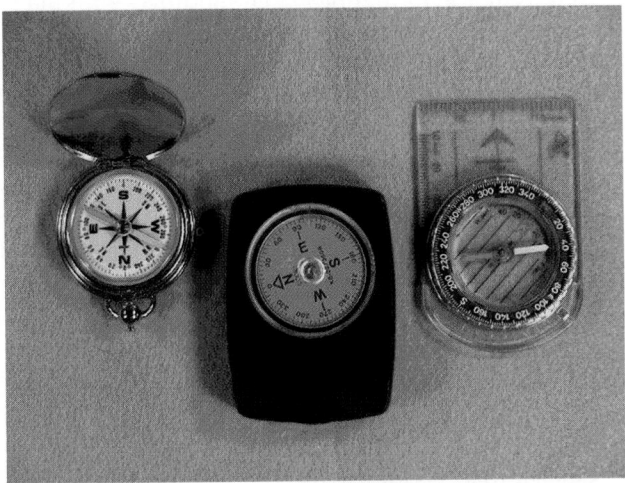

Figure 73-2 The three basic compass types. From left to right: Fixed dial compass, magnetic card compass, baseplate compass. Note the deviation in indicated north resulting from local magnetic influences.

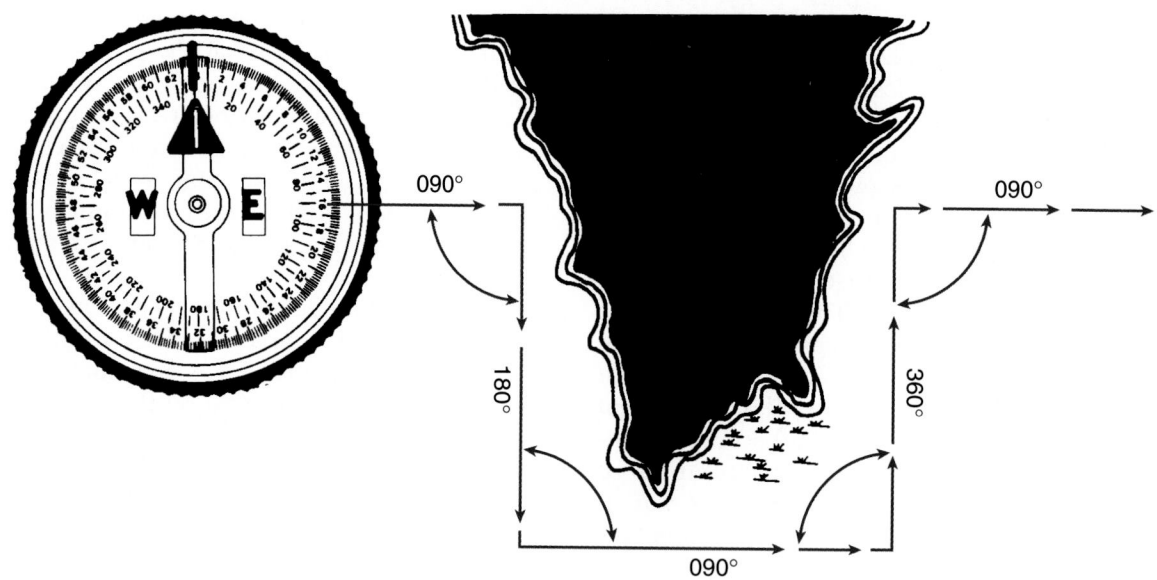

Figure 73-3 Use of the compass to return to an intended route when faced with an obstacle. A course 90° to the intended course is walked for a known number of steps, the obstacle is bypassed, and the original course is regained by walking the reciprocal course of the initial detour for the same distance. (*From Department of the Army:* Map reading and land navigation, Field Manual 21-26, *Washington, DC, 1987, Headquarters, Department of the Army.*)

intended route, the objects forming the natural range will return to alignment.

Use of a compass with a map allows the user to orient the map to the environment and relate bearings taken from the map to bearings measured with the compass. Correction for declination is essential when the compass is used for this task if true bearings are to be used in plotting a route. However, there is no absolute need for the use of true bearings in navigation; it is only important that the map and compass agree. Agreement can be accomplished either by correcting the compass to the map or by correcting the map to the compass. If a baseplate compass with declination adjustment is used, it is simplest to correct the compass to the map and use true bearings for all subsequent travel. With any other type of compass, it may be easier to use magnetic bearings exclusively. If the declination is known or can be determined observationally, magnetic meridians can be drawn on the map to be used in place of the true meridians represented by the map margins. These magnetic meridians will form an angle with the true meridians equal to the declination angle. A map modified in this manner permits magnetic bearings, rather than true, to be taken from the map for use in following a course. The internal consistency of this method is often much less confusing than the method requiring conversion between true bearings and compass bearings. The choice between the use of true or magnetic bearings should be made in advance of travel. Plotting magnetic meridians on a map requires a pencil, straight edge, flat surface, and protractor, items unlikely to be available in a field emergency.[27,28]

To orient a map with a baseplate compass corrected for declination, the compass capsule is rotated such that "N" on the capsule rim is aligned to the direction of travel arrow. An edge of the baseplate parallel to the direction of travel arrow is then placed on one of the vertical borders of the map. The map, with the compass in place, is then rotated until the compass needle is superimposed on the orienting arrow on the base of the capsule. True north on the map is now aligned with true north on the planet.

To orient a map that has been modified with magnetic meridians using an uncompensated baseplate compass, the compass capsule is rotated until "N" on the capsule rim aligns with the direction-of-travel arrow. An edge of the compass parallel to the direction-of-travel arrow is placed on one of the magnetic meridians plotted on the map. The map, with the compass in place, is rotated until the compass needle is superimposed on the orienting arrow. True north on the map now corresponds to true north in the surrounding landscape.[14,25,27,28] If an uncompensated compass of other type is used, the north-south line of the compass face or lubber line is superimposed on a magnetic meridian, and the map and compass are rotated in concert until the indicator needle points to "N."

Once a map is oriented to the environment, back-bearings from landmarks that are visible both on the map and in the landscape can be used to obtain a positional fix by *resection,* or *triangulation.*[25] Each back-

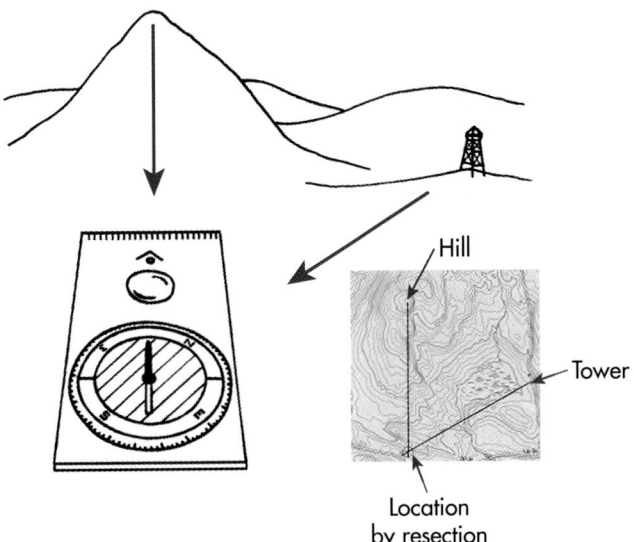

Figure 73-4 Establishing a magnetic fix by crossing the back bearings from two prominent landmarks. This process is known as resection.

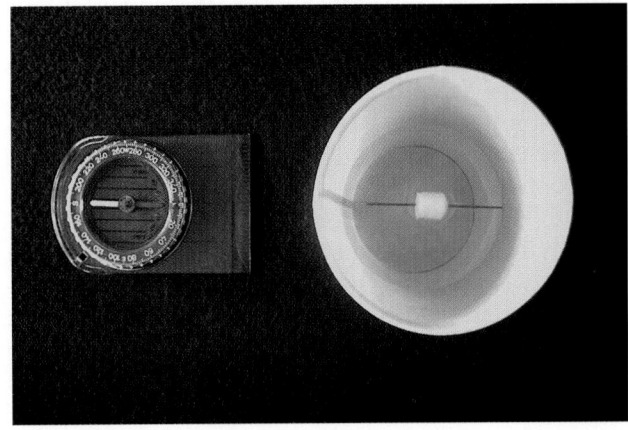

Figure 73-5 Makeshift compass constructed from a plastic cup, straight pin, and foam packing peanut. Note the correspondence between north as indicated by the makeshift device and the commercial compass.

bearing from a landmark represents an LOP that can be plotted on the map. The point of crossing of two or more LOPs fixes the position of the observer (Figure 73-4). Alternatively, the intersection between the LOP represented by a bearing line and a shoreline, riverbank, road, firebreak, or celestial position line can be used to fix position on a map.

Makeshift Compasses

A field-expedient compass can be fabricated with relative ease. Items containing iron, nickel, or cobalt are suitable for use as an indicator needle. Iron in the form of a steel needle, pin, wire, staple, or paper clip is most commonly available. Most of these items are magnetized as purchased. If not, they can be magnetized by stroking them on a magnet salvaged from an electric motor or radio speaker, on a magnetized screwdriver or similar item, on a piece of silk, or on a dry cell battery terminal. A dry cell also can be used to magnetize a needle by wrapping an insulated wire tightly around the needle and connecting the ends of the wire to the battery terminals. Expect sparks and heat. Trial and error will often yield a suitable magnetizer. The indicator needle is floated in water by placing it on a wood chip, leaf, slip of paper, or small piece of cork or closed-cell foam. The container, which may be the cupped palm of the hand or a puddle, should be protected from the wind (Figure 73-5). A compass so constructed will reliably indicate a magnetic north-to-south line. Determination of directions may require external cues, such as the general direction of sunrise or sunset.

CELESTIAL NAVIGATION

Celestial navigation exploits the predictable relationship between the apparent positions of selected celestial bodies and the surface of the earth. The influence of celestial navigation on world history is immense. Millennia before European culture conceived of celestial navigation as a means for facilitating exploration, commerce, and military domination of the seas, the cultures that populated the numerous discreet island archipelagoes of the Pacific Basin were making open ocean voyages over thousands of miles guided by memorized "star paths."[11] The use of simple altitude measuring devices (the Greek gnomon, Arab kamal, and Chinese stretch board) for the qualitative determination of latitude was practiced by mariners in antiquity. As the Age of Exploration dawned, competing governments of Western Europe devoted enormous energy to systematization of celestial navigation, funding legions of astronomers in the development of coordinate systems and accurate tables of stellar, solar, lunar, and planetary positions. Instruments such as the mariner's astrolabe, quadrant, octant, and sextant permitted accurate and reproducible quantitative measurement of the altitude of celestial bodies, and accurate clocks became available to permit the ready determination of longitude.[1,29]

Celestial navigation has its greatest utility and easiest application at sea. Standard celestial practice depends on the availability of a sea horizon as a reference point for the measurement of altitude. The horizon reference for land navigation is necessarily artificial (a plumb bob, bubble level, or level reflective surface). Positions resulting from celestial fixes, even with scrupulous technique, are only approximations of the navigator's actual position. Errors of several miles are common. This is of little consequence in the open ocean, even as landfall approaches; the target destination is generally large enough to be seen from many miles distant. This degree of imprecision may prove troublesome on land, but the accuracy of celestial navigation should still suffice for most wilderness situations.

Although developed for use on trackless seas, celestial navigation has a long and rich tradition of use on land. Lewis and Clark established the positions of landmarks during their exploration of the American West by celestial observation. Various expeditions that led to the discovery of the North and South Poles depended entirely on celestial observations for confirmation of position and direction. Celestial navigation techniques can be applied in a wilderness setting at a variety of levels. Traditional navigation, in which sextant observations lead to the fixing of terrestrial position, can be accomplished with relatively little equipment but requires considerable preplanning. Simplified celestial techniques requiring little or no equipment are well suited to field-expedient navigation and can provide accurate directional information in the absence of a compass. In particular, an understanding of the movement of the sun and several prominent stars can allow accurate route finding without recourse to technology. To understand the relationship between the position of a celestial body and the position of an observer on Earth, it is necessary to discuss the various coordinate systems that are used to describe terrestrial position, celestial position, and the appearance of the sky from the Earth's surface (horizon coordinate system).

Terrestrial Coordinates

In the terrestrial coordinate system, the earth has a North Pole and a South Pole that define its axis of rotation. This axis passes through Earth's center. Any plane that passes through the center of the Earth describes a circle on the surface called a *great circle.* The equator is the great circle described by the plane that passes perpendicular to the earth's axis. The great circle of a plane that contains the Earth's axis is termed a *meridian.* Meridians always run due north and south and converge at the poles. The *Prime Meridian* is the great circle that passes through Greenwich, England. Greenwich was assigned the Prime Meridian by treaty in 1884, in recognition of the work on astronomy and navigation performed at the Greenwich Royal Observatory.

Every point on the Earth's surface lies on a meridian. The angular measurement, or arc, between the Prime Meridian and the meridian of any other point on the planet's surface is the *longitude* (λ) of that point. Longitude is measured in degrees, minutes, and seconds of arc, east or west of the Prime Meridian, from 0° through 180°. The angular measurement between the plane of the equator, as measured north or south from the center of the earth to a point on the surface, is the *latitude* (L) of that point (Figure 73-6). All points at the same latitude form a *parallel* of latitude. Latitude is measured in degrees, minutes, and seconds of arc from 0° through 90° north or south. As such, the latitude of the equator is 0°, whereas that of each pole is 90° north or south, respectively. Every point on the surface of the Earth is defined by a specific longitude and latitude.

A *nautical mile* (1852 m, 6076 feet, or 1.15 statute miles) is the distance on a great circle that subtends an angle of 1 minute of arc as measured from the center of the Earth. A degree of arc (60 minutes of arc) is thus

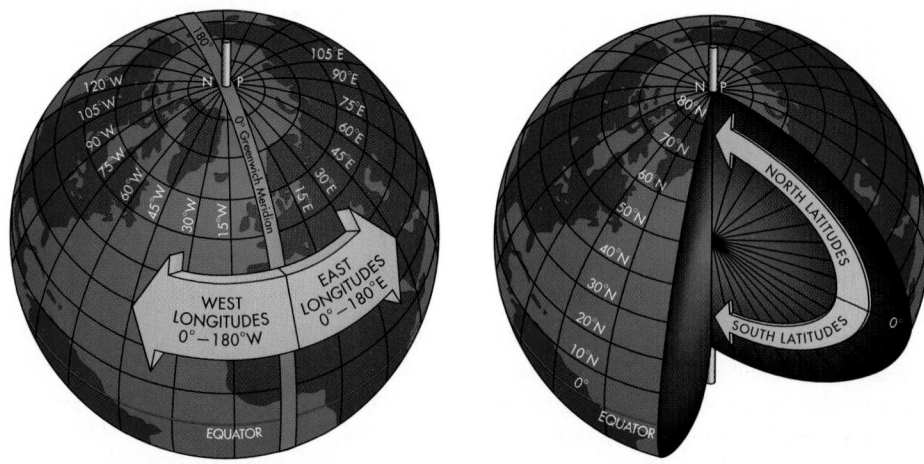

Figure 73-6 Meridians of longitude including the Prime Meridian, and parallels of latitude as measured north and south of the equator in degrees of arc from the center of the Earth. (*From Department of the Air Force:* Survival-training edition, Manual 64-3, *Randolph AFB, Texas, 1969, Air Training Command.*)

60 nautical miles, and 1 second of arc is equal to about 100 feet. It must be recognized that 1 minute of latitude will always equal 1 nautical mile, whereas 1 minute of longitude will only equal 1 nautical mile at the equator. At all points north or south of the equator, 1 minute of longitude will be less than 1 nautical mile, owing to the convergence of the meridians toward the poles.

Longitude bears a special relationship to time. Within reasonable standards of accuracy, the earth rotates once about its axis in 24 hours. As such, our planet moves through 360° of longitude in 24 hours, or 15° each hour, or 1° for every 4 minutes of time. It is this fact that establishes the conventions by which sundials work, clocks run, and time is defined. It also forever links the modern practice of celestial position finding to the accurate keeping of time.

Celestial Coordinates

To a terrestrial observer the sky appears to be an immense hollow sphere with the Earth at its center, and the stars painted on its inner surface. The sphere rotates about the Earth once daily. The sun, moon, and planets wander across the background of stars on concentric spheres of their own. This is exactly the conception of the universe forwarded by Ptolemy in the second century and is termed the *geocentric model*. This theory was highly popular with the Catholic Church; challenging it led to the burning of scores of intellectuals during the Spanish Inquisition. It held sway until the sixteenth century, when it was replaced, gingerly, by an equally incorrect heliocentric (sun-centered) model. The geocentric model, although false, is a useful construct for ordering the heavens and is the model used in the definition of celestial coordinates.

The celestial coordinate system plays off of the terrestrial coordinate system. The terrestrial poles are projected outward to the surface of the imaginary celestial sphere to form the north and south celestial poles. The terrestrial equator is similarly projected outward to form the celestial equator, or *equinoctial*. The celestial correlate to latitude is *declination* (unrelated to magnetic declination in compass use). The declination of a celestial body is the angle measured from the center of the earth (and geocentric universe) north or south of the celestial equator from 0° through 90° of arc. Declinations north of the celestial equator are positive (+), whereas those south of the celestial equator are negative (−). The declinations of the celestial poles are thus +90° and −90°, respectively, whereas that of the celestial equator is 0°. The declinations of the sun, moon, four navigational planets (Venus, Mars, Jupiter, and Saturn), and 57 navigational stars are listed in the daily pages of the *Nautical Almanac*.[7,13]

The celestial correlate to longitude is less intuitive and requires some explanation. Projections of terrestrial meridians onto the celestial sphere form *celestial merid-*

ians. Projection of the Greenwich meridian onto the celestial sphere forms the Greenwich celestial meridian. Projection of an observer's meridian onto the celestial sphere forms the local celestial meridian (Figure 73-7). A meridian on the surface of the celestial sphere that contains a celestial body and the celestial poles and is perpendicular to the celestial equator is termed the *hour circle* of that body. Hour circles converge toward the celestial poles in a manner identical to meridians on Earth. As the celestial sphere rotates about its polar axis, the hour circles of all celestial bodies appear to rotate above a terrestrial observer, rising in the east, sweeping overhead, and setting in the west. A reference hour circle on the celestial sphere called the *first point of Aries,* or the hour circle of Aries, substitutes for the terrestrial Prime Meridian. The first point of Aries is represented by an hour circle that intersects the celestial equator at the point at which the sun crosses it at the moment of the vernal equinox. The angular measurement between the hour circle of a celestial body and the Greenwich celestial meridian is defined as the *Greenwich hour angle* (GHA) of the body. GHA is the celestial equivalent of longitude and is measured westward from the Greenwich celestial meridian from 0° through 360°. The Greenwich hour angle of Aries (GHA^{Aries}) is the angle between the Greenwich celestial meridian and the hour circle of Aries at any given second in time. The GHAs for Aries and for the sun, moon, Venus, Mars, Jupiter, and Saturn are listed for each hour of

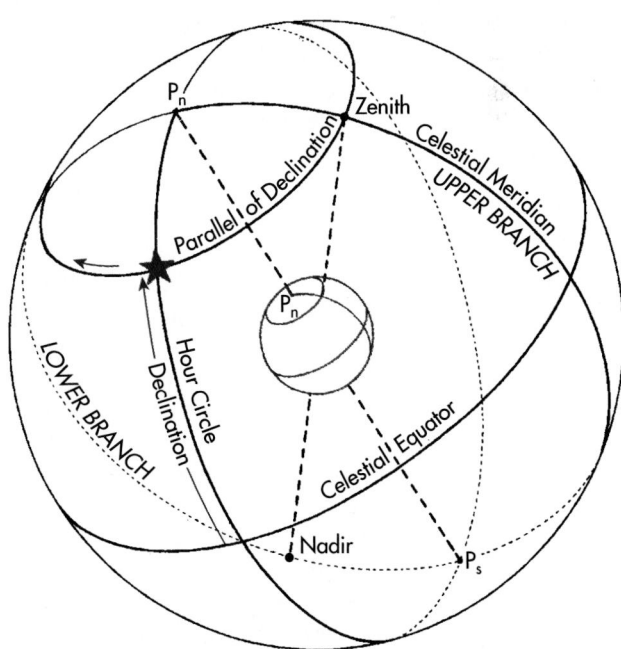

Figure 73-7   Diagram showing the celestial meridian of an observer on the Earth's surface, and the celestial meridian corresponding to the hour circle of an observed star. (*From Bowditch N: The American practical navigator. An epitome of navigation, Washington, DC, 1984,* Defense Mapping Agency Hydrographic/Topographic Center.)

each day of a year in daily pages of the *Nautical Almanac.* Interpolation tables permit determination of hour angles for each second of the year.[13,22]

The GHAs for the 57 navigational stars are defined by their predictable and nearly constant relationship to the hour angle of Aries. The angular measurement between the hour circle of Aries and the hour circle of any of the navigational stars is called the *sidereal hour angle* (SHA) of that star. The GHA of each of the navigational stars is thus equal to the sum of the hour angle of Aries and the SHA of the star in question (GHA^{star} = GHA^{Aries} + SHA^{star}).

In the practice of celestial navigation the hour angle of a celestial body is ultimately defined in reference to the observer's local celestial meridian. The angular measurement between the local celestial meridian and the hour circle of a body is the *local hour angle* (LHA) of that body. LHA, like GHA, is measured westward from the local celestial meridian from 0° through 360°. The LHA of a celestial body equals the GHA of the body plus the observer's longitude if east, or minus the observer's longitude if west (LHA = GHA + east λ; LHA = GHA − west λ). When a celestial body is on an observer's meridian, its GHA equals the longitude of the observer's position.[1]

Horizon Coordinate System

The horizon coordinate system defines celestial position from the point of view of an Earth-bound observer. The point on the celestial sphere directly over the observer's head is the *zenith.* The point on the celestial sphere directly beneath the feet of the observer is the *nadir.* The zenith and nadir lie on a line that includes the observer's terrestrial position and the Earth's center. The plane that passes though the center of the Earth perpendicular to this line is the observer's *celestial horizon.* The celestial horizon lies parallel to the observer's visible horizon. Any great circle on the celestial sphere formed by a plane passing perpendicular to the celestial horizon is termed a *vertical circle* (Figure 73-8). Vertical circles converge at the observer's zenith and nadir in a manner analogous to the convergence of the terrestrial and celestial meridians at their poles. Three of the infinite number of potential vertical circles for any surface position are of particular importance: (1) the *principal vertical,* that vertical circle lying on the observer's celestial meridian; (2) the *prime vertical,* that vertical circle passing through points due east and west of the observer; and (3) the vertical circle containing a celestial body of interest[13] (Figure 73-8).

The angular measurement between an observer's celestial horizon and a celestial body is the *altitude* of that body. Altitudes are expressed in degrees, minutes, and seconds of arc from 0° (the horizon) through 90° (the zenith). In the traditional practice of celestial navigation, altitudes are measured using a sextant, octant, or

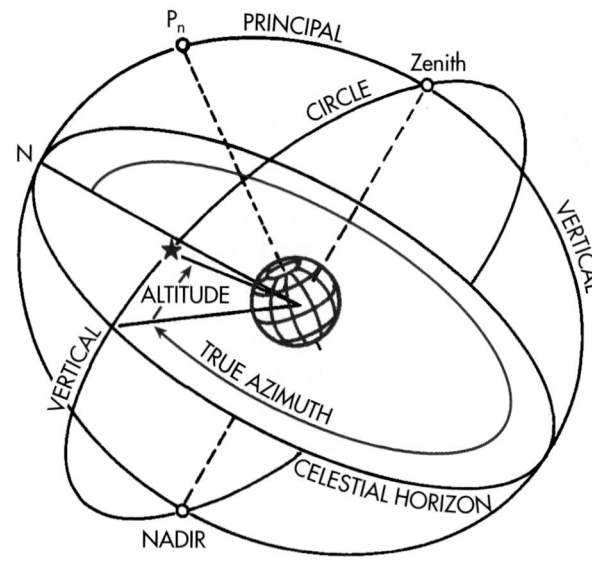

Figure 73-8 Schematic representation of the horizon coordinate system showing the observer's zenith and nadir, the celestial horizon, the prime and principal vertical circles, the elevated pole *(Pn),* and the altitude and azimuth of the body observed. (*From Hobbs RR: Marine navigation: piloting and celestial and electronic navigation, ed 4, Annapolis, Md, 1998, Naval Institute Press.*)

quadrant. Altitude, as measured by an instrument in reference to the horizon, is termed *sextant altitude* (Hs), regardless of the type of instrument used. Hs, once corrected for various atmospheric and geometric factors, is termed *observed altitude* (Ho). The corrections to be applied are tabulated in the *Nautical Almanac.* The true altitude of a body can be calculated for any given terrestrial position at any instant of time through application of spherical trigonometry. This altitude is termed *calculated altitude* (Hc).[1]

The other determinant of the observed position of a celestial body is the angular measurement along the celestial horizon between true north and the vertical circle including the body. This angle is termed the *azimuth* (Zn) of the body and is measured clockwise from 0° through 360° (see Figure 73-8).

CELESTIAL LINES OF POSITION

Celestial Methods for Latitude

The simplest celestial LOP is derived from the *noon sight,* or *meridian altitude of the sun.* This method dominated celestial navigation from the seventeenth century the late 1800s. The noon sight is simple but inflexible. It is very adaptable to wilderness navigation, requiring minimal math and little equipment. The noon sight allows direct determination of latitude by measuring the altitude of the sun at the moment that it passes the observer's meridian. The instant of solar meridian passage is termed *local apparent noon* (LAN), and is that moment when the sun achieves its greatest altitude.

The sun is observed with the sextant for a brief period of time preceding LAN until the altitude ceases to increase and begins to fall. The maximum sextant altitude so determined is corrected using *Almanac* data to yield Ho, which is then converted to *zenith distance* (ZD). Zenith distance is the angular distance between observer's zenith and the body; thus, ZD = 90° − Ho. The algebraic sum of ZD and the declination of the sun (from the *Nautical Almanac*) at the approximate time of observation equals the observer's latitude by the formulas below[7,18]:

1. L = ZD + d, when L and d have the same sign and L > d
2. L = d − ZD, when L and d have the same sign and d > L
3. L = ZD − d, when L and d have different signs

Since the declination of the sun changes very slowly on an hourly basis, accuracy is acceptable if the sun's declination is known for merely the approximate time of observation; exact time is not required. The noon sight requires only the sun's declination and precise altitude. Determination of latitude by meridian passage can be accomplished through observation of any celestial body of known declination, although observation is easiest with the sun.

Another extremely simple observation to determine latitude involves measuring the altitude of Polaris (also known as α-*Ursae Minoris*, the "Pole Star" or "North Star"). Polaris rotates about the true north celestial pole on a very short radius (between 44 and 45 minutes of arc in 1999). At two times each day, the altitude of Polaris will be equal to the altitude of the true pole, and that altitude will equal the latitude of the observer. The altitude of Polaris most closely approximates the altitude of the pole, and thus latitude, when the constellations *Ursae Majoris* (the Big Dipper) and Cassiopeia are positioned as indicated by Figure 73-9. For the remainder of the day, there will be a predictable discrepancy ranging from 0 to 45 minutes of arc between the measured altitude of the star and the latitude of the observer. The *Nautical Almanac* has a brief table that corrects for this discrepancy, allowing an observer to determine accurate latitude by the altitude of Polaris at any time when the star is visible and a suitable horizon is available. The Polaris sight requires GMT to within several minutes, a precise measurement of altitude, and data from the *Nautical Almanac*.[1,7]

The latitude obtained by the noon sight or Polaris sight represents the simplest available celestial LOP. This line can be used to determine a fix if coupled with a sight that yields longitude or with another LOP obtained by any other method. In land navigation, this second LOP might represent a river, shoreline, road, trail, compass bearing, or radio bearing that crosses the determined latitude line at a single point.

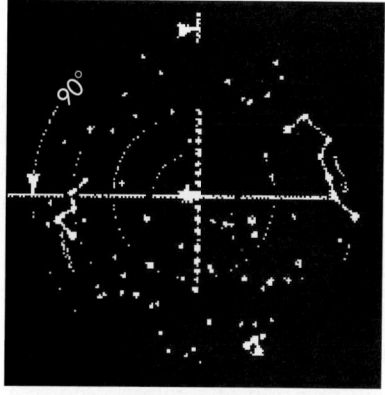

No correction

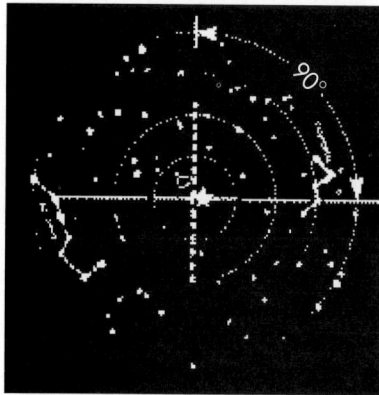

No correction

Figure 73-9 Diagram indicating the appearance of the north circumpolar sky at the two times of day when the observed altitude of Polaris is equivalent to the latitude of the observer. (*From Department of the Air Force:* Survival-training edition, Manual 64-3, *Randolph AFB, Texas, 1969, Air Training Command.*)

Celestial Methods for Longitude

Following invention of the chronometer by John Harrison in 1735, longitude could be directly determined by measuring the altitude of any celestial body of known coordinates at a precisely known instant of time. This method, termed the *time sight*, revolutionized exploration but involves formidable mathematics. A simpler alternative exists that is readily adaptable to the wilderness setting. This traditional technique for establishing longitude is called the *equal altitude method*. The equal altitude method requires accurate timekeeping, the ability to measure altitude with precision, and data from the *Nautical Almanac*. At a convenient interval before the meridian passage of the body (1 to 2 hours), the altitude of the body is taken and the Greenwich Mean Time (GMT) is noted. The sextant is left at the altitude setting of the first observation. After the body passes the meridian, it is observed until it falls to the exact altitude of the first reading. The time is again noted. Meridian passage will have occurred at the midpoint between these two times. The GMT of meridian passage is then known. At the moment of meridian passage, the LHA of the body equals zero, and the GHA of the body (from the *Nautical Almanac*) equals the observer's longitude. In theory, the instant of meridian passage could be found by noting the moment the body reached maximum altitude, achieving the same result. This is highly inaccurate in practice because of the extremely slow rate of change of altitude in the minutes immediately surrounding LAN.[18]

Altitude-Intercept Method

The observed position of a celestial body also can be reconciled with an observer's position on the Earth's surface through the application of spherical trigonometry. A *navigational triangle* can be constructed on the surface of the Earth that has as its vertices the nearest (or elevated) terrestrial pole, the assumed or estimated position of the observer, and the *geographic position* (GP) of the body being observed. The GP is that point on the surface of the earth that lies directly beneath the body at the instant of observation. The body lies at the zenith of an observer at the GP and has a measured altitude of 90°.

A second observer taking a simultaneous measurement of the altitude of the same body from a remote location finds the altitude to be less than 90° to an extent proportional to the distance between the site of observation and the GP. If the altitude of the body from the vantage of the second observer is 50°, that observer's position is 50° × 60 nautical miles per degree, or 3000 nautical miles, from the GP of the body. The second observer's location lies somewhere on a *circle of equal altitude* for the body in question. A small segment of this circle, on a scale of dozens of miles, would appear as a straight line on a chart or map. This line is a celestial line of position.[1,18] The concept of the celestial LOP was developed by Thomas H. Sumner in 1837 in a moment of astonishing intellectual clarity during a gale at sea. Celestial LOPs were originally called "Sumner lines" in recognition.

Before the 1900s, navigational triangles were solved laboriously using logarithmic and trigonometric tables in a process called *sight reduction*. Currently, sight reduction can be accomplished in minutes through the use of published tables of solutions called sight reduction tables. Sight reduction yields the calculated altitude (Hc) and azimuth (Zn) for the observed body as they should appear from the observer's assumed position. Armed with Hc and Zn, the navigator then compares Ho with Hc. If the two are identical, the observer is on the LOP containing the assumed position. When the two altitude values vary, the difference represents the number of nautical miles between the LOP of the assumed position and the LOP of the actual position of the observer. The direction of this difference is given by

Zn. Whether the difference is toward or away from the observed body is neatly summarized in the mnemonics GOAT (greater observed angle, toward), and Coast Guard Academy (calculated greater, away). The results are plotted on a map or plotting sheet. Each observation reduced by this method yields a single, celestial LOP. With two observations of suitable bodies, two LOPs result that will cross. The crossing point is a fix, or the observer's actual position.

This graphical method of navigation is termed the *altitude-intercept method*. It was invented by a French naval officer, Marcq St. Hilaire, in 1875. The logic of the method is beautiful; the navigator assumes that he is somewhere that he knows he is not, then proves how wrong he must be.[2]

Sight reduction tables are published by the governments of the United States and United Kingdom and are available in varying degrees of detail. Inspection tables, such as *Hydrographic Office Publication Numbers 229 and 249 (H.O. 229 and H.O. 249)* allow solutions with minimal recourse to math; all possible solutions are available in the inspection tables, requiring only simple interpolations. Inspection tables tend to be large and bulky, but the few pages covering the latitudes of a planned expedition can be copied and carried with ease. Other tables are quite compact (e.g., *H.O. 211, H.O. 208, the S-Table*), some as few as 9 pages in length, but require serial additions or subtractions to yield a solution, increasing the possibility of error. A compact sight reduction table is included in commercial editions of the *Nautical Almanac*, eliminating the need to purchase and carry additional tables. Solution of the navigational triangle by formula and calculator is possible but beyond the scope of this chapter.

The altitude-intercept method of navigation is highly flexible but not intuitive. The mathematics are daunting, although the method can be used in a "cookbook" manner with success. The interested reader is referred to several of the general references for further details.[1,7,13,18]

Small, military surplus, aeronautical sextants with reliable artificial horizons are readily available and permit very accurate celestial altitude measurements on land. Small box sextants, which fit into a pocket, also can be used to accurately measure altitudes using a dish of water, oil, or mercury to provide a reflective artificial horizon (Figure 73-10). Any quartz wristwatch set to GMT with a known rate of error is sufficient to the task of time keeping. Copies of *Nautical Almanac* pages for the dates of a planned excursion provide all of the needed astronomical data, and other tables from the *Almanac* provide sight corrections and data for interpolation. The *Almanac* itself also can be carried. A map, plotting sheet, or lined paper and a pencil permit the resulting LOPs to be plotted in con-

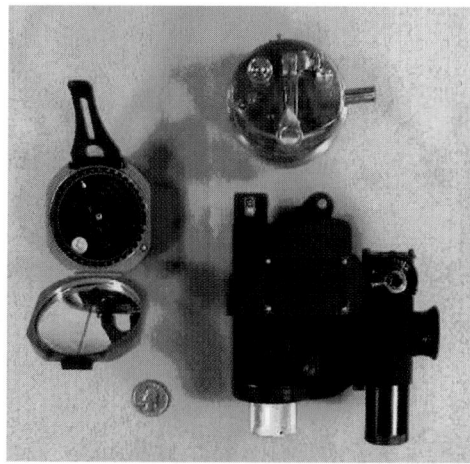

Figure 73-10 A selection of portable altitude measuring devices for celestial navigation. Clockwise from top: box sextant, A-10 aeronautical sextant, pocket transit with clinometer. The box sextant requires a separate artificial horizon such as a reflective dish of water for land use. The A-10 sextant and pocket transit have intrinsic bubble levels. Use of the pocket transit requires averaging of multiple altitude measurements to achieve acceptable accuracy. A quarter is included in the image to provide scale.

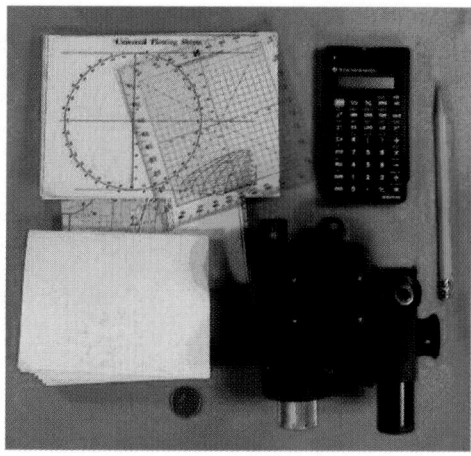

Figure 73-11 A complete portable kit for celestial navigation. Clockwise from upper right: scientific calculator, pencil, A-10 aeronautical sextant, folded copies of almanac daily pages and sight reduction pages from H.O. 249, protractor/straight edge, plotting sheets, and topographic map. The sight reduction pages and calculator can substitute for one another. The topographic map and plotting sheets can substitute for one another, although the map is more useful for land navigation. Not included in the image is an accurate watch set to Greenwich Meridian Time. A quarter is included to provide scale.

text to the area being traveled. The minimum required equipment is surprisingly portable and shown in Figure 73-11.

For practice, I routinely carry the following equipment on trips: (1) aeronautical sextant (the A-10 model, widely available, is the smallest and lightest), (2) the *Nautical Almanac*, (3) photocopies of *H.O. 249* pages covering the latitudes of the planned trip, (4) watch set to GMT, (5) pencil, (6) photocopied plotting sheet, (7) small protractor with a straight edge, and (8) pocket scientific calculator with various formulae on an index card (see Figure 73-11). Although forming the basis for considerable hilarity among companions, this equipment routinely allows determination of direction to within 2° and position to within 2 miles.

The Minimalist Celestial Fix

The training manual published by the U.S. military as *Air Force Manual 64-3*[4] contains detailed instructions for fabrication of a "fishline sextant." This simple device, when used in conjunction with an accurate watch set to GMT, protractor, and limited *Nautical Almanac* information, allows the user to determine latitude by measuring the altitude of Polaris, and longitude by timing the meridian passage of overhead stars. Although I have not tested the accuracy or ease of use of this method, it has the necessary elements required to yield useful positional information and is claimed to allow determination of a fix with an accuracy of 10 miles. The reader is referred to this manual for specifics of the method.

CELESTIAL METHODS FOR DIRECTION FINDING

Shadow Methods

The axis of rotation of the Earth is inclined at about 23.5° from the orbital plane of the solar system. It is this phenomenon that results in the seasons, the variable path of the sun through the sky with each season, and the terrestrial definitions of the tropics, temperate zones, and Arctic and Antarctic zones. The apparent path of the sun is lower in the sky, and shadows cast by the sun are longer, at any given time of day in winter than in summer. A plot of the tips of shadows cast in daylight by a vertical object (a gnomon) on any given date results in a curved line called a *declination curve*. The declination curve is so-named because shadow lengths are proportional to the declination of the sun on the date of the plot. The shadows used in plotting a declination curve will be shortest at noon, when the sun is at its greatest altitude, and longest near sunrise and sunset. A family of declination curves can be plotted empirically for various dates and can then be used in subsequent years to predict shadow lengths for future dates and times. The shadows themselves can be plotted to indicate the direction of the sun, which will give the approximate time of day. This is the principle by which sundials were constructed before the discovery of trigonometry. A family of declination curves will be useful for any point on the Earth's surface near the same latitude as the location where they were plotted. The curves will not be accu-

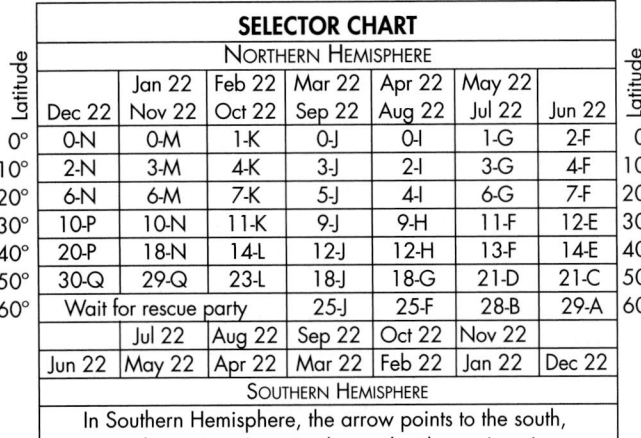

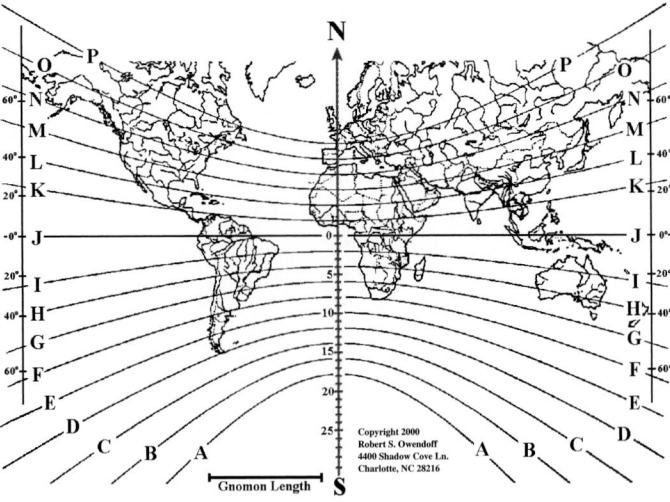

SELECTOR CHART

Latitude	Dec 22	Jan 22 / Nov 22	Feb 22 / Oct 22	Mar 22 / Sep 22	Apr 22 / Aug 22	May 22 / Jul 22	Jun 22	Latitude
0°	0-N	0-M	1-K	0-J	0-I	1-G	2-F	0°
10°	2-N	3-M	4-K	3-J	2-I	3-G	4-F	10°
20°	6-N	6-M	7-K	5-J	4-I	6-G	7-F	20°
30°	10-P	10-N	11-K	9-J	9-H	11-F	12-E	30°
40°	20-P	18-N	14-L	12-J	12-H	13-F	14-E	40°
50°	30-Q	29-Q	23-L	18-J	18-G	21-D	21-C	50°
60°	Wait for rescue party			25-J	25-F	28-B	29-A	60°
	Jun 22	Jul 22 / May 22	Aug 22 / Apr 22	Sep 22 / Mar 22	Oct 22 / Feb 22	Nov 22 / Jan 22	Dec 22	

NORTHERN HEMISPHERE (top) / SOUTHERN HEMISPHERE (bottom)

In Southern Hemisphere, the arrow points to the south, and west (a.m.) is interchanged with east (p.m.)

Figure 73-12 The Universal Pocket Navigator (UPN). Enter the Selector Table with arguments for the approximate date and the approximate latitude as determined from the background map. Stick a pin or toothpick vertically in the center line at the cross mark indicated by the Selector Table to serve as a gnomon. The tip of the gnomon should stand above the figure by the length indicated by the gnomon scale. Hold the figure horizontally, and rotate your body until the shadow of the tip of the gnomon lies on the appropriate lettered curve (from the Selector Table). The arrow now points north. (*From Owendoff RS: Better ways of pathfinding,* Harrisburg, Penn, 1964, The Stackpole Co.)

rate at more distant latitudes because the altitude of the sun changes with the latitude of the observer. This lack of universality can be overcome by moving the gnomon to compensate for changes in latitude. Since the advent of plane and spherical trigonometry, declination curves and gnomon positions can be calculated for any date and location.[26]

The sundial is most commonly used to tell time but also can be used as a sun compass to indicate direction. Shadows cast in the morning hours point westward, whereas those in the afternoon point eastward. The variation between the rising and setting points and due east or west are predictable for any date and latitude (see section on Amplitudes). The shortest shadow cast by the sun occurs at LAN and always lies on a due north-south line. Alternatively, a north-to-south line can be found by bisecting the angle between two points on a declination curve that are at equal distances from the gnomon. Knowing this, a sun compass can be constructed that indicates true direction with a high degree of accuracy whenever the shadow tip of the appropriately positioned gnomon lies on the declination curve for the approximate date of observation. Such a sun compass is included as Figure 73-12.[26] This sun compass has a scale to compensate for the latitude of the user. A copy of this sun compass, a pin or toothpick greater than 1 inch in length, and sunshine are all that are necessary to determine the cardinal directions with an accuracy greater than that commonly achievable with a magnetic compass (Figure 73-13).

In the absence of a copy of Figure 73-12, the same principle can be applied to construct a sun compass on the fly. Any flat surface (e.g., a chip of wood, piece of

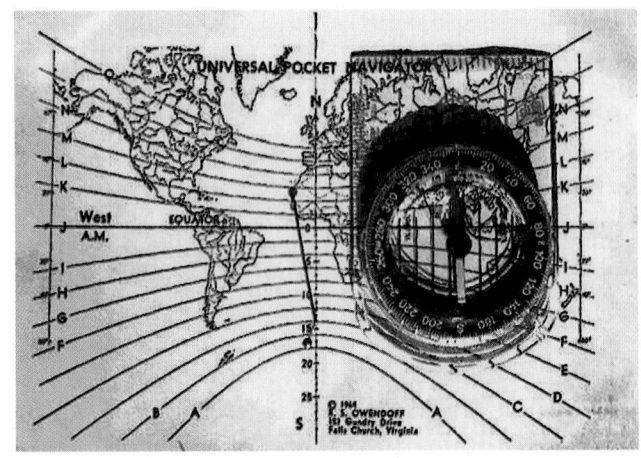

Figure 73-13 Use of the Universal Pocket Navigator to find north. The selector chart was entered with the date of October 25 and the assumed latitude of 40°, yielding declination curve "L" and gnomon position "14." Note the correspondence between magnetic north and north as indicated by the center line of the figure. The magnetic declination at the sight of observation was 4½° west. The UPN reading corresponds to true north.

bark, scrap of paper) is placed horizontally in the sun and a gnomon of convenient length is stuck in the surface in a vertical position. The tip of the shadow cast by the gnomon is marked at various times beginning shortly after sunrise, and a curve is traced between the marks. At some point the sun will pass the meridian, and the shadow will begin to lengthen again. A line between the base of the gnomon and the point of closest approach of the curve represents solar noon and runs due north to due south. Whether the shadow at noon points north or south will depend on whether the ob-

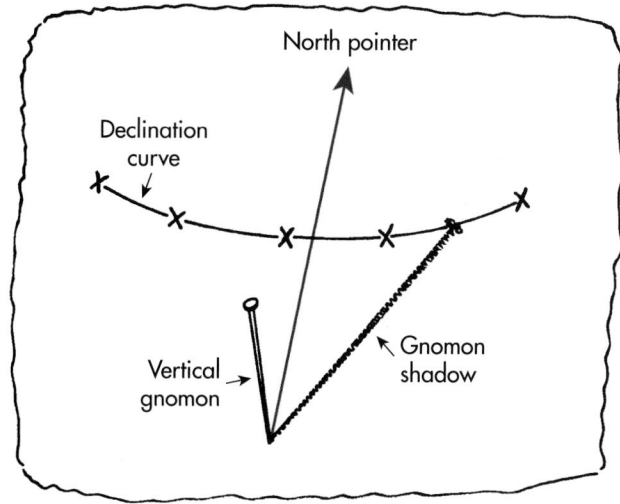

Figure 73-14 A makeshift suncompass inscribed on a scrap of paper. The declination curve has been empirically determined by tracing a line through points representing the tip of the gnomon shadow at various times throughout the day. On subsequent days, rotation of the figure such that the shadow tip touches the curve will orient the line connecting the base of the gnomon to the point of closest approach of the curve to point north. (*From Owendoff RS: Better ways of pathfinding,* Harrisburg, Penn, 1964, The Stackpole Co.)

server is in the Northern Hemisphere, the southern hemisphere, or the tropics. The actual direction indicated by the shadow is easily determined by noting the general direction of sunrise, which is on the eastward side of the sun compass. The remaining afternoon portion of the curve can either be completed freehand as a mirror image of the morning curve, or by continued observation and marking of shadow tips (Figure 73-14). On subsequent days the sun compass is reoriented to true north by rotating the horizontal surface until the tip of the gnomon's shadow touches the curve. A sun compass prepared in this manner is highly portable and remains accurate for many days until there is significant change in the latitude of the traveler or in the declination of the sun. New curves can be prepared on the same compass as needed.

Other methods of direction finding by shadows are significantly less accurate. The direction of travel of a shadow tip over the period of an hour or so will point generally eastward throughout the day.[5] The accuracy of this method is degraded in direct proportion to the length of time before or after noon that the observations take place, and in inverse proportion to the declination of the sun. Errors of greater than 30° are possible when conditions are unfavorable, such as at higher latitudes and during winter when the path of the sun is low in the sky. However, errors incurred during morning hours tend to be canceled by reciprocal errors incurred during afternoon hours as long as the rate of change in latitude while traveling is relatively slow during the period of observation.[26] The shortest shadow cast by a vertical gnomon through the course of the day lies on a north-south line at all latitudes. The point of closest approach of a declination curve to the gnomon may be difficult to accurately determine when the rate of change of the sun's altitude around LAN is slow. As an alternative method, a line bisecting the angle between any two shadows of equal length cast by a vertical gnomon lies on a north-south line at all latitudes.

An ordinary analog wristwatch or pocket watch can be used to give rough north-south direction using the shadow technique. Since a conventional watch has a 12-hour cycle of rotation, the hour hands rotates at 30° per hour, or twice the rate of the apparent angular movement of the sun. Thus, if the hour hand of the watch is aligned with the shadow of a vertical object (i.e., hand is pointing directly at the sun), the bisected angle between the hour hand and 12 o'clock on the dial yields a line that runs generally north to south. At times before 0600 or after 1800, the larger of the two possible angles between the hour hand and 12 o'clock should be used. This method is fraught with errors that increase in magnitude when the sun's altitude is high (tropical or subtropical latitudes; late spring, summer, and early fall months). It is also subject to errors that result from differences between zone time and local time, and from the *equation of time* (the difference between mean solar time and true solar time). However, the watch method can be useful as a direction finder if the potential for inaccuracy is kept in mind, and if techniques are used to reduce avoidable errors. Correspondence between direction determined by the watch method and true direction will be greatest between latitudes of 40° to 60° in the winter months. Accuracy is improved if the watch is set to local solar time at the approximate longitude of observation rather than zone time (local solar time = GMT + east longitude expressed in time; local solar time = GMT − west longitude expressed in time [where 15° of longitude = 1 hour]). Directional errors are further reduced by tilting the watch face to lie in the plane of the sun's apparent path rather than in the horizontal plane.[10,26,27] A digital watch also may be used if the indicated time is drawn as an analog clock face on paper or in the dust.

Direction by Amplitudes

The *amplitude* of a heavenly body is the angular measurement between the body when on the horizon and the observer's prime vertical circle. When the body is rising, the amplitude is reckoned from due east; when the body is setting, the amplitude is reckoned from due west. The amplitude is designated as north or south depending on the relative position of the body on the horizon and the prime vertical circle. The amplitude will always be north when the declination of the body is positive, and vice versa. For objects of constant declination (the "fixed stars"), amplitude is constant. For the sun, moon, and planets, amplitude varies with seasonal variations in the declination of these bodies. Knowledge of the amplitude of the sun for various dates is useful as a means of determining direction at sunrise and sunset. Amplitude of the sun is zero on the dates of the spring and fall equinoxes, and the sun rises due east and sets due west of an observer at any latitude between the Arctic and Antarctic circles on those dates.[1,7] When in the tropics, the amplitude of any body equals its declination. Outside of the tropics, the amplitude of a body is always larger than the declination of the body.[3]

The formula for calculating the amplitude of any body at rising or setting (altitude = 0) is known as Napier's rule[1,19,20]:

Given latitude (L) and declination (d), solve for amplitude (A):

$$A = \sin^{-1}(\sin d/\cos L)$$

The maximum amplitude for the sun at a given latitude is calculated by entering the maximum declinations of the sun occurring at the solstices ($\pm23.5°$) into the formula.[1] The amplitude for any date is calculated by entering the declination of the sun on the date of interest.

For most of the year in most of the world, the sun's amplitude lies within 30° of due east and west. In fall and winter in the Northern Hemisphere, the sun rises and sets south of east and west, whereas in the spring and summer the opposite is true. Maximum amplitudes occur at the solstices, and minimum amplitudes occur at the equinoxes.

A useful table of amplitudes for the sun or other selected celestial body can be easily calculated by Napier's rule and carried on an index card to provide a directional reference in the area of intended travel. The approximate latitude of the area of travel can be determined from a map. The declinations of the body to be used for the dates of travel can be located in the *Nautical Almanac*. A ready-made table of amplitudes covering latitudes from 0 degrees to 77 degrees, and declinations from 0 degrees to 24 degrees, is available in Bowditch's *American Practical Navigator*[1] as Table 27.

Direction by Observation of Circumpolar Stars

Polaris provides the most reliable directional indicator in the night sky. Polaris can be used to indicate direction within a degree of true north at any location above 10° north latitude. Use of the star becomes progressively more difficult as its altitude increases above 60° north because of difficulty relating the star's azimuth to the horizon. A stick with a string tied to the end and weighted with a bolt or washer can be used to find the point on the horizon representing north in this setting. The stick is held such that the string hangs in a line from Polaris to the horizon. The point of intersection of the string with the horizon indicates north.[3]

The Big Dipper (*Ursae Majoris*) can be used to identify Polaris or true north by extending a line from the "Pointers" (α-*Ursae Majoris*, or Dubhe, and β-*Ursae Majoris*, or Merak) toward the north celestial pole. These stars form the leading edge of the Dipper. The distance between them multiplied by 5 indicates the approximate position of Polaris. When the Dipper is low in the sky or below the horizon, a similar process can be followed in identifying north from the constellation Cassiopeia. Cassiopeia has the appearance of a flattened letter "M" when above the pole, and "W" when below. If a line drawn between the stars forming the feet of the "M" (β-*Cassiopeiae*, or Caph, and ϵ-*Cassiopeiae*) is assigned length "X," a perpendicular line of length "2X" extending from the trailing star will indicate approximate north[4] (Figure 73-15).

In the Southern Hemisphere there is no conspicuous star that marks the south celestial pole. However, the distinctive asterism of the Southern Cross can be used to point to the approximate location of the pole and thus to indicate south. The Southern Cross consists of four stars. The declination of the crossbar is approximately $-60°$. The long axis of the cross lies on a line that passes within 3° of the south celestial pole. The distance to the approximate pole from the star forming the base of the cross (α-*Crucis*, or Acrux) is approximately 5 times the length of the long axis of the cross (Figure 73-16). At latitudes where the cross is visible but the south celestial pole is below the horizon, the long axis of the Southern Cross indicates south when the constellation is vertically oriented.[3,4,28]

When the Southern Cross is below the horizon or too low in the sky for reliable observation, the bright stars Canopus (α-*Carinae*) and Achernar (α-*Eridani*) can be used to find south. If a line between these stars is con-

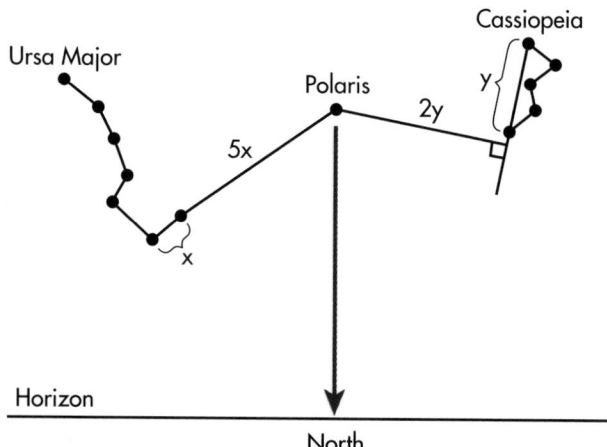

Figure 73-15 The azimuth of Polaris is always within 45 arc minutes of true north. Lines as indicated from "the Pointers" of the constellation Ursa Major, or from the trailing star of the constellation Cassiopeia, also can be used to find north when Polaris is obscured by clouds or below the horizon. (*From Burch D:* Emergency navigation, *Camden, Me, 1986, International Marine Publishing Co.*)

sidered to represent the base of an equilateral triangle, the apex of the triangle points to the approximate location of the south celestial pole[3,4] (see Figure 73-16).

Direction by Observation of Other Stars

It should be clear from the amplitude formula that any object with a known declination of less than plus or minus 5° could be used to give a reasonably accurate indication of east at the time of rising, or west at the time of setting. By virtue of its brightness and of the familiarity of the constellation in which it is located, the star δ-*Orionis* (Mintaka) [declination −0°, 18 minutes] is particularly useful in this regard. Mintaka is the leading star in the belt of the constellation Orion. It rises due east and sets due west at any latitude from which it is observed (Figure 73-17). Unfortunately, the visibility of Mintaka at rising or setting is limited to the months of October through April. When the star is obscured by haze or clouds at rising or the time of rising is missed, the location of the rising can be extrapolated. Within 1 to 2 hours of the rising time, hold a straight edge connecting the star to the horizon at the rising angle of the star, where rising angle = 90° - latitude. The point at which the straight edge touches the horizon indicates the position the star occupied when on the horizon. Because the rising and setting angles of any body are the same, the same technique can be used to determining the point on the horizon where the star will set.[3]

The constellation Scorpius is prominent in the southern sky at mid-northern latitudes during the summer. This constellation contains a distinctive reddish star, Antares (α-*Scorpii*), at the position of the neck of the scorpion. To the east of Antares the tail of the scorpion hangs toward the horizon. Three stars just before the sharp bend in the tail of the figure (ε-, μ-, and ζ-*Scorpii*) form a nearly straight line. The stars comprising the head and claws of the figure (β, δ [Dschubba] and π-*Scorpii*) lie in a fairly straight line located immediately to the west of Antares. The configuration of the constellation is such that the stars forming the linear array of the tail point due south when the line of the head and claws has passed the meridian and is perpendicular to the horizon (Figure 73-18).[3]

In the Carolinas Islands of the South Pacific, the bearings at rising and setting of 32 prominent stars

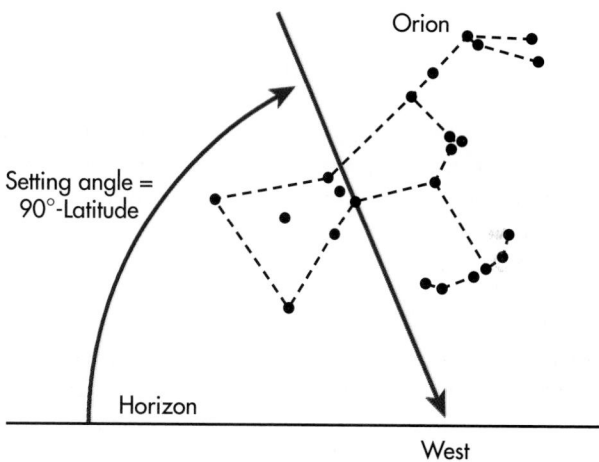

Figure 73-17 Determination of true west by observation of the setting point of the star Mintaka (declination zero) in the belt of the constellation Orion. The rising point of the same star indicates true east. (*From Burch D:* Emergency navigation, *Camden, Me, 1986, International Marine Publishing Co.*)

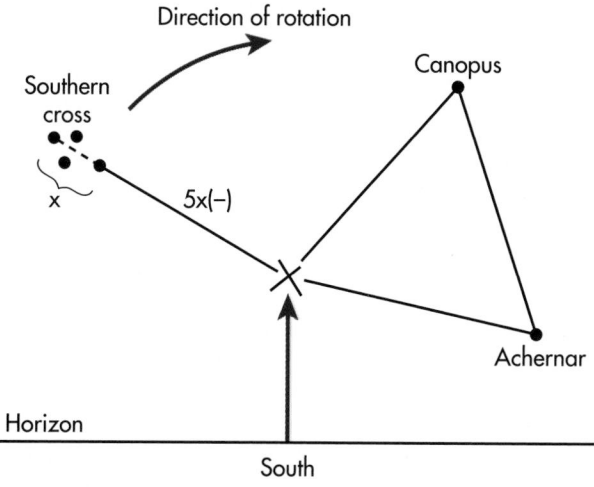

Figure 73-16 Determination of south by circumpolar stars. The long axis of the Southern Cross almost lies along a radius extending from the south celestial pole at the distance indicated in the figure. The apex of an equilateral triangle with the stars Achernar and Canopus forming the vertices of the base also approximates the position of the south celestial pole. (*From Burch D:* Emergency navigation, *Camden, Me, 1986, International Marine Publishing Co.*)

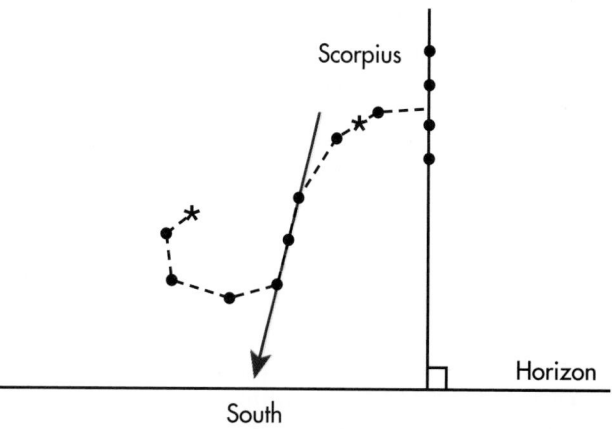

Figure 73-18 Determination of south by observation of the constellation Scorpio. When the best-fit line connecting the stars forming the head and claws of the figure is perpendicular to the horizon, the linear array of stars in the tail of the asterism points south. (*From Burch D:* Emergency navigation, *Camden, Me, 1986, International Marine Publishing Co.*)

are memorized by navigators to permit determination of direction at sea. The fidelity of this "star compass" for direction finding is demonstrated by the ability of these navigators to make successful landfall on minute atolls after open ocean voyages of hundreds of miles.[11] Memorization or recording of the rising or setting azimuths of a few prominent stars at the latitude of a planned trip would afford the same directional reference to the land navigator in case the compass or other navigational aid was lost or damaged. These azimuths could be precalculated in minutes using Napier's rule.

Finally, observation of the movement of any overhead celestial body relative to a fixed reference (e.g., a branch, guy line, the "fishline sextant") over a span of 15 to 20 minutes (4° to 5° of movement) will give a reasonably accurate indication of east and west.

NAVIGATION WITH A POCKET RADIO

Radio transmission and reception are inherently directional. This is particularly evident with reception in the broadcast band (500 to 1600 kHz) and is a principle that is more apparent in inexpensive portable radios than in larger, more expensive models. Radio navigation was used extensively in aviation from the 1930s through the 1950s. There are anecdotal reports of successful sailings from the West Coast of the United States to Hawaii using only an AM radio and jet contrails for navigation.[21]

The internal antenna of the typical pocket AM radio is formed by a ferrite bar wrapped in multiple loops of wire. This ferrite-loop antenna responds most strongly to radio waves when oriented perpendicular to them. Reception is minimized when the antenna is oriented parallel to the transmitted radio waves (i.e., pointed at the transmission tower of the station). The point of minimum radio reception, or *null point,* can be used to find the direction to a source of radio transmission with surprising precision.[3,27] Use of this technique assumes that a broadcast band station is audible, and that the geographic location of the radio transmission can be identified by listening to the station. Once these conditions are met, the procedure for establishing a direction line that runs through the broadcast source and the observer is relatively easy. Radio homing does not determine true direction but can identify the direction to safety. When used in conjunction with a map, radio bearings act as LOPs and multiple bearings to different stations can result in a fix. The procedure for navigation by radio bearings follows:

1. If not known, determine the orientation of the radio's internal antenna. This can be done by opening the case and looking for the antenna (a dark gray or black bar wrapped in fine copper wire), or by rotating the radio while listening to a station and determining the plane of rotation that re-

sults in a null point (rotation about the long axis of the antenna will not change the reception, whereas rotation perpendicular to the long axis will result in nulling).

2. Select an audible AM station and listen until the location of the station is identified. Hold the radio in a manner that allows the long axis of the internal antenna to act as a pointer. Rotate the radio parallel to the ground until the radio signal becomes faintest or disappears. Nulling of the signal can be augmented by tuning to the fringes of the station frequency if the reception is strong.

3. The actual direction to the source of radio transmission will be one of the reciprocal bearings of the LOP connecting the observer and the station location. The bearing that actually points to the radio source can be determined if the observer has even a crude understanding of their position relative to the station (e.g., generally north of, vs. generally south of). The bearing to the broadcast source also can be determined by serially checking the null point of the station while traveling. The angle over which nulling occurs becomes greater as the signal weakens with increasing distance from the source. Thus, if the angle over which the signal nulls is widening as travel progresses, the observer is moving away from the radio source. If the angle over which the station nulls narrows as travel progresses, the observer is moving toward the source.

4. If a compass is available, determine the azimuth of the null point. Keep the compass far enough from the radio to avoid influencing the needle with the radio's metal parts. A compass allows the magnetic bearing to the station to be determined. This bearing can then be followed to safety without further use of the radio.

5. If a map and compass are available, orient the map using the compass and draw a line though the broadcast source on the map at the azimuth of the null point. Extend this line to the edges of the map. Your location is somewhere on or near this line. If you have a map but no compass and can properly orient the map by natural cues, place the radio on top of the broadcast location on the map and rotate it until the signal nulls. Draw a line parallel to the internal antenna through the broadcast location and extend it to the map margins. Again, your position lies somewhere on this line. When two (or more) stations can be tuned and identified, the LOPs connecting the observer to each radio source will cross, and a fix is obtained at the point of crossing. The uncertainty of this fix will be least when the angle between two position lines is close to 90° or when the angles between three position lines are close to 120°.

NAVIGATION WITH THE GLOBAL POSITIONING SYSTEM

The NAVSTAR Global Positioning System exploits the logical framework of celestial navigation in using a predictable extraterrestrial reference for the determination of terrestrial position. In GPS navigation, artificial satellites substitute for celestial bodies as reference points. Calculation of position is based on *circles of equal distance* from the satellites.

The current system consists of a constellation of 27 satellites (24 operational, 3 spares) in six orbital planes (four functioning satellites per orbital plane). The orbital planes are inclined to the earth's equator by 55°. The orbital paths of the satellites are nearly circular and have an altitude of approximately 20,000 km with an orbital period of 11 hours, 58 minutes. At any given time, five to eight satellites are available in line-of-sight to a receiver anywhere on the surface of the earth.[8,15]

The method of position determination using GPS depends on calculation of the range between the satellite and receiver. GPS signals are transmitted on two L-band frequencies by each satellite: L1 (1575.4 MHz) and L2 (1227.6 MHz).[6] Transmitted information includes the precise time as kept onboard the satellite by multiple atomic clocks, a satellite ephemeris (catalog of predicted positions), and data concerning corrections for atmospheric propagation of radio signals and satellite clock errors. The GPS receiver decodes the positional data for each satellite and compares the timing information transmitted by the satellite with time as kept by the receiver's onboard clock. The signal received is in the form of a pseudorandom code. The GPS receiver shifts the code contained in memory to match the received code in phase. The duration of the shift represents the time required for the satellite signal to reach the receiver, usually on the order of 50 to 60 milliseconds. Since distance = speed × time, the transit time of the signal allows a calculation of the distance between receiver and satellite.[12] At any given instant a GPS receiver in contact with a NAVSTAR satellite will lie on the surface of a sphere of equal distance from the satellite. The intersection of this sphere of equal distance with the surface of the Earth forms a circle of equal distance, analogous to the circle of equal altitude in celestial navigation. The intersection of two such circles occurs at two points. The intersection of three such circles occurs at a single point of latitude and longitude on the surface[8,15,16,24] (Figure 73-19). This is the position of the receiver. If the intersection of the sphere of equal distance of a fourth satellite is added, the approximate altitude of the receiver also can be determined. Software allows the GPS receiver to choose the optimal group of four satellites for position determination among the subset of satellites within the line-of-sight of the receiver.

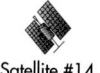

Satellite #14

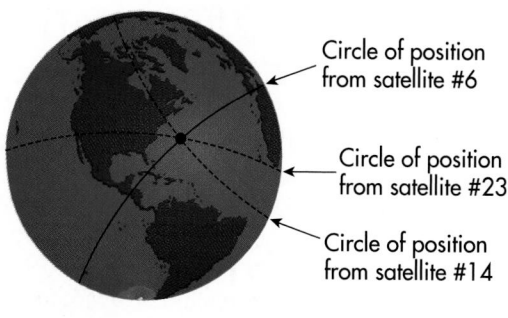

Circle of position from satellite #6

Circle of position from satellite #23

Circle of position from satellite #14

Satellite #6

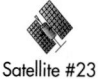

Satellite #23

Figure 73-19 Illustration of a GPS fix from the intersection of three circles of equal distance from three separate satellites. (*From Monahan K, Douglass D:* GPS instant navigation, *Bishop, Calif, 1998, Fine Edge Productions.*)

As currently configured, two levels of service are provided by the GPS system: the Precise Positioning Service (PPS) and the Standard Positioning Service (SPS). Currently, PPS is available only to military users. It provides positional accuracy of 15 m, velocity accuracy of 0.1 m/sec, and time accuracy of 100 nanoseconds. SPS provides civilian users with positional accuracy to 100 m 98% of the time, to 50 m 65% of the time, and to 40 m 50% of the time. Altitude accuracy is relatively poor at 150 m. The relative inaccuracy of the SPS system results from the intentional introduction of timing errors into the broadcast signal from the satellites on frequency L1. The degradation of precise data from the satellites is termed *selective availability* (SA) and is controllable from the ground. One year after public availability of GPS signals was granted in 1994, SA was formally implemented. SA has been turned off periodically since that time for obscure reasons, permitting civilian users to achieve military accuracy with commercial receivers. In the first decade of the twenty-first Century, SA will be phased out and a new frequency (L5) will be added to the signals broadcast by the third generation of NAVSTAR satellites. This will allow even greater accuracy to the civilian user.[8] The limitations in accuracy imposed by SA have been overcome by an in-

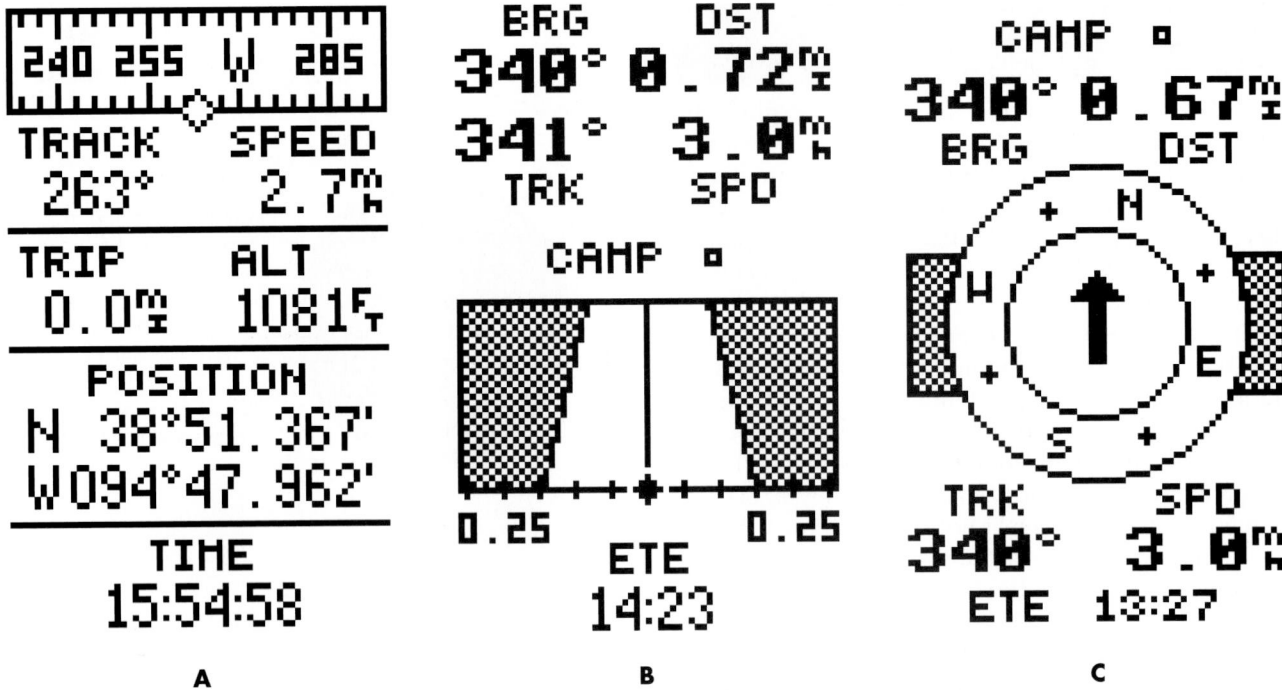

Figure 73-20 Screen images from a common portable GPS receiver showing various navigation screens. *Screen A* displays the time, the terrestrial coordinates and altitude of the observer's position, and the direction and velocity of travel. *Screen B* shows the bearing and distance to a selected waypoint (CAMP), the track made good by the observer, the velocity of travel, and a graphical representation of deviation from the intended course. *Screen C* shows the distance and bearing to the selected waypoint in compass format. *(Courtesy GARMIN International, Olathe, Kan.)*

genious method of error reduction developed by commercial users. This is termed *differential GPS* (DGPS). DGPS utilizes a fixed receiver at a precisely known position that broadcasts corrections between the established position of the fixed receiver and the position as determined by GPS. Specially equipped mobile GPS receivers receive the correction factor from the differential receiver and apply it to their position. DGPS permits 1- to 3-meter positional accuracy, and 3-meter altitude accuracy.

Global Navigation Satellite System (GLONASS), a Soviet-era system, has marginally better satellite coverage in higher northern and southern latitudes (>50°) and no SA. Positional accuracy is 30 meters. GLONASS receivers are not widely available, however, and the system offers no compelling advantages over GPS for the surface navigator.

GPS reaches its greatest utility when used in conjunction with a topographic map and compass. The raw output of the receiver is in latitude and longitude to the nearest second of arc, or in Universal Transverse Mercator (UTM) grid coordinates as used on topographic maps. This information is somewhat abstract in isolation, but software included with the receiver permits the user to understand absolute and relative position and perform sophisticated navigational feats, even in the absence of other aids to navigation. When used with a map, GPS allows the user to plot position

and route at will, determine bearings to landmarks, and enter the locations of landmarks into memory for use as *waypoints*. Even without a map, GPS allows the user to determine precise position, approximate altitude, bearing and linear distance to established waypoints, deviation from the intended course to a waypoint, and velocity of travel.

Waypoint navigation is a feature of particular utility in wilderness navigation. Waypoints can be entered into the GPS receiver manually via a keypad, or current position can be entered and stored as a waypoint with a single key-press. Groups of waypoints can be stored as a route. As a course is walked, waypoints can be stored and labeled with reference to a prominent landmark or terrain feature. On the return route, the receiver sequentially gives the bearing and distance to any waypoint within the stored route and displays a graphical representation of the deviation of the current course from the course needed to reach the waypoint (Figure 73-20). The receiver informs the user that a waypoint has been reached by sounding an alarm. Theoretically, this allows a user to follow a route in white-out conditions or in total darkness, using no visual references other than the display of the GPS receiver. Most current receivers have memory capacity sufficient for the storage of several hundred waypoints. Identification of a large number of waypoints on a complex route essentially allows the user to follow a "breadcrumb route" on return to their objective.[15]

All receivers can calculate the heading of travel and thus provide the user with a method of determining a true bearing and the cardinal directions by walking a brief, straight course. Speed of travel is displayed, and estimated time en route at the current speed is given. Simple moving maps highlighting a desired route are available on many models and permit the user to "walk the line" of a route on the receiver's graphic display. Some newer units incorporate low-resolution, digitized maps and display the user's position on the map image. When applied with common sense and routine awareness of approximate location, GPS renders it virtually impossible to become or remain lost and effectively eliminates much of the pathfinding challenge inherent to wilderness travel.

In practice, GPS should be applied to a wilderness trek in the following manner: Before embarking on a trip, the user should enter into the receiver the precise location of various important landmarks on the intended route of travel. These locations can be obtained from a trail guide or a USGS topographic map. The waypoints obtained in this manner are labeled and stored as a route within the receiver's memory. At the beginning of the trip, the location of the nearest town or source of assistance also is entered as a waypoint, as would the location of the trailhead where the trip is begun. The trip then progresses using map, compass, established trails, or the GPS receiver to follow the intended route. When pausing to camp, the position of the camp would be named and entered as yet another waypoint. At any time the bearing and distance to any waypoint of interest is available to the user. If, in a spasm of self-reliance, the user decides to lay aside the GPS receiver and pursue traditional methods of route finding, and he or she becomes lost, reactivation of the receiver allows the direction and distance to safety to be immediately determined.

GPS suffers from several limitations. Most receivers have a battery life of between 15 and 30 hours. Dead batteries yield a useless receiver. The receivers are relatively fragile, and many are not waterproof or even particularly water-resistant. Obstruction of the sky by terrain features or heavy foliage interferes with the reception of satellite signals and may render the receiver unable to acquire a sufficient number of satellites to provide a fix. Still, GPS is unsurpassed in ease of use, accuracy, and utility for wilderness navigation. Reliance on GPS as the sole navigational resource for any wilderness expedition is a grave error, however. As with all high-tech methodology, a GPS receiver can be easily disabled. The more self-contained methods of navigation discussed in earlier sections should be utilized whenever possible to maintain positional awareness and navigational skill should the GPS receiver fail.

CONCLUSION

The body of literature covering the topic of navigation is immense. Many techniques for determining direction and position exist in addition to those described above. Several of the references[1,3,9,26,27] catalog these methods. It is sufficient to the task of navigation if the above methods are understood in terms of how they work, even if why they work remains obscure. Practice is essential, and the reader is encouraged to increase his or her familiarity with the motion of celestial bodies, the inconstancy of the earth's magnetic field, and the use of a variety of common navigational aids. The study of land navigation should be a routine component of the preparation for any wilderness expedition.

REFERENCES

1. Bowditch N: *The American practical navigator. An epitome of navigation,* Washington, DC, 1984, Defense Mapping Agency Hydrographic/Topographic Center.
2. Buckley WF: Celestial navigation, *Motor Boating and Sailing* 111:68, 1977.
3. Burch D: *Emergency navigation,* Camden, Me, 1986, International Marine Publishing Co.
4. Department of the Air Force: *Survival-training edition. Manual 64-3,* Randolph AFB, Texas, 1969, Air Training Command.
5. Department of the Army: *Map reading and land navigation. Field manual 21-26,* Washington, DC, 1987, Headquarters, Department of the Army.
6. Dixon C: *Using GPS,* Dobbs Ferry, NY, 1999, Sheridan House.
7. Dutton B: *Navigation and nautical astronomy,* Annapolis, Md, 1943, United States Naval Institute.
8. Dye S, Baylin F: *The GPS manual. Principals and applications,* Boulder, Colo, 1997, Baylin Publications.
9. Gatty H: *The raft book,* New York, 1943, George Grady Press.
10. Gatty H: *Nature is your guide,* New York, 1958, Dutton.
11. Gladwin T: *East is a big bird,* Cambridge, Mass, 1970, Harvard University Press.
12. Herring TA: The global positioning system, *Sci Am* Feb 1994, p 44.
13. Hobbs RR: *Marine navigation: piloting and celestial and electronic navigation,* ed 4, Annapolis, Md, 1998, Naval Institute Press.
14. Hodgson M: *Compass and map navigator. The complete guide to staying found,* Merrillville, Tenn, 1997, ICS Books.
15. Hotchkiss NJ: *A comprehensive guide to land navigation with GPS,* ed 2, Herndon, Va, 1995, Alexis Publishing.
16. Hurn J: *GPS. A guide to the next utility,* Sunnyvale, Calif, 1989, Trimble Navigation.
17. Kjellstrom B: *Be expert with map and compass,* New York, 1975, Charles Scribner's Sons.
18. Letcher JS: *Self-contained celestial navigation with H.O. 208,* Camden, Me, 1977, International Marine Publishing.
19. Mills HR: *Positional astronomy and astronavigation: a new approach using the pocket calculator,* Chellenham, UK, 1978, Stanley Thornes, Ltd.
20. Mills HR: *Practical astronomy,* Chichester, UK, 1994, Albion Publishing.
21. Milligan JE: *Celestial navigation by H.O.249,* Centreville, Md, 1974, Cornell Maritime Press,
22. Mixter GW: *A primer of navigation,* ed 7, New York, 1995, WW Norton & Co..
23. Moffit FA, Bouchard H: *Surveying,* ed 6, New York, 1975, Intex Educational Publishers.
24. Monahan K, Douglass D: GPS instant navigation, Bishop, Calif, 1998, Fine Edge Productions.
25. Mooers RL Jr: *Finding your way in the outdoors,* New York, 1972, Outdoor Life Books.
26. Owendoff RS: *Better ways of pathfinding,* Harrisburg, Penn, 1964, The Stackpole Co.
27. Rutstrum C: *The wilderness route finder,* New York, 1967, Macmillan.
28. Seidman D: *The essential wilderness navigator,* Camden, Me, 1995, Ragged Mountain Press.
29. Williams JED: *From sails to satellites. The origin and development of navigational science,* Oxford, UK, 1992, Oxford University Press.

Special Populations and Considerations

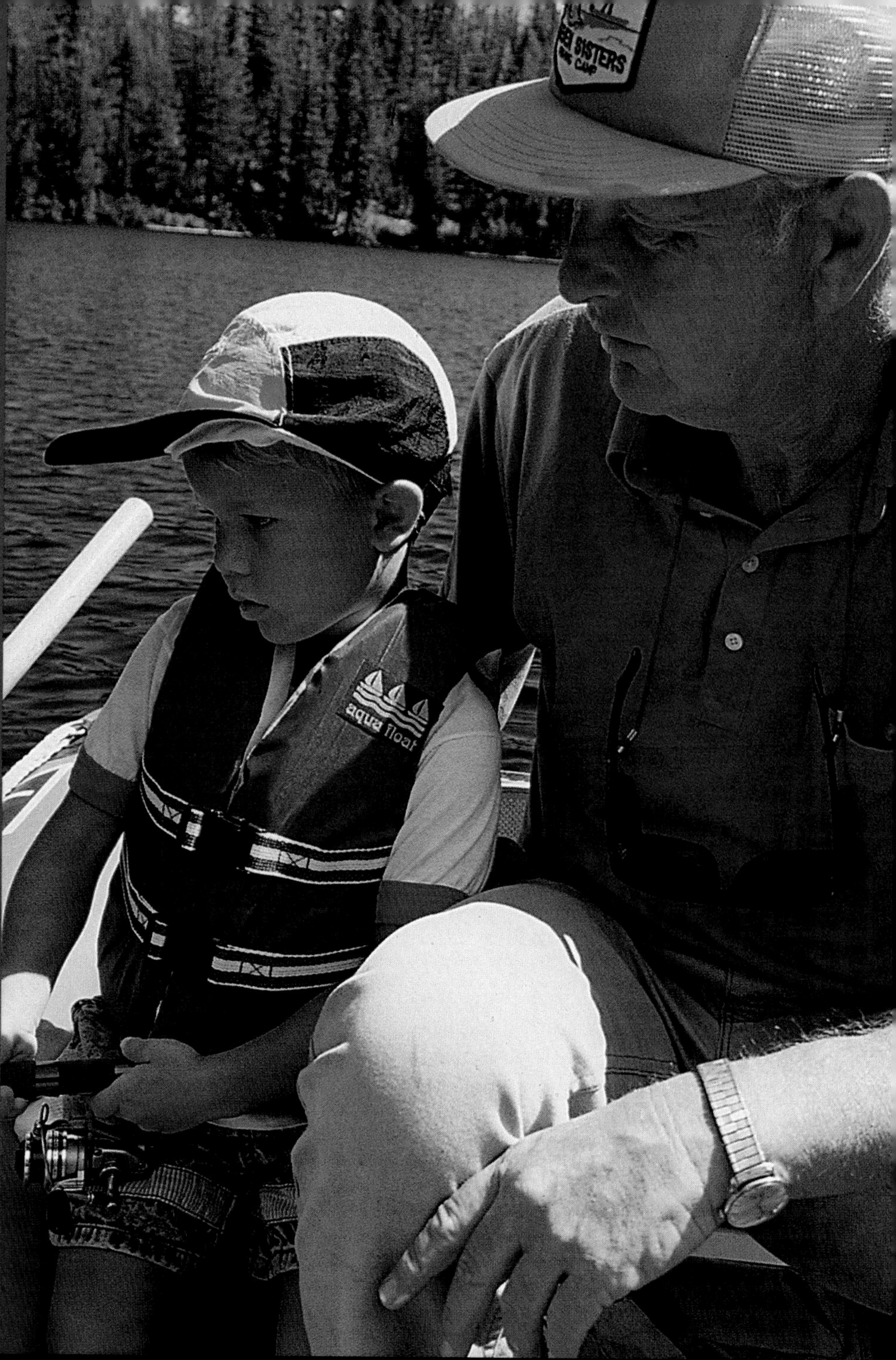

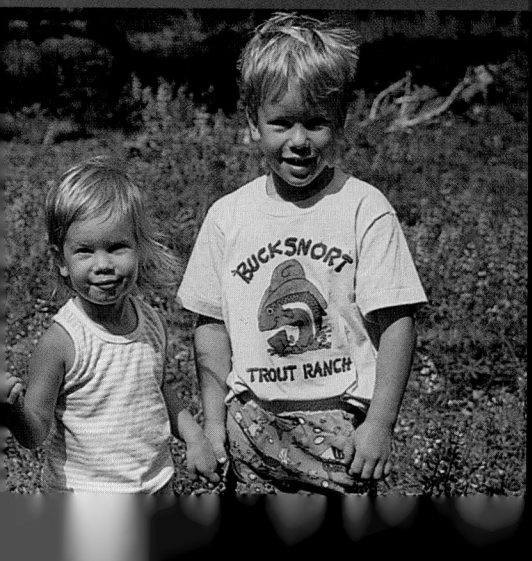

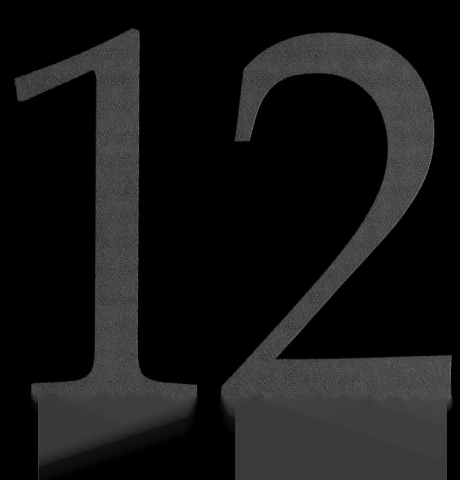

12

74 Children in the Wilderness

Judith R. Klein and Barbara C. Kennedy

Once the realm of a few adventurous individuals, the wilderness today attracts an ever-broadening range of explorers. This includes many in the pediatric age group, as parents seek to share the joys and lessons of wilderness travel with their children. In 1990, of the estimated 11 million people participating in backpacking and wilderness camping, nearly 25% were under 17 years of age.[65] Millions of other children annually visit national parks and recreation areas or travel to developing countries.

Wilderness travel with children requires special preparation and places extra demands on parents. However, it also affords unique opportunities. Parents and children interact in a setting distant from the stresses of work and school. Isolated from the distractions of computers, television, and modern life, children experience new environments, interact with individuals of different cultural heritage, and participate in activities that enrich their lives. These activities bring families together as they learn to rely on one another for support and entertainment.

Physicians and other health care professionals can encourage and facilitate such undertakings by providing preventive health and treatment guidelines for those planning wilderness travel with children. This chapter focuses on how children differ from adults and how to prevent, recognize, and treat the medical problems children are likely to encounter in a wilderness setting. Because wilderness travel may encompass travel to foreign countries, risk avoidance, pediatric travel immunizations and prophylaxis, and common pediatric medical problems associated with travel and developing countries are also reviewed.

WHAT MAKES CHILDREN DIFFERENT

Size and Shape

Children differ from adults in a variety of physical, physiologic, and psychologic ways. The most obvious difference is size. During development, children may grow from the average 7-pound baby to a 140-pound adolescent, a twentyfold difference. Accordingly, medications and fluids must be calculated on an individual basis, based on the weight of the child (Table 74-1).

This variation in size also influences a child's risk of developing serious complications from envenomations. Many snakes, spiders, scorpions, and poisonous marine animals deliver the same unit dose of venom re-gardless of the victim's size. Children often experience greater toxicity because of the increased dose of venom per kilogram of weight.

Children also have a larger body surface area (BSA) to mass ratio than adults. For example, a 7-pound infant has 2.5 times more BSA per unit weight than a 140-pound adult. In addition to the larger BSA, the part of the body most often left exposed, the head, takes up a larger proportion of the body in a young child (Figure 74-1). As a result, children experience greater exposure to environmental factors, such as cold, heat, and solar radiation. They are also more likely to have toxic effects from topical agents, such as insect repellents and medications.

Musculoskeletal System

A child nearly doubles in height between birth and 2 years and again between 2 and 18 years, and bone-remodeling potential is much greater than in adults. Because of the active osteogenic potential of the periosteum, nonunion or permanent angulation deformities at the metaphysis are unusual in children, and fractures heal quite rapidly; a fractured femur typically heals in 3 weeks in a newborn compared with 20 weeks in a 20-year-old. The strong, pliable periosteum also permits the development of greenstick and buckle fractures, which are not seen in the adult population. A fracture with intact periosteum is more stable, with little swelling or crepitus. If nondisplaced, it is often incorrectly dismissed as a sprain.

Children have an open growth plate, or physis, at the ends of long bones that connects the metaphysis to the epiphysis (Figure 74-2). The growth plates consist of soft cartilaginous cells that have the consistency of rubber and act as shock absorbers. They protect the joint surfaces from the grossly comminuted fractures seen in adults. However, because the growth plate is more vulnerable to injury than the strong ligaments or capsular tissues that attach to the epiphysis, a true sprain in a child is rare. Any significant juxtaarticular tenderness in a child should be assumed to be a growth plate injury. Such an injury is most common at the ankle (lateral malleolus), the knee (distal femur), and the wrist (distal radius). Physeal fractures have been classified into five Salter-Harris groups (see Figure 74-2). Salter-Harris I and II fractures generally heal without complications. However, Salter-Harris III and IV fractures often require open reduction of displaced fractures to realign the joint and growth plates and to permit normal growth. A Salter-Harris V fracture has a poor prognosis; the impaction and crushing of some or all of the growth plate may result in a bony bridge that inhibits further growth or causes unequal, angulated growth. Consequently, any significant injury, especially if it involves the growth plate, requires full evaluation in a medical facility.

Cardiovascular and Respiratory Systems

The basic physiologic parameters change greatly during the transition from infancy to childhood to adulthood. These differences are important to recognize to avoid unnecessary and potentially harmful interventions in healthy children but also to intervene when abnormal vital signs are present. For example, a blood pressure of 65/35 mm Hg, pulse rate of 160 beats/min, and respiratory rate of 40 breaths/min are considered ominous vital signs for an adult. How-

ever, these vital signs are normal in a 2-month-old infant.[28] Although blood pressure readings may not be available in a wilderness setting, it is possible to assess the strength of the pulse and determine the pulse and respiratory rate of an ill child. In general, infants and children have greater respiratory and heart rates and lower blood pressure than adults (Table 74-2).

Thermoregulation

Because environmental extremes are often encountered when traveling in wilderness areas, it is important to recognize that thermoregulation is less efficient in children than in adults (see Chapter 4). A number of physiologic and morphologic differences make children more susceptible than adults to heat illness[65] (see Chapters 10 and 11). During exercise, children generate more metabolic heat per unit mass than do adults. Children also have lower cardiac output at a given metabolic rate, resulting in a lower capacity to convey heat from the body core to the periphery. Because of their larger BSA/mass ratio, children also gain heat more rapidly from the environment than do adults when ambient temperature exceeds skin temperature. Under these same conditions, cooling from conduction, convection, and radiation ceases to be effective, leaving evaporation (sweating) as the only effective means of heat dissipation. Unfortunately, children have a lower capacity for evaporative cooling, possibly because of decreased sweat volume, regional differences in sweat patterns, and a higher sweat point (the rectal temperature when sweating starts). Finally, children acclimatize to hot environments at a slower rate than adults.

TABLE 74-1. Average Weights for Age

| AGE (YR) | WEIGHT | |
	kg	lb
1	10	22
3	15	33
6	20	44
8	25	55
9½	30	66
11	35	77

Modified from National Center for Health Statistics: *Am J Clin Nutr* 32:607, 1979.

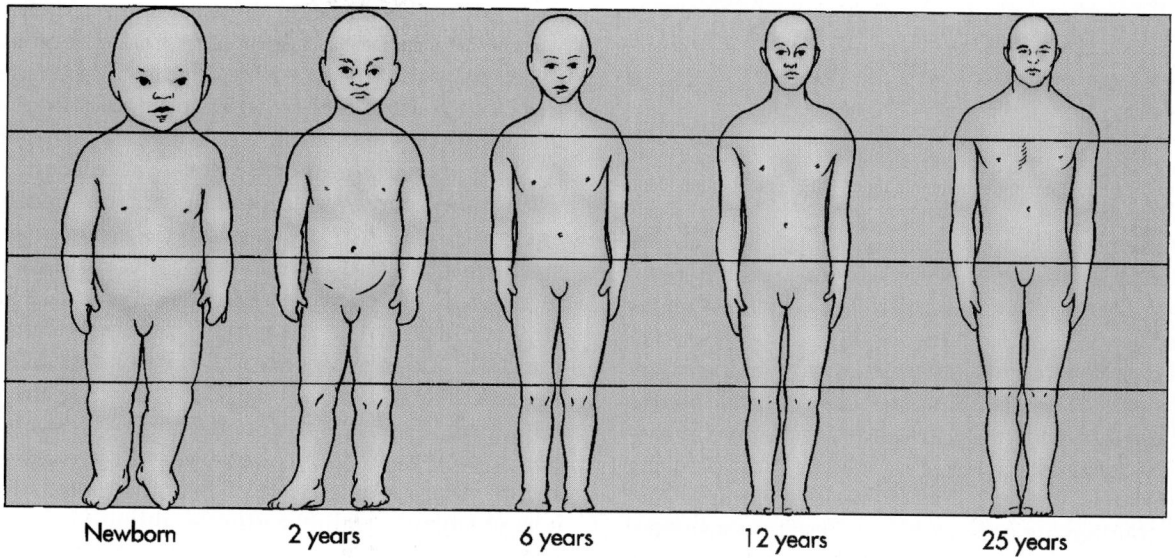

Figure 74-1 Body proportions.

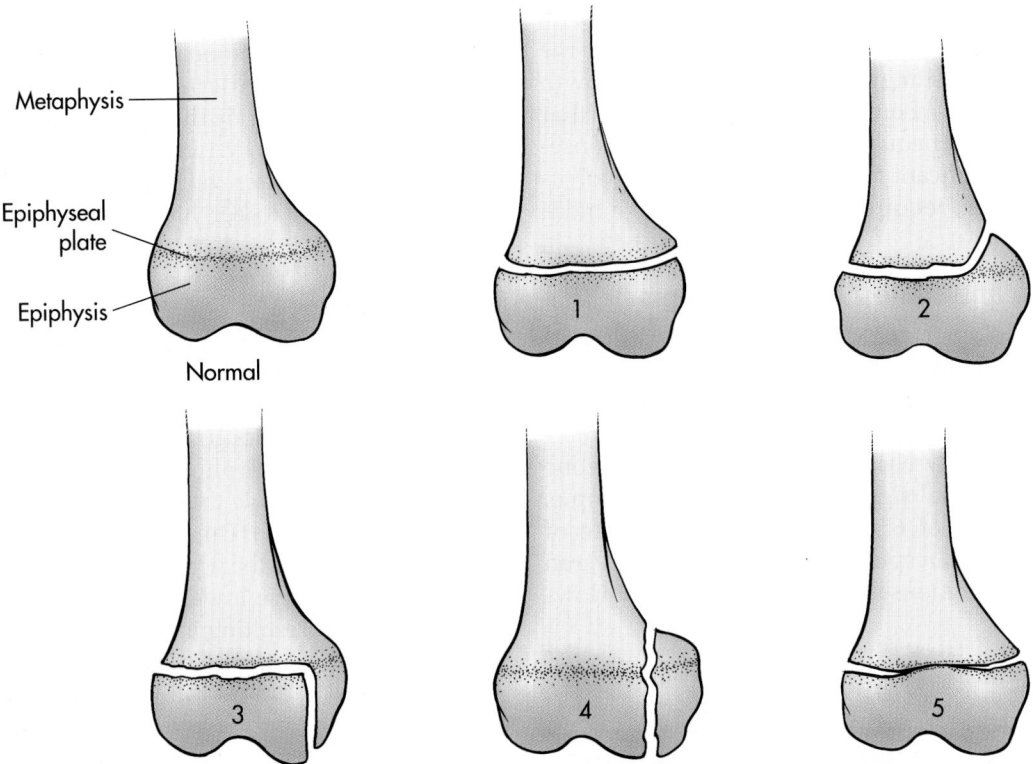

Figure 74-2 Salter-Harris classification of physeal fractures.

TABLE 74-2. Age-Specific Resting Heart Rate and Respiratory Rate*

AGE	HEART RATE (BEATS/MIN)	RESPIRATORY RATE (BREATHS/MIN)
0-5 mo	140 ± 40	40 ± 12
6-11 mo	135 ± 30	30 ± 10
1-2 yr	120 ± 30	25 ± 8
3-4 yr	110 ± 30	20 ± 6
5-7 yr	100 ± 20	16 ± 5
8-11 yr	90 ± 30	16 ± 4
12-15 yr	80 ± 20	16 ± 3

*Mean rate ± 2 SD.

Children are also at greater risk for hypothermia (see Chapter 6). Their larger BSA/mass ratio causes them to cool more rapidly than adults in cold environments. Children have less subcutaneous fat and thus less "natural" insulation. Infants in particular have an inefficient shivering mechanism.[10] Humans are poorly adapted to a cold environment and must rely on adaptive behavioral responses, such as seeking shelter and dressing appropriately, to maintain body heat. Infants and young children are not capable of these responses and must rely on their caregivers to provide shelter and appropriate clothing.

Immunology and Infections

Children experience a greater number of infections than adults. The average 1-year-old has six to eight infections per year, whereas the average adult has only three to four infections per year. Infections in children tend to be more severe. The younger the child, the more likely that a given infection represents a first exposure. A first-exposure infection is more likely to cause fever and produce severe symptoms than a reexposure, in which the infection is modified by the antibodies produced from the first exposure. Young children are also less likely to have cross-reacting antibodies from a previous infection with an antigenically related organism.

Many common respiratory or viral infections produce more severe symptoms in children because of anatomic differences. The pediatric bronchioles, eustachian tubes, and larynx are narrower and therefore more easily obstructed by edema and mucus. This obstruction worsens the symptoms, prolongs clearance of infection, and increases the risk of secondary infection. Pertussis, or whooping cough, is a classic example of the differences in severity of infection between children and adults. Nearly 20% of infants with pertussis have severe complications, such as pneumonia, seizures, or encephalopathy; adult pertussis, although a common cause of chronic cough, is generally indistinguishable from a common cold.[48]

TABLE 74-3. Age-Specific Expectations for Wilderness Travel

AGE	EXPECTATION	SAFETY ISSUES
0-2 yr	Distance traveled depends on the adults; child carriers used	Provide "safe play area," e.g., tent floor, extra tarp laid out; bells on shoes; ipecac syrup
2-4 yr	Difficult age; stop every 10-15 minutes; hike ½-2 miles on own	Dress in bright colors; teach how to use whistle; ipecac syrup
5-7 yr	Hike 1-3 hr/day; cover 3-4 miles over easy terrain; rest every 30-45 minutes	Carry whistle: three blows = "I'm lost"; carry own pack with mini–first-aid kit and water
8-9 yr	Hike a full day with easy pace; cover 6-7 miles over variable terrain; if over 4 feet tall, can use framed pack	As for 5-7 years; teach map use and route finding; precondition by increasing maximum distances by 10%/wk or less; watch for overuse injuries; keep weight of pack 20% or less of body weight
10-12 yr	Hike a full day at moderate pace; cover 8-10 miles over variable terrain	As for 8-9 yr
Teens	Hike 8-12 miles at adult pace; may see a decrease in pace or distance with growth spurt	As for 8-9 yr

GENERAL CONSIDERATIONS AND EXPECTATIONS

Children of different ages have different needs and abilities. Expectations regarding distances of travel, pace, and safety issues vary depending on age (Table 74-3).

First 2 Years

Travel Expectations. Since they are typically carried, children in their first 2 years of life can travel long distances, depending on the adult's hiking abilities. However, they require attention and care almost all their waking hours. Most children are content in front carriers (infants less than 6 months) or back carriers (older infants and toddlers) and can easily travel for hours at a time. Because of their increased risk of illness and limited communication skills, however, infants must be watched closely for signs of infection, hypothermia, hyperthermia, and altitude illness. Parents must be prepared to give prompt treatment or evacuate to seek medical attention should signs of serious illness develop. Evacuation plans should be formulated before departure.

Entertainment in this age group is simple. A few small toys, which can be attached to the carrier on a short string, the natural surroundings, and a little parental attention provide ample amusement. A toddler can spend hours examining rocks, leaves, and sticks and rarely tires of a parent's undivided attention. If a child is comforted by a pacifier, it can be attached to the child's shirt or carrier, with extras packed for emergencies.

Safety. As babies become more active with rolling, crawling, and then walking, they require constant attention. Bells attached to their shoes may function as an alerting device, ringing when they are on the move.

These children are often considered "grazing creatures," putting everything they come across into their mouths. When they are not being carried, it is best to have a child-proofed area for them to play in, such as a tent floor or an extra tarp laid out. Toxic ingestions are common in this age group, and parents should be prepared. Syrup of ipecac should be included in the pediatric first-aid kit to induce emesis after certain toxic ingestions.

Food and Drink. Nourishment in the first 2 years is fairly simple. Infants in their first 4 to 6 months require only breast milk or formula. As long as the mother remains healthy, breast-feeding is the safest and most convenient way to feed an infant. If the mother is not nursing or not available, formula may be used. Formula is most conveniently carried in a powdered form and mixed as needed. The water for formula may be boiled once a day and stored in individual bottles with airtight lids. The powder for the formula is added just before feeding. Any unused, reconstituted formula should be discarded after 2 to 3 hours at room temperature.

Baby cereals can be carried conveniently in a dry form to be mixed with formula or breast milk. Dry cereals mixed with breast milk or formula have a higher nutritional value than ready-to-feed cereals in jars. Jars of commercial pureed foods may be carried, but the empty jars must be packed out. Once a jar of baby food has been opened, it should be used for only that meal. Without refrigeration, opened jars of baby food spoil quickly. Some families prefer to bring a hand grinder and make their own pureed foods (see Suggested Readings).

By 9 to 12 months, many babies are eating finger foods. Parents should be cautioned to avoid any hard round foods, such as peanuts or candies, which may cause choking. Up to 1 year of age, honey should be avoided because of an increased risk of botulism. Parents may also want to avoid citrus foods, which may cause rashes around the mouth and in the diaper area. Any new foods should be tested at home first to be certain the baby will accept it when away from home.

All water for drinking must be disinfected by boiling, iodination, or the use of small-pore filters, depending on the water source. Chronic iodide poisoning and neonatal goiter have been associated with prolonged ingestion of large amounts of iodine; small amounts ingested for water disinfection appear safe. Nonetheless, if both boiled water and iodinated water are available, it is prudent to use boiled water for infants and small children. In addition, infants and small children often reject the taste of iodinated water. Iodine must be kept out of reach of small children; severe acute toxicity can occur with an ingestion of only 2 to 4 g.

Diapers. Most children under age 2 years are in diapers, either disposable or cloth. Soiled diapers in a wilderness environment require special care. Thin paper diaper liners may be purchased to help collect the stool. The stool and liner should be buried in a trench at least 6 inches deep and 200 feet from any water source. If disposable diapers are used, they should be packed out after the stool has been removed and buried. The used disposable diaper should be wrapped and placed in a double bag for packing out. To reduce weight, urine-soaked diapers may be set out in the sun to dry before repacking. Superabsorbent diapers may be left on babies much longer and still keep them dry but cannot be dried out as easily.

On longer trips, some families prefer to use cloth diapers, which may be washed out and reused. Cloth diapers must be changed more frequently, since they are not as absorbent. Washing cloth diapers is labor intensive and requires an abundant supply of water. A washbasin is needed, and the diapers must be washed in hot soapy water. The diapers should be rinsed at least twice to remove irritating soap residue and the wastewater dumped at least 200 feet from a water source.

Equipment. Since infants and young children are not capable of extended hikes, they are typically transported in carriers. Excellent front and back carriers are available. Most front carriers work well from infancy until an age when babies can sit, typically 6 to 9 months (Figure 74-3). A front carrier must extend up high enough in the back to support the baby's head completely. Once a child is sitting well, back carriers are more ideal (Figure 74-4). Back carriers function on the same principle as framed backpacks, redistributing the weight off the shoulders and onto the hips. Many back carriers are able to stand alone and can double as a highchair. Children must be strapped into back carriers, since it is easy for a child to be catapulted out of a carrier if the adult bends over or falls.

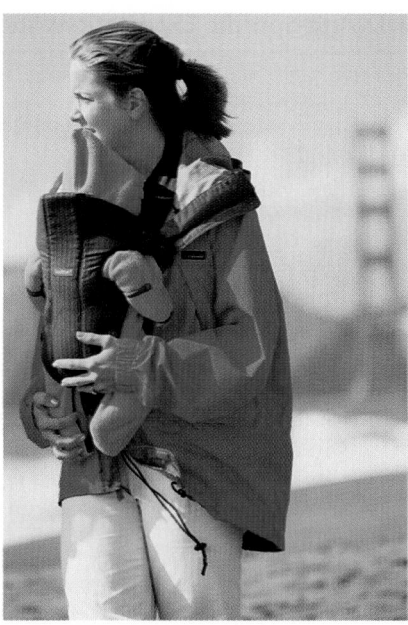

Figure 74-3 Young infant in front carrier.

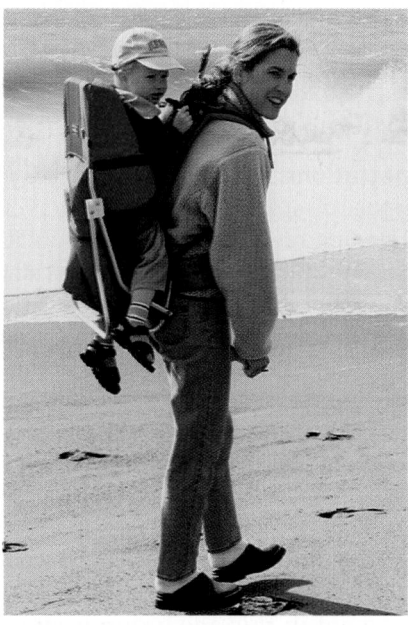

Figure 74-4 Toddler in back carrier.

Sleeping bags are available for infants and toddlers. In a warm climate a few blankets generally suffice, and in a colder climate an insulated snowsuit is often adequate. Children, including young infants, need their own sleeping pads. Such pads protect them from hard, rough ground under the tent and insulate them from the cold ground at night.

Shoes for young children should protect their feet and allow for full range of movement. The best shoes for toddlers are lightweight and flexible. They need shoes that stay on well, since children often flip their shoes off while in a carrier. Velcro-strapped shoes stay on well and are easy to put on and take off. Since children often lose shoes, an extra pair should be included.

Two to 4 Years

Travel Expectations. Children 2 to 4 years old are the most challenging to take into the wilderness. Two-year-olds become easily frustrated and throw temper tantrums. By 2 years of age, children are becoming too heavy to carry for prolonged periods, but they are still incapable of hiking long distances on their own. They are just gaining bladder and bowel control, and accidents are frequent. Despite these difficulties, wilderness trips with this age group can be successful with appropriate planning, preparation, and readjustment of expectations.

A key ingredient to successful wilderness trips with small children is to keep things slow, simple, and flexible. This is the age of independence and assertion. The children need to be given some control and allowed to set a pace. Adults should encourage young children to express their natural curiosity and enthusiasm for the outdoors by letting them stop to explore their surroundings. Parents should expect to stop at least every 15 minutes while hiking. If a diversion or a stimulus is needed to get the children hiking again, parents can begin a story or favorite song and continue it while hiking. With patience and plenty of time, parents can expect children in this age group to travel 1 to 2 miles over easy terrain.

Safety. Unfortunately, 2- to 4-year-olds are notorious for exploring their environment by wandering off or putting objects in their mouths. These young children must be watched closely and cautioned to keep wild mushrooms, plants, stones, and any nonedible item out of their mouths. Parents should continue to carry syrup of ipecac in the first-aid kit for potential toxic ingestions. Children should be kept within sight at all times, since their desire to explore often defies good judgment and exceeds their physical abilities. Although attacks are rare, mountain lions may view small children as easy prey and can strike quickly. Parents should discourage their children from wandering ahead unaccompanied.

When selecting campsites, dangerous features, such as steep drop-offs and fast or deep water, should be avoided. Children should be dressed in brightly colored clothing. Older children may carry a whistle to call for help when they are lost. The standard distress signal is three blows to indicate "I'm lost" or "I need help"; the response is two blows to indicate "help is coming." Parents should teach children to stay put when they discover they are lost and to wait for rescue. If children panic and start running, they increase the chance of being injured and separated farther from the family.

Food. The diet of 2- to 4-year-olds is usually simple but individualized. They tend to have strong prefer-

ences and dislikes. Unfortunately, most children at this age do not care for the convenient "all-in-one-pot" cooking common around campfires. Foods should be tested at home for acceptability. Nutritious snacks, such as raisins, granola bars, bagels, crackers, string cheese, and fruit bars, can be packed. These snacks sometimes become a child's meal. Small children should not be given items that may cause choking, such as peanuts, grapes, hard candies, or hot dogs. Adults should be trained in basic cardiopulmonary resuscitation (CPR) and know how to assist a choking child.

Toileting. Most children become toilet-trained by the end of their third year. Accidents are common, however, and parents need to be prepared with extra dry clothing. Children should be taught correct toileting procedures for the wilderness environment. Stools should be deposited at least 200 feet from a water source, buried in a hole approximately 6 inches deep, and completely covered. Many families carry a special trowel for this purpose. Some groups staying in one location for more than a day dig a specific toileting trench, 12 to 18 inches deep, to be used multiple times. They then add enough dirt after each use to cover all waste. Children need help learning to squat over the trench and to bury their stools.

It may be years before children gain reliable nighttime bladder control, so parents should be prepared for accidents. Cotton and down sleeping bags should be avoided, because they lose their insulating abilities and take a long time to dry when wet. Fortunately, many synthetic bags are available with fills such as Polarguard, Quallofil, and Hollofil, which maintain warmth and loft when wet.

School Age (5 Years and Older)

Travel Expectations. Once children enter the school years, their abilities and attention span increase dramatically. This enables them to participate more actively in many outdoor activities. Children are hungry for knowledge and readily absorb information about nature and outdoor activities. They enjoy being included in the initial planning, as well as in the field activities such as setting up camp, cooking, and cleaning up. School-age children can understand maps and often enjoy following their progress from one point to another. This is an ideal age to explain to them the rules of living in and traveling through wilderness areas. The examples and rules parents set for appropriate wilderness behavior at this age may become lifetime lessons.

When parents are planning for hiking trips, they must have appropriate expectations for children's differing abilities (see Table 74-3). Children enrolled in organized sports activities are likely to have greater endurance in the wilderness. An individual child's hiking ability can be estimated by hikes around the neighborhood or in a local park. If this becomes a routine, the children become preconditioned, increase their endurance, and learn to pace themselves. Parents can test methods for motivating their children. It is better to underestimate than overestimate a child's ability.

Safety. School-age children can learn to become more self-sufficient and in tune with their surroundings. They can be taught to recognize landmarks in their environment and thus are less likely to become lost. Children should be encouraged to view their surroundings from different angles. They should periodically turn around to see where they came from and where they are going. As children advance in the school years, they can learn survival skills, such as how to maintain warmth, build a shelter, secure food and water, and use a signal mirror, map, and compass. They should still carry a whistle and know how to use it appropriately.

Equipment. Children like to feel important, capable, and independent. These feelings are enhanced if they are allowed to carry some of their own gear. Even 5-year-olds like to carry their own soft backpacks. Items they can carry in the packs include snacks, a favorite small toy, tissues or a handkerchief, sunscreen, a small trash bag, and a whistle. As the children grow, the contents of their backpacks should reflect their increasing independence, with more self-care and survival items. In addition to the preceding items, they may carry their own water bottle, a mini–first-aid kit (adhesive bandages, wipes, personal medication), insect repellent, and other survival items as they learn to use them. The maximum weight of these packs should be 20% of the child's body weight until he or she has had significant backcountry experience and has proved that more can be carried comfortably. Once children reach 4 feet in height, they can be fitted for a framed backpack. Internal-framed backpacks tend to be more comfortable than external-framed packs. When a backpack is properly fitted, the waistband should rest at the hips and the shoulder strap adjusted so that the weight is carried on the hips, not the shoulders. With a framed pack, children can carry even more of their gear. The total weight should be gradually increased to allow the child to become comfortable with heavier loads.

ENVIRONMENTAL ILLNESSES

Dehydration

Children are at greater risk of dehydration than are adults. Since BSA/weight ratio of a child is greater than that of an adolescent or adult, insensible fluid losses through the skin account for a larger percentage of total fluid losses as the size of the child decreases. In addition, the sodium concentration of children's sweat is generally less than that of an adult, leading to greater relative free water loss. Infants are unable to report

thirst, an important marker of fluid deficit, increasing their risk of dehydration. Children are often preoccupied and fail to report or meet their need for fluids.

Symptoms. A 2% decrease in body weight through fluid loss results in mildly increased heart rate, elevated body temperature, and decreased plasma volume. Water losses of 4% to 5% of body weight reduce muscular work capacity by 20% to 30%.[66] Symptoms of dehydration include weakness, fatigue, nausea, vomiting, and ultimately lethargy. Dehydration also predisposes a child to other environmental hazards, such as hypothermia, hyperthermia, and acute mountain sickness.

Treatment. Caregivers must provide fluids and coax children to hydrate themselves frequently. For short (less than 2 hours) periods of activity, water is as efficacious a rehydration solution as carbohydrate-electrolyte drinks.[44] A child eating a normal diet does not require electrolyte replacement unless sweating is prolonged or excessive. By closely monitoring a child's urine output, fluid deficits can be recognized and promptly managed. A child with decreased urine output or dark concentrated urine needs extra fluids.

Hypothermia

Children cool more rapidly than adults because of their proportionally large BSA and often lack the knowledge and judgment to initiate responses that will maintain warmth in a cold environment (see Chapter 6). It is also more physiologically difficult for them to maintain their body temperature in cold climates. As a result, parents participating in cold weather recreation with children should be able to recognize, treat, and, preferably, prevent hypothermia and frostbite.

Hypothermia is defined as a core body temperature below 35° C (95° F). At this temperature the body no longer generates enough heat to maintain body functions. The condition is considered mild when the core temperature is 33° C (91.4° F) or above, moderate at temperatures between 28° C (82.4° F) and 32° C (89.6° F), and severe when it is less than 28° C. The signs and symptoms of hypothermia are variable (Table 74-4). The most important clue to significant hypothermia is altered mental status. The child who begins to undress, stumble, or make inappropriate remarks should be evaluated promptly for hypothermia. Shivering is not a reliable marker of the severity of hypothermia. Physicians should caution parents that hypothermia can develop at moderate temperatures if adverse climatic conditions are compounded by illness, fatigue, dehydration, inadequate nutrition, or wet clothing.

Prevention. When preparing for cold weather activities, children should dress in layers to allow clothing to be added or subtracted as necessary (Figure 74-5). This

TABLE 74-4. Signs and Symptoms of Hypothermia*

TEMPERATURE	SIGNS/SYMPTOMS
Mild: 33°-35° C (about 91°-95° F)	Sensation of cold, shivering, increased heart rate, progressive incoordination in hand movements, poor judgment, mild ataxia, slurred speech, confusion
Moderate: 28°-32° C (about 82°-90° F)	Loss of shivering, inability to walk or follow commands, paradoxical undressing, increasing confusion, decreased arrhythmia threshold
Severe: <28° C (<82° F)	Rigid muscles, progressive loss of reflexes and voluntary motion, hypotension, bradycardia, hypoventilation, dilated pupils, increasing risk of fatal arrhythmias, appearance of death

*Data from adult subjects.

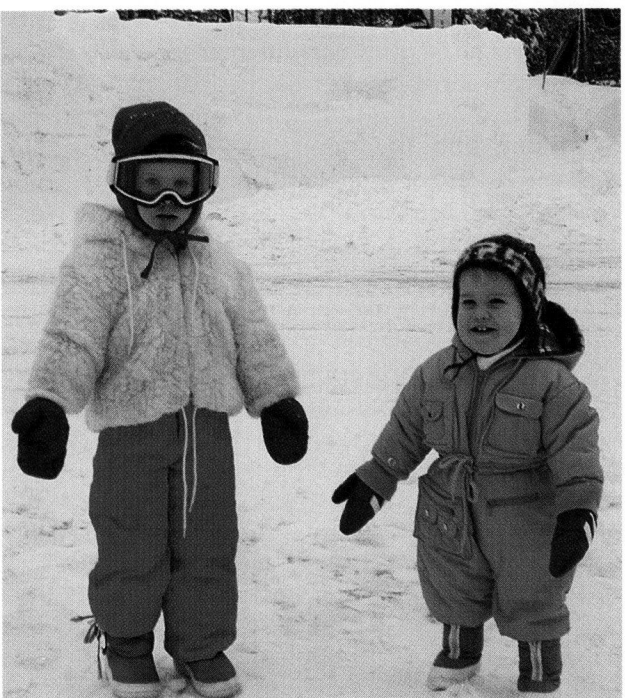

Figure 74-5 Layering of clothing for cold environments.

avoids excessive perspiration while maintaining warmth. An inner, wicking layer should be followed by a middle, insulating layer, and then by an outer, protective layer.

Clothing that maintains low thermal conductance when moist is particularly important. Conductive heat loss may increase fivefold in wet clothing and up to 25-fold if the child is completely immersed in water. Wool retains warmth when wet because of its unique ability to suspend water vapor within the fibers; however, it is heavier than synthetics and takes much longer to dry. Cotton has a high thermal conductance that increases greatly when wet and is therefore a poor choice for wilderness activities in cold weather. Newer synthetic materials (polypropylene, Capilene, Thermax, Coolmax) wick moisture away from the skin and dry quickly, making them ideal for an inner layer. The middle, insulating layer may incorporate wool, polyester pile, Thinsulate, or similar materials. Windproof and water-resistant outer garments (Gore-Tex) decrease heat loss from convection and keep children dry. Hats and mittens are essential; the uncovered head of a child dissipates up to 70% of total body heat production at ambient temperatures of 5° C (41° F).

Treatment. For the hypothermic child, field rewarming begins with limiting further exposure to the cold environment. Wet clothing should be removed, and the child's head and neck should be protected from further heat loss. Placing the child with a normothermic person in a sleeping bag insulated from the ground provides external warming. Hot water bottles, insulated to prevent burns, may also be placed at the axillae, neck, and groin. If the child is alert, oral hydration with warm fluids containing glucose repletes glycogen and corrects dehydration, which frequently accompanies hypothermia. Signs of severe hypothermia dictate immediate evacuation as conditions permit; rescuers should handle the victim gently to prevent arrhythmias.

Frostbite

Localized cold injury results in frostbite (see Chapter 7). Predisposing factors include wet skin, constricting garments that hinder blood circulation, fatigue, contact with cold metal, and windchill. If skin temperature drops below 10° C (50° F), cutaneous sensation is generally abolished, and injury may go unnoticed. Skin cooled to −4° C (24.8° F) freezes.

Frostbite has traditionally been divided into degrees of injury similar to burns. First-degree injury manifests with numbness, erythema, and edema without tissue loss. Second-degree frostbite results in superficial blistering, whereas third-degree injury produces deeper blisters containing bloody fluid. Fourth-degree injury extends through the dermis to subcuticular tissues. In children, frostbite that extends into bone may affect the growth plate and result in skeletal deformities.[34]

Treatment. All wet and constricting clothing should be removed and hypothermia treated aggressively. Rapid rewarming, the primary treatment for frostbite, should be initiated as soon as possible. This is best accomplished by immersion of the frostbitten area in water warmed to 40° to 42° C (104° to 107.6° F). This narrow temperature range maximizes rewarming speed while preventing further injury from a burn wound. Thawing usually takes 30 to 45 minutes and is complete when the skin is soft and pliable. Although field rewarming is indicated unless evacuation occurs quickly, great care should be taken to avoid refreezing. Refreezing causes much more damage than delayed thawing. Vigorous rubbing should also be avoided because it is ineffective and potentially harmful. After thawing, blister fluid should be aspirated to prevent further contact with tissue-damaging prostaglandins and thromboxanes, and a sterile dressing should be applied.

Hyperthermia

Families participating in wilderness activities in hot climates must take special precautions to avoid heat illnesses (see Chapter 10). Children do not tolerate the demands of exercise in the heat as well as adults. They generate more heat per kilogram and are less able to disperse heat from the core to the periphery. Parents planning wilderness ventures with children in hot climates can follow some simple guidelines for avoiding heat illness. The most obvious entails reducing the duration and intensity of activities under conditions of high climatic heat stress, keeping in mind that the risk of heat illness depends on relative humidity, wind velocity, and radiant heat, as well as standard dry bulb thermometer temperature (Figure 74-6).

Prevention. Children should be fully hydrated before prolonged exercise and actively encouraged to drink fluids at regular intervals. Infants and neonates are most vulnerable to heat illness. Under high climatic heat stress, infants fed undiluted cow's milk or formula

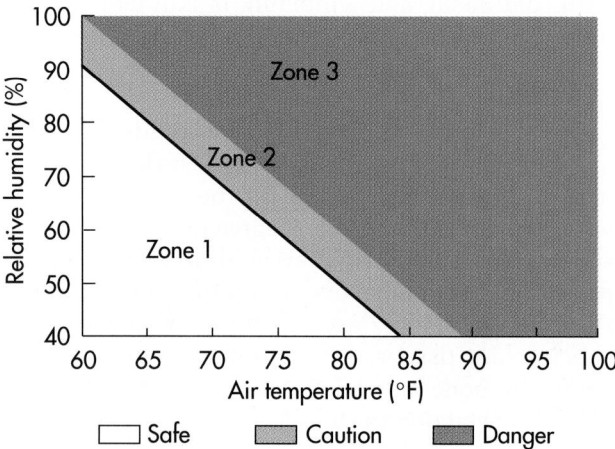

Figure 74-6 Activity levels based on temperature and relative humidity.

may develop marked salt retention and dehydration. They should be given extra water or dilute feedings. The lower osmolar load of breast milk appears to protect against heat illness and hypernatremia.

Since their mechanisms of evaporative heat loss (sweating) are immature relative to those of an adult, children should be encouraged to engage in activities in the shade to maximize other means of dissipating heat, such as radiation (skin-to-air gradient). Also, since sweat evaporated from clothing contributes less to cooling than sweat evaporated from skin, children should remove sweat-soaked clothing and wear dry, lightweight, loose-fitting clothing. Finally, children acclimatize to the heat slower than adults, often taking 10 to 14 days to acclimate fully. The intensity and duration of exercise should be gradually increased over this period.

Symptoms and Treatment. Early signs and symptoms of heat illness include flushing, tachycardia, weakness, mild confusion, headache, and nausea. Vomiting often occurs in children. Sweating may be present or absent and should not be relied on as a clinical indicator of the severity of hyperthermia. If heat illness develops, children should be removed from obvious sources of heat, including direct sunlight, and have their clothing removed. Convective cooling can be increased in the field by vigorous fanning after spraying or sprinkling the victim with water. If available, ice packs or cold compresses placed at the groin, axilla, and scalp will aid cooling. If the child is alert, dehydration may be corrected with oral fluids. Progression of symptoms or failure to respond to treatment mandates immediate evacuation (see Chapter 11).

Sun Damage

The hazards of overexposure to sunlight include sunburn, photoaging, skin cancer, and phototoxic and photoallergic reactions (see Chapter 14). Preventing ultraviolet (UV) damage to the skin should begin in childhood, since 80% of a person's lifetime sun exposure occurs before 21 years of age.[3] Recent evidence suggests that the risk of developing malignant melanoma is at least double if a person has had one or more severe sunburns in childhood. This risk is even higher if a child is light skinned with a propensity to burn rather than tan.[22,51,76] Tolerance to sun exposure is determined by the amount of melanin in the skin and the ability of the skin to produce melanin in response to sunlight. In general, children have lower melanin levels and thinner skin than adults and are at greater risk of sun damage.[35]

The ultraviolet wavelengths UVA and UVB are principally responsible for the harmful effects of solar radiation. UVB is primarily responsible for suntan and sunburn and also promotes the development of skin cancer and aging of the skin. UVB increases 4% for every 305-m (1000-foot) gain in elevation over sea level. Therefore a backpacker at 3050 m (10,000 feet) will have a 40% increase in UVB exposure. UVA, which is 10 to 100 times more abundant than UVB, is only 0.001 as potent at inducing sunburn. It is also less affected than UVB by changes in season or solar zenith angle. UVA is primarily responsible for photosensitivity reactions and solar urticaria. It also contributes to skin cancer and skin aging. A number of drugs often used in adolescence, such as tetracycline, vitamin A derivatives (Retin-A, Accutane), and nonsteroidal antiinflammatory drugs (NSAIDs), increase the risk of photosensitivity reactions and the need for UVA protection. Sunscreens should protect against both UVA and UVB.

The harmful effects of UV radiation from the sun can be reduced if parents are educated regarding the dangers of sun exposure and encouraged to use sun-protective clothing and sunscreens early in their children's lives.[3,77] Studies indicate that regular use of a sunscreen with a sun protection factor (SPF) of at least 15 for the first 18 years of life reduces a person's lifetime risk of developing nonmelanoma skin cancer by 78%.[22]

Prevention. The most effective means of preventing sun damage is avoidance of excessive sun exposure and the use of protective clothing. Midday hours, particularly around bodies of water, at high altitude, and at the equator, are the most dangerous in terms of quantity of UV exposure. Shady areas should be used for activities during these times. Hats with wide brims and neck drapes help to protect the face and neck from sun exposure. Clothing made from tightly woven fabrics is more protective; loosely woven fabrics, such as that in most T-shirts, have an SPF of only 5. Most clothing loses even more of its protective effect when wet. High-SPF (25 to 30) clothing is cool and lightweight, dries quickly, and can maintain its full SPF capabilities even when wet.

Proper eye protection is often overlooked in infants and young children. Excessive UV light, particularly during snow and water activities, can result in UV keratitis and corneal burns with even brief exposures. Properly fitting sunglasses that transmit fewer than 10% of UV rays should be part of a child's outdoor activity armamentarium. Side shields and polarizing lenses are particularly important on the snow.

Sunscreens. Most sunscreens have ingredients such as paraaminobenzoic acid (PABA), PABA esters, cinnamates, salicylates, and anthranilates that protect the skin from sun damage by absorbing primarily UVB. Dibenzoylmethane absorbs only UVA. Benzophenones block UVB and to a lesser degree UVA.[32] Sunscreens that combine ingredients that protect the skin from both UVB and UVA are the most effective. Micronized titanium dioxide, which reflects UV light similar to the sun block zinc oxide, is almost colorless but retains the ability to scatter sunlight.

The SPF is a measure of a sunscreen's effectiveness. It is measured in terms of the minimal dose (in length of time) of UV radiation required to cause skin erythema. Sunscreens with SPF of 30 or higher provide a superior degree of photoprotection and almost completely prevent the cellular changes seen with sunburn.[31]

Water-resistant sunscreens maintain their effectiveness for up to 40 minutes of water immersion, whereas waterproof sunscreens maintain their effectiveness for up to 80 minutes of water immersion.[32] Either should be reapplied if longer times are spent in the water or if the water is turbulent. Excessive sweating and rubbing of the skin are also indications for reapplication.

Treatment. When sunburn occurs, the mainstays of treatment are cool compresses, topical antipruritics, and NSAIDs.[32] A high-potency topical steroid, betamethasone dipropionate, may work synergistically with NSAIDs to reduce the UVB-induced erythema by as much as 42% to 58% if used early in the burning process.[30] Strong topical steroids should be used judiciously, since just a 7-day course may suppress the hypothalamic-pituitary-adrenal axis. As always, the best cure is prevention.

High-Altitude Illness

High-altitude illness comprises a continuum from acute mountain sickness (AMS) to life-threatening conditions such as high-altitude pulmonary edema (HAPE) and high-altitude cerebral edema (HACE). AMS usually develops within 24 hours of ascent. The incidence and severity depend on individual susceptibility, as well as the rate of ascent and the altitude attained. The sleeping altitude is particularly important to the development of symptoms. The true incidence of high-altitude illness is unknown but is probably 10% to 20% at 2500 m (8202 feet) in adults and children (see Chapter 1).

Symptoms. The cardinal symptoms of AMS are a bitemporal, throbbing headache, anorexia, and malaise. Children appear particularly prone to nausea and vomiting. Other symptoms include dizziness, dyspnea on exertion, and fragmented sleep. Infants may display nonspecific findings such as irritability, poor feeding, and sleep disturbance. Manifestations of severe AMS include dyspnea at rest and ataxia, which presage HAPE and HACE, respectively.

Prevention. The best method of preventing high-altitude illness is to allow for acclimatization through a graded ascent (Box 74-1). After day trips to higher altitude, children should return to lower altitude to sleep to aid acclimatization. A high-carbohydrate diet may also help reduce the risk of high-altitude illness.

Acetazolamide reduces the incidence of AMS in adults.[36] Pretreatment mimics the acclimatized state by inducing a hyperchloremic metabolic acidosis, allow-

---

Box 74-1 RECOMMENDATIONS FOR PREVENTING HIGH-ALTITUDE ILLNESS

1. Avoid abrupt ascent to a sleeping altitude higher than 3000 m (9843 feet).
2. Spend 2 or 3 nights at 2500 to 3000 m before going higher.
3. Avoid abrupt increases of greater than 500 m (1640 feet) in sleeping altitude per night.

Modified from Klocke DL, Decker WW, Stepanek J: *Mayo Clin Proc* 73:988, 1998.

---

ing for a compensatory increase in respiration. Clinical experience suggests that it is also beneficial in children. The primary indication for acetazolamide prophylaxis in children is a history of recurrent AMS despite graded ascent.[70] Acetazolamide is given at 5 mg/kg/day, in two divided doses, up to a maximum daily dose of 250 mg. It should be started 24 hours before ascent and continued while at altitude. Side effects include dehydration, nausea, and somnolence; paresthesias may be particularly bothersome in children.

Dexamethasone also prevents or reduces symptoms of AMS in adults, but experience with its use in children is limited.

Treatment. Treatment of mild AMS requires prompt recognition of symptoms, cessation of ascent, and time for acclimatization to occur. *Proceeding to higher altitude in the presence of symptoms is strongly contraindicated and may lead to the life-threatening conditions HAPE and HACE.* Symptomatic therapy includes rest, acetaminophen for headache, and descent. Promethazine (Phenergan) may be used to relieve nausea and vomiting. The dose is 0.2 to 0.5 mg/kg every 6 hours, preferably per rectum. Descent is unequivocally the most successful treatment for AMS and is mandatory if symptoms progress or fail to improve. Although descent should proceed as far as necessary for improvement, 500 to 1000 m (1640 to 3281 feet) is often sufficient. If immediate descent is not possible, oxygen should be administered if available. Limited studies examining dexamethasone and acetazolamide for the treatment of AMS suggest that both are effective.[26] Dexamethasone should probably be reserved for patients with deterioration of consciousness, truncal ataxia, or severe vomiting, the hallmarks of HACE. These symptoms of HACE or any symptoms of HAPE demand immediate descent and possible evacuation.

Bites and Stings

Bites and stings often occur in the pediatric age group. In 1995 the American Association of Poison Control Centers recorded 77,368 calls regarding bites and envenomations; 44% involved patients 17 years of age or

younger.[38] Remarkably, major morbidity occurred in less than 0.1% of cases, with no deaths in patients less than 17 years of age. This emphasizes the need for appropriate triage to determine which children require aggressive therapy. Harmful interactions between children and surrounding fauna can be limited by education and judicious use of protective clothing, sturdy footwear, and appropriate chemical barriers.

Snakes. Most snakebites can be prevented. Children up to 10 years of age are particularly likely to handle snakes and have a higher rate of bites than any other age group.[14] They also have more severe envenomation syndromes than do adults.[74] Children should be instructed not to handle snakes, reach blindly into crevices, or turn over rocks and fallen limbs. A useful adage is that hands and feet should never go where the eyes cannot see. When walking through endemic areas, hikers should stay on trails and wear long, loose pants and boots that extend above the ankle. Campsites should be on open ground, away from woodpiles or rockpiles.

If a bite occurs, the child should back away from the snake and be calmed. Agitation and movement of the bitten extremity will encourage venom circulation. The wound should be cleansed rapidly and any constricting items of clothing or jewelry removed from the extremity. The bitten extremity should be immobilized promptly and positioned below the level of the heart. No incision over the bite should be made. The use of mechanical suction (e.g., Extractor, Sawyer Products, Safety Harbor, Fla.) has been shown in animal studies to safely remove up to 30% of injected venom if applied within 3 minutes for 30 to 60 minutes.[7] However, there is a possibility that its use may worsen local venom effects. Parents traveling to snake-infested areas should consider adding such a product to their medical kit (see Chapters 38 to 40). All pediatric victims of potentially poisonous snakebites should be transported to a medical facility for prompt evaluation.

Hymenoptera. Hymenoptera stings (bees, wasps, hornets, and ants) are the most common cause of envenomation in children. Although Hymenoptera venom possesses intrinsic toxicity, the amount delivered is small, and multiple stings are necessary for significant human morbidity. However, the venom components are potent antigens capable of producing IgE-mediated anaphylaxis in sensitized individuals. Although children appear less susceptible to systemic reactions than adults, physicians should educate parents in the management of Hymenoptera stings, particularly if a child has had a previous severe reaction.

Hymenoptera stings usually produce local pain, swelling, and erythema. A stinger should be removed as quickly as possible by whatever means available, since rapid removal of the stinger is much more important than the method of extraction.[73] Within 20 seconds, 90% of venom sac contents are discharged into

Box 74-2   RECOMMENDATIONS FOR AVOIDING MOSQUITOES AND USING REPELLENTS

1. Wear long-sleeved shirt and pants.
2. Minimize outdoor activities at dusk.
3. Use mosquito netting to cover the heads of infants and children, and in sleeping area.
4. Spray clothing, netting, and screens with permethrin preparations (Permanone, Duranon).
5. Use insect repellents with no more than 35% diethyltoluamide (DEET) on exposed skin only, avoiding children's hands.
6. Apply DEET products over any other creams such as sunscreen to minimize absorption and maximize repellent effect.
7. Keep DEET out of reach of small children.

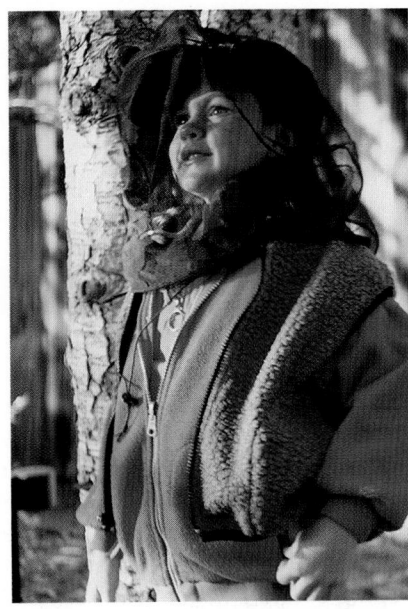

Figure 74-7   Mosquito netting draped over child's hat.

the victim, and within 1 minute, 100%.[62] Applying ice or cool compresses reduces pain and swelling. Elevation and immobilization are indicated for large local reactions on extremities. In older children, oral antihistamines may provide additional symptomatic relief.

Early signs of a systemic reaction include generalized pruritus, urticaria, angioedema, bronchospasm, and laryngeal edema. Their presence mandates medical evaluation. Epinephrine is the drug of choice for systemic sting reactions and should be administered in the field if available (0.01 mg/kg subcutaneously of 1:1000 aqueous concentration). Parents may prefer a spring-loaded automatic injector that delivers 0.3 mg (EpiPen) or 0.15 mg (EpiPen Jr.) of epinephrine subcutaneously when triggered by pressing the device against the thigh. EpiPen Jr. is used for children up to 15 kg and EpiPen for larger children and adults. Since up to half of all patients with anaphylactic reactions have no forewarning, epinephrine belongs in all wilderness medical kits (see Chapters 36 and 37).

Mosquitoes. Mosquitoes are not only a nuisance but also a vector for disease (see Chapter 32). Steps can be taken to avoid mosquitoes (Box 74-2). A proper wardrobe provides an excellent physical barrier to mosquitoes. This should include ankle-high footwear, pants cinched at the ankles or tucked into socks, a long-sleeved shirt, and a full-brimmed hat. Mosquito netting draped over a child's hat will protect the face and neck without the toxic side effects occasionally seen with repellents (Figure 74-7). Mosquito netting, especially in the sleeping area, has been found to reduce the mosquito attack rate by 97%.[75]

Repellents containing diethyltoluamide (DEET) are effective against mosquitoes, ticks, blackflies, and many other arthropods. Although generally of low toxicity, DEET is absorbed cutaneously, and toxic encephalopathy attributed to its use has been reported. Children may be at particular risk because of their greater BSA/mass ratio (see Chapter 65). However, with proper application, it is an excellent repellent. High concentrations of DEET may cause dermatitis with erythema, bullae, skin necrosis, and residual scarring. Although products containing 100% DEET are commercially available, long-acting formulations of 35% DEET appear equally effective in protecting against mosquitoes, with less potential for toxicity. It is prudent to avoid using products containing higher than 35% DEET in children. DEET products can be applied over other creams, such as sunscreen, to minimize absorption and maximize repellent effect. Parents should also be cautioned to keep DEET out of the reach of small children, since ingestions may be fatal.[75]

The pesticide permethrin, available as a 0.5% spray (Permanone, Duranon Tick Repellent), is safe and effective against arthropods, especially ticks. Unlike DEET repellents, these permethrin products are applied to fabric or netting, not to skin. Permethrins as a class have low toxicity in mammals. The combination of DEET applied to exposed skin and permethrin treatment of clothing is particularly effective in protecting against mosquito bites and ticks. The protective effect of mosquito netting is greatly enhanced when the netting is impregnated with permethrin.[75] These effects are longer lasting with permethrin soaks (up to 20 washings) than with permethrin spraying of clothing or netting.

Ticks. As with mosquitoes, ticks serve as vectors for disease, most notably Lyme disease (see Chapter 33). Transmission of the Lyme spirochete, *Borrelia burgdorferi*, typically requires 48 to 72 hours or more of tick contact.[64] Tick checks should be conducted regularly while traveling through wilderness areas. A tick embedded in skin should be grasped with forceps close to the skin surface and gentle traction applied. Use of alcohol or open flames for tick removal is strongly discouraged, because these techniques are unreliable and may induce tick salivation or regurgitation into the wound. A vaccine against Lyme disease is now available for children over age 15 years who have frequent or prolonged exposure to ticks in Lyme-endemic areas.

FOREIGN TRAVEL WITH CHILDREN

Visits to foreign countries provide superb educational, social, and cultural experiences for children. Unfortunately, traveling with children to wilderness or rural areas within developing nations entails the risks of not only wilderness travel but also poor sanitation conditions, with exposure to bacteria, viruses, protozoa, and helminths not usually seen in the developed world. Parents should be aware of the greater risk of traveling to a developing country with a child under 2 years or less than 15 kg.

The physician provides guidance and information to parents planning foreign travel. The Internet provides both physician and traveler with up-to-the-minute information (Table 74-5). Preparation for foreign travel with children includes identification and avoidance of risky endeavors, administration of appropriate immunizations and prophylactic medications, knowledge of common childhood diseases and their treatment, and posttravel follow-up by an informed physician.

General Recommendations

Physicians should emphasize to families that risk avoidance is the most important aspect of safe travel (Box 74-3).[20] Parents should select transport, activity, and overnight settings carefully to avoid unnecessary hazards. Freshwater swimming should be avoided in developing countries to prevent parasitic infections such as schistosomiasis. Where swimming is appropriate, parents should provide close supervision. In one study in Washington state, drowning was the leading cause of pediatric mortality in the wilderness, followed by closed head injury and exposure.[47] Since traumatic injury is the leading cause of morbidity and mortality among children, great effort should be made to prevent it.[56] Protective devices, such as car seats, helmets, personal flotation devices, and protective clothing and pads, should be used as often as possible (Figure 74-8).

Skin protection is vital in the outdoors, particularly in tropical environments. The use of closed shoes can prevent infection with hookworm, *Strongyloides*, the agents of cutaneous larva migrans, and other parasites that enter the skin. Clothing should be selected based on ambient temperature and expected conditions; even in hot, sunny climates, light clothing should cover as much BSA as possible to provide protection from parasites, insects, and UV light. Sunscreen should be used liberally and reapplied every few hours, particularly after swimming.

Parents should take great care in selecting foods and safe drinking water for themselves and their children,

---

Box 74-3 RECOMMENDATIONS FOR AVOIDING RISKS DURING TRAVEL

1. Select appropriate settings: supervised swimming, safe campsites, protective devices.
2. Protect skin: sunscreen, repellents, protective clothing, closed shoes.
3. Eat and drink cleanly: water disinfection, careful food selection.
4. Avoid bugs and wild animals: clothing, netting, repellents, vigilance.

Modified from Fischer PR: *Infect Dis Clin North Am* 12:355, 1998.

TABLE 74-5. Resources for Current Travel Immunizations and Malaria Prophylaxis Recommendations

RESOURCE	COMMENTS
Centers for Disease Control and Prevention (CDC)	General web site: www.cdc.gov cdc.gov/travel/index.htm: index of travel information, vaccines, disease outbreaks; access to "Bluesheet" summary of indicated vaccines and "Yellow Book" online text of health information by destination country cdc.gov/mmwr/international/world.html: *Morbidity and Mortality Weekly Report* online; international bulletin on disease outbreaks cdc.gov/ncidod/ncid/htm: National Center for Infectious Diseases Phone: 404-332-4555
Medical College of Wisconsin International Traveler's Clinic	www.intmed.mcw.edu/travel.html Phone: 414-259-4949
World Health Organization (WHO)	General web site: www.who.int/ith/index.html Phone (in Geneva): (00 41 22) 791 21 11
Malaria Network	www.malarianetwork.org/: information on malaria control for health care workers; organization sponsored by WHO

who are particularly vulnerable to disease and diarrhea (Box 74-4). All foods should be well cooked, canned, or peelable. All milk products should be pasteurized or boiled. Water should never be consumed from the tap; only bottled, 1-minute-boiled, or chemically treated (iodine) *and* microfiltered (0.2 μm pore size) water should be ingested (see Chapter 51). In certain areas, even bottled water is suspect. Breast-feeding is safest for young infants. If formula is used, only properly disinfected water should be used for its preparation. Frequent handwashing, particularly with infants and toddlers and especially around mealtimes, will successfully interrupt the fecal-oral passage of disease.

Parents should also focus their efforts on avoiding contact between children and insects or wild animals. Mosquitoes and ticks can be avoided by avoiding outdoor activities between dusk and dawn and by wearing protective clothing and repellent (see Box 74-2). As mentioned, DEET is an effective repellent but should not be used at concentrations greater than 35% in children because of the probable risk of toxicity.[20] Children's hands should be free of DEET to prevent accidental eye and mouth contact. Outer clothing and bed netting should be treated with permethrin. Parents should check for ticks daily when in tick-infested areas. Children should be warned to watch where they place their hands and feet (in crevices, unattended shoes, sleeping bags) to avoid the unexpected arthropod or snake.

Immunizations

Foreign travel with children requires advance planning because vaccines recommended for travel to certain countries may take up to 6 weeks to complete. The Centers for Disease Control and Prevention (CDC) Internet site (see Table 74-5) provides current information on immunizations and prophylaxis based on the following:

1. Countries of travel
2. Length of time in each country
3. Location of destinations (rural vs. urban)
4. Time of year
5. Type of lodging and eating facilities
6. Previous immunizations
7. Age and weight of the child

Vaccines may be categorized as routine (polio, diphtheria-tetanus-pertussis, *Haemophilus* influenza B, hepatitis B, measles-mumps-rubella, varicella), routine for travel (hepatitis A, immunoglobulin), geographically indicated or required (yellow fever, typhoid, meningococcus, Japanese encephalitis, cholera, Lyme disease), and indicated for extended stay (rabies)[69] (Tables 74-6 and 74-7).

Box 74-4 RECOMMENDATIONS FOR PREVENTING TRAVELER'S DIARRHEA

1. Eat only well-cooked vegetables, meat, and seafood.
2. Eat only fruit that can be peeled.
3. Drink only disinfected or boiled water, carbonated drinks, hot tea, or coffee.
4. Drink or eat only pasteurized dairy products.
5. Avoid ice cubes, or use only those made from disinfected water.
6. Breast-feed infants.
7. Prepare formula with disinfected or boiled water only.
8. Wash hands thoroughly before eating or preparing food.
9. Brush teeth with disinfected water.
10. Beware of food from street vendors.

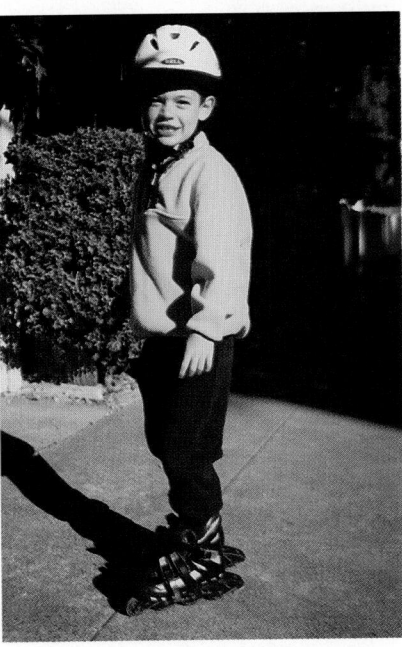

Figure 74-8 Appropriate helmet use.

TABLE 74-6. Categories of Vaccines for Children

TYPE OF VACCINE	EXAMPLES
Routine	Polio, diphtheria-tetanus-pertussis (DTaP), *Haemophilus influenzae* (Hib), measles-mumps-rubella (MMR), varicella-zoster virus (VZV), hepatitis B
Routine for travel (developing countries)	Hepatitis A or immune globulin (IgG)
Required or geographically indicated	Yellow fever, typhoid, meningococcal, Japanese encephalitis, cholera, Lyme disease
Extended stay	Rabies

Modified from Thanassi WT, Weiss EL: *Emerg Med Clin North Am* 15:43, 1997.

TABLE 74-7. Vaccines for Children Who Travel

VACCINE	DESCRIPTION	DOSING	COMMENTS/ CONTRAINDICATIONS	LENGTH OF TRAVEL		
				BRIEF (<2 WK)	INTERMEDIATE (2 WK TO 3 MO)	LONG TERM RESIDENTIAL (>3 MO)
ROUTINE						
Polio*	OPV: live attenuated, oral IPV: inactivated, injection	IPV at 2, 4 mo; OPV at 12-18 mo, 4-6 yr; may accelerate to q 4-8 wk × 3 doses	IPV at 2 and 4 mo decreases risk of polio in undiagnosed immuno-compromised infants; AAP recommendation may change to IPV only	+	+	+
Diphtheria-tetanus-pertussis*	DTP: D, T toxoid + whole cell P DTaP: DT toxoid + acellular P Td: booster	DTaP recommended at 2, 4, 6, 15-18 mo and 4-6 yr; Td booster at age 12, then q 10 yr	May accelerate to dose every 4 wk × 3 doses if necessary; decreased incidence of vaccine-related reactions with DTaP	+	+	+
Haemophilus B*	Hib polysaccharide: protein conjugate	0.5 ml IM at 2, 4, 6, 12-15 mo	Typically given as combination with DTaP	+	+	+
Hepatitis B	Recombivax HB: inactivated viral antigen Engerix-B: same	3 doses: 0, 1, 6 mo <11 yr: 0.25 ml IM >11 yr: 0.5 ml IM 3 doses 0, 1, 6 mo <11 yr: 0.5 ml IM >11 yr: 1.0 ml IM	Some protection after just 1 or 2 doses; may accelerate Engerix-B to 0, 1, 2, 12 mo	+	+	+
Measles-mumps-rubella†	Live attenuated viruses	0.25 ml IM at 12-15 mo, then booster at 4-6 or 11-12 yr	May accelerate to 6-12 mo, repeat 1 mo later, then per usual schedule; give at least 2-3 wk before IgG	+	+	+
Varicella	Live attenuated virus	12 mo-12 yr: 0.5 ml SC as single dose >12 yr: 2 doses 4-8 wk apart	Give at least 2-3 wk before IgG; may be given with MMR using different sites; avoid if immunocompromised	+	+	+
ROUTINE FOR TRAVEL						
Hepatitis A	Havrix: inactive virus (720ELU) Vaqta (24U)	>2 yr: 2 × 0.5 ml doses 6-12 mo apart	Preferred for hepatitis A protection if over age 2 yr Protects in 4 wk after dose 1	+	+	+
Immune globulin (IgG)	Antibodies	<2 yr: 0.02 ml/kg for <3 mo of travel; 0.06 ml/kg q 5 mo and 3 days before travel	Hepatitis A protection for those under age 2 yr; beware of timing with live virus vaccines			+

REQUIRED OR GEOGRAPHICALLY INDICATED

Vaccine	Type	Dose	Comments				
Yellow fever	Live virus	>9 mo: 0.5 ml SC at least 10 days before departure; booster q 10 yr	Required for parts of sub-Saharan Africa, of tropical South America; may give at 4-9 mo if traveling to epidemic area; under 9 mo: risk of vaccine-related encephalitis	+	+	+	+
Typhoid	Heat inactivated	6 mo-2 yr: 2 × 0.25 ml SC 4 wk apart, booster q 3 yr	Fever, pain with heat killed; significantly fewer side effects with ViCPS and Ty21a; important for Latin America, Asia, Africa; vaccine not a substitute for eating and drinking cleanly	±	+	+	+
	ViCPS: polysaccharide Ty21a: oral live attenuated	2-6 yr: 0.5 ml IM × 1 booster q 2 yr >6 yr: 1 capsule q 2 days × 4; booster q 5 yr					
Meningococcal	Serogroups A, C, Y, W-135: polysaccharide	>2 years: 0.5 ml SC; booster in 1 yr if 1st dose after age 4 yr, otherwise in 5 yr	Use for central Africa, Saudi Arabia for the Hajj, Nepal, and epidemic areas; minimal efficacy under age 2 yr	±	±	±	±
Japanese encephalitis	Inactivated virus	1-3 yr: 0.5 ml SC at 0, 7, 14-30 days >3 years: 1.0 ml SC at 0, 7, 14-30 days Last dose > 10 days before travel	Indicated for parts of India and rural Asia if stay > 1 mo; no safety data for under age 1 yr; high rate of hypersensitivity	+	±	±	±
Cholera	Inactivated bacteria	>6 mo: 0.2 ml SC	Vaccine of questionable efficacy; not recommended by CDC or WHO; do not use under 6 mo				
Lyme disease	LYMErix: antigenic protein	>15 yr: 0.5 ml IM at 0, 1, 12 mo	Indicated for frequent, prolonged exposure to Lyme-endemic area, not brief exposures				
EXTENDED STAY							
Rabies	HDCV: human diploid cell	1 ml IM in deltoid muscle at 0, 7, 21-28 days if > 1 mo stay	If exposed and immunized: give vaccine, 1 ml IM at 0, 3 days If exposed and unimmunized: give rabies Ig (RIG), 20 IU/kg half at site and half IM; give vaccine, 1 ml IM at 0, 3, 7, 14, 28 days	+	+	±	+

Consult Centers for Disease Control and Prevention (CDC) for current and specific vaccine recommendations for destination country.

AAP, American Academy of Pediatrics; *IM,* intramuscularly; *SC,* subcutaneously; *q,* every; *WHO,* World Health Organization; +, recommended; ±, consider.

*DtaP, poliovirus vaccine, and *Haemophilus influenzae* type b vaccine may be given at 4-week intervals if necessary to complete the recommended schedule before departure.

† Measles: two additional doses given if younger than 12 months of age at first dose.

TABLE 74-8. Recommended Timing and Sequence of Nonroutine Immunizations for Foreign Travel*

4-6 WEEKS BEFORE DEPARTURE	1 WEEK AFTER INITIAL VISIT	WEEK OF DEPARTURE
Hepatitis A (need second dose 6-12 mo later)		*or* Immune globulin for hepatitis A prevention
Yellow fever		
Typhoid-heat inactivated *or* ViCPS *or* Ty21a (oral, 1 capsule q 2 days × 4)		Typhoid: heat inactivated
Meningococcal		Meningococcal (if not given at initial visit)
Japanese encephalitis	Japanese encephalitis	Japanese encephalitis
Rabies	Rabies	Rabies

*Give only immunizations indicated for area of travel, length of stay, and age of child. Simultaneous administration of routine and travel-related vaccines is acceptable with the exception of yellow fever with cholera (yellow fever at least 3 weeks before cholera) and MMR or VZV with IgG. Administer IgG at least 3 weeks after these live virus vaccines (see Table 74-7).

The risk of acquiring diseases covered by many routine childhood immunizations (diphtheria, pertussis, tetanus, measles, polio, hepatitis B) is greater in developing nations. Consequently, children who have not completed their primary series of immunizations may require an acceleration of the vaccination schedule or extra doses to maximize protection before travel.

Ideally, a visit to the physician to discuss travel plans and begin immunizations should be made 4-6 weeks before travel. Not all immunologic agents recommended for travel are compatible, and some require multiple doses. Therefore the selection of immunizations to be given at any one time and the interval between immunizations are important (Table 74-8). In general, all toxoid, recombinant, inactivated, and live attenuated vaccines may be given simultaneously. Exceptions are those against yellow fever and cholera, which should not be given simultaneously or within 3 weeks of each other. Alternatively, the cholera vaccine can be omitted, since its effectiveness is limited.[54] Live attenuated vaccines should be given either simultaneously or at least 30 days apart to avoid reduced immunoreactivity to each vaccine. Administration of immune globulin interferes with the humoral response to the live attenuated virus vaccines such as measles, mumps, and rubella (MMR) and varicella. If immune globulin is given first, these vaccinations should be delayed by at least 6 weeks, and preferably 3 months, to obtain an adequate immunogenic response. When both are needed for travel, it is best to give MMR or varicella vaccine first; immune globulin can be given closer to the time of travel, at least 2 weeks and preferably 4 weeks later. Immune globulin does not interfere with antibody production induced by live viral vaccines against polio (oral vaccine) or yellow fever and may be given at the same visit. Travel vaccines that require multiple doses or early administration include hepatitis A, inactivated typhoid, Japanese encephalitis, rabies, yellow fever, and MMR (if immune globulin is to be given near the time of departure).

Malaria Prophylaxis

The risk of acquiring malaria during visits to developing countries in the tropics is significant (see Chapter 65). Even areas where the overall risk is relatively low may have foci of intense transmission. Children under 5 years are particularly vulnerable and represent the largest proportion of fatalities from this disease. Of the 30,000 to 50,000 cases of malaria acquired by travelers from Europe and North America per year, most occur among visitors to sub-Saharan Africa (82%) and Asia (8%).[39]

Protective measures to prevent mosquito bites help interrupt the transmission of malaria but are not foolproof (see Box 74-2). Therefore chemoprophylaxis is highly recommended for travelers to countries where malaria is endemic. *Plasmodium vivax* and *P. falciparum* are the two most abundant species responsible for malaria. The most lethal species, *P. falciparum*, has developed widespread resistance to chloroquine and in some areas (rural Thailand, Cameroon, Indonesia) resistance to mefloquine.[6] Therefore the choice of prophylactic agent depends on the presence of resistant malaria in the area of travel.

Chloroquine (Aralen) is the still the drug of choice for travelers to the few areas where chloroquine-resistant strains of *P. falciparum* are not a problem (Central America west of the Panama Canal, Haiti, Dominican Republic, and Middle East) or areas where falciparum malaria does not occur (Egypt). Chloroquine prophylaxis should be given weekly starting 1 week before travel and continued for 4 weeks thereafter. Chloroquine is passed through breast milk, although not in sufficient quantities to protect an infant. Therefore a breast-fed infant should receive chloroquine prophylaxis in the standard recommended doses (Table 74-9). Chloroquine is not readily available in liquid form in the United States. The powder, which is extremely bitter, may be suspended in a syrup or mixed with food. Instant pudding effectively masks the bitter taste and makes the medicine more palatable. An acceptable-tasting syrup (Nivaquine) is available in most developing countries. Chloroquine should be kept out of the reach of children. As little as

TABLE 74-9. Malaria Chemoprophylaxis

MEDICATION	INDICATIONS	DOSING

Mefloquine (Lariam)	Travel to chloroquine-resistant areas
	   Child > 15 kg
	Avoid in child with epilepsy or psychiatric
	   illness
		Given weekly: 1 wk before to 4 wk
		   after travel
		15-19 kg: ¼ tablet
		20-30 kg: ½ tablet
		30-40 kg: ¾ tablet
		>40 kg: 1 tablet (250 mg)

Doxycycline	Alternative to mefloquine in chloroquine-
	   resistant areas if contraindication to
	   mefloquine
	>8 yr of age only
		2 mg/kg/day up to 100 mg/day
		1-2 days preexposure and 4 wk after
		   exposure; photosensitivity possible

Chloroquine (Aralen)
  (liquid: Nivaquine)
	Travel to chloroquine-sensitive areas
	   (Caribbean, Central America north of Panama,
	   Middle East)
	Safe in children under 15 kg
		5 mg/kg/wk up to 500 mg for 1 wk
		   before and 4 wk after exposure;
		10 mg/ml liquid available outside
		   United States

Proguanil (Paludrine)	Take with chloroquine when possible, partic-
	   ularly in Africa
	Not available in United States
		Give daily while taking chloroquine
		   <2 yr: 50 mg/day
		   2-6 yr: 100 mg/day
		   7-10 yr: 150 mg/day
		   >10 yr: 200 mg/day

Pyrimethamine-
  sulfadoxine (Fansidar)
	Prepare for treatment if symptoms develop
	   and medical attention > 24 hr away
	Contraindicated if age < 2 mo or sulfa
	   allergy
		Single dose:
		   2 mo-1 yr: ¼ tablet
		   1-3 yr: ½ tablet
		   4-8 yr: 1 tablet
		   9-14 yr: 2 tablets
		   >14 yr: 3 tablets

Atovaquone (250 mg) +
  proguanil (100 mg)
  (Malarone)
	Prepare for treatment in Fansidar-resistant
	   areas (parts of Southeast Asia, Amazon
	   basin)
	Not available in United States
		Dose per day × 3 days
		   11-20 kg: 1 tablet
		   21-30 kg: 2 tablets
		   31-40 kg: 3 tablets
		   >40 kg: 4 tablets

Primaquine	Prevention of relapse with *Plasmodium vivax*
	   or *P. ovale*
	Use after prolonged stay in malaria-endemic
	   area
	Avoid if glucose-6-phosphate dehydrogenase
	   deficient
		0.3 mg/kg/day for 14 days after
		   leaving area

Data from *Red book: report of the Committee on Infectious Disease*, Elk Grove Village, Ill, 1997, American Academy of Pediatrics.

1 g may be fatal in small children.[49] If a toxic chloroquine ingestion occurs, syrup of ipecac should be administered immediately to provoke emesis, and the child should be transported promptly to a medical facility.

Proguanil (Paludrine) is not available in the United States but is widely available overseas. It is recommended for use with chloroquine, particularly in chloroquine-resistant areas if mefloquine and doxycycline are contraindicated. This would include children less than 15 kg and those under age 8 years with epilepsy or psychiatric disorders. Unfortunately, this regimen is only 40% to 60% effective and should not be used unless alternative therapies are contraindicated.

For children over 15 kg traveling to chloroquine-resistant areas, mefloquine (Lariam) is the preferred agent. It is started 1 week before travel and given weekly during travel and for 4 weeks after return.

Mefloquine should be avoided in children with psychiatric illnesses, epilepsy, or underlying cardiac arrhythmias. Doxycycline may be used in children over age 8 years with contraindications to mefloquine. Unlike mefloquine, however, doxycycline must be given daily. Side effects include diarrhea and photosensitivity. Since neither of these agents can be used in small children (less than 15 kg), parents should seriously consider the risks of acquiring malaria before traveling to a malaria-endemic area with an infant or toddler.

If a child develops an acute febrile illness in a malaria-endemic area where medical care is not immediately available, pyrimethamine with sulfadoxine (Fansidar) may be used as standby treatment.[4] Fansidar is given as a one-time dose. Prophylaxis with this drug is not recommended because of the risk of Stevens-Johnson syndrome. Fansidar should not be given to infants less than 2 months old or to children allergic to sulfa medications. Atovaquone with proguanil (Malarone) is an alternative standby treatment that has been used successfully in Fansidar-resistant areas (parts of Southeast Asia and the Amazon basin).[41,52] Studies have also demonstrated the efficacy of this preparation as prophylaxis against *P. falciparum,* but this use has not yet gained widespread acceptance.[37,63] Malarone is not available in the United States. All patients who take Fansidar or Malarone for presumptive treatment of malaria should be transported to a medical facility as soon as possible for definitive care.

Primaquine is an antimalarial drug used to prevent emergence of *P. vivax* and *P. ovale* after heavy exposure or prolonged (many months) exposure to mosquitoes. Routine chemoprophylaxis does not kill the exoerythrocytic stages of these *Plasmodium* species. Primaquine is taken daily for 2 weeks after leaving a malarial area. Primaquine should not be given to anyone with glucose-6-phosphate dehydrogenase (G6PD) deficiency.

TRAVEL-RELATED PROBLEMS

After boredom and restlessness, motion sickness and eustachian tube dysfunction are the most common problems of children during travel. Parents can minimize the first two problems by preparing small activity packs or bags with paper, pencils, crayons, cards, travel puzzles, or small toys.

Motion Sickness

Motion sickness can occur with air, land, or sea travel, particularly in children ages 2 through 12 years. Emotional upset, noxious odors, and ear infections can make the symptoms worse. Children experiencing motion sickness are often pale and diaphoretic and feel nauseated and weak. They may vomit, but unfortunately this does not provide prolonged relief. Children known to be susceptible to motion sickness should be seated in the middle or near the front of the boat, plane, or car, where motion is minimized. They should be encouraged to look at objects far away and avoid focusing on close objects, such as books. Some children obtain significant relief from using headphones to listen to music or stories.

Dimenhydrinate (Dramamine, 1 to 1.5 mg/kg) administered 1 hour before departure and repeated every 6 hours can help children known to be prone to motion sickness. If dimenhydrinate is not available, diphenhydramine (Benadryl, 1.25 mg/kg every 6 hours) may also be effective. Both medications may cause drowsiness, and diphenhydramine occasionally causes paradoxical hyperexcitability in children. Scopolamine patches should not be used because children are particularly susceptible to the side effects of belladonna alkaloids. Whether patches release too much scopolamine and consequently produce serious side effects in children is not known.[49]

Eustachian Tube Dysfunction

Eustachian tube dysfunction causes discomfort that results from a pressure disequilibrium between the eustachian tube and the surrounding atmospheric pressure. About 15% of children have this problem, particularly during airplane descent. Swallowing often helps relieve the pressure disequilibrium and may be facilitated by drinking or, for the breast-fed infant, by nursing. Older children may chew gum or yawn to equalize middle ear and atmospheric pressure. Contrary to popular belief, decongestants are not useful with eustachian tube dysfunction in children and may cause paradoxical drowsiness.[9]

Most airline cabins are pressurized to provide an oxygen concentration of 17% to 18%, not the 21% of sea-level air. Supplemental oxygen may be necessary for children with congenital heart disease or pulmonary disease (asthma, bronchopulmonary dysplasia) if cyanosis or respiratory distress develops.

Traveler's Diarrhea

Traveling to wilderness areas or developing countries requires leaving behind modern sanitation and reliably disinfected tap water (see Chapter 52). Unfortunately, this places travelers at increased risk for diarrheal illness. Traveler's diarrhea affects 25% to 50% of adult travelers from low-risk to high-risk countries. In one pediatric study, 40% of children under age 2 years developed prolonged diarrhea during travel in tropical or subtropical areas.[50] Young children are at greater risk for traveler's diarrhea and its complications because of relatively poor hygiene, immature immune systems, lower gastric pH, more rapid gastric emptying, and difficulties with adequate hydration.[16]

Traveler's diarrhea has been defined as greater than three unformed stools in a day or any number of such stools when accompanied by symptoms such as fever, abdominal cramping, vomiting, or blood or mucus in the stools.[50] In small children the course tends to be more severe and prolonged, lasting from 3 days to 3 weeks. Traveler's diarrhea can be caused by preformed toxins, viruses, invasive bacteria, or parasites (Table 74-10). Enterotoxigenic *Escherichia coli* is responsible for 50% of traveler's diarrhea. Rotavirus and Norwalk-like viruses account for another 30%.[5] *Shigella* remains the most common cause of invasive diarrhea.

Prevention. Standard recommendations for prevention of traveler's diarrhea are based primarily on known potential vehicles for transmission of the illness (see Box 74-4). Transmission is through fecal-oral contamination, with water, food, and fingers the most common sources. Careful selection and preparation of food and beverages can decrease the risk of acquiring traveler's diarrhea. Washing hands thoroughly before eating decreases bacterial carriage and also reminds children about the need for precautions. According to the

TABLE 74-10. Causes of Traveler's Diarrhea in Children

AGENT	EXAMPLES
Preformed toxin	Enterotoxigenic *Escherichia coli** *Staphylococcus aureus* *Bacillus cereus*
Viral	Rotavirus* Norwalk agent* Adenovirus Enterovirus Influenza Hepatitis
Bacterial	*Shigella** *Campylobacter* *Salmonella* Enteroinvasive *Escherichia coli* *Yersinia enterocolitica* *Vibrio cholera*
Parasitic	*Giardia lamblia* *Entamoeba histolytica* *Cryptosporidium*

Modified from Bonadio WA: *Emerg Med Clin North Am* 13:457, 1995.
*Most common.

Box 74-5 SIGNS OF DEHYDRATION IN CHILDREN

MILD-MODERATE (5%-10%)

Irritability
Sunken eyes
Dry mucous membranes
Extreme thirst

SEVERE (>10%)

Lethargy
Extremely sunken eyes
Extremely dry mucous membranes
Inability to consume oral liquids
Cool, mottled extremities
Rapid thready pulse
Tachypnea

Modified from *Treatment of diarrhoea: manual for physicians and other senior health workers*, Geneva, 1995, World Health Organization.

"boil it, cook it, peel it, or forget it" rule, all raw vegetables and salads should be avoided, meats and seafood well cooked, and fruits properly peeled (see Chapter 51).

Treatment. The major cause of morbidity and mortality in infants and small children with diarrhea is dehydration[1] (Box 74-5). According to the World Health Organization (WHO), dehydration is best categorized as mild-moderate or severe.[72] This distinction is based on changes in behavior and mental state, quality of mu-

Box 74-6 HOMEMADE ORAL REHYDRATION SOLUTION

1 teaspoon (5 g) salt
1 cup (50 g) rice cereal
1 quart (1 L) disinfected water

Data from World Health Organization.

cous membranes, oliguria or anuria, changes in vital signs, and decreasing peripheral perfusion. Children young enough to be wearing diapers should have some urine output at least every 8 hours. If not, they are probably dehydrated.

The cornerstone of therapy is oral rehydration therapy (ORT), which can be used alone successfully in 90% to 95% of cases, especially if instituted early.[23] ORT is as effective as intravenous hydration in mild-moderate dehydration from diarrhea. Parents traveling to developing countries or wilderness areas with children should carry a prepared powdered oral rehydration solution (ORS) or a recipe for a homemade solution (Box 74-6). Powdered ORS is readily available in most developing countries through WHO and may be obtained in the United States from Jianas Brothers, Kansas City, Missouri (816-421-2880). Although earlier studies reported rice-based ORS as more effective in reducing stool output than standard glucose-based ORS,[46,53] more recent studies demonstrated that any advantage from rice-based ORS is lost after 6 hours of rehydration.[18,45] Rice ORS has lower osmolality and higher concentration of organic solutes; therefore the osmotic gradient across the intestinal lumen is lower and intestinal sodium transport decreased, theoretically resulting in less stool water. Because of hydrolysis of its starches, however, rice-based ORS is stable only for 12 hours, after which it must be discarded and a new solution made.[58]

For rapid treatment of mild-moderate dehydration, 50 to 100 ml/kg of ORS should be administered over the first 4-hour period, followed by maintenance solution to provide for basic fluid requirements and to replace ongoing losses.[5,58] Ideal ORS should contain 75 to 90 mEq/L of sodium, 2% to 2.5% carbohydrate, and 20 mEq/L of potassium (Table 74-11). If a solution with more than 3% glucose is used, the osmotic pressure exerted by glucose in the intestinal lumen produces fluid losses greater than fluid absorption, thereby exacerbating diarrhea. Most colas and juices contain nearly 10% to 15% glucose or carbohydrate and are not appropriate rehydration solutions.[25,42] The high sodium concentration in the ORS poses a risk for hypernatremia if the solution is used for maintenance fluids or to prevent dehydration. For maintaining hydration, alternating ORS with a fluid that has less sodium, such as water or breast milk, will avert hy-

TABLE 74-11. Field Treatment of Dehydration in Children

	REHYDRATION SOLUTION	MAINTENANCE SOLUTION
Volume	50-100 ml/kg/4 hr* (1-1.5 oz/lb/4 hr)	75-150 ml/kg/day* (1-2.5 oz/lb/day)
Electrolytes		
Na$^+$ (mEq/L)	75-90	50-60
Glucose (%)	2-2.5	2-2.5
K$^+$ (mEq/L)	20	20
Bicarbonate (mEq/L)	30	30

Modified from Goepp J, Santosham M: *Principles Pract Pediatr Updates* 1:1, 1993.
*Add 10 ml/kg, or about 4 ounces, for each diarrheal stool and 5 ml/kg, or about 2 ounces, for each bout of emesis.

pernatremia. Alternatively, a separate solution containing 50 to 60 mEq/L sodium can be used. Maintenance fluid volumes are 75 to 150 ml/kg/day. An additional 10 ml/kg, or 4 ounces, can be given for each diarrheal stool and 5 ml/kg, or 2 ounces, for each episode of emesis.[35] If vomiting develops, most children will still tolerate ORS if given in small volumes (5 to 10 ml) every 5 minutes. Feeding of solid food, particularly complex carbohydrates, should be continued during and after diarrhea because it promotes enterocyte regeneration.[9,19,57] Severe dehydration requires prompt medical attention and administration of intravenous fluids for rehydration.

Although oral hydration should be the cornerstone of therapy for diarrhea and dehydration, medications may be helpful. Antimotility agents such as loperamide and diphenoxylate are of no proven efficacy, according to the American Academy of Pediatrics (AAP) guidelines for acute gastroenteritis.[1] In general, they should be avoided; however, loperamide may be used with older children if fever, bloody stool, and abdominal distention are absent[17] (see Table 74-12). Other antidiarrheal agents (e.g., bismuth) have not been shown to be effective in children and should be avoided, particularly in those under 2 years.

Antibiotic chemoprophylaxis remains controversial for adults and is not recommended for children.[1] The use of antibiotics should be limited to children with fever, bloody stools, or abdominal distention in whom invasive bacterial diarrhea is suspected.[27] Under age 3 to 6 months, the risk of bacteremia with *Salmonella* infection is significant, so antibiotic treatment is also indicated. With increasing bacterial resistance to trimethoprim-sulfamethoxazole, azithromycin is now the drug of choice for treatment of bacterial diarrhea.[29,67] The dose is 10 mg/kg on day 1, then 5 mg/kg once daily for 5 days. Although quinolones (e.g., ciprofloxacin) can be used in children over age

12 years and perhaps younger, increasing bacterial resistance to quinolones makes azithromycin an even better choice. If symptoms do not improve rapidly, parents should seek immediate medical attention for their children. *Salmonella typhi* infection, or typhoid fever, if suspected, should be managed immediately in a hospital setting with quinolones or third-generation cephalosporins.

Respiratory Infections

Respiratory tract infections are common in the pediatric population. Most infections, such as acute otitis media (AOM), sinusitis, pharyngitis, croup, bronchiolitis, and bronchitis, involve the upper respiratory tract. The majority of these infections are viral in etiology; the remainder are usually the result of infections with *Streptococcus pneumoniae*, *Haemophilus influenzae*, or *Moraxella catarrhalis*. Since definitive diagnoses based on otoscopy and auscultation of the lungs often cannot be made during wilderness travel, parents must rely on symptoms and the presence of fever to determine whether treatment is necessary. The presence of high fever, otalgia, facial pain, sore throat without cough or rhinorrhea, or mucopurulent nasal discharge lasting longer than 10 days likely merits both antimicrobial and symptomatic treatment. However, 20% to 80% of AOM and 50% of streptococcal pharyngitis cases resolve without intervention.[12,13] Furthermore, antibiotic treatment of certain upper respiratory infections, such as bronchitis, bronchiolitis, croup, and most pharyngitis, does not shorten the course, minimize symptoms, or decrease complications.[43]

With increasing use of antibiotics, bacterial resistance to these agents has risen dramatically. From 10% to 30% of *S. pneumoniae* infections are resistant to penicillin and 5% to 20% to macrolides such as erythromycin.[11] Up to 20% of *H. influenzae* and 70% of *M. catarrhalis* infections are resistant to amoxicillin. However, testing has demonstrated sensitivity to high-dose amoxicillin, even among resistant strains. First-line therapy for these infections is therefore high-dose amoxicillin at 60 to 80 mg/kg.[67] Second-line therapy is high-dose amoxicillin-clavulanate (same amoxicillin component dosing), cefuroxime, or ceftriaxone.[43] Uncomplicated AOM in children over 2 years may be treated for 5 to 7 days; otherwise the standard treatment for AOM is 10 days and, for sinusitis, 14 days. Exudative pharyngitis with fever and lymphadenopathy but without cough can be treated for 10 days with penicillin or amoxicillin, or for 5 days with azithromycin.

Fever of Undetermined Origin

High fever that develops in a child during the course of foreign travel may be the result of a common infection (e.g., AOM, pharyngitis) or the manifestation of a tropical disease. If malaria is suspected, the child should immediately be taken to the closest medical facility. If this cannot occur within 24 hours, any child over 2 months old should be given Fansidar as standby treatment (see Table 74-9).

Salmonella typhi infection, more commonly known as typhoid fever, can also present with high fever, paradoxical bradycardia, and at least initially, without diarrhea. Children who appear ill with high fevers may have invasive typhoidal disease and should be treated in a medical facility. *Salmonella* resistance is rising in developing countries, but strains are typically susceptible to quinolones (over age 12 years) and third-generation cephalosporins (e.g., cefixime, ceftriaxone).

Dengue fever, caused by a mosquito-borne arbovirus, can also cause high fever, headaches, and severe myalgias (see Chapter 66). With the exception of recurrent dengue, which can result in hemorrhagic complications, the treatment of dengue fever is purely symptomatic.

Rashes

Identification of rashes in the pediatric population is an art. Although parents cannot be expected to become familiar with all types of rashes, they should learn to distinguish common rashes from potentially dangerous exanthems. Petechial, purpuric, or mucosal lesions are markers for potentially serious disease and should prompt parents to seek medical attention immediately. Standard dermatologic textbooks with photographs can be used to instruct parents to recognize common viral exanthems and rashes caused by varicella, scabies, and contact dermatitides (poison oak, poison ivy). Scabies can be abolished safely with permethrin. Contact dermatitis can be treated with 1% hydrocortisone cream.

Soft Tissue Injuries

Soft tissue injuries are extremely common among children, particularly as they become more ambulatory (see Chapter 18). All wounds sustained in the wilderness should be thoroughly irrigated with clean water and explored to ensure that no foreign bodies remain. In general, lacerations should not be sutured in the backcountry due to the risk of infection. They should be covered with a water-resistant dressing, splinted if located over a joint, and observed. If no evidence of infection develops over 4 to 5 days, the laceration may be repaired by delayed primary closure.

PEDIATRIC WILDERNESS MEDICAL KITS

When a family travels in remote areas, any medical kit must be adapted to meet the special needs of children. Actual items carried vary depending on the ages of the children, preexisting medical conditions, length of travel, specific environmental conditions en-

---

Box 74-7 PEDIATRIC WILDERNESS MEDICAL KIT: BASIC SUPPLIES

1. Identification and basic health information for child: past medical history, medications, allergies, blood type, weight
2. First-aid supplies: adhesive bandages, gauze pads, gauze roll, tape, nonadherent dressings, moleskin/Spenco 2nd skin/Nu Skin, benzoin, alcohol wipes, povidone-iodine solution for dilution and disinfection, safety pins, tweezers, lightweight malleable splint (SAM splint), syringe (20-35 ml), 18-gauge plastic catheter for wound irrigation
3. Oral rehydration salts
4. Sunscreen: SPF of 15 or greater
5. Insect repellent: DEET <35%
6. Whistle for child
7. For infant <3 mo: rectal thermometer, bulb syringe

---

countered, and medical sophistication of the adults. Although individual preference plays a role in assembling a medical kit, certain items are essential for management of common problems during wilderness travel with children (Box 74-7).

To reduce weight and bulk, medications selected for a wilderness medical kit should have multiple uses (Table 74-12). For example, diphenhydramine is effective for allergic symptoms, pruritus, motion sickness, nausea, and insomnia. Desitin, best known for its use in preventing diaper rash, is also an excellent sunscreen, since it contains 40% zinc oxide. A broad-spectrum antifungal cream, such as miconazole or clotrimazole, covers not only tineal infections (ringworm, jock itch, athlete's foot), but also *Candida* infections (diaper rash, vaginitis).

Most children can chew tablets once their first molars are present (about 15 months of age). Before that time, chewable medications or tablets can be crushed between two spoons and mixed with food. Liquid medications add excess weight and the potential for leaks; they should be carried in powder form only for children under 6 months. Medication can be camouflaged in a food such as instant pudding.

Painful musculoskeletal injuries are a potential complication of wilderness activities, and pain medication for children should be included in every medical kit. Acetaminophen not only relieves minor aches and pains but also is effective for fever control. It is well tolerated by most children and available in many pleasant-tasting forms for children unable to swallow pills: chewable 80- or 160-mg tablets, elixir, and concentrated drops. Ibuprofen appears to be more effective than acetaminophen for pain and fever control. Its duration of action is 6 to 8 hours vs. 4 to 6 hours for acetamin-

TABLE 74-12. Pediatric Wilderness Medical Kit: Medications

MEDICATION	INDICATION	DOSE
TOPICAL MEDICATION		
Antibiotic or antiseptic ointment (e.g., bacitracin-polymyxin)	Superficial skin infections	Apply as directed qd-tid
Topical corticosteroid (e.g., 1% hydrocortisone)	Contact or atopic dermatitis, insect bites, sunburn	Apply to affected areas bid-tid (use sunscreen aggressively; avoid >1% on face)
Antifungal cream (e.g., clotrimazole, miconazole)	Yeast at diaper area, groin, scalp, feet; ringworm	Apply bid for 7-10 days and for several days after rash has resolved
Desitin cream	Sunscreen, diaper area erythema	Apply thick coat as sunscreen or thin coat for diaper area
Permethrin (Elimite)	Scabies, lice, treatment for clothing and mosquito netting	Apply 5% cream from chin to soles of feet and wash after 8-14 hr; do not use <2 mo of age or on eyes, nose, or mouth
Anesthetic eye drops (e.g., proparacaine)*†	Removal of superficial ocular foreign body	1 drop in affected eye for removal of foreign body; must patch eye for protection for at least 1 hr
Antibiotic eye ointment (e.g., erythromycin)†	Purulent conjunctivitis, suspected corneal abrasion	Use as directed tid-qid
ORAL MEDICATIONS		
Diphenhydramine 　12.5 mg/5 ml elixir 　25- or 50-mg capsules	Allergic symptoms, pruritus, insomnia, nausea, motion sickness	1.25 mg/kg/dose every 6 hr up to 25-50 mg/dose; may cause paradoxical restlessness in children
Acetaminophen 　80 mg/0.8 ml drops 　160 mg/5 ml elixir 　80- and 160-mg chewable tabs	Fever control, pain	15-20 mg/kg every 4-6 hr up to 650 mg/dose
or Ibuprofen 　40 mg/1 ml drops 　100 mg/5 ml elixir 　50- or 100-mg chewable tabs 　100- or 200-mg caplets	Fever control, pain, antiinflammatory	10 mg/kg/dose every 8 hr up to 600 mg/dose
Acetaminophen with codeine† 　120 mg acetaminophen and 　12 mg codeine/5 ml elixir	Severe pain, severe cough	As for acetaminophen, or 0.5-1 mg/kg of codeine every 4-6 hr
Dimenhydrinate (Dramamine) 　12.5 mg/5 ml elixir 　50-mg chewable tabs	Motion sickness	1-1.5 mg/kg/dose 1 hr before departure and every 6 hr thereafter; may cause drowsiness
ORAL ANTIBIOTICS (CHOOSE APPROPRIATE ACCORDING TO CHILD'S AGE)		
Amoxicillin† 　125- or 250-mg chewable tabs 　250-mg capsules	Otitis media, sinusitis, pharyngitis, pneumonia, urinary tract infection (UTI)	60-80 mg/kg/day for upper respiratory infection (URI) or divided tid for pneumonia
Amoxicillin-clavulanate (Augmentin) 　200- and 400-mg chewable tabs 　200 and 400 mg/5 ml elixir	Resistant acute otitis media (AOM), sinusitis, animal bites, soft tissue infections	Same as amoxicillin dosing divided bid
Azithromycin (Zithromax)† 　125 and 250 mg/5 ml elixir 　250-mg tabs (best)	AOM, sinusitis, pharyngitis, pneumonia, traveler's diarrhea, skin infections, animal bites	10mg/kg on day 1, then 5 mg/kg/day qd × 5 days
Ciprofloxacin (Cipro)† 　100-, 200-, 500-mg tabs	Approved for >8 yr of age: UTI, traveler's diarrhea, aquatic wounds	20-30 mg/kg/day divided bid up to 500 mg bid

qd, Every day; *bid*, twice daily; *tid*, three time daily; *SC*, subcutaneously.
*Administration of this medication by other than trained medical personnel is strongly discouraged given the risk of overuse and subsequent worsening of eye injury; if significant eye irritation persists, medical attention must be sought to evaluate for corneal injury.
†Available by prescription only.

TABLE 74-12. Pediatric Wilderness Medical Kit: Medications—cont'd

MEDICATION	INDICATION	DOSE
OTHER PREPARATIONS		
Epinephrine (premeasured)† 0.15 mg (EpiPen Jr.) 0.3 mg (EpiPen)	Anaphylaxis, severe asthma	0.15 mg SC up to 15 kg; 0.3 mg SC if over 15 kg
Syrup of ipecac	Induce vomiting for noncaustic ingestions in alert child	15 ml followed by 1-2 glasses of water; may repeat in 20 min if no emesis
Oral rehydration packet (ORS)	Dehydration	See Table 74-11
FOREIGN TRAVEL		
Loperamide 1 mg/5 ml 1-mg capsules	Nonbloody, minimally febrile, significant diarrhea over 2 years of age (not recommended by AAP)	13-20 kg: 1 mg tid 20-30 kg: 2 mg bid >30 kg: 2 mg tid
Appropriate malaria prophylaxis if indicated†		See Table 74-9
Pyrimethamine-sulfadoxine (Fansidar)†	Standby treatment for malaria if immediate medical attention unavailable	See Table 74-9
TRAVEL TO HIGH ALTITUDE		
Acetazolamide (Diamox)† 30 or 50 mg/ml suspension 125-mg tabs	Recurrent acute mountain sickness (AMS) despite graded ascent	5 mg/kg/day divided bid up to 250 mg/day
Promethazine (Phenergan)† 12.5 or 25 mg/suppository	Nausea and vomiting associated with AMS	0.25-0.5 mg/kg/dose every 6 hr up to 25 mg/dose
SNAKE-INFESTED AREAS		
Extractor (negative-pressure suction device)‡	Poisonous snakebites	Apply per instructions within 3 min of bite

‡Sawyer Products, Safety Harbor, Fla.

ophen. Ibuprofen is available in many forms: infant drops (40 mg/1 ml), children's elixir (100 mg/5 ml), 50- or 100-mg chewable tablets, and 100- or 200-mg caplets. Tylenol with codeine combines a centrally acting agent, codeine, with a peripherally acting analgesic, acetaminophen. It is indicated for treatment of moderate to severe pain. Acetaminophen has the added effect of fever control, and codeine has antitussive properties. Codeine can cause respiratory depression, particularly in children under 12 months of age, and may elevate intracranial pressure, especially in the presence of head injury; its use should be avoided in these situations. Dosing is based on the codeine component: both the liquid formulation (12 mg/5 ml) and tablets (10, 20, or 30 mg of codeine per tablet) are given at 0.5 to 1 mg/kg up to every 6 hours.

Two or three antibiotics will cover most bacterial infections in children. Age, allergies, intolerance, and past experience must be taken into account when antibiotics are selected. Given increasing bacterial resistance to common antibiotics, antimicrobial choices should be reevaluated periodically to ensure that infections likely to be encountered can be successfully treated with these agents. All oral antibiotics require a prescription. Amoxicillin is available in pleasant-tasting chewable tablets (125 and 250 mg) and in powdered form for suspension (125 and 250 mg/5 ml) Given current resistance patterns, high-dose therapy with 60 to 80 mg/kg divided three times daily is indicated. Amoxicillin is well tolerated by most children. Amoxicillin-clavulanate (Augmentin) provides excellent coverage for recurrent pharyngitis, soft tissue infections, animal bites, and infections when a resistant organism is anticipated. The most common side effect is diarrhea, but this has been reduced with newer formulations, available in 200- and 400-mg (amoxicillin component) chewable tablets and in 200 and 400 mg/5 ml liquid. Dosing is 60 to 80 mg/kg divided twice a day. Azithromycin (Zithromax) is a long-acting macrolide without the gastrointestinal effects of erythromycin. It is effective for treatment of AOM, sinusitis, pharyngitis, lower respiratory infections, traveler's diarrhea, and common animal bites. It is particularly useful in children with penicillin allergy. Dosing is extremely convenient because of azithromycin's long half-life: a 10 mg/kg initial dose on day 1 is followed by 5 mg/kg/day for 5 days. Ciprofloxacin (Cipro) has a broad spectrum of coverage and is useful for treatment of bacterial diarrhea, complex urinary tract infections, and wounds acquired in an aquatic environment. Its use has been discouraged in children under 12 years because of a potential problem with arthropathic effects on weight-bearing joints. However, a study involving more than 600 children found only a 1.3% rate of reversible arthralgia and no evidence of arthropathy.[60] Nonetheless, ciprofloxacin should not be routinely recommended for children under 12 years unless a special situation arises in which the benefits of its use outweigh the risks.

Syrup of ipecac should also be included in every pediatric medical kit. Small children tend to explore their environment with hands and mouths. If toxic ingestions are recognized within 30 minutes and there is no contraindication to induced emesis (caustic agent or solvent, altered mental status, less than 1 year of age), ipecac should be administered immediately. One tablespoon or 15 ml should be given with one or two glasses of water; this dose may be repeated in 20 minutes if emesis does not occur.

Parents of children with special medical conditions should carry a pertinent medical summary and have resources to access specialty physicians in destination countries. A generous supply of necessary medications with instructions for worsening symptoms must be included in the medical kit. An extra supply of all essential medications should be kept with either parents or patient in case the medical kit is lost or separated from the patient when the medication is needed. Some travelers in endemic areas for hepatitis B and acquired immunodeficiency syndrome (AIDS) carry their own needles and syringes for emergency use. The International Association for Medical Assistance to Travelers (417 Center St., Lewiston, NY 14692; 716-754-4883) has a directory of qualified physicians worldwide who speak English.

INFANTS AND YOUNG CHILDREN

A family traveling with an infant must be particularly vigilant in monitoring their child's state of health. Infants become hypothermic, hyperthermic, septic, and dehydrated more rapidly than adults or older children. A thermometer and appropriate lubricant should be included in the medical kit for monitoring rectal temperature. A temperature greater than 38° C (100.4° F) in a child less than 3 months of age requires evacuation for medical evaluation. Digital thermometers are recommended, since they are less likely to break, are easy to read, and are three to four times faster than a glass thermometer. Some emit an audio alarm when the reading is ready.

Infants are less tolerant of problems with excess mucus; a bulb syringe is handy for suctioning mucus from the oropharynx and nasal passages. A few drops of saline solution (¼ tsp of salt in 1 cup of water) instilled into the nares a few minutes before aspiration help to loosen mucus. Nasal aspiration should be reserved for times of most need, such as before feeding and sleep, since the procedure is irritating to the child. Other uses for a clean bulb syringe include flushing foreign bodies from ears and administering enemas.

Away from the conveniences of home, diapers tend to be changed less frequently; consequently, diaper rash may become a problem. A good barrier cream (e.g., Desitin) may be helpful and should be started at the first signs of irritation. If the rash progresses despite appropriate treatment, an antifungal cream (e.g., miconazole, clotrimazole) may be used.

Lost Children

Lost children in the wilderness is a common, preventable problem. Children should be taught to recognize landmarks and to turn around and look backward periodically to familiarize themselves with the terrain. Those who are capable of reading a compass and topographic map should carry these at all times. Young children should wear brightly colored clothing to facilitate a search should they become lost. They should carry a whistle around their necks and should be taught the universal signal for help: three blows in a row. It should be emphasized to the child that the whistle is intended for emergency use only. All children should either know or carry with them a piece of paper with their parents' name, address, and phone number. Older children who venture without their parents should always inform an adult where they are going, with whom, and when they expect to return.

Programs such as "Hug a Tree" instruct children in the basics of survival and orienteering when lost: stay in one place to facilitate any search, take advantage of the natural shelter provided by a tree, and feel the security of a large natural protector. By "hugging a tree" and not wandering, children can make signals from rocks or branches to indicate their location. Children should be taught to avoid becoming wet, to wear a hat, and to stuff pine needles or dry grasses into their clothes to insulate themselves if they are cold. Children can practice making temporary shelters out of logs, branches, and leaves to experience the warmth and protection of these natural features.

Homesickness

Most children will experience some degree of distress when faced with separation from home, particularly when they will not be accompanied by a parent. Predisposing factors to the depression and anxiety referred to as "homesickness" include young age, little prior separation experience, high parental separation anxiety, great perceived distance from home, few initial positive experiences after separation, preexisting anxiety or depression, and little perceived control over the situation.[71] Parents should introduce short periods of separation from home and family that lead up to longer periods. They should discuss the exciting aspects of the adventure to come and encourage active decision making regarding activities and destination. Parents should also alleviate their own separation anxiety and ensure positive early postseparation experiences for their child. The presence of familiar faces, such as friends or favorite playmates, can significantly reduce a child's feeling of homesickness. The child will remember favorite games and meals as fun experiences.

REFERENCES

1. American Academy of Pediatrics: The management of acute gastroenteritis in young children, *Pediatrics* 97:424, 1996.
2. AAP Guidelines: Prevention of rotavirus disease: guidelines for use of rotavirus vaccine, *Pediatrics* 102:1483, 1998.
3. Banks B et al: Attitudes of teenagers toward sun exposure and sunscreen use, *Pediatrics* 89:40, 1992.
4. Barry M: Medical considerations for international travel with infants and older children, *Infect Dis Clin North Am* 6:389, 1992.
5. Bonadio WA: Acute infectious enteritis in children, *Emerg Med Clin North Am* 13:457, 1995.
6. Brasseur P et al: Multi-drug resistant falciparum malaria. In Cameroon 1987-88, *Am J Trop Med Hyg* 46:8, 1992.
7. Bronstein AC, Russell FE, Sullivan JB: Negative pressure suction in the field treatment of rattlesnake bite victims, *Vet Hum Toxicol* 28:485, 1986.
8. Buchanan BJ, Hoagland J, Fischer PR: Pseudoephedrine and air travel–associated ear pain in children. In *Program and abstracts of the 5th International Conference on Travel Medicine*, Geneva, 1997.
9. Claeson M, Merson MH: Global progress in the control of diarrheal diseases, *Pediatr Infect Dis J* 9:345, 1990.
10. Dexter W: Hypothermia, *Postgrad Med* 88:55, 1990.
11. Doern GV et al: Prevalence of antimicrobial resistance among respiratory tract isolates of *Streptococcus pneumoniae* in North America: 1997 results from SENTRY antimicrobial surveillance program, *Clin Infect Dis* 27:764, 1998.
12. Dowell SF, Schwartz B, Phillips WR: Appropriate use of antibiotics for URIs in children. Part I. Otitis media and acute sinusitis, *Am Fam Physician* 58:1113, 1998.
13. Dowell SF, Schwartz B, Phillips WR: Appropriate use of antibiotics for URIs in children. Part II. Cough, pharyngitis and the common cold, *Am Fam Physician* 58:133, 1998.
14. Downey D, Omer G, Moheb M: New Mexico rattlesnake bites: demographic review and guidelines for treatment, *J Trauma* 31:1380, 1991.
15. Duggan C et al: How valid are clinical signs of dehydration in infants? *J Pediatr Gastroenterol Nutr* 22:56, 1996.
16. DuPont HL: Diarrheal disease in the developing world, *Infect Dis Clin North Am* 9:313, 1995.
17. Ericsson CD et al: Treatment of travelers' diarrhea with sulfamethoxazole and trimethoprim and loperamide, *JAMA* 263:257, 1990.
18. Faruque ASG et al: Randomized, controlled, clinical trial of rice versus glucose oral rehydration solutions in infants and young children with acute watery diarrhoea, *Acta Paediatr* 86:1308, 1997.
19. Fayad IM et al: Comparative efficacy of rice-based and glucose-based oral rehydration salts plus early reintroduction of food, *Lancet* 342:772, 1993.
20. Fischer PR: Travel with infants and children, *Infect Dis Clin North Am* 12:355, 1998.
21. Foster JA, Watson B, Bell LM: Travel with infants and children, *Emerg Med Clin North Am* 15:71, 1997.
22. Gallagher R: Suntan, sunburn, and pigmentation factors and the frequency of acquired melanocytic nevi in children, *Arch Dermatol* 126:770, 1990.
23. Gavin N, Merrick N, Davidson B: Efficacy of glucose-based rehydration therapy, *Pediatrics* 98:45, 1996.
24. Gentile DA, Kennedy BC: Wilderness medicine for children, *Pediatrics* 88:967, 1991.
25. Goepp J, Santosham M: Oral rehydration therapy, *Principles Pract Pediatr Updates* 1:1, 1993.
26. Grissom CK et al: Acetazolamide in the treatment of acute mountain sickness: clinical efficacy and effect on gas exchange. Abstract from Sixth Annual Scientific Meeting of the Wilderness Medical Society, 1990, Snowbird, Utah.
27. Guarino A et al: Oral bacterial therapy reduces the duration of symptoms and of viral excretion in children with mild diarrhea, *J Pediatr Gastroenterol Nutr* 25:516, 1997.
28. Guidelines for cardiopulmonary resuscitation and emergency cardiac care, *JAMA* 268:2199, 1992.
29. Hoge CW et al: Trends in antibiotic resistance among diarrheal pathogen isolates in Thailand over fifteen years, *Clin Infect Dis* 26:341, 1998.
30. Hughes G: Synergistic effects of oral nonsteroidal drugs and topical corticosteroids in the therapy of sunburn in humans, *Dermatology* 184:54, 1992.
31. Kaidbey K: The photoprotective potential of the new superpotent sunscreens, *J Am Acad Dermatol* 22:449, 1990.
32. Kaplan LA: Wilderness dermatology: an overview. Abstract from Third Annual Winter Meeting on Wilderness Medicine, 1993, Sun Valley, Idaho.
33. Katsambas A, Nicolaidou E: Cutaneous malignant melanoma and sun exposure: recent developments in epidemiology, *Arch Dermatol* 132:444, 1996.
34. Kelly K et al: Profound accidental hypothermia and freeze injury of the extremities in a child, *Crit Care Med* 18:679, 1990.
35. Kleinman R: We have the solution: now what's the problem? *Pediatrics* 90:113, 1992.
36. Klocke DL, Decker WW, Stepanek J: Altitude-related illness, *Mayo Clin Proc* 73:988, 1998.
37. Lell B et al: Randomised placebo-controlled study of atovaquone plus proguanil for malaria prophylaxis in children, *Lancet* 351:709, 1998.
38. Litovitz TL et al: 1995 annual report of the American Association of Poison Control Centers toxic exposure surveillance systems, *Am J Emerg Med* 14:487, 1996.
39. Lobel HO, Kozarsky PE: Update on the prevention of malaria for travelers, *JAMA* 278:1767, 1997.
40. Longworth DL: Drug-resistant malaria in children and in travelers, *Pediatr Clin North Am* 42:649, 1995.
41. Looareesuwan S et al: Clinical studies of atovaquone alone or in combination with other antimalaria drugs, for treatment of acute uncomplicated malaria in Thailand, *Am J Trop Med Hyg* 54:62, 1996.
42. The management of acute diarrhea in children: oral rehydration, maintenance, and nutritional therapy, *MMWR* 41, 1992.
43. Mason WH: The management of common infections in ambulatory children, *Pediatr Ann* 25:620, 1996.
44. Meyer F et al: Drink composition and the electrolyte balance of children exercising in the heat, *Med Sci Sport Exerc* 27:882, 1995.
45. Molina S et al: Clinical trial of glucose–oral rehydration solution (ORS), rice-dextrin ORS, and rice flour ORS of the management of children with acute diarrhea and mild or moderate dehydration, *Pediatrics* 95:191, 1995.
46. Mota-Hernandez F: Rice solution and World Health Organization solution by gastric infusion for high stool output diarrhea, *Am J Dis Child* 145:937, 1991.
47. Newman LM et al: Pediatric wilderness recreational deaths in western Washington state, *Ann Emerg Med* 32:687, 1998.
48. *Pertussis: report of the Committee on Infectious Disease*, Elk Grove Village, Ill, 1991, American Academy of Pediatrics.
49. *Physicians' desk reference*, ed 46, Montvale, NJ, 1992, Medical Economics Data.
50. Pitzinger B: Incidence and clinical features of traveler's diarrhea in infants and children, *Pediatr Infect Dis J* 10:719, 1991.
51. Pope D et al: Benign pigmented nevi in children, *Arch Dermatol* 128:1201, 1992.
52. Radloff PD et al: Atovaquone and proguanil for *Plasmodium falciparum* malaria, *Lancet* 347:1511, 1996.
53. Rahnan A: Rice-ORS shortens the duration of watery diarrhoeas, *Trop Geogr Med*, 1990, p 230.
54. *Red book: report of the Committee on Infectious Disease*, Elk Grove Village, Ill, 1997, American Academy of Pediatrics.

55. Reyes I, Shoff WH: General medical advice for travelers, *Emerg Med Clin North Am* 15:1, 1997.

56. Rivara FP, Aitken M: Prevention of injuries to children and adolescents, *Adv Pediatr* 45:37, 1998.

57. Salahuddin S: A traditional diet as part of oral rehydration therapy in severe acute diarrhoea in young children, *J Diarrhoeal Dis Res* 9:258, 1991.

58. Santosham M: A comparison of rice-based oral rehydration solution and "early feeding" for the treatment of acute diarrhea in infants, *J Pediatr* 166:868, 1990.

59. Santosham M et al: A double-blind clinical trial comparing World Health Organization oral rehydration solution with a reduced osmolarity solution containing equal amounts of sodium and glucose, *Pediatrics* 128:45, 1996.

60. Schaad U: Role of the new quinolones in pediatric practice, *Pediatr Infect Dis J* 11:1043, 1992.

61. Schaad UB et al: Use of fluoroquinolones in pediatrics: consensus report of the International Society of Chemotherapy commission, *Pediatr Infect Dis J* 14:1, 1995.

62. Schumacher MJ, Tveten MS, Egen NB: Rate and quantity of delivery of venom from honeybee stings, *J Allergy Clin Immunol* 93:831, 1994.

63. Shanks GD, Gordon DM, Klotz FW: Efficacy and safety of atovaquone plus proguanil as suppressive prophylaxis for *Plasmodium falciparum* malaria, *Clin Infect Dis* 27:494, 1998.

64. Sood SK et al: Duration of tick attachment as a predictor of the risk of Lyme disease in an area in which Lyme disease is endemic, *J Infect Dis* 175:996, 1997.

65. *Sports participation in 1990: series 1*, Mt Prospect, Ill, 1990, National Sporting Goods Association.

66. Squire DL: Heat illness: fluid and electrolyte issues for pediatric and adolescent athletes, *Pediatr Clin North Am* 37:1085, 1990.

67. Talan DA: Update on antibiotic treatment of emergency department and outpatient infections. Abstract from Stanford Symposium on Emergency Medicine and Acute Care, 1999, Maui, Hawaii.

68. Talan DA, Citron DM, Abrahamian FM: Bacteriological analysis of infected dog and cat bites: emergency medicine animal bite infection study group, *N Engl J Med* 340:85, 1999.

69. Thanassi WT, Weiss EL: Immunizations and travel, *Emerg Med Clin North Am* 15:43, 1997.

70. Theis MK et al: Acute mountain sickness in children at 2835 meters, *Am J Dis Child* 147:143, 1993.

71. Thurber CA, Sigman MD: Preliminary models of risk and protective factors for childhood homesickness: review and empirical synthesis, *Child Dev* 69:903, 1998.

72. *Treatment of diarrhoea: manual for physicians and other senior health workers*, Geneva, 1995, World Health Organization.

73. Visscher PK, Vetter RS, Camazine S: Removing bee stings, *Lancet* 348:301, 1996.

74. White R, Weber R: Poisonous snakebite in Central Texas, *Ann Surg* 213:466, 1991.

75. Wyler D: Malaria chemoprophylaxis for the traveler, *N Engl J Med* 329:31, 1993.

76. Zanetti R: Cutaneous melanoma and sunburns in childhood in a southern European population, *Eur J Cancer* 28A:1172, 1992.

77. Zinman R et al: Predictors of sunscreen use in childhood, *Arch Pediatr Adolesc Med* 149:804, 1995.

SUGGESTED READINGS

Brody J: *Jane Brody's good food book*, New York, 1987, Bantam.

Castle S: *The complete new guide to preparing baby foods*, New York, 1992, Bantam.

Foster L: *Take a hike!* San Francisco, 1991, Sierra Club.

Hodgson M: *Wilderness with children*, Harrisburg, Pa, 1992, Stackpole Books.

Ross C, Gladfelter T: *Kids in the wild*, Seattle, 1995, Mountaineers.

Silverman G: *Backpacking with babies and small children*, Berkeley, Calif, 1986, Wilderness Press.

75 Women in the Wilderness

Kenneth F. Trofatter, Jr., and Barbara D. Dahl

Problems common and unique to a woman might diminish the wilderness experience or place her at risk. This chapter emphasizes a practical approach to the evaluation, management, and impact assessment of gynecologic and obstetric conditions of women undertaking short-term or long-term wilderness activities. A framework is provided for the diagnosis and the selection of empiric therapy, based on historical and physical observations, under circumstances in which limited medical care and resources are available. Preexisting conditions are also addressed, with consideration of access to a medical facility in the field.

PREPARATION FOR THE WILDERNESS EXPERIENCE

The goal of preparation is to anticipate and recognize problems rather than to address them for the first time under suboptimal circumstances. A high priority is to identify medical problems that could be exacerbated by physical demands and the wilderness setting. These must be evaluated in relation to characteristics of the environment, length of the excursion, additional conditioning and acclimation, and difficulty in accessing more sophisticated medical care. For physically challenging conditions and prolonged stays, women should undergo thorough medical assessment (Box 75-1).

After historical information is collected, a comprehensive physical examination is performed, with special attention to the cardiovascular and respiratory systems, musculoskeletal system, genitourinary tract, and breasts. Other recommended tests include: Pap smear, vaginitis screening, pregnancy test, urinalysis, hemoglobin/hematocrit (Hgb/Hct), and urine culture and screening for sexually transmitted infections (STIs) and hepatitis. Additional screening, as indicated by age, medical status, and risk factors, include electrocardiogram (ECG) with stress testing, pulmonary function tests, mammogram if over age 40 or with strong family history of breast cancer, and thyroid panel. Bone densitometry should be considered in perimenopausal and postmenopausal women and in young women with a history of fractures or abnormal menses consistent with a hypoestrogenic state.

In anticipation of a wilderness trip, supplemental iron, vitamins, and calcium are recommended (Table 75-1). Maintenance medications should provide optimal control of medical conditions and cover planned time, emergency needs, and expected dose adjustments. Contraceptive needs should be reviewed and options explored. Hormonal replacement therapy should be discussed with postmenopausal women at risk for osteoporosis. Box 75-2 lists basic supplies for hygienic and anticipated therapeutic needs. Special considerations for pregnancy are discussed in a separate section.

PHYSIOLOGIC ADAPTATIONS

Women at Altitude

Recent studies have found no difference in the incidence of acute mountain sickness (AMS) in women and men.[57] Differences in how men and women respond to altitude may be hormonally mediated. Adaptation to high altitude involves a series of physiologic responses triggered by hypoxemia. The sigmoidal shape of the oxyhemoglobin dissociation curve prevents a drop in the oxygen saturation below 90% until an altitude of about 2400 m (8000 feet) in healthy individuals. At higher altitudes, hypoxia stimulates respiratory, cardiovascular, and hematologic changes that depend on both degree of hypoxia and time.

The earliest and probably most important response to altitude is an increase in minute ventilation caused by increases in tidal volume and respiratory rate. This hypoxic ventilatory response (HVR) is mediated by chemoreceptors in the carotid bodies, which respond to a decrease in arterial oxygen pressure (PaO_2) and signal the respiratory center in the medulla to increase ventilation.[141] HVR has been closely related to adequacy of acclimatization and the risk of developing AMS.[58,83,135] The degree of HVR to a given PaO_2 varies among individuals and is genetically influenced. The HVR is inhibited by respiratory depressants, such as alcohol and sedatives and stimulated by respiratory stimulants, such as caffeine and cocoa. Progesterone is a potent respiratory stimulant and acts primarily through activation of peripheral arterial chemoreceptors.[26,60,61]

Progesterone is produced by all steroid-forming glands, including the ovaries, testes, and adrenal cortex, and by the corpus luteum and placenta in the pregnant female. Ovariectomy in female cats lowers the carotid sinus nerve response to hypoxia and likewise decreases HVR, although translation of carotid nerve activity in the central nervous system (CNS) into ventilation was similar in ovariectomized and intact animals.[152] Exogenous progesterone and estrogen administration to male rats living at 3600 m (12000 feet)

Box 75-1 ASSESSMENT OF A WOMAN'S HEALTH: SCREENING HIGHLIGHTS

Menstrual history: age of menarche, regularity, characteristics, timing, extent of blood flow (length, amount), intermenstrual bleeding, perimenstrual symptoms (e.g., dysmenorrhea, headache, premenstrual syndrome), plans for managing periods (hygienic, therapeutic)

Sexual history: age of coitarche, number of partners, sexual orientation, sexually transmitted infections, contraceptive history, plans for sexual activity in the wilderness, dyspareunia

Gynecologic history: ovarian cysts, uterine fibroids, endometriosis, cervical dysplasia, surgical history, pelvic pain, vaginal discharge, vaginal infections and treatment, pregnancy and complications

Breast: galactorrhea, discharge, masses, surgery

Gastrointestinal/urinary tract: ulcers, irritable bowel syndrome, gallbladder disease, constipation, urinary tract infections, kidney stones, stress incontinence, urgency incontinence

Musculoskeletal/skin: injuries (exercise related and accidents), limitations, muscle cramps, joint pain and swelling, arthritis, rashes, acne, sun sensitivity, hirsutism, hair loss

Exposure to abuse: battering, sexual harassment, sexual assault

Habits: smoking, alcohol, illicit drug use

Current problems: condition, medications, status of control, complications

Immunizations: measles, mumps, rubella, polio, diphtheria, tetanus, hepatitis, others

Family history: thyroid disease, hypertension, autoimmune disorders, diabetes, breast and gynecologic malignancies, osteoporosis

Allergies: general, drug related, bite and sting sensitivity

Nutritional: eating disorders, weight changes, food sensitivities, dietary preference (e.g., vegetarianism), caloric intake, assessment of mineral and vitamin intake in diet, supplements (e.g., iron, vitamins, calcium) including homeopathic compounds

Box 75-2 BASIC SUPPLIES FOR WOMEN'S HYGIENE

STANDARD

Sanitary napkins or tampons (store in plastic bag)

Toilet paper (store in plastic bag)

Cotton underwear

Matches or cigarette lighter (to burn toilet paper after use)

Plastic trowel (to bury feces)

Toiletries (soap, small towel, toothbrush and paste, dental floss, comb)

Moisturizing lotion (unscented, to prevent skin chapping/cracking)

OPTIONAL

Urinal guide (if long periods of poor weather are anticipated)

Vaginal speculum and gloves (if trained medical professional accompanies expedition)

Premoistened towelettes (convenient for cleaning/ washing when water is limited or weather precludes bathing)

TABLE 75-1. Examples of Medications for Women's Health

INDICATION	MEDICATION*	DOSE
Nutritional supplements	Ferrous sulfate	300 mg qd-tid
	Calcium carbonate	1250 mg qd
	Multivitamin	1 tablet qd
Headache/pain	Acetaminophen	325 mg, 1 or 2 q3-4h
Dysmenorrhea/pain	Ibuprofen	200 mg, 1-4 q4-6h
Nausea/vomiting	Promethazine (tablet or suppository)	25 mg q4-6h
Urinary tract infection	Ampicillin	250-500 mg qid
	Trimethoprim/sulfamethoxazole	160 mg/800 mg bid
Yeast vulvovaginitis	Miconazole (cream or suppository)	One applicator hs × 3-7 days
	Fluconazole	150 mg single dose
Bacterial vaginosis	Metronidazole (tablets)	250-500 mg bid-tid
	Metronidazole or clindamycin (vaginal gel)	One applicator hs × 3-7 days
Urine pregnancy test kit	As needed	
Menstrual regulation or breakthrough bleeding	Conjugated estrogen (Premarin)	2.5 mg qd
	Medroxyprogesterone acetate	5-10 mg qd

qd, Daily; *bid,* twice daily; *tid,* three times daily; *qid,* four times daily; *q,* every; *h,* hour; *hs,* at bedtime.
*Suggested medications or equivalent depending on tolerance, allergy history, and patient preferences.

significantly inhibited norepinephrine and dopamine turnover in the carotid sinus, thus stimulating the afferent chemoreflex.[44] In pregnant females, HVR is enhanced and most likely driven by higher progesterone levels. Mean P_{O_2} value at 4,400 m (14,500 feet) in nonpregnant women is 51 mm Hg (carbon dioxide pressure [P_{CO_2}] 28 mm Hg) vs. 59 mm Hg (P_{CO_2} 23 mm Hg) in pregnant women.[64] Increased ventilation is a key factor in adapting to altitude in pregnancy, as evidenced by the linear correlation between birth weight and maternal ventilatory rate.[110] Despite higher levels of progesterone in women, particularly in the luteal phase of the menstrual cycle, when progesterone levels increase approximately tenfold, no difference has been observed between males and nonpregnant females in the incidence of AMS, although one study has reported a lower incidence of gastrointestinal (GI) and cardiovascular symptoms in females vs. males at altitude.[57,62] To date, no study has been done comparing HVR and the incidence of AMS in premenopausal women in follicular vs. luteal phases.

Cardiovascular adaptations to altitude also occur early and are mediated by release of catecholamines. Hypoxia stimulates a sympathoadrenal release of epinephrine and norepinephrine, resulting in elevated heart rate, cardiac output, and mean arterial pressure (MAP). This catecholamine-mediated response was studied in females at 4300 m (14,000 feet). Norepinephrine levels rose steadily during the initial days at altitude, reached a plateau at 4 to 6 days, and remained elevated for the duration at altitude.[97] Norepinephrine levels correlated with increased heart rate and MAP. This response, previously demonstrated in males, reflects elevation in whole body sympathetic nerve activity at altitude.[95,96] No difference was found in the sympathetic response to hypoxia between follicular-phase and luteal-phase subjects; however, for a given norepinephrine level, heart rates and MAPs were lower for follicular vs. luteal subjects, possibly reflecting effects of hypoxia and ovarian hormones on adrenergic receptors.

Other circulatory changes at altitude include decreased plasma volume from dehydration, increased insensible water loss, and fluid shifts into the extravascular space. Euvolemia is usually regained with adequate hydration and acclimatization.[52] Also, hypoxic pulmonary vasoconstriction results in increased pulmonary vascular resistance and increased pulmonary artery pressure. Cerebral blood flow (CBF) also increases at altitude. Although hypoxic vasodilation and hypocapnic vasoconstriction both contribute to regulating CBF, the hypoxic response is thought to dominate at altitudes over 3800 m (12,500 feet).[71,125]

Hematologic changes occur at altitude in response to hypoxia. Within hours, erythropoietin levels increase, with red blood cell mass increasing a few days later. The higher the altitude, the greater the increase in Hct and blood viscosity, which may actually be detrimental to oxygen transport despite an increase in O_2-carrying capacity.[70] This hypoxia-induced polycythemia is associated with chronic mountain sickness.[150] Recent animal studies suggest that, under hypoxic conditions, female ovarian hormones reduce erythropoietin levels and hypoxic-induced polycythemia.[44] It is not known whether this hormonally mediated effect is significant in human females at altitude.

Hot and Cold Environments

Because of the lower sweat rate in females compared with males, women rely more heavily on dimensional characteristics and circulatory mechanisms for heat dissipation in hot environments.[137,138] Females adapt more easily to hot, wet environments than do males because of this lower sweat rate and decreased risk of dehydration.[9,98] In hot, dry environments, however, a higher sweat rate is advantageous because perspiration decreases the risk of hyperthermia, provided adequate fluid replacement is available. With acclimation to dry heat, women are able to increase the sudorific response to equal that of men.[165] With similar acclimatization and physical training, women tolerate physical activity in hot environments at least as well as men.[51,63,69] Thus women planning wilderness expeditions to hot, dry destinations are advised to plan a 1- to 2-week acclimation period in a hot environment.[10]

Adaptation of females to hot temperatures may also depend on menstrual phases. Some evidence suggests that women in the follicular phase of the menstrual cycle may adapt better to hot environments than women in the luteal phase. The resting core temperature in women is approximately 0.4° C higher during the luteal phase than during the follicular phase.[49] Also, the threshold core temperature for the onset of thermoregulatory responses, such as sweating and vasodilation, is increased during the luteal phase. Therefore women in the luteal phase may have more difficulty in reaching thermal equilibrium in hot environments.[29,122]

In moderately cold environments, women on average adapt better than men, partly because of thicker subcutaneous fat. At extreme cold temperatures, however, women may be at a disadvantage because of the decrease in insulation from lower muscle mass. Although adaptation to cold environments depends more on body size, physical fitness, and degree of acclimation than on gender, exercise performed during cold exposure may be more effective in maintaining body heat in women than men.[55,99]

CONTRACEPTION

Women of reproductive age who anticipate having a heterosexual relationship while in the wilderness should strongly consider a reliable and convenient form of contraception, especially for extended excursions (Box 75-3). Pregnancy is a relative contraindica-

---

Box 75-3 CONTRACEPTIVE OPTIONS

HORMONAL

Oral contraceptives

Monophasic combination pills
Multiphasic combination pills
Monophasic progestin-only pills

Injectable

Depo-Provera (medroxyprogesterone), 150 mg intramuscularly every 3 months

Implantable

Norplant system (levonorgestrel), six Silastic implants subcutaneously

BARRIER

Condom and spermicide
Diaphragm and spermicide
Contraceptive sponge
Cervical cap and spermicide
Female condom

INTRAUTERINE DEVICE (IUD)

ParaGard-T (copper enveloped)
Progestasert system (IUD containing progesterone)

EMERGENCY CONTRACEPTION

Preven (0.05 mg ethinyl estradiol + 0.25 mg levonorgestrel/tablet), two tablets within 72 hours postexposure; repeat dose in 12 hours

---

tion to both brief and prolonged wilderness experiences because of the frequent, inconvenient, and life-threatening complications that can occur. Any form of hormonal contraception or an intrauterine device should be used for at least 3 months before departure to minimize risk of complications.

Hormonal Contraceptives

Combination (estrogen and progestin) oral contraceptives (OCs), either monophasic or multiphasic, offer the most reliable, convenient, cost-effective, and sensible risk/benefit ratio for the healthy reproductive-age woman. Brand selection should be done with a qualified health care professional. Previous experience of use, complications of therapy, menstrual history, and skin type should be considered. For example, women with histories of irregular cycles and polycystic ovary syndrome may be better suited to brands with low androgenic side effects. Failure rates with optimal use are extremely low (1%), but may be worsened by concomitant drug therapy, substance abuse, chronic GI disturbance, and changes in dietary habits or weight.[160] Common side effects include nausea, vomiting, weight gain,

and breakthrough bleeding. Other potential benefits include normalization of cycles, fewer midcycle ovulatory (i.e., mittelschmerz) and perimenstrual (e.g., dysmenorrhea, headaches) symptoms, lighter menstrual flow, suppression of ovarian cyst formation, reduced risk for endometrial cancer, prevention of osteoporosis, and increased bone mass. OCs may decrease the risk of acquiring certain STIs but cannot be relied on for this. Major contraindications include history of thromboembolic disease, certain autoimmune disorders with thromboembolic risk factors, uncontrolled hypertension, hepatic dysfunction, and cigarette smoking.[50,105,164] If a thrombotic or thromboembolic event is suspected in the field, OC use should be suspended and aspirin taken while awaiting evacuation. High altitude is a potential risk factor for thromboembolic events, but increased risk from use of OCs or hormonal replacement therapy has not been systematically studied. As a precaution, women planning high-altitude excursions should consider a combination pill containing the lowest dose of ethinyl estradiol (20 μg) or its equivalent.

Progestin-only OCs are not generally recommended for the wilderness traveler because of higher failure rates (4% to 9%), increased frequency of irregular and unpredictable bleeding, and potentially deleterious effects on bone density over time from suppression of ovarian estrogen production. The progestin-only injectable Depo-Provera (medroxyprogesterone) and the implantable Norplant system (six Silastic capsules containing levonorgestrel, 36 mg/capsule) have similar drawbacks. Although extremely convenient for maintenance contraception, problems include weight gain, irregular bleeding, headache, fatigue, and abdominal pain, especially early in therapy.[129,140] Prolonged use of progestin-only methods may be associated with reduced bone mass, which could be hazardous for women involved in strenuous physical activities.[151]

Depo-Provera (150 mg intramuscularly) is administered every 3 months, so extended wilderness experiences would necessitate transport and storage of the drug in its glass container and syringes for administration. Once Depo-Provera is injected, it cannot be removed. Side effects and complications, such as irregular bleeding, must be dealt with for an indefinite period, possibly a year or longer, until its effects on the hypothalamic-pituitary axis have dissipated. Similarly, once the Norplant system is placed, it cannot be readily removed in a wilderness setting unless a trained health care provider and adequate surgical supplies are available. Furthermore, subcutaneous location of the 34-mm capsules, usually on the inner aspects of the upper arm, could be traumatized by certain strenuous wilderness activities. Once implants are removed, however, cyclic hormonal activity and menstruation return almost immediately.

Irregular bleeding with a long-term progestin-only OC can usually be managed with oral estrogen (e.g., Premarin, 2.5 mg daily) for 21 to 25 days sequentially. Estrogen administration results in rapid cessation of bleeding. Within days after discontinuation, a menstrual-like withdrawal bleed should occur in the continued presence of the progestin. If the withdrawal bleed persists beyond the length of a normal period, or if irregular bleeding recurs and persists, the course of estrogen therapy is simply repeated for another cycle. No withdrawal bleed indicates that progestin has fallen below biologically active levels, with unreliable contraceptive activity.

Barrier Contraceptives

The barrier contraceptive methods have the widest safety profile, excluding latex allergy and method failure resulting in pregnancy, but all have the same disadvantages for regular use in a wilderness setting. Failure rates even under ideal use with a spermicidal foam or gel are relatively high, estimated at 20% with "typical use" and 6% to 9% with "perfect use." The compounds in barrier devices are variably susceptible to extremes of heat or cold, which may compromise their tensile strength and effectiveness. Some couples find these methods inconvenient and messy which might discourage compliance in an environment not conducive to cleanup. Bulk and weight complicate transport of sufficient spermicidal compound. Barrier methods decrease risk of gonorrhea, chlamydial infection, and human immunodeficiency virus (HIV) but offer minimal protection against human papillomavirus (HPV) or genital herpes simplex virus (HSV).

Intrauterine Devices

An intrauterine device (IUD) is a highly effective and convenient form of contraception, especially for the parous woman in a stable relationship.[38,47] Ideally it should be inserted at least 3 months before departure. Complications occur most often within the first month after initial insertion and when the device is replaced. IUDs are occasionally associated with increased menstrual flow, dysmenorrhea, intermenstrual spotting, and expulsion. However, the ParaGard-T copper-enveloped IUD and the Progestasert system, which has a reservoir with 36 mg of progesterone and conforms to the endometrial cavity, carry minimal risk for these side effects. Once inserted, the ParaGard-T is effective for 10 years or longer. The Progestasert system requires annual replacement.

The most serious risk, affecting 1% of IUD users, is acute or indolent pelvic infection that might become clinically significant and even life threatening in the wilderness. The risk for this is greatest within the first month after insertion or replacement and among women at increased risk for STIs. Women with multiple partners, previous pelvic infections, unrecognized chlamydial infection or gonorrhea, recurrent episodes of bacterial vaginosis, or tobacco use are at highest risk.[113] When acute pelvic inflammatory disease (PID) occurs, with lower abdominopelvic pain, peritoneal signs, purulent vaginal discharge, and fever, the IUD should be removed immediately by simple traction on the string protruding from the external cervical os. Broad-spectrum antibiotics should be started. Evacuation is mandatory when the device cannot be removed. Pelvic infection should be suspected, even without fever and peritoneal signs, if irregular bleeding occurs, particularly when accompanied by pelvic discomfort and discharge. When the IUD is removed at this stage, the infection may respond to therapy with oral or simple parenteral antibiotics (see later discussion).

Another potentially serious risk for IUD users is pregnancy, occurring in approximately one of 100 users per year. Both intrauterine and extrauterine (ectopic) pregnancies can occur with an IUD in place. Unfortunately, the latter is more common, but the risk is still only half that in women who use no contraception. Confirmed or suspected pregnancy in a woman with an IUD is an indication for immediate evacuation.

Emergency Contraception

In the event of unanticipated or careless sexual activity, suspected contraceptive failure, or sexual assault, consideration should be given to emergency postcoital contraception.[53,54] In the wilderness setting the only practical approach is hormonal therapy, ideally starting within 72 hours after exposure. Preven and several combination OCs reduce the risk of pregnancy by at least 75%.[157,158] Treatment regimens with standard OC formulations include Ovral (0.05 mg ethinyl estradiol and 0.50 mg norgestrel), two tablets; Lo-Ovral (0.03 mg ethinyl estradiol and 0.30 mg norgestrel), four tablets; and Nordette or Levlen (0.03 mg ethinyl estradiol and 0.15 mg levonorgestrel), four tablets. The dose is repeated 12 hours later. Common side effects include nausea, vomiting, irregular bleeding, cramping, and headache, but these are usually transient and can be managed symptomatically. Administering an antiemetic 1 hour before each dose is recommended.[7]

SEXUAL ASSAULT

Sexual assault of women in the wilderness is fortunately a rare occurrence. Wilderness morbidity and mortality statistics are limited, but one study of eight National Park Service areas in California over 3 years reported only one incident of sexual assault.[108] Many incidents are probably not reported, however, since only 7% of all rapes are reported.[35]

The best defense against sexual assault is not going into the wilderness with unfamiliar people. The chance of meeting an assailant is quite low. A woman traveling into the wilderness alone or with someone she does not know well is advised to tell friends or family exactly where and with whom she is traveling and when she anticipates returning.

If sexually assaulted, the woman is advised to seek medical attention as soon as possible. Most emergency departments are prepared to handle the evaluation and treatment of sexual assault victims. It may be impossible to reach a medical facility for many hours or even days, but an attempt should be made to preserve potential evidence. If a medical facility can be reached in a few hours, the woman should try not to eat, drink, urinate, or defecate. Women are also advised to avoid douching, gargling, brushing teeth, or changing clothes. If clothes are removed, clothes should be placed in a paper bag and brought to the medical facility.

VAGINITIS

Vaginitis is a frequent indication for seeking medical care and a common incidental finding at gynecologic evaluation. Although rarely dangerous in healthy women, vaginitis can compromise the wilderness experience. Environmental conditions and constraints on hygiene can contribute to vaginitis and diminish the efficacy of therapy. Self-diagnosis of vaginitis is often incorrect, leading to inappropriate treatment selection.

In premenopausal women, more than 90% of infectious causes of vaginitis are bacterial vaginosis (40% to 50%), candidiasis (20% to 25%), and trichomoniasis (15% to 20%). Symptoms include vaginal discharge, itching, erythema, and irritation of the vagina, introitus,

and vulva. Therefore most vaginitis of clinical significance is more accurately described as vulvovaginitis. Severe manifestations are intense discomfort, swelling, dyspareunia, dysuria, and urinary retention. The medical history, pelvic examination, and evaluation of vaginal fluid provide the diagnosis of vaginitis (Table 75-2). Recent evidence suggests that accurate diagnosis of the most common causes of vaginitis can often be done without a vaginal speculum.[22] Because diagnostic capabilities in the wilderness are limited, clinical features can help guide diagnosis and treatment of vaginitis and improve the chance of therapeutic success.

Bacterial Vaginosis

Bacterial vaginosis (BV) is the most prevalent cause of vaginitis, affecting as many as two thirds of women attending sexually transmitted disease (STD) clinics and 12% to 25% of premenopausal women undergoing gynecologic evaluation. The most common complaints of women with BV are discharge and odor, itching, and irritation of the vulva and vagina. More than 50% of women with BV do not complain of symptoms or are unaware that symptoms result from a treatable condition.

The cause of BV is uncertain and may be multifactorial. BV is characterized by an overgrowth (100 to 1000-fold) of bacterial species in the vagina and GI tract and a dramatic reduction in lactobacilli, especially the predominant hydrogen peroxide–producing species.[155] The organisms implicated in BV are risk factors for upper genital tract infection, premature labor and delivery, and postoperative wound infections in women.[30]

TABLE 75-2. Differential Diagnosis of Vulvovaginitis

FACTORS	NORMAL	BACTERIAL VAGINOSIS	VULVOVAGINAL CANDIDIASIS	TRICHO-MONIASIS	ATROPHIC VAGINITIS	OTHER
Discharge	White, clear, finely granular	Gray-white, thin, homogenous, adherent, frothy	White, thick, curdlike, adherent	Gray to yellow-green, occasionally frothy, adherent	Thin, clear to serosanguineous	Normal
pH	3.8 to 4.2	>4.5	≤4.5	>4.5	>4.5	3.8 to 4.2
Amine odor	Absent	Present	Absent	Variably present	Usually absent	Absent
Primary complaints	None	Malodorous discharge	Pruritus, irritation	Severe pruritus, discharge, dyspareunia, dysuria	Burning, soreness, dyspareunia	Burning, irritation, swelling, soreness
Microscopic appearance	Normal epithelial cells, lactobacilli	"Clue cells," no WBCs	Budding yeast, hyphae, spores	Trichomonads, many WBCs (PMNs)	Small, round (parabasal) epithelial cells, many PMNs	Normal
Other findings and diagnostic features	None	Minimal vulvar involvement	Vulvar and vaginal erythema, predisposing medical conditions	Intense vulvovaginal erythema, "strawberry cervix," other STIs	Atrophy of vulva and vaginal epithelium	Highly variable

WBCs, White blood cells; *PMNs,* polymorphonuclear neutrophil leukocytes; *STIs,* sexually transmitted infections.

Local defects in host immunity may contribute to recurrent and persistent cases.[31]

The discharge accompanying BV is typically thin, watery, grayish white, frothy, and homogenous (not flocculent), uniformly coating the vaginal walls and introitus. More than 50% of women with BV complain of a fishy odor, particularly during menstruation and immediately after unprotected sexual intercourse. Blood and semen can alkalinize the vagina and volatilize a variety of amines (e.g., cadaverine) produced by anaerobic organisms. The diagnosis of BV is confirmed by the presence of three of the following: (1) discharge, (2) pH greater than 4.5, (3) release of amines (fishy odor) when discharge is exposed to 10% potassium hydroxide (KOH) ("whiff test"), and (4) microscopic detection of "clue cells" (epithelial cells coated with bacteria) in saline solution. Microscopic appearance of pure BV is characterized by few if any leukocytes and few motile, curved rods (lactobacilli).

The antimicrobial agent most successful in treating BV is metronidazole, which can be administered orally (500 mg 2 or 3 times daily for 5 to 7 days) or as a 0.75% vaginal gel (once or twice daily for 5 days).[75] These regimens have initial response rates in excess of 90%. Single-dose oral treatment with metronidazole (2.0 g) yields initial response rates of 80% to 90% but is accompanied by higher recurrence rates within 1 month of treatment. This regimen should be considered when drug supplies are limited or when the GI side effects of oral metronidazole are not well tolerated. Clindamycin (300 to 600 mg orally twice daily for 5 to 7 days or 2% vaginal gel daily for 7 days) has comparable efficacy, but disadvantages are expense, deleterious effects on normal vaginal lactobacilli, and increased risk for pseudomembranous enterocolitis, which could be life-threatening in the wilderness. Cure rates of 67% have been achieved with ampicillin (250 to 500 mg 4 times daily for 7 days) and amoxicillin (250 to 500 four times daily for 7 days), but again, deleterious effects on the normal vaginal flora often are followed by an overgrowth of yeast organisms.

Yeast (Candida) Vaginitis

Symptomatic yeast infections, more often referred to as *vulvovaginal candidiasis* (VVC), are the second most frequent cause of vaginitis and account for about 25% of cases. From 80% to 90% of these result from overgrowth of *Candida albicans*. *C. glabrata* and *C. tropicalis* account for most of the remainder and are of growing concern because of increased resistance to over-the-counter (OTC) antifungal preparations used to treat presumed "yeast infections," an incorrect presumption more than half the time. Risk factors for yeast infections include pregnancy, hormonal therapy, recent antibiotic use, corticosteroid therapy, postovulatory phase of menstrual cycle, frequent coitus, condom use, and intravaginal use of spermicidal compounds.[41,128,142] The presence of gonorrhea, chlamydial infection, and BV are negative risk factors. Recurrent or recalcitrant yeast infections should suggest depressed cell-mediated immunity and frequently affect women with undiagnosed or poorly controlled diabetes, pregnancy, HIV infection, lymphoproliferative disorders, and autoimmune diseases.

The most common complaint of women with VVC is vulvar pruritus or burning, not vaginal discharge.[131] In more severe cases, redness, irritation, burning, soreness, swelling, and external dysuria are variably present. The characteristic white, flocculent ("cottage cheese"), adherent discharge is often diagnostic but is not consistently present or visible externally. The yeast discharge is thicker than that seen with BV or trichomoniasis, is usually not frothy or malodorous, and often has a pH of 4.5 or less, unless a mixed infection is present. About 50% of yeast infections are confirmed by direct microscopic examination of the discharge diluted in saline; however, diagnosis is most reliably accomplished by detection of budding yeast, hyphae, or spores using a slide preparation with 10% KOH added to lyse background epithelial cells and bacteria.

The foundation of treatment for VVC is a variety of azole derivatives, many of which (e.g., butoconazole, clotrimazole, miconazole, tioconazole) are available OTC as topical creams, vaginal tablets, and suppositories. Prescription compounds for local application do not provide a significant advantage over these in most cases. Therapy periods range from 1 to 14 days, depending on the formulation and severity of the infection. Generally a treatment regimen of at least 3 days results in a greater initial response rate and a lesser chance of immediate recurrence. Symptoms related to inflammatory vulvar involvement will respond most rapidly to the topical creams, although their application at first may be accompanied by burning pain. Oral fluconazole (150 mg, single dose) has been approved for VVC and is a convenient therapeutic agent to include in the basic pharmacopoeia of a wilderness expedition. Women with frequent recurrences or predictable outbreaks at specific times in their cycle, most often premenstrually, should consider prophylactic suppressive therapy with fluconazole (150 mg orally) or clotrimazole (500 mg vaginal tablet) weekly.

Trichomonas Vaginitis

Trichomonas vaginalis is a single-celled parasite that causes vaginitis in 2 to 3 million women annually in the United States.[67] It is predominantly sexually transmitted and is found most often in individuals with multiple sexual partners and those with a history of or current STIs. Diagnosis and treatment of a woman and her sexual partner are best accomplished at a screening visit before departure on a wilderness excursion. Unlike BV and yeast vaginitis, detection of *Trichomonas*, even in asymptomatic women, is an indication for treatment and for more complete STI screening.

Symptoms and physical findings accompanying *Trichomonas* infections are highly variable. The organism can be carried asymptomatically for extended periods, but most women will develop clinically significant disease over time, often during or immediately after menstruation. The most common complaints include severe vulvovaginal pruritus, dyspareunia, and dysuria. Physical examination often reveals intense erythema of the vagina and introitus and petechial lesions of the cervix ("strawberry cervix"). The vaginal discharge is typically gray or yellow-green, somewhat cloudy, and variably frothy and malodorous. The presence of the latter two findings frequently indicates a mixed infection with the amine-producing organisms seen in BV.[91] The pH of vaginal fluid is usually above 5.0 and frequently exceeds 6.0.

The clinical features of trichomoniasis overlap sufficiently with those of BV and yeast vaginitis to make them impractical alone for even presumptive diagnosis.[59] The diagnosis is confirmed by microscopic detection of the motile parasites on simple saline wet mount. Polymorphonuclear neutrophil leukocytes (PMNs) are usually present in high concentration and can interfere with microscopic diagnosis when the organisms are nonmotile. Under these circumstances, culture is now recognized as the most sensitive diagnostic technique, although not likely to be available in a wilderness setting.

Because of the diagnostic difficulties, empiric therapy is justified in the wilderness. Metronidazole is the only drug approved for trichomoniasis in the United States. It is administered in a single oral dose (2 g) and in severe cases or single-dose failures for a week (500 mg bid) or longer. For optimal results, sexual partners should be treated simultaneously and sexual activity curtailed during therapy. To minimize GI side effects, metronidazole should be taken with plenty of water. This may not reduce the unpleasant metallic taste but may reduce the risk of nausea, vomiting, and gastric irritation. Because a disulfiram-like effect is possible, alcohol should be avoided while taking metronidazole. At present, metronidazole 0.75% vaginal gel is not appropriate for treatment of trichomoniasis.

Atrophic Vaginitis

Atrophic vaginitis occurs in postmenopausal and hypoestrogenized premenopausal women, such as some amenorrheic athletes and women on ovarian suppressive therapy with gonadotropin-releasing hormone (GnRH) agonists. The presumed etiology is lost estrogen effect on the vaginal epithelium, accompanied by reduction in epithelial cell glycogen, an important substrate for lactobacilli, with subsequent overgrowth of nonacidophilic organisms. Symptoms include burning or soreness, dyspareunia, and vaginal discharge that is often watery or even serosanguineous.[21,120] It should be suspected in women of any age with vulvovaginal atrophy. Typically the vagina is uniformly erythematous

and may have areas of petechial changes. The pH of the vagina usually exceeds 5 (often 6 to 7) and microscopic evaluation of the discharge reveals small, round, immature epithelial cells (parabasal cells), increased PMNs, and a paucity of lactobacilli. Treatment includes the use of topical or oral estrogen replacement therapy.

Noninfectious Vulvovaginitis

Certain noninfectious causes of vulvovaginitis result from environmental exposures that cause local irritative or allergic reactions. These may be of greater significance when attention to personal hygiene is limited.[59] Common causative agents include latex condoms, spermicidal compounds, soaps, detergents, fabric softeners, deodorant products, menstrual pads and tampons, and topical medications such as antimycotics and povidone-iodine. Exclusion of an infectious etiology and identification of the source of the reaction usually make the diagnosis. Once a potentially offending cause, such as a recent change in laundry detergent, is identified, the first step in management is removal from exposure. Treatment is usually symptomatic (pain relief, antihistamines, Sitz baths). Topical corticosteroids are rarely indicated and may initially exacerbate symptoms.

URINARY TRACT INFECTIONS

In sexually active adolescent and adult women, bacterial bladder infections (cystitis) are the most common manifestation of urinary tract infection (UTI) and a frequent source of medical complaints.[16] They occur more frequently in women than men, presumably because of the shorter length of the urethra, its location in proximity to the vagina and enclosed within the introitus, and trauma secondary to sexual activity. Women with recurrent vaginitis, particularly BV; congenital or acquired genitourinary tract abnormalities; diaphragm use and use of spermicidal compounds; poor hygiene; and cigarette abuse are at increased risk for developing UTIs, as are pregnant women.[45,56,120,153] About 5% of pregnant women develop asymptomatic bacteriuria, 20% of whom progress to upper tract disease. Wilderness conditions, with restricted access to fluid, deferred voiding, and less attention to personal hygiene, increase the potential for development of UTIs. Attention to maintenance of urinary tract health should be a primary goal of the female wilderness traveler.

Common symptoms of cystitis include urinary frequency, urgency, dysuria, hematuria, foul-smelling or cloudy urine, and low back discomfort.[68,90] Some women develop UTIs in relation to phase of the menstrual cycle or after sexual activity. Upper tract involvement, or pyelonephritis, should be suspected with accompanying fever, chills, malaise, flank pain, and occasionally, nausea and vomiting. Under wilderness conditions, symptoms, elevated urine pH (7 to 8), and indirect evidence of

TABLE 75-3. Antibiotic Regimens for Urinary Tract Infections

TYPE OF INFECTION	SELECTED ANTIBIOTICS	LENGTH OF TREATMENT
Cystitis (acute)	Ampicillin, 250 to 500 mg qid	3-7 days
	Amoxicillin, 500 mg tid	
	Cephalexin, 500 mg qid	
	Nitrofurantoin,* 100 mg qid	
	Sulfamethoxazole/trimethoprim,* 1 or 2 tablets bid	
Prophylaxis	Any of the above: 1 pill/day or 1 pill after coitus	Indefinitely
Pyelonephritis† (outpatient care)	Amoxicillin, 500 mg tid	10-14 days
	Cephalexin, 500 mg qid	
	Ciprofloxacin,‡ 500 mg bid	
	Sulfamethoxazole/trimethoprim,* 1 or 2 tablets bid	

bid, Twice daily; *tid*, three times daily; *qid*, four times daily.
*Contraindicated for use near term in pregnancy.
†Serious infections require parenteral antibiotics.
‡Contraindicated during pregnancy and lactation.

pyuria (leukocyte esterase) or bacteria (nitrites) on urine dipstick test suggest UTI. Under ideal conditions, microscopic confirmation of pyuria and culture of organisms from a clean urine specimen are still the best methods for confirming the diagnosis and assessing the antibiotic sensitivity of etiologic bacteria.

Management of UTIs includes both prophylactic and therapeutic measures. Women should drink at least six to eight glasses (48 to 64 oz) of noncarbonated fluid per day. Under dehydrating conditions, sufficient fluid should be ingested to generate voiding at least every 3 to 4 hours while awake.[116,145] Women should void when the urge arises or on a regular schedule and not risk bladder overdistention. They should be reminded to wipe from front to back after urination and defecation and to void after sexual intercourse. Treatment of symptomatic cystitis usually requires a 3- to 7-day course of antibiotics (Table 75-3).[73] Treatment of pyelonephritis usually requires a 10- to 14-day course of oral therapy or, when indicated, parenteral antibiotics until symptoms have resolved for 24 hours, followed by oral therapy to complete the 10 to 14 days.[136] Recurrent cystitis should be treated for longer than 3 days, and prophylactic therapy should be considered on an ongoing basis or after precipitating events such as coitus. Persistent problems eventually warrant urologic evaluation.[43] Pregnant women often require longer courses of therapy; pyelonephritis in pregnancy warrants suppressive therapy throughout gestation.

MENSTRUATION

Normal Cycle

Menstrual cycle disturbances are among the most frequent indications for which women seek medical care. Among highly trained female athletes and in environments that impose extreme physical and psychologic demands, such disturbances can be found in as many as 50% of women not taking OCs. Understanding bleeding abnormalities requires a basic understanding of the normal menstrual cycle (Figure 75-1). Normal cycles occur at regular intervals, require ovulation, and typically average 28 days (range 21 to 35 days). By convention the first day of the menstrual cycle corresponds to the first day of the menstrual period, which usually lasts about 4 days (range 3 to 7 days). The onset of menstrual bleeding represents desquamation of the functional endometrium, resulting from progesterone withdrawal in the absence of conception during the previous cycle, and coincides with recruitment of a new group of primordial follicles for maturation. The first stage of the menstrual cycle, up to the time of ovulation, is referred to as the follicular phase, or endometrial proliferative phase. The second stage is the luteal phase, or endometrial secretory phase.

Follicular recruitment depends on the presence of follicle-stimulating hormone (FSH) released from the pituitary as the consequence of pulsatile release of GnRH by the hypothalamus.[46,124] FSH stimulates transformation of a primordial follicle into a primary follicle with a primary oocyte surrounded by a layer of granulosa cells.[88] Under the mitogenic influence of FSH, granulosa cells replicate to several layers, producing the secondary or preantral follicle. The granulosa cell layer is surrounded by a basement membrane that provides clear separation from the stromal theca cells. The theca cells are the primary source of androgens, predominantly androstenedione and testosterone, which are converted to the estrogens estrone and estradiol, respectively, by aromatization in the granulosa cells, an event also stimulated by FSH. Estrogens in turn enhance production of their own receptors and receptors for FSH, further stimulating granulosa cell division, aromatase activity, and more estrogen produc-

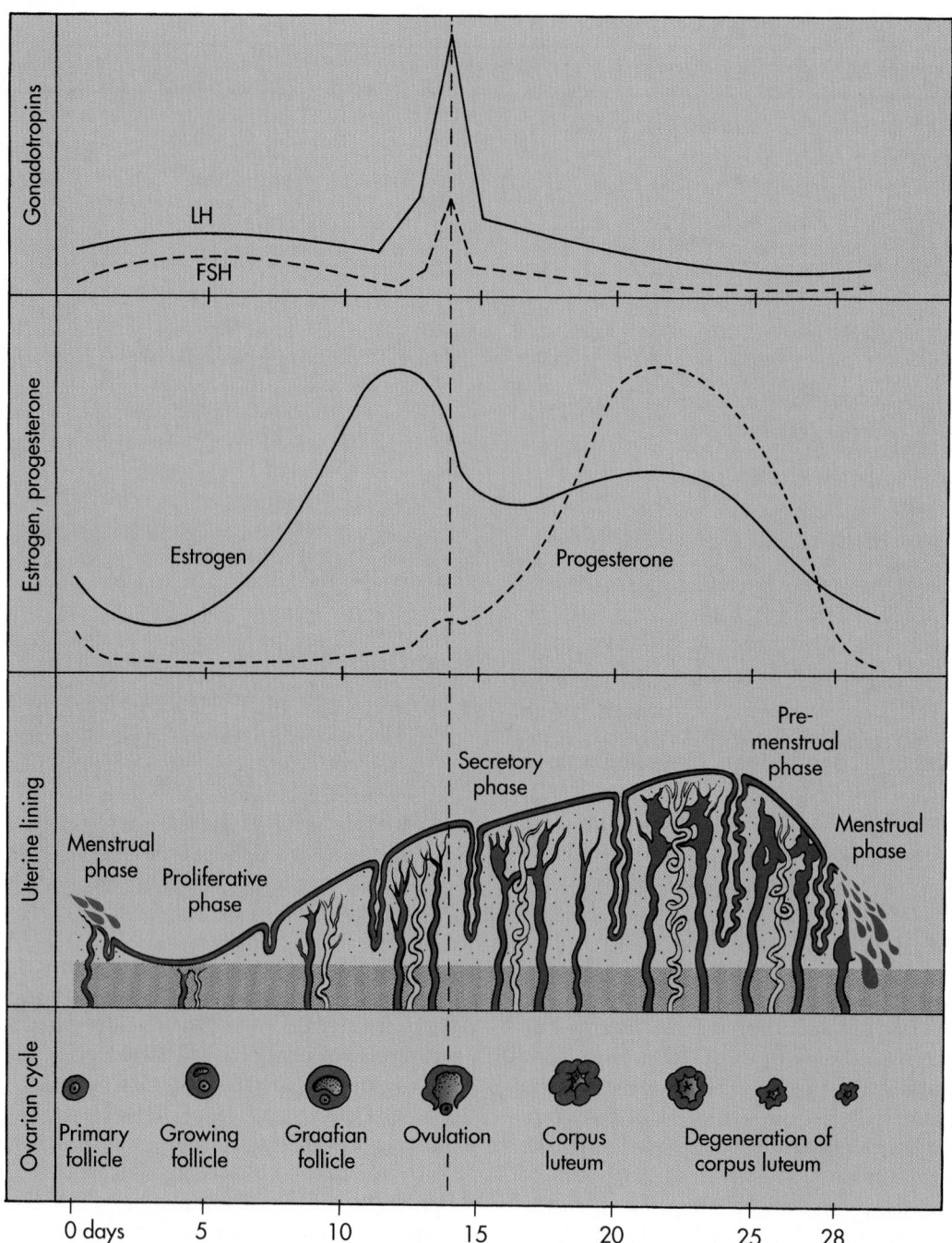

Figure 75-1 Normal human ovarian and endometrial (menstrual) cycle. (*Modified from Shaw ST Jr, Roche PC: Menstruation. In Finn CA, editor: Oxford reviews of reproduction and endocrinology, vol 2, Oxford, UK, 1980, Oxford University Press.*)

tion. With adequate estrogen the follicle secretes and accumulates fluid, displacing the oocyte and surrounding granulosa cells eccentrically, forming the tertiary (antral) or mature follicle.[108] Without sufficient estrogen, androgens arrest maturation of the follicle at the preantral stage and promote its atresia.[66]

In addition to their mitogenic and aromatase-enhancing effects, estrogen and FSH stimulate production of receptors for luteinizing hormone (LH) on the theca cells and on the granulosa cells in the late follic-

ular phase. LH, which is also released from the pituitary in response to pulsatile hypothalamic GnRH, stimulates uptake of cholesterol, a primary precursor of androgens, by the theca cells and is essential for adequate estrogen production. Significant expression of LH receptor on the granulosa cells is not achieved until late in the follicular phase and prepares the dominant follicle to respond to a midcycle surge in release of LH from the pituitary and the subsequent rupture of the follicle and release of the oocyte (ovulation). The events leading up to ovulation itself are complex.[80,89,160] Elevated circulating levels of estrogen, predominantly estradiol, trigger release of both LH and FSH by direct effect on the pituitary, with a rapid drop in circulating estrogen. This event precedes ovulation by 26 to 32 hours, resulting in resumption of meiosis by the oocyte and weakening of the follicular wall.

The preovulatory presence of sufficient LH receptors on the granulosa cell is essential for their next steroidogenic role, the production of progesterone, in the second phase of the menstrual cycle. Their readiness for this role is anticipated by the rise in production of 17-hydoxyprogesterone (17-OHP) just before ovulation.[128] After ovulation, LH stimulates 3β-hydroxysteroid dehydrogenase activity, resulting in production of progesterone from cholesterol-derived pregnenolone at the ovulatory site, now the corpus luteum (CL). This luteinization results in progesterone production that peaks 7 to 8 days after ovulation. Progesterone induces the secretory phase of endometrial development, preparing for implantation of the embryo. With conception and the production of adequate human chorionic gonadotropin (hCG) by embryonic trophoblasts, the CL persists, enlarges, and increases its production of progesterone and estrogen.[2] With no conception the CL loses its sensitivity to LH and FSH, degenerates (luteolysis), and decreases production of progesterone and estrogen.[101] Without hormonal support the functional endometrium degenerates and is again shed with menstruation. The drop in these hormones is also a signal to resume release of FSH and LH from the pituitary with recruitment of more follicles. In normal menstrual cycles the luteal phase (from ovulation to menses) is 14 days (± 2 days).

Although the primary feedback loop for production of reproductive hormones is directly between ovary and pituitary, the hypothalamus plays an integral role in maintaining responsiveness of the pituitary by the pulsatile release of GnRH. Pulsatility maintains pituitary GnRH receptors. Loss of pulsatility results in downregulation of these receptors, with inhibited secretion of FSH and LH. The pulse generator for the rhythmic release of GnRH is located in the arcuate nucleus of the hypothalamus.[32] It is influenced by numerous neurotransmitters and steroid hormones. During the menstrual cycle, pulsatile release of GnRH occurs hourly during the follicular phase and every hour and a half during the luteal phase. Factors that disrupt the normal pulsatile release of GnRH or reduce the ability of the pituitary to respond to it are the major contributors to menstrual cycle abnormalities in premenopausal women.[24]

Abnormal Uterine Bleeding

Abnormal uterine bleeding (AUB) can be loosely defined as any aberration in the normal menstrual bleeding pattern in premenopausal women and as any bleeding episode in postmenopausal women. The most common causes of AUB are problems related to pregnancy and hormonal contraceptive therapy. Initial evaluation of AUB in any premenopausal woman includes a urine or serum screen for hCG, regardless of contraceptive history. Nonpregnancy-related causes of abnormal bleeding can be divided into episodes in ovulatory women, in anovulatory women, and from extrauterine causes, either ovulatory or anovulatory.

Historical information is useful in developing a presumptive etiology and empiric therapeutic approach for AUB, particularly in the absence of laboratory resources. Past history includes age at onset of menses, regularity of menses, usual length of period and blood flow, perimenstrual symptoms, medical problems, pregnancy history, STI history, surgical history, and basic endocrinologic review of systems.[72] The current problem is then characterized by changes in the frequency of bleeding, amount of flow, new symptoms, relationship to activities, recent sexual history, systemic symptoms, weight change, change in medications or use of other health-related products, and change in exercise patterns.

Ovulatory Women. When the premenopausal woman who has consistently had regular cyclic menses presents with a history of progressively increasing amount and duration of menstrual flow, the most common causes are uterine fibroids, particularly submucosal (just beneath the endometrium) fibroids, endometriosis, and adenomyosis (endometriosis of the uterine muscle wall). These conditions are frequently associated with progressive dysmenorrhea and are more likely to occur with advancing age. Occasionally an endometrial polyp or IUD, either of which can be accompanied by endometritis, results in a similar presentation. The use of certain medications (e.g., estrogens, warfarin, nonsteroidal antiinflammatory drugs [NSAIDs]) or homeopathic compounds should always be part of the evaluation of AUB, as well as clues to an acquired blood dyscrasia such as idiopathic thrombocytopenic purpura or leukemia. Otherwise healthy women with a history of heavy menstrual bleeding from the time of menarche should be evaluated for inborn coagulation disorders, most often von Willebrand's disease. An abrupt change in the duration or amount of blood flow should suggest a corpus luteal cyst, often associated with unilateral lower abdominal discomfort, or acute PID, often accompanied by more diffuse abdominal pain and systemic symptoms. Hyperplasia of the endometrium is unusual in ovulating women, and malignancies of the uterus or ovaries (estrogen secreting) are rare. Perimenopausal women who are still ovulatory may have progressively more periods, which may be accompanied by changes in flow and duration, with or without the underlying causes noted.

A regularly cyclic woman with intermenstrual or postcoital bleeding should also be evaluated for cervicovaginal infections, such as BV, yeast, *Trichomonas,* and condylomata. Endocervical polyps, cervical dysplasia, and even invasive cervical carcinoma can occur in this group. When precipitated by coitus, profuse bleeding and dyspareunia can result. Acute pelvic or abdominal pain that accompanies bleeding with coitus should suggest penetrating trauma, an uncommon but potentially life-threatening emergency. Acute pain with coitus and not usually accompanied by bleeding is more likely to be the result of PID, rupture of an ovarian cyst, or torsion of the adnexa.

A clear history and the supportive physical findings limit the differential diagnosis and therapy, although codependent conditions may be present. A synergistic relationship between bleeding and infection is often found in women with prolonged bleeding or short intervals between bleeding episodes. Endometritis can develop from loss of protective cervical mucus and ascending infection by pathogenic organisms that have proliferated in a more alkaline (blood-induced) vaginal environment. Endometritis in turn can precipitate heavier, more frequent, and more symptomatic bleeding. Unfortunately, many women with AUB first present for medical care at this stage. Unless they have been attentive to abnormalities from the onset, a diagnosis based on history alone is difficult. For example, an ovulatory woman with menorrhagia from uterine fibroids may suddenly develop intermenstrual bleeding (from the fibroids or endometritis), which is difficult to distinguish from accompanying chronic anovulation.

Anovulatory Women. Anovulatory AUB is more common than ovulatory abnormalities among women who partake in wilderness experiences. Anovulatory bleeding problems can be divided into those occurring with adequate estrogen production and those accompanied by low estrogen production. The former, often characterized by hypersecretion of gonadotropins and frequent heavy bleeding, is usually seen in women with polycystic ovary syndrome (PCOS). In contrast, anovulation in the absence of normal estrogen production usually results from inadequate release of gonadotropins from the pituitary, often presents with complete amenorrhea, and may result from physical conditioning. Hypoestrogenism can have significant effects on a woman's participation in strenuous wilderness experiences.

Female Athletic Triad. The American College of Sports Medicine first coined the term *female athletic triad* in 1992, but the interrelated components of the triad—disordered eating, amenorrhea, and osteoporosis—had been recognized for many years.[117] The disorder usually begins with either weight control for participation in activities that emphasize physical appearance, such as cheerleading and dance, or weight loss precipitated

by excessive exercise without sufficient caloric or nutritional intake. The eating disorder may evolve into frank anorexia or bulimia and may worsen with starvation, limited variety of nutritional intake, overeating and purging (vomiting, laxatives, enemas), and use of diet pills, appetite suppressants, and diuretics.[36] Unless the syndrome begins before menarche, as usually occurs in female gymnasts or ballet dancers, it is usually preceded by menstrual irregularity before frank amenorrhea. Prolonged amenorrhea usually signals inadequate ovarian estrogen production secondary to deficient gonadotropin secretion. Since estrogen plays an integral role in promoting bone growth, loss of bone density (osteoporosis) can evolve rapidly at this point, particularly if the diet is also deficient in the minerals and vitamins necessary for skeletal integrity and if the exercise program is vigorous. Skeletal stress accompanying physical exertion is usually characterized by high rates of bone turnover.

The consequences of the triad range from impaired performance to life-threatening conditions. Electrolyte imbalances, vitamin and mineral deficiencies, and loss of bone and muscle mass result in loss of strength and endurance. This sets the stage for multiple or recurrent stress fractures and major musculoskeletal injury. Reduced net bone formation can result in failure to achieve optimal growth and peak bone mass, scoliosis, and increased risk for serious osteoporotic complications later in life. Electrolyte imbalances, combined with weight-reducing drugs, can result in lethal arrhythmias and cardiomyopathies. Depression, coupled with an uncompromising and distorted body image, may lead to suicide attempts.

Management of young women with the female athletic triad may be difficult because many of its characteristics are valued and encouraged in the athlete: competitive nature, high self-expectations, obsessive-compulsive or perfectionist tendencies, and self-critical attitudes. The woman must understand the balance between healthy and unhealthy expression of these characteristics in terms of her goals, current well-being, and long-term health consequences. Those at risk for the triad can often be identified by a vigilant health care provider or physical trainer and offered help before full manifestation of the condition.[40] Unfortunately, the condition often goes unrecognized or is ignored until a serious complication has occurred and mandates intervention.

Physically active women and individuals involved in their training and health care should be educated about the female athletic triad. Athletic training should include ongoing assessment of weight, growth, and menstrual history. Women involved in high-risk activities, such as dancing, figure skating, gymnastics, and running, should be considered for baseline and periodic assessment of bone density.[19]

The steps in reversing the condition include temporary reduction in exercise, increased and balanced caloric intake, and a diet rich in calcium (1200 to 1500 mg/day) and vitamins. Counseling should be offered to deal with obstacles to physical and long-term rehabilitation. To reduce their risk of skeletal injury, amenorrheic women with osteoporosis who are unwilling to reduce their physical activity should receive nutritional counseling and hormonal replacement therapy at levels currently recommended to treat postmenopausal women.[34] Recent studies have indicated that the bisphosphonates, such as alendronate (5 to 10 mg daily), and to a lesser degree, selective estrogen receptor modulators (SERMs), such as raloxifene (30 to 150 mg daily), can improve bone density and decrease fracture risks in women not receiving estrogen replacement therapy.[37,42]

Wilderness Risks. The major risks of AUB to the wilderness participant depend on the etiology, severity, and chronicity of the process. Heavy and prolonged bleeding can result in significant blood loss, chronic iron deficiency, and infectious morbidity. These can impair endurance, prolong acclimatization, particularly at altitude, and increase susceptibility to acute cardiopulmonary decompensation. As an aesthetic measure, efforts should be made to maintain personal hygiene, thoroughly wash or not wear bloody clothing, and either store tampons or sanitary napkins in sealed containers or dispose of them away from camp and supply sites. There is no evidence that menstrual blood is an olfactory attractant to bears and sharks. In amenorrheic hypoestrogenized women, nutritional deficiency and osteoporosis can result in impaired endurance and prolonged acclimatization, susceptibility to acute deterioration in electrolyte status, particularly in high temperature and humid or aquatic environments, cardiac decompensation, and complicated musculoskeletal injury at exertional levels below the threshold expected by training.

PREGNANCY AND CHILDBIRTH

Pregnancy is considered a relative contraindication to wilderness activities unless access to medical care is available in the field or provisions are made for rapid evacuation. Even though prior pregnancy experience is a relatively good predictor of outcome after the first trimester, pregnancy is still characterized by its unpredictability. No interval during pregnancy is considered absolutely safe. Mortality rates are currently less than eight per 100,000 live births. Many women with infertility and "high-risk" medical problems (e.g., diabetes, hypertension, autoimmune disorders) are conceiving and carrying pregnancies to viability. These women have become more active wilderness participants, appreciating the benefits of regular exercise in their medical management. Women with chronic medical conditions should discuss the potential consequences of pregnancy in a wilderness setting with their health care providers.

Physiologic Changes Accompanying Pregnancy

Hormonal changes accompanying pregnancy result in physiologic adaptations affecting every organ system within weeks of conception. For example, progesterone has smooth muscle relaxation effects that help to maintain uterine quiescence, but these also contribute to vasomotor instability, hypotension, gastric reflux, and constipation. Estrogens stimulate hepatic production of many hormone binding globulins and of coagulation factors II, V, VII, VIII, IX, X, XII, and fibrinogen, which contribute to the hypercoagulable state of pregnancy. Both estrogen and progesterone stimulate rapid uterine hypertrophy, as well as pancreatic β-cell hyperplasia that leads to hyperinsulinemia, increased peripheral glucose utilization, and susceptibility to hypoglycemia in early pregnancy.

During pregnancy, cardiac output increases 30% to 50%, much by the end of the first trimester, from an increase in stroke volume secondary to an increase in preload. The balance comes from a gradual increase in maternal heart rate that usually peaks between 24 and 28 weeks' gestation. Uterine blood flow increases from 50 to more than 500 ml/min, corresponding to an increase from about 1% to 15% to 20% of total cardiac output. Systemic vascular resistance (SVR) decreases, primarily from the low-resistance placental vascular bed, the equivalent of a large arteriovenous shunt, and also from the peripheral vasodilatory effects of progesterone, estrogen, and other factors. Decreased SVR is reflected by a fall in MAP, with a nadir in the midtrimester. Without this midtrimester pressure drop, placental abnormalities may be manifested later in pregnancy as fetal growth restriction and preeclampsia. Because of the dramatic hemodynamic changes, women with known or unrecognized cardiovascular disease may decompensate under the stress of pregnancy. This is particularly true during labor and in the immediate postpartum period, when cardiac output can increase an additional 20% to 60% because of exertion, pain, and fear. Sudden increases in SVR and intravascular volume resulting from uterine involution and autotransfusion immediately after delivery place further demands on the cardiovascular system.

Healthy women who regularly participate in moderate exercise during pregnancy are usually able to meet cardiovascular demands. The benefits of regular exercise outweigh the risks, except in women who have predisposing risk factors or contraindications, such as incompetent cervix; history of preterm labor, delivery, or premature rupture of membranes; bleeding; cardiac disease; or preeclampsia.[11] Because of the incursions on cardiac reserves demanded by the pregnancy, however, even well-conditioned athletes have limits on strenuous activity.[74,82] Exceeding this limit could have deleterious effects on fetal status because of decreased uterine perfusion, increased uterine contractions, maternal acidosis, and hypoglycemia.[12,143]

Total blood volume increases 40% to 50% during normal pregnancy, most during the first half of pregnancy, from a rapid expansion of plasma volume. Plasma volume peaks at about 32 weeks' gestation, despite high levels of renin, angiotensin, and aldosterone, findings usually associated with hypertension and decreased intravascular volume in the nonpregnant state. The compensatory mechanism appears to be pregnancy-related refractoriness to the vasoconstrictor effects of angiotensin II, an effect mediated by progesterone, perhaps placental-derived prostaglandins, and atrial natriuretic peptide. By 20 weeks' gestation, in response to an increase in plasma erythropoietin, red cell mass continues to expand until term and eventually reaches levels one-third higher than in the nonpregnant state. A disproportionate increase in plasma volume over red cell mass results in the so-called physiologic anemia of pregnancy. Fetal demands in the second half of pregnancy are an additional drain on iron stores and often produce true iron deficiency. Trained athletes may be at greater risk for this because of iron losses from mechanical hemolysis, intestinal bleeding, hematuria, sweating, low intake, or poor intestinal absorption.[33]

Respiratory system changes in normal pregnancy more than compensate for the physiologic anemia to maintain fetal and maternal homeostasis. Progesterone directly stimulates the respiratory center and increases its sensitivity to CO_2, resulting in a 30% to 40% increase in tidal volume (TV). Respiratory rate (RR) does not change significantly, but as a result of TV changes, minute ventilation (TV $\times$ RR) increases 25% to 30%, despite a slight decrease in total lung capacity. A 20% reduction of functional residual capacity, resulting from decreases in both expiratory reserve volume and residual volume, completes the picture of relative hyperventilation with a compensated respiratory alkalosis. Many of these changes are completed by the end of the first trimester; their sum is a dramatic 50% increase in alveolar ventilation, increased Pa_{O_2}, 30% increase in minute O_2 uptake, and significant decrease in Pco_2. The overall effect is to increase the O_2-carrying capacity of maternal blood to accommodate fetal and maternal metabolic needs, while facilitating diffusion of CO_2 from the fetus. For the wilderness traveler, these changes lead to higher O_2 saturation under hypoxic conditions, such as at altitude.

Significant changes in the urinary system account for many of the complaints and complications of pregnancy. Beginning in the first trimester, the ureters become dilated, elongated, and more tortuous, presumably under the influence of progesterone. Further dilation of the proximal ureters occurs when the uterus reaches the level of the pelvic brim at about 20 weeks' gestation and compresses the ureters. Frequently at this stage, women present for the first time with pyelonephritis, more often on the right than on the left due to dextrorotation of the uterus by the descending colon. Contributing to the risk of upper tract infection, vesicoureteral reflux occurs secondary to decreased competency of the ureterovesical junction. This is exacerbated by a progressive decrease in bladder capacity and doubling of intravesicular pressures (from 10 to 20 cm H_2O) during gestation. These factors also contribute to frequent complaints of urinary incontinence that plague pregnant women.

Integumentary and musculoskeletal changes can have a significant impact on the well-being of the pregnant wilderness traveler. Under the influence of estrogen, proliferation and dilation of small arterioles in the skin helps to compensate for increased demands to remove heat generated by maternal and fetal metabolism. Because of these inherent changes, pregnant women have a limited capacity to respond further to heat stress and are at increased risk for hyperthermia in hot and humid environments. Estrogen and other pregnancy-associated hormones also increase sensitivity of the skin to damage by sun exposure, particularly in fair-skinned individuals, and to the risk of pyogenic granulomata of extremities and gums resulting from trauma and inflammation. Some pregnant women have a predisposition to develop skin hyperpigmentation in a nonuniform distribution because of excessive melanin deposition in the dermis and epidermis. This is enhanced by sun exposure; often affects the face (melasma), midline abdomen (linea nigra), nipples, axillae, and perineum; and may require a prolonged period for resolution after delivery. It may never resolve completely.

Striae gravidarum, or "stretch marks," may be the most notorious superficial effects of pregnancy. These result from breaks in dermal collagen and frequently occur on the abdomen, buttocks, thighs, and breasts. Striae are not necessarily associated with skin stretching and may be found before significant uterine growth or weight gain has occurred, reflecting their underlying hormonal basis. Hair loss during pregnancy, as well as nail brittleness and loss of adhesiveness between the nail and nail bed, may also increase the risk of sun exposure and trauma, respectively, for the pregnant wilderness traveler.

Weight gain, weight redistribution, and ligamentous relaxation may pose the greatest risks, even to the well-conditioned pregnant woman.[6] Overall weight gain during pregnancy is usually about 20 to 35 pounds. Some weight gain is important during pregnancy to avoid a catabolic state and may be more important to the highly conditioned athlete who enters pregnancy with limited fat stores. This weight increases stress on the weight-bearing skeleton and ligaments throughout the body and may accumulate more rapidly than conditioning can handle. Much of the weight gain is contributed by uterine and fetal growth, resulting in forward displacement of the center of gravity. This is usually accompanied by progressive lordosis of the lower spine and increased strain on spinal ligaments, disks, and paravertebral muscles. When lumbar lordosis is exaggerated, traction and compression on the sciatic nerves can cause significant pain and weakness in the buttocks and lower extremities. Changes in the lower spine are frequently followed by compensatory flexion of the cervical spine. This in turn can place traction on the median and ulnar nerves, resulting in pain, paresthesias, and weakness of the upper extremities.

The challenges of weight gain are accompanied by dramatic changes in ligamentous support throughout the body. Under the influence of relaxin and other hormones, ligaments become more compliant and hydrophilic. Benefits of this include relaxation in the sacroiliac joints and symphysis pubis to facilitate delivery, but hormonal effects on other ligaments can lead to complications. For example, fluid retention by the flexor retinaculum in the wrist can cause compression of the median nerve, resulting in carpal tunnel syndrome, a common complaint of pregnancy. This may be more than just a nuisance to the wilderness traveler, because pain and hand weakness can compromise activities, such as climbing and canoeing, that require hand strength and endurance. Even more troublesome, pelvic girdle instability, accompanied by weight gain, shift in center of gravity, and spinal lordosis, usually leads to gait and balance disturbances. These not only predispose to more frequent falls during pregnancy under far less strenuous conditions than those encountered in many wilderness settings, but also lead to an increase in the severity of trauma accompanying these falls. The anterior cruciate ligament is especially prone to severe trauma, accounts for 3 to 4 times more injuries in women than men, and is especially susceptible to trauma in the active pregnant woman.[166] Difficult terrain also poses a risk to the pregnant wilderness traveler.

Unless there are other medical or pregnancy-related contraindications (e.g., risk for premature labor, incompetent cervix, multiple gestation, bleeding), exercise and specialized training should be encouraged throughout pregnancy, taking precautions to avoid prolonged exposure to extremes in temperature, dehydration, hypoglycemia, prolonged anaerobic conditions, and excessive skeletal stress.[79,147] Active and physically fit women tolerate labor better than inactive women. A program specifically designed for pregnant women, including exercises to strengthen the abdominal and back muscles, and careful attention to posture may reduce the risks related to changes in skeletal support.

Wilderness Participation. Pregnant women are more susceptible to altitude sickness, more likely to develop severe symptoms, and may require longer periods of adjustment before exertional activities can be undertaken. Gradual progression to higher altitudes and limited activity until completely comfortable will minimize symptoms and allow for fetal compensation. A pregnant woman must maintain adequate fluid intake throughout this process, since reduced O_2 saturation combined with decreased uterine perfusion secondary to dehydration could endanger the fetus. Depending on the altitude, gestational age, maternal Hgb levels, and degree of training, even the well-acclimated pregnant woman may find that endurance and ability to participate in strenuous activity at altitude are limited.[13] When a trip is planned, frequent rest periods should be scheduled. A higher incidence of preeclampsia and fetal growth restriction has been found among women at higher elevations and may reflect the limits of the placenta and fetus to extract O_2 even from well-conditioned individuals.[119,171]

Although swimming is considered an excellent form of exercise for pregnant women, scuba diving is potentially hazardous. The fetus is at risk from nitrogen bubbles in the fetal-placental circulation during decompression on ascent. Most authorities consider pregnancy a contraindication to diving.[23] Diving is compromised by increased abdominal girth, difficulty breathing due to engorgement of the mucous membranes of the nose and oropharynx, and increased buoyancy secondary to fat deposition. Higher levels of body fat also increase the risk of decompression sickness, since nitrogen tends to be retained in these tissues. Dyspnea may be exaggerated and lead to panic, even in the experienced diver who is pregnant.[113] As with exertion at high altitude, the pregnant woman may have limited ability to maintain anaerobic metabolism for prolonged periods because of fetal needs. The pregnant woman should also limit prolonged nondiving immersion in cold water that might lead to hypoventilation and hypothermia.

Acclimation to environments characterized by high temperatures, particularly with high humidity, may be especially difficult for the pregnant woman and even dangerous to the fetus. Hyperthermia has been shown to be teratogenic in various animal models and a higher incidence of birth defects, particularly neural tube defects, have been found among offspring of women who experienced hyperthermia by environmental exposure or febrile illness in the first trimester.[132,210] Later in pregnancy the fetus depends on the woman to eliminate excess heat. Elevation of ambient temperature decreases the heat gradient and the ability of the pregnant woman to dissipate heat. Elevated humidity exacerbates this situation by decreasing the contribution of perspiration to heat loss. This increases the risk of elevated maternal core temperature, which further raises fetal metabolic activity and heat generation. Hyperthermia increases the risk of premature labor, particularly with dehydration and loss of electrolytes. Fetal stress, resulting from decreased uterine perfusion secondary to compensatory peripheral vasodilation and depletion of intravascular volume, further increases the likelihood of preterm labor.

Preparation for Pregnancy

The woman who is pregnant and plans to participate in wilderness activities or who anticipates a wilderness delivery needs thorough medical evaluation and counseling before departure. The evaluation begins with the obstetric history and complications for which she is at high risk for recurrence, including preterm labor, premature rupture of membranes, preeclampsia, gestational diabetes, fetal growth restriction, group B β-hemolytic streptococcal colonization, UTIs, chorioamnionitis, blood group isoimmunization, thromboembolic events, surgical delivery, and postdelivery complications. A complete physical examination should be conducted.

Laboratory evaluation before departure includes standard blood work recommended by the American College of Obstetricians and Gynecologists: complete blood count, blood type and antibody screen (and screen of partner if the woman is Rh negative or isoimmunized), and basic serology (rapid plasma reagin, rubella, hepatitis B, HIV). Serologic screening for HSV-2 should be considered in the woman with no history of genital herpes because of the potential for first-time outbreaks during pregnancy in women with unrecognized infection.[14,104] Individuals at risk and those not previously evaluated should also be offered Hgb electrophoresis to assess for hemoglobinopathies. Urinalysis and urine culture are performed because of the high frequency of asymptomatic infections during pregnancy that complicate outcome. Vaginal fluid should be assessed for BV, since treatment early in pregnancy may prevent premature rupture of membranes and preterm labor. A Pap smear is often done as well. A woman beyond 15 weeks' gestation before departing should be offered biochemical screening (e.g., maternal serum α-fetoprotein, estriol, hCG) to assess for certain congenital and chromosomal abnormalities. Abnormal biochemical markers may indicate complications such as fetal growth restriction and preeclampsia, resulting primarily from early abnormalities in placentation that can become clinically significant later in gestation. These conditions also increase the risk for premature delivery, as well as for maternal and fetal morbidity and mortality.

Since diabetes arises as a complication of the hormonal milieu in at least 3% of all pregnancies, routine screening is indicated in any woman who is not diabetic before pregnancy. Oral administration of a 50-g glucose challenge in the nonfasting state is usually done at 24 to 28 weeks' gestation, followed by a plasma glucose determination 1 hour later. Values of 140 mg/dl or greater (but less than 200 mg/dl) warrant further evaluation with a fasting 3-hour oral glucose tolerance test using a 100-g glucose challenge. If the fasting value before administration of the glucose load is 120 mg/dl or greater, or if the 1-hour challenge is 200 mg/dl or more, the woman is considered diabetic and should not have the 3-hour test done. Otherwise, values of 90 mg/dl or greater while fasting, 190 mg/dl or more at 1 hour, 165 mg/dl or greater at 2 hours, and 145 mg/dl or more at 3 hours are considered abnormal. Two abnormal values or persistent elevation of the fasting level indicate diabetes. If departure is planned before 24 to 28 weeks' gestation, the 1-hour challenge can be done using a portable plasma glucose meter. If the woman has significant risk factors (age 35 or older, obesity, family history, steroid use, PCOS, other endocrinopathy such as thyroid disease) the 1-hour and possibly the 3-hour tests should be administered early, regardless of gestational age.[100] If the woman had gestational diabetes with a previous pregnancy, it is best to assume she will have it again. Proper dietary counseling and regular blood sugar monitoring with a portable plasma glucose monitor should be conducted throughout the pregnancy. Insulin, sufficient syringes, and alcohol wipes should be included with the basic medical supplies in the event glycemic control deteriorates. The goal is to maintain fasting plasma glucose levels at 90 mg/dl or less and lower than 120 mg/dl 2 hours after meals. Physical conditioning reduces but does not eliminate the risk of developing diabetes during pregnancy. Women with pregestational diabetes of any duration should have a baseline ECG and possibly an echocardiogram before participation in any wilderness-related activities.

The pregnant wilderness traveler should have an obstetric sonogram before departure for additional risk assessment. Early in the pregnancy, sonography can accurately confirm gestational age, viability, intrauterine location, and number of babies. It is also useful in ruling out the presence of an ectopic pregnancy, adnexal mass, or molar pregnancy that could lead to life-threatening complications. In midtrimester an ultrasound is useful not only in estimating gestational age, but also in determining the presence of major fetal abnormalities, the location of the placenta in relationship to the cervix, and the cervical length and integrity of the internal cervical os. Beyond 20 weeks' gestation, normal fetal growth and blood flow patterns in the umbilical and middle cerebral arteries can be assessed by

Doppler velocimetry. Normal results indicate lower risk for complications, such as intrauterine growth restriction, preeclampsia, and preterm labor.[38] Any findings that significantly increase maternal or fetal risk are contraindications to elective wilderness travel during pregnancy.

Prolonged wilderness excursions during pregnancy, particularly those extending into late second and third trimesters, should include preparations for ongoing assessment and even emergency delivery. Routine antepartum care usually includes visits to a health care provider at least monthly until 26 to 28 weeks, every 2 weeks thereafter until 36 weeks, then weekly until delivery. Beyond the due date, more frequent visits are often recommended. Routine visits focus on uterine activity, vaginal discharge, abdominopelvic pain, bleeding, headaches, symptoms of UTI, current medications, and fetal activity.

The basic antepartum examination includes measurements of blood pressure, weight, and uterine size (height of uterine fundus above symphysis) and subjective assessments of peripheral edema and reflexes. Urine is tested at each visit with a multitest strip that provides estimates of glycosuria, proteinuria, pH, and presence of nitrites. For the wilderness traveler, elevated pH and presence of nitrites may be associated with UTIs under circumstances that might preclude culture capabilities.[156] In Rh-negative women with Rh-positive partners the antibody screen is often repeated at 26 to 28 weeks, before the administration of Rh-immune globulin for prophylaxis against third-trimester sensitization. If an antibody screen cannot be done, Rh-immune globulin should be administered empirically. Maternal Hgb and Hct are frequently done in each trimester to assess need for iron supplementation. Since many women require supplemental iron during pregnancy, this should be taken prophylactically under circumstances that obviate determination of Hgb levels, unless the woman has a contraindication, such as hemochromatosis.

Basic supplies for the pregnant wilderness traveler might include a diary to record progress, reminders of scheduled testing, and complications; tape measure; stethoscope; sphygmomanometer; urine test strips; and prenatal vitamins and iron. Other supplies include a glucometer with test strips, Rh-immune globulin, a calcium supplement, and basic medications for the most common pregnancy complaints: an antiemetic such as promethazine, prochlorperazine, or chlorpromazine for nausea and vomiting; acetaminophen for headaches and pain; stool softener for constipation; and antibiotics to cover UTIs and vaginitis. In addition to the basic medical supplies, the pregnant woman should have changes in clothing size and possibly shoe size. When delivery in the wilderness is planned or a strong possibility, special preparations need to be made (Box 75-4).

Box 75-4   SUPPLIES FOR MANAGEMENT OF WILDERNESS DELIVERY

STANDARD

Clean towels
Surgical sponges
Surgical gloves
Umbilical cord clamps
Suction bulb
Suture kit
Scalpel
Scissors
Syringes and needles
Local anesthetic
Injectable oxytocin
Injectable and oral methylergonovine
Oral analgesics (e.g., ibuprofen, acetaminophen with codeine)
Oral broad-spectrum antibiotic
Sanitary napkins

OPTIONAL

Injectable magnesium sulfate
Intravenous fluids and administration supplies
Injectable narcotic
Naloxone
Misoprostol
Prostaglandin $F_{2\alpha}$
Injectable antibiotic
Neonatal mask and Ambu bag

Complications

Miscarriage. Women who are pregnant or become pregnant for the first time while in the wilderness are at high risk for complications. Approximately 15% to 25% of all pregnancies abort spontaneously during the first trimester, and this number may exceed 60% to 70% in the true primigravida.[134] Reasons may be related to immunologic naivete to paternal antigens expressed by the fetal tissues. In contrast, isolated miscarriages in women who have successfully carried pregnancies are often the result of chromosomal abnormalities. Pending miscarriage in the first trimester is usually preceded by embryonic demise and accompanied by a reduction or loss in early pregnancy-related symptoms, such as breast tenderness and nausea. Bleeding and uterine contractions eventually occur and accompany expulsion of the products of conception. Under most circumstances, hemorrhage during miscarriage is self-limited and not life-threatening but at times can be heavy, especially if fetal death does not precede the event and occurs late in the first trimester or during the second trimester, or if the expulsion process is prolonged or incomplete. Spontaneous abortion after the first trimester is much riskier but less common. It also can result from chromosomal abnormalities or fetal anomalies but is more likely to be caused by chorioamnionitis, UTIs, severe abnormalities of placentation, poorly controlled maternal medical conditions, or cervical incompetence.

Any acute and significant blood loss in a physiologically hostile environment can compromise the endurance of the most highly trained individual. Under wilderness conditions, control of significant maternal hemorrhage accompanying miscarriage may be difficult unless provisions, facilities, and medicinal supplies are available. Uterine curettage is the method most often used to complete evacuation of the uterus when medical facilities are available. Once empty, uterine involution, spontaneous or aided by uterine massage, is usually sufficient to impede bleeding from the implantation site. In the absence of the ability to perform curettage, treatment with methylergonovine (0.2 mg orally or intramuscularly) can enhance uterine contractions, accelerate expulsion of products of conception, and promote uterine involution to maintain hemostasis. Methylergonovine should not be used in patients with hypertensive disorders, underlying vascular disease, and certain cardiac abnormalities unless the benefits clearly outweigh the risks of acute generalized vasoconstriction. As an alternative, prostaglandin $F_{2\alpha}$ (250 μg intramuscularly) or misoprostol (100 μg orally or vaginally) can be administered with less risk of cardiovascular compromise.

Ectopic Pregnancy. Far more dangerous than miscarriage, ectopic pregnancy must always be considered a life-threatening emergency that requires immediate medical attention. Ectopic pregnancy refers to implantation at any location outside the uterine cavity, most often (more than 95%) the fallopian tube. Hemorrhage resulting from ectopic pregnancy is still the leading cause of death in the first trimester. The incidence of ectopic pregnancy has tripled over the past 30 years and now exceeds one of every 100 pregnancies.[121] This increase is directly proportional to the rise in incidence of acute and chronic PID. The most common predisposing risk factors include a history of infections, multiple sexual partners, early age of onset of sexual activity, delayed childbearing, and previous IUD use. Independent risk factors are a history of abdominal and tubal surgery, including previous tubal sterilization procedures, endometriosis, DES exposure, and pregnancy by assisted reproductive interventions. Regardless of the etiology, an ectopic pregnancy increases the risk for another ectopic pregnancy approximately tenfold. A woman with a history of ectopic pregnancy should not intentionally plan to conceive again in the wilderness and should have her intrauterine pregnancy confirmed sonographically before departure.

Most women with a tubal ectopic pregnancy become symptomatic before 12 weeks' gestation and present with complaints of abdominal pain and altered menses. Early pregnancy symptoms may be minimal or absent. The pain often begins unilaterally with sudden onset and is usually severe, distinguishable from the cramping, intermittent pain accompanying miscarriage by its persistence and intensity. Clinical findings include a tender adnexal mass, nontender cervix, small to slightly enlarged nontender uterus, and absence of high-grade fever. Low-grade temperature elevation to 38° C (100.4° F) may occur in as many as 20% of women with ectopic pregnancy. When intraperitoneal hemorrhage accompanies rupture of the tube, the pain becomes diffuse with peritoneal signs of tenderness, guarding, and rebound. Shoulder pain from diaphragmatic irritation may be present as well. Pelvic examination at this point usually elicits discomfort with movement of the cervix and uterus. Fullness of the cul de sac posterior to the uterus and abdominal distention suggest significant intraperitoneal blood loss.

Vaginal bleeding accompanying an ectopic pregnancy usually follows a variable period of amenorrhea. It often begins with minimal flow of blood darker than that seen during miscarriage and results from inadequate progestational support of the decidualized endometrium. Uterine cramping may ensue, with passage of organized clot and tissue in the form of a decidual cast resembling products of conception, leading to the mistaken diagnosis of spontaneous abortion. However, cessation of pain is typical with completion of miscarriage and quite atypical with passage of a decidual cast concurrent to an ectopic pregnancy. With rupture of an ectopic pregnancy, heavier, bright-red bleeding may occur vaginally and if accompanied by significant intraperitoneal hemorrhage, may rapidly result in hemodynamic decompensation that only can be controlled surgically. The differential diagnosis of ectopic pregnancy includes normal intrauterine pregnancy with a corpus luteal cyst or hemorrhagic corpus luteum, threatened or incomplete abortion, PID, adnexal torsion (usually associated with adnexal enlargement from a benign or neoplastic process), endometriosis, UTI or ureteral stone, degenerating fibroid, and appendicitis. Although simultaneous intrauterine and ectopic pregnancies were once considered to be extremely rare, the incidence is now estimated at one in 6000 in the general population and greater than one in 100 among recipients of assisted reproductive techniques.

The diagnosis of ectopic pregnancy is considered presumptively in any woman with a positive pregnancy test, abnormal bleeding, and abdominal pain. In a full-service medical care facility the first step in management is to assess serum hCG levels and ascertain location of the pregnancy. An intrauterine pregnancy can usually be confirmed by transvaginal sonography once the serum hCG exceeds 1000 mIU/ml, corresponding to 2 to 3 weeks after conception or 4 to 5 weeks from the last normal menstrual period (LMP). In contrast, absence of an intrauterine pregnancy at hCG levels of 1000 mIU/ml or greater suggests ectopic pregnancy. In the absence of sonography, serum progesterone level greater than 25 ng/ml indicates a viable intrauterine pregnancy, greatly reducing the chance of an ectopic pregnancy.[149] Progesterone level less than 25 ng/ml is not diagnostic under these circumstances because it cannot differentiate nonviable intrauterine pregnancy from ectopic pregnancy.

In a wilderness setting that precludes the ability to perform a sonogram and quantitative determinations of hCG and progesterone, plans for evacuation must be made at first suspicion of the diagnosis. In extraordinary circumstances when the diagnosis is questionable, evacuation is not readily possible, and an experienced health care provider is available, the only technique that might offer some reassurance is culdocentesis. Needle aspiration of serous fluid from the posterior cul de sac argues against but does not exclude an ectopic pregnancy, since more than 75% of symptomatic cases with an ectopic pregnancy will have some degree of intraperitoneal hemorrhage. The presence of nonclotting blood confirms intraperitoneal hemorrhage and in approximately 95% of cases indicates ectopic pregnancy. The remainder usually result from bleeding of the corpus luteum.

Treatment options for ectopic pregnancy are not usually available in the wilderness. In the past, management of ectopic pregnancy has been exclusively surgical. Once an ectopic pregnancy is symptomatic, and when peritoneal signs or evidence of hemodynamic instability are present, laparoscopic or open abdominal procedures are still necessary. In recent years, however, medical therapy with methotrexate has proved useful in management of early, unruptured ectopic pregnancies.[148] Women with known risk factors who are attempting to become pregnant are encouraged to be followed proactively. They can often have the diagnosis of ectopic pregnancy confirmed by hCG and transvaginal sonography within 35 days from the LMP and before significant symptoms and tubal rupture. If the adnexal mass is less than 4 cm and the patient is minimally symptomatic and hemodynamically stable, single-dose methotrexate therapy (50 mg/m^2 intramuscularly) is effective and reduces the need for surgical intervention, thereby maximizing the opportunity for preservation of the fallopian tube. The quantitative hCG is followed serially until undetectable. If there is a slow fall or plateau in hCG levels and the woman is still stable, the dose can be repeated, usually no sooner than 1 week after the initial dose. Methotrexate is less likely to be effective when the ectopic mass is more than 4 cm, there is fetal cardiac activity, the woman is symptomatic, or significant free peritoneal fluid is present. Methotrex-

---

Box 75-5 LATER COMPLICATIONS OF PREGNANCY REQUIRING EVACUATION

Placenta previa
Placental abruption
Preterm labor
Premature rupture of membranes
Chorioamnionitis
Preeclampsia/eclampsia/HELLP syndrome

HELLP, Hemolysis, elevated liver function enzymes, and low platelets.

---

ate is contraindicated when the woman is hemodynamically unstable, has active pulmonary disease, or is not willing to return for follow-up.

Later Pregnancy. Common conditions that do not cause problems until 20 weeks' gestation or later cannot be optimally managed in most wilderness settings (Box 75-5). The safest course of action is to make plans for immediate evacuation. Second- and third-trimester bleeding could simply be the result of cervical effacement, labor, cervical polyps, coital trauma, or vaginitis, but it could also be much more dangerous if the source is placenta previa or placental abruption. Historical information and physical findings may suggest an etiology, but a definitive diagnosis is not possible without verification.

PLACENTA PREVIA. When evaluating bleeding, placenta previa always must be given primary consideration. Placenta previa results from implantation of the placenta in the lower uterine segment over or near the internal cervical os. It occurs in approximately one of 200 births. Risk increases with age and parity, multiple gestations, women who have submucosal fibroids or have had multiple dilation and curettage procedures (D&Cs) or cesarean sections, and in cigarette smokers.[1,65] The classic presentation of placenta previa is painless, sudden, heavy, and bright-red vaginal bleeding.[17] It may occur with exertional activity, straining on the toilet, or intercourse but also occurs at rest with no obvious precipitating factor. Many women report awakening at night in a pool of blood as the initial manifestation of a placenta previa, probably the result of stretching of the lower uterine segment and implantation site by a bladder that has become distended while sleeping. Uterine contractions may accompany the bleeding and may be the precipitating cause if they have been significant enough to initiate cervical effacement. Physical examination is limited until the placental location has been ascertained by sonography. The uterus is usually nontender, and the baby is often in a lie well out of the pelvis because the placenta displaces the presenting part. Digital examination of the cervix and simple speculum examination of the vagina are contraindicated, unless capabilities are available for immediate delivery, because they could disrupt the placental interface from the lower uterine segment, resulting in catastrophic hemorrhage. Interestingly, women who bleed for the first time with a placenta previa may have significant blood loss, but the bleeding is often self-limited and rarely compromises fetal well-being. The course of subsequent bleeds is much less predictable. Once a woman with a complete placenta previa has bled significantly, she should probably be hospitalized until delivery. In most instances, cesarean section is required for safe delivery.

PLACENTAL ABRUPTION. Placental abruption is defined as separation of the placenta from the maternal interface before delivery. Risk factors include hypertensive disorders (e.g., preeclampsia, chronic hypertension), other chronic diseases with vascular compromise (e.g., diabetes, renal disease, certain autoimmune disorders), coagulation disorders (presence of lupus anticoagulants or anticardiolipin antibodies, protein S or C deficiencies, factor V Leiden, antithrombin III deficiency), trauma, chorioamnionitis, advanced maternal age, multiparity, and cigarette abuse.[106,123] One of the most common causes of placental abruption in recent years has been cocaine use.

Placental abruption is highly variable in presentation, depending on the location and the extent of the separation and hemorrhage. About 80% of placental abruptions result in visible bleeding accompanying the onset of other symptoms. Twenty percent result in concealed subchorionic hemorrhage that may not become apparent until many days after the event. Unlike placenta previa, abruption is usually accompanied by sudden onset of sharp pain. The pain may be focal and continuous, intermittently intensifying with the frequent uterine contractions and irritability that usually accompany and can extend the placental separation. Severe abruptions may be accompanied by prolonged tetanic contractions with extravasation of hemorrhage into the myometrium (Couvelaire uterus); these may compromise uterine involution after delivery. Fetal compromise is much more common with placental abruption than with placenta previa. Traumatic separation of the placenta results in a greater likelihood of disrupted placental vasculature, resulting in fetal blood loss into the subchorionic clot or into the maternal circulation as a fetal-maternal hemorrhage. This can be a major cause of blood group isoimmunization that can affect future pregnancies.

Diagnosis of placental abruption is usually based on clinical signs and symptoms and maternal history. Standard sonography is not as useful a diagnostic tool as it is with placenta previa, because small abruptions may be difficult to differentiate from placental tissue and normal placental vascular channels. Magnetic resonance imaging (MRI) and Doppler modalities are more useful but are rarely necessary as diagnostic tools. No laboratory tests are diagnostic for placental abruption, but abnormalities of coagulation studies may suggest small abruptions and may help ascertain the extent of consumptive coagulopathy in large abruptions. A Kleihauer-Betke screen should also be done to assess fetal cells in the maternal circulation. Rh-negative unsensitized women should be given Rh-immune globulin when an abruption is suspected or confirmed. In view of the association with cocaine use, urine toxicologic screens are almost routine in the absence of other causes of placental abruption. If delivery is necessary or deemed inevitable, route of delivery is determined by the degree of fetal or maternal compromise and the prospects for vaginal delivery.

PREMATURE LABOR. Despite the advances that have been made in obstetric and neonatal care in the past 50 years, rates of preterm delivery, defined as delivery before 37 completed weeks' gestation, have not changed, persisting in the range of 8% to 10% of all pregnancies in the United States. It is still the leading cause of perinatal morbidity and mortality. Preterm labor, defined as regular uterine contractions resulting in progressive cervical change, as assessed by effacement, dilation, and softening, complicates twice as many pregnancies as actually progress to preterm delivery. Symptoms of preterm labor include mild and menstrual-like to painful uterine contractions, intermittent low back pain or pressure, pelvic pressure, increase in vaginal discharge resulting from effacement with compression of endocervical glands or leaking of amniotic fluid, and bloody "show." The more common risk factors for preterm labor and delivery include premature rupture of membranes, subclinical or overt chorioamnionitis, UTI, substance abuse (tobacco, cocaine, amphetamines), preeclampsia, multiple gestation, hydramnios, dehydration, constipation, chronic stress, and incompetent cervix.[102] The pregnant wilderness traveler is at risk for several of these factors and should strive to reduce their occurrence.

Thorough evaluation and management of preterm labor cannot be done in most wilderness settings. Some empiric measures can be taken, however, based on the woman's symptoms and palpation of uterine contractions alone, while awaiting evacuation or to prepare for delivery if evacuation is delayed or impossible. Pelvic examination should be avoided unless placenta previa has been previously excluded and sterile supplies are available. If done by an experienced person, cervical examination should determine dilation, effacement, and consistency, as well as the station and presentation of the baby. Once it has been concluded that the woman is in preterm labor and evacuation is required, examinations should not be repeated unless delivery appears imminent. If she clearly has ruptured membranes, characteristics of the fluid should be noted (clear, bloody, meconium stained), but no internal vaginal examination should be performed initially to minimize risks of introducing infection.

Interim measures for managing preterm labor include the following: encourage the woman to empty her bladder and rectum; place her at rest on her side; make sure she is kept warm and comfortable; and provide oral hydration with 32 to 64 ounces of fluid over an hour. These measures alone will decrease uterine activity in as many as one third of women having preterm contractions. If available, a broad-spectrum antibiotic, preferably one with coverage of both group B β-hemolytic streptococci and anaerobic organisms, should be given orally or parenterally.[126] Parenteral corticosteroids, if available, are useful in accelerating fetal lung maturity in anticipation of premature delivery. Administration of β-methasone (12 mg intramuscularly; repeat dose in 12 to 24 hours) or dexamethasone (6 mg intramuscularly every 6 hours for four doses) has become an accepted part of empiric therapy when the estimated gestational age is less than 34 weeks. Many common medications have tocolytic activity, but each should be administered only after careful consideration of their potential risks and side effects (Box 75-6). Of these, the prostaglandin synthetase inhibitors are most likely to be part of the routine supplies on a wilderness excursion and are also probably the safest to use in combination with initial measures of rest and hydration. If preterm labor cannot be stopped before evacuation, guidelines exist for management of delivery, as detailed later.

HYPERTENSIVE DISORDERS. Pregnancy-induced hypertensive disorders include preeclampsia, eclampsia, and HELLP syndrome. These disorders complicate 10% or more of all pregnancies and are responsible for 15% to 20% of maternal mortality in the United States. Although guidelines have been put forth for their definition, the etiology of these conditions and the differences between them are unknown. Variability in presentation and unpredictability in course characterize these disorders. All are specific to pregnancy, despite mimicking nonpregnancy-related diseases, and do not begin to resolve until the baby and placenta are delivered. Generalized vasospasm and hypersensitivity to vasoconstrictors are typically present.[86,162] Major risk factors for preeclampsia include nulliparity, obesity, previous history of preeclampsia, underlying hypertension or chronic renal disease, pregestational diabetes, autoim-

---

Box 75-6 MEDICATIONS IN COMMON USE FOR TOCOLYSIS

MAGNESIUM SULFATE

Calcium antagonist ($MgSO_4$), 4-6 g IV over 20-30 min (or IM in split doses to buttocks), followed by continuous infusion of 2-4 g/hr × 12-24 hr.

Interrupt or decrease infusion if deep tendon reflexes cannot be elicited or respiratory compromise develops.

Effects are readily reversible by calcium gluconate in emergency circumstances.

Do not use in combination with nifedipine.

TERBUTALINE SULFATE

β-Sympathomimetic, 0.25 mg SC initially, then every 1-4 hr.

Repeat dosing should be withheld in the presence of maternal hypotension, tachycardia, or chest pain.

Before administration, the woman should be well hydrated, but care must be taken not to fluid overload once therapy has begun because of risk for pulmonary edema.

NIFEDIPINE

Calcium channel blocker, 10 mg SL every 20 min × 1 to 4 doses, then 10-20 mg PO q6h.

Decrease dose or frequency for maternal hypotension.

Do *not* use in combination with $MgSO_4$.

INDOMETHACIN

Prostaglandin synthetase inhibitor, 50-100 mg per rectum initially, then 25-50 mg PO q6h.

Do not use for more than 24 to 48 hours because of effects on fetal urine output (decreased production of amniotic fluid), potential for masking fever, and possible premature closure of the fetal ductus arteriosus.

Safe for use in combination with magnesium, terbutaline, and nifedipine.

IBUPROFEN

Prostaglandin synthetase inhibitor, 600-800 mg PO initially, then 400-800 mg PO q6h.

Appears to have much less effect on fetal urine output and ductus arteriosus than terbutaline but can mask fever.

Safe for use in combination with magnesium, terbutaline, and nifedipine.

IM, Intramuscularly; *IV,* intravenously; *SC,* subcutaneously; *SL,* sublingually; *PO,* orally; *q6h,* every 6 hours.

mune disorders, antiphospholipid antibody syndrome, maternal age over 40, multiple gestation, molar pregnancy, hydrops fetalis, intrauterine growth restriction, and oligohydramnios.[20,39,115,161] Genetic predisposition for preeclampsia is supported by the strong association of family history and identification of certain genetic markers, such as angiotensinogen gene T235, associated with disease expression.[77,111,112]

The diagnosis of preeclampsia is based on the triad of hypertension, proteinuria, and edema. Hypertension is defined as systolic blood pressure of 140 mm Hg and higher or diastolic blood pressure of 90 mm Hg or higher measured on two separate occasions 6 or more hours apart. Proteinuria is defined as 300 mg or greater in 24 hours or the presence of 0.1 g/L (1+ or greater) by dipstick on at least two random urine specimens 6 hours apart. Edema is considered significant to the diagnosis of preeclampsia only if it generalized or if the woman has gained 5 pounds in a week. The strict diagnosis of preeclampsia requires the presence of hypertension with proteinuria, edema, or both. Women meeting these criteria have at least mild preeclampsia.

Diagnostic criteria for severe preeclampsia require only one of the following: blood pressure of 160 mm Hg systolic and higher or 110 mm Hg diastolic and higher on two occasions at least 6 hours apart; proteinuria (5 g/24 hours or higher); oliguria (400 ml/24 hours or higher); persistent epigastric pain; pulmonary edema or cyanosis; impaired liver function of unclear etiology; thrombocytopenia (less than 100,000/mm³); and eclampsia (grand mal seizures). Most cases of severe preeclampsia are associated with intrauterine growth restriction or abnormalities of fetal umbilical (increased resistance) and middle cerebral (decreased resistance) arterial flow consistent with relative placental insufficiency.[18] Eclampsia, as a subset of severe preeclampsia, is a major cause of maternal and fetal morbidity and mortality worldwide, occurring in about one of 2000 pregnancies in the United States. Although difficult to anticipate, the presence of visual disturbances, severe headache, irritability, epigastric or right upper quadrant pain, nausea and vomiting, and cerebral dysfunction must be considered predictors of eclampsia.[92,169] Only about half of women complain of these symptoms before seizure, and as many as one third will not have a seizure until the postpartum period, sometimes as the first significant event suggesting preeclampsia.[15]

The most serious subset of severe preeclampsia, occurring in about 10% of cases, is HELLP syndrome, or *h*emolysis, *e*levated *l*iver function enzymes, and *l*ow *p*latelets.[93,133] Hemolysis is defined as an abnormal peripheral smear consistent with a microangiopathic process, total bilirubin greater than 1.2 mg/dl, and lactic dehydrogenase (LDH) greater than 600 U/L. Elevated liver enzymes include aspartate aminotransaminase greater than 70 U/L and LDH greater than 600 U/L. Low platelets generally refer to levels less than 100,000/mm³, although some women with the other manifestations of the syndrome will maintain platelet counts above 100,000/mm³.[76] Unlike severe preeclampsia/eclampsia, HELLP syndrome tends to affect older, white, and multiparous women. Onset of most cases of HELLP syndrome is before 37 weeks' gestation; as many as 15% of cases present before 26 weeks. Although 80% of women will have the diagnosis of preeclampsia made before delivery, more than 50% will not develop the most severe manifestations of HELLP syndrome until 1 to 2 days postpartum. During this time, mobilization of extracellular tissue fluid can suddenly precipitate pulmonary edema because of delayed renal recovery. Renal failure, disseminated intravascular coagulation, sepsis, hepatic hematoma and rupture, adult respiratory distress syndrome, and retinal detachment have been reported.[139]

If preeclampsia is suspected, plans should be made for immediate evacuation from the wilderness setting. While awaiting evacuation, the woman should be placed at rest and have free access to fluids. If magnesium sulfate is available, it should be administered in the same manner as described for preterm labor (see Box 75-6) to decrease the risk for seizures.[169] Because of the increased likelihood of renal compromise with preeclampsia, magnesium toxicity must be carefully monitored by assessment of deep tendon reflexes. Antihypertensive medications should be administered with great caution or not at all, since preeclampsia is often accompanied by intravascular volume depletion (even with an excess of total body water) by the time the condition is recognized. Antihypertensive agents that cause vasodilation can greatly reduce MAP, placing the baby at risk for acute placental insufficiency when the placental perfusion may already be compromised. Indications for administration of an antihypertensive drug include persistent blood pressure greater than 160 mm Hg systolic or 110 mm Hg diastolic. The goal should not be to normalize blood pressure, but to maintain it in the range of 140/90 mm Hg. The α/β blocking agent labetalol administered in incremental doses (20, 40, and 80 mg intravenously at 10- to 20-minute intervals, up 300 mg) is widely used for this purpose. If a pregnant woman has a seizure, the airway should be maintained, oral cavity protected, woman positioned on her side, and no efforts made to restrain the myoclonic activity. If magnesium sulfate is available, it is still the treatment of choice for eclamptic seizures and should be administered as previously described. Alternatively, a loading dose of diphenylhydantoin (20 mg/kg intravenously no faster than 50 mg/min) or lorazepam (1 to 2 mg intravenously) can be given.

Management

Delivery. For many reasons, a wilderness delivery at term should rarely be "planned." If it is planned, only multiparous women who have had uncomplicated pregnancies, labor and delivery, and postpartum courses and who are willing to accept the risks of unexpected fetal and maternal complications should consider this as an option. A pregnant woman planning a wilderness experience of any duration that will carry beyond 20 weeks' gestation should include emergency provisions and plans. The location, duration of stay, and distance will dictate the extent of these plans from medical care facilities, convenience of evacuation routes, and ease of communication with and availability of evacuation support.

When the woman is in labor preparing for delivery, either a health care provider or the person with the most childbirth experience who is willing to assist in the delivery should be identified as team leader and "midwife." Participatory roles for other members of the party should be defined in cooperation with the pregnant woman. Requests for privacy and intimacy should be respected to the extent possible.

By necessity and practicality, delivery in the wilderness dictates a laissez-faire approach. Excessive intervention (e.g., repeated cervical examinations, artificial rupture of membranes, augmentation of uterine contractions by oxytocin or nipple stimulation, manual cervical dilation) is neither warranted nor appropriate, since delivery cannot be expedited for concerns of fetal distress, and such intervention may increase maternal and fetal risks. To the extent possible, a clean, comfortable, and quiet site is prepared for the delivery. If clean and sterile supplies and medications are available, these should be brought to this location and inventoried by the team leader (see Box 75-3). Otherwise, clean towels, clothing, bedding, soap, and water should be made readily accessible.

Fetal position should be determined. In late third-trimester pregnancies, this can be accomplished by external abdominal palpation using Leopold's maneuvers (Figure 75-2). In preterm pregnancies this may first require internal digital examination, but fetal position is extremely important because the risk of malpresentation (breech, transverse, or compound lie) is inversely proportional to gestational age, as is the disparity between fetal head and abdominal circumferences. At term the incidence of breech presentation is approximately 3%, whereas it may exceed 25% under 30 weeks' gestation. If the woman reports fetal activity, or if this is visible or palpable on abdominal examination, evaluation of fetal heart activity is usually unnecessary. If the woman or the examiner cannot detect fetal activity, and since fetal activity frequently diminishes with onset of labor, viability is assessed by auscultation. A stethoscope or the ear can be positioned over the location of the baby's back and shoulder. A stethoscope bell placed on the abdomen with minimal pressure is usually more sensitive than the diaphragm. Normal fetal heart rate at term usually falls to between 120 and 160 beats/min. Under most wilderness situations, once viability is confirmed, further auscultation is probably unnecessary and may even provoke anxiety because of the inherent difficulties of fetal heart rate detection with unamplified methods, subtle changes in fetal position, descent of the presenting part, and the increasing discomfort of labor as it progresses.

If facilities are available to perform an emergency cesarean section in the wilderness, intermittent fetal heart rate monitoring is done for 1 or 2 minutes every 20 to 30 minutes during the first stage of labor and every 10 to 15 minutes during the second stage. However, even under these highly unlikely circumstances, cesarean section should be considered only with persistent fetal bradycardia or with failure to progress in labor.

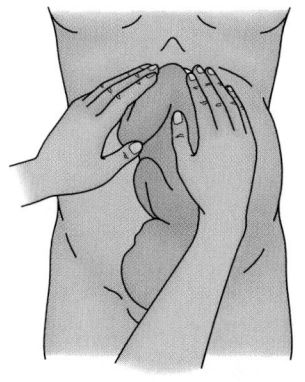 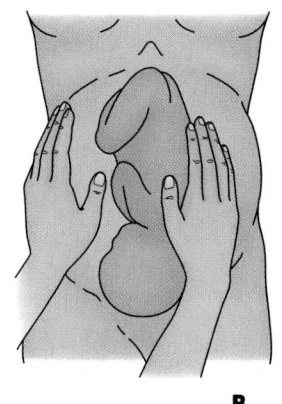 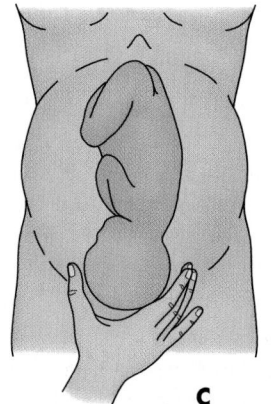 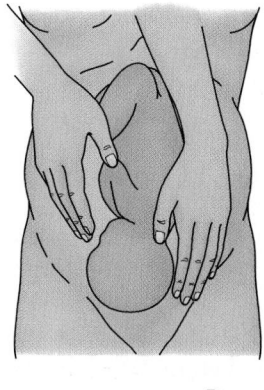

A   B   C   D

Figure 75-2   Ascertaining fetal position by Leopold's maneuvers. **A,** First maneuver. Assess part of fetus in upper uterus. **B,** Ascertain location of fetal back. **C,** Identify presenting part. **D,** Determine descent of presenting part.

In the early stages of labor or with spontaneous rupture of membranes in the absence of regular uterine contractions, rest interspersed with brief periods of ambulation, fluid intake, and frequent light meals should be encouraged. Prophylactic antibiotics should be started, especially when there has been premature rupture of membranes. Antibiotic coverage is the same as that recommended for preterm labor. Digital cervical examination is usually not necessary at this point and is contraindicated with rupture. As labor becomes more active, as gauged by increased frequency, regularity, and strength of uterine contractions, pelvic pressure, and discomfort level, the safest approach is to limit oral intake to clear liquids only. The GI tract becomes quiescent with active labor, and any stomach contents present at the outset will likely be present at the end. Since vomiting is not unusual, especially during the "transition" phase of labor, clear liquids minimize discomfort and decrease risk of aspiration. Intermittent ambulation may also decrease the discomfort associated with contractions and can be continued, if the woman desires, until she feels the need to push. During this time she should also be reminded to empty her bladder because she may not be able to differentiate the sensation to void from that of pressure from the presenting fetal part. A full bladder not only adds to the discomfort of labor but can also impede descent of the baby into the pelvis, prolonging the process.

Although some women become irritable as labor intensifies before complete dilation and do not want to be touched, others appreciate low back or extremity massage between contractions. Assistance with breathing and relaxation techniques to distract, maintain composure, and preserve the energy that will be required during the second stage of labor are also beneficial. During labor, no oral pain medication should be given, and parenteral narcotics, although acceptable, should be administered sparingly (ideally, intravenously with the onset of a contraction) unless naloxone is available to manage the fetal depression that may result. If a skilled health care provider is managing the delivery and pain is intolerable, a paracervical block can be considered once the cervix has reached 7 to 8 cm of dilation. This should only be done if the provider has performed the procedure previously. The cervix is usually completely effaced at this point, so care must be taken not to inject the baby or inject the anesthetic agent intravenously.

When the woman begins to feel involuntary efforts to push with contractions, cervical examination should be performed with a clean or sterile glove or freshly washed hands. At the same time that cervical dilation and effacement are assessed, the presenting fetal body part should be identified, determining its station in relation to the ischial spines in midpelvis. If the cervix is completely dilated and effaced so that no cervical tissue is palpable between the presenting part and the

vaginal wall, the first stage of labor is complete, and the woman can begin pushing with contractions. If the cervix is not completely dilated, the woman should be encouraged not to push with contractions so that she does not become exhausted. She also risks entrapping the cervix between the presenting part and the pelvis, which can lead to cervical edema and thickening, although this usually results from cephalopelvic disproportion. If membranes have ruptured, presence or absence of meconium should be noted. If membranes have not ruptured, they should not be ruptured intentionally, particularly if the baby is premature or in a breech presentation.

Usually, once the cervix is completely dilated, the desire to push is involuntary, and pain is less of an issue until the moment of delivery. Pushing is done only with uterine contractions. At the onset of a contraction the woman takes in a deep breath, expels this, and then taking in another deep breath and holding this, bears down without releasing air as if straining to have a bowel movement. Most contractions are long enough to permit two or three attempts at this maneuver. Proper pushing is evident by expansion of the introitus and rectum during the effort and should not be accompanied by tensing of the extremities. Once the contraction is over, she should expel any held air and begin restful breathing, trying to relax completely to conserve energy and recover for the next contraction. The woman may push in any position in which she feels comfortable. However, she should avoid laying flat on her back because uterine compression of the inferior vena cava can lead to hypotension and decreased uterine perfusion. Common positions include semirecumbent, with back and head elevated and legs drawn up or supported at the knees during contractions; lateral recumbent, with superior leg flexed and supported during contractions; squatting; sitting; kneeling on all fours; and standing while being supported from behind around the torso. These positions can also be used for the actual delivery, as long as the attendant has adequate access. Once the presenting part reaches, distends, and remains at the vaginal introitus between contractions, final preparations are made for the delivery. A delivery position should be selected that allows control of the presenting part, protection of the perineum, and room to accomplish completion of the birth with as little trauma to the baby as possible. Delivery should be performed during a contraction.

Vertex Delivery. The most common fetal presentation is the cephalic (or vertex) presentation, with the fetal head facing the perineum (occiput anterior) (Figure 75-3). When the perineum begins to distend with a contraction, the woman should be instructed to bear down. Intentional cutting of an episiotomy in a wilderness setting is not recommended. Spontaneous lacerations are

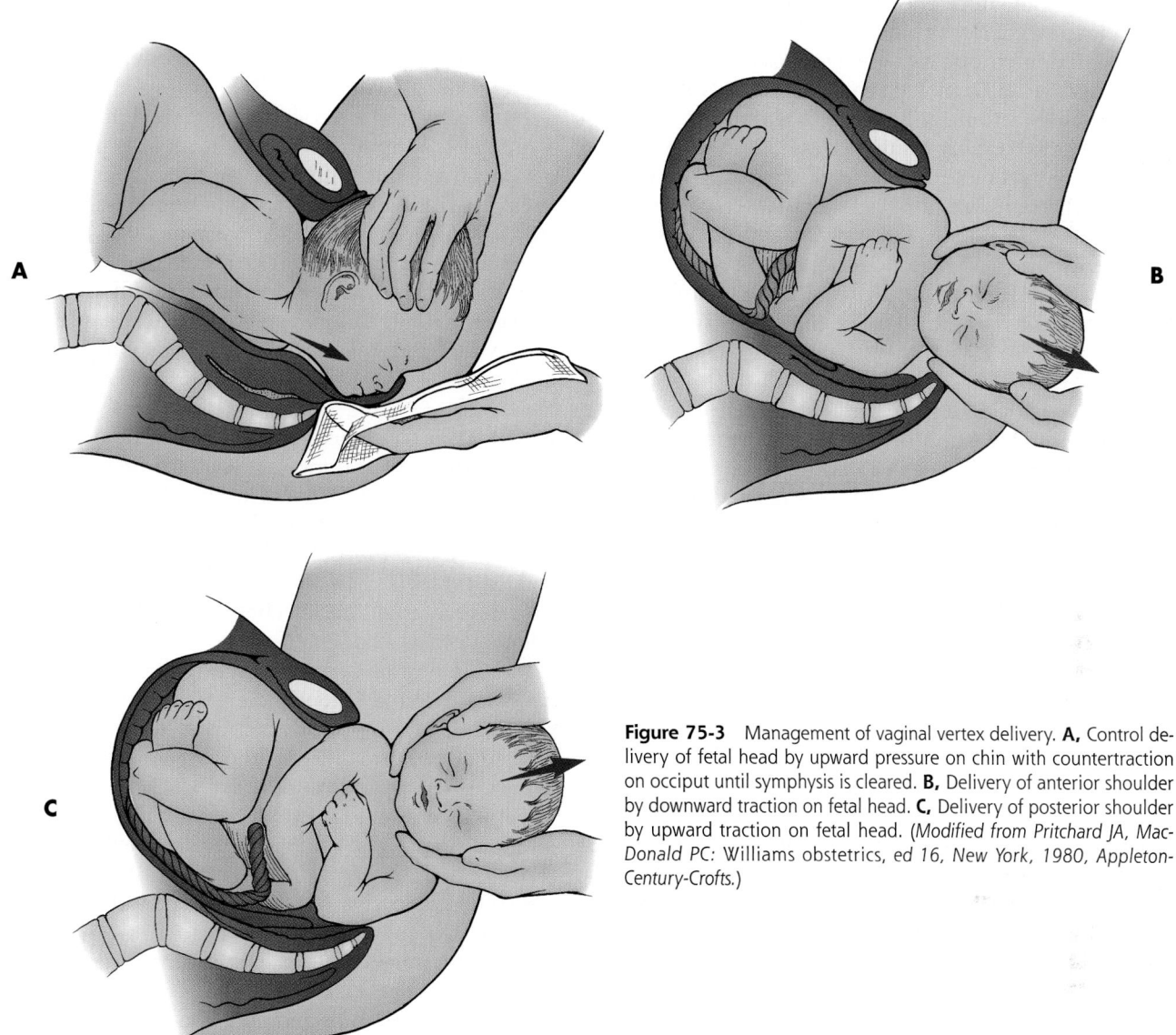

Figure 75-3   Management of vaginal vertex delivery. **A,** Control delivery of fetal head by upward pressure on chin with countertraction on occiput until symphysis is cleared. **B,** Delivery of anterior shoulder by downward traction on fetal head. **C,** Delivery of posterior shoulder by upward traction on fetal head. (*Modified from Pritchard JA, Mac-Donald PC:* Williams obstetrics, *ed 16, New York, 1980, Appleton-Century-Crofts.*)

more likely to occur along tissue planes that are less vascular and less likely to extend into the rectum. The perineum should be supported between the rectum and the introitus by the index finger and thumb of the nondominant hand while the fetal head is maintained in flexion until the crown has just begun to clear the symphysis. The woman stops pushing while the attendant exerts steady inward and upward pressure at the perineum against the fetal chin, thereby extending the head and completing its delivery while protecting the perineum. Once delivered, the fetal head will usually rotate laterally to align itself with the shoulders. The infant's mouth and nose should be cleaned by bulb aspiration or simple swabbing with a clean gauze or cloth. This step is especially important when meconium is present to prevent aspiration of this fluid when the baby is free to take its first breaths. Once the oropharynx is cleaned, the fetal neck should be palpated to ascertain the presence of a nuchal cord. If present, one or more loops of umbilical cord are often loose enough to be slipped over the baby's head before completion of the delivery. If they cannot be slipped over the head but are not tight, the baby can frequently be delivered through the loops. If the cord is tightly applied around the neck, the attendant should doubly clamp or tie a section of one loop, cut between the clamps, and then deliver the baby.

In the final stages of delivery the woman resumes pushing while steady downward (toward the maternal sacrum) traction is applied with hands cupping both sides of the fetal head. When the anterior shoulder has cleared the symphysis, the perineum should again be supported while the head is elevated and the posterior shoulder delivered. The rest of the baby's body usually follows without effort. The baby is held below the perineum (to prevent loss of blood to the placenta from the baby) while the oropharynx is again cleaned and the baby dried. Usually, rubbing the baby dry is sufficient to stimulate breathing and crying. The umbilical cord should then be doubly clamped or tied and then severed. The baby should be thoroughly dried, wrapped in clean, dry, and warm fabric with its head covered and given to the mother if she desires. If the baby does not cry within 10 to 15 seconds after delivery, has obvious airway obstruction, or is premature, the umbilical cord should be cut immediately and resuscitative efforts begun.

Shoulder Dystocia. If there is difficulty delivering the anterior shoulder (shoulder dystocia) by the method outlined, immediate steps should be taken to accomplish this. True shoulder dystocia occurs in less than 1% of deliveries, is rare in uncomplicated labors, but is a substantial cause of fetal and maternal morbidity.[144] Shoulder dystocia is often anticipated when the fetal head snaps back tightly and fails to rotate after its delivery. If available, other individuals can assist. Throughout the steps necessary to accomplish delivery, excessive traction on the fetal head is avoided because it may stretch the brachial plexus, resulting in an Erb's or Klumpke's palsy. The first step is to position the woman so that the buttocks are elevated to allow at least 12 inches of free space beneath the perineum to maneuver. Both legs should then be flexed upward to the chest (McRobert's maneuver) while the woman is supported in a semirecumbent position behind her back. Delivery should then be attempted again by downward traction on the fetal head.

If the shoulder is still impacted against the symphysis, pressure applied with the fist or heel of the hand just above the symphysis in the midline may reduce it sufficiently to accomplish the delivery. The assistants should not push on the uterine fundus because this can further impact the shoulder. If these maneuvers fail, an episiotomy should be cut to admit several fingers or the hand beneath the posterior shoulder. Once the hand has been inserted, the baby should be rotated by applying pressure to the shoulder and scapula (Wood's maneuver). The corkscrew rotation will deliver the posterior shoulder as it turns anteriorly, the anterior shoulder will dislodge, and the baby can be delivered without further difficulty. If this rotational maneuver fails, the posterior arm is delivered by grasping it along the forearm and sweeping it across the chest and out the vagina. This technique may fracture the humerus or the clavicle but is preferable to losing the baby because of inability to complete a delivery. Once the posterior arm is out, the anterior shoulder can usually be displaced downward, or the baby can then be rotated, allowing

completion of the delivery. This approach is preferable to intentionally fracturing the clavicle, which can be technically difficult and does not provide as much room for the delivery.

If the baby is in a vertex presentation but facing the symphysis (occiput posterior), the labor is often more prolonged and uncomfortable, particularly in the lower back. The delivery is basically accomplished as described, however, except the final maneuvers to deliver the fetal head are extension first, then flexion. Perineal and introital trauma is a greater risk with an occiput posterior delivery. Management of this fetal presentation by the wilderness birth attendant should be a minor challenge compared with delivery of a breech baby.

Breech Delivery. Since most wilderness deliveries will be "unexpected" and more likely to be premature, the baby also will more likely be in a breech lie. Other than chance and prematurity, the greatest risk factors for a baby to be in a breech presentation are unsuspected congenital fetal anomalies, chromosomal abnormalities, and maternal uterine abnormalities. Each of these adds a new level of challenge to the birth attendant. Under the best of circumstances, delivery of a breech carries a threefold to fourfold greater risk than a vertex presentation for morbidity resulting from prematurity, congenital abnormalities, and trauma at delivery. The trauma often results from disproportion between the larger fetal head and the smaller body circumference of a premature infant. This disproportion can lead to entrapment of the head and is especially problematic when the fetal body has negotiated an incompletely dilated cervix.

Breech babies come in many forms: frank breech (hips flexed, knees extended, buttocks presenting), complete breech (both hips and both knees flexed, buttocks and feet presenting), incomplete breech (one hip flexed, one hip partially extended, both knees flexed, buttocks and feet presenting), and footling breech (hips and knees extended, feet presenting). Regardless of the form, the approach in a wilderness setting demands patience. No effort should be made to deliver a breech baby until the presenting part is visible at the introitus and the cervix is completely dilated. Membranes should not be artificially ruptured in breech presentations. As the amniotic sac balloons into the birth canal, it helps to dilate the cervix completely. This facilitates descent of the baby, providing a lubricated smooth surface against which the body can freely move, and cushions the umbilical cord against compression in the birth canal.

When the cervix is completely dilated, the woman is instructed to push. Regardless of the type of breech presentation, the safest course is to allow the body to be extruded to at least the level of the umbilicus by maternal efforts alone (Figure 75-4). This increases the

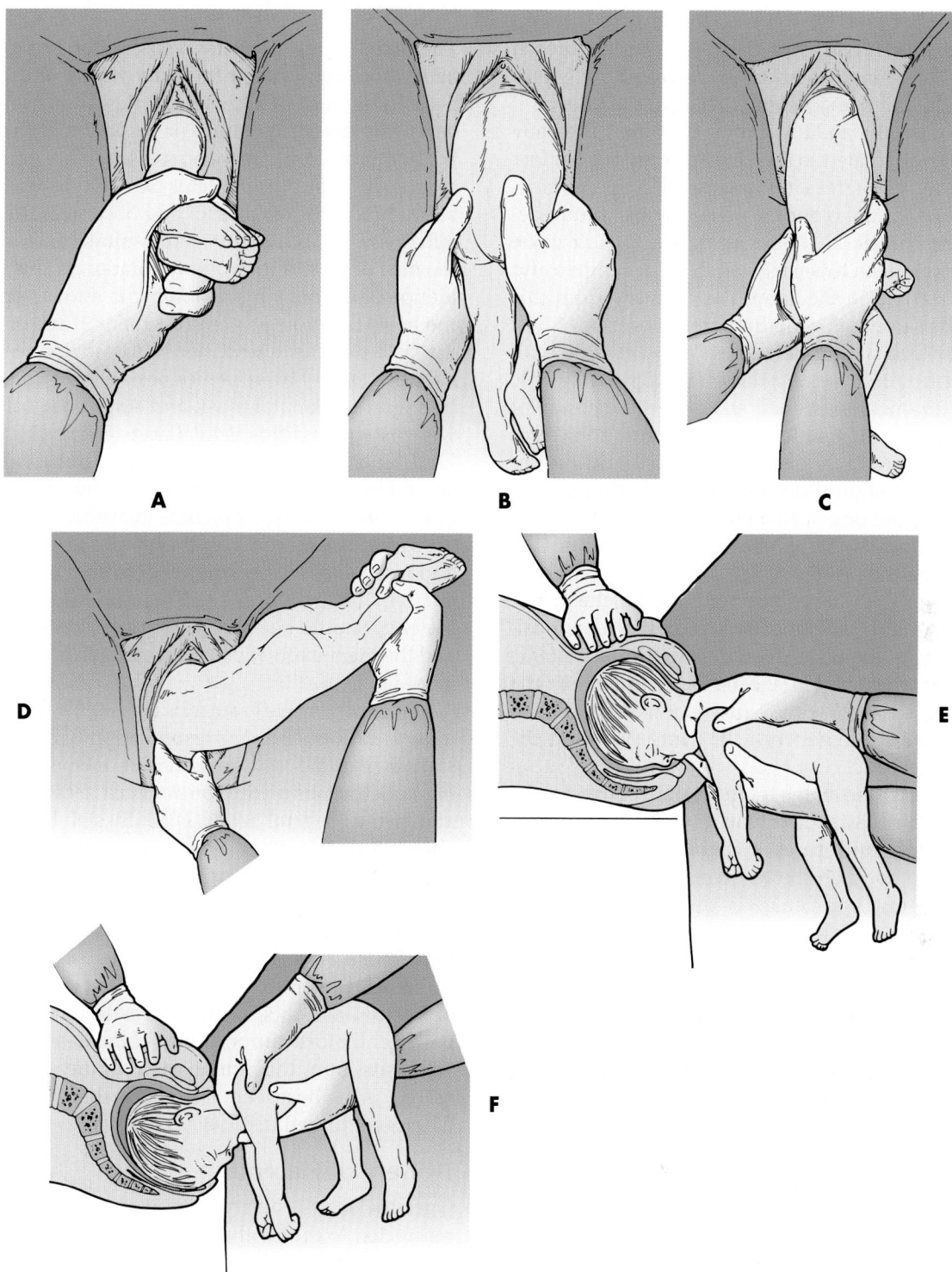

Figure 75-4 Management of vaginal breech delivery. **A,** Downward traction at ankles until buttocks clear the introitus. **B,** Traction on pelvic girdle until an axilla becomes visible. **C,** Delivery of posterior shoulder and arm. **D,** Delivery of anterior shoulder and arm with downward traction. **E,** Cradling the baby on forearm, finger is inserted into mouth or against chin. **F,** Delivery completed by outward traction while maintaining fetal head in flexed position. (*Modified from Pritchard JA, MacDonald PC: Williams obstetrics, ed 16, New York, 1980, Appleton-Century-Crofts.*)

chance that the fetal head has begun to pass through the pelvic inlet. A baby in a frank or complete breech lie should have the posterior leg delivered by gently grasping the thigh and flexing the leg at the knee as it is rotated medially and toward the introitus. The baby should then be rotated to the sacrum anterior position, then another 45 degrees in the same direction to facilitate delivery of the other leg using the technique described for the first. The legs and buttocks can be wrapped in a clean towel to provide a firmer grip and decrease trauma to the baby. The delivery from this point is the same as for footling breech presentations. The upper legs should be grasped on each side with the index fingers crossing the infant's pelvic girdle and both thumbs positioned just above the crease of the buttocks. Using gentle side-to-side rotational motion over an arc of 90 degrees outward and downward, traction should be applied while the mother pushes, until the upper portion of a scapula is visible at the introitus. With the baby's body rotated 45 degrees toward the opposite side, the arm is delivered by flexion and medial rotation across the chest. The baby is rotated to the opposite side in the same position, and the other arm is then delivered. If assistants are present, the woman should be helped into the McRobert's position, with hyperflexion at the hips to maximize the space between the symphysis and the sacrum.

Maintaining the baby in the same plane as the vagina, the birth attendant reaches palm up between the baby's legs and into the vagina, supporting the baby's entire body on the forearm while placing the second and fourth fingers over the infant's maxillae and placing the middle finger into the mouth or on the chin. The other hand is positioned over the infant's upper back so those fingers are overlying each shoulder. If there is sufficient room, the middle fingers can be applied to the fetal occiput. Then with the woman pushing, the baby's head is flexed downward, completing the delivery. Firm suprapubic pressure can help to maintain the head in flexion. During this final stage the baby's body should not be elevated more than 45 degrees above the plane of the vagina to avoid hyperextension of the head. If the fetal head cannot be delivered because the cervix is incompletely dilated, the cervix can be cut at the 2 and 10 o'clock positions (Duhrssen's incisions) to provide sufficient room to complete the delivery. Once delivered, if the baby breathes and cries spontaneously or with minimal stimulation, cutting the umbilical cord can be delayed while the baby is dried. This allows some of the blood retained in the placenta from umbilical vein compression (common with breech deliveries) to return to the baby. On the contrary, if the baby is clearly depressed, the umbilical cord should be immediately clamped and cut and neonatal resuscitation begun.

Neonatal Resuscitation

The first steps in neonatal resuscitation are to dry the baby thoroughly, keep the baby warm, and clear the nose and mouth of excess fluid. Respiratory effort and heart rate (by auscultation or palpation at the base of the umbilical cord) are then assessed. If breathing spontaneously with pulse greater than 100 beats/min, the baby should be kept warm and observed. If the pulse falls below 100 beats/min and respiratory effort is poor, the next step is to improve ventilation. If further stimulation of the baby by rubbing with a towel or flicking the heels fails to elicit improvement in respiratory effort and pulse, the next step is to provide ventilatory support, ideally by applying positive-pressure ventilation with a neonatal mask and Ambu bag (preferably with oxygen). If this is available, gentle (15 to 30 cm H_2O) and rapid (40 to 60 breaths/min) ventilation should be performed for 30 seconds and the heart rate reassessed. If no equipment is available, the resuscitator's mouth is placed over the infant's nose and mouth, and rapid shallow breaths are delivered at a rate of 30-40/min. If this restores heart rate and respiratory effort, the baby should be observed for deterioration in status and the maneuvers repeated as necessary until support is available.

If the baby's heart rate falls below 60 beats/min, full infant cardiopulmonary resuscitation (CPR) should be started. Cardiac compression is performed by (1) placing both thumbs on the sternum just above the xiphoid and facing the fetal head, (2) gently stabilizing this position with the other fingers around the chest, and (3) supplying compressions to a depth of ½ to ¾ inch at a rate of approximately 90/min. Care should be taken not to deliver compression to the baby's ribs. Ventilation should be continued simultaneously as described. If the heart rate after 30 seconds of chest compression is 80 to 100 beats/min, the resuscitator continues with ventilatory support only. If the heart rate is over 100 beats/min, the person discontinues CPR and observes. If the heart rate is still less than 80 beats/min, CPR is continued.

Delivery of Placenta

Once the baby is delivered and stabilized, attention is redirected to the mother. The first step is to assess the status of placental separation. The heel of the nondominant hand is placed just above the symphysis to hold the uterus in position, then the fingers are cupped to apply pressure to the uterine fundus while providing gentle, steady downward traction on the umbilical cord. If this maneuver does not promote placental separation, as indicated by a gush of bleeding, lengthening of the cord, and descent of the placenta into the vagina, efforts should be interrupted until these signs ensue. When the placenta does descend, the mother should be instructed to push once again to complete the third stage of labor. Rotating the placenta several times once it has passed through the introitus will usually result in complete extrusion of the attached chorioamnionic membranes. With signs of placental separation but resistance to extraction, the hand should be placed through the vagina and into the cervix. If the placenta is filling the cervix, it should be grasped and gently extracted. If the placenta does not separate spontaneously or is adherent to the uterine wall (placenta accreta), no effort should be made to separate it manually in a wilderness setting, since this could precipitate uncontrollable hemorrhage. Excessive traction on the umbilical cord also could result in uterine inversion, causing vasomotor collapse and hemodynamic decompensation.

Once placental expulsion has occurred, the uterus can be gently massaged abdominally to promote contraction and involution. Usually this is sufficient to control hemorrhage from the placental bed. If this is ineffective, it may be necessary to explore the uterus manually for retained placenta while compressing the fundus externally until it contracts. Additional measures to aid uterine involution and control bleeding include administration of oxytocin (10 to 40 U intramuscularly), nipple massage to promote endogenous release of oxytocin, methylergonovine (0.2 mg intramuscularly or orally every 2 to 4 hours), prostaglandin $F_{2\alpha}$ (250 µg intramuscularly), misoprostol (100 to 200 µg orally every 4 to 6 hours), and prostaglandin E_2 (20-mg suppository every 2 hours).[6] If none of these measures is successful, and if bleeding from a laceration has been eliminated as a source, the uterus can be packed with clean sponges or towels until additional medical assistance arrives.

Once the placenta is removed and uterine bleeding controlled, maternal damage is assessed and repaired. The most common sites of lacerations are the perineum, periurethral tissues surrounding the external meatus, lower vagina, and cervix. Significant cervical lacerations in unhurried deliveries are rare unless uncontrollable pushing has occurred before complete dilation. Other lacerations from a spontaneous delivery usually occur along tissue planes that do not disrupt vital areas; they will heal naturally or can be repaired later. Significant bleeding at any of these sites can usually be easily controlled by direct pressure. If available, application of ice packs to the perineum for the first 12 to 24 hours after delivery provides relief.

During the postpartum period the woman should be encouraged to drink fluids and void frequently. Bladder overdistention resulting from impaired sensation and pain after delivery is a common cause of permanent bladder dysfunction. It may also contribute to uterine subinvolution and continued blood loss. Once the baby has stabilized after delivery, the mother should begin breast-feeding, which also helps control excessive postpartum blood loss. After a wilderness delivery a broad-spectrum antibiotic, if available, should be continued for 24 to 48 hours. If the mother is Rh negative and the baby's blood type is Rh positive or unknown, Rh-immune globulin should be given within 48 to 72 hours after delivery.

Perimortem Cesarean Section

In the rare event that a pregnant woman with a viable baby sustains a lethal injury while partaking in a wilderness trip, performing a perimortem cesarean section should be considered.[84] Ordinarily this procedure is done in a full-service medical facility when death is imminent and while CPR is being performed on the woman or when skilled medical personnel deem that the pregnancy is interfering with resuscitative efforts. In the wilderness, cesarean section should only be considered at the moment of maternal death, when surgical technique is irrelevant and speed is of the essence.

In skilled hands the entire procedure can be performed in 30 seconds or less. A vertical incision is made in the midline abdomen from the umbilicus to the symphysis. The incision is rapidly extended through subcutaneous tissues and fascia. The rectus muscles are bluntly separated in the midline and the peritoneum entered. The uterus is then incised vertically from fundus to bladder reflection. Once a site of entry into the uterine cavity is obtained, two fingers are inserted and the incision extended by blunt dissection to avoid sharp injury to the baby. Membranes are ruptured, the baby is delivered, and neonatal resuscitative efforts are initiated.

Breast-Feeding

Unless the baby is too premature or too unstable to nurse, breast-feeding should be encouraged as soon as possible after birth. Benefits include promotion of uterine contractions that control hemorrhage at the placental insertion site, encouragement of maternal-newborn bonding, provision of easily digestible and balanced nutritional support for the baby, and transmission of antibodies (IgA) that protect the enteric mucosa against invasion by colonizing bacteria.[94,146] Long-term benefits for the baby include decreased incidence of allergies, enteric infections, UTIs, otitis media, childhood obesity, and diabetes, as well as psychologic and perhaps cognitive advantages.* Benefits for the mother include more rapid return to prepregnancy weight, enhanced bone remineralization, and reduced risk of ovarian cancer and premenopausal breast cancer.[5]

---

*References 85, 87, 130, 132, 154, 167.

During the first 24 hours after delivery, frequent brief feedings are recommended (every 2 to 3 hours; 5 minutes on each breast, alternating first breast). Although a small amount of breast fluid (colostrum) is present initially, it contains electrolytes, minerals, and a high concentration of protein and protective IgA antibodies. The length of time spent at nursing and the interval between feedings can be increased as milk production is established over the next 2 to 3 days. The feeding schedule is typically 10- to 15-minute periods on each breast 8 to 12 times per day. It should be made clear to the mother that babies are not restricted to this regimen. Because babies have an innate urge and ability to suck, and mothers have an innate urge to mother, breast-feeding should require little formal education. However, first-time mothers often think they will not be able to breast-feed, will not provide sufficient nutrition to their babies, or will encounter frustrations and difficulties. Patience, relaxation, simple modifications in technique, and reinforcement of the benefits of nursing are beneficial. Mothers are reassured when they see that their baby is gaining weight and voiding five or six times daily and thus is receiving adequate nutritional and fluid support. Nursing women should be instructed to drink plenty of fluids (2 L/day); increase their caloric intake by 500 to 600 kcal/day, including a total protein intake of 60 to 70 g/day; and consume foods rich in calcium (1200 mg/day).

Several conditions can interfere with breast-feeding or cause maternal frustration. Breast engorgement 48 to 72 hours after delivery, signifying the onset of milk production accompanied by lymphatic obstruction, can cause pain and low-grade fever, interfere with the baby latching on, and inhibit milk letdown. Frequent feedings and warm compresses just before nursing help to stimulate milk letdown. Cool compresses after nursing, a supportive nursing bra, and acetaminophen usually provide symptomatic relief until milk production and newborn consumption are in equilibrium and lymphatic obstruction is resolving. Engorgement usually resolves within 24 to 48 hours.

Sore and cracked nipples are a frequent complaint of woman nursing for the first time.[25,27] Short frequent feedings with several rotations between breasts at each sitting can be beneficial. After each feeding, gently cleansing with water and then applying a small amount of milk, expressed from the breast and spread around the areola to dry, help protect the nipples. Lanolin formulations designed for breast-feeding women can be used as well. Dry absorbent nursing pads should be placed over the nipples between feedings. If contact with clothing or even the nursing pads creates discomfort, breast shells can be used to prevent surface contact. Occasionally, nipple shields can be beneficial, as well as for the infant who has difficulty latching on to the breast.[168]

Mastitis occurs in 2% to 3% of lactating women and should not be confused with breast engorgement since it rarely occurs until at least 3 to 4 weeks postpartum.[81] Unlike breast engorgement, mastitis is usually unilateral and accompanied by localized pain, erythema, brawny edema, fever, and malaise. It is more common among women who report painful and cracked nipples and who participate in vigorous exercise- and work-related upper body activities.[48] These women should be encouraged to empty their breasts by nursing or pumping before these activities and to wear a properly fitting and supportive bra as preventive measures for mastitis. Women who develop mastitis should continue to nurse from the affected breast and may benefit from warm compresses and pumping between nursings. They should be placed on a course of antibiotics (e.g., dicloxacillin 500 mg or cephalexin 500 mg four times daily) for 10 to 14 days, with coverage for *Staphylococcus*, *Streptococcus*, and *Escherichia coli*, the most common isolates from affected breasts. Failure to improve or worsening while on this regimen, as determined by consolidation, widening of erythema and induration, and abscess formation, occurs in 10% to 15% of women. Incision and drainage may be required.[136]

Certain substances, prescription drugs, and maternal medical conditions may affect breast-feeding. Excessive alcohol consumption and cigarette smoking should be avoided because of the deleterious effects on lactation and toxic effects on the baby. Street drugs should always be avoided because of the potentially harmful effects on mother and baby and the unknown chemicals used to prepare the drugs or enhance their effects. Infectious diseases (e.g., HIV, hepatitis B) acquired through intravenous drug use are transmitted in body fluids, including breast milk, and can have devastating effects in a newborn during the first year of life. Women with active tuberculosis should not breast-feed until they have received at least 2 months of therapy.

Few data address the safety of most prescription and OTC drugs in lactating women and their babies. Many new drugs become available each year, but few of these have been systematically evaluated in women, with even fewer tested in pregnant or lactating women because of ethical and liability concerns. In 1994 the American Academy of Pediatrics published a summary of recommendations for the use of drugs by lactating women (Box 75-7).[4] Despite some controversy, this list is an excellent general guideline for drug use in lactating women. When given a choice of agents to prescribe or recommend in pregnancy or during lactation, health care providers should always consider those products with which there is the most clinical experience.

Box 75-7 CATEGORIZATION OF DRUG USE BY LACTATING WOMEN

CONTRAINDICATED

Amphetamines
Aspirin (high dose)
Bromocriptine
Cytotoxic agents
Ergotamine
Lithium
Radiopharmaceuticals

EFFECTS UNKNOWN BUT OF CONCERN

Antianxiety drugs
Antidepressants
Antipsychotics
Metronidazole
Psychotropics

AFFECTING MILK SUPPLY

Decongestants
Diuretics
Combination oral contraceptives

USUALLY CONSIDERED COMPATIBLE WITH BREAST-FEEDING

Analgesics
Antiasthmatics
Antibiotics
Anticoagulants
Anticonvulsants
Antiemetics
Antihistamines
Antihypertensives
Antithyroids
Corticosteroids
Digoxin
Narcotics
Oral contraceptives
Sedatives

REFERENCES

1. Abu-Heija AT, El-Jallad F, Ziadeh S: Placenta previa: effect of age, gravidity, parity and previous caesarean section, *Gynecol Obstet Invest* 47:6, 1999.
2. Alexander H et al: Utero-ovarian interaction in the regulation of reproductive function, *Hum Reprod Update* 4:550, 1998.
3. Alexander JM et al: Efficacy of treatment for syphilis in pregnancy, *Obstet Gynecol* 93:5, 1999.
4. American Academy of Pediatrics, Committee on Drugs: The transfer of drugs and other chemicals into human milk, *Pediatrics* 93:137, 1994.
5. American Academy of Pediatrics Work Group on Breastfeeding: Breast-feeding and the use of human milk, *Pediatrics* 100:1035, 1997.
6. American College of Obstetricians and Gynecologists: Exercise during pregnancy and the postpartum period, *Technical Bulletin* 189, 1994.
7. American College of Obstetricians and Gynecologists: Emergency oral contraception, *Practice Patterns* 2, 1996.
8. American College of Obstetricians and Gynecologist: Postpartum hemorrhage, *Educational Bulletin* 243, 1998.
9. Anderson GS, Ward R, Mekjavic IB: Gender differences in physiological reactions to thermal stress, *Eur J Appl Physiol* 71:95, 1995.
10. Aoyagi Y, McLellan TM, Shephard RJ: Interactions of physical training and heat acclimation: the thermophysiology of exercising in a hot climate, *Sports Med* 23:173, 1997.
11. Artal R: Exercise in pregnancy, *Semin Perinatol* 20:4, 1996.
12. Artal R et al: Exercise in pregnancy: maternal cardiovascular and metabolic responses in normal pregnancy, *Am J Obstet Gynecol* 140:123, 1981.
13. Artal R et al: A comparison of cardiopulmonary adaptations to exercise in pregnancy at sea level and altitude, *Am J Obstet Gynecol* 172:1170, 1995.
14. Ashley RL, Wald A: Genital herpes: review of the epidemic and potential use of type-specific serology, *Clin Microbiol Rev* 12:1, 1999.
15. Atterbury JL et al: Clinical presentation of women readmitted with postpartum severe preeclampsia or eclampsia, *J Obstet Gynecol Neonatal Nurs* 27:134, 1998.
16. Barnett BJ, Stephens DS: Urinary tract infection: an overview, *Am J Med Sci* 314:245, 1997.
17. Baron F, Hill WC: Placenta previa, placenta abruptio, *Clin Obstet Gynecol* 41:527, 1998.
18. Benedetto C et al: A two-stage screening test for pregnancy-induced hypertension and preeclampsia, *Obstet Gynecol* 92:1005, 1998.
19. Bennell KL et al: Skeletal effects of menstrual disturbances in athletes, *Scand J Med Sci Sports* 7:261, 1997.
20. Berkowitz KM: Insulin resistance and preeclampsia, *Clin Perinatol* 25:873, 1998.
21. Bernier F, Jenkins P: The role of vaginal estrogen in the treatment of urogenital dysfunction in postmenopausal women, *Urol Nurs* 17:92, 1997.
22. Blake DR et al: Evaluation of vaginal infections in adolescent women: can it be done without a speculum? *Pediatrics* 102:939, 1998.
23. Bolton ME: Scuba diving and fetal well-being: a survey of 208 women, *Undersea Biomed Res* 7:183, 1980.
24. Bravender T, Emans SJ: Menstrual disorders: dysfunctional uterine bleeding, *Pediatr Clin North Am* 46:545, 1999.
25. Brent N et al: Sore nipples in breast-feeding women, *Arch Pediatr Adolesc Med.* 152:1077, 1998.
26. Brodeur PM et al: Progesterone receptors and ventilatory stimulation by progestin, *J Appl Physiol* 60:590, 1986.
27. Cable B, Stewart M, Davis J: Nipple wound care: a new approach to an old problem, *J Hum Lact* 13:313, 1997.
28. Caforio L et al: Predictive value of uterine artery velocimetry at midgestation in low- and high-risk populations: a new perspective, *Fetal Diagn Ther* 14:201, 1999.
29. Carpenter AJ, Nunneley SA: Endogenous hormones subtly alter women's response to heat stress, *J Appl Physiol* 65:2313, 1988.
30. Carr PL, Felsenstein D, Friedman RH: Evaluation and management of vaginitis, *J Gen Intern Med* 13:335, 1998.
31. Cauci C et al: Impairment of the mucosal immune system: IgA and IgM cleavage detected in vaginal washings of a subgroup of patients with bacterial vaginosis, *J Infect Dis* 178:1698, 1998.
32. Chabbert Buffet N et al: Regulation of the human menstrual cycle, *Front Neuroendocrinol* 19:151, 1998.
33. Chatard JC et al: Anaemia and iron deficiency in athletes: practical recommendations for treatment, *Sports Med* 27:229, 1999.
34. Chen EC, Brzyski RG: Exercise and reproductive dysfunction, *Fertil Steril* 71:1, 1999.
35. Committee on the Judiciary, United States Senate: *Violence against women: the increase of rape in America 1990*, Washington, DC, 1991, Library of Congress.
36. Constantini NW, Warren MP: Special problems of the female athlete, *Baillieres Clin Rheumatol* 8:199, 1994.
37. Cummings SR et al: Effect of alendronate on risk of fracture in women with low bone density but without vertebral fractures, *JAMA* 280:2077, 1998.

38. Dardano KL, Burkman RT: The intrauterine contraceptive device: an often-forgotten and maligned method of contraception, *Am J Obstet Gynecol* 181:1, 1999.

39. Dekker GA, Sibai BM: Etiology and pathogenesis of preeclampsia: current concepts, *Am J Obstet Gynecol* 179:1359, 1998.

40. DiFiori JP: Menstrual dysfunction in athletes. How to identify and treat patients at risk for skeletal injury, *Postgrad Med* 97:143, 1995.

41. Eckert LO et al: Vulvovaginal candidiasis: clinical manifestations, risk factors, management algorithm, *Obstet Gynecol* 92:757, 1998.

42. Ettinger B et al: Raloxifene reduces the risk of incident vertebral fractures: 24-month interim analyses, *Osteoporosis Int* 8(suppl 3):11, 1998.

43. Faro S, Fenner DE: Urinary tract infections, *Clin Obstet Gynecol* 41:744, 1998.

44. Favier R: Differential effects of ventilatory stimulation by sex hormones and almitrine on hypoxic erythrocytosis, *Pflugers Arch* 434:97, 1997.

45. Fihn SD et al: Use of spermicide-coated condoms and other risk factors for urinary tract infection caused by *Staphylococcus saprophyticus, Arch Intern Med* 158:281, 1998.

46. Filicori M et al: Interaction between menstrual cyclicity and gonadotropin pulsatility, *Horm Res* 49:169, 1998.

47. Fortney JA, Feldblum PJ, Raymond EG: Intrauterine devices: the optimal long-term contraceptive method? *J Reprod Med* 44:269, 1999.

48. Foxman B, Schwartz K, Looman SJ: Breastfeeding practices and lactation mastitis, *Soc Sci Med* 38:755, 1994.

49. Frascarolo P, Schutz Y, Jequier E: Decreased thermal conductance during the luteal phase of the menstrual cycle in women, *J Appl Physiol* 69:2029, 1990.

50. Fruzzetti F: Hemostatic effects of smoking and oral contraceptive use, *Am J Obstet Gynecol* 180(suppl 2):S369, 1999.

51. Frye AJ, Kamon E: Sweating efficiency in acclimated men and women exercising in humid and dry heat, *J Appl Physiol* 54:972, 1983.

52. Fusch C et al: Water turnover and body composition during long-term exposure to high altitude (4900-7,600 m), *J Appl Physiol* 80:1118, 1996.

53. Glasier A: Drug therapy: emergency postcoital contraception, *N Engl J Med* 337:1058, 1997.

54. Glasier A: Emergency contraception in a travel context, *J Travel Med* 6:1, 1999.

55. Graham TE: Thermal, metabolic, and cardiovascular changes in men and women during cold stress, *Med Sci Sports Exerc* 20(5 suppl):S185, 1988.

56. Gupta K et al: Inverse association of H_2O_2-producing lactobacilli and vaginal *Escherichia coli* colonization in women with recurrent urinary tract infections, *J Infect Dis* 178:446, 1998.

57. Hackett PH, Rennie D: The incidence, importance, and prophylaxis of acute mountain sickness, *Lancet* 2:1149, 1976.

58. Hackett PH et al: Fluid retention and relative hypoventilation in acute mountain sickness, *Respiration* 43:321, 1982.

59. Haefner HK: Current evaluation and management of vulvovaginitis, *Clin Obstet Gynecol* 42:184, 1999.

60. Hannhart BC, Pickett CK, Moore LG: Effects of estrogen and progesterone on carotid body neural output responsiveness to hypoxia, *J Appl Physiol* 68:1090, 1990.

61. Hannhart BC et al: Influence of pregnancy on ventilatory and carotid body neural output responsiveness to hypoxia in cats, *J Appl Physiol* 67:797, 1989.

62. Harris CW, Shields JL, Hannon JP: Acute altitude sickness in females, *Aerospace Med* 37:1163, 1966.

63. Havenith G, Van Middendorp H: The relative influence of physical fitness, acclimatization state, anthropometric measures and gender on individual reactions to heat stress, *Eur J Appl Physiol* 61:419, 1990.

64. Hellegers A et al: Alveolar PCO_2 and PO_2 in pregnant and nonpregnant women at high altitude, *Am J Obstet Gynecol* 82:241, 1961.

65. Hendricks MS et al: Previous cesarean section and abortion as risk factors for developing placenta previa, *J Obstet Gynaecol Res* 25:137, 1999.

66. Hillier SG, Tetsuka M: Role of androgens in follicle maturation and atresis, *Baillieres Clin Obstet Gynecol* 11:249, 1997.

67. Hook EW III: Trichomonas vaginalis—no longer a minor STD, *Sex Transm Dis* 26:388, 1999.

68. Hooton TM, Stamm WE: Diagnosis and treatment of uncomplicated urinary tract infection, *Infect Dis Clin North Am* 11:551, 1997.

69. Horstman DH, Christensen E: Acclimatization to dry heat: active men vs. active women, *J Appl Physiol* 52:825, 1982.

70. Horstman DW, Weiskopf R, Jackson RD: Work capacity during 3-week sojourn at 4300 meters: effects related to polycythemia, *J Appl Physiol* 49:311, 1980.

71. Huang SY et al: Internal carotid and vertebral arterial flow velocity in men at high altitude, *J Appl Physiol* 63:395, 1987.

72. Iglesis EA, Coupey SM: Menstrual cycle abnormalities: diagnosis and management, *Adolesc Med* 10:255, 1999.

73. Iravani A et al: A trial comparing low-dose, short-course ciprofloxacin and standard 7 day therapy with co-trimoxazole or nitrofurantoin in the treatment of uncomplicated urinary tract infection, *J Antimicrob Chemother* 43(suppl A):67, 1999.

74. Jacque-Fortunato S et al: A comparison of the ventilatory responses to exercise in pregnant, postpartum and nonpregnant women, *Semin Perinatol* 20:263, 1996.

75. Joesoef MR, Schmid GP, Hillier S: Bacterial vaginosis: review of treatment options and potential clinical indications for therapy, *Clin Infect Dis* 28(suppl 1):S57, 1999.

76. Jones SL: HELLP! A cry for laboratory assistance: a comprehensive review of the HELLP syndrome highlighting the role of the laboratory, *Hematopathol Mol Hematol* 11:147, 1998.

77. Kahn SR: Severe preeclampsia associated with coinheritance of factor V Leiden mutation and protein S deficiency, *Obstet Gynecol* 91:812, 1998.

78. Kahsar-Miller M, Azzizz R: The development of the polycystic ovary syndrome: family history as a risk factor, *Trends Endocrinol Metab* 9:55, 1998.

79. Kardel KR et al: Training in pregnant women: effects on fetal development and birth, *Am J Obstet Gynecol* 178:280, 1998.

80. Karsch FJ et al: Gonadotropin-releasing hormone requirements for ovulation, *Biol Reprod* 56:303, 1997.

81. Kaufmann R, Foxman B: Mastitis among lactating women: occurrence and risk factors, *Soc Sci Med* 33:701, 1991.

82. Khodignian N et al: A comparison of cross-sections and longitudinal methods of assessing the influence of pregnancy on cardiac function during exercise, *Semin Perinatol* 20:23, 1996.

83. King AB, Robinson SM: Ventilation response to hypoxia and acute mountain sickness, *Aerospace Med* 43:419, 1972.

84. Lanoix R, Akkapeddi V, Goldfeder B: Perimortem cesarean section: case reports and recommendations, *Acad Emerg Med* 2:1063, 1995.

85. Lanting CI et al: Neurological differences between 9-year-old children fed breast-milk or formula-milk as babies, *Lancet* 344:1329, 1994.

86. Lewinsky RM, Riskin-Mashiah S: Autonomic imbalance in preeclampsia: evidence for increased sympathetic tone in response to the supine-pressor test, *Obstet Gynecol* 91:935, 1998.

87. Lucas A et al: Breast milk and subsequent intelligence quotient in children born preterm, *Lancet* 339:261, 1992.

88. Macklon NS, Fauser BC: Follicle development during the normal menstrual cycle, *Maturitas* 30:181, 1998.

89. Mahesh VB, Brann DW: Regulation of the preovulatory gonadotropin surge by endogenous steroids, *Steroids* 63:616, 1998.

90. Malterud K, Baerheim A: Peeing barbed wire: symptom experiences in women with lower urinary tract infection, *Scand J Prim Health Care* 17:49, 1999.

91. Mardh PA et al: Symptoms and signs in single and mixed genital infections, *Int J Gynaecol Obstet* 63:145, 1998.

92. Martin JN Jr et al: Early risk assessment of severe preeclampsia: admission battery of symptoms and laboratory tests to predict likelihood of subsequent significant maternal morbidity, *Am J Obstet Gynecol* 180:1407, 1999.

93. Martin JN Jr et al: The spectrum of severe preeclampsia: comparative analysis by HELLP (hemolysis, elevated liver enzyme levels, and low platelet count) syndrome classification, *Am J Obstet Gynecol* 180:1373, 1999.

94. Maxson RT, Jackson RJ, Smith SD: The protective role of enteral IgA supplementation in neonatal gut origin sepsis, *J Pediatr Surg* 30:231, 1995.

95. Mazzeo RS et al: Arterial catecholamine responses during exercise with acute and chronic high-altitude exposure, *Am J Physiol* 261 (*Endocrinol Metab* 24):E419, 1991.

96. Mazzeo RS et al: Sympathetic responses during 21 days at high altitude (4300 m) as determined by urinary and arterial catecholamines, *Metabolism* 43:1226, 1994.

97. Mazzeo RS et al: Catecholamine response during 12 days of high altitude exposure (4300 m) in women, *J Appl Physiol* 84:1151, 1998.

98. McArdle WD, Katch FI, Katch VL: *Exercise physiology: energy, nutrition, and human performance*, ed 3, Philadelphia, 1991, Lea & Febiger.

99. McArdle WD et al: Thermal adjustment to cold-water exposure in resting men and women, *J Appl Physiol* 56:1565, 1984.

100. McMahon MJ, Ananth CV, Liston RM: Gestational diabetes mellitus: risk factors, obstetric complications and infant outcomes, *J Reprod Med* 43:372, 1998.

101. Messinis IE: Luteal function—luteolysis, *Ann NY Acad Sci* 816:151, 1997.

102. Mikamo H et al: Bacterial isolates from patients with preterm labor with and without preterm rupture of the fetal membranes, *Infect Dis Obstet Gynecol* 7:190, 1999.

103. Milunsky A et al: Maternal heat exposure and neural tube defects, *JAMA* 268:882, 1992.

104. Mindel A, Estcourt C: Public and personal health implications of asymptomatic viral shedding in genital herpes, *Sex Transm Infect* 74:387, 1998.

105. Mishell DR Jr: Cardiovascular risks: perception versus reality, *Contraception* 59(suppl 1):21S, 1999.

106. Misra DP, Ananth CV: Risk factor profiles of placental abruption in first and second pregnancies: heterogeneous etiologies, *J Clin Epidemiol* 52:453, 1999.

107. Mombelli G et al: Oral vs intravenous ciprofloxacin in the initial empirical management of severe pyelonephritis or complicated urinary tract infections: a prospective randomized clinical trial, *Arch Intern Med* 159:53, 1999.

108. Monniaux D et al: Follicular growth and ovarian dynamics in mammals, *J Reprod Fertil Suppl* 51:3, 1997.

109. Montalvo R et al: Morbidity and mortality in the wilderness, *West J Med* 68:248, 1998.

110. Moore LG et al: Infant birth weight is related to maternal arterial oxygenation at high altitude, *J Appl Phys Respir Environ Exerc Physiol* 53:695, 1982.

111. Morgan T, Ward K: New insights into the genetics of preeclampsia, *Semin Perinatol* 23:14, 1999.

112. Morgan T et al: Angiotensinogen Thr235 variant is associated with abnormal physiologic change of the uterine spiral arteries in first-trimester decidua, *Am J Obstet Gynecol* 180:95, 1999.

113. Morgan WP: Anxiety and panic in recreational scuba divers, *Sports Med* 20:398, 1995.

114. Morrison CS et al: Use of sexually transmitted disease risk assessment algorithms for selection of intrauterine device candidates, *Contraception* 59:97, 1999.

115. Myatt L, Miodovnik M: Prediction of preeclampsia, *Semin Perinatol* 23:45, 1999.

116. Nygaard I, Linder M. Thirst at work—an occupational hazard? *Int Urogynecol J* 8:340, 1997.

117. Otis CL et al: American College of Sports Medicine position stand: the female athlete triad, *Med Sci Sports Exerc* 29:i, 1997.

118. Palmer SK et al: Altered blood pressure course during normal pregnancy and increased preeclampsia at high altitude (3100 meters) in Colorado, *Am J Obstet Gynecol* 180:1161, 1999.

119. Pandit L, Ouslander JG: Postmenopausal vaginal atrophy and atrophic vaginitis, *Am J Med Sci* 314:228, 1997.

120. Patterson TF, Andriloe VT: Detection, significance, and therapy of bacteriuria in pregnancy: update in the managed health care era, *Infect Dis Clin North Am* 11:593, 1997.

121. Pisarska MD, Carson SA: Incidence and risk factors for ectopic pregnancy, *Clin Obstet Gynecol* 42:2, 1999.

122. Pivarnik JM et al: Menstrual cycle phase effects temperature regulation during endurance exercise, *J Appl Physiol* 72:543, 1992.

123. Rana A et al: Abruptio placentae and chorioamnionitis—microbiological and histologic correlation, *Acta Obstet Gynecol Scand* 78:363, 1999.

124. Rebar RW: The normal menstrual cycle. In Keye WR, Chang RJ, Rebar RW, editors: *Infertility: evaluation and treatment,* Philadelphia, 1995, WB Saunders.

125. Reeves JT et al: Headache at high altitude is not related to internal carotid arterial blood velocity, *J Appl Physiol* 59:909, 1985.

126. Reimer T, Ulfig N, Friese K: Antibiotics: treatment of preterm labor, *J Perinat Med* 27:35, 1999.

127. Richards JS et al: Molecular mechanisms of ovulation and luteinization, *Mol Cell Endocrinol* 145:47, 1998.

128. Richardson BA et al: Use of nonoxynol-9 and changes in vaginal lactobacilli, *J Infect Dis* 178:441, 1998.

129. Risser WL et al: Weight change in adolescents who used hormonal contraception, *J Adolesc Health* 24:433, 1999.

130. Rogan WJ, Gladen BC: Breast-feeding and cognitive development, *Early Hum Dev* 31:181, 1993.

131. Ryan CA et al: Risk assessment, symptoms, and signs as predictors of vulvovaginal and cervical infections in an urban U.S. STD clinic: implications for use of STD algorithms, *Sex Transm Infect* 74(suppl 1):S59, 1998.

132. Saarinen VM, Kajosaari M: Breast feeding as prophylaxis against atopic disease: prospective follow-up until 17 years old, *Lancet* 346:1065, 1995.

133. Saphier CJ, Repke JT: Hemolysis, elevated liver enzymes, and low platelets (HELLP) syndrome: a review of diagnosis and management, *Semin Perinatol* 22:118, 1998.

134. Saraiya M et al: Estimates of the annual number of clinically recognized pregnancies in the United States, 1981-1991, *Am J Epidemiol* 149:1025, 1999.

135. Schoene RB et al: The relationship of hypoxic ventilatory response to exercise performance on Mount Everest, *J Appl Physiol* 56:1478, 1984.

136. Scott-Conner CEH, Schorr SJ: The diagnosis and management of breast problems during pregnancy and lactation, *Am J Surg* 170:401, 1995.

137. Shapiro Y et al: Physiological responses of men and women to humid and dry heat, *J Appl Physiol* 49:1, 1980.

138. Shapiro Y et al: Heat balance and transfer in men and women in hot-dry and hot-wet conditions, *Ergonomics* 24:375, 1981.

139. Sheikh RA et al: Spontaneous intrahepatic hemorrhage and hepatic rupture in the HELLP syndrome: four cases and a review, *J Clin Gastroenterol* 28:323, 1999.

140. Singh K, Chye GC: Adverse effects associated with contraceptive implants: incidence, prevention and management, *Adv Contracept* 14:1, 1998.

141. Smith CA et al: Carotid bodies are required for ventilatory acclimatization to chronic hypoxia, *J Appl Physiol* 60:1003, 1986.

142. Sobel JD et al: Vulvovaginal candidiasis: epidemiologic, diagnostic, and therapeutic considerations, *Am J Obstet Gynecol* 178:203, 1998.

143. Soultanakis H, Artal R, Wiswell R: Prolonged exercise in pregnancy: glucose homeostasis, ventilatory, and cardiovascular responses, *Semin Perinatol* 20:315, 1996.

144. Spellacy WN: Shoulder dystocia risks, *Am J Obstet Gynecol* 180:1047, 1999.

145. Stapleton A, Stamm WE: Prevention of urinary tract infection, *Infect Dis Clin North Am* 11:719, 1997.

146. Steinwender G et al: Effect of early nutritional deprivation and diet on translocation of bacteria from the gastrointestinal tract in the newborn rat, *Pediatr Res* 39:415, 1996.

147. Sternfeld B: Physical activity and pregnancy outcome: review and recommendations, *Sports Med* 23:33, 1997.

148. Stovall TG, Ling FW: Single-dose methotrexate: an expanded clinical trial, *Am J Obstet Gynecol* 168:1759, 1993.

149. Stovall TG et al: Serum progesterone and uterine curettage in differential diagnosis of ectopic pregnancy, *Fertil Steril* 57:456, 1992.

150. Sui GJ et al: Subacute infantile mountain sickness, *J Pathol* 155:161, 1988.

151. Tang OS et al: Long-term depot-medroxyprogesterone acetate and bone mineral density, *Contraception* 59:25, 1999.

152. Tatsumi K: Role of endogenous female hormones in hypoxic chemosensitivity, *J Appl Physiol* 83:1706, 1997.

153. Tchoudomirova K et al: History, clinical findings, sexual behavior and hygiene habits in women with and without recurrent episodes of urinary symptoms, *Acta Obstet Gynecol Scand* 77:654, 1998.

154. Temboury MC et al: Influence of breastfeeding on the infant's intellectual development, *J Pediatr Gastroenterol Nutr* 18:32, 1994.

155. Thorsen P et al: Few microorganisms associated with bacterial vaginosis may constitute the pathologic core: a population-based microbiologic study among 3596 pregnant women, *Am J Obstet Gynecol* 178:580, 1998.

156. Tincello DG, Richmond DH: Evaluation of reagent strips in detecting asymptomatic bacteriuria in early pregnancy, *BMJ* 316:435, 1998.

157. Trussell J, Ellertson C, Steward F: The effectiveness of the Yuzpe regimen of emergency contraception, *Fam Plann Perspect* 28:58, 1996.

158. Trussell J, Rodriguez G, Ellertson C: Updated estimates of the effectiveness of the Yuzpe regimen of emergency contraception, *Contraception* 59:147, 1999.

159. Trussell J, Vaughan B: Contraceptive failure, method-related discontinuation and resumption of use: results from the 1995 National Survey of Family Growth, *Fam Plann Perspect* 31:64, 1999.

160. Tsafriri A, Reich R: Molecular aspects of mammalian ovulation, *Exp Clin Endocrinol Diabetes* 107:1, 1999. 9:1328-1322, 1994.

161. Van Pampus MG et al: High prevalence of hemostatic abnormalities in women with a history of severe preeclampsia, *Am J Obstet Gynecol* 180:1146, 1999.

162. Vedernikov Y, Saade GR, Garfield RE: Vascular reactivity in preeclampsia, *Semin Perinatol* 23:34, 1999.

163. Waldenstrom U: Warm tub bath and sauna in early pregnancy: risk of malformation uncertain, *Acta Obstet Gynecol Scand* 73:449, 1994.

164. Walker ID: Factor V Leiden: should all women be screened prior to commencing the contraceptive pill? *Blood Rev* 13:8, 1999.

165. Wells CL: Responses of physically active and acclimated men and women to exercise in a desert environment, *Med Sci Sports Exerc* 12:9, 1980.

166. Wiggins DL, Wiggins ME: The female athlete, *Clin Sports Med* 16:593, 1997.

167. Wilson AC et al: Relation of infant diet to childhood health: seven year follow up of cohort of children in Dundee infant feeding study, *BMJ* 316:21, 1998.

168. Wilson-Clay B: Clinical use of silicone nipple shields, *J Hum Lact* 12:279, 1996.

169. Witlin AG, Sibai BM: Magnesium sulfate therapy in preeclampsia and eclampsia, *Obstet Gynecol* 92:883, 1998.

170. Witlin AG et al: Risk factors for abruptio placentae and eclampsia: analysis of 445 consecutively managed women with severe preeclampsia and eclampsia, *Am J Obstet Gynecol* 180:1322, 1999.

171. Zamudio S et al: Blood volume expansion, preeclampsia, and infant birth weight at high altitude, *J Appl Physiol* 75:1566, 1993.

SUGGESTED READINGS

Arroyo A et al: Inappropriate gonadotropin secretion in polycystic ovary syndrome: influence of adiposity, *J Clin Endocrinol Metab* 82:3728, 1997.

Augenbraun MH, Rolfs R: Treatment of syphilis, 1998: nonpregnant adults, *Clin Infect Dis* 28(suppl 1):S21, 1999.

Baker DA: Antiviral therapy for genital herpes in nonpregnant and pregnant women, *Int J Fertil Womens Med* 43:243, 1998.

Baker DA, Blythe JG, Miller JM: Once-daily valacyclovir hydrochloride for suppression of recurrent genital herpes, *Obstet Gynecol* 94:103, 1999.

Balen AH et al: Polycystic ovary syndrome: the spectrum of the disorder in 1714 patients, *Hum Reprod* 10:2701, 1995.

Benedetti JK. Zeh J, Corey L: Clinical reactivation of genital herpes simplex virus infection decreases in frequency over time, *Ann Intern Med* 131:14, 1999.

Bernardes J: The Jarisch-Herxheimer reaction and fetal monitoring changes in pregnant women treated for syphilis, *Obstet Gynecol* 93:631-632, 1999.

Beutner KR et al: External genital warts: report of the American Medical Association Consensus Conference, AMA Expert Panel on External Genital Warts, *Clin Infect Dis* 27:796, 1998.

Beutner KR et al: Imiquimod, a patient-applied immune-response modifier for treatment of external genital warts, *Antimicrob Agents Chemother* 42:789, 1998.

Beutner KR et al: Genital warts and their treatment, *Clin Infect Dis* 28(suppl 1):S37, 1999.

Bohmer JT et al: Cervical wet mount as a negative predictor for gonococci- and *Chlamydia trachomatis*-induced cervicitis in a gravid population, *Am J Obstet Gynecol* 181:283, 1999.

Centers for Disease Control and Prevention: 1998 guidelines for treatment of sexually transmitted diseases, *MMWR* 47(RR-1):1, 1998.

Chrousos GP, Torpy DJ, Gold PW: Interactions between the hypothalamic-pituitary-adrenal axis and the female reproductive system: clinical implications, *Ann Intern Med* 129:229, 1998.

Crave JC et al: Effects of diet and metformin administration on sex hormone-binding globulin, androgens, and insulin in hirsute and obese women, *J Clin Endocrinol Metab* 80:2057, 1995.

Diamond C et al: Clinical course of patients with serologic evidence of recurrent genital herpes presenting with signs and symptoms of first episode disease, *Sex Transm Dis* 26:221, 1999.

Diaz-Mitoma F et al: Oral famciclovir for the suppression of recurrent genital herpes: a randomized controlled trial. Collaborative Famciclovir Genital Herpes Research Group, *JAMA* 280:887, 1998.

Douchi T et al: Body fat distribution in women with polycystic ovary syndrome, *Obstet Gynecol* 86:516, 1995.

Dunaif A: Insulin resistance and the polycystic ovary syndrome: mechanism and implications for pathogenesis, *Endocr Rev* 18:774, 1997.

Dunaif A et al: The insulin-sensitizing agent troglitazone improves metabolic and reproductive abnormalities in the polycystic ovary syndrome, *J Clin Endocrinol Metab* 81:3299, 1996.

Ehrmann DA et al: Troglitazone improves defects in insulin action, insulin secretion, ovarian steroidogenesis, and fibrinolysis in women with polycystic ovary syndrome, *J Clin Endocrinol Metab* 82:2108, 1997.

Falsetti L et al: Treatment of hirsutism by finasteride and flutamide in women with polycystic ovary syndrome, *Gynecol Endocrinol* 11:251, 1997.

Habel LA et al: Risk factors for incident and recurrent condylomata acuminata among women, *Sex Transm Dis* 25:285, 1998.

Kiddy DS et al: Diet-induced changes in sex hormone binding globulin and free testosterone in women with normal or polycystic ovaries: correlation with serum insulin and insulin-like growth factor-I, *Clin Endocrinol* 31:757, 1989.

Knochenhauer ES et al: Prevalence of the polycystic ovarian syndrome in unselected black and white women of the southeastern United States: a prospective study, *J Clin Endocrinol Metab* 83:3078, 1998.

Koutras DA: Disturbances of menstruation in thyroid disease, *Ann NY Acad Sci* 816:280, 1997.

Langley PC, Tyring SK, Smith MH: The cost effectiveness of patient-applied versus provider-administered intervention strategies for the treatment of external genital warts, *Am J Manag Care* 5:69, 1999.

Legro RS et al: Evidence for a genetic basis for hyperandrogenemia in polycystic ovary syndrome, *Proc Natl Acad Sci USA* 95:14956, 1998.

Legro RS, Finegood D, Dunaif A: A fasting glucose to insulin ratio is a useful measure of insulin sensitivity in women with polycystic ovary syndrome, *J Clin Endocrinol Metab* 83:2694, 1998.

Mardh PA, Arvidson M, Hellberg D: Sexually transmitted diseases and reproductive history in women with experience of casual travel sex abroad, *J Travel Med* 3:138, 1996.

Nelson DB et al: Factors predicting upper genital tract inflammation among women with lower genital tract infection, *J Womens Health* 7:1033, 1998.

Nestler JE et al: Insulin stimulates testosterone biosynthesis by human thecal cells from women with polycystic ovary syndrome by activating its own receptor and using inositol glycan mediators as the signal transduction system, *J Clin Endocrinol Metab* 83:2001, 1998.

Nestler JE et al: Ovulatory and metabolic effects of D-chiro-inositol in the polycystic ovary syndrome, *N Engl J Med* 340:1314, 1999.

Nestler JE et al: A direct effect of hyperinsulinemia on serum sex hormone-binding globulin levels in obese women with the polycystic ovary syndrome, *J Clin Endocrinol Metab* 72:83, 1991.

Rosen T, Brown TJ: Cutaneous manifestations of sexually transmitted diseases, *Med Clin North Am* 82:1081, 1998.

Scott LL: Prevention of perinatal herpes: prophylactic antiviral therapy? *Clin Obstet Gynecol* 42:134, 1999.

Sheffield JS, Wendel GD Jr: Syphilis in pregnancy, *Clin Obstet Gynecol* 42:97, 1999.

Singh AE, Romanowski B: Syphilis: review with emphasis on clinical, epidemiologic, and some biologic features, *Clin Microbiol Rev* 12:187, 1999.

Stanberry L et al: New developments in the epidemiology, natural history and management of genital herpes, *Antiviral Res* 42:1, 1999.

Stanley M: The immunology of genital human papilloma virus infection, *Eur J Dermatol* 8(7 suppl):8, 1998.

Tulppala M et al: Polycystic ovaries and levels of gonadotropins and androgens in recurrent miscarriage: preliminary experience of 500 consecutive cases, *Hum Reprod* 9:1328, 1994.

Van Voorst Vader PC: Syphilis management and treatment, *Dermatol Clin* 16:699, 1998.

Velazquez E, Acosta A, Mendoza SG: Menstrual cyclicity after metformin therapy in polycystic ovary syndrome, *Obstet Gynecol* 90:392, 1997.

Velazquez EM et al: Metformin therapy in polycystic ovary syndrome reduced hyperinsulinemia, insulin resistance, hyperandrogenemia, and systolic blood pressure, while facilitating normal menses and pregnancy, *Metabolism* 43:647, 1994.

Wald A: Herpes: transmission and viral shedding, *Dermatol Clin* 16:795, 1998.

West RV: The female athlete: the triad of disordered eating, amenorrhea, and osteoporosis, *Sports Med* 26:63, 1998.

Xiao E, Ferin M: Stress-related disturbances of the menstrual cycle, *Ann Med* 29:215, 1997.

Yoshimura Y: Insulin-like growth factors and ovarian physiology, *J Obstet Gynaecol Res* 24:305, 1998.

Young H: Syphilis: serology, *Dermatol Clin* 16:691, 1998.

Zawadzki JK, Dunaif A: Diagnostic criteria for polycystic ovary syndrome: towards a rational approach. In Dunaif A et al., editors: Polycystic ovary syndrome, Boston, 1992, Blackwell Scientific.

Zenilman JM: Update of the CDC STD treatment guidelines: changes and policy, *Sex Transm Infect* 74:89, 1998.

76 Elders in the Wilderness

Blair Dillard Erb

Too many people live their lives by the calendar.

John Glenn, senior astronaut[22]

Seniors in our society are encouraged to remain mentally, physically, and socially active. They perceive this recommendation as a welcome invitation to live life to its fullest. In response, elders in increasing numbers have come to enjoy the fellowship, camaraderie, and adventure of wilderness activities. Unfortunately, health risk associated with high-performance activities increases with age because of altered physiologic function, unrecognized impairments, or effects of illnesses and their treatment.

To reduce risk, seniors should be advised to temper their enthusiasm with the caution derived from the wisdom of experience. John Glenn made his second space flight safely at age 77 because of thoughtful planning and training. A maxim from his aeronautical colleagues reminds us, "There are old pilots, and there are bold pilots, but there are no old, bold pilots."

This review examines the risks, pathology, treatment, and, most important, prevention of health problems of elders as they venture into the wilderness.

THE AGING PROCESS

Aging is a natural consequence of life's continuum. It results in anatomic, biochemical, and physiologic alterations in function. Degenerative disorders and diseases occur that include a variety of problems, such as atherosclerotic and cerebrovascular diseases; chronic obstructive pulmonary disease; emphysema; diabetes mellitus; arthritis; emotional, mood, and memory disorders (e.g., depression, Alzheimer's disease); impaired thermoregulation; and increase in medication intake. These may affect individual performance and increase medical risk in the wilderness. The cumulative effect of these changes on elders subjected to stressful environmental factors results in a major increase in health risk and health care demand.[9]

Every organ system of the body is affected to some degree by the aging process. Anatomic changes are usually organ specific, occurring in a way that is unique to the organ and the disease. Organs appear to age independently of each other and not necessarily in a parallel fashion. For example, glomerular filtration rate (GFR) and renal blood flow (RBF) decrease with age, but many elders have normal serum creatinine levels because there is a concomitant loss of muscle mass and creatinine production.

Physical and physiologic alterations may evolve so slowly that they may not be apparent for many years, yet result in functional and anatomic changes. The degree of loss of function in various physiologic systems can be approximated by using the "1% rule," which states that "most organ systems lose function at roughly 1% per year after the age of 30 years."[18] Some age-related morphologic changes and their resulting functional changes include the following:

Cardiovascular system: elongation and tortuosity of aorta and arteries, thickening of arterial intima, fibrosis of arterial media, sclerosis of cardiac valves, especially aortic and mitral

Functional results: decreased cardiac output of 20% to 30% by age 70 years; decreased maximal heart rate of 6 to 10 beats/min/decade

Lung: decreased elasticity, decreased activity of cilia, and reduced volume

Functional results: decreased vital capacity of roughly 30 ml/year after age 30 years

Kidney: increase in number of abnormal glomeruli

Functional results: compensatory reduction in muscle mass neutralizing creatinine elevation; proteinuria

Gastrointestinal tract: decreased gastric hydrochloric acid, reduced salivary flow, and decreased number of taste buds

Functional results: modified appetite, food intake, and motility

Musculoskeletal system: decreased height and weight, loss of skeletal calcium, sarcopenia, increased ratio of fat to muscle mass, reduced elasticity in connective tissue, decreased viscosity of synovial fluid, loss of cartilaginous surfaces, and hypertrophic changes in joints

Functional results: osteoporosis, degenerative joint disease, failure to thrive (FTT) syndrome, loss of muscle mass and strength of 20% by age 65 years

Central nervous system: reduced brain mass, brain weight, decreased cortical cell count

Functional results: impaired cerebral function; decreased nerve conduction; loss of agility; and sensory impairment, including taste, smell, and touch

Eyes: decreased translucency of the lens and decreased size of the pupil, potential increase in intraocular pressure, and arcus senilis

Functional results: decreased vision, including color and night vision, and impaired accommodation

Ears: loss of auditory neurons and atrophy of cochlear hair cells.

Functional results: decrease in hearing, primarily affecting high tones, especially frequencies greater than 2000 Hz

Skin: flattening and atrophy, attenuation of undulations in the dermal rete pegs, loss of cytoplasm of basal keratinocytes, and loss of dermal collagen

Functional results: decreased skin thickness, risk of dermoepidermal separation, decreased resistance to tear, and loss of elasticity

Inasmuch as aging reflects a time dimension, injuries and illnesses that occur along the path of life may produce cumulative anatomic scars, which, when combined with the degenerative changes of aging, may result in a functionally impaired elderly person. The risk may be greatly exaggerated by wilderness ventures. The challenge to health professionals is to determine the extent of that risk and to take appropriate action.

CLASSIFICATIONS OF ELDERS

For purposes of identifying elderly individuals at risk, it is useful to divide them into groups. Barry and Eathorne[3] suggest classifying elders as the *hale* and the *frail.* This is a clever play on words but not very useful from a medical perspective. Smith,[27] as reported by Howley, recommends classifying individuals according to chronologic age: (1) *athletic old* (less than 55 years of age, (2) *young old* (55 to 75 years of age), and (3) *old old* (greater than 75 years). However, this scheme focuses only on chronologic age and implies from a limited perspective that there is uniform functional change that may be quantified by age in years.

I prefer a comprehensive classification that defines three factors: (1) *chronologic:* simple time-based classification in years, (2) *pathologic:* describing morphologic and anatomic changes, and (3) *functional:* defining functional changes that may modify or impair an individual.

ETIOLOGY OF THE AGING PROCESS

Why do some individuals age faster than others? Lifestyle and genetic predisposition are the most commonly incriminated "causes," but this does not explain the biologic basis for aging.[13] Somehow, and often indirectly, genetic events may determine longevity. For example, there is an increased risk of development of Alzheimer's disease in the presence of an allele of apolipoprotein E (ApoE) gene, which encodes a carrier of cholesterol.[2] Support for genetic determination of tissue longevity is scant.

Most biologists believe that the processes of aging are multifactorial. Stochastic theories suggest that deoxyribonucleic acid (DNA) damage and damage to proteins occurs from a variety of sources, such as reactive oxygen species including superoxide, the hydroxyl radical, and hydrogen peroxide. Mitochondria are an important source of reactive oxygen species and a major site of damage.

Other theories on the aging process include cellular changes, autoimmune mechanisms, neuroendocrine factors, and even a "biological clock," but Strehler[30] feels that the cause should explain the progressive deleterious and intrinsic changes universal within the species.

For example, some animals, usually cold-blooded fish or amphibians, which may grow to an indeterminate size, may have an indeterminate lifespan, whereas warm-blooded animals with a limited or fixed size after maturation may die at a more predictable time and at an actuarially determined rate.[31]

Questions concerning the nature and cause of aging include the following:

- Does aging affect everybody? Yes, but with considerable variation.
- Is aging a disease? Are there decrements in or natural losses of function and anatomic content representing "normal aging"? If so, there must be such a thing as "abnormal aging."
- Is aging genetically programmed as a sequence of events? Evidence suggests that genetic events may influence longevity, especially by modifying various influences such as cholesterol and blood sugar.
- Is aging a result of natural selection? Darwin's laws of natural selection and evolution have been considered, but in the 2 to 3 million years of human existence, there have been too few old humans in any generation until recently to provide proof of a selective advantage favoring genetic expressions related to aging.
- Is there a finite number of population doublings of human fibroblasts? Hayflick suggested that there are 50 doublings of fibroblasts during their lifespan. If, for example, the lifespan of fibroblasts is 18 months, 50 doublings would result in a predicted lifespan of approximately 75 years.
- Is an individual responsible for personal longevity? Lifestyle factors, such as lack of exercise, dietary habits, tobacco use, and drug and alcohol use, not only influence anatomic and functional characteristics but may have deleterious effects on health and length of life. In perhaps the clearest summation of these theories, Hayflick suggests that the ultimate effect from the many factors influencing and affecting human life is that we simply exceed our reserve capacity. This lends support to the mountaineering dictum, "Always keep your reserve," which is particularly appropriate for elders.

DEMOGRAPHY OF ELDERS AND THE WILDERNESS

Extended lifespans during the twentieth century have resulted in changes in the composition by age of the populations of Western civilizations. The median age in the United States in 1900 was 23 years, rose to 30 years in 1950, and reached 33 years in 1990. Predictions for changes in life expectancy forecast a median age of 36 years in the year 2000, and 41 years by 2025. Persons over 65 years were the fastest growing segment (22.3%) of the U.S. population between 1980 and 1990, when the total persons over 65 years of age was 35.1 million.[6] Estimates predict that by the year 2030, the number of individuals 65 years and over will reach 70 million in the United States alone.[1]

It is not simply the size and growth of this group of seniors that is responsible for its changing medical needs, but rather changes in the characteristics of the lifestyle and activities adopted by them. Of the 18 million persons between ages 65 and 74, most are retirees, and many devote their new leisure time to outdoor activities. The largest increases in elders between 1980 and 1990 occurred in regions of the United States most commonly associated with an active outdoor lifestyle: mountain states 44%, Pacific states 31%, and southern Atlantic states 34%. By contrast, the population of elders in the north central area increased only 11.4%.[6,11]

Leaf[21] reported three locations in the world, all in relatively remote mountainous areas (the Caucasus Mountains in Georgia, the Andes in Equador, and the Karakoram range in Pakistani-controlled Kashmir), where individuals frequently live to ages beyond 100 years. Speculation suggests that this is due to a combination of factors, including genetic selection and a physically active lifestyle.

WHY ELDERS VENTURE INTO THE WILDERNESS

Most members of Western industrialized cultures adhere to principles of hard work, family and fiscal responsibility, and delayed gratification. As retirement years approach, seniors begin to collect their "rewards." These include the pleasures and benefits of recreational activities. Nash[24] suggests that the personal reasons for elders to venture into the wilderness are for enjoyment of nature, for physical fitness, for tension reduction, for tranquility and solitude away from noise and crowds, for experiences with friends, for enhancement of skill and competency, and for excitement or even risk-taking (Figure 76-1).

As a result, outdoor recreational activities selected in the U.S. National Park System in order of decreasing frequency include: driving for pleasure, sightseeing, walking for pleasure, picnicking, stream/lake/ocean/pool swimming, and motorboating. Less common recreational activities include backpacking, off-road motorcycling, exploration, kayaking, and cross-country skiing.[5] Although the venture frequency of the latter group is much less than the former, the risk per venture is much greater. These ventures often take place in difficult and inaccessible areas under extraordinary environmental circumstances and, in the event of an emergency, may invoke search and rescue services and/or a medical intervention.

ENVIRONMENTAL STRESSES AND ELDERS

Potential physiologic stresses encountered in the great diversity of outdoor wilderness activities are legion. They include extremes of heat and cold, high altitude, water immersion, tropical humidity, and desert aridity. The common denominator in nearly all of these ven-

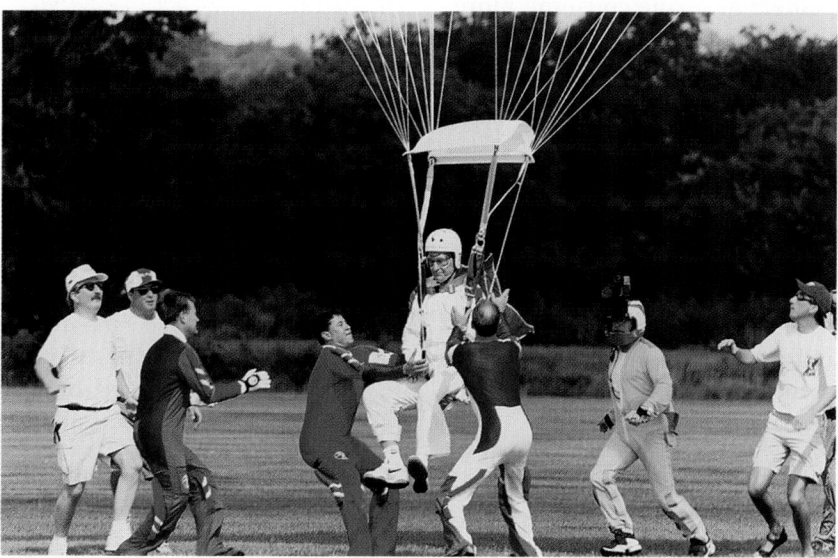

Figure 76-1 President George Bush celebrating his 75th birthday with a parachute jump. He remarked, "Even old guys can still do stuff." *(Newsweek, June 21, 1999. Photo courtesy George Bush Presidential Library.)*

tures is physical activity, often at extreme levels. To compound the complexity, with any environmental stress, the physician may be dealing with an elder afflicted with subclinical disease or manifest disease.

When the physiologic demands from environmental stresses are added to the increase and prevalence of disease associated with aging, risk for illness and injury is multiplied. The complete package of age, conditioning, environment, and nature of the activity must be considered when an elder is advised or treated in the wilderness.

Heat (see Chapter 10)

Tolerance to heat depends on physiologic factors: (1) characteristics of the host, including health status and medications, frequency and duration of exposure, and history of recent acclimatization; and (2) additional environmental factors. Industry has considered levels for permissible exposure limits (PEL), threshold limit values (TLV), and standards for maximal exposure, but there has been no consensus on an exact environmental stress index for heat.

Elders in a hot wilderness setting may have personal host characteristics, in addition to the environment, that further limit tolerance and safety. Weight; fractionated body mass; cardiovascular, renal, or pulmonary problems; and the presence of various medications may influence individual response to heat.

Regulation of body heat may be affected by altered function of the thermoregulatory center located in the anterior preoptic hypothalamic nuclei, by deranged skin sensors, or by medications used to treat various diseases, including anticholinergics, β-blockers, antipsychotic medications, and major tranquilizers. Side effects influence adaptation of sweat mechanisms to thermal stress. Diuretics may produce hypovolemia with loss of adequate subcutaneous circulation for heat dissipation. Because elders as a rule consume more medications than younger persons, it is very important to approach heat injury preventatively rather than after hyperthermia occurs.

The cardiovascular system plays a major role in heat regulation through heat dissipation. Circulatory abnormalities, peripherovascular disease, hypertension, and reduced cardiac output may modify heat dissipation, resulting in vulnerability to heat injury. Functional capacity as measured by maximal O_2 consumption ($\dot{V}O_2$ max) decreases 5% to 15% per decade after age 25 years. β-Blockers and calcium channel blockers may also influence cardiac output by modifying heart rate and myocardial contractility.

To prevent heat-related illness in the elderly, it is prudent to suggest a regular exercise program in heat. A regular program of physical activity consisting of 60 to 100 minutes of low-intensity exercise per day for 7 to 14 days at tolerable heat levels before the planned exposure should result in significant adaptation in nor-

mal individuals. The exercise level should require an oxygen consumption of less than 50% of the individual's $\dot{V}O_2$ max. Experience teaches us that a degree of adaptation results from frequent and extended periods of exposure. Acclimatization to heat yields a more beneficial response to concomitant exercise. This includes lower heart rate, enhanced tolerance to physical activity, predictable core temperature in response to heat stress, increased sweat rate, and decreased sodium loss through sweating.

Additional environmental factors, such as high humidity, high winds, and infrared and ultraviolet radiation exposure, may modify levels of individual tolerance to heat, partly through skin changes. It is valuable to teach individuals to be aware of the environment and whether the skin feels warm, cold, or damp. It also is helpful to advise the prospective wilderness venturer that, as a general rule, it takes a breeze of greater than 5 knots (5.75 mph) to be appreciated against the skin of the face. This may serve as a body signal reflecting one of the features that may add to the process of heat dissipation (see Body Signals, Box 76-2).

Characteristics of Elders Vulnerable to Heat Exposure

1. Host characteristics: obesity, decreased physical functional capacity
2. Infrequent heat exposure
3. Altered thermoregulatory center in the hypothalamus or insensitive skin sensors
4. Metabolic and serum electrolyte abnormalities
5. Heart disease, coronary artery disease, pulmonary disease, diabetes, and renal disease
6. Peripheral vascular disease
7. Multiple medications, often in combination: anticholinergics, antipsychotics, tranquilizers, and β-blockers
8. Alcohol

Prevention of Heat Injury in the Elderly

1. Maintain adequate hydration.
2. Assess the health status, with particular emphasis on history, cardiovascular status, obesity, and previous history of problems associated with heat exposure.
3. Maintain adequate nutritional status—food, fluid, and electrolyte intake.
4. Use estrogen replacement therapy where indicated (see Clinical Medicine, Menopause).
5. Participate in a proper acclimatization program.
6. Avoid the use of superfluous medication.

Cold (see Chapter 6)

Cold exposure is poorly tolerated among the elderly, and body temperature is more difficult to control in elders than in younger people. Peripheral vasoconstrictive response to cold is diminished. Systolic hypertension through stimulation of the sympathetic nervous system is exaggerated in a cold environment. Cardiac workload is increased, and consequently, in the presence of coronary artery disease, angina is frequently precipitated by exertion and cold. Four avoidance factors for persons with coronary artery disease are exertion, exposure to cold, eating excessively, and emotional extremes, any one of which can precipitate angina. These factors are referred to as "the four Es of angina." An elder individual should remember that any one of these can induce angina and should be particularly careful not to combine any two of these potential ischemia-producing factors.

With aging, diminished metabolic rate occurs. When associated with age-related reduction in muscle mass, the shivering response is blunted and there is reduced capacity for heat generation.

Exhaustion added to hypoglycemia and dehydration compounds the problem of impaired metabolic function, making the elder individual more vulnerable to the effects of cold. Adequate food intake is essential for maintaining body heat and may become critical. Other physical environmental influences, such as wind, humidity, ultraviolet and infrared radiation, and altitude, should be factored into the exposure equation. The wind chill index provides a useful teaching device for reminding the explorer about the hazards of combining cold and wind. The classic combination of cold, dampness, wind, and exhaustion may prove fatal, especially in an elder with decreased physical reserve.

Medical conditions may contribute to hypothermia. Cardiovascular disease, metabolic diseases such as hypothyroidism and diabetes, compromised nutritional status, and modified thermoregulatory responses resulting from central nervous system disease or medication may influence heat conservation.

Heat loss may also be increased by damp, wet clothing. All persons should be cautioned to carry ample clothing for changes after saturation with moisture.

The fundamental mechanism for heat conservation, peripheral vasoconstriction, may be enhanced to some small degree by long-term adaptation to cold, resulting in more effective protective function. When an elder recognizes intolerance to cold, he or she may begin a program of gradual increase in exposure to cold. However, prevention of cold injury is best achieved through a learning process derived from experience. Elders should never venture unaccompanied into the cold wilderness. Judgment and independent responsibility may be impaired by elders who find themselves lost or in a rescue situation.

Characteristics of Elders Vulnerable to Cold Exposure, Cold Injury, and Frostbite

1. Peripheral vascular disease (impaired vasoconstriction)
2. Hypertension (cold-induced)
3. Heart disease, including coronary artery disease, decreased cardiac output, congestive heart failure
4. Metabolic diseases (diabetes, obesity, hypothyroidism)
5. Hematologic disorders (anemia, dysproteinemias)
6. Pulmonary disease (cold-induced asthma, chronic obstructive pulmonary disease)
7. Drugs and alcohol
8. Medications, particularly β-blockers and tranquilizers

Prevention of Cold Injury in the Elderly

1. Avoid exhaustion during wilderness ventures.
2. Limit exposure.
3. Carry and wear adequate clothing, including rain gear.
4. Stay dry and avoid damp undergarments from excessive sweating.
5. Maintain adequate nutrition with high carbohydrates and fat. Carry adequate food for the trip.
6. Maintain adequate fluid intake. Do not consume cold ice or snow!
7. Participate in a preexpedition physical training program. Avoid exhaustion.
8. Pay attention to medication effects.
9. Avoid alcohol and illicit drugs.
10. Always maintain access to an adequate shelter.

Altitude

Demographic data for altitude illness among the elderly are limited. Most studies have been on healthy, vigorous young males. However, Houston,[15] Honigman,[14] and others studied the general population at moderate altitude (2000 to 3000 m [6562 to 9843 feet]) elevation at ski resorts in Colorado. Predictors of mountain sickness included chronic residence at altitude greater than 1000 m (3281 feet) before a high-altitude venture, underlying lung problems, previous history of acute mountain sickness ($p < 0.05$) and, surprisingly, age younger than 60 years. This apparent paradox probably is due to natural self selection among the small group of elderly individuals who expose themselves to altitude and activity.

Hackett[12] reported that aging reduces physiologic components of the gas exchange process, such as vital capacity and hypoxic ventilatory drive, that maintain oxygenation. Older persons are known to have a lower arterial PO_2 because of thickening of the pulmonary alveolar-capillary membrane.[19]

Although 25% of visitors to moderate altitude develop some degree of mountain sickness, data reflect a protective effect from living at moderate elevations of 1500 to 2000 m (4921 to 6562 feet), which is consistent with empiric observations that staging of altitude ascent reduces the incidence of acute mountain sickness.

Honigman found that most frequent predictors of acute mountain sickness are: (1) altitude of residence greater than 1000 m, (2) history of previous episode of acute mountain sickness, (3) age less than 60 years, (4) poor or average physical condition, and (5) lung disease.

Decreased fitness, alcohol intake, excessive activity within the first 12 hours after arriving at altitude, pre-existing cardiopulmonary disease, and medication increase the risk of altitude illness among elders. Alcohol tolerance is so variable that total abstinence during a wilderness venture is recommended. It is prudent to avoid sedatives and hypnotics at high altitude.

Characteristics of Elders Vulnerable to Altitude Illnesses

1. Abrupt ascent in altitude from near sea level to 3000 m (9843 feet) or greater, without an extra night for acclimatization for every additional 600 to 900 m (1969 to 2953 feet) of continuing ascent
2. History of previous episode of altitude sickness
3. Preexisting lung disease characterized by decreased capacity and decreased hypoxic ventilatory response
4. Preexisting cardiovascular disease
5. Metabolic abnormalities associated with diabetes and renal disease
6. Medication that influences respiratory drive
7. Low physical functional capacity
8. Obesity

Prevention of Altitude Sickness in Elders

1. Avoid strenuous physical activity at altitude if there is a history of acute mountain sickness.
2. Limit the intensity of physical activity in the presence of cardiovascular disease.
3. Limit physical activity in the presence of pulmonary disease, especially if there is decreased vital capacity.
4. Avoid significant physical activity for at least 12 hours after arrival at an altitude of 2500 m (8202 feet) or more above sea level, and delay physical activity for an additional 24 hours for every 600 to 900 m additional altitude.
5. Be aware of all medications and their effect on hypoxic ventilatory drive.

CLINICAL MEDICINE IN ELDERS

Wilderness medicine can be simply defined as "traditional medicine in a nontraditional setting." Nature of the site, environmental conditions, and type of activity affect care, search and rescue, transportation, and medical support. When elder age is a factor, an additional set of concerns is added, including reduction in physical reserve, increase in rate of physical deterioration during exercise, and therefore reduction in margin of safety. Enhanced skills of analysis, planning, intervention, and action are demanded of the rescuers and medical team.

There are two important occasions when elders and wilderness leaders should consider health/medical evaluation for elderly venturers: (1) during the planning phase before the venture and (2) following symptoms that may occur during or after the venture. Components of the pretrip evaluation are based on the characteristics of the individual and on the nature of the proposed venture. These are discussed in the Medical Examination section. Evaluation after the onset of symptoms and/or for intervention and disposition requires clinical judgment dictated by the specific problem or symptom and is considered in discussions of specific illnesses.

Cardiovascular Disease

Age-related changes in the cardiovascular system affect heart rhythm, myocardial pump function, and afterload. With aging, there is progressive reduction in the number of pacemaker cells in the sinoatrial (SA) node, increase in myocyte cell volume per nucleus in both ventricles, increase in peripheral vascular resistance, and increase in aortic impedance from loss of elasticity. Increased levels of circulating catecholamines are associated with aging, especially with stress, but β-adrenergic vasodilation decreases with age. This is important for exercise tolerance in elders.

Cardiac rhythm disturbances range from the nuisance effect of premature systoles to significant rhythm disturbances, such as atrial fibrillation, to potentially life-threatening ventricular arrhythmias. An elder who is aware of symptoms related to a arrhythmia should seek evaluation by a physician before a wilderness venture. The evaluation should include history of onset of symptoms and initiating factors, physical examination with emphasis on auscultation of the mitral and aortic valves, electrocardiogram, ambulatory monitoring if there is a history of heart disease or light-headedness, and possibly an echocardiogram.

Valvular changes, especially of the aortic and mitral valves, may be recognized by auscultation and confirmed by echocardiography, and perhaps by cardiac catheterization. The subject with a prosthetic cardiac valve may be at risk during prolonged ventures with exposure to inclement weather or infectious diseases among fellow venturers or diseases among the local populace.

The presence of pump failure, either systolic or diastolic, may be indicated by recent weight gain, shortness of breath, orthopnea, or ankle edema. It is confirmed by physical examination, electrocardiography, echocardiography, and chest x-ray. Although digitalis, diuretics, and angiotensin I-converting enzyme (ACE) inhibitors may relieve symptoms of systolic dysfunction, the subject with heart failure should limit remote wilderness ventures to those activities that do not cause excessive shortness of breath, that is, to the point of requiring breathing through the open mouth, or excessive fatigue.

Peripheral vascular disease, claudication, symptomatic carotid disease, and aortic aneurysms warrant caution in regard to the difficulty of return or evacuation in the event of incapacity.

Coronary Artery Disease

A heart attack is the ultimate medical emergency. In the United States, approximately 1.5 million persons sustain myocardial infarctions annually, 30% of whom do not survive. Of these victims, 50% die within the first hour of the onset of chest pain. If a victim survives the first hour, which may be the time required to initiate a search and rescue, there may be approximately an 85% chance of survival expected subsequently.

Only half of persons with myocardial infarction have premonitory symptoms, but interrogation about this during a medical history could alert one to the likelihood of myocardial infarction. The history should include a detailed assessment of risk factors for coronary artery disease. Subsequent physical examination and testing may provide recommendations aimed at reducing life-threatening cardiac events.

Many physiologic stresses related to environmental extremes have as a common denominator an increase in catecholamine output with a concomitant rise in heart rate, blood pressure, and cardiac output. This results in increased cardiac work load and myocardial oxygen demand.

Since the myocardium depends almost entirely on aerobic metabolism, workload is reflected in myocardial oxygen consumption. Delivery of oxygen (O_2) to the myocardium in response to workload demands depends on coronary blood flow. Hence, integrity of the coronary arteries is essential for a viable response to wilderness stresses.

Knowledge of the existence and extent of coronary artery disease will influence physician recommendations for the nature and level of activity, expected tolerance to environmental stresses, and recommendations as to the degree of remoteness, level of exertion, and environmental factors that the individual should consider in the proposed wilderness ventures.

The Preventure Assessment

Since there is no absolutely risk-free activity for a person with significant cardiovascular disease, prevention is the fundamental principle for reducing risk. Before vigorous outdoor activity by an elder, the physician should: (1) question the individual regarding planned activities, (2) have a knowledge of the planned activity and be aware of anticipated exertion and environmental circumstances, (3) have a thorough understanding of previous history of coronary artery disease and other illnesses, and (4) be prepared to make specific recom-

mendations regarding physical activity and exposure (see Medical Examination).

There are currently no published guidelines to aid in advising elderly individuals intending to venture into the wilderness, but the American College of Cardiology 26th Bethesda Conference produced "Recommendations for Determining Eligibility in Competitive Athletes with Cardiovascular Abnormalities." These guidelines divide patients into two categories: (1) those with mildly increased risk, having a left ventricular ejection fraction (LVEF) of greater than 50% (or revascularization of such lesions), and (2) those with a substantially increased risk, having a LVEF of less than 50%, exercise-induced myocardial ischemia, exercise-induced complex ventricular arrhythmias, and occlusive lesions of greater than 50% in one or more coronary arteries.

Transposing the recommendations for athletes to the elderly, persons with mildly increased risk are advised to restrict activities to levels of low dynamic activity, that is, activities requiring an energy expenditure equivalent to walking, and a low moderate static level equivalent to lifting less than 15 to 20 pounds. Those persons with substantially increased risk are advised to participate only in low-level dynamic and static activities.

Persons with atrial fibrillation but without structural heart disease, and who can maintain an appropriate heart rate response to exercise, have no limitations. For persons with atrial fibrillation, structural heart disease, and an appropriate rate response to exercise, activities consistent with the limitations of the structural heart disease are allowed. Persons with atrial fibrillation requiring anticoagulation should not participate in activities risking physical contact and injury.

In considering these recommendations, one must remember that these guidelines were developed for competitive athletes and are not necessarily applicable to recreational activities. Nevertheless, the guidelines provide a framework for an initial evaluation.

A fascinating philosophical discussion dealing with the limitations of wilderness activities in subjects who have undergone cardiac surgery appeared in a series of letter exchanges and editorials in the *Journal of the American Medical Association*. The conclusion returned the decision-making process to the clinical judgment of the cardiologist on a case-by-case basis.[26]

Hypertension

Hypertension, the "silent killer," is an important marker for potential cardiovascular problems among elders. Cardiovascular mortality was shown to be 3 times as high in hypertensive elders compared with those with normal blood pressure. Complications include angina, myocardial infarction, left ventricular hypertrophy, heart failure, stroke (both ischemic and hemorrhagic), and renal failure. The most widely accepted values of blood pressure considered to represent hypertension are systolic above 140 mm Hg or diastolic over 90 mm Hg. In the health survey for England,[25] systolic blood pressure over 160 mm Hg was observed in 35% of men and 37% of women aged 65 to 74, increasing to 41% and 49%, respectively, after age 75 years. Isolated systolic hypertension is almost exclusively a disorder of elders with a prevalence of 0.8% at age 50 years, 12.6% at 70 years, and 23.6% at 80 years.[29]

There is an increased effect of oral sodium intake on blood pressure in the elderly. An increase of 100 mmol/day is associated with a 10- to 15-mm Hg rise in systolic pressure, compared with a 4- to 5-mm Hg rise in younger adults who ingest the same sodium load.[20] In elders, isolated systolic hypertension is recognized as a predictor of stroke.

Treatment of hypertension is mandatory before an elder ventures into the wilderness. Useful medications, however, may cause significant side effects. Diuretics, an integral part of treatment, may deplete volume and electrolytes such as potassium and sodium. β-Blockers, of particular value for the systolic component, may limit heart rate response to activity or modify body temperature control during exposure to heat or cold. Calcium channel blockers are of value in treatment of hypertension, but headache, flushing, and edema are reported in about one third of patients taking them. The least complicated treatment for hypertension is control of obesity and restriction of dietary sodium intake.

Treatment of hypertension in the elderly includes all of the foregoing with the caveat that exertion in the wilderness setting may magnify the physiologic and pharmacologic effects of medications.

Gastrointestinal Disorders

The gastrointestinal tract maintains relatively normal function during the aging process. Constipation, however, is a frequent complaint among 26% of elderly men and 34% of elderly women. There is a difference between the medical definition and elder perception of constipation and their need for laxatives. Normal frequency of bowel movements varies between three defecations per day and three per week. However, laxatives are used by 15% to 30% of elders on a regular basis. When such individuals find themselves in the wilderness, away from the convenience of their bathroom, alteration in bowel habits, even to the point of fecal impaction, may occur. Therefore it is prudent to obtain a detailed history of habits and medication before embarking on a wilderness venture. Dietary fruit, fiber, and grain with stool softeners for elders during a wilderness venture may help avoid impaction, rectal fissure, hemorrhoidal bleeding, leaking incontinence, and chafing.

An increased prevalence of several gastrointestinal disorders is noted among elders. These include malig-

nancies of colon and pancreas, gastric ulceration that may bleed, especially after nonsteroidal antiinflammatory drug (NSAID) ingestion, and *Helicobacter pylori* infection. Prospects for bleeding or obstruction from colon malignancies, bleeding from gastric ulcers, and possible perforation of ulcers should alert the individual or group leader to the seriousness of remote adventures and urgency for medical attention. A surgical emergency may arise from an incarcerated or strangulated inguinal or ventral hernia.

Diarrhea among elders contracted in Third World countries may be severe, leading to dehydration, gastrointestinal bleeding, or perforation of a hollow organ. Exacerbation of diverticulitis or acute cholecystitis, with or without pancreatitis, persistent or unusual abdominal pain, vomiting, bleeding, and worsening dehydration are reasons for ending the venture and initiating evacuation to medical care.

When traveling to remote Third World countries, it is prudent for expeditions to carry intravenous (IV) fluids and to consider appropriate antimicrobial prophylaxis or medications for the presumptive treatment of infectious diarrhea.

Genitourinary Disorders

Elders are particularly vulnerable to urinary tract disorders, including infections, obstructions, and ureteral, renal, or bladder stones. Bladder infections in women are common in remote settings because of dehydration and difficulty with hygiene. Incontinence after hysterectomy is frequent, and discomfort from chafing and bladder infection may be present. It is prudent for women to carry medicated skin pads and cotton diapers. Men may incur bladder infections from benign prostatic hypertrophy with obstruction. Anticholinergic medications may induce bladder relaxation with subsequent retention. Terazosin hydrochloride, an α_1-selective adrenoreceptor blocking agent, may improve urine flow in instances of obstruction resulting from benign prostatic hypertrophy by reducing bladder outlet obstruction without affecting bladder contractility.

Dehydration from fluid loss or inadequate oral replacement may precipitate infection. Adequate fluid intake is the key to genitourinary health in the wilderness, but the participant must be cautioned about water quality.

Menopause

Menopause in women is a normal phenomenon associated with aging. Rather than occurring as a discrete event, the menopause transition may take place over a period of several years beginning around 40 years or as late as 50 to 55 years of age. Also known as the climacteric, this is a time in life when the opportunity for leisure activities may be greatest. Women who participate in wilderness activities must deal with the symptoms and somatic changes of menopause in addition to the physical and environmental stresses of the wilderness.

Symptoms that foretell the onset of menopause include vasomotor flushing, night sweats, insomnia, vaginal dryness, and variation in menstrual cycle and flow. Convention accepts that 12 months of cessation of menses is confirmation of menopause.

As ovarian production of estrogen declines, the androgen/estrogen ratio changes dramatically. Gonadotropin feedback results in increased follicle-stimulating hormone (FSH) in a range of up to 30 MIU/ml. Progesterone secretion is variable and may either increase or decrease.[28] Resulting anatomic changes from these hormonal alterations may affect lipid ratios, the coronary arteries, cortical and trabecular bone, and changes in body fat distribution with a shift in fat towards the center of the body. Changes in cognitive function have also been reported.

Vulnerability to osteoporotic fractures is a serious hazard for the elderly woman in the wilderness. In trabecular bone found in the spinal column, resorption and formation occur 4 to 8 times as fast as that of cortical bone. As a result, there is an increased risk of compression fracture of the spine or fracture of hip in the event of a fall.

Hormonal replacement therapy should be considered for menopausal or postmenopausal women or in those who have had surgical hysterectomy. The three classic indications for hormone replacement therapy are: (1) for symptoms related to estrogen deficiency, such as vasomotor symptoms or genitourinary tissue atrophy; (2) for prevention or treatment of osteoporosis; and (3) for prevention of a cardiovascular morbidity and mortality, all of which may occur in the wilderness setting.

Combinations of estrogens and progestins may be used in treatment.[17] Examples include:

Daily estrogen as 0.625 mg conjugated estrogen or 1 mg micronized estradiol

Daily progestin as 2.5 mg medroxyprogesterone acetate or 0.35 mg norethindrone

Transdermal route of administration may be convenient in the wilderness setting, reducing some of the packing load.

Musculoskeletal Disorders

Musculoskeletal disorders are a leading cause of morbidity among elders. In the wilderness, joint stress associated with extended hiking, injuries from repetitive motion, falls, and other trauma, when superimposed on the aging body, can induce functional impairments. Limitations in mobility and from pain lead to a loss of satisfaction or success or even to significant hazards during wilderness ventures.

Arthritis is among the most common causes of chronic disability in elders. About 15% of the U.S. population in 1990 reported having arthritis. More significant is a reported prevalence of nearly 50% among persons 65 years of age or older.

Musculoskeletal conditions with increased incidence in adults over age 50 years include osteoarthritis, osteoporosis, polymyalgia rheumatica, giant cell arteritis, gout (especially associated with diuretic use), and other crystal-associated arthritides such as calcium pyrophosphate deposition disease, basic calcium phosphate deposition disease, rheumatoid and other inflammatory arthritides, and spinal stenosis.

The aging joint undergoes degenerative changes in its components. Cartilage has very little ability to heal. Therefore injuries to cartilage tend to accumulate with age, leading to irreversible damage and osteophyte formation, developing into hypertrophic osteoarthritic change in joints of the extremities and spine.

Skeletal muscle undergoes specific age-related changes with loss of muscle mass. Changes in hormones, growth hormone/insulin-like growth factor-1 (GH/IGF-1), the androgen/estrogen ratio, cytokines/growth factor, interleukin-6, and free radical production may be related to these atrophic changes.

The syndromes causing loss of muscle mass in elders are either (1) intrinsic: sarcopenia, resulting in diminished reserves of muscle mass, or (2) extrinsic: failure to thrive (FTT) syndrome, from diseases and/or increased metabolic demands.

Prevention and treatment of sarcopenia and FTT include a regimen of regular exercise, including both aerobic training and strength training. Progressive resistance training (PRT) is effective in the treatment of sarcopenia. Lean mass is lost along with bone mass at menopause. Estrogen replacement appears to be helpful in some postmenopausal women. Evidence supporting testosterone replacement for FTT in elderly men is lacking.

A detailed history and physical examination, with emphasis on prior and present symptoms, is of value for an elder contemplating physical activity and essential for an elder planning remote wilderness activities. Although radiologic studies and laboratory tests may help establish a diagnosis, a common tendency is to rely too heavily on the radiograph to explain symptoms. Joint aspiration and synovial fluid analysis helps in the diagnosis of metabolic or inflammatory arthritides.

Treatment of arthritis in a layered stepwise manner begins with rest, acetaminophen, NSAIDs, and topical capsaicin. Elders especially must be cautioned about the gastric irritation from NSAIDs and their danger in the presence of comorbid conditions and anticoagulant therapy.

Intraarticular corticosteroids may help reduce inflammation. Injection serves the extra function of providing access for aspiration of synovial fluid from a joint effusion. Total joint replacement (TJR) for hips and knees has been used with increasing frequency for the management of severe intractable and progressive pain.

Physical therapy before and after the onset of symptoms, including body weight reduction, PRT, aerobic conditioning, and spa therapy, may be effective in treatment or during preparation for a wilderness venture. Corsets, braces, and canes prescribed by the treating specialist should be used, but the layperson is cautioned against self-prescription.

A conditioning program before the venture may help prevent musculoskeletal problems or may precipitate symptoms that alert the individual to a problem not previously recognized. It is better for symptoms to occur at home and serve as a warning for potential future untoward events than to occur in a remote location far from medical care. Since degenerative changes in the dorsolumbar and cervical spine may become symptomatic, it is appropriate to carry a backpack during a conditioning program before a hiking venture. At least one and preferably two hiking sticks are recommended for hiking activities.

Growth Hormone in Elders

With advancing age, there are decreases in lean body mass, body fat, and protein synthesis. GH deficiency is associated with changes in body composition and protein metabolism similar to those of aging. With advancing years, men and women with no clinical evidence of pituitary abnormalities show decreases in GH secretion and serum levels of IGF-1. Administration of recombinant human GH (rhGH) to these GH/IGF-1–deficient elders has been reported to result in improvements in nitrogen balance, increase in lean body mass, and decrease in percent body fat. Studies also suggest that there may be an increase in lumbar vertebral bone density, but no significant change in the mineral density of the radius or proximal femur.

Long-term administration of GH has been reported to cause some side effects, including edema, hypertension, carpal tunnel syndrome, and arthralgia.

Further studies are needed to determine if normalization of GH and IGF-I levels in healthy elders will lead to improvements in the physical and functional quality of their lives. The prospect of improved muscle mass and strength for elders considering wilderness activities should be followed closely by those interested in human performance.

Neurologic Disorders and the Senses

Organic neurologic disorders, clinically apparent or subclinical, are frequent among elders. Symptoms of neurologic problems may be precipitated by minor activities or environmental stresses in the wilderness.

Physical activity to which a participant may be unaccustomed, especially when extreme environmental conditions are superimposed, can make subtle changes more apparent. However, if a victim responds with denial, the result can be devastating.

A history of ischemic or hemorrhagic stroke that in the past resulted in a degree of paresis, especially when accompanied by symptoms such as dizziness, changes in rational thought, or seizure, should alert leaders to potential problems in a wilderness venture.

Altitude, especially above 2500 m (8202 feet), may induce changes in mentation not apparent at lower levels. Leaders should be especially diligent in the assessment of individuals with a previous history of altitude sickness or who are taking medications, including anticoagulants, for cerebrovascular disease.

Our senses are our warning system for hazards in the wilderness. The five classical sensory "instruments" send signals to the central nervous system during interpretation of the physical environment. With age, these sensors undergo functional degeneration. Up to 75% of elders have visual and auditory impairments not reported to their physicians. Changes may be subtle. Again, the aging rule is a 1% loss per year after age 30 years of physiologic function in most organ systems.

Vision. There is decreased visual acuity caused by morphologic changes in the lens, choroid, retina, rods and cones, and other neural elements, and by an increase in intraocular pressure. Night vision and color vision are noticeably decreased after age 50 years. Hypoxia, to which the elder's eye may be sensitive, may cause tunnel vision. This may be a valuable "body signal" indicating an altitude that may be hazardous to the individual.

The most troublesome ophthalmologic effects of age are glaucoma and changes in refractive power. Increased intraocular pressure may be associated with halos and declining vision. This is a serious medical condition warranting continuing care by an ophthalmologist (see Chapter 22). Manifestations and treatment of farsightedness range from purchasing a pair of nonprescription "reading glasses" to elaborate multipower prescription lenses. Negotiating rough terrain may be difficult using bifocals. An older person walking on a wooded trail may be unable to see the roots and rocks in his or her path. The wilderness is no place for a broken hip. Trifocals and various lens designs have been tried, but experience suggests that trail glasses should be configured for distance, with separate reading glasses for close-up work, such as map reading. Decreased tear secretion and "dry eyes" may affect elders in a dusty wilderness environment.

Hearing. Hearing problems are common in elders, affecting 60% of Americans over age 65 years. Presbycusis may be the result of previous middle ear infection, vascular disease, exposure to noise, or the natural loss of sensitivity and distortion of signals associated with advancing age. Acoustical trauma may have caused a permanent reduction in sensitivity to high-frequency sound, and the failure to hear the "click pitch" of consonants may obscure communications. Problems with sound localization may result in loss of directional hearing. Confused sound signals cannot be processed as accurately by an aging brain. Add tinnitus and a hostile environment, and the hearing sense loses its value as an important survival tool.

Taste and Smell. Some lingual papillae are lost because of age, diminishing the ability to taste. Salivary secretion is reduced. Dentures may cover secondary taste sites. Olfactory bulbs also undergo significant atrophy with age. Combined taste and olfactory sensory deprivation may account for decreased "pleasure" of trail food taste.

Touch. In addition to assisting in fine movement needed for technical work, sensitivity of touch against a hostile environment may be lifesaving. For example, conventional wisdom holds that the threshold for feeling a gentle breeze against the cheek is about 5 miles per hour.

Impairment of cold awareness, which originates from stimuli at the end bulbs of Krause in the skin, along with age-attenuated metabolic adaptation to cold, can interfere with signals that trigger an individual to assume cover.

There is a "sixth sense" built into the aging wilderness adventurer derived from years of experience and exposure, study, and review of wilderness activities. This is *wisdom!* As a result of assimilating and processing these data, elders frequently acquire a reputation for survival. One who develops this aura is affectionately known as a "salty dog."

Neuropsychiatric Disorders

Situational stresses are often superimposed on environmental stresses during wilderness ventures. Difficulties with group interaction, changes in rational thought in individuals with organic brain disease, or behavioral upheaval from bipolar states can jeopardize the health and safety not only of the individual but also of an entire group.

Problems associated with drug abuse or alcoholism are a danger to the individual and are potentially devastating to the group. Subtle alcoholism may become full-blown withdrawal psychosis during a hypoxic event or during extreme physical exertion. Drug use in elders may not be "recreational," but withdrawal from ethical drugs may be quite severe. Leaders of wilderness ventures must recognize the danger of disruptive psychiatric problems and attempt to prevent them by careful screening before the venture.

As people age, a variety of cognitive disorders become apparent, including progressive dementia, confusional states, and cognitive disorders resulting from psychiatric syndromes. Symptoms may be precipitated in vulnerable individuals by physical or environmental stresses of the wilderness. The two usual sources of information concerning the status of patients are patients' families and the patients themselves. It is rare for a family member to approach the physician with concerns about the cognitive function of a relative; thus an interview and brief mental status testing should be included in the medical evaluation.

A cognitive examination should provide the examiner with insight into prior cognitive skills and personality traits to serve as a baseline. Included should be the nature of the subject's memory at that time, the interval since onset of symptoms, the nature of onset (slow or sudden), and current state of cognitive function.

Frontotemporal dementia, such as Pick's disease, may manifest itself early with a change in personality with inappropriate and often volatile behavior. Alzheimer's disease is frequently manifested by apathy and decline in ability to learn new information.

Physician assessment of cognitive function and neuropsychiatric disorders may identify potential disaster during wilderness undertakings.

Diabetes Mellitus and Other Metabolic Disorders

Type II ("adult-onset") diabetes mellitus, whether requiring insulin or controlled by oral hypoglycemic medication, is not necessarily a contraindication to wilderness activities; however, other problems related to diabetes may increase risk of medical emergencies. Cardiovascular disorders, coronary artery disease, cerebrovascular disorders, peripheral and autonomic neuropathy, nephropathy, poor wound healing and/or infection, and vulnerability to frostbite and cold injury all may be associated with this metabolic disorder.

Insulin-dependent (type I) diabetes is a very different situation because of the additional problems with caloric intake and energy expenditure. Hypoglycemic episodes may lead to accidents from mental confusion. The vestibular apparatus in elders is particularly sensitive to such episodes. The "buddy system" should be deployed to assist the insulin-dependent diabetic in the wilderness.

Pharmacology, Pharmacokinetics, and Polypharmacy

Older people are the major consumers of all categories of medications. Health status and pharmacokinetics of elders alter drug choices, dosages, prospects for adverse reactions, and even therapeutic goals. Physician assessment of elders before wilderness activities should include careful review of all medications.

Age-related physiologic changes may influence pharmacokinetics: reduced gastric acid production and altered gastric emptying, affecting absorption; reduced splanchnic blood flow, affecting first pass (or presystemic) clearance; reduced body water, serum albumin, body fat, and body mass, affecting protein binding; changes in hepatic size and blood flow, affecting hepatic clearance; and reduced glomerular filtration rate and renal tubular function, affecting renal clearance.

As a result, physicians recognize that it is almost always prudent to begin with a lower starting dose and lower maintenance dose of certain prescribed medications in elderly patients.

Renal clearance of some drugs is reduced as a result of aging. The clinical significance of altered renal clearance resulting in elevated blood levels is, of course, related to the drug. Drugs with a very narrow therapeutic ratio should be carefully monitored. These include antibiotics such as gentamicin, streptomycin, and kanamycin; β-blockers such as atenolol and sotalol; cardiac glycosides such as digoxin; and psychotropic drugs such as lithium.

Hepatic clearance of drugs is of even more concern in the elderly because of a silent reduction in clearance capacity of up to 50% or more in this age group. Causes of reduced hepatic clearance include reduction of absolute liver size, decrease in hepatic blood flow, and perhaps altered enzyme activities. Benzodiazepines, nitrazepam, chlordiazepoxide, midazolam, and colabazepam, eliminated primarily by oxidation, should be reduced in dosage. Oxazepam, eliminated by glucuronidation, also should be given in reduced dosage.

Comorbidity, the presence of multiple pathologic problems, makes drug choice particularly important because of the prospects of worsening a coexisting disease when a prescription is given for another disease condition. For example, thiazide diuretics may worsen control of diabetes; calcium channel blockers may result in ankle edema; β-blockers may increase symptoms of peripheral vascular disease; dopamine blockers given as antiemetics may exacerbate parkinsonism; and NSAIDs may render hypertension, heart disease, or renal failure more difficult to control.

Counseling, packaging labels, diaries, and supervision are important instruments for proper control of toxic and side effects of medications in elders.

Excessive use of medicines is often seen.[26] "Polypharmacy" represents a less-than-desirable state of duplication of medications, failure to recognize potential drug interactions, and inadequate attention to pharmacokinetics and pharmacologic principles.[25] Alcohol abuse frequently compounds the problem of polypharmacy. It is a great help to have each participant carry all presently consumed medications to his or her physician for review before the wilderness venture.

PHYSICAL ACTIVITY AND ELDERS

The common denominator among wilderness ventures is physical activity. For elders, the demands of certain physical activities may be excessive. The physical workload of a wilderness venture depends on its nature and the characteristics of its component parts. For example, is it a walking venture or a climb? What is the nature of the terrain? What is the altitude? What is the environmental temperature? It is prudent for elders to examine plans for a prospective wilderness venture and to select activities consistent with their personal capacity and tolerance.

Wilderness activities can be classified according to their physical, technical, and environmental characteristics. The skill, judgment, and capacity of all participants, elders included, can then be matched with the characteristics of the venture to determine if individual capacity is adequate for the demands.

One classification of wilderness ventures ranges from extreme physical demands to minimal demand and includes:

1. Extreme performance ventures, such as Himalayan trekking or climbing major peaks
2. High-performance ventures, such as remote hunting activity, particularly at high altitude or under stresses of heat, dust, or cold. Jungle trekking is also an environmentally and physically stressful venture.
3. Recreational activities. Trail walking is generally considered recreational but because of endurance and risks may present physiologic hazards. Alpine hiking, National Park trail walking and forest-based orienteering may fit this classification.
4. Therapeutic activities. These may be recommended for persons with illness or disability. For more than a century, physical activity has been recommended for certain individuals with cardiovascular disease and other physical limitations to improve functional capacity.

Although this classification is very general, it can be helpful to match the physical and intellectual demands of specific wilderness ventures with individuals of varied skill, judgment, and physical capacity.

Classification of Participants in Wilderness Ventures

Successful participation by elders in wilderness activities depends on the capacity of the individual to tolerate the physical workload. After examining the nature of the wilderness venture and the characteristics of its environment, each participant should match his or her personal capacity with the characteristics of the venture being considered. Review of the functional capacity and experience of an individual may be used for personal classification. One classification considers:

Group A: Demonstrated high-performance individuals—athletes in training, mountaineers continually active and in training, workers in heavy physical tasks, etc.

Group B: Healthy, vigorous individuals—athletes, active hunting guides, etc.

Group C: Healthy, "deconditioned" individuals—young to middle aged, healthy, business and professional people who are moderately active.

Group D: Those with risk factors—individuals at risk because of age or because of lifestyle, smoking, excessive alcohol, or because of factors not under their control. Most elders are in Group D.

Group E: Those who are manifestly ill—subjects at any age with chronic illness or physical limitations, such as heart disease, diabetes, or neuromuscular or orthopedic problems.

Although this classification is general, it serves as a starting place for more precise recommendations for a specific adventure. The populations presenting to the physician may fit the distribution curve as shown in Box 76-1.

Metabolic Classifications

The workload of the venture and the functional capacity of the individual can be defined with precision by using a metabolic classification. The energy requirement of activities as derived from oxygen consumption studies may be used to match the demands of an activity with the functional capacity of an individual. Energy cost may be defined by oxygen consumption ($\dot{V}O_2$), or calories, or METs. These units are simply different ways of expressing the same data based on oxygen consumption. The term "MET" is useful because it represents the energy cost of an easily definable physical activity, sitting. One MET, the energy cost of sitting quietly, is defined by convention as 3.5 ml/O_2/kg body weight/min. Multiples of the MET may be used to define the energy cost of various activities or tasks. An activity requiring twice the metabolic cost of sitting is a 2 MET activity; a 3 MET activity represents 3 times the energy cost of sitting, or 10.5 ml/O_2/kg/min.

Walking 3 miles per hour on a level surface is a 3 MET activity. Each 2.5% grade increase increases the energy cost one additional MET when walking 3 miles

per hour. Hence, walking up a 2.5% grade at 3 miles per hour is a 4 MET activity. Most activities of daily living (ADLs) are less than 3 METs. Tables of the energy cost of various activities have been established. Components of tasks and activities in the wilderness can be defined in METs.

This unit may also be used to define the functional capacity of the individual. Using the same system of measuring O_2 consumption of an individual on a treadmill or cycle ergometer, the maximal physical work capacity (PWC$_{max}$) may be determined in METs. The average 40-year-old man in the United States has a PWC$_{max}$ of 10 METs, or 35 ml/O_2/kg/min. Hence, this

---

Box 76-1 WILDERNESS VENTURES

CLASSIFICATION OF WILDERNESS VENTURES

1. Extreme-performance ventures: may exceed 12 METs
2. High-performance ventures: up to 10 to 12 METs
3. Recreational activities: up to 8 to 10 METs
4. Therapeutic activities: highly individualized

Ventures are classified according to physical and intellectual difficulty.

Energy cost studies using $\dot{V}O_2$ or MET values help indicate metabolic difficulty.

CLASSIFICATION OF PARTICIPANTS IN WILDERNESS VENTURES

Group A = demonstrated high-performance individuals
Group B = healthy, vigorous individuals
Group C = healthy "deconditioned" individuals
Group D = those with risk factors
Group E = those who are manifestly ill

The functional capacity, also measured in METs of participants in ventures, provides a useful basis for matching participants with appropriate activities and helps determine the extent of a preventure medical examination.

DISTRIBUTION CURVE FOR WILDERNESS ADVENTURERS

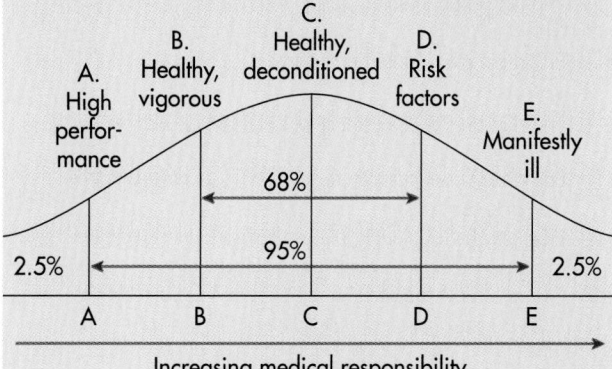

This normal curve may be roughly applied to a classification scheme for grouping wilderness venturers according to their functional characteristics.

provides a useful scale from 1 MET (the energy cost of sitting) to 10 METs (the PWC$_{max}$ of the average 40-year-old male).

As individuals age, they lose about 1 MET of PWC$_{max}$ per decade after 40 years of age, so the average capacity of a 70-year-old man is approximately 7 METs.

Tolerance to physical activity among females has been increasing for two decades and is now accepted as being about 1 to 2 METs less than that of a male of the same age. Physically active and conditioned females, however, are now of approximately the same capacity as males.

Matching Individuals with Activities

An individual who plans to participate in a wilderness venture has often already been through a form of natural selection. For example, one who aspires to participate in an expedition to Mount Everest will in all likelihood have already participated in a similar activity and will have proven his or her capacity to function at an extreme level of performance. This subject would likely be in group A or B. An individual who may not have been involved recently in high level activities or who has become "deconditioned" is in group C. There may still be the desire to participate, perhaps as a reaf-firmation of youth or vigor in some form of exciting or hazardous activity.

Particular attention should be directed toward any individual at risk of illness or injury (group D) even though manifest evidence of disease may not have been displayed. For example, cardiovascular risk factors such as smoking, fat-laden diet, and high blood pressure may warrant a precise medical examination to determine a level of functional capacity considered safe for the individual, even if a symptomatic disease is already present.

Group E includes persons with definite manifestations of illness. Outdoor activities have been used as a form of physical therapy for persons with various illnesses, including cardiovascular diseases. Persons in this category should be individualized as far as assessment is concerned and require a high degree of medical evaluation and supervision.

Elders are encouraged to "read" their personal physiologic responses to activity using "body signals" such as mouth breathing, which occurs at about 60% of maximal capacity, and sweating, which occurs under standard conditions at around 7 METs, depending on the environment. Some "body signals" are listed in Box 76-2.

Box 76-2 BODY SIGNALS

Participants in wilderness activities should learn to read the physiologic "body signals" that help an individual recognize impending medical problems from environmental stresses.

PRIMARY

Cardiovascular
  Heart rate: used to estimate physiologic effect of physical workload
  Pounding in head: possibly related to physiologic or pathologic systolic hypertension
  Chest pain: physiologic or pathologic
  Fluttering in chest: arrhythmia
Respiratory
  Mouth breathing: >60% of maximal physical work capacity
  Breathing too hard to talk: >85% of maximal physical work capacity
  Cough: dry air; early high-altitude pulmonary edema
  Cheyne-Stokes respiration: altitude
  Cyanosis of nailbeds, nose, or ear lobes: consider hypoxia

SECONDARY

Musculoskeletal
  Tremulousness: quadriceps weakness and cramps, consider volume depletion and hyponatremia

Shivering: cooling, body temperature >35.5° C (96° F)
Stopped shivering with confusion: possibly further dangerous cooling, body temperature probably <33.9° C (93° F)
Sweating: air temp/humidity or heavy physical work above 7 METs
Gastrointestinal
  Abdominal distention (with flatus): altitude
  Dry mouth: dehydration
  Loss of appetite: altitude and/or dehydration
Genitourinary
  Urinary frequency: altitude ("hochdiurese" of Alpine mountaineers)
Sensory
  Tubular vision: altitude/hypoxia
  Loss of color discrimination: hypoxia
  Loss of night vision discrimination: hypoxia
  Visual central white spot: hypoxia
  Sense of touch: wind against cheek >5 mph
  Taste: diminished with dehydration and hypoxia
  >Smell: diminished with dehydration and hypoxia
Neurologic
  Headache: altitude, cerebral edema
  Lack of analytic decisiveness: altitude and hypoxia
  Confusion and irrational behavior: altitude, hypoxia, and possible cerebrovascular abnormalities

Physical Conditioning to Prepare Elders for Wilderness Ventures

After an elder considering a wilderness venture determines his or her personal classification, it may be prudent to obtain a medical examination. A physical conditioning program may be recommended to increase individual reserve capacity. As a rule of thumb, an individual considering an 8-hour activity can tolerate an energy cost of approximately one fourth to one third of his or her maximal physical work capacity (PWC_{max}). If the demands for a venture exceed prospective tolerance, PWC_{max} can be enhanced about 15% by a 3- to 6-month graduated conditioning program.

A conditioning program should include flexion and extension exercises during the warm-up, an active aerobic cardiovascular conditioning component, and a cool-down component. The aerobic component should last at least 20 minutes at a level about 50% of individual PWC_{max}. Some persons can learn to count the pulse corresponding to this level of activity. This provides a useful monitoring technique. Mouth breathing is a useful body signal for marking the intensity of activity. Consequently, if the subject keeps the intensity below that requiring mouth breathing, the aerobic activity should be in a range below 60% of the individual maximal capacity. This level of conditioning is helpful and reasonably safe for seniors, although not at a level of intensity sufficient for conditioning competitive athletes.

The American College of Sports Medicine has developed a position paper on exercise and physical activity for older adults that should be reviewed by the serious student of the subject.[1] This includes endurance training to help maintain and improve cardiovascular function, and strength training to help offset loss of muscle mass. Additional benefits from regular exercise include improved bone health, reduction of risk from osteoporosis, improved postural stability, and increased flexibility and range of motion. Psychologic benefits and alleviation of depressive symptoms may also occur.

MEDICAL EXAMINATION

By the time an individual qualifies for the designation "elder," that person has usually made some arrangements for medical care, examination, and advice. However, as an elder considers a venture into the wilderness, there is often confusion, or at least insecurity, over the prospect of developing some form of medical problem. A medical examination may be necessary.

Components of the Medical Examination

A survey of wilderness leaders served as the basis for developing specific components for medical examination for prospective participants in wilderness activities.[8,9]

There are five categories of characteristics included in the health examination:

1. *Personal characteristics*, which provide a profile of the subject regarding age; gender; education; occupation; status as volunteer or recruit; history of a recent or remote similar venture; use of tobacco, alcohol, drugs, or steroids; history of psychological or interpersonal problems especially during wilderness ventures; and history of athletics.

2. *Historical features*, such as illness, with particular emphasis on cardiovascular, pulmonary, musculoskeletal, and neurologic problems; problems associated with a previous venture; history of a successful similar venture; intolerance to altitude, heat, or cold; psychologic problems; accidents; and pertinent family history.

3. *Medical examination* to include examination of heart rate, blood pressure, precise cardiac examination (including auscultation), examination of peripheral pulses and carotid arteries, auscultation of the chest, abdominal palpitation with rectal examination, musculoskeletal system with range of motion of joints and back, and height and weight.

4. *Physiologic examination*, which is only rarely required, depends largely on the nature of the venture and may range from simple simulation of the planned activity to functional aerobic testing for $\dot{V}O_2$ max using a treadmill, cycle, or step ergometry. Functional testing with electrocardiographic monitoring is frequently used for diagnostic testing and for predicting cardiovascular response to exercise. Testing by running for speed or endurance and evaluation of dynamic strength and agility are rarely used but are interesting during skill assessment. Testing for hypoxic ventilatory response (HVR) may be primarily of research interest but nonetheless should be considered if precision is needed for elders going to high altitude.

5. *Psychologic interviews* are largely dependent on the skill and technique of the examiner but should attempt to uncover a history of previous difficulties with group interaction and team activities, or problems with physical and environmental stress or remote adventures.

In the survey of wilderness leaders, the best single predictor of a successful venture was found to be a history of a similar successful venture and the psychologic profile of the individual. The most important part of the medical examination before a wilderness venture was determined to be an in-depth interview by an examiner experienced not only in medical care but also in the nature of the venture. After the interview, appropriate medical, laboratory, radiographic, and physiologic studies may be performed.

TABLE 76-1. Components of Medical Examination for Various Classifications of Participants According to the Nature of the Venture

CLASSIFICATION OF CHARACTERISTICS OF PARTICIPANT	CLASSIFICATION OF WILDERNESS VENTURE			
	EXTREME PERFORMANCE	HIGH PERFORMANCE	RECREATIONAL	THERAPEUTIC
A. Demonstrated high performance	2,3,(5)	2,3,(5)	2	*
B. Healthy, vigorous	2,3,4,(5)	2,3,(5)	(2)	(2)
C. Healthy "deconditioned"	1,2,3,(4),(5)	2,3,(4),(5)	2,(4)	2,(3),(4)
D. Risk factors	1,2,3,(4),(5)	1,2,(3),(4),(5)	2,(3),(4),(5)	2,(3),(4),(5)
E. Illness	*	*	1,2,(3),(4),(5)	1,2,(3),(4),(5)

*Individualized assessment indicated.
Category of component features of medical examination (see text): *1*, personal characteristics; *2*, medical historical features; *3*, medical features; *4*, physiologic studies; *5*, psychologic features. All categories of component features should be considered in the examination of prospective participants, but features enclosed in parentheses are of prime importance.

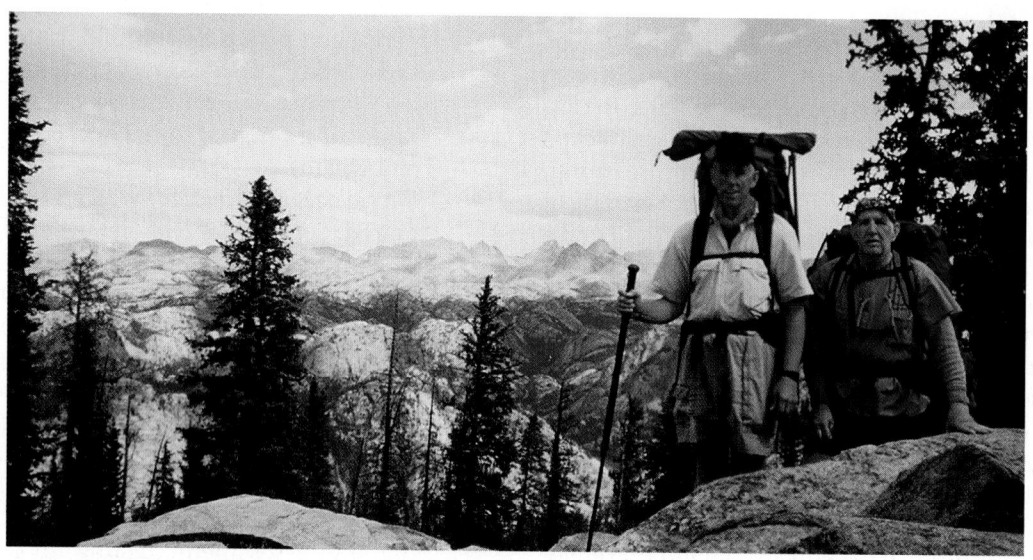

Figure 76-2 A pair of Gray Eagles. *(Courtesy John Duckworth, MD.)*

To assist in determining the content of a medical examination, Table 76-1 matches the individual with the venture and identifies the components of the medical examination that may be needed. Elders are included in their appropriate classification, according to performance characteristics derived from the five categories. Most commonly, they fit in categories D or E.

COUNSELING AND TEACHING ELDERS BEFORE WILDERNESS VENTURES: THE GRAY EAGLES

The drive, determination, and spirit of the individual who loves the wilderness are powerful. Aging seems only to sharpen this desire and to deepen its signifi-

cance. One focused observation of aging individuals in the wilderness was that of the "Gray Eagles," the brainchild of retired Memphis pathologist Dr. John Duckworth and retired Kraft Food executive Mr. John Johnson.[7] Formalized in 1987, the Gray Eagles began taking 10-day cross-country wilderness hiking trips into the mountains of the western United States (Figure 76-2). Their experiences have been invaluable in providing a unique opportunity to learn about groups of elders in the wilderness. Experience emphasizes the need for: (1) preselection based on experience, interviews, and medical history; (2) a stringent 6-month conditioning program with good boots, well "broken in" with 100 miles of use; (3) walking with a backpack, unless contraindicated, weighing one third of total body weight; (4) orientation meetings that include features of safety, review of risk, and recognition of clinical problems, such as the symptoms of hypothermia, hyperthermia, hypoxia, and fatigue; (5) the "three season" principle for packing clothes because of the prospects of weather change; and (6) orientation sessions with officials in the area to determine safety precautions unique to the region and to let the officials know of the presence of the Gray Eagles.

Using a detailed approach to preparation, the Gray Eagles have had very few medical problems. Of interest, however, is the observation that one successful year involving participation by an elderly person does not guarantee that the next year will be uneventful. With increasing age causing reduction of reserve, tolerance may change dramatically, and vascular symptoms may go from tolerable to intolerable with environmental stress.

The most potentially serious problems confronted by the Gray Eagles have been behavioral problems from organic brain syndrome not previously recognized, but precipitated by the environmental and physical stress of the venture.

EPILOGUE

Time is a peculiar dimension. It is difficult to define other than by changes that take place during its passage. Changes in anatomy, physiology, and function take place with time.

Seasons change from the promise of spring, to the full glory of summer, to a time of reflection in fall just before winter, the season of death.

Similarly, there is a time of day at dusk and sunset for reflection on the satisfaction of time well spent. The optimist sees sunset as sunrise in reverse.

Remember, the elderly still climb mountains: it's just that their definition of mountains has changed.[10]

REFERENCES

1. American College of Sports Medicine Position Stand, Exercise and physical activity for older adults, *Med Sci Sports Exerc* 30:992, 1998.
2. Baker AT, Martin GR: Molecular and biologic factors in aging: the origins, causes, and prevention of senescence. In Cassel CK et al, editors: *Geriatric medicine,* ed 3, New York, 1996, Springer.
3. Barry HC, Eathorne SW: Exercise and aging, *Med Clin North Am* 78:357, 1994.
4. Bowman WD: Problems of older people in the wilderness, *Syllabus,* Wilderness Medical Society Winter Meeting, 345-349, Feb 1997.
5. Cordell HK et al: The background and status of an interagency research effort: the Public Area Recreation Visitors Survey (PARVS). In Cordell BM, editor: *Proceedings, Southeastern Recreational Research Conference,* Asheville, NC, Athens, Georgia, 1986, Institute of Community and Area Development, University of Georgia.
6. Decentennial state population changes by age, *Statistical Bulletin* 73:30, 1992.
7. Erb BD: Elderly in the wilderness, the gray eagles, *Wilderness Medicine Letter* 12:8, 1995.
8. Erb BD: Medical selection of participants in wilderness ventures, *Syllabus,* Wilderness Medical Society Annual Meeting, p 489, Aug 1995.
9. Erb BD: Predictors of success in wilderness ventures: physical activity, the environment and fatigue, *Wilderness Medicine Letter* 7:8, 1990.
10. Erb BD: The elderly in the wilderness, *Wilderness Medicine Letter* 12:6, 1995.
11. Geographic profile of the aged, *Statistical Bulletin* 4:2, 1993.
12. Hackett P: New concepts of high altitude cerebral edema: acute mountain sickness, *J Wilderness Med* (in press).
13. Hayflick L: Why do we live so long? *Geriatrics* 43:77, 1988.
14. Honigman B et al: Acute mountain sickness in a general tourist population at moderate altitudes, *Ann Intern Med* 118:587, 1993.
15. Houston CS: Incidence of acute mountain sickness: a study of winter visitors to six Colorado resorts, *Am Alpine J* 27:162, 1985.
16. Jones BA: Decreasing polypharmacy in clients most at risk, *AACN Clinical Issues* 8:627, 1997.
17. Kaiser FE, Wilson M-MG, Morley JE: Menopause/female sexual function. In Cassel CK et al, editors: *Geriatric medicine,* ed 3, New York, 1996, Springer.
18. Kane RL, Ouslander JG, Abrass IB: *Essentials of clinical geriatrics,* ed 3, New York, 1994, McGraw-Hill.
19. Kronenberg RS, Drage CW: Attenuation of the ventilatory and heart rate responses to hypoxia and hypercapnia with aging in normal men, *J Clin Invest* 52:1812, 1973.
20. Law WR, Frost CD, Weld NJ: By how much does dietary salt reduction lower blood pressure. I. Analysis of observational data among populations, *BMJ* 312:811, 1991.
21. Leaf A: Every day is a gift when you are over 100, *Nat Geog* 143:93, 1973.
22. *Meet the Press,* National Broadcasting Company, Inc., 15 Nov 1998.
23. Monane M, Monane S, Semia T: Optimal medication use in elders: key to successful aging, *West J Med* 167:233, 1997.
24. Nash R: *Wilderness and the American mind,* ed 3, New Haven, Conn, 1982, Yale University Press.
25. OPCS, Social survey division: *Health survey for England,* 1993, HMSO, London, 1994.
26. Rennie D: Will mountain trekkers have heart attacks? *JAMA* 261:1045, 1989.
27. Smith EL (reported by Howley EH): Special considerations in developing exercise programs for the older adult. In *Behavioral health: a handbook of environmental enhancement and disease prevention,* New York, John Wiley and Sons.
28. Speroff L: Menopause and hormone replacement therapy, *Clin Geriatr Med* 9:33, 1993.
29. Straessen J, Amery A, Fagard R: Isolated systolic hypertension in the elderly, *J Hypertens* 8:393, 1990.
30. Strehler BL: Concepts and theories in aging. In Viidik A, editor: *Lectures on gerontology,* New York, 1982, Academic Press.
31. Thompson DW: *On growth and form, new edition,* Cambridge, UK, 1942, Cambridge University Press.

77 Medical Liability and Wilderness Medicine

Carolyn S. Langer

The following is an excerpt from the standard "fine print" found on the back of cruise passengers' tickets:

CARRIER NOT LIABLE FOR PASSENGER'S MEDICAL CARE

(a) Medical Services on Vessel. The Carrier does not undertake that a physician or medical personnel will be aboard the Vessel. If the Vessel does carry a physician or medical personnel, then they are independent contractors and work directly for the Passengers.

(b) Consent of Treatment. If, in the opinion of the Carrier, a Passenger in need of medical or surgical services is unable to request it, the Passenger hereby expressly consents to such treatment, if any, and to pay the cost thereof charged by the Vessel's physician or other physician or medical personnel designated by the Carrier who in doing so is acting on behalf of the Passenger.

(c) Treatment at Passenger's Risk. All medicines and all medical or surgical services furnished by the Vessel's physician, if any, or any other physician or medical personnel (all of whom are engaged by the Passenger as independent contractors) or ship's officers, employees or agents of the Carrier, shall be and are accepted by and at the Passenger's sole risk and expense, and the Carrier shall not be responsible for the quality, nature or consequence thereof.

(d) Passenger's Obligation to Report Medical Conditions. Before this Ticket is issued, the Passenger must report to the Carrier or its general agent, all pre-existing illness, disabilities or pregnancy and all other conditions for which the Passenger may require medical attention during the course of the Cruise. If any such condition arises after the Ticket is issued, the Passenger must report all such conditions to the Carrier, Purser or Vessel's Master or physician, if any, before boarding, or if the Passenger has boarded the Vessel, then before the Vessel leaves port. The Carrier, Vessel and the Vessel's physician, if any, shall have no liability in connection with any such condition.

(e) Lack of Obligation to Examine Passenger. Neither the Carrier, nor the Vessel's physician, if any, has any obligation to examine any Passenger for any purpose prior to boarding or sailing.

(f) Refusal of Passage. The Carrier reserves the right to refuse passage to a Passenger who has failed to give proper notice of any disability, illness, pregnancy or other condition requiring special care, attention or treatment or who in the Carrier's sole opinion is physically or mentally unfit for the Cruise. In such event, the Passenger is not entitled to any refund of fare.

From Levinson J, editor, Ger E, medical editor: *Safe passage questioned: medical care and saftey for the polar tourist,* Centreville, Md, 1998, Cornell Maritime Press.

In recent years, personal wealth, general interest, increased leisure time, and sophisticated marketing have led to expanded participation by the general public (with an aging population) in expeditions and cruises to remote environments, including wilderness areas. Such travel poses a higher risk of injury and illness (than does travel in urban areas) and often involves exposure to extreme weather conditions, limited access to medical personnel and supplies, and extended patient management due to scarce medical evacuation capabilities. What are the medical-legal ramifications for tour operators and trip physicians? Historically the probability of a lawsuit was low because participants were younger, more physically fit, and more experienced adventurers who tended to be greater risk takers with an awareness of and a willingness to assume these risks. However, the increased involvement of a less prepared and marginally aware general population in these wilderness pursuits has undoubtedly generated a concomitant increase in exposure to liability. To minimize this liability, tour operators and trip physicians must implement sound risk management strategies for medical clearance, education, and provision of medical services to trip participants.

TORT LAW AND THE DOCTRINE OF NEGLIGENCE

Case Study: Snakebite and Medical Malpractice

On August 11, a victim sustained a rattlesnake bite on the index and middle fingers of his left hand. Suction cups and a tourniquet were immediately applied, and the victim was transported to the hospital within 15 minutes. Another 15 minutes passed before Dr. A arrived. Dr. A proceeded to treat the patient by injecting antivenin into the base of the fingers bitten by the snake and into the left deltoid, despite an instruction sheet accompanying the antivenin that cautioned, "Do not inject serum into a finger or toe." Dr. A packed the patient's hand in ice and admitted him to the hospital. Two days later the patient was sent home with instructions to keep the hand in ice.

Eight days later the victim's two fingers, hand, and arm were edematous, discolored, and odorous from gangrene. Dr. B assumed care of the patient, applying a heating pad and injecting antibiotics. Nevertheless, on

September 9, the two fingers required amputation. Is Dr. A liable for medical malpractice?

In tort law, members of society owe a duty to others to act reasonably and in a way that will not hurt another person or his or her property. In the context of wilderness medicine, redress for a private civil wrong is typically sought under the negligence doctrine. To bring a cause of action under a negligence theory, the plaintiff (the party filing the claim) must establish the following four elements:

1. Duty: The defendant has a duty to use due care as a reasonably prudent person would under similar circumstances. For example, a plaintiff could argue that a trip physician owes the participants a duty to demonstrate the "knowledge, skill, and care customarily exercised by a reasonable and prudent physician under similar circumstances, given the prevailing state of medical knowledge and available resources."[3] To meet this duty, physicians must typically adhere to the standard of care prevailing within the medical community.

2. Breach of duty: Defendants breach their duty when they fail to conform to the duty of care or to act in accordance with norms or standards of practice. This breach may occur either through commission or omission of certain acts. For example, a physician may breach the duty of care by failing to diagnose or treat a condition (omission) or by improperly treating a patient (commission).

3. Causation: The plaintiff must further prove that the defendant's conduct was the direct, foreseeable, and proximate cause of the resulting injury. In other words, absent the defendant's conduct, the harm would not have occurred. Establishing causation is often the most problematic step for plaintiffs. For example, an injured traveler might allege that a trip leader or medical practitioner breached the duty of care by delaying medical evacuation, but the defendant could argue that the injury had already occurred and that any delay in evacuation neither caused nor aggravated the injury.

4. Damages: Finally the plaintiff must demonstrate damages, that is, harm to the individual's person, property, or interests for which the redress is customarily a monetary award. Awards may encompass special damages (e.g., out-of-pocket losses, medical expenses, lost earnings), general damages (pain and suffering), and punitive damages. Punitive damages are rare in the medical context because the plaintiff must prove that the defendant's conduct exceeded simple negligence and was grossly negligent, reckless, or malicious. Nonetheless, physicians should be aware that their insurance policies generally do not provide malpractice coverage for punitive damages.

Medical malpractice is a specific form of negligence occurring during the execution of a physician's professional or fiduciary duties. Medical malpractice can be defined as medical care that falls below the standard of care expected of a reasonably prudent physician under similar circumstances, resulting in foreseeable harm to the patient. In all negligence suits the plaintiff bears the burden of proof in establishing the requisite four elements under a "more probable than not" standard. In other words, the plaintiff must establish that there was a greater than 50% probability that the defendant's breach of duty caused the harm.

In the snakebite case presented earlier the first element is clearly demonstrated. Dr. A's actions established a physician-patient relationship and an acceptance of the duty to render care. Establishing the second and third elements is more problematic. The court held that Dr. A did not breach his duty. The court elaborated, "There are wide variations in accepted methods of treatment of rattlesnake bites. The method of treatment chosen and used by the defendant was an acceptable method of treatment." (This point is debatable, but in general there are frequently "medical experts" who will take a contrary position.) In other words, even though physicians must act with the level of skill and learning possessed by minimally qualified members of the profession, they are judged by reference to the beliefs of the school that they follow, provided that it is a recognized school of practice in the medical community.

The court further held that the plaintiff failed to establish causation. Expert testimony showed that "rattlesnake bites in extremities always present some chance of tissue destruction" and that the most probable cause of tissue death in the two distal phalanges was the rattlesnake venom. Thus Dr. A was found not liable.

Each state has its own body of statutory, regulatory, and case law (in addition to federal law). Thus, although this chapter presents general legal and risk management principles, physicians should always familiarize themselves with the laws and precedents in their own states before implementing policies and procedures related to wilderness or travel medicine.

LIABILITY CONCERNS IN WILDERNESS MEDICINE

The remainder of this chapter examines how the legal doctrines apply in the unique circumstances of wilderness medicine. Not surprisingly, increased participation of the general population in adventure travel has led to higher—and in many cases unrealistic—expectations on the part of the public. Some unseasoned travelers to remote destinations anticipate the same level of medical resources (including personnel, equipment, medications, and evacuation capabilities) to which they have access in their own large, urban tertiary care medical centers. It is therefore vital for tour operators and trip physicians to understand the duty and standard of care to which they must adhere and to educate trip participants regarding the risks of travel.

DUTY TO WARN AND EDUCATE TRIP PARTICIPANTS

Case Study: Duty to Warn

A middle-aged male traveler booked a tour to Bolivia through a travel agent. In the trip brochure the tour operator represented itself as an experienced and reputable company and stated that it researched all locations to which it arranged tours and "would care for participants from 'portal to portal.'"[6] In addition, the travel agent asked both the tour operator and local health agencies about health requirements and necessary precautions. During the trip, the traveler developed high altitude cerebral edema after flying from Chile (at sea level) to La Paz, Bolivia (elevation 3960 m [13,000 feet]), in less than 1 hour. He subsequently sued the travel agent and tour organizer for failure to warn him of the health risks associated with his travel.

In general there is no duty to warn of dangers that are as obvious to the participant as to the organizer. Obvious dangers might include possible seasickness or airsickness, substandard sanitation, and poor environmental conditions. Moreover, travel agents and tour operators have no duty to investigate potential vacation sites (not even those where conditions and terrain are dangerous) or lower standards of medical care in foreign countries. However, they do have a duty to warn travelers of known unreasonable risks or dangers, such as political turmoil and criminal attacks, that are foreseeable or likely to occur. Typically, to incur this duty to warn, the travel agent or tour operator must have actual or constructive notice of the hazardous condition arising from their knowledge of special circumstances (e.g., prior occurrences). In addition, travel agents and tour operators may contractually expand their duty to warn through representations made in brochures or other advertisements. In the case mentioned earlier, for example, the court recognized that tour organizers are not insurers of the safety of tourists with whom they contract and need not warn of obvious hazards. Nonetheless, in this case the travel organizer contractually expanded its obligation through its representations and brochures and created a reasonable expectation on the part of the tourist that it would research the risks of high altitude travel and warn him of accompanying dangers.

Even in the absence of liability, trip organizers and medical practitioners have incentive to prevent travel-associated injury or illness because they suffer financially and ethically when a tourist experiences physical or financial loss, fellow travelers are inconvenienced, or the reputation of the company or medical practice is potentially damaged. Sound risk management principles dictate that travel companies provide as much useful information as feasible to prevent adverse consequences. Companies lacking the wherewithal to research health hazards may benefit from the assistance of a medical adviser. Depending on the nature of the trip, some or all of the following information may be useful to participants:

1. Environmental conditions (e.g., climate, altitude, terrain)
2. Activity level (type, intensity, duration, and frequency of activity or exertion required)
3. Specific health hazards (e.g., tropical diseases, marine envenomation, frostbite, heat injuries)
4. General health information (e.g., safety of local food and water, local medical resources)
5. Known risks (e.g., political unrest, high crime areas)
6. Recommended immunizations

MEDICAL CLEARANCE OF TRIP PARTICIPANTS

Tour operators have no duty to medically screen trip participants. Travelers have a responsibility to exercise due caution for their own safety. Nonetheless, do tour operators have the right or an incentive to screen participants? Medical clearance of travelers may serve several beneficial purposes. It can function to educate participants about potential health hazards, thereby reducing their risk of harm. Medical screening affords the participant's private physician the opportunity to better manage the patient's care. It also may enable a tour operator to arrange accommodations in advance for participants with special needs. Moreover, medical clearance may reduce the tour operator's liability, costs, and inconvenience.

On the other hand, medical screening has certain disadvantages. Some authorities consider medical screening useless because a high-risk patient with a strong desire to go on a trip may ignore the inherent dangers and conceal any significant medical history (or shop around for a physician willing to grant the medical clearance). In addition, since the enactment of the Americans with Disabilities Act (ADA) of 1990, many tour operators fear discrimination suits for medically screening out disabled persons. However, with a proper understanding of the legal issues underlying medical clearance and the ADA, tour operators and physicians can safeguard the interests of all parties involved.

The Americans with Disabilities Act

Title III of the ADA prohibits all places of public accommodation and services operated by private entities from discriminating against the disabled. Furthermore, a public accommodation may not apply eligibility criteria that screen out an individual or any class of individuals with disabilities "unless such criteria can be shown to be necessary for the provision of the goods, services, facilities, advantages, or accommodations."[8] For example, "a cruise line could not apply eligibility criteria to potential passengers in a manner that would screen out individuals with disabilities unless the criteria are 'necessary.'"[9]

A public accommodation is not required to permit an individual to participate in services when the individual poses a direct threat to the health or safety of others. This determination that the participant poses a significant risk must be an individualized assessment using reasonable judgment based on current medical knowledge or the best available objective evidence. Although the "direct threat exception" to the ADA permits exclusion of participants only when they are a threat to others, the "safety exception" may justify excluding individuals when they pose a threat to themselves. The "safety exception" holds that a public accommodation may impose legitimate safety requirements that are necessary for safe operations. As an example, the regulations cite as a valid screening criterion the requirement for all participants in a recreational rafting expedition to meet a necessary level of swimming proficiency.

For screening criteria to be valid, however, they must be uniformly applied to all prospective participants, not merely to those with disabilities. Moreover, they must be based on actual risks, not on mere speculation, stereotypes, or generalizations about a person or class of persons with a particular disability. A tour organizer could not, for example, categorically exclude all persons with a history of angina from a high altitude trip but rather must afford individuals with documented, well-controlled angina an opportunity to establish their fitness and eligibility for the trip.

Even when screening criteria are valid and the prospective participant cannot meet those requirements, a public accommodation must make reasonable modifications in policies and practices or must accommodate the disabled individual unless such modifications would fundamentally alter the nature of the goods, services, or facilities offered. For example, a cruise line could be required (as a reasonable modification) to provide an individual who relies on a wheelchair for mobility with a stateroom on the same level as the restaurant. However, a mountain trek would not be required to transform to a bus tour to accommodate this same individual.

Medical Screening

To minimize the potential for discrimination claims, tour operators should provide physicians granting medical clearance as much information as possible regarding the physical demands of the trip. Tour organizers must provide detailed information concerning environmental conditions, specific health hazards, health and living conditions in the destination site, and availability of local medical resources. Companies should be as specific as possible in describing environmental conditions (e.g., altitude in feet, temperature in degrees). Trip organizers also must delineate the type, intensity, duration, and frequency of activity (e.g., bus tour, mild walking [1.6 to 3 km or 1 to 2 miles per day], vigorous hiking [specify distance and terrain], backpacking [specify weight of gear], trekking to remote areas [e.g., 24 hours from definitive medical care], climbing, swimming, canoeing, etc.).

The health care professional in turn must tailor the medical history and examination to the physical demands of the trip. The physician should become familiar with the patient's medical history, including any medications that could interact with the environment to which the patient is traveling. If applicable, the medical practitioner should advise the patient to bring extra medications or medical equipment (a spare pair of eyeglasses, extra hearing aid batteries, an anaphylaxis kit, etc.) in case complications or exacerbations occur. The physician also should inform the patient of applicable first aid procedures. The physician may need to inform the trip organizer of special needs or accommodations as well.

Because patients and their physicians may be hesitant to disclose confidential medical information to a travel company, medical clearance forms should emphasize functional abilities and limitations rather than diagnoses. If medical clearance forms request sufficiently detailed information about the prospective participant's medical fitness to meet the physical demands of the trip, travel companies frequently do not need to know about specific medical diagnoses. Companies that do request confidential medical information should disclose this information only to employees who have a need to know and should ensure that the company medical adviser or trip physician safeguards this information in a locked file. The company also may want to encourage high-risk patients to share medical information with trip leaders or bring along key medical records. Even though a company-employed medical adviser or private family physician makes determinations about medical fitness and medical clearance, the travel company bears the legal responsibility for excluding disabled participants or for failing to accommodate their needs.

PROFESSIONAL LIABILITY, MEDICAL MALPRACTICE, AND GOOD SAMARITAN LAWS

In addition to those complaints arising from a lack of proper health warnings, injured trip participants commonly base claims on the company's failure to provide adequate medical services and facilities and the negligent delivery of medical care. Historically, tour operators and cruise ships have had no obligation to ensure the health or safety of participants or to provide health care—particularly physicians' services—on trips. Trip organizers should nonetheless ascertain the appropriate standard of care for their particular circumstances by determining the medical resources that other companies have provided on similar expeditions to similar destinations. Companies generally have the duty to staff trips to remote locations with personnel who have "significant training to provide adequate first aid and medical care until evacuation can be arranged."[4] Typically these staff members are emergency medical technicians (EMTs) or laypersons with basic first aid training. Organizers of trips to locales with readily available medical care may have a lesser obligation to furnish staff trained in first aid. In the event of an adverse medical outcome, travel company employees are judged by a "reasonably prudent person" standard; that is, they have the duty to use reasonable care to furnish such aid and assistance as an ordinarily prudent person or trip leader would under similar circumstances.

Several professional medical organizations, such as the American College of Emergency Physicians and the Wilderness Medical Society, are currently seeking to define and establish standards of care for the provision of medical services on cruise ships and expeditions. In the meantime, many companies voluntarily staff physicians on their trips (and publicize that they have done so) for the comfort and convenience of the participants or to provide a competitive marketing advantage. Travel companies that advertise the presence of trip physicians and medical facilities in brochures, contracts, and other correspondence to participants or prospective participants contractually expand their obligation by creating an implied or express contract for the availability of certain medical services. At a minimum, it is expected that trip physicians will have the resources and capability to evaluate and manage emergencies and, when necessary, will arrange for more definitive care for the types of injuries and illnesses that might be reasonably anticipated on these types of trips.[1]

Who, if anyone, is liable when the physician commits medical malpractice? Is the physician protected by Good Samaritan laws? Although Good Samaritan laws vary from state to state, most of these laws generally hold physicians and other personnel free from liability when assisting in an emergency, provided their conduct was not grossly negligent (a higher threshold than simple negligence), wanton, or willful. Other provisions common to many Good Samaritan laws include the requirement to render care in an emergency or at the scene of an emergency, to act in good faith, to provide services gratuitously, and to have no preexisting

duty to the victim to respond or provide aid. For example, if a physician happens upon a stranger in need of emergent care while hiking up a mountain and provides medical care, his or her services would most likely fall within the purview of Good Samaritan laws.

On the other hand, does the physician acting as the "trip physician" lose his or her Good Samaritan protection? A typical custom in the adventure travel industry is to offer physicians generous discounts on trips in exchange for the provision of medical support for fellow participants. Many of these physicians are under the mistaken impression that they are covered by Good Samaritan laws in the event of a malpractice claim. The discounted fee, however, is the equivalent of compensation, and these physicians, along with those on straight salaries, would in all likelihood be considered independent contractors with a preexisting duty to render medical care to fellow participants.

This potential exposure to malpractice claims has two important risk management implications for expedition physicians. First, physicians must familiarize themselves with the medical issues that they are likely to encounter on their trips and must possess the knowledge and skills to diagnose and treat relevant medical disorders. A physician employed on a cruise to known endemic areas, for example, must be familiar with the diagnosis and treatment of tropical diseases. A physician with a mountain trekking group should be able to recognize the signs and symptoms of high altitude sickness and be proficient in the management of this condition. In determining the standard of care, a jury would expect the physician to anticipate foreseeable medical problems, assess the patient, and administer first aid measures as a reasonably prudent physician would under similar circumstances, taking into account the remote location, the extremes of environment, and the limited capability to transport medical equipment on the trip.

Physicians should not assume that their medical malpractice insurance policies cover claims arising out of medical services rendered on trips. Many insurance policies carry limitations on coverage for care delivered outside the scope of a physician's normal practice or beyond a certain geographic area. In these cases trip physicians should seek extended coverage through their own insurance policies or through the tour organizer.

The negligence of a physician generally will not be imputed under a theory of respondeat superior (master-servant relationship) to the tour organizer or carrier. Many courts have noted that the relationship between a trip member and a physician is not a traditional activity over which a cruise ship or tour organizer has control. Moreover, a shipping or travel company is not in the business of providing medical services to participants and does not possess the requisite expertise to supervise a physician brought along for the convenience of the participants. Nonetheless, once the carrier or tour organizer goes about hiring a physician, it owes a duty to participants to exercise reasonable care in the selection of a competent and qualified physician. To the extent that the company fails to discharge this duty, it may be subject to a cause of action for the negligent hiring of an incompetent physician. Therefore cruise lines and tour operators should ensure that trip physicians are proficient in general medical care, emergency treatment, and the medical management of diseases endemic to the destination site.

Furthermore, travel companies and cruise ships should brief trip physicians on available resources, host country medical facilities, and evacuation procedures. Finally, companies should conduct formal credentialing of prospective trip physicians, verifying medical school graduation, board certification, and state licensure and researching any history of disciplinary actions.

DUTY TO RESCUE AND ABANDONMENT DOCTRINE

A physician who is on an expedition to Alaska and approaching the summit of Denali happens upon a trekker with multiple fractures and hypothermia. Does the physician have an obligation to treat the victim or attempt a rescue?

Abandonment is the unilateral termination of the physician-patient relationship by the physician without adequate notice to the patient, despite the need for ongoing medical care. Generally a physician has no legal duty to provide care for or to rescue endangered strangers. "The law imposes no liability upon those who stand idly by and fail to rescue a stranger who is in danger."[5] Moreover, abandonment occurs only in the presence of an established physician-patient relationship. Thus the physician who refuses to enter into a physician-patient relationship and initiate treatment will not be held liable for abandonment.

Traditionally, once an individual initiated a rescue attempt, he or she could abandon rescue efforts at any time. "[The] motives in discontinuing the services are immaterial . . . [The rescuer] may without liability discontinue the services through mere caprice or because of personal dislike or enmity toward the [victim]."[7] However, if by giving aid the rescuer has put the victim in a worse position than before the attempt to aid, the rescuer may be liable. For example, the victim may have relied on the rescuer's efforts to his or her detriment, foregoing other opportunities to obtain assistance during the rescuer's intervention.

The best risk management tool is to assume that physicians who either implicitly or explicitly agree to treat patients create a duty to provide continuity of care. Given these circumstances, physicians can generally avoid liability for abandonment under the following conditions:

1. The physician and patient mutually consent to terminate the relationship.
2. The patient dismisses the physician.
3. The victim no longer requires care, recovers, or dies.
4. The physician dies or is disabled.
5. Further rescue efforts would place the rescuer's life in danger.
6. The physician gives the patient reasonable notice of his or her intent to withdraw from the care of the patient and, particularly in an emergency, continues to treat the patient until another qualified health care provider takes over the case.

Improper termination of the physician-patient relationship may lead to a cause of action for breach of contract or professional negligence, as well as for abandonment.

STANDING ORDERS AND MEDICAL KITS

There is tremendous variability in the medical expertise of trip leaders and participants and in the resources, including medical equipment and supplies, that accompany treks and trips into the wilderness. The delivery of medical care by nonphysicians represents one of the most problematic and controversial issues for trip organizers. Absent any representations to the contrary in travel brochures or other documents sent to participants, there is no implied or express contract to provide medical care to trip participants. Nonetheless, because of the nature of the business proprietor–customer relationship, trip leaders have some preexisting duties, namely, to exercise due care in the performance of their duties and in facilitating evacuations when feasible, as would be considered reasonable under the circumstances. In other words, if they have made no claims to the contrary, trip leaders and staff have no duty to render care beyond basic first aid services that an ordinary layperson could provide.

May a nonmedical trip leader or an EMT, paramedic, or other allied health care provider render medical services beyond the scope of his or her training or certification? One state board of registration in medicine defines the practice of medicine as[10]:

Conduct, the purpose or reasonably foreseeable effect of which is to encourage the reliance of another person upon an individual's knowledge or skill in the maintenance of human health by the prevention, alleviation, or cure of disease and involving or reasonably thought to involve an assumption of responsibility for the other person's physical or mental well being: diagnosis, treatment, use of instruments or other devices, or the prescription or administration of drugs for the relief of diseases or adverse physical or mental conditions.

A person who holds himself out to the public as a physician or surgeon, or with the initials M.D. or D.O. in connection with his name, and who also assumes responsibility for another person's physical or mental well being, is engaged in the practice of medicine. The practice of medicine does not mean conduct . . . engaged in by persons licensed by other boards of registration with authority to regulate such conduct; nor does it mean assistance rendered in emergency situations by persons other than licensees.

Most states require that an EMT or paramedic act under the supervision of a physician. Supervision usually entails direct observation, radio or telephone communication, or written guidelines, protocols, or standing orders (although usually with reasonable access to a physician who can respond to questions and provide requested guidance). These statutes were enacted under the assumption that physician consultation would be fairly accessible. Even with the advent of cellular telephones and telemedicine, however, many trekkers and travelers to remote regions cannot easily obtain physician consultation. In general, trip leaders and staff who practice beyond the scope of their education, training, and certification could be engaging in the unlawful practice of medicine.

Even in an emergency situation, it is unclear whether the Good Samaritan statutes protect trip leaders and staff. As previously discussed, travel companies and their trip leaders are to a certain extent compensated for safeguarding the safety and welfare of participants. Therefore it seems most likely that courts would use a reasonable care standard in determining the negligence of trip leaders. In other words, the court would determine how a reasonable trip leader with similar education, training, and certification would respond in similar circumstances, taking into account the emergent nature of the victim's illness or injury, the remoteness of their location, the scarcity of medical equipment, the limited means of evacuation, and the inaccessibility of definitive medical care.

On many expeditions and treks into the wilderness, medical kits stocked with prescription drugs, including controlled substances, are brought along. Again, failure of nonmedical trip leaders to provide these medications would not be considered negligence when doing so is in violation of the law, particularly when the trip organizer did not create the peril and provided adequate advance warnings to trip participants. If a nonphysician dispenses these drugs, it could very likely constitute the unlawful practice of medicine. Moreover, physicians who do not accompany the travelers but who nonetheless write the initial prescriptions to stock the medical kits expose themselves to lawsuits arising out of any malpractice on the part of the trip leader with regard to use of those medications. For example, a nonmedical trip leader might improperly diagnose and dispense medications or might overlook certain drug interactions. Additionally, physicians who write prescriptions to stock medical kits face the risk of being disciplined by their respective state boards of medicine for inappropriate prescribing practices.

This legal dogma of course is of little comfort to trip leaders who find themselves in emergency situations. In some instances trip leaders on overseas travel have been known to purchase or to recommend that participants purchase medications that would require a prescription in the United States but that are available over the counter in foreign countries. Although the purchase and use of these medications is legal on foreign soil, travelers should be cautioned about the potential lack of guarantees regarding the safety, quality, and efficacy of locally procured drugs. If the nonphysician trip leader chooses to dispense medications, whether originally stocked in the medical kit before departure from the United States or obtained abroad, a court would in all likelihood judge any adverse consequences in accordance with a "due care" standard. That is, a trip leader who dispensed medications with resultant harm to the patient would be expected to demonstrate the due care of a reasonably prudent person under similar circumstances, taking into account the emergent nature of the medical condition, the remoteness of the trip, the availability of definitive medical care, and so forth. To avoid these awkward situations, trip organizers should adhere to the following basic risk management principles:

1. Do not advertise medical capabilities and resources beyond the scope of expertise of trip staff members or those resources readily accessible in the country.
2. Emphasize the need for trip participants to bring along an adequate supply of their own prescription drugs, and even verify that they have done so.
3. Caution trip participants about the lack of safeguards concerning the safety, quality, and efficacy of medications obtained overseas.

If trip organizers choose to equip staff members with medical kits, one expert in wilderness medicine recommends that the contents of the kit be based on the following factors[2]:

- The environmental extremes encountered during the trip
- Endemic diseases
- The medical expertise of the medical officer
- The medical expertise of the expedition members
- The number of people on the trip
- The responsibility for local health care
- The length of the trip
- The distance from definitive medical care
- The availability of rescue (i.e., helicopter)

MEDICAL RECORD KEEPING IN WILDERNESS MEDICINE

Good record keeping is of paramount importance in the practice of wilderness medicine. The medical record is both a health care document and a legal document. Although storage space and the portability of medical records on trips to remote locations are often limited, trip physicians should nonetheless strive to be as thorough as possible in documenting medical care. The medical record functions as a complete, written, and chronological record of a patient's medical history, condition, and treatment. In medical malpractice claims, which are frequently litigated years after the alleged occurrence, these records may be the only written source from which the sequence of events and subsequent treatment can be reconstructed. Moreover, memories fade and witnesses become less available over time. Therefore courts tend to give tremendous weight to the written record and will often assume that documented events occurred and undocumented events did not occur, particularly when the oral testimonies of the litigants conflict.

Although the length and content of entries will vary with the specific circumstances, notes should at a minimum include the patient's chief complaint, the results of the physical examination (including normal findings), an assessment, and a treatment plan. The key point to remember in the creation of medical records is that they may be used to prove or disprove that the medical practitioner adhered to the appropriate standard of care. Therefore physicians should record sufficient details to reflect their thought processes and to justify the care provided under the circumstances. Moreover, physicians should document events chronologically and as soon as feasible after the delivery of medical care. Once notes have been entered into the chart or record, the medical practitioner should never alter or write over the original notes. Pages should not be removed or inserted. If corrections are necessary, the physician should place a single line through the error,

enter the correction, and initial and date the correction. Addenda should be placed after the last entry in the chart. Of course, notes should always be legible, signed, and dated by the health care provider making the entry. Upon completion of the trip, the company should treat these medical records as confidential information and should place them in locked medical files, granting access to designated personnel (company medical advisers or others with a need to know) only. Some states have explicit laws or regulations that dictate the minimum period for retention of medical records. In the absence of such laws, travel companies and cruise lines should store medical records for the period of time corresponding to the statute of limitations for tort claims in their states, which is usually a couple of years.

CONCLUSION

The services of physicians on cruises and expeditions can be invaluable to the safety and welfare of participants. The expanded participation of higher risk individuals on trips to more remote regions of the world increases the liability exposure of health care providers. Legal issues, particularly causation, become more complex when medicine is practiced in these unconventional settings. By following the risk management principles outlined in this chapter, physicians can continue to provide effective care while minimizing their liability.

REFERENCES

1. Backer H: *Wilderness Med Lett* 6:10, 1989.
2. Donner H: *Wilderness Med Lett* 13:8, 1996.
3. Flamm MB: Health care provider as a defendant. In American College of Legal Medicine: *Legal medicine*, ed 3, St Louis, 1995, Mosby.
4. Herr RD: The climb physician: an endangered species? *J Wilderness Med* 1:144, 1990.
5. *Miller v Arnal Corp.*, 632 P.2d 990 (Ariz. App. 1981).
6. *Philippe v Lloyd's Aero Boliviano*, 589 So. 2d 536, 540 (La. App. 1992).
7. *Restatement (Second) of Torts* §323.
8. 28 *Code of Federal Regulations* 36.301.
9. 28 *Code of Federal Regulations* 36, App. B.
10. 243 *Code of Massachusetts Regulations* 2.01.

78 Ethics of Wilderness Medicine

Kenneth V. Iserson

Ethics is the application of rules and principles to guide human action. Bioethics is the area of ethics that applies specifically to health care providers and biomedical researchers. It involves the encounter between the patient and the health care provider, biomedical research, and health care policy. Wilderness medicine, however, is not directly comparable to either the medicine delivered in health care facilities or even the care delivered by urban emergency medical services. Wilderness medicine is unique, and its special attributes provide unique ethical problems (Table 78-1). For example, a hospital's working environment is rarely a factor considered by the hospital-based practitioner in the determination of what medical care to deliver, but the working environment is of major concern in the wilderness. Similarly, whereas patients are usually known to the hospital practitioner and arrive requesting care, neither condition is true in the wilderness setting. Even more striking are the differences between the hospital and the wilderness setting with regard to equipment availability, personnel training, the need for evacuation or rescue, and the provision for the security of those involved. All these differences can lead to unique ethical dilemmas.

This chapter first provides an overview of ethical values in general and the values applied to bioethics. It then describes and provides a model for bioethics decision making. Next is an adaptation of the model for the bioethics of wilderness medicine, which includes the ethics of wilderness health care providers, researchers, and in some cases, makers of health care policy. Finally, unique dilemmas in wilderness medicine are discussed.

APPLICATION OF RULES, PRINCIPLES, AND ACTION GUIDES TO HUMAN ACTIVITIES

Individuals' values, which are acquired throughout life from many sources, develop into their ethical action guides. In everyday situations, some individuals may be unaware that these values are guiding their actions. However, when facing situations that are rarely encountered, often termed *ethical dilemmas*, people may question how they should apply their values to solve practical problems. These situations may often develop in wilderness medicine, since the settings often encompasses scenarios and practitioners who must demonstrate expertise outside the usual scope of their medical specialties.

Both patients' and clinicians' values control patient-clinician encounters. When patients express their values, clinicians can get an impression of the patients' views about necessary treatment, desired quality of life, and other complex attitudes that control the willingness to seek and accept medical care. Whether these expressions are deemed valid is based on the clinicians' "bedside" determination of patients' decision-making capacity. The clinicians' own values, both personal and professional, are also part of the relationship and sometimes conflict with the patients' values.

Ethical discussions often revolve around applying ethical rules in a consistent manner or in a way that could be applied by all practitioners in the same situation *(universalizability)*. Ethical decisions derived from accepted principles, rules, or values should be applied uniformly (consistently) across all scenarios. If an accepted rule is that patients with decision-making capacity may make their own decisions about health care, this rule should be applied to all situations, not just when it is convenient for the health care provider. Likewise, if the rule is truly ethical, all health care providers, not just by a privileged or unique group, must be able to apply it to practice.

Sources of Values

The basic elements of any ethical discussion are personal values. Values are the guideposts used to structure an individual's actions in life. They signify what a person's duties and responsibilities are, what is important to the person, and how the person interacts with others. Thomas Aquinas said that the three vital things for each person are "to know what he ought to believe; to know what he ought to desire; and to know what he ought to do."[1]

Personal values derive from many sources: family, society, school, religion, the media, and professional training and related interactions. Family and religion generally guide the development of values in the formative years. For nearly everyone, these values form the bedrock on which his or her life is structured. Emphasizing the importance of early childhood learning is the maxim, "If you control a child's life until the age of 6 years, he is yours forever." Additional significant influences are the media, schooling, and society. In this electronic age, the media begin to influence an individual's values early in life. Secular education broadens a

TABLE 78-1. Differences Among Hospital Practice, Emergency Medical Services, and Wilderness Medicine

	HOSPITAL PRACTICE	EMERGENCY MEDICAL SERVICES	WILDERNESS MEDICINE*
Environment	Controlled, known, static	Partly controlled, partly known, changeable	Uncontrolled, partly known, changeable
Patient	Known, requests care	Unknown, sometimes requests care	Unknown, sometimes requests care
Equipment	Sophisticated	Adequate	Rudimentary
Security	Safe	Usually safe	Questionable
Personnel	Highly educated, definitive care	Highly educated, basic care	Variable education, basic care
Evacuation	Rare	Built into system	Major concern
Rescue	No	Rare	Common

*Includes search and rescue.

child's experiences and values beyond the small world of the home. Finally, societal pressures continue to influence most individuals' value systems throughout life. Taken as a whole, different individuals' values derived from these multiple sources may conflict, leading to disagreements over which action to take when ethical dilemmas arise.

Professional schooling and interactions often further refine how a person's previously learned values are applied. For example, one reason that medical students take anatomy courses is to destroy an ingrained cultural value against mutilating the dead. This allows them to accept and acquire the values of beneficial mutilation (surgery), handling the dead (resuscitations, pathology, transplants), and invading another's body (every invasive medical procedure).[11] In addition, when exposed to clinical practice, medical students, nurses, medics, and other health care providers learn to adopt the values of their preceptors. In any residency program the majority of trainees behave remarkably like the faculty. Trainees learn intrinsic professional values.

Values in Modern Biomedical Ethics

Another category of values, sometimes referred to as the *Georgetown bioethics catechism,* has emerged as an ideal for modern medicine, especially in the United States. These values include autonomy, beneficence, nonmaleficence, and distributive justice.

For the past 2 decades in the United States, the overriding professional and societal bioethical value has been a patient's autonomy. *Autonomy* recognizes an adult's right to accept or reject recommendations for his or her personal medical care (even to the extent of refusing all care) in the presence of appropriate decision-making capacity (see Decision-Making Capacity and Consent). Current bioethical opinion demands that clinicians respect patient autonomy. This is the counterweight to the long-practiced paternalism

(or parentalism) of the medical profession, wherein what was "good" for the patient was determined solely by the physician. Coupled with paternalism is coercion, the threat or use of violence to influence behavior or choice. The august figure in white (or in a medic's or search-and-rescue uniform) who implies that there will be dire consequences if medical recommendations are not followed remains a potent force against patient autonomy.

At the patient's bedside, *beneficence,* the act of doing good, and *confidentiality,* the holding of information in confidence, have been long-held and nearly universal tenets of the medical profession. Likewise, *personal integrity,* the adherence to one's own moral and professional standards, is basic to thinking and acting ethically. The basic tenet taught to all medical students is *nonmaleficence,* or "First, do no harm." This credo, often stated in the Latin form, *"Primum non nocere,"* derives from the historical knowledge that patients' encounters with physicians can be harmful as well as helpful. It recognizes every physician's fallibility.

The concept of *comparative* or *distributive justice* suggests that comparable individuals and groups in society should share equitably in the benefits and burdens of that society. Many society-wide decisions about the allocation of limited health care resources are based on this principle. Yet it is a fallacy to extrapolate from this valid principle to the idea that simply because a need to limit health care resource expenditures exists, individual clinicians can arbitrarily limit or terminate care on a case-by-case basis for individual patients.[18]

Decision-Making Capacity and Consent

A significant concern in the wilderness setting is whether patients have decision-making capacity, thus retaining their autonomy to make reasonable health care decisions. Many ethical dilemmas in emergency medical care revolve around ascertaining a patient's decision-making capacity, often linked with consent to

---

Box 78-1 COMPONENTS OF DECISION-MAKING CAPACITY

Knowledge of the options
Awareness of the consequences of each option
Appreciation of personal costs and benefits of options
    in relation to relatively stable values and preferences

Modified from Buchanan AE: The question of competence. In Iserson KV et al, editors: *Ethics in emergency medicine,* ed 2, Tucson, Ariz, 1995, Galen Press.

(or more often refusal of) a medical procedure. Since a basic canon of both ethics and law, as stated by Justice Cardozo,[23] is, "Every human being of adult years and sound mind has a right to determine what shall be done with his own body," these decisions about what action to take can often be made clearer by understanding what is meant by *decision-making capacity* and how it relates to consent. (Note that the term *competent* is often used, when *capacity* is really what is meant. *Competent,* meaning "possessing the requisite natural or legal qualifications," is a legal term and can be determined only by the court.[21])

Capacity refers to a patient's decision-making ability as determined by clinicians. Capacity is always decision-specific rather than global. Although an inebriated person, for example, may have the capacity to refuse to have stitches put into a small laceration, especially with evidence that he has previously refused similar treatments without remorse, the same individual may not have the capacity either to accept an elective operation of any sort or to refuse an emergency lifesaving procedure or operation. To have adequate decision-making capacity in any particular circumstance, a person must understand the available options and the consequences of acting on the various options and be able to compare any option he or she chooses against the costs and benefits related to a relatively stable framework of personal values and priorities[3,4] (see Box 78-1). This last requirement is the most difficult to understand and requires a subjective interpretation. The easiest way to assess it is to ask why an individual made such a decision. Disagreement with the physician's recommendation is *not* in itself grounds for determining whether a person is incapable of making his or her own decisions. In fact, even the refusal of lifesaving medical care may not prove the person incapable of making valid decisions, if it is made on the basis of firmly held religious beliefs, as in the case of a Jehovah's Witness refusing a blood transfusion.

A person must be permitted to consent to or refuse any medical intervention (implicitly or explicitly) if he or she has decision-making capacity for that decision and if the clinician respects the patient's autonomy. Three general types of consent exist: presumed, implied, and informed. *Presumed consent,* sometimes called *emergency consent,* covers the necessary lifesaving procedures that any reasonable person would wish to have if lacking decision-making capacity; controlling hemorrhage and securing an airway in an unconscious victim of a fall are common examples. *Implied consent* is when a person with decision-making capacity cooperates with a procedure, such as holding out an arm to donate blood or to allow initiation of an intravenous line. *Informed consent* is when a person who retains decision-making capacity is given all the pertinent facts regarding the risks and benefits of a particular procedure, understands them, and voluntarily agrees to undergo the procedure.[9]

Questions applying to consent in the wilderness setting can be difficult. Does the victim have the capacity to understand the situation? Will decision-making capacity be questioned only if a person refuses "good" medical care? Also, unresolved even in standard medical practice, what procedures require informed, as distinct from implied, consent? The requirement to obtain informed consent varies in practice and law from area to area. This variation stems from differing local practice standards and state law and disparities in physician training. Determining decision-making capacity and providing an opportunity for a victim to consent to a procedure when appropriate are crucial to respecting a patient's autonomy.

Security: Another Value Applicable to Wilderness Medicine

Given the unique setting of wilderness medicine, the value of security must also be applied. *Security* (safety) signifies a measure of responsibility toward oneself, one's companions, and the patient. This responsibility is to avoid risking the wilderness team's safety from the environment, from victims, and from their own poor judgment. This is a concept far removed from normal medical practice. However, this value is of paramount importance in wilderness medicine. Security is the responsibility of any wilderness medical provider, even if he or she is not officially designated a provider but must take over in a medical crisis on the basis of special knowledge or skills. Decisions about rescue, evacuation, stopping of group travel, or even attempts to perform certain medical interventions must include security considerations.

Security is wilderness medicine's controlling value in most circumstances. Concerns about safety are applied in the following order: oneself, other team members, and then the patient. Ethical theory supports this hierarchy. Beneficence by medical personnel does *not* imply a need to endanger oneself. Indeed, if medical skills are to be useful, medical personnel must be able to render care. In addition, inherent in any leadership position is a responsibility to protect one's team. Therefore the team members' safety is the second responsibility. Finally, the patient's security should be ensured but never at the expense of the medical team's safety. This is to say that in unknown or unknowable circumstances, the medical leader may have to weigh potential risks vs. benefits. All risks must be considered in these "calculations," since otherwise, these concerns are often ignored. An example is the case in which a badly injured trekker may survive if evacuated by aeromedical transport. The helicopter team is willing to attempt a pickup, if requested. The wilderness medical care provider must determine whether local conditions are sufficiently safe, balanced against the chance of benefit to the patient, to justify the request.

A unique ethical problem that arises in wilderness settings—and has often led to disasters—is for the team, especially the nonmedical team leader, to ignore or override the medical person's decision. Individual team members have been harmed and multiple team members lost, often because of factors other than team members' safety and well-being.[16,22]

In the language of ethics, utilitarian thinking plays a dominant role in wilderness ethics. Utilitarianism is the philosophy that promotes the greatest good (or happiness) for the greatest number of individuals. In wilderness medicine, it promotes the well-being of the many over the well-being of the individual. This can be defended by simply recognizing the unique aspects of wilderness medical practice, such as the uncontrolled environment, unfamiliarity with the patient, rudimentary equipment, and changeable situations—all contributing to safety concerns. Heeding the value of security is especially important because the majority of people who are in the wilderness have risk-taking personalities, leading them to downplay security in favor of adventure.

Ethical Dilemmas

Health care professionals commonly apply their values without much deliberation. They act instinctively based on their prior behavior and training. Values are constantly (although not necessarily consistently) applied to everyday decisions. Of course, most decisions are not ethical decisions. Ethical dilemmas arise with conflict between two seemingly equivalent values that are represented by different and mutually exclusive possible actions. A graphic depiction of this situation is the practitioner between a rock and a hard place. The practitioner has a profound decision to make. That is where ethical decision making comes into play.

An example of a bioethical dilemma in wilderness medicine may help illustrate ethical decision making. A distress call has been received from anxious relatives or by radio from a plane flying over a wilderness area.

The victim is in a hazardous area (such as on an active volcano) or more commonly, is caught in terrible weather (snow or a thunderstorm). The clinician directing a search-and-rescue team must decide how to respond to the call in a setting that may put the team in danger. The standard bioethical value of beneficence directly competes with the wilderness bioethical value of security. Each has a strong pull on the decision maker, with each value providing good arguments for sending or not sending the rescue team. Although the value of security may often be considered paramount in the wilderness setting, the emotional and altruistic pulls of beneficence make this a difficult choice. Considering this case, a word should first be said about rights and duties in relation to health care.

Although the word *rights* is glibly used in many situations in society, a personal right is present only if another person or society as a whole has an identifiable *duty* to the individual. For example, if all U.S. citizens had a right to health care, the government would have the duty to provide this care. Health care providers would have a corresponding duty to deliver this care. However, except in limited circumstances, such as emergency departments and prisons, no such legal right currently exists. Morally and practically, citizens do not have the right to *health,* and how much health care people are owed is unresolved.[17] Correspondingly, no health care practitioner has a duty to provide all the health care people desire. Practitioners do, however, have a duty to provide security, when possible, for those they direct in wilderness settings. This may provide part of the answer for this case; yet other factors may be involved.

Since the ethical dilemma arises when two or more seemingly "correct" actions appear to have equal benefits, the choice of actions should be examined first. How are these proposed "correct" actions determined in the first place? After that, which of these actions is the more ethically acceptable?

Solving the Bioethical Dilemma

Deciding on an Action in the Standard Setting. Jonsen et al[15] have suggested four groups of factors to consider when determining a course of action in the face of a bioethical dilemma in the standard clinical paradigm. These include the medical indications for the action, the patient's (or surrogate's) preferences, consideration of the quality of life, and other contextual factors. These have been seen as an "ethical square," with the top two boxes weighing more heavily (Figure 78-1).

In a broad sense, *patient wishes* equate to *patient autonomy.* In a growing number of instances, however, especially at the end of life, surrogate decision makers, rather than the patient, may exercise this autonomy. This may also be true in the wilderness setting, albeit with less legal backing. Many critically ill patients in

MEDICAL INDICATION	**PATIENT WISHES**
1. What is the patient's medical problem? Prognosis? 2. Is the problem acute? Chronic? Critical? Emergent? Reversible? 3. What are the goals of treatment? 4. What are the probabilities of treatment success? 5. What are the plans in case of therapeutic failure? 6. In sum, how can this patient be benefited by medical interventions, and how can harm be avoided?	1. What has the patient expressed about treatment preferences? 2. Has the patient been informed of benefits and risks, understood, and given consent? 3. Does the patient have decision-making capacity? What is the evidence of incapacity? 4. Has the patient expressed prior preferences, e.g., advance directives? 5. If the patient is incapacitated, who is the appropriate surrogate? Is the surrogate using appropriate standards? 6. Is the patient unwilling or unable to cooperate with medical treatment? If so, why? 7. In sum, is the patient's right to choose being respected to the best extent possible?
QUALITY OF LIFE	**CONTEXTUAL FEATURES**
1. What are the prospects, with or without treatment, for a return to patients normal life? 2. Are there biases that might prejudice the provider's evaluation of the patient's quality of life? 3. What physical, mental, and social deficits is patient likely to experience if treatment succeeds? 4. Is the patient's present or future condition such that he or she might judge continued life undesirable?	1. SAFETY ISSUES. (In wilderness medicine, these are often the most important considerations.) 2. Are there family issues that might influence treatment decisions? 3. Are there provider (SAR or trip member) issues that might influence treatment decisions? 4. Are there financial and economic factors? (evacuation/rescue costs) 5. Are there problems of allocations of resources? 6. What are legal implications of treatment decisions? 7. Any provider, organization-related, or institutional conflicts of interest?

Figure 78-1 The ethical square. (*Modified from Jonsen AR, Siegler M, Winslade WJ: Clinical ethics, ed 4, New York, 1998, McGraw-Hill.*)

health care facilities have an advance directive (durable power of attorney for health care) naming a surrogate to make health care decisions if they lack decision-making capacity. Finding such advance directives in the wilderness setting would be rare and in emergency situations, may not be valid, especially if the message is in an unusual form, such as a tattoo or MedicAlert jewelry.[8,14] Most people do not have advance directives. Those that do carry them do so only if they believe themselves to be terminally ill. Wilderness patients rarely belong to that group. More frequently, though, people without terminal illnesses wear nonstandard advance directives. Experience has shown that these cannot be relied on to reflect a person's current wishes (e.g., tattoos) or can easily be misinterpreted (e.g., do-not-resuscitate jewelry).[12,14] Furthermore, it is not the wilderness practitioner's job to interpret either nonstandard legal or quasilegal documents that are not part of his or her training. Standard forms, such as area- or state-wide prehospital do-not-resuscitate forms or advance directives, if present, should be followed. Many of these, however, are specifically not applicable after trauma.[9,10]

If a person lacks decision-making capacity, a spouse, close friend, or medical care provider makes critical decisions for the patient, acting in his or her "best interest." Parents normally act as decision makers for minor chil-

dren. Rarely, a court-appointed guardian has been named to replace parents. A child may also be an "emancipated minor," meaning that he or she lives alone and is self-supporting. Two key issues arise in children's medical care. First, children should not be denied emergency care simply because no permission is available. In these cases, *emergency* is defined broadly. Anything that causes pain or that may increase the child's morbidity or mortality should be treated. In wilderness situations, reasonable efforts to get parental consent usually do not apply if they are not already on the scene. They may have given blanket consent to treat their child, but that is not required if an emergency exists. Second, if the child is old enough to understand the situation and cooperate, it is both ethically important and good medical practice to have him or her assent to the proposed treatment. The assent is the agreement but does not constitute legal permission, since the child is under age.[9]

Medical indications are often more straightforward in the wilderness setting than they are in standard health care. In the wilderness, treatment is basic, injuries and illnesses are generally acute, and intervention is normally life preserving rather than death prolonging. Standard clinical algorithms are used by the clinicians for their appropriate level of training and expertise. In remote areas, of course, questions may arise about

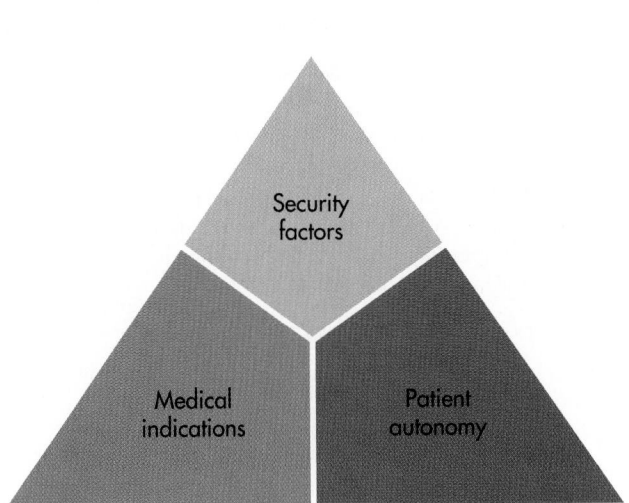

Figure 78-2   *Wilderness medicine's ethical triangle.*

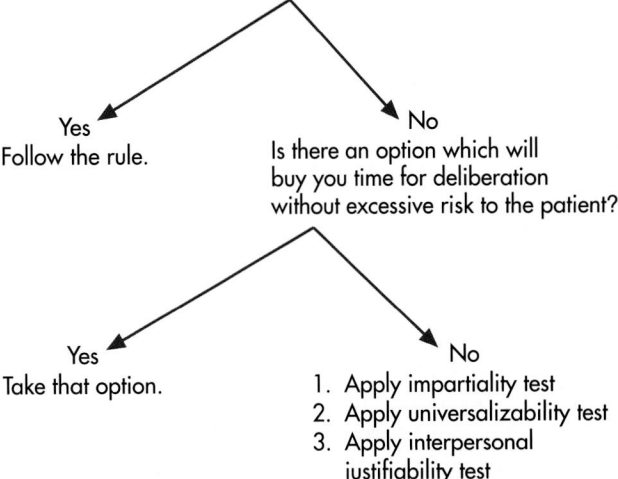

Figure 78-3   A rapid approach to emergency ethical problems. *(Modified from Iserson KV: An approach to ethical problems in emergency medicine. In Iserson KV et al, editors: Ethics in emergency medicine, ed 2, Tucson, Ariz, 1995, Galen Press.)*

whether the ophthalmologist should attempt to reduce a hip dislocation or whether the nurse should attempt to establish a surgical airway. These dilemmas should, when feasible, be decided with input from the patient or surrogate. As a matter of proper planning, behavior in critical scenarios must be decided in advance. Normally, however, medical indications are clear.

Bioethicists normally feel most comfortable helping resolve cases using only the medical indications and patient (or surrogate) wishes, which are all above the double line in Figure 78-1. When these factors are ambiguous, however, two other sets of factors must be considered: contextual factors and quality of life. In the wilderness setting, the primary contextual factor is safety. This may overshadow all other considerations involved in a victim's treatment. Other contextual factors include everything from financial implications of various treatments to the effect of various options on other trip members. In the standard medical situation, this is admittedly a fuzzy area. Related to these, and even more nebulous, are quality-of-life factors. These relate to the nature of a person's current and presumed future existence as viewed by others. If a person has decision-making capacity, his or her own view of life is comfortably built into personal autonomy. In the wilderness setting, time and circumstances usually do not allow clinicians to make quality-of-life judgments.

Deciding on an Action in the Wilderness. The importance of security factors in the wilderness setting leads to the altered diagram of decision making for ethical problems in wilderness medicine (Figure 78-2). This includes three groups of factors to consider when deciding on a course of action in the wilderness setting: patient autonomy, security, and medical indications.

Within this decision model, the security factors must be given the most weight.

Security factors include the safety of the medical and rescue personnel and victim, proposed procedures, and the evacuation method. As mentioned previously, the security of the medical team is a valid consideration because of the inherent risk-taking nature of people in the wilderness. In recent legal actions pertaining to wilderness injuries, the law has recognized a "doctrine of reasonable implied assumption of risk." This implied risk is also part of an acceptable concept of wilderness triage. Wilderness triage takes place when the same injuries or illnesses that would cause minimal morbidity in a medically sophisticated environment inevitably cause death if they occur in the wilderness. A fractured femur in the lone wilderness traveler or an abdominal gunshot wound in a remote area is often a virtual death sentence. This is a risk that wilderness adventurers take, although not always with a clear understanding of the enormity of the risk.

Both standard bioethics and wilderness medical ethics often involve difficult situations with no "correct" answer. Usually, more than two possible actions exist. This is the wilderness ethical and standard bioethical dilemma. What should the practitioner do?

Bioethical Decision-Making Process[13]

Using an Algorithm as a Guide for a Decision. In bioethics, although disagreements may arise regarding the optimal course of action using a specific set of values, general agreement often exists as to what constitutes ethically wrong actions. The method of ethical case analysis described in Figure 78-3 is designed to provide the emergency practitioner with prompt assistance in selecting an ethically correct, although not necessarily a theoretically "best," course of action.[12] This method applies equally well in both the wilderness setting and the normal hospital setting.

The first step in using the algorithm in Figure 78-3 is to use a known precedent. This is the simplest solution to an ethical dilemma but requires planning in advance, including reading and thinking about ethical problems. Many physicians and other health care professionals are not prepared to do this. Just as with any emergency procedure, wilderness medicine physicians and health care professionals should be prepared with a course of action for the most common ethical dilemmas likely to occur in the wilderness setting.

With no precedent, the second step is to "buy time." What action is not harmful to the patient that provides time for the consultation or information gathering needed to refine the action plan? In a wilderness medical setting, this might mean placing a person's arm in a sling for comfort while deciding whether an inexperienced provider should attempt to reduce a dislocation or fracture.

With no precedent on which to rely and no way to "buy time," the health care professional must select a possible course of action and test it for ethical viability. The impartiality test, universalizability test, and interpersonal justifiability test are drawn from three different philosophical theories. First, the impartiality test is applied. The practitioner asks whether he or she would have this action performed if in the patient's place. In essence, this is a form of the Golden Rule, "Do unto others as you would have done unto you." According to John Stuart Mill,[20] this espouses "the complete spirit of the ethics of utility." Second, the universalizability test asks if the health care professional would feel comfortable having all practitioners perform this action in all relevantly similar circumstances. This generalizes the action and asks whether developing a universal rule for the contemplated behavior is reasonable. This is merely a restatement of Kant's categorical imperative ("Act as if the maxim of thy act were to become by thy will a universal law of nature."). Finally, the interpersonal justifiability test asks if the practitioner can supply good reasons to others for his or her action. Will peers, superiors, or the public be satisfied with the action taken and reasons for it? This test uses David Gauthier's basic theory of consensus values as a final screen for a proposed action.[6] If all three tests can be answered in the affirmative, the health care professional can have reasonable assurance that the proposed action falls within the scope of morally acceptable actions. If, however, the proposed action fails any of these tests, the algorithm must be applied to another proposed action.

Box 78-2 ETHICAL DILEMMAS IN WILDERNESS CARE

STANDARD OF CARE DILEMMAS

Limited resources: The standard of care differs. What should be brought into the field? How are resources distributed?

Cultural: Are Western standards of care and attitudes appropriate when treating locals in a foreign country?

Nontrained personnel: How much authority is delegated to nontrained personnel?

PRIORITY IN CARE DILEMMAS

Triage choices: Who should be rescued first? (Those most injured or ill? Injured or ill rescuers? Those with the best chance of survival? Women and children? Those with important information, such as scientists who have collected data? Those who do not volunteer to stay behind?)

Issues of survival

Issues of direct life-threatening situations for the provider or providers

Motorized vehicle restrictions and environmental protection in wilderness areas

DECISION-MAKING DILEMMAS

Unavailability of a surrogate or a family member
Euthanasia
Lack of ethics consultation
Advance directives
No-rescue areas

ETHICAL DILEMMAS IN WILDERNESS MEDICINE

With its unique setting and mode of practice, wilderness medicine provides practitioners with ethical dilemmas that are rarely seen by most other providers. These dilemmas can be grouped into three categories: standards of care, priority in care, and the decision-making process (Box 78-2). As might be expected, some of the issues in each group deal with provider-patient dilemmas, whereas others have more to do with group or governmental policies. Also, the unusual circumstances found in wilderness settings may result in ethical decisions different from those in standard medical settings. The ethical decision-making process used to puzzle through these dilemmas, however, is similar to that used in other settings; wilderness medical care's unique setting and issues sometimes obscure this basic truism.

Application of Values

In wilderness medicine, ethical dilemmas arise, and values must be applied to patient-clinician interactions, group activities, and public wilderness policies. In this setting the unique position of wilderness medical practitioners must be recognized. These dilemmas have few parallels in other areas of medical practice, except perhaps battlefield medical practice or medical care during major, widespread disasters. These dilemmas may include providing euthanasia for potentially nonfatal medical conditions, abandoning patients, and prioritizing medical care between original patients and rescue team members. A limited discussion of the ethical dilemmas involved in each of these follows.

Standard of Care Dilemmas

Limited Resources. In the wilderness setting, resources are limited. Medical equipment is usually confined to supplies that can be carried into the field on foot or in some cases on horseback or by helicopter. Wilderness rescue personnel may have limited medical skills. The combination of limited skills and limited availability of supplies and equipment gives rise to ethical dilemmas. What should be included in wilderness medical kits? Their composition is resource allocation at its most basic. Who decides?

Rarely do people consider advanced decision making a part of medical care. However, it is very much a part of wilderness medicine. For example, decisions regarding the contents of medical kits made well in advance rather than during triage affect the patient's care. Although the individual wilderness traveler usually determines what is carried into the field, he or she generally fails to realize that this decision may set a limit on treatment. Any traveler into a wilderness area must assume that the contents of the medical kit will be the only resources available for medical treatment. When equipment is selected for organized wilderness excursions or search-and-rescue teams, however, the decision may be made by the group, a medical committee, or the medical director or advisor. The selection still limits the medical care that can be given.

Although commercially available standardized medical kits are usually designed on the basis of "medical" criteria, it is vital to recognize that some types of treatment will be implicitly unavailable because of what is excluded from these kits. Decisions must be made concerning what to include in field medical kits, yet no one is expected to carry a fully stocked emergency department into the field. Clearly identifying the ethical dilemmas entailed in compiling these kits helps team members in their decisions. For example, if a decision not to carry antiarrhythmic medications or a defibrillator is made and if a team member suffers a cardiac rhythm abnormality, there will be little that can be done for him or her. Some people may omit medical kit items that will foreseeably be useful, such as intravenous solutions. As the medical person on one doomed expedition to the Himalayan peak Nanda Devi recalled, "[My]

irritation grew as [I] remembered [being] pressured into leaving intravenous fluids behind."[22] This preexpedition resource decision may doom a team member. It helps if team members know in advance that these decisions were made—and even participate in making them.

Explicit triage decisions, although harder to make, are often easier to recognize as ethical dilemmas. These are discussed later in the chapter.

Cultural Differences. Many wilderness emergencies occur in places outside of the United States or other Western countries. Are Western standards of care and attitudes appropriate when treating locals in a foreign country? Whose values control medical treatment and other actions?

Three circumstances may present ethical dilemmas in the delivery of medical care during wilderness expeditions to remote areas. The first is a lack of cultural sensitivity. Aggressive offers to care for disease or injury may frustrate or anger local patients or providers, whose methods of treatment fit within the region's cultural milieu and may be as good as or better than "modern" medicine. Temporarily replacing or upstaging traditional healers and their healing methods may degrade them in the eyes of the local population.

The second situation is when medical problems occur that are beyond the capabilities of an expedition's practitioners. After offering the care for which they are competent, practitioners may feel obligated to attempt treatments beyond their knowledge or abilities. An internist may face treating a gunshot wound to the chest, a psychiatrist may encounter a complicated obstetric emergency, or a paramedic may confront an epidemic. Often without any direction except a moral compass, these caregivers may be tempted to stretch their abilities beyond the limits of patient safety. Cultural ethical concerns should be considered when deciding which course of action to pursue.

The third situation relates to the larger question of the fairness of chance encounters: a woman's life is saved through the luck that a passing trekker could treat her pyelonephritis; after a surgeon relocates a hip, a man will continue to provide for his family; and a paramedic happens to be on hand to intubate a child with epiglottitis. These situations in themselves rarely encompass ethical issues. The larger question, which may be more philosophical than practical, is how these interventions interfere with the balance of life in the area. Are chance encounters an aberration or simply a part of life? One of the most common situations in this category is a wilderness team from a developed country leaving medications behind with individuals who would not normally have access to them. Beyond the questions of the medications' efficacy, continued availability, and safety in inexperienced hands, there are the ethical concerns about interfering and altering the life balance in other cultures. Trekkers who traverse areas that others commonly visit do not face this dilemma, since medications are routinely distributed by the succession of groups. This question arises, however, in expeditions entering rarely visited areas, such as remote areas in Papua-New Guinea or the Amazon basin.

How Much Authority Is Given to Nontrained Personnel? Wilderness travelers face ethical dilemmas when they encounter medical situations for which they are untrained. This is certainly not restricted to laypersons. Medics, physician assistants, nurses, and physicians may quickly find themselves out of their depth in a wilderness setting. This occurs when they treat patients with conditions comfortably treated only in an urban environment or when an illness or injury is beyond the scope of personal experience and knowledge. In deciding whether to intervene in such a situation, the person planning to help must weigh the chance of benefiting the patient (value of beneficence) against the chance of doing the recipient of care harm (nonmaleficence).

The following hypothetical case illustrates both the questions raised in this type of dilemma and the application of the rapid decision-making model (see Figure 78-3). A backcountry excursion sets out with a medical provider who is unprepared for orthopedic emergencies. When a group member dislocates her shoulder, the provider may be unwilling to go beyond his level of training by attempting a shoulder relocation, although the victim (as well as the rest of the party) may encourage the attempt. Another member of the party with even less training volunteers to attempt the maneuver; the clinician is in a double bind, seemingly forced to either overextend his or her skills or to acquiesce to even less knowledgeable medical care for the victim.

How could this dilemma be resolved using the rapid decision-making model? (See Figure 78-3.) The first step would be to anticipate such a situation in advance and plan a course of action. Since orthopedic trauma is common in the wilderness, any medical provider should expect to face such a situation. (Note that planning may obviate this ethical dilemma, as it does in many other situations, since the provider may then learn the requisite orthopedic knowledge and skills in advance or may abandon plans to assume this wilderness medical role.) Whether or not the skill level is unchanged, the provider may also decide on an ethical course of action after discussing in advance the potential problem with knowledgeable peers or acquiring information from other sources. Perhaps the provider decides to act in such a situation (a paradigm or model case). It is reasonable to base intervention on (1) determining whether the patient has decisional capacity, (2) informing the patient fully and honestly of the apparent situation and options, and (3) acquiescing to the patient's desires, whether attempting relocation or simply securing the arm in place. Honest acceptance of the patient's autonomy to control her medical care often resolves a seemingly difficult ethical dilemma. Yet the circumstances in this case may be that the provider believes the "experienced" layman offering to help may actually have no knowledge at all. The provider must then decide whether the paradigm case for which he prepared a response is similar enough to the current circumstances to use that response. If it is, the dilemma is resolved, and that rule should be followed.

If, however, the provider believes that the current situation differs significantly from his paradigm case or if from lack of foresight he simply failed to decide in advance on an ethical course of action, he should go to step two: buying time. In the scenario presented, buying time may consist of making the patient comfortable before contacting help or thinking through the problem. Help may be available to organized wilderness excursions through radio or cellular telephone communication. The assistance may be experienced advice about other actions to resolve the dilemma or orthopedic advice on ways to reduce the shoulder. Sometimes, however, no help is available or not enough time can be bought to secure help. The health care provider must make a decision to act: go to step three.

At this stage, the provider attempts to choose an action (by applying Figure 78-2) that is ethically acceptable, even if it is not the optimal action he might select if more time were available to consider the problem. Possible actions in this case might include attempting a reduction, allowing the lay person to attempt a reduction, simply immobilizing the victim's shoulder, leaving the victim and going for help, or ignoring the situation and leaving the decision to someone else. The provider must first choose a course of action (remembering that not deciding is also a course of action) and then decide whether the choice falls within the scope of ethically acceptable behavior. If, for example, the proposed action is shoulder immobilization, the three tests of impartiality (Golden Rule), universalizability (should every practitioner do as I plan to do?), and interpersonal justifiability (would I be ashamed to have my actions publicized?) should be applied to this action. If the action passes all three tests, it is probably ethically acceptable and may be used. Remember that ethically acceptable actions may differ with the circumstances or the wilderness group involved.

Health care policy is another aspect of this type of ethical dilemma. Restricting medical practitioners from fully using their skills and knowledge may limit wilderness medical care. Paramedics, for example, are told that in some jurisdictions, on penalty of losing their licenses, they may not reduce fractures, perform cricothyrotomies, or in a few locations, perform endotracheal intubations. Emergency medical technicians, first aiders, first responders, and the like are more severely restricted. Nurses may not know what procedures their licenses allow, and physicians are constantly concerned about liability. In general, many practitioners in wilderness settings feel that the laws and administrative policies under which they work restrict their actions. This attitude and their subsequent behavior may lead to substandard care for victims of wilderness injury or illness. The Wilderness Medical Society and other groups have begun working to overcome these limitations. At present, however, an ethical dilemma may exist when practitioners face medical situations in the field that they know how to treat but that exceed their licenses or official certifications. A clear conflict may exist between the law and ethical responsibility. Practitioners have to decide the best course of action, preferably in advance of the problem.

Priority in Care Dilemmas

Triage takes on new dimensions in wilderness settings. Ethical dilemmas easily arise when health care providers face not only triage among victims but also critical decisions about whether to help victims at all. These settings also produce situations in which the rescuers or other members of the party may be placed in danger by helping an injured person.

Triage Choices: Whom to Rescue First and How to Distribute Resources.
Medical practitioners, especially those in fields of surgery and emergency care, are familiar with medical triage in which multiple patients need care and in which patients must be sorted by severity of injury, availability of resources, and possibility of successful treatment. These triage decisions have their own unique set of ethical dilemmas. Wilderness triage is unusual on several counts and may present ethical dilemmas markedly different from those encountered in nonwilderness environments.

Three ethical dilemmas result from wilderness triage questions that are unlikely to occur elsewhere except for battlefield settings.[5] The first dilemma arises when, providing care for a group, the wilderness practitioner knows all the victims and may have personal ties to at least one. This is unlike normal triage scenarios and complicates any decision about who gets treated, especially if resources are limited. For example, in an outbreak of giardiasis in a party of 12, the provider may have only enough metronidazole (Flagyl) to treat 5 people. Another, more serious example would be a lightning strike in the midst of six people, with only one other individual capable of providing assistance. In each case, the medical practitioner applying triage criteria may be torn between medical and personal concerns.

A second ethical triage dilemma arises in what may be termed the "us vs. them" situation. Members of both the wilderness party and local population may be in the victim pool to be triaged. To whom does the provider owe primary responsibility? Some may argue that the implicit or explicit contract between the provider and group members warrants treating group members first. If the battlefield is considered analogous, the same contract exists there. The Geneva Convention specifies that patients are always to be triaged for medical care on the basis of medical need and the ability to treat. Whether military caregivers follow this dictum in practice is moot. The wilderness caregiver must carefully consider this issue before venturing into the field.

Finally, ethical dilemmas arise because not all team members are equal. If triage among team members is necessary, treatment on the basis of pure medical necessity is not always realistic. In the giardiasis example, will the sickest patients be treated or will treatment be given to the less sick guide and translator, who are essential people needed to get the party safely out of the wilderness? The greatest good for the greatest number, or the concept of group safety, must prevail. However, this may be neither a comfortable nor an intuitively obvious decision.

An ethical dilemma also arises when a rescue team member is injured while out in the field. The question is asked whether rescue teams should treat their injured team member before, or instead of, victims. Wilderness rescue is an inherently dangerous operation. Although the safety record of some organized and experienced rescue groups has been excellent, this is not universal, particularly with ad hoc rescue attempts.[7] An ethical dilemma arises when rescuers themselves become victims. Where should the team's priorities lie? Again, an analogy can be drawn with triage parameters in emergency care. The principle of triage is that as long as resources are available, the most seriously injured are treated first. Those that cannot be saved with available resources or evacuated in time to be saved are given only comfort measures. This situation logically and morally prevails in wilderness medical care. However, emotion rather than reason often influences actions, so the wilderness health care provider must ensure that ethical decision making prevails.

Issues of Survival.
In some situations, the lives of expedition members may be put at immediate risk if an injured person receives optimal assistance. One well-known example was the high-altitude climber in the Peruvian Andes, Simon Yates, who, while trying to lower his injured climbing partner, Joe Simpson,[24] down to base camp, found himself in a situation in

which he had to either cut the lowering rope tethering his partner, almost assuredly killing him, or risk also dying himself (unbelievably, Simpson survived):

I couldn't help him, and it occurred to me that in all likelihood he would fall to his death. I wasn't disturbed by the thought. In a way I hoped he would fall. I knew I couldn't leave him while he was still fighting for it, but I had no idea how I might help him. I could get down. If I tried to get him down I might die with him. It didn't frighten me. It just seemed a waste. It would be pointless. . . . The knife! The thought came out of nowhere. Of course, the knife. Be quick, come on, get it. . . . I reached down again, and this time I touched the blade to the rope. It needed no pressure. The taut rope exploded at the touch of the blade, and I flew backwards into the seat as the pulling strain vanished. . . . I was alive, and for the moment that was all I could think about. . . . There was no guilt, not even sorrow. . . . I was actually pleased that I had been strong enough to cut the rope. There had been nothing else left to me, and so I had gone ahead with it. I had done it. . . . I was alive because I had held everything together right up to the last moment. It had been executed calmly. . . . I should feel guilty. I don't. I did right.

In another example, a diver may surface and suffer from an air embolism. Review of the ethical considerations in wilderness medicine's ethical triangle, it is found that both medical indications and possibly the patient (autonomy) influence the decision to transport the victim more rapidly to a recompression chamber. This example demonstrates again that in the wilderness setting, security factors are primary in making ethical decisions. Unless the safety of the other divers can be guaranteed, the boat should not leave the area until the other divers are safely on board.

Issues of Direct Life-Threatening Situations for the Provider. Health care providers in a wilderness setting often have the opportunity to literally rescue others, which directly supports their underlying motivation to be of help to others. However, situations arise in which providing help puts the caregiver (or the entire team) at significant risk. This has already been discussed in Safety: Another Value Applicable to Wilderness Medicine. Wilderness medical leaders commonly decline to enter a dangerous situation to attempt to rescue a patient. However, a more direct and powerful ethical issue arises when the caregiver must directly and explicitly sacrifice the patient for personal or team safety. (This is somewhat analogous to the difference between passive and active euthanasia.) This occurs, for example, when a helicopter hoisting a patient encounters difficulties that endanger the craft. Standard procedure is to cut the hoist line, sacrificing the patient. In the abstract, the safety of the helicopter crew (and possibly rescuers on the ground) outweighs that of the patient. Yet in reality, the conflict between safety and beneficence may not be intrinsically clear to the health care provider; an answer in favor of safety contradicts all professional education and experiences. This conflict must be resolved in advance or within a few seconds during the event if anyone is to survive. In the analogous scenario of the battlefield, the question is raised, "How many medics do you sacrifice to save one infantryman?" So too with rescuers.

Decision-Making Dilemmas

Health care decisions are generally the responsibility of the adult with decision-making capacity. If a patient lacks the ability to make these decisions, health care providers normally seek a surrogate decision maker, an advance directive, or the counsel of a bioethics committee or colleague. These resources are rarely available in the wilderness setting. Health care decisions can therefore become more problematic.

Unavailability of a Surrogate or a Family Member. When a person needing health care in the wilderness lacks decision-making capacity because of illness or injury, the health care provider must make decisions based on knowledge of the patient's values (often from a relatively brief period of interaction), the values of the group, or the provider's own perceptions of what is in the patient's best interest. When family or close friends are present, they may act as surrogates to make decisions for the patient, but this is much less frequent in the wilderness setting than in the urban environment. The wilderness medical provider must therefore be prepared to make difficult decisions without this guidance.

Advance Directives. To allay the problems of the absence of surrogate decision makers or knowledge about a patient's wishes, health care providers for organized expeditions, especially those in which significant risk of danger exists, may want to request that each team member complete an advance directive. However, as explained earlier, the normal forms of advance directive (durable power of attorney for health care and living will) may not suffice in the wilderness setting. Rather, a more specific directive should be used. It should detail how aggressive each individual would want the team to be in trying to extract them from a dangerous situation if the victim (1) had a reasonable chance of survival given available resources, (2) had a reasonable chance of survival but with serious physical disability, (3) had a reasonable chance of survival but with serious brain injury, or (4) had a poor chance of surviving. Any directive given by a team member would of course be tempered by the need to ensure the safety of other team members, but such a directive might give the medical provider a better idea of each team member's desires. Indeed, just discussing these scenarios with the team may be beneficial in elucidating attitudes and health care desires in the wilderness.

Some team members might want to use a durable power of attorney, naming a surrogate within the team, for use with or in place of the more specific directive.

Euthanasia. Controversy continues to rage in society and medicine over the concept of active euthanasia (so-called mercy killing). In wilderness medicine, however, euthanasia may be less ethically problematic, although it is a very sensitive issue to discuss and a devastating event for those involved. Active euthanasia may be an ethically acceptable alternative in the rare situation when a patient will die either because he or she cannot be rescued from the wilderness environment or because the survival of group members would be jeopardized by attempting to evacuate or remain with him or her until help arrives. The seriously injured person on a high-altitude climb with inclement weather quickly approaching and the injured caver in a flooding cave are two examples. In these cases, euthanasia is based on the beneficence of relieving suffering in a doomed individual (although many in the medical profession believe that mercy killing violates professional principles), security for other members of the party (not creating more victims), and perhaps patient autonomy (although some psychiatrists might argue that by asking for death a person demonstrates a lack of decision-making capacity).[2] Indeed, a particularly difficult situation is the psychiatric patient who cannot be made to continue out of the wilderness and who will endanger the group and himself or herself if either remains. This has happened at least once in the dual peril of war and wilderness, when British soldiers of the 111th Indian Infantry Brigade in Burma euthanized their own during World War II.[25] In nonwar situations, however, any episodes of active wilderness euthanasia have gone unreported.

Further complicating the preceding scenarios is the question of whether such patients should be simply left to die (passive euthanasia) or more humanely killed (active euthanasia). This question should be given serious consideration, since many incidents of passive euthanasia in wilderness settings occur, especially in high-risk or remote areas. Passive euthanasia has occurred, for example, at least several times on Everest expeditions when unconscious, hypothermic climbers were left to die when conditions made it difficult or impossible to get them down.[22] The ethical question of what is best for the injured individual almost always comes in direct conflict with other team members' lack of confidence in their (or their medical person's) prognosis and their unwillingness to implement active euthanasia. The lack of certainty about prognosis may sometimes be justified. For example, during a recent disastrous Everest expedition, a physician-climber who was left for dead (active euthanasia was not discussed among team members) survived by eventually making it back to camp on his own.

Dilemmas in Wilderness Policies

Ethical decision making plays a part in policies governing wilderness medicine. The values of beneficence and nonmaleficence make proposed and actual rules for wilderness medical practice untenable. These policies include no-rescue areas, prohibition of motorized vehicles in wilderness areas, prohibition of environmental destruction, and restriction of medical providers' roles (see How Much Authority Is Given to Nontrained Personnel?).

Motorized Vehicle Restrictions and Environmental Protection in Wilderness Areas. A policy occasionally imposed on wilderness medical practice is that of no motorized vehicles in designated wilderness areas. This rule has logical roots but is enforced only intermittently. When it is used to hinder rescue efforts or delay needed medical care, however, it defeats a basic purpose of society: the assurance of citizens' welfare.

A related issue is the basic tenet of wilderness travel that the environment should be left at least as pristine as it was found. Situations arise, however, when preservation of a wilderness area must be weighed against pain and suffering or life and death. Helicopter pads chopped into the forest or a new entryway blasted into a cave are only two examples. The preservation of wilderness areas is an important goal, but so is the preservation of human life and values, and these should not be overridden to reach a symbolic goal. Human life is a priority.

No-Rescue Areas. Perhaps the most pernicious concept proposed to govern wilderness medical care is that of the "no-rescue area," into which adventurers would go with the foreknowledge that no rescue would be available.[19] Akin to playing Russian roulette, people entering these wilderness areas would put life and limb at risk while society condoned and presumably enforced a requirement not to assist those in need. This macho concept disregards patient and societal beneficence and individual autonomy. Those familiar with advance directives, such as health care powers of attorney or living wills, know that patients in extremis often countermand their preconceived instructions. To prevent wilderness trekkers from doing the same to preserve their life contradicts basic ethical values.

REFERENCES

1. Aquinas T: *Two precepts of charity*, 1273.
2. Backer HD: Wilderness medicine. In Iserson KV et al, editors: *Ethics in emergency medicine*, Tucson, Ariz, 1995, Galen Press.
3. Buchanan AE: The question of competence. In Iserson KV et al, editors: *Ethics in emergency medicine*, ed 2, Tucson, Ariz, 1995, Galen Press.
4. Drane JF: Competency to give an informed consent, *JAMA* 252:925, 1984.
5. Frisina ME: Ethical principles and the practice of battlefield health care, *Milit Chaplains Rev* Spring 1991.
6. Gauthier DP: *Morals by agreement*, Oxford, England, 1986, Clarendon Press.

7. Iserson KV: Injuries in search and rescue volunteers: a 30 year experience, *West J Med* 151:352, 1989.

8. Iserson KV: The 'no code' tattoo: ethical dilemma, *West J Med* 156:309, 1992.

9. Iserson KV: Pediatric bioethics. In Reisdorff EJ, Roberts MR, Wiegenstein JG, editors: *Pediatric emergency medicine,* Philadelphia, 1992, WB Saunders.

10. Iserson KV: A simplified prehospital advance directive law: Arizona's approach, *Ann Emerg Med* 22:1703, 1993.

11. Iserson KV: *Death to dust: what happens to dead bodies?* Tucson, Ariz, 1994, Galen Press.

12. Iserson KV: An approach to ethical problems in emergency medicine. In Iserson KV et al, editors: *Ethics in emergency medicine,* Tucson, Ariz, 1995, Galen Press.

13. Iserson KV: Bioethics. In Rosen P, Barkin RM, et al, editors: *Emergency medicine: concepts and clinical practice,* ed 4, St Louis, 1998, Mosby.

14. Iserson KV: Nonstandard advance directives: a pseudoethical dilemma, *J Trauma* 44:139, 1998.

15. Jonsen AR, Siegler M, Winslade WJ: *Clinical ethics,* ed 4, New York, 1998, McGraw-Hill.

16. Kauffman AJ, Putnam WL: *K2: 1939 tragedy—the full story of the ill-fated Wiessner expedition,* Seattle, Wash, 1992, The Mountaineers.

17. Knopp RK et al: An ethical foundation for health care: an emergency medicine perspective, *Ann Emerg Med* 21:1381, 1992.

18. Landesman BM: Physician attitudes toward patients. In Iserson KV et al, editors: *Ethics in emergency medicine,* Tucson, Ariz, 1995, Galen Press.

19. McAvoy L, Dustin D: You're losing your right to be alone, *Backpacker* 12:60, 1984.

20. Mill JS: Utilitarianism, London, 1861. In *The Great Books,* Chicago, 1952, *Encyclopaedia Britannica.*

21. Nolan JR, Connolly MJ: *Black's law dictionary,* ed 5, St Paul, Minn, 1979, West Publishing.

22. Roskelley J: *Nanda Devi: the tragic expedition.* Harrisburg, Penn, 1987, Stackpole Books.

23. *Schloendorff v. Society of New York Hospital,* 105 N.E. 92, 93, 1914.

24. Simpson J: *Touching the void,* London, 1988, Butler & Tanner.

25. Swann SW: Euthanasia on the battlefield, *Milit Chaplains Rev* Spring 1991.

79 The Changing Environment

James K. Mitchell

Three miles southwest of the Kremlin, not far from Moscow's Olympic Stadium, lies the Novodevichiy Cemetery, one of the most celebrated burying places in Russia. Amid ornate memorials to former leaders like Gromyko and Khrushchev, and to giants of the arts, such as Chekhov and Shostakovich, stands a white marble pedestal carrying the sculpted head of Vladimir Illich Vernadsky (1863-1945). Little known in the West, Vernadsky was a prescient observer of the emerging role of humans as makers of the global environment. It was he who first announced that we are living at a time when the power of humankind to change the earth now rivals that of geologic processes.[6] In the past, students of natural history could regard the human life span as a mere blink of a cosmic eye that witnessed little environmental change. Today we are faced with the prospect that the planet may be fundamentally transformed by humans, perhaps within a few decades, but more probably over the space of one or two generations.

This situation has not come about all at once, or equally everywhere. On a global scale, it has gradually built up over centuries, although the local manifestations of increased human agency have been sometimes masked by other processes. For example, conversion of "natural" ecosystems to "managed" ecosystems is a dominant feature on the global scale, but in some parts of the world (especially the United States and Western Europe) managed ecosystems are also being abandoned. Such is the case in New Jersey, where hilltop nineteenth-century farmlands have largely reverted to regrowth forests.[75]

The complications of environmental change might best be appreciated with the aid of a time machine such as the one envisioned by H.G. Wells in 1935. Imagine, for a moment, being in a mature pine forest in southern New England. What might be observed as the machine slips into the past at this location?

The surrounding landscape comes clearly into view. The pine trees shrink slowly down into youth as the years wind back, since most of today's pines trace their origin to the abandonment of farmlands at or near the turn of the century. The pines disappear entirely in the late nineteenth century and are replaced by shrubs and eventually by grasses. By the mid-1800s the local vicinity is completely open and appears as a shifting mosaic of agricultural crops and pasture, rotated in time and space. This is the high tide of farming in New England. Thereafter, the sequence goes into reverse. By the eighteenth century, trees begin to return, connecting the

remnant patches of presettlement vegetation. Gradually the forest closes in and traces of human presence fade. Little breaks the monotony, apart from occasional fires started by lightning or Native Americans clearing seasonal cultivation patches, or major windstorms that topple weaker trees. As the sixteenth century approaches, clearly the landscape is essentially similar from decade to decade.

The time traveler's dominant impression is one of change. The preceding sequence of changes has been documented by many analysts of the New England landscape.[14a,44a,62] The sequence might be different elsewhere but is no less dynamic.[80] Sometimes the changes are sudden and dramatic, and sometimes they are slow and imperceptible.* Sometimes they are "natural" (e.g., storms) and sometimes they are caused by humans (e.g., example, forest clearance). For the bulk of human history, natural changes have seemed to dominate, although in fact people have been major shapers of the environment for millennia.[13a,43,74a,80] A casual observer of the New England landscape might conclude that the well-wooded 1990s scene is more "natural" than the cleared fields of the 1850s. However, today's scene is just as much a product of human choices as that of the nineteenth century, albeit different in composition and appearance.

In any event, deciding whether human or natural factors are responsible for a given environmental change is often difficult; both factors tend to operate interdependently (Figure 79-1). It is widely believed

---

*Arguments between uniformitarians (who give primacy to continuous, small-scale changes) and catastrophists (who favor change as a function of intermittent large-scale events) have continued for more than a century (Oldroyd DR: *Thinking about the earth: A history of ideas in geology*, Cambridge, 1996: 131-144). Although the uniformitarian position has dominated among earth scientists, recent evidence in support of catastrophic explanations is compelling. For example, the fossil record indicates that mass extinctions have occurred throughout the globe at many times in the past. (See Martin PS, Klein RG, editors: *Quaternary extinctions: a prehistoric revolution*, Tucson, 1984, University of Arizona Press.) Some analysts argue that the age of dinosaurs ended 65 million years ago when a massive meteor collided with the earth, perhaps striking the Gulf of Mexico near the Yucatan Peninsula. (See Alvarez W, Asaro F: What caused mass extinction? *Sci Am* 263:78, 1990.) The impact may have thrown sufficient dust into the atmosphere that solar radiation was reflected back into space, causing global temperatures to plummet. A similar although smaller effect was noted in 1992 when volcanic Mt. Pinatubo in the Philippines spewed ash, dust, and gases into the atmosphere and lowered mean global temperature by an estimated 2° C (3.6° F). (See Dutton EC, Christy JR: Solar radiative forcing at selected locations and evidence of global lower troposphere cooling following eruptions of El Chichon and Pinatubo, *Geophys Res Lett* 19:2313, 1992.)

Natural influences

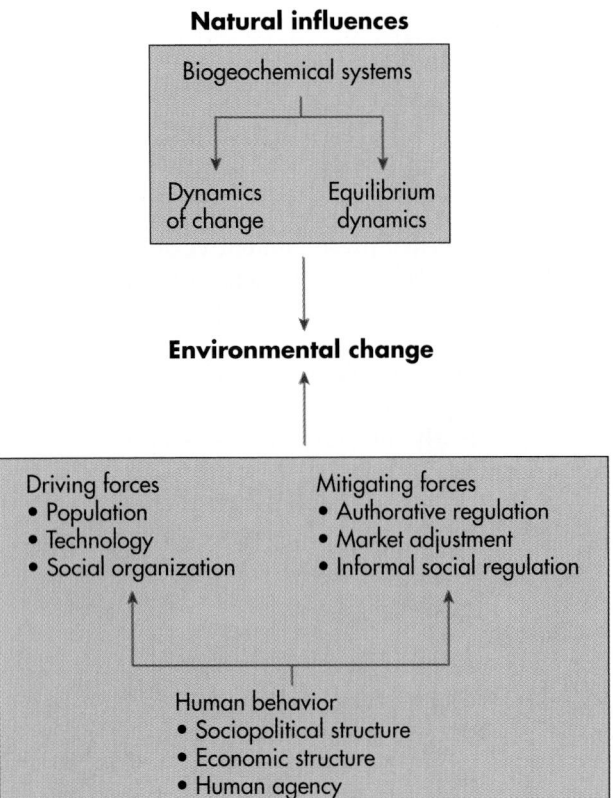

Figure 79-1 Human and natural forces for environmental change. (*Modified from Kates RW, Turner BL II, Clark WC: The great transformation. In Turner BL II, editor:* The earth as transformed by human action, *Cambridge, UK, 1990, Cambridge University Press.*)

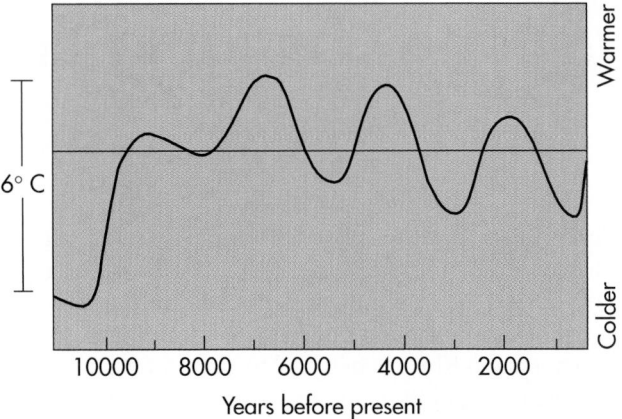

Figure 79-2 Variations of mean global temperature during the past 10,000 years. Horizontal line represents present global average temperature. (*Modified from Henderson-Sellers A, Robinson PJ:* Contemporary climatology, *New York, 1991, Wiley.*)

that people have reached a critical threshold as environmental modifiers; they are able to equal or surpass the effects of nature. Portentous changes are becoming manifest in the entire biosphere. We can at last begin to speak of a human "transformation" of the global environment.[37,75]

This chapter addresses environmental change and its human dimensions, with special attention to implications for environmental and wilderness medicine. What types of changes are likely to occur? How will they affect the natural environment, especially wilderness areas? What will be the consequences for society in general and for medical practitioners in particular? Can anything be done to improve our chances of successfully negotiating this impending time of dislocation and discontinuity?[46]

ISSUES OF ENVIRONMENTAL CHANGE

In recent years a number of environmental change issues have come to prominence. They include climate change, stratospheric ozone depletion, erosion of biodiversity, population growth, and burgeoning pollution. These issues affect all environments, from urban centers

to remote wilderness areas. In the discussion that follows, they are examined on a variety of scales. Although each scale is characterized by different expressions of change, all are interconnected. Local changes can aggregate to produce global effects, and global changes have many different disaggregated local effects.[75]

Climate Change

Weather is the state of the atmosphere at any specific time. Climate is the average weather pattern at a particular location. Weather and climate are usually described by such measures as temperature, precipitation, pressure, humidity, and wind speed and direction. In most parts of the world these measures have been recorded for less than a century, so the actual historical record of direct observations is relatively brief compared with the human tenure of the earth. However, scientists are often able to extend the historical record by constructing synthetic climate data from other evidence, such as tree rings, fossils, concentrations of plankton in ocean sediments, pollen in sedimentary rocks, and isotopes of carbon and oxygen in rocks and glacial ice. For example, narrow intervals between annual growth rings in trees and thin layers of organic material in lake sediments usually indicate cold, dry conditions. Clues like these permit investigators to open a window on past climates.

Figure 79-2 illustrates trends in average global temperature during the past 10,000 years. Note that the global temperature has been in flux throughout this period. Not only has weather varied about long-term average conditions, but the averages themselves have changed over time. For example, during the most recent ice age (about 10,000 years ago), average global temperatures were approximately 6° C (10.8° F) cooler than at present.[25] In other words, a massive environmental change (the Wisconsin ice age) was connected with a relatively small climatic change. It is worthwhile remembering that regional changes in climate may or may not parallel global changes. For example, between 2600 and 2700 years ago—roughly at the time of Socrates and Confucius—North America was colder and wetter than the continental average since the end of the Wisconsin glaciation, whereas conditions in Europe were warmer and drier. Fortunately, the climate has remained within a range that sustains life for most of the earth's history, and the changes have occurred at very slow rates over thousands to millions of years.

Currently a broad consensus exists among atmospheric scientists that global temperatures may rise significantly in coming decades.[44] One indicator of this trend is the fact that 1998 and 1999 are widely believed to have been the two warmest years of this century. Although the global climate system is enormously complex, two factors point toward warming. First, it is known that certain greenhouse gases warm the atmosphere by trapping short-wave radiation reflected from the earth's surface when it is heated by solar radiation. Second, atmospheric concentrations of these gases, which include carbon dioxide, methane, and nitrous oxide, are steadily increasing. Normally the materials in greenhouse gases pass through long biogeochemical cycles between natural sources and natural sinks. For example, sulfur enters the atmosphere as sulfur dioxide from volcanic eruptions and washes back to the oceans in the form of mildly acid rainfall whose constituents are later incorporated into bottom sediments. Human activities can increase source loads (e.g., emissions) and reduce the absorptive capacities of natural sinks. In the case of carbon dioxide, the greenhouse gas about which there is most concern, both processes are at work simultaneously. Emissions of carbon dioxide have been increasing as energy-hungry societies burn petroleum hydrocarbons, coal, and wood. At the same time, forests that usually absorb huge amounts of atmospheric carbon dioxide continue to be cleared—although at rates that are less than predicted a decade ago.

Atmospheric scientists are currently struggling to estimate how climate might change as greenhouse gases accumulate. For this purpose they rely heavily on general circulation models (GCMs) that mathematically simulate the global climate system. The chemistry and physics of climate are complex and the models, although increasingly sophisticated, are still imperfect. Their accuracy is constrained both by the limits of current knowledge about the dynamics of the atmosphere and by the computational power of the most advanced supercomputers. They are also hedged with other limitations. For example, the present generation of GCMs is too coarse to provide more than a broad-gauge portrayal of atmospheric conditions in a lattice of regions over the earth's surface. They do not reveal storm systems that bring most of the weather to middle and high latitudes. They also do not incorporate the role of clouds as reflectors and absorbers of energy. They do

TABLE 79-1. Effects of Global Climate Change in Different Latitudes

	LATITUDINAL ZONES IMPACTED		
INDICATOR	LOW	MIDDLE	HIGH
Biological productivity	−	?	+
Precipitation	+	−	+
Food production	−	+	+
Malaria transmission	0	+	0

Data from references 5, 28, 44, 57, and 79.
+, Increase; −, decrease; 0, no change; ?, uncertain.

not satisfactorily account for all of the carbon dioxide that is believed to have been liberated into the atmosphere through human activities. Nonetheless, many have considerable confidence in the accuracy of GCMs because of their relative success in replicating present and past climates.

The Intergovernmental Panel on Climate Change (IPCC), a joint United Nations–World Meteorological Organization committee of leading earth scientists, has synthesized existing research on climate change. Their initial conclusions pointed to a probable rise in mean global temperatures of about 0.3° C (0.54° F) per decade to 10° C (18° F) above the present value by 2025 and to 30° C (54° F) above the present value by 2100. More recently, these values have been revised downwards to take account of atmospheric aerosol feedback effects that were not included in the original (1990) calculations. The refined estimates are nonetheless still sobering. If nothing is done to alter present patterns of energy use and land use, there will be twice the preindustrial age (mid-eighteenth century) concentration of greenhouse gases in the atmosphere by 2030. This will probably raise mean global temperature about 0.2° C (0.36° F) per decade to 2° C (3.6° F) above the present value by 2100.[27] (See also: http://www.doc.mmu.ac.uk/aric/ace/gcc_10.html.)

Although the IPCC estimates embody a consensus about global warming, the level of agreement declines as researchers attempt to forecast the resulting impacts, especially at regional and local levels. An enhanced greenhouse effect would have a greater effect on the global climate than would temperature alone. Solar radiation provides the energy that drives the climate system. The effects of a warmer atmosphere could produce a cascade of changes in many climate variables. For example, precipitation patterns might change in ways that do not mirror temperature fluctuations.

GCMs generally indicate that lower latitudes and lower elevations will be less affected by anticipated climate changes than will upper latitudes and higher elevations. However, the most recent generation of climate change impact simulations paints no simple pictures.[1,56] Different combinations of effects would be likely at different latitudes (Table 79-1). Probably a mosaic of regional and local changes will occur along a spectrum from strongly positive to strongly negative depending on how, when, and where they occur. For example, tropical islands might experience heavier precipitation combined with more frequent severe storms and rising sea levels. The net impacts of such changes are difficult to assess. For Malé and other heavily populated low-lying islands of the Indo-Pacific Ocean, the results could be disastrous, whereas other places, such as high-standing islands of the Caribbean, could see offsetting agricultural benefits.[58]

More than any other factor, the rate of climate change is of concern to humans. General circulation models indicate that absolute changes in temperature will be smaller than those that have occurred at other times during the earth's history. However, the anticipated climate changes would still occur at a rate and magnitude that are unprecedented in human experience. Whereas past changes usually occurred slowly enough for plants and animals to adapt or migrate, examples of mass extinctions after rapid change exist. Many scientists fear that today and in the future, insufficient time and undeveloped areas will be available for plants and animals to make similar adjustments.

Although changes of average climate would have important long-term consequences, variations in extreme weather might produce the most immediate and significant impacts.[45] Droughts, floods, and tropical cyclones are unusual events in today's climate. If mean climates change, changes in the frequency and severity of these extremes would probably also occur and become manifest well before the permanent shifts could be confirmed.[24] The geographic distribution of such events would also be affected. As a result, natural hazards would be likely to pose increased risks to society. Moreover, exposure and vulnerability to extreme events would probably be exacerbated because populations at risk might respond to the new conditions on the basis of outdated information and assumptions.[17] We might find that our previous experience prepared us to "fight the last war" rather than the new one.

Stratospheric Ozone Depletion

The stratosphere is a distinct layer of the upper atmosphere that occurs between 9 and 35 miles above the ground. It contains significant concentrations of ozone (O_3), a gas that is formed when solar radiation splits ordinary oxygen atoms.* The stratospheric ozone layer absorbs most of the ultraviolet (UV) radiation from

space that would otherwise damage plant and animal species.

During the 1970s and 1980s, researchers discovered that stratospheric ozone was being lost and that the ozone layer was thinning to the point of disappearance, particularly in polar regions.[22a,48] Chlorofluorocarbons (CFCs) were held to be at fault. For decades, these synthetic compounds had been manufactured in large quantities, mainly for use as aerosol propellants and refrigerants. Once CFCs escape into the atmosphere, they remain stable until reaching the stratosphere, where they decompose under the action of UV radiation. Chlorine atoms are released and bond with ozone atoms, breaking them down into oxygen and other products. As a result, the ozone shield is weakened or removed.

If the ozone layer is sufficiently depleted, intensity of UV radiation that reaches the earth's surface could be significantly increased. This could have deleterious consequences for human populations and for plant and animal species. For humans, increased incidence of skin cancer, cataracts, and immune system suppression are three recognized effects of high UV exposure. Although humans might take precautions to protect themselves against UV radiation, such as reducing time spent outdoors or adding sun blocks, glasses, and clothes, nonhuman species may not be able to make the necessary adaptations. Serious disruption of human and agricultural systems is possible.

During their winter seasons, the Antarctic[59] and to a lesser extent the Arctic[42,72a,74] have experienced elevated levels of UV radiation. "Ozone holes" have been clearly traced to CFCs, and an international agreement, the Montreal Protocol, was reached to phase out CFC usage by 1996. Much progress has been made towards that goal, but these compounds are still being produced in some developing countries and the substitute chemicals that were introduced elsewhere may also contribute to global warming.[38] In any case, chlorine atoms are extremely long lived in the stratosphere, perhaps persisting for 100 to 200 years. There will continue to be some potential for additional ozone depletion in the decades to come.

Erosion of Biodiversity

Loss of species or the habitats that support them is a controversial and potentially serious global problem that comes under the heading "erosion of biodiversity." Biodiversity is not an agent of change like greenhouse gas buildup or ozone depletion. It is an index against which environmental changes can be assessed.[26,72] Like climate change and ozone depletion, biodiversity has a range of dimensions from global to local.[30] Two aspects of biodiversity that are of great importance are numbers and interconnections of species.

Estimates of the number of existing species are wide ranging because the state of knowledge about the

---

*Ozone also accumulates near ground level as a by-product of the photochemical modification of exhaust gases from automobiles and other sources of pollution. Concentrations of this type of ozone are sometimes reported in local news media, but the ground-level "ozone problem" should not be confused with the stratospheric one.

planet's biologic resources is both uneven and incomplete.[73] It is estimated that the earth hosts between 5 and 15 million species. About 1.75 million of these have been named.[40] Higher order mammals and birds in temperate ecosystems are well documented, but insects, worms and micro-lifeforms in tropical regions[19] are far less known. In the United States, approximately 100,000 species are recognized,[18] but only about one fifth of these have been surveyed to date.[73]

Paleobiologic research indicates that the number and type of species have varied greatly over time. New species evolve through adaptive genetic mutations, whereas others perish because of competitive pressures of natural selection. Emergence and disappearance rates depend on the speed and direction of environmental change and the ability of species to adjust. What is most troubling about the recent record is the disappearance of so many species. "Between 1600 and 1994, at least 484 species of animals and 654 species of plants (mostly vertebrates and flowering plants) became extinct. The rate of extinction in groups such as birds and mammals also increased dramatically during this period. Nearly three times as many species of birds and mammals became extinct between 1810 and 1994 (112 species) as were lost between 1600 and 1810

TABLE 79-2. Percentage of U.S. Species at Risk

RISK LEVEL	PERCENTAGE
Extinct	1%
Critically imperiled	6.5%
Imperiled	8.8%
Vulnerable	15.4%
Secure	69.3%

From Stein BA, Flack SR, *Environment* 39:6, 1997.

(38 species)."[64] Plant losses are presumed to have been much greater. On some oceanic islands, such as Hawaii, the disappearance of native animal species is almost total. Of 269 extinct Hawaiian species, most were either invertebrates (135) or plants (105). A majority of the rest are birds (15) and land snails (11).[73] Commercial forestry and fishing have proved particularly injurious to biodiversity because they harvest desirable species and destroy undesirable species at the same time.[29] Agriculture and animal husbandry also contribute to species extinctions, especially by modifying the habitats that support biota. Particular concerns have been expressed about threats to tropical forests and the near extinction of some marine species, such as the northern cod and the blue whale. However, the problem is general in scope and may be most important for the "noncelebrity" species that do not elicit much human compassion.

In the United States it is estimated that about 32% of all species are now under serious pressure, sometimes to the point of threatened extinction[73] (Table 79-2). However, the picture varies widely among particular groups of species (Table 79-3). Denizens of freshwater ecosystems, such as shellfish, crustaceans, amphibians, and fish, are far more likely to be in danger than are flowering plants, conifers, mammals and birds. Likewise, on the U.S. mainland, loss of biodiversity is more acute in Sunbelt states and east of the Mississippi River than in states of the northern Great Plains and the northern Rocky Mountains.

For many people, the protection of threatened species is a moral imperative. For others it is a luxury. Quite apart from moral issues, the rising rate of species extinction has practical implications.[65] For example, loss of the planet's genetic stock hampers the search for wild strains of domestic crops that are resistant to pests and diseases that plague high-yield domestic varieties.

TABLE 79-3. U.S. Species Groups at Risk

SPECIES	VULNERABLE	IMPERILED	EXTINCT	SECURE
Freshwater mussels	16.4	39.7	11.8	32.1
Crayfish	17.3	32.8	0.9	49
Amphibians	14	23.9	2.5	59.6
Freshwater fish	14.1	22	2.6	61.3
Flowering plants	16.6	15.8	0.9	66.7
Conifers	12.2	14	0	73.8
Ferns	11.9	8.9	0.7	78.5
Tiger beetles	13.6	6.3	0	80.1
Dragonflies	10.4	7.6	0.4	81.6
Reptiles	11.9	6.1	0	82
Butterflies	12.3	4	0.5	83.2
Mammals	9.1	7.2	0.2	83.5
Birds	5.4	5.8	3.3	85.5

Modified from Stein BA, Flack SR: *Environment* 39:6, 1997.

The so-called Green Revolution, which has helped alleviate world hunger in recent decades, owes much of its success to introduction of resistant wild genetic strains into commercial agriculture.

Biodiversity is also important in the stability of global ecosystems. For example, the extent to which entire species can be eliminated from an ecosystem before it collapses is unknown. Likewise, the extent to which some nominally "wild" species may thrive under human management while others succumb is hotly debated.[21] Most ecologists believe that ecosystems containing a wide diversity of organisms are more resilient to change than those with few species. Regardless of the degree of resilience, biodiversity and environmental change may be connected by negative feedback relationships. Thus, environmental change may lead to loss of biodiversity that in turn produces lowered resistance to pressures for further change.

Despite intuitive, theoretic, and case study arguments in favor of preserving biodiversity, it has been difficult to agree on standardized measures of biodiversity or its loss. Deforestation of South American rainforests is a case in point. The Amazon Basin is one of the world's premier wilderness regions and is also regarded as its most important source of biodiversity. Perhaps impelled by dramatic and widely-publicized reports of forest clearances by ranchers, homesteading farmers, and mineral firms in Brazil during the late 1980s, levels of international concern about the loss of biodiversity in Amazonia have been high. However, as in most developing countries, comprehensive and reliable data on Brazilian deforestation are difficult to secure and interpret.[71,82]

"Up to 1988, the best estimates suggest that 6-7% of the forest has been subject to at least one cutting in the past 30 years. Inclusion of secondary forest, known to have been deforested prior to 1960, but with advanced secondary forest that satellite imagery cannot differentiate from primary forest, raises the estimate by roughly 100,000 km². The latest estimates from INPE, the Brazilian Space Agency, show that deforestation had grown to about 472,000 km² in 1994, including the deforestation that occurred prior to 1960. It should be emphasized that all of this remaining 372,000 km² of deforestation (9% of the total forest) should not be interpreted as land that has been deforested and transferred to agricultural use for ever. Land that has been cleared and later abandoned will often return to forest cover, even if used for pasture, although there is some uncertainty about the length of the process of forest recovery from pasture abandonment to mature forest."[20]

Population Growth

Human population is one of the primary driving forces behind contemporary environmental change. Beginning with the Reverend Thomas Malthus (1766-1834), many people have argued that rising populations must eventually deplete resources and degrade environments because the earth is, for all intents and purposes, a closed system.[36] This does not mean that it will be impossible for the earth to hold additional human populations. If the record of the last four centuries provides a demographic lesson, it is that the global carrying capacity is highly elastic—up to some as yet unreached limit.[13] Leaving aside the argument that human ingenuity can make possible the support for larger populations indefinitely, clearly from the perspective of burdens on the physical environment, how people live is more important than the number of people. All other things being equal, richer societies place heavier burdens on the physical environment than poorer ones. For example, the United States, with just 5% of the global population, consumes approximately 25% of the world's energy resources.[14]

The global population has undergone unprecedented growth in the last several centuries (Figure 79-3). By 1800 the earth's population was approximately 1 billion. By 1920 it had doubled. Three billion was reached in 1960, and the present estimate is over 5 billion. The United Nations estimates that more than 8 billion people will be on Earth by the year 2025.[76] Numbers may level out to between 12 and 15 billion by 2100. Most of the new growth is likely to occur in developing countries of Asia, Africa, and Latin America (Table 79-4). The recent experience of China suggests that the process of development can itself perpetuate or increase historical rates of population growth, at least until economic conditions improve significantly.

The composition of future populations is an increasing concern of governments and individuals. In places like Japan and Eastern Europe, natural increase is now well below the rate necessary to replace existing populations, whereas in the United States, increasing numbers are maintained largely by immigration. As a result, the fraction of national populations that is more than 65 years old is growing rapidly in the more developed world. Meanwhile, increasing expertise in genetic manipulation holds out the prospect of significantly longer lifespans for populations that can afford the kind of scientific research and medical care that will make this possible. In other words, some parts of the world's population will become increasingly healthier and older, and others may remain caught in a cycle of short sickness-prone lives followed by early deaths. Quite apart from the staggering societal impacts that such a change would produce, the implications for wilderness are considerable. For those who can be assured of longer lives, the quality of life experience—including the quality of their environments—may become of foremost importance. Wilderness areas would be among the most cherished places and decisions about their future all the more portentous. Among developing countries, a different future might obtain, perhaps dominated by intense pressure to convert all available resources into supports for survival. Although such scenarios are not difficult to envision, they carry with them a danger of indulging in stereotypical dichotomizations that ignore possibilities for a range of more nuanced outcomes.

Pollution

Unwanted by-products of production and consumption that exceed the absorptive capacity of the environment are known as *pollution*. Pollution comes in many forms, including solid physical materials, liquid chemical compounds, and energy (e.g., thermal pollution). Some pollutants (such as certain isotopes of plutonium) are highly toxic even in small amounts. Many materials that are beneficial in small amounts can be deleterious in large quantities. For example, phosphorus is a nutrient that limits biologic productivity in coastal and marine ecosystems. Small amounts of phosphorus can increase algal growth at the bottom of marine food chains. When larger amounts of phosphorus-rich runoff from fertilizers or septic systems enter these en-

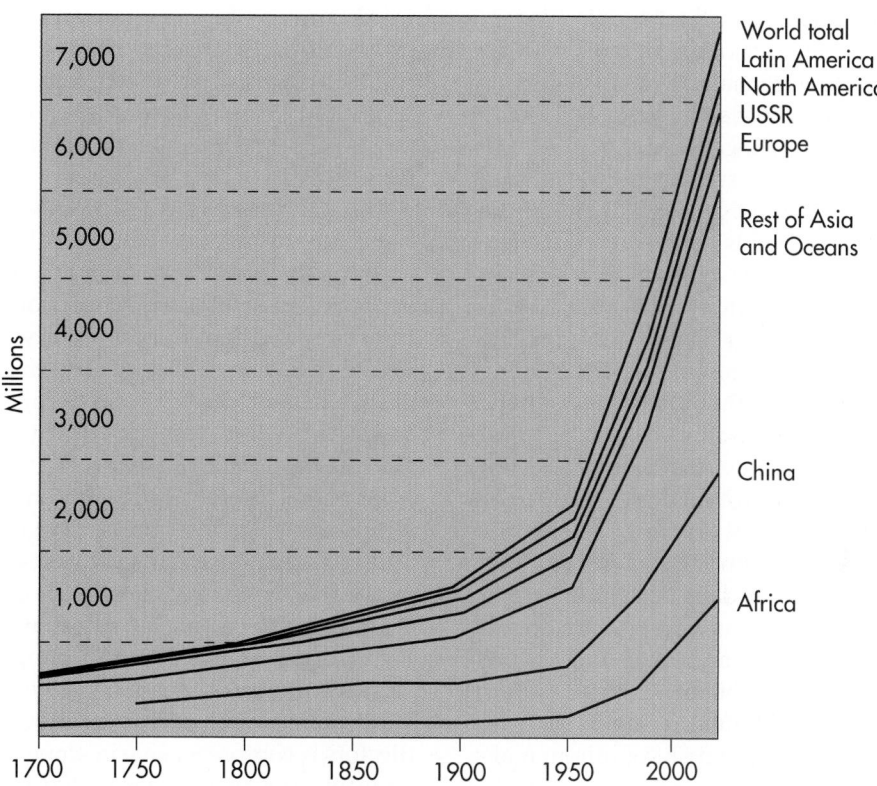

Figure 79-3 Global population (1700-2020). (*Modified from Demeny P: Population. In Turner BL II, editor: The earth as transformed by human action, Cambridge, UK, 1990, Cambridge University Press.*)

TABLE 79-4. Average Annual Percentage Rates of Population Increase

	1700-1750	1750-1800	1800-1850	1850-1900	1900-1950	1950-1985	1985-2020
Africa	0	0	0.1	0.4	1	2.6	2.7
Asia	0.3	0.5	0.5	0.3	0.8	2.1	1.4
Europe	0.3	0.6	0.7	0.7	0.6	0.6	0.1
Russia	0.3	0.7	1	1	0.7	1.2	0.6
North America	0.8	1	3.2	2.6	1.2	1.3	0.6
Latin America	0.8	0.5	1.2	1.6	1.6	2.6	1.6
Oceania	—	—	—	—	1.6	1.9	1.2
WORLD TOTAL	0.25	0.44	0.55	0.54	0.84	1.88	1.45

From Demeny P: Population. In Turner BL II, editor: *The earth as transformed by human action,* Cambridge, UK, 1990, Cambridge University Press.

vironments, the entire population of algae can begin a period of explosive growth ("bloom"). Extensive blooms can produce "red tides" or "brown tides."[12] This occurs when algae prevent light from penetrating coastal waters and the decomposition of dead algae consumes dissolved oxygen. Large fish kills are a frequent result.

The preferences of people for quick and convenient disposal of pollutants into available environmental sinks (e.g., soil, streams, groundwater, oceans, atmosphere) have sometimes been validated by incomplete science. For decades in the United States and elsewhere, scientists advised policymakers that "the solution to pollution is dilution." As a result, physical and chemical wastes have been released into environments that had finite capacities for absorbing them. Once the absorptive capacities were reached, a variety of serious problems occurred. These included biologically "dead" rivers (e.g., Cleveland's Cuyahoga River), "dead" lakes (e.g., Lake Erie), and "dead" seas (e.g., the sewage sludge dumping ground in the New York Bight off the coasts of New Jersey and Long Island). Although some of these conditions can be reversed, the processes are slow, costly, contentious, and often incomplete. Also, a growing body of evidence suggests that the aggregate effect of pollution may be jeopardizing the functioning of fundamental Earth systems. Buildup of atmospheric carbon dioxide is an excellent example of this process.

Despite a large volume of evidence, the effects of pollutants on receiving environments are not fully known.[14] This is partly because of a lack of scientific knowledge about the normal (unpolluted) functioning of some environments, such as deep oceans and tropical forests. The sheer volume and variety of materials released into the environment and their interactions complicate the study of effects of any single pollutant. Sometimes the effects of pollutants are subtle, long delayed, and far removed from the point of origin, making it difficult to connect causes and consequences. Sometimes experts disagree about evidence of pollution impacts collected in the field and evidence acquired from laboratory experiments. Even the impacts of well-studied events, such as the *Exxon Valdez* tanker grounding, are in dispute.[7,55] Nonetheless, there is a broad consensus that the absorptive capacity of receiving media is not inexhaustible and that pollution is a growing world problem that is pushing society against the limits of environmental resilience.

IMPACTS OF ENVIRONMENTAL CHANGE ON WILDERNESS AREAS

The task of assessing environmental change impacts in wilderness areas poses particularly difficult challenges to researchers. To begin with, the term *wilderness* is rarely used by scientists. For example, readers of the voluminous reports of the Intergovernmental Panel on Climate Change[27] might search in vain for references to wilderness impacts. Instead, there are comments about the effects of climate fluctuations on specific types of ecosystems, land covers or land uses—such as forests or nature reserves—some of which may be defined as wildernesses by different interest groups. The lack of references to wilderness in the scientific literature can be explained by the emergence of a widely shared conviction among scientists that no part of the world is now truly "natural." As one prominent ecologist puts it: "Overall, any clear dichotomy between pristine ecosystems and human-altered areas that may have existed in the past has vanished."[78] In other words, our environments are arranged on a continuum from intensely human-constructed places, such as cities, to places where the human presence is small, intermittent, or nonexistent, such as wilderness areas. Most places show evidence of both human and natural influences.

If scientists shy away from the term *wilderness*, the same cannot be said of political leaders and the general public. Unfortunately in this larger arena there is little agreement about meanings of wilderness. "Naturalness" and "remoteness" are two commonly mentioned wilderness attributes, but measures of both can be highly subjective. Depending on the definition adopted, a wilderness area might include some of the world's most biologically productive ecosystems (e.g., tropical forests of the Brazilian Amazon Basin) together with some of its least productive (e.g., Sahara Desert) and some of those that have been thoroughly transformed by human activities (e.g., so-called urban wilderness areas, such as Portland, Oregon's Forest Park). Some analysts have attempted to cut through this Gordian knot by equating wilderness with uninhabited areas or roadless places, but neither of these indicators is comprehensive in scope when it comes to accounting for all the places that humans perceive as "wild."

In view of the potential for confusion that exists in discussions of such a complex concept, it is worthwhile to briefly consider the philosophical and evolutionary background of the term.

The notion of wilderness can be found in several of the world's earliest cultures,[63] but formulation of a powerful philosophical and political movement that espouses the value of unaltered natural areas did not occur until the nineteenth and early twentieth centuries in the United States.[67] Although the wilderness movement subsequently diffused elsewhere, widespread public concern for the preservation of wild lands remains a characteristically American preoccupation,[68] perhaps because the contrast between juxtaposed human-dominated landscapes and ostensibly "natural" ones is so apparent in the United States (e.g., California's Central Valley and Sierra Nevada mountains; Florida's Everglades and Gold Coast). Yet despite the volume of public debate about wilderness, the concept itself remains poorly defined, even in the United States.*

However, most analysts recognize that the term refers to places that have some or all of the following three characteristics: few or no permanent resident human populations, unmanaged biogeochemical systems, and no significant modification by modern technology. Places that meet these criteria might include deep oceans, high mountains, deserts, circumpolar lands, certain oceanic islands, coastal fringes, most areas of active vulcanicity, and some of the world's great forests (e.g., taiga and tropical rainforests).†

The three criteria are best regarded as necessary but not sufficient to identify an area as wilderness. Spatial dimensions must also be taken into account. An acre of wetland that is surrounded by shopping malls would not be considered wilderness even if it is in biologically pristine condition. As a rule of thumb, a wilderness should encompass at least several square miles.

If the foregoing criteria were to be applied to the United States, they would include a great diversity of environments. Most would be marginal lands and waters, that is, beyond the boundaries of areas that are permanently settled at present and perhaps without prospects for human occupancy or use in the long term. Some protected areas within the ecumene (inhabited lands) might also qualify as wilderness because they are administered as such. However, most protected areas, such as national parks, national forests, and national recreational areas, would probably not meet all three major wilderness criteria because they are often subject to intensive management of residual plant and animal populations, as well as to human visitors.[41]

Conversion of Wilderness

In many parts of the world, the frontiers of wilderness areas are being pushed back as land is converted to managed uses. Economic growth and population increases are the ultimate driving forces of this conversion at the global scale. At local and regional levels a variety of conversion processes are apparent. These include resource extraction industries, such as mining and forestry, agriculture, animal husbandry, tourism, and commercial and residential uses.[50] These processes are not confined to land. They also affect freshwater and shallow water marine environments. Tourism is exerting pressure on coral reefs in Belize, Kenya, and many other countries.

Most land conversion is driven by demands for additional cropland. The highest levels of land conversion are found in developing countries with rapidly growing populations (Table 79-5). Most of the world's prime agricultural lands have been brought under cultivation, so attention has turned to other terrains that are spatially and agriculturally marginal.[3] Often these are wilderness areas. For example, during the last four decades, many formerly unpopulated parts of Sumatra and Borneo have been settled by government-sponsored "transmigrants" from the heavily populated Indonesian island of Java.

Land conversion may fragment existing wilderness areas by dividing them into smaller blocks. This process is well advanced in the Amazon rainforest of Brazil, where new long-distance, government-built roads bring settlers.[49] As a result, ecologic "islands" that may not be sustainable are created. Forest edge environments replace deep forest ones. The islands may be too small to retain the previous diversity of species. Governments often attempt to protect such islands by designating them as parks or wilderness areas, but this may be insufficient to prevent further changes. In any case, to be effective, such places often require intensive management of ecosystems and visitors, which defeats the objective of designating them as wilderness in the first instance. Moreover, the management actions may ripple through the ecosystems in unforeseen ways, perhaps contributing to the long-term conversion process.

Human Penetration of Wilderness Areas

Wilderness areas may be degraded without being converted to other uses. This usually occurs in one of three ways: direct impacts from increasing human presence; indirect effects of conventional industrial technologies in adjacent areas, and global effects of innovative, powerful, and often high-risk technologies.

Direct Impacts. Few parts of the planet have not been explored by humans at ground level. Formerly remote areas are being penetrated for a variety of reasons. Canada's James Bay is slowly being altered by a huge hydropower scheme; gold prospecting has intruded into the innermost recesses of Amazonia and Angola;

---

*The definition included in the Wilderness Act (1964) is typically vague: ". . . an area where the Earth and its community of life are untrammeled by man, where man himself is a visitor who does not remain." For practical purposes, "roadless areas" are often used as an indicator of wilderness in North America. Even in a well-researched region like North America, exhaustive inventories of the species present in wilderness areas are generally lacking whereas at the global level only the approximate distribution of wilderness areas has been mapped. See the assessment of McClosky M and Spalding H: A reconnaissance-level inventory of the amount of wilderness remaining in the world, *Ambio* 18:223, 1989.

†How should formerly developed areas that have reverted to unmanaged states be classified? Many such areas can be found in Western Europe and North America (e.g., the Adirondack Mountains of New York). Often, radical differences exist between predevelopment conditions and reverted conditions. For the purposes of this discussion, such areas are considered wilderness.

TABLE 79-5. Global Land Use Changes (1700-1980)

REGION	VEGETATION TYPES	PERCENTAGE CHANGES				
		1700-1850	1850-1920	1920-1950	1950-1980	1700-1980
Tropical Africa	Forests and woodlands	−1.6	−4.6	−6.8	−9.6	−20.9
	Grassland and pasture	0.9	2.8	3.6	2.5	10.1
	Croplands	29.5	54.4	54.5	63.2	404.5
North Africa/Middle East	Forests and woodlands	−10.5	−20.6	−33.3	−22.2	−63.2
	Grassland and pasture	−0.4	−0.6	−1.3	−3.4	−5.6
	Croplands	35	59.3	53.5	62.1	435
North America	Forests and woodlands	−4.4	−2.8	−0.5	0.3	−7.3
	Grassland and pasture	−0.1	−11.3	−2.7	0.1	−13.7
	Croplands	1566.7	258	15.1	−1.5	6666.7
Latin America	Forests and woodlands	−1.7	−3.6	−7	−9.6	−20.3
	Grassland and pasture	2.1	4	8.4	9.6	26.2
	Croplands	157.1	150	93.3	63.2	1928.6
China	Forests and woodlands	−28.9	−17.7	−12.7	−15.9	−57
	Grassland and pasture	−0.7	−0.3	−0.3	−1.6	−2.9
	Croplands	158.6	26.7	13.7	24.1	362.1
South Asia	Forests and woodlands	−5.4	−8.8	−13.1	−28.3	−46.3
	Grassland and pasture	0	0.5	0	−1.6	−1.1
	Croplands	34	38	38.8	54.4	296.2
Southeast Asia	Forests and woodlands	−0.4	−2	−2	−2.9	−7.1
	Grassland and pasture	−1.6	−7.3	−7.9	−12.4	−26.4
	Croplands	75	200	66.7	57.1	1275
Europe	Forests and woodlands	−10.9	−2.4	−0.5	6.5	−7.8
	Grassland and pasture	−21.1	−7.3	−2.2	1.5	−27.4
	Croplands	97	11.4	3.4	−9.9	104.5
Russia	Forests and woodlands	−6.2	−7.5	−3.5	−1.2	−17.3
	Grassland and pasture	0.9	−0.4	−0.4	−0.5	−0.3
	Croplands	184.8	89.4	21.3	7.9	606.1
Pacific developed countries	Forests and woodlands	0	−2.2	−1.1	−4.7	−7.9
	Grassland and pasture	−0.2	−1.3	−0.8	−2.7	−4.9
	Croplands	20	216.7	47.4	107.1	1060
TOTAL	Forests and woodlands	−4	−4.8	−5.1	−6.2	−18.7
	Grassland and pasture	−0.3	−1.3	0.5	0.1	−1
	Croplands	102.6	70	28.1	28.3	466.4

From Richards JF: Land transformation. In Turner BL II, editor: *The earth as transformed by human action*, Cambridge, UK, 1990, Cambridge University Press.

and Philippine coral reefs are subject to cyanide poisoning in pursuit of aquarium fish.[16]

The penetration of wilderness is facilitated by modern industrial technologies, especially transportation technologies. For example, road building encourages invasion of wilderness areas for recreation, resource extraction, or other purposes. The roads themselves have environmental impacts ranging from vegetation clearance to drainage impedance, but their roles as conduits of change are even more significant. They bring new people, exotic materials, and different lifestyles to remote places. Similar inroads are made by boats and aircraft and their support facilities.

As economic gain is an important incentive for wilderness penetration, recreational and esthetic needs are also increasing visitation. Hunting and fishing have long attracted visitors to wilderness areas like the Boundary Waters Canoe Area of northern Minnesota. Such pursuits are being reinforced by "ecotourism." An increasing number of people want to visit remote areas to appreciate pristine beauty. For many people who formerly might have sought out Yellowstone National Park and the Grand Canyon, the destinations of choice include places such as Antarctica, the high Himalaya, Amazonia, and even Siberia. The more remote the destination, the more attractive. Since most ecotourists want to visit the wilderness for only brief periods, they are whisked in and out by the most modern transportation technologies.

Visits from ecotourists can change wilderness environments. Seemingly insignificant impacts that are repeated can eventually become major problems. In the Masai Mara Reserve of Kenya's Serengeti Plains, the savanna ecosystem has been altered by successive photographic safaris. Safari camps require open campfires; fuel wood is scavenged from fallen trees that would otherwise provide important ecologic niches for local plants and animals. Climbing expeditions on Mt. Everest have reported large volumes of garbage left by earlier expeditions. Decomposition is slow in the dry mountain air. The scarring of scientific sites in Antarctica by discarded refuse and vehicle tracks is well known. Even the Galapagos Islands, the one-time archetypical wilderness of Charles Darwin, are succumbing to the effects of their popularity with ecotourists. Geographers from the United States are assisting the government of Ecuador in carrying capacity studies that will be the basis for land use regulations and other development controls to limit further degradation of these internationally valued sites.

Indirect Impacts. One of the most potent indirect impacts on wilderness areas follows the introduction (inadvertent or intentional) of nonnative species. Negative impacts have been demonstrated in the United States countless times, such as after the introduction of English sparrows, Asian gypsy moths, and Africanized "killer" bees. One recent example occurred in Glacier National Park. Pack trips within the park were curtailed because horses were introducing exotic species of grasses picked up from stable feed and passed through the digestive tract within the feces.

The problems of small islands and introduced species are legendary. Guam's experience with the brown tree snake is a good example.[51] These snakes are native to New Guinea, but several managed to travel to Guam on airplanes in 1962. They thrived in the absence of native snakes or predators. Now Guam has as many as 30,000 brown tree snakes per square mile, and they have devastated native bird species. These snakes are beginning to show up in the Hawaiian Islands, where conditions are also favorable for colonization. The potential outcome is discouraging, although efforts to intercept the snakes are being increased.

High-Risk Technologies. Technologic risks are an increasingly familiar threat to modern industrial society. Such risks are usually perceived as limited to accidents in urban industrial zones like Bhopal, India, where more than 3000 people died after the accidental release of methylisocyanate gas in 1984. However, some technologies have the potential to affect very large areas at great distances from the point of origin, up to and including the entire global environment.

Biotechnology exemplifies the powerful, high-risk technologies. Through genetic engineering, new organisms are being created, primarily for agricultural purposes. Nuclear technologies are another example. Like biotechnologies, they are characterized by considerable uncertainty about potential impacts. For decades after World War II, a massive nuclear war between the United States and the Soviet Union was a serious possibility that would have brought catastrophic changes to the earth as a whole.[60] Many military nuclear facilities were located in remote areas throughout the United States and the Soviet Union. With the end of the Cold War, this threat has diminished, although regional nuclear conflicts among lesser powers are still possible. The risks for nuclear weapons accidents still remain. Nuclear bombs have been lost at sea, improperly managed nuclear wastes have exploded in the Ural Mountains and elsewhere, and military nuclear wastes are buried on small Pacific islands, often within reach of rising sea levels. Environmental contamination around nuclear weapons manufacturing plants in the United States has been reported, and nuclear submarine propulsion systems have been discarded into the Arctic Ocean north of Russia.

Civilian uses of nuclear technologies pose risks to wilderness areas. Accidents like the explosion and fire at the Chernobyl nuclear power station have had global repercussions. Deposition of highly radioactive fallout in Arctic areas of Scandinavia demonstrates that no wilderness is immune from the effects of major nuclear accidents.[4] The proposed placement of a repository for high-level nuclear waste in Yucca Mountain in the middle of semiarid Nevada provides another example of the connection between high-risk technologies and wilderness areas.[11]

CONSEQUENCES OF ENVIRONMENTAL CHANGE

Research on global environmental change continues to reveal an ever greater number of connections between human and natural systems. Linkages among species in a given ecosystem, among different ecosystems, and among global biogeochemical systems have been described. Providing details about all vulnerable systems is not possible, but the range of interconnections can be illustrated by a few examples.

Scientists have recently explored the likely impacts of environmental changes on users of wilderness areas in northern Canada. In one case, rising temperatures and increased precipitation were judged likely to pose few problems for rafters and canoeists on the Mackenzie River, but accompanying forest fires were seen as much greater threats. Further north on Bathurst Island, the likelihood of increased winter snowfall combined with larger summer insect populations seemed likely to stress the existing large caribou herds to a point where hunting might be have to be curtailed. Throughout the region, a shift from consumptive uses of wilderness lands (e.g., hunting) to nonconsumptive ones (e.g., scenic tourism) is a potential outcome.[8]

Coral reefs provide a second illustration of environmental change effects. Such reefs are among the most prized wilderness ecosystems. Major reefs, such as the Great Barrier Reef of Australia and the reefs off Belize, are national and international treasures. Coral reefs cover only 0.17% of the ocean floor—an area about the size of Texas.[22,67a,78a] However, the importance of such reefs far exceeds their physical extent. Their biologic diversity is second only to that of tropical forests; their productivity is among the highest in the world; they protect adjacent lands from wave action, nourish valuable fish populations, and generate millions of dollars in tourist revenues.

When subject to physical or chemical stress, coral "bleaches," losing color as a consequence of biochemical changes. Such stresses may be caused by fluctuations in sea level, temperature, or salinity and by pollution. Although reefs sometimes recover, bleaching often leads to death of the coral organisms and decomposition or disintegration of the reefs. In 1987, marine scientists began to notice high levels of coral bleaching and mortality off Puerto Rico. A worldwide pattern of severe coral bleaching began to emerge.[9] Some scientists interpreted the problem as a harbinger of global warming, but it is unclear that this is the case. Nonetheless, coral reefs are vulnerable to temperature changes and sea level increases so that the threat of future damage is considerable. The best estimate now available is that sea level may rise an average of 1 m by 2100. Healthy reefs can grow upward by as much as 10 cm per decade, which may allow some reefs to adjust to rising sea level. However, if reefs are unhealthy—the evidence of bleaching suggests that many are—the rate of inundation may well exceed the coral's ability to keep pace.[70]

Among the stresses that afflict coral reefs are coral mining for cement, dredging for navigation, coral collection for aquariums, and disruption by divers and commercial fishing. Many places also experience significant biochemical effects from coastal pollution and sediment or pollution runoff from land.

The loss of coral reefs is already significant. Estimates suggest that 5% to 10% of the world's living reefs have been destroyed by human activities. An additional 60% are thought to be at risk over the next 20 to 40 years.[81] The consequences for society are potentially enormous. The physical protection of coastlines could be drastically reduced. The locally rich fisheries of coral islands could be diminished to the impover-ished levels that typify deep oceans. Prized tourist attractions would disappear together with the revenues they generate. Opportunities for the recovery of medicinal products from reef organisms could well be lost. Finally, the genetic resources of the planet could be further eroded. These are just some of the consequences of environmental change for one type of wilderness area. Similar, perhaps larger, effects may occur elsewhere.

Environmental Change and Medical Emergencies

The causes and characteristics of many medical emergencies, and perhaps also the appropriate responses, are directly and indirectly connected with the environment in which they occur. This text contains many examples of emergency medicine challenges that are posed by environments in general and wilderness environments in particular. In some cases, an environmental agent causes a medical emergency (e.g., reptile bites, altitude sickness, wild animal attacks). In others, the environment affects the treatment of problems that are not environmentally created (e.g., wilderness trauma and surgical emergencies, hunting injuries, wilderness medical liability). In many cases, the environment serves as both agent and context. Inasmuch as the process of environmental change is global in scope, it probably will also affect emergency medicine. A number of examples follow.

Increasing human penetration of wilderness areas is steadily driving up the number of wilderness emergencies. For example, the number of climbers seeking to scale Mt. McKinley (Denali) has increased by 250% in the 20 years between 1978 and 1998.[77] In 367 U.S. national parks, the number of search and rescue missions per million visits has climbed from 12 (1987) to 19.4 (1991). More than 5000 rescues occurred in 1991—a 78% increase over a 5-year period.[54] The cost of a single rescue in Denali averages about $55,000 and can exceed $100,000; throughout the country the National Park Service spent over $3 million on search and rescue operations in 1991. Personnel from the Park Service, the U.S. military, and volunteers may be exposed to high risk when called on to retrieve inexperienced and underequipped parties. Given the rising cost of such operations, it has been proposed that individuals who participate in risky adventures should post rescue bonds before departing into the wilderness. The combination of increasing populations and projected changes in environmental conditions can only add to the costs and difficulties of search and rescue in wilderness areas in the future.

As settlement advances into wilderness areas, new patterns of disease are likely to form. For example, African land conversion from unmanaged wetlands to irrigated agriculture may spread the range of schisto-somiasis and other water-borne diseases that are associated with drainage canals.[66] Likewise, more people may be exposed to virulent diseases of wilderness ecosystems. Conversion of tropical forest in Africa may increase exposure to malaria carried by mosquitoes, on-chocerciasis (river blindness) carried by simulium flies, and trypanosomiasis (sleeping sickness) carried by tsetse flies.

Pollutants often migrate into wilderness areas ahead of people. Air pollution is particularly mobile. Higher smokestacks have been a common means of diluting airborne pollutants, but they also allow these materials to disperse more widely. Trees and lakes in New York's Adirondack Mountains have been affected by acid rains transported from the Ohio Valley, and once-clear vistas in the Grand Canyon have been obscured by smoke from a distant coal-fired power plant. The growing severity of winter haze in the Arctic is a further problem.[72a,74] Although the Arctic is a remote area, increasing haze has been observed there for almost a century. This smog consists of many different industrial pollutants that originate far to the south in industrial areas, especially the heavy manufacturing industries of Russia. Intense cold is perhaps the most obvious environmental health hazard in the Arctic, but the buildup of industrial air pollutants may also have significant health effects, both directly on the body and indirectly through uptake by food sources in the Arctic environment.

The effect of weather on human mortality has long been a focus of biometeorologic research.[32] A range of medical conditions that are weather related are listed in Box 79-1. For example, well-established linkages exist between high summer temperatures and human mortality, especially among the elderly.[34] Although "global warming" need not mean that all parts of the Earth will experience significantly elevated temperatures, some researchers are convinced that summer heat waves are likely to become more extreme, leading to increased mortality from this cause.[35]

The medical effects of UV radiation have already been noted. Further erosion of the stratospheric ozone layer will undoubtedly increase the likelihood of cataracts, skin cancers, and immune system diseases. Reduction of biodiversity threatens to reduce the availability of natural materials that have medicinal value. Ethnobotanists are currently working with traditional shamans in Amazonia to catalog the medicinal properties of plants in tropical forests. Marine species are also an important source of new medicines. Scientists have recently extracted from sharks a powerful agent against bacteria, fungi, and parasites that may spur research into naturally occurring antibiotics.

The "ozone hole" is a dramatic example of the expanding capacity of humans to modify the biosphere.

Box 79-1 CAUSES OF DEATH CONSIDERED TO BE WEATHER RELATED

Active rheumatic fever
Adverse effect of medicinal agents
Cerebrovascular disease
Complications of medical care
Complications of pregnancy and childbirth
Contusion and crushing of intact skin surface
Diseases of the arteries, arterioles, and capillaries
Diseases of the blood and blood-forming organs
Diseases of the digestive system
Disease of the musculoskeletal system and connective tissue
Diseases of the nervous system and sense organs
Diseases of the skin and subcutaneous tissue
Diseases of the veins and lymphatics
Effects of foreign body entering through orifice
Endocrine, nutritional, and metabolic diseases
Fractures of the skull, spine, trunk, and limbs
Hypertensive disease
Influenza
Injury to nerves and spinal cord
Intracranial injury
Ischemic heart disease
Neoplasms: benign and malignant
Superficial injury
Toxic effects of substances of chiefly nonmedical sources

Modified from Kalk LS, Davis RE: *Ann Assoc Am Geographers* 79:44, 1989.

Usually the process is inadvertent, and wilderness areas are not singled out for attention. Sometimes, however, the very remoteness and isolation of wilderness areas encourages dramatic environmental changes. Such was the case in northwest Alaska in 1962 when the U.S. government buried 15,000 pounds of radioactive soil at Point Hope.[52] The project was conducted by the U.S. Geological Survey acting in conjunction with the Atomic Energy Commission. The intent was to study effects of Arctic environments on radioactive isotopes. However, the burial was illegal; no public hearings were held, no markers were erected, and high-level wastes instead of low-level wastes were included. When the land was returned to the Inupiat (Eskimos) in 1971, they were not informed about the buried soils. They now attribute current elevated cancer rates to living and hunting for many years in a contaminated area. Government officials reject this view. The Point Hope case is not an isolated example. There is significant evidence that metropolitan governments have often tended to regard wilderness peripheries and their populations as dispensable when issues of national security and the welfare of metropolitan residents are at stake.[15]

Complexity and Uncertainty

Although we have ample reason to be concerned about the environmental changes that lie ahead for wilderness areas, the subject is hedged with complexity and uncertainty. The potential for change exists, but it is difficult to be certain how fast and how far such changes will proceed. The following two cases illustrate some of the dimensions of complexity and uncertainty.

The north (Na Pali) coast of the Hawaiian island of Kauai is representative of wilderness areas that are particularly vulnerable to climate change. It is one of the most remote and beautiful places in Hawaii, accessible only on foot, from the ocean, or by air, weather permitting. The potential for increased rainfall, storminess, and sea level rise could radically alter this wilderness. For example, increased rainfall on Kauai's massive central peak, Mount Waialeale ("the wettest place on Earth"), would make hiking on steep Na Pali access trails that are already subject to erosion and landslides difficult. The few available campsites near beaches may be eliminated by rising sea level. Sea caves that can be entered only by inflatable small powerboats during calm conditions may become inaccessible. Flash floods in Na Pali streams may erode archaeologic sites, and increased moisture in the air would add to the mistiness that is now only an occasional feature of the area. Offshore waters host migrating whales that can be seen from the coast, but increased soil erosion might add to sediment loads and discourage these highly valued mammals.

As the Na Pali coast becomes increasingly hazardous to visitors on foot, larger numbers may try to enter by helicopter, with more high technology–dependent visitors and fewer low technology–dependent ones. Health and safety emergencies may increase, or the mix of emergencies may change. Already the skies over Na Pali are crowded with noisy aircraft. Several crashes and deaths occur every year. Leptospirosis from Na Pali streams is now a health hazard and may become worse. The bacteria were introduced from Southeast Asia in imported rats and pigs. In 1989 the Hawaiian Islands reported 66 cases of leptospirosis, with two resulting deaths.[53] Despite the potential for problems, no one can yet say with certainty which, if any, of these changes will come about. Nonetheless, we see strong indications that the Na Pali coast will not remain in its present state.

A second case that illustrates the complex interplay of environmental linkages and the potential for problems is provided by the highlands of Papua New Guinea.[2] Since the sweet potato was introduced to this area in the 1500s, it has become a staple crop for residents of remote mountain valleys. Sweet potatoes are susceptible to frost damage and tend to deplete mountain soils. In response to these constraints, villagers have developed specialized social and agricultural adjustments, including the practice of "mounding" and a complex system of resource exchanges between residents of higher elevations and lower elevations. Global warming might reduce the frost hazard, but increased precipitation or increased UV radiation could also threaten crop survival. There is currently no way of confirming the extent and severity of possible changes. However, a delicately worked out system of human ecology like this one would not remain unaffected by climate changes of the types that are anticipated in the next several decades.

WHAT MIGHT BE DONE ABOUT LIMITING ENVIRONMENTAL CHANGE?

At the beginning of this chapter it was suggested that change is a dominant, perhaps "normal," feature of the world's landscapes and environments. What is different about the present era of environmental change is the extent to which it is directly attributable to human decisions and actions. It seems unlikely that people will stand by and do nothing if the anticipated changes are perceived as threatening, especially if they are also perceived as caused by humans. However, also likely are responses to environmental change that will not be motivated solely by concern about environmental hazards, such as medical emergencies in wilderness areas. Recognition is growing throughout the world that improved environmental quality is an appropriate goal for all countries, not just developed ones. Therefore public policies toward the environment will seek both to mitigate risks such as those connected with environmental emergencies and to secure rewards by safeguarding and enhancing valued resources such as wilderness areas. Let us briefly examine some recent developments that provide clues to future public policies.

Changes in Environmental Science and Policymaking

Traditional conceptions of wilderness have emphasized the value of nature in a pristine condition, a condition that must be protected and preserved against human modifications. As argued herein, such a view does not square with the vast bulk of scientific knowledge that recognizes the pervasiveness of past human impacts on natural systems and looks towards future environments that are even more completely human-dominated. Such recognition implies that science and society might pay attention to both the restoration of degraded environments and the preservation of little disturbed ones. Environmental management policies might focus on the redevelopment of so-called brownfields, as well as development of more familiar greenfield sites. Both of these trends are clearly detectable in practice. Restoration ecology has become a new growth area in the environmental sciences and a new entry in the tool kit of environmental managers.[33] The implications for wilderness areas of such a shift are considerable. On the one hand, a restored watershed is not the same as one that has never been allowed to deteriorate; neither is a hand-reared endangered species the same as one that survives without direct human help. On the other hand, it is possible that environments might be restored to states that are functionally equivalent to wilderness. This raises fascinating—but as yet unanswerable—questions. Would the availability of human-constructed alternatives to natural areas mean a slackening in political pressures to preserve "authentic" wilderness? Would "synthetic wildernesses" contain suites of medical risks similar to other kinds of wilderness? It is simply not possible to answer these questions at present. At this point, we must interpret and manage wilderness as it now exists using a more or less conventional battery of environmental policies, programs, and initiatives.

International Actions

The first Earth Day (April 22, 1970) ushered in an important era of environmental politics in the United States.[10] The immediate result was a striking increase in public awareness of environmental issues. The United Nations Conference on the Human Environment (Stockholm, 1972) played a similar role on the international stage. In June 1992 the United Nations Conference on Environment and Development (UNCED) marked the twentieth anniversary of the Stockholm meeting and focused attention squarely on the global environment and emerging issues of environmental change. Several significant international agreements that addressed the task of slowing environmental change were signed[23]:

1. The Rio Declaration, a broad agreement on principles of environmental management and development
2. The Convention on Climate Change, a nonbinding treaty for industrialized and developing countries that is intended to stabilize and eventually reduce greenhouse gas emissions
3. The Convention on Biodiversity, a nonbinding treaty that establishes a framework to preserve the planet's biologic diversity and to share products derived from genetic stocks

These agreements are unusual because they broadly and directly link issues of environmental management to issues of economic development and because they took place under the glare of international publicity in a global forum. Many other international agreements are more narrowly targeted and have been signed without such fanfare. They include, for example, the Montreal Protocol on CFCs, the Convention on International Trade in Endangered Species of Wild Fauna and Flora

(CITES), the London Dumping Convention, the World Heritage List, and various agreements about the protection of Antarctica. (CITES aims to limit trafficking in endangered species, and the Dumping Convention bans ocean disposal of wastes.)

Important as are agreements among governments, they do not constitute the only kind of international action to limit environmental change. Increasingly, nongovernmental organizations (NGOs) have become significant international policy actors. Such organizations can serve as catalysts for responsible environmental management by marshaling public support for governmental agreements. They can also take action themselves, as in the case of so-called debt-for-nature swaps.

Debt-for-nature swaps were first begun in 1987 as an innovative way to accomplish three goals: to ease the debt burdens of developing countries, to relieve the international banking community of risky development loans, and to protect important environmental resources in debt-ridden developing countries. The mechanism operates as follows. An environmental organization purchases some of the debt of a developing country from a lien-holding institution. Since no one expects the loans to be paid back in the near future, they have lost their luster as financial instruments and can be purchased well below face value. The organization then forgives the debt in return for the debtor country's agreement to undertake environmental protection measures. These may include establishing preservation areas or deferring environmentally destructive development proposals. Debt-for-nature swaps offer one means for private organizations in the developed world to make a direct commitment to limiting unwanted environmental changes in developing countries. However, at present they fall short of being an adequate solution because the amount of debt greatly exceeds the funds that are available for buy-backs.

At the start of the twenty-first century, NGOs have begun to pioneer even more important roles in the shaping of international environmental policy. Perhaps the most potentially far-reaching of these has been the rise of broad-based coalitions of environmental, human rights and labor groups to oppose what they perceive as the hegemony of the World Trade Organization (WTO). The collapse of recent WTO meetings in Seattle (December 1999) as a result of such opposition may be the opening engagement of a much broader global campaign towards striking a better balance between a desire for open markets and a potentially stronger impetus towards environmental protection and social equity. If it develops as forecast, the movement will be complex and changeable. For example, one dimension may involve challenges to scientific protocols, standards, and labels on which many U.S. and international food safety regulations are based, as in the cases of genetically modified foods and "mad cow disease" (spongiform bovine encephalitis). Another form may include wage rates, import quotas, and workplace environmental protections that affect the manufacture of goods in emerging Third World markets. Yet another dimension may be concerned with regulating the differential burden of greenhouse gas contributions to the global atmosphere or the constitutional rights of women and minorities.

National Actions

Because national states retain sovereignty over most of the resources within their borders, they are still the most powerful institutions for managing the global environment. For example, the U.S. government has authority to regulate pollution, manage federal lands, and control waste disposal.[61] It also has important supervisory and review powers over the actions of state governments. Finally, it has strong indirect influence on economic factors that are deeply implicated in environmental issues.

The federal government's record of regulating environmental change in wilderness areas is complex and illustrates both the strengths and limitations of existing national level public initiatives. Approximately 4.5% of U.S. territory (104 million acres) is now included in the National Wilderness System together with about 10,700 miles of free-flowing waters that are part of the Wild and Scenic Rivers system.[14] The purpose of these designations is to protect the relevant areas against significant modification by humans. Most of the designated wildernesses are in Alaska (60%), and the bulk of the rest are in the 11 westernmost coterminous states. Typically, a wilderness area is embedded within—and surrounded by—

other types of public land, such as National Forests, National Parks, or Fish and Wildlife Reserves. Many types of human uses and human activities are permitted in the surrounding lands, which have spillover effects on the wilderness areas. Wilderness management is usually in the hands of the same agencies that administer the surrounding public lands, so management has often been a neglected stepchild of those agencies. Moreover, recent research has disclosed that the boundaries of wilderness areas are often ill-suited to permit the survival of many species that they contain. Especially in the case of migratory animals or those with large territorial ranges, what happens to them outside the wilderness is just as important as what happens within. So it makes little sense to restrict efforts for limiting environmental change to wilderness areas alone. Such efforts usually need to be applied to the private lands and waters that interdigitate with the federally managed wilderness and nonwilderness areas. In other words, holistic management principles that can be applied across governmental boundaries both within and between countries are necessary.

Together with business and industry, environmental interest groups are important nongovernmental participants in shaping U.S. environmental policy. Although direct action groups such as Greenpeace often receive publicity in the mass media, most U.S. environmental groups are political lobbying organizations. As shown in Table 79-6, membership in the major environmental organizations has increased greatly in the last two decades, especially during the Reagan presidency, when environmental issues were widely perceived to have been ignored by the U.S. government.[47]

TABLE 79-6. National Environmental Lobbying Organizations

ORGANIZATION (YEAR FOUNDED)	MEMBERSHIP (IN THOUSANDS)					
	1960	1969	1972	1979	1983	1990
Sierra Club (1892)	15	83	136	181	346	560
National Audubon Society (1905)	32	120	232	300	498	600
National Parks & Conservation Association (1919)	15	43	50	31	38	100
Izaak Walton League (1922)	51	52	56	52	47	50
The Wilderness Society (1935)	10	44	51	48	100	370
National Wildlife Federation (1936)	—	465	525	784	758	975
Defenders of Wildlife (1947)	—	12	15	48	63	80
Environmental Defense Fund (1967)	—	—	30	45	50	150
Friends of the Earth (1969)	—	—	8	23	29	30
Natural Resources Defense Council (1970)	—	—	6	42	45	168
Environmental Action (1970)	—	—	8	22	20	20
TOTAL	123	819	1117	1576	1994	3103

Modified from Mitchell RC, Mertig AG, Dunlap RE: *Soc Nat Resources* 4:219, 1991.

New environmental interest groups are also joining the fray. For example, the American Medical Association has recently formed an Environmental Health Task Force that is charged with studying harmful environmental issues such as waste disposal and ozone depletion. In addition, the National Association of Physicians for the Environment was established in April 1992 to educate physicians about environmental hazards to human health and to develop recommendations for policymakers.[31]

Local Actions

One of the most popular environmental slogans of recent years is "Think Globally, Act Locally." This advice recognizes that most environmental issues need to be addressed at the grassroots level if they are to be resolved successfully. In local communities, the effects of environmental problems are most forcefully felt by individuals, and the "not in my back yard" (NIMBY) syndrome is a powerful deterrent to projects with perceived negative impacts on environment and health.[69] For example, opposition to creating sites for sanitary landfills has raised garbage disposal costs to the point that recycling has become an accepted part of daily activities for many Americans. In other words, the political pressure of the NIMBY syndrome has yielded significant environmental benefits.

Many different kinds of local initiatives can affect the rate at which wilderness areas change. Formal measures such as planning and zoning regulations or restrictions on the availability of public utilities are obvious examples. Less conventional approaches may also be significant. Some local communities in the United States have sought to discourage further development of fragile remote areas by informing prospective newcomers about the discomforts and drawbacks of rural living.*

Nontraditional leaders are an emerging facet of local environmental activism. In the United States, women play key leadership roles in many local environmental groups. The same is true in developing countries such as India (the Chipko Movement) and Kenya (the Greenbelt Movement).[39] Chico Mendes, a Brazilian rubber-tapper who urged a slowdown in clearance of Amazonian forests, is another widely heralded example.

Looking across the range of environmental change issues and responses, new institutions and new philosophies of human-nature relations are emerging and are being linked to a broad range of public concerns. Issues of environmental change are now seen as intertwined with issues of economics and security. In other words, the principle of diversity in natural systems, which imparts resilience in the face of stress, is now being replicated in social systems. This is a hopeful sign at a time when environmental changes are unprecedented in rate and magnitude.

SUMMARY

Environmental change has been a characteristic feature of the earth's history, but today the changes are unprecedented in human experience. Nonetheless, people are capable of taking positive steps to confront and manage anticipated changes, despite the complexity and uncertainty. During the next several decades, wilderness areas will be particularly affected by environmental transformations that occur within and around them—perhaps more so than at any comparable period in the past. Like other sectors of society, emergency medicine and emergency medical systems will face new challenges as a result. Wilderness medical systems may need to be redesigned with particular attention to improving their flexibility.

---

*This strategy is favored by officials in Spokane County, Washington, who point out that in many areas public services are irregular and unreliable, emergency response times for medical emergencies are not guaranteed, perceived amenities such as forested glades can turn into liabilities during wildfire season, and floods, snowstorms, and landslides frequently disrupt transportation and communications (*New York Times*, May 30, 1999).

REFERENCES

1. Alcamo J, Kreileman E, Leemans R, editors: Integrated scenarios of global change: results from the IMAGE 2 model, *Global Environ Change* (special issue) 6:255.1996.
2. Allen BJ: Adaptation to frost and recent political change in highland Papua New Guinea. In Allan NJR, Knapp GW, Stadel C, editors: *Human impacts on mountains*, Totowa, NJ, 1988, Rowman & Littlefield.
3. Allen JC, Barnes DF: The causes of deforestation in developing countries, *Ann Assoc Amer Geographers* 75:163, 1985.
4. Anspaugh LR, Catlin RJ, Goldman M: The global impact of the Chernobyl reactor accident, *Science* 242:1513, 1988.
5. Arnell NW: Climate change and global water resources, *Glob Environ Change* 9(suppl):S31, 1999.
6. Bailes KE: *Science and Russian culture in an age of revolution: V.I. Vernadsky and his scientific school (1863-1945)*, Bloomington, Ind, 1990, Indiana University Press.
7. Birkland TA: In the wake of the Exxon Valdez: how environmental disasters influence policy, *Environment* 40:4, 1998.
8. Brotton J, Staple T, Wall G: Climate change and tourism in the Mackenzie Basin. In Cohen SJ, editor: *Mackenzie Basin Impact Study: final report*, Downsview, Ontario, Canada, 1997, Environment Canada.
9. Bunkley-Williams L, Williams EH: Global assault on coral reefs, *Nat Hist* April 1990, p 46.
10. Cahn R, Cahn P: Did Earth Day change the world? *Environment* 32:16, 1990.
11. Carter LJ: *Nuclear imperatives and public trust: dealing with radioactive waste*, Washington, DC, 1987, Resources for the Future.
12. Cherfas J: The ocean fringe—under siege from the land, *Science* 248:163, 1990.
13. Cohen JE: *How many people can the earth support?* New York, 1995, WW Norton.
13a. Conzen MP, editor: *The making of the American landscape*. New York, 1990, Routledge.
14. Council on Environmental Quality: *Environmental Quality: the 25th anniversary report of the Council on Environmental Quality*, Washington, DC, 1997.
14a. Cronon W: *Changes in the land: Indians, colonists and the ecology of New England*, New York, 1984, Hill and Wang Publishers.

15. Dalby S: Ecopolitical discourse: "environmental security" and political geography, *Prog Human Geogr* 16:503, 1992.

16. Derr M: Raiders of the reef, *Audubon* 92:48, 1992.

17. Dracup JA, Kendall DR: Floods and droughts. In Waggoner PE, editor: *Climate change and U.S. water resources,* New York, 1990, Wiley.

18. Eisner T et al: Building a scientifically sound policy for protecting endangered species, *Science* 268:1231, 1995.

19. Erwin TL: Beetles and other insects of tropical forest canopies at Manaus, Brazil, sampled by insecticidal fogging. In Whitmore TC, Chadwick AC, editors: *Tropical rain forest ecology and management,* Oxford, UK, 1993, Blackwell Scientific.

20. Faminow MD: *Cattle, deforestation and development in the Amazon: an economic, agronomic and environmental perspective,* New York, 1998, CAB International.

21. Freese CH, editor: *Harvesting wild species: implications for biodiversity conservation,* Baltimore, 1997, Johns Hopkins University Press.

22. Goreau TJ: Control of atmospheric carbon dioxide, *Global Environ Change* 2:5, 1992.

22a. Haas PM: Policy responses to stratospheric ozone depletion, *Global Environ Change* 1:224, 1991.

23. Haas PM, Levy MA, Parson EA: How should we judge UNCED's success? *Environment* 34:6, 1992.

24. Hassol SJ, Katzenberger J: 1997. *Elements of change: natural hazards and global change,* Aspen, Colo, 1997, Aspen Global Change Institute.

25. Henderson-Sellers A, Robinson PJ: *Contemporary climatology,* New York, 1991, Wiley.

26. Heywood VH, editor: *Global biodiversity assessment,* Cambridge, UK, 1995, Cambridge University Press.

27. Houghton JT et al, editors: *Climate change 1995: the science of climate change.* Contribution of Working Group I to the second assessment report of the Intergovernmental Panel on climate change. New York, 1996, Cambridge University Press.

28. Hulme M et al: Climate change scenarios for global impacts studies, *Global Environ Change* 9(suppl):S3, 1999.

29. Hunter ML, editor: *Maintaining biodiversity in forest ecosystems,* Cambridge, UK, 1999, Cambridge University Press.

30. Huston MA: *Biological diversity: the coexistence of species on changing landscapes,* Cambridge, UK, 1994, Cambridge University Press.

31. *The Internist,* May 1992 (referenced in Environment 34:21, 1992).

32. Jones TS: Morbidity and mortality associated with the July 1980 heat wave in St. Louis and Kansas City, Missouri, *JAMA* 247:3327, 1982.

33. Jordan WR, Gilpin ME, Aber JB, editors: *Restoration ecology: a synthetic approach to ecological research,* Cambridge, UK, 1987, Cambridge University Press.

34. Kalkstein LS: *The impacts of predicted climate changes upon human mortality,* Publications in Climatology Series XLI (1), Newark, 1988, University of Delaware.

35. Kalkstein LS, Davis RE: Weather and human mortality: an evaluation of demographic and interregional responses in the United States, *Ann Assoc Amer Geographers* 79:44, 1989.

36. Kates RW: The human environment: the road not taken, the road still beckoning, *Ann Assoc Amer Geographers* 77:525, 1987.

37. Kates RW, Turner BL II, Clark WC: The great transformation. In Turner BL II et al, editors: *The earth as transformed by human action: global and regional changes in the biosphere over the past 300 years,* Cambridge, UK, 1990, Cambridge University Press.

38. Krueger JP, Rowlands IH: Protecting the earth's ozone layer, *Global Environ Change* 6:245, 1996.

39. Lake RW: Rethinking NIMBY, *J Am Planning Assoc* 87:97, 1993.

40. Lawton JH, May R: *Extinction rates,* Oxford, UK, 1995, Oxford University Press.

41. Machlis GA, Ticknell TL: *The state of the world's parks: an international assessment of resource management, policy, and research,* Boulder, Colo, 1985, Westview Press.

42. Mahlman JD: Global change: a looming Arctic ozone hole, *Nature* 360:209, 1992.

43. Marsh GP: *Man and nature; or the earth as modified by human action* (orig. 1864), Cambridge, UK, 1965, Belknap Press of Harvard University Press.

44. Martens P et al: Climate change and future populations at risk of malaria, *Global Environ Change* 9(suppl):S89, 1999

44a. Merchant C: *Ecological revolutions: nature, gender, and science in New England,* Chapel Hill, NC, 1989, University of North Carolina Press.

45. Mitchell JK, Ericksen NJ: Effects of climate change on weather-related disasters. In Mintzer IM, editor: *Confronting climate change,* New York, 1991, Cambridge University Press.

46. Mitchell JK, Cutter SL: Hazard continuities and discontinuities in an era of environmental and societal transformation, *Environmental Hazards* 1:1, 1999.

47. Mitchell RC, Mertig AG, Dunlap RE: Twenty years of environmental mobilization: trends among national environmental organizations, *Society Nat Resources* 4:219, 1991.

48. Morrisette PM et al: Prospects for a global greenhouse accord: lessons from other agreements, *Glob Environ Change* 1:209, 1991.

49. Myers N: *The shrinking ark,* Oxford, UK, 1980, Pergamon Press.

50. National Academy of Sciences: *Conversion of tropical moist forests,* Washington, DC, 1980, National Academy Press.

51. *New York Times,* July 14, 1992.

52. *New York Times,* December 12, 1992.

53. *New York Times,* December 29, 1992.

54. *New York Times,* March 28, 1993.

55. *New York Times,* April 30, 1993.

56. Parry M, Livermore M, editors: A new assessment, *Glob Environ Change* 9(suppl):S51, 1999.

57. Parry M et al: Climate change and world food security A new assessment of the global effects of climate change, *Global Environ Change* 9(suppl), 1999.

58. Pernetta JC: Impacts of climate change and sea level rise on small island states: national and international responses, *Global Environ Change* 2:19, 1992.

59. Pitari G, Viscunti G, Verdecchia M: Global ozone depletion and the Antarctic ozone hole, *J Geophys Res* 97:8075, 1992.

60. Pittock AB et al: *Environmental consequences of nuclear war,* SCOPE 28, New York, 1986, Wiley.

61. Platt RH: *Land use and society: geography, law, and public policy,* Washington, DC, 1996, Island Press.

62. Raup H: View from John Saunderson's farm: a perspective for the use of the land, *Forest History* 10:1, 1966.

63. Redman CL: *Human impact on ancient environments.* Tucson, Ariz, 1999, University of Arizona Press.

64. Reid WV: Strategies for conserving biodiversity, *Environment* 39:16, 1997.

65. Reid WV, Miller KR: *Keeping options alive: the scientific basis for conserving biodiversity,* Washington, DC, 1989, World Resources Institute.

66. Rosenfield PL, Bower B: Management strategies for mitigating adverse impacts of water development projects, *Prog Water Technol* 11:285, 1979.

67. Rudzitis G: *Wilderness and the changing American West,* New York, 1996, John Wiley and Sons.

67a. Salvat B: Coral reefs—a challenging ecosystem for human societies, *Global Environ Change* 2:12, 1992.

68. Schmitt PJ: *Back to nature: the Arcadian myth in urban America,* New York, 1989, Oxford University Press.

69. Shiva V: *Staying alive: women, ecology, and development,* Atlantic Highlands, NJ, 1988, Zed Books.

70. Smith SV, Buddemeier RW: Global change and coral reef ecosystems, *Annu Rev Ecol Systematics* 23:89, 1992.

71. Smith ZA: *The environmental policy paradox,* Upper Saddle River, NJ, 2000, Prentice Hall.

72. Solbrig OT: The origin and function of biodiversity, *Environment* 33:16, 1991.

72a. Soroos MS: The odyssey of Arctic haze: toward a global atmospheric regime, *Environment* 34:6, 1992.

73. Stein BA, Flack SR: Conservation priorities: the state of U.S. plants and animals, *Environment* 39:6, 1997.

74. Stonehouse B, editor: *Arctic air pollution,* New York, 1986, Cambridge University Press.

74a. Thomas WL Jr: *Man's role in changing the face of the earth,* Chicago, 1956, University of Chicago Press.

75. Turner BL II et al, editors: *The earth as transformed by human action: global and regional changes in the biosphere over the past 300 years,* Cambridge, UK, 1990, Cambridge University Press.

76. United Nations: *World demographic estimates and projections,* New York, 1988.

77. US Senate, Committee on Energy and Natural Resources: Statement of Stephen C. Saunders, Deputy Assistant secretary, Fish and Wildlife and Parks, Department of the Interior, before the Subcommittee on National Parks, Historic Preservation and Recreation, on S. 698, A Bill to review the suitability and feasibility of recovering costs of high altitude rescues at Denali National Park and Preserve in the State of Alaska, and for other purposes, May 13, 1999.

78. Vitousek PM: Beyond global warming: ecology and global change, *Ecology* 75:1861, 1994.

78a. Weber R: Reviving coral reefs, *State of the world 1993*, Worldwatch Institute, New York, 1993, WW Norton.

79. White A, Cannell MGR, Friend AD: Climate change impacts on ecosystems and the terrestrial carbon sink: a new assessment, *Global Environ Change* 9(suppl):S21, 1999.

80. Wilcove DS: *The condor's shadow: the loss and recovery of wildlife in America*, New York, 1999, WH Freeman.

81. Wilkinson CR: Coral reefs are facing widespread extinctions: can we prevent these through sustainable management practices? Address at International Symposium on Coral Reefs, Guam, 1992.

82. Zuidema PA, Sayer JA, Dijkman W: Forest fragmentation and biodiversity: the case for intermediate-sized conservation areas, *Environmental Conservation* 23:290, 1996.

Appendix: Drug Stability Information

Sarah R. Williams

Stability data on drug products are derived from studies done in controlled environmental conditions. It is often difficult to ascertain whether a drug product can be safely used after storage under conditions other than those specified by the manufacturer. Stability of drug products is also related to the drug's container. If, for example, a parenteral drug packaged in a syringe for ready use is frozen, the drug may be fully potent, but the sterility of the product may be lost. Hairline cracks in the syringe may have resulted from freezing. Thus, for most of the drug products listed, stability and sterility cannot be guaranteed if products are stored under conditions other than those recommended by the manufacturers. Slight variations in packaging and formulation between brands may influence the drug's stability. The following guide should be supplemented with drug packaging information provided by the manufacturer.

Acetaminophen (Elixir, Drops, Tablets)

Store below 40° C (104° F), preferably between 15° and 30° C (59° and 86° F). Avoid freezing. Stability after freezing is unknown.

Acetaminophen with Codeine (Tablets, Elixir)

Store below 40° C (104° F), preferably between 15° and 30° C (59° and 86° F). Protect from light and moisture. Do not refrigerate or freeze.

Acetazolamide (Capsules, Tablets, Oral Solution, Injection)

Capsules and Tablets. Store at room temperature (15° to 30° C [59° to 86° F]).

Oral Solution. An extemporaneous oral formulation of acetazolamide 25 mg/ml in a 1:1 mixture of Ora-Sweet, Ora-Plus, or cherry syrup (diluted 1:4 with simple syrup) was stable at 94% of initial concentration for up to 60 days. Temperatures tested were 5° and 25° C (41° and 77° F), and the solutions were protected from light.

Reconstituted Powder for Injection. Store at room temperature (15° to 30° C [59° to 86° F]). It should be used within 24 hours because it does not contain preservatives. Conservatively, it is stable for 12 hours at room temperature, but if refrigerated, it is stable for 3 days. Other research has demonstrated 90% potency for 1 week at ambient conditions, 4 weeks when refrigerated, and 8 weeks when frozen (admixed with 50 ml dextrose 5% in water [D5W], 100 ml sodium chloride [NaCl] injection, 50 ml lactated Ringer's [LR] injection, or 45 ml LR injection with 5 ml sodium bicarbonate [NaHCO₃] 5%). It should not be frozen if combined with LR or NaHCO₃ because the solution becomes turbid.

Acetic Acid Solution

Store in airtight container, between 20° and 25° C (68° and 77° F).

Albuterol (Tablets, Syrup, Inhaled Formulations)

Tablets and Syrup. Store between 2° and 25° C (36° and 77° F). Protect tablets from excessive moisture.

Aerosol Inhaler. Store between 15° and 30° C (59° and 86° F). Do not expose to excessive temperatures (49° C [120° F]) for more than 1 to 2 days due to explosion danger of the chlorofluorocarbons. Do not puncture or incinerate aerosol containers.

Inhalation Solution and Capsules for Inhalation. Store between 2° and 30° C (36° and 86° F). Inhalation solution is light yellow to clear; discard if discolored.

Aloe (Gel, Ointment, Laxatives)

Topical. *Aloe vera* has been used for burns, wounds, and pruritus. It consists of substances capable of producing topical anesthesia, bactericidal activity, and increased local microcirculation, but actual therapeutic capability is not clear. Lotions are for external use only.

Laxative. Aloe acts as a stimulant laxative if taken internally due to anthraquinone glycosides. Aloe laxatives (Nature's Remedy) should be stored at room temperature. Avoid humidity and temperatures over 38° C (100° F).

Aluminum Acetate (Otic and Topical Preparations)

Otic Solution. A clear colorless liquid comprised of acetic acid 2% in aqueous aluminum acetate solution. Store below 30° C (86° F) and avoid freezing.

Topical Solution. Virtually indefinitely stable. Partially used irrigation solutions have high potential contamination rates. Label extemporaneously prepared solutions with a 7-day expiration date, which is consistent with the shelf life recommended by the manufacturer.

Antacids

Aluminum hydroxide gel suspension should not be frozen. Avoid freezing Milk of Magnesia. On freezing, many antacids separate into water and gel layers, which may not affect therapeutic value but may affect taste and prevent re-formation of the emulsion, even with shaking.

Aspirin (Tablets, Oral Solution, Suppositories)

Tablets. Do not crush. Aspirin is stable in dry air but gradually hydrolyzes to salicylate and acetate and gives off a vinegar odor.

Oral Solution. An extemporaneous oral solution can be made from a commercial buffered effervescent tablet (Alka-Seltzer) with 90 ml of water.

Suppositories. Store between 2° and 15° C (36° and 59° F).

Atropine Injection

Store at room temperature (15° to 30° C [59° to 86° F]). Atropine sulfate 1 mg/ml solution packaged in Tubex (0.5 ml and 1 ml) has been shown to be stable for 3 months. Atropine methylnitrate 10 mg/ml solution is stable for 6 months when stored in dark bottles at room temperature.

Azithromycin (Tablets, Capsules, Suspension, Injection)

Capsules and Tablets. Store below 30° C (86° F).

Suspension. Single-dose packets should be stored at room temperature (5° to 30° C [41° to 86° F]) and, if reconstituted with 60 ml of water, should be used immediately. Discard multiple-dose suspension after 10 days.

Injection. Store under 30° C (86° F). After preparation, it is stable for 24 hours at room temperature and 7 days if refrigerated.

Bacitracin (Topical, Injection)

Topical. If in aqueous solution, must be refrigerated and is stable only 1 week due to oxidation. However, it is stable in anhydrous bases (paraffins, petrolatum, white wax, lanolin). Therefore it is stable in its common ointment form but is rapidly inactivated in water. Calamine, benzocaine, and zinc oxide have been combined with bacitracin without affecting its stability. Store topical lotion between 15° and 30° C (59° and 86° F).

Injection. Store sterile powder for injection between 2° and 15° C (36° and 59° F), and protect from light. If refrigerated, it is stable for 1 week after reconstitution.

Bismuth Subsalicylate (Tablets, Suspension)

Store at room temperature and avoid heat greater than 40° C (104° F). Suspension should not be frozen.

Butorphanol Tartrate (Injection, Nasal Solution)

Store below 30° C (86° F). Inspect parenteral drug for particulate matter or discoloration before use (if container permits). Protect from light and do not freeze.

Calcium Chloride Injection

10% solution. Drug pH is altered significantly if frozen or exposed to temperatures over 40° C (104° F). The product should not be used if either occurs.

Cephalexin (Capsules, Tablets, Oral Suspension)

Store at room temperature (15° to 30° C [59° to 86° F]) in tight containers.

Suspension. Stable after mixing for 2 weeks if refrigerated between 2° and 8° C (36° and 46° F). Keep tightly closed. Shake well before using.

Cetriaxone Injection

Store sterile powder for injection at or below room temperature (25° C [77° F]). Protect from light. The color of solution ranges from light yellow to amber, depending on concentration, length of storage, and diluent. Once mixed, intramuscular (IM) and intravenous (IV) solutions remain greater than 90% potent for up to 10 days if refrigerated at 4° C (39° F). Potency is affected by diluent, concentration, and temperature. IM and IV preparations may maintain greater than 90% stability for as short as 1 to 3 days, respectively, at room temperature. If reconstituted with D5W or 0.9% NaCl solution and then frozen at −20° C (−4° F), preparations have been stable for 26 weeks in polyvinylchloride (PVC) or polyolefin containers. Thaw at room temperature before using. Unused thawed solutions should be discarded. Do not refreeze. Ceftriaxone may be incompatible with other antimicrobials; do not mix.

Charcoal, Activated

Sealed aqueous suspensions may be stored for at least 1 year. Keep in well-sealed metal or glass containers.

Ciprofloxacin (Capsules, Tablets, Injection)

Protect medication from intense ultraviolet light, such as sunlight. Store tablets below 30° C (86° F). Store microcapsules and suspension diluent below 25° C (77° F), but do not freeze.

Injection. Store between 5° and 25° C (41° and 77° F) and IV infusion between 5° and 30° C (41° and 86° F). Avoid temperatures over 40° C (104° F). When medication is diluted for injection, it is stable for 2 weeks at room temperature, below 30° C (86° F) or when refrigerated between 2° and 8° C (36° and 46° F). Do not freeze.

Exposure to excessive sunlight may cause phototoxicity in persons on this medication.

Cyclopentolate Hydrochloride Ophthalmic Solution

Store between 15° and 30° C (59° and 86° F) in airtight containers.

DEET-Containing (Diethyl Methylbenzamide) Insect Repellents

DEET is the best all-purpose insect repellent. It is colorless and has a faint pleasant odor, is practically insoluble in water, but is miscible with alcohol. Store in airtight containers. DEET may be toxic internally. Do not store near fire or open flame. Avoid contact with plastic or rayon. If in a propellant can, avoid temperatures of 49° to 54° C (120° to 130° F) due to explosion danger.

Dermabond (2-Octyl Cyanoacrylate) Topical Skin Adhesive

Should be used immediately after crushing the glass ampule, since it will not flow freely after a few minutes. Store below 30° C (86° F), away from moisture and direct heat.

Dexamethasone Injection

4 mg/ml injection. A clear colorless to light yellow solution that is sensitive to light and extremes of temperature. Do not store at high temperature for long periods. It maintains full potency for 6 months up to 40° C (104° F) and up to 3 months at 50° C (122° F). Do not use after freezing.

Dextroamphetamine (Tablets, Elixir, Capsules)

Tablets. Store in well-sealed containers.

Elixir and Extended-Release Capsules. Store in tight, light-resistant containers, below 40° C (104° F), preferably at 15° to 30° C (59° to 86° F). Do not freeze elixir.

Dextrose (Oral, Injection)

Oral. Store in well-filled airtight containers.

Injection. Store 50% parenteral dextrose below 25° C (77° F). Do not freeze or expose to extreme heat. Do not use if cloudy. Discard unused portions.

Diazepam (Injection, Capsules, Tablets)

Protect from light, and store at a room temperature less than 40° C (104° F), preferably 15° to 30° C (59° to 86° F). Avoid freezing. When frozen, diazepam tends to

flocculate and precipitate. Reheat with warm water; if no precipitate is visible, the product may be used.

Digoxin Injection

Digoxin has been shown to be stable at room temperature for 3 months in Tubex cartridges. Protect from light, and store between 15° and 25° C (59° and 77° F). Use diluted injection immediately. This product is compatible with most IV infusion fluids.

Diltiazem (Capsules, Oral Solution, Injection)

Capsules. Store at room temperature (15° to 30° C [59° to 86° F]). Protect from excess humidity.

Oral Solution. 12 mg/ml solution prepared in Ora-Sweet, Ora-Sweet SF, or Ora-Plus or in a 1:4 mixture of cherry syrup and simple syrup was more than 92% potent for up to 60 days at either 5° or 25° C (41° or 77° F). 1 mg/ml solution prepared from dextrose, fructose, mannitol, and sorbitol (but not lactose) remained potent for a minimum of 50 days at 25° C (77° F).

IV Solution. Should be preferably stored between 2° and 8° C (36° and 46° F), without freezing, but may be stored at room temperature for up to 1 month and then discarded.

Diphenhydramine (Tablets, Elixir, Injection)

Drug in tablet, elixir, and injection (10 mg/ml) form is stable after freezing. Container should be checked for cracks or leakage. Store in light-resistant container, preferably between 15° and 30° C (59° and 86° F).

Domeboro (Astringent and Otic Solutions)

Astringent Solution. Do not cover compress or wet dressing with plastic; allow to breathe.

Otic Solution. A clear colorless liquid. Store below 30° C (86° F). Avoid freezing.

Dopamine Hydrochloride Injection

Protect from light. Do not use if there is yellow, pink, purple, or brown discoloration of the solution, which indicates decomposition. Store at room temperature. Brief exposure to temperatures of 40° C (104° F) is tolerated, but excessive heat should be avoided. Do not freeze. Stable at least 24 hours after diluted for injection.

Doxycycline (Capsules, Tablets, Syrup, Suspension, Injection)

Oral Formulations. Store capsules, tablets, syrup, and suspension below 30° C (86° F), preferably between 15° and 30° C (59° and 86° F). Store delayed release capsules between 15° and 25° C (59° and 77° F). Suspension is stable for 2 weeks after reconstitution at room temperature.

Injection. Frozen, reconstituted 10 mg/ml solution for injection in sterile water is stable for 8 weeks when stored at −20° C (−4° F). After thawing, excess heating is not recommended. Do not refreeze. Protect from light. The infusion should be completed within 6 to 48 hours (brand and diluent dependent) if not refrigerated.

Epinephrine Injection (Salts, Solutions)

Epinephrine darkens on exposure to light and air. Oxidation causes a color change to pink, then brown. Epinephrine should be stored at 25° C (77° F); avoid freezing. Heat above 40° C (104° F) and exposure to light may inactivate the product.

Erythromycin (Tablets, Suspensions, Topical, Injection)

Oral Formulations. Erythromycin estolate and erythromycin ethylsuccinate (EES 200 and 400) liquid suspensions maintain their potency for 14 days at room temperature. Refrigeration maintains optimal taste. Tablets should not be crushed.

Topical. Stable for 2 years stored between 15° and 30° C (59° and 86° F). Store pledgets between 15° and 30° C (59° and 86° F) and ointment under 27° C (81° F). Gel should also be stored at room temperature. An extemporaneous topical solution made from tablets with hydroalcoholic vehicle as a 2% solution was stable for 60 days at 25° C (77° F). A 2.7% preparation in E-Solve was stable for 4 months when refrigerated between 4° and 8° C (39° and 46° F).

Injection. Erythromycin lactobionate injection is stable at room temperature in dry form. After reconstitution a 5% solution is stable for 2 weeks if refrigerated but should be used within 24 hours due to possible contamination. Prepared IV solution should be used within 8 hours.

Estazolam Tablets

Store below 30° C (86° F). Stable for 3 years after date of manufacture.

Fluocinolone Acetonide and Fluocinonide (Ointment, Shampoo)

Ointment. Store in a tight container below 40° C (104° F), preferably between 15° and 30° C (59° and 86° F). Avoid freezing.

Shampoo. Stable for 3 months after extemporaneous formulation.

Furazolidone (Tablets, Liquid)

Store in light-resistant container. Exposure to strong light may cause darkening. Do not expose to excessive heat. May crush tablets and administer in spoonful of corn syrup.

Furosemide (Oral Formulation, Injection)

Furosemide products should be stored at controlled room temperature (15° to 30° C [59° to 86° F]). Discoloration may occur when exposed to light. Do not use if discolored.

Oral Formulations. Tablets and solutions should be stored in tightly closed light-resistant containers. Discard oral solution bottles 60 days after opening.

Injection. Protect containers from light. May be used after refrigeration, barring evidence of cracking, leaking, or other damage to glass. All intact ampules or syringes, when returned to room temperature, should be vigorously shaken to redissolve any constituents that may have crystallized out of solution; stability should not be affected. When packaged in Tubex cartridges (2 ml of 10 mg/ml), potency was retained for 3 months at room temperature.

Gamma Benzene Hexachloride (Lotion, Shampoo)

The lotion and shampoo become thick when frozen but do not lose effect. The effect of high temperatures is unknown. Protect from light. Spray should not be exposed to temperatures below −2° C (28° F) or above 54° C (129° F).

Glucagon Injection

In powder form, glucagon should be refrigerated, but it is stable at room temperature for several weeks. When diluent is added to powder, the resulting solution may be used for up to 3 months, if refrigerated. Thawing will not affect activity. Cloudy or thick diluent should not be used. Do not use if stored at temperatures greater than 35° C (95° F) for an extended period.

Hydrocortisone (Tablets, Suspension, Topical Cream, Injection)

Oral Preparations. Store below 40° C (104° F), preferably 15° to 30° C (59° to 86° F). Protect suspension from light and do not freeze.

Topical. Do not refrigerate.

Injection. Do not freeze. Only use reconstituted solutions if clear, and discard after 3 days.

Hydroxypropyl Methylcellulose Topical Ocular Solution

Store at room temperature (15° to 30° C [59° to 86° F]) in tight containers. Do not freeze.

Ibuprofen Tablets

Store at room temperature (15° to 30° C [59° to 86° F]). Protect from light.

Intravenous Solutions (D5W, D5NS, etc.)

Effects of freezing these solutions are unknown. Incomplete resolubilization, especially with electrolyte solutions, seems a real danger.

Ketoconazole (Shampoo, Tablets)

Shampoo. Should be stored at or below 25° C (77° F). Protect from light.

Oral Tablets. Should be protected from moisture and stored at room temperature (15° to 30° C [59° to 86° F]).

Lidocaine Injection

Lidocaine 1% injection is a relatively stable drug, but excessive heat or cold decreases shelf life. It should be stored between 15° and 40° C (59° and 104° F). It may be used after thawing, provided the container is completely intact and the solution remains clear. Lidocaine with epinephrine exposed to temperatures over 40° C (104° F) for a long period should not be used due to loss of epinephrine effect.

Loperamide Hydrochloride Capsules

Store at room temperature (15° to 30° C [59° to 86° F]). Do not mix oral solution with other solvents.

Lorazepam (Tablets, Injection)

Both oral and parenteral formulations should be protected from light.

Tablets. Should be stored at room temperature (15° to 30° C [59° to 86° F]) in tightly closed bottles.

Injection. IM/IV formulations should be refrigerated and kept in a carton to protect from light. No potency loss occurs through IV tubing.

Mannitol Injection

5% to 25% injection is stable at higher air temperatures. Solutions of 15% or higher crystallize at lower temperatures but will resolubilize when warmed to 80° C (176° F). Sterility cannot be guaranteed if frozen.

Meperidine Hydrochloride (Injection, Oral Solutions)

Injection (100 mg/ml) may be used after thawing if the solution shows no signs of precipitation or cloudiness and if the ampules or vials show no signs of cracking or leaking. It should be stored between 15° and 30° C (59° and 86° F) and protected from light. Neither injection nor oral solutions should be frozen.

Midazolam (Injection, Oral Solution)

Midazolam appears stable over a wide temperature range.

Morphine Sulfate (Injection, Solution, Soluble Tablets)

Exposed to air, morphine sulfate loses its water; it may darken on prolonged exposure to light. Store between 15° and 30° C (59° and 86° F) and avoid freezing. Freezing does not affect potency but may create insoluble particles.

Injection. Store in syringes or glass and protect from light. Parenteral midazolam, 2 mg/ml (hydrochloride salt) in 0.9% NaCl injection, was stable in polypropylene infusion-pump syringes at both 5° and 30° C (41° and 86° F) for 10 days. A 3 mg/ml concentration maintained at least 90% stability for 1 week when stored in disposable polypropylene syringes in 20°, 32° and 60° C (68°, 90°, and 140° F). A 40 mg/L solution in 0.9% NaCl was stable when protected from light at 21° C (70° F) over 24 hours, with no loss in glass or laminate containers and less than 2% loss in PVC bags.

Oral Solution. 2.5 mg/ml of injectable midazolam and flavored dye-free syrup maintained greater than 90% of the original concentration throughout a 56-day trial period at temperatures of 7°, 20°, or 40° C (45°, 68°, or 104° F).

Nalbuphine Hydrochloride Injection

Injection for IM, subcutaneous (SC), or IV use should be protected from light. Store at room temperature (15° to 30° C [59° to 86° F]).

Naloxone Hydrochloride Injection

Should be protected from light during storage (0.4 mg/ml). Should not be used after being frozen. Store between 15° and 30° C (59° and 86° F).

Neosporin Ointment

Store between 15° and 25° C (59° and 77° F).

Nifedipine (Capsules, Tablets, Injection)

All preparations should be protected from light.

Oral Formulations. Protect capsules and tablets from moisture. Store capsules between 15° and 25° C (59° and 77° F) and tablets below 30° C (86° F).

Injection. Store below 25° C (77° F). Ready-to-use infusion retains potency for only 1 hour in daylight and 6 hours in artificial light. Keep in container until absolutely ready to use.

Nitroglycerin (Sublingual Tablets, Spray, Topical, Injection)

Protect from light; do not remove vials from the outer storage carton until use. Store at room temperature (15° to 30° C [59° to 86° F]), unless otherwise specified below. Protect from moisture. Do not freeze. Avoid excessive heat (40° C [104° F]).

Oral Preparations. Keep sublingual (SL) tablets in original glass container, tightly capped. Discard cotton once removed. Store at room temperature (15° to 30° C [59° to 86° F]). Protect from moisture, heat, cold, and humidity. Discard unused SL tablets after 6 months. Translingual spray has guaranteed potency for 4 years from the date of manufacture. Store below 50° C (122° F).

Topical Ointment. Tube should be kept tightly closed and stored at controlled room temperature (15° to 30° C [59° to 86° F]).

Injection. Nitroglycerin solutions (diluted in D5W or 0.9% NaCl solutions in glass containers) are stable for up to 2 days at room temperature and up to 7 days when refrigerated. Extemporaneous solutions of nitroglycerin in concentrations ranging from 0.035 to 1 mg/ml were stable in glass for up to 70 days at room temperature or 6 months when refrigerated. Brief exposure up to 40° C (104° F) does not adversely affect the potency or stability of the solution.

Norfloxacin (Tablets, Ophthalmic Solution)

Tablets. Should be stored in tightly closed containers. Avoid temperatures above 40° C (104° F).

Ophthalmic Solution. Should be protected from light and stored at room temperature (15° to 30° C [59° to 86° F]).

Ofloxacin (Tablets, Otic Solution, Injection)

Tablets. Store below 30° C (86° F) in a well-closed container.

Otic Solution. Store between 15° and 25° C (59° and 77° F).

Injection. Protect from light, freezing, and excessive heat. Store single-use vials and premixed bottles at room temperature (15° to 30° C [59° to 86° F]). Store premixed minibags at or below 25° C (77° F); brief exposure to 40° C (104° F) will not affect it.

Penicillin GK Injection

Stable in powder form for 2 to 3 years if stored at no greater than 30° C (86° F). Higher temperatures cause decreased potency.

Phenobarbital Injection

Not stable in aqueous solutions. Do not use if there is precipitation. Protect from light.

Phenylephrine (Nasal/Ophthalmic Solutions, Injection)

Do not use if brown or if there is precipitation. Store parenteral solution below 40° C (104° F), preferably between 15° and 30° C (59° and 86° F). Protect from light and freezing.

Phenytoin (Tablets, Injection)

Oral Preparations. Store at room temperature (15° to 30° C [59° to 86° F]). Avoid exposure to moisture and light.

Injection. Stable if no precipitation or haziness. A precipitate may form when refrigerated or frozen but will dissolve when warmed to room temperature. A faint yellow color has no effect on potency. More stable in normal saline than in D5W. Infuse within 2 hours of mixing the solution.

Polysporin Ointment

Store between 15° and 25° C (59° and 77° F).

Potassium Permanganate Astringent Solution

Diluted form is used to clean wounds, ulcers, abscesses, and dermatoses. Use 0.1% solution in water diluted 1:10 to provide a 0.01% solution. Undiluted potassium permanganate is composed of dark-purple or near-black crystals or granular powder and is soluble in cold and boiling water. It is incompatible with iodides, reducing agents, and most organic substances and may be explosive if it contacts organic or other oxidizable substances.

Povidone-Iodine Solution

Do not heat because iodine concentration may either decrease due to interaction with dissolved oxygen or increase due to water evaporation. Store below 42° C (108° F). Do not freeze. Protect from light.

Prednisone (Tablets, Oral Solution, Suspension)

Protect from light. Store tablets under 40° C (104° F), preferably between 15° and 30° C (59° and 86° F). Store oral solution and concentrate between 15° and 30° C in a tight container. Suspension prepared using 50 mg of prednisone powder, 100 mg of sodium benzoate, and a sufficient quantity of simple syrup to bring the volume to 100 ml was stable for 12 weeks at room temperature. Shake well.

Procaine Penicillin G Injection

Should be refrigerated but is stable at room temperature for 6 months. Higher temperatures increase hydrolysis and decrease potency. May be frozen and retain potency.

Prochlorperazine (Injection, Solution, Tablets, Capsules)

Store in tight, light-resistant containers. Store between 15° and 30° C (59° and 86° F) and avoid freezing. Discard discolored (nonpotent) solution.

Promethazine (Injection, Tablets, Solution, Suppositories)

Protect from light. Store oral and parenteral products between 15° and 30° C (59° and 86° F). Store suppositories between 2° and 8° C (36° and 46° F). Avoid freezing.

Pseudoephedrine, Pseudoephedrine/Triprolidine (Tablets, Capsules)

Pseudoephedrine Tablets and Capsules. Store between 15° and 25° C (59° and 77° F) in a dry place and protect from light. Should not be crushed.

Triprolidine. Store between 15° and 30° C (59° and 86° F) and protect from light.

Sodium Bicarbonate Injection

Do not freeze. Do not use if product has been frozen.

Sodium Sulfacetamide (Ophthalmic Solution and Ointment)

Ophthalmic Solution. Store in a light-resistant container in a cool place, between 8° and 15° C (46° and 59° F). Discard if solution darkens (brown color).

Ophthalmic Ointment. Do not freeze. Store between 15° and 30° C (59° and 86° F).

Temazepam Capsules

Store in a tight, light-resistant container, between 15° and 30° C (59° and 86° F).

Tetanus Toxoid Injection

Do not use after freezing. Should be refrigerated but remains stable for months when stored at room temperature.

Tetracaine Hydrochloride Ophthalmic Solution and Topical Lidocaine/Epinephrine/Tetracaine (LET)

Ophthalmic solution. Protect ampules from light. Refrigerate between 2° and 8° C (36° and 46° F) to prevent crystallization and oxidation. Stable for a few days at room temperature (15° to 30° C [59° to 86° F]). If returned to cool storage, stability is as labeled by the manufacturer.

Topical LET. Anesthetic solution stored in amber glass containers is stable for 4 weeks at approximately 18° C (65° F) and for 26 weeks if refrigerated (4° C [39° F]).

Tetracycline (Tablets, Topical Solution, Injection)

Outdated products may cause renal tubular disease.

Tablets. Store between 15° and 30° (59° and 86° F). Stable at room temperature; darkens on exposure to moist air or sunlight.

Topical. Solution prepared with diluent from the manufacturer is stable for 2 months at room temperature.

Injection. Reconstituted solutions are stable at room temperature for 12 hours (6 to 12 hours in D5W).

Tolnaftate Topical Antifungal

Store between 2° and 30° C (36° and 86° F). Do not freeze. May solidify at low temperatures but liquefies easily when warmed; its potency is not affected. Aerosol products are under pressure. Do not puncture or place in proximity to heat or flame.

Triazolam Tablets

Store at controlled room temperature (15° to 30° C [59° to 86° F]). Protect from light.

Trimethoprim/Sulfamethoxazole (Tablets, Suspensions, Injection)

Protect from light. Do not refrigerate.

Oral Preparations. Store tablets and suspensions in a dry place, between either 15° and 25° C (59° and 77° F) or 15° and 30° C (59° and 86° F), depending on the formulation.

Injection. Should be used within 4 or 6 hours (depending on dilution in D5W). Injection (16 mg/80 mg per ml) has been shown to maintain greater than 90% stability for over 60 hours when stored in polypropylene syringes. Discard if cloudy or with precipitate. Use within 24 hours if using multiple-use vial for injection.

Zinc Salts

Zinc oxide is practically insoluble in alcohol and water but dissolves in dilute mineral acids. Store zinc acetate in airtight containers and zinc chloride and sulfate in airtight nonmetallic containers. Zinc sulfate ophthalmic solutions should be stored below 40° C (104° F) in tight containers; avoid freezing.

ACKNOWLEDGMENTS

Thanks to Robert J. Matutat, Pharm. D., and Philip E. Johnston, Pharm. D., for their work on a previous version of this appendix.

SUGGESTED READINGS

American Hospital Formulary Service: *Drug information 1999,* Bethesda, Md, 1999, AHFS.

American Pharmaceutical Association: *Handbook of nonprescription drugs,* Washington, DC, 1990, National Association of Pharmacists.

Micromedex healthcare series, Englewood, Colo, 1998, Micromedex.

Parfitt K, editor: *Martindale: the complete drug reference,* London, 1998, Pharmaceutical Press.

Parfitt K, editor: *Martindale: the complete drug reference,* electronic version, Englewood, Colo, 1998, Micromedex.

Physician's desk reference, Montvale, NJ, 1999, Medical Economics.

Physician's desk reference, electronic version, Englewood, Colo, 1998, Micromedex.

Physician's desk reference for nonprescription drugs and dietary supplements, Montvale, NJ, 1999, Medical Economics.

Index